Begin Thinking
LIKE A NURSE
using your
PEARSON
RESOURCES

Simplify your study time by using the resources included with this textbook at **http://www.nursing.pearsonhighered.com**

D0142332

Further enhance your Clinical Reasoning with the additional resources below.
For more information and purchasing options visit **www.mypearsonstore.com**.

Break Through
to improving results
MyNursingLab®

MyNursingLab provides a guided learning path that is proven to help students synthesize vast amounts of information, guiding them from memorization to true understanding through application.

Think Like a Nurse in Clinical

Clinical references across the nursing curriculum available!

Thinking Like a Nurse for NCLEX-RN® Success

ALWAYS LEARNING

PEARSON

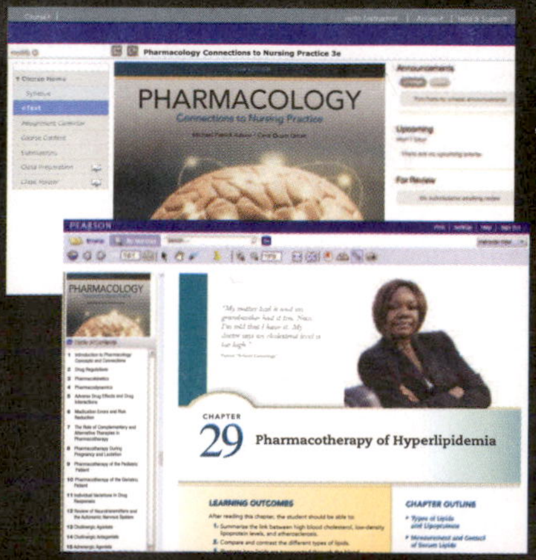

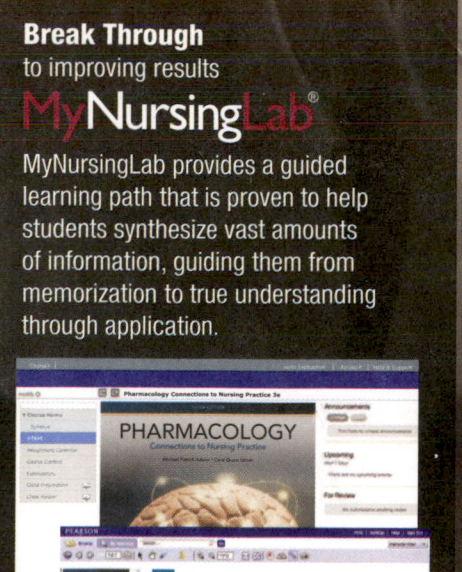

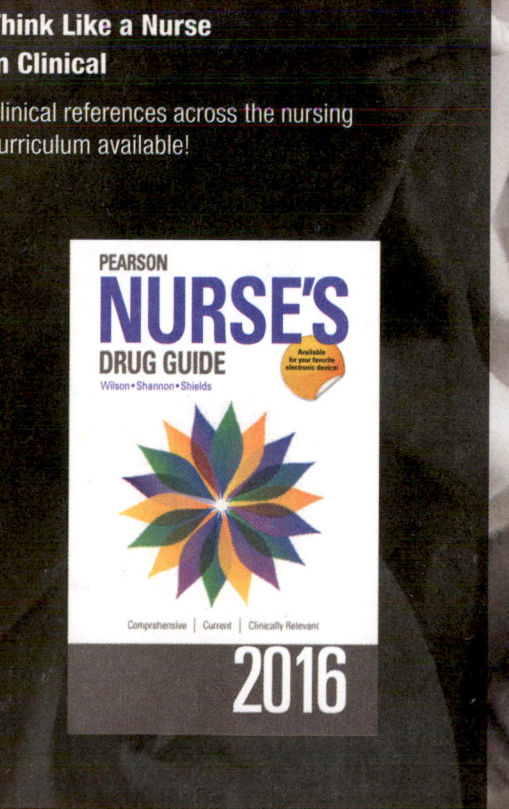

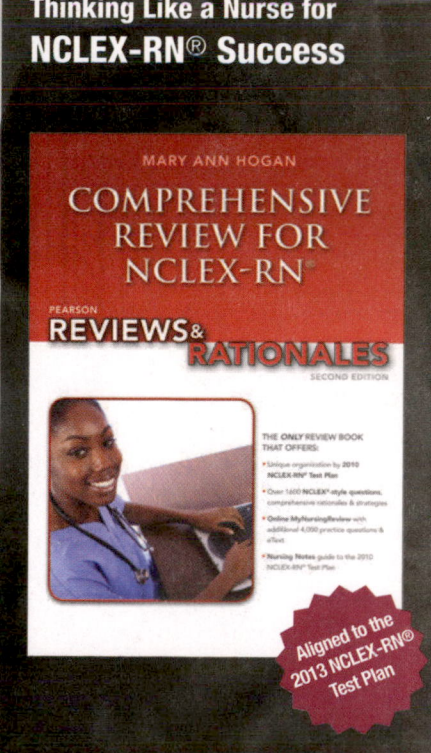

THIRD EDITION

PHARMACOLOGY
Connections to Nursing Practice

Michael Patrick Adams
Professor of Anatomy and Physiology
St. Petersburg College
Formerly Dean of Health Professions
Pasco-Hernando State College

Carol Quam Urban
Director, School of Nursing
Associate Dean, College of Health and Human Services
Associate Professor
George Mason University

PEARSON

Boston Columbus Indianapolis New York San Francisco Hoboken
Amsterdam Cape Town Dubai London Madrid Milan Munich Paris Montréal Toronto
Delhi Mexico City São Paulo Sydney Hong Kong Seoul Singapore Taipei Tokyo

Publisher: Julie Levin Alexander
Publisher's Assistant: Sarah Henrich
Product Manager: Pamela Fuller
Editorial Assistant: Erin Sullivan
Project Manager: Cathy O'Connell
Program Manager: Erin Rafferty
Development Editor: Teri Zak
Production Editor: Mary Tindle, S4Carlisle
    Publishing Services
Manufacturing Buyer: Maura Zaldivar-Garcia
Art Director: Maria Guglielmo
Cover and Interior Designer: Wee Design Group

Vice President of Sales & Marketing: David Gesell
Vice President, Director of Marketing: Margaret Waples
Senior Product Marketing Manager: Phoenix Harvey
Field Marketing Manager: Debi Doyle
Marketing Specialist: Michael Sirinides
Marketing Assistant: Amy Pfund
Media Product Manager: Travis Moses-Westphal
Composition: S4Carlisle Publishing Services
Printer/Binder: RR Donnelley/Owensville
Cover Printer: Phoenix Color/Hagerstown
Cover Image: PM Images/Collection: Iconica/
    Getty Images

Credits and acknowledgments for content borrowed from other sources and reproduced, with permission, in this textbook appear on appropriate page within text (or on page 1362).

Many of the designations by manufacturers and sellers to distinguish their products are claimed as trademarks. Where those designations appear in this book, and the publisher was aware of a trademark claim, the designations have been printed in initial caps or all caps.

Notice: Care has been taken to confirm the accuracy of information presented in this book. The authors, editors, and the publisher, however, cannot accept any responsibility for errors or omissions or for consequences from application of the information in this book and make no warranty, express or implied, with respect to its contents.

The authors and publisher have exerted every effort to ensure that drug selections and dosages set forth in this text are in accord with current recommendations and practice at time of publication. However, in view of ongoing research, changes in government regulations, and the constant flow of information relating to drug therapy and drug reactions, the reader is urged to check the package inserts of all drugs for any change in indications of dosage and for added warnings and precautions. This is particularly important when the recommended agent is a new and/or infrequently employed drug.

Library of Congress Cataloging-in-Publication Data
Adams, Michael, 1951-, author.
  Pharmacology: connections to nursing practice / Michael P. Adams, Carol Urban.—Third edition.
    p.; cm.
  Includes bibliographical references and index.
  ISBN 978-0-13-392361-2 — ISBN 0-13-392361-4
  I. Urban, Carol Q. (Carol Quam), author.   II. Title.
  [DNLM: 1. Drug Therapy—nursing.   2. Drug Administration Schedule.   3. Medication Errors—prevention & control.
    4. Nursing Records.   5. Pharmacology—methods. WY 100.1]
  RM300
  615'.1—dc23
                                                                    2014035797

10 9 8 7 6 5 4 3 2 1

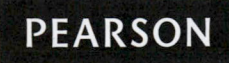

ISBN-10:   0-13-392361-4
ISBN-13: 978-0-13-392361-2

About the Authors

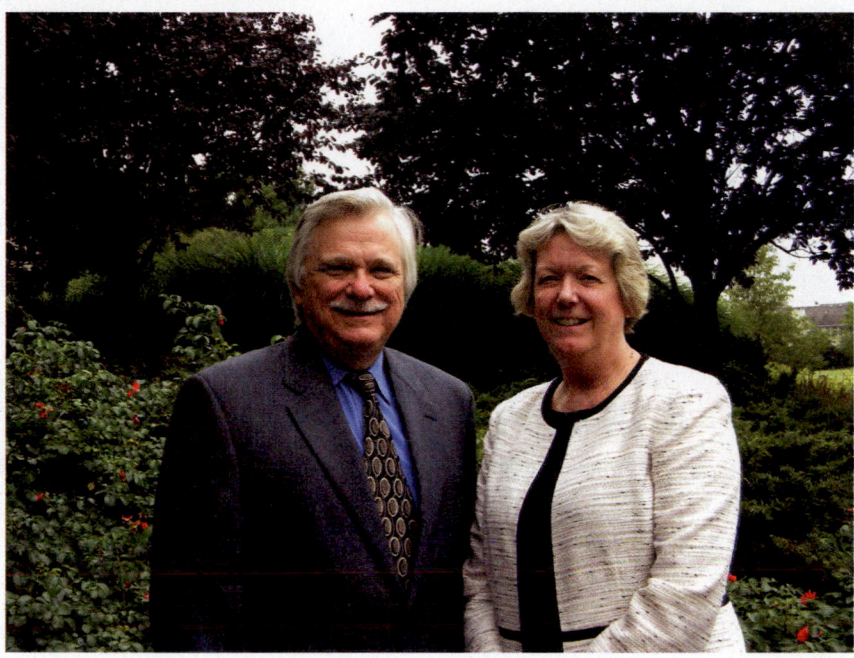

Michael Patrick Adams, PhD, is an accomplished educator, author, and national speaker. The National Institute for Staff and Organizational Development in Austin, Texas, named Dr. Adams a Master Teacher. He has published two other textbooks with Pearson Education: *Core Concepts in Pharmacology* and *Pharmacology for Nurses: A Pathophysiologic Approach*.

Dr. Adams obtained his master's degree in pharmacology from Michigan State University and his doctorate in education from the University of South Florida. Dr. Adams was on the faculty of Lansing Community College and was Dean of Health Professions at Pasco-Hernando State College for over 15 years. He is currently Professor of Anatomy and Physiology at St. Petersburg College.

Carol Quam Urban, PhD, RN, Associate Professor, is the Director of the School of Nursing and an Associate Dean in the College of Health and Human Services at George Mason University in Fairfax, Virginia. She has most recently worked with faculty in the School of Nursing to open three grant-funded nurse-managed health clinics, serving uninsured patients in local counties, and is especially interested in increasing medication health literacy in these populations. She has published the Pearson textbook *Pharmacology for Nurses: A Pathophysiologic Approach* with Dr. Adams and Dr. Holland.

I dedicate this book to nursing educators, who contribute every day to making the world a better and more caring place.

—MPA

To my daughter, Joy, an extraordinary and resilient woman who continues to change the world for the better. And in memory of my son, Keith, the bravest and happiest soul I know.

—CQU

Thank You

First Edition Contributors

We extend a heartfelt thanks to our contributors, who gave their time, effort, and expertise so tirelessly to the development and writing of chapters and resources that helped foster our goal of preparing student nurses for evidence-based practice.

Diane Benson, RN, EdD
Humboldt State University, Arcata, California
Chapter 29

Rebecca Boehne, RN, PhD
Linfield College, Portland, Oregon
Chapter 74

Jacqueline Rosenjack Burchum, APRN, BC
The University of Tennessee Health Science Center, Memphis, Tennessee
Chapter 73

Pamela Evans-Smith, RN, MSN
University of Missouri–Columbia, Columbia, Missouri
Chapter 57

Geralyn Frandsen, RN, MSN, EdD
Maryville University, St. Louis, Missouri
Chapters 26, 27, 28, 30, and 44

Denise Marie McEnroe-Ayers, RN, MSN
Kent State University at Tuscarawas, New Philadelphia, Ohio
Chapters 67, 72, 75, 76, and 77

Mariann Montgomery, RN, MSN
Kent State University at Tuscarawas, New Philadelphia, Ohio
Chapters 66, 67, 68, 75, 76, and 77

Kim Alexander Noble, RN, PhD
Temple University, Philadelphia, Pennsylvania
Chapter 46

G. Elaine Patterson, RNC, MA, FNP-C EdD
Ramapo College of New Jersey, Mahwah, New Jersey
Chapters 10, 11, 12, 70, and 71

Janice Lynn Reilley, RN, C, MSN, EdD
Widener University, Chester, Pennsylvania
Chapter 63

Luann G. Richardson, RN, PhD
Duquesne University, Pittsburgh, Pennsylvania
Chapter 60

Roberta Shea, RN, CCNS, MSN
Indiana University School of Nursing, Bloomington, Indiana
Chapters 9, 66, 67, and 68

Pat Teasley, RN, MSN, APRN, BC
Central Texas College, Killeen, Texas
Chapters 22, 23, 24, 25, 57, and 58

Reviewers

Our heartfelt thanks go out to our colleagues from schools of nursing across the country who have given their time generously to help create this exciting new edition of our pharmacology textbook. These individuals helped us plan and shape our book and resources by reviewing chapters, art, design, and more. *Pharmacology: Connections to Nursing Practice* has reaped the benefit of your collective knowledge and experience as nurses and teachers, and we have improved the materials due to your efforts, suggestions, objections, endorsements, and inspiration. Among those who gave their time generously to help us are the following:

Wanda Barlow, MSN, RN, FNP-BC
Instructor
Winston-Salem State University
Winston-Salem, North Carolina

Carole Berube, MA, MSN, BSN, RN
Professor Emerita
Bristol Community College
Fall River, Massachusetts

Sophia Beydoun, MSN, RN
Instructor
Henry Ford College
Dearborn, Michigan

Staci M. Boruff, PhD, RN
Professor
Walters State Community College
Morristown, Tennessee

Sharon Burke, EdD, MSN, RNC
Assistant Professor
The Pennsylvania State University
Abington, Pennsylvania

Judy Callicoatt, RN, MS, CNS
ADN Instructor
Trinity Valley Community College
Kaufman, Texas

Katrina Coggins, MSN, RN, CEN
Assistant Professor
Western Carolina University
Cullowhee, North Carolina

Tamara Condrey, DNP, RN, ACNS-BC, CCRN, CNE
Assistant Professor
Columbus State University
Columbus, Georgia

Rebecca A. Crane, MSN, RN, CHPN, CLNC
Assistant Professor
Ivy Tech Community College
Bloomington, Indiana

Lynette DeBellis, RN, MA
Assistant Professor
Westchester Community College
Valhalla, New York

Debra Dickman, MS, RN, CNE
Assistant Professor
Blessing-Rieman College of Nursing
Quincy, Illinois

Teresa Dobrzykowski, PhD, APRN, BC
Assistant Professor
Indiana University
South Bend, Indiana

Deborah Dye, RN, MSN
Department Chair and Assistant Professor
Ivy Tech Community College
Lafayette, Indiana

Nancy W. Ebersole, PhD, RN
Direct-Entry MSN Program Coordinator
Salem State University
Salem, Massachusetts

Anita Fitzgerald, RN, A/GNP
Lecturer, Director, Learning Center
California State University
Long Beach, California

Suzanne Franzoni-Kleeman, MSN, RN, CEN
Assistant Professor
American International College
Springfield, Massachusetts

Preface

Pharmacology is one of the most challenging and dynamic subjects for professional nurses. Each month new drugs are being introduced, and new indications are continually being developed for existing medications. Some medications that were considered drugs of choice only a decade ago are now rarely prescribed. Current knowledge of drug actions, mechanisms, interactions, and legislation is mandatory for nurses to provide safe and effective patient care in all health care settings. Pharmacotherapeutics remains a critical and ever-changing component of patient care.

The subtitle of this text, *Connections to Nursing Practice*, has guided its development. At a fundamental level, pharmacology is a series of interrelated essential concepts. Some key concepts are borrowed from, or shared with, the natural and applied sciences. Prediction of drug action requires a thorough knowledge of anatomy, physiology, chemistry, and pathology as well as the social sciences of psychology and sociology. This interdisciplinary nature of pharmacology makes the subject difficult to learn but fascinating to study.

However, the discipline of pharmacology is far more than a collection of isolated facts. To effectively learn this discipline, the student must make connections to nursing practice and, ultimately, connections to patient care. Patients expect to receive effective and safe medication administration from a nurse who is competent in the study of pharmacology. *Pharmacology: Connections to Nursing Practice* identifies key pharmacologic concepts and mechanisms and clearly connects them to current nursing theory and practice for providing optimal patient care.

Pharmacology: Connections to Nursing Practice recognizes that pharmacology is not an academic discipline to be learned for its own sake but is a critical tool to prevent disease and promote healing. This connection to patients, their assessment, diagnoses, and interventions supports basic nursing practice. Like other core nursing subjects, the focus of pharmacology must be to teach and promote wellness for patients.

Structure of the Text

This text is organized according to body systems (units) and diseases (chapters). Unit 1, the first seven chapters, identifies fundamental pharmacologic principles that are applied throughout the text. Although new drugs are constantly being developed, these chapters build the structural framework for understanding the applications of all drugs. The role of complementary and alternative therapies, which are used by many patients, is included in the context of holistic care.

Unit 2 connects pharmacology, the nurse, and the patient, with an emphasis on positive patient outcomes. The four chapters in this unit recognize the essential role of nurse–patient interactions in providing optimum patient care throughout the life span. The fact that individuals vary in their responses to drug action is an important theme introduced in this unit.

Units 3 through 11 provide the concepts and connections that are necessary to understand the actions and adverse effects of individual drugs on different body systems. Many of the units begin with a chapter that briefly reviews relevant anatomy and physiology, which is a useful feature for the student when studying drug actions. Each chapter clearly identifies the concepts and connections necessary for safe and effective pharmacotherapy. Pharmacology is intimately related to the study of disease processes. The connections between pharmacology and pathophysiology are clearly established for each drug class in every chapter.

Resources for Student Success

Online Resources available for download at www.pearsonhighered.com/nursingresources include:

- Making the Patient Connection exercises and answers
- Additional Case Studies and answers
- Suggested answers to Connection Checkpoints, and more!

Resources for Faculty Success

Pearson is pleased to offer a suite of resources to support teaching and learning, including:

- **TestGen Test Bank**
- **Lecture Note PowerPoints**
- **Instructor's Resource Manual**
- **New! Annotated Instructor's eText**—This version of the eText is designed to help instructors maximize their time and resources in preparing for class. The annotated eText contains suggestions for classroom and clinical activities and key concepts to integrate into the classroom in any way imaginable. Additionally, each chapter has recommendations for integrating other digital Pearson Nursing resources, including The Neighborhood 2.0, Real Nursing Skills 2.0, and MyNursingLab.

A Practical Approach to Learning Pharmacology

UNIT 4	Pharmacology of the Central Nervous System
CHAPTER 17	Review of the Central Nervous System 208
CHAPTER 18	Pharmacotherapy of Anxiety and Sleep Disorders 216
CHAPTER 19	Pharmacotherapy of Mood Disorders 239
CHAPTER 20	Pharmacotherapy of Psychoses 264
CHAPTER 21	Pharmacotherapy of Degenerative Diseases of the Central Nervous System 285
CHAPTER 22	Pharmacotherapy of Seizures 309
CHAPTER 23	Pharmacotherapy of Muscle Spasms and Spasticity 334
CHAPTER 24	Central Nervous System Stimulants and Drugs for Attention Deficit/Hyperactivity Disorder 350
CHAPTER 25	Pharmacotherapy of Severe Pain and Migraines 366
CHAPTER 26	Anesthetics and Anesthesia Adjuncts 394
CHAPTER 27	Pharmacology of Substance Abuse 416

◄ **Disease and Body System Approach.** The organization by body systems (units) and diseases (chapters) places the drugs in context with how they are used therapeutically. This organization connects pharmacology and pathophysiology to nursing care.

▶ **Prototype Approach.** The vast number of drugs that the practicing nurse must learn is staggering. To facilitate learning, this text uses a prototype approach in which the most representative medications in each classification are introduced in detail. This edition features 193 prototype drugs that include detailed information on therapeutic effects, mechanism of action, pharmacokinetics, adverse effects, contraindications, drug interactions, pregnancy category, and treatment of overdose.

PROTOTYPE DRUG | **Omeprazole (Prilosec)**

Classification: **Therapeutic:** Antiulcer drug
Pharmacologic: Proton pump inhibitor

Therapeutic Effects and Uses: Omeprazole was the first PPI to be approved in 1989 for PUD and is available by prescription and OTC. By prescription it is approved for the short-term, 4- to 8-week therapy of active duodenal and gastric ulcers, GERD, and maintenance of erosive esophagitis. OTC, it is indicated for the relief of heartburn. Most patients are symptom free after 2 weeks of

---

Adverse Effects: Reported effects after PO dosing include headache, GI upset, paradoxical hypoprothrombinemia (in patients with severe liver disease), severe hemolytic anemia, hyperbilirubinemia, kernicterus, bronchospasm, and dyspnea. Possible pain at the injection site, hematoma and nodule formation, erythematous skin eruptions (with repeated injections), and peculiar taste sensations may occur. **Black Box Warning**: Severe reactions such as shock, anaphylaxis, and cardiac arrest have occurred when vitamin K is given by the IV or IM route. These routes should only be used when subcutaneous or oral routes are not feasible.

◄ **Black Box Warnings.** The Food and Drug Administration requires black box warnings included in the packaging for drugs that have exceptional toxicity. In this edition, these black box warnings are clearly identified for all prototype medications.

▶ **Drug Tables.** Easy-to-understand tables provide average dosages for most medications. Unique to this text is a listing of the most common and the most serious adverse effects for each drug or drug class. This allows the student to immediately recognize important safety information regarding the drug(s) he or she is administering.

TABLE 60.4   Selected Drugs for Inflammatory Bowel Disease and Irritable Bowel Syndrome

Drug	Route and Adult Dose (maximum dose where indicated)	Adverse Effects
First-Line Drugs for Inflammatory Bowel Disease		
balsalazide (Colazal, Giazo)	PO (Colazal): 2.25 g tid for 8–12 weeks PO (Giazo): 3.3 g bid for up to 8 weeks	*Headache, abdominal pain, diarrhea, nausea, vomiting, rash, flulike illness, allergic reactions*
mesalamine (Asacol, Canasa, Lialda, Others)	PO (delayed release tablets): 800 mg tid for 6 weeks PO (delayed release capsules): 1 g qid for 8 weeks	<u>Hepatotoxicity, blood dyscrasias, renal impairment, salicylate hypersensitivity, crystalluria (sulfasalazine)</u>
olsalazine (Dipentum)	PO: 500 mg bid (max: 3 g/day)	
sulfasalazine (Azulfidine)	PO: 1–2 g/day in four divided doses (max: 8 g/day)	
Drugs for Irritable Bowel Syndrome		
alosetron (Lotronex)	PO: Begin with 1 mg daily for 4 weeks; may increase to 1 mg bid (max: 2 mg/day)	*Constipation, abdominal discomfort, nausea, and rash* <u>Ischemic colitis, ileus</u>
dicyclomine (Bentyl)	PO/IM: 20–40 mg qid (max: 160 mg/day PO; 80 mg/day IM)	*Dry mouth, blurred vision, drowsiness, constipation, urinary hesitancy, and tachycardia*
hyoscyamine (Anaspaz, Gastrosed, Levsin)	PO: 0.15–0.3 mg 1–4 times/day	<u>Confusion, paralytic ileus</u>
linaclotide (Linzess)	PO: 145–290 mcg once daily	*Abdominal pain and distention, flatulence* <u>Severe diarrhea</u>
lubiprostone (Amitiza)	Chronic idiopathic constipation: PO: 24 mcg taken twice daily IBS with constipation: PO: 8 mcg taken twice daily (max: 48 mcg/day)	*Nausea, diarrhea, headache, dyspnea* <u>Allergic reactions</u>

Note: Italics indicate common adverse effects. <u>Underline</u> indicates serious adverse effects.

Connections to Nursing Practice

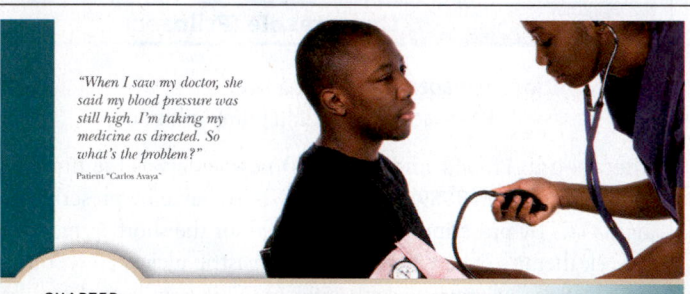

"When I saw my doctor, she said my blood pressure was still high. I'm taking my medicine as directed. So what's the problem?"
Patient "Carlos Avaya"

CHAPTER
31   Drugs Affecting the Renin-Angiotensin-Aldosterone System

LEARNING OUTCOMES

After reading this chapter, the student should be able to:

1. Illustrate the steps in the renin-angiotensin-aldosterone pathway.
2. Identify the primary physiological factors that control renin secretion.
3. Explain the two primary functions of angiotensin-converting enzyme.
4. Describe multiple mechanisms by which angiotensin II raises blood pressure.
5. Explain how the actions of aldosterone can lead to high blood pressure.
6. Identify the specific steps in the renin-angiotensin-aldosterone system that can be blocked by medications.
7. For each of the classes shown in the chapter outline, identify the prototype and representative drugs and explain the mechanism(s) of drug action, primary indications, contraindications, significant drug interactions, pregnancy category, and important adverse effects.
8. Apply the nursing process to care for patients receiving pharmacotherapy with angiotensin-converting enzyme inhibitors and angiotensin receptor blockers.

CHAPTER OUTLINE

▶ Components of the Renin-Angiotensin-Aldosterone System

▶ Physiological Actions of the Renin-Angiotensin-Aldosterone System

▶ Drugs Affecting the Renin-Angiotensin-Aldosterone System
  Angiotensin-Converting Enzyme Inhibitors
  PROTOTYPE Lisinopril (Prinivil, Zestril), *p. 491*
  Angiotensin II Receptor Blockers
  PROTOTYPE Losartan (Cozaar), *p. 493*
  Aldosterone Antagonists

◀ **Making the Patient Connection** is a feature that opens each chapter with a quote and a photo of a patient. It reinforces to the student that the focus of pharmacology must always be on the patient. To drive this important message home, the patient who is introduced at the start of the chapter is revisited at the end with critical thinking exercises. These questions assist the student to apply the content learned in the chapter to a realistic patient scenario. An additional case study is also included for further application of knowledge learned.

Case Study: Making the Patient Connection

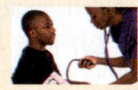

Remember the patient "Carlos Avaya" at the beginning of the chapter? Now read the remainder of the case study. Based on the information presented within this chapter, respond to the critical thinking questions that follow.

Carlos Avaya is a 26-year-old single man who was diagnosed with primary HTN 4 months ago. Carlos has been taking losartan (Cozaar) 50 mg daily PO and has been faithful in taking the medication as prescribed. When Carlos was told that his blood pressure was still elevated during this clinic visit, he was obviously distressed and concerned.

The health care team begins to investigate external factors that may be causing his blood pressure to remain elevated. Carlos has never smoked or used alcohol. He does not like to exercise but participates in a weekly game of soccer at the nearby community center. He denies being overly stressed with work or home life. Furthermore, he claims that he rarely salts his food.

The nurse asks Carlos to describe a typical day. During the description the nurse notices a concerning pattern. Because Carlos lives alone, he frequently cooks for himself. He admits that he enjoys salty foods such as pretzels and popcorn. He denies having consumed either prior to the visit to the clinic. However, to Carlos, cooking a meal involves preparing canned processed foods and frozen dinners. He never reads food labels. Without recording a complete dietary history, the nurse is able to determine that Carlos's intake of sodium-rich foods is quite extensive.

Critical Thinking Questions

1. In your own words, how would you describe how losartan (Cozaar) works to reduce blood pressure?
2. Considering the adverse effects of losartan (Cozaar), when would you instruct Carlos to notify the prescriber?
3. In addition to teaching Carlos about his losartan (Cozaar), what additional health teaching should he receive?

See Answers to Critical Thinking Questions on student resource website.

CONNECTIONS | Treating the Diverse Patient

Global Health Implications of *H. Pylori* Infection

H. pylori occurs worldwide and has a noted association with an increased risk of gastric cancer, particularly in genetically susceptible subgroups. *H. pylori* is also associated with gastritis and PUD. Infection with the bacteria usually occurs in infancy or childhood, years before symptoms of gastric effects may appear, and close contact between family members in crowded housing may be associated with a higher incidence of the infection (Melius et al., 2013). Because gastric cancer is a significant cause of death worldwide, public health measures such as adequate sanitation, drinking water, and nutrition may decrease the risk of transmission and improve the general health of those infected with the disease. The need for these measures takes on special importance in light of the global increase in antibiotic-resistant strains of *H. pylori*, including in the United States (Gatta, Vakil, Vaira, & Scarpignato, 2013).

◄ **Connections: Treating the Diverse Patient** features identify gender, cultural, and ethical influences that are important modifiers of drug action.

► **Connections: Complementary and Alternative Therapies** features present herbal therapies and dietary supplements that may be considered as alternatives to conventional drugs. These features include a description of the herb or supplement, history of use, standardization of dose, and brief description of the scientific evidence supporting (or not supporting) the use of the product.

CONNECTIONS | Complementary and Alternative Therapies

Hawthorn

Description
Hawthorn (*Crataegus*) is a thorny shrub or small tree that is widespread in North America, Europe, and Asia. Leaves, flowers, and berries of the plant are dried or extracted in liquid form.

History and Claims
Hawthorn, sometimes called May bush, was used in ancient Greece. In traditional Chinese medicine, hawthorn is used as a digestive aid. European and American interest in the herb began in the late 1800s. It has been widely used in European countries to treat HTN and HF. The berries may be consumed raw or made into jellies, juices, and alcoholic beverages. Some cultures believe that the shrub is magical, and it is used in religious rites to ward off evil spirits.

Standardization
Active ingredients in hawthorn include flavonoids and procyanidins. A typical dose is 4.5 to 6 g of dried leaves or flowers or 160 to 900 mg of extract per day.

Evidence
Hawthorn has been well studied (National Center for Complementary and Alternative Medicine, 2012). Positive inotropic action, improved exercise tolerance, and vasodilation have been documented. Some studies also report its ability to lower blood lipids. Hawthorn has been used to lower blood pressure but is slow in onset, taking 4 weeks or longer before a small effect is experienced. Hawthorn may work by inhibition of ACE or reduction of cardiac workload. Hawthorn has few adverse effects at normal doses. This product should be used with caution in patients taking cardiac glycosides and other prescription medications for cardiovascular disease. Because hypotension may occur, frequent blood pressure measurements should be taken when using this therapy.

CONNECTIONS: NURSING PRACTICE APPLICATION

Patients Receiving Pharmacotherapy with Angiotensin-Converting Enzyme Inhibitors and Angiotensin Receptor Blockers

Assessment	Potential Nursing Diagnoses
Baseline assessment prior to administration:	• *Decreased Cardiac Output*
• Obtain a complete health history including cardiovascular (MI, HF), diabetes, renal disease, and the possibility of pregnancy. Obtain a drug history including allergies, current prescription and over-the-counter (OTC) drugs, herbal preparations, and alcohol use. Be alert to possible drug interactions.	• *Activity Intolerance* • *Sexual Dysfunction* • *Deficient Knowledge* (Drug Therapy) • *Risk for Decreased Cardiac Tissue Perfusion*, related to adverse drug effects
• Evaluate appropriate laboratory findings, electrolytes, especially potassium level, liver function studies, and lipid profiles.	• *Risk for Falls*, related to adverse drug effects • *Risk for Injury*, related to adverse drug effects
• Obtain baseline weight, vital signs (especially blood pressure and pulse), breath sounds, and cardiac monitoring (e.g., ECG, cardiac output) if appropriate. Assess for location, character, and amount of edema, if present.	
• Assess the patient's ability to receive and understand instructions. Include the family and caregivers as needed.	
Assessment throughout administration:	
• Assess for desired therapeutic effects (e.g., lowered blood pressure within established limits).	
• Continue periodic monitoring of electrolytes, especially potassium.	
• Assess for adverse effects: headache, cough, orthostatic hypotension, fatigue or weakness, lightheadedness or dizziness, symptoms of hyperkalemia, sexual dysfunction, or impotence. Angioedema should be immediately reported to the health care provider.	

◄ **Connections: Nursing Practice Applications** concisely connect the nursing process to the major drug class(es) in each drug chapter and incorporate outcomes from the Quality and Safety Education for Nurses (QSEN) competencies of patient-centered care, teamwork and collaboration, patient safety, and evidence-based practice. Potential nursing diagnoses are included that students can complete to tailor care plans that are unique to the patients under their care. When a nursing diagnosis is directly linked to a drug or drug class used, a "related to" statement is included to highlight that information. Each nursing intervention is patient centered and includes the rationale and associated patient and family teaching. Collaboration with other disciplines, such as social support services or dietary services, is also included in the interventions. Important life span and diverse patient considerations are noted throughout. The Nursing Practice Applications are organized to help students learn to think like a nurse as they take them through the processes of drug administration, nursing care, and teaching that are necessary in pharmacotherapy.

Connections: Patient Safety, a QSEN competency, is a feature that presents a brief patient–nurse scenario that illustrates potential pitfalls encountered by nurses that can lead to medication errors. Most scenarios end with a question asking the student to identify what went wrong, what the nurse should do in the situation, what the nurse should question about the order, or what the nurse should do differently in order to prevent medication administration errors.

CONNECTIONS   Patient Safety

◀ **A Tenfold Error**

The nurse is caring for a 6-year-old boy newly diagnosed with seizures, tonic-clonic type. In reviewing the written orders, valproic acid (Depakene) 150 mg/kg/day is ordered. The pharmacist calls the unit to verify the order and the nurse contacts the prescriber. The order is corrected to 15 mg/kg/day. What could be done to prevent this error from recurring?

See Answer to Patient Safety Question on student resource website.

CONNECTIONS   Evidence-Based Practice

◀ **Use of Proton Pump Inhibitors and Increased Risk of Infections**

Clinical Question
The acidic environment of the stomach is known to be a natural barrier to infection caused by ingested bacteria and it plays a role in the destruction of respiratory pathogens. The long-term effects of decreasing the acidity of the gastric fluid are uncertain. Because PPIs decrease the acidity, is there an association between PPI use and GI or respiratory infections?

Evidence
An increased risk of enteric bacterial infection (such as salmonella) has been demonstrated to exist in patients taking PPIs (Bavishi & Dupont, 2011). Evidence also suggests a link between PPI use and an increased risk of respiratory infections, including pneumonia (Ramsay, Pratt, Ryan, & Roughead, 2013). These effects may be related to the decrease in gastric acidity and the protective mechanism against respiratory bacteria that it provides. Bacterial overgrowth may be of concern in patients who take PPIs and subsequently develop *Clostridium difficile*–associated diarrhea (CDAD). This infection has been associated previously with prior antibiotic use or immunosuppression. Recently, an increased risk for the development of hospital-acquired *C. difficile* colitis in

hospitalized patients who are receiving PPIs has been noted, especially with long-term use (Barletta, El-Ibiary, Davis, Nguyen, & Raney, 2013). The use of PPIs, as well as other gastric acid inhibitors such as H_2-antagonists, has also been shown to increase the risk of pneumonia, sepsis, and GI infections in infants and children (Chung & Yardley, 2013).

Implications
In patients who are receiving PPIs, the nurse should frequently assess for the development of severe diarrhea, especially that which is watery and contains mucus, blood, or pus. Respiratory symptoms such as cough, congestion, adventitious breath sounds, and dyspnea, especially when associated with fever, should also be assessed and reported.

Critical Thinking Question
What categories of patients may be at increased risk for developing infections associated with PPI use?

See Answers to Critical Thinking Questions on student resource website.

◀ **Connections: Evidence-Based Practice**, also a QSEN competency, is a feature that illustrates connections to nursing or pharmacology research and discusses the short- and long-term directions of pharmacotherapeutics. A critical thinking question is presented at the end of each feature to challenge the student to connect scientific evidence to nursing practice.

▶ **Connections: Lifespan Considerations** features clearly identify important considerations to ensure safe and effective pharmacotherapy in the older adult and pediatric populations.

CONNECTIONS   Lifespan Considerations

◀ **Reducing the Cost of Medications for Older Adults**

Because the cost of prescription drugs may be a major cause for nonadherence in the older adult, nurses should explore any cost concerns with these patients as well as discuss ways to cut pharmacy costs. Chan (2010) recommends several strategies that may help to reduce prescription costs, including:

- For a new prescription, do not buy a whole bottle; instead ask for just a few pills. Adverse effects may require a change in medication.
- Ask for generic drugs when receiving a prescription.
- Buy OTC generic drugs when possible.
- Ask if there is a therapeutic generic equivalent in the same class of a brand drug if a generic of that drug is not available. Request available assistance, such as a social worker, or access to a government or community program to reduce medication costs.
- Explore the use of drug "deals" such as the "$4 prescription" or "free antibiotics," which chain pharmacies may offer.
- Request a review of all medications taken so that nonessential drugs are no longer needed.
- Split pills when appropriate, with a higher dosage ordered and split in half, but only if able to follow directions explicitly.

PharmFACT

Off-label prescribing is common practice in pediatrics. One study found that over 90% of prescriptions for antidepressants in children were written for off-label indications (Lee et al., 2012).

▲ **PharmFacts** connect relevant statistics to the presented material. They add interest to the subject and place it in perspective with other nursing concepts.

CONNECTION Checkpoint 31.3

From what you learned in Chapter 28, what effect would you expect angiotensin II formation to have on cardiac output and afterload? *See Answer to Connection Checkpoint 31.3 on student resource website.*

◀ **Connection Checkpoints** ask the student to recall past concepts from previous chapters that are related to current study. Unique to this text, these reinforce material learned in previous chapters that has direct application to the current chapter.

▶ **Connections: Community-Oriented Practice** features provide important information that nurses need to convey to their patients to ensure that they receive effective pharmacotherapy after leaving the hospital or clinical setting.

CONNECTIONS   Community-Oriented Practice

◀ **Maintaining Fluid Balance During Exercise**

Hyponatremia from excessive fluid intake has been noted as a growing problem in athletes, particularly novice athletes who may have heard that they need to "keep drinking" to maintain hydration. Many sports drinks contain some electrolytes but are also high in fructose or other sugars. This creates a hypertonic solution that may paradoxically cause increased water loss. Unless exercise is extreme or prolonged, athletes, especially children, should be encouraged to drink when thirsty and maintain urine at a color of clear yellow, not dark yellow or colorless. Adequate fluid intake to match thirst will help ensure normal hydration and sodium levels and prevent complications such as exercise-associated hyponatremia (EAH).

Nursing Responsibilities:
- Assess for abdominal pain. Determine the type, intensity, and location of pain.
- Assess the patient for pork allergy because the enzymes in pancrelipase come from pork.
- Monitor intake and output ratio and weight. Note the patient's appetite and quality of stools, weight loss, abdominal bloating, polyuria, thirst, hunger, and itching. Pancreatic insufficiency is frequently associated with steatorrhea, bulky stools, and insulin-dependent diabetes. Dose may need to be regulated based on fat intake in the diet.

Lifespan and Diversity Considerations:
- Evaluate the child's or older adult's nutritional status and weigh weekly to ensure that adequate nutritional requirements are being met.

Patient and Family Education:
- Take this drug just before, during, or immediately after meals.

▶ **Nursing Responsibilities** specific to some prototype drugs are provided in a bulleted list format. Nursing Responsibilities include important life span and diversity considerations and patient and family education needs. When a prototype drug does not have a correlating Nursing Practice Application, a more complete Nursing Responsibilities section follows the prototype drug section.

Learning Through Visuals and Media

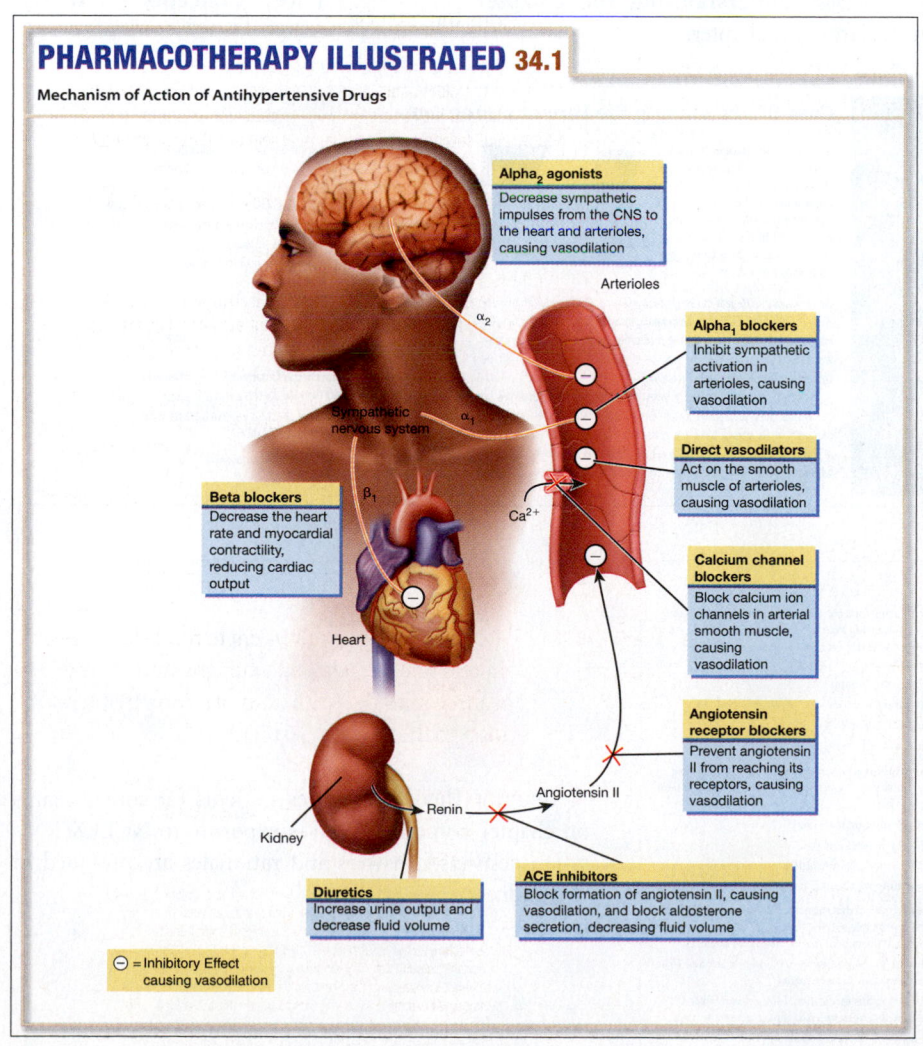

PHARMACOTHERAPY ILLUSTRATED 34.1

Mechanism of Action of Antihypertensive Drugs

Alpha₂ agonists
Decrease sympathetic impulses from the CNS to the heart and arterioles, causing vasodilation

Arterioles

Alpha₁ blockers
Inhibit sympathetic activation in arterioles, causing vasodilation

Direct vasodilators
Act on the smooth muscle of arterioles, causing vasodilation

Sympathetic nervous system

Beta blockers
Decrease the heart rate and myocardial contractility, reducing cardiac output

Heart

Calcium channel blockers
Block calcium ion channels in arterial smooth muscle, causing vasodilation

Angiotensin receptor blockers
Prevent angiotensin II from reaching its receptors, causing vasodilation

Kidney

Renin

Angiotensin II

Diuretics
Increase urine output and decrease fluid volume

ACE inhibitors
Block formation of angiotensin II, causing vasodilation, and block aldosterone secretion, decreasing fluid volume

⊖ = Inhibitory Effect causing vasodilation

◀ **Pharmacotherapy Illustrated** features visually present the mechanism of action for more than 33 of the prototype drugs, showing students specifically how drugs counteract the effects of disease.

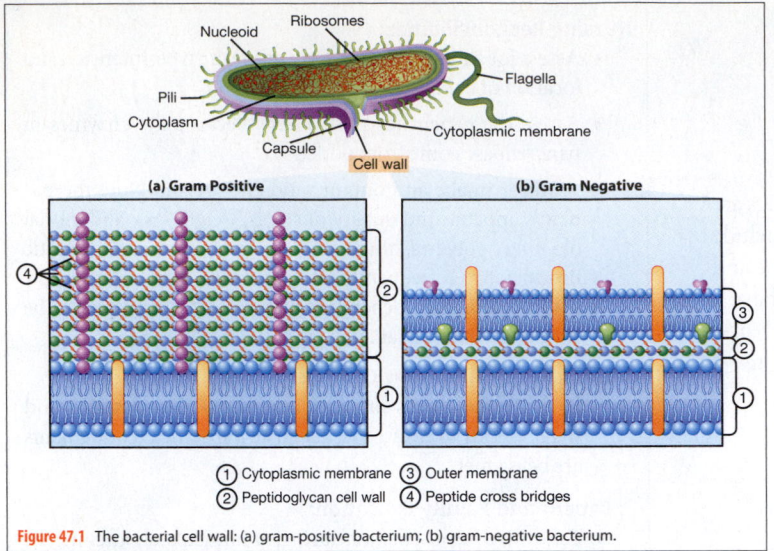

Figure 47.1 The bacterial cell wall: (a) gram-positive bacterium; (b) gram-negative bacterium.

① Cytoplasmic membrane ③ Outer membrane
② Peptidoglycan cell wall ④ Peptide cross bridges

◀ **Vivid, Colorful, and Effective Illustrations** help students review the anatomy, physiology, and pathophysiology of a body system to better understand the impact of disease on that system.

Understanding the Chapter

The most comprehensive chapter review in its class! **Understanding the Chapter** begins with a **Key Concepts Summary**, which quickly identifies the numbered key concepts from the chapter.

▶ **Making the Patient Connection** reconnects the student to the patient presented in the scenario at the chapter opening. The student learns additional details about the patient's health history and participates in critical thinking questions about the scenario. This allows application of knowledge obtained in the chapter.

Case Study: Making the Patient Connection

Remember the patient "Carlos Avaya" at the beginning of the chapter? Now read the remainder of the case study. Based on the information presented within this chapter, respond to the critical thinking questions that follow.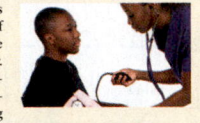

Carlos Avaya is a 26-year-old single man who was diagnosed with primary HTN 4 months ago. Carlos has been taking losartan (Cozaar) 50 mg daily PO and has been faithful in taking the medication as prescribed. When Carlos was told that his blood pressure was still elevated during this clinic visit, he was obviously distressed and concerned.

The health care team begins to investigate external factors that may be causing his blood pressure to remain elevated. Carlos has never smoked or used alcohol. He does not like to exercise but participates in a weekly game of soccer at the nearby community center. He denies being overly stressed with work or home life. Furthermore, he claims that he rarely salts his food.

The nurse asks Carlos to describe a typical day. During the description the nurse notices a concerning pattern. Because Carlos lives alone, he frequently cooks for himself. He admits that he enjoys salty foods such as pretzels and popcorn. He denies having consumed either prior to the visit to the clinic. However, to Carlos, cooking a meal involves preparing canned processed foods and frozen dinners. He never reads food labels. Without recording a complete dietary history, the nurse is able to determine that Carlos's intake of sodium-rich foods is quite extensive.

Critical Thinking Questions

1. In your own words, how would you describe how losartan (Cozaar) works to reduce blood pressure?

2. Considering the adverse effects of losartan (Cozaar), when would you instruct Carlos to notify the prescriber?

3. In addition to teaching Carlos about his losartan (Cozaar), what additional health teaching should he receive?

See Answers to Critical Thinking Questions on student resource website.

Chapter Review

1 The community health nurse teaches a patient at home. Lisinopril (Prinivil) has been prescribed for the patient. Which statement, if made by the patient, indicates that further teaching is necessary?
1. "I should notify my health care provider of symptoms of hypotension such as dizziness or fainting."
2. "I should avoid the use of salt substitutes containing potassium."
3. "If a dose is missed, I will take it as soon as possible but not too close to the next dose."
4. "Too much calcium in my diet will elevate my blood pressure."

2 The patient states, "I always keep my lisinopril (Prinivil) on my kitchen window sill. It helps me to remember to take it." The nurse's response would be based on which pharmacologic concept about heat and moisture?
1. They cause the medicine to break down.
2. They enhance the strength of the drug.
3. They crystallize the medication.
4. They convert the medicine to toxic metabolites.

3 A patient is hospitalized for uncontrolled hypertension and is receiving enalapril (Vasotec). The nurse should notify the health care provider if the patient exhibits:
1. Dry mucous membranes.
2. A decline in systolic blood pressure.
3. Nonproductive cough.
4. A reduction of diastolic blood pressure.

4 The nurse is caring for a patient with chronic hypertension. The patient is receiving losartan (Cozaar) daily. Which patient manifestations would the nurse conclude is an adverse effect of this medication?
1. Irritability and tremors
2. Headache and dizziness
3. Sleepiness and slurred speech
4. Pruritus and rash

5 Irbesartan (Avapro) is prescribed for each of the following patients. A nurse should question the order for which patient? A patient who has:
1. Severe dehydration from diuretic therapy.
2. Long-term diabetes mellitus.
3. A systolic blood pressure of 162.
4. A 5-year history of heart failure.

6 The nurse determines that the patient does not understand an important principle in self-administration of benazepril (Lotensin) when the patient makes which statement?
1. "I will learn to monitor my own blood pressure and write down all my daily measurements."
2. "While taking this medication, I should avoid over-the-counter medications for colds, sinus, or appetite control."
3. "This drug will not impair thinking and reaction time. I don't need to wait to start driving my car."
4. "Drinking alcohol while on this medication can lower my blood pressure and lead to dizziness and faintness."

See Answers to Chapter Review in Appendix A.

◀ **Chapter Review** prepares students for course exams on chapter content and gives exposure to NCLEX-RN®-style questions. Answers and rationales are provided in Appendix A.

► An **Additional Case Study** gives students another opportunity to apply their knowledge to patient care.

Additional Case Study

Sara Gaggi is a 51-year-old overweight white female with HTN who presents for an evaluation of heartburn that has been increasing in both intensity and frequency during the past 18 months. She reports epigastric burning after eating. It is worse after eating spicy foods or drinking red wine. She is occasionally awakened at night with symptoms. OTC antacids and H₂-receptor antagonists relieved her symptoms initially, but lately they have provided only minimal relief. Her only routine medication is amlodipine, a calcium channel blocker for her high blood pressure. Because the symptoms are increasing and her current therapy is not relieving her symptoms, an endoscopy was performed, which revealed the presence of GERD.

1. How would you describe to Sara the dangers of self-medicating GERD symptoms with OTC medications?
2. What three risk factors in this case predispose Sara for the development of GERD?
3. What medications will her health care provider likely prescribe?

See Answers to Additional Case Study on student resource website.

References

Anand, B. S. (2012). *Peptic ulcer disease*. Retrieved from http://emedicine.medscape .com/article/181753-overview#a0101

Barletta, J. F., El-Ibiary, S. Y., Davis, L. E., Nguyen, B., & Raney, C. R. (2013). Proton pump inhibitors and the risk for *Clostridium dificile* infection. *Mayo Clinic Proceedings, 88*, 1085–1090. doi:10.1016/j.mayocp.2013.07.004

Bavishi, C., & Dupont, H. L. (2011). Systematic review: The use of proton pump inhibitors and increased susceptibility to enteric infection. *Alimentary Pharmacology & Therapeutics, 34*, 1269–1281. doi:10.1111/j.1365-2036.2011.04874.x

Chung, E. Y., & Yardley, J. (2013). Are there risks associated with empiric acid suppression treatment in infants and children suspected of having gastroesophageal reflux disease? *Hospital Pediatrics, 3*(1), 16–23. doi:10.1542/peds.2012-0077

Fraser, L. A., Leslie, W. D., Targownik, L. E., Papaioannou, A., & Adachi, J. D. (2013). The effect of proton pump inhibitors on fracture risk: Report from the Canadian multicentre osteoporosis study. *Osteoporosis International, 24*, 1161–1168. doi:10.1007/s00198-012-2112-9

Gatta, L., Vakil, N., Vaira, D., & Scarpignato, C. (2013). Global eradication rates for *Helicobacter pylori* infection: Systematic review and meta-analysis of sequential therapy. *BMJ (Clinical Research Ed.), 347*, f4587. doi:10.1136/bmj.f4587

Gill, J. M., Player, M. S., & Metz, D. C. (2011). Balancing the risks and benefits of proton pump inhibitors. *Annals of Family Medicine, 9*, 200–202. doi:10.1370/afm.1269

Melius, E. J., Davis, S. I., Retid, J. T., Lewin, M., Herlihy, R., Henderson, A., . . . Cheek, J. E. (2013). Estimating the prevalence of active

Helicobacter pylori infection in a rural community with global positioning system technology-assisted sampling. *Epidemiology and Infection, 141*, 472–480. doi:10.1017/S0950268812000714

Patti, M. G. (2014). *Gastroesophageal reflux disease*. Retrieved from http://emedicine .medscape.com/article/176595-overview

Ramsay, E. N., Pratt, N. L., Ryan, P., & Roughead, E. E. (2013). Proton pump inhibitors and the risk of pneumonia: A comparison of cohort and self-controlled case series designs. *BMC Research Methodology, 13*, 82. doi:10.1186/1471-2288-13-82

◄ Detailed **References** and a **Selected Bibliography** provide the foundation for evidence-based nursing practice and support the currency and accuracy of the textbook content.

Selected Bibliography

Ahn, J. S., Eom, C. S., Jeon, C. Y., & Park, S. M. (2013). Acid suppressive drugs and gastric cancer: A meta-analysis of observational studies. *World Journal of Gastroenterology: WJG, 19*, 2560. doi:10.3748/wjg.v19.i16.2560

Gurney, S., Carvalho, L., Gonzalez, C., Galaviz, E., & Sonstein, F. (2014). An efficacious and cost-effective pharmacologic treatment for *Helicobacter pylori*. *The Journal for Nurse Practitioners, 10*, 22–29. doi:10.1016/j.nurpra.2013.09.013

Hart, A. M. (2013). Evidence-based recommendations for GERD treatment. *The Nurse*

Practitioner, 38(8), 26–34. doi:10.1097/01.NPR.0000431881.25363.84

Herdman, T. H., & Kamitsuru, S. (Eds.). (2014). *NANDA International nursing diagnoses: Definitions and classification, 2015–2017*. Oxford, United Kingdom: Wiley-Blackwell.

Hernández-Díaz, S., Martín-Merino, E., & Rodríguez, L. A. G. (2013). Risk of complications after a peptic ulcer diagnosis: Effectiveness of proton pump inhibitors. *Digestive Diseases and Sciences, 58*, 1653–1662. doi:10.1007/s10620-013-2561-9

Marmo, R., Bucci, C., Rea, M., & Rotondano, G. (2013). Treat the patient, not just the source of bleeding. *The American Journal of Gastroenterology, 108*(9), 1533–1534. doi:10.1038/ajg.2013.190

National Center for Complementary and Alternative Medicine. (2012). *Herbs at a glance: Ginger*. Retrieved from http://nccam.nih .gov/health/ginger

New to the Third Edition

• Updated Connections features cover current topics that nurses will face in practice.

• Connections: Nursing Practice Applications include important life span and diverse patient considerations that are needed to ensure effective pharmacotherapy and patient safety.

• NCLEX-RN®-style review questions include an increased number of "select all that apply" to better prepare students for these questions on the actual exam.

• New chapter added on Individual Variations in Drug Responses to reflect some of the factors that affect pharmacotherapeutic outcomes.

• More than 25 new drugs added to update medications approved by the FDA since the previous edition.

• Revised art program: More than 20 figures have been added or revised in this edition to enhance the clarity of difficult pharmacologic concepts.

Contents

UNIT 1 Fundamental Principles of Pharmacology

CHAPTER 1 Introduction to Pharmacology: Concepts and Connections 2
Brief History of Pharmacology 3
Pharmacology: The Study of Medicines 4
Characteristics of an Ideal Drug 5
Classification of Drugs 5
Drug Prototypes 6
Naming Drugs 7
Connecting Pharmacology to Clinical Nursing Practice 8

CHAPTER 2 Drug Regulations 12
Patent Medicines 13
Brief History of Drug Legislation 13
Drug Standards 15
The U.S. Food and Drug Administration 16
Drug Approval 17
Changes to the Drug Approval Process 18
Prescription and Over-the-Counter Drugs 19
Drug Schedules 20
Prescriptive Authority for Nurses 20

CHAPTER 3 Pharmacokinetics 24
Introduction to Pharmacokinetics 25
Primary Processes of Pharmacokinetics 27
   Route of Administration 27 • Drug Concentration and Dose 30 •
   GI Tract Environment 30 • Blood Flow to the Absorption
   Site 31 • Drug Ionization 31 • Drug Interactions 31 •
   Surface Area 31
Time–Response Relationships 36

CHAPTER 4 Pharmacodynamics 42
Interpatient Variability 43
Therapeutic Index 44
Dose–Response Relationship 44
Potency and Efficacy 45
Receptor Theory 46
Agonists and Antagonists 48
Pharmacogenetics 48

CHAPTER 5 Adverse Drug Effects and Drug Interactions 52
Adverse Drug Effects 53
Drug Interactions 58

CHAPTER 6 Medication Errors and Risk Reduction 66
Medication Errors and Their Impact on Health Care 67
Factors Contributing to Medication Errors 67
Drug Names and Medication Errors 70
Reporting Medication Errors 70
Strategies for Reducing Medication Errors 72

CHAPTER 7 The Role of Complementary and Alternative Therapies in Pharmacotherapy 79
Types of Complementary and Alternative Therapies 80
History of Herbal Therapies 81
Standardization of Herbal Products 82
Dietary Supplement Regulation 84
Herb–Drug Interactions 85
Specialty Supplements 87

UNIT 2 Pharmacology and the Nurse–Patient Relationship

CHAPTER 8 Pharmacotherapy During Pregnancy and Lactation 92
Rationale for Drug Use During Pregnancy and Lactation 93
Pharmacotherapy During Pregnancy 93
Pharmacotherapy During Lactation 97

CHAPTER 9 Pharmacotherapy of the Pediatric Patient 103
Testing and Labeling of Pediatric Drugs 104
Pharmacokinetic Variables in Pediatric Patients 106
Pharmacologic Implications Associated with Growth and Development 107
Medication Safety for Pediatric Patients 109
Determining Pediatric Drug Dosages 110
Adverse Drug Reactions in Children and Promoting Adherence 110

CHAPTER 10 Pharmacotherapy of the Geriatric Patient 116
Polypharmacy 117
Physiological Changes Related to Aging 118
Pharmacokinetic and Pharmacodynamic Changes in Older Adults 118
Adherence and Drug Misuse Among Older Adults 120
Adverse Drug Reactions in Older Adults 121

CHAPTER 11 Individual Variations in Drug Responses 126
Psychosocial Influences 127
Cultural and Ethnic Variables 127
Genetic Influences 128
Gender Influences 130

UNIT 3 Pharmacology of the Autonomic Nervous System

CHAPTER 12 Review of Neurotransmitters and the Autonomic Nervous System 136
Overview of the Nervous System 137
Structure and Function of the Autonomic Nervous System 138
Synaptic Transmission 140
Cholinergic Transmission 142
   Cholinergic Receptors and Neurotransmitters 142 •
   Termination of Acetylcholine Action 143
Adrenergic Transmission 144
   Alpha-Adrenergic Receptors 145 • Beta-Adrenergic
   Receptors 145 • Termination of Norepinephrine Action 145
Regulation of Autonomic Functions 146
Classifying Autonomic Drugs 147

CHAPTER 13 Cholinergic Agonists 149

Cholinergic Receptors 150

Muscarinic Agonists 152

> PROTOTYPE DRUG: Bethanechol (Urecholine) 153

Pharmacotherapy of Myasthenia Gravis 155

> PROTOTYPE DRUG: Pyridostigmine (Mestinon, Regonol) 157

Nicotinic Agonists 158

> CONNECTIONS: Nursing Practice Application Patients Receiving Pharmacotherapy with Cholinergic Agonists 159

CHAPTER 14 Cholinergic Antagonists 163

Classification of Cholinergic Antagonists 164

Muscarinic Antagonists 165

> PROTOTYPE DRUG: Atropine (Atropen) 166

Nicotinic Antagonists: Ganglionic Blockers 168

Nicotinic Antagonists: Neuromuscular Blockers 168

> PROTOTYPE DRUG: Succinylcholine (Anectine, Quelicin) 170

> CONNECTIONS: Nursing Practice Application Patients Receiving Pharmacotherapy with Cholinergic (Muscarinic) Antagonists 173

CHAPTER 15 Adrenergic Agonists 177

Actions of Adrenergic Agonists 178

Mechanisms of Action of Adrenergic Agonists 178

Classification of Adrenergic Agonists 179

Nonselective Adrenergic Agonists 180

> PROTOTYPE DRUG: Epinephrine (Adrenalin) 181

Alpha-Adrenergic Agonists 183

> PROTOTYPE DRUG: Phenylephrine (Neo-Synephrine) 184

Beta-Adrenergic Agonists 185

> PROTOTYPE DRUG: Isoproterenol (Isuprel) 186

> CONNECTIONS: Nursing Practice Application Patients Receiving Pharmacotherapy with Adrenergic Agonists 187

CHAPTER 16 Adrenergic Antagonists 192

Actions of Adrenergic Antagonists 193

Alpha-Adrenergic Antagonists 193

> PROTOTYPE DRUG: Prazosin (Minipress) 196

Beta-Adrenergic Antagonists 197

> PROTOTYPE DRUG: Propranolol (Inderal, InnoPran XL) 199

> PROTOTYPE DRUG: Metoprolol (Lopressor, Toprol XL) 201

> CONNECTIONS: Nursing Practice Application Patients Receiving Pharmacotherapy with Adrenergic Antagonists 203

UNIT 4   Pharmacology of the Central Nervous System

CHAPTER 17 Review of the Central Nervous System 208

Scope of Central Nervous System Pharmacology 209

Neurons and Neurotransmission 210

Structural Divisions of the Central Nervous System 211

Functional Systems of the Central Nervous System 213

CHAPTER 18 Pharmacotherapy of Anxiety and Sleep Disorders 216

Anxiety Disorders 217

Sleep Disorders 220

Management of Anxiety and Sleep Disorders 222

Pharmacotherapy of Anxiety and Insomnia 224

> PROTOTYPE DRUG: Lorazepam (Ativan) 226

> PROTOTYPE DRUG: Zolpidem (Ambien, Edluar, Others) 229

> PROTOTYPE DRUG: Phenobarbital (Luminal) 232

> CONNECTIONS: Nursing Practice Application Patients Receiving Pharmacotherapy for Anxiety or Sleep Disorders 234

CHAPTER 19 Pharmacotherapy of Mood Disorders 239

Categories of Mood Disorders 240

Major Depressive Disorder 240

Pathophysiology of Depression 241

Assessment of Depression 242

Nonpharmacologic Therapies for Depression 243

Pharmacotherapy of Depression 244

> *Tricyclic Antidepressants 244*

> PROTOTYPE DRUG: Imipramine (Tofranil) 246

> *Selective Serotonin Reuptake Inhibitors 248*

> PROTOTYPE DRUG: Fluoxetine (Prozac, Sarafem) 248

> *Atypical Antidepressants 250*

> PROTOTYPE DRUG: Venlafaxine (Effexor) 251

> *Monoamine Oxidase Inhibitors 253*

> PROTOTYPE DRUG: Phenelzine (Nardil) 254

> CONNECTIONS: Nursing Practice Application Patients Receiving Pharmacotherapy with Antidepressants 255

Bipolar Disorder 257

Drugs for Bipolar Disorder 257

> PROTOTYPE DRUG: Lithium Carbonate (Eskalith, Lithobid) 258

CHAPTER 20 Pharmacotherapy of Psychoses 264

Characteristics of Psychoses 265

Symptoms of Schizophrenia 265

Etiology of Schizophrenia 267

Management of Psychoses 268

Antipsychotic Drugs 269

> *First-Generation Antipsychotics 270*

> PROTOTYPE DRUG: Chlorpromazine 272

> PROTOTYPE DRUG: Haloperidol (Haldol) 273

> *Second-Generation (Atypical) Antipsychotics 274*

> PROTOTYPE DRUG: Risperidone (Risperdal) 274

> PROTOTYPE DRUG: Aripiprazole (Abilify) 277

> CONNECTIONS: Nursing Practice Application Patients Receiving Pharmacotherapy with Antipsychotics 279

CHAPTER 21 Pharmacotherapy of Degenerative Diseases of the Central Nervous System 285

Degenerative Diseases of the Central Nervous System 286

Parkinson's Disease 286

Pharmacotherapy of Parkinson's Disease 288

> PROTOTYPE DRUG: Levodopa and Carbidopa (Sinemet, Parcopa) 289

> PROTOTYPE DRUG: Pramipexole (Mirapex) 291

> PROTOTYPE DRUG: Benztropine (Cogentin) 294

Alzheimer's Disease 295

Pharmacotherapy of Alzheimer's Disease 296

> PROTOTYPE DRUG: Donepezil (Aricept) 298

Multiple Sclerosis 300

> PROTOTYPE DRUG: Interferon beta-1b (Betaseron, Extavia, Plegridy) 301

Amyotrophic Lateral Sclerosis 304

> CONNECTIONS: Nursing Practice Application Patients Receiving Pharmacotherapy for Neurodegenerative Disorders 304

CHAPTER 22 **Pharmacotherapy of Seizures 309**
Characteristics of Seizure Disorders 310
Classification of Seizure Disorders 313
Generalized Seizures 313 • Partial Seizures 314
Antiepileptic Drugs 317

PROTOTYPE DRUG: Diazepam (Valium) 320

PROTOTYPE DRUG: Phenytoin (Dilantin, Phenytek) 322

PROTOTYPE DRUG: Carbamazepine (Carbatrol, Tegretol, Others) 323

PROTOTYPE DRUG: Ethosuximide (Zarontin) 325

PROTOTYPE DRUG: Gabapentin (Neurontin) 326

PROTOTYPE DRUG: Valproic Acid (Depacon, Depakene, Depakote) 326
Other Miscellaneous Drugs 327

CONNECTIONS: Nursing Practice Application
Patients Receiving Pharmacotherapy for Seizures 329

CHAPTER 23 **Pharmacotherapy of Muscle Spasms and Spasticity 334**
Etiology and Pathophysiology of Muscle Spasms and Spasticity 335
Nonpharmacologic Therapies for Muscle Spasms and Spasticity 336
Pharmacotherapy of Muscle Spasms 337

PROTOTYPE DRUG: Cyclobenzaprine (Amrix, Flexeril) 338
Pharmacotherapy of Muscle Spasticity 341

PROTOTYPE DRUG: Dantrolene (Dantrium, Revonto) 342
Skeletal Muscle Relaxants as Surgical Adjuncts 345

CONNECTIONS: Nursing Practice Application Patients Receiving Pharmacotherapy for Muscle Spasms and Spasticity 345

CHAPTER 24 **Central Nervous System Stimulants and Drugs for Attention Deficit/Hyperactivity Disorder 350**
Characteristics of Central Nervous System Stimulants 351
Etiology and Pathophysiology of Attention Deficit/Hyperactivity Disorder 352
Pharmacotherapy of Attention Deficit/Hyperactivity Disorder 353

PROTOTYPE DRUG: Amphetamine and Dextroamphetamine (Adderall, Adderall XR) 355

PROTOTYPE DRUG: Atomoxetine (Strattera) 357
Pharmacotherapy of Narcolepsy 358

PROTOTYPE DRUG: Modafinil (Provigil) 358
Methylxanthines 359

PROTOTYPE DRUG: Caffeine 359

CONNECTIONS: Nursing Practice Application Patients Receiving Pharmacotherapy with Central Nervous System Stimulants 361

CHAPTER 25 **Pharmacotherapy of Severe Pain and Migraines 366**
General Principles of Pain Management 367
Pain Management with Opioids 372

PROTOTYPE DRUG: Morphine Sulfate (Astramorph PF, Duramorph RF, Roxanol, Others) 376
Pain Management with Nonopioids 379

PROTOTYPE DRUG: Tramadol (Ultram, Others) 379

CONNECTIONS: Nursing Practice Application
Patients Receiving Pharmacotherapy for Pain 380
Pharmacotherapy with Opioid Antagonists 384
Pharmacotherapy of Migraines 385

PROTOTYPE DRUG: Sumatriptan (Imitrex, Others) 387

CONNECTIONS: Nursing Practice Application
Patients Receiving Pharmacotherapy for Migraines 390

CHAPTER 26 **Anesthetics and Anesthesia Adjuncts 394**
Types of Anesthesia 395
Principles of General Anesthesia 395
Intravenous Anesthetics 396

PROTOTYPE DRUG: Fentanyl (Sublimaze) 396

PROTOTYPE DRUG: Midazolam (Versed) 398

PROTOTYPE DRUG: Propofol (Diprivan) 399
Inhalation Anesthetics 401

PROTOTYPE DRUG: Nitrous Oxide 402

PROTOTYPE DRUG: Isoflurane (Forane) 403
Local Anesthetics 404

CONNECTIONS: Nursing Practice Application
Patients Receiving General Anesthesia 407

PROTOTYPE DRUG: Procaine (Novocaine) 408

PROTOTYPE DRUG: Lidocaine (Anestacon, Dilocaine, Xylocaine, Others) 410
Adjuncts to Anesthesia 411

CONNECTIONS: Nursing Practice Application
Patients Receiving Local Anesthesia 412

CHAPTER 27 **Pharmacology of Substance Abuse 416**
Fundamental Concepts of Substance Abuse 417
Legislation of Controlled Substances 418 • Addiction and Dependence 418 • Tolerance 419
Central Nervous System Depressants 420
Sedatives and Antianxiety Drugs 421 • Opioids 421

PROTOTYPE DRUG: Buprenorphine with naloxone (Suboxone, Zubsolv) 422
Alcohol (Ethanol) 423

PROTOTYPE DRUG: Disulfiram (Antabuse) 426
Marijuana and Related Substances 426
Hallucinogens 427
LSD and Similar Hallucinogens 427
Club Drugs and Miscellaneous Hallucinogens 428
Central Nervous System Stimulants 429
Amphetamines and Methylphenidate 429 • Cocaine 430 • Caffeine 431
Nicotine 431

PROTOTYPE DRUG: Varenicline (Chantix) 432
Inhalants 432

CONNECTIONS: Nursing Practice Application Patients Receiving Pharmacotherapy for Substance Abuse Disorders 433
Anabolic Steroids 434

UNIT 5   Pharmacology of the Cardiovascular System

CHAPTER 28 **Review of the Cardiovascular System 440**
Structure and Function of the Cardiovascular System 441
Functions and Properties of Blood 441
Cardiac Structure and Function 444
Hemodynamics and Blood Pressure 448

CHAPTER 29 Pharmacotherapy of Hyperlipidemia 453

Types of Lipids and Lipoproteins 454

Measurement and Control of Serum Lipids 456

Drugs for Dyslipidemias 458

> PROTOTYPE DRUG: Atorvastatin (Lipitor) 462
>
> PROTOTYPE DRUG: Cholestyramine (Questran) 464
>
> PROTOTYPE DRUG: Gemfibrozil (Lopid) 466
> *Miscellaneous Drugs for Dyslipidemias 467*
>
> CONNECTIONS: Nursing Practice Application Patients Receiving Pharmacotherapy for Hyperlipidemia 468

CHAPTER 30 Pharmacotherapy with Calcium Channel Blockers 473

Physiological Role of Calcium Channels in Muscle Contraction 474

Types of Calcium Channels 475

Consequences of Calcium Channel Blockade 475

Classification of Calcium Channel Blockers 476

> PROTOTYPE DRUG: Nifedipine (Adalat CC, Procardia XL) 477
>
> PROTOTYPE DRUG: Verapamil (Calan, Isoptin, Verelan) 480
>
> CONNECTIONS: Nursing Practice Application Patients Receiving Pharmacotherapy with Calcium Channel Blockers 482

CHAPTER 31 Drugs Affecting the Renin-Angiotensin-Aldosterone System 486

Components of the Renin-Angiotensin-Aldosterone System 487

Physiological Actions of the Renin-Angiotensin-Aldosterone System 489

Drugs Affecting the Renin-Angiotensin-Aldosterone System 490

> PROTOTYPE DRUG: Lisinopril (Prinivil, Zestril) 491
>
> PROTOTYPE DRUG: Losartan (Cozaar) 493
>
> CONNECTIONS: Nursing Practice Application Patients Receiving Pharmacotherapy with Angiotensin-Converting Enzyme Inhibitors and Angiotensin Receptor Blockers 496

CHAPTER 32 Diuretic Therapy and the Pharmacotherapy of Renal Failure 501

Review of Renal Physiology 502

Pharmacotherapy for Patients with Renal Failure 504

Diuretic Therapy 505

> *Loop (High-Ceiling) Diuretics 506*
>
> PROTOTYPE DRUG: Furosemide (Lasix) 508
> *Thiazide and Thiazide-Like Diuretics 509*
>
> PROTOTYPE DRUG: Hydrochlorothiazide (Microzide) 510
> *Potassium-Sparing Diuretics 511*
>
> PROTOTYPE DRUG: Spironolactone (Aldactone) 512
> *Osmotic Diuretics 513*
>
> PROTOTYPE DRUG: Mannitol (Osmitrol) 514
> *Carbonic Anhydrase Inhibitors 515*
>
> PROTOTYPE DRUG: Acetazolamide (Diamox) 515
>
> CONNECTIONS: Nursing Practice Application Patients Receiving Pharmacotherapy with Diuretics 516

CHAPTER 33 Pharmacotherapy of Fluid Imbalance, Electrolyte, and Acid–Base Disorders 521

Principles of Fluid Balance 522

Fluid Replacement Agents 523

> PROTOTYPE DRUG: Normal Serum Albumin (Albuminar, Plasbumin, Others) 525
>
> PROTOTYPE DRUG: 5% Dextrose in Water (D_5W) 526
>
> PROTOTYPE DRUG: Dextran 40 (Gentran 40, Others) 527

Physiology of Electrolytes 528

Pharmacotherapy of Electrolyte Imbalances 528

> PROTOTYPE DRUG: Sodium Chloride (NaCl) 530
>
> PROTOTYPE DRUG: Potassium Chloride (KCl) 531
>
> PROTOTYPE DRUG: Magnesium Sulfate ($MgSO_4$) 532

Pharmacotherapy of Acid–Base Imbalances 533

> PROTOTYPE DRUG: Sodium Bicarbonate 534
>
> PROTOTYPE DRUG: Ammonium Chloride 535
>
> CONNECTIONS: Nursing Practice Application Patients Receiving Pharmacotherapy for Fluid and Electrolyte Imbalances 536

CHAPTER 34 Pharmacotherapy of Hypertension 541

Etiology and Pathogenesis of Hypertension 542

Nonpharmacologic Management of Hypertension 543

Guidelines for the Management of Hypertension 543

Pharmacotherapy of Hypertension 544

> *Initial Drug of Choice 544 • Adding Drugs to the Antihypertensive Regimen 544 • Enhancing Patient Adherence 546 • Antihypertensives in African Americans 546*

Drug Classes for Hypertension 546

> PROTOTYPE DRUG: Hydralazine (Apresoline) 551

Management of Hypertensive Emergency 552

> PROTOTYPE DRUG: Nitroprusside Sodium (Nitropress) 552
>
> CONNECTIONS: Nursing Practice Application Patients Receiving Pharmacotherapy with Direct Vasodilators 554

CHAPTER 35 Pharmacotherapy of Angina Pectoris and Myocardial Infarction 559

Pathophysiology of Myocardial Ischemia 560

> *Myocardial Oxygen Supply 560 • Myocardial Oxygen Demand 560*

Etiology of Coronary Artery Disease 560

Pathophysiology of Angina Pectoris 561

Nonpharmacologic Therapy of Coronary Artery Disease 562

Pharmacologic Management of Angina Pectoris 562

Drug Classes for Angina Pectoris 564

> PROTOTYPE DRUG: Nitroglycerin (Nitrostat, Nitro-Bid, Nitro-Dur, Others) 565
>
> PROTOTYPE DRUG: Atenolol (Tenormin) 566

Pathophysiology of Myocardial Infarction 567

Pharmacologic Management of Myocardial Infarction 569

> *Aspirin 569 • Anticoagulants and Antiplatelet Drugs 571 • Nitrates 572 • Beta-Adrenergic Blockers 572 • Angiotensin-Converting Enzyme Inhibitors 572 • Pain Management 572*
>
> CONNECTIONS: Nursing Practice Application Patients Receiving Pharmacotherapy with Organic Nitrates for Angina and Myocardial Infarction 573

CHAPTER 36 Pharmacotherapy of Heart Failure 578

Etiology of Heart Failure 579

Pathophysiology of Heart Failure 579

Ventricular Hypertrophy 579 • Activation of the Sympathetic Nervous System 580 • Increased Plasma Volume and Preload 581 • Natriuretic Peptides and Neurohumoral Factors 581

Pharmacologic Management of Heart Failure 581

Drugs for Heart Failure 582

PROTOTYPE DRUG: Digoxin (Lanoxin, Lanoxicaps) 587

PROTOTYPE DRUG: Milrinone (Primacor) 589

CONNECTIONS: Nursing Practice Application   Patients Receiving Pharmacotherapy for Heart Failure 591

CHAPTER 37 Pharmacotherapy of Dysrhythmias 596

Etiology of Dysrhythmias 597

Phases and Measurement of the Cardiac Action Potential 597

Classification of Dysrhythmias 599

General Principles of Dysrhythmia Management 600

Drugs for Dysrhythmias 601

Sodium Channel Blockers: Class I 601

PROTOTYPE DRUG: Procainamide 604

Beta-Adrenergic Antagonists: Class II 606 • Potassium Channel Blockers: Class III 607

PROTOTYPE DRUG: Amiodarone (Cordarone, Pacerone) 607

Calcium Channel Blockers: Class IV 609 • Miscellaneous Antidysrhythmics 609

CONNECTIONS: Nursing Practice Application   Patients Receiving Pharmacotherapy for Dysrhythmias 610

CHAPTER 38 Pharmacotherapy of Coagulation Disorders 614

Disorders of Hemostasis 615

Overview of Coagulation Modifiers 617

Anticoagulants 617

PROTOTYPE DRUG: Heparin 619

PROTOTYPE DRUG: Warfarin (Coumadin) 621

PROTOTYPE DRUG: Dabigatran (Pradaxa) 623

CONNECTIONS: Nursing Practice Application   Patients Receiving Pharmacotherapy with Anticoagulants 624

Antiplatelet Drugs 626

PROTOTYPE DRUG: Clopidogrel (Plavix) 627

PROTOTYPE DRUG: Abciximab (ReoPro) 629

Drugs for Intermittent Claudication 630

Thrombolytics 631

PROTOTYPE DRUG: Alteplase (Activase) 632

CONNECTIONS: Nursing Practice Application   Patients Receiving Pharmacotherapy with Thrombolytics 633

Hemostatics 635

PROTOTYPE DRUG: Aminocaproic Acid (Amicar) 635

Drugs for Hemophilia 636

von Willebrand's Disease 638

CHAPTER 39 Pharmacotherapy of Hematopoietic Disorders 642

Physiology of Hematopoiesis 643

Hematopoietic Growth Factors 643

PROTOTYPE DRUG: Epoetin Alfa (Epogen, Procrit) 644

PROTOTYPE DRUG: Filgrastim (Neupogen) 646

CONNECTIONS: Nursing Practice Application   Patients Receiving Pharmacotherapy with Erythropoietin 647

CONNECTIONS: Nursing Practice Application   Patients Receiving Pharmacotherapy with Colony-Stimulating Factors 649

PROTOTYPE DRUG: Oprelvekin (Neumega) 651

Classification of Anemias 652

Antianemic Drugs 653

PROTOTYPE DRUG: Ferrous Sulfate (Feosol, Feostat, Others) 655

PROTOTYPE DRUG: Cyanocobalamin (Nascobal) 658

UNIT 6   Pharmacology of Body Defenses

CHAPTER 40 Review of Body Defenses and the Immune System 664

Organization of the Lymphatic System 665

Innate (Nonspecific) Body Defenses 665

Inflammation 667

Specific (Adaptive) Body Defenses 668

Humoral Immune Response 669 • Cell-Mediated Immune Response 670

CHAPTER 41 Pharmacotherapy of Inflammation and Fever 672

Pathophysiology of Inflammation and Fever 673

Pharmacotherapy of Inflammation 673

Nonsteroidal Anti-Inflammatory Drugs 674

Salicylates 674

PROTOTYPE DRUG: Aspirin (Acetylsalicylic Acid) 676

Ibuprofen-Like Drugs 679

PROTOTYPE DRUG: Ibuprofen (Advil, Motrin, Others) 679

Cyclooxygenase-2 Inhibitors 682

PROTOTYPE DRUG: Celecoxib (Celebrex) 682

Antipyretic and Analgesic Drugs 683

PROTOTYPE DRUG: Acetaminophen (Tylenol) 683

CONNECTIONS: Nursing Practice Application   Patients Receiving Pharmacotherapy for Inflammation and Fever 685

CHAPTER 42 Immunostimulants and Immunosuppressants 689

Immunostimulants 690

PROTOTYPE DRUG: Interferon Alfa-2b (Intron A) 691

PROTOTYPE DRUG: Aldesleukin (Proleukin) 694

Immunosuppressants 695

PROTOTYPE DRUG: Cyclosporine (Gengraf, Neoral, Sandimmune) 698

PROTOTYPE DRUG: Azathioprine (Azasan, Imuran) 700

PROTOTYPE DRUG: Basiliximab (Simulect) 703

CONNECTIONS: Nursing Practice Application   Patients Receiving Pharmacotherapy with Immunomodulators 704

CHAPTER 43 Immunizing Agents 709

Discovery of Vaccines 710

Vaccines and the Immune System 710

Types of Vaccines 711

General Principles of Vaccine Administration 712

Active Immunity: Bacterial Immunizations 712

Diphtheria 713 • Pertussis (Whooping Cough) 714 • Tetanus 714 • Pneumococcus 714 • Meningococcus 715

Active Immunity: Viral Immunizations 715

Hepatitis B 715

PROTOTYPE DRUG: Hepatitis B Vaccine (Engerix-B, Recombivax HB) 716

Hepatitis A 717 • Influenza 717 • Rabies 717 • Measles, Mumps, and Rubella 718 • Polio 719 • Varicella Zoster 719 • Human Papillomavirus 720 • Rotavirus 720

Passive Immunity 721

PROTOTYPE DRUG: Rh₀[D] Immune Globulin (RhoGAM) 721

CONNECTIONS: Nursing Practice Application Patients Receiving Immunizations 724

UNIT 7 Pharmacology of the Respiratory System and Allergy

CHAPTER 44 **Pharmacotherapy of Asthma and Other Pulmonary Disorders 730**

Physiology of the Lower Respiratory Tract 731

Pathophysiology of Asthma 732

Administration of Pulmonary Drugs via Inhalation 733

Principles of Asthma Pharmacotherapy 734

PROTOTYPE DRUG: Albuterol (Proventil, Ventolin, VoSpire) 736

PROTOTYPE DRUG: Ipratropium (Atrovent) 739

PROTOTYPE DRUG: Beclomethasone (Beconase AQ, Qvar) 740

PROTOTYPE DRUG: Cromolyn 742

PROTOTYPE DRUG: Zafirlukast (Accolate) 743

PROTOTYPE DRUG: Theophylline (Theo-Dur, Others) 744

Chronic Obstructive Pulmonary Disease 745

CONNECTIONS: Nursing Practice Application Patients Receiving Pharmacotherapy for Asthma and COPD 746

CHAPTER 45 **Pharmacotherapy of Allergic Rhinitis and the Common Cold 752**

Physiology of the Upper Respiratory Tract 753

Pathophysiology of Allergic Rhinitis 754

Pharmacotherapy of Allergic Rhinitis 754

PROTOTYPE DRUG: Fexofenadine (Allegra) 758

CONNECTIONS: Nursing Practice Application Patients Receiving Pharmacotherapy with Antihistamines 760

PROTOTYPE DRUG: Fluticasone (Flonase, Veramyst) 762

Decongestants 763

PROTOTYPE DRUG: Pseudoephedrine (Sudafed) 763

Drugs for the Common Cold 765

Antitussives 765

PROTOTYPE DRUG: Dextromethorphan (Delsym, Robitussin DM, Others) 766

Expectorants and Mucolytics 767

CONNECTIONS: Nursing Practice Application Patients Receiving Pharmacotherapy for Symptomatic Cough and Cold Relief 768

UNIT 8 Pharmacology of Infectious and Neoplastic Diseases

CHAPTER 46 **Basic Principles of Anti-Infective Pharmacotherapy 774**

Pathogenicity and Virulence 775

Describing and Classifying Bacteria 776

Classification of Anti-Infectives 776

Mechanisms of Action of Anti-Infectives 776

Inhibition of Cell Wall Synthesis 778 • Inhibition of Protein Synthesis 778 • Disruption of the Plasma Cell Membrane 778 •

Inhibition of Nucleic Acid Synthesis 778 • Inhibition of Metabolic Pathways (Antimetabolites) 778 • Other Mechanisms of Action 778

Acquired Resistance 779

Mechanisms of Resistance 779 • Promotion of Resistance 780 • Prevention of Resistant Strains 780

Indications and Selection of Specific Anti-Infectives 782

Host Factors Affecting Anti-Infective Selection 783

Host Defenses 783 • Local Tissue Conditions 783 • Allergy History 783 • Other Host Factors 784

Superinfections 784

CHAPTER 47 **Antibiotics Affecting the Bacterial Cell Wall 786**

Structure of Bacterial Cell Walls 787

Penicillins 788

Natural Penicillins 790

PROTOTYPE DRUG: Penicillin G 790

Broad-Spectrum Penicillins (Aminopenicillins) 791

PROTOTYPE DRUG: Ampicillin (Principen) 792

Extended-Spectrum (Antipseudomonal) Penicillins 792 • Penicillinase-Resistant (Antistaphylococcal) Penicillins 793

Cephalosporins 794

PROTOTYPE DRUG: Cefazolin (Ancef, Kefzol) 795

Carbapenems 797

PROTOTYPE DRUG: Imipenem-Cilastatin (Primaxin) 797

Miscellaneous Cell Wall Inhibitors 798

PROTOTYPE DRUG: Vancomycin (Vancocin) 798

CONNECTIONS: Nursing Practice Application Patients Receiving Pharmacotherapy with a Penicillin, Cephalosporin, or Vancomycin Antibiotic 800

CHAPTER 48 **Antibiotics Affecting Bacterial Protein Synthesis 804**

Mechanisms of Antibiotic Inhibition of Bacterial Protein Synthesis 805

Tetracyclines 806

PROTOTYPE DRUG: Tetracycline (Sumycin, Others) 808

Macrolides 809

PROTOTYPE DRUG: Erythromycin (EryC, Erythrocin, Others) 810

Aminoglycosides 812

PROTOTYPE DRUG: Gentamicin (Garamycin, Others) 813

Miscellaneous Inhibitors of Bacterial Protein Synthesis 814

CONNECTIONS: Nursing Practice Application Patients Receiving Pharmacotherapy with a Tetracycline, Macrolide, or Aminoglycoside Antibiotic 816

CHAPTER 49 **Fluoroquinolones and Miscellaneous Antibacterials 821**

Bacterial DNA Replication 822

Inhibition of DNA Replication 822

Fluoroquinolones 823

Adverse Effects 824

PROTOTYPE DRUG: Ciprofloxacin (Cipro) 825

Miscellaneous Antibacterials 827

CONNECTIONS: Nursing Practice Application Patients Receiving Pharmacotherapy with Fluoroquinolones 828

CHAPTER 50 **Sulfonamides and the Pharmacotherapy of Urinary Tract Infections 833**

Pathophysiology of Urinary Tract Infections 834

Pharmacotherapy of Urinary Tract Infections 834
Acute Uncomplicated Cystitis 834 • Complicated Urinary Tract Infection 836 • Infants and Children 836 • Pregnancy 836 • Older Adults 837 • Recurring Urinary Tract Infections 837
Sulfonamides 837
Adverse Effects 839
PROTOTYPE DRUG: Trimethoprim-Sulfamethoxazole (Bactrim, Septra) 839
Urinary Antiseptics 841
PROTOTYPE DRUG: Nitrofurantoin (Furadantin) and Nitrofurantoin Macrocrystals (Macrobid, Macrodantin) 841
CONNECTIONS: Nursing Practice Application Patients Receiving Pharmacotherapy for Urinary Tract Infection 843

CHAPTER 51   Pharmacotherapy of Mycobacterial Infections 848
Types of Mycobacterial Infections 849
Pathogenesis and Diagnosis of Tuberculosis 849
Pharmacotherapy of Tuberculosis 851
Standard Regimen 852 • Patients Who Are HIV Positive 852 • Pregnant Patients 854 • Chemoprophylaxis Patients 854
PROTOTYPE DRUG: Isoniazid (INH) 855
Drugs for Leprosy 859
PROTOTYPE DRUG: Dapsone (DDS) 859
CONNECTIONS: Nursing Practice Application Patients Receiving Pharmacotherapy for Tuberculosis 860
Drugs for *Mycobacterium Avium* Complex Infections 862

CHAPTER 52   Pharmacotherapy of Fungal Infections 866
Characteristics of Fungi and Fungal Infections 867
Drugs for Systemic Fungal Infections 869
PROTOTYPE DRUG: Amphotericin B Deoxycholate (Fungizone) 870
Drugs for Both Systemic and Superficial Fungal Infections 872
PROTOTYPE DRUG: Fluconazole (Diflucan) 873
Drugs for Superficial Fungal Infections 874
PROTOTYPE DRUG: Nystatin (Mycostatin, Nystop, Others) 877
CONNECTIONS: Nursing Practice Application Patients Receiving Pharmacotherapy with Antifungals 879

CHAPTER 53   Pharmacotherapy of Protozoan and Helminthic Infections 884
Classification and Pathogenesis of Protozoan Infections 885
Drugs for Malaria 886
PROTOTYPE DRUG: Chloroquine (Aralen) 887
Drugs for Nonmalarial Protozoan Infections 890
PROTOTYPE DRUG: Metronidazole (Flagyl) 891
PROTOTYPE DRUG: Pyrimethamine (Daraprim) 895
Classification and Pathogenesis of Helminthic Infections 897
Drugs for Helminthic Infections 899
PROTOTYPE DRUG: Mebendazole (Vermox) 899
CONNECTIONS: Nursing Practice Application Patients Receiving Pharmacotherapy for Protozoan and Helminthic Infections 901

CHAPTER 54   Pharmacotherapy of Non-HIV Viral Infections 906
Characteristics of Viruses 907
Pharmacotherapy of Non-HIV Viral Infections 909
Drugs for Herpesviruses 910
PROTOTYPE DRUG: Acyclovir (Zovirax) 911
Drugs for Influenza Viruses 913
PROTOTYPE DRUG: Amantadine (Symmetrel) 914
Drugs for Hepatitis Viruses 915
PROTOTYPE DRUG: Tenofovir (Viread) 919
CONNECTIONS: Nursing Practice Application Patients Receiving Pharmacotherapy with Antivirals for Non-HIV Viral Infections 921

CHAPTER 55   Pharmacotherapy of HIV-AIDS 926
Pathogenesis of HIV Infection 927
General Principles of HIV Pharmacotherapy 929
Classification of Antiretroviral Drugs 931
Antiretroviral Drugs 933
PROTOTYPE DRUG: Zidovudine (Retrovir, AZT) 933
PROTOTYPE DRUG: Efavirenz (Sustiva) 935
PROTOTYPE DRUG: Lopinavir with Ritonavir (Kaletra) 937
Prophylaxis of HIV Infections 939
CONNECTIONS: Nursing Practice Application Patients Receiving Pharmacotherapy with Antiretrovirals 940
Pharmacotherapy of Opportunistic Infections Associated with HIV-AIDS 944

CHAPTER 56   Basic Principles of Antineoplastic Therapy 948
Characteristics of Cancer 949
Etiology of Cancer 950
Detection and Prevention of Cancer 950
Goals of Chemotherapy 951
Staging and Grading of Cancer 952
The Cell Cycle and Growth Fraction 952
Cell Kill Hypothesis 954
Improving the Success of Chemotherapy 955
Combination Chemotherapy 955 • Dosing Schedules 955 • Route of Administration 955
Toxicity of Antineoplastic Agents 956
Hematologic System 957 • Gastrointestinal Tract 957 • Cardiopulmonary System 958 • Urinary System 958 • Reproductive System 958 • Nervous System 958 • Skin and Soft Tissue 958 • Other Effects 958

CHAPTER 57   Pharmacotherapy of Neoplasia 962
Classification of Antineoplastic Drugs 963
Antineoplastic Medications 963
Alkylating Agents 963
PROTOTYPE DRUG: Cyclophosphamide (Cytoxan) 964
Antimetabolites 968
PROTOTYPE DRUG: Methotrexate (MTX, Rheumatrex, Trexall) 969
Antitumor Antibiotics 972
PROTOTYPE DRUG: Doxorubicin (Adriamycin) 973
Hormones and Hormone Antagonists 975
PROTOTYPE DRUG: Tamoxifen 976
Natural Products 980

PROTOTYPE DRUG: Vincristine (Oncovin) 981
Biologic Response Modifiers and Targeted Therapies 983
CONNECTIONS: Nursing Practice Application Patients Receiving Cancer Chemotherapy 983
Miscellaneous Antineoplastics 988
Drugs for Reducing Adverse Effects 991
Preparing and Administering Antineoplastics 992

UNIT 9   Pharmacology of the Gastrointestinal System

CHAPTER 58   Review of the Gastrointestinal System 996
Overview of the Digestive System 997
Physiology of the Upper Gastrointestinal Tract 997
Physiology of the Lower Gastrointestinal Tract 999
Physiology of the Accessory Organs of Digestion 1000
Regulation of Digestive Processes 1001
Nutrient Categories and Metabolism 1002

CHAPTER 59   Pharmacotherapy of Peptic Ulcer Disease 1004
Physiology of the Upper Gastrointestinal Tract 1005
Etiology and Pathogenesis of Peptic Ulcer Disease 1005
Etiology and Pathogenesis of Gastroesophageal Reflux Disease 1008
Pharmacotherapy of Peptic Ulcer Disease and Gastroesophageal Reflux Disease 1008
Pharmacotherapy with Proton Pump Inhibitors 1010
PROTOTYPE DRUG: Omeprazole (Prilosec) 1011
Pharmacotherapy with H$_2$-Receptor Antagonists 1013
PROTOTYPE DRUG: Ranitidine (Zantac) 1014
Pharmacotherapy with Antacids 1015
PROTOTYPE DRUG: Aluminum Hydroxide (AlternaGEL, Others) 1016
Pharmacotherapy of Helicobacter pylori Infection 1017 • Miscellaneous Drugs Used for Peptic Ulcer Disease and Gastroesophageal Reflux Disease 1018
CONNECTIONS: Nursing Practice Application Patients Receiving Pharmacotherapy for Peptic Ulcer Disease 1019

CHAPTER 60   Pharmacotherapy of Bowel Disorders and Other Gastrointestinal Conditions 1023
Pathophysiology of Constipation 1024
Pharmacotherapy with Laxatives 1025
PROTOTYPE DRUG: Psyllium Mucilloid (Metamucil, Others) 1026
Pathophysiology of Diarrhea 1027
Pharmacotherapy of Diarrhea 1028
PROTOTYPE DRUG: Diphenoxylate with Atropine (Lomotil) 1029
CONNECTIONS: Nursing Practice Application Patients Receiving Pharmacotherapy with Laxatives or Antidiarrheals 1030
Pharmacotherapy of Inflammatory Bowel Disease 1030
PROTOTYPE DRUG: Sulfasalazine (Azulfidine) 1033
Pharmacotherapy of Irritable Bowel Syndrome 1035
Pathophysiology of Nausea and Vomiting 1036
Pharmacotherapy of Nausea and Vomiting 1037
PROTOTYPE DRUG: Ondansetron (Zofran, Zuplenz) 1040
Pharmacotherapy of Pancreatitis 1041

PROTOTYPE DRUG: Pancrelipase (Creon, Pancreaze, Zenpep) 1041
CONNECTIONS: Nursing Practice Application Patients Receiving Pharmacotherapy with Antiemetics 1042

CHAPTER 61   Vitamins and Minerals 1047
Role of Vitamins in Health and Disease 1048
Regulation of Vitamins 1049
Recommended Dietary Allowance 1050
Fat-Soluble Vitamins 1051
Vitamin A (Aquasol A) 1051 • Vitamin D (Calcijex, Rocaltrol) 1051 • Vitamin E (Aquasol E, Vita-Plus E, Others) 1052 • Vitamin K (AquaMEPHYTON) 1053
Water-Soluble Vitamins 1053
Thiamine: Vitamin B$_1$ 1053 • Riboflavin: Vitamin B$_2$ 1054 • Niacin: Vitamin B$_3$ 1054 • Pyridoxine: Vitamin B$_6$ 1054 • Folic Acid: Vitamin B$_9$ 1055 • Cyanocobalamin: Vitamin B$_{12}$ 1055 • Vitamin C: Ascorbic Acid 1056
Minerals 1056
CONNECTIONS: Nursing Practice Application Patients Receiving Pharmacotherapy with Vitamin or Mineral Supplements 1058

CHAPTER 62   Enteral and Parenteral Nutrition 1062
Enteral Nutrition 1063
Methods of Administration 1064 • Enteral Formulations 1064 • Elements of Enteral Nutrition 1065 • Complications of Enteral Therapy 1065 • Drug and Food Interactions 1068
Parenteral Nutrition 1069
Components of Total Parenteral Nutrition Solutions 1070 • Complications of Parenteral Therapy 1071 • Drug and Food Interactions 1072
CONNECTIONS: Nursing Practice Application Patients Receiving Pharmacotherapy with Enteral and Parenteral Nutrition 1073

CHAPTER 63   Weight Reduction Strategies and the Pharmacotherapy of Obesity 1078
Etiology of Obesity 1079
Pathogenesis of Obesity 1079
Measurement of Obesity 1080
Nonpharmacologic Therapies for Obesity 1080
Pharmacotherapy of Obesity 1082
PROTOTYPE DRUG: Orlistat (Alli, Xenical) 1082
Adjuncts to Obesity Therapy 1085

UNIT 10   Pharmacology of the Endocrine System

CHAPTER 64   Review of the Endocrine System 1090
Overview of the Endocrine System 1091
Hormone Receptors 1091
Negative Feedback Mechanisms 1091
Hormone Pharmacotherapy 1093

CHAPTER 65   Hypothalamic and Pituitary Drugs 1096
Functions of the Hypothalamus 1097
Functions of the Pituitary Gland 1098
Pharmacotherapy of Growth Hormone Disorders 1098
PROTOTYPE DRUG: Somatropin (Genotropin, Humatrope, Norditropin, Nutropin, Saizen, Serostim, Zorbtive) 1099
PROTOTYPE DRUG: Octreotide (Sandostatin) 1102

Pharmacotherapy of Antidiuretic Hormone
Disorders 1103

CONNECTIONS: Nursing Practice Application Patients
Receiving Pharmacotherapy with Growth Hormone 1104

PROTOTYPE DRUG: Desmopressin (DDAVP) 1106

CONNECTIONS: Nursing Practice Application
Patients Receiving Pharmacotherapy with Antidiuretic
Hormone 1107

CHAPTER 66   Pharmacotherapy of Diabetes Mellitus 1111

Physiology of Serum Glucose Control 1112

Pathophysiology of Diabetes Mellitus: Types
of Diabetes 1113

Symptoms and Diagnosis of Diabetes 1114

Complications of Diabetes Mellitus 1114

PROTOTYPE DRUG: Glucagon (GlucaGen) 1115

Insulin Therapy 1117
Insulin Adjunct 1118

PROTOTYPE DRUG: Human Regular Insulin (Humulin R,
Novolin R) 1119

Antidiabetic Drugs for Type 2 Diabetes 1121

CONNECTIONS: Nursing Practice Application
Patients Receiving Pharmacotherapy with Insulin 1122
Sulfonylureas 1125

PROTOTYPE DRUG: Glyburide (DiaBeta, Glynase,
Micronase) 1125
Biguanides 1126

PROTOTYPE DRUG: Metformin (Glucophage, Glumetza,
Others) 1126
Meglitinides 1127

PROTOTYPE DRUG: Repaglinide (Prandin) 1127
Thiazolidinediones 1128

PROTOTYPE DRUG: Rosiglitazone (Avandia) 1128
Alpha-Glucosidase Inhibitors 1129

PROTOTYPE DRUG: Acarbose (Precose) 1129
Incretin Enhancers 1130

PROTOTYPE DRUG: Sitagliptin (Januvia) 1130

Miscellaneous Antidiabetic Drugs 1131

CONNECTIONS: Nursing Practice Application Patients
Receiving Pharmacotherapy for Type 2 Diabetes 1132

CHAPTER 67   Pharmacotherapy of Thyroid Disorders 1137

Physiology of the Thyroid Gland 1138

Diagnosis of Thyroid Disorders 1139

Hypothyroid Disorders 1140

Pharmacotherapy of Hypothyroid Disorders 1140

PROTOTYPE DRUG: Levothyroxine (Levothroid, Levoxyl,
Synthroid, Unithroid) 1141

Hyperthyroid Disorders 1142

CONNECTIONS: Nursing Practice Application Patients
Receiving Pharmacotherapy with Thyroid Hormone
Replacements 1143

Pharmacotherapy of Hyperthyroid Disorders 1145

PROTOTYPE DRUG: Propylthiouracil (PTU) 1145

CONNECTIONS: Nursing Practice Application Patients
Receiving Pharmacotherapy with Antithyroid Drugs 1147

CHAPTER 68   Corticosteroids and Drugs Affecting the Adrenal
Cortex 1151

Physiology of the Adrenal Gland 1152

Overview of Corticosteroid Pharmacotherapy 1153

Adverse Effects of Corticosteroids 1154

Replacement Therapy with Corticosteroids 1155

PROTOTYPE DRUG: Hydrocortisone (Cortef, Solu-Cortef,
Others) 1157

Corticosteroids for Nonendocrine Conditions 1158

CONNECTIONS: Nursing Practice Application Patients
Receiving Pharmacotherapy with Systemic Corticosteroids
1160

Mineralocorticoids 1162

PROTOTYPE DRUG: Fludrocortisone 1162

Antiadrenal Drugs 1163

CHAPTER 69   Estrogens, Progestins, and Drugs Modifying Uterine
Function 1166

Hormonal Regulation of Female Reproductive
Function 1167

Estrogens 1167

PROTOTYPE DRUG: Conjugated Estrogens (Cenestin, Enjuvia,
Premarin) 1168

Progestins 1171

PROTOTYPE DRUG: Medroxyprogesterone (Depo-Provera,
Depo-SubQ-Provera, Provera) 1171

CONNECTIONS: Nursing Practice Application Patients
Receiving Pharmacotherapy with Estrogen 1172

Hormone Replacement Therapy 1174

CONNECTIONS: Nursing Practice Application Patients
Receiving Pharmacotherapy with Progestin 1175

Uterine Stimulants: Oxytocics 1176

PROTOTYPE DRUG: Oxytocin (Pitocin) 1177

Uterine Relaxants: Tocolytics 1179

CONNECTIONS: Nursing Practice Application Patients
Receiving Pharmacotherapy with Oxytocin (Pitocin) 1180

Pharmacotherapy of Female Infertility 1181

PROTOTYPE DRUG: Clomiphene (Clomid, Serophene) 1183

CHAPTER 70   Drugs for Modifying Conception 1189

Options and Choices for Birth Control 1190

Combination Oral Contraceptives 1190

PROTOTYPE DRUG: Estradiol and Norethindrone (Ortho-
Novum, Others) 1194

Progestin-Only Oral Contraceptives 1195

Adverse Effects of Combined Oral Contraceptives 1196

Drugs for Long-Term Contraception and Newer
Contraceptive Delivery Methods 1197

Spermicides 1199

PROTOTYPE DRUG: Nonoxynol-9 1200

Emergency Contraception 1200

CONNECTIONS: Nursing Practice Application Patients
Receiving Hormonal Contraceptives 1201

Drugs for Pharmacologic Abortion 1202

PROTOTYPE DRUG: Mifepristone (Mifeprex) 1203

CHAPTER 71 Drugs for Disorders and Conditions of the Male Reproductive System 1208

Regulation of Male Reproductive Function 1209

Pharmacotherapy with Androgens 1210

PROTOTYPE DRUG: Testosterone 1211

Anabolic Steroids 1212

CONNECTIONS: Nursing Practice Application
Patients Receiving Pharmacotherapy with Androgens 1213

Etiology of Male Sexual Dysfunction 1214

Pharmacotherapy of Male Infertility 1215

Pharmacotherapy of Erectile Dysfunction 1216

PROTOTYPE DRUG: Sildenafil (Viagra) 1218

Pathophysiology of Benign Prostatic Hyperplasia 1219

Pharmacotherapy of Benign Prostatic Hyperplasia 1220

PROTOTYPE DRUG: Finasteride (Proscar) 1221

CONNECTIONS: Nursing Practice Application Patients Receiving Pharmacotherapy for Benign Prostatic Hyperplasia 1223

UNIT 11 Additional Drug Classes

CHAPTER 72 Pharmacotherapy of Bone and Joint Disorders 1228

Role of Calcium in Body Homeostasis 1229

Regulation of Calcium Balance 1230

Pharmacotherapy of Hypocalcemia 1232

PROTOTYPE DRUG: Calcium Salts 1232

Pathophysiology of Metabolic Bone Disease 1233

CONNECTIONS: Nursing Practice Application Patients Receiving Pharmacotherapy for Osteoporosis 1234

Pharmacotherapy of Metabolic Bone Disease 1237

PROTOTYPE DRUG: Calcitriol (Calcijet, Rocaltrol) 1237

PROTOTYPE DRUG: Alendronate (Fosamax) 1240

PROTOTYPE DRUG: Raloxifene (Evista) 1242

Pathophysiology and Pharmacotherapy of Joint Disorders 1244

PROTOTYPE DRUG: Hydroxychloroquine (Plaquenil) 1249

CONNECTIONS: Nursing Practice Application Patients Receiving Pharmacotherapy for Rheumatoid Arthritis and Osteoarthritis 1251

Pharmacotherapy of Gout and Hyperuricemia 1253

PROTOTYPE DRUG: Colchicine (Colcrys) 1253

PROTOTYPE DRUG: Allopurinol (Lopurin, Zyloprim) 1255

CONNECTIONS: Nursing Practice Application Patients Receiving Pharmacotherapy for Gout 1257

CHAPTER 73 Pharmacotherapy of Dermatologic Disorders 1261

Anatomy of the Integumentary System 1262

Classification of Skin Disorders 1263

Pharmacotherapy of Skin Infections 1264
  Scabicides and Pediculicides 1265

PROTOTYPE DRUG: Permethrin (Acticin, Elimite, Nix) 1265

Pharmacotherapy of Acne and Rosacea 1266
  Acne Vulgaris 1267

CONNECTIONS: Nursing Practice Application
Patients Receiving Pharmacotherapy for Lice or Mite Infestation 1267
  Rosacea 1269

PROTOTYPE DRUG: Tretinoin (Avita, Retin-A, Others) 1269

Pharmacotherapy of Dermatitis 1271

CONNECTIONS: Nursing Practice Application Patients Receiving Pharmacotherapy for Acne and Related Skin Conditions 1271

Pharmacotherapy of Psoriasis 1274
  Topical Drugs 1274
  Systemic Drugs 1275

Pharmacotherapy of Minor Skin Burns 1277

PROTOTYPE DRUG: Benzocaine (Americaine, Anbesol, Others) 1278

Pharmacotherapy of Alopecia 1279

CHAPTER 74 Pharmacotherapy of Eye and Ear Disorders 1283

Anatomy of the Eye 1284

Pathophysiology of Glaucoma 1286

Pharmacotherapy of Glaucoma 1286

PROTOTYPE DRUG: Latanoprost (Xalatan) 1287

PROTOTYPE DRUG: Timolol (Betimol, Timoptic, Others) 1290

CONNECTIONS: Nursing Practice Application Patients Receiving Pharmacotherapy for Glaucoma 1291
  Miscellaneous Drugs for Treating Glaucoma 1292

Pharmacotherapy for Eye Examinations 1292

Pharmacotherapy for Other Eye Conditions 1294

Anatomy of the Ear 1295

Pharmacotherapy with Otic Preparations 1295

CONNECTIONS: Nursing Practice Application Patients Receiving Pharmacotherapy for Otitis 1298

CHAPTER 75 Emergency Preparedness: Bioterrorism and Management of Poisoning 1302

Emergency Preparedness, Bioterrorism, and Nursing 1303

Biologic Agents 1305

Chemical and Physical Agents 1306

Management of Poisoning 1308

PROTOTYPE DRUG: Activated Charcoal (CharcoAid) 1309

PROTOTYPE DRUG: Edetate Calcium Disodium (Calcium EDTA) 1310

PROTOTYPE DRUG: Dimercaprol (BAL in Oil) 1311

CONNECTIONS: Nursing Practice Application
Patients Receiving Pharmacotherapy for Poisoning or Overdose 1312

Appendices

A Answers to Chapter Review 1316

B ISMP List of *High-Alert* Medications in Acute Care Settings 1343

Glossary 1344

Credits 1362

Index 1363

UNIT

1

Fundamental Principles of Pharmacology

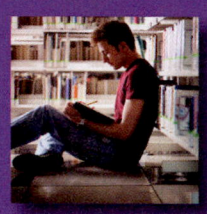 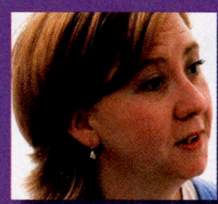 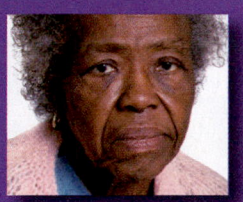 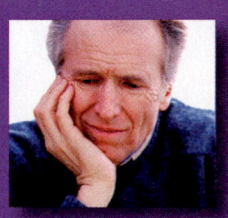

CHAPTER 1 Introduction to Pharmacology: Concepts and Connections / 2

CHAPTER 2 Drug Regulations / 12

CHAPTER 3 Pharmacokinetics / 24

CHAPTER 4 Pharmacodynamics / 42

CHAPTER 5 Adverse Drug Effects and Drug Interactions / 52

CHAPTER 6 Medication Errors and Risk Reduction / 66

CHAPTER 7 The Role of Complementary and Alternative Therapies in Pharmacotherapy / 79

"Wow, I just left my first pharmacology class and my head is swirling. How will I ever remember all this?"

Student "Josh Remming"

CHAPTER

1

Introduction to Pharmacology: Concepts and Connections

LEARNING OUTCOMES

After reading this chapter, the student should be able to:

1. Identify key events in the history of pharmacology.
2. Compare and contrast the terms *drug*, *pharmacology*, and *pharmacotherapy*.
3. Explain the importance of pharmacotherapy to clinical nursing practice.
4. Using specific examples, explain the difference between the pharmacologic and therapeutic methods of classifying drugs.
5. Identify the advantages of using prototype drugs to study pharmacology.
6. Classify drugs by their chemical, generic, and trade names.
7. Compare the advantages and disadvantages of a pharmaceutical company being granted exclusivity for the development of a new drug.
8. Analyze possible differences between generic drugs and their brand-name equivalents.
9. Assess the responsibilities of the nurse in drug administration.

CHAPTER OUTLINE

▸ Brief History of Pharmacology

▸ Pharmacology: The Study of Medicines

▸ Characteristics of an Ideal Drug

▸ Classification of Drugs

▸ Drug Prototypes

▸ Naming Drugs

▸ Connecting Pharmacology to Clinical Nursing Practice

KEY TERMS

bioavailability, 8

chemical names, 7

combination drugs, 7

drug, 4

exclusivity, 7

generic name, 7

indications, 5

pharmacologic classification, 5

pharmacology, 4

pharmacotherapy, 4

prototype drug, 6

therapeutic classification, 5

trade name, 7

More drugs are being administered to consumers than ever before. Over 3.6 billion prescriptions are dispensed each year in the United States, and the number is rapidly approaching 4 billion. Sales of prescription medications at retail pharmacies in the United States exceeded $227 trillion in 2011 (Kaiser Family Foundation, 2012). The applications of pharmacology to medicine have expanded over the centuries and the nurse serves a key role in ensuring the success of pharmacotherapy. The purpose of this chapter is to introduce fundamental concepts of pharmacology and to emphasize the connections between drug therapy and clinical nursing practice.

PharmFACT

According to the National Center for Health Statistics (2013), 48% of Americans have taken a prescription drug in the past 30 days. This percentage increases to 90% for those 65 years and older.

Brief History of Pharmacology

1.1 The practice of applying products to relieve suffering has been recorded throughout history by virtually every culture.

The story of pharmacology is rich and exciting, filled with accidental discoveries and landmark events. Its history likely began when a human first used a plant to relieve symptoms of disease. One of the oldest forms of health care, herbal medicine has been practiced in virtually every culture dating to antiquity. The Babylonians recorded the earliest surviving "prescriptions" on clay tablets in 3000 BC, although magic and the art of reading omens were probably considered just as legitimate to healing as the use of herbal remedies. At about the same time, the Chinese recorded the *Pen Tsao* (Great Herbal), a 40-volume compendium of plant remedies dating to 2700 BC. The Egyptians followed in 1500 BC by archiving their remedies on a document known as the Eber's papyrus, which contains over 700 magical formulas and remedies. Galen, the famous Greek physician, described over 1,000 healing preparations using plant products before his death in AD 201.

Little is known about pharmacology during the Dark Ages. Although it is likely that herbal medicine continued to be practiced, especially in monasteries and in centers of Arabic culture, few historical events related to drug therapy were recorded. Pharmacology, and indeed medicine, could not advance until the discipline of science was eventually viewed differently than magic and superstition.

The first recorded reference to the word *pharmacology* was found in a text titled "Pharmacologia sen Manuductio and Materiam Medicum" by Samuel Dale in 1693. Before this date, the study of herbal remedies was called "Materia Medica." The term *Materia Medica* likely originated from a Latin term meaning "medical matters," although use of this term continued into the early 20th century.

Although the exact starting date is obscure, modern pharmacology is thought to have begun in the early 1800s. At that time, chemists were making remarkable progress in separating specific substances from complex mixtures. This enabled chemists to isolate the active agents morphine, colchicine, curare, cocaine, and other early drugs from their natural plant products. Pharmacologists could then study their effects in animals more precisely, using standardized amounts. Some of the early researchers even used themselves as test subjects. Friedrich Sertürner, who first isolated morphine from opium in 1805, injected himself and three of his friends with a huge dose of 100 mg of his new product. He and his cohorts suffered acute morphine intoxication for several days afterward.

Pharmacology as a distinct discipline was officially recognized when the first Department of Pharmacology was established in Estonia in 1847. John Jacob Abel, who is considered the father of American pharmacology due to his many contributions to the field, founded the first pharmacology department in the United States at the University of Michigan in 1890.

In the 20th century, the pace of change in all areas of medicine became exponential. Pharmacologists no longer needed to rely on the slow, laborious process of isolating active agents from scarce natural products. They could synthesize drugs "from scratch" in the laboratory. Hundreds of new drugs could be synthesized and tested in a relatively short time span. More importantly, it became possible to understand how drugs produced their effects, right down to their molecular mechanism of action.

The current practice of pharmacology is extremely complex and has progressed far beyond its early, primitive history. The nurses and other health professionals who administer medications, however, must never forget the early roots of pharmacology: the application of products to relieve or prevent human suffering. Whether a substance is extracted from the Pacific yew tree, isolated from a fungus, or created in a laboratory, the central purpose of pharmacology is focused on the patient and improving the quality of life.

CONNECTION Checkpoint 1.1

Some modern drugs used in the treatment of diabetes, cardiovascular disorders, and other conditions have unique sources. Using an online dictionary or search engine, what are the natural sources for exenatide (Byetta), captopril (Capoten), and vincristine (Oncovin)? What conditions are they used to treat? *See Answer to Connection Checkpoint 1.1 on student resource website.*

Pharmacology: The Study of Medicines

1.2 Pharmacology is the study of medicines.

The word *drug* has already been used numerous times in this text. What exactly is a drug? Is everything a drug, including water, vitamin C, or perhaps a can of cola? What about substances naturally found in the body, such as estrogen or testosterone? Is it even possible to define a drug?

The definition of a drug is indeed difficult but is nevertheless important to the health care profession. There are many definitions, but perhaps the clearest is that a **drug** is any substance that is taken to prevent, cure, or reduce symptoms of a medical condition. Considering the substances listed earlier, which, then, are drugs? Although it may seem vague, the correct answer is "it depends."

- The caffeine consumed in a cup of coffee is not considered a drug. Yet caffeine is included in several therapies for headache pain, including Excedrin and Fioricet. For the patient trying to get pain relief, caffeine is a drug.

- Vitamin C, if ingested as part of an orange or tomato, is food. Food is not a drug. However, someone with a vitamin C deficiency may be administered vitamin C to cure scurvy. For this patient, vitamin C is then considered a drug.

- A can of cola is certainly not listed in any drug guide. However, if a patient with diabetes is experiencing a hypoglycemic reaction, the glucose in a can of soda may raise the patient's blood sugar and prevent a coma; thus the glucose in the cola may be considered a drug in this example.

- Substances normally found in the body are not considered drugs unless they are administered to treat a condition. For example, the hormone estrogen circulating in the blood is not a drug. However, if it is taken as an oral contraceptive to prevent a condition (pregnancy), estrogen is considered a drug.

Once the meaning of the term *drug* is understood, the next essential term is *pharmacology*. The word *pharmacology* is derived from two Greek words, *pharmakon,* which means "medicine" or "drug," and *logos,* which means "study." Thus, **pharmacology** is most simply defined as the study of medicines. Pharmacology is an expansive subject, ranging from understanding how drugs are administered, to where they travel in the body, to the actual responses they produce. **Pharmacotherapy**, or pharmacotherapeutics, is the application of drugs for the purpose of disease prevention and treatment of suffering.

Drugs are a form of medical intervention given to improve a patient's condition or to prevent harm. Pharmacotherapy often begins when the patient experiences signs or symptoms that cause dissatisfaction with current or future health status. A major role of the nurse is to design interventions that meet the desired health goals of the patient. Pharmacotherapy is a critical intervention for many conditions. The rationale for pharmacotherapy is illustrated in Figure 1.1.

Over 11,000 brand-name and generic drugs and combination agents are currently available for pharmacotherapy. Each

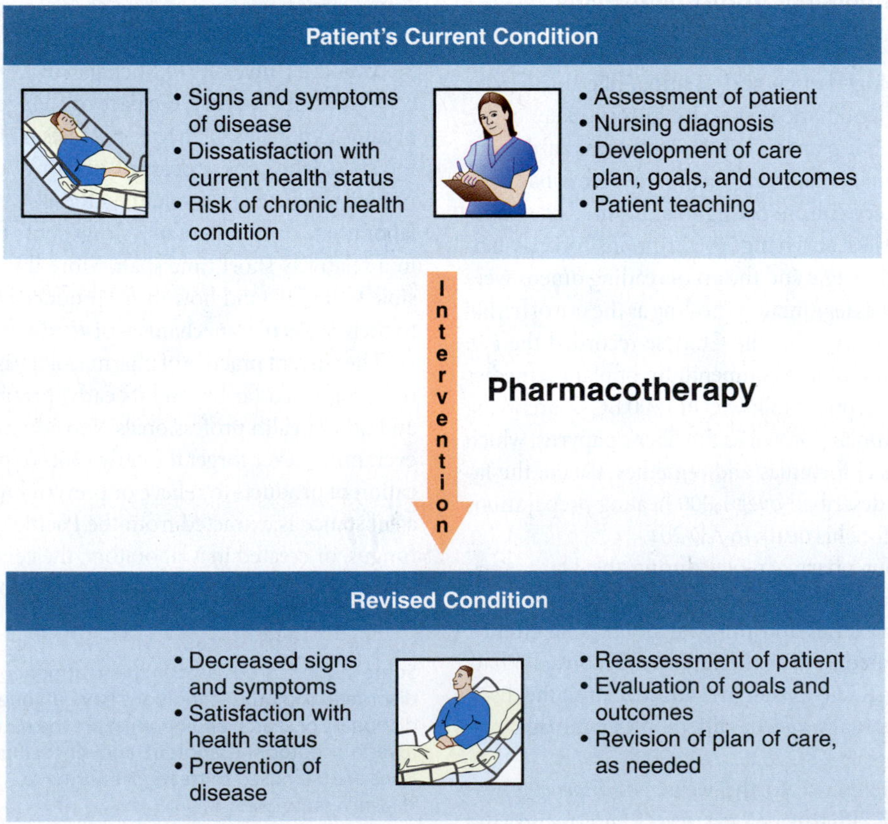

Patient's Current Condition

- Signs and symptoms of disease
- Dissatisfaction with current health status
- Risk of chronic health condition

- Assessment of patient
- Nursing diagnosis
- Development of care plan, goals, and outcomes
- Patient teaching

Intervention

Pharmacotherapy

Revised Condition

- Decreased signs and symptoms
- Satisfaction with health status
- Prevention of disease

- Reassessment of patient
- Evaluation of goals and outcomes
- Revision of plan of care, as needed

Figure 1.1 Rationale for pharmacotherapy: A partnership between the patient and the health care provider.

has its own characteristic set of therapeutic applications, interactions, adverse effects, and mechanism of action. Many drugs are prescribed for more than one disease and most produce multiple effects on the body. Further complicating the study of pharmacology is the fact that drugs may elicit different responses depending on individual patient factors such as age, gender, race, body mass, health status, and genetics. Indeed, learning the applications of existing medications and staying current with new drugs introduced every year are an enormous challenge for the nurse. The task, however, is a critical one for both the patient and the health care provider. If applied properly, drugs can dramatically improve patients' quality of life. If applied improperly, the consequences of drug action can cause permanent disability and even death.

There are important exceptions to the drug definition mentioned earlier. What about crack cocaine, ecstasy, LSD, or the fumes in glues and paint thinners? These are certainly drugs, but they are not taken "to prevent, cure, or reduce symptoms of a medical condition." In fact, they are taken to produce a biologic effect viewed as desirable or pleasurable by the user (see Chapter 27). Other exceptions to this definition of the term "drug" will become apparent as the student studies pharmacology.

Characteristics of an Ideal Drug

1.3 The perfect drug is safe and effective.

As they begin their journey in mastering pharmacology, nursing students should start with a notion of the ideal or "perfect drug." Learning the characteristics of an ideal drug gives a basis for comparison to "real drugs." It is always the goal of pharmacotherapy to select the perfect or ideal drug for the patient. Just what is a perfect drug? It is one that:

- Effectively treats, prevents, or cures the patient's condition.
- Produces a rapid, predictable response at relatively low doses.
- Produces no adverse effects.
- Can be taken conveniently, usually by mouth.
- Can be taken infrequently, usually once a day, and for a short length of time.
- Is inexpensive and easily accessible.
- Is quickly eliminated by the body after it produces its beneficial effect.
- Does not interact with other medications or food.

After reading this description, it should appear clear to the student that there is really no such thing as a perfect drug. Some drugs meet most of the criteria, whereas others meet very few. At the very least, it is expected that all prescription drugs have some degree of effectiveness at treating or preventing a health condition. The conditions for which a drug is approved are its **indications**. Every prescription drug has at least one indication, and most have multiple indications. Some drugs are used for conditions for which they have not been approved; these are called unlabeled or off-label indications.

As a general rule, the more a medicine strays from the perfect drug profile, the less commonly it is used. This is because whenever possible, health care providers strive to prescribe the most effective, safest, and most convenient medication for the patient. In

the home care setting, drugs that cause annoying adverse effects, have inconvenient dosing schedules, or are expensive are often not taken by patients, potentially worsening their condition and causing failure of treatment outcomes. Of course, some essential drugs do produce serious adverse effects or must be given by invasive routes, such as intravenously. In these cases, the drug is either administered in a clinical setting by a nurse, or the patient receives careful instructions and regular monitoring on an outpatient basis.

Classification of Drugs

1.4 Drugs may be organized by their therapeutic classification or pharmacologic classification.

The U.S. Food and Drug Administration (FDA, 2013) document *Approved Drug Products with Therapeutic Equivalence Evaluations*, informally called the "Orange Book," lists over 11,000 approved drugs. With the vast number of drugs available, it is essential that methods be used to group similar agents to aid in their study and understanding. The two basic classifications of drugs are therapeutic and pharmacologic. Both categories are widely used in classifying prescription and nonprescription drugs. The key difference is that the **therapeutic classification** describes what is being treated by the drug, whereas the **pharmacologic classification** describes how the drug acts.

Drugs are placed into therapeutic classes based on their usefulness in treating a specific disease. Table 1.1 shows the method of

TABLE 1.1 Organizing Drug Information by Therapeutic Classification

THERAPEUTIC FOCUS: DRUGS AFFECTING CARDIOVASCULAR DISEASE

Therapeutic Usefulness	Therapeutic Classification
Influence blood clotting	Anticoagulants
Lower blood cholesterol	Antihyperlipidemics
Lower blood pressure	Antihypertensives
Restore normal cardiac rhythm	Antidysrhythmics
Treat angina	Antianginals

TABLE 1.2 **Organizing Drug Information by Pharmacologic Classification**

FOCUS ON HOW A DRUG WORKS: PHARMACOTHERAPY OF HYPERTENSION

Mechanism of Action	Pharmacologic Classification
Lowers plasma volume	Diuretic
Blocks heart calcium channels	Calcium channel blocker
Blocks hormonal activity	Angiotensin-converting enzyme inhibitor
Blocks physiological reactions to stress	Adrenergic antagonist (or blocker)
Dilates peripheral blood vessels	Vasodilator

therapeutic classification, using cardiovascular drugs as an example. Many different types of drugs affect cardiovascular function. Some drugs influence blood coagulation, whereas others lower cholesterol levels or prevent the onset of stroke. Drugs may be used to treat hypertension, heart failure, abnormal cardiac rhythm, chest pain, myocardial infarction (MI), or circulatory shock. Thus, drugs that treat cardiovascular disorders may be placed in several therapeutic classes, for example, anticoagulants, antihyperlipidemics, and antihypertensives. The key to therapeutic classification is to simply state what condition is being treated by the particular drug. Other examples of therapeutic classifications include antidepressants, antipsychotics, drugs for erectile dysfunction, and antineoplastics. Notice how the prefix *anti-* often refers to a therapeutic classification.

The pharmacologic classification addresses a drug's mechanism of action or how a drug produces its effect in the body. Table 1.2 illustrates the use of pharmacologic classification, using hypertension as an example. A diuretic treats hypertension by lowering plasma volume. Calcium channel blockers treat this disorder by decreasing the force of cardiac contractions. Other drugs block components of the renin-angiotensin system. Notice that each example describes how hypertension might be controlled. A drug's pharmacologic classification is more specific than its therapeutic classification and requires an understanding of biochemistry and physiology. Pharmacologic classifications may use a drug's chemical name.

Although classifications help to organize drugs, the process is by no means easy or standardized. Most drugs have multiple classifications. For example, the drug epinephrine is classified as a vasoconstrictor, an autonomic nervous system agent, an adrenergic agonist, a sympathomimetic, a bronchodilator, an agent for anaphylaxis, an ocular mydriatic, an antiglaucoma agent, a catecholamine, and a topical hemostatic. This is clearly a mix of therapeutic (e.g., antiglaucoma) and pharmacologic (e.g., catecholamine) classifications. Which one(s) should the student remember? Unfortunately for nursing students, the answer is all of them. The classification chosen primarily depends on the specific clinical use of the drug (What condition is being treated?). Sometimes the classification of choice is simply a preference of the health care provider. Although challenging, remembering the different classifications will pay dividends as the student's pharmacology course progresses.

CONNECTION Checkpoint 1.2

State whether each of the following classifications for aspirin is therapeutic or pharmacologic: anticoagulant, salicylate, central nervous system agent, analgesic, antipyretic. Use a drug guide, if needed. *See Answer to Connection Checkpoint 1.2 on student resource website.*

Drug Prototypes

1.5 A prototype drug is the agent to which all other medications in a class are compared.

As discussed in Section 1.4 learning thousands of drugs is simplified, at least somewhat, by grouping similar drugs together into broad classifications. Just knowing its therapeutic or pharmacologic classification can reveal important information about a drug. An additional strategy is helpful when learning pharmacology. It is a common and useful practice to select a single drug from a class and compare all other medications in the class to this representative medication. This is called a **prototype drug**. By learning about the prototype drug in depth, the actions and adverse effects of other drugs in the same class may be predicted. For example, by learning the actions and effects of penicillin V, students can extend this knowledge to all other drugs in the penicillin class of antibiotics. In this textbook, the drug prototypes are clearly identified, and detailed information regarding their therapeutic effects, mechanism of action, adverse effects, contraindications, precautions, and nursing responsibilities, including patient and family education, is presented.

Selecting a drug to serve as the prototype for a class is not always a simple matter; health care providers and textbooks sometimes disagree. The traditional prototype approach uses the oldest and best understood drug in the class. For example, atropine has been used for thousands of years and still remains a drug prototype for certain indications (see Figure 1.2). Sometimes, however, newer drugs are developed in the same class that are more effective or have a more favorable safety profile. Over time, an older prototype drug may be infrequently prescribed and a different, more clinically useful prototype may be chosen for the class. This textbook uses a practical approach to drug prototypes, selecting a combination of traditional drugs and those most widely used. Regardless of the approach, the student must remember that the prototype is the drug to which all others in a class are compared.

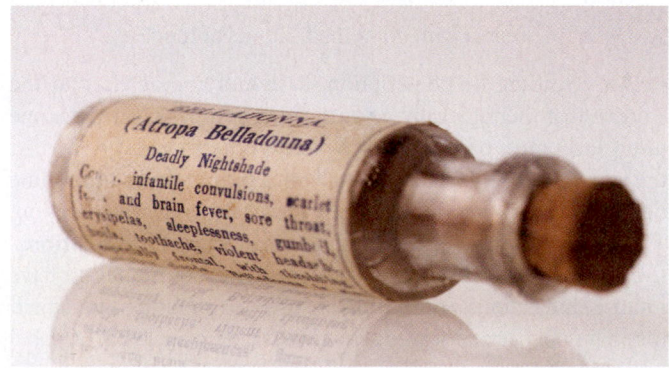

Figure 1.2 Obtained from the deadly nightshade plant *Atropa belladona*, atropine remains a traditional drug prototype.

Courtesy of Darren Falkenberg/Fotolia.

Naming Drugs

1.6 Drugs have chemical, generic, and trade names.

Despite the utility of using drug classes and prototypes when studying pharmacology, learning thousands of drug names remains a challenge. Adding to this difficulty is that most drugs have multiple names. The three basic types of drug names are chemical, generic, and trade names.

Chemical names are assigned using standard nomenclature established by the International Union of Pure and Applied Chemistry (IUPAC). A drug has only one chemical name. This chemical name is sometimes helpful in predicting a drug's physical and chemical properties. Although chemical names convey a clear and concise meaning about the nature of a drug to the chemist, these names are often complicated and difficult to remember or pronounce. For example, it is unlikely that the nurse would remember that the chemical name for alprazolam (Xanax) is 8-chloro-1-methyl-6-phenyl-4H-5-triazolo[4,3-α][1,4]-benzodiazepine. In only a few cases, usually when the name is brief and easily remembered, will nurses use chemical names. Examples of easy to remember chemical names of common drugs include lithium carbonate, calcium gluconate, and sodium chloride.

Drugs are sometimes named and classified by a portion of their chemical structure, known as the chemical group name. In the Xanax example, a portion of the chemical name, benzodiazepine, is used as a drug class. Other examples include the fluoroquinolones, aminoglycosides, phenothiazines, and thiazides. Although these names may seem complicated when first encountered, knowledge of chemical group names will become invaluable as the nursing student begins to learn and understand the actions of the drugs in the major drug classes.

The **generic name** of a drug is assigned by the United States Adopted Name Council. With few exceptions, generic names are less complicated and easier to remember than chemical names. Many organizations, including the FDA, the *United States Pharmacopeia*, and the World Health Organization, routinely describe a medication by its generic name. Because there is only one generic name for each drug, health care providers often use this name, and students must memorize it. Fortunately, sometimes components of a generic name can help a student recognize other drugs in that same class. For example, the ending *-lol* is used in the generic name of beta-adrenergic blockers and the ending *-statin* denotes a lipid-lowering drug.

A drug's **trade name**, sometimes called the proprietary, product, or brand name, is assigned by the pharmaceutical company marketing the drug. The trade name is intentionally selected to be short and easy to remember so that patients will remember it (and ask for it by name). The term *proprietary* suggests ownership. In the United States, the FDA grants the pharmaceutical company exclusive rights to name and market a drug for a certain number of years after it approves a new drug application. During the period of **exclusivity**, competing companies are not allowed to market generic versions of the product. The rationale for exclusivity is that the developing pharmaceutical company needs sufficient time to recoup the millions of dollars in research and development costs involved in designing and testing the new drug. Without the guarantee of exclusivity, there is little incentive to pharmaceutical companies to develop new and unique drugs. When exclusivity expires,

TABLE 1.3 Examples of Generic Drugs Contained in Brand-Name Products	
Generic Drugs	**Brand Names**
Aspirin	Acetylsalicylic Acid, Acuprin, Anacin, Aspergum, Bayer, Bufferin, Ecotrin, Empirin, Excedrin, Maprin, Norgesic, Salatin, Salocol, Salsprin, Supac, Talwin, Traphen-10, Vanquish, Verin, ZORprin
Diphenhydramine	Allerdryl, Benadryl, Benahist, Bendylate, Caladryl, Compoz, Diahist, Diphenadril, Eldadryl, Fenylhist, Fynex, Hydramine, Hydril, Insomnal, Noradryl, Nordryl, Nytol, Tusstat, Wehdryl
Ibuprofen	Advil, Amersol, Apsifen, Brufen, Haltran, Medipren, Midol 200, Motrin, Nuprin, Pamprin-IB, Rufen, Trendar

competing companies may sell a generic equivalent drug, sometimes using a different name, which the FDA must approve. The typical length of exclusivity for a new drug is 5 years; however, this may be extended by 3 additional years if the drug is determined to have a new indication, can be delivered by a different route, or is made available in a different dosage form. If, for example, the pharmaceutical company completes pediatric studies and determines the dosage and safety of a drug in this population, the FDA adds 6 months of exclusivity. Orphan drugs (see Chapter 2) have 7 years of exclusivity. Pharmaceutical companies can make millions of dollars in sales from exclusivity; thus they usually make great efforts to receive extensions from the FDA. Expiration dates for the exclusivity of specific drugs are listed by the FDA in the *Approved Drug Products with Therapeutic Equivalence Evaluations*.

Trade names are a challenge for students to learn because there may be dozens of product names containing the same drug. In addition, many products contain more than one active ingredient. Drugs with more than one active generic ingredient are called **combination drugs**. This poses a problem in trying to match one generic name with one product name. As an example, refer to Table 1.3 and consider the drug diphenhydramine (generic name), also called Benadryl (one of many trade names). Low doses of diphenhydramine may be purchased over the counter (OTC). Higher doses require a prescription. If the nurse is looking for diphenhydramine, it may be listed under many trade names such as Benadryl, Nytol QuickCaps, Sominex, and Unisom, formulated alone or in combination with other active ingredients. Acetaminophen and aspirin are additional examples of agents that appear in many combination drugs with dozens of different trade names. To avoid this confusion, generic names should be used when naming the active ingredients in a combination drug. When referring to a drug, it is conventional to write the generic name in lowercase first, followed by the trade name in parentheses with the first letter capitalized. Examples include alprazolam (Xanax) and acetaminophen (Tylenol).

1.7 Generic drugs are less expensive than brand-name drugs, but they may differ in bioavailability.

During the years of exclusivity for a new drug, the pharmaceutical company determines the price of the medication. Because there is no competition, the price is relatively high. Once the exclusive rights end, competing companies market the generic equivalent drug for less money, and consumer savings may be considerable. In some states, pharmacists may routinely substitute a generic drug when the prescription calls for a brand name. In other states, the pharmacist must dispense drugs directly as written by a health care provider or obtain approval before providing a generic substitute.

PharmFACT

In a recent study, almost 50% of the physicians surveyed expressed negative perceptions about the quality of generic drugs, and more than a quarter preferred not to use generics as first-line drugs for themselves or their family (Shrank et al., 2011).

Pharmaceutical companies marketing brand-name drugs often lobby aggressively against laws that might restrict the routine use of certain brand-name drugs. The lobbyists claim that there are significant differences between a trade-name drug and its generic equivalent and that switching to the generic drug may be harmful for the patient. Consumer advocates on the other hand argue that generic substitutions should always be permitted because of the cost savings to patients.

Are there really significant differences between a brand-name drug and its generic equivalent? The answer is unclear. Despite the fact that the dosages may be identical, drug formulations are not always the same. The two drugs may have different inert ingredients. If in tablet form, the active ingredients may be more tightly compressed in one of the preparations. Liquid drugs may use different solvents such as water or alcohol.

The key to comparing brand-name drugs and their generic equivalents lies in measuring the **bioavailability** of the two agents. Bioavailability is defined by the Federal Food, Drug, and Cosmetic Act (see Chapter 2) as the rate and extent to which the active ingredient is absorbed from a drug product and becomes available at the site of drug action to produce its effect. Bioavailability may be affected by many factors, including inert ingredients and tablet compression. Anything that affects the absorption of a drug or its travel to the target cells can certainly affect drug action. Measuring how long a drug takes to exert its effect (onset time) gives pharmacologists a crude measure of bioavailability. If the trade and generic products have the same rate of absorption and have the same onset of therapeutic action, they are said to be bioequivalent.

The importance of bioavailability differences between a trade name drug and its generic equivalent depends on the specific circumstances of pharmacotherapy. For example, if a patient is in circulatory shock and the generic equivalent drug takes 5 minutes longer to produce its effect, that may indeed be significant. However, if a generic medication for arthritis pain relief takes 45 minutes to act, compared to the brand-name drug, which takes 40 minutes, it probably does not matter which drug is used, and the inexpensive product should be prescribed to provide cost savings to the consumer. As a general rule, bioavailability is of most concern when using critical care drugs and those with a narrow safety margin. In these cases, the patient should continue taking the brand-name drug and *not* switch to a generic equivalent, unless approved by the health care provider. For most other drugs, the generic equivalent may be safely substituted for the trade name drug.

In the age of Internet pharmacies, the issue of exclusive marketing rights has drastically changed. Other countries are not bound by U.S. drug laws, and it is easy for patients to obtain brand-name drugs through the mail at a fraction of what they cost in the United States. For example, a pharmaceutical company may have exclusivity for selling Cialis in the United States but companies in India and China sell the identical drug through Internet pharmacies and ship it to customers in the United States. In some cases, they even sell the drug to consumers without a prescription. Other countries do not have the same quality control standards as the United States, and the patient may be purchasing a useless or even harmful product. Furthermore, although Internet sites may appear to be based in the United States, they may instead be based in other countries and obtaining their medications from unreliable sources. Nurses must strongly urge their patients not to purchase drugs from overseas pharmacies because there is no assurance that the drugs are safe or effective.

Connecting Pharmacology to Clinical Nursing Practice

1.8 **Pharmacology is intimately connected to nursing practice and is a key intervention in relieving and preventing human suffering.**

The importance of pharmacology to nursing clinical practice cannot be overstated. As nursing students progress toward their chosen specialty, knowledge of pharmacology is at the core of patient care and is integrated into the nursing process. The connection between pharmacology and clinical nursing practice is emphasized throughout this entire textbook. Indeed, pharmacology would not be an important science without its connections to patient care and nursing practice.

Whether administering medications or supervising drug use, the nurse is expected to understand the pharmacotherapeutic principles for all medications received by each patient. Given the large number of different drugs and the potential consequences of medication errors, this is indeed an enormous task. A major goal of this textbook is to prepare the nurse for the responsibilities of drug administration. Chapters 2 through 4 of this textbook provide the legal and scientific bases for pharmacotherapeutics. The nurse's responsibilities include knowledge and understanding of the following:

- What drug is ordered:
  - Name (generic and trade) and drug classification
  - Intended or proposed use
  - Effects on the body
  - Contraindications
  - Special considerations, such as how age, gender, weight, body fat distribution, genetic factors, and pathophysiologic states affect pharmacotherapeutic response
  - Expected and potential adverse events
- Why the drug has been prescribed for this particular patient
- How the drug is supplied by the pharmacy
- How the drug is to be administered, including dose ranges
- What nursing process considerations related to the drug apply to this patient

A major goal in studying pharmacology is to eliminate medication errors and to limit the number and severity of adverse drug events. Many adverse effects are preventable. Professional nurses can routinely avoid many serious adverse drug effects in their patients by applying their experience and knowledge of pharmacotherapeutics to clinical practice. Some adverse effects, however, are not preventable. It is vital that the nurse be prepared to recognize and respond to potential adverse effects of medications. The nursing management of adverse effects and medication errors are discussed in Chapters 5 and 6, respectively.

Before any drug is administered, the nurse must obtain and process pertinent information regarding the patient's medical history, physical assessment, disease processes, and learning needs and capabilities. Growth and developmental factors must always be considered. It is important to remember that a large number of variables influence a patient's response to drugs throughout the life span. Having a firm understanding of these variables can increase treatment success. Chapters 8 through 11 of this textbook address these aspects of pharmacotherapy. For a nurse, knowledge of pharmacology is an ongoing, lifelong process that builds as a nurse is in practice and chooses specific clinical areas. It may seem daunting at first, but learning prototypes, recognizing key similarities in generic names, and always looking up unknown or new drugs will help build this knowledge base.

Despite its essential nature, the study of pharmacology should be viewed in the proper perspective. Drugs are just one of many tools available to the nurse for preventing or treating human suffering. Although pharmacology is a key intervention in many cases, nurses must use all the healing sciences in treating their patients. The effectiveness of a drug in treating disease can never substitute for skilled, compassionate nursing care. Too much reliance on drug therapy can diminish the importance of the nurse–patient relationship.

CHAPTER
1
Understanding the Chapter

Key Concepts Summary

1.1 The practice of applying products to relieve suffering has been recorded throughout history by virtually every culture.

1.2 Pharmacology is the study of medicines.

1.3 The perfect drug is safe and effective.

1.4 Drugs may be organized by their therapeutic classification or pharmacologic classification.

1.5 A prototype drug is the agent to which all other medications in a class are compared.

1.6 Drugs have chemical, generic, and trade names.

1.7 Generic drugs are less expensive than brand-name drugs, but they may differ in bioavailability.

1.8 Pharmacology is intimately connected to nursing practice and is a key intervention in relieving and preventing human suffering.

Case Study: Making the Patient Connection

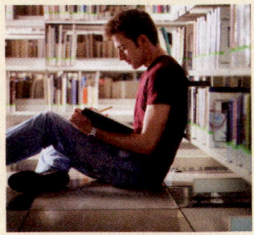

Remember the student "Josh Remming" at the beginning of the chapter? Now read the remainder of the case study. Based on the information presented within this chapter, respond to the critical thinking questions that follow.

Josh Remming, a 23-year-old student, is in his first semester of nursing school. He thought that nursing would provide him with a great career and lots of opportunity. He enjoys helping people and has always been fascinated with health care. However, after the first pharmacology class, Josh is worried because there seems to be an overwhelming amount of content to learn in just one semester.

At the end of the class, Josh talks with other students who are concerned and a bit anxious. Much of the conversation centers around lecture content provided by the professor. Following are some of the questions from Josh's classmates. How would you respond?

Critical Thinking Questions

1. What is the difference between therapeutic classification and pharmacologic classification?
2. What classification is a barbiturate? macrolide? birth control pills? laxatives? folic acid antagonist? antianginal agent?
3. What is a prototype drug, and what advantages does a prototype approach to studying pharmacology offer?
4. Why do nurses need to know all this pharmacology?

See Answers to Critical Thinking Questions on student resource website.

Additional Case Study

Sarah Hawkins, an elderly woman who lives on a fixed income, is on multiple medications. She says that all her friends are taking the generic form of their medications. While you are visiting her, she asks you, "What do you think of generic medicines? Are they safe? Are they as good? Are they worth it?"

1. How do generic equivalent drugs differ from a proprietary (trade name) drug?
2. What would you recommend that Sarah do about accepting generic drugs?

See Answers to Additional Case Study on student resource website.

Chapter Review

1 The nurse is using a drug handbook to determine the indications for the drug furosemide (Lasix). The term *indications* is defined as the:
   1. Way a drug works on the target organs.
   2. Amount of the drug to be administered.
   3. Conditions for which a drug is approved.
   4. Reason that the drug should not be given.

2 While completing the health history, the nurse asks the patient, "What medications do you take regularly?" Which drug name would the nurse expect the patient to use in providing the answer?
   1. Chemical
   2. Generic
   3. Trade
   4. Standard

3 When providing nursing care for the patient, the nurse understands that drugs are:
   1. One of many tools available to prevent or treat human suffering.
   2. The most important part of the therapeutic treatment plan.
   3. Primarily the concern of the health care provider and not included in nursing care.
   4. Substances that should be relied on for health and wellness.

4 Which patient characteristics, if noted in the patient's medical record, would the nurse consider important information that may affect the physiological response to various types of drug therapy? Select all that apply.
   1. 82-year-old and female
   2. Asian and obese
   3. Past medical history of kidney disease
   4. Mother and sister with diabetes
   5. Has no medical insurance

5 The nurse is looking up a drug that has been prescribed and wants to know the therapeutic classification for the drug. Which of the following would indicate a therapeutic classification?

1. Beta-adrenergic antagonist
2. Antihypertensive
3. Diuretic
4. Calcium channel blocker

6 The nurse is asked by a family member: "They're giving mom Motrin and she takes Advil. Hasn't the wrong drug been ordered?" The nurse will respond, knowing that:

1. There has been an error in the order and the nurse will contact the health care provider.
2. There may be a reason for the health care provider to order a different drug.
3. Not all health care agencies buy the same generic drugs and that may account for the difference.
4. Motrin and Advil are trade names for the same generic drug, ibuprofen.

See Answers to Chapter Review in Appendix A.

References

Kaiser Family Foundation. (2012). *Total retail sales for prescription drugs filled at retail pharmacies.* Retrieved from http://kff.org/other/state-indicator/total-sales-for-retail-rx-drugs/

National Center for Health Statistics. (2013). *Health, United States, 2012: With special feature on emergency care.* Retrieved from http://www.cdc.gov/nchs/data/hus/hus12.pdf#091

Shrank, W. H., Liberman, J. M., Fischer, M. A., Girdish, C., Brennan, T. A., & Choudry, N. K. (2011). Physician perceptions about generic drugs. *The Annals of Pharmacotherapy, 45,* 31–38. doi:10.1345/aph.1P389

U.S. Food and Drug Administration. (2013). *Electronic orange book: Approved drug products with therapeutic equivalence evaluations.* Washington, DC: U.S. Department of Health and Human Services. Retrieved from http://www.accessdata.fda.gov/scripts/cder/ob/default.cfm

Selected Bibliography

Allam, A. N., El gamal, S. S., & Naggar, V. F. (2011). Bioavailability: A pharmaceutical review. *International Journal of Pharmacy and Biotechnology, 1,* 80–96.

Duncan, D. (2010). Generic prescribing and substitution: The big issues. *British Journal of Community Nursing, 15*(5), 248–249.

Howland, R. H. (2010). Are generic medications safe and effective? *Journal of Psychosocial Nursing Mental Health Services, 48*(3), 13–16. doi:10.3928/02793695-20100204-01

Newman, D. J., & Cragg, G. M. (2012). Natural products as sources of new drugs over the 30 years from 1981 to 2010. *Journal of Natural Products, 75,* 311–335. doi:10.1021/np200906s

U.S. Food and Drug Administration. (2012). *Facts about generic drugs.* Retrieved from http://www.fda.gov/drugs/resourcesforyou/consumers/buyingusingmedicinesafely/understandinggenericdrugs/ucm167991.htm

U.S. Food and Drug Administration. (2012). *Frequently asked questions on patents and exclusivity.* Retrieved from http://www.fda.gov/Drugs/DevelopmentApprovalProcess/ucm079031.htm

U.S. Government Accountability Office. (2012). *Drug pricing: Research on savings from generic drug use GAO-12-371R.* Retrieved from http://www.gao.gov/products/GAO-12-371R

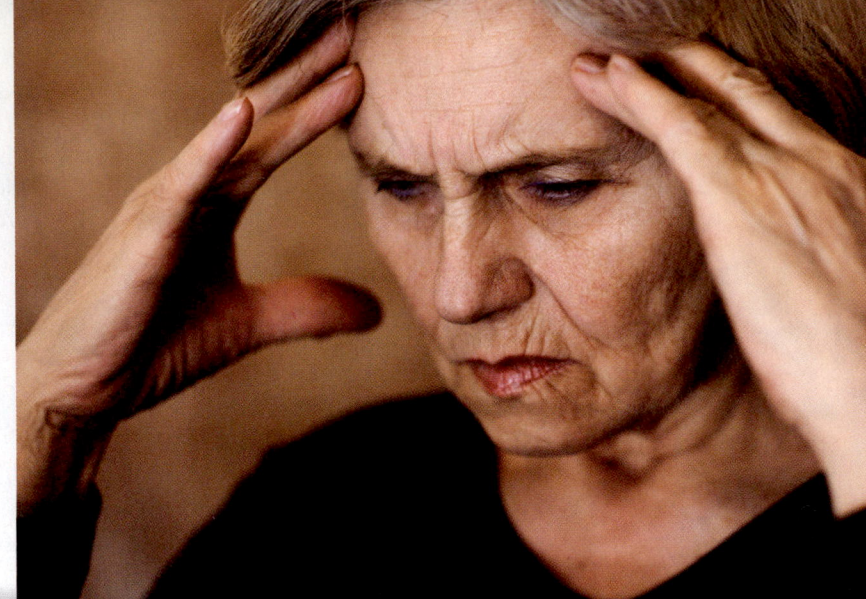

"This headache medicine I bought at the grocery store must be safe because I didn't need a prescription."

Patient "Gertrude Stone"

2

Drug Regulations

LEARNING OUTCOMES

After reading this chapter, the student should be able to:

1. Explain the role of patent medicines in the history of pharmacology and the legislation of drugs.
2. Outline the key U.S. drug regulations and explain how each has contributed to the safety and effectiveness of medications.
3. Describe how the *United States Pharmacopeia-National Formulary* (USP-NF) controls drug purity and standards.
4. Evaluate the role of the U.S. Food and Drug Administration in the drug approval process.
5. Categorize the four stages of new drug approval.
6. Explain the role of a placebo in new drug testing.
7. Discuss how changes to the approval process have increased the speed at which new drugs reach consumers.
8. Compare and contrast prescription and over-the-counter drugs.
9. Explain how scheduled drugs are classified and regulated.
10. Discuss the requirements and regulations needed for nurses to have the ability to prescribe drugs.

CHAPTER OUTLINE

▸ Patent Medicines

▸ Brief History of Drug Legislation

▸ Drug Standards

▸ The U.S. Food and Drug Administration

▸ Drug Approval

▸ Changes to the Drug Approval Process

▸ Prescription and Over-the-Counter Drugs

▸ Drug Schedules

▸ Prescriptive Authority for Nurses

KEY TERMS

clinical phase trials, 17

controlled substances, 20

dependence, 20

formulary, 15

Investigational New Drug (IND), 17

New Drug Application (NDA), 18

new molecular entities, 18

orphan disease, 14

patent medicines, 13

pharmacopeia, 15

placebo, 17

postmarketing surveillance, 18

preclinical research, 17

scheduled drugs, 20

U.S. Food and Drug Administration (FDA), 16

Laws govern all aspects of the drug approval, labeling, marketing, manufacturing, and distribution process. The purpose of this legislation is to inform the public and to protect it from unsafe and ineffective products. This chapter examines standards and legislation regulating drugs in the United States.

Patent Medicines

2.1 Early American history saw the rise of patent medicines and the lack of adequate drug regulations.

People have an expectation that the drug they are taking is effective at treating their condition, whether it is asthma, diabetes, or a headache. They expect the label to contain clear and accurate instructions on how the product should be taken. They expect that the drug will be safe if the instructions are correctly followed. Are these reasonable assumptions? In the United States and Canada, the answer is yes. But Americans have not always had this reassurance. Although drugs have been used for thousands of years, it was not until the 20th century that extensive standards and regulations were developed to protect the public from unsafe and ineffective products.

In early America, there were few attempts to regulate drugs. This period saw the rise of **patent medicines**. Although the term *patent* implies a legal right to manufacture or sell a drug, this was not the case. Patent medicines contained a brand name that clearly identified the product, such as William Radam's Microbe Killer, Stanley's Snake Oil, Dr. Kilmer's Swamp Root, or Dr. Moore's Indian Root Pills. Because there were no laws to the contrary, these products claimed to cure just about any symptom or disease. Dr. William's Pink Pills for Pale People, which contained iron oxide and magnesium sulfate, claimed to cure rheumatism, nervous headache, palpitations, grippe, neuralgia, locomotor ataxia, partial paralysis, sallow complexion, and all forms of weakness in men or women. A typical advertisement from this era is shown in Figure 2.1.

Patent medicines were often harmless (and ineffective), containing coloring, flavoring, and an aromatic substance that "smelled like medicine." At their worst, some contained hazardous levels of dangerous or addictive substances. In fact, cocaine, heroin, and morphine were freely distributed in patent medicines; some elixirs contained up to 50% morphine, which indeed caused many painful disorders to "disappear." Addictive ingredients were purposely added to guarantee repeat customers for their products. (Note the similarity with nicotine added to tobacco and caffeine added to soft drinks.) In the late 1800s, the familiar Coca-Cola soft drink was a patented beverage that contained an estimated 9 mg of cocaine per serving and was claimed to cure headache, dyspepsia,

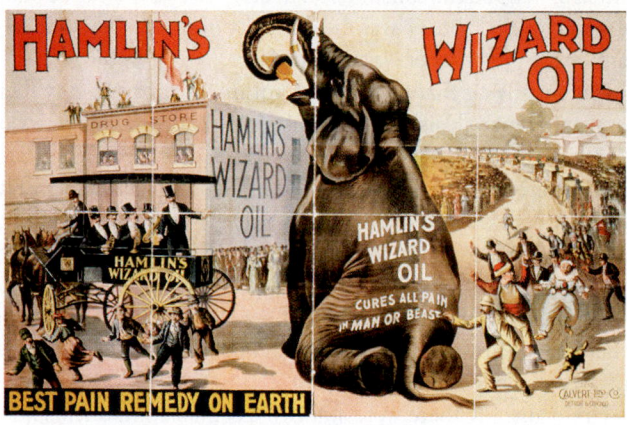

Figure 2.1 Patent medicines contained a name brand that clearly identified the product and claimed to cure just about any symptom or disease.
Courtesy of Fine Art/Corbis.

hysteria, morphine addiction, and impotence. The need for stricter regulation became more apparent in the 1860s as cocaine was synthesized, and the use of opiates as painkillers during the Civil War caused thousands of soldiers to become addicted.

Although the marketing and use of patent medicines may seem humorous and even unbelievable to modern consumers, a few of these products are still available over the counter (OTC). Examples of patent medicines that survived the drug regulations of the 1900s include Smith Brothers Throat Drops, Fletcher's Castoria, Doan's Pills, Vick's VapoRub, and Phillip's Milk of Magnesia. Of course, the ingredients of these products have changed over time so that they conform to modern regulations regarding labeling, safety, and effectiveness.

Brief History of Drug Legislation

2.2 In the 1900s, drug legislation was enacted to make drugs safer and more effective.

Although individual states attempted to regulate drugs, the first national law was the Drug Importation Act, passed in 1848, which attempted to stop the entry of unsafe drugs into the United States. In the early 1900s, the United States began to develop and enforce tougher drug legislation to protect the public. This was, in part, spurred by the tragic deaths of 13 children in St. Louis in 1901 who were given diphtheria antitoxin that was contaminated with tetanus. In 1902, the Biologics Control Act was passed to standardize the quality of sera, antitoxins, and other blood-related products. Passed shortly thereafter, the Pure Food and Drug Act (PFDA) of

1906 was a significant and powerful piece of drug legislation that gave the government authority to control the labeling of medicines. Essentially, this law required that drug labels accurately reflect the contents. Prior to this date, many labels did not contain any indication of the active ingredient within the bottle or its amount. Although the ingredients had to be accurately labeled, a drug could still be marketed for any disease.

In 1912, the Sherley Amendment to the PFDA prohibited the sale of drugs labeled with false therapeutic claims that were intended to defraud the consumer. A major weakness, as borne out in subsequent legal battles, was the difficulty of proving that the false claim made by the seller was intentional.

It is surprising that up to this point in American history there was no attempt to legislate the use of addictive drugs. The Harrison Narcotic Act of 1914 was passed to require prescriptions for high doses of narcotic drugs and to mandate that pharmacists and health care providers keep narcotic records. Since 1914, hundreds of additional state and federal laws have been passed to regulate drugs with abuse potential, including the landmark Comprehensive Drug Abuse Prevention and Control Act (see Section 2.8). Additional details on the history of the regulation of controlled substances are included in Chapter 27.

Unfortunately there were still two essential components missing from the regulation of drugs in the early 20th century. Although the PFDA and other legislation required that ingredients be listed on the label and prohibited intentional false claims, manufacturers did not have to prove that the drug was effective. Furthermore, product safety did not have to be tested before the drug was marketed. Bringing the issue to the forefront was an incident in 1937 in which an elixir of sulfanilamide containing a poisonous chemical (diethylene glycol) killed 107 persons, mostly children.

In 1938, Congress passed the landmark Food, Drug, and Cosmetic Act (FDCA), which corrected certain loopholes in previous laws. This was the first law preventing the sale of newly developed drugs that had not been thoroughly tested for safety. Drug labels were required to contain instructions for safe use. The FDCA was also the first attempt at regulating cosmetics and medical devices. Unfortunately, the FDCA did not clearly define "prescription" or specify which drugs required a prescription. Most drugs, including many addictive and harmful substances, were sold by the corner druggist, sometimes legally, other times illegally. In 1951, the Durham-Humphrey Amendment to the FDCA delineated the difference between safer drugs, which may be sold OTC, and more dangerous drugs, which require prescriptions.

In the late 1950s, the drug thalidomide was found to produce severe birth defects in the children of women taking the drug as a sleeping pill and to treat morning sickness during pregnancy. Although the drug was not approved in the United States, it is estimated that over 20,000 Americans received the drug, because it was widely distributed to health care providers without FDA approval. As with other drug legislation, it took a tragedy to convince Congress to pass tougher regulations. Passage of the Kefauver-Harris Amendment to the FDCA in 1962 mandated that manufacturers prove their drugs were effective for specific purposes, as well as safe, through the conduct of "adequate and well-controlled" studies. This law was applied retroactively to all drugs introduced since the passage of the FDCA. This amendment also required all significant adverse reactions to be reported to the FDA and that complete information about adverse effects be included in literature distributed to health care providers. For the first time, informed consent was required from patients participating in experimental drug research.

The emphasis on effectiveness continued as the FDA contracted with the National Academy of Sciences and the National Research Council in 1966 to evaluate the effectiveness of 4,000 drugs that were approved between 1938 and 1962 based only on their safety. Approximately 40% of all drugs introduced between 1938 and 1962 were found to be ineffective and were subsequently removed from the market. In 1972, a review of OTC drugs began to examine the safety and effectiveness of these products.

In the 1980s, the public placed considerable political pressure on the FDA to find drugs to treat rare or unusual disorders. Pharmaceutical companies were reluctant to develop drugs for these disorders because there would not be enough sales to recoup their research and development costs. To encourage development of such drugs, the Orphan Drug Act became law in 1983. An **orphan disease** is defined as a serious, although rare, disease that affects fewer than 200,000 people in the United States. With the passage of this legislation, drug manufacturers are now offered development grants, tax credits for clinical investigation expenses, and 7 years of exclusivity to market an orphan drug. Over 700 medications have been approved as orphan drugs since the passage of this act.

A major focus in the 1990s was to speed the drug approval process, which could be prolonged for many years. The Prescription Drug User Fee Act (PDUFA) of 1992 assessed fees from drug manufacturers to be used specifically for reducing the review time for new drug applications. From 1992 to 2002, the number of full-time equivalent employees examining new drug applications at the FDA increased from 1,277 to 2,337. The PDUFA was reauthorized in 1997 with the passage of the Food and Drug Administration Modernization Act, which also included provisions to accelerate the review of medical devices, regulate the advertising of unapproved uses of drugs, and regulate health claims for foods. The PDUFA continued to be reauthorized in 2012, with an added goal to improve communication between the FDA and new drug sponsors. From 2014 to 2016, the PDUFA is expected to generate $3 billion annually in revenue.

In reaction to the rising popularity of dietary supplements, Congress passed the Dietary Supplement Health and Education Act of 1994 to control misleading industry claims. Due in part to intense lobbying from the dietary supplement industry, the regulation of these products remains less stringent than that for prescription or OTC drugs. The regulation of herbal products and dietary supplements is discussed in detail in Chapter 7.

In early 2000, the focus of drug regulation turned to access. Advocacy groups claimed that the high cost of drugs caused unequal access to adequate health care for the poor, the uninsured/underinsured, and the elderly. In 2003, the Medicare Prescription Drug Improvement and Modernization Act was passed, which provides a benefit that pays 75% of prescription drug spending up to the first $2,250. Those qualifying for the low-income criteria may have their premiums and cost subsidized by the government. Participants are protected against catastrophic costs at $3,600 per year with most beneficiaries paying a 5% copay amount. A brief time line of major events in U.S. drug regulation is shown in Table 2.1.

TABLE 2.1 Historical Time Line of Regulatory Acts, Standards, and Organizations

Year	Regulatory Acts, Standards, and Organizations
1820	Physicians establish the first comprehensive publication of drug standards, the *United States Pharmacopeia* (USP).
1848	The Drug Importation Act requires that all drugs (as defined by the newly established pharmacopeia) entering the United States be inspected and analyzed for "quality, purity, and fitness for medical purposes."
1852	Pharmacists found the American Pharmaceutical Association (APhA). The APhA establishes the *National Formulary* (NF), a standardized publication focusing on pharmaceutical ingredients. The USP continues to catalog all drug-related substances and products.
1862	The Federal Bureau of Chemistry, established under the administration of President Lincoln, eventually becomes the Food and Drug Administration (FDA).
1902	The Biologics Control Act controls the quality of sera and other blood-related products.
1906	The Pure Food and Drug Act prohibits the manufacture and sale of adulterated or misbranded foods, drugs, and medications.
1912	The Sherley Amendment makes medicines safer by prohibiting the sale of drugs labeled with false therapeutic claims.
1914	The Harrison Narcotics Act requires those who dispense opium, cocaine, and related substances to keep records of the drugs they dispense and makes it illegal to possess narcotics without a prescription. This act allows physicians to prescribe narcotics only for treatment, not to addicts.
1938	The Food, Drug, and Cosmetic Act is the first law preventing the marketing of drugs not thoroughly tested.
1944	The Public Health Service Act is enacted and covers many health issues, including biologic products and the control of communicable diseases.
1970	The Comprehensive Drug Abuse Prevention and Control Act (also known as the Controlled Substances Act) organizes regulated drugs (including opiates, cocaine, cannabis, stimulants, depressants, and hallucinogens) into five schedules and imposes restrictions and penalties.
1975	The *United States Pharmacopeia* and *National Formulary* become a single standardized publication, the USP-NF.
1986	The Anti-Drug Abuse Act increases sentences and imposes mandatory minimum sentences for those convicted of illegal drug activity based on the type and quantity of drug involved.
1986	The Childhood Vaccine Act authorizes the FDA to acquire information about patients taking vaccines, to recall biologics, and to recommend civil penalties if guidelines regarding biologic use were not followed.
1988	The FDA is officially established as an agency of the U.S. Department of Health and Human Services.
1992	The Prescription Drug User Fee Act requires that nongeneric drug and biologic manufacturers pay fees to be used for improvements in the drug review process.
1994	The Dietary Supplement Health and Education Act requires clear labeling of dietary supplements and gives the FDA the power to remove supplements that cause a significant public risk.
1997	The FDA Modernization Act reauthorizes the Prescription Drug User Fee Act, representing the largest reform effort of the drug review process since 1938.
2002	The Best Pharmaceuticals for Children Act improves the safety and efficacy of medicines for children and continues the exclusivity provisions for pediatric drugs as mandated under the Food and Drug Administration Modernization Act of 1997.
2003	The Medicare Prescription Drug Improvement and Modernization Act provides seniors and those with disabilities a prescription drug benefit and better benefits under Medicare.
2007	The Food and Drug Administration Amendments Act (FDAAA) of 2007 reauthorizes and expands the Prescription Drug User Fee Act, the Modernization Act, the Best Pharmaceuticals for Children Act, and the Pediatric Research Equity Act.
2012	The Food and Drug Administration Safety and Innovation Act (FDASIA) of 2012 reauthorizes the Prescription Drug User Fee Act (PDUFA). Requires the FDA to implement a structured benefit-risk framework in the new drug approval process.

Drug Standards

2.3 The standardization of drug purity and strength is specified by the *United States Pharmacopeia-National Formulary.*

Until the 1800s, drugs were prepared from plants that were available in the natural environment. The strength and purity of the products varied considerably because they were entirely dependent on the experience (and integrity) of the druggist preparing the product and the quality of the local ingredients. Potency and safety varied from region to region and, indeed, from batch to batch. Consider the simple analogy of baking. If 100 people across the world were asked to bake a loaf of bread, the final products would vary considerably in size, taste, and nutritional value. It is likely that no two loaves would be the same. It is obvious that a standard recipe must be followed. Similarly, to obtain consistency in the preparation and potency of drugs, standards (recipes) are needed.

Among the first standards used by pharmacists was the **formulary**, or list of pharmaceutical products and drug recipes. In the United States, the first comprehensive publication of drug standards, the *United States Pharmacopeia* (USP), was established in 1820. A **pharmacopeia** is a medical reference summarizing standards of drug purity, strength, and directions for synthesis. From 1852 until 1975, two major compendia maintained drug standards in the United States, the USP and the *National Formulary* (NF), which were established by the American Pharmaceutical Association (APhA). All drug products were covered in the USP, whereas the NF focused on nondrug ingredients. In 1975, the two were merged into a single publication named the *United States*

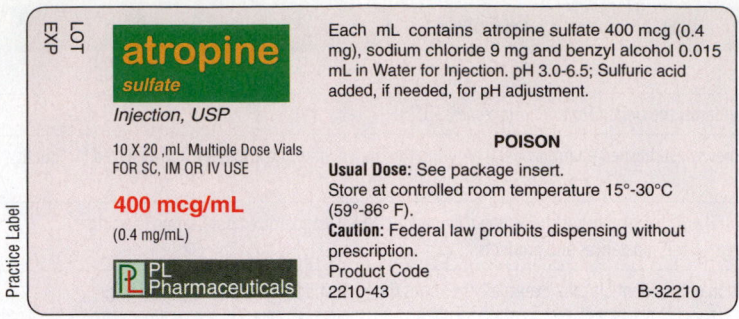
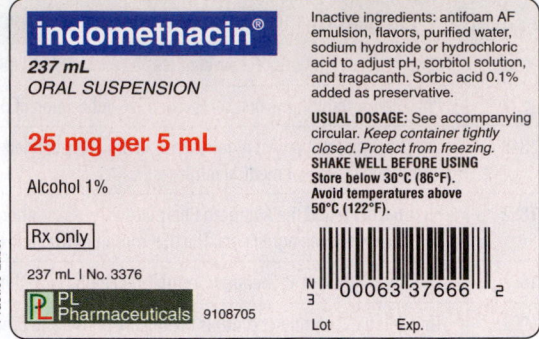

For educational purposes only

Figure 2.2 Medication with the USP label (left) and without USP label (right). Practice Label "for educational purposes only."

Pharmacopeia-National Formulary (USP-NF). The current document consists of more than 270 chapters and 4,700 drug monographs. The USP-NF is published annually, with two supplements being issued throughout the year. Today, the USP label can be found on many medications verifying the purity and exact amounts of ingredients found within the container. Drugs marketed in the United States must conform to USP-NF standards to avoid possible charges of adulteration and misbranding. Sample labels are illustrated in Figure 2.2. The USP also provides a voluntary program for verifying the label accuracy of dietary supplements (see Chapter 7).

The U.S. Food and Drug Administration

2.4 **The regulatory agency responsible for ensuring that drugs and medical devices are safe and effective is the U.S. Food and Drug Administration.**

The establishment of a regulatory agency for food and drugs in the United States began with a single chemist appointed by President Lincoln in 1862. The **U.S. Food and Drug Administration (FDA)** was established by the PFDA of 1906 and later expanded to carry out the provisions of the FDCA of 1938. It is one of the oldest drug regulatory agencies in the world. The FDA states its mission as follows:

- Protecting the public health by ensuring the safety, efficacy, and security of human and veterinary drugs, biologic products,

medical devices, the nation's food supply, cosmetics, and products that emit radiation

- Advancing the public health by helping to speed innovations that make medicines and foods more effective, safer, and more affordable

- Helping the public get the accurate, science-based information they need to use medicines and foods to improve their health

With such an important and vast mission, the FDA is organized around seven branches, as shown in Figure 2.3. The Center for Drug Evaluation and Research (CDER) states its mission as facilitating the availability of safe, effective drugs; keeping unsafe or ineffective drugs off the market; improving the health of Americans; and providing clear, easily understandable drug information for safe and effective use. All new drugs must be approved by the CDER before they can be marketed. This includes prescription drugs, OTC drugs, and all generic equivalents. After marketing, the CDER is responsible for continued monitoring of safety and may issue additional warnings to health care providers or consumers as additional information becomes available.

The Center for Biologics Evaluation and Research (CBER) regulates the use of biologics (drugs derived from living sources), including sera, vaccines, and blood products. One historical achievement involving biologics is the 1986 Childhood Vaccine Act. This act authorizes the FDA to acquire information about patients taking vaccines, to recall biologics, and to recommend civil penalties if guidelines regarding biologics are not followed. The mission of

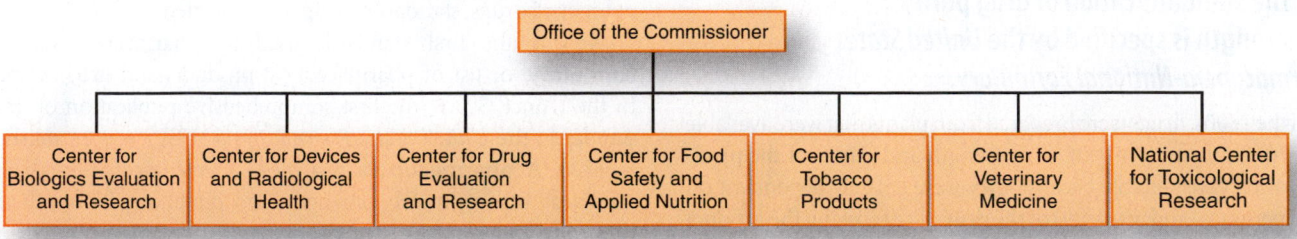

Figure 2.3 Organization of the Food and Drug Administration showing the seven centers that regulate human and veterinary drugs, biologic products, medical devices, the nation's food supply, cosmetics, tobacco, and products that emit radiation.

the CBER was recently expanded to include the regulation of gene therapy and treatment with human cells or tissue-based products.

The FDA also oversees the administration of herbal products, dietary supplements, and cosmetics through the Center for Food Safety and Applied Nutrition (CFSAN). Although it does not require testing of herbal or dietary supplements prior to marketing, the CFSAN is responsible for taking action against any supplement that is deemed to be unsafe.

The CFSAN also regulates cosmetics, which are legally defined by the FDCA of 1938 as "articles intended to be rubbed, poured, sprinkled, or sprayed on, introduced into, or otherwise applied to the human body . . . for cleansing, beautifying, promoting attractiveness, or altering the appearance." Examples of products considered cosmetics are skin moisturizers, perfumes, lipsticks, fingernail polishes, eye and facial makeup preparations, shampoos, toothpastes, and deodorants. Can a product be both a cosmetic and a drug? In most cases, cosmetics are not drugs; however, it depends on a product's intended use. For example, if a shampoo is marketed to treat a condition such as dandruff, the active ingredient is considered a drug. If a skin cream claims to provide sunscreen protection, it may be considered a drug. Cosmetics do not require approval by the CFSAN prior to marketing, and regulations are much less restrictive compared to drug approval. Manufacturers of cosmetics are generally careful not to promote unwarranted therapeutic claims, such as that a product prevents or treats a condition or disease. This would cause the product to be considered a drug by the FDA, and it would be subject to tighter regulations.

In 2009, the FDA was given the authority to regulate the manufacture, marketing, and distribution of tobacco products. To carry out this legislative mandate, the FDA created a seventh branch, the Center for Tobacco Products.

Drug Approval

2.5 The drug approval process established by the Food and Drug Administration ensures that drugs sold in the United States are safe and effective.

Drugs are discovered in any number of ways. Penicillin was discovered purely by accident while the scientist was studying an unrelated topic. Many drugs have been isolated from natural substances, including plants and bacteria. Some drugs are "me too" drugs, whereby the pharmacologist simply took a well-known drug and slightly modified the chemical structure to produce a very similar agent. As molecular biology and genetics have progressed into the modern era, drugs have been purposefully designed to fit into specific receptor sites on enzymes or cells.

Regardless of the path to discovery, all drugs must be approved by the FDA before they can be sold in the United States. (Medical marijuana, discussed in Chapter 27, has become an exception to this approval process). The FDA drug review and approval process follows a well-developed and organized plan, as summarized in Figure 2.4.

The first stage of drug development is **preclinical research**, which involves extensive laboratory testing by the pharmaceutical company. Scientists perform testing on human and microbial cells cultured in the laboratory. Studies are performed in several species of animals to examine the drug's effectiveness at different doses and to look for adverse effects. The goals of this extensive testing on cultured cells and in animals are to determine drug action and to predict whether the drug will cause harm to humans. Because laboratory tests do not accurately reflect the precise way the human body will respond to the drug, preclinical research results are always inconclusive. Most drugs do not proceed past the preclinical research stage because they are either too toxic or simply not effective. The FDA does not regulate preclinical testing.

If a drug appears promising, the pharmaceutical company submits an **Investigational New Drug (IND)** application to the FDA that contains all the animal and cell testing data. Scientists at the FDA study the data and must be convinced that the drug is safe enough to allow human testing. Approval from the FDA is necessary before the next stage can begin.

Clinical investigation, the second stage of drug testing, takes place in three different stages termed **clinical phase trials**. These clinical trials are the longest part of the drug approval process and occur in sequential stages.

- **Phase 1.** Testing is conducted on 20 to 80 healthy volunteers for several months to determine proper dosage and to assess for adverse effects. The focus of the phase 1 trial is on safety. If unacceptable levels of toxicity are noted, the clinical trials are stopped.

- **Phase 2.** Several hundred patients with the disease to be treated are given the drug. The primary focus of the phase 2 trial is on effectiveness, although safety data continue to be recorded. In most cases, the effectiveness of the new drug is compared to an inert substance, or **placebo**, which serves as a control "nontreatment" group. In other cases the new drug is compared to a standard drug used for the same condition. For example, a new drug for reducing fever may be compared to acetaminophen

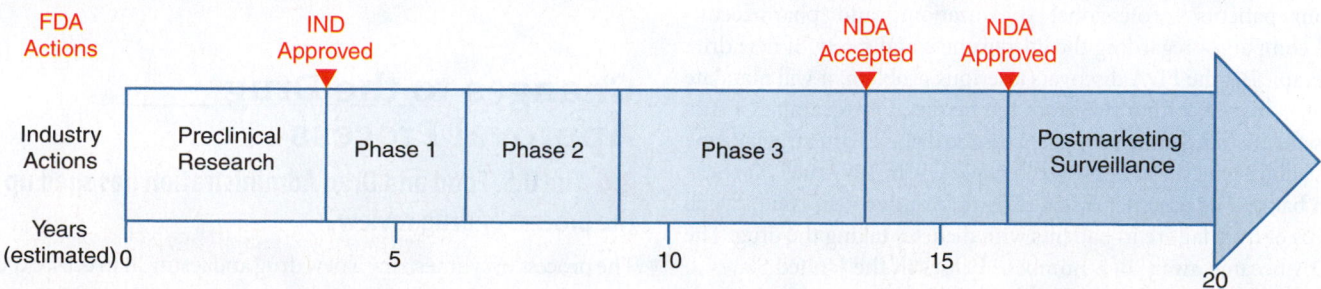

Figure 2.4 Drug development time line.

(Tylenol). If the new drug is found to have the same (or less) effectiveness and safety profile compared to the standard drug, the pharmaceutical company may stop the clinical trials. This phase may take several years.

- **Phase 3.** Large numbers of patients with the disease are given the drug to determine patient variability. Potential drug–drug interactions are examined. Patients with chronic conditions such as cardiac, renal, or hepatic impairment are given the drug to determine safety in these important populations. Assessment of effectiveness and safety continues for several years, and thousands of patients may be given the new drug during phase 3.

If the drug continues to show promise through the clinical phase trials, a **New Drug Application (NDA)** is submitted to the FDA. The NDA signals that the pharmaceutical company is ready to sell the new drug. During the NDA review, the FDA examines all preclinical and clinical data to assess whether the proposed new drug is safe and effective. By law, the CDER is obligated to act on at least 90% of the NDAs for standard drugs within 10 months of submission. For priority drugs, the benchmark is 6 months. If the NDA is approved, the manufacturer may begin selling the new drug. If the NDA is rejected, the FDA indicates whether the drug is "approvable" or "not approvable." "Approvable" means that the drug will likely be approved if the pharmaceutical company conducts additional testing or addresses specific issues identified by the FDA. A designation of "not approvable" indicates that the drug has significant barriers to approval.

The number of new drugs approved each year during the past decade has ranged from 78 to 101. Many of the new drugs, however, closely resembled existing medications. A better way to track advances in drug therapy is to monitor how many of the approved drugs are **new molecular entities**, those medications that are truly unique and structurally different from existing drugs. The number of new molecular entities has ranged from 20 to 30 per year.

Postmarketing surveillance, stage 4 of the drug approval process, begins after the NDA review has been completed. The purpose of stage 4 testing is to survey for harmful drug effects in a larger population. Some adverse effects are very subtle, take longer to appear, and are not identified until a drug is prescribed for large numbers of people. Adverse drug reactions are reported by the manufacturers, health care providers, and patients to the Adverse Event Reporting System (FAERS), a computerized database designed to support the FDA's postmarketing surveillance program.

The FDA holds public meetings annually to receive comments from patients, professional organizations, and pharmaceutical companies regarding the effectiveness and safety of new drug therapies. If the FDA discovers a serious problem, it will mandate that a drug be withdrawn from the market. One example of successful postmarketing surveillance is the diabetes drug troglitazone (Rezulin), which was approved by the FDA in 1997. In 1998, Britain banned its use after discovering at least one death and several cases of liver failure in patients with diabetes taking the drug. The FDA became aware of a number of cases in the United States in which Rezulin was linked with liver failure. Consumer advocates also claimed that the drug caused several cases of heart failure. Rezulin was recalled in March 2000 after health professionals asked the FDA to reconsider its therapeutic benefits versus its identified

risks. The FDA withdrew 15 prescription drugs from the market from 2001 to 2010.

The drug approval process has several important limitations. Historically, drug trials have used Caucasian males as their test population. Because gender and racial differences may affect how drugs are handled by the body, data obtained during clinical trials may not be representative of the population as a whole. Pharmaceutical companies are now including a more diverse population in their clinical trials. Most drugs have not been tested in children: Pediatric doses and responses are often based on experience rather than research data. Although clinical trials test drugs in pregnant laboratory animals and examine for possible birth defects, these data may not be representative of how drugs affect pregnant women or their fetuses. Finally, adverse effects may occur at such a low level that they are statistically insignificant in clinical trials using a few thousand patients. Several million patients may need to take the drug before these effects can be identified.

Another limitation of the drug approval process relates to off-label uses. When a new drug is tested by a pharmaceutical company it is for a specific indication; FDA approval is based on this indication. After several years of clinical experience, however, health care providers may find that the drug is also useful for indications not approved by the FDA. Or, the prescriber may find that the drug works better at a different dosage level or by a different route of administration. Once initially approved by the FDA for any indication, health care providers may legally prescribe the drug for other indications they feel are appropriate, despite the fact that the drug was never tested or approved for these additional conditions. How widespread is off-label prescribing? It is estimated that over 20% of prescriptions are for indications not approved by the FDA. The use of off-label drugs is particularly prevalent in cancer treatment and in pediatric patients. Although the FDA does not regulate off-label uses of drugs, laws prohibit pharmaceutical companies from advertising or promoting their drugs for off-label uses. It has not been clearly established whether or not off-label prescriptions increase risks to patients.

PharmFACT

It takes about 12 years of research and development, costing about $350 million, before a drug is submitted to the FDA for review (Drug Information Online, n.d.).

CONNECTION Checkpoint 2.1

In 2013, oxcarbazepine (Oxtellar), an antiseizure drug, and ponatinib (Iclusig), a monoclonal antibody for treating leukemia, were approved. Are these considered therapeutic or pharmacologic classifications? *See Answer to Connection Checkpoint 2.1 on student resource website.*

Changes to the Drug Approval Process

2.6 The U.S. Food and Drug Administration has sped up the process of drug review.

The process of synthesizing a new drug and testing it in cells, experimental animals, and humans takes many years. The NDA can include dozens of volumes of experimental and clinical data that must be examined during the FDA drug review process. Some NDAs contain over 100,000 pages of data. Even after all experiments have been concluded and clinical data have been gathered, the FDA review process can take several years.

Expenses associated with development of a new drug can cost the drug developer millions of dollars. Some studies estimate the cost of bringing a new drug to market at up to $1.8 billion (Morgan, Grootendorst, Lexchin, Cunningham, & Greyson, 2011). Pharmaceutical companies are often critical of the regulatory process and are anxious to get the drug marketed to recoup their high research and development expenses. The public is also anxious to receive new medications, particularly for diseases that have a high mortality rate. Although the criticisms of government regulatory agencies are certainly understandable, and sometimes justified, the fundamental priority of the FDA is to ensure the safety of medications. Without an exhaustive review of scientific data, the public could be exposed to dangerous or ineffective drugs.

In the early 1990s, due to pressures from consumer groups and various drug manufacturers, government officials began to plan how to speed up the drug review process. Reasons identified for the delay in the FDA drug approval process included outdated guidelines, poor communication, and not enough staff to handle the workload.

In 1992, the PDUFA was passed, requiring drug and biologic manufacturers to provide yearly product user fees. This added revenue allowed the FDA to hire more employees and to restructure its organization to more efficiently handle the processing of a greater number of drug applications. The result of restructuring was a resounding success. The average time for NDA review for new medications was cut in half.

As part of the FDA modernization, priority drugs now receive accelerated approval. These are drugs intended to treat serious and life-threatening conditions, such as cancer and AIDS, that lack effective treatments. In some cases, the FDA may grant accelerated approval before the drug has completed phase 3 trials. The FDA usually requires the pharmaceutical company to file subsequent reports confirming the effectiveness of the drug.

PharmFACT

The number of new molecular entities approved in 2012 was 39. The largest single indication was for the chemotherapy of cancer (FDA, 2013).

Prescription and Over-the-Counter Drugs

2.7 Over-the-counter drugs are usually safe and effective when used according to label instructions.

The 1951 Durham-Humphrey Amendment to the FDCA clearly established the difference between prescription and OTC drugs. To obtain a prescription drug, an order must be given authorizing the patient to receive the medication. Prescription medications are judged by the FDA to be potentially addictive or too harmful for self-administration. In some cases, they are used to treat conditions too complex for self-diagnosis by the consumer or the drug may require a skilled nurse or health care provider to administer it.

The advantages of requiring a prescription are numerous. The health care provider has an opportunity to examine the patient and determine a specific diagnosis. The prescriber can maximize therapy by ordering the proper drug for the patient's condition and by controlling the amount and frequency of the drug to be dispensed. In addition, the health care provider has an opportunity to teach the patient proper use of the drug and its expected adverse effects.

In contrast to prescription drugs, OTC drugs do not require an order from a health care provider. In most cases, patients may treat themselves safely if they carefully follow instructions included with the medication. A key point to remember is that no drug is without risk; if patients do not follow the guidelines on the label, serious adverse effects may result.

Patients prefer to take OTC medications for many reasons. OTC drugs may be obtained more easily than prescription drugs. No appointment with a health care provider is required, thus saving time and money. Without the assistance of a health care provider, however, choosing the proper medication for a specific problem can be challenging for a patient. OTC drugs may interact with foods, herbal products, prescription drugs, or other OTC drugs. Patients may not be aware that some OTC medications can impair their ability to function safely. Self-treatment is sometimes ineffective, and the potential for harm may increase if the disease is allowed to progress.

During the past decade, consumer groups have pushed for the reclassification of certain drugs from prescription to OTC in cases whereby a high margin of safety exists with the medicines. For example, prior to 1996, substances that were used to assist in smoking cessation, such as nicotine patches and gum, were available by prescription only but are now available OTC. Other switches from prescription to OTC include famotidine (Pepcid AC), cimetidine (Tagamet HB), omeprazole (Prilosec), cetirizine (Zyrtec), and loratadine (Claritin). Over the past 25 years, 700 products have been changed from prescription to OTC. The decision to reclassify a drug may be initiated by the manufacturer or mandated by the FDA during its review process.

CONNECTIONS | Lifespan Considerations

Reducing the Cost of Medications for Older Adults

Because the cost of prescription drugs may be a major cause for nonadherence in the older adult, nurses should explore any cost concerns with these patients as well as discuss ways to cut pharmacy costs. Chan (2010) recommends several strategies that may help to reduce prescription costs, including:

- For a new prescription, do not buy a whole bottle; instead ask for just a few pills. Adverse effects may require a change in medication.
- Ask for generic drugs when receiving a prescription.
- Buy OTC generic drugs when possible.
- Ask if there is a therapeutic generic equivalent in the same class of a brand drug if a generic of that drug is not available. Request available assistance, such as a social worker, or access to a government or community program to reduce medication costs.
- Explore the use of drug "deals" such as the "$4 prescription" or "free antibiotics," which chain pharmacies may offer.
- Request a review of all medications taken so that nonessential drugs are no longer needed.
- Split pills when appropriate, with a higher dosage ordered and split in half, but only if able to follow directions explicitly.

Herbal products and dietary supplements are also widely available OTC. Herbal products and dietary supplements are not considered drugs; they are not marketed to treat any disease, and they are not subject to the same regulatory process as drugs. Some of these products can, however, cause adverse effects and interact with medications. Nurses should always inquire about their patients' use of herbal products and dietary supplements and caution them that the FDA has not tested these products for effectiveness or safety. In some cases, herbal products are contraindicated. For example, St. John's wort should not be taken concurrently with antidepressant medications.

PharmFACT

Over 1,200,000 emergency department visits each year involve the nonmedical use of prescription or OTC pharmaceuticals. About half of these visits involve multiple drugs, and about 20% involve alcohol (Substance Abuse and Mental Health Services Administration, 2013).

Drug Schedules

2.8 Drugs with a potential for abuse are categorized into schedules.

Dependence is a powerful physiological or psychological need for a substance. Some drugs are frequently abused or have a high potential for dependence; thus the selling and distribution of these drugs are highly restricted. Drugs that have a significant potential for abuse are placed into five categories called *schedules*. These **scheduled drugs** are classified and regulated according to their potential for abuse, as shown in Table 2.2. Concepts of dependence and drug schedules are discussed in detail in Chapter 27.

In the United States, **controlled substances** are drugs whose use is restricted by the Comprehensive Drug Abuse Prevention and Control Act of 1970 and its later revisions. Hospitals and pharmacies must register with the Drug Enforcement Administration (DEA) and use their registration numbers to purchase scheduled drugs. They must maintain complete records of all quantities purchased and sold. Drugs with the highest abuse potential have additional restrictions. For example, providers must use a special order form to obtain Schedule II drugs, and orders must be written and

signed by the provider. Telephone orders to a pharmacy are not permitted. Refills for Schedule II drugs are not permitted; patients must visit their health care provider first. Health care providers convicted of unlawful manufacturing, distributing, and dispensing of controlled substances face severe penalties.

CONNECTION Checkpoint 2.2

Once a new drug is approved, it is assigned names. What are the two basic types of drug names and who assigns them? *See Answer to Connection Checkpoint 2.2 on student resource website.*

Prescriptive Authority for Nurses

2.9 Advanced practice nurses are allowed to prescribe drugs under state regulations.

Historically, prescribing drugs was the responsibility of the physician or dentist. With the growth of advanced nursing degrees at the master's and doctoral levels, nurses began to specialize and to obtain certification as certified nurse midwives (CNMs), certified registered nurse anesthetists (CRNAs), nurse practitioners (NPs), and clinical nurse specialists (CNSs). These advanced practice registered nurses (APRNs) complete graduate-level education that includes advanced pharmacology content and they obtain certification by exam in one of the four above specialties.

The ability to prescribe drugs is regulated by state law, and each state has different requirements for prescriptive authority. In some states, APRNs are authorized to prescribe drugs independently of physician collaboration, delegation, or supervision. In others, the APRN must have some level of physician collaboration or delegation and may not prescribe independently (Phillips, 2012). The specialty of the APRN may also affect prescriptive authority and there may be additional requirements for a CRNA rather than an NP, as an example. Controlled substance prescriptive authority may also vary from state to state. With the growth of Internet and mail-order prescriptions, problems still remain to be worked out on interstate acceptance of APRN prescriptions, especially for controlled substances, when laws vary across state borders.

TABLE 2.2 U.S. Drug Schedules and Examples

Drug Schedule	Abuse Potential	Examples	Therapeutic Use
I	Highest	Heroin, GHB, LSD, marijuana, MDMA, mescaline, methaqualone, methcathinone, peyote, and psilocybin	No currently acceptable medical use; no prescriptions may be written
II	High	Potent opioids (such as codeine in high doses, fentanyl, methadone, morphine, oxycodone, meperidine), amphetamine, cocaine, methamphetamine, methylphenidate, PCP, short-acting barbiturates	Have currently accepted medical use but use may be severely restricted; normally no refills are permitted (but there are exceptions)
III	Moderate	Anabolic steroids, buprenorphine ketamine, codeine (lower doses compounded with aspirin or acetaminophen), hydrocodone (lower doses compounded with aspirin or acetaminophen), and intermediate-acting barbiturates	Have currently accepted medical use; less stringent controls than Schedule II drugs; five refills allowed in a 6-month period
IV	Low	Benzodiazepines (such as alprazolam, diazepam, midazolam, temazepam), long-acting barbiturates, meprobamate, pentazocine, tramadol, and zolpidem	Have currently accepted medical use; similar controls to Schedule III drugs; five refills allowed in a 6-month period
V	Lowest	Cough medicines with codeine, antidiarrheal medicines with small amounts of opioids	Have currently accepted medical use; similar controls to Schedule III and IV drugs

From *Controlled Substance Schedules, U. S. Department of Justice,* n.d. Retrieved from http://www.deadiversion.usdoj.gov/schedules/.

In 2008, a joint task force of APRNs and members of the National Council of State Boards of Nursing began work on a consensus model to define APRN practice and education requirements and to develop standards that would ensure uniform regulation of practice (APRN Joint Dialogue Group, 2008). The consensus model has not yet been implemented in all states, but it has helped to standardize the scope of practice for these nurses, including prescriptive authority, and to improve the inclusion of APRNs in direct reimbursement plans by health insurance companies.

With the passage of the Patient Protection and Affordable Care Act (ACA) in 2010, it is estimated that an additional 32 million Americans who previously had limited access to health care or were uninsured will gain health care coverage (Osborne, 2011). The APRN is viewed as an essential member of the health care system's ability to deliver affordable care. The ability to prescribe drugs, a key component of most treatment plans, will ensure that these patients are provided the best and cost-effective care possible by all APRNs and other health care providers.

CHAPTER

2

Understanding the Chapter

Key Concepts Summary

2.1 Early American history saw the rise of patent medicines and the lack of adequate drug regulations.

2.2 In the 1900s, drug legislation was enacted to make drugs safer and more effective.

2.3 The standardization of drug purity and strength is specified by the *United States Pharmacopeia-National Formulary*.

2.4 The regulatory agency responsible for ensuring that drugs and medical devices are safe and effective is the U.S. Food and Drug Administration.

2.5 The drug approval process established by the Food and Drug Administration ensures that drugs sold in the United States are safe and effective.

2.6 The U.S. Food and Drug Administration has sped up the process of drug review.

2.7 Over-the-counter drugs are usually safe and effective when used according to label instructions.

2.8 Drugs with a potential for abuse are categorized into schedules.

2.9 Advanced practice nurses are allowed to prescribe drugs under state regulations.

Case Study: Making the Patient Connection

Remember the patient "Gertrude Stone" at the beginning of the chapter? Now read the remainder of the case study. Based on the information presented within this chapter, respond to the critical thinking questions that follow.

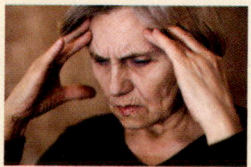

Gertrude Stone lives alone in the same house she has owned for 46 years. Although she is seldom sick, when she needs to see a health care provider she must ride the public bus system. The trip requires two bus transfers and can be tiring.

Because Gertrude lives only one block from a grocery store, she often self-medicates using OTC drugs. She strongly believes in the use of herbs, vitamins, and home remedies.

As a parish nurse, you assist with the health fair at a church where Gertrude is an active member.

Critical Thinking Questions

1. How would you respond to Gertrude about the safety of OTC drugs?
2. What are the advantages and disadvantages of OTC medications?
3. How can Gertrude be certain that OTC medications are safe for her?

See Answers to Critical Thinking Questions on student resource website.

Additional Case Study

Your 12-year-old nephew is preparing a report for school about the FDA and the drug approval process. You, the nurse in the family, are often called on by family members to answer questions about anything health related. Below are his questions. How would you respond?

1. What is the role of the FDA?

2. What role does the FDA play in regulating herbal and dietary supplements?

3. How quickly can a new drug be approved by the FDA?

See Answers to Additional Case Study on student resource website.

Chapter Review

1 The nurse knows that governmental drug legislation requires the drug manufacturer to prove that a drug is both safe and:

1. Free of adverse effects and potential reactions.
2. Effective for a specified purpose.
3. Reasonable in cost and easily accessible.
4. Beneficial to various population groups.

2 The drug research participant with a particular disease is taking part in an investigative study to examine the effects of a new drug. Previously, this drug was tested using healthy volunteers. The next phase of the clinical trial investigation in which the patient will be participating is:

1. Phase 1
2. Phase 2
3. Phase 3
4. Phase 4

3 When considering various drug therapies, the nurse knows that most drug testing and approval occurs with which population?

1. Multiple population types and is usually safe for all patients
2. Caucasian males and may not be safe for other populations
3. Older adults, and may be harmful to children and adolescents as well
4. Animals, which verifies the drug's effectiveness in humans

4 The patient requests that a refill prescription of a Schedule II controlled substance be telephoned to the drug store. When responding to the patient, the nurse would consider which factor? Refills of Schedule II drugs:

1. Are less costly than the original prescription.
2. Must be listened to by at least two people.
3. Are verified through the local DEA office.
4. Are not permitted under federal law.

5 The nurse knows that drugs that are subject to stricter regulations are those:

1. With a high potential for abuse or dependency.
2. That are most costly and difficult to produce.
3. With adverse effects and high occurrence of drug or food interactions.
4. That have taken years to be proven effective in the laboratory.

6 A nurse notes that multiple patients had a reaction to the same medication, a drug that has been available for several years. Which action should the nurse take? Select all that apply.

1. File an Adverse Event Report with the FDA.
2. Note the reaction in the patient's chart.
3. Notify the health care provider who ordered the drug.
4. Wait until the FDA sends a notification of the drug's recall before informing the patient.
5. Compare each patient's reaction to determine if it is the same.

See Answers to Chapter Review in Appendix A.

References

APRN Joint Dialogue Group. (2008). *Consensus model for APRN licensure, accreditation, certification, and education.* Retrieved from https://www.ncsbn.org/Consensus_Model _for_APRN_Regulation_July_2008.pdf

Chan, M. (2010). Reducing cost-related medication nonadherence in patients with diabetes. *Drug Benefit Trends, 22,* 67–71. Retrieved from http://dbt.consultantlive.com/ diabetes-management/content/article/1145628/ 1554670

Drug Information Online. (n.d.). *New drug approval process.* Retrieved from http://www .drugs.com/fda-approval-process.html

Morgan, S., Grootendorst, P., Lexchin, J., Cunningham, C., & Greyson, D. (2011). The cost of drug development: A systematic review. *Health Policy, 100,* 4–17. doi:10.1016/ j.healthpol.2010.12.002

Osborne, K. (2011). Regulation of prescriptive authority for certified nurse-midwives and certified midwives: A national overview. *Journal of Nurse Midwifery & Women's Health, 56,* 543–556. doi:10.1111/j.1542-2011 .2011.00123x

Phillips, S. J. (2012). APRN consensus model implementation and planning. *The Nurse Practitioner, 37*(1), 22–45. doi:10.1097/01 .NPR.0000408277.35639.0b

Substance Abuse and Mental Health Services Administration. (2013). *Drug abuse warning network, 2011: National estimates of drug-related emergency department visits.* Retrieved from http://www.samhsa.gov/data/2k13/ DAWN2k11ED/DAWN2k11ED.htm

U.S. Food and Drug Administration. (2013). *New molecular entity approvals for 2012.* Retrieved from http://www.fda.gov/Drugs/ DevelopmentApprovalProcess/DrugInnovation/ ucm336115.htm

Selected Bibliography

Berger, M. M., Eck, S., & Ruberg, S. J. (2010). Raising the bar of efficacy for drug approval requires an understanding of patient diversity. *Journal of Clinical Oncology, 28*(20), e343–e344. doi:10.1200/JCO.2010.28.2475

Buppert, C. (2012). The perils of off-label prescribing. *Journal for Nurse Practitioners, 8*, 567–568.

Daggumalli, J. S., & Martin, I. G. (2012). Are pharmaceutical market withdrawals preventable? A preliminary analysis. *Therapeutic Innovation & Regulatory Science, 46*, 694–700. doi:10.1177/0092861512458776

DiMasi, J. A., Feldman, L., Seckler, A., & Wilson, A. (2010). Trends in risks associated with new drug development: Success rates for investigational drugs. *Clinical Pharmacology & Therapeutics, 87*, 272–277. doi:10.1038/clpt.2009.295

Goldberg, N. H., Schneeweiss, S., Kowai, M. K., & Gagne, J. J. (2010). Availability of comparative efficacy data at the time of drug approval in the United States. *Journal of the American Medical Association, 305*, 1786–1789. doi:10.1001/jama.2011.539

Lowes, R. (2010). *FDA vows to bring its "regulatory science" into 21st century.* Retrieved from http://www.medscape.com/viewarticle/730061

Marshall, V., & Baylor, N. W. (2011). Food and drug administration regulation and evaluation of vaccines. *Pediatrics, 127*, S23–S30. doi:10.1542/peds.2010-1722E

O'Malley, P. G. (2012). What does off-label prescribing really mean? *Archives of Internal Medicine, 172*, 759–760. doi:10.1001/archinternmed.2012.789.

U.S. Department of Justice. (n.d.). *Controlled substance schedules.* Retrieved from http://www.deadiversion.usdoj.gov/schedules/

U.S. Food and Drug Administration. (2013). *FDA organization.* Retrieved from http://www.fda.gov/AboutFDA/CentersOffices/default.htm

U.S. Food and Drug Administration. (2013). *Prescription drug user fee act (PDUFA).* Retrieved from http://www.fda.gov/ForIndustry/UserFees/PrescriptionDrugUserFee/default.htm

Wellman-Labadie, W. (2010). The U.S. Orphan Drug Act: Rare disease research stimulator or commercial opportunity? *Health Policy, 95*, 216–228. doi:10.1016/j.healthpol.2009.12.001

Wertheimer, A. (2011). Off label prescribing of drugs for children. *Current Drug Safety, 6*(1), 46–48. doi:10.2174/157488611794479973

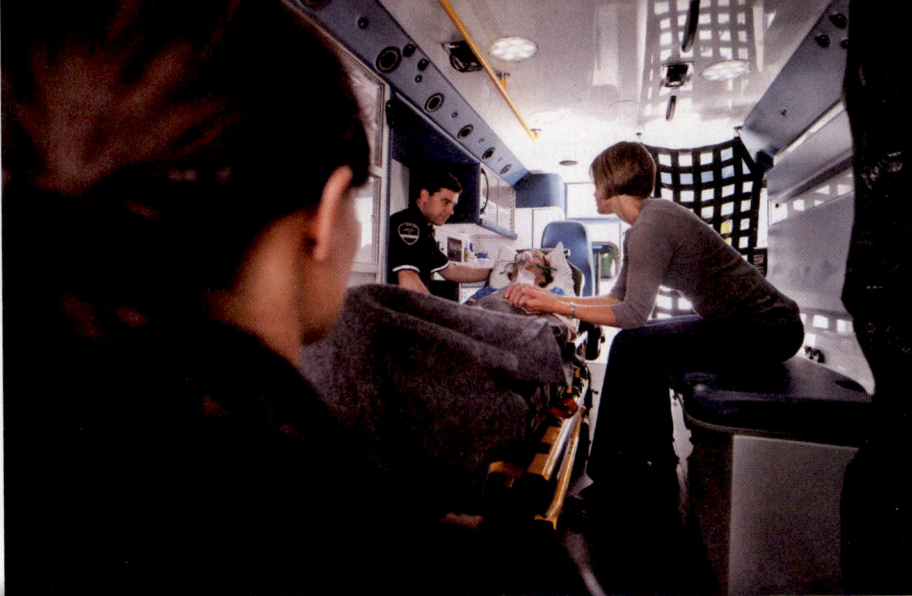

"I'm terribly worried about my father, John Kessler. He's been so ill for so long. I don't know if his body can take much more."

Patient's daughter, "Emily Kessler Myers"

CHAPTER

3

Pharmacokinetics

LEARNING OUTCOMES

After reading this chapter, the student should be able to:

1. Identify the four primary processes of pharmacokinetics.
2. Explain mechanisms by which drugs cross plasma membranes.
3. Discuss factors affecting drug absorption.
4. Discuss how drugs are distributed throughout the body.
5. Describe how plasma proteins affect drug distribution.
6. Explain the metabolism of drugs and its applications to pharmacotherapy.
7. Identify major processes by which drugs are excreted.
8. Explain how enterohepatic recirculation affects drug activity.
9. Explain how a drug reaches and maintains its therapeutic range in the plasma.
10. Explain the applications of a drug's plasma half-life ($t_{1/2}$) to pharmacotherapy.
11. Differentiate between loading and maintenance doses.

CHAPTER OUTLINE

▸ Introduction to Pharmacokinetics

▸ Primary Processes of Pharmacokinetics
  Absorption
  Distribution
  Metabolism
  Excretion

▸ Time–Response Relationships
  Drug Plasma Levels
  Drug Half-Life
  Loading and Maintenance Doses

KEY TERMS

absorption, 27

affinity, 32

blood–brain barrier, 32

diffusion, 26

distribution, 31

drug-protein complexes, 32

enteral route, 27

enteric-coated, 28

enterohepatic recirculation, 36

enzyme induction, 34

excretion, 35

extended release, 28

fetal–placental barrier, 32

first-pass effect, 28

hepatic microsomal enzyme system, 33

isozymes, 33

loading dose, 39

maintenance doses, 39

metabolism, 33

minimum effective concentration, 37

pharmacokinetics, 25

plasma half-life ($t_{1/2}$), 38

prodrugs, 33

substrate, 34

therapeutic drug monitoring, 37

therapeutic range, 37

topical route, 29

toxic concentration, 37

transdermal patches, 29

Most drugs produce their effects by causing a physiological or chemical change in specific target cells in the body. To produce a therapeutic effect, a drug must reach its target cells in sufficient quantities. For many medications, such as topical agents used to treat superficial skin conditions, this is an easy task. For most medications, however, the process of reaching target cells to cause a physiological change is challenging. Drugs are exposed to a myriad of different barriers and destructive processes after they enter the body. The purpose of this chapter is to examine factors that act on the drug as it attempts to reach its target cells and to provide examples of how the nurse can use this information to improve the success of drug therapy.

Introduction to Pharmacokinetics

3.1 Pharmacokinetics focuses on what the body does to drugs after they are administered.

The term **pharmacokinetics** is derived from the root words *pharmaco*, which refers to medicines, and *kinetics*, which means "movement" or "motion." Pharmacokinetics is thus the study of drug movement throughout the body. In practical terms, it describes what the body does to the medication after it is administered. Pharmacokinetics is a core subject in pharmacology, and a firm grasp of this topic allows nurses to better understand and predict the actions and adverse effects of medications in their patients.

Drugs face numerous obstacles in reaching their target cells. For most medications, the greatest barrier is crossing the many membranes that separate the drug from its target cells. A drug taken by mouth, for example, must cross the plasma membranes of the mucosal cells of the gastrointestinal (GI) tract and the endothelial cells of the capillaries to enter the bloodstream. To leave the bloodstream, it must again cross capillary cells, travel through interstitial fluid, and perhaps enter target cells by passing through their plasma membranes. Depending on the mechanism of action, the drug may also need to enter cellular organelles such as nuclei, which are surrounded by additional membranes. Some of the membranes and barriers that many drugs must successfully penetrate before they can elicit a response are illustrated in Figure 3.1.

While seeking their target cells and attempting to pass through the various membranes, drugs are subjected to numerous physiological

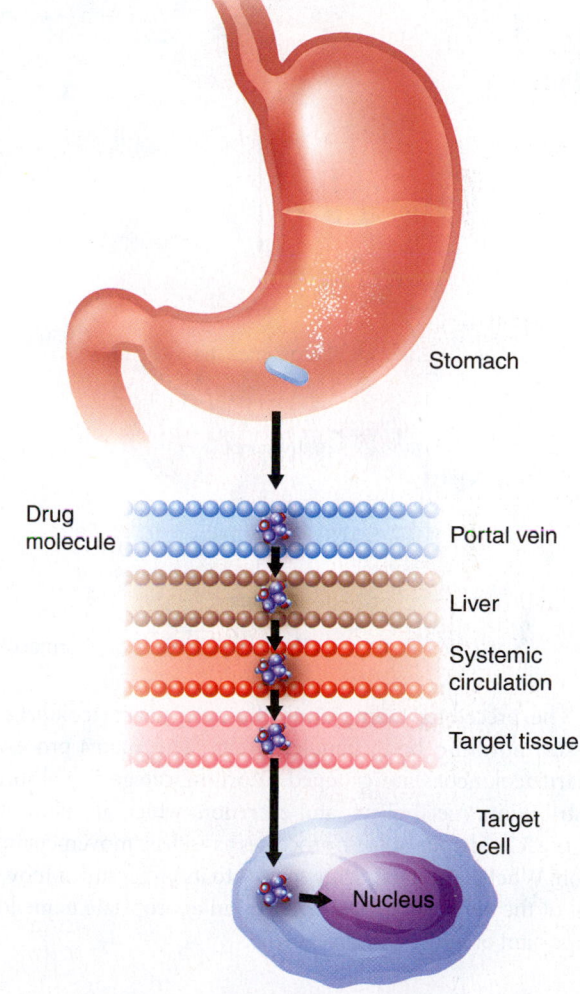

Figure 3.1 Barriers that a drug administered by the oral route must cross before interacting with a target cell.

processes. For medications given by the oral route, stomach acid and digestive enzymes often break down the drug molecules. Enzymes in the liver and other organs may chemically change the drug molecule, making it less active. If seen as foreign by the body, phagocytes may attempt to remove the drug, or an immune response may be triggered. The kidneys, large intestine, and other organs attempt to rapidly excrete the drug from the body.

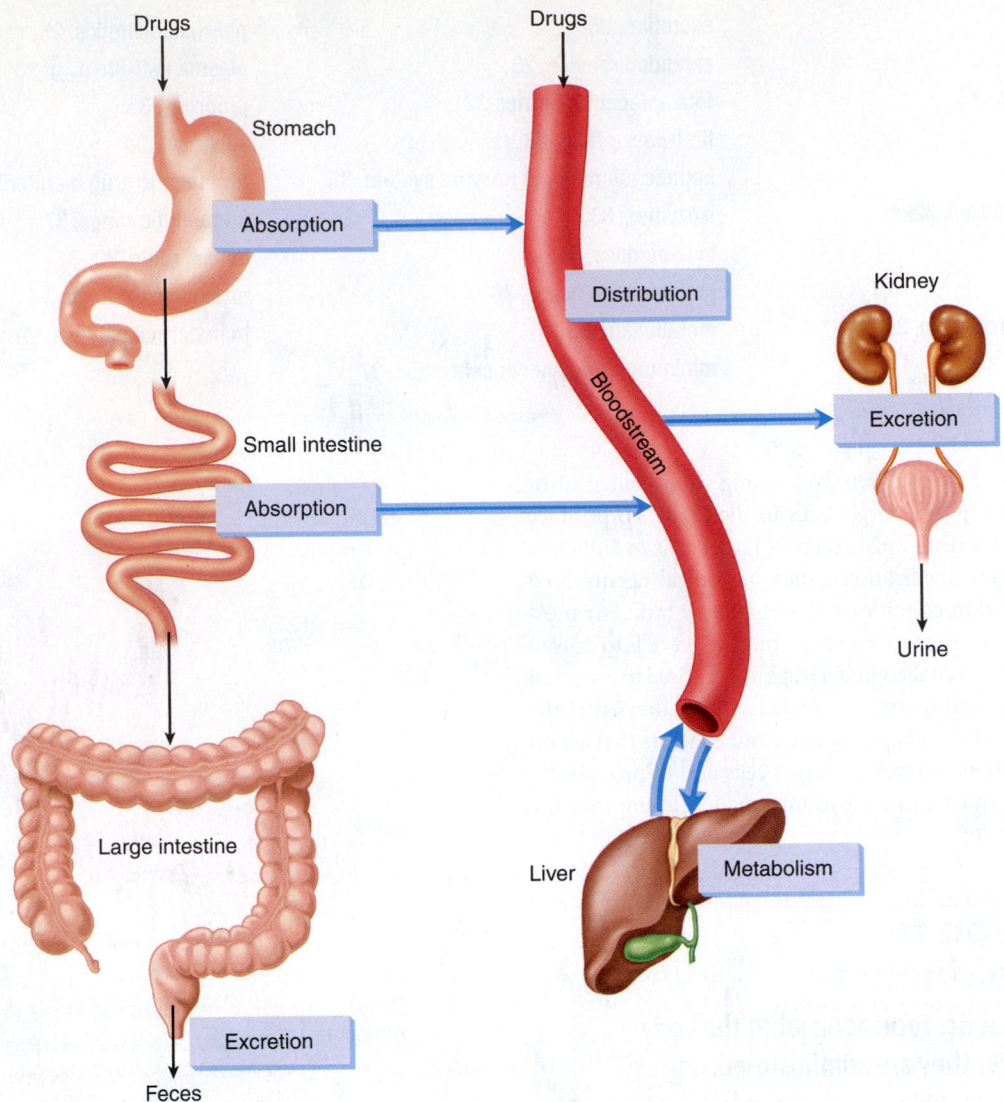

Figure 3.2 The four processes of pharmacokinetics: absorption, distribution, metabolism, and excretion.

The preceding examples all illustrate pharmacokinetic processes: how the body handles drugs. The many processes of pharmacokinetics are grouped into four categories: absorption, distribution, metabolism, and excretion, which are illustrated in Figure 3.2. All four of these processes have drug movement in common. Whether it involves movement to its target site or movement out of the body, kinetics is certainly an appropriate name for this important branch of pharmacology.

3.2 Drugs use diffusion and active transport to cross plasma membranes to reach their target cells.

With few exceptions, drugs must cross plasma membranes and enter cells to produce their effects. Plasma membranes are composed of a lipid bilayer, with proteins and other molecules interspersed in the membrane. Like other chemicals, drugs use two primary processes to cross membranes: diffusion and active transport.

Simple **diffusion** or passive transport is the movement of a chemical from an area of higher concentration to an area of lower concentration. This is best explained by the use of an example. When first administered, a drug given by the intravenous (IV)

route is in high concentration in the blood but has not yet entered the tissues. The drug will move quickly by passive diffusion from its region of high concentration (blood) to a region of low concentration (tissues) to produce its action. With time the drug will be inactivated (metabolized) by the tissue and more doses of the drug may be administered, creating a continual concentration gradient from blood to tissue.

Diffusion assumes that the chemical is able to freely cross the plasma membrane. This, however, is not the case for all drugs. Passage across the lipid-rich plasma membrane is dependent on the physical characteristics of the drug molecule. Drug molecules that are small, nonionized, and lipid soluble will usually pass through plasma membranes by simple diffusion and easily reach their target cells. This process is illustrated in Figure 3.3. Drugs may also enter through open channels in the plasma membrane; however, the molecule must be very small, such as urea, alcohol, and water.

Large molecules, ionized drugs, and water-soluble agents have difficulty crossing plasma membranes by simple diffusion. These agents may require carrier, or transport, proteins to cross membranes. A drug that moves into a cell along its concentration gradient utilizing a membrane carrier protein is using the process of

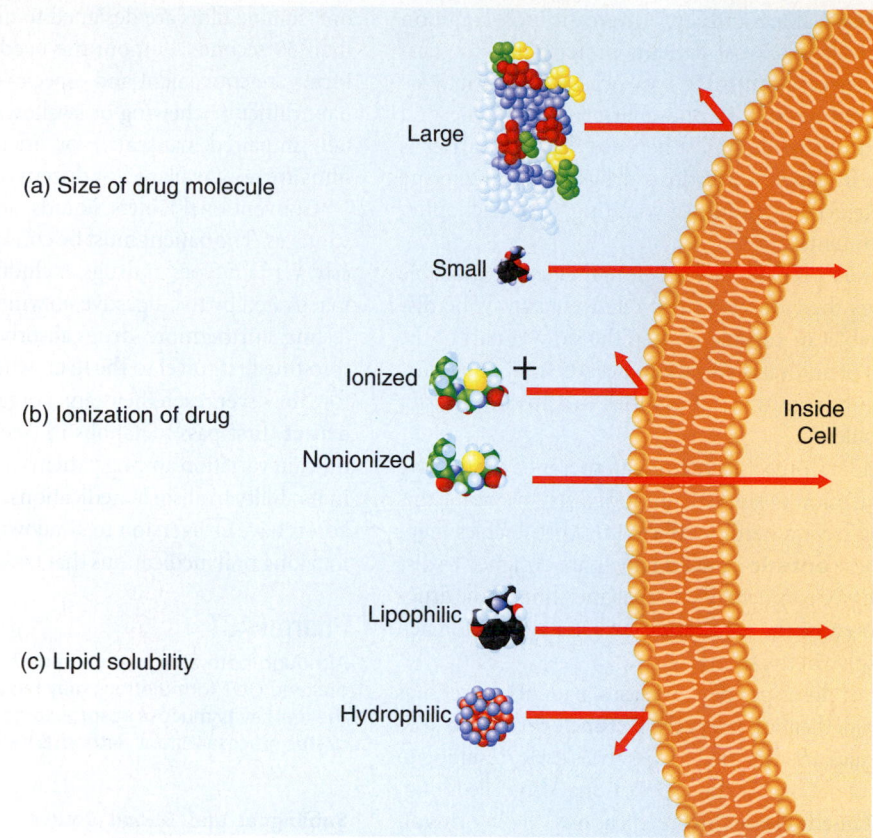

Figure 3.3 Passage of drugs across plasma membranes: (a) small drugs; (b) nonionized drugs; and (c) lipophilic drugs are more likely to cross membranes.

facilitated diffusion. This process does not require energy expenditure from the cell, but it does require that a specific carrier protein be present on the plasma membrane. Transport proteins are selective and only carry molecules that have specific structures.

Some drugs cross membranes against their gradient, from low concentration to high concentration, through the process of active transport. This requires expenditure of energy on the part of the cell and a carrier protein. Carrier proteins that assist in active transport are sometimes called pumps.

Primary Processes of Pharmacokinetics

3.3 Absorption is the process of moving a drug from the site of administration to the bloodstream.

For most medications the first step toward reaching target cells is **absorption**, the process by which drug molecules move from their site of administration to the blood. With the exception of a few topical medications, local anesthetics, anti-infectives for intestinal parasites, and some radiologic contrast agents, the majority of drugs must be absorbed in order to produce an effect. Of course, drugs administered directly into blood vessels by IV or intra-arterial routes are not absorbed because they are placed directly in the bloodstream.

Absorption is the primary pharmacokinetic factor determining the onset of drug action—the length of time it takes a drug to produce its effect. In general, the more rapid the absorption,

the faster the onset of drug action. Drugs used in critical care are designed to be absorbed within seconds or minutes, or they are given intravenously. At the other extreme are drugs such as the contraceptive Mirena, which is a polyethylene tube placed in the uterus. The drug inside Mirena, levonorgestrel, is absorbed slowly from the tube and provides contraceptive protection for up to 5 years.

In addition to onset time, absorption determines the intensity of drug action. For any given drug, a specific percentage of the drug is absorbed, ranging from 0% to 100%. Everything else being equal, drugs with higher absorption rates produce a more effective response than those with lower absorption rates. The degree of absorption is conditional on many factors.

Route of Administration

The route of administration is one of the most important variables affecting drug absorption. The three broad categories of routes of drug administration are enteral, topical, and parenteral. Each route has characteristics that offer both advantages and disadvantages. Whereas some drugs are formulated to be given by several routes, others are specific to only one route.

Enteral route: The **enteral route** includes drugs delivered to the GI tract, either orally (PO) or through nasogastric or gastrostomy tubes. Most medications administered by the enteral route are intended for absorption to the general circulation, taking advantage of the combined absorptive surfaces of the oral mucosa, stomach, and small intestine. A few enteral medications are administered for local effects, such as infections of the GI tract.

Tablets and Capsules: Tablets and capsules are the most common forms of oral medications. Most patients prefer tablets or capsules because of their ease of use. In some cases, tablets may be scored, allowing for one-half or one-quarter dosing. The oral route is considered one of the safest because the skin barrier is not compromised. In cases of overdose, drugs remaining in the stomach can be retrieved by inducing vomiting or by suctioning out the stomach contents.

Tablets and capsules must dissolve before the drug is available for absorption; thus their onset time is relatively slow. The dissolution rate of a tablet or capsule is often the slowest part of the absorption process of an oral medication. Because oral liquid formulations do not undergo dissolution, they are absorbed faster than tablets or capsules.

The strongly acidic stomach contents can present a destructive obstacle to the absorption of some medications. To overcome this barrier, tablets may have a hard, waxy coating that enables them to resist acidity. These **enteric-coated** tablets are designed to dissolve in the alkaline environment of the small intestine. Some drugs are enteric coated because the medications will irritate the stomach mucosa if they dissolve in the stomach.

As the number of doses per day increases, patients sometimes forget to take their medication properly. **Extended release** (XR, XL) tablets or capsules are designed to dissolve slowly, resulting in a longer duration of action for the medication. Also called long-acting (LA) or sustained release (SR) medications, these forms allow for the convenience of once or twice a day dosing.

Some patients, particularly children, have difficulty swallowing tablets and capsules. Crushing tablets or opening capsules and sprinkling the medication over food or mixing it with juice may make the drug more palatable and easier to swallow. The nurse should not crush tablets or open capsules, however, unless the manufacturer specifically states that this is permissible. In general, the following types of drugs should not be chewed, crushed, or opened:

- **Extended release formulations.** These drugs contain a high amount of medication that is intended to be released over an extended period. Opening the capsule or crushing the tablet will release the entire drug immediately, possibly resulting in a toxic effect.

- **Enteric-coated drugs.** When crushed or opened, these drugs are exposed to stomach acid, which may destroy them. In addition, the drugs may irritate the stomach mucosa and cause nausea or vomiting.

- **Oral cavity effects.** Drugs that have a bitter taste are often coated with a thin layer of glucose or inert material to mask their taste. If crushed or opened, the bitter taste is experienced. Other drugs stain the teeth or cause an anesthetic-like effect on the tongue if crushed and exposed to the oral cavity. In addition, some drugs irritate the oral mucosa.

As an alternative to crushing, some drugs are available in liquid form for patients who have difficulty swallowing tablets or capsules. Liquid forms include elixirs, syrups, and suspensions. Liquid drugs are usually heavily flavored and sweetened to mask their bitter taste.

In recent years, two alternatives to tablets, capsules, and liquids have been developed. Orally disintegrating tablets (ODTs) and the oral soluble films are designed to dissolve in the oral cavity in less than 30 seconds, without the need to drink water. These dosage forms are convenient and especially appropriate for patients who have difficulty chewing or swallowing and patients who are mentally impaired, nauseated, or uncooperative. ODTs and soluble films are now available for dozens of medications.

Conventional tablets, liquids, and capsules have certain disadvantages. The patient must be conscious and able to swallow properly. Certain types of drugs, including proteins such as insulin, are inactivated by the digestive enzymes in the stomach and small intestine. Furthermore, drugs absorbed from the stomach and small intestine first travel to the liver, where they may be inactivated before they ever reach their target organs—a process called **first-pass effect** (first-pass metabolism) (see Section 3.5). There is also significant variation among patients in the motility of the GI tract and in its ability to absorb medications. In addition, children and some adults have an aversion to swallowing large tablets and capsules or to taking oral medications that taste bad.

PharmFACT

Although both are given by mouth, the same drug administered in oral and ODT formulations may have different doses. This is because the oral cavity mucosa absorbs some drugs at a different rate than the gastric mucosa (Hirani, Rathod, & Vadalia, 2009).

Sublingual and Buccal Routes: Sublingual and buccal administrations are enteral routes in which the medications are not swallowed but instead are kept in the mouth. The mucosa of the oral cavity contains extensive capillaries that provide an excellent absorptive surface for certain drugs. Medications given by this route are not subjected to destructive stomach acid, and they do not undergo the hepatic first-pass effect. Medications administered by the sublingual or buccal routes include small tablets, ODTs, and soluble films.

For the sublingual route, the medication is placed under the tongue and allowed to slowly dissolve. Because of the rich blood supply to the region under the tongue, the sublingual route results in a rapid onset of drug action. Sublingual dosage forms are most often formulated as ODTs or as soft gelatin capsules filled with liquid drug.

When multiple medications are ordered, the sublingual preparations should be administered after oral medications have been swallowed. After moistening the oral cavity, the patient should be instructed not to move the drug with the tongue or to eat or drink anything until the medication has completely dissolved. The sublingual mucosa is not suitable for extended release formulations because it is a relatively small area and is constantly being bathed by a substantial amount of saliva that will remove these drugs from the region.

To administer drugs by the buccal route, the tablet is placed in the oral cavity between the gum and cheek. The patient should be instructed not to manipulate the drug with the tongue; otherwise it could get displaced to the sublingual area, where it will be more rapidly absorbed, or to the back of the throat, where it could be swallowed. The buccal mucosa is thicker and less permeable to medications than the sublingual area, providing for slower absorption. The buccal route is preferred over the sublingual route for sustained release delivery because of its greater mucosal surface area. For example, testosterone, a drug normally given by injection, is available in a buccal form (Striant). Buccal testosterone releases the drug over 12 hours and gives a more consistent, sustained drug level than does the transdermal patch delivery system for testosterone (see Chapter 71). Drugs formulated for buccal administration generally do not cause irritation and are small enough to not cause discomfort to the patient. Like the sublingual route, drugs administered by the buccal route avoid the first-pass effect by the liver as well as the destructive enzymes of the stomach and small intestine.

Nasogastric and Gastrostomy Tubes: Patients with a nasogastric (NG) tube or an enteral feeding mechanism, such as a gastrostomy (G) tube, may have their medications administered through these devices. Drugs administered through these tubes are usually in liquid form. Although solid drugs can be crushed or dissolved, they tend to clog the tubes. Sustained release medications should not be crushed and administered through NG or G tubes. Drugs administered by these routes are exposed to the same physiological processes as those given PO.

Topical route: The **topical route** of drug administration includes medications applied to the skin or mucous membranes. The skin is the topical route most commonly used. Topical medications applied to the skin are absorbed very slowly because the drug must penetrate the thick, keratin layer of the epidermis.

Topical drugs are also applied to mucous membranes of the eye, ear, nose, respiratory tract, urinary tract, vagina, or rectum. Some of these medications are absorbed very rapidly because these membranes are relatively thin and have a rich blood supply.

Many drugs are applied topically to produce a local effect. For example, antibiotics are applied topically to treat skin infections. Antineoplastic agents may be instilled into the urinary bladder via catheter to treat localized tumors of the bladder mucosa. Corticosteroids are sprayed into the nostrils to reduce inflammation of the nasal mucosa due to allergic rhinitis. Topical delivery produces fewer adverse effects compared to the same drug given PO or parenterally. This is because, when given topically, drugs are absorbed more slowly and the amount of the drug reaching the general circulation is minimal. The most common adverse events resulting from topical administration are transient burning, stinging, or redness of the area where the medications are applied.

Some drugs are given topically to provide for slow release and absorption of the drug to the general circulation. These medications are given for their systemic, rather than local, effects. For example, a nitroglycerin patch is not applied to the skin to treat a local skin condition but to treat coronary artery disease. Likewise, prochlorperazine (Compazine) suppositories are inserted rectally not to treat a disease of the rectum but to alleviate nausea.

The distinction between topical drugs given for local effects and those administered for systemic effects is an important one for the nurse. In the case of local drugs, absorption is undesirable and may result in adverse effects if the drug reaches the systemic circulation. For systemic drugs, absorption across the skin or mucous membrane is essential for the therapeutic action of the drug. Neither type of topical agent should be applied to abraded or denuded skin because it could affect drug absorption.

The use of **transdermal patches** provides an effective means of delivering certain medications. Examples include nitroglycerin to treat angina pectoris, testosterone for hypogonadism, and scopolamine (Transderm Scop) for motion sickness. Transdermal patches contain a specified amount of medication, although the rate of delivery and the actual dose received can vary. Patches are changed on a regular dosing schedule, often daily or weekly, depending on the medication. Medications administered by this route avoid the first-pass effect in the liver and bypass digestive enzymes.

The ophthalmic route is used to treat local conditions of the eye and surrounding structures. Common indications include excessive dryness, eye infections, glaucoma, and dilation of the pupil during eye examinations. Ophthalmic drugs are absorbed into the systemic circulation via drainage of the drug into the nasolacrimal ducts and subsequently to the nasopharynx and the GI tract. Generally this is a slow process and only small amounts reach the general circulation; thus ophthalmic drugs cause few systemic adverse effects. Infants are an exception. The concentration of drugs reaching the systemic circulation is higher than in an adult, giving a greater chance for adverse drug events.

The otic route is used to treat local conditions of the ear, including infections and accumulations of earwax in the auditory canal. Otic medications should always be brought to room temperature before administration because cold medications may cause dizziness or nausea. Systemic adverse effects from otic preparations are not observed unless the drug is applied to areas of open abrasions or injury, such as a ruptured tympanic membrane.

Drugs are applied by the intranasal route for their local effects on the nasal mucosa or for systemic absorption. Advantages of this route include convenience and rapid onset of action. Local indications include the application of drops or sprays for shrinking swollen nasal mucous membranes or for loosening secretions and facilitating drainage. For example, decongestant nasal sprays bring immediate relief from the nasal congestion caused by the common cold (see Chapter 45). Intranasal formulations of corticosteroids have revolutionized the treatment of allergic rhinitis due to their effectiveness and high safety margin.

The nasal mucosa also provides an excellent absorptive surface for certain medications to produce systemic actions. Advantages of this route include avoidance of the first-pass effect and digestive enzymes. For example, an intranasal form of vitamin B_{12} is available that is used for patients lacking intrinsic factor, a substance required for the absorption of this vitamin in the GI tract. Intranasal calcitonin is available to treat osteoporosis. Being a protein, calcitonin would be destroyed by stomach enzymes if given PO (see Chapter 72).

Although the nasal mucosa provides an excellent surface for drug delivery, there is a potential for damage to the ciliated cells within the nasal cavity and mucosal irritation is common. Mucus secretion is unpredictable and may inhibit drug absorption from this site.

The vaginal route is used to treat local conditions such as vaginal infections, pain, and itching. The vagina has a rich blood supply, and drugs inserted into it may be absorbed across the mucosa and produce systemic effects. For example, vaginal creams containing estrogen not only produce local effects on the vagina but also result in significant levels of this hormone in the circulation. The contraceptive NuvaRing, inserted into the vagina, contains estrogen and progestin, which are absorbed and provide contraception protection for a month.

The rectal route may be used for either local or systemic drug delivery. It is a safe and effective means of delivering medications to comatose patients or to those who are experiencing nausea and vomiting. Rectal medications are normally in suppository form, although a few laxatives and diagnostic agents are given via enema. Although absorption is slower than by other routes, the rectal route is steady and reliable provided the medication can be retained by the patient. Venous blood from the lower rectum is not transported to the circulation by way of the liver; thus the first-pass effect is avoided as are the digestive enzymes of the upper GI tract.

Parenteral route: The parenteral route refers to the administration of drugs by routes other than enteral or topical. A needle is used to deliver drugs into the skin layers, subcutaneous tissue, muscles, or veins. Less common parenteral delivery methods include administration into arteries (intra-arterial), bone (intraosseous), body cavities (intrathecal), or organs (intracardiac). Parenteral drug administration is more invasive than topical or enteral because of the potential for introducing pathogenic microbes directly into the blood or body tissues. The nurse must know the correct anatomic locations for parenteral administration, proper administration technique, and safety procedures regarding disposal of hazardous equipment.

Intradermal and Subcutaneous Administration: Injection into the skin delivers drugs to the blood vessels that supply the various layers of the skin. Medications may be injected either intradermally or subcutaneously. The major difference between these methods is the depth of injection. An advantage of both methods is that they offer a means of administering drugs to patients who are unable to take medications PO. Drugs administered by these routes avoid digestive enzymes and the hepatic first-pass effect. However, only small volumes can be administered by these routes, and injections can result in pain and swelling at the injection site.

The intradermal (ID) route administers drugs into the dermis layer of the skin. Because the dermis contains more blood vessels than the deeper subcutaneous layer, drugs are more readily absorbed. This route is usually employed for allergy and disease screening or for local anesthetic delivery prior to venous cannulation. ID injections are limited to very small volumes of medication, usually only 0.1 to 0.2 mL.

The subcutaneous route delivers drugs to the deepest layers of the skin. Insulin, heparin, vitamins, some vaccines, and other medications are given in this area because the sites are easily accessible and provide for rapid absorption. Subcutaneous doses are small in volume, usually ranging from 0.5 to 1 mL. It is important to rotate injection sites in an orderly and documented manner to promote absorption, lessen tissue damage, and minimize discomfort.

Intramuscular Administration: The intramuscular (IM) route delivers drugs directly into large muscles. Because muscle tissue has a rich blood supply, drug molecules quickly move into blood vessels to produce a more rapid onset of action than with oral, ID, or subcutaneous administration. In a few cases, the drug is formulated in an oily, viscous base that promotes slow and continuous absorption from the muscle.

The anatomic structure of muscle permits this tissue to receive a larger volume of drug than the subcutaneous region. Adults with well-developed muscles can tolerate up to 3 mL in the gluteus maximus and gluteus medius muscles. In the deltoid muscle, volumes of 0.5 to 1 mL are recommended.

Intravenous Administration: The intravenous (IV) route delivers drugs and fluids directly into the bloodstream, which immediately distributes them throughout the body. The IV route is used when a very rapid onset of action is desired. Unlike other routes in which absorption may be unpredictable, an exact level of drug in the bloodstream can be attained by fine adjustments to the IV flow rate. Like other parenteral routes, IV drugs bypass the enzymatic processes of the alimentary canal and avoid the first-pass effect of the liver. The IV route is useful for patients who are comatose or otherwise unable to take oral medications. The three basic types of IV administration include large-volume infusion, intermittent infusion, and IV bolus (push) administration.

Although the IV route offers the fastest onset of drug action, it is also the most dangerous. Once injected, the medication cannot be retrieved. If the drug solution or the needle is contaminated, pathogens have a direct route to the bloodstream and body tissues. Patients receiving IV injections must be closely monitored for adverse reactions. Although some adverse reactions occur immediately after injection, others may take hours or days to appear. Antidotes for drugs that can cause potentially dangerous or fatal reactions must always be readily available.

CONNECTION Checkpoint 3.1

Pharmaceutical companies are always exploring novel methods of drug delivery, such as soluble films, so that the period of exclusivity of a medication can be extended. From what you learned in Chapter 1, why is exclusivity important to a pharmaceutical company? *See Answer to Connection Checkpoint 3.1 on student resource website.*

Drug Concentration and Dose

For almost all drugs, higher doses produce a faster and greater response. This is because a higher dose produces a greater concentration gradient for diffusion. As an example, consider the antihypertensive drug diltiazem (Cardizem) given as a 100-mg tablet, which is about 50% absorbed. Half of the drug (50 mg) will reach the bloodstream for distribution to target cells. If the dose of diltiazem is doubled to 200 mg, greater amounts of the drug (100 mg) will be absorbed in the bloodstream. Although the percentage absorbed remains the same (50%), the higher dose results in a greater quantity of drug in the blood and, subsequently, more drug is available to produce an action at its target cells. This concept is further explained in Chapter 4.

GI Tract Environment

For drugs given by mouth, the physical and chemical conditions within the GI tract play a significant role in drug absorption. Most absorption occurs in the small intestine, because this portion of the GI tract is longer, and the absorptive surfaces of the microvilli are much more extensive as compared to the stomach. Furthermore the time spent by food and drugs in the stomach is brief, and the thick mucus layer in the organ discourages absorption.

Digestive motility is variable among patients; very rapid motility may speed the drug through the GI tract before complete absorption occurs. Abnormally slow motility may cause the drug to be retained in the stomach, where it is exposed for a longer time to destructive enzymes and high acidity. Fatty foods in the stomach nearly always slow drug absorption. With few exceptions, absorption is most complete when the drug is taken between meals; the presence of food in the stomach may lessen the incidence of nausea and vomiting, but it also slows absorption. All these factors contribute to wide patient variability with regard to absorption and onset of drug action when drugs are administered PO.

Blood Flow to the Absorption Site

For a drug to be absorbed, there must be adequate blood flow to the site of administration; thus drugs are absorbed faster from areas of the body where blood flow is high. IM injections are placed into large muscles because they have a high blood flow that maximizes absorption. During heart failure or shock, the amount of blood flow to certain tissues is reduced and absorption from the GI tract or IM sites may be diminished. Topical drugs placed on the skin have slow absorption due to the poor blood supply to the upper layers of the skin.

In some circumstances blood flow can be manipulated to purposely slow absorption. For example, local anesthetics can be toxic if absorbed too quickly. To purposely slow absorption, a vasoconstrictor (epinephrine) is sometimes added to local anesthetics to reduce blood flow to the treated region. As another example, applying ice packs to the site can slow the absorption of a drug to the region; adding heat can cause the opposite effect.

Drug Ionization

Ionized molecules are those that carry a positive or a negative charge. Most drugs can exist in either a charged or an uncharged state, depending on the pH of the surrounding fluid. The ionization of a drug affects its ability to cross plasma membranes and to be excreted by the body (see Section 3.6). Aspirin, or acetylsalicylic acid, provides an example of the effects of ionization on absorption, as depicted in Figure 3.4. In the highly acidic environment of the stomach, aspirin is in its nonionized form and is thus readily absorbed and distributed in the bloodstream. As aspirin enters the alkaline environment of the small intestine, however, it becomes ionized. In its ionized form, the aspirin molecule is less likely to be absorbed and distributed to target cells. Unlike acidic drugs such as aspirin, medications that are weakly basic are in their nonionized form in an alkaline environment; therefore, basic drugs are much more likely to be absorbed in alkaline environments such as the small intestine. In simplest terms, it may help the student to remember the following:

- Acids are absorbed in acids because they are nonionized.
- Bases are absorbed in bases because they are nonionized.

Drug Interactions

Drug–drug and food–drug interactions have the potential to affect absorption. For example, administering oral tetracyclines with food or drugs containing calcium, iron, or magnesium can significantly delay absorption of the antibiotic. High-fat meals can slow stomach motility significantly and delay the absorption of oral medications taken with the meal. The mechanisms and types of drug interactions are presented in detail in Chapter 5.

Surface Area

Other factors being equal, drugs will be absorbed faster when applied to regions of the body having a larger surface area. This is one reason why the small intestine is such an important organ for drug

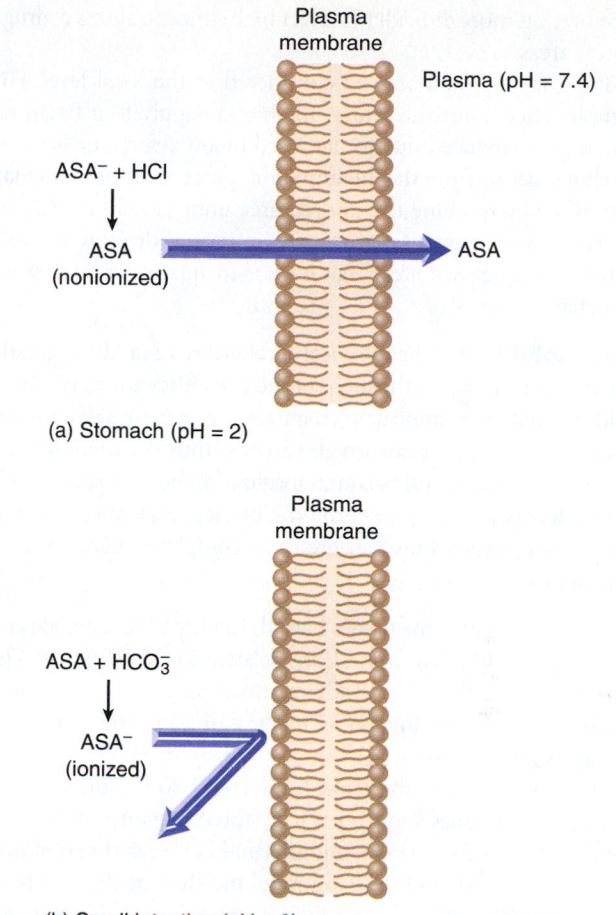

Figure 3.4 Effect of pH on drug absorption: (a) A weak acid such as aspirin (ASA) is in a nonionized form in an acidic environment and absorption occurs. (b) In a basic environment, aspirin is mostly in an ionized form and absorption is prevented.

absorption. Relative to the oral cavity and stomach, the microvilli of the small intestine provide a vast surface area that is richly supplied with blood vessels. Another region with an enormous surface area is the lung. Inhaled substances such as bronchodilators or crack cocaine act almost instantaneously due to the large absorptive surface provided by terminal bronchioles and alveoli.

3.4 Distribution describes how drugs are transported throughout the body.

Distribution is the phase of pharmacokinetics describing the *movement* of medications throughout the body after they are absorbed. Drugs are not simply passive agents, being swept along an inert path to their target tissues. Rather, drugs may interact with blood components and may be chemically and physically changed before they reach their targets. Like absorption, several key factors influence drug distribution.

Blood flow to tissues: The simplest factor determining drug distribution is the amount of blood flow to body tissues. Because the heart, liver, and kidneys receive a great percentage of the blood supply, these organs receive the highest exposure to absorbed drugs. Skin, bone, and adipose tissue receive a meager blood flow;

therefore, it is more difficult to deliver high concentrations of drugs to these areas.

Blood flow should also be considered at the local level. For example, after traumatic injury, the blood supply to a fractured bone may be reduced due to damaged blood vessels, or blocked by cellular debris from the inflammatory process. Antibiotics may have difficulty reaching the injured area until blood flow can be restored. The delivery of high concentrations of drugs to injured, necrotic, or abscessed areas that have inadequate perfusion is always challenging.

Drug solubility: The physical properties of a drug greatly influence how it moves throughout the body after administration. Lipid solubility is an important characteristic because it determines how quickly a drug is absorbed, mixes within the bloodstream, crosses membranes, and becomes localized in body tissues. Lipid-soluble agents are not limited by the barriers that normally stop water-soluble drugs; thus they are more completely distributed to body tissues.

Tissue storage: Some tissues have the ability to accumulate and store drugs in high concentrations relative to other tissues. The bone marrow, teeth, eyes, and adipose tissue have an especially high **affinity**, or attraction, for certain medications. Examples of agents that are stored in adipose tissue are diazepam (Valium), lipid-soluble vitamins, and tetracycline, which binds to calcium salts and accumulates in bones and teeth. Once stored in tissues, drugs may remain in the body for many months and be released very slowly back to the circulation. For example, the therapeutic effects of alendronate (Fosamax), a drug for osteoporosis, will continue for 4 to 7 months after the drug is discontinued.

Drug-protein binding: Many drugs bind reversibly to plasma proteins, particularly albumin, to form **drug-protein complexes**. These complexes are too large to cross capillary membranes; the drugs continue circulating in the bloodstream and are unavailable for distribution to their site of action. Medications will remain trapped in the bloodstream bound to plasma proteins until they are released or displaced from the drug-protein complex. Only unbound, or free, drugs can reach their target cells or be excreted by the kidneys. This concept is illustrated in Figure 3.5. Some drugs, such as the anticoagulant warfarin (Coumadin), are highly bound; 99% of the drug in the plasma exists in drug-protein complexes, and only 1% exists as a free drug available to reach target cells.

The number of binding sites on a plasma protein such as albumin is limited. What happens when two or more drugs compete for the same binding sites? The drug that has the greater affinity (attraction) for these binding sites binds first. This competition for binding sites may result in drug–drug and drug–food interactions when one medication displaces another from plasma proteins. The displaced medication can quickly reach high levels in the blood and produce adverse effects. This is especially important for drugs such as warfarin that have a narrow margin of safety. Most drug guides give the percentage of the drug bound to plasma proteins; when giving multiple medications that are highly bound, the nurse should monitor for potential adverse effects. This topic is further discussed in Chapter 5.

Special barriers to drug distribution: Most capillaries in the body are relatively porous due to spaces between the endothelial

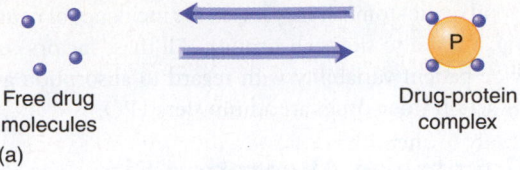

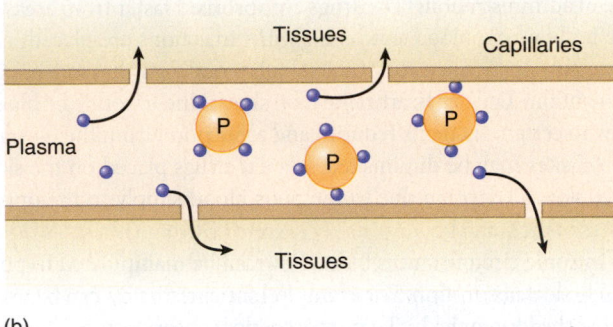

(b)

Figure 3.5 Plasma protein binding and drug availability: (a) The drug exists in a free state or is bound to plasma protein. (b) Drug-protein complexes are too large to cross membranes.

cells. Many drugs can exit the bloodstream by traveling through the spaces and enter the interstitial fluid with relative ease. The brain and placenta, however, possess special anatomic barriers that inhibit many chemicals and drugs from exiting the blood. These barriers are referred to as the **blood–brain barrier** and **fetal–placental barrier**.

Unlike other capillaries, those in the brain have endothelial cells that are sealed by tight junctions and a thick basement membrane. Brain cells known as astrocytes press firmly against the basement membrane, secreting chemicals that adjust the capillary permeability. The purpose of the blood–brain barrier is obvious: to protect the brain from pathogens and toxic substances. Some highly lipid-soluble agents such as general anesthetics, sedatives, antianxiety agents, and anticonvulsant drugs readily cross the blood–brain barrier to produce their actions on the central nervous system (CNS). In contrast, most antitumor medications and antibiotics do not easily cross this barrier, making brain cancers and infections difficult to treat. The blood–brain barrier becomes more permeable when it is inflamed due to infections such as meningitis. In neonates, the blood–brain barrier is not fully developed, allowing many drugs to readily cross the barrier.

The series of membranes that separate the maternal blood from the fetal blood serves as a fetal–placental barrier that prevents potentially harmful substances from passing from the mother's bloodstream to the fetus. In reality, the placenta is an inefficient barrier because substances such as alcohol, cocaine, caffeine, and certain prescription medications can easily cross the placental barrier and cause potential harm to the fetus. Consequently, no prescription medication, over-the-counter (OTC) drug, or herbal therapy should be taken by a pregnant woman without first consulting a health care provider. The nurse should always question women of childbearing age regarding their pregnancy status before a drug is prescribed. Substances that cause birth defects, or teratogens, are presented in Chapter 5. Chapter 8 presents special concerns related to pharmacotherapy of pregnant and lactating patients.

3.5 Metabolism is a process that changes the activity of a drug and makes it more likely to be excreted.

Drug **metabolism**, also called biotransformation, is the process used by the body to chemically change a drug molecule. Metabolism involves hundreds of complex biochemical pathways and reactions that alter the structure and function of drugs, nutrients, vitamins, and minerals. The liver is the primary site of drug metabolism, although the kidneys and cells of the intestinal tract also have high metabolic rates. To survive, all cells must undergo metabolism to some extent. The types of metabolic reactions, however, are specific to each type of cell: Reactions occurring in liver cells are very different from those in skin cells or brain cells.

In most cases, metabolic reactions change the structure of a drug so that it can be more easily excreted by the body. This often changes the drug from lipid soluble (easily absorbed and distributed) to water soluble, which is more easily excreted by the kidneys. In addition, once the molecule has been changed to water soluble, it is less able to enter tissues. The products of drug metabolism, or metabolites, usually have less pharmacologic activity than the original molecule. In this way, metabolism provides an essential detoxifying effect for drugs and other substances entering the body.

On some occasions a metabolite may exhibit a *greater* therapeutic action than the original drug. This is the case for codeine. Although 90% of codeine is changed to inactive metabolites by the liver, 10% is converted to morphine, which has significantly greater ability to relieve severe pain. In a few cases, the metabolite has greater toxicity than the original drug. Probably the most common example of this is acetaminophen (Tylenol), which is converted to a metabolite that is highly toxic to the liver.

CONNECTION Checkpoint 3.2

Both codeine and morphine are scheduled drugs. From Chapter 2, which law was enacted to control the distribution of these drugs? *See Answer to Connection Checkpoint 3.2 on student resource website.*

In a few cases, the drug administered to the patient has no pharmacologic activity at all until it undergoes metabolism. Medications that require metabolism to produce their therapeutic actions are called **prodrugs**. For example, the antihypertensive enalapril (Vasotec) is converted in the liver to a metabolite called enaliprat, which has considerably more ability to lower blood pressure than the original drug. Examples of other prodrugs include benazepril (Lotensin) and losartan (Cozaar).

Hepatic microsomal enzymes: Most metabolism in the liver is accomplished by the **hepatic microsomal enzyme system**. This enzyme complex is known as the P450 system, named after cytochrome P450 (CYP), which is a key component of the system. Although this system is complex, a key point to remember is that CYP is simply an enzyme that metabolizes drugs as well as nutrients and other endogenous substances. Although the liver is the major site for CYP activity, nearly every tissue in the body has some CYP enzymes.

It was once thought that a single CYP enzyme was responsible for all drug metabolism, but scientists have since identified more than 50 CYPs. These different forms are called **isozymes** of cytochrome P450. Although very similar, each isozyme performs slightly different metabolic functions. CYPs are named by assigning numbers to indicate their subfamily, such as CYP1, CYP2, CYP3, and so on. Additional letters and numbers are added to further identify the specific gene, such as CYP1A1, CYP3A4, and CYP26C1. Fortunately for nursing students, only a handful of the 50-plus isozymes are responsible for the majority of drug metabolism, as shown in Table 3.1. Indeed, a single isozyme, CYP3A4, is responsible for about 50% of all drug metabolism in the liver.

The CYPs are important to pharmacotherapy because they determine the speed at which most drugs are metabolized and they contribute significantly to drug–drug interactions. Changes in hepatic microsomal enzyme activity have the potential to alter drug action. These effects may either increase or decrease drug

TABLE 3.1	Isozymes of Cytochrome P450: Selected Substrates, Inducers, and Inhibitors		
Isozyme	**Substrates**	**Inducers**	**Inhibitors**
CYP1A2	acetaminophen, amitriptyline, caffeine, dantrolene, diazepam, estradiol, haloperidol, imipramine, lidocaine, methadone, ondansetron, ritonavir, tacrine, tamoxifen, verapamil, warfarin	omeprazole, phenobarbital, phenytoin, rifampin, ritonavir	cimetidine, ciprofloxacin, erythromycin, isoniazid, ketoconazole, levofloxacin, paroxetine
CYP2C9	amiodarone, amitriptyline, dapsone, ethosuximide, ibuprofen, imipramine, naproxen, nifedipine, omeprazole, phenytoin, progesterone, propranolol, ritonavir, sulfonamides, tamoxifen, testosterone, tricyclic antidepressants, valproic acid, warfarin	barbiturates, carbamazepine, ethanol, phenobarbital	cimetidine, disulfiram, fluconazole, fluoxetine, fluvastatin, ketoconazole, omeprazole, ritonavir, sertraline
CYP2C19	diazepam, escitalopram, omeprazole, pentamidine, sertraline	carbamazepine, phenytoin, rifampin, St. John's wort	cimetidine, clopidogrel, fluconazole, fluvoxamine, isoniazid
CYP2D6	amitriptyline, captopril, chlorpromazine, citalopram, codeine, fluoxetine, haloperidol, imipramine, lidocaine, loratadine, meperidine, methamphetamine, metoprolol, mexiletine, ondansetron, oxycodone, paroxetine, propranolol, ritonavir, tamoxifen, tramadol, trazodone, venlafaxine	carbamazepine, phenobarbital, phenytoin, rifampin, ritonavir	amiodarone, cimetidine, citalopram, fluoxetine, haloperidol, methadone, paroxetine, ritonavir, sertraline
CYP3A4	alprazolam, amiodarone, carbamazepine, chlorpromazine, cocaine, cortisol, cyclosporine, diltiazem, erythromycin, ketoconazole, lidocaine, lovastatin, nifedipine, omeprazole, prednisone, ritonavir, sertraline, tamoxifen, venlafaxine, verapamil	dexamethasone, ethosuximide, nevirapine, phenobarbital, phenytoin, prednisone	clotrimazole, diltiazem, erythromycin, fluconazole, fluoxetine, grapefruit juice, ketoconazole, metronidazole, nifedipine, norfloxacin, omeprazole, fluoxetine, ritonavir, sertraline, verapamil, zafirlukast

action, depending on the specific interaction. There are three major consequences of the CYP system that have importance to pharmacotherapy:

- **Drugs as substrates.** When a drug is metabolized by a CYP, it is said to be a **substrate** for the enzyme. For example, naproxen and warfarin are substrates for CYP2C9. Codeine and amphetamine are substrates for a different isozyme, CYP2D6. Each isozyme of CYP can metabolize many different drugs, and a drug may be metabolized by multiple CYPs. Because of this overlap, two drugs that are administered concurrently may compete for binding sites on the same CYP isozyme, resulting in a drug–drug interaction.

- **Drugs as enzyme inhibitors.** Some drugs are able to inhibit the action of CYP isozymes. The inhibition may affect all hepatic microsomal enzymes or it may be specific to a single isozyme. Inhibiting a CYP enzyme could affect the amount of active drug available. For example, ciprofloxacin (Cipro) inhibits CYP1A2. Administering Cipro concurrently with naproxen (a substrate for CYP1A2) could result in less metabolism of naproxen, higher amounts of naproxen in the blood, and a prolonged drug effect. Because naproxen is a relatively safe drug, this higher level may not produce noticeable toxicity. However, giving

Cipro with a more toxic drug such as warfarin (also a substrate for CYP1A2) has the potential to increase levels of warfarin and cause a serious drug interaction. The dose of warfarin would need to be adjusted downward to avoid toxicity. It is important to note that CYP enzyme inhibition can occur after a single dose of an inhibitor.

- **Drugs as enzyme inducers.** A few drugs have the ability to increase metabolic activity in the liver, a process called **enzyme induction**. For example, phenobarbital causes the liver to synthesize greater amounts of microsomal enzymes, including CYP3A4, CYP2C19, and CYP2C9. By doing so, phenobarbital accelerates the metabolism (inactivation) of most drugs metabolized in the liver. In fact, with continued therapy phenobarbital increases the rate of its own destruction. In these patients, because drugs will be inactivated at a much faster rate, higher doses may be required to achieve an optimum therapeutic effect. Unlike CYP inhibition, which can occur after a single dose, enzyme induction generally takes from days to weeks of pharmacotherapy.

Metabolism has a number of additional therapeutic consequences. As shown in Pharmacotherapy Illustrated 3.1, drugs absorbed from the stomach or small intestine cross directly into the

PHARMACOTHERAPY ILLUSTRATED 3.1

FIRST-PASS EFFECT: Oral Drug Is Metabolized to an Inactive Form Before It Has an Opportunity to Reach Target Cells

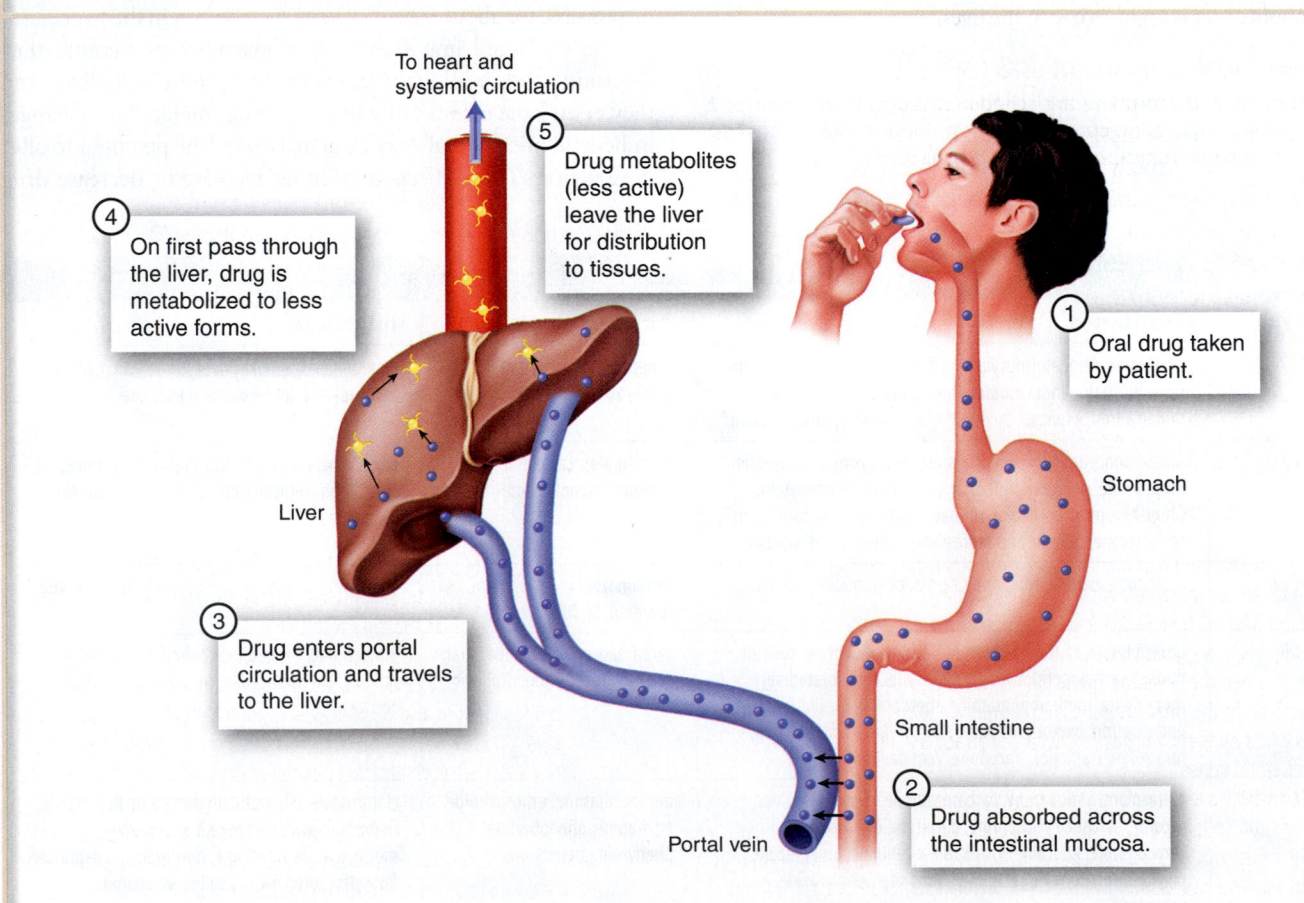

To heart and systemic circulation

⑤ Drug metabolites (less active) leave the liver for distribution to tissues.

④ On first pass through the liver, drug is metabolized to less active forms.

Liver

③ Drug enters portal circulation and travels to the liver.

① Oral drug taken by patient.

Stomach

Small intestine

② Drug absorbed across the intestinal mucosa.

Portal vein

hepatic-portal circulation, which carries blood to the liver before it is distributed to other body tissues. Some drugs can be completely metabolized to an inactive form on their first trip through the liver *before they even reach the general circulation.* This first-pass effect is important to pharmacology, because a large number of oral drugs can be rendered inactive by hepatic metabolic reactions. Alternate routes of delivery, such as the sublingual, rectal, or parenteral routes that bypass the first-pass effect, may need to be considered for these drugs. Remember, however, that even drugs administered by parenteral routes may be rapidly inactivated when passing through the liver.

Patient variation in metabolism: Certain patients have diminished hepatic metabolic activity, which may result in altered drug action. Infants do not develop a mature microsomal enzyme system until at least 1 year of age. Hepatic enzyme activity is generally reduced in older adults; thus these patients may require lower doses. Patients with liver impairment will require reductions in drug dosage because of the decreased metabolic activity. The nurse should pay careful attention to laboratory values that may indicate liver disease so that drug doses may be adjusted accordingly.

The baseline level of hepatic microsomal enzyme function is genetically determined. Genetic differences in the function of CYP enzymes may cause people to metabolize drugs at widely different rates. Some patients metabolize at a faster rate, others at a slower rate. Certain genetic disorders have been recognized in which patients lack specific metabolic enzymes. In these "slow metabolizers" normal drug doses may cause toxicity. Genetic differences are not always predictable, although some occur at a higher rate in certain ethnic populations (see Chapter 4).

Certain lifestyle factors also affect CYP enzyme activity and thus may influence response to medications. Chronic alcohol consumption and tobacco use induce certain CYP enzymes. St. John's wort, a popular herbal remedy for depression, is an enzyme inducer and can affect the therapeutic response to certain medications. On the other hand, grapefruit juice is an inhibitor of CYP3A4 activity. These examples underscore the importance of obtaining a thorough patient history prior to initiating drug therapy.

3.6 Excretion processes remove drugs from the body.

Drugs will continue to act on the body until they are either metabolized to an inactive form or removed from the body by **excretion**. The rate at which a drug is excreted determines its concentration in the blood and, ultimately, its duration of action. Pathologic states, especially liver or kidney disease, often increase the duration and intensity of drug action in the body because they interfere with natural excretion mechanisms.

Renal excretion: Although drugs are removed from the body by numerous organs and tissues, the primary site of excretion is the kidney. In an average size person, the kidneys filter approximately 180 L of blood each day. Unbound (free) drugs, water-soluble agents, electrolytes, and small molecules easily pass through the pores of the glomerulus and enter the filtrate in the renal tubule. Proteins, blood cells, and drug-protein complexes are not filtered because of their large size.

After filtration at the renal corpuscle, drugs may undergo reabsorption in the renal tubule. Mechanisms of reabsorption are the same as absorption elsewhere in the body. Nonionized and lipid-soluble drugs cross renal tubular membranes more easily and return to the circulation; ionized and water-soluble drugs generally remain in the filtrate.

Drug-protein complexes and other substances too large to be filtered at the glomerulus are sometimes secreted into the distal tubule of the nephron. For example, only 10% of a dose of penicillin G is filtered; 90% is secreted into the renal tubule. As with metabolic enzyme activity, secretion mechanisms are less active in infants and in older adults.

The renal excretion of drugs is greatly influenced by the pH of the filtrate in the renal tubule. Weak acids like aspirin are excreted more efficiently when the filtrate is slightly alkaline. This is because aspirin is ionized in an alkaline environment, and the ionized drug will remain in the filtrate to be excreted in the urine. Weakly basic drugs such as diazepam (Valium) are excreted more quickly if the filtrate is slightly acidic because they are ionized in that environment. The pH of the filtrate may be intentionally manipulated to speed up renal excretion. For example, following an overdose of

---

CONNECTIONS   Treating the Diverse Patient

One Size Does Not Fit All

One of the challenges of modern pharmacology is to develop medications that produce an optimal result with minimal adverse effects for all users. Although humans vary in their individual response to medications, drugs have traditionally been designed to target the "average" person, a one-size-fits-all approach, when the "average" person does not exist. A solution to this dilemma may come in the near future with pharmacogenomics, the science that predicts when a patient will have a positive or an adverse response to a drug based on inherited genes.

Scientists have determined that the way a person responds to a medication depends on certain traits found in the genes: small variations in the sequence of their nucleotide bases. Without knowing the specific genes involved in the drug response, one cannot predict the individual response to a medication.

Gene variation diagnostic tools called single nucleotide polymorphisms (SNPs [pronounced snips]) are expensive to access. However, DNA microarrays (DNA chips) are part of an evolving technology that will open the door to a targeted drug response for a group of patients. Review of gene susceptibility prior to prescribing the drug may be a possibility in the future.

This technology would also be beneficial in clinical trials. By predetermining patients' responses, those with known adverse reaction to a drug would be excluded. Clinical trials would be conducted with smaller groups, resulting in less expense and, ultimately, in reduced cost of drugs to the consumer. The health care provider could prescribe in confidence, unlike the current method in which the prescriber gives the patient a medication that may or may not be effective or have adverse effects based on the individual response.

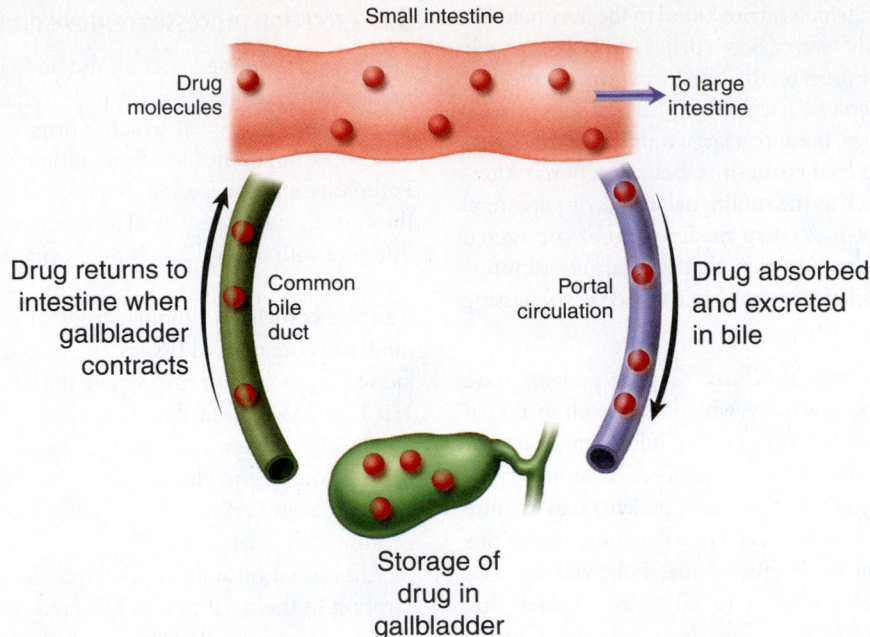

Figure 3.6 Enterohepatic recirculation of a drug can increase its half-life in the body and prolong its duration of action.

an acidic drug such as aspirin, nurses may administer sodium bicarbonate. Sodium bicarbonate makes the urine more basic, which ionizes the aspirin molecule, facilitating its urinary excretion. The excretion of diazepam, on the other hand, can be enhanced by giving a drug such as ammonium chloride, which acidifies the filtrate and ionizes the diazepam molecule.

Impairment of kidney function can dramatically affect pharmacokinetics. Patients with renal failure will have diminished ability to excrete medications and may retain drugs for extended periods. Doses for these patients must be reduced to prevent drug toxicity. Because small to moderate changes in renal function can cause rapid increases in serum drug levels, kidney function must be constantly monitored in patients receiving nephrotoxic drugs or medications that have a narrow margin of safety.

Pulmonary excretion: Drugs delivered by gaseous or volatile liquid forms are especially suited for excretion by the respiratory system. The rate of respiratory excretion is dependent on factors that affect gas exchange, including diffusion, gas solubility, and blood flow to the lungs. The elimination of gaseous and volatile anesthetics following surgery is primarily dependent on respiratory activity: The faster the breathing rate, the more rapid the excretion. On the other hand, the respiratory removal of water-soluble agents such as alcohol is more dependent on blood flow to the lungs. The greater the blood flow through lung capillaries, the greater the pulmonary excretion. In contrast with other methods of excretion, the lungs excrete most drugs in their original unmetabolized form.

Glandular secretion: Glandular activity is another elimination mechanism. Water-soluble drugs may be secreted into the saliva, sweat, or breast milk. The "funny taste" that patients experience when given certain drugs is an example of the secretion of medications into saliva. Another example is the garlic smell that can be detected when standing next to a perspiring person who has recently eaten garlic. Excretion into breast milk is of considerable

importance for basic drugs such as morphine or codeine, because these can achieve high concentrations and potentially affect the nursing infant. Lactating women should always check with their health care provider before taking any prescription medication, OTC drug, or herbal supplement. Drugs of special concern to the pregnant or breast-feeding patient are discussed in Chapter 8.

Fecal and biliary excretion: Certain oral drugs travel through the GI tract without being absorbed and are excreted in the feces. Examples include mebendazole (Vermox), a drug used to kill intestinal worms, and barium sulfate, a radiologic contrast agent.

Some drugs are secreted in bile, a process known as biliary excretion. Drugs secreted into bile will enter the duodenum and eventually leave the body in the feces. However, some substances in bile are reabsorbed and circulated back to the liver by **enterohepatic recirculation**, as illustrated in Figure 3.6. This is a normal physiological mechanism for salvaging and reusing useful substances.

Drugs or their metabolites may participate in this process and recirculate numerous times with the bile. This has the result of extending their half-life in the body and possibly prolonging drug action. This is an important route of excretion for tamoxifen, barbiturates, carbamazepine, rifampicin, and oral contraceptives. Recirculated drugs are eventually metabolized by the liver and may be excreted by the kidneys. Recirculation and elimination of drugs through biliary excretion may continue for several weeks after therapy has been discontinued.

Time–Response Relationships

3.7 The therapeutic response of most drugs depends on their concentration in the plasma.

The therapeutic response from most drugs is directly related to their concentration in the plasma. Although the concentration of the drug at its target tissue is more predictive of drug action, this quantity is impossible to measure. For example, although it is possible to conduct a laboratory test that measures the serum level of lithium carbonate (Eskalith) by taking a blood sample, it is a far different matter to measure the quantity of this drug in neurons within the brain.

It is common practice to monitor the plasma levels of drugs that have a low safety margin and to use these data to predict drug action or toxicity. Results of **therapeutic drug monitoring** are used by the health care provider to keep the drug dose within a predetermined therapeutic range. For example, the therapeutic range for the antibiotic vancomycin (Vancocin) is 20 to 40 mcg/mL and the toxic level is considered to be greater than 80 mcg/mL. For patients with severe infections, the nurse would carefully monitor the laboratory results for vancomycin to be certain that serum levels fall within the therapeutic range. Dosages would be adjusted upward or downward based on therapeutic drug monitoring and the patient responses. The nurse should always remember, however, that individual responses to drugs are highly variable and patients may experience toxic effects (or no effects) even if the serum concentration of the drug lies in the normal range.

A number of important pharmacokinetic principles can be illustrated by measuring the drug plasma level following a single dose administered PO. These pharmacokinetic values for a hypothetical drug are shown graphically in Figure 3.7. In this example, the plasma drug level slowly increased and took about 2 hours before the **minimum effective concentration** was reached. The minimum effective drug plasma concentration, that amount of drug required to produce a therapeutic effect, is 6 mcg/mL. The level

of drug then entered the **therapeutic range**, which for this drug lies between 6 and 12 mcg/mL. In this range, the drug produced its desired therapeutic action. After peaking, the drug plasma level slowly began to fall out of the therapeutic range due to excretion processes. A higher dose might have caused the drug plasma level to reach a **toxic concentration**, the level of drug that results in serious adverse effects. The goal of pharmacotherapy is to reach and maintain a plasma drug level in the therapeutic range while avoiding the toxic concentration.

These values have great clinical significance. For example, if the patient has a severe headache and is given half of an aspirin tablet, the plasma drug level will likely remain below the minimum effective concentration, and the patient will not experience pain relief. Two or three tablets will increase the plasma level of aspirin into the therapeutic range, and the pain will subside. Taking six or more tablets may result in adverse effects, such as GI bleeding or tinnitus. For each drug administered, the nurse's goal is to keep its plasma concentration in the therapeutic range. For some drugs, this therapeutic range is quite wide. For other medications, the difference between a minimum effective dose and a toxic dose can be extremely narrow.

3.8 The drug half-life estimates the duration of action for most medications.

In the example illustrated in Figure 3.7, the serum concentration of the drug reached a peak and then fell back below the therapeutic range. The length of time a drug concentration remains in the

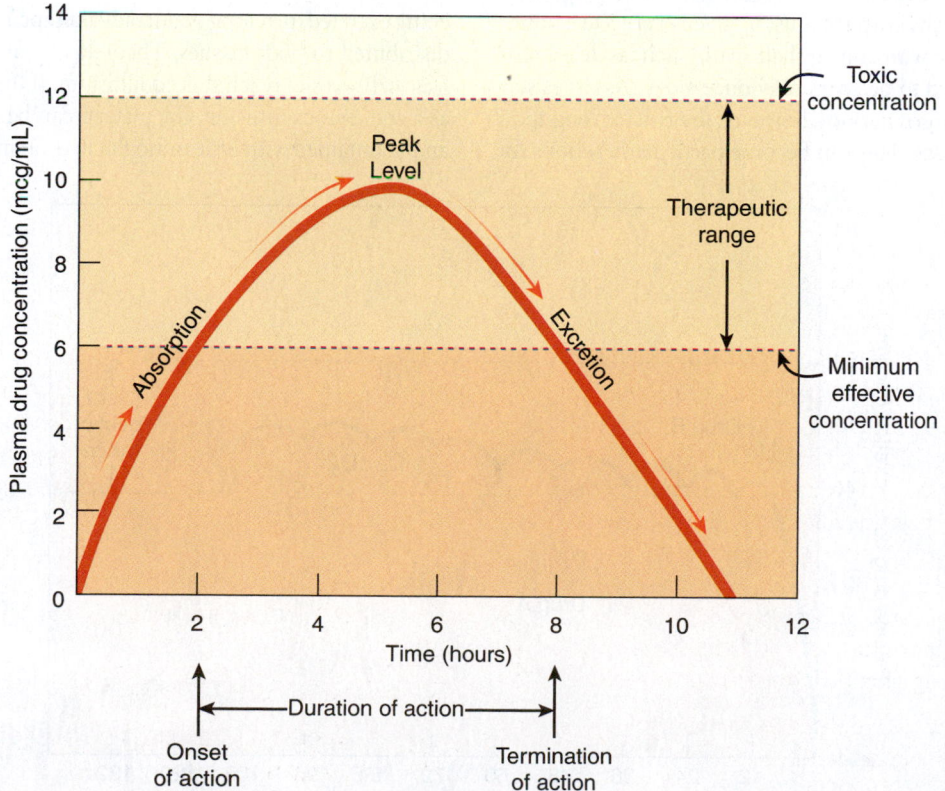

Figure 3.7 Single-dose drug administration. Pharmacokinetic values for this drug are as follows: onset of action = 2 hours; duration of action = 6 hours; termination of action = 8 hours after administration; peak plasma concentration = 10 mcg/mL; time to peak drug effect = 5 hours; $t_{1/2}$ = 4 hours.

therapeutic range is its *duration of action*. In this example, the duration of action was 6 hours. The duration of action is an important pharmacokinetic variable that is determined by how rapidly the drug is metabolized and excreted.

The most common description of a drug's duration of action is its **plasma half-life (t₁/₂)**: the length of time required for the plasma concentration of a drug to decrease by one half after administration. Some drugs have a half-life of only a few minutes, whereas others have a half-life of several hours or days. A few drugs have exceptionally long half-lives; for example, amiodarone (Cordarone) has a $t_{1/2}$ of 40 to 55 days.

Is it better to administer a drug with a short or long half-life? The answer depends on the patient's condition and the treatment goal. Drugs with short half-lives are ideal for conditions and procedures having a brief duration. For example, during a dental procedure, local anesthesia may only be needed for 15 to 20 minutes; thus procaine (Novocain), with a half-life of 8 minutes, may be sufficient. Giving a drug with a long duration of action could cause adverse effects after the patient leaves the office. As another example, a simple headache can be relieved with a short-acting drug such as aspirin ($t_{1/2}$ = 15 to 20 minutes), rather than a drug with a 10- or 12-hour duration. Because short-acting drugs are rapidly excreted, the risk of long-term adverse effects is reduced.

Long-duration drugs do have certain advantages. In the preceding example, procaine would not be suitable for a dental procedure that lasts 2 hours because multiple injections would be necessary. Long-duration drugs are beneficial in treating chronic conditions such as heart failure or hypertension and for the prevention of conditions such as migraine headaches, seizures, or pregnancy. Short-acting drugs such as aspirin must be given every 3 to 4 hours, whereas medications with longer half-lives, such as felodipine ($t_{1/2}$ = 10 hours), need to be given only once a day. As drugs stay in the body for prolonged periods, however, the risk for long-term adverse effects increases. This can become particularly serious for patients with significant renal or hepatic impairment; diminished metabolism and excretion will cause the plasma half-life of a drug to increase, and the concentration may reach toxic levels. In these patients, medications must be given less frequently, or the dosages must be reduced.

As a rule of thumb, when a drug is discontinued it takes approximately four half-lives before the agent is considered "functionally" eliminated. After four half-lives, 94% of the drug has been eliminated. In the case of procaine with a half-life of only 8 minutes, the drug is considered eliminated in 32 minutes. Although some drug remains, the amount is too small to produce any beneficial or toxic effect. In the example of felodipine ($t_{1/2}$ = 10 hours), the drug would take 40 hours to be eliminated. Note, however, that this "rule of thumb" does not apply to all drugs; it certainly does not apply to medications administered to patients with renal or hepatic impairment.

3.9 Repeated dosing allows a plateau drug plasma level to be reached.

Few drugs are administered as a single dose. When multiple doses are administered over an extended period, the goal is to keep the drug plasma level *continuously* within the therapeutic range. In other words, the next dose should be administered before the drug plasma level falls below the minimum effective concentration.

Multiple doses result in an accumulation of drug in the bloodstream, as shown in Figure 3.8. If doses are timed correctly, a plateau drug plasma level will be reached and maintained within the therapeutic range. From a pharmacokinetic perspective, at the plateau level the amount of drug absorbed equals the amount of drug being excreted, resulting in a steady therapeutic level of drug being distributed to body tissues. Theoretically, it takes approximately four half-lives to reach this equilibrium. If the medication is given as a continuous infusion, the plateau can be reached very quickly and maintained with little or no fluctuation in drug plasma levels.

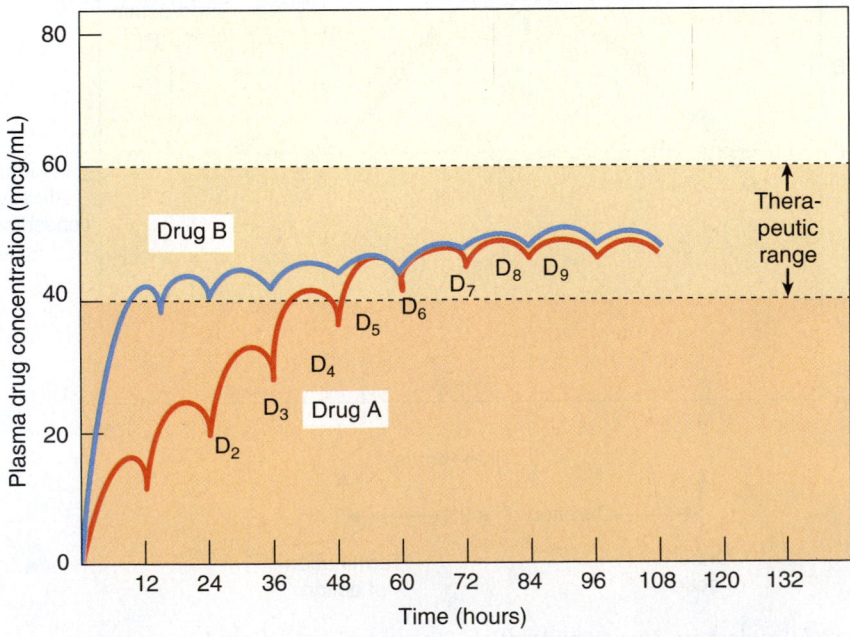

Figure 3.8 Multiple-dose drug administration. Drug A and drug B are administered every 12 hours. Drug B reaches the therapeutic range faster, because the first dose is a loading dose.

Note that in Figure 3.8, plasma drug levels are not necessarily smooth and continuous: There are peaks as well as troughs. When giving oral drugs, there is always some degree of fluctuation in peak concentration and trough concentration levels. A key point is that the peak should not rise into the toxic range, nor should the trough fall below the therapeutic range. Sustained or extended release formulations are designed to slowly release the drug so peak and trough fluctuations are minimized. Changing the dosing schedule can also reduce fluctuations. For example, rather than giving 60 mg of codeine once daily, it may be given 30 mg bid or 20 mg tid to reduce wide variation in the peak and trough levels.

The plateau may be reached faster by administration of loading doses followed by regular maintenance doses. A **loading dose** is a higher amount of drug, often given only once or twice, that is administered to "prime" the bloodstream with a level sufficient to quickly induce a therapeutic response. Before plasma levels drop back toward zero, intermittent **maintenance doses** are given to keep the plasma drug concentration in the therapeutic range. Although blood levels of the drug fluctuate with this approach, the equilibrium state can be reached almost as rapidly as with a continuous infusion. Loading doses are particularly important for drugs with prolonged half-lives and for situations in which it is critical to raise drug plasma levels quickly, as might be the case when administering an antibiotic for a severe infection. In Figure 3.8, it took almost five doses (48 hours) before a therapeutic level was reached using a routine dosing schedule. With a loading dose, a therapeutic level was reached within 12 hours.

CHAPTER

3 Understanding the Chapter

Key Concepts Summary

3.1 Pharmacokinetics focuses on what the body does to drugs after they are administered.

3.2 Drugs use diffusion and active transport to cross plasma membranes to reach their target cells.

3.3 Absorption is the process of moving a drug from the site of administration to the bloodstream.

3.4 Distribution describes how drugs are transported throughout the body.

3.5 Metabolism is a process that changes the activity of a drug and makes it more likely to be excreted.

3.6 Excretion processes remove drugs from the body.

3.7 The therapeutic response of most drugs depends on their concentration in the plasma.

3.8 The drug half-life estimates the duration of action for most medications.

3.9 Repeated dosing allows a plateau drug plasma level to be reached.

Case Study: Making the Patient Connection

Remember the patient "John Kessler" at the beginning of the chapter? Now read the remainder of the case study. Based on the information presented within this chapter, respond to the critical thinking questions that follow.

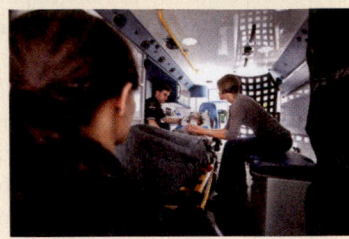

John Kessler has been ill for a long time and his prognosis is poor. He is 84 years old with multiple debilitating and chronic conditions. He has had uncontrolled diabetes for more than 20 years and has experienced many complications due to this condition. Three years ago, he developed chronic renal failure and requires dialysis three times a week. To further complicate his condition, John has continued to consume alcohol every day and smokes one pack of cigarettes per day. He has a long history of both alcohol and tobacco use.

Five days ago, his daughter noticed that he was becoming increasingly weak and lethargic. Last night when his temperature reached 38.8°C (102°F)

and he became confused, his daughter took him to the emergency department, and he was admitted to the medical unit. A chest x-ray this morning revealed bilateral pneumonia. John is receiving multiple medications through both the intravenous and inhalation routes.

Critical Thinking Questions

1. What factors may influence drug metabolism or excretion in this patient?

2. Discuss why drug elimination for this patient may complicate the pharmacotherapy.

3. How will the IV or inhalation drug therapy affect the absorption of his medications?

4. John will receive a loading dose of IV antibiotic and then be placed on maintenance doses every 6 hours. What is the purpose of this regimen? Why would this patient be a candidate for a loading dose?

See Answers to Critical Thinking Questions on student resource website.

Additional Case Study

Janice Albertson is a student nurse caring for a patient on the unit in which you are the RN. She has researched every drug her patient will be receiving and is familiar with the dose, mechanism of action, and possible adverse effects. Now she comes to you and asks, "Why is the drug's plasma half-life listed in the drug reference book? What is the value of this information?"

1. How would you respond to Janice's questions?

2. When is the use of drugs with short half-lives indicated?

3. List the indications for the use of a drug with a long half-life.

See Answers to Additional Case Study on student resource website.

Chapter Review

1 The nurse is teaching the patient about a newly prescribed medication. Which statement made by the patient would indicate the need for further medication education?

1. "The liquid form of the drug will be absorbed faster than the tablets."

2. "If I take more, I'll have a better response."

3. "Taking this drug with food will decrease how much drug gets into my system."

4. "I can consult my health care provider if I experience unexpected adverse effects."

2 The nurse is caring for several patients. Which patient will the nurse anticipate is most likely to experience an alteration in drug metabolism?

1. A 3-day-old premature infant

2. A 22-year-old pregnant female

3. A 32-year-old man with kidney stones

4. A 50-year-old executive with hypertension

3 The patient is receiving multiple medications, including one drug specifically used to stimulate gastric peristalsis. The nurse knows that this drug could have what influence on additional oral medications?

1. Increased absorption

2. Reduced excretion

3. Decreased absorption

4. Enhanced distribution

4 A patient is being discharged from the hospital with a nebulizer for self-administration of inhalation medication. Which statement made by the patient indicates to the nurse that patient education has been successful?

1. "Inhaled medications should only be taken in the morning."

2. "Doses for inhaled medication are larger than those taken orally."

3. "Medicines taken by inhalation produce a very rapid response."

4. "Inhaled drugs are often rendered inactive by hepatic metabolic reactions."

5 The nurse is caring for a patient with hepatitis and resulting hepatic impairment. The nurse would expect the duration of action for most medications to:

1. Decrease.
2. Improve.
3. Be unaffected.
4. Increase.

6 The nurse is monitoring the therapeutic drug level for a patient on vancomycin (Vancocin) and notes that the level is within the accepted range. What does this indicate to the nurse? Select all that apply.

1. The drug should cause no toxicities or adverse effects.
2. The drug level is appropriate to exert therapeutic effects.
3. The dose will not need to be changed for the duration of treatment.
4. The nurse will need to continue monitoring because each patient response to a drug is unique.
5. This drug will effectively treat the patient's condition.

See Answers to Chapter Review in Appendix A.

References

Hirani, J. J., Rathod, D. A., & Vadalia, K. R. (2009). Orally disintegrating tablets: A review. *Tropical Journal of Pharmaceutical Research, 8,* 161–172.

Selected Bibliography

Allen, L. V., Popovich, N. V., & Ansel, H. C. (2010). *Ansel's pharmaceutical dosage forms and drug delivery systems* (9th ed.). Baltimore, MD: Lippincott Williams & Wilkins.

Amur, S., Zineh, I., Abernethy, D. R., Huang, S., & Lesko, L. J. (2010). Pharmacogenomics and adverse drug reactions. *Personalized Medicine, 7,* 633–642. doi:10.2217/pme.10.63

Bauer, L. A. (2011). Clinical pharmacokinetics and pharmacodynamics. In J. T. DiPiro, R. L. Talbert, G. C. Yee, G. R. Matzke, B. G. Wells, & L. M. Posey (Eds.), *Pharmacotherapy: A pathophysiology approach* (8th ed., pp. 12–35). New York, NY: McGraw-Hill.

Buxton, I. L., & Benet, L. Z. (2011). Pharmacokinetics: The dynamics of drug absorption, distribution, action and elimination. In L. L. Brunton, B. A. Chabner, & B. C. Knollman (Eds.), *The pharmacological basis of therapeutics* (12th ed., pp. 17–40). New York, NY: McGraw-Hill.

Hoffman, E. M., Breitenbach, A., & Breitkreutz, J. (2011). Advances in orodispersible films for drug delivery. *Expert Opinion in Drug Delivery, 8,* 299–316. doi:10.1517/17425247.2011.553217

Khan, E. U. (2011). The basics of pharmacokinetics in prescribing and clinical practice. *Nurse Prescribing, 9,* 557–566.

Papadopoulos, J., & Smithburger, P. L. (2010). Common drug interactions leading to adverse drug events in the intensive care unit: Management and pharmacokinetic considerations. *Critical Care Medicine, 38,* S126–S135. doi:10.1097/CCM.0b013e3181de0acf

Ranade, V. V., & Cannon, J. B. (2011). *Drug delivery systems* (3rd ed.). Boca Raton, FL: Taylor and Francis.

Rosenbaum, S. E. (2011). *Basic pharmacokinetics and pharmacodynamics: An integrated textbook and computer simulations.* Hoboken, NJ: John Wiley & Sons.

Shargell, L., Yu, A., & Wu-Pong, S. (2012). *Applied biopharmaceutics & pharmacokinetics* (6th ed.). Blacklick, OH: McGraw-Hill.

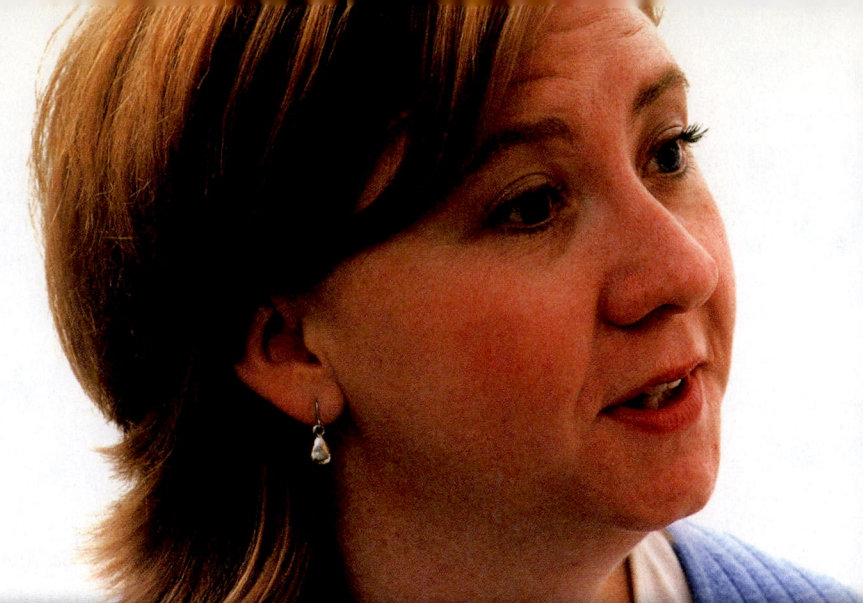

CHAPTER

4 Pharmacodynamics

LEARNING OUTCOMES

After reading this chapter, the student should be able to:

1. Apply frequency distribution curves to explain interpatient variability in medication response.
2. Explain the importance of the median effective dose (ED_{50}) to clinical practice.
3. Compare and contrast median lethal dose (LD_{50}) and median toxicity dose (TD_{50}).
4. Relate a drug's therapeutic index to its margin of safety.
5. Identify the significance of the dose–response relationship to clinical practice.
6. Compare and contrast the terms *potency* and *efficacy*.
7. Describe the relationship between receptors and drug action.
8. Distinguish between an agonist, partial agonist, and antagonist.
9. Explain possible future developments in the field of pharmacogenetics.

CHAPTER OUTLINE

▶ Interpatient Variability

▶ Therapeutic Index

▶ Dose–Response Relationship

▶ Potency and Efficacy

▶ Receptor Theory

▶ Agonists and Antagonists

▶ Pharmacogenetics

KEY TERMS

agonist, 48

antagonist, 48

dose–response relationship, 45

efficacy, 45

frequency distribution curve, 43

intrinsic activity, 47

margin of safety (MOS), 44

median effective dose (ED$_{50}$), 43

median lethal dose (LD$_{50}$), 44

median toxicity dose (TD$_{50}$), 44

partial agonist, 48

pharmacodynamics, 43

pharmacogenetics, 48

potency, 45

receptor, 47

second messenger, 47

therapeutic index (TI), 44

The term *pharmacodynamics* comprises the root words *pharmaco*, which refers to medicines, and *dynamics*, which means "change." In simplest terms, pharmacodynamics refers to how a drug changes the body. A more complete definition explains **pharmacodynamics** as the branch of pharmacology concerned with the mechanisms of drug action and the relationships between drug concentration and responses in the body. This chapter examines the mechanisms by which drugs affect patients, and how the nurse can apply these principles to clinical practice.

Interpatient Variability

4.1 Patients have widely different responses to drugs, which can be depicted on a frequency distribution curve.

The principles of pharmacodynamics have important clinical applications. Health care providers must be able to predict whether a given dose of medication will produce a therapeutic change in their patients. Why does the "average" dose obtained from a drug guide sometimes produce a hyperresponse and at other times no response at all? Knowledge of dose–response relationships, therapeutic indexes, and drug–receptor interactions—all topics of pharmacodynamics—can help nurses provide safer and more effective treatment.

The interpatient variability observed during drug therapy can be illustrated by examining a frequency distribution curve. Shown in Figure 4.1, a **frequency distribution curve** is a graphic representation of the number of patients responding with a particular drug action at different doses. On the horizontal axis, notice the wide range in doses that produced the patient responses shown on the curve. A few patients responded to the drug at very low doses (10 to 20 mg). As the dose was increased, more and more patients responded. The peak of the curve (50 mg) indicates the largest number of patients responding to the drug. Some patients required very high doses (80 to 90 mg) to elicit the desired response. The curve does not show the magnitude of the response, only whether or not a measurable response occurred among the patients. As an example, think of the given response to an antihypertensive drug as defined by a reduction of 20 mm in systolic blood pressure. A few patients experienced the desired 20-mm reduction at a drug dose of only 10 mg; a 50-mg dose gave the largest number of patients the 20-mm reduction in blood pressure. However, a few patients needed as much as 90 mg of the drug to produce the same 20-mm reduction.

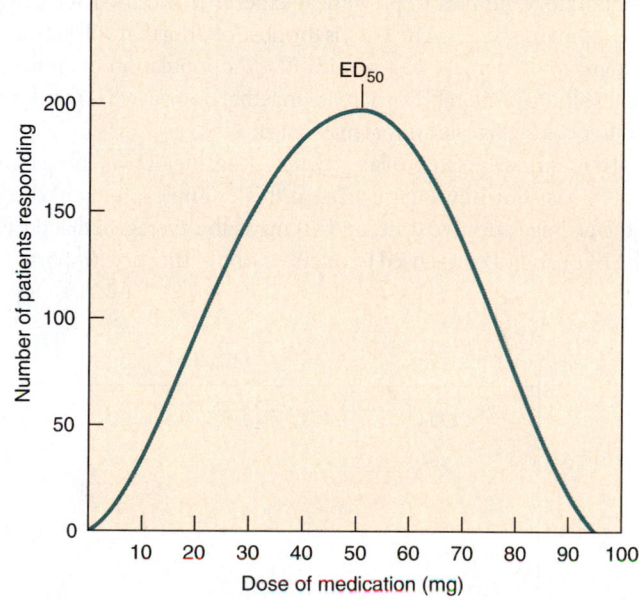

Figure 4.1 Frequency distribution curve: interpatient variability in drug response.

The dose in the middle of the frequency distribution curve represents the drug's **median effective dose (ED$_{50}$)**. The ED$_{50}$ is the dose required to produce a specific therapeutic response in 50% of a group of patients. Drug guides usually use the ED$_{50}$ as the "average" or standard dose for a drug.

The interpatient variability shown in Figure 4.1 has important clinical implications. First, the nurse should realize that the standard or average dose predicts a satisfactory therapeutic response for only half the population. But what about responses in the rest of the patients? Many patients will require more or less than the average dose for optimum pharmacotherapy. Using the systolic blood pressure example, assume that a large group of patients is given the average dose of 50 mg. Some of these patients will experience toxicity at this level because they only need 10 mg to achieve blood pressure reduction. A few patients in this group will probably have no reduction in blood pressure at all. By monitoring the patient, taking vital signs, and interpreting any associated laboratory data, the nurse is key in determining whether the average dose is effective for the patient. *It is not enough to simply memorize an average dose for a drug; the nurse must have the skills to know when and how to adjust this dose to obtain the optimum therapeutic response.*

Therapeutic Index

4.2 The therapeutic index describes a drug's margin of safety.

Selecting a dose that produces an optimum therapeutic response for each individual patient is certainly important, but the nurse must also be able to predict whether that dose is safe for that patient. Frequency distribution curves can also be used to illustrate the safety of a drug.

The **median lethal dose (LD$_{50}$)** is a value often determined in laboratory animals in preclinical experiments during the drug development process. The LD$_{50}$ is the dose of drug that will kill 50% of a group of animals. Just as with ED$_{50}$, a population of animals will exhibit considerable variability in lethal dosage; what may be a nontoxic dose for one animal may kill another.

To examine the safety of a particular drug, the LD$_{50}$ is compared to ED$_{50}$, as shown in Figure 4.2a. In this example, 10 mg of drug is the average effective dose, and 40 mg is the average lethal dose. The ED$_{50}$ and LD$_{50}$ are used to calculate one of the most important

values in pharmacology, a drug's therapeutic index. The **therapeutic index (TI)** is defined as the ratio of a drug's LD$_{50}$ to its ED$_{50}$.

$$\text{Therapeutic index} = \frac{\text{median lethal dose (LD}_{50})}{\text{median effective dose (ED}_{50})}$$

The larger the difference between the two doses, the greater the TI. In Figure 4.2a, the TI is 4 (40 mg ÷ 10 mg). Essentially, this means that it would take an error in magnitude of approximately four times the average dose to be lethal to a patient. In terms of dosage, this is a relatively safe drug, and small to moderate medication errors or changes in the drug's bioavailability would likely not be fatal. Thus, the TI is a measure of a drug's safety margin: the higher the value, the safer the medication. Drugs exhibit a wide range of TIs, from 1 to 2 to greater than 100.

As another example, the TI of a second drug is shown in Figure 4.2b. Drug Z has the same ED$_{50}$ as drug X but shows a different LD$_{50}$. The TI for drug Z is only 2 (20 mg ÷ 10 mg). The difference between an effective dose and a lethal dose is very small for drug Z; thus the drug has a narrow safety margin. Small medication errors or changes in the drug's metabolism or excretion could have lethal consequences. The TI offers the nurse practical information on the safety of a drug and a means to compare one drug to another.

In Figure 4.2b, notice that the two curves overlapped. Some patients required a dose of 15 to 20 mg to produce the desired effect, yet this same dose was lethal in other patients. This type of drug would require careful assessment of hepatic and renal function prior to the initiation of therapy. With drugs exhibiting a low TI, it is prudent to begin with the lowest dose possible, then increase the amount of drug with careful monitoring.

Because the LD$_{50}$ cannot be experimentally determined in humans, other estimates of drug safety are available. The **median toxicity dose (TD$_{50}$)** is the dose that will produce a given toxicity in 50% of a group of patients. The TD$_{50}$ value may be extrapolated from animal data or based on adverse effects recorded in patient clinical trials.

The **margin of safety (MOS)** is another index of a drug's effectiveness and safety. The MOS is calculated as the amount of drug that is lethal to 1% of animals (LD$_1$) divided by the amount of drug that produces a therapeutic effect in 99% of the animals (ED$_{99}$). In general, the higher the MOS value, the safer the medication. Of course this considers only the lethality of the drug and does not account for non-lethal, though serious, adverse effects that may occur at lower doses.

CONNECTION Checkpoint 4.1

From what you learned in Chapter 2, before a pharmaceutical company tests a drug in patients after preclinical trials have been completed, what document must be submitted to the FDA? *See Answer to Connection Checkpoint 4.1 on student resource website.*

Dose–Response Relationship

4.3 The dose–response relationship describes how the actions of a drug change with increasing dose.

In the preceding section, frequency distribution curves were used to graphically visualize interpatient differences in responses to medications in a *population*. Pharmacodynamics is also used to study the variability in responses in a *single patient*.

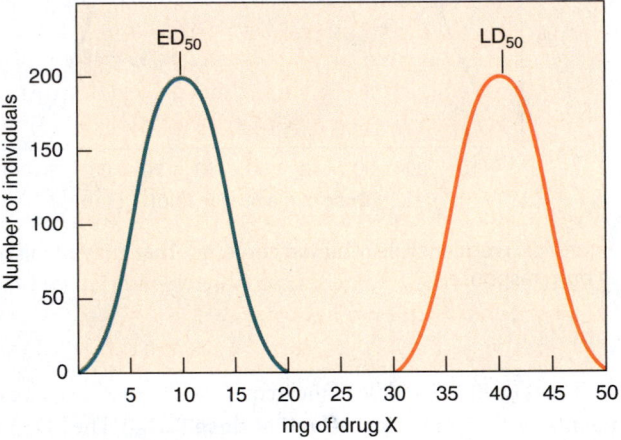

(a) Drug X : TI = $\dfrac{LD_{50}}{ED_{50}} = \dfrac{40}{10} = 4$

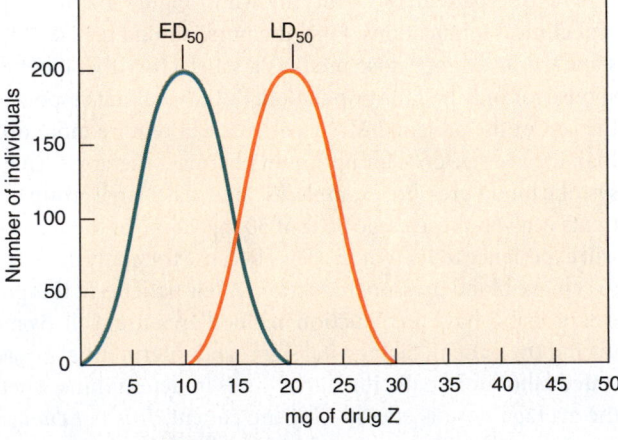

(b) Drug Z : TI = $\dfrac{LD_{50}}{ED_{50}} = \dfrac{20}{10} = 2$

Figure 4.2 Therapeutic index: (a) Drug X has a therapeutic index of 4. (b) Drug Z has a therapeutic index of 2.

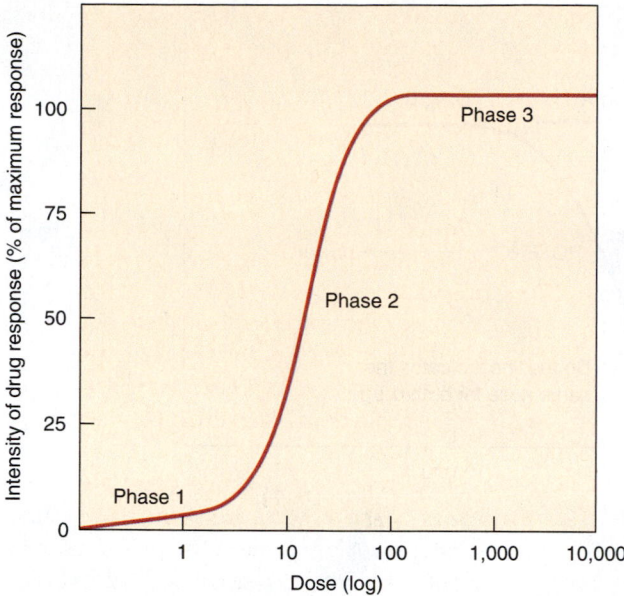

Figure 4.3 Dose–response relationship.

How does a patient respond to varying doses of a drug? Common sense would suggest that a larger dose would produce more drug effect. For example, an antibiotic would kill more bacteria if the dose was increased from 10 to 20 mg. An antihypertensive drug would cause a greater reduction in blood pressure if the dose was increased from 50 to 100 mg. These simple examples describe the **dose–response relationship**, one of the most fundamental concepts in pharmacology. A graphic representation of this relationship, the dose–response curve, is illustrated in Figure 4.3. Examining and comparing dose–response curves can yield a large amount of information about a drug.

A dose–response curve plots the drug dose administered to the patient versus the intensity or degree of response obtained. There are three distinct phases of a dose–response curve that indicate essential pharmacodynamic principles. Phase 1 occurs at the lowest doses. The flatness of this portion of the curve indicates that few target cells have been affected by the drug; doses that are too small will not produce a therapeutic effect. Phase 2 is the rising, straight line portion of the curve. In this portion, there is a linear relationship between the amount of drug administered and the degree of response obtained from the patient. For example, if the dose is doubled, twice as much response may be obtained. This is the most desirable range of doses for pharmacotherapeutics, because giving more drug results in proportionately more effect; a lower drug dose gives less effect. In phase 3 increasing the drug dose produces no additional therapeutic response—a plateau has been reached. This may occur for a number of reasons. One possible explanation is that all the target receptors for the drug are occupied. It could also mean that the drug has brought 100% relief, such as when a migraine headache has been terminated; giving higher doses produces no additional relief. Although increasing the dose during phase 3 does not result in additional therapeutic effects, the nurse should be mindful that increasing the dose may produce more adverse effects.

The dose–response curve in Figure 4.3 is smooth and continuous; thus it is sometimes called a graded dose–response curve. This is important to pharmacotherapeutics because, by adjusting the

dose in small increments, the prescriber is able to attain virtually any degree of therapeutic response (0% to 100%) within the linear range of drug doses. This is especially true when using the intravenous (IV) route, during which the nurse can adjust the infusion rate in very small increments.

Many types of adverse effects also follow a graded dose–response relationship: the higher the dose, the more intense the adverse effect. By adjusting the dose lower, while still keeping it within the therapeutic range, adverse effects may be lessened. Some adverse effects, such as anaphylaxis, are independent of dose in that even the smallest amount of drug may trigger a serious adverse response (see Chapter 5).

Potency and Efficacy

4.4 Potency and efficacy are fundamental concepts of pharmacodynamics that describe a drug's activity.

Within a pharmacologic class, not all drugs are equally effective at treating a disorder. For example, some antineoplastic drugs kill more cancer cells than others; some antihypertensive medications lower blood pressure to a greater extent than others; and some analgesics are more effective at relieving severe pain than others in the same class. Furthermore, drugs in the same class are effective at different doses: One antibiotic may be effective at a dose of 1 mg/kg, whereas another is most effective at 100 mg/kg. Nurses need a method to compare one drug to another so that they can administer treatment effectively.

There are two fundamental ways to compare medications within therapeutic and pharmacologic classes. First is the concept of **potency**, which is the amount of drug needed to produce a specified effect. A drug that is more potent will produce its therapeutic effect at lower doses, compared to another drug in the same class. As an example, consider two calcium channel blockers used for hypertension: amlodipine (Norvasc) and nifedipine (Procardia). Amlodipine produces its decrease in blood pressure at 10 mg/day and nifedipine at 60 mg/day. Amlodipine is clearly more potent than nifedipine because it takes a lower dose (6 times less) to produce its antihypertensive effect.

Thus, potency is a way to compare the doses of two independently administered drugs in terms of how much is needed to produce a particular response. A useful way to visualize the concept of potency is by examining dose–response curves. When comparing the two drugs shown in Figure 4.4a, drug A is more potent because it requires a lower dose to produce the same response.

A second method used to compare drugs is called **efficacy**, which is defined as the maximum response that can be produced from a particular drug. In the example in Figure 4.4b, drug A has greater efficacy because it produces a higher maximal response.

Which is more important to the outcomes of pharmacotherapy: potency or efficacy? Perhaps the best way to understand these important concepts is to use the specific example of headache pain. Two common over-the-counter (OTC) analgesic therapies are ibuprofen, 200 mg, and aspirin, 650 mg. The fact that ibuprofen relieves pain at a lower dose indicates that this agent is more potent than aspirin. At the given doses, however, both are equally effective at relieving headaches; thus they have the same efficacy. If the patient is experiencing severe pain, however, neither aspirin nor ibuprofen has sufficient

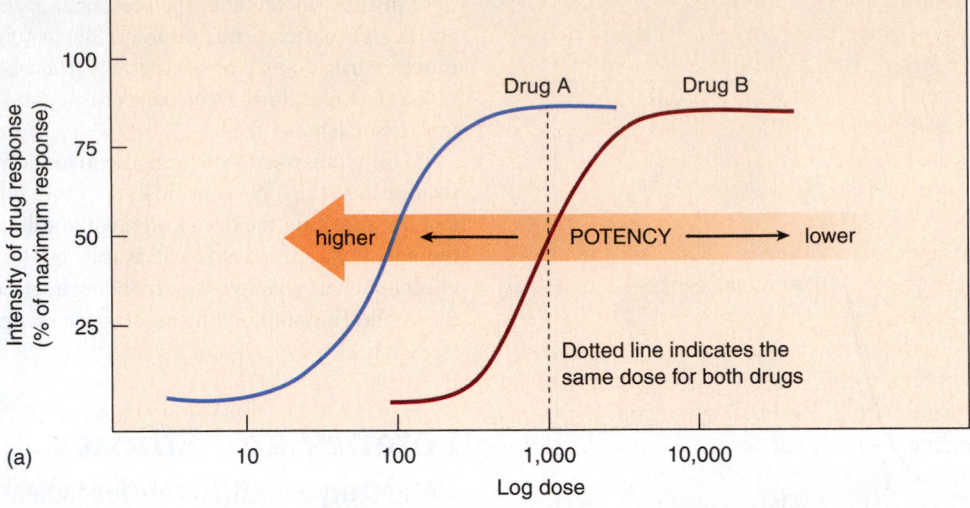

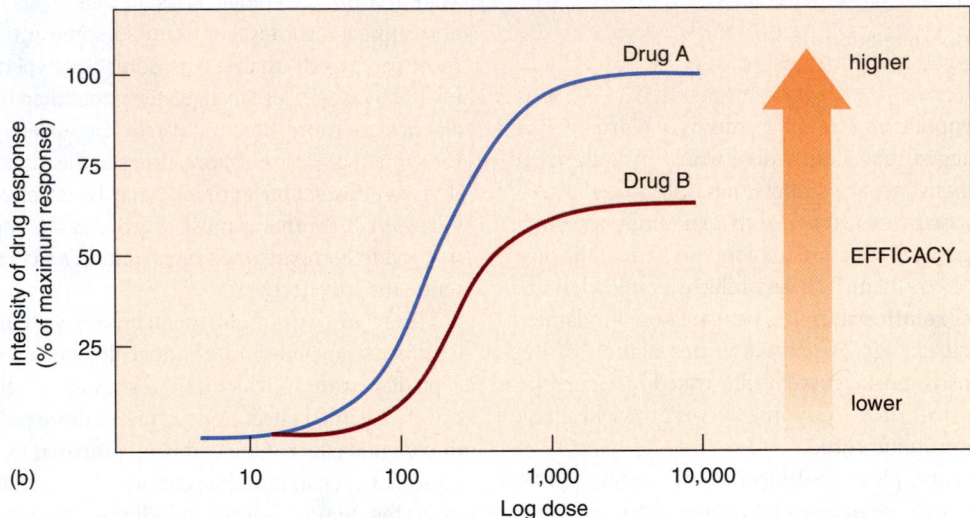

Figure 4.4 Potency and efficacy: (a) Drug A has a higher potency than drug B. (b) Drug A has a higher efficacy than drug B.

efficacy to bring relief. Narcotic analgesics, such as morphine, have a greater efficacy than aspirin or ibuprofen and could effectively treat this type of pain. From a pharmacotherapeutic perspective, efficacy is almost always more important than potency. In the preceding example, the average dose is unimportant to the patient, but headache relief is essential. As another comparison, the patient with cancer is much more concerned with how many cancer cells have been killed (efficacy) than with the dose the nurse administered (potency). In the comparison of Norvasc to Procardia, although Norvasc is clearly more potent, both drugs reduce blood pressure to the same degree; thus they have the same efficacy. Although the nurse will often hear claims that one drug is more potent than another, a more compelling concern is which drug has greater efficacy.

A word of caution is necessary at this point. In Section 4.3, it is stated that many adverse effects are related to dose—that higher doses produce more intense adverse effects. This is true only when comparing doses of the same drug. For example, a therapeutic dose for amlodipine is 10 mg/day. Giving 20 or 30 mg of amlodipine will most certainly increase the risk of experiencing an adverse effect.

Can the dose of amlodipine be compared to a dose of nifedipine, which is 60 mg/day? The answer is absolutely not. In fact, 10 mg of amlodipine gives the same risk of adverse effects as 60 mg of nifedipine. *The point is that when two different drugs are compared, one cannot assume that the drug with the lower dose gives fewer adverse effects.*

An additional word of caution is necessary. In clinical practice the term *potency* is often misused to indicate a more effective drug. The nurse should remember the correct definitions of the words *potency* and *efficacy* and try to incorporate them into clinical practice.

Receptor Theory

4.5 Most drugs produce their actions by activating or inhibiting specific cellular receptors.

Drugs rarely create new actions in the body; instead, they enhance or inhibit existing physiological and biochemical processes. To cause such changes, the drug must interact with specific chemicals that are normally found in the body. A cellular molecule to which a medication binds to produce its effects is called a **receptor**. A receptor may be thought of as the drug's specific target. The concept of a drug binding to a receptor and causing a change in physiology is a fundamental concept in pharmacology. Receptor theory predicts that the response of a drug is proportional to the concentration of receptors that are bound or occupied by the drug. Receptor theory explains the mechanisms by which most drugs produce their effects.

It is important to understand, however, that receptors do not exist in the body solely to bind drugs; their normal function is to bind endogenous molecules such as hormones, neurotransmitters, and growth factors. The drug simply uses existing targets to cause its effects. When drugs bind to the receptor they either enhance or inhibit a normal cellular function. The binding is usually reversible and the action of the drug is terminated once the drug leaves its receptor. In a few cases, binding of the drug is irreversible. Drugs that have the ability to bind to a receptor and produce a strong action are said to have high **intrinsic activity**. Intrinsic activity and efficacy are related. Drugs that have high intrinsic activity have high efficacy.

Although a drug receptor can be any type of molecule, the vast majority are proteins. As shown in Figure 4.5, a receptor may be depicted as a three-dimensional protein spanning across the plasma membrane. The extracellular component of a receptor often consists of subunits arranged in a specific shape that will bind the specific drug or endogenous chemical (sometimes called a ligand). The receptor may form a membrane channel that regulates substances entering and leaving the cell.

A drug binds to its receptor in a very selective manner, much like a lock and key. Once the receptor is occupied, a series of **second messenger** events is triggered within the cell such as the conversion of adenosine triphosphate (ATP) to cyclic adenosine monophosphate (cyclic AMP), the release of intracellular calcium, or the activation of specific G proteins and associated enzymes. These cascades of biochemical events initiate the drug's action by either stimulating or inhibiting the normal activity of the cell. Small changes to the structure of a drug, or its receptor, may weaken or even eliminate binding between the two molecules, rendering the drug ineffective.

Not all receptors are proteins bound to the plasma membrane: Some are intracellular molecules such as DNA or enzymes in the cytoplasm. By interacting with these types of receptors, medications are able to inhibit protein synthesis or regulate events such as cell division and metabolism. Examples of agents that bind intracellular components include steroid hormones and certain vitamins.

Receptor subtypes have been discovered that permit the "fine-tuning" of pharmacotherapy. For example, the first drugs affecting the autonomic nervous system affected all types of autonomic receptors. These agents were not very useful because they produced such a broad range of therapeutic and adverse effects. Later, it was discovered that two basic receptor types existed in the body, alpha and beta, and drugs were then developed that were selective for only one type. This permitted more specific drug therapy (and fewer adverse effects). Still later, several subtypes of alpha and beta receptors, including alpha-1, alpha-2, beta-1, and beta-2, were discovered that allowed even more specificity in pharmacotherapy. In recent years, researchers have further divided and refined various drug receptor subtypes. It is likely that research will continue to result in the development of new medications that activate very specific receptors to cause therapeutic responses while avoiding some adverse effects.

Some drugs act independently of cellular receptors. These agents are associated with other mechanisms, such as changing the permeability of cellular membranes, depressing membrane

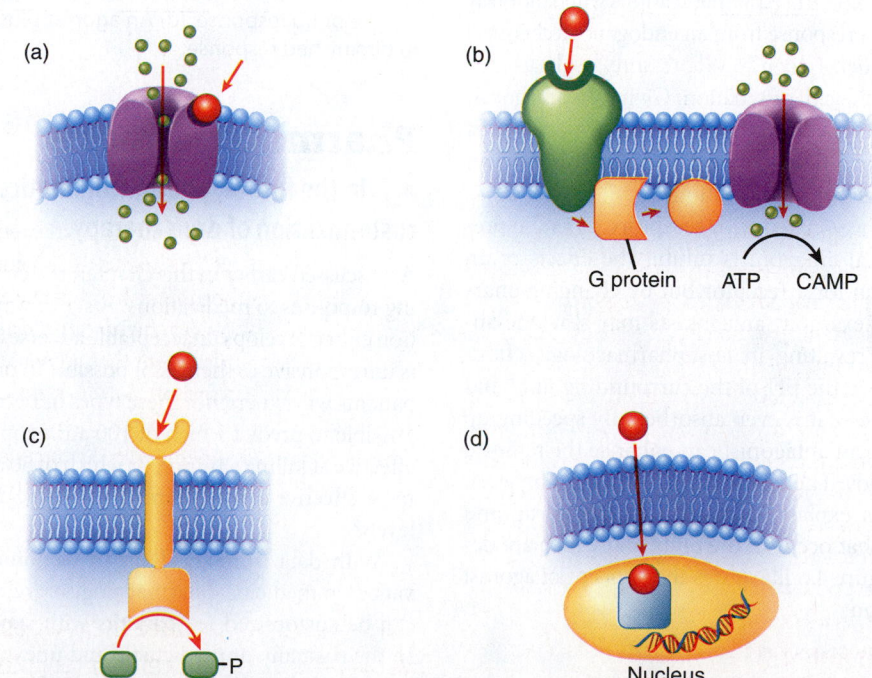

Figure 4.5 Types of cellular receptors: (a) Drug binds to the receptor opening channel. (b) Drug binds to the receptor, causing a G protein–mediated reaction in the cell. (c) Drug binds to the transmembrane receptor to signal a change inside the cell. (d) Drug enters the cell nucleus to increase synthesis of specific proteins.

excitability, or altering the activity of cellular pumps. Actions such as these are often described as nonspecific cellular responses. Ethyl alcohol, general anesthetics, and osmotic diuretics are examples of agents that act by nonspecific mechanisms.

Agonists and Antagonists

4.6 Agonists, partial agonists, and antagonists compete for cellular receptors and can modify drug action.

When a drug binds to a receptor, several possible consequences can result. In simplest terms, some specific action in the cell is either enhanced or inhibited. The actual biochemical mechanism underlying the therapeutic effect, however, may be extremely complex. In some cases, the mechanism of action is not known.

When a drug binds to its receptor, it may produce a response that mimics the effect of the endogenous regulatory molecule. For example, when the drug bethanechol is administered, it binds to acetylcholine receptors in the autonomic nervous system and produces the same actions as acetylcholine. A drug that activates a receptor and produces the same type of response as the endogenous substance is called an **agonist**. Agonists sometimes produce a greater maximal response than the endogenous chemical. The term **partial agonist** is used to describe a medication that produces a weaker, or less efficacious, response than an agonist.

A second possibility is that a drug will occupy a receptor and prevent the endogenous chemical from binding to produce its action. This type of drug, an **antagonist**, often competes with agonists for receptor binding sites. For example, the drug atropine competes with acetylcholine for certain receptors in the autonomic nervous system. If the dose is high enough, atropine may completely block the effects of acetylcholine because acetylcholine cannot reach its receptors. Antagonists may be used as medications when the body is producing too much of a response from an endogenous chemical or from a drug overdose, such as high blood pressure, fast heart rate, secretion of excess stomach acid, or sedation. Giving an antagonist in these situations may reverse the adverse effects. An antagonist has no intrinsic activity; the actions observed after administering an antagonist are caused by lack of agonist action.

Not all antagonism is associated with receptors, as in the previous example. Functional antagonists inhibit the effects of an agonist, not by competing for a receptor but by changing pharmacokinetic factors. For example, antagonists may slow the absorption of an agonist, resulting in less pharmacologic effect. An antagonist may change the pH of the surrounding fluid and neutralize the agonist before it is even absorbed. By speeding up metabolism or excretion, an antagonist can enhance the removal of an agonist from the body. The relationships that occur between agonists and antagonists explain many of the drug–drug and drug–food interactions that occur in the body and which are described in Chapter 5. Figure 4.6 illustrates the concept of agonist and antagonist drug action.

CONNECTION Checkpoint 4.2

From what you learned in Chapter 3, phenytoin is an inducer of CYP1A2, the enzyme that metabolizes acetaminophen. Would phenytoin be considered a functional agonist or an antagonist to acetaminophen? *See Answer to Connection Checkpoint 4.2 on student resource website.*

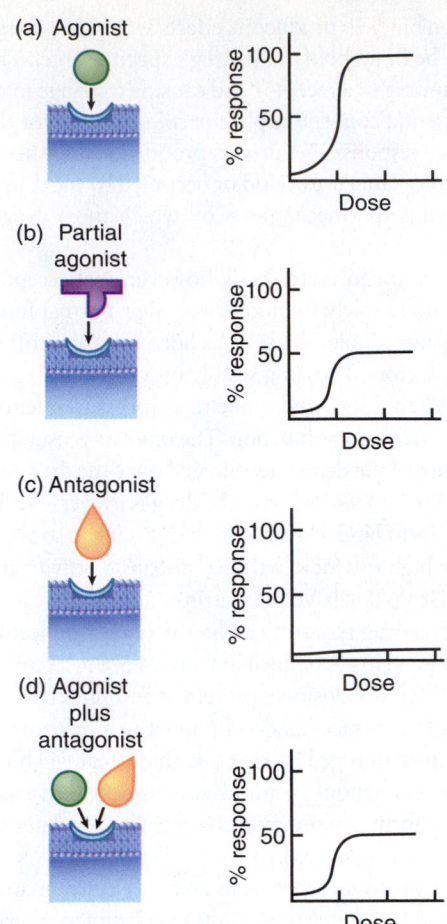

Figure 4.6 Agonists, partial agonists, and antagonists: (a) An agonist results in maximum response. (b) A partial agonist results in less than maximum response. (c) An antagonist results in little or no response. (d) An agonist plus antagonist results in diminished response.

Pharmacogenetics

4.7 In the future, pharmacogenetics may allow customization of drug therapy.

As discussed earlier in this chapter, patients can have widely differing responses to medications. A significant portion of the population either develops unacceptable adverse effects to certain drugs or is unresponsive to them. Is it possible to predict, in advance, which patients will experience these types of responses? For example, is it possible to predict which of 100 antineoplastic drugs will be most effective at killing a tumor, or which of 50 antidiabetic drugs will be most effective at maintaining a particular patient's blood glucose levels?

With data from the Human Genome Project and other advances in medicine, pharmacologists are hopeful that future drugs can be customized for patients with specific genetic similarities. In the past, any unpredictable and unexplained drug reaction has been labeled idiosyncratic response. It is hoped that, by analyzing a DNA test before prescribing a drug, these idiosyncratic adverse effects can someday be avoided.

Pharmacogenetics is the branch of pharmacology that studies the role of genetic variation in drug responses. The most important advances in pharmacogenetics so far have been the identification of subtle genetic differences in drug-metabolizing enzymes. Genetic differences in these enzymes are responsible for a significant portion of drug-induced toxicity. It is hoped that the use of pharmacogenetic information may someday allow for drug therapy that is customized to a patient's individual molecules. Although therapies based on a patient's genetically based response may not be widespread at this time, pharmacogenetics may radically change the way pharmacotherapy will be practiced in the future.

CONNECTIONS | Treating the Diverse Patient

◖ Enzyme Deficiencies in Ethnic Populations

Pharmacogenetics has identified ethnic populations of people, such as males of Mediterranean and African descent, who are deficient in glucose-6-phosphate dehydrogenase (G6PD), an enzyme that is essential in carbohydrate metabolism. As reviewed by Carter (2012), G6PD deficiency is the most common enzyme deficiency, with about 400 million people affected worldwide. Over 60 different mutations that encode for G6PD have been identified. When certain oxidative drugs are given, such as primaquine, sulfonamides, or nitrofurantoin (Macrobid), an acute hemolysis of red blood cells (RBCs) occurs due to the breaking of chemical bonds in the hemoglobin molecule, with large numbers of circulating RBCs being destroyed. Genetic typing does not always predict toxicity. Patients may not realize they carry a genetically linked trait and may report a history of "severe allergy" to fava beans for example, which induced the hemolytic symptoms in the past. The role of the nurse is critical in observing patients carefully for 24 to 72 hours following administration of these medications. Prevention is the best treatment.

CHAPTER

4

Understanding the Chapter

Key Concepts Summary

4.1 Patients have widely different responses to drugs, which can be depicted on a frequency distribution curve.

4.2 The therapeutic index describes a drug's margin of safety.

4.3 The dose–response relationship describes how the actions of a drug change with increasing dose.

4.4 Potency and efficacy are fundamental concepts of pharmacodynamics that describe a drug's activity.

4.5 Most drugs produce their actions by activating or inhibiting specific cellular receptors.

4.6 Agonists, partial agonists, and antagonists compete for cellular receptors and can modify drug action.

4.7 In the future, pharmacogenetics may allow customization of drug therapy.

Case Study: Making the Patient Connection

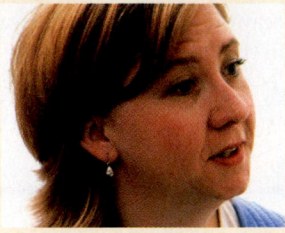

Remember the patient "Katherine Hunter" at the beginning of the chapter? Now read the remainder of the case study. Based on the information presented within this chapter, respond to the critical thinking questions that follow.

Katherine Hunter prides herself on being a wise consumer and cautiously examines the claims by manufacturers for all her purchases. She researches everything she buys, such as automobiles, household appliances, and medications. Recently, she has begun to seriously consider assertions made by the advertisements for various types of antacids. Most brands claim to be the most efficient in relieving the symptoms of indigestion. Others say that their brand is the most potent antacid available without a prescription.

Some products claim that they not only relieve heartburn, but also supply the body with needed vitamins and minerals. When purchasing an OTC medication, all Katherine wants is something that will work quickly with few adverse effects.

Critical Thinking Questions

1. How would you teach Katherine the difference between potency and efficacy?
2. Which of the two concepts (potency and efficacy) would be most important for selecting a drug? Why?
3. What are the drawbacks of comparing two different medications?

See Answers to Critical Thinking Questions on student resource website.

Additional Case Study

As the nurse practicing in a middle school, you have been asked to speak to the eighth-grade pre-health professionals' class. The topic for today's discussion is "how drugs work in the body." The teacher has provided you with an outline of concepts that you will need to address.

1. Describe the link between a drug's action and drug receptors.
2. Why do people respond differently to medication?
3. What are drug agonists and drug antagonists?

See Answers to Additional Case Study on student resource website.

Chapter Review

1 What parameters would the nurse use to determine whether the average dose of a medication is effective for a patient? Select all that apply.

　1. Physical examination
　2. Vital signs
　3. Laboratory values
　4. Dosage time
　5. Efficacy

2 The nurse knows that a drug with a high therapeutic index is:

　1. Probably safe.
　2. Often dangerous.
　3. Frequently risky.
　4. Most likely effective.

3 While reviewing a drug manufacturer's package insert, the nurse reads about the dose–response curve. The purpose of the dose–response curve is to illustrate the relationship between:

　1. The amount of a drug administered and the degree of response it produces.
　2. The prevalence of toxic effects in a given population.
　3. The degree of response and the total duration of action of the drug.
　4. The peak serum drug level when half the dose is administered.

4 A research nurse is discussing the TD_{50} of a drug with the other members of the investigation team. On which of the following would the discussion focus?

　1. Effectiveness
　2. Dose response
　3. Receptor subtypes
　4. Toxicity

5 A patient with myasthenia gravis has been receiving neostigmine, a cholinergic agonist, for the past 2 years. The nurse is ready to administer benztropine, a cholinergic antagonist. Which result will likely occur when these drugs are combined?

1. Neostigmine will exhibit a greater effect.
2. Neostigmine will exhibit a lesser effect.
3. Neostigmine will not be affected by the administration of benztropine.
4. Neostigmine will first exhibit a greater effect, followed by a lesser effect.

6 When considering pharmacodynamic principles for a patient's drug therapy, the nurse is aware that affinity for a receptor is most closely associated with a drug's:

1. Potency.
2. Efficacy.
3. Metabolism.
4. First-pass effect.

See Answers to Chapter Review in Appendix A.

References

Carter, S. M. (2012). *Glucose-6-phosphate dehydrogenase deficiency*. Retrieved from http://emedicine.medscape.com/article/200390-overview

Selected Bibliography

Bauer, L. A. (2011). Clinical pharmacokinetics and pharmacodynamics. In J. T. DiPiro, R. L. Talbert, G. C. Yee, G. R. Matzke, B. G. Wells, & L. M. Posey (Eds.), *Pharmacotherapy: A pathophysiology approach* (8th ed., pp. 15–37). New York, NY: McGraw-Hill.

Blumenthal, D. K., & Garrison, J. C. (2011). Pharmacodynamics: Molecular mechanisms of drug action. In L. L. Brunton, B. A. Chabner, & B. C. Knollman (Eds.), *The pharmacological basis of therapeutics* (12th ed., pp. 41–72). New York, NY: McGraw-Hill.

Copeland, R. A. (2010). The dynamics of drug-target interactions: Drug-target residence time and its impact on efficacy and safety. *Expert Opinion on Drug Discovery, 5*(4), 305–310. doi:10.1517/17460441003677725

Howland, R. H. (2009). Effects of aging on pharmacokinetic and pharmacodynamic drug processes. *Journal of Psychosocial Nursing and Mental Health Services, 47*(10), 15–18. doi:10.3928/02793695-20090902-06

Kudzma, E. C., & Carey, E. T. (2009). Pharmacogenomics: Personalizing drug therapy. *American Journal of Nursing, 109*(10), 50–57.

Weng, L., Zhang, L., Peng, Y., & Huang, R. S. (2013). Pharmacogenetics and pharmacogenomics: A bridge to individualized cancer therapy. *Pharmacogenomics, 14*(3), 15–24. Retrieved from http://www.medscape.com/viewarticle/779255

Whitley, H., & Lindsey, W. (2009). Sex-based differences in drug activity. *American Family Physician, 80*, 1254–1258.

Zopf, Y., Rabe, C., Neubert, A., Hanson, C., Brune, K., Hahn, E. G., & Dormann, H. (2009). Gender-based differences in drug prescription: Relation to adverse drug reactions. *Pharmacology, 84*, 333–339. doi:10.1159/000248311

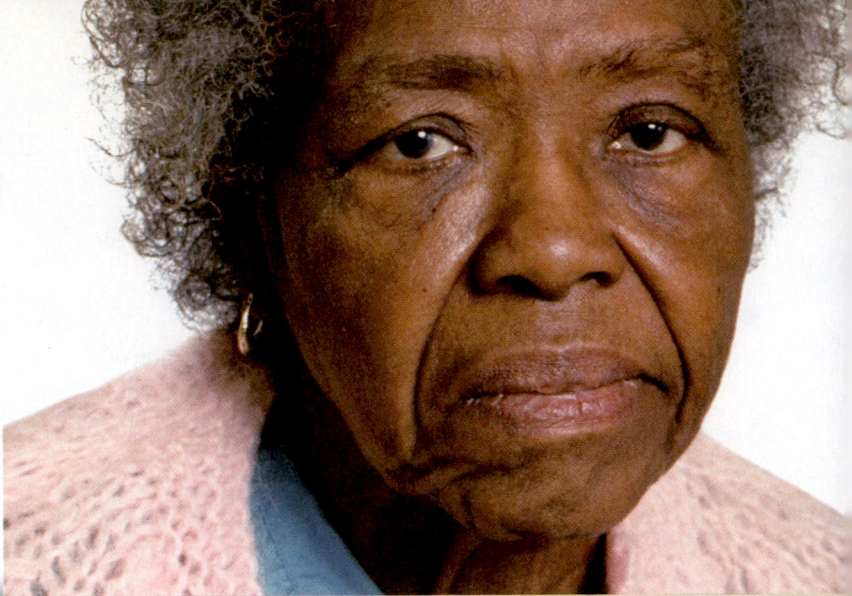

"I was told to watch for drug reactions. But with all the drugs I take, how would I ever know if I'm having a reaction or not?"

Patient "Elizabeth Washington"

CHAPTER

5

Adverse Drug Effects and Drug Interactions

LEARNING OUTCOMES

After reading this chapter, the student should be able to:

1. Differentiate between adverse effects and side effects.

2. Create a plan to minimize or prevent adverse drug events in patients.

3. Explain the advantages and disadvantages of the Adverse Event Reporting System.

4. Describe the incidence and characteristics of drug allergies.

5. Explain how idiosyncratic reactions differ from other types of adverse effects.

6. Explain why certain drugs with carcinogenic or teratogenic potential are used in pharmacotherapy.

7. Report the characteristic signs, symptoms, and treatment for each of the following organ-specific adverse events: nephrotoxicity, neurotoxicity, hepatotoxicity, dermatologic toxicity, bone marrow toxicity, cardiotoxicity, and skeletal muscle toxicity.

8. Use examples to explain the importance of drug interactions to pharmacotherapy.

9. Describe the mechanisms of drug interactions that alter absorption, distribution, metabolism, or excretion.

10. Differentiate among additive, synergistic, and antagonistic drug interactions.

11. Identify examples of drug–food interactions that may impact pharmacotherapeutic outcomes.

CHAPTER OUTLINE

▶ Adverse Drug Effects

  The Role of the Nurse in Managing Adverse Effects

  Allergic Reactions

  Idiosyncratic Responses

  Carcinogenicity and Teratogenicity

  Organ-Specific Drug Toxicity

▶ Drug Interactions

  Pharmacokinetic Drug Interactions

  Pharmacodynamic Drug Interactions

  Drug Interactions with Food and Dietary Supplements

KEY TERMS

additive effect, 60

adverse drug effect, 53

FDA Adverse Event Reporting System (FAERS), 54

antagonistic effect, 61

black box warning, 54

drug allergies, 54

drug interaction, 58

idiosyncratic response, 55

ototoxicity, 57

risk–benefit ratio, 55

side effects, 53

synergistic effect, 61

teratogens, 56

Drugs are administered with the goal of producing a therapeutic effect. All drugs, however, produce both intended therapeutic effects as well as unintended effects. An **adverse drug effect** is an undesirable and potentially harmful action caused by the administration of medication. Adverse effects, also called adverse events, are a significant component of pharmacotherapy and, when severe, may cause treatment to be discontinued or result in permanent harm to the patient. The purpose of this chapter is to examine the different types of adverse effects and drug interactions, so that the nurse can minimize their impact on treatment outcomes.

Adverse Drug Effects

5.1 The nurse plays a key role in preventing and managing adverse drug effects.

Although every drug has the *potential* to produce adverse events, most pharmacotherapy can be conducted without significant undesirable effects. Indeed, drugs that produce serious adverse effects are screened and removed from consideration during the drug development and approval process or are restricted for treating serious health conditions such as cancer. Patients expect that their drugs, including over-the-counter (OTC) medications, herbal products, and dietary supplements, will be free from serious adverse effects when taken as directed. Although the majority of drugs are very safe, adverse effects cannot be entirely avoided.

Side effects are types of drug effects that are predictable and which may occur even at therapeutic doses. Side effects are less serious than adverse effects. Patients are often willing to tolerate annoying side effects if they believe the drug will improve their condition or prevent a disease. The distinction between an adverse effect and a side effect, however, is often unclear. For example, is headache a side effect or an adverse effect? What about nausea? The answer lies in the severity of the symptoms. Headache or nausea may be minor (side effects), or they may become intense and disabling (adverse effects). The U.S. Food and Drug Administration (FDA) defines serious drug effects as those that:

- Result in a patient's death, hospitalization, or disability
- Cause a congenital abnormality
- Cause a life-threatening event
- Require an intervention to prevent permanent damage

Adverse drug events may be specific to a single type of tissue or affect multiple organ systems. The most common adverse events are nausea and vomiting, which may occur when drugs are administered by any route. Headache and changes in blood pressure are also very common adverse drug events. Some adverse effects, though rare, are serious enough to warrant regular or continuous monitoring. Examples of serious events include impairment or failure of entire organs, such as cardiac, hepatic, or renal failure or loss of vision or hearing. Anaphylaxis, Stevens–Johnson syndrome (SJS), cancer, and birth defects are additional rare, adverse drug events that occur with certain drugs.

Many adverse effects are extensions of a drug's pharmacologic actions. These types of events are considered dose dependent: As the drug dose increases, the risk for adverse effects also increases. For example, antihypertensive drugs are given to lower blood pressure, but high doses cause hypotension, which may manifest as dizziness or fainting. Drugs for treating insomnia or anxiety may depress brain activity too much at higher doses, resulting in drowsiness or daytime sedation. Knowing the therapeutic actions of the drug enables the nurse to predict the signs and symptoms of many of the adverse effects that occur during treatment. It is important for nurses and their patients to understand that the difference between a drug being a beneficial medication or a toxic substance is often simply a matter of dose.

Can adverse effects be prevented? Although nurses play a key role in minimizing the number and severity of adverse events in their patients, some adverse effects simply cannot be predicted or prevented. Skilled health care providers including nurses, however, have multiple ways to minimize or prevent adverse effects, from having expert knowledge of how a drug acts to obtaining a comprehensive medical history from their patients. The following are means that health care providers use to minimize or prevent adverse drug events in their patients:

- **Obtain a thorough medical history.** The medical history of the patient may reveal drug allergies or conditions that contraindicate the use of certain drugs. The history may also identify prescription drugs, OTC drugs, dietary supplements, and herbal products taken by the patient that could negatively interact with the prescribed medication.

- **Thoroughly assess the patient and all diagnostic data.** Assessment may reveal underlying hepatic or renal impairment that will affect the way the drug is handled by the body. The very young and the elderly are most susceptible to drug reactions because metabolism and excretion of drugs in these populations are less predictable. To prevent adverse effects, average drug doses should be adjusted based on careful patient assessment.

- **Prevent medication errors.** Administering the incorrect dose or giving the drug to the wrong patient may cause unnecessary adverse effects. Methods of preventing medication errors are described in detail in Chapter 6.

- **Monitor pharmacotherapy carefully.** Monitor patient signs and symptoms regularly after initial drug doses or when doses are increased. This is especially critical when caring for patients who are very ill or when giving parenteral agents. Patients receiving drugs that have frequent or potentially severe adverse effects should be monitored continuously until the baseline effects of the drug have been established.

- **Know the drugs.** It is essential for nurses to know the most frequent and most serious adverse effects for every drug administered. A comprehensive knowledge of the drugs, herbal products, and supplements taken by their patients helps nurses to monitor for and identify adverse effects and provide the necessary interventions before they become serious.

- **Be prepared for the unusual.** Anaphylaxis may occur immediately and unpredictably (see Section 5.3). Other adverse effects may be delayed, occurring days, weeks, or months after therapy is initiated. Some drugs produce actions opposite to those expected (see Section 5.4). Patients may be reluctant to report certain adverse effects (such as impotence) without prompting by the nurse.

- **Question unusual orders.** If the nurse suspects that the wrong dose has been ordered or the pharmacy has filled the order incorrectly, the drug should not be administered until the prescriber or the pharmacy has been contacted.

- **Teach patients about adverse effects.** The patient is the nurse's ally in identifying and preventing adverse effects. Teaching patients what therapeutic and adverse effects to expect from the drug and which types of symptoms to report to their health care provider are important in self-management and preventing serious adverse events. Furthermore, inadequate teaching may result in poor patient adherence to the drug regimen and suboptimal treatment outcomes.

PharmFACT

According to Davies et al. (2009), approximately one in seven hospitalized patients experiences an adverse drug reaction. The drugs most frequently associated with these adverse events are diuretics, opioid analgesics, and anticoagulants.

5.2 The FDA continues to monitor for new adverse events after a drug is approved and marketed.

Before approving a drug, the FDA carefully examines all clinical information supplied by the manufacturer regarding drug effectiveness and safety. Although extensive testing may have been conducted, clinical research has certain limitations and the FDA's decision is based on a relatively small number of clinical trials. Once marketed, the drug is disseminated to a larger and more diverse patient population, at which point adverse effects that were not discovered during clinical trials may begin to surface. For this reason, the FDA continues to monitor the safety of drugs after they are approved.

Established in 1993, the FDA's MedWatch Safety Information and **Adverse Event Reporting System (FAERS)** is a voluntary program that encourages health care providers and consumers to report suspected adverse effects directly to the FDA or the product manufacturer. By law, reports received by the manufacturers are forwarded to the FDA to be added to the computerized information database.

The number of adverse events reported to the FDA has steadily grown every year. In 2000, the FDA received 266,866 adverse event reports. More than 800,000 events are now reported annually: approximately 60% by health care providers and 40% by consumers.

Data from the FAERS are analyzed by clinical reviewers, usually a physician, pharmacist, or nurse, at the Center for Drug Evaluation and Research of the FDA. If a potential safety concern is identified, the FDA may take one of the following actions:

- Conduct additional epidemiologic studies to determine the validity or extent of the safety concern.

- Require changes to a product's labeling information.

- Require a **black box warning** in the drug insert that warns prescribers that the drug carries a risk for a serious or even fatal adverse effect.

- Restrict the use of the drug in specific populations.

- Communicate safety information to health care providers and consumers.

- Recall a product that may have quality or performance concerns.

- Remove the product from the market.

The FDA disseminates changes in safety information through its MedWatch website. Interested parties may subscribe to podcasts, electronic newsletters, and even cell phone text message alerts giving them the latest drug safety information.

The FAERS provides a national database for making safety decisions about drugs, but it does have limitations. Because the system relies on voluntary reports, not all adverse events are reported. The FDA does not attempt to prove causation, which is whether the adverse event was caused by the drug or by some other factor involved in treatment. Reports sometimes do contain insufficient or vague details regarding the incident.

A word of caution is necessary regarding the reporting of adverse drug events. The placebo effect predicts that a certain percentage of patients will respond with positive therapeutic outcomes to a treatment, even if the substance is inert and has no pharmacologic properties (essentially a "sugar pill"). The same holds true for side and adverse effects. A certain percentage of patients will experience headache, nausea and vomiting, rash, changes in blood pressure, or pain following the administration of a placebo. Thus when examining drug information, the nurse should always examine the incidence of adverse effects that occur over and above that caused by a placebo. It is important to understand that the patient is not faking symptoms that result from placebo administration; they truly believe, and may be visibly experiencing, side effects. However, the drug itself may not be responsible for the self-reported effects.

5.3 Allergic reactions are caused by a hyperresponse of the immune system.

Drug allergies are common events, comprising 6% to 10% of all adverse drug effects. Although drug allergies may elicit a diverse range of patient symptoms, all are caused by a hyperresponse of body defenses. Depending on the type of allergic response, basophils, mast cells, eosinophils, or lymphocytes secrete chemical mediators that trigger the allergic response. Specific chemical mediators of allergy include histamine, serotonin, leukotrienes, prostaglandins, and complement.

Several characteristics define a drug allergy. Allergies typically occur with very small amounts of drug; the severity of allergy symptoms is usually not proportional to the dose. The symptoms of allergy are unrelated to the pharmacologic actions of the drug; anaphylaxis has the same symptoms regardless of the drug that induces it. Patients often exhibit cross-allergy, an allergic reaction to drugs with a similar structure, such as those from the same pharmacologic class. Drug allergies require a previous exposure to the drug (or a very similar drug). This sensitizes the patient to subsequent exposures, during which a hyperresponse of body defenses is rapidly mounted upon reexposure to the drug.

The signs and symptoms of drug allergy are variable and range from minor to life threatening. Symptoms may appear within minutes after the drug is administered or they may develop after prolonged pharmacotherapy. Because the signs and symptoms of drug allergy are nonspecific, it is sometimes difficult to attribute an allergy symptom to any given drug, especially in patients receiving multiple drugs. Complicating an accurate diagnosis is that symptoms of drug allergy are the same as those of allergy to other substances, such as certain foods, or environmental triggers, such as insect stings, animal dander, or dust mites. It is important to determine the source of allergy, especially in patients with severe reactions, so that the offending drug or environmental substance can be avoided in the future. The pharmacologic treatment of allergy is presented in Chapter 45.

Although allergic reactions are possible with most drugs, some medications exhibit a relatively higher incidence. The drugs or drug classes most likely to cause allergic reactions include penicillins and related antibiotics (monobactams and cephalosporins); radiologic contrast media containing iodine; insulin; nonsteroidal anti-inflammatory drugs (NSAIDs), including aspirin; sulfonamides; cancer chemotherapy agents; preservatives (sulfites and paraben); and certain antiseizure drugs.

Patients are usually unaware of the true definition of allergy and often report any adverse effect they experience as a drug allergy. For example, many patients experience acute nausea and vomiting with narcotic analgesics such as codeine and will report that they have an allergy to codeine during a drug history. In fact, these symptoms are not caused by an overactive immune response and are thus not a true allergy. Inaccurate reporting of allergies may lead to the health care provider avoiding the use of entire drug classes and prescribing more expensive second-line medications that could be less effective or produce more adverse effects.

5.4 Idiosyncratic reactions are unusual drug responses often caused by genetic differences among patients.

An **idiosyncratic response** is an adverse drug effect that produces unusual and unexpected symptoms that are not related to the pharmacologic action of the drug. Idiosyncratic reactions are not classified as allergies because they are not immune related. They are rare, unpredictable, and vary from patient to patient.

Many, though not all, idiosyncratic reactions are due to unique, individual genetic differences among patients. For example, mutations involving specific metabolic enzymes may cause certain patients to be extremely sensitive to the effects of a drug or to be resistant. The drug may be handled by a different metabolic pathway, resulting in the accumulation of a metabolite that gives a different and unexpected response from the original drug.

Historically, the term *idiosyncratic* has been used to denote any drug effect that could not be explained. With advances in the understanding of drug mechanisms, more and more drug responses are now understood. With improved reporting of adverse drug events, rare "unexpected" events are now documented and may be "expected." Thus use of the term *idiosyncratic*, although still common in clinical practice, will likely continue to diminish with time.

PharmFACT

Death rates from adverse drug reactions are associated with age, race, gender, and urbanization. Highest death rates are experienced by persons older than age 55, blacks, males, and those residing in rural areas (Shepherd, Mohorn, Yacoub, & May, 2012).

5.5 Some drugs have the ability to induce cancer or cause birth defects.

Most adverse effects occur within minutes or hours after a drug is administered; some develop after several days or weeks of pharmacotherapy. In a few instances, the adverse effect may occur years or even decades after the drug was administered. Such is the case with drug-induced cancer.

Why would a drug be approved by the FDA if it was known to cause cancer in humans? In most cases, drugs that produce cancer in laboratory animals during preclinical trials are not submitted for approval to the FDA. However, there are a few conditions that may warrant the approval of a drug with carcinogenic potential. The answer lies in the **risk–benefit ratio**. If a patient has a condition that is likely to cause premature death if left untreated, the benefits of taking a drug with carcinogenic potential may outweigh the long-term risks. This assumes, of course, that effective, safer alternatives are not available.

Of the thousands of drugs and drug combinations approved for pharmacotherapy, only a few increase the risk of acquiring cancer. Most of these drugs, shown in Table 5.1, fall into three primary classes: antineoplastics, immunosuppressants, and hormonal agents.

TABLE 5.1   Selected Drugs Suspected of Causing Cancer in Humans

Class	Drug	Type of Cancer
Antineoplastic	adriamycin chlorambucil cisplatin cyclophosphamide dacarbazine doxorubicin etoposide metronidazole nitrosoureas phenytoin propylthiouracil teniposide	Leukemia, urinary bladder
Hormones and hormone antagonists	anabolic steroids estrogen replacement therapy and oral contraceptives progesterone tamoxifen	Uterus, breast, hepatic
Immunosuppressants	azathioprine cyclosporine	Lymphoma, skin

Some of the antineoplastics are known chemical carcinogens. With the goal of eliminating cancer cells, some of these drugs cause molecular damage or mutations in deoxyribonucleic acid (DNA). Although much of the DNA damage in normal cells is repaired by enzymes, some mutations persist and accumulate in cells as a person ages, increasing cancer risk. The initial damage done by the drug may take decades to manifest as cancer. Leukemia is the type of cancer with the greatest cancer risk from antineoplastic therapy. However, the patient may never develop cancer as a result of these medications; indeed, the majority of patients receiving antineoplastic drugs do not develop the disease. Furthermore, if the cancer treatment was successful, the patient may have benefited from additional years of life due to pharmacotherapy with these drugs. Because pharmacotherapy combined with surgery and radiation therapy can result in a total cure for some patients, the benefit of drug therapy outweighs the small risk of developing cancer later in life.

The second class of drugs that can induce cancer are the immunosuppressants. These medications are administered to dampen the immune system of patients receiving transplanted tissues or who have serious inflammatory disorders. Because a natural function of the immune system is to remove cancer cells that form in the body, any drug that inhibits this system would be expected to have some degree of cancer risk. Lymphoma is the most frequent type of cancer resulting from immunosuppressant use. Again, the risk is small, compared to the benefits provided by these drugs.

The third group that may cause cancer consists of hormones or hormone antagonists. Little is known about the mechanisms by which hormone imbalances lead to cancer, and the topic is a subject of ongoing research. In some cases, hormones protect the patient from cancer, or they may reduce the incidence of one type of cancer but increase the risk of another type. Probably the best studied of the hormone mechanisms is how estrogen binds to its intracellular receptors. About 70% of patients with breast cancer are estrogen receptor (ER)-positive: THE hormone promotes tumor formation in the mammary gland. Cancers caused by hormones or hormone antagonists tend to affect reproductive organs, such as the vagina, uterus, or breast.

A similar question might be asked regarding drugs that cause birth defects, or **teratogens**. Why would a drug be approved by the FDA if it was shown to produce birth defects in laboratory animals during the preclinical stage of drug testing? The answer to this question is very different from that for cancer-inducing drugs.

Teratogens affect a small percentage of the overall population: those who are pregnant. In most cases these drugs are safe to use in males and in adults outside their childbearing years. Thus, known teratogens may be approved for indications in patients who do not have the potential to become pregnant. When approved for females with reproductive potential, however, these drugs have increased risks. Although a pregnancy test may be performed prior to pharmacotherapy and the nurse may warn the patient to discontinue the drug if pregnancy is suspected, the potential still remains for exposing an embryo or fetus to a toxic agent. In females with reproductive potential, teratogenic drugs are not used unless they have clear benefits that outweigh the possible risk of birth defects. All health care providers must carefully assess patient compliance with instructions against this potential risk. In extreme cases, such as with the drug isotretinoin (Amnesteem, others), women of reproductive

potential must provide two negative pregnancy tests prior to receiving the drug and one each month the prescription is refilled.

The nurse should remember that drugs are not tested in pregnant humans before FDA approval, and that animal testing cannot predict with great accuracy the effects on the human fetus. In some cases, the risks to a human embryo or fetus have been determined after a drug has been approved. The FDA has established pregnancy categories, which gauge the risk of a drug causing birth defects (see Chapter 8). All drug use should be assumed dangerous during pregnancy, unless data have otherwise demonstrated the drug to be safe. No woman should take a drug, herbal product, or dietary supplement during pregnancy unless approved by the patient's health care provider.

5.6 Drug toxicity may be specific to particular organs.

Very few drugs produce adverse effects in every organ system; these agents would be too toxic for safe pharmacotherapy. Instead, adverse effects are often organ specific, targeting one or a few organs. It is important for the nurse to learn these specific toxicities so that appropriate signs, symptoms, and diagnostic tests can be carefully monitored. Selected organ-specific toxicities are summarized in Table 5.2.

Nephrotoxicity: The kidneys are one of the most common organs affected by drugs. This is because these organs filter large volumes of blood, and most drugs are excreted by the renal route. Some drugs are reabsorbed or secreted by the kidney, exposing renal tubule cells to high concentrations of these agents. A few obstruct the urinary system by causing crystalluria in the urinary tract. Drug nephrotoxicity may manifest as acute symptoms that appear after one or several doses, or as chronic symptoms that appear after several months of pharmacotherapy.

TABLE 5.2	Organ-Specific Toxicity
Toxicity	**Example Drugs and Classes**
Bone marrow	ACE inhibitors, antimalarials, antineoplastics, antiseizure drugs (carbamazepine, phenytoin), antithyroid drugs, cephalosporins, chloramphenicol, chlorpromazine, chlorpropamide, cimetidine, furosemide, methyldopa, NSAIDs, phenylbutazone, sulfonamides
Cardiotoxicity	anthracycline antineoplastics (daunorubicin, doxorubicin, epirubicin, idarubicin, mitoxantrone)
Dermatologic	antiseizure drugs (carbamazepine, phenobarbital, phenytoin), cephalosporins, erythromycin, NSAIDs, penicillin, radiologic contrast media, sulfonamides, tetracyclines
Hepatotoxicity	carbamazepine, chlorpromazine, statins (HMG CoA reductase inhibitors)
Nephrotoxicity	ACE inhibitors, acyclovir, aminoglycosides, amphotericin B, cisplatin and other platinum-based antineoplastics, cocaine, cyclosporine, NSAIDs, radiologic contrast media, sulfonamides, tacrolimus
Neurotoxicity	aminoglycosides, cisplatin, ethanol, loop diuretics, methyldopa, salicylates, vincristine
Skeletal muscle and tendon toxicity	fluoroquinolone antibiotics, statins

It is critical for the health care provider to identify at-risk patients and attempt to prevent drug-induced nephrotoxicity. Means for prevention include providing proper hydration, monitoring urinary lab values, and adjusting doses appropriately for patients with renal impairment. Patients with serious renal impairment should not receive nephrotoxic drugs unless other therapeutic options have been exhausted.

Neurotoxicity: Although the blood–brain barrier prevents many drugs from reaching the brain, neurotoxicity is a relatively common adverse effect of certain drug classes. This is because the brain receives a large percentage of the blood supply and is especially sensitive to small amounts of toxic substances. For sedatives, antidepressants, antianxiety drugs, antiseizure drugs, and antipsychotics, the difference between a therapeutic dose and one that produces adverse effects may be very small. Indeed, drowsiness is seen in a majority of patients receiving these drugs when therapy is initiated. Signs and symptoms of toxicity in the central nervous system (CNS) include depression, mania, sedation, behavioral changes, suicidal feelings, hallucinations, and seizures. The special senses may be affected, including visual changes, loss of balance, and hearing impairment. Hearing impairment, or **ototoxicity**, can result from drug-induced damage to the eighth cranial nerve.

Effective teaching is essential when patients are beginning therapy with potentially neurotoxic drugs. The nurse should warn patients not to drive vehicles or perform other hazardous tasks until they are familiar with the effects of these drugs. Caregivers should be taught to report changes in patient behavior, because the person receiving the medication may have difficulty recognizing these signs. The nurse should be aware that neurotoxic drugs can significantly worsen preexisting mental health disorders. Serious symptoms such as seizures, delirium, suicidal ideation, or significant visual or hearing impairment should be immediately reported to the prescriber.

Hepatotoxicity: The liver receives all drugs absorbed in the stomach and intestinal mucosa via the hepatic-portal vein. A major function of the liver is to metabolize and detoxify drugs and other chemicals that enter the body; thus it should not be surprising that hepatotoxicity is one of the most common adverse drug effects. Effects of hepatotoxic drugs range from minor, transient increases in liver enzyme values to fatal hepatitis.

The nurse should regularly monitor liver enzyme tests when administering hepatotoxic drugs, because changes in these laboratory values are early signs of liver toxicity. Symptoms of liver impairment are vague and nonspecific and include right upper quadrant pain, anorexia, bloating, fatigue, and nausea or vomiting. During chronic hepatotoxicity, jaundice, itching, and easy bruising are evident. In serious cases, the liver will be unable to metabolize other drugs, resulting in high serum drug levels. Extreme care must be taken when administering potentially hepatotoxic drugs to patients with preexisting liver disease.

Dermatologic toxicity: Drug reactions affecting the skin are some of the most common types of adverse effects. These reactions may be caused by a hypersensitivity response or by nonimmune-type responses. Rash, the most common cutaneous drug reaction, usually occurs within 1 to 2 weeks of initiation of drug therapy and resolves without serious complications. Drug-induced rash is sometimes accompanied by itching (pruritus). Although almost any drug can cause rash, antibiotics are the most frequent drug class causing this condition. Urticaria (hives) are raised welts that are often accompanied by intense pruritus and, although less common than rash, are a symptom of a potential allergic reaction that could lead to anaphylaxis.

Serious and even fatal dermatologic toxicity can occur. In angioedema, swelling occurs in the dermis, periorbital region, and around the mouth and throat. Angioedema is a severe drug reaction because the swelling may impair breathing and may be fatal. SJS is another drug-induced condition that can be fatal. This syndrome causes severe blistering of the skin, usually accompanied by mucous membrane involvement and fever.

Phototoxicity is a type of drug-induced dermatologic toxicity in which certain drugs cause the skin to absorb excess ultraviolet radiation from the sun or heat lamps. Symptoms resemble sunburn and are best prevented by advising patients to avoid direct sunlight. Phototoxicity resolves when the drug is discontinued.

Most types of drug-induced dermatologic toxicity do not require pharmacologic treatment. If pruritus is prominent, an antihistamine or a corticosteroid may be administered. In all cases of serious drug-induced hypersensitivity, the nurse should discontinue the drug until the cause of the skin condition can be diagnosed.

Bone marrow toxicity: Drugs affecting the bone marrow are of great concern due to the possibility of serious and perhaps fatal outcomes. The bone marrow serves as a nursery for the production of red blood cells, white blood cells, and platelets. Drugs may affect only one of these types of cells or all three. When all three groups are affected, drug-induced pancytopenia or aplastic anemia occurs, and the patient is at great risk for serious illness. Loss of white blood cells may cause agranulocytosis or neutropenia, which places the patient at risk for serious infections. The drug class most likely to cause bone marrow toxicity is the antineoplastics. Bone marrow toxicity is the dose-limiting factor with these drugs (see Chapter 57).

The role of the nurse in preventing bone marrow toxicity is to carefully monitor laboratory data and recognize changes that suggest impending toxicity, such as decreases in red cells, white cells, or platelets. In many cases, bone marrow toxicity can be quickly reversed if the condition is recognized early and the drug is discontinued. Furthermore, the nurse should carefully monitor the therapeutic regimen of patients who have preexisting blood cell disorders because adding a drug with bone marrow toxicity may worsen these conditions.

Cardiotoxicity: Some drugs damage cardiac muscle cells, affecting the ability of the heart to effectively pump blood to the tissues. The most common cardiotoxic drugs belong to a chemical class called the anthracyclines, which include daunorubicin (Cerubidine, DaunoXome), doxorubicin (Adriamycin), epirubicin (Ellence), idarubicin (Idamycin), and mitoxantrone (Novantrone). These are all antineoplastic medications. The cardiotoxicity of these drugs can be severe and lead to bradycardia, tachycardia, heart failure, and acute left ventricular failure. The nurse administering cardiotoxic drugs must be vigilant in observing for signs of cardiotoxicity such as excessive fatigue, cough, shortness of breath (especially when recumbent), weight gain, or peripheral edema.

A second type of cardiotoxicity is manifested as prolongation of the QT interval on the electrocardiogram (ECG). The QT interval represents the time needed to depolarize and repolarize the cardiac ventricles. Lengthening of the QT interval is associated with a rare type of ventricular tachycardia called torsade de pointes, which can cause sudden cardiac death. More than a hundred drugs have been shown to cause QT prolongation and several have been removed from the market because of this adverse effect. Because the QT interval represents the dysrhythmia potential of a drug, the FDA now requires all new medications to be tested for QT prolongation prior to approval. When administering drugs that prolong the QT interval, nurses should carefully monitor cardiac function, especially in patients with preexisting cardiac disease.

Skeletal muscle and tendon toxicity: Skeletal muscle is relatively resistant to the effects of drugs, despite its extensive blood supply. In skeletal muscle the incidence of drug-induced myopathy is low but may be serious when it does occur. The most severe myopathy is rhabdomyolysis, a syndrome characterized by extensive muscle necrosis with the release of muscle enzymes and other constituents into the circulation. Rhabdomyolysis is a rare, though serious adverse effect of statins, common medications used to treat excessive lipid levels in the blood.

Some of the fluoroquinolone antibiotics exhibit toxicity to cartilage and tendons. This is most often manifested as rupture of the Achilles tendon, which is most apparent in adults over age 65. Patients under age 18 should not take these medications because they may interfere with cartilage growth.

To prevent skeletal muscle or tendon toxicity, the nurse should assess for unexplained muscle or joint soreness or pain during therapy. Laboratory tests such as creatine kinase (CK) should be evaluated regularly during therapy with drugs that have muscle toxicity.

Drug Interactions

5.7 Drug interactions may significantly affect pharmacotherapeutic outcomes.

A **drug interaction** occurs when a substance increases or decreases a drug's actions. The substance causing the interaction may be another drug, a dietary supplement, an herbal product, or a food. The substance participating in the drug interaction must be external to the body and is usually taken concurrently with the medication. Although substances that are naturally found in the body (endogenous substances) routinely interact with drugs, these are not considered drug interactions because they are part of the body's normal response to the drug.

Because patients often take multiple drugs concurrently, drug interactions occur continually. Even if only one drug is taken, the potential for a drug–food interaction still exists. Although drug interactions are impossible to totally eliminate, most interactions go unnoticed and treatment outcomes are rarely affected. Indeed, it is likely that most drug interactions have yet to be documented or researched because they do not cause clinically noticeable effects or harm to the patient.

Some drug interactions are important to pharmacology because they are known to cause adverse effects or otherwise affect treatment

outcomes. By studying the mechanisms of potential drug interactions, the nurse can prevent certain adverse effects and optimize treatment outcomes. For example, if the patient is receiving gentamicin, the nurse should use caution when administering acyclovir, because the drug combination can cause higher than normal levels of acyclovir in the blood. The prescriber should reduce the dose of acyclovir or substitute a different drug. Understanding drug interactions can directly affect the success of pharmacotherapy.

Drug interactions occur by dozens of different mechanisms. To simplify their study, it may be helpful to remember that drug interactions can have three basic effects on the action of a drug:

- The actions of the drug can be *inhibited*, resulting in less therapeutic action. For example, milk interferes with the absorption of tetracycline, causing a lower serum level of antibiotic, thus diminishing its therapeutic effects.

- The actions of the drug may be *enhanced*, causing a greater therapeutic response. For example, coadministration of the two antiviral drugs lopinavir and ritonavir causes a greater reduction in levels of HIV than occurs when either drug is used alone.

- The drug interaction may produce a totally *new and different response*. For example, when used alone disulfiram (Antabuse) has no pharmacologic effects. When taken with alcohol, however, the combination produces dramatic, new actions such as severe headache, flushing, dyspnea, palpitations, and blurred vision (see Chapter 27).

5.8 Pharmacokinetic drug interactions include changes in the absorption, distribution, metabolism, or excretion of medications.

Recall from Chapter 3 that pharmacokinetics is the branch of pharmacology dealing with how the body acts on a drug after it is administered. Many drug interactions involve some aspect of the pharmacokinetics of the medication. When studying drug interactions, it is convenient to use the same categories for pharmacokinetics that are presented in Chapter 3. The general types of pharmacokinetic interactions are illustrated in Figure 5.1.

Absorption: Most drugs need to be absorbed to produce their actions. Any substance that affects absorption has the potential to influence drug response. In fact, this is one of the most common mechanisms of drug interactions. By interfering with normal absorption, drug action may be inhibited or enhanced. Increasing absorption will raise drug serum levels and produce an enhanced effect; substances inhibiting absorption have the opposite effect.

The simplest way to affect absorption is to change the speed of substances moving through the gastrointestinal (GI) tract. Opioids such as morphine or heroin will slow peristalsis, giving drugs additional time for absorption. Laxatives and drugs that stimulate the parasympathetic nervous system will speed substances through the GI tract, diminishing the absorption time of other drugs. The bile acid resins such as cholestyramine (Questran) bind other drugs and prevent their absorption.

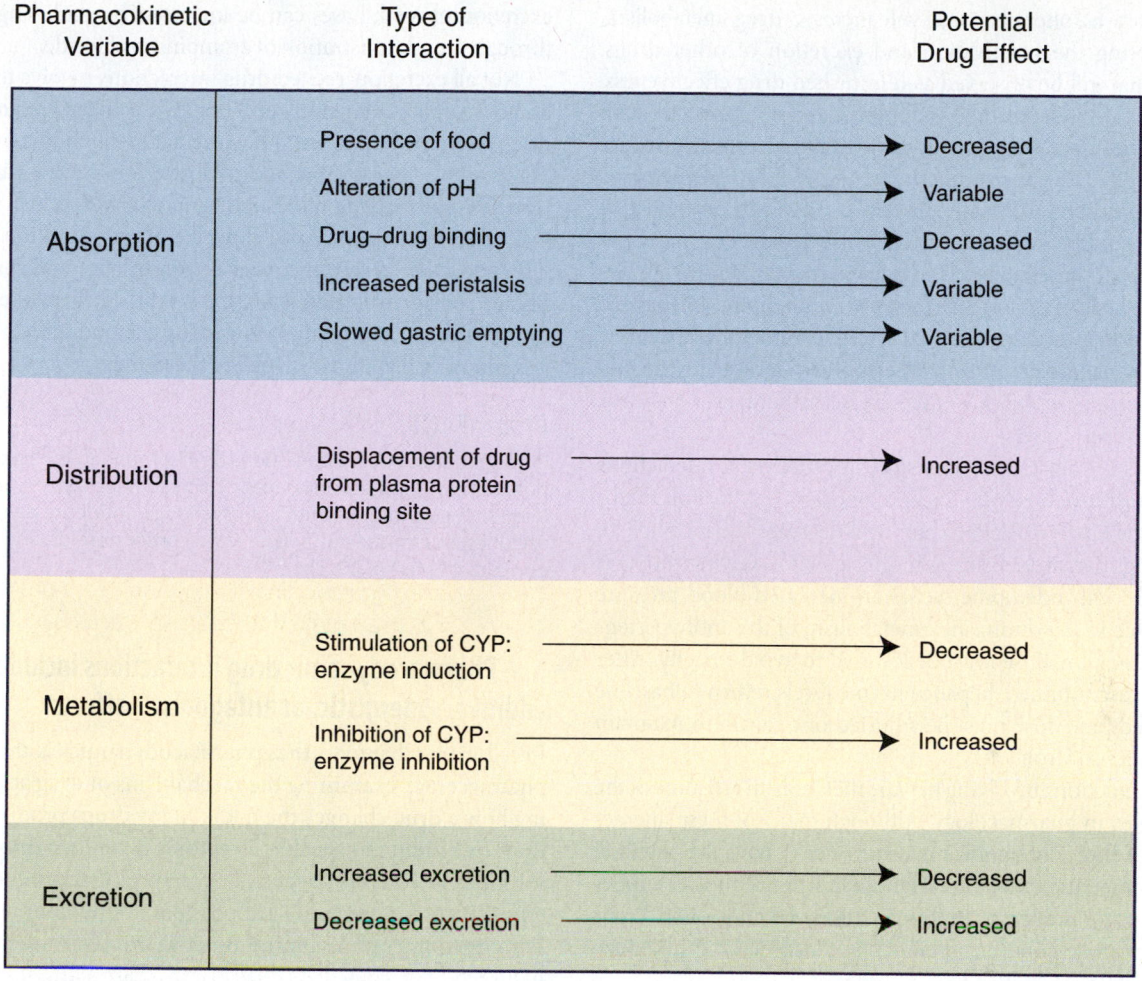

Pharmacokinetic Variable	Type of Interaction	Potential Drug Effect
Absorption	Presence of food	Decreased
	Alteration of pH	Variable
	Drug–drug binding	Decreased
	Increased peristalsis	Variable
	Slowed gastric emptying	Variable
Distribution	Displacement of drug from plasma protein binding site	Increased
Metabolism	Stimulation of CYP: enzyme induction	Decreased
	Inhibition of CYP: enzyme inhibition	Increased
Excretion	Increased excretion	Decreased
	Decreased excretion	Increased

Figure 5.1 Types of pharmacokinetic drug–drug interactions.

Many drug–drug interactions caused by changes in absorption may be prevented by taking the two drugs at least 2 to 3 hours apart. In the case of drug–food interactions, the interacting food should be avoided, or the drug may be taken on an empty stomach. Taking drugs on an empty stomach, however, may increase the incidence of nausea or vomiting, which could result in loss of the drug before complete absorption occurs. The nurse must teach patients with drug-induced nausea not to take drugs with antacids or milk unless approved by the prescriber. Antacids are alkaline (basic) substances that raise the pH of the GI contents and have the potential to change the percentage of ionized drug. Ionized forms of drugs are less able to cross the intestinal mucosa than nonionized forms.

Distribution: Distribution is the movement of a drug from its site of absorption to its site of action. Many drugs travel through the blood bound to plasma proteins and, when bound, the drug is unable to leave the blood to reach its target. Drugs may compete for available binding sites on plasma proteins; one drug may prevent another from binding to plasma proteins or may displace a drug from its binding sites. If this occurs, the amount of unbound or free drug increases, potentially raising the drug serum concentration to toxic levels. For example, diazepam displaces phenytoin

from plasma proteins, causing a rapid increase in the plasma concentration of free phenytoin and an increased risk of adverse effects. Drugs that have a high potential for displacing other drugs from protein binding sites include aspirin and other NSAIDs, phenylbutazone, and sulfonamides.

A second potential drug–drug interaction involving distribution can occur if the pH of the plasma is altered by a drug. For example, when an alkaline substance such as sodium bicarbonate is infused, the pH of plasma increases, causing acidic drugs to become ionized. The ionized acidic drugs are less able to cross membranes and they accumulate in the extracellular spaces, creating an ionization (pH) gradient. The pH gradient moves acidic drugs from inside cells to the extracellular spaces, thus altering distribution.

Metabolism: A large number of drugs are metabolized by hepatic enzymes. Drug metabolites generally have less activity than the original drug and are more readily excreted by the kidneys. Any drug-induced change in the activity of hepatic enzymes has the potential to cause drug–drug interactions.

As discussed in Chapter 4, certain drugs have the ability to increase (induce) or decrease (inhibit) hepatic enzyme activity.

Inducers such as phenobarbital will increase drug metabolism, thus promoting the inactivation and excretion of other drugs. Clinically, this will be observed as diminished drug effectiveness. For example, if phenobarbital is administered concurrently with the antihypertensive drug nifedipine, less blood pressure reduction will result. The dose of nifedipine will need to be increased to produce an optimal therapeutic effect. However, care must be taken if the inducer is discontinued because hepatic enzyme activity will return to baseline levels in a few days or weeks. Once hepatic enzymes return to normal, the dose of nifedipine will have to be adjusted downward to avoid toxicity. Also, remember that a few drugs (prodrugs) are *activated* by metabolism. Increasing the metabolism of prodrugs will cause an increase, rather than a decrease, in therapeutic response.

Inhibitors of hepatic metabolism will cause drug interactions that are opposite to those of inducers. For example, ritonavir inhibits the hepatic enzyme CYP3A4 and will decrease the metabolism of other drugs that are substrates for this enzyme. Giving ritonavir concurrently with nifedipine causes an increased blood pressure reduction due to the diminished metabolism of the antihypertensive. The nifedipine dose must be lowered to avoid toxicity. After ritonavir is discontinued, hepatic enzyme levels return to baseline and the nifedipine dose must be adjusted once again to maintain blood pressure control.

Drug interactions involving hepatic metabolism are some of the most complex in pharmacology. Although many of these interactions are not clinically significant, others clearly have the potential to affect therapeutic outcomes. The nurse will need to remember which drugs are inducers, inhibitors, and substrates of CYP enzymes to optimize pharmacotherapeutic outcomes and minimize adverse effects (see Chapter 3).

CONNECTION Checkpoint 5.1

From what you learned in Chapter 3, explain the significance of the first-pass effect on pharmacotherapy. *See Answer to Connection Checkpoint 5.1 on student resource website.*

Excretion: Most drugs are eliminated from the body through renal excretion. A drug interaction may occur if a substance changes the glomerular filtration rate (GFR), the amount of fluid filtered (mL) by the kidney per minute. The higher the GFR, the more rapid will be the excretion of other drugs.

A second type of excretion-related interaction may occur if one drug changes the secretion or reabsorption of another drug in the renal tubule. For example, methotrexate competes with NSAIDs for the same secretion mechanism. If taken concurrently, NSAIDs will block the renal secretion of methotrexate, thus raising drug serum levels and increasing the potential for methotrexate toxicity.

Renal elimination may also be affected by drugs that change the pH of the filtrate in the renal tubules. Changing the pH causes drugs to become more (or less) ionized. The excretion of weak acids can be significantly increased by alkalinizing the urine through the administration of sodium bicarbonate. This drug interaction may be used therapeutically to promote more rapid excretion of acidic drugs such as aspirin during overdose situations. Similarly,

excretion of weak bases can be increased by acidifying the urine through the administration of ammonium chloride.

Not all excretion-related drug interactions involve the kidneys. Some drugs are extensively excreted by the biliary system and two drugs excreted in this way may interact through this mechanism. For example, pravastatin and cyclosporine use the same carrier protein to move drug molecules from the liver to bile. Giving the two drugs concurrently will slow the biliary excretion of pravastatin and raise its serum concentration to potentially toxic levels. Because biliary excretion is not the dominant form of elimination for most drugs, this type of drug–drug excretion interaction is far less common than those involving the kidneys.

PharmFACT

Polycyclic aromatic hydrocarbons (PAHs) found in tobacco smoke are potent inducers of several hepatic microsomal enzymes. Smoking has been shown to interact with antipsychotics, antidepressants, benzodiazepines, oral contraceptives, inhaled corticosteroids, and beta blockers (Lucas & Martin, 2013).

5.9 Pharmacodynamic drug interactions include additive, synergistic, or antagonistic effects.

Recall from Chapter 4 that pharmacodynamics is the branch of pharmacology examining the mechanisms of drug action, meaning how a drug changes the body. Many drugs produce their actions by binding to specific receptors. When two drugs compete for the same receptor, or activate receptors that produce opposite effects, drug interactions are possible. Many common interactions encountered in clinical practice are pharmacodynamic in nature.

During a pharmacodynamic drug interaction, drug action may be either enhanced or inhibited. The result of the interaction may be desirable (increased therapeutic response/decreased adverse effect) or undesirable (decreased therapeutic response/increased adverse effect). The basic pharmacodynamic drug–drug interactions are illustrated in Figure 5.2.

The pharmacodynamic drug interaction that is easiest to visualize is the **additive effect**. In this interaction, two drugs from a similar therapeutic class produce a combined summation response. This is used extensively in treating hypertension. For example, a diuretic may be used to lower systolic blood pressure by 10 mmHg, and a beta blocker may be added to the regimen to produce another 15-mmHg reduction. Combined, the two drugs produce a 25-mmHg reduction. Why would two drugs be prescribed (with more expense to the patient), rather than a single drug? There are two rationales. First, to produce a 25-mmHg reduction using only the diuretic, the dose would have to be increased. Keeping the doses of both the diuretic and beta blocker low and taking advantage of their additive effect reduces the potential for adverse drug events caused by higher medication doses. Second, some drugs have low efficacy and it may not be possible to achieve a 25-mmHg reduction with a single drug. The maximum effect from the diuretic may have been a 10-mmHg reduction, and another drug would need to be added to the regimen to achieve a greater response. In this example, the two drugs act at

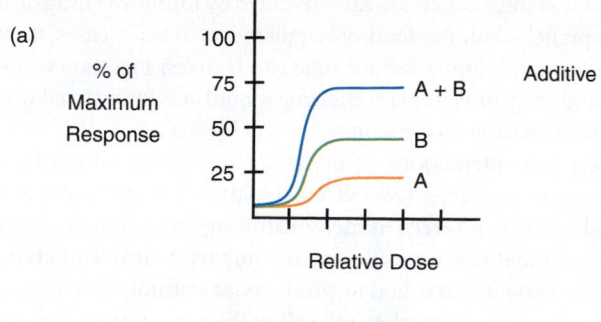

(a)

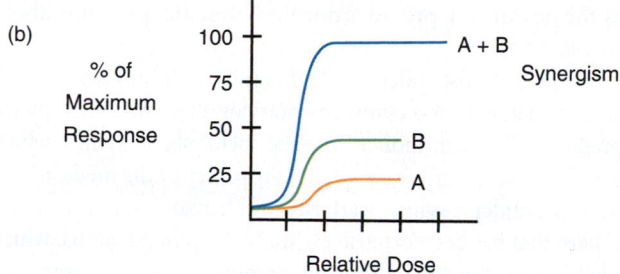

(b)

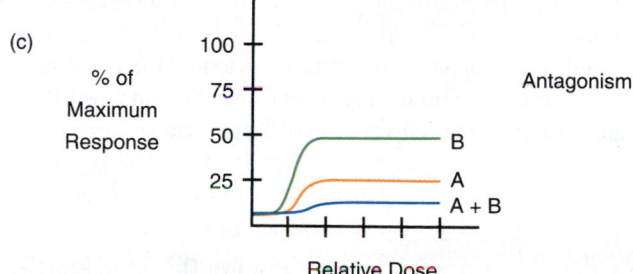

(c)

Figure 5.2 Additive, synergistic, and antagonistic drug interactions: (a) additive response; (b) synergistic response; (c) antagonistic response.

very different types of receptors to produce the additive therapeutic response: beta blockers in cardiac muscle and diuretics in the renal tubules.

It should be remembered that additive effects also apply to adverse effects. This is seen frequently in drugs that affect the CNS. For example, narcotic analgesics, antidepressants, antiseizure drugs, and antianxiety drugs all may cause sedation as a side effect. When taken concurrently, drugs from these classes can cause additive sedation that could profoundly affect the ability to safely operate a vehicle. Caution must always be used when administering multiple medications that have similar adverse effects such as nephrotoxicity, hepatotoxicity, or bone marrow toxicity.

Another pharmacodynamic drug interaction that produces an enhanced response is a **synergistic effect**. In this interaction, the effect of the two drugs is greater than would be expected from simply adding the two individual drugs' responses. This type of interaction is used extensively in treating infections. For example, Synercid is a combination drug that contains quinupristin and dalfopristin, two antibiotics that are effective against resistant *Staphylococcus* infections. Both drugs bind to

the bacterial ribosome and produce greater killing than would be predicted from adding the two individual drugs' effects. Another example is the combination antibiotic Bactrim, which combines trimethoprim and sulfamethoxazole to produce a synergistic effect on bacterial cell killing.

A third type of pharmacodynamic interaction occurs when adding a second drug results in a diminished pharmacologic response. This **antagonistic effect** can result in drug actions being "cancelled." For example, drugs activating the sympathetic nervous system, such as epinephrine, will increase the heart rate and dilate the bronchi. A drug such as carvedilol (Coreg) will have the opposite effects: slowed heart rate and bronchoconstriction. Thus, carvedilol is considered an antagonist to epinephrine and may cancel its actions, depending on the doses of the two drugs. Why would a nurse administer drugs with opposite actions? This is generally done to reduce the adverse effects of a drug. For example, if a drug given to treat hypertension has a potential adverse effect of increasing heart rate, an antagonist may be given to slow the heart rate, keeping it within normal limits. When given intentionally, an antagonist does not necessarily reverse all actions of the first drug: It may selectively inhibit an undesirable action.

In some cases, antagonists are used to treat symptoms of drug overdose. For example, patients taking an overdose of narcotics, such as morphine or heroin, experience coma and life-threatening CNS depression. The administration of naloxone (Narcan), a specific narcotic antagonist, can quickly reverse some of the serious adverse effects of morphine.

Pharmacodynamic interactions can be indirect and complex. The well-documented drug interaction between digoxin (Lanoxin) and diuretics, such as furosemide (Lasix), is an excellent example of an indirect effect. Furosemide enhances the excretion of potassium ion (hypokalemia), which increases the cardiotoxicity of digoxin. This can be a life-threatening interaction. Another example is the inhibition of vitamin K production in the intestine caused by antibiotics. If the patient is also taking warfarin (Coumadin), bleeding may occur because the liver is prevented from producing certain clotting factors. Again, the antibiotic did not directly interact with warfarin, yet the combination produced a serious adverse effect.

CONNECTION Checkpoint 5.2

The types of curves shown in Figure 5.2 are called dose–response curves. From what you learned in Chapter 4, explain the three phases of these curves. *See Answer to Connection Checkpoint 5.2 on student resource website.*

5.10 Food, nutrients, and dietary supplements may interact with medications and affect their actions.

Historically, interactions between drugs and food, dietary supplements, and herbal products have been largely dismissed as clinically unimportant. Although a few interactions, such as tetracyclines with calcium products, have been documented for decades, only since the late 1980s have drug–food interactions been recognized as important to maximizing pharmacotherapeutic outcomes. The interaction that prompted the increased interest in this topic was that of a benign and healthy substance: grapefruit juice. The interaction was discovered by chance in a research study designed to examine the effects of alcohol on felodipine, a calcium channel blocker. The researchers used grapefruit juice incidentally to disguise the taste of the alcohol.

Patients often take medications with juice because it covers up the bitter taste of a drug and provides a plentiful source of vitamins and minerals. Unfortunately, grapefruit juice also contains substances that increase the absorption of certain oral drugs. This occurs because grapefruit juice inhibits the enzyme CYP3A4 in the wall of the intestinal tract. As drugs are absorbed, they are not inactivated by CYP3A4, and higher amounts reach the circulation. Surprisingly, the inhibition from grapefruit juice may last up to 3 days after drinking the juice. The substances in the juice inhibiting CYP3A4 enzymes are called furanocoumarins. Fortunately, only a few drug classes interact with grapefruit juice. Examples include benzodiazepines, certain calcium channel blockers, and statins (HMG CoA reductase inhibitors).

Most of the drug–food interactions discovered thus far act by either increasing or decreasing the absorption or bioavailability of the drug. Some of these interactions are shown in Table 5.3.

TABLE 5.3 Selected Drug–Food and Drug–Herbal Interactions

Drug	Interaction
antiplatelet and anticoagulant drugs	Garlic can increase the risk of bleeding.
atovaquone (Malarone)	Fatty food enhances absorption.
azithromycin (Zithromax)	Food reduces absorption.
calcium channel blockers and cyclosporine	Grapefruit juice enhances absorption.
cholestyramine (Questran)	Drug binds iron, folic acid, and vitamin A to decrease their absorption.
CNS depressants	Valerian can increase drowsiness and sedation.
etidronate (Didronel)	Milk, calcium, and iron bind the drug and decrease absorption.
fluoroquinolones	Calcium, iron, and other metal ions bind the drug and decrease absorption.
lovastatin (Mevacor)	Food increases absorption.
MAO inhibitors	Foods containing tyramine can cause hypertensive crisis.
NSAIDs	Food reduces the incidence of side effects.
penicillin G	Food (milk) and metal ions reduce absorption.
selective serotonin reuptake inhibitors (SSRIs)	St. John's wort and grapefruit juice increase risk of adverse effects (serotonin syndrome).
sucralfate (Carafate)	Food protein binds the drug to decrease absorption.
tetracyclines	Dairy products and iron reduce absorption.
warfarin (Coumadin)	Vitamin K antagonizes the action of warfarin; ginkgo, garlic, and St. John's wort may increase risk of bleeding.
zidovudine (AZT)	Food reduces bioavailability.

Drug–food interactions are easily avoided by timing the drug dose appropriately with the food or supplement. In most cases, there should be a minimum 2-hour time gap between ingestion of the food and drug. In a few cases, the drug should be administered with food to increase its absorption.

Very few interactions of drugs with herbal products have been clearly documented. As more patients take these products, however, research is demonstrating that certain drug–herb combinations may significantly impact pharmacotherapy. Because patients view herbal products as natural, they do not usually mention them when recording their medication history; thus the health care provider must ask specific questions about their use.

Perhaps the most widely studied herb is St. John's wort, which is taken by patients as a complementary or alternative therapy for depression. The herb induces hepatic metabolic enzymes, which can reduce the effectiveness of certain prescription medications, including antidepressants, warfarin, and benzodiazepines. A second herb that has been extensively studied is ginkgo biloba, which is taken to improve circulation and memory. Ginkgo may produce additive anticoagulant effects when taken with warfarin or antiplatelet drugs. It can also antagonize the effects of antiseizure drugs, thus increasing the risk for seizures. Because both St. John's wort and ginkgo can significantly affect drug action, the nurse should assess for the use of these substances when obtaining the patient's health history. Other effects of herbal products are presented in Chapter 7.

CONNECTIONS Community-Oriented Practice

◄ Food–Drug Interactions

The nurse has a critical role in patient education related to food–drug interactions. One of the common questions a patient will ask is "Do I take this drug with food?" Most medications can be administered with food, so of greater importance is what foods the patient should avoid when taking the drug.

Foods may contain naturally occurring substances or be fortified with vitamins that do not mix well with medications. The drug ingredients may not work as well as they should when certain foods are taken concurrently. Food nutrients can affect absorption, metabolism, or elimination of the drug by binding with ingredients in the medication. And as more is learned about the active compounds in foods such as phytochemicals, more study is needed to predict when significant food–drug interactions may occur.

As mentioned in this chapter, a common food–drug interaction may occur when a patient eats grapefruit or drinks grapefruit juice with select medications. However, other compounds in food or beverages may also significantly alter pharmacokinetic processes and, thus, drug effects. Other juices such as apple, orange, pomegranate, and tomato and other foods including teas, chocolate, and cruciferous vegetables have compounds that may also impact pharmacokinetic processes or the way in which the drugs work in the body, and not as much is known yet about these interactions or how to predict them (Won, Oberlies, & Paine, 2012). Because research into the influence of foods and juices other than grapefruit is limited, unless ordered otherwise, the safest way to take a medication is with a glass of water.

CHAPTER

5

Understanding the Chapter

Key Concepts Summary

5.1   The nurse plays a key role in preventing and managing adverse drug effects.

5.2   The FDA continues to monitor for new adverse events after a drug is approved and marketed.

5.3   Allergic reactions are caused by a hyperresponse of the immune system.

5.4   Idiosyncratic reactions are unusual drug responses often caused by genetic differences among patients.

5.5   Some drugs have the ability to induce cancer or cause birth defects.

5.6   Drug toxicity may be specific to particular organs.

5.7   Drug interactions may significantly affect pharmacotherapeutic outcomes.

5.8   Pharmacokinetic drug interactions include changes in the absorption, distribution, metabolism, or excretion of medications.

5.9   Pharmacodynamic drug interactions include additive, synergistic, or antagonistic effects.

5.10   Food, nutrients, and dietary supplements may interact with medications and affect their actions.

Case Study: Making the Patient Connection

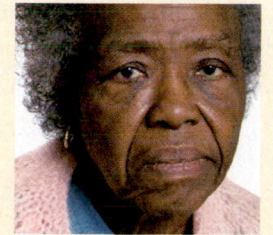

Remember the patient "Elizabeth Washington" at the beginning of the chapter? Now read the remainder of the case study. Based on the information presented within this chapter, respond to the critical thinking questions that follow.

The more medication an individual takes, the more likely it is that an adverse reaction may occur. For Elizabeth Washington this is a real possibility because she takes multiple medications for various physical problems. Elizabeth is a 77-year-old African American woman with several chronic conditions that require pharmacotherapy, including diabetes, heart failure, arthritis, and depression. She has been wheelchair bound since her stroke 2 years ago and has lost functional ability of her left side.

Unfortunately, she does not have a regular health care provider. Elizabeth obtains all her health care from a clinic operated for lower income individuals. The primary health care providers in the clinic are medical residents and interns who rotate every month as part of their medical training. Therefore, it is unlikely that she will see the same prescriber more than a couple of times. Her medical record is quite extensive and spans her health history for the last 15 years. Because her medical history record is so lengthy, Elizabeth fears that the new doctors will not take the time to read the entire chart before prescribing the newest treatment or therapy.

Critical Thinking Questions

1. Identify ways that you can minimize or prevent adverse drug events in this patient.
2. What existing conditions make Elizabeth more susceptible to a drug reaction?
3. Discuss how drug reactions can affect pharmacokinetics.
4. Differentiate among additive, synergistic, and antagonist drug effects.

See Answers to Critical Thinking Questions on student resource website.

Additional Case Study

As the triage nurse in the emergency department, you determine the patient's chief complaint, obtain vital signs, collect past medical history information, and ask about drug and food allergies. While assessing a patient with a suspected ankle fracture, she tells you that she is allergic to codeine because it makes her nauseated and sleepy.

1. What further questions would you ask the patient about drug allergies?
2. Differentiate among an adverse effect, a side effect, and drug allergy.
3. Is this patient experiencing an idiosyncratic reaction? Explain.

See Answers to Additional Case Study on student resource website.

Chapter Review

1 Prior to the administration of an antibiotic, the patient informs the nurse that 4 years ago the patient experienced an allergic reaction. Based on this information what should the nurse do first?

1. Ask the patient to describe the reaction further.
2. Notify the health care provider on call about the patient's statements.
3. Administer the dose and observe the patient for a reaction.
4. Check the medical administration record for documented allergies.

2 The nurse is researching a new drug prior to administration. The drug handbook states that the adverse effects are "dose related," which means that:

1. As the dose increases, the risk of adverse effects also increases.
2. The adverse effects should be expected after the first dose.
3. Oral preparations will produce the most adverse effects.
4. The timing of each dose should be correlated with the presence of adverse effects.

3 The patient is receiving a medication that may cause nephrotoxicity. To decrease the risk of this adverse reaction, the nurse should encourage the patient to:

1. Avoid sunbathing and exposure to direct sunlight.
2. Increase the intake of potassium-enriched foods.
3. Abstain from alcoholic beverages.
4. Increase fluid intake to promote adequate hydration.

4 On physical examination, the nurse observes raised hive-like welts covering the patient's trunk and arms. The patient also reports intense itching after receiving a new medication. The nurse will suspect what dermatologic adverse effect?

1. Angioedema
2. Stevens–Johnson syndrome
3. Urticaria
4. Photosensitivity

5 When observing a patient for bone marrow toxicity, the nurse would monitor for:

1. Increased complaints of muscle and bone pain in the lower extremities.
2. Decrease in red blood cells, white blood cells, and platelets.
3. Decrease in the range of motion of the upper and lower extremities.
4. Increase in hepatic enzymes.

6 The patient is receiving a medication that causes hepatotoxicity. What symptoms would alert the nurse that this drug-related toxicity has occurred?

1. Black furry tongue and vaginal yeast infection
2. A sudden reduction in blood pressure on rising
3. Right upper quadrant pain and anorexia
4. Uncontrollable movements in the face, arms, and legs

See Answers to Chapter Review in Appendix A.

References

Davies, E. C., Green, C. F., Taylor, S., Williamson, P. R., Mottram, D. R., & Pirmohamed, M. (2009). Adverse drug reactions in hospital in-patients: A prospective analysis of 3695 patient-episodes. *PLoS ONE, 4*(2), e4439. doi:10.1371/journal.pone.0004439

Lucas, C., & Martin, J. (2013). Smoking and drug interactions. *Australian Prescriber, 36,* 102–104.

Shepherd, G., Mohorn, P., Yacoub, K., & May, D. W. (2012). Adverse drug reaction deaths reported in United States vital statistics, 1999–2006. *The Annals of Pharmacotherapy, 46,* 169–175. doi:10.1345/aph.1P592

Won, C. S., Oberlies, N. H., & Paine, M. F. (2012). Mechanisms underlying food–drug interactions: Inhibition of intestinal metabolism and transport. *Pharmacology & Therapeutics, 136,* 186–201. doi:10.1016/j.pharmthera.2012.08.001

Selected Bibliography

Bilyeu, K. M., Gumm, C. J., Fitzgerald, J. M., Fox, S. W., & Selig, P. (2011). Cultivating quality: Reducing the use of potentially inappropriate medications in older adults. *American Journal of Nursing, 111*(1), 47–52. doi:10.1097/01.NAJ.0000393060.94063.15

Boullata, J. I., & Armenti, V. T. (Eds.). (2010). *Handbook of drug-nutrient interactions* (2nd ed.). New York, NY: Humana Press.

Chen, X. W., Sneed, K. B., Pan, S. Y., Cao, C., Kanwar, J. R., Chew, H., & Zhou, S. F. (2012). Herb–drug interactions and mechanistic and clinical considerations. *Current Drug Metabolism, 13,* 640.

George, E. L., Henneman, E. A., & Tasota, F. J. (2010). Nursing implications for prevention of adverse drug events in the intensive care unit. *Critical Care Medicine, 38*(Suppl. 6), S136–S144. doi:10.1097/CCM.0b013e3181de0b23

Jordan, S. (2011). Adverse events: Expecting too much of nurses and too little of nursing research. *Journal of Nursing Management, 19,* 287–292. doi:10.1111/j.1365-2834.2011.01265.x

Lund, B. C., Carnahan, R. M., Chrischilles, E. A., & Kaboli, P. J. (2010). What types of inappropriate prescribing predict adverse drug events in older adults. *The Annals of Pharmacotherapy, 44,* 957–963. doi:10.1345/aph.1P182

Magro, L., Moretti, U., & Leone, R. (2012). Epidemiology and characteristics of adverse drug reactions caused by drug–drug interactions. *Expert Opinion on Drug Safety, 11,* 83–94. doi:10.1517/14740338.2012.631910

Posadzki, P., Watson, L., & Ernst, E. (2013). Herb–drug interactions: An overview of systematic reviews. *British Journal of Clinical Pharmacology, 75,* 603–618. doi:10.1111/j.1365-2125.2012.04350.x

Pronsky, Z., & Crowe, S. R. (2012). *Food–medication interactions* (17th ed.). Pottstown, PA: Food Medication Interactions.

Tsai, H.-H., Lin, H.-W., Simon Pickard, A., Tsai, H.-Y., & Mahady, G. B. (2012). Evaluation of documented drug interactions and contraindications associated with herbs and dietary supplements: A systematic literature review. *International Journal of Clinical Practice, 66,* 1056–1078. doi:10.1111/j.1742-1241.2012.03008.x

U.S. Department of Health and Human Services, National Toxicology Program. (2011). *Report on carcinogens, twelfth edition.* Retrieved from http://ntp.niehs.nih.gov/ntp/roc/twelfth/roc12.pdf

Valente, S., & Murray, L. P. (2011). Creative strategies to improve patient safety: Allergies and adverse drug reactions. *Journal for Nurses in Staff Development, 27*(1), E1–E5. doi:10.1097/NND.0b013e31819b5f0b

Wilmer, A., Louie, K., Dodek, P., Wong, H., & Ayas, N. (2010). Incidence of medication errors and adverse drug events in the ICU: A systematic review. *Quality and Safety in Health Care, 19*(5), 1–9. doi:10.1136/qshc.2008.030783

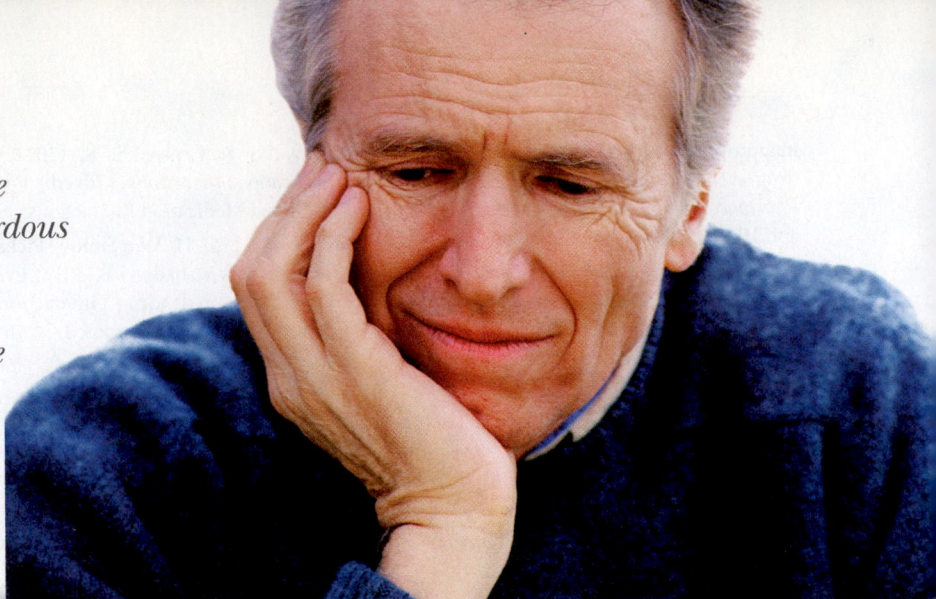

"He was always so cautious about everything. Isn't it amazing . . . he survived a war, worked in a hazardous occupation, and never even got a traffic ticket. Yet all it took was one trip to the hospital for a simple procedure. Now, it's all over."

Friend of "Ross Holland"

CHAPTER

6 Medication Errors and Risk Reduction

LEARNING OUTCOMES

After reading this chapter, the student should be able to:

1. Critique the following statement: "All medication errors can be prevented."
2. Describe the impact of a medication error on all aspects of health care delivery, including patients, nurses, and health care agencies.
3. Using specific examples, analyze major types of medication errors and how they can be prevented.
4. Describe procedures for reporting and documenting medication errors and incidents.
5. Explain how rules, policies, and procedures can help prevent medication errors.
6. Develop a list of strategies that the nurse can implement in practice to reduce medication errors.
7. Explain how medication reconciliation can lead to a reduction in medication errors.
8. Design patient teaching information that can be used to reduce medication errors.
9. Identify strategies that health care agencies use to prevent medication errors.

CHAPTER OUTLINE

▶ Medication Errors and Their Impact on Health Care

▶ Factors Contributing to Medication Errors

▶ Drug Names and Medication Errors

▶ Reporting Medication Errors

▶ Strategies for Reducing Medication Errors

KEY TERMS

adherence, 73

health care failure mode and effect
    analysis (HFMEA), 74

high-alert medications, 70

medication administration record
    (MAR), 71

medication error, 67

medication error index, 67

medication reconciliation, 72

polypharmacy, 73

risk management, 74

root-cause analysis (RCA), 74

sentinel event, 67

In their clinical practice, nurses must maximize patient safety by striving to be 100% accurate when administering medications. Drug administration, however, requires multiple complex steps to be accomplished by physicians, pharmacists, nurses, and patients and can never be 100% error free. Occasionally, medication errors are made that can significantly impact treatment outcomes. The purpose of this chapter is to examine the reasons for medication errors and explore strategies that nurses may use to prevent them.

PharmFACT

Most people think of a medication error as a one-time event in a patient. However, repeating the same error in the same patient (such as the wrong dose) occurs frequently and is associated with greater harm to the patient (Crespin et al., 2010).

Medication Errors and Their Impact on Health Care

6.1 Medication errors are preventable events that may significantly impact treatment outcomes.

According to the National Coordinating Council for Medication Error Reporting and Prevention (NCC MERP, 2013), a **medication error** is:

> any preventable event that may cause or lead to inappropriate medication use or patient harm while the medication is in the control of the health care professional, patient, or consumer. Such events may be related to professional practice, health care products, procedures, and systems, including prescribing; order communication; product labeling, packaging, and nomenclature; compounding; dispensing; distribution; administration; education; monitoring; and use.

The NCC MERP has developed a **medication error index** that categorizes medication errors by evaluating the extent of harm an error can cause, as shown in Figures 6.1 and 6.2.

Whereas most medication errors do not result in patient harm, when they do, it may be devastating to the patient and to those health care providers involved in the error. Kuo, Touchette, and Marinac (2013) studied medication errors identified by clinical pharmacists and submitted in error reports. While 95% of the errors did not result in harm, 4% of the errors were serious enough to require treatment or medical intervention. Common classifications of drugs that resulted in drug errors included anti-infectives, hematologic drugs, and cardiovascular drugs. An accrediting body for health care agencies, The Joint Commission, considers certain categories of risk to patients to be "sentinel events." A **sentinel event** is "an unexpected death or injury, or the risk of these types of death or injury" (The Joint Commission, 2013). Whereas reporting sentinel events to The Joint Commission is currently voluntary for health care agencies, 4% of reported sentinel events in 2012 were related to medication error (The Joint Commission, n.d.). The Joint Commission disseminates "Sentinel Event Alerts" to all agencies it has accredited and publishes the alerts on its website. The alerts are meant to trigger a review of policies, procedures, or processes by the health care agency to prevent a future event from occurring, or to take corrective action if an error has occurred. The alerts remain in a permanent database maintained by The Joint Commission.

Medication errors may have significant impact beyond the patient involved. Errors may extend the length of hospitalization, which increases medical costs for the patient and agency. Undue harm to the patient due to medication errors is a cause of expensive legal challenges for the health care industry, physicians, and nurses. If frequent medication errors occur, the accreditation of the facility may be scrutinized and revoked. The agency also suffers loss of reimbursement as well as being perceived by the public as unsafe or delivering substandard care.

There is no acceptable occurrence rate for medication errors. The goal of every health care organization should be to improve medication administration systems to prevent harm to patients due to medication errors. All errors, whether or not they affect the patient, should be investigated with the goal of identifying policies and procedures that can improve the medication administration process to prevent future errors. The investigation of errors should be conducted in a nonpunitive manner that encourages staff to report errors, thereby building a culture of safety within an organization. Medication errors, especially those types that occur repeatedly, can alert nurses and health care administrators that a new policy, procedure, or process needs to be implemented to maximize patient safety.

Factors Contributing to Medication Errors

6.2 Medication errors may be caused by human factors, inadequate communication, or confusing labels, packaging, or drug names.

Many different factors contribute to medication errors. When considering the number of health care personnel involved, from medication order to administration, patient-related factors, packaging, and other non–human-related elements, there are many opportunities for a medication error to occur. It is not surprising that research into the causes of medication errors has found that the majority stem from human factors, such as deficient knowledge, prescribing or administration errors, and errors of omission, regardless of the type of health care setting (Crespin et al., 2010;

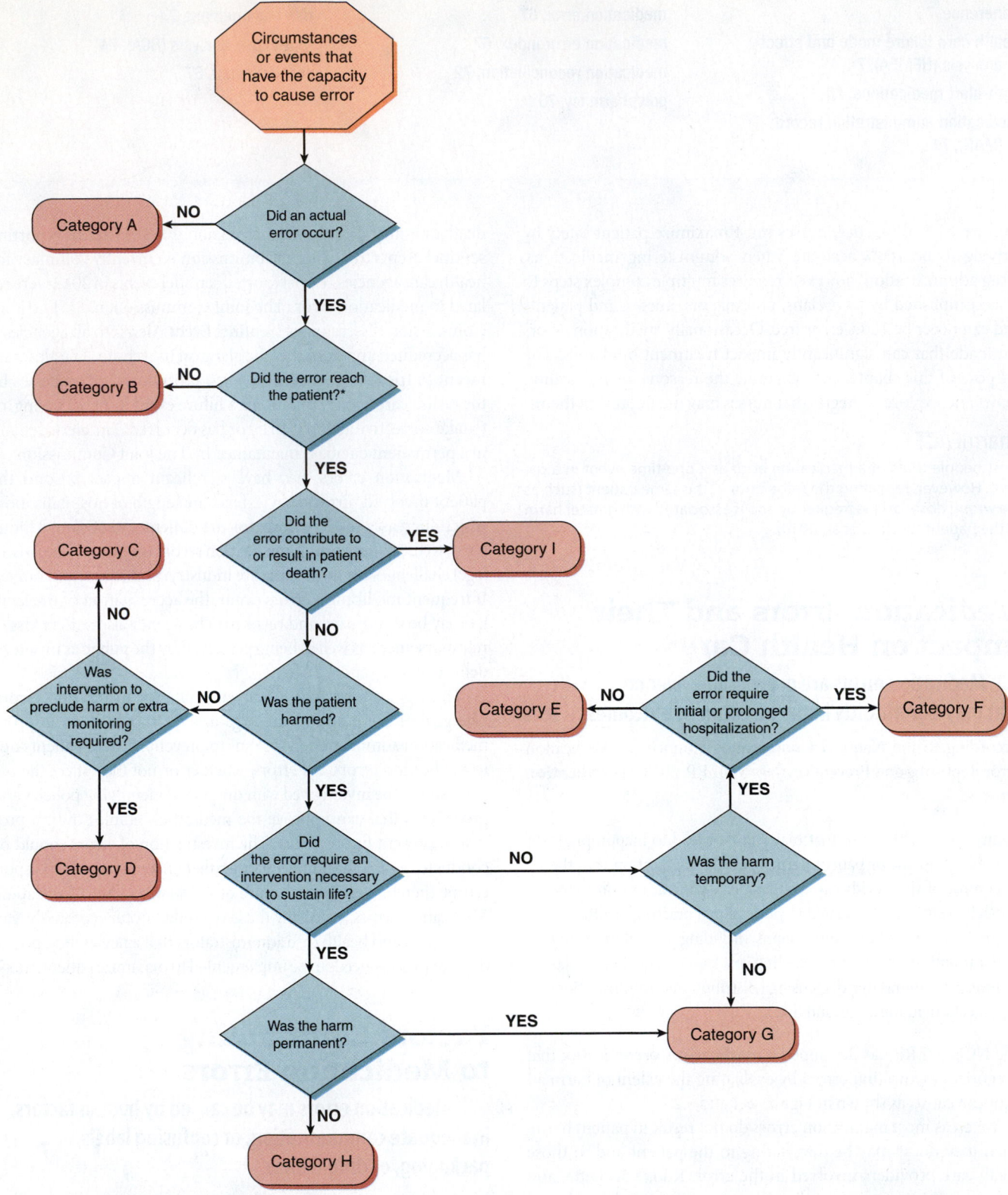

*An error of omission does reach the patient.

Figure 6.1 NCC MERP Index for categorizing medication errors algorithm.
From National Coordinating Council for Medication Error Reporting and Prevention, © 2001b. All Rights Reserved.

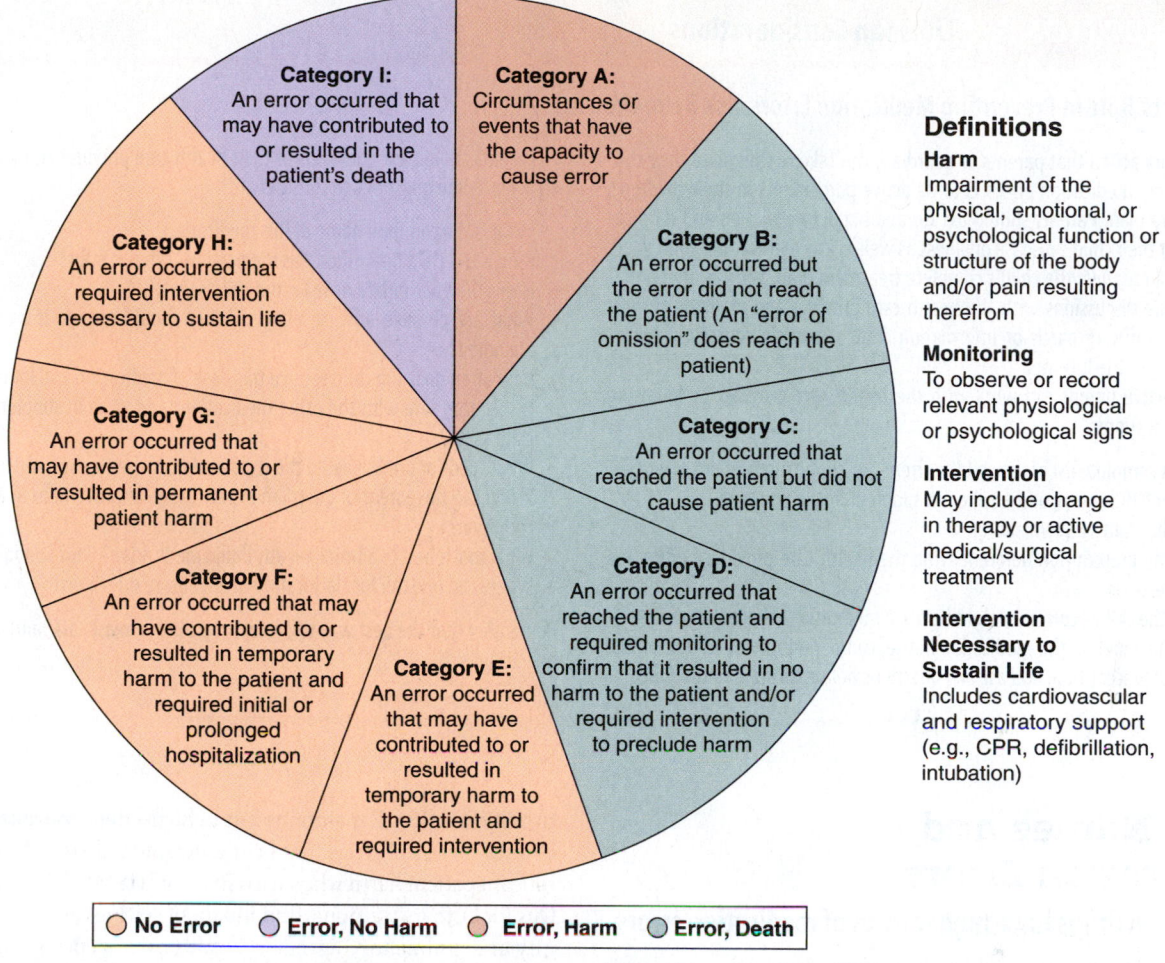

Definitions

Harm
Impairment of the physical, emotional, or psychological function or structure of the body and/or pain resulting therefrom

Monitoring
To observe or record relevant physiological or psychological signs

Intervention
May include change in therapy or active medical/surgical treatment

Intervention Necessary to Sustain Life
Includes cardiovascular and respiratory support (e.g., CPR, defibrillation, intubation)

Figure 6.2 NCC MERP Index for categorizing medication errors.
From National Coordinating Council for Medication Error Reporting and Prevention, © 2001a. All Rights Reserved.

Kuo et al., 2013; Latif, Rawat, Pustavoitau, Pronovost, & Pham, 2013). The most frequent categories of errors include the following.

- Errors in patient assessment (e.g., inadequate medication history, incomplete physical assessment)
- Inaccurate prescribing (e.g., wrong drug, incorrect dose)
- Errors in administration (e.g., route or time of administration, omissions)

Most medication errors involve a breach of one of the cardinal "5 rights" of medication administration: the right patient, drug, dosage, route, and time. Labeling designs, changes in packaging, and problems with dispensing devices are other factors contributing to errors. In many settings, the nurse remains the last line of defense to prevent a medication error from occurring.

Studying the types and causes of medication errors allows agencies and facilities to design ways to prevent them. Once a common source of error is identified, the U.S. Food and Drug Administration (FDA) works with health care agencies to determine changes that may be made to prevent that error in the future. For example, if two drug names sound too similar and are causing medication errors, the FDA may mandate a change in name. The FDA may also request pharmaceutical companies to more clearly label or package

a drug to avoid confusion. Other forms of intervention include educating health care professionals and consumers about common errors and how to prevent them.

The Institute for Safe Medication Practices (ISMP) is a non-profit agency comprising 23 national health care organizations. It was founded in 1994 to help standardize medication error reporting systems, examine interdisciplinary causes of medication errors, and promote medication safety. ISMP offers many informational brochures and tools that assist in error avoidance. An example of a tool that has decreased error rates related to unclear medication orders is the ISMP's list of error-prone abbreviations, symbols, and dose designations (ISMP, 2013b). In 2001, The Joint Commission issued a specific Sentinel Event Alert addressing the need to avoid using these error-prone abbreviations. Appendix B of this text includes a list of these abbreviations and symbols. With the rise of the electronic health record (EHR), more abbreviations have been standardized or are now issued in fully written form.

CONNECTION Checkpoint 6.1

From what you learned in Chapter 5, describe the similarities and differences between a synergistic effect and an additive effect and how they might contribute to a medication error. *See Answer to Connection Checkpoint 6.1 on student resource website.*

Parents' Role in Preventing Medication Errors: Ask Before You Act

The primary action that parents or guardians can take to safeguard their children against medication errors is to be active participants in their children's health care plan. Parents should ask for additional information and clarification about their child's disease or illness as well as any medications prescribed. They should request the child's complete treatment plan. Sources of information include discussions with the health care provider and readings of most recent scientific research or information from reputable sources in books, magazines, or the Internet.

A proactive parent can work with the health care provider by following these suggestions:

- Make a complete list of the child's current prescribed medications, over-the-counter (OTC) drugs, and any herbal supplements or vitamins.
- Note the child's known allergies.
- Read the prescription before leaving the health care provider's office and ask questions.
- Know the child's current weight because medication is based on weight.
- Read the label on the medication bottle, comparing it with what is on the original prescription, and ask any questions before giving it to the child.

Parents should ask questions of their health care provider and write down answers. Some questions to consider are:

- What is the common name of this medication?
- Why is the child prescribed this medication? What is it for?
- Is this the appropriate dose for the child's weight?
- What are possible adverse effects? What should one do if any of these are noted?
- How often does the child receive this dose of medication and for how long?
- Is this drug safe with the other medications and vitamin supplements the child takes?
- What foods or drinks should the child avoid to have the best outcome?
- When can the parent or guardian expect to see improvement in the child's condition?
- What tool is best to administer any liquid medication? Cup? Spoon? Syringe?
- Where can one call for clarification of any future questions?

Remember that the best way to protect the child is to ask, ask, and ask before one acts.

Drug Names and Medication Errors

6.3 Certain drugs have higher rates of medication errors.

Some types of medication errors are independent of the drug being administered. For example, failure to perform adequate medication order checks, forgetting to give a dose, or administering the medication to the wrong patient can occur with any medication. Some drugs, however, have higher error rates than others. Furthermore, when an error does occur, certain medications have greater potential to cause harm. Learning which drugs have the highest error rates and produce the most serious consequences can help the nurse to be more vigilant when administering these agents.

With thousands of generic and brand names for drugs, it is inevitable that some will look or sound similar; for example, *hydroxyzine* and *hydralazine* or *Novalin* and *NovoLog*. It is easy to understand how a verbal order given in a hurry over a cell phone could result in the wrong drug. It is likely that hundreds of medication errors occur each year because of look-alike or sound-alike drugs. This is a primary reason why verbal drug orders should always be confirmed in writing before being administered. The ISMP publishes a list of confused drug names and recommends the use of "Tall Man Letters" as a method to reduce the chance that one drug will be mistaken for another (ISMP, 2011). For example, "hydroxyzine" would be written as hydrOXYzine to avoid confusion with hydralazine (which is recommended as "hydrALAZINE"). A selection of look-alike or sound-alike drug names is included in Table 6.1.

Drugs that have a narrow therapeutic index are more likely to cause serious consequences should a medication error occur. These drugs are not necessarily more error prone than others, but the nurse should give extra care when administering them due to their

toxicity. The ISMP maintains lists of **high-alert medications** and defines these as "drugs that bear a heightened risk of causing significant patient harm when used in error" (ISMP, 2013a). There are lists for both institutional and inpatient settings as well as community and ambulatory agencies. Health care agencies may build in additional safeguards with these medications such as independent double-checks or automated alerts. Each patient care unit may include its own, additional list of high-alert medications. For example, high-alert drugs on cancer units or a pediatric unit may differ from those on a medical–surgical unit. A selected list of high-alert drugs is included in Appendix B.

PharmFACT

In a study of pediatric patients, 38% of the documented drug errors involved an incorrect dose, 20% a drug omission, and 14% a wrong drug. It is estimated that 2.5% of the pediatric medication errors resulted in harm to a child (The Joint Commission, 2008).

Reporting Medication Errors

6.4 Medication errors must be properly documented and reported.

Although some medication errors go unreported, it is always the nurse's legal and ethical responsibility to document all occurrences. In severe cases, adverse reactions caused by medication errors may require the initiation of lifesaving interventions for the patient, including available antidotes. After such an incident, the patient may require close supervision, and additional medical treatments may be warranted.

The FDA has coordinated the reporting of medication errors at the federal level. The FDA Safety Information and Adverse Event Reporting Program, known as MedWatch, provides important

TABLE 6.1   Look-Alike and Sound-Alike Drug Names

acetazolamide	acetohexamide
AcipHex	Aricept
Adderall	Inderal
bupropion	buspirone
carboplatin	cisplatin
Celebrex	Cerebyx
chlorpromazine	chlorpropamide
cycloserine	cyclosporine
daunorubicin	doxorubicin
dimenhydramine	diphenhydramine
Diprivan	Ditropan
dobutamine	dopamine
ephedrine	epinephrine
Humalog	Humulin
hydromorphone	morphine
infliximab	rituximab
isotretinoin	tretinoin
Kaletra	Keppra
Lamisil	Lamictal
lamivudine	lamotrigine
leucovorin	Leukeran
Lexapro	Loxitane
MS Contin	OxyContin
Neulasta	Neumega
oxycodone	OxyContin
paroxetine	fluoxetine
Retrovir	ritonavir
Seroquel	Sinequan
sumatriptan	zolmitriptan
Tiagabine	tizanidine
TobraDex	Tobrex
Tramadol	trazodone
Trental	tegretol
valacyclovir	valganciclovir
vinblastine	vincristine
Viracept	Viramune
Zantac	Zyrtec
Zestril	Zetia
Zyprexa	Celexa

and timely clinical information about safety issues involving medical products, including prescription and over-the-counter (OTC) drugs, biologics, medical- and radiation-emitting devices, and special nutritional products. The FDA encourages nurses and other health care providers to report medication errors to its database, which is used to assist other professionals in avoiding similar mistakes. Medication errors, or situations that can lead to errors, may be reported anonymously directly to the FDA by telephone or online. Since 1992, the FDA has received over 30,000 reports of medication errors. The number of actual errors is likely much higher.

In conjunction with the *United States Pharmacopeia* (USP), the ISMP operates the voluntary National Coordinating Council for Medication Error Reporting Program (NCC MERP), which accepts reports from consumers and health care professionals related to medication safety. Medication errors from the NCC MERP voluntary reporting system are shared with the FDA. The NCC MERP has resulted in dozens of medication-related patient safety changes, including nationwide hazard alerts; packaging, labeling, and nomenclature changes; and health care system changes.

The USP also offers MEDMARX, a national, Internet-accessible database that hospitals and health care systems use to track adverse drug events and medication errors. Agencies participate in MEDMARX voluntarily and subscribe to it on an annual basis. MEDMARX is operated as a quality improvement tool, which facilitates productive and efficient documentation, reporting, analysis, tracking, trending, and prevention of adverse drug events.

All medical facilities have policies and procedures that provide guidance to the nurse on reporting medication errors. Documentation of the error should occur in a factual manner and must include specific nursing interventions that were implemented following the error to protect patient safety, such as monitoring vital signs and assessing the patient for possible complications. Documentation does not simply record that a medical error occurred. Failure to document nursing actions taken related to the error could be interpreted as either negligence or failure to acknowledge that the incident occurred. The nurse should record the names of all individuals who were notified of the error and any follow-up monitoring or treatment prescribed or needed. The patient's **medication administration record (MAR)**, whether in print form or part of an electronic health record, should also contain information about what medication was given or omitted. The nurse who made or observed the medication error should complete a written occurrence report. The occurrence report allows the nurse an opportunity to identify factors that contributed to the medication error. The occurrence report is not usually included in the patient's health record and the nurse should learn the specific policies applicable to the agency of employment about the methods used to report errors.

Accurate documentation in the health record and on the occurrence report is essential for legal reasons. These documents verify that the patient's safety was protected and serve as a tool to improve medication administration processes. Legal issues may arise or worsen if there is an attempt to hide a mistake or delay corrective action, or if the nurse forgets to document interventions in the patient's chart.

CONNECTION Checkpoint 6.2

Additional important functions of the *United States Pharmacopeia* are presented in Chapter 2. What is the role of the USP in drug regulation?
See Answer to Connection Checkpoint 6.2 on student resource website.

Strategies for Reducing Medication Errors

6.5 Nurses use multiple strategies for reducing medication errors.

What can the nurse do in the clinical setting to avoid medication errors and promote safe drug administration? The nurse can begin by adhering to the four steps of the nursing process:

1. **Assessment.** Obtain a thorough medication history every time the patient enters the health care setting or transfers to another unit or agency. Ask the patient about food or medication allergies, current health concerns, and use of OTC medications and herbal supplements. Assess renal and hepatic functions, and determine if other body systems are impaired and could affect pharmacotherapy. Identify areas of needed patient education with regard to medications.

2. **Planning.** Minimize factors that contribute to medication errors: Avoid using abbreviations that could be misunderstood, question unclear orders, do not accept verbal orders, and follow specific facility policies and procedures related to medication administration. Be aware of situations or settings that may increase the risk of errors, such as a busy environment.

3. **Implementation.** When engaged in a medication-related task, focus entirely on the task. Noise, other events, and talking coworkers can distract the nurse's attention and result in a medication error. Keep the following points in mind as well:

   • Positively verify the identity of each patient before administering the medication, according to facility policy and procedures. Never bypass safeguards when checking for identification such as barcoded patient ID bands, which require scanning at the bedside.

   • Use the correct procedures and techniques for all routes of administration. Use sterile materials and techniques when administering parenteral medications.

   • Calculate medication doses correctly and measure liquid drugs carefully. Some medications, such as heparin, have a narrow safety margin for producing serious adverse effects. When giving these medications, ask a colleague or a pharmacist to check the calculations to make certain the dosage is correct and follow any agency-required nomograms as appropriate. Always double-check pediatric calculations prior to administration.

   • Open medication packages or bottles immediately prior to administering the drug and in the presence of the patient.

   • Record the medication and all dosing information on the MAR immediately after administration.

   • Always confirm that the patient has swallowed an oral medication. Do not leave the medication at the bedside unless there is a specific order that it may be left there.

   • Be alert for long-acting oral dosage forms with indicators such as SR, LA, XL, and XR. These tablets or capsules usually must remain intact for the extended release feature to remain effective. Instruct the patient not to crush, chew, or break the medication in half, because doing so could cause an overdose.

4. **Evaluation.** Assess the patient for expected therapeutic outcomes and determine if any adverse effects have occurred. The nurse should be especially vigilant in observing for adverse effects if this is the first time the patient has ever taken the drug, or if the dosage is being increased. Because antibiotics have the highest rate of drug allergy, the nurse must be especially observant for signs and symptoms of allergy following administration of these agents. All adverse effects noted should be reported to the health care provider, documented in the health care record, and reported to the next shift's nurse along with any additional orders from the provider. Have the patient restate information about the drug and dosing directions, including the correct dose of medication and the right time to take it. Asking the patient to demonstrate an understanding of the goals of pharmacotherapy assists the nurse in determining whether additional patient education is necessary.

Nurses must be motivated and determined to stay current on pharmacotherapeutics and should never administer a medication unless they are familiar with its uses and adverse effects. There are many venues by which nurses can obtain updated medication knowledge. Each nursing unit should have current drug references available. Nurses can also call the pharmacy to obtain information about the drug or, if available, look it up on the Internet using reliable sources. Many nurses are now relying on pharmacology and medical-related applications for handheld devices such as cell phone applications to provide current information. These devices can be updated daily or weekly by downloading the most current data. A word of caution is necessary: Drug references may sometimes give incorrect information. Nurses must rely on common sense and good judgment. If a dose appears to be inaccurate in a reference source, nurses should always check with the prescriber or pharmacist before administering. In addition, some electronic health records may have an automated drug reference available which may be accessed directly from the administration record. Whenever errors in drug references are encountered, nurses have a duty to contact the publisher of the inaccurate data, so that future medication errors may be prevented.

6.6 Thorough medication reconciliation is an important means of reducing medication errors.

Recent research has suggested that inadequate medication reconciliation is a primary cause for many medication errors. **Medication reconciliation** is the "process of comparing a patient's medication orders to all of the medications that the patient has been taking" (The Joint Commission, 2006). Medication reconciliation should occur anytime there is a change in the site of the patient's care: admission, transfer, or discharge from a health care facility, and with more care being given in community settings, any time the patient seeks care from a provider. Patients should keep a detailed list of their drugs, the dose, and how often they take them. Unfortunately, sometimes patients arrive in the provider's office or health care agency with a medication history that ranges from a sketchy memory recall to a bag of pills or dated pillbox, or a list of medications that may or may not be the actual drugs or dosages that the patient is on. A thorough assessment of the medication history during medication reconciliation, comparing the patient's recall against any provided lists, has been a significant factor in decreasing medication errors on admission to the health care setting (Gardella, Cardwell, & Nnadi, 2012; Gleason et al., 2010).

Many older adults have several chronic medical disorders concurrently, each of which may be treated by individual specialists. It is common for patients to receive multiple prescriptions, sometimes for the same condition, that have conflicting pharmacologic actions, a condition termed **polypharmacy**. Although not unique to older patients, polypharmacy is most often seen in the older age group. Keeping track of multiple medications, their doses, indications, routes, and frequency of administration is a major challenge for both patients and health care providers. Failure to properly record medication information, and to communicate that information to health care providers, is a potential cause of medication errors.

In 2004, The Joint Commission identified hundreds of serious medication errors attributed to the lack of medication reconciliation and developed recommendations for their prevention. In 2006, The Joint Commission recommendations included the following:

- Implement a process for obtaining and documenting a complete list of the patient's current medications on the patient's admission. This process includes a comparison of the medications the organization provides to those on the list. Medications should include prescription medications, OTC medications, vitamins, and herbal products.

- Communicate a complete list of the patient's medications to the next provider of service when a patient is referred or transferred to another setting, service, practitioner, or level of care within or outside the organization.

- On discharge from the facility, provide the patient with the complete list of medications to be taken as well as instructions on how to take any newly prescribed medications.

6.7 Adequate patient education and adherence are essential strategies for safe medication usage.

In the hospital setting, the physician, nurse, and pharmacist are largely responsible for preventing medication errors, and they collaborate to ensure that the patient is receiving the correct drug in the manner designated by the prescriber. In the home setting, this responsibility relies on proper patient adherence to drug therapy. For prescription drugs, health care providers provide the patients with verbal and written instructions on how and when to take the medication. Labels for over-the-counter (OTC) medications, herbal products, and dietary supplements indicate the correct method of taking the agent; however, patients do not always read or understand the information given.

Adherence is a major factor affecting pharmacotherapeutic outcomes and for increasing the risk of medication errors. As it relates to pharmacotherapy, **adherence**, or compliance, is defined as taking medications in the manner prescribed by the health care provider. In the case of OTC products, adherence means correctly following the instructions on the label. Patient nonadherence (noncompliance) ranges from not taking the medication at all to taking it at the wrong time or at the wrong dose. It is estimated that approximately 50% of patients with chronic illnesses do not take their medications as prescribed, leading to increased complications, death, and additional costs estimated at $100 billion per year (Brown & Bussell, 2011).

Many factors can influence patient adherence with pharmacotherapy. One of the most common sources of nonadherence is simply forgetting a dose of medication. This occurs frequently when the drug must be taken more than twice daily. Another source of nonadherence is that the drug may be too expensive or not approved by the patient's health insurance plan. Patients often discontinue the use of drugs that have annoying adverse effects or those that impair major lifestyle choices. Adverse effects that often prompt nonadherence are headache, dizziness, nausea, diarrhea, and impotence.

Patients often take medications in an unexpected manner, sometimes self-adjusting their doses. Some feel that if one tablet is good, two must be better. Others believe that they will become dependent on the medication if it is taken as prescribed; thus they only take half the necessary dose. Still others simply stop taking the medication when they start feeling better. Patients are usually reluctant to admit or report nonadherence to the nurse for fear of being reprimanded or feeling embarrassed.

In a study of low-income patients with multiple chronic conditions, Mishra, Gioia, Childress, Barnet, and Webster (2011) determined that whereas factors such as complex medication regimens affected a patient's ability to understand and take the medications, participants also felt that they lacked a role in the decision-making process with their providers about how to manage their conditions. Patients who decided to stop taking a drug, or to take less than the prescribed amount, did so because they had just "reached a limit" on how many more pills they could take (Mishra et al., 2011, p. 253).

Because reasons for nonadherence are many and varied, the nurse must be vigilant in questioning patients about taking their medications. When pharmacotherapy fails to produce the expected treatment outcomes, nonadherence should always be considered as a possible explanation. There are steps that the nurse can take to increase the potential for patient adherence to the therapeutic regimen. All of these steps focus on effective teaching. Knowing that patients often feel overwhelmed with the amount of information provided and that they perceive they lack a voice in the decision-making process, the nurse can discuss the prescription routine with the patient and ask questions: Will the patient be able to fill the prescription? How will it fit into the patient's usual routine or with other medications? Listening for clues that suggest the patient is overwhelmed by the routines, the nurse can ask further questions about what suggestions the patient might have to make the routine workable. Patients may be reluctant to discuss these suggestions with their provider but may feel comfortable in doing so with the nurse because of the nurse–patient relationship.

In the plan of care, it is important to address essential information that the patient must know regarding the prescribed medications. This includes factors such as the name of the medication, why it has been ordered, expected drug actions, associated adverse effects, and information regarding interactions with other medications, foods, herbal supplements, or alcohol. Patients should be encouraged to take an active role in ensuring the effectiveness of their medication and their own safety. It is important to remember that, unless diagnosed as mentally incompetent, a well-informed adult always has the legal option of refusal to take any medication. It is the nurse's responsibility, however, to ensure that the patient has all the necessary information to make an informed decision.

For patients receiving outpatient therapy or those being released from a hospital, the nurse must carefully assess their ability to take their medications in a safe and effective manner. If the nurse believes that a patient may have difficulty in properly administering the medications, caregivers should be consulted and other arrangements made to ensure that the patient receives the correct drugs using the proper dosing schedule. With each successive health care visit, the nurse can review the medication history, asking questions about the prescribed medications. Being alert to reports that the patient is not taking, or is not taking correctly, the prescribed drugs may suggest an overwhelming, complex medication routine that needs to be reassessed if it is to be successful. Economic conditions sometimes result in difficult choices for patients between obtaining medications and other required necessities. Nurses provide medication education and follow-up that will result in positive health outcomes and the prevention of negative health effects and even larger expenditures as a result of poor medication adherence. Special considerations related to drug administration to pediatric and geriatric patients are presented in greater detail in Chapters 9 and 10, respectively.

PharmFACT

Approximately 75% of adults do not follow their provider's directions for their medications, including failure to fill the prescription, not taking the medicine for the prescribed amount of time, or stopping the drug without notifying their provider. (PhRMA, 2011)

6.8 Health care agencies are actively involved in reducing medication errors.

Most health care agencies use automated, computerized, locked cabinets for medication storage on patient care units. Each nurse on the unit has a code for accessing the cabinet and removing a medication dose. These automated systems also maintain an inventory of drug supplies. These systems are not foolproof, however, and the nurse must always perform system checks to ensure that the proper medication is in the correct patient drawer.

Larger health care agencies often have **risk management** departments to examine risks and minimize the number of medication errors. Risk management personnel investigate incidents, track data, identify problems, and provide recommendations for improvement. Nurses collaborate with risk management committees to seek means of reducing medication errors by modifying policies and procedures within the institution. Examples of institutional policies and procedures include the following:

- Store medications under proper conditions (light and temperature control) and separate medications that have look-alike names or packaging.

- Read the drug label to avoid the administration of time-expired medications.
- Avoid the transfer of doses from one container to another.
- Avoid overstocking of medications.
- Monitor adherence to avoiding the use of prohibited prescription abbreviations.
- Remove outdated reference books.

6.9 Analytical tools may be used to identify risk and analyze errors.

Health care agencies use analytical tools to assess for the likelihood of errors and to analyze errors once they have occurred. Two such tools are the health care failure mode and effect analysis (HFMEA) and root-cause analysis (RCA). These tools help agencies identify how errors occur and how to take steps to prevent them from occurring again.

In the case of medication administration, **health care failure mode and effect analysis (HFMEA)** identifies processes where errors may occur related to prescription, dispensing, and administration. Each process at risk for failure is analyzed and the severity and probability of each is determined. For example, when prescribing, an inaccurate assessment of the patient may occur. The level of the patient's pain may not be adequately assessed or the wrong analgesic may be chosen because of an inadequate consideration of all factors that may affect the use of that medication. The effects of these failures, if they occurred, might include poor pain control or the wrong drug or dose being prescribed. The severity of the failure may be estimated—catastrophic, major, moderate, or minor—and a severity score established. Catastrophic failures would rank as "4," while minor failures would rank as "1." The probability of a failure may also be ranked with possibilities ranging from frequent to remote. A "hazard score" is assigned, which is the severity score multiplied by the probability score (Cheng et al., 2012). In the above example of patient pain and the process of choosing (prescribing) an analgesic, the severity score for selecting an inappropriate analgesic for a patient with undiagnosed hepatic insufficiency may be catastrophic (ranked 4) and the probability of that occurring may be occasional (ranked 3). This would result in a hazard score of 12. The higher the hazard score, the more critical it is to identify strategies to prevent such a failure from occurring. Health care organizations use HFMEA as a risk management strategy to prevent health system errors of any kind from occurring.

Once an error has occurred, it is essential to analyze why it happened so that steps can be taken to prevent its recurrence. **Root-cause analysis (RCA)** attempts to focus attention on the causes of the error, rather than on the person responsible for the error, so that patient harm can be reduced or eliminated through investigating system vulnerabilities (U.S. Department of Veterans Affairs, 2013). An analysis of what happened, why it occurred, and how to prevent it from happening again is conducted. RCA of medication errors is often interdisciplinary because there are many opportunities for errors to occur in various departments. An analysis of people, equipment or supplies, policies and procedures, and environmental

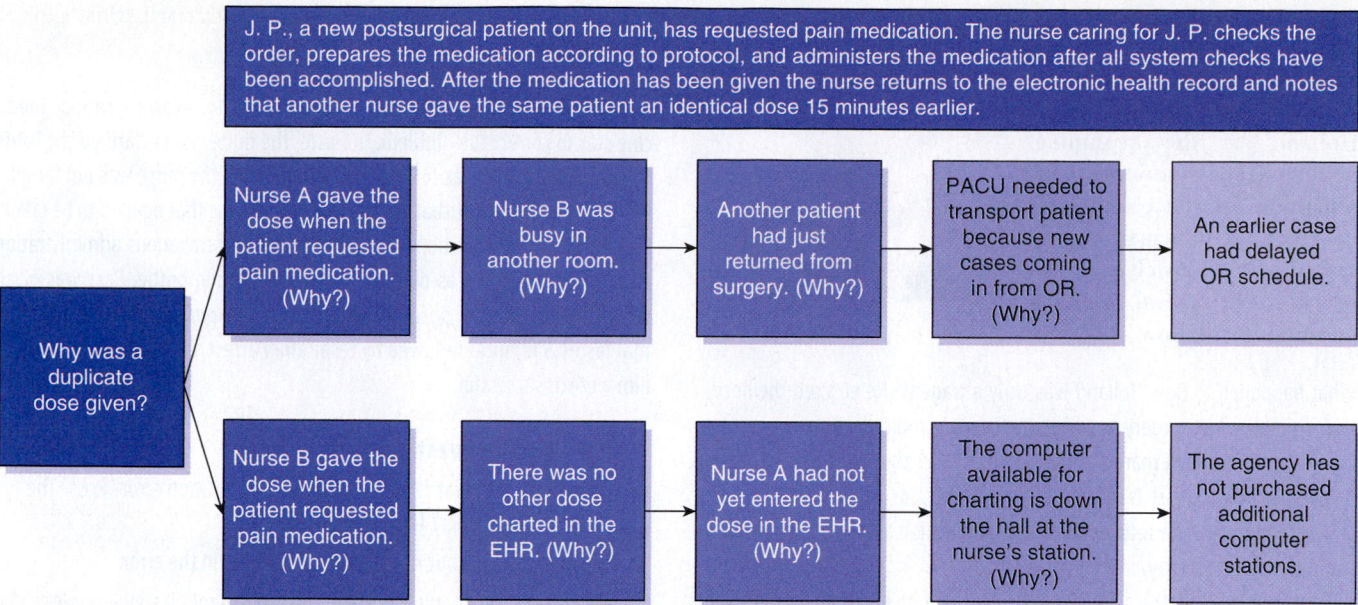

Figure 6.3 Sample root cause analysis: Duplicate dose of a narcotic analgesic.

factors involved in the error is included. For each category, "why did the error occur?" is asked, with each question's answer prompting a further "why?" question. This technique is sometimes called the "5 Whys" for this reason (iSixSigma, n.d.). There are many ways to diagram the analysis, and the nurse should utilize the tool(s) used in the specific health care agency. Figure 6.3 illustrates the beginning of a diagram for an error in which a duplicate dose of a narcotic analgesic was given after the patient returned from the recovery unit (PACU) from surgery (OR). Note that after asking "why" questions, causes are identified that involve equipment, procedures, and other

departments. Each of those causes would also be examined to determine all possible remedies to prevent a recurrence.

Nurses aim to maximize patient safety by striving to be 100% accurate when administering medications. Drug administration, however, requires multiple complex steps accomplished by the entire health care team and can never be 100% error free. Being aware of potential areas that may increase medication errors, and employing strategies to mitigate risk, are integral components of the nursing role to ensure that pharmacotherapy provides maximum therapeutic effects with minimal harm.

CHAPTER

Understanding the Chapter

Key Concepts Summary

6.1 Medication errors are preventable events that may significantly impact treatment outcomes.

6.2 Medication errors may be caused by human factors, inadequate communication, or confusing labels, packaging, or drug names.

6.3 Certain drugs have higher rates of medication errors.

6.4 Medication errors must be properly documented and reported.

6.5 Nurses use multiple strategies for reducing medication errors.

6.6 Thorough medication reconciliation is an important means of reducing medication errors.

6.7 Adequate patient education and adherence are essential strategies for safe medication usage.

6.8 Health care agencies are actively involved in reducing medication errors.

6.9 Analytical tools may be used to identify risk and analyze errors.

Case Study: Making the Patient Connection

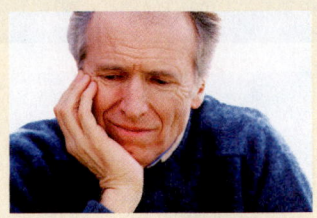

Remember the patient "Ross Holland" at the beginning of the chapter? Now read the remainder of the case study. Based on the information presented within this chapter, respond to the critical thinking questions that follow.

What happened to Ross Holland was truly a tragedy. He entered the hospital for simple sinus surgery and never recovered. Ironically, Ross was a super vigilant man. As a Vietnam veteran, he had seen the worst of combat for 4 years. During the last 6 months of the conflict, he survived in a prisoner of war camp. When he returned home, he took a job as a safety inspector in the automobile industry.

From a previous physical exam, Ross knew that he had a slightly irregular heartbeat, but he never really took it seriously. In fact, he never mentioned it when the nurse was admitting him to the hospital. However, the condition became a problem soon after surgery. The nurse caring for him noticed a series of cardiac irregularities on the monitor and contacted the health care provider. The health care provider ordered Ross to receive a cardiac medicine stat to correct the problem. In haste, the nurse never clarified the route that the medication was to be given. Additionally, the nurse was not familiar with the medication's usual dose or any precautions that needed to be taken. As a result, the medication was given by direct intravenous administration without being diluted as directed on the medication bottle. Ross was given 100 times the normal dose. Consequently, he experienced seizure activity that lasted 5 minutes followed by respiratory arrest. All efforts to resuscitate him were unsuccessful.

Critical Thinking Questions

1. Ultimately, who was responsible for this medication error? Ross? The health care provider? The nurse? Why?

2. Identify the contributing factors that resulted in the error.

3. What strategies should a nurse use to prevent medication errors?

4. What policy could health care facilities implement to avoid medication errors?

See Answers to Critical Thinking Questions on student resource website.

Additional Case Study

You are the health nurse in an elementary school. One day, a student's mother tells you, "Medications frighten me. Both my children have asthma and frequently require medications. When I give any of my children medications, I worry that I will make an error. There is so much that can go wrong."

1. How would you respond to this mother's concern?

2. Create a list of strategies that parents can use to prevent medication errors.

3. What referral resources could help reduce her anxiety?

See Answers to Additional Case Study on student resource website.

Chapter Review

1 It is 2:45 a.m. and the nurse has telephoned the prescriber to report that the patient is experiencing an acute episode of postoperative pain. How can the nurse avoid medication errors when receiving a telephone order from a prescriber?

1. Decline to accept the telephone order.
2. Refuse to call the prescriber but attempt to comfort the patient.
3. Instruct the patient's family to call the prescriber.
4. Repeat the order verbally to ensure accuracy.

2 The nurse cannot read the number of milligrams (mg) to be administered in a drug order written by the health care provider. It is questionable whether 125 mg, 1.25 mg, or 12.5 mg should be administered. What action would be most appropriate to prevent a medication error?

1. Telephone the health care provider about the illegible medication order.
2. Ask another nurse to read the questionable medication order.
3. Contact the pharmacist about the medication order.
4. Consult a drug handbook and administer the normal dose.

3 The nurse is counseling the patient on a medication taken daily. Which is a strategy that the nurse should include in this teaching session that might prevent a medication error?

1. Insist on brand-name drugs rather than generic drugs.
2. Have all prescriptions filled at one pharmacy.
3. Request all prescriptions be placed in easily opened containers.
4. Consult the Internet about possible adverse effects.

4 When given a medication, the patient tells the nurse, "I've never seen this pill before. It's not like the others I take." Which would be the most appropriate action for the nurse to take?

1. Instruct the patient that different brands are frequently used.
2. Administer the medication in the existing form.
3. Verify the order and double-check the drug label.
4. Advise the patient to talk with the health care provider and give the drug.

5 While administering medication to several patients, the nurse suddenly realizes that the wrong medication has been given to a patient. Which would be the *first* priority action taken by the nurse?

1. Assess the patient in order to monitor for adverse effects.
2. Call the health care provider and report the error.
3. Complete the hospital's drug error form.
4. Report the medication error to the FDA.

6 As the nurse enters the room to administer medication, the patient states, "I'm in the bathroom. Please leave the medication on my bedside table, and I will take it when I come out." Which would be the appropriate response by the nurse?

1. "I will leave the medication and follow up with you in 30 minutes."
2. "You must take the medication now or refuse the dose."
3. "Let me know when you are ready, and I will then return with your medicine."
4. "I've given the drug to your visitors. Take it when you come out of the bathroom."

See Answers to Chapter Review in Appendix A.

References

Brown, M. T., & Bussell, J. K. (2011). Medication adherence: WHO cares? *Mayo Clinic Proceedings, 86,* 304–314. doi:10.4065/mcp.2010.0575

Cheng, C. H., Chou, C. J., Wang, P. C., Lin, H. Y., Kao, C. L., & Su, C. T. (2012). Applying HFMEA to prevent chemotherapy errors. *Journal of Medical Systems, 36,* 1543–1551. doi:10.1007/s10916-010-9616-7

Crespin, D. J., Modi, A. V., Wei, D., Williams, C. E., Greene, S. B., Pierson, S. J., & Hansen, R. A. (2010). Repeat medication errors in nursing homes: Contributing factors and their association with patient harm. *The American Journal of Geriatric Pharmacotherapy, 8,* 258–270. doi:10.1016/j.amjopharm.2010.05.005

Gardella, J. E., Cardwell, T. B., & Nnadi, M. (2012). Improving medication safety with accurate preadmission medication lists and postdischarge education. *Joint Commission Journal on Quality and Patient Safety, 38*(10), 452–458.

Gleason, K. M., McDaniel, M. R., Feinglass, J., Baker, D. W., Lindquist, L., Liss, D., & Noskin, G. A. (2010). Results of the medications at transitions and clinical handoffs (MATCH) study: An analysis of medication reconciliation errors and risk factors at hospital admission. *Journal of General Internal Medicine, 25,* 441–447. doi:10.1007/s11606-010-1256-6

Institute for Safe Medication Practices. (2011). *FDA and ISMP lists of look-alike drug names with recommended tall man letters.* Retrieved from http://www.ismp.org/Tools/tallmanletters.pdf

Institute for Safe Medication Practices. (2013a). *ISMP high-alert medications.* Retrieved from http://www.ismp.org/Tools/highAlertMedicationLists.asp

Institute for Safe Medication Practices. (2013b). *ISMP's list of error-prone abbreviations, symbols, and dose designations.* Retrieved from http://www.ismp.org/Tools/errorproneabbreviations.pdf

iSixSigma. (n.d.). *Determine the root cause: 5 whys.* Retrieved from http://www.isixsigma.com/tools-templates/cause-effect/determine-root-cause-5-whys/

The Joint Commission. (n.d.). Summary data of sentinel events reviewed by The Joint Commission. Retrieved from http://www.jointcommission.org/assets/1/18/2004_4Q_2012_SE_Stats_Summary.pdf

The Joint Commission. (2001). Medication errors related to potentially dangerous abbreviations. *Sentinel Event Alert, 23.* Retrieved from http://www.jointcommission.org/assets/1/18/SEA_23.pdf

The Joint Commission. (2006). Using medication reconciliation to prevent errors. *Sentinel Event Alert, 35.* Retrieved from http://www.jointcommission.org/assets/1/18/SEA_35.PDF

The Joint Commission. (2008). Preventing pediatric medication errors. *Sentinel Event Alert, 39.* Retrieved from http://www.jointcommission.org/assets/1/18/SEA_39.PDF

The Joint Commission. (2013). Infection control related sentinel events. *Sentinel Event Alert, 28.* Retrieved from http://www.jointcommission.org/topics/hai_sentinel_event.aspx

Kuo, G. M., Touchette, D. R., & Marinac, J. S. (2013). Drug errors and related interventions reported by United States clinical pharmacists: The American College of Clinical Pharmacy Practice-Based Research Network medication error detection, amelioration and prevention study. *Pharmacotherapy, 33,* 253–265. doi:10.1002/phar.1195

Latif, A., Rawat, N., Pustavoitau, A., Pronovost, P. J., & Pham, J. C. (2013). National study on the distribution, causes, and consequences of voluntary reported medication errors between the ICU and non-ICU settings. *Critical Care Medicine, 41,* 389–398. doi:10.1097/CCM.0b013e318274156a

Mishra, S. I., Gioia, D., Childress, S., Barnet, B., & Webster, R. L. (2011). Adherence to medication regimens among low-income patients with multiple comorbid chronic conditions. *Health & Social Work, 36,* 249–258. doi:10.1093/hsw/36.4.249

National Coordinating Council for Medication Error Reporting and Prevention. (2001a). *NCC MERP Index for Categorizing Medication Errors.* Retrieved from http://www.nccmerp.org/pdf/indexColor2001-06-12.pdf

National Coordinating Council for Medication Error Reporting and Prevention (2001b). *NCC MERP Index for Categorizing Medication Errors Algorithm.* Retrieved from http://www.nccmerp.org/sites/default/files/algorColor2001-06-12.pdf

National Coordinating Council for Medication Error Reporting and Prevention. (2013). *About medication errors: What is a medication error?* Retrieved from http://www.nccmerp.org/aboutMedErrors.html

PhRMA. (2011). *Improving prescription medicine adherence is key to better health care.* Retrieved from http://www.phrma.org/sites/default/files/pdf/PhRMA_Improving%20Medication%20Adherence_ExecSummary.pdf

U.S. Department of Veterans Affairs. (2013). *Culture change: Prevention, not punishment.* Retrieved from http://www.patientsafety.va.gov/vision.html#rca

Selected Bibliography

Etchells, E. (2010). Admitting medication errors: Five critical concepts. *Quality and Safety in Health Care, 19*, 369–370. doi:10.1136/qshc.2010.041020

Jones, J. H., & Treiber, L. (2010). When the 5 rights go wrong: Medication errors from the nursing perspective. *Journal of Nursing Care Quality, 25*, 240–247. doi:10.1097/NCQ.0b013e3181d5b948

Kaboli, P. J., Glasgow, J. M., Jaipaul, C. K., Barry, W. A., Strayer, J. R., Mutnick, B., & Rosenthal, G. E. (2010). Identifying medication misadventures: Poor agreement among medical record, physician, nurse, and patient reports. *Pharmacotherapy, 30*, 529–538. doi:10.1592/phco.30.5.529

Kane-Gill, S. L., Kowiatek, J. G., & Weber, R. J. (2010). A comparison of voluntarily reported medication errors in intensive care and general care units. *Quality and Safety in Health Care, 19*, 55–59. doi:10.1136/qshc.2008.027961

Peron, E. P., Marcum, Z. A., Boyce, R., Hanion, J. T., & Handler, S. M. (2010). Year in review: Medication mishaps in the elderly. *The American Journal of Geriatric Pharmacotherapy, 9*(1), 1–10.

Sauer, B. C., & Hepler, C. D. (2013). Application of system-level root cause analysis for drug quality and safety problems: A case study. *Research in Social and Administrative Pharmacy, 9*(1), 49–59. doi:10.1016/j.sapharm.2012.02.005

Seidl, K. L., & Newhouse, R. P. (2012). The intersection of evidence-based practice with 5 quality improvement methodologies. *Journal of Nursing Administration, 42*(6), 299–304. doi:10.1097/NNA.0b013e31824ccdc9

Spath, P. L. (2011). *Error reduction in health care: A systems approach to improving patient safety* (2nd ed.). San Francisco, CA: Jossey-Bass.

Wierenga, P. C., Lie-A-Huen, L., De Rooif, S. E., Klazinga, N. S., Guchelaar, H. J., & Smorenburg, S. M. (2009). Application of the bow-tie model in medication safety risk analysis: Consecutive experience in two hospitals in the Netherlands. *Drug Safety, 32*, 663–673. doi:10.2165/00002018-200932080-00005

Wilmer, A., Louie, K., Dodel, P., Wong, H., & Ayas, N. (2010). Incidence of medication errors and adverse drug events in the ICU: A systematic review. *Quality and Safety in Health Care, 19*, 1–9. doi:10.1136/qshc.2008.030783

Wright, K. (2010). Do calculation errors by nurses cause medication errors in clinical practice? A literature review. *Nurse Education Today, 1*, 85–97. doi:10.1016/j.nedt.2009.06.009

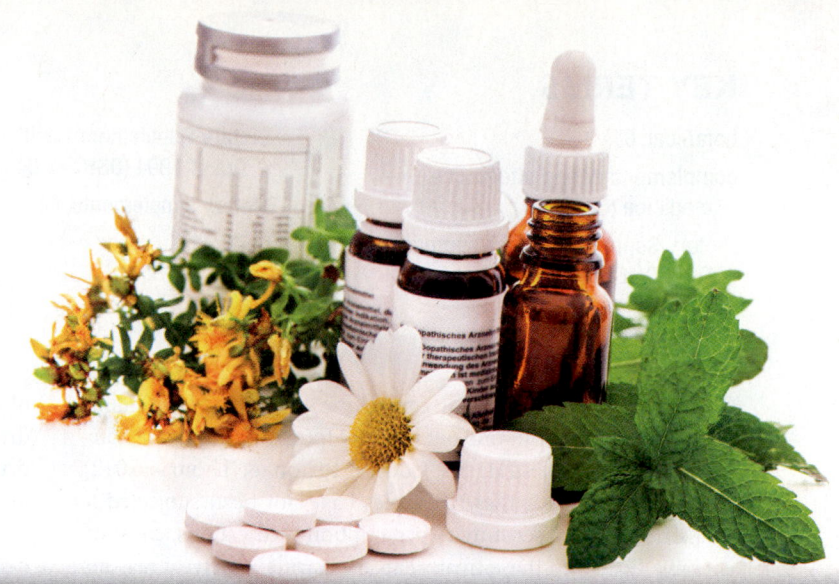

"My daughter is getting so frustrated with me. It seems that I can't remember anything. Just last week I forgot to take my medications twice and failed to pick up my grandson at his weekly tae kwon do lesson."

Patient "Larry Bunch"

CHAPTER 7

The Role of Complementary and Alternative Therapies in Pharmacotherapy

LEARNING OUTCOMES

After reading this chapter, the student should be able to:

1. Identify specific types of complementary and alternative therapies that are used by patients to promote wellness.
2. Analyze why herbal and dietary supplements have steadily increased in popularity.
3. Explain why it is important to standardize herbal products based on specific active ingredients.
4. Describe legislation that governs the use of herbal and dietary supplements.
5. Describe drug interactions and adverse effects that may be caused by herbal preparations.
6. Distinguish between an herbal product and a specialty supplement.
7. Discuss the role of the nurse in teaching patients about complementary and alternative therapies.

CHAPTER OUTLINE

▶ Types of Complementary and Alternative Therapies

▶ History of Herbal Therapies

▶ Standardization of Herbal Products

▶ Dietary Supplement Regulation

▶ Herb–Drug Interactions

▶ Specialty Supplements

KEY TERMS

botanical, 81

complementary and alternative
  medicine (CAM), 80

Dietary Supplement and Nonprescription
  Drug Consumer Protection Act, 84

Dietary Supplement Health and Education
  Act of 1994 (DSHEA), 84

dietary supplements, 84

herb, 81

polyherbacy, 85

specialty supplements, 87

USP Verification Program, 85

Complementary and alternative medicine represents a multibillion dollar industry. About one out of every four Americans use complementary therapies (Harris, Cooper, Relton, & Thomas, 2012). Despite the fact that these therapies have not been subjected to the same scientific scrutiny as prescription medications, consumers have turned to these treatments for a wide variety of reasons. The availability of herbal and dietary supplements at a reasonable cost has convinced many consumers to try them, sometimes in lieu of prescription medications. This chapter focuses on the role of complementary and alternative therapies in the prevention and treatment of disease.

Types of Complementary and Alternative Therapies

7.1 Complementary and alternative therapies are used by a large number of people to prevent and treat disease.

Complementary and alternative medicine (CAM) comprises an extremely diverse set of therapies and healing systems thatare considered to be outside of mainstream health care. Although diverse, the major CAM systems have certain common characteristics:

- Focus on treating the individual
- Consideration of the health of the whole person
- Emphasis on the integration of mind and body
- Emphasis on disease prevention, self-care, and self-healing
- Recognition of the role of spirituality in health and healing

Because of its popularity, the scientific community has begun to examine the effectiveness, or lack of effectiveness, of CAM therapies. Although research into these alternative systems has been conducted, few CAM therapies have been subjected to rigorous, controlled clinical studies. It is likely that some of these therapies will be found ineffective, whereas others will become mainstream treatments. The definition of a complementary therapy as being "outside the mainstream" is somewhat ambiguous because the line between an alternative therapy and a conventional therapy is constantly changing. Increasing numbers of health care providers are now recommending CAM therapies to their patients. Table 7.1 lists the most common CAM therapies.

Nurses have long known the value of CAM in preventing and treating disease. Prayer, meditation, massage, and yoga have been used to treat both body and spirit for centuries. From a pharmacologic perspective the value of CAM therapies lies in their ability to reduce the need for medications. For example, if a patient can find anxiety relief through massage or biofeedback therapy, the use of antianxiety drugs may be reduced or eliminated. Reduction of drug dose leads to fewer adverse effects and better compliance with drug therapy. This chapter focuses on two types of CAM therapies: herbs and specialty supplements.

The nurse should be sensitive to the patient's beliefs about and need for alternative treatment and not be judgmental. The advantages and the limitations of the CAM should be presented to patients so they may make rational and informed decisions about their treatment. Pharmacotherapy and CAM can play complementary roles in patient wellness.

TABLE 7.1 Complementary and Alternative Therapies

Healing Method	Examples
Biologic-based therapies	Herbal therapies
	Nutritional supplements
	Special diets
Alternative health care systems	Naturopathy
	Homeopathy
	Chiropractic
	Native American medicine (e.g., sweat lodges, medicine wheel)
	Chinese traditional medicine (e.g., acupuncture, Chinese herbs)
Manual healing	Massage
	Pressure-point therapies
	Hand-mediated biofield therapies
Mind–body interventions	Yoga, Pilates
	Meditation
	Hypnotherapy
	Guided imagery
	Biofeedback
	Movement-oriented therapies (e.g., music, dance)
Spiritual	Shamans
	Faith and prayer
Others	Bioelectromagnetics
	Detoxifying therapies
	Animal-assisted therapy

History of Herbal Therapies

7.2 Natural products from plants have been used as medicines for thousands of years.

An **herb** is technically a **botanical** (plant-based substance) that does not have any woody tissue such as stems or bark. In common usage, however, consumers tend to use "herb" to refer to a wide variety of products including substances such as ginkgo biloba (which is a tree) and chondroitin (which is derived from animals). Over time, the term *herb* has come to refer to any plant product with some useful application either as a food enhancer, such as flavoring, or as a medicine.

The use of herbs has been recorded for thousands of years. One of the earliest recorded uses of plant products was a prescription for garlic written in 3000 BC. Eastern and Western medicine have recorded thousands of herbs and herb combinations reputed to have therapeutic value. Over time, the popularity of specific herbs and remedies has varied, depending on the availability of the botanical (i.e., geographical region) and perceived effectiveness. The most popular herbals and their primary uses are shown in Table 7.2.

With the birth of the pharmaceutical industry in the late 1800s, the interest in herbal medicine began to wane. Synthetic drugs could be standardized and produced more cheaply than natural herbal products. Regulatory agencies required that products be safe and effective. The focus of health care was on diagnosing and treating specific diseases, rather than promoting wellness and holistic care. Most alternative therapies were no longer taught in medical or nursing schools. These healing techniques were criticized as being unscientific relics of the past.

TABLE 7.2 Popular Herbal Supplements

Herb	Medicinal Part	Primary Use(s)	Herb Feature (Chapter)
Acai	Berries	Vitamin and mineral supplement, antioxidant, possible weight loss	—
Aloe vera	Leaves	Topical application for minor skin irritations and burns	73
Bilberry	Berries and leaves	Terminate diarrhea, improve and protect vision, antioxidant	74
Black cohosh	Roots	Relief of menopausal symptoms	70
Chlorophyll/chlorella	Leaves	Improve digestion, vitamin and mineral supplement	—
Cranberry	Berries/juice	Prevent urinary tract infection	50
Echinacea	Entire plant	Enhance immune system, treat the common cold	42
Elderberry	Berries and flowers	Congestion in respiratory system due to colds and flu	—
Evening primrose	Oil extracted from seeds	Source of essential fatty acids, relief of premenstrual or menopausal symptoms, relief of rheumatoid arthritis and other inflammatory symptoms	—
Flaxseed (ground) and/or oil	Seeds and oil	Reduce blood cholesterol, laxative	35
Garlic	Bulbs	Reduce blood cholesterol, reduce blood pressure, anticoagulation	38
Ginger	Root	Antiemetic, antithrombotic, diuretic, promote gastric secretions, anti-inflammatory, increase blood glucose, stimulation of peripheral circulation	59
Ginkgo	Leaves and seeds	Improve memory, reduce dizziness	21
Ginseng	Root	Relieve stress, enhance immune system, decrease fatigue	—
Grape seed	Seeds/oil	Source of essential fatty acids, antioxidant, restore microcirculation to tissues	34
Green tea	Leaves	Antioxidant; lower LDL cholesterol; prevent cancer; relieve stomach problems, nausea, vomiting	63
Horny goat weed	Leaves and roots	Enhance sexual function	—
Milk thistle	Seeds	Antitoxin, protection against liver disease	—
Red rice yeast extract	Dried in capsules	Reduce blood cholesterol	—
Saw palmetto	Berries	Treatment of benign prostatic hyperplasia	71
Soy	Beans	Source of protein, vitamins, and minerals; relief of menopausal symptoms, prevent cardiovascular disease, anticancer	69
Stevia	Leaves	Natural sweetener	—
St. John's wort	Flowers, leaves, stems	Reduce depression, reduce anxiety, anti-inflammatory	19
Valerian	Roots	Relieve stress, promote sleep	—
Wheat or barley grass	Leaves	Improve digestion, vitamin and mineral supplement	—

Beginning in the 1970s and continuing to current times, alternative therapies and herbal medicine have experienced a remarkable resurgence, such that the majority of adult Americans are either currently taking herbal therapies on a regular basis or have taken them in the past. Why would people turn to folk remedies and products with uncertain effectiveness when effective prescription medications are available? This increase in popularity has been due to a number of factors:

- Herbal products and dietary supplements were once available only in specialty health food stores but can now be purchased in virtually all supermarkets and pharmacies.

- Complementary therapies are aggressively marketed by the supplement industry as viable and natural alternatives to conventional medicine. The increased availability of the Internet as a marketing tool has led to sites with misleading information about the effectiveness of herbal and dietary supplements.

- The baby-boom generation has demonstrated a renewed interest in natural alternatives and preventive medicine.

- The gradual aging of the population has led people to seek therapeutic alternatives for chronic conditions such as pain, arthritis, anxiety, depression, hormone-replacement therapy, and prostate difficulties.

- People have the impression that natural substances are safer than synthetic pharmaceuticals.

- The high cost of prescription medicines has driven people to seek less expensive alternatives.

- Nurses and other health care providers have been more proactive in promoting self-care and recommending CAM for their patients.

Numerous surveys have been conducted to determine the extent of alternative therapy use in the United States. Results of these studies agree that there is widespread and progressively increasing use of these therapies. One of the largest studies of Americans' use of complementary therapies conducted by the National Center for Complementary and Alternative Medicine (NCCAM) surveyed over 23,000 people (Barnes, Bloom, & Nahin, 2008). Findings of this study included the following:

- Thirty-eight percent of adults and about 12% of children are currently using CAM.

- Women and those with higher educational levels are most likely to use CAM.

- Of those who take natural products, the most commonly used are fish oil (37%), glucosamine (20%), echinacea (20%), flaxseed (16%), ginseng (14%), ginkgo biloba (11%), chondroitin (11%), garlic (11%), and coenzyme Q (9%).

- The most frequent conditions treated with CAM are back pain (17%), head or chest cold (10%), joint pain/arthritis (5%), neck pain (5%), and anxiety or depression (5%).

- People are more likely to use CAM when they are unable to afford conventional health care.

This pharmacology text emphasizes CAM by the use of "Connection" features appearing throughout the chapters. The inclusion of these therapies is not an endorsement, nor does it imply their effectiveness.

They are included because the nurse will frequently need to teach specific natural therapies, and because some of them have the potential to impact pharmacotherapy (see Section 7.5). The student should refer to the current medical literature for complete dosing and safety information. Several excellent sources of reliable information are available. The National Center for Complementary and Alternative Medicine (NCCAM) is a branch of the National Institutes of Health (NIH). It offers current information on research involving these products.

PharmFACT

According to Broussard, Louik, Honein, and Mitchell (2010), 9.4% of women take herbal products during pregnancy, with ginger and ephedra being the most frequently consumed. Potentially, this results in as many as 395,000 births in the United States in which the fetus received prenatal exposure to herbal products.

Standardization of Herbal Products

7.3 Herbal products are available in a variety of formulations, some containing standardized extracts and others containing whole herbs.

The pharmacologically active chemicals in an herbal product may be present in only one specific part or in all parts of the plant. For example, the active chemicals in chamomile are in the aboveground portion such as the leaves, stems, or flowers. For other herbs, such as ginger, the underground roots are used for their healing properties. It is, therefore, essential to know which portion of the plant contains the active chemicals if growing or collecting herbs for home use.

Most prescription drugs contain only one active chemical. This chemical can be standardized and measured, so that the amount of drug received by the patient is precisely known. Herbs, however, may contain dozens of active chemicals, many of which have not yet been isolated, studied, or even identified. It is possible that some of these substances work together synergistically and may not have the same activity if isolated. Furthermore, the strength of an herbal preparation can vary from batch to batch, depending on where it was grown and how it was collected, stored, and preserved. How is it possible, then, for consumers to know the strength of an herbal product, given so much potential variability in ingredients?

To achieve consistency in the strength or dose of an herbal product, scientists have attempted to standardize herbal products. This standardization is based on one of the following methods.

- Active ingredient extracts: These standardize the amount of biologically active substances in the herb. For example, the active ingredient in saw palmetto has been determined to be fatty acids; therefore, these are used to standardize extracts of this herb.

- Marker extracts: These standardize the potency of the herb based on a common substance in the whole herb that may not be the active ingredient. For example, ginseng is standardized on the percent of ginsenosides in the extract.

Regardless of which method is used, standardization allows the consumer to compare products and know the strength of the herb. Some of these standardizations are shown in Table 7.3. It should be understood that the active ingredient in an herb is not always

TABLE 7.3   Standardization of Selected Herbal Products

Herb	Standardization	Percent
Black cohosh rhizome	Triterpene glycosides	2.5
Cascara sagrada bark	Anthocyanosides	25
Echinacea purpurea, whole herb	Echinacosides	4
Ginger rhizome	Pungent compounds (gingerols)	>10
Ginkgo leaf	Flavone glycosides	24–25
	Lactones	6
Ginseng root	Ginsenosides	5–15
Milk thistle root	Silymarin	80
St. John's wort, whole herb	Hypericins	0.3–0.5
	Hyperforin	3–5
Saw palmetto berries	Fatty acids and sterols	80–90

TABLE 7.4   Liquid Formulations of Herbal Products

Product	Description
Tea	Fresh or dried herbs are soaked in hot water for 5–10 min before ingestion; convenient
Infusion	Fresh or dried herbs are soaked in hot water for long periods, at least 15 min; stronger than teas
Decoction	Fresh or dried herbs are boiled in water for 30–60 min until much of the liquid has boiled off; very concentrated
Tincture	Active ingredients are extracted using alcohol by soaking the herb; alcohol remains as part of the liquid
Extract	Active ingredients are extracted using organic solvents to form a highly concentrated liquid or solid form; solvent may be removed or be part of the final product

known and there may be more than one. Furthermore, the active ingredient may be different, depending on the indication for which the herb is being used. Until science can better characterize these substances, it is best to conceptualize the active ingredient of an herb as being the entire herb. An example of the ingredients and standardization of ginkgo biloba using a marker substance is shown in Figure 7.1. As explained in Section 7.4, it should not be assumed that an herb is safe or effective simply because it contains the standard amount of extract.

The two basic formulations of herbal products are solid and liquid. Solid products include pills, tablets, and capsules made from the dried herbs. Other solid products are salves and ointments that are administered topically. Liquid formulations are made by extracting the active chemicals from the plant using solvents such as water, alcohol, or glycerol. The liquids are then

concentrated in various strengths and ingested. The types of liquid herbal formulations are described in Table 7.4. Figure 7.2 illustrates some of the formulations of ginkgo biloba, one of the most popular herbals.

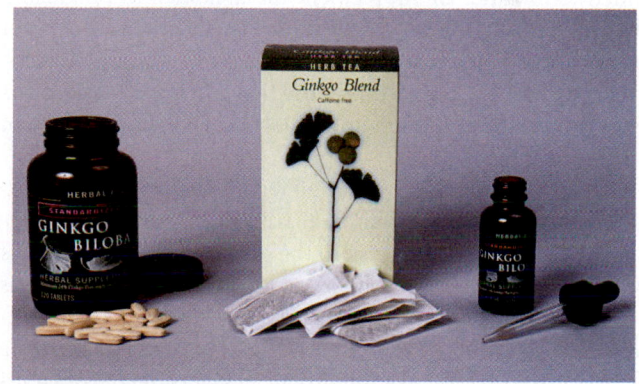

Figure 7.2 Three different ginkgo formulations: tablets, tea bags, and liquid extract.

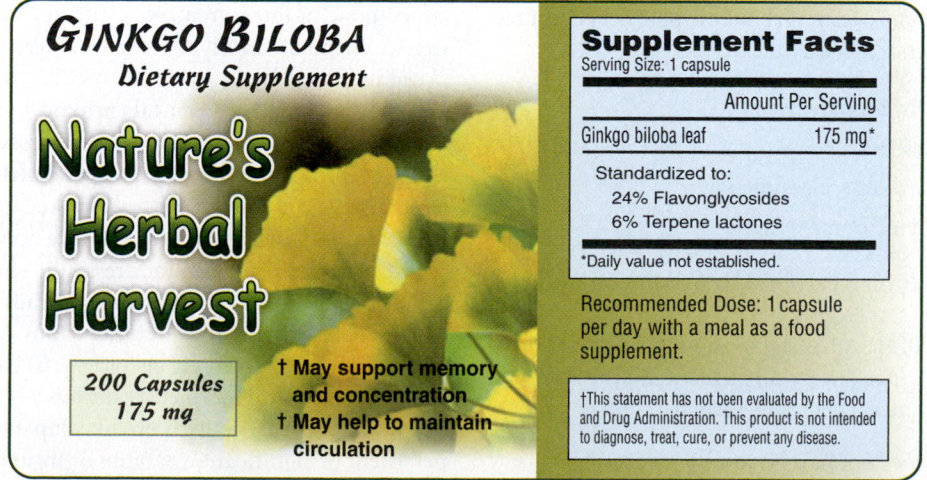

Figure 7.1 Ginkgo Biloba label. The label indicates the product is standardized to percentages of the two active ingredients, flavonglycosides and terpenes, that are found in the ginkgo leaf. Also note the health claims on the label, which have not been evaluated by the FDA.

Dietary Supplement Regulation

7.4 Herbal products and dietary supplements are not regulated in the same manner as prescription medications.

Since the passage of the Food, Drug, and Cosmetic Act in 1936, Americans have come to expect that all approved prescription and over-the-counter (OTC) drugs have passed rigid standards of safety prior to being marketed. Furthermore, it is expected that these drugs have been tested for effectiveness and that they truly provide the medical benefits claimed by the manufacturer. Indeed, most people would be outraged if they found out that the drug they purchased for pain relief or to cure an infectious disease was totally ineffective. For herbal products and specialty supplements, however, Americans cannot and should not expect the same quality standards. These products are regulated by a far less rigorous law, the **Dietary Supplement Health and Education Act of 1994 (DSHEA)**.

The DSHEA exempts dietary supplements from the Food, Drug, and Cosmetic Act, the legislation that regulates prescription drugs. **Dietary supplements** are defined as products intended to enhance or supplement the diet such as botanicals, vitamins, minerals, or any other extract or metabolite that is not already approved as a drug by the U.S. Food and Drug Administration (FDA) as of 1994. Because they are not considered as drugs by the FDA, they are not subjected to the same degree of scrutiny as drugs.

A strength of the DSHEA is that it gives the FDA the authority to remove from the market any product that poses a "significant or unreasonable" risk to the public. The FDA used this legislative authority when the dietary supplement ephedra was removed from the market because of reported serious side effects in some patients. However, it took 7 years from the time the FDA first warned consumers of the dangers of ephedra until it was removed.

The DSHEA requires these products to be clearly labeled as "dietary supplements." The product label must state that the product is not intended to diagnose, treat, cure, or prevent any disease. However, the label may make claims about the product's effect on body structure and function, such as the following:

- Helps promote healthy immune systems
- Reduces anxiety and stress
- Helps to maintain cardiovascular function
- May reduce pain and inflammation

An example of an herbal label for L-carnitine is shown in Figure 7.3.

Unfortunately, the DSHEA has significant flaws that lead to a lack of standardization in the dietary supplement industry and less protection for the consumer. These flaws include:

- The manufacturer does not have to test the safety of a dietary supplement prior to marketing. If it is to be removed from the market, the FDA has the burden of proving that the dietary supplement is harmful.

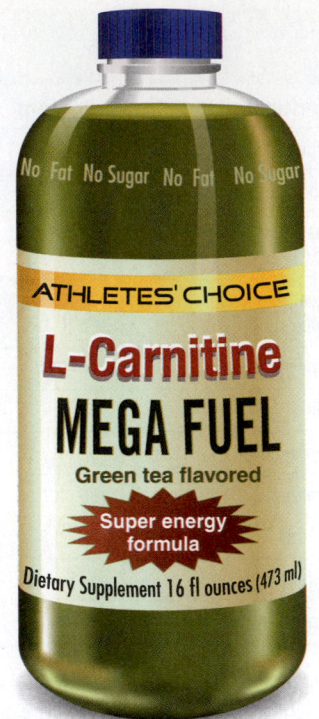
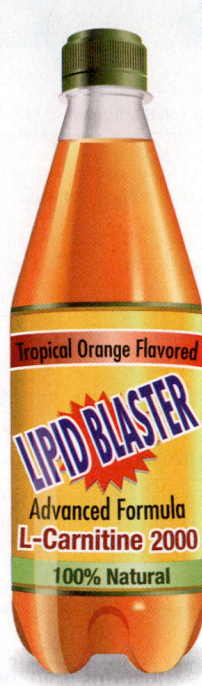

Figure 7.3 L-carnitine is a popular dietary supplement. Notice the claims of improving athletic performance and weight loss, neither of which have been supported by the scientific literature.

- Effectiveness does not have to be demonstrated by the manufacturer.
- The accuracy of the label is not regulated; the product may or may not contain the product listed in the amounts claimed.

Lax government oversight has resulted in a lack of quality and sometimes blatant mislabeling of herbal and supplement products. For example, testing of more than 1,200 dietary supplement products has determined that 25% did not contain the correct amount of labeled ingredients. In some cases, the products contained none of the ingredients claimed on the label, and others were contaminated with potentially dangerous heavy metals such as cadmium and lead.

Several steps have been taken to address the lack of purity and mislabeling of herbal and dietary supplements. In 2007, Congress passed the **Dietary Supplement and Nonprescription Drug Consumer Protection Act**. Companies that market herbal and dietary supplements are now required to include their contact information (address and phone number) on the product labels so consumers can report adverse events. Companies must notify the FDA of any serious adverse event reports within 15 days of receiving such reports. Under this act, a "serious adverse event" is defined as any adverse reaction resulting in death, a life-threatening experience, inpatient hospitalization, a persistent or significant disability or incapacity, or a congenital anomaly or birth defect, as well as any event requiring a medical or surgical intervention to prevent one of these conditions based on reasonable medical judgment. Companies must keep records of such events for at least 6 years, and the records are subject to inspection by the FDA.

Also in 2007, the FDA announced a final rule that requires the manufacturers of dietary supplements to evaluate the identity, purity, potency, and composition of their products. The labels must accurately reflect the content of the products, which must be free of contaminants such as pesticides, toxins, glass, or heavy metals. The rule was phased in over a 3-year period.

The United States Pharmacopeia (USP) is a nonprofit public health organization that has attempted to raise the standards and quality of pharmaceuticals and dietary supplements (see Chapter 1). The USP has developed a voluntary process by which a manufacturer may submit a product for the **USP Verification Program**. Using a multistep approach, the USP examines the manufacturing processes used to create a supplement and tests the product to see if it contains the ingredients specified on the label and whether the product will break down and release its ingredients in the body (bioavailability). If the product meets the stringent standards of the USP, it may then carry the USP verified dietary supplement mark on the label. The verification mark indicates to consumers that the product has been manufactured under acceptable standards of purity, has been tested for active ingredients stated on the label, and is free of harmful contaminants. However, it does not indicate that the product is safe or effective.

CONNECTION Checkpoint 7.1

From what you learned in Chapter 2, what is a pharmacopeia? What function does it serve in the United States? *See Answer to Connection Checkpoint 7.1 on student resource website.*

Herb–Drug Interactions

7.5 Natural products may have pharmacologic actions and can interact with conventional drugs.

A key concept to remember when learning about alternative therapies is that "natural" is not synonymous with "better" or "safe." It is likely that some botanicals do indeed contain active chemicals that are as powerful as, and perhaps more effective than, some currently approved medications. Thousands of years of experience, combined with current scientific research, have shown that some of these herbal remedies have therapeutic actions. Just because a substance comes from a natural product, however, does not make it safe or effective. For example, poison ivy is natural but it certainly is not safe or therapeutic. The dried seed pods of the poppy plant yield opium, which has therapeutic effects but can also kill if taken inappropriately. Some natural products may not offer an improvement over conventional therapy in treating certain disorders and, indeed, may be of no value whatsoever. Furthermore, a patient who substitutes an unproven alternative therapy for an established, effective medical treatment may delay healing and cause irreparable harmful effects.

Some herbal products contain ingredients that may cause additive, synergistic, or antagonistic interactions with prescription or OTC drugs. For example, ginkgo biloba and ginger have the ability to increase bleeding time. If used concurrently with anticoagulants, these herbs may increase the potential for adverse bleeding events. St. John's wort, kava, and valerian cause relaxation and may result in excessive sedation if taken concurrently with central nervous system (CNS) depressants. A few herbals have organ-specific toxicity. The herb comfrey given concurrently with large doses of acetaminophen may increase the patient's risk of hepatotoxicity. Herbals such as psyllium, aloe, and flaxseed may bind to drugs in the gastrointestinal (GI) tract, thus slowing their absorption.

The true extent of herb–drug interactions is unknown. Most reports in the medical literature are anecdotal, often given as a case report on a single patient. It is often impossible to know the exact amount of herb taken because there is such a wide variation in the quality of products on the market or even to know what chemical within the herb (either active ingredients or contaminants) may have caused the reported interaction. Relatively few controlled scientific studies of herb–drug or dietary supplement–drug interactions have been conducted. The majority of the information regarding these interactions is theoretical, rather than clinically based.

Questions on the use of herbal and dietary supplements are important because these products are contraindicated for certain patients. Patients taking medications with potentially serious adverse effects such as insulin, warfarin (Coumadin), antiepileptic drugs, antineoplastic agents, or digoxin (Lanoxin) should be warned to never take any herbal product or dietary supplement without first discussing their needs with a health care provider. Pregnant or lactating women should not take these products

---

CONNECTIONS | Lifespan Considerations

◀ Older Adults at Risk for Polyherbacy

One of the most important health issues affecting older adults is the excessive or inappropriate use of medications. Although health care providers assess for polypharmacy, elderly patients may not divulge the use of herbs and supplements when talking to health care providers. With the increased use of herbs and supplements by older adults, a new health care dilemma has developed—**polyherbacy**, the use of multiple herbs or other supplements.

There are many issues related to the use of herbals and nutritional supplements that should be considered with older adults. For example, there may be:

- Inadequate data that examine the effects and impact that supplements have on the natural physiological changes that occur during the aging process. Because older adults experience diminished kidney and liver function, they may be at greater risk for toxicity.
- Altered pharmacokinetic processes that would increase the older adult's incidence of serious adverse effects.
- Unknown chemicals in the preparation that could interact with other medications.

Health care providers should always inquire about herbal use as part of a comprehensive medication history and should also be aware of the adverse effects that may result from such products.

without approval of their health care provider. The nurse should also remember that the potential for any drug interaction increases in older adults, especially those with hepatic or renal impairment. Potential drug interactions with selected herbs are shown in Table 7.5.

Another warning that must be heeded with natural products is to beware of allergic reactions. It is not unusual to find dozens of different chemicals in teas and infusions made from the flowers, leaves, or roots of a plant. Patients who have known allergies to food products or medicines should

TABLE 7.5 Documented Herb–Drug Interactions

Common and (Scientific) Name	Interacts with	Effects of Interaction
Echinacea (*Echinacea purpurea*)	amiodarone, anabolic steroids, ketoconazole, methotrexate	May increase hepatotoxicity
Feverfew (*Tanacetum parthenium*)	aspirin and other NSAIDs; heparin; warfarin	Increases bleeding risk
Flaxseed (*Linum usitatissimum*)	most drugs	Binds to drugs; decreases absorption
Garlic (*Allium sativum*)	aspirin and other NSAIDs; warfarin	Increases bleeding risk
	insulin; oral antidiabetic agents	Has additive hypoglycemic effects
	saquinavir	Induces CYP3A4 enzymes; decreases drug effectiveness
Ginger (*Zingiber officinale*)	aspirin and other NSAIDs; heparin; warfarin	Increases bleeding risk
Ginkgo (*Ginkgo biloba*)	anticonvulsants	Decreases drug effectiveness
	tricyclic antidepressants	May decrease seizure threshold
	omeprazole	Induces CYP2C19 enzymes; decreases drug effectiveness
	trazodone	Increases drug effects
Ginseng (*Panax quinquefolius/ Eleutherococcus senticosus*)	CNS depressants	Potentiates sedation
	digoxin	Increases toxicity
	diuretics	May attenuate diuretic effects
	insulin; oral antidiabetic agents	Increases hypoglycemic effects
	MAO inhibitors	May cause hypertension, manic symptoms, headaches, nervousness
	warfarin	Decreases anticoagulant effects
Goldenseal (*Hydrastis canadensis/ Eleutherococcus senticosus*)	diuretics	May attenuate diuretic effects
Green tea	warfarin	Decreases anticoagulant effects
Kava kava (*Piper methysticum*)	barbiturates; benzodiazepines; alcohol and other CNS depressants	Potentiates sedation
	levodopa/carbidopa	Worsens Parkinson's symptoms
	phenothiazines	Increases risk and severity of dystonic reactions
St. John's wort (*Hypericum perforatum*)	opioids, alcohol, and other CNS depressants	Potentiates sedation
	cyclosporine	May decrease cyclosporine levels
	efavirenz, indinavir	Decreases antiretroviral activity
	MAO inhibitors	May cause hypertensive crisis
	oral contraceptives	Decreases drug effectiveness
	selective serotonin reuptake inhibitors; tricyclic antidepressants	Increases risk of serotonin syndrome
	warfarin	Decreases anticoagulant effects
Soy	warfarin	Decreases anticoagulant effects
Valerian (*Valeriana officinalis*)	barbiturates; benzodiazepines and other CNS depressants	Potentiates sedation

seek medical advice before taking a new herbal product. It is always wise to take the smallest amount possible when starting herbal therapy, even less than the recommended dose, to see if allergies or other adverse effects occur.

Nurses have an obligation to seek the latest medical information on herbal products, because there is a good possibility that their patients are using them to supplement traditional medicines. Each patient who takes an herbal product does so for a reason. The nurse needs to listen, assess, and understand the patient's goals for taking the supplement. Does the patient have an accurate understanding of the actions of the herb? Are there more effective therapies, either pharmacologic or nonpharmacologic, for the patient's condition? Is there a potential for harmful effects from the product due to high doses or herb–drug interactions? Establishing a supportive attitude toward the use of CAM is important. Nurses often need to educate their patients on the role of alternative therapies in the treatment of their disorder and discuss which treatment or combination of treatments will best meet their patients' health goals. Patients should be advised to be skeptical of marketing claims for herbal products and to seek health information from reputable sources.

CONNECTION Checkpoint 7.2

St. John's wort induces hepatic CYP metabolic enzymes. From what you learned in Chapter 5, how could this herb affect therapy with antidepressants or benzodiazepines that are substrates for CYP enzymes? *See Answer to Connection Checkpoint 7.2 on student resource website.*

Specialty Supplements

7.6 Specialty supplements are nonherbal dietary products that are widely used to promote wellness.

Specialty supplements are nonherbal dietary products used to enhance a wide variety of body functions. These supplements form a diverse group of products obtained from plant and animal sources. They are more specific in their action than herbal products and are generally targeted for one condition or a smaller group of related conditions. The most popular specialty supplements are listed in Table 7.6.

In general, specialty supplements have a legitimate rationale for their use. For example, chondroitin and glucosamine are natural substances in the body necessary for cartilage growth and maintenance. Amino acids are natural building blocks of muscle protein. Flaxseed and fish oils contain omega fatty acids that have been shown to reduce the risk of heart disease in certain patients.

As with herbal products, the link between most specialty supplements and their claimed benefits is unclear. In most cases, the body already has sufficient quantities of the substance; thus taking additional amounts may be of no benefit. In other cases, the supplement is marketed for conditions for which the supplement has no proven effect. The good news is that these substances are generally not harmful unless taken in large amounts. The bad news, however, is that they can give patients false hopes of an easy cure for chronic conditions such as heart disease or the pain of arthritis. As with herbal products, the health care provider should advise patients to be skeptical about any health claims regarding the use of these supplements.

TABLE 7.6 Selected Specialty Supplements		
Name	**Primary Uses**	**Supplement Feature (Chapter)**
Amino acids	Build protein, muscle strength, and endurance	—
Carnitine	Enhance energy and sports performance, heart health, memory, immune function, and male fertility	36
Chromium	Treatment of diabetes; hyperglycemia	66
Coenzyme Q10	Prevent heart disease, provide antioxidant therapy	29
DHEA	Boost immune and memory functions	—
Fish oil	Reduce cholesterol levels, enhance brain function and increase visual acuity	68
Glucosamine and chondroitin	Alleviate arthritis and other joint problems	72
Lactobacillus acidophilus	Maintain intestinal health	60
Melatonin	Reduce sleeplessness and jet-lag during travel	18
Methyl sulfonyl methane (MSM)	Reduce allergic reactions to pollen and foods, relieve pain and inflammation of arthritis	—
Selenium	Reduce the risk of certain types of cancer	—
Vitamin C	Prevent colds	45

CHAPTER

7

Understanding the Chapter

Key Concepts Summary

7.1 Complementary and alternative therapies are used by a large number of people to prevent and treat disease.

7.2 Natural products from plants have been used as medicines for thousands of years.

7.3 Herbal products are available in a variety of formulations, some containing standardized extracts and others containing whole herbs.

7.4 Herbal products and dietary supplements are not regulated in the same manner as prescription medications.

7.5 Natural products may have pharmacologic actions and can interact with conventional drugs.

7.6 Specialty supplements are nonherbal dietary products that are widely used to promote wellness.

Case Study: Making the Patient Connection

Remember the patient "Larry Bunch" at the beginning of the chapter? Now read the remainder of the case study. Based on the information presented within this chapter, respond to the critical thinking questions that follow.

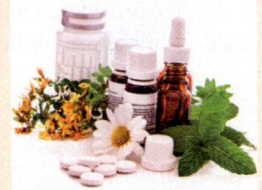

Sixty-nine-year-old Larry Bunch was not only frustrating his daughter, but his forgetfulness was annoying him as well. Since the death of his wife 2 years ago, his forgetfulness seemed to be worsening. To remedy the situation, he purchased a bottle of ginkgo biloba at the health food store and began taking the supplement about 6 months ago.

Larry was hospitalized 3 years ago for a cardiac condition (atrial fibrillation). When he was discharged from the hospital, he was placed on an anticoagulant therapy to prevent blood clots from forming in his heart. Today, Larry comes to his health care provider's office for a scheduled blood test to determine the effectiveness of his anticoagulant.

When the results from the blood test return, it is noted that Larry's coagulation time is abnormally high. Based on the test, Larry is at high risk of hemorrhaging. As the nurse, you note that his vital signs are within normal limits, and he states he feels well. However, you also observe some large bruises on Larry's arms, which he cannot explain.

Critical Thinking Questions

1. What is the relationship between this patient's use of ginkgo and the laboratory results?

2. What instructions should this patient receive about taking the supplement?

3. Discuss the hazards that patients face when using complementary and alternative therapies.

4. What should the health care provider do concerning Larry's forgetfulness?

See Answers to Critical Thinking Questions on student resource website.

Additional Case Study

"It must be safe, after all, it is sold in the grocery store!" exclaimed Linda. As you, the nurse, talk with the patient, Linda Thomas, she explains to you that she takes multiple OTC dietary supplements. Because the bottle states that the ingredients are "all natural," she knows it must be good for her.

1. What are the hazards associated with believing that all medication-type substances sold in the supermarket are safe?

2. Discuss how the words "all natural ingredients" can be confusing.

3. Identify the nurse's role in working with patients who participate in complementary and alternative therapies.

See Answers to Additional Case Study on student resource website.

Chapter Review

1 A patient asks why all health care providers do not rely on complementary and alternative medicine. When talking to this patient the nurse knows that many complementary and alternative therapies:

1. Have not been subjected to rigorous clinical studies.
2. Consist only of old wives' tales and fables.
3. Only provide a placebo effect.
4. Are costly and not worth the risk.

2 Which health teaching concept should be included in the instructions for a patient taking echinacea?

1. Dosage can be doubled if symptoms fail to resolve in 48 hours.
2. Limit fluid intake while taking this supplement.
3. Take the smallest amount possible when starting herbal therapy.
4. Allergic reactions are not possible with natural supplements.

3 Which patient is most likely to experience drug toxicity while taking herbal supplements?

1. An 80-year-old female with cirrhosis
2. A 58-year-old male with cardiac irregularities
3. A 30-year-old female with pneumonia
4. An 18-year-old male with chronic acne

4 The patient asks the nurse, "Why are herbal supplements so popular?" The nurse's answer is based on which factors? (Select all that apply.) Herbal supplements:

1. Can now be purchased in virtually all supermarkets.
2. Are aggressively marketed by the herbal and supplement industry.
3. Cost less than prescription medicines.
4. Are safer than synthetic pharmaceuticals.
5. Appeal to the aging population.

5 The nurse is teaching at a community wellness seminar when one participant asks, "How can I be sure that my herbal supplement is pure?" Which of the following labeling marks indicates that the product meets acceptable standards of purity?

1. USP verified dietary supplement mark
2. DEA prescriber number
3. FDA identification and regulation code
4. U.S. Customs Service integers

6 Polyherbacy may be of concern in the older adult population. A pharmacokinetic factor for this concern is that the older adult:

1. Is more likely to have difficulty using herbal products correctly.
2. May spend too much on herbal products rather than prescriptions.
3. May hold unrealistic expectations for the outcomes of herbal therapy.
4. May have age-related changes in liver or kidney function.

See Answers to Chapter Review in Appendix A.

References

Barnes, P. M., Bloom, B., & Nahin, R. L. (2008). *Complementary and alternative medicine use among adults and children: United States, 2007* (CDC National Health Statistics Reports No. 12). Retrieved from http://nccam.nih.gov/news/camstats/2007

Broussard, C. S., Louik, C., Honein, M. A., & Mitchell, A. A. (2010). Herbal use before and during pregnancy. *American Journal of Obstetrics & Gynecology, 202,* 443.e1–443.e6. doi:10.1016/j.ajog.2009.10.865

Harris, P. E., Cooper, K. L., Relton, C., & Thomas, K. J. (2012). Prevalence of complementary and alternative medicine (CAM) use by the general population: A systematic review and update. *The International Journal of Clinical Practice, 66,* 924–939. doi:10.1111/j.1742-1241.2012.02945.x

Selected Bibliography

Anastasi, J. K., Chang, M., & Capilli, B. (2011). Herbal supplements: Talking with your patients. *The Journal for Nurse Practitioners, 7*, 29–35. doi:10.1016/j.nurpra.2010.06.004

Anderson, E. (2009). Complementary therapies and older adults. *Topics in Geriatric Rehabilitation, 25*, 320–328. doi:10.1097/TGR.0b013e3181bdd560

Barnes, J. (2012). Adverse drug reactions and pharmacovigilance of herbal medicines. In J. Talbott & J. K. Aronson (Eds.), *Stephens' detection and evaluation of adverse drug reactions: Principles and practice* (6th ed., pp. 645–683). Chichester, United Kingdom: John Wiley & Sons. doi:10.1002/9780470975053

Booth-LaForce, C., Scott, C. S., Heitkemper, M. M., Cornman, B. J., Lan, M. C., Bond, E. F., & Swanson, K. M. (2010). Complementary and alternative medicine (CAM) attitudes and competencies of nursing students and faculty: Results of integrating CAM into the nursing curriculum. *Journal of Professional Nursing, 26*, 293–300. doi:10.1016/j.profnurs.2010.03.003

DerMarderosian, A., and Beutler, J. A., (2012). *The review of natural products* (7th ed.). St. Louis, MO: Wolters Kluwer.

Fontaine, K. L. (2014). *Complementary and alternative therapies for nursing practice* (4th ed.). Upper Saddle River, NJ: Prentice Hall.

Hung, S. K., & Ernst, E. (2010). Herbal medicine: An overview of the literature from three decades. *Journal of Dietary Supplements, 7*, 217–226. doi:10.3109/19390211.2010.487818

Izzo, A., & Edzard, E. (2009). Interactions between herbal medicines and prescribed drugs: An updated systematic review. *Drugs, 69*, 1777–1798. doi:10.2165/11317010-000000000-00000

Kennedy, D. A., & Seely, D. (2010). Clinically based evidence of drug–herb interactions: A systematic review. *Expert Opinion on Drug Safety, 9*, 79–124. doi:10.1517/14740330903405593

Kunle, O. F., Egharevba, H. O., & Ahmadu, P. O. (2012). Standardization of herbal medicines—A review. *International Journal of Biodiversity and Conservation, 4*, 101–112. doi:10.5897/IJBC11.163

Lapenna, S., Gemen, R., Wollgast, J., Worth, A., Maragkoudakis, P., & Caldeira, S. (2013). Assessing herbal products with health claims. *Critical Reviews in Food Science and Nutrition* (Published online April 1, 2013). doi:10.080/10408398.2012.726661

Prieto-Gracia, J. M. (2013). Common herbal-drug and food-drug interactions. *Nurse Prescribing, 11*, 241.

UNIT

2

Pharmacology and the Nurse–Patient Relationship

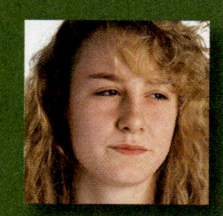 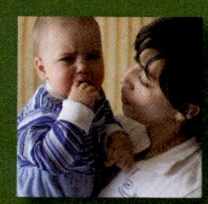 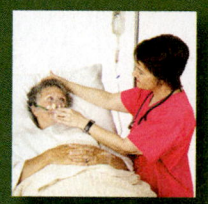 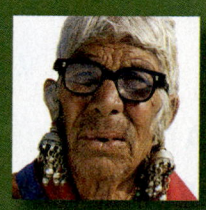

CHAPTER 8   Pharmacotherapy During Pregnancy and Lactation / 92

CHAPTER 9   Pharmacotherapy of the Pediatric Patient / 103

CHAPTER 10   Pharmacotherapy of the Geriatric Patient / 116

CHAPTER 11   Individual Variations in Drug Responses / 126

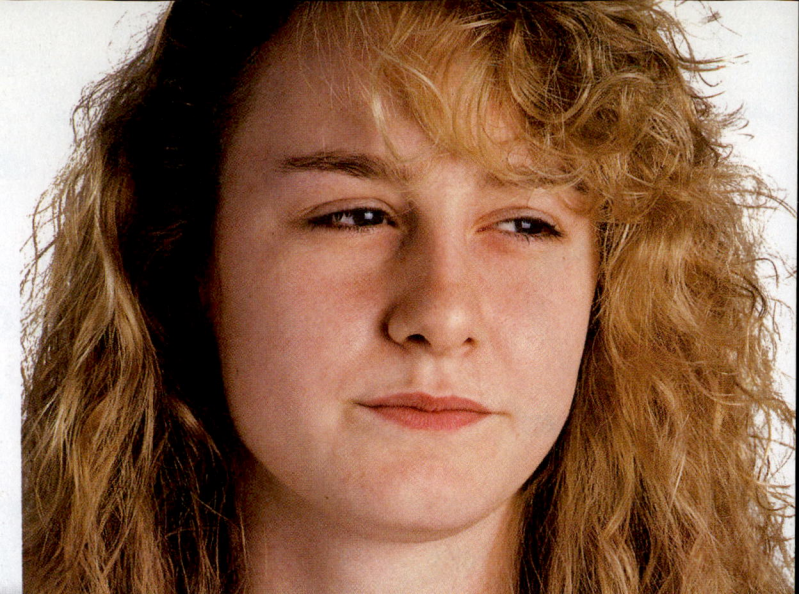

"I've been so nauseated every morning during the past 3 weeks and I'm late with my period. Please tell me I'm not pregnant. I just can't deal with a child right now."

Patient "May David"

CHAPTER

8 Pharmacotherapy During Pregnancy and Lactation

LEARNING OUTCOMES

After reading this chapter, the student should be able to:

1. Discuss the rationale for using drugs during pregnancy and lactation.
2. Describe physiological changes during pregnancy that may affect the absorption, distribution, metabolism, and excretion of drugs.
3. Describe the placental transfer of drugs from mother to infant.
4. Differentiate among the U.S. Food and Drug Administration pregnancy risk categories.
5. Explain how drugs administered during the different stages of fetal development affect the potential for teratogenic effects.
6. Identify factors that influence the transfer of drugs into breast milk.
7. Describe signs of adverse drug reactions in the breast-feeding infant.
8. Outline important points in patient and family education regarding drug use during pregnancy and lactation.

CHAPTER OUTLINE

▶ Rationale for Drug Use During Pregnancy and Lactation

▶ Pharmacotherapy During Pregnancy

    Changes in Pharmacokinetic Variables During Pregnancy

    Placental Transfer of Drugs from Mother to Infant

    FDA Fetal Risk Categories

    Adverse Drug Effects During Pregnancy

▶ Pharmacotherapy During Lactation

    Transfer of Drugs into Breast Milk

    Adverse Drug Effects During Lactation

Administering medications to pregnant women requires special precautions. The nurse must be aware of the physiological changes occurring in the pregnant woman along with the developmental stage of the fetus. The nurse must also be able to identify potential adverse drug events occurring in both the mother and the fetus. This chapter describes the pharmacokinetic changes that occur during pregnancy and explains the importance of carefully monitoring the pharmacotherapy of pregnant and lactating women. Emphasis is placed on drugs to avoid or use cautiously, efforts to prevent adverse effects, and the importance of patient and family education.

Rationale for Drug Use During Pregnancy and Lactation

8.1 Women frequently use drugs during pregnancy and lactation.

The nurse caring for the pregnant or lactating woman faces the challenge of concurrently being responsible for the health and safety of two persons, knowing that most medications cross the placenta and are secreted in breast milk. Despite potential risks to the fetus, first-trimester use of prescription drugs has increased by more than 60% in the past 30 years (Mitchell et al., 2011). Approximately 90% of pregnant women report taking at least one medication, with an estimated 70% taking at least one prescription medication (Centers for Disease Control and Prevention [CDC], 2013b). With the availability of the Internet, women may choose to search for drug information online, but Peters et al. (2013) found that even lists of "safe" drugs found in web-based information were inadequate and might provide false reassurance to women about the adverse effects posed by drugs taken during pregnancy.

Health care providers always exercise great caution when initiating pharmacotherapy during pregnancy or lactation. Drug therapy is often postponed until after delivery and lactation, and if that is not possible, safer nonpharmacologic alternatives may be implemented. Certain acute and chronic conditions, however, must be managed with medications during pregnancy. These include the following:

- **Treatment of certain preexisting illnesses.** If the patient has preexisting epilepsy, asthma, hypertension, or a psychiatric disorder, it would be unwise to discontinue pharmacotherapy during pregnancy or lactation.

- **Treatment of complications related to pregnancy.** Thromboembolic disorders, gestational diabetes, and gestational hypertension may occur during pregnancy and must be treated for the safety of both the mother and growing fetus.

- **Treatment of conditions unrelated to pregnancy.** Antibiotics may be necessary to treat infections acquired during pregnancy. Acute urinary tract infections and sexually transmitted infections have the potential to harm the mother or fetus if undetected or inadequately treated.

The goal of pharmacotherapy in pregnant patients is to treat the mother without causing ill effects for the fetus. Often, pharmacotherapy can be safely conducted with the same drugs and dosage levels as in nonpregnant patients. In other cases, a medication may need to be discontinued, changed to a lower dose, or replaced with a safer drug. In all pregnant patients, health care providers must carefully consider the therapeutic value of a given medication against its potential adverse effects.

Pharmacotherapy During Pregnancy

8.2 Physiological changes during pregnancy can alter normal pharmacokinetic responses.

Most body systems in a woman undergo predictable changes during pregnancy. Some organs increase in size. Some physiological activities speed up while others slow down, altering the pharmacokinetic responses to drugs. The health care provider must understand these changes in maternal physiology when prescribing drugs for the pregnant woman (Figure 8.1).

Absorption: During pregnancy, increased levels of progesterone cause a decrease in gastric tone and intestinal motility, resulting in delayed gastric emptying. Drugs remain longer in the gastrointestinal (GI) tract, leading to extended time for absorption of oral drugs. High estrogen levels in the pregnant woman cause increased hydrochloric acid production in the stomach, which may affect the absorption of certain acid labile drugs. Furthermore, as the enlarging uterus rises into the abdomen it presses up against the stomach, leading to slower gastric emptying. Medications may take a longer time to be absorbed and distributed, thus prolonging their onset and durations of action. Some women experience nausea and vomiting and are unable to take oral medications during early pregnancy.

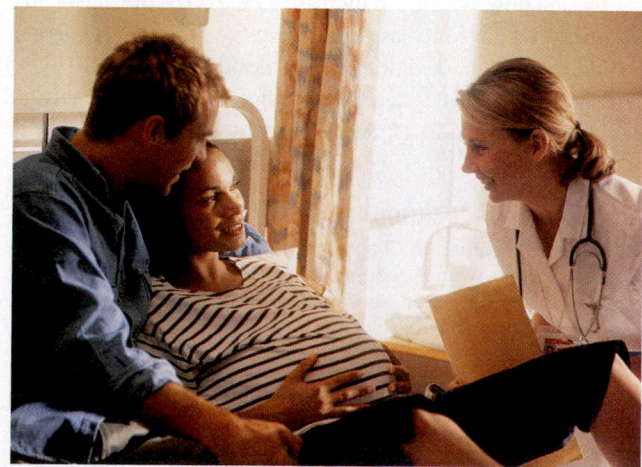

Figure 8.1 Teaching women about the safety of drug use during pregnancy is an essential component of nursing care.
Courtesy of Flying Colors/Photodisc/Getty.

Progesterone also increases pulmonary blood flow, respiratory tidal volume, and minute volume by 40%. As a result, respiratory agents such as cromolyn (Intal) are absorbed in larger quantities, leading to higher serum drug levels.

Distribution: Distribution of drugs during pregnancy is affected by changes in total body water, which may increase by over 50%. This increase leads to greater hemodilution of plasma proteins and drugs. Because the plasma proteins are diluted, fewer are available to bind with drugs, thus causing a higher concentration of "free" drug in the plasma. This results in more drug molecules being available for transfer across the placenta or to be secreted in breast milk. Highly lipophilic drugs are distributed into the lipid-rich breast milk and are ultimately passed to the breast-feeding infant. A woman's heart rate may increase up to 15 beats per minute during pregnancy, leading to greater drug distribution.

Metabolism: It was originally thought that metabolism was the pharmacokinetic process least affected by pregnancy. There is a growing body of evidence that suggests metabolism is significantly altered throughout pregnancy (Giaginis, Theocharis, & Tsantili-Kakoulidou, 2012; Isoherranen & Thummel, 2013; Jeong, 2010; Shea, Oberlander, & Rurak, 2012). Some of the cytochrome P450 enzymes increase, noticeably CYP2D6 and 3A4, whereas others such as CYP1A2 decrease. Researchers have also found that a single CYP enzyme system may have multiple alleles, different genetic forms of the same enzyme. Because of these unique differences among individuals, even knowing the pathway through which a drug is metabolized will not always accurately predict how that drug will be metabolized. The fetal liver is still developing throughout this time and lacks the ability to metabolize most drugs received from the mother's system. Lifestyle factors, such as smoking and eating broccoli or other cruciferous vegetables, may also alter how an enzyme system metabolizes a drug. Until more is learned about how drug metabolism is affected during pregnancy, providers use caution when prescribing any drug during this time and limit prescriptions to those drugs known to have demonstrated a low-risk safety profile.

Excretion: Excretion of drugs during pregnancy is enhanced by renal plasma flow, which can increase 50% to 70% during the first two trimesters. This increased flow leads to a higher glomerular filtration rate and marked decreases in blood urea nitrogen (BUN) and creatinine levels. Because these changes result in the increased renal elimination of drugs, doses of many medications must be adjusted.

CONNECTION Checkpoint 8.1

From what you learned in Chapter 3, what effects on drug metabolism may occur if a woman required any of the following drugs during pregnancy: acetaminophen, sertraline, or propranolol? (See Table 3.1 for specific CYP450 enzymes listings.) *See Answer to Connection Checkpoint 8.1 on student resource website.*

8.3 Many drugs pass from mother to infant via the placenta.

The **placenta** is a temporary organ that allows for nutrition and gas exchange between the mother and fetus. As much as 10% of the mother's cardiac output circulates through the placenta.

Although the blood of the mother does not circulate through the fetus, capillary-like structures in the placenta allow an extensive exchange of substances. The placenta offers a degree of protective filtration of the maternal blood, preventing certain harmful substances from reaching the fetus. Nutritional substances such as vitamins, fatty acids, glucose, and electrolytes freely pass from mother to fetus.

Most drugs cross the placenta and pass from mother to fetus by simple diffusion. A few drugs cross by way of active transport. The role the placenta plays in drug metabolism is under study. It is known that metabolic enzymes are present in the placenta and likely contribute to drug metabolism. What is not known with certainty is how a particular drug is metabolized through the placenta. Some drugs may be metabolized extensively and presumably have little or no effect on the developing fetus, whereas other drugs may be altered to become toxic metabolites capable of harm. It should be understood that drugs may cause fetal harm without crossing the placenta or entering the fetal blood. For example, certain drugs may cause constriction of placental blood vessels, impairing nutrient exchange. Other drugs can alter maternal physiology to such an extent that the fetus is affected.

Multiple factors impact the transfer of drugs across the placenta. These variables are the same as those affecting the movement of substances across other biologic membranes (see Chapter 3).

- **Plasma drug level in the mother.** In general, the higher the dose taken by the mother, the greater the amount of drug available to cross the placenta and affect the fetus. This is the rationale for prescribing the lowest effective doses of drugs during pregnancy.

- **Solubility of the drug.** Highly lipid-soluble drugs will cross the placental barrier more easily than water-soluble drugs.

- **Molecular size.** Small molecules such as alcohol with molecular weights (MW) less than 300 easily cross the placental barrier; those with MW greater than 500 are slower to cross. Large drugs such as heparin, with MW greater than 1,000, do not generally cross the placenta to the fetus.

- **Protein binding.** When a drug is bound to maternal plasma proteins, the drug–protein complex is too large to cross the placental membrane. Thus drugs that are highly protein bound are more likely to cross the placenta more slowly and in lower doses compared to nonbound drugs.

- **Drug ionization.** Nonionized drugs cross the placenta more easily than ionized drugs. The maternal serum pH is slightly higher than that of the fetus. Upon reaching the relatively acidic environment of the fetus, drugs that are weak bases become ionized. This effectively traps them on the fetal side of the placenta, because ionized drugs cannot recross the placental membrane back to the mother (ion trapping). An example is nicotine (a weak base), which can appear in higher concentrations in the fetus than in the mother due to ion trapping.

- **Blood flow to the placenta.** Decreased uterine blood flow may cause drugs to remain trapped in the fetus for extended periods, resulting in fetal adverse effects. During labor the patient is usually instructed to remain in the lateral position during active uterine contractions to prevent pressure on the aorta and vena cava. Pressure on these vessels will obstruct uterine blood flow and may cause drug accumulation in the fetus.

The most common antidepressants, the selective serotonin reuptake inhibitors (SSRIs), when taken by pregnant women, may increase the risk of preterm labor and may cause withdrawal symptoms in newborns that include agitation, irritability, trouble feeding, sleep disturbances, and convulsions (Hayes et al., 2012). Health care providers have been advised to taper dosages of SSRIs during the third trimester so that the fetus receives no drug through the placenta for at least 7 to 10 days prior to birth.

8.4 The U.S. Food and Drug Administration pregnancy risk categories are used as guides in prescribing medications during pregnancy.

In an effort to protect an unborn child from negative drug effects, the U.S. Food and Drug Administration (FDA) has developed drug **pregnancy categories** that rate medications as to their risks during pregnancy. Table 8.1 shows the five pregnancy categories, which guide the health care team and the patient in selecting drugs that are least hazardous for the fetus. Nurses who treat pregnant women must be knowledgeable of the drug pregnancy categories for all medications commonly prescribed for their patients.

Testing drugs in humans to determine their ability to cause birth anomalies is unethical and prohibited by law. Although drugs are tested in pregnant laboratory animals, the structure of the human placenta is unique among mammals. The FDA pregnancy drug categories are extrapolated from these animal data and may only be crude approximations of the actual risk to a human fetus. In a few cases, human data are available to show pregnancy risks. Regardless of the pregnancy category, no prescription drug, over-the-counter (OTC) medication, or herbal product should be taken during pregnancy unless the health care provider verifies that the therapeutic benefits to the mother clearly outweigh the potential risks for the unborn.

In a few cases, drugs are encouraged during pregnancy because they improve the health of the mother. For example, women are encouraged to take multivitamins and iron due to the increased metabolic demands placed on the mother during pregnancy. Vitamin B_9 (folic acid) has been found to prevent fetal spinal cord defects. These agents are designated as pregnancy category A drugs and are safe for use during pregnancy. The category B agents are also considered safe. For example, the penicillin and macrolide antibiotics are category B agents that can be safely used to treat infections during pregnancy.

The category C drugs make up to two thirds of all prescription medications. The primary reason for a category C designation is that sufficient data are simply not available to decide whether the drug is safe or whether it may cause birth defects. Category C agents should be avoided during pregnancy because there is a possibility they may cause fetal abnormalities.

All category D and X drugs should be avoided during pregnancy because they have the potential to cause birth defects. For example, angiotensin-converting enzyme (ACE) inhibitors, a class of antihypertensive drugs, are known to impede intrauterine growth and increase the risk of fetal demise. Use of certain other antihypertensive drugs can result in renal atrophy. Certain antibiotics such as tetracyclines cause permanent staining of deciduous teeth. A category X drug such as isotretinoin (Accutane), which is used for serious acne, can cause fetal brain damage. Other category X drugs such as misoprostol (Cytotec), a GI protective agent, may lead to abortion, and thalidomide (Thalomid), an immunosuppressant, has been known to cause fetal limb abnormalities. Additionally, alcohol, nicotine,

TABLE 8.1	**Current FDA Pregnancy Category Ratings with Examples**	
Risk Category	**Interpretation**	**Drugs**
A	Adequate, well-controlled studies in pregnant women have not shown an increased risk of fetal abnormalities to the fetus in any trimester of pregnancy.	Prenatal multivitamins, insulin, thyroxine, folic acid
B	Animal studies have revealed no evidence of harm to the fetus; however, there are no adequate and well-controlled studies in pregnant women. OR Animal studies have shown an adverse effect, but adequate and well-controlled studies in pregnant women have failed to demonstrate risk to the fetus in any trimester.	Penicillins, cephalosporins, azithromycin, acetaminophen, ibuprofen in the first and second trimesters
C	Animal studies have shown an adverse effect and there are no adequate and well-controlled studies in pregnant women. OR No animal studies have been conducted and there are no adequate and well-controlled studies in pregnant women.	Most prescription medicines; antimicrobials such as clarithromycin, fluoroquinolones, and Bactrim; selective serotonin reuptake inhibitors (SSRIs); corticosteroids; and most antihypertensives
D	Adequate well-controlled or observational studies in pregnant women have demonstrated a risk to the fetus. However, the benefits of therapy may outweigh the potential risk. For example, the drug may be acceptable if needed in a life-threatening situation or serious disease for which safer drugs cannot be used or are ineffective.	ACE inhibitors, alcohol, alprazolam, angiotensin receptor blockers (ARBs) in the second and third trimesters, carbamazepine, cyclophosphamide, gentamicin, lithium carbonate, methimazole, mitomycin, nicotine, nonsteroidal anti-inflammatory drugs (NSAIDs) in the third trimester, penicillamine, phenytoin, propylthiouracil, streptomycin, tetracyclines, and valproic acid
X	Adequate well-controlled or observational studies in animals or pregnant women have demonstrated positive evidence of fetal abnormalities or risks. The use of the product is contraindicated in women who are or may become pregnant. There is no indication for use in pregnancy.	Clomiphene, fluorouracil, isotretinoin, leuprolide, menotropins, methotrexate, misoprostol, nafarelin, oral contraceptives, raloxiphene, ribavirin, statins, temazepam, testosterone, thalidomide, and warfarin

TABLE 8.2 Street Drugs and Their Potential Effects During Pregnancy

Drug	Potential Effects
Amphetamines/methamphetamine	Increased risk of pregnancy complications, such as premature birth and placental problems Possible birth defects, including heart defects and cleft lip or palate After birth, the infant may have withdrawal-like symptoms such as jitteriness, drowsiness, and breathing problems
Cannabis/marijuana	Reduced fertility in both men and women Slowed fetal growth Slightly decreased length of pregnancy After birth, the infant may have withdrawal-like symptoms such as excessive crying and trembling
Club drugs such as PCP, ketamine, and LSD	After birth, the infant may have withdrawal symptoms Increased risk of learning and behavioral problems
Cocaine	Increased risk of miscarriage or premature birth Low birth weight with increased risk of health problems such as mental retardation and cerebral palsy, and even death Increased risk of birth defects involving the urinary tract and possibly other birth defects May cause an unborn baby to have a stroke, which can result in irreversible brain damage or a heart attack, and sometimes death Placental problems, including placental abruption, which can lead to heavy bleeding that can be life threatening for both mother and baby After birth, the infant may have mild behavioral disturbances, jitteriness, and irritability; may startle and cry at the gentlest touch or sound Increased risk of sudden infant death syndrome (SIDS)
Heroin	Increased risk of serious pregnancy complications, including poor fetal growth, premature rupture of the membranes, premature birth, and stillbirth Low birth weight often combined with breathing problems and possibility of lifelong disabilities Increased risk of birth defects After birth, the infant may have withdrawal symptoms such as fever, sneezing, trembling, irritability, diarrhea, vomiting, continual crying, and, occasionally, seizures Increased risk of SIDS
Inhalants, glues, and solvents	Miscarriage, slow fetal growth, preterm birth, and birth defects

Adapted from "Street Drugs and Pregnancy," March of Dimes, 2013.

and certain illicit drugs such as cocaine may negatively affect the unborn child. Selected abused substances and their effects on the fetus are listed in Table 8.2.

There are several limitations of the current drug classification system used to assess drug safety in the pregnant patient. For example, the current A, B, C, D, and X pregnancy labeling system gives no specific clinical information to help guide nurses or their patients as to whether a medication is truly safe. Furthermore, the system does not indicate how the dose should be adjusted during pregnancy or lactation. To address these issues, the FDA is updating these categories to provide more descriptive information on the risks and benefits of taking each medication. The new labels will include pharmacokinetic and pharmacodynamic information that will suggest optimum doses for the childbearing patient (FDA, 2008). To gather this information, the FDA is encouraging all pregnant women who are taking medications to join a pregnancy registry that will survey drug effects on both the patient and the fetus or newborn. Evaluation of a large number of pregnancies is needed to determine the effects of medicine on babies.

8.5 The stage of development has an important influence on adverse drug effects in the embryo and fetus.

The effects of drugs on the fetus depend on the stage of fetal development and the dosage received by the fetus. For the vast majority of medications, very little scientific data are available on the effects of drugs on the human fetus. Lack of knowledge does not mean they are safe; these drugs have the potential for causing adverse drug reactions in the fetus and, in some cases, may cause fetal malformations.

A **teratogen** is any substance, organism, or physical agent that interferes with growth or development of the embryo or fetus and produces a permanent abnormality or death. The word derives from the Greek "gennan" (to produce) and "terata" (monster). The baseline incidence of teratogenic events is approximately 3% of all pregnancies. Potential fetal consequences of drug use include intrauterine fetal death, physical malformations, growth impairment, behavioral abnormalities, and neonatal toxicity.

There are no "absolute" teratogens. Whether or not a drug produces a teratogenic effect depends on multiple, complex factors. Like other effects of drugs, there is a dose–response relationship, with risk increasing with higher doses. The timing of drug therapy and the stage of fetal development critically affect the risk for possible fetal consequences. Because of the constant changes that occur during fetal development, the specific risk is dependent on when during gestation the drug is administered. A well-known example is the drug thalidomide, which causes its fetal effects from day 35 to day 48 after the last menstrual period. The specific malformation is linked to the time of exposure: 35 to 37 days, no ears; 39 to 41 days, no arms; 41 to 43 days, no uterus; 45 to 47 days, no tibia; and 47 to 49 days, triphalangeal thumbs.

Preimplantation period: Weeks 1 to 2 of the first trimester are known as the preimplantation phase. Before implantation, the developing embryo has not yet established a blood supply with the mother. This is sometimes called the "all-or-none" period because exposure to a teratogen either causes death of the embryo or has no effect. Drugs are less likely to cause congenital malformations during this period because the baby's organ systems have not yet begun to form. Drugs such as nicotine, however, can create a negative environment for the embryo and potentially cause intrauterine growth retardation.

Embryonic period: During the embryonic period, from 3 to 8 weeks postconception, internal structures develop rapidly. This is the period of maximum sensitivity to teratogens. Teratogenic agents taken during this phase can lead to structural malformation and spontaneous abortion. The specific abnormality depends on which organ is forming at the time of exposure.

Fetal period: The fetal phase is from 9 to 40 weeks postconception or until birth. During this time there is continued growth and maturation of the baby's organ systems. Blood flow to the placenta increases and placental vascular membranes become thinner. Such alterations maximize the transfer of substances from the maternal circulation to the fetal blood. As a result, the fetus may receive larger doses of medications and other substances taken by the mother. Because the fetus lacks mature metabolic enzymes and efficient excretion mechanisms, medications will have a prolonged duration of action within the unborn child. Exposure to teratogens during the fetal period is more likely to produce slowed growth or impaired organ function, rather than gross structural malformations.

The nurse caring for the pregnant woman must differentiate adverse drug effects from the normal symptoms of pregnancy. Nausea, vomiting, abdominal cramps, flushed skin, or diaphoresis may indeed be either normal symptoms of pregnancy or adverse drug effects. Fetal tachycardia may be due to drugs being taken by the mother or a fetal cardiac anomaly. During all stages of pregnancy, the nurse should help the mother assess medications and dietary supplements to determine if they are necessary and if adjustments are required. Impairments in the functioning of the mother's liver or kidneys may have a profound impact on maternal and fetal safety. Health care providers must consider these factors, so as to minimize the risk of toxicity to the mother and child. Through careful assessments, the nurse contributes greatly to this risk–benefit analysis, which is essential for protecting both the mother and her baby.

CONNECTION Checkpoint 8.2

From what you learned in Chapter 5, explain why the FDA might approve a drug, even though it is a known teratogen and can cause fetal abnormalities. *See Answer to Connection Checkpoint 8.2 on student resource website.*

Pharmacotherapy During Lactation

8.6 Transfer of drugs from mother to infant may occur through breast milk.

According to the Breastfeeding Report Card 2013 by the CDC (2013a), 77% of mothers breast-feed their infants and about 49% continue to breast-feed for at least 6 months. Breast-feeding is

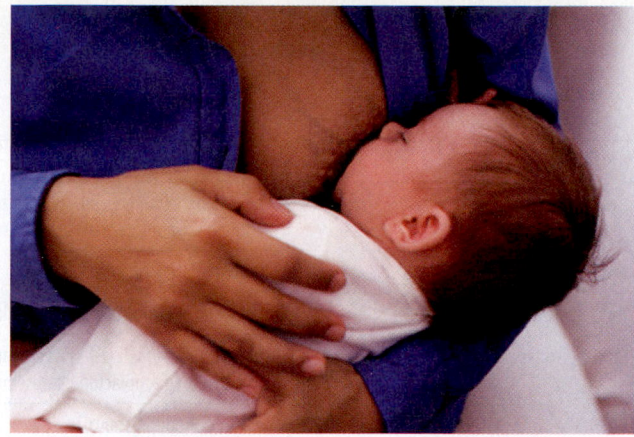

Figure 8.2 Nurses should teach lactating women to avoid all drugs, herbal products, or dietary supplements unless approved by their health care provider.
Courtesy of Dorling Kindersley, Inc.

highly recommended as a means of providing nutrition, emotional bonding, and immune protection to the neonate (Figure 8.2).

The majority of drugs are secreted into breast milk to some extent. Fortunately, there are relatively few instances in which breast-feeding must be discontinued due to medication use. For the few drugs that are absolutely contraindicated during lactation, equally effective, safer alternatives are usually available. Some of these agents are shown in Table 8.3. Although most medications probably cause no harm to the breast-feeding baby, their effects have not been fully studied.

Drugs enter breast milk primarily by passive diffusion. In the first week of life, the alveolar cells in the breast have large gaps between them, allowing drugs and other substances to penetrate the milk. By the second week of life the alveolar cells swell, closing the intracellular gaps and limiting the drug's access to the milk.

PharmFACT

Because the negative effects of tobacco smoking on the fetus are well documented, many women convert to nicotine-replacement therapy (NRT) during pregnancy. However, studies clearly demonstrate that many of the negative effects on the fetus are due to nicotine alone, and NRT may not be a safe alternative (Bruin, Gerstein, & Holloway, 2010).

It is important for the nurse to understand factors that influence the amount of drug secreted into breast milk. This allows the nurse to aid the patient in making responsible choices regarding lactation and in reducing exposure of her newborn to potentially harmful substances. The amount of drug that passes to the infant during lactation depends on multiple factors:

- **Plasma drug level in the mother.** The higher the dose of drug taken by the mother, the more will be secreted into breast milk. It is therefore standard practice that if a drug must be prescribed for a lactating patient, the lowest effective dose should be ordered.

- **Solubility of the drug.** Highly lipid-soluble drugs enter the milk at higher concentrations. Milk at the end of a feed contains

TABLE 8.3   Selected Drugs Compatible with Breast-Feeding

Class	Compatible Drugs	Drugs to Be Avoided
Analgesics (opioids)	codeine and morphine in occasional doses	—
Analgesics (nonopioid)	acetaminophen, aspirin, ibuprofen	—
Anti-infectives	penicillins, trimethoprim, sulfisoxazole (over 1 month of age), macrolides, aminoglycosides, cephalosporins, isoniazid, fluconazole, acyclovir	chloramphenicol, ciprofloxacin, tetracyclines, metronidazole
Antimigraine agents	propranolol	ergotamine
Antiseizure agents	carbamazepine, diazepam (single dose), valproic acid, phenytoin	ethosuximide
Cardiovascular agents	iron salts, heparin, warfarin, verapamil, lidocaine, digoxin, prazosin, nifedipine, spironolactone, furosemide	atenolol, ACE inhibitors, statins, hydrochlorothiazide
Central nervous system agents	tricyclic antidepressants	lithium carbonate
Cytotoxic agents and immunosuppressants	—	all drugs in this class should be avoided
Gastrointestinal agents	aluminum hydroxide, magnesium hydroxide, promethazine (single dose)	cimetidine, metoclopramide
Hormones	prednisone, hydrocortisone (single dose), insulin, thyroid hormone, oxytocin (short term)	oral contraceptives, estrogens, testosterone

Adapted from "Breastfeeding and Maternal Medication: Recommendations for Drugs in the Eleventh WHO Model List of Essential Drugs." Copyright © 2002 World Health Organization. Retrieved from http://whqlibdoc.who.int/hq/2002/55732.pdf

considerably more fat and may have a higher concentration of lipid-soluble drugs. Furthermore the percentage of lipids in milk increases progressively from day 1 to day 84 of lactation. Drugs that act on the central nervous system (CNS) are usually lipophilic and have a tendency to penetrate milk at higher concentrations.

- **Molecular size and protein binding.** Some drugs, such as heparin and insulin, are simply too large to pass through membranes by passive diffusion. In addition when drugs are highly protein bound, they are less likely to enter the milk than those that are free. The health care provider may choose drugs with greater protein binding capacity for the lactating mother to limit the amount secreted in milk.

- **Drug ionization.** Milk is slightly more acidic than plasma; the pH of milk is 7.2 and plasma 7.4. This pH gradient allows weakly basic drugs to transfer more readily into breast milk and accumulate due to ion trapping (see Chapter 4).

- **Drug half-life.** Drugs with short half-lives will be metabolized and eliminated quickly by the mother. This results in smaller amounts being secreted into milk.

Once ingested by the infant, a drug is subjected to the usual pharmacokinetic influences. The infant's stomach content is quite acidic; therefore, some drugs may be destroyed and have reduced bioavailability. Additionally some drugs are inactivated when ingested with calcium and protein-rich nutrients in the mother's milk. Some drugs by their nature are likely removed by the infant's liver during first-pass metabolism and never get to the plasma. It is important to remember that the baby's organs responsible for metabolizing and eliminating medications are immature and are not able to perform all the functions of adult organs.

Considering the many variables, it is not surprising that it is difficult to accurately predict the amount of maternal drug that will transfer to the infant plasma during lactation. Estimates of drug transference to breast milk range from less than 1% to 3%. Regardless of the amount, it is imperative for the nurse to teach the mother that many prescription medications, OTC drugs, and herbal products are secreted in breast milk and have the potential to affect her child. The same guidelines for drug use during pregnancy apply during lactation—drugs should only be taken if the benefits to the mother clearly outweigh the potential risks to the infant.

8.7 Drugs present in breast milk may cause adverse effects in the breast-feeding infant.

Although the concentration of drugs in breast milk is often very low (less than 3%), their effects on the infant can be serious. Common drug effects seen in breast-feeding infants are nonspecific and include diarrhea, constipation, sedation, and irritability. The nurse has an important responsibility to monitor for adverse drug effects in breast-feeding infants and to teach new mothers to do the same. Selected drugs that enter the breast milk and have been shown to produce adverse effects are shown in Table 8.4.

The nurse must inform the mother that all drugs of abuse are contraindicated during both pregnancy and breast-feeding. If she takes such drugs, her infant may experience withdrawal symptoms and test positive for the drug for several weeks to months following exposure.

In general, topical medications applied to the mother's skin are safe to use during lactation. The nurse must remind the mother, however, that the breast-feeding infant may ingest substances like vitamins E, A, or D in creams that are rubbed on her nipples to soften them.

CONNECTIONS (Complementary and Alternative Therapies

◖ Herbal Remedies as Galactagogues

Breast-feeding has been associated with improved infant outcomes but women who breast-feed may be concerned about whether or not they have an adequate supply of milk for their infant. A real or perceived inadequate milk supply may be a reason to stop breast-feeding, and women may consider the use of galactagogues, substances used to initiate or augment a mother's milk supply. Galactagogues include both prescribed drugs and herbal preparations. Because herbal preparations may be easily obtained over the counter, women may turn to these preparations when they are concerned about having an adequate milk supply.

Fenugreek, galega or goat's rue, and silymarin or milk thistle have all been used as herbal galactagogues. Studies have shown that substances such as fenugreek do have a positive effect on milk supply and may facilitate weight gain in infants (Turkyilmaz et al., 2011). However, herbal products have not been subjected to rigorous clinical trials and insufficient information is available about the amount of the herb product that crosses into the breast milk. Because of this, they should not be used as first-choice preparations when the milk supply is inadequate (Zuppa et al., 2010).

Other measures such as working with a lactation consultant to improve breast-feeding technique, improved maternal nutrition and fluid intake, and manually expressing milk are possible solutions that are low-risk options. If it is determined that a drug or herbal preparation may be advised, the woman should consult with her health care provider to determine the best choice.

TABLE 8.4 Classes of Medications that May Cause Serious Effects in a Baby Following Breastfeeding

Drug Class	Potential Adverse Effect
Antiepileptics (e.g. phenobarbitol, ethosuximide)	Sedation
Antineoplastics	Neutropenia
Beta-blockers	Lethargy, cyanosis and bradycardia
Benzodiazepines	Sedation and weight loss
Ergot alkaloids	Vomiting and diarrhea
NSAIDs	Increased bleeding
Opioids	Sedation and withdrawal symptoms
Phenothiazines	Sedation
Pseudoephedrine	Inhibition of milk production

Lactation risk categories have been developed that serve as guidelines for the health care provider to identify safe and contraindicated drugs during lactation. Table 8.5 summarizes these lactation categories.

CONNECTION Checkpoint 8.3

From what you learned in Chapter 3, how long would it take a 600-mg dose of a drug with a $t_{1/2}$ of 8 hours to reach five half-lives and be safe for a lactating patient concerned about passing the drug through her breast milk? How much drug would be left at that time? *See Answer to Connection Checkpoint 8.3 on student resource website.*

TABLE 8.5 Summary of Hale's Lactation Risk Categories

Category	Explanation	Examples
L1 Safest	Controlled studies in breast-feeding women demonstrate remote possibility of harm to the infant.	Acetaminophen, penicillins, Depo-Provera greater than 1 month after birth
L2 Safer	Studies in limited number of breast-feeding women show no increased adverse effect in the infant. Risk to the infant is remote.	Macrolides, cephalosporins, second-generation antihistamines, prednisone, SSRIs
L3 Moderately Safe	No controlled studies are available; risk to the infant is possible. Drugs should be prescribed only if the benefit outweighs the risk to the infant.	Bactrim, first-generation antihistamines, doxycycline
L4 Possibly Hazardous	Positive evidence of risk to the infant exists. Benefits of the drug to the mother may be acceptable despite the risk to the infant. May be needed in a life-threatening situation for a serious disease for which no other drug can be used.	Lithium, ergot preparations, high-dose corticosteroids
L5 Contraindicated	Documentation of significant risk or potential for risk to the infant. The risk of using the drug far outweighs the benefit from breast-feeding. The drug is contraindicated in the breast-feeding woman.	Radioactive isotopes, cocaine, heroin

From *Medications and Mother's Milk*, 14th ed., by T. W. Hale, 2010, Amarillo, TX: Hale Publishing Co. Adapted with permission.

CHAPTER

8

Understanding the Chapter

Key Concepts Summary

8.1 Women frequently use drugs during pregnancy and lactation.

8.2 Physiological changes during pregnancy can alter normal pharmacokinetic responses.

8.3 Many drugs pass from mother to infant via the placenta.

8.4 The U.S. Food and Drug Administration pregnancy risk categories are used as guides in prescribing medications during pregnancy.

8.5 The stage of development has an important influence on adverse drug effects in the embryo and fetus.

8.6 Transfer of drugs from mother to infant may occur through breast milk.

8.7 Drugs present in breast milk may cause adverse effects in the breast-feeding infant.

Case Study: Making the Patient Connection

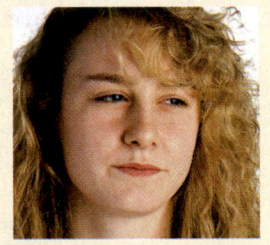

Remember the patient "May David" at the beginning of the chapter? Now read the remainder of the case study. Based on the information presented within this chapter, respond to the critical thinking questions that follow.

May David, a 22-year-old woman, comes to the clinic to obtain a pregnancy test. She has not had her menstrual period for the past 6 weeks but claims that infrequent menses are not unusual for her. She feels nauseous in the mornings but the feeling is only temporary. You ask May, "Is it possible that you might be pregnant?" May's response is "I doubt it, since we have always used a condom during intercourse." She goes on to explain that she has been taking an antiseizure medication for several years to control her epilepsy and is taking some herbal medicines for a feeling of well-being.

May's vital signs are: temperature, 36.7°C (98°F); pulse, 68 beats/minute; respiration, 18 breaths/minute; and blood pressure, 110/70 mmHg. She is 1.7 m (5 feet 6 inches) tall and is surprised that she has gained 2.3 kg

(5 lb) in the past 4 weeks, bringing her weight to 65.8 kg (145 lb). A urine specimen is sent to the laboratory for human chorionic gonadotropin (HCG). A complete physical examination is performed, followed by a vaginal examination via speculum. All physical findings were within normal limits except for the urine qualitative HCG, which is positive and quantitative HCG = 550, indicating pregnancy. May smokes approximately a half pack of cigarettes per day.

Critical Thinking Questions

1. What are some key points the nurse will discuss with May regarding her condition and the medication she is taking?

2. What education should the nurse provide for May regarding the use of medication during pregnancy?

3. While caring for May, the nurse must consider FDA pregnancy risk categories. In your own words explain these categories.

4. What effect does May's tobacco use possibly have on her unborn baby?

See Answers to Critical Thinking Questions on student resource website.

Additional Case Study

You are caring for Irina, an 18-year-old mother of a 6-month-old baby boy. She confides in you that she has experienced postpartum depression since her child was born. She tries to take care of herself but just does not feel very good most of the time. Her husband insists that she continue breast-feeding, but she is now having doubts. After a lengthy discussion Irina states, "The only time I feel good is when I smoke a 'joint' (marijuana) before feeding my son."

1. How should the nurse respond to Irina?

2. What teaching should the nurse carry out at this time?

See Answers to Additional Case Study on student resource website.

Chapter Review

1 A patient in her first trimester of pregnancy asks the nurse which medications should be avoided during pregnancy. The nurse's response is based on the knowledge that during pregnancy:

1. Most over-the-counter medications are safe.
2. When possible, drug therapy is postponed until after pregnancy and lactation.
3. It is wise to discontinue all drugs used in treating medical conditions.
4. The decision whether or not to take medication is the responsibility of the woman.

2 The nurse is preparing to discuss drug use during pregnancy with a group of nursing students. The main topic is the FDA drug classifications. Which of the following drugs should the nurse inform the students are the most detrimental to the fetus?

1. Category A
2. Category B
3. Category C
4. Category X

3 A pregnant patient asks the nurse what factors determine if a drug will cross the placenta. The nurse's response will be based on which of the following principles?

1. Highly lipid-soluble drugs cross the placental membrane more easily than low lipids.
2. The lower the lipid content, the easier it crosses the placental membrane.
3. Drugs with large molecular weight pass rapidly through the placental membrane.
4. Highly protein-bound drugs pass rapidly through the placental membrane.

4 The nurse is administering medication to a group of pregnant women. At which stage of fetal development will congenital malformations *least* likely occur?

1. 1 to 2 weeks
2. 3 to 4 weeks
3. 5 to 6 weeks
4. 7 to 8 weeks

5 The community health nurse is visiting a postpartum mother who is breast-feeding her 3.2 kg (7 lb) infant daughter. Which of the following statements, if made by the mother, indicates that further teaching is necessary? Select all that apply.

1. "When using over-the-counter medication, I should take only the lowest effective dose."
2. "The higher the dose of medication, the more likely it will be secreted into breast milk."
3. "I shouldn't take any drug during breast-feeding, even my prescriptions."
4. "Medication in liquid form should be avoided since it more readily enters the breast milk."
5. "Now that I'm no longer pregnant, I don't need to worry about the medicines affecting my baby."

6 The nurse is administering medications to a patient who is 32 weeks pregnant. Which of the following normal physiological principles associated with pregnancy will affect drug absorption?

1. Medications are absorbed and distributed more quickly in pregnant women.
2. There is greater hemoconcentration of drugs in pregnant patients.
3. Drugs remain longer in the gastrointestinal tract, leading to extended time for absorption.
4. Drug metabolism is highly affected by pregnancy.

See Answers to Chapter Review in Appendix A.

References

Bruin, J. E., Gerstein, H. C., & Holloway, A. C. (2010). Long-term consequences of fetal and neonatal nicotine exposure: A critical review. *Toxicological Sciences, 116,* 364–374. doi:10.1093/toxsci/kfq103

Centers for Disease Control and Prevention. (2013a). *Breastfeeding report card—United States 2010.* Retrieved from http://www.cdc.gov/breastfeeding/data/reportcard.htm

Centers for Disease Control and Prevention. (2013b). *Use of medications in pregnant women.* Retrieved from http://www.cdc.gov/pregnancy/meds/data.html

Giaginis, C., Theocharis, S., & Tsantili-Kakoulidou, A. (2012). Current toxicological aspects on drug and chemical transport and metabolism across the human placental barrier. *Expert Opinion on Drug Metabolism & Toxicology, 8,* 1263–1275. doi:10.1517/17425255.2012.699041

Grant, E., & Golightly, P. (2010). Safe use of medications in breastfeeding mothers. *Prescriber, 21,* 70–73. doi:10.1002/psb.681

Hale, T. W. (2010). *Medications and mother's milk* (14th ed.). Amarillo, TX: Hale.

Hayes, R. M., Wu, P., Shelton, R. C., Cooper, W. O., Dupont, W. D., Mitchel, E., & Hartert, T. V. (2012). Maternal antidepressant use and adverse outcomes: A cohort study of 228,876 pregnancies. *American Journal of Obstetrics and Gynecology, 207,* 49.e1–49.e9. doi:10.1016/j.ajog.2012.04.028

Isoherranen, N., & Thummel, K. E. (2013). Drug metabolism and transport during pregnancy: How does drug disposition change during pregnancy and what are the mechanisms that cause such changes? *Drug Metabolism and Disposition, 41,* 256–262. doi:10.1124/dmd.112.050245

Jeong, H. (2010). Altered drug metabolism during pregnancy: Hormonal regulation of drug-metabolizing enzymes. *Expert Opinion on Drug Metabolism & Toxicology, 6,* 689–699. doi:10.1517/17425251003677755

March of Dimes. (2013). *Street drugs and pregnancy.* Retrieved from http://www.marchofdimes.com/pregnancy/illicit-drug-use-during-pregnancy.aspx

Mitchell, A. A., Gilboa, S. M., Werler, M. M., Kelley, K. E., Louik, C., & Hernandez-Diaz, S. (2011). Medication use during pregnancy, with particular focus on prescription drugs: 1976–2008. *American Journal of Obstetrics and Gynecology, 205,* 51.e1–51.e8. doi:10.1016/j.ajog.2011.02.029

Peters, S. L., Lind, J. N., Humphrey, J. R., Friedman, J. M., Honein, M. A., Tassinari, M. S., … Brousard, C. S. (2013). Safe lists for medication in pregnancy: Inadequate evidence base and inconsistent guidance from Web-based information, 2011. *Pharmacoepidemiology and Drug Safety, 22,* 324–328. doi:10.1002/pds.3410

Shea, A. K., Oberlander, T. F., & Rurak, D. (2012). Fetal serotonin reuptake inhibitor exposure: Maternal and fetal factors. *Canadian Journal of Psychiatry, 57*(9), 523–529.

Turkyilmaz, C., Onal, E., Hirfanoglu, I. M., Turan, O., Koç, E., Ergenekon, E., & Atalay, Y. (2011). The effect of galactagogue herbal tea on breast milk production and short-term catch-up of birth weight in the first week of life. *Journal of Alternative and Complementary Medicine, 17,* 139–142. doi:10.1089/acm.2010.0090

U.S. Food and Drug Administration. (2008). *Content and format of labeling for human prescription drug and biological products:* *Requirements for pregnancy and lactation labeling.* Retrieved from http://www.regulations.gov/#!documentDetail;D=FDA-2006-N-0515-0001

World Health Organization. (2002). *Breastfeeding and maternal medication: Recommendations for drugs in the eleventh WHO model list of essential drugs.* Retrieved from http://whqlibdoc.who.int/hq/2002/55732.pdf

Zuppa, A. A., Sindico, P., Orchi, C., Carducci, C., Cardiello, V., Romagnoli, C., & Catenazzi, P. (2010). Safety and efficacy of galactagogues: Substances that induce, maintain, and increase breast milk production. *Journal of Pharmacy and Pharmaceutical Sciences, 13,* 162–174.

Selected Bibliography

The Academy of Breastfeeding Medicine Protocol Committee. (2011). ABM Clinical Protocol #9: Use of galactagogues in initiating or augmenting the rate of maternal milk secretion (First Revision January 2011). *Breastfeeding Medicine, 6*(1), 41–49. doi:10.1089/bfm.2011.9998

Briggs, G. G., Freeman, R. K., & Yaffe, S. J. (2014). *Drugs in pregnancy and lactation* (10th ed.). Philadelphia, PA: Lippincott Williams & Wilkins.

Cabbage, L. A., & Neal, J. L. (2011). Over-the-counter medications and pregnancy: An integrative review. *Nurse Practitioner, 36*(6), 22–28. doi:10.1097/01.NPR.0000397910.59950.71

Centers for Disease Control and Prevention. (2010). *Folic acid data and statistics.* Retrieved from http://www.cdc.gov/ncbddd/folicacid/data.html

Henderson, E., & Mackillop, L. (2011). Prescribing in pregnancy and during breast feeding: Using principles in clinical practice. *Postgraduate Medical Journal, 87,* 349–354. doi:10.1136/pgmj.2010.103606

Rowe, H., Baker, T., & Hale, T. W. (2013). Maternal medication, drug use, and breastfeeding. *Pediatric Clinics of North America, 60,* 275–294. doi:10.1016/j.pcl.2012.10.009

Thorpe, P. G., Gilboa, S. M., Hernandez-Diaz, S., Lind, J., Cragan, J. D., Briggs, G., … Honein, M. A. (2013). Medications in the first trimester of pregnancy: Most common exposures and critical gaps in understanding fetal risk. *Pharmacoepidemiology & Drug Safety, 22,* 1013–1018. doi:10.1002/pds.3495

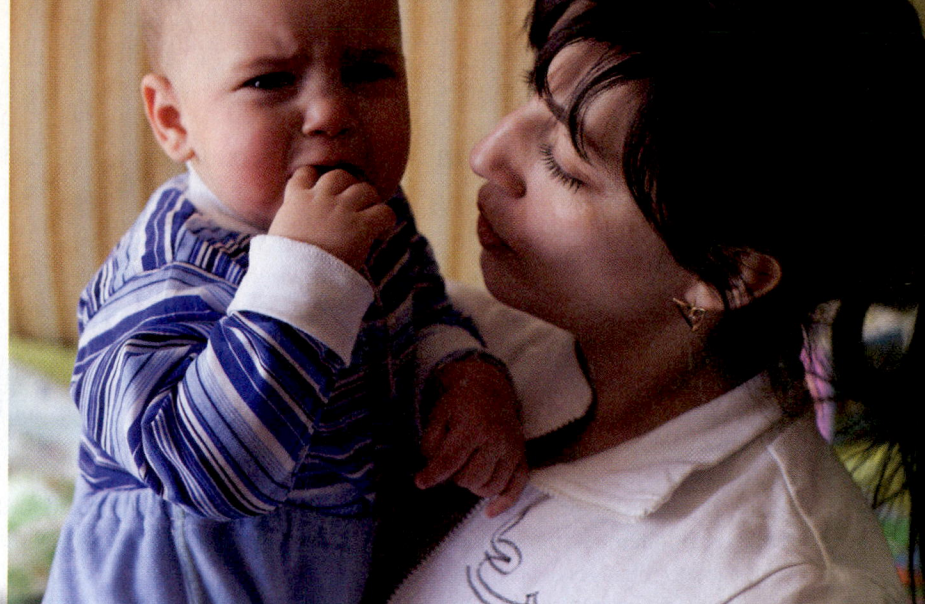

"Last evening my Timmy suddenly started vomiting and refused to eat. This morning he had two large, loose, green stools. Please help him."

Patient "Timmy's" mother, Ms. Thomas

CHAPTER

9

Pharmacotherapy of the Pediatric Patient

LEARNING OUTCOMES

After reading this chapter, the student should be able to:

1. Identify the purposes of the Food and Drug Administration Modernization Act of 1997, the Best Pharmaceuticals for Children Act of 2002, and the Pediatric Research Equity Act of 2003.

2. Explain how differences in pharmacokinetic variables can impact drug response in pediatric patients.

3. Discuss the nursing and pharmacologic implications associated with each of the pediatric developmental age groups.

4. Describe safe methods and techniques appropriate for administering medications to pediatric patients.

5. Explain several methods for accurately calculating drug doses in pediatric patients.

6. Describe nursing interventions for minimizing adverse effects during pediatric pharmacotherapy.

7. Propose appropriate teaching strategies to enhance medication adherence in pediatric patients.

CHAPTER OUTLINE

▸ Testing and Labeling of Pediatric Drugs

▸ Pharmacokinetic Variables in Pediatric Patients

▸ Pharmacologic Implications Associated with Growth and Development

▸ Medication Safety for Pediatric Patients

▸ Determining Pediatric Drug Dosages

▸ Adverse Drug Reactions in Children and Promoting Adherence

KEY TERMS

Best Pharmaceuticals for Children Act (BPCA), 105

body surface area (BSA) method, 110

body weight method, 110

directly observed therapy (DOT), 113

Food and Drug Administration (FDA) Modernization Act, 104

nomogram, 110

Pediatric Research Equity Act of 2003, 105

Beginning with conception, and continuing throughout the lifespan, the organs and systems within the body undergo predictable physiological changes that influence the absorption, metabolism, distribution, and elimination of medications. A child's body systems are in a constant state of development; therefore, the effects of drugs can often be unpredictable. Health care providers must recognize such changes to ensure that drugs are delivered in a safe and effective manner to children and patients of all ages.

The purpose of this chapter is to examine how principles of developmental physiology and lifespan psychology apply to drug administration. Emphasis is placed on drug dosage determination, maximizing therapeutic effects, and minimizing adverse effects. There is strong focus on patient and family education as well as on the importance of promoting adherence with pharmacotherapy.

Testing and Labeling of Pediatric Drugs

9.1 Legislation has attempted to improve the testing and labeling of pediatric drugs.

Pediatric patients receive large numbers of drugs, nearly all of which are the same as those given to adult patients. The distribution of the drug classes, however, is different in children. Cardiovascular drugs are the most commonly prescribed class in adults, whereas children are more likely to receive respiratory drugs and anti-infectives due to the high incidence of infectious diseases in this population. Table 9.1 provides a summary of the top drug prescriptions by age given to patients by outpatient providers (Chai et al., 2012). Antibiotics are the most commonly prescribed drugs,

followed by drugs for asthma. As the child's age increases, prescriptions for drugs used for attention deficit/hyperactivity disorder (ADHD) also increase.

Until the 1990s very little drug information was specifically targeted for the pediatric patient. Drug trials with pediatric patients were virtually unheard of, and data regarding the pharmacokinetics and adverse effects of most drugs were not well documented in this population. Most pediatric drugs were not available in dosage and delivery forms compatible with neonates or infants. Few drugs contained labeling information specifically for pediatric patients. Drugs that were found to be effective in adults were assumed to also be effective in children.

In 1997, the **Food and Drug Administration (FDA) Modernization Act** was passed, which gave financial incentives for pharmaceutical companies to conduct pediatric research in pharmacology. In exchange for providing pediatric labeling, the legislation provided drug companies with an additional 6 months of exclusivity, giving them the ability to market the drug with no competition. It is estimated that the additional 6 months of exclusivity has generated $14 billion for pharmaceutical companies conducting the pediatric studies (Pasquali, Burstein, Benjamin, Jr., Smith, & Li, 2010). From 1998 to 2011, 182 drugs were granted pediatric exclusivity by the FDA. The most frequent drug classes were antidepressants and mood stabilizers, angiotensin-converting enzyme (ACE) inhibitors, lipid-lowering preparations, HIV antivirals, nonsteroidal anti-inflammatory drugs (NSAIDs), and antirheumatic drugs.

Several flaws in the FDA Modernization Act were quickly noted. Many of the medications studied by the drug companies were chosen not for their potential value in children, but instead to extend their exclusivity and generate higher profits. The act

TABLE 9.1 Top Prescriptions for Children under 17 Years of Age (2002–2010)				
DRUG	**USE**	**RANKING BY PERCENTAGE OF PRESCRIPTIONS BY AGE**		
		0–23 Months	**2–11 Years**	**12–17 Years**
albuterol (Proventil)	Asthma	4	3	2
amoxicillin (Amoxil)	Antibiotic	1	1	4
amoxicillin/clavulanate (Augmentin)	Antibiotic	7	10	12
azithromycin (Zithromax, Zmax)	Antibiotic	2	2	3
cefdinir (Omnicef)	Antibiotic	5	8	No ranking
cephalexin (Keflex)	Antibiotic	15	9	15
fluticasone (Flonase)	Allergies	No ranking	6	9
methylphenidate (Ritalin)	ADHD	No ranking	5	1
montelukast (Singulair)	Asthma	20	4	6
prednisolone	Allergies, Inflammation	6	7	19

gave no incentives for studying off-patent (generic) drugs or those that have smaller markets. In 2002, Congress passed the **Best Pharmaceuticals for Children Act (BPCA)**, which authorized the FDA to contract for the testing of already approved pediatric drugs or when the pharmaceutical company declines the option of exclusivity. This act was reauthorized by Congress in 2007 with several new provisions. The **Pediatric Research Equity Act of 2003** (PREA) authorized the FDA to require research of pediatric uses for new drugs when an approved use includes a condition or conditions applicable to pediatric patients (Vernon, Shortenhaus, Mayer, Allen, & Golec, 2012). In addition to studying drugs, this mandate was extended to biologics in 2010, recognizing the increased development and use of these therapeutic agents in recent years.

The increased emphasis on pediatric drugs has led to more than 500 pediatric labeling changes associated with studies directly associated with the BPCA and PREA (National Research Council, 2012). Table 9.2 shows some of the changes that resulted from research studies conducted under these acts.

A concern is that the majority of the pediatric clinical trials are being conducted overseas, with many using children in underdeveloped countries. Presumably, the studies can be conducted more cheaply overseas due to fewer regulations. Questions have been raised about whether the children or their families understood the risks of participating (National Research Council, 2012).

Despite the limitations of current research, more information is available to guide the pharmacotherapy of the pediatric patient than previously. Drugs such as vaccines and antibiotics have adequate pediatric labeling. Unfortunately, the amount of information about the use of steroids and drugs for treating HIV, gastrointestinal (GI) disorders, pain, and hypertension in children is still minimal.

TABLE 9.2 Examples of Labeling Changes

Potential Risks or Hazards	Drug Name	Disease or Condition Treated	Summary of New Information Contained in Drug Labeling
Unnecessary exposure to ineffective therapies	sumatriptan (Imitrex)	Migraines	Five studies did not establish safety and effectiveness, and postmarketing experience showed that children were having serious adverse effects, such as stroke and vision loss. The product is not recommended for children under 18 years old.
	tolterodine (Detrol)	Overactive bladder and urge incontinence	The drug was not shown to be effective for children and appeared to show a possible increase in aggressive, hyperactive, and abnormal behavior.
	irinotecan (Camptosar)	Tumors	Children had more rapid disease progression and died more quickly. The labeling states that the drug should not be used to treat children with a particular kind of tumor.
	temozolomide (Temodar)	Astrocytoma	Effectiveness in children is not demonstrated.
Ineffective dosing	oxcarbazepine (Trileptal)	Partial seizures	Dose for children ages 2 to 4 and weighing less than 44 pounds is twice the dose per body weight compared to adults.
	methylphenidate (Ritalin)	Attention deficit/hyperactivity disorder	Children ages 13 to 17 eliminated the drug from their bodies faster than the comparison age group. Therefore, the dosing regimen may be increased to prevent ineffective dosing.
Overdosing	leflunomide (Arava)	Juvenile rheumatoid arthritis	Children weighing less than 88 pounds require a lower-than-expected dose. Overdosing on leflunomide, which has significant toxicity, could make the drug's risks to children outweigh its benefits.
Previously unlabeled adverse effects, including effect on growth and development	venlafaxine (Effexor)	Depression; generalized anxiety disorder	This drug is associated with an increased risk of suicidal thinking and behavior.
	ciprofloxacin (Cipro)	Complicated urinary tract infection or kidney infection	This drug is associated with increased adverse effects to joints or surrounding tissues for children.
	fentanyl (Duragesic)	Chronic pain	This drug should be used only by children age 2 or older who are opioid tolerant. Use by others can lead to life-threatening respiratory depression and death.
	budesonide (Pulmicort Respules)	Asthma	This drug is now labeled with safety information in patients as young as 6 months. Drug can cause growth suppression and pneumonia.
	fluoxetine (Prozac)	Depression, obsessive-compulsive disorder (OCD)	Effectiveness established in ages 7 to 17 with OCD and ages 8 to 17 with depression. Drug can cause height and weight suppression. It also has a possible link to suicide ideation.
	fluticasone	Flonase: Allergic rhinitis Intranasal	Effectiveness and safety have been established in ages 3 to 9 years with no effect on bone function.
		Cutivate: Dermatoses Topical	Subnormal adrenal function was noted. Drug is not recommended for children.

From *Pediatric Drug Research: Studies Conducted Under Best Pharmaceuticals for Children Act,* from the U. S. Government Accountability Office, 2007. Retrieved from http://www.gao.gov/new.items/d07557.pdf

Pharmacokinetic Variables in Pediatric Patients

9.2 Pharmacokinetic responses in children differ from those in adults.

As discussed in Chapters 3 and 4, drugs must reach their target cells in sufficient quantities to produce therapeutic effects. This depends on what the body does to the medication after it is administered (pharmacokinetics) and the mechanisms by which a drug changes the body (pharmacodynamics). The normal physiological changes of growth and development markedly affect pharmacokinetics and pharmacodynamics. The nurse must understand the unique actions of drugs in their pediatric patients to deliver safe and effective pharmacotherapy.

Absorption: Two primary factors have the potential to influence the oral absorption of drugs in pediatric patients: increased gastric pH and delayed gastric emptying. Low gastric acid production may enhance the absorption of acid-labile drugs such as ampicillin and penicillin and slow the absorption of weak acids like phenobarbital. This is especially true for premature infants and neonates. Gastric acid production may not reach adult levels until age 2 or 3.

Slowed gastric motility in very young children will keep the drug in the stomach longer. This will increase the absorption of drugs that are absorbed across the stomach mucosa, but slow the rate of drug absorption for drugs that rely on the intestine for absorption. The rate of bile salt secretion is diminished in premature infants and neonates, which will delay the absorption of lipid-soluble drugs and vitamins.

In the infant, relatively low blood flow to skeletal muscles leads to slow and erratic absorption of drugs administered by the intramuscular (IM) and subcutaneous routes. Weak muscle contractions may also contribute to the delayed absorption and distribution of IM drugs. IM injections are generally avoided due to their unpredictable absorption rates and their associated pain.

The skin of infants is thin and highly permeable, allowing lotions and topical drugs to be absorbed at a more rapid rate than adults. For example, use of topical corticosteroids in infants has been found to cause systemic effects such as adrenal insufficiency, hyperglycemia, and glaucoma. Care must be taken to prevent accidental overdose.

CONNECTION Checkpoint 9.1

From what you learned in Chapter 3, what effect does food in the stomach have on drug absorption? What effect might this have on neonates who are given frequent feedings? *See Answer to Connection Checkpoint 9.1 on student resource website.*

Distribution: Three main factors affecting drug distribution in children are the proportion of water to fat, immature liver function, and the underdeveloped blood–brain barrier.

Approximately 80% of a newborn's body weight is due to water. This gradually decreases to 60%, that of an adult, during the first year. The higher proportion of water dilutes water-soluble drugs such as furosemide (Lasix). In addition, water-soluble drugs will move out of the serum to other areas of the infant's body where water concentration is high. The overall effect is lower serum drug levels; higher doses may be needed to maintain adequate serum levels of the drug.

What about lipid-soluble drugs? Infants have a low percentage of body fat compared to adults. Lipid-soluble drugs that would normally be distributed to fat tend to stay in the blood, raising serum drug levels.

Prior to age 6 months, the child's immature liver produces very small amounts of plasma proteins. Drugs that normally bind to plasma proteins will now be present as "free" drugs in the serum. Drugs and endogenous substances such as bilirubin compete for the few available protein-binding sites. In some cases, previously bound substances or drugs may be displaced into the serum, leading to potential toxicity. Drugs with high levels of protein binding include ampicillin, morphine, phenytoin (Dilantin), and propranolol (Inderal).

The blood–brain barrier is a network of capillaries in the central nervous system (CNS) that form tight junctions, which prevent the passage of certain medications into the brain. Because the child's blood–brain barrier is not fully developed at birth, drugs and other chemicals can easily penetrate the CNS, resulting in heightened responses. The nurse caring for neonates taking drugs such as barbiturates that affect CNS functions should assess for potential toxicity. It is also possible that some drugs not intended for CNS penetration may access the brain, causing adverse CNS effects such as seizures, drowsiness, or dizziness.

Metabolism: The rate at which drugs are metabolized in children is impacted by the immaturity of the hepatic cytochrome P450 (CYP450) enzyme system. Metabolism is significantly slower in children, leading to reduced clearance rates and extended half-lives for drugs extensively metabolized by the liver. To avoid toxicity, drug doses must be accurately determined and administered at adequately spaced intervals to allow sufficient time for metabolic handling of the drug. The metabolic rate reaches adult levels by ages 3 to 5 years. Until then, the nurse should remain vigilant for signs of toxicity in patients taking drugs such as salicylates that are metabolized primarily in the liver.

The enzyme alcohol dehydrogenase is markedly reduced at birth, gradually increasing until age 5. This enzyme is responsible for detoxifying benzyl alcohol, a preservative found in parenteral drug formulations. Newborns are especially sensitive to the effects of benzyl alcohol and can develop "gasping syndrome," which can lead to respiratory and cardiovascular failure. The nurse must ensure that neonates do not receive products containing benzyl alcohol.

Excretion: The child's ability to effectively excrete most drugs depends on the maturity and function of the kidneys. For drugs to be excreted efficiently, the kidneys must have an adequate glomerular filtration rate and active tubular secretion and reabsorption functions. Young children have immature renal systems with slower renal clearance, resulting in accumulation of drugs excreted by the kidneys. Signs of nephrotoxicity include oliguria, urinary frequency, hematuria, cloudy urine, rising blood urea nitrogen (BUN) and creatinine, and fever. Although standard pediatric doses can be administered at approximately 3 to 5 months of age when the infant is able to concentrate urine, serum levels of nephrotoxic drugs such as gentamicin must be monitored closely to prevent adverse reactions.

Pharmacologic Implications Associated with Growth and Development

9.3 The role of the nurse in administering medications changes with each developmental age group.

The nurse responsible for administering pediatric medications must take into consideration the age, weight, and developmental level of the child. For the purposes of medication administration, the pediatric patient is defined as being any age from birth to 16 years and weighing less than 50 kg (110 lb). Additionally, children are classified as neonates, infants, toddlers, preschoolers, school-age children, and adolescents.

Growth is a term that characterizes the progressive increase in physical (body) size. *Development* refers to the functional evolution of the physical, psychomotor, and cognitive capabilities of a living being. Stages of growth and physical development usually go hand in hand in a predictable sequence, whereas psychomotor and cognitive development have a tendency to be more variable in nature.

From birth through adolescence, the growth and development of the pediatric patient mandate adjustments in pharmacotherapeutics above and beyond the calculation of doses. The child's ability to become an active (and willing) partner in his or her own wellness has important implications to nursing care and pharmacotherapeutics.

Pharmacotherapy of the infant: Infancy is the period from birth to 12 months of age. The first 28 days of life are referred to as the neonatal period. During this time, nursing care and pharmacotherapy are directed toward safety of the infant, proper dosing of prescribed drugs, and teaching parents how to administer medications properly. A primary goal is to have the child ingest the entire dose of medication without spitting it out because it is difficult to estimate the amount lost. If the child vomits immediately after taking the drug, the dose may be reordered. The following nursing interventions and parental teaching points are important for this age group:

- The infant should be held and cuddled while administering medications and offered a pacifier if the infant is on fluid restrictions caused by vomiting or diarrhea.

- Medications are often administered to infants via droppers into the eyes, ears, nose, or mouth. Oral medications should be directed to the inner cheek and the child given time to swallow the drug to avoid aspiration. If rectal suppositories are administered, the buttocks should be held together for 5 to 10 minutes to prevent expulsion of the drug before absorption has occurred.

- Special considerations must be observed when administering IM or intravenous (IV) injections to infants. Unlike adults, infants lack well-developed muscle masses, so the smallest needle appropriate for the drug should be used. For volumes less than 1 mL a tuberculin syringe is appropriate. The vastus lateralis is a preferred site for IM injections, because it has few nerves and is relatively well developed in infants. The gluteal site is usually contraindicated because of potential damage to the sciatic nerve, injury to which may result in permanent disability.

- Because of the lack of choices for injection sites, the nurse must rotate injection sites from one leg to the next to avoid overuse and to prevent inflammation and excessive pain.

- For IV sites, the feet and scalp veins may provide good venous access.

Pharmacotherapy of the toddler: Toddlerhood ranges from 1 to 3 years of age. By age 1 most of the pharmacokinetic responses are similar to that of the adult. The 2-year-old is able to metabolize drugs at a very rapid rate; therefore, the health care provider must adjust drug doses accordingly to maintain therapeutic levels.

During this period, a toddler displays a tremendous sense of curiosity. The child begins to explore, wants to try new things, and tends to place everything in the mouth. This becomes a major concern for medication and household product safety. Toddlers can swallow liquids and may be able to chew solid medications. When prescription drugs are supplied as flavored elixirs, it is important to teach parents that the child not be given access to the medications. Poisoning is extremely common at this age. Some of the most common poisonous substances involved in the exposure of children less than 6 years are analgesics, cough and cold preparations, topical ointments, and vitamins.

Administering medications to toddlers can be challenging for the nurse. At this stage, the child is rapidly developing increased motor ability and learning to assert independence but has extremely limited ability to reason or understand the relationship of medicines to health. Giving long, detailed explanations to the toddler will prolong the procedure and create additional anxiety. Short, concrete explanations followed by immediate drug administration are best for this age group. Physical comfort in the form of touching, hugging, or verbal praise following drug administration is important.

- Pharmaceutical companies often formulate pediatric medicines in sweet syrups to facilitate drug administration. Extra caution should be observed when medications are flavored. Toddlers may not differentiate between a food product and the medication and may ingest an overdose if the medication is not kept in a child-safe location.

- The nurse should mix unpleasant tasting oral medications with more appetizing food such as jam, syrup, or fruit puree, if possible. The medication may be followed with a carbonated beverage or mint-flavored candy. Nurses should teach parents to avoid placing medicine in milk, orange juice, or cereals because children may associate these healthy foods with unpleasant tasting medications in the future.

- IM injections for toddlers may be given into the vastus lateralis muscle. For IV medications, the nurse may choose to access the scalp or feet veins. Additional peripheral site options become available in late toddlerhood.

- Suppositories may be difficult to administer due to the child's resistance. For these invasive administration procedures, having a parent close by will usually reduce the toddler's anxiety and increase cooperation.

Pharmacotherapy of preschoolers: The preschool child ranges in age from 3 to 5 years. In general, principles of medication administration that pertain to the toddler also apply to this age group. Preschoolers tend to cooperate better in taking oral medications if they are crushed or mixed with food or flavored beverages.

- After a child has been walking for about a year, the ventrogluteal site may be used for IM injections because it causes less pain than the vastus lateralis site. Use of the dorsogluteal site has declined due to the risk of affecting the sciatic nerve. The scalp veins can no longer be used for IV access; peripheral veins are used for IV access.

- Like the toddler, the preschooler often physically resists medication administration. A brief explanation followed immediately by medication administration is usually the best method. Uncooperative children may need to be restrained, and patients over 4 years of age may require two adults to administer the medication.

- Before and after medication procedures, the child may benefit from opportunities to play-act troubling experiences with dolls. When the child plays the role of doctor or nurse by giving a "sick" doll a pill or injection, comforting the doll, and explaining that the doll will now feel better, the little actor feels safer and more in control of the situation.

Pharmacotherapy of the school-age child: The school-age child is between 6 and 12 years of age. Some refer to this period as the middle childhood years. Rapid physical, mental, and social development occur and early ethical–moral development begins

to take shape. During this time, most children remain relatively healthy, with respiratory infections and GI upsets being the most common complaints. When serious illness occurs at this age, the child may become confused and depressed because it is important for the child to be like his peers during this developmental age. When caring for an ill child, the nurse must be aware of possible nonadherence to treatment regimens.

The nurse is usually able to gain considerable cooperation from school-age children. Detailed explanations of the effects and importance of medications in maintaining wellness may be of value, because the child has developed some reasoning ability and can understand the relationship between receiving the medicine and feeling better. When children are old enough to welcome choices, they can be offered limited dosing alternatives to provide a sense of control and encourage cooperation. The option of taking one medication before another or the chance to choose which drink will follow a chewable tablet helps to distract children from the issue of whether they will take the medication at all. It also makes an otherwise strange or unpleasant experience a little more tolerable.

- Allowing children to feel that they are willing participants, rather than victims, in medication administration is an important foundation for adherence.

- Praise for cooperation is appropriate for any pediatric patient and will set the stage for successful medication administration in the future.

- School-age children can take chewable tablets and may be able to swallow tablets or capsules. Many still resist injections;

CONNECTIONS **Evidence-Based Practice**

◖ Acute Otitis Media vs. Otitis Media with Effusion

Clinical Question
What are the guidelines for treating AOM and OME?

Acute otitis media (AOM) is an inflammatory or infective process of the middle ear that may be bacterial, fungal, or viral in origin and is often associated with upper airway infection. It is common among young children, especially those exposed to cigarette smoke. Otitis media with effusion (OME) is fluid in the middle ear space without signs or symptoms of inflammation. AOM and OME may be concurrent, and together they represent one of the most common reasons to seek treatment for children in the United States. Eighty percent of all children will experience at least one episode of AOM by age 3 (Natal, 2011). Persistent OME without AOM may lead to hearing loss and language difficulties, and, although rare, AOM may lead to complications such as acute mastoiditis or localized brain abscess. In 2004, the American Association of Family Physicians conducted a systematic review of practices in the diagnosis and treatment of AOM and OME and developed evidence-based practice guidelines.

Evidence
Children with structural differences in the ear or eustachian tubes (e.g., children under 6 months of age, Down syndrome, cleft palate) are at risk for developing OME and AOM. In children without structural differences, the presence of OME was often treated even when AOM was not present, possibly representing inappropriate treatment with unnecessary antibiotics. Pneumatic otoscopy (i.e.,

using a small puff of air against the tympanic membrane while observing for movement) assists in determining the presence of fluid accumulation in the middle ear and should be part of the exam of any child brought in to the health care provider for ear complaints. The use of antimicrobials, antihistamines, decongestants, and corticosteroids was not found to be helpful in cases of OME.

Implications
For patients without structural differences in the ear or eustachian tubes who are not at risk for developing OME with AOM, nurses should educate patients and families that a period of watchful waiting is appropriate if an ear infection is suspected. Increasing fever, changes in the child's behavior suggesting the presence of pain, or concerns that a child's hearing is affected should be evaluated by the health care provider. Antihistamines and decongestants were not proven to be effective for OME and should be avoided unless recommended by the provider. Any child with a history of OME lasting longer than 3 months should also receive follow-up hearing and/or language testing.

Critical Thinking Questions
How should a nurse respond to a parent's request for antibiotics to treat their child's AOM symptoms? Based on the research, when would antibiotics be indicated for treatment of AOM?

See Answers to Critical Thinking Questions on student resource website.

however, an experienced pediatric nurse can usually administer parenteral medications quickly and compassionately without the need for restraining the child.

- The ventrogluteal site is preferred for IM injections, although the muscles of older children are developed enough for the nurse to use other sites.

Pharmacotherapy of the adolescent: Adolescence occurs between ages 13 and 16 years. Rapid physical growth and psychological maturation have a great impact on personality development. The adolescent strongly relates to peers, wanting and needing their support, approval, and presence. Physical appearance and conformity with peers in terms of behavior, dress, and social interactions is important. The strong sense of independence leads teens to self-medicate, either with or without their parents' knowledge. Treatment objectives for the nurse should include teaching parents to keep their medications safely stowed out of sight from inquisitive, experiment-minded adolescents. Parents should also be taught the signs and symptoms of drugs commonly abused by teens such as marijuana, inhalants, and methamphetamine.

The most common needs for the pharmacotherapy of teens are for skin problems, headaches, menstrual symptoms, sex-related concerns, eating disorders, contraception, alcohol and tobacco use, and sports-related injuries.

- Of primary concern to the adolescent are the initiation of sexual intercourse and the avoidance of pregnancy and sexually transmitted infections. The nurse must be prepared to address a variety of topics related to sexuality, including the importance of responsible sexual practices, condom use, and other contraceptive methods.

- Eating disorders commonly occur in this population. The nurse should carefully question adolescents about their eating habits and their use of over-the-counter (OTC) appetite suppressants or laxatives that may be contributing to bulimia or anorexia.

- Alcohol, tobacco use, and other illicit drug experimentation are prevalent in this population. Teenage athletes may use amphetamines to delay the onset of fatigue as well as anabolic steroids to enhance performance. The nurse assumes a key role in educating adolescent patients about the hazards of tobacco use and illicit drugs.

- The adolescent has a need for privacy and control in drug administration. The nurse should communicate with the teen more in the manner of an adult rather than as a child. Teens usually appreciate thorough explanations of their treatment, and ample time should be allowed for them to ask questions.

- Despite their need to have independence and the desire to self-medicate, teens have a very poor understanding of medication information. Adolescents are reluctant to admit their lack of knowledge, so the nurse should carefully explain important information regarding their medications and expected adverse effects, even if these patients claim to understand.

CONNECTION Checkpoint 9.2

The nurse educator is teaching a group of new graduate nurses about the use of the anticoagulant heparin in pediatric patients admitted to the ICU. From what you learned in Chapter 6, what should the nurse include in her instructions about the necessary precautions for this type of drug? *See Answer to Connection Checkpoint 9.2 on student resource website.*

Medication Safety for Pediatric Patients

9.4 The nurse is a key member of the health care team in ensuring medication safety in pediatric patients.

The nurse is often responsible for administering medications to children. The importance of accurate drug dosage calculations, proper administration techniques, proper efforts to minimize adverse effects, and the need for overall safety cannot be overemphasized.

Principles of safe medication practice for pediatric patients are identical to those of adult patients. Medication safety is a team approach. Every level of responsibility is involved, including hospital-wide (or corporation-wide) policies, prescriber actions, pharmacy guidelines, nursing interventions, and patient and family adherence. Responsibility for preventing medication errors in pediatric patients is shared by every member of the team.

The safety and effectiveness of a medication regimen depends on proper procurement, storage, and administration of the drug. In the hospital setting, nurses are responsible for adherence to the basic rules of drug administration: right patient, right drug, right route, right dose, at the right time. Younger pediatric patients may not be able to accurately identify themselves; thus it is imperative that the nurse use precautions to ensure that the right child receives the prescribed medication. The nurse must check the child's identification band against the medication record. Most hospitals' policies require that drugs such as digoxin, heparin, insulin, chemotherapeutic agents, opioid analgesics, and barbiturates be double-checked with another nurse prior to administration. If the nurse suspects that a dose of medication ordered by the prescriber is outside the normal range, it is the nurse's responsibility to question the order because some drugs can be lethal to pediatric patients. The nurse should regularly check reputable online drug information sources for the most recent information on pediatric drugs and their adverse effects.

The American Academy of Pediatrics established guidelines in 2007 to prevent pediatric medication errors in the inpatient setting. Since that time, computerized physician order entry programs, electronic health records, programmable infusion pumps, and other technologies have been implemented. Because no system is fail-safe, the nurse should always follow the guidelines for safe medication practice as follows:

Nursing Actions and Guidelines

- Check medication calculations with another professional member of the health care team.

- Confirm patient identity before administration of each dose.

- Be familiar with medication ordering and dispensing systems.
- Verify drug orders before medication administration.
- Verify unusually large or small volumes or dosage units for a single patient dose.
- When a patient, a parent, or a caregiver questions whether a drug should be administered, listen attentively, answer questions, and double-check the medication order.
- Remain familiar with the operation of medication administration devices and the potential for errors with such devices, particularly patient-controlled analgesia (PCA) or infusion pumps.

Nursing Education and Communication

- Develop and maintain continuous education programs for nursing competencies in devices used for pediatric medication administration, particularly PCA and infusion pumps.
- Develop and maintain a pediatric medications knowledge base.
- Discuss medication orders with the prescriber whenever possible.
- Integrate and provide education for the patient and caregiver regarding the medication regimen.
- Record and verify patient identity, weight, allergies, and previous medication use.
- Be aware of and be involved in ongoing error-tracking systems and pharmacy programs. Encourage blame-free error reporting. Ensure that all staff members understand the method of reporting and are knowledgeable about the health care agency's system for reporting errors.

Determining Pediatric Drug Dosages

9.5 The nurse must be accurate when calculating drug dosages of pediatric patients.

Nurses must consistently update their skills in calculating pediatric doses because errors in drug administration may have serious consequences. Drug dosage calculation for pediatric patients should be individualized and nurses should take into consideration the child's age, height, weight, maturational state, and body surface area (BSA). All drug calculations for pediatric patients in critical care settings should be double-checked by the pharmacist and another nurse prior to administration.

Two common procedures of calculating pediatric dosages are the body weight method and body surface area method. Utilization of the **body weight method** requires a calculation of the number of milligrams of drug, based on the child's weight in kilograms (mg/kg). A unit of time is usually included; for example, gentamicin 5 mg/kg/24 h. The body weight method is simple and a dose can be calculated quickly. However, the serum concentrations of many drugs are not proportional to body weight, and body weight does not take into consideration pharmacokinetic variables such as changes in metabolism and elimination rates, as discussed in Section 9.2.

The **body surface area (BSA) method** uses an estimate of the child's BSA. This method is believed to be the most valid basis

for dosage, because it is related to certain physiological functions that account for the pharmacokinetic differences in pediatric patients. The BSA method better estimates blood volume, metabolism, and the effects of drugs. Measurements of the fluid volume compartment and the serum concentrations of drugs also correlate well with the BSA.

Using the BSA method, the child's height and weight are plotted on a **nomogram** (Figure 9.1) and a line is drawn between the two points. The point at which the line intersects the surface area line is the child's BSA. The dose is calculated as BSA ÷ 1.73 × adult dose × pediatric dose.

Other methods, including electronic calculators, are used to estimate pediatric doses. Each method has specific advantages and disadvantages. The student should refer to a medication mathematics text for practice calculation examples.

Adverse Drug Reactions in Children and Promoting Adherence

9.6 Pediatric patients are more susceptible than adults to adverse drug effects.

Because of their smaller size and immature or developing organ systems, pediatric patients are more susceptible to adverse effects. The nurse may find it challenging to identify adverse effects because infants and young children often do not have the maturity or verbal skills to accurately describe their feelings following the medication administration. Identifying pediatric adverse effects will depend on the skill and ability of the nurse in assessing subtle changes in patient response. For example, a child on diuretics should have strict intake and output measurements to help determine if the drug is working properly. Excessive weight gain could be caused by edema resulting from poor kidney excretion, or weight loss might be due to excessive diuresis. Signs of ototoxicity may go unnoticed for a long time unless someone checks that the child no longer responds to verbal commands. It may be necessary to consult a psychologist to identify signs of suicidal ideation from antidepressant use in adolescents.

Most types of adverse effects that occur in children age 1 or older are the same as those in adults. Like adults, the majority of adverse effects are dose related; thus the nurse must pay close attention to the proper dose and frequency of drug administration.

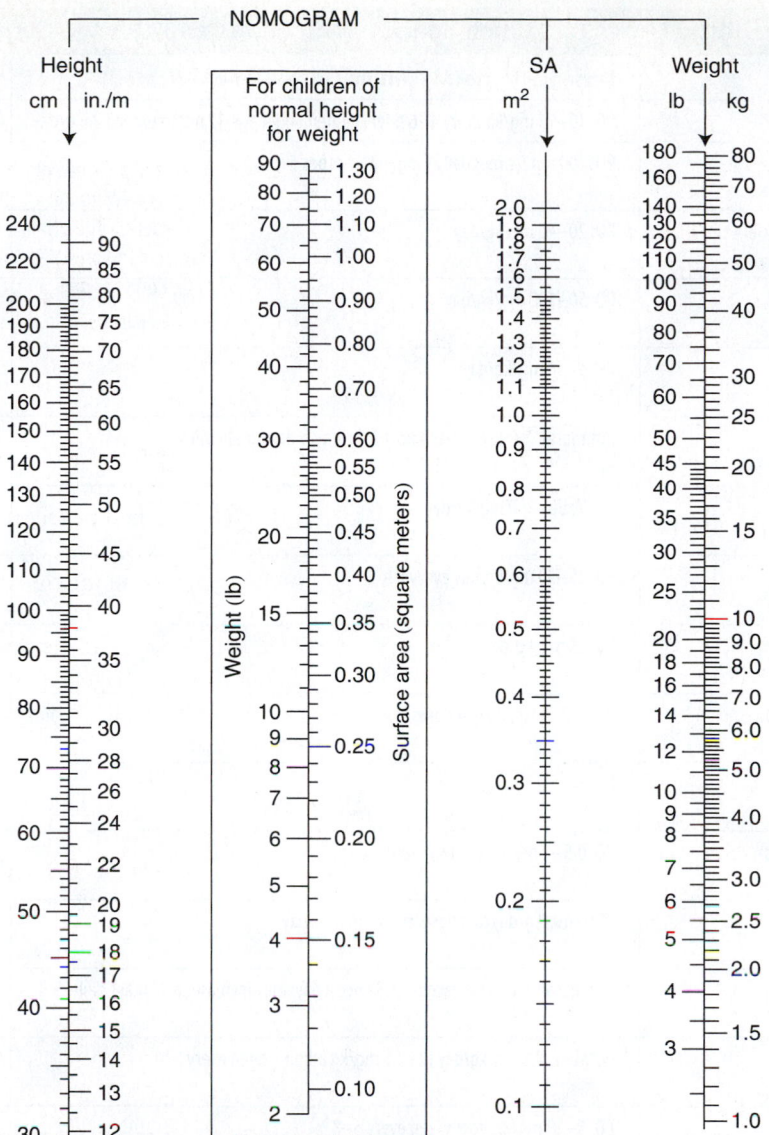

Figure 9.1 West nomogram for estimation of surface areas.

Adapted from "Figure 715.1" from Nelson Textbook of Pediatrics, 18E by R. M. Kliegman, R. E. Behrman, H. B. Jenson, and B. M. D. Stanton. Copyright © 2007 by Saunders, an imprint of Elsevier Inc. Used by permission of Elsevier, Inc.

Knowing specific drugs and their adverse effects in the adult population will help the nurse quickly identify signs and symptoms in pediatric patients. For example, antibiotics such as amoxicillin frequently result in diarrhea in both adults and children. Anti-anxiety agents, antidepressants, and antipsychotic drugs that cause CNS depression will likely cause drowsiness in both adults and children.

A few types of adverse effects are specific to children due to their immature or developing organs and tissues. For example, tetracycline must be avoided in the neonate because of the potential for permanent staining of the teeth. Sulfonamides can cause jaundice in neonates, and aspirin is contraindicated in children with fever due to the potential for Reye's syndrome. Glucocorticoids can inhibit growth. Table 9.3 illustrates a list of commonly used drugs and their adverse effects on the pediatric patient.

CONNECTION Checkpoint 9.3

The nurse gives a preschooler a sedative but, rather than sleep, the child becomes excited and experiences insomnia. From what you learned in Chapter 5, this is most likely classified as what type of effect? *See Answer to Connection Checkpoint 9.3 on student resource website.*

Like adults, children may also experience drug interactions. Drugs that are most likely to contribute to drug interactions in pediatric patients are those with high potency, narrow therapeutic index, and extensive protein binding, and those that affect vital organ functions or hepatic metabolism.

Often parents' first response to their child's illness is to provide home remedies. OTC and herbal treatments are extremely common in some households, and research suggests that they are on the rise among a large segment of the population. The nurse must

TABLE 9.3   **Selected Pediatric Drugs for Which Specific Indications and Dosage Guidelines Exist**

Drug	Dosage/Route (Maximum Dose Where Indicated)	Adverse Effects
acetaminophen (Tylenol)	PO: 10–15 mg/kg every 4–6 h for children under age 12 not to exceed 2.6 g/day	Methemoglobinemia, hepatotoxicity
acyclovir (Zovirax)	PO: 200 mg 5 times daily for genital herpes	*Diarrhea, nausea* Renal failure, seizures
amoxicillin (Amoxil, Trimox) or amoxicillin/clavulanate (Augmentin)	PO: 20–40 mg/kg/day	*Diarrhea* Anaphylaxis
ampicillin (Principen)	PO: 50–100 mg/kg/day	*Diarrhea* Anaphylaxis
azithromycin (Zithromax)	PO: 5–10 mg/kg/day	*Diarrhea* Hepatotoxicity
budesonide (Rhinocort)	Intranasal: 2 sprays in each nostril 2 times a day for allergies	*Headache, fatigue* Paresthesia
ceftriaxone (Rocephin)	IV/IM: 50–100 mg/kg/day	*Diarrhea* Colitis
cephalexin (Keflex)	PO: 25–50 mg/kg/day every 6 h	*Diarrhea* Anaphylaxis, angioedema
clarithromycin (Biaxin)	PO: 15 mg/kg/day	*Vomiting, diarrhea* Colitis
diphenoxylate and atropine (Lomotil)	PO: 1/2–1 tsp, up to 4 doses/day	*Dizziness, sedation* Paralytic ileus
erythromycin (EryC, Erythrocin)	PO: 30–50 mg/kg/day	*Nausa, vomiting* Hepatotoxicity
ferrous sulfate (Feosol, Fergon, others)	PO: 0.5–1 mg/kg/day maintenance	*Nausea, black stools* Shock
fluconazole (Diflucan)	PO: 6 mg/kg/day first dose, then 3 mg/kg/day	*Headache, nausea* Hepatotoxicity
fluticasone (Flonase)	Intranasal: 1 spray in each nostril once a day; may increase to 2 sprays daily	*Nasal dryness* Epistaxis
gentamicin (Garamycin)	IV/IM: 6–7.5 mg/kg/day (2–2.5 mg/kg administered every 8 h)	*Pain at injection site* Neurotoxicity, nephrotoxicity
ibuprofen (Advil, Motrin)	PO: 5–10 mg/kg/dose given every 6–8 h	*Nausea, heartburn* GI bleeding
imipramine (Tofranil)	PO: 25–50 mg/day for nocturnal enuresis	*Urinary retention* Angioedema
loracarbef (Lorabid)	PO: 15–30 mg/kg/day	*Nausea, rash*
methylphenidate (Ritalin)	PO: 5–10 mg/day (dose not to exceed 60 mg/day, depending upon brand name)	*Nervousness, insomnia* Palpitations
minocycline (Minocin)	4 mg/kg/day bid	*Dizziness, nausea*
nystatin (Mycostatin)	PO: 1–6 mL (100,000–600,000 units) qid	*Nausea, vomiting* Diarrhea
oxcarbazepine (Trileptal)	PO: 8–10 mg/kg/day not to exceed 600 mg/day	*Fatigue* Somnolence
penicillin G	PO: 25–50 mg/kg/day every 3–4 h	*Diarrhea* Anaphylaxis
trimethoprim-sulfamethoxazole (Bactrim, Septra)	8 mg/kg/day trimethoprim–40 mg/kg/day sulfamethoxazole every 12 h	*Nausea, rash, anemia* Exfoliative dermatitis
valproic acid (Depakene, Depakote)	PO: 10–15 mg/kg/day initially (dose not to exceed 60 mg/kg/day)	*Drowsiness, nausea* Bone marrow suppression

Note: Italics indicate common adverse effects. Underline indicates serious adverse effects.

become aware of commonly used OTC and herbal remedies in order to advise the families about the pros and cons. Parents must understand that OTC and herbal therapies may have adverse effects of their own and may interact with prescription medications. Herbal remedies commonly used in homes include St. John's wort, echinacea, ginseng, licorice, and sassafras.

PharmFACT

Adult medication use in the home is closely associated with poisonings in children. The most frequent classes involving emergency department (ED) visits are hypoglycemics and beta blockers. The most serious ED visits in children were due to exposure to opioids (Burghardt et al., 2013).

A drug will fail to achieve optimum therapeutic outcomes if it is not taken properly. Adherence, also called compliance, is taking the drug according to the instructions on the label or as provided by the prescriber. Maximizing adherence to the medication regimen is a major goal of the pediatric nurse. The nurse must assess the patient and family to determine factors that could affect the family's ability to assist the child with the medication regimen and develop strategies that will enhance medication adherence. The more complex, expensive, and inconvenient the medication regimen, the less likely the child and family will adhere. Children are most likely to adhere to their medication regimen if the following conditions exist:

- High expectations of successful outcomes of the therapy
- Supportive family members who are able to communicate with the prescriber
- Positive interactions with the nurse and caregivers
- Minimal adverse effects from the medications
- Simple, short-term, inexpensive regimen with minimum disruption to daily routine

The nurse works with the child and family to enhance adherence by applying direct measures. The patient and family should be asked directly whether or not they have doubts about their ability to adhere to the regimen. If there is doubt, the nurse should explore the areas of concerns with the family and start by teaching the importance of the drug, route of administration, expected outcomes, and possible adverse effects. In long-term drug therapy the nurse may have to arrange for follow-up appointments to assess drug responses or to administer the oral drug(s) to the child and observe the drug being swallowed. This technique is known as **directly observed therapy (DOT)**. In extreme cases when the child does not appear to be responding appropriately to the prescribed regimen, periodic measurement of plasma drug levels can help determine the amount of drug ingested and whether it has been taken as prescribed.

CHAPTER

9 Understanding the Chapter

Key Concepts Summary

9.1 Legislation has attempted to improve the testing and labeling of pediatric drugs.

9.2 Pharmacokinetic responses in children differ from those in adults.

9.3 The role of the nurse in administering medications changes with each developmental age group.

9.4 The nurse is a key member of the health care team in ensuring medication safety in pediatric patients.

9.5 The nurse must be accurate when calculating drug dosages of pediatric patients.

9.6 Pediatric patients are more susceptible than adults to adverse drug effects.

Case Study: Making the Patient Connection

Remember 11-month-old "Timmy," the patient introduced at the beginning of the chapter? Now read the remainder of the case study. Based on the information presented within this chapter, respond to the critical thinking questions that follow.

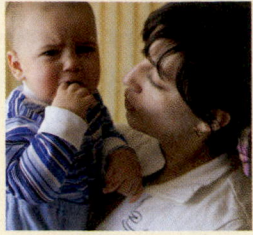

Ms. Thomas reports that Timmy has not been eating well for the past 72 hours. Last night he vomited three times after drinking sips of water and also had several very loose, green foul-smelling bowel movements. He voided only once in the past 12 hours. For the past 5 days Timmy has been taking amoxicillin for an ear infection. Timmy lies still on the examination table but responds to his mother's commands. The nurse prepares Timmy for examination.

Timmy's preliminary diagnosis is gastroenteritis with mild dehydration. His vital signs are as follows: temperature, 38.5°C (101.4°F); heart rate, 160 beats/min; respiration, 38 breaths/min; blood pressure, 100/57 mmHg; and weight, 8.6 kg (19 lb). His skin is dry and warm to touch, and there is slight tenting. The following laboratory studies were performed: serum electrolytes, complete blood count, blood urea nitrogen, creatinine, urinalysis, and stool for culture and sensitivity. Electrolytes were as follows: sodium, 136 mEq/L; potassium, 4.2 mEq/L; chloride, 114 mEq/L; bicarbonate, 9 mEq/L.

An IV line was inserted immediately and a solution of D_5W in 1/3 NSS was started to infuse at 30 mL/h. Timmy was placed on NPO.

Critical Thinking Questions

1. What primary factors are contributing to this risk for deficient fluid balance?
2. What are some physical signs to assess when evaluating dehydration in this infant?
3. What would best explain the cause for diarrhea in this patient?
4. What are some key points to focus on when monitoring the infant's IV fluid intake?

See Answers to Critical Thinking Questions on student resource website.

Additional Case Study

Sinead, a 3-year-old girl, arrives at the emergency department in status asthmaticus. Her mother informs you that she was diagnosed with asthma 9 months ago and since then has been back to the emergency department for treatment twice. Two hours prior to admission, Sinead started coughing and wheezing and then an hour ago started having difficulty breathing. Her mother attempted to relieve the symptoms by giving steam and fluids but the condition only worsened. Sinead has audible expiratory wheeze, nasal flaring, and inter- and substernal retractions.

1. What nursing actions would take priority?
2. What nursing assessment should the nurse carry out immediately?
3. What immediate outcomes could be expected from treatment?

See Answers to Additional Case Study on student resource website.

Chapter Review

1 The nurse is preparing to administer medication to the pediatric patient. Which factor(s) is/are true regarding the pharmacokinetics in the pediatric population? Select all that apply.

1. Slower gastric motility in young children will keep the drug in the stomach longer.
2. Before 6 months of age, there is greater plasma protein binding of drugs and drug distribution will be lower in this age group.
3. Before age 5, the liver may not metabolize drugs as readily as an adult's liver and doses must be adjusted accordingly.
4. Drug excretion by the kidneys will not equal an adult's until the child is at least 2 years of age.
5. Drugs with central nervous system effects have little to no effect in infants and very young children.

2 The nurse is preparing to give an intramuscular injection to a 7-month-old infant. Which is the preferred site?

1. Vastus lateralis
2. Deltoid
3. Dorsogluteal
4. Ventrogluteal

3 The experienced pediatric nurse is teaching a new nursing student about injections in the pediatric population. Which statement by the student would indicate that teaching was effective?

1. "Intramuscular (IM) injections in infants are absorbed slowly."
2. "Children experience rapid absorption of IM medications."
3. "IM injections are encouraged due to their predictable absorption rate."
4. "Strong muscle contractions result in delayed absorption of IM medication."

4 It is time to give a 3-year-old oral medication. Which comment by the nurse is most therapeutic?

1. "This is the medicine that makes you better."

2. "If you don't take your medicine you can't go home."

3. "Would you like to take your medicine with water or juice?"

4. "See how easily your roommate has taken his medicine?"

5 Drugs that are most likely to create drug interactions in pediatric patients are those with:

1. Low potency.

2. Wide therapeutic index.

3. Extensive protein binding.

4. Effects on the skin.

6 The health care provider knows that the pediatric patient and parents will most likely adhere to the medication regimen if the:

1. Regimen is simple and inexpensive.

2. Medications are costly but well known.

3. Medications are prescribed for a long period.

4. Medications are taken at different times each day.

See Answers to Chapter Review in Appendix A.

References

American Academy of Pediatrics. (2007). AAP Publications Reaffirmed, January 2007. Policy statement: Prevention of medication errors in the pediatric inpatient setting. *Pediatrics, 119*(5), 1031. doi:10.1542/peds.2007-0471

American Association of Family Physicians. (2004).*Clinical practice guideline: Otitis media with effusion.* Retrieved from http://www.aafp.org/patient-care/clinical-recommendations/all/otitis-media-effusion.html

Burghardt, L. C., Ayers, J. W., Brownstein, J. S., Bronstein, A. C., Ewald, M. B., & Bourgeois, F. T. (2013). Adult prescription drug use and pediatric medication exposures and poisonings. *Pediatrics, 132,* 18–27. doi:10.1542/peds.2012-2978

Chai, G., Governale, L., McMahon, A. W., Trinidad, J. P., Staffa, J., & Murphy, D. (2012). Trends in outpatient prescription drug utilization in US children, 2002–2010. *Pediatrics, 130,* 23–31. doi:10.1542/peds.2011-2879

Kliegman, R. M., Stanton, B., St. Geme, J., Schor, N., & Behrman, R. E. (Eds.). (2011). *Nelson textbook of pediatrics* (19th ed.). Philadelphia, PA: W. B. Saunders.

Lee, E., Teschemaker, A. R., Johann-Liang, R., Bazemore, G., Yoon, M., Shim, K. S., … Wutoh, A. K. (2012). Off-label prescribing patterns of antidepressants in children and adolescents. *Pharmacoepidemiology and Drug Safety, 21,* 137–144. doi:10.1002/pds.2145

Natal, B. L. (2011). *Emergent management of acute otitis media.* Retrieved from http://emedicine.medscape.com/article/764006-overview#a0199

National Research Council. (2012). *Safe and effective medicines for children: Pediatric studies conducted under the Best Pharmaceuticals for Children Act and the Pediatric Research Equity Act.* Washington, DC: The National Academies Press.

Pasquali, S. K., Burstein, D. S., Benjamin, Jr., D. K., Smith, B., & Li, J. S. (2010). Globalization of pediatric research: Analysis of clinical trials completed for pediatric exclusivity. *Pediatrics, 126,* e687–e692. doi:10.1542/peds.2010-0098

U.S. Government Accountability Office. (2007). *Pediatric drug research: Studies conducted under Best Pharmaceuticals for Children Act.* Retrieved from http://www.gao.gov/new.items/d07557.pdf

Vernon, J. A., Shortenhaus, S. H., Mayer, M. H., Allen, A. J., & Golec, J. H. (2012). Measuring the patient health, societal and economic benefits of US pediatric therapeutics legislation. *Paediatric Drugs, 14,* 283–294. doi:10.2165/11633590-000000000-00000

Selected Bibliography

Bazzano, A. T., Manglone-Smith, R., Schonlau, M., Suttorp, M. J., & Brook, R. H. (2009). Off-label prescribing to children in the United States outpatient setting. *Academic Pediatrics, 9*(2), 81–88. doi:10.1016/j.acap.2008.11.010

Budnitz, D. S., Lovegrove, M. C., & Rose, K. O. (2014). Adherence to label and device recommendations for over-the-counter pediatric liquid medications. *Pediatrics, 133*(2), e283–e290. doi:10.1542/peds.2013-2362

Doherty, C., & McDonnell, C. (2012). Tenfold medication errors: 5 years' experience at a university-affiliated pediatric hospital. *Pediatrics, 129,* 916–924. doi:10.1542/peds.2011-2526

Rodriguez, W., & Maldonado, S. (2010). United States paediatric legislation impact on paediatric drug studies. In K. Rose & J. N. van der Anker (Eds.), *Guide to paediatric drug development and clinical research.* Basel, Switzerland: Karger.

U.S. Food and Drug Administration. (2013). *2013 safety alerts for human medical products, drugs and therapeutic biological products, medical devices, and special nutrition and cosmetic products.* Retrieved from http://www.fda.gov/Safety/MedWatch/SafetyInformation/SafetyAlertsforHumanMedicalProducts/ucm333878.htm

Yaffe, S. J., & Aranda, J. V. (2010). *Neonatal and pediatric pharmacotherapy: Therapeutic principles in practice* (4th ed.). Philadelphia, PA: Lippincott Williams & Wilkins.

Zajicek, A., & Barrett, J. S. (2013). The grand challenges in obstetric and pediatric pharmacology. *Frontiers in pharmacology, 4,* 170. doi:10.3389/fphar.2013.00170

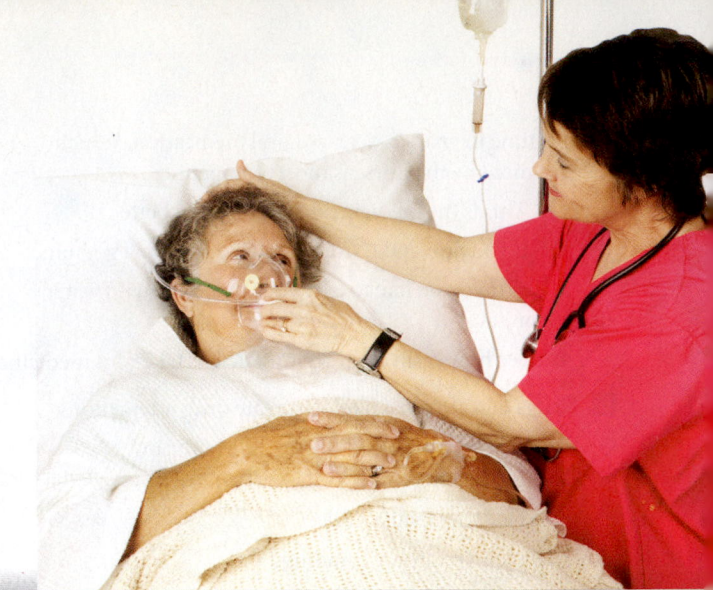

Mary Smith, 80 years old, is being transported via ambulance to the emergency department. She looks pale and thin with sunken eyes and chapped, dry lips. "I'm so relieved my neighbor came by to check on me. I have not been able to get out of bed for 2 days."

Patient "Mary Smith"

LEARNING OUTCOMES

After reading this chapter, the student should be able to:

1. Describe factors that lead to polypharmacy in older adults.

2. Identify age-related physiological changes in the older adult.

3. Explain how age-related physiological changes alter pharmacokinetics and pharmacodynamics and affect drug response in older adults.

4. Explain strategies that the nurse may implement to improve adherence with drug therapy in geriatric patients.

5. Explain why older adults are more likely to experience adverse drug reactions and interactions.

6. Identify specific drugs that are particularly hazardous for use in older patients.

7. Differentiate medication responses that result from age-related alterations in specific body systems from those that occur in younger individuals.

8. Develop nursing interventions that maximize pharmacotherapeutic outcomes in older adults.

9. Generate key points for family and patient education regarding drug pharmacotherapy for older adults.

CHAPTER OUTLINE

▸ Polypharmacy

▸ Physiological Changes Related to Aging

▸ Pharmacokinetic and Pharmacodynamic Changes in Older Adults

▸ Adherence and Drug Misuse Among Older Adults

▸ Adverse Drug Reactions in Older Adults

Beers criteria, 121

drug misuse, 120

polypharmacy, 117

potentially inappropriate medications
(PIMs), 121

Older adults are 65 years of age and older. Of this age group, those older than 84 years are the fastest growing segment of the population. The average age of the population has increased significantly during the past few decades because of improved access to health care, people choosing healthier lifestyles, and more effective treatment of chronic diseases. With the increase in lifespan, however, has come an increased reliance on medications to maintain health. This chapter focuses on aspects of pharmacology unique to geriatric patients and provides steps that the nurse can take to provide safe, effective pharmacotherapy for this population.

PharmFACT

By 2030, projections estimate that there will be more than 72 million adults over age 65 in the United States, more than twice the number living in 2000. This population represented about 12% of the population in the year 2000 but will comprise 19% of the population by 2030 (Department of Health & Human Services, Administration on Aging, 2010).

Polypharmacy

10.1 Older adults take more medications than any other segment of the population.

The pharmacotherapy of older adults is more challenging than that of their middle-age or younger counterparts. To deliver safe and effective pharmacotherapy for patients in this age group, the nurse must consider many age-related variables that affect pharmacotherapy. In addition, the older adult generally experiences more chronic conditions than their younger counterparts. Most of these conditions require drug therapy to treat and prevent complications. Finally, many older adults self-medicate for minor conditions that do not require prescription drug therapy.

Longevity inevitably leads to increased illnesses, which, in turn, necessitate the use of increased numbers of medications. Comorbidity, the presence of several chronic medical disorders concurrently, is common among older adults. By about age 65, half the older population has two or more chronic disorders, the most prevalent being a combination of hypertension and arthritis. Other comorbidities that occur in a significant number of older adults are heart disease with arthritis, hypertension with diabetes, and depression with nearly any other chronic disorder.

Comorbidities often result in the need for multiple drugs, a condition termed **polypharmacy**. Although not unique to older patients, polypharmacy is prevalent in this age group because of these comorbidities. The higher the number of drugs taken by a patient, the greater the possibility of experiencing adverse effects and drug interactions. As presented in Chapter 5, drugs that may be safe when used as monotherapy can have additive adverse effects when combined with other drugs. For example, taking multiple drugs that

cause central nervous system (CNS) depression can lead to excessive sedation, thus increasing the risk for accidents or injury due to falls. Taking two or more drugs that cause renal or liver impairment can result in additive organ damage in older adults who may already have some degree of impaired function due to normal aging processes.

Polypharmacy may also occur when the patient takes over-the-counter (OTC) drugs, herbal products, and dietary supplements in conjunction with prescribed medications. For example, older adults frequently seek OTC medications to treat constipation and minor aches and pains. Many also take vitamins, alternative therapies, and dietary supplements. Most patients are unaware that these agents can interact with prescription medications.

Patients who visit multiple health care providers and use different pharmacies may experience polypharmacy because each provider or pharmacist may not be aware of all the drugs ordered by other prescribers. Nurses should urge patients to report all prescription and OTC products at each office visit and teach them to use one pharmacy for their prescription needs.

CONNECTIONS | Community-Oriented Practice

Reducing Medication Errors in Older Adults

Most older adults take multiple prescription drugs. It is common for older adults with some degree of cognitive impairment to forget to take medicines or to take double doses. In the home setting, certain strategies should be implemented to avoid these types of medication errors. Nurses should teach geriatric patients (or their caregivers) to follow some or all of the following strategies:

- Set a schedule whereby medicines are taken at the same time each day. Unless contraindicated, taking medications around mealtimes may assist the patient to remember to take them.
- Keep a written daily record of drugs taken that includes drug name, dose, date, and time taken.
- Use a memory aid such as pill holders that have compartments for each day of the week and each time of day (morning, noon, or night).
- For patients with visual impairments, clearly color-code the medication bottles so they are easily recognized and request large-print labeling when possible.
- Keep an up-to-date written record of all drugs taken, the doses, and the prescriber's name. Bring this information to all health care provider appointments.
- When possible, request that a once-daily medication be prescribed, if available, to decrease the number of medications taken throughout the day.
- Keep a record of all OTC drugs, herbal products, dietary supplements, and vitamins taken. Bring this record to all health care provider appointments.
- Whenever possible, learn medicines by name, and understand why each is being prescribed.
- Use one pharmacy to fill all prescriptions.

In addition to polypharmacy, many other factors can alter a geriatric patient's response to medication. These include physiological changes associated with aging, changes in pharmacokinetics and pharmacodynamics, and patient adherence with the therapeutic regimen.

CONNECTION Checkpoint 10.1

From what you learned in Chapter 5, state the differences among additive, synergistic, and antagonistic effects. *See Answer to Connection Checkpoint 10.1 on student resource website.*

Physiological Changes Related to Aging

10.2 Anatomic and physiological changes associated with aging may alter the patient's response to medications.

With advancing age, certain anatomic and physiological changes occur. These predictable changes should be considered a normal part of the aging process, rather than as diseases or pathologic conditions. Awareness of the physiological changes that occur during the lifespan is critically important in properly assessing and caring for the older adult (Figure 10.1). Failure to recognize these changes may lead to less than optimal therapeutic outcomes and may endanger patient safety.

Giving an "average dose" of a drug to an older adult may produce a very different response compared to the same dose given to a younger patient, even if the two patients weigh the same. The pharmacologic action of the drug in older adults may be enhanced or diminished. The adverse effects may be more severe or entirely different from those observed in younger patients. The older patient may experience more drug interactions. What factors are responsible for this wide variation in drug response in the geriatric population?

In general, physiological processes slow down with advancing age. For example, the rate of absorption of nutrients from the

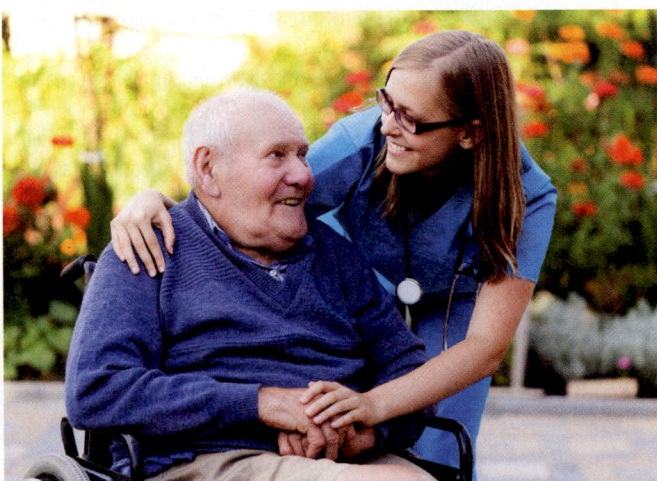

Figure 10.1 Pharmacology of the older adult can be challenging due to physiological changes that occur with aging.
Courtesy of © Barabas Attila/Fotolia.

gastrointestinal (GI) system tends to slow due to the decrease in GI motility and reduced GI blood flow. Metabolism also diminishes due to decreased liver size and reduced blood flow to this organ. Additionally, as a person ages the production of serum albumin by the liver declines. The older adult has a decreased volume of total body water, leading to higher concentrations of substances in the serum.

Cardiovascular system changes in the older adult are related to changes in cardiac muscle and increased peripheral resistance (hypertension). These physiological changes lead to decreased contractile force, which diminishes cardiac output and slows the circulation of nutrients and drugs.

In the nervous system, conduction velocity slows and sensory functions such as vision, hearing, and smell begin to diminish. Brain mass begins to decline, resulting in a progressive loss of cognitive ability. Additionally, as an adult ages the efficiency of the blood–brain barrier declines, allowing more substances to enter the CNS and affect the brain.

Older adults undergo a progressive decline in renal function as a result of decreased renal blood flow, decreased glomerular filtration rate, and decreased numbers of nephrons. The kidneys begin to lose their ability to effectively excrete creatinine and other wastes from the body. The body retains drugs and other substances for longer periods.

Normal, age-related physiological changes in organ systems can greatly affect responses to medications. Selected changes, and their effects on drug response, are shown in Table 10.1.

Pharmacokinetic and Pharmacodynamic Changes in Older Adults

10.3 Normal aging processes can alter pharmacokinetic and pharmacodynamic responses to drugs.

To produce therapeutic effects, most drugs must reach their target cells in sufficient quantities. To a large extent, this depends on what the body does to the medications after they are administered, a process known as pharmacokinetics. Drug response is also dependent on pharmacodynamic factors: the mechanisms by which drugs change the body. The normal physiological changes of aging affect pharmacokinetics and pharmacodynamics. Knowing about these changes when administering medications to the older adult helps the nurse to understand the unique actions of drugs in these patients and to predict and prevent adverse effects.

Absorption: Overall, absorption of nutrients and drugs tend to slow with aging. Fortunately, although the rate slows, absorption is usually complete because most drugs are absorbed by passive diffusion.

Because of the increased gastric pH in older adults, oral tablets and capsules that require high levels of acid for absorption may dissolve more slowly and take longer to reach their target tissues. Furthermore, decreased blood flow to and from the GI tract in the older adult delays the absorption and subsequent distribution of medications. Slowed motility allows drugs to remain longer in the GI tract, increasing the length of time for absorption and raising the risk for adverse effects such as nausea and vomiting. Physiological

TABLE 10.1 Physiological Factors Affecting Medication Responses in Older Adults

Body System	Changes in Physiological Factors	Effect on Medication Response
Cardiovascular system	• Decreased force of contraction and stroke volume • Decreased oxygen uptake by tissues • Decreased serum albumin and serum-binding capacity	• Reduced cardiac output and slowed distribution • Decreased metabolism • Changed drug distribution, producing unpredictable and toxic levels of highly protein-bound drugs such as phenytoin
Central nervous system	• Decreased brain size, number of neurons, and peripheral nerve function • Declining efficiency of blood–brain barrier	• Decreased drug distribution • Increased penetration of drug in the brain
Endocrine system	• Alterations in carbohydrate metabolism • Decreased growth hormone production and altered corticosteroid activity, leading to increased body fat, decreased muscle, and decreased bone mass	• Reduced insulin secretion and increased insulin resistance, manifesting as type 2 diabetes mellitus • Increased absorption of fat-soluble drugs
Gastrointestinal system	• Decreased GI motility • Decreased emptying of gastric contents • Reduced gastric acid production • Increased gastric pH • Decreased blood flow to the GI tract • Decreased thirst perception, leading to risk for dehydration, electrolyte imbalance, and poor nutritional intake	• Slowed rate of absorption • Increased potential for adverse effects
	• Decreased liver size • Decreased blood flow to the liver • Decreased ability of the liver to metabolize drugs	• Slowed metabolism • Prolonged drug half-life, increasing the potential for adverse effects
Musculoskeletal system	• Decreased lean muscle mass and increased and redistributed body fat	• Extended and increased effect of fat-soluble drugs such as diazepam
Respiratory system	• Decreased muscle strength and endurance	• Decreased chest and lung expansion and response to hypoxia, resulting in altered rate of absorption and excretion of some respiratory drugs
Urinary system	• Decreased total fluid volume • Decreased renal blood flow, glomerular filtration, and tubular secretory function • Decreased creatinine clearance	• Higher concentrations of water-soluble drugs • Reduced rate of excretion and decreased drug clearance • Decreased drug excretion

changes that lead to alterations in the rate and quantity of drug absorption are listed in Table 10.1.

Distribution: The extent to which drug distribution is affected in the older adult depends on whether the drug is fat soluble or water soluble. Age-related increases in fat storage cause lipid-soluble drugs such as diazepam (Valium), phenobarbital (Luminal), and haloperidol (Haldol) to be stored in the body for extended periods, leading to lower plasma levels and increased drug concentrations in the tissues. The longer a drug remains in the tissues, the more significant the response to the drug will be and the greater the potential for adverse effects. Age-related decreases in total body water result in water-soluble drugs such as gentamicin (Garamycin) and hydrochlorothiazide (Microzide) having less total body fluid for dilution. Therefore, water-soluble drugs have higher serum concentrations and may produce more intense actions. To prevent toxicity, the peak and trough levels of drugs with a low safety index such as gentamicin are checked periodically, and drug dosages are adjusted accordingly.

Because of declining liver function, plasma protein levels are reduced up to 13% in the older adult. This decrease results in fewer binding sites for certain drugs, and higher concentrations of free drugs, which may lead to toxicity. In older adults taking highly protein-bound drugs such as phenytoin (Dilantin) and warfarin (Coumadin), the nurse must carefully assess for signs of toxicity, even when the patient is receiving therapeutic doses.

Higher levels of drugs are able to enter the brain in older adults due to the inefficient blood–brain barrier. Patients taking drugs such as benzodiazepines, antipsychotic agents, antiepileptic drugs, or tranquilizers that affect the CNS must be assessed for signs of adverse effects that often manifest as reduced cognitive function, drowsiness, confusion, and even hallucinations and psychoses.

Metabolism: Although most tissues metabolize drugs to some extent, the liver is by far the most important organ performing this function. Age-related changes in the liver include reduced hepatic function, decreased liver mass, diminished blood flow, and alteration in the activity of some hepatic enzymes.

The liver is a complex organ, and age-related changes are often unpredictable. The level of some metabolic enzymes may be reduced with aging, whereas others remain unchanged. In general, reduced metabolism means that drugs will have extended durations of action. Drugs with a long half-life such as gentamicin, digoxin (Lanoxin), and acetaminophen (Tylenol) remain longer in the body with the potential for accumulation in tissues. Such drugs should be prescribed with longer intervals between doses or in reduced dosages, and the patient should be monitored closely.

CONNECTIONS | **Lifespan Considerations**

◀ **Drug Monitoring in the Older Adult**

To avoid toxicity, a number of drug dosage changes should be made for the older adult:

- The older adult should be started on the smallest effective dose of medication and then be titrated upward.
- Observe the older patient for signs of drug accumulation about 3 to 5 days after new drug initiation. Consider any change in physical or emotional behavior as possible drug intoxication.
- Monitor hydration and nutritional status, especially among older patients, because dehydration and low protein in the diet are primary causes of drug toxicity in this age group.

CONNECTION Checkpoint 10.2

From what you learned in Chapter 3, what are CYP enzymes? State the differences between a substrate and an inducer of CYP enzymes. *See Answer to Connection Checkpoint 10.2 on student resource website.*

Excretion: The kidneys excrete the majority of drugs. The rate of drug clearance in older adults decreases proportionately to age-related decrease in renal function. The half-life of drugs is increased and the dosages or frequency of administration should be decreased to avoid toxicity due to drug accumulation. Patients who are taking drugs that are excreted primarily by the kidneys should receive periodic serum creatinine tests to assess renal function. Creatinine clearance levels tend to decrease from about 140 mL/minute at ages 17 to 24 years to around 96 mL/minute at ages 75 to 84. Dosages of drugs must be carefully adjusted in patients with impaired renal function.

Pharmacodynamic changes: Pharmacodynamic changes are usually associated with drug receptors. Evidence suggests that older adults have decreased numbers of receptors and, possibly, changes in receptor sensitivity. In assessing the older adult, the nurse will find that there is a decreased response to beta-adrenergic agonists and antagonists and, at the same time, an increased response to anticholinergics, CNS depressants, and drugs such as warfarin. There is limited information on how pharmacodynamic alterations actually occur in older adults.

Adherence and Drug Misuse Among Older Adults

10.4 Adherence with the therapeutic regimen is a major challenge for many older adults.

Drug adherence or compliance is the willingness and ability to take medications as instructed on the label or by the health care provider. Health care providers often assume that patients leaving the clinic or hospital will be adherent, fill their prescriptions, and take their medicines as directed. It may be surprising to learn that over a third of patients report they are often nonadherent with drug therapy. Reasons for nonadherence are many and varied but include the following patient responses (Martin et al., 2010):

- Didn't have the medicine on hand when it was time to take the dose (31%)
- Ran out of medicine (29.5%)
- Bothered by side effects (22.4%)
- Change in daily routine (21.4%)
- Felt better (16.4%)

Although nonadherence is not unique to older adults, this population is especially vulnerable. Older adult patients are more likely to have visual impairment, functional disabilities, and cognitive dysfunction that may be sources of medication errors and nonadherence. Functional hearing loss can prevent older adults from understanding the verbal instructions given by the health care provider. The large number of drugs taken by some older adults makes for a complicated dosing schedule that can be confusing for patients of any age.

Successful management of medical problems depends on a patient's adherence with the regimen. One of the main responsibilities of the nurse is to assess barriers to medication adherence in the older adult. Studies suggest that nonadherence is affected by three factors: the individual patient, the health care provider, and the patient's social support network.

Adherence at the patient level requires the patient's comprehension and commitment to the treatment. The patient must be able to afford the medication, believe in its efficacy, appropriately self-administer, and adjust to lifestyle changes that may be required. The health care provider must be able to effectively instruct the patient regarding a medication's efficacy, prescribe cost-effective medication, decrease the complexity of the regimen, and provide manageable and understandable instructions. Nurses play a key role in assessing the patient's understanding of the medications that have been ordered and for assessing patient concerns with cost or effects.

The nurse should provide the older adult's spouse or caregiver with adequate information regarding the patient's medication regimen, expected lifestyle changes, and the need for emotional support and monitoring. Table 10.2 lists reasons that patients give for nonadherence and provides suggestions for the nurse to promote adherence.

Drug misuse is a specific form of nonadherence that is common among older adults. Misuse includes overuse, underuse, or, in some cases, erratic use. This misuse may be accidental or deliberate. Self-adjusting the medication dose is a common practice: Patients change their dose level depending on how they feel. Some believe that taking extra doses will speed their recovery. Uninsured or underinsured patients who cannot afford their medications may try to make the medications last longer by splitting doses. Patients rarely report such practices to their health care provider. Drug misuse may have serious consequences: Many older adult visits to emergency departments are drug related, with nonadherence accounting for a substantial percentage.

CONNECTION Checkpoint 10.3

From what you learned in Chapter 2, describe some of the benefits to older adults created by the Medicare Prescription Drug Improvement and Modernization Act of 2003. *See Answer to Connection Checkpoint 10.3 on student resource website.*

TABLE 10.2	Promoting Adherence in the Older Adult Patient
Reasons for nonadherence	• Unpleasant adverse effects • Forgetfulness • Cognitive or physical impairment • Poor or misunderstood instructions • Complicated regimens • Inability or refusal to purchase the medication • Health beliefs about medications
Ways the nurse can promote adherence	• Assist the older adult in comprehending and committing to the drug treatment regimen. • Communicate the instructions in such a manner that the older patient fully understands the purpose of the treatment. • Provide the older patient with social support services to obtain the medications. • Work with a pharmacist to ensure that the medication is dispensed in containers that are easily opened and in formulations that are easily taken. • Make sure all drugs are clearly labeled with instructions. • Simplify the regimen to reduce the number of drugs and doses per day. • Suggest that the older patient use a daily or weekly pill counter. • Provide the patient with a check-off calendar to document each time a medication is taken. • Engage family members or friends in supporting the older patient in efforts to comply. • Encourage the older patient to report signs of adverse effects. • Schedule periodic tests to determine plasma drug levels. • Place follow-up calls to high-risk patients.

Adverse Drug Reactions in Older Adults

10.5 Older adults are at high risk for experiencing adverse drug reactions and interactions.

An adverse effect is an undesirable and potentially harmful action caused by the administration of medications (see Chapter 5). Although older adults have many factors that predispose them to an increased risk of adverse effects, the number of drugs prescribed is probably the most important. The risk of an adverse effect greatly increases with the number of drugs taken. People over age 65 account for approximately 13% of the population but consume 34% of the total number of prescriptions. The average senior takes 14 prescription medications per year and persons age 80 to 84 take 18 prescriptions per year (American Society of Consultant Pharmacists, 2013). To minimize adverse effects, prescribers should order drugs only when they are needed and for the shortest length of time necessary to produce a therapeutic effect. Medications and doses should be reviewed on a regular basis to ensure that the intervention is still necessary.

Age-related physiological changes in renal and hepatic function are often responsible for placing older patients at greater risk for adverse effects. As the ability of the kidney to excrete drugs diminishes, serum drug levels may rise to cause toxicity. Loss of the ability of the liver to metabolize drugs can also raise serum drug levels and cause adverse effects. The nurse must be vigilant in assessing laboratory results of renal and hepatic function in older adult patients. Doses of most drugs must be adjusted with renal or hepatic impairment to prevent adverse effects.

As a person ages it often becomes difficult for the nurse to differentiate between behaviors that may be a natural part of aging and symptoms caused by adverse effects. For example, a frail older person who walks with an ataxic gait might be wrongly suspected of having an adverse effect from benzodiazepines or phenytoin, although the condition might be caused by normal aging. Older adults are more likely to experience CNS drug adverse effects such as dizziness and drowsiness, which are also symptoms that are often associated with normal aging processes. Medications should be considered as an underlying cause of the following symptoms in older patients:

• Sudden change in mental status
• Rapid weight loss
• Dehydration
• Restlessness
• Falls
• Anorexia
• Urinary retention or fluid retention
• Change in bowel habits
• Major change in functional status of any organ system

Combining a thorough literature review with expert consensus, health care providers have compiled a list of drugs of special concern for older adults. These are sometimes referred to as **potentially inappropriate medications (PIMs)**. Known as the **Beers criteria** or Beers list, health care providers should avoid prescribing PIMs to older adults because they have been found to produce a high incidence of adverse effects in this population. In 2012, the Beers criteria were updated following a systematic review and grading of the evidence (American Geriatrics Society, 2012). The Beers criteria have limitations because they do not consider all patient-related factors, and they do not address duplicate drug class prescriptions, drug–drug interactions, or inappropriate length of therapy (Corsonello et al., 2012). The updated Beers list incorporates evidence-based practice and research to establish three categories of drugs: drugs or classes to avoid, potentially inappropriate drugs or classes to avoid in older adults with certain diseases that the drugs may exacerbate, and drugs to be used with caution (American Geriatrics Society, 2012). Table 10.3 provides a list of PIMs and their specific adverse effects of concern for older adults.

A drug interaction occurs when a medication interacts with another substance and the drug's actions are affected. The "other substance" causing the drug interaction may be another drug, a dietary supplement, an herbal product, or a food (see Chapter 5). The large number of prescription drugs and OTC products taken by older adults predisposes this population to a high risk for drug interactions.

Another factor contributing to the increased risk for drug interactions is the presence of comorbidities (see Section 10.2). For example, the patient with both arthritis and heart disease may be

TABLE 10.3   Selected High-Risk Drugs for Older Adults

Drug	Adverse Response
antihistamines (e.g., chlorpheniramine, diphenhydramine, hydroxyzine, promethazine)	Sedation, confusion, anticholinergic effects
benzodiazepines (e.g., alprazolam, lorazepam, oxazepam)	Confusion, depression, anticholinergic effects
digoxin (Lanoxin)	Reduced renal clearance can cause serious toxicity
GI drugs (e.g., ranitidine, cimetidine)	Liver dysfunction, blood dyscrasias (ranitidine)
	Confusion, depression (cimetidine)
muscle relaxants (e.g., carisoprodol, cyclobenzaprine, oxybutynin)	Sedation, weakness, anticholinergic effects
nonsteroidal anti-inflammatory drugs (NSAIDs) (e.g., naprosyn, naproxen, oxaprozin)	Photosensitivity, nephrotoxicity, fluid retention
opioid analgesics (e.g., meperidine, pentazocine)	Sedation, confusion
phenytoin (Dilantin)	Confusion, ataxia, slurred speech, diplopia
psychotropic drugs and other CNS depressants (e.g., chlordiazepoxide, thioridazine, barbiturates, meprobamate)	Sedation, confusion
skeletal muscle relaxants (e.g., carisoprodol, methocarbamol, cyclobenzaprine)	Sedation, confusion
tricyclic antidepressants (e.g., amitriptyline, doxepin, imipramine)	Hallucinations, confusion, anticholinergic effects

using nonsteroidal anti-inflammatory drugs (NSAIDs) for pain and warfarin (Coumadin) to prevent blood clots. The NSAID may increase the effect of the warfarin, thus raising the potential for bleeding. The patient with both diabetes and hypertension may be taking thiazides and insulin. The thiazides reduce the effectiveness of insulin, thus affecting glycemic control.

The nurse plays a key role in optimizing pharmacotherapy outcomes in older adult patients, including addressing adverse effects, drug interactions, and issues of polypharmacy. One of the primary nursing responsibilities is to make a connection between the patient and family and the medication regimens. This entails assessing the level of comprehension, cultural beliefs, dietary practices, and physiological conditions of the patient and family. Advanced age does not negate the patient's right to know the names of the prescribed medications, the reasons they are being prescribed, and the potential adverse effects. Table 10.4 highlights nursing responsibilities and rationales regarding adverse effects and drug–drug interactions in older patients.

PharmFACT

In one study, older adults taking one or more of the drugs on the Beers criteria PIMs list were 25% more likely to have a hospital admission. The risk increased proportionately with the number of inappropriate drugs taken (Sehgal et al., 2013).

TABLE 10.4   Nursing Responsibilities Related to Adverse Drug Reactions and Drug Interactions in Older Adults

Nursing Responsibilities	Rationales
• Review the patient's medications to determine the potential for adverse effects and drug interactions. Consider cultural and dietary issues.	• Adverse effects are common in older patients because of physiological changes in body composition, multiple illnesses, polypharmacy, and nonadherence. • Some dietary practices may lead to adverse effects and interactions (e.g., low-salt intake may lead to lithium toxicity).
• Instruct the patient about potential adverse effects.	• A well-informed patient is better able to notify the health care provider as early as possible to minimize adverse effects.
• Assess the patient's fluid volume.	• Alteration in fluid volume could lead to increased sensitivity to alpha antagonists and other drugs with effects on blood pressure.
• Instruct the patient about the proper time to administer medications.	• Taking medications at the proper time will ensure optimum effectiveness and lower the chance for adverse effects.
• Ensure that the fewest number and lowest doses of medications with the simplest regimens have been prescribed for the patient.	• Polypharmacy may lead to drug toxicity.
• Monitor the patient for expected responses and any changes from normal.	• Adverse effects may not always be predictable because they may arise from sudden changes in the patient's condition.
• Discard all unused and expired medications, and instruct the patient to do the same.	• Drug effects diminish after the expiration date and some drugs can become toxic over time.
• Assess and monitor the patient's mental status for any alterations that may be caused by adverse effects.	• Delirium or confusion may be caused by adverse effects of psychoactive drugs.
• Periodically review the patient's OTC medications, nutritional supplements, and prescribed medications.	• Review of all drugs and alternative therapies can reduce the chances of adverse effects.

CHAPTER

10 Understanding the Chapter

Key Concepts Summary

10.1 Older adults take more medications than any other segment of the population.

10.2 Anatomic and physiological changes associated with aging may alter the patient's response to medications.

10.3 Normal aging processes can alter pharmacokinetic and pharmacodynamic responses to drugs.

10.4 Adherence with the therapeutic regimen is a major challenge for many older adults.

10.5 Older adults are at high risk for experiencing adverse drug reactions and interactions.

Case Study: Making the Patient Connection

Remember the patient "Mary Smith" at the beginning of the chapter? Now read the remainder of the case study. Based on the information presented within this chapter, respond to the critical thinking questions that follow.

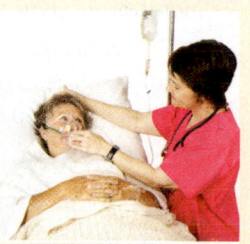

Mary has an IV solution of normal saline infusing in her left arm and oxygen by mask at 2 L/minute. Last week she heard that her older cousin had passed away, and since then she has become extremely depressed. She refuses to eat or drink but continues to take her medications on a regular basis. This 80-year-old woman is dehydrated and somewhat confused. Her neighbor provides the history. The nurse finds that Mary has been taking a diuretic (hydrochlorothiazide), an antihypertensive (atenolol), and multivitamins daily.

Vital signs are as follows: temperature, 38.6°C (101.4°F); apical pulse, 100 beats/min; respiratory rate, 32 breaths/min; and blood pressure, 92/62 mmHg. Her skin is dry and warm to the touch, and her lips are pale, dry, and chapped. She weighs 51.3 kg (113 lb) and her height is 1.7 m (5'7"). Her speech is quiet and slurred. Mary has not eaten anything during the past

24 hours and has only taken sips of water during the past 12 hours. She has voided once in 12 hours.

The following laboratory tests are completed: urinalysis, blood urea nitrogen (BUN)/creatinine, CBC, and basal metabolic panel (BMP). Mary is prescribed IV rehydration fluid and is stabilized in the emergency department before being admitted to the hospital unit.

Critical Thinking Questions

1. What are some potential predisposing factors that could lead to this patient's condition? (The student may need to consult later chapters or a drug reference book for the drugs included.)

2. What are the most immediate patient care priorities for the nurse to address at this time?

3. What priority areas will the nurse assess?

4. What are some of the expected patient outcomes following management of dehydration?

See Answers to Critical Thinking Questions on student resource website.

Additional Case Study

Ms. Haynes, 88 years of age, is fiercely independent and lives in an assisted-living facility in her own apartment with meals taken in a group dining room, which she clearly enjoys. She has a history of diabetes controlled with an oral antidiabetic drug, hypertension controlled with an antihypertensive drug and a mild diuretic, and occasional stomach upset for which she takes antacids. Her daughter suspects that her mother has not been taking any of her medications regularly because her blood sugar and blood pressure have been extremely variable lately and she asks the nurse for assistance.

1. What should the nurse do to assess whether Ms. Haynes is taking her medications regularly?

2. If Ms. Haynes is not taking her medications, what would the nurse's next action be?

3. What follow-up should be recommended to Ms. Haynes's daughter?

See Answers to Additional Case Study on student resource website.

Chapter Review

1 In general, drug absorption in the older adult is somewhat slowed. What physiological changes may account for this? Select all that apply.

1. Increased gastric pH
2. Decreased rate of blood flow to the GI tract
3. Increased gastrointestinal motility
4. Increased body surface area
5. Decreased cardiac output

2 The nurse completes an initial home assessment of an independent 82-year-old woman recently diagnosed with type 2 diabetes mellitus managed with insulin injections. What is the most appropriate nursing action for insulin administration for this patient?

1. Teach the daughter how to administer the insulin to her mother.
2. Instruct the patient how to administer the insulin.
3. Recommend daily visits by a home health aide to give the insulin.
4. Ask the health care provider to change the order to an oral antidiabetic medication.

3 Which age-related change in the older patient makes it necessary to reduce drug dosages?

1. Decrease in total body fat
2. Decrease in renal blood flow
3. Increase in plasma protein levels
4. Increase in total body water

4 Older adults experience adverse effects more frequently than young adults due to which of the following? Select all that apply.

1. Excessive prescribing
2. Multiple-drug therapy
3. Increased drug sensitivity
4. Increased body mass
5. Lack of consistent exercise

5 One third of older adult patients report that they are often nonadherent with drug therapy. Which response is given most frequently for nonadherence?

1. "The drugs prevented me from doing other things I wanted to do."
2. "I didn't have my medicine with me."
3. "I wanted to save money."
4. "I didn't believe the drugs were effective."

6 Which statement by the patient would inform the nurse that more teaching is necessary prior to discharge?

1. "It doesn't matter if the medication works as long as the doctor prescribed it."
2. "This medication is fully covered by my health insurance."
3. "I have been taking my medications by myself all my life."
4. "I don't mind making changes to my lifestyle while I am on this drug."

See Answers to Chapter Review in Appendix A.

References

American Geriatrics Society. (2012). American Geriatrics Society updated Beers criteria for potentially inappropriate medication use in older adults. *Journal of the American Geriatrics Society, 60,* 616–631. doi:10.1111/j.1532-5415.2012.03923.x

American Society of Consultant Pharmacists. (2013). *ASCP fact sheet.* Retrieved from https://www.ascp.com/articles/about-ascp/ascp-fact-sheet

Corsonello, A., Onder, G., Abbatecola, A. M., Guffanti, E. E., Gareri, P., & Lattanzio, F. (2012). Explicit criteria for potentially inappropriate medications to reduce the risk of adverse drug reactions in elderly people. *Drug Safety, 35*(Suppl. 1), 21–28. doi:10.1007/BF03319100

Department of Health & Human Services, Administration on Aging. (2010). *Aging statistics.* Retrieved from http://www.aoa.gov/aoaroot/aging_statistics/index.aspx

Martin, M., Kohler, C., Kim, Y., Kratt, P., Schoenberger, Y., Litaker, M., . . . Pisu, M. (2010). Taking less than prescribed: Medication nonadherence and provider–patient relationships in lower-income, rural minority adults with hypertension. *Journal of Clinical Hypertension, 12,* 706–713. doi:10.1111/j.1751-7176.2010.00321.x

Sehgal, V., Bajwa, S. J., Sehgal, R., Bajaj, A., Khaira, U., & Kresse, V. (2013). Polypharmacy and potentially inappropriate medication use as the precipitating factor in readmissions to the hospital. *Journal of Family Medicine and Primary Care, 2,* 194–199. doi:10.4103/2249-4863.117423

Selected Bibliography

Albert, S. M., Colombi, A., & Hanlon, J. (2010). Potentially inappropriate medications and the risk of hospitalization in retirees: Analysis of a US retiree health claims database. *Drugs and Aging, 27*, 407–415. doi:10.2165/11315990-000000000-00000

Fialová, D., & Onder, G. (2009). Medication errors in elderly people: Contributing factors and future perspectives. *British Journal of Clinical Pharmacology, 67*, 641–645. doi:10.1111/j.1365-2125.2009.03419.x

Hanlon, J. T., Schmader, K. E., & Semla, T. P. (2013). Update of studies on drug-related problems in older adults. *Journal of the American Geriatrics Society, 61*, 1365–1368. doi:10.1111/jgs.12354

Hutchison, L. C., & Sleeper, R. B. (2010). *Fundamentals of geriatric pharmacotherapy: An evidence-based approach.* Bethesda, MD: American Society of Health-Systems Pharmacists.

Kanaan, A. O., Donovan, J. L., Duchin, N. P., Field, T. S., Tjia, J., Cutrona, S. L., . . . Gurwitz, J. H. (2013). Adverse drug events after hospital discharge in older adults: Types, severity, and involvement of Beers criteria medications. *Journal of the American Geriatrics Society, 61*, 1894–1899. doi:10.1111/jgs.12504

Koper, D., Kamenski, G., Flamm, M., Böhmdorfer, B., & Sönnichsen, A. (2013). Frequency of medication errors in primary care patients with polypharmacy. *Family Practice, 30*, 313–319. doi:10.1093/fampra/cms070

Maher, R. L., Hanlon, J., & Hajjar, E. R. (2014). Clinical consequences of polypharmacy in elderly. *Expert Opinion on Drug Safety, 13*, 57–65. doi:10.1517/14740338.2013.827660

Mazer, M., Bisgaier, J., Dailey, E., Srivastava, K., McDermoth, M., Datner, E., & Rhodes, K. V. (2011). Risk for cost-related medication nonadherence among emergency department patients. *Academic Emergency Medicine, 18*, 267–272. doi:10.1111/j.1553-2712.2011.01007.x

McLachlan, A. J., Hilmer, S. N., & Le Couteur, D. G. (2010). Dosing errors: Age-related changes in pharmacokinetics. In S. Koch, F. M. Gloth, & R. Nay (Eds.), *Medication management in older adults* (pp. 53–68). New York: NY: Springer. doi:10.1007/978-1-60327-457-9_12

Meeks, T. W., Culberson, J. W., & Horton, M. S. (2011). Medications in long-term care: When less is more. *Clinics in Geriatric Medicine, 27*(2), 171–191. doi:10.1016/j.cger.2011.01.003

Planton, J., & Edlund, B. J. (2010). Strategies for reducing polypharmacy in older adults. *Journal of Gerontological Nursing, 36*, 8–12. doi:10.3928/00989134-20091204-03

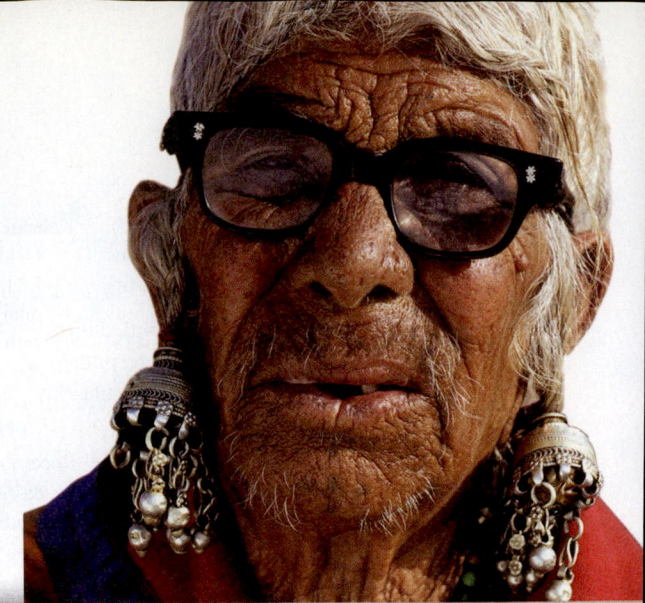

"It was so humiliating. When I was in the hospital, no one ever called me by name. I overheard someone refer to me as the Indian woman in room 425. No one really tried to communicate with me."

Patient "Aponi Nampeyo"

11 Individual Variations in Drug Responses

LEARNING OUTCOMES

After reading this chapter, the student should be able to:

1. Describe the fundamental concepts underlying a holistic approach to patient care and their importance to pharmacotherapy.
2. Identify psychosocial and spiritual factors that can affect pharmacotherapeutics.
3. Explain how ethnicity can affect pharmacotherapeutic outcomes.
4. Identify examples of how cultural values and beliefs can influence pharmacotherapeutic outcomes.
5. Convey how genetic polymorphisms can influence pharmacotherapy.
6. Explain how pharmacogenomics may lead to customized drug therapy.
7. Explain how gender can influence the actions of certain drugs.

CHAPTER OUTLINE

▸ Psychosocial Influences

▸ Cultural and Ethnic Variables

▸ Genetic Influences

▸ Gender Influences

KEY TERMS

culture, 127

ethnicity, 127

genetic polymorphism, 129

pharmacogenetics, 130

psychosocial, 127

Pharmacotherapy would indeed be simplified if the "average" dose given in a drug guide produced the same response in every patient. However, as presented in Chapter 4, patients can respond very differently to drug administration. For example, the same dose of an antihypertensive drug can result in a desired therapeutic effect in one patient and produce no effect or profound hypotension in other patients. The purpose of this chapter is to examine some of the factors that may cause this variability, including psychosocial influences, culture and ethnicity, gender, and genetics. Knowledge of these factors can contribute to safer and more effective pharmacotherapy.

Psychosocial Influences

11.1 Many psychosocial influences impact pharmacotherapy.

The term **psychosocial** is used in health care to describe the interaction between one's psychological development and one's social environment. Psychosocial nursing is part of a holistic model that includes the examination of patients' social roles, environmental stressors, culture, values, and family, all of which contribute to health and wellness.

Psychosocial also includes the spiritual nature of a person. *Psycho-social-spiritual* is a term that appears in the health care literature. Studies have established that these factors have a tremendous impact on health and well-being. Health care providers recognize that the close relationship among the psychological, social, and spiritual nature of individuals strongly influences their illness and wellness.

The psychosocial history of the patient, which is often collected during the initial assessment between the patient and the nurse, can influence the success of pharmacotherapy. Important assessment data include developmental needs, environmental stressors, and life transitions that could require major adaptations by the patient. The nurse also considers the patient's level of motivation to correct the health issue, because nonadherence to medication regimens and recommended lifestyle adjustments could impede the success of pharmacotherapy. For example, a highly stressed, middle-aged patient who is struggling with a new business might find it difficult to focus on wellness goals such as maintaining normal blood pressure and cholesterol levels.

A thorough psychosocial assessment should provide the health care provider with a clear picture of the patient's living arrangements, family involvement and interaction, financial resources, emotional condition, physical condition, and cognitive functioning. For example, does the patient have a trusting and empathetic relationship with their family? Would the family be able and willing to help the patient through some difficult challenges with adverse effects or long-term therapy? Is the patient emotionally stable enough to receive prescription drugs that have a possible suicidal risk? All of this information is important to developing effective health goals and pharmacotherapeutic outcomes.

In some cases the patient assessment may indicate a need to address psychosocial interventions before pharmacotherapy is begun. Behavioral or cognitive therapies may be employed to reduce negative thoughts and behaviors that could impact therapy. In children or adolescents, attempts at psychosocial therapies may be a prerequisite to initiating pharmacotherapy for conditions such as attention deficit/hyperactivity disorder, major depressive disorder, or bipolar disorder. The integrated use of pharmacologic and psychosocial therapies is believed to increase therapeutic success in addiction treatment.

CONNECTION Checkpoint 11.1

The frequency dose–response curve can be used to depict interpatient variability to drug response. From what you learned in Chapter 4, draw a typical frequency dose–response curve, labeling the axes and the median effective dose (ED_{50}). *See Answer to Connection Checkpoint 11.1 on student resource website.*

Cultural and Ethnic Variables

11.2 Cultural and ethnic variables can influence pharmacotherapy.

Although they are sometimes used interchangeably, culture and ethnicity differ in their exact definitions. An ethnic group is a community of people who share a common ancestry and similar genetic heritage. **Ethnicity** implies that people have biologic and genetic similarities. **Culture** is a set of beliefs, values, and norms that provide meaning for an individual or group. People within a culture have common rituals, religious beliefs, language, and certain expectations of behavior. Cultural and ethnic variables are important aspects of patient care that directly relate to pharmacotherapy. Both can influence the occurrence of specific drug effects and patient treatment outcomes.

For most of the history of pharmacology, the impact of cultural and ethnic variables was unknown or largely ignored. This was primarily caused by a lack of diversity in the conduct of clinical trials and follow-up reporting. For example, until relatively recently, clinical trials have included mostly Caucasians although non-Caucasians comprise about 25% of the U.S. population. Little attention was focused on identifying differences in pharmacologic effects in diverse ethnic or cultural groups. Indeed, the large majority of clinical trials even excluded females.

The protocol for many clinical trials now includes participants of different ages, genders, and ethnic groups whenever possible. Indeed, much research specifically examines differences among these populations. This type of research has confirmed that there is

CONNECTIONS   Treating the Diverse Patient

◀ Medication Refusal on Religious Grounds

One of the "rights" of medication administration is refusal. Patients have the right to refuse their medications due to religious or other objections. Perhaps most familiar is a refusal to accept blood or blood products by a Jehovah's Witness member because of religious beliefs. Less familiar is medication refusal due to the fact that the medication or treatment contains animal-derived products. For example, acceptance or refusal of porcine (pork) and bovine (beef) drugs or surgical products by members of the Jewish, Muslim, and Hindu faiths may also vary among members of the faith. Hoesli and Smith (2011) reported that more than 1,000 medications contain animal-based products, including the use of inactive ingredients such as gelatin. Depending on the religious tradition, beef, pork, chicken, fish, shellfish, or all meat may be refused on religious or moral grounds. They recommend that, when possible, a compounding laboratory be approached about making a comparable product for the patient that does not contain the offending product. That option should be explored if other formulations are not available for use. In the case of an animal-derived drug such as heparin, the provider should discuss the medication with the patient and explore alternative therapies if possible. Informed consent prior to surgery should include the disclosure of an animal-based product such as a porcine heart valve. Overall, sensitivity to a patient's religious beliefs and traditions should be maintained for medication administration. When a patient questions whether or not a drug or treatment should be used, nurses should encourage further discussion with informed religious leaders.

a biologic basis for variations or differences in metabolic response to drugs among various ethnic groups (see Section 11.4).

Certainly there are many more cultures and subcultures than ethnic groups. To have complete knowledge about the many variations in culture among a population of patients is impossible. However, nurses can strive to understand the significance of the cultural traditions and their potential impact on patients' pharmacologic regimens. Patients bring cultural beliefs (religious or ideological) that may challenge or conflict with what the health care provider believes to be in their best interests. How illness is defined is sometimes based on the cultural beliefs of an individual. One example that illustrates this point is the difference in belief systems between age groups—each with its own unique culture.

PharmFACT

Native Americans and Alaska Natives have an infant death rate almost double the rate of Caucasians. They are twice as likely to have diabetes as Caucasians (U.S. Department of Health and Human Services, 2011).

The nurse must keep in mind the following variables when treating patients from different cultural and ethnic groups.

- **Dietary considerations.** Cultures vary in their dietary preferences and practices, with diets that include some foods and exclude others. Patients need to understand that foods can increase or decrease the effectiveness of certain medications. Spices and herbs can be important to a patient's culture but may affect pharmacologic therapies. For example, some cultures include a diet high in foods such as cheese, pickled fish, or wine that can interact with medications to cause adverse events. Certain herbs can affect anticoagulants, beta blockers, and antidepressants. Assessing the primary foods of a patient's culture is an important component of the patient's psychosocial history.
- **Alternative therapies.** Various cultural groups use alternative therapies, such as vitamins, herbs, or acupuncture, either along with or in place of modern medicines. Some folk remedies and traditional treatments have existed for thousands of years and helped form the foundation for modern medical practice. For example, Chinese patients may consult with herbalists to treat diseases, whereas Native Americans may collect, store, and use herbs to treat and prevent disease. Certain Hispanic cultures use spices and herbs to maintain a balance of hot and cold to promote wellness. The nurse can assess the treatments used and interpret the effect of these herbal and alternative therapies on the prescribed medications to maximize positive outcomes. The nurse can explain that certain herbs or supplements may cause potential health risks when combined with prescribed drugs.
- **Beliefs about health and disease.** Cultures view health and illness in different ways. Individuals may seek assistance from people in their own community whom they believe have healing powers. Native Americans may consult with a tribal medicine man, whereas Hispanics seek a folk healer. African Americans sometimes practice healing through the gift of laying-on-of-hands. The nurse's understanding of the patient's trust in alternative healers is important. The more nurses know about the various cultural beliefs, the better support and guidance they can provide to patients.

PharmFACT

Ethnic and racial minorities represent one third of the U.S. population but more than half of uninsured U.S. citizens are from ethnic minorities. This lack of access to health care causes a large health disparity gap. The rate of preventable hospitalizations for minorities is more than double the rate for Caucasians ("Ending Racial and Ethnic Health Disparities," 2011).

Genetic Influences

11.3 Genetic polymorphisms can affect drug action.

Scientists have identified specific regions on various chromosomes that influence hepatic metabolism. For example, certain drugs, such as antidysrhythmics, antidepressants, and opioids, are metabolized differently in individuals of African, Native American, and Asian descent. As technology advances, nurses will likely begin to see variations in the prescribed amounts and forms of medication based on the ethnicity of the patient.

Humans of all races and cultures share remarkable deoxyribonucleic acid (DNA) similarities: 99.8% of our DNA sequences are identical. However, the remaining 0.2% may result in significant differences in patients' ability to handle medications. Some of these differences arise when a mutation occurs in the DNA that encodes for a certain protein. This creates a **genetic polymorphism**—two or more versions of the same protein. In pharmacology, the best characterized genetic polymorphisms have been discovered in the hepatic CYP 450 enzymes that metabolize drugs and in proteins that serve as receptors for drugs.

How can a genetic polymorphism affect drug action? In the case of enzymes, the altered "mutated" form of the enzyme has a changed structure. The structure of an enzyme is intimately related to its function; even a single base mutation in DNA can cause an amino acid change in the enzyme, altering its function. The mutated version of the enzyme may increase or decrease the speed of drug metabolism and excretion, depending on the specific genetic polymorphism. In some cases, the enzyme becomes totally non-functional. This concept is illustrated in Figure 11.1.

As a specific example, genetic polymorphism has been discovered in the enzyme acetyltransferase, which metabolizes (deactivates) isoniazid (INH), a drug prescribed for tuberculosis. The altered form of the enzyme performs its metabolic process, known as acetylation, more slowly because of the mutation. The reduced acetylation and diminished clearance by the kidney can cause INH to accumulate in the blood to toxic levels. These patients, who are usually Caucasians or African Americans, are known as slow acetylators. In contrast, mutations in many patients of Japanese descent result in *rapid* acetylation. These patients will inactivate the drug so quickly that it will not produce a therapeutic effect. Procainamide, hydralazine, sulfonamide antibiotics, and dapsone are other medications that are metabolized by acetylation.

Several other enzyme polymorphisms have importance to pharmacotherapy. Asian Americans and certain other ethnic groups are slow metabolizers of codeine and morphine due to an inherent absence of the enzyme CY2D6 (debrisoquine hydroxylase). This genetic polymorphism can lead to higher than normal plasma drug levels and adverse effects. Some African Americans have decreased effects from beta-adrenergic antagonist drugs such as propranolol (Inderal) because of genetically influenced variances in plasma renin levels. Another set of oxidation enzyme polymorphisms has been found that alters the response to drugs such as warfarin (Coumadin) and diazepam (Valium).

A second type of genetic polymorphism affects protein receptors. Receptors are proteins that have a specific structure that accepts the drug (or other endogenous molecule) in a lock-and-key-type

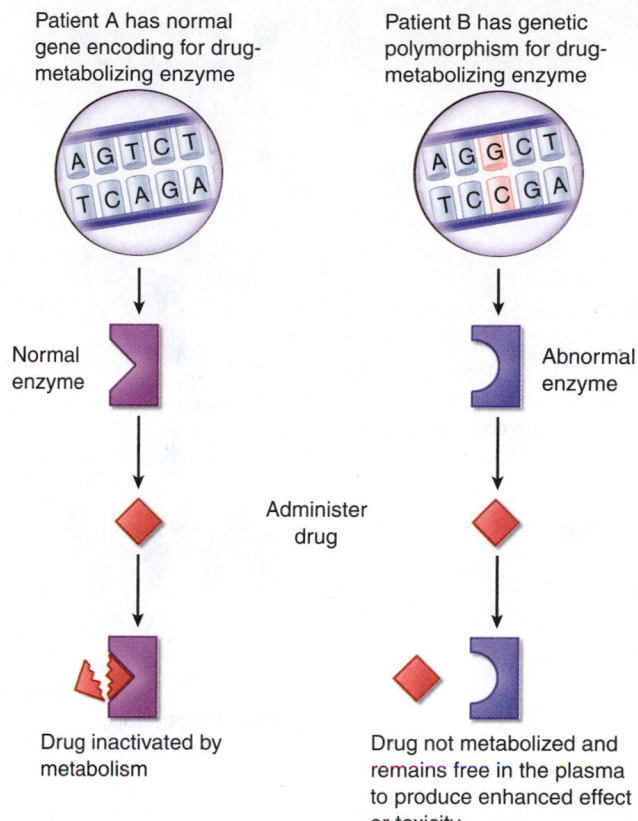

Figure 11.1 Consequences of genetic polymorphisms.

interaction. Small changes in the structure of the protein may result in a defective receptor that no longer "accepts" the drug. An active area of current research, receptor polymorphisms have been associated with an increased risk of schizophrenia, prostate cancer, breast cancer, and many other disorders. Relative to drug therapy, a few receptor polymorphisms have been shown to impact drug action, as shown in Table 11.1.

Genetic polymorphisms often occur in specific ethnic groups because members have settled in the same geographic area and have married mates within the same ethnic group for hundreds of generations. This practice results in amplified genetic polymorphisms being expressed within that specific group.

TABLE 11.1	Polymorphisms of Importance to Pharmacotherapy	
Type	**Result of Polymorphism**	**Drugs Affected**
Enzymes		
Acetyltransferase	Slow acetylation in African Americans and Caucasians; fast acetylation in Japanese and Eskimos	Hydralazine, isoniazid, and procainamide, sulfonamide antibiotics
Debrisoquin hydroxylase (CYP2D6)	Poor metabolism in Asians and African Americans	Codeine, haloperidol, metoprolol, morphine, perphenazine, propranolol, tricyclic antidepressants
Mephenytoin hydroxylase (CYP2C19)	Poor metabolism in Asians and African Americans	Barbiturates, diazepam, imipramine, warfarin
Receptors or Drug Targets		
Angiotensinogen	Blood pressure reduction	Angiotensin-converting enzyme (ACE) inhibitors
Dopamine receptor	Dyskinesias	Levodopa, antipsychotics
Beta$_2$-adrenergic receptor	Bronchodilation	Beta$_2$ agonists

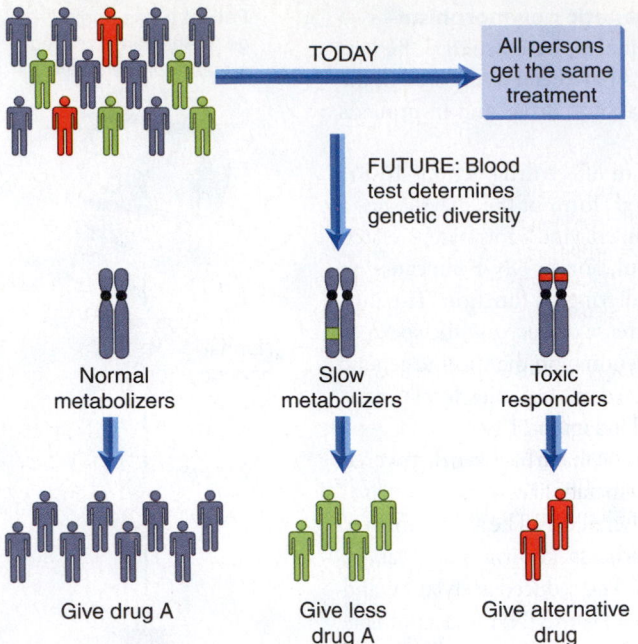

Figure 11.2 Pharmacogenomics and the future of pharmacotherapy.

Pharmacogenetics is the study of specific genetic variations that alter patients' responses to medications. *Pharmacogenomics* is a related term that is more general in scope, referring to the network of genes that govern a person's response to drug therapy. Both pharmacogenetics and pharmacogenomics attempt to identify genetic differences in metabolism or receptor targets that affect individual drug responses, with the ultimate goal of improving the safety and effectiveness of drug therapy through use of genetically guided treatment. It is expected that these fields will reveal data that will someday allow drug therapy that is customized for each individual patient based on his or her genetic profile, as illustrated in Figure 11.2.

CONNECTION Checkpoint 11.2

The best known genetic polymorphisms are those involving hepatic CYP enzymes. From what you learned in Chapter 3, explain the type of drug–drug interaction that might occur if Drug A induced CYP enzymes and Drug B was inactivated by the same enzymes. *See Answer to Connection Checkpoint 11.2 on student resource website.*

Gender Influences

11.4 Males and females may respond differently to drugs.

There are well-established differences in the patterns of disease between males and females. Women tend to pay more attention to changes in health patterns and seek health care earlier than their male counterparts. However, many women do not seek medical attention for potential cardiac problems, because heart disease has traditionally been considered to be a "man's disease." Alzheimer's disease affects both men and women, but studies in various populations have shown that 1.5 to 3 times as many women have the disease. Alzheimer's disease is now recognized as a primary "woman's health issue," along with osteoporosis, breast cancer, and fertility disorders.

Adherence to the medication regimen of a particular drug class may be influenced by gender because the adverse effects affect only one gender. A common example is certain antihypertensive drugs that produce male impotence. Males can experience strokes if they abruptly stop taking their medication to avoid impotence. Some drugs can cause gynecomastia, an increase in breast size, which can be embarrassing for males. Similarly, certain drugs can cause masculine adverse effects such as increased hair growth, which can be a cause of nonadherence in women taking these medications. Also in females, the estrogen contained in oral contraceptives causes an elevated risk of thromboembolic disorders.

Research has found many examples of differences in drug response between men and women. If males and females contain nearly all the same genes, how can these differences be explained? Although they may have identical genes, the "expression" of the genes differs greatly. For example, both males and females possess the same genes for hepatic metabolic enzymes, but one gender may produce more of a certain enzyme, thus producing a different degree of drug action. An example of a gender difference in a pharmacologic outcome is aspirin, which is more effective at preventing heart attacks in men than in women.

Some of the gender differences in drug response may be explained by differences in body composition, such as the fat-to-muscle ratio. Cerebral blood flow variances in genders can alter patient response to specific analgesics. An example is the benzodiazepines

CONNECTIONS   Treating the Diverse Patient

◖ Personalized Medicine in the Era of BiDil

BiDil, a fixed-dose combination of hydralazine and isosorbide dinitrate, became available in 2005 and was marketed to African Americans after research demonstrated that it was particularly effective in treating hypertension (HTN) in that population. Since that time, many articles have been written, research conducted, and questions raised about the efficacy, ethics, and legality of marketing a medication strictly to one population, especially based on race or ethnicity.

The incidence of HTN is higher in African Americans than other populations, and not all antihypertensive drugs work as well in all populations. Prior to the release of BiDil, some health care providers recommended initiating therapy with two drugs to ensure adequate response. The combination of a thiazide diuretic and calcium channel blocker seems to provide adequate control of HTN in African Americans. Therefore, was a "new and improved" fixed-combination medication needed? Postmarketing research suggested that BiDil was indeed an effective method of controlling HTN in its target population but the additional cost of the fixed-combination pill was a hindrance to its success as cheaper generic brands of hydralazine and isosorbide continued to be prescribed separately and more cheaply than the brand-name drug.

The questions raised by the approval of a "race-based drug" have advanced the era of pharmacogenomics. Recognizing that "race" or outward appearance are not sensitive indicators of genotype and ancestry has highlighted the need to recruit more diverse patients into clinical drug trials. It has also raised important questions about how genotypes can be identified and how those affect pharmacodynamics. BiDil has proven its clinical effectiveness and has also launched an era of more personalized medicine and how that may be achieved.

given for anxiety. Women experience slower elimination rates and this difference becomes more significant if a woman is concurrently taking oral contraceptives.

In the past, the majority of drug research studies were conducted using only male subjects. These studies assumed that there were no differences between genders and conclusions would apply to both males and females. Current research, however, recognizes that gender differences in drug response may exist, and new drug development research now includes both males and females, as appropriate. Gender consideration is necessary in the analyses of clinical data and assessment of potential pharmacokinetic and pharmacodynamic differences.

CHAPTER

11 Understanding the Chapter

Key Concepts Summary

11.1 Many psychosocial influences impact pharmacotherapy.

11.2 Cultural and ethnic variables can influence pharmacotherapy.

11.3 Genetic polymorphisms can affect drug action.

11.4 Males and females may respond differently to drugs.

Case Study: Making the Patient Connection

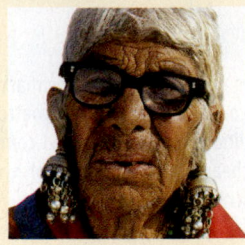

Remember the patient "Aponi Nampeyo" at the beginning of the chapter? Now read the remainder of the case study. Based on the information presented within this chapter, respond to the critical thinking questions that follow.

While traveling out of state with her husband to visit her children and grandchildren, Aponi Nampeyo became ill and was hospitalized. After being examined in the emergency department, she was diagnosed with appendicitis and underwent an emergency appendectomy. Aponi is a native of the United States and has lived most of her life in Arizona. She is well educated but she is not overly talkative and is comfortable with silence.

Aponi willingly accepts Western medical treatments. However, she also relies on traditional herbs and remedies from her youth. As the nurse caring for this patient, you are curious about her culture and health practices. However, you do not want to appear nosy or intrusive.

Critical Thinking Questions

1. Should nurses discuss cultural beliefs with patients? Explain your answer.
2. Describe how the nurse could learn about Mrs. Nampeyo's culture.
3. Are most health care workers culturally competent? Why? Why not?

See Answers to Critical Thinking Questions on student resource website.

Additional Case Study

Marjorie, a 30-year-old woman, is a single parent with three small children. She works as a self-employed housekeeper and earns minimum wage. Her annual income is $15,600, which pays for her family's housing, groceries, bus transportation, and clothing. Marjorie needs a job that pays benefits such as medical insurance. However, she fears that she will not be able to secure one because she never finished high school. She is constantly trying to save money. She has just been diagnosed with diabetes and requires insulin therapy.

1. Is it likely that Marjorie will be able to adequately care for her diabetes?
2. List the psychosocial factors that will influence this patient's ability to adhere to the therapy for her diabetes.
3. What can the nurse do to help this patient?

See Answers to Additional Case Study on student resource website.

Chapter Review

1 In initiating holistic care with a patient who has chronic headaches, which action would the nurse take?

1. Tell the patient to take Tylenol as directed on the label.
2. Ask the patient what he or she believes may be contributing to the problem.
3. Monitor the patient's pupil response to light.
4. Refer the patient to an ophthalmologist for an eye exam.

2 Various psychosocial variables may influence nonadherence to pharmacotherapy. An example of this would occur when the patient reports that the prescribed drug:

1. Produces an unpleasant aftertaste.
2. Is a very large tablet and difficult to swallow.
3. Is too expensive for the patient to afford.
4. Potentially causes hepatotoxicity.

3 A Native American patient states, "I will only take medications that are approved by the Shaman." The nurse understands that this statement reflects the patient's:

1. Ethnicity.
2. Cultural belief.
3. Genetic polymorphisms.
4. Health-related bias.

4 The nurse knows that patients characterized as slow acetylators:

1. Are more prone to drug toxicity.
2. Require more time to absorb enteral medications.
3. Must be given liquid medications only.
4. Should be advised to decrease protein intake.

5 Which of the following is considered a gender factor that may influence effective pharmacotherapy? Select all that apply.

1. Fat-to-muscle ratio
2. Cerebral blood flow
3. Limited drug research on females
4. Health beliefs
5. Dietary considerations

6 Which is the most effective method for a nurse to recognize patient-specific genetic influences?

1. Ask the patient if there have been drug-dose–related problems in the past.
2. Consult reference books and the Internet for information.
3. Observe the effects with other patients of similar racial-ethnic background.
4. Be cautious with all drugs and observe for individual patient responses.

See Answers to Chapter Review in Appendix A.

References

Ending racial and ethnic health disparities in the USA. (2011). *The Lancet, 377*(9775), 1379. doi:10.1016/S0140-6736(11)60556-4

Hoesli, T. M., & Smith, K. M. (2011). Effects of religious and personal beliefs on medication regimen design. *Orthopedics, 34,* 292–295. doi:10.3928/01477447-20110228-17

U.S. Department of Health and Human Services, Office of Minority Health. (2011). *American Indian, Alaska Native profile.* Retrieved from http://minorityhealth.hhs.gov/templates/ browse.aspx?lvl=2&lvlID=52

Selected Bibliography

Alfirevic, A., & Pirmohamed, M. (2010). Drug-induced hypersensitivity reactions and pharmacogenomics: Past, present, and future. *Pharmacogenomics, 11,* 497–499.

American Psychological Association. (2011). Practice guidelines regarding psychologists' involvement in pharmacological issues. *American Psychologist, 66*(9), 835–849. doi:10.1037/a0025890

Cheek, D. J. (2013). What you need to know about pharmacogenomics. *Nursing 2013, 43*(3), 44–48. doi:10.1097/01.NURSE.0000426621.59131.e5

Dawson, L. J. (2010). Promoting cultural competence in advanced pharmacology for nurse practitioner students. *Nursing Education Perspectives, 31,* 189–190. doi.org/10.1043/1536-5026-31.3.189

Ellison, G. T., Kaufman, J. S., Head, R. F., Martin, P. A., & Kahn, J. D. (2008). Flaws in the U.S. Food and Drug Administration's rationale for supporting the development and approval of BiDil as a treatment for heart failure only in black patients. *The Journal of Law, Medicine & Ethics, 36,* 449–457. doi:10.1111/j.1748-720x.2008.290.x

Grabenstein, J. D. (2013). What the world's religions teach, applied to vaccines and immune globulins. *Vaccine, 31*(16), 2011–2023. doi:10.1016/j.vaccine.2013.02.026

Hall-Lipsey, E. A., & Chisholm-Burns, M. A. (2010). Pharmacotherapeutic disparities: Racial, ethnic, and sex variations in medication treatment. *American Journal of Health-System Pharmacy, 67,* 462–468. doi:10.2146/ajhp090161

Johansson, I., & Ingelman-Sundberg, M. (2010). Genetic polymorphism and toxicology: With an emphasis on cytochrome P450. *Toxicological Sciences, 120,* 1–13. doi:10.1093/toxsci/kfq374

Ma, Q., & Lu, A. Y. (2011). Pharmacogenetics, pharmacogenomics, and individualized medicine. *Pharmacological Reviews, 63,* 437–459. doi:10.1124/pr.110.003533

Narayan, M. C. (2010). Culture's effects on pain assessment and management. *American Journal of Nursing, 110*(4), 38–47. doi:10.1097/01.NAJ.0000370157.33223.6d

O'Malley, P. (2011). Pharmacogenomics for the clinical nurse specialist—genetics, prescribing, and outcomes. *Clinical Nurse Specialist, 25*(3), 110–112. doi:10.1097/NUR.0b013e3182170fc2

Pestka, E. L., Burbank, K. F., & Junglen, L. M. (2010). Improving nursing practice with genomics. *Nursing Management, 41*(3), 40–44. doi:10.1097/01.NUMA.0000369499.99852.c3

Phan, V. H., Moore, M. M., McLachlan, A. J., Piquette-Miller, M., Xu, H., & Clarke, S. J. (2009). Ethnic differences in drug metabolism and toxicity from chemotherapy. *Expert Opinion on Drug Metabolism and Toxicology, 5,* 243–257. doi:10.1517/17425250902800153

Regitz-Zagrosek, V. (Ed.). (2012). *Sex and gender differences in pharmacology.* Berlin, Germany: Springer.

Rusert, B. M., & Royal, C. D. M. (2011). Grassroots marketing in a global era: More lessons from BiDil. *The Journal of Law, Medicine & Ethics, 39,* 79–90. doi:10.1111/j.1748-720X.2011.00552.x

Shah, R. R., & Shah, D. R. (2012). Personalized medicine: Is it a pharmacogenetic mirage? *British Journal of Clinical Pharmacology, 74,* 698–721. doi:10.1111/j.1365-2125.2012.04328.x

Soldin, O. P., Chung, S. H., & Mattison, D. R. (2011). Sex differences in drug disposition. *Journal of Biomedicine and Biotechnology, 2011.* doi:10.1155/2011/187103

UNIT

3

Pharmacology of the Autonomic Nervous System

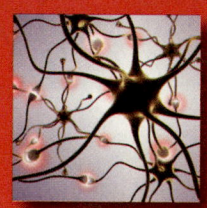 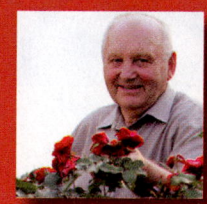 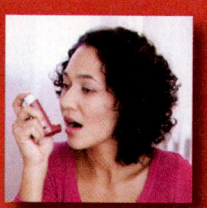 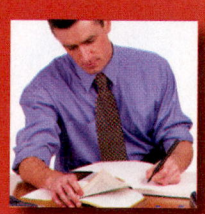

CHAPTER 12   Review of Neurotransmitters and the Autonomic Nervous System / 136

CHAPTER 13   Cholinergic Agonists / 149

CHAPTER 14   Cholinergic Antagonists / 163

CHAPTER 15   Adrenergic Agonists / 177

CHAPTER 16   Adrenergic Antagonists / 192

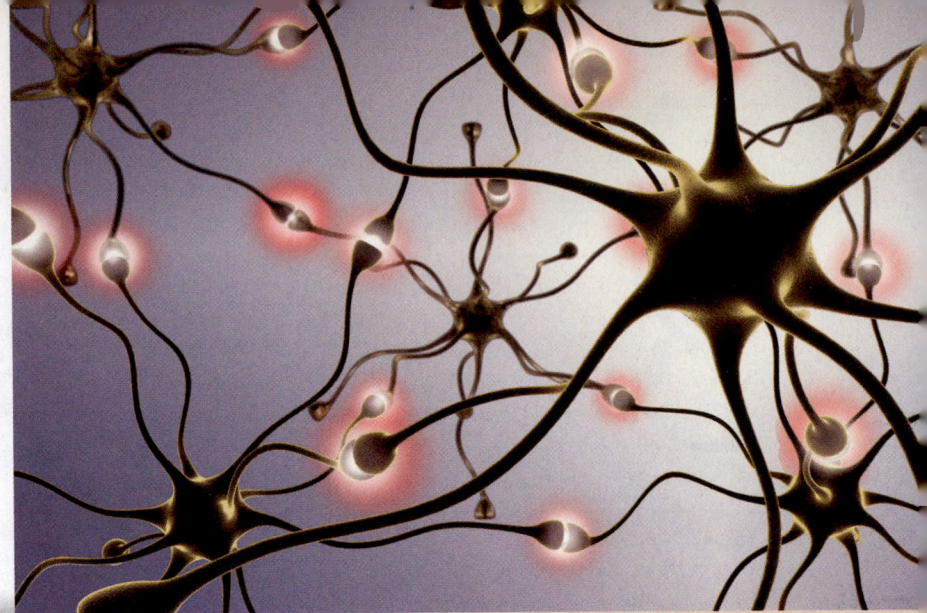

LEARNING OUTCOMES

After reading this chapter, the student should be able to:

1. Distinguish between the functions of the central and peripheral nervous systems.

2. Compare and contrast the two divisions of the peripheral nervous system.

3. Compare and contrast the actions of the sympathetic and parasympathetic divisions of the autonomic nervous system.

4. Explain the process of synaptic transmission.

5. Explain mechanisms by which drugs affect synaptic transmission.

6. Describe the actions of acetylcholine at cholinergic synapses.

7. Describe the actions of norepinephrine at adrenergic synapses.

8. Compare the actions of the adrenal medulla with those of other sympathetic effector organs.

9. Explain how higher centers in the brain can influence autonomic function.

10. Design a method for classifying autonomic drugs based on which receptors are affected.

CHAPTER OUTLINE

▸ Overview of the Nervous System

▸ Structure and Function of the Autonomic Nervous System

▸ Synaptic Transmission

▸ Cholinergic Transmission
  Cholinergic Receptors and Neurotransmitters
  Termination of Acetylcholine Action

▸ Adrenergic Transmission
  Alpha-Adrenergic Receptors
  Beta-Adrenergic Receptors
  Termination of Norepinephrine Action

▸ Regulation of Autonomic Functions

▸ Classifying Autonomic Drugs

KEY TERMS

acetylcholine (Ach), 140	cholinergic, 142	norepinephrine (NE), 140
acetylcholinesterase (AchE), 143	fight-or-flight response, 138	parasympathetic nervous system, 138
adrenergic, 144	ganglia, 140	rest-and-digest response, 138
autonomic nervous system (ANS), 137	monoamine oxidase (MAO), 145	somatic nervous system, 137
autonomic tone, 139	muscarinic, 143	sympathetic nervous system, 138
catecholamines, 144	neuroeffector junction, 140	synapse, 140
catechol-O-methyltransferase (COMT), 145	neurotransmitters, 140	synaptic cleft, 140
	nicotinic, 142	

Neuropharmacology represents one of the largest, most complicated, and least understood branches of pharmacology. Nervous system drugs are used to treat a large and diverse set of conditions, including pain, anxiety, depression, schizophrenia, insomnia, and seizures. Through their action on nerves, these medications are used to treat disorders affecting other body systems such as abnormalities in heart rate and rhythm, hypertension, glaucoma, asthma, and even a runny nose.

Traditionally, the study of neuropharmacology begins with the autonomic nervous system. This is because autonomic physiology lays the foundation for understanding nervous, cardiovascular, and respiratory pharmacology. This chapter serves two purposes. First, it provides a comprehensive review of autonomic nervous system physiology, a subject that is sometimes covered superficially in anatomy and physiology classes. Second, it introduces the four fundamental classes of autonomic medications, which are presented in depth in Chapters 13 through 16.

Overview of the Nervous System

12.1 The two major subdivisions of the nervous system are the central nervous system and the peripheral nervous system.

The nervous system is the master controller of most activities occurring within the body. Compared to the other major regulator, the endocrine system, the nervous system acts instantaneously to make adjustments that maintain vital functions. The brain, spinal cord, and peripheral nerves act as a smoothly integrated whole to accomplish minute-to-minute changes in essential functions such as heart rate, blood pressure, pupil size, and intestinal movement. The basic functions of the nervous system are to:

- Monitor the internal and external environment of the body and alert the brain of important changes.

- Process and integrate the environmental changes that are perceived and determine an appropriate response.

- Respond to the environmental changes by producing an action or a response.

The nervous system has two major divisions: the central nervous system (CNS) and the peripheral nervous system. The CNS is made up of the brain and spinal cord, whereas the peripheral division consists of nerves that carry messages to and from the CNS. Drugs used to treat disorders and conditions of the CNS are discussed in Chapters 17 through 26. The functional divisions of the nervous system are illustrated in Figure 12.1.

12.2 The peripheral nervous system is divided into somatic and autonomic components.

With its immense potential and complexity, the human brain requires a continuous flow of information to accomplish its functions. In addition, the brain would be useless without a means to carry out its commands. The peripheral nervous system provides the brain the means to communicate with and receive sensory messages from the outside world.

Neurons in the peripheral nervous system *recognize* changes to the environment (sensory division) and *respond* to those changes by moving muscles or secreting chemicals (motor division). The sensory division consists of specialized nerves that recognize touch, pain, heat, body position, light, or specific chemicals in body fluids. These sensory neurons send their messages to the spinal cord. Based on this information, the brain determines what messages are important, determines whether an action is needed, and plans an appropriate response.

The motor division is divided into two components. The **somatic nervous system** consists of nerves that provide for the voluntary control of skeletal muscle. The nerves of the **autonomic nervous system (ANS)** provide for the involuntary control of vital functions of the cardiovascular, digestive, respiratory, and genitourinary systems. The ANS controls vital life activities without people being aware of its functions. The three main activities of the ANS are:

- Contraction of smooth muscle of the bronchi, blood vessels, gastrointestinal (GI) tract, eye, and genitourinary tract

- Contraction of cardiac muscle

- Secretion of salivary, sweat, gastric, and bronchial glands

The ANS is particularly important to pharmacology because a large number of medications affect autonomic nerves. Some of these drug actions produce desirable, therapeutic effects, whereas others produce adverse effects. The remainder of this chapter reviews the structure and function of this complex system.

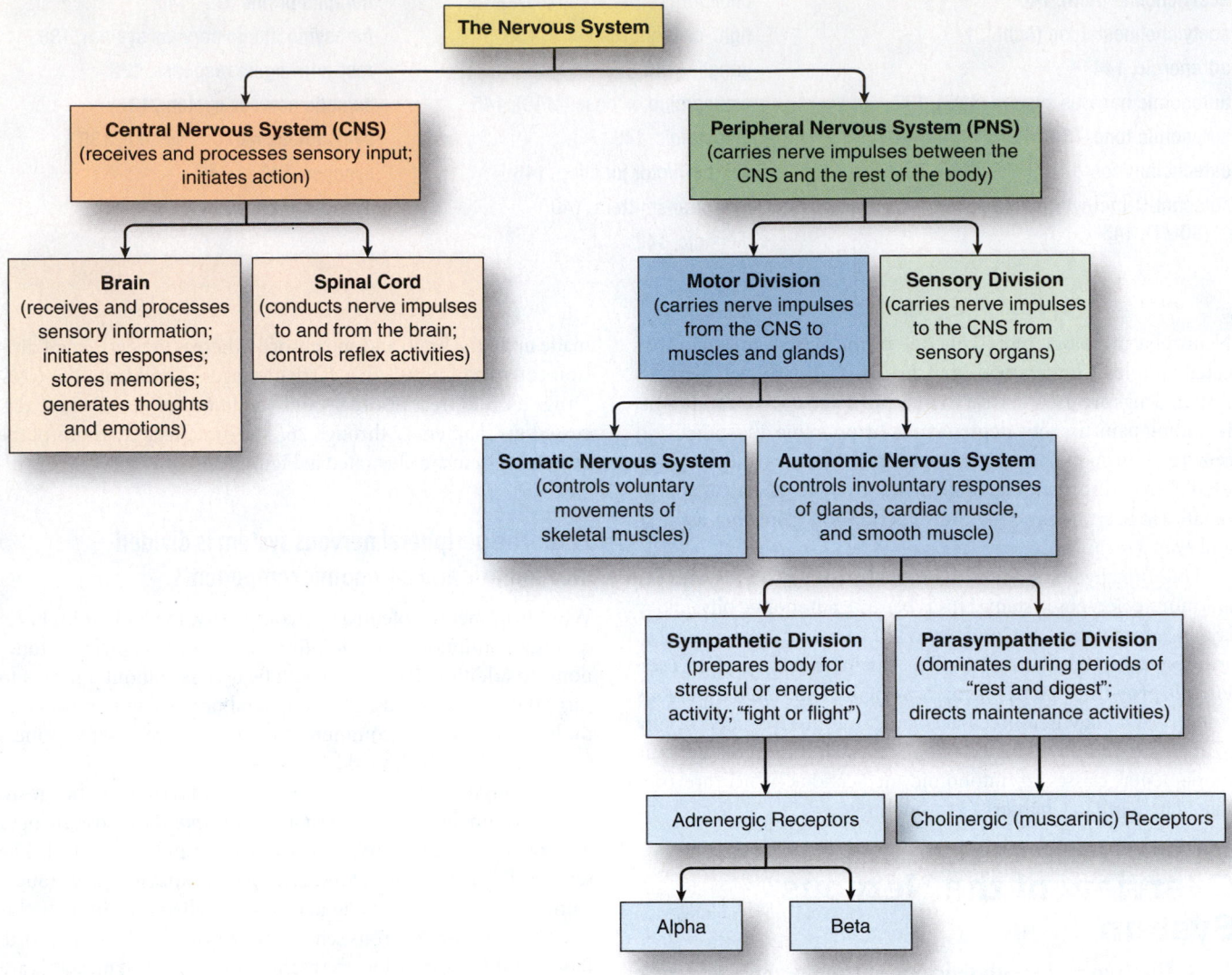

Figure 12.1 Functional divisions of the nervous system.

Structure and Function of the Autonomic Nervous System

12.3 The autonomic nervous system is divided into two mostly opposing components: the sympathetic and parasympathetic branches.

The ANS has two distinct divisions: the *sympathetic* nervous system and the *parasympathetic* nervous system. Most organs and glands receive nerves from both branches, and the two divisions have opposing actions. For example, one branch causes cardiac muscle to contract faster and with greater force; the other causes it to relax. The ultimate action of the cardiac muscle, smooth muscle, or gland depends on which branch is sending the most signals at any given time. The major actions of the two divisions are shown in Figure 12.2. It is essential for the student to learn these actions early in the study of pharmacology because knowledge of autonomic effects is used to predict the actions and adverse effects of many drugs.

The **sympathetic nervous system** is activated under emergency conditions or stress and produces a set of actions called the **fight-or-flight response**. Activation of this branch prepares the body for heightened activity and for an immediate response to a threat. The brain experiences an increase in alertness and readiness. Heart rate and blood pressure increase and blood is shunted to skeletal muscles, thus preparing the body for sudden, intense physical activity. The liver immediately produces more glucose for energy. The bronchi dilate to allow maximum airflow into the lungs, and breathing becomes faster and deeper. The pupils dilate to provide better vision for dealing with the emergency. The body warms and perspiration increases. At the same time the body is preparing for the threat, nonemergency maintenance functions such as peristalsis and urine formation are temporarily suspended.

The **parasympathetic nervous system** is activated under nonstressful conditions and produces a set of symptoms known as the **rest-and-digest response**. These nerves promote relaxation and body maintenance activities. Digestive secretions

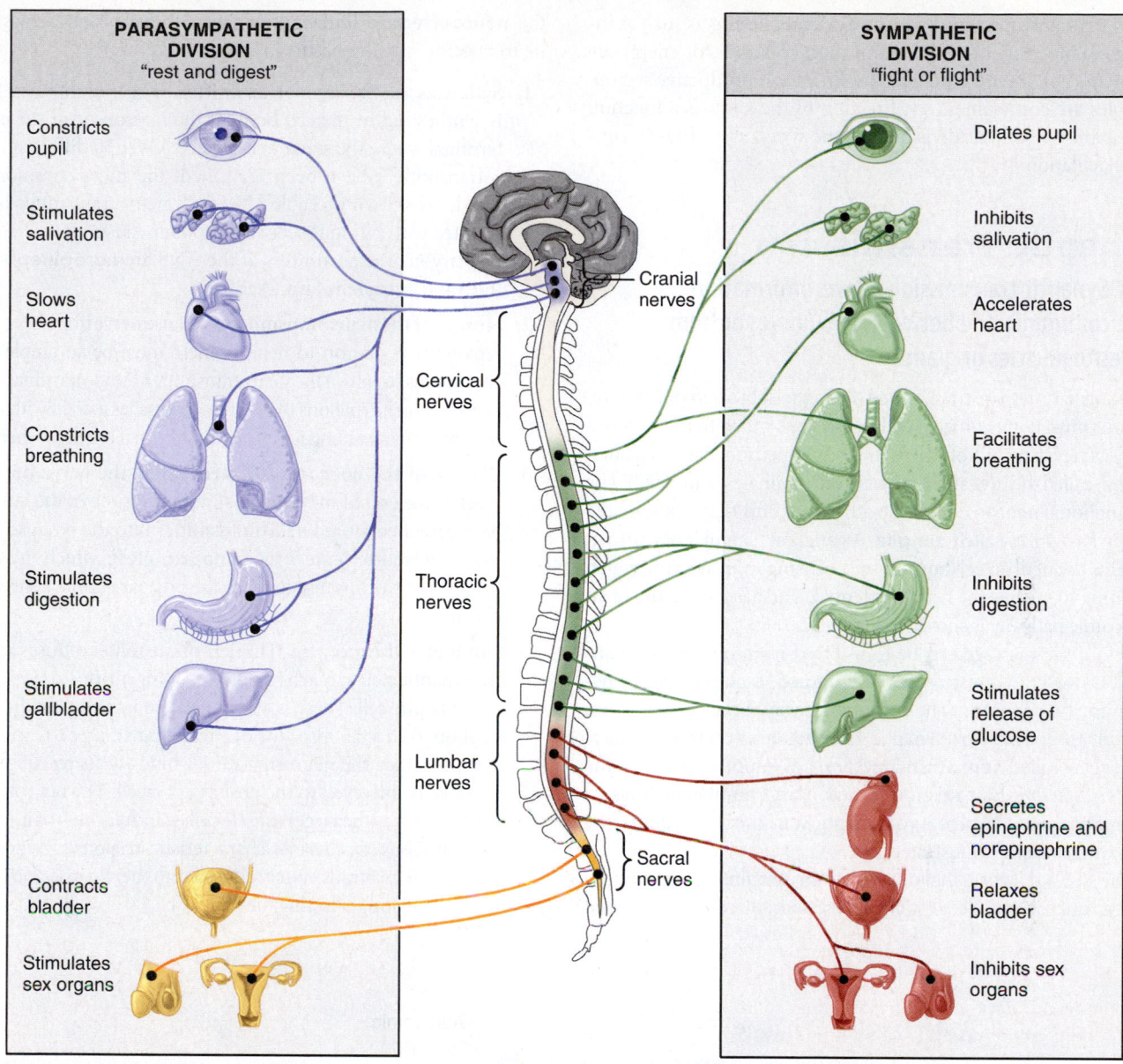

PARASYMPATHETIC DIVISION
"rest and digest"

Constricts pupil

Stimulates salivation

Slows heart

Constricts breathing

Stimulates digestion

Stimulates gallbladder

Contracts bladder

Stimulates sex organs

Cranial nerves

Cervical nerves

Thoracic nerves

Lumbar nerves

Sacral nerves

SYMPATHETIC DIVISION
"fight or flight"

Dilates pupil

Inhibits salivation

Accelerates heart

Facilitates breathing

Inhibits digestion

Stimulates release of glucose

Secretes epinephrine and norepinephrine

Relaxes bladder

Inhibits sex organs

Figure 12.2 Effects of the sympathetic and parasympathetic nervous systems.
From *Biology: A Guide to the Natural World* (5th ed., Figure 27.8), by D. Krogh, © 2011. Reprinted and electronically reproduced by permission of Pearson Education, Inc., Upper Saddle River, New Jersey.

increase, peristalsis propels substances along the alimentary canal, and defecation is promoted. Heart rate and blood pressure decline. Because less air is needed, the bronchi constrict and respiration slows. The student should notice that the actions of the parasympathetic division are opposite to those of the sympathetic division.

Under most conditions, the two branches of the ANS cooperate to achieve a balance of readiness and relaxation. Because they have opposite effects, homeostasis may be achieved by changing one or both branches. For example, heart rate can be increased by either increasing the firing of sympathetic nerves or by decreasing the firing of parasympathetic nerves. This allows the body to fine-tune its essential organ systems.

There is always some degree of autonomic activity even in the absence of stimuli. This background level of activity is known as **autonomic tone**. For example, sympathetic nerves

are constantly firing, keeping arterioles in a constant state of constriction. This sympathetic tone allows for faster changes in blood pressure because the vessels are in a constant state of readiness. On the other hand, parasympathetic tone on the smooth muscle of the alimentary and urinary tracts maintains continuous contractions and keeps intestinal peristalsis and urine flow steady. With the important exception of the vascular system, the predominant tone of autonomic tissues is from the parasympathetic nervous system.

The sympathetic and parasympathetic divisions do not always have opposite effects. For example, the constriction of arterioles is controlled entirely by the sympathetic branch. Sympathetic stimulation causes constriction of arterioles, whereas lack of stimulation causes vasodilation. Only sympathetic nerves control the adrenal medulla and the sweat glands. The sympathetic division is also solely responsible for the release of renin by the kidneys, an action that increases blood pressure. Metabolic effects such as increases in blood glucose and mobilization of lipids for energy are uniquely sympathetic functions. In the male reproductive system, the roles are complementary. Erection of the penis is a function of the parasympathetic division, and the sympathetic branch controls ejaculation.

Synaptic Transmission

12.4 Synaptic transmission allows information to be communicated between two nerves or from nerves to muscles or glands.

For information to be transmitted throughout the nervous system, neurons must communicate with each other and with muscles and glands. The basic unit of the ANS is a two-neuron chain. The first neuron, called the preganglionic neuron, originates in the CNS. The preganglionic neuron connects with the second nerve outside the CNS in structures called **ganglia**. A ganglion (singular of *ganglia*) contains the neuron cell body of the postganglionic neuron, which is waiting to receive the action potential. The basic structure of an autonomic pathway is shown in Figure 12.3.

Before the message can be transferred from one nerve to another, however, it must cross the **synapse**, a physical space between the two neurons. The communication of the message from one cell to another, or synaptic transmission, utilizes chemical messengers called **neurotransmitters**. It is important to study the details of synaptic transmission because a large number of drugs affect this process. The process of synaptic transmission is illustrated in Pharmacotherapy Illustrated 12.1.

The second (postganglionic) neuron terminates on smooth muscle, cardiac muscle, or a gland at a specialized synapse called the **neuroeffector junction**. Synaptic transmission across the neuroeffector junction occurs in several steps.

1. **Synthesis of the neurotransmitter.** The neurotransmitter is synthesized in the cell body of the neuron or in the axon terminal where the synapse is located. Over 50 different neurotransmitters have been identified, the most common of which are shown in Table 12.1. Each neurotransmitter is associated with a unique set of functions and responses. The two primary neurotransmitters of the ANS are **norepinephrine (NE)** and **acetylcholine (Ach)**.

2. **Storage of the neurotransmitter.** Because nerve impulses travel rapidly from neuron to neuron, there must be an ample and continuous supply of the neurotransmitter. At the terminal ends of each axon lie millions of granules or vesicles loaded with neurotransmitters, waiting for an action potential to release them.

3. **Release of the neurotransmitter.** When the nerve impulse reaches the end of the axon, it stimulates some of the vesicles to release their stored neurotransmitter into the synapse. The neurotransmitter enters the **synaptic cleft**, which must be bridged for the impulse to reach the postganglionic neuron or organ.

4. **Binding to the receptor.** The neurotransmitter diffuses across the synaptic cleft to reach receptors waiting on the surface of the postsynaptic cell. There is a brief delay in impulse conduction of about 0.2 to 0.5 msec for the neurotransmitter to cross the synapse. Once the neurotransmitter binds to its receptor, the message is conveyed to the postsynaptic cell. The neurotransmitter induces the target muscle cell, glandular cell, or another neuron tissue to elicit its characteristic response. Generally, the more neurotransmitter released into the synapse, the more intense and longer lasting the response.

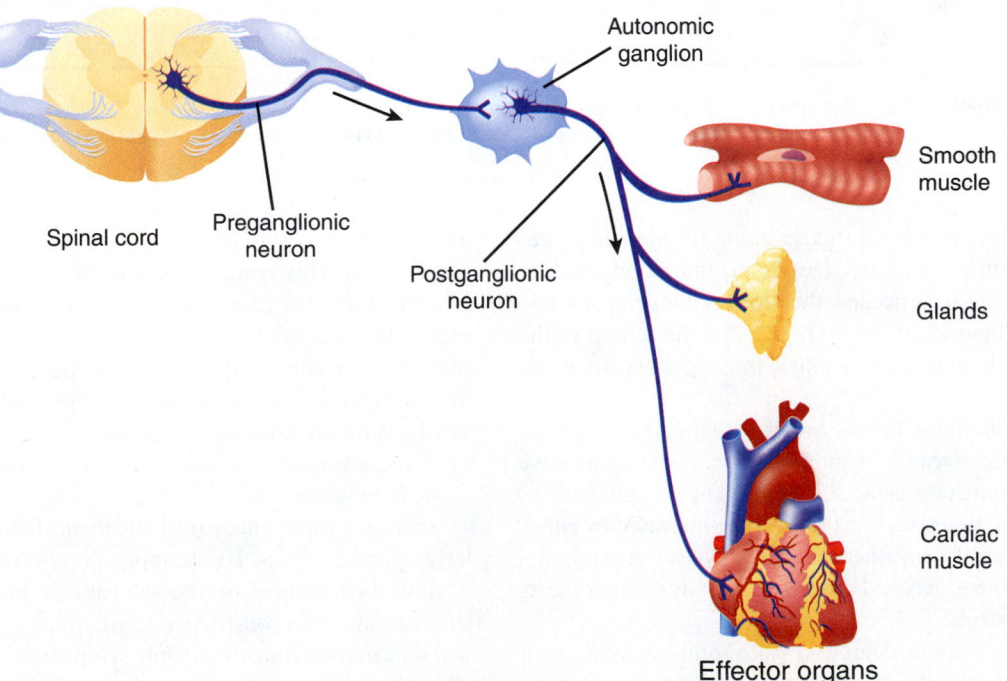

Figure 12.3 Basic structure of an autonomic pathway.

PHARMACOTHERAPY ILLUSTRATED 12.1

Synaptic Transmission

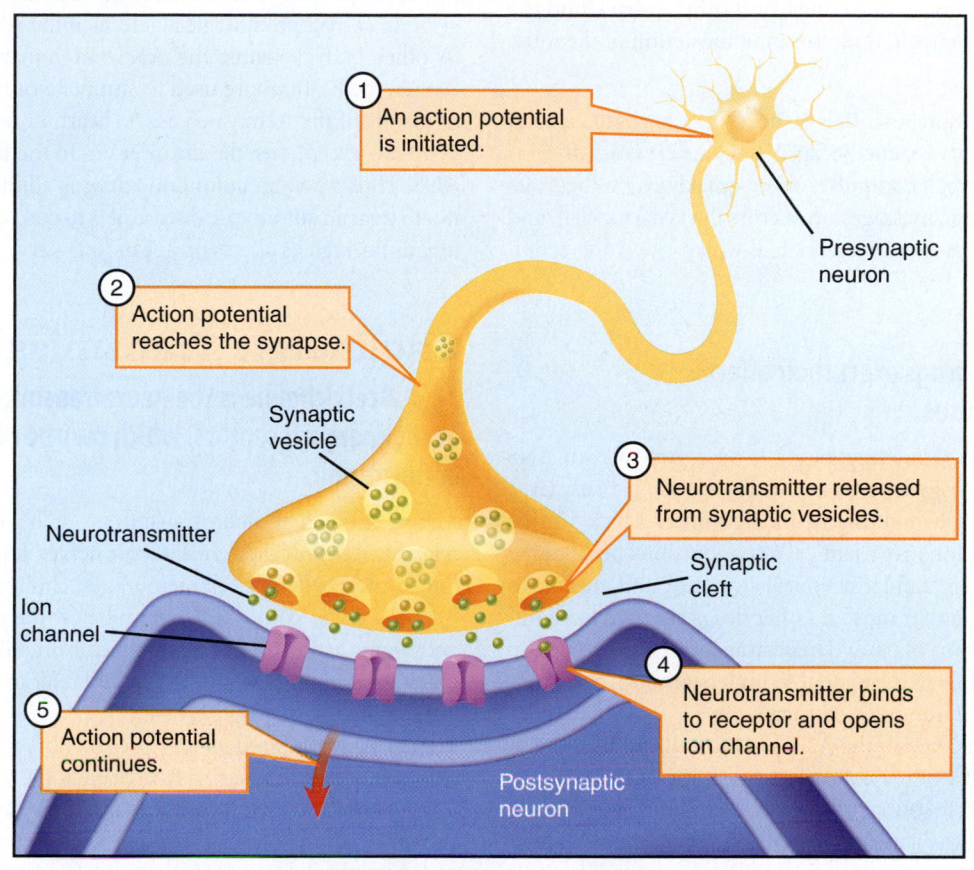

1. An action potential is initiated.

Presynaptic neuron

2. Action potential reaches the synapse.

Synaptic vesicle

Neurotransmitter

Ion channel

3. Neurotransmitter released from synaptic vesicles.

Synaptic cleft

4. Neurotransmitter binds to receptor and opens ion channel.

5. Action potential continues.

Postsynaptic neuron

TABLE 12.1	Selected Neurotransmitters: Effects and Clinical Applications	
Neurotransmitter	**Primary Location**	**Clinical Application (Chapter Number)**
Acetylcholine	Synapses throughout the CNS; preganglionic neurons ending in the ganglia in both the sympathetic and parasympathetic nervous systems (nicotinic); postganglionic neurons ending in neuroeffector target tissues in the parasympathetic nervous system (muscarinic)	Alzheimer's disease (21); Myasthenia gravis (13)
Dopamine	Limbic system and hypothalamus; some sympathetic ganglia	Attention deficit/hyperactivity disorder (24); Parkinson's disease (21); psychoses (20)
Gamma aminobutyric acid (GABA)	Cerebellum, cerebral cortex; interneurons throughout the CNS	Anxiety (18); seizures (22)
Glutamate	Throughout the CNS	Seizures (22)
Nitrous oxide	CNS, adrenal gland, and nerves to the penis	Impotence (71)
Norepinephrine	Throughout the CNS; most neuroeffector target junctions in the sympathetic nervous system	Attention deficit/hyperactivity disorder (24); cocaine and amphetamine abuse (27); depression (19)
Serotonin (5-HT)	Limbic system and hypothalamus; primary neurotransmitter in the extrapyramidal system; GI tract	Anxiety (18); depression (19); nausea and vomiting (60); psychoses (20)
Substance P	Pain pathways in the spinal cord; brain and sensory neurons	Analgesia (25)

5.   **Termination of neurotransmitter action.** Once the message is transmitted, the neuron and the effector cell must return to baseline conditions and ready themselves for future messages. This is accomplished by removal of the neurotransmitter. The neurotransmitter is either degraded in the synaptic cleft by enzymes, or it diffuses back into the preganglionic neuron, thus stopping the action of the muscle or gland.

Conduction of action potentials in the ANS is much slower than in the somatic nervous system. Because somatic nerves are myelinated and have no ganglia, impulses more quickly reach their target tissues. Autonomic messages must cross the synaptic cleft, and postganglionic nerves are unmyelinated, which slows the action potential.

12.5 Autonomic drugs exert their effects by acting at synapses.

The student may be wondering why it is necessary to learn ANS anatomy and physiology in such depth. The reason is that a large number of drugs act by altering neurotransmitter activity in the ANS. Some medications are identical to endogenous neurotransmitters, or have a very similar chemical structure, and are able to directly activate a gland or muscle. Other drugs are used to stimulate or block the actions of natural neurotransmitters. A firm grasp of autonomic physiology is essential to understanding the actions and adverse effects of hundreds of drugs.

The two-neuron chain of the ANS allows multiple locations at which drugs can act. Some medications affect the outflow of nervous impulses at their source—the CNS. A second potential site for drug action is at the ganglia, the synapse where the preganglionic and postganglionic neurons meet. Yet a third possible site is at the end of the chain, at the neuroeffector junction of the target organs.

Although complex, actions of drugs affecting this ANS can be grouped into just a few categories. The five general mechanisms by which drugs affect synaptic transmission in the ANS are as follows:

*   Medications may affect the *synthesis* of the neurotransmitter in the preganglionic nerve. Drugs that decrease neurotransmitter synthesis inhibit autonomic responses. Those that increase neurotransmitter synthesis have the opposite effect.

*   Medications can prevent the *storage* of the neurotransmitter in vesicles within the preganglionic nerve. Prevention of neurotransmitter storage inhibits autonomic actions.

*   Medications can influence the *release* of the neurotransmitter from the preganglionic nerve. Promoting neurotransmitter release stimulates autonomic responses, whereas preventing neurotransmitter release has the opposite effect.

*   Medications can bind to the *neurotransmitter receptors* on the postganglionic cell. Drugs that bind to receptors and stimulate the cell will increase autonomic responses. Those that attach to the postganglionic cell and prevent the natural neurotransmitter from reaching its receptors will inhibit autonomic actions.

*   Medications can *prevent the destruction or reuptake* of the neurotransmitter. These drugs cause the neurotransmitter to remain in the synapse for a longer time and will stimulate autonomic actions.

It is important to understand that autonomic drugs are rarely given to correct physiological defects in the ANS itself. Compared to other body systems, the ANS has remarkably little disease. Rather, medications are used to stimulate or inhibit target organs or glands of the ANS, such as the heart, lungs, or digestive tract. With few exceptions, the disorder lies in the target organ, not the ANS. Thus when an autonomic drug is administered, the goal is not to treat an autonomic disease; it is to correct disorders of target organs through its effects on autonomic nerves.

Cholinergic Transmission

12.6 Acetylcholine is the neurotransmitter released at cholinergic receptors, which may be nicotinic or muscarinic.

Ach was the first neurotransmitter to be identified. Neurons releasing Ach are called **cholinergic** nerves. Located on postganglionic or neuroeffector cell membranes, cholinergic receptors bind Ach and either continue the impulse (at the ganglia) or cause an autonomic action (at the neuroeffector organ). When reading the following sections, the student should refer to the sites of Ach and NE action shown in Figure 12.4.

Ach is synthesized in the preganglionic nerve terminal and stored in synaptic vesicles. A preganglionic neuron may contain 300,000 vesicles, each housing as many as 50,000 Ach molecules. When an action potential reaches the nerve terminal, a brief burst of Ach is released into the synaptic cleft, where it diffuses across to attach to its receptors on the postganglionic cell.

PharmFACT

Sir Henry Dale identified acetylcholine as a neurotransmitter in 1914, and Otto Loewi demonstrated its physiology. The pair was awarded the Nobel Prize in Physiology or Medicine in 1936 for their work (Nobelprize.org, 2011).

Cholinergic Receptors and Neurotransmitters

Two types of cholinergic receptors bind Ach. These are named after certain chemicals that bind to them:

*   **Nicotinic receptors.** Located at preganglionic neurons ending in the ganglia in both the sympathetic and parasympathetic nervous systems

*   **Muscarinic receptors.** Located at postganglionic neurons ending in neuroeffector target tissues in the parasympathetic nervous system

Early research on laboratory animals found that the actions of Ach at the ganglia resembled those of nicotine, the active chemical in tobacco products. Because of this similarity, receptors for Ach in the ganglia are called **nicotinic** receptors. Nicotinic receptors are also found in skeletal muscle, which is controlled by

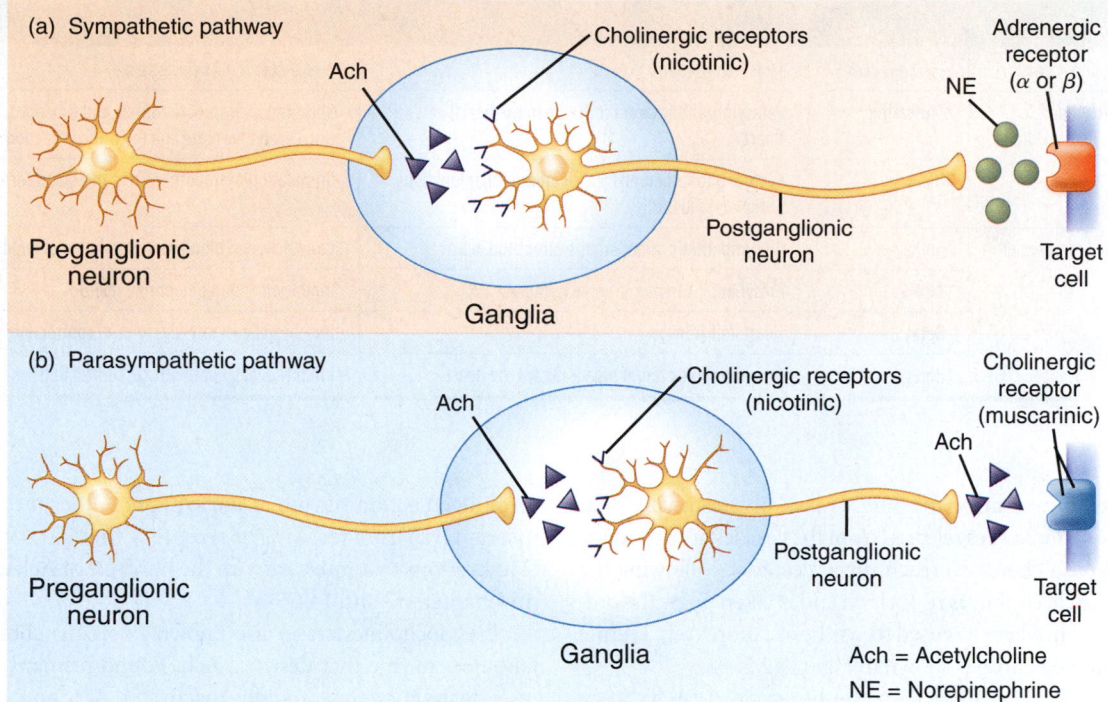

Figure 12.4 Receptors in the autonomic nervous system: (a) Sympathetic pathway: Ach is released at the ganglia (nicotinic receptor) and NE at the effector organ (adrenergic receptor). (b) Parasympathetic pathway: Ach is released at both the ganglia (nicotinic receptor) and effector organ (cholinergic receptor).

the somatic nervous system, and in the adrenal medulla. Because nicotinic receptors are present in so many locations, drugs affecting these receptors produce profound effects on both the ANS and somatic nervous system. Activation of Ach nicotinic receptors always produces stimulatory actions. Nicotinic actions include increased sweat production, increased release of adrenal medullary hormones, and enhanced nerve conduction in the ganglia; and tachycardia, hypertension, and increased tone and motility in the digestive tract. Although nicotinic receptor blockers were some of the first drugs used to treat hypertension, they are rarely used for this purpose today due to the discovery of safer drugs. The primary current therapeutic application of these drugs is to produce skeletal muscle relaxation (a somatic effect) during surgical procedures. A complete discussion of nicotinic blockers can be found in Chapter 14.

CONNECTION Checkpoint 12.1

Nicotine induces hepatic microsomal enzymes. From what you learned in Chapter 5, how can this induction affect the actions of medications? *See Answer to Connection Checkpoint 12.1 on student resource website.*

Activation of Ach receptors at postganglionic nerve endings in the parasympathetic nervous system results in the classic symptoms of parasympathetic stimulation shown in Figure 12.2. Early research determined that these actions closely resembled those produced after eating the poisonous mushroom *Amanita muscaria*. The active substance in this mushroom is the

chemical muscarine; thus, these Ach receptors were named **muscarinic** receptors. Muscarinic receptors are also found in most sweat glands and in blood vessels serving skeletal muscles. The locations of nicotinic and muscarinic receptors are illustrated in Figure 12.4.

Unlike the actions of Ach at nicotinic receptors, which are always stimulatory, Ach action at muscarinic receptors may be stimulatory or inhibitory, depending on the target organ. For example, activation of muscarinic receptors in the heart will *decrease* the heart rate, but activation of muscarinic receptors in the intestine will *increase* peristalsis. Drugs that affect muscarinic receptors have more pharmacologic applications than those affecting nicotinic receptors. Medications that block muscarinic receptors are used during ophthalmic procedures, as preanesthetic drugs, and in the pharmacotherapy of asthma and bradycardia (see Chapter 16).

Although Ach itself can stimulate both muscarinic and nicotinic receptors, some drugs are selective to only one type. Table 12.2 summarizes the types of responses produced by activation of the two types of Ach receptors.

Termination of Acetylcholine Action

The goal of nerve transmission is to produce an immediate, though transient, response. To accomplish this, Ach must be rapidly removed from the synaptic cleft after producing its effect. The enzyme that resides in the synaptic cleft and catalyzes the destruction of Ach is called **acetylcholinesterase (AchE)**, or cholinesterase (*Note*: The suffix *-erase* can be thought of as "wiping out" the Ach.)

TABLE 12.2 Types of Autonomic Receptors

Neurotransmitter	Receptor	Primary Locations	Selected Responses
Acetylcholine (cholinergic)	Muscarinic	Parasympathetic target (other than the heart) Heart	Stimulation of smooth muscle and exocrine gland secretions Decreased heart rate and force of contraction
	Nicotinic	Postganglionic neurons and neuromuscular junctions of skeletal muscle	Stimulation of smooth muscle and gland secretions
Norepinephrine (adrenergic)	Alpha$_1$	All sympathetic target organs except the heart	Constriction of blood vessels; dilation of pupils
	Alpha$_2$	Presynaptic adrenergic nerve terminals	Inhibition of norepinephrine release
	Beta$_1$	Heart and kidneys	Increased heart rate and force of contraction; release of renin
	Beta$_2$	All sympathetic target organs except the heart	Inhibition of smooth muscle contraction

AchE is quite efficient at performing its task. It is estimated that over half the Ach molecules released from the vesicles are destroyed before they have a chance to reach their receptors. Following the breakdown of Ach, choline is re-formed and is taken up by the preganglionic neuron, where it is used to synthesize more Ach. The life cycle of Ach in the neuron is shown in Figure 12.5.

Medications can interfere with the life cycle of Ach. Some drugs (and poisons) can prevent the inactivation of Ach by blocking the acetylcholinesterase enzyme. These drugs will cause a prolonged action of Ach at the synapse. Other medications will prevent Ach from reaching its receptors, thus blocking its actions. Medications that interfere with the life cycle of Ach are presented in Chapters 13 and 14.

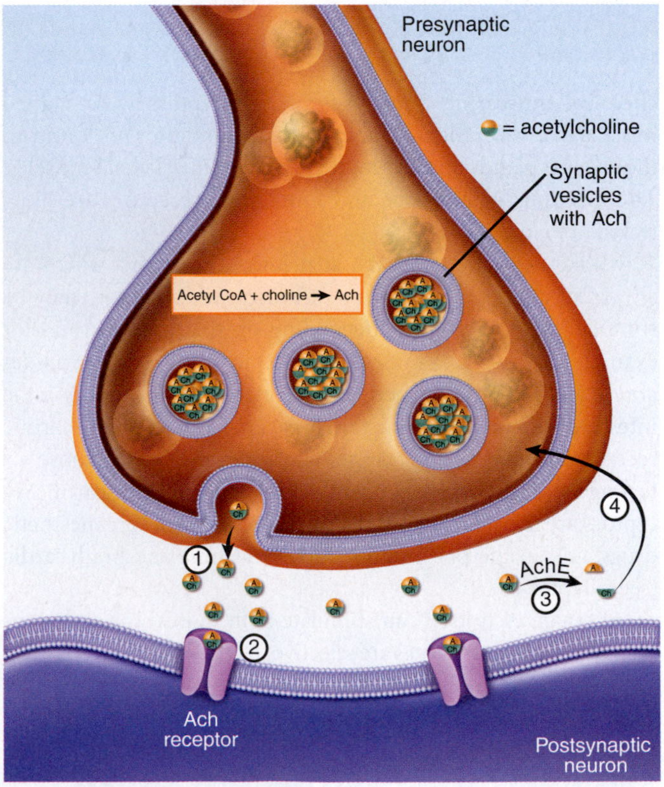

Pseudocholinesterase, also known as plasma cholinesterase, is another enzyme that destroys Ach. Found primarily in the liver, pseudocholinesterase rapidly inactivates Ach and drugs with a chemical structure similar to Ach as they circulate in the plasma. Some people are born with a genetic deficiency of this enzyme and are unable to inactivate succinylcholine, a surgical drug structurally similar to Ach. These patients are particularly sensitive to the effects of succinylcholine (see Chapter 26).

Adrenergic Transmission

12.7 Norepinephrine is the primary neurotransmitter released at adrenergic receptors, which may be alpha or beta.

In the sympathetic nervous system, NE is the neurotransmitter released at almost all postganglionic nerves. NE belongs to a class of hormones called **catecholamines**, all of which are involved in neurotransmission. Other endogenous catecholamines include epinephrine (adrenalin) and dopamine. The receptors at the ends of postganglionic sympathetic neurons are called **adrenergic**, which is derived from the word *adrenaline.*

NE is synthesized in the nerve terminal and stored in vesicles until an action potential triggers its release into the synaptic cleft. NE then diffuses across the cleft to bind to its receptors on the effector cell.

Adrenergic receptors are of two basic types: alpha (α) and beta (β). These receptors are further divided into the subtypes beta$_1$, beta$_2$, alpha$_1$, and alpha$_2$. Activation of each type of subreceptor results in a characteristic set of physiological responses, which are summarized in Table 12.2.

Figure 12.5 Life cycle of acetylcholine (Ach): (1) Ach is released into the synaptic cleft; (2) Ach binds to receptors on the postsynaptic membrane; (3) Ach is broken down into acetate and choline. (4) Choline is returned to the presynaptic neuron and recycled to make additional Ach.

PharmFACT

According to Aronson (2000), adrenaline was isolated and identified by John Jacob Abel in 1897, who founded the very first Department of Pharmacology at the University of Michigan. The name was changed to "epinephrine" in the United States because Parke, Davis, and Co. owned the trademark rights to the word *adrenalin* (without a final "e"). It is still known as adrenaline in the rest of the world.

Alpha-Adrenergic Receptors

When alpha receptors are stimulated, enzymes on the inside of the plasma membrane are activated and a cascade of changes occurs within the cell. These changes occur due to the production of a second messenger, the G-protein, which initiates the cascade. In alpha$_1$ receptors intracellular calcium stores are released, causing excitatory effects such as smooth muscle contraction or sphincter closure. Drugs affecting alpha$_1$ receptors are primarily used for their effects on vascular smooth muscle in the treatment of hypertension (see Chapters 16 and 34). Drugs that block the alpha$_1$ receptor are used to treat benign prostatic hyperplasia (see Chapters 14 and 71).

Stimulation of alpha$_2$ receptors causes different effects due to the activation of a separate cascade of events in the target cells. By increasing cyclic adenosine monophosphate (cAMP) within the cell, activation of alpha$_2$ receptors inhibits NE release from sympathetic nerve endings, causing mostly *inhibitory* actions. In addition, activation of alpha$_2$ receptors in the CNS can suppress the outflow of sympathetic activity from the brain. Indeed, as will be discussed in Chapter 15, drugs that affect alpha$_2$ receptors are usually used for their ability to decrease blood pressure due to their effects on the CNS, not the ANS.

Beta-Adrenergic Receptors

Three subtypes of beta-adrenergic receptors have been identified, although only beta$_1$ and beta$_2$ have pharmacologic importance. Beta receptors act by increasing the second messenger cAMP in target cells. The specific response caused by activation of the beta receptor depends on its location.

The primary tissues served by beta$_1$ receptors are the heart, coronary vessels, and kidneys. Activation of these receptors increases the heart rate and strength of contraction and dilates the coronary arteries, thus preparing the heart for fight or flight. Beta$_1$ receptors in the kidney respond by releasing renin, which helps to maintain (increase) blood pressure.

Beta$_2$ receptors are more widely distributed than beta$_1$ receptors, with locations in the smooth muscle in arterioles, the GI tract, and the lungs. Activation of these receptors will dilate arteries to skeletal muscles, dilate bronchioles, slow peristalsis, and decrease urine production.

The significance of adrenergic receptor subtypes to pharmacology cannot be overstated. Some drugs are selective and activate only one type of adrenergic receptor, whereas others affect all of them. Furthermore, a drug may activate one type of receptor at low doses and begin to affect other receptor subtypes as the dose is increased. Committing the receptor types and their responses to memory is an essential step in learning autonomic pharmacology.

Other types of adrenergic receptors exist. Although the functional role of dopamine was once thought to be only a chemical precursor to NE, research has determined that this agent serves a larger role as a neurotransmitter. Five dopaminergic receptors (D1 through D5) have been discovered in the CNS. Dopaminergic receptors are important to the action of certain antipsychotic medicines (see Chapter 20) and in the treatment of Parkinson's disease (see Chapter 21). Dopamine receptors in the peripheral nervous system are located in the arterioles of the kidney and other viscera. Although these receptors likely have a role in autonomic function, their therapeutic importance has yet to be discovered.

Termination of Norepinephrine Action

The termination of NE action occurs through mechanisms different from those of Ach. The majority of the NE (50% to 80%) is taken back into the nerve terminal, a process known as *reuptake*. Following its reuptake, NE is repackaged in vesicles for future use or destroyed enzymatically by **monoamine oxidase (MAO)**. NE entering the circulation, such as that secreted by the adrenal glands or given as medication, is destroyed by the enzyme **catechol-O-methyltransferase (COMT)** in kidney and liver cells. Many drugs affect autonomic function by influencing the synthesis, storage, release, reuptake, or destruction of NE. The life cycle of NE is shown in Figure 12.6.

Activation of the sympathetic division produces longer lasting effects than those of parasympathetic activation. This is because NE acts *indirectly* through a second messenger mechanism. Its effects are produced more slowly than Ach, which acts directly at cholinergic sites. Furthermore, the primary means of inactivation of NE is through reuptake, which is a slower process than the direct enzymatic destruction of Ach.

CONNECTION Checkpoint 12.2

The herb St. John's wort is believed to inhibit the reuptake of serotonin into presynaptic nerve terminals in the CNS. From what you learned in Chapter 7, what is the most common indication for using this herb? *See Answer to Connection Checkpoint 12.2 on student resource website.*

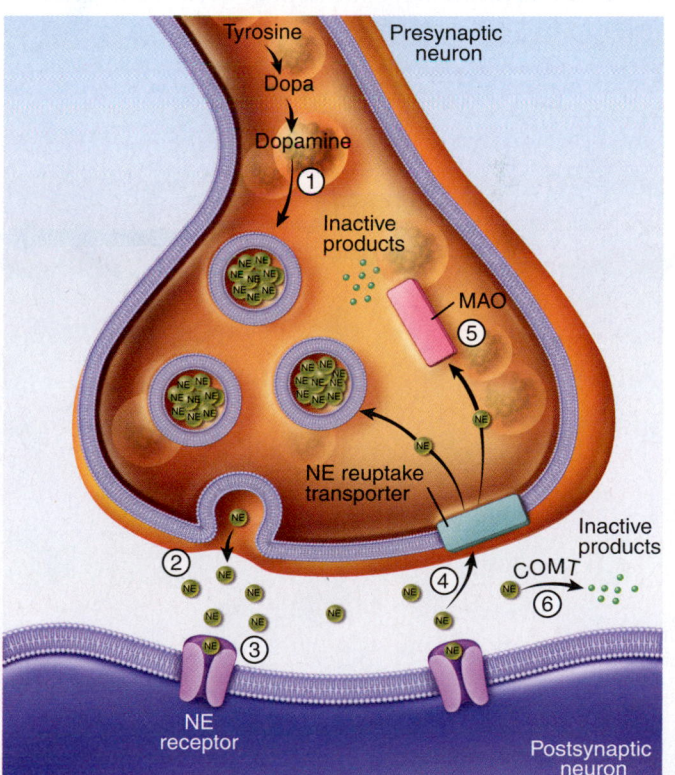

Figure 12.6 Life cycle of norepinephrine (NE): (1) NE is synthesized from the amino acid tyrosine; (2) NE is released into the synaptic cleft; (3) NE binds to receptors on the postsynaptic membrane; (4) NE is taken back into the presynaptic neuron; (5) NE is degraded by MAO; (6) Small amounts of NE are degraded by COMT.

12.8 The adrenal medulla is a specialized type of sympathetic nervous system tissue that secretes epinephrine and norepinephrine.

Lying in the inner portion of each adrenal gland, the adrenal medulla is closely associated with the sympathetic nervous system but has a different anatomic and physiological arrangement than the rest of the sympathetic branch. Early in embryonic life, the adrenal medulla is part of the neural tissue that is destined to become the sympathetic nervous system. This primitive tissue splits, however, and the adrenal medulla becomes its own functional division. Preganglionic neurons from the spinal cord terminate in the adrenal medulla and release the neurotransmitters epinephrine and NE *directly* into the blood. Approximately 80% of the secretion is epinephrine, with the other 20% being NE. Once released, these agents are widely distributed to target organs, where they elicit the classic fight-or-flight symptoms.

Once released into the systemic circulation by the adrenal gland, epinephrine and NE produce more diffuse and longer lasting effects than those produced by activation of sympathetic neurons in the ANS. In addition, the bloodstream distributes these agents to all body cells, not just those innervated by the ANS. Significant concentrations of epinephrine and NE may persist for as long as 30 seconds, and their effects on tissues may continue for several minutes until the liver eventually deactivates the hormones. It is estimated that 25% to 50% of all sympathetic nervous system responses at any given time are due to circulating hormones from the adrenal medulla.

Regulation of Autonomic Functions

12.9 The autonomic nervous system is influenced by higher levels of control in the cerebral cortex and hypothalamus.

Although it is often stated that control of the ANS is involuntary, this is an oversimplification. For example, strong emotions such as rage are seated in the brain, but they trigger the heart to race, the blood pressure to rise, and the respiration rate to increase. Mental depression can have the opposite effects. The smell of steak or chicken cooking on the grill can increase peristalsis, resulting in "grumbling" of the stomach and increased salivation. Clearly, autonomic actions can be modified by higher brain centers.

The roles of higher centers in regulating the ANS are shown in Figure 12.7. The hypothalamus is thought to be the main integration center of the ANS. This tissue receives signals from the cerebrum and sensory input, such as emotions, from the limbic system of the brain. The hypothalamus interprets the information and responds by sending messages to the various portions of the ANS, such as increasing peristalsis and salivation when the sights, sounds, and smells of the grilled steak are experienced. Messages from the hypothalamus travel along the medulla oblongata, the brainstem, and the spinal cord.

Drugs can affect the ANS by influencing these higher centers. For example, drugs that decrease anxiety or diminish the incidence

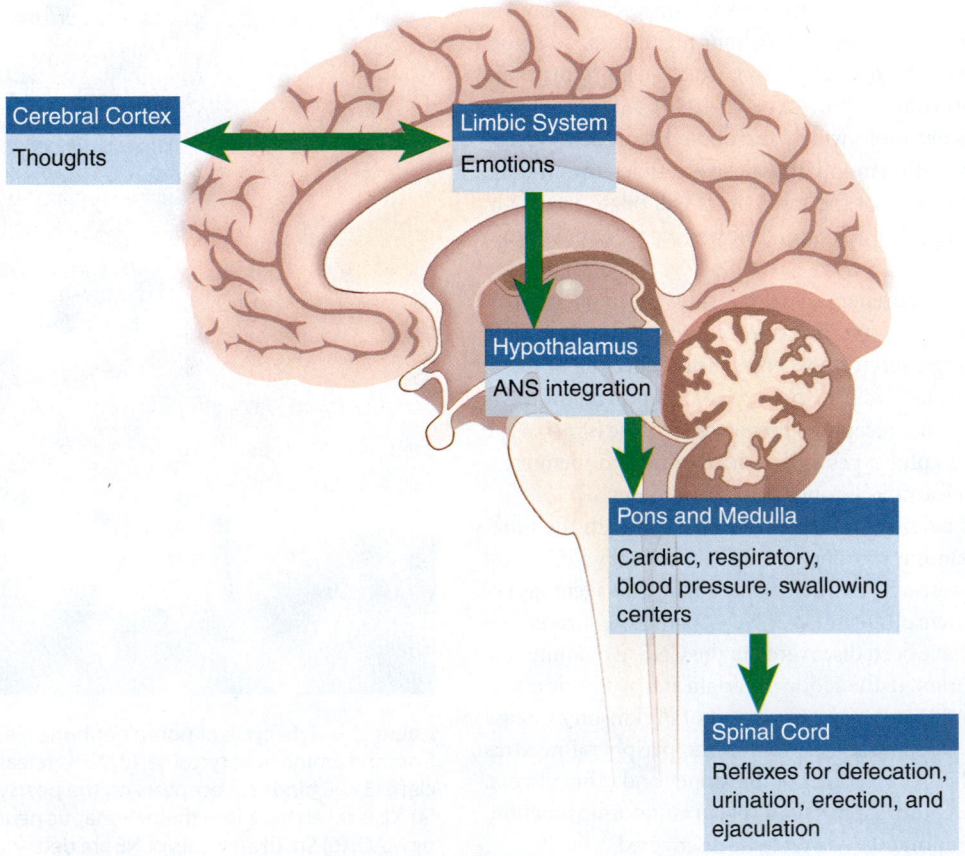

Figure 12.7 Higher centers influencing autonomic function.

of panic attacks can slow the heart rate and lower blood pressure through their ability to affect conscious thought. It is important to understand that these drugs do not necessarily act on autonomic receptors. Nor do patients consciously lower their blood pressure or heart rate. The autonomic effect is indirect, caused by a reduction of stress, and it is at a subconscious level. Controlling autonomic activity through conscious thought is the principle underlying biofeedback therapy.

Classifying Autonomic Drugs

12.10 Autonomic drugs are classified by which receptors they stimulate or block.

At this point of the chapter, it is normal for students to feel overwhelmed by the complexity of the various autonomic receptors and their actions. It is the existence of these different receptors, however, that allows drugs to cause very specific therapeutic actions. For example, it is desirable to have drugs that affect blood pressure without increasing heart rate, or drugs that dilate bronchi without causing hypertension. At this stage in the study of pharmacology, the student can just memorize the receptor types and actions, because applications in the coming chapters will provide clarity to this subject.

Given the opposite actions of the sympathetic and parasympathetic nervous systems, autonomic drugs are classified based on one of four possible actions:

1. **Stimulation of the sympathetic nervous system.** These drugs are called sympathomimetics or adrenergic agonists and they produce the classic symptoms of the fight-or-flight response.

2. **Stimulation of the parasympathetic nervous system.** These drugs are called parasympathomimetics or muscarinic agonists and they produce the characteristic symptoms of the rest-and-digest response.

3. **Inhibition of the sympathetic nervous system.** These drugs are called adrenergic antagonists or adrenergic blockers and they produce actions opposite to those of the sympathomimetics.

4. **Inhibition of the parasympathetic nervous system.** These drugs are called anticholinergics, parasympatholytics, or muscarinic blockers and they produce actions opposite to those of the parasympathomimetics.

There is a method for simplifying the learning of autonomic pharmacology. On examining the preceding four drug classes, it is evident that only one group need be learned because the others are logical extensions of the first. If the fight-or-flight symptoms of the sympathomimetics are learned, the other three groups are either the same or opposite. For example, both the sympathomimetics and the anticholinergics increase heart rate and dilate the pupils. The other two groups, the parasympathomimetics and the adrenergic antagonists, have the opposite effects of slowing heart rate and constricting the pupils. Although this is an oversimplification and exceptions exist, it is a time-saving means of learning the basic actions and adverse effects of dozens of drugs affecting the ANS. It should be emphasized again that mastering the actions and terminology of autonomic drugs early in the study of pharmacology will reap rewards later in the course when these drugs are applied to various systems. Table 12.3 shows the many applications of autonomic drugs in medicine and the chapter in this text in which each is covered.

TABLE 12.3	Indications for Autonomic Drugs	
Indication	**Autonomic Class**	**Chapter**
Allergic rhinitis and the common cold	Alpha$_2$-adrenergic agonists	45
Alzheimer's disease	Cholinergic agonists	21
Angina pectoris	Beta-adrenergic blockers	35
Asthma and COPD	Beta-adrenergic agonists Anticholinergics	44
Benign prostatic hyperplasia	Alpha-adrenergic blockers	71
Dysrhythmias	Beta-adrenergic blockers	37
Eye examinations	Anticholinergics	74
Glaucoma	Alpha-adrenergic blockers Beta-adrenergic blockers Cholinergic agonists	74
Heart failure	Beta-adrenergic blockers Beta-adrenergic agonists	36
Hypertension	Alpha$_1$-adrenergic blockers Alpha$_2$-adrenergic agonists Beta-adrenergic blockers	34
Hypotension and shock	Beta-adrenergic agonists	15
Myasthenia gravis	Cholinergic agonists	13
Myocardial infarction	Beta-adrenergic blockers	35
Parkinson's disease	Anticholinergics	21
Peptic ulcer disease	Anticholinergics	59
Thyroid crisis (storm)	Beta-adrenergic blockers	67

CHAPTER

12   Understanding the Chapter

Key Concepts Summary

12.1   The two major subdivisions of the nervous system are the central nervous system and the peripheral nervous system.

12.2   The peripheral nervous system is divided into somatic and autonomic components.

12.3   The autonomic nervous system is divided into two mostly opposing components: the sympathetic and parasympathetic branches.

12.4   Synaptic transmission allows information to be communicated between two nerves or from nerves to muscles or glands.

12.5   Autonomic drugs exert their effects by acting at synapses.

12.6   Acetylcholine is the neurotransmitter released at cholinergic receptors, which may be nicotinic or muscarinic.

12.7   Norepinephrine is the primary neurotransmitter released at adrenergic receptors, which may be alpha or beta.

12.8   The adrenal medulla is a specialized type of sympathetic nervous system tissue that secretes epinephrine and norepinephrine.

12.9   The autonomic nervous system is influenced by higher levels of control in the cerebral cortex and hypothalamus.

12.10   Autonomic drugs are classified by which receptors they stimulate or block.

References

Aronson, J. K. (2000). Where name and image meet—the argument for "adrenaline." *British Medical Journal, 320*, 506–509. doi:10.1136/bmj.320.7233.506

Krogh, D. (2011). *Biology: A guide to the natural world* (5th ed.). San Francisco, CA: Benjamin Cummings.

Nobelprize.org. (2011). *The Nobel Prize in physiology or medicine 1936*. Retrieved from http://nobelprize.org/nobel_prizes/medicine/laureates/1936

Selected Bibliography

Martini, F. H., Nath, J. L., & Bartholomew, E. F. (2012). *Fundamentals of human anatomy and physiology* (9th ed.). San Francisco, CA: Benjamin Cummings.

Parati, G., & Esler, M. (2012). The human sympathetic nervous system: Its relevance in hypertension and heart failure. *European Heart Journal, 33*, 1058–1066. doi:10.1093/eurheartj/ehs041

Silverthorn, D. U. (2013). *Human physiology: An integrated approach* (6th ed.). Upper Saddle River, NJ: Pearson /Benjamin Cummings.

Squire, L. R., Berg, D., Bloom, F. E., Du Lac, S., & Ghosh, A. (Eds.). (2012). *Fundamental neuroscience*. Waltham, MA: Academic Press.

Westfall, T. C., & Westfall, D. P. (2011). Neurotransmission: The autonomic and somatic motor nervous systems. In L. L. Brunton, B. A. Chabner, & B. C. Knollman (Eds.), *Goodman and Gilman's the pharmacological basis of therapeutics* (12th ed., pp. 171–218). New York, NY: McGraw-Hill.

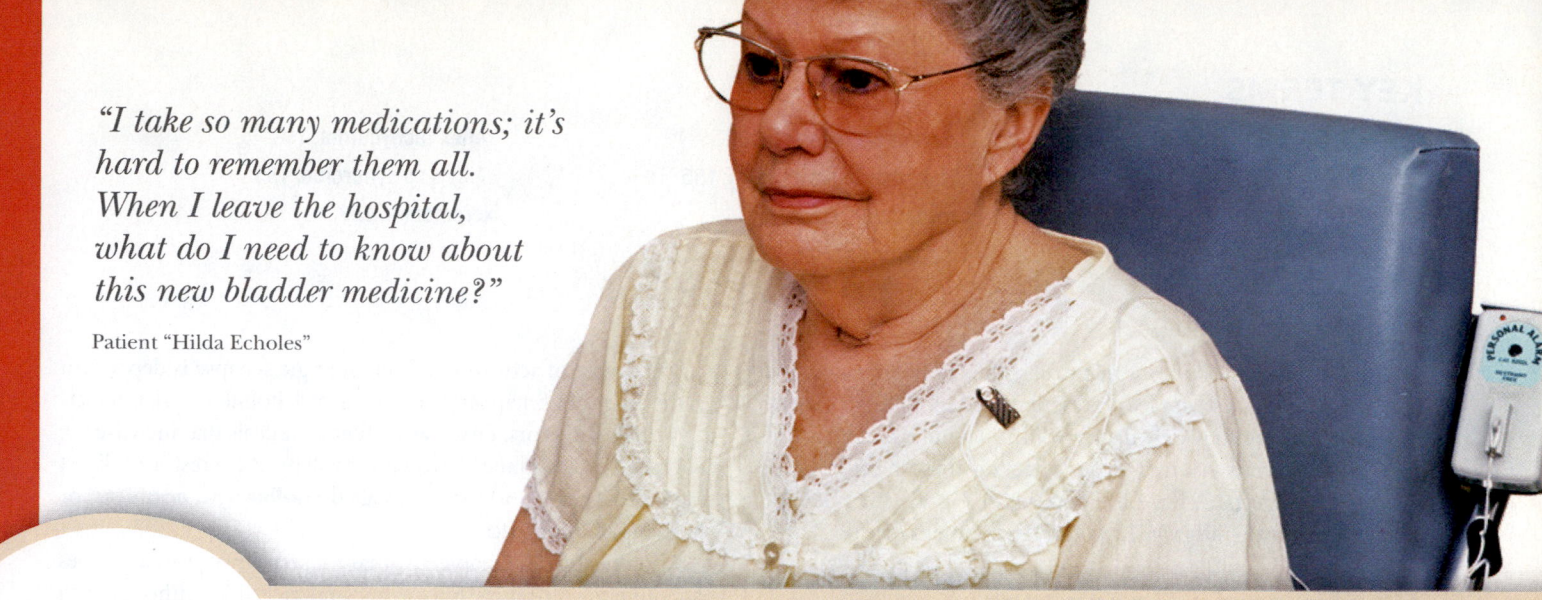

"I take so many medications; it's hard to remember them all. When I leave the hospital, what do I need to know about this new bladder medicine?"

Patient "Hilda Echoles"

CHAPTER

13

Cholinergic Agonists

LEARNING OUTCOMES

After reading this chapter, the student should be able to:

1. Compare and contrast the mechanisms of action for direct- and indirect-acting cholinergic agonists.
2. Identify the actions of muscarinic agonists and their pharmacologic uses.
3. Describe the pharmacotherapy of myasthenia gravis.
4. Differentiate between the treatment of cholinergic crisis and myasthenic crisis.
5. Explain the actions and pharmacologic applications of nicotine.
6. For each of the classes shown in the chapter outline, identify the prototype and representative drugs and explain the mechanism(s) of drug action, primary indications, contraindications, significant drug interactions, pregnancy category, and important adverse effects.
7. Apply the nursing process to care for patients receiving pharmacotherapy with cholinergic agonists.

CHAPTER OUTLINE

▶ **Cholinergic Receptors**

▶ **Muscarinic Agonists**
   Direct-Acting Muscarinic Agonists
   PROTOTYPE Bethanechol (Urecholine), *p. 153*

   Indirect-Acting Muscarinic Agonists (acetylcholinesterase inhibitors)

▶ **Cholinergic Crisis**

▶ **Pharmacotherapy of Myasthenia Gravis**
   PROTOTYPE Pyridostigmine (Mestinon, Regonol), *p. 157*

▶ **Nicotinic Agonists**

KEY TERMS

acetylcholinesterase (AchE)
  inhibitors, 154
cholinergic agonists, 150
cholinergic crisis, 155

muscarinic agonist, 150
myasthenia gravis (MG), 155
myasthenic crisis, 156
nicotinic agonist, 150

reflex tachycardia, 153
Sjögren's syndrome, 153
xerostomia, 153

Of the four classes of autonomic drugs, the cholinergic agonists comprise the smallest and least prescribed group. Because cholinergic synapses are so widely dispersed throughout the central and peripheral nervous systems, drugs affecting these receptors will have diverse effects. A few have applications in the treatment of glaucoma, myasthenia gravis, and early Alzheimer's disease.

Cholinergic Receptors

13.1 Drugs can activate cholinergic receptors either directly or indirectly.

Recall from Chapter 12 that cholinergic receptors are located throughout the peripheral nervous system. To understand the effects of cholinergic drugs, it is important to review these locations. In the autonomic nervous system:

- At the neuroeffector junctions in the parasympathetic division.
- At the ganglia in both the parasympathetic and sympathetic divisions.

In the somatic nervous system:

- At the neuromuscular junctions, which result in skeletal muscle contraction.

In addition, cholinergic synapses are present throughout the central nervous system (CNS). These locations are summarized in Figure 13.1.

The degree of activation at a cholinergic synapse is dependent on the amount of neurotransmitter, acetylcholine (Ach), interacting with its receptors. Drugs and other chemicals that increase the action of Ach at cholinergic receptors will promote rest-and-digest responses. These substances are called **cholinergic agonists**, or parasympathomimetics.

Also recall from Chapter 12 that there are two primary types of cholinergic receptors: muscarinic and nicotinic. Although Ach itself stimulates both types of receptors, drugs may be selective for only one type. For example, bethanechol is selective for muscarinic receptors and thus it is called a **muscarinic agonist**. On the other hand, nicotine is selective for nicotinic receptors and therefore is classified as a **nicotinic agonist**. Note that both bethanechol and nicotine are considered cholinergic agonists: The terms *muscarinic* and *nicotinic* are used to specify which cholinergic synapses are activated. If the student has not yet learned the differences between muscarinic and nicotinic receptors, then Section 12.6 should be reviewed before continuing. A summary of the differences is provided in Table 13.1.

Cholinergic agonists can activate cholinergic receptors directly or indirectly. Direct-acting drugs, such as bethanechol, enter the synaptic cleft and bind to Ach receptors to produce typical rest-and-digest responses. Some of these direct-acting drugs cause the release of additional Ach into the synaptic cleft, thus enhancing the normal physiological responses caused by Ach. The direct-acting cholinergic

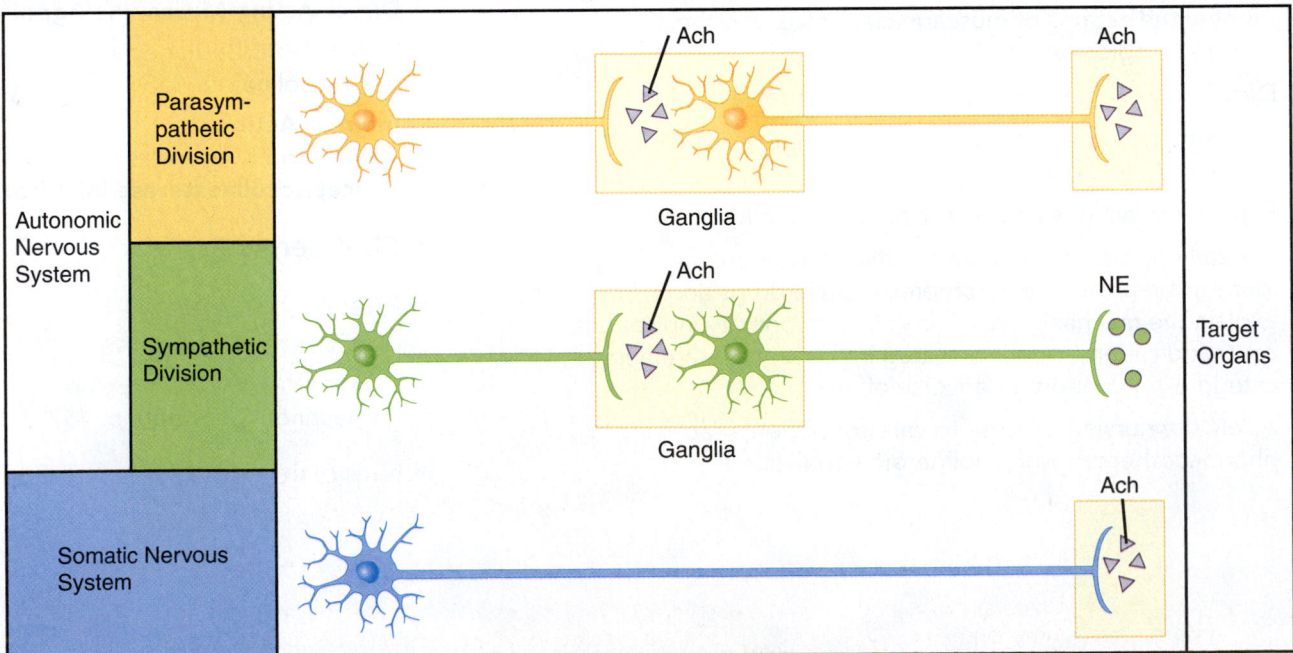

Figure 13.1 Locations of cholinergic synapses. Acetylcholine is released at the ganglia in both the parasympathetic and sympathetic divisions, at the neuroeffector junctions in the parasympathetic division, and in the somatic nervous system at neuromuscular synapses.

TABLE 13.1 Types of Cholinergic Receptors and Their Actions

	Muscarinic	Nicotinic
Receptor location	Glands, smooth muscle, cardiac muscle	Skeletal muscle, autonomic ganglia, brain, adrenal gland*
General actions	Pupil constriction Decreased accommodation of the eye Increased GI motility Decreased heart rate Decreased blood pressure Increased glandular secretions (salivary, lacrimal, and sweat) Constriction of bronchial smooth muscle	Skeletal muscle contraction Initial stimulation of glandular secretion, followed by inhibition Increased heart rate Increased blood pressure
Antagonists	Atropine, scopolamine	Mecamylamine, succinylcholine, tubocurarine

*Some effects of nicotinic activation are caused by the release of epinephrine from the adrenal gland. The epinephrine subsequently activates the adrenergic receptors.

agonists essentially act by the same mechanism as Ach itself. Direct mechanisms of cholinergic activation are shown in Figure 13.2.

Indirect-acting drugs inhibit acetylcholinesterase (AchE) (also called cholinesterase), the enzyme in cholinergic synapses that destroys Ach. By blocking the destruction of Ach, the neurotransmitter accumulates and remains in the synaptic cleft for a longer time to produce enhanced rest-and-digest responses. Some indirect drugs such as neostigmine (Prostigmin) bind only briefly to AchE and exhibit short durations of action. These drugs are called *reversible* cholinesterase inhibitors.

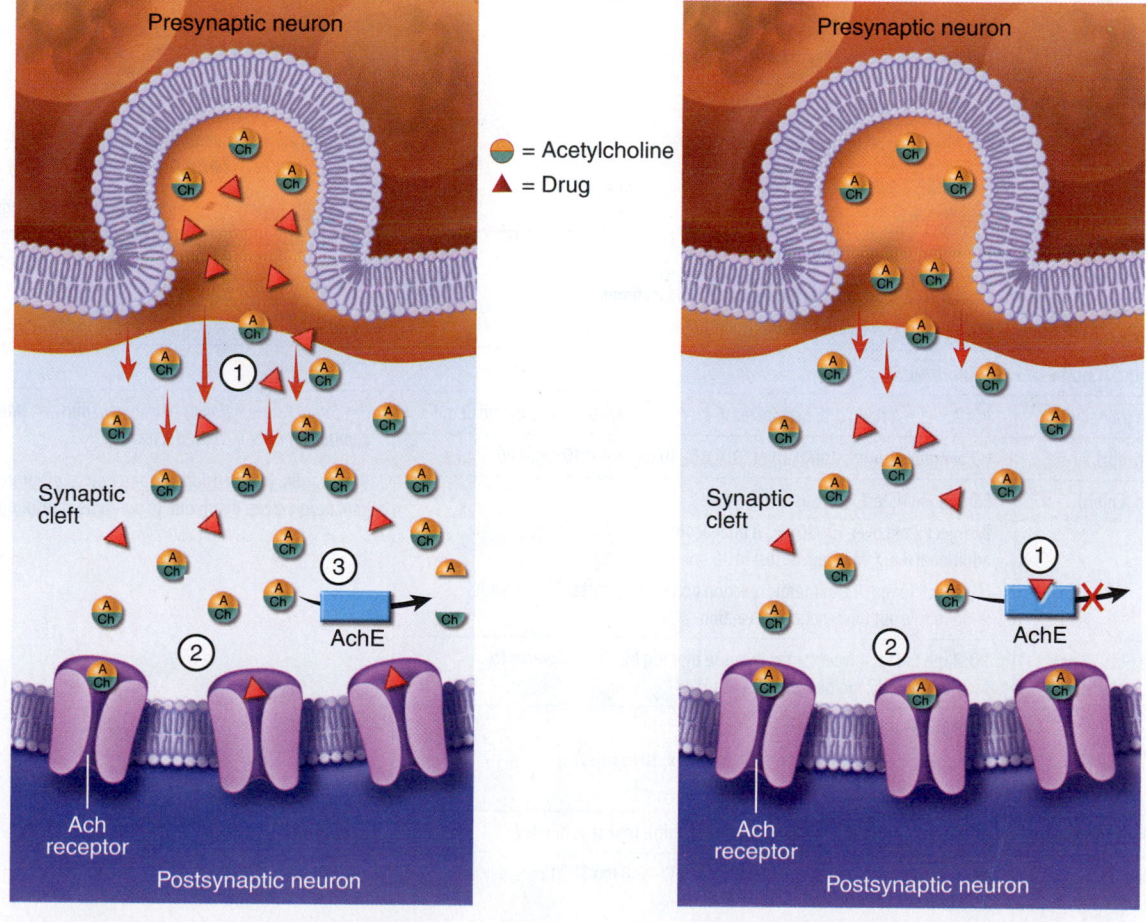

(a) Direct Cholinergic Agonist   (b) Indirect Cholinergic Agonist

Figure 13.2 (a) Mechanisms of action for direct cholinergic agonists. Direct cholinergic agonists can act by two mechanisms: (1) drug causes more acetylcholine (Ach) to be released into the synaptic cleft, resulting in additional Ach to occupy Ach receptors; (2) drug binds to Ach receptors, enhancing the action potential on the postsynaptic neuron. (3) drug is inactivated by acetylcholinesterase (AchE). (b) Mechanism of action for indirect cholinergic agonists: (1) drug binds the enzyme (AchE), which prevents the Ach from being destroyed. This increases the amount of Ach remaining in the synaptic cleft, (2) thus enhancing the action potential on the postsynaptic neuron.

There are certain chemicals that bind *irreversibly* to AchE. For example, certain insecticides and nerve gas agents bind to AchE for prolonged periods and can cause significant mortality if ingested or absorbed. Because of the hazardous nature of these chemicals, irreversible cholinesterase inhibitors are not widely used in medicine.

Note that physiologically it does not matter whether the cholinergic synapse was activated directly or indirectly: The parasympathetic responses are the same. There are some important differences, however, as will be discussed in Section 13.3. Indirect mechanisms are shown in Figure 13.2.

Muscarinic Agonists

13.2 Muscarinic agonists produce their effects by directly stimulating cholinergic receptors.

Muscarinic agonists are drugs that activate cholinergic receptors located at the neuroeffector junctions in the parasympathetic nervous system. Although Ach itself is a muscarinic agonist, it has little therapeutic value as a drug because it is rapidly destroyed both in the bloodstream and in synapses (by AchE) and produces many adverse effects. Muscarinic agonists used as medications are relatively resistant to destruction by AchE and exhibit a longer duration of action than Ach. Muscarinic agonists are poorly absorbed across the gastrointestinal (GI) tract and generally do not cross the blood–brain barrier. They have minimal effects on Ach nicotinic receptors in the ganglia. Because of the potential for serious adverse effects, few muscarinic agonists are widely used in pharmacotherapy. Available drugs are listed in Table 13.2.

Muscarinic agonists have widespread effects on the body, nearly all of which are due to parasympathetic activation. All of these drugs can increase the degree of smooth muscle tone and contractions of the GI tract. When administered before meals, stomach emptying is promoted due to increased peristalsis of the alimentary canal. Muscarinic agonists should never be administered to patients with suspected obstructive disease of the GI tract because the

TABLE 13.2	Cholinergic Agonists	
Drug	**Route and Adult Dose (Maximum Dose Where Indicated)**	**Adverse Effects**
Direct Acting (Muscarinic Agonists)		
bethanechol (Urecholine)	PO: 10–50 mg tid or qid (max: 200 mg/day)	*Increased salivation, abdominal cramping, sweating, flushing of the skin, miosis, blurred vision, nausea, vomiting*
carbachol (Isopto Carbachol, Miostat)	Topical: 1–2 drops of 0.75–3% solution tid in lower conjunctival sac every 4–8 h	<u>Orthostatic hypotension with possible syncope, bradycardia, reflex tachycardia, complete heart block, acute bronchospasm</u>
cevimeline (Evoxac)	PO: 30 mg tid (max: 90 mg/day)	
pilocarpine (Isopto-Carpine, Salagen)	Topical: 1–2 drops in affected eye tid or qid for chronic glaucoma PO: 5–10 mg tid for xerostomia (max: 10 mg/dose, 30 mg/day)	
Indirect Acting (Cholinesterase Inhibitors)		
ambenonium (Mytelase)	PO: 2.5–5 mg tid or qid; may increase every 1–2 days to 50–75 mg tid or qid	*Involuntary contraction or twitching of muscles, nausea, vomiting, miosis, increased salivation*
donepezil (Aricept)	PO or orally disintegrating tablet (ODT): 5–10 mg (max: 10 mg/day)	<u>Bradycardia, hypotension, dyspnea, seizures, bronchospasm, cholinergic crisis, death due to paralysis of respiratory muscles</u>
edrophonium (Enlon)	Edrophonium test for myasthenia gravis IV: Inject 2 mg over 15–30 sec; if no reaction after 45 sec, inject additional 8 mg. May repeat test in 30 min IM: Inject 10 mg; if cholinergic reaction occurs, retest after 30 min with 2 mg to rule out false-negative reaction	
galantamine (Razadyne)	PO: 4 mg bid for 4 weeks; may increase by 4 mg bid every 4 weeks to target dose of 12 mg bid (max: 24 mg/day)	
neostigmine (Bloxiverz, Prostigmin)	PO: 15–375 mg/day IM/subcutaneous: 0.5–2.5 mg q1–3 h (max: 10 mg/day) IV: 0.5–2.5 mg (max: 5 mg/day)	
physostigmine (Antilirium)	IM/IV: 0.5–2 mg (IV not faster than 1 mg/min); repeat as needed	
pyridostigmine (Mestinon, Regonol)	PO: 60 mg–1.5 g/day; sustained release: 180–540 mg 1–2 times/day at intervals of at least 6 h IV: 0.1 to 0.25 mg/kg	
rivastigmine (Exelon)	PO: Start with 1.5 mg bid; may increase to target dose of 3–6 mg bid (max: 12 mg/day) Transdermal: Start with one 4.6-mg patch daily (max: one 9.5-mg patch daily)	
tacrine (Cognex)	PO: 10 mg qid; increase in 40 mg/day increments not sooner than every 4 weeks (max: 160 mg/day)	

Note: Italics indicate common adverse effects. <u>Underline</u> indicates serious adverse effects.

increased peristaltic contractions could lead to injury or rupture to the mucosa.

CONNECTION Checkpoint 13.1

From what you learned in Chapter 12, would you expect the cholinergic agonists to have similar or opposite effects to the following: adrenergic agonists, adrenergic antagonists, cholinergic antagonists? *See Answer to Connection Checkpoint 13.1 on student resource website.*

Muscarinic agonists also stimulate the smooth muscle of the urinary tract, increasing ureteral peristalsis and promoting emptying of the bladder. These are considered therapeutic actions in patients with urinary retention. Care must be taken not to administer muscarinic agonists when obstructive uropathy is present, however, because the increased smooth muscle contractions of the ureters and bladder could aggravate pain and bleeding.

Muscarinic agonists stimulate most exocrine glands, increasing lacrimal, sweat, digestive, and salivary secretions. This action has been used to advantage in treating patients with **xerostomia** (dry mouth) or those with **Sjögren's syndrome**, a chronic autoimmune disorder characterized by excessive dryness of mucous membranes, which is associated with rheumatoid arthritis in menopausal women. In addition to creating discomfort for the patient, xerostomia can promote dental caries, periodontal disease, oral ulcers, and candidiasis.

In the eye, muscarinic agonists cause the muscles of the iris to contract and produce pupillary constriction, or miosis. Miosis has no therapeutic application and is considered an adverse effect of muscarinic agonists. A second effect on the eye is contraction of the ciliary muscle, which causes loss of ability to focus for near vision. Although this action may cause blurred vision, ciliary muscle contraction has an indirect, beneficial effect: It allows fluid to drain from the anterior chamber of the eye, reducing intraocular pressure. When applied topically to the eye, cholinergic agonists, such as pilocarpine, can be of value in treating glaucoma. Cholinergic agonists are considered second-line drugs for glaucoma therapy, having been replaced by safer, more effective alternatives (see Chapter 74).

Muscarinic agonists contract bronchial smooth muscle, causing the airways to narrow. In patients with respiratory disease, bronchoconstriction may trigger episodes of breathlessness or an asthma attack. This is why muscarinic agonists are contraindicated in patients with a history of asthma.

When activated, muscarinic receptors in the cardiovascular system slow the heart rate and lower blood pressure. Baroreceptors in the carotid arteries and aortic arch, however, recognize the falling blood pressure and signal the vasomotor center in the medulla to increase the heart rate. This phenomenon, known as **reflex tachycardia**, is not unique to the cholinergic agonists; it can occur with any drug that causes blood pressure to fall. When administering cholinergic agonists by the oral (PO) or parenteral routes, the patients' heart rate must be closely monitored to avoid bradycardia. Blood pressure must also be monitored to prevent serious hypotension, particularly in those with preexisting cardiovascular disease. Patients with hyperthyroidism may experience atrial fibrillation. Serious heart disease is a contraindication to therapy with cholinergic agonists.

Occasionally, patients experience acute poisoning from eating certain species of mushrooms containing high amounts of muscarine, the original cholinergic agonist isolated from the mushroom *Amanita muscaria*. *A. muscaria* itself has only small amounts of muscarine, but several other species of fungi possess significant amounts of this toxin that can cause severe illness if ingested. Symptoms of acute poisoning appear 30 to 90 minutes after ingestion and resemble an overdose of cholinergic agonists: an exaggerated parasympathetic response. Symptoms may persist for 24 hours. *Amanita* species are sometimes intentionally ingested to obtain psychotic effects, reportedly to expand or alter spatiotemporal awareness.

PharmFACT

Muscarinic receptors are named after muscarine, which is obtained from the mushroom *Amanita muscaria*. The actual chemical that causes poisoning in patients eating this mushroom, however, is primarily ibotenic acid, which causes excitement, hallucinations, and confusion. Death from *Amanita* mushroom poisoning is rare (Mechem, 2014).

Symptoms of parasympathetic stimulation, whether caused by medications or poisoning, may be reversed by administering an anticholinergic drug. Atropine is considered the specific antidote for these conditions. Acute symptoms of parasympathetic stimulation will begin to resolve within minutes after a subcutaneous injection of atropine. Atropine is a prototype cholinergic antagonist presented in Chapter 14.

PROTOTYPE DRUG	Bethanechol (Urecholine)

Classification: Therapeutic: Drug to treat urinary retention
Pharmacologic: Cholinergic agonist, muscarinic agonist (direct acting)

Therapeutic Effects and Uses: Approved in 1948, bethanechol is an older drug that is available in tablet form. Effects of bethanechol are most noted in the digestive and urinary tracts, where it stimulates smooth muscle contraction. In the urinary tract, bethanechol relaxes the sphincters and causes the detrusor muscle of the bladder to contract. These combined actions result in voiding; thus it is used to treat nonobstructive urinary retention in patients with atony of the bladder. Off-label uses include the treatment of adynamic ileus and gastric atony.

Mechanism of Action: Structurally similar to Ach, bethanechol interacts directly with muscarinic receptors to cause body responses typical of parasympathetic stimulation. This drug is selective for muscarinic receptors. Bethanechol is not destroyed by AchE; therefore, its actions are more prolonged than those of Ach.

Pharmacokinetics:

Route(s)	PO
Absorption	Poorly absorbed PO
Distribution	Widely distributed; does not cross the blood–brain barrier
Primary metabolism	Unknown
Primary excretion	Renal
Onset of action	30 min
Duration of action	1–6 h

Adverse Effects: The adverse effects of bethanechol are predictable knowing its parasympathetic actions. Common adverse effects include increased salivation, abdominal cramping, sweating, flushing of the skin, miosis, blurred vision, nausea, and vomiting. Serious effects include orthostatic hypotension with possible syncope, bradycardia, reflex tachycardia, complete heart block, and acute bronchospasm.

Contraindications/Precautions: Bethanechol should be used with extreme caution in patients with disorders that could be aggravated by increased contractions of the GI tract, such as suspected bowel obstruction, recent GI surgery, an active ulcer, or an inflammatory disease. Patients with suspected urinary obstruction or those who have had recent bladder surgery should not receive this drug, because the increased smooth muscle contractions could worsen these conditions. Patients with cystitis should not be given bethanechol because contractions of the bladder may force urine up the ureters to the kidneys if the sphincter fails to open. Because of the possibility of bronchoconstriction, administration of bethanechol to patients with asthma or chronic obstructive pulmonary disease (COPD) is contraindicated. Muscarinic agonists such as bethanechol can slow the heart rate; thus they are contraindicated in patients with recent myocardial infarction (MI), severe bradycardia, hypotension, or hypertension. Patients with hyperthyroidism can experience dysrhythmias with bethanechol use. Other contraindications include peritonitis, epilepsy, and Parkinson's disease.

Drug Interactions: Concurrent therapy with AchE inhibitors should be avoided because this class also stimulates muscarinic receptors, and excessive parasympathetic activity will result. Procainamide, quinidine, atropine, and epinephrine antagonize the effects of bethanechol. Concurrent administration of bethanechol with ganglionic blockers may result in a rapid fall in blood pressure. **Herbal/Food:** Unknown.

Pregnancy: Category C.

Treatment of Overdose: Overdose will result in serious cholinergic symptoms such as nausea, vomiting, abdominal cramping, diarrhea, salivation, and hypotension. Administration of subcutaneous atropine quickly reverses most symptoms.

Nursing Responsibilities: Key nursing implications for patients receiving bethanechol are included in the Nursing Practice Application for Patients Receiving Pharmacotherapy with Cholinergic Agonists.

Drugs Similar to Bethanechol (Urecholine)

Other direct-acting cholinergic agonists include carbachol, cevimeline, and pilocarpine.

Carbachol (Isopto Carbachol, Miostat): Carbachol is a direct-acting cholinergic agonist. Carbachol intraocular (Miostat) is a solution for injection into the anterior chamber of the eye to promote miosis during surgery. Carbachol topical (Isopto Carbachol) is an ophthalmic solution used to lower intraocular pressure in certain types of glaucoma. Vision may be clouded due to pupillary constriction. Should absorption occur, adverse effects would be those of parasympathetic stimulation. This drug is pregnancy category C.

Cevimeline (Evoxac): Cevimeline is a newer, direct-acting cholinergic drug whose only indication is the treatment of xerostomia in patients with Sjögren's syndrome. Given orally, cevimeline increases saliva flow, relieving dry mouth. The most common adverse effect is excessive sweating, although this occurs less frequently than with

pilocarpine. Other signs of parasympathetic stimulation are possible, such as diarrhea, runny nose, miosis, and bradycardia. This drug is pregnancy category C.

Pilocarpine (Isopto-Carpine, Salagen): Pilocarpine is a direct cholinergic agonist that is administered orally or as an ophthalmic solution. Salagen is an oral preparation of pilocarpine given for xerostomia due to its ability to stimulate salivary flow. When given orally, the adverse effects of pilocarpine are those expected of parasympathetic stimulation, which include diarrhea, runny nose, miosis, and bradycardia. Excessive sweating occurs in 30% to 60% of the patients taking oral pilocarpine.

Pilocarpine is also used in the pharmacotherapy of certain types of glaucoma and to counteract the effects of mydriatics and cycloplegics following eye examinations. This drug is pregnancy category C.

13.3 Acetylcholinesterase inhibitors may be used to treat Alzheimer's disease, glaucoma, or myasthenia gravis.

The indirect-acting cholinergic agonists inhibit the enzymatic destruction of Ach, allowing the neurotransmitter to remain on cholinergic receptors for a longer time. Like the direct-acting agonists, these drugs essentially prolong the actions of Ach. Unlike the direct-acting (muscarinic) agonists, however, the **acetylcholinesterase (AchE) inhibitors** are nonselective and affect Ach synapses located at the autonomic ganglia, muscarinic receptors, neuromuscular junctions, and Ach synapses in the CNS.

The muscarinic actions of the AchE inhibitors are identical to those described for the direct-acting drugs in Section 13.2. As such, these drugs would be expected to increase peristalsis in the GI and urinary tracts, and some can decrease intraocular pressure.

The AchE inhibitors have some additional nonautonomic indications due to their actions in the CNS and on motor nerve endings in skeletal muscle. These other indications include Alzheimer's disease, the prophylaxis of nerve gas poisoning, and myasthenia gravis.

Alzheimer's disease: AchE inhibitors used to treat mild to moderate Alzheimer's disease include galantamine (Reminyl), donepezil (Aricept), rivastigmine (Exelon), and tacrine (Cognex). These drugs increase the amount of Ach in cholinergic synapses in the brain, which improves memory and cognitive function. The AchE inhibitors do not cure or slow the progress of Alzheimer's disease: Improvement is limited and short lived. Donepezil is presented as a prototype drug for Alzheimer's disease in Chapter 21.

Glaucoma: Physostigmine (Antilirium) and echothiophate (Phospholine Iodide) have been used as ophthalmic solutions to cause pupillary constriction. They reduce intraocular pressure in the eye by contracting the ciliary muscle; thus they were once used to treat glaucoma. The ophthalmic AchE inhibitors have been replaced by safer and more effective antiglaucoma drugs (see Chapter 74).

Prophylaxis of nerve gas poisoning: A relatively new use of the AchE inhibitors is to protect military and public service personnel in the event of a bioterrorist attack with nerve gases. In the U.S.–Iraq Persian Gulf War in 1990, American soldiers were given 30 mg tid of oral pyridostigmine for several weeks. Theoretically, the pyridostigmine would cover the active site of AchE so that a toxic nerve agent would be unable to bind to the enzyme. Fortunately, no troops were exposed to these toxic nerve gases, so the effectiveness of prophylaxis with pyridostigmine remains unproven.

13.4 A cholinergic crisis may develop with overdoses of AchE inhibitors or with certain toxins.

When cholinergic receptors are overstimulated, a medical emergency known as a **cholinergic crisis** may result. Overdoses of AchE inhibitors, or exposure to toxic nerve gases (such as Sarin) or organophosphate insecticides (such as Malathion), may cause an acute accumulation of Ach at cholinergic synapses. The use of nerve gases as a bioterrorist threat is discussed in Chapter 75.

A cholinergic crisis is recognized by signs of intense parasympathetic stimulation such as miosis, nausea, vomiting, urinary incontinence, increased exocrine secretions, abdominal cramping, and diarrhea. As the crisis progresses, signs of sympathetic and nicotinic stimulation appear, including tachycardia, hyperglycemia, and muscle twitching, with progressive muscle weakness and possibly flaccid paralysis. In massive overdoses, mechanical ventilation may be required and paralysis of respiratory muscles may cause death. CNS effects are prominent with the organophosphates and include headache, blurred vision, anxiety, delirium, convulsions, and coma. In general, overdose with AchE drugs produces less severe and shorter duration effects than does poisoning with organophosphates.

The treatment of cholinergic crisis includes administration of atropine, the specific antidote that reverses muscarinic effects. Subcutaneous atropine can act within minutes. Because some insecticides have long-lasting effects, atropine therapy may continue for several weeks.

Pralidoxime (Protopam) is a cholinergic agonist that has primarily antinicotinic action, which can reverse muscle twitching and increase muscle strength. It is a specific antidote for poisoning by organophosphate insecticides and is used to control overdoses of the AchE inhibitors used to treat myasthenia gravis. In acute poisoning, pralidoxime is administered by IV infusion over 15 to 30 minutes. To be most effective, pralidoxime must be given as soon as possible after the suspected poisoning or overdose. Furthermore, it should always be administered concurrently with atropine. Duodote is a drug that contains both pralidoxime and atropine combined in a single intramuscular (IM) injection.

Pharmacotherapy of Myasthenia Gravis

13.5 Acetylcholinesterase inhibitors are used in the pharmacotherapy of myasthenia gravis to increase the strength of muscular contraction.

Myasthenia gravis (MG), which literally means "grave muscular weakness," first appeared in medical reports in 1672 and afflicts about 125 per million people in the United States. It is one of the best understood autoimmune diseases of the nervous system. The disease occurs when antibodies attack nicotinic synapses on skeletal muscles, resulting in symptoms of extreme fatigue, double vision, speech impairment, and difficulty chewing or swallowing. The most visible symptom is an obvious drooping of the eyelids (ptosis) due to muscular weakness. The ocular muscles may become so fatigued that the patient is unable to open the eyelids. Muscle fatigue worsens after exercise, or late in the day. MG is considered a progressive disease, although the severity of symptoms fluctuates over time.

PharmFACT

Myasthenia gravis most commonly affects young adult women (under 40 years) and older men (over 60 years). A baby born to a mother with MG may acquire antibodies from the mother and show temporary symptoms of the disorder, but these disappear in 2 to 3 months (National Institutes of Health, 2010).

MG is diagnosed by the anti–acetylcholine receptor (AChR) antibody test. A person without MG should have virtually no antibodies to the acetylcholine receptor. In a patient with MG, the body forms antibodies to the Ach receptor, and these can be measured in the blood with an accuracy of almost 100%. If the diagnosis is unclear, the edrophonium test may be performed. A small amount of edrophonium (Enlon), an anticholinesterase inhibitor, is administered by rapid IV infusion. An immediate, dramatic improvement in muscle strength, posture, and respiratory function following the injection supports a diagnosis of MG. The most useful measurement is the degree of ptosis of the eyelids. If ptosis diminishes or a completely closed eyelid opens after the edrophonium injection, diagnosis of MG is confirmed. Patients often exhibit adverse effects from the edrophonium injection, including bradycardia, bronchospasm, or lightheadedness; however, they resolve within a few minutes due to the very short half-life of the drug. Atropine should be available as an antidote in the event that more severe symptoms develop.

For patients with suspected MG, it is important to perform an accurate baseline physical assessment of neuromuscular and respiratory function. The patient's swallowing ability should be assessed prior to medication administration due to decreased muscle strength caused by the disease process. Subsequent assessments are important for monitoring the progress of pharmacotherapy.

Management of MG is divided into symptomatic control and immunosuppression as shown in Pharmacotherapy Illustrated 13.1. In the early stages of the disease, symptoms can be controlled successfully with AchE inhibitors, usually pyridostigmine. These drugs are effective for mild symptoms, act rapidly, and produce few serious adverse effects at low to moderate doses. Muscarinic side effects such as diarrhea and abdominal cramps are common, and muscle twitching can occur. High doses should not be used because AchE inhibitors can begin to affect Ach nicotinic receptors, worsening the degree of muscle weakness.

As MG progresses, immunosuppressant drugs such as corticosteroids are added to the regimen to bring additional relief to these patients. Corticosteroids such as prednisone reduce AchE receptor antibody levels and result in symptomatic improvement. Care must be taken when initiating corticosteroid therapy because patient symptoms may dramatically worsen during the first few days of therapy. Doses of prednisone are gradually increased until the desired therapeutic effect is obtained. Unfortunately, improvement may take weeks or even months, and corticosteroids can

PHARMACOTHERAPY ILLUSTRATED 13.1

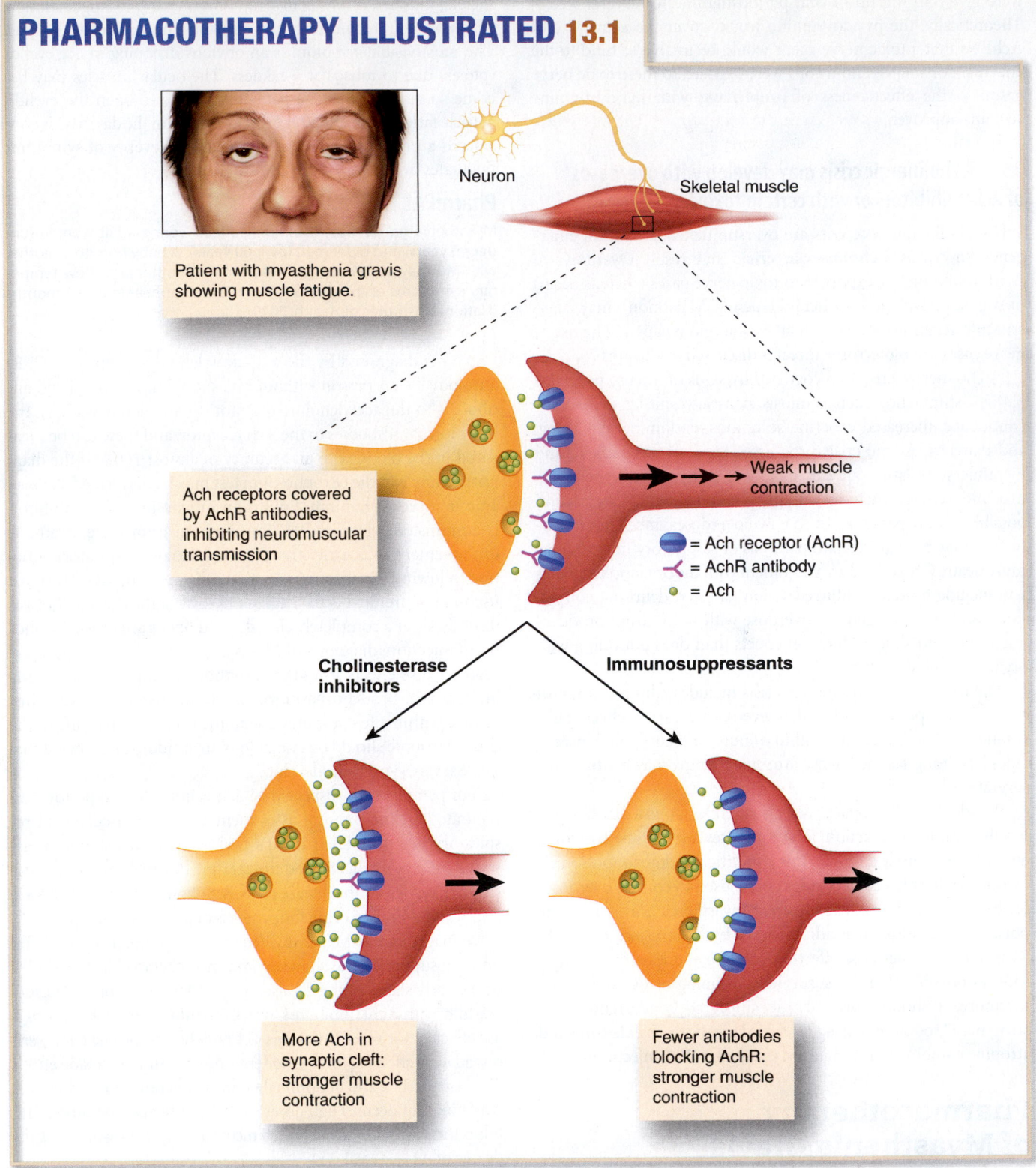

Patient with myasthenia gravis showing muscle fatigue.

Neuron

Skeletal muscle

Ach receptors covered by AchR antibodies, inhibiting neuromuscular transmission

Weak muscle contraction

= Ach receptor (AchR)

= AchR antibody

= Ach

Cholinesterase inhibitors

Immunosuppressants

More Ach in synaptic cleft: stronger muscle contraction

Fewer antibodies blocking AchR: stronger muscle contraction

exhibit considerable toxicity when given on a long-term basis (see Chapter 68). Therapy with corticosteroids is limited to the shortest time necessary, although some patients may require these drugs for the rest of their life.

Other immunosuppressants such as azathioprine (Imuran), cyclosporine (Sandimmune), or mycophenolate mofetil (CellCept)

may be administered as alternatives to corticosteroids. Occasionally, these alternatives are administered concurrently with prednisone to allow for lower doses of the corticosteroid. Immunosuppressants are discussed in Chapter 42.

A **myasthenic crisis** may occur if a patient with MG abruptly discontinues the medication. This leads to extreme muscular weakness and symptoms similar to those of a cholinergic crisis. Rapid, correct diagnosis is essential, however, because antidotes for the myasthenic crisis and the cholinergic crisis are very different. Weakness that appears approximately 1 hour after drug administration that is accompanied by signs of muscarinic overstimulation suggests cholinergic crisis (overdose) and is treated by prompt withdrawal of neostigmine and immediate administration of atropine. Weakness that occurs 3 hours or more after drug administration without muscarinic overstimulation is more likely due to myasthenic crisis (underdose, abrupt discontinuation or drug resistance) and is treated by more intensive AchE therapy.

To more clearly distinguish between a cholinergic and myasthenic crisis, the edrophonium test may be used, administering the smallest amount possible. If symptoms improve, it indicates that the patient is experiencing a myasthenic crisis, and AchE inhibitor therapy is indicated. If symptoms worsen after giving edrophonium, it indicates a cholinergic crisis; pharmacotherapy with an anticholinergic such as atropine is immediately initiated.

It should be clearly understood that MG is a disease affecting skeletal muscle; it is not a disorder of the autonomic nervous system. It is presented in this chapter dealing with the autonomic nervous system because the primary pharmacotherapy for the disease is AchE inhibitors. Although these drugs provide symptomatic relief, they do not cure or slow the progression of MG. With treatment, however, patients may experience a near-normal life expectancy.

| PROTOTYPE DRUG | **Pyridostigmine (Mestinon, Regonol)** |

Classification: **Therapeutic:** Drug for MG
Pharmacologic: Indirect-acting cholinergic agonist, AchE inhibitor

Therapeutic Effects and Uses: Approved in 1955, pyridostigmine is available by both oral and parenteral routes for the symptomatic treatment of MG. Affecting the neuromuscular synapses, pyridostigmine increases the strength of skeletal muscle contraction and delays fatigue. An average dose is ten 60-mg tablets per day, spaced apart to provide for maximum muscle strength. The sustained release form (Mestinon Timespan) consists of 180-mg tablets that are taken once or twice daily.

Pyridostigmine is also approved for military personnel with potential exposure to certain nerve gases. Pyridostigmine is only effective if administered several hours prior to nerve gas exposure. If exposure occurs, pyridostigmine is discontinued and the antidotes (atropine and pralidoxime) are administered.

The intravenous (IV) form of pyridostigmine (Regonol) is administered to reverse the neuromuscular blocking action of nondepolarizing muscle relaxants. When given by the IV route, extreme caution should be used to avoid overdosage, which can worsen neuromuscular blockade.

Mechanism of Action: Pyridostigmine reversibly inhibits the action of AchE at cholinergic synapses, which allows Ach to accumulate and cause a greater effect. Its use in treating MG is due to its effects on nicotinic Ach receptors in skeletal muscle.

Pharmacokinetics:

Route(s)	PO and IV
Absorption	PO: only 1–2% is absorbed; the oral dose is much higher than the parenteral dose
Distribution	Distributed to most tissues; crosses the placenta; does not cross the blood–brain barrier
Primary metabolism	Hepatic and plasma, by cholinesterases
Primary excretion	Kidneys
Onset of action	PO: 15–30 min; IV: 2–5 min
Duration of action	3–6 h (regular), 6–12 h (extended release)

Adverse Effects: In addition to its effects on nicotinic receptors, pyridostigmine also affects muscarinic receptors. At muscarinic synapses, pyridostigmine will enhance the parasympathetic response, resulting in increased peristalsis, bronchoconstriction, bradycardia, and hypotension. Common adverse effects include involuntary contraction or twitching of muscles, nausea, vomiting, miosis, and increased salivation. Potentially serious adverse effects include those of cholinergic crisis.

Contraindications/Precautions: Pyridostigmine should be used with caution in patients with disorders that could be aggravated by increased contractions of the GI tract, such as suspected bowel obstruction or active ulcers. Patients with suspected urinary obstruction should not receive this drug because the increased smooth muscle contractions could worsen this condition. Because of the potential for bronchoconstriction, patients with asthma or COPD should be treated cautiously with cholinergic agonists. Cholinergic agonists such as pyridostigmine can cause bradycardia; thus they are used cautiously in patients with recent MI or heart failure.

Drug Interactions: Because of the potential for additive effects, other cholinergic agonists should not be administered concurrently with pyridostigmine. Drugs that interfere with neuromuscular transmission such as local anesthetics, some general anesthetics, and antidysrhythmic drugs should be used cautiously in patients with MG because severe muscular weakness may result. If administered to patients with MG, the dose of pyridostigmine should be increased. Cholinergic drugs increase gastric acid secretion and should be used with caution with other ulcer-promoting drugs such as corticosteroids or nonsteroidal anti-inflammatory drugs (NSAIDs). **Herbal/Food**: Unknown.

Pregnancy: Category C.

Treatment of Overdose: Overdose with pyridostigmine may be life threatening because the drug can cause a cholinergic crisis leading to respiratory failure. The administration of atropine reverses most overdose symptoms.

Nursing Responsibilities: Key nursing implications for patients receiving pyridostigmine are included in the Nursing Practice Application for Patients Receiving Pharmacotherapy with Cholinergic Agonists.

Drugs Similar to Pyridostigmine (Mestinon, Regonol)

Other AchE inhibitors for MG include ambenonium, edrophonium, and neostigmine.

Ambenonium (Mytelase): Ambenonium is an older oral drug approved in 1956. Its only indication is in the pharmacotherapy of MG. It is not a first-line medication for this disorder because it tends to produce more muscarinic adverse effects than other drugs. Ambenonium must be used with caution because there is a very narrow margin between the first appearance of side effects and subsequent toxic effects. This drug is pregnancy category C.

Edrophonium (Enlon): The primary use of edrophonium is to diagnose MG, although it may be used to periodically assess the progress of AchE therapy (see discussion of the edrophonium test earlier in this section). It was approved in 1951. This drug is pregnancy category C.

Neostigmine (Bloxiverz, Prostigmin): Approved in 1939, neostigmine is available by the parenteral route for the symptomatic treatment of MG when treatment with pyridostigmine has been unsuccessful. Neostigmine increases the strength of skeletal muscle contraction and delays fatigue. It is also indicated for the prevention and treatment of postoperative distention and urinary retention and for the reversal of effects of nondepolarizing neuromuscular blocking drugs after surgery.

Neostigmine has a shorter duration of action than pyridostigmine and causes a higher frequency of adverse effects. The adverse effects result from its ability to stimulate the parasympathetic nervous system. Common adverse effects include involuntary contraction or twitching of muscles, nausea, vomiting, miosis, and increased salivation. Potentially serious adverse effects include those of cholinergic crisis. If using large doses of neostigmine to treat MG, atropine (an anticholinergic) is sometimes administered concurrently to reverse the muscarinic adverse effects of neostigmine.

Patients with obstructive disorders of the GI or urinary tracts should not receive this drug because the increased smooth muscle contractions could worsen these conditions. This drug should be used with caution in patients with asthma, bradycardia, recent MI, or heart failure. This drug is pregnancy category C.

CONNECTION Checkpoint 13.2

Ambenonium is six times more potent than neostigmine. Does this mean it is six times more effective? From what you learned in Chapter 4, clearly explain the difference between efficacy and potency. *See Answer to Connection Checkpoint 13.2 on student resource website.*

Nicotinic Agonists

13.6 Nicotine acts by activating Ach receptors at the ganglia.

Very few drugs are used for their effects on Ach nicotinic receptors located in the autonomic ganglia. These ganglia synapse with neurons leading to skeletal muscles (nicotinic receptors) as well as those leading to effector organs (muscarinic receptors). Drugs affecting the ganglia have the potential to produce widespread, nonselective effects on the autonomic nervous system.

The only drug in widespread use that activates ganglionic receptors is nicotine. The most active component of tobacco smoke, nicotine is well absorbed from the GI and respiratory mucosa as well as from the skin. Because nicotine acts at the ganglia, both parasympathetic and sympathetic responses are stimulated. Stimulation of organ activity generally occurs with low doses, such as those acquired by cigarette smoking. Within seconds after smoking, activation of the CNS increases alertness. The heart rate and blood pressure increase, although these parameters may subsequently decrease due to the baroreceptor reflex. The emetic center in the CNS is triggered, causing a feeling of nausea. As the level of nicotine in the blood falls, these same organ systems become depressed. Nicotine is pregnancy category D.

Nicotine is an extremely dangerous substance. Acute toxicity, which can occur due to the accidental ingestion of insecticides containing nicotine, may cause death due to paralysis of the respiratory muscles. The chronic effects of nicotine in tobacco smokers such as lung cancer and emphysema are well documented and presented in Chapter 27.

As a drug, nicotine is used as nicotine replacement therapy (NRT) in tobacco cessation programs. Delivery systems include chewing gum (Nicorette), transdermal patches (Habitrol, NicoDerm), and nasal spray (Nicotrol). Use of these products reduces the uncomfortable symptoms of nicotine withdrawal, such as difficulty sleeping, lack of concentration, depression, headaches, and food cravings. As tobacco use diminishes over an 8- to 12-week period, these products are gradually withdrawn.

CONNECTIONS Community-Oriented Practice

◀ Myasthenia Gravis: Medications and Nutrition

Although everyone needs good nutrition for optimal health, patients with chronic diseases may have special needs. People with MG may face certain nutritional challenges due to difficulty related to fatigue, chewing, swallowing, and adverse effects of medications.

If possible, meals should be planned for times when the patient's strength is best. If the patient becomes fatigued later in the day, smaller, more frequent feedings may help or the dosage amount taken may be adjusted by the provider. Modifications such as the consistency of food or body position at meals can help improve tolerance of meals.

Sometimes these drugs can cause diarrhea or cramping. The patient should notify the health care provider and not take over-the-counter (OTC) medications. Foods with high-fat content, spicy foods, or dairy products can aggravate diarrhea. Coffee, tea, or chocolate can stimulate the intestinal system because they contain caffeine.

Diarrhea can result in loss of body fluid and minerals. Therefore, easy-to-digest foods that are high in minerals should be added to the patient's diet. Foods such as applesauce, ripe bananas, white rice, and baked or broiled chicken or fish may help. Light nutritious soups are good choices as well.

When a person takes corticosteroids such as prednisone for an extended time, bone thinning may result. Taking adequate amounts of calcium and vitamin D is important. Foods to include are milk products, cooked dark green vegetables, salmon, dried beans, and calcium-fortified juices and cereals. Because corticosteroids can cause fluid retention, salt substitutes or spices may be healthy alternatives to table salt. Avoid cured or smoked meats, canned vegetables and soups, salty snacks, and pickled foods.

CONNECTIONS: NURSING PRACTICE APPLICATION

Patients Receiving Pharmacotherapy with Cholinergic Agonists

Assessment	Potential Nursing Diagnoses*
Baseline assessment prior to administration: • Obtain a complete health history including cardiovascular, cerebrovascular, respiratory, musculoskeletal or thyroid diseases, GI or genitourinary obstruction, or diabetes. Obtain a drug history including allergies, current prescription and OTC drugs, and herbal preparations. Be alert to possible drug interactions. • Evaluate appropriate laboratory findings such as hepatic or renal function studies. • Obtain baseline vital signs, bowel sounds, urinary output, muscle strength, and mental status as appropriate. Assess the patient's ability to swallow. • Assess the patient's ability to receive and understand instructions. Include patient, family, and caregiver as needed.	• *Ineffective Airway Clearance* • *Impaired Physical Mobility* • *Urinary Retention* • *Impaired Urinary Elimination* • *Incontinence* • *Deficient Knowledge* (Drug Therapy) • *Risk for Injury*, related to adverse effects of drug therapy
Assessment throughout administration: • Assess for desired therapeutic effects dependent on the reason for the drug (e.g., increased ease of urination, improved muscle strength and coordination, lessened ptosis, and improved swallowing). • Continue frequent and careful monitoring of vital signs, mental status, bowel sounds, urinary output, and musculoskeletal function, including swallowing ability as appropriate. • Assess for and promptly report adverse effects: bradycardia, hypotension, dysrhythmias, tremors, dizziness, headache, dyspnea, decreased urinary output, abdominal pain, or changes in mental status.	

Implementation

Interventions and (Rationales)	Patient-Centered Care
Ensuring therapeutic effects: • Continue frequent assessments as above for therapeutic effects dependent on the reason the drug therapy is given. (Ability to carry out ADLs has improved; urinary elimination and output are improved; musculoskeletal weakness, ptosis, diplopia, chewing, and swallowing are improved. A larger percentage of the dose may be needed at times of greater fatigue such as late afternoon and at mealtimes or during periods of increased stress. A decrease in dosage during remission may be needed.) **Lifespan:** Assess for subtle changes in muscle strength or voice quality or slurred speech in the older adult. (Subtle changes that occur during the day, especially if timed around drug peaks or troughs, may indicate underdosage rather than age-related changes.)	• Encourage the patient, family, or caregiver to practice supportive measures along with drug therapy to maximize therapeutic effects (e.g., adequate rest periods in MG). • Have the patient, family, or caregiver maintain a diary of variations in muscle strength, particularly periods of weakness, to assist the provider in appropriate dosage. • Instruct the patient not to self-regulate the dosage to avoid over- or underdosage. If periods of weakness occur, the provider will adjust the dosage after determining the cause (e.g., under- vs. overdosage). • **Lifespan:** Teach the patient, family, or caregiver the importance of noting even subtle changes in the diary and the timing of doses taken.
• Continue frequent monitoring of bowel sounds and urine output if drugs are given postoperatively or postpartum. (Assessments will detect early signs of adverse effects as well as monitoring for therapeutic action. Drug onset is in approximately 60 min with increased urination and peristalsis following. Drugs are not given if a mechanical obstruction is known or suspected. **Lifespan:** Be aware that the male older adult is at higher risk for mechanical obstruction due to an enlarged prostate.)	• Instruct the patient to have bathroom facilities nearby after taking the drug. The patient may need assistance to the toilet or commode if dizziness occurs.
• Provide supportive nursing measures; e.g., regular toileting schedule, safety measures, etc. (Nursing measures such as assisting the patient to normal voiding position will supplement therapeutic drug effects and optimize outcome. **Lifespan:** A home assessment is especially important for the older adult. The presence of throw rugs and other hazards that obstruct mobility increase the risk for falls.)	• Assess ability of the patient, family, or caregiver to perform ADLs at home, and explore the need for additional health care referrals. Evaluate home safety needs.
• Schedule activities and allow for adequate periods of rest to avoid fatigue. (Excess fatigue can lead to either a cholinergic or a myasthenic crisis in patients with MG.)	• Instruct the patient to plan activities according to muscle strength and fatigue and to allow for frequent and adequate rest periods. • Instruct the patient to report extreme fatigue immediately.

(continued)

CONNECTIONS: NURSING PRACTICE APPLICATION (continued)

• Follow appropriate administration techniques for ophthalmic doses. Sustained release tablets should not be crushed or chewed. Administer the drug with food, milk, or small snack. (Administering with food helps to minimize adverse effects. Sustained release tablets must be swallowed whole and a change of dosage form may be needed if dysphagia is present.)	• Instruct the patient in proper administration techniques, followed by a teach-back. • Have the patient report any difficulty in swallowing if sustained release tablets are used.
Minimizing adverse effects: • Monitor for signs of excessive ANS stimulation and notify the health care provider if pulse is less than 60 beats/min or BP is below established parameters. (Cholinergic agonists decrease heart rate and BP. Atropine may be ordered to counteract drug effects.)	• Instruct the patient to promptly report tremors, palpitations, changes in blood pressure, dizziness, urinary retention, abdominal pain, or changes in behavior (e.g., confusion, depression, or drowsiness). Instruct the patient to report dyspnea, salivation, sweating, or extreme fatigue immediately, because these are signs of a potential overdose.
• Help the patient to rise from lying or sitting to standing until drug effects are assessed. (Direct-acting cholinergic agonists may cause significant orthostatic hypotension. **Lifespan:** Be aware that dizziness may increase the risk of falls in the older adult.)	• Instruct the patient to rise from lying or sitting to standing slowly, and to avoid prolonged standing in one place to avoid dizziness or falls.
• Report periods of muscle weakness and association to dosage time to the provider promptly. (Muscle weakness occurring within 1 h of dose may indicate overdosage or cholinergic crisis. Weakness occurring 3 h or longer after dose may indicate underdosage, drug resistance, or myasthenic crisis.)	• Instruct the patient to report any severe muscle weakness that occurs 1 h after taking the drug or if it occurs 3 or more hours after taking the medication. • Assist the patient, family, or caregiver to record variations of muscle strength, particularly periods of weakness, and associated dose times to assist the provider in appropriate dosage.
• Continue to monitor hepatic function laboratory values. (Cholinergic agonists may cause liver toxicity, and liver enzymes may be monitored weekly for up to 6 weeks.)	• Teach the patient, family, or caregiver about the importance of returning for follow-up laboratory studies.
• Provide for eye comfort such as an adequately lighted room and appropriate safety measures. (Cholinergic agonists cause miosis with difficulty seeing in low-light levels and blurred vision.)	• Caution the patient about driving in low-light conditions, at night, or if vision is blurred. Night-light use at home and safety measures may be needed to prevent falls.
• Carefully calculate and monitor doses. (Careful calculation will avoid overdosage.)	• Ensure that the patient, family, or caregiver is administering the correct dose by observing teach-back.
Patient understanding of drug therapy: • Use opportunities during administration of medications and during assessments to discuss the rationale for drug therapy, desired therapeutic outcomes, commonly observed adverse effects, parameters for when to call the health care provider, and any necessary monitoring or precautions. (Using time during nursing care helps to optimize and reinforce key teaching areas.)	• The patient, family, or caregiver should be able to state the reason for the drug; appropriate dose and scheduling; what adverse effects to observe for and when to report them; equipment needed as appropriate and how to use that equipment; and the required length of medication therapy needed with any special instructions regarding renewing or continuing the prescription as appropriate. • Instruct the patient to wear a medic-alert bracelet or other device describing the disease and the medications used.
Patient self-administration of drug therapy: • When administering the medications, instruct the patient, family, or caregiver in proper self-administration of drugs and ophthalmic drops. (Utilizing time during nurse-administration of these drugs helps to reinforce teaching.)	• Instruct the patient in proper administration techniques, followed by teach-back. • The patient, family, or caregiver is able to discuss appropriate dosing and administration needs.

*Nursing Diagnoses—Definitions and Classification 2015–2017. Copyright © 2014, 1994–2014 by NANDA International. Used by arrangement with John Wiley & Sons Limited.

The goal of NRT is to gradually reduce the patient's physical dependence on nicotine. The nurse should remember, however, that psychological dependence also occurs with nicotine and that most successful smoking cessation programs include behavioral modification therapy such as self-help groups. The consistent use of NRT roughly doubles a patient's chances of quitting smoking, but a great deal of persistence and motivation is required.

CONNECTION Checkpoint 13.3

Some cholinergic agonists activate both muscarinic and nicotinic receptors. From what you learned in Chapter 12, give the locations where each of these receptors may be found. *See Answer to Connection Checkpoint 13.3 on student resource website.*

CHAPTER

13

Understanding the Chapter

Key Concepts Summary

13.1 Drugs can activate cholinergic receptors either directly or indirectly.

13.2 Muscarinic agonists produce their effects by directly stimulating cholinergic receptors.

13.3 Acetylcholinesterase inhibitors may be used to treat Alzheimer's disease, glaucoma, or myasthenia gravis.

13.4 A cholinergic crisis may develop with overdoses of AchE inhibitors or with certain toxins.

13.5 Acetylcholinesterase inhibitors are used in the pharmacotherapy of myasthenia gravis to increase the strength of muscular contraction.

13.6 Nicotine acts by activating Ach receptors at the ganglia.

Case Study: Making the Patient Connection

Remember the patient "Hilda Echoles" at the beginning of the chapter? Now read the remainder of the case study. Based on the information presented within this chapter, respond to the critical thinking questions that follow.

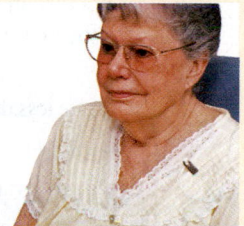

Hilda Echoles is an 82-year-old patient who lives alone in a two-story house. Recently, she fell down her front door steps and fractured her right femur. She was taken to the nearest hospital and underwent a total hip replacement 2 weeks ago. As she nears the time for her discharge, the urinary catheter, which was inserted during surgery, was removed. Since that time, Hilda has experienced urinary retention and required intermittent catheterization.

To aid in urinary elimination, the health care provider has ordered bethanechol (Urecholine) 20 mg three times per day. Because the medication

has demonstrated some effectiveness in achieving bladder emptying, Hilda will be discharged on this medication until she sees the health care provider 2 weeks after discharge.

Critical Thinking Questions

1. As Hilda's nurse, you will be reviewing her discharge medications before she leaves the hospital. What pertinent information should she receive about bethanechol?

2. Hilda states, "Sometimes, my memory is not so good and I forget to take my medication." What should she do if she forgets a dose? List suggestions that you could provide this patient to help remember her medication times and to ensure safe and effective administration.

3. What parameters would you use to determine the effectiveness of this drug therapy?

See Answers to Critical Thinking Questions on student resource website.

Additional Case Study

The patient has smoked cigarettes for the past 25 years. She tells the nurse that she has been using nicotine replacement therapy (Nicorette) as prescribed, for the past week. However, she continues to think about and crave cigarettes, especially when she is with a group of her coworkers who smoke.

1. What should the nurse tell this patient about her continued thoughts and cravings for cigarettes?

2. Identify two websites with helpful tips that might aid this patient with smoking cessation.

See Answers to Additional Case Study on student resource website.

Chapter Review

1 The nurse is discussing the adverse effects associated with a muscarinic agonist. The nurse knows that reflex tachycardia may occur with this drug because:

1. Baroreceptors acknowledge transient hypotension and signal the medulla to increase the heart rate.
2. This drug stimulates the sinoatrial node in the right atrium.
3. Aortic receptors identify episodes of systolic hypertension and stimulate heart rhythms.
4. This drug stimulates bronchial smooth muscle contraction and a narrowing of the airway.

2 The nurse is preparing a plan of care for a patient with myasthenia gravis. Which of the following outcome statements would be appropriate for a patient receiving a cholinergic agonist such as pyridostigmine (Mestinon) for this condition? The patient will exhibit:

1. An increase in pulse rate, blood pressure, and respiratory rate.
2. Enhanced urinary elimination.
3. A decrease in muscle weakness, ptosis, and diplopia.
4. Prolonged muscle contractions and proprioception.

3 The nurse is discussing the therapeutic effects of bethanechol (Urecholine) with a patient who is receiving this drug for urinary retention. The nurse understands that bethanechol:

1. Changes the diameter of the urethral opening.
2. Increases the amount of urine made in the kidneys.
3. Improves blood flow to the kidney.
4. Increases the contractions of the bladder and structures that promote urination.

4 The nurse is monitoring the patient for which of the common adverse effects associated with bethanechol (Urecholine)? Select all that apply.

1. Abdominal discomfort
2. Sweating
3. Flushed skin
4. Constipation
5. Blurred vision

5 A health care provider has ordered neostigmine (Prostigmin) for each of these patients. A nurse should question the order for which patient?

1. A patient with postoperative abdominal distention
2. A patient who is experiencing urinary retention
3. A patient who has chronic obstructive pulmonary disease
4. A patient who has received nondepolarizing muscle relaxants

6 The provider orders neostigmine (Prostigmin) for a patient who has not urinated in the past 16 hours. The nurse collaborates with the prescriber about which data related to this drug therapy?

1. Heart rate less than 60 beats per minute
2. Change in pupillary size from 3 mm to 1 mm
3. Increased salivation
4. Respiratory rate of 16 breaths per minute

See Answers to Chapter Review in Appendix A.

References

Mechem, C. C. (2014). *Hallucinogenic mushroom toxicity*. Retrieved from http://emedicine.medscape.com/article/817848-overview

National Institutes of Health. (2010). *Myasthenia gravis fact sheet*. Retrieved from http://www.ninds.nih.gov/disorders/myasthenia_gravis/detail_myasthenia_gravis.htm

Selected Bibliography

Anderson, P. D. (2012). Emergency management of chemical weapons injuries. *Journal of Pharmacy Practice, 25*, 61–68. doi:10.1177/0897190011420677

Brown, J. H., & Laiken, N. (2011). Muscarinic receptor agonists and antagonists. In L. L. Brunton, B. A. Chabner, & B. C. Knollman (Eds.), *The pharmacological basis of therapeutics* (12th ed., pp. 219–238). New York, NY: McGraw-Hill.

Chaplin, S., & Hajek, P. (2010). Nicotine replacement therapy for smoking cessation. *Prescriber, 21*(19), 62–65. doi:10.1002/psb.679

Diaz-Manera, J., Rojas Garcia, R., & Illa, I. (2012). Treatment strategies for myasthenia gravis: An update. *Expert Opinion on Pharmacotherapy, 13*, 1873–1883. doi:10.1517/14656566.2012.705831

Herdman, T. H., & Kamitsuru, S. (Eds.). (2014). NANDA International nursing diagnoses: Definitions and classification, 2015–2017. Oxford, United Kingdom: Wiley-Blackwell.

Moss, J. I. (2012). Gulf War illnesses are autoimmune illnesses caused by reactive oxygen species which were caused by nerve agent prophylaxis. *Medical Hypotheses, 79*, 283–284. doi:10.1016/j.mehy.2012.04.043

Sadeghian, H. (2010). Therapy update in nerve, neuromuscular junction and myopathic disorders. *Current Opinion in Neurology, 23*, 496–501. doi:10.1097/WCO.0b013e32833d7367

Shah, A. K. (2014). *Myasthenia gravis*. Retrieved from http://emedicine.medscape.com/article/1171206-overview

Taylor, P. (2011). Anticholinesterase agents. In L. L. Brunton, B. A. Chabner, & B. C. Knollman (Eds.), *The pharmacological basis of therapeutics* (12th ed., pp. 239–254). New York, NY: McGraw-Hill.

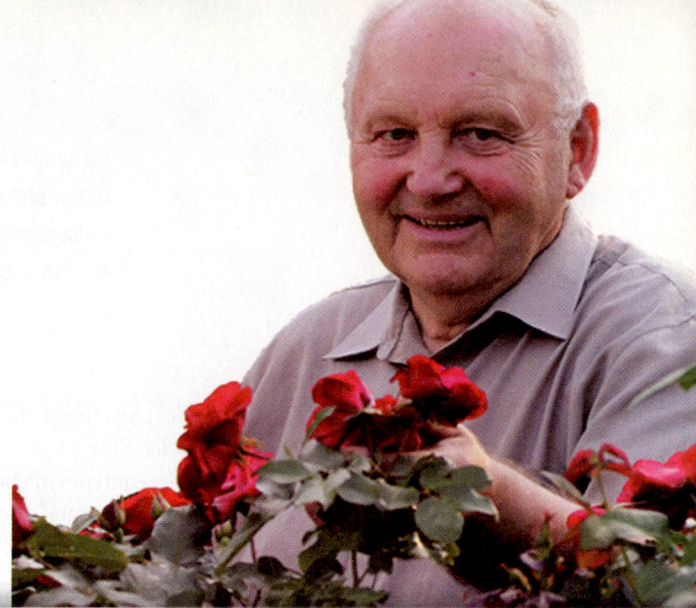

"I felt fine 2 days ago while working in the garden. How did I end up in this emergency room?"

Patient "Pete Elbertson"

CHAPTER 14

Cholinergic Antagonists

LEARNING OUTCOMES

After reading this chapter, the student should be able to:

1. Identify the physiological responses produced when a drug blocks cholinergic receptors.
2. Differentiate among the following terms: *cholinergic antagonists, muscarinic antagonists, nicotinic antagonists, ganglionic blockers,* and *neuromuscular blockers.*
3. Explain how the therapeutic actions and adverse effects of the cholinergic antagonists can be explained by their blockade of muscarinic or nicotinic receptors.
4. Identify symptoms of anticholinergic syndrome.
5. Compare and contrast the actions of the depolarizing and nondepolarizing neuromuscular blockers.
6. Compare and contrast the indications for drugs that block nicotinic receptors at the ganglia versus those that block nicotinic receptors at the neuromuscular junction.
7. For each of the classes shown in the chapter outline, identify the prototype and representative drugs and explain the mechanism(s) of drug action, primary indications, contraindications, significant drug interactions, pregnancy category, and important adverse effects.
8. Apply the nursing process to care for patients receiving pharmacotherapy with cholinergic antagonists.

CHAPTER OUTLINE

▸ **Classification of Cholinergic Antagonists**

▸ **Muscarinic Antagonists**
   PROTOTYPE Atropine (Atropen), *p. 166*

▸ **Nicotinic Antagonists**
   Ganglionic Blockers
   Neuromuscular Blockers (depolarizing type)
   PROTOTYPE Succinylcholine (Anectine, Quelicin), *p. 170*
   Neuromuscular Blockers (nondepolarizing type)

KEY TERMS

anticholinergic
  syndrome, 166
belladonna, 165
curare, 172
ganglionic blockers, 165

malignant hyperthermia, 171
motor end plate, 168
muscarinic antagonists, 164
neuromuscular blockers, 165

nicotinic antagonists, 164
nondepolarizing neuromuscular blockers
  (NDNBs), 172
pseudocholinesterase, 170

Cholinergic antagonists (anticholinergics) are drugs that inhibit the action of the neurotransmitter acetylcholine (Ach) at cholinergic synapses. Because there are two different types of cholinergic synapses, muscarinic and nicotinic, the actions and therapeutic uses of these drugs are dependent on their specific site of action. Though not as widely used as the adrenergic antagonists, several anticholinergics are important to pharmacotherapy.

Classification of Cholinergic Antagonists

14.1 Cholinergic antagonists act by blocking the effects of acetylcholine at muscarinic or nicotinic receptors.

As discussed in Chapter 13, cholinergic receptors in the autonomic nervous system are found in three anatomic locations, illustrated in Figure 14.1. This results in two primary classes of cholinergic antagonists:

- **Muscarinic antagonists** are drugs that block receptors at cholinergic synapses in the parasympathetic nervous system and at a few target organs in the sympathetic nervous system.
- **Nicotinic antagonists** are drugs that block receptors at cholinergic synapses in the ganglia or in the somatic nervous system at the neuromuscular junction.

Drugs that block the action of Ach at muscarinic receptors have more therapeutic applications than those that block nicotinic receptors. These drugs are known by a number of names, including anticholinergics, cholinergic blockers, muscarinic antagonists, and parasympatholytics. Although the term *anticholinergic* is commonly used in clinical practice, the most accurate term for this group of drugs is *muscarinic antagonists*. This is because these drugs are selective for Ach muscarinic receptors at therapeutic doses and have little effect on nicotinic receptors. The muscarinic antagonists are shown in Table 14.1.

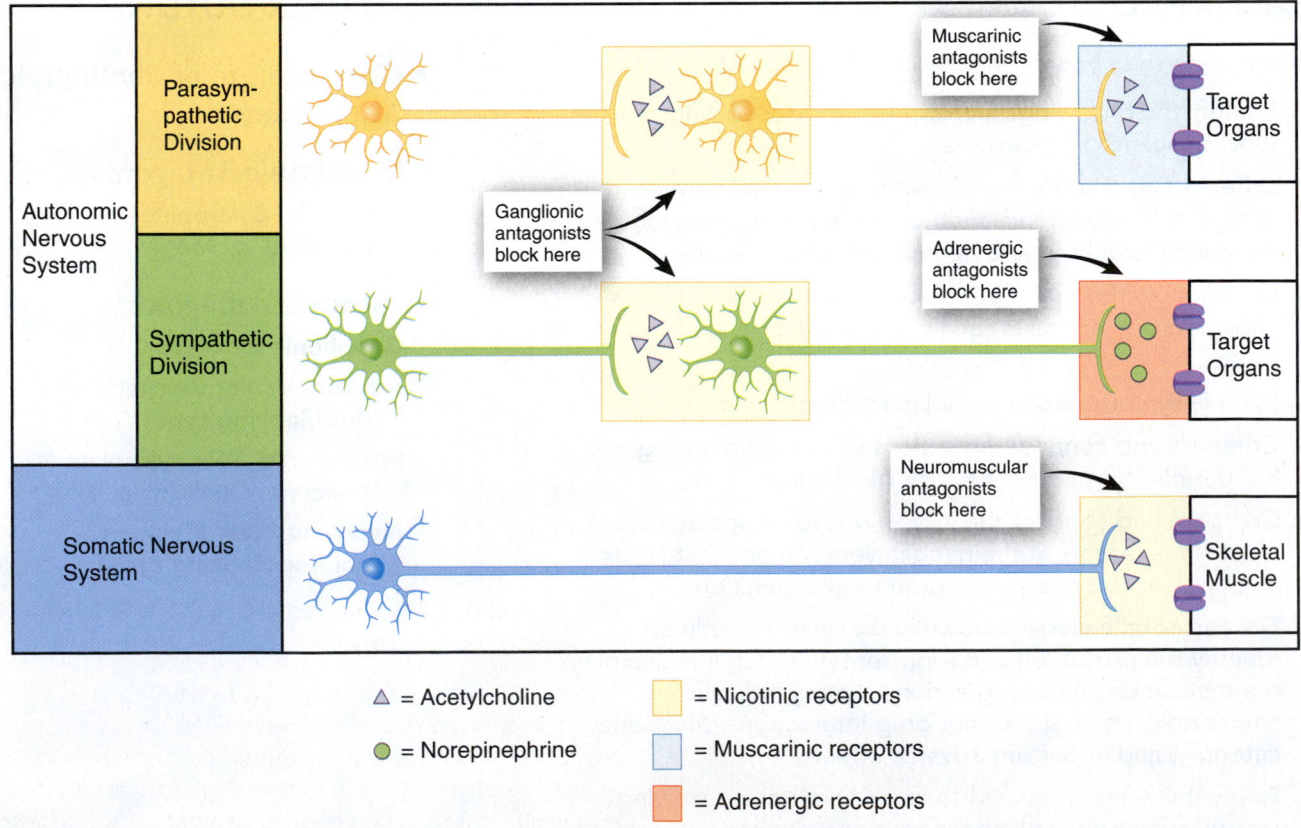

Figure 14.1 Sites of cholinergic antagonist actions. Muscarinic antagonists block cholinergic receptors in the parasympathetic nervous system. Nicotinic antagonists block cholinergic receptors at ganglia, or in the somatic nervous system at the neuromuscular junction.

TABLE 14.1 Muscarinic Antagonists (Anticholinergics)

Drug	Route and Adult Dose (Maximum Dose Where Indicated)	Adverse Effects
aclidinium (Tudorza Pressair)	Inhalation: one inhalation (400 mcg) twice daily	*Headache, cough, dry mouth, blurred vision, mydriasis, constipation, insomnia, urinary retention, burning, nasopharyngitis (inhalation forms), or stinging (eyedrop forms)*
atropine	Preanesthesia: IV/IM/subcutaneous: 0.4–0.6 mg 30–60 min before surgery Dysrhythmias: IV/IM: 0.5–1 mg every 1–2 h prn (max: 3 mg) Cholinergic crisis: IV: 1–2 mg, repeated every 20–30 min	<u>Worsening of glaucoma, tachycardia, paradoxical bradycardia, dysrhythmias, paralytic ileus, urinary retention; inhalation forms may cause sinusitis, paradoxical bronchospasm (inhalation forms), and oropharyngeal candidiasis</u>
benztropine (Cogentin)	PO: 0.5–1 mg/day (max: 6 mg/day) IM: 1–4 mg once or twice daily	
cyclopentolate (Cyclogyl)	Topical: 1 drop of 0.5–2% solution in the eye 40–50 min before the procedure, followed by 1 drop in 5 min	
dicyclomine (Bentyl)	PO: 20–40 mg qid IM: 10–20 mg qid	
glycopyrrolate (Cuvposa, Robinul)	PO for peptic ulcer: 1–2 mg tid–bid (max: 8 mg/day) PO for excessive drooling: 0.02 mg/kg tid (max: 0.1 mg/kg tid) IM/IV: 0.1–0.2 mg tid–qid	
hyoscyamine (Anaspaz, Levsin, others)	PO: 0.0625–0.125 mg 3–4 times daily IV/IM/subcutaneous: 0.25–0.5 mg every 4 h	
ipratropium (Atrovent)	Metered-dose inhaler (MDI): 2 inhalations qid (max: 12 inhalations/day) Nebulizer: 500 mcg every 6–8 h	
mepenzolate (Cantil)	PO: 25–50 mg qid	
methscopolamine (Pamine)	PO: 2.5 mg tid	
oxybutynin (Ditropan, Oxytrol)	PO: 5 mg bid–tid (max: 20 mg/day) or 5 mg sustained release daily (max: 30 mg/day) Transdermal: 1 patch twice weekly	
propantheline (Pro-Banthine)	PO: 7.5–15 mg tid–qid	
scopolamine (Transderm-Scop)	Preanesthetic: PO: 0.4–0.8 mg Transdermal: 1 patch every 72 h starting 12 h before travel	
tiotropium (Spiriva)	Inhalation/HandiHaler: 1 capsule inhaled/day	
tolterodine (Detrol)	PO: 2 mg bid (regular release), or 4 mg once daily (sustained release)	
trihexyphenidyl	PO: 1 mg/day gradually increased to 6–10 mg/day (max: 15 mg/day)	
tropicamide (Mydriacyl)	Topical: 1–2 drops of 0.5–1% solution in each eye	

Note: *Italics* indicate common adverse effects. <u>Underline</u> indicates serious adverse effects.

The muscarinic antagonists compete with Ach for binding to muscarinic receptors. When Ach is prevented from binding, parasympathetic responses are diminished at the neuroeffector organs. Suppressing the effects of Ach at muscarinic receptors will allow symptoms of sympathetic nervous system activation to predominate (fight-or-flight response). Most therapeutic uses of the muscarinic antagonists are predictable extensions of their parasympathetic-blocking actions: dilation of the pupil, increase in heart rate, drying of secretions, and bronchodilation. Note that these are the same symptoms as fight-or-flight sympathetic activation; thus blocking the parasympathetic division causes actions similar to those that result when activating the sympathetic division. Their actions are also *opposite* those of the cholinergic agonists discussed in Chapter 13.

Nicotinic antagonists can act at two locations. **Ganglionic blockers** inhibit transmission at the ganglia in the sympathetic and parasympathetic nervous systems, thus affecting both autonomic divisions. **Neuromuscular blockers** do not act on the autonomic nervous system at all but instead inhibit transmission at the neuromuscular junctions on skeletal muscles in the somatic nervous system. The therapeutic uses of nicotinic antagonists are more limited than those of muscarinic antagonists due to their widespread and diverse actions on body function. The specific sites of action of the ganglionic and nicotinic blockers are shown in Figure 14.1.

Muscarinic Antagonists

14.2 Muscarinic antagonists have been used for a diverse number of conditions, but they are rarely drugs of choice due to their adverse effects.

Anticholinergics are very old drugs that have been used for a large number of disorders over many centuries. The deadly nightshade plant, *Atropa belladonna*, grows throughout the world and has been a natural source of alkaloids with anticholinergic activity. References to the use of **belladonna** date back to the ancient Hindus, the Roman Empire, and the Middle Ages. The name *belladonna* is Latin for "pretty woman." Roman women applied extracts of belladonna to the face and to the eyes to create the preferred female attributes of that era—pink cheeks and dilated doe-like eyes. Because of its extreme toxicity, extracts of belladonna were sometimes used for intentional poisoning, including suicide.

Although once widely prescribed, the development of safer and more effective medications has greatly decreased the current usage of muscarinic antagonists. Most muscarinic antagonists are now prescribed as alternative medications when the preferred drug is contraindicated or not well tolerated. Potential therapeutic applications of these drugs include the following:

- **Gastrointestinal (GI) disorders.** Muscarinic antagonists suppress the secretion of gastric acid and can be used to treat peptic ulcer disease (see Chapter 59). These drugs also slow intestinal motility and can reduce cramping and diarrhea associated with irritable bowel syndrome (IBS) (see Chapter 60).

- **Ophthalmic procedures.** Topical application of muscarinic antagonists to the eye causes pupil dilation (mydriasis) and paralysis of accommodation (cycloplegia), actions that are beneficial during ophthalmic examinations (see Chapter 74).

- **Cardiac rhythm abnormalities.** Muscarinic antagonists accelerate the heart rate, which is beneficial for patients experiencing bradycardia.

- **Adjuncts to anesthesia.** Combined with drugs from other classes, muscarinic antagonists can decrease excessive salivary and respiratory secretions and reverse the bradycardia caused by general anesthetics (see Chapter 26).

- **Asthma and chronic obstructive pulmonary disease (COPD).** The muscarinic antagonists ipratropium (Atrovent), tiotropium (Spiriva), and aclidinium (Tudorza Pressair) are useful in treating asthma and COPD due to their ability to dilate the bronchi (see Chapter 44).

- **Antidotes for poisoning or overdose.** These drugs are specific antidotes for overdoses with muscarinic agonists or for poisoning with muscarinic mushrooms or organophosphate insecticides (see Chapter 13).

- **Urge incontinence (overactive bladder).** A few muscarinic antagonists such as oxybutynin (Ditropan, Oxytrol) are used to prevent involuntary voiding due to their antispasmodic effects on the smooth muscle of the bladder and detrusor muscle.

- **Parkinson's disease.** Muscarinic antagonists such as benztropine (Cogentin) are used for their effects on the central nervous system (CNS) and are prescribed to treat mild symptoms of Parkinson's disease (see Chapter 21).

CONNECTION Checkpoint 14.1

From what you learned in Chapter 13, describe the symptoms of a cholinergic crisis and explain why muscarinic antagonists are drugs of choice in reversing this condition. *See Answer to Connection Checkpoint 14.1 on student resource website.*

Muscarinic antagonists exhibit a relatively high incidence of adverse effects, most of which are predictable because they are associated with inhibition of the parasympathetic nervous system. Adverse effects that limit their usefulness include tachycardia and CNS stimulation. Men with prostate disorders should avoid muscarinic antagonists due to the increased risk of urinary retention. Adverse effects such as xerostomia (dry mouth) and dry eyes occur in many patients due to the blockade of muscarinic receptors on the salivary glands and lacrimal glands, respectively. Blockade

of muscarinic receptors can inhibit sweating, which may lead to hyperthermia. In the eye, muscarinic antagonists can paralyze the ciliary muscle and the sphincter of the iris. These ocular effects can cause photophobia (sensitivity to bright light) and increase intraocular pressure; therefore, these drugs are usually avoided in patients with glaucoma.

Overdose with anticholinergic substances produces a set of symptoms known as **anticholinergic syndrome**. Symptoms of anticholinergic syndrome include dry mouth, blurred vision, photophobia, visual changes, difficulty swallowing, agitation, and hallucinations. Although uncommon, death may result with high doses. Drugs from several other classes have cholinergic-blocking effects, including antihistamines, antipsychotics, and tricyclic antidepressants, and can trigger these same symptoms. Certain plant substances (including belladonna) also trigger anticholinergic syndrome. Children sometimes eat the colorful, purple berries of the deadly nightshade plant, mistaking them for cherries. Plants such as henbane and angel's trumpet are sometimes intentionally ingested for their hallucinogenic effects.

The specific antidote for anticholinergic toxicity is physostigmine, a reversible cholinesterase inhibitor. Because physostigmine is capable of inducing a cholinergic crisis with high doses, it is generally only administered to patients showing severe symptoms of anticholinergic syndrome such as seizures or psychoses.

PharmFACT

- Well known in antiquity as a poison, atropine derives its name from Greek mythology: Atropos was the fiercest of the three Fates who chose how a person was to die.
- From about 1850 to 1950 atropine was incorporated into liniments and plasters, which could be purchased at the corner apothecary or pharmacy to cure neuralgia, tuberculosis, mastitis, pleurisy, and rheumatism (Lee, 2007).

PROTOTYPE DRUG	Atropine (Atropen)

Classification: Therapeutic: Drug for treatment of bradycardia, antidote for cholinergic agonist overdose
Pharmacologic: Anticholinergic, muscarinic antagonist

Therapeutic Effects and Uses: Atropine has been used for centuries for a wide variety of disorders; however, it remains a drug of choice for very few conditions because adverse effects are so common. The actions of atropine are predictable based on its ability to block muscarinic receptors.

One of the most important actions of atropine is to increase the heart rate, which can be used to advantage when the drug is administered to patients with bradycardia. However, this increase in heart rate is considered an adverse effect when atropine is administered for other indications. The drug should be used with caution in patients with dysrhythmias because it can cause tachycardia.

Like other muscarinic antagonists, atropine can relax smooth muscle in the GI, genitourinary (GU), and respiratory tracts. This action has led to its use in treating hypermotility or spastic disorders of the GI tract including dysentery, abdominal cramping, and IBS. Slowing peristalsis too much, however, can lead to constipation. In the urinary tract, decreased smooth muscle tone can lead to urinary retention.

Because atropine decreases the quantity of exocrine secretions, the drug has been used to suppress secretions of the salivary glands and respiratory tract during surgical procedures. Excessive drying and thickening of bronchial secretions, however, can worsen asthma. Once widely used to produce bronchodilation in patients with asthma, atropine is now rarely prescribed for this disorder due to the development of safer drugs.

Topical administration of atropine to the eye will cause mydriasis and paralyze the ciliary muscle, causing cycloplegia. This may be used to advantage in ophthalmic examinations. When used for other indications, however, these actions on the eye are considered adverse effects and can result in blurred vision and photophobia.

Atropine is an antidote used to reverse symptoms of toxicity due to overdose of cholinergic agonists, including organophosphate insecticides and ingestion of mushrooms containing muscarine. AtroPen is an intramuscular (IM) autoinjection delivery system for poisonings due to toxic nerve agents or insecticides. Improvement in symptoms is usually noted within minutes.

Mechanism of Action: By occupying muscarinic receptors, atropine blocks the parasympathetic activation by Ach and induces symptoms of the fight-or-flight response. At therapeutic doses, atropine is specific for muscarinic receptors. At high doses, the drug may block nicotinic receptors in the ganglia and on skeletal muscle.

Pharmacokinetics:

Route(s)	PO, IV, IM, subcutaneous, inhalation, or ophthalmic
Absorption	Well absorbed by all routes
Distribution	Completely distributed; crosses the blood–brain barrier and placenta; small amounts are secreted in breast milk
Primary metabolism	Hepatic
Primary excretion	Renal
Onset of action	Subcutaneous/IM: 15 min; PO: 30 min; IV: 2–4 min
Duration of action	Half-life: 2–3 h

Adverse Effects: Common adverse effects include drying of the oral and nasal mucosa, constipation, urinary retention, increased heart rate, blurred vision, and photophobia. Serious adverse effects include ventricular fibrillation, delirium, and coma.

Contraindications/Precautions: Atropine is contraindicated in patients with acute angle-closure glaucoma because the drug may cause paralysis of the iris muscle, which can increase intraocular pressure. Safety has not been established for pregnancy and lactating mothers. Anticholinergics may cause fetal tachycardia.

Atropine should be used with caution in patients with chronic obstructive pulmonary disease (COPD) because drying of the bronchial mucosa can cause viscous mucous plugs. Blockade of cardiac muscarinic receptors can accelerate heart rate and exacerbate pre-existing cardiovascular pathology. Patients with hyperthyroidism should not be given atropine because the heart rate in these patients is generally high and administration of anticholinergics can cause dysrhythmias. Atropine is contraindicated for patients with serious GI conditions such as ulcerative colitis and ileus because blockade of muscarinic receptors can decrease the tone and motility of intestinal smooth muscle, which can exacerbate intestinal conditions. Patients with gastroesophageal reflux disease (GERD) and hiatal hernia experience decreased muscle tone in the lower esophageal sphincter and delayed stomach emptying. Atropine exacerbates

these symptoms, increasing the risk of esophageal injury and aspiration. Patients with Down syndrome are more sensitive to the effects of atropine due to structural differences in the CNS caused by the trisomy chromosomal abnormality. Patients with Down syndrome also tend to have disorders such as GERD and heart disease, which may be adversely affected by anticholinergics.

Drug Interactions: Care must be taken when administering atropine concurrently with other drugs with anticholinergic actions, such as antihistamines, tricyclic antidepressants, quinidine, and phenothiazines, because their anticholinergic effects will be additive. Because atropine slows GI motility, the absorption of orally (PO) administered drugs may be altered. **Herbal/Food:** Some herbal supplements have atropine-like effects that potentiate the medication and can be harmful to the patient. For example, aloe, senna, buckthorn, and cascara sagrada may increase the effect of atropine, particularly if the herbs are used chronically.

Pregnancy: Category C.

Treatment of Overdose: Overdose with atropine is serious, with signs of parasympathetic blockade that include respiratory depression and circulatory collapse. Central signs such as hallucinations, seizures, and mania may be evident. Treatment is mostly supportive and may include drugs to control seizures and to increase respirations and heart rate.

Nursing Responsibilities: Key nursing implications for patients receiving atropine are included in the Nursing Practice Application for Patients Receiving Pharmacotherapy with Cholinergic (Muscarinic) Antagonists.

Drugs Similar to Atropine (Atropen)

Other muscarinic antagonists include aclidinium, benztropine, cyclopentolate, dicyclomine, glycopyrrolate, ipratropium, mepenzolate, methscopolamine, oxybutynin, propantheline, scopolamine, tolterodine, trihexyphenidyl, and tropicamide.

Antisecretory drugs: Glycopyrrolate (Cuvposa, Robinul), mepenzolate (Cantil), methscopolamine (Pamine), and propantheline (Pro-Banthine) are called antisecretory drugs because they reduce gastric acid secretions in patients with peptic ulcer disease. Drugs with greater effectiveness and fewer adverse effects have replaced the anticholinergics for the first-line therapy of peptic ulcer disease. Rarely, some of these drugs may be used off-label to treat IBS. An IV form of glycopyrrolate is available to reverse neuromuscular blockade following surgery. In 2010, an oral form of glycopyrrolate (Cuvposa) was approved to reduce excessive drooling in children age 3 to 16 years with certain neurologic conditions.

Antispasmodic drugs: Although all anticholinergics slow motility in the GI tract, only dicyclomine is U.S. Food and Drug Administration (FDA) approved for slowing GI motility. Hyoscyamine (Anaspaz, Levsin, others) has potent antispasmodic activity that is used for hypermotility disorders including IBS, spastic colitis, infant colic, renal and biliary colic, and spastic bladder. Dicyclomine (Bentyl) is given for its ability to relax bowel spasms in patients with IBS. Hyoscyamine and dicyclomine should never be administered to patients with suspected obstructive disease of the GI or GU tracts because the decreased motility and tone caused by the drugs can worsen these conditions.

Bronchodilation drugs: Aclidinium (Tudorza Pressair), ipratropium (Atrovent, Combivent), and tiotropium (Spiriva) are used for patients with COPD. The primary action of these drugs is relaxation of bronchial smooth muscle, which dilates the airways. Delivered via inhalation, these drugs produce more localized action with fewer systemic adverse effects than atropine.

Centrally acting drugs: Benztropine (Cogentin) and trihexyphenidyl are prescribed to reduce the muscular tremor and rigidity associated with Parkinson's disease. They may be used alone for mild forms of the disease or in combination with other drugs to reduce symptoms of advanced Parkinson's. Benztropine tends to produce less CNS stimulation than does trihexyphenidyl. A parenteral form of benztropine is available for treating symptoms of acute parkinsonism associated with the use of certain antipsychotic medications. Their use is limited by adverse effects such as sedation and confusion.

Ophthalmic drugs: Anticholinergics may be applied topically to the eye to produce cycloplegia and mydriasis during ophthalmic procedures. Drugs used for this purpose include tropicamide (Mydriacyl), cyclopentolate (Cyclogyl), and scopolamine (Isopto Hyoscine).

Scopolamine (Hyoscine, Transderm-Scop): Scopolamine is very similar to atropine, although scopolamine crosses the blood–brain barrier and is more likely to cause sedation at therapeutic doses. Scopolamine is very effective for preventing motion sickness. For this indication, a transdermal patch containing scopolamine is applied to the skin, usually behind the ear, for slow release of the drug. The most common adverse effect from the transdermal product is dry mouth, although sedation may be a problem in some patients. This drug is pregnancy category C.

Urge incontinence (overactive bladder) drugs: Fesoterodine (Toviaz), oxybutynin (Ditropan), and tolterodine (Detrol) are anticholinergics used for their ability to relax smooth muscle in the urinary bladder. In patients with urge incontinence, this action limits smooth muscle spasms in the bladder, thus diminishing incidences of involuntary voiding. Oxybutynin is a first-line drug for this condition. Formulations include immediate release and extended release (XL) tablets and a transdermal patch (Oxytrol). The slower release formulations tend to cause fewer autonomic-related adverse effects. Tolterodine is an alternative to oxybutynin and is also available in an extended release (LA) formulation.

CONNECTION Checkpoint 14.2

From what you learned in Chapter 12, which of the following classes would give physiological responses similar to the muscarinic antagonists: adrenergic agonists, adrenergic antagonists, or cholinergic agonists? *See Answer to Connection Checkpoint 14.2 on student resource website.*

Nicotinic Antagonists: Ganglionic Blockers

14.3 Ganglionic blockers act at the autonomic ganglia to lower blood pressure in emergency situations.

Ganglionic blockers are drugs that interrupt the transmission of nerve impulses at nicotinic receptors at the autonomic ganglia. As discussed in Chapter 12, both the sympathetic and parasympathetic nervous systems have ganglia. This means that, unlike the muscarinic antagonists that selectively block parasympathetic actions, nicotinic antagonists nonselectively inhibit the entire autonomic nervous system. If parasympathetic and sympathetic actions are both inhibited, what types of effects will be observed?

In most cases, inhibiting the ganglia in both systems will affect the parasympathetic system more than the sympathetic. This is because the predominant, baseline autonomic tone to most organs is from the parasympathetic nervous system. When ganglionic blockers slow parasympathetic nerve impulses, symptoms characteristic of anticholinergic drugs, such as urinary retention, constipation, blurred vision, increased heart rate, and dry mouth, occur.

Although they affect all autonomic organs, the ganglionic blockers' only action that has therapeutic usefulness is vasodilation. By reducing sympathetic vasomotor tone at the arterioles, ganglionic blockers are capable of causing profound hypotension. Emergency kits must be readily available so that a vasoconstrictor such as epinephrine may be administered if blood pressure falls to a dangerous level.

Because of their potential toxicity only one ganglionic blocker, mecamylamine (Inversine, Vecamyl), is approved for use. Mecamylamine is a potent, long-acting nicotinic receptor antagonist that was originally used to reduce blood pressure in patients with severe hypertension (HTN). This drug is rarely prescribed for this purpose today due to the development of safer antihypertensives. However, two other indications for mecamylamine emerged in the late 1990s. Mecamylamine was approved by the FDA as an orphan drug for the treatment of nicotine dependence. It is thought to reduce the psychological rewarding effects of nicotine through its central actions in the brain. It has also been approved as an orphan drug to treat Tourette's syndrome that is unresponsive to other medications. Common adverse effects include weakness, fatigue, sedation, headache, mydriasis, blurred vision, decreased libido, impotence, and urinary retention. Serious adverse effects include orthostatic hypotension, precipitation of angina, choreiform movement, and adynamic ileus. Dosage information for mecamylamine is given in Table 14.2.

Nicotinic Antagonists: Neuromuscular Blockers

14.4 Muscle contraction occurs when the motor end plate is depolarized.

The neuromuscular junction is a specialized cholinergic synapse that allows for communication between the nervous system and skeletal muscle. This synapse on the muscle, known as a **motor end plate**, receives an action potential from the axon of a motor neuron. Like other cholinergic synapses, the action potential causes the release of Ach, which travels across the synaptic cleft to its receptors on skeletal muscle. Anatomically, the neuromuscular junction is part of the somatic nervous system (not the autonomic).

Binding of Ach to its receptors changes the permeability of the muscle cell membrane and opens sodium channels, allowing sodium ions to rush in. Being a positive ion, sodium causes the inside of the muscle cell to depolarize and acquire a positive charge. This depolarization at the motor end plate triggers the release of calcium

TABLE 14.2 Nicotinic Antagonists

Drug	Route and Adult Dose (Maximum Dose Where Indicated)	Adverse Effects
Ganglionic Blocker		
mecamylamine (Inversine)	PO: 2.5 mg, increased by increments of 2.5 mg until desired blood pressure response is attained	*Orthostatic hypotension, blurred vision, anorexia, nausea, vomiting, constipation, diarrhea, dry mouth* <u>Adynamic ileus</u>
Neuromuscular Blockers		
Ultrashort Acting		
succinylcholine (Anectine, Quelicin)	IV: 0.3–1.1 mg/kg over 10–30 sec	*Transient flushing of the face, neck, or chest; rash, weakness, increased salivation* <u>Respiratory depression, anaphylaxis, prolonged apnea, cardiac arrest, bradycardia, dysrhythmias, hypotension, increases and decreases in heart rate, malignant hyperthermia, muscle paralysis</u>
Short Acting		
mivacurium (Mivacron)	IV loading dose: 0.15 mg/kg given over 5–15 sec IV maintenance dose: 0.1 mg/kg generally every 15 min IV continuous infusion: initial infusion of 9–10 mcg/kg/min, then 6–7 mcg/kg/min	
Intermediate Acting		
atracurium (Tracrium)	IV: 0.4–0.5 mg/kg initial dose, then 0.08–0.1 mg/kg 20–45 min after the first dose if necessary; reduce doses if used with general anesthetics	
cisatracurium (Nimbex)	IV: 0.15 or 0.20 mg/kg for intubation; 0.03 mg/kg every 20 min prn or 1–2 mcg/kg/min for maintenance	
pancuronium (Pavulon)	IV: 0.04–0.1 mg/kg initial dose, may give additional doses of 0.01 mg/kg at 30- to 60-min intervals	
rocuronium (Zemuron)	IV: 0.6 mg/kg initially followed by continuous infusion of 0.01–0.012 mg/kg/min	
vecuronium (Norcuron)	IV: 0.04–0.1 mg/kg initially, then after 25–40 min, 0.01–0.15 mg/kg every 12–15 min or 0.001 mg/kg/min by continuous infusion	
Long Acting		
tubocurarine	IV: 6–9 mg followed by 3–4.5 mg in 3–5 min if necessary	

Note: *Italics* indicate common adverse effects. <u>Underline</u> indicates serious adverse effects.

ions from internal storage areas within the muscle cell. The intense, though brief, release of calcium is quickly followed by skeletal muscle contraction.

As presented in Chapter 12, destruction of Ach by the enzyme acetylcholinesterase (AchE) removes the neurotransmitter from the motor end plate, allowing the muscle cell membrane to repolarize. Calcium returns to its internal storage depots, and muscle relaxation occurs. This process by which the action potential causes muscular contraction is known as *excitation-contraction coupling.*

When multiple action potentials arrive at a specific motor end plate, the muscle cell undergoes a series of repeated depolarizations and repolarizations. This causes a continuous depolarized state in which calcium does not return to its storage depots, and a *sustained* muscle contraction is achieved. This contraction, however, can only be sustained by a continuous cycle of depolarizations and repolarizations. If the cell is simply depolarized (without undergoing repolarization), calcium will return to its storage areas and contraction will totally cease, resulting in a flaccid muscle. This paralyzed condition is necessary when performing certain surgical procedures. The depolarization of the motor end plate is illustrated in Figure 14.2.

14.5 Depolarizing neuromuscular blockers are given to produce muscle paralysis during short medical–surgical procedures.

The nicotinic synapse at the neuromuscular junction can be affected by drugs that can act by either a depolarizing or nondepolarizing mechanism. These depolarizing and nondepolarizing neuromuscular blockers produce the same result: total skeletal muscle relaxation or muscle paralysis.

Succinylcholine is the sole member of the depolarizing neuromuscular blocker class of drugs. This drug competes with Ach for nicotinic receptors on the motor end plates of skeletal muscle. Once bound to Ach receptors, succinylcholine produces muscle contraction by the same mechanism as Ach. However, succinylcholine is not destroyed by AchE, and the drug causes a prolonged and continuous depolarization of the muscle cell. Without repolarization, calcium returns to its internal storage depots and the muscle relaxes. The mechanism of action of succinylcholine is illustrated in Figure 14.3a.

It is important to note that succinylcholine does not enter the CNS. Although the drug causes muscle paralysis, it does not produce anesthesia or loss of consciousness. The patient is still able to

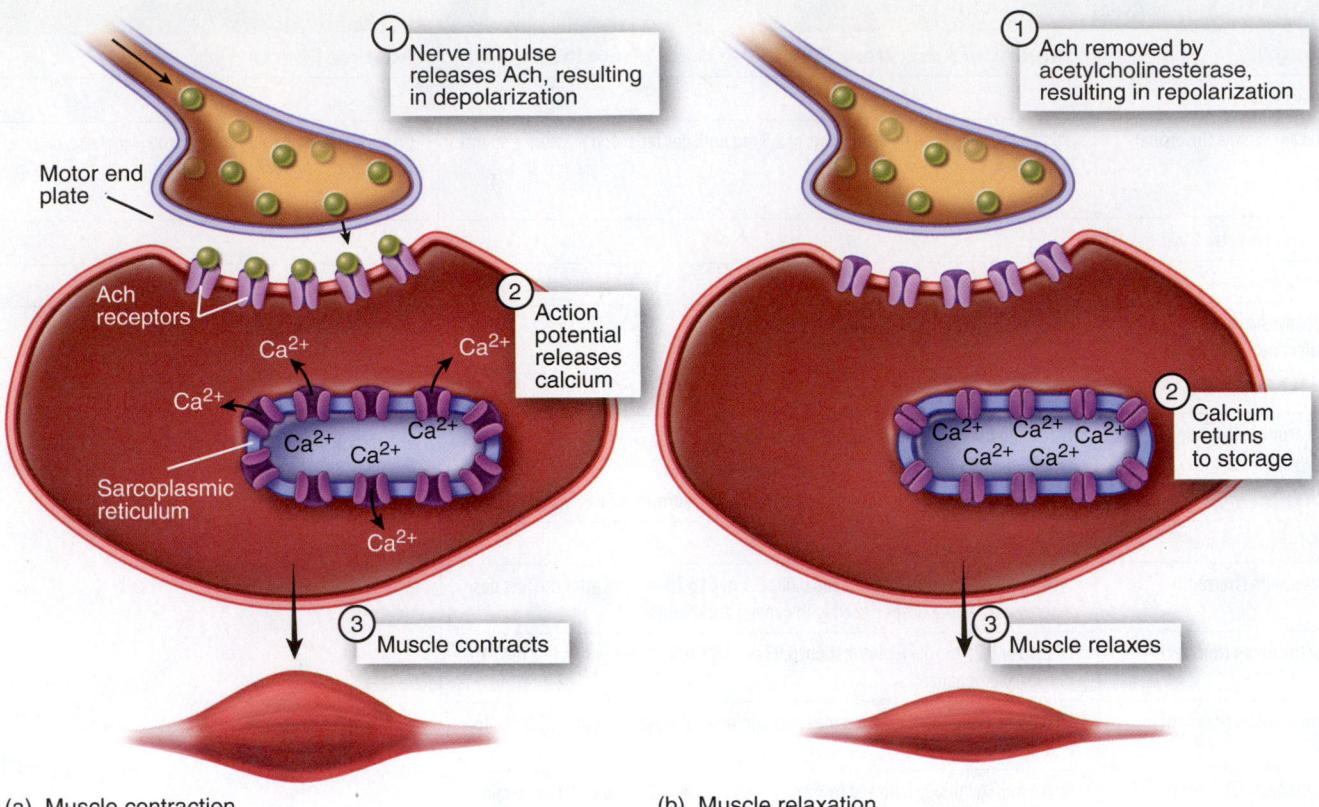

(a) Muscle contraction

(b) Muscle relaxation

Figure 14.2 Normal depolarization of the motor end plate: (a) Depolarization: Ach causes calcium to be released from storage, resulting in muscle contraction. (b) Repolarization: Ach is destroyed by acetylcholinesterase, calcium returns to storage, and muscle relaxation results.

feel pain and is aware of his or her surroundings. Thus succinylcholine is only one component of balanced anesthesia, as discussed in Chapter 26.

CONNECTION Checkpoint 14.3

Pyridostigmine also affects nicotinic receptors in skeletal muscle. From what you learned in Chapter 13, would you expect this drug to interact with neuromuscular blockers? What is the primary indication for pyridostigmine? *See Answer to Connection Checkpoint 14.3 on student resource website.*

PROTOTYPE DRUG	Succinylcholine (Anectine, Quelicin)

Classification: Therapeutic: Skeletal muscle relaxant
Pharmacologic: Neuromuscular blocker (depolarizing type)

Therapeutic Effects and Uses: Effects of succinylcholine are first noted as muscle weakness and muscle spasms. Eventually muscle paralysis occurs. The drug is primarily used as an adjunct to surgical anesthesia to cause complete skeletal muscle relaxation of the abdominal muscles. It may also be used to relax muscles during the insertion of an endotracheal tube and to assist in the management of mechanical ventilation. Administration of succinylcholine reduces the amount of general anesthetic needed for surgical procedures.

When given IV, succinylcholine induces muscle relaxation in less than a minute. When the infusion is discontinued, muscle control returns in a few minutes, because the drug is rapidly destroyed in the plasma by the enzyme plasma cholinesterase (**pseudocholinesterase**). This makes the drug ideal for very short procedures, such as intubation or electroconvulsive shock therapy.

Some patients have a genetic deficiency in plasma cholinesterase. In these patients, succinylcholine will have an unusually prolonged duration of action, and paralysis may persist for hours. Because there is no specific antidote for succinylcholine overdose, the patient must receive supportive treatment until the drug is metabolized and removed by the body. This adverse effect may be avoided by assessing plasma cholinesterase levels prior to surgery. If low, succinylcholine may be contraindicated, or the dose lowered to prevent prolonged muscle paralysis.

In addition to genetic deficiency, pseudocholinesterase levels may be decreased during therapy with cholinesterase inhibitors such as pyridostigmine, which is a drug of choice for myasthenia gravis (see Chapter 13). These patients will exhibit a prolonged duration of muscle paralysis if given succinylcholine.

Mechanism of Action: Like endogenous Ach, succinylcholine binds to cholinergic receptor sites at neuromuscular junctions (nicotinic). After repeated contractions the skeletal muscle membranes are unable to repolarize as long as the drug stays on the receptor. The result is total muscle relaxation or paralysis.

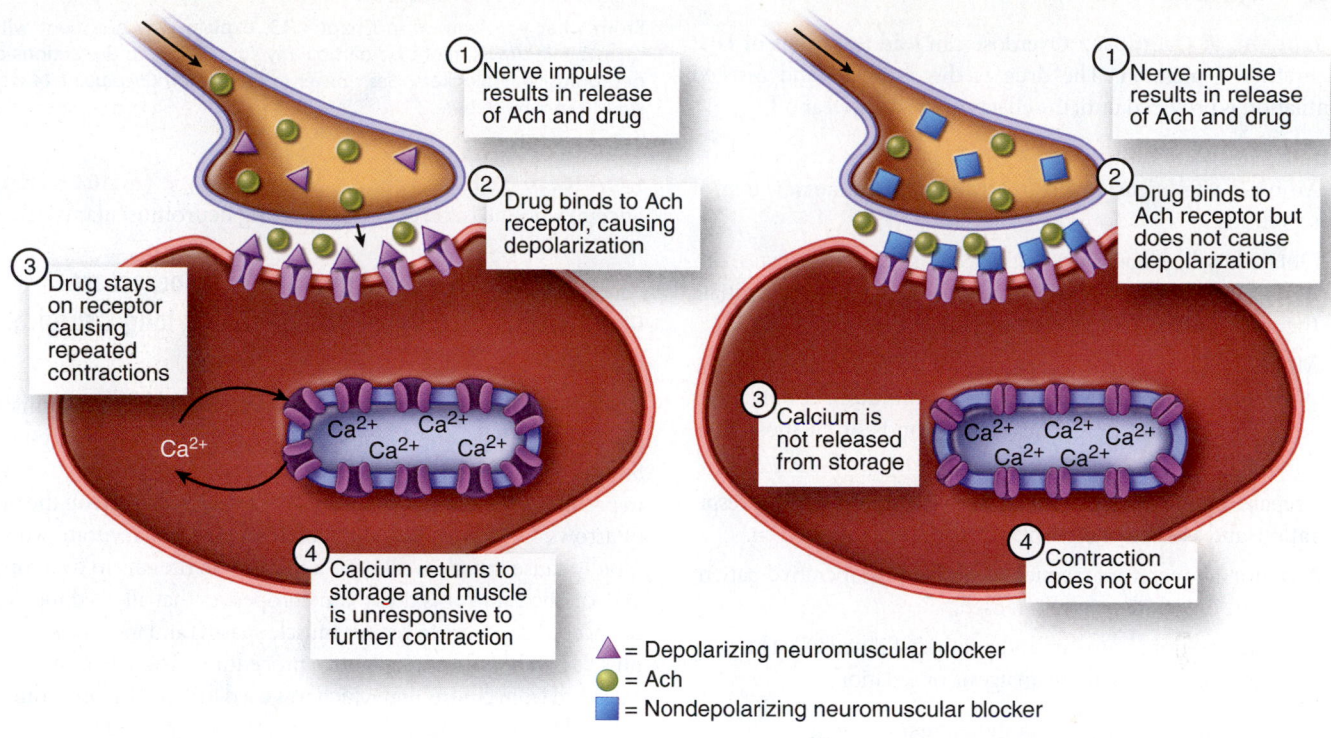

Figure 14.3 Mechanism of action of neuromuscular blockers: (a) Depolarizing neuromuscular blocker occupies Ach receptors and causes depolarization and muscle paralysis. (b) Nondepolarizing neuromuscular blocker occupies Ach receptors and causes muscle paralysis without depolarization.

Pharmacokinetics:

Route(s)	IM, IV
Absorption	Well-absorbed IM
Distribution	Completely, including crossing the placenta
Primary metabolism	Plasma by pseudocholinesterase
Primary excretion	Renal
Onset of action	IV: less than 1 min; IM: 2–3 min
Duration of action	IV: 2–3 min; IM: 10–30 min

Adverse Effects: Succinylcholine can cause complete paralysis of the diaphragm and intercostal muscles; thus mechanical ventilation is necessary during surgery. If doses are high, succinylcholine will also inhibit nerve transmission at the ganglia, causing tachycardia, hypotension, and urinary retention. In certain susceptible patients, a rapid onset of extremely high fever with muscle rigidity may occur, a serious condition known as **malignant hyperthermia**. The high temperature is caused by excessive metabolic activity in muscles, triggered by the drug. Although rare, malignant hyperthermia may be fatal. Other serious adverse effects include respiratory depression, apnea, and dysrhythmias. **Black Box Warning**: Children with certain congenital musculoskeletal diseases (e.g., Duchenne's muscular dystrophy) are at greater risk for cardiac arrest when this drug is used and should be monitored especially closely. Since there is no way to predict which patients are at risk, the use of succinylcholine in children should be reserved for emergency intubation or instances where immediate securing of the airway is necessary.

Contraindications/Precautions: Because succinylcholine is an essential component of balanced surgical anesthesia, there are few absolute contraindications. Patients with a personal or family history of malignant hyperthermia should not receive this drug. Succinylcholine should be used cautiously in patients with preexisting electrolyte imbalances or heart failure because this drug can cause a sudden release of intracellular potassium, resulting in hyperkalemia. Patients with pulmonary or metabolic disorders should be monitored carefully because succinylcholine can cause respiratory depression and acidosis. Due to its renal excretion, succinylcholine should be used cautiously in patients with kidney disease. Because the drug can increase intraocular pressure, it is contraindicated in patients with glaucoma.

Drug Interactions: Additive skeletal muscle inhibition will occur if succinylcholine is given concurrently with clindamycin, phenothiazine, aminoglycosides, furosemide, lithium, quinidine, or lidocaine. If succinylcholine is given concurrently with the anesthetics halothane or nitrous oxide, the risk of dysrhythmias, sinus arrest, apnea, and malignant hyperthermia is increased. Use with digoxin can increase the risk of dysrhythmias due to the hyperkalemia caused by the neuromuscular blocker. If opioid analgesics are given concurrently with succinylcholine, there is an increased risk of bradycardia and sinus arrest. **Herbal/Food**: Melatonin may increase the neuromuscular blocking action of succinylcholine.

Pregnancy: Category C.

Treatment of Overdose: Overdose can lead to serious or fatal respiratory depression. The drug is discontinued and assisted ventilation is provided until the effects of the drug wear off.

Nursing Responsibilities:

- Monitor vital signs frequently and keep the airway free of secretions.
- Obtain baseline laboratory tests such as serum electrolytes. Imbalances in potassium, calcium, and magnesium can potentiate the actions of neuromuscular blockers.
- Monitor for transient apnea, which usually occurs at the point of maximal drug effect (1 to 2 minutes); spontaneous respiration should return in a few seconds or, at most, 3 or 4 minutes.
- Prepare for emergency endotracheal intubation, artificial respiration, and assisted or controlled respiration with oxygen.
- Monitor temperature frequently in the postoperative patient when succinylcholine has been used.
- Provide emotional support and pain relief if needed. The drug will cause paralysis without analgesia or sedation.

Lifespan and Diversity Considerations:

- Because of postprocedural stiffness or muscle weakness, extra caution should be exercised when assisting the older patient with ambulation or activities of daily living (ADLs) to prevent falls or injury.
- When used in children, monitor vital signs, especially heart rate and rhythm frequently due to increased risk of cardiac arrest related to certain congenital musculoskeletal diseases. The existence of these diseases may not always be known and the drug is usually avoided in children when possible.

Patient and Family Education:

- Muscle stiffness and pain that may last for as long as 24 to 30 hours may occur after the procedure.
- Understand that sore throat and hoarseness are common even when the pharyngeal airway has not been used.
- Report persistent muscle weakness.

CONNECTIONS Patient Safety

◀ Medication Errors

Lee et al. (2010) reported that medication errors are frequent during interunit hospital transfers. Most errors involved medication omission, and one third or more of all errors resulted in adverse patient effects. Factors increasing the risk of errors included lack of a complete medication history including home medications and incomplete transfer orders, regardless of whether a paper chart, computerized medical record, or hybrid chart was used. As a nurse working in the postanesthesia care unit (PACU), how could the chance for a medication error be decreased when transferring a patient from the PACU to a surgical unit?

See Answer to Patient Safety Questions on student resource website.

CONNECTION Checkpoint 14.4 _____

From what you learned in Chapter 13, explain why a patient with myasthenia gravis might be particularly susceptible to the actions of neuromuscular blockers. *See Answer to Connection Checkpoint 14.4 on student resource website.*

Drugs Similar to Succinylcholine (Anectine)

Succinylcholine is the only depolarizing neuromuscular blocker.

14.6 Nondepolarizing neuromuscular blockers are given to produce muscle paralysis during longer surgical procedures.

The first neuromuscular blocker was **curare**, which was initially extracted from different plant species native to the rain forests of South America. Indians of the region cooked the roots and stems to produce a thick, tarry substance that could be rubbed on the tips of arrows. Once shot into the muscle of an animal, curare would rapidly cause muscle weakness, allowing the Indians to overcome and kill the game. It is these same properties that allowed medical science to use curare to reduce muscle spasms and to cause skeletal muscle paralysis during operative procedures. The active chemical extracted from curare, and which was used for medical procedures, is called tubocurarine. Tubocurarine is no longer used for medical procedures, but there are six **nondepolarizing neuromuscular blockers (NDNBs)** that have similar uses, actions, and adverse effects (see Table 14.2).

Like succinylcholine, the NDNBs are nicotinic antagonists that bind to Ach receptors at motor end plates in skeletal muscle. However, the NDNBs do not cause depolarization of the muscle cell; they act by preventing Ach from reaching its receptors. The mechanism of action of the NDNBs is illustrated in Figure 14.3b.

All NDNBs have identical actions, with their primary application being to relax skeletal muscles during operative procedures. These drugs may also be used to facilitate management of mechanical ventilation by suppressing contractions of respiratory muscles, thus eliminating resistance to mechanical ventilation. Suppressing muscular reflexes allows smoother insertion of an endotracheal tube, which is an additional indication for the use of these drugs. For patients undergoing electroconvulsive shock therapy or those who have tetanus, neuromuscular blockers can reduce the intensity and pain of severe muscle contractions.

The NDNBs are charged molecules that do not readily cross membranes. Thus, they are almost always administered IV. Because they do not cross the blood–brain barrier, they do not induce sedation, analgesia, or loss of consciousness. This allows for complete skeletal muscle paralysis without loss of consciousness. Administration of an anesthetic is necessary when diminished consciousness or analgesia is desired, such as during surgical anesthesia.

The NDNBs differ in their durations of action. This is a critical difference because the muscular relaxation induced by the drug must last long enough to complete the specific surgical procedure. The shortest acting drug, mivacurium, lasts only 12 to 18 minutes, whereas the longer acting agents may last up to 3 hours. All NDNBs have a very rapid onset of action, inducing paralysis within 1 to 2 minutes.

The most serious concern when using NDNBs is paralysis of respiratory muscles leading to apnea and possible respiratory arrest. Excessive respiratory depression caused by NDNBs can be treated by administration of an AchE inhibitor such as neostigmine (Prostigmin). In this respect, the NDNBs differ from succinylcholine. Administration of an AchE inhibitor will not reverse the respiratory depression caused by succinylcholine.

Hypotension is another potentially serious adverse effect of NDNBs. Hypotension results when these drugs trigger the release of histamine and at higher doses when nicotinic receptors at the ganglia are activated. Some neuromuscular blockers such as pancuronium and vecuronium cause less histamine release and have little effect on the ganglia; thus these drugs pose less risk of hypotension. An antihistamine may be administered to lessen the hypotension caused by NDNBs.

Short-acting drug: Mivacurium (Mivacron) is the shortest acting nondepolarizing blocker. Its duration of action is 15 to 20 minutes. A continuous infusion may be used to maintain the neuromuscular block. Rocuronium (Zemuron) has a duration of about 30 minutes.

Intermediate-acting drugs: Atracurium (Tracrium), cisatracurium (Nimbex), and vecuronium (Norcuron) have durations of action of 20 to 45 minutes. Cisatracurium and atracurium are not eliminated by the liver or kidneys and may be better choices for patients with hepatic or renal disease. Vecuronium has the advantage of causing no histamine release.

Long-acting drugs: Pancuronium (Pavulon) has a duration of 60 to 90 minutes.

CONNECTIONS: NURSING PRACTICE APPLICATION

Patients Receiving Pharmacotherapy with Cholinergic (Muscarinic) Antagonists

Assessment	Potential Nursing Diagnoses*
Baseline assessment prior to administration: • Obtain a complete health history including cardiovascular, cerebrovascular, or respiratory disease, for acute (narrow-angle) glaucoma, and the possibility of pregnancy. Assess usual elimination patterns, tearing, and salivation. Obtain a drug history including allergies, current prescription and over-the-counter (OTC) drugs, and herbal preparations. Be alert to possible drug interactions. • Evaluate appropriate laboratory findings such as hepatic or renal function studies. • Obtain baseline vital signs, urinary output, bowel sounds, and cardiac rhythm if appropriate. • Assess the patient's ability to receive and understand instruction. Include family and caregivers as needed.	• *Decreased Cardiac Output* • *Urinary Retention* • *Constipation*, related to adverse effects of drug therapy • *Impaired Oral Mucous Membranes,* related to adverse effects of drug therapy • *Deficient Knowledge* (Drug Therapy) • *Risk for Imbalanced Body Temperature* • *Risk for Injury*, related to adverse effects of drug therapy
Assessment throughout administration: • Assess for desired therapeutic effects dependent on the reason for the drug (e.g., increased ease of breathing, cardiac rhythm stable, and blood pressure [BP] within normal range). • Continue frequent and careful monitoring of vital signs and urinary output and cardiac monitoring as appropriate. • Assess for and promptly report adverse effects: tachycardia, hypertension, dysrhythmias, tremors, dizziness, headache, decreased urinary output. Seizures or ventricular tachycardia may signal drug toxicity and are immediately reported.	

Implementation

Interventions and (Rationales)	Patient-Centered Care
Ensuring therapeutic effects: • Continue frequent assessments as above for therapeutic effects dependent on the reason the drug therapy is given. (Pulse, BP, and respiratory rate should be within normal limits or within parameters set by the health care provider. Gastric motility and cramping have slowed.)	• Teach the patient, family, or caregiver how to monitor pulse and BP. Ensure proper use and functioning of any home equipment obtained.
• Provide supportive nursing measures; e.g., proper positioning for dyspnea; ice chips, fluids, or hard candy for dry mouth. (Nursing measures such as raising the head of the bed during dyspnea will supplement therapeutic drug effects and optimize outcome.)	• Instruct the patient that sips of water, ice chips, oral rinses free of alcohol, or hard candies may ease mouth dryness. (Alcohol-based rinses will worsen mouth dryness.)
• Follow appropriate administration techniques for inhalant or ophthalmic doses.	• Instruct the patient in proper administration techniques, followed by teach-back.
Minimizing adverse effects: • Monitor for signs of excessive ANS stimulation such as anxiety, blurred vision, tachycardia, dry mouth, urinary hesitancy, and decreased sweating. (Adverse effects are due to the blockade of muscarinic receptors. Anticholinergics are contraindicated in patients with acute/narrow-angle glaucoma because mydriasis will increase intraocular pressure. **Lifespan:** Children and older adults may be more sensitive to the effects of anticholinergic drugs and require frequent monitoring.)	• Instruct the patient to report palpitations, shortness of breath, dizziness, dysphagia, or syncope immediately to the health care provider. • **Lifespan:** Older and debilitated patients should report excessive drowsiness or CNS stimulation, even at usual doses of anticholinergics.

(continued)

CONNECTIONS: NURSING PRACTICE APPLICATION (continued)

• Notify the health care provider if BP or pulse exceeds established parameters. Continue frequent cardiac monitoring as appropriate (e.g., ECG) and urine output. (Anticholinergics must be closely monitored because they increase heart rate and the risk for dysrhythmias. External monitoring devices will detect early signs of adverse effects as well as therapeutic effects.)	• To allay possible anxiety, teach the patient about the rationale for all equipment used, and the need for frequent monitoring as applicable.
• Monitor the patient for abdominal distention and auscultate for bowel sounds. Palpate for bladder distention and monitor output. (Anticholinergics may decrease tone and motility of intestinal and bladder smooth muscle. **Lifespan:** The older adult is also at increased risk of constipation due to slowed peristalsis. Be aware that the male older adult is at higher risk for mechanical obstruction due to an enlarged prostate.)	• Teach the patient about the importance of drinking extra fluids and increasing fiber intake. Instruct the patient to notify the health care provider if difficulty with urination occurs or if constipation is severe.
• Minimize exposure to heat and strenuous exercise. (Anticholinergics can inhibit sweat gland secretions. Sweating is necessary for patients to cool down, so the drug can increase their risk for heat exhaustion and heatstroke. **Lifespan:** "Atropine fever"—hyperpyrexia due to suppression of perspiration and heat loss—increases the risk of heatstroke in young children and older adults.)	• Instruct the patient to avoid prolonged or strenuous activity in warm or hot environments, especially on humid days. Extra-hot showers and hot tubs should also be avoided. Dizziness, change in mental status, pale skin, muscle cramping, and nausea are signs of an impending heat exhaustion or stroke and should be reported immediately. Children and older adults should be monitored frequently.
• Provide for eye comfort such as darkened room, soft cloth over eyes, sunglasses, or lubricating eyedrops. (Anticholinergic drugs cause mydriasis, dry eyes, and photosensitivity to light.)	• Instruct the patient that photosensitivity may occur and sunglasses may be needed in bright light or for outside activities. Lubricating eyedrops may soothe dryness. Caution should be taken with driving until drug effects are known.
Patient understanding of drug therapy: • Use opportunities during administration of medications and during assessments to discuss the rationale for drug therapy, desired therapeutic outcomes, commonly observed adverse effects, parameters for when to call the health care provider, and any necessary monitoring or precautions. (Using time during nursing care helps to optimize and reinforce key teaching areas.)	• The patient, family, or caregiver should be able to state the reason for the drug, appropriate dose, and scheduling; what adverse effects to observe for and when to report them; equipment needed as appropriate and how to use that equipment; and the required length of medication therapy needed with any special instructions regarding renewing or continuing the prescription as appropriate.

Patient self-administration of drug therapy:
 	
• When administering the medication, instruct the patient, family, or caregiver in proper self-administration of an inhaler or ophthalmic drops. (Utilizing time during nurse-administration of these drugs helps to reinforce teaching.)
 	
  • Childhood fatalities have occurred from systemic absorption of anticholinergic eyedrops. (Accidental ingestion of a parent's, family member's, or caregiver's eyedrops may be fatal.)
	• Instruct the patient in proper administration techniques, followed by teach-back.
	• The patient, family, or caregiver is able to discuss appropriate dosing and administration needs.
	  • Instruct parents of young children to keep eyedrops and all medications secured and out of the reach of children.

*Nursing Diagnoses—Definitions and Classification 2015–2017. Copyright © 2014, 1994–2014 by NANDA International. Used by arrangement with John Wiley & Sons Limited.

CHAPTER

14   Understanding the Chapter

Key Concepts Summary

14.1 Cholinergic antagonists act by blocking the effects of acetylcholine at muscarinic or nicotinic receptors.

14.2 Muscarinic antagonists have been used for a diverse number of conditions, but they are rarely drugs of choice due to their adverse effects.

14.3 Ganglionic blockers act at the autonomic ganglia to lower blood pressure in emergency situations.

14.4 Muscle contraction occurs when the motor end plate is depolarized.

14.5 Depolarizing neuromuscular blockers are given to produce muscle paralysis during short medical–surgical procedures.

14.6 Nondepolarizing neuromuscular blockers are given to produce muscle paralysis during longer surgical procedures.

Case Study: Making the Patient Connection

Remember the patient "Pete Elbertson" at the beginning of the chapter? Now read the remainder of the case study. Based on the information presented within this chapter, respond to the critical thinking questions that follow.

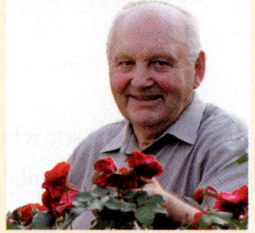

Pete Elbertson is a 60-year-old man who enjoys working in his large vegetable garden. Two days ago, while working with his tomatoes, Pete noticed that insects had infested the plants. To avoid further damage, he powdered the plants with an insecticide. In his rush to finish, he accidentally contaminated himself with the insecticide and kept working for several hours before showering.

Now, Pete presents to the local emergency department with nausea, dizziness, sweating, excessive salivation, weepy eyes, and a runny nose. He reports intermittent twitching of his upper extremities and uncoordinated movement.

His initial assessment reveals an 84-kg (185-lb) Caucasian male with a past medication history of HTN diagnosed 5 years ago. He is married and has two adult children. He smokes one pack of cigarettes per day and does not use alcohol. His vital signs are blood pressure, 158/94 mmHg; heart rate, 58; respiratory rate, 30; and temperature, 37.3°C (99.2°F). His skin is pale and moist. He exhibits copious lacrimation and rhinorrhea. Both pupils are constricted. Crackles are heard bilaterally in all lung fields on inspiration. Since admission to the emergency department he has vomited twice and had one large diarrhea stool.

Pete is diagnosed with acute organophosphate poisoning. The patient is started on oxygen therapy, and the nurse will observe him closely for further respiratory distress. Atropine 2 mg is administered IV every 15 minutes over the next hour.

Critical Thinking Questions

1. Discuss the mechanism of action associated with atropine.
2. Why is this drug being given to Pete?
3. What adverse effects should you expect for the patient from the administration of atropine?

See Answers to Critical Thinking Questions on student resource website.

Additional Case Study

You are caring for Nick, a 56-year-old man, in the intensive care unit. During the past 2 hours, you have been closely monitoring him due to increased respiratory distress. When the health care provider arrives, he informs you that Nick will need to be placed on a mechanical ventilator. The patient will be given a neuromuscular blocking drug to assist with the insertion of an endotracheal tube.

1. Describe the mechanism of action associated with this drug classification.
2. What is the rationale for the administration of neuromuscular blocking drugs for this patient?
3. Identify the problems associated with the administration of neuromuscular blocking drugs.

See Answers to Additional Case Study on student resource website.

Chapter Review

1 Which health teaching concept should the nurse review with a patient receiving tolterodine (Detrol) for urge incontinence?

1. Exercise daily to avoid muscle atrophy.
2. Increase dietary fiber and water intake to avoid constipation.
3. Consume foods high in iron to increase red blood cell production.
4. Monitor the heart rate for bradycardia.

2 The nurse is aware that the therapeutic uses for cholinergic antagonists include (select all that apply):

1. Ophthalmic procedures.
2. Cardiac rhythm abnormalities.
3. Asthma.
4. Poisonings.
5. Urinary retention.

3 Which factor in the patient's history would cause the nurse to question a medication order for atropine?

1. A 42-year-old woman with a history of drug abuse
2. An 85-year-old man with benign prostatic hyperplasia
3. An 18-year-old man with irritable bowel syndrome
4. A 22-year-old woman on the second day of her menstrual cycle

4 Muscarinic antagonists, such as benztropine (Cogentin), are most often contraindicated in glaucoma because these drugs can:

1. Increase intraocular pressure.
2. Promote ocular infections.
3. Cause miosis, which leads to blindness.
4. Detach the retina.

5 The patient will be taking cholinergic antagonists following discharge from the acute care hospital. Which statement, made by the patient, would indicate that additional teaching is needed?

1. "To relieve dry mouth, I should drink plenty of water."

2. "I will avoid activities requiring mental alertness until I know the effects of this drug."

3. "The use of lubricating eyedrops should be avoided. I should see an eye doctor for dry eyes."

4. "I will not breastfeed while taking this drug without consulting my health care provider."

6 The nurse administering succinylcholine knows that this drug causes:

1. Muscle paralysis; it does not produce anesthesia or loss of consciousness.

2. Loss of consciousness, along with muscle paralysis and anesthesia.

3. Deep muscle relaxation and relief from pain.

4. Increased mental alertness with muscle paralysis.

See Answers to Chapter Review in Appendix A.

References

Lee, J. Y., Leblanc, K., Fernandes, O. A., Huh, J. H., Wong, G. G., Hamandi, B., . . . Harrison, J. (2010). Medication reconciliation during internal hospital transfer and impact of computerized prescriber order entry. *Annals of Pharmacotherapy, 44,* 1887–1895. doi:10.1345/aph. 1P314

Lee, M. R. (2007). Solanaceae IV: Atropa belladonna, deadly nightshade. *Journal-Royal College of Physicians of Edinburgh, 37*(1), 77.

Selected Bibliography

Bacher, I., Wu, B., Shytle, D. R., & George, T. P. (2009). Mecamylamine—a nicotinic acetylcholine receptor antagonist with potential for the treatment of neuropsychiatric disorders. *Expert Opinion on Pharmacotherapy, 10,* 2709–2721. doi:10.1517/14656560903329102

Dmochowski, R. R., & Gomelsky, A. (2011). Update on the treatment of overactive bladder. *Current Opinion in Urology, 21*(4), 286–290. doi:10.1097/MOU.0b013e3283468da3

Drag, L. L., & Wright, S. (2012). Prescribing practices of anticholinergic medications and their association with cognition in an extended care setting. *Journal of Applied Gerontology, 31,* 239–259. doi:10.1177/0733464810384592

Ellsworth, P., & Kirshenbaum, E. (2010). Update on the pharmacologic management of overactive bladder: The present and the future. *Urologic Nursing, 30*(1), 29–39.

Herdman, T. H., & Kamitsuru, S. (Eds.). (2014). *NANDA International nursing diagnoses: Definitions and classification, 2015–2017.* Oxford, United Kingdom: Wiley-Blackwell.

Hibbs, R. E., & Zambon, A. C. (2011). Agents acting at the neuromuscular junction and autonomic ganglia. In L. L. Brunton, B. A. Chabner, & B. C. Knollman (Eds.), *The pharmacological basis of therapeutics* (12th ed., pp. 255–276). New York, NY: McGraw-Hill.

Katz, K. D. (2010). *Organophosphate toxicity.* Retrieved from http://www.emedicine.com/med/TOPIC1677.HTM

Naguib, M., Kopman, A. F., Lien, C. A., Hunter, J. M., Lopez, A., & Brull, S. J. (2010). A survey of current management of neuromuscular block in the United States and Europe. *Anesthesia and Analgesia, 111*(1), 110–119. doi:10.1213/ANE.0b013e3181c07428

Warr, J., Thiboutot, Z., Rose, L., Mehta, S., & Burry, L. D. (2011). Current therapeutic uses, pharmacology, and clinical considerations of neuromuscular blocking agents for critically ill adults. *The Annals of Pharmacotherapy, 45,* 1116–1126. doi:10.1097/CND.0b013e3181b5e14d

Westfall, T. C., & Westfall, D. P. (2011). Neurotransmission: The autonomic and somatic motor nervous systems. In L. L. Brunton, B. A. Chabner, & B. C. Knollman (Eds.), *The pharmacological basis of therapeutics* (12th ed., pp. 171–218). New York, NY: McGraw-Hill.

Wilson, J., Collins, A. S., & Rowan, B. O. (2012). Residual neuromuscular blockade in critical care. *Critical Care Nurse, 32*(3), e1–e10. doi:10.4037/ccn2012107

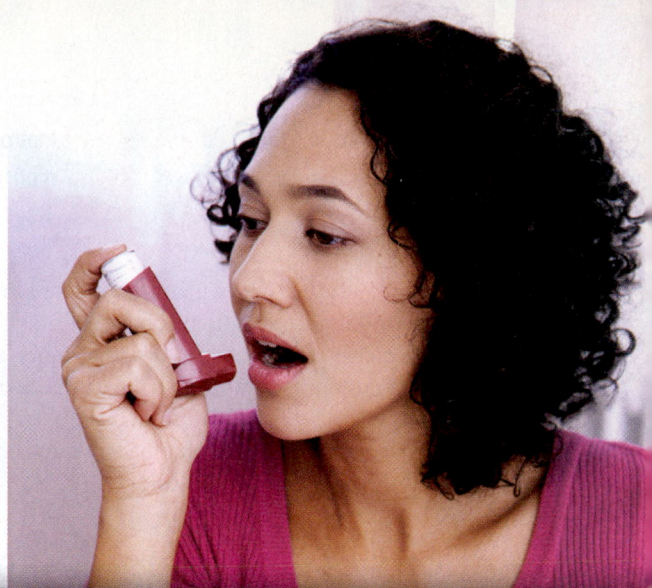

> *"I woke up this morning having difficulty breathing. I think my asthma is acting up again."*
>
> Patient "Alexia Howard"

Adrenergic Agonists

LEARNING OUTCOMES

After reading this chapter, the student should be able to:

1. Identify the physiological responses produced when a drug activates adrenergic receptors.

2. Explain the direct and indirect mechanisms by which adrenergic agonists act.

3. Compare and contrast the characteristics of catecholamines and noncatecholamines.

4. Identify indications for pharmacotherapy with adrenergic agonists.

5. Compare and contrast the types of responses that occur when a drug activates alpha$_1$-, alpha$_2$-, beta$_1$-, or beta$_2$-adrenergic receptors.

6. For each of the classes shown in the chapter outline, identify the prototype and representative drugs and explain the mechanism(s) of drug action, primary indications, contraindications, significant drug interactions, pregnancy category, and important adverse effects.

7. Apply the nursing process to care for patients receiving pharmacotherapy with adrenergic agonists.

CHAPTER OUTLINE

▶ **Actions of Adrenergic Agonists**

▶ **Mechanisms of Action of Adrenergic Agonists**

▶ **Classification of Adrenergic Agonists**

▶ **Nonselective Adrenergic Agonists**
   PROTOTYPE Epinephrine (Adrenalin), *p. 181*

▶ **Alpha-Adrenergic Agonists**
   PROTOTYPE Phenylephrine (Neo-Synephrine), *p. 184*

▶ **Beta-Adrenergic Agonists**
   PROTOTYPE Isoproterenol (Isuprel), *p. 186*

adrenergic agonists, 178

cardiotonic drugs, 185

inotropic drugs, 185

monoamine oxidase (MAO), 179

sympathomimetics, 178

tocolytics, 186

Adrenergic agonists are drugs that activate the sympathetic nervous system and induce symptoms of the fight-or-flight response. The pharmacology of adrenergic drugs is more complex than their cholinergic counterparts due to the existence of the receptor subtypes alpha and beta. Drugs that activate these subtypes have widespread applications to the pharmacotherapy of shock, hypotension, asthma, and the common cold.

Actions of Adrenergic Agonists

15.1 Adrenergic agonists activate the sympathetic nervous system to produce fight-or-flight symptoms.

Adrenergic agonists, also called **sympathomimetics**, are agents that activate adrenergic receptors in the sympathetic nervous system. Drugs in this class include naturally occurring (endogenous) substances such as norepinephrine (NE), epinephrine, and dopamine. NE is the major neurotransmitter in the sympathetic nervous system, whereas epinephrine is the primary hormone released by the adrenal medulla. Dopamine is the immediate biochemical precursor to NE and is a key neurotransmitter in certain regions of the central nervous system (CNS). In addition to their natural physiological roles in the body, NE, epinephrine, and dopamine are available as prescription drugs. A number of synthetic adrenergic agonists that mimic the effects of these natural neurotransmitters are also available.

When administered as drugs, the adrenergic agonists induce symptoms of the fight-or-flight response. Their most important therapeutic actions are on the cardiovascular and respiratory systems. Activation of adrenergic receptors in the myocardium increases the heart rate (positive chronotropic effect) and the force of contraction (positive inotropic effect). Cardiac output increases. Constriction of vascular smooth muscle causes a rapid increase in blood pressure. Administration by the parenteral or inhalation routes immediately relaxes bronchial smooth muscle, resulting in bronchodilation. Activation of adrenergic receptors in the smooth muscle of the gastrointestinal (GI) and urinary tracts slows peristalsis and may cause constipation and urine retention. Metabolic effects include increased oxygen consumption and increased blood glucose and lactate levels. Other adrenergic actions include reduction of glandular secretory activity and mydriasis.

It is important to remember that the symptoms of the fight-or-flight response elicited by the adrenergic agonists may be considered as therapeutic or adverse, depending on the condition of the patient and the goals of pharmacotherapy. For example, if the patient is in shock, increased blood pressure is a key therapeutic effect. However, if the patient is taking an adrenergic agonist to treat nasal congestion, an increase in blood pressure is an adverse effect. Furthermore a therapeutic effect may become an adverse effect if taken to extreme, such as raising blood pressure too much or causing excessive drying of the nasal or oral mucosa.

As discussed in Chapter 14, the actions produced by cholinergic (muscarinic) antagonists are similar to those of adrenergic agonists. This is because blocking muscarinic receptors in the parasympathetic nervous system allows sympathetic nerve impulses to predominate. However, because the sympathetic nervous system has alpha- and beta-receptor subtypes, the actions of many adrenergic agonists are more specific, which allows for wider therapeutic applications due to a lower incidence of adverse effects.

CONNECTION Checkpoint 15.1

From what you learned in Chapter 12, where are most dopaminergic receptors located? Dopaminergic drugs would most likely be prescribed for what disorders? *See Answer to Connection Checkpoint 15.1 on student resource website.*

PharmFACT

Pheochromocytomas are tumors of the adrenal medulla that secrete large amounts of adrenergic agonists including dopamine, epinephrine, and norepinephrine. As expected, signs and symptoms are those of sympathetic nervous system hyperactivity: increased heart rate and blood pressure and anxiety resembling that of a panic attack. Treatment includes pharmacotherapy with antihypertensives until surgery can be performed to remove the tumor (Blake, 2013).

Mechanisms of Action of Adrenergic Agonists

15.2 Adrenergic agonists may act directly by binding to adrenergic receptors, or indirectly by increasing the amount of norepinephrine at synapses.

Sympathomimetics exert their effects by two distinct mechanisms. Most act *directly* by binding to and activating adrenergic receptors. Examples include the three endogenous hormones epinephrine, NE, and dopamine.

Some adrenergic agonists act *indirectly* by increasing the amount of NE available at adrenergic synapses. Any substance that increases the amount of NE in the synaptic cleft will produce a more intense and prolonged fight-or-flight response. A few drugs, such as ephedrine, act by both direct and indirect mechanisms. The mechanisms of indirect-acting agents are shown in Figure 15.1. The three means by which NE can be increased at the synapse include the following:

- **Stimulating the release of NE from its storage vesicles on the presynaptic neuron.** Drugs that act by this mechanism include ephedrine and amphetamine.

- **Inhibiting the reuptake of NE from the synaptic cleft back to the presynaptic neuron.** Examples of drugs that inhibit reuptake of NE include the antidepressant imipramine (Tofranil) and cocaine.

- **Inhibiting the destruction of NE by the enzyme monoamine oxidase (MAO).** Phenelzine (Nardil) is an example of a MAO inhibitor (MAOI).

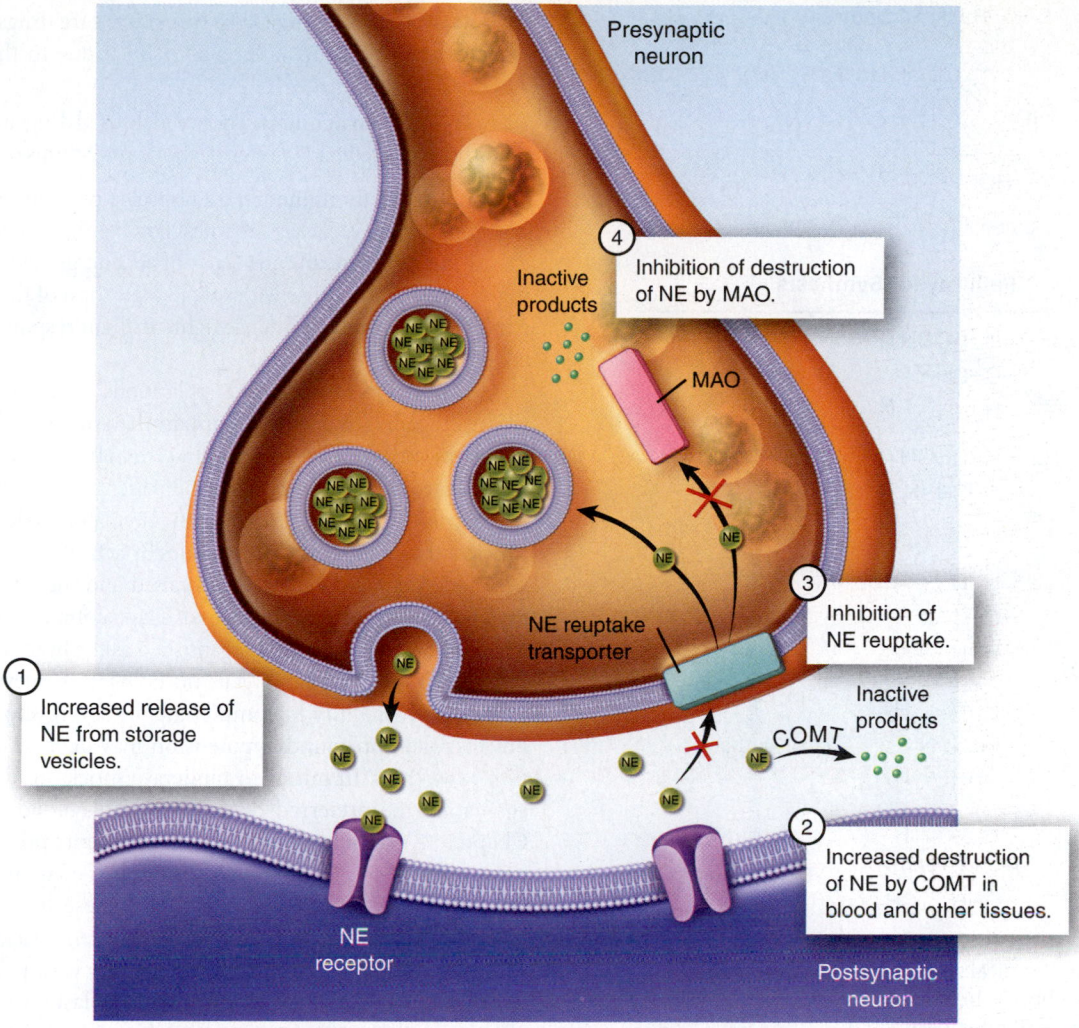

Figure 15.1 Mechanisms of action of adrenergic agonists: (1) stimulation of the release of NE; (2) increased destruction of NE by COMT; (3) inhibition of the reuptake of NE; (4) inhibition of the destruction of NE by MAO.

Indirect adrenergic agonists are less commonly prescribed than the direct agents due to a higher incidence of serious adverse effects. Some indirect-acting agents such as amphetamine and cocaine are drugs of abuse that are used for their central effects on the brain rather than their autonomic effects.

Classification of Adrenergic Agonists

15.3 Adrenergic agonists may be classified as catecholamines or noncatecholamines.

The first adrenergic agonist to be identified, epinephrine, was isolated from extracts of the adrenal gland in the late 1890s. The chemical structure of epinephrine was found to have an aromatic ring with two OH groups, similar to a common organic chemical known as catechol. Because the molecule also has an NH or amino group, the term *catecholamine* was assigned to epinephrine by physiologists. Several other adrenergic agonists share this core chemical structure, including NE, dopamine, isoproterenol, and dobutamine. This has led to a simple chemical classification of adrenergic agonists as catecholamines or noncatecholamines. Examples of noncatecholamines

include phenylephrine, terbutaline, and ephedrine. The fundamental chemical structure of a catecholamine is shown in Figure 15.2.

There are important pharmacokinetic differences between catecholamines and noncatecholamines. Catecholamines have a short duration of action because they are destroyed rapidly by the enzymes **monoamine oxidase (MAO)** and catechol-O-methyltransferase (COMT) (see Figure 15.1). Because these destructive enzymes are active in the mucosa of the intestinal tract, catecholamines cannot be given orally (PO) and must be administered parenterally or by inhalation. Furthermore, the OH groups on the catechol portion of the molecule make these drugs polar and prevent them from crossing the blood–brain barrier.

On the other hand, the noncatecholamines may be taken PO because they are not destroyed as readily by MAO or COMT. This also extends their duration of action. These drugs are less polar than the catecholamines; thus they are better able to enter the brain and affect the CNS.

CONNECTION Checkpoint 15.2

From what you learned in Chapter 3, how does the polarity of a drug molecule affect its absorption? How does it affect its distribution to tissues? *See Answer to Connection Checkpoint 15.2 on student resource website.*

Basic Structure

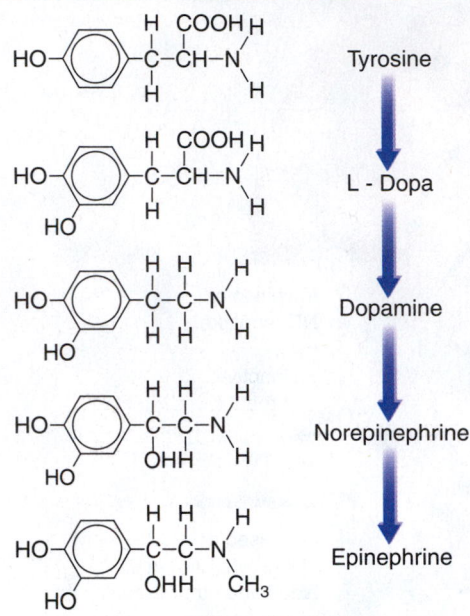

catechol   amine

Pathway for Synthesis

Tyrosine

L - Dopa

Dopamine

Norepinephrine

Epinephrine

Figure 15.2 Basic chemical structure and synthesis of catecholamines. The synthesis of norepinephrine occurs in the neuron near the neuroeffector junction.

Nonselective Adrenergic Agonists

15.4 The nonselective adrenergic agonists activate both alpha and beta receptors and are used to treat bronchospasm, cardiac arrest, and hypotension.

Although the general actions of adrenergic agonists are predictable, based on their activation of the sympathetic nervous system, the specific effects of each drug are dependent on which receptor subtypes are stimulated. As discussed in Chapter 12, adrenergic receptors include alpha$_1$, alpha$_2$, beta$_1$, and beta$_2$ subtypes. Because the receptor responses are very different and critical to understanding drug action, the student will need to remember the specific subclass(es) of receptors activated by each adrenergic agonist drug. Therapeutic applications for the different receptor activations are summarized as follows:

- **Alpha$_1$-receptor agonists.** Generally prescribed for the pharmacotherapy of nasal congestion and hypotension. These drugs may also be used to produce dilation of the pupil (mydriasis) during ophthalmic examinations.
- **Alpha$_2$-receptor agonists.** These drugs are prescribed for the treatment of hypertension (HTN). They act through nonautonomic (centrally acting) mechanisms.

- **Beta$_1$-receptor agonists.** These critical care drugs are used for cardiac arrest, heart failure, and shock due to their powerful effects on the heart.
- **Beta$_2$-receptor agonists.** These widely used drugs are for treating asthma and reducing preterm labor contractions of the uterus.

Some sympathomimetics are nonselective, stimulating two or more adrenergic receptor subtypes. For example, epinephrine and ephedrine stimulate all four types of adrenergic receptors. In doing so, these drugs cause widespread activation of the sympathetic nervous system and an intense fight-or-flight response (and many adverse effects).

One of the most important applications of the nonselective adrenergic agonists is for the pharmacotherapy of shock and other life-threatening cardiac disorders. In certain types of shock, the most serious medical challenge facing the patient is hypotension, which may become so severe as to collapse the circulatory system. In the early stages of shock, the body compensates by activating the sympathetic nervous system; blood pressure is raised and the rate and force of myocardial contraction is increased. These compensatory measures maintain blood flow to vital organs such as the heart and brain, and decrease flow to "less vital" organs, including the kidneys and liver.

The body's ability to compensate for severe shock is limited, however, and profound hypotension may develop as the condition progresses. In minor to moderate shock, fluid replacement agents are the preferred drugs for raising blood pressure (see Chapter 33). Should fluid replacement agents prove ineffective, however, adrenergic agonists are administered to maintain blood pressure. When given intravenously (IV) these drugs immediately increase blood pressure. Because rapid, intense vasoconstriction can cause serious hypoperfusion of tissues with potential organ damage, these drugs are generally used as a last resort, when safer alternatives have failed to produce the desired therapeutic outcome. Epinephrine, NE, and dopamine are nonselective drugs for shock or anaphylaxis when blood pressure and heart rate need to be quickly restored to normal levels. The nonselective adrenergic agonists are shown in Table 15.1.

The nonselective adrenergic agonists cause more autonomic-related adverse effects than the selective drugs. Most of these adverse effects are extensions of their autonomic actions. Cardiovascular effects such as tachycardia, HTN, and dysrhythmias are particularly troublesome and may limit therapy. Blood pressure and heart rate must be monitored continuously during parenteral administration of these drugs. Large doses can induce CNS excitement and seizures. Patients with diabetes may experience a significant increase in blood glucose levels due to an increased breakdown of glycogen in the liver and skeletal muscle. Care must be taken to avoid extravasation because this can cause severe tissue injury. Should extravasation occur, the antidote is phentolamine, an alpha-adrenergic blocker, which will help to counteract the vasoconstriction caused by the catecholamine at the site. Other adverse effects associated with sympathetic activation include dry mouth, nausea, and vomiting.

Amphetamine is a nonselective adrenergic agonist with a marked CNS stimulant effect. Amphetamine also causes anorexia, which has led to its historical use as an appetite suppressant. Because of prominent cardiovascular adverse effects, nervous system effects such as paranoia and psychosis, and the risk of physical dependence, the drug is no longer prescribed for weight loss. Additional details on amphetamine may be found in Chapters 24 and 27.

TABLE 15.1	Selected Adrenergic Agonists	
Drug	**Route and Adult Dose (Maximum Dose Where Indicated)**	**Adverse Effects**
albuterol (Proventil, Ventolin, VoSpire)	Metered-dose inhaler (MDI): 2 inhalations every 4–6 h as needed Nebulizer: 1.25–5 mg every 4–8 h as needed PO: 2–4 mg tid–qid; 8 mg bid for extended release tabs	*Headache, dizziness, tremor, nervousness, throat irritation, drug tolerance* <u>Tachycardia, dysrhythmias, hypokalemia, hyperglycemia</u>
dobutamine (Dobutrex)	IV: Infused at a rate of 2.5–40 mcg/kg/min for a max of 72 h	*Headache, palpitations, nausea, vomiting, increased heart rate and blood pressure, anginal pain* <u>Dysrhythmias, gangrene, severe HTN</u>
dopamine (Dopastat, Intropin)	IV: 2–5 mcg/kg/min initial dose; may be increased to 20–50 mcg/kg/min	*Headache, palpitations, nausea, vomiting, changes in blood pressure (hypo- or hypertension)* <u>Dysrhythmias, gangrene, severe HTN</u>
ephedrine	PO: 12.5–25 mg qid (max: 150 mg/24 h) IM/IV/subcutaneous: 12.5–25 mg	*Headache, nervousness, palpitations, nausea, vomiting* <u>Dysrhythmias, severe HTN, decreased urine output</u>
epinephrine (Adrenalin)	Subcutaneous: 0.1–0.5 mL of 1:1,000 every 10–15 min prn IV: 0.1–0.25 mL of 1:1,000 every 10–15 min	*Headache, palpitations, nausea, vomiting, tremors, changes in blood pressure (hypo- or hypertension)* <u>Dysrhythmias, gangrene, severe HTN, pulmonary edema</u>
indacaterol (Arcapta Neohaler)	Inhalation: 75 mcg once daily	*Cough, oropharyngeal pain, nasopharyngitis, headache, nausea* <u>Hypersensitivity, bronchospasm</u>
isoproterenol (Isuprel)	IV: 0.01–0.02 mg prn	*Headache, nervousness, palpitations, tachycardia* <u>Ventricular dysrhythmias, unstable blood pressure</u>
levalbuterol (Xopenex)	Nebulizer: 0.63 mg tid MDI: 90 mcg (2 inhalations) every 4–6 h	*Headache, dizziness, tremor, nervousness, throat irritation, drug tolerance* <u>Tachycardia, dysrhythmias, hypokalemia, hyperglycemia</u>
midodrine (ProAmatine)	PO: 10 mg tid (max: 20 mg/dose)	*Paresthesia, pruritus* <u>HTN, urinary retention</u>
mirabegron (Myrbetriq)	PO: 25–50 mg q8h	*Paresthesia, nasopharyngitis, urinary tract infection, pruritus* <u>HTN, urinary retention</u>
norepinephrine (Levophed)	IV: Initially 0.5–1 mcg/min, titrate slowly to therapeutic response; usual range 8–30 mcg/min	*Restlessness, anxiety, palpitations, nausea, vomiting, headache* <u>Tachycardia or bradycardia (overdose), severe HTN, hepatic necrosis, cerebral hemorrhage</u>
phenylephrine (Neo-Synephrine)	IV: 0.1–0.18 mg/min until blood pressure stabilizes, then 0.04–0.06 mg/min for maintenance	*Palpitations, tingling or coldness of extremities, nervousness* <u>Severe peripheral vasoconstriction, tachycardia or bradycardia (overdose), HTN, dysrhythmias, necrosis at injection site</u>

Note: Italics indicate common adverse effects. <u>Underline</u> indicates serious adverse effects.

PROTOTYPE DRUG Epinephrine (Adrenalin)

Classification: Therapeutic: Antishock and antianaphylaxis drug, bronchodilator
Pharmacologic: Nonselective adrenergic agonist, catecholamine

Therapeutic Effects and Uses: Epinephrine has several therapeutic applications, all of which are the result of adrenergic receptor activation. It can be administered parenterally, topically, by inhalation, or by instillation.

Epinephrine is a preferred drug for cardiac arrest after cardiopulmonary resuscitation (CPR) has failed. Given as an IV infusion or by intracardiac injection, the drug has the potential to immediately restore cardiac rhythm. Epinephrine also constricts arterioles, raising cerebral and cardiac perfusion pressure, which discourages cardiovascular collapse. The intracardiac route is used only under extreme conditions, usually during open cardiac massage, or when no other route is possible.

Epinephrine can reverse many of the distressing symptoms of anaphylaxis within minutes. Almost immediately after injection, blood pressure increases due to stimulation of alpha$_1$ receptors. Activation of beta$_2$ receptors in the bronchi dilates the airways to relieve shortness of breath. Epinephrine can also be administered by inhalation, which has the potential to immediately terminate acute bronchospasm.

Epinephrine is sometimes added to cartridges of local anesthetics to cause vasoconstriction of local vessels. This forces the anesthetic to remain localized in the tissues for a longer period, prolonging analgesia and slowing the absorption of anesthetic. Epinephrine can also be applied topically to control superficial bleeding along a surgical incision. Repeated injection or application to the same site can result in tissue necrosis due to the diminished blood supply to the area.

Ophthalmic administration of epinephrine causes mydriasis and the outflow of fluid from the anterior chamber of the eye, making the drug an adjunct to the pharmacotherapy of open-angle glaucoma. Intranasal administration can be used to reduce nasal congestion.

Mechanism of Action: Epinephrine is a nonselective adrenergic agonist, stimulating both alpha- and beta-adrenergic receptors throughout the body. Actions typical of the fight-or-flight response are induced.

Pharmacokinetics:

Route(s)	Subcutaneous, IV, intramuscular (IM), inhalation, topical, ophthalmic
Absorption	Not absorbed PO; minimal absorption by inhalation; rapidly absorbed by IM and subcutaneous routes
Distribution	Widely distributed; does not cross the blood–brain barrier; crosses the placenta; secreted in breast milk
Primary metabolism	Rapidly metabolized by MAO and COMT in the liver and most tissues
Primary excretion	Small amount excreted unchanged in the kidneys
Onset of action	Subcutaneous: 3–5 min; IM: 5–10 min; inhalation: 1 min (for local respiratory effects); IV: immediate onset
Duration of action	1–4 h

Adverse Effects: The most common adverse effects of epinephrine are nervousness, tremors, palpitations, tachycardia, dizziness, headache, and stinging at the site of application. Serious adverse effects include HTN, dysrhythmias, pulmonary edema, and cardiac arrest. Intense CNS stimulation including hallucinations, panic attacks, and aggression may occur, especially in patients with preexisting psychiatric disorders. Extravasation of epinephrine can produce an injection site reaction, causing severe tissue damage and necrosis.

Contraindications/Precautions: Contraindications for epinephrine include hypersensitivity to other adrenergic agonists, closed-angle glaucoma, severe shock (other than anaphylaxis), and dysrhythmias. The drug should be used with caution in patients with coronary artery disease because intense angina symptoms may result. Due to its ability to relax uterine smooth muscle, epinephrine will delay labor. Patients with hyperthyroidism or HTN are more sensitive to the effects of administered epinephrine (and other catecholamines). In life-threatening conditions such as anaphylaxis or cardiac arrest, there are no absolute contraindications for the use of epinephrine.

Drug Interactions: Additive cardiovascular effects will occur if epinephrine is used concurrently with other sympathomimetics or antihypotensive drugs. MAO inhibitors block the destruction of catecholamines and will intensify the effects of epinephrine. Tricyclic antidepressants block the reuptake of catecholamines, which is the primary way by which epinephrine is inactivated; thus doses of epinephrine should be lowered in patients using these depressants. Alpha- and beta-adrenergic antagonists inhibit the actions of epinephrine. Epinephrine will decrease the effects of beta blockers. Digoxin and some general anesthetics may sensitize the heart to the effects of epinephrine. Two drugs used for Parkinson's disease, entacapone and tolcapone, are inhibitors of COMT, the enzyme that degrades epinephrine; concurrent use may cause increased effects of epinephrine on the heart and blood pressure. **Herbal/Food**: Caffeine and ephedra should be avoided because they may increase blood pressure and heart rate.

Pregnancy: Category C.

Treatment of Overdose: Overdose of epinephrine is life threatening and the immediate administration of an alpha- or beta-adrenergic blocker is indicated. If blood pressure remains high, a direct vasodilator may be administered.

Nursing Responsibilities: Key nursing implications for patients receiving epinephrine are included in the Nursing Practice Application for Patients Receiving Pharmacotherapy with Adrenergic Agonists.

Drugs Similar to Epinephrine (Adrenalin)

Other nonselective adrenergic agonists include dopamine, droxidopa, ephedrine, and NE.

Dopamine (Dopastat, Intropin): Approved as a drug in 1974, dopamine is a naturally occurring catecholamine that has both alpha- and beta-agonist activity. It is administered by the IV route and has a brief 10-minute duration of action. Doses are slowly increased until the desired therapeutic effects have been achieved. Vital signs should be monitored continuously during the infusion.

Dopamine is primarily used to treat hypovolemic and cardiogenic shock. Whenever possible, hypovolemia is corrected with fluid-expanding agents before starting a dopamine infusion. At low doses (1–5 mcg/kg/minute), the drug selectively stimulates dopaminergic receptors, especially in the kidneys, leading to vasodilation, thus increasing renal blood flow and enhancing urine output. This helps to prevent renal failure, which can occur during shock conditions. At higher doses (more than 10 mcg/kg/minute), dopamine stimulates beta$_1$-adrenergic receptors, causing the heart to beat more forcefully, thus increasing cardiac output. Also at higher doses, dopamine stimulates alpha$_1$-adrenergic receptors, thus causing vasoconstriction and increased blood pressure.

Headache, nausea, and vomiting are common adverse effects. High doses can produce ventricular tachycardia. Severe necrosis or gangrene can result if extravasation occurs; thus phentolamine should be readily available. Dopamine is pregnancy category C.

Droxidopa (Northera): Approved in 2014, droxidopa is a prodrug that is metabolically converted to NE after oral administration. As such, it shares the same vasoconstrictor action as NE. The drug is approved to treat orthostatic hypotension that is associated with neurogenic disorders such as Parkinson's disease. The most common adverse events of droxidopa include headache, dizziness, nausea, HTN, and fatigue. The drug carries a black box warning that the patient should be monitored carefully for supine hypertension during therapy because this increases the risk for serious cardiovascular events. Droxidopa is pregnancy category C.

Ephedrine (Efedron): Ephedrine is a noncatecholamine, originally obtained from the ephedra plant species, that activates both alpha and beta receptors. Although ephedrine was approved by the U.S. Food and Drug Administration (FDA) in 1939, extracts from the ephedra plant have been used to treat various ailments for thousands of years. In Chinese medicine, the herb ma huang contains ephedrine as one of its active ingredients.

Ephedrine acts by two mechanisms: directly, by binding to adrenergic receptors, and indirectly, by causing the release of NE from storage vesicles in the nerve terminals. Ephedrine has been used for its ability to relieve respiratory congestion caused by allergies and to prevent bronchospasm in patients with asthma. It is available by the PO and parenteral routes, is readily absorbed from the GI tract, and crosses the blood–brain barrier. Once in the brain, ephedrine exhibits prominent stimulatory effects, keeping patients alert and awake. It was once used as an over-the-counter appetite suppressant, but this indication is not legal in the United States. The CNS stimulation has also been used to alleviate the CNS depression caused by opioid or barbiturate overdose. This stimulatory effect of ephedrine is also the cause of the major adverse effects of the drug such as nervousness, insomnia, palpitations, and tachycardia. Like the closely related drug pseudoephedrine, ephedrine is highly regulated because it can be used to make methamphetamine. This drug is pregnancy category C.

Norepinephrine (Levophed): Approved in 1938, NE is a nonselective catecholamine that has actions similar to epinephrine, except that is does not activate beta$_2$ receptors. Approved to treat shock and hypotension, NE acts directly on alpha-adrenergic receptors in vascular smooth muscle to immediately raise blood pressure. It also stimulates beta$_1$ receptors in the heart to increase cardiac output. It is given by the IV route and has a duration of only 1 to 2 minutes after the infusion is terminated. Because NE is a powerful vasoconstrictor, continuous monitoring of blood pressure is required to avoid HTN. When first administered, reflex bradycardia is sometimes experienced, and the drug has the ability to produce various dysrhythmias. Blurred vision and photophobia are signs of overdose. Like other drugs in this class, NE produces symptoms of CNS stimulation such as nervousness, insomnia, and confusion. Severe tissue necrosis can result if extravasation occurs; thus phentolamine should be readily available. The primary indications for NE are acute shock and cardiac arrest. This drug is pregnancy category C.

Alpha-Adrenergic Agonists

15.5 Alpha-adrenergic agonists are used to relieve nasal decongestion and elevate blood pressure.

Activation of alpha-adrenergic receptors causes a number of important physiological responses, most of which relate to contraction of vascular smooth muscle. Like the nonselective adrenergic agonists, several of the selective alpha agonists are used to treat hypotension associated with shock and other critical care conditions. Alpha agonists may also be administered to treat patients who are susceptible to orthostatic hypotension.

A second application of alpha-adrenergic agonists is for the treatment of nasal congestion. During upper respiratory infections or allergic rhinitis, arterioles in the nose dilate and produce excess mucus. Alpha$_1$ agonists relieve nasal congestion by causing vasoconstriction of vessels serving the nasal mucosa. Intranasal drugs such as phenylephrine work within minutes and are highly effective at clearing the nasal passages. The intranasal route causes few systemic side effects because absorption is limited. Oral decongestants such as phenylephrine take longer to act and the risk for systemic side effects is higher; however, they are less damaging to the nasal mucosa than the intranasal drugs. The pharmacotherapy of upper respiratory congestion is presented in Chapter 45.

Topical instillation of alpha$_1$ agonists to the eye has two applications. Alpha$_1$-adrenergic receptors are present on the radial muscle of the iris. When these receptors are activated, the radial muscle contracts and the pupil dilates, allowing the health care provider to better examine the interior structures of the eye. Although the alpha$_1$ agonists are effective at producing mydriasis, they are generally second-line drugs for ophthalmic exams. Another ophthalmic application of alpha$_1$ agonists is to relieve conjunctival congestion and redness. The mechanism behind this effect is through alpha$_1$-receptor activation of arterioles in the eye, causing vasoconstriction. Tetrahydrozoline (Tyzine) is widely used for minor eye irritation and redness and is available over the counter (OTC). The pharmacotherapy of ophthalmic conditions is discussed in detail in Chapter 74.

Most adverse effects of the alpha$_1$-adrenergic agonists are logical extensions of their autonomic actions. Their intense vasoconstrictive effect can lead to HTN. This increase in blood pressure can activate the baroreceptor reflex, causing reflex bradycardia. Because of the potential for cardiovascular adverse effects, patients should be continuously monitored when receiving high doses or infusions of these drugs. Should extravasation occur, the intense local vasoconstriction caused by these drugs can lead to tissue necrosis. Major adverse effects or overdose with drugs in this class may be treated by administering a specific alpha-adrenergic antagonist such as phentolamine. Bradycardia can be prevented or reversed by administration of an anticholinergic drug such as atropine. In low doses, many of the alpha agonists can be safely used as OTC drugs for symptoms of the common cold, minor allergies, or ophthalmic conditions.

Activation of alpha$_2$-adrenergic receptors produces very different responses than alpha$_1$ activation. The most important responses to alpha$_2$-receptor agonists occur in the brain rather than the peripheral nervous system. Unlike alpha$_1$ agonists, which increase sympathetic nervous system activity, alpha$_2$ agonists act in the CNS to *decrease* sympathetic activity. Methyldopa (Aldomet) and clonidine (Catapres, Duraclon) are two drugs in this class. Because they decrease blood pressure, their primary therapeutic application is for the treatment of HTN (see Chapter 34).

PROTOTYPE DRUG | **Phenylephrine (Neo-Synephrine)**

Classification: Therapeutic: Nasal decongestant, vasoconstrictor
Pharmacologic: Alpha-adrenergic agonist

Therapeutic Effects and Uses: Approved in 1938, the actions and indications of phenylephrine are predictable extensions of its sympathetic activation. Its most frequent application is for the relief of congestion associated with the common cold and allergies. In the past, pseudoephedrine was the drug of choice for these indications. One advantage of phenylephrine, however, is that it cannot be used by illicit drug dealers to synthesize methamphetamine. Because of this, phenylephrine has largely replaced pseudoephedrine in OTC multisystem cold, allergy, and sinus remedies. Formulations containing phenylephrine are exempt from regulations in most states that require pseudoephedrine products to be kept behind the pharmacy counter. For congestion, phenylephrine is available via oral and intranasal routes. When applied intranasally by spray or drops, it reduces nasal congestion by constricting small blood vessels in the nasal mucosa.

Parenteral administration of phenylephrine causes systemic vasoconstriction that can prevent or reverse acute hypotension caused by spinal anesthesia or vascular shock. Its long duration of activity and lack of significant cardiac adverse effects gives phenylephrine advantages over epinephrine or NE in treating acute hypotension. Unlike epinephrine, which markedly increases the heart rate, phenylephrine tends to slow the heart rate probably due to reflex bradycardia. In situations in which reflex bradycardia is undesirable, this action may be blocked by the administration of atropine.

Phenylephrine is also available for topical use. Applied topically to the eye during ophthalmic examinations, phenylephrine can dilate the pupil, without causing significant cycloplegia. Applied to swollen hemorrhoidal tissue, the drug can relieve itching and burning associated with hemorrhoids.

Mechanism of Action: Phenylephrine directly activates alpha$_1$-adrenergic receptors in the peripheral nervous system. It has weak beta-adrenergic activity at high doses, but this is usually not of clinical significance.

Pharmacokinetics:

Route(s)	PO, IM, subcutaneous, IV, intranasal, and ophthalmic solutions
Absorption	Readily absorbed in the GI tract; well absorbed when given IM or subcutaneously
Distribution	Widely distributed; does not cross blood–brain barrier or enter breast milk in significant amounts
Primary metabolism	Intestinal and hepatic by MAO
Primary excretion	Unknown
Onset of action	Oral: peaks in 1–2 h; subcutaneous/IM: 10–15 min; IV: immediate
Duration of action	Oral: 3 h; subcutaneous/IM: 30–120 min; IV: 15–20 min

Adverse Effects: Phenylephrine causes few serious adverse effects when taken by the PO, intranasal, or ophthalmic routes. Common adverse effects with intranasal phenylephrine use include stinging of the nasal mucosa, sneezing, and rebound congestion. Ophthalmic use can cause narrow-angle glaucoma or photophobia. Parenteral use can lead to symptoms of CNS stimulation such as anxiety, restlessness, and tremor. Serious adverse effects include reflex bradycardia and reduced blood flow to peripheral tissues due to severe vasoconstriction. OTC cough and cold products containing phenylephrine or pseudoephedrine should not be given to children under age 2 years because overdose has caused serious illness and several infant deaths.

Contraindications/Precautions: Phenylephrine is contraindicated in patients with severe HTN, because the drug will raise blood pressure to dangerous levels. Because it causes reflex bradycardia, patients with preexisting bradycardia should not receive phenylephrine. Phenylephrine causes vasoconstriction, which can reduce coronary blood flow in patients with advanced coronary artery disease, causing angina attacks. Phenylephrine also reduces the effectiveness of nitrates such as nitroglycerin that are taken to prevent anginal episodes. Because of its effects on the eye, it should not be administered to patients with narrow-angle glaucoma. Phenylephrine should be used with caution in patients with hyperthyroidism or diabetes because these patients are more sensitive to the potential cardiac adverse effects.

Drug Interactions: Phenylephrine will reduce the effectiveness of antihypertensive medications. A hypertensive crisis may occur in patients receiving MAOIs; phenylephrine should not be administered within 21 days of a MAOI. Increased effects of phenylephrine may occur in patients taking ergot alkaloids and tricyclic antidepressants. Additive effects may occur if phenylephrine is given concurrently with other adrenergic agonists, including amphetamines or cocaine. Concurrent administration with oxytocin during the postpartum period may cause persistent HTN. Concurrent use with halothane or digoxin may increase the risk of dysrhythmias. **Herbal/Food:** Phenylephrine should be used with caution with St. John's wort because this combination may result in HTN. Ingestion of substances with high amounts of caffeine will worsen the CNS stimulation caused by phenylephrine.

Pregnancy: Category C.

Treatment of Overdose: When given by the parenteral route, overdose will result in HTN and possible dysrhythmias. Phentolamine is a specific alpha antagonist that can be used to lower blood pressure, and antidysrhythmic drugs may be indicated.

Nursing Responsibilities: Key nursing implications for patients receiving phenylephrine are included in the Nursing Practice Application for Patients Receiving Pharmacotherapy with Adrenergic Agonists.

Drugs Similar to Phenylephrine (Neo-Synephrine)

Most drugs with predominant alpha-adrenergic agonist activity can be grouped into subclasses based on their indications: intranasal or ocular decongestants. Another drug in this class, methoxamine (Vasoxyl), is no longer available in the United States.

Intranasal decongestants: Oxymetazoline (Afrin), pseudoephedrine (Sudafed), xylometazoline (Neo-Synephrine II, Long-Acting), and tetrahydrozoline (Tyzine) are given by the intranasal route to diminish nasal congestion caused by allergies or the common cold. Use of these medications is generally limited to 3 to 5 days. If the drug is abruptly discontinued, congestion may worsen, a phenomenon known as *rebound congestion*. Although these drugs may also have some beta-adrenergic activity, they are only used for their effects on alpha-adrenergic receptors in the nasal mucosa. The pharmacotherapy of nasal decongestants is presented in Chapter 45.

Pseudoephedrine is an intranasal decongestant that deserves special attention because of its potential for misuse. Pseudoephedrine is the starting chemical for the synthesis of illegal methamphetamine by drug traffickers. Most states have enacted laws to regulate the sale of solid tablet formulations containing pseudoephedrine, requiring that pseudoephedrine be placed behind the pharmacy counter so that only pharmacists can provide the product. Most states also require the pharmacist to record the name and address of the buyer. Note that these precautions are not being taken because pseudoephedrine itself is a dangerous drug, but to limit the availability of the drug to illicit makers of methamphetamine. A prototype feature for pseudoephedrine can be found in Chapter 45.

Ocular decongestants: Naphazoline (Naphcon, Clear Eyes), oxymetazoline (Afrin 12 hour), and tetrahydrozoline (Visine) are available as ophthalmic solutions to relieve redness due to minor eye irritations, such as those caused by the common cold, swimming, allergies, or contact lenses. These drugs act by constricting arteries in the conjunctiva. Other than local stinging, they rarely cause adverse effects. The pharmacotherapy of ocular medications is presented in Chapter 74.

Midodrine (ProAmatine): Approved in 1996, midodrine is converted into an active metabolite that has alpha$_1$-agonist actions. It is given PO for the symptomatic treatment of orthostatic hypotension. The drug increases standing, sitting, and supine systolic and diastolic blood pressure. Because marked elevation of supine blood pressure occurs in as many as 13% of the patients taking the drug, it carries a black box warning that supine and sitting blood pressures should be monitored during therapy and that it should not be used in patients with an initial supine systolic pressure greater than 180 mmHg. Signs of supine HTN include pounding sensations in the ears or chest, blurred vision, and headache. The most common adverse effects are paresthesia, goosebumps, dysuria, and pruritus of the scalp. Midodrine is contraindicated in patients with heart failure, severe cardiac disease, or excessive supine HTN. The drug is pregnancy category C.

CONNECTION Checkpoint 15.3

Parenteral phenylephrine can cause reflex bradycardia. From what you learned in Chapter 14, would the administration of an anticholinergic such as atropine improve or worsen this condition? *See Answer to Connection Checkpoint 15.3 on student resource website.*

Beta-Adrenergic Agonists

15.6 Beta-adrenergic agonists are used to treat asthma, shock, heart failure, and other cardiac disorders.

Activation of beta-adrenergic receptors can produce a wide variety of physiological responses, depending on the location of the receptor and which subtype is stimulated. Some beta-adrenergic agonists are more selective for beta$_1$ receptors, whereas others affect primarily beta$_2$. The indications for the beta$_1$ activators are very different from those of the beta$_2$ activators:

- **Beta$_1$ applications:** cardiac arrest, heart failure, atrioventricular (AV) heart block, and shock
- **Beta$_2$ applications:** asthma and delay of preterm labor

Beta$_1$-adrenergic agonists: Pharmacologically, the most significant site having beta$_1$ receptors is cardiac muscle. Activation of beta$_1$ receptors results in cardiac actions typical of the fight-or-flight response: increased heart rate (positive chronotropic effect), force of contraction (positive inotropic effect), and velocity of impulse conduction across the myocardium (positive dromotropic effect). These cardiac effects may be considered beneficial or adverse, depending on the condition of the patient and the therapeutic goals.

Drugs used for their beta$_1$-agonist actions are sometimes called **cardiotonic drugs** because they increase the force of contraction of the heart. In the treatment of heart failure or shock, they are administered to increase cardiac output. Another name applied to these drugs is **inotropic drugs**, because they reverse the cardiac symptoms of shock by increasing the strength of myocardial contraction. The use of beta$_1$ agonists in treating heart failure is presented in Chapter 36.

Most drugs used for their strong beta$_1$-agonist activity are nonselective and activate other receptor subtypes. For example, although epinephrine is often used for its beta$_1$ activation of the heart following cardiac arrest, the drug has effects on all receptor subtypes. Similarly, although NE is used for its beta$_1$-agonist actions during cardiac arrest, the drug also activates alpha receptors. Dopamine is somewhat unique in that at low doses the drug activates dopamine receptors, and at moderate doses it stimulates both beta$_1$ and dopamine receptors. At high doses dopamine activates all three receptor types: dopamine, alpha, and beta$_1$. Dobutamine is selective for beta$_1$ receptors and isoproterenol activates both beta$_1$ and beta$_2$ receptors.

Beta$_2$-adrenergic agonists: Beta$_2$-adrenergic receptors are more widely distributed than beta$_1$ receptors. Pharmacologically, the most important site is in the lung, where activation of beta$_2$ receptors leads to relaxation of bronchial smooth muscle. Beta$_2$-adrenergic agonists, commonly referred to as bronchodilators, are used extensively in the treatment of asthma and other pulmonary disorders. The following discussion is limited to autonomic bronchodilators; information on other classes of drugs used in the pharmacotherapy of asthma is presented in Chapter 44.

Autonomic drugs used as bronchodilators include nonselective adrenergic agonists as well as those that are selective for beta$_2$ receptors. Epinephrine is the best example of a nonselective drug that is an effective bronchodilator. Unfortunately, epinephrine exhibits a high incidence of adverse effects, such as HTN and dysrhythmias, due to its stimulation of multiple receptor subtypes throughout the body. Likewise, isoproterenol is an effective bronchodilator; however, it also affects beta$_1$ receptors, which increases its potential for producing cardiovascular adverse effects. Selective beta$_2$ agonists were developed to minimize these adverse effects. Selective beta$_2$ agonists such as albuterol have become first-line drugs in the pharmacotherapy of asthma and other conditions characterized by bronchospasm. A drug prototype feature for albuterol can be found in Chapter 44.

When given for asthma, beta$_2$ agonists are administered by either the inhalation or PO route. Inhalation administration of these medications relieves acute bronchospasm within minutes. Some of the inhaled beta$_2$ agonists, such as albuterol (Proventil, Ventolin, VoSpire) and pirbuterol (Maxair), have a rapid onset; however, their duration of action is only 3 to 5 hours. Others, such as formoterol (Xopenex), have longer onsets of action, but their effects can last up to 12 hours. The drug of choice and dosage schedule are individualized for the particular pattern of asthma exhibited by each patient.

Only two beta$_2$ agonists, albuterol and terbutaline, are available by the PO route. An extended release form of albuterol (Proventil Repetabs) allows for the convenience of twice a day dosing. Terbutaline (Brethine) is given 3 or 4 times per day. Because the oral (PO) forms take up to 30 minutes to act, they are not indicated for the relief of acute bronchospasm.

A second therapeutic application of beta$_2$ agonists is for the treatment of preterm labor contractions. Activation of beta$_2$ receptors in the uterus relaxes uterine smooth muscle, leading to a delay in labor. This delay allows for additional maturation of the organ systems of the fetus, which increases the probability of neonatal survival. Terbutaline is the only beta agonist used for this purpose. The FDA has discouraged the off-label use of this drug because it is mostly ineffective at delaying labor and poses a risk for adverse effects. A second beta$_2$ receptor in this class, ritodrine (Yutopar), was removed from the U.S. market. Drugs used to delay preterm labor are called **tocolytics** and are discussed in Chapter 69.

Adverse effects of the beta$_2$ agonists are predictable extensions of their autonomic activation. Tachycardia, palpitations, flushing, insomnia, and tremor are possible adverse effects with all beta$_2$

agonists. The oral forms have some beta$_1$ activity; thus systemic adverse effects are more common than the inhaled drugs, which act locally and produce few systemic adverse effects. Beta agonists should be used cautiously in patients with dysrhythmias or heart failure. These drugs will antagonize the actions of beta-adrenergic blockers.

PROTOTYPE DRUG | Isoproterenol (Isuprel)

Classification: Therapeutic: Bronchodilator, cardiac stimulator
Pharmacologic: Nonselective beta-adrenergic agonist

Therapeutic Effects and Uses: Isoproterenol is a catecholamine that has been available as a drug for over 50 years. Isoproterenol activates both beta$_1$- and beta$_2$-adrenergic receptors but has little effect on alpha receptors. Given by the IV route, isoproterenol immediately activates beta$_1$ receptors to increase the strength of myocardial contraction and improve cardiac output. The cardiac actions of isoproterenol are used to advantage in the pharmacotherapy of cardiogenic or bacteremic shock, cardiac arrest, Adams-Stokes syndrome, and certain types of ventricular dysrhythmias. Dobutamine has largely replaced isoproterenol as a cardiac drug, because it is more specific to beta$_1$ receptors in the heart.

Isoproterenol was once available by inhaler for asthma pharmacotherapy and was a drug of choice due to its bronchodilation effects caused by activation of beta$_2$ receptors in the airways. The development of selective beta$_2$ agonists with fewer cardiac adverse effects, however, led to a significant decline in the use of isoproterenol as an antiasthmatic drug. This drug is no longer available via inhalation devices. Other types of acute bronchospasm, such as that caused by anesthesia, may be reversed by IV isoproterenol.

Mechanism of Action: Isoproterenol is a potent activator of both beta$_1$- and beta$_2$-adrenergic receptors throughout the body.

Pharmacokinetics:

Route(s)	IV
Absorption	N/A
Distribution	Distributed to most tissues; it is unknown if it crosses the placenta or is secreted in breast milk
Primary metabolism	Hepatic by COMT
Primary excretion	Renal: 40–50% unchanged
Onset of action	Immediate
Duration of action	Less than 1 h

Adverse Effects: Adverse effects of isoproterenol are predictable based on its activation of beta-adrenergic receptors. Common adverse effects include headache, nausea, vomiting, and symptoms of CNS stimulation such as tremors, anxiety, and insomnia. Adverse effects affecting the heart include serious dysrhythmias.

Contraindications/Precautions: Because isoproterenol increases the myocardial workload, it should be used with extreme caution in patients with severe cardiac disease, dysrhythmias, or HTN. The drug should be used with caution in patients with hyperthyroidism or diabetes because these patients are more sensitive to the potential cardiac adverse effects.

Drug Interactions: Concurrent administration with a beta-adrenergic blocker diminishes the bronchodilation effect of isoproterenol and may induce bronchospasm in patients with asthma. Use with other bronchodilators or adrenergic agonists such as epinephrine or dopamine may result in additive effects. MAOIs and tricyclic antidepressants should be discontinued at least 2 weeks prior to isoproterenol therapy to avoid possible hypertensive crisis. Isoproterenol should not be concurrently administered with potassium-wasting diuretics because hypokalemia may result. Isoproterenol may lower serum levels of digoxin and induce dysrhythmias.

Pregnancy: Category C.

Treatment of Overdose: Overdose with isoproterenol will cause tachycardia and other dysrhythmias. Blood pressure usually falls. Due to the relatively short half-life of the drug, discontinuing the infusion is often enough to reverse symptoms, although supportive cardiac drugs may be necessary.

Nursing Responsibilities: Key nursing implications for patients receiving isoproterenol are included in the Nursing Practice Application for Patients Receiving Pharmacotherapy with Adrenergic Agonists.

Drugs Similar to Isoproterenol (Isuprel)

Beta-adrenergic agonists may be grouped into two primary subclasses: bronchodilators and tocolytics.

Bronchodilators: Albuterol (Proventil, Ventolin, VoSpire ER), levalbuterol (Xopenex), and pirbuterol (Maxair) are short-acting beta-adrenergic agonists given by inhalation to terminate acute bronchospasm. They are preferred drugs for terminating acute asthma attacks. Patients can be dosed every 20 to 30 minutes until control is achieved. Arformoterol (Brovana), formoterol (Foradil, Performist), indacaterol (Arcapta Neohaler), and salmeterol (Serevent) are also given by inhalation, but the long onset of action of these drugs makes them unsuitable for relieving acute asthma attacks. The longer acting drugs are used in combination with inhaled corticosteroids in the pharmacotherapy of chronic asthma.

Albuterol and terbutaline (Brethaire) are available in tablet form. Because the PO route results in more delayed onset of action, these drugs should not be used to terminate an asthma attack in progress. When given 15 minutes before exercise, albuterol may be used for the prophylaxis of exercise-induced bronchospasm. A complete discussion of bronchodilators may be found in Chapter 47.

Dobutamine (Dobutrex): Dobutamine is a selective beta$_1$-adrenergic agonist that has value in the short-term treatment of certain types of shock due to its ability to cause the heart to beat more forcefully. Dobutamine is especially beneficial in cases where the primary cause of shock is related to heart failure, not hypovolemia. In fact, hypovolemia should be corrected before administering adrenergic agonists such as dobutamine. The resulting increase in cardiac output assists in maintaining blood flow to vital organs; renal blood flow is enhanced, and urine output increased. Dobutamine has a brief half-life of 2 minutes and is only given as an IV infusion. The patient should be monitored continuously during the infusion for abnormal changes in heart rate or rhythm. Dobutamine is a pregnancy category C drug.

Tocolytics: Terbutaline is a beta$_2$ agonist that relaxes uterine smooth muscle. Although not approved by the FDA as a tocolytic, terbutaline may be used off-label for this purpose. It is administered as an IV infusion, subcutaneous injection, or by a portable infusion pump programmed to deliver small amounts of the drug at prescribed intervals. Tocolytics may cause the fetus to experience transient tachycardia. Tocolytics are presented in greater detail in Chapter 69.

Beta$_3$-adrenergic agonists: The beta$_3$-adrenergic receptor has been known for about a decade but has largely been ignored as a pharmacologic target. This receptor is primarily located in adipose tissue and skeletal muscle, though it has subsequently been found in the gallbladder and the urinary bladder. The first drug acting on the beta$_3$ receptor, mirabegron (Myrbetriq), is an oral drug approved in 2012 for the treatment of overactive bladder. The most commonly observed side effects are HTN, nasopharyngitis, urinary tract infection, and headache. This drug is pregnancy category C.

CONNECTION Checkpoint 15.4

A patient has severe bronchoconstriction due to an acute allergic attack. From what you learned in Chapter 3, which route of administration—oral, subcutaneous, or inhalation—would likely give the fastest onset of drug action for this patient? *See Answer to Connection Checkpoint 15.4 on student resource website.*

CONNECTIONS: NURSING PRACTICE APPLICATION

Patients Receiving Pharmacotherapy with Adrenergic Agonists

Assessment	Potential Nursing Diagnoses*
Baseline assessment prior to administration: • Obtain a complete health history including cardiovascular, cerebrovascular, respiratory disease, or diabetes. Obtain a drug history including allergies, current prescription and OTC drugs, and herbal preparations. Be alert to possible drug interactions. • Evaluate appropriate laboratory findings such as hepatic or renal function studies. • Obtain baseline vital signs, weight, ECG, and urinary and cardiac output as appropriate. • For treatment of nasal congestion, assess the nasal mucosa for excoriation or bleeding prior to beginning therapy. • Assess the patient's ability to receive and understand instructions. Include family and caregiver as needed.	• *Decreased Cardiac Output* • *Impaired Gas Exchange* • *Ineffective Airway Clearance* • *Disturbed Sleep Pattern*, related to adverse drug effects • *Deficient Knowledge* (Drug Therapy) • *Risk for Injury*, related to adverse effects of drug therapy or administration

(continued)

CONNECTIONS: NURSING PRACTICE APPLICATION (continued)

Assessment throughout administration:

- Assess for desired therapeutic effects dependent on the reason for the drug (e.g., increased ease of breathing, blood pressure [BP] within normal range, nasal congestion improved).
- Continue frequent and careful monitoring of vital signs, and urinary and cardiac output as appropriate, especially if IV administration is used.
- Assess for and promptly report adverse effects: tachycardia, HTN, dysrhythmias, tremors, dizziness, headache, or decreased urinary output. Severe HTN, seizures, or angina may signal drug toxicity and are immediately reported.

Implementation

Interventions and (Rationales)	Patient-Centered Care
Ensuring therapeutic effects: • Continue frequent assessments as above for therapeutic effects dependent on the reason the drug therapy is given. (Pulse, BP, and respiratory rate should be within normal limits or within the parameters set by the health care provider. Nasal congestion should be decreased, and reddened, irritated sclera improved.)	• Teach the patient, family, or caregiver how to monitor pulse and BP as appropriate. Ensure proper use and functioning of any home equipment obtained using return demonstration or teach-back.
• Provide supportive nursing measures, e.g., proper positioning for dyspnea or shock. (Nursing measures such as raising the head of the bed during dyspnea will supplement therapeutic drug effects and optimize the outcome.)	• Teach the patient to report increasing dyspnea despite medication therapy, and to not take more than the prescribed dose unless instructed otherwise by the health care provider.
Minimizing adverse effects: • Monitor for signs of excessive autonomic nervous system (ANS) stimulation and notify the health care provider if BP or pulse exceeds established parameters. Continue frequent cardiac monitoring (e.g., ECG, cardiac output) and urine output if IV adrenergic agonists are given. (Because adrenergic drugs stimulate heart rate and raise BP, they must be closely monitored to avoid adverse effects. External and invasive monitoring devices will detect early signs of adverse effects as well as monitor for therapeutic effects. **Lifespan:** The older adult may be at greater risk due to previously existing cardiovascular disease. **Diverse Patients:** Research suggests African Americans may experience an impaired [diminished] vascular response to isoproterenol and vital signs should be monitored frequently during administration.)	• Instruct the patient to report palpitations, shortness of breath, chest pain, excessive nervousness or tremors, headache, or urinary retention immediately. • Teach the patient to limit or eliminate the use of caffeine-containing foods and beverages because these may cause excessive nervousness, insomnia, and tremors.
• Closely monitor the IV infusion site when using IV adrenergic agonists. All IV adrenergic drips should be given via infusion pump. (Blanching at the IV site is an indicator of extravasation with intense vasoconstriction. The IV infusion should be immediately stopped and the provider contacted for further treatment orders. Infusion pumps will allow precise dosing of the medication.)	• To allay possible anxiety, teach the patient the rationale for all equipment used and the need for frequent monitoring.
• Monitor oral and nasal mucosa and breath sounds in patients taking inhaled adrenergic drugs. (Inhaled epinephrine and other adrenergic drugs may reduce bronchial secretions, making removal of mucus more difficult.)	• Teach the patient to increase fluid intake to moisten airways and assist in the expectoration of mucus, unless contraindicated.
• Continue to monitor blood glucose level and appropriate laboratory values. (Adrenergic agonists affect a wide range of body systems. Patients with diabetes may need a change in diabetic medication or dosing if glucose remains elevated.)	• Teach patients with diabetes to monitor their blood glucose level more frequently and to notify the health care provider if a consistent increase is noted.
• Provide for eye comfort such as a darkened room, soft cloth over eyes, or sunglasses. Transient stinging after instillation of eyedrops may occur. (Adrenergic agonists can cause mydriasis and photosensitivity to light. Localized vasoconstriction may cause stinging of the eyes.)	• Instruct the patient that photosensitivity may occur and sunglasses may be needed in bright light or for outside activities. The provider should be notified if irritation or sensitivity occurs beyond 12 h after the drug has been discontinued. Soft contact lens users should check with the provider before using, as some solutions may stain lenses. • **Lifespan:** Assist the older adult with ambulation if blurred vision or light-sensitivity occurs, to prevent falls.
• Inspect nasal mucosa for irritation, rhinorrhea, or bleeding after nasal use. Avoid prolonged use of adrenergic nasal sprays. (Vasoconstriction may cause transient stinging, excessive dryness, or bleeding. Rebound congestion with chronic rhinorrhea may result after prolonged treatment.)	• Instruct the patient not to use nasal spray longer than 3–5 days without consulting the provider. OTC saline nasal sprays may provide comfort if mucosa is dry and irritated. Increasing oral fluid intake may also help with hydration. • **Lifespan:** Teach the family or caregiver that adrenergic nasal sprays and other decongestants are not recommended in children and should be used only under a provider's supervision.

CONNECTIONS: NURSING PRACTICE APPLICATION (continued)

Patient understanding of drug therapy: • Use opportunities during administration of medications and during assessments to discuss the rationale for drug therapy, desired therapeutic outcomes, commonly observed adverse effects, parameters for when to call the health care provider, and any necessary monitoring or precautions. (Using time during nursing care helps to optimize and reinforce key teaching areas.)	• The patient, family, or caregiver should be able to state the reason for the drug; appropriate dose and scheduling; what adverse effects to observe for and when to report them; equipment needed as appropriate and how to use that equipment; and the required length of medication therapy needed, with any special instructions regarding renewing or continuing the prescription as appropriate.
Patient self-administration of drug therapy: • When administering medications, instruct the patient, family, or caregiver in proper self-administration of an inhaler, epinephrine autoinjector, nasal spray, or ophthalmic drops. (Utilizing time during nurse-administration of these drugs helps to reinforce teaching.)	• Instruct the patient in proper administration techniques, followed by teach-back. Inhalation forms should only be dispensed when the patient is upright to properly aerosolize the drug and prevent overdosage from excessively large droplets.
	• Teach the patient, family, or caregiver proper technique for the autoinjection epinephrine device and to have on hand for emergency use at all times. If the autoinjector is needed and used, 911 and the health care provider should be called immediately after use. • Teach the patient, family, or caregiver to not share nasal sprays with other people to prevent infection. • The patient, family, or caregiver is able to discuss appropriate dosing and administration needs.

*Nursing Diagnoses—Definitions and Classification 2015–2017. Copyright © 2014, 1994–2014 by NANDA International. Used by arrangement with John Wiley & Sons Limited.

CHAPTER

15   Understanding the Chapter

Key Concepts Summary

15.1 Adrenergic agonists activate the sympathetic nervous system to produce fight-or-flight symptoms.

15.2 Adrenergic agonists may act directly by binding to adrenergic receptors, or indirectly by increasing the amount of norepinephrine at synapses.

15.3 Adrenergic agonists may be classified as catecholamines or noncatecholamines.

15.4 The nonselective adrenergic agonists activate both alpha and beta receptors and are used to treat bronchospasm, cardiac arrest, and hypotension.

15.5 Alpha-adrenergic agonists are used to relieve nasal decongestion and elevate blood pressure.

15.6 Beta-adrenergic agonists are used to treat asthma, shock, heart failure, and other cardiac disorders.

Case Study: Making the Patient Connection

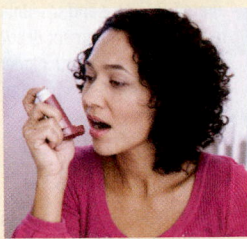

Remember the patient "Alexia Howard" at the beginning of the chapter? Now read the remainder of the case study. Based on the information presented within this chapter, respond to the critical thinking questions that follow.

Alexia Howard is a 22-year-old woman with a history of asthma since childhood. She is presently a student at the local university where she lives in a dormitory. Since the beginning of the semester, Alexia has experienced tremendous stress trying to manage school and part-time employment. Her roommate, an animal lover, has brought stray dogs and cats into their room several times during the past few months until she could find them good homes.

Today Alexia arrives at the University Health Center with tachypnea and acute shortness of breath with audible wheezing. She has not consistently taken her prescribed medications to avoid asthma attacks. A physical exam revealed a heart rate of 110 beats/min and a respiratory rate of 40 breaths/min with signs of accessory muscle use. Auscultation revealed decreased breath sounds with inspiratory and expiratory wheezing. The patient was coughing up small amounts of white sputum. Her saturated oxygen is 93% on room air.

An aerosol treatment with albuterol (Proventil) was ordered, using a small-volume nebulizer for 15 min. Peak flow measures after the treatment showed marked improvement of airflow. On auscultation there was clearing of bilateral breath sounds. Alexia's respiratory rate at the time of discharge was 20 and her heart rate was 108. The patient verbalized that she felt much better but a little nervous.

Alexia was discharged from the University Health Center. She was given a prescription for inhaled steroids and instructed to resume her home medications and use them consistently.

Critical Thinking Questions

1. Discuss the mechanism of action associated with albuterol (Proventil).
2. Why is albuterol being given to Alexia, and why is this route of administration being used?
3. What adverse effects is Alexia demonstrating as a result of the administration of albuterol (Proventil)?

See Answers to Critical Thinking Questions on student resource website.

Additional Case Study

Bill Jennings, a 55-year-old man, has been using an epinephrine inhaler for asthma for several months. He is attending a community health fair at a local church, and you are the nurse screening his blood pressure.

When you take Bill's blood pressure, you discover it is 172/94 mmHg. As you talk with him, the patient reveals that he is also self-medicating with OTC pseudoephedrine 60 mg three times per day for seasonal allergies. Bill says his blood pressure is usually 120/80 mmHg.

1. Explain why the increased blood pressure might be related to the drug combination.
2. What patient teaching should occur in this situation?

See Answers to Additional Case Study on student resource website.

Chapter Review

1 A patient who uses over-the-counter phenylephrine (Neo-Synephrine) nasal spray asks the nurse how the medication works. The nurse's response would be:
1. It helps to shrink the swelling in your nose by tightening the blood vessels there.
2. It works to locally destroy invading organisms that cause colds and flu.
3. It coats the nasal passages to reduce swelling.
4. It is absorbed after you swallow it to act as a decongestant.

2 The nurse is teaching the patient about the use of an adrenergic agonist nasal spray at home. What patient teaching is needed related to this medication? (Select all that apply.)
1. Do not share the nasal spray with another person.
2. Only use this drug for 3 to 5 days unless directed by a health care provider.
3. Symptoms of excessive use of this drug will result in lethargy and fatigue.
4. Infants and children should not use this medication unless directed by a health care provider.
5. This drug can be safely used by individuals with diabetes.

3 The health care provider prescribes epinephrine (adrenalin) to a patient who was stung by several wasps 30 minutes ago. The nurse knows that the primary purpose of this medication for this patient is to:

1. Stop the systemic release of histamine produced by the mast cells.

2. Counteract the formation of antibodies in response to an invading antigen.

3. Increase the number of white blood cells produced to fight the primary invader.

4. Increase a declining blood pressure and dilate constricting bronchi associated with anaphylaxis.

4 A patient takes a dose of albuterol (Ventolin) prior to bedtime. Which effect would the nurse consider normal for this drug?

1. Insomnia

2. Sleepiness

3. Urticaria

4. Tinnitus

5 To evaluate the effectiveness of high-dose dopamine (Intropin, DopaStat), the nurse would assess the:

1. Pupillary response.

2. Blood pressure.

3. Level of consciousness.

4. Gag reflex.

6 A beta-adrenergic agonist is prescribed for each of the following conditions. A nurse would question the order for which patient? Select all that apply.

1. Hyperthyroidism

2. Asthma

3. Shock

4. Dysrhythmias

5. Heart failure

See Answers to Chapter Review in Appendix A.

References

Blake, M. A. (2013). *Pheochromocytoma.* Retrieved from http://emedicine.medscape.com/article/124059-overview

Boyce, J. A., Assa'ad, A., Burks, A. W., Jones, S. M., Sampson, H. A., Wood, R. A., . . . Schwaninger, J. M. (2010). Guidelines for the diagnosis and management of food allergy in the United States: Report of the NIAID-sponsored expert panel. *Journal of Allergy and Clinical Immunology and Allergy, 126*(Suppl. 6), S1–58.

Campbell, R. L., Manivannan, V., Hartz, M. F., & Sadosty, A. T. (2012). Epinephrine auto-injector pandemic. *Pediatric Emergency Care, 28,* 938–942. doi:10.1097/PEC.0b013e318267f689

Mehr, S., Robinson, M., & Tang, M. (2007). Doctor—how do I use my EpiPen? *Pediatric Allergy and Immunology, 18,* 448–452. doi:10.1111/j.1399-3038.2007.00529.x

Selected Bibliography

Bose, D. A., Assel, B. G., Hill, J. B., & Chauhan, S. P. (2011). Maintenance tocolytics for pre-term symptomatic placenta previa: A review. *American Journal of Perinatology, 28,* 45–50. doi:10.1055/s-0030-1262510

Chen, W. L., Tsai, T. H., Yang, C. C. H., & Kuo, T. B. J. (2010). Acute effects of ephedra on autonomic nervous modulation in healthy young adults. *Clinical Pharmacology & Therapeutics, 88,* 39–44. doi:10.1038/clpt.2010.66

Colbert, B. J., Gonzales, L. S., & Kennedy, B. J. (2012). *Integrated cardiopulmonary pharmacology* (3rd ed.). Upper Saddle River, NJ: Pearson.

Havel, C., Arrich, J., Losert, H., Gamper, G., Müllner, M., & Herkner, H. (2011). Vasopressors for hypotensive shock. *Cochrane Database of Systematic Reviews 2011, 5,* CD003709. doi:10.1002/14651858.CD003709.pub3

Herdman, T. H., & Kamitsuru, S. (Eds.). (2014). *NANDA International nursing diagnoses: Definitions and classification, 2015–2017.* Oxford, United Kingdom: Wiley-Blackwell.

Judd, E., & Calhoun, D. A. (2012). Hypertension and orthostatic hypotension in older patients. *Journal of Hypertension, 30,* 38–39. doi:10.1097/HJH.0b013e32834ed663

Kalil, A. (2013). *Septic shock.* Retrieved from http://emedicine.medscape.com/article/168402-overview

Leone, M., & Martin, C. (2008). Vasopressor use in septic shock: An update. *Current Opinion in Anaesthesiology, 21,* 141–147. doi:10.1097/ACO.0b013e3282f46d20

Ortega, V. E., & Peters, S. P. (2010). Beta-2 adrenergic agonists: Focus on safety and benefits versus risks. *Current Opinions in Pharmacology, 10,* 246–253. doi:10.1016/j.coph.2010.04.009

Suffredini, A. F., & Munford, R. S. (2011). Novel therapies for septic shock over the past 4 decades. *Journal of the American Medical Association, 306,* 194–199. doi:10.1001/jama.2011.909

Westfall, T. C., & Westfall, D. P. (2011). Adrenergic agonists and antagonists. In L. L. Brunton, B. A. Chabner, & B. C. Knollman (Eds.), *The pharmacological basis of therapeutics* (12th ed., pp. 277–334). New York, NY: McGraw-Hill.

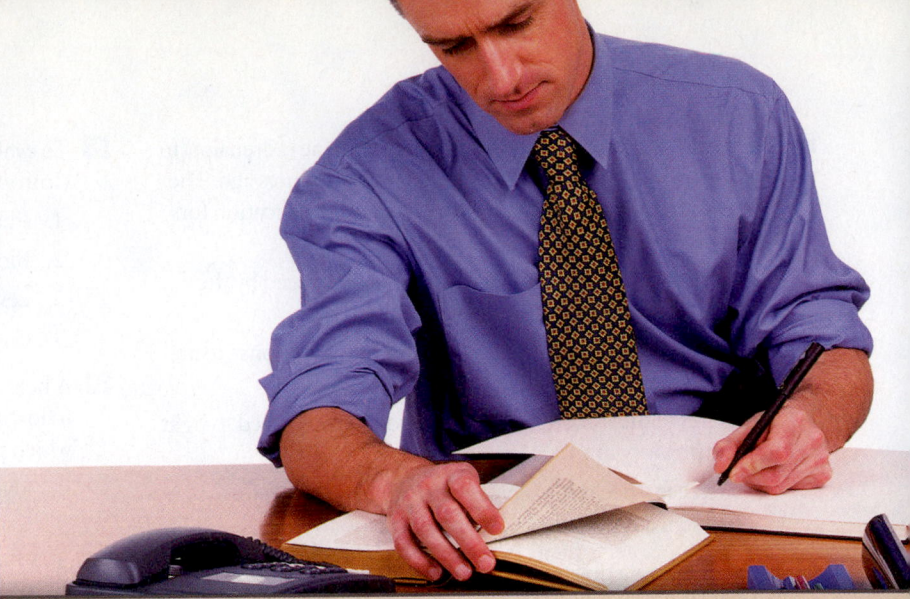

> *"I have all these reports to finish by Friday. I just don't have time to deal with high blood pressure."*
>
> Patient "Amos Tucker"

LEARNING OUTCOMES

After reading this chapter, the student should be able to:

1. Identify the physiological responses produced when a drug blocks adrenergic receptors.

2. Compare and contrast the types of physiological responses that occur when a drug blocks alpha$_1$-, alpha$_2$-, beta$_1$-, and beta$_2$-adrenergic receptors.

3. Identify indications for pharmacotherapy with adrenergic antagonists.

4. Describe the first-dose phenomenon and how it may be prevented.

5. Explain the advantages of selective beta antagonists versus nonselective beta antagonists.

6. Explain why beta-adrenergic antagonists should never be abruptly discontinued.

7. For each of the classes shown in the chapter outline, identify the prototype and representative drugs and explain the mechanism(s) of drug action, primary indications, contraindications, significant drug interactions, pregnancy category, and important adverse effects.

8. Apply the nursing process to care for patients receiving pharmacotherapy with adrenergic antagonists.

CHAPTER OUTLINE

▶ **Actions of Adrenergic Antagonists**

▶ **Alpha-Adrenergic Antagonists**

  PROTOTYPE Prazosin (Minipress), *p. 196*

▶ **Beta-Adrenergic Antagonists**

  Nonselective Beta-Adrenergic Antagonists

  PROTOTYPE Propranolol (Inderal, InnoPran XL), *p. 199*

  Selective Beta$_1$-Adrenergic Antagonists

  PROTOTYPE Metoprolol (Lopressor, Toprol XL), *p. 201*

KEY TERMS

adrenergic antagonists, 193

alpha-adrenergic
antagonists, 193

beta-adrenergic antagonists, 197

first-dose phenomenon, 195

intrinsic sympathomimetic activity (ISA), 197

orthostatic hypotension, 195

pheochromocytoma, 193

Raynaud's disease, 195

Adrenergic antagonists inhibit the sympathetic nervous system and produce many of the same rest-and-digest symptoms as the cholinergic agonists. They have wide therapeutic applications in the management of hypertension (HTN), angina pectoris, myocardial infarction, and heart failure (HF). They also serve limited roles in the pharmacotherapy of benign prostatic hyperplasia, thyroid crisis, and glaucoma.

Actions of Adrenergic Antagonists

16.1 Adrenergic antagonists act by blocking the effects of norepinephrine at adrenergic receptors.

As discussed in Chapter 12, when the adrenergic receptor binds, norepinephrine (NE) symptoms typical of the fight-or-flight response are induced. Drugs that activate these receptors are used to treat shock, cardiac arrest, nasal congestion, and asthma (see Chapter 15). If the student is not yet thoroughly familiar with the actions at the adrenergic receptor, Chapters 12 and 15 should be reviewed before continuing.

Adrenergic antagonists are drugs that compete with NE for adrenergic receptors, as shown in Figure 16.1. By blocking NE from reaching its receptors, symptoms of the fight-or-flight response are *prevented*. With reduced sympathetic activation, nerve impulses from the parasympathetic nervous system will predominate. In fact, most of the symptoms produced by adrenergic antagonists are those of parasympathetic activation. In other words, adrenergic antagonists and cholinergic agonists result in many of the same actions.

CONNECTION Checkpoint 16.1

Although cholinergic agonists and adrenergic antagonists may produce similar physiological actions, their indications are very different. From what you learned in Chapter 13, what are the primary indications for pharmacotherapy with cholinergic agonists? *See Answer to Connection Checkpoint 16.1 on student resource website.*

The presence of the alpha- and beta-adrenergic receptor subtypes in the sympathetic nervous system allows for more specific pharmacologic responses. For example, with the adrenergic agonists, epinephrine activates both alpha and beta receptors, whereas albuterol activates only beta$_2$ receptors. The same type of division occurs with adrenergic antagonists. Actions of these drugs are specific to either alpha blockade or beta blockade. Beta blockade is further divided into those drugs that inhibit both beta$_1$ and beta$_2$ receptors and those that selectively inhibit only beta$_1$ receptors. The therapeutic uses and adverse effects of each drug are dependent on which receptor subtype is activated.

Adrenergic antagonists have wide therapeutic application. They are the most frequently prescribed class of autonomic drugs. Most of their therapeutic applications relate to the cardiovascular system.

Alpha-Adrenergic Antagonists

16.2 Alpha$_1$-adrenergic antagonists are used to treat hypertension and benign prostatic hyperplasia.

Alpha-adrenergic receptors are primarily located on smooth muscle, and their activation results in contraction. Most blood vessels, including those serving the myocardium, genitourinary (GU) system, gastrointestinal (GI) system, and brain, have alpha receptors. Because of their key locations on arterial smooth muscle, the most important effects of **alpha-adrenergic antagonists**, or alpha blockers, are on the cardiovascular system. Blockade of alpha receptors will dilate blood vessels, thus lowering blood pressure.

The specific actions of each alpha-adrenergic antagonist depend on its degree of selectivity for alpha$_1$ or alpha$_2$ receptors. Drugs selective for alpha$_1$ receptors have greater therapeutic application and are listed in Table 16.1. The selective alpha$_1$ blockers doxazosin (Cardura), prazosin (Minipress), and terazosin (Hytrin) have very similar actions, indications, and adverse effects.

Phentolamine (Regitine) and phenoxybenzamine (Dibenzyline) are the only alpha blockers that are nonselective, activating both alpha$_1$ and alpha$_2$ receptors. These drugs have very limited usefulness because they exhibit a high incidence of adverse effects, such as hypotension, tachycardia, nausea, vomiting, and diarrhea.

Selective alpha$_1$ antagonists are primarily used to treat HTN. Their most significant action is blocking vasoconstriction in arterioles and veins, which results in decreased peripheral resistance. Their ability to block alpha$_1$ receptors on arterial smooth muscle lowers blood pressure directly. Their ability to dilate veins lowers blood pressure indirectly by decreasing venous return to the heart. This reduces cardiac output, which results in a reduction in systemic blood pressure. When used to treat HTN, the alpha blockers are often administered concurrently with other classes of antihypertensives, such as diuretics (see Chapter 32).

In addition to dilating vascular smooth muscle, alpha$_1$ blockers relax smooth muscle in the trigone and sphincter muscles at the base of the urinary bladder and in the prostate. Relaxation of these muscles promotes an increase in urine flow in patients who have difficulty voiding due to strictures in this region. This action has resulted in the use of alpha blockers in the treatment of benign prostatic hyperplasia (BPH), a nonmalignant condition in which the prostate gland enlarges to restrict urine flow through the urethra. These drugs increase urine flow and decrease residual urine volume in patients with BPH. Four selective alpha$_1$ antagonists, alfuzosin (Uroxatral), doxazosin (Cardura), silodosin (Rapaflow), and tamsulosin (Flomax), are approved only for BPH. Alpha$_1$ blockers do not cure this disorder, and patients with moderate to severe BPH usually require surgery to correct the restriction in urinary flow. A complete discussion on the pharmacotherapy of BPH is found in Chapter 71.

Alpha$_1$ antagonists are occasionally used to treat pheochromocytoma and Raynaud's disease. **Pheochromocytoma** is a tumor, usually benign, arising from the adrenal medulla that is

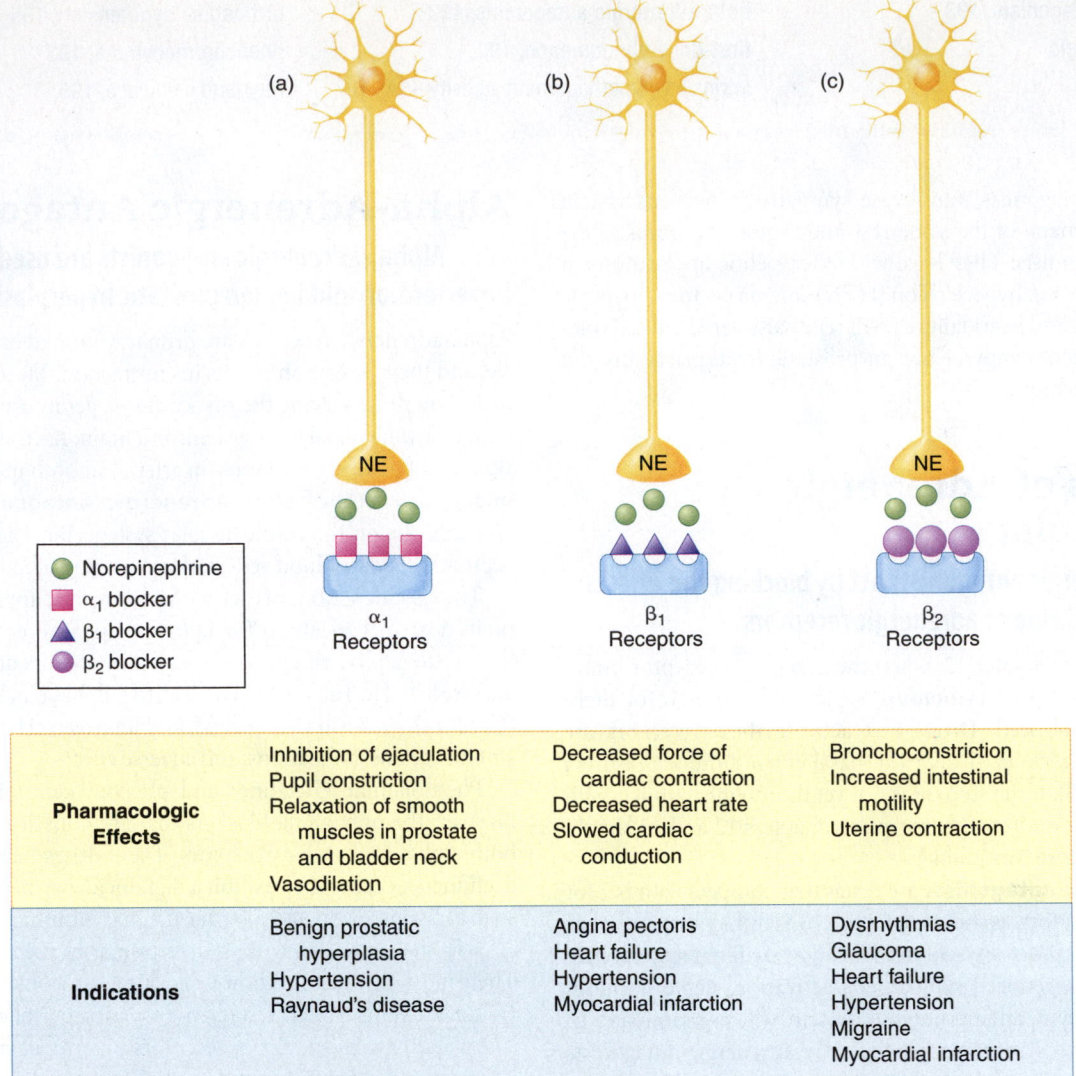

Figure 16.1 Pharmacologic effects and indications of adrenergic antagonists: (a) blockade of alpha₁ receptors; (b) blockade of beta₁ receptors; (c) blockade of beta₂ receptors.

TABLE 16.1	Alpha-Adrenergic Antagonists	
Drug	**Route and Adult Dose (Maximum Dose Where Indicated)**	**Adverse Effects**
alfuzosin (Uroxatral)	PO: 10 mg once daily	*Orthostatic hypotension, dizziness, headache, fatigue*
doxazosin (Cardura)	PO: 1 mg/day; may increase to 16 mg/day in one to two divided doses (max: 16 mg/day)	
phenoxybenzamine (Dibenzyline)	PO: Initially 10 mg bid, may increase by 10 mg at 4-day intervals to 20–40 mg bid or tid	<u>First-dose phenomenon,</u> <u>tachycardia, dyspnea</u>
phentolamine (Regitine)	IV/IM: 5 mg 1–2 h prior to surgery; repeat as needed Intradermal: 5–10 mg diluted in 10 mL of normal saline injected into the affected area within 12 h of catecholamine extravasation	
prazosin (Minipress)	PO: 1 mg/day; may increase to 1 mg bid–tid (max: 20 mg/day)	
silodosin (Rapaflo)	PO: 8 mg once daily	
tamsulosin (Flomax)	PO: 0.4–0.8 mg/day after a meal (max: 0.8 mg/day)	
terazosin (Hytrin)	PO: 1 mg/day; may increase 1–5 mg/day (max: 20 mg/day)	

Note: *Italics* indicate common adverse effects. <u>Underline</u> indicates serious adverse effects.

characterized by excessive secretion of catecholamines. A patient with a pheochromocytoma will exhibit extreme HTN, palpitations, dyspnea, anxiety, and profuse sweating. All are signs of excessive amounts of catecholamines. Although surgical removal is the usual treatment, alpha$_1$-receptor antagonists can be administered to block the peripheral vascular effects of natural (endogenous) catecholamines. This reduces the profound HTN in patients who are high surgical risks.

In **Raynaud's disease**, vasospasms of vessels serving the fingers and toes can lead to intermittent pain and cyanosis of the digits. Emotional stress or cold temperatures usually exacerbate the disorder. The primary treatment is nonpharmacologic: warming techniques and avoidance of cold. For those who require pharmacotherapy, administration of alpha$_1$ antagonists can diminish the vasospasm and bring symptomatic relief to patients. Long-acting calcium channel blockers (see Chapter 30) such as nifedipine (Procardia XL) are also used to relieve Raynaud's vasospasms.

PharmFACT

Raynaud's disease is more common in women and can occur secondary to other diseases, usually autoimmune disorders. For example, 90% of individuals with scleroderma also develop Raynaud's disease. Systemic lupus erythematosus may also occur concurrently with Raynaud's phenomenon (Hansen-Dispenza, 2013).

The adverse effects of alpha$_1$ antagonists are predictable based on their mechanism of action. When the sympathetic nervous system is blocked, parasympathetic tone will predominate; thus most of the significant adverse effects of alpha blockers are due to increased parasympathetic activity.

The limiting adverse effect of pharmacotherapy with alpha$_1$ antagonists is hypotension. The vasodilation caused by alpha$_1$ blockers is more intense when the patient is upright, as compared to recumbent. Significant **orthostatic hypotension** can occur when the patient abruptly changes from a recumbent to an upright position, resulting in diminished blood flow to the brain. Much of this effect is caused by blockade of alpha$_1$ receptors in the veins. As the patient moves to an upright position, blood accumulates in the veins, cardiac output decreases, and blood pressure falls. Orthostatic hypotension is especially pronounced at the beginning of pharmacotherapy and when increasing the dose. This adverse effect is called the **first-dose phenomenon**. Because the first-dose phenomenon can cause syncope due to reduced blood flow to the brain, initial therapy is begun with low doses, usually administered at bedtime.

The fall in blood pressure during alpha$_1$-antagonist therapy may be accompanied by reflex tachycardia, which occurs when the baroreceptor reflex is triggered. Reflex tachycardia can be particularly troublesome in patients who are susceptible to dysrhythmias. A beta-adrenergic antagonist is sometimes administered concurrently with alpha blockers to reduce the risk of reflex tachycardia. A less serious, though annoying, adverse effect of alpha antagonists is nasal congestion, which is caused by vasodilation of blood vessels serving the nasal mucosa.

A number of noncardiovascular adverse effects may also occur during alpha$_1$ blocker pharmacotherapy. Because smooth muscle contraction is inhibited in the vas deferens and ejaculatory ducts, these drugs can cause an inability to ejaculate during intercourse. This is a major cause for discontinuation of alpha-antagonist therapy in sexually active men. Increased smooth muscle activity in the GI tract may cause nausea, vomiting, or abdominal cramping. Incontinence or increased urinary frequency may occur due to more active smooth muscle contractions in the urinary tract. These medications cross the blood–brain barrier and can cause central nervous system (CNS) effects such as depression, lethargy, and vivid dreams. Alpha blockers increase urinary metabolites of vanillylmandelic acid (VMA) and NE, which can result in false-positive test results for pheochromocytoma.

Although a few drugs selectively block alpha$_2$-adrenergic receptors, they are used for research purposes and have no clinical application. Yohimbine is the only drug believed to selectively block alpha$_2$ receptors. Approved in 1938 for the treatment of erectile dysfunction, this drug is not prescribed for this purpose today due to the availability of safer and more effective drugs. Yohimbe (converted to yohimbine in the body) is a natural product obtained from the bark of a West African tree and may be purchased by patients over the counter (OTC) as an herbal supplement. Claims that this herb is a sexual stimulant or aphrodisiac have not been supported by controlled research studies.

CONNECTIONS | Community-Oriented Practice

◀ Lifestyle Modifications for Hypertension

Hypertension is prevalent in the United States and Canada and is treatable with medications. However, patients should be encouraged to adopt healthy lifestyle changes to assist in management of this disease. Changing some basic daily habits can help control HTN and improve quality of life. Nurses can play a major role in helping patients to manage their HTN. Following are some ideas that the nurse should discuss with patients with HTN, including recommendations from the DASH (Dietary Approaches to Stop Hypertension) diet (U.S. Department of Health and Human Services, 2006):

- Begin a weight loss program if overweight.
- Limit alcohol intake to no more than two average drinks per day for men, one for women (an average drink is 12 oz of beer, 5 oz of wine, or 1 oz of hard liquor).
- Participate in physical activity for 30 to 45 minutes, 4 to 6 days per week.
- Eat a balanced diet with fruits, vegetables, grains and grain products, and low-fat or nonfat dairy foods.
- Lower the amount of sodium ingested. Avoid adding salt to foods and minimize eating salty and processed foods.
- Monitor and reduce saturated fat and cholesterol in the diet.
- Stop smoking or using tobacco products.
- Have blood pressure checked regularly, at least once every year.
- Monitor blood pressure at home and record daily to track your progress.
- Take the prescribed medicine every day.
- Talk to your health care provider if you are concerned about your progress. Communication is the key to success.
- Make and keep appointments every 3 to 6 months with the health care provider even if your blood pressure is under control.

PROTOTYPE DRUG	Prazosin (Minipress)

Classification: Therapeutic: Antihypertensive
Pharmacologic: Selective alpha$_1$-adrenergic antagonist

Therapeutic Effects and Uses: The primary therapeutic action of prazosin is a rapid decrease in peripheral resistance that reduces blood pressure. The drug has very little effect on cardiac output or heart rate and it causes less reflex tachycardia than some other drugs in this class. Approved in 1976, its most common use is in combination with other agents, such as beta blockers or diuretics, in the pharmacotherapy of HTN. Optimum therapeutic effects may require 4 to 6 weeks of therapy. Off-label indications include symptomatic BPH, treatment of Raynaud's disease, and hypertensive emergencies associated with pheochromocytoma. An additional off-label use of prazosin is to treat sleep disturbances and nightmares related to post-traumatic stress disorder. Prazosin has a relatively short half-life that requires it to be administered two to three times per day.

Mechanism of Action: Prazosin competes with NE at alpha-adrenergic receptors on vascular smooth muscle in arterioles and veins. It is selective for alpha$_1$-adrenergic receptors and has no activity at alpha$_2$- or beta-adrenergic receptors.

Pharmacokinetics:

Route(s)	PO
Absorption	Well absorbed
Distribution	Completely distributed; small amounts secreted in breast milk
Primary metabolism	Hepatic
Primary excretion	Primarily bile and feces, with small amounts by the kidneys
Onset of action	2 h
Duration of action	Less than 24 h

Adverse Effects: The most common adverse effects of prazosin include dizziness, drowsiness, fatigue, weakness, palpitations, orthostatic hypotension, and headache. Nausea, vomiting, and other GI effects occur in about 5% of patients. Most patients develop tolerance to these adverse effects as therapy progresses. The first-dose phenomenon may cause syncope. Erectile dysfunction, including priapism, is rare but can present a barrier to patient adherence.

Contraindications/Precautions: The only contraindication to the use of prazosin is prior sensitivity to the drug. The drug should be used with caution in older patients and those with renal impairment because these groups tend to exhibit more pronounced orthostatic hypotension and syncope. Patients with coronary artery disease should be treated with caution because prazosin may worsen angina symptoms in these patients.

Drug Interactions: Additive hypotensive effects may occur when prazosin is used concurrently with other antihypertensives and diuretics. This additive effect is used to advantage in the pharmacotherapy of HTN, in which the dose of each individual agent may be lower than if a single drug were used as monotherapy. Ingestion of alcohol or use with erectile dysfunction drugs such as sildenafil (Viagra) may cause increased hypotension. Use with sympathomimetics having alpha-agonist activity will antagonize the therapeutic effects of prazosin. **Herbal/Food**: Hawthorn may cause an additive drop in blood pressure when used with antihypertensive drugs such as prazosin.

Pregnancy: Category C.

Treatment of Overdose: Overdose will lead to hypotension and possibly sudden loss of consciousness; thus it is important to keep the patient supine. Fluid expanders may be administered to raise blood pressure, and renal function should be monitored. Vasopressors such as levarterenol or dopamine may be necessary to increase blood pressure. Drowsiness may also be prominent.

Nursing Responsibilities: Key nursing implications for patients receiving prazosin are included in the Nursing Practice Application for Patients Receiving Pharmacotherapy with Adrenergic Antagonists.

Drugs Similar to Prazosin (Minipress)

Other alpha-adrenergic blockers used for HTN include doxazosin, phenoxybenzamine, phentolamine, and terazosin. Two alpha-adrenergic blockers, alfuzosin and tamsulosin, are indicated only for BPH.

Alfuzosin (Uroxatral): Approved in 2003, alfuzosin is approved to treat BPH as an extended release tablet that permits once-daily dosing. Both tamsulosin and alfuzosin relax smooth muscle in the bladder and prostate gland, which reduces pressure on the urethra, thus enhancing urine flow. The drug is well tolerated, with the most common adverse effects being dizziness, fatigue, headache, and upper respiratory infection. Hypotension may be a serious problem in patients taking antihypertensive drugs or erectile dysfunction agents such as sildenafil (Viagra). Caution should be used in patients with moderate or severe hepatic or renal impairment. This drug is rated as pregnancy category B.

Doxazosin (Cardura): Approved in 1990, doxazosin is an oral drug approved for both HTN and BPH. It has the longest duration of action of the selective alpha$_1$ blockers, allowing for once-daily dosing. The most frequent adverse effects are dizziness, fatigue, headache, and edema. Orthostatic hypotension occurs in about 10% of patients taking the drug, especially when therapy is initiated or with changes in dose. Patients who ingest alcohol or use this drug with erectile dysfunction agents such as sildenafil (Viagra) may experience increased hypotension. The drug should be used cautiously in older adults because they tend to experience more hypotension-related adverse effects. Doxazosin should be taken at bedtime to avoid the first-dose phenomenon. This drug is pregnancy category B.

Phenoxybenzamine (Dibenzyline): Phenoxybenzamine is an older drug, approved in 1954, that blocks both alpha$_1$- and alpha$_2$-adrenergic receptors. The drug has a very prolonged duration of action, and its effects may last up to a week after the drug is discontinued. Because it has the potential to cause extended alpha blockade and serious cardiovascular adverse effects, its use is limited to managing the HTN caused by pheochromocytoma. Off-label indications include symptomatic BPH, Raynaud's disease, and frostbite. The drug is pregnancy category C.

Phentolamine (Regitine): Like phenoxybenzamine, phentolamine blocks both alpha$_1$ and alpha$_2$ receptors. Approved in 1952, it is the only alpha blocker that is given parenterally. Phentolamine may be administered to treat or prevent hypertensive crises during surgical removal of pheochromocytomas. Phentolamine is considered an antidote for treating hypertensive emergencies caused by catecholamine overdose. The drug may be injected subcutaneously to prevent or treat dermal necrosis or sloughing caused by extravasation of catecholamines such as NE and dopamine. Although the drug has been used in the past to diagnose pheochromocytoma, safer measures such as urinary or blood assays of catecholamine levels are more accurate indicators of this disease. This drug is pregnancy category C.

Silodosin (Rapaflo): Approved in 2008, silodosin is a selective alpha$_1$-adrenergic antagonist that is indicated for the management of BPH. The most common adverse effects are retrograde ejaculation, dizziness, diarrhea, orthostatic hypotension, headache, nasopharyngitis, and nasal congestion. It should be taken with food to lessen the risk of adverse effects. Silodosin is not indicated for use in women. This drug is pregnancy category B.

Tamsulosin (Flomax): Like alfuzosin and silodosin, tamsulosin has only one indication: BPH. It is administered orally (PO) and should always be taken with food to reduce the incidence of orthostatic hypotension. The drug is generally well tolerated and exhibits adverse effects similar to other alpha blockers. It is extensively metabolized by hepatic CYP enzymes and may interact with drugs that are inducers or substrates of these enzymes. This drug is pregnancy category B.

Terazosin (Hytrin): Approved in 1987, terazosin has a longer duration of action than prazosin and is approved for both HTN and symptomatic BPH. Given orally, its prolonged half-life permits once-daily dosing. Approximately 16% of the patients taking terazosin will experience headache. Other common adverse effects include dizziness and fatigue. Tolerance develops to most of these adverse effects as therapy progresses. Like other drugs in this class, terazosin should be taken at bedtime to avoid the first-dose phenomenon. Older adults are more sensitive to the hypotensive and adverse effects of terazosin, such as dry mouth and drowsiness. The drug is pregnancy category C.

Beta-Adrenergic Antagonists

16.3 Nonselective beta-adrenergic antagonists affect both beta$_1$ and beta$_2$ receptors and are prescribed for HTN, angina, and other cardiovascular disorders.

Beta-adrenergic antagonists, or beta blockers, are classified as nonselective or selective. Nonselective beta-adrenergic antagonists, such as propranolol, block both beta$_1$ and beta$_2$ receptors. Selective drugs that block only beta$_1$ receptors are sometimes called cardioselective agents and are discussed in Section 16.4. Some beta blockers, such as carvedilol (Coreg), also have some alpha-antagonist activity, which adds to their ability to lower blood pressure.

A few beta blockers such as pindolol (Visken) exhibit mixed beta-antagonist and beta-agonist activity. This low level of beta-agonist activity is called **intrinsic sympathomimetic activity (ISA)**. Theoretically, the agonist action of these drugs may result in fewer adverse effects in patients who have bradycardia, HF, or compromised pulmonary function. Regardless of their receptor specificity, most therapeutic applications of the beta blockers relate to their effects on the cardiovascular system (Table 16.2).

Because their mechanism of action is to antagonize the effects of endogenous catecholamines, all beta blockers have the potential to reduce the heart rate (negative chronotropic effect), decrease the force of myocardial contraction (negative inotropic effect), and slow conduction velocity through the atrioventricular node (negative dromotropic effect). These effects are modest when the heart is at rest. During periods of stress or exercise, however, beta blockers tend to prevent the normal increase in sympathetic stimulation to the heart, which is supposed to bring more blood flow to this organ. In some cases, this results in an undesirable short-term decrease in cardiac output, and the sympathetic nervous system responds by activating alpha receptors and raising blood pressure. In time, peripheral resistance returns to normal or below-normal levels, particularly in patients with HTN, and blood pressure falls.

The primary use of beta-adrenergic antagonists is the treatment of HTN. The following multiple mechanisms are believed to contribute to their antihypertensive effect:

- Diminished myocardial contractility decreases cardiac output.
- The release of renin by the kidney, normally stimulated by catecholamines, is prevented.
- The nonselective adrenergic antagonists block alpha$_1$-adrenergic receptors, relaxing arteriolar smooth muscle.
- Central actions reduce sympathetic output from the vasomotor center in the brain.

The student should refer to Chapter 34 for additional details on the use of beta blockers in HTN management.

Beta-adrenergic antagonists have several other important applications, although they are not always first-line drugs for these conditions. By decreasing cardiac workload and oxygen demand,

TABLE 16.2 Beta-Adrenergic Antagonists

Drug	Route and Adult Dose (Maximum Dose Where Indicated)	Adverse Effects
Selective Beta₁-Adrenergic Antagonists		
acebutolol (Sectral)	PO: 200–800 mg/day in divided doses (max: 1,200 mg/day)	*Fatigue, insomnia, diarrhea, constipation, drowsiness, impotence or decreased libido, hypotension, bradycardia, confusion*
atenolol (Tenormin)	PO: 25–50 mg daily (max: 100 mg/day)	
betaxolol (Kerlone)	PO: 10–20 mg daily (max: 40 mg/day)	Bronchospasm, Stevens-Johnson syndrome, anaphylaxis, worsening of HF; if the drug is abruptly withdrawn, palpitations, rebound, HTN, dysrhythmias, MI
bisoprolol (Zebeta)	PO: 2.5–5 mg once daily (max: 20 mg/day)	
esmolol (Brevibloc)	IV: 500 mcg/kg loading dose followed by 50 mcg/kg/min, may increase dose every 5–10 min (max: 200 mcg/kg/min)	
metoprolol (Lopressor, Toprol XL)	PO: 12.5–20 mg once daily (max: 200 mg/day for HF; 400 mg/day for HTN or angina)	
nebivolol (Bystolic)	PO: 5 mg once daily (max: 40 mg)	
Alpha₁ and Beta Blockers (Centrally Acting)		
nadolol (Corgard)	PO: 40 mg/day, may increase by 40–80 mg every 3–7 days (max: 240–320 mg/day)	*Headache, dizziness, fatigue, drowsiness, anxiety, depression, lethargy, impotence, peripheral vascular insufficiency, hypoglycemia*
penbutolol (Levatol)	PO: 10–20 mg/day (max: 80 mg/day)	
pindolol (Visken)	PO: 5 mg bid, may increase by 10 mg/day every 2–3 weeks (max: 60 mg/day)	Bradycardia, bronchospasm, laryngospasm, respiratory disturbances, may worsen HF and mask symptoms of hypoglycemia, Stevens-Johnson syndrome (propranolol), toxic epidermal necrolysis (propranolol), exfoliative dermatitis (propranolol), dysrhythmias (sotalol)
propranolol (Inderal, InnoPran XL)	PO (extended release): 80–120 mg once daily at bedtime IV: 0.5–3 mg every 4 h prn for dysrhythmias	
sotalol (Betapace, Sorine)	PO: Initial dose of 80–160 mg/day, may increase every 3–4 days in 40–160 mg increments (max: 640 mg/day for life-threatening dysrhythmias)	
timolol (Blocadren, Timoptic)	PO: 10 mg bid (max: 60 mg/day for HTN)	
Mixed Alpha₁- and Beta-Adrenergic Antagonists		
carvedilol (Coreg)	PO (Immediate release): start with 3.125 mg bid (max: 50 mg/day) PO (Extended release): start with 10–20 mg once daily (max: 80 mg/day)	Same as the above two classes
labetalol (Trandate)	PO: 100 mg bid; may increase to 200–400 mg bid (max: 2,400 mg/day)	

Note: *Italics* indicate common adverse effects. <u>Underline</u> indicates serious adverse effects.

beta blockers can ease the acute chest pain characteristic of angina pectoris (see the prototype feature for atenolol in Chapter 35). Because they slow cardiac conduction, beta blockers are used in the pharmacotherapy of certain types of dysrhythmias (see Chapter 37). Some nonselective beta blockers have the ability to reduce intraocular pressure when given as ophthalmic solutions in the pharmacotherapy of glaucoma (see Chapter 74). Other therapeutic uses include the treatment of HF (see Chapter 36), myocardial infarction (MI) (see Chapter 35), and migraine prophylaxis (see Chapter 25). Beta blockers such as propranolol have been used off-label to treat the anxiousness, sweating, and tachycardia associated with stage fright and post-traumatic stress disorder (PTSD).

Pharmacotherapy with nonselective beta antagonists usually produces more adverse effects than treatment with selective beta₁ antagonists. Because of this, the use of the nonselective drugs has been declining. One of the more serious adverse effects with the nonselective beta blockers is that inhibition of beta₂ receptors in the lung can cause bronchoconstriction, which can result in acute shortness of breath, in patients with chronic obstructive pulmonary disease (COPD) or asthma.

The metabolic effects of beta-adrenergic antagonists can be important for patients with diabetes mellitus. Under normal conditions, catecholamines break down glycogen, which frees glucose to enter the blood to be used as an energy source. Many body tissues, particularly skeletal muscles, must receive a continuous source of glucose, especially during prolonged physical activity such as running or heavy exercise. Beta blockers prevent this hyperglycemic effect of the catecholamines and patients with diabetes may develop hypoglycemia. In addition, beta blockers will prevent tachycardia, an important warning sign of impending hypoglycemia. Beta-blocker therapy in patients with diabetes must be carefully monitored.

A second metabolic effect of nonselective beta-adrenergic antagonists relates to lipid metabolism. Catecholamines normally stimulate lipolysis, the breakdown of stored lipid in adipose tissue, resulting in the release of free fatty acids into the blood. Like glucose, these fatty acids serve as an essential energy source for skeletal muscle. By blocking the actions of catecholamines, beta antagonists decrease the amount of free fatty acids available during periods of metabolic stress. Nonselective beta blockers may also increase serum triglycerides and decrease high-density lipoproteins. During the course of therapy with beta blockers, patients with preexisting lipid disorders should have their lipid profiles monitored periodically to prevent hyperlipidemia.

Overdoses with nonselective beta blockers are potentially serious and treatment involves maintaining or restoring cardiovascular function. An anticholinergic such as atropine or a beta-adrenergic agonist such as isoproterenol may be administered to reverse severe bradycardia and cause bronchodilation. Cardiac failure caused by beta-antagonist overdose may be treated by administering digoxin (Lanoxin) or diuretics. Severe hypotension may require the administration of a vasopressor such as epinephrine or NE.

Beta blockers should always be withdrawn gradually over several weeks. If withdrawn abruptly, the heart displays hypersensitivity to catecholamines, and sweating, palpitations, headache, and tremors may occur. This phenomenon is called *rebound cardiac excitation*. Some of the beta blockers have a black box warning to discontinue the drug gradually because patients with coronary artery disease may experience a worsening of angina symptoms, or MIs may occur.

PROTOTYPE DRUG	Propranolol (Inderal, InnoPran XL)

Classification: **Therapeutic:** Antihypertensive, antidysrhythmic
Pharmacologic: Nonselective beta-adrenergic blocker

Therapeutic Effects and Uses: Approved in 1967, propranolol reduces heart rate and slows conduction velocity through the AV node by blocking beta$_1$ receptors in cardiac muscle. The decrease in cardiac output, as well as its suppression of renin activity, results in a reduction in blood pressure. Cardiac workload and myocardial oxygen demand are decreased due to the slower heart rate and decreased cardiac output. Propranolol is prescribed for a wide variety of indications (some off-label), including the following:

- **Hypertension.** For the treatment of HTN, propranolol has largely been replaced by angiotensin-converting enzyme (ACE) inhibitors and calcium channel blockers, which have been found to be more effective at preventing the long-term consequences of HTN such as stroke and MI. It is still widely used in patients with HTN who have angina, prior MI, or heart failure.

- **Angina pectoris.** Beta blockers are the preferred drugs for treating chronic angina. The nonselective drugs such as propranolol are less frequently used than the cardioselective agents.

- **Dysrhythmias.** Propranolol is one of the few beta-adrenergic antagonists approved to treat dysrhythmias. As an antidysrhythmic, propranolol is most effective against tachycardia caused by excessive sympathetic stimulation.

- **Migraine prophylaxis.** Propranolol has been one of the most frequently prescribed drugs for the prevention of migraines.

- **Prophylaxis of MI.** When given following an MI, propranolol has been found to reduce cardiovascular mortality and the risk of reinfarction.

Propranolol has a number of other indications. By lowering venous pressure, it may be useful in reducing portal HTN and bleeding due to esophageal varices. Propranolol is sometimes used to reduce the tachycardia, palpitations, tremor, and nervousness associated with thyroid crisis (storm). It has been used to treat panic attacks, PTSD, chronic agitation, and aggressive behavior. Lastly, it has been used to manage involuntary, rhythmic movements of essential tremor.

Both immediate release and extended release forms of propranolol are available. InnoPran XL has a timed delivery system that is designed for bedtime dosing, with a peak effect in the morning.

Mechanism of Action: Propranolol is a nonselective beta-adrenergic antagonist, affecting both beta$_1$ receptors in the heart, and beta$_2$ receptors in the lung and other locations throughout the body. It has no ISA.

Pharmacokinetics:

Route(s)	Usually PO; IV for severe dysrhythmias
Absorption	Completely absorbed
Distribution	Widely distributed, including the CNS and placenta; secreted in breast milk; 90% bound to plasma protein
Primary metabolism	Hepatic
Primary excretion	90–95% renal
Onset of action	PO: 1–2 h; IV: immediate
Duration of action	Half-life: 3–5 h

Adverse Effects: Propranolol is well tolerated and common adverse effects, such as nausea, vomiting, and diarrhea, generally diminish as therapy progresses. Other frequent adverse effects include fatigue, insomnia, drowsiness, bradycardia, and confusion. Impotence or loss of libido occurs in a small percentage of patients. Serious adverse effects include agranulocytosis, bronchospasm, Stevens-Johnson syndrome, and anaphylaxis. If the drug is abruptly withdrawn, palpitations, rebound HTN, life-threatening dysrhythmias, or myocardial ischemia may occur. **Black Box Warning**: Abrupt withdrawal is not advised in patients with angina or heart disease. Dosage should gradually be reduced over 1 to 2 weeks and the drug should be reinstituted if angina symptoms develop during this period.

Contraindications/Precautions: Because of its depressive effects on the heart, propranolol is contraindicated in cardiogenic shock, sinus bradycardia, greater than first-degree heart block, and severe HF. Patients with cardiac impairment must be monitored carefully to prevent worsening of their condition. Due to its constriction of smooth muscle in the airways, the drug is contraindicated in patients with COPD or asthma. Propranolol should be used cautiously in patients with diabetes because it interferes with glucose metabolism and can cause hypoglycemia. The drug can also mask signs of impending hypoglycemia such as tachycardia and tremors. Propranolol should be used with caution in patients with reduced renal output, because the drug may accumulate to toxic levels in the blood and cause dysrhythmias.

Drug Interactions: Propranolol interacts with many other drugs. When given with other beta blockers, effects on the cardiovascular system may be additive and bradycardia or hypotension may result. Because both propranolol and calcium channel blockers such as verapamil (Calan) and diltiazem (Cardizem) suppress myocardial contractility, concurrent use may lead to additive bradycardia. Use with antidysrhythmic drugs that slow conduction through the AV node such as amiodarone may lead to AV block. Phenothiazines can add to the hypotensive effects of propranolol. Because monoamine oxidase (MAO) inhibitors deplete endogenous catecholamines, concurrent administration with propranolol could result in severe bradycardia and hypotension.

Use of ethanol or antacids containing aluminum hydroxide gel will slow the absorption of propranolol and reduce its therapeutic effects. Administration of beta-adrenergic agonists such as albuterol (Proventil) will antagonize the antihypertensive action of propranolol. **Herbal/Food**: Hawthorn may cause an additive drop in blood pressure when used with antihypertensive drugs such as propranolol. Large doses of vitamin C may reduce the absorption of propranolol.

Pregnancy: Category C.

Treatment of Overdose: Overdose will cause bradycardia, hypotension, and bronchospasm. Treatment may require the use of plasma volume expanders or vasopressors to raise blood pressure to normal levels and atropine to counteract the bradycardia. Isoproterenol (a beta agonist) may be administered to reverse bronchospasm.

Nursing Responsibilities: Key nursing implications for patients receiving propranolol are included in the Nursing Practice Application for Patients Receiving Pharmacotherapy with Adrenergic Antagonists.

Drugs Similar to Propranolol (Inderal, InnoPran XL)

Many beta blockers are available. All nonselective beta-adrenergic blockers have the same actions but differ in their pharmacokinetics and therapeutic applications. Those prescribed exclusively for glaucoma, including betaxolol (Betoptic), carteolol (Ocupress), levobunolol (Betagan), and metipranolol (OptiPranolol), are discussed in Chapter 77.

Carvedilol (Coreg): Approved in 1995, carvedilol is an oral medication approved for the management of HTN and HF and to reduce mortality in patients who have survived the acute phase of an MI. It may be used off-label to treat angina. In addition to being a nonselective beta-receptor blocker, carvedilol blocks alpha₁-adrenergic receptors. Because of its alpha-antagonist action, carvedilol shares similar adverse effects, such as orthostatic HTN, with the alpha₁ blockers. Like most beta blockers, fatigue and dizziness are common adverse effects. Patients with asthma or chronic lung disorders may experience dyspnea or wheezing due to the bronchoconstriction effects of the drug. This drug is pregnancy category C.

Labetalol (Normodyne, Trandate): Like carvedilol, labetalol has nonselective beta-blocking action as well as the ability to selectively block alpha₁-adrenergic receptors. Approved in 1984, it is available by both the oral and IV routes for the therapy of HTN. When treating HTN, the drug may be given concurrently with a thiazide diuretic. The most common adverse effects are generally mild and include insomnia, drowsiness, fatigue, decreased libido, and tingling of the scalp. Orthostatic hypotension is greatest 2 to 4 hours after the drug is administered. When given by the IV route for hypertensive emergencies, as many as 60% of patients will experience orthostatic hypotension. This drug is pregnancy category C.

Nadolol (Corgard): Approved in 1989, nadolol is a nonselective beta-adrenergic blocker that is used to treat HTN and for the long-term management of angina. Off-label uses of nadolol include suppression of ventricular dysrhythmias, migraine prophylaxis, treatment of essential tremor, and anxiety. Given by the oral route, it has a long half-life of 20 to 24 hours, which offers the benefit of once-daily dosing. Unlike many beta blockers, it is not metabolized by the liver and is excreted mostly unchanged by the kidneys. Adverse effects are generally mild and similar to those of propranolol and include drowsiness, fatigue, and decreased libido. This drug is pregnancy category C.

Penbutolol (Levatol): Penbutolol is a nonselective beta-adrenergic antagonist that has a long duration of action, which offers the benefit of once-daily dosing. Approved in 1987, it is used in the pharmacotherapy of HTN as monotherapy, or in combination with other antihypertensives. Treatment of chronic stable angina is an off-label use of penbutolol. Penbutolol has higher lipid solubility than most other drugs in its class and thus has a greater potential for causing CNS adverse effects such as dizziness and fatigue. Other common adverse effects include nausea, vomiting, and diarrhea. The drug is pregnancy category C.

Pindolol (Visken): Approved in 1982, pindolol is an oral, nonselective beta blocker that is used in the pharmacotherapy of HTN, usually in combination with a thiazide diuretic. It is used off-label for the management of chronic stable angina. Pindolol has the highest degree of ISA of any beta blocker, which gives it some beta-agonist action in addition to antagonist activity. Adverse effects are generally mild and temporary and include nausea, vomiting, insomnia, fatigue, and dizziness. Maximum antihypertensive action may take up to 2 weeks to achieve. This drug is pregnancy category B.

Sotalol (Betapace, Sorine): Although all nonselective beta blockers affect heart rate and rhythm, sotalol is one of the few drugs in this class used exclusively as an antidysrhythmic. By slowing the action potential crossing the myocardium, the heart is able to regain normal rhythm. Therapy with sotalol is always begun in a setting where the electrocardiogram (ECG) can be continuously monitored for a minimum of 3 days because this drug can cause or worsen certain dysrhythmias. Adverse effects are those typical of beta blockers but they occur more frequently. For example, fatigue may occur in 20% of patients, dyspnea in 21%, and sinus bradycardia in 16%. Patients with a history of dysrhythmias are more likely to experience serious adverse effects. Abrupt discontinuation of the drug can cause dysrhythmias and MI. Other adverse effects include insomnia, nausea, vomiting, and drowsiness. Approved in 1992, the role of sotalol in the pharmacotherapy of dysrhythmias is presented in Chapter 37. This drug is pregnancy category B.

Timolol (Blocadren, Timoptic): In its oral formulation, timolol (Blocadren) is indicated for HTN, migraine prophylaxis, and reduction of mortality following an acute MI. Chronic, stable angina is an off-label indication for the drug. Timolol (Timoptic) is available as a 0.25% and 0.5% ophthalmic solution to treat glaucoma. Systemic adverse effects are generally mild and transient and include nausea, vomiting, diarrhea, bradycardia, fatigue, and dizziness. Abrupt discontinuation of timolol can cause dysrhythmias and MI. Approved in 1978, timolol (Timoptic) is presented as a prototype for glaucoma in Chapter 74.

16.4 Beta₁-adrenergic antagonists are selective for beta₁ receptors in the myocardium and are used to treat HTN and other cardiovascular disorders.

Because of their specificity for beta₁ receptors in the myocardium, the beta₁-adrenergic antagonists exert fewer noncardiac adverse effects than nonselective agents such as propranolol. This selectivity is not absolute, however; some of these drugs affect beta₂ receptors at higher doses, and a few have intrinsic sympathomimetic activity.

The primary indication for selective beta₁ antagonists is HTN. Some are also used in the pharmacologic management of chronic angina pectoris and HF. Although used for the same indications as the nonselective agents, the beta₁ blockers have certain advantages. The major advantage is that they have little effect on beta₂ receptors in bronchial smooth muscle. This allows the beta₁ blockers to be administered to patients with asthma or COPD with a lower risk of bronchospasm. Because their selectivity for beta₁ receptors is not absolute, bronchospasm is still a potential adverse effect in susceptible patients. The beta₁ blockers also have less effect on glucose and lipid metabolism than the nonselective drugs.

Beta blockers must be used with great caution in patients with a history of HF because both the nonselective and selective beta₁ blockers depress the speed of impulse conduction across the myocardium. In patients with healthy hearts, this effect is a clinical problem only at high doses. In patients with diseased hearts, however, this depression can worsen cardiac impairment and lead to HF. This cardiac impairment may develop gradually in patients taking beta blockers for prolonged periods; therefore, the patient should receive regular assessments of cardiac function during therapy. Generally, beta blockers are discontinued or their doses adjusted as soon as HF is suspected.

Overdose with beta₁ antagonists is treated in a manner similar to the nonselective beta blockers. An anticholinergic drug such as atropine or a beta agonist such as isoproterenol may be given to promote bronchodilation and increase the heart rate. Digoxin (Lanoxin) or diuretics may be indicated if HF develops. Severe hypotension may require the administration of an emergency vasopressor such as dopamine (a beta agonist).

CONNECTION Checkpoint 16.2

Dopamine is a catecholamine. From what you learned in Chapter 15, identify other catecholamines that are used to quickly raise blood pressure in acute care situations. *See Answer to Connection Checkpoint 16.2 on student resource website.*

PROTOTYPE DRUG	**Metoprolol** **(Lopressor, Toprol XL)**

Classification: Therapeutic: Antihypertensive
Pharmacologic: Selective beta₁-adrenergic antagonist

Therapeutic Effects and Uses: Approved in 1978, the primary indication for metoprolol is HTN, as monotherapy or in combination with other antihypertensives. It is also indicated for angina and for the treatment of stable, symptomatic HF.

The therapeutic actions of metoprolol include decreases in heart rate (both resting and during exercise), cardiac output, and blood pressure (both systolic and diastolic). Fixed-dose combination formulations are available for HTN: Lopressor HCT combines metoprolol with the diuretic hydrochlorothiazide in a single tablet. Because it slows the rate and force of myocardial contraction, metoprolol can reduce oxygen demands on the heart and benefit patients with angina and stable HF. Off-label uses include essential tremor, migraine prophylaxis, and the control of heart rate in patients with atrial dysrhythmias.

Recent research has determined that metoprolol reduces the mortality associated with recent MI. Following an acute MI, metoprolol is infused slowly until a target heart rate between 60 and 90 beats per minute is reached. This reduces myocardial oxygen demand at a time when the heart is at great risk for a subsequent MI or life-threatening dysrhythmias. On hospital discharge, patients continue metoprolol therapy by switching to the PO form of the drug.

Mechanism of Action: Metoprolol is a selective beta₁-adrenergic antagonist that competes with endogenous catecholamines at adrenergic receptors in cardiac muscle. At high doses, it may affect beta₂ receptors in bronchial smooth muscle.

Pharmacokinetics:

Route(s)	Usually PO; IV for MI
Absorption	Well absorbed
Distribution	Completely, including CNS and placenta; secreted in breast milk; 12% bound to plasma protein
Primary metabolism	Hepatic
Primary excretion	Renal
Onset of action	PO: 15 min; IV: immediate
Duration of action	13–19 h

Adverse Effects: Metoprolol is well tolerated and adverse effects generally diminish as therapy progresses. Nausea and vomiting are the most common adverse effects. Other common adverse effects include dizziness, fatigue, insomnia, bradycardia, heartburn, and dyspnea. Serious adverse effects include agranulocytosis, laryngospasm, complete heart block, and thyroid storm in patients with thyrotoxicosis. Bronchospasm and dyspnea are rare because the drug has little effect on beta₂ receptors in bronchial smooth muscle. Dysrhythmias, severe HTN, or MI may occur if the drug is abruptly withdrawn. **Black Box Warning**: Abrupt withdrawal is not advised in patients with angina or heart disease. Dosage should gradually be reduced over 1 to 2 weeks and the drug should be reinstituted if angina symptoms develop during this period.

Contraindications/Precautions: Because of its multiple effects on the heart, patients with preexisting cardiac disease such as HF should be carefully monitored. This drug is contraindicated in cardiogenic shock, severe bradycardia, and heart block greater than first degree. Metoprolol should be used with caution in patients with severe hepatic disease because its major route of excretion is the liver. Metoprolol should be used with caution in patients with asthma and those with a history of bronchospasm because the drug may affect beta₂ receptors at high doses.

Drug Interactions: Beta₁ blockers such as metoprolol have the potential to interact with many different drugs. The nurse should always be cautious when administering a beta blocker with any other medication that affects the heart, particularly those that depress AV node conduction. Because certain calcium channel blockers such as verapamil suppress myocardial contractility, concurrent use with metoprolol can lead to additive bradycardia and even heart block. Use with other antihypertensive drugs may cause additive hypotension. Certain drugs, including cimetidine and oral contraceptives, can also add to the hypotensive effect of metoprolol. Metoprolol should not be given with sympathomimetics because the actions of the drugs will cancel each other. Metoprolol can reduce the clearance of lidocaine and cause lidocaine toxicity.

Pregnancy: Category C.

Treatment of Overdose: Overdose of metoprolol will cause bradycardia, hypotension, and bronchospasm. Treatment may require the use of plasma volume expanders or vasopressors to raise blood pressure to normal levels and atropine to counteract the bradycardia. Isoproterenol may be administered for bronchospasm.

Nursing Responsibilities: Key nursing implications for patients receiving metoprolol are included in the Nursing Practice Application for Patients Receiving Pharmacotherapy with Adrenergic Antagonists.

Drugs Similar to Metoprolol (Lopressor, Toprol)

Other beta$_1$-adrenergic antagonists include acebutolol, atenolol, betaxolol, bisoprolol, esmolol, and nebivolol. The beta$_1$-adrenergic antagonists are very similar but differ in their pharmacokinetics and specific indications.

Acebutolol (Sectral): Approved in 1984, acebutolol is an oral cardioselective beta$_1$ antagonist similar to metoprolol that is used for HTN and recurrent ventricular dysrhythmias. An off-label indication is chronic stable angina. In addition to being a selective beta$_1$ blocker, it has mild intrinsic sympathomimetic activity. Because of its 3- to 4-hour half-life, it is usually administered twice daily. Common adverse effects include CNS effects such as fatigue, dizziness, and headache. Higher doses can produce hypotension and bradycardia. Like other beta blockers, care must be taken when using acebutolol with other drugs that depress myocardial conduction because bradycardia and hypotension may result. This drug is pregnancy category B.

Atenolol (Tenormin): Approved in 1981, atenolol is available by the oral route for HTN and for the long-term management of chronic stable angina. It is also given by the IV route to reduce the risk of sudden death in patients with an acute MI. Off-label indications include migraine prophylaxis and the prevention of symptoms in patients undergoing ethanol withdrawal. Atenolol has a long half-life, which allows for once-daily dosing. Common adverse effects are the same as those of other drugs in this class, such as nausea, vomiting, fatigue, dizziness, and headache. The risk of bradycardia is low at normal doses. Like other beta blockers, care must be taken to avoid abrupt discontinuation of therapy, especially in patients with coronary artery disease. Tenoretic is a combination of atenolol and the diuretic chlorthalidone that is approved for HTN. Atenolol is presented as a prototype drug for angina in Chapter 35. This drug is pregnancy category D and is not recommended during pregnancy or lactation.

Betaxolol (Betoptic, Kerlone): Approved in 1985, betaxolol (Kerlone) is available in tablet form for the pharmacotherapy of HTN, sometimes given concurrently with thiazide diuretics. The drug is one of the most potent and selective of the beta blockers; it is nine times more potent than atenolol. It has no ISA, and it inhibits beta$_2$-adrenergic receptors in the lung only at very high doses. When given PO, adverse effects such as nausea, vomiting, dizziness, fatigue, and headache are typical of the beta blockers. The risk of bradycardia increases with higher doses. Like other beta blockers, care must be taken to avoid abrupt discontinuation of therapy, especially in patients with coronary artery disease, because myocardial ischemia, MI, HTN, or dysrhythmias may result.

Betaxolol (Betoptic) is also available as a 0.25% ophthalmic suspension for chronic open-angle glaucoma. Like other beta blockers, Betoptic reduces intraocular pressure. Adverse effects are limited to the eye and include burning and transient blurred vision. This drug is pregnancy category C.

Bisoprolol (Zebeta): Approved in 1992, bisoprolol is approved only for HTN, although HF and chronic stable angina are off-label indications. Given orally, bisoprolol has a longer half-life than metoprolol, which allows for less frequent dosing. The cardioselective nature of bisoprolol action only applies to low doses; at higher doses it also blocks beta$_2$ receptors to cause dyspnea and wheezing. Common adverse effects are the same as those of other drugs in this class, such as fatigue, dizziness, and headache. Like other beta blockers, care must be taken to avoid abrupt discontinuation of therapy, especially in patients with coronary artery disease. Ziac combines bisoprolol with the diuretic hydrochlorothiazide in a single tablet. The drug is pregnancy category C.

Esmolol (Brevibloc): Approved in 1986, esmolol is very different from other beta$_1$-adrenergic blockers. It is administered by continuous IV infusion in emergency situations, usually postoperative or perioperative, to rapidly correct supraventricular tachycardia or severe HTN. It has a very short half-life of only 8 minutes, and the patient must be monitored for hypotension and bradycardia during the infusion. Although it has the same actions and adverse effects as other beta blockers, the actions of esmolol begin to diminish within minutes after discontinuation of the infusion. Esmolol should be used with extreme caution in patients with severe bradycardia, AV block, or cardiogenic shock. Hypotension occurs in about 40% of patients receiving the drug but resolves quickly following completion of the infusion. The drug is pregnancy category C.

Nebivolol (Bystolic): Approved in 2007, nebivolol is a selective beta$_1$-adrenergic blocker that is indicated for the treatment of HTN, either as monotherapy or in combination with other antihypertensives. Nebivolol is highly cardioselective but may activate beta$_2$ receptors at higher doses. It has no ISA activity. Nebivolol has equal effectiveness to other drugs in its class, but it appears to produce fewer adverse effects. The drug is well tolerated, with the most frequently observed adverse effects being headache, fatigue, paresthesia, dizziness, hypotension, and bradycardia. Like other beta blockers, care must be taken to avoid abrupt discontinuation of therapy, especially in patients with coronary artery disease. This drug is pregnancy category C.

CONNECTIONS: NURSING PRACTICE APPLICATION

Patients Receiving Pharmacotherapy with Adrenergic Antagonists

Assessment	Potential Nursing Diagnoses*
Baseline assessment prior to administration: • Obtain a complete health history including cardiovascular, cerebrovascular, or respiratory disease, or diabetes. Obtain a drug history including allergies, current prescriptions and OTC drugs, herbal preparations, and alcohol use. Be alert to possible drug interactions. • Evaluate appropriate laboratory findings including electrolytes, glucose, and hepatic and renal function studies. • Obtain baseline weight, vital signs, and cardiac monitoring (e.g., ECG, cardiac output as appropriate). • For treatment of BPH, assess urinary output. • Assess the patient's ability to receive and understand instructions. Include family and caregivers as needed.	• *Decreased Cardiac Output* • *Impaired Gas Exchange* • *Ineffective Airway Clearance* • *Impaired Urinary Elimination* • *Activity Intolerance* • *Sexual Dysfunction*, related to adverse effects of drug therapy • *Disturbed Sleep Pattern*, related to adverse effects of drug therapy • *Deficient Knowledge* (Drug Therapy) • *Risk for Falls*, related to adverse effects of drug therapy • *Risk for Injury*, related to adverse effects of drug therapy
Assessment throughout administration: • Assess for desired therapeutic effects dependent on the reason for the drug (e.g., blood pressure [BP] within normal range, dysrhythmias/palpitations relieved, greater ease in urination). • Continue frequent and careful monitoring of vital signs, daily weight, and urinary and cardiac output as appropriate, especially if IV administration is used. • Assess for and promptly report adverse effects: bradycardia, hypotension, dysrhythmias, reflex tachycardia (from too rapid decrease in BP or hypotension), dizziness, headache, or decreased urinary output. Severe hypotension, seizures, dysrhythmias, or palpitations may signal drug toxicity and are immediately reported.	

Implementation

Interventions and (Rationales)	Patient-Centered Care
Ensuring therapeutic effects: • Continue frequent assessments as above for therapeutic effects dependent on the reason the drug therapy is given. Daily weights should remain at or close to baseline weight. (Pulse, BP, and respiratory rate should be within normal limits or within the parameters set by the health care provider. Urinary hesitancy or frequency should be decreased and urine output improved. An increase in weight over 1 kg [2 lb] per day may indicate excessive fluid gain. **Diverse Patients:** Research indicates differing responses to antihypertensive therapy, including with adrenergic-blocking drugs, in ethnically diverse populations compared to non-Hispanic whites.)	• Teach the patient, family, or caregiver how to monitor pulse and BP as appropriate. The pulse rate should be taken for one full minute at a pulse point most easily felt. Ensure proper use and functioning of any home equipment obtained. • Have the patient weigh self daily along with BP and pulse measurements, ideally at the same time each day. Report weight gain or loss of more than 1 kg (2 lb) in a 24-hour period.
• Follow appropriate administration techniques for ophthalmic doses.	• Instruct the patient, family, or caregiver in proper administration techniques, followed by teach-back.
Minimizing adverse effects: • Continue to monitor vital signs. Take BP lying, sitting, and standing to detect orthostatic hypotension. Notify the health care provider if BP or pulse decreases beyond the established parameters or if hypotension is accompanied by reflex tachycardia. (Adrenergic antagonists decrease heart rate and cause vasodilation, resulting in lowered BP. Orthostatic hypotension may increase the risk of falls. **Lifespan:** Be aware that dizziness may increase the risk of falls in the older adult. Reflex tachycardia may signal that the BP has dropped too quickly or too substantially.)	• Teach the patient to rise from lying to sitting or standing slowly to avoid dizziness or falls. If dizziness occurs, the patient should sit or lie down and not attempt to stand or walk until the sensation passes. • Instruct the patient to stop taking medication if BP is 90/60 mmHg or below, or below the parameters set by the health care provider, and immediately notify the provider.
• Continue cardiac monitoring (e.g., ECG) as ordered for dysrhythmias in the hospitalized patient. (External monitoring devices will detect early signs of adverse effects as well as monitor for therapeutic effect.)	• Instruct the patient to report palpitations, chest pain, or dyspnea immediately.
• Weigh patient daily and report weight gain or loss. (Daily weight is an accurate measure of fluid status and takes into account intake, output, and insensible losses. Weight gain or edema may signal BP has lowered too quickly, stimulating renin release, or is an adverse effect.)	• Have the patient weigh self daily, ideally at the same time of day, and record weight along with BP and pulse measurements. Have the patient report weight gain or loss of more than 1 kg (2 lb) in a 24-hour period.
• Monitor for breath sounds and for increasing dyspnea or adventitious breath sounds. (Nonselective beta-adrenergic blockers may cause bronchoconstriction.)	• Instruct the patient to immediately report any increasing or severe shortness of breath.

(continued)

CONNECTIONS: NURSING PRACTICE APPLICATION (continued)

• Monitor urine output and symptoms of dysuria such as hesitancy or retention when given for BPH. (Alpha$_2$- and beta-adrenergic blockers may impair urinary sphincter function. Alpha$_1$ blockers given for BPH cause bladder and urinary sphincter relaxation. **Lifespan**: Be aware that the male older adult is at higher risk for mechanical obstruction due to an enlarged prostate.)	• Have the patient report urinary hesitancy, feelings of bladder fullness, or difficulty starting urinary stream promptly.
• Give the first dose of the drug at bedtime. (A first-dose response may result in a greater initial drop in BP than subsequent doses.)	• Instruct the patient to take the first dose of medication immediately before going to bed, and to avoid driving for 12 to 24 hours after the first dose or when the dosage is increased until the effects are known.
• Continue to monitor blood glucose levels and appropriate laboratory work. (Adrenergic antagonists affect a wide range of body systems. They may also interfere with some oral diabetic drugs or change the way a hypoglycemic reaction is perceived.)	• Teach patients with diabetes to monitor their blood sugar more frequently and to be aware of subtle signs of possible hypoglycemia (e.g., nervousness, irritability). Patients on oral antidiabetic drugs should report any consistent changes in their blood sugar levels to the health care provider promptly.
• Assess the patient's mental status and mood. (Adrenergic antagonists may cause depression or dysphoria.)	• Teach the patient to report unusual feelings of sadness, despondency, apathy, or depression that may warrant a change in medication.
• Provide for eye comfort such as adequately lighted room. (Adrenergic antagonists can cause miosis and difficulty seeing in low-light levels.)	• Caution the patient about driving or other activities in low-light conditions or at night until the effects of the drug are known.
• Assess for cold, painful, or tender feet or hands or other symptoms of Raynaud's disease such as cyanosis, intermittent pallor, redness, or paresthesia. (These symptoms may accompany Raynaud's disease or suggest that treatment is not effective. Alternate drug therapy may be required.)	• Teach the patient to report any hand or feet pain, pallor, coldness, numbness, or cyanosis to the health care provider.
• Do not abruptly stop the medication. (Rebound HTN and tachycardia may occur.)	• Teach the patient, family, or caregiver not to stop the medication abruptly and to call the health care provider if the patient is unable to take medication for more than one day due to illness.
Patient understanding of drug therapy: • Use opportunities during administration of medications and during assessments to discuss the rationale for drug therapy, desired therapeutic outcomes, commonly observed adverse effects, parameters for when to call the health care provider, and any necessary monitoring or precautions. (Using time during nursing care helps to optimize and reinforce key teaching areas.)	• The patient, family, or caregiver should be able to state the reason for the drug; appropriate dose and scheduling; what adverse effects to observe for and when to report them; equipment needed as appropriate and how to use that equipment; and the required length of medication therapy needed with any special instructions regarding renewing or continuing the prescription as appropriate.
Patient self-administration of drug therapy: • When administering medications, instruct the patient, family, or caregiver in proper self-administration of drugs and ophthalmic drops. (Utilizing time during nurse-administration of these drugs helps to reinforce teaching.)	• Instruct the patient in proper administration techniques, followed by teach-back. • The drug should be taken at the same time each day when possible. • The patient, family, or caregiver is able to discuss appropriate dosing and administration needs.

*Nursing Diagnoses—Definitions and Classification 2015–2017. Copyright © 2014, 1994–2014 by NANDA International. Used by arrangement with John Wiley & Sons Limited.

CHAPTER

16 Understanding the Chapter

Key Concepts Summary

16.1 Adrenergic antagonists act by blocking the effects of norepinephrine at adrenergic receptors.

16.2 Alpha$_1$-adrenergic antagonists are used to treat hypertension and benign prostatic hyperplasia.

16.3 Nonselective beta-adrenergic antagonists affect both beta$_1$ and beta$_2$ receptors and are prescribed for HTN, angina, and other cardiovascular disorders.

16.4 Beta$_1$-adrenergic antagonists are selective for beta$_1$ receptors in the myocardium and are used to treat HTN and other cardiovascular disorders.

Case Study: Making the Patient Connection

Remember the patient "Amos Tucker" from the beginning of the chapter? Now read the remainder of the case study. Based on the information presented within this chapter, respond to the critical thinking questions that follow.

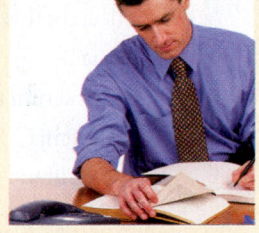

Amos Tucker is a 48-year-old executive who lives a very active life. He has a wife and two teenage children. His job requires frequent travel for up to 2 weeks at a time. Every year, Amos's company recommends a complete health physical as part of the executive benefits package. Amos has not taken advantage of this opportunity in the past. However, this year his wife has insisted that he have a checkup.

Amos arrives at the employee health clinic for the physical exam. On arrival he is visibly anxious and has accepted three calls on his cell phone since entering the clinic. During the initial health history session, Amos reveals that he smokes one pack of cigarettes per day and does not drink alcohol. He states that he has no time for exercise and has gained weight during the past year. Most nights Amos sleeps 4 to 6 hours. He states that he frequently wakes up during the night with thoughts of what he needs to do the next day. He finds it difficult to return to sleep after waking.

His past medical and family history indicate that both of his parents died within the past 10 years. His father died of a stroke and his mother died of a heart attack. Amos states that he has been prescribed prazosin (Minipress) in the past but he stopped taking it. When questioned about why he chose not to take the medication, Amos reluctantly confides in you that he suspected that the medication was causing sexual adverse effects.

The physical examination reveals that Amos is 1.9 m (6'2'') tall and weighs 119 kg (262 lb). His body temperature is 37°C (98.6°F), heart rate is 88 beats/min, respiratory rate is 18 breaths/min, and blood pressure is 160/90 mmHg. During the examination an ECG and laboratory test results were all within normal limits.

Critical Thinking Questions

1. Identify the mechanism of action associated with prazosin (Minipress).
2. Discuss the physiology of sexual disorders associated with alpha-adrenergic antagonists.
3. As this patient's nurse, how would you approach the topic of medication-induced sexual dysfunction?

See Answers to Critical Thinking Questions on student resource website.

Additional Case Study

Richard Perry is a 64-year-old patient who has been successfully treated for HTN for over 15 years with propranolol (Inderal). Mr. Perry is allergic to cats. However, he recently visited his grandson who has a new kitten. He now has weepy eyes and a running nose. He is considering taking the OTC medication pseudoephedrine (Sudafed) to relieve the allergic symptoms.

1. Is it safe for Mr. Perry to take this OTC medication? Why or why not?
2. Is there another OTC medication that would be safer for this patient?

See Answers to Additional Case Study on student resource website.

Chapter Review

1 The patient is started on propranolol (Inderal). Which is the most important action to be included in the plan of care for this patient related to this medication?
1. Monitor apical pulse and blood pressure.
2. Elevate the head of the bed during meals.
3. Take the medication after meals.
4. Consume foods high in potassium.

2 Which of the following should the nurse instruct a patient with diabetes who is prescribed a beta-adrenergic blocker for the treatment of hypertension to do?
1. Increase insulin intake by 2 to 3 units daily each morning.
2. Decrease the intake of carbohydrates while on the antihypertensive medications.
3. Elevate the lower extremities to promote venous drainage.
4. Monitor blood glucose levels frequently and report hypoglycemia.

3 To avoid the first-dose phenomenon, the nurse knows that the initial dose of prazosin (Minipress) should be:
1. Very low and given at bedtime.
2. Doubled and given before breakfast.
3. The usual dose and given before breakfast.
4. Doubled and given immediately after breakfast.

4 A patient who is taking an adrenergic antagonist for hypertension reports being dizzy when first getting out of bed in the morning. The nurse should advise the patient to:
1. Move slowly from the recumbent to the upright position.
2. Drink a full glass of water before rising to increase vascular circulatory volume.
3. Avoid sleeping in a prone position.
4. Stop taking the medication.

5 A health care provider has ordered an alpha$_1$-adrenergic antagonist for each of these patients. A nurse should question the order for the patient with which disorder?

1. Benign prostatic hyperplasia
2. Pheochromocytoma
3. Raynaud's disease
4. Tachycardia

6 The nurse is caring for a patient with chronic hypertension. The patient is receiving a beta-adrenergic blocker daily. Which patient manifestations would the nurse conclude are adverse effects of this medication? Select all that apply.

1. Anorexia
2. Increased serum triglycerides
3. Hypoglycemia
4. Decreased libido
5. Thrombocytopenia

See Answers to Chapter Review in Appendix A.

References

Gupta, N. R., Poulter, J. D., Eldridge, S., Cappuccio, F. P., Caulfield, M., Collier, D. J., … Fedre, G., on behalf of ASCOT investigators. (2010). Ethnic differences in blood pressure response to first- and second-line antihypertensive therapies in patients randomized in the ASCOT Trial. *American Journal of Hypertension, 23,* 1023–1030. doi:10.1038/ajh.2010.105

Hansen-Dispenza, H. (2013). *Raynaud phenomenon.* Retrieved from http://emedicine.medscape.com/article/331197-overview

U.S. Department of Health and Human Services, National Institutes of Health, National Heart, Lung and Blood Institute. (2006). *Your guide to lowering your blood pressure with DASH.* (NIH Publication No. 06-4082). Retrieved from http://www.nhlbi.nih.gov/health/public/heart/hbp/dash/new_dash.pdf

Selected Bibliography

Al-Gobari, M., El Khatib, C., Pillon, F., & Gueyffier, F. (2013). Beta-blockers for the prevention of sudden cardiac death in heart failure patients: A meta-analysis of randomized controlled trials. *BMC Cardiovascular Disorders, 13,* 52. doi:10.1186/1471-2261-13-52

Chen, J. M., Heran, B. S., Perez, M. I., & Wright, J. M. (2010). Blood pressure lowering efficacy of beta-blockers as second-line therapy for primary hypertension. *Cochrane Database of Systematic Reviews, 1,* CD007185. doi:10.1002/14651858.CD007185.pub2

Coons, J. C., McGraw, M., & Murali, S. (2011). Pharmacotherapy for acute heart failure syndromes. *American Journal of Health-System Pharmacy, 68,* 21–35. doi:10.2146/ajhp100202

Herdman, T. H., & Kamitsuru, S. (Eds.). (2014). *NANDA International nursing diagnoses: Definitions and classification, 2015–2017.* Oxford, United Kingdom: Wiley-Blackwell.

McHugh, J., Pokhrel, P., Barber, K., & Guozhen, L. (2010). Beta-blockers in the management of cardiovascular diseases. *Osteopathic Family Physician, 2,* 131–138. doi:10.1016/j.osfp.2010.03.001

Ruz, M. E., Lennie, T. A., & Moser, D. K. (2010). Effects of β-blockers and anxiety on complication rates after acute myocardial infarction. *American Journal of Critical Care, 20,* 67–74. doi:10.4037/ajcc2010216

Self, T. H., Wallace, J. L., & Soberman, J. E. (2012). Cardioselective beta-blocker treatment of hypertension in patients with asthma: When do benefits outweigh risks? *Journal of Asthma, 49,* 947–951. doi:10.3109/02770903.2012.719252

Sharma, A. (2013). *Beta-blocker toxicity.* Retrieved from http://emedicine.medscape.com/article/813342-overview

Stephens, S. (2010). State of the science: β-Blockers and reduction of perioperative cardiac events. *Critical Care Nursing Clinics of North America, 22*(2), 209–215. doi:10.1016/j.ccell.2010.03.013

Westfall, T. C., & Westfall, D. P. (2011). Adrenergic agonists and antagonists. In L. L. Brunton, B. A. Chabner, & B. C. Knollman (Eds.), *The pharmacological basis of therapeutics* (12th ed., pp. 277–334). New York, NY: McGraw-Hill.

Wiysonge, C. S., Bradley, H. A., Volmink, J., Mayosi, B. M., Mbewu, A., & Opie, L. H. (2012). Beta-blockers for hypertension. *Cochrane Database of Systematic Reviews, 11,* CD002003. doi:10.1002/14651858.CD002003.pub4

UNIT

4

Pharmacology of the Central Nervous System

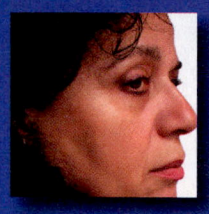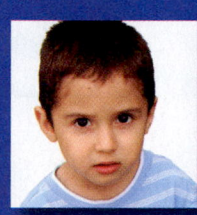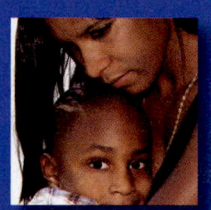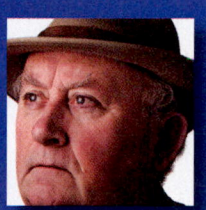

CHAPTER 17   Review of the Central Nervous System / 208

CHAPTER 18   Pharmacotherapy of Anxiety and Sleep Disorders / 216

CHAPTER 19   Pharmacotherapy of Mood Disorders / 239

CHAPTER 20   Pharmacotherapy of Psychoses / 264

CHAPTER 21   Pharmacotherapy of Degenerative Diseases of the Central Nervous System / 285

CHAPTER 22   Pharmacotherapy of Seizures / 309

CHAPTER 23   Pharmacotherapy of Muscle Spasms and Spasticity / 334

CHAPTER 24   Central Nervous System Stimulants and Drugs for Attention Deficit/Hyperactivity Disorder / 350

CHAPTER 25   Pharmacotherapy of Severe Pain and Migraines / 366

CHAPTER 26   Anesthetics and Anesthesia Adjuncts / 394

CHAPTER 27   Pharmacology of Substance Abuse / 416

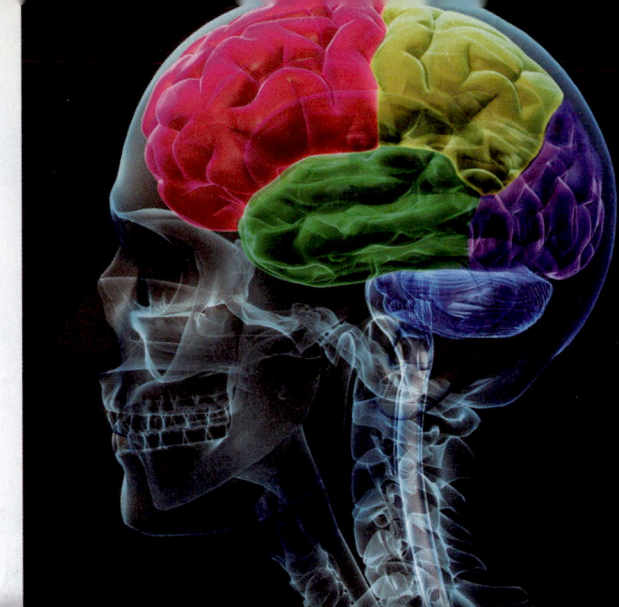

17 Review of the Central Nervous System

LEARNING OUTCOMES

After reading this chapter, the student should be able to:

1. Identify disorders for which central nervous system medications are prescribed.
2. Illustrate the major components of a synapse within the central nervous system.
3. Identify the major neurotransmitters in the central nervous system and their functions.
4. Describe the major structural regions of the brain and their primary functions.
5. Explain the major functional systems of the brain and their primary functions.

CHAPTER OUTLINE

▸ Scope of Central Nervous System Pharmacology

▸ Neurons and Neurotransmission

▸ Structural Divisions of the Central Nervous System

▸ Functional Systems of the Central Nervous System

KEY TERMS

basal nuclei, 214

dopamine, 211

extrapyramidal system, 214

gamma aminobutyric acid (GABA), 211

glutamate, 211

limbic system, 213

neuron, 210

reticular activating system (RAS), 214

serotonin, 211

synapses, 210

Chapters 12 through 16 introduced the autonomic nervous system (ANS)—the system that provides involuntary control over vital functions of the cardiovascular, digestive, respiratory, and genitourinary systems. This chapter launches Unit 4, which examines the pharmacology of the central nervous system (CNS). The two components of the CNS, the brain and spinal cord, are collectively responsible for interpreting sensory information and formulating appropriate responses. Typical responses may include thinking (deciding if the sensory information is harmful or pleasurable), emotions (anger, depression, euphoria), or movement (running away, pounding a fist, or hugging). The purpose of this chapter is to provide a brief review of concepts of CNS anatomy and physiology that are relevant to neuropharmacology.

Scope of Central Nervous System Pharmacology

17.1 Medications affect the central nervous system by stimulating or suppressing the firing of specific neurons.

CNS pharmacology is one of the largest and most important divisions in medicine, encompassing 11 chapters in this textbook. Medications may be administered to treat specific neurologic or psychiatric disorders of the CNS. Many drugs cause CNS adverse effects during pharmacotherapy, whereas some are self-administered to produce pleasurable psychoactive effects. At high doses, a large number of drugs affect the brain, and CNS toxicity is a dose-limiting factor in the pharmacotherapy of many diseases.

Of all divisions of pharmacology, CNS drug mechanisms are probably the least understood. For some medications, pharmacologists only know that the drug acts on the CNS and produces a therapeutic effect, but its mechanism of action remains largely unknown. There are two primary reasons for this lack of understanding about how CNS drugs produce their effects: the uniqueness of the human brain and the complexity of the disorders affecting it.

The human brain is truly unique, with no other species having the same complexity. It is not known if animals experience the same types of mental disorders as humans, and measurement of hallucinations, euphoria, or depression is difficult, if not impossible, in most species. If a drug does induce changes in animal behavior such as depression or anxiety, it is not known whether these data apply to humans because of the enormous differences in brain physiology as well as human social networks that can profoundly influence mental health conditions. Pharmacologists are certainly able to measure changes in brain activity or in the amounts of neurotransmitters in specific regions of the brain,

but these do not adequately explain complex changes in thinking, mood, or behavior. Without good animal models, pharmacologists must rely largely on empirical observations—evidence derived from giving the drugs to patients and determining what works rather than how it works.

Also complicating the study of CNS pharmacology is that mental disorders themselves are incompletely understood. The physiological basis for disorders such as schizophrenia, major depression, bipolar disorder, panic attacks, or post-traumatic stress disorder is not well established. There is great patient variability in symptoms and disease progression with these disorders, and social factors play important roles. Without a complete understanding of the etiology and pathophysiology of mental disorders, pharmacotherapy of these conditions and the development of new drug therapies for CNS disorders will remain challenging.

The next nine chapters present the major classes of drugs whose pharmacotherapeutic goal is to modify the activity of some portion of the CNS. A 10th chapter examines substances that are abused for their effects on the CNS. In a few cases, CNS drugs affect the function of very specific regions of the brain. Most CNS drugs, however, are nonspecific and affect multiple brain regions.

In simplest terms, CNS drugs have two basic actions: They either stimulate (activate) or suppress (inhibit) the firing of neurons. In some cases, CNS drugs may have both actions: activation of some neurons and inhibition of others. The pharmacologic effects of a CNS drug observed in a patient are the result of precisely which neurons are changed, and how many are affected. As a result of neuron modification, the following beneficial effects of CNS drugs are observed and are studied in this unit.

- Reduction in anxiety
- Improved sleep patterns
- Elevated mood
- Management of psychotic symptoms
- Slowing the progression of chronic degenerative diseases of the brain
- Termination and prevention of seizures
- Reduction in muscle spasms and spasticity
- Reduction of hyperactivity and mania
- Reduction in pain
- Induction of anesthesia

CONNECTION Checkpoint 17.1

From what you learned in Chapter 12, what are the two divisions of the peripheral nervous system and what are their primary functions? *See Answer to Connection Checkpoint 17.1 on student resource website.*

Neurons and Neurotransmission

17.2 Neurons in the central nervous system communicate with each other and with body tissues, using neurotransmitters.

The **neuron** is the primary functional cell in all portions of the nervous system. The function of the 100 billion neurons making up the nervous system is to communicate messages through conduction of an action potential. In the CNS, the vast majority of neurons are communicating with other neurons. These neuronal pathways or circuits are extremely complex and provide the basis for the higher level functions of the brain such as thinking, memory, and intelligence. Although a single neuron in the CNS serves no practical function, the interconnections among 100 billion neurons are a major part of what distinguishes the human brain from that of all other species.

Communication between neurons in the brain, as well as that between the brain and other organs, is provided through **synapses**. Synapses are junctions between two neurons, or between a neuron and a muscle or gland. Synapses in the ANS are presented in detail in Chapter 12. The student should review that chapter before proceeding.

Synapses within the CNS operate by the same basic principles as those in the ANS. An action potential from the presynaptic neuron releases a neurotransmitter that moves across the synaptic cleft to activate receptors on the postsynaptic neuron, as illustrated in Figure 17.1a. In some cases, the neuron may be excitatory, enhancing neural transmission (Figure 17.1b). In other cases the impulse inhibits a neurotransmitter from being released, or it causes the release of an inhibitory neurotransmitter that suppresses neuronal conduction (Figure 17.1c). All interconnections in the CNS depend on transmission of the action potential from one neuron to another neuron, or to multiple neurons at synapses.

In the ANS only two neurotransmitters account for nearly all synaptic transmission: acetylcholine (Ach) and norepinephrine (NE). Although these two chemicals also are found in the CNS, more than

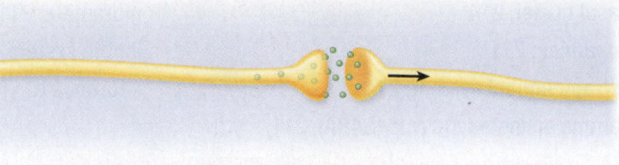

(a) Normal transmission

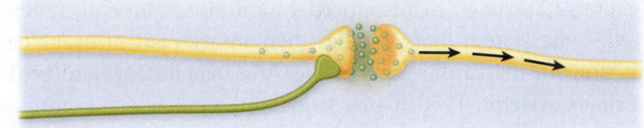

(b) Enhanced transmission due to an excitatory neuron

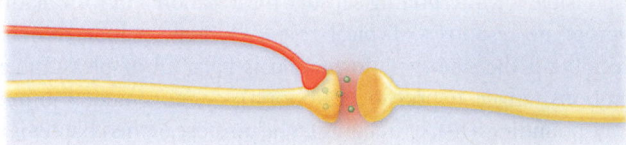

(c) Suppressed transmission due to an inhibitory neuron

Figure 17.1 Modification of neural transmission in the central nervous system: (a) normal transmission; (b) enhanced transmission; (c) suppressed transmission.

30 additional substances have been identified as neurotransmitters in the brain, making the study of neuronal communication in this organ very complex. Some neurotransmitters such as glutamate are primarily stimulatory, whereas others such as gamma aminobutyric acid (GABA) inhibit neuronal activity. NE can activate or inhibit neuronal activity, depending on its location in the brain. A summary of relevant brain neurotransmitters is shown in Table 17.1.

PharmFACT

The characteristic loss of cognitive function that occurs during Alzheimer's disease is directly related to a progressive loss of synapses in the cerebral cortex (Isik, 2010).

TABLE 17.1	Selected Central Nervous System Neurotransmitters and Their Functions		
Neurotransmitter	**Abundance**	**Effect**	**Clinical Significance**
Acetylcholine (Ach)	Widely distributed in the CNS; a major transmitter in the ANS	CNS: May be excitatory or inhibitory; controls voluntary skeletal muscle movement ANS: Activates the parasympathetic nervous system	Myasthenia gravis, Alzheimer's disease
Dopamine	Basal ganglia and limbic system	Usually excitatory; locomotion, attention, learning, and the reinforcing effects of abused drugs	Parkinson's disease; psychoses; motivation, pleasure
Endorphins and enkephalins	Widely distributed in the CNS and peripheral nervous system (PNS)	Usually inhibitory; reduction of pain	Opioids bind to endorphin receptors
Gamma aminobutyric acid (GABA)	Widely distributed in the CNS	Most common inhibitory CNS neurotransmitter	Seizure and anxiety disorders
Glutamate	Widely distributed in the CNS	Most common excitatory CNS neurotransmitter	Memory
Norepinephrine (NE)	Widely distributed in the CNS; a major transmitter in the ANS	CNS: May be excitatory or inhibitory ANS: Activates the sympathetic nervous system	Depression, memory, panic attacks
Serotonin	Common in the brainstem but also found in the limbic system, gastrointestinal tract, and platelets	Usually inhibitory	Anxiety, bipolar disorder, and depression

Adrenergic synapses: Adrenergic synapses utilize NE as the neurotransmitter. Adrenergic synapses in the CNS are abundant in the hypothalamus, the limbic system, and the reticular activating system (RAS). NE activates parts of the brain to heighten alertness and is prominent during waking hours. Adrenergic neurons likely play a role in mood disorders such as depression and anxiety. Drugs used to modify adrenergic synapses in the CNS include caffeine, amphetamines, and tricyclic antidepressants.

Cholinergic synapses: Cholinergic synapses utilize Ach as the neurotransmitter. In the brain, these synapses are most often stimulatory. Cholinergic synapses are abundant in the motor cortex and basal ganglia but are uncommon in other areas. Cholinergic synapses are especially important in the pathophysiology of Parkinson's disease and Alzheimer's disease. Ach is also a major neurotransmitter in the ANS.

Dopaminergic synapses: These synapses utilize dopamine as the neurotransmitter. **Dopamine** is a chemical precursor in the synthesis of NE and, like epinephrine and NE, is classified chemically as a catecholamine. Dopaminergic synapses are generally excitatory and affect arousal and wakefulness. However, two major receptor subtypes exist: D1 is stimulatory, and D2 is inhibitory. Cocaine and amphetamines produce their stimulatory actions by affecting dopamine receptors; marijuana is also thought to exert some of its psychoactive effects by increasing dopaminergic activity. Dopamine receptors are important in the pharmacotherapy of psychosis and Parkinson's disease.

CONNECTION Checkpoint 17.2

The neurotransmitter dopamine is also available as a drug. From what you learned in Chapter 15, what are the indications for dopamine therapy? *See Answer to Connection Checkpoint 17.2 on student resource website.*

Endorphins and enkephalins: Endorphins and enkephalins are small peptides secreted by neurons in the hypothalamus, pituitary, limbic system, and spinal cord. The receptor for these molecules is the opioid receptor, which is involved in pain transmission. Endorphins and enkephalins are sometimes called natural opiates because they produce effects very similar to those of morphine and other opioid drugs. Drugs used to modify the types of synapses in the CNS include opioids such as codeine and morphine.

Gamma aminobutyric acid synapses: These synapses utilize **gamma aminobutyric acid (GABA)** as a neurotransmitter. GABA synapses are the second most common type in the CNS, accounting for 30% to 40% of all brain synapses. GABA is the primary inhibitory neurotransmitter in the CNS and is found throughout the brain, with greatest abundance in the basal ganglia and hypothalamus. Several GABA receptor subtypes have been identified. GABA receptors are the primary site of action for several classes of drugs, including the benzodiazepines and barbiturates.

Glutamate synapses: Glutamate synapses utilize the amino acid **glutamate** (glutamic acid) as a neurotransmitter. Glutamate is the most common neurotransmitter in the CNS, and its synapses are always excitatory in nature. It is found in nearly all regions of the brain. Several glutamate receptor subtypes have been identified, with the N-methyl-D-aspartate (NMDA) receptor being particularly important to memory and learning. In addition to glutamate, zinc, magnesium, glycine, and even phencyclidine (a hallucinogen) bind to the NMDA receptor, thus modulating neuronal activity. High amounts of glutamate can cause neuron death and may be the mechanism responsible for certain types of neurotoxicity.

Serotonergic synapses: Serotonergic synapses utilize **serotonin**, also known as 5-hydroxytryptamine (5-HT), as a neurotransmitter. Although some serotonergic synapses are located in the CNS, 98% of the serotonergic receptors are found outside the CNS in platelets, mast cells, and other peripheral cells. Serotonergic receptors are found throughout the limbic (emotional) system of the brain, often in close association with adrenergic synapses. Serotonin is used by the body to synthesize the hormone melatonin in the pineal gland. Low serotonin levels in the CNS are associated with anxiety and impulsive behavior, including suicidal ideation. Serotonergic receptors play an important role in the mechanism of action of antidepressant drugs.

PharmFACT

Conduction of nerve impulses in large-diameter myelinated neurons can reach speeds up to 268 miles/h (120 m/s) (Silverthorn, 2012).

Structural Divisions of the Central Nervous System

17.3 The central nervous system is divided into several major structural components.

The brain consists of dozens of structural divisions that serve common functions. Identification of the many anatomic components in the CNS is complex and beyond the scope of this text. This section focuses on regions of the CNS that have applications to neuropharmacology. For a more complete discussion of CNS anatomy, the student should consult anatomy and physiology textbooks. Basic brain structures are illustrated in Figure 17.2.

Cerebrum: The cerebrum is the "thinking" part of the brain responsible for perception, speech, conscious motor movement, movement of skeletal muscles, memory, and smell. It is the largest part of the brain, by weight, and the most advanced. Portions of the cerebrum are organized for specialized functions. For example, the occipital lobe is associated with vision and the frontal lobes are concerned with reasoning and planning. Other areas are specific to language, hearing, motor, or sensory functions.

Disorders of the cerebrum may be focal or generalized. Focal abnormalities, often the result of a stroke, occur in specific regions and may affect a single brain function such as vision, hearing, or movement of a particular limb. Generalized disorders of the cerebrum affect widespread areas or multiple regions and can produce drowsiness, coma, hallucinations, depression, or generalized anxiety.

Thalamus: The thalamus is the major relay center in the brain that sends sensory information such as sounds, sights, pain, touch, and temperature to the cerebral cortex for analysis. To reach the cerebrum, all sensory information must travel through the thalamus. Portions of the thalamus comprise the limbic system, an area that controls mood and motivation. Abnormalities of the thalamus have been associated with diverse mood disorders such as obsessive–compulsive disorder, bipolar disorder, anxiety, and panic disorder.

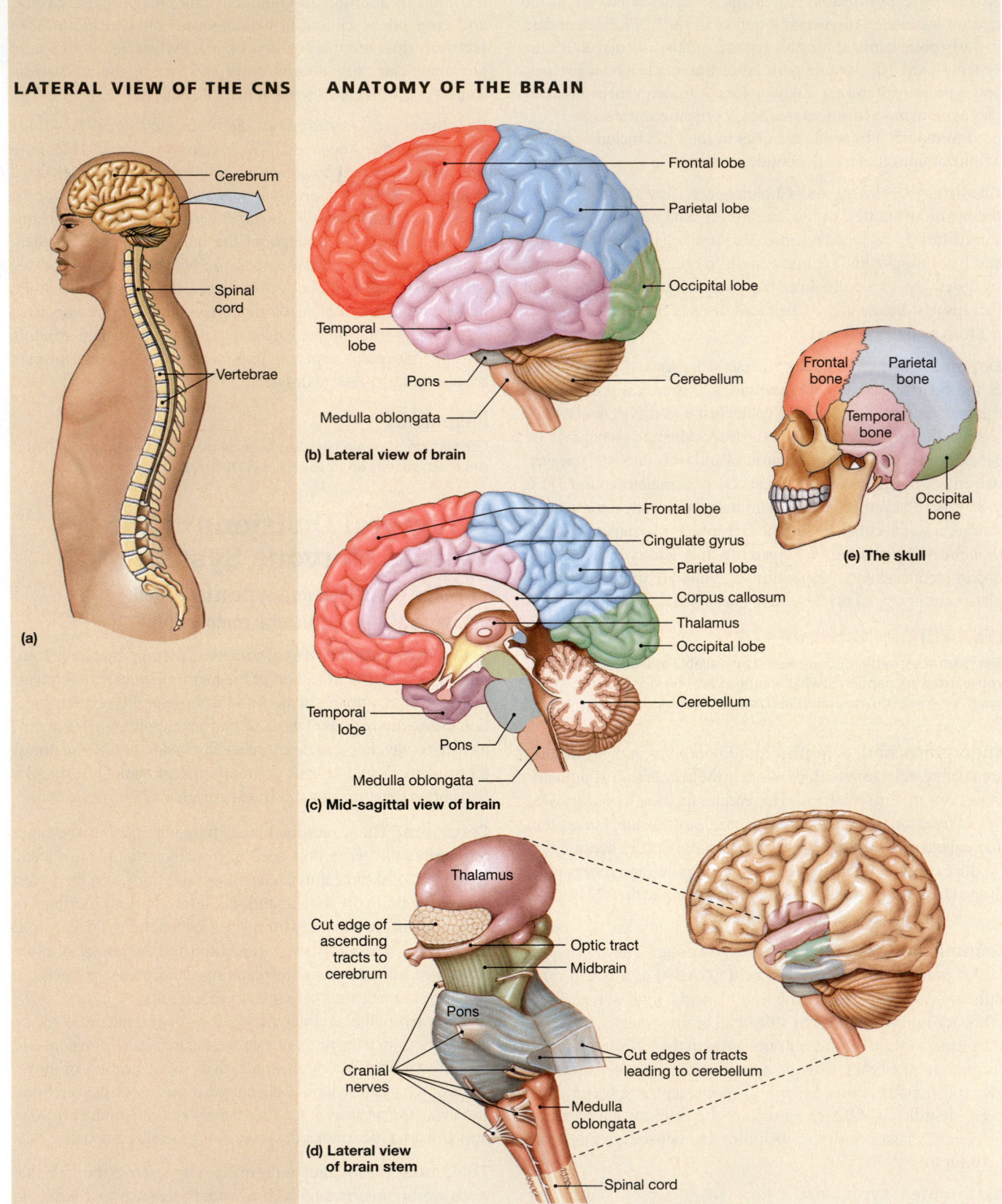

Figure 17.2 Basic anatomy of the brain.

From *Human Physiology: An Integrated Approach* (2nd ed.) by D. U. Silverthorn, 2001. Reprinted and electronically reproduced by permission of Pearson Education, Inc., Upper Saddle River, NJ.

Hypothalamus: The hypothalamus is the major visceral control center in the body. Regulation of hunger, thirst, water balance, and body temperature are functions of this region. The hypothalamus is also part of the limbic system, which is associated with emotional balance. Some neurons in the hypothalamus connect to the brainstem to affect vital centers such as heart rate, respiratory rate, blood pressure, and pupil size. These responses are associated with the fight-or-flight response of the ANS. The many endocrine functions of the hypothalamus are discussed in Chapter 65. Disorders of the hypothalamus may affect some or all of these essential functions.

CONNECTION Checkpoint 17.3

From what you learned in Chapter 12, describe the symptoms of the fight-or-flight response. *See Answer to Connection Checkpoint 17.3 on student resource website.*

Cerebellum: The cerebellum controls muscle movement, balance, posture, and tone. It is involved in learning fine motor skills that make muscular movements smooth and continuous. The cerebellum receives sensory information, including vision, position, equilibrium, and touch, and calculates the strength and extent of muscle movement needed to maintain posture and coordinate complex tasks such as walking, driving, or playing a musical instrument. Injury or disease in this region results in uncoordinated, jerky body movements.

Brainstem: The brainstem, consisting of the medulla oblongata, pons, and midbrain, connects the spinal cord to the brain. Because of its critical location, it serves as the major relay center for messages traveling to and from the brain. In addition, it contains major reflex and control centers involving breathing, heart rate, vision, swallowing, coughing, and vomiting. Injury to the brainstem can be fatal if vital centers are disrupted. The brainstem contains clusters of scattered neurons known as the reticular formation, which help maintain alertness.

Spinal cord: The spinal cord is essentially a conduction pathway to and from the brain. Disruptions of these pathways will prevent transmission of nerve impulses and cause loss of sensory (paresthesia) or motor (paralysis) function.

Blood–brain barrier: The brain must receive a continuous supply of oxygen and glucose; interruptions for even brief periods may cause loss of consciousness. At the same time it needs large quantities of nutrients, the brain must also protect itself from pathogens or toxins that may have entered the blood. Capillaries in most regions of the brain are not as porous as those in other organs; the endothelial cells form tight junctions, creating a seal or barrier to many substances. This is important to pharmacology because CNS drugs must have the capability of penetrating the blood–brain barrier to produce their effects. The blood–brain barrier is illustrated in Figure 17.3.

Functional Systems of the Central Nervous System

17.4 Several functional divisions of the central nervous system are important to pharmacotherapy.

Functional brain systems are clusters of neurons that work together to perform a common function. These clusters may be located far apart from each other in the CNS but they form a network that acts

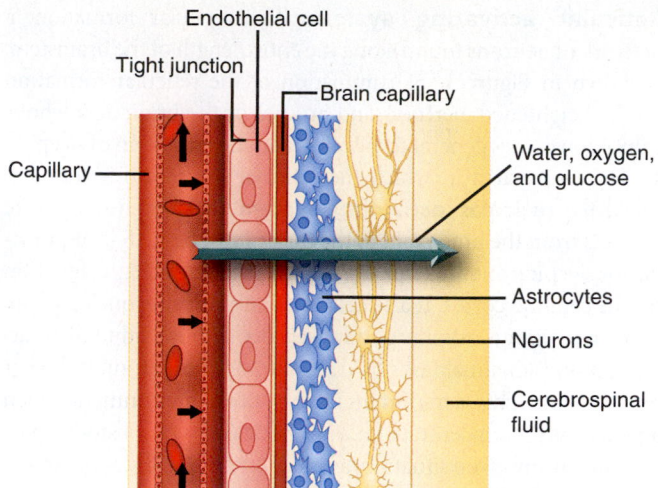

Figure 17.3 Blood–brain barrier.

as a coordinated unit. Some CNS drugs produce their effects by modifying the functions of these systems.

Limbic system: The **limbic system** is a group of structures deep in the brain that are responsible for emotional expression, learning, and memory. Emotional states associated with this system include anxiety, fear, anger, aggression, remorse, depression, sexual drive, and euphoria. Signals routed through the limbic system ultimately connect with the hypothalamus (see Section 17.3). Through its connection with the hypothalamus, autonomic actions such as rapid heart rate, high blood pressure, or peptic ulcers are associated with intense emotional states. The limbic system also communicates with the cerebrum, which allows people to think and reflect on their emotional states. The connection to the cerebrum allows one to use logic to "override" emotional reactions that might be inappropriate or harmful. Parts of the limbic system also allow one to remember emotional responses. The components of the limbic system are illustrated in Figure 17.4.

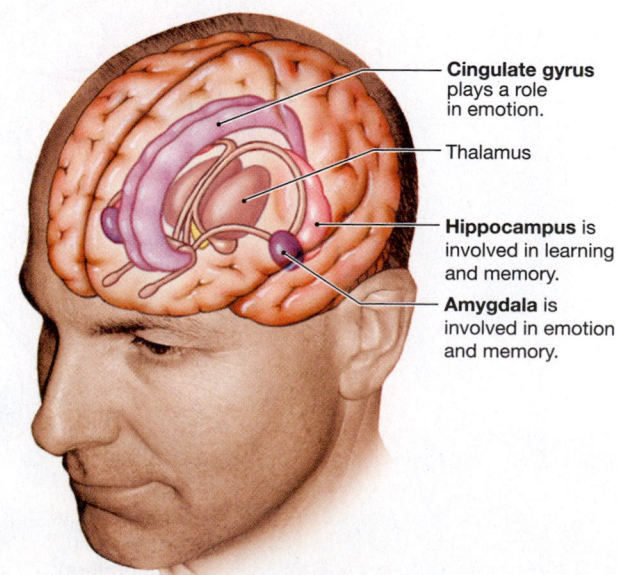

Figure 17.4 Limbic system.
From *Human Physiology: An Integrated Approach* (4th ed.), by D. U. Silverthorn, 2007. Reprinted and electronically reproduced by permission of Pearson Education, Inc., Upper Saddle River, NJ.

Reticular activating system: The reticular formation, a network of neurons found along the entire length of the brainstem, is shown in Figure 17.5. Stimulation of the reticular formation causes heightened alertness and arousal of the brain as a whole. Inhibition causes general drowsiness and the induction of sleep.

The larger area in which the reticular formation is found is called the **reticular activating system (RAS)**. This structure projects from the brainstem to the thalamus. The RAS is responsible for sleeping and wakefulness and performs an alerting function for the cerebral cortex. It also acts as a filter, allowing one to ignore weak, repetitious, or unimportant sensory stimuli and to focus attention on individual tasks by transmitting information to higher brain centers. This is important in busy, noisy environments when a person must concentrate on a specific task, such as studying or reading. In any given situation, as much as 99% of all sensory information may be filtered and never reach consciousness.

The RAS has particular importance to pharmacology because many drugs act by decreasing neuronal activity in this system to cause drowsiness or sleep. Examples include alcohol and sedative–hypnotics. Lysergic acid diethylamide (LSD) interferes with portions of the RAS, causing unusual sensory experiences such as seeing odors or hearing colors.

Basal nuclei: The **basal nuclei**, also called basal ganglia, are a cluster of neurons in the brain that help regulate the initiation and termination of skeletal muscle movement. They also help initiate and terminate certain cognitive functions such as memory, learning, planning, and attention. Connections between the basal ganglia and the limbic system are thought to be associated with psychoses, attention deficit/hyperactivity disorder, and obsessive–acompulsive disorder. Reduced dopaminergic transmission through the basal ganglia is the most common etiology for Parkinson's disease. The basal ganglia are illustrated in Figure 17.6.

Extrapyramidal system: Messages controlling the voluntary movement of skeletal muscle originate in the cerebrum and travel down the CNS in tracts or pathways. The two motor pathways, traveling through the brain, brainstem, and spinal cord, are called pyramidal (direct) and extrapyramidal (indirect). The pyramidal tracts are voluntary tracts involved with the movement of skeletal muscles. The **extrapyramidal system** controls locomotion, complex muscular movements, and posture. The extrapyramidal system has particular importance to pharmacology because it is adversely affected by certain medications, especially the conventional antipsychotic agents (see Chapter 20). Adverse extrapyramidal symptoms include jerking motions, muscular spasms of the head, face, and neck, and akathisia, an inability to remain at rest. Some extrapyramidal symptoms resemble those of Parkinson's disease (see Chapter 21).

PharmFACT

Some of the postsynaptic neurons connect with and receive information from as many as 150,000 presynaptic neurons (Silverthorn, 2012).

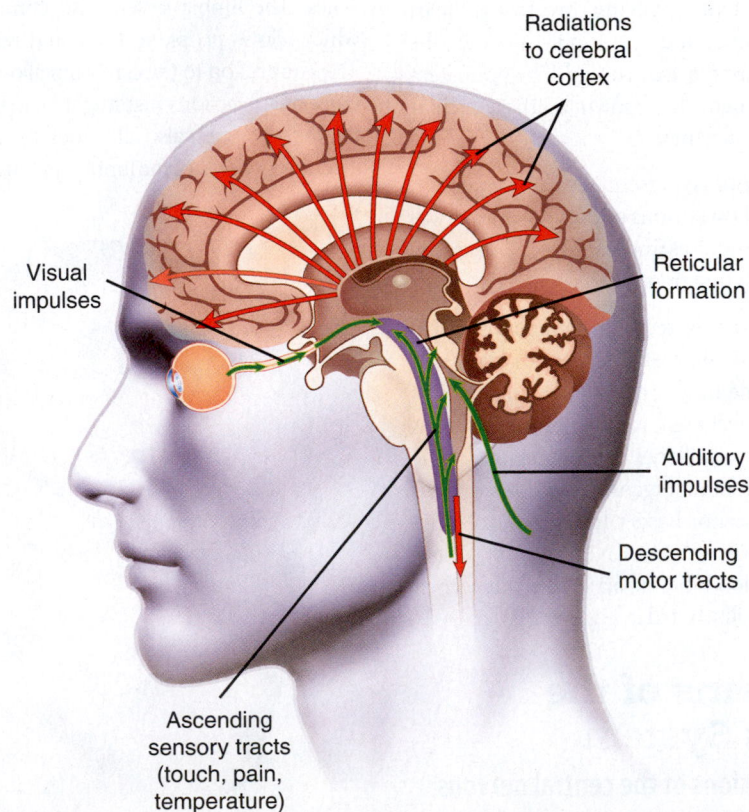

Figure 17.5 With input from sensory neurons, activation of the reticular activating system causes arousal of the cerebral cortex, thus maintaining the awake-and-alert state.

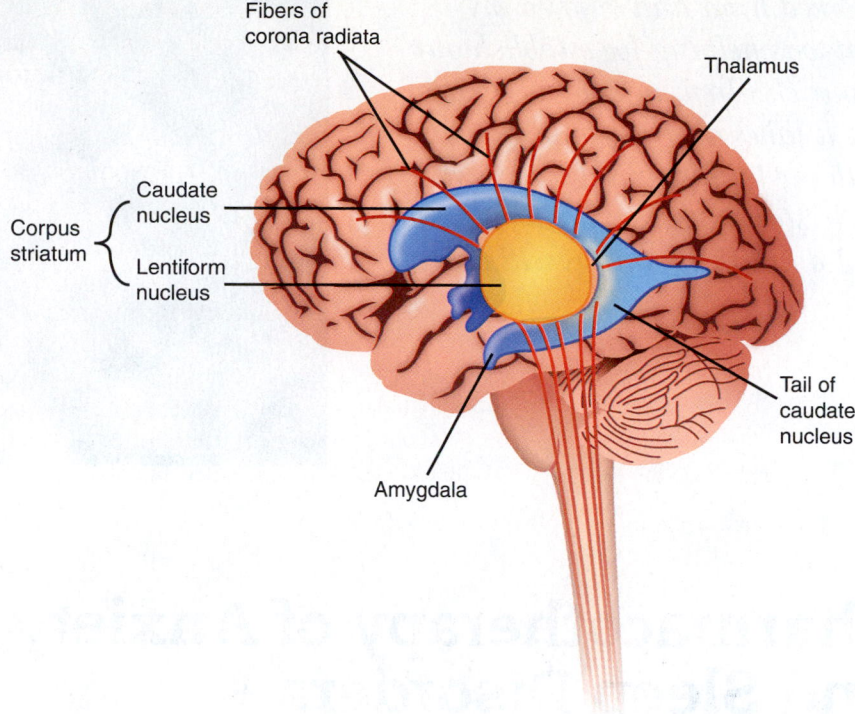

Figure 17.6 The basal ganglia are clusters of gray matter that control learned movement and are involved with the subconscious control of skeletal muscle tone.

Understanding the Chapter

Key Concepts Summary

17.1 Medications affect the central nervous system by stimulating or suppressing the firing of specific neurons.

17.2 Neurons in the central nervous system communicate with each other and with body tissues, using neurotransmitters.

17.3 The central nervous system is divided into several major structural components.

17.4 Several functional divisions of the central nervous system are important to pharmacotherapy.

References

Isik, A. T. (2010). Late onset Alzheimer's disease in older people. *Clinical Interventions in Aging, 5,* 307–311. doi:10.2147/CIA.S11718

Silverthorn, D. U. (2012). *Human physiology: An integrated approach* (6th ed.). San Francisco, CA: Benjamin Cummings.

Selected Bibliography

Krogh, D. (2011). *Biology: A guide to the natural world* (5th ed.). San Francisco, CA: Benjamin Cummings.

Marieb, E. N., & Hoehn, K. (2013). *Human anatomy and physiology* (9th ed.). San Francisco, CA: Benjamin Cummings.

Martini, F. H., Nath, J. L., & Bartholomew, E. F. (2012). *Fundamentals of human anatomy and physiology* (9th ed.). San Francisco, CA: Benjamin Cummings.

Westfall, T. C., & Westfall, D. P. (2011). Neurotransmission: The autonomic and somatic

motor nervous systems. In L. L. Brunton, B. A. Chabner, & B. C. Knollman (Eds.), *The pharmacological basis of therapeutics* (12th ed., pp. 171–218). New York, NY: McGraw-Hill.

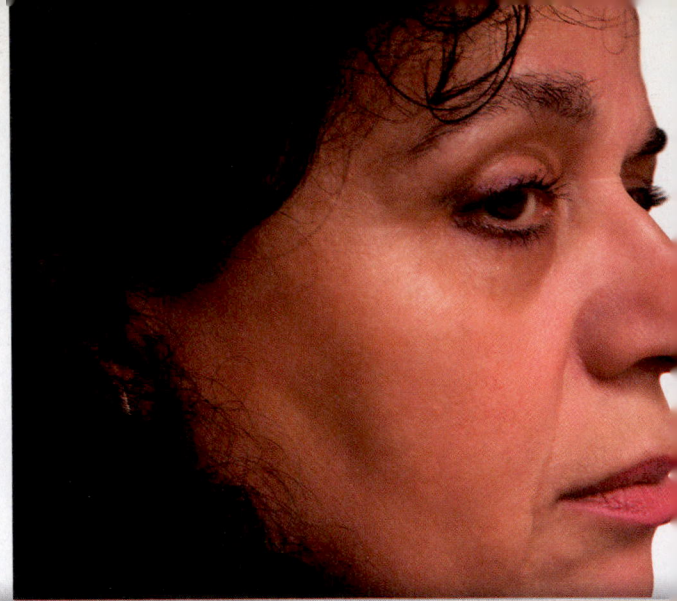

"I've always worked hard and enjoyed my work, whether it was helping Joe establish our home, raising our children, or teaching school. Lately, though, it takes all I've got to get out of bed, deal with my family, and get to work. I just don't understand why my life has taken this turn, and I don't think things will ever improve."

Patient "Seraphina Alvarez"

CHAPTER 18

Pharmacotherapy of Anxiety and Sleep Disorders

LEARNING OUTCOMES

After reading this chapter, the student should be able to:

1. Explain why it is important to obtain an accurate diagnosis of anxiety.
2. Compare and contrast the five major categories of anxiety disorders.
3. Identify the regions and systems of the brain associated with anxiety, sleep, and wakefulness.
4. Describe the normal stages of sleep and explain how they are affected by anxiety and stress.
5. Identify sleep disorders that may benefit from pharmacotherapy.
6. Explain the association between insomnia and anxiety.
7. Describe nonpharmacologic methods for managing anxiety and sleep disorders.
8. Identify the major classes of medications used to treat anxiety and sleep disorders.
9. Describe the nurse's role in the pharmacologic and nonpharmacologic management of anxiety and sleep disorders.
10. For each of the classes shown in the chapter outline, identify the prototype and representative drugs and explain the mechanism(s) of drug action, primary indications, contraindications, significant drug interactions, pregnancy category, and important adverse effects.
11. Develop a plan of care for patients receiving pharmacotherapy for anxiety and sleep disorders.

CHAPTER OUTLINE

▶ Anxiety Disorders

▶ Sleep Disorders

▶ Management of Anxiety and Sleep Disorders

▶ Pharmacotherapy of Anxiety and Insomnia

Benzodiazepines

PROTOTYPE Lorazepam (Ativan), *p. 226*

Nonbenzodiazepine Anxiolytics and Miscellaneous Drugs

PROTOTYPE Zolpidem (Ambien, Edluar, Others), *p. 229*

Antidepressants

Barbiturates

PROTOTYPE Phenobarbital (Luminal), *p. 232*

KEY TERMS

agoraphobia, 218

amygdala, 220

anxiety, 217

anxiolytic, 224

cataplexy, 222

circadian rhythm, 221

generalized anxiety disorder
   (GAD), 218

hypnagogic hallucinations, 222

insomnia, 221

locus coeruleus, 220

narcolepsy, 222

non–rapid eye movement
   (NREM) sleep, 220

obsessive–compulsive disorder
   (OCD), 218

panic disorder, 218

phobia, 218

post-traumatic stress disorder (PTSD), 219

rapid eye movement (REM) sleep, 220

rebound insomnia, 223

sedative–hypnotic, 224

situational anxiety, 218

social anxiety disorder, 218

Anxiety is a generalized feeling of worry, fear, or uneasiness over a perceived threat. This threat, such as an upcoming divorce or pharmacology test, may be clearly identifiable, or it may be an unfocused, general feeling of worry or dread. Anxiety is a normal, adaptive response to stress that prepares a person to deal, both physically and emotionally, with the perceived threat. However, when the anxiety is excessive or irrational, the patient's quality of life may become seriously affected and there will be an increased risk of developing chronic gastrointestinal (GI) and cardiovascular disorders. Anxiety disorders are the most common mental health illnesses encountered in clinical practice. This chapter deals with medications that treat anxiety, cause sedation, or help patients sleep.

Anxiety Disorders

18.1 Proper diagnosis of anxiety disorders is important to identifying the most effective treatment option.

In the clinical setting, most patients with anxiety will present with multiple symptoms and describe their condition in diverse ways. Patients often describe their feelings using terms such as *apprehension, dread, fear,* or *worry*. Anxiety activates the sympathetic nervous system and triggers symptoms of the flight-or-fright response such as rapid heart rate, shortness of breath, hypertension, pounding in the ears, excessive sweating, or dry mouth. Most patients readily admit that their feelings of anxiety are disproportionate to any real threats or dangers. A diagram of how people typically deal with stressful events is shown in Figure 18.1.

It is often challenging for the nurse to sort through the many diverse and subjective patient symptoms to determine the etiology of the anxiety. Patients may be unclear as to why they are feeling anxious, or they may be reluctant to discuss the causes because they may be deeply personal. The health care provider must accurately diagnose the condition, however, because treatment differs among the various types of anxiety disorders. In some cases pharmacotherapy may not be the best option. Anxiety is a disorder that responds well to complementary and alternative medicine (CAM), and the nurse is a key person to recommend and teach patients nonpharmacologic stress-reduction techniques. Some patients benefit from individual or group psychotherapy, which can help to identify and overcome the root causes of their worry and fear. Some anxiety disorders, however, are debilitating and require effective pharmacotherapy.

When obtaining a comprehensive medication history during the initial patient assessment, the nurse should note any

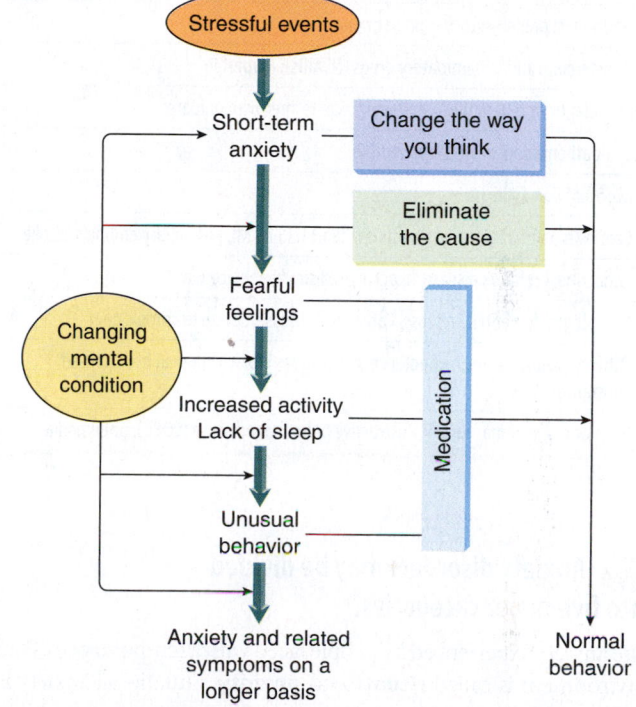

Figure 18.1 Anxiety model. Stressful events lead to symptoms of anxiety, which can be resolved by coping mechanisms or medication.

substances that the patient is taking that may worsen or cause anxiety symptoms. Sometimes discontinuing or substituting alternate drugs for these "anxiety-promoting" medications can lessen patient symptoms. A simple example is substituting decaffeinated beverages for those containing caffeine. In addition, many medical conditions are associated with anxiety symptoms. For example, knowing that one has cancer or has a high risk for myocardial infarction (MI) certainly creates high stress for a patient. In these cases, the anxiety is considered secondary and may resolve once the underlying medical condition is treated. Drugs and medical conditions associated with anxiety disorders are shown in Table 18.1.

CONNECTION Checkpoint 18.1

From what you learned in Chapter 12, which classes of autonomic drugs would be most likely to cause anxiety as a side effect: sympathomimetics, parasympathomimetics, adrenergic blockers, or cholinergic blockers? *See Answer to Connection Checkpoint 18.1 on student resource website.*

TABLE 18.1 Medications and Medical Conditions Associated with Anxiety

Medications

Antibiotics: isoniazid, fluoroquinolones

Antidepressants: bupropion, selective serotonin reuptake inhibitors (SSRIs), tricyclic antidepressants (TCAs)

Antihypertensives: felodipine, methyldopa

Antiseizure drugs: carbamazepine

Bronchodilators: albuterol, theophylline

Hallucinogens: ecstasy, LSD

Hormones: prednisone, thyroid hormone

Nonsteroidal anti-inflammatory drugs (NSAIDs): ibuprofen

Stimulants: amphetamines, caffeine, cocaine, methylphenidate

Sympathomimetics: pseudoephedrine

Medical Conditions

Cardiovascular: angina, dysrhythmias, heart failure, MI, pulmonary embolus, stroke

Endocrine: Cushing's disease, hyperthyroidism, hypoglycemia

Neurologic: dementia, epilepsy, Parkinson's disease, severe or chronic pain

Others: anemias, cancer, impotence, nausea, vertigo, withdrawal from abused substances

Respiratory: asthma, chronic obstructive pulmonary disease (COPD), pneumonia

18.2 Anxiety disorders may be divided into five major categories.

The anxiety experienced by people faced with a temporary stressful environment is called **situational anxiety**. Situational anxiety is not considered a major anxiety disorder because it is not disabling or persistent. To a degree, situational anxiety is beneficial because it motivates people to accomplish tasks in a prompt manner—if for no other reason than to eliminate the source of nervousness. All persons experience situational stress at some time in their lives and, although it may be intense, it does not generally require pharmacotherapy.

Anxiety requires treatment when it becomes chronic and interferes with activities of daily living (ADLs) or begins to result in long-term physical damage such as heart disease. Anxiety disorders may be divided into several major categories: generalized anxiety disorder, panic disorder, social anxiety disorder, obsessive–compulsive disorder, and post-traumatic stress disorder. Not all anxiety experienced by patients is easily classified, and it is common for people to present with multiple types of anxiety, such as generalized anxiety disorder along with panic attacks.

PharmFACT

About 40 million Americans, or 18% of the population, are affected by anxiety disorders. Illnesses that commonly coexist with anxiety include depression, eating disorders, and substance abuse (Anxiety and Depression Association of America, n.d.).

Generalized anxiety disorder (GAD) is excessive anxiety that persists for 6 months or longer. GAD has a gradual onset and is most prevalent in the 20- to 35-year-old age group. The characteristic feature of GAD is excessive worry or fear regarding life events or activities, frequently focusing on family, money, or health. Symptoms include restlessness, fatigue, muscle tension, nervousness, inability to focus or concentrate, an overwhelming sense of dread, and sleep disturbances. Signs of sympathetic nervous system activation that accompany GAD include blood pressure elevation, heart palpitations, varying degrees of respiratory change, and dry mouth. Parasympathetic responses may consist of abdominal cramping, diarrhea, fatigue, and urinary urgency. Some patients experience symptoms for over a decade before seeking help for their condition.

Panic disorder is a type of anxiety characterized by intense feelings of immediate apprehension, fearfulness, terror, or impending doom, accompanied by increased autonomic nervous system activity such as sweating, racing heart rate, shortness of breath, and trembling. To be diagnosed with panic disorder, the patient must present with at least 1 month of ongoing concern or worry about experiencing subsequent episodes. Panic attacks typically last only 1 to 10 minutes, although one attack may quickly follow another and patients may describe the episode as seemingly endless. Up to 5% of the population will experience one or more panic attacks during their lifetime, with women being affected about twice as often as men. Patients with panic disorder usually modify their behavior to try to avoid another attack. Some develop **agoraphobia**, an extreme avoidance of closed places where a panic attack might occur such as airplanes, public meetings, or elevators. Panic attacks are often associated with major depression.

Social anxiety disorder, also called social phobia, is an unreasonable and persistent fear of being judged, ridiculed, or embarrassed by others. Performing and speaking in public are two common examples of activities that may trigger social anxiety disorder. Patients will either avoid the situation entirely or tolerate it with great discomfort. Symptoms include sweating, blushing, tachycardia, trembling, and bowel cramping or diarrhea. The average age of onset is the midteens, and the disorder may persist for decades before the person seeks treatment. Social anxiety disorder is a type of **phobia**, a fearful feeling attached to situations or objects. In addition to social anxiety disorder, specific phobias include fear of snakes, spiders, high altitudes, or exposure to blood. Panic attacks may occur when the person encounters his or her specific phobia; for example, when the person sees blood or is forced to speak or perform in public.

Obsessive–compulsive disorder (OCD) involves recurrent, intrusive thoughts or repetitive behaviors. To be diagnosed with OCD, the behavior or thought must occupy more than 1 hour each day and negatively impact the patient's normal daily activities or relationships. The obsession portion of this behavior involves thoughts, whereas the compulsion portion involves actions. Most patients with this disorder have both obsessions and compulsions. One common example is repetitive thoughts about the fear of exposure to germs. The patient may think about the presence of germs constantly and what can be done to decrease exposure (obsession). The person may engage in repetitive hand washing, possibly to the point of doing damage to the skin of the hands (compulsion). This repetitive activity can occur so frequently that it severely intrudes on the person's ability to do any other activity during the day, including work or school. Other obsessions or compulsions include viewing sexually explicit pictures, doubting whether the iron or stove was turned off, repeating the same words silently, or repetitive counting. Most commonly, the age of onset is the teen years or early adulthood.

Post-traumatic stress disorder (PTSD) is a type of situational anxiety that develops in response to reexperiencing a previous life event. Witnessing or experiencing traumatic events such as combat, physical or sexual abuse, torture, natural disasters, or murder may lead to a sense of helplessness and reexperiencing of the event. The reexperience may take the form of nightmares, hallucinations, or flashbacks, accompanied by uncomfortable physical signs such as tachycardia and extreme nervousness or panic attacks. If the reaction occurs immediately and resolves within 1 month of the event, it is classified as acute stress disorder. To be diagnosed with PTSD the patient must experience distressing symptoms for more than 1 month. Approximately 30% of men and women who have spent time in a war zone experience PTSD (Gore, 2013). The risk of suicide attempts among those diagnosed with PTSD is six times greater than in the general population and even higher among war veterans with PTSD (Sher, 2009).

PharmFACT

For three anxiety disorders, women are twice as likely to be affected as men. These disorders include GAD, panic disorder, and specific phobias (Anxiety and Depression Association of America, n.d.).

18.3 Specific regions of the brain have been identified that are responsible for anxiety.

Research has clearly demonstrated that the modulation of anxiety is accomplished in specific brain regions and by multiple neurotransmitter systems. Neuroimaging studies show that the different types of anxiety disorders activate distinct areas of the brain. Neural pathways associated with GAD, social anxiety disorder, and panic disorder are different.

Neural systems in the brain that are associated with anxiety include the limbic system and the reticular activating system. These are shown in Pharmacotherapy Illustrated 18.1. The student should read Section 17.4 in Chapter 17 for a brief review of these two systems before proceeding.

The limbic system is a cluster of structures in the middle of the brain that is responsible for governing emotions, behavior, and

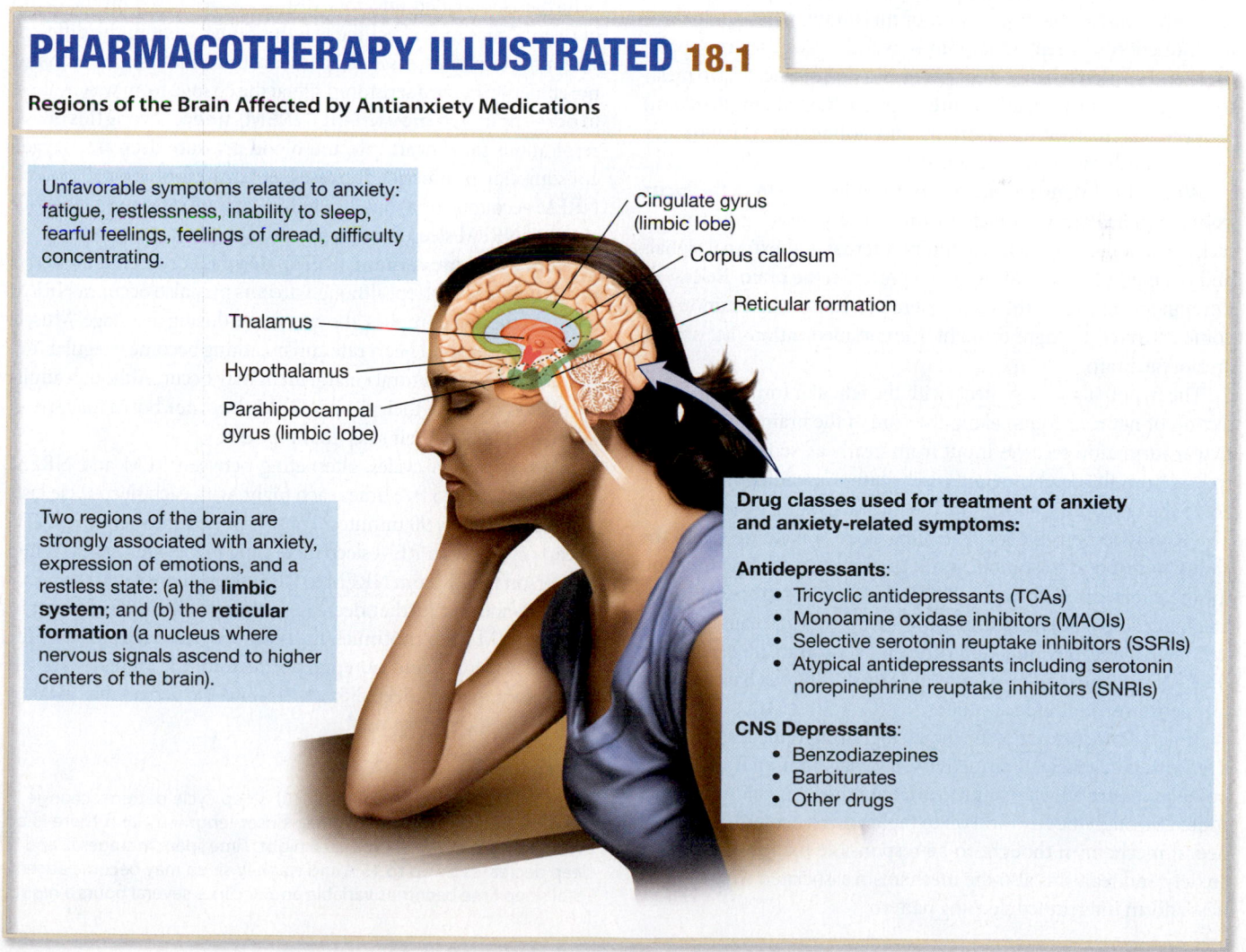

PHARMACOTHERAPY ILLUSTRATED 18.1

Regions of the Brain Affected by Antianxiety Medications

Unfavorable symptoms related to anxiety: fatigue, restlessness, inability to sleep, fearful feelings, feelings of dread, difficulty concentrating.

Cingulate gyrus (limbic lobe)

Corpus callosum

Reticular formation

Thalamus

Hypothalamus

Parahippocampal gyrus (limbic lobe)

Two regions of the brain are strongly associated with anxiety, expression of emotions, and a restless state: (a) the **limbic system**; and (b) the **reticular formation** (a nucleus where nervous signals ascend to higher centers of the brain).

Drug classes used for treatment of anxiety and anxiety-related symptoms:

Antidepressants:
- Tricyclic antidepressants (TCAs)
- Monoamine oxidase inhibitors (MAOIs)
- Selective serotonin reuptake inhibitors (SSRIs)
- Atypical antidepressants including serotonin norepinephrine reuptake inhibitors (SNRIs)

CNS Depressants:
- Benzodiazepines
- Barbiturates
- Other drugs

long-term memory. A key part of the limbic system that is involved in the pathogenesis of anxiety is the **amygdala**, the center of human emotions. The amygdala helps determine the emotional significance of the conscious and subconscious signals received from the cerebral cortex. Once activated the amygdala generates feelings of anxiety and fear and stimulates several regions of the brain that begin the stress response. For example, the midbrain and brainstem may be activated, resulting in stress symptoms related to the autonomic nervous system, such as high blood pressure, elevated breathing rate, and dilated pupils.

Signals routed through the amygdala ultimately connect with the hypothalamus, an important center responsible for modulating the fight-or-flight response of the autonomic nervous system. Emotional states associated with this connection include anxiety, fear, anger, aggression, remorse, depression, sexual drive, and euphoria. The hypothalamus may respond by secreting corticotropin-releasing factor (CRF), which causes the release of corticosteroids from the adrenal glands. Corticosteroids are major modulators of the long-term stress response (see Chapter 68). The hypothalamus also regulates essential somatic functions, including sleep, appetite, and body temperature.

An area in the anterior hypothalamus, called the suprachiasmatic nucleus, receives input from the retina, providing information about the amount of ambient (environmental) light. This structure controls the production of melatonin, which influences the induction of sleep. Melatonin is available as a dietary supplement and is often taken to treat jet lag and sleeplessness. Two melatonin agonists are available by prescription. Ramelteon (Rozerem) is approved for treating insomnia and tasimelteon (Hetlioz) for sleep–wake disorder (see Section 18.9).

Within the brainstem, an area in the pons known as the **locus coeruleus** has been associated with fear responses and panic attacks. The locus coeruleus monitors internal and external signals and is a major location for norepinephrine in the brain. Release of norepinephrine from the locus coeruleus causes the brain to become activated for fight or flight. Certain medications act on this area of the brain.

The hypothalamus connects with the reticular formation, a collection of neurons found along the core of the brainstem. The reticular formation receives input from nearly all sensory organs as well as from the cerebrum and cerebellum. Ascending fibers project to the cerebrum to form the reticular activating system (RAS). The RAS is responsible for regulating sleep, wakefulness, and the ability to respond to stimuli, and it performs an alerting function for the entire cerebral cortex. Drugs that stimulate the RAS cause heightened alertness and arousal; inhibitory drugs cause general drowsiness and the induction of sleep. Neurotransmitters within the RAS regulate the sleep–wake cycle by shifting the balance from one neurotransmitter to another.

If signals are prevented from passing through the RAS, there is a reduction in general brain activity. If signals coming from the hypothalamus are allowed to proceed, then those signals are further routed through the RAS and on to higher brain centers. This is the neural mechanism thought to be responsible for feelings such as anxiety and fear. It is also the mechanism associated with restlessness and an interrupted sleeping pattern.

Sleep Disorders

18.4 Sleep occurs in distinct stages.

The process of sleep has been well studied. It has been established that all people need an adequate amount of sleep to function optimally, although the amounts change throughout the lifespan. For middle-aged adults, 7 to 8 hours of sleep appear to be adequate. Most older adults sleep less than 8 hours, and infants and babies require much more sleep. Although it is known that sleep is essential for wellness, scientists are unsure of its function or how much is needed to maintain optimum health. Following are some theories:

1. Inactivity during sleep gives the body time to repair itself.

2. Sleep is a function that evolved as a protective mechanism. Throughout history, nighttime was the safest time of day for resting.

3. Sleep involves "electrical" charging and discharging of the brain. The brain needs time for processing and filing new information collected throughout the day. When this is done without interference from the outside environment, these vast amounts of data can be retrieved later through memory.

Sleep occurs in two basic phases: rapid eye movement (REM) sleep and non–rapid eye movement (NREM) sleep. NREM sleep is further subdivided into four distinct stages based on the depth of sleep. Drugs may affect the length of time spent in the different stages of sleep. Decreases in the neurotransmitters acetylcholine, norepinephrine, and serotonin signal the change from wakefulness to **non–rapid eye movement (NREM) sleep**. During this phase, respirations slow, heart rate and blood pressure decrease, oxygen consumption by muscles decreases, and urine formation decreases. NREM accounts for about 75% to 85% of total sleep time. The four stages of NREM sleep are described in Table 18.2.

Rapid eye movement (REM) sleep is considered the active dreaming stage of sleep, although dreams may also occur in NREM sleep. As the name implies, the eyes move during this stage. Muscle tone diminishes and heart rate and breathing become irregular. Penile erections and clitoral enlargement may occur. Although adults spend about 25% of their sleep in REM sleep, newborns may spend as much as 80% of their sleep in this phase.

Sleep occurs in cycles, alternating between REM and NREM sleep about four to five times each night, with each sleep cycle lasting approximately 90 minutes. There is more time spent in NREM in early cycles, with REM sleep increasing in the later cycles. When the person moves from NREM to REM sleep, there is an increase of acetylcholine and further decreases in serotonin and norepinephrine. As REM sleep continues, the body progressively increases the levels of serotonin and norepinephrine until the amounts are adequate to stop REM sleep. For a brief time, the person may awaken until the next cycle begins.

PharmFACT

According to Reeve and Balles (2010), sleep cycle patterns change in the older adult. The time for sleep onset lengthens, and there is an average of eight awakenings each night. Time spent in stages III and IV sleep decreases by up to 15% and stage IV sleep may become absent. Total sleep time becomes variable and declines several hours a night.

TABLE 18.2	Stages of Sleep
Stage of Sleep	**Description**
NREM stage I	At the onset of sleep, the patient experiences drowsiness for 1 to 7 min. During this time, the patient can be easily awakened. This stage of sleep is so light that when awakened from it, persons often deny that they were asleep. Respirations slow, muscles relax. This stage lasts for about 4–5% of total sleep time.
NREM stage II	Although deeper than stage I, the patient can still be easily awakened. This stage constitutes the greatest amount of total sleep time, 45–55%.
NREM stage III	This is the period in which a person may experience nightmares, bedwetting, or sleep walking. Heart rate and blood pressure fall; GI activity rises. This stage lasts for about 4–6% of total sleep time.
NREM stage IV	The deepest stage of sleep, this comprises about 12–15% of total sleep time. Dreams that occur are usually thoughtlike and revolve around current concerns or recent events with little story line. This is the stage during which nightmares occur in children. Sleepwalking is also a common behavior for this stage. Heart rate and blood pressure remain low; GI activity remains high.
REM sleep	This stage is characterized by eye movement and a loss of muscle tone. Eye movement occurs in bursts of activity. Dreaming takes place in this stage; dreams are vivid, emotional, storylike, and frequently bizarre. The mind is very active and resembles a normal waking state.

CONNECTIONS Community-Oriented Practice

◀ Residual Sedative Effects of Antihistamines

Antihistamines, particularly the older first-generation "sedating" forms such as diphenhydramine (Benadryl, Sominex, others), are commonly found in over-the-counter (OTC) sleep remedies. While the drowsiness and sedation caused by these drugs may be an annoying side effect when the drugs are used for allergies, it is this property that helps to induce sleep when used for nighttime sedation. Concerns about residual daytime sleepiness and effects on cognitive function, a so-called hangover effect, have been hard to quantify by subjective measures such as patient self-reported sleepiness. In a research study using positron-emission tomography (PET) scanning, which measures functional activity in the brain, Zhang et al. (2010) measured brain binding ratios of diphenhydramine, a newer "nonsedating" antihistamine (bepotastine), and a placebo. For as long as 12 hours after the nighttime dose of diphenhydramine, significant amounts of the drug remained bound to brain receptors, unlike the nonsedating drug or placebo. There was no statistical significance noted in any of the subjective sleepiness ratings as reported by the subjects. The length of binding, and the potential for causing even subtle changes in cognitive functioning, raises concerns.

Antihistamines, particularly older first-generation drugs, are known to reduce REM sleep, have cognitive effects on learning, and are of particular concern in the older adult (Church et al., 2010). Patients who use OTC antihistamine sleep aids should be cautioned about the potential for daytime drowsiness but should also be taught that more subtle effects may occur, such as slowed reaction time, impaired cognitive function, and other systemic effects, even when daytime drowsiness is not evident.

Patients who are deprived of stage IV NREM experience depression and a feeling of apathy and fatigue. Stage IV NREM sleep appears to be linked to repair and restoration of the physical body, whereas REM sleep is associated with learning, memory, and the capacity to adjust to changes in the environment. The body requires the dream state associated with REM sleep to keep the psyche functioning normally. When deprived of REM sleep, people experience a sleep deficit and become frightened, irritable, paranoid, and even emotionally disturbed. Judgment is impaired, and reaction time is slowed. It is speculated that to make up for their lack of dreaming, these persons experience far more daydreaming and fantasizing throughout the day. The stages of sleep are shown in Table 18.2.

There is a wide variation in sleep patterns among adults. Some people do very well with less sleep, whereas others require above-average amounts to feel refreshed and mentally alert. Most people, even young adults, awaken at least once during the night; the elderly awaken more frequently. The nurse can be a valuable ally to the patient experiencing sleep disturbances by explaining these normal variations and by assisting the patient to reach a desirable sleep pattern.

The acts of sleeping and waking are synchronized with many different bodily functions. Body temperature, blood pressure, hormone levels, and respiration all fluctuate on a cyclic basis throughout the 24-hour day, known as the **circadian rhythm**. Even without realizing it, people who are "day persons" or "night persons" structure their activities, even their occupations, around what they recognize as their best individual pattern of sleep and wakefulness. *Circadian dysrhythm* refers to the psychological and biologic stress a person undergoes when traveling rapidly through several time zones, such as during a long airplane journey. "Jet lag" is a very real, and sometimes disabling, phenomenon, although not a permanent dysfunction. When this cycle becomes impaired, pharmacologic or other interventions may be needed to readjust it. Circadian rhythms are based on many complex variables, including light–dark cycles and secretion of hormones such as melatonin. Biologic rhythms likely exist in all living things and have even been identified in bacteria.

18.5 Sleep disorders affect a large percentage of the population.

A sleep disorder is a disturbance in the normal pattern, quality, or quantity of sleep. It is estimated that 40 million Americans experience sleep disorders. Although about 70 specific types of sleep-related disorders have been identified, pharmacotherapy is beneficial in treating only a few of them. Examples of common sleep disorders are shown in Table 18.3.

Insomnia is the most common sleep disorder and the one that is the most frequent indication for pharmacotherapy. Insomnia can be simply defined as the lack of adequate sleep; however, the disorder can be better explained by the following terms:

- **Sleep-onset insomnia.** Inability to fall asleep within a reasonable time, usually more than 30 minutes

TABLE 18.3 Examples of Sleep Disorders

Type	Example(s)
Circadian rhythm sleep disorders	Time zone syndrome (jet lag), shift work sleep disorder
Hypersomnias of central origin	Narcoplexy (with or without cataplexy)
Insomnia	Acute, chronic, transient
Parasomnias	Sleepwalking, sleep terrors, nightmares
Sleep-related breathing disorders	Sleep apnea
Sleep-related movement disorders	Restless leg syndrome

- **Sleep-maintenance insomnia.** Frequent awakenings during the night or the inability to fall back asleep
- **Sleep-offset insomnia.** Premature, early morning awakenings
- **Nonrestorative sleep.** Persistent sleepiness during the day, despite adequate sleep duration

The diagnosis of chronic insomnia is determined by its duration (at least 30 days or more) and the degree to which it affects ADLs. The most frequent symptom reported by patients is excessive daytime drowsiness.

Insomnia has multiple causes and often presents secondary to an underlying disorder. Examples of conditions causing secondary insomnia are shown in Table 18.4. The best approach to resolving secondary insomnia is to treat the underlying disorder. Insomnia not associated with another medical, psychiatric, or medication-related cause is considered to be *primary*.

A thorough medical history can sometimes distinguish between primary and secondary insomnia; however, for objective testing patients are referred to sleep disorder specialists for polysomnography and actigraphy. Polysomnography is a series of tests that record physiological changes occurring during sleep, including eye movement, muscle tension, respiration, cardiac rhythm, and brain wave activity. Polysomnography can also determine the amount of REM and NREM sleep. Brain wave activity is measured using an electroencephalogram (EEG). Actigraphy is another frequently used diagnostic test that measures the motor activity of a patient during waking and sleeping hours. The results of these comprehensive tests can be used to diagnose most sleep disorders.

TABLE 18.4 Causes of Secondary Insomnia

Cause	Description
Drugs	Amphetamines, cocaine, caffeinated beverages, corticosteroids, sympathomimetics, antidepressants, alcohol use, nicotine or tobacco use
Medical disorder	Dementia, anxiety disorder, epilepsy, Parkinson's disease, Tourette's syndrome, psychosis, mania, migraines, asthma, sleep apnea, chronic or severe pain, COPD, gastroesophageal reflux, hyperthyroidism
Poor sleep hygiene	Noisy environment; too much light in the bedroom; large meals; working or exercising just prior to sleeping; partner who snores, talks, or moves frequently during sleep
Stressful situation	Major life event such as marriage, divorce, death of a loved one, chronic or terminal disease, stressful job

In addition to insomnia, **narcolepsy** is a sleep disorder that may respond to pharmacotherapy. Narcolepsy is characterized by severe daytime sleepiness such that the patient is unable to stay awake and may fall asleep quickly and at inappropriate times. An episode of narcolepsy, called a "sleep attack," may last from a few seconds to about 30 minutes. The disorder may start anytime between ages 5 and 50. In addition to the sleep attack, the following four "classic" symptoms are often observed in patients with narcolepsy.

- **Cataplexy** is a sudden loss of muscle strength manifested as slurred speech, sagging of the jaw, head nodding, or even complete collapse of the body. The condition is triggered by strong emotions.
- **Hypnagogic hallucinations** are vivid, fearful sensory illusions that may be experienced at the onset of sleep or on awakening.
- Muscular paralysis may result in the temporary inability to move or speak on awakening.
- Automatic behavior may include actions such as talking or repetitive movements during the sleep episode. The person has no memory of the behavior on awakening.

Pharmacologic treatment for narcolepsy includes stimulants such as amphetamines, methylphenidate, and modafinil (Provigil), which is considered a preferred drug for the disorder. Modafinil is well tolerated and adverse effects such as headache, nausea, nervousness, and anxiety are generally mild. This drug is a Schedule IV controlled substance due to its stimulant properties.

Stimulants such as modafinil are not effective for cataplexy symptoms. Older therapies for cataplexy include antidepressants such as tricyclic antidepressants (TCAs) or selective serotonin reuptake inhibitors (SSRIs). A more recent therapy utilizes sodium oxybate (gamma hydroxybutyrate [GHB], Xyrem). This drug appears to be effective in managing symptoms of both narcolepsy and cataplexy. This substance is very unusual because (as GHB) it has been used illegally to produce euphoria and to enhance sexual stimulation. GHB can cause amnesia and has been implicated in sexual assaults as a "date-rape" drug. Because of these abuses, GHB is listed as a Schedule I drug. However, the same chemical substance, marketed as Xyrem to treat narcolepsy, is a Schedule III drug. It is only available using the Xyrem Success Program, which requires the patient to obtain the drug through a central pharmacy, have regular office visits, and demonstrate understanding about the safety and proper use of the drug. Common adverse effects include headache, nausea, dizziness, and somnolence.

Management of Anxiety and Sleep Disorders

18.6 There is a link between insomnia and anxiety.

The student may be wondering why two seemingly different conditions, anxiety and insomnia, are being presented in the same chapter. There are two fundamental reasons. First, there is a pathophysiologic link between sleep and anxiety, and, second, many of the drugs used to treat anxiety are also effective for treating insomnia.

Research has shown a high incidence of serious insomnia in patients with comorbid mental health conditions such as depression and anxiety. Patients with insomnia are likely to report symptoms of nervousness and anxiety. But which comes first, the anxiety or insomnia? In some patients, insomnia can lead to anxiety and worry about lack of restful sleep. In other patients, anxiety and worry can cause someone to lie awake and experience insomnia. Thus, it is not a matter of which came first or which caused the other. Anxiety and insomnia should be recognized as a continuous, destructive cycle with each "feeding" on the other. Recognizing this link makes insomnia therapy more than just a nighttime problem. It involves treating anxiety during the day while improving sleep at night. The nurse should assess patients for anxiety when they report sleeplessness, and vice versa.

Three classes of drugs contain the drugs of choice for treating both anxiety and insomnia: benzodiazepines, nonbenzodiazepine antianxiety drugs, and antidepressants. The benzodiazepines are used for the short-term therapy of anxiety and for the treatment of patients who are unable to fall asleep due to excessive worrying at bedtime. Some of the nonbenzodiazepines and the newer antidepressants are effective for the longer term therapy of insomnia and anxiety. A second approach is to use combined therapy for the two disorders. Treating both conditions concurrently may result in better sleep outcomes than treating insomnia only.

Long-term use of sleep medications is likely to worsen insomnia, and many of these medications cause physical or psychological dependence. Patients may experience a phenomenon referred to as **rebound insomnia**. This condition occurs when a sedative drug is discontinued abruptly after it has been taken for several months or longer. Symptoms of sleeplessness, anxiety, and daytime drowsiness become markedly worse for a few days before the original insomnia symptoms return.

PharmFACT

A study of more than 1,800 university students by King (2010) found that 27% were at risk for a sleep disorder, most commonly narcolepsy and insomnia. The grade point average for students with sleep disorders (2.65) was significantly lower than that for students not experiencing these types of disorders (2.82).

18.7 Management of anxiety and sleep disorders utilizes a combination of pharmacologic and nonpharmacologic therapies.

There are a variety of possible treatments for anxiety and insomnia, and choice of therapy depends primarily on the severity of the symptoms. In some cases, several therapies may be combined to achieve optimum results. The three types of therapies include complementary and alternative therapies, nonprescription drugs, and prescription drugs.

Complementary and alternative therapies: In mild cases of anxiety or insomnia, patients should be encouraged to explore and develop nonpharmacologic coping strategies to deal with the underlying causes. Such strategies may include cognitive–behavioral therapy, counseling, biofeedback techniques, yoga, and meditation. Complementary and alternative treatments that may be useful in reducing anxiety and enhancing sleepiness are listed in Table 18.5.

Many natural products and supplements are claimed to promote relaxation and sleep. The best studied natural remedy is

TABLE 18.5 Complementary and Alternative Treatments for Anxiety and Insomnia*

Alternative therapies	Acupuncture, aromatherapy, yoga, prayer, massage, meditation, biofeedback therapy, hypnosis, guided imagery, music therapy
Exercise and nutrition	Exercise therapy, nutrition therapy, deep breathing
Herbal therapies	Kava, valerian, chamomile, catnip, ginseng, lemon balm, passionflower, hops, lavender

*Safety and effectiveness have not been demonstrated for most complementary and alternative therapies.

melatonin. Research studies have demonstrated that melatonin supplementation may improve both sleep onset and sleep duration. Melatonin is a natural hormone; however, taking too much can disrupt homeostasis and cause adverse effects such as headaches, mental impairment, and nightmares.

Two herbal products with demonstrated efficacy in promoting relaxation are valerian and kava. Although research has confirmed their effectiveness at promoting sleep, high doses of kava can damage the liver and the herb has the potential to interact with prescription sleep medications. Kava should not be used unless recommended by a health care provider. Valerian is effective at producing drowsiness and is a safer alternative than kava because it has not been shown to cause liver damage. Other herbs are claimed to have relaxation and sleep-promoting properties (often by those marketing the products), but research has not proved their validity or safety in treating anxiety or insomnia.

Nonprescription drugs: Antihistamines are drugs used to treat cold or allergy symptoms. One of the side effects of antihistamines is drowsiness. This is used to advantage in over-the-counter (OTC) sleep aid products such as Sominex and Nytol. In addition, products indicated as "p.m." or "night-time" contain antihistamines that promote sleep. The two antihistamines most frequently used to produce drowsiness are diphenhydramine and doxylamine.

Antihistamines can have a long duration of action (up to 12 hours) and may leave the patient feeling drowsy the next day. They also cause drying of the nose and mouth, which is the reason they are included in cold and flu remedies. Some patients experience dizziness and blurred vision. Antihistamines should not be taken for prolonged periods for insomnia because patients become tolerant to the drowsiness effect of the drugs. The use of antihistamines in treating allergic rhinitis and the common cold is presented in Chapter 45.

Prescription drugs: The remainder of this chapter examines the classes of prescription drugs used to treat anxiety and insomnia. These medications are used when the anxiety or sleep disorder is severe or when the condition is unresponsive to nonpharmacologic therapies.

The first drugs used to treat anxiety and insomnia were *general* central nervous system (CNS) depressants. Ethanol and opium were the two CNS depressants most widely used for treating these disorders until the discovery of the barbiturates in the early 1900s. Other nonselective CNS depressants such as chloral hydrate, methaqualone (Quaalude), and meprobamate (Miltown) were also widely prescribed in the mid-20th century. Because general CNS depressants suppress most neuronal functions, they have serious adverse effects and are very dangerous in overdose situations. Methaqualone was removed from the U.S. market in 1984 because of its addictive potential and widespread illegal use in the 1960s and 1970s. Starting in the 1960s and continuing until present day, more *selective* CNS depressants have been developed that target specific areas of the brain controlling anxiety and sleep, without causing the serious adverse effects of the older drugs.

The terminology used to describe these drugs can be confusing. An **anxiolytic** is any drug that has the ability to relieve anxiety. In the broadest definition, anxiolytics include drugs from a large number of different pharmacologic classes. In clinical practice, however, the term *anxiolytic* is often more narrowly defined to include just the benzodiazepine and nonbenzodiazepine antianxiety drugs.

A *sedative* is a CNS depressant that produces relaxation, calmness, and a reduction in anxiety and excitement. *Tranquilizer* is an older term, though still often used, to describe a sedative. A *hypnotic* is a drug that produces sleep. A sedative is most often administered during the day to induce a feeling of calm or relaxation without causing sleep, whereas hypnotics are used during the night to induce sleep. The term **sedative–hypnotic** is used to describe a drug with the ability to produce a calming effect at lower doses and sleep at higher doses. Very high doses of sedative–hypnotics may produce coma and death due to respiratory failure. All of these drugs—anxiolytics, tranquilizers, sedatives, and hypnotics—are classified more broadly as CNS depressants.

The overlap in meaning can easily be seen with the preceding definitions. Some medications may be used as an anxiolytic, a sedative, or a hypnotic, depending on the dose administered. This is because CNS depression is a continuum ranging from relaxation to sedation to the induction of sleep and anesthesia. To avoid this confusion in terminology, drugs for anxiety and insomnia are usually referred to by their chemical or pharmacologic classifications. The four general classifications of drugs used for patients experiencing anxiety or sleep disorders are as follows:

- Benzodiazepines
- Nonbenzodiazepine anxiolytics
- Antidepressants
- Barbiturates

Many CNS depressants have the potential to cause physical and psychological dependence and nearly all of them are controlled substances. The withdrawal syndrome for some CNS depressants such as the barbiturates can cause life-threatening neurologic reactions (see Chapter 27). Drugs for treating anxiety and insomnia are listed in Table 18.6.

CNS depressants are very effective drugs. If a patient does not respond to these medications with improved relaxation or sleep, it suggests a serious underlying psychiatric or medical condition that requires further assessment by behavioral specialists. This is especially true if the drug worsens insomnia or produces bizarre thinking or unusual behaviors. Examples of such behaviors that should be immediately reported to the health care provider include aggressiveness, hallucinations, suicidal thinking, and unusual extroversion or depersonalization.

Pharmacotherapy of Anxiety and Insomnia

18.8 Benzodiazepines are preferred drugs for generalized anxiety disorder and the short-term therapy of insomnia.

The benzodiazepines are versatile drugs used for a diverse collection of medical conditions, including anxiety, seizure disorders, muscle spasms, premedication for medical procedures and anesthesia, and alcohol withdrawal. Diazepam (Valium) is featured as a prototype drug in Chapter 22 for its use in treating acute seizure disorders.

The benzodiazepines are preferred drugs for GAD and for the short-term management of insomnia. Since the introduction of the first benzodiazepines—chlordiazepoxide (Librium) and diazepam (Valium)—in the 1960s, the class has become one of the most widely prescribed in medicine. Benzodiazepines account for approximately three fourths of all prescriptions for anxiety because they are effective, have a low incidence of drug interactions, and have less abuse potential compared to the older sedative–hypnotic drugs. There is a relatively wide margin of safety between therapeutic and lethal doses.

CONNECTIONS ❯ Complementary and Alternative Therapies

◀ Melatonin

Description
Melatonin is a natural hormone (N-acetyl-5-methoxytryptamine) produced during the night by the pineal gland.

History and Claims
The secretion of melatonin is stimulated by darkness and inhibited by light. As melatonin production rises, alertness decreases, and body temperature starts to fall, both of which make sleep more inviting. Melatonin production is related to age. Children manufacture more melatonin than older adults; however, melatonin production begins to drop at puberty. Supplemental melatonin, 0.5 to 3 mg at bedtime, is alleged to decrease the time required to fall asleep and to produce a deep and restful sleep.

Standardization
Melatonin is commonly marketed as 1- to 3-mg tablets. Melatonin is one of only two hormones not regulated by the FDA and sold over the counter without a prescription (dehydroepiandrosterone [DHEA] is the other).

Evidence
Melatonin appears to help people, particularly the older adult, to fall asleep faster. The National Center for Complementary and Alternative Medicine (2010) cites evidence that melatonin also appears to be useful in people with insomnia related to disrupted circadian rhythm cycles. It is believed that melatonin helps to reset the circadian rhythm for these patients, rather than cause drowsiness. Melatonin appears to be safe for short-term use.

TABLE 18.6 Benzodiazepines and Nonbenzodiazepine Anxiolytics

Drug	Route and Adult Dose (Maximum Dose Where Indicated)	Adverse Effects
Benzodiazepines for Anxiety		
alprazolam (Xanax)	Anxiety: PO (immediate release): 0.25–0.5 mg tid (max: 4 mg/day) Panic disorder: PO (extended release): 3–6 mg once daily in the morning (max: 10 mg/day)	*Drowsiness, lethargy, ataxia, confusion, dizziness, headache, blurred vision, slurred speech* Physical dependence, seizures (following abrupt withdrawal of high doses), birth defects, suicidal ideation, sleepwalking or sleep-driving (with insomnia therapy). With overdose: coma, respiratory depression, paradoxical anxiety, hypotension, dyspnea, cardiac arrest (IV forms)
chlordiazepoxide (Librium)	PO: 5–25 mg tid or qid IM/IV: 50–100 mg 1 h before a medical procedure	
clonazepam (Klonopin)	PO: 1–2 mg/day in divided doses (max: 4 mg/day)	
clorazepate (Tranxene)	PO: 15 mg/day at bedtime (max: 60 mg/day in divided doses)	
diazepam (Valium)	PO: 2–10 mg bid to qid or 15–30 mg/day sustained release IM/IV: 2–10 mg, repeat if needed in 3–4 h	
lorazepam (Ativan)	PO: 2–6 mg/day in divided doses (max: 10 mg/day)	
oxazepam	PO: 10–30 mg tid or qid	
Benzodiazepines for Insomnia		
estazolam	PO: 0.5–1 mg at bedtime (max: 2 mg/day)	
flurazepam (Dalmane)	PO: 15–30 mg at bedtime	
quazepam (Doral)	PO: 7.5–15 mg at bedtime	
temazepam (Restoril)	PO: 7.5–30 mg at bedtime	
triazolam (Halcion)	PO: 0.125–0.25 mg at bedtime (max: 0.5 mg/day)	
Nonbenzodiazepine Anxiolytics		
buspirone (BuSpar)	PO: 7.5–15 mg in divided doses; may increase by 5 mg/day every 2–3 days if needed (max: 60 mg/day)	*Dizziness, headache, nausea, vomiting, drowsiness, fatigue, dry mouth, headache, dream disturbances, unpleasant taste (eszopiclone, ramelteon), decreased testosterone and increased prolactin levels (ramelteon)* Paradoxical excitation, mood changes, tachycardia, blurred vision, confusion, myalgia
eszopiclone (Lunesta)	PO: 2–3 mg/day at bedtime	
ramelteon (Rozerem)	PO: 8 mg/day at bedtime (max: 8 mg/day)	
suvorexant (Belsomra)	PO: 5–20 mg once daily 30 minutes before bedtime	
tasimelteon (Hetlioz)	PO: 20 mg/day at bedtime	
zaleplon (Sonata)	PO: 5–10 mg at bedtime (max: 20 mg/day)	
zolpidem (Ambien, Edluar, others)	PO: immediate release: 5–10 mg at bedtime for 7–10 days (max: 10 mg/day); 12.5 mg extended release at bedtime SL: 1.75–3.5 mg (Intermezzo) or 5–10 mg (Edluar) once per night	

Note: Italics indicate common adverse effects. Underline indicates serious adverse effects.

Although about 15 benzodiazepines are available, all have very similar actions and adverse effects; the various benzodiazepines differ primarily in their onset and duration of action. Some, such as midazolam (Versed), have a rapid onset time of 15 to 30 minutes; others, such as halazepam (Paxipam), take 1 to 3 hours to reach peak serum levels. Although their actions are similar, drugs in this class have different indications, which are shown in Table 18.7.

Benzodiazepines bind to the gamma-aminobutyric acid (GABA) receptor and intensify the effect of GABA, the natural inhibitory neurotransmitter found throughout the brain. Most are metabolized in the liver to active metabolites and are excreted primarily in urine. One major advantage of the benzodiazepines is that they do not produce respiratory depression when taken in therapeutic doses. Death due to overdose is unlikely unless the benzodiazepines are taken in extreme quantities in combination with other CNS depressants, or if the patient has sleep apnea.

The benzodiazepines are categorized as Schedule IV drugs; their use may lead to physical and psychological dependence. The risk of dependence increases with higher doses and more prolonged therapy. Abrupt termination of treatment can result in withdrawal symptoms that include headaches, confusion, irritability, insomnia, and restlessness. Preexisting mental health conditions such as depression or suicidal tendencies may emerge or worsen during benzodiazepine therapy.

Most benzodiazepines are given orally (PO). Those that can be given parenterally, such as diazepam (Valium) and lorazepam (Ativan), the prototype drug in this category, should be monitored

TABLE 18.7   Indications for Benzodiazepines

Drug	GAD	Panic Disorder	Insomnia	Seizures	Alcohol Withdrawal	Preanesthetic Medication	Other
alprazolam (Xanax)	A	A	O				Premenstrual dysphoric disorder
chlordiazepoxide (Librium)	A				A	A	
clonazepam (Klonopin)	O	A	O	A			
clorazepate (Tranxene)	A		O	A	A		
diazepam (Valium)	A		O	A	A	A	Muscle spasms
estazolam	O		A				
flurazepam (Dalmane)	O		A				
lorazepam (Ativan)	A	O	O	A (IV form)	O	A (IV form)	
midazolam (Versed)				O		A	Conscious sedation
oxazepam	A		O		A		
quazepam (Doral)	O		A				
temazepam (Restoril)			A				
triazolam (Halcion)			A				

Note: A = FDA approved for this indication; O = Off-label use.

Note: Off-label uses are highly dependent on the prescriber and change frequently. The student should refer to current reference sources for updated information on approved and off-label indications.

carefully due to their rapid onset of CNS effects and possible hypotension and respiratory depression. Benzodiazepines are given parenterally for conditions such as status epilepticus or severe symptoms of acute schizophrenia. Midazolam (Versed) is administered parenterally because it can act within minutes to produce conscious sedation in patients undergoing minor medical–surgical procedures.

The benzodiazepines have replaced the barbiturates for the short-term treatment of insomnia caused by anxiety because of their greater margin of safety. Benzodiazepines shorten the length of time it takes to fall asleep and reduce the frequency of interrupted sleep. Initially, patients will report an increase in refreshed, deep sleep. Although most benzodiazepines increase total sleep time, some reduce stage IV sleep, and some affect REM sleep. With chronic use, the patient will experience a gradual increase of REM sleep as tolerance develops to the REM-suppressant effects of the medication.

The benzodiazepines approved to treat short-term insomnia are different from those indicated for GAD (see Table 18.6). These anti-insomnia benzodiazepines are administered as hypnotics to induce sleep. Like other benzodiazepines tolerance develops to their therapeutic effects, and all have the potential for physical and psychological dependence. Most produce excessive daytime drowsiness, although this diminishes after a few days of therapy. They are indicated for short-term therapy of insomnia, approximately 4 weeks, although in clinical practice they may be used for longer periods. Rebound insomnia may be significant if these drugs are used for prolonged therapy.

Sedative–hypnotic medications such as the benzodiazepines have the potential to cause sleep-related behaviors that the patient does not remember. These include sleepwalking, sleep-eating, and even making phone calls or driving a car (sleep-driving) while not fully awake. Patients often deny that these events occurred.

Flumazenil (Romazicon) is an antidote for benzodiazepine overdose. Given by rapid IV injection, flumazenil competes with benzodiazepines for the GABA receptor and reverses benzodiazepine-induced sedation within minutes. It has a very short duration of action and multiple doses, given every 30 to 45 seconds, may be necessary. If there is no response after the maximum dose (3 mg/h) has been administered, the patient's sedation was likely caused by a drug other than a benzodiazepine. Flumazenil must be used cautiously because the patient may awaken abruptly with dysphoria, agitation, and even seizures. Flumazenil does not reverse the depressed respiration characteristic of benzodiazepine overdose and it is not an antidote for the serious CNS depression caused by barbiturates or opioids. It does, however, reverse the CNS effects of some of the nonbenzodiazepine drugs such as zolpidem and eszopiclone.

PROTOTYPE DRUG   Lorazepam (Ativan)

Classification: Therapeutic: Antianxiety drug, sedative–hypnotic, antiseizure drug
Pharmacologic: Benzodiazepine, GABA receptor agonist

Therapeutic Effects and Uses: Approved in 1977, lorazepam is administered as oral tablets, concentrated oral solution, or by the intramuscular (IM) or intravenous (IV) routes. It is well absorbed by all routes. Lorazepam is approved for the routine management of GAD and to reduce anxiety prior to surgical or medical procedures. As a preanesthetic drug, it is administered by the IV route 15 to 20 minutes prior to surgery or by the IM route 2 hours prior to the procedure. Mechanically ventilated patients may receive lorazepam infusions to manage excessive anxiety and agitation that commonly occur while connected to this device.

Lorazepam is also used for several off-label indications, including insomnia, seizures, and the prevention or control of acute symptoms associated with ethanol withdrawal. Although used off-label for this indication, it is a preferred drug for treating life-threatening status epilepticus. For this indication it is administered by slow IV injection over a 2- to 4-minute period.

Mechanism of Action: Lorazepam potentiates the actions of GABA, an inhibitory neurotransmitter in the CNS. It is capable of causing all levels of CNS depression, from simple relaxation, to the induction of sleep, to coma.

Pharmacokinetics:

Route(s)	PO, IM, IV
Absorption	Readily absorbed
Distribution	91% bound to plasma proteins; widely distributed, including crossing the placenta; secreted in breast milk
Primary metabolism	Hepatic
Primary excretion	Renal
Onset of action	Peak effect: PO: 1–6 h; IM: 1–1.5 h; IV: 1–5 min
Duration of action	12–24 h

Adverse Effects: The most frequently reported adverse effects, such as dizziness, ataxia, drowsiness, blurred vision, vertigo, sedation, and confusion, are CNS related. These effects are dose related and tolerance to them may develop as therapy progresses. Less common adverse effects include hepatotoxicity (including jaundice), alopecia, anaphylaxis, orthostatic hypotension, cardiac changes (tachycardia, hypotension, cardiac arrest following rapid IV administration), constipation, dry mouth, nausea, vomiting, and anorexia. Paradoxical CNS stimulation can occur in psychiatric patients, the elderly, and hyperactive children. Patients may experience nightmares, talkativeness, mania, sleep disorders, acute rage reactions, anxiety, restlessness, and euphoria.

Contraindications/Precautions: Like other benzodiazepines, use of lorazepam may cause fetal malformations; thus this drug is contraindicated during pregnancy unless the patient's condition is life threatening. It is also contraindicated in lactating women because the drug is secreted in breast milk. Those with a hypersensitivity to benzodiazepines or who have narrow-angle glaucoma, psychosis, or chronic obstructive pulmonary disease (COPD) should not take lorazepam. Precautions must be taken in older adults, those who are debilitated, or those who have hepatic or renal dysfunction. Safe use in children has not been established. Lorazepam is a Schedule IV controlled substance and can cause both physical and psychological dependence. Those with a history of drug abuse should be monitored carefully.

Drug Interactions: There are many potential drug interactions with lorazepam. Most notably additive CNS depression will occur if the drug is given concurrently with other CNS depressants, such as alcohol, opiates, or other sedative–hypnotics. Oral contraceptives inhibit the metabolism of benzodiazepines that undergo oxidation (alprazolam, chlordiazepoxide, diazepam, and others); thus the effectiveness of these antianxiety drugs may be increased. On the other hand, oral contraceptives increase the metabolism of benzodiazepines that undergo conjugation (e.g., lorazepam, oxazepam, and temazepam); thus the antianxiety effects of these drugs may be reduced. There may be increased sedation if lorazepam is taken concurrently with disulfiram. Valproic acid may decrease the effects of lorazepam. **Herbal/Food**: Kava, melatonin, and valerian may cause excessive drowsiness if taken with lorazepam. Excessive ingestion of caffeinated food and drinks may decrease the effectiveness of lorazepam.

Pregnancy: Category D.

Treatment of Overdose: Overdose will cause sedation, lethargy, and coma. Supportive care should be provided while the patient is recovering. Gastric lavage and activated charcoal may be administered. The benzodiazepine antagonist flumazenil may be administered to reverse sedation.

Nursing Responsibilities: Key nursing implications for patients receiving lorazepam are included in the Nursing Practice Application for Patients Receiving Pharmacotherapy for Anxiety or Sleep Disorders.

Drugs Similar to Lorazepam (Ativan)

Benzodiazepines for anxiety: Benzodiazepines that are primarily used to treat anxiety are discussed next and include alprazolam, chlordiazepoxide, clorazepate, diazepam, and oxazepam. Benzodiazepines that are primarily indicated for seizures (clonazepam, clorazepate, diazepam, and lorazepam) are presented in Chapter 22. Midazolam is used as an adjunct to anesthesia and is presented in Chapter 26.

Alprazolam (Xanax):   Approved in 1981, alprazolam is available in several oral formulations and is indicated for the management of GAD and panic disorder. It is used off-label for the short-term treatment of insomnia and for premenstrual dysphoric disorder that is unresponsive to nonpharmacologic therapies. An extended release form (Xanax XR) is administered once daily. An orally disintegrating tablet (ODT) form is also available (Niravam). The drug is well tolerated, with drowsiness being the most common adverse effect. Patients are encouraged to refrain from consuming grapefruit and grapefruit juice while taking alprazolam, because the combination may inhibit the metabolism of the drug. Older adults should receive a small dose, which can then be gradually increased as indicated, to prevent ataxia or excessive sedation. Care must be taken when treating women of childbearing age because alprazolam is a pregnancy category D drug.

Chlordiazepoxide (Librium):   Chlordiazepoxide is a long-acting benzodiazepine that has been available for almost 50 years. It is available as capsules for oral administration; the parenteral formulations are no longer marketed in the United States. It is approved to manage GAD, acute anxiety situations, and symptoms associated with acute alcohol withdrawal. Off-label uses include treatment of panic disorder, tremors, and tension headaches. The use of chlordiazepoxide has markedly declined in favor of the shorter acting drugs in this class such as lorazepam and alprazolam. Drowsiness is the most common adverse effect. Precautions should be used in those with impaired hepatic or renal function. Children and older adults are more likely to experience adverse effects and should be started with a low dose, which may then be gradually increased as needed. Chlordiazepoxide is a pregnancy category D drug and is secreted in breast milk.

Clorazepate (Tranxene): Approved in 1972, clorazepate is available by the oral route to treat GAD, partial seizures, and symptoms associated with ethanol withdrawal. It may be used off-label for the short-term management of insomnia. Clorazepate is essentially a prodrug that is converted into the same active metabolites as diazepam; thus these drugs share the same actions and adverse effects. They are both pregnancy category D drugs.

Diazepam (Valium): Diazepam is an older benzodiazepine that is available for PO, IM, and IV administration. It is FDA approved to treat GAD, seizures, and muscle spasms and for the relief of symptoms associated with acute alcohol withdrawal. It is also approved to produce relaxation or sedation prior to medical procedures. Off-label uses include reduction of agitation, treatment of acute chloroquine overdose, and treatment of withdrawal symptoms associated with benzodiazepine abuse. Diazepam has the same actions and adverse effects as other drugs in its class.

Oxazepam: Approved in 1965, oxazepam is approved to manage the symptoms of acute alcohol withdrawal and for the treatment of mild to moderate GAD associated with depression. It may be used off-label for the short-term management of insomnia associated with situational anxiety. It is available only by the oral route. Actions and adverse effects are the same as other benzodiazepines. This is a pregnancy category D drug.

Benzodiazepines primarily for insomnia: Benzodiazepines primarily used as hypnotics to treat insomnia include estazolam, flurazepam, quazepam, temazepam, and triazolam.

Estazolam: Approved in 1990, estazolam is an intermediate-duration benzodiazepine approved as a hypnotic in the short-term management of insomnia. This drug should be given at bedtime because it causes significant drowsiness and promotes sleep. The most common adverse effects are somnolence, hypokinesia, abnormal coordination, and dizziness. After several weeks of therapy, patients may exhibit tolerance to the sedative effects of the drug and will experience difficulty sleeping during the early morning hours. Estazolam is a pregnancy category X drug.

Flurazepam (Dalmane): Flurazepam, the oldest benzodiazepine hypnotic, was approved in 1970. This drug is only available PO and should be taken at bedtime because it quickly produces significant drowsiness. Flurazepam has a longer duration of action than some drugs in this class because it is converted to long-acting active metabolites in the liver. Its longer duration has the potential to extend drowsiness into the morning hours. Because of the development of tolerance to the sedative effects of this drug and the potential for physical and psychological dependence, therapy is usually limited to 4 weeks. Flurazepam is a pregnancy category X drug.

Quazepam (Doral): Approved in 1985, quazepam is a benzodiazepine hypnotic drug available only by the oral route. It is administered just before bedtime because it quickly produces significant drowsiness. This drug has a long duration of action because it is converted to several active metabolites in the liver that extend the drug's half-life. Patients may experience daytime sedation, although tolerance develops to this adverse effect after a few days. Therapy is usually limited to 4 weeks because of the development of tolerance and the potential for dependence. Quazepam is a pregnancy category X drug.

Temazepam (Restoril): Approved in 1981, temazepam is indicated for the short-term therapy (7–10 days) of insomnia. It is administered PO and should be taken at bedtime due to its rapid onset of action. Unlike flurazepam and quazepam, the metabolism of temazepam does not result in active metabolites; thus the drug may be safer for use in patients with hepatic impairment. Like the other benzodiazepine hypnotics, however, temazepam is a pregnancy category X drug.

Triazolam (Halcion): Approved in 1982, triazolam is very similar to other benzodiazepine hypnotics. Because of its rapid onset, it must be taken immediately prior to sleep. It has a relatively short half-life and has no active metabolites. Daytime drowsiness is less of a problem with triazolam because of its relatively short half-life. It is approved for the short-term therapy (7–10 days) of insomnia. Anterograde amnesia may occur more frequently with triazolam than with other benzodiazepine hypnotics. Triazolam is a pregnancy category X drug.

CONNECTION Checkpoint 18.2

Differences in sleep patterns and ability to sleep may be apparent in different age groups. From what you learned in Chapter 8, should sleeping difficulties in the pregnant or lactating woman be treated with medications? *See Answer to Connection Checkpoint 18.2 on student resource website.*

18.9 Nonbenzodiazepine anxiolytics have become popular choices for treating anxiety and sleep disorders.

Several CNS depressants are used for anxiety and sleep disorders that are chemically unrelated to benzodiazepines. These drugs come from multiple classes and are grouped together as nonbenzodiazepine anxiolytics.

Older CNS depressants, such as paraldehyde (Paracetaldehyde), ethchlorvynol (Placidyl), chloral hydrate, meprobamate (Equanil), and glutethimide (Doriglute), have only historic interest because they are so rarely prescribed due to their potential for serious adverse effects. The student should refer to drug guides or older pharmacology references for information on these medications.

A few nonbenzodiazepine drugs have antianxiety properties but their primary use is for indications other than anxiety. For example, valproic acid (Depakote) is a commonly prescribed antiseizure medication that is used off-label to treat agitation in older adults or anxiety in patients with bipolar disorder. Atenolol (Tenormin), metoprolol (Toprol), and propranolol (Inderal) are beta blockers that reduce the autonomic nervous system symptoms of anxiety such as nervousness, tremor, and tachycardia. Similarly, clonidine (Catapres) is an adrenergic antagonist that can block the autonomic symptoms that accompany anxiety. Diphenhydramine (Benadryl) and hydroxyzine (Vistaril) are antihistamines that produce drowsiness and may be beneficial in calming patients. They offer the advantage of not causing dependence, although their use is often limited by their anticholinergic adverse effects. Diphenhydramine is a common component of OTC sleep aids and medications used to treat seasonal allergies. Because anxiety is a secondary indication for these drugs, they are discussed in other sections of this text.

The most frequently prescribed nonbenzodiazepine anxiolytics are newer drugs that produce more selective CNS depression. Buspirone (BuSpar) is commonly prescribed for its anxiolytic effect. Zolpidem (Ambien), ramelteon (Rozerem), zaleplon (Sonata), suvorexant (Belsomra), and eszopiclone (Lunesta) are used for their hypnotic effects. Other than their use in treating anxiety or insomnia, these drugs share little in common with each other and are discussed individually next.

PROTOTYPE DRUG	Zolpidem (Ambien, Edluar, Others)

Classification: **Therapeutic:** Sedative–hypnotic
Pharmacologic: Nonbenzodiazepine anxiolytic, miscellaneous CNS depressant

Therapeutic Effects and Uses: Approved in 1992, zolpidem is approved for the short-term (7–10 days) treatment of insomnia. Zolpidem decreases sleep-onset time and the number of nighttime awakenings and improves the length and quality of sleep. Muscle relaxation and anticonvulsant effects occur at doses much higher than the hypnotic dose. Immediate release (Ambien), extended release (Ambien CR), oral spray (Zolpimist), and sublingual (Edluar, Intermezzo) forms are available. The sublingual and oral spray forms have a more rapid onset than tablets and eliminate the requirement for water or the need to swallow.

Zolpidem should be administered just prior to expected sleep due to its rapid onset of action. Its lack of active metabolites and short half-life reduce the incidences of excessive daytime drowsiness and rebound insomnia.

Mechanism of Action: Zolpidem has a similar mechanism of action as the benzodiazepines: enhancing the action of GABA, the inhibitory neurotransmitter. Whereas the benzodiazepines bind nonselectively to all three known subtypes of the GABA receptors, zolpidem only binds to one specific type (omega-1). This explains why the drug shares some actions of the benzodiazepines, such as antianxiety and hypnotic effects, but has no effects on muscle relaxation or reducing seizures.

Pharmacokinetics:

Route(s)	PO
Absorption	70% absorbed
Distribution	Widely distributed; unknown if it crosses the placenta; small amounts are secreted in breast milk; 92% bound to plasma protein
Primary metabolism	Hepatic
Primary excretion	Renal, small amounts in bile and feces
Onset of action	7–27 minutes; peak effect: 90 minutes
Duration of action	Duration: 6–8 h; half-life: 1.4–4.5 h

Adverse Effects: Adverse reactions to zolpidem are usually mild and include dizziness, diarrhea, and daytime drowsiness. Other adverse effects include nausea, vomiting, depression, confusion, and amnesia. As with other hypnotic drugs, a small percentage of patients experience abnormal thinking, behavioral changes, and complex behaviors such as sleep-eating, sleep-driving, and hallucinations. Very high doses may cause severe ataxia, bradycardia, altered vision, severe nausea, vomiting, drowsiness, difficulty breathing, and coma. Abrupt withdrawal after long-term use may result in asthenia, diaphoresis, vomiting, tremor, or facial flushing. **Black Box Warning:** Zolpidem is a Schedule IV controlled substance that can be abused and lead to dependency. Store in a safe place to prevent misuse and abuse. Tell your doctor if you have ever abused or been dependent on alcohol, prescription drugs, or street drugs.

Contraindications/Precautions: Other than hypersensitivity to zolpidem, there are no contraindications to the use of this drug. As with other CNS depressants it should be used cautiously in patients with respiratory impairment and in older adults, who are generally more sensitive to the depressive effects of the drugs; lower dosages may be necessary. Because zolpidem is metabolized in the liver and excreted by the kidneys, impaired liver or kidney function can increase serum drug levels and doses should be lowered. Zolpidem should be used with caution in individuals with depression and suicidal ideation because there is a potential for intentional overdose in these patients. The safety and effectiveness in patients under age 18 have not been established.

Drug Interactions: Zolpidem is a substrate for hepatic CYP3A4 enzymes and thus may interact with drugs that induce or inhibit this enzyme system. Concurrent use with other CNS depressants, including alcohol, will cause additive sedation. When given concurrently with certain SSRIs, disorientation or worsening of depression may occur. **Herbal/Food:** The presence of food will reduce absorption of the drug; thus it should be taken on an empty stomach. St. John's wort may cause confusion and, rarely, hallucinations. Valerian, kava, and melatonin supplements may cause additive sedation.

Pregnancy: Category B (immediate release) or C (extended release).

Treatment of Overdose: Overdose with zolpidem can cause serious impairment of consciousness and may be fatal. The benzodiazepine antagonist flumazenil will reverse the sedative effects of zolpidem but may precipitate seizures. Other treatment involves supportive care, such as gastric lavage.

Nursing Responsibilities: Key nursing implications for patients receiving zolpidem are included in the Nursing Practice Application for Patients Receiving Pharmacotherapy for Anxiety or Sleep Disorders.

Drugs Similar to Zolpidem (Ambien, Edluar, Others)

Other drugs in this category include buspirone, eszopiclone, ramelteon, tasimelteon, and zaleplon.

Buspirone (BuSpar): Buspirone is a nonbenzodiazepine anxiolytic approved in 1986 for the short-term management (up to 1 month) of GAD. Available as an oral tablet, it should be taken consistently either with or without food because food affects its absorption. Grapefruit juice may increase the effects of the drug and should be avoided. The mechanism of action for buspirone is unclear but appears to involve two pathways: enhancing dopamine (D_2) receptors and suppressing serotonin receptors in the brain. It is less likely to affect cognitive and motor performance than benzodiazepines and rarely interacts with other CNS depressants. The most common adverse effects include dizziness, drowsiness, nausea, vomiting, and headache. When switching from a benzodiazepine to buspirone, the patient may experience withdrawal symptoms or anxiety; therefore, the dose of benzodiazepine should be gradually tapered while buspirone is increased. Safety and efficacy have not been established in children. Unlike other CNS depressants, buspirone does not cause dependence or have withdrawal symptoms. Therapy may take several weeks to achieve optimal results. Buspirone is sometimes used off-label to treat symptoms of nicotine withdrawal and premenstrual syndrome. It is a pregnancy category B drug.

Eszopiclone (Lunesta): Although not structurally related to other sedative–hypnotics, eszopiclone shares certain properties with zolpidem and the benzodiazepines. Approved in 2004, eszopiclone has a long elimination half-life, about twice as long as that of zolpidem, which offers an advantage in maintaining sleep and decreasing early-morning awakening. On the other hand, the long half-life is more likely to cause sleepiness to carry over into the morning hours and result in daytime sedation. Adverse effects are mild and include headache, dizziness, dry mouth, and an unpleasant taste that may persist into the following day. It is only available PO and should be taken immediately before bedtime due to its rapid onset of action. Eszopiclone is metabolized by hepatic CYP3A4 enzymes; thus potential drug–drug and drug–herb interactions exist for substances that induce or inhibit these enzymes. The onset of action may be reduced if taken with or immediately following a high-fat meal. Older adults with impaired hepatic or renal function may need a lower dose. Eszopiclone may be used for the long-term treatment of insomnia. However, tolerance develops to the sedative effects after a few weeks of therapy and rebound insomnia may occur on withdrawal. Eszopiclone is a Schedule IV controlled substance. It is a pregnancy category C drug.

Ramelteon (Rozerem): Approved in 2005, ramelteon is approved to treat chronic insomnia in people who have problems falling asleep. It appears to be safe for long-term use. Ramelteon has a unique mechanism of action: It activates melatonin receptors, specifically MT1 and MT2, which are mediators of the normal sleep–wake cycle. With an onset of action of 30 minutes and a short duration of action, it is helpful in treating sleep onset but it does not maintain sleep. It is less effective if taken with or immediately after a high-fat meal. There is little next-day residual drowsiness owing to its short half-life. Adverse effects of ramelteon are mild and include dizziness, fatigue, and somnolence. Ramelteon can affect the levels of sex hormones in the body, so the patient may experience amenorrhea, decreased libido, galactorrhea, and problems with fertility. Alcohol should be avoided because it may cause additive CNS depression. Fluvoxamine (Luvox) can greatly increase (more than 50 times) the levels of ramelteon so it should not be used concurrently. Ramelteon is a pregnancy category X drug.

Suvorexant (Belsomra): Approved in 2014 to treat insomnia, suvorexant is the first in a new class of drugs called orexin receptor antagonists. Orexin is a neurotransmitter found in the brain that helps regulate sleep-wake cycles by maintaining wakefulness. Loss of orexin neurons is associated with narcolepsy. By blocking orexin receptors, suvorexant promotes drowsiness and sleep. Caution must be used when combining suvorexant with alcohol or other CNS depressants due to additive sedation. The primary side effect is daytime drowsiness. This drug is pregnancy category C.

Tasimelteon (Hetlioz): One of the newest drugs in this class, tasimelteon was approved in 2014 for non–24-hour sleep–wake disorder. This is a condition that occurs in people who are totally blind. Because no light is perceived, these patients are unable to synchronize the timing of sleep to a 24-hour light–dark cycle. This may result in the patient being active when others are sleeping or drowsy when others are awake. Several weeks or months of therapy may be needed to improve the sleep–wake cycle. The most common adverse effects are headache, elevated ALT, and nightmares. This drug is pregnancy category C.

Zaleplon (Sonata): Approved in 1999, zaleplon is an oral nonbenzodiazepine sedative–hypnotic whose only indication is for the short-term treatment (7–10 days) of insomnia. It is the first drug in a class called pyrazolopyrimidines. Like zolpidem, it binds specifically to the omega-1 GABA receptor but it has a faster onset and shorter duration of action than zolpidem. Zaleplon decreases sleep-onset time and may be useful for patients who awaken early in the morning, for example, 2:00 a.m. or 3:00 a.m. It is sometimes used for treatment of jet lag and has been advertised by pharmaceutical companies for this purpose. Zaleplon should be taken immediately before bedtime due to its rapid onset of action. Administration immediately following a high-fat meal slows the absorption of zaleplon and reduces its effectiveness. The drug is well tolerated and causes few adverse effects. High doses produce symptoms characteristic of other sedative–hypnotics such as drowsiness, confusion, dizziness, and lethargy. Long-term use does not result in tolerance and, although it is a Schedule IV drug, dependence potential appears to be low. It is a pregnancy category C drug.

PharmFACT

Chronic lack of sleep may make people more prone to developing type 2 (non–insulin-dependent) diabetes. Healthy adults who average about 5 hours of sleep per night for eight consecutive nights secrete 50% more insulin than those who average 8 hours of sleep per night. Those who sleep less than 8 hours per night are 40% less sensitive to insulin than those who get more sleep (Chandola, Ferrie, Perski, Akbaraly, & Marmot, 2010).

18.10 Antidepressants are widely prescribed for anxiety disorders.

Until the 1980s, antidepressants were used mainly to treat major depressive disorder, a condition characterized by chronic low mood and loss of interest or pleasure in activities that were previously enjoyable. During the past 20 years, however, pharmacologists have discovered the value of these drugs in treating other disorders, including anxiety. Today, antidepressants are frequently used to treat various anxiety disorders and are the drugs of choice in some cases. Given the effectiveness of antidepressants for these conditions, many believe that in the future, anxiolytics and antidepressants will eventually merge into a single drug class.

Antidepressants act by altering the levels of two important neurotransmitters in the brain: norepinephrine and serotonin.

TABLE 18.8 Indications for Antidepressants Used for Anxiety or Insomnia

Drug	GAD	Panic Disorder	Social Anxiety Disorder	OCD	PTSD	Insomnia
Atypical Antidepressants, Including the SNRIs						
duloxetine (Cymbalta)	A					
trazodone (Oleptro)	0	0				0
venlafaxine (Effexor)	A		A	0		
Selective Serotonin Reuptake Inhibitors (SSRIs)						
citalopram (Celexa)	0	0	0	0	0	
escitalopram (Lexapro)	A	0	0			
fluoxetine (Prozac)	0	A		A	0	
fluvoxamine (Luvox)	0	0	A	A	0	
paroxetine (Paxil)	A	A	A	A	A	
sertraline (Zoloft)	0	A	A	A	A	
Tricyclic Antidepressants (TCAs)						
amitriptyline (Elavil)		0	0			0
clomipramine (Anafranil)				A		
desipramine (Norpramin)	0	0				
doxepin (Silenor)	A					A
imipramine (Tofranil)		0	0			
nortriptyline (Aventyl, Pamelor)		0	0			

Note: A = FDA approved for this indication; O = Off-label use.

Note: Off-label uses are highly dependent on the prescriber and change frequently. The student should refer to current reference sources for updated information on approved and off-label indications.

Restoration of normal neurotransmitter balances reduces symptoms associated with depression, panic attacks, obsessive–compulsive behavior, PTSD, and phobias. A more detailed treatment of these drugs and their use in treating depression is presented in Chapter 19. The following section focuses on their applications to treating anxiety disorders and insomnia.

For most patients, panic attacks and other intense anxiety symptoms come in two stages. The first stage is termed anticipatory anxiety in which the patient begins to think about an upcoming challenge and starts to experience feelings of dread. The second stage is when physical symptoms such as shortness of breath, accelerated heart rate, and muscle tension start to emerge as a consequence of activation of the autonomic nervous system. For panic attacks or phobias, the most useful therapy is to help motivate the patient to face his or her fear and to suppress symptoms in one or both of these stages. If drugs can reduce the negative thoughts associated with the anticipatory component of panic, then there is less likelihood that the patient will become stressed. Drugs can also be used to reduce neuronal activity and suppress the autonomic nervous system, helping the patient to remain calm. The patient can then use self-help coping skills to control the negative behavior.

The antidepressants used to reduce symptoms of panic and anxiety are usually the SSRIs and atypical antidepressants. Older classes such as the TCAs and monoamine oxidase inhibitors (MAOIs) are less commonly employed due to a greater potential for adverse effects. The SSRIs treat symptoms of panic attacks,

OCD, and phobias. Indications for these medications are shown in Table 18.8. Following is a brief summary of additional important considerations for each antidepressant class. Individual drug information, patient teaching, and nursing responsibilities are presented in Chapter 19.

Selective serotonin reuptake inhibitors: This is the most widely prescribed antidepressant class because these drugs are safer than those from other classes and cause fewer sympathomimetic effects (increased heart rate and hypertension) and anticholinergic effects. Some SSRIs can, however, cause weight gain and sexual dysfunction. Overdoses can cause confusion, anxiety, restlessness, hypertension, tremors, sweating, fever, and lack of muscle coordination.

Five SSRIs are approved for anxiety disorders although other drugs in this class are often used off-label. The indications for each drug are given in Table 18.8.

- **Generalized anxiety disorder.** Paroxetine (Paxil) and escitalopram (Lexapro) are drugs of choice for patients with GAD and anxiety that is associated with depressive disorders. Unlike the benzodiazepines that act immediately, onset for the antianxiety effects of the SSRIs may take several weeks.

- **Panic disorder.** The three SSRIs approved for panic disorder, fluoxetine (Prozac), paroxetine (Paxil), and sertraline (Zoloft), are drugs of choice for this disorder. Both frequency and intensity of panic attacks are reduced.

- **Obsessive–compulsive disorder.** Four SSRIs are approved to treat OCD, although others in this class may be used off-label. Paroxetine (Paxil), fluvoxamine (Luvox), fluoxetine (Prozac), and sertraline (Zoloft) are drugs of choice for this disorder. Optimum therapeutic effects may take several months to achieve.

- **Social anxiety disorder.** Paroxetine (Paxil), fluvoxamine (Luvox), and sertraline (Zoloft) are SSRIs approved for the long-term therapy of social anxiety disorder. Because several months may be necessary for optimum therapeutic benefit, the benzodiazepines are better choices for acute symptoms of social anxiety disorder.

- **Post-traumatic stress disorder.** Paroxetine (Paxil) and sertraline (Zoloft) are the two SSRIs approved for the therapy of PTSD. Therapy should be initiated as soon after the traumatic event as possible, and several months may be necessary for optimum results.

Atypical antidepressants: These include serotonin–norepinephrine reuptake inhibitors (SNRIs). Adverse effects are similar to those of the SSRIs and include insomnia, abnormal dreams, sweating, constipation, dry mouth, loss of appetite, weight loss, tremor, abnormal vision, headaches, nausea, vomiting, dizziness, and loss of sexual desire. Two atypical antidepressants are used for anxiety disorders:

- **Duloxetine (Cymbalta).** Approved in 2007 for GAD, duloxetine has the potential to become a first-line drug for this disorder due to its safety and effectiveness, especially in patients with accompanying major depression. It is also approved to treat fibromyalgia, chronic musculoskeletal pain, and diabetic neuropathic pain.

- **Venlafaxine (Effexor).** The extended release form of venlafaxine was the first antidepressant approved for GAD. It is also beneficial in treating panic attacks and social anxiety disorder. It is widely used for anxiety disorders that are accompanied by depression.

Tricyclic antidepressants (TCAs): TCAs are older drugs that, although effective, generally produce more adverse effects than SSRIs. Patients often have annoying anticholinergic effects such as dry mouth, blurred vision, urine retention, and hypertension (see Chapter 14). They are not recommended for patients with a history of heart attack, heart block, or dysrhythmia. Concurrent use with alcohol or other CNS depressants should be avoided, and patients with asthma, GI disorders, alcoholism, schizophrenia, or bipolar disorder should take TCAs with extreme caution. Most TCAs are pregnancy category C or D. Although several drugs in this class are used off-label, only two TCAs are approved for anxiety disorders:

- **Clomipramine (Anafranil).** The only drug in this class approved for OCD, clomipramine is very effective but tends to cause more adverse effects than SSRIs. It is considered an alternative for patients who are unable to tolerate SSRIs.

- **Doxepin (Silenor).** Approved for anxiety associated with depressive disorders, doxepin produces a rapid antianxiety effect. However, because of significant anticholinergic adverse effects, it is not a drug of first choice for anxiety. In 2010, this drug was approved to treat insomnia characterized by difficulty with sleep maintenance (staying asleep).

Monoamine oxidase inhibitors (MAOIs): Once commonly prescribed, it is rare to find these drugs used today due to their high incidence of potential adverse effects. No MAOIs are FDA approved for anxiety disorders, although some may be occasionally used off-label when other therapies fail to produce satisfactory results. The student should refer to Chapter 19 for more information on drugs in this class.

CONNECTION Checkpoint 18.3

Fluvoxamine, fluoxetine, and duloxetine have similar sounding names and may look alike when written as prescriptions. From what you learned in Chapter 6, describe means that you should implement to avoid these types of medication errors. *See Answer to Connection Checkpoint 18.3 on student resource website.*

18.11 Barbiturates are effective sedative–hypnotics but have potentially serious adverse effects that limit their use.

Barbiturates are powerful CNS depressants prescribed for their sedative, hypnotic, and antiseizure effects that have been employed in pharmacotherapy since the early 1900s. Until the discovery of the benzodiazepines, barbiturates were the drugs of choice for patients with anxiety and insomnia. They are now rarely prescribed for anxiety or insomnia because of their significant adverse effects and because of the availability of more effective medications. The risk of psychological and physical dependence is high—several are Schedule II drugs. If a patient does become physically dependent on barbiturates, the withdrawal syndrome is extremely severe and can be fatal. Overdose results in profound respiratory depression, hypotension, and shock. Barbiturates have frequently been used to commit suicide, and death due to overdose was common when these drugs were frequently prescribed in the 1960s and 1970s.

Barbiturates are capable of depressing CNS function at all levels. Like benzodiazepines, barbiturates act by binding to GABA receptor–chloride channel molecules, intensifying the effect of GABA throughout the brain. At low doses they reduce anxiety and cause drowsiness. At moderate doses they inhibit seizure activity (see Chapter 22) and promote sleep by inhibiting brain impulses traveling through the limbic system and the RAS. At higher doses, some barbiturates can induce anesthesia (see Chapter 26). Barbiturates are classified by their duration of action: short acting, intermediate acting, or long acting. Selected barbiturates used to treat sleep disorders are shown in Table 18.9.

When taken for prolonged periods, barbiturates induce the synthesis of hepatic CYP450 enzymes and can stimulate their own metabolism as well as that of hundreds of other drugs that use these enzymes for their breakdown. This significantly increases the risk for drug–drug interactions. After 2 weeks, tolerance begins to develop to the sedative effects of barbiturates; this includes cross-tolerance to other CNS depressants such as the opioids. Tolerance does not develop, however, to the respiratory depressant effects. Thus the patient may take higher and higher doses to produce sleep while approaching dangerous and even lethal dosage levels.

| PROTOTYPE DRUG | Phenobarbital (Luminal) |

Classification: **Therapeutic:** Sedative–hypnotic, antiepileptic drug
Pharmacologic: Barbiturate, GABA receptor agonist

Therapeutic Effects and Uses: A Schedule IV drug, phenobarbital is available as tablets or elixir for PO doses and as injection for IM or IV administration. By the IV route, phenobarbital is reserved for emergency situations such as status epilepticus. It is effective

TABLE 18.9	Selected Barbiturates for Insomnia	
Drug	**Route and Adult Dose (Maximum Dose Where Indicated)**	**Adverse Effects**
butabarbital (Butisol)	Sedative: PO: 15–30 mg tid or qid Hypnotic: PO: 50–100 mg at bedtime	*Somnolence, hangover, confusion, nausea, vomiting, rebound insomnia*
pentobarbital	Preoperative sedation: IM: 150–200 mg in two divided doses Hypnotic: IM: 150–200 mg; IV: 100 mg every 1–3 min up to 500 mg dose	<u>CNS depression, coma, death, bradycardia, liver damage, hypocalcemia, Stevens–Johnson syndrome, severe respiratory depression, birth defects</u>
phenobarbital (Luminal)	Sedative: PO: 30–120 mg/day IV/IM/subcutaneous: 100–320 mg/day	
secobarbital (Seconal)	Sedative: PO: 100–300 mg/day in three divided doses Hypnotic: PO: 100–200 mg	

Note: Italics indicate common adverse effects. Underline indicates serious adverse effects.

for treating generalized and partial seizures, which are likely the most common indications for the use of the drug. The drug is FDA approved for the short-term treatment of insomnia, although there are many safer and equally effective medications available for this indication. Therapeutic serum phenobarbital concentrations range from 15 to 40 mcg/mL.

As a sedative–hypnotic, phenobarbital decreases time to sleep onset and lengthens total sleep time. The number of nighttime awakenings diminishes. Significant rebound insomnia occurs when the drug is discontinued.

Mechanism of Action: Phenobarbital binds to GABA receptors, where it enhances the activity of GABA.

Pharmacokinetics:

Route(s)	PO, IM, and IV
Absorption	Well absorbed by all routes
Distribution	Rapidly and widely distributed; may cross the placenta; secreted in breast milk; 20–45% bound to protein
Primary metabolism	Hepatic
Primary excretion	Renal
Onset of action	IV: 5 min; PO: 8–12 h
Duration of action	Half-life: 53–118 h

Adverse Effects: Many adverse effects are reported with phenobarbital. Serious ones include coma, Stevens–Johnson syndrome, angioedema, and thrombophlebitis. Adverse reactions related to CNS depression include oversedation, "hangover" effect, lethargy, and hallucinations. Other adverse effects can include blood dyscrasias, hypocalcemia, hepatic disease, nausea, vomiting, diarrhea, or constipation. Deficiency in folic acid, calcium, and vitamin D may result in osteomalacia. Phenobarbital can cause paradoxical excitation in older adults or children, especially during the first 2 weeks of treatment. If abruptly discontinued after prolonged use, the patient may experience nightmares, insomnia, tremor, hallucinations, nausea, and vomiting.

Contraindications/Precautions: Phenobarbital is contraindicated in patients with hypersensitivity to barbiturates, suicidal ideation or previous suicide attempt, preexisting CNS depression, severe respiratory disease, severe pain, or hyperthyroidism. Patients with impaired hepatic, renal, and cardiovascular function should not receive phenobarbital, or the dose should be lowered to prevent toxicity. Patients with COPD may experience profound respiratory depression, even at therapeutic doses, and should not receive phenobarbital. A patient who has a familial history of porphyria should not be administered phenobarbital. Porphyria is a metabolic disorder in which neurologic disturbances are noted. Phenobarbital should be used cautiously in patients with hyperthyroidism, diabetes mellitus, and severe anemia. Phenobarbital can cause birth defects and physical dependence in the neonate, and thus it is contraindicated during pregnancy. Phenobarbital is secreted in breast milk and can cause profound effects on the neonate; thus it should not be administered during lactation.

Drug Interactions: Phenobarbital induces CYP450 enzymes and has the potential to interact with drugs that are metabolized by the liver such as corticosteroids, oral contraceptives, and anticonvulsants. Use with other CNS depressants, including alcohol, will cause additive sedation. Valproic acid may increase the risk of phenobarbital toxicity. Phenobarbital may decrease the effectiveness of digoxin, TCAs, metronidazole, quinidine, or oral anticoagulants. **Herbal/Food:** St. John's wort may lead to decreased barbiturate effect. Use of kava, chamomile, eucalyptus, lemon balm, or valerian may increase additive CNS depression.

Pregnancy: Category D.

Treatment of Overdose: Overdosage of phenobarbital is a medical emergency and may be fatal. Activated charcoal is administered followed by gastric lavage. Alkalinization of the urine with sodium bicarbonate increases the renal elimination of phenobarbital.

Nursing Responsibilities: Key nursing implications for patients receiving phenobarbital are included in the Nursing Practice Application for Patients Receiving Pharmacotherapy for Anxiety or Sleep Disorders.

Drugs Similar to Phenobarbital (Luminal)

The barbiturates are classified by duration of action, and all have the same actions and adverse effects as phenobarbital. None are in common use.

Ultra-short acting: With a half-life of less than 10 minutes, methohexital (Brevital) is administered by the IV route to induce or maintain anesthesia, as preoperative sedation, or in the emergency management of seizures.

Short acting: With half-lives of 15 to 40 minutes, secobarbital (Seconal) and pentobarbital are oral drugs that have been used to

CONNECTIONS | Lifespan Considerations

◀ Treating Childhood Anxiety Disorders

Children and adolescents may experience intense fear and worry that can lead to the same types of anxiety disorders experienced by adults. Signs may include excessive worrying about ordinary school activities; physical symptoms such as sweating, headaches, trembling, and palpitations; or social withdrawal. If not recognized and treated, childhood anxiety disorders may lead to low self-esteem, poor interpersonal relationships, drug or alcohol use, or repeated school absences. The incidence is believed to be 13% of all children ages 9 to 17, with girls being affected more than boys.

Treatment of childhood anxiety usually begins with cognitive–behavioral therapy and relaxation techniques. If medication is indicated, the SSRIs are the

drugs of choice for children (Connolly, Suarez, & Sylvester, 2011). The use of antidepressants in children must be carefully monitored and the risk versus the benefit weighed before they are prescribed. In 2007, the U. S. Food and Drug Administration (FDA) issued a black box warning, citing an increased risk of suicide in children, adolescents, and young adults up to age 24. Although recent research has shown that the actual increase in risk may be very small, caregivers must be diligent in monitoring for signs of potential suicidal thoughts in children taking antidepressants, including unusual changes in behavior, sleeplessness, agitation, or social withdrawal, and report any such changes to the health care provider immediately.

treat insomnia and as preoperative medications. These are Schedule II drugs and have been the most widely abused barbiturates.

Intermediate acting: With slightly longer half-lives, amobarbital (Amytal) and butabarbital (Butisol) are oral drugs that have been used as sedative–hypnotics and to provide preanesthesia sedation.

Long acting: Mephobarbital (Mebaral) and phenobarbital are the two long-acting drugs. Mephobarbital is metabolized to phenobarbital in the liver and may be used as a sedative–hypnotic or, rarely, for seizures.

CONNECTIONS: NURSING PRACTICE APPLICATION

Patients Receiving Pharmacotherapy for Anxiety or Sleep Disorders

Assessment	Potential Nursing Diagnoses*
Baseline assessment prior to administration: • Obtain a complete health history including hepatic, renal, respiratory, cardiovascular or neurologic disease, mental status, narrow-angle glaucoma, pregnancy, or breast-feeding. Obtain a drug history including allergies, current prescription and OTC drugs, herbal preparations, and caffeine and alcohol use. Be alert to possible drug interactions. • Assess stress and coping patterns (e.g., existing or perceived stress, duration, coping mechanisms, or remedies). • Obtain a sleep history (e.g., quality and quantity of sleep, restlessness or frequent wakefulness, snoring or apnea, remedies used for sleep, concerns). • Evaluate appropriate laboratory findings (e.g., hepatic or renal function studies). • Obtain baseline vital signs and weight. Assess fall risk. • Assess the patient's ability to receive and understand instructions. Include family and caregivers as needed.	• *Anxiety* • *Disturbed Sleep Pattern,* related to adverse effects of drug therapy • *Fatigue* • *Ineffective Coping* • *Activity Intolerance,* related to sedative effects of medication • *Deficient Knowledge* (Drug Therapy) • *Risk for Injury, Risk for Falls,* related to adverse effects of drug therapy
Assessment throughout administration: • Assess for desired therapeutic effects (e.g., statements of improvement in anxiety, appetite, ability to carry out ADLs, and sleep patterns normalize). • Continue periodic monitoring of liver and renal function studies. • Assess vital signs and weight periodically or if symptoms warrant. • Assess for and promptly report adverse effects: excessive dizziness, drowsiness, lightheadedness, confusion, agitation, palpitations, tachycardia, or musculoskeletal weakness.	

Implementation

Interventions and (Rationales)	Patient-Centered Care
Ensuring therapeutic effects: • Continue assessments as above for therapeutic effects. (If the drug is given for anxiety, the patient reports decreased anxiety, improved sleep and eating habits, improved coping, and ability to carry out ADLs without anxiety. If the drug is given for sleep, the patient reports being able to fall and remain asleep; improved daytime wakefulness.) **Diverse Patients:** Barbiturates induce P450 enzymes and may interact with other drugs. Ethnically diverse populations may also experience less than optimal effects of the drug. Nonbenzodiazepine sedative–hypnotic drugs are also metabolized through the P450 pathways. Women may metabolize some sublingual drugs (e.g., zolpidem [Edluar, Intermezzo]) more slowly, and dosage may need to be halved by the provider.	• Assist the patient in developing healthy coping strategies and sleep habits with referral to appropriate health care providers as needed. • Encourage the patient to keep a sleep diary of bedtime, time involved trying to fall asleep, quality and quantity of sleep, daytime sleepiness. • **Diverse Patients:** Teach ethnically diverse patients to observe for either excessive or less than optimal therapeutic effects and report promptly.

CONNECTIONS: NURSING PRACTICE APPLICATION (continued)

Minimizing adverse effects:

- Continue to monitor vital signs, mental status, coordination, and balance periodically. **Lifespan:** Be particularly cautious with older adults who are at increased risk for falls. Many benzodiazepines and all barbiturates are included on the Beers List of potentially inappropriate drugs for older adults and warrant careful monitoring. (Drugs used for anxiety and sleep may cause excessive drowsiness and dizziness, increasing the risk of falls and injury.)

- Teach the patient to rise from lying or sitting to standing slowly to avoid dizziness or falls. If dizziness occurs, the patient should sit or lie down and not attempt to stand or walk until the sensation passes.

- Ensure patient safety, especially of older adults. Observe for lightheadedness or dizziness. Monitor ambulation until effects of the drug are known. (Dizziness and drowsiness for a prolonged period may occur, depending on the drug's half-life. Daytime drowsiness may impair walking or the ability to carry out usual ADLs. Subtle changes in mental alertness and cognitive functioning may occur, even in the absence of sleepiness.)

- Instruct the patient to call for assistance prior to getting out of bed or attempting to walk alone, and to avoid driving or other activities requiring mental alertness or physical coordination until the effects of the drug are known.

- Assess for changes in level of consciousness, disorientation or confusion, or agitation. (Neurologic changes may indicate overmedication or effects of sleep deprivation.)

- Instruct the patient or caregiver to report increasing lethargy, disorientation, confusion, changes in behavior or mood, slurred speech, or ataxia immediately.
- Have caregivers observe for nighttime behavioral activities such as sleepwalking, sleep-eating, or sleep-driving if nonbenzodiazepine sedative–hypnotic drugs are given, and report immediately. The patient may not remember or be aware of these activities.

- Assess for changes in visual acuity, blurred vision, loss of peripheral vision, seeing rainbow halos around lights, acute eye pain, or any of these symptoms accompanied by nausea and vomiting and report immediately. (Increased intraoptic pressure in patients with narrow-angle glaucoma may occur in patients taking benzodiazepines.)

- Instruct the patient to report any visual changes or eye pain immediately.

- Monitor affect and emotional status. (Drugs may increase the risk of mental depression, especially in patients with suicidal tendencies. Concurrent use of alcohol and other CNS depressants increases the effects and the risk.)

- Instruct the patient to report significant mood changes, especially depression, and to avoid alcohol and other CNS depressants while taking the drug.
- Teach the patient about the need for continued monitoring, especially if preexisting depression is present.

- Encourage appropriate lifestyle changes: lowered caffeine intake including OTC medications that contain caffeine, increased exercise during the day but not immediately before bedtime, limited or no alcohol intake, and smoking cessation. (Healthy lifestyle changes will support and minimize the need for drug therapy. Caffeine and nicotine may decrease the effectiveness of the drugs. Alcohol and other CNS depressants may increase the adverse effects of the drugs.)

- Encourage the patient to adopt a healthy lifestyle of decreased use of or abstinence from caffeine, nicotine, and alcohol, and increased exercise. Avoiding caffeine, decreasing stimulation (e.g., TV, Internet use) before bedtime, and regular bedtime habits help to promote sleep.
- Advise the patient to discuss all OTC medications with the health care provider to ensure caffeine or alcohol is not included in the formulation.

- Avoid abrupt discontinuation of therapy. (Withdrawal symptoms, including rebound anxiety and sleeplessness, are possible with abrupt discontinuation after long-term use.)

- Instruct the patient to take the drug exactly as prescribed and to not stop it abruptly.

- Assess home storage of medications and identify risks for corrective action. (Overdosage may occur if the patient takes additional doses when drowsy or disoriented from medication effects.)

- Instruct the patient that these drugs should not be kept at the bedside to avoid taking additional doses when drowsy.

- Assess prior methods of stress reduction or sleep hygiene. Reinforce previously used effective methods and teach new coping skills. (Drug therapy is used for the shortest amount of time possible. Developing other coping skills or improved sleep hygiene may lessen the need for drug therapy.)

- Teach the patient nonpharmacologic methods for stress relief and for improved sleep hygiene. Refer to appropriate health care providers or support groups as needed.

Patient understanding of drug therapy:

- Use opportunities during administration of medications and during assessments to discuss the rationale for drug therapy, desired therapeutic outcomes, commonly observed adverse effects, parameters for when to call the health care provider, and any necessary monitoring or precautions. (Using time during nursing care helps to optimize and reinforce key teaching areas.)

- The patient should be able to state the reason for the drug, appropriate dose, and scheduling; what adverse effects to observe for and when to report them; and the anticipated length of medication therapy.

Patient self-administration of drug therapy:

- When administering the medication, instruct the patient, family, or caregiver in proper self-administration of the drug, e.g., taking only the amount prescribed. (Utilizing time during nurse-administration of these drugs helps to reinforce teaching.)

- The patient is able to discuss appropriate dosing and administration needs.
- Teach patients to not open, chew, or crush extended release tablets (e.g., zopidem [Ambien]); to swallow them whole with plenty of water. Sublingual forms of the drug (e.g., zolpidem [Edluar, Intermezzo]) should be allowed to dissolve under the tongue; water should not be taken.

*Nursing Diagnoses—Definitions and Classification 2015–2017. Copyright © 2014, 1994–2014 by NANDA International. Used by arrangement with John Wiley & Sons Limited.

CHAPTER

18

Understanding the Chapter

Key Concepts Summary

18.1 Proper diagnosis of anxiety disorders is important to identifying the most effective treatment option.

18.2 Anxiety disorders may be divided into five major categories.

18.3 Specific regions of the brain have been identified that are responsible for anxiety.

18.4 Sleep occurs in distinct stages.

18.5 Sleep disorders affect a large percentage of the population.

18.6 There is a link between insomnia and anxiety.

18.7 Management of anxiety and sleep disorders utilizes a combination of pharmacologic and nonpharmacologic therapies.

18.8 Benzodiazepines are preferred drugs for generalized anxiety disorder and the short-term therapy of insomnia.

18.9 Nonbenzodiazepine anxiolytics have become popular choices for treating anxiety and sleep disorders.

18.10 Antidepressants are widely prescribed for anxiety disorders.

18.11 Barbiturates are effective sedative–hypnotics but have potentially serious adverse effects that limit their use.

Case Study: Making the Patient Connection

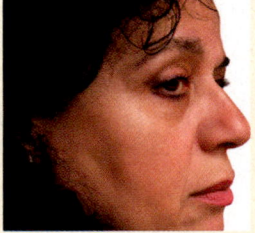

Remember the patient "Seraphina Alvarez" at the beginning of the chapter? Now read the remainder of the case study. Based on the information presented within the chapter, respond to the critical thinking questions that follow.

Seraphina Alvarez, age 55, is an elementary school teacher who has planned on retiring at the end of this academic year. She is the married mother of seven adult children, six of whom live within a 15-mile radius and see her often. Her husband, Joe, has been retired for 3 years. He receives Social Security and a small pension from his former employment as a construction worker. Seraphina and Joe's oldest daughter's two children and two dogs came to live with them approximately 10 months ago because their daughter is unable to provide a home for them. The children, Joseph, age 15, and Mariah, age 12, are "good kids." They are good students who are active in school and church activities. They resent having to move from their long-time home and school and are acting-out some. Seraphina also resents having to raise her grandchildren. It interferes with plans that she and her husband had made to travel after she retired. In fact, she may not be able to retire as planned because they need the extra income to meet the children's needs. She loves the children and tries very hard not to let her resentment show. She also has guilt feelings that she did not do all she could or should have done to raise her daughter to be a responsible parent. As a result, she is unable to sleep well and reports having anxiety. Seraphina first turned to herbal remedies

common in her culture and to prayer. Neither of these interventions has helped, but she is reluctant to discuss her problems with anyone else. She sees her parish priest on a regular basis. He is very supportive of her and understanding of her feelings of resentment but does not realize that she is experiencing anxiety and insomnia.

Seraphina, whose health has always been good, has begun having some health issues, including hypertension, diarrhea, and weight loss. She finds herself becoming more anxious, and her family has noticed that she is decreasing time spent with family and friends and does not leave her home other than to go to work and to go to church. She has lost 16 kg (35 lb) in 2 months and appears to have lost her "zest" for living. Her diet consists of black coffee and fresh fruit. Joe frequently finds her sitting in a rocking chair on their front porch during the night, rather than being in bed. She also has begun missing work, saying "I just don't feel up to facing the kids today."

Critical Thinking Questions

1. What current factors in Seraphina's life are interfering with her ability to get a good night's sleep?

2. What medications may Seraphina's health care provider order on a short-term or longer term basis?

3. What part do herbal remedies play in anxiety control and sleep induction in the Latino culture? What specific herbs is Seraphina probably using?

See Answers to Critical Thinking Questions on student resource website.

Additional Case Study

Craig Edwards is a 46-year-old salesman working at a respected car dealership in the community. With the economy, his income has dropped significantly because it is partially based on commission and he is worried that he is not able to provide for his family. He begins to experience insomnia, difficulty concentrating, and other symptoms related to his anxiety. His health care provider prescribes a short-term course of lorazepam (Ativan) to help him through this difficult period.

1. What adverse effects are associated with this drug therapy?
2. What information should Craig receive about this medication?
3. What nonpharmacologic measures can the nurse recommend to Craig to assist him in feeling better about his current situation?

See Answers to Additional Case Study on student resource website.

Chapter Review

1 A nurse should advise a patient who is receiving lorazepam (Ativan) about the adverse effects of this medication, which include:

1. Tachypnea.
2. Astigmatism.
3. Ataxia.
4. Euphoria.

2 The patient with insomnia is being treated with temazepam (Restoril). The nurse monitors for therapeutic effectiveness by noting which of the following?

1. Sleeping in 3-hour intervals, awaking for a short time, and then returning to sleep
2. Feeling less anxiety during activities of daily living
3. Having fewer episodes of panic attacks when stressed
4. Sleeping 7 hours without awakening

3 Which of these statements, if made by a patient, would indicate that further instruction is needed about alprazolam (Xanax)?

1. "I will stop smoking by undergoing hypnosis."
2. "I will not drive immediately after I take this medication."
3. "I will stop the medicine when I feel less anxious."
4. "I will take my medication with food if my stomach feels upset."

4 The nurse should question a health care provider's order of phenobarbital for the patient with which condition?

1. Seizure disorder
2. Panic disorder
3. Prior to a bronchoscopy
4. Prior to receiving a general anesthetic

5 The nurse is caring for a patient receiving a sedative–hypnotic. Which adverse effect associated with this drug therapy is the highest priority for the nurse?

1. Urinary incontinence
2. Activity intolerance
3. Risk for falls
4. Poor nutritional intake

6 The patient, who is receiving benzodiazepines, is a two-pack per day cigarette smoker. The nurse expects to administer a/an _____ dose of this medication.

1. Larger
2. Smaller
3. Extra
4. Half

See Answers to Chapter Review in Appendix A.

References

Anxiety and Depression Association of America. (n.d.). *Facts & statistics.* Retrieved from http://www.adaa.org/about-adaa/press-room/facts-statistics

Chandola, T., Ferrie, J. E., Perski, A., Akbaraly, T., & Marmot, M. G. (2010). The effect of short sleep duration on coronary heart disease risk is greatest among those with sleep disturbance: A prospective study from the Whitehall II cohort. *Sleep, 33*(6), 739–744.

Church, M. K., Maurer, M., Simons, F. E. B., Bindslev-Jensen, C., van Cauwenberge, P., Bousquet, J., . . . Zuberbier, T. (2010). Risk of first-generation H1-antihistamines: A GA²LEN position paper. *Allergy, 65,* 459–466. doi:10.1111/j.1398-9995.2009.02325.x

Connolly, S. D., Suarez, L., & Sylvester, C. (2011). Assessment and treatment of anxiety disorders in children and adolescents. *Current Psychiatric Reports, 13,* 99–110. doi:10.1007/s11920-010-0173-z

Gore, T. A. (2013). *Posttraumatic stress disorder.* Retrieved from http://emedicine.medscape.com/article/288154-overview

King, J. (2010). *Sleep disorders frequent in college students; linked to poor academic performance.* Retrieved from http://www.medscape.com/viewarticle/723798

National Center for Complementary and Alternative Medicine. (2010). Sleep disorders and CAM: What the science says. *NCCAM Clinical Digest.* Retrieved from http://nccam.nih.gov/health/providers/digest/sleepdisorders-science.htm

Reeve, K., & Balles, B. (2010). Insomnia in adults: Etiology and management. *Journal for Nurse Practitioners 6,* 53–60. doi:10.1016/j.nurpra.2009.09.013

Sher, L. (2009). Suicide in war veterans: The role of comorbidity of PTSD and depression. *Expert Review of Neurotherapeutics, 9,* 921–923. doi:10.1586/ern.09.61

Zhang, D., Tashiro, M., Shibuya, K., Okamura, N., Funaki, Y., Yoshikawa, T., . . . Yanai, K. (2010). Next-day residual sedative effect after nighttime administration of an over-the-counter antihistamine sleep aid, diphendydramine, measured by positron emission tomography. *Journal of Clinical Psychopharmacology, 30,* 694–701. doi:10.1097/JCP.0b013e3181fa8526

Selected Bibliography

Abramowitz, J. S., & Deacon, B. (2010). Anxiety and its disorders: Implications for pharmacotherapy. *Clinical Psychology: Science and Practice, 17,* 104–106. doi:10.1111/j.1468-2850.2010.01199.x

Foral, P., Dewan, N., & Malesker, M. (2011). Insomnia: A therapeutic review for pharmacists. *The Consultant Pharmacist, 26,* 332–341. doi:10.4140/TCP.n.2011.332

Herdman, T. H., & Kamitsuru, S. (Eds.). (2014). *NANDA International nursing diagnoses: Definitions and classification, 2015–2017.* Oxford, United Kingdom: Wiley-Blackwell.

Lie, D. A. (2013). *Sleep disorders: Can CAM help?* Retrieved from http://www.medscape.com/viewarticle/803722

Mihic, S. J., & Harris, R. A. (2011). Hypnotics and sedatives. In L. L. Brunton, B. A. Chabner, & B. C. Knollman (Eds.), *The pharmacological basis of therapeutics* (12th ed., pp. 457–480). New York, NY: McGraw-Hill.

Muris, P. (2012). Treatment of childhood anxiety disorders: What is the place for antidepressants? *Expert Opinion on Pharmacotherapy, 13*(1), 43–64. doi:10.1517/14656566.2012.642864

O'Donnel, J. M., & Shelton, R. C. (2011). Drug therapy of depression and anxiety disorders. In L. L. Brunton, B. A. Chabner, & B. C. Knollman (Eds.), *The pharmacological basis of therapeutics* (12th ed., pp. 397–416). New York, NY: McGraw-Hill.

Roth, T., & Roehrs, T. (2010). Pharmacotherapy for insomnia. *Sleep Medicine Clinics, 5,* 529–539. doi:10.1016/j.jsmc.2010.09.002

Sarris, J., Moylan, S., Camfield, D. A., Pase, M. P., Mischoulon, D., Berk, M., . . . Schweitzer, I. (2012). Complementary medicine, exercise, meditation, diet, and lifestyle modification for anxiety disorders: A review of current evidence. *Evidence-Based Complementary and Alternative Medicine, 2012,* Article ID 809653. doi:10.1155/2012/809653

Stein, M. B., & Steckler, T. (Eds.). (2010). *Behavioral neurobiology of anxiety and its treatment.* Heidelberg, Germany: Springer-Verlag.

Townsend-Roccichelli, J., Sanford, J. T., & VandeWaa, E. (2010). Managing sleep disorders in the elderly. *Nurse Practitioner, 35*(5), 30–37. doi:10.1097/01.NPR.0000371296.98371.7e

Yates, W. R. (2012). *Anxiety disorders.* Retrieved from http://emedicine.medscape.com/article/286227-overview

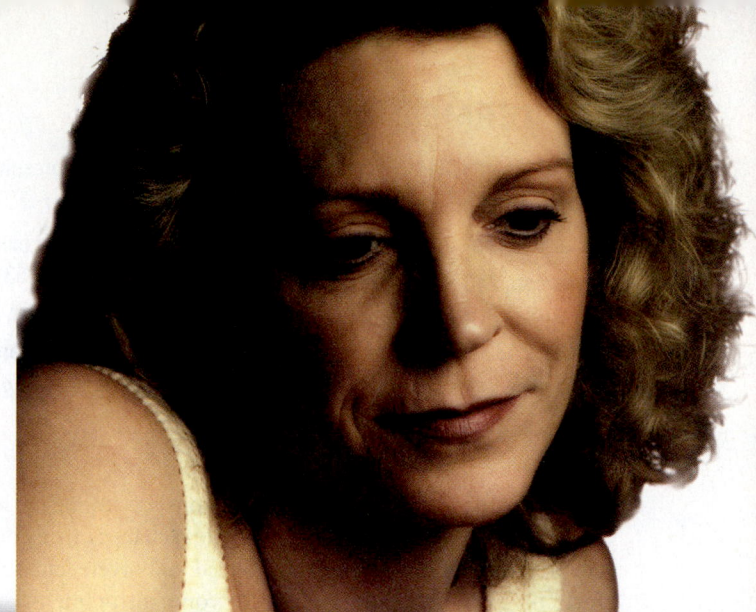

"For the past 4 to 5 weeks my wife, Jane, has been having problems. She doesn't get up to see that the children are off to school, dinner is not started when I get home from work at 6:00 p.m., no housework or laundry has been done, she is frequently still in pajamas with her hair uncombed, and obviously has not showered or brushed her teeth. Her friends say that Jane has not returned their calls in weeks."

"Charlie Albright," Jane's husband

19 Pharmacotherapy of Mood Disorders

LEARNING OUTCOMES

After reading this chapter, the student should be able to:

1. Compare and contrast the major categories of mood disorders and their symptoms.
2. Explain the pathophysiology of major depression and bipolar disorder.
3. Discuss the nurse's role in the assessment of patients with mood disorders.
4. Identify the relationship between suicide and depression.
5. Describe the nurse's role in the pharmacologic and nonpharmacologic management of mood disorders.
6. For each of the classes shown in the chapter outline, identify the prototype and representative drugs and explain the mechanism(s) of drug action, primary indications, contraindications, significant drug interactions, pregnancy category, and important adverse effects.
7. Apply the nursing process to care for patients receiving pharmacotherapy for mood disorders.

CHAPTER OUTLINE

▸ Categories of Mood Disorders

▸ Major Depressive Disorder

▸ Pathophysiology of Depression

▸ Assessment of Depression

▸ Nonpharmacologic Therapies for Depression

▸ Pharmacotherapy of Depression

Tricyclic Antidepressants

PROTOTYPE Imipramine (Tofranil), *p. 246*

Selective Serotonin Reuptake Inhibitors

PROTOTYPE Fluoxetine (Prozac, Sarafem), *p. 248*

Atypical Antidepressants

PROTOTYPE Venlafaxine (Effexor), *p. 251*

Monoamine Oxidase Inhibitors

PROTOTYPE Phenelzine (Nardil), *p. 254*

▸ Bipolar Disorder

▸ Drugs for Bipolar Disorder

PROTOTYPE Lithium Carbonate (Eskalith, Lithobid), *p. 258*

KEY TERMS

antidepressants, 244

atypical antidepressants, 250

bipolar disorder, 257

depression, 240

electroconvulsive therapy
   (ECT), 243

hypomania, 257

major depressive disorder, 240

mania, 257

monoamine oxidase inhibitors
   (MAOIs), 253

mood disorder, 240

mood stabilizers, 257

phototherapy, 243

postpartum depression, 241

seasonal affective disorder, 241

serotonin, 248

serotonin syndrome (SES), 248

suicide, 242

tricyclic antidepressants (TCAs), 244

tyramine, 253

Inappropriate or unusually intense emotions are among the leading mental health disorders. Although mood changes are a normal part of life, when they become prolonged and severe and impair functioning within the family, work environment, or interpersonal relationships, a patient may be diagnosed as having a mood disorder. The purpose of this chapter is to explain the role of pharmacotherapy in treating the two primary categories of mood disorders: major depression and bipolar disorder.

PharmFACT

Clinical depression affects more than 19 million Americans each year and is estimated to be associated with about half of all suicides (Dryden-Edwards, 2011).

Categories of Mood Disorders

19.1 The two primary categories of mood disorders are depression and bipolar disorder.

Mood disorders form a cluster of mental health conditions that occur frequently in the population. They affect all cultures and people of all ages, from children to older adults. Mood disorders are a major cause of disability and can significantly strain social relationships. They are a leading cause of absenteeism and diminished productivity in the workplace.

The diagnosis of mood disorders is often challenging; the line between normal emotion and a mood disorder is sometimes unclear. Because health care providers see patients for such brief periods, they must rely on patient self-reports or caregiver information, both of which are often unreliable. A **mood disorder** can be broadly defined as a persistent disturbance in mood that impairs a person's ability to effectively deal with normal activities of daily living (ADLs).

Mood disorders can present with a wide range of symptoms, which has resulted in classification of the disorder into the following categories.

- **Major depressive disorder.** When people use the word *depression*, they are most often referring to major depressive disorder. This is sometimes called clinical depression.
- **Dysthymic disorder.** This is mild, chronic depression that persists for at least 2 continuous years.
- **Bipolar disorder.** Formerly called manic depression, the patient alternates between intense excitement (mania) and major depressive disorder.
- **Manic and hypomanic episodes.** Include mania symptoms that last for at least 1 week and significantly impact social

functioning. Hypomania is less intense, lasting only 4 days and has less impact on social or work functioning.
- **Cyclothymic disorder.** A mild form of bipolar disorder in which the patient alternates between hypomania and mild depression. Largely undiagnosed, 33% of these patients will eventually develop bipolar disorder.

Mood disorders often coexist with other conditions. For example, about 50% of patients diagnosed with major depression also meet the criteria for an anxiety disorder (see Chapter 18). Of those patients with mood disorder 25% to 40% have a comorbid substance abuse condition. Those with chronic medical conditions such as hypertension (HTN) or arthritis have a higher incidence of depression. The most serious of the comorbid conditions is completed or attempted suicide.

Major Depressive Disorder

19.2 Major depressive disorder is characterized by a depressed mood, with accompanying symptoms, that lasts at least 2 weeks.

Depression is a disorder characterized by a sad or despondent mood that becomes out of proportion to actual life events. Depression can manifest as an extremely diverse set of symptoms, including lack of energy, sleep disturbances, abnormal eating patterns, or feelings of despair, guilt, and hopelessness. Depression is the most common mental health disorder, affecting approximately 10% to 20% of the population. Although women between the ages of 25 and 45 are more likely to have a depressive disorder than any other group, depression in men more frequently results in suicide. Many persons who are depressed never seek or receive care for their depression.

Major depressive disorder is diagnosed when the patient has a depressed mood that lasts for a minimum of 2 weeks and which is present for most of the day, every day, or almost every day. In addition, at least five of the symptoms shown in Table 19.1 must be present. Depressed moods caused by general medical conditions or by substances such as alcohol or other central nervous system (CNS) depressants do not warrant a diagnosis of major depressive disorder. For the purposes of this text, the terms *depression* and *major depressive disorder* are considered interchangeable unless otherwise specified.

Once a diagnosis of a mood disorder is made, additional details about the condition may be provided by the health care provider in the form of "specifiers." The use of specifiers gives mental health professionals additional information about the disorder and its

TABLE 19.1	Symptoms of Depression	
CNS Symptoms	**Behavioral Symptoms**	**General Symptoms**
Feelings of despair, lack of self-worth, guilt, and misery	Staying in bed most of the day and night	Extremely tired; without energy
Obsessed with death; expresses desire to die or to commit suicide	Neglecting usual household chores	Vague physical symptoms (GI pain, joint or muscle pain, or headaches)
Delusions or hallucinations	Not going to work, or unable to function effectively at work	Physiological depression (constipation, sleep disorders, or decreased heart rate)
	Abnormal eating patterns (eating too much or not enough)	
	Lack of interest in personal appearance or sex	
	Avoiding psychosocial and interpersonal interactions	

treatment. Specifiers are best thought of as subcategories of major depressive disorder and bipolar disorder. Some of the specifiers used with depression include with or without psychotic features, single episode or recurrent, melancholic features, atypical features, and catatonic features. Two additional important specifiers are postpartum onset and seasonal onset.

Up to 80% of new mothers experience brief "baby blues" or **postpartum depression** during the first 2 weeks after the birth of a baby. About 10% to 15% of these women will experience major depression within the first 6 months postdelivery, which is likely related to the dramatic hormonal shifts that occur during that period. Along with the hormonal changes, additional situational stresses such as changing responsibilities at work and at home, single parenthood, and caring for children and for aging parents may contribute to the onset of symptoms. Because of the potentially serious consequences of postpartum onset depression, some states mandate that all new mothers receive information about these mood disorders prior to their discharge after giving birth. All levels of health care providers treating new mothers are encouraged to conduct routine screening for symptoms of perinatal mood disorders.

During the dark winter months, some patients experience a type of depression known as **seasonal affective disorder**. Seasonal affective disorder is more common in areas such as Alaska, where the days are very short during the winter months and there is little natural sunlight. This type of depression is associated with a reduced release of the hormone melatonin from the pineal gland. The condition is generally self-limiting and resolves when spring arrives. Exposing patients on a regular basis to specific wavelengths of light may relieve this type of depression and prevent future episodes.

PharmFACT

Pathophysiology of Depression

19.3 The pathophysiology of depression has biologic, genetic, and environmental components.

Depression is one of the oldest known mental health conditions and one of the most frequently diagnosed. Despite this, the etiology of depression is not well understood. Several theories have been proposed to explain the causes of depression and why some people are predisposed to developing the disease. The etiology and pathogenesis are likely influenced by multiple, complex variables.

Research attempting to identify the biologic causes of depression has focused on the levels and function of neurotransmitters in the limbic system of the brain. The limbic system is the region that regulates emotions (see Chapters 17 and 18). Major depression has been associated with abnormally low levels of neurotransmitters such as norepinephrine, serotonin, and dopamine in this region. Although it is well known that some of the antidepressant medications act by increasing the levels of these neurotransmitters, scientists have yet to discover what role each specific neurotransmitter plays in the development of major depressive disorder. Does having depression deplete the brain of these neurotransmitters, or does a loss of neurotransmitters cause depression? The answers remain elusive.

Certain hormonal abnormalities are associated with depression, suggesting that the endocrine system also plays an important role in the pathogenesis of the disease. About half of persons who are depressed have abnormally high serum cortisol levels. Cortisol mobilizes the body for stress situations and is thought to reduce serotonin levels in the brain, bringing about symptoms of depression. Hypothyroidism is also associated with depression. In some patients, therapy with thyroid hormone (T_3) results in a marked improvement in mood.

It is well established that depression has a genetic component. Major depression is 1.5 to 3 times more common in persons who have a first-degree relative (parent or sibling) with depression compared to the general population. In identical twins, when one twin is diagnosed with depression, the other twin has a 50% probability of acquiring the disorder. This relationship holds true whether the twins were raised together or separately. Even fraternal twins have a 19% chance of developing depression when the other twin is diagnosed, which is a percentage higher than that of the general population.

Environmental causes of depression include prolonged stress at work or at home, loss of a loved one, and other traumatic life events. Various childhood events have been associated with an increased risk of adult depression, including sexual or physical abuse, and death of, separation from, or mental illness of a parent.

CONNECTION Checkpoint 19.1

From what you learned in Chapter 17, what are the connections between the limbic system, the hypothalamus, and the cerebrum, and how can these connections be used to explain symptoms of depression? *See Answer to Connection Checkpoint 19.1 on student resource website.*

Assessment of Depression

19.4 Assessment and diagnosis of depression are a collaborative effort among health care providers.

For proper diagnosis and treatment to occur, the recognition of depression must be a collaborative effort among health care providers. Because people who are depressed are present in multiple settings and in all areas of practice, every nurse should be proficient in the assessment and nursing care of patients afflicted with this disorder.

The first step in implementing appropriate treatment for depression is a complete medical examination, because the diagnosis of depression begins by ruling out other medical conditions. Certain medications such as corticosteroids, beta blockers, levodopa, antipsychotic agents, oral contraceptives, and CNS depressants can cause symptoms of clinical depression. Depression may be mimicked by a variety of medical and neurologic disorders, ranging from B-vitamin deficiencies to thyroid gland malfunction to early Alzheimer's disease. If medical causes for the depression are discovered, proper treatment of the underlying disorder may be sufficient to resolve symptoms of depression. If causes for the depression cannot be identified, a psychiatrist or psychologist may be consulted to perform a comprehensive psychological evaluation to confirm the diagnosis.

Because they are comorbid with depression in a significant number of patients, inquiries should be made about alcohol and drug use and any thoughts about suicide. The initial exam should also include questions about any family history of depressive illness. The manifestation of depression that is most obvious to those surrounding a person who is depressed is a change in attitude toward usual daily activities. The patient loses interest in work, school, or other hobbies or activities that he or she previously enjoyed.

Severe depressive illness, particularly that which is recurrent, will require both medication and psychotherapy to achieve optimum outcomes. Daily outpatient visits to a treatment facility may be necessary when beginning treatment, then tapered to a less frequent schedule as improvement is noted. Some patients, especially those at high risk for suicide, will require an initial period of hospitalization where continuous monitoring is provided.

Depression remains greatly underdiagnosed among older adults despite the fact that as many as 6 million Americans over the age of 65 have this disorder. Of this group, only about 10% receive treatment. Elderly patients may be reluctant to admit to depression, seeing this as a sign of weakness or an inability to continue to care for themselves. Depression in the older adult may be manifested as difficulty making decisions and as a growing reluctance to leave the home. Feelings of despair, lack of self-worth, and guilt are common.

Factors that contribute to depression in the older adult include loss of spouse or children; the need to move from a long-term residence to a smaller home or in with other family or to assisted living; loss of friends and other support systems; being unmarried; living alone; having multiple health challenges; the expense of polypharmacy; decreased finances; and worry about end-of-life issues.

CONNECTIONS   **Lifespan Consideration**

◀ Insomnia, Depression, and Suicide Risk in Older Adults

While depression and suicide risk are often viewed as health issues affecting the adolescent, young, or middle adult populations, suicide in the adult age 70 to 74 approximates the rate in the 25–29 age group (crude death rates of 15.16/1,000 and 15.56/1,000, respectively) and for the oldest adults over age 80 (crude death rate of 18.26/1,000), only the suicide rate in adults age 45 to 54 is higher (19.98/1,000) (CDC, 2011b). It is known that insomnia may occur in up to 80% of patients diagnosed with depression, a problem that may be compounded if drugs used for the treatment of depression worsen insomnia (Luca, Luca, & Calandra, 2013). Recent research has demonstrated that insomnia may be a precursor to the development of depression and increases the risk of suicidal ideation (Baglioni et al., 2011; Nardorff, Fiske, Sperry, Petts, & Gregg, 2013). Because the older adult is often at greater risk for insomnia and may attribute sleep disturbances as a normal fact of aging, health care providers should include an assessment of sleep patterns and insomnia as part of the older adult's health screening. When insomnia is noted, appropriate treatment may improve sleep quality and also decrease the risk of depression and suicide.

19.5 The majority of patients who attempt suicide have major depression.

Suicide is defined as the intentional act of ending one's life. The Centers for Disease Control and Prevention (CDC, 2013) lists suicide as the 10th cause of death in the United States; about 35,000 people every year take their own lives. No age group, income level, educational level, race, religion, or other demographic group is exempt from it. About 90% of all persons who turn to suicide, whether successful or not, have a diagnosed mental health or substance abuse disorder (National Institute of Mental Health [NIMH], n.d.). Comorbid conditions include mood disorders, psychoses, personality disorder, anxiety disorders, severe insomnia, chronic alcohol or substance use, chronic disabling or painful disease, and family history, especially in the same-sex parent.

The majority of persons who commit suicide have been diagnosed with major depression. Unfortunately, depending on the drug and the individual patient's response, 3 or more weeks of antidepressant pharmacotherapy may be required before the patient's mood begins to improve. Suicide may occur early in treatment, when a patient is being stabilized on the antidepressant. Some theories have proposed that antidepressant medications actually increase the risk of suicide. This prompted the U.S. Food and Drug Administration (FDA) to issue a black box warning in 2004 indicating that antidepressant medications are associated with an increased risk of suicidal thinking and behavior in children and adolescents (U.S. Food and Drug Administration, 2004). This black box warning was expanded in 2007 to include young adults 18 to 24 years of age.

Researchers have continued to monitor the proposed link between antidepressant medications and suicide rate. Subsequent studies have found that antidepressant use reduces overall suicide attempts and deaths due to suicide in patients who are depressed (Leon et al., 2011). Risks of attempted suicide are highest in the month before pharmacotherapy, and attempts decline after pharmacotherapy begins. The relationship between antidepressants and suicide will likely be a continuing topic of research.

So what interventions can the nurse implement to reduce the potential for suicidal behavior during antidepressant therapy? Careful monitoring of the patient is the simplest yet most important intervention. Weekly and even daily patient contact may be necessary until the antidepressant begins to effectively elevate mood, which could be as long as 12 weeks. A patient who has had a previous suicide attempt is at higher risk and must be more carefully monitored. If a person verbalizes about committing suicide, the talk must be taken seriously. It is a myth that a person who talks about suicide will not actually act. The person may be so depressed that suicide seems like the only option, and talking about it to a friend or nurse may be a last attempt at getting help or having someone intercede. The nurse must judiciously monitor all prescribed drugs because suicidal patients often take overdoses of their medications (including those prescribed to treat the depression!). Therapy with multiple CNS depressants such as for pain, anxiety, insomnia, and depression is strongly discouraged because these drugs produce additive sedation. Worsening symptoms of depression must be reported immediately because these may indicate that the drug is not working or that the patient is not compliant with pharmacotherapy. Switching to a different antidepressant or even hospitalization may be necessary.

Nonpharmacologic Therapies for Depression

19.6 Depression is sometimes treated with nonpharmacologic therapies.

Although pharmacotherapy is the standard treatment for patients with major depression, other therapies may be beneficial for patients with mild to moderate depression or for those whose condition is refractory to conventional treatment. Indeed, psychotherapy may be the treatment of choice if the patient is willing to participate and the depressive state is mild to moderate in intensity. Other nonpharmacologic therapies for depression are shown in Table 19.2.

Older nonpharmacologic treatments include cognitive–behavioral therapies to help patients change negative styles of thought and behavior that are often associated with their depression. These therapies focus on resolving the patients' internal conflicts by looking at the influence of past experiences on current behavior and how behavior is influenced by emotional factors. These therapies are sometimes postponed until the acute depressive symptoms have improved. Light therapy or **phototherapy** is another type of therapy especially useful for people with seasonal affective disorder, using artificial lighting approximately 5 to 20 times brighter than normal indoor lighting. Normal activities can be pursued during the treatment, which can be conducted in the patient's home.

In patients with serious and life-threatening mood disorders that are unresponsive to pharmacotherapy and psychotherapy, **electroconvulsive therapy (ECT)** continues to be a useful treatment. ECT induces a brief convulsion (grand mal seizure) by passing an electric current into the brain through electrodes applied to one or both temples while the patient is anesthetized. A muscle relaxant is given prior to the treatment and the patient is unaware of the treatment or convulsion. Typically, 6 to 12 treatments are needed to relieve depression: In severe, refractory cases ECT may be continued for several of years.

Transcranial magnetic stimulation (TMS) is an emerging therapy for major depression. TMS is a noninvasive procedure that passes a high electric current through a wire stimulation coil placed on or close to a specific area of the head. Treatments are generally administered daily; the length of treatment varies according to patient response. TMS has minimal effects on memory, does not require general anesthesia, and produces its effects without a generalized seizure. Further research is needed to confirm its effectiveness at relieving depression.

Another somatic therapy currently under investigation is vagus nerve stimulation (VNS). VNS involves the surgical implantation of a small generator, about 3 to 4 inches in diameter, into the patient's chest. An electrode is threaded through the subcutaneous tissue from the generator to the vagus nerve on the left side of the patient's neck. The left vagus connects to the brainstem and deep brain structures thought to be involved in epilepsy and some

TABLE 19.2 Nonpharmacologic Therapies for Major Depression	
Type	**Definition**
Cognitive–behavioral therapy	Therapy that helps patients change the negative styles of thought and behavior that are often associated with their depression.
Electroconvulsive therapy (ECT)	The induction of a brief convulsion by passing an electric current through the brain as therapy for affective disorders, especially in patients who have not responded to pharmacotherapy.
Interpersonal therapy	Therapy focusing on the patient's disturbed personal relationships that both cause and exacerbate the depression.
Light therapy or phototherapy	Therapy that uses artificial lighting that is 5 to 20 times brighter than usual indoor lighting; it is used to simulate natural sunlight in areas where there is little natural sunlight for several months of the year, such as Alaska and other areas near the North Pole.
Psychodynamic therapy	Therapy focusing on resolving a patient's internal conflicts.
Repetitive transcranial magnetic stimulation (rTMS) therapy	An effective somatic therapy, experimental in the United States, that involves a device that administers a train of multiple stimuli per second. The device is a metal coil that is placed on or near the patient's head, allowing the magnetic field to pass through the skull and into specific targeted areas of the brain.
Vagus nerve stimulation (VNS)	Somatic therapy that involves placing a small generator into the patient's chest; it is attached to an electrode with ends wrapped around the left vagus nerve on the patient's neck; the generator is programmed for frequency and intensity of stimulus. The electrical current stimulates the vagus nerve.

psychiatric disorders. Stimulating these fibers affects the concentration of the neurotransmitter gamma aminobutyric acid (GABA) and other neurotransmitters in that area. VNS is approved in the United States for treating epilepsy and for the adjunctive treatment of chronic depression for adult patients who are experiencing a major depressive episode and have not had an adequate response to multiple antidepressant medications.

PharmFACT
Approximately 16% of the students in grades 9 through 12 seriously consider suicide each year. Over 8% state that they actually attempted suicide. Although girls most often report attempting suicide, 81% of the suicide deaths from age 10 to 24 are males (CDC, 2014).

Pharmacotherapy of Depression

19.7 The mechanism of action of antidepressants involves modulation of neurotransmitter levels in the brain.

Antidepressants are drugs used to enhance, elevate, or stabilize mood. In the treatment of depression they are used to treat all symptoms of major depressive disorder as well as the depressive phases of bipolar disorder. They are ineffective against the manic phases of bipolar disorder, and other drugs must be used to control those symptoms (see Section 19.12).

The antidepressants act by restoring normal neurotransmitter balances in specific regions of the brain. Depending on the medication, the primary neurotransmitters affected are norepinephrine, serotonin, and, to a lesser degree, dopamine. The two basic mechanisms of action of antidepressants are blocking the enzymatic breakdown of norepinephrine and slowing the reuptake of serotonin into neurons. Although antidepressants may not completely restore chemical balance, they help to manage depressive symptoms while the patient develops effective strategies for coping.

In addition to elevating mood, changing the neurotransmitter balance has a number of other effects on the brain. Some of the antidepressants have become major drugs in the treatment of anxiety disorders such as phobia, obsessive–compulsive behavior, panic disorder, and generalized anxiety disorder, as presented in Chapter 18. Certain antidepressants are also beneficial as adjuvant analgesics in the pharmacotherapy of pain (see Chapter 25). Antidepressants are beneficial in treating depression that is often associated with painful, chronic conditions such as fibromyalgia or muscle spasticity (see Chapter 23).

Once patients begin to "feel better" they sometimes want to discontinue drug therapy due to the expense of the medication or because they are experiencing uncomfortable adverse effects. Nurses must be aware that many patients taking antidepressants stop taking their medication without notifying their health care provider. Unfortunately, about half of these patients will relapse within 6 months of discontinuing antidepressant therapy; the percentage increases to 85% after 3 years. It is important to teach patients that daily antidepressant dosing is required and that adherence to the health care provider's instructions is essential for the long-term maintenance of mental health.

When administered at therapeutic doses, all antidepressants have similar effectiveness; therefore, the choice of drug is not usually based on this factor. The treatment of depression, however, is highly individualized and patients who are unresponsive to one class of medications may respond favorably to drugs from a different class. In fact, patients may respond differently to drugs within the *same* class. Furthermore, the spectrum of adverse effects differs among the classes, and patients may find that drugs from one class are more tolerable than another. Overall, about 65% of patients will respond favorably to antidepressant pharmacotherapy. Success rates improve to 85% when psychotherapy or alternative or adjunctive medicine is used along with antidepressant medications. The four primary classes of antidepressants, shown in Table 19.3, are as follows:

- Tricyclic antidepressants (TCAs)
- Selective serotonin reuptake inhibitors (SSRIs)
- Atypical antidepressants
- Monoamine oxidase inhibitors (MAOIs)

Therapy with antidepressants is generally begun with low doses, usually with a drug from the SSRI class. If no improvement in mood is noted after 2 to 4 weeks, the dose of the drug is increased. Continued lack of response may indicate that the patient is not taking the medication as prescribed, or that a drug from a different class should be used, such as a TCA or an atypical antidepressant. It is important that patients understand that antidepressant therapy may extend for many years. In general, antidepressant therapy should continue for a minimum of 6 months after the depressive symptoms resolve to prevent uncomfortable withdrawal symptoms and the potential for rebound depression.

Tricyclic Antidepressants

19.8 Tricyclic antidepressants were once the mainstay for the treatment of depression but they have many adverse effects.

The **tricyclic antidepressants (TCAs)** have been available in the United States for more than 50 years. Although newer antidepressant classes have been discovered, the TCAs are still prescribed for many patients with major depressive disorder. This group of medications is named after its molecular structure, which has a three-ring core. Because this molecular arrangement is very similar to the structure of the phenothiazine antipsychotics, these two classes of drugs share similar adverse effects (see Chapter 20). Several of the TCAs are also prescribed to treat the depressive stage of bipolar disorder, chronic insomnia, obsessive–compulsive disorder (OCD), neuropathic pain, and fibromyalgia.

The TCAs act by blocking the reuptake transport of norepinephrine and serotonin at synapses, as shown in Figure 19.1. This blockade results in a greater quantity of neurotransmitters available in the synaptic space, leading to a more intensified action. Some TCAs such as desipramine, maprotiline, and protriptyline are specific to blocking the reuptake of norepinephrine, whereas the other drugs in this class affect both norepinephrine and serotonin. In general, all TCAs have similar effectiveness in treating depression and exhibit the same spectrum of adverse effects.

The advantages of TCAs are that they are inexpensive and their effectiveness in treating depression has been well established for many decades. They are rapidly absorbed when given orally (PO) and widely distributed throughout the body. Frequent adverse effects, however, have limited their use in recent years. Most health

TABLE 19.3 Antidepressant Drugs

Drug	Route and Adult Dose (Maximum Dose Where Indicated)	Adverse Effects
Tricyclic Antidepressants (TCAs)		
amitriptyline (Elavil)	PO: 75–100 mg/day (max: 300 mg/day)	*Drowsiness, sedation, dizziness, orthostatic hypotension, dry mouth, constipation, urinary retention, blurred vision, mydriasis, tachycardia* <u>Bone marrow depression, seizures, dysrhythmias, heart block, MI, hepatitis, acute renal failure</u>
clomipramine (Anafranil)	PO: 25 mg once daily (max: 250 mg/day)	
desipramine (Norpramin)	PO: 75–100 mg/day; may increase to 150–300 mg/day	
doxepin (Silenor)	PO (generic for depression or anxiety): 25–150 mg/day in divided doses (max: 300 mg/day)	
	PO (Silenor for insomnia): 3–6 mg at bedtime	
imipramine (Tofranil)	PO: 75–150 mg/day (max: 300 mg/day)	
	IM: 50–100 mg/day in divided doses	
maprotiline (Ludiomil)	PO: 75–150 mg/day in divided doses (max: 225 mg/day)	
nortriptyline (Aventyl, Pamelor)	PO: 25 mg tid or qid (max: 150 mg/day)	
protriptyline (Vivactil)	PO: 15–40 mg/day in divided doses (max: 60 mg/day)	
trimipramine (Surmontil)	PO: 50–100 mg/day in divided doses (max: 300 mg/day)	
Selective Serotonin Reuptake Inhibitors (SSRIs)		
citalopram (Celexa)	PO: start at 20 mg once daily; may increase to 40 mg after 1 week (max: 40 mg/day)	*Nausea, vomiting, dry mouth, insomnia, somnolence, headache, nervousness, anxiety, diarrhea, dizziness, anorexia, fatigue, sexual dysfunction, weight changes* <u>Stevens–Johnson syndrome (SJS), serotonin syndrome, suicidal ideation in children and young adults</u>
escitalopram (Lexapro)	PO: 10 mg once daily; may increase to 20 mg after 1 week (max: 20 mg/day)	
fluoxetine (Prozac)	PO: 20 mg/day (max: 80 mg/day); when stable may switch to 90-mg sustained release capsule once weekly (max: 90 mg/week)	
fluvoxamine (Luvox)	PO (extended release): 100 mg once daily at bedtime (max: 300 mg/day)	
paroxetine (Paxil, Pexeva)	PO (immediate release): start with 20 mg once daily and increase by 10 mg each week as needed (max: 60 mg/day)	
	PO (sustained release): 25 mg daily and increase by 12.5-mg intervals (max: 62.5 mg/day)	
sertraline (Zoloft)	PO: start with 50 mg once daily and increase at weekly intervals as needed (max: 200 mg/day)	
vortioxetine (Brintellix)	PO: 5–20 mg once daily (max: 20 mg/day)	
Serotonin–Norepinephrine Reuptake Inhibitors (SNRIs)		
desvenlafaxine (Pristiq)	PO: 50 mg once daily (max: 100 mg/day)	*Nausea, dry mouth, constipation, sweating, agitation, somnolence, decreased appetite, changes in weight (loss or gain), increased blood glucose level (duloxetine)* <u>Suicidal ideation, hepatotoxicity, syncope, neuroleptic malignant syndrome, abnormal bleeding, HTN (desvenlafaxine, venlafaxine), seizures</u>
duloxetine (Cymbalta)	PO: 40–60 mg/day in 1–2 divided doses (max: 60 mg/day)	
venlafaxine (Effexor)	PO: start with 75 mg/day and increase slowly at 4- to 7-day intervals as needed (max: 375 mg/day for regular release; 225 mg/day for extended release)	
Atypical Antidepressants		
amoxapine	PO: start with 50 mg bid–tid and increase to 100 mg bid–tid by the end of the first week (max: 400 mg/day)	*Insomnia, nausea, dry mouth, constipation, increased blood pressure and heart rate, dizziness, sweating, agitation, blurred vision, headache, tremor, vomiting, drowsiness, somnolence, increased appetite, orthostatic hypotension* <u>SJS, seizures, vaginal, uterine, or anal hemorrhage, suicidal ideation, priapism, neuroleptic malignant syndrome (amoxapine), parkinsonism (amoxapine), elevated hepatic enzymes (mirtazapine), bone marrow suppression (mirtazapine), liver failure (nefazodone)</u>
bupropion (Wellbutrin, Zyban, others)	PO: 100 mg tid (immediate release) or 150 mg bid (sustained release) or 300 mg once daily (extended release) (max: 450 mg/day)	
mirtazapine (Remeron)	PO: 15 mg/day in a single dose at bedtime (max: 45 mg/day)	
nefazodone	PO: 50–100 mg bid (max: 600 mg/day)	
trazodone (Oleptro)	PO: 150 mg/day (max: 600 mg/day for immediate release and 375 mg/day for extended release)	
vilazodone (Viibryd)	PO: begin with 10 mg once daily and gradually increase to 40 mg once daily	
MAO Inhibitors (MAOIs)		
isocarboxazid (Marplan)	PO: 10–30 mg/day (max: 30 mg/day)	*Drowsiness, insomnia, orthostatic hypotension, blurred vision, nausea, constipation, anorexia, dry mouth, urinary retention, sexual dysfunction, overactivity* <u>Hypertensive crisis, circulatory collapse, dysrhythmias</u>
phenelzine (Nardil)	PO: 15 mg tid rapidly increase to at least 60 mg/day tid or qid (max: 90 mg/day)	
selegiline (Emsam)	Transdermal: one patch (6 mg/day)	
tranylcypromine (Parnate)	PO: 30 mg/day; may increase by 10 mg/day at 3-week intervals (max: 60 mg/day)	

Note: *Italics* indicate common adverse effects. <u>Underline</u> indicates serious adverse effects.

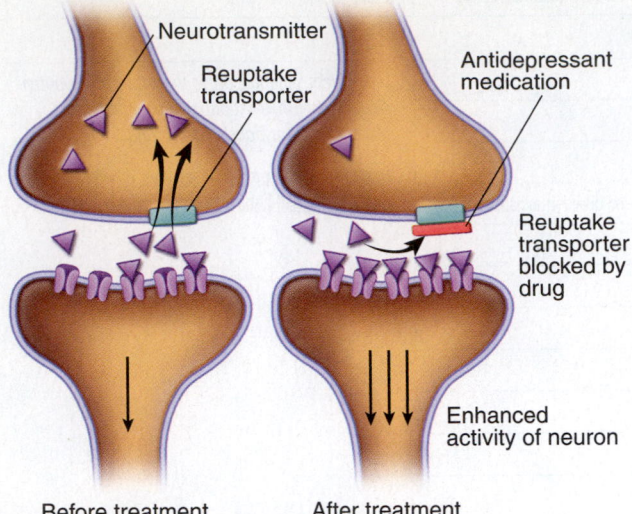

Before treatment   **After treatment**

Figure 19.1 Mechanisms of action of antidepressants: (a) In adrenergic and serotonergic neurons the activity of the neurotransmitter is terminated by reuptake. (b) Tricyclic antidepressants and SSRIs produce their effects by inhibiting the reuptake of neurotransmitters. The neurotransmitter accumulates in the synaptic cleft and activates more receptors, thus causing an enhanced effect at the synapse.

care providers now prefer to prescribe drugs in the SSRI class because they are better tolerated by most patients.

Blockade of muscarinic receptors by TCAs is responsible for causing a high incidence of anticholinergic adverse effects with symptoms such as dry mouth, blurred vision, constipation, urinary retention, and tachycardia. Orthostatic hypotension is common and may be serious enough to cause injury due to falls. Although rare, the most serious adverse effect is the ability of TCAs to cause life-threatening cardiac dysrhythmias, especially if the patient receives an overdose of the medication.

A few of the TCAs have central effects that cause sedation, which can usually be managed by taking the drugs at bedtime. Sedation is worsened by the concurrent use of other CNS depressants such as alcohol. Confusion, dizziness, and fatigue are other possible dose-limiting effects of TCAs. At high doses some cause seizures.

Compared to other classes of antidepressants, TCAs exhibit a relatively high incidence of sexual dysfunction, including impotence and delayed ejaculation in men, and breast enlargement and impaired orgasm in women. Weight gain is possible. In addition, some patients quickly change mood from depression to hypomania or mania and may begin to display symptoms of bipolar disorder. These patients require a dosage adjustment or a change to a different antidepressant.

Tolerance and psychological dependence are usually not major problems with TCAs. Once stabilized, therapy may often be conducted for years without requiring a dosage adjustment. Unlike many CNS depressants, antidepressants such as the TCAs are not drugs of abuse. Patients on high doses for prolonged periods, however, may exhibit a mild withdrawal syndrome on discontinuation and experience symptoms such as irritability, nausea, sleep impairment, muscle aches, and fatigue. To avoid these symptoms, and to

ensure that rebound depression does not occur, it is best that these drugs be withdrawn gradually.

CONNECTION Checkpoint 19.2

Anticholinergic effects are common with TCAs and some other antidepressants. From what you learned in Chapter 14, name the prototype anticholinergic drug. If anticholinergic effects become prominent in a patient, what class of drugs can be used to counteract the cardiovascular adverse effects? *See Answer to Connection Checkpoint 19.2 on student resource website.*

PROTOTYPE DRUG	Imipramine (Tofranil)

Classification: Therapeutic: Tricyclic antidepressant
Pharmacologic: Norepinephrine reuptake inhibitor

Therapeutic Effects and Uses: Approved in 1959 as the first TCA, imipramine is effective in treating major depressive disorder. Like other TCAs, it is given PO and is well absorbed from the gastrointestinal (GI) tract. A drawback to the use of imipramine is that it takes 2 weeks or longer to achieve full therapeutic effect. During the initial weeks of therapy, when blood levels of imipramine have not yet produced their full therapeutic effects, suicide risks may increase, especially in children, adolescents, and young adults. Although it is not a preferred therapy for the disorder, imipramine is one of only two drugs approved for nocturnal enuresis, or bedwetting, in children. The urge to urinate is diminished by the anticholinergic (urinary retention) effects of the drug. A newer form of the drug, imipramine pamoate (Tofranil PM) is only approved for major depression and has different dosage forms.

Like other TCAs, imipramine has a number of off-label indications. These include the adjuvant treatment of cancer or neuropathic pain, overactive bladder, attention deficit/hyperactivity disorder (ADHD), insomnia, and bulimia nervosa. The use of TCAs in treating social anxiety disorder (social phobia) and panic disorder is presented in Chapter 18. The active metabolite of imipramine is desipramine, which is marketed separately as Norpramin.

Mechanism of Action: Imipramine blocks the reuptake of norepinephrine and serotonin into presynaptic nerve terminals. This results in an increased action of both neurotransmitters in neurons. Imipramine also blocks acetylcholine receptors, which is likely responsible for its effectiveness in treating enuresis.

Pharmacokinetics:

Route(s)	PO, IM (rare)
Absorption	Completely absorbed from the GI tract
Distribution	Widely distributed; crosses the placenta; secreted in breast milk; 85–95% bound to plasma protein
Primary metabolism	Hepatic; metabolized to the active metabolite desipramine
Primary excretion	Renal; small amounts in bile and feces
Onset of action	1–2 h for peak serum level; mood elevation requires 2–3 weeks
Duration of action	Not known

Adverse Effects: Frequent adverse reactions with imipramine include orthostatic hypotension (the most common adverse effect), dizziness, confusion, drowsiness, diarrhea, dry mouth, increased appetite, jaundice, urinary retention, rash, pruritus, and photosensitivity. Serious adverse reactions include seizures, hepatitis, acute renal failure, paralytic ileus, leukopenia, agranulocytosis, thrombocytopenia, or eosinophilia. Serious adverse reactions occur with acute doses when imipramine accumulates in cardiac tissue; dysrhythmias, heart failure, or myocardial infarction (MI) can occur. **Black Box Warning**: Antidepressants increase the risk of suicidal thinking and behavior in children, adolescents, and young adults. Patients of all ages should be monitored and observed closely during therapy for clinical worsening, suicidality, or unusual changes in behavior.

Contraindications/Precautions: Imipramine should not be used by patients with seizure disorders because it lowers the seizure threshold. It must be used with caution in persons with suicidal tendencies, urinary retention, prostatic hyperplasia, cardiac or hepatic disease, increased intraocular pressure, or hyperthyroidism. Use in patients with Parkinson's disease will induce or worsen parkinsonism symptoms. Patients with cardiac disease such as heart failure, QT prolongation, or history of MI should be carefully monitored during therapy; use in patients recovering from MI has resulted in sudden death. Imipramine should not be used during pregnancy or lactation.

Drug Interactions: Like other TCAs, imipramine is metabolized by hepatic P450 enzymes and is highly protein bound; thus there is a high potential for drug–drug interactions. Increased sedation can occur when imipramine is given concurrently with alcohol, barbiturates, benzodiazepines, direct-acting sympathomimetics, and other CNS depressants. Drug interactions causing decreased effects of imipramine include oral contraceptives, clonidine, carbamazepine, and indirect-acting sympathomimetics. Concurrent use with thyroid hormone may induce dysrhythmias. Imipramine should not be given concurrently with other drugs that prolong the QT interval, such as the Class IA antidysrhythmics, because of the potential for serious cardiac toxicity. Phenothiazines and TCAs are structurally very similar and concurrent use will likely cause additive anticholinergic adverse effects. Concurrent use of MAOIs must be avoided because this combination may cause hypertensive crisis, seizures, or hyperpyretic crisis. SSRIs must not be used concurrently; this can cause increased toxicity of TCAs. **Herbal/Food**: Several commonly used herbal products may lead to increased imipramine effects, including kava, hops, lavender, valerian, skullcap, and chamomile. An increased anticholinergic effect can occur with the use of belladonna, jimsonweed, or henbane. Serotonin syndrome may occur with the use of St. John's wort.

Pregnancy: Category C.

Treatment of Overdose: Overdoses with TCAs may be life threatening with symptoms that include mixed mania and depression followed by coma. Medical management includes treating possible seizures, hypotension, and dysrhythmias.

Nursing Responsibilities: Key nursing implications for patients receiving imipramine are included in the Nursing Practice Application for Patients Receiving Pharmacotherapy with Antidepressants.

Drugs Similar to Imipramine (Tofranil)

Nine TCAs are available. Desipramine is an active metabolite of imipramine, and the two drugs have the same actions and adverse effects, as previously described.

Amitriptyline (Elavil) and nortriptyline (Aventyl, Pamelor): Amitriptyline has been available by the PO route since 1961 for the therapy of major depression. It has been used for a large number of off-label indications, including neuropathic pain syndromes such as fibromyalgia, and for nocturnal enuresis, social anxiety disorder, ADHD, migraines, persistent hiccups, insomnia, and bulimia nervosa. It produces more sedation than most other TCAs and is thus taken at bedtime. It is metabolized in the liver to nortriptyline, which is marketed as a separate drug. Both amitriptyline and nortriptyline produce significant anticholinergic adverse effects. Like other TCAs, cardiac toxicity is a concern at high doses. These drugs are pregnancy category D.

Clomipramine (Anafranil): Approved in 1991, the only FDA-approved indication for clomipramine is OCD. Depression is an off-label indication. Other off-label uses are premature ejaculation and childhood autism. Because the drug produces significant anticholinergic effects and orthostatic hypotension, it is not a first-line drug for depression. This drug is pregnancy category C.

Doxepin (Silenor): Approved in 1969 to treat major depression, doxepin is also FDA approved to treat insomnia and anxiety. Doses used to treat depression (25–150 mg/day) are much higher than those used for insomnia (3–6 mg). When given PO for depression or anxiety, the most common side effect is sedation. Other adverse effects include nausea and upper respiratory tract infection. A topical form of doxepin (Zonalon) is available for pruritus associated with atopic dermatitis. Because doxepin is absorbed through the skin, topical applications can cause systemic adverse effects. This drug is pregnancy category C.

Maprotiline (Ludiomil): Maprotiline does not have a tricyclic chemical structure but it is included with the TCAs because it has very similar therapeutic and adverse effects. It was approved to treat major depression in 1980. Off-label indications include bulimia nervosa, neuropathic pain, panic attacks, and enuresis. It has the same adverse effects as other drugs in this class and offers no specific advantages over other TCAs. This drug is pregnancy category D.

Protriptyline (Vivactil): Protriptyline is an oral antidepressant that was approved in 1967. It has the same adverse effects as other TCAs except that it tends to produce CNS stimulation rather than sedation. It is the only TCA that has respiratory stimulant activity. These respiratory effects have led to its occasional off-label use for treating chronic obstructive pulmonary disease or sleep apnea. This drug is pregnancy category C.

Trimipramine (Surmontil): Trimipramine was approved in 1979 for major depression. Off-label indications include anxiety, schizophrenia, and rheumatoid arthritis. Drowsiness is a serious problem; however, the incidence of anticholinergic effects is one of the lowest of any drug in its class. It offers no major benefits over other TCAs. This drug is pregnancy category C.

Selective Serotonin Reuptake Inhibitors

19.9 Selective serotonin reuptake inhibitors are the drugs of choice for treating depression due to their low incidence of serious adverse effects.

Serotonin is a natural neurotransmitter in the CNS that is found in high concentrations in certain neurons in the hypothalamus, limbic system, medulla, and spinal cord. It is essential for several body activities, including the cycling between non–rapid eye movement (NREM) and rapid eye movement (REM) sleep (see Chapter 18), pain perception, and emotions. Lack of adequate serotonin in the limbic regions of the CNS can lead to depression. The actions of serotonin are terminated when it is metabolized to a less active substance by the enzyme monoamine oxidase (MAO). This process is illustrated in Figure 19.2. In the scientific literature, serotonin is commonly referred to by its chemical name, 5-hydroxytryptamine (5-HT).

In the 1970s, it became increasingly clear that serotonin had a more substantial role in depression than initially thought. Clinicians knew that the TCAs altered the sensitivity of serotonin to certain receptors in the brain, but they did not know how this chemical change connected to symptoms of depression. Ongoing efforts to find antidepressants with fewer adverse effects than TCAs and monoamine oxidase inhibitors (MAOIs) led to the development of the selective serotonin reuptake inhibitors (SSRIs), which were first introduced in 1987. Whereas the TCAs inhibit the reuptake of both norepinephrine and serotonin into presynaptic nerve terminals, the SSRIs *selectively* target serotonin. Increased levels of serotonin in the synaptic spaces induce complex neurotransmitter changes in presynaptic and postsynaptic neurons in the brain. Essentially, presynaptic receptors become less sensitive, and postsynaptic receptors become more sensitive.

SSRIs are as effective in treating depression as the TCAs but exhibit fewer significant adverse effects. Sympathomimetic effects (increased heart rate and HTN) and anticholinergic effects (dry mouth, blurred vision, urinary retention, and constipation) are less common with this drug class. Sedation occurs less frequently, and cardiotoxicity is not observed. The greater safety profile of the SSRIs has led to their current status as drugs of choice for depression.

One of the most common adverse effects of SSRIs relates to sexual dysfunction. Up to 70% of both men and women can experience decreased libido and inability to reach orgasm. In men, delayed ejaculation and impotence may occur. For patients who are sexually active, these adverse effects may be serious enough to cause nonadherence with pharmacotherapy, and a different antidepressant may be indicated. The SSRIs can cause weight gain, which may also lead to discontinuation. Other common adverse effects include nausea, headache, nervousness, and insomnia.

All drugs in the SSRI class have equal effectiveness and similar adverse effects. In general, SSRIs elevate mood more quickly than TCAs, which is a major advantage when treating serious depression disorders. Like the TCAs, the SSRIs are used for a wide variety of other mental health disorders, including OCD, social anxiety disorder, panic disorder, generalized anxiety disorder, PTSD, and premenstrual dysphoric disorder. They are one of the most widely prescribed drug classes in the United States.

Serotonin syndrome (SES) is a serious medical condition that can occur when a patient is taking multiple medications that affect the metabolism, synthesis, or reuptake of serotonin, causing this neurotransmitter to accumulate in neurons in the CNS. These drugs include SSRIs, MAOIs, TCAs, lithium, St. John's wort, opioids, and triptans. SES sometimes occurs as a result of illicit drug use because amphetamines, cocaine, MDMA or ecstasy, and opioids also affect serotonin levels. Symptoms of SES include mental status changes (confusion, anxiety, restlessness, agitation), HTN, tremors or muscle rigidity, sweating, hyperpyrexia, and ataxia. Symptoms may begin as early as 2 hours after taking the first dose or be delayed for several weeks. Conservative treatment is to discontinue all serotonergic drugs and provide supportive care that stabilizes vital signs; the condition usually resolves in 24 hours. In severe cases, mechanical ventilation and administration of muscle relaxants such as benzodiazepines may be necessary. Agitated patients may require sedation and in severe cases a serotonin antagonist such as cycloheptadine (Periactin) or olanzapine (Zyprexa) may be administered.

PROTOTYPE DRUG	**Fluoxetine (Prozac, Sarafem)**

Classification: **Therapeutic:** Antidepressant, antianxiety drug
Pharmacologic: Selective serotonin reuptake inhibitor (SSRI)

Therapeutic Effects and Uses: Approved in 1987, fluoxetine was the first SSRI marketed to treat major depressive disorder in the United States. Fluoxetine was subsequently approved to treat bulimia nervosa, the first medication ever approved for

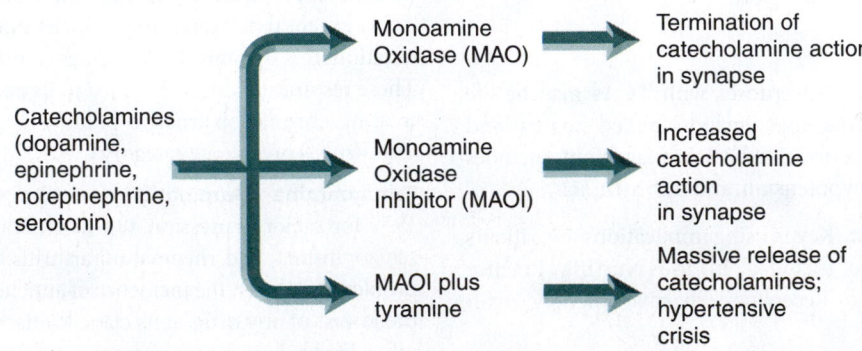

Figure 19.2 Catecholamines and monoamine oxidase.

this condition. It was the first SSRI approved for the treatment of pediatric depression. It is approved for the treatment of OCD in both adults and children, panic disorder, and premenstrual dysphoric disorder.

Fluoxetine is available as tablets, capsules, oral solution, and delayed release capsules. Sarafem is a formulation of fluoxetine specifically marketed for premenstrual dysphoric disorder in a pulvule—a gelatin-based capsule. It is taken daily or for just the 2 weeks prior to an expected menses. Prozac Weekly is a capsule containing enteric-coated granules that allows for only one dose each week. Patients who have stabilized on daily fluoxetine can be switched to Prozac Weekly, which offers the convenience of once-a-week dosing. Symbyax is a fixed-dose combination of fluoxetine and olanzapine that is indicated for bipolar disorder. Olanzapine, an antipsychotic agent, is marketed by itself as Zyprexa for schizophrenia and the manic phase of bipolar disorder.

Fluoxetine is used off-label to treat many other disorders involving multiple body systems. Off-label indications include anorexia nervosa, obesity, alcohol dependence in patients with alcoholism, fibromyalgia, autism, refractory orthostatic hypotension, premature ejaculation, and menopausal hot flashes. Although patients gradually begin to feel less depressed after about 2 weeks of therapy, optimal response may take 8 weeks or longer.

Fluoxetine is extensively metabolized in the liver to norfluoxetine, which has about the same pharmacologic activity as the parent drug. Fluoxetine and norfluoxetine have long half-lives; it takes 30 to 60 days after discontinuing the drug for them to be eliminated by the body. This duration is even more prolonged in patients with liver disease.

Mechanism of Action: As with other serotonin reuptake inhibitors, fluoxetine blocks the uptake of the neurotransmitter serotonin (but not norepinephrine) at the neuronal presynaptic membrane. This increases the amount of neurotransmitter available at the postsynaptic receptor sites, thus enhancing the actions of serotonin.

Pharmacokinetics:

Route	PO
Absorption	Readily absorbed
Distribution	Widely distributed, including the cerebrospinal fluid; likely crosses the placenta; secreted in breast milk; 94% bound to plasma protein
Primary metabolism	Metabolized in the liver to norfluoxetine, an active metabolite
Primary excretion	Renal, small amounts in feces
Onset of action	Peak plasma level: 6–8 h
Duration of action	Half-life: 2–3 days

Adverse Effects: Fluoxetine is better tolerated than drugs from either the TCA or the MAOI classes. The most common adverse effects are nausea and vomiting, which diminish as therapy progresses. Other common GI effects include diarrhea, anorexia, cramping, and flatulence. Fluoxetine does not cause sedation; in fact, insomnia may occur in as many as 25% of patients receiving the drug. Fluoxetine also does not cause the serious cardiotoxicity, orthostatic hypotension, or anticholinergic effects seen with the TCAs. Fluctuations in weight are common. Significant anorexia and weight loss occur in 10% to 15% of patients, whereas others

experience a weight gain of as much as 20 pounds or more. Patients may experience various types of sexual dysfunction, including delayed ejaculation, impotence, anorgasmia, decreased libido, and priapism. The drug may induce seizures in patients with preexisting seizure disorders or during overdoses. Other adverse effects include cramping, constipation, poor concentration, diarrhea, hot flashes, palpitations, and nervousness. Serotonin syndrome can occur. Pediatric patients may experience personality disorders or hyperkinesia. **Black Box Warning**: Antidepressants increase the risk of suicidal thinking and behavior in children, adolescents, and young adults. Patients of all ages should be monitored and observed closely during therapy for clinical worsening, suicidality, or unusual changes in behavior.

Abrupt withdrawal of fluoxetine or other SSRIs can result in a withdrawal syndrome; the patient may experience dizziness, headache, tremor, anxiety, dysphoria, and sensory disturbances. These symptoms usually begin 1 to 7 days after the last dose and may continue for 1 to 3 weeks. Because fluoxetine has an extended half-life and serum levels diminish gradually, withdrawal symptoms are generally less serious than those of the shorter acting SSRIs. Tapering the dose over 2 weeks or longer can prevent withdrawal symptoms.

Contraindications/Precautions: Hypersensitivity to fluoxetine is a contraindication to using the drug. The drug should not be administered to patients with bipolar disorder because it may precipitate a manic episode. It must be used cautiously in persons with cardiac dysfunction, diabetes, or seizure disorders. Children or young adults with a history of attempted suicide should not receive fluoxetine. There are no known age-related precautions for use in the elderly, but children may experience more behavioral adverse effects such as restlessness and insomnia.

Caution must be used when fluoxetine is administered late in pregnancy. The neonate may exhibit symptoms of withdrawal, including irritability, respiratory distress, tremors, abnormal crying, and, possibly, seizures. With supportive care, symptoms of withdrawal in the neonate will disappear in a few days. In most cases, the benefits of treating pregnant women who have major depression with fluoxetine are greater than the potential risks to the neonate.

Drug Interactions: Fluoxetine inhibits multiple CYP450 isozymes and has the potential to interact with many other drugs and herbal products. Drugs that are metabolized by CYP450 may build to toxic levels due to their impaired metabolism. Some drugs affected by diminished metabolism include TCAs, phenothiazines, most atypical antipsychotics, certain antidysrhythmics, and benzodiazepines. Excessive sedation may occur if fluoxetine is given concurrently with other CNS depressants, including opioids, sedative–hypnotics, or alcohol. Taken concurrently with or within 14 days of MAOIs can result in serotonin syndrome or neuroleptic malignant syndrome (NMS). Concurrent use with warfarin, aspirin, or other nonsteroidal anti-inflammatory drugs (NSAIDs) may increase the risk of bleeding. Fluoxetine may cause an increased risk of toxicity to phenytoin, digoxin, or carbamazepine. Concurrent use with certain antipsychotics may lead to increased extrapyramidal symptoms such as akathisia, dystonia, tardive dyskinesia, and pseudoparkinsonism. Fluoxetine can increase the half-life of diazepam. Caution must also be used if the patient is taking lithium because fluoxetine may increase plasma levels of the drug. **Herbal/**

Food: Increased CNS effects may occur if fluoxetine is given concurrently with lavender, kava, or hops. There is an increased risk of serotonin syndrome with the concurrent use of St. John's wort. Increased anticholinergic effects may result from the use of jimsonweed or corkwood. Because grapefruit juice may cause elevated serum levels of fluoxetine, it should be avoided during therapy.

Pregnancy: Category C.

Treatment of Overdose: Overdose can result in seizures, tachycardia, somnolence, and, rarely, death. Supportive treatment is indicated, including gastric lavage and activated charcoal. With intentional overdose, the possibility of multiple drug involvement should always be considered.

Nursing Responsibilities: Key nursing implications for patients receiving fluoxetine are included in the Nursing Practice Application for Patients Receiving Pharmacotherapy with Antidepressants.

Drugs Similar to Fluoxetine (Prozac, Sarafem)

Other SSRIs include citalopram, escitalopram, fluvoxamine, paroxetine, sertraline, and vortioxetine.

Citalopram (Celexa): Citalopram was approved by the FDA in 1998 for the treatment of major depressive disorder in adults. Its antianxiety uses are off-label. These include all five major antianxiety categories: generalized anxiety disorder, social anxiety disorder, OCD, panic disorder, and post-traumatic stress disorder (PTSD). Other off-label uses include schizophrenia, premenstrual dysphoric disorder, and menopausal hot flashes. Citalopram is available as regular tablets, as oral disintegrating tablets, or as an oral solution. It is almost identical structurally to escitalopram but is very different from other SSRIs. Older adults are more susceptible to the anticholinergic effects of citalopram than to other SSRIs. There are fewer drug interactions than with fluoxetine. All other actions and adverse effects are the same as those of fluoxetine and escitalopram. This drug is pregnancy category C.

Escitalopram (Lexapro): Since its approval in 2002, escitalopram has become one of the most frequently prescribed drugs in the United States. Approved indications include major depressive disorder in adults and in adolescents age 12 to 17 years, and generalized anxiety disorder. It is used off-label to treat social anxiety disorder and panic attacks. It is nearly identical structurally to citalopram although it is more potent; 20 mg of escitalopram is bioequivalent to 40 mg of citalopram. It is available as a tablet or solution. Escitalopram has the same spectrum of adverse effects as fluoxetine and other SSRIs. It appears to elevate mood relatively quickly, in 1 to 2 weeks. Its safety and effectiveness in children younger than 12 years have not been established. This drug is pregnancy category C.

Fluvoxamine (Luvox): Approved in 1994, fluvoxamine is an oral SSRI approved to treat OCD and social anxiety disorder. It is the only SSRI not FDA approved to treat major depression, although it is prescribed off-label for that indication. Other off-label uses include anxiety disorders in children, generalized anxiety disorder, PTSD, and panic disorder. It is available as regular release tablets and extended release capsules (Luvox CR). Adverse reactions are the same as with fluoxetine except that fluvoxamine causes sedation rather than CNS excitement. This drug is pregnancy category C.

Paroxetine (Paxil, Pexeva): Approved in 1992, paroxetine is available as oral tablets, oral suspension, or controlled release tablets (Paxil CR). It is approved to treat a large number of mental health conditions, including major depression, OCD, social anxiety disorder, panic disorder, generalized anxiety disorder, PTSD, and premenstrual dysphoric disorder. Off-label indications include hot flashes, fibromyalgia, bipolar disorder (with lithium), and premature ejaculation. Adverse effects are generally mild, dose dependent, and similar to those of other SSRIs. These effects usually diminish or disappear completely in time. A lower starting dosage is recommended for older adults. Precautions are similar to those for other SSRIs except that paroxetine is a pregnancy category D drug.

Sertraline (Zoloft): Approved in 1991, sertraline is one of the most frequently prescribed SSRIs. It is available as tablets or as an oral concentrate that must be diluted before use. Approved indications include major depressive disorder, OCD, PTSD, social anxiety disorder, and premenstrual dysphoric disorder. It may be used off-label to treat generalized anxiety disorder and eating disorders. Contraindications and precautions are the same as with escitalopram. The main difference between sertraline and fluoxetine is that sertraline blocks the uptake of dopamine in addition to blocking the uptake of serotonin. Adverse effects, uses, and drug interactions are the same as those of fluoxetine. The oral concentrate contains 12% alcohol, which is contraindicated in patients taking disulfiram (Antabuse). This drug is pregnancy category C.

Vortioxetine (Brintellix): The newest of the SSRIs, vortioxetine, was approved in 2013 for the treatment of major depression. It has a complex mechanism that enhances serotonin activities in some regions of the brain, while inhibiting that neurotransmitter in other regions. It has the same spectrum of adverse effects as other drugs in this class and is pregnancy category C.

Atypical Antidepressants

19.10 Atypical antidepressants are alternatives to the selective serotonin reuptake inhibitors for depression and anxiety disorders.

Atypical antidepressants are a diverse class of newer drugs that act by mechanisms other than those of the SSRIs, TCAs, and MAOIs. In effect, this is a "miscellaneous" class of drugs because they have very little in common with each other except their ability to alleviate symptoms of depression. They act by preventing the reuptake of specific neurotransmitters in the CNS or by blocking neurotransmitter receptors. Mechanisms include the following:

- Serotonin–norepinephrine reuptake inhibitors (SNRIs): desvenlafaxine (Pristiq), venlafaxine (Effexor), and duloxetine (Cymbalta)

- Norepinephrine and dopamine reuptake inhibitors (NDRIs): bupropion (Wellbutrin)

- Norepinephrine reuptake inhibitors (NRIs): reboxetine (Edronax, Vestra)

- Combined reuptake inhibitor and receptor blocker: trazodone (Desyrel), nefazodone, and mirtazapine (Remeron)

As a group, the atypical antidepressants have similar pharmacologic actions to the SSRIs and exhibit fewer adverse effects than the TCAs and MAOIs. Each drug in the class has certain specific adverse effects, as described next. Some are widely used for indications other than depression, such as neuropathic pain and anxiety disorders. Although the atypical antidepressants are effective, they are generally not superior to other, well-established drugs for the treatment of depression.

PROTOTYPE DRUG	**Venlafaxine (Effexor)**

Classification: **Therapeutic:** Atypical antidepressant
Pharmacologic: Serotonin–norepinephrine reuptake inhibitor (SNRI)

Therapeutic Effects and Uses: Venlafaxine is an atypical antidepressant approved by the FDA in 1993 to treat major depression. Later, its approved indications were extended to include panic disorder, generalized anxiety disorder, and social anxiety disorder. It has been used off-label to treat a large number of other conditions, including neuropathic pain, premenstrual dysphoric disorder, menopausal hot flashes, migraines, OCD, and fibromyalgia. Venlafaxine XR is an extended release capsule that permits once-daily dosing. It is metabolized to an active metabolite in the liver. Venlafaxine has pharmacologic effects, drug interactions, and adverse effects very similar to those of the SSRIs.

Like other antidepressants, there is little potential for psychological dependence with venlafaxine—it is not a drug of abuse. Abrupt discontinuation, however, can cause mild to moderate withdrawal symptoms such as nervousness, headache, agitation, fatigue, drowsiness, tremor, and sweating. Gradual tapering of the dose is a means of preventing withdrawal symptoms.

Mechanism of Action: Venlafaxine inhibits the presynaptic neuronal reuptake of both norepinephrine and serotonin in the CNS.

Pharmacokinetics:

Route(s)	PO
Absorption	92% absorbed from the GI tract
Distribution	Widely distributed; crosses the placenta; secreted in breast milk; 27% bound to plasma protein
Primary metabolism	Metabolized in the liver to desmethylvenlafaxine, an active metabolite; substantial first-pass effect
Primary excretion	Renal
Onset of action	Peak serum level: 5.5 h but the antidepressant action may take 2–3 weeks
Duration of action	Half-life: 5–7 h (9–11 h for the active metabolite)

Adverse Effects: The most common adverse effect of venlafaxine is nausea, which can occur in a large number of patients. Tolerance may develop to the nausea as therapy progresses. The nausea, combined with anorexia, sometimes leads to weight loss. Pediatric patients taking venlafaxine have been shown to have a decrease in overall height as well as weight. Venlafaxine has structural similarities to amphetamines and can cause CNS stimulation, nervousness, and insomnia. Other patients, however, exhibit sedative

effects from the drug. Other CNS adverse effects include headache, emotional lability, dizziness, and asthenia. Sustained elevations, 10 to 15 mmHg, of blood pressure may occur. Types of sexual dysfunction seen with venlafaxine include impotence, abnormal ejaculation, and delayed or absent orgasm in women. Rare, life-threatening adverse reactions include rectal, vaginal, or uterine hemorrhage. **Black Box Warning**: Antidepressants increase the risk of suicidal thinking and behavior in children, adolescents, and young adults. Patients of all ages should be monitored and observed closely during therapy for clinical worsening, suicidality, or unusual changes in behavior.

Contraindications/Precautions: Venlafaxine is contraindicated if the patient has hypersensitivity to venlafaxine or an SSRI, if a MAOI is being used concurrently, or during lactation. Caution must be used when administered to patients with cardiac, hepatic, or renal impairment; recent MI; seizure disorder; anorexia; or suicidal ideation. Venlafaxine is not administered to patients with bipolar disorder or with a history of mania because it can trigger manic episodes. Safety in children under age 18 has not been established. Patients with hepatic impairment may require as much as a 50% reduction in dose.

Drug Interactions: Venlafaxine is primarily metabolized by the hepatic CYP2D6 isozyme; drugs that inhibit CYP2D6 may cause venlafaxine serum levels to rise. Serotonin syndrome may occur if venlafaxine is given concurrently with SSRIs, MAOIs, lithium, or other drugs that act by increasing serotonin levels. If switching from venlafaxine to a MAOI, venlafaxine must be withdrawn at least 7 days before beginning the MAOI. Alcohol, opioids, sedatives, hypnotics, or antihistamines can cause additive CNS depression. Cimetidine, haloperidol, fluoxetine, sertraline, or phenothiazine can lead to increased toxicity. **Herbal/Food**: No food interactions have been reported, but there are several possible interactions with herbal products. St. John's wort and SAM-e may increase the risk of SES. CNS depression may occur with concurrent use of chamomile, kava, hops, lavender, valerian, or skullcap. Jimsonweed or corkwood may cause increased anticholinergic effects. Yohimbe may increase the risk for HTN.

Pregnancy: Category C.

Treatment of Overdose: Overdoses are generally not fatal but can cause serious symptoms such as CNS depression, seizures, altered level of consciousness, hypotension, and dysrhythmias. General measures include inducing emesis and administering activated charcoal and gastric lavage. The ECG must be monitored and antiseizure drugs administered as necessary.

Nursing Responsibilities: Key nursing implications for patients receiving velafaxine are included in the Nursing Practice Application for Patients Receiving Pharmacotherapy with Antidepressants.

Drugs Similar to Venlafaxine (Effexor)

Other atypical antidepressants include amoxapine, bupropion, desvenlafaxine, duloxetine, mirtazapine, nefazodone, trazodone, and vilazodone.

Amoxapine (Asendin): Approved in 1980, amoxapine is chemically related to older TCAs and phenothiazines. The drug exhibits potentially serious adverse effects, which limit its use to patients who have major depression accompanied by psychotic symptoms such as agitation. Adverse effects resemble those of TCAs (blood dyscrasias, orthostatic hypotension, sedation, anticholinergic effects, sexual dysfunction, and cardiac toxicity) and phenothiazines (neuroleptic malignant syndrome and parkinsonism symptoms). There is cross hypersensitivity between amoxapine and TCAs. Amoxapine must be used cautiously in those with suicidal ideation. This drug is pregnancy category C.

Bupropion (Wellbutrin, Zyban, Others): Approved in 1985, bupropion has a chemical structure similar to that of amphetamine. It is approved to treat major depression as well as being the first approved therapy for persistent seasonal affective disorder. Bupropion is also marketed as Zyban and Buproban for the management of nicotine withdrawal during smoking cessation. Off-label uses include neuropathic pain and ADHD.

The naming of bupropion has resulted in medication errors. It is available as immediate release tablets (100 mg, 3 times daily), and as extended release formulations, Wellbutrin SR (150 mg, twice daily) and Wellbutrin XL (300 mg, once daily). In pharmacology, the terms *sustained release* (SR) and *extended release* (XL or XR) are usually used interchangeably, but this is not the case for bupropion. Further confusing the naming is that the U.S. Pharmacopeia requires that all generic versions of prolonged release medications be labeled "extended release." In 2008 a new salt form, bupropion hydrobromide (Aplenzin), was approved as a once-daily tablet (348 mg, once daily) for depression. Caution must be used when dispensing bupropion to be certain the correct salt and dosing schedule is used.

Bupropion not only inhibits the reuptake of serotonin, but it may also affect the activity of norepinephrine and dopamine. Like amphetamine, bupropion has stimulant actions and suppresses the appetite. It does not cause weight gain or sexual dysfunction, which makes it appealing to women who are experiencing hypoactive sexual disorder. Indeed, it is sometimes used to counteract the sexual dysfunction that occurs in patients taking SSRIs. Antidepressant action begins in 1 to 3 weeks and is equal to that of the TCAs. Because bupropion has a greater potential for causing seizures than other antidepressants, it should be used with caution in patients with seizure disorders. The risk for seizures is dose dependent and increases for patients drinking alcohol or taking other drugs that lower the seizure threshold. Seizures have been reported in infants receiving breast milk from mothers taking bupropion. Common adverse reactions include CNS stimulation (agitation, insomnia, and restlessness), weight loss, headache, dry mouth, constipation, and GI upset. About 20% of patients taking this drug will develop tremors. Because of its potential adverse effects, bupropion is usually considered an alternative antidepressant for patients who do not respond to SSRIs. This drug is pregnancy category C.

Desvenlafaxine: Desvenlafaxine (Pristiq) is an SNRI approved in 2008 for the treatment of major depressive disorder. It is available as an extended release tablet that is taken once daily. Common adverse effects include nausea, dizziness, excessive sweating, constipation, somnolence, anxiety, male function disorders, and decreased appetite. Because this drug can raise blood pressure, preexisting HTN should be corrected before starting therapy. Desvenlafaxine should be discontinued gradually to prevent the appearance of withdrawal symptoms. This drug is pregnancy category C.

Duloxetine (Cymbalta): Like venlafaxine, duloxetine is an atypical antidepressant that is classified as an SNRI. First approved for major depression in 2004, it has since received FDA approval to treat neuropathic pain in people with diabetes, fibromyalgia, and generalized anxiety disorder. Stress urinary incontinence is an off-label indication. Abnormal vision is the most frequently reported adverse effect, and nausea is a common reason for discontinuation of therapy. Other adverse events include photosensitivity, bruising, anorexia, thrombophlebitis, constipation, diarrhea, dry mouth, insomnia, and anxiety. No life-threatening adverse effects have been identified. Postmarketing incidences of liver injury suggest that the drug should be used with great caution in patients with preexisting hepatic impairment or in alcoholics. Caution must be exercised when administered to persons with mania, seizures, HTN, cardiac, renal or hepatic disease, the elderly, children, or lactating women. When discontinuing therapy, the dose should be tapered slowly to prevent withdrawal symptoms. Patients may begin feeling the antidepressant effects of duloxetine within 2 weeks of beginning treatment. This drug is pregnancy category C.

Mirtazapine (Remeron): Classified as a tetracyclic compound, this drug was approved in 1996 for major depression in adults. It blocks presynaptic serotonin and norepinephrine receptors, thereby enhancing release of these neurotransmitters from nerve terminals. Unlike the TCAs, it has few anticholinergic actions. It does carry a higher risk of seizure activity in patients with no previous seizure history. Serious adverse reactions include acute renal failure, hepatitis, jaundice, thrombocytopenia, leukopenia, eosinophilia, or agranulocytosis. Other adverse reactions include dizziness, orthostatic hypotension, ECG changes, sedation (which may be a positive effect in those having insomnia secondary to depression), tachycardia, HTN, or extrapyramidal symptoms in the elderly. Mirtazapine should not be used in patients with hypersensitivity to TCAs, seizure disorders, prostatic hypertrophy, serious hepatic or renal impairment, or those who are recovering from MI. Mirtazapine usually elevates mood within 2 to 4 weeks after the initiation of therapy. This drug is pregnancy category C.

Nefazodone: Chemically similar to trazodone, nefazodone causes minimal cardiovascular effects, fewer anticholinergic effects, less sedation, and less sexual dysfunction than some of the other antidepressants. The most common adverse effects are xerostomia, drowsiness, nausea, vomiting, dizziness, and constipation. Although FDA approved only for major depression, the medication is used off-label to treat anxiety, panic attacks, premenstrual dysphoric disorder, PTSD, and social anxiety disorder. Nefazodone acts by blocking serotonin receptors and inhibiting serotonin reuptake. It also has some blocking effect on norepinephrine reuptake. Originally approved in 1994, a brand name form of the drug, Serzone, was removed from the market in 2004 due to a possibility of liver damage; generic nefazodone is still available. A black box warning indicates that the drug should not be used in patients with acute liver impairment, and that hepatic laboratory values should be regularly monitored during therapy.

The drug should be withdrawn if the patient develops signs of hepatic injury such as increased serum AST or serum ALT levels greater than three times normal. This drug is pregnancy category C.

Trazodone (Oleptro): Approved in 1981, trazodone works by producing a moderate, selective blockade of serotonin reuptake. It is not very effective when used alone as an antidepressant, but its sedative properties are especially useful in patients who have antidepressant-induced insomnia. In fact, trazodone is most frequently used off-label as a sleep aid, rather than as an antidepressant. Other off-label indications include generalized anxiety disorder, panic disorder, and as an adjuvant to reduce cravings for alcohol in patients with alcohol dependency. It causes little cardiac toxicity and few anticholinergic effects so it may be useful for older adults and other persons for whom either of these may be intolerable. Common adverse effects include orthostatic hypotension, nausea, sedation, and dry mouth. Reported sexual effects include priapism, anorgasmia, and ejaculation dysfunctions. Overdose with trazodone is considered to be safer than overdose from MAOIs or TCAs, and there have been no reports of death from trazodone use alone. However, death can occur from overdose when the patient combines trazodone with other CNS depressants. In 2010, the FDA approved Oleptro, a controlled release form of trazodone that is taken once daily. This drug is pregnancy category C.

Vilazodone (Viibryd): Approved in 2011, vilazodone is one of the newest drugs for treating major depressive disorder in adults. The drug acts by blocking serotonin reuptake and by demonstrating partial agonist action at serotonin receptors. It appears to have equivalent effectiveness to other drugs in this class. One advantage of vilazodone is that clinical improvement is noted after 7 days of therapy, compared to the 4 to 6 weeks required for some of the other antidepressants. In addition, the drug has only minor adverse effects, with GI-related symptoms being the most common. Like other antidepressants, the drug carries a black box warning about possible increased suicidality in adolescents and young adults. This drug is pregnancy category C.

CONNECTION Checkpoint 19.3

Atypical antidepressants are sometimes used to treat anxiety when drugs from other classes are not effective. From what you learned in Chapter 18, what class of drugs is the traditional choice for the short-term therapy of generalized anxiety disorder? *See Answer to Connection Checkpoint 19.3 on student resource website.*

Monoamine Oxidase Inhibitors

19.11 Monoamine oxidase inhibitors are effective antidepressants but are seldom used due to potentially serious adverse effects.

MAO is a key enzyme located in the liver, intestinal wall, and adrenergic neurons. It is responsible for inactivating monoamines: substances that contain one $-NH_2$ (amine) group. Not only does MAO inactivate natural monoamines such as norepinephrine, dopamine, and serotonin, but it also acts on those present in food and drugs. The **monoamine oxidase inhibitors (MAOIs)** are antidepressants that block the actions of MAO.

In adrenergic neurons, MAOIs slow the destruction of norepinephrine, dopamine, and serotonin. This creates higher levels of these neurotransmitters and enhances their activity in the brain. Through mechanisms incompletely understood, this increase in neurotransmitters creates an antidepressant action.

Although they are as effective in treating depression as the SSRIs or TCAs, serious adverse reactions limit their use. Because of their low safety margin, these drugs are reserved for patients with refractory depression that has not responded to TCAs, atypical antidepressants, or SSRIs. They are rarely used in clinical practice.

A serious adverse reaction with MAOIs is their ability to cause a hypertensive crisis if combined with foods that contain **tyramine**. Widely found in nature, tyramine is a type of monoamine that is formed by the metabolism of tyrosine, an amino acid. When a patient is taking an MAOI, the drug blocks the breakdown of dietary tyramine, causing it to accumulate to high levels. In turn, tyramine causes the release of norepinephrine stored in adrenergic neurons. Rapid vasoconstriction occurs with a potential rise of blood pressure of 30 mmHg or more. Table 19.4 contains a list of tyramine-rich foods that must be avoided by patients taking MAOIs. Products containing tyramine are sometimes marketed as dietary supplements to increase fat loss from the body. There is no valid scientific evidence to support this claim, and these supplements must be strictly avoided by patients taking MAOIs.

TABLE 19.4	Foods High in Tyramine
Category of Food	**Specific Foods**
Meats	Beef or chicken liver, pate
	Hot dogs, bologna
	Pepperoni, salami, sausage
Dairy products	Aged cheese
	Sour cream
	Yogurt
Fruits	Avocados
	Bananas, in large amounts
	Canned figs
	Papaya products, including meat tenderizers
	Raisins
Vegetables	Pods of fava beans
	Fermented soybeans, soybean paste
Fish	Dried or cured fish
	Fermented, smoked, aged fish
	Pickled or kippered herring
Alcohol	Beer
	Wine, especially red wine
Miscellaneous	Protein dietary supplements
	Soups (may contain protein extract)
	Shrimp paste
	Soy sauce
	Yeast, brewer's or extracts

CONNECTIONS Complementary and Alternative Therapies

◀ St. John's Wort for Depression

Description
St. John's wort (*Hypericum perforatum*) is an herb found throughout Great Britain, Asia, Europe, and North America.

History and Claims
The herb gets its name from a legend that red spots once appeared on its leaves on the anniversary of St. John's beheading. The word *wort* is a British term for "plant." Use of the plant dates to ancient Greece, and Native Americans used the herb as an antiseptic or anti-inflammatory agent. Modern uses have focused on the antidepressant properties of the herb.

Standardization
The active substances in St. John's wort are believed to be hyperforin and hypericin. There is no standard dosage; however, some manufacturers are beginning to report dose by the percentage of hypericin in the extract. For example, one commonly used dose is 300 mg tid of St. John's wort standardized to 0.3% hypericin. Some studies use 5% hyperforin.

Evidence
Scientists once thought that St. John's wort produced its effects via the same mechanism as MAOIs, by increasing the levels of serotonin, norepinephrine, and dopamine in the brain. More recent evidence suggests that it may selectively inhibit serotonin reuptake. Newer research by the National Center for Complementary and Alternative Medicine (2012) states that the effectiveness of St. John's wort for minor depression is no better than a placebo. St. John's wort induces hepatic P450 enzymes and has been reported to interact with many medications, including oral contraceptives, warfarin, digoxin, and cyclosporine. It should not be taken concurrently with antidepressant medications.

An active ingredient in St. John's wort is a photoactive compound that when exposed to light produces substances that can damage myelin. Patients have reported feeling stinging pain on the hands after sun exposure while taking the herbal remedy. Patients who take this herb should be advised to apply sunscreen or wear protective clothing when outdoors.

PROTOTYPE DRUG   Phenelzine (Nardil)

Classification: Therapeutic: Antidepressant
Pharmacologic: Monoamine oxidase inhibitor

Therapeutic Effects and Uses: An older drug approved in 1959, phenelzine was once widely used to treat major depression. It has also been used off-label to treat OCD, panic disorder, and social anxiety disorder and for migraine prophylaxis. Although very effective in treating these disorders, phenelzine interacts with tyramine in foods and with many other drugs to produce potentially serious interactions.

Like other antidepressants, phenelzine may take up to 4 to 8 weeks to produce a maximum antidepressant response. This drug is changed to active metabolites in the liver.

Mechanism of Action: Phenelzine produces its effects by binding irreversibly to MAO. This intensifies the actions of endogenous epinephrine, norepinephrine, serotonin, and dopamine in the CNS. Increased concentrations of these neurotransmitters result in elevated mood.

Pharmacokinetics:

Route(s)	PO
Absorption	Well absorbed
Distribution	Widely distributed; crosses the placenta
Primary metabolism	Hepatic
Primary excretion	Renal
Onset of action	Peak level: 2–4 h (antidepressant action takes 2–8 weeks)
Duration of action	Half-life: 11 h

Adverse Effects: The most serious adverse effect of phenelzine is hypertensive crisis precipitated by foods containing tyramine, which can induce fatal intracranial bleeding. Dizziness and orthostatic hypotension are common during therapy. Other frequent adverse reactions include drowsiness, sexual dysfunction, and anorexia. Life-threatening adverse reactions include dysrhythmias and a syndrome of inappropriate antidiuretic hormone-like symptoms. **Black Box Warning**: Antidepressants increase the risk of suicidal thinking and behavior in children, adolescents, and young adults. Patients of all ages should be monitored and observed closely during therapy for clinical worsening, suicidality, or unusual changes in behavior.

Contraindications/Precautions: Patients with schizophrenia, cardiovascular or cerebrovascular disease, hepatic or renal impairment, or pheochromocytoma should not take phenelzine. Caution should be used when prescribing phenelzine to a person with epilepsy, severe or frequent headaches, HTN, dysrhythmias, or suicidal tendencies.

Drug Interactions: Phenelzine interacts with many other drugs. The nurse should consult a current drug guide for a comprehensive list of drug–drug interactions. Other CNS depressants, including alcohol, may lead to additive CNS depression. Concurrent administration with buspirone may increase blood pressure. Use with opioid analgesics may lead to immediate excitation, severe HTN or hypotension, and, occasionally, severe respiratory distress, vascular collapse, seizures, coma, and death. CNS stimulants and sympathomimetics may increase the cardiac stimulant and vasopressor effects of phenelzine. SES may occur if phenelzine is administered with other drugs such as SSRIs, lithium, or dextromethorphan that potentiate the actions of serotonin. **Herbal/Food**: Patients who are taking phenelzine or any MAOI must avoid tyramine-containing foods (see Table 19.4) because these foods may precipitate a hypertensive crisis. Medications containing caffeine, including OTC products, should be avoided because they may increase the risk of HTN and dysrhythmias. An increased sympathomimetic effect may occur when phenelzine is combined with capsicum peppers or large amounts of green tea. Ginkgo, nutmeg, and yohimbe use can result in increased effects. Ginseng use can lead to irritability, hallucinations, mania, and increased tension headaches. Decreased effects can occur with the use of valerian. Serotonin syndrome may occur with the use of St. John's wort.

Pregnancy: Category C.

Treatment of Overdose: Overdosage with phenelzine is serious and can result in death if untreated. Symptoms may include either CNS stimulation (seizures) or depression (coma). Induction of gastric lavage with activated charcoal may be beneficial. Electrolytes and vital signs must be monitored and the appropriate intervention administered to keep values within normal ranges.

Nursing Responsibilities: Key nursing implications for patients receiving phenelzine are included in the Nursing Practice Application for Patients Receiving Pharmacotherapy with Antidepressants.

Drugs Similar to Phenelzine (Nardil)

The other MAOIs that are available include isocarboxazid, selegiline, and tranylcypromine.

Isocarboxazid (Marplan): Like phenelzine, isocarboxazid was initially approved by the FDA for depression in the 1950s. Off-label indications include refractory panic disorder and social anxiety disorder. It is only used when other therapies have failed to produce satisfactory outcomes. The drug has the same precautions and potential interactions as phenelzine, including the possibility of a hypertensive crisis occurring when taken with tyramine-containing products. This drug is pregnancy category C.

CONNECTIONS: NURSING PRACTICE APPLICATION

Patients Receiving Pharmacotherapy with Antidepressants

Assessment	Potential Nursing Diagnoses*
Baseline assessment prior to administration: • Obtain a complete health history including hepatic, renal, urologic, cardiovascular, or neurologic disease, current mental status, narrow-angle glaucoma status, and pregnancy or breast-feeding status. Obtain a drug history including allergies, current prescription and OTC drugs, and herbal preparations. Be alert to possible drug interactions. • Obtain a history of depression or mood disorder, including a family history of same and severity. Use objective screening tools when possible (e.g., Beck Depression Inventory or Geriatric Depression Scale). • Obtain baseline vital signs and weight. • Evaluate appropriate laboratory findings (e.g., CBC, electrolytes, glucose, hepatic and renal function studies). • Assess the patient's ability to receive and understand instructions. Include the family and caregivers as needed.	• Ineffective Coping • Powerlessness • Anxiety • Disturbed Sleep Pattern • Self-Care Deficit (Bathing, Dressing, Feeding) • Imbalanced Nutrition: Less Than Body Requirements • Complicated Grieving • Social Isolation • Impaired Social Interaction • Interrupted Family Processes • Urinary Retention, related to anticholinergic side effects of drug therapy • Noncompliance, related to adverse drug effects of decreased sexual libido or weight gain • Deficient Knowledge (Drug Therapy) • Risk for Self-Directed Violence • Risk for Self-Mutilation • Risk for Suicide • Risk for Injury
Assessment throughout administration: • Assess for desired therapeutic effects (e.g., increased mood, lessening depression, increased activity level, return to normal ADLs, appetite, and sleep patterns). • Continue periodic monitoring of CBC, electrolytes, glucose, and hepatic and renal function studies. • Assess vital signs and weight periodically or as symptoms warrant. • Assess for and promptly report adverse effects: dizziness or lightheadedness, drowsiness, confusion, agitation, suicidal ideations, palpitations, tachycardia, blurred or double vision, skin rashes, bruising or bleeding, abdominal pain, jaundice, change in color of stool, flank pain, or hematuria.	

Implementation

Interventions and (Rationales)	Patient-Centered Care
Ensuring therapeutic effects: • Continue assessments as above for therapeutic effects. (Drugs used for depression may take 2 to 8 weeks before full effects are realized. Use objective measures, e.g., Beck Depression Inventory, when possible to help quantify therapeutic results. For outpatient therapy, prescriptions may be limited to 7 days' supply of medication. Have patient sign "No Harm/No Suicide" contract as appropriate.)	• Teach the patient that full effects may not occur for a prolonged period, but that some improvement should be noticeable after beginning therapy. • Encourage the patient to keep all appointments with the therapist and to discuss ongoing symptoms of depression, reporting any suicidal ideations immediately.

(continued)

CONNECTIONS: NURSING PRACTICE APPLICATION (continued)

Minimizing adverse effects:

- Continue to monitor vital signs, mental status, coordination, and balance periodically. Ensure patient safety; monitor ambulation until the effects of the drug are known. **Lifespan:** Be particularly cautious with the older adult who is at increased risk for falls. (Antidepressant drugs may cause drowsiness and dizziness, hypotension, or impaired mental and physical abilities, increasing the risk of falls.)

- Teach the patient to rise from lying or sitting to standing slowly to avoid dizziness or falls. If dizziness occurs, the patient should sit or lie down and not attempt to stand or walk until the sensation passes.
- Instruct the patient to call for assistance prior to getting out of bed or attempting to walk alone, and to avoid driving or other activities requiring mental alertness or physical coordination until the effects of the drug are known.

- Continue to monitor CBC, electrolytes, and renal and hepatic function. (Some antidepressant drugs may cause hepatotoxicity as an adverse effect. **Diverse Patients:** SSRIs are metabolized through the P450 system and may result in less than optimal therapeutic results based on differences in enzymes. Monitor ethnically diverse patients more frequently in the early stages of drug therapy.)

- Instruct the patient on the need to return periodically for laboratory work.
- Teach the patient to promptly report any abdominal pain, particularly in the upper quadrants, changes in stool color, yellowing of sclera or skin, or darkened urine.
- **Diverse Patients:** Teach ethnically diverse patients to observe for less than optimal therapeutic effects and report promptly.
- Teach the patient to wear or carry medical identification stating the type of drug therapy used, especially if MAOIs are given.

- Assess for changes in level of consciousness, disorientation or confusion, or agitation. (Neurologic changes may indicate under- or overmedication, exacerbation of other psychiatric illness, or adverse drug effects.)

- Instruct the patient or caregivers to report increasing lethargy, disorientation, confusion, changes in behavior or mood, agitation or aggression, slurred speech, or ataxia immediately.

- Assess for changes in visual acuity, blurred vision, loss of peripheral vision, seeing rainbow halos around lights, or acute eye pain, especially if accompanied by nausea and vomiting, and report immediately. (Increased intraocular pressure in patients with narrow-angle glaucoma may occur in patients taking TCAs.)

- Instruct the patient to report any visual changes or eye pain immediately.

- Monitor cardiovascular status. (Early signs of SES include rapid increases in blood pressure and pulse. Headache, palpitations, fever, and neck stiffness may signal a life-threatening hypertensive crisis in a patient taking MAOIs.)

- Instruct the patient to immediately report severe headache, dizziness, paresthesia, palpitations, tachycardia, chest pain, nausea, vomiting, diaphoresis, or fever.

- Assess for bruising, bleeding, or signs of infection. (TCAs may cause blood dyscrasias and increased chances of bleeding or infection.)

- Teach the patient to report any signs of increased bruising, bleeding, or infections (e.g., sore throat, fever, or skin rash) promptly.

- Assess for dry mouth, blurred vision, urinary retention, constipation, and sexual dysfunction. (Anticholinergic-like effects and sexual dysfunction, including loss of libido and impotence, are common antidepressant adverse effects. **Lifespan:** Be aware that the older male adult with an enlarged prostate is at higher risk for mechanical obstruction. Tolerance to anticholinergic effects usually develops in 2 to 4 weeks.)

- Teach the patient to use ice chips, frequent sips of water, chewing gum, or hard candy to alleviate dry mouth, and to avoid alcohol-based mouthwashes, which may increase dryness.
- Use of "dry eye" drops and resting the eyes periodically may help decrease dry eye feeling. Teach the patient to report any feelings of scratchiness or eye pain immediately.
- Instruct the patient to report difficulty with urination, hesitancy, or dysuria promptly.
- Encourage the patient to discuss concerns about sexual functioning and refer to the health care provider if concerns affect medication adherence.

- Continue weekly weights and report gain or loss above 2 kg (5 lb). (Weight gain may be a reason for nonadherence with drug therapy. Adolescents and older adults may be at risk for anorexia and weight loss.)

- Have the patient weigh self weekly and report significant weight gain or loss to the provider.

- Avoid abrupt discontinuation of therapy. (Profound depression, seizures, or withdrawal symptoms may occur with abrupt discontinuation.)

- Instruct the patient to take the drug exactly as prescribed and to not discontinue it abruptly.

Patient understanding of drug therapy:

- Use opportunities during administration of medications and during assessments to discuss the rationale for drug therapy, desired therapeutic outcomes, commonly observed adverse effects, parameters for when to call the health care provider, and any necessary monitoring or precautions. (Using time during nursing care helps to optimize and reinforce key teaching areas.)

- The patient should be able to state the reason for the drug, appropriate dose, scheduling, and what adverse effects to observe for and when to report them.
- Patients taking MAOIs should be given explicit instructions, written as well as verbal, on foods and beverages that must be avoided while taking the medication.

Patient self-administration of drug therapy:

- When administering the medication, instruct the patient, family, or caregiver in proper self-administration of the drug, e.g., take the drug as prescribed and do not substitute brands. (Utilizing time during nurse-administration of these drugs helps to reinforce teaching.)

- Teach the patient to take the medication:
  - Exactly as ordered and the same manufacturer's brand each time the prescription is filled. (Switching brands may result in differing pharmacokinetics and alterations in therapeutic effect.)
- Take a missed dose as soon as it is noticed but do not take double or extra doses to "catch up."
- Take with food to decrease GI upset.
- If the medication causes drowsiness, take at bedtime. If the medication causes insomnia, take the last dose before 4 p.m.
- Do not abruptly discontinue the medication.
- Do not take other drugs, including OTC, herbal products, grapefruit juice, or dietary supplements, while taking the antidepressant.

Selegiline (Emsam): Approved in 2006 for major depression, selegiline is a transdermal patch that delivers a controlled amount of the MAOI over 24 hours. Absorption across the skin bypasses MAO in the intestine; thus there is less risk of a hypertensive crisis when eating foods containing tyramine. The drug is also indicated for the treatment of Parkinson's disease by capsule (Eldepryl) or orally disintegrating tablets (Zelapar). The various forms of this drug should not be administered concurrently due to the risk of hypertensive crisis caused by drug overdose. Common adverse effects include skin irritation at the site of the patch application, headache, sleep disorders, diarrhea, and dry mouth. This drug is pregnancy category C.

Tranylcypromine (Parnate): Tranylcypromine was approved in 1961 for the therapy of depression. Off-label indications include refractory panic disorder and social anxiety disorder. The drug binds reversibly to MAO. This results in a more rapid onset of antidepressant action than phenelzine or isocarboxazid and a more rapid return to normal MAO levels after the drug is discontinued. However, it has the same precautions and potential interactions as phenelzine and is rarely used due to its adverse effects. This drug is pregnancy category C.

Bipolar Disorder

19.12 Bipolar disorder is a serious psychiatric disorder characterized by extreme mood swings from depression to euphoria.

Bipolar disorder, once known as manic-depression, is a relatively common and serious psychiatric disorder. Suicide risk is high and many patients stop taking their medication during the course of pharmacotherapy. The etiology of the disorder is unknown, and symptoms may persist throughout the patient's life span.

Mania is characterized by symptoms that are generally the opposite of depressive symptoms. The excessive CNS stimulation that is characteristic of mania can be recognized by the following symptoms:

- Inflated self-esteem or grandiosity; the belief that one's ideas are far superior to anyone else's
- Decreased need for sleep or food
- Distractibility; racing thoughts with attention too easily drawn to irrelevant external stimuli
- Increased psychomotor or goal-directed activity (either socially, at work or school, or sexually)
- Excessive pursuit of pleasurable activities without consideration of the negative consequences, such as shopping sprees, sexual indiscretions, or unsound business investments
- Increased talkativeness or pressure to keep talking
- With severe disease, delusions, paranoia, hallucinations, and bizarre behavior

To be diagnosed with bipolar disorder, these symptoms must persist for at least 1 week and evidence of impaired functioning must be present. Suicide is a major risk in patients who have bipolar disorder; up to 50% of these patients attempt suicide, and 10% to 20%

succeed in taking their lives. **Hypomania** is characterized by the same symptoms, but they are less severe and do not cause impaired functioning. In some cases, patients may experience a mixed episode where depression and mania are experienced simultaneously.

Although the pathophysiology of bipolar disorder is incompletely understood, mania and hypomania likely result from abnormal functioning of neurotransmitters in the brain. Mania may involve an excess of excitatory neurotransmitters (such as glutamate or norepinephrine) or a deficiency of inhibitory neurotransmitters (such as GABA). It is important to distinguish bipolar disorder from drug abuse, severe anxiety disorders, schizophrenia, dementia, or electrolyte disturbances, which can all produce symptoms similar to those of bipolar disorder.

Nonpharmacologic interventions play important roles in the treatment of patients with bipolar disorder. Lack of sleep, excessive stress, and poor nutrition are triggers for manic episodes and should be addressed in the plan of care. Support groups and psychotherapy are helpful for many patients. ECT is very effective at treating acute manic and depressive episodes.

Pharmacotherapy of bipolar disorder is highly individualized and dependent on the severity of the condition and whether depression or mania is the predominant symptom. For patients with mild symptoms that cause only slight functional disruption, monotherapy with low doses of a mood stabilizer is indicated. More severely affected patients usually require combination therapy with a mood stabilizer plus an atypical antipsychotic. If the patient is on antidepressant medications, these are usually tapered or discontinued because they can worsen mania or hypomania. Caution must be used in female patients of childbearing potential because some drugs used for bipolar disorder cause fetal malformations.

Like the treatment of major depression, nonadherence with drug therapy is a serious problem in patients with bipolar disorder. As many as 50% of patients discontinue their medication during the first year of therapy. Lack of awareness is the single most common reason for nonadherence; mania is simply not viewed as abnormal by the person experiencing it. In fact, people with mania are often able to work tirelessly on projects and accomplish many work- and home-related tasks. Surprisingly, the second most common reason for nonadherence is the presence of a comorbid substance abuse disorder, usually alcoholism. Psychotherapy and family support may be necessary to achieve proper adherence.

Drugs for Bipolar Disorder

19.13 Lithium is the conventional therapy for the treatment of bipolar disorder.

Drugs for bipolar disorder are called **mood stabilizers**, because they have the ability to moderate extreme shifts in emotion and relieve symptoms of mania and depression during acute episodes. The traditional treatment for bipolar disorder is lithium carbonate (Eskalith), a mood stabilizer prescribed as monotherapy or in combination with other drugs. In recent years, valproic acid/divalproex (Depakene) has begun to replace lithium as the first-line therapy for bipolar disorder due to its improved safety profile. Valproic acid and other miscellaneous drugs for bipolar disorder are discussed in Section 19.14. Drugs used to treat bipolar disorder are shown in Table 19.5.

CONNECTIONS Evidence-Based Practice

◀ Treatment of Bipolar Disorder in Children

Finding appropriate pharmacotherapy for the treatment of mental illnesses such as bipolar disorder is difficult, and patient response to the various treatment options may vary. The presence of comorbid symptoms, especially in children, further complicates the choice of medication. Connor and Doerfler (2012) found that children diagnosed with bipolar disorder differed little from children with disruptive behavior disorders (e.g., ADHD, oppositional defiant disorder) on measures of aggressive behavior. They found that clinicians should consider diagnoses other than, or in addition to, bipolar disorder if aggressive behaviors were present. Prior research has also suggested that post-traumatic stress disorder (PTSD) may be a risk factor for the development of bipolar disorder and may be prevalent in children with bipolar disorder

(Alvarez et al., 2011; Strawn et al., 2010). The importance of determining a diagnosis can direct the choice of drug therapy and bipolar disease is often under-responsive to treatment (West, Weinstein, Celio, Henry, & Pavuluri, 2011).

Research studies have noted that risperidone (Risperdal) seems to be more effective than lithium or divalproex (Depakote) for the initial treatment of bipolar disorder in children (Geller et al., 2012; West et al., 2011). However, the presence of other symptoms or conditions such as disruptive behavioral disorders may require combination therapy. Because risperidone has significant metabolic adverse effects such as increases in body mass index (BMI) and adverse changes in lipid levels, relatively lower doses than previously thought may allow more conservative but effective treatment (Geller et al., 2012).

TABLE 19.5   Drugs for Bipolar Disorder

Drug	Route and Adult Dose (Maximum Dose Where Indicated)	Adverse Effects
lithium carbonate (Eskalith, Lithobid)	PO: initially 600 mg tid or 900 mg sustained release bid or 30 mL (48 mEq) of solution tid Maintenance: 300 mg tid or qid or 15–20 mL (24–32 mEq) in two to four divided doses (max: 2.4 g/day)	*Headache, lethargy, fatigue, recent memory loss, nausea, vomiting, anorexia, abdominal pain, diarrhea, dry mouth, muscle weakness, nephrogenic diabetes insipidus, fine hand tremors, reversible leukocytosis* Peripheral circulatory collapse, neurotoxicity, seizures, coma
Antiseizure Drugs		
carbamazepine (Tegretol)	PO: 200 mg bid, gradually increased to 800–1,200 mg/day in three to four divided doses	*Dizziness, ataxia, somnolence, headache, nausea, diplopia, blurred vision, sedation, drowsiness, vomiting, prolonged bleeding time, transient leukopenia* Heart block, aplastic anemia, agranulocytosis, respiratory depression, exfoliative dermatitis, SJS, toxic epidermal necrolysis, deep coma, death (with overdose), liver failure, pancreatitis, bone marrow depression
lamotrigine (Lamictal)	PO: 50 mg/day for 2 weeks, then 50 mg bid for 2 weeks; may increase gradually up to 300–500 mg/day in two divided doses (max: 700 mg/day)	
valproic acid/divalproex (Depakene)	PO: 250–750 mg/day in divided doses (max: 60 mg/kg/day)	
Atypical Antipsychotic Drugs		
aripiprazole (Abilify)	PO: 30 mg daily; may decrease to 15 mg (max: 30 mg daily)	*Tachycardia, sedation, dizziness, headache, lightheadedness, somnolence, anxiety, nervousness, agitation, hostility, insomnia, nausea, vomiting, transient fever, constipation, akathisia, parkinsonism, gynecomastia (risperidone)* Agranulocytosis, neuroleptic malignant syndrome (risperidone, rare), risk of stroke in elderly with dementia-related psychosis (aripiprazole)
asenapine (Saphris)	SL: 5–10 mg bid (max: 20 mg/day)	
olanzapine (Zyprexa)	PO: start with 10 mg once daily; may increase or decrease in 5 mg/day increments	
quetiapine (Seroquel)	PO: start with 25 mg bid and increase by 25–50 mg bid to tid to target dose of 300–400 mg/day divided bid or tid (max: 800 mg/day)	
risperidone (Risperdal)	PO: start with 2–3 mg daily, may increase dose at intervals of 1 mg/day (max: 6 mg/day)	
ziprasidone (Geodon)	PO: 40 mg bid with food, may increase every 2 days up to 80 mg bid	

Note: *Italics* indicate common adverse effects. <u>Underline</u> indicates serious adverse effects.

PROTOTYPE DRUG	Lithium Carbonate (Eskalith, Lithobid)

Classification: Therapeutic: Antimanic, drug for bipolar disorder
Pharmacologic: Alkali metal ion salt

Therapeutic Effects and Uses: Lithium was approved for use in 1970. Its benefit in treating bipolar disorder has been established since the 1950s, but its therapeutic safety has not been proved. Lithium is a simple inorganic element that is found in the same group as sodium and potassium. It is available for PO administration as tablets, syrup, and controlled release and slow release tablets. Onset of action may take 1 to 3 weeks. Dosing is highly individualized and is based on serum drug levels and clinical response. Lithium has a short half-life and must be taken in multiple doses each day.

Lithium is an effective drug for controlling acute manic episodes and for preventing the recurrence of mania or depression. In the patient with mania, lithium decreases euphoria, hyperactivity, and other symptoms without causing sedation. Previously lithium was used for all patients with mania; at the present time it is used primarily for those patients with classic euphoric mania. Lithium, rather than valproic acid, appears to be more effective in reducing suicide risk in persons diagnosed with bipolar disorder. Lithium may also be used for off-label indications, including alcoholism, bulimia, neutropenia, schizophrenia, prevention of vascular headaches, and hyperthyroidism.

Mechanism of Action: The precise mechanism of action of lithium is not known. It likely acts by changing neurotransmitter balance in specific brain regions. Lithium increases the synthesis of serotonin.

Pharmacokinetics:

Route(s)	PO
Absorption	Completely absorbed
Distribution	Distributed to all tissues and body fluids; crosses the blood–brain barrier and placenta; secreted in breast milk; not bound to plasma protein
Primary metabolism	Not metabolized
Primary excretion	Renal
Onset of action	Peak levels: 4–12 h (tablets) or 15–60 minutes (solutions)
Duration of action	Unknown

Adverse Effects: Many possible adverse effects are associated with the use of lithium. These are sometimes divided into those that occur at the initiation of therapy and those that occur with long-term therapy. Initial adverse effects are muscle weakness, lethargy, nausea, vomiting, polyuria, nocturia, headache, dizziness, drowsiness, tremors, and confusion. Many of the initial adverse effects are transient or may be easily managed. Long-term therapy can produce serious toxicity, including kidney impairment (proteinuria, albuminuria, or glycosuria), dysrhythmias, circulatory collapse, and leukocytosis. Lithium interferes with the synthesis of thyroid hormone and can cause hypothyroidism and goiter. **Black Box Warning**: Toxicity from lithium is closely related to serum concentrations and may occur at doses close to therapeutic levels. Facilities should be available to provide prompt and accurate serum concentration data. Serum lithium levels are monitored regularly during therapy and should be maintained within the narrow range of 0.8 to 1.4 mEq/L at the start of therapy and 0.4 to 1 mEq/L during maintenance therapy.

Contraindications/Precautions: Contraindications to the use of lithium include serious cardiovascular or renal impairment and severe dehydration or sodium depletion. Older adults and debilitated patients must be carefully monitored. Caution must be used when the drug is given to patients with cardiovascular disease, thyroid disease, history of a seizure disorder, diabetes, urinary retention, or a systemic infection. Lithium produces an increased incidence of congenital defects, especially those involving the heart, and is normally not used during pregnancy. Its use should be discouraged during lactation.

Drug Interactions: There are many potential drug interactions, some of which can be serious. Diuretics can increase the risk of lithium toxicity by promoting sodium loss; the body replaces lost sodium with lithium, which is also a salt. NSAIDs and thiazide diuretics can increase lithium levels by increasing the renal reabsorption of lithium. Lithium may cause an increased hypothyroid effect of antithyroid drugs or drugs containing iodine. Concurrent administration with haloperidol may cause increased neurotoxicity. SES may result if lithium is administered with other drugs, such as SSRIs or dextromethorphan, or MAOIs that potentiate the actions of serotonin. **Herbal/Food**: An increased lithium effect may occur with the use of dandelion, goldenrod, juniper, parsley, nettle, or horsetail. Black or green tea, cola nut, or plantain may lead to a decreased lithium effect. Significant changes in sodium intake from foods will alter lithium excretion.

Pregnancy: Category D.

Treatment of Overdose: Overdose of lithium is treated with supportive measures such as emesis or lavage, maintaining airway and respiratory function, and dialysis, if lithium intoxication is severe.

Nursing Responsibilities:

- Obtain a complete health history and history of depression and mania symptoms. Obtain a medication history, particularly other medications used for depression or bipolar disorder.

- Assess baseline vital signs, weight, and laboratory studies, especially serum sodium, CBC, hepatic, and renal values. Monitor drug levels, weight, CBC, electrolytes, and urinalysis for protein, albumin, and glucose periodically during therapy.

- Report thirst, dizziness, lethargy or confusion, muscle weakness, or polyuria to the provider immediately after the early period of therapy as possible toxic effects.

Lifespan and Diversity Considerations:

- Carefully assess the older adult for signs of sodium imbalance or dehydration and for therapeutic and adverse effects. Monitor the older adult frequently because lithium toxicity may occur at lower therapeutic levels than in a younger patient.

- Monitor ethnically diverse patients closely for signs of lithium toxicity. Evaluate normal diet routines for high-sodium content foods or beverages that may affect the therapeutic range of the drug.

Patient and Family Education:

- The full therapeutic effects of lithium may take 2 to 3 weeks or more to appear. Monitor the patient more closely during the early stages of therapy.

- Return regularly for laboratory work. Weigh self weekly and report a gain or loss of 1 kg (2 lb) in a day or 2 kg (5 lb) in a week.

- Maintain a normal-sodium diet and fluid intake without unusual or dramatic increases or decreases, which can affect drug level. Be cautious with exercising or on hot days because excessive sweating will lead to water and sodium loss. Avoid caffeine and alcohol.

- Report excessive thirst, urination, dizziness, muscle weakness, tachycardia, palpitations, or confusion promptly to the health care provider.

- Do not abruptly discontinue the drug. If discontinuation of the drug is desired, it should be discussed with the health care provider and alternative therapy considered.

Drugs Similar to Lithium Carbonate (Eskalith, Lithobid)

There are no drugs similar to lithium carbonate.

19.14 Antiseizure and atypical antipsychotic drugs are used to control symptoms of bipolar disorder.

Although lithium is well established as an effective treatment for bipolar disorder, pharmacologists have found several safe alternatives. Some of these have received FDA approval and others are prescribed off-label for bipolar disorder. All of these medications have additional primary indications and are presented in other chapters of this textbook. The other classes include antiseizure drugs, atypical antipsychotics, and antidepressants.

Antiseizure drugs: The antiseizure drugs for bipolar disorder are classified as mood stabilizers. These medications have pharmacologic actions similar to lithium: relieving symptoms and preventing the recurrence of mania and depression.

Valproic acid (Depakene) and divalproex sodium (Depakote ER) are FDA approved for mood stabilization and mania suppression. Valproic acid has replaced lithium as a preferred drug for many patients because it has far fewer adverse effects, a higher therapeutic index, and a more rapid onset of action. The only area in which it does not compare as favorably with lithium is in the ability to prevent suicide. Valproic acid is well tolerated in most patients but can occasionally cause serious toxicity. Rare cases of thrombocytopenia, pancreatitis, and liver failure have occurred and signs of any of these adverse events require immediate withdrawal of the drug. As with lithium, valproic acid is teratogenic and should not be used during pregnancy. It is secreted in breast milk and therefore should not be used during lactation. A prototype feature for this drug is included in Chapter 22.

Carbamazepine (Tegretol) was one of the initial drugs studied as a lithium alternative, but it was not until 2005 that it was approved for that indication. It reduces the symptoms of both manic and depressive phases of bipolar disorder and can reduce recurrence of the condition. It is preferred over lithium for patients who have mixed mania or rapid-cycling bipolar disorder. Neurologic adverse effects such as vertigo, headache, unsteadiness, and ataxia are common during early therapy but usually subside with continued use. Oral contraceptives may be less effective, and pregnant women should not take carbamazepine because this drug is pregnancy category D. Increased CNS toxicity can result if carbamazepine is used concurrently with lithium. Carbamazepine is one of the most frequently prescribed antiseizure drugs, and a prototype feature is included in Chapter 22.

The antiepileptic drug lamotrigine (Lamictal) is indicated for long-term maintenance therapy to prevent or delay relapses. It may be used alone or in combination with other mood stabilizers. The drug is well tolerated by most patients, with the most common adverse events being drowsiness, dizziness, ataxia, headache, diplopia, blurred vision, nausea, vomiting, and rash. Because rare cases of Stevens–Johnson syndrome (SJS) have been documented, any appearance of rash calls for discontinuation of the drug. To minimize the risk of serious skin rashes, the dose of lamotrigine is increased gradually. Lamotrigine is a pregnancy category C drug and should be used cautiously in lactating women.

Other antiseizure drugs have been used off-label for bipolar disorder but they do not appear to be more effective than existing medications. These include oxcarbazepine (Trileptal), gabapentin (Neurontin), and topiramate (Topamax). Clonazepam (Klonopin) and lorazepam (Ativan) are benzodiazepines used for seizures that have been used off-label for bipolar disorder in combination with other agents.

Atypical antipsychotics: The primary use of antipsychotic drugs is to manage symptoms of severe psychosis, such as those found in patients with schizophrenia (see Chapter 20). Some of the antipsychotic medications are also effective in controlling acute symptoms of mania and as long-term mood stabilizers in bipolar disorder. These drugs are usually used in combination with lithium or valproic acid, but they are also effective as monotherapy. The atypical antipsychotics are preferred over the conventional antipsychotics such as chlorpromazine because of a much lower incidence of extrapyramidal adverse effects. Atypical antipsychotics approved for use in treating bipolar disorder include aripiprazole (Abilify), asenapine (Saphris), olanzapine (Zyprexa), quetiapine (Seroquel), risperidone (Risperdal), and ziprasidone (Geodon). All of these drugs are effective in treating manic episodes, but only olanzapine is approved for long-term maintenance therapy. For specific information on typical and atypical antipsychotics, refer to Chapter 20.

Antidepressants: Antidepressants may be used to treat the depression stage of bipolar disorder. These medications must be used with caution because they have a tendency to cause hypomania or mania in depressed patients with bipolar disorder. Because of this potentially serious adverse effect, antidepressants are usually administered concurrently with a mood stabilizer. The antidepressants of choice for treating patients with bipolar disorder are the SSRIs, venlafaxine (Effexor), and bupropion (Wellbutrin). The antidepressant medications are discussed earlier in this chapter.

CHAPTER

19

Understanding the Chapter

Key Concepts Summary

19.1 The two primary categories of mood disorders are depression and bipolar disorder.

19.2 Major depressive disorder is characterized by a depressed mood, with accompanying symptoms, that lasts at least 2 weeks.

19.3 The pathophysiology of depression has biologic, genetic, and environmental components.

19.4 Assessment and diagnosis of depression are a collaborative effort among health care providers.

19.5 The majority of patients who attempt suicide have major depression.

19.6 Depression is sometimes treated with nonpharmacologic therapies.

19.7 The mechanism of action of antidepressants involves modulation of neurotransmitter levels in the brain.

19.8 Tricyclic antidepressants were once the mainstay for the treatment of depression but they have many adverse effects.

19.9 Selective serotonin reuptake inhibitors are the drugs of choice for treating depression due to their low incidence of serious adverse effects.

19.10 Atypical antidepressants are alternatives to the selective serotonin reuptake inhibitors for depression and anxiety disorders.

19.11 Monoamine oxidase inhibitors are effective antidepressants but are seldom used due to potentially serious adverse effects.

19.12 Bipolar disorder is a serious psychiatric disorder characterized by extreme mood swings from depression to euphoria.

19.13 Lithium is the conventional therapy for the treatment of bipolar disorder.

19.14 Antiseizure and atypical antipsychotic drugs are used to control symptoms of bipolar disorder.

Case Study: Making the Patient Connection

Remember the patient "Jane Albright" at the beginning of the chapter? Now read the remainder of the case study. Based on the information presented within this chapter, respond to the critical thinking questions that follow.

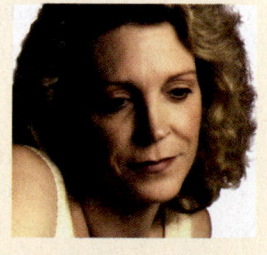

Jane is a 42-year-old mother of three young children. Before the children were born she was employed as a corporate attorney, but she and her husband decided prior to the birth of their first child that she would stay at home until the children completed high school. They are financially stable. Jane has been a soccer coach, Boy Scout leader, president of the ladies' group at her church, and involved in various other community organizations. Within the past month, she has not participated in any of her previous activities and she has not explained why. Jane is in good physical health and had her annual physical exam the previous month. She takes no routine medications or herbal products.

Critical Thinking Questions

1. What first step must Charlie take to aid his wife with her depression?

2. When Jane is evaluated by a mental health professional, they begin talking about how antidepressant drug therapy works. Provide a brief explanation of antidepressant therapy.

3. How can a nurse determine if a therapeutic effect from the antidepressant medication is being achieved with Jane?

See Answers to Critical Thinking Questions on student resource website.

Additional Case Study

Andrew Phillips, age 17, was diagnosed with bipolar illness with acute mania at age 15. He was stabilized with lithium for the manic periods and is also taking valproic acid. This fall, he played football and is looking forward to playing baseball this spring and summer. Although they have a close relationship, his parents have concerns about his dietary habits and post-game festivities, especially now that he is driving and they are not available to monitor the situation.

1. Considering Andrew's activities and eating habits, what risks are possible and what assessments would the nurse make to ensure Andrew's lithium dosage remains effective and within a therapeutic range?

2. What suggestions could the nurse make that would help Andrew participate fully in his sports interests and post-game festivities?

3. What strategies might the nurse suggest for helping Andrew's parents participate in his activities and care?

See Answers to Additional Case Study on student resource website.

Chapter Review

1 A health care provider has ordered imipramine (Tofranil) for each of these patients. A nurse would question the order for the patient with:

1. Seizure disorders.
2. Depression.
3. Enuresis.
4. Neuropathic pain.

2 The nurse determines that the patient understands an important principle in self-administration of fluoxetine (Prozac) when the patient makes which statement?

1. "I should not decrease my sodium or water intake."
2. "This drug can be taken concurrently with a monoamine oxidase inhibitor."
3. "It may take up to 1 month to reach full therapeutic effects."
4. "There are no problems associated with concurrent use of other central nervous system depressants."

3 The nurse is monitoring the patient for early lithium carbonate (Eskalith) toxicity. Which symptoms, if manifested by the patient, would indicate that toxicity may be developing? Select all that apply.

1. Persistent gastrointestinal upset
2. Confusion
3. Polyuria
4. Convulsions
5. Ataxia

4 Which statement made by the patient who is taking lithium carbonate (Eskalith) indicates that further teaching is necessary?

1. "I will be sure to remain on a low-sodium diet."
2. "I will have blood levels drawn every 2 to 3 months, even when I have no symptoms."
3. "Lithium has a narrow margin of safety, so toxicity is a very real concern."
4. "I will not be able to breast-feed my baby."

5 The patient who has been taking venlafaxine (Effexor) for 2 weeks calls the nurse to report that there is no improvement in the depression. The nurse's best response is:

1. "Call your health care provider and see if he or she will change the order to a different medication."
2. "Are you sure that you are taking it as it is ordered? Perhaps you should consider increasing the dosage gradually."
3. "The medication may take up to 3 weeks or longer to be effective. Continue taking the medication as ordered."
4. "Add an over-the-counter antianxiety agent to your daily medications."

6 A 17-year-old patient is started on fluoxetine (Prozac) for treatment of depression. When teaching the patient and his family, what would the nurse include? Select all that apply.

1. Report any sedation to the provider and exercise caution with activities requiring mental alertness.
2. Fluctuations in weight may be managed with a healthy diet and adequate amounts of exercise.
3. Report any thoughts of suicide to the provider immediately, especially during early initiation of the drug.
4. The drug may be safely stopped if unpleasant side effects occur and reported to the provider at the next scheduled visit.
5. The drug may cause excessive thirst but dramatic increase in fluid intake should be avoided.

See Answers to Chapter Review in Appendix A.

References

Alvarez, M. J., Roura, P., Osés, A., Foguet, Q., Solà, J., & Arrufat, F. X. (2011). Prevalence and clinical impact of childhood trauma in patients with severe mental disorders. *Journal of Nervous and Mental Disease, 199,* 156–161. doi:10.1097/NMD.0b013e31820c751c

Baglioni, C., Battagliese, G., Feige, B., Spiegelhalder, K., Nissen, C., Voderholzer, U., . . . Riemann, D. (2011). Insomnia as a predictor of depression: A meta-analytic evaluation of longitudinal epidemiological studies. *Journal of Affective Disorders, 135*(1–3), 10–19. doi:101016/j.jad.2011.01.011

Centers for Disease Control and Prevention. (2011a). *An estimated 1 in 10 U.S. adults report depression.* Retrieved from http://www.cdc.gov/features/dsdepression/

Centers for Disease Control and Prevention. (2011b). *Injury prevention and control: Data and statistics (WISQARS).* Retrieved from http://www.cdc.gov/injury/wisqars/nvdrs.html

Centers for Disease Control and Prevention. (2013). *National suicide statistics at a glance.* Retrieved from http://www.cdc.gov/violenceprevention/suicide/statistics/leading_causes.html

Centers for Disease Control and Prevention. (2014). *Suicide prevention: Youth suicide.* Retrieved from http://www.cdc.gov/violenceprevention/pub/youth_suicide.html

Connor, D. F., & Doerfler, L. A. (2012). Characteristics of children with juvenile bipolar disorder or disruptive behavior disorders and negative mood: Can they be distinguished in the clinical setting? *Annals of Clinical Psychiatry, 24*(4), 261–270.

Dryden-Edwards, R. (2011). *Depression.* Retrieved from http://www.onhealth.com/depression_health/article.htm

Geller, B., Luby, J. L., Joshi, P., Wagner, K. D., Emslie, G., Walkup, J. T., . . . Lavori, P. (2012). A randomized controlled trial of risperidone, lithium, or divalproex sodium for initial treatment of bipolar I disorder, manic or mixed phase, in children and adolescents. *Archives of General Psychiatry, 69,* 515–528. doi:10.1001/archgenpsychiatry.2011.1508

Leon, A. C., Solomon, D. A., Li, C., Fiedorowicz, J. G., Coryell, W. H., Endicott, J., & Keller, M. B. (2011). Antidepressants and risks of suicide and suicide attempts: A 27-year observational study. *The Journal of Clinical Psychiatry, 72,* 580–586. doi: 10.4088/JCP.10m06552

Luca, A., Luca, M., & Calandra, C. (2013). Sleep disorders and depression: Brief review of literature, case report, and nonpharmacologic interventions for depression. *Clinical Interventions in Aging, 8,* 1033–1039. doi:10.2147/CIA.S47230

Nardorff, M. R., Fiske, A., Sperry, J. A., Petts, R., & Gregg, J. J. (2013). Insomnia symptoms, nightmares, and suicidal ideation in older adults. *The Journals of Gerontology, Series B, Psychological Sciences and Social Sciences, 68*(2), 145–152. doi:10.1093/geronb/gbs061

National Center for Complementary and Alternative Medicine. (2012). *Herbs at a glance: St. John's wort.* Retrieved from http://nccam.nih.gov/health/stjohnswort/ataglance.htm

National Institute of Mental Health. (n.d.). *Suicide in the U.S.: Statistics and prevention.* Retrieved from http://www.nimh.nih.gov/health/publications/suicide-in-the-us-statistics-and-prevention/index.shtml

Strawn, J. R., Adler, C. M., Fleck, D. E., Hanseman, D., Maue, D. K., Bitter, S., . . . DelBello, M. P. (2010). Post-traumatic stress symptoms and trauma exposure in youth with first episode bipolar disorder. *Early Intervention in Psychiatry, 4,* 169–173. doi:10.1111/j.1751-7893.2010.00173.x

U.S. Food and Drug Administration. (2004). *FDA launches a multi-pronged strategy to strengthen safeguards for children treated with antidepressant medications* (FDA Publication No. P04-97). Washington, DC: U.S. Government Printing Office.

West, A. E., Weinstein, S. M., Celio, C. I., Henry, D., & Pavuluri, M. N. (2011). Co-morbid disruptive behavior disorder and aggression predict functional outcomes and differential response to risperidone versus divalproex in pharmacotherapy for pediatric bipolar disorder. *Journal of Child and Adolescent Psychopharmacology, 21,* 545–553. doi:10.1089/cap.2010.0140

Selected Bibliography

Barbui, C., Esposito, E., & Cipriani, A. (2009). Selective serotonin reuptake inhibitors and risk of suicide: A systematic review of observational studies. *Canadian Medical Association Journal, 180,* 291–297. doi:10.1503/cmaj.081514

Connolly, K. R., & Thase, M. E. (2011). The clinical management of bipolar disorder: A review of evidence-based guidelines. *The Primary Care Companion to CNS Disorders, 13*(4). doi:10.4088/PCC.10r01097

Herdman, T. H., & Kamitsuru, S. (Eds.). (2014). *NANDA International nursing diagnoses: Definitions and classification, 2015–2017.* Oxford, United Kingdom: Wiley-Blackwell.

Juckett, G., & Rudolph-Watson, L. (2010). Recognizing mental illness in culture-bound syndromes. *American Family Physician, 81,* 206–210.

Maskill, V., Crowe, M., Luty, S., & Joyce, P. (2010). Two sides of the same coin: Caring for a person with bipolar disorder. *Journal of Psychiatric and Mental Health Nursing, 17,* 535–542. doi:10.1111/j.1365-2850.2010.01555.x

Rocha, F. L., Fuzikawa, C., Riera, R., & Hara, C. (2012). Combination of antidepressants in the treatment of major depressive disorder: A systematic review and meta-analysis. *Journal of Clinical Psychopharmacology, 32,* 278–281. doi:10.1097/JCP.0b013e318248581b

Sherrod, T., Quinlan-Colwell, A., Lattimore, T. B., Shatell, M. M., & Kennedy-Malone, L. (2010). Older adults with bipolar disorder: Guidelines for primary care providers. *Journal of Gerontological Nursing, 36*(5), 20–27. doi:10.3928/00989134-20100108-05

U.S. Food and Drug Administration Center for Drug Evaluation and Research. (2006). *Clinical review: Relationship between antidepressant drugs and suicidality in adults.* Retrieved from http://www.fda.gov/ohrms/dockets/ac/06/briefing/2006-4272b1-01-FDA.pdf

Van Lieshout, R. J., & MacQueen, G. M. (2010). Efficacy and acceptability of mood stabilizers in the treatment of acute bipolar depression: Systematic review. *British Journal of Psychiatry, 196,* 266–273. doi:10.1192/bjp.bp.108.057612

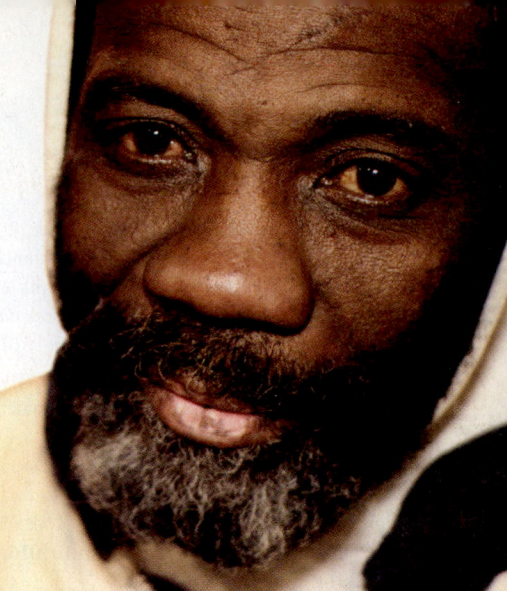

"It started when I was a teenager. I hear voices when there is nobody there. Sometimes, I can ignore them, but other times the voices get louder. You have to watch out because the neighbors may try to steal your soul. You can't let that happen to you. That's not going to happen to me. Don't let it happen to you."

Patient "George Watkins"

CHAPTER

20 Pharmacotherapy of Psychoses

LEARNING OUTCOMES

After reading this chapter, the student should be able to:

1. Describe the general symptoms of psychosis.
2. Compare and contrast the positive and negative symptoms of schizophrenia.
3. Explain theories for the etiology of schizophrenia.
4. Describe the initial treatment and maintenance pharmacotherapy of schizophrenia.
5. Explain the importance of patient drug adherence in the pharmacotherapy of psychoses.
6. Explain how antipsychotic drugs are classified.
7. Discuss the rationale for selecting a specific antipsychotic drug for the treatment of schizophrenia.
8. Identify the extrapyramidal adverse effects of antipsychotic drugs.
9. Describe the nurse's role in the pharmacologic management of schizophrenia.
10. For each of the classes shown in the chapter outline, identify the prototype and representative drugs and explain the mechanism(s) of drug action, primary indications, contraindications, significant drug interactions, pregnancy category, and important adverse effects.
11. Apply the nursing process to care for patients receiving pharmacotherapy for psychosis.

CHAPTER OUTLINE

▶ **Characteristics of Psychoses**

▶ **Symptoms of Schizophrenia**

▶ **Etiology of Schizophrenia**

▶ **Management of Psychoses**

▶ **Antipsychotic Drugs**
First-Generation Antipsychotics
PROTOTYPE Chlorpromazine, *p. 272*
PROTOTYPE Haloperidol (Haldol), *p. 273*
Second-Generation (Atypical) Antipsychotics
PROTOTYPE Risperidone (Risperdal), *p. 274*
Dopamine System Stabilizers (DSSs)
PROTOTYPE Aripiprazole (Abilify), *p. 277*

acute dystonia, 270

akathisia, 270

delusions, 265

dopamine system stabilizers
  (DSSs), 277

dopamine type 2 (D_2)
  receptors, 267

extrapyramidal symptoms (EPS), 269

hallucinations, 265

negative symptoms, 266

neuroleptic malignant syndrome
  (NMS), 270

parkinsonism, 270

positive symptoms, 266

psychosis, 265

schizoaffective disorder, 266

schizophrenia, 265

tardive dyskinesia (TD), 270

Severe mental illness can be incapacitating for the patient and intensely frustrating for caregivers and the health care providers treating the patient. Prior to the 1950s, patients with severe mental illness were institutionalized as soon as symptoms appeared, and often remained that way for their entire lives, with little or no hope of ever improving to the point of being able to function in society. The introduction of chlorpromazine (Thorazine) in the 1950s, and the subsequent development of newer drugs, revolutionized the treatment of mental illness. Many people with schizophrenia and other mental illnesses can now lead normal or near-normal lives as functioning members of society, as long as their health care provider is able to successfully manage their condition. This chapter examines the nature and pharmacotherapy of psychotic illness.

Characteristics of Psychoses

20.1 Psychoses are severe mental disorders characterized by the inability to recognize reality.

Psychosis is a general term used in medicine to describe a loss of contact with reality. A psychosis is a symptom of a mental illness and is not considered a disease in itself. Characteristics of psychosis are relatively easy to recognize and include the following:

- **Delusions. Delusions** are firm ideas and beliefs that are false and not founded in reality. Delusions sometimes are religious in nature, with the individual believing he is a higher power, or a messenger of a higher power. Delusions may be grandiose, with the person believing he is a king or great leader. Some patients with psychosis exhibit paranoid delusions, an extreme suspicion that they are being followed and that others are trying to harm them.

- **Hallucinations. Hallucinations** involve seeing, hearing, or feeling something that is not really there. Hallucinations most often are auditory; patients may hear voices telling them to harm themselves or others, that they are worthless or ugly, or that their behavior is unacceptable. Some patients may have visual hallucinations, seeing persons or objects that are not present.

- **Lack of insight and judgment.** Patients are often unaware of their bizarre behavior and truly believe that the voices they hear and the delusions they experience are real.

- **Mood and affect.** During psychotic episodes, the patient's mood and affect may vary widely and be socially inappropriate. The patient may laugh at sad events or show no emotion at all. The patient may rapidly shift between happy and sad moods for no apparent reason.

Psychotic behavior ranges from total inactivity to extreme agitation and combativeness. Because patients are unable to distinguish what is real from what is illusion, they are often labeled as insane.

Psychoses are classified as acute or chronic. Acute psychotic episodes occur over hours or days, whereas chronic psychoses develop over months or years. Sometimes a specific cause may be attributed to the psychosis, such as brain tumors, overdoses of certain medications, extreme depression, electrolyte disorders, chronic alcoholism, or psychoactive drugs. Treating the underlying disorder may cause the psychosis to disappear.

Unfortunately, the vast majority of psychoses have no identifiable cause. These include psychoses associated with schizophrenia, bipolar disorder, and severe clinical depression.

PharmFACT

Approximately 2.4 million Americans have schizophrenia, or about 1 of every 1,000 adults over age 18 (National Institutes of Health, n.d.).

To function in society, patients with chronic psychoses require long-term pharmacotherapy. Patients must see their health care provider at regular intervals, and medication must be taken for life. Family members and social support groups are important sources of help for patients who cannot function normally in society without continuous drug therapy. One major difficulty is that family relationships may be fractured secondary to the symptoms of psychosis, the length of time symptoms have been evident, and the tendency for the patients to become nonadherent to drug therapy. If these patients stop taking the antipsychotic medications, then symptoms of psychosis will most assuredly promptly reappear.

Symptoms of Schizophrenia

20.2 Schizophrenia, the most common psychosis, has both positive and negative symptoms.

Schizophrenia is the most common psychotic disorder. Symptoms generally begin to appear in early adulthood, with a peak incidence in men 15 to 24 years of age and women 25 to 34 years of age. It is present in all cultures and ethnic groups.

Patients with schizophrenia experience a variety of diverse symptoms that may change over time. The disorder is characterized by abnormal thoughts and thought processes, disordered communication, withdrawal from people and the outside environment, an inability to independently perform activities of daily living (ADLs), and a high risk for suicide. Patients have a marked impairment in their ability to work or attend school. Many people with schizophrenia demonstrate all of these symptoms at some

TABLE 20.1 Common Symptoms of Schizophrenia

Mental Symptoms	Behavioral Symptoms	Interpersonal Symptoms
Hallucinations	Strange behavior, such as communicating in rambling statements or made-up words	Marked withdrawal from social interactions and interpersonal relationships
Delusions	Irrational distrust of others	Difficulty maintaining relationships because they believe friends or partners are unfaithful or persecuting them.
Illusions	Strange or irrational actions; deterioration of personal hygiene and job or academic performance	Stopping attendance at work or school
Paranoia	Constant hypervigilance, worry, and vocalizations that everyone is "out to get me"	Obvious lack of trust in anyone, even those persons with whom the patient has a positive relationship when disease is under control
Indifference or detachment toward life activities	Not appearing to care if someone else (or self) is in danger; not moving to help in a crisis situation; not moving self out of harm's way	Showing a complete lack of concern for self or another's well-being or even safety

time during their illness, whereas others exhibit only one or two. Several subtypes of schizophrenia have been identified based on clinical presentation. Table 20.1 gives examples of symptoms frequently observed in patients with schizophrenia.

Symptoms of schizophrenia are classified as either positive or negative. **Positive symptoms** are those associated with an excess or a distortion of normal function. These include hallucinations, delusions, disorganized thought or speech pattern, and movement disorders. **Negative symptoms** are those associated with a loss of normal functioning. These symptoms include a lack of interest in social activities, reduced or repetitive speech, loss of desire to perform personal hygiene measures, lack of emotion, unresponsiveness, or lack of pleasure in daily activities. Negative symptoms are characteristic of the indifferent personality exhibited by many patients with schizophrenia. Negative symptoms are harder to associate with schizophrenia and may be mistaken for depression or even laziness. Table 20.2 lists the different categories of schizophrenia symptoms.

Proper diagnosis of positive and negative symptoms is important for selection of the appropriate antipsychotic drug. Positive symptoms are easily recognized and more likely to motivate the patient or caregiver to seek treatment. Indeed, the positive symptoms respond more favorably to pharmacotherapy with antipsychotic drugs. The negative symptoms, however, often prevent a patient

with schizophrenia from living independently, holding down a job, and enjoying life. When selecting outcomes for pharmacotherapy, the health care provider must address both positive and negative symptoms.

A third and more recently recognized category of symptoms exhibited during schizophrenia is called cognitive symptoms. These include thinking difficulties, decreased attentiveness or ability to concentrate, and significant learning and memory problems. A retrospective look at the patient diagnosed with schizophrenia will usually reveal that these cognitive symptoms were present for some time but were not recognized as part of schizophrenia until the more obvious positive and negative symptoms appeared.

Schizoaffective disorder is a condition in which the patient exhibits symptoms of both schizophrenia and mood disorder. An acute schizoaffective reaction may include distorted perceptions, hallucinations, and delusions, followed by extreme depression. Over time both positive and negative psychotic symptoms usually appear.

Many conditions can cause bizarre behavior, and these should be distinguished from schizophrenia. Chronic use of amphetamines or cocaine can create a paranoid syndrome. Certain complex partial seizures can cause unusual symptoms that are sometimes mistaken for psychosis. Brain neoplasms, infections, or hemorrhage can also cause bizarre, psychotic-like symptoms.

TABLE 20.2 Categories of Symptoms of Schizophrenia

Positive Symptoms	Negative Symptoms	Cognitive Symptoms
Hallucinations	Apathy	Deficits in long-term memory
Delusions	Withdrawal from other persons and the social environment	Inability to focus attention
Illusions	Lack of ability to perform ADLs	Diminished "working memory": an inability to remember recently learned information and use it right away
Paranoia	Diminished or missing affect	Difficulty following instructions
Agitation, anxiety	Poor judgment	Difficulty following the thread of a conversation
Disorganized thoughts and speech	Lack of awareness or insight	Difficulty in identifying the steps needed to complete a task and placing them in the proper sequence
Aggressiveness, combativeness	Little or no functional speech	

Etiology of Schizophrenia

20.3 The precise etiology of schizophrenia remains unknown.

The etiology and pathogenesis of schizophrenia are complex and likely involve multiple factors. Schizophrenia is best understood as a cluster of distinct disorders, each having a different etiology, rather than as a single disease.

Early theories of the etiology of schizophrenia focused on specific disturbances in child rearing, such as poor communication between parents and offspring with schizophrenia. This view has been rejected in favor of biologic theories. It should be understood, however, that environmental factors such as family dynamics can affect coping skills, which can influence the onset of psychosis, drug response, and adherence to treatment.

There is a definite genetic component to schizophrenia. People have a 5 to 10 times greater risk of getting schizophrenia if they have a first-degree relative with the disorder. In identical twins, if one twin has schizophrenia, the other has nearly a 50% risk of having the disorder. If both parents have schizophrenia, there is a 40% risk that their offspring will have the disorder.

Whether caused by genetics or the environment, schizophrenia is likely the result of neurotransmitter imbalances in specific areas of the brain. This theory suggests the possibility of overactive dopaminergic pathways in the basal nuclei (basal ganglia), an area of the brain responsible for starting and stopping synchronized motor activity such as leg and arm motions during walking. Symptoms of schizophrenia seem to be associated with **dopamine type 2 (D$_2$) receptors**. The basal nuclei are particularly rich in D$_2$ receptors, whereas the cerebrum contains very few. Most antipsychotic drugs act by entering dopaminergic synapses and competing with dopamine for receptors. By blocking D$_2$ receptors, antipsychotic drugs reduce the symptoms of schizophrenia. Pharmacotherapy Illustrated 20.1 shows antipsychotic drug action at the dopaminergic receptor.

PHARMACOTHERAPY ILLUSTRATED 20.1

Mechanism of Action of Antipsychotic Drugs

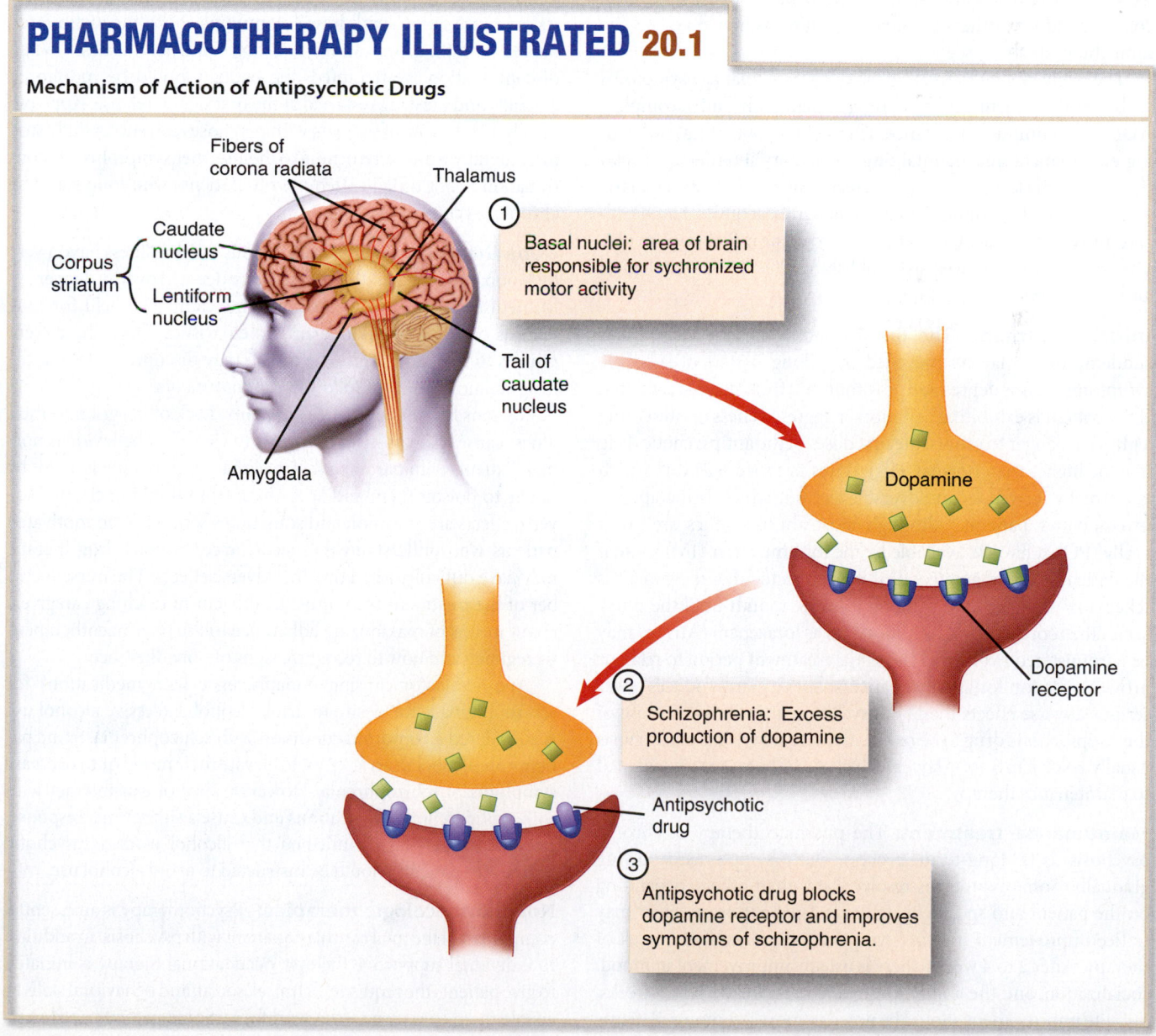

Fibers of corona radiata

Thalamus

Caudate nucleus

Corpus striatum

Lentiform nucleus

Amygdala

Tail of caudate nucleus

① Basal nuclei: area of brain responsible for sychronized motor activity

Dopamine

Dopamine receptor

② Schizophrenia: Excess production of dopamine

Antipsychotic drug

③ Antipsychotic drug blocks dopamine receptor and improves symptoms of schizophrenia.

Management of Psychoses

20.4 Medical management of psychosis is challenging because patients often lack insight into their disease and believe their behavior is normal.

The medical management of severe mental illness is extremely challenging. Many patients do not view their behavior as abnormal and have difficulty understanding the need for drug therapy. When a medication produces undesirable adverse effects, such as severe muscle twitching or sexual dysfunction, patients stop taking it and relapse to experience their former symptoms. Agitation, distrust, and extreme frustration are common because patients cannot comprehend why others are unable to think as they do or see the same things that they see.

The primary goal in treating psychosis is to manage symptoms such that the patient can function independently and accomplish ADLs with minimum assistance. This includes obtaining and holding employment and maintaining satisfactory interpersonal relationships. This level of success in treatment requires setting many small, realistic benchmarks that the patient, caregiver, and health care provider can achieve. These subgoals nearly always involve pharmacotherapy as well as establishing effective psychological and social support.

Initial treatment: The first psychotic episode may occur suddenly or it may be preceded by a long period of subacute symptoms such as depression or withdrawal from normal activities. If the patient is exhibiting agitation or aggressiveness or presenting a physical danger to others, the first doses of the antipsychotic drug may be higher than normal. High doses produce sedation, which is normally viewed as an adverse effect but which is therapeutic in combative patients. Although most antipsychotics are given orally (PO), a few are available by the intramuscular (IM) route if the patient is uncooperative or if it is suspected that the patient is "cheeking" the medicine—hiding it in the mouth until the nurse leaves the room. Benzodiazepines such as lorazepam (Ativan) may be administered IM during the initial treatment period to relax or provide sedation for agitated patients. Lorazepam produces fewer serious adverse effects than antipsychotics and allows the dose of the antipsychotic drug to be reduced. Acute symptoms of psychosis usually resolve in 3 to 7 days, at which time the patient is switched to maintenance therapy.

Maintenance treatment: The pharmacotherapy of chronic psychosis is a long-term process, with symptoms resolving gradually. Some symptoms resolve faster than others, depending on the patient and specific drug used. A patient or caregiver may notice improvement in acute symptoms after less than a week of therapy. After 2 to 4 weeks, there is usually improvement in mood, socialization, and the ability to provide self-care. By 6 to 8 weeks, definite improvement should be noted in most symptoms. Patients

who have experienced untreated schizophrenia for many years are slower to respond than those experiencing their first episode. As long as symptoms continue to gradually improve, the patient is maintained on a stable dosage.

If substantial improvement is not observed after 8 to 12 weeks of therapy, the health care provider must explore reasons for the lack of response. For example, the patient may not be taking the medication, or the original diagnosis may have been incorrect. If the patient has been taking the medication at average doses or higher, the health care provider will generally not increase the dose because doing so increases the potential for serious adverse effects. Instead of increasing the dosage, a different antipsychotic drug may be substituted. The nurse, patient, and caregivers must understand that drug therapy is not a cure; in some cases, medications simply are not able to eliminate all psychotic symptoms.

How long does drug maintenance therapy continue? The answer to this is highly individualized, but the most common answer is for the lifetime of the patient. In patients experiencing their first acute episode, health care providers may slowly taper the dose after a year of successful therapy. Abrupt cessation of some antipsychotics can cause serious withdrawal symptoms, including nightmares, nausea, vomiting, salivation, sweating, and nervousness. When discontinuation is attempted, the patient should be monitored carefully and the drug restarted at the first sign of relapse. Approximately 15% to 25% of patients with psychoses can successfully stop drug therapy without returning to their former symptoms. Discontinuation is not usually attempted in patients with long-standing chronic psychosis.

Nonadherence: Patients with serious mental illness have a very high nonadherence rate. Unless they are deemed overtly dangerous to themselves or other people, patients cannot be held for long periods of hospitalization against their wishes. Once the patient returns to the community, he or she may discontinue taking the drug and not return for follow-up appointments.

Reasons for nonadherence are many. Lack of insight into their illness causes patients with psychosis to view their behavior as normal. Patients with paranoia may feel that drug therapy is a plot by others to poison them and keep them from thinking clearly. Adverse effects are common and sometimes serious. Even motivated patients who understand the need for continuous drug therapy may have difficulty tolerating the adverse effects. The nurse member of the treatment team must be diligent in teaching caregivers about means of maximizing adherence to the pharmacotherapeutic regimen and how to recognize signs of nonadherence.

Another factor causing nonadherence with medications for schizophrenia is the desire to drink alcohol. Excessive alcohol use is considered a comorbid condition with schizophrenia. Some patients use alcohol in an attempt to elevate their mood or to decrease symptoms of schizophrenia. However, alcohol can interact with some antipsychotic medications and cause a suboptimal response. Because studies have confirmed that alcohol worsens psychotic symptoms, patients should be instructed to avoid alcohol use.

Nonpharmacologic therapies: Psychotherapy is an essential component of the total care of the patient with psychosis. In addition to individual supportive therapy, occupational therapy is initiated to give patients the requisite technical, social, and behavioral skills to enable them to return to the workforce. Some patients need skills in performing ADLs such as cooking, cleaning, and dressing. Family and caregiver training are included in the plan of care for the treatment of patients with schizophrenia whenever feasible.

Prognosis: Although there is no cure, schizophrenia can be successfully managed in a significant number of patients. Strong family and caregiver support, combined with pharmacotherapy, can decrease hospitalization and relapse rates and increase the potential for recovery. According to the World Fellowship for Schizophrenia and Allied Disorders (n.d.) the prognosis for schizophrenia after 10 years of the disease is as follows:

- 25% completely recovered
- 25% much improved, relatively independent
- 25% improved, but require extensive support network
- 15% hospitalized, unimproved
- 10% deceased (mostly suicide)

Antipsychotic Drugs

20.5 Selection of an antipsychotic drug depends on its spectrum of adverse effects and the experience of the health care provider.

The pharmacotherapy of psychosis has undergone two major "generations." The first generation appeared in the early 1950s when the original drugs for treating severe mental illnesses were discovered. These drugs include conventional antipsychotics such as chlorpromazine. This essentially ended the era of placing all patients in insane asylums for their lifetimes. Unfortunately, first-generation drugs came with adverse effects that were sometimes as serious as the symptoms of the patient's original disorder.

The second-generation or *atypical* antipsychotic drugs were discovered in the 1970s and 1980s. "Atypical" refers to several characteristics of these drugs compared to the conventional agents:

- Significantly fewer adverse effects related to the extrapyramidal system
- Better patient adherence due to reduced adverse effects and less cognitive impairment
- More effective at resolving negative psychotic symptoms

Two older terms are occasionally used to describe antipsychotic drugs. *Major tranquilizer* was the term used following the introduction of the first-generation drugs because sedation is a prominent action of them. *Neuroleptic* is a term used to denote drugs that have effects on the nervous system, especially those that have Parkinson's-like adverse effects on posture and body movement. Although the student will still encounter reference sources that refer to these drugs as tranquilizers or neuroleptics, *antipsychotic* is more accurate and is the preferred term.

Classification of antipsychotics: There are two means of classifying antipsychotic medications. The older system uses the conventional versus atypical distinction. The conventional group is further subdivided by chemical classes into phenothiazines and nonphenothiazines. This older classification scheme has flaws because there is not always a clear distinction between a drug that is "conventional" and one that is "atypical." Furthermore, some antipsychotics have an adverse effect profile that appears as if it is atypical at low doses but becomes conventional at high doses.

In recent years, a new system for classification has emerged. This system divides these medications by potency levels: low potency (drugs that require higher doses), moderate potency (drugs that require middle range dosing), and high potency (drugs able to control symptoms of schizophrenia with low doses). This categorization was made based on the amount of medication necessary to produce an equivalent effect as compared to other drugs in the same category. As an example, 100 mg of chlorpromazine is approximately equivalent to 2 mg of haloperidol (Haldol). According to the categories, haloperidol is a high-potency drug, whereas chlorpromazine is a low-potency drug (although both are conventional antipsychotics). The nurse must not confuse potency with efficacy or effectiveness. Potency refers to a quantity, whereas efficacy refers to therapeutic response. Unfortunately, the potency classification method does not give any indication of a drug's effectiveness, mechanism of action, or chemical class.

So for the antipsychotic drugs, which classification should the student learn and use? Because the conventional and atypical and potency methods of drug classification are used in clinical practice, the student must be aware of both schemes.

Drug selection: In terms of effectiveness, there is no single drug of choice for the long-term therapy of schizophrenia. Selection of a specific drug is based on clinician experience, the occurrence of adverse effects, and the therapeutic response of each individual patient. For example, patients with both psychosis and Parkinson's disease need an antipsychotic with minimal extrapyramidal symptoms. Those who operate machinery need a drug that does not cause sedation. Men who are sexually active may adhere better to a regimen with a drug that does not cause sexual dysfunction.

Clearly, the second-generation atypical antipsychotics result in a lower incidence of serious adverse effects and have become preferred drugs for psychosis. They are also considerably more expensive. The experience and skills of the health care provider and mental health nurse are particularly valuable in achieving successful psychiatric pharmacotherapy.

Several long-acting IM depot preparations are available for patients who exhibit chronic nonadherence to the therapeutic regimen. For example, risperidone (Risperdal Consta), paliperidone (Invega Sustenna), and fluphenazine decanoate last 2 to 6 weeks, depending on the dose and patient response.

CONNECTION Checkpoint 20.1

From what you learned in Chapter 4, explain why it is more important to receive an antipsychotic drug that has greater effectiveness versus one that has higher potency. *See Answer to Connection Checkpoint 20.1 on student resource website.*

Managing adverse effects: Although antipsychotic drug therapy clearly results in significant improvement in clinical symptoms, adverse effects are common and often serious. An important component of successful antipsychotic pharmacotherapy is managing these adverse effects.

Extrapyramidal symptoms (EPS) are a particularly serious set of adverse reactions to antipsychotic drugs. The term *extrapyramidal* refers to locations in the central nervous system (CNS) outside the cerebrospinal pyramidal tracts of the brain. Whereas the pyramidal system controls visible, voluntary movements, the extrapyramidal system is associated with postural and automatic movements that are not usually noticeable. EPS include the following:

- **Acute dystonia** occurs early in the course of pharmacotherapy with antipsychotics and involves severe muscle spasms, particularly of the back, neck, tongue, and face. In rare cases, acute dystonia can be so severe as to dislocate joints and impair respiration due to laryngospasm. The risk of acute dystonia is greater with high-potency antipsychotics. Administration of drugs with anticholinergic properties such as diphenhydramine (Benadryl) or benztropine (Cogentin) can reverse acute dystonia symptoms within minutes when administered parenterally. For dystonia refractory to anticholinergic drugs, diazepam (Valium) may be administered.

- **Akathisia**, the most common EPS, is an inability to rest or relax. The patient paces, has trouble sitting or remaining still, and has difficulty sleeping. Repetitive movements such as rocking while standing or sitting and crossing and uncrossing legs may be evident. Akathisia can even be mistaken for anxiety and agitation, possibly resulting in an increase in antipsychotic dose, which will exacerbate these adverse effects. In some cases, akathisia may require symptom management with beta-adrenergic blockers, anticholinergics, or benzodiazepines.

- **Parkinsonism** induced by antipsychotic drugs may include tremor, loss of fine motor skills, muscle rigidity, stooped posture, and a shuffling gait. The treatment of antipsychotic drug-induced parkinsonism includes anticholinergic drugs and amantadine (Symmetrel) (see Chapter 21).

- **Tardive dyskinesia (TD)** is characterized by involuntary, unusual tongue and face movements such as lip smacking, rapid eye blinking, and wormlike motions of the tongue. They generally occur during long-term therapy, and symptoms may persist for months or years after the drug is discontinued. Symptoms of TD may worsen when the antipsychotic drug is withdrawn or even become permanent. Because there are no established medicines to treat TD, the best approach is prevention.

When EPS are reported early, the drug is usually withdrawn or the dosage reduced so that the symptoms can be reversed. If the symptoms are allowed to continue for prolonged periods, EPS may become permanent. The nurse must be vigilant in observing and reporting EPS, because prevention is the best treatment. Table 20.3 contains further information on the EPS of antipsychotic medications.

A potentially fatal adverse reaction to antipsychotic medications is **neuroleptic malignant syndrome (NMS)**. Symptoms include high fever, diaphoresis, muscle rigidity, tachycardia, and blood pressure fluctuations. Although rare, without quick, aggressive treatment the condition can rapidly deteriorate to stupor or coma. The most immediate intervention is to discontinue all antipsychotics. Supportive treatment includes antipyretics, electrolytes, and muscle relaxants.

Adverse effects on the reproductive system are a major cause of nonadherence to the drug regimen in some patients. Up to 50% to 60% of men taking antipsychotics may experience ejaculation disorders and erectile dysfunction. In women, decreased libido and inability to achieve orgasm may occur. Many antipsychotics increase serum levels of the hormone prolactin, which can cause secretion of breast milk (galactorrhea) and breast enlargement (gynecomastia). These events may occur in both men and women. Most women will also experience menstrual dysfunction due to the high prolactin levels.

Unlike many CNS drugs, antipsychotic medications do not cause physical or psychological dependence. They also have a wide safety margin between a therapeutic and a lethal dose; deaths due to overdoses of antipsychotic drugs are uncommon. They should be gradually discontinued, however, to avoid withdrawal symptoms.

First-Generation Antipsychotics

20.6 The phenothiazines are effective at treating schizophrenia symptoms but exhibit a high incidence of adverse effects.

The first-generation or conventional antipsychotics form two subclasses: the phenothiazines and nonphenothiazines. *Phenothiazine* is a chemical term that refers to compounds with three rings that are

TABLE 20.3 Extrapyramidal Symptoms of Antipsychotic Medications

Type of Symptom	Time of Onset	Manifestations	Treatment
Acute dystonia	Several hours to 5 days	Severe spasms of the muscles of the tongue, face, neck, or back; involuntary upward deviation of the eyes; arching forward of the trunk while the head and legs are thrust backward	Immediately administer an anticholinergic such as diphenhydramine or benztropine IV or IM. Symptoms usually resolve within 5–20 min.
Akathisia	Within first 2 months of treatment	Pacing, squirming, inability to sit still, uncontrollable need to be moving	Anticholinergics (diphenhydramine, etc.), benzodiazepines (diazepam, alprazolam, etc.), or beta blockers (atenolol, labetalol, etc.).
Antipsychotic-induced parkinsonism	5–30 days	Tremor, rigidity, shuffling gait, masklike facies, drooling, cogwheeling, stooped posture, bradykinesia. Symptoms cannot be distinguished from true Parkinson's disease.	Anticholinergics (benztropine, diphenhydramine, etc.), amantadine. Treatment should not need to be continued for more than a few months, because symptoms should resolve.
Tardive dyskinesia	During long-term therapy	Involuntary, unusual movements of the tongue and face and lip-smacking movements; may include involuntary movements of the arms and legs, fingers, toes, and trunk. Incidence is very high in elderly patients.	For some patients, decreased doses of antipsychotics, administration of benzodiazepines, or gradual withdrawal of anticholinergics may help. Some patients may benefit from switching to an atypical antipsychotic.

TABLE 20.4 First-Generation Antipsychotic Drugs

Drug	Route(s) and Adult Dose (Maximum Dose Where Indicated)	Adverse Effects
Phenothiazines		
chlorpromazine	PO: Hydrochloride: 25–100 mg tid or qid (max: 1,000 mg/day) IM/IV: 25–50 mg (max: 600 mg every 4–6 h) Subcutaneous/IM: Decanoate 12.5–25 mg every 1 to 4 weeks	*Sedation, drowsiness, dizziness, EPS, constipation, photosensitivity, orthostatic hypotension, anticholinergic effects, seizures* <u>Agranulocytosis, pancytopenia, anaphylaxis, TD, NMS, hypothermia, adynamic ileus, sudden unexplained death</u>
fluphenazine	PO: 0.5–10 mg/day in one to four divided doses (max: 20 mg/day)	
perphenazine	PO: 8–16 mg bid to qid (max: 64 mg/day)	
prochlorperazine (Compazine)	PO: 5–10 mg tid or qid IM: 10–20 mg, may repeat every 1–4 h	
thioridazine (Mellaril)	PO: 50–100 mg tid (max: 800 mg/day)	
trifluoperazine	PO: 1–2 mg bid (max: 20 mg/day)	
Nonphenothiazines		
haloperidol (Haldol)	PO: 0.2–5 mg bid or tid IM: 2–5 mg every 4 h prn	*Akathisia, sedation, transient drowsiness, EPS, tremor, orthostatic hypotension, weight changes, anticholinergic effects* <u>TD, NMS, acute renal failure, respiratory depression, laryngospasm, hepatotoxicity, sudden unexplained death, agranulocytosis</u>
loxapine (Loxitane)	PO: start with 20 mg/day and increase to 60–100 mg/day in divided doses (max: 250 mg/day)	
pimozide (Orap)	PO: 1–2 mg/day (max: 10 mg/day)	
thiothixene (Navane)	PO: 2 mg tid (max: 60 mg/day)	

Note: Italics indicate common adverse effects. <u>Underline</u> indicates serious adverse effects.

joined together by nitrogen and sulfur atoms. Originally developed as a yellow dye in the 1800s, phenothiazine became the starting molecule for a series of drugs, which are recognized by the "-zine" suffix. The student will encounter the term *phenothiazine* in other chapters because several drug classes produce "phenothiazine-like" adverse effects. The phenothiazines are listed in Table 20.4.

At equivalent doses, all phenothiazines have the same effectiveness in treating psychoses, and all produce a similar spectrum of adverse effects. Selection of a specific phenothiazine is determined by the severity and extent of expected adverse effects. For example, if EPS are a major concern, thioridazine may be selected because it gives the lowest incidence of EPS in the class. If the patient is driving or working, fluphenazine may be selected because it produces less sedation and fewer anticholinergic effects than other phenothiazines.

It should be clearly understood at the outset of conventional antipsychotic therapy that it is not always possible to control the disabling symptoms of schizophrenia without producing some degree of EPS or anticholinergic adverse effects. Adjunct drug therapy may be warranted to treat expected adverse effects. For example, concurrent pharmacotherapy with an anticholinergic drug may prevent some of the EPS. For acute dystonias, benztropine (Cogentin) may be given parenterally. Levodopa (Dopar, Larodopa) is usually avoided because its ability to increase dopamine function antagonizes the mechanism of action of the phenothiazines. Beta-adrenergic blockers and benzodiazepines are sometimes given to reduce signs of akathisia.

Some phenothiazines have indications beyond psychiatry. These indications include:

- **Nausea and vomiting.** The phenothiazines reduce nausea and vomiting by blocking dopamine receptors in the chemoreceptor trigger zone in the medulla. Although effective, the use of phenothiazines in treating nausea and vomiting has declined due to the discovery of serotonin antagonists such as ondansetron (Zofran).

- **Cold and allergy symptoms.** Promethazine has antihistamine properties that are of benefit for treating serious cough and symptoms of the common cold. For this indication, promethazine is combined with other medications such as codeine or dextromethorphan.

- **Tourette's syndrome.** This condition is characterized by tics: sudden, loud vocalizations, often cursing, and muscle movements such as twitches, kicking, or hitting. The patient feels a premonitory urge, a type of warning, that a tic is forthcoming, and the tics may be consciously suppressed for limited periods. Drugs from a large number of classes have been used to suppress tics, including phenothiazines such as fluphenazine. There is no cure for Tourette's syndrome but the symptoms can be managed in many patients.

- **Organic brain syndrome (OBS).** *Organic brain syndrome* is a general term that refers to decreased mental function due to physical disorders rather than psychiatric illness. OBS can cause symptoms similar to those of schizophrenia, including delirium, amnesia, and agitation. OBS is a common diagnosis in older adults and is associated with a large number of conditions, including head trauma, brain tumors, stroke, shock, drug interactions, adverse effects, and renal or hepatic failure. Chronic OBS is known as dementia. Historically, the phenothiazines were drugs of choice for treating symptoms of OBS; however, atypical antipsychotics such as risperidone (Risperdal) are now more commonly prescribed for this condition.

Classification: Therapeutic: Antipsychotic (first generation)
Pharmacologic: Phenothiazine, dopamine (D_2) receptor antagonist

Therapeutic Effects and Uses: Approved in 1954, chlorpromazine is a low-potency antipsychotic that blocks several types of receptors within and outside the CNS, including dopamine, histamine, norepinephrine, and acetylcholine receptors. The therapeutic effects in a patient with schizophrenia appear to be due to the blocking of dopamine receptors. Peak antipsychotic effects may take as long as 6 weeks to several months. IM dosing is available for acutely agitated patients. Thorazine was once a popular brand name for this drug, but chlorpromazine is now only available in generic form.

The major use of chlorpromazine is to treat the symptoms of schizophrenia and other psychotic disorders. The drug can effectively suppress symptoms of acute psychotic episodes and can greatly decrease the incidence of relapse if it is used consistently. Although once widely prescribed for psychosis, chlorpromazine is rarely used today because of the potential for serious adverse effects. Other approved uses for chlorpromazine include treating schizoaffective disorder, the manic phase of bipolar disorder, as an antiemetic, as an adjunct in the treatment of tetanus, and for intractable hiccups. It is important to understand that chlorpromazine, and the other phenothiazines, do not change the underlying pathology of psychotic disease, but rather deal only with the symptoms.

Mechanism of Action: Chlorpromazine acts by blocking postsynaptic dopamine receptors. Decreases in the function of this neurotransmitter are associated with diminished psychotic symptoms. Decreased dopamine in the chemoreceptor trigger zone in the medulla results in an antiemetic effect.

Pharmacokinetics:

Route(s)	PO, rectal, IM, intravenous (IV) (only for severe conditions)
Absorption	20% absorbed PO; well absorbed IM
Distribution	Widely distributed; crosses the placenta; secreted in breast milk; 92–97% bound to plasma protein
Primary metabolism	Hepatic; some active metabolites
Primary excretion	Renal
Onset of action	1/2–12 h, depending on route; optimum results will take several months
Duration of action	Half-life: 30 h

Adverse Effects: Common adverse effects of chlorpromazine include headache, anticholinergic symptoms (dry mouth, anorexia, nausea, vomiting, and constipation), weight gain, anemia, phototoxicity, blurred vision, dry eyes, and glaucoma. Of all the antipsychotics, phenothiazines are the most likely to produce EPS. Serious or life-threatening adverse effects include tachycardia, cardiac arrest, laryngospasm, respiratory depression, seizures, agranulocytosis, leukopenia, leukocytosis, and NMS. Abrupt withdrawal can induce symptoms such as nausea, vomiting, and tremors. **Black Box Warning**: This drug is not indicated for the treatment of dementia-related psychosis. Older adults with dementia-related psychosis treated with antipsychotic drugs are at increased risk of death compared to placebo.

Contraindications/Precautions: There are many contraindications to the use of chlorpromazine; these are coronary artery disease, severe hypertension or hypotension, blood dyscrasias, coma, brain damage, bone marrow depression, alcohol or barbiturate withdrawal, glaucoma, hepatic dysfunction, and children under age 6 months. The drug should be used with caution in patients with cardiovascular disease because it may cause orthostatic hypotension (especially in older adults), increase the heart rate, and prolong the QT interval on the electrocardiogram (ECG). Patients with severe hepatic impairment may experience excessive CNS depression. The drug decreases the seizure threshold; thus patients with preexisting epilepsy must be carefully monitored. Chlorpromazine may produce drowsiness and lethargy in breastfeeding newborns; thus use is not recommended during lactation. The elderly are very sensitive to the EPS effects of phenothiazines; thus the drug must be used with caution in this population. Patients with benign prostatic hyperplasia (BPH) should use this drug with caution because it may cause urinary retention.

Drug Interactions: Many drug interactions are possible with chlorpromazine. Use with other CNS depressants, including alcohol, will cause additive sedation. Use with tricyclic antidepressants or anticholinergic drugs will result in additive anticholinergic adverse effects. Decreased absorption and thus lower serum levels of chlorpromazine will occur if used with antacids, barbiturates, or lithium. Increased serum levels and possible hypotension may occur if administered concurrently with epinephrine. Use with warfarin can lead to decreased anticoagulant effects. Phenothiazines inhibit the therapeutic effects of levodopa and may cause excessive sedation if used concurrently. **Herbal/Food**: Increased action of chlorpromazine may occur with nutmeg, hops, nettle, and cola tree. Increased anticholinergic effects can occur with henbane leaf, kava, and betel palm.

Pregnancy: Category C.

Treatment of Overdose: Overdose will cause profound CNS depression, seizures, hypotension, and EPS. Treatment is supportive and may include vasopressors and antiseizure drugs. Airway and gastric lavage are provided if taken PO. Epinephrine should not be administered and vomiting should not be induced.

Nursing Responsibilities: Key nursing implications for patients receiving chlorpromazine are included in the Nursing Practice Application for Patients Receiving Pharmacotherapy with Antipsychotics.

Drugs Similar to Chlorpromazine

Similar drugs include fluphenazine, perphenazine, prochlorperazine, thioridazine, and trifluoperazine. Mesoridazine (Serentil), thiethylperazine (Torecan), and promazine (Sparine) are first-generation phenothiazines that have been discontinued in the United States. Promethazine (Phenergan) is chemically classified as a phenothiazine but the drug has no antipsychotic action and its primary use is as an antihistamine (see Chapter 45). All first-generation phenothiazines carry black box warnings that they are not to be used to treat dementia-related psychosis.

Fluphenazine: Approved in 1959, fluphenazine is a high-potency phenothiazine approved to treat psychotic disorders, including schizophrenia. The drug is most often given as fluphenazine decanoate, a long-acting depot formulation that is given either subcutaneously or IM. Administered at 1- to 4-week intervals, fluphenazine decanoate is advantageous for those patients who are not adherent to taking their PO medications daily. Oral and injectable preparations (fluphenazine hydrochloride) are also available. A stable dose of PO fluphenazine is generally achieved before placing the patient on the depot preparation. The injectable preparations are not recommended for children under age 12. Fluphenazine produces less sedation and fewer anticholinergic effects than chlorpromazine, but EPS are a major concern. This drug is pregnancy category C.

Perphenazine: Approved in 1959, perphenazine is a medium-potency agent used to treat schizophrenia, nausea, and vomiting. EPS are prominent. The drug has the same actions and adverse effects as chlorpromazine. This drug is pregnancy category C.

Prochlorperazine (Compazine): Approved in 1956, prochlorperazine (Compazine) is a phenothiazine rarely used as an antipsychotic. Its primary use is for the management of severe nausea and vomiting. For this purpose, it may be administered PO, rectally, IM, or IV. When used as an antiemetic, doses are low and phenothiazine-like adverse effects are rare. Pharmacotherapy with antiemetics is presented in Chapter 60. This drug is pregnancy category C.

Thioridazine (Mellaril): Thioridazine, a low-potency phenothiazine, is approved to treat psychotic disorders, including schizophrenia, behavioral problems in children, major depression, anxiety, and organic brain syndrome, or as an adjunct in the treatment of alcohol withdrawal. Because of the possibility of fatal dysrhythmias (black box warning), thioridazine should be used only to treat conditions that have not responded to safer drugs. Approved in 1959, thioridazine is available PO and has one of the lowest incidences of EPS of the phenothiazines. This drug is pregnancy category C.

Trifluoperazine: Trifluoperazine is a high-potency phenothiazine approved to treat psychotic disorders. Approved in 1958, it is available in PO form. Trifluoperazine causes less sedation than chlorpromazine but EPS is prominent. All other information is the same as with chlorpromazine, except that it cannot be used in children under age 6. Trifluoperazine was formerly available as Stelazine, but this brand name is no longer marketed. This drug is pregnancy category C.

20.7 The nonphenothiazine first-generation antipsychotics have the same therapeutic applications and similar adverse effects as the phenothiazines.

The nonphenothiazine conventional antipsychotic class consists of drugs whose chemical structures are dissimilar to the phenothiazines. Introduced shortly after the phenothiazines, the nonphenothiazines were initially expected to produce fewer serious adverse events. Unfortunately, this is not the case. The spectrum of adverse effects for the nonphenothiazines is identical to that for the phenothiazines, although the degree to which a particular effect occurs depends on the drug utilized.

In general, the nonphenothiazine drugs cause less sedation and fewer anticholinergic adverse effects than chlorpromazine but exhibit an equal or greater incidence of EPS. Concurrent therapy with other CNS depressants must be carefully monitored because of potential additive sedation.

Drugs in the nonphenothiazine class have the same therapeutic effects and efficacy as the phenothiazines. They are also believed to act by the same mechanism as the phenothiazines; that is, by blocking postsynaptic D_2 dopamine receptors. As a class, they offer no significant advantages over phenothiazines in the treatment of schizophrenia and have largely been replaced by the second-generation, atypical antipsychotics. Doses of the nonphenothiazine antipsychotics are shown in Table 20.4.

PROTOTYPE DRUG	Haloperidol (Haldol)

Classification: Therapeutic: Antipsychotic (first generation)
Pharmacologic: Nonphenothiazine, dopamine (D_2) receptor antagonist

Therapeutic Effects and Uses: Haloperidol, a high-potency antipsychotic approved in 1967, is effective in treating both acute and chronic psychotic disorders. It may also be used off-label to treat Tourette's syndrome, persistent hiccups, autism, children with severe behavioral problems (short term) and OBS with psychotic features, and for the emergency sedation of severely agitated or delirious patients. It may be administered PO or IM but should not be given IV due to the potential for dysrhythmias.

Haloperidol decanoate (Haldol LA) is a long-acting IM formulation that is administered once a month. This is an excellent formulation for patients who cannot be independent in their drug regimen, who may become nonadherent to the drug regimen, or who have no family members to assist them in taking their medication on a regular basis. The medication can be administered either in a clinic setting or by a home health nurse.

Mechanism of Action: Haloperidol depresses the cerebral cortex, hypothalamus, and limbic system, which are parts of the brain that control activity and aggression. It blocks neurotransmission at postsynaptic dopamine D_2 receptors and exhibits alpha$_1$-adrenergic blocking and anticholinergic effects.

Pharmacokinetics:

Route(s)	PO, IM
Absorption	Variable PO; well absorbed IM
Distribution	Widely distributed; may cross the placenta; secreted in breast milk and 92% bound to plasma protein
Primary metabolism	Hepatic; significant first-pass metabolism
Primary excretion	Renal; small amounts biliary with extensive enterohepatic recycling
Onset of action	Erratic if given PO; 15–30 minutes IM; decanoate form reaches peak plasma level in 7 days
Duration of action	Half-life: 24 h (PO); 21 h (IM); 3 wk (decanoate)

Adverse Effects: Haloperidol exhibits an adverse effect profile similar to that of other first-generation antipsychotics. Common adverse effects include drowsiness and EPS. Life-threatening adverse effects include TD, NMS, agranulocytosis, respiratory depression, and laryngospasm. Like chlorpromazine, thioridazine, and pimozide, haloperidol increases the QT interval and can pose a risk for dysrhythmias. **Black Box Warning**: This drug is not indicated for the treatment of dementia-related psychosis. Older adults with dementia-related psychosis treated with antipsychotic drugs are at increased risk of death compared to placebo.

Contraindications/Precautions: Contraindications for use of haloperidol include Parkinson's disease, seizure disorders, coma, alcoholism, severe mental depression, CNS depression, or lactation. Elderly or debilitated patients or those with urinary retention, glaucoma, or severe cardiovascular disorders must be given haloperidol cautiously. The drug lowers the seizure threshold; thus patients with preexisting epilepsy must be carefully monitored.

Drug Interactions: Haloperidol is metabolized by hepatic CYP enzymes and can inhibit some isozymes (CYP2D6). Thus interactions are possible with other drugs affecting these enzymes. For example, carbamazepine, an inducer of CYP enzymes, can reduce the serum level of haloperidol by up to 50%. Increased CNS depression can occur if given concurrently with other CNS depressants, including alcohol, tricyclic antidepressants, or opioids. Anticholinergics that are given concurrently may increase intraocular pressure. Use with methyldopa may precipitate dementia. Haloperidol may increase the QT interval and should be used with caution with other drugs that increase this interval due to the potential for additive cardiotoxicity. A few patients who were taking haloperidol and lithium concurrently experienced irreversible brain damage; thus the two drugs should not be combined. Haloperidol inhibits the therapeutic effects of levodopa and may cause excessive sedation if used concurrently. **Herbal/Food**: Increased action of haloperidol may occur if chamomile, hops, kava, nutmeg, skullcap, or valerian is used concurrently. An antagonist action may occur with the use of scopolia or jimsonweed. Increased EPS may occur if betel palm or kava is used concurrently.

Pregnancy: Category C.

Treatment of Overdose: Overdose will result in sedation, respiratory depression, coma, hypotension, and severe EPS. Treatment is supportive. Antidysrhythmic and vasopressor drugs may be necessary to maintain cardiovascular function.

Nursing Responsibilities: The phenothiazine and nonphenothiazine drug classes are both first-generation antipsychotics with very similar pharmacologic actions and adverse effects. Key nursing implications for patients receiving these drugs are included in the Nursing Practice Application for Patients Receiving Pharmacotherapy with Antipsychotics.

Drugs Similar to Haloperidol (Haldol)

Similar drugs include loxapine, pimozide, and thiothixene. Molindone (Moban) was discontinued in 2010. All first-generation nonphenothiazines carry black box warnings that they are not to be used to treat dementia-related psychosis.

Loxapine (Loxitane): Approved in 1975, loxapine is a medium-potency antipsychotic given by the PO route. It is approved to treat schizophrenia, psychotic depression, and other psychotic disorders, and it is used off-label to treat severe behavioral disturbances associated with Parkinson's and Alzheimer's diseases. Use of loxapine is restricted to treating mental illness refractory to treatment from safer drugs. The adverse effect profile of loxapine is the same as that of haloperidol, and EPS frequently occur during therapy. An active metabolite of loxapine is amoxapine, a drug marketed separately as an antidepressant. This drug is pregnancy category C.

Pimozide (Orap): Approved in 1984, pimozide is a PO, high-potency medication used for treating motor and vocal tics associated with Tourette's syndrome. Although not a true antipsychotic medication, it may be used off-label to treat schizophrenia. The drug has little sedative action and should not be used to control acute psychosis characterized by agitation or hyperexcitability. EPS occur frequently with pimozide. Although effective, the drug exhibits a higher degree of cardiotoxicity than others in its class and is thus only used when other therapies fail to achieve their designated outcomes. This drug is pregnancy category C.

Thiothixene (Navane): Thiothixene, a high-potency antipsychotic, is approved to treat psychotic disorders, including schizophrenia, and acute agitation. Approved in 1967, it is available as a PO preparation and has adverse effects that are characteristic of those of other first-generation antipsychotics. It is not a first-line drug for psychosis. This drug is pregnancy category C.

Second-Generation (Atypical) Antipsychotics

20.8 Second-generation antipsychotics have become drugs of choice for the treatment of schizophrenia.

The second-generation, or atypical, antipsychotics have become preferred drugs for the pharmacotherapy of severe mental illness. Available since the early 1990s, the members of this group are diverse and have little in common with each other, except that they all cause a lower incidence of adverse effects, especially EPS, than the first-generation drugs.

The exact mechanisms of action of the various second-generation antipsychotics are mostly unknown. It is known that atypical antipsychotics bind less tightly to dopamine (D2) receptors than the first-generation drugs, which may explain the relatively low incidence of EPS with these drugs. Some inhibit different subtypes of dopamine receptors, D_1 and D_4, which are especially prominent in the limbic system of the brain. Some also inhibit serotonin (5-HT) receptors in the CNS. Like the first-generation drugs, some atypical antipsychotics have prominent anticholinergic adverse effects. Doses of the second-generation antipsychotics are listed in Table 20.5.

PROTOTYPE DRUG | **Risperidone (Risperdal)**

Classification: Therapeutic: Antipsychotic (second-generation, atypical), Antimanic drug
Pharmacologic: Dopamine (D_2) receptor antagonist

Therapeutic Effects and Uses: Risperidone is an atypical antipsychotic available for PO or IM use that has become one of the most frequently prescribed drugs in this class. It was initially

TABLE 20.5 Second-Generation (Atypical) Antipsychotics

Drug	Route and Adult Dose (Maximum Dose Where Indicated)	Adverse Effects
aripiprazole (Abilify)	PO: 10–15 mg/day (max: 30 mg/day) IM: 400 mg once monthly	*Sedation, headache, akathisia, confusion, insomnia, depression, tachycardia, dizziness, lightheadedness, anxiety, nervousness, hostility, nausea, vomiting, constipation, somnolence, EPS, asthenia, dry mouth, weight gain, tremor, restlessness, sleep disorders*
asenapine (Saphris)	Sublingual: 5–10 mg bid	
clozapine (Clozaril, FazaClo)	PO: start with 12.5–25 mg/day and gradually increase to 300–450 mg/day (max: 900 mg/day)	<u>Agranulocytosis (clozapine), NMS, bone marrow suppression, seizures, suicidal tendencies, TD, diabetes mellitus, ischemia, prolonged QT interval, hypotension, acute dystonia (risperidone)</u>
iloperidone (Fanapt)	PO: initial dose 1 mg bid then increased gradually over 1 week to 12 mg/day (max: 24 mg/day)	
lurasidone (Latuda)	PO: 40 mg once daily	
olanzapine (Zyprexa)	PO: start with 5–10 mg/day and gradually increase to 10–20 mg/day (max: 20 mg/day) IM (extended release): 150–405 mg every 2–4 wk	
paliperidone (Invega, Invega Sustenna)	PO: 6 mg/day (max: 12 mg/day) IM: 39–234 mg monthly	
quetiapine (Seroquel)	PO (immediate release): start with 25 mg bid; increase gradually to 300–400 mg/day (max: 800 mg/day) PO (extended release): 300–450 mg/day (max: 800 mg/day)	
risperidone (Risperdal, Risperidol Consta)	PO: start with 1–2 mg/day then increase by 0.5–1 mg/day every 3–7 days (max: 8 mg/day) IM: 12.5–50 mg once every 2 wk (max 50 mg)	
ziprasidone (Geodon)	PO: 20 mg bid (max: 80 mg bid) IM: 10 mg every 2 h or 20 mg every 4 h (max: 40 mg/day)	

Note: Italics indicate common adverse effects. Underline indicates serious adverse effects.

CONNECTIONS Treating the Diverse Patient

◀ Genetic Lack of Enzyme

Many Asian patients have a genetic lack of the enzyme debrisoquine hydroxylase, which is used by the body to metabolize certain antipsychotic drugs and antidepressants. People who lack this enzyme, sometimes called "poor metabolizers," may have up to 50% higher serum levels of haloperidol and other drugs than Caucasians. The initial dose of an antipsychotic or antidepressant may need to be lower than the usual dose in Asian patients who lack this enzyme in order to decrease the chances of serious adverse reactions.

approved in 1993 to treat negative psychotic symptoms in persons with schizophrenia and related psychoses. In subsequent years, approved indications were extended to include acute mania associated with bipolar disorder. In 2006, risperidone became the first drug approved to treat irritability associated with autism in pediatric patients. Off-label uses include the pharmacotherapy of Tourette's syndrome, attention deficit/hyperactivity disorder, severely disruptive behavior in children with developmental disabilities, dementia, and psychotic depression. The IM depot form of Risperdal (Risperdal Consta) requires 3 weeks to produce a therapeutic response; the patient is usually placed on PO antipsychotics during this 3-week period. Subsequent IM injections are administered every 2 weeks. Risperidone is also available as oral disintegrating tablets (Risperdal M-TAB), which are especially beneficial when treating patients suspected of "cheeking" the drug.

Mechanism of Action: The precise mechanism for risperidone is unknown. It is believed that the drug acts by blocking the binding of dopamine to its receptors in various brain regions. It has highest affinity for type D_2 and has less effect on D_1 receptors. It also blocks 5-HT receptors, alpha$_1$-adrenergic receptors, and histaminergic receptors.

Pharmacokinetics:

Route(s)	PO, IM
Absorption	70% absorbed PO; slowly absorbed IM
Distribution	Widely distributed; crosses both the blood–brain and placental barriers; secreted in breast milk; 90% bound to plasma protein
Primary metabolism	Extensive hepatic metabolism by CYP2D6; changed to the active metabolite 9-hydroxyrisperidone
Primary excretion	Renal, with small amounts in feces
Onset of action	Peak action: 1–3 h (optimum antipsychotic effects may take several months)
Duration of action	Half-life: 20 h

Adverse Effects: The adverse effects of risperidone therapy are similar to those of other atypical antipsychotics. Gastrointestinal (GI) effects such as drowsiness, nausea, vomiting, constipation, and increased salivation are common. Symptoms of parkinsonism may occur in 5% to 10% of patients. The incidence of anticholinergic adverse effects is low, and agranulocytosis is very rare. Risperidone elevates serum prolactin levels, which can result in galactorrhea, impotence, gynecomastia, and menstrual irregularities. Hyperglycemia, including some rare cases of diabetic ketoacidosis, has been reported in patients taking this drug. Orthostatic hypotension is common at the initiation of therapy. Excessive weight gain occurs in children taking risperidone. Adverse effects for the PO and IM depot formulations are the same, except the parenteral form may cause pain and local injection-site reactions. **Black Box Warning**: This drug is not indicated for the treatment of dementia-related psychosis. Older adults with dementia-related psychosis treated with atypical antipsychotics are at increased risk of death compared to placebo.

Contraindications/Precautions: Hypersensitivity to risperidone is a contraindication. The drug should be used with caution in patients with severe CNS depression, seizures, dysrhythmias, hypotension, diabetic ketoacidosis, and suicidal ideation. Patients with renal impairment should be treated with caution. Use during lactation is contraindicated because the drug and its active metabolite are secreted in breast milk.

Drug Interactions: Risperidone is a substrate for hepatic CYP2D6 enzymes; thus it may interact with drugs that inhibit or induce these enzymes. For example, many of the selective serotonin reuptake inhibitors (SSRIs) inhibit CYP2D6, which reduces the metabolism of risperidone and raises serum drug levels. Concurrent use with alcohol, benzodiazepines, or other CNS depressants can cause severe CNS depression. Antihypertensives and nitrates may potentiate hypotension. Decreased risperidone levels may occur with the use of phenobarbital, rifampin, omeprazole, or carbamazepine. Increased risperidone levels may occur with the use of verapamil, azole antifungals, and lamotrigine. Risperidone antagonizes the actions of levodopa and dopamine agonists. Risperidone should be used with caution with drugs known to prolong the QT interval, such as amiodarone, droperidol, and pimozide. **Herbal/Food**: Increased CNS depression may occur if used with St. John's wort or valerian. Food does not affect the absorption of risperidone.

Pregnancy: Category C.

Treatment of Overdose: Symptoms of overdose include confusion, sedation, hypotension, and dysrhythmias. Treatment is supportive and includes gastric lavage and maintenance of cardiovascular function.

Nursing Responsibilities: Key nursing implications for patients receiving risperidone are included in the Nursing Practice Application for Patients Receiving Pharmacotherapy with Antipsychotics.

Drugs Similar to Risperidone (Risperdal)

Other drugs classified as atypical antipsychotics include asenapine, clozapine, iloperidone, lurasidone, olanzapine, paliperidone, quetiapine, and ziprasidone. Aripiprazole (Abilify) is an atypical antipsychotic that is a prototype for a different pharmacologic class (see Section 20.9).

Asenapine (Saphris): One of the newer atypical antipsychotics, asenapine was approved in 2009. Like risperidone, asenapine is a dopamine antagonist that also blocks 5-HT receptors. One unique feature of asenapine is that it is approved to treat both schizophrenia and manic or mixed episodes associated with bipolar disorder. A second advantage is that it is administered by the sublingual route, which bypasses hepatic first-pass metabolism. The types and incidences of adverse effects appear to be similar to those of other drugs in this class. The most common adverse effects include akathisia, oral hypoesthesia, somnolence, dizziness, weight gain, and EPS. This drug is pregnancy category C.

Clozapine (Clozaril, FazaClo): In 1989, clozapine (Clozaril) was the first atypical antipsychotic approved for use in the United States. Clozapine is approved for the management of schizophrenia in patients resistant to standard therapies and to reduce the risk of recurrent suicidal behavior in patients with schizophrenia. Off-label indications include treatment of bipolar disorder, severe obsessive–compulsive disorder, and dementia-related behavioral disorders. Clozapine is available as regular tablets or as oral disintegrating tablets (FazaClo).

Because of potentially severe adverse effects, it is generally reserved for schizophrenia symptoms that have not responded favorably to other drugs. The most serious and limiting adverse effect of clozapine is agranulocytosis, a white blood cell (WBC) count below $500/mm^3$. Although it occurs in less than 1% of patients taking the drug, agranulocytosis can be fatal. To avoid toxicity, clozapine therapy requires special monitoring and surveillance requirements. WBC and absolute neutrophil counts (ANCs) are performed weekly for the first 6 months of treatment and reduced in frequency to every 2 weeks for the next 6 months. CNS effects such as sedation, dizziness, confusion, fatigue, and headache are common at the initiation of therapy but may diminish with continued therapy. Clozapine lowers the seizure threshold and can precipitate seizures in 5% of patients taking high doses. Although the incidence of EPS is less than with first-generation drugs, akathisia, tremor, and agitation can still occur. Orthostatic hypotension is common at the initiation of therapy and during dosage changes. Other warnings on the drug label include an increased risk of hyperglycemia leading to diabetic ketoacidosis, increased risk of fatal myocarditis, and a public health advisory stating that the unapproved use of atypical antipsychotics in older adults has been associated with a higher death rate compared to a placebo. This drug is pregnancy category B.

Iloperidone (Fanapt): One of the newer antipsychotics, iloperidone was approved to treat acute schizophrenia in 2009. Like risperidone, iloperidone is a dopamine antagonist that also blocks 5-HT receptors. Iloperidone is not a drug of first choice because it prolongs the QT interval, which is associated with dysrhythmia and sudden death. The drug should be administered with caution when used in combination with other medications that prolong the QT interval. Another disadvantage is that iloperidone requires a week of gradually increasing the dose before the target drug level is reached. This is because the drug can cause orthostatic hypotension and possible syncope with the first few doses. Other common adverse effects include dry mouth, dizziness, fatigue, nasal congestion, somnolence, tachycardia, and weight gain. This drug is pregnancy category C.

Lurasidone (Latuda): Approved in 2010, lurasidone is one of the newer atypical antipsychotics approved to treat patients with schizophrenia. Lurasidone blocks dopamine receptors and its effectiveness is similar to that of other atypical antipsychotics.

Common adverse effects are typical of other drugs in this class: somnolence, akathisia, nausea, agitation, and parkinsonism. Significant hypotension may occur early in treatment. This drug is pregnancy category B.

Olanzapine (Zyprexa): Approved in 1996, olanzapine is a second-generation antipsychotic available as regular tablets, oraldisintegrating tablets, and IM (both immediate release and extended release forms). It is used to treat both the positive and negative symptoms of schizophrenia, and it is also approved to treat acute agitation and mania associated with bipolar disorder (see Chapter 19). A single IM dose can usually calm patients presenting with acute agitation in about 15 minutes. Off-label, it is used to treat severe behavioral symptoms associated with the dementia of Alzheimer's disease. It is also being used experimentally to treat nausea and vomiting in patients with cancer.

Like other second-generation antipsychotics, the incidence of EPS with olanzapine is low, with drowsiness being the most frequent adverse effect. Weight gain has been reported in up to 25% of patients and is a frequent cause of discontinuation of the drug. Other common adverse effects include dizziness, nervousness, insomnia, headache, and hostility. Use with other CNS depressants may cause additive CNS depression. The risk of patients developing type 2 diabetes mellitus is greater with the use of olanzapine than with other atypical antipsychotics. A major advantage of olanzapine is that it rarely causes neutropenia or agranulocytosis, which are major drawbacks to clozapine therapy. Safety and effectiveness in children under age 18 has not been established. This drug is pregnancy category C.

Paliperidone (Invega): Approved in 2006, paliperidone is approved for the acute and maintenance therapy of schizophrenia. Paliperidone can improve both the positive and negative symptoms of schizophrenia. It is available as an extended release tablet and as an IM depot injection (Invega Sustenna), administered once monthly. Paliperidone is the principal active metabolite of risperidone, which is the prototype antipsychotic for this class.

The incidence of serious adverse events with paliperidone is low. The drug is not extensively metabolized in the liver; thus it has less potential for drug–drug interactions than many other antipsychotics. The most common reported adverse effects include restlessness, akathisia, tachycardia, orthostatic hypotension, syncope, increased sensitivity to environmental heat, and sleepiness. The IM form of the drug can cause injection-site reactions. NMS or TD may occur with the use of paliperidone. Like olanzapine, increased appetite and weight gain are possible. It does not cause neutropenia or agranulocytosis and does not appear to lower the seizure threshold. Like other drugs in this class, paliperidone should not be used to treat dementia-related psychosis in elderly patients because it increases the risk of death due to stroke, heart failure, or infections, especially pneumonia. This drug is pregnancy category C.

Quetiapine (Seroquel): Approved to treat both positive and negative symptoms of schizophrenia in 1997, indications were later extended to include the short-term therapy of acute mania associated with bipolar disorder (in combination with lithium or valproic acid). The drug is also approved to treat major depression and depression associated with bipolar disorder. It is sometimes used off-label to treat obsessive–compulsive disorder that is unresponsive to other therapies. Quetiapine is available only in tablet form. An extended release formulation (Seroquel XR) is available.

Like other atypical antipsychotics, the incidence of EPS and other serious adverse effects with quetiapine is low. Unlike clozapine, agranulocytosis has not been reported. Sedation is commonly experienced during the initial stages of therapy. Cautious use is recommended in patients who have a history of cardiovascular disease or seizures, persons with Alzheimer's disease, those who are taking other CNS depressants, and those who are elderly or debilitated. Lens changes have occurred during quetiapine use; thus baseline and 6-month eye examinations are recommended. Other common adverse reactions include weight gain, constipation, postural hypotension, dyspepsia, and xerostomia. Quetiapine carries a black box warning that it may cause increased mortality in elderly patients with dementia-related psychosis and that it may increase the risk of suicidal thinking in younger patients. This drug is pregnancy category C.

Ziprasidone (Geodon): Approved in 2001, ziprasidone is available in PO or IM formulations to treat schizophrenia and acute mania associated with bipolar disorder. The IM formulation is used to treat acute episodes of agitation or psychosis because it can reduce major symptoms in 15 minutes. Ziprasidone may be used off-label to treat Tourette's syndrome. Ziprasidone causes fewer EPS than most other antipsychotics but has the possibility of prolonging the QT interval and thereby causing potentially fatal dysrhythmias; it should not be administered concurrently with other medications that increase the QT interval. It must also be used cautiously in patients with seizure history, Alzheimer's disease, cardiovascular or hepatic disease, or who are being treated with antihypertensives. Additive CNS depression will occur if used concurrently with antianxiety drugs, sedative–hypnotics, alcohol, or opiate preparations. Ziprasidone causes less weight gain than other atypical antipsychotics and does not cause agranulocytosis. This drug is pregnancy category C.

CONNECTION Checkpoint 20.2

When atypical antipsychotic drugs are used to treat bipolar disorder, they are usually combined with drugs from other classes. From what you learned in Chapter 19, what two drugs are usually combined with the atypical antipsychotics? *See Answer to Connection Checkpoint 20.2 on student resource website.*

20.9 Dopamine system stabilizers are a newer class of atypical antipsychotics.

Dopamine system stabilizers (DSSs) are so named because they exhibit both antagonist and partial agonist activities on dopamine receptors. The balance between these two activities appears to account for the decrease in observed adverse effects, relative to other antipsychotics. Aripiprazole (Abilify) is the only approved drug in this class at the current time. It is hoped that this new class will have the same efficacy as other antipsychotic classes, with fewer serious adverse effects.

PROTOTYPE DRUG | **Aripiprazole (Abilify)**

Classification: **Therapeutic:** Atypical antipsychotic
Pharmacologic: Dopamine system stabilizer (DSS)

Therapeutic Effects and Uses: First approved in 2002, aripiprazole controls both the positive and negative symptoms of schizophrenia and improves cognition with only minimal risk of EPS. Aripiprazole is generally classified with the atypical antipsychotics because of its ability to control both negative and positive symptoms. Abilify DISCMELT is administered as oral disintegrating tablets. In 2013 an extended release form of the drug (Abilify Maintena) was approved that permits once-monthly injections.

Aripiprazole appears to have the same level of effectiveness as other atypical antipsychotics but with a lower incidence of adverse effects. An advantage over other atypical drugs is that there is little or no weight gain, hypotension, dysrhythmias, anticholinergic effects, or prolactin release with aripiprazole. It does not appear to lower the seizure threshold.

Since its initial approval, a number of other indications have been added. An IM formulation was approved in 2006 for the treatment of schizophrenia and for manic or mixed episodes associated with bipolar disorder. In 2007, the drug received approval as an add-on for major depressive disorder in patients whose symptoms were not relieved by antidepressants alone. In 2009, aripiprazole was approved to treat irritability associated with autism spectrum disorder in children. The drug is approved for pediatric patients age 13 to 17 for schizophrenia, age 10 to 17 for bipolar disorder, and age 6 to 17 for autism.

Mechanism of Action: Aripiprazole is thought to act through a combination of partial agonist activity at dopamine type 2 (D_2 and D_3) and serotonin type 2 ($5\text{-}HT_{1A}$) receptors and antagonist activity at $5\text{-}HT_{2A}$ receptors.

Pharmacokinetics:

Route(s)	PO, IM
Absorption	Well absorbed PO and IM
Distribution	Widely distributed; unknown if crosses the placenta or is secreted in breast milk
Primary metabolism	Hepatic; metabolized to active metabolite
Primary excretion	Feces, some in urine
Onset of action	Peak effect: 3–5 h (PO); 1–3 h (IM)
Duration of action	Half-life: 75–146 h

Adverse Effects: Frequently reported adverse effects include drowsiness, insomnia, agitation, hyper- or hypotension, lightheadedness, anxiety, headache, restlessness, EPS, akathisia, nausea, vomiting, or constipation. Life-threatening adverse effects include seizures, NMS, and tachycardia. **Black Box Warning**: This drug is not indicated for the treatment of dementia-related psychosis. Older adults with dementia-related psychosis treated with atypical antipsychotics are at increased risk of death compared to placebo. Antidepressants increase the risk of suicidal thinking and behavior in children, adolescents, and young adults. Patients of all ages should be monitored and observed closely during therapy for clinical worsening, suicidality, or unusual changes in behavior.

Contraindications/Precautions: Lactation, seizure disorders, or hypersensitivity are contraindications to the use of aripiprazole. Precautions must be taken when administering aripiprazole to persons with cardiovascular or cerebrovascular disease or any condition that predisposes them to hypotension.

CONNECTIONS   Evidence-Based Practice

◀ Weight Gain in Children and Adolescents Prescribed Atypical Antipsychotics

Clinical Question

What is the effect of atypical (second-generation) antipsychotics on weight gain and other cardiometabolic parameters in children and adolescents prescribed these drugs?

Evidence

Previous research has indicated that children and adolescents prescribed antipsychotic medication may be more prone to weight gain, obesity, hypertension, and diabetes than children who are not on these drugs. In the clinical study SATIETY (Second-generation Antipsychotic Treatment Indications, Effectiveness, and Tolerability in Youth), Correll et al. (2009) investigated the effects of four atypical antipsychotics on the cardiometabolic parameters of weight, glucose, and lipid profiles in children and adolescents age 4 to 19. Children and adolescents who had not been treated previously with any antipsychotic drug, or had not had over 1 week total lifetime treatment, were included in the study. Measurements of weight, body mass index (BMI), fat mass, waist circumference, fasting glucose and insulin levels, and cholesterol and lipid profiles were measured over a 12-week period. The drugs used in the study were olanzapine (Zyprexa), quetiapine (Seroquel), risperidone (Risperdal), and aripiprazole (Abilify). At the end of 12 weeks, a statistically significant difference in weight and lipid profiles was noted. Weight increased by 4.4 to 8.5 kg (9.68 to 18.7 lb) and total cholesterol increased by 9.7 to 15.6 mg/dL on average with significant changes in lipid profiles as well. There was no difference in these changes related to age; all groups experienced significant changes. The changes in lipid profiles were also found to be greater than changes in glucose,

and diabetes or metabolic syndrome was rarely noted during the period of the study. In a systematic review of research, Pringsheim, Panagiotopoulos, Davidson, and Ho (2011) found a greater risk for weight gain, increased BMI, and abnormal lipid panels with olanzapine, clozapine, and quetiapine.

Implications

With the rise in childhood obesity rates and the increase in associated adverse effects such as diabetes, metabolic syndrome, hypertension, and lipid-associated cardiovascular risk, any drug that increases the risk of adverse effects on these parameters must be carefully considered when weighing treatment options. Atypical antipsychotic drugs provide benefit to patients diagnosed with psychiatric illness and may be a required component of treatment for children and adolescents who have debilitating illnesses. Research suggests that the atypical antipsychotics may increase the risk of cardiometabolic effects and the nurse plays a pivotal role in patient and family education about these risks and strategies to minimize these effects. Frequent monitoring of metabolic panels, weight, BMI, and blood pressure is critical to early treatment of any adverse effects and may lead to a reevaluation of lower-risk drugs when possible (Ronsley, Rayter, Smith, Davidson, & Panagiotopoulos, 2012).

Critical Thinking Questions

What education can the nurse provide the child or adolescent and his or her family to decrease the risk of developing adverse cardiometabolic effects when an atypical antipsychotic drug has been prescribed?

See Answers to Critical Thinking Questions on student resource website.

Drug Interactions: Aripiprazole is a substrate for several hepatic CYP enzymes and induces others; thus it may interact with drugs that undergo hepatic metabolism. For example, many of the SSRIs inhibit CYP2D6, which can cause reduced metabolism of aripiprazole, raised serum levels, and possible toxicity. Concurrent use of other antipsychotics or lithium may increase the incidence of EPS. Alcohol and other CNS depressants will cause increased CNS depression. Decreased excretion of aripiprazole may occur with the use of drugs such as fluoxetine or paroxetine. **Herbal/Food:** Grapefruit juice may increase the serum levels of aripiprazole and cause toxicity.

Pregnancy: Category C.

Treatment of Overdose: Overdose can cause vomiting, tremor, and drowsiness, but fatalities have not been reported. There is no specific treatment for overdose.

Nursing Responsibilities: Key nursing implications for patients receiving aripiprazole are included in the Nursing Practice Application for Patients Receiving Pharmacotherapy with Antipsychotics.

Drugs Similar to Aripiprazole (Abilify)

There are no other dopamine system stabilizers.

CONNECTIONS: NURSING PRACTICE APPLICATION

Patients Receiving Pharmacotherapy with Antipsychotics

Assessment	Potential Nursing Diagnoses*
Baseline assessment prior to administration: • Obtain a complete health history including hepatic, renal, urologic, cardiovascular, respiratory, or neurologic disease (especially Parkinson's disease or seizures), current mental status, pregnancy, or breast-feeding. Obtain a drug history including allergies, current prescription and OTC drugs, alcohol use, smoking, and herbal preparations. Be alert to possible drug interactions. • Obtain a history of depression or mental disorders, including a family history of same and severity. • Assess for disturbances in thought processes, perception, verbal communication, affect, behavior, interpersonal relationships, and self-care. Use objective screening tools of the health care agency. • Obtain baseline vital signs and weight. • Evaluate appropriate laboratory findings (e.g., CBC, electrolytes, glucose, hepatic and renal function studies, drug screening). • Assess the patient's ability to receive and understand instructions. Include family and caregivers as needed.	• Disturbed Personal Identity • Anxiety • Impaired Verbal Communication • Impaired Social Interaction • Ineffective Health Maintenance • Impaired Home Maintenance • Noncompliance • Deficient Knowledge (Drug Therapy) • Caregiver Role Strain • Risk for Self-Directed Violence • Risk for Other-Directed Violence • Risk for Self-Mutilation
Assessment throughout administration: • Assess for desired therapeutic effects (e.g., normalizing thought processes, lessening delusions, lessening hallucinations, improvement in positive or negative symptoms, ability to return to normal ADLs, appetite and sleep patterns; if used for other conditions, e.g., severe hiccups, assess for appropriate therapeutic effects). • Continue periodic monitoring of CBC, electrolytes, glucose, hepatic and renal function studies, lipid levels, therapeutic drug levels. • Assess vital signs, especially orthostatic blood pressure, and weigh periodically. • Assess for and promptly report adverse effects: dizziness or lightheadedness, confusion, agitation, suicidal ideations, hypotension, tachycardia, increase in temperature, blurred or double vision, skin rashes, bruising or bleeding, abdominal pain, jaundice, change in color of stool, flank pain, or hematuria. • Assess for and promptly report EPS symptoms including parkinsonism, acute dystonia, akathisia, and TD. • Immediately report signs and symptoms of NMS: unstable blood pressure, elevated temperature, diaphoresis, dyspnea, or muscle rigidity.	

Implementation

Interventions and (Rationales)	Patient-Centered Care
Ensuring therapeutic effects: • Continue assessments as above for therapeutic effects. (Drugs used for psychoses and schizophrenia do not cure the underlying disorder but improve positive and negative symptoms of the disorder. Gradual improvement over several weeks to months should be noted.)	• Teach the patient, family, or caregivers that full effects may not occur immediately, but that some improvement should be noticeable after beginning therapy. • Supportive, inpatient care may be required during the acute, early period of therapy.

(continued)

• Monitor patient adherence to the drug regimen. (Presence of severe mental disorders may result in nonadherence with medications. Regular, consistent dosing is essential to correcting the underlying disorder. Because the drugs do not cure the underlying disorder, if regular administration is disrupted, symptoms may return abruptly. Alternative drug forms such as PO disintegrating tablets or IM depot injections may need to be considered if chronic nonadherence continues.)	• Involve the family or caregiver to the extent possible in ensuring that the patient remains on regular medication routines. • Ensure that the patient takes the medication as prescribed. Never leave medications at the bedside. • Question the possibility of nonadherence if original symptoms or adverse effects suddenly increase in frequency or severity.
Minimizing adverse effects: • Continue to monitor vital signs periodically, especially orthostatic blood pressure, and for tachycardia. Ensure patient safety; monitor ambulation until the effects of the drug are known. **Lifespan:** Be particularly cautious with the older adult who is at increased risk for falls. (Antipsychotic drugs may cause hypotension, increasing the risk of falls and injury.)	• Have the patient rise from lying or sitting to standing slowly to avoid dizziness or falls. If dizziness occurs, the patient should sit or lie down and not attempt to stand or walk, until the sensation passes. • Instruct the patient to call for assistance prior to getting out of bed or attempting to walk alone. For patients who are taking the medications at home or at an outpatient clinic, avoid driving or other activities requiring mental alertness or physical coordination until the effects of the drug are known.
• Continue to monitor motor activity, coordination, and balance, and for EPS symptoms. • Ensure adequate nutrition and fluid intake if TDs are present. (Severe choreoathetoid tongue movement may significantly hinder or prevent adequate nutrition.) • Ensure patient safety if parkinsonism affects gait or if akathisia is present. Acute dystonias may require treatment with other medications to halt spasms. (Bradykinesias, slow to start ambulation, and slow, shuffling gait, may predispose the patient to falls. Akathisia with pacing may significantly impair the patient's ability to rest and sleep; additional medications may be required to treat it. Anticholinergics or other drugs may be required to stop spasms.)	• Instruct the patient, family, or caregiver to immediately report EPS symptoms for additional treatment. • Encourage the patient, family, or caregiver to obtain and record a weight weekly to ensure that dietary needs are being met if TDs are present.
• Monitor for and immediately report signs and symptoms of NMS: unstable blood pressure, elevated temperature, diaphoresis, muscle rigidity. (NMS is a rare but potentially fatal syndrome that must be recognized and treated immediately.)	• Instruct the patient, family, or caregiver to immediately report any changes in level of consciousness, elevated temperature, excessive sweating, severe muscle rigidity, increased respirations, shortness of breath, or incontinence.
• **Lifespan:** Monitor cardiovascular and respiratory function more frequently, particularly in the older adult with existing disease or dementia. (An increased risk of death from cardiovascular events [e.g., heart failure, sudden cardiac death], or from respiratory infection has been noted in some patients, particularly those taking atypical antipsychotic drugs.)	• Instruct the patient, family, or caregiver to immediately report dizziness, palpitations, tachycardia, chest pain, cough, chest congestion, fever, or breathing difficulties.
• Continue to monitor CBC, electrolytes, glucose, renal and hepatic function, lipid levels, and therapeutic drug levels. (Antipsychotic drugs may cause bone marrow depression, hepatotoxicity, increased glucose levels, or hyperlipidemia as adverse effects. **Diverse Patients:** Most antipsychotic drugs are metabolized through the P450 system and may result in different effects based on differences in enzymes. Monitor ethnically diverse patients more frequently to ensure optimal therapeutic effects and minimal adverse effects, especially in early stages of drug therapy.)	• Instruct the patient on the need to return periodically for laboratory work. • Teach the patient, family, or caregiver to promptly report any abdominal pain, particularly in the upper quadrants, changes in stool color, yellowing of sclera or skin, darkened urine, skin rashes, low-grade fevers, general malaise or changes in behavior or activity level, or redness or swelling around sites of injury. • Teach the patient, family, or caregiver to promptly report excessive thirst, urination, hunger, unusual weight loss or gain, or other symptoms of diabetes. • **Diverse Patients:** Teach ethnically diverse patients to observe for appropriate effects, especially in early drug therapy, and promptly report less than optimal or adverse effects.
• Monitor for anticholinergic effects, including dry mouth, drowsiness, blurred vision, constipation, and urinary retention. Provide symptomatic treatment to ease effects. (Anticholinergic symptoms are common adverse effects of antipsychotic drugs. Tolerance to anticholinergic effects usually develops over time. **Lifespan:** Be aware that older men with enlarged prostates are at higher risk for mechanical obstruction.)	• Encourage sips of water, ice chips, hard candy, or chewing gum to ease mouth dryness. Avoid alcohol-based mouthwashes, which are drying to the mucosa and which the patient may drink. • Increase dietary fiber intake and adequate fluid intake. • Promptly report urinary frequency, hesitancy, or retention to the health care provider.
• Monitor for weight gain, gynecomastia (breast enlargement and tenderness in either sex), and changes in secondary sexual characteristics (e.g., amenorrhea, impotence). (Some antipsychotic drugs may cause weight gain and have pituitary effects. Impotence and weight gain may be significant reasons for nonadherence.)	• Teach the patient, family, or caregiver to weigh the patient daily and report a significant weight gain of 2 kg (5 lb) per week to the health care provider. • Encourage a healthy diet of increased fruits and vegetables, adequate protein intake, and increased exercise. • Address sexual concerns in a matter-of-fact manner and refer as appropriate to the health care provider.

CONNECTIONS: NURSING PRACTICE APPLICATION (continued)

- **Lifespan:** Monitor for the possibility of pregnancy in women of childbearing age. (Most antipsychotic drugs are Category C and the benefits of the use of any particular drug must be weighed against possible fetal effects.)
- Monitor adolescents under 24 and older adults for unusual symptoms or expressed thoughts of suicide. (Children and adolescents younger than 24, and the older adult, particularly with dementia, are at greater risk for suicide than other patients.)

- Encourage the patient, family, or caregiver to discuss family planning with the health care provider.
- Teach the patient, family, or caregiver to promptly report a positive pregnancy test or suspicion of pregnancy to the provider.
- Encourage the patient, family, or caregiver to keep all appointments with the health care provider and to promptly report overt symptoms of depression, suicidal ideations, or other unusual behaviors.

- Monitor for alcohol and illegal drug use. (Used concurrently, these cause an increased CNS depressant effect or an exacerbation in psychotic symptoms.)

- Instruct the patient to avoid alcohol and illegal drug use. Refer the patient to community support groups such as AA or NA as appropriate.

- Monitor caffeine use. (Use of caffeine-containing substances may negate the effects of antipsychotics.)

- Teach the patient, family, or caregiver to avoid caffeine-containing beverages, foods, and over-the-counter (OTC) medications, and to read food labels when in doubt about whether a product contains caffeine.

- Monitor for smoking. (Heavy smoking may decrease metabolism of some antipsychotics such as haloperidol, leading to decreased efficacy.)

- Instruct the patient to stop or decrease smoking. Refer the patient to smoking cessation programs, if indicated.

Patient understanding of drug therapy:
- Use opportunities during administration of medications and during assessments to discuss the rationale for drug therapy, desired therapeutic outcomes, commonly observed adverse effects, parameters for when to call the health care provider, and any necessary monitoring or precautions. Use brief explanations during times of delusions or hallucinations. (Using time during nursing care helps to optimize and reinforce key teaching areas. Brief, consistent explanations assist to interrupt delusional periods.)

- The patient, family, or caregiver should be able to state the reason for the drug, appropriate dose and scheduling, and what adverse effects to observe for and when to report them.

Patient self-administration of drug therapy:
- When administering the medication, instruct the patient or caregivers in proper self-administration of the drug, e.g., take the drug as prescribed and do not substitute brands. (Utilizing time during nurse-administration of these drugs helps to reinforce teaching.)

- Teach the patient, family, or caregiver to take the medication:
  - Exactly as ordered and the same manufacturer's brand each time the prescription is filled. (Switching brands may result in differing pharmacokinetics and alterations in therapeutic effect.)
- Ensure that all medication is taken exactly when as ordered. Use of a calendar to track doses may be helpful.
- Unless otherwise directed, mix liquid drug solutions with water, milk, or non-grapefruit juices. Do not mix with cola, tea, or caffeine-containing beverages.
- Administer IM injections by deep gluteal injection using enclosed diluent and safety needle if provided by the manufacturer. Check the enclosed directions about refrigerating dosages.
- If medication causes drowsiness, take at bedtime. Tolerance to anticholinergic effects such as drowsiness usually develops over time.
- Do not abruptly discontinue the medication.

*Nursing Diagnoses—Definitions and Classification 2015-2017. Copyright © 2014, 1994–2014 by NANDA International. Used by arrangement with John Wiley & Sons Limited.

Understanding the Chapter

Key Concepts Summary

20.1 Psychoses are severe mental disorders characterized by the inability to recognize reality.

20.2 Schizophrenia, the most common psychosis, has both positive and negative symptoms.

20.3 The precise etiology of schizophrenia remains unknown.

20.4 Medical management of psychosis is challenging because patients often lack insight into their disease and believe their behavior is normal.

20.5 Selection of an antipsychotic drug depends on its spectrum of adverse effects and the experience of the health care provider.

20.6 The phenothiazines are effective at treating schizophrenia symptoms but exhibit a high incidence of adverse effects.

20.7 The nonphenothiazine first-generation antipsychotics have the same therapeutic applications and similar adverse effects as the phenothiazines.

20.8 Second-generation antipsychotics have become drugs of choice for the treatment of schizophrenia.

20.9 Dopamine system stabilizers are a newer class of atypical antipsychotics.

Case Study: Making the Patient Connection

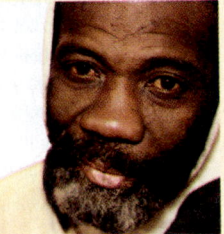

Remember the patient "George Watkins" at the beginning of the chapter? Now read the remainder of the case study. Based on the information presented within this chapter, respond to the critical thinking questions that follow.

George Watkins is a 47-year-old African American male who was admitted to the psychiatric unit this morning. He was diagnosed with schizophrenia at age 20. He is disheveled looking, with long, dirty, stringy hair. His clothes are mismatched and dirty. Although it is summer, he is wearing an overcoat and a winter hat pulled down over his ears. This is George's fourth hospitalization for out-of-control schizophrenia. The last severe episode occurred 4 years ago.

Sheri Watkins, George's wife, states that he quit his job as an assembly line supervisor about 2 weeks ago. He has also quit coaching softball and soccer games. Sheri and George have been married since they were both 18. Their marriage is basically strong but has had its difficult times, especially when George's schizophrenia is active. About 3 to 4 weeks before each hospitalization for psychosis, he stopped taking his antipsychotic medication. He has taken different antipsychotic medications over the course of his schizophrenia, but none has proved to be successful over a long period.

George and Sheri have two children: Toby, who is 14, and Felecia, who is 10. Both children do well in school, have many friends, and are active in

several organizations and sports. As the children get older, they realize that "something is not quite right" with their father. They have never been told of their father's mental illness. The children worry that they will catch whatever it is that causes their father's erratic behavior. George's parents and four siblings live in the same town. George, his father, and his two brothers worked at the same manufacturing plant. His other two siblings are teachers in the local school system, as is Sheri.

Mr. and Mrs. Watkins, George's parents, tell you that their son had a "normal" childhood. He was active in sports, starred on the high school football team, was an honor student, was a Boy Scout, and had many friends. They have always enjoyed many social occasions with their large extended family. George is always welcome at family gatherings, but relatives tend to avoid him when his behavior becomes bizarre. They all know he has schizophrenia but do not fully understand the implications of the diagnosis.

Critical Thinking Questions

1. What are the most likely reasons George gives for discontinuing his medication?

2. What clues do his family and friends have that would indicate that his schizophrenia may be getting out of control?

3. What can be done to prevent George's schizophrenia from getting out of control in the future?

See Answers to Critical Thinking Questions on student resource website.

Additional Case Study

Suzette Anderson is a 19-year-old patient who has been admitted to the psychiatric unit with newly diagnosed schizophrenia. She is agitated and paces back and forth in the day room until she is called for dinner. She is heard muttering to herself, "I don't know why they put me here. They just don't want me to get my inheritance. Maybe it's because they know I'll leave them all when I get the money. I'll be real rich and can start a new life for myself." She demonstrates no overt threatening behavior toward any of the other patients or toward the staff. Her agitation escalates until she cannot calm herself down and will not listen to staff. She begins hitting her fist into the wall and shouting. There is an order for haloperidol (Haldol), 4 mg IM every 1 to 4 hours prn for agitation.

1. What is the main use of haloperidol (Haldol) in this situation?

2. As the nurse caring for Suzette, what adverse effects would you monitor for?

3. How long would you expect Suzette to remain hospitalized? Why?

See Answers to Additional Case Study on student resource website.

Chapter Review

1 The patient states that he has not taken his antipsychotic drug for the past 2 weeks because it was causing sexual dysfunction. The nurse is aware that the name *antipsychotic* indicates that continuing the medication as prescribed is important because:

1. Hypertensive crisis may occur with abrupt withdrawal.
2. Muscle twitching may occur with abrupt withdrawal.
3. Parkinson-like symptoms will occur with withdrawal.
4. Symptoms of psychosis are likely to return if the medication is withdrawn.

2 Prior to discharge, the nurse provides teaching related to adverse effects of phenothiazines to the patient and caregivers. Which of the following should be included?

1. The patient may experience social withdrawal and slowed activity.
2. Severe muscle spasms may occur early in therapy.
3. Tardive dyskinesia is likely early in therapy.
4. Medications should be taken as prescribed to prevent adverse effects.

3 The nurse expects that the patient experiencing extrapyramidal symptoms during therapy with phenothiazines will be prescribed:

1. Benztropine (Cogentin).
2. Diazepam (Valium).
3. Haloperidol (Haldol).
4. Lorazepam (Ativan).

4 Nursing implications of the administration of haloperidol (Haldol) to a patient exhibiting psychotic behavior include which of the following? Select all that apply.

1. Take 1 hour before or 2 hours after antacids.
2. The incidence of extrapyramidal symptoms is high.
3. It is therapeutic if ordered on an as-needed basis.
4. Haldol is contraindicated in Parkinson's disease, seizure disorders, alcoholism, and severe mental depression.
5. Crush the sustained release form for easier swallowing.

5 Which statement made by the patient who is taking risperidone (Risperdal) indicates that further teaching is necessary?

1. "I'll monitor my weight every month."
2. "I can increase my intake of fluids and fiber if I have any gastrointestinal problems."
3. "I'll have my blood pressure monitored regularly."
4. "There is no problem if I want to drink alcohol on the weekends."

6 The development of which symptom(s) in a patient taking an antipsychotic must be reported immediately?

1. Fever, tachycardia, stupor, and incontinence
2. Suddenly occurring muscle spasms, especially in the neck and back
3. Sexual dysfunction
4. Leg pains, pacing, an inability to sit still

See Answers to Chapter Review in Appendix A.

References

Correll, C. U., Manu, P., Olshanskiy, V., Napolitano, B., Kane, J. M., & Malhotra, A. K. (2009). Cardiometabolic risk of second-generation antipsychotic medications during first-time use in children and adolescents. *Journal of the American Medical Association, 302,* 1765–1773. doi:10.1001/jama.2009.1549

Loth, A. K. (2012). *Childhood-onset schizophrenia.* Retrieved from http://emedicine.medscape.com/article/914840-overview

National Institutes of Health. (n.d.). *The numbers count: Mental health disorders in America.* Retrieved from http://www.nimh.nih.gov/health/publications/the-numbers-count-mental-disorders-in-america/index.shtml

Pringsheim, T., Panagiotopoulos, C., Davidson, J., & Ho, J. (2011). Evidence-based recommendations for monitoring safety of second generation antipsychotics in children and youth. *Journal of the Canadian Academy of Child and Adolescent Psychiatry, 20*(3), 218–233.

Ronsley, R., Rayter, M., Smith, D., Davidson, J., & Panagiotopoulos, C. (2012). Metabolic monitoring training program implementation in the community setting was associated with improved monitoring in second-generation antipsychotic-treated children. *Canadian Journal of Psychiatry, 57*(5), 292–299.

World Fellowship for Schizophrenia and Allied Disorders. (n.d.). *Schizophrenia.* Retrieved from http://www.world-schizophrenia.org/disorders/schizophrenia.html

Selected Bibliography

Ardizzone, I., Nardecchia, F., Marconi, A., Ferrara, M., & Carratelli, T. I. (2010). Antipsychotic medication in adolescents suffering from schizophrenia: A meta-analysis of randomized controlled trials. *Psychopharmacology Bulletin, 43*(2), 45–66.

Chen, J., Gao, K., & Kemp, D. E. (2011). Second-generation antipsychotics in major depressive disorder: Update and clinical perspective. *Current Opinion in Psychiatry, 24,* 10–17. doi:10.1097/YCO.0b013e3283413505

Feetham, C. L., & Roberts, H. (2010). Medicine-taking behaviour in schizophrenia—part 1. *Progress in Neurology and Psychiatry, 14*(4), 15–18. doi:10.1002/pnp.167

Feetham, C. L., & Roberts, H. (2010). Medicine-taking behaviour in schizophrenia—part 2. *Progress in Neurology and Psychiatry, 14*(5), 9–14. doi:10.1002/pnp.172

Herdman, T. H., & Kamitsuru, S. (Eds.). (2014). *NANDA International nursing diagnoses: Definitions and classification, 2015–2017.* Oxford, United Kingdom: Wiley-Blackwell.

Kowalski, J. M. (2012). *Medication-induced dystonic reactions.* Retrieved from http://emedicine.medscape.com/article/814632-overview

Leucht, S., Cipriani, A., Spineli, L., Mavridis, D., Örey, D., Richter, F., . . . Davis, J. M. (2013). Comparative efficacy and tolerability of 15 antipsychotic drugs in schizophrenia: A multiple-treatments meta-analysis. *The Lancet, 382,* 951–962. doi.org/10.1016/S0140-6736(13)60733-3

Mattal, A. K., Hill, J. L., & Lenroot, R. K. (2010). Treatment of early onset schizophrenia. *Current Opinion in Psychiatry, 23,* 304–310. doi:10.1097/YCO.0b013e32833b027e

Meyer, J. M. (2011). Pharmacotherapy of psychosis and mania. In L. L. Brunton, B. A. Chabner, & B. C. Knollman (Eds.), *The pharmacological basis of therapeutics* (11th ed., pp. 417–457). New York, NY: McGraw-Hill.

Yoshida, T., Iyo, M., & Hashimoto, K. (2012). Recent advances in potential therapeutic drugs for cognitive impairment in schizophrenia. *Current Psychiatry Reviews, 8,* 140–150. doi.org/10.2174/1573400511208020140

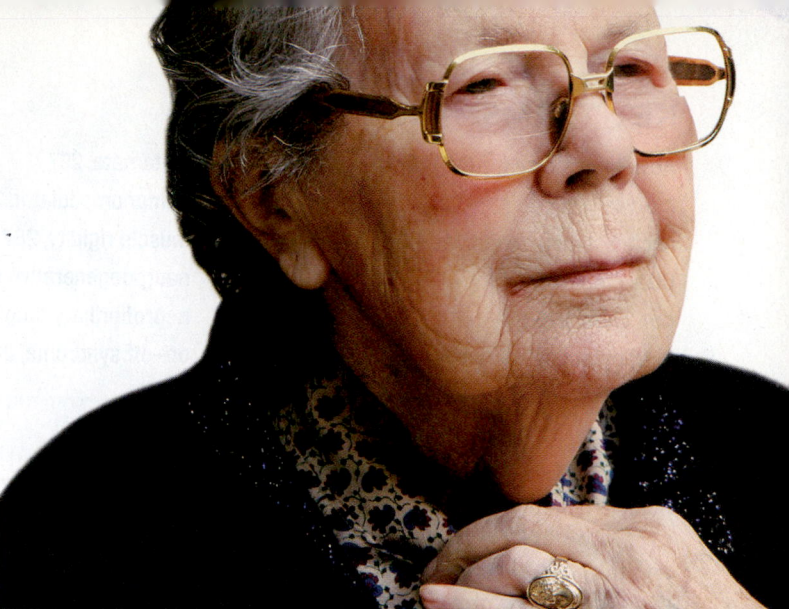

"I just don't understand what's happening. I drove to my hairdresser—it's only three blocks—but forgot I had driven there, and walked home. I walked around and around, until I finally saw our house. Then I couldn't get in because my key wouldn't work, so I paced around the yard until Robert got home. Why did he change the lock on the front door?"

Patient "Mary Lee"

CHAPTER 21

Pharmacotherapy of Degenerative Diseases of the Central Nervous System

LEARNING OUTCOMES

After reading this chapter, the student should be able to:

1. Identify the most common degenerative diseases of the central nervous system.
2. Distinguish between idiopathic Parkinson's disease and secondary Parkinson's disease.
3. Describe symptoms of Parkinson's disease.
4. Explain the neurochemical basis for Parkinson's disease, focusing on the roles of dopamine and acetylcholine in the brain.
5. Describe symptoms of Alzheimer's disease and explain theories about why these symptoms develop.
6. Describe the nurse's role in the pharmacologic management of Parkinson's disease and Alzheimer's disease.
7. Discuss the pharmacologic goals for the management of Parkinson's disease, Alzheimer's disease, and other neurodegenerative disorders.
8. For each of the classes shown in the chapter outline, identify the prototype and representative drugs and explain the mechanism(s) of drug action, primary indications, contraindications, significant drug interactions, pregnancy category, and important adverse effects.
9. Apply the nursing process to care for patients receiving pharmacotherapy for degenerative diseases of the central nervous system.

CHAPTER OUTLINE

▸ Degenerative Diseases of the Central Nervous System

▸ Parkinson's Disease

   Etiology and Pathogenesis of Parkinson's Disease

▸ Pharmacotherapy of Parkinson's Disease

   Dopamine Replacement Therapy

   PROTOTYPE Levodopa and Carbidopa (Sinemet, Parcopa), *p. 289*

   Dopamine Agonists

   PROTOTYPE Pramipexole (Mirapex), *p. 291*

   Miscellaneous Dopaminergic Drugs

   Anticholinergic Drugs

   PROTOTYPE Benztropine (Cogentin), *p. 294*

▸ Alzheimer's Disease

▸ Pharmacotherapy of Alzheimer's Disease

   Cholinesterase Inhibitors

   Reversible Cholinesterase Inhibitors

   NMDA Receptor Antagonist

   PROTOTYPE Donepezil (Aricept), *p. 298*

▸ Multiple Sclerosis

   PROTOTYPE Interferon beta-1b (Betaseron, Extavia, Plegridy), *p. 301*

▸ Amyotrophic Lateral Sclerosis

Alzheimer's disease (AD), 295

bradykinesia, 287

cholinesterase inhibitors, 296

COMT inhibitors, 293

dementia, 295

extrapyramidal symptoms (EPS), 288

glutamate, 297

immunomodulator, 301

muscle rigidity, 287

neurodegenerative diseases, 286

neurofibrillary tangles, 295

on—off syndrome, 288

Parkinson's disease (PD), 286

pill rolling, 287

striatum, 287

substantia nigra, 287

wearing-off effect, 288

Degenerative diseases of the central nervous system (CNS) are difficult to treat pharmacologically. In nearly all cases, medications are unable to cure or reverse the progressive nature of these disorders, and the symptomatic relief provided by the drugs is only temporary. The focus of this chapter is on four debilitating and progressive conditions categorized as degenerative diseases of the CNS: Parkinson's disease, Alzheimer's disease, multiple sclerosis, and amyotrophic lateral sclerosis.

Degenerative Diseases of the Central Nervous System

21.1 Degenerative diseases of the central nervous system are characterized by irreversible and progressive loss of neuronal function.

Degenerative diseases of the CNS (**neurodegenerative diseases**) include a diverse set of disorders that differ in their causes and outcomes. Each involves a progressive and irreversible loss of neuron function in the brain or spinal cord, or both. Neuron loss is sometimes isolated to specific regions of the CNS, and symptoms will vary by the region(s) most affected by the disorder.

Alzheimer's disease and Parkinson's disease are neurodegenerative disorders that present major health care challenges for older adults as well as for the health care industry, which must provide services for the vast numbers of patients with these disorders. Although less common, Huntington's disease, multiple sclerosis, and amyotrophic lateral sclerosis are equally devastating to patients and their families. These disorders are described in Table 21.1.

The etiology of most neurodegenerative diseases is unknown, although the loss of neurons appears to have both genetic and environmental components. Huntington's disease is clearly the result of an autosomal dominant genetic defect. Alzheimer's disease and Parkinson's disease also tend to occur more commonly within families but this does not account for the majority of cases. It is likely that exposure of neurons to various toxins, genetic predisposition, and normal aging processes all have important roles in the etiology of these disorders.

Most neurodegenerative diseases of the CNS progress from subtle signs and symptoms early in the course of the disease to profound neurologic and cognitive deficits. Because of this, neurodegenerative disorders are quite difficult to diagnose in their early stages. With some of them, diagnosis is made only after other neurologic, infectious, cardiovascular, or traumatic etiologies have been ruled out.

With the exception of Parkinson's disease, pharmacotherapy provides only minimal benefit to patients with neurodegenerative disease. Currently, medications are unable to cure or significantly alter the clinical course of any of the degenerative diseases of the CNS.

PharmFACT

About 1 million Americans have Parkinson's disease. Approximately 60,000 new cases are diagnosed each year (National Parkinson Foundation, n.d.).

Parkinson's Disease

21.2 Parkinson's disease is a progressive neurodegenerative disorder characterized by abnormal motor movement.

Named after British physician James Parkinson who identified the condition in 1817, **Parkinson's disease (PD)** is the second most common degenerative disease of the nervous system and the third

TABLE 21.1 Major Degenerative Diseases of the Central Nervous System

Disease	Description
Alzheimer's disease	A chronic, progressive disease that profoundly diminishes memory, reasoning ability, and thinking skills and leaves the patient totally dependent on others for all aspects of care; usually affects persons over age 60.
Amyotrophic lateral sclerosis (Lou Gehrig's disease)	A degenerative disease of the motor neurons characterized by weakness and atrophy of the muscles of the hands, forearms, and legs, spreading to involve most of the body and face; symptoms usually begin during the middle years, with death occurring within 2–5 years.
Huntington's disease (formerly called Huntington's chorea)	A rare hereditary condition characterized by progressive chorea and mental deterioration resulting in dementia; symptoms usually begin in the 30s–50s with death occurring within 15 years.
Multiple sclerosis	A chronic debilitating autoimmune disease characterized by fatigue, muscle weakness, difficulty with balance and walking, and vision, hearing, and speech abnormalities; symptomatic periods alternate with remissions; symptoms vary depending upon which portion of the nervous system is experiencing inflammation.
Parkinson's disease	A debilitating disease characterized by resting tremor, muscle rigidity, hypokinesia, masklike faces, and a slow, shuffling gait. Symptoms usually appear in the 60s.

most common neurologic disorder of older adults. The usual age of onset is 40 to 70, with a peak between 58 and 62 years of age; however, even teenagers can develop the disorder. Men are affected 1.5 times more often than women. The disease is progressive, with the expression of full symptoms developing over many years.

The two etiologies of PD are called idiopathic and secondary. Idiopathic PD, the most common type, has no known cause and is characterized by a progressive destruction of neurons in specific regions of the brain. Some patients with idiopathic parkinsonism have a family history of the disorder, and a genetic link is highly probable.

Secondary Parkinsonism is caused by medical conditions such as head trauma, brain infections, brain tumors, and exposure to neurotoxins. The most frequent cause of secondary Parkinsonism is treatment with antipsychotic drugs (see Chapter 20). Once a patient on antipsychotic therapy shows signs of parkinsonism, the drug is normally discontinued. Symptoms of drug-induced PD are usually reversible but may become permanent if pharmacotherapy is prolonged.

PD begins with subtle symptoms. The patient reports feeling tired and seems to move more slowly, often demonstrating a slight tremor along with fatigue. There are no definitive tests for PD; diagnosis is based on clinical findings after the presence of other neurologic diseases has been ruled out. Once the disease progresses, the symptoms of PD are quite characteristic and can be easily recognized. The four cardinal signs of PD, or parkinsonism, are summarized as follows:

- **Tremor.** The hands and head develop a palsy-like, continuous motion or shaking when at rest. The tremors may be so pronounced that the person cannot hold a glass or eating utensils and successfully bring them to his or her mouth. **Pill rolling** is a common behavior in progressive states, in which patients rub the thumb and forefinger together in a circular motion, resembling the motion of rolling a tablet between two fingers.

- **Muscle rigidity.** Resistance to passive movements of the arms and legs develops. The **muscle rigidity** or stiffness may resemble symptoms of arthritis. Patients often have difficulty bending over and moving limbs. Changes in facial expression, or a lack of facial expression, are due to rigidity of the facial muscles. This rigidity can lead to chewing and swallowing difficulties if the pharyngeal muscles are involved. Uncontrollable drooling may also be evident. A noticeable symptom of PD is a lack of arm swinging while walking; the patient walks with the arms close to the side. Muscle rigidity is present early in the disease process. Although the symptoms may be less noticeable at first, they progress and become obvious in later years.

- **Bradykinesia.** An involuntary slowness of voluntary movement and speech, **bradykinesia** is one of the most noticeable of all symptoms and is marked by difficulty chewing, swallowing, or speaking. Patients with PD have difficulties initiating movement and controlling fine muscle movements. Patients shuffle their feet without taking normal strides, making walking difficult.

- **Postural instability.** Patients may be stooped over and easily lose their balance. Stumbling results in frequent falls with associated injuries.

Although PD is a progressive neurologic disorder primarily affecting muscle movement, other health problems often develop in these patients, including anxiety, sleep disturbances, dementia, and disturbances of the autonomic nervous system such as difficulty urinating and sexual dysfunction. Over half of these patients present with clinical depression. Many develop thought disturbances, and dementia may occur, especially in those over age 70. These associated health problems often require pharmacologic intervention, which increases the possibility of drug interactions and adverse effects in these patients.

21.3 Parkinson's disease is caused by a lack of sufficient amounts of dopamine produced by the substantia nigra.

Although the precise etiology of PD is incompletely understood, much is known about the effects of the disease on the CNS. Neurotransmitter deficiencies in specific regions of the brain are closely associated with the disease.

Involuntary muscle movements are controlled by the basal nuclei (also called basal ganglia), which are clusters of interconnected neurons in several distinct regions of the brain. The basal nuclei are responsible for regulating the flow of information from the cerebral cortex to the motor neurons in the spinal cord. This region helps to synchronize stopping and starting activity such as that which occurs during walking. Two portions of the basal nuclei that are important to the pathogenesis of PD are the substantia nigra and the striatum. The student should review the functions of the basal nuclei and associated structures in Chapter 17.

The **substantia nigra**, a dark band of gray matter in the midbrain, is a primary producer of the neurotransmitter dopamine. The dopamine travels through axons along the nigrostriatal pathway to the **striatum** (also called corpus striatum), where the neurotransmitter is released. In the striatum, dopamine encounters its receptors and produces multiple actions. One function that is important to the pathogenesis of PD is the planning and modulation of motor pathways responsible for unconscious muscle movement. Dopamine serves an inhibitory function, slowing the flow of impulses down spinal neurons.

When dopamine is present, the normal flow of motor impulses from the striatum helps to produce coordinated, unconscious muscle movement. Should levels of dopamine fall because of the loss of dopamine-producing neurons in the substantia nigra, symptoms of parkinsonism may develop. Remarkably, the body can function normally even when as many as 50% of the neurons stop producing dopamine. When 60% to 80% lose their function, however, symptoms of parkinsonism are observed.

A second neurotransmitter modulates the effects of neuronal outflow from the striatum. Acetylcholine (Ach) serves an excitatory function. Under normal conditions, the inhibitory effects of dopamine and the excitatory effects of Ach balance one another to produce smooth, coordinated muscle movement. If dopamine levels decline, Ach has a more dramatic stimulatory effect in this area and the abnormal muscular movements characteristic of PD are observed.

CONNECTION Checkpoint 21.1

Dopamine belongs to a class of natural hormones called catecholamines. From what you learned in Chapter 12, what are the other two major catecholamines found in the nervous system? *See Answer to Connection Checkpoint 21.1 on student resource website.*

Pharmacotherapy of Parkinson's Disease

21.4 The drugs used for Parkinson's disease help to alleviate symptoms but do not cure the disease.

Antiparkinson medications are given to restore the balance between dopamine and Ach in specific regions of the brain. The balance between the two neurotransmitters, dopamine and Ach, offers several means by which drug therapy may be used to manage the symptoms of PD.

- **Dopamine agonists.** These drugs increase the levels of dopamine in the striatum. This may be accomplished by directly replacing dopamine, decreasing the breakdown of dopamine, increasing the release of dopamine from neurons, or activating dopamine receptors.

- **Anticholinergic drugs.** These agents block the excitatory actions of Ach in the striatum.

The goal of pharmacotherapy for PD is to increase the ability of the patient to perform normal activities of daily living (ADLs) such as eating, walking, dressing, and bathing, and decrease the chances of falls that could cause serious injury. Pharmacotherapy is an essential part of the management of PD; drugs decrease symptoms and allow the patient to provide at least some self-care, have some degree of self-worth, and improve his or her quality of life. Although pharmacotherapy does not cure this disorder, symptoms are dramatically reduced in many patients.

Patients receiving prolonged antiparkinson pharmacotherapy may periodically experience a loss of drug effect. This **wearing-off effect** appears gradually near the end of a dosing interval. Symptoms worsen at this time because the concentration of the drug has fallen below the therapeutic level. Adjusting the dosing interval to provide for more frequent dosing may help to reduce this effect.

Another type of loss of drug effect occurs abruptly. The **on–off syndrome** occurs when the patient alternates between symptom-free periods (on) and times when the drugs stop working and symptoms abruptly reappear (off). The on–off time intervals range from just a few minutes to several hours. Off periods may occur even when the serum level of the drug is high. The on–off syndrome is difficult to control. Scheduling doses closer together or using a second, adjunct medication during the off period are strategies used to reduce the on–off syndrome.

Symptoms of parkinsonism are major adverse effects of several classes of antipsychotic drugs. These dyskinesias are referred to as **extrapyramidal symptoms (EPS)**. The term *extrapyramidal* refers to locations in the CNS that contain neurons associated with postural and automatic movements. Recall from Chapter 20 that antipsychotic drugs act through a blockade of dopamine receptors. Thus EPS develop for the same neurochemical reasons as PD: deficiency of dopamine in the striatum. Antiparkinson drugs may be used to treat these symptoms.

If drug therapy becomes ineffective, alternative treatments can be tried. Again, these treatments may help control symptoms, but they will not cure or prevent the disease from progressing. There are four accepted nonmedication treatments for PD: deep brain stimulation (DBS), fetal tissue transplantation, pallidotomy, and thalamotomy. Table 21.2 describes each of these nonpharmacologic therapies.

21.5 Replacement therapy with levodopa is the most effective therapy for treating Parkinson's disease.

Drug therapy for PD attempts to restore the functional balance of dopamine and Ach in the striatum of the brain. Dopamine replacement agents are used to directly increase dopamine levels in this region. Dopamine itself cannot be used for this purpose because it is unable to cross the blood–brain barrier after it is administered. Doses for these drugs are listed in Table 21.3.

Levodopa is a dopaminergic drug that has been prescribed more extensively than any other medication for this disorder. As shown in Pharmacotherapy Illustrated 21.1, levodopa is a precursor in the

---

TABLE 21.2 Nondrug Treatments for Parkinson's Disease

Name of Treatment	Type of Treatment	Procedure
Deep brain stimulation (DBS)	Electrical stimulation	An electrode is implanted in the thalamus or subthalamus. It is connected to a pacemaker-like device that delivers electric currents to interfere with cells that cause tremors. An implantable generator is inserted under the patient's skin in much the same way as a cardiac pacemaker. The patient can adjust the settings by using a special magnet placed over the implanted generator. DBS is used when medications are no longer controlling symptoms.
Fetal tissue transplantation	Surgical	Fetal tissue from either humans or pigs is transplanted into the caudate nucleus of the brain. Expected outcome is that the patient will show a substantial decrease of motor symptoms. This is very controversial and considered experimental at this time. No long-term results are available.
Pallidotomy	Surgical and electrical stimulation	The target area is identified with a computed tomography (CT) scan or magnetic resonance imaging (MRI). When the patient has been sedated, a burr hole is made into the target area and an electrode is inserted. A mild electrical current is passed through the electrode. The patient is closely observed for the desired effects of decreased tremor and rigidity. If the desired effect is not seen, or if untoward effects occur, the probe is repositioned until desired effects occur. A temporary lesion is made. If it is successful, a permanent lesion is made.
Thalamotomy	Surgical	Lesions are surgically produced within the thalamus, which are thought to decrease tremor and rigidity. This is done only to benefit the side of the body that is most affected because there have been surgical complications from bilateral thalamotomy.

PHARMACOTHERAPY ILLUSTRATED 21.1

ANTIPARKINSON DRUGS FOCUS ON RESTORING DOPAMINE FUNCTION AND BLOCKING CHOLINERGIC ACTIVITY IN THE NIGROSTRIATAL PATHWAY

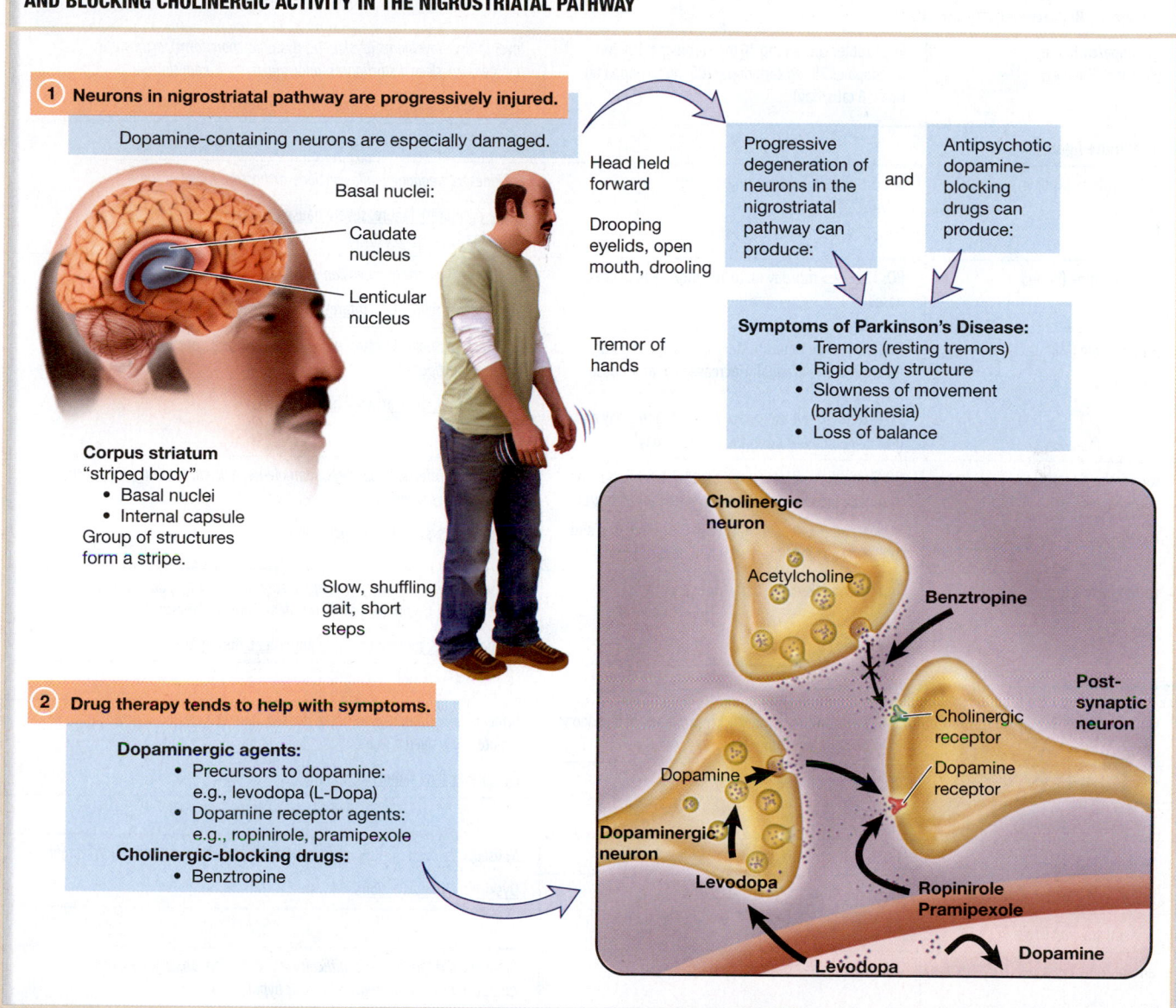

synthesis of dopamine. Unlike dopamine, however, levodopa easily crosses the blood–brain barrier to reach the affected region. Administration of levodopa directly leads to increased biosynthesis of dopamine within the nerve terminals. Carbidopa is nearly always administered with levodopa. Carbidopa increases the plasma levels and half-life of levodopa.

Two to three weeks of therapy are needed before improvement is observed, and many patients require several months of therapy for optimum therapeutic outcomes to be achieved. Dramatic improvement in symptoms is often noted early in therapy. As therapy progresses, however, the beneficial effects of the drug tend to diminish. In addition, the on–off syndrome tends to worsen with continued use of the drug.

PROTOTYPE DRUG | **Levodopa and Carbidopa (Sinemet, Parcopa)**

Classification: Therapeutic: Antiparkinson drug
Pharmacologic: Dopamine replacement agent

Therapeutic Effects and Uses: Approved in 1970, levodopa is an oral (PO) drug indicated for the treatment of idiopathic and secondary PD. The drug restores normal dopamine levels in the striatum of the brain. Levodopa is also used to treat symptoms of PD that occur in patients with manganese and carbon monoxide poisoning. Some symptoms of PD, such as tremor, bradykinesia, gait, and muscle rigidity, respond well to levodopa treatment.

TABLE 21.3	Drugs for Parkinson's Disease	

Drug	Route and Adult Dose (Maximum Dose Where Indicated)	Adverse Effects
Dopamine Replacement Agent		
levodopa/carbidopa (Parcopa, Sinemet)	PO: 1 tablet containing 10 mg carbidopa/100 mg levodopa or 25 mg carbidopa/100 mg levodopa tid (max: 6 tabs/day)	*Involuntary movements (dyskinetic, dystonic, choreiform), orthostatic hypotension, sleep disturbances, anorexia, nausea, vomiting* <u>NMS, hallucinations, agranulocytosis, depression with suicidal ideation</u>
Dopamine Agonists		
apomorphine (Apokyn)	Subcutaneous: 2–4 mg (max: 4 mg)	*Dyskinesias, frequent penile erections, orthostatic hypotension* <u>Acute circulatory failure, severe nausea and vomiting, syncope, hallucinations, sleep attacks</u>
bromocriptine (Parlodel)	PO: 1.25–2.5 mg/day up to 100 mg/day in divided doses	*Nausea, orthostatic hypotension* <u>Shock, acute myocardial infarction (MI), sleep attacks</u>
pramipexole (Mirapex)	PO (immediate release): start with 0.125 mg tid for 1 week and gradually increase to a target dose of 1.5 mg tid PO (extended release): start with 0.375 mg/day and gradually increase dose (max: 4.5 mg/day)	*Dizziness, somnolence, insomnia, dyskinesia, orthostatic hypotension, nausea, constipation* <u>EPS, asthenia, sleep attacks, hallucinations</u>
ropinirole (Requip)	PO (immediate release): start with 0.125 mg tid; and gradually increase to a maximum dose of 4.5 mg/day PO (extended release): start with 0.375 mg/day; and gradually increase to a maximum dose of 4.5 mg/day	*Fatigue viral infection, dizziness, somnolence, nausea, vomiting, dyspepsia, orthostatic hypotension* <u>Sleep attacks, syncope, hallucinations</u>
rotigotine (Neupro)	Transdermal: 2–8 mg daily (one patch)	*Nausea, vomiting, somnolence, application site reactions, dizziness, anorexia, hyperhidrosis, insomnia, peripheral edema, and dyskinesia* <u>Hallucinations, hypertension, falling asleep during ADLs</u>
COMT Inhibitors		
entacapone (Comtan)	PO: 200 mg administered with each dose of levodopa/carbidopa up to 8 times/day	*Urine discoloration, hyperkinesia, nausea, diarrhea, dystonia, orthostatic hypotension, sleep disorder* <u>Dyskinesia, liver failure (tolcapone)</u>
tolcapone (Tasmar)	PO: 100 mg tid (max: 600 mg/day)	
Monoamine Oxidase-B Inhibitors		
rasagiline (Azilect)	PO: 0.5–1 mg once daily	*Nausea, dizziness, confusion, depression, orthostatic hypotension, arthralgia* <u>Dyskinesia, hallucinations</u>
selegiline (Eldepryl, Zelapar)	PO: 5 mg/dose bid (max: 10 mg/day)	
Miscellaneous Drug		
amantadine (Symmetrel)	PO: 100 mg 1–2 times/day	*Dizziness, lightheadedness, difficulty concentrating, anxiety, headache, fatigue, nausea, vomiting, orthostatic hypotension* <u>Dysrhythmias, leukopenia (rare), heart failure</u>

Note: Italics indicate common adverse effects. <u>Underline</u> indicates serious adverse effects.

Others, such as imbalance, sensory problems, sexual dysfunction, and constipation, do not respond as well. Dosing is highly individualized to deliver the least amount of drug that will resolve the patient's symptoms.

The addition of carbidopa boosts the effectiveness of levodopa. Carbidopa itself has no therapeutic effects of its own because it cannot cross the blood–brain barrier. Instead, carbidopa inhibits the breakdown of levodopa in the intestine and peripheral tissues, which makes more levodopa available to reach the CNS. Without carbidopa, only 1% of the dose of levodopa reaches the CNS. The combination of the two drugs allows for much lower doses of levodopa to be prescribed than when levodopa is used alone; 25 mg of levodopa is used as a combination drug versus 125 mg of levodopa when delivered as monotherapy. Carbidopa also decreases dopamine production in peripheral tissues, leading to reduced nausea and vomiting as well as fewer cardiovascular responses to levodopa.

Sinemet is available as an immediate release tablet or a sustained release tablet. Parcopa is a preparation of levodopa and carbidopa that dissolves on the tongue and is swallowed with saliva, which is a distinct advantage for patients with swallowing difficulties. Stalevo is a combination of levodopa, carbidopa, and the COMT inhibitor, entacapone (see Section 21.7). The addition of entacapone is believed to create a more consistent level of levodopa in the blood, which can minimize the extent and duration of the wearing-off effect.

Mechanism of Action: Levodopa is a metabolic precursor of dopamine. When metabolized through decarboxylation to dopamine, dopamine levels in the brain increase. If given alone, 99% of a dose is decarboxylated to dopamine before it ever enters the CNS.

Pharmacokinetics (Levodopa):

Route(s)	PO
Absorption	Well absorbed from the gastrointestinal (GI) tract; absorption is decreased when given with meals
Distribution	Widely distributed throughout the body
Primary metabolism	Stomach, intestines, and liver
Primary excretion	Renal
Onset of action	1–3 h
Duration of action	Half-life: 1 h

Adverse Effects: The adverse effects of this combination of drugs are due to the levodopa component; carbidopa has no significant adverse effects. Common adverse effects include orthostatic hypotension, nausea, vomiting, anorexia, flatulence, dysphagia, abdominal distress, choreiform and involuntary movements, hand tremors, fatigue, headache, anxiety, twitching, numbness, confusion, agitation, nightmares, and insomnia. Life-threatening adverse effects include agranulocytosis, leukopenia, and hemolytic anemia. Other potential adverse effects are related to the anticholinergic properties of levodopa, including urinary retention and dry mouth. Psychosis develops in up to 20% of patients taking levodopa, and drug therapy with an antipsychotic such as clozapine (Clozaril) or quetiapine (Seroquel) may be necessary to control hallucinations and paranoid feelings. **Black Box Warning**: At least 12 hours should elapse between the last dose of levodopa and initiation of therapy with the carbidopa-levodopa combination drug.

Although the dystonias characteristic of PD are treated with levodopa and carbidopa, this drug combination also has the potential to cause dystonias. Some dystonias such as head bobbing or jaw clenching may be minor side effects of levodopa therapy, whereas others such as quick jerking movements may be serious. These dystonias may occur just as the optimum dosage level of levodopa is reached, which is extremely discouraging for patients and their caregivers. To reduce the severity of these dystonias, the dose of levodopa and carbidopa must be reduced. This, of course, causes the symptoms of PD to return.

Contraindications/Precautions: Levodopa is contraindicated in persons with hypersensitivity to the drug and those with narrow-angle glaucoma, undiagnosed skin lesions, acute psychoses, severe psychoneuroses, or within 2 weeks of use of a monoamine oxidase inhibitor (MAOI). Caution must be taken if administering levodopa to persons with cardiac, respiratory, endocrine, renal, or hepatic disease; myocardial infarction (MI) with dysrhythmias; seizure disorder; lactation; peptic ulcer; psychiatric disorders; or hypertension. The drug should not be abruptly discontinued due to the possibility of the development of neuroleptic malignant syndrome (NMS), such as tachycardia, muscular rigidity, fever, mental status changes, diaphoresis, and tachypnea.

Drug Interactions: Although antipsychotic drugs may be used to control psychosis associated with parkinsonism, conventional antipsychotic drugs block dopamine receptors in the brain and can decrease the therapeutic effects of levodopa. MAOIs can lead to a hypertensive crisis. Increased postural hypotension may occur if used with tricyclic antidepressants. Concurrent use with antihypertensives may cause additive hypotension. Decreased levodopa effects can occur with use of anticholinergics, hydantoins, papaverine, or pyridoxine. Antacids may increase the effects of levodopa. **Herbal/Food**: Food, especially high-protein foods and vitamin-fortified foods containing vitamin B_6, decreases the rate and extent of levodopa absorption; however, many persons must take levodopa with food to decrease the nausea and vomiting that may occur. Kava may worsen symptoms of PD. Indian snakeroot will decrease levodopa action while increasing EPS.

Pregnancy: Category C.

Treatment of Overdose: No specific treatment.

Nursing Responsibilities: Key nursing implications for patients receiving levodopa and carbidopa are included in the Nursing Practice Application for Patients Receiving Pharmacotherapy for Neurodegenerative Disorders.

21.6 Dopamine agonists may be used as monotherapy for early symptoms of Parkinson's disease or as adjuncts to levodopa in patients with advanced disease.

Dopamine agonists (also called dopaminergic agonists) directly activate dopamine receptors in the CNS. They are less effective than levodopa at reducing symptoms of PD. They are used as monotherapy for patients with mild to moderate symptoms of PD and may be used in combination with levodopa in patients with advanced disease. Doses of these drugs are listed in Table 21.3.

Dopamine agonists have certain advantages over levodopa. The drugs do not have to be metabolized to be effective and they are not converted to potentially toxic metabolites. Dietary protein does not interfere with their absorption, so a low-protein diet is not necessary. They exhibit a lower incidence of the wearing-off effect and are less likely to cause dyskinesias in patients younger than age 60.

Certain adverse effects of dopamine agonists may be more serious than those of levodopa. These include postural hypotension, unexpected sleep attacks, and hallucinations. This group of drugs is generally reserved for younger patients, who tend to tolerate adverse effects better than older adult patients.

The dopamine agonists are divided into two subclasses: ergot alkaloids and nonergot drugs. Bromocriptine (Parlodel) is an ergot alkaloid derived from the ergot fungus that grows on rye wheat. Another use of ergot alkaloids is in the treatment of migraine headaches. The nonergot alkaloids include apomorphine (Apokyn), pramipexole (Mirapex), ritogitine (Neupro), and ropinirole (Requip).

PROTOTYPE DRUG	Pramipexole (Mirapex)

Classification: **Therapeutic:** Antiparkinson drug
Pharmacologic: Dopamine receptor agonist, nonergot

Therapeutic Effects and Uses: Pramipexole is an oral drug indicated for the treatment of idiopathic PD. It is used as monotherapy in early PD and in combination with levodopa in advanced stages of the disease. It can produce significant motor improvement in early PD and decreases fluctuations in motor performance in late disease. Many patients are able to lower their doses of levodopa when they take pramipexole concurrently. It is also approved for treating moderate to severe symptoms of restless leg syndrome. Several weeks of therapy are necessary for the patient to obtain maximum benefits from pramipexole. An extended duration form of the drug, Mirapex ER, permits a convenient once-daily dosing schedule.

Mechanism of Action: Pramipexole is a selective agonist of the D_2 subfamily of dopamine receptors at both presynaptic and postsynaptic sites in the striatum. The binding helps to restore the balance of dopaminergic effects in the striatum. Binding at D_3 receptors may also contribute to the antiparkinson effects.

Pharmacokinetics:

Route(s)	PO
Absorption	90% absorption
Distribution	Widely distributed, especially to red blood cells; 15% bound to plasma proteins
Primary metabolism	Hepatic (minimal)
Primary excretion	Renal, mostly unchanged
Onset of action	2 h
Duration of action	Half-life: 8 h; in the elderly, 12–14 h

Adverse Effects: Pramipexole has many possible adverse effects. The most common are hallucinations, dizziness, drowsiness, and nausea. The incidence of hallucinations increases with age and may cause discontinuation of therapy in older patients. Orthostatic hypotension occurs in over half the patients taking the drug and may contribute to injury due to falls. Life-threatening adverse effects include sleep attacks, hemolytic anemia, agranulocytosis, and leukopenia. Sleep attacks can occur without warning, regardless of current activity level, and cause accidents. Agitation, insomnia, hypotension, constipation, anorexia, and dyskinesias are other adverse effects. In 2012 the FDA issued a safety alert that pramipexole is associated with new-onset heart failure.

Contraindications/Precautions: Pramipexole should not be used in a person who has hypersensitivity to the drug or to ropinirole. The drug should be used cautiously if the patient has renal, hepatic, or cardiac disease; is taking CNS depressants; or has psychosis, dyskinesia, or affective disorders.

Drug Interactions: Dopamine antagonists that may decrease pramipexole levels include phenothiazines, metoclopramide, and some antipsychotic drugs. Drugs that may increase pramipexole levels include levodopa, cimetidine, ranitidine, diltiazem, verapamil, and quinidine. Pramipexole may worsen dyskinesias when used concurrently with levodopa. **Herbal/Food:** Kava may decrease the effects of pramipexole.

Pregnancy: Category C.

Treatment of Overdose: No specific treatment is available for overdose. General supportive measures should be implemented.

Nursing Responsibilities: Key nursing implications for patients receiving pramipexole are included in the Nursing Practice Application for Patients Receiving Pharmacotherapy for Neurodegenerative Disorders.

Drugs Similar to Levodopa and Pramipexole (Mirapex)

Other dopamine agonists used to treat PD include apomorphine, bromocriptine, and ropinirole. Pergolide (Permax) is a dopamine agonist that was discontinued in the United States due to the possible development of valvular heart disease.

Apomorphine (Apokyn): Apomorphine, available as a subcutaneous injection, is a nonergot dopamine agonist used as a single dose to treat severe "off" episodes in patients who have advanced PD. It is not intended for use as routine management of PD symptoms. Apomorphine is structurally related to morphine, but it does not bind to opioid receptors or cause morphine-like effects (see Chapter 25). Life-threatening adverse effects include sleep attacks or acute circulatory failure. Sleep attacks are more serious than the general drowsiness or sleepiness that occurs frequently with dopaminergic agonists. They can occur during any activity, including driving and other potentially dangerous activities. The drug causes significant nausea and vomiting, and the manufacturer recommends the administration of trimethobenzamide (Tigan), an antiemetic drug, 3 days prior to the apomorphine injection. The antiemetic ondansetron (Zofran) is contraindicated because it may result in severe hypotension and loss of consciousness. Common adverse effects are orthostatic hypotension, anorexia, and agitation. The drug can produce erections and is approved to treat erectile dysfunction in some countries (but not in the United States). This drug is pregnancy category C.

Bromocriptine (Parlodel): Approved in 1978, bromocriptine, available as a tablet, is an ergot alkaloid that has a variety of uses. In addition to being a dopamine agonist used for adjunctive treatment with levodopa for PD, it is approved for pituitary adenoma, acromegaly, and for women with amenorrhea and infertility caused by excessive prolactin secretion. Off-label indications include alcoholism, cocaine withdrawal, mastalgia, NMS, and premenstrual syndrome.

When used concurrently, bromocriptine allows a significant dose reduction of levodopa. Life-threatening adverse reactions may be seizures, shock, or MI. The most common dose-limiting adverse effects are psychological reactions, including confusion, agitation, hallucinations, paranoid delusions, or nightmares. Other adverse effects include orthostatic hypotension, headache, nausea, vomiting, anorexia, or rash on the face and arms. This drug is pregnancy category B.

Ropinirole (Requip): Approved for PD in 1997, ropinirole is an oral nonergot dopamine receptor agonist used as monotherapy for the treatment of early PD, or in combination with levodopa in more advanced disease. The most common adverse effects are syncope, fatigue, drowsiness, nausea and vomiting, and viral infections. A major advantage of ropinirole is that it causes a much lower rate of dyskinesias than levodopa. In addition, the patient taking ropinirole rarely experiences sleep attacks. In 2005, the U.S. Food and Drug Administration (FDA) approved ropinirole to treat restless leg syndrome. This drug is pregnancy category C.

Rotigotine (Neupro): Rotigotine is the only transdermal patch available for treating PD. Initially approved in 2007 for PD, it was subsequently pulled from the market in 2008 due to manufacturing issues. It has been reapproved and is now available to treat early and late stage PD as well as restless leg syndrome. The patch provides for ease of use and is changed daily. Rotigotine can reduce the on–off periods experienced during levodopa therapy. Nausea, vomiting, and drowsiness are common during therapy. Care must be taken to prevent accidents due to falling asleep during ADLs. This drug is pregnancy category C.

21.7 Several miscellaneous dopaminergic agents are used as adjuncts to levodopa therapy.

In addition to levodopa and dopaminergic agonists, several other drugs may be used to increase dopamine levels in the striatum. These drugs act on neurons by either increasing the release of dopamine or by reducing its destruction. Doses of these drugs are listed in Table 21.3.

Amantadine (Symmetrel): Amantadine is the only FDA-approved drug for PD that acts by increasing the release of dopamine from storage sites in the presynaptic neurons. It also blocks the reuptake of dopamine into the presynaptic neurons. Both of these mechanisms result in increased dopamine action. Given PO, the drug produces a rapid reduction in parkinsonism symptoms but its effects begin to diminish after several months of therapy. Adverse effects are primarily CNS related and include confusion, dizziness, irritability, and headache. Amantadine should be used with caution in patients with mental illness because it can exacerbate psychoses and cause hallucinations and suicidal ideation. Amantadine is an antiviral drug used for the prophylactic and symptomatic treatment of influenza A virus infections. A prototype feature may be found in Chapter 54. This drug is pregnancy category C.

Catechol-O-methyltransferase inhibitors: Catechol-O-methyltransferase, or COMT, is the enzyme responsible for metabolizing levodopa to its inactive intermediate 3-O-methyldopa. The **COMT inhibitors** are drugs that prevent the destruction of levodopa in peripheral tissues, thus increasing the amount of levodopa available to enter the brain. This results in a longer half-life and more consistent serum levels of levodopa. The COMT inhibitors have no therapeutic effects on their own; their beneficial effects are entirely the result of increased levodopa levels.

Only two drugs in this category are used in the United States. Approved in 1999, entacapone (Comtan) is available as a tablet and is recommended as an adjunct to levodopa/carbidopa. Entacapone can significantly reduce the "off" time experienced during levodopa therapy. It is contraindicated for pregnant patients (this drug is pregnancy category D) and during lactation. Approved in 1998, tolcapone (Tasmar) is also available as a tablet as an adjunct to levodopa and carbidopa. Tolcapone has a longer duration of action than entacapone and acts on COMT both peripherally and centrally. Tolcapone is a pregnancy category C drug.

Most adverse effects observed during therapy with the COMT inhibitors are those of excessive amounts of levodopa: nausea, vomiting, dyskinesias, postural hypotension, and psychiatric symptoms. Entacapone itself can cause nausea, diarrhea, abdominal pain, and urine discoloration. The most serious adverse effect of tolcapone is liver failure, which may be fatal. Regular monitoring of hepatic status must be performed during tolcapone therapy.

CONNECTIONS Evidence-Based Practice

◖ Preventing Neurodegeneration in Parkinson's Disease

Clinical Question
Can the neurodegeneration that occurs in Parkinson's disease be prevented by drug therapy?

Evidence
Exenatide (Byetta), a glucagon-like peptide-1 (GLP-1), is approved for the treatment of type 2 diabetes mellitus. GLP-1 receptors have been identified throughout the brain and in peripheral tissues. In animal studies, it appears that exenatide may have neuroprotective and neurorestorative effects (Harkavyi & Whitton, 2010; McIntyre et al., 2013). A growing body of research evidence suggests that these effects may prevent apoptosis (programmed cell death) and may restore nerve function (Li et al., 2009; Salcedo, Tweedie, Li, & Greig, 2012).

Aviles-Olmos et al. (2013) conducted a single-blind, randomized study on the use of exenatide in 45 patients with moderate PD. Using both motor and nonmotor rating scales, measurements were taken at baseline after an overnight withdrawal of anti-Parkinson's medications at 6 and 12 months and again at 14 months after a 2-month period of having PD therapy stopped. At the conclusion of the study, patients treated with exenatide exhibited improvements in motor function and on a dementia rating scale compared to the control group. The control group demonstrated varying levels of declines in function on all rating scales. Weight loss, constipation, and nausea were the most common adverse effects reported in the exenatide group, whereas an increase in dyskinesias in some members of the treatment group necessitated a change in their PD drug therapy. The results of this study support the need for a larger, double-blind randomized trial of exenatide use in patients with PD.

Implications
Current drug therapy in Parkinson's disease has been aimed at enhancing the effects of the remaining dopamine in the brain or as replacement therapy once dopamine levels decline. Treatment with exenatide and other GLP-1 agonists may change the focus on treatment to a focus on prevention. By preventing apoptosis and protecting nerve cells from inflammation and oxidative stress that occurs, neurodegeneration may be prevented. In PD, this would prevent cellular decline to the point where PD symptoms occur and replacement therapy is needed. Exenatide and other GLP-1 agonists may also encourage neurogenesis and reverse neurodegeneration (Fan, Li, Gu, Chan, & Xu, 2010), suggesting that the PD process could be reversed. Further studies are needed, but the potential to prevent decline and reverse the neurodegeneration that occurs holds great promise in the treatment of PD and other neurodegenerative disorders.

Critical Thinking Questions
What other neurodegenerative disorders might also benefit from the use of exenatide and other GLP-1 agonists?

See Answer to Critical Thinking Question on student resource website.

TABLE 21.4 Anticholinergic Drugs and Drugs with Anticholinergic Activity Used for Parkinsonism

Drug	Route and Adult Dose (Maximum Dose Where Indicated)	Adverse Effects
benztropine (Cogentin)	PO: 0.5–1 mg/day; gradually increase as needed (max: 6 mg/day)	*Nausea, constipation, dry mouth, blurred vision, drowsiness, dizziness, tachycardia, hypotension, nervousness*
biperiden (Akineton)	PO: 2 mg 1–4 times/day	
diphenhydramine (Benadryl)	PO: 25–50 mg tid–qid (max: 300 mg/day)	Paralytic ileus, cardiovascular collapse, anaphylactic shock (diphenhydramine)
trihexyphenidyl (Artane)	PO: 1 mg on day 1; 2 mg on day 2; then increase by 2 mg every 3–5 days up to 6–10 mg/day (max: 15 mg/day)	

Note: Italics indicate common adverse effects. Underline indicates serious adverse effects.

Monoamine oxidase-B inhibitors: Monoamine oxidase (MAO) is an enzyme found in synaptic spaces that metabolizes catecholamines to inactive compounds. MAO-A acts on norepinephrine and serotonin, whereas MAO-B inactivates dopamine. Although MAOs are distributed throughout the body, most of the MAO in the brain is type B.

Selegiline was the first selective MAO-B inhibitor approved for PD in 1989. Selegiline is available as a tablet or capsule (Eldepryl) and as an orally disintegrating tablet (Zelapar). A selegiline transdermal patch (Emsam) was approved by the FDA in 2006 for the treatment of major depression. Selegiline is used off-label to treat Alzheimer's disease. A second MAO-B inhibitor, rasagiline (Azilect), was approved in 2006 and offers the convenience of once-daily dosing.

By inhibiting MAO-B these drugs increase the level of dopamine in the striatum, resulting in greater dopaminergic activity in this region. These drugs may be prescribed as monotherapy for PD or used concurrently with levodopa or levodopa/carbidopa.

The most frequent adverse effects during MAO-B therapy are those that are also associated with levodopa: nausea, vomiting, confusion, orthostatic hypotension, and dyskinesias. Minor adverse effects include insomnia, headache, arthralgia, and dyspepsia. With most MAOIs, the patient must strictly avoid food containing tyramine and certain medications that could result in hypertensive crisis. Because these drugs selectively inhibit MAO-B, this is not a major concern. With high doses, however, selegiline and rasagiline lose their selectivity for MAO-B, and they begin to affect MAO-A, thus increasing the risk of a hypertensive crisis when high-tyramine foods are eaten. There is a risk of severe CNS toxicity (serotonin syndrome) if MAO-B inhibitors are used concurrently with antidepressants. Rasagiline should not be administered to patients with moderate or severe hepatic impairment. Both of the MAO-B inhibitors are pregnancy category C.

21.8 Anticholinergic drugs are the oldest of the antiparkinson agents and are effective at reducing tremor.

Anticholinergic drugs comprise the oldest category of drugs used to treat PD, having been used for over 150 years. They help to restore the balance between Ach and dopamine by blocking Ach (muscarinic) receptors in the striatum of the brain. This inhibits the effects of Ach, allowing dopamine to have greater influence.

Anticholinergics are of most benefit to the patients whose primary symptom is tremor; they are less effective at reducing bradykinesia. Overall, they exhibit fewer serious adverse effects than levodopa but they are less effective. Anticholinergics are not recommended for older adults because this population often has difficulty with the CNS adverse effects, including confusion, delusion, and hallucinations. The two anticholinergic drugs used most often to treat PD are benztropine (Cogentin) and trihexyphenidyl (Artane). The student should refer to Chapter 14 for a complete discussion on the indications, actions, and adverse effects of this class of medications. Doses of selected anticholinergics used to treat Parkinson's disease are listed in Table 21.4.

CONNECTION Checkpoint 21.2

From what you learned in Chapter 19, what is the other major indication for MAO inhibitors? What food nutrient must be strictly avoided in patients taking these drugs? *See Answer to Connection Checkpoint 21.2 on student resource website.*

PROTOTYPE DRUG   **Benztropine (Cogentin)**

Classification: Therapeutic: Antiparkinson drug
Pharmacologic: Cholinergic antagonist

Therapeutic Effects and Uses: Benztropine is used as combination therapy with trihexyphenidyl or levodopa/carbidopa in the management of PD symptoms. It is also used to treat drug-induced EPS. Although it suppresses tremor and rigidity, it is not effective at alleviating tardive dyskinesia. The patient may notice decreased symptoms after only 2 to 3 days of therapy with benztropine. It is an older medication approved in 1954 that is available by PO and parenteral routes. An off-label indication is to treat hypersalivation in patients who have developmental disabilities.

Mechanism of Action: Benztropine acts by reducing the excess cholinergic effect associated with dopamine deficiency and restores neurotransmitter balance in the striatum.

Pharmacokinetics:

Route(s)	PO, intramuscular (IM), intravenous (IV)
Absorption	Rapidly absorbed
Distribution	Wide distribution; 95% bound to plasma proteins
Primary metabolism	Hepatic
Primary excretion	Renal
Onset of action	1–2 h PO; 15 minutes if given IM or IV
Duration of action	Half-life: 6–10 h

Adverse Effects: Common adverse reactions to benztropine are related to its anticholinergic effects and include sedation, constipation, blurred vision, dry mouth, decreased sweating, urinary retention, and confusion. Paralytic ileus is the only identified life-threatening adverse reaction.

Contraindications/Precautions: Contraindications to the use of benztropine include closed-angle glaucoma, myasthenia gravis, tardive dyskinesia, GI or urinary obstruction, prostatic hypertrophy, peptic ulcers, tachycardia, and children under age 3. Caution must be taken when benztropine is given to persons with psychiatric diagnoses because it may worsen these conditions.

Drug Interactions: Additive toxicity can occur when benztropine is taken with other drugs that exhibit anticholinergic effects, including antihistamines, tricyclic antidepressants, phenothiazines, MAOIs, or quinidine. Alcohol and other CNS depressants will have an additive sedative effect. Antidiarrheals will slow GI motility and decrease absorption of the medication. **Herbal/Food:** Kava will cause a decreased benztropine effect. Jimsonweed or butterbur may lead to increased benztropine effects.

Pregnancy: Category C.

Treatment of Overdose: Overdose can cause circulatory collapse, respiratory depression, shock, and coma. Physostigmine, 1–2 mg subcutaneous or IV, will reverse symptoms of anticholinergic intoxication. If needed, it may be repeated in 2 hours. Other treatment is supportive, according to symptoms being experienced.

Nursing Responsibilities: Key nursing implications for patients receiving benztropine are included in the Nursing Practice Application for Patients Receiving Pharmacotherapy for Neurodegenerative Disorders in this chapter and in the Nursing Practice Application for Patients Receiving Pharmacotherapy with Cholinergic (Muscarinic) Antagonists in Chapter 14.

Drugs Similar to Benztropine (Cogentin)

The only other anticholinergic widely used for PD is trihexyphenidyl (Artane). Biperiden (Akineton) has weak anticholinergic effects and exhibits the same basic actions and adverse effects as trihexyphenidyl. Procyclidine (Kemadrin) was discontinued in 2008.

Trihexyphenidyl (Artane): Approved in 1949, trihexyphenidyl is available in several PO formulations in both regular and extended release forms. It is indicated for both idiopathic and drug-induced PD and its actions and adverse effects are similar to those of benztropine. It is useful in decreasing involuntary movements and salivation, which are two problems experienced by patients with PD. The only life-threatening adverse effect is paralytic ileus. Other adverse effects include typical anticholinergic effects such as constipation, dryness of the mouth, nausea, blurred vision, urinary retention, dizziness, and nervousness. In patients over age 60, the dose must be increased gradually to prevent serious side effects. It must not be given to patients with hypersensitivity to the drug, closed-angle glaucoma, severe cardiac impairment, myasthenia gravis, or GI or urinary obstruction. In addition, this drug should be used with caution in older males due to the potential for developing prostatic hyperplasia. This drug is pregnancy category C.

Alzheimer's Disease

21.9 Alzheimer's disease, the most common dementia, leads to a progressive loss of cognitive function.

Dementia is a chronic, degenerative disorder characterized by progressive memory loss, confusion, and inability to think or communicate effectively. It is usually associated with cerebral atrophy or other degenerative structural changes within the brain. Loss of short-term memory is an early sign. Patients have difficulty finding their way around familiar places and forget where they leave items. Mood swings and changes in behavior or personality eventually develop as patients become angry and frustrated with their condition. They forget how to perform normal ADLs such as bathing, cooking, or toileting and may not comprehend instructions. They often have an altered sense of time and place. Psychosis occurs in about 10% of patients and 15% to 20% develop major depression as comorbid conditions. Late changes include the inability to walk or feed themselves, incontinence, and inability to swallow.

PharmFACT

More than 5 million Americans have Alzheimer's disease. Every 67 seconds, someone in the United States develops Alzheimer's disease (Alzheimer's Association, 2014).

The etiology of most dementia is unknown. Known causes of dementia include multiple small cerebral infarcts (vascular dementia), toxins (lead), severe infections, metabolic disorders (hypothyroidism and vitamin B_{12} deficiency), and brain tumors. Infection with the human immunodeficiency virus (HIV) causes dementia late in the progress of the disease. Alzheimer's disease is the most common type of dementia.

It should be clearly understood that dementia is not a normal consequence of aging. Although cognitive changes such as memory impairment and a decline in the speed of information recall do occur with aging, these rarely interfere with ADLs and are not considered dementia.

Alzheimer's disease (AD) is a neurodegenerative disease that involves a chronic, progressive loss of cognitive function. The disorder generally begins after age 60 and affects as many as 50% of the population over age 85. The patient generally lives 5 to 10 years following diagnosis. AD is the sixth leading cause of death. A summary of the major symptoms of AD is shown in Table 21.5.

AD leads to loss of productivity and wages (both for the patient and the caregivers), and often the patient must be placed in a long-term care facility. It is the third most expensive disease in the United States. In addition to the economics of caring for a person with AD, there are the psychological and emotional costs to families and caregivers. Pharmacotherapy has limited success in improving the cognitive function of patients with AD.

Despite many attempts at identifying the etiology of AD, the causes remain largely unknown. Although the cause has been elusive, structural damage in the brains of patients with AD has been well documented. Beta-amyloid protein and **neurofibrillary tangles** are found at autopsy in the brains of nearly all patients with AD. The neurofibrillary tangles are composed of insoluble proteins (Figure 21.1) and their abundance is proportional to the amount of cognitive impairment observed in the patient. It is suspected

TABLE 21.5	Symptoms of Alzheimer's Disease	
Early (2–4 Years Duration)	**Middle (2–12 Years Duration)**	**Late (2–4 Years Duration and Longer)**
Depression	Lack of ability to recall names of acquaintances	Lack of ability to recognize family members
Loss of ability to concentrate	Recent memory loss	Loss of ambulation ability
Increased anxiety and agitation	Loss of orientation to time, person, or place	Loss of ability to perform any ADLs
Irritability	Changes in personal habits (may become loud, use profane language; undesirable personality characteristics may become pronounced)	Loss of sphincter control
Weight loss	Increasing difficulty with self-care	Loss of ability to recognize self (e.g., does not recognize self in the mirror)
Forgetting the location of common items (car keys, home, etc.); blaming others for moving or stealing items	—	"Sundowning" syndrome (worsening of symptoms in the evening)
Forgetting important dates (family birthdays, health care provider appointments, etc.)	—	—
Not paying bills	—	—

that these structural changes are caused by chronic inflammatory or oxidative cellular damage to the surrounding neurons. Environmental, immunologic, and nutritional factors, as well as viruses, are considered possible sources of brain damage. There are losses in both the numbers and functions of neurons.

In addition to structural changes, there are abnormalities in the balance of neurotransmitters in the brains of patients with AD. The best documented change is a deficiency of Ach, which is likely caused by brain atrophy and destruction of neurons. This loss of cholinergic activity is thought to be responsible for decreased cognition, loss of recent memory, and the inability to retain new information. Deficiencies in other brain neurotransmitters are also likely to contribute to the complex symptoms of AD.

Genetic factors likely contribute to the development of AD; genetic defects on chromosomes 14, 19, and 21 have been identified and may be factors leading to the development of the neurofibrillary tangles. About 5% to 15% of patients with AD show a family history of the disorder.

It is important to assess the degree of cognitive impairment in patients with dementia. Various assessment tools are used to determine a baseline degree of cognition to make decisions on whether pharmacotherapy should be implemented. During pharmacotherapy, these tools are used to determine the progression of dementia and to gauge the effectiveness (or ineffectiveness) of therapy. Tools for assessing the progress of Alzheimer's include periodic magnetic resonance imaging (MRI) and cognitive tests for memory such as the Mini-Mental State Exam (MMSE), which takes only 5 to 10 minutes to administer.

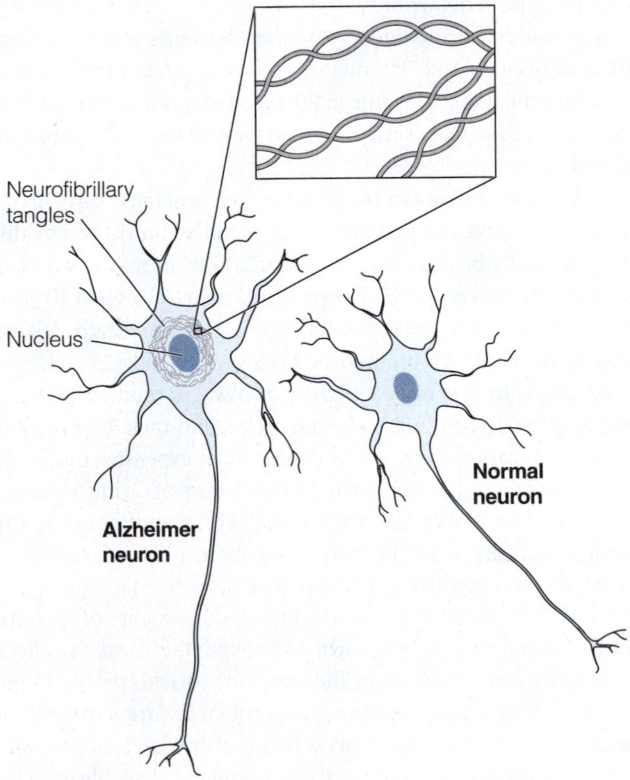

Pharmacotherapy of Alzheimer's Disease

21.10 Pharmacotherapy of Alzheimer's disease produces only modest results and is ineffective at stopping the progression of the disorder.

Drugs are used to slow memory loss and other progressive symptoms of dementia. In most cases, the pharmacologic treatment of dementia is the same regardless of its cause. In addition, pharmacotherapy is often required to treat common comorbid conditions such as depression, anxiety, or psychosis.

The FDA has approved only a few drugs for AD. These medications, listed in Table 21.6, do not cure or prevent AD; at best, they may slow progression of memory loss. The pharmacotherapy of AD is shown in Pharmacotherapy Illustrated 21.2.

The reversible **cholinesterase inhibitors** are the most widely prescribed drug class for treating AD. Donepezil (Aricept),

Figure 21.1 Neuron with neurofibrillary tangles seen in Alzheimer's disease.

TABLE 21.6	Drugs to Treat Alzheimer's Disease	
Drug	**Route and Adult Dose (Maximum Dose Where Indicated)**	**Adverse Effects**
memantine (Namenda)	PO (regular release): initiate with 5 mg once daily and gradually increase to a target dose of 10 mg bid PO (extended release): initiate with 7 mg once daily and gradually increase to a target dose of 28 mg once daily	*Headache, confusion, dizziness, cough, hypertension* Renal failure
Cholinesterase Inhibitors		
donepezil (Aricept)	PO: 5–10 mg at bedtime	*Nausea and vomiting, anorexia, diarrhea, abdominal pain, dizziness, headache, weight loss, muscle cramps* Hallucinations, depression, confusion, hepatotoxicity, increased mortality in patients with mild cognitive impairment (galantamine)
galantamine (Razadyne)	PO (regular release): initiate with 4 mg bid, and gradually increase to target dose of 12 mg bid PO (extended release): initiate with 8 mg once daily and gradually increase to 16–24 mg/day	
rivastigmine (Exelon)	PO: initiate with 1.5 mg bid and gradually increase to a target dose 3–6 mg bid (max: 12 mg bid) Transdermal: initiate with 4.6 mg (one patch) daily and gradually increase to one 9.5 mg patch and then one 13.3 mg patch daily	

Note: *Italics* indicate common adverse effects. <u>Underline</u> indicates serious adverse effects.

a popular first-line therapy because it can be taken once daily, is well tolerated by most patients and is effective at all stages of the disease. Higher doses for severe disease produce GI adverse effects that can limit drug therapy

Ach is naturally degraded in the synaptic cleft by the enzyme cholinesterase. When cholinesterase is inhibited, Ach levels become elevated and produce a more profound effect on Ach receptors. They are similar to the peripheral cholinesterase inhibitors such as neostigmine but demonstrate greater CNS activity.

The goal of pharmacotherapy with reversible cholinesterase inhibitors is to improve function in three domains: ADLs, behavior, and cognition. Although the cholinesterase inhibitors improve all three domains, their effectiveness is modest at best. Therapy is begun as soon as the diagnosis of AD is established. These medications are less effective in treating the severe stages of this disorder, probably because too many neurons have died; increasing the level of Ach is effective only if functioning neurons are present. As the disease progresses and fewer neurons are present, drug effects diminish and the cholinesterase inhibitors are discontinued; their therapeutic benefit may not outweigh their expense or the risks of adverse effects.

All cholinesterase inhibitors used to treat AD have equivalent efficacy. Adverse effects are those expected of drugs that enhance the parasympathetic nervous system (see Chapter 13). The GI system is most often affected, with nausea, vomiting, and diarrhea being frequent adverse events. Rivastigmine (Exelon) is associated with weight loss, which is a potentially serious adverse effect in some older adults. When therapy is discontinued, doses of the cholinesterase inhibitors should be tapered gradually.

CONNECTION Checkpoint 21.3

The cholinesterase inhibitors for Alzheimer's disease are used for their central actions. From what you learned in Chapter 13, what are the indications for cholinesterase inhibitors that act peripherally? What drug is the prototype peripheral cholinesterase inhibitor? *See Answer to Connection Checkpoint 21.3 on student resource website.*

Memantine (Namenda) was approved in 2003 for the treatment of patients with moderate to severe AD. It acts by a different mechanism than the centrally acting cholinesterase inhibitors. Memantine reduces the abnormally high levels of **glutamate**, which is the major

excitatory neurotransmitter of the CNS. Chronic, high levels of brain glutamate have been associated with the progression of AD and cell death. Glutamate exerts its neural effects through interaction with the N-methyl-D-aspartate (NMDA) receptor. Memantine binds to the NMDA receptor, preventing glutamate from causing its excitatory actions and, theoretically, slowing nerve damage.

The only contraindication to the use of memantine is renal failure. Caution is indicated when given to older adults or those with renal impairment or seizure disorder. No life-threatening adverse effects have been identified. Occasional adverse effects have been reported, including dizziness, confusion, vomiting, headache, cough, and hypertension. Because memantine and cholinesterase inhibitors act by different mechanisms, they may be taken in combination. When taken together, these drugs do not interfere with each other's absorption, distribution, metabolism, or elimination. In 2013 an extended release form (Namenda XR) was approved that offers the convenience of once-daily dosing.

Several other drugs have been investigated for their possible benefit in delaying the progression of AD, including various vitamins, statins, nonsteroidal anti-inflammatory drugs (NSAIDs), estrogen, and ginkgo biloba. These agents have not been found to produce any significant reduction in the progression of memory loss.

Other medication classes frequently prescribed for symptoms associated with AD include antipsychotics, antidepressants, and antianxiety drugs. Agitation occurs in the majority of patients with AD, which may be accompanied by delusions, paranoia, hallucinations, or other psychotic symptoms. Atypical antipsychotics such as risperidone (Risperdal) and olanzapine (Zyprexa) may be used to control these episodes. Conventional antipsychotics such as haloperidol (Haldol) are occasionally prescribed, although EPS often limit their use. The antipsychotic medications are presented in Chapter 20.

Although not as common as agitation, anxiety and depression occur in many patients with AD. Anxiolytics such as buspirone (BuSpar) or benzodiazepines are used to control anxiety. Mood stabilizers such as sertraline (Zoloft), citalopram (Celexa), or fluoxetine (Prozac) are given when major depression interferes with daily activities. The student should refer to Chapters 18 and 19 for information on these drugs.

PHARMACOTHERAPY ILLUSTRATED 21.2

ALZHEIMER'S DRUGS WORK BY INTENSIFYING THE EFFECT OF ACETYLCHOLINE AT THE RECEPTOR

① Alzheimer's disease

Characterized by abnormal structures in the brain:
- Neurons die
- The brain shrinks
- Memory is lost

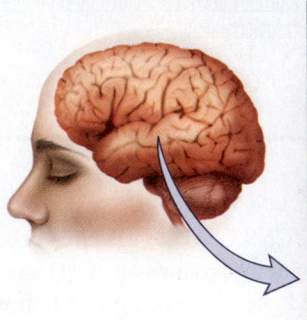

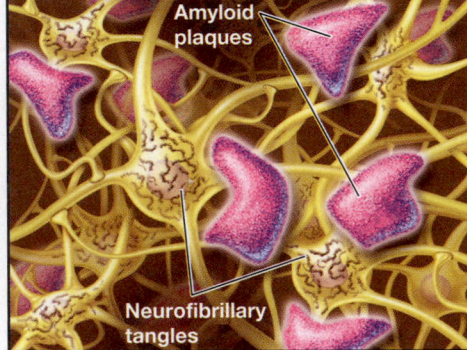

Amyloid plaques

Neurofibrillary tangles

Unhealthy neuronal structure

Healthy neuronal structure

② Drug therapy focuses on restoring or enhancing acetylcholine's role in the brain

- Cholinesterase inhibitors
  e.g., donepezil

③ Factors responsible for brain cell death include excessive transmission of glutamate

Drug therapy:
- N-methyl-D-aspartate (NMDA) receptor agents
  e.g., memantine

Combination drug therapy:
- Donepezil and memantine

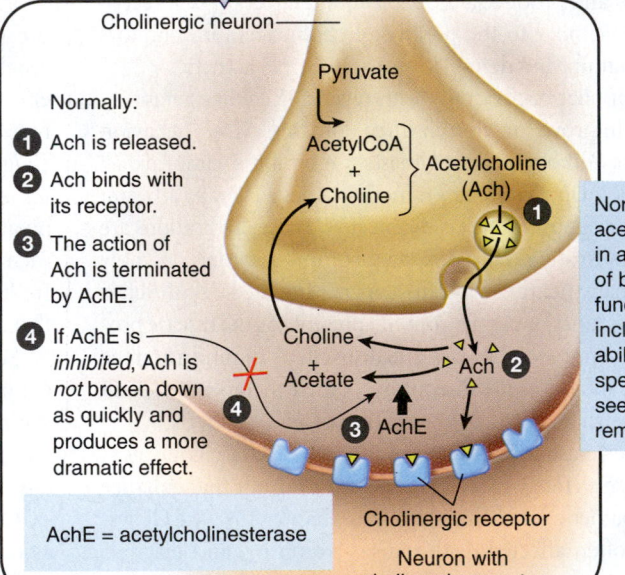

Cholinergic neuron

Pyruvate

AcetylCoA + Choline

Acetylcholine (Ach)

Normally:

① Ach is released.

② Ach binds with its receptor.

③ The action of Ach is terminated by AchE.

④ If AchE is *inhibited*, Ach is *not* broken down as quickly and produces a more dramatic effect.

AchE = acetylcholinesterase

Choline + Acetate

Ach

AchE

Normal role of acetylcholine in a vast array of brain functions, including the ability to speak, move, see, think, and remember.

Cholinergic receptor

Neuron with cholinergic receptor

PROTOTYPE DRUG | **Donepezil (Aricept)**

Classification: Therapeutic: Anti-Alzheimer's drug
Pharmacologic: Reversible cholinesterase inhibitor

Therapeutic Effects and Uses: Originally approved to treat mild to moderate symptoms of AD in 1996, the indication was extended to the treatment of severe AD in 2006. The drug is available in tablet, PO solution, and PO disintegrating tablet (Aricept ODT) forms. It has an extended duration of action that allows for once-daily dosing. Donepezil is the most frequent drug prescribed for Alzheimer's disease.

There is no evidence that donepezil stops the destruction of neurons or that it alters the course of the underlying dementia. It may, however, prolong the time between diagnosis and the institutionalization of the patient. A caregiver must be present to assist the patient in adhering to the medication regimen.

Mechanism of Action: Donepezil raises Ach concentrations in the brain. Because the drug is moderately selective for cholinesterase

CONNECTIONS Complementary and Alternative Therapies

◀ Ginkgo Biloba for Treatment of Dementia

Description
Ginkgo biloba is one of the oldest species of trees in the world, with fossils of the tree dating back to the dinosaurs. Ginkgo seeds and leaves have been used in traditional Chinese medicine for thousands of years. The tree is now planted throughout the world, including the United States.

History and Claims
In Chinese medicine, ginkgo was used to treat asthma, tinnitus, hypertonia, and angina. In Western medicine, the focus has been on treating depression and memory loss. In Germany, an extract of ginkgo biloba is approved for the treatment of dementia.

Standardization
Ginkgo biloba extract is often standardized to contain 24% ginkgo flavonoids and 6% terpenoids. A typical dose is 120 mg/day.

Evidence
In U.S. studies, 120 mg of ginkgo taken daily has been shown to improve mental functioning and stabilize AD. The mechanism of action seems to be related to increasing the blood supply to the brain by dilating blood vessels, decreasing the viscosity of the blood, modifying the neurotransmitter system, and decreasing the density of oxygen-free radicals (Birks & Evans, 2009). Studies concluded that cognitive performance and behavior stabilized or improved for a period of 6 to 12 months in patients with uncomplicated AD. However, not all evidence for ginkgo has been positive. A 6-year study involving over 3,000 older adults concluded that the administration of ginkgo does not delay or prevent the progression of AD (DeKosky et al., 2008). Patients should consult with their health care provider before taking this herb. Although most persons can take ginkgo without problems, those persons who are also taking anticoagulants, aspirin, or NSAIDs may have an increased risk for bleeding. Because the FDA does not approve herbal products, ginkgo and other herbs have not undergone the same scrutiny given to newly developed medications.

---

in the CNS, it produces fewer peripheral adverse effects than other drugs in this class.

Pharmacokinetics:

Route(s)	PO
Absorption	Completely absorbed
Distribution	Well distributed; crosses the blood–brain barrier; 96% bound to plasma proteins
Primary metabolism	Hepatic; metabolized to active metabolites
Primary excretion	Primarily renal; some feces
Onset of action	3–4 h
Duration of action	Half-life: 10 h, if single dose; 70 h if multiple dose

Adverse Effects: Common adverse effects of donepezil that cause discontinuation of therapy are diarrhea, nausea, and vomiting. Donepezil exhibits typical cholinergic effects such as diaphoresis, bradycardia, salivation, and muscle weakness. Other possible adverse effects are anorexia, muscle cramps, fatigue, arthralgia, abnormal dreams, and headache. Many of these adverse events will diminish with continued therapy or by using a lower dose of the drug. Potential life-threatening adverse effects include atrial fibrillation, sinus bradycardia, and seizures. Unlike tacrine (which was removed from the market in 2013), donepezil is not associated with hepatotoxicity. Abrupt discontinuation of the drug results in a sudden decline of cognitive function and an increase in behavioral disturbances.

Contraindications/Precautions: The only contraindication to the use of donepezil is hypersensitivity to the drug. There is a risk of GI bleeding, especially in patients with a history of peptic ulcers or NSAID use. It should be used with caution in patients with hyperthyroidism or hepatic dysfunction, or those who are lactating. Increased numbers of seizures have been recorded in patients taking donepezil, especially in those patients with a history of seizures.

Drug Interactions: Donepezil is metabolized by CYP 450 enzymes (CYP2D6 and CYP3A4), and drugs that enhance or inhibit these enzymes have the potential to interact with donepezil. Decreased effects of donepezil will occur with concurrent administration of phenytoin, phenobarbital, rifampin, dexamethasone, and carbamazepine. Concurrent use of NSAIDs may lead to GI ulceration and bleeding. Synergistic effects will occur with cholinergic agonists, cholinesterase inhibitors, and succinylcholine. Because it is a cholinergic agonist, donepezil will decrease the effects of anticholinergic drugs. Metabolism of donepezil may be inhibited by quinidine and ketoconazole. **Herbal/Food**: None known.

Pregnancy: Category C.

Treatment of Overdose: Overdosage will result in signs of cholinergic crisis, such as nausea, vomiting, bradycardia, respiratory depression, hypotension, and seizures. Anticholinergic drugs such as 1 to 2 mg IV atropine may be administered to reverse some of the overdose symptoms.

Nursing Responsibilities: Key nursing implications for patients receiving donepezil are included in the Nursing Practice Application for Patients Receiving Pharmacotherapy for Neurodegenerative Disorders.

Drugs Similar to Donepezil (Aricept)

Other cholinesterase inhibitors used to treat the symptoms of AD are galantamine and rivastigmine. Tacrine was discontinued in 2013 due to concerns regarding liver toxicity.

Galantamine (Razadyne): Galantamine is an oral cholinesterase inhibitor that has the same uses and actions as donepezil. Approved

◀ NSAIDS for Alzheimer's Disease

The use of NSAIDs for the prevention or treatment of AD has been under study for many years. As more is learned about how AD develops and progresses, therapies may be evaluated based on what is known about the disease. It is known that the development of amyloid deposits in the brain follows inflammation, and amyloid plaques have been a target for research in AD. NSAIDs such as aspirin, naproxen, and ibuprofen, as well as corticosteroids such as prednisone, may significantly decrease inflammation. However, it has been shown that they are not effective in treating AD and may be detrimental in later stages of the disease (Jaturapatporn, Isaac, McCleery, & Tabet, 2012). Recent research suggests that NSAIDs given *before* clinical symptoms develop may halt or slow the progression of the disease, though these drugs may need to be taken long-term, 2 years or longer, to achieve these effects (Breitner et al., 2011; Hoozemans, Veerhuis, Rozemuller, & Eikelenboom, 2011). Because AD symptoms do not develop until significant brain changes have occurred, it is difficult to determine when these drugs should be started; in addition, they have significant adverse effects, especially when given long-term.

　　AD is a devastating disease for the patient as well as the family and caregivers. Patients and their families may be desperate to try any possible method that holds promise of preventing or treating the disease. Because many NSAIDs are available over the counter (OTC), patients or family members may try them as a treatment therapy. Nurses should encourage patients and families to discuss this treatment with the health care provider before starting it. NSAIDs have significant adverse effects, such as GI bleeding and renal damage, and should not be taken for AD unless recommended by the provider.

in 2001, it is indicated for mild to moderate symptoms of dementia. Like other AD medications, it does not alter the progression of the disease. It is available in immediate and extended release (ER) forms. This drug was originally named Reminyl, but to avoid prescribing errors with the drug Amaryl (an antidiabetic drug), the FDA ordered the name changed to Razadyne.

The most frequent adverse effects are nausea and vomiting: The drug may be administered with food or with an antiemetic to reduce this effect. Other adverse reactions include diarrhea, bradycardia, chest pain, fatigue, anemia, syncope, vertigo, headache, insomnia, or tremor. Anorexia and weight loss are possible and may be serious effects in debilitated patients. In addition, it is not recommended for use in persons with severe hepatic or renal dysfunction or in children or a lactating woman. It must be used cautiously in persons with respiratory disease, bradycardia, cardiac conduction disorders, seizure history, history of GI bleeding, peptic ulcer disorder, or asthma. It is a pregnancy category C drug.

Rivastigmine (Exelon): Like other drugs in this class, rivastigmine inhibits brain cholinesterase more than heart or skeletal muscle cholinesterase. Approved in 2000, it is used to treat mild to moderate symptoms of dementia associated with AD and PD. It has similar effectiveness to donepezil. Rivastigmine is given PO with food to prevent nausea and vomiting, which frequently occur with this medication. Liquid preparations should be mixed only with water, soda, or juice. In 2007, a once-daily transdermal patch of rivastigmine was approved by the FDA for moderate to severe AD.

Rivastigmine is contraindicated in patients with hypersensitivity to rivastigmine or carbamate. Nausea, vomiting, anorexia, and diarrhea occur in a significant number of patients. The transdermal patch form of the drug causes a lower incidence of GI adverse effects. Other common adverse effects include headache, vertigo, abdominal pain, and confusion. Cautious use is indicated when given to patients with a hypersensitivity to cholinesterase inhibitors; cardiac, pulmonary, renal, or hepatic disease; diabetes; GI disorders; concurrent use of other cholinergic or anticholinergic drugs; PD; seizure history; or concurrent use of NSAIDs. No potential life-threatening adverse effects have been identified. It is a pregnancy category B drug.

Multiple Sclerosis

21.11 Multiple sclerosis is a chronic, neurodegenerative disease that is treated with immunomodulator drugs.

Multiple sclerosis (MS) is a neurodegenerative disease characterized by demyelination, the destruction or removal of the myelin sheath from a nerve or nerve fiber. The destruction is secondary to an inflammatory response that leads to random areas of demyelination, known as plaques, in the white matter of the CNS. The exact cause of MS is unknown. It is believed that a pathogen, such as a latent virus, may trigger an abnormal autoimmune response in patients who are genetically susceptible. MS is a leading cause of neurologic disability in the 20- to 40-year-old age group, although it may affect persons of any age (Figure 21.2).

MS has a typical pattern of progression that is characterized by periods of symptom exacerbation alternating with periods of remission during which symptoms completely disappear. Remissions may last several months or even years. Less commonly, progression may be continuous without any clear remission periods.

Diagnosis of MS is often difficult because its symptoms mimic those of other neurologic disorders. The early symptoms are frequently vague and nonspecific and include weakness, visual disturbances, paresthesias, mild affective disturbances, and difficulty with bladder control. Cognitive impairment is common. It should be determined if the symptoms are worsening or are intermittent. Also of note is whether the activity level of the patient has decreased, along with worsening fatigue, things that aggravate the symptoms (e.g., hot showers or baths, overexertion, stress), and any changes in personality or behavior. A diagnosis is made after other neurologic disorders have been ruled out. Imaging studies such as magnetic resonance imaging are useful in identifying the areas of demyelination in the brain.

Like other neurodegenerative disorders, there are no drugs available that can cure MS or reverse the progressive demyelination of nerves. Existing drugs for MS are only partially effective and some have serious adverse effects. In general, pharmacotherapy has the following three goals:

- Modify the progression of the disease.
- Treat acute exacerbations.
- Manage symptoms.

Drugs for modifying the progression of MS: Although the exact etiology of MS remains unknown, it is considered an autoimmune disease. The body has mounted an immune attack against its own tissues, in this case, the myelin surrounding nerves. Strategies for slowing the progression of MS have therefore focused on modifying the abnormal immune response of these patients through the

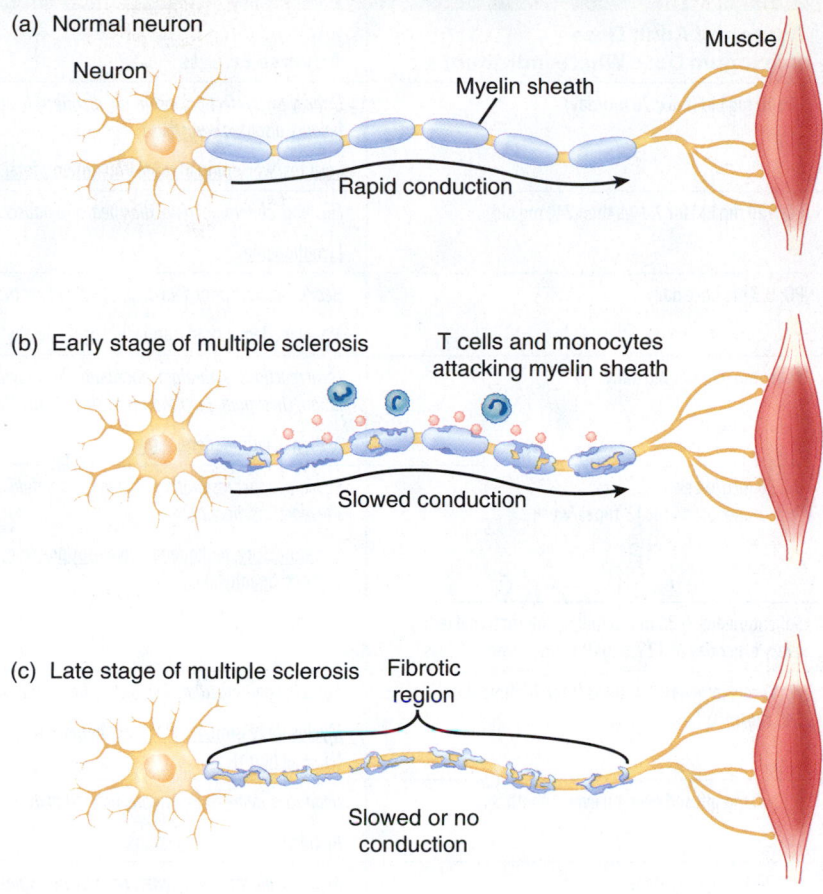

(a) Normal neuron

Neuron

Myelin sheath

Muscle

Rapid conduction

(b) Early stage of multiple sclerosis

T cells and monocytes
attacking myelin sheath

Slowed conduction

(c) Late stage of multiple sclerosis

Fibrotic
region

Slowed or no
conduction

Figure 21.2 Multiple sclerosis.

application of immunomodulators. **Immunomodulator** is a general term that refers to drugs that affect body defenses. There are two basic types of immunomodulators: those that stimulate or boost the immune response and those that suppress some aspect of immune function. Both types are used in MS pharmacotherapy. For detailed information on the immunomodulators, the student should refer to Chapter 42.

The immunomodulators are used to prevent exacerbations in patients with MS. They can decrease the number of new plaques being formed within the CNS, delay future disability, and help patients maintain their present quality of life. Immunomodulators are initiated soon after the diagnosis of MS is confirmed. The earlier treatment is begun, the better chance the patient has of avoiding or delaying permanent neurologic deficits. Treatment should continue indefinitely and only be stopped if toxicity develops or there is no apparent benefit. Doses of these drugs are listed in Table 21.7. The immunomodulators have equal efficacy in treating MS. Selection is frequently based on the clinical experiences of the health care provider and patient tolerance. They all are expensive, with monthly costs exceeding $2,000. Interferon beta-1a (Avonex, Rebif), interferon beta-1b (Betaseron, Extavia, Plegridy), and glatiramer (Copaxone) are immunomodulators used as first-line therapy to modify the progression of MS. All of these drugs require frequent self-administration, which increases the risk for injection-site reactions or abscess formation. The recent development of oral

drugs for MS will likely lead to additional first-line drugs that slow the progression of the disease.

PROTOTYPE DRUG	Interferon beta-1b (Betaseron, Extavia, Plegridy)

Classification: **Therapeutic:** Drug for relapsing forms of multiple sclerosis
Pharmacologic: Immunomodulator

Therapeutic Effects and Uses: Approved in 1993, interferon (IFN) beta-1b is produced by recombinant DNA technology and is very similar to natural IFN. It was one of the first drugs developed that was found to slow the progression of MS. Patients taking IFN beta-1b experience fewer relapses and a reduction in brain lesions characteristic of MS. This drug is available by subcutaneous injection for the treatment of patients with relapsing MS. In 2014, peginterferon beta-1b was approved, which extends the half-life of the drug such that it may be given once every 2 weeks.

Mechanism of Action: The mechanism of action of IFN beta-1b is unknown. It is believed to act by suppressing the activity of T cells and reducing the inflammatory actions of cytokines, which are substances secreted by activated T cells.

TABLE 21.7 Drugs Used to Treat Multiple Sclerosis

Drug	Route and Adult Dose (Maximum Dose Where Indicated)	Adverse Effects
dalfampridine (Ampyra)	PO: 10 mg bid (max: 20 mg/day)	*Urinary tract infection, insomnia, dizziness, headache, nausea, back pain, balance disorder, paresthesia* Seizures, worsening of renal impairment, fetal effects
dimethyl fumarate (Tecfidera)	PO: 120 mg bid for 7 days then 240 mg bid	*Flushing, abdominal pain, diarrhea, and nausea* Lymphopenia
fingolimod (Gilenya)	PO: 0.5 mg once daily	*Headache, back pain, diarrhea, elevated liver transaminase* Macular edema, bradycardia and other dysrhythmias
glatiramer (Copaxone)	Subcutaneous: 20 mg daily	*Local reactions, arthralgia, back pain, flulike symptoms, infection, anxiety, vasodilation, chest pain, palpitations, rash, pruritus, diarrhea, nausea, dyspnea, rhinitis* Asthenia, lymphadenopathy
interferon beta-1a (Avonex, Rebif)	IM: 30 mcg/week Subcutaneous: 44 mcg 3 times/week	*Myalgia, upper respiratory tract infection, flulike symptoms, injection-site reactions, headache* Hepatotoxicity, leukopenia, myelosuppression, severe depression (suicide risk), seizures, anaphylaxis
interferon beta-1b (Betaseron, Extavia, Plegridy)	Subcutaneous: 0.25 mg (8 million international units) every other day or 125 mcg (Plegridy) every 14 days	
mitoxantrone (Novantrone)	IV: 12 mg/m² every 3 months (max: lifetime dose 140 mg/m²)	*Nausea, vomiting, diarrhea, cough, headache, abdominal pain, fever, alopecia* Myelosuppression, renal failure, hepatotoxicity, cardiotoxicity (heart failure, MI, fetal harm)
natalizumab (Tysabri)	IV: 300 mg infused over 1 h every month	*Headache, depression, fatigue, menstrual dysfunction* Anaphylaxis (rare), infections
teriflunomide (Aubagio)	PO: 7–14 mg once daily	*Alopecia, diarrhea, influenza, nausea, paresthesia* Severe hepatotoxicity, teratogenicity, leukopenia, severe skin reactions

Note: Italics indicate common adverse effects. Underline indicates serious adverse effects.

Pharmacokinetics:

Route(s)	Subcutaneous
Absorption	50% absorbed
Distribution	Crosses the blood–brain barrier poorly; crosses placenta and enters breast milk
Primary metabolism	Rapidly metabolized in body tissues
Primary excretion	Unknown
Onset of action	6–12 h
Duration of action	Half-life: 8 min–4 h

Adverse Effects: Adverse effects are very common with IFN beta-1b. Most patients taking interferon beta-1b will experience transient flulike symptoms: Analgesics and antipyretics may be premedicated on injection days to reduce these symptoms. Injection-site reactions also occur in the majority of patients. Patients should be monitored closely for depression and suicidal ideation. Injection-site inflammation occurs in most patients and may progress to necrosis. Other common adverse effects include leukopenia, headache, insomnia, asthenia, increased liver enzymes, rash, peripheral edema, and malaise.

Contraindications/Precautions: The only contraindication is history of hypersensitivity to interferon beta, albumin, or mannitol.

Drug Interactions: Zidovudine (AZT) levels may increase to toxic levels during therapy. **Herbal/Food**: None known.

Pregnancy: Category C.

Treatment of Overdose: Treatment for overdose of this drug has not been documented.

Nursing Responsibilities: Key nursing implications for patients receiving interferon beta-1b are included in the Nursing Practice Application for Patients Receiving Pharmacotherapy for Neurodegenerative Disorders.

Drugs Similar to Interferon Beta-1b (Betaseron, Extavia, Plegridy)

Other drugs used to treat the relapsing symptoms of MS are dimethyl fumarate (Tecfidera), fingolimod (Gilenya), glatiramer (Copaxone), interferon beta-1a, mitoxantrone (Novantrone), natalizumab (Tysabri), and teriflunomide (Aubagio).

Dimethyl fumarate (Tecfidera): Approved in 2013, dimethyl fumarate is one of the newest drugs for treating relapsing forms of MS. Given PO, its mechanism of action is unknown. Adverse effects include mild to moderate flushing, abdominal pain, diarrhea, and nausea. Lymphocyte counts should be monitored during therapy because dimethyl fumarate can cause significant reductions in lymphoctyes. This drug is pregnancy category C.

Fingolimod (Gilenya): Approved in 2010, fingolimod has a unique mechanism of action in that it blocks the capacity of lymphocytes to exit lymph nodes. Because they remain in the nodes, there are fewer lymphocytes in peripheral tissues, including the CNS. The drug can reduce lymphocyte counts to 60% of baseline values within 4 to 6 hours after a single dose. Fingolimod is approved for the treatment of patients with relapsing forms of MS to reduce the annual relapse rate and to delay the accumulation of physical disability. A major advantage is that the drug is given PO with once-daily dosing. Unfortunately the drug has the potential to cause serious dysrhythmias: Patients must be carefully monitored for bradycardia and other cardiac rhythm abnormalities during therapy. Due to the diminished lymphocyte count, patients are at risk for infections. Macular edema is an adverse effect that is especially troublesome in patients with a history of uveitis or diabetes. The most common adverse effects are headache, influenza, diarrhea, back pain, cough, and elevated liver transaminase levels. Fingolimod is pregnancy category C.

Glatiramer (Copaxone): Approved in 1996, glatiramer is one of several first-line drugs in the treatment of relapsing MS, including patients who have experienced their initial clinical episode of the disease. The drug reduces the annual relapse rate for MS and the generation of new lesions in the brain. It is believed to activate suppressor T cells, which dampen the immune response. It is administered daily by the subcutaneous route. The most common adverse effects are injection-site reactions, vasodilation, weakness, dyspnea, and chest pain, which are usually transient. The drug is pregnancy category B.

IFN beta-1a (Avonex, Rebif): Approved in 1996, IFN beta-1a is made through recombinant DNA technology to be structurally identical to the natural IFN produced by the body. IFN beta-1a decreases the frequency of clinical exacerbations and slows the progression to physical disability, which is characteristic of MS. The drug acts by inhibiting the release of proinflammatory cytokines that initiate the autoimmune reaction leading to MS. IFN beta-1a also changes the blood–brain barrier and reduces T-lymphocyte migration into the brain, thereby reducing inflammation. It is available by the subcutaneous (Rebif) and IM (Avonex) routes. Adverse effects are similar to those of other IFNs, with flulike symptoms being observed in the majority of patients. Patients should be monitored for depression and suicidal ideation. Decreased peripheral blood counts, including thrombocytopenia and leukopenia, have been reported. Rare cases of severe hepatotoxicity, including some cases requiring liver transplantation, have been reported in patients taking IFN beta-1a. This drug is pregnancy category C.

Mitoxantrone (Novantrone): Mitoxantrone is an immuno-modulator that is primarily used to treat acute myelogenous leukemia and prostate cancer. In 2000, indications for the drug were extended to include MS but only for patients with chronic, progressive relapses. In treating MS, mitoxantrone acts by suppressing certain cells of the immune system, which can slow the progressive disability associated with MS. Fatigue and GI-related adverse effects are common. The most serious toxicities are myelosuppression and cardiotoxicity. The drug carries a black box warning that it may result in potentially fatal heart failure as long as several years after therapy is discontinued. It is only administered by IV infusion. This drug is pregnancy category D.

Natalizumab (Tysabri): Natalizumab is a monoclonal antibody that acts by preventing white blood cells from migrating to the CNS. This inhibition reduces the inflammation and demyelination of nerves in the brain. It is administered by IV infusion. Although effective for treating MS, its use is severely restricted due to a small risk of progressive multifocal leukoencephalopathy (PML), a rare and sometimes fatal demyelinating disease of the CNS. Natalizumab was briefly removed from the market in 2005 but has since been reapproved with restrictions that limit the prescribers to those who have special training in PML. Only patients of these "approved" health care providers may take the drug. In addition, only certain pharmacies can distribute the drug. The drug carries a black box warning for its risk of producing PML. Additional details on the monoclonal antibody class of drugs may be found in Chapter 42. Natalizumab is pregnancy category C.

Teriflunomide (Aubagio): Approved in 2012, teriflunomide is an oral drug for treating relapsing forms of MS. It is an active metabolite of leflunomide (Arava), an FDA-approved drug for treating rheumatoid arthritis. Teriflunomide acts by suppressing the division of B and T cells. Therapy with the drug reduces the incidences of annual relapse rates and the development of MS lesions in the brain. Teriflunomide is generally well tolerated; however, there are some serious toxicities associated with the drug. It carries a black box warning that severe, and sometimes fatal, liver injury may occur. In addition, the drug may cause birth defects and is Pregnancy Category X. This drug is eliminated very slowly and may take 8 to 24 months to be completely excreted from the body.

Drugs for treating acute exacerbations of MS: Acute exacerbations of the disease are treated with high-dose corticosteroid therapy with prednisone or methylprednisolone. The recommended length of treatment is no longer than 3 weeks and no more than three times a year. Although very high doses are administered, the short-term use of corticosteroids does not usually cause significant adverse effects (see Chapter 68). Another drug that can be used to treat an acute exacerbation is IV gamma globulin. This has proven to be a successful treatment for patients who are unresponsive or unable to tolerate corticosteroids.

Drugs for managing symptoms of MS: Many classes of medications may be ordered to manage symptoms of MS including antianxiety drugs, antidepressants, antipsychotics, or sedative–hypnotics. These symptomatic medications are used to treat other conditions and are discussed in other chapters of this text. The patient may experience physical symptoms such as muscle spasticity or bladder or bowel dysfunction. Depression is very common; it may be the emotional response to a diagnosis of a chronic, progressive, potentially debilitating disease, or it may be secondary to damage to mood-regulating neurons as the disease progresses. Chronic pain may require the use of analgesics. Approved in 2010, dalfampridine (Ampyra) is specifically indicated to improve walking in patients with MS.

Pain is experienced in up to 86% of patients with MS but it is not always well-classified. Research is ongoing to develop a classification system (O'Connor, Schwid, Herrmann, Markman, & Dworkin, 2008; Truini, Barbanti, Pozzilli, & Cruccu, 2013). Determining the cause of pain leads to more effective treatment strategies. For example, neuropathic pain caused by plaques in the spinal cord may respond to drugs such as amitriptyline or carbamazepine. Pain due to muscle spasms related to MS may be treated with baclofen and gabapentin. Because many patients with MS have mixed types of pain, thorough assessment is needed in order to determine the most effective therapy.

PharmFACT

Although it most commonly occurs in adults, it is estimated that 8,000 to 10,000 children have MS in the United States. Children have symptoms similar to those of adults but present with a higher incidence of seizures and mental status changes (National Multiple Sclerosis Society, n.d.).

Amyotrophic Lateral Sclerosis

21.12 The pharmacotherapy of amyotrophic lateral sclerosis is limited to a single drug.

Amyotrophic lateral sclerosis (ALS), commonly known as Lou Gehrig's disease, is the most common degenerative disease of the motor neurons. Its symptoms include weakness and atrophy of the muscles of the legs, hands, and forearms that spread to all muscles of the body. Sensory and cognitive functions are not affected. It usually occurs in middle age and progresses rapidly to death in 2 or 3 years due to respiratory failure or pneumonia. There is no known cause or curative treatment for the disease. About 10% of cases have a familial history of the disorder.

Only one drug has FDA approval for treating patients with ALS. Approved in 1995, riluzole (Rilutek) cannot cure the disease, but it has been proven to extend survival by reducing the degeneration of neurons. It is estimated that survival is prolonged by only 3 months. Riluzole is a tablet that is given every 12 hours on an empty stomach. The patient should avoid high-fat meals immediately before or after taking riluzole because it interferes with medication absorption. Seizures are the only life-threatening adverse effect. Common adverse effects include headache, dizziness, poor concentration, confusion, anxiety, hypotension, and edema.

The patient with ALS experiences painful muscle spasticity. Treatment with muscle relaxants such as baclofen (Lioresal) may bring some relief (see Chapter 23). Anticholinergic drugs such as trihexyphenidyl or benztropine may be administered to decrease saliva production. RimabotulinumtoxinB (Myobloc) may be used off-label to reduce saliva secretion for up to 3 months. Opioids may be necessary to treat severe pain late in the progress of the disease.

CONNECTIONS: NURSING PRACTICE APPLICATION

Patients Receiving Pharmacotherapy for Neurodegenerative Disorders

Assessment	Potential Nursing Diagnoses*
Baseline assessment prior to administration: • Obtain a complete health history including cardiovascular, musculoskeletal diseases, or glaucoma. Obtain a drug history including allergies, current prescription and OTC drugs, and herbal preparations. Be alert to possible drug interactions. • Obtain a history of the current disease and symptoms, exacerbating conditions, and ability to carry out ADLs, particularly mobility and eating. Consider safety concerns and whether alternative care environments are needed. • Evaluate appropriate laboratory findings such as hepatic or renal function studies. • Obtain baseline vital signs, bowel sounds, urinary output, muscle strength, and mental status as appropriate. • Assess for disturbances in thought processes, perception, verbal communication, affect, behavior, interpersonal relationships, and self-care. Use objective screening tools such as the Movement Disorders Society Unified Parkinson's Disease Rating Scale (MDS-UPDRS) or the Mini-Mental State Examination (MMSE) or as per health care agency. • Obtain a history of depression or sleep disorders and current treatments used. • Assess the patient's ability to receive and understand instructions. Include family or caregivers as needed.	• *Impaired Physical Mobility* • *Impaired Swallowing* • *Impaired Verbal Communication* • *Constipation* • *Self-Care Deficit: Bathing, Dressing, Feeding, Toileting* • *Disturbed Sleep Pattern* • *Ineffective Health Maintenance* • *Ineffective Family Health Management* • *Caregiver Role Strain* • *Deficient Knowledge* (Drug Therapy) • *Risk for Injury*, related to disease or adverse effects of drug therapy • *Risk for Falls*, related to disease or adverse effects of drug therapy
Assessment throughout administration: • Assess for desired therapeutic effects dependent on the reason for the drug (e.g., decreased tremors, bradykinesia, or rigidity, decreased agitation, fearfulness, and maintenance of current functioning level). • Continue periodic monitoring of vital signs, mental status, motor function, and the ability to carry out ADLs. • Assess for and promptly report adverse effects: hypotension, increasing tremors, dizziness, salivation, anorexia, dysphagia, nausea, vomiting, diarrhea, changes in heart rate or rhythm, or changes in mental status, including agitation or confusion.	

Implementation

Interventions and (Rationales)	Patient-Centered Care
Ensuring therapeutic effects: • Continue frequent assessments as above for therapeutic effects. Drug therapy may take several weeks or months to have full effect. Support the patient in self-care activities as necessary until improvement is observed. (The ability to carry out ADLs gradually improves with consistent usage of drug therapy in PD. Continued tremors, rigidity, or other symptoms may require dosage adjustment. Symptoms help determine the stage of the disease in AD and whether the medication remains therapeutic.)	• Teach the patient, family, or caregivers that gradual improvement in PD symptoms may be noted. The patient should report continued or increasing symptoms similar to those noted before drug therapy was initiated. • In AD, teach the patient, family, or caregivers that these drugs delay the progression of symptoms but do not treat or cure the underlying disease process. Increasing symptoms or decreasing the ability to perform self-care activities should be reported.

CONNECTIONS: NURSING PRACTICE APPLICATION (continued)

Minimizing adverse effects:

- Ensure patient safety; monitor motor coordination and ambulation, eating, or other essential motor activities. **Lifespan:** Be particularly cautious with older adults who are at increased risk for falls. (Gradual improvement in symptoms may be noticed over time, but the drug does not cure the underlying disorder, and symptoms may wax and wane over the course of the drug regimen. Particular care with ambulation is required in PD because bradykinesia and rigidity may increase the risk of falls.)

- Instruct the patient with PD to call for assistance prior to getting out of bed or attempting to walk alone if bradykinesia, rigidity, or tremors are particularly severe.
- Assess the ability of the patient, family, or caregivers to safely carry out ADLs at home, including previously safe activities such as cooking, walking alone, and living alone. Report changes that may require early intervention to the provider. Explore the need for additional health care referrals.

- Continue to monitor vital signs. Take blood pressure lying, sitting, and standing to detect orthostatic hypotension. **Lifespan:** Be particularly cautious with older adults who are at increased risk for hypotension. Notify the health care provider if blood pressure decreases beyond established parameters or if hypotension is accompanied by reflex tachycardia. (Orthostatic hypotension is a common adverse effect and may increase the risk of falls or injury.)

- Teach the patient to rise from lying to sitting or standing slowly to avoid dizziness or falls. If dizziness occurs, the patient should sit or lie down and not attempt to stand or walk until the sensation passes.

- Monitor for behavioral changes. (Drug therapy may increase the risk of agitation, confusion, depression, or suicidal thoughts, and may cause other mood disturbances such as aggressive behavior.)

- Teach the patient, family, or caregivers to watch for and report immediately any signs of changes in behavior or mood such as increased aggression or confusion. Provide additional health care referrals as required for a support group, counseling, or respite care.

- Carefully evaluate and report dose-related symptoms such as increased tremors and rigidity before the next dose is due or greatly increased symptoms unrelated to the timing of dose. (In PD, the return or gradual increase of symptoms as the next dose comes due may signal a wearing-off time and the dose may need to be increased, the interval of dosage adjusted, or an adjunctive drug added. A significant and sudden increase in symptoms may signal an overdose or on–off syndrome where symptoms dramatically increase. If symptoms are significant, hospitalization may be required to assess for the reason behind the exacerbation.)

- Instruct the patient, family, or caregivers to be aware of newly occurring muscle twitching, including blepharospasm (in the muscles of the eyelids), greatly increasing tremors, rigidity, sweating, or other symptoms, and to report them immediately.
- Encourage the patient, family, or caregivers to maintain a symptom diary if effects seem to diminish as the next dose is due. Review the diary with the patient on each health care visit.

- Evaluate nutritional intake. (Absorption of levodopa taken for PD decreases with high-protein meals or high consumption of foods or vitamins that contain vitamin B_6 [pyridoxine]. Symptoms may dramatically increase if absorption is impaired because the dose does not adequately absorb during the expected time. Patients with neurodegenerative disease may eventually experience difficulty in feeding themselves or with swallowing. Weigh the patient weekly to assess the effects of dietary intake.)

- Teach the patient to take medication for PD on an empty stomach or to avoid taking it with a high-protein meal. Avoid excessive consumption of vitamin B_6-rich foods such as bananas, wheat germ, fortified cereals, green vegetables, meat, and legumes, and avoid multivitamins that contain vitamin B_6.
- Teach the family or caregivers to assist the patient with AD with eating and to offer fluids on a regular basis.

- Monitor hepatic and renal function laboratory values periodically. (A decrease in these functions may slow metabolism and excretion of the drug, possibly leading to overdose or toxicity.)

- Teach the patient, family, or caregivers about the importance of returning for follow-up laboratory studies.

- Monitor for other drug-related changes. (PD replacement drug therapy may cause darkening of urine and perspiration.)

- Advise the patient that urine or sweat may darken and that undershirts or dress shields may help to avoid staining of clothing.

- Evaluate the family or caregivers for signs of stress, fatigue, or other effects related to caring for the patient with a neurodegenerative disease. (Caring for a patient with neurodegenerative disease is challenging and difficult. Additional social and financial resources may be needed, including alternative care environments.)

- Encourage the family or caregivers to discuss concerns related to their own health, financial status, or other issues.
- Provide additional health care referrals as required for a support group, counseling, or respite care.

Patient understanding of drug therapy:

- Use opportunities during administration of medications and during assessments to discuss the rationale for the drug therapy, desired therapeutic outcomes, commonly observed adverse effects, parameters for when to call the health care provider, and any necessary monitoring or precautions. (Using time during nursing care helps to optimize and reinforce key teaching areas.)

- The patient, family, or caregivers should be able to state the reason for the drug, appropriate dose and scheduling, and what adverse effects to observe for and when to report them.

Patient self-administration of drug therapy:

- When administering the medications, instruct the patient, family, or caregiver in proper self-administration of the drugs and the need for regular, consistent dosing. (Utilizing time during nurse-administration of these drugs helps to reinforce teaching.)

- Instruct the patient in proper administration guidelines. Encourage the patient, family, or caregivers to maintain a medication log, noting symptoms or adverse effects along with the dose and timing of medications.
- Patients taking injectable drug forms for the treatment of MS (e.g., interferon beta-1b [Betaseron]) should report increasing redness, pain, or blackening of the injection site, which may indicate that tissue necrosis is occurring.

*Nursing Diagnoses—Definitions and Classification 2015–2017. Copyright © 2014, 1994–2014 by NANDA International. Used by arrangement with John Wiley & Sons Limited.

Understanding the Chapter

Key Concepts Summary

21.1 Degenerative diseases of the central nervous system are characterized by irreversible and progressive loss of neuronal function.

21.2 Parkinson's disease is a progressive neurodegenerative disorder characterized by abnormal motor movement.

21.3 Parkinson's disease is caused by a lack of sufficient amounts of dopamine produced by the substantia nigra.

21.4 The drugs used for Parkinson's disease help to alleviate symptoms but do not cure the disease.

21.5 Replacement therapy with levodopa is the most effective therapy for treating Parkinson's disease.

21.6 Dopamine agonists may be used as monotherapy for early symptoms of Parkinson's disease or as adjuncts to levodopa in patients with advanced disease.

21.7 Several miscellaneous dopaminergic agents are used as adjuncts to levodopa therapy.

21.8 Anticholinergic drugs are the oldest of the antiparkinson agents and are effective at reducing tremor.

21.9 Alzheimer's disease, the most common dementia, leads to a progressive loss of cognitive function.

21.10 Pharmacotherapy of Alzheimer's disease produces only modest results and is ineffective at stopping the progression of the disorder.

21.11 Multiple sclerosis is a chronic, neurodegenerative disease that is treated with immunomodulator drugs.

21.12 The pharmacotherapy of amyotrophic lateral sclerosis is limited to a single drug.

Case Study: Making the Patient Connection

Remember the patient "Mary Lee" at the beginning of the chapter? Now read the remainder of the case study. Based on the information presented within this chapter, respond to the critical thinking questions that follow.

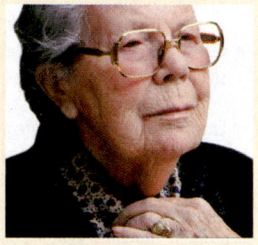

Mary Lee is a 73-year-old retired high school principal with a PhD in educational administration. She has been married to Robert for almost 50 years, and they have three grown children who live within 25 miles of them. Mary's physical health has been good. She has mild hypertension and had colon cancer successfully removed 20 years ago. She has an annual physical and cancer screenings as recommended for her age. Robert makes an appointment

with Mary's health care provider, because he has noticed signs of decreasing mental acuity over the past year. Mary's physical exam is negative, but the health care provider suspects that she is experiencing the early stage of AD. Mary is started on donepezil (Aricept), 5 mg at bedtime.

Critical Thinking Questions

1. What information should be included in the initial assessment in order to determine a diagnosis for Mary?

2. What recommendations will the health care provider most likely make to Mary and her husband?

3. What should Robert be alert for with regard to the donepezil?

See Answers to Critical Thinking Questions on student resource website.

Additional Case Study

Michael, at 45 years of age, could not believe his ears when the health care provider told him he had PD. "Isn't that an old person's disease?" he asked. However, he knew something had been very wrong for about 3 months. At first he felt more tired than usual, and he noticed a slight tremor, especially when he became fatigued. Michael's wife pointed out that his "hand shakes" were getting worse. Like many people first diagnosed with a degenerative nervous system disease, Michael has many questions and concerns. Following are just a few of his questions. As his nurse, how would you respond?

1. What physiological problem causes PD and what is the etiology of this disease? How could a nurse describe this etiology to Michael?

2. Eventually, Michael is prescribed levodopa/carbidopa (Sinemet) for his parkinsonism. How does this medication work? What is the advantage of combining the two medications?

3. What drug-related adverse effects would you discuss with Michael?

See Answers to Additional Case Study on student resource website.

Chapter Review

1 The patient is receiving levodopa/carbidopa for parkinsonism. Which drug would the nurse expect to be added to the patient's drug regimen to help control tremors?
1. Amantadine (Symmetrel)
2. Benztropine (Cogentin)
3. Haloperidol (Haldol)
4. Donepezil (Aricept)

2 Which statement, if made by the patient, would alert the nurse that the antiparkinson medication is effective?
1. "I'm sleeping a lot more, especially during the day."
2. "My appetite has improved."
3. "I'm able to shower by myself."
4. "My skin doesn't itch anymore."

3 The nurse is counseling the caregivers of a patient with Alzheimer's disease. Which statement, if made by a caregiver, would indicate that the session had been effective?
1. "I should give this medication as symptoms of AD become noticeable."
2. "If constipation occurs, I will notify the health care provider immediately."
3. "The medication may improve symptoms but will not cure the disease."
4. "I will take the patient's vital signs before every dose of the medication."

4 The nurse knows that which of the following is a major disadvantage for the use of donepezil (Aricept) to treat the symptoms of early Alzheimer's disease? Select all that apply.
1. Must be administered four times per day
2. Causes constipation
3. May cause vision difficulties
4. May cause potentially life-threatening cardiac dysrhythmias
5. Can be purchased over the counter

5 The nurse knows an advantage to rivastigmine (Exelon) over other cholinesterase inhibitors is that it:
1. Has no significant drug interactions.
2. Does not cause cholinergic adverse effects.
3. Is absorbed best on an empty stomach.
4. Does not alter glucose control in patients with diabetes.

6 Interferon beta-1b (Betaseron) has been ordered for the patient for treatment of MS. The nurse will instruct the patient on possible adverse effects that may be managed symptomatically by the patient. These include (select all that apply):
1. Flulike symptoms.
2. Insomnia.
3. Depression.
4. Rashes.
5. Pain at the injection site and blackening of the surrounding skin.

See Answers to Chapter Review in Appendix A.

References

Alzheimer's Association. (2014). *2014 Alzheimer's disease facts and figures.* Retrieved from http://www.alz.org/downloads/facts_figures_2014.pdf

Aviles-Olmos, I., Dickson, J., Kefalopoulou, Z., Djamshidian, A., Ell, P., Soderlund, T., . . . Foltynie, T. (2013). Exenatide and the treatment of patients with Parkinson's disease. *Journal of Clinical Investigation, 123,* 2730–2736. doi:10.1172/JCI68295

Birks, J., & Evans, J. G. (2009). Ginkgo biloba for cognitive impairment and dementia. *Cochrane Database of Systematic Reviews, 1,* CD003120. doi:10.1002/14651858.CD003120.pub3

Breitner, J. C., Baker, L. D., Montine, T. J., Meinert, C. L., Lyketsos, C. G., Ashe, K. H., . . . Tariot, P. N. (2011). Extended results of the Alzheimer's disease anti-inflammatory prevention trial. *Alzheimer's & Dementia, 7,* 402–411. doi:10.1016/j.jalz.2010.12.014

DeKosky, S. T., Williamson, J. D., Fitzpatrick, A. L., Kronmal, R. A., Ives, R. G., Saxton, J. A., . . . Furberg, C. D. (2008). Ginkgo biloba for prevention of dementia: A randomized controlled trial. *Journal of the American Medical Association, 300*(19), 2253–2262. doi:10.1001/jama.2008.683

Fan, R., Li, X., Gu, X., Chan, J. C., & Xu, G. (2010). Exendin-4 protects pancreatic beta cells from human islet amyloid polypeptide-induced cell damage: Potential involvement of AKT and mitochondria biogenesis. *Diabetes, Obesity & Metabolism, 12*, 815–824. doi:10.111/j.1463-1326.2010.01238.x

Harkavyi, A., & Whitton, P. S. (2010). Glucagon-like peptide 1 receptor stimulation as a means of neuroprotection. *British Journal of Pharmacology, 159*, 495–501. doi:10.1111/j.1476-5381.2009.00486.x

Hoozemans, J. J., Veerhuis, R., Rozemuller, J. M., & Eikelenboom, P. (2011). Soothing the inflamed brain: Effect of non-steroidal anti-inflammatory drugs on Alzheimer's disease. *CNS & Neurological Disorders Drug Targets, 10*(1), 57–67. doi:10.2174/187152711794488665

Jaturapatporn, D., Isaac, M. G., McCleery, J., & Tabet, N. (2012). Aspirin, steroidal and non-steroidal anti-inflammatory drugs for the treatment of Alzheimer's disease. *Cochrane Database of Systematic Reviews, 2*, CD006378. doi:10.1002/14651858.CD006378.pub2

Li, Y., Perry, T., Kindy, M. S., Harvey, B. K., Tweedie, D., Holloway, H. W.,… Greig, N. H. (2009). GLP-1 receptor stimulation preserves primary cortical and dopaminergic neurons in cellular and rodent models of stroke and parkinsonism. *Proceedings of the National Academy of Sciences of the United States of America, 106*, 1285–1290. doi:10.1073/pnas.0806720106

McIntyre, R. S., Powell, A. M., Kaidanovich-Beilin, O., Soczynska, J. K., Alsuwaidan, M., Woldeyohannes, H. O.,… Gallaugher, L. A. (2013). The neuroprotective effects of GLP-1: Possible treatments for cognitive deficits in individuals with mood disorders. *Behavioral Brain Research, 237*, 164–171. doi:10.1016/j.bbr.2012.09.021

National Multiple Sclerosis Society. (n.d.). *Pediatric (child) MS*. Retrieved from http://www.nationalmssociety.org/about-multiple-sclerosis/pediatric-ms/index.aspx

National Parkinson Foundation. (n.d.). *Statistics on Parkinson's*. Retrieved from http://www.pdf.org/en/parkinson_statistics

O'Connor, A. B., Schwid, S. R., Herrmann, D. N., Markman, J. D., & Dworkin, R. H. (2008). Pain associated with multiple-sclerosis: Systematic review and proposed classification. *Pain, 137*, 96–111. doi:10.1016/j.pain.2007.08.024

Salcedo, I., Tweedie, D., Li, Y., & Greig, N. H. (2012). Neuroprotective and neurotrophic actions of glucagon-like peptide-1: An emerging opportunity to treat neurodegenerative and cerebrovascular disorders. *British Journal of Pharmacology, 166*, 1586–1599. doi:10.1111/j.1476-5381.2012.01971.x

Truini, A., Barbanti, P., Pozzilli, C., & Cruccu, G. (2013). A mechanism-based classification of pain in multiple sclerosis. *Journal of Neurology, 260*(2), 351–367. doi:10.1007/s00415-012-6579-2

Selected Bibliography

Alzheimer's Association. (n.d.). *Treatments for sleep changes*. Retrieved from http://www.alz.org/alzheimers_disease_10429.asp#top

Corbett, A., Pickett, J., Burns, A., Corcoran, J., Dunnett, S. B., Edison, P., . . . Ballard, C. (2012). Drug repositioning for Alzheimer's disease. *Nature Reviews Drug Discovery, 11*, 833–846. doi:10.1038/nrd3869

Herdman, T. H., & Kamitsuru, S. (Eds.). (2014). *NANDA International nursing diagnoses: Definitions and Classification, 2015–2017*. Oxford, United Kingdom: Wiley-Blackwell.

Miller, C. E., & Umhauer, M. A. (2011). Emerging oral therapies for multiple sclerosis. *Journal of Neuroscience Nursing, 43*, 3–14. doi:10.1097/JNN.0b013e31820297a9

Ontaneda, D., Hyland, M., & Cohen, J. A. (2012). Multiple sclerosis: New insights in pathogenesis and novel therapeutics. *Annual Review of Medicine, 63*, 389–404. doi:10.1146/annurev-med-042910-135833

Piau, A., Nourhashémi, F., Hein, C., Caillaud, C., & Vellas, B. (2011). Progress in the development of drugs in Alzheimer's disease. *Journal of Nutritional Health and Aging, 15*, 45–57. doi:10.1007/s12603-011-0012-x

Querfurth, H. W., & LaFerla, F. M. (2010). Alzheimer's disease. *New England Journal of Medicine, 362*, 329–344. doi:10.1056/NEJMra0909142

Smith, B., Carson, S., Fu, R., McDonagh, M. S., Dana, T., Chan, B., . . . Gibler, A. (2010). *Drug class review: Disease-modifying drugs for multiple sclerosis. Final Update 1*. Retrieved from http://www.ncbi.nlm.nih.gov/books/NBK50570

Varanese, S., Birnbaum, Z., Rossi, R., & Di Rocco, A. (2010). Treatment of advanced Parkinson's disease. *Parkinson's Disease, 2010* (Article ID 480260, 9 pages). doi:10.4061/2010/480260

Wipfler, P., Harrer, A., Pilz, G., Oppermann, K., Trinka, E., & Kraus, J. (2011). Recent developments in approved and oral multiple sclerosis treatment and an update on future treatment options. *Drug Discovery Today, 16*, 8–21. doi.org/10.1016/j.drudis.2010.10.011

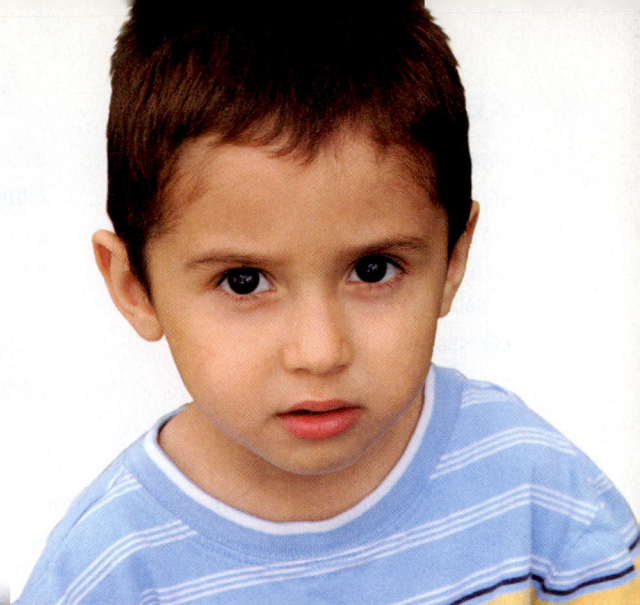

"I'm not sure I can cope with my child having a seizure disorder. The schedule for giving the medicines seems daunting to me. I am not sure I will remember all of the steps to watch for when he has a seizure. Also, I am not sure I understand all the aspects of the medications and how they work."

Patient "Jorge Alvarez's" mother

CHAPTER 22

Pharmacotherapy of Seizures

LEARNING OUTCOMES

After reading this chapter, the student should be able to:

1. Understand the causes of epilepsy.
2. Differentiate among the following terms: *epilepsy*, *seizures*, and *convulsions*.
3. Describe how the presentation and pharmacotherapy of epilepsy change throughout the lifespan.
4. Differentiate the signs, symptoms, and treatment of the different types of seizure disorders.
5. Compare and contrast the pharmacotherapy of generalized and partial seizures.
6. Identify factors that influence the selection of a specific antiepileptic drug by the health care provider.
7. Describe the nurse's role in the pharmacologic management of seizures.
8. For each of the classes shown in the chapter outline, identify the prototype and representative drugs and explain the mechanism(s) of drug action, primary indications, contraindications, significant drug interactions, pregnancy category, and important adverse effects.
9. Apply the nursing process to care for patients receiving antiseizure drugs.

CHAPTER OUTLINE

▶ Characteristics of Seizure Disorders

▶ Classification of Seizure Disorders
Generalized Seizures
Partial Seizures

▶ Antiepileptic Drugs
Barbiturates
Benzodiazepines
PROTOTYPE Diazepam (Valium), *p. 320*
Hydantoins
PROTOTYPE Phenytoin (Dilantin, Phenytek), *p. 322*
Dibenzazepines
PROTOTYPE Carbamazepine (Carbatrol, Tegretol, Others), *p. 323*
Succinimides
PROTOTYPE Ethosuximide (Zarontin), *p. 325*
Miscellaneous Antiepileptics
PROTOTYPE Gabapentin (Neurontin), *p. 326*
PROTOTYPE Valproic Acid (Depacon, Depakene, Depakote), *p. 326*
Other Miscellaneous Drugs

KEY TERMS

absence seizures, 313

atonic seizures, 313

automatisms, 314

complex partial
seizures, 314

convulsions, 310

eclampsia, 311

epilepsy, 310

febrile seizures, 314

generalized seizures, 313

infantile spasm, 315

Lennox-Gastaut syndrome, 315

myoclonic seizures, 314

partial (focal) seizures, 314

postictal state, 313

preeclampsia, 311

seizure, 310

simple partial seizures, 314

status epilepticus, 315

tonic–clonic seizures, 313

The word *epilepsy* is derived from the Greek word "epilepsia," meaning to take hold or seize. Epilepsy is a neurologic condition characterized by recurrent seizures that affects approximately 2 million Americans. Research in the past two decades has resulted in the development of new drugs to treat epilepsy and other seizure disorders. In this chapter the student will study the current medications for seizures and understand the nurse's role in the administration and patient education associated with the medication regimen.

Characteristics of Seizure Disorders

22.1 Epilepsy is characterized by recurrent seizures caused by disturbances in the electrical activity of the brain.

Epilepsy is a disruption of the activity of clusters of neurons in the brain that is characterized by two or more seizures. A **seizure** is a disturbance of the brain's electrical activity that may result in loss of consciousness, sensory malfunction, and an alteration in motor activity. The many diverse symptoms of seizure are caused by abnormal neuronal discharges within the different regions of the brain. Abnormal neuronal discharges can be measured as sharp spikes or waves on an electroencephalogram (EEG), which is a valuable tool in diagnosing seizure disorders.

When a patient presents with symptoms of a seizure, it is important to identify the cause of seizure activity so that the appropriate treatment regimen can be implemented. Epileptic seizures are sometimes symptoms of an underlying disorder such as a brain tumor, head trauma, brain aneurysm, stroke, alcoholism, or infectious disease of the brain. The diagnosis of epilepsy always begins with a search for an underlying disorder that could explain the seizures. Table 22.1 lists common etiologies for seizure disorders. Successful treatment of the underlying condition often eliminates the seizure activity. If a brain abnormality remains after the acute seizure has resolved, recurrent seizures are likely.

In 50% to 70% of cases, the etiology of a seizure is idiopathic; no specific cause can be identified. These patients may have a lower tolerance to environmental triggers, and seizures may occur when they are sleep deprived, are exposed to strobe or flickering lights, or have a fluid and electrolyte imbalance. Diagnostic tests such as complete blood count (CBC), serum lead levels, and blood glucose are important in excluding the systemic causes of seizures. Virtually anything that changes the homeostatic environment of neurons in the brain has the potential to cause seizures, thus complicating the diagnosis and treatment of epilepsy.

It is important to distinguish between the terms *convulsion* and *seizure*. Most often, patients associate epilepsy with **convulsions**, which are involuntary, violent spasms of the large skeletal muscles of the face, neck, arms, and legs. Convulsions are a characteristic

TABLE 22.1	Etiology of Seizure Disorders
Etiology	**Pathophysiology**
Fever	Rapid increase in body temperature may result in febrile seizure. This is particularly noted in infants and toddlers.
Infectious disease	Meningitis and encephalitis, which are infections of the brain, result in brain inflammation and seizure development.
Metabolic disorders	Alteration in the fluid and electrolyte levels can result in seizure development. Hypoglycemia, hyponatremia, and water intoxication contribute to the alteration in electrical impulse transmission at the cellular level.
Miscellaneous causative agents	Medication used to treat mood disorders and psychotic episodes and local anesthetics produce increased levels of stimulatory neurotransmitters or toxicity. Drug abuse, such as cocaine addictions, alters the neurotransmitters in the brain and produces seizures. Alcohol and sedative–hypnotic drug withdrawal can result in seizure activity.
Neoplastic disorders	Both benign and malignant brain lesions, particularly those that grow rapidly, prevent adequate oxygenated blood supply to the brain tissue and contribute to increased intracranial pressure, which results in seizure development.
Trauma	Head injuries may result in increased intracranial pressure, which results in seizure development. Exposure to toxic fumes or substances, or ingestion of poisons, can result in trauma to brain tissue and resultant seizures.
Vascular disorders	Hypoxia of brain tissue disrupts the electrical transmission of impulses contributing to seizure development. Carbon monoxide poisoning reduces the oxygen-carrying ability of the blood and results in cerebral hypoxia. The related ischemia of brain tissue alters the electrical transmission of impulses and contributes to seizure development. Other vascular causes of seizures include hypotension, stroke, shock, and cardiac dysrhythmias.

sign of tonic–clonic seizures. Many forms of epilepsy, however, do not involve convulsions. For example, absence seizures do not involve any dramatic movement of the limbs and may be barely noticeable by those observing the affected person. Thus, it may be stated that all convulsions are seizures, but not all seizures are convulsions. Because of this difference, drugs used to treat epilepsy are best described as antiepileptic drugs (AEDs) or antiseizure medications, rather than anticonvulsants.

PharmFACT

Adults with early Alzheimer's disease who have epilepsy present with cognitive decline almost 7 years earlier (age 64) than those who do not have epilepsy (age 71). The start of seizure activity coincides with the beginning of cognitive decline (Vossel et al., 2013).

Seizures have the potential to significantly impact one's quality of life. They may cause serious injury if they occur while a person is driving a vehicle or performing a potentially hazardous activity. Without pharmacotherapy, epilepsy can severely limit participation in school, employment, and social activities and affect self-esteem. Chronic depression may accompany poorly controlled seizures. Proper treatment, however, can reduce or completely eliminate seizures in many patients. Important considerations in nursing care include identifying patients at risk for seizures, documenting the pattern and type of seizure activity, and implementing safety precautions. In collaboration with the patient, health care provider, and pharmacist, the nurse is instrumental in achieving positive therapeutic outcomes during AED therapy. The nurse must educate patients that effective seizure control is usually achieved through a combination of pharmacotherapy and support from family and caregivers.

22.2 Seizure disorders differ throughout the lifespan.

Seizure disorders occur throughout the lifespan. Of those who experience seizures, about half will experience their first seizure before age 10. Because of this, epilepsy is considered a major disorder of childhood. Fortunately, many patients who have childhood epilepsy experience a reduction in symptoms as they age, and some will no longer require pharmacotherapy as adults. In addition to childhood, epilepsy manifests with higher frequency during pregnancy and in older adults. Treatment of epilepsy differs throughout the lifespan.

Women, pregnancy, and lactation: The pharmacotherapy of epilepsy in women with childbearing potential can be challenging. These patients require special education to prevent conception during AED pharmacotherapy or to safely prevent seizures during pregnancy.

Some AEDs interact with oral contraceptives, diminishing the effectiveness of birth control pills. AEDs that are inducers of hepatic CYP450 enzymes will increase the metabolism of contraceptive hormones, thus decreasing their effectiveness in preventing conception. Antiseizure drugs that induce CYP450 include phenobarbital, carbamazepine, oxcarbazepine, topiramate, and phenytoin. To prevent an unplanned pregnancy, the patient should receive a higher dose of oral contraceptive and be instructed to use a backup method of birth control such as condoms. Therapy with antiseizure drugs that do not induce CYP450 enzymes, such as valproic acid or gabapentin, should be considered for these women.

Pregnancy is a major concern for women with seizure disorders. Women with epilepsy have a higher risk for delivering a child with congenital abnormalities, and many of the AEDs have the potential to produce teratogenic effects. The risk of birth defects is further increased because some AEDs cause folic acid (folate) deficiency, a condition that has been associated with increased risk of neural tube defects in the embryo. Folic acid supplements (0.4 to 4 mg per day) should always be recommended for women who are considering pregnancy and those who become pregnant. The use of vitamin supplementation will also reduce the risk of developing cardiac abnormalities and cleft lip or palate. Single drug therapy should be used whenever possible because therapy with multiple AEDs results in a higher risk of birth defects. Doses are reduced to the lowest possible level that effectively controls the seizures. Newer AEDs such as lamotrigine, gabapentin, and zonisamide should be considered because they appear to have less teratogenicity.

Women who have epilepsy have a reduced fertility rate. Epilepsy and AEDs can disrupt the hypothalamus–pituitary axis, causing menstrual irregularities. The length of the menstrual cycle in these patients may vary from 23 to 35 days, and 40% of women with epilepsy have polycystic ovaries. Many women who have epilepsy do not ovulate. Genital blood flow is diminished and libido is reduced, contributing to a reduction in the frequency of intercourse.

Vitamin K deficiency in neonates has been noted as a result of AED therapy during pregnancy. According to the American Academy of Neurology (2008), it is recommended that prenatal vitamin K be prescribed to women who are taking AEDs during pregnancy to prevent hemorrhagic disease in the newborn; 10 mg of vitamin K should be administered daily beginning on the 36th week of gestation and continuing until delivery.

Gestational epilepsy is a rare condition in which the patient experiences her first seizure during pregnancy. Seizures in a pregnant patient who has never been diagnosed with epilepsy may indicate the development of preeclampsia or eclampsia. **Preeclampsia** usually begins after the 20th week of pregnancy and is diagnosed by blood pressure of 140/90 mmHg or higher on two separate occasions, and 300 mg of protein is found in the urine over a 24-hour period. The rate of preeclampsia in the United States is approximately 5% to 7% of all pregnancies, affecting about 1 in every 2,000 to 3,000 deliveries.

Eclampsia occurs if hypertension (HTN) continues to worsen during pregnancy. Eclampsia is associated with seizures and a high risk of cerebral edema, which can result in coma. If the baby is of proper gestational age, delivery is the treatment of choice for eclampsia. When the pregnant woman is diagnosed with preeclampsia or eclampsia and delivery is not imminent, intravenous (IV) magnesium sulfate may be administered to prevent or terminate seizures. Magnesium sulfate acts by decreasing the amount of acetylcholine liberated from the motor nerve terminals and produces a peripheral neuromuscular blockade. It also has the therapeutic effect of increasing uterine blood flow. Because seizures may extend beyond labor and delivery, magnesium sulfate therapy may continue for 24 hours postpartum or until the HTN resolves.

Because the amounts of AEDs secreted in breast milk are low, breast-feeding may be allowed during AED therapy. The benefits of breast-feeding outweigh the potential adverse effects caused by

CONNECTIONS   Complementary and Alternative Therapies

◀ The Ketogenic Diet

Description
The ketogenic diet is used when seizures cannot be controlled through pharmacotherapy or when the adverse effects of an AED medication are unacceptable. Before antiepileptic drugs were developed, this diet was a primary treatment for epilepsy.

History and Claims
The ketogenic diet may be used for babies, children, or adults. With adults, however, it is harder to develop the ketones that are necessary for the diet.

Standardization
The ketogenic diet is a stringently calculated diet that is high in fat and low in carbohydrates and protein. It limits water intake to avoid ketone dilution and carefully controls caloric intake. Each meal has the same ketogenic ratio of 4 g of fat to 1 g of protein and carbohydrate. Extra fat is usually given in the form of cream.

Evidence
Research suggests that the diet produces a success rate, in some cases, that is equivalent to that of modern antiepileptic drugs (Levy, Cooper, Giri, & Pulman, 2012). The diet appears to be equally effective for every seizure type, although those with drop attacks (atonic seizures) may be the most rapid responders. It also helps children with Lennox-Gastaut syndrome and shows promise in babies with infantile spasms. Adverse effects include hyperlipidemia, constipation, vitamin deficiencies, kidney stones, acidosis, and, possibly, slower growth rates. Those interested in trying the diet must consult with their health care provider. This is not a do-it-yourself diet and may be harmful if not carefully monitored by skilled professionals. Recent studies have examined the possibility that the ketogenic diet could provide benefit for patients with other neurologic disorders such as Alzheimer's disease, Parkinson's disease, and amyotrophic lateral sclerosis (Stafstrom & Rho, 2012).

the drugs (American Academy of Neurology, 2008). Later research confirms that breast-feeding does not affect the cognitive development of children exposed to AEDs in breast milk (Meador et al., 2010). AEDs that have the most protein binding are least likely to appear in high concentration in breast milk. Those with the highest degree of protein binding include phenytoin, tiagabine, and valproic acid. The nurse should instruct mothers taking sedating antiepileptic drugs how to monitor neonates for sedation.

CONNECTION Checkpoint 22.1

From what you learned in Chapter 8, how does each of the following affect the amount of drug that passes to the infant during lactation: lipid solubility of the drug, drug ionization, and drug half-life? *See Answer to Connection Checkpoint 22.1 on student resource website.*

Childhood: Seizures in children are either idiopathic or acquired. Children with idiopathic seizures often have a family history of epilepsy or have an associated serious neurologic abnormality, such as mental retardation or cerebral palsy. Febrile seizures are another form of idiopathic seizure that occurs in children under the age of 2 years. Seizures represent the most common serious neurologic problem affecting children, with an overall incidence of approximately 1% for idiopathic epilepsy.

Acquired seizure disorders may result from injury to the brain during the prenatal, antenatal, or postpartum periods. Infants whose mothers have been exposed to cytomegalovirus during pregnancy are at increased risk of developing an acquired seizure disorder. Other causes of acquired seizures include head trauma, metabolic imbalances, exposure to toxins, and infection.

Seizure treatment for infants and children is usually accomplished with pharmacotherapy. The most commonly prescribed pediatric AEDs include phenobarbital, valproic acid, phenytoin, carbamazepine, felbamate, lamotrigine, and topiramate. To maintain optimum seizure control, the dosage of AEDs should be increased during periods of rapid growth and development.

Nonpharmacologic treatments for epilepsy are available. One such alternative therapy is the ketogenic diet. The beneficial effects of this diet occur when ketones are eliminated from the body,

thus decreasing seizure activity. Other forms of seizure treatment include surgical intervention with an excision of a circumscribed area of the brain affected by the seizure activity. The implantation of a vagal nerve stimulator in the brain is a type of therapy that delivers electrical signals to the vagus nerve to reduce the frequency of seizures.

Older adults: Seizure disorders in the older adult are often idiopathic or associated with an underlying comorbid condition. Stroke accounts for one third of new-onset cases and is the most common risk factor for the development of epilepsy after age 60. Other conditions associated with epilepsy in the aging patient include progressive Alzheimer's disease, subdural hematoma from a head injury due to falling, central nervous system (CNS) infection, and brain tumors.

Older adults often take multiple medications that can contribute to seizure activity. It is vital to regularly monitor the liver and kidney functions of the elderly patient when administering multiple medications because impairment may lead to toxic serum drug levels and possible seizures.

The nurse needs to assess the patient's therapeutic response to the AEDs as well as monitor the serum drug level. The clinical response should be used to guide the needed dosage changes. When possible, only a single AED is prescribed because the use of multiple AEDs increases the risk of adverse drug events. In most patients, therapy with AEDs begins with low doses followed by careful monitoring for drug effectiveness. Gradual dosage changes are made based on clinical outcomes.

Older patients with memory deficits may have difficulty remembering to take their AEDs. The nurse should teach these patients and their caregivers that these medicines must be taken on a regular basis, at the same time each day, for the most effective seizure prevention. If a dose is forgotten, the nurse should teach these patients not to take a double dose of an AED because this could cause serious CNS toxicity. Furthermore, patients need to understand that waiting until the first sign of a seizure before taking their AED is ineffective at stopping the seizure because the drug will not be absorbed quickly enough.

Classification of Seizure Disorders

22.3 Most seizures are classified as generalized or partial.

Seizures begin with the firing of hyperexcitable neurons in the brain. The area where the abnormal electrical activity starts is known as an abnormal focus (plural = foci). As these neurons discharge impulses, the patient begins to exhibit the characteristic signs and symptoms of epilepsy. The specific symptoms depend on the nature of the discharge: the location of the abnormal focus in the brain and the extent of the discharge. Because symptoms vary widely from patient to patient, there are many ways to classify seizures. It is important to identify and classify the type of seizure experienced by the patient because this determines which drugs will be prescribed. There are two broad categories of seizure activity: generalized and partial. Preferred drugs for the management of seizures are shown in Table 22.2.

Generalized Seizures

In **generalized seizures**, multiple foci spread abnormal neuronal discharges across both hemispheres of the brain simultaneously. The patient often experiences loss of consciousness, and the seizure may occur with or without convulsions. The four primary types of generalized seizures are tonic–clonic seizures, absence seizures, atonic seizures, and myoclonic seizures.

Tonic–clonic seizures, also referred to as grand mal seizures, are the type of seizure most associated by the public with epilepsy. It is the most common type of seizure in every age group. The seizure may be preceded by an aura, a warning that a seizure is imminent, that some patients describe as a spiritual feeling, flash of light, or special noise. Neurologists consider the aura to be part of the actual seizure. Loss of consciousness and intense muscle contractions indicate the tonic phase. A hoarse cry may occur at the onset of the seizure due to air being forced out of the lungs, and patients may temporarily lose bladder or bowel control. Breathing may become shallow and even stop momentarily. The clonic phase is characterized by alternating contraction and relaxation of muscles that are characteristic of convulsions. The seizure usually lasts 1 to 2 minutes, after which the patient becomes drowsy and disoriented and sleeps deeply. The period following the seizure is known as the **postictal state**.

Absence seizures, formerly known as petit mal seizures, most often occur in children and last only a few seconds. Approximately half of the patients with absence seizures may also experience at least one tonic–clonic seizure. Absence seizures involve a reduction of normal brain activity. Staring and transient loss of responsiveness are the most common signs, but there may be slight motor activity with eyelid fluttering or muscular jerking movements. These episodes are subtle and can be mistaken for daydreaming or inattention, such as is seen in attention deficit/hyperactivity disorder (ADHD). Children with absence seizures may experience poor academic performance because these episodes can occur several times per day. Most children who experience absence seizures will "outgrow" the disorder and become seizure free in adulthood.

Atonic seizures are sometimes known as drop attacks, due to the fact that the patient will stumble and fall for no apparent reason. The episode is short and lasts only a few seconds. The patient loses control of muscle function throughout the body. During the episode of weakness, the patient's head will droop forward or the trunk muscles will not support the patient, thus causing the drop

TABLE 22.2   Drugs Used for the Management of Seizures

Type of Seizure	First-Line Drugs*	Alternative Drugs
Generalized Seizures		
Absence	ethosuximide, lamotrigine, valproic acid	clonazepam
Atonic	clonazepam, valproic acid	lamotrigine, levetiracetam, topiramate
Myoclonic	valproic acid	clonazepam, lamotrigine, phenobarbital, topiramate
Tonic–Clonic	carbamazepine, lamotrigine, valproic acid	clonazepam, diazepam, levetiracetam, oxcarbazepine, phenobarbital, phenytoin, topiramate, zonisamide
Partial Seizures		
Complex partial	carbamazepine, lamotrigine, phenytoin	gabapentin, oxcarbazepine, phenobarbital, pregabalin, tiagabine, topiramate, zonisamide
Simple partial	carbamazepine, lamotrigine, phenytoin, valproic acid	clorazepate, diazepam, felbamate, gabapentin, levetiracetam, oxcarbazepine, phenobarbital, pregabalin, tiagabine, topiramate, zonisamide
Other Seizures		
Alcohol withdrawal	lorazepam or diazepam	carbamazepine
Febrile	acetaminophen for prophylaxis	diazepam, phenytoin
Infantile spasms	adrenocorticotropic hormone (ACTH)	none
Lennox-Gastaut	benzodiazepines, valproic acid	felbamate, rufinamide
Status epilepticus	lorazepam	diazepam, phenobarbital, phenytoin, valproic acid

*Drugs of choice vary according to patient age and comorbid conditions, prescriber experiences, institution, and geographical region.

CONNECTIONS Evidence-Based Practice

Seizures in the Older Adult

Clinical Question

How is epilepsy different in the older adult population?

Evidence

The incidence of epilepsy over a lifetime has the highest frequency in the very young and the very old (Beghi, Savica, Beghi, Nobili, & Garattini, 2009). In the older adult, stroke, Alzheimer's disease, and head trauma are common causes (Epilepsy Foundation of America, n.d.a). Other factors contributing to the development of seizures in the older adult include malignant and benign brain tumors, metabolic disorders such as electrolyte imbalances, diabetes, renal failure, and psychiatric illness (Acar & Salinsky, 2010).

The diagnosis and treatment of seizure disorders in the older adult is complicated by the existence of comorbidities. For example, diagnosis may be delayed when confusion, behavior changes, dysphagia, weakness, or other symptoms are present and could be explained by another disease process. All older adults found either unconscious or confused on the floor should have an EEG performed with follow-up monitoring, and a seizure disorder suspected until ruled out. Older adults are more susceptible to the adverse effects of AED therapy. Older AEDs have been shown to treat seizures in the older adult successfully, but new drugs such as lamotrigine (Lamictal) and gabapentin

(Neurontin) may have the added benefits of a reduced incidence of adverse effects. In the older adult population, cost must be considered when a newer drug is prescribed (Beghi et al., 2009).

Implications

The nurse caring for older adult patients should always be alert to the possibility of an underlying seizure disorder, particularly when a patient is admitted who has fallen or has been found unconscious. If a seizure disorder is confirmed, the nurse should be cautious in administering and monitoring AEDs because changes in metabolism and excretion related to aging, and the existence of other disease conditions, may increase the risk of adverse effects. If a newer AED is prescribed, the nurse should discuss any concerns about cost with the patient and provide appropriate referrals to social service assistance as needed.

Critical Thinking Questions

What role does the nurse play in the assessment and treatment of the older adult with a suspected seizure disorder?

See Answer to Critical Thinking Question on student resource website.

attack. Although the seizure itself causes no serious harm, the patient is at risk of injury due to falls.

Myoclonic seizures are generalized seizures characterized by jerking body movements, usually involving the muscles of the neck, shoulders, and upper arms. Major muscle groups contract quickly, usually for only a few seconds, and patients appear unsteady and clumsy. These patients do not lose consciousness but may fall or drop whatever they might be holding. Most patients with myoclonic seizures also exhibit tonic–clonic or absence seizures, or both. Myoclonic seizures usually begin around puberty and comprise 5% to 10% of all epilepsies. Although these seizures continue for the life of the patient, they can be controlled with pharmacotherapy. Valproic acid has been the traditional drug of choice for myoclonic seizures but newer AEDs such as topiramate and lamotrigine are being increasingly prescribed.

Partial Seizures

Partial (focal) seizures involve a limited portion of the brain, with the abnormal neuronal discharges starting on one side and traveling only a short distance before they stop. Many partial seizures do not involve loss of consciousness or convulsions, although discharge may begin as a partial seizure and become a generalized seizure. Some symptoms are subtle and reflect the simple nature of neuronal misfiring in limited areas of the brain, whereas other symptoms may be more complex.

Simple partial seizures have an onset that begins at a small, regional focus. Patients with simple partial seizures experience a wide array of symptoms depending on the specific region of the brain affected. If the motor cortex is affected, jerky, rhythmic contractions of a specific muscle group are noted. Seizures affecting the sensory cortex are less noticeable to an observer. Patients may feel for a brief moment that their precise location is vague, they may hear or see things that are not present, or they may have an upset

stomach. Senses of hearing, taste, smell, or sensation may be affected. Other patients become emotional and experience a sense of joy, fear, or grief. Consciousness is retained during the seizure, although the patient may express amnesia about the event. Numerous AEDs are available to treat simple partial seizures.

Complex partial seizures (formerly known as psychomotor or temporal lobe seizures) originate from a single focus, usually in the temporal lobe of the brain. Patients exhibit sensory, motor, or autonomic symptoms with some degree of altered or impaired consciousness. Total loss of consciousness may not occur during a complex partial seizure, but a brief period of somnolence or confusion may follow the episode. Complex partial seizures are usually preceded by an aura that may be described as an unpleasant odor or taste, colored spots, unexplained fear, or tingling. Seizures may start with a blank stare and proceed to repetitive arm movements, leg movements, head rolling, chewing, lip-smacking, or swallowing. These repetitive movements are called **automatisms**. Most patients will be unresponsive to verbal commands and act as if they are having hallucinations. Complex partial seizures occur in about 35% of patients with epilepsy. Numerous AEDs are available to treat complex partial seizures.

22.4 Some types of seizures are called special epileptic seizures or are unclassified.

Not all seizure disorders can be classified neatly into the two broad categories of generalized and partial. These "other" types of seizures are referred to as special or unclassified epileptic seizures.

Febrile seizures are most likely to occur in the 3-month to 5-year age group. As many as 5% of children experience febrile seizures. These seizures are associated with high fever and are characterized by tonic–clonic motor activity lasting 1 to 2 minutes with rapid return of consciousness. They usually occur only once during any given illness. Febrile seizures may be generalized (occur once and quickly resolve) or complex partial (occur multiple times in 24 hours and are prolonged). Pharmacotherapy with AEDs is not necessary with most febrile seizures. Prevention of the onset of fever with acetaminophen is the best method for controlling this disorder.

Status epilepticus is a medical emergency that occurs when a seizure continues for more than 30 minutes or when two or more sequential seizures occur without full recovery of consciousness between seizures. Status epilepticus is sometimes classified as a generalized form of epilepsy because tonic–clonic symptoms are usually exhibited. However, some forms of this disorder do not involve convulsions and may resemble simple partial or complex partial seizures. When generalized tonic–clonic seizures are prolonged or continuous, the time in which breathing is affected by muscle contraction is lengthened and hypoxia may develop. The continuous muscle contraction also can lead to hypoglycemia, acidosis, and hypothermia due to increased metabolic needs, lactic acid production, and heat loss during contraction. If untreated, status epilepticus could lead to brain damage and death. Medical treatment involves administration of AEDs by the IV route. In the home setting, valproic acid or diazepam can be administered by the rectal route.

Infantile spasm, also called West syndrome, usually occurs in the first year of life and is characterized by a sudden bending forward, body stiffening, or arching of the torso. Infantile spasms may occur in clusters, often with several dozen separated by 5 to 30 seconds. Infants who experience infantile spasms often have some degree of mental and developmental delays. Adrenocorticotropic hormone (ACTH) and prednisone are drugs of choice in the treatment of infantile spasms.

Lennox-Gastaut syndrome is considered a mixed seizure that has characteristics of tonic–clonic, atonic, and atypical absence seizures. The cause of this syndrome is unknown. This seizure disorder has a mean age of onset of 26 to 28 months and is often associated with mental retardation and mood instability. In older children, this type of epilepsy is associated with personality disorders and psychotic episodes. The preferred drugs for Lennox-Gastaut syndrome include benzodiazepines and valproic acid, although newer AEDs such as rufinamide are being increasingly prescribed. Seizures associated with Lennox-Gastaut syndrome are often resistant to pharmacotherapy.

22.5 The selection of antiepileptic drug therapy is dependent on seizure type and characteristics.

The choice of AED medication is highly individualized for each patient and is dependent on many factors, including the type of seizure; the patient's medical history, including the characteristics and length of the seizure; the results of the EEG and other diagnostic laboratory studies; and the presence of comorbid medical conditions. To prevent adverse drug effects, the prescriber initially chooses the lowest, effective dose of an AED and increases it as necessary. Serum drug levels may be obtained to assist the health care provider in determining the most effective drug concentration. To prevent adverse effects and possible seizure onset, the discontinuation of an AED or significant dose reductions are extended over 6 to 12 weeks. Drugs for the different types of seizures are listed in Table 22.2.

In most cases, effective seizure management can be obtained by using a single AED. If seizure activity continues, the initial drug is gradually discontinued and replaced by a medication from a different class. Some patients require multiple AEDs for effective seizure control. However, certain AED drug combinations have the potential to increase the incidence of seizures; thus it is important for the nurse to consult current literature for drug compatibility and administration guidelines. At the initiation of pharmacotherapy, the patient must be carefully assessed for adverse effects, particularly increased CNS depression, and advised not to drive or engage in hazardous activities until drug levels have stabilized.

Patients who remain symptom free for prolonged periods often believe that they have "outgrown" their seizures and therefore no longer require medication. Although this may indeed be the case, the nurse should teach patients to never stop taking AEDs without the guidance of their health care provider. In general, withdrawal of antiepileptic medications is attempted only after the patient has been seizure free for at least 3 years. The withdrawal of medications requires close monitoring by the patient's health care provider, and doses must be reduced slowly, one medication at a time, over a period of several months. If seizures recur during the withdrawal process, pharmacotherapy is resumed with the same medication previously prescribed. The nurse must educate the patient and family to maintain strict adherence to the pharmacotherapy regimen. Periodic serum drug levels can assist the nurse in assessing adherence: Low serum drug levels in a patient claiming to be taking his or her medication may indicate nonadherence to therapy.

Approximately 24% to 44% of patients with epilepsy attempt some sort of nondrug treatment, with stress management techniques and prayer being the most common alternative therapies (McElroy-Cox, 2009). Other therapies utilized to manage epilepsy include herbal supplements, chiropractic care, acupuncture, and yoga. The implementation of the ketogenic diet can produce positive effects in some patients by decreasing seizure activity. However, the use of alternative therapies alone for the management of epilepsy is not considered effective and should be discouraged by the nurse.

PharmFACT

Contrary to popular belief, it is impossible to swallow the tongue during a seizure, and one should never force an object into the mouth of someone who is having a seizure (Epilepsy Foundation of America, n.d.b).

22.6 Antiepileptic drugs act by suppressing abnormal neuronal discharges.

All antiepileptic medications suppress neuron discharges, thus preventing the abnormal focus from forming or spreading across the cerebrum. There are at least four mechanisms by which AEDs suppress abnormal discharges. The study of AEDs is complicated because some of these drugs act through multiple mechanisms, and a few have unknown mechanisms. These mechanisms are shown in Pharmacotherapy Illustrated 22.1. The basic mechanisms are:

- Electrolyte movement
  Inhibition of the influx of sodium into neurons
  Inhibition of the influx of calcium in neurons

- Neurotransmitter balance
  An increase in the activity of GABA in the brain
  Blocking of glutamate receptors in the brain

PHARMACOTHERAPY ILLUSTRATED 22.1

MECHANISMS OF ACTION OF ANTIEPILEPTIC DRUGS

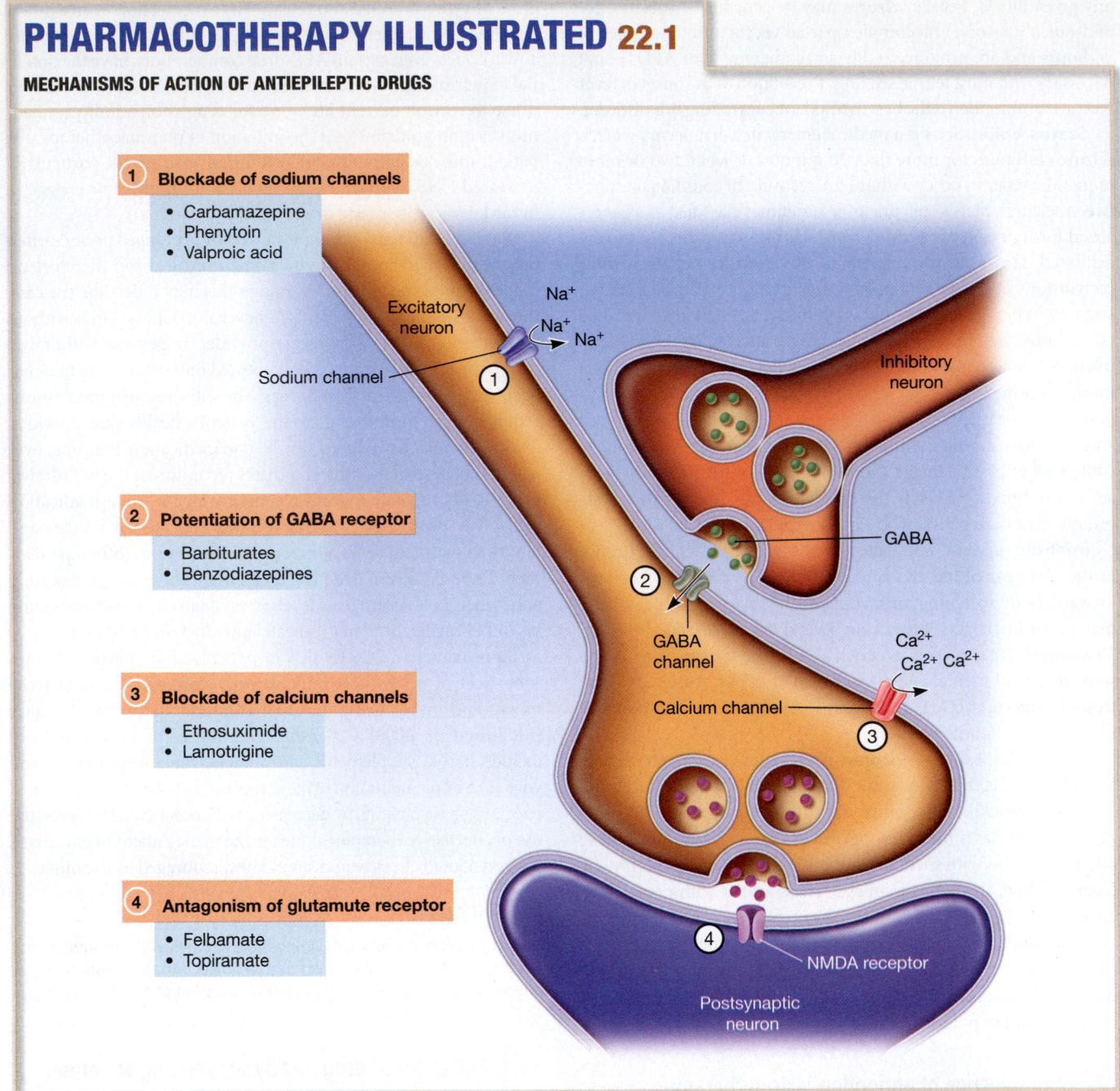

1 Blockade of sodium channels
- Carbamazepine
- Phenytoin
- Valproic acid

2 Potentiation of GABA receptor
- Barbiturates
- Benzodiazepines

3 Blockade of calcium channels
- Ethosuximide
- Lamotrigine

4 Antagonism of glutamute receptor
- Felbamate
- Topiramate

Excitatory neuron

Sodium channel

Na+
Na+ Na+

Inhibitory neuron

GABA

GABA channel

Ca²⁺
Ca²⁺ Ca²⁺

Calcium channel

NMDA receptor

Postsynaptic neuron

Control of electrolyte movement: In their resting state, neurons are surrounded by a high extracellular concentration of sodium, calcium, and chloride ions. Potassium levels are higher inside the cell. An influx of sodium or calcium into the neuron enhances neuronal activity, whereas an influx of chloride ions has an inhibitory effect. This affords several mechanisms to dampen abnormal neuronal activity.

The primary target for many AEDs is the *sodium* channel. The sodium channel on the neuronal plasma membrane must open, allowing sodium to rush into the cell, for an action potential to be generated and propagated. Phenytoin, lamotrigine, and carbamazepine bind to the sodium channel, inactivating it and preventing the passage of sodium ion into the neuron. This slows the excitability of neurons, dampening the flow of abnormal, repetitive discharges.

Calcium channels are found at the synaptic terminals. When opened, calcium enters the presynaptic neuron, causing the release of stored neurotransmitter into the synaptic cleft. Blocking calcium channels prevents the release of the neurotransmitter and dampens impulse conduction. The AEDs believed to block calcium channels include ethosuximide, gabapentin, pregabalin, and lamotrigine.

Neurotransmitter balance: Drugs that enhance or inhibit neurotransmitter activity in the CNS will affect neuronal firing. The neurotransmitter most affected by AEDs is gamma aminobutyric acid (GABA), the primary *inhibitory* neurotransmitter in the brain. Increasing the activity of GABA in the CNS will decrease neuronal firing, thus suppressing seizure activity. There are several

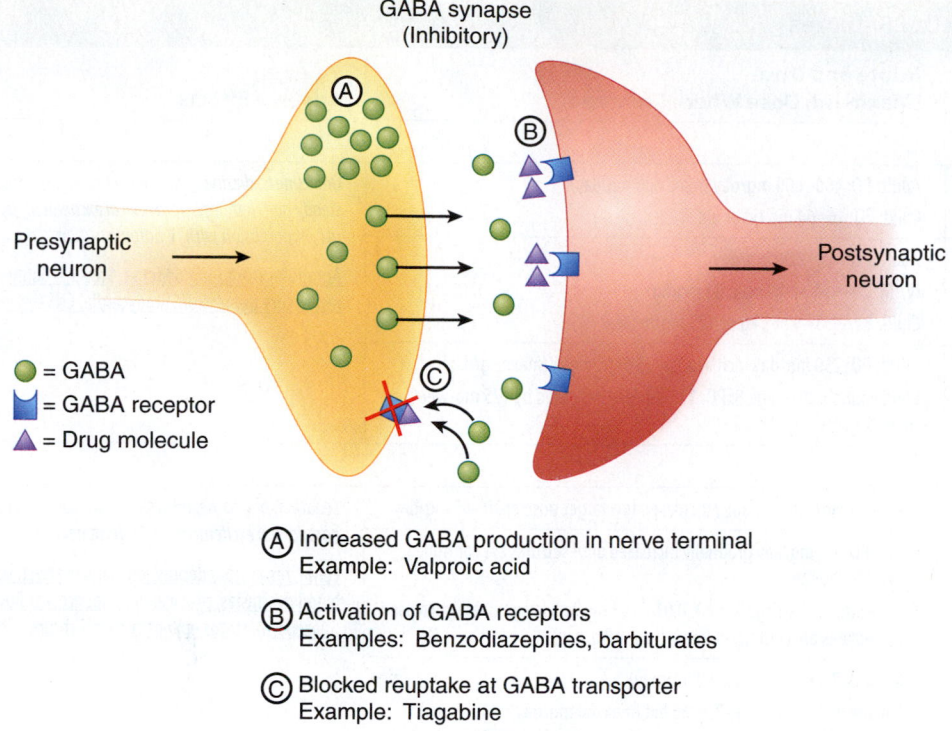

GABA synapse
(Inhibitory)

Presynaptic
neuron

Postsynaptic
neuron

○ = GABA
▢ = GABA receptor
▲ = Drug molecule

Ⓐ Increased GABA production in nerve terminal
　Example: Valproic acid

Ⓑ Activation of GABA receptors
　Examples: Benzodiazepines, barbiturates

Ⓒ Blocked reuptake at GABA transporter
　Example: Tiagabine

Figure 22.1 Mechanisms of action of antiepileptic drugs that affect GABA.

mechanisms by which this may be accomplished by AEDs, as illustrated in Figure 22.1.

- **Increased synthesis or amount of GABA in the presynaptic nerve terminal.** Some drugs block the metabolic breakdown of GABA or enhance its formation. An example is valproic acid.

- **Blocked reuptake of GABA.** After GABA produces its action at the synapse, it is normally pumped back into the presynaptic neuron, which terminates its action. Drugs that block this reuptake will keep GABA on its receptors for a longer time, thus causing more neuronal inhibition. An example is tiagabine.

- **Activation of GABA receptors.** Some drugs mimic GABA and occupy its receptor on the postsynaptic membrane, causing the same inhibitory effect as GABA. This is achieved by stimulating an influx of chloride ion, which causes the neuron to have greater difficulty achieving an action potential. Examples include barbiturates, benzodiazepines, topiramate, and felbamate.

A second neurotransmitter affected by AEDs is glutamate, the primary *excitatory* neurotransmitter in the brain. By blocking glutamate receptors (known as N-methyl-D-aspartate [NMDA] receptors), these drugs serve as antagonists to glutamate and suppress neuronal firing. Examples include topiramate and felbamate.

Antiepileptic medications are difficult to classify. One method is by mechanism of action; however, many AEDs act by multiple means and a few have unknown mechanisms. Another classification scheme groups these drugs into "newer" and "older" generations, but there is no clear distinction between the groups. Grouping by type of seizure is not possible because most of these medications are useful against more than one type. This textbook uses a combination of chemical classes and mechanisms of action.

The student should be aware, however, that other classifications will be encountered in clinical practice. The AEDs are listed in Table 22.3.

Antiepileptic Drugs

22.7 Barbiturates are traditional drugs for tonic–clonic seizures that have been replaced by newer and safer medications.

The barbiturates have been used to treat seizures for almost 100 years. Barbiturates act biochemically in the brain by enhancing the inhibitory action of GABA, the neurotransmitter responsible for suppressing abnormal neuronal discharges.

Although barbiturates are still prescribed for epilepsy, newer drugs have largely replaced them as first-line drugs for this indication. Barbiturates have several major disadvantages. As a class, they have a low margin of safety and can cause profound CNS depression, including sedation, coma, and death. Barbiturates will yield significant sedation when combined with alcohol, antidepressants, and other CNS depressants. Children may exhibit hyperkinesis rather than sedation. Cardiovascular and respiratory adverse effects include respiratory depression, bradycardia, syncope, and hypotension. Patients with impaired hepatic, respiratory, renal, and cardiovascular function should not receive barbiturates, or the doses should be lowered to prevent toxicity. Barbiturates also possess a high potential for drug dependence, and the nurse must be certain that this factor is included as part of patient and caregiver teaching.

This section highlights only the antiseizure properties of barbiturates. These drugs are also classified as sedative–hypnotics, and a prototype feature for phenobarbital can be found in Chapter 18.

TABLE 22.3 Drugs for Seizures

Drug	Route and Dose (Maximum Dose Where Indicated)	Adverse Effects
Barbiturates		
mephobarbital (Mebaral)	Adult: PO: 400–600 mg/day (max: 600 mg/day) Child: PO: 16–64 mg tid or qid	*Drowsiness, dizziness, nausea, vomiting, sedation, confusion, unsteady gait, lethargy, paradoxical excitement, pain at the injection site, hypotension with IV administration*
phenobarbital	Adult: PO: 100–300 mg/day IV/IM: 200–600 mg (max: 20 mg/kg) Child: PO/IV: 3–8 mg/kg or 125 mg/m²/day	Agranulocytosis, angioedema, Stevens–Johnson syndrome (SJS), respiratory depression, bradycardia, CNS depression, coma
primidone (Mysoline)	Adult: PO: 250 mg/day increased by 250 mg/week (max: 2 g/day) Child younger than age 8: PO: 125 mg/day increased by 125 mg/week (max: 2 g/day)	
Benzodiazepines		
clobazam (Onfi)	PO: 5–10 mg/day gradually increased to a target dose of 20–40 mg/day	*Sedation, headache, drowsiness, weakness, vertigo, ataxia, paradoxical excitement, short-term amnesia*
clonazepam (Klonopin)	Adult: PO: 1.5 mg/day gradually increased until seizures are controlled (max: 20 mg/day) Child younger than age 10: PO: 0.01–0.03 mg/kg/day gradually increased until seizures are controlled (max: 0.2 mg/kg/day)	Coma, respiratory depression, cardiac arrest, suicidal ideation, blood dyscrasias, physical dependence, cardiovascular collapse (diazepam), status epilepticus with abrupt withdrawal
clorazepate (Tranxene)	Adult: PO: 7.5 mg tid (max: 90 mg/day) Child age 9–12: PO: 3.75–7.5 mg bid (max: 60 mg/day)	
diazepam (Valium)	Status epilepticus: Adult: IV/IM: 5–10 mg, repeat if needed at 10- to 15-min intervals up to 30 mg Child: IV/IM: 0.2–1 mg slowly every 2–5 min up to 5–10 mg	
lorazepam (Ativan)	Adult: IV: 4 mg injected slowly at 2 mg/min; may repeat dose once after 10 min (max: 8 mg during any 12-h period) Status epilepticus: Child: IV: 0.1 mg/kg slowly over 2–5 min; may repeat with 0.05 mg in 10–15 min (max: 4 mg/dose)	
Hydantoins		
fosphenytoin (Cerebyx)	Adult: IV loading dose: 10–20 mg phenytoin equivalents/kg administered at 100–150 mg phenytoin equivalents/min Maintenance IV dose: 4–6 mg PE/kg/day	*Hypotension, nystagmus, ataxia, lethargy, confusion, slurred speech, dizziness, nervousness, headache, nausea, vomiting, gingival hyperplasia, rash, somnolence*
phenytoin (Dilantin, Phenytek)	Adult: PO (extended release): Initiate with 100 mg tid then adjust for seizure control IV: 10–15 mg/kg loading dose then 100 mg tid Child: PO (extended release): 5 mg/kg/day	Seizures, dysrhythmias, blood dyscrasias, systemic lupus erythematosus, cardiac arrest, cardiovascular collapse, coma, toxic epidermal necrolysis, SJS, osteomalacia
Dicarbazepines		
carbamazepine (Carbatrol, Tegretol)	Adult: PO: 200 mg bid gradually increased to 800–1,200 mg/day Child younger than age 6: PO: 10–20 mg/kg/day gradually increased weekly (max: 35 mg/kg/day) Child age 6–12: PO: 100 mg, gradually increased to 400–800 mg	*Dizziness, headache, ataxia, fatigue, rash, pruritus, dry mouth, nausea, vomiting, diplopia, abnormal gait*
eslicarbazepine (Aptiom)	PO: 400 mg once daily gradually increased to 1,200 mg once daily	SJS, aggravated absence seizures, hallucinations, aplastic anemia, agranulocytosis, heart block, respiratory depression, exfoliative dermatitis, suicidal ideation, status epilepticus (with abrupt withdrawal)
oxcarbazepine (Oxtellar XR, Trileptal)	Adult: PO: 300 mg gradually increased to 2,400 mg/day when used for monotherapy, 1,200 mg/day with other AEDs Child age 4–16: PO: 8–10 mg/kg/day (max: 600 mg/day)	
Succinimides		
ethosuximide (Zarontin)	Adult and child older than age 6: PO: 250 mg bid gradually increased to 1.5 g/day Child age 3–6: PO: 250 mg/day gradually increased to 1.5 g/day	*Drowsiness, headache, euphoria, restlessness, irritability, anxiety, hyperactivity, aggressive behavior, inability to concentrate, night tremors, abdominal pain, epigastric distress*
methsuximide (Celontin)	PO: 150–300 mg/day (max: 1.2 g/day)	Anorexia, SJS, weight loss, blood dyscrasias, systemic lupus erythematosus, suicidal ideation

TABLE 22.3 Drugs for Seizures (continued)

Drug	Route and Dose (Maximum Dose Where Indicated)	Adverse Effects
Miscellaneous Antiepileptic Drugs		
ezogabine (Potiga)	Adult: PO: 100 mg tid gradually increased to 200–400 mg tid	*Dizziness, fatigue, blurred vision, diplopia, vertigo, tremor* Retinal abnormalities, confusion, memory impairment, urinary retention, psychosis, prolongation of QT interval
felbamate (Felbatol)	Adult: PO: 1,200 mg/day gradually increased to 3,600 mg/day Child age 2–14: PO: 15 mg/kg/day (max: 45 mg/kg/day)	*Headache, dizziness, blurred vision, nausea and vomiting, anorexia* Liver failure, aplastic anemia
gabapentin (Neurontin)	Adult and child older than 12 years: PO: 300 mg tid gradually increased to 1,800–2,400 mg/day Child age 3–12: PO: 10–15 mg/kg/day gradually increased to 40 mg/kg/day	*Dizziness, drowsiness, fatigue, weight gain, ataxia, diplopia, nystagmus, tremor, peripheral edema, impaired concentration, dry mouth, flulike syndrome* Increased frequency of partial seizures, blurred vision, accidental injury
lacosamide (Vimpat)	Adult: PO: 50 mg bid gradually increased to 200–400 mg/day	*Dizziness, headache, diplopia, nausea* Suicidal ideation, prolongation of QT interval, syncope, hypersensitivity reactions
lamotrigine (Lamictal)	Adult: PO: 25–50 mg/day gradually increased to 150–500 mg/day (max: 700 mg/day without concurrent valproic acid, 200 mg/day with valproic acid) Child age 2–16: PO: 0.2–1 mg/kg/day gradually increased to 1–5 mg/kg/day (max: 15 mg/kg/day without valproic acid; 5 mg/kg/day or 250 mg/day with concurrent valproic acid)	*Dizziness, headache, ataxia, drowsiness, insomnia, tremor, rash, diplopia, blurred vision, flulike symptoms, infection, nausea, vomiting, back pain* SJS, toxic epidermal necrolysis, emotional lability (children), suicidal ideation
levetiracetam (Keppra)	Adult (regular release): PO: 500 mg bid; gradually increased to 3 g/day Child age 4–16: PO: 20 mg/kg/day; gradually increased to 60 mg/kg/day PO (extended release): 1,000–3,000 mg once daily	*Drowsiness, headache, dizziness, nervousness, flulike symptoms, vomiting, anorexia, asthenia* Emotional lability and personality disorder (children), accidental injury, suicidal ideation, blood dyscrasias
pregabalin (Lyrica)	PO: 150 mg/day gradually increased to 600 mg/day	*Dizziness, confusion, drowsiness, fatigue, weight gain, ataxia, diplopia, nystagmus, tremor, impaired concentration, dry mouth* Increased frequency of partial seizures, blurred vision, accidental injury, angioedema, suicidal ideation
rufinamide (Banzel)	Adult: PO: 400–800 mg/day gradually increased to 3,200 mg/day Child age 4 and older: PO: 10 mg/kg/day gradually increased to 45 mg/kg/day or 3,200 mg/day, whichever is less	*Dizziness, headache, somnolence, nausea, fatigue* Suicidal ideation, shortening of QT interval, hypersensitivity reactions
tiagabine (Gabitril)	Adult: PO: 4 mg/day gradually increased to 56 mg/day Age 12–18: PO: 4 mg/day gradually increased to 32 mg/day	*Dizziness, asthenia, tremor, somnolence, nervousness, difficulty concentrating* Vasodilation, HTN, palpitations, tachycardia, syncope, peripheral edema
topiramate (Topamax, Trokendi XR, Others)	PO: 50 mg/day gradually increased to 400 mg/day	*Paresthesia, anorexia, weight loss, fatigue, dizziness, somnolence, nervousness, psychomotor slowing, difficulty with memory or concentration, confusion* Acute myopia with angle closure glaucoma, oligohidrosis and hyperthermia, suicidal ideation, hyperammonemia with encephalopathy
valproic acid (Depakene, Depakote, Depacon)	Adult/child: PO/IV: 10–15 mg/kg/day gradually increased to 60 mg/kg/day	*Nausea, vomiting, abdominal cramps, anorexia, dyspepsia, drowsiness, dizziness, asthenia, insomnia, weight gain* Deep coma, hallucinations, hyperammonemia, thrombocytopenia, blurred vision, hepatotoxicity, pancreatitis, bone marrow depression, prolonged bleeding time
vigabatrin (Sabril)	Adult: PO: 500 mg bid gradually increased to 1,500 mg/day	*Fatigue, somnolence, nystagmus, tremor, vision changes, memory impairment, weight gain, arthralgia, abnormal coordination* Depression, psychosis, confusion, severe rash, anemia, suicidal ideation
zonisamide (Zonegran)	Adult: PO: 100 mg/day gradually increased to 200–400 mg/day	*Dizziness, ataxia, drowsiness, fatigue, anorexia, speech abnormalities and difficulty in concentrating or remembering, flulike symptoms, headache, abnormal gait, gingivitis, rhinitis* Severe rash including SJS, kidney stones, depression, psychosis

Note: Italics indicate common adverse effects. Underline indicates serious adverse effects.

Nursing responsibilities, lifespan and diversity considerations, and patient and family education for this drug class may also be found in Chapter 18.

Mephobarbital (Mebaral): Mephobarbital is a long-acting antiepileptic drug administered orally for preventing tonic–clonic and absence seizures. It is also approved for preoperative sedation induction. Mephobarbital produces adverse hematologic effects such as agranulocytosis, leukopenia, and thrombocytopenia. This drug should be administered cautiously, and the patient should be assessed for signs and symptoms of hypotension and CNS depression. Mephobarbital is converted to phenobarbital in the liver and offers no significant advantages over phenobarbital. It is pregnancy category D.

Phenobarbital: For epilepsy, phenobarbital is effective for long-term management of tonic–clonic seizures and partial seizures. It can be administered in patients with status epilepticus or febrile seizures or to treat eclampsia. It is relatively ineffective in treating absence seizures. It has largely been replaced by safer AEDs, although it is still considered an important drug for neonatal seizures.

Oral (PO) administration of phenobarbital may take several weeks for an optimal level of antiseizure activity to be achieved. The advantages of phenobarbital are that it is relatively inexpensive and long acting, and it can suppress seizures without causing major sedation with careful selection of dosage. The sedation effect of the drug is prominent at the initiation of therapy but often diminishes as treatment progresses.

Phenobarbital is a major inducer of hepatic CYP450 enzymes and will markedly increase the metabolism of other drugs metabolized by these enzymes. This results in a significant potential for drug interactions with other medications metabolized in the liver. Phenobarbital also increases its own metabolism, which leads to significant tolerance as therapy progresses. Phenobarbital is pregnancy category D. Women of childbearing potential who are taking barbiturates should use two methods of birth control.

Primidone (Mysoline): Primidone is a barbiturate that is metabolized in the liver to phenobarbital, which is responsible for many of its pharmacologic effects. It is effective for treating all types of seizures except absence seizures. It has no approved indications other than seizure. The actions and adverse effects of primidone are equivalent to those of phenobarbital. It is pregnancy category D.

PharmFACT

Twenty to thirty percent of patients with epilepsy also have psychiatric disturbances, the most common of which is mood or anxiety disorder. The risk of suicide in patients with epilepsy is about 25%, which is almost twice that of the general population (Algreeshah, 2013).

22.8 Benzodiazepines are important drugs in the treatment of status epilepticus.

Benzodiazepines are the first-line drugs for the treatment of certain anxiety disorders and are one of the most widely prescribed drug classes in the United States. Detailed information about the benzodiazepines used for anxiety and a prototype feature for lorazepam (Ativan) are included in Chapter 18. The remainder of this section focuses on the antiseizure properties of drugs in this class.

Benzodiazepines control seizures by acting in the limbic, thalamic, and hypothalamic regions of the CNS. All drugs in this class act by enhancing the inhibitory action of GABA. They accomplish this by increasing the affinity of GABA for its receptors.

The applications of benzodiazepines in the treatment of seizure disorders are limited. The parenteral benzodiazepines diazepam (Valium) and lorazepam are utilized in the treatment of status epilepticus. Clonazepam (Klonopin) and clorazepate (Tranxene) are used for specific types of seizures, usually when other drugs have not proven effective.

When giving these medications by the IV route, the patient is administered oxygen, and resuscitation equipment should be readily available. IV administration of diazepam or lorazepam for status epilepticus should be given in a large vein and they should not be mixed with other drugs or IV fluid additives. These drugs have a tendency to precipitate from solution and are irritating to veins. Close monitoring of the respiratory and cardiovascular systems is necessary for the early recognition of adverse effects associated with respiratory depression or cardiovascular collapse. Benzodiazepines should never be discontinued abruptly because status epilepticus may result.

PROTOTYPE DRUG	**Diazepam (Valium)**

Classification: **Therapeutic:** Antiepileptic drug, antianxiety drug, skeletal muscle relaxant
Pharmacologic: Benzodiazepine, GABA receptor agonist

Therapeutic Effects and Uses: Diazepam was originally approved in 1963. In antiseizure therapy, the primary indication for diazepam is status epilepticus. It may also be used to prevent seizures in patients who have received toxic substances or during the acute phase of alcohol or benzodiazepine withdrawal. Oral diazepam may be combined with other AEDs in the treatment of refractory seizures. A newer indication for diazepam is the oral prophylaxis of febrile seizures in children age 6 months to 5 years.

Diazepam has a large number of other indications. It was once widely prescribed for the management of anxiety disorders, although it has largely been replaced by other drugs such as alprazolam (Xanax). It is administered prior to procedures such as cardioversion or endoscopy to provide relaxation or sedation. Oral or parenteral diazepam may be administered for muscle relaxation in patients with acute inflammation, trauma, tetanus, or spasticity.

Mechanism of Action: Diazepam enhances the action of GABA in the brain, thus inhibiting the abnormal neuronal discharges characteristic of seizures.

Pharmacokinetics:

Route(s)	IV, IM, PO, rectal
Absorption	Rapidly absorbed by the GI tract; erratic absorption with IM administration
Distribution	Widely distributed; crosses the blood–brain barrier and the placenta; 99% bound to protein
Primary metabolism	Hepatic
Primary excretion	Renal
Onset of action	IV: 1–5 min; IM: 15–30 min; PO: 30–60 min
Duration of action	Half-life: 20–50 h

Adverse Effects: The most serious adverse effect of diazepam is cardiovascular collapse. The nurse should assess for hypotension, tachycardia, and edema, which are precursors to cardiovascular collapse. CNS adverse effects include drowsiness, fatigue, ataxia, dizziness, and vertigo. Diazepam can cause urinary retention and menstrual irregularities. The major respiratory adverse effect is laryngeal spasm and cough. Benzodiazepines are Schedule IV drugs and possess a risk for substance abuse in susceptible individuals (see Chapter 27).

Contraindications/Precautions: Diazepam should not be administered to patients with depressed vital signs, those in shock, or those with acute alcohol intoxication. It is also contraindicated in the presence of narrow-angle glaucoma because it can increase intraocular pressure. Diazepam should be used cautiously in patients with depression and myasthenia gravis, and a reduced dose should be administered in patients with impaired hepatic or renal function. Patients who have respiratory disorders such as chronic obstructive pulmonary disease (COPD) should be monitored closely due to the risk of respiratory depression. After prolonged therapy, abrupt discontinuation of diazepam may precipitate withdrawal symptoms, including seizures in patients with epilepsy. The drug can cause birth defects and should not be administered to pregnant patients unless benefits clearly outweigh the potential risks. Diazepam is not recommended during lactation because the drug is secreted in breast milk and may cause CNS depression in the neonate.

Drug Interactions: Diazepam is metabolized by hepatic CYP450 enzymes and may interact with drugs that inhibit these enzymes. Other CNS depressants, including alcohol, will intensify the sedative effects of diazepam. Concurrent administration with cimetidine will increase the plasma levels of diazepam. Administration of diazepam with antiparkinsonism medications may worsen the severity of Parkinson's disease symptoms. Diazepam when administered with phenytoin will result in increased phenytoin levels and possible toxicity. Diazepam should never be administered within 14 days of a monoamine oxidase inhibitor (MAOI) due to the risk of hypertensive crisis. **Herbal/Food**: Kava and valerian administered with diazepam will result in additive sedative effects. Echinacea may lower the serum levels of diazepam. Grapefruit juice increases the peak serum concentrations of diazepam by as much as two times.

Pregnancy: Category D.

Treatment of Overdose: Flumazenil (Romazicon) is administered for overdosage of diazepam. This medication is a specific benzodiazepine receptor antagonist that reverses the CNS depression from diazepam.

Nursing Responsibilities: Key nursing implications for patients receiving diazepam are included in the Nursing Practice Application for Patients Receiving Pharmacotherapy for Seizures and in the Nursing Practice Application for Patients Receiving Pharmacotherapy for Anxiety or Sleep Disorders in Chapter 18.

Drugs Similar to Diazepam (Valium)

Clobazam (Onfi), clonazepam, clorazepate, and lorazepam are benzodiazepine antiepileptic medications.

Clobazam (Onfi): Available in Europe for almost 40 years, clobazam was approved for the U.S. market in 2013. It is available in tablet or oral suspension form for one specific indication: seizures associated with Lennox-Gastaut syndrome in patients 2 years of age or older. The drug exhibits the adverse effects typical of benzodiazepines, especially sedation, which can be profound when the drug is used with alcohol or other CNS depressants. Stevens–Johnson syndrome is a serious, though rare, adverse effect. Tolerance to the sedation effect, as well as the antiepileptic effect, occurs with continued therapy. Clobazam is pregnancy category C and a Schedule IV controlled substance.

Clonazepam (Klonopin): Approved in 1975, clonazepam is an oral benzodiazepine with strong antiseizure properties. It is approved for the prophylaxis of absence seizures, Lennox-Gastaut syndrome, akinetic and myoclonic seizures, and nocturnal myoclonus. Its primary use as an AED is to treat refractory myoclonic seizures. Clonazepam is also approved for the treatment of panic disorder, with or without agoraphobia. It is occasionally prescribed off-label for other anxiety disorders, insomnia, and restless leg syndrome.

Like other drugs in the class, the most common adverse effect is sedation. Hyperactivity, restlessness, irritability, and cardiovascular or respiratory depression are possible. If given for an extended period, the patient may require an increase in dose due to the development of tolerance. Tolerance also develops to the sedative side effects of the drug. Therapeutic serum levels are 20 to 80 mg/mL. Clonazepam is pregnancy category C and a Schedule IV controlled substance.

Clorazepate (Tranxene): Approved in 1972, clorazepate is approved for the pharmacotherapy of anxiety, partial seizures, and seizures associated with acute ethanol withdrawal. It may be used off-label to treat insomnia. Clorazepate is only administered PO, is rapidly absorbed, and has a long duration of action. The actions of clorazepate are the same as those of diazepam because the two drugs share the same active metabolite. It is not a first-line drug for epilepsy but it may be used as an adjunct to control partial seizures. Most adverse effects are CNS related and include mental depression, confusion, fatigue, tremor, and vertigo. Like diazepam, clorazepate is a Schedule IV drug and is pregnancy category D.

Lorazepam (Ativan): Approved in 1977, lorazepam is a preferred drug for treating status epilepticus because it persists in the cerebrospinal fluid (CSF) longer than diazepam. Whereas diazepam remains active in the brain for 30 to 60 minutes, lorazepam may prevent seizures for up to 12 hours. It is also used to prevent or treat seizures associated with acute ethanol withdrawal. When given orally, lorazepam is indicated for the short-term management of anxiety disorders or anxiety associated with depressive symptoms. It is the most potent of the benzodiazepines and has the ability to produce skeletal muscle relaxation, sedation, and a hypnotic state. Oral, IM, and IV forms are available. Lorazepam is pregnancy category D and a Schedule IV controlled substance. A prototype feature for lorazepam is presented in Chapter 18.

CONNECTION Checkpoint 22.2

In addition to epilepsy, what are other indications for benzodiazepines? *See Answer to Connection Checkpoint 22.2 on student resource website.*

22.9 Hydantoins are effective in the management of most types of seizures but have many adverse effects.

First used in 1938, phenytoin (Dilantin) became a drug of choice for many types of epilepsy because it provided effective seizure prevention without the serious CNS depression and abuse potential associated with barbiturates such as phenobarbital. Despite having many drawbacks, phenytoin remains an important drug in the pharmacotherapy of seizures.

Hydantoins act by delaying the influx of sodium ions across neuronal membranes in the brain. Sodium ion movement is the major factor determining the initiation and propagation of a neuron action potential. Hydantoin medications do not block the sodium channels but instead desensitize them. Total blockage of sodium channels would cause neuronal activity to cease as is seen with the administration of local anesthetics. At high doses, the hydantoins begin to exert excitatory CNS effects and can induce seizures.

PROTOTYPE DRUG	Phenytoin (Dilantin, Phenytek)

Classification: **Therapeutic:** Antiepileptic drug
Pharmacologic: Hydantoin, neuronal sodium channel modulator

Therapeutic Effects and Uses: Phenytoin is approved for the prophylactic therapy of all types of seizures except absence seizures. Phenytoin has been used to prevent seizures that might occur during neurosurgery or eclampsia. The IV form of phenytoin is effective in treating generalized convulsions due to status epilepticus. The action of IV phenytoin is not immediate; therefore, an IV benzodiazepine should be administered prior to, or concurrently with, IV phenytoin to achieve faster seizure control. Phenytoin injections must always be performed slowly (not to exceed 50 mg/min in adults) to prevent cardiovascular collapse. Phenytoin (Phenytek) is an extended release form of the drug that allows once-daily dosing.

Patients taking phenytoin must be monitored very closely and the dosage adjusted based on clinical response and laboratory results. The therapeutic serum range is narrow, 10 to 20 mcg/mL, and small increases in dose can produce large changes in the serum concentration. Thus, the patient should be educated on the importance of maintaining a strict schedule for administration of the medication and for keeping all laboratory appointments. The brand of phenytoin should not be changed without approval of the health care provider because differences in bioavailability among brands have been noted.

Phenytoin is a Class 1B antidysrhythmic and may be used to treat ventricular tachycardia (especially those induced by digoxin) or paroxysmal atrial tachycardia, although it is not approved for these indications (see Chapter 37). Other off-label indications for phenytoin include the treatment of migraine headaches, diabetic neuropathy, and neuropathic pain.

Mechanism of Action: Phenytoin inhibits seizure activity by delaying the influx of sodium ions in neurons, thus slowing the propagation and spread of abnormal discharges. Unlike some AEDs, phenytoin does not elevate the seizure threshold.

Pharmacokinetics:

Route(s)	PO, IV
Absorption	Slowly but completely absorbed in the GI tract
Distribution	Enters the CSF; crosses the placenta; secreted in breast milk; 95% bound to protein
Primary metabolism	Hepatic
Primary excretion	Renal
Onset of action	PO (with loading dose): 30–120 min
Duration of action	Half-life is highly variable, ranging from 7 to 42 h with an average of 24 h

Adverse Effects: Phenytoin can be a very toxic drug and patients must be monitored carefully during therapy. CNS adverse effects are relatively common and include lethargy, headache, drowsiness, and dizziness. High doses can cause nystagmus, confusion, ataxia, coma, and seizures. Cardiovascular adverse effects include bradycardia, ventricular fibrillation, hypotension, and phlebitis. Gastrointestinal (GI) adverse effects include gingival hyperplasia (swelling of the gums), weight loss, and liver necrosis. Hematologic adverse effects include agranulocytosis, leukopenia, thrombocytopenia, and aplastic anemia. Rashes and serious dermatologic conditions occur in 5% to 10% of patients taking the drug. Abrupt discontinuation of phenytoin can induce status epilepticus. **Black Box Warning**: When IV infusion rates exceed 50 mg/min in adults the patient is at risk for hypotension and dysrhythmias. Careful cardiovascular monitoring is necessary.

Contraindications/Precautions: Patients who have developed a rash, sore throat, fever, oral ulcers, or other hypersensitivity reactions to a hydantoin should not receive phenytoin. This medication is contraindicated in patients who have experienced seizures caused by hypoglycemia. Phenytoin should be administered cautiously to patients with impaired liver or kidney function because these may increase the serum concentration of phenytoin to toxic levels. Patients with serious cardiovascular signs and symptoms such as dysrhythmias, bradycardia, and heart failure must be monitored carefully during therapy. Patients with blood dyscrasias should not receive phenytoin because this drug can worsen these conditions. Phenytoin is a known teratogen and should not be administered to pregnant patients unless the seizures cannot be managed by safer drugs. The drug is secreted in breast milk, although it may be used during lactation, if necessary, to control serious seizures.

Drug Interactions: Because phenytoin strongly induces CYP450 enzymes, the metabolism of many other drugs will be affected, and drug–drug interactions are common. Phenytoin increases the metabolism of corticosteroids, warfarin, and oral contraceptives, thus rendering these drugs less effective. Chronic alcohol ingestion, carbamazepine, and barbiturates can increase the metabolism of phenytoin, thus decreasing the antiseizure effects of phenytoin. Amiodarone, chloramphenicol, diazepam, valproic acid, isoniazid, omeprazole, and ticlopidine will increase phenytoin levels when administered concurrently. **Herbal/Food**: The administration or consumption of foods that contain folic acid, calcium, and vitamin D will decrease the absorption of phenytoin. Ginkgo may decrease the antiseizure effectiveness of phenytoin.

Pregnancy: Category D.

Treatment of Overdose: Overdoses of phenytoin are treated with activated charcoal with gastric lavage.

Nursing Responsibilities: Key nursing implications for patients receiving phenytoin are included in the Nursing Practice Application for Patients Receiving Pharmacotherapy for Seizures.

Drugs Similar to Phenytoin (Dilantin, Phenytek)

Fosphenytoin is the only other hydantoin. A third drug in this class, mephenytoin (Mesantoin), was removed from the market due to an unacceptable incidence rate of fatal blood dyscrasias.

Fosphenytoin (Cerebyx): Approved in 1996, fosphenytoin is a prodrug that is converted to phenytoin following metabolism. Given only by the parenteral route, it is considered functionally equivalent to phenytoin; their actions and adverse effects are the same. Doses on the label are indicated as phenytoin equivalents (PE). Indications for fosphenytoin include tonic–clonic seizures, status epilepticus, and seizure prophylaxis during neurosurgery. Because the drug is converted to phenytoin, therapeutic serum levels of phenytoin may be monitored during therapy. Advantages of fosphenytoin over phenytoin include more rapid IV administration (important during status epilepticus), ability to be administered by the IM route, and less pain and phlebitis at the injection site. The adverse effects are the same as IV phenytoin, except that fosphenytoin may cause intense burning, itching, and paresthesia (not at the site of injection) for several minutes to hours following the IV dose. Fosphenytoin carries the same black box warning as phenytoin. The drug is pregnancy category D.

22.10 Carbamazepine is a drug of choice for treating many tonic–clonic and partial seizures.

The dibenzazepines are a small class of drugs that have important applications to seizure management. These drugs have three rings in their structures, which makes them chemically related to the tricyclic antidepressants (see Chapter 19). The drugs in this class, carbamazepine (Carbatrol, Tegretol), eslicarbazepine (Aptiom), and oxcarbazepine (Oxtellar XR, Trileptal), have similar pharmacologic activity.

The mechanisms of action of the dicarbazepines are incompletely understood. Like phenytoin, they affect the sodium channels in cortical neurons, slowing the propagation and spread of repetitive action potentials. These drugs have other actions, however, that are unexplained by the sodium channel mechanism, including analgesic, anticholinergic, antidysrhythmic, antidepressant, and sedative effects. They also have muscle relaxant and neuromuscular-blocking properties. Doses for the dicarbazepines are listed in Table 22.3.

PROTOTYPE DRUG	Carbamazepine (Carbatrol, Tegretol, Others)

Classification: Therapeutic: Antiepileptic drug
Pharmacologic: Dibenzazepine, neuronal sodium channel modulator

Therapeutic Effects and Uses: Approved by the U.S. Food and Drug Administration (FDA) in 1968, carbamazepine is one of the most widely prescribed AEDs in the world because of its effectiveness and relative safety. It is indicated for the management of generalized tonic–clonic, for partial seizures with complex symptomatology, and for mixed seizure patterns. It is ineffective against absence seizures. Carbamazepine may be administered as monotherapy or in combination with other AEDs. Carbamazepine is also approved for the treatment of acute mania associated with bipolar disorder, either as monotherapy or in combination with lithium (see Chapter 19). Carbamazepine is available as an extended release form (Tegretol XR and Carbatrol CR), and as a multiphasic extended release form (Equetro).

Prior to its use as an AED, carbamazepine was approved to treat pain associated with trigeminal neuralgia. It remains one of the most effective drugs for this condition. Off-label uses of

CONNECTIONS	Treating the Diverse Patient

◖ **Post-Traumatic Epilepsy in Veterans with Traumatic Brain Injury**

Epilepsy occurring after any form of head trauma is a possibility, and soldiers returning from war and conflict have experienced seizures and epilepsy related to closed and open head wounds. Chen, Ruff, Eavey, and Wasterlain (2009) investigated the incidence of post-traumatic epilepsy (PTE) in veterans returning from Iraq. As many as 53% of soldiers returning from World War II and the Korean and Vietnam Wars experienced PTE after a penetrating brain injury. Using modern imaging techniques such as magnetic resonance imaging (MRI) and computed tomography (CT) scans, the authors estimated the risk of PTE at between 10% and 25% if brain injury is noted on imaging. The estimate may be higher due to symptoms that may be diagnosed as post-traumatic stress disorder (PTSD) but that may actually be caused by partial complex seizures. PTE may develop after a seizure-free period and, while usually occurring within 5 years after brain injury, may not occur until as long as 20 years later. The authors of this study support early short-term treatment with antiepileptic drugs (AEDs) after injury, follow-up imaging and EEG monitoring for 2 years, and continuing AED therapy for patients with symptoms of PTE.

PTE in the wounded veteran population significantly affects their ability to re-enter civilian life as productive members of society. Depending on whether the PTE is controlled or not, normal life activities such as driving and employment using skills learned in the armed services, for example, automotive or aviation jobs, may be difficult or impossible to obtain or maintain. Nurses should be aware of the stigma of epilepsy in all patients, but especially for veterans returning from combat with head wounds. Reentry into society may be difficult for any veteran with wounds related to combat. However, when a closed head injury has resulted in PTE and negatively affects the ability to function normally in society, the veteran, who may look normal, has suffered a significant wound that cannot be seen. By providing teaching and care, and by working with veterans' support groups, nurses can help ease the transition for these veterans when they return home.

carbamazepine include the treatment of neuropathic pain associated with diabetic neuropathy and postherpetic pain. The drug is also used off-label to treat hiccups and for the management of severe symptoms of dementia such as aggression and agitation, which are seen in some patients with Alzheimer's disease.

Although carbamazepine is structurally similar to the tricyclic antidepressants it does not produce the antidepressant effects of drugs in that class (see Chapter 19). The medication is metabolized in the liver to an active metabolite and is a potent inducer of CYP450 enzymes that will increase its own metabolism. Long-term administration of carbamazepine will result in the need to increase the dose because its half-life becomes shortened.

For all indications, therapy with carbamazepine must be monitored carefully and the dosage adjusted based on clinical outcomes and drug serum levels. The therapeutic serum concentrations usually range from 4 to 12 mcg/mL. Several weeks of therapy may be required before the optimum dose is determined and the effective plasma drug concentration is achieved.

Mechanism of Action: Carbamazepine inhibits sodium channels, blocking the repetitive, sustained firing of neurons that is characteristic of epilepsy. Other mechanisms are likely but are incompletely understood.

Pharmacokinetics:

Route(s)	PO
Absorption	Slowly absorbed through the GI tract
Distribution	Widely distributed; enters the CSF; crosses the placenta; secreted in breast milk; 75–85% bound to proteins
Primary metabolism	Hepatic (induces CYP enzymes)
Primary excretion	Primarily renal with some in feces
Onset of action	Slow and variable
Duration of action	Half-life: 14–16 h; 35–40 h for extended release

Adverse Effects: Carbamazepine is well tolerated; adverse effects are usually transient and diminish as therapy progresses. The most frequently observed effects include drowsiness, dizziness, ataxia, and nausea and vomiting. Transient sedation is common at the onset of therapy or after dosage increases. Other CNS effects include confusion, blurred vision, lethargy, and visual disturbances, although the patient usually develops tolerance to these effects. Other possible adverse effects include myalgia, leg cramps, carbamazepine-induced systemic erythematosus, heart block, aplastic anemia, respiratory depression, phototoxicity, urticaria, and alopecia. Elevated hepatic enzymes occur during therapy, although the patient is usually asymptomatic for hepatic disease. A few rare cases of serious hepatic impairment have been documented. Some patients have reported urinary retention and frequency, and male patients may experience impotence. **Black Box Warning**: Aplastic anemia and agranulocytosis have been reported with this drug. Serious and sometimes fatal dermatologic reactions, including toxic epidermal necrosis and SJS, have also occurred with carbamazepine. Patients testing positive for the HLA-B 1502 gene (usually found in people of Asian ancestry) are at higher risk for severe dermatologic reactions and should not receive this drug unless the benefit clearly outweighs the risk.

Contraindications/Precautions: Patients who are hypersensitive to tricyclic antidepressants should not take carbamazepine. Patients who have been diagnosed with increased intraocular pressure, systemic lupus erythematosus, cardiac disease, hepatic disease, and liver disease should not take carbamazepine. This medication is contraindicated with HTN. Older adults should be monitored closely if they possess a history of cardiac disease because a major adverse effect is heart block. Carbamazepine causes multiple birth defects in laboratory animals. If used during pregnancy, monotherapy is recommended because the use of two or more AEDs increases the risk of teratogenesis.

Drug Interactions: Carbamazepine has the ability to increase the activity of hepatic CYP450 enzymes, which can result in decreased serum concentrations of AEDs and other drugs metabolized by the liver. Increased carbamazepine levels have been noted when the drug is administered with verapamil, erythromycin, ketoconazole, or nefazodone. Patients who take carbamazepine with anticoagulants will experience decreased hypoprothrombinemic effects. Carbamazepine may decrease the effectiveness of oral contraceptives. **Herbal/Food**: Ginkgo may decrease the antiepileptic effectiveness of carbamazepine. Grapefruit juice and St. John's wort induce CYP enzymes and can decrease serum carbamazepine levels.

Pregnancy: Category D.

Treatment of Overdose: Activated charcoal and gastric lavage are administered with carbamazepine overdose.

Nursing Responsibilities: Key nursing implications for patients receiving carbamazepine are included in the Nursing Practice Application for Patients Receiving Pharmacotherapy for Seizures.

Drugs Similar to Carbamazepine (Carbatrol, Tegretol)

Other dibenzazepines include eslicarbazepine and oxcarbazepine.

Eslicarbazepine (Aptiom): One of the newest AEDs, eslicarbazepine was approved in 2013 for the treatment of partial onset seizures. It is usually used as an add-on treatment to therapy with other drugs in this class. It has a long half-life that allows for once-daily dosing. Eslicarbazepine and oxcarbazepine have very similar actions and adverse effects because both are converted to the same active metabolite. Common adverse effects include dizziness, somnolence, nausea, headache, vomiting, blurred vision, and tremor. This drug is pregnancy category C.

Oxcarbazepine (Oxtellar XR, Trileptal): Like carbamazepine, oxcarbazepine is similar to the tricyclic antidepressants and does not possess antidepressant activity. The two drugs act by the same mechanism and have similar actions. Approved in 2000, oxcarbazepine can be administered as monotherapy or in combination with other medications in the treatment of partial seizures, with or without secondary generalization. Off-label uses include the treatment of neuropathic pain and bipolar disorder. A major advantage of oxcarbazepine over carbamazepine is that drug interactions appear less significant and monitoring of drug plasma levels and hematologic values is generally not necessary. Although it induces CYP450 enzymes, it is not as strong an inducer as carbamazepine and it does not induce its own metabolism. In 2013, an extended release form of the drug (Oxtellar XR) was approved for once-daily dosing.

For checking adherence with the drug regimen or in overdose situations, the therapeutic serum concentration of the drug is 12 to 30 mcg/mL. Adverse effects are similar to those of carbamazepine, with dizziness, drowsiness, headache, and ataxia being the most common effects. It is important to monitor renal function when administering this medication because it is excreted through the kidneys. In addition, significant hyponatremia can develop during therapy, thus serum sodium levels should be regularly monitored. Oxcarbamazepine is pregnancy category C, although caution should be used during pregnancy because this drug is closely related structurally to carbamazepine, which is category D.

22.11 Succinimides are often the drugs of choice for the pharmacotherapy of absence seizures.

Succinimides form a small group of AEDs that suppress the influx of calcium into neurons during neuronal transmission. This is believed to increase the electrical threshold of the neuron, which reduces the likelihood of abnormal action potentials. Recent research has questioned this mechanism of action, and the actual mechanism of antiepileptic activity of this group remains largely unknown. Despite the small size of the class and their unknown mechanism of action, these drugs have important roles in the pharmacotherapy of absence seizures.

PROTOTYPE DRUG   Ethosuximide (Zarontin)

Classification: **Therapeutic:** Antiepileptic drug
Pharmacologic: Succinimide, neuronal calcium channel modulator

Therapeutic Effects and Uses: Ethosuximide is the only drug in this class that is commonly prescribed. Approved in 1960, it is a preferred drug for managing absence seizures. Because ethosuximide is ineffective in treating simple or complex partial seizures and tonic–clonic seizures, combination pharmacotherapy is needed to manage mixed seizures.

Ethosuximide is only administered by the oral route. Therapeutic serum concentrations range from 40 to 100 mcg/mL, although dosing is usually based on clinical response rather than serum levels. It may take 4 to 7 days before optimum therapeutic levels are attained.

Mechanism of Action: Ethosuximide depresses the motor cortex by delaying the calcium influx into the neuron.

Pharmacokinetics:

Route(s)	PO
Absorption	Readily and completely absorbed
Distribution	Widely distributed; very small amounts bound to proteins; crosses the placenta and is secreted in breast milk
Primary metabolism	Hepatic
Primary excretion	Primarily renal, with some in feces and bile
Onset of action	Peak: 4 h
Duration of action	Half-life: 30 h in children; 60 h in adults

Adverse Effects: The most common adverse effects of ethosuximide are GI related, including anorexia, nausea, vomiting, abdominal pain, and diarrhea. Adverse CNS events include drowsiness, dizziness, ataxia, confusion, aggressiveness, and night terrors. Hematologic toxicity may include agranulocytosis, pancytopenia, and aplastic anemia. Dermatologic effects include rash, pruritus, and exfoliative dermatitis. Like most AEDs, this drug may increase the risk of suicidal ideation.

Contraindications/Precautions: Ethosuximide is contraindicated in patients who have a known sensitivity to succinimides. It should be administered with caution to patients with liver or kidney impairment. Administration of ethosuximide may increase the frequency of tonic–clonic seizures. Patients with blood dyscrasias or bone marrow suppression should not receive this drug because it can worsen these conditions. Safety has not been established for the administration of this medication during pregnancy. Although small amounts of the drug are secreted in breast milk, the American Academy of Pediatrics (2001) considers the use of the drug compatible with breast-feeding.

Drug Interactions: Ethosuximide can participate in many drug–drug interactions. When used in combination therapy with other AEDs, serum drug levels should be regularly monitored. CNS depressants and ethanol may cause additive sedation. Use of ethanol may also reduce the effectiveness of the antiseizure medication. Ethosuximide administered concurrently with phenobarbital, phenothiazines, or tricyclic antidepressants can increase seizure frequency. Isoniazid administered in combination with ethosuximide can result in increased serum ethosuximide levels. Carbamazepine will cause a decrease in ethosuximide serum levels. Concurrent use of valproic acid will inhibit the metabolism of ethosuximide, leading to possible toxicity. **Herbal/Food**: Unknown.

Pregnancy: Category C.

Treatment of Overdose: Activated charcoal and gastric lavage are administered with ethosuximide overdose.

Nursing Responsibilities: Key nursing implications for patients receiving ethosuximide are included in the Nursing Practice Application for Patients Receiving Pharmacotherapy for Seizures.

Drugs Similar to Ethosuximide (Zarontin)

Methsuximide is the only other drug in this class. Another succinimide, phensuximide (Milontin), is no longer marketed in the United States.

Methsuximide (Celontin): Like ethosuximide, methsuximide is indicated for the management of absence seizures. This drug is rarely used in clinical practice because it is less effective and more toxic than ethosuximide. It has the same indications and adverse effects as ethosuximide. This drug is pregnancy category C.

22.12 Several miscellaneous drugs are important in treating epilepsy.

As explained in Section 22.6, it is difficult to classify AEDs because many act by multiple mechanisms, whereas others are unique and are the only drug in a class. Several of these "miscellaneous" drugs are widely used. Following the discussion of the two prototypes, other miscellaneous drugs and their indications are described.

PROTOTYPE DRUG **Gabapentin (Neurontin)**

Classification: **Therapeutic:** Antiepileptic drug
Pharmacologic: GABA analog

Therapeutic Effects and Uses: Gabapentin consists of a molecule of the neurotransmitter GABA with an attached side chain. The side chain makes the molecule lipid soluble so that it readily crosses the blood–brain barrier. Approved in 1993, gabapentin is used in combination with other AEDs to control partial seizures with or without secondary generalization. Doses are based on therapeutic response, making it unnecessary to measure serum drug levels during therapy. It is available as capsules, as tablets, and as an oral solution.

Therapy with gabapentin has been found to benefit a number of other conditions. Gabapentin (Gralise) is approved for the treatment of postherpetic neuralgia and gabapentin (Horizont) for restless-leg syndrome (Horizont). Gabapentin is used off-label for other conditions with neuropathic pain such as diabetic neuropathy. In fact, the drug is probably prescribed more often for the treatment of neuropathic pain than for epilepsy. Hot flashes are reduced in approximately 50% of the women taking the drug. It has been designated as an orphan drug for the treatment of amyotrophic lateral sclerosis (ALS). Some research has suggested that gabapentin is useful in treating trigeminal neuralgia, paresthesia, spasticity, and ocular ataxia in patients with multiple sclerosis.

Mechanism of Action: The exact mechanism of anticonvulsant action for gabapentin is unknown. Although closely related structurally to GABA, it does not appear to bind to GABA receptors or to prevent endogenous GABA from binding. It does not appear to affect the binding of other neurotransmitters such as serotonin, dopamine, glutamate, or histamine. It likely affects calcium channels but its exact mechanism has not been determined.

Pharmacokinetics:

Route(s)	PO
Absorption	50–60% is absorbed from the GI tract
Distribution	Crosses the blood–brain barrier and the placenta; readily passes into the CSF; secreted in breast milk; very small amounts bound to proteins
Primary metabolism	Not metabolized
Primary excretion	Excreted unchanged by the kidneys
Onset of action	1 h
Duration of action	Half-life: 5–6 h

Adverse Effects: Gabapentin is well tolerated, with CNS symptoms such as drowsiness, fatigue, nystagmus, and dizziness being the primary adverse effects. The administration of gabapentin can lead to increased frequency of viral infections, weight gain, and gastric upset. Behavioral problems such as hostility, emotional lability, impaired cognition, aggressiveness,

and hyperkinesia have been reported in the pediatric population age 3 to 12.

Contraindications/Precautions: Gabapentin should not be administered during pregnancy or lactation unless the benefits of pharmacotherapy outweigh the risks. It should not be administered in patients who have experienced a hypersensitivity reaction to GABA-related medications. It should be used cautiously with status epilepticus, renal impairment, and with older adults. Gabapentin should be used with caution in patients with renal impairment because the drug could accumulate to toxic levels. The drug should be discontinued gradually to prevent withdrawal-associated seizures.

Drug Interactions: A major advantage of gabapentin is that it does not induce CYP450 enzymes, and thus it exhibits fewer drug interactions than many other AEDs. No interactions with carbamazepine, phenobarbital, phenytoin, or valproic acid have been observed. Morphine and hydrocodone may cause additive CNS depression when administered with gabapentin. **Herbal/Food:** The administration of ginkgo with gabapentin may result in decreased anticonvulsant effects.

Pregnancy: Category C.

Treatment of Overdose: Overdose results in dyspnea, sedation, double vision, and slurred speech. Renal dialysis can be utilized to treat gabapentin overdose.

Nursing Responsibilities: Key nursing implications for patients receiving gabapentin are included in the Nursing Practice Application for Patients Receiving Pharmacotherapy for Seizures.

PROTOTYPE DRUG **Valproic Acid (Depacon, Depakene, Depakote)**

Classification: **Therapeutic:** Antiepileptic drug, antimanic drug
Pharmacologic: GABA agonist

Therapeutic Effects and Uses: Valproic acid has been an important drug in treating epilepsy since 1978. Valproic acid has several trade names and formulations, which sometimes causes confusion when studying this drug.

- Valproic acid (Depakene) is the standard form of the drug given by the oral route.
- Valproate sodium is the sodium salt of valproic acid given orally or IV (Depacon).
- Divalproex sodium (Depakote ER) is a sustained release combination of valproic acid and its sodium salt in a 1:1 mixture. It is given orally and is available in an enteric-coated form.

All three formulations of the drug form valproate after absorption or on entering the brain. The pharmacokinetics of each form varies, and they are not interchangeable. In this text, the name "valproic acid" is used to describe all forms of the drug, unless specifically stated otherwise.

Valproic acid is administered as monotherapy or in combination with other AEDs to treat absence seizures and complex partial seizures. It is also approved for the prevention of migraine headaches and mania associated with bipolar disorder. Off-label indications include severe behavioral disturbances such as agitation due to dementia, Alzheimer's disease, or explosive temper in patients with ADHD; persistent hiccups; and status epilepticus refractory to IV diazepam. Dosage adjustments for valproic acid are usually based on patient response; normal serum drug levels for epilepsy are 50 to 100 mcg/mL. In 2007, the FDA approved Stavzor, a soft gelatin capsule of valproic acid. The capsule dissolves in the small intestine, rather than the stomach, thus reducing nausea and vomiting, which are common adverse effects of the drug.

Mechanism of Action: Valproic acid increases concentrations of the inhibitory neurotransmitter GABA in the brain. Abnormal neuron discharges are suppressed, leading to decreased seizure activity.

Pharmacokinetics:

Route(s)	IV, PO
Absorption	Rapidly absorbed in the GI tract
Distribution	Crosses the placenta and is secreted in breast milk; 80–90% bound to protein
Primary metabolism	Hepatic
Primary excretion	Renal and GI tract
Onset of action	15–30 min
Duration of action	Half-life: 5–20 h

Adverse Effects: Valproic acid is well tolerated in most patients and adverse effects rarely cause discontinuation of therapy. The most common adverse effects are GI related, such as nausea, vomiting, diarrhea, abdominal pain, and diminished appetite. An enteric-coated formulation of valproic acid can be used to reduce these uncomfortable effects. These effects are usually transient and not severe. CNS adverse effects such as headache, tremor, dizziness, and sedation occur in about 25% of patients. High doses of valproic acid cause diminished platelet aggregation, which can result in prolonged bleeding and clotting times. Bone marrow depression, photosensitivity, and pulmonary edema are rare potential adverse effects. Valproic acid may cause hyperammonemic encephalopathy, especially in combination with topiramate, which requires discontinuation of valproic acid therapy. **Black Box Warning:** Serious hepatotoxicity has been reported in infants younger than age 2 taking valproic acid. Life-threatening pancreatitis has occurred as a result of valproic acid administration. When given during pregnancy, valproic acid can produce neural tube defects and children exposed while in utero demonstrate lower cognitive scores.

Contraindications/Precautions: Patients with hypersensitivity to any formulation of valproic acid should not be administered this drug. Other contraindications include bleeding disorders, cirrhosis, congenital metabolic disorders, and autoimmune deficiency syndrome. Patients with known or suspected pancreatitis should not receive this drug because life-threatening pancreatitis has been reported. Valproic acid should be administered cautiously in patients with a low serum albumin and renal impairment. Extreme caution should be used in treating patients under age 2 because fatal hepatotoxicity has been reported. The drug should not be administered to patients with known hepatic impairment. Abrupt discontinuation may cause status epilepticus. This drug is a known

teratogen and should only be used during pregnancy when benefits of therapy clearly outweigh the risk of birth defects.

Drug Interactions: Valproic acid inhibits CYP enzymes, which can result in many drug–drug interactions. Valproic acid administered concurrently with alcohol and other CNS depressants may result in additive sedation. Patients taking enzyme-inducing AEDs such as carbamazepine, phenytoin, and phenobarbital will metabolize valproic acid more rapidly, and dosage adjustment will be necessary. Valproic acid may increase the serum levels of tricyclic antidepressants, requiring a reduction in antidepressant dosage. Aspirin increases the serum drug levels of valproic acid and should not be administered concurrently. Isoniazid will elevate serum valproic acid levels. Cholestyramine will decrease absorption of valproic acid. Cimetidine will increase valproic acid levels and will place the patient at risk for hepatotoxicity. Valproic acid should not be administered with topiramate due to an increased risk of hyperammonemic encephalopathy. **Herbal/Food:** Ginkgo may decrease the antiepileptic effects of valproic acid.

Pregnancy: Category D.

Treatment of Overdose: The effects from overdose of valproic acid may be serious and include sedation, heart block, deep coma, and death. Naloxone (Narcan) is utilized to reverse the CNS depression, and hemodialysis can lower drug serum levels. Caution must be used when administering naloxone because this drug may also reverse the antiseizure action of valproic acid.

Nursing Responsibilities: Key nursing implications for patients receiving valproic acid are included in the Nursing Practice Application for Patients Receiving Pharmacotherapy for Seizures.

Other Miscellaneous Drugs

Ezogabine (Potiga): One of the newer AEDs, ezogabine was approved in 2011 for the adjunctive treatment of partial onset seizures in adults. The drug acts by stabilizing potassium channels in the brain, which reduces brain excitability. The drug should be used with caution in patients with benign prostatic hyperplasia because it may cause urinary retention. Dizziness, somnolence, and fatigue are common side effects during therapy. Ezogabine carries a black box warning that the drug may cause retinal abnormalities and vision loss. All patients should receive baseline and periodic ophthalmic examinations while taking this drug. Ezogabine is a Schedule V drug and is pregnancy category C.

Felbamate (Felbatol): Approved in 1993, felbamate is an oral drug that is effective against most types of seizures. Serious adverse effects, however, limit its use to severe partial seizures and the treatment of partial and generalized seizures associated with Lennox-Gastaut syndrome in children who have not responded to other therapies. Although the incidence of these adverse effects is rare, they may be serious or fatal. More common adverse effects include nausea, vomiting, anorexia, drowsiness, dizziness, insomnia, and vision changes. This drug carries a black box warning that fatal aplastic anemia and fatal hepatic failure have been associated with felbamate use. Baseline and periodic hematologic and hepatic laboratory tests should be conducted. This drug is pregnancy category C.

Lamotrigine (Lamictal): Approved in 1994, lamotrigine is an oral drug indicated for the adjunctive therapy of partial seizures,

Lennox-Gastaut syndrome, absence seizures, and tonic–clonic seizures in adults and pediatric patients 2 years of age or older. It is also used in the maintenance therapy of bipolar disorder. The mechanism of antiseizure action is largely unknown but likely relates to this drug's ability to inhibit flow through sodium ion channels and probably calcium channels as well. Lamotrigine is rapidly absorbed, 55% bound to plasma proteins, and almost entirely excreted by the kidneys.

Lamotrigine does not induce or inhibit hepatic metabolic enzymes. It is metabolized by CYP450 enzymes, however, and patients who are taking potent inducers of CYP450 enzymes (e.g., carbamazepine, phenytoin, and phenobarbital) will metabolize the drug more rapidly. Doses of lamotrigine will need to be increased in these patients to produce an optimal antiseizure response. On the other hand, valproic acid will reduce the elimination of lamotrigine, and the dose of lamotrigine should be reduced to prevent toxicity. Oral contraceptives reduce serum levels of lamotrigine, and the dosage of the AED will need to be adjusted when therapy with the hormones is initiated or discontinued and during the "pill-free" week of the month. Lamotrigine is one of the preferred drugs for managing epilepsy in pregnant women.

Lamotrigine is generally well tolerated by patients. The most common adverse effects are drowsiness, dizziness, ataxia, headache, diplopia, blurred vision, nausea, vomiting, and rash. Patients should be monitored for the development of suicidal ideation. Over 10% of patients taking this AED will develop a rash, which normally occurs during the first 2 to 8 weeks of therapy. This drug carries a black box warning that serious dermatologic toxicity, including SJS, has been reported, especially in children. Lamotrigine should be discontinued at the first sign of any type of rash. This drug is pregnancy category C.

Levetiracetam (Keppra): Levetiracetam is available for both PO and IV routes and is utilized in the therapy of the following seizures: adjunctive therapy for partial seizures in adults and children age 4 years and older, adjunctive therapy for myoclonic seizures in adults and adolescents age 12 years and older, and adjunctive therapy of primary generalized tonic–clonic seizures in adults and children age 6 years and older. Approved in 1999, the mechanism of its antiseizure activity is unknown. Levetiracetam is excreted unchanged by the kidneys; thus dosage should be reduced in patients with renal impairment. Few significant drug interactions have been recorded. In 2008, an extended release form of the drug (Keppra XR) was approved to treat partial onset seizures.

Levetiracetam is well tolerated, with the most common adverse effects being drowsiness, dizziness, infections, headache, and asthenia. The nurse must teach the patient to exercise care in performing tasks because an increase in accidental injuries is associated with levetiracetam use. Pediatric patients exhibit a relatively high incidence of behavioral effects, including agitation, nervousness, hyperkinesia, hostility, depression, and emotional lability. Levetiracetam is pregnancy category C.

Pregabalin (Lyrica): Approved in 2004, pregabalin is an oral AED that is very similar to gabapentin. Pregabalin is indicated for the adjunctive therapy of adult patients with partial onset seizures. Like gabapentin, it is used more often for its other approved indications: the management of neuropathic pain associated with diabetic peripheral neuropathy, postherpetic neuralgia, and fibromyalgia.

Off-label uses include the therapy of anxiety and social phobia. The safety of pregabalin in pediatric patients has not been established. Although its mechanism of action has not been clearly demonstrated, it is thought to act by increasing GABA levels by reducing the calcium channel function of neurons in the brain. This drug does not affect CYP450 enzymes; thus it has fewer drug–drug interactions than many other AEDs. Pregabalin is not bound to plasma proteins and is excreted in an unmetabolized form by the kidneys. Dose reduction in patients with renal impairment is necessary to avoid toxicity.

Pregabalin is well tolerated by most patients. Dizziness and drowsiness are the most common adverse effects and these may affect 20% to 40% of patients taking pregabalin, especially at high doses. Other common adverse effects of pregabalin are blurred vision, lethargy, dry mouth, peripheral edema, weight gain, and difficulty with concentration or attention. Concurrent administration with other CNS depressants can lead to increased sedation. Because pregabalin is a Schedule V controlled substance that may cause physical and psychological dependence, it should be used with caution in patients with a known or suspected history of substance abuse. Pregabalin is pregnancy category C.

Rufinamide (Banzel): Rufinamide is an oral drug approved in 2008 for the adjunctive treatment of seizures associated with Lennox-Gastaut syndrome in children 4 years and older, and in adults. The drug is well tolerated, with dizziness, headache, and fatigue being common adverse effects. The drug acts by regulating the activity of sodium channels in the brain. The drug is contraindicated in patients with familial short ST syndrome. Rufinamide is pregnancy category C.

Tiagabine (Gabitril): Tiagabine is given by the oral route for the adjunctive treatment of partial seizures in patients who have not responded to therapy with other AEDs. Safety in patients under age 12 has not been established. Approved in 1997, it acts by inhibiting GABA reuptake into the presynaptic neuron. Tiagabine is extensively metabolized by CYP3A enzymes. Patients who are taking potent inducers of CYP450 enzymes (e.g., carbamazepine, phenytoin, and phenobarbital) will metabolize tiagabine more rapidly. Doses of tiagabine will need to be increased in these patients to produce an optimal antiseizure response. Tiagabine itself does not induce CYP enzymes; thus it has fewer drug–drug interactions than many other AEDs. Tiagabine is 98% bound to plasma proteins and is eliminated in both the urine and feces.

Approximately 10% to 20% of patients taking tiagabine experience adverse effects that require discontinuation of therapy. The most common adverse effects are dizziness, lethargy, confusion, somnolence, nausea, irritability, tremor, asthenia, abdominal pain, and difficulty with concentration or attention. As with other AEDs the nurse should teach patients to avoid injury due to possible sedative effects. Although tiagabine suppresses seizures in patients with epilepsy, it has been found to increase new-onset seizures when given to patients without epilepsy (for off-label indications). Because of this, the FDA and the manufacturer have advised prescribers not to administer tiagabine for any indication other than partial seizures in patients 12 years and older. An additional FDA warning advises health care providers to monitor carefully for any increase in suicidal behavior or ideation. Tiagabine is pregnancy category C.

Topiramate (Topamax, Trokendi XR, others): Approved in 1996, topiramate has become an important medication in treating a broad range of seizure types in adults and children. It may be used as monotherapy or in combination with other AEDs. The drug is usually well tolerated, with the most frequent adverse effects being dizziness, fatigue, paresthesia, anorexia, weight loss, and psychomotor slowing. Newer, extended release forms (Qudexy XR, Trokendi XR) offer the convenience of once-daily dosing. During therapy, patients should be monitored for visual changes, glaucoma, metabolic acidosis, cognitive dysfunction, and suicidal behavior. Adequate fluid intake should be encouraged to prevent kidney stone formation. Because this drug can decrease sweating, the patient may be susceptible to hyperthermia during hot weather. Topiramate is pregnancy category D and may increase the risk of oral clefts in children exposed to the drug while in utero.

Vigabatrin (Sabril): Available PO, vigabatrin was approved in 2009 for adjunctive therapy of refractory complex partial seizures in adults. Because of potential serious adverse effects, vigabatrin is available in a restricted distribution program and is only prescribed when patients have not responded adequately to other medications. This drug contains a black box warning that permanent vision loss can occur during therapy. Other serious adverse effects include anemia, confusion, and memory impairment. Vigabatrin is pregnancy category C.

Zonisamide (Zonegran): Approved in 2000, zonisamide (Zonegran) is an oral sulfonamide that is effective in combination with other AEDs for partial seizures in adults. Safety in patients under age 16 has not been established although the drug is sometimes used off-label in children. It produces antiepileptic effects by inhibiting sodium and calcium channels in brain neurons. Zonisamide has a long half-life and 2 weeks may be required before optimum antiseizure activity is achieved.

Zonisamide is well tolerated by most patients. The most common adverse effects are dizziness, ataxia, drowsiness, fatigue, anorexia, speech abnormalities, and difficulty in concentrating or remembering. Because many patients are allergic to sulfonamides, it is important to assess these patients for sulfonamide hypersensitivity prior to the administration of the medication. Sulfonamides can cause fatal skin reactions, including SJS. The medication should be administered cautiously in patients who are receiving drugs that inhibit or reduce CYP3A4 enzymes; phenytoin, carbamazepine, phenobarbital, and valproic acid will decrease the half-life of zonisamide. Doses of zonisamide will need to be increased in these patients to produce an optimal antiseizure response. Zonisamide itself does not induce CYP enzymes; thus it has fewer drug–drug interactions than many other AEDs. Zonisamide is pregnancy category C.

CONNECTIONS: NURSING PRACTICE APPLICATION

Patients Receiving Pharmacotherapy for Seizures

Assessment	Potential Nursing Diagnoses*
Baseline assessment prior to administration: • Obtain a complete health history including hepatic, renal, cardiovascular, or neurologic disease, mental status, narrow-angle glaucoma, pregnancy, or breast-feeding. Obtain a drug history including allergies, current prescription and OTC drugs, and herbal preparations. Be alert to possible drug interactions. • Obtain a seizure history (e.g., frequency, duration, physical symptoms, preseizure symptoms that occur, and length of postictal period). • Obtain baseline vital signs, weight, and, in pediatric patients, height. • Obtain a developmental history in pediatric patients (e.g., DDST-II level of growth and development, and school performance). • Evaluate appropriate laboratory findings (e.g., CBC, electrolytes, hepatic or renal function studies). • Assess the patient's ability to receive and understand instructions. Include the family and caregivers as needed.	• *Situational or Chronic Low Self-Esteem* • *Impaired Social Interaction* • *Deficient Knowledge* (Drug Therapy) • *Risk for Injury*, related to seizures or adverse drug effects
Assessment throughout administration: • Assess for desired therapeutic effects (e.g., diminished or absence of seizure activity). • Continue periodic monitoring of CBC and liver and renal function studies. • Assess vital signs and weight periodically or if symptoms warrant. Assess height and weight in all pediatric patients. • Assess for and promptly report adverse effects: excessive dizziness, drowsiness, lightheadedness, confusion, agitation, palpitations, tachycardia, blurred or double vision, continuous seizure activity, skin rashes, bruising or bleeding, abdominal pain, jaundice, change in color of stool, flank pain, and hematuria.	

Implementation

Interventions and (Rationales)	Patient-Centered Care
Ensuring therapeutic effects: • Continue assessments as above for therapeutic effects. (Antiseizure drugs may not completely resolve symptoms but frequency and severity of seizures should be diminished.)	• Teach the patient, family, or caregiver to keep a seizure diary of frequency, type, length, preseizure symptoms, and postictal period.

(continued)

CONNECTIONS: NURSING PRACTICE APPLICATION *(continued)*

Minimizing adverse effects:

- Continue to monitor vital signs, mental status, coordination, and balance periodically. Ensure patient safety; monitor ambulation until effects of the drug are known. **Lifespan:** Be particularly cautious with the older adult who is at increased risk for falls. (Antiseizure drugs may cause drowsiness and dizziness, hypotension, or impaired mental and physical abilities, increasing the risk of falls and injury.)

- Teach the patient to rise from lying or sitting to standing slowly to avoid dizziness or falls. If dizziness occurs, the patient should sit or lie down and not attempt to stand or walk, until the sensation passes. **Lifespan:** Teach the patient, family, or caregiver to be especially cautious with the older adult who is at greater risk for falls.
- Instruct the patient to call for assistance prior to getting out of bed or attempting to walk alone, and to avoid driving or other activities requiring mental alertness or physical coordination until the effects of the drug are known.

- **Lifespan:** Continue to monitor height, weight, and developmental level in pediatric patients. In the school-age child, assess school performance. (Adverse effects of antiseizure drugs or unresolved seizures may hinder normal growth and development.)

- Teach the patient's family or caregiver to keep regularly scheduled appointments with the health care provider and report any developmental lags or concerns.

- Continue to monitor drug levels, CBC, renal and hepatic function, and pancreatic enzymes.
- **Diverse Patients:** Some antiseizure drugs induce or inhibit P450 enzymes and may interact with other drugs. Ethnically diverse populations may also experience less than optimal effects of the drug. (Antiseizure drugs require periodic evaluation of drug levels to correlate level with symptoms. Antiseizure drugs may cause hepatotoxicity and valproic acid may cause pancreatitis as an adverse effect.)

- Instruct the patient on the need to return periodically for laboratory work.
- **Diverse Patients:** Teach all patients, but especially ethnically diverse patients, to observe for less than optimal effects and report promptly.
- Instruct the patient to carry a wallet identification card or wear medical identification jewelry indicating a seizure disorder and antiseizure medication.
- Teach the patient to promptly report any abdominal pain, particularly in the upper quadrants, changes in stool color, yellowing of sclera or skin, or darkened urine.

- Assess for changes in level of consciousness, disorientation, confusion, or agitation. (Neurologic changes may indicate overmedication or adverse drug effects.)

- Instruct the patient, family, or caregiver to report increasing lethargy, disorientation, confusion, changes in behavior or mood, slurred speech, or ataxia immediately.

- Assess for changes in visual acuity, blurred vision, loss of peripheral vision, seeing rainbow halos around lights, acute eye pain, accompanied by nausea and vomiting, and report immediately. (Increased intraoptic pressure in patients with narrow-angle glaucoma may occur in patients taking benzodiazepines.)

- Instruct the patient to report any visual changes or eye pain immediately.

- Assess for bruising, bleeding, or signs of infection. (Antiseizure drugs may cause blood dyscrasias and increased chances of bleeding or infection.)

- Teach the patient to report any signs of increased bruising, bleeding, or infections (e.g., sore throat and fever, or skin rash) promptly.

- Monitor for dermatologic effects including red or purplish skin rash, blisters, and sunburn. Immediately report severe rashes, especially associated with blistering. (Carbamazepine may cause significant dermatologic effects including SJS.)

- Teach the patient to wear sunscreens and use protective clothing for sun exposure and to avoid tanning beds. Immediately report any sunburn or rashes.

- Monitor affect and emotional status. (Antiseizure drugs may increase the risk of mental depression and suicide. Concurrent use of alcohol or other CNS depressants increases the effects and the risk.)

- Instruct the patient, family, or caregiver to report significant mood changes, especially depression, and to avoid alcohol and other CNS depressants while taking the drug.

- Assess the condition of gums and oral hygiene measures. (Hydantoins and phenytoin-like drugs may cause gingival hyperplasia, increasing the risk of oral infections.)

- Instruct the patient to maintain excellent oral hygiene and keep regularly scheduled dental appointments.

- Encourage appropriate lifestyle and dietary changes: increased intake of foods that are rich in vitamins K, D, and B, and folic acid, lowered caffeine intake including OTC medications that contain caffeine, and limited or no alcohol intake. (Caffeine and nicotine may decrease the effectiveness of the benzodiazepines. Barbiturates, drugs with GABA action, and hydantoins and phenytoin-like drugs affect the absorption of vitamins K, D, and B, and folic acid. Alcohol and other CNS depressants may increase the adverse effects of antiseizure drugs.)

- Encourage the patient to decrease or abstain from caffeine, nicotine, and alcohol, and to increase the intake of foods that are rich in vitamins K, D, and B, and folic acid.
- Advise the patient to discuss all OTC medications with the health care provider to ensure that caffeine or alcohol is not included in the formulation.

- **Lifespan:** Monitor children for paradoxical response to barbiturates. (Hyperactivity may occur.)

- Instruct the patient, family, or caregiver to notify the health care provider if the patient exhibits hyperactive behavior.

- **Lifespan:** Assess women of childbearing age for the possibility of pregnancy, and plans for pregnancy, breast-feeding, and contraceptive use. (Antiseizure medications are category D in pregnancy. AEDs are known to decrease the effectiveness of oral contraceptives and additional forms of contraception should be used.)

- Discuss pregnancy and family planning with women of childbearing age. Explain the effect of medications on pregnancy and breast-feeding and the need to discuss any pregnancy plans with the health care provider. Discuss the need for additional forms of contraception, including barrier methods.

- Avoid abrupt discontinuation of therapy. (Status epilepticus may occur with abrupt discontinuation.)

- Instruct the patient to take the drug exactly as prescribed and to not stop it abruptly.

- Provide emotional support and appropriate referrals as needed. (Treatment with antiseizure drugs may require using combinations of drugs, and seizure activity may diminish but may not be resolved. Social isolation and low self-esteem may occur with continued seizure disorder.)

- Teach the patient, family, and caregiver about support groups, and make appropriate referrals as needed.

CONNECTIONS: NURSING PRACTICE APPLICATION (continued)

• Closely monitor the IV infusion site when using IV antiseizure drugs. All IV drips should be given via infusion pump. (Benzodiazepines, hydantoins, and barbiturates are irritating to the vein. Blanching and pain at the IV site are an indicator of extravasation; the IV infusion should be immediately stopped and the provider contacted for further treatment orders. Infusion pumps will allow precise dosing of the medication.)	• Teach the patient to report pain or burning at the IV site or in the extremity with the IV immediately.
Patient understanding of drug therapy: • Use opportunities during administration of medications and during assessments to discuss the rationale for drug therapy, desired therapeutic outcomes, commonly observed adverse effects, parameters for when to call the health care provider, and any necessary monitoring or precautions. (Using time during nursing care helps to optimize and reinforce key teaching areas.)	• The patient should be able to state the reason for the drug, appropriate dose and scheduling, what adverse effects to observe for and when to report them, and the anticipated length of medication therapy.
Patient self-administration of drug therapy: • When administering the medication, instruct the patient, family, or caregiver in proper self-administration of the drug, e.g., take the drug as prescribed and do not substitute brands. (Utilizing time during nurse-administration of these drugs helps to reinforce teaching.)	Teach the patient to take the medication: • Exactly as ordered and the same manufacturer's brand each time the prescription is filled. (Switching brands may result in differing pharmacokinetics and alterations in seizure control.) • Read label directions for how to take the medication. Some forms may not be opened or chewed; others require chewing thoroughly. When in doubt, consult a pharmacist or other health care provider. • Take a missed dose as soon as it is noticed but do not take double or extra doses to "catch up." • Take with food to decrease GI upset. • Do not abruptly discontinue the medication.

*Nursing Diagnoses—Definitions and Classification 2015–2017. Copyright © 2014, 1994–2014 by NANDA International. Used by arrangement with John Wiley & Sons Limited.

CHAPTER 22

Understanding the Chapter

Key Concepts Summary

22.1 Epilepsy is characterized by recurrent seizures caused by disturbances in the electrical activity of the brain.

22.2 Seizure disorders differ throughout the lifespan.

22.3 Most seizures are classified as generalized or partial.

22.4 Some types of seizures are called special epileptic seizures or are unclassified.

22.5 The selection of antiepileptic drug therapy is dependent on seizure type and characteristics.

22.6 Antiepileptic drugs act by suppressing abnormal neuronal discharges.

22.7 Barbiturates are traditional drugs for tonic–clonic seizures that have been replaced by newer and safer medications.

22.8 Benzodiazepines are important drugs in the treatment of status epilepticus.

22.9 Hydantoins are effective in the management of most types of seizures but have many adverse effects.

22.10 Carbamazepine is a drug of choice for treating many tonic–clonic and partial seizures.

22.11 Succinimides are often the drugs of choice for the pharmacotherapy of absence seizures.

22.12 Several miscellaneous drugs are important in treating epilepsy.

Case Study: Making the Patient Connection

Remember the patient "Jorge Alvarez" at the beginning of the chapter? Now read the remainder of the case study. Based on the information presented within this chapter, respond to the critical thinking questions that follow.

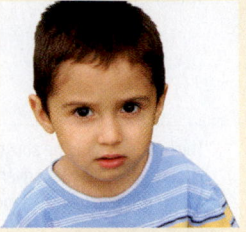

Jorge Alvarez is a 3-year-old boy who has been hospitalized following his seizure. Since being admitted 2 days ago he has experienced three subsequent tonic–clonic seizures lasting 2 to 2 1/2 minutes each. Prior to having a seizure Jorge notices a flash of light. He then loses consciousness, emits a hoarse cry, and has intense muscle contractions. During the clonic phase he is incontinent of bowel and bladder. His postictal phase is characterized by drowsiness, disorientation, and deep sleep.

On admission Jorge was scheduled for a sleep-and-awake EEG. His EEG revealed a high-voltage spike discharge, which is diagnostic of a tonic–clonic seizure. The laboratory studies performed on Jorge included a serum lead level to rule out lead intoxication and a serum glucose level to rule out hypoglycemia. Both the lead level and blood glucose were in the normal range.

Jorge has been started on the following medications to assist in controlling his tonic–clonic seizures: carbamazepine (Tegretol) 300 mg PO tid and phenytoin (Dilantin) 120 mg PO tid.

Critical Thinking Questions

1. Jorge's mother expresses concern about what to do if he has a seizure. Create a list of home safety tips that could be given to her.

2. What will you instruct Jorge's mother with regard to his medication administration?

See Answers to Critical Thinking Questions on student resource website.

Additional Case Study

Matt has had epilepsy since childhood. It seems that his current medications are no longer keeping him seizure free. Valproic acid (Depakene) is being added to Matt's medication regimen. How would you respond to the following questions from Matt about this new medication?

1. How does valproic acid (Depakene) work to prevent seizures?

2. What adverse effects are associated with this drug?

3. Why should Matt inform his dentist that he is now on valproic acid?

See Answers to Additional Case Study on student resource website.

Chapter Review

1 A 10-year-old child has been evaluated for a learning disability and has been diagnosed with absence seizures. Ethosuximide (Zarontin) has been ordered and the nurse is teaching the patient and family about the drug. Because of the patient's age, it is important to include instructions to:

1. Curtail after-school sports activities because the drug's metabolism may be increased with physical activity.

2. Increase intake of calcium-rich foods and vitamin D to prevent bone loss.

3. Monitor height and weight weekly to be sure GI side effects are not hindering nutrition and normal growth.

4. Increase fluid intake to avoid dehydration caused by the drug.

2 The nurse is caring for a 42-year-old patient who was recently diagnosed with partial seizures and has been prescribed oxcarbazepine (Trileptal). Which laboratory study would the nurse expect to be ordered?

1. CBC with differential

2. Serum albumin and glucose levels

3. Sedimentation rate and platelet count

4. Serum sodium and renal function studies

3 An 80-year-old patient is prescribed carbamazepine (Tegretol) for a newly diagnosed seizure disorder. The nurse will implement safety measures because this patient is at an increased risk for which adverse effects with the administration of this drug?

1. Dementia and confusion

2. Insomnia and forgetfulness related to sleep deprivation

3. Stroke and decreased motor function

4. Sedation and falls

4 A 23-year-old patient has been taking gabapentin (Neurontin) for control of partial seizures. He is admitted to the emergency department with slurred speech, dyspnea, reports of double vision, and sedation. The admitting nurse suspects the patient has:

1. Not taken his drug for several days.

2. Taken an overdose of the drug, either accidentally or deliberately.

3. Taken the drug with grapefruit or grapefruit juice.

4. Continued to smoke despite prior patient education that smoking interacts with the drug.

5 The nurse, who is monitoring a patient taking phenytoin (Dilantin), has noted symptoms of nystagmus, confusion, and ataxia. Considering these findings, the nurse would suspect that the dose of the drug should be:

1. Reduced.
2. Increased.
3. Maintained.
4. Discontinued.

6 Carbamazepine (Tegretol) has been prescribed for a 24-year-old patient for the control of partial seizures. The nurse will teach the patient to immediately report:

1. Blurred vision.
2. Leg cramps.
3. Blister-like rash.
4. Lethargy.

See Answers to Chapter Review in Appendix A.

References

Acar, G., & Salinsky, M. C. (2010). Demographic and historical backgrounds of the elderly with nonepileptic seizures: A comparative study. *Neurology India, 58*, 48–52. doi:10.4103/0028-3886.60396

Algreeshah, F. S. (2013). *Psychiatric disorders associated with epilepsy.* Retrieved from http://emedicine.medscape.com/article/1186336-overview#a1

American Academy of Neurology. (2008). *Breastfeeding while taking seizure medicine does not appear to harm children.* Retrieved from https://www.aan.com/PressRoom/Home/PressRelease/603

American Academy of Pediatrics. (2001). The transfer of drugs and other chemicals into human milk. *Pediatrics, 108*, 776–789.

Beghi, M., Savica, R., Beghi, E., Nobili, A., & Garattini, L. (2009). Utilization and costs of antiepileptic drugs in the elderly: Still an unsolved issue. *Drugs and Aging, 26*(2), 157–168. doi:10.2165/0002512-200926020-00007

Chen, J. W. Y., Ruff, R. L., Eavey, R., & Wasterlain, C. G. (2009). Posttraumatic epilepsy and treatment. *Journal of Rehabilitation Research & Development, 46*, 685–695. doi:10.1682/JRRD.2008.09.0130

Epilepsy Foundation of America. (n.d.a). *Causes of epilepsy.* Retrieved from http://www.epilepsyfoundation.org/aboutepilepsy/causes/index.cfm

Epilepsy Foundation of America. (n.d.b). *First aid.* Retrieved from http://www.epilepsyfoundation.org/aboutepilepsy/firstaid/index.cfm

Levy, R. G., Cooper, P. N., Giri, P., & Pulman, J. (2012). Ketogenic diet and other dietary treatments for epilepsy. *Cochrane Database of Systematic Reviews, 3*, CD001903. doi:10.1002/14651858.CD001903.pub2

McElroy-Cox, E. (2009). Alternative approaches to epilepsy treatment. *Current Neurology and Neuroscience Reports, 9*(4), 313–318. doi:10.1007/s11910-009-0047-0

Meador, K. J., Baker, G. A., Browning, N., Clayton-Smith, J., Combs-Cantrell, D. T., Cohen, M., . . . Loring, D. W. (2010). Effects of breastfeeding in children of women taking antiepileptic drugs. *Neurology, 75*, 1954–1960. doi:10.1212/WNL.0b013e3181ffe4a9

Stafstrom, C. E., & Rho, J. M. (2012). The ketogenic diet as a treatment paradigm for diverse neurological disorders. *Frontiers in Pharmacology, 3*, 59.

Vossel, K. A., Beagle, A. J., Rabinovici, G. D., Shu, H., Lee, S. E., Naasan, G., . . . Mucke, L. (2013). Seizures and epileptiform activity in the early stages of Alzheimer disease. *JAMA Neurology, 70*, 1158–1166. doi:10.1001/jamaneurol.2013.136

Selected Bibliography

Chong, D. J., & Bazil, C. W. (2010). Update on anticonvulsant drugs. *Current Neurology and Neuroscience Reports, 10*(4), 308–318. doi:10.1007/s11910-010-0120-8

Guerrini, R., Zaccara, G., la Marca, G., & Rosati, A. (2012). Safety and tolerability of antiepileptic drug treatment in children with epilepsy. *Drug Safety, 35*, 519–533. doi:10.2165/11630700-000000000-00000

Herdman, T. H., & Kamitsuru, S. (Eds.). (2014). *NANDA International nursing diagnoses: Definitions and classification, 2015–2017.* Oxford, United Kingdom: Wiley-Blackwell.

Leppik, I. E., Walczak, T. S., & Birnbaum, A. K. (2012). Challenges of epilepsy in elderly people. *The Lancet, 380*(9848), 1128–1130. doi:10.1016/S0140-6736(12)61517-7

Ochoa, J. G., & Riche, W. (2013). *Antiepileptic drugs.* Retrieved from http://emedicine.medscape.com/article/1187334-overview

Sander, J. W., Ryvlin, P., Stefan, H., Booth, D. R., & Bauer, J. (2010). Generic substitution of antiepileptic drugs. *Expert Review of Neurotherapeutics, 10*, 1887–1898. doi:10.1586/ern.10.163

Verrotti, A., Loiacono, G., Coppola, G., Spalice, A., Mohn, A., & Chiarelli, F. (2011). Pharmacotherapy for children and adolescents with epilepsy. *Expert Opinion on Pharmacotherapy, 12*, 175–194. doi:10.1517/14656566.2010.517194

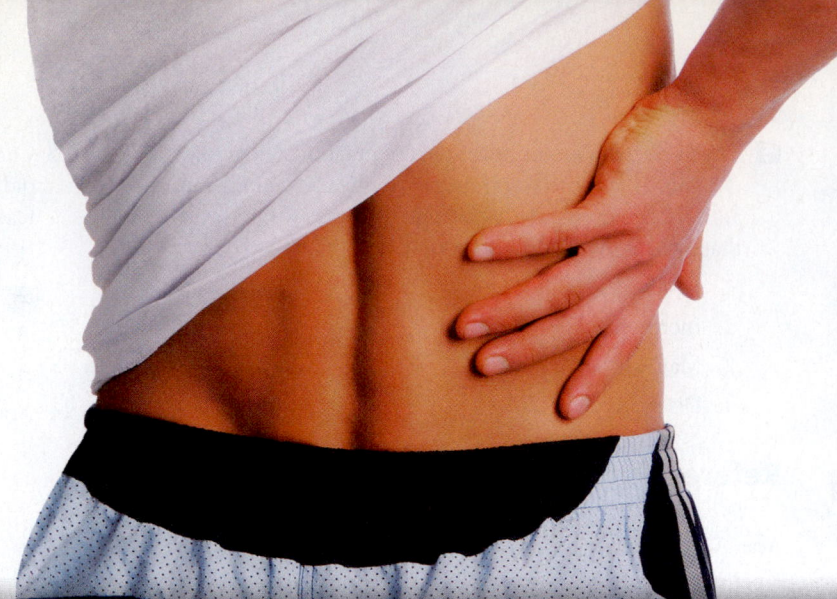

"I was lifting concrete blocks to build a landscaping wall in my front yard yesterday. When I woke up this morning, I couldn't bend down to put on my pants after my shower. My back hurts so bad I can hardly walk."

Patient "Andrew Eskew"

CHAPTER

23 Pharmacotherapy of Muscle Spasms and Spasticity

LEARNING OUTCOMES

After reading this chapter, the student should be able to:

1. Compare and contrast the etiology and pathophysiology of muscle spasm and muscle spasticity.
2. Describe the nonpharmacologic management of muscle spasms and muscle spasticity.
3. Identify drug classes used to treat muscle spasms and spasticity.
4. Compare and contrast the actions of the centrally acting and direct-acting skeletal muscle relaxants.
5. Explain the role of skeletal muscle relaxants as surgical adjuncts.
6. Describe the nurse's role in the pharmacologic management of muscle spasms and muscle spasticity.
7. For each of the classes shown in the chapter outline, identify the prototype and representative drugs and explain the mechanism(s) of drug action, primary indications, contraindications, significant drug interactions, pregnancy category, and important adverse effects.
8. Apply the nursing process to care for patients receiving pharmacotherapy for muscle spasms and spasticity.

CHAPTER OUTLINE

▶ Etiology and Pathophysiology of Muscle Spasms and Spasticity

▶ Nonpharmacologic Therapies for Muscle Spasms and Spasticity

▶ Pharmacotherapy of Muscle Spasms

Centrally Acting Skeletal Muscle Relaxants

PROTOTYPE Cyclobenzaprine (Amrix, Flexeril), *p. 338*

▶ Pharmacotherapy of Muscle Spasticity

Direct-Acting Skeletal Muscle Relaxants

PROTOTYPE Dantrolene (Dantrium, Revonto), *p. 342*

▶ Skeletal Muscle Relaxants as Surgical Adjuncts

dystonia, 336

malignant hyperthermia, 342

muscle spasms, 335

muscle spasticity, 335

The administration of drugs to relieve muscle spasms and musculoskeletal pain dates back to the early 19th century when scientists discovered curare, a substance used for hundreds of years by Amazon Indians as a poison on arrows. Although everyone suffers from muscle aches and pains from time to time, these symptoms often resolve without pharmacotherapy. There are some conditions, however, where medications may be used to relieve painful muscle pain, spasm, or spasticity. This chapter examines how these drugs produce their actions and their applications to the pharmacotherapy of muscle conditions.

Etiology and Pathophysiology of Muscle Spasms and Spasticity

23.1 Whereas muscle spasms are often caused by overuse of skeletal muscle, muscle spasticity involves damage to motor nerves.

Intense skeletal muscle contractions can cause severe pain and disability. Abnormal contractions may be classified as spasms or spasticity. Although both may occur in the same patient, the etiology, pathogenesis, and treatment strategies differ for the two conditions.

Muscle spasms: **Muscle spasms** are involuntary contractions of skeletal muscles that are usually localized to a specific muscle group. As the affected muscles strongly contract and tighten, the spasm causes sudden, intense pain, which gradually diminishes after a few minutes. Patients may refer to the condition as a charley horse or cramp. In addition to causing intense pain, chronic or severe spasms can impair joint mobility.

When treating a patient with muscle spasms, it is important to identify their cause. The etiology of muscle spasms may involve many body systems, including the nervous, musculoskeletal, endocrine, and cardiorespiratory systems. The most common etiology of muscle spasm is overuse of a skeletal muscle. When subjected to trauma or overexertion, the muscle may spasm. If the history does not reveal muscle overuse or injury, the health care provider will need to assess for possible metabolic or electrolyte imbalances such as hypocalcemia, hypokalemia, or dehydration. Poor blood circulation to the legs, known as claudication, is a common cause of muscle cramping.

Some medications may cause muscle spasms, muscle weakness, and other types of myopathy as adverse effects, as shown in Table 23.1. Signs of drug-induced myopathy usually develop slowly after several months of drug therapy. The most important class causing this pathology is the statins, which are widely used to lower blood cholesterol levels. Statins can cause a severe form of myopathy called rhabdomyolysis that may cause significant disability and morbidity. Most drug-induced myopathies are reversible in their early stages. If a medication is suspected of causing myopathy, the dose is lowered or the drug is discontinued.

Muscle spasticity: Muscle spasticity has a different etiology than muscle spasm. **Muscle spasticity** is a condition caused

TABLE 23.1 Medications That May Cause Myopathy as an Adverse Effect

Drug Class	Example(s)
Alzheimer's drug	donepezil (Aricept)
Antihyperlipidemics	statins (Crestor, Lipitor, Zocor), niacin, red yeast rice
Antineoplastics	cisplatin (Platinol), imatinib (Gleevec), vincristine
Antiulcer drugs: proton pump inhibitors	esomeprazole (Nexium), omeprazole (Prilosec)
Asthma drugs	albuterol (Proventil, Ventolin), terbutaline (Brethine)
Antifungals	fluconazole (Diflucan), ketoconazole (Nizoral)
Calcium channel blockers	nifedipine (Procardia)
Diuretics	furosemide (Lasix), hydrochlorothiazide (Microzide)
Immunosuppressants	corticosteroids, leflunomide (Arava)

by damage to upper motor neurons in the central nervous system (CNS), which causes certain muscle groups to remain in a continuous state of contraction. The patient may experience irritable deep tendon reflex activity, muscle spasms, involuntary jerking, and scissoring movements of the lower extremities. Patients with muscle spasticity are unable to voluntarily relax their limbs. Spasticity, also referred to as hypertonia, causes pain that is more intense than muscle spasm and produces greater impairment of mobility.

Whereas muscle spasms occur most often with overexertion, muscle spasticity is associated with neuromuscular diseases that are the result of damage to neurons in the region of the cerebral cortex that controls muscle movements. Conditions most commonly associated with muscular spasticity include severe head or spinal cord trauma, multiple sclerosis (MS), stroke, cerebral palsy (CP), trauma, and amyotrophic lateral sclerosis (ALS).

Under normal conditions a muscle receives a balance of both excitatory and inhibitory signals from motor neurons. When a muscle needs to contract, an impulse is sent from the brain or spinal cord down an excitatory motor neuron. When a muscle needs to relax, the brain sends a signal to the muscle through an inhibitory motor neuron. As a simple example, consider flexion and extension of the elbow. Forearm flexion occurs when the biceps receives an excitatory impulse: At the same time its antagonist, the triceps, receives an inhibitory impulse. On extension, the opposite occurs: The biceps receives the inhibitory message while the triceps contracts after receiving the excitatory message. Proper contraction of skeletal muscle thus involves a balance of signals from the CNS through both excitatory and inhibitory motor neurons.

Muscle spasticity from a spinal cord injury occurs when there is an imbalance of excitatory and inhibitory signals. The area that is distal to the spinal cord injury or lesion becomes disassociated from the inhibitory area of the brain, and the excitatory impulses dominate at the affected muscles. The muscles may go into spastic paralysis; flexor muscles become tight, and the muscles can be extended only with great difficulty. Once extended, the muscles tend to immediately flex back. It is important to understand that although the obvious symptoms appear to be muscle related, the cause of the spasticity is actually neurologic injury. Neuromuscular diseases that exhibit muscle spasticity include MS, stroke, CP, and ALS.

In the advanced stages of MS, muscle spasticity is caused by destruction of the myelin sheath, which interrupts the main motor pathways from the spinal cord to the muscles. Spasticity results in a stiff, unbalanced gait and may eventually confine these patients to a wheelchair. Patients with MS are treated with a combination of medications including muscle relaxants, corticosteroids, and immunosuppressants (see Chapter 21).

Approximately 35% of patients experience spasticity following a stroke. If the brain area affected by the stroke is able to reestablish communication with the muscle, the spasticity may be reversible and voluntary movement may be restored. In many cases, however, the spasticity becomes permanent and can be recognized by a clenched fist, permanently flexed elbow, or pointed toes.

Cerebral palsy is a neurologic disorder that results in severe muscular spasticity, which can affect facial muscles, cause an unsteady, scissoring gait, and result in painful joint contractures and deformities. The primary cause of spasticity associated with CP is congenital trauma to the brain or spinal cord. Pharmacologic options for treating CP are limited. Intrathecal baclofen may be beneficial in reducing severe spasticity.

Muscle spasms, spasticity, and twitching are also characteristic of ALS, also known as Lou Gehrig's disease. ALS is caused by the degeneration and loss of lower and upper motor neurons in the CNS. The disorder is progressive and fatal. Muscle relaxants may bring some pain relief during periods of intense muscle spasticity.

Dystonia is a chronic neurologic disorder that is characterized by involuntary muscle contraction that forces body parts into abnormal, painful movements or postures. The condition may affect the entire body (generalized dystonia), or it may be localized to a single body region (focal dystonia) such as the arms, legs, trunk, neck, eyelids, face, or vocal cords. Dystonia may occur secondary to other neurologic disorders such as MS, stroke, or CP. The impairment in mobility and intense pain produced by muscle spasms and spasticity inhibits the patient's ability to perform activities of daily living (ADLs). Generalized dystonias are treated with high doses of anticholinergic drugs such as benztropine, benzodiazepines, and baclofen. Patients with focal dystonia may obtain some relief with botulinum toxin type A.

Dupuytren's contracture is a condition of the hand in which a thick cord of connective tissue forms in the palm, causing the fingers to curl inward. Although not usually painful, the curling is progressive and can restrict motion and use of the hand. This disorder is not caused by muscles; therefore, traditional muscle relaxants and antispasmodics are ineffective. For severe cases, surgical removal of the connective tissue cord is performed. In 2010 an enzyme medication, collagenase (Xiaflex), was approved to treat this disorder. This enzyme is injected multiple times into the affected cord, over a 4-week interval. The most frequently reported adverse effects are swelling of the affected hand, contusion, injection-site reaction or hemorrhage, and localized pain.

PharmFACT

Dystonia affects about 300,000 people in the United States and is the third most common movement disorder, following essential tremor and Parkinson's disease. It can affect someone at any stage of the lifespan (American Dystonia Society, n.d.).

Nonpharmacologic Therapies for Muscle Spasms and Spasticity

23.2 Nonpharmacologic interventions for treating muscle spasms and spasticity are limited.

The therapeutic goals for treating muscle spasms or spasticity are to decrease discomfort and enhance mobility so that the patient is better able to perform ADLs. Nonpharmacologic complementary and alternative therapies (CAT) are sometimes implemented to achieve these goals. When the spasms or spasticity are prolonged or disabling, pharmacotherapy is initiated. A combination of CAT and drug therapy is often the most effective treatment.

Nonpharmacologic interventions that sometimes benefit patients with muscle spasm or spasticity include the application of heat or cold, massage, traction, and manipulation. The application of heat or cold to the affected site will reduce or relieve the muscle spasm and pain. If the spasm has occurred due to overexertion, application of heat to the area can reduce cramping and relieve localized pain. If the spasms persist after 3 to 5 days, the application of cold packs to the site may be used to slow the transmission of pain impulses. The application of touch, massage, and gentle pressure are sometimes effective at promoting musculoskeletal relaxation. Other nonpharmacologic techniques that may be useful include acupuncture, sensory nerve stimulation, and ankle splints for leg pain.

The implementation of physical therapy is sometimes effective for treating muscle spasticity. Routine and consistent physical therapy exercises provide the patient with increased muscle movement and decreased severity of symptoms. Effective physical therapy exercises include muscle stretching, which assists in the prevention of contractures (permanent shortening of muscles). The implementation of muscle group strengthening and repetitive motion exercises may allow for safer ambulation. In extreme cases, surgery may be necessary to release tendons or to sever the nerve–muscle pathway.

Herbal remedies are occasionally used to treat patients with muscle spasms. Black cohosh, first used for neuralgia and muscular pain in the 1840s, may be applied topically to produce relaxation of muscles. Castor oil packs can be applied to the site of pain and muscle spasm. The castor oil should be warmed, soaked into a flannel, wool, or cotton cloth, and then applied to the tonic muscle. Capsaicin, derived from cayenne pepper, is applied topically as a cream four times per day to increase mobility and reduce pain. It is important to instruct the patient to wear gloves while applying capsaicin cream to prevent irritation of the skin on the hands and to avoid introducing the capsaicin to the eyes or other parts of the body not under treatment. A high potency, prescription drug containing 8% capsaicin (Qutenza) was approved in 2010.

CONNECTIONS   Evidence-Based Practice

◀ Treating Spastic Cerebral Palsy in Children with Intrathecal Baclofen

Clinical Question
Can children with cerebral palsy with spasticity be safely and effectively treated with intrathecal baclofen?

Evidence
Between 70% and 90% of patients with CP have spasticity along with other motor disorders. Prior treatment for CP patients with spasticity has included diazepam (Valium), dantrolene (Dantrium), and oral baclofen (Lioresal). Because these drugs are given PO, they may cause significant systemic adverse effects such as drowsiness, confusion, behavior changes, and hypotension. In the early 2000s, the American Academy for Cerebral Palsy and Developmental Medicine (AACPDM) performed a systematic review of treatment and noted beneficial effects of continuous intrathecal baclofen in patients with spastic CP, but noted that no well-controlled studies in children had been conducted (Butler et al., 2000). It was known that many children with spastic CP did not respond well or at all to traditional medications.

Early studies in the use of intrathecal baclofen (ITB) determined that ITB was a safe and effective method to manage the spasticity, pain, and startle response in CP; increase the ease of care and other measures of improvement with fewer systemic adverse effects; and was a cost-effective treatment with a significant gain in quality of life indicators (deLissovoy, Matza, Green, Werner, & Edgar, 2007; Hoving et al., 2007). Additional studies have continued to demonstrate that ITB is an effective treatment measure for spastic and dystonic CP, especially for children younger than 18 and for children with extreme spasticity and dystonia (Motta, Antonello, & Stignani, 2011), which does not carry an increased risk of mortality (Krach, Kriel, Day, & Strauss, 2010). Because ITB has not been in use long term, Vles et al. (2013) conducted a study into the long-term effects of ITB. Significant and continued positive impacts on pain, ease of care, quality of life, and parental satisfaction with the treatment were noted.

Implications
Based on these findings, ITB may offer improved and targeted treatment of the spasticity, pain, loss of ADL ability, and other effects of CP in children, especially for those who have not responded well or at all to traditional oral (PO) medications or surgery. Nurses often provide the most direct support and connection to families dealing with the long-term implications of CP. They can provide education on the use and care of the ITB pump, site care, and drug effects to monitor for those families choosing this option. Nurses may also help educate school staff and nurses on the use and care of the pump and the monitoring required for adverse effects.

Critical Thinking Questions

1. What are some common adverse effects of baclofen?
2. Considering the method of delivery (intrathecal), what other aspects of care should the nurse be concerned about?

See Answers to Critical Thinking Questions on student resource website.

A final nonpharmacologic therapy for muscle spasm is treatment with B complex vitamins, specifically pyridoxine (B_6). In an assessment of therapies for muscle cramps, the American Academy of Neurology found vitamin B complex to be the only effective nonpharmacologic therapy supported by research evidence (Katzberg, Khan, & So, 2010). The B complex vitamins can reduce both the intensity and duration of leg cramps.

PharmFACT
After spinal cord injury 40% to 67% will experience muscle spasticity and a large number of these patients will require pharmacotherapy (Brashear & Elovic, 2011).

Pharmacotherapy of Muscle Spasms

23.3 Nonsteroidal anti-inflammatory drugs and skeletal muscle relaxants are used to treat muscle spasms.

Muscle spasms, especially those caused by injury, are painful and sometimes associated with inflammation. Nonsteroidal anti-inflammatory drugs (NSAIDs) such as aspirin, naproxen, and ibuprofen are usually the first-line drugs for treating minor to moderate pain due to muscle overexertion. These drugs have the ability to relieve muscle pain and reduce inflammation around the injury site, which can take pressure off the surrounding nerves and enhance mobility. The pharmacology of NSAIDs is presented in Chapter 41.

Muscle relaxants are prescribed for moderate to severe muscle spasms. Although these drugs are not analgesics, they can promote pain relief by relaxing tight, contracted muscles without interfering with normal muscle function. When skeletal muscle relaxants are used in combination with NSAIDs, pain relief is greater than when either agent is used alone.

The centrally acting skeletal muscle relaxants relieve muscle spasms by their actions in the CNS. They do not directly affect the neuromuscular junction or muscles themselves. The precise mechanism of action of centrally acting skeletal muscle relaxants is unclear but it is believed they help to restore the balance of excitatory and inhibitory impulses from motor neurons in the CNS. Like the benzodiazepines, they can produce significant drowsiness, especially if combined with alcohol or other CNS depressants. The sedative effects may be beneficial in helping patients with muscle spasms or spasticity to obtain needed sleep. The centrally acting skeletal muscle relaxants include cyclobenzaprine (Amrix, Flexeril), baclofen (Lioresal), and tizanidine (Zanaflex). Some drugs in this class are used for both muscle spasms and spasticity. Mechanisms of action are shown in Pharmacotherapy Illustrated 23.1. Doses of the centrally acting muscle relaxants are listed in Table 23.2.

Drugs from a number of other classes have been used to treat and prevent muscle spasms. Calcium channel blockers including diltiazem (Cardizem, Dilacor) and verapamil (Calan) may be used off-label to prevent muscle cramps. The mechanism for this action is unknown but may be related to the drugs' ability to dilate arteries and bring additional oxygen to muscles. The American Academy of Neurology found calcium channel blockers to be the only

PHARMACOTHERAPY ILLUSTRATED 23.1

MECHANISM OF ACTION OF DRUGS USED TO TREAT MUSCLE SPASMS AND SPASTICITY

Sensory perception of pain

Motor response to muscle: Spasm due to pain

Cerebral cortex

Centrally-acting drugs act in the CNS by
- Reducing excitability
  - Tizanidine
- Enhancing inhibition
  - Baclofen

Spinal cord

Sensory

Motor

Neuromuscular junction

Neuromuscular blockers
- Succinylcholine

Direct-acting drugs
- Dantrolene
- Botulinum

Skeletal muscle

Stretch and pain receptors

pharmacologic therapy for muscle spasms supported by research evidence (Katzberg et al., 2010).

Benzodiazepines such as diazepam (Valium) are occasionally prescribed to relax skeletal muscle. Diazepam may be used as an adjunct to relieve skeletal muscle spasms associated with CP, paraplegia, and tetanus. Diazepam is a featured prototype drug for seizures in Chapter 22.

Quinine is one of the oldest and most effective drugs for relieving nocturnal leg cramping. However, this medication is rarely used for this indication. In 2010, the U.S. Food and Drug Administration (FDA) issued a black box warning that the drug should not be used to treat muscle cramps due to the risk for life-threatening hematologic toxicity. The drug may still be used to treat resistant malarial infections (see Chapter 53).

CONNECTION Checkpoint 23.1

Benzodiazepines are some of the most widely prescribed drugs. From what you learned in Chapter 18, what are the major indications for drugs in this class? *See Answer to Connection Checkpoint 23.1 on student resource website.*

PROTOTYPE DRUG	Cyclobenzaprine (Amrix, Flexeril)

Classification: **Therapeutic:** Skeletal muscle relaxant
Pharmacologic: Centrally acting antispasmodic

Therapeutic Effects and Uses: Cyclobenzaprine is indicated for the short-term therapy of acute musculoskeletal conditions that are unrelated to CNS disease. Cyclobenzaprine is not effective for

TABLE 23.2	**Centrally Acting Skeletal Muscle Relaxants**	
Drug	**Route and Adult Dose (Maximum Dose Where Indicated)**	**Adverse Effects**
baclofen (Lioresal)	PO: Start with 5 mg tid and increase gradually to 40–80 mg/day to control spasms (max: 80 mg/day) Intrathecal: 50-mcg bolus	*Drowsiness, dizziness, weakness, fatigue, confusion, altered mental status, nausea, vomiting, constipation, urinary frequency* QT prolongation, dysrhythmias
carisoprodol (Soma)	Adult: PO: 350 mg tid	*Drowsiness, confusion, postural hypotension, nausea, vomiting, hiccups, vertigo, ataxia, tremor, syncope* Anaphylactic shock, physical dependence, profound sedation
chlorzoxazone (Paraflex, Parafon Forte)	PO: 250–500 mg tid or qid (max: 3 g/day)	*Drowsiness, dizziness, anorexia, heartburn, nausea, vomiting, diarrhea, abdominal pain, lightheadedness, overstimulation, rash, pruritus, urticaria, discoloration of urine* Hepatotoxicity, jaundice, anemia, neutropenia
cyclobenzaprine (Amrix, Flexeril)	PO: 5–10 mg tid for tablets; 15 mg once daily for extended release capsules (max: 30 mg/day)	*Drowsiness, xerostomia, dizziness, fatigue, nausea, constipation, dyspepsia* Tongue edema, potential for QT prolongation, hallucinations, serotonin syndrome
metaxalone (Skelaxin)	PO: 800 mg tid–qid	*Nausea, vomiting, GI upset, drowsiness, dizziness, headache, anxiety* Hemolytic anemia, jaundice, hepatotoxicity, anaphylaxis
methocarbamol (Robaxin)	PO: 1.5 g qid for 2–3 days then 4–4.5 g/day in divided doses IV/IM: 1–3 g once daily for 3 days; repeat after a drug-free interval of 48 h if necessary; do not exceed 3 mL/min	*Drowsiness, dizziness, lightheadedness, fever, pruritus, rash, syncope, thrombophlebitis, pain, blurred vision, headache, tachycardia, syncope* Anaphylactic shock, sloughing of skin with extravasation
orphenadrine (Norflex)	PO: 100 mg bid IM/IV: 60 mg every 12 h (max: 250 mg/day)	*Dry mouth, drowsiness, weakness, dizziness, agitation, tachycardia, syncope, palpitations, increased ocular tension, blurred vision, nausea, vomiting, abdominal cramps, pruritus, urticaria* Anaphylactic shock, hallucinations
tizanidine (Zanaflex)	PO: 4–8 mg every 6–8 h as needed (max: 36 mg/day)	*Dry mouth, somnolence, asthenia, fatigue, back pain, dizziness, flulike symptoms* Hepatotoxicity, hypotension, bradycardia, hallucinations

Note: Italics indicates common adverse effects. Underline indicates serious adverse effects.

treating muscle spasm due to spinal cord injury or CP. The drug promotes skeletal muscle relaxation, thus decreasing muscle spasms and increasing joint mobility. The manufacturer recommends that treatment not extend beyond 3 weeks. Fibromyalgia is an off-label indication for the drug.

Cyclobenzaprine is chemically related to the tricyclic antidepressants (TCAs) and it exhibits some antidepressant effects. The drug is available by immediate release tablet or extended release capsule. Cyclobenzaprine is occasionally abused as a recreational drug due to its sedative actions.

Mechanism of Action: The action of cyclobenzaprine is thought to occur at the brainstem and spinal cord levels. The drug increases norepinephrine activity by blocking its synaptic reuptake to produce an anticholinergic effect. Cyclobenzaprine acts centrally and thus has no direct action on skeletal muscle.

Pharmacokinetics:

Route(s)	PO
Absorption	Well absorbed in the gastrointestinal (GI) tract
Distribution	It is unknown whether the drug crosses the placenta or is secreted in breast milk; 93% bound to protein
Primary metabolism	Extensive hepatic metabolism via CYP enzymes to inactive metabolites
Primary excretion	Renal
Onset of action	1 h
Duration of action	12–24 h

Adverse Effects: The commonly reported adverse effects of cyclobenzaprine are drowsiness, dizziness, and xerostomia. Sedation can be a limiting effect with the first few doses. Other adverse effects of cyclobenzaprine include edema of the tongue and face with sweating, myalgia, hepatitis, and alopecia. Potential cardiovascular adverse events include orthostatic hypotension, tachycardia, syncope, palpitations, and vasodilation. The patient may report having an unpleasant taste, a coated tongue with discoloration, vomiting, anorexia, diarrhea with flatulence, or paralysis.

Contraindications/Precautions: Cyclobenzaprine should be used with great caution in patients older than age 65 because this population is more likely to experience confusion, hallucinations, and adverse cardiac events from the drug. Cyclobenzaprine also should be used cautiously in patients who have increased intraocular pressure, prostatic hyperplasia, urinary retention, and seizures. Patients with hypersensitivity to TCAs should not receive this drug. Like the TCAs, cyclobenzaprine can adversely affect the heart and therefore should be used with caution in patients with cardiovascular disease, including those with heart failure or dysrhythmias with heart block. It is contraindicated in patients who have QT interval prolongation on the electrocardiogram (ECG), or who are in the recovery phase of a myocardial infarction (MI). The drug is metabolized in the liver and thus should be administered cautiously to patients with hepatic impairment. Patients with a history of hyperthyroidism should not be administered cyclobenzaprine.

Drug Interactions: Cyclobenzaprine should not be administered with alcohol, opioids, barbiturates, or any other CNS depressants because significant sedation may occur. Phenothiazines and anticholinergic drugs will enhance the anticholinergic adverse effects and are contraindicated with cyclobenzaprine. Use with TCAs may result in additive CNS depression and increased anticholinergic effects. A potentially fatal hypertensive crisis can occur if cyclobenzaprine is used within 14 days of a monoamine oxidase inhibitor. Serotonin syndrome has been reported when cyclobenzaprine is coadministered with other drugs that increase serotonin such as SSRIs, SNRIs, TCAs, tramadol, bupropion, meperidine or verapamil. **Herbal/Food**: Additive CNS depression may occur if cyclobenzaprine is administered concurrently with valerian or kava.

Pregnancy: Category B.

Treatment of Overdose: Signs of overdose include CNS depression and tachycardia. Physostigmine (Antilirium) may be administered to reverse serious anticholinergic adverse effects. Overdose is generally not fatal.

Nursing Responsibilities: Key nursing implications for patients receiving cyclobenzaprine are included in the Nursing Practice Application for Patients Receiving Pharmacotherapy for Muscle Spasms and Spasticity.

Drugs Similar to Cyclobenzaprine (Amrix, Flexeril)

The following medications are other centrally acting skeletal muscle relaxants: baclofen, carisoprodol, chlorzoxazone, metaxalone, methocarbamol, orphenadrine, and tizanidine. Chlorphenesin (Maolate) is a centrally acting muscle relaxant that was removed from the market in the United States.

Baclofen (Lioresal): Approved in 1977, baclofen is used to reduce muscle spasticity in patients with injury or disease of upper motor neurons such as that associated with MS, CP, ALS, and spinal cord trauma. Off-label indications include the treatment of tardive dyskinesia related to long-term pharmacotherapy with antipsychotic agents, persistent hiccups, and for management of neuropathic pain. The drug resembles the inhibitory neurotransmitter GABA and acts by inhibiting neuronal activity within the brain and spinal cord. Baclofen is usually administered PO, but it can be administered by infusion delivered directly into the intrathecal space, using a small catheter and a pump. This provides a direct route for the baclofen to reach its target sites in the spinal cord and brain. Because the baclofen is delivered continuously at its site of action, very small amounts are needed to produce a therapeutic effect. The health care provider determines the amount of drug to be released by the pump and the dosing schedule. The pump must be refilled every 1 to 3 months and the battery lasts 5 to 7 years. Several months of therapy may be required to achieve full therapeutic benefit from baclofen.

Adverse effects related to the administration of baclofen include drowsiness, dizziness, weakness, and fatigue. Abrupt discontinuation following prolonged therapy may cause high fever, seizures, severe rebound muscle spasticity, and hallucinations. This drug is pregnancy category C.

Carisoprodol (Soma): An older drug approved by the FDA in 1959, carisoprodol is administered PO for the short-term therapy (up to 3 weeks) of acute, painful musculoskeletal conditions. It is effective in relieving the pain, muscle spasms, and spasticity associated with CP. The drug produces significant sedation in 40% of patients taking it and may cause significant CNS and respiratory depression if taken with alcohol or other CNS depressants. The general sedative nature of the drug is likely responsible for its ability to relieve the pain associated with muscle spasms. Although not a controlled substance, carisoprodol can cause physical dependence and has been abused by recreational drug users. The active metabolite of carisoprodol is meprobamate, a rarely used antianxiety agent and a Schedule IV drug. The drug should be used with caution in patients with a history of drug abuse. The development of newer drugs and increased levels of carisoprodol abuse in recent years has led to less frequent prescribing of the drug. This drug is pregnancy category C.

Chlorzoxazone (Paraflex, Parafon Forte): Chlorzoxazone is an oral centrally acting skeletal muscle relaxant administered for the symptomatic treatment of discomfort associated with acute, painful musculoskeletal conditions. It is ineffective in the treatment of spasticity related to neurodegenerative disorders such as CP. The actions of the drug may be largely due to its sedative effects. It should not be combined with alcohol or other CNS depressants. Chlorzoxazone is hepatotoxic and should not be used in patients with liver impairment. Other adverse effects include anorexia, nausea, vomiting, rash, and red-orange discoloration of urine. Older adults may experience more adverse CNS effects than younger patients. This drug is pregnancy category C.

Metaxalone (Skelaxin): Approved in 1962, metaxalone is administered PO and is indicated for the symptomatic relief of muscle spasm and pain related to musculoskeletal conditions. It is ineffective in the treatment of spasticity-related neurologic disorders. The therapeutic effects of metaxalone are likely due to its ability to depress the CNS. Like chlorzoxazone, metaxalone may cause liver injury and is contraindicated in patients with hepatic impairment. It should not be administered to patients over age 65 due to significant anticholinergic effects. Drowsiness, nausea and vomiting, and anxiety are common adverse effects. This drug is pregnancy category C.

Methocarbamol (Relaxin, Robaxin): Approved in 1957, methocarbamol has central sedative effects that likely are responsible for its ability to reduce muscle spasms. It is used as an adjunct to physical therapy interventions. It can be administered intravenously (IV) for the treatment of tetanus or other acute musculoskeletal conditions. Methocarbamol may cause significant dizziness and sedation and should not be taken with alcohol or other CNS depressants. It is contraindicated in patients with significant renal impairment. It should not be administered to patients over age 65 due to significant anticholinergic effects. This drug is pregnancy category C.

Orphenadrine (Norflex): Orphenadrine is an older drug that was approved in 1959. It is administered PO or parenterally to relax skeletal muscles and reduce pain. The drug has analgesic properties and may be administered parenterally to produce local anesthetic effects. It may be used off-label as an adjunct in the treatment of the muscular rigidity associated with Parkinson's disease. The most common side effect of orphenadrine is xerostomia. Orphenadrine is structurally very similar to diphenhydramine (Benadryl) and can cause prominent anticholinergic effects: It should not be used with other anticholinergic drugs due to the risk for additive toxicity. Orphenadrine produces a mild to moderate euphoric effect that has led to its abuse. This drug is pregnancy category C.

Tizanidine (Zanaflex): Approved in 1996, tizanidine is a centrally acting alpha$_2$-adrenergic agonist that inhibits motor neurons mainly at the spinal cord level. It has no direct effect on muscle fibers. Approved for the management of muscle spasticity, tizanidine is most effective in patients who have significantly diminished muscle tone, including spasticity related to brain or spinal cord injury or MS. Tizanidine is as effective as baclofen in treating muscle spasticity and is considered a first-line drug. One disadvantage of tizanidine is that it has a short duration of action that requires dosing every 6 to 8 hours.

The most common adverse effects of tizanidine include xerostomia, fatigue, weakness, dizziness, and drowsiness. Hypotension is common at higher doses; the drug is closely related to clonidine (Catapres), which is an antihypertensive agent. Hallucinations are uncommon but patients with a history of psychosis should be carefully monitored for this adverse effect. Tizanidine is hepatotoxic and should not be used in patients with liver impairment. Older adults, especially those with some degree of renal impairment, may experience frequent adverse effects such as drowsiness, dizziness, dry mouth, and asthenia. This drug is pregnancy category C.

CONNECTION Checkpoint 23.2

Cyclobenzaprine is very similar to the TCAs. From what you learned in Chapter 19, describe the major indications (approved and off-label) for the TCAs. *See Answer to Connection Checkpoint 23.2 on student resource website.*

PharmFACT

The brain lesions of CP occur in the fetus and through age 3, but the diagnosis may not be made until age 5 or later (Abel-Hamid, 2013).

Pharmacotherapy of Muscle Spasticity

23.4 Direct-acting skeletal muscle relaxants are often used to relieve muscle spasticity.

Medications effective in the treatment of spasticity include muscle relaxants that act at the level of the CNS, neuromuscular junction, or muscle tissue. Some of the centrally acting medications used to treat muscle spasms, such as baclofen (Lioresal) and tizanidine (Zanaflex), are also effective in treating spasticity.

Dantrolene (Dantrium, Revonto) and the botulinum toxins act directly on skeletal muscle to relieve spasticity. These are called direct-acting muscle relaxants or antispasticity agents. Dantrolene is the prototype for direct-acting agents. Doses of these drugs are listed in Table 23.3. The mechanisms of action of direct-acting antispasmodics are shown in Pharmacotherapy Illustrated 23.2.

TABLE 23.3 Direct-Acting Muscle Relaxants

Drug	Route and Dose (Maximum Dose Where Indicated)	Adverse Effects
abobotulinumtoxinA (Dysport)	Cervical dystonia: IM: 500 units, in divided doses Glabellar lines: IM: 50 units given in 5 equal doses	*Injection reactions, headache, dysphagia, muscle weakness, pain, tenderness, bruising, flulike symptoms, dry mouth, ptosis of eyelids*
incobotulinumtoxinA (Xeomin)	Cervical dystonia: IM: 120 units Blepharospasm: IM: 10–50 units per eye in 6 injections (max: 50 units per eye)	Spread of toxin to surrounding muscles, anaphylaxis and other hypersensitivity reactions, difficulty swallowing or breathing (cervical dystonia therapy), corneal ulceration (blepharospasm therapy)
onabotulinumtoxinA (Botox)	Cervical dystonia: IM: 198–300 units in divided doses (max: 50 units per site) Upper limb spasticity: 75–360 units in divided doses (max: 50 units/site) Axillary hyperhidrosis: IM: 50 units per site Migraines: IM: 155 units in divided doses across specific head/neck regions (max: 5 units per site) Overactive bladder: 100–200 units across 20–30 injections sites in the detrusor muscle	
onabotulinumtoxinA (Botox Cosmetic)	Glabellar lines: IM: 20 units divided among affected muscles	
rimabotulinumtoxinB (Myobloc)	Cervical dystonia: IM: 2,500–5,000 units divided among affected muscles	
dantrolene (Dantrium, Revonto)	Spasticity: PO: 25 mg once daily; may increase to 25 mg bid–qid (max: 100 mg bid–qid) Malignant hyperthermia: IV push: 1 mg/kg; repeat as needed (max: 10 mg/kg); may continue PO at 1–2 mg/kg qid for 1–3 days	*Hypersensitivity, drowsiness, dizziness, lightheadedness, fatigue, speech disturbance, insomnia, mental depression, blurred vision, diplopia, photophobia, vomiting, anorexia, GI upset, crystalluria, urinary frequency, urinary retention, nocturia, enuresis, difficult erection* Muscle weakness, diarrhea, hepatic necrosis

Note: Italics indicates common adverse effects. Underline indicates serious adverse effects.

PHARMACOTHERAPY ILLUSTRATED 23.2

MECHANISM OF ACTION OF DIRECT-ACTING ANTISPASMODICS

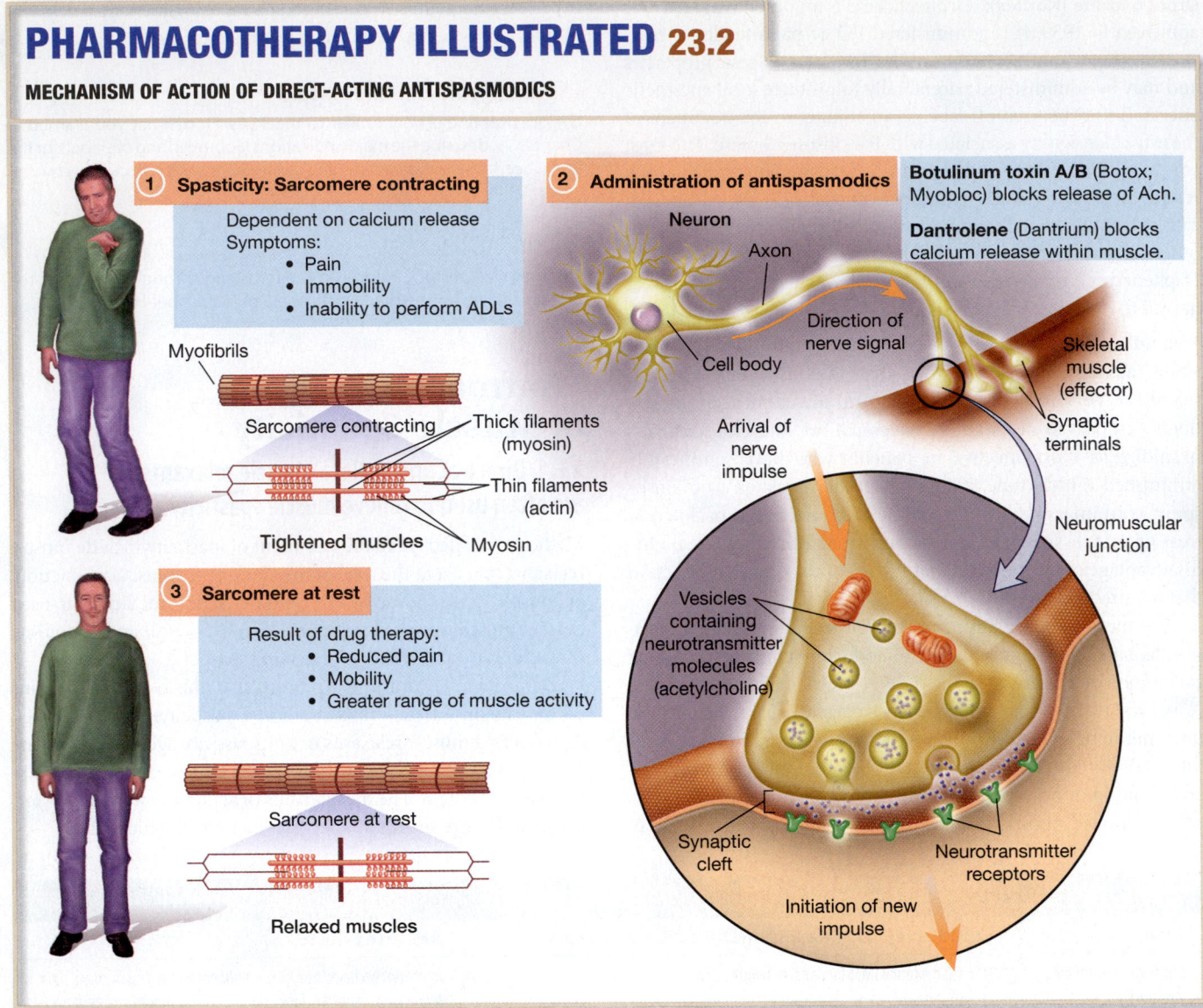

1   Spasticity: Sarcomere contracting

Dependent on calcium release
Symptoms:
- Pain
- Immobility
- Inability to perform ADLs

Myofibrils

Sarcomere contracting

Thick filaments (myosin)

Thin filaments (actin)

Myosin

Tightened muscles

3   Sarcomere at rest

Result of drug therapy:
- Reduced pain
- Mobility
- Greater range of muscle activity

Sarcomere at rest

Relaxed muscles

2   Administration of antispasmodics

Botulinum toxin A/B (Botox; Myobloc) blocks release of Ach.

Dantrolene (Dantrium) blocks calcium release within muscle.

Neuron

Axon

Direction of nerve signal

Cell body

Arrival of nerve impulse

Skeletal muscle (effector)

Synaptic terminals

Neuromuscular junction

Vesicles containing neurotransmitter molecules (acetylcholine)

Synaptic cleft

Neurotransmitter receptors

Initiation of new impulse

PROTOTYPE DRUG	**Dantrolene (Dantrium, Revonto)**

Classification: Therapeutic: Direct-acting skeletal muscle relaxant, antispasticity agent
Pharmacologic: Calcium release blocker (skeletal muscle cells)

Therapeutic Effects and Uses: Approved in 1974, dantrolene is a direct-acting skeletal muscle relaxant indicated for spasticity, especially for spasms of the head and neck muscles following a spinal cord injury, stroke, and in cases of CP or MS. When administered PO (Dantrium), the drug induces relaxation of the skeletal muscles. It may be used off-label to treat malignant neuroleptic syndrome or for the treatment of pain following heavy exercise.

When administered IV, Revonto is a preferred drug for treating **malignant hyperthermia**, a rare condition that is an

adverse effect of succinylcholine (Anectine) and some general anesthetics. A patient with malignant hyperthermia will experience a sudden onset of tachycardia, ventricular dysrhythmia, and hypotension. This is due to the rapid release of calcium ions in muscle cells, which produces hypermetabolism and intense muscle rigidity. The muscle metabolic rate becomes so elevated that it quickly raises the body temperature to a dangerous level. There is a strong genetic predisposition to malignant hyperthermia, and patients with a family history of the disorder should not receive drugs that have the potential to cause this adverse effect. It is important for the anesthesia provider and circulating nurse to have phentolamine (Regitine) available in the event of extravasation of dantrolene.

Mechanism of Action: Dantrolene is related to phenytoin (Dilantin), an antiepileptic drug. Dantrolene directly relaxes spastic muscles by interfering with the release of calcium ions that have been stored in the sarcoplasmic reticulum of skeletal muscle.

Pharmacokinetics:

Route(s)	PO, IV
Absorption	Approximately 35% is slowly and incompletely absorbed from the GI tract
Distribution	Crosses the placenta; highly bound to plasma protein
Primary metabolism	Hepatic
Primary excretion	Renal and feces
Onset of action	Peak concentration: 5 h
Duration of action	Half-life: 8.7 h (PO) or 4–8 h (IV)

Adverse Effects: Muscle weakness and drowsiness are the most common adverse effects of dantrolene therapy. Other adverse effects include xerostomia, dizziness, nausea, photosensitivity, diarrhea, tachycardia, erratic blood pressure, and urinary retention. **Black Box Warning**: Dantrolene is hepatotoxic and deaths due to liver failure have occurred in patients taking this drug. Baseline and periodic hepatic function tests should be conducted during therapy. The lowest possible effective dose should be used to avoid hepatotoxicity and the drug should be discontinued if no therapeutic effect is noted after 45 days of treatment.

Contraindications/Precautions: There are no contraindications to the use of dantrolene in treating malignant hyperthermia because this is a fatal condition if left untreated. For spasticity, dantrolene is contraindicated in patients with preexisting hepatic disease. Because it can cause muscle weakness, dantrolene should not be used when spasticity is necessary to sustain an upright position or balance when standing or walking. Dantrolene should be used cautiously in the presence of impaired cardiac or pulmonary function. The risk of dantrolene-induced hepatotoxicity is greatest in women over the age of 35; thus it should be administered cautiously in these patients.

Drug Interactions: Dantrolene interacts with other CNS depressants, including alcohol, to cause additive sedation. The combination of estrogen and dantrolene in women can result in hepatotoxicity. Calcium channel blockers such as verapamil (Calan) place the patient at increased risk of ventricular fibrillation and cardiovascular collapse when dantrolene sodium is administered intravenously. **Herbal/Food**: Use of kava or valerian may result in additive sedation.

Pregnancy: Category C.

Treatment of Overdose: Overdose with dantrolene results in muscle weakness, lethargy, and coma. General supportive measures are administered until the effects of the drug diminish.

Nursing Responsibilities: Key nursing implications for patients receiving dantrolene are included in the Nursing Practice Application for Patients Receiving Pharmacotherapy for Muscle Spasms and Spasticity.

Drugs Similar to Dantrolene (Dantrium)

Botulinum toxins are also direct-acting muscle relaxants.

Botulinum toxin (Botox, Botox Cosmetic, Dysport, Myobloc, Xeomin): Botulinum toxin is a natural substance obtained from *Clostridium botulinum*, the gram-positive bacterium responsible for botulism. The drug blocks neuromuscular transmission by binding to motor nerve terminals and inhibiting the release of acetylcholine. Without sufficient amounts of acetylcholine, the muscle is unable to contract and flaccid paralysis occurs.

Since its initial approval by the FDA in 1989, several forms of botulinum toxin have been developed and marketed. Each of the formulations differs in potency and they may not be interchanged or substituted for each other. To avoid medication errors, the FDA renamed the various products in 2009. The botulinum products are listed in Table 23.3. Table 23.4 gives the approved indications for the products.

The first botulinum product approved in 1989 was onabotulinumtoxin A (Botox). This formulation is approved for all indications: blepharospasm, cervical dystonia, glabellar lines (facial wrinkles; Figure 23.1), severe axillary hyperhidrosis (axillary perspiration), upper limb spasticity, strabismus, and chronic migraines. For each of these indications, small doses are injected into the affected muscles. The dose differs for the specific indication.

One of the newer indications for Botox is for the treatment of overactive bladder or urinary incontinence in patients with an associated neurologic condition such as MS. For these indications, the drug is injected directly into the detrusor muscle of the bladder

TABLE 23.4 Indications for Botulinum Toxin

	Axillary Hyperhidrosis	Blepharospasm	Cervical Dystonia	Glabellar Lines	Overactive Bladder	Chronic Migraine	Strabismus	Upper Limb Spasticity
abobotulinumtoxinA (Dysport)			X	X				
incobotulinumtoxinA (Xeomin)		X	X	X				
onabotulinumtoxinA (Botox)	X	X	X	X	X	X	X	X
onabotulinumtoxinA (Botox Cosmetic)				X				
rimabotulinumtoxinB (Myobloc)			X					

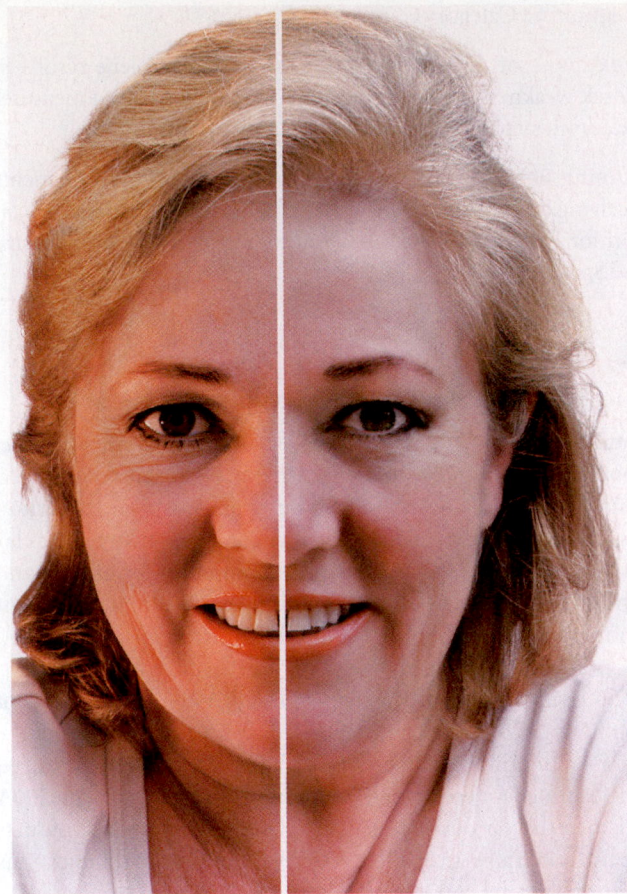

Figure 23.1 Botox therapy: (left) before treatment; (right) after treatment.
Courtesy of Jo Ann Snover/Shutterstock.

through a cystoscope. A single administration of Botox requires injections at 20 to 30 sites in the detrusor muscle, which may be repeated every 6 to 12 weeks. This therapy is only approved if therapy with an anticholinergic drug has been unsuccessful.

Because of the extreme weakness associated with botulinum, therapies may be needed to improve muscle strength. To circumvent major problems with mobility or posture, administration of botulinum toxin is often limited to the small muscle groups. Sometimes this drug is administered with centrally acting PO medications to increase the functional mobility range of muscle groups.

In general, botulinum therapy is well tolerated and adverse effects are related to the dose injected in each muscle. The drug can cause significant pain when it is injected into the muscle. The severity of pain experienced can be blocked by the administration of a local anesthetic. The therapeutic effects of botulinum therapy are effective within 6 weeks and last for 3 to 6 months. All botulinum toxin formulations carry a black box warning that the drug may spread to distant muscles, resulting in a risk for asthenia, generalized muscle weakness, diplopia, blurred vision, dysphagia, dysphonia, urinary incontinence, and breathing difficulties. Swallowing and breathing difficulties can be life threatening. These effects

---

Botox: Beyond Wrinkles

Botox (botulinum toxin type A) has received tremendous media attention as public figures confess to using, or are suspected of using, the drug to reduce the appearance of aging. The drug continues to be used cosmetically to enhance appearance, and there are other clinical conditions where it has demonstrated effectiveness. It is also being used to study how the nerves and brain communicate, potentially leading to new treatments for brain and other disorders.

Besides treating wrinkles and signs of aging, Botox has clinical indications for treating blepharospasm, cervical dystonia, and axillary hyperhidrosis, as well as migraines, Parkinson's disease, chronic pain, overactive bladder, and CP. By blocking nerve transmission, spasticity and resulting symptoms, including pain, may be alleviated. Researchers are also using Botox to study how nerve cells use neurotransmitters in the synaptic cleft. By studying how Botox disrupts the processes of neurotransmitters by affecting specific proteins needed for their release and reuptake, new treatments for psychiatric and other disorders where these proteins also work to signal cell response may be possible (Xu et al., 2013).

There is another, darker side to Botox that often goes unreported in the media, and the FDA has issued a black box warning about Botox and botulinum toxins. The FDA (2008, 2009) reported that the most notable adverse effects related to Botox and botulinum toxins have occurred in children with spastic CP and have included effects ranging from muscle flaccidity to system-wide symptoms of botulism with respiratory distress and death. Effects noted in adults have included weakness, dysphagia, dysphonia, dyspnea, and respiratory distress.

The FDA black box warning includes the following:

- Be aware of possible systemic spread of the drug beyond the regional area of injection. These effects may occur within hours as well as weeks to months after the injection.
- Symptoms of botulinum toxin effects include dysphagia, dysphonia, diplopia, blurred vision, ptosis, urinary incontinence, generalized muscle weakness, and respiratory distress.
- The effects above may be observed at both low and higher doses of the drug. While the most frequent incidence of toxicity occurred in children with spastic CP, they also occurred in adults.
- Difficulty swallowing or breathing is potentially life threatening and requires immediate reporting.

Botox and botulinum toxins have earned a place in the treatment of cosmetic conditions as well as more serious medical concerns such as cervical dystonia. The drug is not without risk despite its popularity. Health care providers should continuously monitor the patient postadministration, and the patient should be educated about the possibility of adverse effects and when to seek emergency care.

---

may occur hours or weeks after treatment. The risk is highest for children. Botulinum toxin is pregnancy category C.

CONNECTION Checkpoint 23.3

Myasthenia gravis is a serious skeletal muscular disorder, but it does not result in spasticity. From what you learned in Chapter 13, what are the symptoms of this disorder and what is the primary pharmacotherapy?
See Answer to Connection Checkpoint 23.3 on student resource website.

Skeletal Muscle Relaxants as Surgical Adjuncts

23.5 Skeletal muscle relaxants are administered during surgery in combination with anesthetic agents.

During certain surgical procedures it is necessary to produce total skeletal muscle relaxation in the patient. Skeletal muscle relaxants such as succinylcholine (Anectine) and tubocurarine are administered in combination with general anesthetics to induce skeletal muscle relaxation, which aids in intubation and other invasive procedures. These drugs are also administered to facilitate endoscopy, to enhance the management of mechanical ventilation, and to control the severity of muscle contractions resulting from electroshock therapy.

The skeletal muscle relaxants used as surgical adjuncts have the ability to produce complete muscle paralysis; thus mechanical ventilation may be necessary. Continuous monitoring is required. Most of these drugs have very rapid onsets of action and brief half-lives; drug effects rapidly diminish following the surgical procedure.

The skeletal muscle relaxants used as surgical adjuncts are presented in Chapter 14. A prototype feature for succinylcholine can be found in that chapter.

CONNECTIONS: NURSING PRACTICE APPLICATION

Patients Receiving Pharmacotherapy for Muscle Spasms and Spasticity

Assessment	Potential Nursing Diagnoses*
Baseline assessment prior to administration:	• *Pain: Acute, Chronic*
• Obtain a complete health history including cardiovascular, respiratory, hepatic, renal, or musculoskeletal diseases. Obtain a drug history including allergies, current prescription and OTC drugs, and herbal preparations. Be alert to possible drug interactions.	• *Impaired Physical Mobility*
	• *Self-Care Deficit: Bathing, Feeding, Dressing, Toileting*
• Obtain a history of the current condition and symptoms, exacerbating conditions, and ability to carry out ADLs, particularly related to mobility.	• *Disturbed Body Image*
	• *Fatigue*
• If present, assess the level of pain. Use objective screening tools when possible (e.g., FLACC [face, limbs, arms, cry, consolability] for infants or very young children, Wong-Baker FACES scale for children, numerical rating scale for adults). Assess the history of pain associated with muscle spasms and what has worked successfully or not for the patient in the past.	• *Deficient Knowledge* (Drug Therapy)
	• *Risk for Injury,* related to disease condition, adverse drug effects
• Evaluate appropriate laboratory findings such as hepatic or renal function studies.	
• Obtain baseline vital signs, muscle strength, and presence of muscle spasms.	
• Assess the patient's ability to receive and understand instruction. Include the family or caregivers as needed.	
Assessment throughout administration:	
• Assess for desired therapeutic effects dependent on the reason for the drug (e.g., decreased muscle spasm, rigidity, decreased pain).	
• Continue periodic monitoring of vital signs and motor function.	
• Assess for and promptly report adverse effects: fatigue, drowsiness, dizziness, dry mouth, orthostatic hypotension, tachycardia, palpitations, swelling of tongue or face, diplopia, urinary retention, diarrhea, or constipation.	

Implementation

Interventions and (Rationales)	Patient-Centered Care
Ensuring therapeutic effects:	• Teach the patient that gradual improvement may be noted over several days and full therapeutic effects may take 1 week or longer. Nonpharmacologic measures may be needed until the full medication effect is noted.
• Continue assessments as above for therapeutic effects. Drug therapy may take several days to have the full effect with lessening pain and tenderness, increased range of motion (ROM), and increased ability to complete ADLs noted. Support the patient in self-care activities as necessary until improvement is observed. (Ability to carry out ADLs gradually improves with consistent usage.)	
Minimizing adverse effects:	• Instruct the patient to call for assistance prior to getting out of bed or attempting to walk alone if pain, spasms, or rigidity are particularly severe.
• Ensure patient safety; monitor motor coordination and ambulation or other essential motor activities. **Lifespan:** Be cautious with older adults who are at increased risk for falls. (Gradual improvement in symptoms may be noticed over several days but pain or spasms may affect motor skills. Particular care with ambulation is required because pain, spasms, or rigidity may increase the risk of falls. Cyclobenzaprine is included in the Beers List of potentially inappropriate drugs for older adults and warrants careful monitoring.)	• Assess the ability of the patient, family, or caregiver to carry out ADLs at home, and explore the need for additional health care referrals if disability will require long-term physical therapy (e.g., CP). Evaluate home safety needs.
	• Instruct the patient to avoid driving or other activities requiring mental alertness or physical coordination until the effects of the drug are known.

(continued)

CONNECTIONS: NURSING PRACTICE APPLICATION (continued)

- Continue to monitor vital signs, particularly blood pressure. Take the blood pressure lying, sitting, and standing to detect orthostatic hypotension. **Lifespan:** Be cautious with older adults who are at increased risk for hypotension. Notify the health care provider if the blood pressure decreases beyond established parameters, or if hypotension is accompanied by reflex tachycardia. (Orthostatic hypotension is a possible adverse effect and, in addition to muscle spasms, pain, or rigidity, may increase the risk of falls or injury. Cyclobenzaprine may cause tachycardia and palpitations.)

- Teach the patient to rise from lying to sitting or standing slowly to avoid dizziness or falls if hypotension is noted. If dizziness occurs, the patient should sit or lie down and not attempt to stand or walk, until the sensation passes.
- Have the patient immediately report dizziness, lightheadedness, rapid heart rate, palpitations, or syncope.

- Monitor muscle tone, ROM, and degree of muscle spasm. (Improvement should be observed over the first week or two of therapy. Increased ROM and decreased muscle tenderness and rigidity help to determine the effectiveness of the drug therapy.)

- Teach the patient how to perform gentle ROM exercises and to exercise only to the point of mild physical discomfort but never pain, throughout the day.

- Provide additional pain relief measures such as positional support, gentle massage, and moist heat or ice packs. (Supportive nursing measures may increase pain relief and supplement drug therapy.)

- Teach the patient complementary pain interventions such as positioning, gentle massage, application of heat or cold to the painful area, distraction with television or music, or guided imagery.

- Continue to monitor renal and hepatic function periodically if the patient is on long-term use of the drug. (Muscle relaxants and antispasmodic drugs may cause hepatotoxicity as an adverse effect. **Lifespan:** Women over the age of 35 taking are at greater risk for hepatotoxicity and should be monitored more frequently.)

- Instruct the patient on the need to return periodically for laboratory work.

- Assess bowel sounds periodically if constipation or diarrhea is problematic. Increase fluid and dietary fiber intake to prevent GI effects and to ease dry mouth effects. (Muscle relaxant drugs may decrease peristalsis as an adverse effect. Significantly diminished or absent bowel sounds are immediately reported to the health care provider. **Lifespan:** The older adult is at increased risk of constipation due to slowed peristalsis. Additional fluids and fiber may ease constipation and prevent diarrhea, but additional medications such as MiraLAX or Colace may be required if constipation is severe.)

- Teach the patient to increase fluids to 2 L per day and increase intake of dietary fiber such as fruits, vegetables, and whole grains.
- Instruct the patient to report severe constipation to the health care provider for additional advice on laxatives or stool softeners.

- Assess for tongue or facial swelling. (While rare, cyclobenzaprine may cause swelling of the tongue or face and should be reported immediately.)

- Instruct the patient to immediately report any swelling of the tongue, face, or throat.

- Avoid the use of other CNS depressants, including alcohol, and use with caution with antihypertensive medications given concurrently. (CNS depressants and alcohol may increase sedative properties of the drug. Antihypertensive medication may increase risk of hypotension.)

- Teach the patient to avoid or eliminate alcohol while on the drug. If other sedatives or antihypertensives are ordered, have the patient consult with the health care provider about dose and sequencing. Immediately report any dizziness, palpitations, or syncope.

- Assess for urinary retention periodically. (Muscle relaxants and antispasmodics may cause urinary retention as an adverse effect. **Lifespan:** Be aware that older men with an enlarged prostate are at higher risk for mechanical obstruction.)

- Instruct the patient to immediately report an inability to void, increasing bladder pressure, or pain.

- **Lifespan:** Patients who are breast-feeding should talk with their provider about the need to stop nursing and pump breasts, discarding the milk and using alternative feedings while on these drugs. (It is unknown whether these drugs are secreted in breast milk.)

- Instruct patients who are pregnant or breast-feeding and on these drugs that the provider may recommend discontinuing breast-feeding while on the drug. If so, alternative feeding plans may be discussed.

Patient understanding of drug therapy:
- Use opportunities during administration of medications and during assessments to discuss the rationale for drug therapy, desired therapeutic outcomes, commonly observed adverse effects, parameters for when to call the health care provider, and any necessary monitoring or precautions. (Using time during nursing care helps to optimize and reinforce key teaching areas.)

- The patient should be able to state the reason for the drug, appropriate dose, scheduling, and adverse effects to observe for and when to report them.

Patient self-administration of drug therapy:
- When administering the medication, instruct the patient, family, or caregiver in proper self-administration of the drug, e.g., take the drug as prescribed when needed. (Utilizing time during nurse-administration of these drugs helps to reinforce teaching.)

- Instruct the patient in proper administration guidelines. Dose should be taken consistently and not prn for best results unless otherwise ordered. Encourage the patient to maintain a medication log, noting symptoms along with dose and timing of medications and bring the log to each health care visit.
- Teach patients to not open, chew, or crush extended release tablets (e.g., cylcobenzaprine [Amrix, Flexeril]); swallow them whole with plenty of water.
- Take the drug with food or milk if stomach upset occurs.

*Nursing Diagnoses—Definitions and Classification 2015–2017. Copyright © 2014, 1994–2014 by NANDA International. Used by arrangement with John Wiley & Sons Limited.

CHAPTER

23

Understanding the Chapter

Key Concepts Summary

23.1 Whereas muscle spasms are often caused by overuse of skeletal muscle, muscle spasticity involves damage to motor nerves.

23.2 Nonpharmacologic interventions for treating muscle spasms and spasticity are limited.

23.3 Nonsteroidal anti-inflammatory drugs and skeletal muscle relaxants are used to treat muscle spasms.

23.4 Direct-acting skeletal muscle relaxants are often used to relieve muscle spasticity.

23.5 Skeletal muscle relaxants are administered during surgery in combination with anesthetic agents.

Case Study: Making the Patient Connection

Remember the patient "Andrew Eskew" at the beginning of the chapter? Now read the remainder of the case study. Based on the information presented within this chapter, respond to the critical thinking questions that follow.

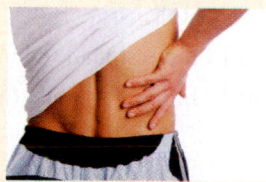

Andrew is a 27-year-old landscaper who was building a landscaping wall yesterday. His job requires lifting, bending, and twisting. On arising today he stated that his back hurts and he cannot move from side to side. The nurse has performed a physical assessment on Andrew, which revealed tightened muscles in the lumbosacral region and limited mobility. The patient describes his pain as a level 7 on a scale of 1 to 10.

Critical Thinking Questions

1. What are the etiology and pathophysiology of Andrew's muscle spasms? What are other possible causes of muscle spasms?

2. Andrew has been prescribed cyclobenzaprine (Flexeril) to relieve his back spasms. What is the action of this medication and why has it been prescribed?

3. What should Andrew be instructed regarding the administration of this medication?

See Answers to Critical Thinking Questions on student resource website.

Additional Case Study

A 46-year-old woman is diagnosed with cervical dystonia. She has difficulty maintaining normal head position and reports neck pain. She is to start on botulinum therapy.

1. What is the action of and rationale for administering botulinum toxin type A?

2. Create a list of adverse effects that this patient may experience due to botulinum therapy.

See Answers to Additional Case Study on student resource website.

Chapter Review

1 A 67-year-old patient experienced a severe back strain while lifting groceries from his car. He is given a prescription for cyclobenzaprine (Flexeril). The nurse will include what precautions in the teaching plan for this patient? Select all that apply.

1. Report any palpitations or rapid pulse rate immediately.
2. Take frequent walks throughout the day to relieve soreness.
3. Rinse the mouth frequently with an alcohol-based mouthwash to relieve excess secretions.
4. Be cautious with driving or other activities requiring alertness.
5. Immediately report any facial or tongue swelling.

2 A patient with spastic cerebral palsy is being treated with oral baclofen (Lioresal). Which patient statement indicates the need for more teaching?

1. "I will be cautious about activities because I may feel weak."
2. "It may take several months before I experience full effects of the drug."
3. "If I experience unpleasant side effects, I can stop taking the drug."
4. "I will be sure to get enough fluid and fiber in my diet."

3 A patient has been taught to apply capsaicin to increase mobility and relieve pain. Which instruction is most important for the nurse to give to this patient?

1. Apply the medication liberally above and below the site of pain.
2. Apply with a gloved hand only to the site of pain.
3. Apply to areas of redness and inflammation.
4. Apply liberally with a bare hand.

4 A patient has been treated for cervical dystonia with an injection of botulinum toxin type A (Botox). Which of the following will the nurse teach the patient to immediately report?

1. Fever, aches, or chills
2. Difficulty swallowing, blurred vision, or ptosis
3. Moderate levels of muscle weakness on the affected side
4. Continuous spasms and pain on the affected side

5 A patient has been taking cyclobenzaprine (Amrix, Flexeril) for muscle spasms. The patient is admitted to the emergency department with severe central nervous system depression. Which medication will the nurse expect to be ordered and administered?

1. Naloxone (Narcan)
2. Meperidine (Demerol)
3. Diazepam (Valium)
4. Physostigmine (Antilirium)

6 A female patient, age 45, is receiving dantrolene (Dantrium) for treatment of painful muscle spasms associated with multiple sclerosis. What will the nurse teach the patient? Select all that apply.

1. Increase fluid and fiber intake to prevent constipation.
2. Inform the health care provider if she is taking estrogen products.
3. Sip water, ice, or suck on hard candy to relieve xerostomia.
4. Be sure to obtain 20 minutes of sun exposure per day to boost vitamin D levels.
5. Return periodically to the provider to monitor her liver function.

See Answers to Chapter Review in Appendix A.

References

Abel-Hamid, H. Z. (2013). *Cerebral palsy.* Retrieved from http://emedicine.medscape.com/article/1179555-overview#aw2aab6b2b2

American Dystonia Society. (n.d.). *About dystonia.* Retrieved from http://www.dystonia.us/dystonia.htm

Brashear, A., & Elovic, E. (2011). *Spasticity: Diagnosis and management.* New York, NY: Demos Medical.

Butler, C., Campbell, S., Adams, R., Abel, M., Chambers, H., Goldstein, M., . . . O'Donnell, M. (2000). Evidence of the effects of intrathecal baclofen for spastic and dystonic cerebral palsy. *Developmental Medicine and Child Neurology, 42,* 634–645. doi:10.1111/j.1469-8749.2000.tb00371.x

deLissovoy, G., Matza, L. S., Green, H., Werner, M., & Edgar, T. (2007). Cost-effectiveness of intrathecal baclofen therapy for the treatment of severe spasticity associated with cerebral palsy. *Journal of Child Neurology, 22,* 49–59. doi:10.1177/0883073807299976

Hoving, M. A., vanRaak, E. P., Spincemaille, G. H., Palmans, L. J., Sleypen, F. A., & Vies, J. S. (2007). Intrathecal baclofen in children with spastic cerebral palsy: A double-blind, randomized, placebo-controlled, dose-finding study. *Developmental Medicine and Child Neurology, 49,* 654–659. doi:10.1111/j.1469-8749.2007.00654.x

Katzberg, H. D., Khan, A. H., & So, Y. T. (2010). Assessment: Symptomatic treatment for muscle cramps (an evidence-based review): Report of the Therapeutics and Technology Assessment Subcommittee of the American Academy of Neurology. *Neurology, 74,* 691–696. doi:10.1212/WNL.0b013e3181d0ccca

Krach, L. E., Kriel, R. L., Day, S. M., & Strauss, D. J. (2010). Survival of individuals with cerebral palsy receiving continuous intrathecal baclofen treatment: A matched-cohort study. *Developmental Medicine and Child Neurology, 52,* 672–676. doi:10.1111/j.1469-8749.2009.03473.x

Motta, F., Antonello, C. E., & Stignani, C. (2011). Intrathecal baclofen and motor function in cerebral palsy. *Developmental Medicine and Child Neurology, 53,* 443–448. doi:10.1111/j.1469-8749.2010.03904.x

U.S. Food and Drug Administration. (2008). *FDA issues statement about dangers of Botox and botulinum toxin products.* Retrieved from http://www.usrecallnews.com/2008/02/fda-issues-statement-about-dangers-of-botox-and-botulinum-toxin-products.html

U.S. Food and Drug Administration. (2009). *FDA gives updates on botulinum toxin safety warnings; established names of drugs changed.* Retrieved from http://www.fda.gov/NewsEvents/Newsroom/PressAnnouncements/2009/ucm175013.htm

Vles, G. F., Soudant, D. L., Hoving, M. A., Vermeulen, R. J., Bonouvrié, L. A., van

Oostenbrugge, R. J., & Vles, J. S. (2013). Long-term follow-up on continuous intrathecal Baclofen therapy in non-ambulant children with intractable spastic cerebral palsy. *European Journal of Paediatric Neurology, 17,* 639–644. doi:10.1016/j.ejpn.2013.06.003

Xu, J., Luo, F., Zhang, Z., Xue, L., Wu, X. S., Chiang, H. C., . . . Wu, L. G. (2013). SNARE proteins synaptobrevin, SNAP-25, and syntaxin are involved in rapid and slow endocytosis at synapses. *Cell Reports, 3,* 1414–1421. doi:10.1016/j.celrep.2013.03.010

Selected Bibliography

Amatya, B., Khan, F., La Mantia, L., Demetrios, M., & Wade, D. T. (2013). Non pharmacological interventions for spasticity in multiple sclerosis. *Cochrane Database of Systematic Reviews, 2,* CD009974. doi:10.1002/14651858.CD009974.pub2

Bhimani, R. H., Anderson, L. C., Henly, S. J., & Stoddard, S. A. (2011). Clinical measurement of limb spasticity in adults: State of the science. *Journal of Neuroscience Nursing, 43,* 104–115. doi:10.1097/JNN.0b013e31820b5f9f

Blyton, F., Chuter, V., Walter, K. E. L., & Burns, J. (2012). Non-drug therapies for lower limb muscle cramps. *Cochrane Database of Systematic Reviews, 1,* CD008496. doi:10.1002/14651858.CD008496.pub2

Carlson, H., & Carlson, N. (2011). An overview of the management of persistent musculoskeletal pain. *Therapeutic Advances in Musculoskeletal Disease, 3,* 91–99. doi:10.1177/1759720X11398742

Darlington, A. B. (2011). The Botox phenomenon. *Plastic Surgical Nursing, 30,* 22–26. doi:10.1097/PSN.0b013e3181cfe65c

Delgado, M. R., Hirtz, D., Aisen, M., Ashwal, S., Fehlings, D. L., McLaughlin, J., . . . Vargus-Adams, J. (2010). Practice parameter: Pharmacologic treatment of spasticity in children and adolescents with cerebral palsy (an evidence-based review): Report of the Quality Standards Subcommittee of the American Academy of Neurology and the Practice

Committee of the Child Neurology Society. *Neurology, 74,* 336–343.

Herdman, T. H., & Kamitsuru, S. (Eds.). (2014). *NANDA International nursing diagnoses: Definitions and classification, 2015–2017.* Oxford, United Kingdom: Wiley-Blackwell.

Lemone, P., & Burke, K. (2012). *Medical surgical nursing: Critical thinking in client care* (5th ed.). Upper Saddle River, NJ: Pearson.

Valiyil, R., & Christopher-Stine, L. (2010). Drug-related myopathies of which the clinician should be aware. *Current Rheumatology Reports, 12,* 213–220. doi:10.1007/s11926-010-0104-3

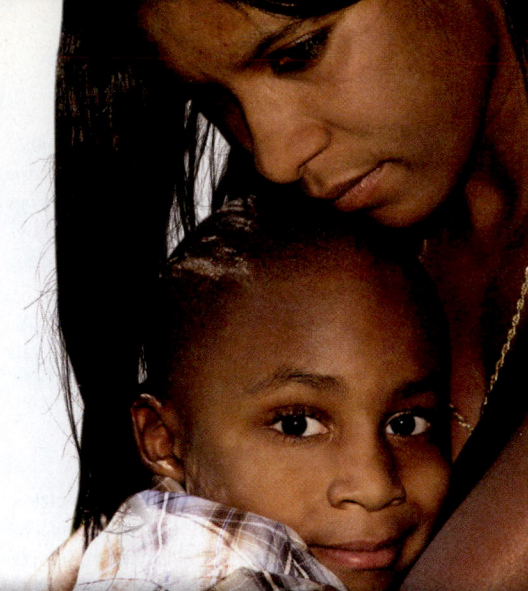

"The school nurse recommended we consider Adderall for Jonathon. He's just doing poorly in school and hates to do his homework. Why would he need a drug for that?"

Patient "Jeanine Hogan," mother of Jonathon

CHAPTER

24 Central Nervous System Stimulants and Drugs for Attention Deficit/Hyperactivity Disorder

LEARNING OUTCOMES

After reading the chapter, the student should be able to:

1. Describe the general actions and pharmacotherapeutic applications of central nervous system stimulants.

2. Identify the signs and symptoms of attention deficit/hyperactivity disorder and narcolepsy.

3. Compare and contrast the central nervous system stimulants and nonstimulants in treating attention deficit/hyperactivity disorder.

4. Compare and contrast the different pharmacotherapies available for narcolepsy.

5. Describe the nurse's role in the pharmacologic management of attention deficit/hyperactivity disorder and narcolepsy.

6. For each class shown in the chapter outline, identify the prototype and representative drugs and explain the mechanism(s) of drug action, primary indications, contraindications, significant drug interactions, pregnancy category, and important adverse effects.

7. Apply the nursing process to care for patients receiving pharmacotherapy with central nervous system stimulants.

CHAPTER OUTLINE

▶ **Characteristics of Central Nervous System Stimulants**

▶ **Etiology and Pathophysiology of Attention Deficit/ Hyperactivity Disorder**

▶ **Pharmacotherapy of Attention Deficit/ Hyperactivity Disorder**

Psychostimulants

PROTOTYPE Amphetamine and Dextroamphetamine (Adderall, Adderall XR), *p. 355*

Nonstimulants

PROTOTYPE Atomoxetine (Strattera), *p. 357*

▶ **Pharmacotherapy of Narcolepsy**

PROTOTYPE Modafinil (Provigil), *p. 358*

▶ **Methylxanthines**

PROTOTYPE Caffeine, *p. 359*

KEY TERMS

anorexiants, 353

attention deficit/hyperactivity
disorder (ADHD), 352

cataplexy, 358

central nervous system (CNS)
stimulants, 351

euphoria, 351

hypnagogic hallucinations, 358

methylxanthines, 359

narcolepsy, 358

sleep attacks, 358

sleep paralysis, 358

The central nervous system (CNS) stimulants are a small group of drugs that have limited pharmacotherapeutic applications. Attention deficit/hyperactivity disorder (ADHD) and narcolepsy are conditions that diminish mental alertness and that may benefit from treatment with these medications. Some of the CNS stimulants such as cocaine and methamphetamine are widely abused. The purpose of this chapter is to examine the actions and pharmacotherapeutic applications of the CNS stimulants.

Characteristics of Central Nervous System Stimulants

24.1 Central nervous system stimulants increase alertness, enhance the ability to concentrate, and delay the symptoms of fatigue.

The **central nervous system (CNS) stimulants** are a diverse group of pharmacologic agents. The stimulants range from widely accessible agents (caffeine) to Schedule I controlled substances (ecstasy). All CNS stimulants have the common action of raising the general alertness level of the brain. Wakefulness and the ability to focus or concentrate are increased. Mood is often elevated, and the person may temporarily become unaware of physical fatigue. For some of the controlled substances, mood elevation may progress to **euphoria**, an intense sense of happiness and well-being.

Because people generally view the sensations associated with CNS stimulation as desirable, many are driven to repeat the pleasurable experience. With continued use, physical and psychological dependence occur. Because of this, many CNS stimulants are highly regulated as scheduled drugs (Table 24.1).

Not all effects of these drugs on the CNS are pleasurable. Stimulants have the potential to cause adverse effects due to excessive excitation. Nervousness, dizziness, and irritability are common, and convulsions may occur at higher doses. Most of the stimulants also affect the cardiovascular system and can increase heart rate and cause dysrhythmias. Loss of appetite, or anorexia, occurs with some of the CNS stimulants.

Some medications produce CNS excitation as an adverse effect. For example, antihistamines are prescribed to treat allergy symptoms but may cause CNS stimulation and insomnia in some patients. Albuterol (Proventil) inhalers are used for asthma but the drug may cause nervousness, tremors, and anxiety. Drugs that normally cause CNS depression, such as antidepressants, may cause paradoxical CNS excitement, especially in the very young or very old. Occasionally, drugs are purposefully taken in large amounts for their CNS stimulation adverse effects. For example, the primary over-the-counter (OTC) drug for treating cough, dextromethorphan, is abused by teenagers and can cause dizziness, restlessness, hallucinations, and seizures when taken in very high amounts. Additional information on the substance abuse aspects of the CNS stimulants is presented in Chapter 27.

The therapeutic applications of the CNS stimulants are limited. These include the following:

- ADHD
- Narcolepsy
- Weight management
- Stimulation of respiration
- Migraine headaches

If CNS stimulants elevate mood, why are they not used to treat major depressive disorder? In fact, CNS stimulants have been used in the past to treat major depression. CNS stimulants, however, are nonselective in their CNS actions; the excitement produced by these drugs affects all parts of the brain. They produce many potentially serious adverse effects, including physical and psychological dependence. The tricyclic antidepressants and the selective serotonin reuptake inhibitors (SSRIs) have been demonstrated to be more effective and safer than stimulants in the treatment of depression. These drugs are able to elevate mood without causing CNS excitation.

TABLE 24.1	Central Nervous System Stimulants That Are Scheduled Drugs
Schedule	**Central Nervous System Stimulants**
I	3,4-methylenedioxymethamphetamine (MDMA, ecstasy), aminorex, cathinone, fenethylline, mephedrone, methcathinone, methaqualone (Quaalude), methylaminorex
II	amphetamine (Adderall, Dexedrine), cocaine, lisdexamfetamine (Vyvanse), methamphetamine (Desoxyn), methylphenidate (Concerta, Ritalin), phenmetrazine (Preludin)
III	benzphetamine (Didrex), chlorphentermine, clortermine (Voranil), dronabinol (Marinol), phendimetrazine (Plegine, Prelu 2)
IV	cathine (norpseudoephedrine), diethylpropion (Tenuate), fencamfamin, fenproporex, mazindol (Sanorex), mefenorex, modafinil (Provigil), phentermine (Adipex, Fastin), pipradrol
V	pyrovalerone

From *Lists of: Scheduling Actions, Controlled Substances and Regulated Chemicals, Drug Enforcement Administration*, 2014. Retrieved from http://www.deadiversion.usdoj.gov/schedules/orangebook/orangebook.pdf.

Etiology and Pathophysiology of Attention Deficit/Hyperactivity Disorder

24.2 Attention deficit/hyperactivity disorder is characterized by inattention, hyperactivity, and impulsive behavior.

Attention deficit/hyperactivity disorder (ADHD) is a neuropsychiatric condition that presents in children before age 7 and can extend into adulthood. It is characterized by symptoms of impulsive behavior, lack of attention, and hyperactivity. The patient diagnosed with ADHD must exhibit symptoms of inattention and hyperactivity, as shown in Table 24.2 (American Psychiatric Association, 2013).

ADHD occurs in approximately 11% of all children, age 4 to 17. The condition is more common in males: 13% of males versus 6% of females. The overall incidence of ADHD has increased an average of 5% per year from 2003 to 2011 (Centers for Disease Control and Prevention [CDC], 2013).

Symptoms of ADHD such as impulsive behavior, distractibility, lack of attention, and hyperactivity during the school-age years can lead to poor performance and lack of interest in school activities. The symptoms of inattention and hyperactivity also contribute to difficulty with peer and family relationships. Hyperactive children usually have increased motor activity with impulsivity and a tendency to interrupt at inappropriate times. This behavior can result in disciplinary action by teachers and parents. Some additional symptoms noted include difficulty remembering details and the placement of personal items, changing tasks without completing prior tasks, and disturbances in sleep.

Symptoms continue into adulthood in 35% to 55% of persons diagnosed with childhood ADHD. Symptoms in adults include workaholic tendencies, being overwhelmed, talking excessively, low tolerance for frustration, chronic boredom, short temper, quitting jobs abruptly, personal relationship problems, and multiple driving violations. Adults with ADHD are more likely to have an "addictive" personality, which may be exhibited in behavior that includes smoking and using illegal substances. Adult ADHD is treated with the same therapies as childhood ADHD.

Considerable attention has focused on the causes of ADHD, and it is clear that the etiology is complex and involves multiple variables. Studies on twins have indicated that genetics is an important contributor to the development of ADHD. An identical twin has a 92% probability of presenting with ADHD if his or her twin has been diagnosed with the disorder and about 25% of families with a member diagnosed with ADHD will have other relatives also diagnosed. This percentage is significantly higher than the general population, which is approximately 5%.

Brain injury has been studied as a contributing factor in the development of ADHD because some children who experience head trauma will exhibit symptoms of the disorder. The percentage of brain injuries that lead to a diagnosis of ADHD is small but remains relevant in assessing for the condition as the patient ages.

Environmental agents such as lead can contribute to the development of ADHD in children. Children living in buildings built prior to 1972 have a higher risk of developing lead poisoning. Other environmental agents that contribute to the development of ADHD include alcohol and cigarette smoking by the mother during pregnancy. Food additives and sugar intake by the child have been implicated as causes of ADHD, but research studies have failed to find a strong link.

There are differences in the anatomy and physiology of children with ADHD and control subjects. Children with a known diagnosis of ADHD possess a smaller brain volume in the frontal lobes, temporal gray matter, caudate nucleus, and cerebellum. Children who are affected by ADHD have a deficiency in the catecholamines dopamine and norepinephrine. The brain of a child with ADHD also has decreased development in the area of self-regulation. This factor yields the development of symptoms such as irritability, aggression, learning disability, and motor disorders when the child is stimulated.

TABLE 24.2 Symptoms That May Lead to a Diagnosis of Attention Deficit/Hyperactivity Disorder

Inattention

1. Often does not give close attention to details or makes careless mistakes in schoolwork, work, or other activities.
2. Often has trouble keeping attention on tasks or play activities.
3. Often does not seem to listen when spoken to directly.
4. Often does not follow instructions and fails to finish schoolwork, chores, or duties in the workplace (not due to oppositional behavior or failure to understand instructions).
5. Often has trouble organizing activities.
6. Often avoids, dislikes, or does not want to do things that take a lot of mental effort for a long period of time (such as schoolwork or homework).
7. Often loses things needed for tasks and activities (e.g., toys, school assignments, pencils, books, or tools).
8. Is often easily distracted.
9. Is often forgetful in daily activities.

Hyperactivity/Impulsivity

1. Often fidgets with hands or feet or squirms in seat.
2. Often gets up from seat when remaining in seat is expected.
3. Often runs about or climbs when and where it is not appropriate (adolescents or adults may feel very restless).
4. Often has trouble playing or enjoying leisure activities quietly.
5. Is often "on the go" or often acts as if "driven by a motor."
6. Often talks excessively.
7. Often blurts out answers before questions have been finished.
8. Often has trouble waiting one's turn.
9. Often interrupts or intrudes on others (e.g., butts into conversations or games).

CONNECTIONS Treating the Diverse Patient

◀ Attention Deficit/Hyperactivity Disorder Increase in Girls

ADHD occurs in both boys and girls, but significantly more attention and research has been given to boys with the disorder. This is beginning to change, and it is clear that there are differences in the presentation of ADHD symptoms as well as when the diagnosis is made. ADHD in girls tends to be diagnosed later than in boys (after age 7), symptoms tend to differ, and treatment may need to take into consideration the natural premenstrual hormone fluctuations that occur.

Similar to boys with ADHD, girls do not tend to outgrow symptoms of ADHD after childhood (Mick et al., 2011). Teachers were found to notice ADHD symptoms in girls but tended to consider boys as being more symptomatic and having more problems than girls (Evans et al., 2013). Medication has been found to be effective for girls as well as boys, but the traditional stimulants such as methylphenidate and amphetamine were found to cause increased premenstrual stimulating effects.

The symptoms of ADHD can cause functional impairment in children and be challenging for parents and teachers. The goal of pharmacotherapy for ADHD is to reduce inattention and promote the child's ability to focus and concentrate on tasks.

Pharmacotherapy of Attention Deficit/Hyperactivity Disorder

24.3 Psychostimulants are central nervous system stimulants indicated for the treatment of ADHD and narcolepsy.

Medications used to treat patients with ADHD are classified as stimulants or nonstimulants. Stimulants account for 70% to 80% of drugs taken for this disorder. The nonstimulants were not developed until 2003 and generally have a longer duration of action with fewer adverse effects. Successful treatment of ADHD usually requires a combination of pharmacotherapy and behavioral therapies.

The most frequently prescribed medications for ADHD are CNS stimulants: amphetamines and amphetamine-like drugs. During the 1920s, amphetamines were used to treat asthma, hay fever, and the common cold. Amphetamine use became widespread in World War II because these drugs were able to keep soldiers alert and delay fatigue during combat. Amphetamines were not listed as scheduled substances until 1970. Amphetamine sulfate has been used to make several other salts that have psychoactive properties, including methamphetamine and ecstasy (methylenedioxymethamphetamine or MDMA), an illegal substance used to induce euphoria.

CONNECTION Checkpoint 24.1

The older adult may experience different responses to drugs related to the aging process or to adverse effects of drug therapy. From what you learned in Chapter 10, what symptoms might be anticipated in an older adult taking CNS stimulants and what should the nurse do if they occur? *See Answer to Connection Checkpoint 24.1 on student resource website.*

Amphetamine exists in two closely related but distinct chemical forms: d-amphetamine (dextroamphetamine) and l-amphetamine (levoamphetamine). When using the term *amphetamine* it is understood that the drug is a mixture of the d- and l-forms. To be more precise, this mixture is sometimes called racemic amphetamine. The d-form, dextroamphetamine, is marketed separately as Dexedrine. The psychostimulants approved for ADHD include methylphenidate, dextroamphetamine, dexmethylphenidate, and lisdexamfetamine. Doses of these drugs are listed in Table 24.3.

Despite the name *psychostimulant*, these drugs do not act by stimulating the brain in a person with ADHD. Instead, these drugs increase attention and enhance the child's ability to focus on tasks and improve learning. Significant improvement in academic performance and in peer and family relationships is common. When used appropriately for ADHD, these drugs do not cause euphoria, and dependence has not been a serious problem. Psychostimulants are the most effective drugs for this disorder, reducing the symptoms of ADHD in 70% to 80% of the treated children.

The stimulants have actions on both the autonomic nervous system and the CNS. Amphetamines are sympathomimetics and activate alpha- and beta-adrenergic receptors by promoting the release of norepinephrine in the autonomic nervous system (see Chapter 15). Typical symptoms of sympathetic activation caused by amphetamines include vasoconstriction, hypertension (HTN), and tachycardia.

In people with no ADHD, the CNS stimulant actions of amphetamines are the result of increased release of dopamine due to inhibition of the reuptake of this neurotransmitter in presynaptic neurons. At very high doses, amphetamines enhance the release of the neurotransmitter serotonin (5-hydroxytryptamine or 5-HT) in the brain, which is responsible for serious psychotic behaviors. Amphetamines also are **anorexiants**, which means that they diminish the appetite. This effect is produced by direct inhibition of the appetite center in the hypothalamus. The application of the amphetamines to the pharmacotherapy of obesity is presented in Chapter 63.

Almost from the time they were discovered, amphetamines have been abused for their stimulant effects. These drugs are often abused by those who wish to delay fatigue, for example, truck drivers, students, and health care workers working long shifts. Athletes may take amphetamines to increase their energy level and enhance performance. Long-term amphetamine abuse may lead to tolerance, dependence, and serious adverse effects. Amphetamine and methamphetamine are Schedule II drugs.

Cocaine is an illicit drug that has similar sympathomimetic, CNS stimulant, and anorexiant effects to amphetamine. In fact, the

TABLE 24.3	Central Nervous System Stimulants and Drugs for Attention Deficit/Hyperactivity Disorder and Narcolepsy

Drug	Route and Dose (Maximum Dose Where Indicated)	Adverse Effects
Amphetamines and Amphetamine-Like Drugs		
amphetamine and dextroamphetamine (Adderall, Adderall XR)	3–5 years old: PO: 2.5 mg one to two times/day, may increase by 2.5 mg at weekly intervals 6 years old: PO: 5 mg daily to bid, may increase by 5 mg at weekly intervals (max: 40 mg/day) Adult: 10 mg extended release, once daily (max: 30 mg/day)	*Irritability, dizziness, palpitations, euphoria, insomnia, tachycardia, weight loss, application site reactions (Daytrana)* Sudden death, dependence, psychosis
dexmethylphenidate (Focalin, Focalin XR)	PO: 2.5 mg bid; may gradually increase for desired effect (max: 20 mg/day); extended release is 5 mg/day	
lisdexamfetamine (Vyvanse)	PO: 30 mg once daily (max: 70 mg/day)	
methylphenidate (Concerta, Daytrana, Metadate, Methylin, Ritalin, Quillivant XR)	Narcolepsy: Adult: PO: 10 mg bid–tid ADHD: Child: PO: 5–10 mg; gradually increase to desired effect (max: 60 mg/day) Adult: 20–30 mg; gradually increase to desired effect (max: 60 mg)	
Nonstimulants for ADHD		
atomoxetine (Strattera)	Child less than 70 kg: PO: start with 0.5 mg/kg/day; may increase after 3 days to target dose of 1.2 mg/kg/day (max: 1.4 mg/kg or 100 mg) Adult: PO: start with 40 mg; may increase after 3 days to target dose of 80 mg/day (max: 100 mg/day)	*Headache, palpitations, decreased appetite, insomnia, irritability, fatigue, somnolence, dry mouth, upper abdominal pain, nausea, vomiting, constipation, urinary retention, cough* Suicidal ideation, severe liver injury
clonidine (Kapvay)	Child age 6–17: PO: Start with 0.1 mg/day and gradually increase to desired response (max: 4 mg/day)	*Somnolence, fatigue, upper respiratory tract infection, irritability, sore throat, insomnia, nightmares, emotional disorder, constipation, increased body temperature* Bradycardia, syncope, serious sedation, severe hypotension
guanfacine (Intuniv)	Child age 6–17: PO: Start with 1 mg/day and gradually increase to desired response (max: 4 mg/day)	*Sedation, abdominal pain, dizziness, mild hypotension, dry mouth, constipation* Bradycardia, syncope, serious sedation, severe hypotension
Drugs for Narcolepsy		
armodafinil (Nuvigil)	PO: 150–250 mg/day given as a single dose in the morning or 1 h prior to the start of the work shift	*Dizziness, nausea, insomnia, headache, anxiety* Stevens–Johnson syndrome (SJS), hypersensitivity, mania
modafinil (Provigil)	PO: 200 mg once daily in the morning or 1 h prior to the start of the work shift	*Headache, nausea, nervousness, rhinitis, diarrhea, back pain, anxiety, insomnia, dizziness, dyspepsia* Hypersensitivity reaction, SJS
sodium oxybate (Xyrem)	PO: Two doses of 2.25 g, the first given at bedtime, the second given 2.5–4 h later (max: 9 g/day)	*Headache, nausea, dizziness, nasopharyngitis, drowsiness, disorientation, irritability* Seizures, respiratory depression, decreased level of consciousness, coma, psychosis
Methylxanthine		
caffeine	Neonatal apnea: PO or IV: 20–30 mg/kg as a loading dose; maintenance dose: 5 mg/kg for 10–12 days Mental alertness: PO: 100–200 mg tid–qid as needed	*Tachycardia, flushing, restlessness, insomnia, irritability, tremor, palpitations, polyuria* Kernicterus in neonates, seizures

Note: Italics indicate common adverse effects. Underline indicates serious adverse effects.

signs and symptoms of cocaine abuse are indistinguishable from those of amphetamine abuse. Cocaine has a much shorter half-life, which leads to more frequent repeated doses. Additional details regarding cocaine dependence are included in Chapter 27.

Overall, drugs in the psychostimulant class have equivalent effectiveness and very similar adverse effect profiles. For unknown reasons, however, some patients respond more favorably to one drug over another. Thus the choice of psychostimulant and the dose are

CONNECTIONS | Evidence-Based Practice

◖Assessing Cardiovascular Risk of Attention Deficit/Hyperactivity Disorder Medications

Clinical Question
Should cardiovascular risk influence the decision to use medications for ADHD?

Evidence
The most common drugs used to treat ADHD are CNS stimulants and, as such, they may raise the heart rate and blood pressure. In children and adults with underlying cardiovascular disorders, ADHD medications have been associated with an increase in adverse cardiac events including dysrhythmias and sudden cardiac death. Although these events are rare, the FDA has recognized the increased risk and requires their citation in a black box warning in the drug literature for ADHD medications. Elia and Vetter (2010) investigated the risk and also the availability of screening tools for detecting cardiac disease. Their study suggested that the highest risk is associated with performing exercise, and that ECG monitoring prior to and during drug therapy may detect cardiac disease in previously asymptomatic patients. While not every case of cardiac disease was detected through ECG monitoring, and a normal ECG did not guarantee safety in taking the drugs, the ECG was noted to be a cost-effective screening tool that providers could use before ordering more expensive diagnostic screenings.

Implications
The patient history is a crucial assessment tool that nurses use to assess cardiovascular risk. A personal or family history of murmurs or cardiac defects at birth, or current history of cardiac problems or palpitations may suggest the need for ECG monitoring. Genetic syndromes such as Marfan and Turner syndromes have also been linked to a high incidence of cardiovascular disease and should be assessed during the initial patient history. Blood pressure and pulse rate should be assessed prior to medication therapy and at each office visit thereafter.

Critical Thinking Questions
Methylphenidate (Concerta, Daytrana, Metadate, Methylin, Ritalin, Quillivant XR) is used in the treatment of ADHD. What are some of the adverse effects noted with this medication? What education should be provided to the patient prescribed this medication?

See Answers to Critical Thinking Questions on student resource website.

---

largely determined individually, by therapeutic response. Therapy is always begun with a low dose, which is gradually increased until the desired therapeutic effect is attained. Another consideration is the dosing schedule for the medication. Older preparations must be taken every 4 hours, which is inconvenient for the school-age child. Extended duration products are now available that last 10 to 12 hours and provide a consistent therapeutic level throughout the day. For children who have difficulty taking medication by mouth, a transdermal patch is now available. Regardless of the medication taken, it is important for the nurse and caregiver to understand that drugs are used to control but not cure the disorder. Approximately 60% of children with the disorder will continue to need medication into their adult years.

PROTOTYPE DRUG	Amphetamine and Dextroamphetamine (Adderall, Adderall XR)

Classification: Therapeutic: Drug for ADHD
Pharmacologic: CNS stimulant, anorexiant, sympathomimetic

Therapeutic Effects and Uses: Adderall is a combination drug containing four different salts of amphetamine and dextroamphetamine. Amphetamine was approved in 1939, Adderall in 1996 and Adderall XR, an extended duration form, in 2001.

Adderall increases motor activity, alertness, and wakefulness and elevates the patient's mood. In children with ADHD the medication produces a paradoxical sedation effect. The mechanism of this effect is unclear. The drug affects the satiety center in the hypothalamus, causing anorexiant effects that lead to loss of appetite and weight.

Amphetamines are used to treat ADHD and narcolepsy. Although an effective appetite suppressant, amphetamine is rarely used for weight loss therapy because its inhibition of appetite is short term, and dependence results from long-term use. Illegal forms of amphetamine may be smoked, inhaled, or injected.

Mechanism of Action: Adderall produces sympathomimetic effects as well as central stimulation actions on the cerebral cortex and the reticular activating system (RAS). The actions of the medication are due to the release of norepinephrine and dopamine. The benefits of the drug in treating ADHD may also be due to its effects on the neurotransmitter serotonin in the brain.

Pharmacokinetics:

Route(s)	Oral (PO)
Absorption	Rapidly absorbed
Distribution	Widely distributed to all tissues, including the CNS; secreted in breast milk
Primary metabolism	Hepatic
Primary excretion	Renal
Onset of action	30–60 min
Duration of action	Up to 10 h

Adverse Effects: Symptoms of excessive CNS and peripheral stimulation by Adderall include irritability, insomnia, nervousness, palpitations, elevated blood pressure, and tachycardia. Weight loss is noted with the medication. Impotence and change in libido may occur with high doses. Long-term use of amphetamines has been reported to cause growth inhibition in children; however, discontinuation of the drug often results in rebound growth. Psychiatric symptoms associated with amphetamine abuse include euphoria, hallucinations, delusions, paranoia, delirium, and depression.

Long-term users of amphetamine will experience tolerance to the mood-elevating effects of the drug. This results in abusers requiring increasingly higher doses to achieve the same stimulant effect. **Black Box Warning**: All amphetamine-containing products, including Adderall, have a high potential for abuse, and administration for prolonged periods may lead to drug dependence. In addition, amphetamines may cause sudden death due to serious cardiac events. This has occurred primarily in children with preexisting cardiac abnormalities.

Contraindications/Precautions: Patients with hypersensitivity to sympathomimetic amines (e.g., epinephrine or norepinephrine) or who have a history of drug abuse should not be prescribed Adderall. Because the conditions may worsen, Adderall is contraindicated in patients with the following disorders: diabetes, glaucoma, hyperthyroidism, moderate to severe HTN, cardiac disorders, and Tourette's syndrome. Patients with bipolar disorder may exhibit signs of mania when administered amphetamines. Amphetamines should be discontinued gradually to prevent withdrawal symptoms such as severe depression, anxiety, agitation, hypersomnia, dysphoric mood, or suicidal ideation.

Drug Interactions: Alkaline drugs such as acetazolamide and sodium bicarbonate decrease the elimination of Adderall from the body and prolong its half-life. On the other hand, acidic drugs such as ammonium chloride and ascorbic acid increase the elimination of Adderall from the body. The administration of Adderall with furazolidone can cause an increase in blood pressure effects. Selegiline administered with amphetamines can precipitate hypertensive crisis, which may be fatal. **Herbal/Food**: Foods and fluids containing caffeine can cause additive CNS stimulation and increase insomnia, nervousness, and anxiety. Melatonin should be avoided because it may enhance the CNS stimulation from Adderall.

Pregnancy: Category C.

Treatment of Overdose: The treatment of overdosage of amphetamine and amphetamine-related medications includes gastric lavage and the administration of chlorpromazine. Chlorpromazine contains strong alpha-adrenergic blocking actions that counteract the effects of amphetamine. In the event that overdosage results in severe HTN, phentolamine is administered intravenously (IV). Acidification of the urine can speed the renal elimination of the drug.

Nursing Responsibilities: Key nursing implications for patients receiving amphetamine and dextroamphetamine are included in the Nursing Practice Application for Patients Receiving Pharmacotherapy with Central Nervous System Stimulants.

Drugs Similar to Amphetamine and Dextroamphetamine (Adderall, Adderall XR)

Other psychostimulants for ADHD include dexmethylphenidate, lisdexamfetamine, and methylphenidate. Benzphetamine (Didrex) is an amphetamine indicated for obesity (see Chapter 63). Pemoline (Cylert), an amphetamine-like drug used for ADHD and narcolepsy, was removed from the market in 2005 due to incidences of fatal hepatic failure.

Dexmethylphenidate (Focalin, Focalin XR): Approved in 2001, dexmethylphenidate has effects identical to methylphenidate and the amphetamines. The drug blocks the reuptake of norepinephrine and dopamine in presynaptic neurons. It is used to manage symptoms of ADHD. In 2005, a once-daily extended release capsule (Focalin XR) was approved by the FDA. The most common adverse effects are abdominal pain, nausea, fever, and decreased appetite. Although not common, twitching (vocal or motor tics) is a reported reason for discontinuation of therapy. Inhibition of growth is a potential long-term adverse effect of the use of stimulants in children. Dexmethylphenidate should not be administered to patients who have primary psychiatric disorders because the drug may worsen these conditions. The drug has a high potential for dependence and is a Schedule II substance. This drug is pregnancy category C.

Lisdexamfetamine (Vyvanse): Approved in 2007, lisdexamfetamine is a prodrug of dextroamphetamine approved for the treatment of ADHD. Because the drug is rapidly metabolized to dextroamphetamine, the actions and adverse effects are identical to those of other psychostimulants. This drug is a Schedule II controlled substance and is pregnancy category C.

Methylphenidate (Concerta, Daytrana, Metadate, Methylin, Ritalin, Quillivant XR): Although structurally dissimilar to amphetamine, methylphenidate shares the same mechanism of action, pharmacologic actions, and adverse effects. Methylphenidate is approved for the treatment of ADHD and narcolepsy. Rarely, it may be used off-label for major depression refractory to more traditional therapies. In treating ADHD, it is as effective as the amphetamines. The patient's condition should be regularly assessed and drug-free periods may be ordered during prolonged therapy. The drug is available in several extended release forms for once-daily dosing. A transdermal patch (Daytrana) was approved by the FDA in 2006 for children age 6 to 12. The patch is generally worn for 9 hours. The extended duration forms benefit children because they do not require the school nurse to administer a dose during the school day. It is important to note that this medication is contraindicated in children under the age of 6. Like other amphetamine-like drugs, methylphenidate is a schedule II controlled substance.

Methylphenidate is well tolerated and produces fewer peripheral adverse effects than amphetamine. Physical dependence is uncommon at therapeutic doses, although it may occur with the illicit parenteral or inhaled forms of the drug. Withdrawal symptoms are uncommon when the drug is discontinued. Nervousness, loss of appetite, and insomnia are the most common adverse effects. Methylphenidate should not be used in patients with severe anxiety, psychoses, or bipolar disorder because it may worsen these conditions. Sudden unexplained cardiac death has occurred in some people taking this drug; therefore, all patients should be screened for preexisting cardiac disease, especially structural abnormalities or ventricular dysrhythmias. In 2013, the FDA issued a safety announcement that all forms of methylphenidate may cause priapism, a prolonged and painful penile erection. In addition a warning was added that the drug is associated with an increased risk for peripheral vasculopathy, specifically Raynaud's disease. This drug is pregnancy category C.

24.4 Several nonstimulants are effective in treating symptoms of attention deficit/hyperactivity disorder.

Nonstimulants have been used off-label to manage ADHD since 2003. Atomoxetine (Strattera) was the first nonstimulant approved for the treatment of ADHD. Clonidine and guanfacine were approved in 2010 and 2006, respectively. The three nonstimulants do not have any abuse potential and are not controlled substances.

These drugs offer alternatives for parents who are hesitant to place their children on CNS stimulants. The doses for these agents are listed in Table 24.3.

Tricyclic antidepressants (TCAs) that have been used off-label for ADHD include imipramine (Tofranil), desipramine (Norpramin), and nortriptyline (Aventyl). The TCAs are less effective than the psychostimulants, can cause significant anticholinergic adverse effects such as dry mouth and constipation, and are cardiotoxic when taken in high doses. Bupropion (Wellbutrin) is another antidepressant that has been used off-label for treating ADHD. Antidepressants are considered second-line therapy for ADHD and are usually only used when the patient has not responded adequately to psychostimulants or has a comorbid condition such as depression or anxiety.

CONNECTION Checkpoint 24.2

From what you learned in Chapter 19, what class of antidepressants contains the drugs of choice for major depressive disorder? To what antidepressant class does bupropion belong? *See Answer to Connection Checkpoint 24.2 on student resource website.*

PROTOTYPE DRUG	Atomoxetine (Strattera)

Classification: **Therapeutic:** Drug for ADHD
Pharmacologic: Nonstimulant, norepinephrine reuptake inhibitor

Therapeutic Effects and Uses: Atomoxetine is administered to improve attentiveness and the ability to follow tasks in patients with ADHD. The medication decreases distraction and forgetfulness. It has the ability to diminish symptoms of ADHD in children and adults, and it is approved for patients age 6 years and older. Unlike the stimulants that have an onset of action of 1 hour, atomoxetine takes 2 to 4 weeks for optimal reduction of ADHD symptoms.

Mechanism of Action: Atomoxetine is a selective norepinephrine reuptake inhibitor (SNRI), which allows for increased concentration of the neurotransmitter in the prefrontal cortex. This region of the brain is associated with control of social behavior, personality expression, and short-term memory.

Pharmacokinetics:

Route(s)	PO
Absorption	Rapidly absorbed
Distribution	Distributed to most tissues; unknown if secreted in breast milk; 98% bound to protein
Primary metabolism	Hepatic, by CYP2D6
Primary excretion	Renal; small amounts in feces
Onset of action	2–4 weeks for ADHD symptoms
Duration of action	Half-life: 5.2 h

Adverse Effects: Common adverse effects with atomoxetine include xerostomia, headache, decreased appetite, and insomnia. CNS adverse effects include mood swings, irritability, and agitation. Because rare incidences of liver injury have been reported, patients with elevated hepatic enzymes or symptoms such as jaundice, nausea, vomiting, or anorexia should immediately discontinue the drug. Cardiovascular adverse effects include orthostatic hypotension, tachycardia, HTN, and palpitations. The patient may experience cough due to rhinorrhea, nasal congestion, and sinusitis. Weight loss and anorexia, along with urinary retention, urinary hesitancy, impotence, delayed menses, and menstrual irregularities, have been reported. **Black Box Warning**: Atomoxetine has been associated with a small increased risk for suicidal ideation. Caregivers should immediately report suicidal thoughts or unusual behavioral changes to their health care provider.

Contraindications/Precautions: If the patient has received a monoamine oxidase inhibitor (MAOI) in the last 14 days the administration of atomoxetine should be delayed due to the risk of neuroleptic malignant syndrome or hypertensive crisis. Administration of the medication to any patient who has jaundice or elevated liver enzymes should be delayed until enzyme levels are in the normal range. Atomoxetine is also contraindicated in those diagnosed with narrow-angle glaucoma because the drug is associated with an increased risk of mydriasis in some patients. It is important to administer atomoxetine cautiously in patients with HTN, tachycardia, moderate to severe hepatic insufficiency, and cardiovascular disease.

Drug Interactions: The elimination of atomoxetine is prolonged if it is administered with fluoxetine, paroxetine, or quinidine. Concurrent administration of albuterol with atomoxetine can result in increased heart rate and HTN. Drugs that activate the sympathetic nervous system should be used cautiously with atomoxetine due to the possibility of HTN. Some common sympathomimetics include amphetamines, pseudoephedrine, ephedrine, phenylephrine, dopamine, and norepinephrine. **Herbal/Food**: It is recommended that the patient not consume any herbal supplements while taking atomoxetine.

Pregnancy: Category C.

Treatment of Overdose: Overdose with atomoxetine will cause agitation, abnormal behavior, and signs of sympathetic stimulation such as mydriasis, dry mouth, and tachycardia. The patient should receive supportive treatment for cardiopulmonary effects. Gastric lavage and repeated applications of activated charcoal may prevent systemic absorption.

Nursing Responsibilities: Key nursing implications for patients receiving atomoxetine are included in the Nursing Practice Application for Patients Receiving Pharmacotherapy with Central Nervous System Stimulants.

Drugs Similar to Atomoxetine (Strattera)

Other nonstimulant drugs approved for ADHD include clonidine and guanfacine (Intuniv).

Clonidine (Kapvay): Clonidine, an older drug that was originally approved to treat HTN in 1974, was approved in 2010 to treat ADHD. In addition, it has been used off-label to treat a number of conditions, including pain, hot flashes, Tourette's syndrome, and withdrawal symptoms from alcohol, opioids, and nicotine. Clonidine is a centrally acting alpha$_2$-adrenergic agonist but it is not known how this mechanism improves the clinical symptoms of ADHD. It is not a psychostimulant and there is no risk of physical dependence. The extended release tablet offers the advantage of once-daily dosing. The tablets should not be crushed, chewed, or broken. Kapvay is not interchangeable with other forms of clonidine. Kapvay can cause sedation and fatigue, especially during the early stages of therapy.

Blood pressure should be monitored during therapy because the drug can cause hypotension, syncope, and bradycardia. Clonidine should be discontinued gradually to prevent rebound hypotension. Caution should be used if other antihypertensives or CNS depressants are concurrently administered. Drugs that affect sinus node function may interact with clonidine to cause bradycardia and AV block. The drug has not been approved to treat adult patients with ADHD. This drug is pregnancy category C.

Guanfacine (Intuniv): Originally approved in 1986 for the treatment of HTN, the indication for ADHD was added for guanfacine in 2009. Guanfacine may be used as monotherapy, or in combination therapy with stimulant-type ADHD medications. Like clonidine, guanfacine is an alpha$_2$-adrenergic agonist. It is not a psychostimulant, and it does not cause dependence. The extended release tablet offers the advantage of once-daily dosing. The tablets should not be crushed, chewed, or broken. Because the drug is a known antihypertensive, blood pressure should be monitored during therapy; some patients have experienced bradycardia and syncope due to reduced blood pressure. The drug should not be abruptly discontinued because transient rebound HTN may result. Sedation and lethargy are common, especially at the start of therapy. Caution should be used if other antihypertensives or CNS depressants are concurrently administered. Guanfacine is pregnancy category B.

Pharmacotherapy of Narcolepsy

24.5 Narcolepsy is characterized by excessive daytime sleepiness and is treated with central nervous system stimulants and antidepressants.

Narcolepsy is a chronic neurologic disorder in which the patient experiences excessive daytime sleepiness. The disorder affects 1 in 2,000 Americans and usually begins in childhood, although it may not be diagnosed until adulthood. Narcolepsy is caused by a deficiency in certain neurotransmitters in the neurons in the hypothalamus, a region responsible for controlling sleep patterns. The patient experiences an abnormal pattern of rapid eye movement (REM) sleep during the night, which causes the patient to have a "deficit" of restful sleep. There is a genetic predisposition to acquiring the disorder.

Narcolepsy is characterized by four symptoms, which separate it from other types of sleep disorders. Patients with narcolepsy may not experience all four symptoms:

- **Sleep attacks. Sleep attacks** are sudden bouts of sleep that last 10 to 30 minutes and may occur during the daytime without warning.

- **Cataplexy.** Approximately 90% of patients who have narcolepsy experience **cataplexy**, a bilateral loss of muscle tone and emotion. The cataplexy may last from several seconds to minutes, and symptoms range from clumsiness to complete collapse.

- **Sleep paralysis.** Approximately 60% of patients diagnosed with narcolepsy experience **sleep paralysis**, which is the temporary inability to move after waking up from sleep.

- **Hypnagogic hallucinations. Hypnagogic hallucinations** are vivid, dreamlike sensations, sometimes of a frightening nature, that occur with sleep paralysis.

Severe narcolepsy can be disabling and interfere with normal activities such as employment or success at school. To accommodate the disorder, the patient may require a schedule that includes several 15-minute daytime naps.

PharmFACT

After obstructive sleep apnea and restless leg syndrome, narcolepsy is the third most frequently diagnosed primary sleep disorder found in patients seeking treatment at sleep clinics. Up to 10% of patients diagnosed with narcolepsy and cataplexy together report having a close relative with the same symptoms (National Institute of Neurological Disorders and Stroke, 2013).

The goal of narcolepsy pharmacotherapy is to reduce the incidence of daytime drowsiness and other symptoms associated with the disorder. Traditional therapies have focused on CNS stimulants. Dextroamphetamine and methylphenidate are approved to treat narcolepsy (see Section 24.3). The CNS stimulants are effective at reducing daytime drowsiness but may cause nervousness, insomnia, and dependence. A newer stimulant, modafinil, has become widely used in the treatment of narcolepsy and is the prototype for this disorder.

CNS stimulants are not effective at treating cataplexy. Antidepressants such as selegiline (Eldepryl), imipramine (Tofranil), and fluoxetine (Prozac) have been used off-label to treat cataplexy and provide symptomatic relief in about 80% of patients. The only drug specifically approved by the FDA for treating cataplexy is sodium oxybate (gamma-hydroxybutyrate [GHB], Xyrem). Sodium oxybate reduces daytime sleepiness as well as episodes of cataplexy, sleep paralysis, and hypnagogic hallucinations.

PROTOTYPE DRUG	Modafinil (Provigil)

Classification: Therapeutic: Drug for narcolepsy
Pharmacologic: CNS stimulant

Therapeutic Effects and Uses: Approved in 1998, modafinil is an oral drug used to treat patients with narcolepsy and to treat the excessive sleepiness associated with shift work (circadian rhythm disruption). The drug increases daytime alertness and locomotor activity. Modafinil may also be prescribed to treat fatigue related to Parkinson's disease, obstructive sleep apnea, and multiple sclerosis.

Similar to amphetamines, modafinil can induce euphoria and psychoactive symptoms. Although the abuse potential for modafinil is less than that of other CNS stimulants, it is still classified as a Schedule IV controlled substance. It does not appear to suppress appetite or promote weight loss.

Mechanism of Action: The mechanism by which modafinil exerts its wake-promoting effects is unknown. The drug increases dopamine levels in the brain by inhibiting dopamine uptake.

Pharmacokinetics:

Route(s)	PO
Absorption	Rapidly absorbed
Distribution	Distributed to most tissues; unknown if secreted in breast milk; 60% bound to protein
Primary metabolism	Hepatic by multiple CYP enzymes
Primary excretion	Renal
Onset of action	Peak: 2–4 h
Duration of action	Half-life: 15 h

Adverse Effects: Serious adverse effects from modafinil are infrequent. The primary CNS adverse effects are headache, nervousness, insomnia, cataplexy, and paresthesia. Cardiovascular adverse effects include increased and decreased blood pressure, vasodilation, and syncope. Nausea, vomiting, diarrhea, and dry mouth are frequent gastrointestinal (GI) adverse effects. Pulmonary effects include pharyngitis, rhinitis, and dyspnea. Serious rashes, including cases of Stevens–Johnson syndrome (SJS), requiring hospitalization and discontinuation of treatment, have been reported with the use of modafinil. Modafinil can be abused or lead to dependence. This drug should be stored in a safe place to prevent misuse and abuse.

Contraindications/Precautions: Modafinil should not be administered to patients who have had an acute myocardial infarction (MI) or those with valvular heart disease or a hypersensitivity to modafinil. The safety of the medication has not been established in patients younger than age 16. The drug should be discontinued at the first sign of rash because SJS has been reported with the use of modafinil. The drug should be used with caution in patients with schizophrenia because it may worsen symptoms of patients with psychotic disorders and may cause suicidal ideation. The drug should be used with caution in those with a history of substance abuse. Severe hepatic impairment may increase serum modafinil levels as much as 50%; doses in these patients must be reduced to prevent toxicity. This drug is not approved for use in children for any indication.

Drug Interactions: CYP450 enzymes metabolize modafinil, and the drug can inhibit and induce different isozymes. For example, modafinil inhibits CYP2C19, the primary metabolic enzyme for phenytoin, diazepam, and propranolol; levels of these drugs increase when given concurrently with modafinil. When modafinil is administered with cyclosporine, the therapeutic levels of cyclosporine decrease. Modafinil may increase the levels of clomipramine and warfarin. TCA levels increase with modafinil. Modafinil may decrease the effectiveness of oral contraceptives and cause unplanned pregnancies. **Herbal/Food**: Foods and beverages containing caffeine may worsen insomnia.

Pregnancy: Category C.

Treatment of Overdose: Overdose causes agitation, insomnia, anxiety, aggressiveness, palpitations, and confusion. Overdoses are usually not fatal. The patient should receive supportive treatment and gastric lavage.

Nursing Responsibilities: Key nursing implications for patients receiving modafinil are included in the Nursing Practice Application for Patients Receiving Pharmacotherapy with Central Nervous System Stimulants.

Drugs Similar to Modafinil (Provigil)

Antidepressants used to treat narcolepsy are presented in Chapter 19, and the amphetamines are discussed in Section 24.3. Armodafinil and sodium oxybate are other drugs specifically indicated for narcolepsy.

Armodafinil (Nuvigil): Approved in 2007, armodafinil is closely related to modafinil and exhibits the same actions and adverse effects. It is approved to treat narcolepsy and shift work sleep disorder

and to improve wakefulness in patients with obstructive sleep apnea who often experience daytime drowsiness. Like modafinil serious rashes, including cases of Stevens–Johnson syndrome (SJS), have been reported with the use of the drug. Armodafinil is a Schedule IV controlled substance and is pregnancy category C.

Sodium oxybate (Xyrem): Sodium oxybate is a very unusual drug because it is the sodium salt of GHB, a Schedule I controlled substance. GHB can produce euphoria, sedation, and amnesia and is known as a "date rape" drug (see Chapter 27). Classified as a Schedule III controlled substance, sodium oxybate is only available from a centralized pharmacy to approved health care providers due to its abuse potential. It has strong hypnotic effects and is given in two doses: one at bedtime and one 4 hours later. It is approved for excessive daytime sleepiness associated with narcolepsy and for symptoms of cataplexy. The drug is sometimes administered with CNS stimulants in the management of narcolepsy. The most frequently reported adverse effects are headache, nausea, vomiting, dizziness, depression, and drowsiness. Sodium oxybate carries a black box warning that the drug is associated with adverse CNS events that include seizures, respiratory depression, profound decreases in level of consciousness, coma, and death. This drug is pregnancy category C.

CONNECTION Checkpoint 24.3

From what you learned in Chapter 18, during which stage of sleep does most of a person's active dreaming occur? *See Answer to Connection Checkpoint 24.3 on student resource website.*

Methylxanthines

24.6 Methylxanthines are central nervous system stimulants used for their ability to increase alertness or their effects on the respiratory system.

Methylxanthines are substances similar to xanthine, a chemical produced during the breakdown of deoxyribonucleic acid (DNA). Unlike the other CNS stimulants discussed in this chapter, the methylxanthines are not used for their effects on the brain. Instead, the methylxanthines are associated with treating patients with chronic obstructive pulmonary disease (COPD), asthma, and other restrictive lung diseases due to their ability to relax bronchial smooth muscle. The methylxanthines include caffeine, theophylline, and theobromine. Caffeine is the prototype drug for the methylxanthines. The dose of caffeine is listed in Table 24.3.

Theophylline and theobromine are formed by the metabolic breakdown of caffeine in the liver. Although rarely used, theophylline is still available as a drug to treat asthma that is resistant to other therapies. Theobromine is a natural substance found in chocolate that once was used as a drug to treat HTN and other vascular disorders. Although similar to caffeine, it has very little CNS stimulant activity.

PROTOTYPE DRUG	Caffeine

Classification: **Therapeutic:** CNS and respiratory stimulant
Pharmacologic: Methylxanthine

Therapeutic Effects and Uses: Caffeine is a methylxanthine naturally found in over 60 plant species. Most consumption in the United States is from coffee, tea, soft drinks, chocolate, and energy beverages. Caffeine has potent psychoactive properties. When taken PO it quickly restores mental alertness and aids in wakefulness. In addition to its consumption in beverages and food, caffeine is also available in OTC products designed to increase alertness and delay fatigue.

The only FDA-approved indication for caffeine is as a respiratory stimulant in the management of apnea in premature infants. For this indication, caffeine (Cafcit) may be administered IV or PO (e.g., added to formula feedings).

Caffeine also has a number of off-label indications. In patients with asthma, orally administered caffeine will produce bronchodilation and smooth muscle relaxation. Caffeine produces a mild diuresis due to increased blood flow to the glomerulus and has been used as an OTC diuretic product. Caffeine can be administered IV to relieve headache associated with lumbar puncture.

Caffeine itself has no analgesic properties. However, it enhances pain relief when administered with a narcotic analgesic. Caffeine is also combined with ergotamine (Cafergot) in the treatment of migraine headaches. It may be administered parenterally in emergency situations to treat circulatory collapse.

Mechanism of Action: Caffeine is metabolized in the liver to theobromine and theophylline, both of which are active metabolites that enhance the CNS and respiratory stimulant effects of caffeine. When higher doses are administered, the medulla, respiratory center, and vagus nerve are stimulated and produce a relaxation of smooth muscle, which is particularly evident in the bronchi and coronary and systemic blood vessels.

Pharmacokinetics:

Route(s)	PO, intramuscular (IM), IV
Absorption	Rapidly absorbed
Distribution	Widely distributed; crosses the blood–brain barrier and the placenta; secreted in breast milk; 36% bound to plasma proteins
Primary metabolism	Hepatic
Primary excretion	Renal
Onset of action	15–45 min
Duration of action	Half-life: 3–5 h in adults; 36–144 h in neonates

Adverse Effects: Caffeine may cause adverse effects at therapeutic doses, many of which are extensions of its pharmacologic actions. Excessive CNS stimulation may cause nervousness, insomnia, tremors, and restlessness. The cardiovascular effects of caffeine include tingling of the face, palpitations, tachycardia, bradycardia, and ventricular ectopic beats. GI effects noted with the administration of caffeine are related to the stimulation of the vagus nerve and include nausea, vomiting, epigastric pain, hematemesis, and kernicterus in neonates. Clonic seizures can result in rare instances. Caffeine withdrawal can produce symptoms of irritability, headache, lethargy, or anxiety.

Contraindications/Precautions: Caffeine should not be administered during acute MI or to patients with cardiac dysrhythmias because the drug increases the workload of the heart. Caffeine increases the secretion of gastric acid; therefore, patients who have peptic ulcer disease should limit their caffeine intake. Patients with anxiety disorders, insomnia, or panic attacks should not be administered caffeine because it may worsen these conditions. It should be used cautiously in patients with diabetes mellitus, hiatal hernia, HTN, and heart disease. Patients with hepatic or renal impairment should receive lower doses because the drug may accumulate to toxic levels.

Drug Interactions: Caffeine administered with cimetidine will increase the effect of cimetidine. Beta-adrenergic agonists administered with caffeine will result in increased cardiovascular stimulation. Additive effects are likely if the drug is taken concurrently with other CNS stimulants. Patients taking drugs for insomnia or anxiety should limit their intake of caffeine. Caffeine is a substrate of hepatic cytochrome CYP1A2. Drugs that enhance or inhibit this enzyme may interact with caffeine. **Herbal/Food:** Food and fluids that contain caffeine will increase the insomnia or restlessness that is normally noted with methylxanthines.

Pregnancy: Category B (Cafcit is labeled as category C).

Treatment of Overdose: Caffeine overdose can potentially cause dysrhythmias, insomnia, delirium, and seizures. The patient is supported through symptom management. High serum levels of caffeine can be dialyzed with peritoneal or hemodialysis.

Nursing Responsibilities: Key nursing implications for patients receiving caffeine are included in the Nursing Practice Application for Patients Receiving Pharmacotherapy with Central Nervous System Stimulants.

Drugs Similar to Caffeine

Theophylline is the only other methylxanthine used as a drug.

Theophylline: Theophylline is not used to treat ADHD, but it is administered to produce bronchodilation in patients with acute bronchospasm. It decreases wheezing and obstructed airways in asthma and bronchitis. It is important to note that the medication is a CNS stimulant that can produce restlessness, insomnia, and irritability. Close monitoring is required to prevent drug toxicity. Once widely prescribed, theophylline use has declined due to the development of safer drugs for patients with asthma (see Chapter 44).

PharmFACT

Pregnant women should limit their caffeine intake to 200 mg per day, the equivalent of a 12-ounce cup of coffee. Women who consume more than 500 mg per day may be more likely to have infants with a faster breathing rate, higher heart rate, and insomnia for the first few days of life (March of Dimes, 2012).

CONNECTIONS: NURSING PRACTICE APPLICATION

Patients Receiving Pharmacotherapy with Central Nervous System Stimulants

Assessment	Potential Nursing Diagnoses*
Baseline assessment prior to administration: • Obtain a complete health history including hepatic, renal, cardiovascular, or neurologic disease, including epilepsy, and neonatal or previously existing symptoms of cardiac problems. Obtain a drug history including allergies, current prescription and OTC drugs, and herbal preparations. Be alert to possible drug interactions. • Obtain a social and behavioral history. Use objective screening tools when possible. • Obtain a nutritional history and assess normal sleep patterns. • Obtain baseline vital signs, height, and weight. • Evaluate appropriate laboratory findings (e.g., electrolytes, CBC, hepatic, and renal function studies). • Assess the patient's ability to receive and understand instructions. Include the family and caregiver as needed.	• *Imbalanced Nutrition: Less than Body Requirements*, related to adverse effects of drug therapy • *Disturbed Sleep Pattern* • *Urinary Retention* • *Interrupted Family Processes* • *Deficient Knowledge* (Drug Therapy) • *Risk for Delayed Growth and Development*, related to adverse drug effects • *Risk for Social Isolation*
Assessment throughout administration: • Assess for desired therapeutic effects (e.g., increased ability to focus, normalized activity levels with lessened impulsivity, maintenance of normal appetite and sleep patterns). • Continue periodic monitoring of electrolytes, CBC, and hepatic and renal function studies. • Continue to monitor vital signs, especially pulse, blood pressure, and height and weight weekly. **Lifespan:** Be aware that the child, adolescent, or older adult is at greater risk for cardiovascular effects and may be more likely to experience adverse effects related to anorexia from the drug. • Assess for and promptly report adverse effects: dizziness, lightheadedness, anxiety, agitation, excessive physical activity, tachycardia, increased blood pressure, HTN, palpitations.	

Implementation

Interventions and (Rationales)	Patient-Centered Care
Ensuring therapeutic effects: • Continue assessments as above for therapeutic effects. (Therapeutic effects of ADHD drugs include the ability to focus and stay on task, lessened impulsivity, and improved social interactions.)	• Teach the patient, family, or caregiver to keep a social/behavioral diary. Involve school faculty and other caregivers (e.g., after-school care).
Minimizing adverse effects: • Continue to monitor pulse and blood pressure on health care visits. (Tachycardia, increased blood pressure, or HTN may occur if dose is excessive. An increased risk of dysrhythmias and sudden death has been noted with some drugs.)	• Teach the patient, family, or caregiver to take the pulse along with weekly height and weight, or any time symptoms warrant (e.g., child reports chest discomfort or palpitations). Assist the patient, family, or caregiver to find the pulse location most easily felt and have the patient, family, or caregiver return demonstrate pulse taking before going home.
• Weigh the patient weekly and obtain height. Report any weight loss or failure to gain weight during expected growth periods. Assess nutrition and use of other stimulating products (e.g., energy drinks and caffeinated beverages). (Diminished appetite or anorexia from stimulating effects of the drug, or use of other stimulants, may impair normal nutrition needed for growth and development. **Lifespan:** Children, adolescents, and older adults are more likely to experience adverse effects related to anorexia from the drug.)	• Teach the patient, family, or caregiver to obtain height and weight weekly and to report any loss of weight or lack of expected growth. Ensure proper use and functioning of any home equipment used (e.g., electronic scale). • Discuss the need to avoid or eliminate all foods, beverages, or OTC drugs that contain caffeine or other stimulants.
• Continue to monitor sleep patterns. (Stimulatory effects of the drug may affect normal sleeping patterns and may indicate excessive dosage.)	• Instruct the patient, family, or caregiver to inform the provider of disruption to sleep, increased agitation during the day (possible effect from lack of sleep), or excessive sleepiness during the day. • Have the patient take the dose early in the day and before 4 p.m. to help alleviate insomnia unless extended release formulation is used. Take extended release formulations in the morning.

(continued)

CONNECTIONS: NURSING PRACTICE APPLICATION (continued)

• Assess for excessive stimulatory effects: agitation, aggression, tremors, or seizures and report immediately. (Excessive CNS stimulation may cause seizures as an adverse effect.)	• Instruct the patient, family, or caregiver to report tremors or seizures to the health care provider immediately.
• Assess for urinary retention periodically. (Atomoxetine [Straterra] and other norepinephrine reuptake inhibitors may cause urinary retention as an adverse effect. **Lifespan:** Be aware that the older male adult with an enlarged prostate is at higher risk for mechanical obstruction.)	• Instruct the patient to immediately report an inability to void, increasing bladder pressure, or pain.
• Continue to monitor for dermatologic effects including red or purplish skin rash, blisters, or sunburn. (Armodafinil and methylphenidate have been associated with severe skin effects including SJS and exfoliative dermatitis. Sunscreen and protective clothing should be used.)	• Teach the patient to wear sunscreen and protective clothing for sun exposure and to avoid tanning beds. Immediately report any severe sunburn or rashes.
• Assess the need for continuous medication or the need for drug holidays with the patient, family, caregiver, and the health care provider based on social/behavioral diary findings. (Dependent on the degree of behavior, drug holidays on nonschool days or vacation periods may be recommended.)	• Teach the patient, family, or caregiver about the use of drug holidays and explore options. If the drug dose is at the upper range, consider tapering the dose prior to beginning the drug holiday to avoid rebound hyperactivity or agitation.
• Assess the home environment for medication safety and need for appropriate interventions. Advise the family on restrictions of prescription renewal. (Some of these drugs are scheduled drugs and may not be used by any person other than the patient. Safeguard the medication in the home to prevent overdose.)	• Instruct the patient, family, or caregiver in proper medication storage and the need for the drug to be used by the patient only. • Teach the family or caregiver about prescription renewal restrictions (i.e., new prescription each time, no refills, and prescription may not be called in) and explore school policies regarding in-school use (e.g., single dose sent each day, and secured blister-pack used if multiple doses are sent).
• Assess for increasing depression, agitation, delusional thoughts, or expressions of suicide or self-harm. Promptly refer any of these symptoms to the provider. (Atomoxetine has been associated with an increased risk of suicide. Modafinil and armodafinil have been associated with an increased risk of psychiatric symptoms, including paranoia and suicidal ideations.)	• Teach the family or caregiver to be alert for signs of increased depression, confusion, paranoia, or expressions of suicide. Promptly notify the provider if symptoms are noted.
Patient understanding of drug therapy: • Use opportunities during administration of medications and during assessments to discuss the rationale for the drug therapy, desired therapeutic outcomes, commonly observed adverse effects, parameters for when to call the health care provider, and any necessary monitoring or precautions. (Using time during nursing care helps to optimize and reinforce key teaching areas.)	• The patient, family, and caregiver should be able to state the reason for the drug, appropriate dose and scheduling, what adverse effects to observe for, and when to report them.

Patient self-administration of drug therapy:
• When administering the medication, instruct the patient, family, or caregiver in proper self-administration of the drug (e.g., take the drug as prescribed and do not substitute brands). (Utilizing time during nurse-administration of these drugs helps to reinforce teaching.)
	• Teach the patient to take the medication:
	  • Exactly as ordered and in the morning to prevent insomnia.
	  • Do not take double or extra doses to increase mental focus or to prevent sleepiness. The drug will not achieve these effects but will increase the adverse effects of the drug.
	  • Do not abruptly discontinue the medication without consulting the health care provider.
	  • Do not open, chew, or crush extended release tablets; swallow them whole with plenty of water.

*Nursing Diagnoses—Definitions and Classification 2015–2017. Copyright © 2014, 1994–2014 by NANDA International. Used by arrangement with John Wiley & Sons Limited.

CHAPTER
24
Understanding the Chapter

Key Concepts Summary

24.1 Central nervous system stimulants increase alertness, enhance the ability to concentrate, and delay the symptoms of fatigue.

24.2 Attention deficit/hyperactivity disorder is characterized by inattention, hyperactivity, and impulsive behavior.

24.3 Psychostimulants are central nervous system stimulants indicated for the treatment of ADHD and narcolepsy.

24.4 Several nonstimulants are effective in treating symptoms of attention deficit/hyperactivity disorder.

24.5 Narcolepsy is characterized by excessive daytime sleepiness and is treated with central nervous system stimulants and antidepressants.

24.6 Methylxanthines are central nervous system stimulants used for their ability to increase alertness or their effects on the respiratory system.

Case Study: Making the Patient Connection

Remember the patient "Jonathon Hogan" at the beginning of the chapter? Now read the remainder of the case study. Based on the information presented within this chapter, respond to the critical thinking questions that follow.

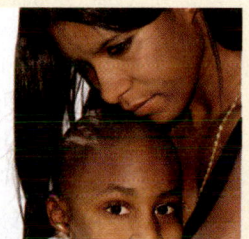

Jonathon Hogan has had trouble at school beginning in kindergarten and for the past year. His teachers have consistently reported that he is easily distracted and wanders around the classroom even during a lesson. Getting him to do his homework after school has been a struggle. Jonathon loves art and does well at video games. Because he is a happy-go-lucky child, his parents have assumed that it is Jonathon's right-brain dominance that has created trouble with left-brain logical work. With more homework now in second

grade, Jonathon is struggling to keep up in school. The school nurse suspects he may have ADHD. She has recommended an appointment with Jonathon's health care provider and told his parents that Adderall may help Jonathon focus on his schoolwork.

Critical Thinking Questions

1. What is ADHD and why would Jonathon be experiencing more difficulty as he becomes older?

2. How might amphetamine sulfate and dextroamphetamine (Adderall) help Jonathon with his ADHD?

3. What caregiver education would be appropriate regarding dextroamphetamine and amphetamine sulfate (Adderall)?

See Answers to Critical Thinking Questions on student resource website.

Additional Case Study

Anna Steinmetz has graduated from nursing school and is working nights. She is having difficulty adjusting to her night schedule. Her health care provider suggested she utilize a medication to assist with her adjustment to shift work. She has been prescribed modafinil (Provigil).

1. What effect does modafinil (Provigil) have on the patient's ability to maintain alertness during shift work?

2. What teaching will you provide to the patient regarding this medication?

3. The patient reports feelings of lightheadedness with position changes. What interventions will assist in maintaining patient safety?

See Answers to Additional Case Study on student resource website.

Chapter Review

1 An elementary school nurse is providing education to the faculty on the use of central nervous system stimulants used to treat attention deficit/hyperactivity disorder. Of the following, which is most important for the nurse to convey to the faculty?

1. Have the child bring the drug dose in a lunch bag and come to the office to take it to avoid being teased.
2. Request that the parents leave an extra copy of the prescription at the school in case the dose runs out.
3. Suggest that the parents have two prescriptions filled, one for home and one to keep at school.
4. Keep the drugs in a locked drawer, clearly labeled with the student's name and only the number of doses allowed by school policy.

2 Which therapeutic outcome would the nurse consider most significant in evaluating a patient who started atomoxetine (Strattera) 6 months ago?

1. Decrease in attention
2. Decrease in hyperactivity
3. Development of mydriasis
4. Elevated liver enzymes

3 A patient who has overdosed on amphetamine sulfate and dextroamphetamine (Adderall XR) is admitted to the emergency department. The nurse would anticipate which medications to be administered to assist in counteracting the effects of the overdosage?

1. Chlorpromazine (Thorazine)
2. Phenytoin (Dilantin)
3. Propofol (Diprivan)
4. Dexamethasone (Decadron)

4 A high school student taking atomoxetine (Strattera) for attention deficit/hyperactivity disorder visits the school nurse's office and confides, "I am so depressed. The world would be better off without me." Which action would the nurse take for this patient?

1. Tell the patient to stop taking atomoxetine immediately and not to take it until checking with the provider.
2. Assure the patient that these are normal symptoms because the drug may take 3 or 4 weeks to work.
3. Alert the family or caregiver that immediate attention and treatment are needed for these symptoms.
4. Have the patient increase intake of caffeine by consuming cola products, coffee, or tea to counteract the depressive effect.

5 An office worker has made an appointment with the provider for heart palpitations, dysrhythmias, and facial tingling. The nurse is taking the patient's history. Which of the following does the nurse note may explain the symptoms?

1. The patient takes zolpidem (Ambien) for occasional insomnia.
2. The patient has been working late frequently and has relied on coffee to maintain alertness.
3. The patient is taking gabapentin (Neurontin) for pain associated with herpes zoster.
4. The patient has been under stress at work and has switched to using herbal teas.

6 A patient who is taking methylphenidate (Concerta, Metadate, Ritalin) for attention deficit/hyperactivity disorder reports having insomnia. Which intervention will assist in the promotion of sleep?

1. Have a glass of wine with dinner.
2. Eat a chocolate bar at bedtime.
3. Take the drug before 4 p.m.
4. Switch to decaffeinated coffee.

See Answers to Chapter Review in Appendix A.

References

American Psychiatric Association. (2013). *Diagnostic and statistical manual of mental disorders* (5th ed.). Washington, DC: Author.

Centers for Disease Control and Prevention (CDC). (2013). *Attention deficit/hyperactivity disorder (ADHD) data and statistics in the United States.* Retrieved from http://www.cdc.gov/ncbddd/adhd/data.html

Drug Enforcement Administration. (2014). *Lists of: Scheduling actions, controlled substances and regulated chemicals.* Retrieved from http://www.deadiversion.usdoj.gov/schedules/orangebook/orangebook.pdf

Elia, J., & Vetter, V. L. (2010). Cardiovascular effects for the treatment of attention-deficit hyperactivity disorder: What is known and how should it influence prescribing in children? *Pediatric Drugs, 12,* 165–175. doi:10.2165/11532570-000000000-00000

Evans, S. W., Brady, C. E., Harrison, J. R., Bunford, N., Kern, L., State, T., & Andrews, C. (2013). Measuring ADHD and ODD symptoms and impairment using high school teachers' ratings. *Journal of Clinical Child & Adolescent Psychology, 42,* 197–207. doi:10.1080/15374416.2012.738456

March of Dimes. (2012). *Caffeine in pregnancy.* Retrieved from http://www.marchofdimes.com/pregnancy/caffeine-in-pregnancy.aspx

Mick, E., Byrne, D., Fried, R., Monuteaux, M., Faraone, S. V., & Biederman, J. (2011). Predictors of ADHD persistence in girls at 5-year follow-up. *Journal of Attention Disorders, 15,* 183–192. doi:10.1177/1087054710362217

National Institute of Neurological Disorders and Stroke. (2013). *Narcolepsy fact sheet.* Retrieved from http://www.ninds.nih.gov/disorders/narcolepsy/detail_narcolepsy.htm

Selected Bibliography

Charach, A., & Fernandez, R. (2013). Enhancing ADHD medication adherence: Challenges and opportunities. *Current Psychiatry Reports, 15*(7), 1–8. doi:10.1007/s11920-013-0371-6

Chirdkiatgumchai, V., Xiao, H., Fredstrom, B. K., Adams, R. E., Epstein, J. N., Shah, S. S., . . . Froehlich, T. E. (2013). National trends in psychotropic medication use in young children: 1994–2009. *Pediatrics, 132,* 615–623. doi:10.1542/peds.2013-1546

Cortese, S., Holtmann, M., Banaschewski, T., Buitelaar, J., Coghill, D., Danckaerts, M., . . . Sergeant, J. (2013). Practitioner review: Current best practice in the management of adverse events during treatment with ADHD medications in children and adolescents. *Journal of Child Psychology and Psychiatry, 54,* 227–246. doi:10.1111/jcpp.12036

Dopheide, J. A., & Pliszka, S. R. (2009). Attention-deficit–hyperactivity disorder: An update. *Pharmacotherapy, 29,* 656–679. doi:10.1592/phco.29.6.656

Elia, J., Sackett, J., Turner, T., Schardt, M., Tang, S. C., Kurtz, N., . . . Borgmann-Winter, K. (2012). Attention-deficit/hyperactivity disorder genomics: Update for clinicians. *Current Psychiatry Reports, 14,* 579–589. doi:10.1007/s11920-012-0309-4

Herdman, T. H., & Kamitsuru, S. (Eds.). (2014). *NANDA International nursing diagnoses: Definitions and classification, 2015–2017.* Oxford, United Kingdom: Wiley-Blackwell.

National Institute of Mental Health. (2012). *Attention deficit hyperactivity disorder.* Retrieved from http://www.nimh.nih.gov/health/publications/attention-deficit-hyperactivity-disorder/index.shtml

Preda, A. (2013). Stimulants. *Medscape reference.* Retrieved from http://emedicine.medscape.com/article/289007-overview

Ryan, J. B., Katsiyannis, A., & Hughes, E. M. (2011). Medication treatment for attention deficit hyperactivity disorder. *Theory into Practice, 50*(1), 52–60. doi:10.1080/00405841.2010.534939

Schweitzer, J. B., & McBurnett, K. (2012). New directions for therapeutics in ADHD. *Neurotherapeutics, 9,* 487–489. doi:10.1007/s13311-012-0137-6

Sonuga-Barke, E. J., Brandeis, D., Cortese, S., Daley, D., Ferrin, M., Holtmann, M., . . . Sergeant, J. (2013). Nonpharmacological interventions for ADHD: Systematic review and meta-analyses of randomized controlled trials of dietary and psychological treatments. *American Journal of Psychiatry, 170,* 275–289. doi:10.1176/appi.ajp.2012.12070991

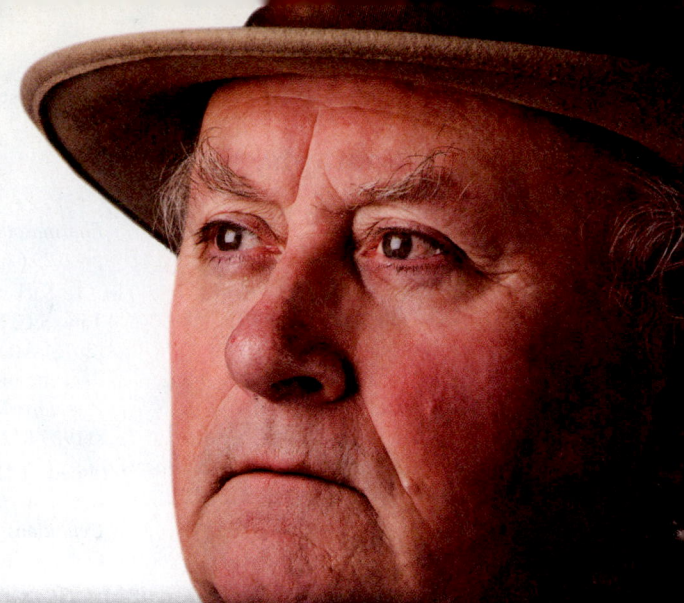

"I'm having urological surgery tomorrow and I am worried about pain. I've taken pain medicine daily for years because of chronic pain from back problems and numerous back surgeries. Will I experience severe pain after this procedure?"

Patient "Larry Smith"

CHAPTER

25 Pharmacotherapy of Severe Pain and Migraines

LEARNING OUTCOMES

After reading this chapter, the student should be able to:

1. Identify key principles of pain management.
2. Describe the assessment and classification of pain.
3. Refute the common pain myths, using objective evidence.
4. Explain the phases of pain physiology: transduction, transmission, perception, and modulation.
5. Describe pharmacologic and nonpharmacologic therapies used in pain management.
6. Describe the types of opioid receptors in the central nervous system.
7. Identify the classes of drugs used for minor, moderate, and severe pain.
8. Compare and contrast the actions of opioid agonists, mixed opioid agonists-antagonists, and opioid antagonists.
9. Describe the use of nonopioids and adjuvant analgesics in the treatment of pain.
10. Compare and contrast the actions and adverse effects of the opioids and nonopioids for analgesia.
11. For each of the classes shown in the chapter outline, identify the prototype and representative drugs and explain the mechanism(s) of drug action, primary indications, contraindications, significant drug interactions, pregnancy category, and important adverse effects.
12. Explain the role of opioid antagonists in the diagnosis and treatment of acute opioid toxicity.
13. Compare the types of drugs used for preventing migraines to those for terminating migraines.
14. Apply the nursing process to care for patients receiving pharmacotherapy for pain and for migraines.

CHAPTER OUTLINE

▸ **General Principles of Pain Management**

▸ **Pain Management with Opioids**
  Opioid Analgesics
  PROTOTYPE Morphine Sulfate (Astramorph PF, Duramorph RF, Roxanol, Others), *p. 376*
  Mixed Agonist-Antagonist Opioids

▸ **Pain Management with Nonopioids**
  Nonopioid Analgesics
  Nonsteroidal Anti-Inflammatory Drugs (NSAIDs) and Acetaminophen
  Centrally Acting Analgesics
  PROTOTYPE Tramadol (Ultram, Others), *p. 379*
  Adjuvant Analgesics

▸ **Pharmacotherapy with Opioid Antagonists**

▸ **Pharmacotherapy of Migraines**
  PROTOTYPE Sumatriptan (Imitrex, Others), *p. 387*

KEY TERMS

addiction, 369

adjuvant analgesics, 383

analgesics, 368

auras, 385

endorphins, 370

gate control theory, 369

kappa receptors, 372

migraine, 385

mu receptors, 372

narcotic, 372

neuropathic pain, 368

nociceptor pain, 368

nociceptors, 368

nonopioid analgesics, 379

opiates, 372

opioid, 372

opium, 372

tension headache, 385

Pain is a subjective experience that has both physiological and emotional components. Usually associated with trauma or disease, pain may be viewed as a natural defense mechanism that helps people avoid potentially damaging situations and encourages them to seek medical help. Pain medications are some of the most frequently prescribed drugs in medicine. This chapter examines the drug classes used in pain management and for the pharmacotherapy of migraines.

General Principles of Pain Management

25.1 The primary goal of pain management is to reduce pain to a level that allows the patient to continue normal daily activities.

Pain management is one of the most important tasks for health care providers. It is also one of the most difficult because the experience of pain by the patients and its assessment by the health care provider are subjective. The perception of pain can clearly be influenced by comorbid conditions such as anxiety, fatigue, and depression. For example, knowing that health care providers and caregivers are attentive and actively engaged in pain management may lower patients' anxiety, thus reducing pain perception and increasing pain tolerance. Listening carefully, showing respect, and helping patients to understand their treatment options are important steps to attaining optimum pain relief.

The immediate goal of pain management is to reduce pain to a level that allows the patient to perform reasonable activities of daily living (ADLs) such as sleeping, eating, and normal physical activities. For some disorders, the patient should understand that the total elimination of pain may not be a realistic goal, or that the pain may require a long period of treatment. Several key principles underlie the nursing management of pain:

- The patient should be considered the expert on his or her own pain; the nurse should always believe the patient's self-assessment of pain.

- Pain management is a patient right and should be based on the patient's goals. The patient should be screened for pain during an initial assessment and periodically thereafter. If pain cannot be effectively managed, then a pain management specialist should be consulted.

- Nonpharmacologic interventions such as massage or the application of heat or cold should be encouraged in pain management.

A combination of therapies is optimum because different modalities work by different mechanisms, thus improving the effectiveness of pain management.

- Dosing should be individualized and adjusted to produce the established pain management goal in each patient.

- Adverse effects from pain medications should be anticipated and prevented whenever possible. Should they appear, adverse effects should be immediately addressed.

- Around-the-clock dosing for moderate to severe pain should be implemented because it is much easier to *maintain* a pain-free level than to *eliminate* existing or escalating pain.

25.2 Proper assessment and classification of pain guides its treatment.

Pain assessment includes documenting the location, intensity, and quality (sharp, dull, burning) of the pain and any precipitating or relieving factors. For most adults, the 0-to-10 numerical rating scale is the standard for rating pain intensity, with 0 being no pain and 10 being the greatest pain imaginable. The pain rating is used as a reference point, initially as a baseline level of pain and later as an indicator of effectiveness as to how well the treatment is achieving the patient's goals.

Pain may be classified as acute or chronic. Acute pain has an abrupt onset but brief duration; it subsides as healing takes place or the pain stimulus ceases. Examples of acute pain include that associated with surgical incisions, labor and delivery, sprained joints, or myocardial infarction (MI). Although it may be severe, acute pain is often self-limiting; high doses of pain medication may be necessary, but therapy is usually of short duration. There is little risk of chronic drug adverse effects or dependence because of the relatively brief treatment period.

Chronic pain is that which persists longer than 6 months, can interfere with ADLs, and is sometimes associated with feelings of helplessness or hopelessness. Chronic pain can be further grouped as either nonmalignant or malignant (cancer) pain. Chronic nonmalignant pain is not life threatening and usually responds favorably to a consistent, stable dose of pain medication as part of a treatment regimen. The most common example is low back pain. Cancer pain ends with control of the disease or death. Although the majority of patients with cancer experience pain during the advanced stages of the disease, 90% of the cancer pain can be controlled with oral (PO) drugs, using around-the-clock dosing, with as-needed (prn) doses for breakthrough pain.

CONNECTIONS Evidence-Based Practice

◀ Opioids for Chronic Noncancer Pain Management

Clinical Question
Are opioids appropriate for the management of chronic noncancer pain?

Evidence
Opioids for acute pain and pain associated with cancer are accepted treatments but the use of chronic opioid therapy (COT) for chronic noncancer pain (CNCP) is controversial. Many diseases lead to chronic pain including osteoarthritis, fibromyalgia, and back pain. In addition, current drug therapy and other nondrug treatments result in large health care costs. Any decisions to use COT must be balanced against the very real concerns of abuse, diversion (use for recreational purposes, especially by persons not prescribed the drug), and addiction. The American Pain Society and American Academy of Pain Management sought to develop recommendations for the use of opioids for pain management in chronic noncancer pain.

After systematic review of over 8,000 studies by Chou et al. (2009), recommendations were established for the use of COT for CNCP, including:

- A thorough health history should be conducted including assessment of risk for substance abuse or addiction. The impact of pain on the patient's quality of life should be considered, and benefits and risks of COT should be evaluated.
- Patients should discuss benefits and risks of COT with their provider, sign an informed consent document, and a written plan of care should be established with the patient.

- A trial of opioids over several weeks to months should be tried to determine whether COT is appropriate. Drug type and dosing (short- versus long-acting opioids, around-the-clock versus as-needed dosing) may be evaluated during this period. Adverse effects or substance abuse or diversion during this period should be evaluated before continuing the COT plan of care.
- Patients on COT require frequent ongoing assessments, including for therapeutic and adverse effects as well as substance abuse, addiction, or diversion. Escalating doses and high-dose opioid use may suggest the need to consider options such as opioid rotation to different drugs.
- Any patient exhibiting substance abuse behaviors or intolerable adverse effects should be tapered off COT.
- Nondrug therapies such as cognitive–behavioral therapy should be considered along with COT.

Implications
Opioid therapy for chronic noncancer pain is an effective method for pain relief for select patients, but a thorough health history, continuous monitoring, and a consideration of nondrug therapies to supplement the opioid therapy should be part of the drug regimen.

Critical Thinking Question
Select two of the preceding recommendations and develop strategies that the nurse can incorporate in the care of a patient with chronic noncancer pain.

See Answers to Critical Thinking Questions on student resource website.

PharmFACT

Low Back Pain in America
- Low back pain is the most common cause of job-related disability in adults.
- Low back pain most often occurs between the ages of 30 to 50 due to the aging process and too little exercise.
- Heavy backpacks can cause muscle strains and low back pain and are responsible for thousands of medical visits by preteens each year (National Institute of Neurological Disorders and Stroke, 2013).

Another useful method for classifying pain is according to its source: nociceptor or neuropathic. **Nociceptors** are the sensory nerve receptors located throughout the body that initiate pain transmission when stimulated. For example, a needlestick will activate receptors in the finger, producing **nociceptor pain**. This type of pain may be further subdivided into somatic pain, which produces sharp, localized sensations usually experienced in muscles and joints, or visceral pain, which is described as a generalized dull, throbbing, or aching pain usually located in internal organs. Nociceptor pain responds quite well to **analgesics**, which are medications that relieve pain.

In contrast, **neuropathic pain** is caused by injury or irritation to nerve tissue and typically is described as burning, shooting, or numbing pain. The cause of neuropathic pain is sometimes difficult to determine. Analgesic treatment of neuropathic pain is often unsuccessful or high doses may be required. Neuropathic pain responds well to adjuvant analgesics such as antiseizure drugs and antidepressants (see Section 25.11).

25.3 Health care providers and patients sometimes hold myths about pain that impede optimum pain management.

Commonly held but untrue beliefs by both patients and health care providers may interfere with effective pain management. For example, health care providers may undertreat pain because of common misconceptions about pain. Furthermore, patients may not report their pain accurately or may refuse pain medications because of similar misconceptions.

A pervasive myth is that health care professionals can successfully recognize pain, independent of the patient's report. The nurse must understand that patients are the authorities on their own pain. Pain is whatever the patient says it is, existing whenever the patient says it does. Patient self-report of pain is sufficient for a nursing diagnosis of pain.

A closely related myth is that a person in pain must look and act like he or she is in pain. Some patients do not show or report pain accurately because they feel it is a sign of weakness. In addition, vital signs are sometimes unreliable indicators of pain. Although they may be elevated during the initial experience of acute pain owing to sympathetic arousal, vital signs return to normal as the body adapts. A related misconception is the belief that if a person is able to sleep, he or she must not be experiencing much pain. Although it is certainly true that pain can interfere with sleep quality and quantity, social withdrawal and excessive sleep may be indicators of coping mechanisms for some people with severe or chronic pain.

Both patients and health care providers may share the myth that the use of potent analgesics inevitably leads to addiction. **Addiction** is the continued use of a substance despite serious health and social consequences (see Chapter 27). The incidence of addiction to opioids, which are used in the treatment of severe pain, is less than 1% in patients with no previous history of drug abuse. Related to this myth is the belief that patients experiencing chronic pain overreport pain because they are addicted to opioids.

Another contradictory myth is the belief that the more pain a person experiences, the more he or she is likely to tolerate it. In fact, the opposite is more likely to occur. Unrelieved pain creates anxiety and fatigue, both of which increase pain perception and decrease tolerance. A related myth is that there is no physiological basis for the moderating effects of emotions on pain perception.

25.4 Pain transmission processes allow multiple targets for pharmacologic intervention.

Pain physiology may be divided into four phases: transduction, transmission, perception, and modulation. These phases are illustrated in Figure 25.1.

Pain transduction: Pain transduction begins when nociceptor nerve endings in the peripheral nervous system are stimulated.

This occurs when local tissue injury causes the release of chemical mediators of inflammation, including prostaglandins, leukotrienes, histamine, bradykinin, and substance P. These substances sensitize peripheral nociceptors, making them easier to activate.

Pain transmission: The nerve impulse signaling the pain travels from the nociceptor to the spinal cord along two types of sensory neurons called A and C fibers. A fibers are wrapped in myelin, a lipid substance that speeds nerve transmission, and carry signals for intense, well-defined pain. On the other hand, C fibers are unmyelinated and thus carry information more slowly and conduct poorly localized pain, which is often perceived as burning or a dull ache.

A fibers have three subtypes: alpha (α), beta (β), and delta (Δ). Aα fibers have the fastest transmission and respond to touch and pressure on muscle; Aβ fibers are slower and respond to touch and pressure on skin. Finally, AΔ fibers are the slowest of the A fibers and respond to tissue injury, producing the sensation of sharp pain.

The sensory nerve fibers enter the dorsal horn of the spinal cord and have adjacent synapses in an area called the substantia gelatinosa. The **gate control theory** proposes a gating mechanism for the transmission of pain in the spinal cord. Signals from faster Aα or Aβ fibers reach the spinal cord and close the gate before those of C fibers reach the region (or gate), in effect blocking the transmission of these

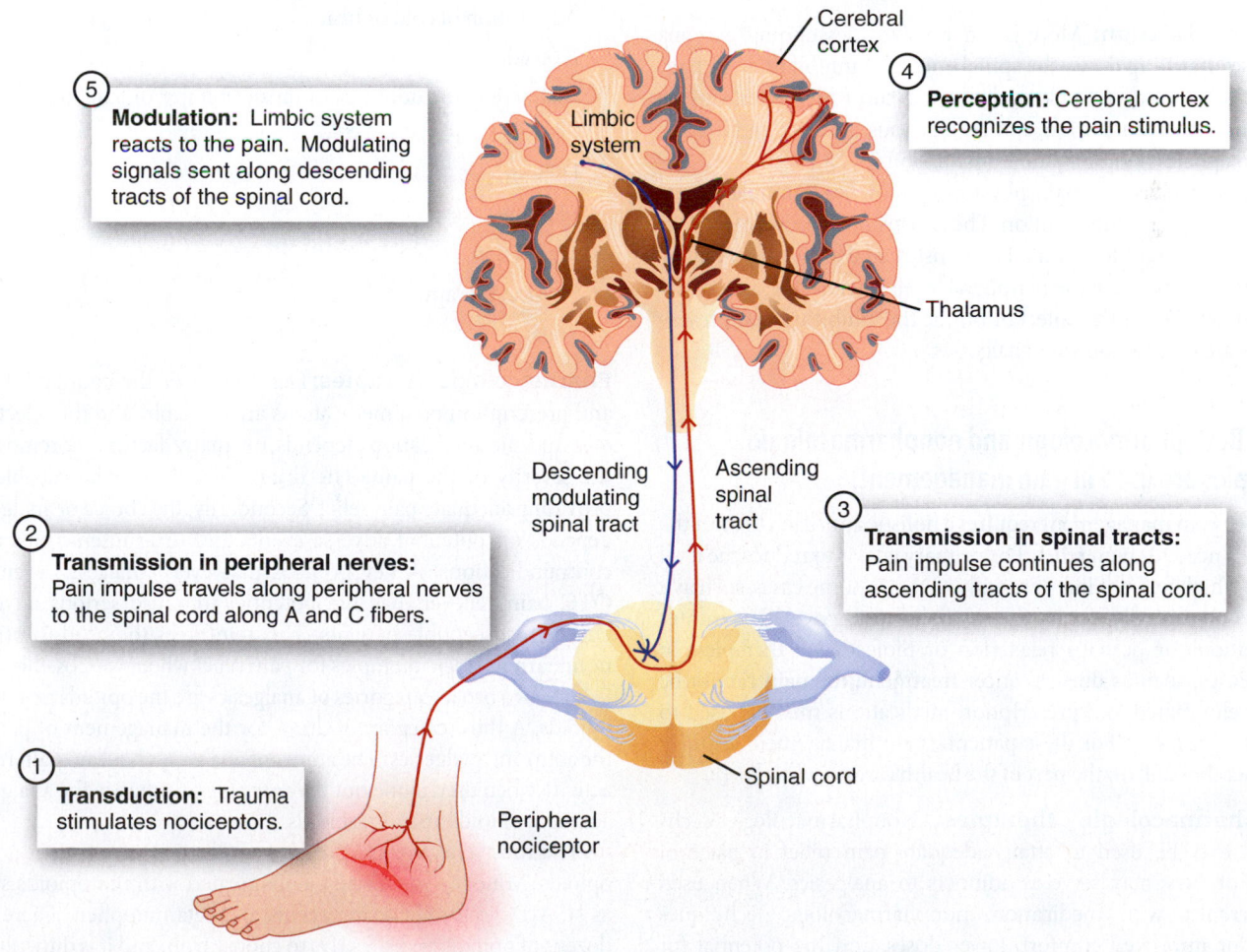

⑤ Modulation: Limbic system reacts to the pain. Modulating signals sent along descending tracts of the spinal cord.

④ Perception: Cerebral cortex recognizes the pain stimulus.

Cerebral cortex

Limbic system

Thalamus

Descending modulating spinal tract

Ascending spinal tract

② Transmission in peripheral nerves: Pain impulse travels along peripheral nerves to the spinal cord along A and C fibers.

③ Transmission in spinal tracts: Pain impulse continues along ascending tracts of the spinal cord.

Spinal cord

① Transduction: Trauma stimulates nociceptors.

Peripheral nociceptor

Figure 25.1 Phases of pain physiology.

types of pain impulses. The gate control theory, proposed in 1965, has withstood the test of time and has been found to be more complex than originally proposed. The "gates" can also be closed when flooded with nonnociceptor impulses. Gate control explains the effectiveness of massage, transcutaneous electrical nerve stimulation, and, possibly, acupuncture in reducing pain.

Once a pain impulse reaches the spinal cord, neurotransmitters are responsible for passing the message along to the next neuron. At the spinal cord level, glutamate is the neurotransmitter for A fibers, whereas both glutamate and substance P are neurotransmitters for C fibers. Impulse transmission from the spinal cord to the brain is moderated by both excitatory and inhibitory neurotransmitters. The activity of substance P may be affected by other neurotransmitters released from neurons in the central nervous system (CNS). One group of neurotransmitters functions as endogenous opioids, or natural pain modifiers; these include **endorphins** and enkephalins.

Pain perception: Perception, the conscious experience of pain, occurs in the brain. Numerous cortical structures and pathways are involved in perception, including the reticular activating system, the somatosensory system, and the limbic system (see Chapter 17). When the pain impulse reaches the brain, it may respond to the sensation with a wide variety of possible actions, ranging from signaling the skeletal muscles to jerk away from a sharp object to mental depression in those experiencing chronic pain.

Pain modulation: Modulation involves descending nervous impulses traveling down the spinal cord that inhibit afferent pain transmission via a feedback mechanism. Neurotransmitters such as serotonin, norepinephrine, and endogenous opioids (endorphins and enkephalins) inhibit pain transmission.

The four phases of pain physiology allow for multiple targets for pharmacologic intervention. The two primary classes of analgesics act at different locations: The nonsteroidal anti-inflammatory drugs (NSAIDs) act at the peripheral level, whereas the opioids act on the CNS. Drugs that affect or mimic the inhibitory neurotransmitters are used as adjuvant analgesics.

25.5 Both pharmacologic and nonpharmacologic therapies are used in pain management.

Effective pain management requires a holistic approach to meet the patient's need for pain relief. The primary goal is to reduce the level to that which will not interfere with ADLs. In some cases, such as a headache, pain relief is easy to accomplish using over-the-counter medications or perhaps relaxation or biofeedback therapies. In other cases, such as during cancer treatment, the pain cannot be totally eliminated and prescription medications must be used to reduce pain levels. For these patients, pain management requires considerable skill on the part of the health care provider.

Nonpharmacologic therapies: Nonpharmacologic techniques may be used to attain adequate pain relief in place of drugs, or they may serve as adjuncts to analgesics. When used concurrently with medication, nonpharmacologic techniques allow for improved comfort, lower doses, and the potential for

---

CONNECTIONS | **Lifespan Considerations**

◀ **Pain Assessment in the Very Young**

According to Voepel-Lewis, Zanotti, Danmeyer, and Merkel (2010), behavioral rating scales such as the FLACC scale have been used with children as young as 3 months to 7 years of age. Developed by the University of Michigan Health System, FLACC stands for the five categories assessed: face, legs, activity, cry, and consolability. Each category is scored 0 to 2 and then added to get a 0-to-10 rating. For example, an infant with a pain rating of 0 would have no particular facial expression (F), legs relaxed (L), be lying quietly (A), without crying (C), and relaxed (C). On the other extreme, a rating of 10 would be seen as an infant crying steadily, with a rigid body and drawn up or kicking legs, clenched jaw or quivering chin, and who is difficult to console or comfort. The scale has undergone extensive testing for construct validity and reliability over the years since it was developed and is now used for assessing pain in nonverbal patients of all ages.

---

fewer drug-related adverse events. Nondrug interventions should routinely be considered in the nursing plan of care for patients with pain. Some complementary and alternative therapies used for reducing pain include the following:

- Acupressure and acupuncture
- Application of cold or heat
- Biofeedback therapy
- Distraction, including art or music therapy, or laughter
- Electrical nerve stimulation
- Hypnosis
- Massage
- Meditation
- Physical therapy
- Yoga

Pharmacologic therapies: Dozens of over-the-counter (OTC) and prescription pain medications are available, and the selection of a specific medication depends on many factors. Foremost is the severity of the pain. The drug selected must be capable of providing adequate pain relief. Secondarily, the choice of analgesic depends on potential adverse events and drug interactions and contraindications. A key point is that every analgesic, even an OTC pain reliever, has the potential to cause serious adverse effects in susceptible patients. This reinforces the need to utilize nonpharmacologic therapies for pain relief whenever possible.

The two broad categories of analgesics are the opioids and nonopioids. A third category of drugs for the management of pain is the adjuvant analgesics. The adjuvant analgesics have no pain relief activity when used alone but they are able to enhance the analgesic action of opioids and nonopioids.

The most effective drug class for relieving severe pain is the opioids. Minor to moderate pain is treated with nonopioids such as NSAIDs, centrally acting agents, or acetaminophen. There are dozens of opioids and NSAIDs to choose from and it is difficult for

PHARMACOTHERAPY ILLUSTRATED 25.1

SITES OF ANALGESIC ACTION

Cerebral cortex

④ Perception
- opioids
- alpha$_2$-adrenergic agonists

⑤ Modulation
- antidepressants
- antiepileptic agents

Limbic system

Thalamus

Descending modulating spinal tract

Ascending spinal tract

③ Transmission in spinal tracts
- opioids
- alpha$_2$-adrenergic agonists
- NSAIDs

② Transmission in peripheral nerves
- local anesthetics

① Transduction
- NSAIDs

Spinal cord

Peripheral nociceptor

---

beginning students, and even experienced health care providers, to learn the subtle differences of drugs within each class. Although the large number of analgesics appears overwhelming, many of them are quite similar and prescribers most often use only a few drugs in each class. The various drugs used for analgesia and the levels at which they act are shown in Pharmacotherapy Illustrated 25.1.

The pharmacologic management of acute and chronic pain is based on the analgesic ladder proposed by the World Health Organization. Pain ratings of less than 4 are treated with nonopioid analgesics, complementary and alternative therapies (CATs), or a combination of the two. When pain ratings become moderate (4 to 6), PO opioids are added to the baseline treatment. When pain is severe (7 to 10), parenteral opioids are used. If chronic pain has neuropathic qualities, adjuvant analgesics are added.

Combination drugs: It is common practice to use opioid and nonopioid analgesics concurrently in the pharmacotherapy of pain. For convenience, these combinations are available as fixed-dose tablets or capsules. The two classes of analgesics work synergistically to relieve pain, and the dose of opioid can be lowered to avoid dependence and opioid-related adverse effects. Use of these combinations in chronic pain management has a dose ceiling due to the toxicities of the nonopioid analgesic. For example, patients taking a combination product containing acetaminophen need to be aware of the risk of acute liver failure with high doses. Liver enzyme levels should be monitored regularly, and care must be taken not to exceed the maximum daily dosages for acetaminophen. It is important to note that the FDA requested that manufacturers limit the dose of acetaminophen in prescription products to a maximum of 325 mg per dosage unit. However, the maximum daily dose of acetaminophen remains at 4,000 mg/day. Therefore, the healthcare provider can still prescribe 12 dosage units per day of the drug and remain below the maximum. Common combination analgesics include:

- Endocet (oxycodone, 5–10 mg; acetaminophen, 325 mg)
- Norco (hydrocodone, 7.5–10 mg; acetaminophen, 325 mg)
- Percocet (oxycodone, 2.5–10 mg; acetaminophen, 325 mg)
- Percodan (oxycodone, 4.8355 mg; aspirin, 325 mg)
- Lortab 5 (hydrocodone, 5 mg; acetaminophen, 300 mg)
- Vicodin HP (hydrocodone, 10 mg; acetaminophen, 300 mg)

Management of cancer pain: Patients with intractable cancer pain require more invasive techniques because rapidly growing tumors often press on vital tissues and nerves. Furthermore, chemotherapy and surgical treatments for cancer can cause severe pain. Radiation therapy may provide pain relief by shrinking solid tumors that may be pressing on nerves. Surgery may be used to reduce pain by removing part of or the entire tumor. Injection of alcohol or another neurotoxic substance into neurons is occasionally performed to cause nerve blocks. Nerve blocks irreversibly stop impulse transmission along the treated nerves and have the potential to provide total pain relief. Injection of local anesthetics or steroid hormones as nerve blocks provide relief for months and is used for pain resulting from pressure on spinal nerves.

Patient-controlled analgesia: Patient-controlled analgesia (PCA) is a method of drug delivery that uses an infusion pump to deliver a prescribed amount of opioid by patient self-administration. By pressing a button, the patient can self-administer the opioid, thus relieving the anxiety of waiting for a prn drug administration. The patient does not have unlimited access to the drug; the infusion pump is programmed by the nurse to deliver a prescribed amount of drug over a designated time period. If the patient attempts to self-administer the drug too often, the patient is locked out until the next dose interval. The program is adjusted depending on the patient's response to the drug. Morphine is the opioid usually used for PCA; however, fentanyl or ketamine may be used.

PCA allows patients to participate in their own care. Frequent, small doses of analgesics give a more consistent serum drug level than would be obtained by administering larger doses three to four times per day. PCA requires that the patient be conscious and capable of understanding the operation of the pump. Patients should be taught not to be overly concerned about activating the pump because the program is set to prevent the possibility of overdose. Nurses, family members, or visitors should not use the device to give the patient more medication, but should consult with the health care provider if they feel that the patient's pain is not relieved.

Pain Management with Opioids

25.6 Opioid analgesics exert their effects by interacting with specific receptors in the central nervous system.

Opium is one of the oldest known natural remedies; it has been used to relieve pain for thousands of years. Extracted from the unripe seeds of the poppy plant, *Papaver somniferum*, **opium** is a milky substance that contains over 20 different chemicals having pharmacologic activity. Opium contains 9% to 14% morphine and 0.8% to 2.5% codeine. Natural substances obtained from opium (such as morphine and codeine) are called **opiates**.

In the late 1800s, scientists began to create synthetic and semisynthetic substances with morphine-like properties. There are now over a dozen different synthetic drugs with morphine-like activity. **Opioid** is a general term referring to any of these substances, natural or synthetic, and is often used interchangeably with the term *opiate*.

Pharmacotherapy with opioids is predominantly used to relieve moderate to severe pain. With proper dosing, opioids can relieve any degree of pain; they are most effective in treating constant, dull types of pain. In large quantities opioids produce euphoria and severe CNS depression that can lead to stupor, coma, or death. When used for prolonged periods at high doses, opioids cause physical and psychological dependence.

Narcotic is a term commonly used to describe certain medications. In the context of law enforcement, *narcotic* is used to describe a broad range of abused illegal drugs such as hallucinogens, cocaine, amphetamines, and marijuana. In medical settings, however, narcotic is more restrictively defined as a morphine-like drug used to alleviate pain. To avoid confusion, it is best to use the combined term *narcotic analgesic* rather than simply *narcotic*. In clinical practice, a narcotic analgesic is the same as an opioid, and the terms may be used interchangeably.

Opioids exert their actions by interacting with at least six types of receptors in the CNS: mu, kappa, and delta are the three major receptor types. From the perspective of pain management, the **mu** and **kappa receptors** are the most important, as shown in Figure 25.2. Activation of the mu receptor is responsible for the analgesic properties of the opioids as well as some of the adverse effects such as respiratory depression and physical dependence (see Chapter 27). Drugs that activate opioid receptors are called opioid agonists; those that block these receptors are called opioid antagonists. Because there are multiple opioid receptors, three general types of drug–receptor interactions are possible:

- **Opioid agonist.** Drugs that activate both mu and kappa receptors; for example, morphine and codeine (see Section 25.7)
- **Mixed opioid agonist-antagonist.** Drugs that occupy one receptor and block (or have no effect) on the other; for example, pentazocine (Talwin), butorphanol (Stadol), and buprenorphine (Buprenex) (see Section 25.8)
- **Opioid antagonist.** Drugs that block both mu and kappa receptors; for example, naloxone (Narcan) (see Section 25.12)

The types of agonist actions produced by activating the mu and kappa receptors are shown in Table 25.1. Analgesia is obviously the desired response in pain management. The other responses constitute adverse effects of opioid therapy and must be assessed, prevented, or managed as part of the plan of care for a patient receiving opioid therapy (see Nursing Practice Application for Patients Receiving Pharmacotherapy for Pain).

Opioids do not lower the threshold for pain at the nociceptor level and they do not slow or block the transmission of the pain impulse. It is the perception and emotional response to pain that is

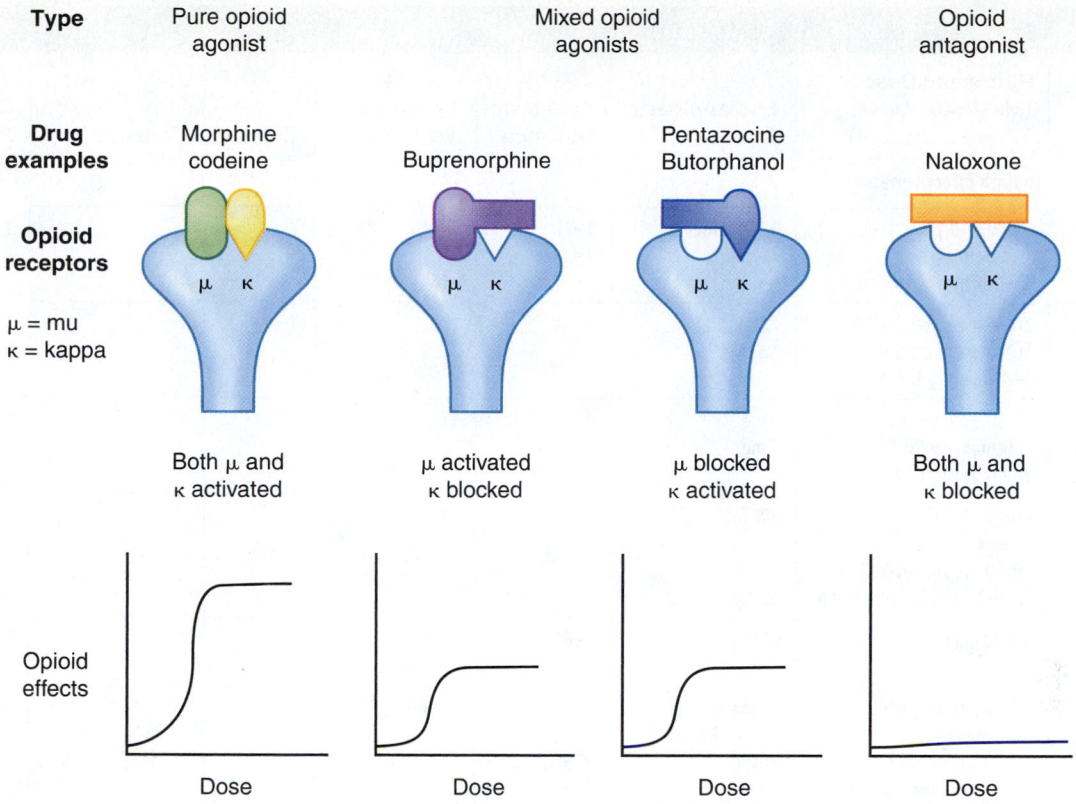

Figure 25.2   Types of opioid receptors.

TABLE 25.1 Responses Produced by Activation of Specific Opioid Receptors		
Response	**Mu Receptor**	**Kappa Receptor**
Analgesia	Yes	Yes
Decreased GI motility	Yes	Yes
Euphoria	Yes	No
Miosis	No	Yes
Physical dependence	Yes	No
Respiratory depression	Yes	No
Sedation	Yes	Yes

altered. Essentially the patient knows that the pain still exists, but it does not cause concern or anxiety.

25.7 Opioids are the drugs of choice for moderate to severe pain that cannot be controlled with other classes of analgesics.

Over 20 different opioids are available as medications. This large group is split into subclasses by similarities in their chemical structures, mechanisms of action, and effectiveness. Each classification is useful in explaining some of the similarities and differences among the opioids. The most basic classification is by effectiveness, which

places opioids into the two basic categories of strong or moderate analgesic activity. The opioids are listed in Table 25.2. The opioids that have very short durations of action are used primarily as anesthesia adjuncts and are presented in Chapter 26.

Opioids produce many important physiological actions in addition to analgesia. They are effective at suppressing the cough reflex and at slowing the motility of the gastrointestinal (GI) tract in patients with severe diarrhea. Opioids are powerful CNS depressants and can cause sedation, which may be considered a therapeutic effect or an adverse effect, depending on the patient's disease state. Some patients experience euphoria and intense relaxation, which are reasons why these drugs are frequently abused.

Opioids have the potential to produce many serious adverse effects, including respiratory depression, sedation, nausea, vomiting, and constipation. Table 25.2 compares the major adverse effect potentials of the individual opioids.

Management of opioid adverse effects is summarized in Table 25.3. Through activation of primarily the mu receptors, opioids can cause profound respiratory depression, which is the most serious adverse effect of drugs in this class. Respiratory depression is most problematic during the initial period of drug administration and with patients who have not previously taken these drugs (opiate naïve). Patients at greatest risk include those with preexisting respiratory impairment or those concurrently taking other respiratory depressant drugs. A current medication history is very important, especially alcohol use and other CNS depressants, because these drugs will cause additive respiratory depression and

TABLE 25.2   Selected Opioid Analgesic Comparison

Drug	Route and Dose (Maximum Dose Where Indicated)	Equianalgesic Dose*	Analgesic Duration	Respiratory Depression	Emesis	Constipation	Dependence Potential
Opioid Agonists with High Effectiveness							
fentanyl (Sublimaze)	IM: 0.05–0.1 mg Transdermal: 25–100 mcg every 72 h	0.1–0.2 mg 25 mcg/h	1–2 h 3 days	Y	Y	?	Y
hydromorphone (Dilaudid)	PO: 1–4 mg every 4–6 h Subcutaneous/IM/IV: 1–4 mg every 4–6 h	7.5 mg 1.5 mg	4–5 h	YY	Y	Y	YYY
levorphanol (Levo-Dromoran)	PO: 2–3 mg tid/qid Subcutaneous/IV: 1–2 mg every 6–8 h	4 mg 2 mg	4–8 h	YY	Y	YY	YY
meperidine (Demerol)	PO: 50–150 mg every 3–4 h IM: 50–100 mg every 3–4 h IV: 1–1.5 mg/kg every 3–4 h	300 mg 75 mg 50 mg	2–4 h	YY		Y	YYY
methadone (Dolophine)	PO: 20 mg every 6–8 h	20 mg	4–8 h	YY	Y	YY	Y
morphine	PO: 30 mg every 4 h Sustained release IM: 10 mg every 4 h IV: 2–10 mg every 2–4 h; 0.1–1 mg/mL continuous	30 mg 30 mg SR 10 mg 10 mg	4–5 h 8–12 h 4–5 h 4–5 h	YY	YY	YY	YYYY
oxymorphone (Opana)	Subcutaneous: 1.0–1.5 mg every 4–6 h Rectal: 1 suppository (5 mg) every 4–6 h PO (extended release): 5–20 mg bid	1 mg 10 mg 1 mg	3–6 h 36 h 12 h	YY	YY	YY	YYY
Opioids with Moderate Effectiveness							
codeine	PO: 15–60 mg qid IM: 15–30 mg every 4–6 h	200 mg 120 mg	4–6 h				
hydrocodone (Hycodan)	PO: 5–10 every 4–6 h	30 mg	4–6 h	Y		Y	Y
oxycodone (OxyContin)	PO: 5–10 mg qid Controlled release: 10–20 mg every 12 h	20 mg 20 mg	4–6 h 8–12 h	YY	YY	YY	YY
Opioids with Mixed Agonist-Antagonist Effects							
buprenorphine (Buprenex)	IM/IV: 0.3 mg every 6 h	0.3 mg	6 h	YY	Y		YY
butorphanol (Stadol)	IM: 1–4 mg every 3–4 h IV: 0.5–2 mg IV every 3–4 h	2 mg 1 mg	3–4 h	YYY	Y		YY
nalbuphine (Nubain)	Subcutaneous/IM/IV: 10–20 mg every 3–6 h	10 mg	3–6 h	Y	Y		YY
pentazocine (Talwin)	PO: 50–100 every 3–4 h Subcutaneous/IM: 30 mg every 3–4 h	25 mg 30 mg	4–6 h	Y	YY		YY

* Dose in milligrams that produces the same degree of analgesia as that produced by 10 mg of morphine.

Y = low incidence, YY = moderate incidence, YYY = high incidence, YYYY = highest incidence.

TABLE 25.3 Management of Opioid Adverse Effects

Adverse Effect	Management
Constipation	Assume it will occur and initiate preventive measures: Increase dietary fiber and fluid intake; use stool softeners and mild laxatives if needed.
Nausea	Usually transient. Antiemetics are administered, as needed.
Orthostatic hypotension	Assess blood pressure before ambulation; change positions slowly; assist with ambulation if needed.
Respiratory depression	Monitor respiratory status frequently—especially initially and with dosage increases. Avoid other CNS depressants that could have additive effects such as alcohol, antidepressants, and barbiturates. Use coughing, deep breathing, and incentive spirometry. If the patient is unresponsive and the respiratory rate is less than 12 breaths/min, administer naloxone per protocol.
Sedation	Common with initiation of therapy or during dosage increase. Tolerance develops in several days. Use safety precautions, especially with ambulation.
Urinary retention	Monitor for bladder distention. More common in elderly men. Tolerance usually develops with long-term dosing. Monitor; if receiving epidural administration, use an indwelling catheter.

sedation. Tolerance to respiratory depression usually occurs within 48 to 72 hours of initiation of therapy.

Respirations should be monitored before initiating therapy and regularly throughout opioid pharmacotherapy. The drugs should be withheld if respirations fall below 12 per minute. Narcotic antagonists such as naloxone (Narcan) should be readily available if respirations fall below 10 per minute (see Section 25.12). If opioids are administered by continuous epidural or intravenous (IV) routes, interventions should be taken to reduce the risk of respiratory depression. These include frequent monitoring of vital signs, level of consciousness, and pain rating as well as proper body positioning. Airway equipment and narcotic antagonists are usually kept at the bedside.

Opioids can cause orthostatic hypotension by inhibiting the baroreceptor reflex and by causing peripheral vasodilation. Dizziness and fainting are possible; assistance may therefore be needed with ambulation. Hydromorphone and meperidine are especially prone to causing hypotension. Patients with hypovolemia are more sensitive to this hypotensive effect; therefore, volume deficiencies should be corrected before initiating opioid therapy.

Increased intracranial pressure (ICP) is a severe adverse reaction that can occur as an indirect result of respiratory depression. When respiration is suppressed, the CO_2 content of the blood increases. The result is vasodilation of cerebral blood vessels and rising ICP. This is of particular concern in patients with conditions that might cause elevated ICP, such as those with head injury, intracranial bleeding, or brain tumors. Narcotic analgesics are usually contraindicated in these patients.

Opioids promote urinary retention by increasing the tone in the bladder sphincter and through suppression of stimuli that normally signal bladder fullness. If the patient has not voided within 6 hours, especially after surgery, insertion of a urinary catheter may be necessary. Patients prone to urinary hesitancy, such as those with benign prostatic hyperplasia, must be carefully monitored.

Constipation, nausea, and vomiting frequently occur during opioid administration. Constipation occurs because the drugs suppress intestinal peristalsis, increase the tone of the anal sphincter, and inhibit secretion of fluids into the intestine. Bowel function should be closely monitored, especially after surgery or with long-term use. The plan of care for these patients should include a bowel program to prevent or manage constipation. A baseline program would include increased dietary fiber, adequate fluid intake, and a stool softener such as docusate sodium. More active interventions are implemented if the patient does not resume or maintain normal bowel elimination. The constipation-promoting effect of the opioids is used to advantage in the treatment of severe diarrhea (see Chapter 60).

Opioids directly stimulate the chemoreceptor trigger zone in the medulla to cause intense nausea and vomiting in certain patients. An antiemetic such as promethazine (Phenergan) or ondansetron (Zofran) may be indicated. Orders for prn antiemetics should be made available whenever parenteral opioids are used.

Prolonged use of opioids results in tolerance. Typically, tolerance is noted when patients report that the duration of analgesia is decreasing or admit to taking the drug more frequently as therapy progresses. Increasingly higher doses will be needed to produce the same degree of analgesia. Tolerance does not develop equally for all opioid actions. Whereas tolerance to respiratory depression, sedation, and euphoria develops rapidly, tolerance never develops to the constipation or miosis effects. It should be remembered that as doses of opioids are increased to more effectively manage pain, the incidence of adverse effects will also increase.

All of the narcotic analgesics have the potential to cause physical and psychological dependence (see Chapter 27). Dependence is most likely to occur when high doses are taken for extended periods. Health care providers and nurses are sometimes hesitant to administer the proper amount of opioid analgesics for fear of causing patient dependence or of producing serious adverse effects such as sedation or respiratory depression. Undermedication, however, results in patients not receiving adequate pain relief. When used according to accepted medical practice, patients can, and indeed should, receive the pain relief they need without fear of dependence or serious adverse effects.

Opioids are frequently abused for nonmedical purposes. The risk of abuse is especially high in patients with a history of substance abuse. Opioids are frequently diverted from medical sources (e.g., patients, pharmacies, hospitals), either stolen or sold for criminal intent. Opioids are even stolen from family members, especially the elderly. Illicit users may "doctor shop" and obtain opioids from different prescribers and then sell the pills for profit.

Many patients who experience an adverse reaction to an opioid will report that they are allergic to these drugs. For example, patients who experience nausea, vomiting, or severe dizziness will often state they are allergic to narcotics. True allergic (Type I hypersensitivity) reactions to opioids, however, are actually rare. Although some of the opioids do indeed cause direct histamine release from mast cells, these types of idiosyncratic reactions do not result in the classic signs of anaphylaxis; thus they are not true allergic reactions. Morphine, codeine, and meperidine have the highest potential for nonimmune histamine release. When a real immune hypersensitivity reaction does occur, it may extend to other drugs in the opioid class.

Equianalgesic use in pain management: Table 25.2 includes a column labeled "Equianalgesic Dose." It is often necessary to change the route of a patient's pain medication or even the drug itself. One of the most frequently occurring examples that a nurse may encounter is the transition a patient makes from IV medications after surgery to PO analgesics prior to discharge. Using relative potency information (equivalent dose), the primary health care provider can determine the appropriate new dose. Following surgery, it is not unusual to have orders for a parenteral opioid for severe pain, an oral opioid for moderate pain, and a combination opioid and nonopioid for mild pain. The nurse can use these same equivalencies in choosing the drug and dose when a range of analgesic options is ordered.

CONNECTION Checkpoint 25.1

A common abbreviation for morphine sulfate is MS or MSO$_4$. From what you learned in Chapter 6, why should this abbreviation be avoided and what can you do to prevent this type of medication error? *See Answer to Connection Checkpoint 25.1 on student resource website.*

PROTOTYPE DRUG	**Morphine Sulfate (Astramorph PF, Duramorph RF, Roxanol, Others)**

Classification: Therapeutic: Narcotic analgesic
Pharmacologic: Opioid agonist

Therapeutic Effects and Uses: Morphine sulfate is the narcotic analgesic of choice for the management of most types of acute and severe chronic pain. Morphine is a drug of choice for relieving acute chest pain associated with MI. The drug was in use for thousands of years prior to its approval by the U.S. Food and Drug Administration (FDA) in 1939 and is still obtained from unripe seeds of the poppy plant.

In addition to relieving severe pain, morphine is used off-label to treat several other conditions. Its CNS depressant action may be used to provide preanesthetic sedation and to calm severely agitated patients. In patients who are terminally ill, its respiratory depressant action may be used to relieve the shortness of breath associated with end-stage cancer, heart failure, or pulmonary edema.

The advantages of morphine therapy, especially in the treatment of chronic cancer pain where dosing increases over time, are that morphine has no upper end dose limit, and that patients develop tolerance to all the adverse effects except constipation. Extended release tablets (MS Contin, Oramorph SR) or capsules (Avinza, Kadian) are available. Initiation of therapy is usually begun with shorter acting agents. Once the correct dose has been titrated, the patient may be switched to extended release formulations. In 2004, the FDA approved an extended release liposome injection (DepoDur), which is given by a single epidural injection for postsurgical pain.

Mechanism of Action: Morphine occupies mu and kappa receptor sites in the brain and dorsal horn of the spinal cord that alter the release of afferent neurotransmitters. The dominant effect alters the perception of and emotional response to pain, producing analgesia and euphoria. The drug mimics the actions of endogenous endorphins.

Pharmacokinetics:

Route(s)	PO, IV, subcutaneous, intramuscular (IM), rectal, epidural, intrathecal
Absorption	PO variable, 30%; subcutaneous or IM may be erratic or delayed
Distribution	Widely distributed; crosses the placenta; is secreted in breast milk
Primary metabolism	Hepatic; significant first-pass metabolism
Primary excretion	Renal; 7–10% in bile and feces
Onset of action	PO: 30–60 min; IV: rapid; epidural: 15–30 min
Duration of action	PO: 4–7 h; IV: 4–5 h; epidural: 4–24 h

Adverse Effects: Morphine depresses the CNS, causing sedation, dizziness, anxiety, and a feeling of floating or disorientation. Tolerance often develops to these CNS effects after a few days of therapy. Hallucinations and seizures may occur at high doses. Morphine reduces the sensitivity of the respiratory center to CO$_2$, thus decreasing tidal volume and rate and producing respiratory depression. The resulting increase in CO$_2$ produces cerebral vasodilation and increases cerebrospinal fluid (CSF) pressure. Morphine stimulates the chemoreceptor trigger zone in the medulla, producing nausea and vomiting, which may require the administration of an antiemetic drug during the first few days of therapy. The drug delays digestion, increases smooth muscle tone in the intestinal tract, and slows peristalsis in the colon, leading to constipation. Morphine also causes spasm of the sphincter of Oddi, which can result in intense pain (biliary colic) and potential obstruction of bile flow. Urinary retention may occur due to increasing bladder sphincter tone. Peripheral vasodilation may cause orthostatic hypotension. Pruritus is more common when morphine is given by the IV and epidural routes and is not considered a sign of hypersensitivity in the absence of skin rash. **Black Box Warnings**: Morphine is a Schedule II controlled substance with a high potential for physical and psychological dependence. The extended release forms are prescribed for opioid-tolerant patients only and are not intended for prn use. The extended release forms should never be opened, chewed, dissolved, or crushed because this can lead to fatal overdose. Alcohol and products containing alcohol should never be consumed when taking Avinza.

Contraindications/Precautions: Morphine is contraindicated in patients with hypersensitivity to opioids. Premature infants are especially sensitive to the effects of morphine; thus the drug should not be used during pregnancy or during the delivery of premature infants. It should be used with caution in the elderly and in those with undiagnosed abdominal pain, hepatic or renal impairment, shock, CNS depression, head injury or increased ICP, chronic obstructive pulmonary disease (COPD), or other conditions with decreased respiratory reserve, including severe obesity. Mothers should wait 4 to 6 hours after a dose of morphine before breast-feeding; withdrawal symptoms have been noted in nursing infants whose mothers abruptly discontinue opioid use. Morphine should never be withdrawn abruptly because this will precipitate symptoms of acute opioid withdrawal. Discontinuation should be conducted gradually over several days.

Drug Interactions: When morphine is used with other CNS depressants, including alcohol, skeletal muscle relaxants, and monoamine oxidase inhibitors (MAOIs), increased sedation will result. Administration of an opioid antagonist such as naloxone will reverse the effects of morphine and may produce immediate withdrawal symptoms. Concurrent use with antidiarrheal drugs such as loperamide will cause additive constipation. **Herbal/Food**: Use of kava, valerian, or chamomile can increase CNS depression. St. John's wort may decrease the analgesic action of morphine.

Pregnancy: Category C.

Treatment of Overdose: Morphine overdose can cause coma and life-threatening respiratory depression and requires immediate treatment. Naloxone is a specific antidote for morphine intoxication (see Section 25.12).

Nursing Responsibilities: Key nursing implications for patients receiving morphine are included in the Nursing Practice Application for Patients Receiving Pharmacotherapy for Pain.

Drugs Similar to Morphine Sulfate (Astramorph PF, Duramorph RF, Roxanol, Others)

Other opioids used for pain management are shown in Table 25.2. Propoxyphene (Darvon, Darvocet), once a widely used opioid, was removed from the U.S. market in 2010 due to an unacceptable risk of cardiac rhythm abnormalities. The following are descriptions of opioids with pure agonist activity. All these agents have the same actions and adverse effects as morphine. All are controlled substances.

Codeine: Approved by the FDA in 1939, codeine can be administered by the PO, subcutaneous, or IM routes. Because it has stronger antitussive action than morphine, it is often used for suppression of severe cough. At the low doses needed for cough suppression, codeine does not produce the serious adverse effects characteristic of morphine. When used to treat cough and other severe cold symptoms, low doses are usually combined with guaifenesin (a nonnarcotic antitussive), promethazine (a phenothiazine with antihistamine action), phenylephrine (a decongestant), or brompheniramine (an antihistamine). Doses required to produce analgesia are much higher than those needed for cough suppression. When prescribed for analgesia, it is usually in combination with acetaminophen and its use is often limited by nausea and vomiting. During the metabolism of codeine in the CNS, about 10% is converted to morphine, which is responsible for its analgesic effects. Codeine may also be used off-label to treat serious diarrhea. This drug is pregnancy category C; the category changes to D if used in high doses or close to term.

Fentanyl (Abstral, Actiq, Duragesic, Fentora, Onsolis, Sublimaze): Originally approved in 1968 as an IV anesthetic (Sublimaze) for short-term surgical procedures, fentanyl has since been introduced in multiple formulations. These include oral tablets (Fentora), buccal film (Onsolis), sublingual tablets (Abstral), oral transmucosal lozenges (Actiq), and transdermal patches (Duragesic).

All the nonanesthetic formulations of fentanyl are restricted to the management of breakthrough pain in patients who are already receiving and who are tolerant to around-the-clock opioid therapy for their chronic, persistent pain. This includes intractable cancer pain. Giving these formulations to patients who are opioid naïve can result in serious or fatal respiratory depression. Generally, the initial dose depends on how much morphine the patient has been receiving, that is, how tolerant the patient has become to the effects of opioids. Doses are gradually increased until the breakthrough pain is relieved. The buccal, transdermal, and transmucosal forms of fentanyl have black box warnings regarding the dependence potential for this drug and the serious adverse effects that can occur if the drug is misused.

Several other opioids, for example, remifentanil (Ultiva), alfentanil (Alfenta), and sufentanil (Sufenta), are closely related to fentanyl and are used as IV anesthetics. These drugs and a prototype feature for fentanyl are presented in Chapter 26.

Hydrocodone (Hycodan, others): Approved in 1957, hydrocodone is used for analgesia, most often combined with acetaminophen, aspirin, or ibuprofen in fixed dose combinations such as Vicodin, Lortab, and Norco. Acetaminophen has a dose ceiling that limits the use of such combinations in chronic pain management. Hydrocodone is an effective antitussive and is combined with decongestants or antihistamines for severe cold and flu symptoms. Although it is slightly more effective than codeine as an antitussive, it causes more sedation. This drug is pregnancy category C; the category changes to D if used in high doses or close to term.

Hydromorphone (Dilaudid, Exalgo): Approved in 1984, hydromorphone is available by the PO, rectal, and parenteral routes. Its primary application is analgesia, including PCA. Hydromorphone produces less nausea but more orthostatic hypotension than morphine. It has a more rapid onset of action and a shorter duration of activity than morphine, requiring PO dosing every 3 to 6 hours. An extended duration formulation of the drug (Exalgo) was approved in 2010. Hydromorphone has black box warnings regarding the dependence potential for this drug and the serious adverse effects that can occur if the drug is misused. This drug is pregnancy category C.

Levorphanol (Levo-Dromoran): Approved in 1953, levorphanol is a pure opioid agonist available by the PO and parenteral routes for severe pain. At equianalgesic doses, levorphanol exhibits the same actions and adverse effects as morphine. It offers no advantages over the use of other drugs in this class. This drug is pregnancy category B; the category changes to D if used in high doses or close to term.

Meperidine (Demerol): Approved in 1942, meperidine is available by both the PO and parenteral routes for the treatment of severe pain. Toxicity can occur due to its active metabolite, called normeperidine, which is a CNS stimulant with a half-life of 15 to 30 hours. Accumulation of this metabolite can result from doses greater than 400 to 600 mg per day or administration longer than 48 hours. Normeperidine can cause tremors and seizures, which are not reversed with narcotic antagonists (naloxone). For this reason, meperidine is not recommended for use longer than 48 hours, for chronic pain, or for use in PCA. When meperidine is used in high doses or longer than 48 hours, the nurse needs to consult with the prescriber and report any incidences of tremors and irritability before giving the next dose. Because of these adverse effects, meperidine is considered a second-line agent that is used when other opioids are contraindicated. An off-label use for meperidine is for the management of shivering, a common complication in the postoperative period. The drug has a short half-life that requires dosing every 3 to 4 hours. This drug is pregnancy category C; the category changes to D if used in high doses or close to term.

Methadone (Dolophine): Approved in 1947, methadone is an oral preparation with pharmacologic effects similar to those of morphine; adverse effects are similar with lower incidence. Methadone is frequently prescribed in the management of opiate dependency (see Chapter 27) and is increasingly used for management of chronic pain. Methadone has a long duration of action and can be dosed once daily. Oral liquid (Methadose) and dispersible tablets (Diskets) are available for treating opiate withdrawal symptoms because they offer less risk for abuse than regular tablets. IV methadone is used for the short-term therapy of hospitalized patients. A black box warning indicates that when converting from other analgesics to methadone particular diligence is necessary because deaths have been reported during the conversion period. The deaths were likely due to raising the dose of methadone too quickly, resulting in cardiac and respiratory failure. This drug is pregnancy category C.

Oxycodone (OxyContin, others): Approved in 1976, oxycodone is an oral opioid that is often combined with acetaminophen (Endocet, Percocet) or with aspirin (Percodan) for the management of moderate to severe pain. The drug is used when around-the-clock analgesia is needed for an extended period of time. It is not indicated for short-term or prn use. Oxycodone causes less nausea, vomiting, and hallucinations than morphine. The immediate release forms of this drug have a short duration of action, requiring dosing every 3 to 4 hours. The extended release form (OxyContin) can be dosed twice a day. OxyContin has become a popular drug of abuse (see Chapter 27). A black box warning states that all patients receiving oxycodone should be routinely monitored for signs of misuse, abuse, and addiction. Breaking, cutting, chewing, crushing, or dissolving the extended release tablets may result in a potentially fatal overdose. This drug is pregnancy category B; the category changes to D if used in high doses or close to term.

Tapentadol (Nucynta): One of the newer drugs in this class, tapentadol was approved in 2008 and is indicated for moderate to severe pain. The immediate release form (Nucynta) is for acute pain, whereas the extended release form (Nucynta ER) is for chronic pain and pain associated with diabetic neuropathy. Tapentadol acts by dual mechanisms: It is used as a mu-receptor agonist and blocks the reuptake of norepinephrine. It has the same abuse potential (Schedule II) as other drugs in this class and has the same spectrum of adverse effects. The most common adverse effects include nausea, constipation, dizziness, headache, and somnolence. The incidence of GI-related adverse effects may be lower with tapentadol than with other drugs in this class. This drug is pregnancy category C.

25.8 Mixed agonist and antagonist opioids exhibit moderate analgesia with less risk of dependence than morphine.

The mixed agonist-antagonist opioids are narcotic analgesics that were developed with the intention of producing drugs with strong analgesia that have fewer adverse effects than morphine and other pure opioid agonists. The four drugs in this class are used to treat moderate pain but are not as effective as morphine in treating severe pain. Their advantage is that they cause less respiratory depression and have a lower potential for dependence. These drugs have some abuse potential but less so than the pure opioid agonists. The types of adverse effects, contraindications, and nursing responsibilities are similar to those of the pure opioid agonists (see Section 25.7).

With both agonist and antagonist actions, what would happen if a person addicted to morphine or heroin took one of the drugs in this class? Blocking opioid receptors would cause the patient to experience opioid withdrawal symptoms. In fact, some of the mixed agonist-antagonist drugs are indicated for the induction of opioid withdrawal and the maintenance of opioid dependence (see Chapter 27).

Buprenorphine (Buprenex, Butrans, Suboxone): Originally approved in 1981, buprenorphine is a partial agonist at the mu receptors and an antagonist at the kappa receptors. It is indicated for the relief of moderate to severe pain when given by the parenteral route (Buprenex). Sublingual (Suboxone) and orally disintegrating tablet (Zubsolv) forms combine buprenorphine with naloxone for the management of opioid withdrawal and dependence. In 2010, a transdermal patch system (Butrans) was approved that provides 7 days of analgesia. Abuse of buprenorphine has been reported but is less common because the drug does not produce the same degree of euphoria observed with the pure opioid agonists. Furthermore, withdrawal symptoms from this drug are generally mild and its onset may be delayed 1 to 2 weeks. Buprenorphine is a Schedule III drug. Respiratory depression can be a serious adverse effect at high doses. A black box warning states that when using the transdermal form of the drug, a dose of 20 mcg/h (the highest dose patch, worn for 7 days) should not be exceeded due to a risk of QT interval prolongation. The patch application site should not be subjected to high external temperatures because this increases drug release and can cause overdose or death. This drug is pregnancy category C. A prototype drug feature for buprenorphine with naloxone (Suboxone, Zubsolv) can be found in Chapter 27.

Butorphanol (Stadol): Approved in 1978, butorphanol is an agonist at the kappa receptors and is a weak antagonist at the mu receptors. Delivered by the IV or IM route, it is approved for moderate to severe pain and as a preanesthetic medication that supplements general anesthesia. A nasal spray form of the drug (Stadol NS) has a fast onset of 20 to 40 minutes but it must be repeated every 4 to 6 hours for continuous pain control. Drowsiness and dizziness are experienced by a large number of patients, and the intranasal form can cause nasal congestion. Like buprenorphine, the drug is not commonly abused and withdrawal symptoms are mild. Butorphanol is a Schedule III drug. This drug is pregnancy category C.

Nalbuphine (Nubain): Approved in 1979, nalbuphine is an agonist at the kappa receptors and a weak antagonist at the mu receptors. Given by the IV, IM, or subcutaneous route, it is approved for moderate to severe pain and as a preanesthesia or general anesthesia adjunct. Drowsiness is the most common adverse effect. The risk for dependence is low, and nalbuphine is not a scheduled drug. Abrupt discontinuation, however, can precipitate mild opioid withdrawal symptoms. This drug is pregnancy category B (category D with prolonged use or high doses at term).

Pentazocine (Talwin): Approved in 1967, pentazocine was the first of the agonist-antagonist opioids marketed. Available by both the

PO and parenteral routes, it is approved to treat moderate to severe pain and as a supplement to general anesthesia. The drug is available in combination tablets with acetaminophen and naloxone. The drug acts as an agonist at the kappa receptors and a weak antagonist at the mu receptors. Pentazocine causes less nausea, vomiting, and respiratory depression than morphine. Like other drugs in this class, drowsiness and dizziness are common adverse effects. Also like other mixed agonists-antagonists, pentazocine does not produce euphoria and has a low potential for abuse (Schedule IV). Withdrawal symptoms are similar to those of other opioids but milder. A major advantage is that overdose with pentazocine does not result in the high mortality observed with morphine. This drug is pregnancy category C.

Pain Management with Nonopioids

25.9 Nonsteroidal anti-inflammatory drugs are the medications of choice for mild to moderate pain.

The **nonopioid analgesics** include NSAIDs, acetaminophen, and a few centrally acting agents. NSAIDs, such as aspirin and ibuprofen, are the drugs of choice for mild to moderate pain, especially for pain associated with inflammation. Nonopioids have many advantages over the opioids. Acetaminophen, aspirin, and many NSAIDs are available OTC and are inexpensive. They are available in many different formulations, including those designed for pediatric patients. For most patients, they are safe and produce adverse effects only at high doses. NSAIDs have antipyretic and anti-inflammatory actions as well as analgesic properties. Indeed, some NSAIDs are used primarily for their anti-inflammatory effects. The doses and roles of NSAIDs in the treatment of inflammation and fever are discussed in Chapter 41. Prototype features for ibuprofen and aspirin are also included in Chapter 41. Nursing practice applications for the nonopioid analgesics are similar to those for the opioid analgesics and are presented in the Nursing Practice Application for Patients Receiving Pharmacotherapy for Pain. Additional nursing responsibilities for the nonopioids can be found with the prototype drugs and the Nursing Practice Application for Patients Receiving Pharmacotherapy for Inflammation and Fever in Chapter 41.

NSAIDs act at peripheral sites by inhibiting pain mediators at the nociceptor level. When tissue is damaged, chemical mediators, including histamine, potassium ion, hydrogen ion, and bradykinin,

are released locally. Also released during tissue damage is arachidonic acid, which is metabolized into chemical mediators of inflammation and pain such as prostaglandins. Prostaglandins can induce pain through the formation of free radicals.

NSAIDs inhibit cyclooxygenase, an enzyme responsible for the formation of prostaglandins. Because they act by a different mechanism than opioids, NSAIDs do not produce the severe adverse effects observed with the narcotic analgesics. The most prominent effects are GI related and include nausea, vomiting, anorexia, dyspepsia, and ulceration of the GI mucosa. At high doses, the ulceration can be severe, resulting in bleeding and even perforation. In 2010 a fixed combination of naproxen and omeprazole (Vimovo) was approved to reduce the risk of developing NSAID-induced gastric ulcers. Other common NSAID adverse events include dizziness, headache, and rash. These drugs do not cause physical or psychological dependence. When combined with opioids in fixed dose combinations, NSAIDs produce a synergistic analgesic effect that allows the dose of opioid to be lowered.

Acetaminophen is an important nonopioid analgesic that is not classified as an NSAID. Its effectiveness in relieving pain and reducing fever is equal to aspirin and ibuprofen. Acetaminophen is featured as a prototype antipyretic in Chapter 41.

25.10 A few miscellaneous analgesics reduce pain by acting on the central nervous system.

Two analgesics suppress pain by acting on the CNS but are not classified as opioids. Clonidine (Catapres, Duroclon) and ziconotide (Prialt) act by unique mechanisms in the CNS. Tramadol (Ultram) has mixed opioid-nonopioid analgesic actions. Of the three miscellaneous analgesics, only tramadol is widely prescribed. The doses of these centrally acting medications are listed in Table 25.4.

PROTOTYPE DRUG	**Tramadol (Ultram, Others)**

Classification: Therapeutic: Analgesic
Pharmacologic: Mixed opioid-nonopioid analgesic

Therapeutic Effects and Uses: Tramadol was approved for the treatment of moderate pain in 1995. The immediate release formulations are indicated for short-term (5 days or less) relief of acute pain, whereas the extended release products (Conzip, Ryzolt, Tramadol ER) are approved to treat moderate to moderately severe

TABLE 25.4   Nonopioid Centrally Acting Analgesics

Drug	Route and Adult Dose for Pain (Maximum Dose Where Indicated)	Adverse Effects
clonidine (Catapres, Duraclon)	Epidural: 30–40 mcg/h by continuous infusion or 100–900 mcg bolus	*Drowsiness, orthostatic hypotension, dry mouth, anxiety, constipation* <u>Severe hypotension, dysrhythmias</u>
tramadol (Ultram)	PO (immediate release): 25–100 mg every 4–6 h prn (max: 400 mg/day) PO (extended release): 100 mg once daily (max: 300 mg/day)	*Dizziness, nausea, vomiting, constipation, lethargy* <u>Hallucinations, emotional lability, respiratory depression</u>
ziconotide (Prialt)	Intrathecal: 0.1 mcg/h via infusion; may increase as needed up to 0.1 mcg/h no more than every 2–3 days (max: 0.8 mcg/h)	*Dizziness, nausea, diarrhea, somnolence, asthenia* <u>Confusion, memory impairment, hallucinations</u>

Note: Italics indicate common adverse effects. <u>Underline</u> indicates serious adverse effects.

CONNECTIONS: NURSING PRACTICE APPLICATION

Patients Receiving Pharmacotherapy for Pain

Assessment	Potential Nursing Diagnoses*
Baseline assessment prior to administration: • Obtain a complete health history including cardiovascular, neurologic, respiratory, hepatic, renal, cancer, gallbladder or urologic disease, pregnancy, or breast-feeding. Note recent surgeries or injuries. Obtain a drug history including allergies, current prescription and OTC drugs, and herbal preparations. Be alert to possible drug interactions. • Assess the level of pain. Use objective screening tools when possible (e.g., FLACC for infants or very young children, Wong-Baker FACES scale for children, numerical rating scale for adults). Assess pain history and what has worked or not for the patient in the past. • Obtain baseline vital signs and weight. • Evaluate appropriate laboratory findings (e.g., CBC, hepatic and renal function studies). • Assess the patient's ability to receive and understand instructions. Include family and caregivers as needed.	• *Acute Pain* • *Chronic Pain* • *Ineffective Breathing Pattern* • *Constipation*, related to adverse drug effects • *Deficient Knowledge* (Drug Therapy) • *Risk for Injury*, related to adverse drug effects • *Risk for Falls*, related to adverse drug effects
Assessment throughout administration: • Assess for desired therapeutic effects (e.g., absent or greatly diminished pain, ability to move more easily without pain or carry out postoperative treatment care). Continue to use pain rating scale to quantify level of improvement. • Continue periodic monitoring of CBC, hepatic and renal function studies. • Assess vital signs, especially blood pressure, pulse, and respiratory rate. • Assess for and report adverse effects: excessive dizziness, drowsiness, confusion, agitation, hypotension, tachycardia, bradypnea, pinpoint pupils.	

Implementation

Interventions and (Rationales)	Patient-Centered Care
Ensuring therapeutic effects: • Continue assessments as above for therapeutic effects. Give the drug before the start of acute pain and encourage regularly scheduled doses for the first 24 to 48 hours postoperatively for adequate postoperative pain relief. Provide additional comfort measures to supplement drug therapy. (Consistent use of a pain rating scale by all providers will help quantify level of pain relief and leads to better pain control. Watch for subtle signs of pain: hesitancy to move, shallow breaths to avoid increasing pain, grimacing on movement. Encouraging the patient to maintain regular doses around the clock during the acute postoperative or pain period may provide better relief than giving prn doses on request when pain has increased to the point medication is needed.)	• Teach the patient that pain relief, rather than merely control, is the goal of therapy. • Encourage the patient to take the drug consistently during the acute postoperative or procedure period rather than requesting only when pain is severe. • Explain the rationale behind the pain rating scale (i.e., it allows consistency among all providers). • Encourage the patient, family, or caregiver to use additional, nonmedicinal pain relief techniques (e.g., distraction with television or music, massage, or guided imagery).
Minimizing adverse effects: • Continue to monitor vital signs, especially respirations and pulse oximetry as ordered, postoperatively and in patients with acute pain. For terminal cancer pain, obtain instructions from the oncologist or hospice provider on any dose restrictions. (Respiratory depression is most common with the first dose of an opioid and when given in the presence of other CNS depressants, e.g., postoperatively when the patient may still be experiencing the effects of general anesthesia agents. Count respirations before giving the opioid drug, and contact the provider before giving if the respirations are below 12 per minute in the adult patient, or as ordered in the child. Continue to assess the respiratory rate every 15 to 30 minutes for the first 4 hours. For terminal cancer pain, the drug might not be withheld regardless of respiratory rate, dependent on the provider.)	• Encourage the patient to take deep breaths in the postoperative period. • Encourage consistent pain medication usage to increase activity tolerance. • Encourage patients with terminal cancer to take the dose consistently around the clock with prn doses as required. Advise the family or caregiver of the provider's instructions for adequate pain relief and to contact the provider if any pain remains.
• Monitor blood pressure and pulse periodically or if symptoms warrant. Ensure patient safety; monitor ambulation until the effects of the drug are known. **Lifespan:** Be particularly cautious with older adults who are at increased risk for falls. (Opioids may cause hypotension as an adverse effect and increase the risk of falls.)	• Teach the patient to rise from lying or sitting to standing slowly to avoid dizziness or falls. If dizziness occurs, the patient should sit or lie down and not attempt to stand or walk until the sensation passes. • Instruct the patient to call for assistance prior to getting out of bed or attempting to walk alone, and to avoid driving or other activities requiring mental alertness or physical coordination until the effects of the drug are known.
• Continue to assess bowel sounds. Increase fluid intake and dietary fiber intake. (Decreased peristalsis is an adverse effect of opioid drugs. **Lifespan:** The older adult is at increased risk of constipation due to slowed peristalsis as a result of the aging process. Significantly diminished or absent bowel sounds should be reported to the health care provider immediately. Additional fluids and fiber may ease constipation but additional medications such as MiraLAX or Colace may be required.)	• Teach the patient to increase fluids to 2 L per day and increase intake of dietary fiber such as fruits, vegetables, and whole grains. • Instruct the patient to report severe constipation to the health care provider for additional advice on laxatives or stool softeners.

CONNECTIONS: NURSING PRACTICE APPLICATION (continued)

• Monitor for itching or reports of itching. (Opioids may cause histamine release with itching or a sensation of itching. In severe cases, antihistamines may be required. Assess for itching as an expected side effect versus signs and symptoms of true allergy or anaphylaxis: changes in vital signs, especially hypotension, tachycardia, dyspnea, or urticaria.)	• Teach the patient to report itching to the health care provider, especially if severe or increasing. • Instruct the patient to immediately report any itching associated with dizziness or lightheadedness, difficulty breathing, palpitations, or significant hives.
• Assess for changes in level of consciousness, disorientation or confusion, agitation, headache, sluggish or pinpoint pupils, or seizures immediately. (Neurologic changes may indicate overmedication, increased intracranial pressure, or adverse drug effects. **Lifespan:** Older adults may be at risk for confusion and falls.)	• Instruct the patient, family, or caregiver to immediately report increasing lethargy, disorientation, confusion, changes in behavior or mood, agitation or aggression, slurred speech, ataxia, or seizures. • Ensure patient safety if disorientation is present.
• Assess for urinary retention, especially in the postoperative period. (Opioids may cause urinary retention as an adverse effect. **Lifespan:** Be aware that the older male adult with an enlarged prostate is at higher risk for mechanical obstruction.)	• Encourage the patient to move about in bed and to start early ambulation as soon as allowed postoperatively. Assist to normal voiding position if unable to use the bathroom or commode. • Instruct the patient to immediately report the inability to void, increasing bladder pressure, or pain.
• Administer antiemetics 30 to 60 minutes before opioid dose in patients who have a history of nausea and vomiting. (Nausea and vomiting are common adverse effects.)	• Encourage the patient to report nausea if it occurs. Small amounts of food intake (e.g., dry crackers) and sips of carbonated beverages (e.g., ginger ale) may help if the patient is not NPO.
• Monitor pain relief in the patient on a PCA pump. If a basal dose is not given continuously, assess that pain relief is adequate and contact the provider if pain remains present. Teach and encourage the patient to use the self-medication control button whenever pain is present or increasing, or before activities. (PCA-administered pain control has greatly improved pain relief for patients with regular dosing but is only effective when taken as needed. Review dosage history and patient symptoms to ensure adequate pain relief. Contact the provider if dose, frequency, or basal dose seems inadequate for relief.)	• Instruct the patient, family, or caregiver on the use of the PCA pump. Encourage use on an as-often-as-needed basis, and emphasize the limitations present to protect the patient (i.e., overdose is not possible).
• For IV push administration, dilute the drug with 4 to 5 mL of sterile normal saline and administer over 4 to 5 minutes unless otherwise ordered. The patient should remain supine to prevent dizziness or hypotension. Monitor blood pressure, pulse rate, and respiratory rate before and after the dose. (Opioids may cause hypotension and significant dizziness. Keeping the patient supine will limit these effects.)	• Explain the rationale to the patient for the need to remain flat during the drug administration and for 15 to 30 minutes after the dose, and to call for assistance before getting out of bed.
• Assess the home environment for medication safety and need for appropriate interventions. Advise the family on restrictions of prescription renewal and use. (Opioids are Scheduled drugs and may not be used by any person other than the patient. Safeguard medication in the home to prevent overdose.)	• Instruct the patient, family, or caregiver in proper medication storage and need for the drug to be used by the patient only. • Teach the family or caregiver about prescription renewal restrictions (i.e., new prescription each time, no refills, prescription may be called in) as appropriate for the Schedule of the drug.
Patient understanding of drug therapy: • Use opportunities during administration of medications and during assessments to discuss the rationale for drug therapy, desired therapeutic outcomes, commonly observed adverse effects, parameters for when to call the health care provider, and any necessary monitoring or precautions. (Using time during nursing care helps to optimize and reinforce key teaching areas.)	• The patient should be able to state the reason for the drug, appropriate dose and scheduling, what adverse effects to observe for, and when to report them.
Patient self-administration of drug therapy: • When administering the medication, instruct the patient, family, or caregiver in the proper self-administration of the drug (e.g., take the drug as prescribed when needed). (Utilizing time during nurse-administration of these drugs helps to reinforce teaching.)	Teach the patient to take the medication: • Before the pain becomes severe and, for cancer pain, as consistently as possible. • If using a PCA pump, use the self-dosage button whenever pain begins to increase or before activities such as sitting at the bedside. • Teach patients to not open, chew, or crush extended release tablets (e.g., oxycodone [OxyContin]); swallow them whole with plenty of water. • Take with food to decrease GI upset. • Because opioids are Scheduled drugs (most often C-II through IV), federal law restricts the sale and use of the drug to the person receiving the prescription only. Additional prescriptions may be necessary if the drug is continued beyond the first prescription (e.g., phone-in refills are not allowed for C-II drugs). Do not share with any other person and do not discard the unused drug down drains or in the garbage or flush it down the toilet. Return the drug to the pharmacy or health care provider for proper disposal.

*Nursing Diagnoses—Definitions and Classification 2015–2017. Copyright © 2014, 1994–2014 by NANDA International. Used by arrangement with John Wiley & Sons Limited.

chronic pain that requires round-the-clock analgesia. An orally disintegrating tablet (Rybix ODT, Ultram ODT) is available for patients who have difficulty swallowing tablets. Ultracet is a fixed dose combination of tramadol and acetaminophen. Off-label uses of tramadol include treatment of neuropathic pain and restless leg syndrome.

Mechanism of Action: Tramadol has a unique mechanism that involves both opioid and nonopioid actions. The drug and one of its metabolites bind to the opioid mu receptor. This opioid agonist activity is weak: approximately 10 times less than that of codeine. In addition to its central opioid action, tramadol inhibits norepinephrine and serotonin reuptake in spinal neurons, which inhibits the transmission of pain impulses.

Pharmacokinetics:

Route(s)	PO
Absorption	75% absorbed
Distribution	Widely distributed; crosses the placenta; small amounts secreted in breast milk; 20% bound to protein
Primary metabolism	Hepatic by CYP enzymes to an active metabolite; significant first-pass metabolism
Primary excretion	Renal
Onset of action	30–60 min
Duration of action	9 h

Adverse Effects: Tramadol is well tolerated, and its most common adverse effects are vertigo, dizziness, headache, nausea, vomiting, constipation, and lethargy. Because it acts centrally, symptoms of CNS stimulation such as nervousness, tremor, anxiety, agitation, confusion, visual impairment, and hallucinations are possible. Some patients experience drowsiness or depression rather than CNS excitation. Seizures have been reported, especially in patients who are concurrently taking antidepressants. Although respiratory depression can occur, it is not as severe as that caused by opioids. Physical dependence is possible although at much less risk than morphine; tramadol is not a controlled substance. Symptoms of opioid withdrawal, such as anxiety, sweating, tremors, panic attacks, and paresthesias, may occur if the drug is abruptly discontinued.

Contraindications/Precautions: Patients with a history of hypersensitivity to tramadol should not be given the drug. Caution should be exercised in patients allergic to codeine and other opioid agonists because cross-hypersensitivity has been reported. Although the risk for dependence is low, the drug should be used with caution in patients with a history of substance abuse. Tramadol should not be administered to patients with a history of depression or suicidal ideation because the drug can be fatal in overdose situations, especially if combined with alcohol or other CNS depressants. Because tramadol causes some degree of respiratory depression, it should be used cautiously in patients with COPD. The drug should be used with caution in patients with renal or hepatic impairment or in those with increased ICP. Because tramadol lowers the seizure threshold, it should be used with caution in patients with a history of seizures. Tramadol should be avoided during pregnancy and lactation because its chronic use can cause physical dependence and postpartum withdrawal symptoms in the newborn.

Drug Interactions: Use of tramadol concurrently with carbamazepine or certain antidepressants increases the risk of seizures. Carbamazepine also has additive CNS depressant effects and may reduce the analgesic activity of tramadol. Ethanol combined with tramadol may result in death. When used with other CNS depressants, the dose of tramadol should be reduced. Concurrent use of tramadol with MAOIs can result in seizures or serotonin syndrome. Procarbazine, rasagiline, and selegiline should not be given concurrently with tramadol because these drugs all increase serotonin levels and may result in serotonin syndrome. Tramadol is changed to an active metabolite by the hepatic CYP2D6 enzyme. If inhibitors of this enzyme (e.g., amiodarone, chloroquine, haloperidol, ritonavir, quinidine) are given concurrently with tramadol, a reduced analgesic effect may result. **Herbal/Food**: Food significantly affects the absorption of the extended release form of tramadol. St. John's wort is contraindicated due to the possibility of serotonin syndrome. Caution should be observed when using herbs such as valerian or kava that may have an additive CNS depressant effect.

Pregnancy: Category C.

Treatment of Overdose: Overdose with tramadol can result in serious CNS depression, respiratory depression, and death. Administration of naloxone will reduce some, but not all, of the symptoms of tramadol overdose and may precipitate convulsions.

Nursing Responsibilities: Key nursing implications for patients receiving tramadol are similar to those for opioid agents and are included in the Nursing Practice Application for Patients Receiving Pharmacotherapy for Pain.

CONNECTIONS **Lifespan Considerations**

◀ **Influence of Increasing Age on Pain Expression and Perception**

Pain control in the older adult can be challenging. Knowledge of the aging process, behavioral cues, subtle signs of discomfort, and verbal and non-verbal responses to pain is a must when it comes to effective pain management. Older patients may have a decreased perception of pain or simply ignore pain as a natural consequence of aging. Because these patients frequently go undermedicated, a thorough assessment is a necessity. Older adults may have difficulty with numerical rating scales and may respond more appropriately to the Wong-Baker Faces scale. When administering opioids for pain relief, the nurse should always monitor older adult patients closely. Aging decreases both hepatic metabolism and renal excretion; smaller doses are usually indicated and adverse effects may be heightened. Initial doses should be 25% to 50% lower with frequent reassessment. The nurse should closely monitor decreased respirations, level of consciousness, and dizziness. Body weight should be taken prior to the start of opioid administration and doses calculated accordingly. Bed rails should be kept raised and the bed in a low position at all times to prevent injury from falls. Some opioids, such as meperidine (Demerol) or hydromorphone (Dilaudid), should be used cautiously due to orthostatic hypotension. Many older adults take multiple drugs (polypharmacy); therefore, it is important to obtain a complete list of all medications taken and to check for interactions.

Drugs Similar to Tramadol (Ultram)

The two other centrally acting analgesics are clonidine and ziconotide. These drugs act by very different mechanisms than tramadol and are less frequently prescribed.

Clonidine (Catapres, Duraclon): Originally approved as an oral drug for hypertension (Catapres) in 1974, clonidine has been used off-label for a large number of other indications, including hot flashes, Tourette's syndrome, attention deficit/hyperactivity disorder (ADHD), and withdrawal from ethanol, nicotine, and opioids. It has a very limited role in treating severe, intractable cancer pain that is refractory to other drugs, including opioids. For this indication, it is administered as an epidural infusion, usually in combination with opioids. Clonidine activates alpha$_2$-adrenergic receptors in the spinal cord, resulting in decreased pain signals reaching the brain. Because this drug is absorbed into the circulation, the most serious adverse effects from the epidural use of clonidine are the same as those from PO administration: severe hypotension and bradycardia. When given by epidural infusion, clonidine carries a black box warning that it should not be used for obstetrical, postpartum, or perioperative pain management. Clonidine is also available as a transdermal patch (clonidine TTS), which releases the drug over 7 days. Clonidine (Kapvay) was approved by the FDA to treat ADHD in 2010 (see Chapter 24). The antihypertensive actions of clonidine are discussed in Chapter 34. Clonidine is pregnancy category C.

Ziconotide (Prialt): Ziconotide, approved in 2004, is unusual in that it was originally obtained from a species of saltwater snail. Like clonidine, its use is limited to patients whose pain is refractory to all other analgesics, including morphine. It is only administered by intrathecal infusion. An off-label use is for severe muscle spasticity due to spinal cord injury. The drug provides analgesia by blocking N-type calcium channels at the presynaptic nerve terminals in the spinal cord. This prevents neurotransmitter release, thus blocking pain transmission. Ziconotide has the potential for frequent and serious adverse effects. The drug carries a black box warning regarding the potential for severe psychiatric symptoms and neurologic impairment, including impaired cognition, decreased consciousness, and hallucinations. Dizziness, nausea, and vomiting occur in about half the patients receiving the drug. Although these adverse effects are serious, the student should remember that patients with cancer receiving this agent are terminally ill, and pain relief is often the primary therapeutic goal. This drug is pregnancy category C.

25.11 Adjuvant analgesics have primary indications other than pain control but can enhance analgesia.

Some types of pain are not adequately relieved by analgesics alone. **Adjuvant analgesics** are a diverse group of drugs that are used to enhance analgesia for specific indications. All of these drugs have other primary classifications, such as antidepressant, antiseizure, tranquilizer, or anti-inflammatory. The use of adjuvant analgesics includes two primary indications:

- Pain that is refractory to opioids, such as intractable cancer pain
- Neuropathic pain, which is caused by damage to the nerve itself, and pain caused by swelling in the CNS, which puts pressure on nerves.

In patients with intractable cancer pain, adjuvant analgesics are used in combination with analgesics to enhance the level of pain relief. It is important to understand that these agents supplement pain relief; they do not substitute for proper dosing of opioid analgesics in patients with severe pain. Adjuvant analgesics are generally not used if the pain is well managed with opioids, because these drugs have additional adverse effects and drug interactions that can complicate therapy.

Neuropathic pain is difficult to control with analgesics. The most common cause of neuropathic pain is diabetes, but herpes zoster infections, acute trauma, cancer, and certain autoimmune conditions can also cause this type of pain. Neuropathic pain is commonly described as steady burning, electric shock, or "pins and needles" sensations. Rather than treat with high doses of opioids, several adjuvant analgesics have been found to be effective at relieving neuropathic pain. These drugs may be used alone or in combination with opioids.

Adjuvant analgesics can be added at any step in the pain management ladder; they are usually dosed on a regular schedule as opposed to prn. The use of specific adjuvant analgesics and their doses are often guided by experience, rather than controlled clinical trials, and the majority of these drugs are prescribed off-label for their analgesic effects. Table 25.5 summarizes the effects and uses of selected adjuvant analgesics.

Antidepressants: Some of the most commonly prescribed adjuvant analgesics come from the antidepressant drug class. Both of the common classes of antidepressants, tricyclics and selective serotonin reuptake inhibitors (SSRIs), are used as adjuncts in the management of neuropathic pain. Although the tricyclics seem to be more effective, the SSRIs cause fewer serious adverse effects. These drugs increase the levels of the inhibitory neurotransmitters serotonin and norepinephrine in the CNS, resulting in increased pain modulation and decreased pain perception. Patients experiencing neuropathic pain may need trials with different antidepressants until the right combination of effectiveness and tolerable adverse effects is found. Doses of these drugs are generally lower than those used to treat depression, and the drugs act to relieve pain within 5 to 7 days. If improvement in pain relief is not noted within 1 week, the drug is discontinued. Duloxetine (Cymbalta) was the first of the antidepressants to receive approval for the treatment of diabetic peripheral neuropathic pain, chronic musculoskeletal pain, and fibromyalgia pain. Other drugs used for this purpose include amitriptyline (Elavil), imipramine (Tofranil), doxepin (Sinequan), paroxetine (Paxil), and venlafaxine (Effexor).

CONNECTION Checkpoint 25.2

Use of tricyclic antidepressants has declined in recent decades due to a higher incidence of adverse effects compared to drugs in the SSRI class, but they are useful in the treatment of neuropathic pain. From what you learned in Chapter 19, what type of adverse effects would likely be observed in patients taking tricyclics for migraines? *See Answer to Connection Checkpoint 25.2 on student resource website.*

Antiseizure drugs: Antiseizure drugs commonly prescribed for neuropathic pain include gabapentin (Neurontin), valproic acid (Depakene), phenytoin (Dilantin), and carbamazepine (Tegretol). The antiseizure drugs act by suppressing neuronal discharges and reducing the hyperexcitability that occurs after nerve injury. These drugs may cause nausea, vomiting, sedation, confusion, or

TABLE 25.5 Adjuvant Analgesics

Drug Class	Examples	Effect	Use
Antiseizure drugs	carbamazepine (Tegretol) clonazepam (Klonopin) gabapentin (Gralise, Neurontin)	Decrease nerve impulse transmission and spontaneous neuron firing.	Reduce peripheral nerve pain in diabetic neuropathy, post-herpetic neuralgia, and trigeminal neuralgia.
Benzodiazepines	diazepam (Valium) lorazepam (Ativan)	Potentiate effects of gamma aminobutyric acid (GABA) and other inhibitory neurotransmitters.	Relax skeletal muscle in muscle spasm; reduce anxiety in terminal dyspnea.
Bisphosphonates	pamidronate (Aredia) zoledronate (Reclast, Zometa)	Inhibit bone resorption.	Reduce cancer-related bone pain.
Corticosteroids	dexamethasone (Decadron) prednisone (Deltasone, others)	Reduce cerebral and spinal edema via various mechanisms in prostaglandin cascade.	Reduce swelling and pain in CNS cancer, spinal cord compression, postspinal surgery.
Selective serotonin reuptake inhibitors (SSRIs)	citalopram (Celexa) fluoxetine (Prozac) fluvoxamine (Luvox) sertraline (Zoloft)	Increase concentrations of inhibitory neuro-transmitters (serotonin and norepinephrine) in the CNS.	Reduce neuropathic pain.
Tricyclic antidepressants	amitriptyline (Elavil) amoxapine desipramine (Norpramin) doxepin (Sinequan) imipramine (Tofranil) nortriptyline (Aventyl) protriptyline (Vivactil)	Increase concentrations of inhibitory neuro-transmitters (serotonin and norepinephrine) in the CNS.	Reduce neuropathic pain.

dizziness. Gabapentin is considered a first-line drug for treating neuropathic pain, and an extended release tablet form of the drug (Gralise) was approved to treat postherpetic neuralgia in 2011.

Corticosteroids: Corticosteroids are used as adjuvants in pain management because they reduce inflammatory swelling and pressure on the brain, spinal cord, and spinal nerves. Dexamethasone (Decadron) is a drug of choice when given parenterally to reduce either cerebral or spinal cord edema; oral prednisone (Deltasone) may follow for a period of time. Steroids can also be injected directly into joints in refractory arthritis, or epidural/spinal tracts for chronic musculoskeletal pain. Their effects are discussed in Chapter 68.

Local anesthetics: Mexiletine (Mexitil) is a Class IB antidysrhythmic drug with anesthetic properties that is given PO for neuropathic pain refractory to other analgesics. Caution must be used when giving this drug to patients with heart disease or dysrhythmias. Short IV infusions of lidocaine (Xylocaine) may also provide temporary relief for some patients. A 5% lidocaine patch is approved for postherpetic neuralgia.

Muscle relaxants: Muscle relaxants such as the benzodiazepines may be used effectively as adjuvant an algesics when muscle spasm is a component of the pain. Muscle spasm can be present following orthopedic injury or with musculoskeletal disease or degenerative nervous system conditions. Benzodiazepines can also be used to reduce anxiety in the terminal dyspnea of heart failure or end-stage respiratory disease. Examples include diazepam (Valium), lorazepam (Ativan), and oxazepam (Serax).

Bone-specific agents: Patients with bone cancer or metastases may experience severe pain. For palliative care, the administration of calcitonin, either subcutaneously or intranasally, may provide some relief for bone pain. The adjuvant analgesic activity of the bisphosphonates such as pamidronate (Aredia) and zolendronate (Reclast, Zometa) has been well established. The use of calcitonin and bisphosphonates in treating bone disorders is presented in Chapter 72.

Miscellaneous agents: Capsaicin is a product obtained from chili peppers that is available as a cream to treat minor musculoskeletal pain. A prescription patch containing 8% capsaicin (Qutenza) was approved in 2010 for the relief of pain associated with postherpetic neuralgia. Milnacipran (Savella) is a serotonin and norepinephrine reuptake inhibitor (SNRI) approved in 2009 for the treatment of fibromyalgia. Although the exact mechanism by which milnacipran acts is unknown, it is believed that pain relief occurs through regulation of abnormal serotonergic and noradrenergic pathways.

Pharmacotherapy with Opioid Antagonists

25.12 The primary indication for an opioid antagonist is opioid-induced respiratory depression.

Opioid overdose can result from excessive doses during pain therapy, or from attempted suicide or substance abuse. Any opioid may be abused for its psychoactive effects; however, morphine, meperidine, and heroin are preferred by abusers due to their potency. Although heroin is currently available as a legal analgesic in many countries, it is deemed too dangerous for therapeutic use by the FDA, and it is a major drug of abuse. Once injected or inhaled, heroin rapidly crosses the blood–brain barrier to enter the brain, where it is metabolized to morphine. Thus, the effects of heroin administration are actually caused by activation of the mu and kappa receptors from its morphine metabolite. The initial effect is an intense euphoria, or rush, followed by several hours of deep relaxation.

In recent years, OxyContin has become a major drug of abuse. Because this long-acting form of oxycodone is especially beneficial to patients with chronic pain who need around-the-clock relief, it has become a first-line drug in pain management. Abusers use the drug either for its effective pain relief action or for its side effects such as relaxation or euphoria. Many of the opioid drugs are given in combination with aspirin or acetaminophen, which causes dose-limiting adverse effects. OxyContin, however, only contains oxycodone and it could be crushed by abusers and injected or snorted for an even greater drug experience. In response to the widespread abuse, the manufacturer of OxyContin reformulated the drug so that it is highly resistant to crushing, breaking, or dissolving. OxyContin is a frequent target for "doctor shoppers" who visit multiple health care providers, often reporting fictitious symptoms to obtain prescriptions. It is a potent and dangerous drug that can cause death when misused or abused.

Acute opioid intoxication is a medical emergency, with respiratory depression being the most serious medical challenge. Infusion with the opioid antagonist naloxone (Narcan) may be used to reverse respiratory depression and other acute symptoms. In administering naloxone, small doses are used and repeated until the respiratory depression is reversed and the patient begins to exhibit opioid withdrawal symptoms. The patient must be constantly monitored to ensure that the effects of the drug are sufficiently long to outlast the respiratory depression caused by the opioid overdose; IV doses of naloxone only last 1 hour. Maintenance of a patent airway is essential and resuscitation equipment should be immediately available. It is important to understand that naloxone will reverse both the toxic and therapeutic effects of opioids. Thus if the patient was using the opioid for analgesia, naloxone will reverse this effect and pain will quickly return.

In 2014, the FDA approved Evzio, a hand-held autoinjector containing naloxone. This device is designed to be used by family members or caregivers to treat a person with a known or suspected opioid overdose. Once turned on, the device gives verbal instructions for injecting the drug by either the IM or subcutaneous route. A training device is included with the packaging.

If an opioid antagonist fails to quickly reverse the acute symptoms, the overdose was likely due to a nonopioid substance. Doses for the opioid antagonists are listed in Table 25.6. The fixed dose combination of naloxone and buprenorphine (Suboxone, Zubsolv) has become a first-line therapy for the maintenance treatment of opioid dependence. Naloxone with buprenorphrine is a prototype drug in Chapter 27.

When abusing an opioid, the user usually develops tolerance to the euphoric effects of the drug and quickly escalates the dose.

Following therapy with an opioid antagonist, however, the patient will become much more sensitive to the effects of opioids. If the patient returns to drug-taking behavior at the same dose used prior to opioid antagonist therapy, death may result.

Another indication for opioid antagonists is for the treatment of opioid-induced constipation or postoperative ileus. Alvimopan (Entereg) and methylnaltrexone (Relistor), both approved in 2008, act as mu receptors in the GI tract. Because they do not cross the blood–brain barrier, these drugs do not interfere with the central effects of opioids such as analgesia.

CONNECTION Checkpoint 25.3

Prochlorperazine (Compazine) is an antiemetic drug in the phenothiazine class that may be prescribed to decrease the nausea and vomiting caused by opioids. From what you learned in Chapter 20, what conditions are drugs in the phenothiazine class used to treat? Considering the adverse effects of the phenothiazines, what additive effects are more likely to occur when taking a phenothiazine and an opioid analgesic together? *See Answer to Connection Checkpoint 25.3 on student resource website.*

Pharmacotherapy of Migraines

25.13 Migraines are a severe type of headache related to specific triggers.

Headaches are some of the most common complaints of patients. The pain and inability to concentrate causes a significant number of work-related absences and can interfere with activities of daily life. When the headaches are persistent, or manifest as migraines, drug therapy is warranted.

Why does a headache hurt? Although the skull and the brain lack pain receptors, the muscles of the scalp, face, and neck are abundantly supplied with nociceptors. These receptors can be stimulated by muscle tension, dilated blood vessels, and other headache triggers.

Of the several varieties of headaches, the most common type is the **tension headache**. This occurs when muscles of the head and neck become tight due to stress, causing a steady and lingering pain. Although quite painful, tension headaches are self-limiting and more of an annoyance than an emergency. Tension headaches can be effectively treated with OTC analgesics such as aspirin, acetaminophen, or ibuprofen. Table 25.7 differentiates the two common types of headaches.

The most painful type of headache is the **migraine**, which is characterized by throbbing or pulsating pain, sometimes preceded by an aura. **Auras** are sensory warnings of an imminent migraine attack. Examples include flashing lights, visual blind spots, and arm or leg tingling. Nausea, vomiting, and extreme sensitivity to light and sound accompany most migraines. A positive family history is present in the majority of people who experience migraines.

TABLE 25.6 Opioid Antagonists

Drug	Route and Adult Dose (Maximum Dose Where Indicated)	Adverse Effects
naloxone (Narcan)	IV: 0.4–2 mg; may be repeated every 2–3 min up to 10 mg if necessary	*Muscle and joint pains, difficulty sleeping, anxiety, headache, nervousness, withdrawal symptoms, vomiting*
naltrexone (ReVia, others)	PO: 25 mg followed by another 25 mg in 1 h if no withdrawal response (max: 800 mg/day)	Hepatotoxicity

Note: *Italics* indicate common adverse effects. <u>Underline</u> indicates serious adverse effects.

TABLE 25.7 Differentiation of Major Headache Types

Characteristics	Vascular (Migraine) Headache	Tension Headache
Pain quality	Pulsating or throbbing	Steady pressure or tightness
Pain location	Unilateral (more often) or bilateral	Bilateral (head-band or ice tongs) pattern
Pain severity	Moderate to severe	Mild to moderate
Duration	4–72 h	Usually several hours
Precursors or triggers	Hormonal changes in women; stress or heightened emotions; bright or flickering lights; change in weather or altitude Foods: alcohol, aged cheeses, chocolate, caffeine, fermented or pickled foods, aspartame, MSG	Stress or anxiety
Associated symptoms	May be preceded by aura, nausea, vomiting, extreme sensitivity to light or sound; aggravated by physical activity	Uncommon

Patients who get migraines appear to have blood vessels that overreact to various triggers. Triggers for migraines include foods containing nitrates or MSG, alcohol (especially red wine), perfumes, food additives, caffeine, chocolate, aspartame, and hormonal and environmental changes. Some patients can prevent or reduce the frequency of migraine attacks by avoiding known triggers.

The neurotransmitter serotonin (5-hydroxytryptamine or 5-HT) appears to be a key factor (although not the only factor) in the pathogenesis and treatment of migraines. What is the connection between serotonin levels and migraines? During a migraine, the amount of serotonin in the brain declines, causing the vessels to dilate. Nerves surrounding the dilated vessels become inflamed, resulting in pain. As neurons in the brain generate additional serotonin, or serotonin agonist drugs are administered, the vessels dilate and pain diminishes.

PharmFACT

Migraine Statistics

- About 70% of patients with migraines have a first-degree relative with a history of migraine.
- Before puberty, more boys have migraines than girls; after puberty, women are three times more likely to have migraines than men.
- History of migraine is associated with an increased incidence of major cardiovascular disease, especially if the patient experiences migraines with aura.
- Migraines are rare after age 50 (Chawla, 2013).

25.14 Analgesics and triptans are the primary classes of drugs used to abort acute migraine pain.

The two primary goals of migraine pharmacotherapy are to terminate an acute migraine in progress and to prevent or reduce the frequency of the disorder. Drugs used to stop a migraine in progress are different from those used for prophylaxis. The prophylactic agents are discussed in Section 25.15.

Migraine pharmacotherapy is most effective if begun before the pain has reached a severe level. Drug therapy is conducted in stages based on the severity of the migraine.

- **Mild migraine (occasional headaches with no other functional impairment).** NSAIDs offer the safest and least expensive therapy; thus they are tried initially. Acetaminophen is generally not effective alone but offers additive pain relief when combined with an NSAID and caffeine. Oral serotonin (5-HT)

agonists (triptans or ergot alkaloids) are initiated in persistent mild migraines that are refractory to NSAIDs.

- **Moderate migraine (moderate pain, nausea, and some functional impairment).** Oral, intranasal, or subcutaneous serotonin (5-HT) agonists are the drugs of choice. If serotonin agonists are contraindicated or ineffective, dopamine agonists such as metoclopramide (Reglan) or prochlorperazine (Compazine) may be prescribed.

- **Severe migraine (severe pain more than three times per month, marked nausea or vomiting, and functional impairment).** Subcutaneous, IM, or IV serotonin agonists may be indicated. A secondary choice would be a parenteral dopamine agonist, either as monotherapy or in combination with a serotonin agonist. Narcotic analgesics are effective at terminating pain from migraines that have proven to be refractory to other therapies.

The two major drug classes used to terminate migraines, the triptans and the ergot alkaloids, are both serotonin receptor agonists. About 90% of the serotonin receptors (also called serotonergic) are found in the intestine, with the remaining 10% occurring throughout the CNS and in platelets. In the CNS, serotonin is responsible for moderating diverse responses such as anger, anxiety, depression, sleep, appetite, and vomiting. At least seven serotonin receptor subtypes have been identified. Other drugs acting at serotonin receptors include certain antianxiety agents, antidepressants, antiemetics, and various hallucinogens. Doses for the triptans and ergot alkaloids are listed in Table 25.8.

Triptans: The first of the triptans, sumatriptan (Imitrex), was marketed in the United States in 1992. This drug was quickly followed by the introduction of the "second-generation" triptans with improved pharmacokinetic profiles: more thorough absorption, faster onset of action, and longer duration. Although all triptans have very similar actions and adverse effects, individual patients may respond more favorably, and with fewer adverse effects, to one triptan over another. The longer duration triptans are believed to be better at preventing the headache from recurring following its termination.

Triptans are selective for the 5-HT_1 receptor subtype, and they are thought to act by constricting certain intracranial vessels. They are effective in aborting migraines with or without auras. Although the PO forms of the triptans are most convenient, patients who experience nausea and vomiting during the migraine may require

TABLE 25.8	Drugs Used to Terminate Acute Migraines	
Drug	**Route and Adult Dose (Maximum Dose Where Indicated)**	**Adverse Effects**
Triptans		
almotriptan (Axert)	PO: 6.25–12.5 mg, may repeat in 2 h (max: 2 doses/24 h)	*Paresthesia, tingling, dry mouth, warming sensation, dizziness, vertigo* Coronary artery vasospasm, MI, cardiac arrest
eletriptan (Relpax)	PO: 20–40 mg, may repeat in 2 h (max: 80 mg/24 h)	
frovatriptan (Frova)	PO: 2.5 mg, may repeat in 2 h (max: 3 doses/24 h)	
naratriptan (Amerge)	PO: 1–2.5 mg, may repeat in 4 h (max: 5 mg/24 h)	
rizatriptan (Maxalt)	PO: 5–10 mg, may repeat in 2 h (max: 30 mg/24 h)	
sumatriptan (Imitrex, others)	PO: 25–100 mg, may repeat in 2 h (max: 200 mg/24 h) Nasal: 5–20 mg, may repeat once (max: 40 mg/24 h) Subcutaneous: 6 mg, may repeat in 1 h, once in 24 h	
zolmitriptan (Zomig, Zomig ZMT)	PO: 2.5 mg or less, may repeat in 2 h (max: 10 mg/24 h) PO (orally disintegrating tablet): 1.25–2.5 mg (max: 5 mg) Nasal: 5 mg, may repeat once after 2 h (max: 10 mg/24 h)	
Ergot Alkaloids		
dihydroergotamine (DHE 45, Migranal)	Nasal: 1 spray (0.5 mg) each nostril, may repeat once in 15 min (max: 3 mg/24 h, 4 mg/week) IM/subcutaneous: 1 mg, repeat at 1 h intervals for total 3 mg (max: 6 mg/week)	*Weakness, nausea, vomiting, abnormal pulse, throat irritation, nasal irritation, or dysgeusia (distorted sense of taste)*
ergotamine (Ergostat; with caffeine: Cafergot; with caffeine, belladonna, pentobarbital: Cafergot P-B)	Sublingual: 2 mg, may repeat in 30 min for total 3 doses/24 h or 5 doses/week PO: 2 tablets (2 mg), 1 additional tablet repeated every 30 min (max: 6 mg/attack or 10 mg/week) Rectal: 2 mg, may repeat once in 1 h	Delirium, seizures, cerebrovascular events (hemorrhage), intermittent claudication, birth defects, inhibition of lactation or cause of infant vomiting, physical dependence, withdrawal resembles migraine

Note: Italics indicate common adverse effects. <u>Underline</u> indicates serious adverse effects.

an alternate dosage form. Intranasal formulations are available and prefilled syringes of triptans may be used for patients who are able to self-administer the medication.

Triptans are not effective at preventing migraines. Other drugs, accompanied by lifestyle changes, must be used for prophylaxis (see Section 25.15).

Ergot alkaloids: For patients who are unresponsive to triptans, the ergot alkaloids may be used to abort migraines. They should be separated from triptan use by at least 24 hours. The first purified alkaloid, ergotamine (Ergostat), was isolated from the ergot fungus in 1920, although the actions of the ergot alkaloids had been known for thousands of years. Ergotamine is an inexpensive drug that is available in PO, sublingual, and suppository forms. Modification of the original molecule has produced a number of other pharmacologically useful drugs, such as dihydroergotamine (Migranal), which is available parenterally and as a nasal spray. Because the ergot alkaloids interact with adrenergic, dopaminergic, and serotonergic receptors, they produce multiple actions and adverse effects. The ergot alkaloids promote vasoconstriction, which terminates a migraine in progress. Adverse effects may include nausea, vomiting, weakness in the legs, myalgia, numbness and tingling in fingers and toes, angina-like pain, and tachycardia. Toxicity may be evidenced by constriction of peripheral arteries: cold, pale, numb extremities and muscle pain. Other possible adverse effects include dizziness, drowsiness, vasoconstriction, warming sensations, tingling, lightheadedness, weakness, and neck stiffness.

Ergot alkaloids, which constrict both arteries and veins, are contraindicated in peripheral vascular disease, coronary artery disease, and severe hypertension because they decrease blood flow. Metoclopramide or prochlorperazine may be administered concurrently with ergot alkaloids to reduce or prevent nausea and vomiting. Many ergot alkaloids are pregnancy category X drugs and should not be used by women who may become pregnant. These drugs may inhibit lactation or cause vomiting in breast-fed infants. Regular daily use can cause physical dependence. Withdrawal symptoms of headache, nausea, and vomiting resemble the symptoms of migraines. Dosing and duration of use need to be restricted. Dangers of overuse and dependence should be included in patient and family teaching.

PROTOTYPE DRUG	Sumatriptan (Imitrex, Others)

Classification: **Therapeutic:** Antimigraine agent
Pharmacologic: Serotonin (5-HT$_1$) receptor agonist

Therapeutic Effects and Uses: Available by the PO, intranasal, and subcutaneous routes, sumatriptan is used to relieve acute migraine headaches. It was the first triptan approved by the FDA in 1992. It is not effective for long-term prophylaxis of migraines; other drugs must be used for this purpose. Sumavel DosePro and Alsuma are systems that consist of a subcutaneous dose of sumatriptan with an autoinjector pen. Treximet is a fixed dose combination of sumatriptan and naproxen that was approved in 2008 for the treatment of acute migraines.

Mechanism of Action: Sumatriptan is structurally similar to serotonin. Sumatriptan activates the 5-HT$_1$ serotonin receptors on intracranial and extracerebral blood vessels, resulting in vasoconstriction and reduced transmission in trigeminal pain pathways. It has no intrinsic analgesic activity.

Pharmacokinetics:

Route(s)	PO, intranasal, subcutaneous
Absorption	15% PO; 97% subcutaneous
Distribution	Widely distributed; crosses the placenta; secreted in breast milk; less than 21% bound to plasma protein
Primary metabolism	Hepatic
Primary excretion	60% renal; 40% feces
Onset of action	PO: 30–60 min; intranasal: 15–20 min; subcutaneous: 10–15 min
Duration of action	PO: 6–8 h; intranasal: unknown; subcutaneous: 4–6 h

Adverse Effects: Sumatriptan has infrequent adverse effects that include mild and transient dizziness or nausea, diarrhea, myalgia, and inflammation and pain at the subcutaneous injection site. Headache recurrence occurs in a large percentage of patients taking sumatriptan. Although rare, serious cardiac events have been documented with sumatriptan use. These events include coronary artery vasospasm, myocardial ischemia, dysrhythmias, and MI. These serious events are more likely to occur in patients with preexisting cardiac disease.

Contraindications/Precautions: Sumatriptan is contraindicated in patients with coronary artery disease, cerebrovascular disease, or peripheral vascular disease. This drug is not recommended for patients with uncontrolled hypertension, hypercholesterolemia, or those who have a strong family history of cardiovascular disease. Sumatriptan is contraindicated in patients with serious renal or hepatic impairment. Patients with a history of epilepsy have an increased risk for seizures when taking sumatriptan. The drug is associated with fetal deformities and demise in animal studies; it should be avoided in pregnant women. Overuse of abortive therapies for migraine headaches can lead to rebound headaches.

Drug Interactions: Sumatriptan is metabolized by monoamine oxidase and should not be used within 2 weeks of MAOIs or SSRIs. Use of sumatriptan should be avoided within 24 hours of ergot alkaloids or any other 5-HT$_1$ agonist due to risk of vasospastic reactions. Serotonin syndrome is possible when giving sumatriptan with other drugs that increase serotonin levels or activity, including buspirone (BuSpar), other triptans, amphetamines, sibutramine, trazodone, tricyclic antidepressants (TCAs), lithium, duloxetine, venlafaxine, or meperidine. **Herbal/Food**: St. John's wort and feverfew should be avoided during therapy with sumatriptan.

Pregnancy: Category C.

Treatment of Overdose: Few overdoses have been recorded. Treatment of overdose is supportive.

Nursing Responsibilities: Key nursing implications for patients receiving sumatriptan are included in the Nursing Practice Application for Patients Receiving Pharmacotherapy for Migraines.

Drugs Similar to Sumatriptan (Imitrex)

Other triptans include almotriptan, eletriptan, frovatriptan, naratriptan, rizatriptan, and zolmitriptan. All of the triptans have the same therapeutic effects and spectrum of adverse effects. All of the drugs in this class are pregnancy category C.

Almotriptan (Axert): Almotriptan was approved as an oral antimigraine drug in 2001. The drug is well absorbed and has an onset of action of 1 to 3 hours. The drug is extensively metabolized to inactive metabolites by CYP450 enzymes, and 75% is excreted via the kidneys. Drug–drug interactions with agents metabolized in the liver may occur.

Eletriptan (Relpax): Approved in 2002, eletriptan is a newer triptan with improved GI absorption and a more rapid onset of action than sumatriptan. It also has a longer duration. Less than 10% is excreted via the kidneys, making the drug safe to use in patients with renal impairment. The drug is extensively metabolized by CYP450 enzymes and thus has the potential for drug–drug interactions with agents metabolized in the liver.

Frovatriptan (Frova): Approved in 2001, frovatriptan has the same effects as sumatriptan but has a slow onset and a very long duration. The 26-hour half-life results in less headache recurrence with this drug. This drug is extensively metabolized by hepatic CYP450 enzymes, and the majority is eliminated in the feces.

Naratriptan (Amerge): Approved in 1998, this drug has a relatively slow onset of action (3 to 4 hours) but with a longer duration of action than sumatriptan. This drug is extensively metabolized to inactive metabolites by CYP450 enzymes and is excreted by the kidneys.

Rizatriptan (Maxalt): Approved in 1998, rizatriptan is absorbed more quickly than sumatriptan, with an onset of 60 to 90 minutes. It is available as PO disintegrating tablets (Maxalt-MLT), which are allowed to dissolve on the tongue and be swallowed with saliva. Hepatic CYP450 enzymes do not significantly metabolize the drug. The most common adverse effects include asthenia, fatigue, somnolence, pain or pressure sensation, and dizziness.

Zolmitriptan (Zomig): Zolmitriptan is an oral drug that has the same effects as sumatriptan but is available in additional formulations as a nasal spray and as orally disintegrating tablets (Zolmig ZMT). This drug is metabolized to an active metabolite in the liver, which is responsible for some of its antimigraine activity. The most common adverse effects include neck/throat/jaw pain, dizziness, paresthesia, somnolence, warm or cold sensation, nausea, and dry mouth. Zolmitriptan should not be used to treat cluster headaches.

25.15 Drugs from many different classes are used for migraine prophylaxis.

Prior to initiation of migraine prophylaxis, patients should attempt lifestyle changes and nonpharmacologic therapies to reduce the frequency of migraines. First and foremost, the patient needs to identify personal triggers for migraines. The nurse can help by guiding the patient through the process of assessing and identifying those personal migraine triggers. Foods are a common culprit, especially those containing nitrates or MSG. Omitting common migraine triggers from the diet is a first step in migraine prophylaxis. Other lifestyle changes that may help include adopting regular sleep patterns and meals, participating in aerobic exercise (start slowly because sudden intense activity may cause headaches), avoiding alcohol (especially red wine), and smoking cessation. Other helpful self-care measures include keeping a diary that notes when headaches start, how long they last, what provides relief, what the response is to the medication, and food intake or stress in the past 24 hours. Relaxation exercises, meditation, yoga, or progressive muscle relaxation may help. Nontraditional therapies may also be useful in preventing migraines in some patients.

Drugs for migraine prophylaxis include various classes of drugs that are discussed in other chapters of this textbook. These include beta-adrenergic blockers, calcium channel blockers, antidepressants, and antiseizure drugs. Because all of these drugs have the potential to produce adverse effects, prophylaxis is only initiated if the incidence of migraines is high and the patient is unresponsive to the drugs used to abort migraines. Example prophylactic antimigraine agents are shown in Table 25.9. Doses for these drugs are found in the chapters where their primary indication is presented.

Preventive treatment is recommended for headaches that occur three or more times a month. Of the various drugs, the beta-adrenergic blocker propranolol (Inderal) is one of the most commonly prescribed, although other drugs in this class have similar effectiveness. The use of beta blockers is particularly beneficial in patients with comorbid conditions such as hypertension or angina.

TCAs, especially amitriptyline (Elavil), have been used for decades to prevent migraines and are preferred for patients who may have a mood disorder or insomnia in addition to their migraines. The antimigraine action of these drugs is independent of their antidepressant action. SSRIs such as fluoxetine (Prozac) have been prescribed off-label for migraines because they exhibit fewer adverse effects than the tricyclics.

Other classes of drugs used for migraine prevention include calcium channel blockers, certain antiseizure drugs, estrogens for menstrual migraines, and miscellaneous agents such as methysergide (Sansert). An extended release form of valproic acid (Stavzor) was approved for migraine prophylaxis in 2008. Onabotulinum-toxinA (Botox), a drug often used to erase facial wrinkles, was approved to treat chronic migraines in 2010 (see Chapter 23).

TABLE 25.9   Drugs Used for Migraine Prophylaxis

Drug Class	Examples
Antiseizure drugs	gabapentin (Neurontin)
	topiramate (Topamax)
	valproic acid (Depakene, Depakote)
Beta-adrenergic blockers	atenolol (Tenormin)
	metoprolol (Lopressor)
	propranolol (Inderal)
	timolol (Blocadren)
Calcium channel blockers	nifedipine (Procardia)
	nimodipine (Nimotop)
	verapamil (Isoptin)
Tricyclic antidepressants	amitriptyline (Elavil)
	imipramine (Tofranil)
	protriptyline (Vivactil)
Miscellaneous	methysergide (Sansert)

CONNECTIONS | Complementary and Alternative Therapies

Natural Therapies for Migraines

- Acupuncture has been found to be helpful for headache pain in clinical trials. A trained acupuncturist uses thin, disposable needles at specific points on the body to treat the pain.
- Biofeedback and relaxation training can be learned and used to stop or relieve migraine pain. Biofeedback is a relaxation technique that uses monitors to teach the patient how to respond to stress by controlling responses such as muscle tension.
- Massage and chiropractic therapy may be useful in reducing tension headaches. As stress reduction techniques, they may be useful for migraine prevention, especially by improving sleep quality.

- Riboflavin (vitamin B_2) may reduce the frequency of migraine attacks, but effects develop slowly, up to 3 months for maximum effect. Doses of 400 mg per day produce few adverse effects.
- Coenzyme Q10 may also reduce the frequency of attacks.
- Magnesium supplements may be useful in preventing migraines, especially in people who have low serum magnesium levels.

Used with permission from Mayo Foundation for Medical Education & Research. All Rights Reserved.

CONNECTIONS: NURSING PRACTICE APPLICATION

Patients Receiving Pharmacotherapy for Migraines

Assessment	Potential Nursing Diagnoses*
Baseline assessment prior to administration: • Obtain a complete health history including cardiovascular, neurologic, hepatic, or renal disease, pregnancy, or breast-feeding. Obtain a drug history including allergies, current prescription and OTC drugs, herbal preparations, caffeine, nicotine, and alcohol use. Be alert to possible drug interactions. • Obtain baseline vital signs, apical pulse, level of consciousness, and weight. • Assess level of pain. Use objective screening tools when possible (e.g., Wong-Baker FACES scale for children, numerical rating scale for adults). Assess history of pain and what has worked successfully or not for the patient in the past. • Evaluate appropriate laboratory findings (e.g., CBC, hepatic or renal function studies). • Assess the patient's ability to receive and understand instructions. Include family and caregivers as needed.	• *Acute Pain* • *Ineffective Health Maintenance* • *Ineffective Coping* • *Deficient Knowledge* (Drug therapy)
Assessment throughout administration: • Assess for desired therapeutic effects (e.g., headache pain is decreased or absent). • Continue monitoring level of consciousness and neurologic symptoms (e.g., numbness or tingling). • Assess vital signs, especially blood pressure and pulse, periodically. • Continue periodic monitoring of hepatic and renal function studies. • Assess stress and coping patterns for possible symptom correlation (e.g., existing or perceived stress, duration, coping mechanisms, or remedies). • Assess for and promptly report adverse effects: chest pain or tightness, palpitations, tachycardia, hypertension, dizziness, lightheadedness, confusion, numbness, or tingling in extremities.	

Implementation

Interventions and (Rationales)	Patient-Centered Care
Ensuring therapeutic effects: • Continue assessments as above for therapeutic effects. Give the drug before the start of acute pain when possible. (Consistent use of a pain rating scale by all providers will help quantify the level of pain relief and leads to better pain control. Encourage the patient to start medication before the headache becomes severe for better control. Pain relief begins within several minutes after administration.)	• Teach the patient that pain relief, rather than merely control, is the goal of therapy. • Encourage the patient to take the drug before a headache becomes severe and to take it consistently as ordered. • Explain the rationale behind the pain rating scale (i.e., it allows consistency among all providers). • Encourage the patient to use additional, nonmedicinal pain relief techniques (e.g., quiet, darkened, cool room).
Minimizing adverse effects: • Monitor blood pressure and pulse periodically, especially in patients at risk for undiagnosed cardiovascular disease. Cardiovascular status should be monitored frequently following the first dose given. (Triptans and ergot alkaloids cause vasoconstriction. **Lifespan:** Postmenopausal women, men over age 40, smokers, and people with other known coronary artery disease risk factors may be at greatest risk. Older adults may have undetected cardiovascular disease, placing them at greater risk for adverse effects.)	• Instruct the patient to immediately report any chest pain or tightness or throat pain that is severe or continues following drug dosage.
• Observe for changes in severity, character, or duration of headache. (Sudden severe headaches of "thunderclap" quality can signal subarachnoid hemorrhage. Headaches that differ in quality and are accompanied by such signs as fever, rash, or stiff neck may herald meningitis.)	• Instruct the patient to immediately report changes in character or duration of headache or if accompanied by additional symptoms such as fever, rash, or stiff neck.
• Continue to monitor neurologic status periodically. (Dizziness or lightheadedness may be related to headache, an adverse drug effect, or may signal cerebral ischemia.)	• Instruct the patient to immediately report increasing dizziness, lightheadedness, or blurred vision.
• Monitor dietary intake of foods that contain tyramine, caffeine, alcohol, or other food triggers. (Some foods or beverages may trigger an acute migraine. Correlating symptoms with food or beverages assists in avoiding the cause of the headache.)	• Encourage the patient to keep a food diary and correlate symptoms with specific foods or beverages. Teach the patient to avoid or limit foods containing tyramine, such as pickled foods, beer, wine, and aged cheeses, which are often known triggers for migraines.

CONNECTIONS: NURSING PRACTICE APPLICATION (continued)

• Encourage the patient to discuss other methods of migraine control if ergot alkaloids are required for more than short-term use. (Ergot alkaloids cause significant vasoconstriction and cause dependence. Other, safer drugs may be needed for long-term relief of migraines.)	• Instruct the patient to discuss treatment options for long-term migraine relief with the health care provider.
• **Lifespan:** Women who are planning pregnancy, are pregnant, or are breast-feeding should discuss the use of drug therapy and alternative treatment before using antimigraine drugs. (Triptans are known to cause birth defects in animals. Ergotamine and other ergot alkaloids are category X drugs.)	• Teach women of childbearing age to discuss the use of antimigraine drugs before planning pregnancy and to discontinue use if pregnant or breast-feeding unless directed otherwise by the health care provider.
Patient understanding of drug therapy: • Use opportunities during administration of medications and during assessments to discuss the rationale for drug therapy, desired therapeutic outcomes, commonly observed adverse effects, parameters for when to call the health care provider, and any necessary monitoring or precautions. (Using time during nursing care helps to optimize and reinforce key teaching areas.)	• The patient should be able to state the reason for the drug, appropriate dose and scheduling, what adverse effects to observe for, and when to report them.
Patient self-administration of drug therapy: • When administering the medication, instruct the patient, family, or caregiver in the proper self-administration of the drug (e.g., take the drug as prescribed when needed). (Utilizing time during nurse-administration of these drugs helps to reinforce teaching.)	• Teach the patient to take the medication before the pain becomes severe or at the first symptoms of a migraine if possible. • Use the drug exactly as prescribed; overuse can lead to rebound headaches. • Teach the patient the proper administration of subcutaneous medication and have the patient or caregiver return demonstrate the technique. (Pain or redness at the injection site is common but usually disappears within an hour after the dose is taken.) • Instruct the patient that the appropriate intranasal dose is one spray into one nostril unless otherwise ordered by the health care provider.

*Nursing Diagnoses—Definitions and Classification 2015–2017. Copyright © 2014, 1994–2014 by NANDA International. Used by arrangement with John Wiley & Sons Limited.

CHAPTER 25

Understanding the Chapter

Key Concepts Summary

25.1 The primary goal of pain management is to reduce pain to a level that allows the patient to continue normal daily activities.

25.2 Proper assessment and classification of pain guides its treatment.

25.3 Health care providers and patients sometimes hold myths about pain that impede optimum pain management.

25.4 Pain transmission processes allow multiple targets for pharmacologic intervention.

25.5 Both pharmacologic and nonpharmacologic therapies are used in pain management.

25.6 Opioid analgesics exert their effects by interacting with specific receptors in the central nervous system.

25.7 Opioids are the drugs of choice for moderate to severe pain that cannot be controlled with other classes of analgesics.

25.8 Mixed agonist and antagonist opioids exhibit moderate analgesia with less risk of dependence than morphine.

25.9 Nonsteroidal anti-inflammatory drugs are the medications of choice for mild to moderate pain.

25.10 A few miscellaneous analgesics reduce pain by acting on the central nervous system.

25.11 Adjuvant analgesics have primary indications other than pain control but can enhance analgesia.

25.12 The primary indication for an opioid antagonist is opioid-induced respiratory depression.

25.13 Migraines are a severe type of headache related to specific triggers.

25.14 Analgesics and triptans are the primary classes of drugs used to abort acute migraine pain.

25.15 Drugs from many different classes are used for migraine prophylaxis.

Case Study: Making the Patient Connection

Remember the patient "Larry Smith" at the beginning of the chapter? Now read the remainder of the case study. Based on the information presented within this chapter, respond to the critical thinking questions that follow.

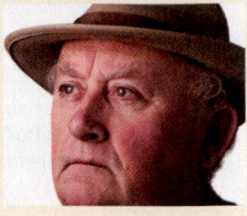

Larry Smith was being seen for an outpatient presurgery work-up the evening before scheduled urologic surgery. The nurse conducts a thorough history and examination related to his back pain and current pain management. His anticipated hospital stay is 2 days postsurgery.

Larry Smith is a 64-year-old male. Vital signs are blood pressure, 108/64 mmHg; pulse, 88 beats/min; respirations, 16 breaths/min. He has a well-healed midline scar on his back from lumbar vertebrae surgery, with a shorter scar over his right iliac crest. He moves a bit slowly with some limited lumbar range of motion. He also uses a cane for ambulating any distance. He describes his pain as a constant dull ache in the lower back that increases with prolonged standing or walking. Mr. Smith also reports a feeling of "cold electricity" down both legs, with the left greater than the right, which increases with standing and walking, as well as numbness of the middle toes on his left foot. He has been using mixed opioid and nonopioid analgesics for the past 8 years and previously had used SSRI antidepressants as adjuvant for his pain. His current health care provider weaned him off Vicodin ES about a year ago. He now takes methadone 20 mg twice a day. When the pain is not relieved he uses Norco for breakthrough pain. His use of Norco is 1 to 2 per day. Constipation is an ongoing problem, requiring stool softeners and occasional laxatives.

Critical Thinking Questions

1. How should Larry's postoperative pain be managed? Is there a referral the nurse can make to facilitate effective pain management?

2. How could the nurse best communicate Larry's needs to the postoperative nursing staff?

3. What should be included in the care plan for postoperative management of analgesic adverse effects?

See Answers to Critical Thinking Questions on student resource website.

Additional Case Study

Rita Manson presents to the emergency department with vomiting, severe abdominal and back pain, and jaundice. Her jaundice is recent but the pain and vomiting have continued for a couple of months. Her diagnostic work-up reveals advanced pancreatic cancer with metastasis to the spine.

1. What is the drug of choice for Rita's pain management? Which route of administration would be expected initially?

2. Her prescribed pain medication is morphine sulfate 2 to 10 mg IV every 2 hours as needed for pain. Outline a nursing approach to pain management for the first 24 hours.

3. What adverse effects would the nurse expect?

4. As part of the patient's pain management, dexamethasone (Decadron) 5 mg IV is prescribed every 6 hours for 2 days. Explain the use of corticosteroids in pain management.

5. After several days, Rita expresses her concern about "becoming hooked on that narcotic." How would the nurse respond?

See Answers to Additional Case Study on student resource website.

Chapter Review

1 The nurse is monitoring the patient for adverse effects associated with morphine. Which adverse effects would be expected? Select all that apply.

1. Respiratory depression
2. Hypertension
3. Urinary retention
4. Constipation
5. Nausea

2 Several days postoperative bowel surgery, the patient is eating soft food, ambulating regularly, and using hydrocodone (Vicodin) for pain. What should the nursing care plan include?

1. Monitoring vital signs for respiratory depression
2. Inserting a urinary catheter for urinary retention
3. Weaning pain medication to prevent addiction
4. Increasing dietary fiber and fluids and administering a stool softener if needed

3 A patient who has migraines self-administered sumatriptan (Imitrex) for the first time yesterday. Today, the patient informs the nurse that after taking the medication, the patient began to experience chest pain. The patient further states that the drug was effective in relieving the headache. The nurse should:

1. Encourage the patient to continue using the drug because it was effective.

2. Advise the patient to tell the health care provider about the chest pain at the next visit.

3. Instruct the patient to contact the health care provider to report the chest pain today and to not use the sumatriptan until talking to the health care provider.

4. Encourage the patient to lie down in a quiet room and use cold packs during the next migraine.

4 A patient with diabetes reports increasing pain and numbness in his legs. "It feels like pins and needles all the time, especially at night." Which drug would the nurse expect to be prescribed for this patient?

1. Ibuprofen (Motrin)

2. Gabapentin (Neurontin)

3. Naloxone (Narcan)

4. Methadone

5 The emergency department nurse is caring for a patient with a migraine. Which drug would the nurse anticipate administering to abort the patient's migraine?

1. Morphine

2. Dihydroergotamine (Migranal)

3. Propranolol (Inderal)

4. Ibuprofen (Motrin)

6 The nurse is caring for several patients who are receiving opioids for pain relief. Which patient is at the highest risk of developing hypotension, respiratory depression, and mental confusion?

1. A 23-year-old female, postoperative ruptured appendix

2. A 16-year-old male, post–motorcycle injury with lacerations

3. A 54-year-old female, post–myocardial infarction

4. An 86-year-old male, postoperative femur fracture

See Answers to Chapter Review in Appendix A.

References

Chawla, J. (2013). *Migraine headache*. Retrieved from http://emedicine.medscape.com/article/1142556-overview

Chou, R., Fanciullo, G. J., Fine, P. G., Adler, J. A., Ballantyne, J. C., Davies, P., . . . Miaskowski, C., American Pain Society-American Academy of Pain Medicine Opioids Guidelines Panel. (2009). Clinical guidelines for the use of chronic opioid therapy in chronic noncancer pain. *The Journal of Pain, 10*, 113–130. doi:10.1016/j.pain.2008.10.008

Mayo Clinic. (2011). *Migraine*. Retrieved from http://www.mayoclinic.org/diseases-conditions/migraine-headache/basics/alternative-medicine/CON-20026358

National Institute of Neurological Disorders and Stroke. (2013). *Low back pain fact sheet*. Retrieved from http://www.ninds.nih.gov/disorders/backpain/detail_backpain.htm#250353102

Voepel-Lewis, T., Zanotti, J., Danmeyer, J. A., & Merkel, S. (2010). Reliability and validity of face, legs, activity, cry, consolability behavioral tool in assessing acute pain in critically ill patients. *American Journal of Critical Care, 19*, 55–62. doi:10.4037/ajcc2010624

Selected Bibliography

Abdulla, A., Adams, N., Bone, M., Elliott, A., Gaffin, J., Jones, D., . . . Schofield, P. (2013). Evidence-based clinical practice guidelines on the management of pain in older people: Executive summary. *British Journal of Pain, 7*, 152–154. doi:10.1177/2049463713495669

Bozoghlanian, M., & Vasudevan, S. V. (2012). Overview of migraine treatment. *Pain Management, 2*, 399–414. doi:10.2217/pmt.12.29

Chaparro, L. E., Wiffen, P. J., Moore, R. A., & Gilron, I. (2012). Combination pharmacotherapy for the treatment of neuropathic pain in adults. *Cochrane Database of Systematic Reviews, 7*, CD008943. doi:10.1002/14651858.CD008943.pub2

Dworkin, R. H., O'Connor, A. B., Audette, J., Baron, R., Gourlay, G. K., Haanpää, M. L., . . . Wells, C. D. (2010, March). Recommendations for the pharmacological management of neuropathic pain: An overview and literature update. *Mayo Clinic Proceedings, 85*(Suppl. 3), S3–S14. doi:10.4065/mcp.2009.0649

Francis, G. J., Becker, W. J., & Pringsheim, T. M. (2010). Acute and preventive pharmacologic treatment of cluster headaches. *Neurology, 75*, 463–473. doi:10.1212/WNL.0b013e3181eb58c8

Friedberg, F., Williams, D. A., & Collinge, W. (2012). Lifestyle-oriented non-pharmacological treatments for fibromyalgia: A clinical overview and applications with home-based technologies. *Journal of Pain Research, 5*, 425. doi:10.2147/JPR.S35199

Gordon, A. (2012). The five pillars of pain management. *Pain Management, 2*, 335–344. doi:10.2217/pmt.12.31

Herdman, T. H., & Kamitsuru, S. (Eds.). (2014). *NANDA International nursing diagnoses: Definitions and classification, 2015–2017*. Oxford, United Kingdom: Wiley-Blackwell.

Meeker, M. A., Finnell, D., & Othman, A. K. (2011). Family caregivers and cancer pain management: A review. *Journal of Family Nursing, 17*, 29–60. doi:10.1177/1074840710396091

Minozzi, S., Amato, L., & Davoli, M. (2013). Development of dependence following treatment with opioid analgesics for pain relief: A systematic review. *Addiction, 108*, 688–698. doi:10.1111/j.1360-0443.2012.04005.x

O'Connor, L. (2013). Understanding individual reactions to opioids in pain management. *Nurse Prescribing, 11*, 233.

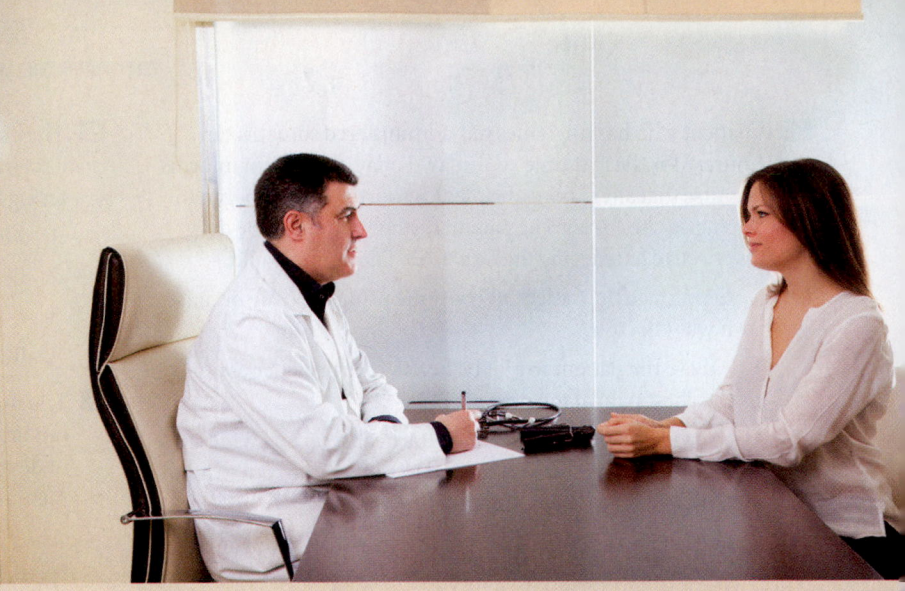

CHAPTER

26 Anesthetics and Anesthesia Adjuncts

LEARNING OUTCOMES

After reading this chapter, the student should be able to:

1. Compare and contrast the four basic types of anesthesia.
2. Explain the five general purposes of balanced anesthesia.
3. Compare and contrast the four stages of general anesthesia.
4. Identify drug classes used to produce general anesthesia.
5. For each of the classes shown in the chapter outline, identify the prototype and representative drugs and explain the mechanism(s) of drug action, primary indications, contraindications, significant drug interactions, pregnancy category, and important adverse effects.
6. Describe the nursing care associated with the administration of regional and general anesthesia.
7. Explain the rationale for using adjunct agents during general anesthesia.
8. Apply the nursing process to care for patients receiving local or general anesthesia.

CHAPTER OUTLINE

▶ Types of Anesthesia

▶ Principles of General Anesthesia

▶ Intravenous Anesthetics
   Opioid Anesthetics
   PROTOTYPE Fentanyl (Sublimaze), *p. 396*
   Benzodiazepine Anesthetics
   PROTOTYPE Midazolam (Versed), *p. 398*
   Miscellaneous Intravenous Anesthetics
   PROTOTYPE Propofol (Diprivan), *p. 399*

▶ Inhalation Anesthetics
   PROTOTYPE Nitrous Oxide, *p. 402*
   PROTOTYPE Isoflurane (Forane), *p. 403*

▶ Local Anesthetics
   Classification of Local Anesthetics
   Esters
   PROTOTYPE Procaine (Novocaine), *p. 408*
   Amides
   PROTOTYPE Lidocaine (Anestacon, Dilocaine, Xylocaine, Others), *p. 410*

▶ Adjuncts to Anesthesia

KEY TERMS

amide, 409

balanced anesthesia, 395

dissociative anesthesia, 400

esters, 408

general anesthesia, 395

local anesthesia, 395

minimum alveolar concentration, 401

monitored anesthesia care (MAC), 395

neurolept analgesia, 396

regional anesthesia, 395

surgical anesthesia, 395

Throughout history, the application of anesthesia has allowed patients to experience a temporary loss of sensation, resulting in comfort during surgical intervention. The use of opium as an anesthetic was recorded as far back as 4200 BC, and the ancient Chinese recorded acupuncture as a form of anesthesia. The modern implementation of anesthesia dates back to 1856 when Dr. John C. Warren performed a surgical procedure using ether. Modern anesthesia now offers safer and more effective drugs. This chapter introduces drugs used for general and local anesthesia along with the adjuvant medications administered during surgical procedures.

Types of Anesthesia

26.1 Anesthesia is used to produce a controlled loss of sensation during a diagnostic or surgical procedure.

Certain medical procedures produce a significant degree of pain and would not be possible without anesthesia. There are four types of anesthesia. The type of anesthesia selected depends on the degree of sedation and analgesia needed to conduct the procedure.

General anesthesia is the loss of sensation throughout the entire body, accompanied by loss of consciousness (LOC). General anesthesia is necessary for major surgical procedures.

The application of **local anesthesia** results in loss of sensation to a limited body region without LOC. It affects only the immediate area that surrounds where the anesthetic is administered. **Regional anesthesia** is similar, except that it encompasses a larger body area, such as an entire limb. Local and regional anesthesias produce fewer adverse effects than general anesthesia and are thus the methods of choice where applicable.

A fourth type of anesthesia is **monitored anesthesia care (MAC)**, which uses sedatives, analgesics, and other low-dose drugs that allow patients to remain responsive and breathe without assistance during the medical procedure. This type of anesthesia is used during diagnostic procedures and minor surgeries to supplement local and regional anesthesias. Subtypes of MAC are based on the degree of sedation produced:

- **Minimal sedation (anxiolysis).** Patients respond to verbal commands. Airway, ventilation, and cardiovascular functions are normal.
- **Moderate (conscious) sedation.** Patients respond to verbal or light tactile prompting. Airway, ventilation, and cardiovascular functions are usually adequate.
- **Deep sedation/analgesia.** Patients are aroused by repeated or painful stimulation. Airway and ventilation intervention may be required. Cardiovascular functions are usually adequate.

Principles of General Anesthesia

26.2 Balanced anesthesia uses multiple drugs to provide for the safe induction and maintenance of general anesthesia.

General anesthesia is accomplished by the administration of a variety of drugs. The purposes of general anesthesia include the following:

- Analgesia: blocking the sensation of pain
- Relaxation: relieving the intense anxiety associated with medical procedures
- Hypnosis: producing unconsciousness to block awareness of the procedure
- Amnesia: blocking memory of the events associated with the procedure
- Loss of reflexes: blocking autonomic and other reflexes that may be affected by the procedure

Because no single drug can safely accomplish all five purposes, a pharmacologic approach called balanced anesthesia is used. **Balanced anesthesia** is the use of a combination of medications to produce general anesthesia. Drugs administered to achieve balanced anesthesia include neuromuscular blockers, short-acting benzodiazepines, opioids, and general anesthetics. The purpose of the combination of these medications is to provide sedation, rapid induction of unconsciousness, muscle relaxation, and analgesia. The use of multiple drugs reduces the need for large amounts of inhaled anesthetics, which increases patient safety.

Balanced anesthesia involves the administration of intravenous (IV) medications prior to the general anesthetic. The IV medications produce muscle relaxation, diminish pain, and promote sleep. After the patient loses consciousness, inhaled general anesthetics are administered to maintain the anesthetized state. For short procedures, lower amounts of anesthesia are administered, or parenteral agents alone may be sufficient.

General anesthesia is a progressive process that occurs in distinct phases, which are described in Table 26.1. The most effective medications can quickly induce all four stages, whereas others are able to induce only stage 1. Major surgical procedures require the patient to be maintained in stage 3, which is referred to as **surgical anesthesia**. The patient should progress from stage 2 to stage 3 rapidly because stage 2 produces excitement, hyperactivity, and a feeling of panic. During stage 2 the patient is monitored closely for heart rate irregularities and increases in blood pressure. During recovery from general anesthesia, the patient moves in reverse order back up through the four stages.

TABLE 26.1 **Stages of General Anesthesia**

Stage	Characteristics
1	*Analgesia:* The patient loses general sensation but may remain awake. This stage progresses until the patient loses consciousness.
2	*Excitement and hyperactivity:* The patient may become delirious and attempt to resist treatment. The heart rate and respiratory rate may become irregular. The patient's blood pressure may increase. The administration of IV agents may calm the patient.
3	*Surgical anesthesia:* The patient's skeletal muscles become relaxed and delirium stabilizes. The cardiopulmonary effects stabilize. The patient becomes still with diminished eye movements. The surgical procedure is begun. The patient remains in stage 3 until the procedure ends.
4	*Paralysis of the medulla:* If breathing and cardiac function cease, death could result. This stage of general anesthesia is avoided.

PharmFACT

About 60% of women giving birth in hospitals receive epidural anesthesia. Women with higher educational attainment (master's/doctoral degrees) were more likely to have epidural anesthesia than those having lower degrees or no degrees (Osterman & Martin, 2011).

Intravenous Anesthetics

26.3 Intravenous anesthetics include opioids, benzodiazepines, and several miscellaneous agents.

IV anesthetics are important components of balanced anesthesia. After a single IV bolus, these drugs enter the brain, allowing the patient to quickly progress through stages 1 and 2. They are occasionally used alone for minor diagnostic and surgical interventions. Concurrent administration of IV and inhaled anesthetics allows the dose of the inhaled anesthetic to be reduced. The lower dosage of inhaled anesthetic produces a better surgical outcome and lowers the risk of serious adverse effects from the anesthesia. The combined use of IV and inhaled anesthesia also allows for a greater degree of analgesia and muscle relaxation than when inhalation anesthetics are used alone.

Less than a dozen drugs are used as IV anesthetics. Some of these drugs also have nonanesthetic indications. Drugs from the following classes are used for IV anesthesia:

- Benzodiazepines
- Opioids
- Miscellaneous agents

PharmFACT

Certified registered nurse anesthetists administer about 34 million anesthetics each year. Nurse anesthetists are the primary providers of anesthesia care for the United States armed forces (American Association of Nurse Anesthetists, 2014).

26.4 Opioids are used as intravenous anesthetics to provide analgesia and to accomplish neurolept anesthesia.

As presented in Chapter 25, the opioids, or narcotic analgesics, are the most effective drugs available for pain relief, including perioperative pain management. To produce deep anesthesia, however, opioids must be combined with other anesthetics. Combinations allow lower doses to be used and provide the necessary analgesia for painful procedures.

Alfentanil (Alfenta), fentanyl (Sublimaze), remifentanil (Ultiva), and sufentanil (Sufenta) are opioids used as IV anesthetics. These medications are opioid receptor agonists that provide a rapid onset of action with a short duration of 10 to 30 minutes. Their primary disadvantage is respiratory depression. Muscle rigidity may occur, which can impair ventilation further. A complete discussion of the mechanisms, actions, and adverse effects of the opioids is included in Chapter 25. A prototype feature for morphine can be found in that chapter. Doses for the opioid anesthetics are listed in Table 26.2.

The combination of droperidol and fentanyl produces a type of anesthesia called **neurolept analgesia**. Neurolept analgesia produces feelings of indifference to the patient's surroundings. The patient appears to be asleep but does not lose consciousness. Fentanyl is a potent opioid agonist with pharmacologic action that is similar to that of morphine. Droperidol is an antipsychotic drug related to haloperidol. It has the ability to reduce the nausea and vomiting adverse effects of opioids and produces sedation by reducing anxiety and motor activity.

PROTOTYPE DRUG **Fentanyl (Sublimaze)**

Classification: **Therapeutic:** Analgesic, anesthetic
Pharmacologic: Opioid agonist

Therapeutic Effects and Uses: Fentanyl is an opioid analgesic that is administered IV for short-duration analgesia as part of premedication, balanced anesthesia, induction and maintenance of anesthesia, and for postoperative pain. When given IV, it has an immediate onset of action, and its analgesic effects last about 60 minutes. It may be administered with droperidol to produce neurolept analgesia. As an anesthetic it may be administered with oxygen in high-risk patients, such as those undergoing open heart surgery or certain complicated neurologic or orthopedic procedures.

Since its approval in 1968 as an IV anesthetic, fentanyl has been introduced in multiple formulations, including oral (PO) tablets (Fentora), buccal film (Onsolis), sublingual tablets (Abstral), transmucosal lozenges (Actiq), and transdermal patches (Duragesic). All of these nonanesthetic formulations of fentanyl are prescribed for the management of breakthrough pain in patients who are already receiving and who are tolerant to around-the-clock opioid therapy for their chronic, persistent pain. Opioids such as fentanyl will result in tolerance if taken in high drug dosages over an extended time. Doses need to be adjusted periodically for adequate pain management. Physical and psychological dependence may occur with continued use. Abrupt discontinuation of the drug may cause intense withdrawal symptoms (see Chapter 27). Fentanyl is a Schedule II controlled substance. When taken illegally, fentanyl gives the same effects as heroin.

Mechanism of Action: Fentanyl is an opioid agonist at the mu and kappa receptors. The mechanism of action is the same as that of morphine and other opioids. Fentanyl has a more rapid onset of action than morphine.

TABLE 26.2 Intravenous Anesthetics

Drug	Route and Adult Dose (Maximum Dose Where Indicated)	Adverse Effects
Opioids		
alfentanil (Alfenta)	IV: 8–20 mcg/kg for surgery lasting longer than 30 min Maintenance anesthesia: 3–5 mcg/kg in incremental doses Continuous infusion: 0.5–1 mcg/kg/min Total dose: 8–40 mcg/kg	*Skeletal muscle rigidity, nausea, vomiting, postoperative drowsiness, shivering, HTN, bradycardia, prolonged QT interval, constipation* <u>Apnea, respiratory depression, laryngospasm, bronchospasm, circulatory depression, cardiac arrest, respiratory depression, respiratory arrest, anaphylactoid reaction</u>
fentanyl with droperidol	Droperidol: 2.5 mg IV; additional doses of 1.25 mg as needed Fentanyl: 2–20 mcg/kg IV; additional doses of 25–100 mcg as needed	
remifentanil (Ultiva)	IV: 0.5 mcg/kg/min or 1 mcg/kg IV bolus	
sufentanil (Sufenta)	IV: 1–8 mcg/kg; may give additional doses of 10–50 mcg if needed Primary anesthetic: 1–30 mcg/kg IV administered with 100% oxygen	
Benzodiazepines		
diazepam (Valium)	IV: 5–10 mg, repeat every 10–15 min as needed	*Drowsiness, hypotension, tachycardia, retrograde amnesia* <u>Cardiovascular collapse, respiratory arrest, laryngospasm</u>
midazolam (Versed)	Premedication: 0.15–0.25 mg/kg IV over 20–30 sec Nonpremedicated: 0.3–0.35 mg/kg IV over 20–30 sec	
Miscellaneous IV Anesthetics		
etomidate (Amidate)	IV: 0.2–0.6 mg/kg over a period of 30–60 sec for induction	*Pain on injection, transient skeletal muscle movements* <u>Changes in ventilation (hyper or hypo) and blood pressure (hyper or hypo)</u>
fospropofol (Lusedra)	IV: 6.5 mg/kg followed by supplemental doses of 1.6 mg/kg as needed	*Paresthesia, pruritus* <u>Respiratory depression, hypoxemia, hypotension</u>
ketamine (Ketalar)	IV: 1–4 mg/kg IM: 6.5–13 mg/kg	*Respiratory depression, laryngospasm, apnea, nausea, vomiting* <u>HTN, tachycardia, vivid dreams, hallucinations, delirium</u>
methohexital (Brevital)	IV: For induction: 1–1.5 mg/kg at a rate of 1 mL every 5 sec	*Postoperative psychomotor impairment, retrograde amnesia, hypothermia, sloughing with extravasation, skeletal muscle hyperactivity* <u>Circulatory depression, respiratory depression, respiratory arrest, apnea, anaphylaxis</u>
propofol (Diprivan)	IV: 2–2.5 mg/kg every 10 sec until induction onset	*Pain at injection site, skeletal muscle movements* <u>Dysrhythmias, hypotension</u>

Note: Italics indicate common adverse effects. <u>Underline</u> indicates serious adverse effects.

Pharmacokinetics:

Route(s)	IV, intramuscular (IM), transdermal, transmucosal, epidural
Absorption	Rapid
Distribution	Crosses the placenta; secreted in breast milk; 80% bound to protein
Primary metabolism	Hepatic (CYP3A4)
Primary excretion	Renal
Onset of action	IV: immediate; IM: 7–15 min; transdermal: 24–72 h peak; transmucosal: 20–30 min peak; epidural: 10–15 min
Duration of action	IV: 0.5–1 h; IM: 1–2 h; transdermal: 17-h half-life; transmucosal: unknown; epidural: 2–3 h

Adverse Effects: The most common adverse effects of fentanyl include respiratory depression, apnea, skeletal muscle rigidity, and bradycardia. The peak respiratory depression occurs 5 to 15 minutes after an IV dose. The respiratory depression, however, will continue postoperatively and outlast the analgesic effects of the drug. Nausea, vomiting, and constipation are common adverse effects produced by most opioids. Transdermal patches can cause localized pain, irritation, ulceration, and bleeding. **Black Box Warning:** Fentanyl has significant abuse potential and should not be prescribed to patients with a high risk for misuse, abuse, or diversion. The drug carries a high risk for death due to overdose or respiratory depression.

Contraindications/Precautions: Patients with respiratory impairment should be administered fentanyl with caution due to the respiratory depression caused by the drug. Patients with hepatic or renal impairment should receive lower doses. The drug may worsen bradydysrhythmia. Patients with head trauma should not receive fentanyl because intracranial pressure may increase. Fentanyl is secreted in breast milk and can cause sedation and respiratory depression in the neonate; thus it should not be administered during lactation.

Drug Interactions: Caution should be used when administering fentanyl with other central nervous system (CNS) depressants due to additive sedation. Fentanyl is metabolized by CYP450 enzymes (CYP3A4) in the liver and intestinal mucosa and has the potential to interact with other drugs that induce or inhibit this enzyme. Cardiovascular depression may occur if nitrous oxide is used with high doses of fentanyl. **Herbal/Food:** St. John's wort may intensify or prolong the effects of fentanyl anesthesia and may induce the metabolism of fentanyl via CYP3A4. Use of valerian or kava may cause additive CNS depression.

Pregnancy: Categories B (parenteral) and C (transdermal and transmucosal forms).

Treatment of Overdosage: In the event of overdosage, the patient is supported with mechanical ventilation until the drug is metabolized and the effects diminish. The patient may be administered a narcotic antagonist such as naloxone (Narcan) to reverse serious respiratory depression.

Nursing Responsibilities: Key nursing implications for patients receiving fentanyl are included in the Nursing Practice Application for Patients Receiving General Anesthesia in this chapter and in the Nursing Practice Application for Patients Receiving Pharmacotherapy for Pain in Chapter 25.

Drugs Similar to Fentanyl (Sublimaze)

Additional opioid IV general anesthetics include alfentanil, remifentanil, and sufentanil.

Alfentanil (Alfenta): Approved in 1996, alfentanil is an opiate agonist that has a more rapid onset and a shorter duration of action than fentanyl. It is administered IV to provide analgesia as a component of balanced anesthesia. Uses include assisting in intubation, promoting the induction of anesthesia, and as an infusion for the maintenance of anesthesia. A labeled indication is for the management of severe postoperative pain when given by the epidural route. The most common adverse effects are respiratory depression, nausea, vomiting, and muscle rigidity. Respiratory depression may be delayed; thus the patient should be monitored for some time after surgery. Alfentanil must be used with caution with other CNS depressants. Other actions and adverse effects are the same as those for fentanyl.

Remifentanil (Ultiva): Approved in 1996, remifentanil is an IV opioid that is similar to fentanyl. It is rapidly metabolized, which allows for a shorter duration of respiratory depression than fentanyl. Recovery from anesthesia occurs 5 to 10 minutes after discontinuation of the drug. This agent is administered during the induction and maintenance of general anesthesia to provide analgesia during the postoperative period. Although it does not produce deep anesthesia, remifentanil may be used alone or in combination with midazolam in monitored anesthesia care. Hypotension is greater with remifentanil than with fentanyl. Respiratory depression, pruritus, sweating, nausea, and vomiting

are other adverse effects. Other actions and adverse effects are the same as those for fentanyl.

Sufentanil (Sufenta): Approved in 1984, sufentanil is an IV opioid used as a component of balanced anesthesia or as a primary anesthetic agent. As a primary anesthetic the patient should be administered 100% oxygen. During IV use, the onset of action is immediate and recovery time is comparable to that of fentanyl. It is sometimes administered with bupivacaine as an epidural anesthesia adjunct during labor and delivery. During epidural use, the onset of action is about 10 minutes and recovery time is 1.7 hours. Sufentanil is 5 to 10 times more potent than fentanyl. The most common adverse effects are respiratory depression and muscle rigidity, and the drug must be used with caution with other CNS depressants.

CONNECTION Checkpoint 26.1

In pain management, opioids are often available in fixed dose combinations with nonopioids. From what you learned in Chapter 25, what is the rationale for using a nonopioid analgesic with an opioid? What specific nonopioid analgesic is most frequently found in these combination drugs? *See Answer to Connection Checkpoint 26.1 on student resource website.*

26.5 Benzodiazepines are used in anesthesia to produce relaxation, sedation, and amnesia.

The primary indication for benzodiazepine use is to treat symptoms of anxiety (see Chapter 18). For anesthesia, drugs in this class are used at high doses to cause sedation and induce unconsciousness. Benzodiazepines are a component of balanced anesthesia, most often administered in combination with inhalation anesthetics to allow the patient to feel less anxiety and experience amnesia. They may be administered PO as a premedication to relax the patient prior to minor medical procedures. The most commonly utilized benzodiazepine for surgical procedures is midazolam (Versed). Diazepam (Valium) and lorazepam have a slower onset and longer duration than midazolam and are occasionally used as anesthesia adjuncts. A detailed discussion of benzodiazepines is found in Chapter 22, along with a prototype feature for diazepam. Doses for the two benzodiazepines used as IV anesthetics are listed in Table 26.2.

PROTOTYPE DRUG | **Midazolam (Versed)**

Classification: **Therapeutic:** IV anesthetic
Pharmacologic: Benzodiazepine, gamma aminobutyric acid (GABA) receptor agonist

Therapeutic Effects and Uses: Approved in 1985, midazolam is administered to reduce the anxiety and stress associated with surgery. It is approved by the U.S. Food and Drug Administration (FDA) for the induction of amnesia, induction and maintenance of general anesthesia, and sedation prior to short diagnostic procedures such as an endoscopy. Off-label uses include status epilepticus that is refractory to other drugs and for sedation of mechanically ventilated patients. Midazolam syrup is indicated for use in children to produce sedation, anxiolysis, and amnesia prior to minor medical procedures or induction of anesthesia.

Induction of anesthesia occurs in 1 to 2 minutes following an IV bolus of midazolam. If the patient has received an opioid premedication, induction is even more rapid. Awakening and complete recovery of memory occurs in about 2 hours but may extend to 6 hours in older adults or those with heart failure or hepatic impairment.

Midazolam is a Schedule IV controlled substance. It has abuse potential similar to that of other benzodiazepines.

Mechanism of Action: Midazolam acts at the limbic, thalamic, and hypothalamic regions of the brain to produce CNS depression and skeletal muscle relaxation. This is the same mechanism of action as other benzodiazepines.

Pharmacokinetics:

Route(s)	IV, IM, PO
Absorption	Rapid absorption
Distribution	Widely distributed; crosses the blood–brain barrier and the placenta; secreted in breast milk; 97% protein bound
Primary metabolism	Hepatic
Primary excretion	Renal
Onset of action	IV: 1.5 min; IM: 5–15 min; PO: 10–30 min
Duration of action	IV/IM/PO: 2–6 h

Adverse Effects: Respiratory depression and apnea are potentially serious adverse events. CNS adverse effects include drowsiness, fatigue, ataxia, slurred speech, and tremor. Potentially serious cardiovascular effects include hypotension, tachycardia, and cardiovascular collapse. Laryngospasm is the most severe pulmonary complication noted with the administration of midazolam. Paradoxical reactions such as hyperactivity or aggressive behavior have been reported in pediatric patients and in those with preexisting psychiatric disorders. **Black Box Warning:** Respiratory depression and arrest have occurred with midazolam use. Respiratory status must be continuously monitored and resuscitative equipment must be readily available.

Contraindications/Precautions: Patients who have acute, narrow-angle glaucoma should not be administered midazolam because the drug may increase intraocular pressure. Patients experiencing shock, coma, or depressed vital signs should not be administered benzodiazepines because the drug may worsen these conditions.

Drug Interactions: The administration of benzodiazepines with any medication that depresses the CNS, including alcohol, increases the patient's risk for sedation. Use of benzodiazepines and phenytoin (Dilantin) will result in an increased serum phenytoin level and additive CNS depression. Midazolam is metabolized by hepatic CYP3A4 enzyme, and inhibitors or inducers of this enzyme may interact with midazolam. **Herbal/Food:** Increased sedation may occur if benzodiazepines are administered with kava or valerian. Grapefruit juice may increase the serum concentration of midazolam. Melatonin should be avoided because it may increase the actions of benzodiazepines.

Pregnancy: Category D.

Treatment of Overdose: Overdose with midazolam causes sedation, confusion, diminished reflexes, and coma. General supportive measures should be taken, and the patient may be treated with flumazenil (Romazicon), which is a specific benzodiazepine antagonist. Flumazenil acts within minutes but may induce seizures with rapid reversal.

Nursing Responsibilities: Key nursing implications for patients receiving midazolam are included in the Nursing Practice Application for Patients Receiving General Anesthesia in this chapter and in the Nursing Practice Application for Patients Receiving Pharmacotherapy for Anxiety or Sleep Disorders in Chapter 18.

Drugs Similar to Midazolam (Versed)

The only other benzodiazepine administered to produce anesthesia is diazepam.

Diazepam (Valium): Diazepam has been widely prescribed for anxiety and as an adjunct in seizure management. In the surgical suite diazepam is used as a premedication (by the IM route) for relief of anxiety associated with the surgical procedure. It is used by the IV route prior to cardioversion for the relief of anxiety and tension and to produce amnesia. When administered parenterally, it has an onset of action of 1 to 5 minutes and produces short-acting effects. Diazepam decreases the patient's anxiety and relaxes the skeletal muscles. Diazepam impairs the patient's ability to remember the perioperative events. A prototype feature for diazepam may be found in Chapter 22.

CONNECTION Checkpoint 26.2

Benzodiazepines are sometimes used for seizure control. From what you learned in Chapter 22, what are the indications for lorazepam and diazepam in treating seizures? *See Answer to Connection Checkpoint 26.2 on student resource website.*

26.6 Propofol and ketamine are widely used intravenous drugs for inducing and maintaining anesthesia.

Several miscellaneous drugs are used as parenteral anesthetics. Propofol (Diprivan) and ketamine (Ketalar) are two of the widely used IV anesthetics. The two drugs are not related chemically, but both have short durations and can induce anesthesia rapidly. Fospropofol (Lusedra) is a newer IV anesthetic with actions nearly identical to those of propofol. Etomidate (Amidate) and methohexital (Brevital) are much less frequently used in balanced anesthesia. Doses for these drugs are listed in Table 26.2.

PROTOTYPE DRUG	Propofol (Diprivan)

Classification: **Therapeutic:** IV anesthetic, sedative–hypnotic drug
Pharmacologic: N-methyl-D-aspartate (NMDA) receptor agonist

Therapeutic Effects and Uses: Approved in 1989, propofol has become the most widely used IV anesthetic due to its effectiveness and relative safety profile. It is indicated for the induction and maintenance of general anesthesia. In the intensive care unit (ICU), the drug may be administered to intubated, mechanically ventilated adult patients to provide continuous sedation and control of stress responses. It has an almost immediate onset of action and is used effectively for conscious sedation. Emergence from anesthesia is rapid, and few adverse effects occur during recovery. Unlike other anesthetics that cause nausea and vomiting, propofol has an antiemetic effect that can prevent nausea and vomiting in patients receiving chemotherapy. Off-label uses include refractory migraines, refractory status epilepticus, and the treatment of agitation associated with alcohol withdrawal.

Mechanism of Action: The exact mechanism by which propofol produces anesthesia is not clear. It is believed to act by activating GABA receptors, which causes a general inhibition of CNS activity.

Pharmacokinetics:

Route(s)	IV
Absorption	Rapid
Distribution	Widely distributed to body tissues; highly protein bound
Primary metabolism	Hepatic
Primary excretion	Renal
Onset of action	Immediate
Duration of action	IV: 10–15 min

Adverse Effects: Injection site pain, apnea, respiratory depression, and hypotension are common adverse effects. Propofol has been associated with a collection of metabolic abnormalities and organ system failures, referred to as propofol infusion syndrome (PIF). The syndrome is characterized by severe metabolic acidosis, hyperkalemia, lipemia, rhabdomyolysis, hepatomegaly, and cardiac and renal failure. PIF is usually associated with prolonged, high-dose infusions of the drug. Deaths have resulted from this syndrome.

Contraindications/Precautions: Propofol is contraindicated in patients who have a known hypersensitivity reaction to the medication or its emulsion, which contains soybean and egg products. The emulsion supports rapid microorganism growth; unused portions must be discarded. Obstetric patients and those with increased intracranial pressure should not be administered propofol. The drug should be used with caution in patients with cardiac or respiratory impairment. It is not recommended for induction of anesthesia in children younger than 3 years. Although not a controlled substance, incidences of propofol abuse have occurred, including the high profile case of Michael Jackson, a famous musician, who used this medication (among others) to induce sleep.

Drug Interactions: The dose of propofol should be reduced in patients receiving preanesthetic medications such as opioids or benzodiazepines. Use with other CNS depressants can cause additive CNS and respiratory depression. **Herbal/Food:** Unknown.

Pregnancy: Category B.

Treatment of Overdose: Overdosage will produce cardiac and respiratory depression. The treatment includes mechanical ventilation of the patient, increasing the flow rate of IV fluids, and administering vasopressor agents as needed to maintain blood pressure.

Nursing Responsibilities: Key nursing implications for patients receiving propofol are included in the Nursing Practice Application for Patients Receiving General Anesthesia.

Drugs Similar to Propofol

Other miscellaneous IV anesthetics include etomidate, ketamine, and methohexital. Thiopental sodium (Pentothal) was the gold standard for IV anesthetics for over 70 years. The sole U.S. manufacturer of this drug decided to discontinue the drug in the United States in 2010, likely because of the popularity, effectiveness, and relative safety of propofol.

Etomidate (Amidate): Approved in 2007, etomidate is a hypnotic drug indicated for the IV induction of general anesthesia for short medical–surgical procedures such as cardioversion, endotracheal intubation, or reduction of dislocations. It is also approved to supplement anesthesia produced by low-potency drugs such as nitrous oxide. It has a very rapid onset of action and hypotension is uncommon. It provides only 5 to 10 minutes of anesthesia. A major adverse effect is that it suppresses corticosteroid synthesis and can cause dangerous adrenal insufficiency if used for long periods. Concurrent use of opioids or benzodiazepines can worsen this suppression. This drug is pregnancy category C.

Fospropofol (Lusedra): Fospropofol was approved in 2008 for use as a sedative–hypnotic in patients undergoing diagnostic or surgical procedures. Fospropofol is a prodrug: It is immediately converted into propofol following IV injection. As such, the two drugs have nearly identical actions. Fospropofol has an onset of action of about 4 minutes, compared to propofol, which is nearly immediate. It also has a more prolonged time to awakening. The most common adverse effects are pruritus and paresthesia. Fospropofol is a Schedule IV controlled substance. This drug is pregnancy category B.

Ketamine (Ketalar): Approved in 1970, ketamine is an IV anesthetic that was initially used in veterinary medicine. It is a rapid-acting drug that produces a trance-like feeling of being separated from the environment called **dissociative anesthesia**. When used alone, ketamine is indicated during surgeries and brief diagnostic procedures that do not require skeletal muscle relaxation. It is also used prior to the administration of other general anesthetic agents. Ketamine is used with pediatric patients due to its rapid induction of general anesthesia and the fact that it lasts up to 25 minutes. Ketamine has strong analgesic actions and immediately increases blood pressure and skeletal muscle tone. The patient's eyes may be open during the surgical procedure.

Ketamine is a common drug of abuse that is known under the names of jet, super acid, Special K, green K, and cat Valium. It is a club drug that is similar to phencyclidine (PCP), which is popular among teens and young adults. It is easily added to drinks or administered through injection to cause temporary amnesia and is sometimes referred to as a date rape drug (see Chapter 27). Potentially serious cardiovascular adverse effects of ketamine include hypertension (HTN) and tachycardia. Respiratory depression occurs with the administration of IV ketamine. The most serious neurologic adverse effect is emergence phenomena in adult patients, which can occur for 24 hours postoperatively. Emergence phenomena include delirium, hallucinations, confusion, excitement, and irrational behavior.

Methohexital (Brevital): Approved in 2001, methohexital is a barbiturate general anesthetic agent that can be used to induce general anesthesia or administered as a continuous IV infusion. It is also approved to supplement anesthesia produced by low-potency drugs such as nitrous oxide. Like other IV anesthetics, it has a rapid onset, a short duration of action, and a relatively fast recovery period. IM and rectal forms are available for use in children. Severe adverse reactions include respiratory depression, laryngospasm, and hypotension. Adverse CNS effects may persist for 24 hours and include confusion, delirium, somnolence, anxiety, and seizures. Other adverse events include shivering, nausea, vomiting, and anaphylaxis. Methohexital is a Schedule IV controlled substance. Details on the mechanisms of action of barbiturates and their applications as sedatives may be found in Chapter 18. This drug is pregnancy category B.

Inhalation Anesthetics

26.7 Inhalation anesthetics used to produce loss of consciousness are classified as gases or volatile liquids.

Following the administration of IV agents, inhalation anesthetics are given to rapidly produce unconsciousness and total analgesia. Inhalation anesthetics are supplied as gases or volatile liquids. These drugs produce their effects on the CNS by inhibiting the flow of sodium into neurons, which delays the nerve impulses and dramatically reduces the activity of the neurons. Although the mechanism of action is incompletely understood, inhibitory GABA receptors in the brain become active and are thought to be responsible for the anesthetic action. This action is similar to that of the antiepileptic medications described in Chapter 22. Other CNS neurotransmitters likely contribute to the sedative effects of the inhalation anesthetics.

The first general anesthetic was the gas diethyl ether, which was discovered in the 1840s. Although popular for over 100 years, gaseous anesthetics were explosive and presented a danger to the surgical team members, who were exposed to fumes from the drugs. Furthermore, the gases produced a very high incidence of nausea and vomiting following the procedure. The only gaseous anesthetic in use today is nitrous oxide.

The potency of inhalation anesthetics is described by the **minimum alveolar concentration**: the concentration of drug vapor in the alveoli that prevents a motor response in 50% of subjects when exposed to a painful stimulus. A low value of minimum alveolar concentration indicates that a very small amount of anesthetic is needed to immobilize the patient. Inhalation anesthetics have low minimum alveolar concentrations and are thus very potent. The exception is nitrous oxide, which is a low-potency anesthetic with a high minimum alveolar concentration value. The minimum alveolar concentration changes with the age of the patient. It is lowest in newborns, peaks in infants, and gradually declines with age.

Inhalation anesthetics are rapidly absorbed from the alveoli into the general circulation. The anesthesiologist controls the length and depth of anesthesia by delivering the exact concentration of drug needed to maintain a desirable degree of immobility. These drugs are very lipid soluble and quickly cross the blood–brain barrier to produce sedating effects. Metabolism of inhalation anesthetics is minimal, and elimination of the drug is mostly by exhalation. Modern anesthetics are designed to have a fast recovery time so that the patient regains consciousness soon after the infusion is stopped. Because anesthetics are lipid soluble, they are stored in fat and slowly released, which explains why obese patients may take longer to recover from anesthesia.

CONNECTIONS | **Evidence-Based Practice**

◀ Malignant Hyperthermia and Anesthetic Agents

Clinical Question
Can a risk for malignant hyperthermia be predicted?

Evidence
Malignant hyperthermia is a rare but potentially fatal condition that occurs when a susceptible individual receives certain "triggering" medications (e.g., succinylcholine) during anesthesia. A genetic predisposition to malignant hyperthermia has been discovered. Patients with preexisting musculoskeletal conditions, especially those that are genetically linked, may be at greater risk, even if the true incidence of malignant hyperthermia occurring in these populations is unknown. Researchers are also beginning to investigate the existence of specific genes that could then be used to develop testing for susceptibility, rather than utilize patient history or muscle-core biopsy. Because there may be several or many different gene variants involved, DNA testing is not yet definitive (Stowell, 2014). It has also been noted that the onset of malignant hyperthermia is different for different anesthetic agents. Patients given the anesthetic halothane had earlier onset of malignant hyperthermia than those given other anesthetics when succinylcholine was used concurrently (Visolu, Young, Wieland, & Brandom, 2014).

Implications
The nurse plays a key role in assessing a patient for possible malignant hyperthermia risk during the preoperative period. Existing myopathies or unusual heat-associated illnesses in a child or adult should be noted and

the anesthesiologist or anesthetist alerted. A personal or immediate-family history of problems with previous anesthetic use should also be noted. Symptoms of malignant hyperthermia often begin with unexplained tachycardia. Jaw muscle spasms and rigidity may occur, followed by a dramatic increase in body temperature, rhabdomyolysis indicated by dark brown-colored urine, dysrhythmias, and potential death.

Any patient experiencing mild spasms in the jaw muscles must be observed more closely for development of malignant hyperthermia for at least 10 hours postprocedure. Fevers that occur in the postanesthesia care unit (PACU) or after the patient is discharged are not usually associated with malignant hyperthermia, especially if more than 2 hours have elapsed since the anesthetic was given. Patients with darkened urine or with severe jaw rigidity should be hospitalized overnight postoperatively to observe for the development of malignant hyperthermia.

Critical Thinking Questions
1. Why is it important for the nurse to ask about a patient's family surgical history before the administration of anesthesia?
2. What symptoms would concern the nurse if they develop in the immediate postoperative period?

See Answers to Critical Thinking Questions on student resource website.

PROTOTYPE DRUG	Nitrous Oxide

Classification: Therapeutic: Gaseous general anesthetic
Pharmacologic: GABA-receptor agonist, opioid agonist

Therapeutic Effects and Uses: Nitrous oxide is an odorless, nonirritating, inorganic gas used for a large number of medical and surgical procedures. When administered alone it is one of the least potent anesthetics and is unable to induce deep anesthesia at therapeutic doses. Because of its low potency, the use of nitrous oxide is either limited to minor surgical procedures or combined with the IV anesthetic agents for more complex procedures. The majority of patients requiring sedation for dental, diagnostic, and surgical procedures are administered nitrous oxide.

One major advantage of nitrous oxide is that it has strong analgesic properties. At a concentration of 20%, nitrous oxide delivers analgesic efficiency equaling that of morphine. This agent has a low potency and does not produce loss of consciousness or profound skeletal muscle relaxation.

Nitrous oxide is always combined with oxygen (25% to 30%) and is administered in a semiclosed method. The patient may be administered an IV anesthetic to produce sedation. When drowsy or asleep, the patient inhales the nitrous oxide through a tube or by mask. Nitrous oxide is also used for dental procedures in which the mask is placed over the nose. Other procedures in which nitrous oxide is administered include those related to obstetrics and surgery. Nitrous oxide lowers the minimum alveolar concentration of other anesthetics, essentially making them more potent. This permits a decrease in the dosages required for IV and inhalation anesthetics.

Nitrous oxide has been used illegally to produce relaxation, euphoria, and hallucinations. Abusers may steal the nitrous oxide tanks from medical facilities. The gas has also been used as a propellant in whipped cream canisters and cooking sprays, and abusers can obtain small amounts from those sources. Long-term abuse can lead to anemia, depletion of vitamin B_{12}, tinnitus, and peripheral neuropathy.

Mechanism of Action: The mechanism of action of nitrous oxide is not fully known. Its analgesic effects are believed to be due to activation of opioid receptors in the midbrain. The relaxation properties of the drug are likely due to activation of GABA receptors, which inhibits neuronal firing.

Pharmacokinetics:

Route(s)	Inhalation
Absorption	Rapid
Distribution	Crosses the blood–brain barrier to concentrate in the nerve cells
Primary metabolism	Not metabolized
Primary excretion	100% through the lungs, unchanged
Onset of action	2–5 min
Duration of action	Half-life is variable; peak effect: less than 10 min

Adverse Effects: When administered in low to moderate doses, nitrous oxide produces few adverse effects. When administered in higher doses, patients exhibit some adverse effects of stage 2 anesthesia such as anxiety, excitement, and combativeness. Lowering the inhaled dose quickly reverses these adverse effects. Because nitrous oxide is exhaled, the patient may temporarily have some difficulty breathing at the end of the procedure.

Rapid diffusion of the gas from the bloodstream back into the lungs causes alveolar hypoxia, with symptoms that include nausea, vomiting, lethargy, and dizziness. Some patients describe these symptoms as equivalent to a "hangover" from too much alcohol consumption. Alveolar hypoxia can be prevented by breathing 100% oxygen for several minutes following the conclusion of nitrous oxide therapy.

Contraindications/Precautions: Because patients must be awake and follow the instructions of the physician or dentist, nitrous oxide is contraindicated in those with an impaired level of consciousness or an inability to comply with instructions. Because the diffusion of nitrous oxide may lead to expansion of closed spaces, its use in patients with conditions such as undiagnosed abdominal pain, abdominal distention, bowel obstruction, head injury, and pneumothorax is contraindicated. Patients who have hypotension, shock, chronic obstructive pulmonary disease, cyanosis, or chest pain should not be administered nitrous oxide.

Drug Interaction: The administration of adrenergic agonists (such as epinephrine) or caffeine with nitrous oxide may exacerbate dysrhythmias. Use with CNS depressants may cause additive sedation and respiratory depression. Excessive hypotension may result if amiodarone or antihypertensive drugs are used concurrently with nitrous oxide. **Herbal/Food:** Milk thistle taken before and after anesthesia may lower the potential risk of liver damage. St. John's wort should be discontinued 2 to 3 weeks prior to administration of general anesthetics due to possible hypotension risk.

Pregnancy: Category C.

Treatment of Overdose: Effects of the drug usually diminish quickly after the gas is discontinued. Metoclopramide (Reglan) or another antiemetic agent may be administered to reduce the nausea and vomiting associated with nitrous oxide.

Nursing Responsibilities: Key nursing implications for patients receiving nitrous oxide are included in the Nursing Practice Application for Patients Receiving General Anesthesia.

Drugs Similar to Nitrous Oxide
Nitrous oxide is the sole gaseous general anesthetic.

26.8 Volatile liquid general anesthetics are used to induce and maintain deep anesthesia.

The volatile liquids form a second class of inhalation anesthetics. The volatile liquid drugs have a low vapor pressure that allows them to vaporize (form a gas) at low temperatures and pressures. An anesthesia machine is used to vaporize the liquid, mix the vapors with oxygen and air, and deliver them to patients in precisely controlled amounts. The anesthesia machine also establishes a partial pressure gradient that ensures the anesthetic will continue to flow from the machine to the alveoli, to the blood, and eventually to the brain. Like the gases, the volatile liquid anesthetics are

TABLE 26.3 Inhalation Anesthetics

Drug	Adult Concentration	Adverse Effects
Gas		
nitrous oxide	70% with 30% oxygen	*Anxiety*
		Malignant hyperthermia, nausea, vomiting
Volatile Liquids		
desflurane (Suprane)	7.3% concentration	Laryngospasm, hypotension, apnea, increased secretions, vasodilation, respiratory depression, tachycardia, malignant hyperthermia, nausea, vomiting
enflurane (Ethrane)	0.5–3% concentration	
isoflurane (Forane)	0.1–2% concentration	
sevoflurane (Ultane)	0.5–3% concentration	

Note: *Italics* indicate common adverse effects. Underline indicates serious adverse effects.

lipid soluble and rapidly cross the blood–brain barrier to cause sedation.

Desflurane (Suprane), isoflurane (Forane), and sevoflurane (Ultane) are the most widely used of the volatile liquid anesthetics. All of these drugs have a rapid onset of action.

The minimum alveolar concentrations of the volatile liquid anesthetics are very low, making them very potent. This factor contributes to the ability of these drugs to rapidly produce unconsciousness at low doses. Although they have the ability to produce deep anesthesia, they produce little analgesia and are usually used in combination with nitrous oxide and opioids as part of balanced anesthesia.

Some volatile liquid anesthetics sensitize the heart to the action of catecholamines such as epinephrine, norepinephrine, and dopamine and can cause serious dysrhythmias. These drugs also depress cardiovascular and pulmonary function, placing the patient at risk for laryngospasm or respiratory arrest. The gaseous and volatile liquid anesthetics are listed in Table 26.3.

PROTOTYPE DRUG | Isoflurane (Forane)

Classification: **Therapeutic:** Inhaled general anesthetic
Pharmacologic: GABA and glutamate receptor agonist

Therapeutic Effects and Uses: Approved in 1979, isoflurane has become a preferred inhalation anesthetic due to its effectiveness and favorable safety profile. Isoflurane provides smooth and rapid induction of general anesthesia with a low degree of metabolism by the body. It is almost entirely eliminated through respirations. The drug provides excellent muscle relaxation. It is FDA approved for the induction and maintenance of general anesthesia and may be used off-label as adjuvant therapy in the treatment of status asthmaticus.

Isoflurane does not sensitize the myocardium for dysrhythmias, and it produces fewer cardiovascular effects than other general anesthetics. Isoflurane does not cause the hepatotoxicity observed with halothane.

Mechanism of Action: The exact mechanism of action of isoflurane is unknown. It interacts with multiple receptors in the brain, including glutamate and GABA receptors.

Pharmacokinetics:

Route(s)	Inhalation
Absorption	Rapidly absorbed by the lungs
Distribution	Crosses the blood–brain barrier to concentrate in neurons; unknown if it is secreted in breast milk
Primary metabolism	Minimal metabolism
Primary excretion	95% pulmonary
Onset of action	7–10 min for surgical anesthesia
Duration of action	Patient begins to regain consciousness less than 1 h after drug is discontinued

Adverse Effects: Mild nausea, vomiting, and tremor are common adverse effects. The drug produces a dose-dependent respiratory depression and a reduction in blood pressure. Malignant hyperthermia with elevated temperature and unstable blood pressure has been reported, although the incidence is rare.

Contraindications/Precautions: Patients with a known history or genetic predisposition to malignant hyperthermia should not use isoflurane. Caution should be used when treating patients with head trauma or brain neoplasms due to possible increases in intracranial pressure. Safety has not been established in patients under age 18. Elderly patients are more susceptible to the cardiovascular effects of the drug. Patients with a prolonged QT interval should be administered isoflurane with caution.

Drug Interactions: Coughing, breath holding, or laryngospasm may occur when used concurrently with nitrous oxide. Skeletal muscle weakness, respiratory depression, or apnea may occur if isoflurane is administered concurrently with systemic polymyxin or aminoglycosides. Additive effects can occur if isoflurane is administered with other skeletal muscle relaxants. Additive hypotension may result if used concurrently with antihypertensive medications such as beta-adrenergic blockers. Epinephrine, norepinephrine, dopamine, and other adrenergic agonists should be administered with caution because of the possibility of dysrhythmias. Levodopa should be discontinued 6 to 8 hours before isoflurane administration. Isoflurane should be administered with caution with other drugs that prolong the QT interval, such as amiodarone, ibutilide, droperidol, and phenothiazines.
Herbal/Food: St. John's wort should be discontinued 2 to 3 weeks

prior to administration of general anesthetics due to possible hypotension risk.

Pregnancy: Category C.

Treatment of Overdose: Isoflurane causes profound respiratory depression. The patient is treated symptomatically until the effects of the drug diminish.

Nursing Responsibilities: Key nursing implications for patients receiving isoflurane are included in the Nursing Practice Application for Patients Receiving General Anesthesia.

Drugs Similar to Isoflurane (Forane)

Volatile liquid anesthetics similar to isoflurane include desflurane, enflurane, and sevoflurane. Halothane (Fluothane), the historical prototype for this drug class, was voluntarily removed from the market due to a small incidence of fatal hepatitis associated with the drug.

Desflurane (Suprane): Desflurane, approved in the 1990s, produces a rapid induction of general anesthesia. It is administered to induce and maintain anesthesia in adults. When administered to children it is used to maintain anesthesia. Adverse effects of desflurane are laryngospasm, apnea, and increased pulmonary secretions. The drug produces a dose-dependent reduction in blood pressure, and malignant hyperthermia has been reported. Desflurane must be used with IV anesthetics because it may cause coughing and excitation during induction. It does not sensitize the myocardium for dysrhythmias. This is a pregnancy category B drug.

Enflurane (Ethrane): Approved in 1972, enflurane is administered for induction and maintenance of general anesthesia, usually in conjunction with other agents as a component of balanced anesthesia. It is approved for obstetric anesthesia. It has strong muscle relaxant properties. It does not sensitize the myocardium for dysrhythmias, and postanesthesia nausea, vomiting, and CNS stimulation are uncommon. When administered in high concentrations, however, it can cause seizures and is thus contraindicated in patients with a history of seizure disorders. Rare cases of malignant hyperthermia have been reported, and enflurane is contraindicated in patients with a history of this disorder. This is a pregnancy category B drug.

Sevoflurane (Ultane): Approved in 1995, sevoflurane is a volatile liquid general anesthetic agent that is administered to induce and maintain sedation. It has a faster uptake, distribution, and elimination than isoflurane. It also does not cause the cardiovascular reactions commonly encountered with some of the other general anesthetics, and it is safer to use in patients with coronary artery disease. Sevoflurane does not cause respiratory irritation and is safe for administration with children. Furthermore, this drug does not cause coughing and excitation during induction and can thus be used without IV anesthetics. Sevoflurane produces a dose-dependent reduction in blood pressure, and malignant hyperthermia has been reported. This is a pregnancy category B drug.

PharmFACT

Each year in the United States, anesthesia is reported as the underlying cause of death in approximately 34 patients. The greatest cause of death is attributed to overdose of anesthetic (Li, Warner, Lang, Huang, & Sun, 2009).

Local Anesthetics

26.9 Local anesthetic agents block pain transmission in peripheral nerves and are grouped in two major classes.

Local anesthesia results in the loss of sensation to a small, limited area of the body. The primary advantage of local anesthesia is that pain relief can be provided without causing generalized depression of the CNS and respiratory systems. The nausea, vomiting, tremors, and anxiety associated with general anesthetic recovery are avoided. The types of adverse events associated with local anesthesia are relatively minor relative to the potential risks of general anesthesia.

Several techniques are used to deliver local and regional anesthesia. The method employed is dependent on the location and extent of the desired anesthesia (Figure 26.1):

- **Topical (surface) anesthesia.** The drug is applied or sprayed directly on the surface of the skin or mucous membrane. The anesthesia does not penetrate into deeper skin layers. This is used to provide relief for minor skin irritations or prior to needlesticks.

- **Infiltration anesthesia.** The drug is injected into deeper skin layers and travels to surrounding regions. This provides pain relief during minor skin surgeries or dental procedures, or prior to deep needlesticks.

- **Nerve block.** The drug is injected surrounding a peripheral nerve and all regions innervated by the nerve lose sensation. This is used for dental procedures or for regional anesthesia.

- **Epidural anesthesia.** The drug is injected into the epidural space surrounding the spinal cord. The anesthetic blocks sensation to multiple nerve roots supplying limited regions of the chest, pelvis, abdomen, or limbs. It is used for urologic and obstetric procedures.

- **Spinal anesthesia.** The drug is injected into the cerebrospinal fluid, usually in the lumbar region. This procedure is used to block sensation to larger areas of the lower abdomen or pelvis.

Although safer than general anesthetics, the health care provider has less control over the onset and duration of drug action with local anesthetics. The onset of local anesthesia is dependent on the drug's ability to diffuse from the application site to the surrounding nerves. In general, local anesthetics are small, lipid-soluble molecules that can move quickly through tissues and spaces to enter neurons. Local anesthetics are nonselective; they will block transmission at all types of sensory nerves. The sense of sharp pain is usually affected first, followed by other senses such as warmth, cold, touch, and pressure. Motor fibers are also affected by local anesthetics.

Termination of local anesthetic action depends on blood flow to the region. Local blood vessels carry the drug away from the application site to the systemic circulation, where it is metabolized and excreted. Usually only minimal systemic effects are observed because absorption into the general circulation is slow and the drug is sufficiently diluted by the blood.

The duration of anesthetic action may be extended by injecting a vasoconstrictor such as epinephrine in combination with the local anesthetic. The epinephrine reduces blood flow to the region and slows absorption of the anesthetic. This not only extends the

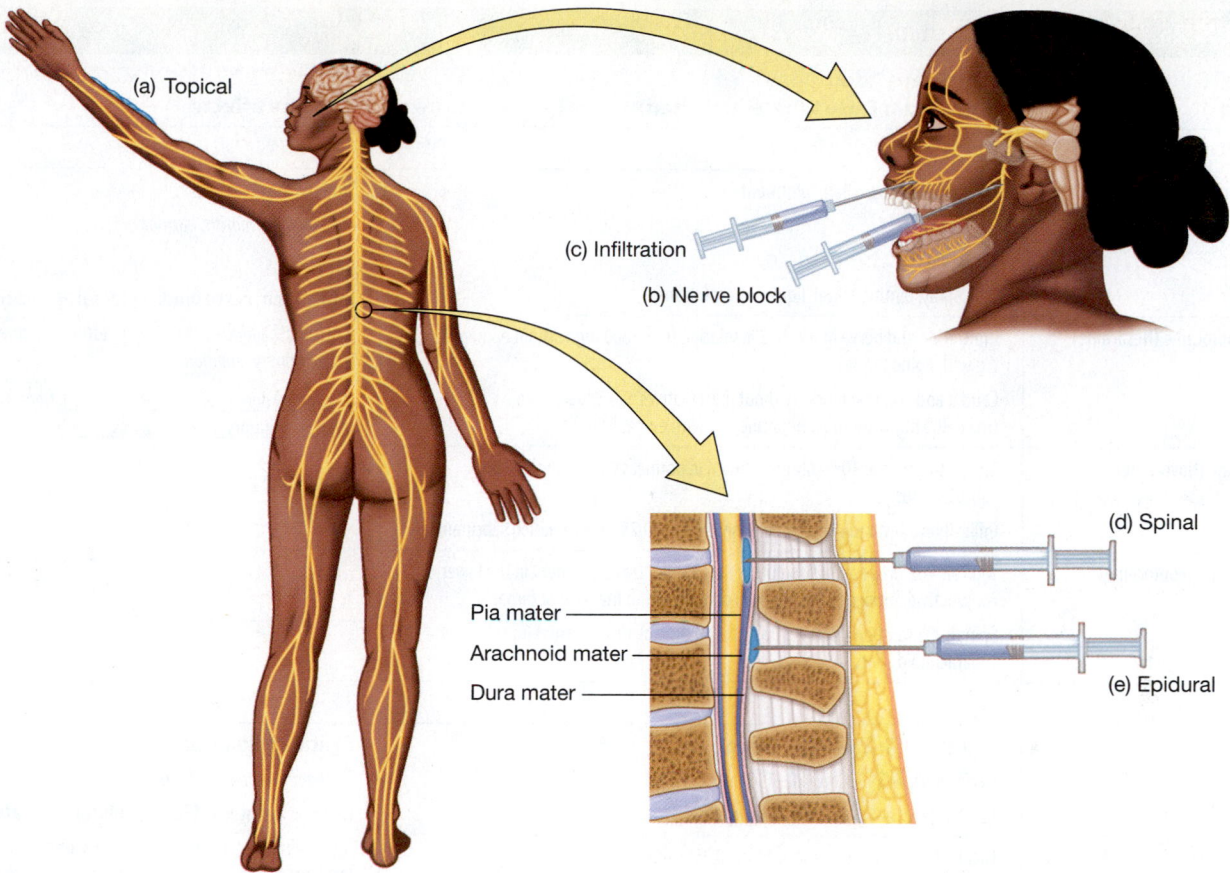

Figure 26.1 Techniques for applying local anesthesia: (a) topical; (b) nerve block; (c) infiltration; (d) spinal; (e) epidural.

duration of anesthesia, it also prevents the anesthetic from reaching the circulation too quickly, which could result in systemic toxicity. The amount of epinephrine used in local anesthesia is very small and it is released very slowly into the systemic circulation; therefore, adverse effects from the epinephrine are rare.

The two major classes of local anesthetics are named by their chemical structures: esters and the amides. The two classes differ primarily by their incidence of allergic reactions, with the amide type having the lower incidence. Although they vary in time of onset and duration of action, most local anesthetics have equivalent effectiveness. The local anesthetics are listed in Table 26.4.

26.10 Ester-type local anesthetics have been widely used for topical and spinal anesthesia.

Cocaine was the first local anesthetic to be widely used for medical procedures. Cocaine is a natural ester found in the leaves of the *Erythroxylum coca*, a plant native to the Andes Mountains in Peru. Cocaine was discovered by a German chemist in 1855 and ultimately used in 1884 as a topical eye anesthetic. Although still approved by the FDA as a local anesthetic, cocaine is a Schedule II controlled substance and is rarely used because of its high potential for abuse. In 1904 a German chemist named Einhorn discovered

---

CONNECTIONS Treating the Diverse Patient

◖ Postoperative Cognitive Dysfunction After Noncardiac Surgery

Postoperative cognitive dysfunction (POCD) has been noted after cardiac surgery. Symptoms include transient confusion and declines in cognitive skills such as word recall, word learning, and memory. POCD also occurs after other types of surgeries as well. Evered, Scott, Silbert, and Maruff (2011) conducted a study of patients undergoing coronary artery bypass graft (CABG) and total hip joint replacement (THJR), then followed these patients over the next 3 months. At 7 days postoperative, older adult patients had a higher incidence of POCD after CABG than THJR, but at 3 months postoperative, there was no significant difference noted and the incidence of POCD seemed to be independent of type of surgery. Cardiovascular risk factors in either group were not found to be predictive of POCD. These findings support previous studies such as by Monk et al. (2008), which concluded that advancing age is a risk factor for POCD and may have an impact on surgical mortality in the first postoperative year.

Monitoring brain function during surgery may help prevent POCD by allowing for lower doses of anesthetic. Chan, Cheng, Lee, and Gin (2013) found that intraoperative monitoring and analyzing of brain function by EEG allowed for titration of anesthetic agents to maintain a constant level of brain function, and lower rates of POCD were noted. The use of anesthetic agents was able to be reduced by up to 27%.

TABLE 26.4   Local Anesthetics

Drug	Route and Adult Dose (Maximum Dose Where Indicated)	Adverse Effects
Ester Type		
benzocaine (Americaine, Anbesol, Solarcaine, others)	Topical: 5% spray, cream, ointment 6% cream 8% lotion 20% spray, ointment, gel, liquid, otic solution	**Topical applications:** *erythema, dermatitis, burning* Anaphylaxis **Infiltration, nerve block, epidural applications:** *Postspinal headache, sedation, paresthesia, blurred vision, urinary retention* Myocardial depression, anaphylactic reactions, cardiac arrest, respiratory arrest, seizures, fetal bradycardia
chloroprocaine (Nesacaine)	Infiltration and nerve block: 1–2% solution (max: 800 mg without epinephrine, 1 g with epinephrine) Caudal and epidural block (without preservatives): 2–3% solution (max: 800 mg without epinephrine, 1 g with epinephrine)	
procaine (Novocaine)	Spinal anesthesia: 10% solution diluted in normal saline at 1 mL/5 sec subcutaneous Infiltration anesthesia or peripheral nerve block: 0.25–0.5% solution subcutaneous	
tetracaine (Pontocaine)	Topical: 1–2 drops of 0.5% solution or 1.25–2.5 cm of ointment in the lower conjunctival fornix or 0.5% solution or ointment to the nose or throat Spinal: 1% solution diluted with equal volume of 10% dextrose injected in the subarachnoid space	
Amide Type		
articaine (Septocaine, Zorcaine)	Infiltration: 0.5–2.5 mL (20–100 mg) Nerve block: 0.5–3.4 mL (20–136 mg) Oral surgery: 1–5.1 mL (40–204 mg)	**Topical applications:** *Erythema, dermatitis, burning* **Infiltration, nerve block, epidural applications:** *Hypersensitivity, dizziness, drowsiness, urinary retention, fecal incontinence, slowing of labor, numbness of lips or tongue, hypotension, blurred or double vision* Laryngeal edema, bradycardia, anaphylactoid reaction, respiratory arrest, seizures, rectal bleeding (dibucaine)
bupivacaine (Exparel, Marcaine, Sensorcaine)	Local infiltration, sympathetic block: 0.25% solution Epidural, caudal, or retrobulbar block: 0.25%–0.75% solutions Liposomal (Exparel): 8–20 mL of 1.3% solution	
dibucaine (Nupercainal)	Topical: Apply to skin 1 ounce every 24 h	
lidocaine (Anestacon, Dilocaine, Xylocaine, others)	Infiltration: 0.5–1% solution Nerve block: 1–2% solution Epidural: 1–2% solution Caudal: 1–1.5% solution Spinal: 5% solution with dextrose Saddle block: 1.5% with dextrose Topical: 2.5–5% jelly, ointment, cream, or solution	
mepivacaine (Carbocaine, Isocaine, Polocaine)	Subcutaneous: 1–5 cartridges, each containing approximately 1.8 mL (54 mg) of a 3% solution	
prilocaine	Subcutaneous: 1–2 mL (40–80 mg) of a 4% solution	
ropivacaine (Naropin)	Surgical anesthesia: Intrathecal administration: Epidural: 25–200 mg (0.5–1% solution) Nerve block: 5–250 mg (0.5–0.75% solution) Labor pain: 20–40 mg (0.2% solution) Postoperative pain management: Epidural: 12–20 mg/h (0.2% solution) Infiltration: 2–200 mg (0.2–0.5% solution)	

Note: Italics indicate common adverse effects. Underline indicates serious adverse effects.

Patients Receiving General Anesthesia

Assessment	Potential Nursing Diagnoses*
Baseline assessment prior to administration: • Obtain a complete health history including cardiovascular, respiratory, hepatic, renal, or neurologic disease, pregnancy, or breast-feeding. Obtain a drug history including allergies, current prescription and OTC drugs, herbal preparations, caffeine, nicotine, and alcohol use. Be alert to possible drug interactions. • Assess for previous history of anesthesia and note any significant reactions. Obtain family history of anesthesia problems, particularly related to use of neuromuscular blockers (e.g., succinylcholine), or any unusual effects related to surgery. • Obtain baseline vital signs, height, and weight. Note day/hour the patient last ate or drank. • Evaluate laboratory findings appropriate to the procedure (e.g., CBC, electrolytes, hepatic or renal function studies, MRI or CT scan results). • Obtain required preoperative paperwork (e.g., informed consent, completed history and physical). • Administer any preoperative adjunctive drugs (e.g., sedative, analgesic) as ordered. • Assess the level of anxiety, and any concerns or questions the patient, family, or caregiver may have. Reinforce preoperative teaching, including deep-breathing exercises. Provide the family or caregiver with information on the anticipated length of the procedure, the waiting room area, and telephone and cafeteria or food availability. • **Lifespan:** For pediatric patients, allow the parents or caregiver to stay with the child as long as agency policy permits to decrease patient anxiety. Provide a simple explanation of the procedure appropriate for the age of the child. • **Lifespan:** When working with older adults, note assistive devices (e.g., glasses, hearing aids) and remove only when necessary. Give to the family, caregiver, or provide for safekeeping. Ensure that devices are available in the postoperative period. • Initiate IV access site if required for the procedure. • Assess the patient's ability to receive and understand instructions. Include the family and caregiver as needed.	• *Anxiety* • *Impaired Gas Exchange* • *Ineffective Breathing Pattern*, related to drug effects • *Decreased Cardiac Output* • *Disturbed Sensory Perception* • *Nausea*, related to adverse drug effects • *Deficient Knowledge* (Drug Therapy) • *Risk for Injury*, related to adverse drug effects or diminished sensation and sensorium from the drug • *Risk for Infection*, related to adverse drug effects or contaminated drug solution (e.g., propofol)
Assessment throughout administration: • Assess for desired therapeutic effects (e.g., diminished level of consciousness). • Assess vital signs, especially blood pressure and pulse, frequently. Report blood pressure less than 90/60 mmHg, pulse above 100 beats/min, or per the parameters as ordered by the health care provider. • Maintain operative sterility throughout the procedure. • Assess level of consciousness in the postoperative period. Continue frequent monitoring of vital signs and pulse oximetry. • Assess for and promptly report adverse effects: bradycardia or tachycardia, hypotension or HTN, dysrhythmias, dyspnea, jaw muscle rigidity, or dark brown-colored urine.	

Implementation

Interventions and (Rationales)	Patient-Centered Care
Ensuring therapeutic effects: • Continue assessments as above for therapeutic effects. Provide for patient safety during preoperative and operative periods, and assess level of consciousness, vital signs, and return of motor and sensory sensation postoperatively. (Duration of anesthetic action will depend on the drugs used and adjunctive or reversal agents used.)	• Provide a quiet environment postoperatively, and frequently orient the patient to the PACU.
• Assess for shivering in the postoperative period and provide additional blankets or warmth as needed. (General anesthetics depress the CNS and some autonomic activity. As autonomic activity returns, shivering is common. Warm blankets provide comfort during this period.)	• Continue to orient the patient in the postoperative period, and allay anxiety about shivering.
Minimizing adverse effects: • Continue to monitor vital signs frequently, including temperature. Report blood pressure below 90/60 mmHg or per the parameters as ordered by the health care provider, tachycardia or significant bradycardia, dysrhythmias, or dyspnea. Report any jaw muscle rigidity or cola-colored urine and fever immediately. (CNS depression will cause decreases in all vital signs but significant bradycardia, hypotension, decreased respiratory rate, or dyspnea should be reported promptly. **Lifespan:** The older adult is more sensitive to the effects of anesthesia and may be more likely to experience adverse effects such as hypotension and delirium. Malignant hyperthermia associated with succinylcholine and some anesthetics is a rare but potentially fatal adverse effect. Early symptoms include unexplained tachycardia, jaw muscle spasms or rigidity, and cola-colored urine.)	• Explain all procedures and monitoring to the patient. Continue to reorient the patient to surroundings frequently in the postoperative period.

(continued)

• Provide adequate pain relief in the immediate postoperative period. (General anesthetics do not necessarily provide analgesia, dependent on the agent. Adequate pain relief begins ideally in the preoperative period. Assess for nonverbal signs of pain such as restlessness or grimacing as the patient regains consciousness.)	• Provide the rationale for pain relief preoperatively and encourage the patient to request pain medication as able. Assure the patient, family, or caregiver that pain needs will be frequently monitored.
• Encourage the patient to take deep breaths and move lower extremities frequently in the postoperative period. (General anesthetics given by inhalation are excreted via the lungs. Deep breathing assists in removing remaining anesthetic. Early range-of-motion exercises may help prevent venous thrombosis and complications.)	• Teach the patient deep-breathing exercises in the preoperative period, and that early movement of legs will be encouraged in the early postoperative period, unless otherwise ordered by the provider.
• Ensure patient safety in the postoperative period. Frequently orient the patient to surroundings, day, and time and maintain a safe environment. (During the period of anesthesia, consciousness is lost along with the ability to orient to day, time, and person. Confusion related to these effects in the postoperative period is common. Use of safety measures such as side rails may be necessary until the patient regains consciousness.)	
• For patients receiving ketamine and other drugs causing neurolept analgesia, provide a quiet, calm environment postprocedure. Avoid overstimulating the patient while taking vital signs. Use a soft touch and voice to explain all procedures performed. (During recovery from neurolept analgesia drugs, confusion and misinterpretation of sensory stimulation may cause extreme anxiety, fear, or paranoia. Keep all stimuli to a minimum until the patient regains full consciousness.)	• Explain the full procedure and required postprocedural care to the patient, family, or caregiver. Alert the family or caregiver that visiting may be restricted during the immediate recovery period in order to minimize sensory stimulation.
• **Lifespan and Diverse Patients:** Continue to monitor hepatic function. (Lifespan: Normal physiologic changes related to aging may increase the risk of toxicity in the older adult requiring drugs with hepatic metabolism. Diverse Patients: Because drugs such as fentanyl and midazolam are metabolized through the P450 system, they may result in less than optimum results based on differences in enzymes.)	• **Lifespan:** Monitor hepatic laboratory values pre- and postoperatively and report abnormalities. • **Diverse Patients:** Monitor for therapeutic and adverse effects frequently in ethnically diverse patients.
Patient understanding of drug therapy: • Use opportunities during the preoperative period to discuss the rationale for the drug therapy, desired therapeutic outcomes, commonly observed adverse effects, and any necessary monitoring or precautions. (Using time during nursing care helps to optimize and reinforce key teaching areas.)	• The patient should be able to state the reason for the drug(s), anticipated sensations, and adverse effects to observe for, and when to report them.
Patient self-administration of drug therapy: • When administering fentanyl for analgesia, instruct the patient, family, or caregiver in the proper self-administration of the drug. (Utilizing time during nurse-administration of these drugs helps to reinforce teaching.)	Teach the patient to take the medication: • Remove old fentanyl patches and dispose them safely because these may still contain some medications. • Apply the new fentanyl patch to clean, dry skin. Press firmly on the patch for 30 seconds to ensure proper skin contact. • Do not split, chew, or swallow the transmucosal or buccal forms of fentanyl.

*Nursing Diagnoses—Definitions and Classification 2015–2017. Copyright © 2014, 1994–2014 by NANDA International. Used by arrangement with John Wiley & Sons Limited.

procaine (Novocaine), which soon came into widespread use, especially in dental offices.

Esters act by decreasing the amount of sodium that enters the neuron, thereby depressing depolarization and preventing conduction of the pain impulse. Esters may be administered with epinephrine as a vasoconstrictor to limit blood loss at the surgical site and to decrease the amount of anesthetic absorbed systemically. The local anesthetic effect of an ester is rapid, occurring in 1 to 8 minutes. The duration ranges from 15 to 60 minutes.

Ester-type anesthetics are generally safe when applied as directed. All can cause serious CNS and cardiac toxicity, however, if they reach the blood in high concentrations. The first CNS symptoms may be stimulatory: anxiety, nervousness, dizziness, tremor, or seizures. Subsequent CNS depression may cause the patient to become drowsy, experience respiratory depression, and enter a coma. High amounts can cause dysrhythmias, QT prolongation, hypotension, and cardiac arrest. Care must be taken that the drug is administered correctly to prevent serious adverse effects.

<table>
<tr><td>PROTOTYPE DRUG</td><td>Procaine (Novocaine)</td></tr>
</table>

Classification: Therapeutic: Local anesthetic
Pharmacologic: Ester, sodium channel blocker

Therapeutic Effects and Uses: Procaine is used for spinal, epidural, and peripheral nerve blocks through injection or infiltration. It produces local anesthesia with loss of sensation close to the injection or application site. It has a short duration of action. An off-label use is for the treatment of severe pain due to cancer, herpes, or burns. Once used widely in dentistry, it has largely been replaced by other local anesthetics.

Procaine causes vasodilation, which could potentially increase its rate of absorption from tissues and cause systemic toxicity. Some procaine solutions contain small amounts of epinephrine, which constricts arteries to keep the procaine localized and prolong the anesthetic effect. The drug is rapidly metabolized to inactive metabolites by esterase, an enzyme found in the plasma. Once it reaches the plasma, the half-life of procaine is only 40 seconds.

Mechanism of Action: Procaine decreases the influx of sodium into the neuron, which increases the threshold for depolarization and prevents the conduction of the nerve impulse.

Pharmacokinetics:

Route(s)	Subcutaneous
Absorption	Rapid
Distribution	Not distributed; highly bound to plasma proteins
Primary metabolism	Metabolized by plasma esterase
Primary excretion	Renal: 80% as metabolites
Onset of action	2–5 min
Duration of action	1 h

Adverse Effects: With therapeutic doses, adverse effects are rare. Adverse events may occur, however, if multiple doses of procaine are administered or if it is injected intravascularly. The most severe adverse effects include respiratory arrest and anaphylaxis. A patient who has experienced an allergic reaction to procaine will likely be allergic to other esters. Myocardial depression may result in atrioventricular (AV) block dysrhythmias or cardiac arrest. CNS effects are stimulatory and usually transient; nervousness, dizziness, confusion, and tremor may occur. Spinal anesthesia with procaine can cause headache, palsies, spinal nerve paralysis, and meningism (nuchal rigidity, photophobia, and headache). Cutaneous lesions can occur in a delayed time frame. The caudal or epidural administration of procaine in the obstetric patient can result in urinary incontinence, loss of perineal sensation, slowing of labor, and increased incidence of forceps delivery.

Contraindications/Precautions: Patients who have experienced hypersensitivity to any ester anesthetic or agent containing para-aminobenzoic acid (PABA) should not receive procaine. Patients with generalized septicemia, inflammation, or sepsis should not be injected with procaine. It is also contraindicated in patients with heart block, hypotension, HTN, or altered coagulation. It should be used cautiously in elderly and acutely ill patients. Patients who have increased abdominal pressure should be administered procaine cautiously.

Drug Interactions: Ester anesthetics such as procaine may antagonize the antimicrobial effects of sulfonamides. There is an increased risk of hypotension when administered with antihypertensives. Procaine is incompatible with aminophylline, chlorothiazide, magnesium sulfate, phenobarbital, phenytoin, secobarbital, and sodium bicarbonate. **Herbal/Food:** Unknown.

Pregnancy: Category C.

Treatment of Overdose: The effects of procaine overdosage are treated symptomatically. Rapid systemic absorption will affect the cardiovascular system and could require cardiopulmonary resuscitation.

Nursing Responsibilities: Key nursing implications for patients receiving procaine are included in the Nursing Practice Application for Patients Receiving Local Anesthesia.

Drugs Similar to Procaine (Novocaine)

Other local anesthetic esters include benzocaine, chloroprocaine, and tetracaine.

Benzocaine (Americaine, Anbesol, others): Approved in 1938, benzocaine is an over-the-counter (OTC) local anesthetic ester applied topically as a lotion, cream, ointment, spray, gel, or otic solution. Chemically it is almost identical to procaine, but it has a prolonged duration of anesthetic action. It provides temporary relief of pain and discomfort due to sunburn, minor wounds, pruritus, serous otitis media, swimmer's ear, otitis externa, canker sores, sore throat, hemorrhoids, and anal fissures. It can be applied to the penis as a male desensitizer to slow the onset of ejaculation. Benzocaine preparations are commonly used as an anesthetic for the passage of catheters and endoscopic tubes. Onset of anesthetic action occurs in less than a minute and because absorption of benzocaine is minimal, systemic effects are rare. Contact dermatitis can occur and is more common with benzocaine than with some of the other topical anesthetics. Although rare, benzocaine sprays have been associated with serious methemoglobinemia, a condition in which hemoglobin is unable to bind sufficient oxygen. This drug is pregnancy category C.

Chloroprocaine (Nesacaine): Approved in 1957, chloroprocaine is a short-acting local anesthetic ester that is used for infiltration, epidural, and caudal anesthesia. It is not effective as a topical agent. Anesthesia occurs in 6 to 12 minutes and can last up to 90 minutes if epinephrine is added to the injection. A test dose is given before epidural use to assess for intravascular or subarachnoid injection. In the event of intravascular injection, the patient would experience an epinephrine response with tachycardia, circumoral pallor, palpitations, and nervousness. Signs of subarachnoid injection include motor paralysis and extensive sensory anesthesia. Like other ester anesthetics, allergic reactions such as rash, pruritus, and anaphylaxis are possible. This drug is pregnancy category C.

Tetracaine (Pontocaine): Tetracaine is a local anesthetic ester that is used in spinal anesthesia and topically. It may be used to anesthetize the conjunctiva during eye surgery and in the nose and throat to eliminate the laryngeal and esophageal reflexes. It is administered on the skin to relieve pruritus, pain, and burning. An OTC preparation (Viractin) is available for topical treatment of pain associated with cold sores and fever blisters. Onset of action is rapid for topical use (3 to 10 minutes) but longer following spinal administration (15 minutes). Of the topical anesthetics, tetracaine is the most likely to cause skin sensitivity, including rash, erythema, pruritus, burning, and edema. Systemic absorption can cause significant CNS and cardiac toxicity. Tetracaine is contraindicated in patients who are hypersensitive to ester-type anesthetics, sulfites, or PABA. This drug is pregnancy category C.

26.11 Local anesthetics from the amide class have a lower incidence of adverse effects than those from the ester class.

Amide-type local anesthetics have largely replaced the administration of drugs from the ester class. The amides produce less effect on myocardial contractility, and the incidence of allergic reactions is lower. Amides and esters have the same mechanism of action: decreasing the sodium flux into the neuron, thus inhibiting the initial depolarization and conduction of the nerve impulse. Whereas the esters are inactivated by the enzyme esterase in the plasma, the amides are metabolized by hepatic CYP450 enzymes. Caution should be exercised when administering large amounts of amide anesthetics to patients with hepatic impairment.

PROTOTYPE DRUG | **Lidocaine (Anestacon, Dilocaine, Xylocaine, Others)**

Classification: Therapeutic: Local anesthetic
Pharmacologic: Amide, sodium channel blocker

Therapeutic Effects and Uses: Lidocaine is a local anesthetic that has a prompt onset of action of 2 to 5 minutes. It has a longer duration of action than procaine, lasting 10 to 90 minutes, depending on its route of administration. It may be administered as a surface and infiltration anesthetic agent to block the nerve. It is also used in caudal and spinal block anesthesia to relieve local discomfort of the skin and mucous membranes. Lidocaine patches are administered to relieve pain related to postherpetic neuralgia (Lidoderm) or dental procedures (DentiPatch). Parenteral lidocaine is administered to treat life-threatening ventricular dysrhythmias (see Chapter 37). In 2007 the FDA approved Zingo (lidocaine hydrochloride monohydrate), which is a needle-free intradermal injection system. Zingo is indicated for rapid local anesthesia for procedures such as IV insertions or blood draws.

Mechanism of Action: Lidocaine blocks the conduction of action potentials by reducing the sodium permeability, thus decreasing the action potential and slowing nerve conduction.

Pharmacokinetics:

Route(s)	Subcutaneous, IM, IV, IV bolus; topical
Absorption	Topical absorption: 3% through intact skin
Distribution	Crosses the blood–brain barrier and the placenta; secreted in breast milk
Primary metabolism	Hepatic via CYP3A4 and 2D6
Primary excretion	Renal
Onset of action	IV: 45–90 sec; IM: 5–15 min; topical: 2–5 min
Duration of action	IV: 10–20 min; IM: 60–90 min; topical: 30–60 min
	Half-life: 1.5–2 h

Adverse Effects: When used topically, adverse reactions to lidocaine are uncommon. Mild and transient reactions at the site of application include erythema, pruritus, dermatitis, and burning. The transoral DentiPatch may cause alterations in taste, headache, and gingivitis. Should the drug be accidentally injected intravascularly, CNS adverse effects will be those of stimulation (anxiety, tremors, shivering, and seizures) followed by depression (drowsiness, respiratory depression, and coma). Cardiovascular effects include hypotension, dysrhythmias, cardiovascular collapse, and cardiac arrest.

Contraindications/Precautions: Patients who have experienced a hypersensitivity reaction to amide-type local anesthetics should not be administered lidocaine. Topical lidocaine should not be applied to seriously damaged skin from trauma, burns, or eczema.

Other precautions apply to patients receiving parenteral lidocaine, although these also apply to situations in which the drug is accidentally injected intravascularly. Patients who have been diagnosed with Stokes-Adams syndrome, untreated sinus bradycardia, or sinoatrial, AV, or intraventricular heart block should not be administered lidocaine. The medications should be used cautiously in the presence of liver or kidney disease, myasthenia gravis, and hypovolemia as well as in debilitated patients and the elderly or when there is a family history of malignant hyperthermia.

Drug Interactions: Lidocaine patches can cause toxic effects with tocainide and mexiletine. Barbiturates decrease lidocaine activity. Increased pharmacologic effects of lidocaine will be noted if it is administered with cimetidine, beta blockers, or quinidine. **Herbal/Food:** After receiving transoral lidocaine, patients should not eat or drink until the effects of the anesthesia have worn off.

Pregnancy: Category B.

Treatment of Overdose: Overdose may occur if the drug is injected intravascularly. The patient is treated through symptom management.

Nursing Responsibilities: Key nursing implications for patients receiving lidocaine are included in the Nursing Practice Application for Patients Receiving Local Anesthesia.

Drugs Similar to Lidocaine (Anestacon, Dilocaine, Xylocaine, Others)

Other local anesthetic amides include articaine, bupivacaine, dibucaine, mepivacaine, prilocaine, and ropivacaine. The amides levobupivacaine (Chirocaine) and etidocaine (Duranest) have been removed from the U.S. market.

Articaine (Septocaine, Zorcaine): Approved in 2000, articaine is approved for administration by infiltration or by nerve block for dental procedures. It is unique because it has both an amide and an ester group. Anesthesia is rapid, occurring in 1 to 6 minutes, and lasts up to an hour. Articaine appears to diffuse through soft tissue and bone better than other local anesthetics. It is combined with epinephrine, which provides vasoconstriction and prolongs the duration of action. The adverse effects are the same as those of other amide anesthetics. This drug is pregnancy category C.

Bupivacaine (Exparel, Marcaine, Sensorcaine): Approved in 1972, bupivacaine is an amide local anesthetic that is used for infiltration anesthesia, peripheral sympathetic nerve, and epidural block. Bupivacaine in dextrose solution is administered for spinal anesthesia. Its 3- to 9-hour duration of action is one of the longest of any local anesthetic. In 2011 a liposomal form (Exparel) was developed that provides analgesia for up to 72 hours. The anesthetic is injected into the surgical area for procedures such as bunionectomy and hemorrhoidectomy. Adverse effects are similar to those of other amide anesthetics. This drug is pregnancy category C.

Dibucaine (Nupercainal): Approved in 1947, dibucaine is administered to relieve pain and itching related to hemorrhoids and other anorectal disorders. It is also administered to relieve discomfort from insect bites, sunburn, minor burns, cuts, and scratches. It is a long-acting amide anesthetic that inhibits the initiation and conduction of nerve impulses by reducing the permeability of nerve cells to sodium ions. It is available OTC. This drug is pregnancy category C.

Mepivacaine (Carbocaine, Isocaine, Polocaine): Approved in 1960, mepivacaine is an amide anesthetic used for infiltration, transtracheal anesthesia, and epidural nerve blocks in surgical and dental procedures. Onset of action is very rapid—less than a minute for the upper and lower jaws. Epidural onset is 7 to 15 minutes. This drug has an intermediate duration of action of 60 to 100 minutes for soft tissue and 115 to 150 minutes for epidural. Mepivacaine is sometimes combined with levonordefrin, a vasoconstrictor that prolongs the duration of action of the local anesthetic. The adverse effects are the same as those of other amide anesthetics. This drug is pregnancy category C.

Prilocaine (Citanest): Approved in 1965, prilocaine is used primarily for dental anesthesia via infiltration or nerve block. Onset of action is 2 minutes and its duration is 1 to 2 hours. The adverse effects are the same as those of other amide anesthetics. This drug is pregnancy category B.

Ropivacaine (Naropin): Ropivacaine is a newer local anesthetic agent approved in 1996 that is used in epidural anesthesia and postoperative pain management. It has an onset of action of 1 to 30 minutes and a duration of anesthetic action of 2 to 6 hours. It is important that disinfecting agents with heavy metal content not be used to disinfect the skin prior to the insertion of the epidural catheter because these have been associated with swelling and edema. Also, the container of ropivacaine should not be cleaned with a heavy metal disinfecting agent. Unlike most local anesthetics, the presence of epinephrine does not affect the systemic absorption of ropivacaine. Like other amide anesthetics, high serum concentrations may cause serious CNS and cardiac toxicity; care must be taken not to accidentally inject the drug intravascularly or intrathecally. This drug is pregnancy category B.

Adjuncts to Anesthesia

26.12 Adjunctive agents are used during the perioperative phase to enhance anesthesia or to treat the potential adverse effects of the anesthetics.

Surgery is often a stressful and painful procedure for patients. In addition, anesthetics dampen vital reflexes, which can lead to aspiration pneumonia. Diminished autonomic function can have serious adverse effects on the cardiovascular and gastrointestinal (GI) systems. Adjunctive medications are those used to enhance anesthesia or to make the procedure safer and less unpleasant for patients.

Preoperative medications: The most common preoperative symptom is anxiety. Oral benzodiazepines may be given for several days prior to a major procedure to lessen anxiety. Just prior to surgery, midazolam (Versed) may be administered parenterally to sedate the patient and to cause perioperative amnesia (see Section 26.5).

Aspiration pneumonia is a potentially serious problem during a surgical procedure because the patient may lose protective airway reflexes. Histamine (H_2) receptor antagonists such as ranitidine (Zantac) or famotidine (Pepcid) can reduce the possibility of aspiration pneumonia by decreasing gastric fluid volume and reducing acidity. For aspiration prophylaxis, the H_2 receptor antagonist may be given PO the night prior to surgery and by IV infusion an hour before the procedure. A drug prototype feature for ranitidine is found in Chapter 59.

Anticholinergics such as atropine may be administered prior to surgery to reduce salivary and airway secretions. Atropine also blocks the bradycardia caused by some anesthetics. The drug is given by the IM route 45 to 60 minutes prior to anesthesia. A prototype feature for atropine is presented in Chapter 14.

Pain management: Pain reduction is an important component of preanesthesia and postanesthesia care. Opioids are used when the pain is expected to be severe, but these drugs can cause significant respiratory depression. If the pain level is moderate or mild, nonsteroidal anti-inflammatory drugs (NSAIDs) are administered because they cause fewer serious adverse reactions than the opioids. Clonidine (Catapres, Duraclon) is a centrally acting alpha$_2$-adrenergic agonist that has been used to reduce severe pain associated with surgery. When administered epidurally Duraclon allows the dosages of the anesthetic and opioids to be reduced. The primary indication of clonidine is HTN (Catapres), but it has largely been replaced by safer antihypertensives (see Chapter 34).

Neuromuscular blockers: Skeletal muscle relaxation is an important component of general anesthesia. Insertion of an endotracheal tube would be difficult and painful without muscle relaxation, and contraction or spasticity of muscles during a surgical procedure could render some operations impossible. Complete paralysis of muscle is necessary for major surgical procedures. Although some of the general anesthetics do have mild to moderate ability to relax skeletal muscles, most are incapable of causing the degree of relaxation necessary for surgery.

It is important to note that neuromuscular blockers do not enter the CNS. Although these drugs cause muscle paralysis, they do not induce unconsciousness or provide analgesia. The patient is still able to feel pain and is aware of his or her surroundings.

The nondepolarizing neuromuscular blocking agents such as atracurium (Tracrium) and cisatracurium (Nimbex) have a short duration of action and bind competitively with acetylcholine to produce skeletal muscle relaxation. The depolarizing neuromuscular blocking agents such as succinylcholine (Anectine) are ultra-short acting and possess a high affinity for the acetylcholine receptor sites.

The neuromuscular blocking agents are very dangerous; the diaphragm and intercostal muscles are paralyzed and breathing requires a mechanical ventilator. Serious cardiovascular adverse effects are possible. Details of the actions, indications, and adverse effects of the neuromuscular blockers are included in Chapter 14. A prototype feature for succinylcholine is included in that chapter.

CONNECTION Checkpoint 26.3

Atropine and succinylcholine are both cholinergic blockers but they produce very different effects. From what you learned in Chapter 14, explain the mechanisms for the differences in pharmacologic actions. (*Hint:* One drug affects the muscarinic receptor and the other the nicotinic receptor.) *See Answer to Connection Checkpoint 26.3 on student resource website.*

CONNECTIONS: NURSING PRACTICE APPLICATION

Patients Receiving Local Anesthesia

Assessment	Potential Nursing Diagnoses*
Baseline assessment prior to administration: • Obtain a complete health history including cardiovascular, hepatic, renal, respiratory, or neurologic disease, pregnancy, or breast-feeding. Obtain a drug history including allergies, current prescription and OTC drugs, herbal preparations, caffeine, nicotine, and alcohol use. If the patient reports allergy to "caine" drugs, note the specific drug and reactions the patient experienced. Be alert to possible drug interactions. • Obtain baseline vital signs and weight. • Assess for areas of broken skin, abrasions, burns, or other wounds in the area to be treated with a local anesthetic. • Evaluate laboratory findings appropriate to the procedure (e.g., CBC, electrolytes, hepatic, or renal function studies). • Assess the patient's ability to receive and understand instructions. Include the family and caregivers as needed.	• *Acute Pain* • *Deficient Knowledge* (Drug Therapy) • *Risk for Aspiration*, related to drug effects • *Risk for Infection*, related to adverse drug effects • *Risk for Injury*, related to loss of sensation and function of anesthetized area or region from drug effects
Assessment throughout administration: • Assess for desired therapeutic effects (e.g., local or regional area numbness). • Assess vital signs, especially blood pressure and pulse, if regional block is used. Report a blood pressure less than 90/60 mmHg, pulse above 100 beats/min, or per the parameters as ordered by the health care provider. • Assess the local or regional area blocked. Expect blanching in the localized area if the local anesthetic contained epinephrine. If a regional area was blocked, periodically assess the patient's ability to move limbs distal to the block. • Assess level of consciousness if a large regional block was given. Report any increasing drowsiness, dizziness, lightheadedness, confusion, or agitation immediately. • Assess for and promptly report adverse effects: bradycardia or tachycardia, hypotension or HTN, or dyspnea.	

Implementation

Interventions and (Rationales)	Patient-Centered Care
Ensuring therapeutic effects: • Continue assessments as above for therapeutic effects. Assess the localized area for numbness and blanching if the local anesthetic included epinephrine. Assess the patient's ability to move limbs distal to the regional anesthetic. (Duration of anesthetic action will depend on the solution used and whether epinephrine is included in the solution. If a large regional area is blocked [e.g., epidural], the patient may regain some motor ability before sensation returns and the return of motor activity signals decreasing levels of anesthesia. An ability to perceive pressure-type sensations may remain during anesthesia and may be alarming to the patient. Epinephrine in the anesthetic solution will constrict localized blood vessels and result in blanching of the area.)	• Teach the patient that the area may be numb for several hours after the procedure is completed. • Teach the patient that it is normal that a slight pressure sensation may remain during anesthesia (e.g., sensation of "tugging" during suturing) but that no pain should be felt. Have the patient alert the health care provider if more than slight pressure sensation or any pain is noticed during anesthesia. • Teach the patient that it is normal to regain some ability to move limbs (e.g., after epidural anesthetic), and movement may return before the ability to feel the movement.
Minimizing adverse effects: • Continue to monitor vital signs, especially blood pressure and pulse, for patients given regional anesthesia. Report blood pressure below 90/60 mmHg or per the parameters as ordered by the health care provider, tachycardia, bradycardia, changes in level of consciousness, dyspnea, or decrease in respiratory rate, immediately. (Adverse effects of local anesthesia are rare. Regional blocks may cause hypotension with the possibility of reflex tachycardia. Be particularly cautious with older adults who are at increased risk for hypotension due to physiological changes related to aging or concurrent vasoactive drug use. Bradycardia, hypotension, decreased level of consciousness, decreased respiratory rate, and dyspnea may signal that the anesthesia has entered the systemic circulation and is acting as a general anesthetic.)	• Instruct the patient to report any increasing nausea, drowsiness, dizziness, light-headedness, confusion, or anxiety immediately. If dizziness occurs, the patient should sit or lie down and not attempt to stand or walk until the sensation passes.
• **Diverse Patients:** Continue to monitor hepatic function and drug effects. (Because amide anesthetics such as lidocaine are metabolized through the P450 system, they may result in less than optimum results based on differences in enzymes.)	• Teach ethnically diverse patients to observe and report effects of local anesthetic use to ensure therapeutic results.
• Caution the patient not to eat, chew gum, or drink until mouth sensation has returned if local (dental) or oral/throat anesthesia has been used. If throat anesthesia is used, assess gag reflex before eating. (Local anesthetics are effective for up to 3 h or more. Biting injuries to oral mucous membranes may occur while tissue is numb. Aspiration of food or liquids is possible until swallowing sensation and gag reflex return.)	• Instruct the patient to refrain from eating or drinking for 1 h or more post-anesthesia, or until sensation has completely returned to the oral cavity or throat.

CONNECTIONS: NURSING PRACTICE APPLICATION *(continued)*

• Ensure patient safety; monitor motor coordination and ambulation post-regional block until certain that motor movement is unaffected. **Lifespan**: Be particularly cautious with older adults who are at increased risk for falls. (Numbness or effects on motor ability post-regional anesthetic may impair movement and increase the risk of falls or injuries.)	• Instruct the patient to call for assistance prior to getting out of bed or attempting to walk alone post-epidural block, and to avoid driving or other activities requiring physical coordination (e.g., regional upper limb block) until residual effects of the drug are known.
• Assess areas of abrasion, burns, or open wounds if a local anesthetic is applied to area. (Large open or denuded areas may increase the amount of drug absorption into the general circulation. Use sterile technique to apply the drug to open areas.)	• Instruct the patient to report increased redness, swelling, or drainage from open areas under treatment.
• Read all labels carefully before using parenteral solutions. (Solutions containing epinephrine must *never* be used IV or for local anesthesia in areas of decreased circulation [e.g., fingertips, toes, earlobes, tip of nose, penile tissue] due to vaso-constrictive effects.)	• Provide an explanation of desired effects of the local anesthetic and the need for postprocedure monitoring.
• Monitor pain relief in patients post-regional block (e.g., epidural). (Pain sensation will increase as the regional block wears off. Additional pain relief may be required.)	• Teach the patient to report any discomfort or pain as anesthesia wears off.
Patient understanding of drug therapy: • Use opportunities during administration of medications and during assessments to discuss the rationale for the drug therapy, desired therapeutic outcomes, commonly observed adverse effects, parameters for when to call the health care provider, and any necessary monitoring or precautions. (Using time during nursing care helps to optimize and reinforce key teaching areas.)	• The patient should be able to state the reason for the drug, anticipated sensations, adverse effects to observe for, and when to report them.
Patient self-administration of drug therapy: • When administering the medication, instruct the patient, family, or caregiver in proper self-administration of drug, e.g., take the drug as prescribed when needed. (Utilizing time during nurse-administration of these drugs helps to reinforce teaching.)	• Teach the patient to take oral medication (e.g., lidocaine viscous) by swishing and spitting if used for oral cavity, or by gargling, and do not swallow unless directed by the health care provider. Apply topical medication in a thin layer to the skin area as directed.

*Nursing Diagnoses—Definitions and Classification 2015–2017. Copyright © 2014, 1994–2014 by NANDA International. Used by arrangement with John Wiley & Sons Limited.

Postoperative medications: Because many anesthetics induce severe nausea and vomiting in the postanesthesia phase, the administration of antiemetic drugs is indicated for prophylaxis in high-risk patients or for treatment. Several drugs have been used as antiemetics. Promethazine (Phenergan) is an older antiemetic that may be administered pre- or postoperatively. It has the advantage of also being a sedative; thus it can be used in the induction phase of anesthesia. Also an older medication, metoclopramide (Reglan), may be administered near the end of the surgical procedure for prophylaxis of postanesthetic nausea and vomiting. A newer and very effective antiemetic is ondansetron (Zofran, Zuplenz), a 5-HT$_3$ antagonist. Commonly used to prevent the acute nausea and vomiting caused by cancer chemotherapeutic agents, ondansetron may be injected just prior to chemotherapy or 30 minutes before the end of the surgical procedure.

CHAPTER
26 Understanding the Chapter

Key Concepts Summary

26.1 Anesthesia is used to produce a controlled loss of sensation during a diagnostic or surgical procedure.

26.2 Balanced anesthesia uses multiple drugs to provide for the safe induction and maintenance of general anesthesia.

26.3 Intravenous anesthetics include opioids, benzodiazepines, and several miscellaneous agents.

26.4 Opioids are used as intravenous anesthetics to provide analgesia and to accomplish neurolept anesthesia.

26.5 Benzodiazepines are used in anesthesia to produce relaxation, sedation, and amnesia.

26.6 Propofol and ketamine are widely used intravenous drugs for inducing and maintaining anesthesia.

26.7 Inhalation anesthetics used to produce loss of consciousness are classified as gases or volatile liquids.

26.8 Volatile liquid general anesthetics are used to induce and maintain deep anesthesia.

26.9 Local anesthetic agents block pain transmission in peripheral nerves and are grouped in two major classes.

26.10 Ester-type local anesthetics have been widely used for topical and spinal anesthesia.

26.11 Local anesthetics from the amide class have a lower incidence of adverse effects than those from the ester class.

26.12 Adjunctive agents are used during the perioperative phase to enhance anesthesia or to treat the potential adverse effects of the anesthetics.

Case Study: Making the Patient Connection

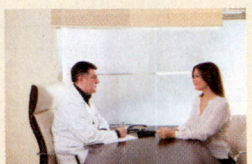

Remember the patient "Elena Moore" at the beginning of the chapter? Now read the remainder of the case study. Based on the information presented within this chapter, respond to the critical thinking questions that follow.

Elena is a 37-year-old woman who is scheduled for a vaginal hysterectomy after a positive Pap smear returned with results suggestive of cancer. While in the holding area of the operating room suite, she states that she is fearful of general anesthesia. The preoperative nurse caring for this patient notices that she is very anxious. Upon further assessment and conversation, she states that her mother died of breast cancer when she was young.

The patient's vital signs are as follows: blood pressure 138/88 mmHg, temperature 36.3°C (97.4°F), pulse 94 beats/min, and respiration 20 breaths/min. She denies pain and states that she is concerned she will wake up during the surgery. She is to receive balanced anesthesia.

Critical Thinking Questions

1. In your own words, how would you describe balanced anesthesia to Elena?

2. How does nitrous oxide differ from IV anesthetic agents?

3. How should the nurse educate a patient regarding the use of IV propofol?

See Answers to Critical Thinking Questions on student resource website.

Additional Case Study

Anthony Holiday is a 28-year-old steelworker for a heating and cooling company. While on the job he cut his right hand with a piece of steel for an air-conditioning vent. He is admitted to the emergency department for sutures to the right middle finger and palm. The laceration will be anesthetized with lidocaine prior to suturing.

1. What is the action of lidocaine?

2. Why is lidocaine preferred over procaine?

See Answers to Additional Case Study on student resource website.

Chapter Review

1 The surgical nurse becomes alerted that the patient who is receiving general anesthesia has become excitable and hyperactive with irregular heart and respiratory rates. The nurse knows that the patient has entered which stage of general anesthesia?

1. Stage 1
2. Stage 2
3. Stage 3
4. Stage 4

2 The nurse should question the administration of propofol (Diprivan) for which patient? An individual with:

1. Allergy to eggs or soy products.
2. Allergy to iodine.
3. Kidney disease.
4. Addison's disease.

3 During the administration of nitrous oxide, the patient develops anxiety, excitement, and combativeness. The nurse would anticipate what change in the patient's anesthesia is needed?

1. The nitrous oxide dose will be increased.
2. Propofol (Diprivan) will be given along with the nitrous oxide.
3. Succinylcholine (Anectine) will be given to the patient.
4. The nitrous oxide dose will be decreased.

4 The nurse is providing the patient, who will be receiving ketamine (Ketalar), with preoperative instructions. Which statement, if made by the patient, indicates that teaching is successful?

1. "The medication will decrease anxiety during surgery."

2. "I will experience increased energy due to this drug."

3. "I may experience a feeling of being separated from the environment."

4. "The drug will cause me to have dry mouth after the operation."

5 The patient who is having a scalp laceration sutured will be receiving local anesthesia with lidocaine (Xylocaine) that contains epinephrine. The nurse knows that the purpose of this drug combination is to:

1. Increase the duration of the anesthetic action.

2. Increase vasodilation at the site of the laceration.

3. Decrease blood pressure in individuals who are hypertensive.

4. Ensure that infection at the wound site will not occur.

6 Identify the general anesthetic agents that are parenteral opioid agents. Select all that apply.

1. Nitrous oxide

2. Alfentanil (Alfenta)

3. Sufentanil (Sufenta)

4. Regimental (Ultiva)

5. Succinylcholine (Anectine)

See Answers to Chapter Review in Appendix A.

References

American Association of Nurse Anesthetists. (2014). *Certified registered nurse anesthetists at a glance.* Retrieved from http://www.aana.com/ceandeducation/becomeacrna/Pages/Nurse-Anesthetists-at-a-Glance.aspx

Chan, M. T. V., Cheng, B. C. P., Lee, T. M. C., & Gin, T. (2013). BIS-guided anesthesia decreases postoperative delirium and cognitive decline. *Journal of Neurosurgical Anesthesiology, 25*(1), 33–42. doi:10.1097/ANA.0b013e3182712fba

Evered, L., Scott, D. A., Silbert, B., & Maruff, P. (2011). Postoperative cognitive dysfunction is independent of type of surgery and anesthetic.

Anesthesia & Analgesia, 112, 1179–1185. doi:10.1213/ANE. 0b013e318215217e

Li, G., Warner, M., Lang, B., Huang, L., & Sun, L. S. (2009). Epidemiology of anesthesia related mortality in the United States, 1999–2005. *Anesthesiology, 110,* 759–765. doi:10.1097/ALN.0b013e31819b5bdc

Monk, T. G., Weldon, B. C., Garvan, C. W., Dede, D. E., van der Aa, M. T., Hellman, K. M., & Gravenstein, J. S. (2008). Predictors of cognitive dysfunction after major noncardiac surgery. *Anesthesiology, 108,* 18–30. doi:10.1097/01.anes.0000296071.19434.1e

Osterman, M. J., & Martin, J. A. (2011). Epidural and spinal anesthesia use during labor: 27-state reporting area, 2008. *National Vital Statistics Reports, 59*(5), 1–16.

Stowell, K. M. (2014). DNA testing for malignant hyperthermia: The reality and the dream. *Anesthesia & Analgesia, 118,* 397–406. doi:10.1213/ANE.0000000000000063

Visolu, M., Young, M. C., Wieland, K., & Brandom, B. W. (2014). Anesthetic drugs and onset of malignant hyperthermia. *Anesthesia & Analgesia, 118,* 388–396. doi:10.1213/ANE.0000000000000062

Selected Bibliography

Bosslet, G. T., Devito, M. L., Lahm, T., Sheski, F. D., & Mathur, P. N. (2010). Nurse-administered propofol sedation: Feasibility and safety in bronchoscopy. *Respiration, 79*(4), 315–321. doi:10.1159/000271604

Burns, S. M. (2010). Local anesthetic toxicity. *Nursing 2011, 40*(2), 72. doi:10.1097/01.NURSE.0000367875.25886.c7

Dillane, D., & Finucane, B. T. (2010). Local anesthetic systemic toxicity. *Canadian Journal of Anesthesia/Journal canadien d'anesthésie, 57,* 368–380. doi:10.1007/s12630-010-9275-7

Herdman, T. H., & Kamitsuru, S. (Eds.). (2014). *NANDA International nursing diagnoses: Definitions and classification, 2015–2017.* Oxford, United Kingdom: Wiley-Blackwell.

Kuehn, B. M. (2011). FDA considers data on potential risks of anesthesia use in infants, children. *Journal of the American Medical Association, 305,* 1749–1753. doi:10.1001/jama.2011.546

Mayo Clinic. (2013). *Anesthesia.* Retrieved from http://www.mayoclinic.com/health/anesthesia/MY00100

Press, C. D. (2013). *General anesthesia.* Retrieved from http://emedicine.medscape.com/article/1271543-overview

Rooks, J. P. (2011). Safety and risks of nitrous oxide labor analgesia: A review. *Journal of Midwifery & Women's Health, 56,* 557–565. doi:10.1111/j.1542-2011.2011.00122.x

U.S. Drug Enforcement Administration. (2013). *Ketamine.* Retrieved from http://www.deadiversion.usdoj.gov/drug_chem_info/ketamine.pdf

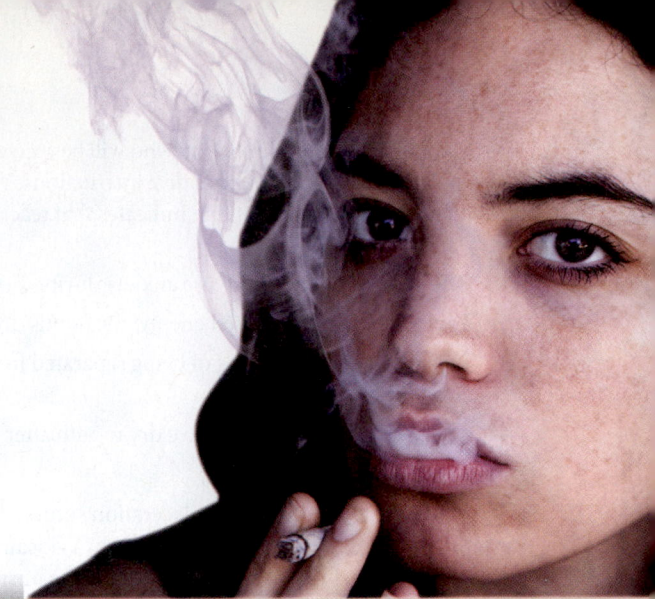

"I have been getting high since I was 14 years old. Do I need to stop just because I am pregnant?"

Patient "J. C. Wilkins"

LEARNING OUTCOMES

After reading this chapter, the student should be able to:

1. Describe the types of substances abused by individuals.

2. Identify the five drug schedules of controlled substances and give examples of drugs in each schedule.

3. Explain major legislation regulating controlled substances in the United States.

4. Identify factors contributing to addiction.

5. Compare and contrast physical and psychological dependence.

6. Compare and contrast withdrawal syndromes for the different classes of abused substances.

7. Discuss the significance of drug tolerance to pharmacology.

8. Explain the major characteristics of abuse, dependence, and tolerance resulting from use of the following substances: sedatives, opioids, alcohol, marijuana, hallucinogens, club drugs, amphetamines, methylphenidate, cocaine, caffeine, nicotine, inhalants, and anabolic steroids.

9. Identify the role of the nurse in recognizing, preventing, and treating substance abuse.

CHAPTER OUTLINE

▶ **Fundamental Concepts of Substance Abuse**
  Legislation of Controlled Substances
  Addiction and Dependence
  Tolerance
▶ **Central Nervous System Depressants**
  Sedatives and Antianxiety Drugs
  Opioids
  PROTOTYPE Buprenorphine with naloxone (Suboxone, Zubsolv), *p. 422*
  Alcohol (Ethanol)
  PROTOTYPE Disulfiram (Antabuse), *p. 426*
▶ **Marijuana and Related Substances**
▶ **Hallucinogens**
  LSD and Similar Hallucinogens
  Club Drugs and Miscellaneous Hallucinogens
▶ **Central Nervous System Stimulants**
  Amphetamines and Methylphenidate
  Cocaine
  Caffeine
▶ **Nicotine**
  PROTOTYPE Varenicline (Chantix), *p. 432*
▶ **Inhalants**
▶ **Anabolic Steroids**

KEY TERMS

addiction, 418

anterograde amnesia, 421

club drug, 428

controlled substances, 418

cross-tolerance, 420

delirium tremens, 425

hallucinogens, 427

opioids, 421

physical dependence, 419

psychological dependence, 419

rebound effects, 419

reticular formation, 429

sedatives, 421

substance abuse, 417

tachyphylaxis, 420

tetrahydrocannabinol (THC), 426

tolerance, 419

withdrawal syndrome, 419

Throughout history individuals have consumed both natural substances and therapeutic drugs to increase performance, assist with relaxation, induce spiritual visions, or to simply fit in with their peer group. **Substance abuse** is the self-administration of a drug in a manner that does not conform to the norms within the person's given culture or society. The term *substance abuse* is preferred over the term *drug abuse*, because some of these agents are not considered to be drugs by the users. With the 2013 publication of the *Diagnostic and Statistical Manual of Mental Disorders,* 5th edition ("DSM-5"), a newer term was introduced to describe this condition to avoid the term *abuse* entirely: *substance use disorder* (American Psychiatric Association, 2013). Because most nurses are still familiar with the term *substance abuse*, that term will continue to be used in this chapter for clarity.

This chapter introduces the types of drugs commonly abused by patients and the pharmacologic management of withdrawal syndromes.

Fundamental Concepts of Substance Abuse

27.1 A wide variety of different substances may be abused by patients.

Characteristics of substance abuse vary widely from drug to drug and person to person. Diagnosis of this disorder is often difficult, even for experienced health care providers. Recognition of abuse is relatively easy for substances such as heroin, cocaine, or hallucinogens. However, what about legal substances such as alcohol, tobacco or marijuana (in some states)? How many beers must one drink or cigarettes must one smoke before it is labeled as substance abuse? And with legal prescription drugs is it considered substance abuse if a patient continues to refill prescriptions, such as oxycodone, even after symptoms have resolved? It is apparent that, with the exception of certain illegal substances, there is often not a clear distinction among proper use, misuse, and substance abuse.

There are certain characteristics, however, that assist in the proper diagnosis of substance abuse. Nurses should be aware of these characteristics because they may be the first to recognize the following when obtaining a patient history.

- Craving for a specific substance despite an understanding that the substance is lowering the patient's quality of life (physical dependence)

- Failure to maintain normal work or home relationships because a substance is being used repeatedly

- Recognition that, over time, increased amounts of the substance are needed to produce the desired effect (tolerance)

- Repeated, unsuccessful attempts have been made to discontinue using the substance

- Recognition that behavioral changes occur when the substance is discontinued, such as agitation, drowsiness, anxiety, pain, etc. (withdrawal syndrome)

- Increased amount of time is devoted to obtaining or using the substance, which reduces time available for work, home, or leisure activities

Abused substances belong to a large number of diverse chemical classes. Although they have few structural similarities, most have in common the ability to affect the brain. In some cases, illicit drugs are taken to stimulate the brain, while others use drugs to sedate the brain or dull the sensation of pain. Still other substances, such as lysergic acid diethylamide (LSD), and club drugs, such as ecstasy, are used to provide alternative psychoactive experiences such as visions or hallucinations. An important exception is the anabolic steroids, which are used for their effects on the muscular system rather than the nervous system.

Although the public associates substance abuse with illegal drugs, this is not necessarily the case. Alcohol and nicotine are the two most commonly abused substances and both are legal for adults. In addition, legal prescription drugs, such as oxycodone (OxyContin), methylphenidate (Adderall), and alprazolam (Xanax), are frequent drugs of abuse. Marijuana is a frequently used drug, despite the fact it is illegal in most states.

Several drugs that were once used therapeutically are now illegal due to their high potential for abuse. Cocaine was once used as a local anesthetic, but today all the cocaine acquired by users is obtained illegally from South America. LSD is now illegal although it was briefly used in psychotherapy in the 1940s and 1950s. Phencyclidine (PCP) was popular back in the early 1960s as an anesthetic but was withdrawn from the market in 1965 due to patients reporting serious adverse effects while recovering from anesthesia. Many amphetamines once used for bronchodilation were discontinued in the 1980s after psychotic episodes were reported.

PharmFACT

As encouraging trends, the use of inhalants and cocaine among teens has been steadily declining and alcohol use is at historically low levels. However, marijuana use remains high, with 6.5% of 12th graders reporting daily use (National Institute on Drug Abuse, 2014).

Legislation of Controlled Substances

27.2 Drugs with a potential for abuse are restricted by the Controlled Substances Act and are categorized into schedules.

It is not surprising that drugs and other substances with abuse potential are highly regulated. Many of these substances can cause significant harm to the user and those surrounding the user when memory or performance becomes impaired. A significant percentage of motor vehicle and other accidents result from substance abuse. The government clearly has a role in protecting individuals and the public from such dangerous drugs. The Controlled Substances Act (CSA), the primary legislation establishing scheduled drugs, was presented in Chapter 2.

Diversion from legal medical use is a source of some of the abused drugs. Because of this, legislation has been enacted to closely track potential drugs of abuse from manufacturer to consumer. Prescription drugs may be stolen from pharmacies, health care provider offices, or patients, and sold illegally, sometimes at a very high profit. In some cases, health care workers who have the responsibility of dispensing or administering the medications conduct the theft.

Patients contribute to the diversion by faking or exaggerating their symptoms to obtain prescriptions for pain medication or sedatives. Some patients obtain the same prescription from several health care providers, commonly referred to as "doctor shopping," and sell their pills to substance abusers. Because of the multitude of ways that legal drugs can be diverted to abusers, the tracking of drugs with abuse potential must be closely monitored.

In the United States, **controlled substances** are classified according to their potential for abuse and toxicity. This classification uses five schedules, with Schedule I drugs having the highest potential for abuse (see Chapter 2). In recent years, a few exceptions have been made to the placement of drugs in the schedules. For example, gamma hydroxybutyrate (GHB) is used illegally as a club drug as a stimulant or aphrodisiac and is classified as a Schedule I drug that has "no therapeutic use." However, this same substance is approved to treat narcolepsy because the drug Xyrem is a Schedule III drug. As another example, marijuana is a Schedule I agent, yet several states have legalized its use for specific medical indications.

CONNECTION Checkpoint 27.1

Prior to the CSA, other attempts were made to legislate narcotics. From what you learned in Chapter 2, name the first major law in the United States that was passed in 1914 to control narcotic use and explain its major provisions. *See Answer to Connection Checkpoint 27.1 on student resource website.*

Addiction and Dependence

27.3 Addiction is an overwhelming compulsion to continue repeated drug use.

Addiction is an overwhelming compulsion that drives someone to repeat drug-taking behavior, despite serious health and social consequences. Why would someone continue to abuse drugs even when he or she is aware of its compelling negative consequences? The drug experience is highly personal for each user, and it is difficult to generalize reasons for continued substance abuse. It may be summarized that the drug experience brings some degree of pleasure or satisfaction to the user. Whether it be euphoria, sedation, hallucinations, or feelings of well-being or excitement, the substance abuser finds the drug experience reinforcing and worth repeating.

Addiction depends on multiple, complex, and interacting variables. These variables focus on the following categories:

- **Agent or drug factors.** Cost, availability, dose, mode of administration (e.g., oral [PO], intravenous [IV], inhalation), speed of onset, duration of drug action, and length of drug use
- **User factors.** Genetic factors (e.g., metabolic enzymes, innate tolerance), risk-taking behavior, prior experiences with drugs, pathologic state (such as severe pain) that may indicate a drug with abuse potential
- **Environmental factors.** Social and community norms, role models, peer influences, educational opportunities

In the case of legal prescription drugs, addiction may begin with a legitimate need for pharmacotherapy. For example, narcotic analgesics may be indicated for pain relief or sedatives for a sleep disorder. These drugs may result in a favorable experience, such as pain relief or sleep, and patients will want to repeat these positive experiences. If pharmacotherapy is not carefully monitored, patients may take these drugs at high doses for prolonged periods, thus increasing the risk of addiction.

It is a common misunderstanding, even among some health care providers, that the therapeutic use of scheduled drugs creates large numbers of addicted patients. In fact, prescription drugs infrequently cause addiction when used according to accepted medical protocols. The risk of addiction for prescription medications is primarily a function of the dose and the length of therapy. Because of this, medications having a potential for abuse are prescribed at the lowest effective dose and for the shortest time necessary to treat the medical problem. Nurses should administer these medications as prescribed for the relief of patient symptoms without undue fear of producing dependency.

PharmFACT

In 2012, almost 24 million Americans age 12 years old or older were current (past month) illicit drug users. This estimate represents 9.2% of the population age 12 years old or older (Substance Abuse and Mental Health Services Administration [SAMHSA, 2013]).

27.4 Physical and psychological dependence lead to continued drug-seeking behavior despite negative health and social consequences.

Whether or not a drug is addictive is related to how easily an individual can stop taking the substance on a repetitive basis. Substance dependence occurs when a person has an overwhelming craving to take a drug and cannot stop. Substance dependence is classified by two distinct categories: physical dependence and psychological dependence.

Physical dependence occurs when the body adapts to repeated use of the substance by altering normal physiology. Essentially, the cells adapt and view the medication-altered environment as normal. These changes in physiology are reversible and when the agent is discontinued, uncomfortable symptoms known as withdrawal result (see Section 27.5). Opioids, such as morphine and heroin, may produce physical dependence relatively quickly with repeated doses, particularly when taken IV. Alcohol, central nervous system (CNS) depressants, some stimulants, and nicotine are other examples of substances that may produce physical dependence relatively easily with extended use.

It is important to understand that physical dependence is not the same as addiction. Physical dependence may occur during the normal course of therapy, such as in patients receiving high doses of narcotic analgesics during cancer treatment. A patient with cancer may be physically dependent, that is, withdrawal symptoms may occur on discontinuing the drug. However, withdrawal from a medication taken under medical supervision such as analgesics, antidepressants, or antianxiety drugs should not be considered as evidence that the patient has a substance use disorder. Addiction implies destructive, compulsive substance use. Although physical dependence does indeed occur in patients who are addicted, it is important to understand that the two terms have different meanings.

In contrast, **psychological dependence** produces no signs of physical discomfort after the agent is discontinued. The user, however, has an intense emotional desire to continue despite obvious negative economic, physical, or social consequences. This intense craving may become worse if the patient has an unsupportive home environment or social contacts who have substance use disorders. Strong psychological craving for a substance is responsible for relapses during substance abuse therapy and often causes a return to drug-seeking behavior. The development of psychological dependence usually requires the use of relatively high doses for a prolonged time, such as with marijuana and antianxiety drugs. However, psychological dependence may also develop quickly, perhaps after only one use, such as with crack cocaine. Whereas physical dependence is often overcome within a few days or weeks after discontinuing the drug, psychological dependence may persist for months, years, or even an entire lifetime.

27.5 A withdrawal syndrome is a set of characteristic symptoms that occurs when an abused substance is discontinued.

Once a patient becomes physically dependent and the substance is abruptly discontinued, a **withdrawal syndrome** will occur. Some substances exhibit severe and prolonged withdrawal symptoms, whereas others produce barely noticeable symptoms. Because the withdrawal syndrome may be particularly acute for patients dependent on alcohol and sedatives, the process of withdrawal from these agents is best accomplished in a substance

abuse treatment facility. Examples of the types of withdrawal syndromes experienced with the different abused substances are shown in Table 27.1. In a medical setting a withdrawal syndrome may be induced by a rapid dosage reduction or by the administration of an antagonist drug in patients who are physically dependent.

In general, symptoms of withdrawal are opposite to those of the drug's effects. For example, a person may use alprazolam to *reduce* anxiety, but withdrawal may *cause* intense anxiety symptoms. A person may abuse methamphetamine as a stimulant to stay awake, but during withdrawal the person will experience lethargy and fatigue. Once these **rebound effects** become intense, the person is driven to take additional doses of the abused substance because that will cause the withdrawal symptoms to disappear. For some patients, avoidance of withdrawal symptoms is the major motivator for continuing drug use. Thus, the cycle of continued substance abuse is perpetuated.

Prescription drugs may be used to reduce the severity of withdrawal symptoms. For example, alcohol withdrawal can be treated with a short-acting benzodiazepine such as oxazepam (Serax), and opioid withdrawal can be treated with methadone. Symptoms of nicotine withdrawal may be relieved by nicotine replacement therapy in the form of patches or chewing gum. No specific pharmacologic intervention is indicated for withdrawal from CNS stimulants, hallucinogens, marijuana, or inhalants.

With chronic substance abuse, a patient will often associate the drug use with his or her surroundings, including social contacts with other users. Users tend to revert back to drug-seeking behavior when they return to the company of other substance abusers. Counselors often encourage users to refrain from associating with past social contacts or relationships with other substance abusers to lessen the possibility for relapse. The formation of new social contacts, including association with self-help groups such as Alcoholics Anonymous, helps some patients transition to a drug-free lifestyle.

Tolerance

27.6 Tolerance occurs when the body adapts to a drug and larger doses are needed to produce a therapeutic effect.

Tolerance is a biologic condition that occurs when the body adapts to a substance after repeated administration. Over time, larger doses of the drug are required to produce the same initial effect. For example, at the start of pharmacotherapy a patient may find that 2 mg of a sedative is effective at inducing sleep. After taking the medication for several months, the patient may require 4 or perhaps 6 mg to fall asleep. Development of drug tolerance is common for drugs that affect the nervous system. Tolerance should be considered a natural consequence of continued drug use: Development of tolerance is not evidence of addiction or drug abuse. Indeed, tolerance is an expression of natural homeostasis—the body's attempt to return systems to normal.

Tolerance does not develop at the same rate for all actions of a drug. For example, patients usually develop tolerance to the nausea and vomiting produced by narcotic analgesics after only a few

TABLE 27.1 **Withdrawal Symptoms and Treatment for Selected Drugs of Abuse**

Drug Class	Symptoms	Treatment
Alcohol	Tremors, fatigue, anxiety, abdominal cramping, hallucinations, confusion, seizures, delirium	Benzodiazepines, antiseizure drugs; disulfiram and naltrexone after withdrawal is over
Anabolic steroids	Mood swings, fatigue, restlessness, anorexia, insomnia, reduced sex drive, depression, and psychological craving for steroids	Behavioral therapy, symptomatic treatment such as antidepressants
Barbiturates and other sedative–hypnotics	Insomnia, anxiety, weakness, abdominal cramps, tremor, anorexia, seizures, hallucinations, and delirium	Same as alcohol
Benzodiazepines	Insomnia, irritability, abdominal pain, nausea, sensitivity to light and sound, headache, fatigue, and tremors	Gradual tapering of dosage over several weeks or months; for acute benzodiazepine intoxication, flumazenil (Romazicon) is administered by rapid IV infusion (15–20 sec)
Cocaine and amphetamines	Mental depression, anxiety, agitation, irritability, extreme fatigue, hunger, disturbed sleep, psychological craving	Behavioral therapy; no specific pharmacologic treatment available
Hallucinogens	Dependent on the specific drug; may include anxiety, mental depression, insomnia, paranoid delusions, panic attacks, lethargy	Treatment usually is not necessary; symptoms resolve in about 12 h; PCP excretion is very pH dependent and acidification of the urine increases the clearance rate of PCP by about 100-fold.
Marijuana	Irritability, restlessness, insomnia, tremor, chills, weight loss	No treatment
Nicotine	Irritability, anxiety, restlessness, headaches, increased appetite, insomnia, inability to concentrate, decrease in heart rate and blood pressure	Nicotine replacement therapy, varenicline (Chantix) or bupropion (Zyban)
Opioids	Excessive sweating, restlessness, dilated pupils, agitation, goose bumps, tremor, violent yawning, increased heart rate and blood pressure, nausea, vomiting, abdominal cramps and pain, muscle spasms with kicking movements, weight loss	Methadone maintenance; buprenorphine therapy; clonidine reduces anxiety, agitation, cramping, and sweating; oxazepam reduces muscle spasms and insomnia; antiemetics for nausea and vomiting; detoxification can be completed in 2–3 days; withdrawal may be done more rapidly using naltrexone in combination with propofol anesthetic, the antiemetic ondansetron, the antidiarrheal octreotide, and clonidine and benzodiazepines for other symptoms

doses. Tolerance to the mood-altering effects of these drugs and to their ability to reduce pain develops more slowly but eventually may be complete. Tolerance never develops to the drug's ability to constrict the pupils. Patients will often endure annoying side effects of drugs, such as the sedation caused by antihistamines, if they know that tolerance to these effects will develop quickly. Thus knowing details regarding the development of tolerance helps the nurse to deliver essential patient information that may enhance adherence.

Tolerance may lead to serious consequences for those patients abusing hazardous substances. As a patient self-administers higher and higher doses to obtain a desired effect such as euphoria or sedation, the risk of overdose escalates. In some cases, the drug abuser may reach a daily dose that would be lethal for a nonaddicted person. Tolerance fades after the patient discontinues the abused drug, often after 10 to 14 days. If the patient should return to drug-taking behavior with the same high dose, the results may be fatal.

The rapid development of tolerance after only a couple of doses, called **tachyphylaxis**, occurs with drugs such as cocaine, LSD, and amphetamines but is not unique to abused substances. For example, patients with coronary artery disease will exhibit acute tachyphylaxis to the therapeutic effects of nitroglycerin. Tachyphylaxis can occur to virtually any action of a drug, adverse effects as well as therapeutic effects. Tachyphylaxis is beneficial when it occurs to an adverse effect of a drug, such as nausea, vomiting, or dizziness.

Cross-tolerance occurs between closely related drugs. The more two drugs are similar chemically, the greater the possibility

of cross-tolerance between them. This occurs frequently between drugs in the same class, such as among different barbiturates or among various opioids. It sometimes occurs between dissimilar drugs that have the same pharmacologic action. For example, patients who are physically dependent on ethanol exhibit cross-tolerance to other CNS depressant drugs such as benzodiazepines and barbiturates. Ethanol-dependent patients will require higher doses of these drugs to produce a therapeutic effect. Ethanol does not exhibit cross-tolerance to drugs in very different pharmacologic classes, such as amphetamines or LSD.

The term *resistance* is often confused with tolerance. Resistance, however, refers to microorganisms and infections and should not be used interchangeably with tolerance. For example, microorganisms may become resistant to the effects of an antibiotic; they do not become tolerant. Patients may become tolerant to the effects of pain relievers; they do not become resistant.

Central Nervous System Depressants

27.7 **Central nervous system depressants, which include sedatives, opioids, and alcohol, decrease the activity of the central nervous system.**

CNS depressants form a diverse group of drugs that cause patients to feel sedated or relaxed (see Chapters 18 and 25). Drugs in this group include sedatives, antianxiety drugs, opioids, and alcohol. Although the majority are legal substances, these classes of drugs are strictly controlled due to their abuse potential.

PharmFACT

In 2012, 19.9 million people used marijuana. Almost 9 million additional persons age 12 years old or older (3.4% of the population) were current users of illicit drugs other than marijuana (SAMHSA, 2013).

Sedatives and Antianxiety Drugs

Sedatives, also known as sedative–hypnotics and tranquilizers, are primarily prescribed for sleep disorders and certain forms of epilepsy. The two general classes of sedatives are the barbiturates and the nonbarbiturate sedative–hypnotics. The safety profiles and addictive potential of the two classes are roughly equivalent.

Physical and psychological dependence develop when high doses of barbiturates are taken for extended periods. Doses may be three or more times above normal due to the development of tolerance. Abusers often combine sedatives with other substances, such as stimulants or alcohol. Addicts often alternate between amphetamines (uppers), which keep them awake for several days, and sedatives (downers), which are needed to relax and fall asleep.

Sedative users appear dull or apathetic and exhibit signs similar to alcohol intoxication such as slurred speech and motor incoordination. The medical use of barbiturates and nonbarbiturate sedative–hypnotics has declined markedly over the past two decades because safer alternatives such as the benzodiazepines are available. With the decline in therapeutic use, fewer cases of illicit barbiturate use have been reported. The use of the barbiturates in treating sleep disorders was discussed in Chapter 18, and their use in epilepsy was presented in Chapter 22.

Overdoses of sedatives are extremely dangerous because the drugs suppress the respiratory centers in the brain: Very high doses are often fatal. In the 1960s to 1970s, barbiturates were the drugs most commonly used to commit suicide. The withdrawal syndrome from these drugs resembles that of alcohol and may be life threatening.

Starting in the 1970s, the benzodiazepine class of CNS depressants began to replace barbiturates because they exhibited an improved safety profile. Rather than considered sedatives, benzodiazepines are more accurately called antianxiety drugs. They are one of the most widely prescribed classes of drugs, and a drug class commonly abused among teens and college students. Although their primary indication is anxiety, they may be used to treat seizures, sleep disorders, and muscle spasms. Benzodiazepines include alprazolam (Xanax), clonazepam (Klonopin), diazepam (Valium), temazepam (Restoril), triazolam (Halcion), and midazolam (Versed).

Flunitrazepam (Rohypnol) is an infamous benzodiazepine of abuse because it causes **anterograde amnesia**, a type of short-term memory loss where the user cannot remember events that occur while under the influence of the drug. Effects begin 30 minutes after PO administration and last for 8 hours or longer. The abuser is conscious during this time but is unable to transfer thoughts from short-term to long-term memory. Flunitrazepam is called a "date-rape" drug because sexual predators can expose an unknowing person to the drug and perform a physical assault with the likelihood that the victim will not remember the event. Flunitrazepam is not approved by the U. S. Food and Drug Administration (FDA) for any medical condition. Most of the drug in the United States originates from Mexico, although it can be obtained legally in several other countries.

Patients on high doses of antianxiety drugs appear detached, sleepy, or disoriented. Often, patients will appear carefree and without worry. Despite their enormous popularity, however, benzodiazepines are not frequently abused in high doses. Users sometimes combine these drugs with alcohol, cocaine, or heroin to augment their drug experience. In terms of acute toxicity, benzodiazepines are safer than barbiturates and other sedatives. Serious respiratory depression is rare and death due to overdose usually only occurs with extremely high doses. However, if combined with alcohol, cocaine, or heroin, overdose may be lethal. Withdrawal symptoms are less severe than with barbiturates.

Another popular abused CNS depressant is a substance that occurs naturally in the body called gamma-hydroxybutyric acid (GHB). The drug is approved by the FDA as sodium oxybate (Xyrem) to treat patients with narcolepsy who experience excessive daytime sleepiness or cataplexy (weak or paralyzed muscles). Although Xyrem is regulated as a Schedule III drug, its active ingredient GHB is classified as Schedule I. It is very unusual for the FDA to classify a drug in two schedules. It is distributed to prescribers and patients only through a single centralized pharmacy.

Once sold in health food stores as a dietary supplement to enhance athletic performance, GHB is now abused by recreational users for its ability to produce euphoria at low doses. Like flunitrazepam, GHB is called a date-rape drug because it induces retrograde amnesia in the user and has been used in sexual assaults. Most illegal GHB is obtained through home laboratories in the United States, with batches varying widely in purity and potency. The drug is usually dissolved in liquid and doses are difficult to estimate. The same enzyme that metabolizes ethanol also metabolizes GHB; concurrent use, which is common, leads to prolonged effects of GHB and an increased risk of overdose. Overdose causes severe respiratory depression, seizures, and coma. Death from GHB overdose is sometimes caused by the aspiration of vomitus, because the patient may experience coma, vomiting, and seizures simultaneously. There is no antidote for overdose with GHB.

Opioids

Opioids, also known as opiates or narcotic analgesics, are morphine-like substances prescribed for severe pain, anesthesia, persistent cough, and life-threatening diarrhea. The opioid class includes morphine, codeine, meperidine (Demerol), oxycodone (OxyContin), fentanyl (Duragesic, Sublimaze), methadone, and heroin. The therapeutic effects of the opioids are discussed in detail in Chapter 25.

The effects of oral opioids begin within 30 minutes and may last over a day. Injecting or smoking opium produces immediate effects, including the brief, intense rush of euphoria sought by heroin addicts. Individuals experience a range of emotions from extreme pleasure to slowed body activities and profound sedation. Other symptoms include slurred speech, constricted pupils (miosis), an increase in the pain threshold, and respiratory depression. Tolerance develops rapidly to most effects of opioids, and the addicted patient may eventually require 10 times the initial dose to achieve the desired effects.

Opioid dependence can occur rapidly and withdrawal produces very intense and unpleasant symptoms that start within a few hours after discontinuation of parenteral agents and within 3 to 5 days for those dependent on oral opiates. Withdrawal symptoms include dysphoria, diaphoresis, violent yawning, lacrimation, rhinorrhea, pupil dilation (mydriasis), fever, diarrhea, goose bumps, and muscle cramping and tremor. Although extremely unpleasant, withdrawal from opioids is not life threatening, compared to barbiturate or alcohol withdrawal, and the person is not delirious. The withdrawal syndrome is self-limiting, peaking within 36 to 72 hours after discontinuation of parenteral opioids, and individual symptoms are treated as necessary. For patients dependent on low to moderate doses, withdrawal symptoms are relatively mild and resemble a case of the flu. Babies born to pregnant opioid users will experience withdrawal symptoms following birth.

Oxycodone is an opioid that deserves special attention because the incidence of substance abuse of this drug has escalated in the past decade. Oxycodone was approved by the FDA in 1976 and has been widely prescribed for moderate pain when combined with aspirin (Percodan) and acetaminophen (Percocet). In 1995, oxycodone (OxyContin) was formulated in a timed release preparation for the purpose of bringing long-duration relief from chronic pain. Whereas Percocet and Percodan contain only 2.5 to 10 mg per tablet, OxyContin contains 10 to 160 mg per tablet. Drug abusers soon discovered that when OxyContin tablets are crushed, dissolved, and injected, the drug delivers a rush of euphoria similar to that of morphine or heroin.

In 2010, the manufacturer of OxyContin developed a reformulated form that is highly resistant to crushing, breaking, or dissolving. If it is extracted, the drug forms an insoluble gel when dissolved in water for injection or snorting. This tamper-resistant form has greatly reduced OxyContin abuse. Unfortunately, those who abuse this class of medications are switching to other opiates, including heroin.

Treatment of opioid addiction: Methadone has been the conventional treatment of choice for opioid addiction. Although methadone has addictive properties of its own, it does not produce the same degree of euphoria as other opioids; it may be taken PO and its effects last 24 hours. Heroin addicts are switched to methadone during the detoxification phase of treatment to prevent unpleasant withdrawal symptoms. If the patient decides to take heroin during methadone therapy, most of the euphoric rush will be blocked because most of the opiate receptors are already occupied by methadone. During maintenance therapy, patients must report to the methadone clinic daily for their dose and to receive counseling. In some cases, patients who have remained heroin-free may be trusted with several doses for home administration. Patients sometimes remain on methadone maintenance the remainder of their lives, although most patients eventually choose to detoxify and discontinue methadone use altogether. Gradual dose reduction occurs over a period of about 6 months. Withdrawal from methadone is more prolonged than with heroin or morphine, but the symptoms are less intense.

For many health care providers, buprenorphine has become an important alternative to methadone therapy. Options include buprenorphine (Subutex) as monotherapy or buprenorphine combined with naloxone (Suboxone, Zubsolv). These are Schedule III drugs intended for the office management of opioid dependence. Naloxone is also used alone for the emergency treatment of severe opioid-induced respiratory depression (see Chapter 25).

PROTOTYPE DRUG	**Buprenorphine with naloxone (Suboxone, Zubsolv)**

Classification: **Therapeutic:** Drug for treating opioid addiction, narcotic analgesic

Pharmacologic: Opioid agonist-antagonist

Therapeutic Effects and Uses: Buprenorphine is a Schedule III narcotic analgesic that produces analgesia when given by the IM/IV (Buprenex) or transdermal (Butrans) routes for moderate to severe pain. The combination of buprenorphine with naloxone, a narcotic antagonist, is given by the sublingual route three to four times per week for the management of opioid dependence. When taken as directed, the combination drug reduces craving in opioid-dependent patients and prevents the unpleasant symptoms of withdrawal.

While methadone maintenance has been the traditional treatment of choice for opioid addicts, buprenorphine with naloxone offers certain advantages. It is unlikely that the combination drug will be abused because the presence of naloxone would cause unpleasant effects identical to withdrawal symptoms. Detoxification can be more rapid and the maintenance can be conducted through office environments, rather than a daily visit to a methadone clinic.

Mechanism of Action: Buprenorphine produces its analgesic effects by occupying mu receptors in the brain and dorsal horn of the spinal cord in a manner similar to that of other opioid agonists. Because buprenorphine exhibits some opioid antagonist activity at the kappa receptor, it is considered a mixed opioid agonist-antagonist. Naloxone competes with opioid agonists for the mu and kappa receptors, thus antagonizing the effects of morphine and other opioids.

Pharmacokinetics:

Route(s)	Sublingual; tablets or oral film
Absorption	Variable (buprenorphine well absorbed; naloxone poorly absorbed)
Distribution	Bound to plasma protein (96% buprenorphine, 45% naloxone); crosses the placenta; secreted in breast milk
Primary metabolism	Hepatic
Primary excretion	Renal (30%) and feces (69%)
Onset of action	Approximately 45 min
Duration of action	8–12 h (may be as long as 72 h at high doses)

Adverse Effects: Buprenorphine with naloxone is a relatively safe drug that produces mild and transient side effects. The most frequently reported adverse events include headache, nausea, vomiting, hyperhidrosis, constipation, insomnia, pain, and peripheral edema. Abrupt discontinuation of the drug will precipitate immediate opioid withdrawal symptoms. Respiratory depression and death have occurred with high doses, although these have been with the IV route.

Buprenorphine is an opioid and thus can produce dependence when taken on a chronic basis. Although Suboxone and Zubsolv are both sublingual forms of the drug, they are not dose equivalent and care must be taken when switching between products.

Contraindications/Precautions: Buprenorphine with naloxone is contraindicated in patients with hypersensitivity to either drug. This combination may induce withdrawal in patients who have chronic physical dependence on opioids. Naloxone should be used with caution in patients with cardiovascular disease. Naloxone may precipitate seizures in patients with seizure disorders.

Drug Interactions: Caution should be used when taking buprenorphine with other narcotic analgesics and CNS depressants because additive sedation will occur. Deaths have occurred when taking very high doses of buprenorphine concomitantly with benzodiazepines. The use of buprenorphine is contraindicated with alvimopan (Entereg).

Pregnancy: Category C.

Treatment of Overdose: Buprenorphine overdose can cause coma, hypotension, and life-threatening respiratory depression, and requires immediate treatment. Additional naloxone doses are indicated to reverse the opioid intoxication.

Nursing Responsibilities: Key nursing implications for patients receiving buprenorphine are included in the Nursing Practice Application for Patients Receiving Pharmacotherapy for Substance Abuse Disorders.

Drugs Similar to Buprenorphine with Naloxone (Suboxone, Zubsolv)

Naltrexone is an opioid antagonist that exhibits actions similar to those of naloxone. It is presented later in this chapter as a treatment for alcohol dependence.

Alcohol (Ethanol)

One of the most commonly abused drugs is alcohol, the pharmacologically active agent in beer, wine, and liquor. Although there are many types of alcohol, the only one having widespread medical significance is ethanol or ethyl alcohol. Therefore, in this text, the terms *ethanol* and *alcohol* are used interchangeably. The economic, social, and health consequences of alcohol abuse are staggering. Small quantities of alcohol consumed on a daily basis, however, have been found to reduce the risk of stroke and heart attack.

Alcohol is readily absorbed across the gastrointestinal (GI) tract, primarily from the small intestine. Food slows the absorption of alcohol by prolonging gastric emptying time and diluting the alcohol, thus delaying its onset of action. Once it has entered the blood, alcohol is immediately distributed to the tissues. The drug easily crosses the blood–brain barrier so its effects on the brain are observed quickly, within 5 to 30 minutes after consumption.

Alcohol is metabolized and excreted at a constant rate, depending on the activity of two hepatic enzymes, alcohol dehydrogenase and aldehyde dehydrogenase. Metabolism is a two-step process, first yielding acetaldehyde and then acetic acid, or acetate, as shown in Pharmacotherapy Illustrated 27.1. There is wide genetic variability in the amounts and activity of these enzymes. For example, a significant number of Asians have a deficiency of aldehyde dehydrogenase, resulting in an accumulation of acetaldehyde and severe flushing and other uncomfortable symptoms when consuming alcohol. Patients who are alcohol dependent and those who drink alcoholic beverages regularly have higher amounts of these enzymes and thus are able to drink greater quantities of alcohol without becoming intoxicated.

The elimination of alcohol from tissues occurs at a constant rate, which is independent of the concentration of alcohol in the blood. The blood alcohol level declines at about 15 mg/hour; no food or drug can speed up the rate of alcohol excretion once it has reached the blood. Eating pizza or drinking strong coffee following an alcohol binge does nothing to speed up excretion of the drug. It is a simple fact that if one drinks alcohol at a faster rate than it can be metabolized, intoxication will occur and will continue until the body eventually metabolizes the alcohol that has accumulated in the blood. The "average" rate of metabolism is one alcoholic drink per hour. Because alcohol is vaporized and excreted by the lungs, breath testing can be used to estimate the amount of alcohol in the blood, a common practice in law enforcement.

Alcohol is classified as a CNS depressant because it has the ability to slow the region of the brain controlling alertness and wakefulness. Effects of alcohol include sedation, relaxation, loss of motor coordination, reduced judgment, and decreased inhibition. Alcohol intoxication may cause partial or total amnesia, resulting in an inability to remember details that occurred during an alcohol binge. Alcohol also increases blood flow in certain areas of the skin, causing a flushed

PHARMACOTHERAPY ILLUSTRATED 27.1

METABOLISM OF ALCOHOL

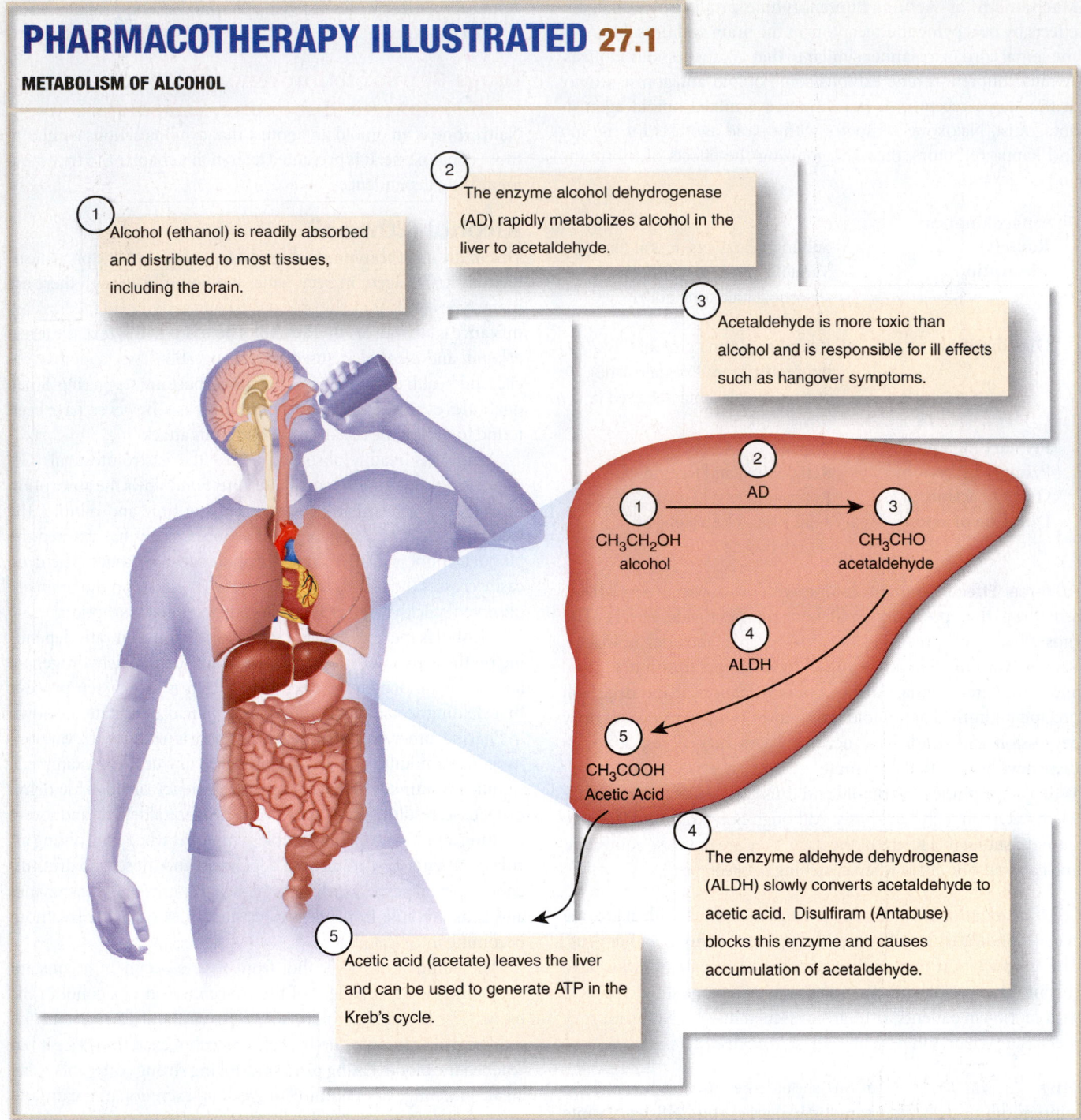

1. Alcohol (ethanol) is readily absorbed and distributed to most tissues, including the brain.

2. The enzyme alcohol dehydrogenase (AD) rapidly metabolizes alcohol in the liver to acetaldehyde.

3. Acetaldehyde is more toxic than alcohol and is responsible for ill effects such as hangover symptoms.

4. The enzyme aldehyde dehydrogenase (ALDH) slowly converts acetaldehyde to acetic acid. Disulfiram (Antabuse) blocks this enzyme and causes accumulation of acetaldehyde.

5. Acetic acid (acetate) leaves the liver and can be used to generate ATP in the Kreb's cycle.

$$\underset{\text{alcohol}}{\overset{1}{CH_3CH_2OH}} \xrightarrow{\overset{2}{AD}} \underset{\text{acetaldehyde}}{\overset{3}{CH_3CHO}}$$

$$\overset{4}{ALDH}$$

$$\underset{\text{Acetic Acid}}{\overset{5}{CH_3COOH}}$$

face, pink cheeks, or red nose. Like most drugs, the effects of alcohol are directly related to the amount consumed. Acute overdoses of alcohol produce vomiting, severe hypotension, respiratory failure, and coma. Death due to alcohol poisoning is not uncommon.

Chronic alcohol consumption produces both psychological and physiological dependence and directly leads to a large number of adverse health effects. Not surprisingly, the organ most affected by chronic alcohol abuse is the liver, which is responsible for metabolizing and detoxifying alcohol. Hepatitis occurs in up to 90% of heavy users. Alcoholism is a common cause of cirrhosis, a debilitating and often fatal failure of the liver to perform its vital functions. Liver impairment results in abnormalities in blood clotting and

nutritional deficiencies and makes the patient very sensitive to the effects of medications. Chronic alcohol use also damages the brain, impairing memory and cognitive function.

Drug doses for patients with alcoholism should be decreased to avoid toxicity because such patients are more susceptible to adverse drug effects and drug interactions. Combining alcohol with nonsteroidal anti-inflammatory drugs (NSAIDs) such as aspirin can promote serious GI bleeding. Combining alcohol with acetaminophen can increase the risk of fatal hepatic injury. Alcohol should never be combined with other CNS depressants, because their effects are cumulative and profound sedation or coma may result. Combining alcohol with sedatives, benzodiazepines, or opioids may be fatal. Selected drug interactions involving alcohol are shown in Table 27.2.

CONNECTION Checkpoint 27.2

Alcohol induces CYP3A and increases the formation of a toxic metabolite of acetaminophen. From what you learned in Chapter 3, what is CYP3A and what is its importance to pharmacotherapy? *See Answer to Connection Checkpoint 27.2 on student resource website.*

One of the major adverse effects of alcohol consumption occurs not in the patient, but in the fetus of a pregnant alcohol user. These effects, known as fetal alcohol syndrome, include birth defects and major health challenges for the child. There is no safe "dose" for alcohol consumption during pregnancy; thus use of this drug must be strictly avoided. Additional details on alcohol as a teratogen are presented in Chapter 8.

Alcohol withdrawal is severe and may be life threatening. About 5% to 10% of withdrawal cases proceed to **delirium tremens**, a syndrome of intense agitation, confusion, terrifying hallucinations, uncontrollable tremors, panic attacks, and paranoia. Without treatment, 35% of the patients with delirium tremens will die. Prevention of seizures and delirium tremens is a top priority and may be accomplished by administering a benzodiazepine such as lorazepam (Ativan) or diazepam (Valium). Hallucinations may require the administration of an antipsychotic drug such as risperidone (Risperdal).

Long-term therapy for alcohol dependence includes behavioral counseling and self-help groups such as Alcoholics Anonymous. Pharmacologic management of alcohol dependence includes disulfiram and naltrexone. Disulfiram (Antabuse) is given to discourage relapses.

TABLE 27.2 Drug–Drug Interactions with Alcohol

Class	Example Drug(s)	Interaction	Consequences
Acetaminophen	—	Increased acetaminophen metabolism to toxic metabolites	Severe, possibly fatal liver damage
Anesthetics	propofol (Diprivan) and enflurane (Ethrane)	Cross-tolerance	Larger anesthetic doses needed to induce anesthesia
		Additive hepatic toxicity	Increased risk of liver damage
Antianginal medications	nitroglycerin, isosorbide dinitrate (Isordil)	Additive effects on blood pressure	Hypotension, dizziness, possible fainting
Antibiotics	furazolidone (Furoxone), griseofulvin, and metronidazole (Flagyl)	Additive toxicity	Nausea, vomiting, headache, possible seizures, reduced antibiotic effectiveness
Anticoagulants	warfarin (Coumadin)	Acute consumption enhances warfarin bioavailability; chronic consumption reduces its availability	Modification of coagulation: bleeding disorders, hemorrhage
Antidepressants	amitriptyline (Elavil), paroxetine (Paxil), sertraline (Zoloft), fluoxetine (Prozac)	Additive CNS depression/sedation	Drowsiness, lethargy
Antihistamines	diphenhydramine (Benadryl and others), loratadine (Claritin), cetirizine (Zyrtec)	Additive CNS depression	Drowsiness, lethargy, dizziness
Antipsychotics	chlorpromazine (Thorazine)	Additive CNS depression	Drowsiness, lethargy
		Additive hepatotoxicity	Increased risk of liver damage
Antiseizure medications	phenytoin (Dilantin)	Chronic alcohol use may decrease phenytoin bioavailability	Increased risk of seizures
Antituberculars	isoniazid and rifampin	Decreased bioavailability	Decreased effectiveness in eliminating tuberculosis
Beta blockers	propranolol (Inderal)	Additive effects on blood pressure	Hypotension, dizziness, possible fainting
HMG-CoA reductase inhibitors (statins)	atorvastatin (Lipitor), simvastatin (Zocor)	Additive hepatotoxicity	Liver damage
NSAIDs	aspirin, ibuprofen, naproxen, others	Additive GI toxicity	Increased risk of GI bleeding
Opioids	morphine, codeine, and meperidine (Demerol)	Additive CNS depression and sedation	Drowsiness, lethargy
Sedatives and antianxiety drugs	diazepam (Valium), lorazepam (Ativan), alprazolam (Xanax), phenobarbital (Luminal)	Additive CNS depression and sedation	Drowsiness, lethargy
Miscellaneous	sulfonylureas, metronidazole (Flagyl), isoniazid (INH)	Disulfiram-like reaction	Facial flushing, nausea, vomiting

PROTOTYPE DRUG	Disulfiram (Antabuse)

Classification: Therapeutic: Drug for treating alcohol abuse
Pharmacologic: Alcohol antagonist; acetaldehyde dehydrogenase inhibitor

Therapeutic Effects and Uses: By itself, disulfiram produces few effects. If alcohol is consumed while taking disulfiram, however, the patient becomes violently ill in a syndrome called the disulfiram–alcohol reaction. The only indication for disulfiram is for the management of chronic alcohol abuse.

This drug should only be administered to patients who are fully informed of its effects and who are motivated to maintain sobriety. It should never be administered to a patient who is experiencing current alcohol intoxication. The use of disulfiram does not cure alcohol abuse: It only prevents impulsive drinking as long as the patient chooses to take it. The protective action of disulfiram may last for 2 weeks after the drug is discontinued.

Mechanism of Action: Disulfiram irreversibly inhibits the enzyme acetaldehyde dehydrogenase, causing toxic acetaldehyde to build up in the blood. Acetaldehyde is sometimes called the "hangover" chemical because it is responsible for causing miserable symptoms following a night of high alcohol consumption.

Pharmacokinetics:

Route(s)	PO
Absorption	Rapidly absorbed
Distribution	Crosses the placenta; secreted in breast milk
Primary metabolism	Hepatic
Primary excretion	Lung and feces
Onset of action	12 h
Duration of action	1–2 weeks

Adverse Effects: At therapeutic doses, disulfiram produces few adverse effects, unless ingested with alcohol. At extreme doses, the drug itself can cause neurologic toxicity, psychosis, hepatotoxicity, and blood dyscrasias.

Because the disulfiram–alcohol reaction can be serious and even fatal, disulfiram therapy should not be initiated in patients at high risk for returning to alcohol abuse. Disulfiram is contraindicated in patients who are receiving metronidazole because acute psychosis may occur. All products containing alcohol must be strictly avoided, including cough syrups, mouthwashes, or liquid vitamins. Even topical products containing alcohol should be avoided because the alcohol may be absorbed across the skin. Disulfiram is also contraindicated in patients with severe heart disease and psychoses.

Drug Interactions: Ingestion of even small amounts of alcohol will immediately result in headache, palpitations, chest pain, dyspnea, nausea, violent vomiting, and, sometimes, bizarre behaviors. Severe respiratory depression may occur. Symptoms begin within 5 to 10 minutes after alcohol consumption and may continue for several hours.

Pregnancy: Category C.

Treatment of Overdose: No specific treatment for disulfiram overdose is available.

Nursing Responsibilities: Key nursing implications for patients receiving disulfiram are included in the Nursing Practice Application for Patients Receiving Pharmacotherapy for Substance Abuse Disorders.

Drugs Similar to Disulfiram (Antabuse)

Naltrexone (ReVia, Vivitrol, Others): Approved in 1984, naltrexone is an opioid antagonist that reduces the psychological craving for alcohol. Why does a drug that blocks opiate receptors have an effect on alcohol dependence? Although the mechanism is unclear, endogenous opioids appear to be involved in "reward pathways" for alcohol. Blocking the reward pathways with naltrexone affects the psychological experience or craving characteristic of alcohol dependence. Naltrexone does not produce a "hangover" reaction when a person consumes alcohol, as does disulfiram. Oral naltrexone may be given once daily for several months up to a year. An intramuscular (IM) suspension of naltrexone (Vivitrol) offers the convenience of once-a-month injections. Naltrexone is also approved to treat opiate dependence. Successful use of naltrexone in alcohol or opioid rehabilitation programs is entirely dependent on patient adherence; if the patient stops taking naltrexone, the CNS effects of alcohol or opioids will return. Severe opioid withdrawal may occur if the drug is administered to a patient who has received opioids within 5 to 7 days prior to naltrexone dosing; thus the drug is contraindicated in these patients.

Naltrexone may be used off-label to treat nicotine withdrawal. Naltrexone has been awarded orphan drug status by the FDA to treat symptoms of childhood autism. In 2009, a fixed dose combination of naltrexone with morphine (Embeda) was approved to treat moderate to severe pain. Morphine is used to provide effective analgesia, and naltrexone is included to block some of the side effects of morphine and to prevent product misuse. Patients with serious hepatic impairment should not receive naltrexone. This drug is pregnancy category C.

Marijuana and Related Substances

27.8 Marijuana is the most frequently abused illicit substance.

Cannabinoids are natural products obtained from the hemp plant *Cannabis sativa,* which thrives in tropical climates. Cannabinoids include marijuana, hashish, and hash oil. Hashish is a solid, dried resin of the plant that is extremely potent. Hash oil is made by dissolving hashish or marijuana in a solvent such as alcohol, then allowing the liquid to evaporate to form a thick, oily concentrated form of cannabis.

Although more than 70 natural cannabinoid substances have been identified, the ingredient responsible for most of the psychoactive properties is **tetrahydrocannabinol (THC)**. Selective breeding and cultivation of *Cannabis* has produced varieties of the plant that produce much higher concentrations of THC than in previous decades. The THC content of marijuana varies from 5% to 25%; hashish from 20% to 60%; and hash oil from 30% to 80%.

Humans, as well as many other mammals, fish, and birds, produce small amounts of endogenous cannabinoids. These substances, known as endocannabinoids, are types of internal messengers that allow for intercellular communication. The exact purpose of the endocannabinoids has yet to be discovered, although they have some of the same characteristics as neurotransmitters and can modulate neuronal function. The endocannabinoids have some structural similarities to THC and bind to the same receptors, known as CB1 and CB2 receptors. Agonists and antagonists to CB1 and CB2 have been discovered, with the hope that the research may lead to new pharmacologic agents.

Marijuana, also known as grass, pot, weed, reefer, or dope, is the most commonly used illicit drug in the United States; more than 40% of the population age 12 or older has used the drug at least once. Marijuana is usually smoked as cigarettes (joints), but it may be used in pipes, brewed as teas, or added to food. Oral absorption results in a lower serum blood level of the drug than does inhalation.

When inhaled, marijuana produces effects that occur within minutes and last 1 to 3 hours. Use of marijuana slows motor activity, decreases coordination, and causes disconnected thoughts and euphoria. The experience is nearly always pleasant and involves laughter and an increase in the subjective perception of sounds, colors, and thoughts. The subjective experience is dependent on the social surroundings during drug use. Positive, friendly, happy surroundings produce a more favorable drug experience than taking the drug alone. Time appears to pass more slowly. It increases thirst and a craving for food, particularly chocolate and other sweets. One hallmark symptom of marijuana use is red or bloodshot eyes, caused by dilation of blood vessels.

Following feelings of euphoria, the person may become sleepy or depressed or experience paranoia. Driving is sometimes impaired, particularly when the drug is combined with alcohol. Because marijuana smoke is inhaled more deeply and held within the lungs for a longer period than cigarette smoke, marijuana smoke introduces four times more particulates (tar) into the lungs than does tobacco smoke. Smoking marijuana on a daily basis may increase the risk of lung cancer and other respiratory disorders. Chronic use is associated with apathy and a lack of motivation in achieving or pursuing life goals, and very high doses may cause hallucinations. THC accumulates in reproductive tissues, particularly the gonads, and has been reported to cause amenorrhea and decreased spermatogenesis.

Marijuana produces less physical dependence or tolerance than many other abused substances. At usual doses, withdrawal symptoms are mild, if they are experienced at all. After chronic abuse of high doses, patients may experience irritability, restlessness, and insomnia. Psychological dependence occurs when the drug is taken on a chronic basis. Metabolites of THC remain in the body for months to years, allowing laboratory specialists to easily determine whether someone has taken marijuana. For 3 to 5 days after a single use, THC can be detected in the urine.

Medical marijuana is a controversial topic; many health care providers and politicians are reluctant to endorse a drug that impairs judgment and may harm users. THC appears to reduce the pressure in the eyeball, a condition called glaucoma. Patients receiving antineoplastic drugs have reported that THC reduces the severe nausea and vomiting associated with these drugs. The ability of THC to reduce muscle spasticity may lead to applications for patients with multiple sclerosis and other spasticity disorders. In most cases, current drugs for these conditions have been demonstrated to be more effective and safer. Although the medical value of the drug remains to be conclusively proven, several states have approved the medical use of marijuana, despite its being a Schedule I drug.

Hallucinogens

27.9 Hallucinogens and club drugs cause an altered state of thought and perception.

Hallucinogens are a diverse class of chemicals that have in common the ability to produce an altered, dreamlike state of consciousness. These drugs sometimes produce a profound emotional experience, allowing the user to feel enhanced interconnectedness with others and experience a higher, spiritual plane of consciousness. Sometimes called "psychedelics," the prototype drug for this class is lysergic acid diethylamide (LSD). More recently, some drugs in this class have become closely associated with the nightclub scene and are abused by those seeking a drug-induced experience from the music, dancing, and social contact; thus the name "club drugs."

For nearly all drugs of abuse, predictable symptoms occur in every user. Effects from hallucinogens, however, are highly variable and depend on the mood and expectations of the user and the surrounding environment in which the substance is used. Two patients taking the same agent will report completely different experiences, and the same patient may report different symptoms with each use. All hallucinogens are Schedule I drugs: They have no medical use.

LSD and Similar Hallucinogens

LSD, also called acid, the beast, blotter acid, and California sunshine, is derived from a fungus that grows on rye and other grains. LSD is nearly always administered PO and can be manufactured in capsule, tablet, or liquid form. A common and inexpensive method for distributing LSD is to place drops of the drug on paper, often containing the images of cartoon characters or graphics related to the drug culture, as shown in Figure 27.1. After drying, the paper is then cut into small squares to be ingested, with each square representing a "dose." The drug is extremely potent, with doses as low as 25 mcg producing an effect.

Immediately after use, LSD is widely distributed throughout the body, including the brain. Effects begin within an hour and may last from 6 to 12 hours. Although the exact mechanism of action of the drug is unclear, it affects the central and autonomic nervous systems, increasing blood pressure, elevating body temperature, dilating pupils, causing dry mouth, and increasing the heart rate.

LSD and other hallucinogens are used for their psychoactive, rather than their physical, effects. LSD users may experience symptoms such as laughter, visions, religious revelations, or deep personal insights. Common occurrences are hallucinations and after-images being projected onto people as they move. Users also report extremely bright lights and vivid colors. Some users hear voices; others report seeing sounds and hearing colors. Many experience a profound sense of truth and deep directed thoughts. The user's sense of time is altered.

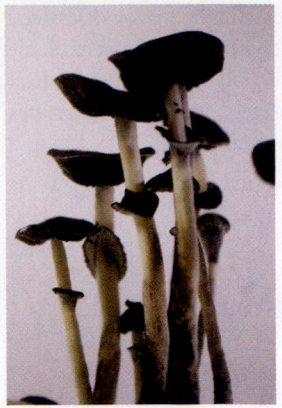 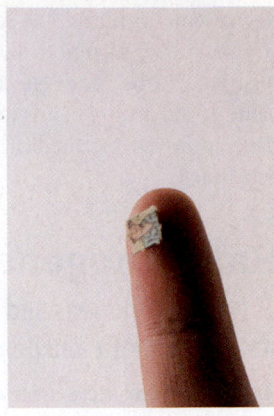

Figure 27.1 Psychoactive substances: (left) Psilocybin is obtained from a species of mushroom; (right) LSD is often blotted on paper before ingesting.
Courtesy of © cbaloga/fotolia (left); © Joe Bird/Alamy (right).

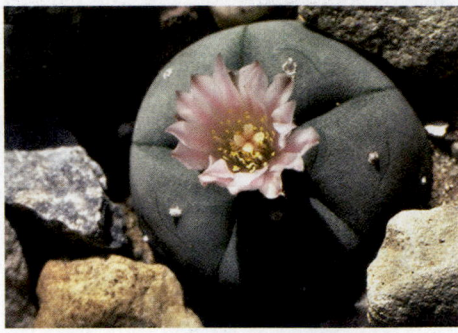

Mescaline

Figure 27.2 The chemical structure of mescaline, derived from the peyote cactus.
Courtesy of R. Konig/Jacana/Science Source.

Unpleasant experiences with LSD, known as "bad trips," can be terrifying and may include acute anxiety, panic attacks, confusion, severe depression, and paranoia. Repeated use may impair memory and the ability to reason. In extreme cases, patients may develop psychoses. One common adverse effect is flashbacks, in which the user experiences the effects of the drug again, sometimes weeks, months, or years after the drug was initially taken. Flashbacks may occur without warning.

LSD is considered a recreational drug: Users rarely become dependent on the drug, and there are no withdrawal symptoms. Continuous users will experience tolerance very quickly, sometimes after only 2 to 3 days.

The following drugs are considered similar to LSD and produce equivalent psychoactive effects.

- **Psilocybin.** The primary psychoactive substance in over 100 species of psilocybin mushrooms found in Mexico and Central America (see Figure 27.1). Known as "magic mushrooms" or "shrooms," psilocybin is a prodrug that is metabolized to its active metabolite psilocin. Possession of these mushroom species is illegal. Psilocybin and psilocin are listed as Schedule I drugs. The drug is taken by eating fresh psilocybin mushrooms or by ingesting dried extracts.

- **Mescaline.** Found in the peyote cactus and several other cacti species of Mexico and Central America, as shown in Figure 27.2. The drug is usually taken in capsules consisting of dried cactus. The cactus, which grows very slowly, has become quite rare due to overharvesting. In the United States, peyote use is illegal for all but members of the Native American Church, who use the drug in religious ceremonies.

- **Dimethyltryptamine (DMT).** A natural substance found in many species of plants in Central and South America and the Caribbean Islands. Like some of the other hallucinogens, DMT was used by native cultures in their spiritual ceremonies to induce visions. The drug is usually smoked but may be snuffed (snorted through the nostrils), injected, or taken PO.

Club Drugs and Miscellaneous Hallucinogens

Club drug is a relatively new term that refers to substances taken by people at dance clubs, all-night parties, and raves. It is a vague term that refers to a diverse group of abused substances that includes ecstasy, GHB, methamphetamine, Rohypnol, ketamine, and other agents, usually ingested with alcohol. Not all club drugs are hallucinogens, and some of these are covered in other sections of this chapter. The following are descriptions of several major club drugs and some miscellaneous hallucinogens:

- **MDMA (3, 4-methylenedioxymethamphetamine, XTC, or ecstasy).** An amphetamine originally synthesized for research purposes that has since become popular among teens and young adults. Taken PO, its effects last 3 to 6 hours. The drug is unique because it produces both stimulant and hallucinogenic effects simultaneously. MDMA enhances emotions and awareness, increases social and extroversion behaviors, and allows the user to stay awake and physically active for long periods. Chronic users exhibit behavioral disorders such as depression, anxiety, sleeplessness, and hostility. It has a narrow therapeutic index and overdoses may be fatal.

- **MDA (3, 4-methylenedioxyamphetamine).** Called the "love drug" due to a belief that it enhances sexual desires. This drug is sometimes a component of ecstasy.

- **DOM (2, 5 dimethoxy-4-methylamphetamine).** A recreational drug often linked with rave parties as a drug of choice having the name STP. The drug has effects similar to LSD but with a longer duration.

- **Phencyclidine (PCP, crystal, angel dust).** Produces a trance-like state without loss of consciousness that may last for days. Once available as an anesthetic, the substance was removed from the market in 1965 because patients experienced delirium

◖ Drug and Alcohol Use in Middle-Aged, Older, and Ethnically Diverse Adults

Although surveillance, understanding, and treatment options for substance abuse have increased during the last few decades, there are still populations in which substance abuse is not fully researched or understood. Substance abuse in the adult over age 65 and in ethnically and racially diverse patients has not been studied extensively. A full understanding of the extent of substance abuse in these populations and whether standard treatment options are effective have yet to be determined.

As the baby boom generation ages, older adults who may have experienced drug or alcohol abuse in their teenage and young adult years during the 1960s and 1970s may have similar problems in their middle and older adult years. There is little research to suggest whether these problems continue or will be experienced again as they enter into their older adult years. Blazer and Wu (2009) conducted a 2-year study on substance abuse among middle-aged and older adults. Overall, alcohol use was common, with 60% reporting alcohol use during the past year, but drug abuse or dependence was very low (0.33% for any drug) in all adults age 50 or over. Marijuana was the most common drug used in the 50–64 age group, with approximately 4% of the study population reporting use, compared to less than 1% (0.7%) in the 65 or older population. The 50–64 age group had higher alcohol and drug use than the over-65 population, prompting the researchers to raise a concern that in the near future, more of these adults may need treatment for abuse.

Recent research challenges health care providers' beliefs about substance use in different racial and ethnic groups; among rural, small, and large metropolitan counties; and even between inner-city and metropolitan areas. Current research suggests that even among a traditionally identified racial or ethnic group (e.g., black, Hispanic, Asian, Caucasian), there are multiple variations related to subgroups and cultures and country of origin. The same is true for geographic location and proximity to an inner-city environment. Large metropolitan areas do not necessarily equate with higher substance abuse problems as has been traditionally defined, depending on the racial or ethnic group studied.

Nurses can play a key role in the identification and referral for substance abuse treatment by conducting thorough health histories, assessing for co-existing conditions that often accompany substance abuse (e.g., signs of frequent falls, absences from work, health conditions such as TB or HIV/AIDS), and, above all, establishing a trusting relationship with patients so that open communication can assist them in making appropriate health care decisions for the treatment of a substance abuse problem. For the overlooked populations of the older adult and patients from diverse racial and ethnic backgrounds with substance use, the nurse's role becomes even more crucial to ensure appropriate care.

---

and panic attacks as they recovered from anesthesia. The powdered drug is sometimes sprinkled on marijuana and smoked, or it may be snorted or taken as tablets. Typical effects include slurred speech, detachment from reality, time distortion, and a sensation of floating in space. It does not produce the same types of hallucinations seen with LSD. Phencyclidine is probably the most dangerous of the hallucinogens because high doses can cause severe and violent panic attacks, seizures, coma, and death.

- **Ketamine (K, kitkat, or special K).** Closely related to phencyclidine, ketamine has been used historically as an anesthetic but is now rarely used for that purpose. The most common source of the drug is diversion from veterinary offices. Liquid ketamine may be added to drinks, injected, or evaporated to a solid form, which is snorted or taken as pills. Effects are similar to those of phencyclidine, although they only last 35 to 40 minutes. Unconsciousness and amnesia may occur at high doses, and psychoses can be induced with continued use.

- **Dextromethorphan (DXM, robo).** A substance included in over-the-counter (OTC) cold remedies for its cough suppressant properties. Of the drugs of abuse, it is the only substance that can be readily and legally purchased by teens. Abusers will purchase extra-strength remedies and consume large quantities to achieve dissociative effects similar to those of phencyclidine and ketamine. Effects include slurred speech, dizziness, drowsiness, euphoria, and lack of motor coordination. Overdose can cause brain damage, seizures, stroke, hypothermia, and death. Because cold medicines also contain ingredients such

as antihistamines, aspirin, or acetaminophen, abusers of dextromethorphan may experience toxicity due to overdose from these agents. Pure dextromethorphan is also available on the black market in high-dosage tablet form.

Central Nervous System Stimulants

27.10 Stimulants such as amphetamines and cocaine increase the activity of the central nervous system.

The stimulants include a diverse family of drugs with the ability to excite the CNS. Some are prescription drugs used to treat narcolepsy and attention deficit/hyperactivity disorder (ADHD). As drugs of abuse, stimulants are taken to produce a sense of exhilaration, improve mental and physical performance, reduce appetite, or prolong wakefulness. Stimulants include the amphetamines, methylphenidate, and cocaine. Some CNS stimulants are club drugs. Caffeine is also included as a CNS stimulant although it does not have the same negative health characteristics as the other drugs in this group.

Amphetamines and Methylphenidate

Amphetamines produce their effects by increasing the activity of the endogenous neurotransmitters norepinephrine, serotonin (5-HT), and dopamine. Norepinephrine affects awareness and wakefulness by activating neurons in a part of the brain called the **reticular formation**. High doses of amphetamines give the user a feeling of self-confidence, elevated mood, euphoria, and empowerment. Fatigue is diminished and the person can perform at a high level of alertness for an extended time. Appetite is suppressed.

By increasing the activity of norepinephrine, many physiological actions of amphetamines resemble those of sympathetic nervous system activation (see Chapter 15). Cardiovascular and respiratory activities are significantly affected, resulting in increased heart rate, high blood pressure, and increased breathing rate. Other symptoms include dilated pupils, sweating, and tremors. Overdoses of some stimulants lead to seizures, dysrhythmias, stroke, and cardiac arrest.

Although short-term use of amphetamines induces pleasurable feelings, long-term use causes restlessness, anxiety, defensiveness, and fits of rage, especially when the user is coming down from a prolonged drug experience. Chronic use can lead to a psychosis that closely resembles paranoid schizophrenia, although this condition usually resolves within several days after discontinuation of the drug. Tolerance to the pleasurable effects of amphetamines occurs very quickly, especially if the drugs are injected.

Amphetamines and dextroamphetamines were once widely prescribed to treat depression, weight loss, drowsiness, and congestion. Because of their ability to enhance alertness, pilots, students, and health care workers on long shifts have historically abused amphetamines. In the 1970s it was recognized that the adverse effects and abuse potential of amphetamines outweighed their legitimate medical uses. Current therapeutic applications of these drugs are extremely limited. Most substance abusers obtain these agents from illegal laboratories, which can produce some of the amphetamines using readily available chemicals and make tremendous profits. Physical dependence to amphetamines is unusual, and withdrawal symptoms are not life-threatening. The only potentially serious symptom of amphetamine withdrawal is depression.

Dextroamphetamine (Dexedrine) may be used for short-term weight loss, when all other attempts to reduce weight have been exhausted, and to treat narcolepsy, a rare disease in which patients fall asleep unexpectedly. Methamphetamine, commonly called *ice*, is often used as a recreational drug for users who like the rush of euphoria that it gives them. It is usually administered in powder or crystal form (crystal meth) but it may also be smoked. Methamphetamine is a Schedule II drug marketed under the trade name Desoxyn, although most abusers obtain it from illegal methamphetamine laboratories. Methamphetamine can be easily synthesized from pseudoephedrine, a common OTC decongestant. This has led to states placing pseudoephedrine behind the pharmacist counter and motivated pharmaceutical manufacturers to find a replacement drug for pseudoephedrine in their cold and flu remedies. A structural analog of methamphetamine, methcathinone (street name Cat), is made illegally and snorted, taken PO, or injected IV. Methcathinone is a Schedule I agent.*

Methylphenidate (Ritalin) is a CNS stimulant widely prescribed for children diagnosed with attention deficit/hyperactivity disorder (ADHD) because the drug exerts a calming effect in children who are inattentive or hyperactive. The drug stimulates the alertness center in the brain and the child is able to focus on complex tasks for longer periods. The therapeutic applications of methylphenidate are discussed in Chapter 24.

Methylphenidate is a Schedule II drug that has many of the same pharmacologic actions as cocaine and amphetamines. It is sometimes abused by adolescents and adults seeking euphoria, increased alertness, or appetite suppression. Tablets are crushed and snorted or dissolved in liquid and injected IV. Ritalin is sometimes mixed with heroin, a combination called a "speedball." Most Ritalin is obtained by diversion from legal prescriptions, by theft, or by patients selling or sharing their drugs.

Cocaine

Cocaine is a natural substance obtained from leaves of the coca plant, which grows in the Andes Mountains of South America. Natives in this region chew the coca leaves, or make teas of the substance. Much of the cocaine entering the United States comes from Colombia and other South American countries. It was once used as an anesthetic for eye, nose, and throat surgery but is no longer used for this purpose.

Cocaine is a Schedule II drug that produces psychoactive and physiological actions similar to the amphetamines, although its effects can be much more rapid and intense. It is the second most commonly used illicit drug in the United States. Routes of administration include snorting, smoking, inhaling vapors, and injecting. Injection or inhalation of cocaine produces an instantaneous euphoria that lasts 10 to 20 seconds. In small doses, cocaine produces feelings of intense euphoria, a decrease in hunger and pain, illusions of physical strength, and increased sensory perception. Larger doses will increase these effects and cause rapid heartbeat, dysrhythmias, sweating, dilation of the pupils, and an elevated body temperature. The half-life of cocaine is short, 60 to 90 minutes when injected, and tolerance rapidly develops to the pleasurable aspects of the drug. Because of the short half-life, addicts may take cocaine at intervals of 10 to 45 minutes, sometimes for several consecutive days. Unfortunately, tolerance develops slowly to the cardiovascular actions of cocaine. As the abuser escalates the doses to produce a desired level of euphoria, cardiovascular damage may be progressive.

Cocaine readily crosses the placenta to produce marked effects on the fetus. Because the fetus does not have the hepatic enzymes necessary to metabolize cocaine, drug effects are prolonged. Reports of cocaine-related changes include increased risk of miscarriage, preterm labor, low birth weight, and, possibly, birth defects. Newborns have increased irritability, feeding difficulties, and are easily startled.

The adverse effects of cocaine use are essentially the same as those for amphetamines. Metabolism by the liver forms an active metabolite that is more toxic than cocaine itself. After the feelings of euphoria diminish, the cocaine user may be left with a sense of irritability, exhaustion, insomnia, depression, and extreme distrust. Some users report the sensation that insects are crawling under the skin. Users who snort cocaine develop a runny nose, a crusty redness around the nostrils, and deterioration of the nasal cartilage. Overdose can result in dysrhythmias, seizures, stroke, or death due to respiratory arrest. Psychological dependence often leads to intense craving for the drug.

Caffeine

Caffeine is a natural substance found in the seeds, leaves, or fruits of more than 63 plant species throughout the world. Significant amounts of caffeine are consumed in chocolate, coffee, tea, soft drinks, and ice cream. Caffeine is sometimes added to OTC pain relievers and stimulants because it has been shown to increase the effectiveness of these medications. Caffeine is rapidly distributed to almost all parts of the body after ingestion, and several hours are needed to metabolize and eliminate the drug. Caffeine has a pronounced diuretic effect.

Caffeine is considered a CNS stimulant because it produces increased mental alertness, restlessness, nervousness, irritability, and insomnia. The physical effects of caffeine include dilation of the respiratory passages, increased blood pressure, increased production of stomach acid, and changes in blood glucose levels. Repeated use of caffeine may result in physical dependence and tolerance. Withdrawal symptoms include severe headaches, fatigue, depression, and impaired performance of daily activities.

Nicotine

27.11 Nicotine is a powerful and highly addictive cardiovascular and central nervous system stimulant.

Although nicotine is sometimes considered a CNS stimulant because it enhances alertness, its actions and long-term consequences place it into a class by itself. Nicotine is unique among abused substances in that it is legal, strongly addictive, and highly carcinogenic. Furthermore, tobacco use can cause harmful effects to those in the immediate area due to secondhand smoke. Patients often do not consider tobacco use to be substance abuse. It is the most common form of chemical dependence in the United States. Tobacco use among young people has been declining: The rate of smoking among youths age 12 to 17 in 2012 was half of the rate reported in 2002.

PharmFACT

In 2012, an estimated 69.5 million Americans age 12 years old and older were current users of a tobacco product. This represents 26.7% of the population in that age range (SAMHSA, 2013).

The most common method by which nicotine enters the body is through the inhalation of cigarette, pipe, or cigar smoke. Tobacco smoke contains several thousand chemicals, a significant number of which are carcinogens. The primary addictive drug present in cigarette smoke is nicotine, which reaches the brain in only 15 seconds, with effects that last from 30 minutes to several hours. Although nicotine has a half-life of only 2 to 3 hours, it accumulates in the body and is slowly released from the tissues, giving the patient virtually a 24-hour exposure to the drug.

Nicotine affects many body systems, including the nervous, cardiovascular, and endocrine systems. Nicotine promotes the release of epinephrine and has a direct stimulatory effect on the reticular activating system of the brain, causing symptoms that range from increased alertness and ability to focus to feelings of relaxation or lightheadedness. The psychoactive effects of smoking are generally described as pleasurable. The cardiovascular effects of nicotine include an accelerated heart rate and increased blood pressure, caused by activation of nicotinic receptors located throughout the autonomic nervous system (see Chapter 12). The cardiovascular effects of nicotine are particularly serious in smokers who are taking oral contraceptives—their risk of a fatal heart attack is five times greater than that of nonsmokers. Muscular tremors may occur with moderate doses of nicotine, and convulsions result from very high doses. Nicotine produces lower body weight by reducing appetite and increasing body metabolism. Chronic use leads to emphysema, heart disease, and lung cancer. There is clear evidence that tobacco use affects the reproductive system. Smokers are much more likely to be infertile, and smoking during pregnancy can cause birth defects and lower birth weight.

Both psychological and physical dependence occur relatively quickly with nicotine. Patients tend to continue their drug use for many years, despite overwhelming medical evidence that the quality of their life will be adversely affected and their lifespan shortened. Furthermore, a large majority of smokers try to quit each year and are unsuccessful and state that they wish they had never started the habit. Only 25% of those who attempt to stop smoking remain tobacco-free 1 year later.

Discontinuation of tobacco results in a withdrawal syndrome that includes agitation, impaired concentration, weight gain, anxiety, headache, and an extreme craving for the drug. The syndrome peaks at 24 to 48 hours after the last dose and may continue over several weeks. Symptoms vary in intensity among patients and are not related to dose or duration of use; those who are light smokers or who have smoked for a shorter length of time do not necessarily have less intense withdrawal symptoms. Approximately 90% of individuals who successfully stop smoking do so without any treatment.

Nicotine replacement therapy (NRT) is based on the assumption that the blood level of nicotine is what drives people to continue smoking. When blood nicotine levels fall, the person begins to experience early symptoms of withdrawal, which are quickly eliminated by smoking another cigarette. Indeed, blood nicotine levels have clearly been shown to influence smoking behavior. For example, if a smoker is switched to low-nicotine cigarettes, he or she will take longer and more frequent puffs. NRT delivery systems include transdermal patches (Figure 27.3), nasal sprays, and chewing gum that raise serum nicotine levels and help patients to

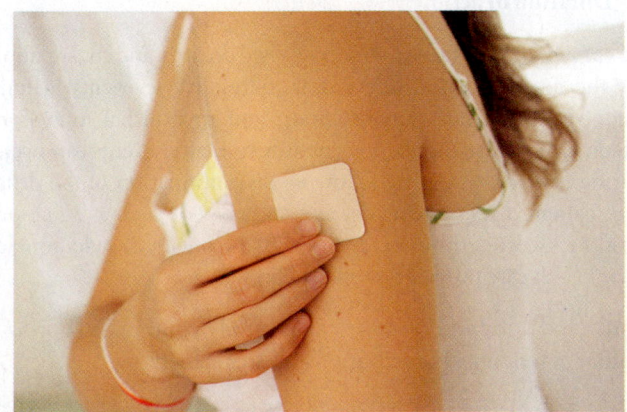

Figure 27.3 Nicotine replacement therapy: transdermal patch.
Courtesy of Ruth Jenkinson/Dorling Kindersley.

deal with the unpleasant withdrawal symptoms. Tobacco use, however, has a strong psychological component and simply replacing nicotine with patches or gum is ineffective for a large number of patients.

Recently, prescription medications have been used to promote smoking cessation. Bupropion (Zyban), a drug classified as an antidepressant, reduces cravings for nicotine and has been found to double the likelihood of becoming tobacco-free if it is taken for 3 to 6 months. Therapy generally begins 1 to 2 weeks before smoking cessation to lessen the severity of withdrawal symptoms. Bupropion is sometimes given concurrently with NRT. When used for depression, bupropion is marketed by the trade name of Wellbutrin. Varenicline (Chantix) is a newer drug approved by the FDA to manage nicotine withdrawal in patients seeking smoking cessation. Both bupropion and varenicline carry a black box warning that advises patients of serious neuropsychiatric events that can occur during therapy or shortly following discontinuation of the drug.

PROTOTYPE DRUG | **Varenicline (Chantix)**

Classification: **Therapeutic:** Drug for smoking cessation
Pharmacologic: Nicotinic receptor agonist

Therapeutic Effects and Uses: Doses are gradually increased over an 8-day period and maintained for 12 to 24 weeks to reduce withdrawal symptoms and cravings for smoking. It also prevents nicotine from reaching its receptors, thus blocking some of the pleasurable sensations should the person relapse and start smoking again.

Mechanism of Action: Varenicline activates nicotinic acetylcholine receptors in the brain and blocks nicotine from reaching the brain's receptors.

Pharmacokinetics:

Route(s)	PO
Absorption	Completely absorbed
Distribution	Bound to plasma protein (20%)
Primary metabolism	Mostly unmetabolized
Primary excretion	Renal
Onset of action	3–4 h
Duration of action	24 h

Adverse Effects: Nausea, vomiting, vivid dreams, and constipation are the most common side effects. Rare adverse events include angioedema, serious skin reactions, and myocardial infarction. **Black Box Warning:** Serious neuropsychiatric events can occur during therapy or shortly following discontinuation of the drug. Any patients experiencing changes in behavior such as agitation, hostility, depressed mood, or thoughts of suicide should contact their health care provider immediately.

Contraindications/Precautions: The only contraindication is a history of serious skin reactions with varenicline.

Drug Interactions: When used in combination with NRT, varenicline causes an increased incidence of nausea, vomiting, headache, dizziness, and fatigue, which may result in a premature termination of therapy.

Pregnancy: Category C.

Treatment of Overdose: No specific treatment for varenicline overdose is available.

Nursing Responsibilities: Key nursing implications for patients receiving varenicline are included in the Nursing Practice Application for Patients Receiving Pharmacotherapy for Substance Abuse Disorders.

Drugs Similar to Varenicline (Chantix)

There are no drugs similar to varenicline.

Inhalants

27.12 Inhalant abuse occurs when patients breathe the fumes of vaporized substances.

Inhalants are a diverse group of substances that have in common the ability to vaporize or form a gas at room temperature. Some are already in gaseous form, whereas others are liquids that have the property of volatility—rapid evaporation when exposed to air. Sometimes the liquids are heated to increase the speed or extent of vaporization. Most drugs in this class are placed in a paper or plastic bag or soaked on a cloth and deeply inhaled. Inhaling the fumes is known as huffing.

Inhalants differ greatly in their chemical structures and include nearly any chemical that can be vaporized. Products abused as inhalants include adhesives and glues, aerosols, cleaning agents, solvents, and fuels. These products are readily available and can be purchased at hardware or office supply stores. The highest use of inhalants is found among teens and preteens, probably because these agents can be found in nearly every household. Legal anesthetics such as nitrous oxide that are sometimes abused by medical personnel are also classified as inhalants and are discussed in Chapter 26.

The inhalation route affords almost instantaneous drug action and, because most of the inhalants are lipid soluble, the substances quickly enter the brain. The specific psychoactive effects depend on the inhalant used but generally include lightheadedness, drowsiness, exhilaration, and euphoria. Hallucinations are common. Symptoms of inhalant abuse often resemble alcohol intoxication. Because most psychoactive effects of inhalants are transient and disappear within minutes, the user may repeat the drug use multiple times over a period of several hours. Coma and death are possible with repeated exposure or high doses.

Because most inhalant abuse is sporadic, physical dependence is not observed, and it is unknown whether tolerance develops. Some of the inhalants cause hangover-like symptoms after the psychoactive effects wear off. When chronic abuse does occur, it is generally in adult males. Chronic effects can be serious and permanent, with the most obvious effects on the nervous system. Cognitive impairment, tremors, loss of coordination, hallucinations, psychosis, and dementia may be observed. Nephrotoxicity is common with certain inhalants. The breathing reflex may be diminished and patients may suffocate from placing a plastic bag over their heads.

Treatment for inhalant abuse is symptomatic. Long-term behavioral therapy may be needed to reinforce to the patient that permanent damage will result from chronic, continued abuse.

Patients Receiving Pharmacotherapy for Substance Abuse Disorders

Assessment	Potential Nursing Diagnoses*
Baseline assessment prior to administration: • Obtain a complete health history including cardiovascular, neurologic, respiratory, or hepatic disease, pregnancy, or breast-feeding. Obtain a drug history including allergies, substance used in disorder, current prescription and OTC drugs, and herbal preparations. Be alert to possible drug interactions. • Obtain a dietary history, especially noting possible vitamin deficiencies. • Assess for the presence and level of pain. • Obtain baseline vital signs and weight. • Evaluate appropriate laboratory findings (e.g., hepatic function studies, CBC). • Assess the patient's commitment to treatment and the ability to receive and understand instructions. Include family and caregivers as needed.	• *Anxiety* • *Ineffective Coping* • *Compromised Family Coping* • *Diarrhea*, related to excess alcohol intake, adverse drug effects • *Imbalanced Nutrition,* less than body requirements • *Impaired Memory* • *Insomnia* • *Social Isolation* • *Deficient Knowledge* (Drug Therapy) • *Risk for Injury*, related to substance use disorder, adverse drug effects
Assessment throughout administration: • Assess for desired therapeutic effects (e.g., decreased use or abstinence from the substance). • Continue periodic monitoring of hepatic function studies, CBC. • Assess vital signs, especially blood pressure and pulse. • Assess for and report adverse effects: headache, nausea, vomiting, insomnia, constipation, pain, skin rashes, excessive dizziness, drowsiness, confusion, agitation, thoughts of suicide, seizures.	

Implementation

Interventions and (Rationales)	Patient-Centered Care
Ensuring therapeutic effects: • Continue assessments as above for therapeutic effects. Substance use treatment requires commitment and continuing treatment and follow-up. (Nonpharmacologic measures such as group therapy may assist the patient in maintaining a substance-free state. Regularly scheduled visits with the health care provider provide opportunities to evaluate the success of treatment and for relapse.)	• Teach the patient that maintaining consistency of treatment to decrease substance use and eventual abstinence is the goal of therapy.
Minimizing adverse effects: • Continue to monitor vital signs, including respiratory rate, pulse, and blood pressure as ordered in patients receiving buprenorphine and disulfiram. (Buprenorphine (Suboxone, Zubsolv) is an opioid and may cause opioid-related adverse effects in higher dosages. Disulfiram (Antabuse) may cause intense reactions when alcohol is ingested or absorbed through the skin and may cause cardiovascular effects such as dysrhythmias, chest pain, and respiratory depression.)	• Teach the patient receiving buprenorphine to maintain the dosage as prescribed and to not increase the dose. • Teach the patient receiving disulfiram that all forms of alcohol must be avoided, including skin preparations that contain alcohol and mouth rinses. A reaction may occur up to 14 days after the last dose.
• Monitor for changes in behavior, including depression, hostility, agitation, or thoughts of suicide in patients taking varenicline (Chantix). (The drug carries a black box warning for serious neuropsychiatric events.)	• Instruct the patient, family, or caregiver to immediately report any unusual changes in mood or behavior.
• Monitor for skin rashes and facial or throat edema in patients taking varenicline. (Serious dermatologic reactions including angioedema have been noted.)	• Instruct the patient to immediately report any unusual rashes, changes in skin condition, or swelling of the tongue, face, or throat.
• Additional NRT should not be used during smoking cessation therapy with varenicline (Chantix). (Additional NRT will increase the incidence of adverse drug effects and may lead to early cessation of therapy.)	• Teach the patient that other NRT, including OTC patches and gum, should not be used while taking varenicline.
• Provide referrals to supportive therapies as an adjunct to substance use treatment. (Nonpharmacologic measures such as group therapy may be beneficial during therapy and to assist in maintaining a substance-free state after treatment.)	• Provide referral to supportive therapies such as Alcohol or Narcotics Anonymous and smoking cessation groups.
Patient understanding of drug therapy: • Use opportunities during administration of medications and during assessments to discuss the rationale for drug therapy, desired therapeutic outcomes, commonly observed adverse effects, parameters for when to call the health care provider, and any necessary monitoring or precautions. (Using time during nursing care helps to optimize and reinforce key teaching areas.)	• The patient should be able to state the reason for the drug, appropriate dose and scheduling, what adverse effects to observe for, and when to report them.
Patient self-administration of drug therapy: • When administering the medication, instruct the patient, family, or caregiver in the proper self-administration of the drug (e.g., take the drug exactly as prescribed). (Utilizing time during nurse-administration of these drugs helps to reinforce teaching.)	• The patient is able to discuss appropriate dosing and administration needs. • Teach the patient taking buprenorphine (Suboxone, Zubsolv) to take the medication sublingually by placing the tablet under the tongue and allowing it to dissolve. Do not chew or swallow the tablet. If more than one tablet is used, place all tablets under the tongue at the same time.

*Nursing Diagnoses—Definitions and Classification 2015–2017. Copyright © 2014, 1994–2014 by NANDA International. Used by arrangement with John Wiley & Sons Limited.

Anabolic Steroids

27.13 Anabolic steroids are abused for their ability to increase muscle strength.

All of the drugs presented thus far in this chapter have in common the ability to affect the CNS and produce psychoactive effects. Many produce euphoria, some induce relaxation, whereas others enhance alertness. In most cases, the user views the drug experience as pleasurable and the drug effects are experienced soon after it is taken, sometimes within seconds. Anabolic steroids, however, are not taken for their CNS actions, and their desirable effects may be delayed for weeks or months. In this respect they are different from other abused substances.

Anabolic steroids are very similar to testosterone, the primary male sex hormone or androgen. The term *anabolic* means growth or building up. Because these substances can add to skeletal muscle mass and increased strength, they are usually abused in an attempt to enhance athletic performance. Do these drugs actually boost performance? The answer is a qualified yes. The most important aspects of athletic performance are skill, training, and confidence. If these factors are equal among performers, anabolic steroids may indeed provide an extra boost in performance, which is all important in a competitive sport such as track, downhill skiing, or swimming where a few hundredths of a second can mean the difference between first and sixth place. On the other hand, no amount of steroid is able to overcome lack of athletic skill or inadequate training. Most sports organizations have banned the use of these drugs and athletes may be eliminated from competition if they test positive for anabolic steroids. Some abusers take anabolic steroids to enhance their appearance and self-confidence, rather than for athletic competition.

Anabolic steroids have legitimate medical uses as replacement therapy for men who secrete deficient quantities of testosterone and they are occasionally used to treat certain cancers. Doses used by abusers, however, are 10 to 100 times higher than those required for therapeutic use.

Anabolic steroids may be taken as tablets, as IM injections, or applied as ointments or as a transdermal patch. Abusers may take two or more different types of steroids concurrently, sometimes by different routes, a practice called "stacking." The drugs may be taken in a cyclic pattern called "pyramiding" in which the dose is progressively increased over 6 to 12 weeks, then slowly decreased to zero. Abusers believe that this is a safer and more effective way to obtain benefits from the drugs.

One of the ironies of steroid abuse is that the very drug that is being taken to enhance appearance and performance eventually produces serious consequences that have the opposite effect. Men may believe that anabolic steroids make them appear more masculine, but the drugs can cause infertility, impotence, testicular atrophy, and breast enlargement (gynecomastia). Women taking anabolic steroids will develop masculine characteristics, excessive growth of body hair (hirsutism), shrinking of breast size, menstrual irregularities, and deepening of the voice. The most serious adverse effects, in both men and women, include hepatic cysts, elevated cholesterol, myocardial infarction, and stroke. Personality changes include aggression, violent behavior, depression, insomnia, anorexia, and decreased libido.

Anabolic steroids are classified as Schedule II drugs due to their abuse potential. In an attempt to stem the rising abuse of these drugs, Congress passed the Anabolic Steroid Control Act of 2004 to control 26 different steroid precursors, such as androstenedione (Andro). Some companies were legally selling these precursors as dietary supplements, despite the fact that these agents are metabolized to steroids in the body and essentially carry the same risks. It is interesting to note that one of the most popular supplements, dehydroepiandrosterone (DHEA), was specifically and intentionally omitted from that list and remains legal. DHEA is a natural steroid precursor secreted by the adrenal gland that is claimed to have antiaging and performance-enhancing properties.

27.14 The nurse has a pivotal role in recognizing and treating substance abuse.

The nurse serves a key role in the prevention, diagnosis, and treatment of substance abuse. During assessment, nurses may be the first members of the health care team to recognize symptoms and signs of substance abuse. Patients are often reluctant to report their drug use for fear of embarrassment or being arrested. In known IV drug users, the nurse must consider the possibility of HIV infection, hepatitis, tuberculosis, and associated diagnoses. The nurse must be knowledgeable about the signs and symptoms of substance abuse and develop a keen sense of perception during the assessment process. In their role as educators, nurses distribute important information on substance abuse prevention and the proper use of prescription drugs. A trusting nurse–patient relationship is essential to helping patients deal with their dependence.

It is often difficult for a practitioner not to condemn or stigmatize a patient for his or her substance abuse. Nurses, especially those in large cities, are all too familiar with the devastating medical, economic, and social consequences of drug abuse. The nurse must be firm in disapproving substance abuse, yet compassionate in trying to help the patient receive treatment. A list of social agencies dealing with dependency should be readily available to provide to patients. Whenever possible, the nurse should attempt to involve family members and other close contacts in the treatment regimen.

CHAPTER

27 Understanding the Chapter

Key Concepts Summary

27.1 A wide variety of different substances may be abused by patients.

27.2 Drugs with a potential for abuse are restricted by the Controlled Substances Act and are categorized into schedules.

27.3 Addiction is an overwhelming compulsion to continue repeated drug use.

27.4 Physical and psychological dependence lead to continued drug-seeking behavior despite negative health and social consequences.

27.5 A withdrawal syndrome is a set of characteristic symptoms that occurs when an abused substance is discontinued.

27.6 Tolerance occurs when the body adapts to a drug and larger doses are needed to produce a therapeutic effect.

27.7 Central nervous system depressants, which include sedatives, opioids, and alcohol, decrease the activity of the central nervous system.

27.8 Marijuana is the most frequently abused illicit substance.

27.9 Hallucinogens and club drugs cause an altered state of thought and perception.

27.10 Stimulants such as amphetamines and cocaine increase the activity of the central nervous system.

27.11 Nicotine is a powerful and highly addictive cardiovascular and central nervous system stimulant.

27.12 Inhalant abuse occurs when patients breathe the fumes of vaporized substances.

27.13 Anabolic steroids are abused for their ability to increase muscle strength.

27.14 The nurse has a pivotal role in recognizing and treating substance abuse.

Case Study: Making the Patient Connection

Remember the patient "J. C. Wilkins" at the beginning of the chapter? Now read the remainder of the case study. Based on the information presented within this chapter, respond to the critical thinking questions that follow.

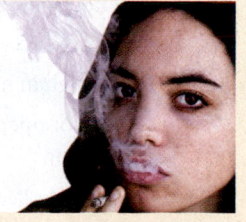

J. C. Wilkins has come to the counseling clinic to get information and advice about her pregnancy and drug use. She is a 19-year-old woman who has been living with her boyfriend for the past 18 months. Since she moved in, she has been a daily user of heroin.

J. C. has a long history of substance abuse. When she was 14 years old, her stepfather sexually abused her on a regular basis. To cope with the guilt and shame, she began using alcohol and marijuana. On her 16th birthday, J. C. ran away from home and never returned. Since then she has done anything and everything possible to survive, including selling herself for sex.

To support herself and her heroin addiction, J. C. has become a prostitute. She states that she usually drinks at least four to five beers before she walks the streets at night. If she cannot score enough heroin, she will smoke crack or take Valium just to "mellow out." J. C. says that her drug abuse is only to calm her nerves and get her through the night. In periods when she was not able

to obtain drugs, she states she felt sick with trembling and perfuse sweating. However, she is convinced that she can stop any time she wishes.

J. C. reports that she has not had a menstrual period in 2 months and her breasts are swollen and tender. She is certain she is pregnant, although she has not been tested, and is confused about what to do. She is hopeful that her unemployed boyfriend is the father but is not totally sure. She believes that if she stops working, he will abandon her, and there will be no means to support herself or a baby.

Critical Thinking Questions

1. How would you classify J. C.'s substance abuse? Physical dependence or psychological dependence, or both? Explain.

2. Create a list of abused substances reported by J. C. What symptoms of withdrawal would you expect with each?

3. What effect will J. C.'s substance abuse have on her unborn baby? Should J. C. stop using drugs while pregnant? Why or why not?

4. As the nurse, describe your approach in dealing with this patient.

5. Addiction depends on multiple variables such as drug factors, user factors, and environmental factors. Considering the case study, describe how each variable attributes to J. C.'s substance abuse.

See Answers to Critical Thinking Questions on student resource website.

Additional Case Study

A neighbor reports that patient Martin Thomas was discovered wandering the halls in his apartment building in a confused state. The neighbor states that Martin called him by the wrong name even though they have known each other for several years. Martin was agitated about not being able to find the bus stop. In the emergency department, Martin appears apprehensive, diaphoretic, and trembling. His nose and cheeks are red with spider veins, and his abdomen is noticeably distended. He tells you that up until 3 days ago, he consumed alcohol daily. However, because he has no money, he cannot buy any liquor and has not been drinking.

1. Define *delirium tremens*. What is the treatment priority for this condition?

2. Discuss how food or beverages can increase the excretion rate of alcohol.

3. Describe the effects of alcohol on the central nervous system. Is alcohol a stimulant or a depressant?

See Answers to Additional Case Study on student resource website.

Chapter Review

1 The patient returned from major surgery 3 hours ago and requests medication for pain. In considering the best action for this patient, the nurse knows that:

1. Prescription drugs rarely cause addiction when used according to accepted medical protocol.

2. All drugs should be withheld until the patient's past substance abuse history is evaluated.

3. It is best to wait until the patient can no longer tolerate the pain to avoid addiction problems.

4. Patients often request analgesia when it is not really needed.

2 Which of the following statements made by the patient recovering from a substance use disorder would indicate high potential for relapse?

1. "I need the help of a support system to stop using."

2. "After I stop using, I will no longer have a desire to use drugs."

3. "Whom I hang out with doesn't make any difference in whether or not I use drugs."

4. "Talking with other recovering addicts will help me cope."

3 A nurse is teaching a patient who will begin varenicline (Chantix) for smoking cessation. Which of the following instructions will the nurse give the patient? Select all that apply.

1. Doses will be increased over a week's period and the drug used for up to 6 months.

2. Smoking may continue because the drug blocks the harmful effects of nicotine.

3. The drug is not known to cause any adverse effects and has an excellent safety profile.

4. Any unusual rashes, skin reactions, or facial edema should be reported immediately.

5. Any unusual changes in behavior including depression, hostility, or thoughts of suicide should be reported immediately.

4 Which parameter is most critical when a nurse is assessing a patient with an overdose of sedatives?

1. Cardiac stimulation

2. Respiratory suppression

3. Hepatic dysfunction

4. Depression of consciousness

5 A 22-year-old heroin addict is exhibiting withdrawal symptoms. Which symptoms of withdrawal does the nurse expect?

1. Somnolence, lethargy, and fatigue

2. Dry skin, rash, and itching

3. Paranoia, hallucinations, and delusions

4. Chills, runny nose, and muscle spasms

6 While teaching the patient about disulfiram (Antabuse), which of the following should the nurse instruct the patient to avoid?

1. Mouthwash, alcoholic beverages, and over-the-counter cold medications

2. Dairy products such as milk, cream, and yogurt

3. Foods high in iron such as green leafy vegetables

4. Driving or operating machinery while taking this medication

See Answers to Chapter Review in Appendix A.

References

American Psychiatric Association. (2013). *Diagnostic and statistical manual of mental disorders* (5th ed.). Washington, DC: Author.

Blazer, D., & Wu, L. T. (2009). The epidemiology of substance use and disorders among middle aged and elderly community adults: National survey on drug use and health. *American Journal of Geriatric Psychiatry, 17,* 237–245. doi:10.1097/JGP.0b013e318190b8ef

Criss, E. (2009). Huffing: Prehospital identification & treatment of inhalant abuse. *JEMS, 34*(5), 42–43, 45, 47.

National Institute on Drug Abuse. (2014). *Drug facts: High school and youth trends.* Retrieved from http://www.drugabuse.gov/publications/drugfacts/high-school-youth-trends

Substance Abuse and Mental Health Administration. (2011). *Results from the 2010 national survey on drug use and health: Summary of national findings* (NSDUH Series H-41, HHS Publication No. [SMA] 11-4658). Retrieved from http://oas.samhsa.gov/NSDUH/2k10NSDUH/2k10Results.htm

Substance Abuse and Mental Health Services Administration. (2013). *Results from the 2012 national survey on drug use and health; summary of national findings* (NSDUH Series H-46, HHS Publication No. [SMA] 13-4795). Retrieved from http://www.samhsa.gov/data/NSDUH/2012SummNatFindDetTables/NationalFindings/NSDUHresults2012.htm#ch2

Selected Bibliography

Akerman, S. C., Hammel, J. L., & Brunette, M. F. (2010). Dextromethorphan abuse and dependence in adolescents. *Journal of Dual Diagnosis, 6,* 266–278. doi:10.1080/15504263.2010.537515

Alameida, M. D., Harrington, C., LaPlante, M., & Kang, T. (2010). Factors associated with alcohol use and its consequences. *Journal of Addictions Nursing, 21,* 194–206. doi:10.3109/10884602.2010.515692

Cahill, K., Stead, L. F., & Lancaster, T. (2012). Nicotine receptor partial agonists for smoking cessation. *Cochrane Database of Systematic Reviews, 4,* CD006103. doi:10.1002/14651858.CD006103.pub5

Ciketic, S., Hayatbakhsh, M. R., Doran, C. M., Najman, J. M., & McKetin, R. (2012). A review of psychological and pharmacological treatment options for methamphetamine dependence. *Journal of Substance Use, 17,* 363–383. doi:10.3109/14659891.2011.592900

Cohen, L. M., Collins, F. L., Jr., Young, A. M., McChargue, D. E., Leffingwell, T. R., & Cook, K. L. (2009). *Pharmacology and treatment of substance abuse.* New York, NY: Taylor & Francis.

Conca, A. J., & Worthen, D. R. (2012). Nonprescription drug abuse. *Journal of Pharmacy Practice, 25,* 13–21. doi:10.1177/0897190011431148

Fornili, K., & Burda, C. (2010). Overview of current federal policy for substance abuse disorders. *Journal of Addictions Nursing, 21,* 247–251. doi:10.3109/10884602.2010.525788

Hasin, D. S., O'Brien, C. P., Auriacombe, M., Borges, G., Bucholz, K., Budney, A., . . . Grant, B. F. (2013). DSM-5 criteria for substance use disorders: Recommendations and rationale. *The American Journal of Psychiatry, 170,* 834–851. doi:10.1176/appi.ajp.2013.12060782

Herdman, T. H., & Kamitsuru, S. (Eds.). (2014). *NANDA International nursing diagnoses: Definitions and classification, 2015–2017.* Oxford, United Kingdom: Wiley-Blackwell.

Howard, M. O., Bowen, S. E., Garland, E. L., Perron, B. E., & Vaughn, M. G. (2011). Inhalant use and inhalant use disorders in the United States. *Addiction Science & Clinical Practice, 6*(1), 18.

O'Malley, P. (2010). Prescription and over-the-counter drug and substance abuse: Something available for every age, anytime and anywhere: Update for the clinical nurse specialist. *Clinical Nurse Specialist, 24,* 286–288. doi:10.1097/NUR.0b013e3181fbf1b5

Soghoian, S. (2013). *Disulfiram toxicity.* Retrieved from http://emedicine.medscape.com/article/814525-overview

UNIT
5

Pharmacology of the Cardiovascular System

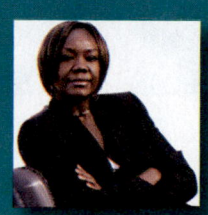 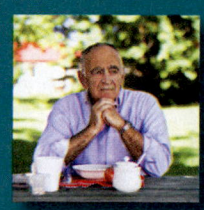 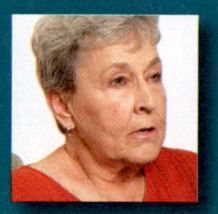 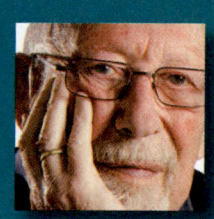

CHAPTER 28   Review of the Cardiovascular System / 440

CHAPTER 29   Pharmacotherapy of Hyperlipidemia / 453

CHAPTER 30   Pharmacotherapy with Calcium Channel Blockers / 473

CHAPTER 31   Drugs Affecting the Renin-Angiotensin-Aldosterone System / 486

CHAPTER 32   Diuretic Therapy and the Pharmacotherapy of Renal Failure / 501

CHAPTER 33   Pharmacotherapy of Fluid Imbalance, Electrolyte, and Acid–Base Disorders / 521

CHAPTER 34   Pharmacotherapy of Hypertension / 541

CHAPTER 35   Pharmacotherapy of Angina Pectoris and Myocardial Infarction / 559

CHAPTER 36   Pharmacotherapy of Heart Failure / 578

CHAPTER 37   Pharmacotherapy of Dysrhythmias / 596

CHAPTER 38   Pharmacotherapy of Coagulation Disorders / 614

CHAPTER 39   Pharmacotherapy of Hematopoietic Disorders / 642

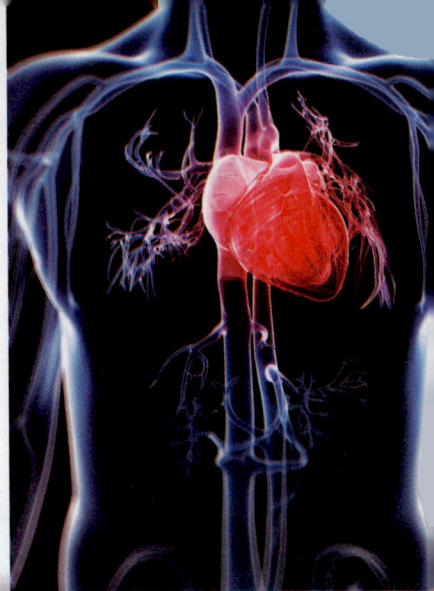

CHAPTER

28

Review of the Cardiovascular System

LEARNING OUTCOMES

After reading this chapter, the student should be able to:

1. Describe the major structures of the cardiovascular system.
2. Identify the components of blood and their functions.
3. Construct a flowchart diagramming the primary steps of hemostasis.
4. Describe the structure of the heart and the function of the myocardium.
5. Describe the role of the coronary arteries in supplying the myocardium with oxygen.
6. Illustrate the flow of electrical impulses through the normal heart.
7. Explain the major factors affecting cardiac output.
8. Explain the effects of cardiac output, peripheral resistance, and blood volume on hemodynamics.
9. Discuss how the vasomotor center, baroreceptors, chemoreceptors, and hormones regulate blood pressure.

CHAPTER OUTLINE

▶ **Structure and Function of the Cardiovascular System**

▶ **Functions and Properties of Blood**
   Components of Blood
   Hemostasis

▶ **Cardiac Structure and Function**
   Cardiac Muscle
   Coronary Arteries
   Cardiac Conduction System
   Cardiac Output

▶ **Hemodynamics and Blood Pressure**
   Hemodynamic Factors Affecting Blood Pressure
   Neural Regulation of Blood Pressure
   Hormonal Influences on Blood Pressure

KEY TERMS

afterload, 448	erythropoietin, 441	prothrombin, 444
antidiuretic hormone (ADH), 450	extrinsic pathway, 443	reflex tachycardia, 449
atrial natriuretic peptide (ANP), 451	fibrin, 444	renin-angiotensin-aldosterone
atrial reflex, 450	fibrinogen, 444	system (RAAS), 451
automaticity, 445	hemopoiesis, 442	sinus rhythm, 445
baroreceptors, 449	hemostasis, 443	stroke volume, 447
cardiac output (CO), 447	inotropic drugs, 448	thrombin, 444
chemoreceptors, 449	intrinsic pathway, 443	thrombopoietin, 442
coagulation, 443	myocardium, 444	vasomotor center, 449
contractility, 447	peripheral resistance, 449	venous return, 447
ectopic foci, 445	preload, 447	

It is likely that the nurse will administer more cardiovascular drugs than any other class of medications. Why is this the case? First, health care providers have discovered the huge benefits of keeping blood pressure and blood lipid values within normal limits and how to prevent heart attacks and strokes. Second, the heart and vessels weaken over time and, as the average lifespan of the population increases, more pharmacotherapy will be needed to treat the chronic cardiovascular diseases of older adults.

A comprehensive knowledge of cardiovascular anatomy and physiology is essential to understanding cardiovascular pharmacology, which encompasses the next 11 chapters of this book. The purpose of this chapter is to offer a brief review of the components of the structure and function of the cardiovascular system that are important to pharmacotherapy. For more comprehensive treatments of these topics, the student should refer to an anatomy and physiology textbook.

Structure and Function of the Cardiovascular System

28.1 The cardiovascular system consists of the blood, heart, and blood vessels.

The three major components of the cardiovascular system are the blood, heart, and blood vessels, as shown in Figure 28.1. These three components work as an integrated whole to transport the essential oxygen, nutrients, and other substances that keep the body in homeostasis. Disruption of this flow for even brief periods can have serious, if not mortal, consequences. The functions of the cardiovascular system are diverse and include the following:

- Transport of nutrients and wastes
- Pumping of blood
- Regulation of blood pressure
- Regulation of acid–base balance
- Regulation of fluid balance
- Regulation of body temperature
- Protection against invasion by microbes

The cardiovascular system can only function with the cooperation of other body systems. For example, the role of the autonomic nervous system in controlling heart rate and blood vessel diameter is presented in Chapter 12. The kidneys are intimately involved in assisting the cardiovascular system with fluid and acid–base balance, as discussed in Chapter 33. The respiratory system must bring oxygen to the blood and remove carbon dioxide from it. The student should view the cardiovascular system as an important part of the body's ability to maintain overall homeostasis.

Functions and Properties of Blood

28.2 Blood consists of formed elements and plasma.

Blood is a liquid connective tissue that consists of formed elements suspended in plasma. The solid, formed elements of the blood are the erythrocytes, leukocytes, and platelets. When combined, the formed elements comprise about 45% of the composition of blood.

The most numerous blood cells are erythrocytes, which comprise 99.9% of the formed elements. Carrying the iron-containing protein hemoglobin, the erythrocytes are responsible for transporting oxygen to the tissues and carbon dioxide from the tissues to the lungs. A single erythrocyte can carry as many as one billion molecules of oxygen. Erythrocyte homeostasis is controlled by **erythropoietin**, a hormone secreted by the kidney in response to low oxygen levels in the blood. Once secreted, erythropoietin stimulates the body's production of erythrocytes. Insufficient numbers of erythrocytes or structural defects such as sickle shapes lead to anemia, which is a common indication for pharmacotherapy (see Chapter 39).

Although small in number, leukocytes serve an essential role in the body's defense against infection. Unlike erythrocytes, which are all structurally identical, there are several types of leukocytes, each serving a different function. For example, neutrophils are the most common leukocyte and they respond to bacterial infections through phagocytosis of the microbes. The second most common leukocyte, the lymphocyte, is the key cell in the immune response that responds by secreting antibodies (B lymphocytes) or secreting cytokines (T lymphocytes) that rid the body of the microbe. A review of body defenses and the immune system is presented in Chapter 40.

The final formed elements of the blood are thrombocytes or platelets, which are actually fragments of larger cells called

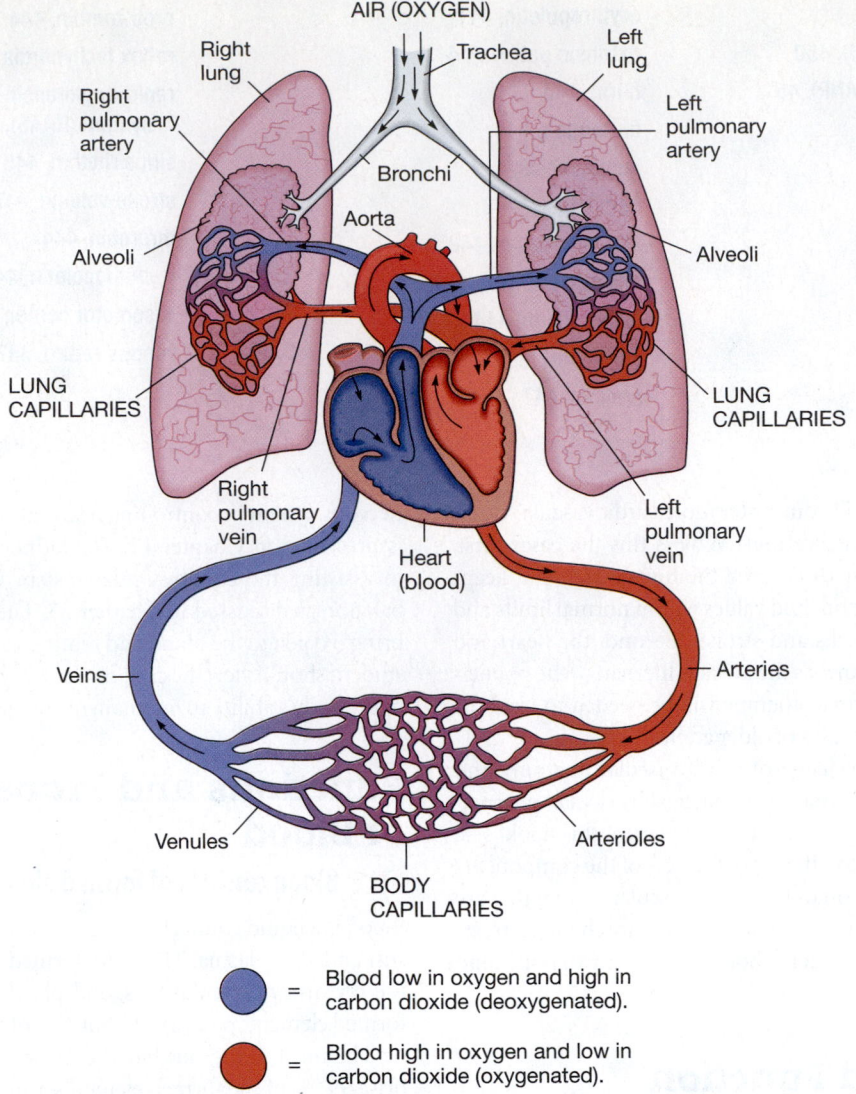

AIR (OXYGEN)

Right lung

Trachea

Left lung

Right pulmonary artery

Left pulmonary artery

Bronchi

Aorta

Alveoli

Alveoli

LUNG CAPILLARIES

LUNG CAPILLARIES

Right pulmonary vein

Left pulmonary vein

Heart (blood)

Veins

Arteries

Venules

Arterioles

BODY CAPILLARIES

= Blood low in oxygen and high in carbon dioxide (deoxygenated).

= Blood high in oxygen and low in carbon dioxide (oxygenated).

Figure 28.1 The cardiovascular system.

megakaryocytes. Platelets stick to the walls of damaged blood vessels to begin the process of blood coagulation, which prevents excessive bleeding from sites of injury. Abnormally low numbers of platelets, or thrombocytopenia, can result in serious delays in blood clotting. Platelet homeostasis is controlled by the hormone **thrombopoietin**, which promotes the formation of additional platelets. The role of platelets and thrombopoietin in blood coagulation is a major topic in Chapter 38, which discusses the pharmacotherapy of blood coagulation.

The production and maturation of blood cells, called **hemopoiesis** or hematopoiesis, occurs in red bone marrow. It is here that primitive stem cells of the blood become committed to forming erythrocytes, leukocytes, or platelets. This process occurs continuously throughout the lifespan and is subject to various homeostatic controls as well as certain drugs and physical agents. For example, ionizing radiation and a large number of drugs have the potential to adversely affect bone marrow and cause myelosuppression. Myelosuppression is a very serious adverse effect that reduces the number of erythrocytes, leukocytes, and thrombocytes, leaving patients susceptible to anemia, infection, and bleeding. Many

drugs used to treat cancer and those given to reduce the possibility of transplant rejection can produce profound myelosuppression as a dose-limiting adverse effect.

Plasma is the fluid portion of blood that consists of water, proteins, electrolytes, lipoproteins, carbohydrates, and other regulatory substances. The primary proteins in plasma are albumins (54%), globulins (38%), and fibrinogen (7%). Albumin is the primary regulator of blood osmotic pressure (also called oncotic pressure), which determines the movement of fluids among the vascular, interstitial, and cellular compartments or spaces. Globulins, also known as immunoglobulins or antibodies, are important in protecting the body from foreign agents such as bacteria or viruses. Fibrinogen is a critical protein in the coagulation of blood. The liver synthesizes over 90% of the plasma proteins; therefore, patients with serious hepatic impairment will have deficiencies in coagulation and in maintaining body defenses.

Serum is a term closely related to plasma. Serum contains all the components of plasma, except clotting factors such as fibrinogen have been removed. Serum is often used for blood typing and for determining blood levels of substances such as cholesterol, glucose, and hormones.

Fluid balance in the body is achieved by maintaining the proper amount of plasma in the blood. Too little water in plasma results in dehydration, whereas too much causes edema and hypertension (HTN). Various organs help to maintain normal fluid balance, including the kidneys, gastrointestinal (GI) tract, and skin. The pharmacotherapy of fluid and electrolyte imbalances is an important topic in pharmacology and is discussed in Chapter 33.

CONNECTION Checkpoint 28.1

From what you learned in Chapter 3, what role does plasma protein play in the distribution of drugs? *See Answer to Connection Checkpoint 28.1 on student resource website.*

PharmFACT

To maintain homeostasis, the body must make 3 million erythrocytes every second. Red blood cells are so numerous that they comprise approximately one third of all cells in the body (Martini, Nath, & Bartholomew, 2012).

28.3 Hemostasis is a complex process involving multiple steps and a large number of enzymes and factors.

The process of **hemostasis** is complex, involving 13 different clotting factors that contribute to the stoppage of blood flow. Hemostasis occurs in a series of sequential steps, sometimes referred to as a cascade. Hemostasis is an essential mechanism that the body uses to prevent excessive bleeding following injury. Medications can be used to modify several of these steps, either to speed up or delay the clotting process (see Chapter 38).

Injury to a blood vessel triggers the clotting process. The vessel spasms, causing constriction, which slows blood flow to the injured area. Platelets have an affinity for the damaged vessel: They become sticky and adhere to each other and to the injured area. The clumping of platelets, or aggregation, is facilitated by adenosine diphosphate (ADP), the enzyme thrombin, and thromboxane A_2. Platelet receptor sites and von Willebrand's factor make adhesion possible. The aggregated platelets disintegrate to initiate a platelet binding cascade. Blood flow is further slowed, thus allowing the process of **coagulation**, which is the formation of an insoluble clot, to occur. The basic steps of hemostasis are shown in Figure 28.2.

When collagen is exposed at the site of vessel injury, the damaged cells initiate the coagulation cascade. Coagulation itself occurs when fibrin threads create a meshwork that fortifies the blood constituents so that clots can develop. During the cascade, various plasma proteins that are circulating in an inactive state are converted to their active forms. Two separate pathways, along with numerous biochemical processes, lead to coagulation. The **intrinsic pathway** is activated in response to injury and takes several minutes to complete. The **extrinsic pathway** is activated when blood leaks out of a vessel and enters tissue spaces. The extrinsic pathway is less complex and is completed within seconds. The two pathways share some common steps and the outcome is the same—the formation of the fibrin clot. The steps in each pathway are shown in Figure 28.3.

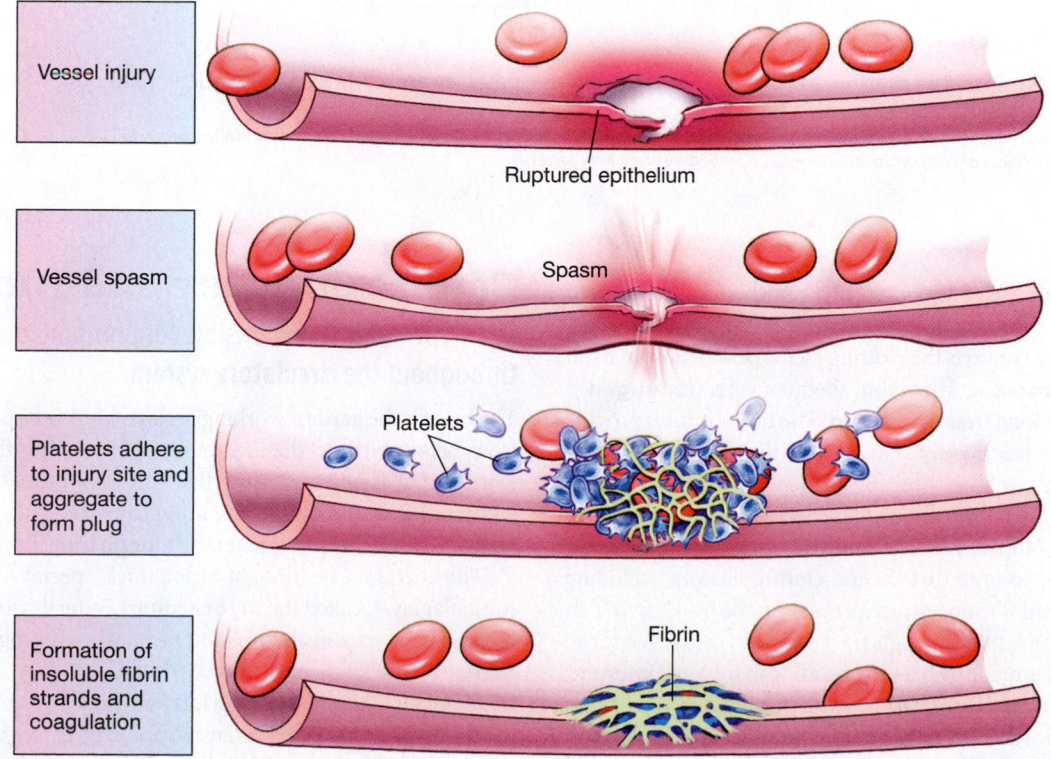

Figure 28.2 The basic steps in hemostasis.

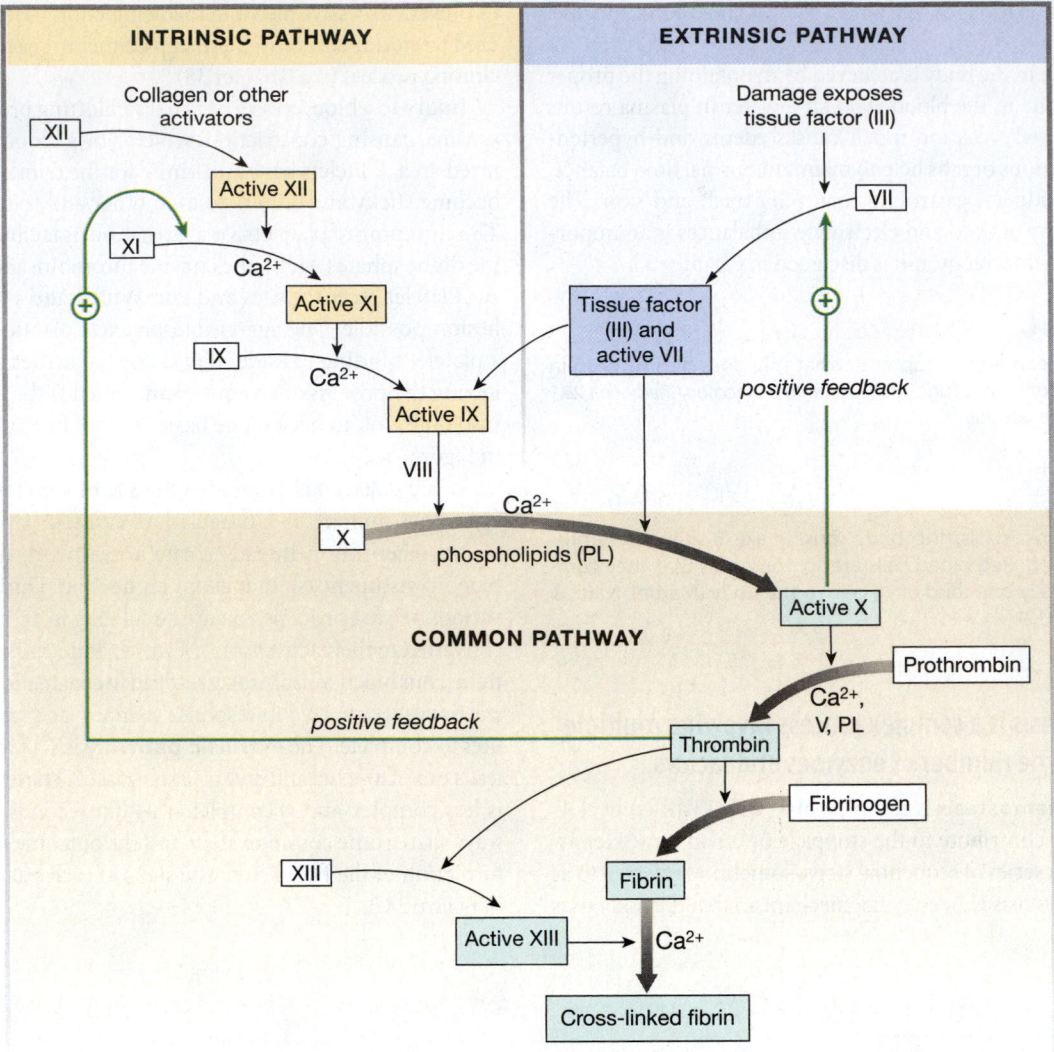

Figure 28.3 The coagulation cascade. Both the intrinsic pathway and extrinsic pathway lead to a common pathway and eventually a dense fibrin clot.
From *Human Physiology: An Integrated Approach*, 5th ed., by D. U. Silverthorn, 2010. Reprinted and electronically reproduced by permission of Pearson Education, Inc., Upper Saddle River, New Jersey.

Near the end of the common pathway, a chemical called prothrombin activator (see Active X in Figure 28.3) is formed. The prothrombin activator converts the clotting factor **prothrombin** to an enzyme called **thrombin**. Thrombin then converts **fibrinogen**, a plasma protein, to long strands of **fibrin**. The fibrin strands provide a framework to anchor the clot. Thus two of the factors essential to clotting, thrombin and fibrin, are only formed after injury to the vessels. The fibrin strands form an insoluble web over the injured area to stop blood loss. Normal blood clotting occurs in about 6 minutes.

It is important to note that several clotting factors, including thromboplastin and fibrinogen, are proteins made by the liver that are constantly circulating through the blood in an inactive form. Vitamin K, which is made by bacteria residing in the large intestine, is required for the liver to make four of the clotting factors. Because of the crucial importance of the liver in creating these clotting factors, patients with serious hepatic impairment often have abnormal coagulation.

Cardiac Structure and Function

28.4 The heart is responsible for pumping blood throughout the circulatory system.

The heart is the hardest working organ in the body, pumping blood from before birth to the last minute of life. With the continuous workload, it is not surprising that this organ eventually weakens and that heart disease is the leading cause of death in the United States. The heart is a frequent target for pharmacotherapy.

The heart may be thought of as a thick, specialized muscle. The muscular layer, called the **myocardium**, is the thickest of the heart layers and is responsible for the physical pumping action of the heart. The thickness of the myocardium is greatest in the left ventricle because this chamber performs the greatest amount of work. Cardiac muscle contains extensive branching networks of cellular structures that connect cardiac muscle cells to each other, allowing the entire myocardium to contract as a coordinated whole.

Should myocardial cells (myocytes) die, the body is unable to replace them because cardiac muscle cells do not undergo mitosis. If a large area of cardiac muscle becomes deprived of oxygen and undergoes necrosis, the myocytes are replaced by fibrotic scar tissue and heart function becomes impaired. The different regions of the heart may not contract in a coordinated manner because conduction of the electrical potential may skip over areas of necrosis on the myocardium. This can result in heart failure or dysrhythmias, which are frequent indications for pharmacotherapy (see Chapters 36 and 37).

The heart has four chambers that receive blood prior to being pumped, as illustrated in Figure 28.4b. These chambers differ in size, depending on their function. The left ventricle is the largest, because it must hold enough blood to pump to all body tissues. During heart failure, the size of the left ventricle and the thickness of the myocardial layer in this chamber can increase in size in patients, which is a condition known as left ventricular hypertrophy.

PharmFACT

The heart pumps about 8,000 liters of blood every day, which is enough to fill forty, 55-gallon drums or 8,800 quart-size containers (Martini et al., 2012).

28.5 The coronary arteries bring essential nutrients to the myocardium.

Working continuously around the clock, the heart requires a bountiful supply of oxygen and other nutrients. These are provided by the right and left coronary arteries and their branches, as shown in Figure 28.4a. The coronary arteries have the ability to rapidly adapt to the heart's needs for oxygen. For example, during exercise the heart rate and strength of contraction markedly increase, and healthy coronary arteries quickly dilate to provide oxygen to meet this increased workload on the myocardium.

The coronary arteries are subject to atherosclerosis, a buildup of fatty plaque, which narrows the lumen and restricts the blood supply reaching myocytes. If allowed to progress, the narrowing results in chest pain, a condition known as angina pectoris. The first sign of angina is pain upon exercise or exertion, since this is when the workload on the heart is increased. Continued narrowing increases the risk of a myocardial infarction.

The coronary arteries are important targets for pharmacotherapy. Chapter 29 explains how reducing lipid levels in the blood can decrease the risk of atherosclerosis of the coronary arteries (and other arteries). Chapter 35 discusses how drugs can be used to reduce angina pain and decrease the risk of mortality following a heart attack. Chapter 36 introduces drugs that reduce the cardiac workload in patients with heart failure so that the heart does not require as much oxygen from the coronary arteries.

28.6 The cardiac conduction system keeps the heart beating in a synchronized manner.

For the heart to function properly, the atria must contract simultaneously, sending their blood into the ventricles. Following atrial contraction, the right and left ventricles then must contract simultaneously. Lack of synchronization of the atria and ventricles or of the right and left sides of the heart may have profound consequences. Proper timing of chamber contractions is made possible by the cardiac conduction system, a branching network of specialized cardiac muscle cells that sends a synchronized, electrical signal across the myocardium. These electrical impulses, or action potentials, carry the signal for the cardiac muscle cells to contract and must be coordinated precisely for the chambers to beat in a synchronized manner. The cardiac conduction system is illustrated in Figure 28.5.

Control of the cardiac conduction system begins in a small area of tissue in the wall of the right atrium known as the sinoatrial (SA) node or cardiac pacemaker. Cells in the SA node have the property of **automaticity**, the ability to spontaneously generate action potentials without an outside signal from the nervous system. The SA node generates a new action potential approximately 75 times per minute under resting conditions. This is referred to as the normal **sinus rhythm**. The SA node is greatly influenced by the activity of the sympathetic and parasympathetic divisions of the autonomic nervous system.

Upon leaving the SA node, the action potential travels quickly across both atria and through internodal pathways to the atrioventricular (AV) node. Myocytes in the AV node also have the property of automaticity, although less so than the SA node. Should the SA node malfunction, the AV node has the ability to spontaneously generate action potentials and continue the heart's contraction at a rate of 40 to 60 beats per minute. Compared to other areas in the heart, impulse conduction through the AV node is slow. This allows the atria sufficient time to completely contract and empty their blood before the ventricles receive their signal to contract. If the ventricles should contract prematurely, the AV valves will close and the atria will be prevented from completely emptying their contents.

As the action potential leaves the AV node, it travels rapidly to the AV bundle or bundle of His. The pathway between the AV node and the bundle of His is the only electrical connection between the atria and the ventricles. The impulse is conducted down the right and left bundle branches to the Purkinje fibers, which rapidly carry the action potential to all regions of the ventricles almost simultaneously. Should the SA and AV nodes become nonfunctional, cells in the AV bundle and Purkinje fibers can continue to generate myocardial contractions at a rate of about 30 beats per minute.

Although action potentials normally begin at the SA node and spread across the myocardium in a coordinated manner, other regions of the heart may also initiate beats. These **ectopic foci**, or ectopic pacemakers, may send waves of depolarization across the myocardium that compete with those from the normal conduction pathway. The timing and synchronization of atrial and ventricular contractions may be affected. Although healthy hearts occasionally experience an extra beat without incident, ectopic foci in diseased hearts have the potential to cause dysrhythmias, or disorders of cardiac rhythm. The events associated with the cardiac conduction system are recorded on an electrocardiogram (ECG).

It is important to understand that the underlying purpose of the cardiac conduction system is to keep the heart beating in a regular, synchronized manner so that cardiac output can be maintained. Dysrhythmias that profoundly affect cardiac output have the potential to produce serious, if not mortal, consequences. These types of dysrhythmias require pharmacologic intervention, as discussed in Chapter 37.

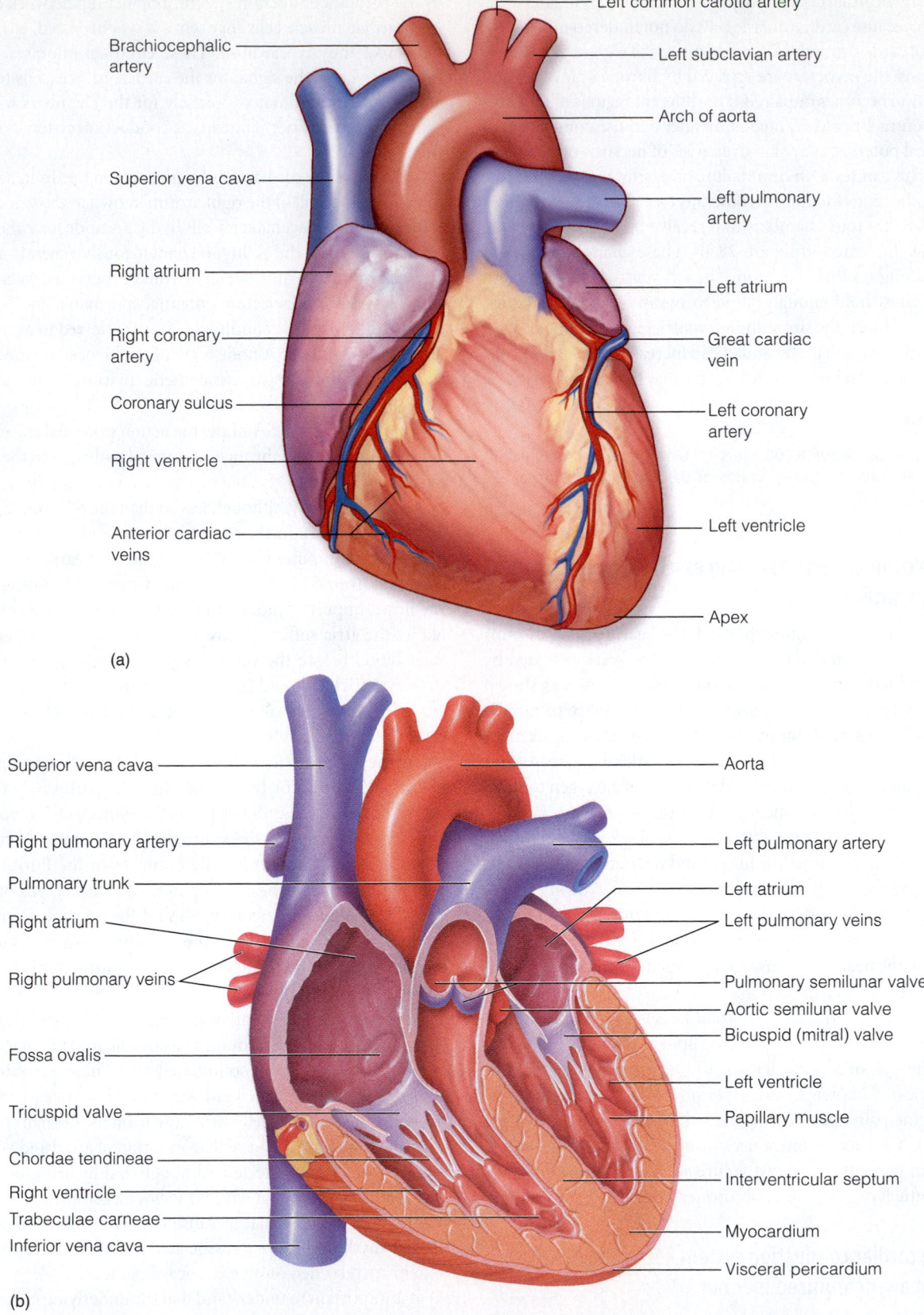

Left common carotid artery

Brachiocephalic artery

Left subclavian artery

Arch of aorta

Superior vena cava

Left pulmonary artery

Right atrium

Left atrium

Right coronary artery

Great cardiac vein

Coronary sulcus

Left coronary artery

Right ventricle

Anterior cardiac veins

Left ventricle

Apex

(a)

Superior vena cava

Aorta

Right pulmonary artery

Left pulmonary artery

Pulmonary trunk

Left atrium

Right atrium

Left pulmonary veins

Right pulmonary veins

Pulmonary semilunar valve

Aortic semilunar valve

Bicuspid (mitral) valve

Fossa ovalis

Left ventricle

Tricuspid valve

Papillary muscle

Chordae tendineae

Right ventricle

Interventricular septum

Trabeculae carneae

Myocardium

Inferior vena cava

Visceral pericardium

(b)

Figure 28.4 The heart: (a) coronary arteries and veins; (b) chambers and valves.

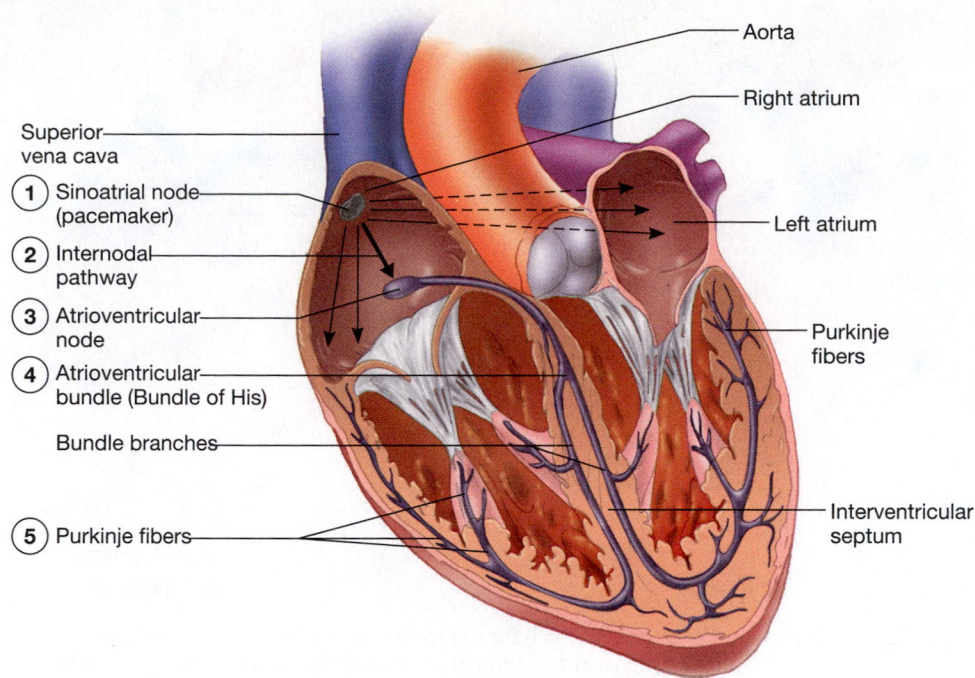

Superior
vena cava

① Sinoatrial node
(pacemaker)

② Internodal
pathway

③ Atrioventricular
node

④ Atrioventricular
bundle (Bundle of His)

Bundle branches

⑤ Purkinje fibers

Aorta

Right atrium

Left atrium

Purkinje
fibers

Interventricular
septum

1. The sinoatrial (SA) node fires a stimulus across the walls of both
   left and right atria causing them to contract.

2. The stimulus arrives at the atrioventricular (AV) node.

3. The stimulus is directed to follow the AV bundle (Bundle of His).

4. The stimulus now travels through the apex of the heart through
   the bundle branches.

5. The Purkinje fibers distribute the stimulus across both ventricles
   causing ventricular contraction.

Figure 28.5 The cardiac conduction system.

28.7 Cardiac output is determined by stroke volume and heart rate.

To understand how medications act on the heart and to predict the consequences of pharmacotherapy, it is essential to have a comprehensive knowledge of normal cardiac physiology. This includes a thorough understanding of factors that determine the amount of blood pumped by the heart and the forces acting on the chambers.

The amount of blood pumped by each ventricle per minute is the **cardiac output (CO)**. The CO is essentially a measure of how effectively the heart is performing as a pump. The average CO is 5 L/minute. CO can be calculated by multiplying stroke volume by the heart rate.

CO = stroke volume (mL/beat) × heart rate (beats/minute)

Stroke volume: Stroke volume is the amount of blood pumped by a ventricle in a single contraction. What types of factors might cause a ventricle to eject more blood during a contraction? To understand these factors, a simple comparison to a rubber band is useful. If you stretch a small rubber band 2 inches, it will snap back with a certain force. Stretching the band 4 inches will cause it to snap back with greater force. The force of the snap will continue to increase up to a certain limit, after which the rubber band

has been stretched as far as possible and has reached maximum force (or it breaks!).

Cardiac muscle fibers are analogous to rubber bands. If you fill the chambers with more blood, the fibers will have more stretch and will "snap back" with greater force. This is known as Starling's law of the heart: The strength (force) of contraction, or **contractility**, is proportional to the muscle fiber length (stretch). The contractility determines the amount of blood ejected per beat, or the stroke volume. The degree to which the ventricles are filled with blood and the myocardial fibers are stretched just prior to contraction is called **preload**. Up to a physiological limit, drugs that increase preload and contractility will increase the CO. In addition to preload, the force of contraction can be increased by activation of beta₁-adrenergic receptors in the autonomic nervous system.

What causes the chambers to fill up with more blood, become stretched (more preload), and contract with greater force? Although several factors affect preload, the most important is **venous return**: the volume of blood returning to the heart from the veins. Giving a drug that constricts veins will increase venous return to the heart, as will simply increasing the total amount of blood in the vascular system (increased blood volume). Drugs or other mechanisms that constrict veins or increase blood volume will therefore

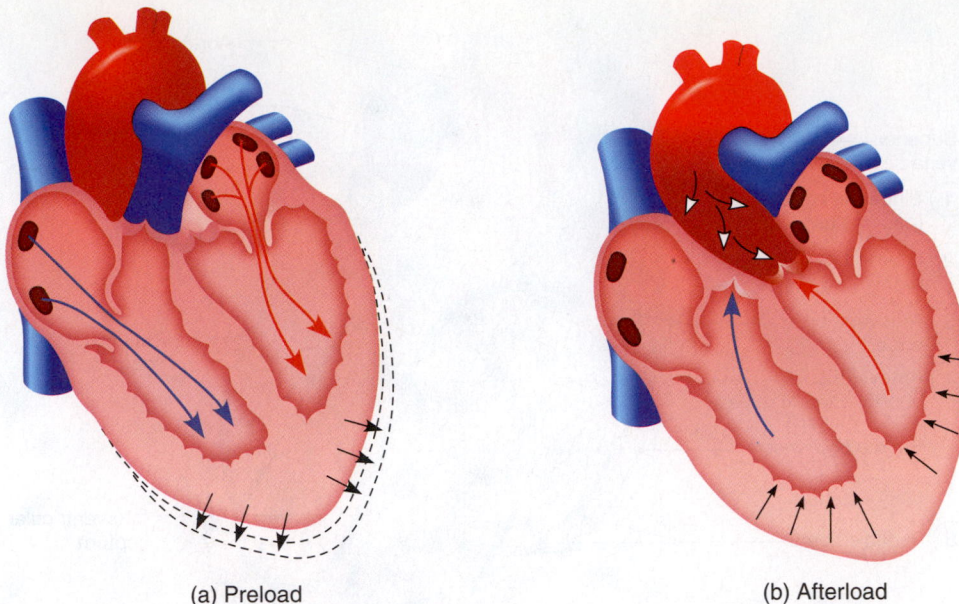

(a) Preload   (b) Afterload

Figure 28.6 (a) Preload is the degree to which the ventricles are filled with blood and the myocardial fibers are stretched just prior to contraction. (b) Afterload is the systolic pressure in the aorta that must be overcome for blood to be ejected from the left ventricle.

increase stroke volume and CO. Conversely, drugs that dilate veins or reduce blood volume will lower CO.

Factors that increase cardiac contractility are called positive **inotropic drugs**. Examples of positive inotropic drugs include epinephrine, norepinephrine, thyroid hormone, and dopamine. Factors that decrease cardiac contractility are called negative inotropic drugs. Examples include quinidine and beta-adrenergic antagonists such as propranolol.

A second primary factor affecting stroke volume is afterload. In order for the left ventricle to pump blood out of the heart, it must overcome a substantial "back pressure" in the aorta. **Afterload** is the systolic pressure in the aorta that must be overcome for blood to be ejected from the left ventricle. As afterload increases, the heart pumps less blood, and stroke volume (and thus CO) decreases. The most common cause of increased afterload is an increase in systemic blood pressure, or HTN. HTN creates an increased workload on the heart, which explains why patients with chronic HTN are more likely to experience heart failure. Antihypertensive drugs create less afterload, increase stroke volume, and result in less workload for the heart. Preload and afterload are illustrated in Figure 28.6.

Heart rate: Heart rate is the second primary factor determining CO. Heart rate is generally controlled by the autonomic nervous system, which makes the minute-by-minute adjustments demanded by the circulatory system. Both sympathetic and parasympathetic fibers are found in the SA node, and heart rate is determined by which fibers are firing at a greater rate at any given moment. Circulating hormones such as epinephrine and thyroid hormone also affect heart rate. In theory, drugs that increase heart rate will increase CO, although compensatory mechanisms may prevent this effect (see Section 28.8). In addition, a very rapid heart rate may not give the chambers sufficient time to completely fill, thus reducing CO.

CONNECTION Checkpoint 28.2

From what you learned in Chapter 12, predict what effect the following would have on heart rate: sympathomimetics, parasympathomimetics, adrenergic agonists, and anticholinergics. *See Answer to Connection Checkpoint 28.2 on student resource website.*

Hemodynamics and Blood Pressure

28.8 The primary factors responsible for blood pressure are cardiac output, peripheral resistance, and blood volume.

The homeostatic regulation of blood pressure is a key topic in pharmacology because HTN is so prevalent in the population. Regulation of blood pressure is complex with many diverse factors, both local and systemic, interacting to maintain adequate blood flow to the tissues. The three primary factors that regulate arterial blood pressure—CO, peripheral resistance, and blood volume—are shown in Figure 28.7. The following simple formula should be memorized (as well as understood) because it will help in predicting the actions and adverse effects of many classes of cardiovascular medications:

$$\text{Blood pressure} = \text{CO} \times \text{peripheral resistance}$$

CO is determined by heart rate and stroke volume as discussed in Section 28.7. From the preceding equation, it is easy to see that as CO increases, blood pressure also increases. This is important to pharmacology because medications that change the CO, stroke volume, or heart rate have the potential to influence a patient's blood pressure.

As blood speeds through the vascular system, it exerts force against the walls of the vessels. Although the lining of the blood vessel is extremely smooth, friction reduces the velocity of the blood. Further friction is encountered as the stream of fast-moving

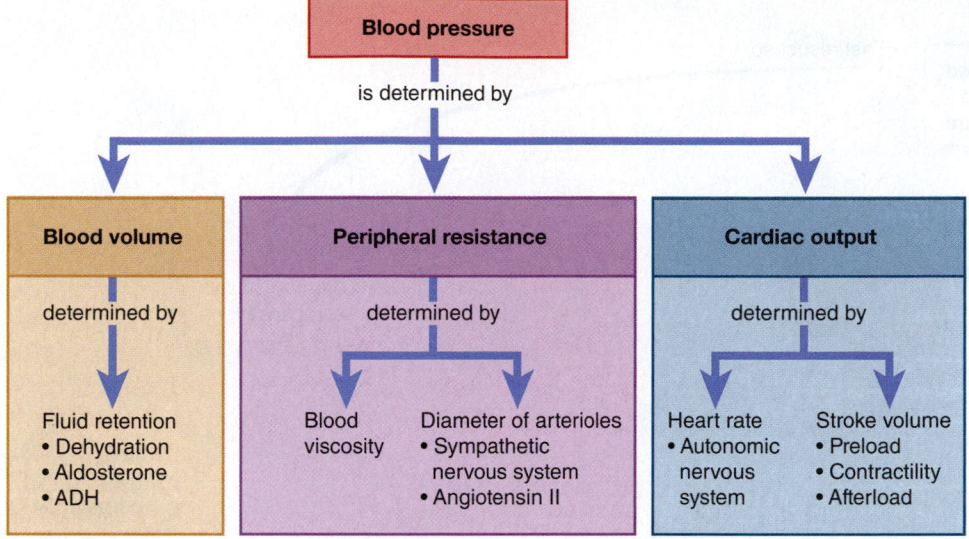

Figure 28.7 The primary factors affecting blood pressure.

blood narrows to enter smaller vessels, divides into two channels (arteries), or encounters fatty deposits on the vessel walls (plaque). Blood flow may exhibit turbulence, a chaotic, tumbling motion that greatly increases friction. The friction that blood encounters in the arteries is called **peripheral resistance**. Arteries have smooth muscle in their walls, which controls the total peripheral resistance. For example, if the smooth muscle constricts, the inside diameter or lumen of the arteries will become smaller and create more resistance and higher blood pressure. A large number of medications affect vascular smooth muscle. Some of these drugs cause vessels to constrict, thus raising blood pressure, whereas others relax smooth muscle, thereby opening the lumen and lowering blood pressure.

An additional factor responsible for blood pressure is the total amount of blood in the vascular system, or blood volume. Although the average person maintains a relatively constant blood volume of approximately 5 L, this can be changed by endogenous regulatory factors, certain disease states, and pharmacotherapy. More fluid in the vascular system increases venous pressure and venous return to the heart, thus increasing CO and arterial blood pressure. Drugs are frequently used to adjust blood volume. For example, infusion of intravenous (IV) fluids quickly increases blood volume and raises blood pressure. This is used to advantage when treating hypotension due to shock. On the other hand, diuretics cause fluid loss through urination, thus decreasing blood volume and lowering blood pressure.

PharmFACT

It is estimated that all the blood vessels in an adult stretch through about 60,000 miles of internal body landscape (Marieb & Hoehn, 2013).

28.9 Neural regulation of blood pressure includes baroreceptor and chemoreceptor reflexes.

It is critical for the body to maintain a normal range of blood pressure and for it to be able to safely and rapidly change pressure as it proceeds through daily activities such as sleep and exercise. Hypotension can cause dizziness and lack of adequate urine

formation, whereas extreme HTN can cause vessels to rupture and result in ischemia of critical organs. Figure 28.8 illustrates how the body maintains homeostasis during periods of blood pressure change.

The central and autonomic nervous systems are intimately involved in regulating blood pressure. On a minute-to-minute basis, blood pressure is regulated by a cluster of neurons in the medulla oblongata called the **vasomotor center**. Sensory receptors in the aorta and the internal carotid artery provide the vasomotor center with vital information on conditions in the vascular system. **Baroreceptors** have the ability to sense pressure within large vessels, whereas **chemoreceptors** recognize levels of oxygen, carbon dioxide, and the acidity or pH in the blood. The vasomotor center reacts to information from baroreceptors and chemoreceptors by raising or lowering blood pressure accordingly. Nerve fibers travel from the vasomotor center to the arteries, where the smooth muscle is directed to either constrict (raise blood pressure) or relax (lower blood pressure). As discussed in Chapter 16, sympathetic outflow from the vasomotor center stimulates alpha$_1$-adrenergic receptors on arterioles, causing vasoconstriction. Alpha$_2$-adrenergic agonists can also decrease blood pressure by their central effects on the vasomotor center.

The baroreceptor reflex is an important mechanism used by the body for making rapid adjustments to blood pressure. If pressure in the vascular system increases, the baroreceptors in the aortic arch and carotid sinus trigger reflexes that constrict the arterioles and veins and accelerate the heart rate. Together, these actions return blood pressure to normal levels within seconds.

Drugs that raise or lower blood pressure can trigger the baroreceptor reflex. For example, antihypertensives administered by the IV route cause an immediate reduction in blood pressure that is recognized by the baroreceptors. The baroreceptors respond by attempting to return blood pressure back to the original levels. The resulting accelerated heart rate, or **reflex tachycardia**, may cause the patient to experience palpitations. The baroreceptors are not able to offer a continuous or sustained reduction in blood pressure. Continued administration of an antihypertensive

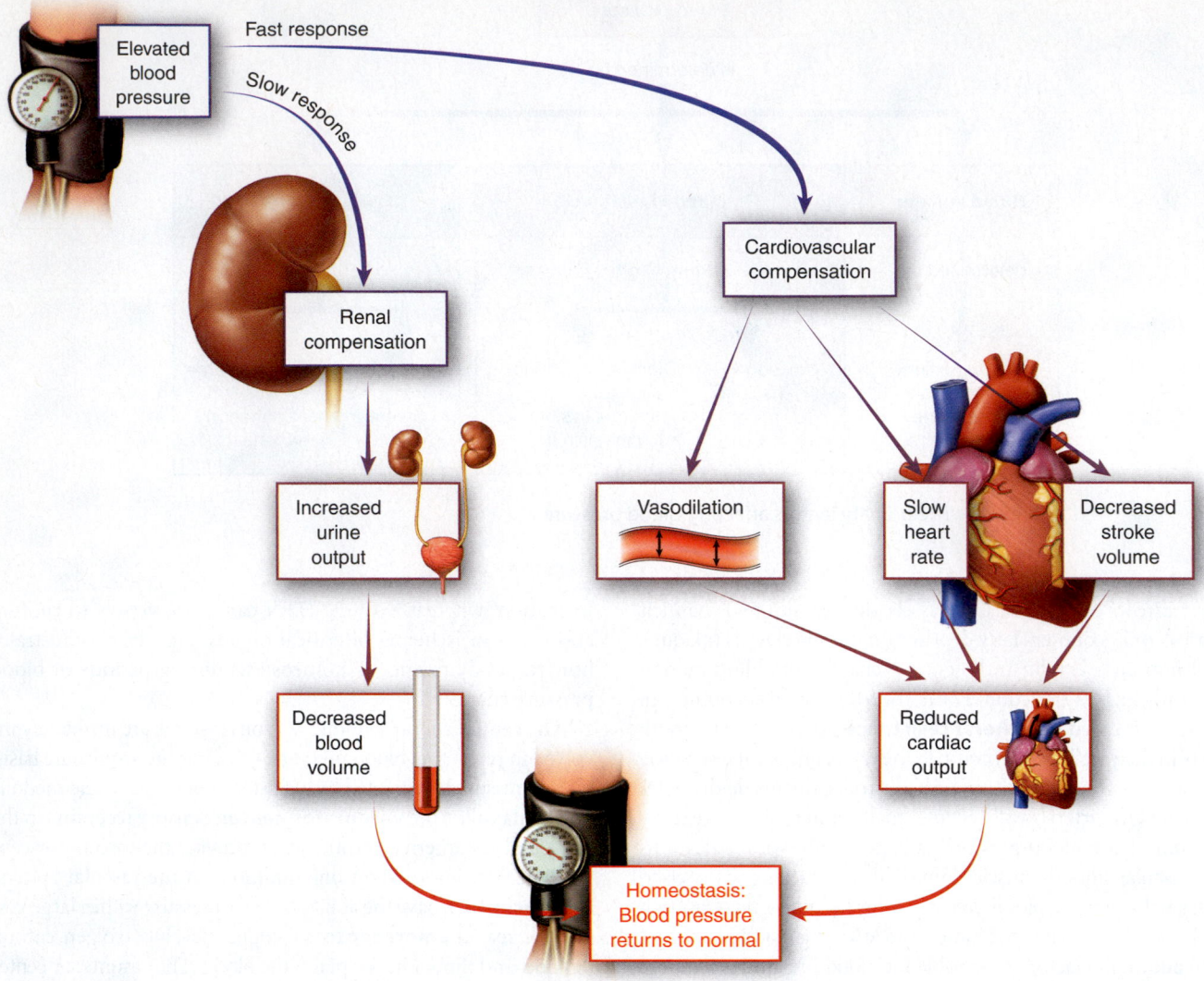

Figure 28.8 Cardiovascular and renal control of blood pressure.

drug will "overcome" the reflex. In addition, with aging or certain disease states such as diabetes, the baroreceptor response may be diminished.

Another example of the baroreceptor reflex occurs when baroreceptors in the right atrium are triggered. These receptors recognize excess stretching of the right atrium, such as might occur when large amounts of IV fluids are administered. The **atrial reflex** causes the heart rate and CO to increase until the backlog of venous blood (or IV fluid) is distributed throughout the body.

The chemoreceptor reflex can also significantly affect blood pressure. Sensors in the carotid sinus and near the aortic arch recognize levels of oxygen and carbon dioxide and the acidity (pH) in the blood. Triggering these chemoreceptors activates the sympathetic nervous system and causes heart rate and CO to increase. The purpose of this reflex is to circulate blood faster so that the respiratory system can remove excess carbon dioxide (which returns pH to normal levels) and add more oxygen to the blood.

CONNECTION Checkpoint 28.3 _____

Many autonomic drugs dilate or constrict blood vessels. From what you learned in Chapter 12, which class of autonomic drugs is most commonly prescribed for HTN? *See Answer to Connection Checkpoint 28.3 on student resource website.*

28.10 Hormones may have profound effects on blood pressure.

Several hormones affect blood pressure, and certain classes of medications are given to either enhance or block the actions of these hormones. For example, injection of the catecholamines epinephrine or norepinephrine will immediately raise blood pressure, which is essential for patients experiencing shock.

Antidiuretic hormone (ADH) is a hormone released by the posterior pituitary gland when blood pressure falls or when the osmotic pressure of the blood increases. ADH, also known as vasopressin, is a potent peripheral vasoconstrictor that quickly increases blood pressure. The hormone also acts on the kidneys to

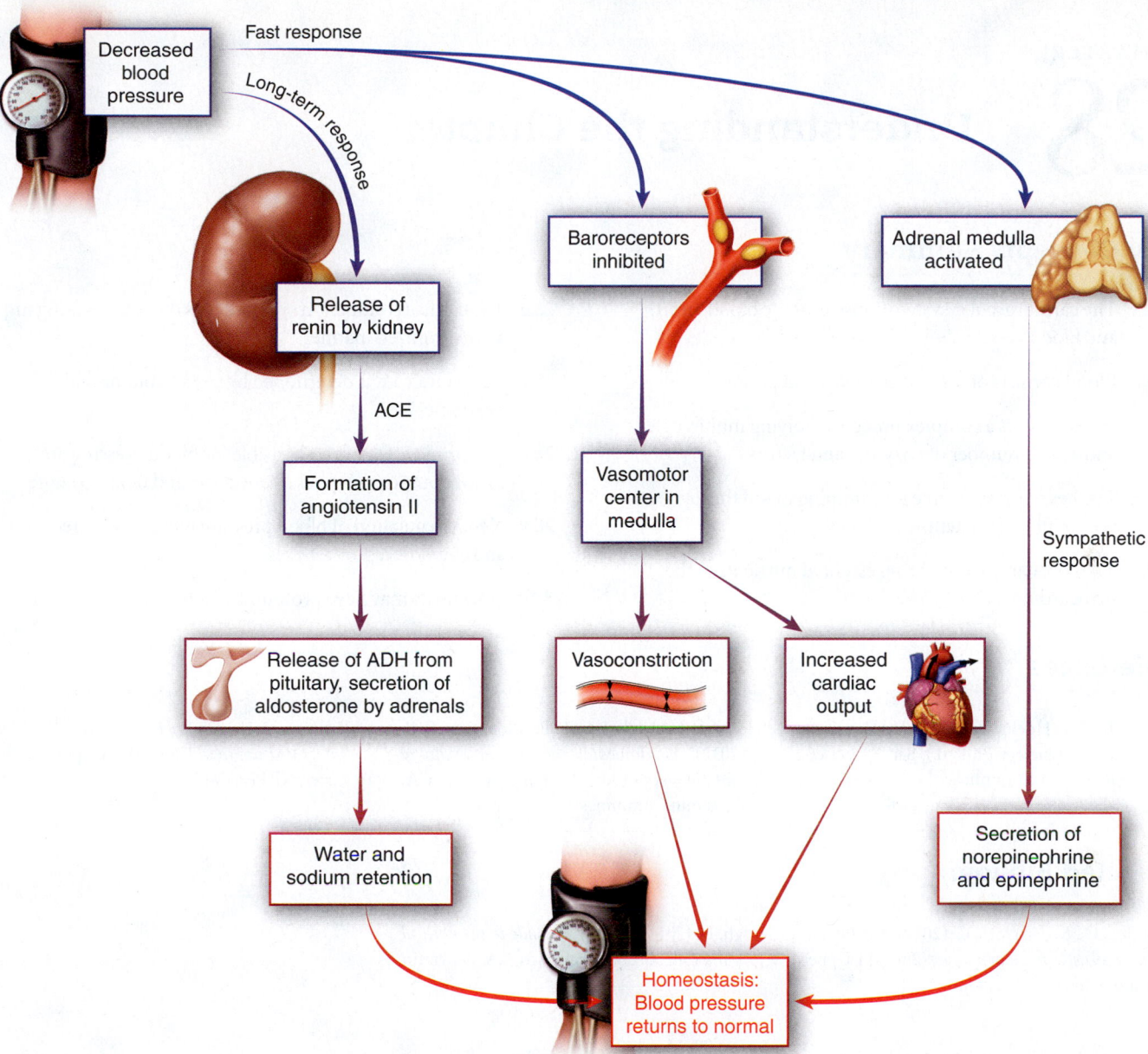

Figure 28.9 Endocrine and nervous control of blood pressure.

conserve water and increase blood volume, thereby causing blood pressure to increase. The pharmacotherapy of ADH and related hormones is discussed in Chapter 65.

The **renin-angiotensin-aldosterone system (RAAS)** is particularly important in the drug therapy of HTN. As blood pressure falls, the enzyme renin is released by the kidneys. Through a two-step pathway, angiotensin II is formed, which subsequently increases CO and constricts arterioles to return blood pressure to original levels. Angiotensin II also promotes the release of aldosterone from the adrenal gland, which causes sodium and water retention. Drugs that block the RAAS are key drugs in the treatment of HTN and heart failure.

Atrial natriuretic peptide (ANP) is a hormone that is secreted by specialized cells in the right atrium when large increases in blood volume produce excessive stretch on the atrial wall. ANP has multiple effects, all of which attempt to return blood pressure to original levels. Sodium ion transport in the kidney is affected, resulting in enhanced sodium and water excretion. The release of ADH and aldosterone is suppressed by ANP. In addition, ANP reduces sympathetic outflow from the central nervous system, resulting in dilation of peripheral arteries. A summary of the various nervous and hormone factors influencing blood pressure is shown in Figure 28.9.

CHAPTER

28

Understanding the Chapter

Key Concepts Summary

28.1 The cardiovascular system consists of the blood, heart, and blood vessels.

28.2 Blood consists of formed elements and plasma.

28.3 Hemostasis is a complex process involving multiple steps and a large number of enzymes and factors.

28.4 The heart is responsible for pumping blood throughout the circulatory system.

28.5 The coronary arteries bring essential nutrients to the myocardium.

28.6 The cardiac conduction system keeps the heart beating in a synchronized manner.

28.7 Cardiac output is determined by stroke volume and heart rate.

28.8 The primary factors responsible for blood pressure are cardiac output, peripheral resistance, and blood volume.

28.9 Neural regulation of blood pressure includes baroreceptor and chemoreceptor reflexes.

28.10 Hormones may have profound effects on blood pressure.

References

Marieb, E. N., & Hoehn, K. (2013). *Human anatomy and physiology* (9th ed.). San Francisco, CA: Benjamin Cummings.

Martini, F. H., Nath, J. L., & Bartholomew, E. F. (2012). *Fundamentals of human anatomy and physiology* (9th ed.). San Francisco, CA: Benjamin Cummings.

Silverthorn, D. U. (2013). *Human physiology: An integrated approach* (6th ed.). Upper Saddle River, NJ: Pearson.

Selected Bibliography

D'Amico, D., & Barbarito, C. (2012). *Health and physical assessment in nursing* (2nd ed.). Upper Saddle River, NJ: Pearson.

Krogh, D. (2011). *Biology: A guide to the natural world* (5th ed.). San Francisco, CA: Benjamin Cummings.

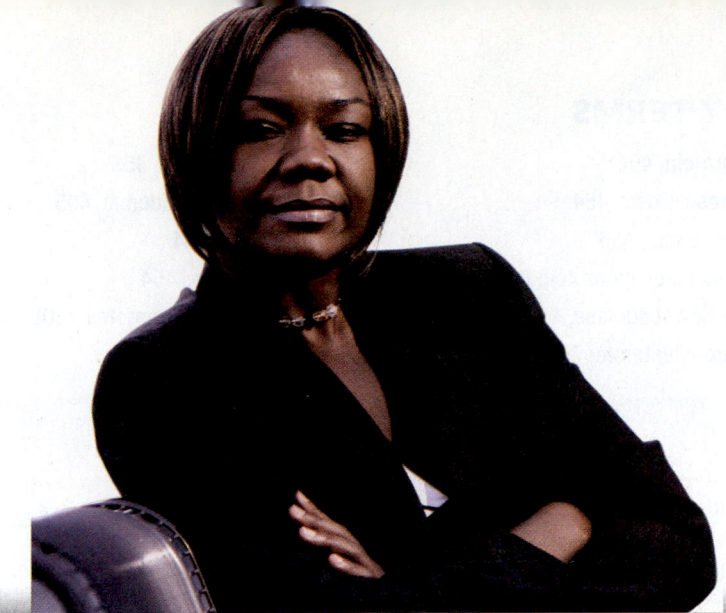

"My mother had it and my grandmother had it too. Now, I'm told that I have it. My doctor says my cholesterol level is too high."

Patient "Belinda Cummings"

Pharmacotherapy of Hyperlipidemia

LEARNING OUTCOMES

After reading this chapter, the student should be able to:

1. Summarize the link between high blood cholesterol, low-density lipoprotein levels, and atherosclerosis.
2. Compare and contrast the different types of lipids.
3. Illustrate how lipids are transported through the blood.
4. Compare and contrast the clinical importance of the different types of lipoproteins.
5. Give examples of how cholesterol and low-density lipoprotein levels can be controlled with nonpharmacologic means.
6. For each of the classes shown in the chapter outline, identify the prototype and representative drugs and explain the mechanism(s) of drug action, primary indications, contraindications, significant drug interactions, pregnancy category, and important adverse effects.
7. Categorize antihyperlipidemic drugs based on their classification and mechanism of action.
8. Explain the nurse's role in the safe administration of drugs for lipid disorders.
9. Apply the nursing process to care for patients receiving pharmacotherapy for lipid disorders.

CHAPTER OUTLINE

▶ Types of Lipids and Lipoproteins

▶ Measurement and Control of Serum Lipids

▶ Drugs for Dyslipidemias
  HMG-CoA Reductase Inhibitors
  PROTOTYPE Atorvastatin (Lipitor), *p. 462*
  Bile Acid Sequestrants
  PROTOTYPE Cholestyramine (Questran), *p. 464*
  Niacin
  Fibric Acid Drugs
  PROTOTYPE Gemfibrozil (Lopid), *p. 466*
  Miscellaneous Drugs for Dyslipidemias

KEY TERMS

apoprotein, 454

atherosclerosis, 454

dyslipidemia, 455

high-density lipoprotein (HDL), 454

HMG-CoA reductase, 458

hypercholesterolemia, 455

hyperlipidemia, 455

hypertriglyceridemia, 455

lecithins, 454

lipoproteins, 454

low-density lipoprotein (LDL), 454

phospholipids, 454

reverse cholesterol transport, 454

rhabdomyolysis, 460

steroids, 454

sterol nucleus, 454

triglycerides, 454

very low-density lipoprotein (VLDL), 454

Research during the 1970s and 1980s brought about a nutritional revolution as new knowledge about lipids and their relationships to obesity and cardiovascular disease allowed people to make more intelligent lifestyle choices. Since then advances in the diagnosis of lipid disorders have helped to identify those people at greatest risk for cardiovascular disease and those most likely to benefit from pharmacologic intervention. As a result of this knowledge and from advancements in pharmacology, the incidence of death due to most cardiovascular diseases has been declining, although they remain the leading cause of death in the United States.

Types of Lipids and Lipoproteins

29.1 Lipids are classified as triglycerides, phospholipids, or sterols.

There are three types of lipids that are important to human physiology, as illustrated in Figure 29.1. The most common types are **triglycerides** or neutral fats, which consist of three fatty acids attached to a chemical backbone of glycerol. Triglycerides are the major storage form of fat in the body and the only type of lipid that serves as an important energy source. They account for 90% of the total lipids in the body.

A second class, the **phospholipids**, is formed when a phosphorous group replaces one of the fatty acids in a triglyceride. This class of lipids is essential to building plasma membranes. The best known phospholipids are **lecithins**, which are found in high concentration in egg yolks and soybeans. Once promoted as a natural treatment for high cholesterol levels, controlled studies have not shown lecithin to be of benefit for this disorder.

The third class of lipids, the **steroids**, is a diverse group of substances having a common **sterol nucleus** or ring structure. Cholesterol is the most widely known of the steroids, and its role in promoting **atherosclerosis** has been clearly demonstrated. Atherosclerosis is the presence of plaque—a fatty, fibrous material within the walls of the arteries. Unlike the triglycerides that provide fuel for the body, cholesterol is a vital component of plasma membranes and serves as a building block for essential biochemicals, including vitamin D, bile acids, cortisol, estrogen, and testosterone. Although clearly essential for life, the body needs only minute amounts of cholesterol because the liver is able to synthesize adequate amounts from other chemicals. It is not necessary, nor desirable, to provide excess cholesterol in the diet. The dietary sources of cholesterol are obtained solely from animal products; humans do not absorb the sterols produced by plants.

29.2 Lipoproteins are important predictors of cardiovascular disease.

Because lipid molecules are not soluble in plasma, they must be specially packaged for transport through the blood. To accomplish this, the body forms complexes called **lipoproteins**, which consist of various amounts of cholesterol, triglycerides, and phospholipids bound to carrier proteins. The protein component is called an **apoprotein** (*apo-* means "separated from" or "derived from"). The four apoproteins important to lipid transport are known as A-I, A-II, A-IV, and B-100.

Lipoproteins are classified according to their composition, size, and weight or density, which come primarily from the amount of apoprotein present in the complex. Each type varies in lipid and apoprotein makeup and serves a different function in transporting lipids from the sites of synthesis and absorption to the sites of utilization. For example, **high-density lipoprotein (HDL)** contains the most apoprotein, up to 50% by weight. The highest amount of cholesterol is carried by **low-density lipoprotein (LDL)**. Figure 29.2 illustrates the three basic lipoproteins and their compositions.

To understand the pharmacotherapy of lipid disorders, it is important to know the functions of the major lipoproteins and their roles in transporting cholesterol. LDL transports cholesterol from the liver to the tissues and organs, where it is used to build plasma membranes or to synthesize other steroids. Once in the tissues it can also be stored for later use. Storage of cholesterol in the lining of blood vessels, however, is not desirable because it contributes to plaque buildup. LDL is often called "bad" cholesterol because this lipoprotein contributes significantly to plaque deposits and coronary artery disease (CAD). Sixty to seventy percent of the cholesterol circulating in the blood is found in LDL.

Very low-density lipoprotein (VLDL) is the primary carrier of triglycerides in the blood. VLDLs account for virtually all triglycerides being transported from the liver to storage in adipose tissue. Through a series of steps, VLDL is reduced in size to become LDL. Lowering LDL levels in the blood has been shown to decrease the incidence of CAD.

HDL is manufactured in the liver and small intestine and assists in the transport of excess cholesterol away from the body tissues and back to the liver for metabolism in a process known as **reverse cholesterol transport**. The cholesterol component of the HDL is then broken down to unite with bile, which is subsequently excreted in the feces. Excretion via bile is the only route the body uses to remove cholesterol. Because HDL transports cholesterol for destruction and removes it from the body, it is considered "good" cholesterol. Patients with insufficient

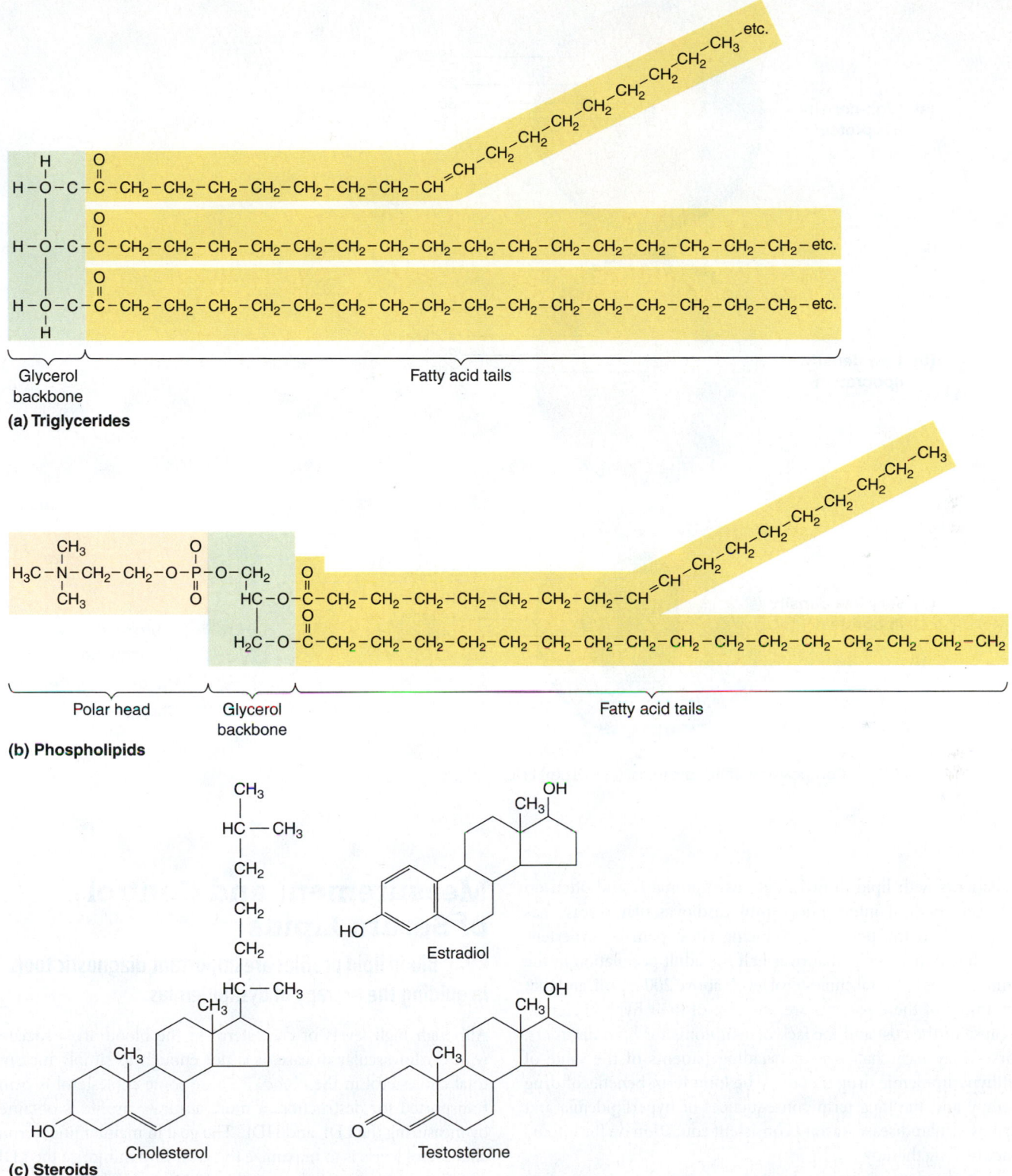

Figure 29.1 Chemical structure of lipids.

amounts of HDL are at risk for atherosclerosis, even if their total cholesterol levels are normal.

Several terms are used to describe lipid disorders. **Hyperlipidemia** is the general term meaning high levels of lipids in the blood. The term *hyperlipidemia*, however, does not specify which lipid is elevated. Elevated blood cholesterol, or **hypercholesterolemia**, is the type of hyperlipidemia that is most familiar to the general public. **Dyslipidemia** is the term that refers to abnormal (excess or deficient) levels of lipoproteins. Some patients exhibit an increase in triglyceride levels known as **hypertriglyceridemia**.

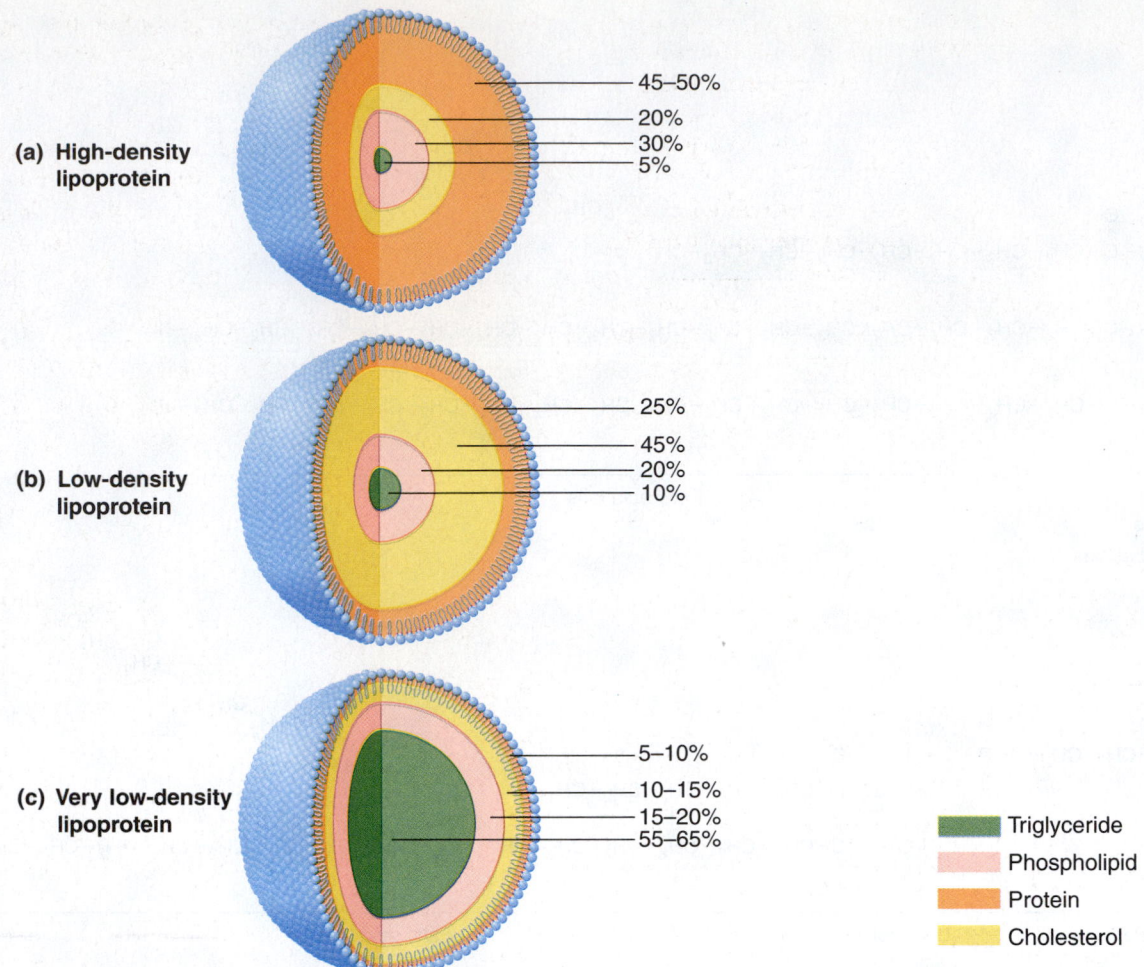

Figure 29.2 Composition of lipoproteins: (a) HDL; (b) LDL; (c) VLDL.

Patients with lipid disorders are asymptomatic and often do not seek medical intervention until cardiovascular disease has progressed to the point of producing chest pain or hypertension. Research suggests that over half the adult population in the United States has total cholesterol levels above 200 mg/dL and that two thirds of these patients are unaware of their hyperlipidemia. Because of the cost and the lack of symptoms for lipid disorders, nurses may face challenges persuading patients of the value of antihyperlipidemic drug therapy. The long-term benefits of drug therapy and the long-term consequences of hyperlipidemia and cardiovascular disease warrant consistent education on the importance of drug therapy.

Hyperlipidemia may be inherited or acquired. Certainly, diets high in saturated fats and lack of exercise contribute greatly to the development of hyperlipidemia and resulting cardiovascular diseases. However, genetics determines one's ability to metabolize lipids and contributes to high lipid levels in substantial numbers of patients. Some genetic dyslipidemias can be so severe as to cause CAD and death due to myocardial infarction (MI) in childhood (Citkowitz, 2013). For most patients, dyslipidemias are the result of a combination of genetic and environmental (lifestyle) factors.

Measurement and Control of Serum Lipids

29.3 Blood lipid profiles are important diagnostic tools in guiding the therapy of dyslipidemias.

Although high levels of cholesterol in the blood are associated with cardiovascular disease, it is not enough to simply measure total cholesterol in the blood. Because some cholesterol is being transported for destruction, a more accurate profile is obtained by measuring the LDL and HDL. The goal in maintaining normal cholesterol levels is to maximize the HDL and minimize the LDL. This is sometimes stated as a ratio of LDL to HDL. If the ratio is greater than 5 (five times more LDL than HDL), the male patient is considered at risk for cardiovascular disease. The normal ratio in women is slightly lower at 4.5.

Scientists have further divided LDL into subclasses of lipoproteins. For example, one variety found in LDL, called *lipoprotein (a)*, has been strongly associated with plaque formation and heart disease. It is likely that further research will find other varieties with the expectation that drugs will be designed to be more selective

TABLE 29.1 Standard Laboratory Lipid Profiles

Type of Lipid	Laboratory Value (mg/dL)	Standard
Total cholesterol	Less than 200	Desirable
	200–240	Borderline high
	Greater than 240	High
Low-density lipoproteins (LDLs)	Less than 100	Optimal
	100–129	Near or above optimal
	130–159	Borderline high
	160–189	High
	Greater than 189	Very high
High-density lipoproteins (HDLs)	Less than 40 (men) or 50 (women)	Low
	Greater than 60	Desirable
Serum triglycerides	Less than 150	Normal
	150–199	Borderline high
	200–499	High
	Greater than 500	Very high

From "Executive Summary of the Third Report of the National Cholesterol Education Program (NCEP) Expert Panel on Detection, Evaluation, and Treatment of High Blood Cholesterol in Adults (Adult Treatment Panel III), by Expert Panel on Detection," 2001, *JAMA: The Journal of the American Medical Association*, *285*(19), 2486–2497.

toward the "bad" lipoproteins. Table 29.1 gives the desirable, borderline, and high laboratory values for each of the major lipids and lipoproteins. These values change periodically as additional research becomes available on the association between heart disease and lipid levels.

Establishing treatment guidelines for dyslipidemia has been difficult because the condition itself has no symptoms and the progression to cardiovascular disease may take decades. In the late 1980s, guidelines were developed regarding the diagnosis and treatment of cholesterol disorders. Until 2013, the guidelines focused on determining levels of LDL and HDL that could prevent the development of coronary heart disease (CHD). Essentially, if a patient exhibited laboratory values shown to be at high risk (see Table 29.1), pharmacotherapy was initiated and continued until these values returned to the normal range.

In 2013, major revisions were made to these guidelines by the American College of Cardiology (ACC) and the American Heart Association (AHA). The 2013 ACC/AHA guidelines (Stone et al., 2013) no longer stress specific target goals for LDL levels. Four treatment categories were established for the prevention of CHD.

1. Adults with atherosclerotic cardiovascular disease
2. Adults with diabetes, age 40 to 75 years with LDL levels between 70 and 189 mg/dL
3. Adults with LDL cholesterol levels of 190 mg/dL or higher

4. Adults age 40 through 75 years who have LDL levels 70 through 189 mg/dL and 7.5% or greater 10-year risk of atherosclerotic cardiovascular disease.

Based on the results of hundreds of clinical trials over many years, the ACC/AHA guidelines also recommended specific medication classes for treating patients in these categories. The statins are the recommended first-line therapy for all categories. Unlike previous guidelines, the goal is no longer to use medications to achieve a target LDL goal. Follow-up measures of LDL are still recommended to determine adherence to the drug regimen.

The fourth category of the ACC/AHA guidelines, which bases pharmacotherapy on a 7.5% or greater risk of atherosclerotic cardiovascular disease, has been controversial. The calculation of risk gives heavy emphasis to age, which suggests that most of the population over age 60 should be on statin medications. The guidelines, however, should be viewed as recommendations meant to generate conversations about wellness between patients and their health care providers.

Blood lipid profiles are used to classify the different patterns of hyperlipidemias observed in clinical practice. These patterns are shown in Table 29.2. The specific type of dyslipidemia exhibited by patients is considered when planning therapy. For example, Type I requires dietary restrictions and does not respond well to pharmacotherapy. Whereas the remaining types respond to the statins, the hypertriglyceridemias may respond better to therapy with fibric acid drugs (fibrates).

29.4 Lipid levels can often be controlled through therapeutic lifestyle changes.

Therapeutic lifestyle changes (TLCs) should always be included in any plan for treating or preventing cardiovascular disease. Many patients with borderline high-risk laboratory values can control their dyslipidemia entirely through nonpharmacologic means.

Patients should be taught that all drugs used for hyperlipidemia have adverse effects and that preventing atherosclerotic cardiovascular disease without pharmacotherapy should be a therapeutic goal. Following are the most important lipid-reduction lifestyle interventions:

- Monitor blood lipid levels regularly, as recommended by the health care provider.
- Maintain weight at an optimal level.
- Implement a medically supervised exercise plan.
- Reduce dietary saturated fats and cholesterol.
- Increase soluble fiber in the diet, as found in oat bran, apples, beans, grapefruit, and broccoli.
- Eliminate tobacco use.

The single most important lifestyle factor contributing to dyslipidemia is a high amount of saturated fat in the diet. Nutritionists recommend that the intake of dietary fat be limited to less than 30% of the total caloric intake and that cholesterol intake be reduced as much as possible. It is interesting to note that restriction of dietary cholesterol alone will not result in a significant reduction in blood cholesterol levels. In fact, cutting back on cholesterol

TABLE 29.2 Types of Dyslipidemias

Name	Laboratory Findings	Features
Type I Exogenous hyperlipidemia	Triglycerides increased three times Chylomicrons increased Cholesterol normal	Rare condition, usually occurring in childhood
Type IIa Familial hypercholesterolemia	LDL and cholesterol increased Triglycerides and VLDL normal	Common condition, may occur at any age
Type IIb Combined familial hyperlipidemia Carbohydrate-induced hypertriglyceridemia	LDL, VLDL, cholesterol, and triglycerides increased	May occur at any age but more commonly in adults
Type III Dysbetalipoproteinemia	Chylomicrons, VLDL, cholesterol, and triglycerides increased	Uncommon condition, occurs in middle-aged adults
Type IV Endogenous hyperlipidemia Carbohydrate-induced hypertriglyceridemia	VLDL and triglycerides increased Cholesterol normal or elevated Glucose intolerance Hyperuricemia	Most common dyslipidemia, occurs in middle-aged adults; associated with obesity, excessive alcohol intake, tobacco use, and other lifestyle factors
Type V Mixed hyperlipidemia Carbohydrate- and fat-induced hypertriglyceridemia	LDL, VLDL, cholesterol, and chylomicrons increased Triglycerides increased three times Glucose intolerance Hyperuricemia	Uncommon type, may begin in childhood and manifest in adults

consumption may actually increase the amount of circulating cholesterol. How is this possible? The liver reacts to a low-cholesterol diet by making more cholesterol and by inhibiting its excretion whenever saturated fats are present. Saturated fats are the building blocks that the liver uses for making cholesterol. The 2013 ACC/AHA guidelines call for a reduction of saturated fat in the diet to 5% to 6% of total calories. In addition, levels of trans fatty acids from meat and dairy products should be reduced.

Nutritionists also recommend increased dietary intake of plant sterols as a means to reduce blood cholesterol levels. Plant sterols, also called phytosterols or stanols, are lipids used by plants to construct their cell membranes. The structure of plant sterols is very similar to that of cholesterol. When ingested, however, the plant sterols compete with cholesterol for absorption in the digestive tract. When the body absorbs the plant sterols, cholesterol is excreted from the body, less cholesterol is delivered to the liver, and serum LDL (the "bad" cholesterol) levels fall. Rich, natural sources of plant sterols include wheat, corn, rye, oats, and rice, as well as nuts and olive oil. In recent years, plant sterols have been added to commercial products such as margarines, salad dressings, certain cereals, and some fruit juices.

Drugs for Dyslipidemias

29.5 The statins are the most effective drugs for reducing blood lipid levels.

In the late 1970s substances were isolated from various species of fungi that were found to inhibit cholesterol production in human cells in the laboratory. This class of drugs, known as the statins, has revolutionized the treatment of lipid disorders. Statins can produce a dramatic reduction in LDL cholesterol levels, lower triglyceride and VLDL levels, and raise the level of "good" HDL cholesterol. High-intensity statin therapy is able to lower LDL levels by more than 50% and reduce the incidence of serious cardiovascular-related adverse events by 25% to 30%. This means that about one in every three or four heart attacks, strokes, or blood clots can be prevented with appropriate statin therapy.

Cholesterol is manufactured in the liver by a series of more than 25 metabolic steps, beginning with acetyl CoA, a two-carbon unit that is produced from the breakdown of fatty acids (Figure 29.3). Of the many enzymes involved in this complex pathway, **HMG-CoA reductase** (3-hydroxy-3-methylglutaryl

CONNECTIONS | **Lifespan Considerations**

❮ **Pediatric Dyslipidemias and Lipid-Lowering Drugs**

Many people consider dyslipidemia to be a condition that occurs with advancing age. Dyslipidemias are also a concern for some pediatric patients, and multiple research studies have demonstrated that the early stages of atherosclerosis begin in childhood. With the increasing childhood obesity epidemic, there is concern that dyslipidemias, cardiovascular disease, and metabolic syndrome will occur at younger and younger ages. Risk factors for dyslipidemias in children are similar to those in adults and include overweight or obesity, family history of dyslipidemias or premature cardiovascular disease, hypertension, smoking or passive smoke exposure, and known genetic lipid disorders. The AHA worked to develop guidelines for the use of statin drugs for select children at risk for hyperlipidemia. Statins may be considered for pediatric patients after age 10 or after menarche in girls. Recently, drug therapy for pediatric dyslipidemias has been recommending statin use only for select children, with diet and lifestyle changes remaining the treatment of choice for the majority of children. For children with LDL levels above 190 mg/dL, or above 160 mg/dL with the presence of two or more cardiovascular risk factors, being overweight or obese, or a family history of coronary artery disease before age 50, drug therapy may be considered for children older than 8 years of age (Cook & Kavey, 2011; Eiland & Luttrell, 2010; Jellinger et al., 2012).

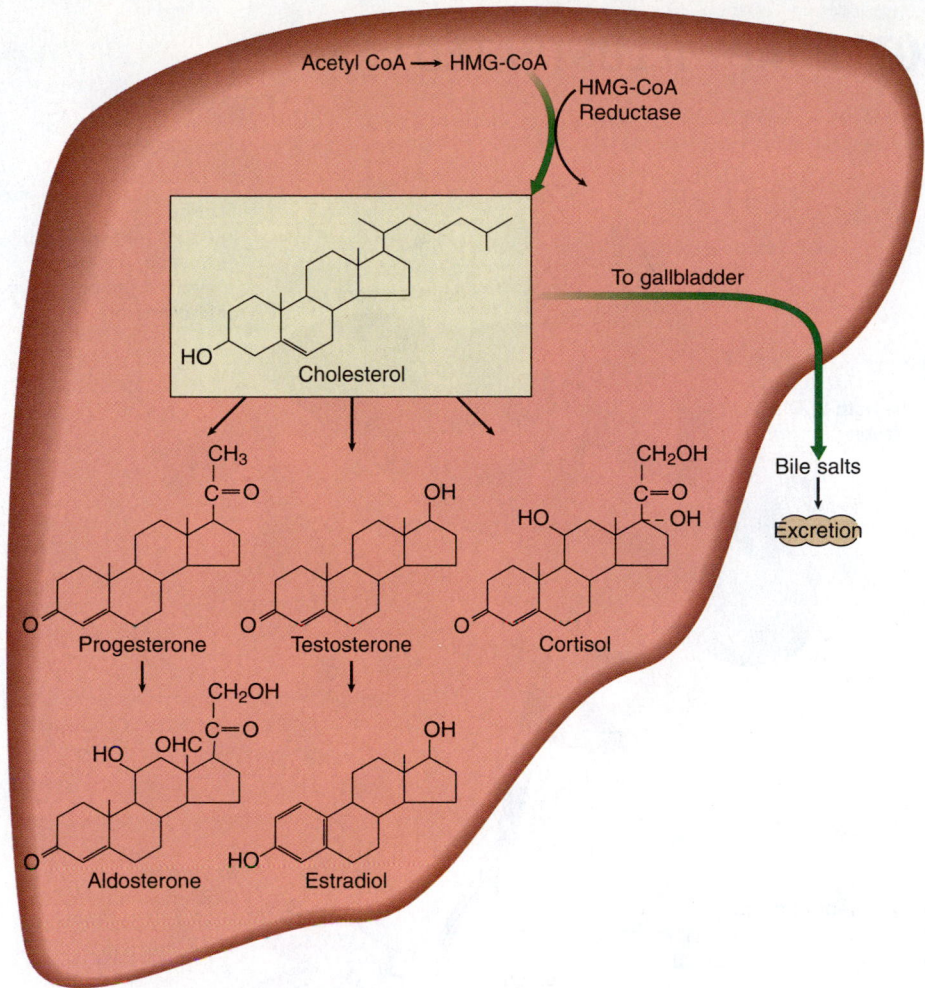

Figure 29.3 Cholesterol biosynthesis and excretion.

coenzyme A reductase) serves as the primary regulatory enzyme for cholesterol biosynthesis. Under normal conditions, this enzyme is controlled through negative feedback. High levels of LDL cholesterol in the blood will shut down production of HMG-CoA reductase, thus turning off the cholesterol synthesis pathway. Pharmacotherapy Illustrated 29.1 shows some of the steps in the biosynthesis of cholesterol and the importance of HMG-CoA reductase.

The statins act by inhibiting HMG-CoA reductase, resulting in less cholesterol biosynthesis. As the liver makes less cholesterol, it responds by making more LDL receptors on the surface of liver cells. The greater number of LDL receptors on liver cells removes additional LDL from the blood. Blood levels of both LDL and cholesterol are reduced. The drop in lipid levels is not permanent, however, so patients must continue these drugs for the remainder of their lives or until their hyperlipidemia can be controlled through dietary or lifestyle changes.

Statins clearly slow the progression of CHD and reduce mortality in patients with a history of cardiovascular disease. This type of therapy is called *secondary* prevention, because the patient is already at risk for increased mortality. *Primary* prevention is the administration of statins to patients with no history of cardiovascular disease. The evidence for a reduction in cardiovascular adverse events with statin therapy is clear for adults with diabetes, age 40 to 75 years with LDL levels between 70 and 189 mg/dL, and for adults with LDL cholesterol levels of 190 mg/dL or higher. The 2013 ACC/AHA guidelines also include statin therapy for adults age 40 through 75 years who have LDL levels 70 through 189 mg/dL and 7.5% or greater 10-year risk of atherosclerotic cardiovascular disease (Stone et al., 2013).

Currently, seven statins are available for treating various types of dyslipidemias, and these are listed in Table 29.3. Although differences among the statins exist, their actions and adverse effects are similar. Lovastatin, pravastatin, and simvastatin are natural substances derived from fungi and have a different chemical structure than the synthetic statins. There are also differences in potency among the drugs. For example, the maximum daily dose for pitavastatin is only 4 mg, whereas the dose is 80 mg for atorvastatin. The half-lives of the statins vary from 20 hours (rosuvastatin) to less than an hour (fluvastatin). Whereas pravastatin is eliminated by the renal route, the other statins are metabolized by hepatic P450 enzymes. In patients with renal disease, dosage adjustment is required for lovastatin, pravastatin, simvastatin, and rosuvastatin but not for fluvastatin or atorvastatin. Research evidence for

PHARMACOTHERAPY ILLUSTRATED 29.1

Mechanisms of Action of Lipid-Lowering Drugs

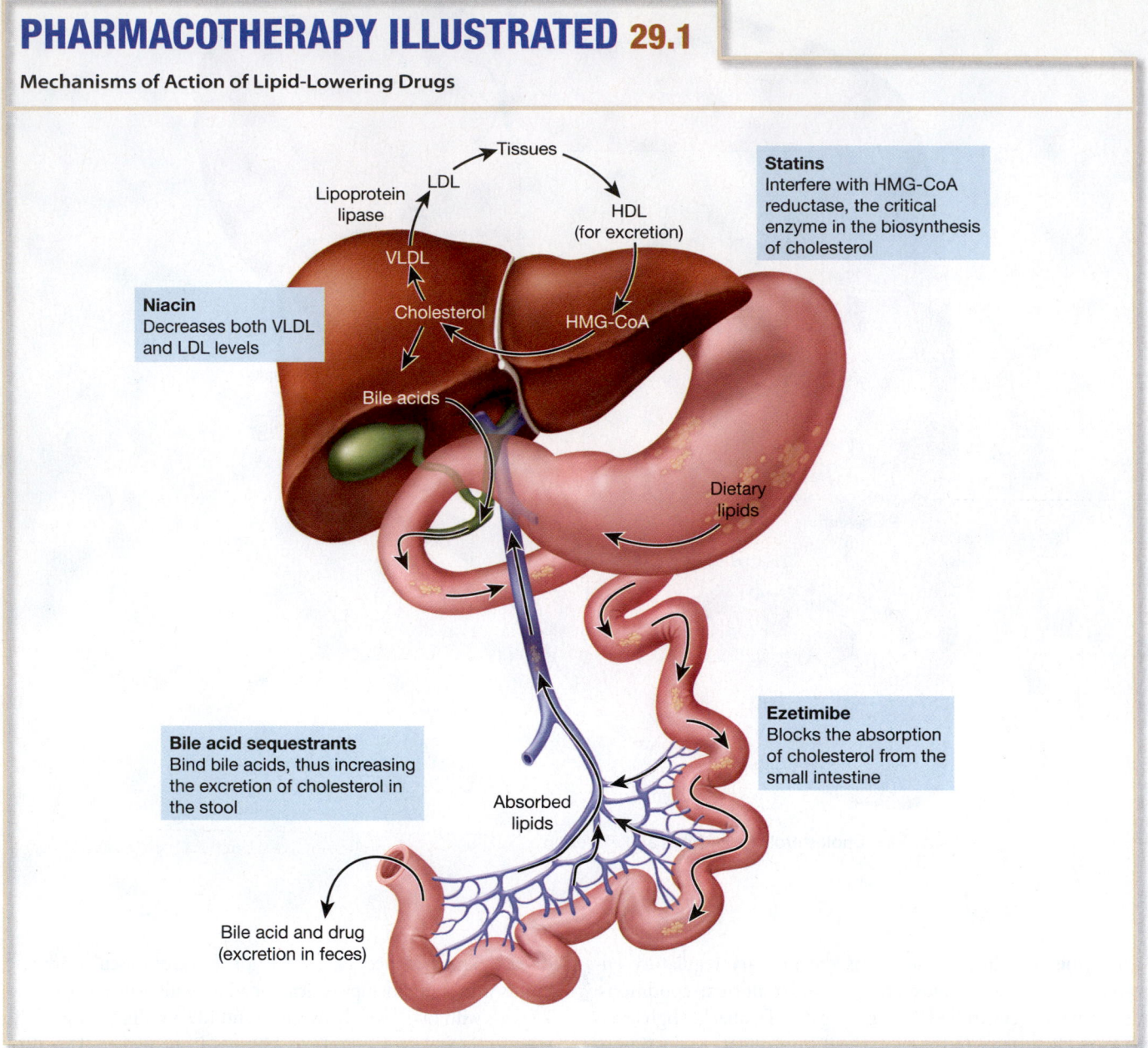

Statins
Interfere with HMG-CoA reductase, the critical enzyme in the biosynthesis of cholesterol

Niacin
Decreases both VLDL and LDL levels

Ezetimibe
Blocks the absorption of cholesterol from the small intestine

Bile acid sequestrants
Bind bile acids, thus increasing the excretion of cholesterol in the stool

cardiovascular adverse event prevention is greatest for atorvastatin and rosuvastatin. However, in clinical practice the choice of statin is often guided by the experience of the prescriber and the response of each individual patient.

All the statins are given orally (PO) and are tolerated well by most patients. Adverse effects are rarely severe enough to cause discontinuation of therapy. Minor adverse effects include headache, abdominal cramping, diarrhea, muscle or joint pain, and heartburn.

Severe myopathy and rhabdomyolysis are rare, although serious adverse effects of the statins. **Rhabdomyolysis** is a breakdown of muscle fibers usually due to muscle trauma or ischemia. The mechanism by which statins cause this disorder is unknown. During rhabdomyolysis, the contents of muscle cells spill into the systemic circulation, causing potentially fatal acute renal failure. Macrolide antibiotics such as erythromycin, azole antifungals, fibric acid

drugs, and certain immunosuppressants should be avoided during statin therapy, because these interfere with statin metabolism and increase the risk of severe myopathy. Levels of creatine kinase (CK), an enzyme released during muscle injury, should be obtained if myopathy is suspected. If CK levels become elevated during therapy, the drug should be immediately discontinued. Statins may be discontinued if muscle weakness persists even without CK elevation. Nurses should urge all patients who develop unexplained muscle or joint pain during statin therapy to immediately report this to the prescriber.

Statins are pregnancy category X drugs because teratogenic effects have been reported in laboratory animals exposed to these drugs. Statins should not be used in patients who may become pregnant, are pregnant, or who are breast-feeding.

Because cholesterol biosynthesis in the liver is higher at night, statins with short half-lives such as lovastatin should be

TABLE 29.3 Drugs for Dyslipidemias

Drug	Route and Adult Dose (Maximum Dose Where Indicated)	Adverse Effects
HMG-CoA Reductase Inhibitors		
atorvastatin (Lipitor)	PO: 10–20 mg once daily (max: 80 mg/day)	*Headache, dyspepsia, abdominal cramping, myalgia, back pain, rash, pruritus* Rhabdomyolysis, severe myositis, elevated hepatic enzymes
fluvastatin (Lescol)	PO: 20 mg daily (max: 80 mg/day)	
lovastatin (Altoprev, Mevacor)	PO: 10–60 mg once daily (max: 80 mg/day immediate release; 60 mg/day extended release)	
pitavastatin (Livalo)	PO: 1–4 mg daily (max: 4 mg/day)	
pravastatin (Pravachol)	PO: 10–40 mg daily (max: 80 mg/day)	
rosuvastatin (Crestor)	PO: 5–40 mg daily (max: 80 mg/day)	
simvastatin (Zocor)	PO: 5–40 mg daily (max: 80 mg/day)	
Bile Acid Sequestrants		
cholestyramine (Questran)	PO: 4–8 g bid–qid (max: 32 g/day)	*Constipation, nausea, vomiting, abdominal pain, bloating, dyspepsia* Gastrointestinal (GI) tract obstruction, vitamin deficiencies due to poor absorption
colesevelam (WelChol)	PO: 1.875 g bid (max: 3.75 g/day)	
colestipol (Colestid)	PO: 5–20 g/day in divided doses (30 g/day granules or 16 g/day tablets)	
Fibric Acid Drugs		
fenofibrate (Lofibra, TriCor, Triglide, Others)	PO: Initial dosing 50–160 mg/day depending on brand name	*Myalgia, flulike symptoms, nausea, vomiting, increased serum transaminase and creatinine levels* Rhabdomyolysis, cholelithiasis, pancreatitis
fenofibric acid (Fibricor, Trilipix)	PO (Fibricor: regular release): 35–105 mg once daily PO (Triplex: delayed release): 45–135 mg once daily	
gemfibrozil (Lopid)	PO: 600 mg bid (max: 1,500 mg/day)	
Other Drugs for Dyslipidemia		
ezetimibe and simvastatin (Vytorin)	PO: 10 mg/10 mg or 10 mg/20 mg every evening (max: 10 mg/80 mg)	*Arthralgia, fatigue, abdominal pain, diarrhea* Anaphylaxis, rhabdomyolysis
ezetimibe (Zetia)	PO: 10 mg daily (max: 10 mg/day)	*Nasopharyngitis, myalgia, upper respiratory tract infection, arthralgia, diarrhea* Anaphylaxis, rhabdomyolysis
icosapent (Vascepa)	PO: 4 g/day	*Arthralgia* Hypersensitivity
lomitapide (Juxtapid)	PO: 5–60 mg once daily	*Abdominal pain, diarrhea, nausea, vomiting, dyspepsia, reduced absorption of fat-soluble vitamins and fatty acids* Fetal toxicity, hepatotoxicity
mipomersen (Kynamro)	Subcutaneous: 200 mg once weekly	*Injection-site reactions, flulike symptoms, nausea, headache, and elevations in serum transaminases*
niacin (Niaspan, Niacor)	Hyperlipidemia: PO: 250 mg regular release or 500 mg extended release daily (max: 6 g/day regular release or 1–2 g/day extended release) Niacin deficiency: PO: 50–100 mg q6–8 h	*Flushing, nausea, pruritus, headache, bloating, diarrhea* Dysrhythmias
omega-3-acid ethyl esters (Lovaza)	PO: 4 g/day	*Belching, dyspepsia, fishy taste* Hypersensitivity

Note: *Italics* indicate common adverse effects. <u>Underline</u> indicates serious adverse effects.

administered in the evening. The other statins have longer half-lives and are effective regardless of the time of day they are taken.

Much research is ongoing to determine the other therapeutic effects of the drugs in the statin class. For example, statins block the vasoconstrictive effect of the A-beta protein, a significant chemical associated with Alzheimer's disease. Cholesterol and A-beta protein had very similar effects on blood vessels, both causing vasoconstriction. Preliminary research suggests that the statins may protect against dementia by inhibiting this protein, thus slowing dementia caused by blood vessel constriction. Research also suggests that the statins may have the ability to lower the incidence of colorectal cancer. The mechanism of this effect is unknown. Several attempts have been made to move low doses of certain statins to over-the-counter (OTC) status; however, the U.S. Food and Drug Administration (FDA) has not approved these applications.

PROTOTYPE DRUG	**Atorvastatin (Lipitor)**

Classification: **Therapeutic:** Antihyperlipidemic
Pharmacologic: HMG-CoA reductase inhibitor, statin

Therapeutic Effects and Uses: Approved in 1996, atorvastatin was initially approved to treat hypercholesterolemia. Following several years of use, it became evident that the drug also prevents adverse cardiovascular events in high-risk patients. After 2 to 4 weeks of therapy, atorvastatin lowers LDL and VLDL cholesterol as well as triglycerides. It appears to lower LDL cholesterol levels greater than most other statins—as much as 60%. Atorvastatin may also be prescribed for the treatment of familial hypercholesterolemia. All patients receiving this drug should be placed on a cholesterol-lowering diet, because this will enhance the drug's therapeutic effects. The primary goal in atorvastatin therapy is to reduce the risk of MI and stroke.

To decrease gastrointestinal (GI) discomfort, atorvastatin may be administered with food. It produces the same degree of LDL cholesterol reduction regardless of the time of day it is taken. Because atorvastatin is not excreted by the kidneys, no adjustment in dosage is necessary in patients with renal impairment. Extensive metabolism to active metabolites gives atorvastatin a long duration of action.

Mechanism of Action: Atorvastatin acts by inhibiting HMG-CoA reductase, the primary regulatory enzyme in cholesterol biosynthesis. As the liver makes less cholesterol, it responds by making more LDL receptors, removing LDL cholesterol from the blood. Blood levels of both LDL and cholesterol are reduced.

Pharmacokinetics:

Route(s)	PO
Absorption	Rapidly absorbed but only 30% reaches the circulation; food reduces absorption
Distribution	Widely distributed; crosses the placenta and is secreted in breast milk; 98% bound to plasma proteins
Primary metabolism	Hepatic; extensively metabolized to active metabolites
Primary excretion	Biliary
Onset of action	2 weeks for lipid-lowering effect; peak plasma level: 1–2 h
Duration of action	Half-life: 14 h (20–30 h for active metabolites)

Adverse Effects: Most patients tolerate atorvastatin well and only 2% or fewer discontinue the drug due to adverse effects. Common adverse effects include headache, intestinal cramping, diarrhea, and constipation. The most serious adverse effect is rhabdomyolysis. Therapy is generally discontinued in patients reporting unexplained muscle pain, weakness, fever, or fatigue due to the potential for rhabdomyolysis.

Contraindications/Precautions: Patients with hepatic impairment should be monitored carefully, because the liver extensively metabolizes atorvastatin and the drug has been associated with a small risk of liver failure. Liver enzyme tests may become elevated during therapy, although this does not necessarily indicate liver damage. Because atorvastatin is pregnancy category X, pregnancy testing should be conducted prior to treatment in women of childbearing years, and these patients should be advised to take precautions to prevent pregnancy during therapy. Atorvastatin is contraindicated during lactation because the drug is secreted in breast milk.

Drug Interactions: Because atorvastatin is a substrate for hepatic CYP3A4, it has the potential to interact with many other drugs. For example, it may increase digoxin levels by 20% as well as increase levels of norethindrone and ethinyl estradiol (oral contraceptives). Erythromycin may increase atorvastatin levels by as much as 40%. Risk of rhabdomyolysis increases with concurrent administration of atorvastatin with macrolide antibiotics, cyclosporine, and azole antifungals. The risk of myopathy increases when atorvastatin is administered concurrently with fibric acid drugs or niacin. Atorvastatin may increase serum transaminases and CK levels. **Herbal/Food:** Grapefruit juice inhibits the metabolism of statins, allowing them to reach high serum levels. Because HMG-CoA reductase inhibitors decrease the synthesis of Coenzyme Q10 (CoQ10), patients may benefit from CoQ10 supplements. Red rice yeast should not be taken with statins because it increases their toxicity.

Pregnancy: Category X.

Treatment of Overdose: No specific therapy is available; patients are treated symptomatically.

Nursing Responsibilities: Key nursing implications for patients receiving atorvastatin are included in the Nursing Practice Application for Patients Receiving Pharmacotherapy for Hyperlipidemia.

Drugs Similar to Atorvastatin (Lipitor)

Other statins include fluvastatin, lovastatin, pitavastatin, pravastatin, rosuvastatin, and simvastatin.

Fluvastatin (Lescol): Approved in 1993, fluvastatin is a synthetic statin that has the shortest half-life of all the drugs in this class. Because the kidneys excrete less than 5% of a PO dose, dosage adjustment for patients with renal impairment is not necessary. Fewer drug interactions are expected with fluvastatin because it is not metabolized through the hepatic P450 system. It is approved for hypercholesterolemia and several other types of dyslipidemia. In 2003, the indications were expanded to include prevention of major cardiac events such as cardiac death and nonfatal MI. An extended release formulation, called Lescol-XL, is available. The drug may be administered without regard to meals. Fluvastatin is well tolerated and its adverse effects are similar to those of atorvastatin. It is contraindicated in patients with severe hepatic impairment and in patients who are pregnant. Fluvastatin is a pregnancy category X drug.

Lovastatin (Altoprev, Mevacor): Approved in 1987, lovastatin, a natural substance derived from fungi, was the first HMG-CoA reductase inhibitor marketed. Lovastatin is a prodrug with no intrinsic activity of its own, but the liver converts it to several active metabolites. This drug may achieve a 20% to 40% reduction in LDL cholesterol. Lovastatin is more effective if administered in the evening and should be taken on an empty stomach to maximize absorption. Although only 10% of this drug is excreted by the kidneys, dosage adjustment for patients with renal impairment is recommended. Lovastatin was originally approved for hypercholesterolemia; however, its indications have been expanded to include slowing the progression of CHD and prevention of MI and stroke. An extended release form is available (Altoprev) as is a fixed-dose combination product with lovastatin and niacin (Advicor). Adverse effects are the same as those of other drugs in this class. It is contraindicated in patients with severe hepatic impairment and in patients who are pregnant. Lovastatin is a pregnancy category X drug.

Pitavastatin (Livalo): Approved in 2009, pitavastatin is one of the newest drugs in the statin class. It is indicated for patients with primary hyperlipidemia and mixed dyslipidemia as an adjunctive therapy to diet to reduce elevated total cholesterol, LDL, apolipoprotein B, and triglycerides, and to increase HDL. It may be administered with or without food and without regard to the time of day. It has similar effectiveness and adverse effects as other statins. Because it is only minimally metabolized by CYP enzymes, it may exhibit fewer drug–drug interactions than some of the other statins. However, like other drugs in this class, hepatic enzymes should be evaluated regularly and there is a small risk of myopathy. This drug is pregnancy category X and patients should be advised not to breast-feed during pitavastatin therapy.

Pravastatin (Pravachol): Like lovastatin, pravastatin is a natural substance derived from fungi. Twenty percent of the drug is excreted by the kidneys, and dosage adjustment for patients with renal impairment is recommended. Like fluvastatin, it is not metabolized through the hepatic P450 system; thus fewer drug interactions are expected. The drug may be taken without regard to meals and is slightly more effective if administered in the evening. Approved in 1991, pravastatin is approved for primary hypercholesterolemia, slowing the progression of coronary atherosclerosis and the prevention of MI and stroke. Unlabeled uses include other types of dyslipidemias. Pravigard PAC is a copackage that contains separate aspirin and pravastatin tablets in various dosage strengths. Adverse effects are the same as those of other drugs in this class. It is contraindicated in patients with hepatic impairment and in those who are pregnant. Pravastatin is a pregnancy category X drug.

Rosuvastatin (Crestor): Approved in 2003, rosuvastatin is a second-generation statin that contains a sulfur group. This drug is the most potent, has the longest half-life in its class (20 hours), and is capable of lowering LDL cholesterol by as much as 65%. Rosuvastatin is not a prodrug and it undergoes minimal hepatic metabolism. This drug may be administered with or without food and without regard to time of day. It is approved for hypercholesterolemia, hypertriglyceridemia, and for slowing the progression of coronary atherosclerosis. Adverse effects are the same as those of other drugs in this class. Rosuvastatin is a pregnancy category X drug.

Simvastatin (Zocor): Approved in 1991, simvastatin is a natural substance derived from fungi. Like lovastatin, simvastatin is an inactive prodrug that is changed to active metabolites by the liver. The drug can lower LDL cholesterol levels by as much as 47%. Although the kidneys excrete only 13% of the drug, dosage adjustment for patients with significant renal impairment is recommended. The drug may be taken with or without food but should be administered in the evening for maximum effectiveness. It is approved for hypercholesterolemia, for hypertriglyceridemia, slowing the progression of coronary atherosclerosis, and prevention of MI and stroke. Adverse effects are the same as those of other drugs in this class. Simvastatin is contraindicated in patients with hepatic impairment and in those who are pregnant. This is a pregnancy category X drug.

CONNECTION Checkpoint 29.1

Several of the statins are prodrugs. From what you learned in Chapter 4, what type of dosage adjustment should be made if these statin prodrugs are prescribed for a patient with hepatic cirrhosis? If a dosage adjustment is not made, what types of adverse effects might you observe? *See Answer to Connection Checkpoint 29.1 on student resource website.*

PharmFACT

The American Academy of Pediatrics recommends that all children undergo cholesterol screening once between the ages of 9 and 11 years and again from age 17 to 21 years. The goal of the screening is to identify the presence of familial hypercholesterolemia, which can occur in one in every 300–500 children (de Ferranti & Washington, 2012).

29.6 Bile acid sequestrants are often combined with statins to reduce LDL cholesterol levels.

Bile acids contain a high concentration of cholesterol and are secreted by the liver to emulsify fats in the small intestine. After performing their digestive function, bile acids are reabsorbed in the ileum and sent back to the liver to again become part of bile. This mechanism is known as enterohepatic circulation. In effect, the cholesterol in bile acids is recycled, with only small amounts leaving the body in the feces.

Prior to the discovery of the statins, the primary means of lowering blood cholesterol was through the use of bile acid sequestrants or resins. The bile acid sequestrants bind to bile acids, forming a large complex that cannot be reabsorbed from the small intestine. The enterohepatic circulation of cholesterol is interrupted and the bound bile acids and cholesterol are eliminated in the feces. The liver responds to the loss of cholesterol by making more LDL receptors, which removes LDL cholesterol from the blood in a mechanism similar to that of the statins.

The bile acid resins are capable of producing a 20% drop in LDL cholesterol, which is generally less response than can be obtained from the statins. They are no longer considered first-line drugs for dyslipidemia, although they are sometimes combined with statins for patients who have contraindications or intolerance to statins.

The bile acid sequestrants tend to cause more frequent adverse effects than statins. Because they are not absorbed into the systemic circulation, adverse effects are limited to the GI tract, causing symptoms such as abdominal pain, bloating, diarrhea, steatorrhea, and constipation. In addition to binding bile acids, these agents can bind drugs such as digoxin and warfarin and increase the potential for drug–drug interactions. Bile acid sequestrants also interfere with the absorption of vitamins and minerals, and nutritional

CONNECTIONS | Complementary and Alternative Therapies

◀ Coenzyme Q10

Description

Coenzyme Q10 (CoQ10) is a lipid-soluble vitamin-like substance found in most animal cells. It is an essential component in the cell's mitochondria for producing adenosine triphosphate (ATP) energy. Because the heart requires high levels of ATP, a sufficient level of CoQ10 is especially important to that organ.

History and Claims

The applications of CoQ10 to treating disease are relatively recent, with the agent being claimed to be an antioxidant and having benefited patients with heart failure in the mid-1960s. Subsequent reports have claimed that CoQ10 may be beneficial in angina pectoris, dysrhythmias, periodontal disease, immune disorders, neurologic disease, obesity, diabetes mellitus, and cancers.

Standardization

The dose of CoQ10 varies widely. Typical doses range from 100 to 200 mg/day.

Evidence

As with most dietary supplements, controlled research studies with CoQ10 are often lacking and give conflicting results. Supplementation with CoQ10 may be important to patients taking the HMG-CoA reductase inhibitors (statins) because these drugs significantly lower blood levels of CoQ10 (Suzuki et al., 2008). Coenzyme Q10 and cholesterol share the same metabolic pathways. Inhibition of the enzyme HMG-CoA reductase by statins decreases CoQ10 levels. Many of the adverse effects of statins, including muscle weakness and rhabdomyolysis, may be due to the decrease in CoQ10 levels; supplementation with CoQ10 may improve myopathy symptoms.

Foods richest in this substance are pork, sardines, beef heart, salmon, broccoli, spinach, and nuts. Older adults appear to have an increased need for CoQ10. Although CoQ10 can be synthesized by the body, many amino acids and other substances are required for this synthesis; thus patients with nutritional deficiencies may need supplementation.

---

deficiencies may occur with extended use. Other medications and vitamins should be taken at least 1 hour before or 4 hours after taking a bile acid sequestrant to avoid drug interactions.

Bile acid sequestrants may cause a transient increase in triglyceride levels. This effect is particularly prominent and often sustained in patients with preexisting hypertriglyceridemia. Because of this, the bile acid sequestrants are generally not prescribed for patients with elevated triglycerides.

PROTOTYPE DRUG | Cholestyramine (Questran)

Classification: **Therapeutic:** Antihyperlipidemic
Pharmacologic: Bile acid sequestrant

Therapeutic Effects and Uses: Approved in 1966, cholestyramine is indicated for the reduction of elevated serum cholesterol in patients with primary hypercholesterolemia (elevated LDL) who do not respond adequately to dietary modifications alone. Cholestyramine monotherapy slows the progression and increases the rate of regression of coronary atherosclerosis. A secondary indication is to relieve pruritus associated with partial biliary obstruction. It is available as a powder that is mixed with fluid before being taken once or twice daily. The drug should be mixed with 60 to 180 mL of water, noncarbonated beverages, highly liquid soups, or pulpy fruits (applesauce, crushed pineapple) to prevent esophageal irritation. The patient should swallow the medication immediately after stirring. If taken with too small a fluid volume or if not completely swallowed, the drug can swell in the throat or esophagus to cause an obstruction.

It may take 30 days or longer for cholestyramine to produce its maximum effect. To avoid interference with absorption, cholestyramine should not be taken at the same time as vitamins or other medications. An off-label indication for cholestyramine is diarrhea caused by *Clostridium difficile*, although antibiotics are the drugs of first choice.

Mechanism of Action: Cholestyramine binds to bile acids, forming an insoluble complex containing cholesterol that is excreted in the feces. Cholestyramine lowers LDL cholesterol levels by increasing LDL receptors on hepatocytes.

Pharmacokinetics:

Route(s)	PO
Absorption	Not absorbed
Distribution	Not distributed; acts locally in the alimentary canal
Primary metabolism	Not metabolized
Primary excretion	Feces
Onset of action	1–2 days
Duration of action	2–4 weeks

Adverse Effects: Cholestyramine is not absorbed or metabolized once it enters the intestine; thus it does not produce systemic adverse effects. Common GI-related adverse effects include constipation, bloating, belching, and nausea. Serious adverse effects include obstruction of the GI tract, hyperchloremic acidosis, and malabsorption syndrome. Chronic use may cause increased bleeding due to hypoprothrombinemia associated with vitamin K deficiency.

Contraindications/Precautions: Cholestyramine should be used cautiously in patients with GI disorders such as peptic ulcer disease, hemorrhoids, inflammatory bowel diseases, or chronic constipation, because bile acid sequestrants may worsen or aggravate these conditions. This drug should not be used in patients with complete biliary obstruction. Bile acid resins should be used with caution in patients with hypertriglyceridemia because they may increase serum triglyceride concentrations. They are absolutely contraindicated if serum triglycerides rise above 400 mg/dL. Although cholestyramine use is safe during pregnancy because it is not absorbed, precautions must be taken to ensure that this drug is not interfering with vitamin absorption, especially folic acid.

Drug Interactions: Cholestyramine can bind to other drugs and interfere with their absorption, causing reduced effects. This interaction has been reported for digoxin, penicillins, iron supplements, thyroid hormone, and thiazide diuretics, although it has the potential to occur with any drug administered PO. Cholestyramine may indirectly increase the effects of warfarin by binding to vitamin K, decreasing its absorption and lowering the levels of vitamin K in the body. The absorption of raloxifene can be reduced as much as 60% if coadministered with cholestyramine. To reduce the possibility of absorption interference, cholestyramine should be administered 1 hour before or 4 hours after other PO medications. **Herbal/Food:** Cholestyramine may block the absorption of iron and fat-soluble vitamins in food.

Pregnancy: Category B.

Treatment of Overdose: No specific therapy is available; patients are treated symptomatically.

Nursing Responsibilities: Key nursing implications for patients receiving cholestyramine are included in the Nursing Practice Application for Patients Receiving Pharmacotherapy for Hyperlipidemia.

Drugs Similar to Cholestyramine (Questran)

Other bile acid sequestrants include colesevelam and colestipol.

Colesevelam (WelChol): Approved in 2000, colesevelam is a bile acid-binding drug that is claimed to have more bile acid-binding capacity than the older resins. The drug has the capacity to reduce LDL cholesterol by as much as 20%. It may be administered as monotherapy or concurrently with statins to achieve greater efficacy. At least 2 weeks of therapy may be necessary before maximum therapeutic response is achieved. In 2008, colesevelam was approved as an adjunct to diet, exercise, and antidiabetic drugs to improve glycemic control in patients with type 2 diabetes. It is not approved for patients with type 1 diabetes. The most common adverse reactions with colesevelam are constipation, dyspepsia, and nausea. Colesevelam can interfere with the absorption of other medications and should be administered 4 hours after other PO drugs. Like cholestyramine, colesevelam can increase serum triglyceride levels and is contraindicated in patients with triglyceride levels greater than 500 mg/dL. The large tablets can cause dysphagia or esophageal obstruction; thus this drug should be used with caution in patients with swallowing disorders. An oral suspension, dissolved in 4 to 8 ounces of water, is available for patients who have difficulty swallowing the tablets. This drug is pregnancy category B.

Colestipol (Colestid): Approved in 1977, colestipol acts by the same mechanism as cholestyramine, has the same effectiveness in lowering LDL cholesterol, and exhibits the same adverse effects. Other drugs should be administered at least 1 hour before or 4 to 6 hours after a dose of colestipol to prevent interference with absorption. Maximum therapeutic effects may take as long as a month to appear. Because the drug can increase serum triglycerides, it should not be administered to patients with hypertriglyceridemia. Colestipol is rarely used as monotherapy. In addition to its use in treating elevated HDL cholesterol, colestipol may be used off-label to treat digoxin overdose, diarrhea, and pruritus associated with biliary obstruction. This drug is pregnancy category B.

PharmFACT
Familial hypercholesterolemia affects 1 in 500 people and is a genetic disease that predisposes people to premature CAD (Citkowitz, 2013).

29.7 Niacin can reduce triglycerides and LDL cholesterol levels, but adverse effects limit its usefulness.

Niacin, also called nicotinic acid, is a B-complex vitamin (B3). Its ability to lower lipid levels, however, is unrelated to its role as a vitamin because much higher doses are needed to produce its antihyperlipidemic effects. For lowering cholesterol, the usual dose is 2 to 3 g per day. When taken as a vitamin, the dose is only 25 mg per day.

The primary action of niacin (Niaspan) is to decrease the production of VLDL, which lowers serum triglyceride levels. Because LDL is synthesized from VLDL, the patient also experiences a reduction in LDL cholesterol levels. Niacin also has the desirable effect of increasing HDL levels, although this effect does not appear to be significant in reducing mortality from cardiovascular disease. As with other lipid-lowering drugs, maximum therapeutic effects may take a month or longer to achieve.

Although effective at reducing LDL cholesterol by 20%, niacin produces more adverse effects than the statins. Intense flushing and hot flashes occur in almost every patient. Taking one aspirin tablet 30 minutes prior to niacin administration can reduce uncomfortable flushing in many patients. In addition, a variety of uncomfortable GI effects such as nausea, excess gas, and diarrhea are commonly reported. Paresthesias, such as tingling in the extremities, may also occur.

More serious adverse effects such as hepatotoxicity and gout are possible but uncommon. Patients with elevated liver enzymes or a history of liver disease should use an alternate drug to lower lipids. In patients predisposed to gout, niacin may increase uric acid levels and precipitate acute gout.

Niacin is not usually prescribed for patients with diabetes mellitus because the drug can raise fasting glucose levels. When beginning therapy, patients with diabetes should monitor their blood glucose levels more frequently until the effect of niacin is determined.

Because of the high incidence of adverse effects, niacin is most often used in lower doses in combination with a statin or bile acid sequestrant; the beneficial effects of these drugs are additive. Combining niacin with lovastatin can reduce LDL cholesterol by as much as 45%. The two drugs are combined in a fixed-dose formulation marketed as Advicor. Simcor is a combination of niacin and simvastatin, which is used to lower LDL levels.

Because supplemental niacin is available without a prescription, patients should be instructed not to attempt self-medication with this drug. One form of niacin that is available OTC as a vitamin supplement, called nicotinamide, has no lipid-lowering effects. If niacin is to be used to lower cholesterol, it should be done under medical supervision.

29.8 Fibric acid drugs lower triglyceride levels but have little effect on LDL cholesterol.

Three fibric acid drugs are sometimes used for patients with high triglyceride levels: fenofibrate (Antara, Lofibra, TriCor, Triglide), fenofibric acid (Fibricor, Trilipix), and gemfibrozil (Lopid). They are preferred drugs for treating severe hypertriglyceridemia

---

CONNECTIONS | Patient Safety

◄ Concurrent Medication Administration

The nurse administers the following oral medications ordered for a 64-year-old man: tetracycline 500 mg bid, digoxin (Lanoxin) 0.25 mg/day, and cholestyramine (Questran) 4 g bid ac and at bed time. At 8:00 a.m., before breakfast, the nurse administers tetracycline 500 mg, digoxin 0.25 mg, and cholestyramine 4 mg. What should the nurse have done differently?

See Answer to the Patient Safety Question on student resource website.

(Types IV and V hyperlipidemia), although they have little effect on LDL cholesterol. Fibric acid drugs activate the enzyme lipoprotein lipase, which increases the breakdown and elimination of triglyceride-rich particles from the plasma. In most patients, combining a fibric acid drug with a statin results in greater decreases in triglyceride levels than either drug used alone. This combination is not recommended for patients with type 2 diabetes because it has not been shown to have cardiovascular benefits in these patients. Doses for the fibric acid drugs are listed in Table 29.3.

The most common adverse effects of the fibrates relate to the GI system: dyspepsia, diarrhea, abdominal pain, nausea, and vomiting. Taking these medications with meals usually diminishes GI distress. Drugs in this class are generally not used in patients with hepatic impairment or gallbladder disease.

PROTOTYPE DRUG | Gemfibrozil (Lopid)

Classification: **Therapeutic:** Antihyperlipidemic
Pharmacologic: Fibric acid drug (fibrate)

Therapeutic Effects and Uses: Approved in 1981, gemfibrozil lowers serum triglycerides and LDL cholesterol. It is most effective in patients who present with hypertriglyceridemia and VLDL. Effects of gemfibrozil include up to a 50% reduction in VLDL with an increase in HDL. It is less effective than the statins at lowering LDL; thus it is not used as monotherapy. It is considered a second-line therapy that is used when statins are ineffective or not well tolerated.

Mechanism of Action: The exact mechanism of action of gemfibrozil is unknown. The drug inhibits the breakdown of stored fat, or lipolysis, in adipose tissue. By inhibiting the uptake of free fatty acids by the liver, hepatic production of triglycerides is decreased. The drug may also increase the excretion of cholesterol in the feces.

Pharmacokinetics:

Route(s)	PO
Absorption	Well absorbed
Distribution	Unknown; distribution across the placenta or secretion in breast milk is unknown; 99% bound to plasma protein
Primary metabolism	Hepatic; undergoes enterohepatic recirculation
Primary excretion	Primarily renal, 6% in feces
Onset of action	1–2 h
Duration of action	Half-life: 1.5 h

Adverse Effects: The most common adverse effects of gemfibrozil are GI related, such as abdominal cramping, diarrhea, nausea, and dyspepsia. Nervous system effects include headache, dizziness, peripheral neuropathy, and diminished libido. Serious adverse effects include cholelithiasis, anemia, and eosinophilia.

Contraindications/Precautions: Gemfibrozil may worsen or cause biliary disease; thus it is contraindicated in patients with preexisting gallbladder disease or serious liver impairment. Because it is excreted by the kidneys, the drug should be used cautiously in patients with renal impairment.

Drug Interactions: Although antihyperlipidemic agents from different drug classes are sometimes combined to produce an enhanced effect, the use of gemfibrozil with statins increases the risk of myositis and rhabdomyolysis. CK levels should be regularly monitored during combined therapy and the combination immediately discontinued if myopathy is suspected. In most cases the risk of rhabdomyolysis, which may be fatal, outweighs the potential benefits of combined statin and gemfibrozil therapy.

Concurrent use of gemfibrozil with PO anticoagulants may increase the risk of bleeding because the fibrate displaces warfarin from its plasma protein binding sites. If a patient is taking warfarin, dosages should be lowered. More frequent monitoring of prothrombin time (PT) and international normalized ratio (INR) is necessary until stabilization occurs.

Gemfibrozil may enhance the hypoglycemic effects of antidiabetic drugs. Serum glucose levels must be carefully monitored because the dosage of the antidiabetic drug may require adjustment. **Herbal/Food:** No significant interactions.

Pregnancy: Category C.

Treatment of Overdose: No specific therapy is available; patients are treated symptomatically.

Nursing Responsibilities: Key nursing implications for patients receiving gemfibrozil are included in the Nursing Practice Application for Patients Receiving Pharmacotherapy for Hyperlipidemia.

Drugs Similar to Gemfibrozil (Lopid)

Drugs similar to gemfibrozil include fenofibrate and fenofibric acid.

Fenofibrate (Antara, Lofibra, TriCor, Triglide) and fenofibric acid (Fibricor, Trilipix): Once absorbed, fenofibrate is quickly converted to fenofibric acid, its active metabolite. Thus the actions and adverse effects of the two drugs are the same. Fenofibrate is indicated as supplemental therapy to diet to reduce elevated LDL, total cholesterol, triglycerides, and apo B and to increase HDL in patients with primary hypercholesterolemia, hypertriglyceridemia, and mixed dyslipidemia. Approved in 1993, fenofibrate may reduce serum triglycerides by as much as 30%. One advantage of the fenofibrate formulations over gemfibrozil is that they may be taken once daily rather than twice a day. The different formulations of fenofibrate and fenofibric acid vary in strength, bioavailability, and whether the drug should be administered with a meal. These forms are not interchangeable. One of the forms, Trilipix, is approved for concurrent therapy with statins. The most frequent adverse effects are GI related, such as nausea, vomiting, dyspepsia, constipation, flatulence, and abdominal pain. Liver function tests should be performed periodically to monitor for elevated serum transaminases. Myopathy and rhabdomyolysis have been reported, and the risks for these adverse effects are increased when coadministered with a statin. Rash and photosensitivity are other adverse effects. These drugs are pregnancy category C.

CONNECTION Checkpoint 29.2

From what you learned in Chapter 10, what changes in physiology occur with aging that may require decreased starting dosages for antihyperlipidemic drugs? *See Answer to Connection Checkpoint 29.2 on student resource website.*

Miscellaneous Drugs for Dyslipidemias

29.9 Newer strategies have been developed to treat dyslipidemias.

The large numbers of people with elevated lipid values has encouraged the pharmaceutical industry to investigate new drugs for controlling LDL cholesterol and triglycerides. The search for new and improved antilipidemics has resulted in several new drugs for this condition.

Ezetimibe (Zetia): Ezetimibe (Zetia) is the only drug in a class called the cholesterol absorption inhibitors. Cholesterol is absorbed from the intestinal lumen by cells in the jejunum of the small intestine. Ezetimibe blocks this absorption by as much as 50%, causing less cholesterol to enter the blood. Unlike the statins, the drug does not inhibit cholesterol biosynthesis in the liver or increase the excretion of bile acid.

When given as monotherapy, ezetimibe produces a modest reduction in LDL of about 20%. Adding a statin to the therapeutic regimen reduces LDL by an additional 15% to 20%. The drug produces a slight drop in serum triglycerides. Ezetimibe is available as a single tablet with a once-daily dosing regimen. Vytorin is a fixed-dose combination tablet containing ezetimibe and simvastatin, and Liptruzet combines ezetimibe with atorvastatin.

Nasopharyngitis, myalgia, upper respiratory tract infection, arthralgia, and diarrhea are the most common adverse effects of ezetimibe, although these rarely require discontinuation of therapy. Because bile acid sequestrants inhibit the absorption of ezetimibe, these drugs should not be taken together. In addition, ezetimibe and statins should not be given concurrently to patients with serious hepatic impairment or with elevated serum transaminase levels. Ezetimibe is pregnancy category C.

Omega-3 fatty acids: Nutritionists have long reported the benefits of eating fish rich in omega-3 fatty acids such as tuna, salmon, and halibut. The two principal omega-3 fatty acids are eicosapentaenoic acid (EPA) and docosahexaenoic acid (DHA). Vegetarian sources of omega-3 fatty acids include flaxseed oil, soybeans, walnuts, and pumpkin seeds.

The role of omega-3 fatty acids in preventing cardiovascular disease is well established. When taken as dietary supplements, the omega-3 fatty acids are usually marketed as fish oil. Fish oil supplementation has been shown to decrease mortality due to MI and stroke. A typical dose of omega-3 fatty acids in fish oil capsules is 180 mg of EPA and 120 mg of DHA.

Two prescription formulations of omega-3 fatty acids are available: omega-3-acid ethyl esters (Lovaza) and icosapent (Vascepa). Both drugs are approved as an adjunct to diet in the treatment of severe hypertriglyceridemia. Adverse effects are minor and include belching, fishy taste, and arthralgia. The drugs should be used with caution in patients who are allergic to seafood, especially shellfish.

Drugs for familial hypercholesterolemia: Two drugs were approved in 2013 for a very narrow indication: as an adjunct to lowering LDL in patients with homozygous familial hypercholesterolemia (HoFH). HoFH is a genetic disorder in which the body has such high levels of cholesterol and LDL that cardiovascular disease begins in childhood and results in death by the mid-30s. Many of these patients have a diminished response to therapy with statins and other antihyperlipidemics. The two new drugs, lomitapide (Juxtapid) and mipomersen (Kynamro), act by very different and unique mechanisms. Therapy is very costly and will likely limit their widespread use.

The primary protein that composes particles of LDL is called apolipoprotein B (apo B). When assembling the lipoprotein, lipid molecules are transported and loaded onto the apo B. Upon completion, the lipoprotein is assembled and leaves the intestine or liver as chylomicrons or VLDL, which eventually raises blood LDL levels. Lomitapide and mipomersen interfere with different aspects of this genesis of lipoprotein.

Lomitapide is classified as a microsomal triglyceride transfer protein (MTP) inhibitor. Inhibition of MTP interferes with the transfer of lipids to apo B, thus lowering plasma levels of LDL. The drug is given PO and is indicated only for HoFH. GI adverse effects such as diarrhea, nausea, vomiting, dyspepsia, and abdominal pain occur in almost all patients. Drug interactions may be serious with medications that inhibit hepatic CYP3A4, including ketoconazole, clarithromycin, lopinavir/ritonavir, or telithromycin. These drugs will markedly increase levels of lomitapide. Lomitapide is contraindicated during pregnancy (category X).

Mipomersen is classified as an inhibitor of apo B synthesis. The message for making apo B leaves the DNA as a strip of messenger RNA (mRNA). Mipomersen is a huge molecule that has mRNA complementary to apo B (called an antisense message). The antisense message binds to the apo B strip of RNA, preventing the synthesis of the apo B protein. Mipomersen is given as once-weekly subcutaneous injection. The drug is pregnancy category B.

Mipomersen and lomitapide carry identical black box warnings that the drugs can cause elevations in transaminases and may increase hepatic fat (hepatic steatosis). The drugs are contraindicated in patients with active hepatic disease, and transaminases (ALT and AST) must be measured prior to and during therapy. The drugs are only available in restricted use programs that require prescribers and pharmacists to be certified through special training.

CONNECTIONS: NURSING PRACTICE APPLICATION

Patients Receiving Pharmacotherapy for Hyperlipidemia

Assessment	Potential Nursing Diagnoses*
Baseline assessment prior to administration: • Obtain a complete health history including cardiovascular, musculoskeletal (preexisting conditions that might result in muscle or joint pain), GI (peptic ulcer disease, hemorrhoids, inflammatory bowel disease, chronic constipation, gallbladder disease, dysphagia or esophageal strictures), and the possibility of pregnancy. Obtain a drug history including allergies, current prescription and OTC drugs, herbal preparations, and alcohol use. Be alert to possible drug interactions. • Evaluate appropriate laboratory findings, especially liver function studies, lipid profiles, and CK. • Assess the patient's ability to receive and understand instructions. Include the family or caregiver as needed.	• *Overweight* • *Obesity* • *Ineffective Health Maintenance* (Individual or Family) • *Chronic Pain*, related to adverse drug effects • *Deficient Knowledge* (Drug Therapy)
Assessment throughout administration: • Assess for desired therapeutic effects (e.g., lowered total cholesterol and LDL levels, increased HDL levels). • Continue periodic monitoring of lipid profiles, liver function studies, CK, and uric acid levels. • Assess for adverse effects: musculoskeletal discomfort, nausea, vomiting, abdominal cramping, or diarrhea. Immediately report any severe musculoskeletal pain, unexplained muscle tenderness accompanied by fever, inability to perform activities of daily living (ADLs) due to musculoskeletal weakness or pain, unexplained numbness or tingling of extremities, yellowing of the sclera or skin, severe constipation, straining with passing of stools, or tarry stools.	

Implementation

Interventions and (Rationales)	Patient-Centered Care
Ensuring therapeutic effects: • Follow appropriate administration guidelines. (Many of the lipid-lowering drugs have specific administration requirements. For best results, they should be taken at night when cholesterol biosynthesis is at its highest.)	• Teach the patient to take the drug following appropriate guidelines (see Patient self-administration of drug therapy).
• Encourage appropriate lifestyle changes: lowered fat intake, increased exercise, limited alcohol intake, and smoking cessation. Provide for dietitian consultation as needed. (Healthy lifestyle changes will support and minimize the need for drug therapy.)	• Encourage the patient and family to adopt a healthy lifestyle of low-fat food choices, increased exercise, decreased alcohol consumption, and smoking cessation. • Encourage increased intake of foods rich in omega-3 and coenzyme Q10: fish such as salmon and sardines, nuts, extra-virgin olive and canola oils, beef, chicken, and pork. Supplementation may be needed; instruct the patient to seek the advice of a health care provider before taking supplements.
Minimizing adverse effects: • Continue to monitor periodic liver function tests and CK levels. (Abnormal liver function tests or increased CK levels may indicate drug-induced adverse hepatic effects or myopathy and should be reported. **Lifespan:** Monitor the older adult frequently because age-related physiological changes may affect the drug's metabolism or excretion. **Diverse Patients:** Because statins metabolize through the P450 system pathways, monitor ethnically diverse patients to ensure optimal therapeutic effects and to minimize adverse effects.)	• Instruct the patient on the need to return periodically for laboratory work.

CONNECTIONS: NURSING PRACTICE APPLICATION (continued)

- Continue to assess for drug-related symptoms, which may indicate that adverse effects are occurring. (Lipid-lowering drugs often adversely affect the liver but may also cause drug-specific adverse effects.)
- Assess for the possibility of increased adverse effects when a combination of lipid-lowering agents is used. (Lipid-lowering agents may be combined for better effects, but this increases the risk of adverse effects.)

- Teach the patient the importance of reporting signs or symptoms related to adverse drug effects as follows:
  - **Statins:** Report unusual or unexplained muscle tenderness, increasing muscle pain, numbness or tingling of extremities, or effects that hinder normal ADLs. **Lifespan:** The drug should not be taken during pregnancy, or if pregnancy is suspected, or while breast-feeding.
  - **Bile acid resins:** Report severe nausea, heartburn, constipation, or straining with passing stools. Any tarry stools or yellowing of the sclera or skin should also be reported. **Lifespan:** The older adult may have an increased risk of bleeding due to drug-related changes with vitamin K synthesis.
  - **Niacin:** Report flank, joint, or stomach pain, or yellowing of the sclera or skin.
  - **Fibric acid drugs:** Report unusual bleeding or bruising, right upper quadrant pain, muscle cramping, or changes in the color of the stool. Patients with diabetes on PO medications may need a change in their dosage and should monitor their glucose more frequently in early therapy. **Lifespan:** Monitor the older adult for dizziness and assist with ambulation to prevent falls. **Diverse Patients:** Research has indicated that Hispanics and Native Americans may have a greater risk for development of gallbladder disease than other ethnic groups.
- Instruct patients taking a combination of lipid-lowering drugs to be alert to symptoms related to adverse effects of *both* drugs, as above.

- If long-term therapy is used, ensure adequate intake of fat-soluble vitamins (A, D, E, K) and folic acid in the diet or consider supplementation. (Lipid-lowering drugs may cause depletion or diminished absorption of these nutrients.)

- Instruct the patient, family, or caregiver about foods high in folic acid and fat-soluble vitamins, and about the need to consult with the health care provider about the need for vitamin and folic acid supplementation while on long-term therapy.

Patient understanding of drug therapy:
- Use opportunities during administration of medications and during assessments to discuss the rationale for drug therapy, desired therapeutic outcomes, commonly observed adverse effects, parameters for when to call the health care provider, and any necessary monitoring or precautions. (Using time during nursing care helps to optimize and reinforce key teaching areas.)

- The patient, family, or caregiver should be able to state the reason for the drug, appropriate dose and scheduling, what adverse effects to observe for and when to report them, and the anticipated length of medication therapy.

Patient self-administration of drug therapy:
- When administering the medication, instruct the patient, family, or caregiver in proper self-administration of the drug, e.g., during the evening meal. (Utilizing time during nurse-administration of these drugs helps to reinforce teaching.)

- The patient, family, or caregiver is able to discuss appropriate dosing and administration needs.
- The patient takes the drug following appropriate guidelines:
  - **Statins:** Most are taken with the evening meal; avoid grapefruit and grapefruit juice, which could inhibit the drug's metabolism, leading to toxic levels.
  - **Bile acid resins:** Take before meals with plenty of fluids, mixing powders or granules thoroughly with liquid. Take other medications 1 h before or 4 h after the bile acid resin is taken.
  - **Niacin:** Take with cold water to decrease the sensation of flushing associated with the drug. Take one adult-strength (325-mg) aspirin 30 min before the niacin dose.
  - **Fibric acid drugs:** Take with a meal.

*Nursing Diagnoses—Definitions and Classification 2015–2017. Copyright © 2014, 1994–2014 by NANDA International. Used by arrangement with John Wiley & Sons Limited.

29

Understanding the Chapter

Key Concepts Summary

29.1 Lipids are classified as triglycerides, phospholipids, or sterols.

29.2 Lipoproteins are important predictors of cardiovascular disease.

29.3 Blood lipid profiles are important diagnostic tools in guiding the therapy of dyslipidemias.

29.4 Lipid levels can often be controlled through therapeutic lifestyle changes.

29.5 The statins are the most effective drugs for reducing blood lipid levels.

29.6 Bile acid sequestrants are often combined with statins to reduce LDL cholesterol levels.

29.7 Niacin can reduce triglycerides and LDL cholesterol levels, but adverse effects limit its usefulness.

29.8 Fibric acid drugs lower triglyceride levels but have little effect on LDL cholesterol.

29.9 Newer strategies have been developed to treat dyslipidemias.

Case Study: Making the Patient Connection

Remember the patient "Belinda Cummings" at the beginning of the chapter? Now read the remainder of the case study. Based on the information presented within this chapter, respond to the critical thinking questions that follow.

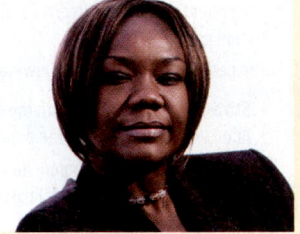

Belinda Cummings is a 39-year-old black female who feels fine. However, she recently had her cholesterol level checked at her church's health fair where she was told that it exceeded the normal value. As directed, she made an appointment and saw her health care provider for a checkup.

During the office visit, the nurse collects Belinda's social and health history. Belinda's vital signs are within normal limits, except her blood pressure is elevated (142/90 mmHg). She is also slightly overweight and has been on a low-carbohydrate diet for 1 week. Her favorite foods are potato chips and all dairy products, especially cheese. She admits to smoking less than a pack of cigarettes per day and occasionally drinks a glass of wine with dinner. Belinda is divorced and has one teenage son.

A series of laboratory tests is completed during the visit. Belinda's physical exam is normal, and there are no ECG abnormalities. The blood tests are unremarkable with the exception of the lipid profile.

	Patient Value	Normal Range
Total Cholesterol	240 mg/dL	Less than 200
Triglycerides	199 mg/dL	Less than 150
HDL Cholesterol	30 mg/dL	Greater than 60
LDL Cholesterol	184	Less than 100
Cholesterol-to-HDL Ratio	6.6	Less than 4.5

The patient is placed on a standard cholesterol-lowering diet and prescribed atorvastatin (Lipitor) 10 mg daily. Belinda is instructed to return to the office in 1 month for a follow-up visit.

Critical Thinking Questions

1. How would you respond to Belinda when she asks you, "Is high cholesterol due to heredity or from what I eat?"

2. What health teaching should you provide the patient about ways to reduce high blood lipid levels?

3. Create a list of potential adverse effects that this patient should be taught to watch for related to the medication.

See Answers to Critical Thinking Questions on student resource website.

Additional Case Study

David Hamilton has been taking cholestyramine (Questran) for elevated blood lipid levels for 2 years. He presents today in your clinic for a routine follow-up visit that will include a lipid profile test. He states that he has been somewhat consistent with his cholesterol-lowering diet and attempting to get "a little more" exercise. You are the nurse caring for David.

1. Outline key concepts related to health promotion activities that you would want to be sure David understands.

2. What adverse effects related to Questran should David watch for?

3. If David's triglyceride levels increase or remain consistently high, what drug group(s) might be prescribed?

See Answers to Additional Case Study on student resource website.

Chapter Review

1 The patient taking atorvastatin (Lipitor) reports weakness and fatigue, pain in the shoulders, and aching joints. The nurse initially assesses the patient for which condition?

1. Rhabdomyolysis
2. Renal failure
3. Rheumatoid arthritis
4. Hepatic insufficiency

2 A patient is receiving cholestyramine (Questran) for elevated low-density lipoprotein levels. Which adverse effect should the nurse include in the care plan to monitor the patient?

1. Orange-colored urine
2. Abdominal pain
3. Sore throat and fever
4. Decreased capillary refill

3 The provider orders colestipol (Colestid) in combination with atorvastatin (Lipitor) for a patient with elevated low-density lipoprotein levels. The nurse collaborates with the prescriber about which data related to the patient?

1. Past history of peptic ulcer disease
2. Recent myocardial infarction
3. Laboratory value for serum sodium of 136 mEq/L
4. Allergies to foods high in tyramine

4 Which assessment findings discovered by the nurse would be an expected adverse effect associated with niacin therapy? Select all that apply.

1. Fever and chills
2. Intense flushing and hot flashes
3. Tingling of the fingers and toes
4. Dry mucous membranes
5. Hypoglycemia

5 The community health nurse visits a patient who has been prescribed lovastatin (Mevacor). Which statement, if made by the patient, indicates that further teaching is necessary concerning this drug therapy?

1. "I should try to maintain my body weight at an optimal level."
2. "Most patients with lipid disorders don't have any symptoms."
3. "The best time for me to take this medication is before I go to bed."
4. "I will take my drug with beverages that contain grapefruit juice."

6 The nurse is caring for a patient receiving gemfibrozil (Lopid) for hyperlipidemia. The nurse would validate the order with the prescriber if the patient reported a history of which of the following? Select all that apply.

1. Gallbladder disease
2. Angina
3. Hypertension
4. Diabetes
5. Renal disease

See Answers to Chapter Review in Appendix A.

References

Citkowitz, E. (2013). Familial hypercholesterolemia. *Medscape Reference*. Retrieved from http://emedicine.medscape.com/article/121298-overview

Cook, S., & Kavey, R. E. (2011). Dyslipidemia and pediatric obesity. *Pediatric Clinics of North America, 5*, 1363–1373. doi:10.1016/j.pcl.2011.09.003

de Ferranti, S., & Washington, R. L. (2012). NHLBI guidelines on cholesterol in kids: What's new and how does this change practice? *AAP News, 33*(2), 1–1. doi:10.1542/aapnews.2012332-1b

Eiland, L. S., & Luttrell, P. K. (2010). Use of statins for dyslipidemia in the pediatric population. *Journal of Pediatric Pharmacology and Therapeutics, 15*, 160–172.

Expert Panel on Detection. (2001). Executive summary of the third report of the National Cholesterol Education Program (NCEP) Expert Panel on Detection, Evaluation, and Treatment of High Blood Cholesterol in Adults (Adult Treatment Panel III). *JAMA: The Journal of the American Medical Association, 285*, 2486–2497. doi:10.1001/jama.285.19.2486

Jellinger, P. S., Smith, D. A., Mehta, A. E., Ganda, O., Handelsman, Y., Rodbard, H. W., . . . Seibel, J. A. (2012). American Association of Clinical Endocrinologists' guidelines for management of dyslipidemia and prevention of atherosclerosis. *Endocrine Practice, 18*(2), 269–293.

Stone, N. J., Robinson, J., Lichtenstein, A. H., Merz, C. N. B., Lloyd-Jones, D. M., Blum, C. B., . . . Wilson, P. W. F. (2013). 2013 ACC/AHA guideline on the treatment of blood cholesterol to reduce atherosclerotic cardiovascular risk in adults: A report of the American College of Cardiology/American Heart Association Task Force on Practice Guidelines. *Journal of the American College of Cardiology*. Online First: November 2013. doi:10.1016/j.jacc.2013.11.002

Suzuki, T., Nozawa, T., Sobajima, M., Igarashi, N., Matsuki, A., Fujii, N., & Inoue, H. (2008). Atorvastatin-induced changes in plasma coenzyme Q10 and brain natriuretic peptide in patients with coronary artery disease. *International Heart Journal, 49*(4), 423–433.

Selected Bibliography

American Heart Association. (2013). *Youth and cardiovascular diseases—Statistics.* Retrieved from http://www.heart.org/idc/groups/heart-public/@wcm/@sop/@smd/documents/downloadable/ucm_319577.pdf

Berglund, L., Brunzell, J. D., Goldberg, A. C., Goldberg, I. J., Sacks, F., Murad, M. H., & Stalenhoef, A. F. (2012). Evaluation and treatment of hypertriglyceridemia: An Endocrine Society clinical practice guideline. *Journal of Clinical Endocrinology & Metabolism, 97*(9), 2969–2989. doi:10.1210/jc.2011-3213

Bersot, T. P. (2011). Drug therapy for hypercholesterolemia and dyslipidemia. In L. L. Brunton, B. A. Chabner, & B. C. Knollman (Eds.), *The pharmacological basis of therapeutics* (12th ed., pp. 877–908). New York, NY: McGraw-Hill.

Herdman, T. H., & Kamitsuru, S. (Eds.). (2014). *NANDA International nursing diagnoses: Definitions and classification, 2015–2017.* Oxford, United Kingdom: Wiley-Blackwell.

Jellinger, P. S., Smith, D. A., Mehta, A. E., Ganda, O., Handelsman, Y., Rodbard, H. W., . . . & Seibel, J. A. (2012). American Association of Clinical Endocrinologists' guidelines for management of dyslipidemia and prevention of atherosclerosis. *Endocrine Practice, 18*, 1–78.

Oldways. (n.d.). *Heritage pyramids and total diet.* Retrieved from http://www.oldwayspt.org/eating-well/introduction-traditional-diet-pyramids

Psaty, B. M., & Weiss, N. S. (2014). 2013 ACC/AHA guideline on the treatment of blood cholesterol: A fresh interpretation of old evidence. *JAMA: The Journal of the American Medical Association, 311*, 461–462. doi:10.1001/jama.2013.284203

Ray, K. K., Seshasai, S. R., Erqou, S., Sever, P., Jukema, J. W., Ford, I., & Sattar, N. (2010). Statins and all-cause mortality in high-risk primary prevention: A meta-analysis of 11 randomized controlled trials involving 65,229 participants. *JAMA Internal Medicine, 170*, 1024–1031. doi:10.1001/archinternmed.2010.182

Smith, R. J., & Hiatt, W. R. (2013). Two new drugs for homozygous familial hypercholesterolemia: Managing benefits and risks in a rare disorder. *JAMA Internal Medicine, 173*, 1491–1492. doi:10.1001/jamainternmed.2013.6624

Spratt, K. A. (2010). Treating dyslipidemia: Re-evaluating the data using evidence-based medicine. *The Journal of the American Osteopathic Association, 110*(4, Suppl. 5), 6–11.

Taylor, F., Ward, K., Moore, T. H. M., Burke, M., Davey-Smith, G., Casas, J. P., & Ebrahim, S. (2011). Statins for the primary prevention of cardiovascular disease. *Cochrane Database of Systematic Reviews, 1*, CD004816. doi:10.1002/14651858.CD004816.pub4

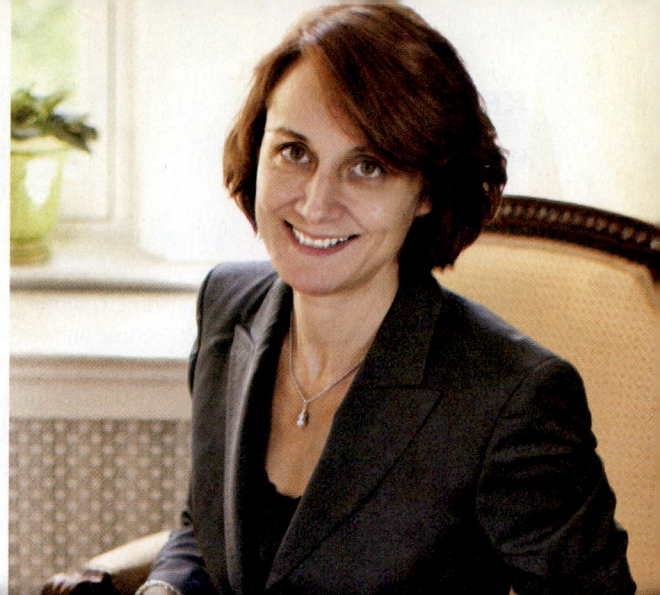

"My friends all take diuretics for their hypertension, but my provider is giving me something called a 'calcium channel blocker.' Would someone please tell me what calcium has to do with high blood pressure?"

Patient "Elise Freeman"

CHAPTER
30 Pharmacotherapy with Calcium Channel Blockers

LEARNING OUTCOMES

After reading this chapter, the student should be able to:

1. Describe the role of calcium ions in the contraction of smooth and cardiac muscle.
2. Explain why the actions of the $beta_1$-adrenergic antagonists are similar to those of the calcium channel blockers.
3. Describe how calcium channel blockers interact with the L-type calcium channel.
4. Identify the physiological effects of calcium channel blockers on arterial smooth muscle and cardiac muscle.
5. Explain the classification of calcium channel blockers.
6. Compare and contrast the actions of dihydropyridine versus nondihydropyridine calcium channel blockers.
7. For each of the classes shown in the chapter outline, identify the prototype and representative drugs and explain the mechanism(s) of drug action, primary indications, contraindications, significant drug interactions, pregnancy category, and important adverse effects.
8. Apply the nursing process to care for patients receiving calcium channel blockers.

CHAPTER OUTLINE

▸ **Physiological Role of Calcium Channels in Muscle Contraction**

▸ **Types of Calcium Channels**

▸ **Consequences of Calcium Channel Blockade**

▸ **Classification of Calcium Channel Blockers**

Dihydropyridines

PROTOTYPE Nifedipine (Adalat CC, Procardia XL), *p. 477*

Nondihydropyridines

PROTOTYPE Verapamil (Calan, Isoptin, Verelan), *p. 480*

KEY TERMS

calcium channel, 474

dihydropyridine, 476

negative chronotropic effect, 476

negative inotropic effect, 476

sarcolemma, 474

sarcoplasmic reticula, 474

Since the approval of the first calcium channel blocker (CCB) 30 years ago, this class of drugs has become one of the most widely prescribed in medicine. One reason for their widespread use is that these drugs treat two chronic diseases that affect millions of people: hypertension (HTN) and coronary artery disease (CAD). Their success is also related to their effectiveness and a highly favorable safety profile.

CCBs are also known as calcium channel antagonists. These drugs do not physically block calcium channels; therefore, *antagonist* is a more accurate term than *blocker*. Because both terms are used interchangeably in clinical practice, they are used as synonyms throughout this text.

Physiological Role of Calcium Channels in Muscle Contraction

30.1 Calcium channels facilitate contraction in cardiac and smooth muscles.

Recall from muscle physiology that the signal for contraction is an action potential traveling across the muscle plasma membrane, or **sarcolemma**. The action potential causes a depolarization that opens voltage-gated channels in the sarcolemma, allowing ions to enter and leave the muscle cell. In skeletal muscle, as in nervous tissue, the primary ion channels facilitate Na^+ and K^+ movement. In cardiac and smooth muscle a third type of voltage-gated channel, the **calcium channel**, is of particular importance to cardiovascular physiology and pharmacotherapy. Contraction of these muscle types requires the movement of calcium ions (Ca^{2+}).

Under resting conditions, the concentration of free Ca^{2+} in the cytoplasm of a muscle cell is very low. Depolarization of the sarcolemma, however, changes the amount of free Ca^{2+} in two ways. First, calcium channels in the sarcolemma open, allowing extracellular calcium to rush into the cell. Secondly, depolarization releases large amounts of calcium ions stored in cellular structures called **sarcoplasmic reticula**. This huge increase in cytoplasmic Ca^{2+} removes the inhibition of actin and myosin filaments by the proteins calmodulin (smooth muscle) or troponin C (cardiac muscle) through a cascade of complex reactions. Actin and myosin are then free to slide, and muscle contraction occurs. This process is illustrated in Figure 30.1.

Muscle contraction is terminated when the amount of free cytoplasmic Ca^{2+} is reduced, by either pumping to the outside of the cell or by returning the Ca^{2+} to storage in the sarcoplasmic reticulum.

Recall from Chapter 15 that activation of beta$_1$-adrenergic receptors in cardiac muscle increases heart rate and contractility. This is because, in myocardial cells, the signal for opening calcium channels is linked to activation of the sympathetic nervous system. In effect, calcium channels open when the sympathetic nervous system supplies the action potential, depolarizing the sarcolemma.

This has important implications to pharmacology. Blocking cardiac beta$_1$ receptors with adrenergic antagonists will *prevent* the opening of calcium channels. Thus the cardiac effects of beta$_1$-adrenergic blockers, and their pharmacotherapeutic indications and adverse effects, are similar to those of CCBs.

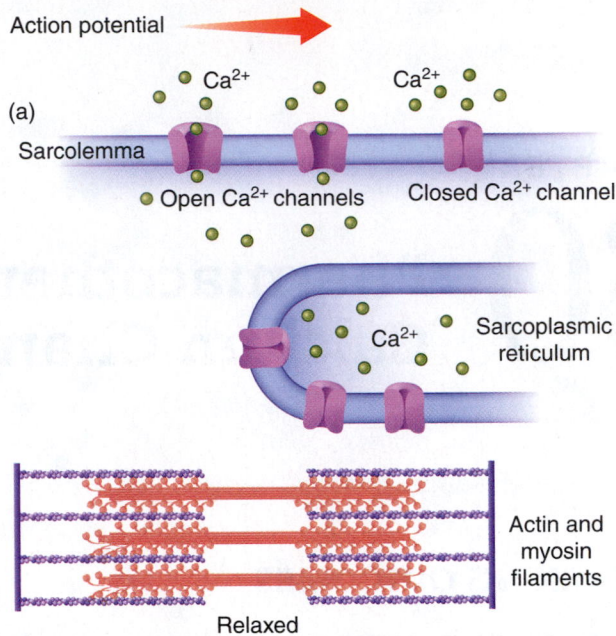

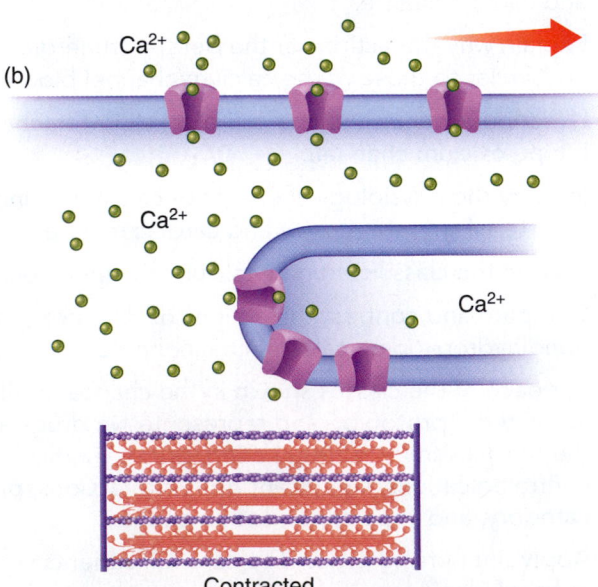

Figure 30.1 Calcium channels and muscle contraction: (a) Calcium channels open as the action potential travels along the sarcolemma. (b) Large amounts of calcium are released from storage in the sarcoplasmic reticula, causing actin and myosin filaments to slide and muscle contraction to occur.

CONNECTION Checkpoint 30.1

From what you learned in Chapters 15 and 16, what type of drug–drug interaction would you expect between a CCB and (a) a beta-adrenergic antagonist such as propranolol (Inderal) and (b) a sympathomimetic such as epinephrine? *See Answer to Connection Checkpoint 30.1 on student resource website.*

Types of Calcium Channels

30.2 The calcium channel consists of multiple subunits and is present in many tissues.

Research has discovered different types of calcium ion channels, which are named by the letters *L*, *T*, and *N*. Differences in the structures and locations of the channels are important to drug action.

Pharmacologically, the most important calcium channels are the L type, because they are the ones that bind CCBs. L-type calcium channels are found on the sarcolemma of cardiac and smooth muscles. The channel spans across the membrane and consists of three main parts. An extracellular portion serves as a receptor to bind CCBs. A central portion serves as a pore through which calcium ions travel. An intracellular portion serves as a second messenger capable of initiating a cascade of events that signal the cell to perform specific functions.

The L-type calcium channel is regulated by voltage changes across the sarcolemma. When an action potential depolarizes the membrane the channel opens, allowing Ca^{2+} to rush in. The L-type channels are relatively slow, which allows for a sustained flow of Ca^{2+} into the cell. When a CCB medication is present, the channel changes shape. Although the drug does not physically block the opening, the change in shape of the channel is enough to prevent Ca^{2+} from entering the muscle cell. The L-type calcium channel is illustrated in Figure 30.2.

L-type calcium channels are widespread in the cardiovascular system, and these channels bind all current CCBs. L-type calcium channels are also present in other tissues, particularly in neurons and endocrine and sensory cells. This leads to other potential uses of these drugs, a topic discussed later in this chapter.

T-type calcium channels are present in vascular smooth muscle as well as the sinoatrial (SA) node where they are involved in pacemaker functions of the heart. Like the L-type channels, they are also located in other tissues throughout the body. The drug mibefradil was developed as a selective T-channel blocker but was removed from the market after serious drug interactions were discovered. At this time, there are no drugs approved by the U.S. Food and Drug Administration (FDA) that act by blocking T-type calcium channels.

N-type calcium channels are found throughout the nervous system. Their primary role appears to be to control neurotransmitter release at synapses. They also are involved in the transmission of pain impulses in the spinal cord. Although a great deal of research is currently being conducted on drugs that target N-type channels in the nervous system, none are currently approved for use in the United States.

Consequences of Calcium Channel Blockade

30.3 Blocking calcium channels has significant physiological effects on the heart and vascular smooth muscle.

The therapeutic applications of CCBs are the result of actions of the drugs on vascular smooth muscle, cardiac muscle, and the conduction system in the heart. Some CCBs have greater actions on the heart, whereas others have more effect on arteriolar smooth muscle. None of the CCBs affect serum calcium levels.

Effects on vascular smooth muscle: The influx of calcium ions into smooth muscle cells is essential for contraction. Because

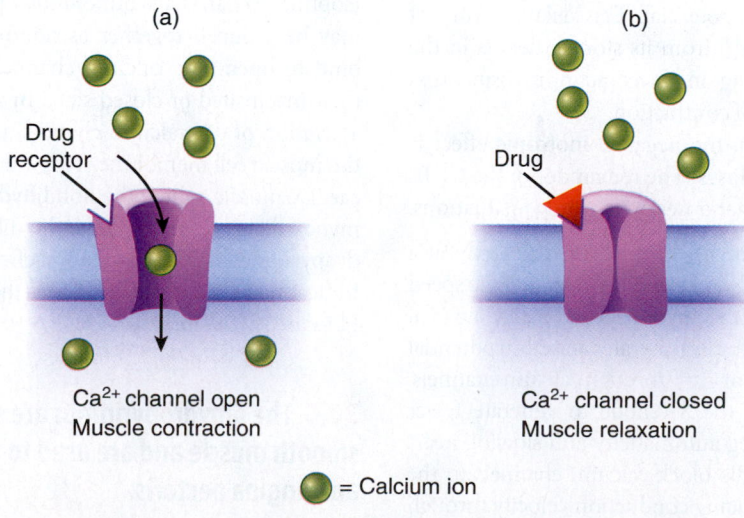

= Calcium ion

Figure 30.2 L-type calcium channel: (a) Calcium channel opens when an action potential passes across the sarcolemma. Calcium enters the cell and muscle contraction occurs. (b) Calcium channel antagonist binds to the receptor, changing its shape; channel closes and muscle relaxation occurs.

the degree of contraction of arterioles controls peripheral resistance, the blockade of calcium channels has significant physiological effects on blood pressure. All CCBs dilate peripheral arterioles, resulting in a decrease in systemic blood pressure. Afterload is reduced, resulting in lower myocardial oxygen demand and less workload for the heart. This is particularly important for patients with angina, who will experience less chest pain due to the decrease in cardiac workload (see Chapter 35).

Another important group of vessels affected by CCBs are the coronary arteries. Dilation of the coronary arteries by the CCBs brings more blood to the myocardium, which is beneficial for patients with myocardial ischemia. Veins and cardiac preload are not affected by drugs in this class.

Effects on the myocardium: Most CCBs reduce the force of myocardial contraction. This **negative inotropic effect** occurs because these drugs reduce the inward movement of Ca^{2+} during the plateau phase of the action potential. This delayed entry of Ca^{2+} prevents the release of Ca^{2+} from its storage depots in the sarcoplasmic reticulum, resulting in fewer actin–myosin cross bridges and a diminished force of contraction.

For verapamil and diltiazem, the negative inotropic effect is clearly apparent at therapeutic doses. The remainder of the CCBs will only exhibit this effect at higher doses or in overdose situations.

Effects on cardiac conduction: In general, CCBs exhibit a **negative chronotropic effect**: the property of slowing the speed of electrical conduction across the myocardium. Under normal conditions, the SA node automatically generates an action potential because of an inward movement of Ca^{2+} through calcium channels. Blocking calcium entry causes the SA node to generate fewer action potentials, thus decreasing automaticity and slowing heart rate. Similarly, some of the CCBs block calcium channels in the atrioventricular (AV) node, reducing conduction velocity through this region of the heart and further slowing the spread of the action potential across the myocardium. Because of these actions on the cardiac conduction system, the CCBs are sometimes used to correct certain rhythm abnormalities of the heart (see Chapter 37).

Not all CCBs affect cardiac conduction to the same degree. Verapamil and diltiazem exhibit this effect at therapeutic doses, whereas the remainder of the CCBs exhibit a negative chronotropic effect only at high doses, or not at all.

CONNECTION Checkpoint 30.2

From what you learned in Chapter 28, define afterload. If a drug increases afterload, what effect would this likely have on cardiac output? *See Answer to Connection Checkpoint 30.2 on student resource website.*

Classification of Calcium Channel Blockers

30.4 Calcium channel blockers are classified by their chemical structures as dihydropyridines or nondihydropyridines.

Despite the fact that all CCBs affect L-type calcium channels, there are differences in actions and adverse effects among the specific drugs. This is because the drugs interact with different subunits of the calcium channel. This gives rise to a classification of calcium channel antagonists based on their chemical structures.

The **dihydropyridines** are the largest class of CCBs. They include amlodipine (Norvasc), felodipine (Plendil), isradipine (DynaCirc), nicardipine (Cardene), nifedipine (Adalat CC, Procardia XL), nimodipine, and nisoldipine (Nisocor). The dihydropyridines bind reversibly to closed-type (inactivated) calcium channels, changing the channels' structure and making them unresponsive to depolarization. Because closed-type channels are found in greater numbers in vascular smooth muscle than in cardiac muscle, dihydropyridines are primarily used for their vasodilation effect on arterial smooth muscle.

The remaining CCBs are chemically dissimilar to the dihydropyridines and bind to different subunits of the L-type calcium channel. Although they are chemically different from each other, diltiazem (Cardizem, Dilacor, Tiazac) and verapamil (Calan, Isoptin, Verelan) have quite similar pharmacologic properties and may be grouped together as nondihydropyridines. These drugs bind to open-type calcium channels, causing them to revert to their inactivated or closed state. In addition these drugs delay reactivation of the calcium channel, thus slowing repolarization of the muscle cell membrane. This effect is particularly noticeable in cardiac muscle, where the nondihydropyridines slow the speed of myocardial conduction. Like the dihydropyridines, the nondihydropyridines have a vasodilation effect on vascular smooth muscle. Indications for the various CCBs that have been approved by the FDA are shown in Table 30.1.

30.5 The dihydropyridines are selective for vascular smooth muscle and are used to treat hypertension and angina pectoris.

All dihydropyridines have very similar actions and adverse effects. All except clevidipine are well absorbed after oral (PO) administration, and most are highly protein bound, excreted by the liver, and undergo extensive first-pass metabolism. Because of this,

TABLE 30.1 FDA-Approved Indications for Calcium Channel Blockers

Drug	Hypertension	Chronic Stable Angina	Vasospastic Angina	Unstable Angina	Dysrhythmias	Subarachnoid Hemorrhage
Dihydropyridines						
amlodipine (Norvasc)	X	X	X			
clevidipine (Cleviprex)	X					
felodipine (Plendil)	X					
isradipine (DynaCirc)	X					
nicardipine (Cardene)	X	X				
nicardipine (Cardene SR)	X					
nifedipine (Adalat, Procardia XL)	X	X	X			
nimodipine						X
nisoldipine (Sular)	X					
Nondihydropyridines						
diltiazem (Cardizem, Dilacor)		X	X			
diltiazem extended release (Cartia XT, Dilt-CD)	X	X	X			
diltiazem extended release (Cardizem LA, Dilacor XR, Taztia XT, Tiazac)	X	X				
diltiazem injection (Cardizem)					X	
verapamil (Calan, Verelan)	X	X	X	X	X	
verapamil injection (Isoptin)					X	

dosage adjustments are necessary in patients with significant hepatic impairment.

Drugs in this class are highly selective for calcium channels located in vascular smooth muscle. At high doses, however, the dihydropyridines lose their selectivity and also affect calcium channels in the heart. All dihydropyridines are equivalent in effectiveness for treating HTN and angina. Some are available in extended release formulations that allow for once-daily dosing. Doses for the dihydropyridines are listed in Table 30.2.

The dihydropyridines are well tolerated in most patients. Common adverse effects include flushed skin, headache, dizziness, peripheral edema, lightheadedness, nausea, and diarrhea, although these are usually not severe enough to warrant discontinuation of therapy. The vasodilation caused by the blockade of calcium channels in vascular smooth muscle may cause reflex tachycardia. This is generally transient and clinically important only in patients with preexisting myocardial ischemia or dysrhythmias. If a CCB must be used for these patients, extended release formulations are selected because they produce a more gradual change in blood pressure with less reflex tachycardia.

PROTOTYPE DRUG   **Nifedipine (Adalat CC, Procardia XL)**

Classification: **Therapeutic:** Antihypertensive
Pharmacologic: Calcium channel blocker, dihydropyridine type

Therapeutic Effects and Uses: Approved in 1981, nifedipine is a CCB with several indications. For HTN it may be given alone or in combination with drugs from other antihypertensive classes. Its ability to dilate the coronary arteries makes it an important drug in

TABLE 30.2 Calcium Channel Blockers

Drug	Route and Adult Dose (Maximum Dose Where Indicated)	Adverse Effects
Dihydropyridines		
amlodipine (Norvasc)	PO: 5–10 mg once daily (max: 10 mg/day)	*Flushed skin, hypotension, headache, dizziness, peripheral edema, lightheadedness, nausea, diarrhea, constipation*
clevidipine (Cleviprex)	IV: 1–2 mg/h initial dose, gradually increased until goal blood pressure is reached (max: 16 mg/h)	<u>Hepatotoxicity, MI, HF, confusion, mood changes, gingival hyperplasia</u>
felodipine (Plendil)	PO: 5–10 mg once daily (max: 10 mg/day)	
isradipine (DynaCirc)	PO (controlled release): 5 mg once daily (max: 20 mg/day)	
nicardipine (Cardene, Cardene SR)	PO: 20–40 mg tid or 30–60 mg bid (Cardene SR) (max: 120 mg/day)	
nifedipine (Adalat CC, Procardia XL)	PO: 30–60 mg once daily	
nimodipine	PO: 60 mg qid for 21 consecutive days	
nisoldipine (Sular)	PO: 17–34 mg once daily (max: 34 mg/day)	
Nondihydropyridines		
diltiazem (Cardizem, Dilacor, Taztia XT, others)	PO: 30 mg 4 times daily (max: 480 mg/day) Extended release forms: 120–240 mg once daily	
verapamil (Calan, Isoptin, Verelan)	PO: 80–160 mg tid (max: 480 mg/day) PO (Verelan, Calan SR): 100–200 mg once daily	

Note: Italics indicate common adverse effects. <u>Underline</u> indicates serious adverse effects.

the treatment of chronic stable or variant angina (see Chapter 35). When used as an antianginal, a beta-adrenergic blocker may be administered concurrently to prevent reflex tachycardia. Nifedipine may be used off-label to treat hypertensive emergency, persistent hiccups, or premature labor contractions, or to prevent migraines.

Nifedipine is usually prescribed as extended release tablets because this allows for once-daily dosing. At high doses, the immediate release form of nifedipine should be used with great caution because its use has been associated with an increased risk for myocardial infarction (MI).

Mechanism of Action: Nifedipine acts by selectively blocking calcium channels in vascular smooth muscle, including those in the coronary arteries, causing a decrease in the amount of intracellular calcium available for muscle contraction. This results in a fall in blood pressure and a diminished myocardial oxygen demand due to the reduced afterload. Nifedipine has no effect on myocardial conduction except at toxic doses.

Pharmacokinetics:

Route(s)	PO
Absorption	Well absorbed (90%)
Distribution	Widely distributed; secreted in breast milk; 92–98% bound to plasma protein
Primary metabolism	Hepatic; extensive first-pass metabolism
Primary excretion	Renal (80%) with small amounts in feces (15%)
Onset of action	30–60 min (immediate release capsules); 6 h (extended release tablet)
Duration of action	4–8 h (24 h for extended release); half-life: 2–5 h

Adverse Effects: Nifedipine is well tolerated and serious adverse effects are not common. Most adverse effects such as hypotension, dizziness, headache, and flushing are related to the vasodilation action of the drug. The most common cardiovascular-related adverse effect is peripheral edema, which occurs more frequently with nifedipine than with other CCBs. Other severe, though rare, adverse effects include hepatotoxicity, MI, heart failure (HF), severe hypotension, and confusion.

Contraindications/Precautions: The only contraindication is hypersensitivity to nifedipine or other dihydropyridines. Caution must be observed when using nifedipine in patients with bradycardia or HF because this drug has negative inotropic effects that can worsen these conditions. The immediate release form is contraindicated in patients with acute MI or cardiogenic shock. Because nifedipine causes blood pressure to fall, it should be used cautiously in patients with preexisting hypotension. Any signs of worsening pulmonary edema call for discontinuation of the drug. Patients with significant hepatic impairment are at risk for drug accumulation and toxicity. Older adults are at much greater risk of nifedipine toxicity and experience a higher overall mortality when treated with this drug.

Drug Interactions: Nifedipine is a substrate for hepatic CYP3A4 and may interact with drugs that induce or inhibit this enzyme. When given concurrently with nifedipine, other antihypertensive drugs have additive effects on blood pressure. These additive hypotensive effects are used to advantage in the pharmacotherapy of HTN (see Chapter 34). Concurrent use of nifedipine with a beta-adrenergic blocker increases the risk of HF due to additive negative inotropic and chronotropic effects. Nifedipine may increase the serum levels of digoxin by as much as 45%, leading to bradycardia and digoxin toxicity. Alcohol potentiates the vasodilation action of nifedipine and could lead to syncope caused by a rapid drop in blood pressure. **Herbal/Food**: Grapefruit juice may enhance the absorption of nifedipine. Melatonin may reduce the effectiveness of nifedipine by increasing blood pressure and heart rate. St. John's wort can induce CYP3A4 and increase the metabolism of nifedipine and reduce the plasma level of this drug.

Pregnancy: Category C.

Treatment of Overdose: Overdosage may result in pronounced hypotension, which is treated with rapid-acting vasopressors such as dopamine or dobutamine. Calcium infusions may also be indicated.

Nursing Responsibilities: Key nursing implications for patients receiving nifedipine are included in the Nursing Practice Application for Patients Receiving Pharmacotherapy with Calcium Channel Blockers.

Drugs Similar to Nifedipine (Adalat CC, Procardia XL)

Other dihydropyridines include amlodipine, clevidipine, felodipine, isradipine, nicardipine, nimodipine, and nisoldipine.

Amlodipine (Norvasc): Amlodipine is indicated for the treatment of HTN, chronic stable angina, and Prinzmetal's variant angina. Approved in 1992, amlodipine has the longest half-life (35 hours) of the dihydropyridines, which allows for once-daily dosing. Like other dihydropyridines, amlodipine affects mainly arteriolar smooth muscle, including that in the coronary arteries, and has no significant effect on cardiac conduction. The drug is well tolerated, with headache, dizziness, and dose-dependent peripheral edema being frequent adverse effects. Reflex tachycardia rarely occurs because the drug has a very gradual onset. In the treatment of HTN, several weeks may be required to achieve optimal outcomes. Amlodipine is used in many fixed-dose combination products with valsartan (Exforge), valsartan and hydrochlorothiazide (Exforge HCT), atorvastatin (Caduet), aliskiren (Amturnide, Tekamlo), olmesartan (Azor), olmesartan and hydrochlorothiazide (Tribenzor), benazepril (Lotrel), and telmisartan (Twynsta). This drug is pregnancy category C.

Clevidipine (Cleviprex): Approved in 2008, clevidipine is an injectable emulsion that is approved for the treatment of HTN when rapid control of blood pressure is desirable. The dose is doubled every 90 seconds until the blood pressure approaches the goal, then the infusion is slowed, with dose adjustments every 5 to 10 minutes. Blood pressure falls within minutes and must be monitored continuously during the infusion. With such rapid titration, hypotension and reflex tachycardia may occur. The most common adverse effects are nausea, vomiting, and headache. Patients with HF must be monitored carefully because clevidipine may worsen this condition. This drug is pregnancy category C.

Felodipine (Plendil): Approved in 1991, felodipine is a dihydropyridine that has greater selectivity for vascular smooth muscle than nifedipine and is approved only for the pharmacotherapy of HTN. It exerts no significant effects on the heart. Its elimination half-life of 11 to 16 hours allows for once-daily dosing. Typical adverse effects are facial flushing, headache, peripheral edema, and reflex tachycardia. Lexxel is a fixed-dose combination of felodipine with enalapril. This drug is pregnancy category C.

Isradipine (DynaCirc): Approved in 1990, isradipine is the most potent of the dihydropyridines and is approved for the pharmacotherapy of HTN, either alone or in combination with a thiazide diuretic. Chronic stable angina is an off-label indication for the drug. The physiological actions of isradipine are selective to arterioles, and the drug has no appreciable effect on the heart. Reflex tachycardia is usually not significant. A sustained release form (DynaCirc CR) is available for once-daily dosing. Optimum response may require 2 to 4 weeks of therapy. Headache, facial flushing, and dizziness are the most common adverse effects. This drug is pregnancy category C.

Nicardipine (Cardene): Approved in 1988, nicardipine is indicated for the pharmacotherapy of chronic stable angina and HTN. Beta-adrenergic blockers or sublingual nitrates may be administered concurrently to reduce the possibility of reflex tachycardia in patients with angina pectoris. A sustained release form (Cardene SR) allows for once-daily dosing, and an intravenous (IV) form (Cardene IV) is available for initiation of therapy in patients with severe HTN. An off-label use of nicardipine is for migraines. The actions, contraindications, and adverse effects are similar to those of nifedipine. Peripheral edema, dizziness, headache, and facial flushing are the most common adverse effects. This drug is pregnancy category C.

Nimodipine: Approved in 1988, nimodipine is an oral calcium channel blocker with one very specific indication: to reduce the incidence and severity of ischemic deficits in patients with subarachnoid hemorrhage from ruptured intracranial berry aneurysms. The drug prevents vasospasm of the injured vessel and reduces the severity of the resulting neurologic deficit. Nimodipine appears to have a greater smooth muscle relaxation effect on cerebral arteries than arteries in other areas of the body. The most frequent adverse effects are hypotension, edema, and headache. This drug carries a black box warning that it should never be given by the parenteral route because life-threatening adverse events have occurred when administered by this route. This drug is pregnancy category C.

Nisoldipine (Sular): Approved in 1995, nisoldipine is selective for vascular smooth muscle and has no significant effect on the myocardium. It is approved only for HTN but may be used off-label for angina. The extended release form, Sular, allows for once-daily dosing. Peripheral edema and headache are relatively common in patients taking this drug. Reflex tachycardia may cause angina pain in patients with myocardial ischemia. Like other CCBs, it should be used with caution in patients with hypotension, peripheral edema, or HF. This drug is pregnancy category C.

PharmFACT

It is estimated that 10% to 20% of patients taking calcium channel antagonists will develop gingival hyperplasia. This condition can be successfully managed by professional dental care and oral antiseptic rinses such as chlorhexidine (Peridex) (Mejia, 2012).

30.6 The nondihydropyridines act on both vascular smooth muscle and the myocardium.

The nondihydropyridine group of CCBs consists of two drugs, verapamil (Calan, Isoptin, Verelan) and diltiazem (Cardizem, Dilacor, Tiazac). Although the two drugs are chemically dissimilar, they share common physiological actions, adverse effects, and indications.

Like the dihydropyridines, drugs in this class block L-type calcium channels in vascular smooth muscle, causing vasodilation. As expected from this physiological action, the nondihydropyridines are used in the pharmacotherapy of HTN and angina. Thus the dihydropyridines and nondihydropyridines share these two indications. Doses for the nondihydropyridines are listed in Table 30.2.

It is important to note that verapamil and diltiazem have actions on the heart that the dihydropyridines do not possess. These drugs block calcium channels in the myocardium, causing a negative inotropic effect. In addition, the nondihydropyridines decrease the speed of myocardial conduction, resulting in a slower heart rate.

These cardiac effects of the nondihydropyridines may be viewed as therapeutic or adverse, depending on the patient and the reasons for administering the drugs. For example, by slowing conduction across the heart, verapamil and diltiazem can suppress abnormal cardiac rhythms. They are indicated for specific types of dysrhythmias, such as atrial flutter or fibrillation (see Chapter 37). In certain patients, however, slowing the speed of conduction may result in serious adverse effects. For example, slowing the heart rate can diminish cardiac output in patients with moderate or severe HF and worsen this condition. Slowing impulse conduction may cause partial or complete heart block in patients with bradycardia or second-degree or third-degree AV block. Concurrent treatment with a beta-adrenergic agonist may be necessary to counteract these adverse cardiac effects.

Other adverse effects from the nondihydropyridines include constipation, flushed skin, headache, dizziness, edema of the ankles and feet, and lightheadedness. Gingival hyperplasia is an uncommon adverse effect that occurs with long-term therapy and usually reverses after the drugs are discontinued. Most patients tolerate the nondihydropyridine CCBs well and experience few serious adverse effects.

CONNECTIONS Lifespan Considerations

High Blood Pressure in Children

Hypertension is often perceived as an adult health problem, but children and even babies can have high blood pressure. The American Heart Association recommends that all children age 3 and older have their blood pressure taken yearly. A diagnosis of HTN is based on an average systolic and/or diastolic blood pressure at or above the 95th percentile for blood pressure, as determined by age, height, and gender, on three or more occasions. A diagnosis of prehypertension is based on an average at or above the 90th percentile for age, height, and gender (Expert Panel on Integrated Guidelines for Cardiovascular Health and Risk Reduction in Children and Adolescents, 2011; Moyer, 2013; Riley & Bluhm, 2012).

While lifestyle modifications such as weight reduction, increased exercise, and diet modification are the preferred therapies for childhood HTN, drug therapy may be indicated. Antihypertensive therapy should begin with a single antihypertensive at the lowest recommended dose and the choice of CCBs, angiotensin-converting enzyme (ACE) inhibitors, angiotensin receptor blockers, or beta blockers may be determined by concurrent conditions (e.g., calcium channel blockers may be useful for hypertensive children with migraines; ACE inhibitors or angiotensin receptor blockers for children with diabetes or renal disease). Ongoing therapy should include monitoring for end-organ damage, appropriate laboratory values, and continued emphasis on the need for non-pharmacologic measures (Falkner, Lurbe, & Schaefer, 2010).

PROTOTYPE DRUG | Verapamil (Calan, Isoptin, Verelan)

Classification: Therapeutic: Antihypertensive, antianginal, antidysrhythmic
Pharmacologic: Calcium channel blocker; phenylalkylamine type

Therapeutic Effects and Uses: Verapamil was the first CCB approved by the FDA in 1981. The drug is a class IV antidysrhythmic (see Chapter 37) because it slows myocardial conduction velocity, especially through the AV node, and stabilizes certain types of abnormal heart rhythms. In the vasculature, calcium channel blockade causes vasodilation of arterioles, which lowers blood pressure and reduces cardiac workload. Verapamil also dilates the coronary arteries, an action that is important when the drug is used to treat angina. It is approved to treat variant, unstable, and chronic angina (see Chapter 35). Off-label indications include migraine prophylaxis and acute mania.

Verapamil is available in PO, oral extended release, and IV formulations. Covera-HS is a unique formulation that delays the release of verapamil until 4 to 5 hours after ingestion and then releases it slowly. Covera-HS should be taken at night so that the drug is in the bloodstream on awakening. The inert shell of the drug is sometimes found in the stool. The therapeutic serum level of verapamil is 0.08 to 0.3 mcg/mL. Tarka is a fixed-dose combination of verapamil with trandolapril for HTN.

Mechanism of Action: Verapamil acts by inhibiting the flow of calcium ions into both cardiac muscle cells and vascular smooth muscle cells. Blocking calcium entry causes vasodilation of peripheral arterioles and reduced contractility of the myocardium.

Pharmacokinetics:

Route(s)	PO and IV
Absorption	Well absorbed
Distribution	Widely distributed; crosses the placenta; secreted in breast milk
Primary metabolism	Hepatic; extensive first-pass metabolism
Primary excretion	Renal (70%) with small amounts in feces (16%)
Onset of action	PO: 1–2 h; IV: 1–5 min
Duration of action	PO: 3–7 h (extended release: 24 h); IV: 2 h
	Half-life: 2–8 h

Adverse Effects: Most adverse effects of verapamil are extensions of its actions on the cardiovascular system. Peripheral vasodilation may cause flushed skin, headache, dizziness, lightheadedness, and peripheral edema. High doses and IV administration may cause serious hypotension. The most serious adverse effects of verapamil are cardiac related, including worsening of HF, bradycardia, reflex tachycardia, and AV block. Constipation is relatively common. Central nervous system (CNS) effects such as confusion, drowsiness, and mood changes have been reported, though they are uncommon. Elevated hepatic enzymes and rare cases of liver damage have been reported.

Contraindications/Precautions: Verapamil is contraindicated in patients with AV heart block, sick sinus syndrome, severe hypotension, bleeding aneurysm, or those undergoing intracranial surgery. Because verapamil can cause bradycardia and pulmonary edema, patients with HF should be carefully monitored, especially when the drug is administered IV. The drug should be used with caution in patients with renal or hepatic impairment because this can delay clearance of verapamil and its metabolites.

Drug Interactions: Verapamil is metabolized by hepatic P450 enzymes and exhibits many drug–drug interactions. Verapamil has the ability to elevate blood levels of digoxin. Because digoxin and verapamil both slow conduction through the AV node, their concurrent use must be carefully monitored to avoid bradycardia. Use with other antihypertensive drugs, including ACE inhibitors or beta-adrenergic blockers, may cause additive hypotension or bradycardia. Concurrent administration of verapamil with buspirone can triple the plasma concentration of buspirone. Verapamil should not be administered with statins because the risk of myopathy increases significantly. Carbamazepine serum concentration may increase during concurrent therapy with verapamil, causing adverse effects such as diplopia, ataxia, or dizziness. Use with alcohol can raise serum levels of the CCB and prolong its effects. **Herbal/Food**: Grapefruit juice may increase verapamil levels. Use with caution with herbal supplements, such as hawthorn, which may have additive hypotensive effects. High doses of calcium supplements may diminish the effects of CCBs and should not be used without consulting the health care provider.

Pregnancy: Category C.

Treatment of Overdose: Treatment of overdose is aimed at reversing hypotension with vasopressors such as dopamine or norepinephrine. Atropine, levarterenol, or isoproterenol may be administered to treat bradycardia. Calcium salts may be administered to increase calcium available to the myocardium and arterioles.

Nursing Responsibilities: Key nursing implications for patients receiving verapamil are included in the Nursing Practice Application for Patients Receiving Pharmacotherapy with Calcium Channel Blockers.

Drugs Similar to Verapamil (Calan, Isoptin, Verelan)

The only other nondihydropyridine is diltiazem. A third drug in this class, bepridil (Vascor), is no longer available in the United States because it was found to produce dysrhythmias.

Diltiazem (Cardizem, Dilacor, Taztia XT, Tiazac): Like other nondihydropyridines, diltiazem has the ability to relax both coronary and peripheral blood vessels. Approved in 1982, diltiazem reduces heart rate, blood pressure, and cardiac workload. The drug slows electrical conduction through the AV node. It is useful in the treatment of atrial dysrhythmias and HTN as well as stable and vasospastic angina. Migraine prophylaxis is an off-label indication. When given as extended release capsules (Cardizem LA, Dilacor XR, Taztia XT), it is administered once daily. An IV formulation is available to treat atrial fibrillation. The drug is well tolerated and serious adverse effects are uncommon and similar to those of verapamil. Like verapamil, diltiazem should be used cautiously in patients with bradycardia, AV block, HF, or serious hypotension.

There are several formulations of diltiazem and not all are approved for the same indications (see Table 30.1). The doses among the forms are not always equivalent. Even more confusing is that generics are labeled as "diltiazem extended release," which does not tell the prescriber which brand name product the generic is equivalent to. Caution must always be used when administering this drug to ensure that the patient is receiving the correct dose and form of diltiazem.

CONNECTIONS Evidence-Based Practice

◖ Calcium Channel Blockers and Heart Failure

Clinical Question

Do calcium channel blockers increase the risk of heart failure in patients with hypertension?

Evidence

CCBs are a commonly used treatment for HTN. Because they exert negative inotropic effects, they may cause or worsen HF in susceptible patients. In a meta-analysis of clinically randomized studies of over 150,000 patients performed by Shibata and colleagues (2010), a higher incidence of HF was found in patients taking CCBs, regardless of whether MI was also present. Patients with diabetes taking CCBs were found to have the highest incidence with a higher risk also observed in patients with isolated systolic HTN. When comparing CCBs to other antihypertensive medications, CCBs were found to have the highest incidence of HF over ACE inhibitors, angiotensin receptor blockers, beta blockers, and diuretics. There was no significant difference noted whether dihydropyridines or nondihydropyridine CCBs were used.

Implications

CCBs are widely used for treatment and control of HTN but are not without risks. Because of the negative inotropic effects on the myocardium, CCBs should be used with extreme caution in patients with a history of HF, and in patients with diabetes or isolated systolic HTN. Patients taking CCBs should be monitored frequently for the development of HF, and evaluation of ventricular function before starting therapy with CCBs may be advised.

Critical Thinking Questions

1. What are the signs and symptoms of HF?
2. What should the nurse teach the patient if a CCB is prescribed?

See Answers to Critical Thinking Questions on student resource website.

Patients Receiving Pharmacotherapy with Calcium Channel Blockers

Assessment	Potential Nursing Diagnoses*
Baseline assessment prior to administration: • Obtain a complete health history including cardiovascular (MI or HF), musculoskeletal (preexisting conditions that might result in fatigue, weakness, muscle or joint pain), and the possibility of pregnancy. Obtain a drug history including allergies, current prescription and OTC drugs, herbal preparations, and alcohol use. Be alert to possible drug interactions. • Evaluate appropriate laboratory findings: electrolytes, especially potassium level, liver function studies, and lipid profiles. • Obtain baseline weight, vital signs (especially blood pressure and pulse), breath sounds, and cardiac monitoring (e.g., ECG, cardiac output) if appropriate. Assess for location, character, and amount of edema, if present. • Assess the patient's ability to receive and understand instructions. Include the family or caregiver as needed.	• *Decreased Cardiac Output* • *Fatigue* • *Activity Intolerance* • *Deficient Knowledge* (Drug Therapy) • *Risk for Decreased Cardiac Tissue Perfusion*, related to adverse drug effects • *Risk for Falls*, related to adverse effects • *Risk for Injury*, related to hypotension, dizziness associated with adverse drug effects
Assessment throughout administration: • Assess for desired therapeutic effects (e.g., lowered blood pressure within established limits; lessened or absent angina and dysrhythmias if present). • Continue periodic monitoring of electrolytes, especially potassium. • Assess for adverse effects: nausea, headache, constipation, musculoskeletal fatigue or weakness, flushing, lightheadedness or dizziness, sexual dysfunction, or impotence. Myalgia, arthralgia, peripheral edema, facial edema, significant constipation, inability to maintain activities of daily living (ADLs) due to musculoskeletal weakness or pain, or unexplained numbness or tingling of extremities should be reported immediately to the health care provider.	

Implementation

Interventions and (Rationales)	Patient-Centered Care
Ensuring therapeutic effects: • Continue frequent assessments as above for therapeutic effects dependent on the reason the drug therapy is given. (Blood pressure and pulse should be within normal limits or within parameters set by the health care provider. If the drug is given for angina or dysrhythmias, significant improvement in reports of pain, palpitations, or ECG demonstrates improvement.)	• Teach the patient, family, or caregiver how to monitor pulse and blood pressure. Ensure proper use and functioning of any home equipment obtained.
• Encourage appropriate lifestyle changes: lowered fat intake, increased exercise, limited alcohol intake, and smoking cessation. Provide for dietitian consultation as needed. (Healthy lifestyle changes will support and minimize the need for drug therapy.)	• Encourage the patient, family, or caregiver to adopt a healthy lifestyle of low-fat food choices, increased exercise, decreased alcohol consumption, and smoking cessation.
Minimizing adverse effects: • Continue to monitor vital signs. Take the blood pressure lying, sitting, and standing to detect orthostatic hypotension. **Lifespan:** Be particularly cautious with older adults who are at increased risk for hypotension. Ensure patient safety. (CCBs cause vasodilation, resulting in lowered blood pressure. Orthostatic hypotension may increase the risk of falls and injury. **Diverse Patients:** Because CCBs metabolize through the P450 system pathways, monitor ethnically diverse patients to ensure optimal therapeutic effects and minimize adverse effects.)	• Teach the patient to rise from lying or sitting to standing slowly to avoid dizziness or falls. If dizziness occurs, the patient should sit or lie down and not attempt to stand or walk, until the sensation passes. • Instruct the patient to stop taking the medication if the blood pressure is 90/60 mmHg or below, or per parameters set by the health care provider, and promptly notify the provider. • Instruct the patient to call for assistance prior to getting out of bed or attempting to walk alone, and to avoid driving or other activities requiring mental alertness or physical coordination until the effects of the drug are known.
• Continue to monitor periodic electrolyte levels, especially potassium, ECG as appropriate, and hepatic and renal function laboratory values. (Hypokalemia may increase the risk for dysrhythmias.)	• Instruct the patient on the need to return periodically for laboratory work or ECGs. • Advise the patient to carry a wallet identification card or wear medical identification jewelry indicating CCB therapy. • **Lifespan:** The drug should not be taken during pregnancy, if pregnancy is suspected, or while breast-feeding.
• Weigh the patient daily and report weight gain or loss of 1 kg (2 lb) or more in a 24-h period or 2 kg (5 lb) per week. (Daily weight is an accurate measure of fluid status and takes into account intake, output, and insensible losses. Weight gain or edema may signal blood pressure has lowered too quickly, stimulating renin release or is an adverse effect.)	• Have the patient weigh self daily, ideally at the same time of day, and record weight along with blood pressure and pulse measurements. Have the patient report weight loss or gain of more than 1 kg (2 lb) in a 24-h period.

CONNECTIONS: NURSING PRACTICE APPLICATION (continued)

• Observe for paradoxical increase in chest pain or angina symptoms. (Severe hypotension may cause this and may indicate blood pressure has decreased too quickly or too substantially.)	• Instruct the patient to report chest pain or other angina-like symptoms, especially if increasing.
• Monitor for signs of HF (e.g., increasing dyspnea or postural nocturnal dyspnea, rales or crackles in the lungs, and frothy pink-tinged sputum). (CCBs are negative inotropes and can decrease myocardial contractility, increasing the risk of, or precipitating HF.)	• Instruct the patient to immediately report any severe shortness of breath, frothy sputum, profound fatigue, or swelling of extremities because they are possible signs of HF.
• Observe for hypersensitivity reaction or angioedema, especially of the facial area.	• Instruct the patient to immediately seek medical attention for difficulty breathing, throat tightness, hives or rash, muscle cramps, or tremors. Promptly report any angioedema around the facial area.
• Observe for constipation. (CCBs may cause constipation due to decreased peristalsis. **Lifespan:** The older adult is at increased risk of constipation due to slowed peristalsis.)	• Instruct the patient to increase fluid and fiber intake to facilitate stool passage. • If constipation persists, consider use of stool softener or laxative (such as MiraLAX) or as recommended by the health care provider.
• Assess the condition of gums and oral hygiene measures. (While uncommon, CCBs may cause gingival hyperplasia, increasing the risk of oral infections.)	• Instruct the patient to maintain excellent oral hygiene and keep regularly scheduled dental appointments.
• Monitor patient diet and medications for concurrent use of alcohol, grapefruit or grapefruit juice, herbal supplements, and alternative medications. (Alcohol and melatonin use may increase risk for hypotension, drowsiness, and dizziness. Grapefruit juice may increase drug levels with increased adverse effects.)	• Provide the patient with information on products to avoid while taking CCBs, specific to the drug ordered.
Patient understanding of drug therapy: • Use opportunities during administration of medications and during assessments to discuss the rationale for drug therapy, desired therapeutic outcomes, commonly observed adverse effects, parameters for when to call the health care provider, and any necessary monitoring or precautions. (Using time during nursing care helps to optimize and reinforce key teaching areas.)	• The patient, family, or caregiver should be able to state the reason for the drug, appropriate dose and scheduling, what adverse effects to observe for and when to report them, and the anticipated length of medication therapy.
Patient self-administration of drug therapy: • When administering the medication, instruct the patient, family, or caregiver in proper self-administration of the drug. (Utilizing time during nurse-administration of these drugs helps to reinforce teaching.)	• The patient, family, or caregiver is able to discuss appropriate dosing and administration needs.

*Nursing Diagnoses—Definitions and Classification 2015–2017. Copyright © 2014, 1994–2014 by NANDA International. Used by arrangement with John Wiley & Sons Limited.

CHAPTER
30   Understanding the Chapter

Key Concepts Summary

30.1 Calcium channels facilitate contraction in cardiac and smooth muscles.

30.2 The calcium channel consists of multiple subunits and is present in many tissues.

30.3 Blocking calcium channels has significant physiological effects on the heart and vascular smooth muscle.

30.4 Calcium channel blockers are classified by their chemical structures as dihydropyridines or nondihydropyridines.

30.5 The dihydropyridines are selective for vascular smooth muscle and are used to treat hypertension and angina pectoris.

30.6 The nondihydropyridines act on both vascular smooth muscle and the myocardium.

Case Study: Making the Patient Connection

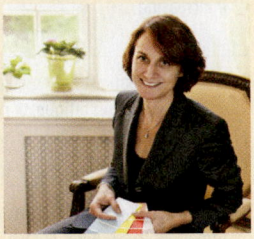

Remember the patient "Elise Freeman" at the beginning of the chapter? Now read the remainder of the case study. Based on the information presented within this chapter, respond to the critical thinking questions that follow.

Elise Freeman, a 40-year-old interior designer, had no idea that her blood pressure was elevated. One day at the shopping mall she saw an automatic blood pressure machine and thought she would try it. She could hardly believe the machine's reading when it revealed her blood pressure was 150/92 mmHg. She was certain that there must be something wrong with the machine. After all, she felt fine. In fact, she is rarely ill and never misses work due to illness.

Just to be certain, Elise made an appointment with her doctor for a checkup. During her first clinic visit, her blood pressure was 146/90 mmHg, heart rate was 78 beats/min, respiratory rate was 16 breaths/min, and temperature was 36.8°C (98.2°F). Elise was instructed on lifestyle modifications for HTN and

told to return to the clinic in 1 month. The next month, Elise's blood pressure remained elevated. Multiple diagnostic studies, which included an ECG and blood chemistry levels, were completed. Her health care provider prescribed amlodipine (Norvasc) and instructed her to return in 1 week.

All of this has caused Elise to be concerned and worried about her health. She has accessed the Internet to learn as much about HTN as possible and amlodipine in particular. With all the information about high blood pressure, she is even more confused and anxious.

Critical Thinking Questions

1. Describe how calcium channel blockers control HTN.

2. Elise asks you, the nurse, if calcium channel blockers can cure HTN. How would you respond?

3. What adverse effects are associated with calcium channel blockers?

See Answers to Critical Thinking Questions on student resource website.

Additional Case Study

Mabel Hillside was prescribed amlodipine (Norvasc) 5 mg once daily. However, Mabel's health insurance does not cover prescription drug costs and she will be required to self-pay for the drug. As you are talking with this patient, she says, "Why should I take this medicine? After all, I feel just fine and it is very expensive. Plus I keep forgetting to take it."

1. How would you respond to Mabel's remark about feeling "just fine"?

2. What adverse effects related to amlodipine might cause the patient to stop taking the medication?

3. List strategies that Mabel can use to remember to take her hypertensive medication.

See Answers to Additional Case Study on student resource website.

Chapter Review

1 Nifedipine (Procardia) is being initiated for a patient with elevated blood pressure. What health teaching would be most appropriate? The patient should:

1. Weigh daily at the same time each day.
2. Avoid crowds while taking this medication.
3. Increase intake of calcium-containing foods.
4. Take this medication only when feeling that blood pressure is elevated.

2 A patient is receiving felodipine for hypertension. In the care plan the nurse includes the need to monitor the patient for which adverse effect?

1. Rash and chills
2. Increased urinary output
3. Weight loss
4. Reflex tachycardia

3 A patient with primary hypertension has started therapy with verapamil (Calan). The nurse performs what important intervention during the initial course of this treatment?

1. Uses an electric razor to shave the patient
2. Monitors the patient for increased thrombocyte levels
3. Administers the medication only during waking hours
4. Measures intake and output ratio and daily weight

4 The nurse determines that the patient understands an important principle in self-administration of nifedipine (Procardia) when the patient makes which statement?

1. "The use of antacids when taking the medication will enhance absorption."
2. "Grapefruit juice may enhance the absorption of nifedipine."
3. "If I miss a dose, I should take two nifedipine capsules when I remember."
4. "This drug will make my birth control pills ineffective."

5 What health teaching should the nurse provide for a patient receiving diltiazem (Cardizem)? Select all that apply.

1. Avoid driving or performing other activities requiring mental alertness until the effects of the drug are known.

2. Maintain adequate fluid and fiber intake to facilitate stool passage.

3. Report weight gain of 2 kg per week.

4. Rise slowly from prolonged periods of sitting or lying down.

5. Immediately stop taking the medication if sexual dysfunction is noted.

6 A health care provider has ordered nifedipine (Procardia XL) for each of these patients. A nurse will most closely monitor which patient for drug-related problems?

1. A patient who is admitted for an appendectomy in the morning

2. A patient who is receiving renal dialysis three times per week

3. A patient who develops pulmonary edema in the intensive care unit

4. A patient who receives psychotropic drugs for bipolar disease

See Answers to Chapter Review in Appendix A.

References

Expert Panel on Integrated Guidelines for Cardiovascular Health and Risk Reduction in Children and Adolescents. (2011). Expert panel on integrated guidelines for cardiovascular health and risk reduction in children and adolescents: Summary report. *Pediatrics, 128*(Suppl. 5), S213–S256. doi:10.1542/peds.2009-2107C

Falkner, B., Lurbe, E., & Schaefer, F. (2010). High blood pressure in children: Clinical health policy implications. *Journal of Clinical Hypertension, 12*(4), 261–276. doi:10.1111/j.1751-7176.2009.00245.x

Mejia, L. M. (2012). *Drug-induced gingival hyperplasia*. Retrieved from http://emedicine.medscape.com/article/1076264-overview

Moyer, V. A. (2013). Screening for primary hypertension in children and adolescents: U.S. Preventive Services Task Force recommendation statement. *Annals of Internal Medicine, 159*, 613–619. doi:10.7326/0003-4819-159-9-201311050-00725

Riley, M., & Bluhm, B. (2012). High blood pressure in children and adolescents. *American Family Physician, 85*, 693–700.

Shibata, M. C., Leon, H., Chatterley, T., Dorgan, M., & Vandermeer, B. (2010). Do calcium channel blockers increase the diagnosis of heart failure in patients with hypertension? *American Journal of Cardiology, 106*, 228–235. doi:10.1016/j.amjcard.2010.02.031

Selected Bibliography

Cain, S. M., & Snutch, T. P. (2011). Voltage-gated calcium channels and disease. *BioFactors, 37*, 197–205. doi:10.1002/biof.158

Catterall, W. A. (2011). Voltage-gated calcium channels. *Cold Spring Harbor Perspectives in Biology, 3*(8). doi:10.1101/cshperspect.a003947

Chrysant, S. G. (2010). The role of angiotensin receptor blocker and calcium channel blocker combination therapy in treating hypertension: Focus on recent studies. *American Journal of Cardiovascular Drugs, 10*, 315–320. doi:10.2165/11538850-000000000-00000

Elliott, W. J., & Ram, C. V. S. (2011). Calcium channel blockers. *The Journal of Clinical Hypertension, 13*, 687–689. doi:10.1111/j.1751-7176.2011.00513.x

Herdman, T. H., & Kamitsuru, S. (Eds.). (2014). *NANDA International nursing diagnoses: Definitions and classification, 2015-2017*. Oxford, United Kingdom: Wiley-Blackwell.

Izzo, J. L. (2010). Are there benefits of antihypertensive therapy beyond blood pressure lowering? *Current Hypertension Reports, 12*, 440–447. doi:10.1007/s11906-010-0160-0

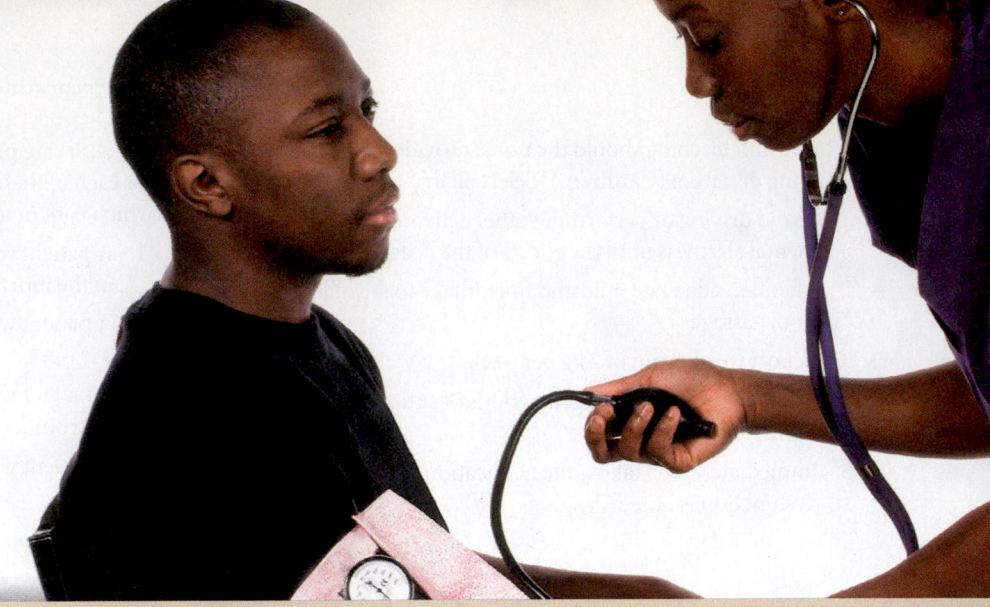

"When I saw my doctor, she said my blood pressure was still high. I'm taking my medicine as directed. So what's the problem?"

Patient "Carlos Avaya"

CHAPTER

31

Drugs Affecting the Renin-Angiotensin-Aldosterone System

LEARNING OUTCOMES

After reading this chapter, the student should be able to:

1. Illustrate the steps in the renin-angiotensin-aldosterone pathway.
2. Identify the primary physiological factors that control renin secretion.
3. Explain the two primary functions of angiotensin-converting enzyme.
4. Describe multiple mechanisms by which angiotensin II raises blood pressure.
5. Explain how the actions of aldosterone can lead to high blood pressure.
6. Identify the specific steps in the renin-angiotensin-aldosterone system that can be blocked by medications.
7. For each of the classes shown in the chapter outline, identify the prototype and representative drugs and explain the mechanism(s) of drug action, primary indications, contraindications, significant drug interactions, pregnancy category, and important adverse effects.
8. Apply the nursing process to care for patients receiving pharmacotherapy with angiotensin-converting enzyme inhibitors and angiotensin receptor blockers.

CHAPTER OUTLINE

▶ **Components of the Renin-Angiotensin-Aldosterone System**

▶ **Physiological Actions of the Renin-Angiotensin-Aldosterone System**

▶ **Drugs Affecting the Renin-Angiotensin-Aldosterone System**

Angiotensin-Converting Enzyme Inhibitors

PROTOTYPE Lisinopril (Prinivil, Zestril), *p. 491*

Angiotensin II Receptor Blockers

PROTOTYPE Losartan (Cozaar), *p. 493*

Aldosterone Antagonists

The **renin-angiotensin-aldosterone system (RAAS)** is a key homeostatic mechanism controlling blood pressure and fluid balance. The RAAS is presented early in the study of cardiovascular pharmacology because the drugs affecting this pathway are frequently used to treat hypertension (HTN) and heart failure (HF). This chapter examines components of the RAAS and describes how drugs affecting this system are used for therapeutic benefit.

Components of the Renin-Angiotensin-Aldosterone System

31.1 The formation of angiotensin II requires two enzymatic steps.

In the mid-1900s, scientists discovered a peptide circulating in the blood that caused profound vasoconstriction. Named angiotensin (*angio* = blood vessel; *tensin* = pressure), high levels of this substance were found in people with HTN. Thus began the search for components of what is now called the renin-angiotensin-aldosterone system.

We now know that there are several forms of angiotensin. **Angiotensin II** is the vasopressor substance originally isolated by scientists in the 1900s. The formation of angiotensin II requires two key enzymatic steps, and an understanding of these steps is critical to learning the pharmacology of drugs affecting the RAAS. The RAAS is illustrated in Figure 31.1.

Step 1—Formation of angiotensin I: **Angiotensinogen** is a protein synthesized by the liver that is continuously circulating in the bloodstream. In the blood, angiotensinogen is split by the enzyme renin to form **angiotensin I**. Neither angiotensinogen nor angiotensin I has any significant physiological actions; they simply serve as precursors to angiotensin II.

Step 2—Formation of angiotensin II: Angiotensin I travels through the circulation until it encounters angiotensin-converting enzyme (ACE), which cleaves two amino acids to form angiotensin II. ACE is located on the membrane surface of the blood vessel endothelium. Because the lung possesses such an extensive number of capillaries, it is the primary organ responsible for converting angiotensin I to angiotensin II. Angiotensin II is one of the most potent natural vasoconstrictors known; it is approximately 40 times more potent at raising blood pressure than norepinephrine.

31.2 Renin secretion is controlled by the juxtaglomerular cells of the kidney and the sympathetic nervous system.

Because renin is responsible for the first step in the RAAS pathway, it is a major factor in determining the amount of angiotensin II produced in the body. Therefore, factors affecting the secretion of renin are important to understanding the pharmacotherapy associated with this system.

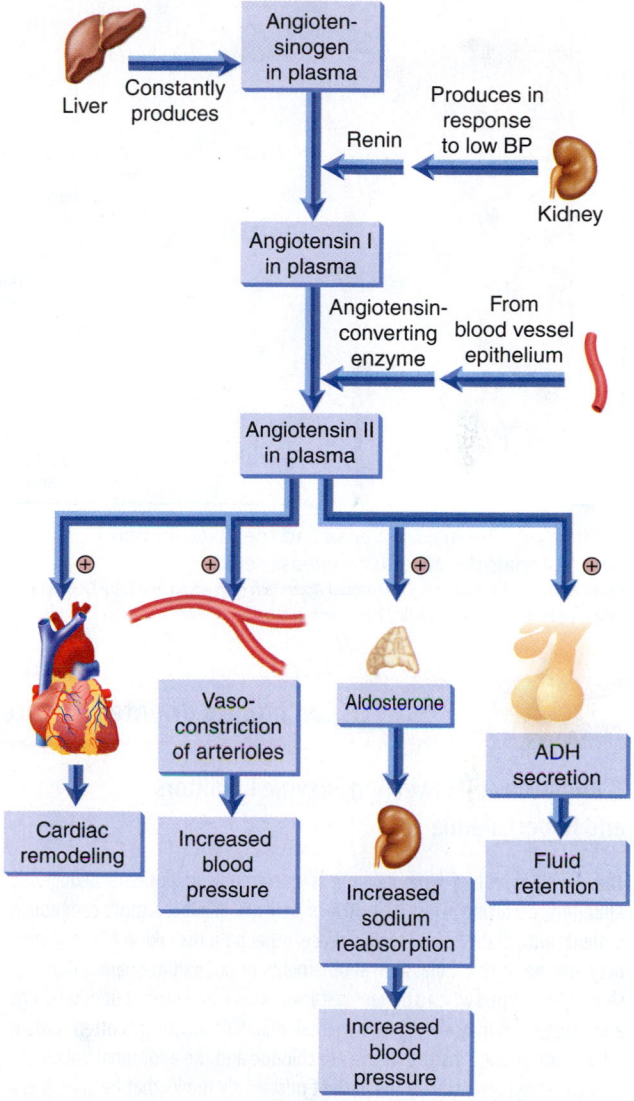

Figure 31.1 The renin-angiotensin-aldosterone pathway.

Renin is an enzyme that is synthesized, stored, and secreted by specialized cells in the kidney known as **juxtaglomerular (JG) cells** (also called granular cells). Found in the afferent arteriole that supplies blood to the glomerulus, JG cells are specialized smooth muscle cells that act as pressure sensors. As blood pressure falls, there is less pressure on the JG cells, which respond by releasing renin to the circulation. The increase in renin ultimately leads to larger amounts of circulating angiotensin II, which returns blood pressure to normal. The release of renin is caused by factors that lower blood pressure, such as a loss of blood volume due to dehydration or hemorrhage. Through negative feedback, increased blood pressure is sensed by the JG cells, which then turn off renin secretion.

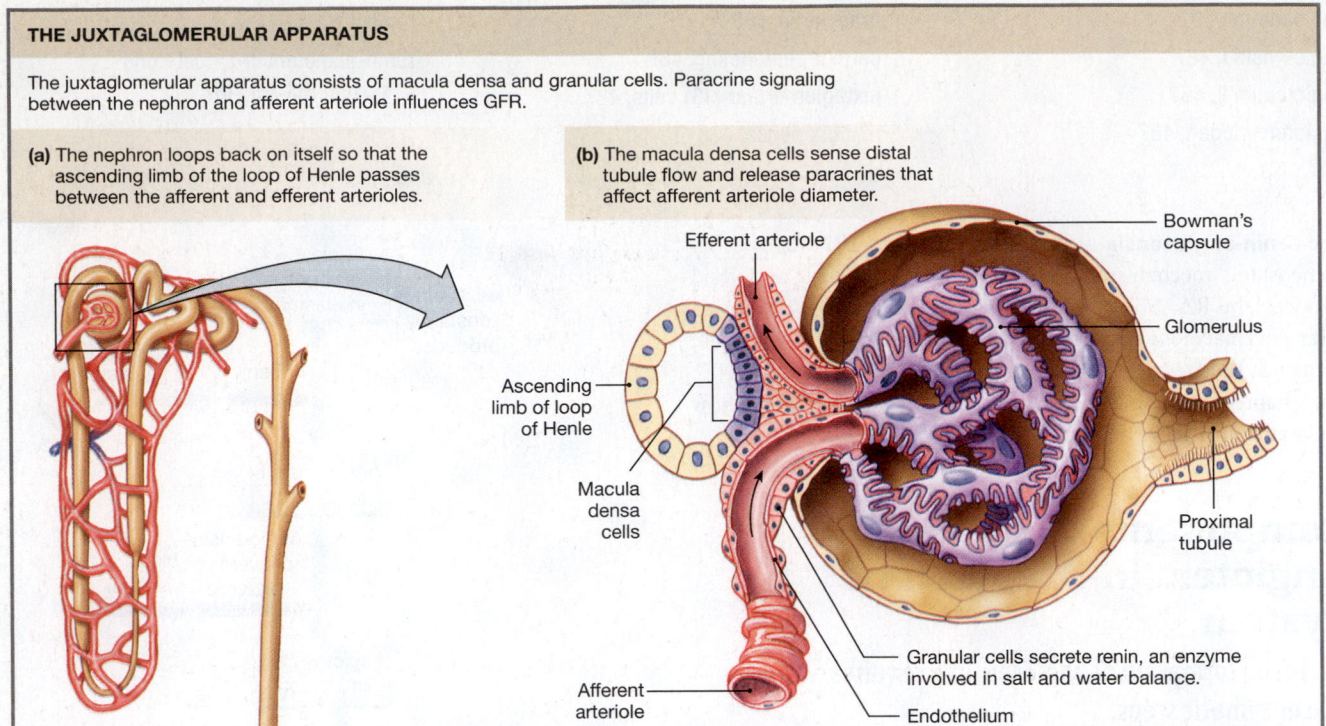

THE JUXTAGLOMERULAR APPARATUS

The juxtaglomerular apparatus consists of macula densa and granular cells. Paracrine signaling between the nephron and afferent arteriole influences GFR.

(a) The nephron loops back on itself so that the ascending limb of the loop of Henle passes between the afferent and efferent arterioles.

(b) The macula densa cells sense distal tubule flow and release paracrines that affect afferent arteriole diameter.

Efferent arteriole

Bowman's capsule

Glomerulus

Ascending limb of loop of Henle

Macula densa cells

Proximal tubule

Granular cells secrete renin, an enzyme involved in salt and water balance.

Afferent arteriole

Endothelium

Figure 31.2 The macula densa and the juxtaglomerular (JG) cells. Osmoreceptors in the macula densa sense low sodium levels, which signals the JG cells to release renin.
From *Human Physiology: An Integrated Approach* (6th ed., p. 639), by D. U. Silverthorn, © 2013. Reprinted and electronically reproduced by permission of Pearson Education, Inc., Upper Saddle River, New Jersey.

◀ **Angiotensin-Converting Enzyme Inhibitors and Hyperkalemia**

The development of hyperkalemia is uncommon in patients taking ACE inhibitors, occurring in less than 30% of patients. While it is more common in patients with diabetes and renal disease, other patients taking ACE inhibitors may also be at risk. Potassium supplements or potassium-sparing diuretics should be stopped when a patient is started on ACE inhibitors, but other drugs and substances may also cause hyperkalemia. Salt substitutes often contain potassium chloride instead of sodium chloride and the additional potassium may cause hyperkalemia if the patient mistakenly thinks that because it is a salt substitute, it can be used liberally as a healthy replacement to table salt.

Other drugs that have been known to increase the risk of hyperkalemia when given concurrently with ACE inhibitors include NSAIDs, beta blockers, heparin, ketoconazole, trimethoprim, pentamidine, and immunosuppressants such as cyclosporine and tacrolimus. In addition to diabetes or renal disease, severe HF, volume depletion, or advanced age also place the patient at risk. Prior to starting ACE inhibitors, a thorough personal and drug history should be taken to screen for any condition or medication that may lead to hyperkalemia development. Frequent testing for potassium levels may be necessary if the patient is taking concurrent medications that raise the risk for hyperkalemia. The patient should be educated to avoid salt substitutes that contain potassium chloride.

Several other important factors control the release of renin. Adjacent to the JG cells in the distal convoluted tubule of the nephron is a specialized cluster of cells called the macula densa. The macula densa is in a perfect location to sense the flow rate and the concentration of sodium ions (osmolality) in the urinary filtrate.

As blood pressure falls, blood flow through the kidney diminishes and the flow rate of renal tubular filtrate slows. The **macula densa** recognizes the decreased flow rate (and less sodium) and sends a chemical message to the JG cells to release more renin. The renin release forms more angiotensin II and blood pressure rises.

Anatomically, the JG cells and the macula densa are in proximity, as shown in Figure 31.2. The JG cells and the macula densa are sometimes considered a single anatomic unit called the juxtaglomerular complex.

CONNECTION Checkpoint 31.1

Substances that lower blood pressure may trigger reflex tachycardia. From what you learned in Chapter 28, explain the mechanism involved in this reflex. *See Answer to Connection Checkpoint 31.1 on student resource website.*

A third mechanism for controlling the release of renin is more direct: activation of the sympathetic nervous system. JG cells contain beta₁-adrenergic receptors, which are activated by the classic fight-or-flight response of the sympathetic nervous system (see Chapter 12). The release of renin helps to raise blood pressure when dealing with a stressful or harmful situation.

To summarize, factors that promote the release of renin by JG cells will raise blood pressure. The three primary factors causing an increase are decreased pressure in blood flowing through the kidney, decreased tubular flow rate (or fewer sodium ions) sensed by the macula densa, and activation of the sympathetic nervous system. Conversely, the factors that decrease renin secretion lower blood pressure. These factors are illustrated in Figure 31.3.

Increasing renin secretion will not always cause an increase in blood pressure. Remember that RAAS is a two-step pathway, and both steps are essential to produce a physiological response. Section 31.3 examines this second step.

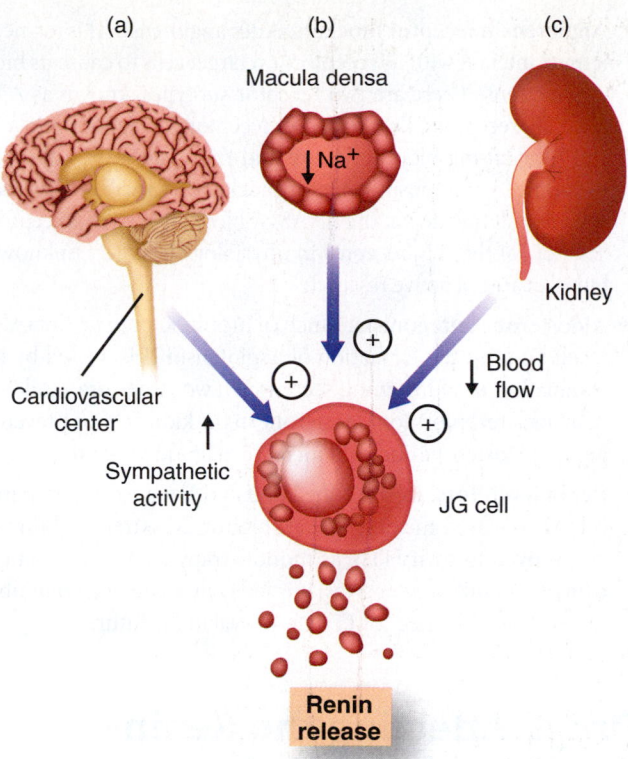

(a) (b) (c)

Macula densa

↓Na⁺

Kidney

Cardiovascular center

↑ Sympathetic activity

+

+

+

+

↓ Blood flow

JG cell

Renin release

Figure 31.3 Overview of factors affecting renin release: (a) activation of the sympathetic nervous system; (b) low osmolarity in the macula densa; (c) low blood flow through the kidney.

CONNECTION Checkpoint 31.2

From what you learned in Chapter 12, other than JG cells, in what organ are beta₁-adrenergic receptors predominantly located? What is the response of that organ when these receptors are activated? *See Answer to Connection Checkpoint 31.2 on student resource website.*

31.3 Angiotensin-converting enzyme is responsible for the formation of angiotensin II.

Once angiotensin I is formed, its conversion to angiotensin II by ACE is almost instantaneous. This is because ACE lies on the membranes of blood vessels and has immediate access to angiotensin I as soon as it is formed. A single pass of the blood through lung capillaries converts most of the circulating angiotensin I to angiotensin II.

In addition to its role in the formation of angiotensin II, ACE has a second function important to homeostasis and pharmacotherapy. ACE is one of several enzymes that break down **bradykinin**, a natural mediator of inflammation and pain. Bradykinin has many of the same effects as histamine (see Chapter 44), including increasing arteriolar vasodilation and vascular permeability, and is likely responsible for some of the adverse effects of the ACE inhibitor medications. When referring to its actions on bradykinin, ACE is sometimes called kininase II; *kininase* is the general term for an enzyme that breaks down kinins. ACE and kininase II refer to the identical enzyme.

Pharmacologically, ACE is an important enzyme in the RAAS because it serves as a target molecule for drugs in the ACE inhibitor class of medications. Inhibition of ACE will prevent the formation of angiotensin II, thus interrupting the RAAS pathway.

These medications also inhibit kininase II, thus preventing the breakdown of bradykinin. Accumulation of bradykinin in certain tissues can cause several adverse effects of ACE inhibitors, such as angioedema and cough.

Physiological Actions of the Renin-Angiotensin-Aldosterone System

31.4 Angiotensin II has multiple effects on the cardiovascular system that raise blood pressure and affect cardiac function.

The final product of the two-step renin-angiotensin pathway is angiotensin II. Angiotensin II has several important physiological effects important to homeostasis and to pharmacotherapy.

Direct vasoconstriction: Angiotensin II acts directly on vascular smooth muscle to cause vasoconstriction and increased systemic blood pressure. This effect is rapid; formation of angiotensin II results in a nearly instantaneous increase in blood pressure. This vasopressor action of angiotensin II is much greater on arterioles compared to veins; arterioles serving the kidneys are especially sensitive to this vasopressor action.

Increased sympathetic nervous system activity: Angiotensin II activates the sympathetic nervous system by causing the release of norepinephrine from sympathetic nerve terminals. The adrenal medulla is also affected by angiotensin II, which responds by releasing additional epinephrine to the circulation. Furthermore, through largely unknown mechanisms, angiotensin II increases sympathetic outflow from the brain. All three of these actions increase peripheral resistance and raise blood pressure.

Alteration of cardiovascular structure: The long-term presence of angiotensin II can also cause hypertrophy of myocardial cells (myocytes) and promote collagen deposits in the cardiac matrix, essentially forming scar-like tissue in the heart. These changes are known as **cardiac remodeling**. The hypertrophy, fibrosis, and remodeling of cardiac structure have been correlated with increased morbidity and mortality associated with HF. In blood vessels, angiotensin II causes the release of multiple chemical mediators of atherosclerosis, accelerating the deposition of fatty plaque on the walls of the vessels. Increased plaque deposits lead to an increased risk for myocardial infarction (MI) and stroke.

CONNECTION Checkpoint 31.3

From what you learned in Chapter 28, what effect would you expect angiotensin II formation to have on cardiac output and afterload? *See Answer to Connection Checkpoint 31.3 on student resource website.*

Release of aldosterone and effects on the renal tubule: Angiotensin II has two primary effects on the kidney that promote an increase in blood pressure. First, angiotensin II has a direct effect on the nephron that increases Na⁺ and Cl⁻ reabsorption in the proximal tubule. Second, angiotensin II indirectly affects sodium reabsorption by stimulating the adrenal cortex to synthesize and secrete additional amounts of the hormone aldosterone. Aldosterone acts on the distal and collecting tubules of the nephron to increase Na⁺ reabsorption and K⁺ and H⁺ excretion.

The enhanced sodium reabsorption from both direct and indirect actions of angiotensin II causes the body to retain water, thus increasing blood volume and raising blood pressure. Aldosterone is a key component of the RAAS.

Unlike its immediate and direct effects on sympathetic nerves, the actions of angiotensin II on the kidney develop more slowly. This slow vasopressor response is believed to be responsible for producing a sustained elevation of blood pressure and a gradual decline of renal function.

Students often think of angiotensin II as a "bad actor" because it can create HTN and cause the damaging effects of cardiac remodeling. Remember, however, that the cardiovascular and renal effects of angiotensin II serve an essential homeostatic function. Should blood pressure fall, the increased synthesis and production of angiotensin II help return blood pressure to normal levels to maintain blood flow to vital organs. When the body is subjected to chronically elevated levels of angiotensin II, however, the once vital reflex pathway becomes a detriment to the body.

31.5 The renin-angiotensin-aldosterone pathway offers multiple points for drug intervention.

Having learned details of the different components in the short pathway leading from angiotensinogen to angiotensin II, the student should recognize several potential mechanisms by which drugs could intervene:

- **ACE inhibitors.** These are the largest and most important class of drugs modifying the RAAS. ACE inhibitors block the conversion of angiotensin I to angiotensin II.

- **Angiotensin receptor blockers.** After angiotensin II is formed, it must interact with its receptors on target cells to cause its biologic actions. There are two receptor subtypes, known as AT_1 and AT_2 receptors. Blocking AT_1 receptors prevents angiotensin from raising blood pressure and from causing cardiac remodeling. Angiotensin receptor blockers are medications that intervene at this step in the RAAS by blocking the AT_1 receptor. The role of the AT_2 receptor in physiology is largely unknown but is an area of active research.

- **Aldosterone antagonists.** Much of the blood pressure increase resulting from the formation of angiotensin II is caused by its stimulation of aldosterone secretion. Two drugs are available that block receptors for aldosterone in the kidney, thus preventing the aldosterone-induced increase in blood pressure.

- **Renin inhibitors.** In 2007, the Food and Drug Administration (FDA) approved the first renin inhibitor. Aliskiren (Tekturna) is approved to treat HTN as monotherapy or in combination with other antihypertensives. It is likely that other renin inhibitors will be submitted for FDA approval in the future.

Drugs Affecting the Renin-Angiotensin-Aldosterone System

31.6 ACE inhibitors are key drugs in the pharmacotherapy of hypertension and heart failure.

First detected in the venom of pit vipers in the 1960s, inhibitors of ACE have been approved for HTN since the 1980s. Since then drugs in this class have become first-line drugs in the treatment of HTN and HF. Doses for the ACE inhibitors are listed in Table 31.1.

ACE inhibitors block the conversion of angiotensin I to angiotensin II. The decline in angiotensin II levels causes blood pressure to decrease because there is less sympathetic activation and, thus, lower peripheral resistance. In addition, the decreased aldosterone secretion reduces blood volume, which also contributes to blood pressure reduction.

Research studies have clearly demonstrated that ACE inhibitors can slow the progression of HF and reduce mortality from this disease. This is likely due to both the reduction in systemic blood pressure and a reversal of the angiotensin II-induced structural changes in the heart. Because of their relative safety, they have replaced digoxin (Lanoxin) as the first-line drugs for the treatment of chronic HF. Indeed, unless specifically contraindicated, all patients with HF usually receive an ACE inhibitor, as discussed in Chapter 36.

Research has also indicated a clear benefit for administering ACE inhibitors to patients who have experienced a recent MI. If therapy is begun immediately after the infarction and continued for several weeks, these drugs lower the mortality associated with an acute MI. The mechanism by which these drugs improve the outcome following an acute MI involves reduced peripheral vascular resistance, improved perfusion, and a direct action on the myocardium that reduces the cardiac workload.

ACE inhibitors may also be prescribed as prophylaxis therapy in patients at high risk for an adverse cardiovascular event. ACE inhibitors can reduce the incidence of a stroke or MI in these

TABLE 31.1 ACE Inhibitors

Drug	Route and Adult Dose (Maximum Dose Where Indicated)	Adverse Effects
benazepril (Lotensin)	PO: 10–40 mg in one to two divided doses (max: 40 mg/day)	*Headache, dry cough, dizziness, orthostatic hypotension, rash*
captopril (Capoten)	PO: 6.25–25 mg tid (max: 450 mg/day)	
enalapril (Vasotec)	PO: 5–40 mg in one to two divided doses (max: 40 mg/day)	<u>Angioedema, acute renal failure, first-dose phenomenon, fetal toxicity</u>
fosinopril (Monopril)	PO: 5–40 mg once daily (max: 40 mg/day)	
lisinopril (Prinivil, Zestril)	PO: 5–10 mg daily (max: 80 mg/day)	
moexipril (Univasc)	PO: 7.5–30 mg once daily (max: 30 mg/day)	
perindopril (Aceon)	PO: 4 mg once daily (max: 16 mg/day for HTN; 4 mg/day for HF)	
quinapril (Accupril)	PO: 10–20 mg once daily (max: 80 mg/day)	
ramipril (Altace)	PO: 2.5–20 mg daily (max: 20 mg/day)	
trandolapril (Mavik)	PO: 1–4 mg once daily (max: 8 mg/day)	

Note: *Italics* indicate common adverse effects. <u>Underline</u> indicates serious adverse effects.

high-risk patients. They may also prevent or delay the progression of renal disease and retinopathy in patients with diabetes.

All ACE inhibitors have very similar indications and adverse effect profiles. All drugs in this class are approved to treat HTN, and a few are approved for HF and acute MI and for prophylaxis of cardiovascular disease. With the exception of enalaprilat, ACE inhibitors are administered orally (PO), and nearly all offer the convenience of once-daily dosing. Many of the ACE inhibitors are prodrugs, which are converted to active metabolites by enzymes in the liver. Most ACE inhibitors are excreted by the kidneys; thus dose reductions may be required in patients with significant renal impairment.

The low incidence of serious adverse effects is a major contributing factor to the widespread use of the ACE inhibitors. Orthostatic hypotension following the first few doses of the drug can be severe in patients who are on low-sodium diets or who have HF. Drug therapy is sometimes begun with very low doses and increased gradually to avoid orthostatic hypotension. Hyperkalemia may occur during ACE inhibitor therapy; however, this is predominantly a major concern only for patients with diabetes, those with renal impairment, and those who are taking potassium supplements or potassium-sparing diuretics. Persistent, dry cough is an annoying adverse effect that occurs in 5% to 20% of patients taking ACE inhibitors. This adverse effect is likely due to a buildup of bradykinin in the lungs. Drugs in this class have minimal or no effect on serum glucose or uric acid levels.

Though rare, the most serious adverse effect of ACE inhibitors is the development of **angioedema**, a rapid swelling of the throat, face, larynx, and tongue that can lead to airway obstruction and death. When it does occur, angioedema most often develops within a few hours after the first dose, although it may occur after several days of ACE inhibitor therapy. Accumulation of bradykinin is thought to be responsible. Treatment of angioedema is to discontinue the drug immediately and maintain the airway until the effects of the drug wear off.

All the ACE inhibitors carry a black box warning regarding the risk for major congenital defects if the drugs are taken during pregnancy. This risk for fetal kidney malformation is well documented for the second and third trimesters, which has resulted in a

pregnancy category D rating during these pregnancy periods. The risk for other congenital defects such as heart and neural tube defects during the first trimester is not as clear, causing some of the drugs to be rated category C during this period. Most health care providers will discontinue ACE inhibitors as soon as pregnancy is determined. Women with HTN should be advised not to discontinue these drugs during pregnancy without health care provider knowledge because HTN itself is a risk factor for congenital defects.

PharmFACT

ACE inhibitors are especially useful in patients with diabetes. Although these drugs do not directly lower blood glucose, they do increase the body's sensitivity to insulin by increasing insulin release and improving glucose uptake in peripheral tissues. Because of this action, ACE inhibitors are sometimes used off-label to prevent new-onset type 2 diabetes (Tocci et al., 2011).

PROTOTYPE DRUG | Lisinopril (Prinivil, Zestril)

Classification: Therapeutic: Antihypertensive
Pharmacologic: ACE inhibitor

Therapeutic Effects and Uses: Approved for the treatment of HF, HTN, and acute MI, lisinopril is one of the most frequently prescribed medications. Approved in 1987, it may be used as monotherapy or combined with other drugs: Fixed-dose combinations of lisinopril and hydrochlorothiazide (a diuretic) are marketed for HTN as Prinzide and Zestoretic. Unlike many drugs in this class, lisinopril is active itself; it is not a prodrug. Treatment of migraines is an off-label indication for lisinopril.

Although captopril was the first drug that was marketed in this class, lisinopril is more widely prescribed because it has a longer duration of action that allows for once-daily dosing. Like other ACE inhibitors, 2 to 3 weeks of therapy may be required to achieve maximum therapeutic outcomes.

Mechanism of Action: Lisinopril binds to and inhibits the action of ACE, thus preventing the conversion of angiotensin I to angiotensin II. The decrease in serum angiotensin II reduces aldosterone secretion, which results in less sodium and water retention. In patients with HTN, blood pressure is reduced with minimal effect on heart rate, stroke volume, or cardiac output.

Pharmacokinetics:

Route(s)	PO
Absorption	25–30% absorbed from the gastrointestinal (GI) tract
Distribution	Small amount crosses the blood–brain barrier; crosses the placenta; limited amounts are secreted in breast milk; not bound to plasma protein
Primary metabolism	Not metabolized
Primary excretion	Renal
Onset of action	1 h; peak effect: 6–8 h
Duration of action	24 h; half-life: 12 h

Adverse Effects: Lisinopril is well tolerated and adverse effects are uncommon and transient. The most common adverse effects are cough, headache, dizziness, orthostatic hypotension, and rash. Hyperkalemia occurs in about 2% to 5% of patients taking ACE inhibitors, although this usually resolves during therapy. Patients with HF or renal impairment or who are taking potassium supplements or potassium-sparing diuretics are at highest risk for hyperkalemia. Rare, though serious adverse effects include angioedema, agranulocytosis, and hepatotoxicity. **Black Box Warning**: Fetal injury and death may occur when ACE inhibitors are taken during pregnancy. When pregnancy is detected, they should be discontinued as soon as possible.

Contraindications/Precautions: Lisinopril should be used with extreme caution in patients with hyperkalemia because they may experience serious and even fatal dysrhythmias. Patients with a history of angioedema should not receive lisinopril. Caution should be used in treating patients with serious renal impairment: Dosage should be reduced. Lisinopril is contraindicated during pregnancy.

Drug Interactions: Indomethacin and other nonsteroidal anti-inflammatory drugs (NSAIDs) interact with lisinopril to decrease antihypertensive activity. The combination of lisinopril and NSAIDs may also worsen preexisting renal disease. Because of synergistic hypotensive action, concurrent therapy with diuretics and other antihypertensives such as ACE inhibitors should be carefully monitored. When taken with potassium supplements or potassium-sparing diuretics, hyperkalemia may result. Lisinopril may increase lithium levels and toxicity. **Herbal/Food**: Hawthorn should not be taken concurrently with lisinopril due to the possibility of additive hypotensive action.

Pregnancy: Categories C (first trimester) and D (second and third trimesters).

Treatment of Overdose: Overdose will cause hypotension, which may be treated with normal saline or a vasopressor. The drug may also be removed by hemodialysis.

Nursing Responsibilities: Key nursing implications for patients receiving lisinopril are included in the Nursing Practice Application for Patients Receiving Pharmacotherapy with Angiotensin-Converting Enzyme Inhibitors and Angiotensin Receptor Blockers.

Drugs Similar to Lisinopril (Prinivil, Zestril)

In addition to lisinopril, there are nine other ACE inhibitors on the market. All have very similar actions and adverse effects.

Benazepril (Lotensin): Approved in 1991, benazepril is approved only for HTN, although an off-label indication is HF. It is a prodrug that is metabolized by hepatic enzymes to its active form, benazeprilat. It has a long duration of action that allows for once-daily dosing and is excreted by the kidneys. Orthostatic hypotension is the most common adverse effect, especially after the first dose. Other adverse effects, contraindications, and indications are the same as those of lisinopril. Lotensin HCT is a fixed-dose combination of benazepril and hydrochlorothiazide. Lotrel is a combination of benazepril with amlodipine. This drug is pregnancy category C (first trimester) and D (second and third trimesters).

Captopril (Capoten): Captopril, the first ACE inhibitor marketed in 1981, is approved for HTN, HF, left ventricular dysfunction after an acute MI, and diabetic nephropathy. It has a short half-life, which requires multiple daily doses for some patients. The drug should be taken on an empty stomach, because food reduces its bioavailability. Neutropenia and agranulocytosis have occurred during captopril use. Other adverse effects, contraindications, and indications are the same as those of lisinopril. Capozide is a fixed-dose combination of captopril and hydrochlorothiazide. This is a pregnancy category D drug.

Enalapril (Vasotec): Approved in 1985, enalapril is indicated for HTN, HF, and asymptomatic left ventricular dysfunction in post-MI patients. Like most drugs in this class, it has an extended half-life and is excreted by the kidneys. It has a shorter half-life than some other ACE inhibitors and may require twice-daily dosing. Enalapril is a prodrug, being converted by hepatic enzymes to enalaprilat, which is its active form. The most frequent adverse effect is hypotension, which can be especially troublesome in patients with HF. Adverse effects, contraindications, and indications are the same as those of lisinopril. Enalaprilat (Vasotec IV) is available as a drug for severe HTN and is the only ACE inhibitor administered parenterally. Vaseretic is a fixed-dose combination of enalapril and hydrochlorothiazide. Both enalapril and enalaprilat are pregnancy category D drugs.

Fosinopril (Monopril): Approved in 1991, fosinopril is approved for HTN and HF. It is a prodrug that is metabolized by hepatic enzymes to its active form, fosinoprilat. An extended half-life allows for once-daily dosing, and it may be taken without regard to meals. It is excreted by both the liver and kidneys and does not require a dosage adjustment in patients with renal impairment. The most common adverse effects of fosinopril are orthostatic hypotension, dizziness, and headache. Monopril HCT is a fixed-dose combination of Monopril and hydrochlorothiazide. This drug is pregnancy category C (first trimester) and D (second and third trimesters).

Moexipril (Univasc): Approved in 1995, moexipril is indicated only for HTN. It is a prodrug that is metabolized to its active form, moexiprilat, by hepatic enzymes. An extended half-life allows for once-daily dosing. This drug should be taken on an empty stomach, because food reduces its bioavailability by 40% to 50%. It is excreted by the kidneys, and dosage should be reduced in patients with renal impairment. Dizziness is one of the most common adverse effects. Adverse effects, contraindications, and indications are the same as those of lisinopril. Uniretic is a fixed-dose combination of moexipril and hydrochlorothiazide. Moexipril is a pregnancy category D drug.

Perindopril (Aceon): Approved in 1993, perindopril is approved for HTN and the prophylaxis of cardiovascular events such as MI in patients with coronary artery disease. HF is an off-label use. It is a prodrug that is metabolized by hepatic enzymes to its active form, perindoprilat. It is excreted by the kidneys, and its long half-life allows for once- or twice-daily dosing. Food may reduce the bioavailability of the drug by as much as 35%. Cough and dizziness are the most frequent adverse effects of perindopril. Other adverse effects, contraindications, and indications are the same as those of lisinopril. This is a pregnancy category D drug.

Quinapril (Accupril): Approved in 1991, quinapril is indicated for HTN and as adjunctive therapy for HF in combination with diuretics or digoxin. It is a prodrug that is metabolized by hepatic enzymes to its active form, quinaprilat, and may be dosed either once or twice daily. Because the kidney contributes to about 96% of the excretion of the drug, doses should be reduced in patients with renal impairment. Adverse effects are generally mild and transient and include dizziness, cough, and diarrhea. Other adverse effects, contraindications, and indications are the same as those of lisinopril. Accuretic is a fixed-dose combination of quinapril and hydrochlorothiazide. This is a pregnancy category D drug.

Ramipril (Altace): Approved in 1991, ramipril is indicated for HTN, HF following an MI, and to reduce mortality and stroke in high-risk patients with left ventricular dysfunction after an acute MI. It is a prodrug that is metabolized by hepatic enzymes to its active form, ramiprilat. Excretion is predominantly renal, and dosage should be reduced in patients with serious renal impairment. It may be administered without regard to meals. The most common adverse effects are orthostatic hypotension, dizziness, and headache. Other adverse effects, contraindications, and indications are the same as those of lisinopril. This is a pregnancy category D drug.

Trandolapril (Mavik): Approved in 1996, trandolapril is indicated for HTN and HF following an MI and to reduce the mortality in high-risk patients with left ventricular dysfunction after an acute MI. It is a prodrug that is metabolized by hepatic enzymes to trandolaprilat, its active form. It has an extended half-life that permits once-daily dosing and may be administered without regard to meals. Unlike other ACE inhibitors, a large amount of trandolapril (66%) is excreted in the feces. Dosages should be lowered in patients with hepatic or renal impairment. The most common adverse effects are cough, dizziness, and fatigue. Other adverse effects, contraindications, and indications are the same as those of lisinopril. Tarka is a fixed-dose combination of trandolapril and the calcium channel blocker verapamil SR, which is prescribed for HTN. This is a pregnancy category D drug.

CONNECTION Checkpoint 31.4

ACE inhibitors decrease sympathetic activation. From what you learned in Chapters 15 and 16, what type of interactions (additive or antagonistic) would you expect from the autonomic drugs epinephrine and propranolol? *See Answer to Connection Checkpoint 31.4 on student resource website.*

31.7 Angiotensin II receptor blockers act by inhibiting the AT_1 receptor and are used for hypertension and heart failure.

While pharmacologists were examining the mechanism of action of the ACE inhibitors in the 1980s and developing new drugs in this class, research continued on the other enzymes and components of the RAAS. The receptors for angiotensin II in smooth muscle, known as AT_1 and AT_2, were discovered, and a new class of drugs, the angiotensin II receptor blockers (ARBs), was developed. The ARBs are selective for AT_1-type receptors. Unlike the ACE inhibitors, ARBs do not prevent the formation of angiotensin II, but they do effectively block it from activating their target receptors. Doses for the ARBs are listed in Table 31.2.

The ARBs cause vasodilation, with a resultant reduction in peripheral resistance and fall in blood pressure, by blocking angiotensin II receptors in arteriolar smooth muscle. The blockade of AT_1 receptors in the adrenal gland prevents secretion of aldosterone and promotes increased Na^+ and excretion of water by the kidneys. Blockade of AT_1 receptors in the heart prevents the destructive effects of angiotensin-induced cardiac remodeling. Although they act by a different mechanism, ARBs essentially produce the same pharmacologic actions as the ACE inhibitors.

The indications for ARBs are the same as those for the ACE inhibitors. All are approved to treat HTN, and they are often combined with drugs from other classes. Valsartan (Diovan) and candesartan (Atacand) were subsequently approved to treat HF. Some are approved to treat MI and are used for the prophylaxis of stroke. All are administered orally and have prolonged half-lives that permit once-daily dosing. A few are prodrugs, and most are extensively bound to plasma proteins.

Are the ARBs identical to the ACE inhibitors? Not exactly. Unlike the ACE inhibitors, they do not cause cough, and angioedema is less common. This is because ARBs do not promote the accumulation of bradykinin, as do the ACE inhibitors. ARBs can, however, cause dizziness, hypotension, and hyperkalemia, especially in patients with renal impairment or who are concurrently taking potassium supplements or potassium-sparing diuretics.

If ARBs have the same pharmacologic actions and an improved safety profile, why have they not replaced the ACE inhibitors? The answer is because the ACE inhibitors are generally less expensive, and health care providers have much more clinical experience prescribing them. Because the ARBs are newer, a significant body of research has not yet accumulated that demonstrates clear benefits over the ACE inhibitors. Because of these factors, the ARBs are usually reserved for patients unable to tolerate the adverse effects of ACE inhibitors.

PROTOTYPE DRUG   **Losartan (Cozaar)**

Classification: **Therapeutic:** Antihypertensive

Pharmacologic: Angiotensin II receptor blocker

Therapeutic Effects and Uses: Approved for the treatment of HTN, stroke prophylaxis in patients with left ventricular hypertrophy, and the prevention of type 2 diabetic nephropathy, losartan was the first ARB marketed in 1995. An off-label use is for HF. Although losartan undergoes extensive first-pass

TABLE 31.2 Angiotensin II Receptor Blockers, Aldosterone Antagonists, and Renin Inhibitors

Drug	Route and Adult Dose (Maximum Dose Where Indicated)	Adverse Effects
Angiotensin II Receptor Blockers		
azilsartan (Edarbi)	PO: 40–80 mg once daily	*Headache, dizziness, orthostatic hypotension, fatigue, diarrhea, upper respiratory infection*
candesartan (Atacand)	PO: Start at 16 mg/day for HTN and 4 mg/day for HF (max: 32 mg/day)	
eprosartan (Teveten)	PO: 600 mg/day or 400 mg PO: qid–bid (max: 800 mg/day)	Angioedema, acute renal failure, first-dose phenomenon, fetal toxicity and neonatal mortality
irbesartan (Avapro)	PO: 150–300 mg/day (max: 300 mg/day)	
losartan (Cozaar)	PO: 25–50 mg in one to two divided doses (max: 100 mg/day)	
olmesartan medoxomil (Benicar)	PO: 20–40 mg/day	
telmisartan (Micardis)	PO: 40 mg/day (max: 80 mg/day)	
valsartan (Diovan)	PO: 80 mg/day (max: 320 mg/day)	
Aldosterone Antagonists		
eplerenone (Inspra)	PO: Start with 25–50 mg/day (max: 100 mg/day for HTN; 50 mg/day for HF)	*Minor hyperkalemia, headache, fatigue, gynecomastia (spironolactone)*
spironolactone (Aldactone)	PO: 50–100 mg/day in single or divided doses (max: 400 mg/day)	Dysrhythmias (from hyperkalemia), dehydration, hyponatremia, agranulocytosis and other blood dyscrasias
Renin Inhibitor		
aliskiren (Tekturna)	PO: 150 mg/day (max: 300 mg/day)	*Diarrhea, hypotension, cough* Angioedema

Note: Italics indicate common adverse effects. Underline indicates serious adverse effects.

metabolism and has a short half-life, it is metabolized to an active intermediate that exerts more prolonged action, allowing for once-daily dosing. Two daily doses may be necessary in some patients. Its actions include vasodilation and reduced blood volume, due to the drug blocking the release of aldosterone by angiotensin II. Hyzaar is a fixed-dose combination of losartan and hydrochlorothiazide.

Mechanism of Action: Losartan selectively blocks angiotensin AT_1 receptors, resulting in a decline in blood pressure. The blockade of angiotensin II receptors prevents cardiac remodeling and deterioration of renal function in patients with diabetes.

Pharmacokinetics:

Route(s)	PO
Absorption	Well absorbed from the GI tract
Distribution	Does not appear to cross the blood–brain barrier or the placenta, or to be secreted in breast milk; approximately 99% bound to protein
Primary metabolism	Hepatic: extensive first-pass metabolism; converted to active metabolite
Primary excretion	35% renal, 60% in feces
Onset of action	6 h
Duration of action	Half-life: 1.5–2 h (losartan), 6–9 h (highly active metabolite)

Adverse Effects: The incidence of adverse effects of losartan is very low. The most common adverse effects are headache, dizziness, nasal congestion, fatigue, and insomnia. Serious adverse effects include angioedema and acute renal failure. **Black Box Warning**: Fetal injury and death may occur when ARBs are taken during pregnancy. When pregnancy is detected, they should be discontinued as soon as possible.

Contraindications/Precautions: Losartan is contraindicated in patients with prior hypersensitivity to the drug. Because ARBs exhibit the same teratogenic effects as ACE inhibitors, they should not be used during pregnancy and lactation. Caution should be used in treating patients with serious renal or hepatic impairment and dosage may need to be reduced. Patients with a history of angioedema should be monitored carefully. Patients with hypovolemia are at high risk of symptomatic hypotension during therapy. Hypovolemia should be corrected prior to administration of losartan.

Drug Interactions: The drug interactions of losartan and other ARBs are similar to those of the ACE inhibitors. Indomethacin and other NSAIDs may decrease the antihypertensive activity of losartan. When taken concurrently with potassium supplements or potassium-sparing diuretics, care must be taken to avoid hyperkalemia. Concurrent use of losartan with diuretics and other antihypertensives may cause additive hypotensive effects. Use with alcohol may also add to the hypotensive effects of losartan. Losartan may increase lithium levels and toxicity. **Herbal/Food**: Hawthorn should not be taken concurrently with losartan due to the possibility of additive hypotensive action.

Pregnancy: Categories C (first trimester) and D (second and third trimesters).

Treatment of Overdose: Overdose will cause hypotension, which may be treated with an infusion of normal saline or a vasopressor. The drug is not removed by hemodialysis.

Nursing Responsibilities: Key nursing implications for patients receiving losartan are included in the Nursing Practice Application for Patients Receiving Pharmacotherapy with Angiotensin-Converting Enzyme Inhibitors and Angiotensin Receptor Blockers.

Drugs Similar to Losartan (Cozaar)

In addition to losartan, seven other ARBs are available. They all have similar indications, actions, and adverse effects.

Azilsartan medoxomil (Edarbi): The newest of the ARBs, azilsartan was approved in 2011 for the treatment of HTN, either as monotherapy or in combination with other antihypertensives. Azilsartan medoxomil is a prodrug that is converted to its active form (azilsartan) when it is absorbed across the GI tract. It appears to lower blood pressure faster than other drugs in its class. The drug is well tolerated, with diarrhea being the most frequent adverse effect. Caution should be used in treating volume or salt-depleted patients because transient hypotension may occur. Edarbyclor is a fixed-dose combination of azilsartan with chlorthalidone approved to treat HTN. This drug is pregnancy category C (first trimester) and D (second and third trimesters).

Candesartan (Atacand): Approved in 1998, candesartan is indicated for HTN and HF in patients with left ventricular dysfunction. It is a prodrug that is metabolized to its active form during its absorption from the GI tract. Optimal therapeutic effects may take up to 4 weeks. The drug is 99% protein bound and is primarily excreted in the bile (66%). Adverse effects are generally mild and include headache and dizziness. Other adverse effects, contraindications, and indications are the same as those of losartan. Atacand HCT is a fixed-dose combination of candesartan and hydrochlorothiazide. This drug is pregnancy category D.

Eprosartan (Teveten): Approved in 1997, eprosartan is indicated only for HTN. It is mostly unmetabolized and primarily excreted in the feces (90%). Optimum blood pressure reduction may require 2 to 3 weeks of therapy. The most common adverse effects are upper respiratory infection, cough, abdominal pain, and fatigue. Other adverse effects, contraindications, and indications are the same as those of losartan. Teveten HCT is a fixed-dose combination of eprosartan and hydrochlorothiazide. This drug is pregnancy category D.

Irbesartan (Avapro): Approved in 1997, irbesartan is indicated for HTN and type 2 diabetic nephropathy. The drug is 90% protein bound and is primarily excreted in the feces (80%). Adverse effects are generally mild and include dizziness, upper respiratory infection, orthostatic hypotension, diarrhea, dyspepsia, and fatigue. Hyperkalemia may occur in 19% of patients taking this medication. Other adverse effects, contraindications, and indications are the same as those of losartan. Avalide is a fixed-dose combination of irbesartan and hydrochlorothiazide. This drug is pregnancy category D.

Olmesartan medoxomil (Benicar): Approved in 2002, olmesartan is indicated only for HTN. It is a prodrug that is metabolized to its active form during its absorption from the GI tract. Olmesartan is 99% protein bound and excreted equally in urine and the feces.

The drug is administered once daily and optimal blood pressure reduction may require 2 weeks of therapy. The drug exhibits few adverse effects, with dizziness being the most common complaint. Other adverse effects, contraindications, and indications are the same as those of losartan. There are three fixed-dose combinations of olmesartan: Benicar HCT (with hydrochlorothiazide), Azor (with amlodipine), and Tribenzor (with amlodipine and hydrochlorothiazide). This drug is pregnancy category D.

Telmisartan (Micardis): Approved in 1998, telmisartan is indicated for HTN and for cardiovascular risk reduction in patients unable to take ACE inhibitors. An off-label use is for the treatment of renal dysfunction in patients with diabetic nephropathy. It is mostly unmetabolized, 99% protein bound, and excreted primarily in the feces. Initial doses should be reduced in patients with hepatic impairment. The drug is well tolerated and serious adverse effects are uncommon. Adverse effects, contraindications, and indications are the same as those of losartan. Fixed-dose combinations include Micardis HCT (with hydrochlorothiazide) and Twynsta (with amlodipine). This drug is pregnancy category D.

Valsartan (Diovan): Approved in 1996, valsartan is indicated for HTN, HF, and MI when the patient is unable to tolerate an ACE inhibitor. It undergoes hepatic metabolism, is 95% protein bound, and is eliminated in the feces. Because food can reduce drug absorption by as much as 40%, the drug should be given on an empty stomach. Headache and dizziness are the two most common adverse effects. Other adverse effects, contraindications, and indications are the same as those of losartan. Fixed-dose combinations include Diovan HCT (with hydrochlorothiazide), and Exforge (with amlodipine). This drug is pregnancy category D.

31.8 Aldosterone antagonists block the biologic effects of aldosterone in the renal tubule.

As described in Section 31.3, angiotensin II causes the release of aldosterone, which subsequently contributes to increased blood pressure due to sodium and water retention. Receptors for aldosterone are located in the distal tubule and collecting ducts of the nephron. Two drugs are available that block these receptors in the kidney, thus inhibiting the physiological actions of aldosterone. Both spironolactone (Aldactone) and eplerenone (Inspra) are used to treat edema and HTN. Doses for these drugs are listed in Table 31.2.

Spironolactone is an aldosterone antagonist that has been used for its diuretic action for many decades. By binding to aldosterone receptors, spironolactone produces a mild diuresis by promoting Na^+ and Cl^- excretion. Because it has little or no effect on the excretion of potassium, spironolactone is also classified as a potassium-sparing diuretic and is featured as a prototype diuretic in Chapter 32. Spironolactone produces only a mild diuresis; it is often combined with drugs from other diuretic classes when used for HTN. It is also useful in treating primary aldosteronism, a rare condition in which the body produces an overabundance of aldosterone, usually due to a tumor of the adrenal gland. Spironolactone has been shown to reduce morbidity, mortality, and dysrhythmias associated with HF.

The primary concern with spironolactone is potassium retention, which can result in serious hyperkalemia. Some patients

CONNECTIONS Complementary and Alternative Therapies

◀ Hawthorn

Description

Hawthorn (*Crataegus*) is a thorny shrub or small tree that is widespread in North America, Europe, and Asia. Leaves, flowers, and berries of the plant are dried or extracted in liquid form.

History and Claims

Hawthorn, sometimes called May bush, was used in ancient Greece. In traditional Chinese medicine, hawthorn is used as a digestive aid. European and American interest in the herb began in the late 1800s. It has been widely used in European countries to treat HTN and HF. The berries may be consumed raw or made into jellies, juices, and alcoholic beverages. Some cultures believe that the shrub is magical, and it is used in religious rites to ward off evil spirits.

Standardization

Active ingredients in hawthorn include flavonoids and procyanidins. A typical dose is 4.5 to 6 g of dried leaves or flowers or 160 to 900 mg of extract per day.

Evidence

Hawthorn has been well studied (National Center for Complementary and Alternative Medicine, 2012). Positive inotropic action, improved exercise tolerance, and vasodilation have been documented. Some studies also report its ability to lower blood lipids. Hawthorn has been used to lower blood pressure but is slow in onset, taking 4 weeks or longer before a small effect is experienced. Hawthorn may work by inhibition of ACE or reduction of cardiac workload. Hawthorn has few adverse effects at normal doses. This product should be used with caution in patients taking cardiac glycosides and other prescription medications for cardiovascular disease. Because hypotension may occur, frequent blood pressure measurements should be taken when using this therapy.

---

experience GI-related adverse effects such as nausea, vomiting, and diarrhea. Because spironolactone has a similar chemical structure to steroid hormones, it sometimes causes endocrine adverse effects in males, such as gynecomastia and erectile dysfunction. Females may experience menstrual irregularities and breast tenderness.

Eplerenone (Inspra) is a newer aldosterone antagonist that has a very different chemical structure than spironolactone. It is more selective for aldosterone receptors and has a very low incidence of endocrine-related adverse effects. Like spironolactone, hyperkalemia is a potentially serious adverse effect. Headache and dizziness are common adverse effects. Eplerenone is approved to treat HTN and HF and to reduce morbidity and mortality associated with post-MI in patients with left ventricular dysfunction.

For additional information on aldosterone antagonists, see Chapter 32.

CONNECTIONS: NURSING PRACTICE APPLICATION

Patients Receiving Pharmacotherapy with Angiotensin-Converting Enzyme Inhibitors and Angiotensin Receptor Blockers

Assessment	Potential Nursing Diagnoses*
Baseline assessment prior to administration:	• *Decreased Cardiac Output*
• Obtain a complete health history including cardiovascular (MI, HF), diabetes, renal disease, and the possibility of pregnancy. Obtain a drug history including allergies, current prescription and over-the-counter (OTC) drugs, herbal preparations, and alcohol use. Be alert to possible drug interactions.	• *Activity Intolerance*
	• *Sexual Dysfunction*
	• *Deficient Knowledge* (Drug Therapy)
• Evaluate appropriate laboratory findings, electrolytes, especially potassium level, liver function studies, and lipid profiles.	• *Risk for Decreased Cardiac Tissue Perfusion,* related to adverse drug effects
• Obtain baseline weight, vital signs (especially blood pressure and pulse), breath sounds, and cardiac monitoring (e.g., ECG, cardiac output) if appropriate. Assess for location, character, and amount of edema, if present.	• *Risk for Falls,* related to adverse drug effects
	• *Risk for Injury,* related to adverse drug effects
• Assess the patient's ability to receive and understand instructions. Include the family and caregivers as needed.	
Assessment throughout administration:	
• Assess for desired therapeutic effects (e.g., lowered blood pressure within established limits).	
• Continue periodic monitoring of electrolytes, especially potassium.	
• Assess for adverse effects: headache, cough, orthostatic hypotension, fatigue or weakness, lightheadedness or dizziness, symptoms of hyperkalemia, sexual dysfunction, or impotence. Angioedema should be immediately reported to the health care provider.	

Implementation

Interventions and (Rationales)	Patient-Centered Care
Ensuring therapeutic effects: • Continue frequent assessments as above for therapeutic effects. (Blood pressure and pulse should be within normal limits or within parameters set by the health care provider.)	• Teach the patient, family, or caregiver how to monitor pulse and blood pressure. Ensure proper use and functioning of any home equipment obtained.
• Encourage appropriate lifestyle changes: lowered fat intake, increased exercise, limited alcohol intake, and smoking cessation. Provide for dietitian consultation as needed. (Healthy lifestyle changes will support and minimize the need for drug therapy.)	• Encourage the patient to adopt a healthy lifestyle of low-fat food choices, increased exercise, decreased alcohol consumption, and smoking cessation.
Minimizing adverse effects: • Continue to monitor vital signs. Take the blood pressure lying, sitting, and standing to detect orthostatic hypotension. **Lifespan:** Be particularly cautious with the first few doses of the drug and with older adults who are at increased risk for hypotension. Ensure patient safety. (ACE inhibitors and ARBs cause vasodilation, resulting in lowered blood pressure. A first-dose effect may occur with a significant drop in blood pressure with the first few doses. Orthostatic hypotension may increase the risk of falls and injury.)	• Instruct the patient to take the first dose of the new prescription in the evening before bed and to be cautious during the next few doses until drug effects are known. • Teach the patient to rise from lying or sitting to standing slowly to avoid dizziness or falls. If dizziness occurs, the patient should sit or lie down and not attempt to stand or walk, until the sensation passes. • Instruct the patient to stop taking the medication if the blood pressure is 90/60 mmHg or below, or per parameters set by the health care provider, and promptly notify the provider. • Instruct the patient to call for assistance prior to getting out of bed or attempting to walk alone, and to avoid driving or other activities requiring mental alertness or physical coordination until the effects of the drug are known.
• Continue to monitor periodic electrolyte levels, especially potassium, hepatic and renal function laboratory values, and ECG as appropriate. (Hyperkalemia may occur and may increase the risk of dysrhythmias.)	• Instruct the patient on the need to return periodically for laboratory work. • Advise the patient to carry a wallet identification card or wear medical identification jewelry indicating ACE inhibitor/ARB therapy.
• Monitor for persistent dry cough or increasing cough severity. (ACE inhibitors increase bradykinin levels, which results in a dry cough. A change in the severity of the cough may indicate another disease process or may result in the need to consider other medications.)	• Teach the patient to anticipate a dry cough that may persist and to use nonmedicinal measures to treat (e.g., OTC cough lozenges or hard candy or increased fluid intake). • Instruct the patient that if the cough becomes troublesome when in a supine position, sleep with the head elevated on additional pillows. • Advise the patient to consult with the health care provider about the use of antihistamines to treat a persistent cough unrelieved by nonmedicinal measures. • Instruct the patient to promptly report any change in the severity or frequency of a cough. Any cough accompanied by shortness of breath, fever, or chest pain should be reported immediately because it may indicate more severe pathologic conditions.
• Monitor for hyperkalemia. (Reduced aldosterone levels may cause hyperkalemia, especially in patients with diabetes or impaired kidney function. **Lifespan:** The older adult may be at greater risk for hyperkalemia related to renal effects of aging.)	• Instruct the patient on the signs of hyperkalemia (nausea, irregular heartbeat, profound fatigue or muscle weakness, and slow or faint pulse), and to report them immediately. • Teach the patient to avoid salt substitutes containing potassium chloride, consuming snacks advertised as "electrolyte-fortified," specialized sports drinks that contain high levels of potassium, or excessive intake of foods high in potassium different from their normal diet.
• Monitor for the development of angioedema. (**Lifespan and Diverse Patients:** The older adult and patients of African American heritage are at higher risk for the development of angioedema.)	• Teach the patient to observe for and immediately report swelling of the mouth, lips, tongue, or throat, hoarseness, or sudden difficulty with breathing.
• Assess for the possibility of pregnancy or breast-feeding. (**Lifespan:** The drugs may cause birth defects if taken during pregnancy and may have adverse effects on the breast-feeding child.)	• **Lifespan:** The drug should not be taken during pregnancy, if pregnancy is suspected, or while breast-feeding.
Patient understanding of drug therapy: • Use opportunities during the administration of medications and during assessments to discuss the rationale for the drug therapy, desired therapeutic outcomes, commonly observed adverse effects, parameters for when to call the health care provider, and any necessary monitoring or precautions. (Using time during nursing care helps to optimize and reinforce key teaching areas.)	• The patient, family, or caregiver should be able to state the reason for the drug, appropriate dose and scheduling, what adverse effects to observe for and when to report them, and the anticipated length of medication therapy.
Patient self-administration of drug therapy: • When administering the medication, instruct the patient, family, or caregiver in proper self-administration of the drug, e.g., take the first dose of the new prescription at bedtime. (Utilizing time during nurse-administration of these drugs helps to reinforce teaching.)	• The patient, family, or caregiver is able to discuss appropriate dosing and administration needs.

CHAPTER

31   Understanding the Chapter

Key Concepts Summary

31.1 The formation of angiotensin II requires two enzymatic steps.

31.2 Renin secretion is controlled by the juxtaglomerular cells of the kidney and the sympathetic nervous system.

31.3 Angiotensin-converting enzyme is responsible for the formation of angiotensin II.

31.4 Angiotensin II has multiple effects on the cardiovascular system that raise blood pressure and affect cardiac function.

31.5 The renin-angiotensin-aldosterone pathway offers multiple points for drug intervention.

31.6 ACE inhibitors are key drugs in the pharmacotherapy of hypertension and heart failure.

31.7 Angiotensin II receptor blockers act by inhibiting the AT_1 receptor and are used for hypertension and heart failure.

31.8 Aldosterone antagonists block the biologic effects of aldosterone in the renal tubule.

Case Study: Making the Patient Connection

Remember the patient "Carlos Avaya" at the beginning of the chapter? Now read the remainder of the case study. Based on the information presented within this chapter, respond to the critical thinking questions that follow.

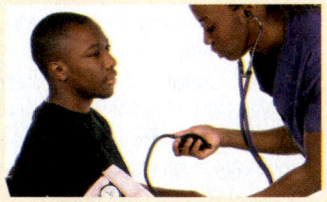

Carlos Avaya is a 26-year-old single man who was diagnosed with primary HTN 4 months ago. Carlos has been taking losartan (Cozaar) 50 mg daily PO and has been faithful in taking the medication as prescribed. When Carlos was told that his blood pressure was still elevated during this clinic visit, he was obviously distressed and concerned.

The health care team begins to investigate external factors that may be causing his blood pressure to remain elevated. Carlos has never smoked or used alcohol. He does not like to exercise but participates in a weekly game of soccer at the nearby community center. He denies being overly stressed with work or home life. Furthermore, he claims that he rarely salts his food.

The nurse asks Carlos to describe a typical day. During the description the nurse notices a concerning pattern. Because Carlos lives alone, he frequently cooks for himself. He admits that he enjoys salty foods such as pretzels and popcorn. He denies having consumed either prior to the visit to the clinic. However, to Carlos, cooking a meal involves preparing canned processed foods and frozen dinners. He never reads food labels. Without recording a complete dietary history, the nurse is able to determine that Carlos's intake of sodium-rich foods is quite extensive.

Critical Thinking Questions

1. In your own words, how would you describe how losartan (Cozaar) works to reduce blood pressure?

2. Considering the adverse effects of losartan (Cozaar), when would you instruct Carlos to notify the prescriber?

3. In addition to teaching Carlos about his losartan (Cozaar), what additional health teaching should he receive?

See Answers to Critical Thinking Questions on student resource website.

Additional Case Study

Ella Daniels, a middle-aged African American woman, takes spironolactone (Aldactone) for HTN. As the nurse responsible for providing her with health information, you plan to talk with her about this drug.

1. How does the mechanism of action of spironolactone differ from that of lisinopril (Prinivil, Zestril)?

2. What are the main precautions specific to spironolactone that should be included in the teaching plan?

See Answers to Additional Case Study on student resource website.

Chapter Review

1 The community health nurse teaches a patient at home. Lisinopril (Prinivil) has been prescribed for the patient. Which statement, if made by the patient, indicates that further teaching is necessary?

1. "I should notify my health care provider of symptoms of hypotension such as dizziness or fainting."

2. "I should avoid the use of salt substitutes containing potassium."

3. "If a dose is missed, I will take it as soon as possible but not too close to the next dose."

4. "Too much calcium in my diet will elevate my blood pressure."

2 The patient states, "I always keep my lisinopril (Prinivil) on my kitchen window sill. It helps me to remember to take it." The nurse's response would be based on which pharmacologic concept about heat and moisture?

1. They cause the medicine to break down.

2. They enhance the strength of the drug.

3. They crystallize the medication.

4. They convert the medicine to toxic metabolites.

3 A patient is hospitalized for uncontrolled hypertension and is receiving enalapril (Vasotec). The nurse should notify the health care provider if the patient exhibits:

1. Dry mucous membranes.

2. A decline in systolic blood pressure.

3. Nonproductive cough.

4. A reduction of diastolic blood pressure.

4 The nurse is caring for a patient with chronic hypertension. The patient is receiving losartan (Cozaar) daily. Which patient manifestations would the nurse conclude is an adverse effect of this medication?

1. Irritability and tremors

2. Headache and dizziness

3. Sleepiness and slurred speech

4. Pruritus and rash

5 Irbesartan (Avapro) is prescribed for each of the following patients. A nurse should question the order for which patient? A patient who has:

1. Severe dehydration from diuretic therapy.

2. Long-term diabetes mellitus.

3. A systolic blood pressure of 162.

4. A 5-year history of heart failure.

6 The nurse determines that the patient does not understand an important principle in self-administration of benazepril (Lotensin) when the patient makes which statement?

1. "I will learn to monitor my own blood pressure and write down all my daily measurements."

2. "While taking this medication, I should avoid over-the-counter medications for colds, sinus, or appetite control."

3. "This drug will not impair thinking and reaction time. I don't need to wait to start driving my car."

4. "Drinking alcohol while on this medication can lower my blood pressure and lead to dizziness and faintness."

See Answers to Chapter Review in Appendix A.

References

National Center for Complementary and Alternative Medicine. (2012). *Herbs at a glance: Hawthorn.* Retrieved from http://nccam.nih.gov/health/hawthorn

Silverthorn, D. U. (2013). *Human physiology: An integrated approach* (6th ed.). San Francisco, CA: Pearson/Benjamin Cummings.

Tocci, G., Paneni, F., Palano, F., Sciarretta, S., Ferrucci, A., Kurtz, T., & Volpe, M. (2011). Angiotensin-converting enzyme inhibitors, angiotensin II receptor blockers and diabetes: A meta-analysis of placebo-controlled clinical trials. *American Journal of Hypertension, 24*(5), 582–590. doi:10.1038/ajh.2011.8

Selected Bibliography

Azizi, M., & Ménard, J. (2013). Renin inhibitors and cardiovascular and renal protection: An endless quest? *Cardiovascular Drugs and Therapy, 27,* 145–153. doi: 10.1007/s10557-012-6380-6.

Benjamin, R., Szwejkowski, B. R., Rekhraj, S., Hj Elder, D., & Struthers, A. D. (2011). Update on heart failure. *British Journal of Diabetes and Vascular Disease, 11,* 25–30. doi:10.1177/1474651410397246

Cokkinos, D. V., & Pantos, C. (2011). Myocardial remodeling, an overview. *Heart Failure Reviews, 16,* 1–4. doi:10.1007/s10741-010-9192-4

Fitzgerald, M. A. (2011). Hypertension treatment update: Focus on direct renin inhibition. *Journal of the American Academy of Nurse Practitioners, 23,* 239–248. doi:10.1111/j.1745-7599.2010.00589.x

Herdman, T. H., & Kamitsuru, S. (Ed.). (2014). *NANDA International nursing diagnoses: Definitions and classification, 2015–2017.* Oxford, United Kingdom: Wiley-Blackwell.

Holdiness, A., Monahan, K., Minor, D., & de Shazo, R. D. (2011). Renin angiotensin aldosterone system blockade: Little to no rationale for ACE inhibitor and ARB combinations. *The American Journal of Medicine, 124,* 15–19. doi:10.1016/j.amjmed.2010.07.021

Izzo, J. L., Jr., & Weir, M. R. (2011). Angiotensin-converting enzyme inhibitors. *The Journal of Clinical Hypertension, 13,* 667–675. doi:10.1111/j.1751-7176.2011.00508.x

Kohlwes, J. (2012). ACE inhibitors versus ARBs versus DRIs: A systematic update. *Journal of General Internal Medicine, 27,* 1585. doi:10.1007/s11606-012-2212-4

Miller, N. H. (2010). Cardiovascular risk reduction with renin-angiotensin aldosterone system blockade. *Nursing Research and Practice, 2010,* Article ID 101749, 7 pages. doi:10.1155/2010/101749

Powers, B. J., Coeytaux, R. R., Dolor, R. J., Hasselblad, V., Patel, U. D., Yancy W. S., Jr., . . . Sanders, G. D. (2012). Updated report on comparative effectiveness of ACE inhibitors, ARBs, and direct renin inhibitors for patients with essential hypertension: Much more data, little new information. *Journal of General Internal Medicine, 27,* 716–729. doi:10.1007/s11606-011-1938-8

Siragy, H. M. (2011). A current evaluation of the safety of angiotensin receptor blockers and direct renin inhibitors. *Vascular Health and Risk Management, 7,* 297. doi:10.2147/VHRM.S15541

White, C. M. (2012). Comparative effectiveness of renin-angiotensin system inhibitors in hypertension. *Journal of Comparative Effectiveness Research, 1*(2), 125–127. doi:10.2217/cer.12.2

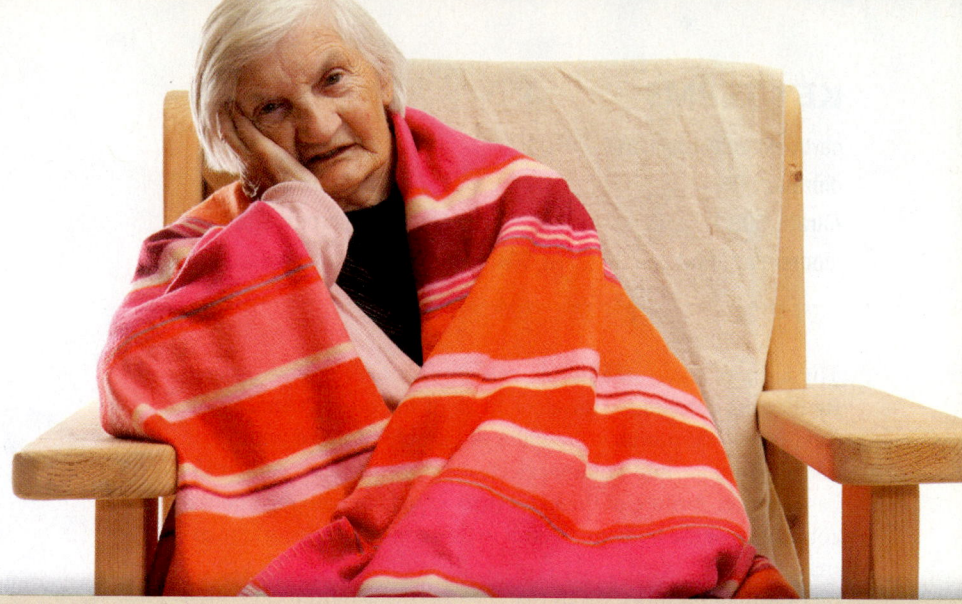

"I feel terrible. I have no energy and I feel as weak as a kitten. Lately, I don't even feel like getting out of bed in the mornings. I try to take my medications just as I was told to do."

Patient "Katherine Crosland"

CHAPTER

32

Diuretic Therapy and the Pharmacotherapy of Renal Failure

LEARNING OUTCOMES

After reading this chapter, the student should be able to:

1. Explain the role of the urinary system in maintaining fluid, electrolyte, and acid–base homeostasis.

2. Explain the physiological processes that change the composition of filtrate as it travels through the nephrons.

3. Describe the adjustments in pharmacotherapy that must be considered in patients with renal failure.

4. Identify indications for diuretics.

5. Compare and contrast the loop, thiazide, potassium-sparing, osmotic, and carbonic anhydrase inhibitor diuretics.

6. Describe the nurse's role in the pharmacologic management of renal failure and in diuretic therapy.

7. For each of the classes shown in the chapter outline, identify the prototype and representative drugs and explain the mechanism(s) of drug action, primary indications, contraindications, significant drug interactions, pregnancy category, and important adverse effects.

8. Apply the nursing process to care for patients who are receiving pharmacotherapy with diuretics.

CHAPTER OUTLINE

▸ Review of Renal Physiology

▸ Pharmacotherapy for Patients with Renal Failure

▸ Diuretic Therapy

Loop (High-Ceiling) Diuretics

PROTOTYPE Furosemide (Lasix) *p. 508*

Thiazide and Thiazide-Like Diuretics

PROTOTYPE Hydrochlorothiazide (Microzide) *p. 510*

Potassium-Sparing Diuretics

PROTOTYPE Spironolactone (Aldactone), *p. 512*

Osmotic Diuretics

PROTOTYPE Mannitol (Osmitrol), *p. 514*

Carbonic Anhydrase Inhibitors

PROTOTYPE Acetazolamide (Diamox), *p. 515*

KEY TERMS

carbonic anhydrase, 515

diuretic, 505

filtrate, 502

glomerular filtration rate (GFR), 504

glomerulus, 502

natriuresis, 505

nephrons, 502

osmotic pressure, 513

reabsorption, 503

renal failure, 504

secretion, 503

symporter, 506

The kidneys serve an amazing role in maintaining homeostasis. By filtering a volume equivalent to all of the body's extracellular fluid every 100 minutes, the kidneys are able to make immediate adjustments to fluid volume, electrolyte composition, and acid–base balance. Failure of the kidneys to adjust to changing internal conditions of the body may result in dire consequences, and pharmacotherapy is often used to correct these imbalances. This chapter examines diuretics, drugs that increase urine output, and other medications used to treat patients with renal dysfunction.

PharmFACT

More than 16,000 kidney transplants are performed annually. Approximately 10,500 of these patients receive organs from deceased donors, and 6,000 receive organs from living donors. Over 80,500 people are on the waiting list for kidney transplants (Axelrod et al., 2010).

Review of Renal Physiology

32.1 The kidneys are major organs of excretion and body homeostasis.

When most people think of the kidneys, they think of excretion. Although this is certainly true, the kidneys have many other essential homeostatic functions. The kidneys are the primary organs for regulating fluid balance, electrolyte composition, and the pH of body fluids. They also secrete the enzyme renin, which helps to regulate blood pressure (see Chapter 31), and erythropoietin, a hormone that stimulates red blood cell production (see Chapter 39). In addition, the kidneys are responsible for the production of calcitriol, the active form of vitamin D, which helps maintain bone homeostasis (see Chapter 72). It is not surprising that our overall health is strongly dependent on the proper functioning of the kidneys.

The urinary system consists of two kidneys, two ureters, one urinary bladder, and a urethra. Blood enters the kidneys through the large renal arteries, bringing 25% of the total cardiac output to the kidneys each minute. After a series of branches, blood enters the **nephrons**, the functional units of the kidney. Each kidney contains over 1 million nephrons.

In the nephron, blood travels at high pressure through the **glomerulus**, a specialized capillary containing pores. The fluid portion of the blood is filtered through the glomerular pores and collected by Bowman's capsule, the first portion of the collecting system of the nephron. Together, the glomerulus and Bowman's capsule are called the renal corpuscle. During filtration, not all substances in the blood reach Bowman's capsule. Plasma proteins and the formed elements of the blood—the erythrocytes, leukocytes, and platelets—are too large to pass through the pores of the glomerulus and thus continue circulating through the bloodstream. Water and other small molecules in plasma, however, readily pass through the glomerular pores and enter the next section of the nephron.

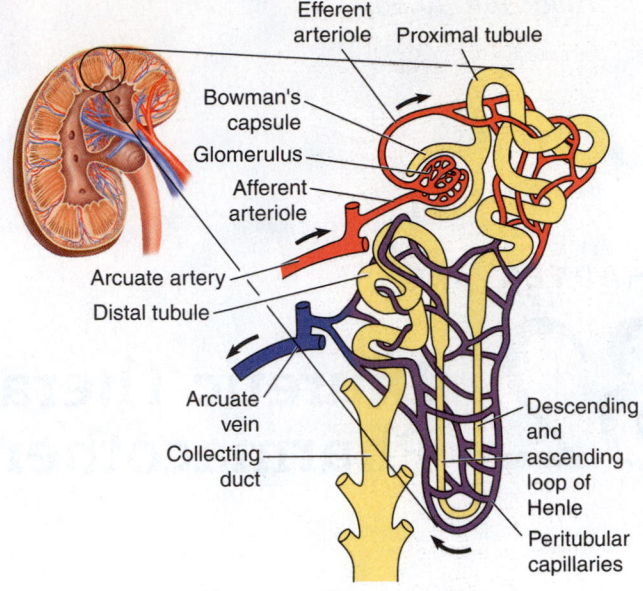

Figure 32.1 The nephron.

The fluid filtered into Bowman's capsule is called **filtrate**. Essentially, the initial composition of filtrate may be thought of as plasma minus proteins. After leaving Bowman's capsule, the filtrate enters the proximal tubule, travels through the loop of Henle and, subsequently, the distal tubule. The proximal and distal tubules are twisted and highly convoluted, which greatly increases the length of the nephron, allowing for enhanced processing of substances in the filtrate. The filtrate eventually reaches common collecting ducts, which empty into increasingly larger collecting structures inside the kidney. Fluid leaving the collecting ducts and entering subsequent portions of the kidney is called urine. Approximately 1 mL of urine is produced each minute. Parts of the nephron and their functions are illustrated in Figure 32.1.

Many drugs are small enough to pass through the glomerulus and enter the filtrate. If the drug is bound to a plasma protein, however, the drug–protein complex will be too large to be filtered and will continue circulating in the blood. Plasma proteins such as albumin are also too large to pass through the filter and will not be present in the filtrate or in the urine of healthy patients. The appearance of excess plasma proteins in urine (proteinuria or albuminuria) is a sign of kidney pathology. For example, during glomerulonephritis the glomeruli become inflamed and the size of the pores increases, allowing larger substances such as proteins to enter the filtrate.

CONNECTION Checkpoint 32.1

From what you learned in Chapter 3, explain how plasma protein binding markedly affects the excretion of a drug. *See Answer to Connection Checkpoint 32.1 on student resource website.*

32.2 The composition of filtrate changes dramatically as a result of the processes of reabsorption and secretion.

The filtrate's composition changes dramatically as it makes its long journey through the nephron. Some substances in the filtrate cross the tubule walls to reenter the blood; this process is known as tubular **reabsorption**. Water is the most important molecule reabsorbed in the tubule. For every 180 L of water entering the filtrate each day, approximately 178.5 L are reabsorbed, leaving only 1.5 L to be excreted in the urine. Over 65% of the filtered sodium is reabsorbed in the proximal tubule, and 25% in the loop of Henle. Glucose, amino acids, and essential ions such as chloride, calcium, and bicarbonate are also reabsorbed.

Hormones can markedly affect the degree of reabsorption in the renal tubule. Aldosterone, for example, exerts a major effect on the tubule by stimulating sodium reabsorption in the distal portions of the nephron. Under the influence of aldosterone, potassium excretion is increased because this ion is "exchanged" for sodium ions, which are reabsorbed. Antidiuretic hormone (ADH) also affects kidney function, increasing water reabsorption by making the collecting ducts become more permeable to water. The formation of urine is indeed a dynamic process that undergoes continuous modification as the filtrate travels down the tubule. Many drugs have the ability to either enhance or block the effects of hormones on tubular processes.

Certain ions and molecules too large to pass through Bowman's capsule may still enter the urine by crossing from the blood to the filtrate using a process known as tubular **secretion**. The tubule contains molecular pumps for organic acids and bases. Acidic drugs secreted in the proximal tubule include penicillin G, ampicillin, sulfisoxazole, nonsteroidal anti-inflammatory drugs (NSAIDs), and furosemide. Basic drugs include procainamide, epinephrine, dopamine, neostigmine, and trimethoprim. Potassium, phosphate, hydrogen, and ammonium ions also enter the filtrate through active secretion. The amounts of selected substances reabsorbed, secreted, and excreted are shown in Table 32.1.

Reabsorption and secretion are critical to the pharmacokinetics of drugs. Some drugs are reabsorbed, whereas others are secreted into the filtrate. For example, approximately 90% of a dose of penicillin G enters the urine through secretion. When the kidney is diseased, reabsorption and secretion mechanisms are impaired and serum drug levels may be dramatically affected. Figure 32.2 illustrates the possible fates of drugs entering the glomerulus.

CONNECTION Checkpoint 32.2

From what you learned in Chapter 31, explain the relationship between angiotensin II and the release of aldosterone by the adrenal gland and its significance to pharmacology. *See Answer to Connection Checkpoint 32.2 on student resource website.*

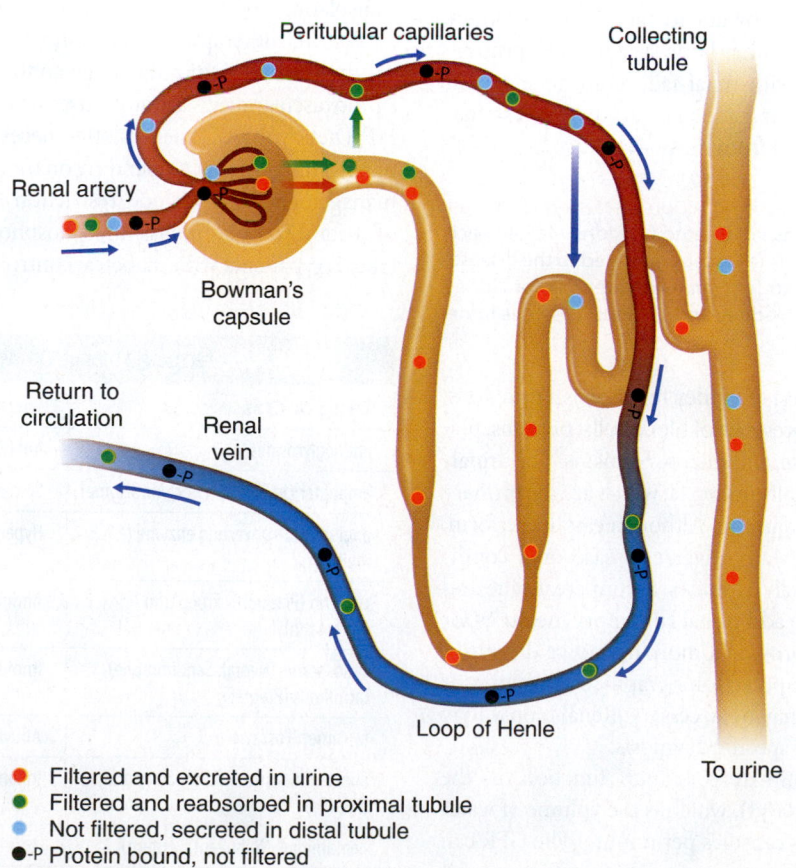

- 🔴 Filtered and excreted in urine
- 🟢 Filtered and reabsorbed in proximal tubule
- 🔵 Not filtered, secreted in distal tubule
- ⚫-P Protein bound, not filtered

Figure 32.2 Fates of drugs entering the glomerulus: filtration, reabsorption, secretion, and excretion.

TABLE 32.1 Substances Filtered, Reabsorbed, and Excreted by the Kidneys

Substance	Filtered	Reabsorbed	Excreted
Water	180 L	178–179 L	1–2 L
Glucose	162 g	162 g	0 g
Proteins	2 g	1.9 g	0.1 g
Ions			
Sodium	579 g	575 g	4 g
Potassium	29.6 g	29.6 g	2 g
Bicarbonate	275 g	274.97 g	0.03 g
Metabolic Waste Products			
Creatine	1.6 g	0 g	1.6 g
Urea	54 g	24 g	30 g
Uric acid	8.5 g	7.7 g	0.8 g

Pharmacotherapy for Patients with Renal Failure

32.3 Renal failure may significantly impact the success of pharmacotherapy.

Renal failure is a condition characterized by a decrease in the kidneys' ability to maintain electrolyte and fluid balance and excrete waste products. Renal failure may be due to damage to the kidney itself or result from disorders of other body systems. The primary treatment goals for a patient with renal failure are to maintain blood flow through the kidneys and adequate urine output so that metabolic wastes can be removed from the body.

PharmFACT

Approximately 400,000 Americans are treated for kidney failure each year, and about 90,000 die annually from causes related to the disease. African Americans have a three to four times greater risk for kidney failure than Caucasians (National Kidney and Urologic Diseases Information Clearinghouse, 2012).

The most basic diagnostic test of kidney function is a urinalysis, which examines urine for the presence of blood cells, proteins, pH, specific gravity, ketones, glucose, and microorganisms. The urinalysis can detect proteinuria and albuminuria, which are the primary measures of structural kidney damage. Although easy to perform, the urinalysis is nonspecific: Many diverse diseases and conditions can cause abnormal urinalysis values. Serum creatinine and blood urea nitrogen (BUN) are additional laboratory measures for detecting kidney disease. To provide a more definitive diagnosis, diagnostic imaging such as computed tomography, sonography, or magnetic resonance imaging may be necessary. Renal biopsy may be performed to obtain a more specific diagnosis.

The best marker for estimating kidney function is the **glomerular filtration rate (GFR)**, which is the volume of water filtered through the Bowman's capsules per minute. The GFR can be used to predict the onset and progression of kidney failure and it indicates the ability of the kidneys to excrete drugs from the body. With normal values ranging from 90–120 mL/min, a progressive

decline in GFR indicates a reduction in the number of functioning nephrons. As nephrons "die," however, the remaining healthy ones have the ability to compensate by increasing their filtration capacity. Because of this, patients with significant kidney damage may be asymptomatic until 50% or more of the nephrons have become nonfunctional and the GFR has fallen to less than half its normal value.

Renal failure may be classified as acute or chronic, depending on its onset. Acute renal failure requires immediate treatment because retention of nitrogenous waste products in the body such as urea and creatinine can result in death if left untreated. The most common cause of acute renal failure is renal hypoperfusion, the lack of sufficient blood flow through the kidneys. Hypoperfusion can lead to permanent destruction of kidney cells and nephrons. To correct this type of renal failure, the cause of the hypoperfusion must be quickly identified and corrected. Potential causes include heart failure (HF), dysrhythmias, hemorrhage, toxins, and dehydration. Pharmacotherapy with nephrotoxic drugs can also lead to either acute or chronic renal failure. It is good practice for the nurse to remember common nephrotoxic drugs, which are listed in Table 32.2, so that kidney function may be continuously monitored during therapy with these drugs.

Chronic renal failure occurs over a period of months or years. Over half of the patients with chronic renal failure have long-standing hypertension (HTN) or diabetes mellitus. Due to the long, gradual development of chronic renal failure and its nonspecific symptoms, the condition may go undetected for many years. By the time the disease is diagnosed, the renal impairment may be irreversible. In end-stage renal disease (ESRD), dialysis and kidney transplantation become treatment alternatives.

Pharmacotherapy of renal failure attempts to cure the cause of the dysfunction. Diuretics are given to increase urine output, and cardiovascular drugs are administered to treat underlying HTN or HF. Dietary management is often necessary to prevent worsening of renal impairment. Depending on the stage of the disease, dietary management may include restriction of protein and reduction of dietary sodium, potassium, phosphorous, and magnesium intake. For patients with diabetes, control of blood glucose through

TABLE 32.2 Nephrotoxic Drugs

Drug or Class	Indication/Classification
aminoglycosides	Antibiotics
amphotericin B (Amphotec, AmBisome)	Systemic antifungal
angiotensin-converting enzyme (ACE) inhibitors	Hypertension, HF
cisplatin (Platinol), carboplatin (Paraplatin)	Antineoplastic
cyclosporine (Neoral, Sandimmune), tacrolimus (Prograf)	Immunosuppressant
foscarnet (Foscavir)	Antiviral
nonsteroidal anti-inflammatory drugs (NSAIDs)	Inflammation and pain
pentamidine (NebuPent, Pentam)	Anti-infective (*Pneumocystis*)
radiographic intravenous (IV) contrast agents	Diagnosis of kidney and vascular disorders

TABLE 32.3 Pharmacologic Management of Renal Failure

Complication	Pathogenesis	Selected Therapies
Anemia	Kidneys are unable to synthesize sufficient erythropoietin for red blood cell production.	epoetin alfa (Procrit, Epogen)
Hyperkalemia	Kidneys are unable to adequately excrete potassium.	Dietary restriction of potassium; polystyrene sulfate (Kayexalate) with sorbitol
Hyperphosphatemia	Kidneys are unable to adequately excrete phosphate.	Dietary restriction of phosphate; phosphate binders such as calcium carbonate (Os-Cal 500, others), calcium acetate (Calphron, PhosLo), lanthanum carbonate (Fosrenol), sucroferric oxyhydroxide (Velphoro), or sevelamer (Renagel)
Hypervolemia	Kidneys are unable to excrete sufficient sodium and water, leading to water retention.	Dietary restriction of sodium; loop diuretics in acute conditions, thiazide diuretics in mild conditions
Hypocalcemia	Hyperphosphatemia leads to loss of calcium.	Usually corrected by reversing the hyperphosphatemia, but additional calcium supplements may be necessary
Metabolic acidosis	Kidneys are unable to adequately excrete metabolic acids.	Sodium bicarbonate or sodium citrate

intensive insulin therapy may reduce the risk of renal damage. See Table 32.3 for a summary of selected medications used to prevent and treat the complications of renal failure.

The nurse serves a key role in assessing and providing interventions for patients with renal failure. Once a diagnosis has been established, all nephrotoxic medications should be either discontinued or used with extreme caution. Because the kidneys excrete most drugs or their metabolites, many medications will require a significant dosage reduction in patients with moderate to severe renal failure. The importance of this cannot be overemphasized: Administering the "average" dose to a patient in severe renal failure can have fatal consequences.

Diuretic Therapy

32.4 Diuretics are used to treat hypertension, heart failure, accumulation of edema fluid, and renal failure.

By simple definition, a **diuretic** is a drug that increases the rate of urine flow. These drugs are administered to treat a large number of disorders, including HTN, HF, renal failure, or removal of edema fluid. Diuretics do more than increase urine flow; they also change the rate of excretion of specific electrolytes, most importantly sodium and potassium. The goal of most diuretic therapy is to reduce extracellular fluid volume, so that abnormal fluid retention by the body may be reversed. Excretion of excess fluid in the body is particularly important in the following conditions:

- HTN
- Heart failure
- Renal failure
- Liver failure or cirrhosis
- Pulmonary edema

The most common mechanism by which diuretics act is by blocking sodium ion (Na^+) reabsorption in the nephron, thus sending more Na^+ to the urine (**natriuresis**). The human body is particularly sensitive to sodium imbalances; dietary intake must be balanced with excretion mechanisms. For example, a 1% increase in sodium reabsorption (retention) could potentially cause a 1.8-L net gain of water each day, which is equivalent to 4 lb of body weight. On the other hand, even small decreases in sodium reabsorption can cause net losses of sodium from the body, resulting in volume depletion and circulatory collapse. These examples illustrate the need for patients to monitor their weight daily when taking diuretics.

Natriuresis results in two other important effects. Chloride ions (Cl^-) follow sodium, potentially causing a net loss of chloride from the body and possible hypochloremia. In addition, because water molecules travel passively with sodium ions, blocking the reabsorption of Na^+ increases the total volume of urination, or diuresis. The amount of diuresis produced by a diuretic is directly related to the amount of sodium reabsorption that is blocked: Those that block the most sodium are the most effective at increasing urine output. Diuretics also affect the renal excretion of ions such as magnesium, potassium, phosphate, calcium, and bicarbonate. It is important to remember that imbalances may occur in virtually any electrolyte during diuretic therapy.

Diuretics are classified into five major groups, based on differences in their chemical nature and mechanism of action. The sites in the nephron at which the various diuretics act are shown in Pharmacotherapy Illustrated 32.1.

- **Loop or high-ceiling.** These drugs prevent the reabsorption of Na^+ in the loop of Henle; thus, they are called loop diuretics. Because there is an abundance of Na^+ in the filtrate within the loop of Henle, drugs in this class are capable of producing large increases in urine output.

- **Thiazides.** The largest diuretic class, the thiazides act by blocking Na^+ in the distal tubule. Because most Na^+ has already been reabsorbed from the filtrate by the time it reaches this part of the nephron, the thiazides produce less diuresis than loop diuretics.

- **Potassium-sparing.** The third major class is named potassium-sparing diuretics, because they have minimal effect on potassium ion (K^+) excretion. These drugs produce a mild diuresis.

- **Osmotic.** These drugs are relatively inert drugs that change the osmolality of filtrate, causing water to remain in the nephron for excretion. These drugs are very effective but are rarely prescribed because they can produce potentially serious adverse effects.

- **Carbonic anhydrase inhibitors.** These drugs block the enzyme in the nephron responsible for bicarbonate reabsorption. They produce a weak diuresis and are rarely used.

It is common practice to combine two or more drugs in the pharmacotherapy of HTN and fluid retention disorders. Diuretics are often a component of fixed-dose combinations with drugs

PHARMACOTHERAPY ILLUSTRATED 32.1

SITES OF ACTION OF THE DIURETICS

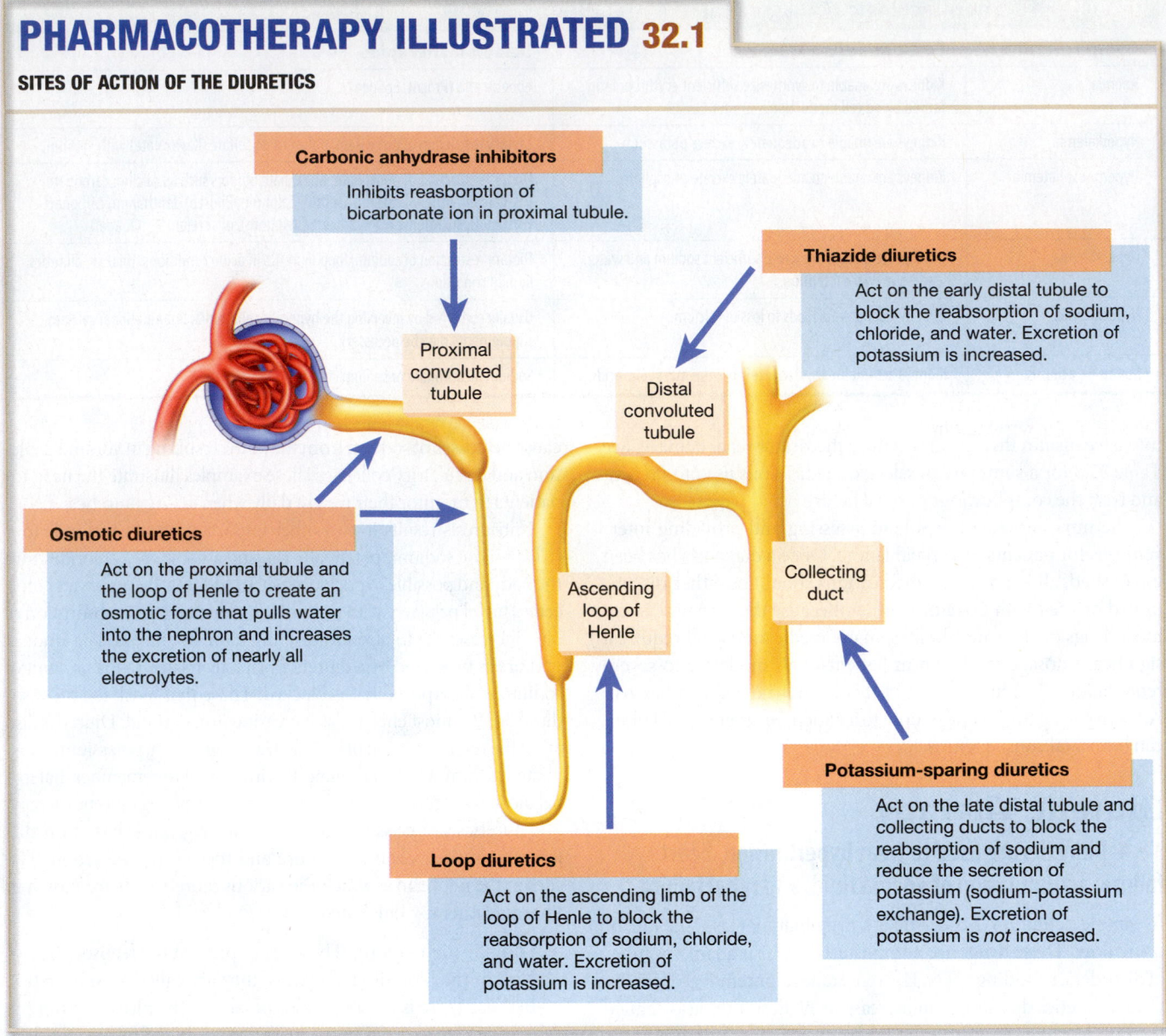

Carbonic anhydrase inhibitors

Inhibits reasborption of bicarbonate ion in proximal tubule.

Thiazide diuretics

Act on the early distal tubule to block the reabsorption of sodium, chloride, and water. Excretion of potassium is increased.

Proximal convoluted tubule

Distal convoluted tubule

Osmotic diuretics

Act on the proximal tubule and the loop of Henle to create an osmotic force that pulls water into the nephron and increases the excretion of nearly all electrolytes.

Collecting duct

Ascending loop of Henle

Potassium-sparing diuretics

Act on the late distal tubule and collecting ducts to block the reabsorption of sodium and reduce the secretion of potassium (sodium-potassium exchange). Excretion of potassium is *not* increased.

Loop diuretics

Act on the ascending limb of the loop of Henle to block the reabsorption of sodium, chloride, and water. Excretion of potassium is increased.

---

from other classes. The primary rationales for combination therapy are that the incidence of adverse effects is decreased and the pharmacologic effects (such as diuresis or blood pressure reduction) may be enhanced. For patient convenience, some of these drugs are available in single-tablet formulations. Examples of single-tablet diuretic combinations include the following:

- **Aldactazide.** Hydrochlorothiazide and spironolactone
- **Apresazide.** Hydrochlorothiazide and hydralazine
- **Dyazide.** Hydrochlorothiazide and triamterene
- **Moduretic.** Hydrochlorothiazide and amiloride

Loop (High-Ceiling) Diuretics

32.5 The most effective diuretics are the loop diuretics that block sodium reabsorption in the loop of Henle.

The most effective diuretics, the loop or high-ceiling diuretics, act by blocking the reabsorption of sodium and chloride in the loop of Henle. This occurs when the drug inhibits the molecule responsible

for transporting sodium and chloride from the filtrate to the blood, known as the Na^+-K^+-$2Cl^-$ symporter. A **symporter** is a membrane protein that transports two molecules at the same time. When the loop diuretics block this symporter, sodium and chloride are prevented from being reabsorbed, and diuresis is increased. All loop diuretics have an additional action that is responsible for a major adverse effect of drugs in this class: increasing potassium excretion. An illustration showing the effects caused when this symporter is inhibited is shown in Figure 32.3.

All loop diuretics are available for either oral (PO) or parenteral administration and are extensively bound to plasma proteins. They have relatively short half-lives, and extended release preparations are not available. When given intravenously (IV), loop diuretics have the ability to cause large amounts of fluid to be excreted by the kidney in a very short time. Loop diuretics are used to reduce the edema associated with HF, hepatic cirrhosis, or chronic renal failure. Furosemide and torsemide are also approved for HTN, although their short half-lives make them less suitable for this indication than thiazide diuretics. Occasionally, loop diuretics are given

CONNECTIONS | Evidence-Based Practice

◀ Diuretic Use as a Risk for Falls in the Older Adult

Clinical Question
Does diuretic use contribute to the risk of falls in the older adult?

Evidence
Falls are a known health problem for older adults and result in increased hospitalizations and adverse outcomes. The cause of a fall is not always evident when a patient is brought to an emergency department. Mussi et al. (2009) sought to determine whether syncope related to orthostatic hypotension may have been the causative factor for a fall in adults older than 65 admitted to an emergency department. Orthostatic hypotension was found in up to 12.4% of patients tested for syncope using ECG and positional blood pressure monitoring. Vasoactive drugs, including diuretics, were associated with a significantly higher risk of orthostatic hypotension-related syncope, regardless of daily dose. Other drug classifications such as opioids, benzodiazepines, and antipsychotic medications all contribute to an increased risk of falls in the older adult population (Huang et al., 2012).

Thiazide diuretics, one of the most widely used diuretic classes, may contribute to falls through several mechanisms. Hypovolemia may occur as diuresis ensues, and hypokalemia may develop if potassium intake is inadequate. Glover and Clayton (2012) propose that thiazide-induced hyponatremia (TIH) may occur more often than suspected, and there may be a genetic component that makes some patients more susceptible to TIH. These patients may have an increased risk of subsequent adverse effects such as hypovolemia and hypotension and, thus, increased risk for falls. The authors propose that finding a genetic predisposition to TIH would lead to pharmacogenetic profiling and safer diuretic use. Whereas diuretics are well-established as treatments for many chronic diseases, Wehling (2013) suggests that they are overused, especially in the absence of evidence-based studies of their use in the older adult. He proposes that because of significant adverse effects such as falls, confusion, and the development of diabetes, as well as higher mortality rates associated with diuretic use in the older adult, other drug classes such as renin-angiotensin inhibitors and calcium channel blockers should be used before diuretics are considered.

Implications
Older adult patients receiving diuretic therapy need frequent and careful monitoring for the development of orthostatic hypotension that may cause syncope, including the use of postural blood pressure monitoring. Frequent monitoring of electrolyte levels, especially sodium and potassium, may detect early depletion that increases the risk of hypotension and falls. Assisting the patient with ambulation after ensuring that blood pressure is stable; teaching the patient, family members, or caregivers to monitor the blood pressure before activities; and ensuring that the patient remains adequately but not overly hydrated are safety measures that may prevent falls related to syncope caused by a drop in blood pressure. If significant changes in postural blood pressure readings are noted, the nurse should consult with the health care provider and a change in medication strategies may be warranted.

Critical Thinking Questions
Many older adults have concurrent medical conditions that increase their risk of polypharmacy and for developing hypotension and complications from diuretic therapy. List at least five drug classifications that may be used to treat other conditions in the older adult, increasing fall risk.

See Answer to Critical Thinking Questions on student resource website.

to speed the renal excretion of a drug that has been overdosed or a toxin that has been accidentally ingested. Doses of the loop diuretics are listed in Table 32.4.

The rapid excretion of large amounts of fluid has the potential to produce serious adverse effects, including dehydration and electrolyte imbalances. Signs of dehydration include thirst, dry mouth, weight loss, and headache. Dizziness and fainting can result from the fall in blood pressure caused by the rapid fluid loss. Potassium depletion can be serious and result in dysrhythmias. Potassium supplements are often prescribed concurrently with these diuretics to prevent hypokalemia. Potassium loss is of particular concern to those concurrently taking digoxin (Lanoxin), because hypokalemia predisposes these patients to dysrhythmias. With large doses, significant loss of sodium, magnesium, and calcium is possible. Continuous use of loop diuretics in postmenopausal women may affect bone metabolism due to excessive calcium loss. Loop diuretics can cause gout in some patients due to hyperuricemia—the accumulation of uric acid in the blood.

Although rare, loop diuretics may cause ototoxicity, which may manifest as tinnitus, vertigo, or deafness. Use of other ototoxic drugs such as the aminoglycoside antibiotics should be avoided during loop diuretic therapy due to the potential for additive

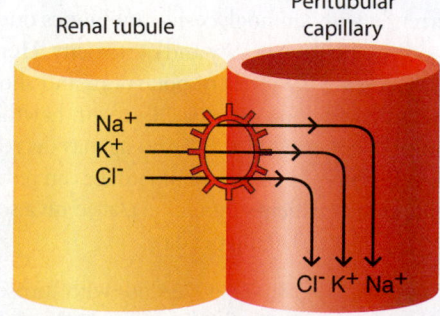

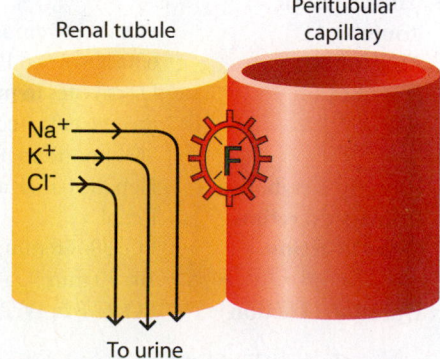

Figure 32.3 Symporter protein in the loop of Henle: (a) normal reabsorption of inhibition of the Na⁺, K⁺, and Cl⁻; (b) inhibition of symporter by furosemide causes excretion of Na⁺, K⁺, and Cl⁻.

TABLE 32.4 Loop Diuretics

Drug	Route and Adult Dose (Maximum Dose Where Indicated)	Adverse Effects
bumetanide (Bumex)	PO: 0.5–2 mg/day, may repeat at 4- to 5-h intervals if needed (max: 10 mg/day) IV/IM: 0.5–1 mg over 1–2 min, repeated every 2–3 h prn (max: 10 mg/day)	*Minor hypokalemia, orthostatic hypotension, tinnitus, nausea, diarrhea, dizziness, fatigue* <u>Serious hypokalemia, blood dyscrasias, dehydration, ototoxicity, electrolyte imbalances, circulatory collapse</u>
ethacrynic acid (Edecrin)	PO: 50–100 mg one to two times/day; may increase by 25–50 mg prn (max: 400 mg/day) IV: 0.5–1 mg/kg or 50 mg (max: 100 mg/dose)	
furosemide (Lasix)	PO: 20–80 mg in one or more divided doses (max: 600 mg/day) IV/IM: 20–40 mg in one or more divided doses (max: 600 mg/day)	
torsemide (Demadex)	PO/IV: 10–20 mg/day (max: 200 mg/day)	

Note: *Italics* indicate common adverse effects. <u>Underline</u> indicates serious adverse effects.

hearing impairment. Due to the risk for serious adverse effects, loop diuretics are normally prescribed for patients with moderate to severe fluid retention such as acute pulmonary edema, or when thiazide diuretics have failed to achieve therapeutic goals.

PROTOTYPE DRUG | **Furosemide (Lasix)**

Classification: **Therapeutic:** Antihypertensive
Pharmacologic: Loop- or high-ceiling-type diuretic

Therapeutic Effects and Uses: An established diuretic approved in 1966, furosemide is frequently used in the treatment of acute edema associated with liver cirrhosis, renal impairment, or HF because it has the ability to remove large amounts of edema fluid from the patient in a short time. When given IV, diuresis begins within 5 minutes, providing rapid relief from distressing symptoms such as dyspnea. Unlike the thiazide diuretics, furosemide is able to increase urine output even when blood flow to the kidneys is diminished, which makes it of particular value in patients with low cardiac output or renal failure. It is also approved for HTN, although it is not a preferred drug for this indication because of its short half-life and potential for serious adverse effects.

Mechanism of Action: Furosemide prevents the reabsorption of sodium and chloride by blocking the Na^+-K^+-$2Cl^-$ symporter in the loop of Henle. Because this is the region of the nephron that normally filters the bulk of sodium, furosemide can exert a profound diuresis. The extensive diuresis results in the increased urinary excretion of sodium, chloride, potassium, and hydrogen ions.

Pharmacokinetics:

Route(s)	PO, IV, intramuscular (IM)
Absorption	60% absorbed PO
Distribution	Distributes to most tissues; crosses the placenta; secreted in breast milk; 95% bound to plasma protein
Primary metabolism	Hepatic (small amounts)
Primary excretion	Renal
Onset of action	PO: 30–60 min; IV: 5 min; IM: 10–30 min
Duration of action	PO: 6–8 h; IV: 2 h; IM: 4–8 h

Adverse Effects: The greatest concerns during furosemide therapy are excessive fluid loss and electrolyte imbalances. Hypovolemia may cause orthostatic hypotension and syncope. Imbalances may occur in any or all electrolytes, causing symptoms such as tachycardia, dysrhythmias, nausea, and vomiting. Ototoxicity is rare but may result in permanent hearing deficit. Hyperuricemia caused by the drug may cause exacerbations of gout. In patients with hypokalemia and hypochloremia, furosemide may induce metabolic alkalosis. **Black Box Warning:** Furosemide is a potent diuretic that, if given in excessive amounts, may lead to profound diuresis with water and electrolyte depletion. Careful medical supervision is required.

Contraindications/Precautions: Contraindications include hypersensitivity to furosemide or sulfonamide antibiotics, anuria, hepatic coma, or severe fluid or electrolyte depletion. Due to its high potency, fluid loss must be carefully monitored to avoid possible dehydration and hypotension. Any preexisting hypovolemia or hypotension should be corrected before furosemide therapy is initiated. Because loop diuretics can increase blood glucose, serum glucose levels should be assessed in patients with diabetes mellitus.

Drug Interactions: Hypokalemia from the use of furosemide may cause dysrhythmias in patients taking digoxin; therefore, combination therapy with furosemide and digoxin should be avoided or carefully monitored. Concurrent use with corticosteroids, amphotericin B, or other potassium-depleting drugs can result in hypokalemia. When given with lithium, elimination of lithium is decreased, causing a higher risk of toxicity. Furosemide may diminish the hypoglycemic effects of sulfonylureas and insulin. Concurrent use with NSAIDs can result in a diminished diuretic effect. Additive hypotension will occur if furosemide is given concurrently with antihypertensives, including other diuretics. Use of ethanol should be restricted because it may add to the hypotensive and diuretic actions of furosemide. Furosemide should not be used concurrently with aminoglycoside antibiotics due to the possibility of additive nephrotoxicity and ototoxicity. **Herbal/Food:** Oral aloe can decrease the levels of potassium and should not be used concurrently with loop diuretics. Use with hawthorn could result in additive hypotensive effects. Ginseng may decrease the effectiveness of loop diuretics. High sodium intake can reduce the effectiveness of diuretics; patients should be placed on a sodium-restricted intake of 1,500 to 2,300 mg per day.

Treatment of Overdose: Overdose with furosemide can result in serious hypotension, fluid loss, and electrolyte imbalances. Treatment is supportive with replacement of fluids and electrolytes and the possible administration of a vasopressor.

Pregnancy: Category C.

Nursing Responsibilities: Key nursing implications for patients receiving furosemide are included in the Nursing Practice Application for Patients Receiving Pharmacotherapy with Diuretics.

Drugs Similar to Furosemide (Lasix)

Furosemide is the most commonly prescribed drug in this class. Other loop diuretics include bumetanide, ethacrynic acid, and torsemide.

Bumetanide (Bumex): Approved in 1983, bumetanide is indicated for ascites and the treatment of peripheral edema, usually associated with HF or renal failure. This drug is available by the PO, IV, and intramuscular (IM) routes and is 40 times more potent than furosemide but has a shorter duration of action. It may be used in acute clinical situations when furosemide has proven ineffective in patients with severe renal impairment. Like furosemide, bumetanide can cause electrolyte imbalances, hypotension, and dehydration. Unlike furosemide and torsemide, bumetanide is not approved for HTN, although it may be used off-label for that indication. This drug is pregnancy category C.

Ethacrynic acid (Edecrin): Approved in 1967, ethacrynic acid is indicated for the treatment of edema, usually associated with heart, liver, or renal failure. Given by either the oral or IV route, ethacrynic acid is the only loop diuretic that does not contain a sulfur group in its structure; thus it can safely be used in patients allergic to sulfonamides. Of the loop diuretics, ethacrynic acid causes the most severe hearing loss, which may be irreversible. The patient must be carefully monitored to prevent excessive electrolyte and fluid losses. Although ethacrynic acid is not approved for HTN, it may be prescribed off-label for this indication. This drug is pregnancy category B.

Torsemide (Demadex): Approved in 1993, torsemide is indicated for the treatment of HTN and edema, usually associated with heart, liver, or renal failure. Given by either the oral or IV route, torsemide is twice as potent as furosemide and has a longer half-life, which offers the advantage of once-a-day dosing. The incidence of ototoxicity with torsemide is very low, and the risk of hypokalemia is less than that of other drugs in this class. At higher doses, however, torsemide carries the same potential risks as furosemide and other loop diuretics, including electrolyte imbalances and hypovolemia. Torsemide is contraindicated in patients with sensitivity to sulfonylureas. This drug is pregnancy category B.

Thiazide and Thiazide-Like Diuretics

32.6 The thiazides are the most commonly prescribed class of diuretics.

The thiazides comprise the largest and most commonly prescribed class of diuretics. Like the loop diuretics, the thiazides block a symport protein in the renal tubule wall that is responsible for reabsorbing sodium and chloride ions from the filtrate. However, the thiazides block a different symport protein and in a different location than the loop diuretics. The thiazides act on the Na^+Cl^- symporter in the distal tubule to block Na^+ reabsorption and increase K^+ and water excretion. The thiazides are less effective than the loop diuretics because over 90% of the Na^+ has already been reabsorbed by the time the filtrate reaches the distal tubule. There are simply fewer Na^+ to block; thus the maximum diuresis produced by thiazides is less than the loop diuretics.

The primary indication for thiazide diuretics is the treatment of mild to moderate HTN. Mild HTN can often be controlled with only a thiazide diuretic, whereas moderate to severe HTN requires two or more antihypertensive agents. Thiazides are also indicated for edema due to mild to moderate heart, liver, and renal failure. They are not effective in patients with severe organ impairment because their ability to produce a diuresis diminishes as blood flow through the kidneys is reduced. Doses of the thiazide diuretics are listed in Table 32.5.

Thiazides are available only by the PO route with the exception of chlorothiazide (Diuril, Diurigen), which may be administered parenterally. All the thiazide diuretics have equivalent effectiveness and safety profiles. They differ, however, in their potency and duration of action. For example, metolazone (Zaroxolyn) is 10 times more potent than hydrochlorothiazide (Microzide). At therapeutic doses all thiazides produce the same level of diuresis.

Three drugs in Table 32.5, chlorthalidone (Hygroton), indapamide (Lozol), and metolazone (Zaroxolyn), are not true thiazides because they do not contain the two-ring structure that chemically defines a thiazide. However, these drugs block the same symport protein and have the same pharmacologic effects as thiazides. They are sometimes called "thiazide-like" and are always considered along with the true thiazides because of their similar mechanism of action, indications, and adverse effects.

The adverse effects of thiazides are similar to those of the loop diuretics, though their frequency is less and they do not cause ototoxicity. Dehydration and excessive loss of sodium, potassium, or chloride ions may occur with overtreatment: Hypokalemia and hypochloremia can cause metabolic alkalosis. Concurrent therapy with digoxin requires careful monitoring to avoid dysrhythmias caused by excessive potassium loss. Potassium supplements are sometimes prescribed during thiazide therapy to prevent hypokalemia. Patients with diabetes should be aware that thiazide diuretics sometimes increase blood glucose levels. Like the loop diuretics, thiazides can increase serum levels of uric acid, although this is only clinically significant in patients with a history of gout.

CONNECTIONS ‹ Community-Oriented Practice

‹ Diuretics: A Banned Substance?

Diuretics are included in the banned substance list by the International Olympic Committee (IOC) and the World Anti-Doping Agency (WADA, 2014) except under highly regulated use for clinical conditions. Elite athletes seeking a competitive edge may use diuretics to help achieve rapid weight loss to meet specific weight categories in some sports and to mask the presence of other banned substances by reducing their concentration in urine by increasing urine volume, or to alter urine pH and inhibiting urinary excretion of acidic or basic drugs. Hydrochlorothiazide and furosemide are the most commonly detected diuretics, although all classifications have also been detected (Cadwallader, de la Torre, Tieri, & Botrè, 2010).

TABLE 32.5   Thiazide and Thiazide-Like Diuretics

Drug	Route and Adult Dose (Maximum Dose Where Indicated)	Adverse Effects
Short Acting		
chlorothiazide (Diuril)	PO: 250 mg–1 g/day once or twice daily in divided doses IV: 250 mg–1 g/day in one to two divided doses (max: 2 g/day)	*Minor hypokalemia, fatigue* Serious hypokalemia, electrolyte depletion, dehydration, hypotension, hyponatremia, hyperglycemia, coma, blood dyscrasias
hydrochlorothiazide (Microzide)	PO: 25–100 mg/day as single or divided dose (max: 50 mg/day for HTN; 100 mg/day for edema)	
Intermediate Acting		
bendroflumethiazide and nadolol (Corzide)	PO: 1 tablet/day (40–80 mg nadolol and 5 mg bendroflumethiazide)	
metolazone (Zaroxolyn)	PO: 2.5–10 mg once daily (max: 20 mg/day)	
Long Acting		
chlorthalidone (Hygroton)	PO: 50–100 mg/day (max: 50 mg/day for HTN; 200 mg/day for edema)	
indapamide (Lozol)	PO: 1.25–2.5 mg once daily (max: 5 mg/day)	
methyclothiazide (Enduron)	PO: 2.5–5 mg once daily (max: 5 mg/day for HTN; 10 mg/day for edema)	

Note: Italics indicate common adverse effects. Underline indicates serious adverse effects.

PROTOTYPE DRUG   Hydrochlorothiazide (Microzide)

Classification: Therapeutic: Antihypertensive
Pharmacologic: Thiazide-type diuretic

Therapeutic Effects and Uses: Approved in 1959, hydrochlorothiazide (sometimes abbreviated HCTZ) is the most widely prescribed diuretic for HTN. Like many diuretics, it produces few adverse effects and is effective at producing a 10- to 20-mmHg reduction in blood pressure. Patients with severe HTN or a compelling condition such as HF, postmyocardial infarction (post-MI), high risk for coronary artery disease, diabetes, chronic kidney disease, or recurrent stroke prevention may require the addition of a second drug from a different class to control the disease.

Hydrochlorothiazide is approved to treat ascites, edema, HF, HTN, and nephrotic syndrome. Off-label indications include premenstrual syndrome (PMS), diabetes insipidus, hypercalciuria, and nephrolithiasis. Hydrochlorothiazide is the most common agent found in fixed-dose combination drugs for HTN.

Mechanism of Action: Hydrochlorothiazide acts on the distal tubule to decrease the reabsorption of Na^+. This results in less water reabsorption, increased diuresis, and removal of edema fluid. Blood volume decreases and blood pressure falls. Increasing the amount of sodium in the distal tubule also increases potassium excretion via a sodium–potassium exchange mechanism.

Pharmacokinetics:

Route(s)	PO
Absorption	Variable; incompletely absorbed
Distribution	Distributed to most tissues; crosses the placenta and is secreted in breast milk
Primary metabolism	Not metabolized
Primary excretion	Renal
Onset of action	2 h; peak effect: 4 h
Duration of action	6–12 h; half-life: 45–120 min

Adverse Effects: Hydrochlorothiazide is generally well tolerated and exhibits few serious adverse effects. Hypotension may cause dizziness or headache. Electrolyte imbalances such as hypochloremia, hypomagnesemia, hypokalemia, and hyponatremia may occur. Dysrhythmias due to hypokalemia may be serious if not prevented by maintaining normal serum potassium levels, usually by the administration of potassium supplements during therapy. Hydrochlorothiazide may precipitate gout attacks due to its tendency to cause hyperuricemia. Blood dyscrasias such as leukopenia, agranulocytosis, and aplastic anemia are rare, though serious, adverse effects.

Contraindications/Precautions: Contraindications include anuria and prior hypersensitivity to thiazide diuretics or sulfonamide antibiotics. Because hydrochlorothiazide can cause glycosuria and hyperglycemia, serum glucose levels must be carefully monitored in patients with diabetes. Preexisting hypovolemia or hypotension should be corrected before thiazide therapy is initiated because diuretics can worsen these conditions. Hydrochlorothiazide should not be used in neonates with jaundice because it can cause hyperbilirubinemia.

Drug Interactions: When given concurrently with other antihypertensives, additive effects on blood pressure usually occur. Thiazides may reduce the effectiveness of anticoagulants, sulfonylureas, and antidiabetic drugs, including insulin. Cholestyramine and colestipol bind to and decrease the absorption of HCTZ, thus reducing its effectiveness. Hydrochlorothiazide increases the risk of renal toxicity from NSAIDs. Corticosteroids and amphotericin B increase potassium loss when given with HCTZ. Hypokalemia caused by HCTZ may increase digoxin toxicity and the possibility of dysrhythmias. Hydrochlorothiazide decreases the excretion of lithium and can lead to lithium toxicity. Because thiazides decrease the renal excretion of calcium, concurrent administration with calcium supplements may lead to hypercalcemia. **Herbal/Food**: Ginkgo biloba may produce a paradoxical increase in blood pressure. Oral aloe can decrease levels of potassium and should not be used concurrently with thiazide diuretics. Use with hawthorn could result in additive hypotensive effects. High sodium intake can reduce the effectiveness of diuretics; patients should be placed on a sodium-restricted diet of 1,500 to 2,300 mg per day.

Treatment of Overdose: Overdose is manifested as electrolyte depletion, which is treated with infusions of fluids containing electrolytes. Infusion of fluids also prevents dehydration and hypotension.

Pregnancy: Category B.

Nursing Responsibilities: Key nursing implications for patients receiving hydrochlorothiazide are included in the Nursing Practice Application for Patients Receiving Pharmacotherapy with Diuretics.

Drugs Similar to Hydrochlorothiazide (Microzide)

Many thiazide and thiazide-like diuretics are available. They may be grouped into subclasses based on their relative duration of action.

Short-acting thiazides: This group includes chlorothiazide (Diuril) and hydrochlorothiazide (Microzide). These drugs have a rapid onset of 1 to 2 hours with a duration of action of 6 to 12 hours. Chlorothiazide is available by the IV route for patients who are unable to take PO thiazides.

Intermediate-acting thiazides: This group includes metolazone (Zaroxolyn) and Corzide, a fixed-dose combination of bendro-flumethiazide (a thiazide) with nadolol (a beta-adrenergic blocker). These drugs have an onset time of about 2 hours with a duration of action of 12 to 24 hours.

Long-acting thiazides: This group includes chlorthalidone (Hygroton), indapamide (Lozol), and methyclothiazide (Enduron). These drugs have a 2-hour onset with a duration of action ranging from 24 to 72 hours.

CONNECTION Checkpoint 32.3

The use of lithium is often contraindicated when a patient is taking diuretics. From what you learned in Chapter 19, identify the indications for lithium and explain how the use of a diuretic can lead to lithium toxicity. *See Answer to Connection Checkpoint 32.3 on student resource website.*

Potassium-Sparing Diuretics

32.7 Potassium-sparing diuretics have low effectiveness but can help prevent hypokalemia.

As discussed in Sections 32.5 and 32.6, hypokalemia is a potentially serious adverse effect of the loop and thiazide diuretics. The therapeutic advantage of the potassium-sparing diuretics is that increased diuresis can be obtained without lowering blood potassium levels. The potassium-sparing diuretics are listed in Table 32.6. There are two distinct subclasses of potassium-sparing diuretics: sodium ion channel inhibitors and aldosterone antagonists.

Sodium ion channel inhibitors: In the distal tubule, Na^+ is reabsorbed from the filtrate through sodium ion channels. As the sodium ion in the filtrate travels across the renal tubule cell and returns to the bloodstream, potassium ion moves in the opposite direction. In other words, as sodium ion is reabsorbed, potassium ion is secreted.

Triamterene (Dyrenium) and amiloride (Midamor) block the Na^+ channel, causing sodium to stay in the filtrate. Because water always follows sodium ions, additional water remains in the filtrate and ultimately leaves in the urine. When the sodium ion channel is blocked, another important action occurs: Potassium ion is not secreted to the filtrate. The body, therefore, does not lose potassium, as is the case with the thiazide and loop diuretics. Because most of the sodium ion has already been removed before the filtrate reaches the distal tubule, these potassium-sparing diuretics produce only a mild diuresis. Drugs in this class are rarely prescribed alone, but they may be used in combination with thiazide or loop diuretics to minimize loss of potassium ions in the pharmacotherapy of HTN or edema.

Aldosterone antagonists: Aldosterone is the primary mineralocorticoid hormone secreted by the adrenal gland. The physiological targets, or membrane receptors (MRs), for aldosterone are located in the distal tubule and collecting ducts of the nephron. Once bound to its receptors, the MR–aldosterone complex causes the renal tubule cells to synthesize more Na^+ channels, thereby allowing for more reabsorption of Na^+ from the filtrate. Simply stated, aldosterone increases sodium reabsorption.

Spironolactone (Aldactone) and eplerenone (Inspra) prevent the formation of the MR–aldosterone complex and are called aldosterone antagonists. By blocking the actions of aldosterone,

TABLE 32.6 Potassium-Sparing Diuretics		
Drug	**Route and Adult Dose (Maximum Dose Where Indicated)**	**Adverse Effects**
Sodium Channel Inhibitors		
amiloride (Midamor)	PO: 5–10 mg/day (max: 20 mg/day)	*Minor hyperkalemia, headache, fatigue, gynecomastia (spironolactone)*
triamterene (Dyrenium)	PO: 50–100 mg bid (max: 300 mg/day)	
Aldosterone Antagonists		<u>Dysrhythmias (from hyperkalemia), dehydration, hyponatremia, agranulocytosis, and other blood dyscrasias</u>
eplerenone (Inspra)	PO: 25–50 mg once daily (max: 100 mg/day for HTN; 50 mg/day for HF)	
spironolactone (Aldactone)	PO: 25–100 mg one to two times/day (max: 400 mg/day)	

Note: Italics indicate common adverse effects. <u>Underline</u> indicates serious adverse effects.

these drugs enhance the excretion of sodium and the retention of potassium. Like the sodium ion channel inhibitors, spironolactone and eplerenone produce only a weak diuresis, and they are normally combined with drugs from other classes when treating HTN or edema. Spironolactone has also been found to significantly reduce mortality in patients with HF and, because of this important beneficial effect, its use has increased. The aldosterone antagonists are also used to treat hyperaldosteronism, a rare disorder in which a tumor of the adrenal gland secretes large amounts of aldosterone.

Using potassium supplements or adding potassium-rich foods to the diet when taking these medications may lead to life-threatening hyperkalemia. Signs and symptoms of hyperkalemia include muscle weakness, ventricular tachycardia, or fibrillation. Other minor adverse effects of the drugs include headache, dizziness, nausea, and vomiting. Spironolactone binds to progesterone and androgen receptors, resulting in a small incidence of gynecomastia, menstrual abnormalities, and impotence. Gynecomastia, abnormal enlargement of the breasts in males, appears to be related to dosage level and duration of therapy; it may persist after the drug is discontinued. The incidence of adverse reproductive system effects is lower with eplerenone.

PROTOTYPE DRUG	Spironolactone (Aldactone)

Classification: **Therapeutic:** Antihypertensive
Pharmacologic: Potassium-sparing diuretic/aldosterone antagonist

Therapeutic Effects and Uses: Approved in 1960, spironolactone is the most frequently prescribed potassium-sparing diuretic. The most common indication for spironolactone is mild HTN. Because it does not cause potassium depletion, the drug is particularly useful in patients who are at high risk for hypokalemia. However, spironolactone does such an efficient job of retaining potassium that hyperkalemia may develop, especially if the patient is taking potassium supplements or is receiving angiotensin-converting enzyme (ACE) inhibitors. When serum potassium levels are monitored carefully and maintained within normal values, serious adverse effects from spironolactone are uncommon.

Spironolactone is approved for the management of edema and sodium retention associated with HF, nephrotic syndrome, and liver disease. It is particularly useful in treating edema or ascites in patients with hepatic cirrhosis, because it counteracts the large amount of aldosterone secreted by these patients. Spironolactone may also be used for the short-term, preoperative treatment of primary hyperaldosteronism. An off-label indication is to improve survival and reduce hospitalizations in patients with severe HF. Other off-label indications include treatment of minor edema associated with PMS, polycystic ovary, and hirsutism in females. Aldactazide is a fixed-dose combination of spironolactone with hydrochlorothiazide.

Mechanism of Action: Spironolactone acts by inhibiting the actions of aldosterone in the distal tubule and collecting ducts of the nephron. When the actions of aldosterone are blocked by spironolactone, sodium, chloride, and water excretion are increased and the body retains potassium.

Pharmacokinetics:

Route(s)	PO
Absorption	Rapid absorption; 73% absorbed
Distribution	Distributed to most tissues; crosses the placenta; secreted in breast milk; more than 90% bound to plasma protein
Primary metabolism	Hepatic and renal; converted to active metabolites
Primary excretion	Renal (40–57%) and feces (35–40%)
Onset of action	2–3 days; may take 2 weeks for maximum effect
Duration of action	2–3 days; half-life: 1.3–2.4 h for parent compound, and 18–23 h for active metabolites

Adverse Effects: Hyperkalemia induced by spironolactone can cause life-threatening cardiac dysrhythmias. Signs and symptoms associated with spironolactone-induced hyperkalemia include muscle weakness, paresthesia, fatigue, bradycardia, flaccid paralysis of the extremities, and shock. In men, spironolactone can cause gynecomastia, impotence, and diminished libido. Women may experience menstrual irregularities, hirsutism, and breast tenderness. Fertility may decrease during therapy. Agranulocytosis and other blood dyscrasias are rare adverse effects. **Black Box Warning**: Spironolactone produces tumors in laboratory animals; unnecessary use of the drug should be avoided.

Contraindications/Precautions: Contraindications include anuria, severe renal impairment, pregnancy, and hyperkalemia. Older patients and those with renal insufficiency or diabetes mellitus are at greatest risk for hyperkalemia. At high doses, spironolactone produces teratogenic effects in laboratory animals; thus it should not be used during pregnancy. A major metabolite of spironolactone is secreted in breast milk; thus this drug should not be given to lactating patients.

Drug Interactions: When combined with ammonium chloride, acidosis may occur. Aspirin and other salicylates may decrease the diuretic effect of the medication. Concurrent use with digoxin may decrease the effects of digoxin. When taken with potassium supplements, ACE inhibitors, angiotensin receptor blockers (ARBs), or the potassium salts of other drugs (such as penicillin G potassium), severe hyperkalemia and possible dysrhythmias may result. Concurrent use with other antihypertensives will result in an additive hypotensive effect. **Herbal/Food:** Licorice extract contains a substance with aldosterone-like actions and should be avoided. Use with hawthorn may result in hypotension.

Treatment of Overdose: Acute overdoses produce drowsiness, mental confusion, rash, nausea, vomiting, dizziness, or diarrhea. The most serious symptoms of spironolactone overdose are related to hyperkalemia. If severe, therapies are administered to counteract the hyperkalemia. These include IV calcium chloride, calcium gluconate, sodium bicarbonate, or the administration of glucose with rapid-acting insulin. Cationic exchange resins such as sodium polystyrene sulfonate (Kayexalate) may be administered.

Pregnancy: Category D.

Nursing Responsibilities: Key nursing implications for patients receiving spironolactone are included in the Nursing Practice Application for Patients Receiving Pharmacotherapy with Diuretics.

Drugs Similar to Spironolactone (Aldactone)

The three other potassium-sparing diuretics include amiloride, eplerenone, and triamterene.

Amiloride (Midamor): Approved in 1981, amiloride is an oral Na$^+$ channel inhibitor with weak diuretic activity whose major indication is HTN. It is also used to treat peripheral edema due to HF and to reverse thiazide-induced hypokalemia. When combined with a thiazide diuretic, additive hypotensive action is achieved, and potassium balance is maintained. It should not be used as monotherapy or in combination with other potassium-sparing diuretics because hyperkalemia may develop. Contraindications and adverse effects are similar to those of spironolactone, including a black box warning for the risk of severe hyperkalemia in patients receiving other potassium-containing drugs. Moduretic is a fixed-dose combination of amiloride and hydrochlorothiazide. Amiloride is pregnancy category B.

Eplerenone (Inspra): Approved in 2002, eplerenone is an aldosterone antagonist administered by the oral route that was initially approved for HTN. Later, post-MI management of HF was added as an indication. Two to four weeks of therapy are required to achieve maximum therapeutic effects. Eplerenone is more selective for the aldosterone receptor than spironolactone, and it has the advantage of producing a lower incidence of endocrine-related adverse effects such as gynecomastia, impotence, or menstrual irregularities. Like other drugs in this class, however, the development of hyperkalemia is a potentially serious adverse effect, especially if the drug is used concurrently with ACE inhibitors. Eplerenone is sometimes referred to as a selective aldosterone receptor antagonist. This drug is pregnancy category B.

Triamterene (Dyrenium): Approved in 1964, triamterene is an oral drug that acts by the same mechanism as amiloride and has the same indications and adverse effects. It is a relatively weak diuretic and is sometimes used to manage hypokalemia in patients who are unable to tolerate potassium supplements. Triamterene is rarely used as monotherapy and should not be used concurrently with other potassium-sparing diuretics due to the potential for hyperkalemia. Dyazide is a fixed-dose combination of triamterene and hydrochlorothiazide. This drug is pregnancy category C.

CONNECTION Checkpoint 32.4

From what you learned in Chapter 31, explain why patients who are taking an ACE inhibitor should probably not receive an aldosterone antagonist. *See Answer to Connection Checkpoint 32.4 on student resource website.*

Osmotic Diuretics

32.8 Osmotic diuretics cause diuresis by increasing the osmolality of the filtrate.

The osmotic diuretics, shown in Table 32.7, are a small class of drugs that are reserved for very specific indications. Unlike the thiazides and loop diuretics that block transport proteins, osmotic diuretics are mostly inert and act by raising the osmolality, which is a measure of the amount of dissolved particles, or solutes in a solution. This in turn increases the **osmotic pressure**, which creates a force that moves substances between compartments. Osmotic diuretics cause water to shift compartments by creating a difference in osmotic pressure across a membrane or between two body compartments.

When given IV, osmotic diuretics are filtered at the glomerulus and readily enter the renal filtrate. Once in the tubule, they remain unchanged. As normal sodium and water reabsorption progresses in the proximal tubule, the diuretic remains behind, and its concentration in the tubule begins to increase. The osmolality of the filtrate increases due to the presence of the osmotic diuretic in the tubule. This osmotic force draws water into the filtrate, resulting in increased diuresis. The influence of osmotic pressure on water movement is presented in greater detail in Chapter 33.

A second action of osmotic diuretics is their ability to raise the osmolality of the plasma. This creates an osmotic force that moves water from the intracellular and extravascular spaces to the plasma. The increased volume of water in the plasma is filtered by the kidney, resulting in enhanced diuresis. This action is

TABLE 32.7 **Miscellaneous Diuretics**		
Drug	**Route and Adult Dose (Maximum Dose Where Indicated)**	**Adverse Effects**
Carbonic Anhydrase Inhibitors		
acetazolamide (Diamox)	PO: 250–375 mg/day (max: 1,500 mg/day) IM/IV: 250–375 mg/day	*Electrolyte imbalances, fatigue, nausea, vomiting, dizziness*
methazolamide (Neptazane)	PO: 50–100 mg bid–tid (max: 300 mg/day)	<u>Dehydration, blood dyscrasias, pancytopenia, flaccid paralysis, hemolytic anemia, aplastic anemia</u>
Osmotic Diuretics		
glycerin	PO: 1–1.8 g/kg, 1–2 h before ocular surgery	*Electrolyte imbalances, fatigue, nausea, vomiting, dizziness*
mannitol (Osmitrol)	IV: 100 g infused over 2–6 h	<u>Hyponatremia, edema, convulsions, tachycardia</u>
urea (Ureaphil)	IV: 1–1.5 g/kg over 1–2.5 h	

Note: Italics indicate common adverse effects. <u>Underline</u> indicates serious adverse effects.

used to advantage in the treatment of two conditions where fluid has accumulated in extravascular spaces. For example, following a traumatic head injury, fluid accumulates in the brain, causing dangerously high intracranial pressure. Osmotic diuretics create an osmotic force that promotes the fluid to leave the brain and enter the blood, thus reducing cerebral edema. A second example is high intraocular pressure caused by excess fluid accumulation in the eye (glaucoma). Osmotic diuretics can cause the fluid to leave the eye and enter the blood, thus relieving the high intraocular pressure.

Osmotic diuretics are rarely the drugs of first choice due to their potential toxicity. Mannitol and urea are given by the IV route under controlled conditions where the patient can be closely monitored. Although as diuretics they are useful in increasing urine output, they are contraindicated in patients with severe renal impairment. The rapid movement of water from the extravascular spaces to the blood can result in severe dehydration in the tissues and cause a serious fluid overload in patients with severe HF. Electrolyte imbalances, especially hyponatremia, may occur with these agents.

| PROTOTYPE DRUG | Mannitol (Osmitrol) |

Classification: Therapeutic: Drug for renal failure
Pharmacologic: Osmotic diuretic

Therapeutic Effects and Uses: Approved in 1944, mannitol is a parenteral diuretic primarily used to increase urine output in patients experiencing oliguria from acute renal failure. In addition, by its ability to increase the osmolality of plasma, this drug is able to "pull" fluid out of extravascular spaces; thus it is used to reduce intracranial pressure following head trauma and to lower intraocular pressure in patients with acute glaucoma. Reduction in the amount and pressure of cerebrospinal fluid can occur as quickly as 15 minutes after initiating the infusion; intraocular pressure reduction may take up to an hour. Mannitol may be administered concurrently with nephrotoxic drugs such as cisplatin (an antineoplastic drug) to speed them through the kidney and reduce damage to the walls of the renal tubules.

Mannitol has nondrug uses as a sweetener and food stabilizer. When taken orally, it is absorbed so slowly that it has no effect on insulin levels, making it an alternative sweetener in foods for patients with diabetes. The drug has a laxative effect when taken in large quantities.

Mechanism of Action: Administered by the IV route, mannitol is filtered by the glomerulus of the kidney but is incapable of being reabsorbed from the renal tubule. This creates an osmotic gradient, resulting in decreased water and Na^+ reabsorption and increased diuresis.

Pharmacokinetics:

Route(s)	IV
Absorption	Does not cross biologic membranes
Distribution	Remains in extracellular space; does not cross the blood–brain barrier
Primary metabolism	Hepatic (small amounts)
Primary excretion	Renal
Onset of action	1–3 h
Duration of action	4–6 h; half-life: 100 min

Adverse Effects: Electrolyte imbalances, either deficiencies or excesses, can occur during mannitol therapy. For example, as mannitol draws fluid from the intravascular spaces, hyperkalemia or hypernatremia may occur. However, mannitol also increases the excretion of sodium and potassium ions, which can result in hypokalemia or hyponatremia. The same holds true for fluid balance. As mannitol draws fluid into the extracellular spaces, peripheral edema, HF, or pulmonary edema may occur. As diuresis progresses, the patient may become hypovolemic and dehydrated. Other adverse effects include fatigue, nausea, vomiting, dizziness, convulsions, and tachycardia.

Contraindications/Precautions: Contraindications include anuria, severe HF, organic central nervous system (CNS) disease or intracranial bleeding, severe dehydration, and shock. A test dose may be given to patients with oliguria to determine renal function. Function is considered satisfactory if urine flow is at least 30 to 50 mL/h over 2 to 3 hours following an IV test dose of 0.2 g/kg. If this response is not achieved, the kidneys are too impaired to administer a full dose of mannitol.

There is evidence that high doses of mannitol may open the blood–brain barrier by temporarily shrinking the endothelial cells that line the barrier. Should this happen, mannitol will enter the brain (bringing water with it) and increase intracranial pressure. Extreme precautions must be taken when treating patients with high intracranial pressure. Experimentally, mannitol is used to intentionally open the blood–brain barrier to deliver higher doses of various drugs, such as antineoplastic agents, directly to the brain.

Drug Interactions: Because of its intense diuretic effect, mannitol can increase the excretion of many drugs. This results in a decreased effect for drugs such as lithium, imipramine, salicylates, barbiturates, and potassium supplements. **Herbal/Food**: Unknown.

Pregnancy: Category C.

Treatment of Overdose: Overdose will result in a shift of fluid to the vascular compartment, resulting in HF and pulmonary edema. Intense diuresis may cause significant electrolyte imbalances, especially hyponatremia. There is no specific antidote and treatment is supportive to the presenting symptoms.

Nursing Responsibilities: Key nursing implications for patients receiving mannitol are included in the Nursing Practice Application for Patients Receiving Pharmacotherapy with Diuretics.

Drugs Similar to Mannitol (Osmitrol)

Other osmotic diuretics include glycerin and urea. Drugs in this class are infrequently used.

Glycerin: Also known as glycerol, glycerin is an osmotic diuretic given for a large number of indications. When given by the oral route, glycerin creates an osmotic gradient like mannitol that can reduce intraocular and intracranial pressure. As a laxative suppository, glycerin draws water into the colon, creating more bulk and promoting defecation. It is used in a variety of over-the-counter (OTC) products as an emollient or lubricant, including toothpaste, shaving cream, hair products, soaps, and skin care products. Like mannitol, it tastes sweet and is used as a food additive to sweeten and keep products moist. Contraindications for oral use include hypovolemia, HF, or intestinal obstruction. This drug is pregnancy category C.

Urea (Ureaphil): Urea is a small molecule that is a natural waste product of nitrogen metabolism in the body. Approved in 1966 as a drug, it is given IV to create an osmotic gradient that reduces cerebral edema and intraocular pressure. Contraindications and adverse effects are similar to those of mannitol. It is also available topically to rehydrate the skin or to remove excess keratin. Urea has a large number of industrial uses, including its use in fertilizer, hair products, deicing agents, and bath oils, and even as a flavor enhancer in cigarettes. This drug is pregnancy category C.

Carbonic Anhydrase Inhibitors

32.9 Carbonic anhydrase inhibitors are weak diuretics that have specific indications.

Carbonic anhydrase is an essential enzyme that helps regulate acid–base balance in the body. Carbonic anhydrase converts CO_2 to carbonic acid (H_2CO_3), which immediately dissociates to bicarbonate ion (HCO_3^-). Note that these reactions are reversible.

$$CO_2 + H_2O \longleftrightarrow H_2CO_3 \longleftrightarrow HCO_3^- + H^+$$

Carbonic acid is present in multiple tissues. In red blood cells, it converts CO_2 (an acidic, poorly soluble gas) to bicarbonate, which can be transported to the lungs, reconverted to CO_2, and exhaled. In the mucosa of the stomach, carbonic anhydrase is responsible for forming gastric acid (H^+). For this chapter, the most important action of carbonic anhydrase occurs in the renal tubule cells.

In the kidney tubules, carbonic anhydrase is necessary for the formation and reabsorption of bicarbonate ion, which is essential for maintaining proper acid–base balance. Sodium ions are reabsorbed with bicarbonate ion in the proximal tubule using a symporter protein.

Several drugs that inhibit carbonic anhydrase are available. Blocking carbonic anhydrase prevents bicarbonate formation and reabsorption in the renal tubule. Without bicarbonate ion, sodium reabsorption does not occur, more water remains in the filtrate, and diuresis is promoted. The reduction in plasma bicarbonate eventually causes metabolic acidosis, which tends to reverse the diuretic action of this drug.

Although once used as diuretics, the carbonic anhydrase inhibitors are now rarely prescribed for that purpose because they produce only a weak, short-lived diuresis and can contribute to metabolic acidosis. Carbonic anhydrase inhibitors that are given by the oral route include acetazolamide (Diamox) and methazolamide (Neptazane). Methazolamide is only approved for reducing intraocular pressure in patients with open-angle glaucoma. Acetazolamide (Diamox), also used to decrease intraocular fluid pressure, has several other indications. Two drugs in this class, dorzolamide (Trusopt) and brinzolamide (Azopt), are administered topically to the eye for open-angle glaucoma. The antiglaucoma drugs in this class are discussed in Chapter 74.

PROTOTYPE DRUG	Acetazolamide (Diamox)

Classification: Therapeutic: Drug for edema, antiglaucoma drug
Pharmacologic: Carbonic anhydrase inhibitor

Therapeutic Effects and Uses: Given by either the oral or parenteral route, acetazolamide produces a mild diuresis and

is occasionally used to reduce edema fluid in patients with HF. An older drug approved in 1953, it has largely been replaced by thiazide diuretics.

Acetazolamide also has applications as an anticonvulsant for treating absence seizures and in treating motion sickness. It has been used to acclimatize people to high altitudes to prevent or treat acute mountain sickness. It accomplishes this by increasing the renal excretion of bicarbonate, which accumulates in the body because of the hyperventilation that occurs at high altitude. Acetazolamide is effective in treating open-angle glaucoma and for preoperative treatment of acute closed-angle glaucoma, although it is not a preferred drug for these disorders.

Mechanism of Action: Acetazolamide produces its diuretic effect by inhibiting carbonic anhydrase activity in the proximal renal tubule, causing increased excretion of sodium and bicarbonate. In the eye, the inhibition of carbonic anhydrase reduces the rate of aqueous humor formation and consequently lowers intraocular pressure.

Pharmacokinetics:

Route(s)	PO, IV
Absorption	75% absorbed when given with food
Distribution	Distributed to most tissues; crosses the placenta and is secreted in breast milk
Primary metabolism	Not metabolized
Primary excretion	Renal
Onset of action	PO: 90 min; IV: 2 min
Duration of action	PO: 8–12 h; PO extended release: 18–24 h; IV: 15 min; half-life: 2.4–5.8 h

Adverse Effects: Acetazolamide can cause various electrolyte imbalances, including hyperchloremia and hypokalemia. Gastrointestinal adverse effects include nausea, vomiting, diarrhea, and anorexia. CNS effects may occur, such as dizziness, fatigue, and numbness in the extremities, lips, or facial muscles. Metabolic acidosis may result from excess bicarbonate loss.

Contraindications/Precautions: Acetazolamide is contraindicated in patients who have hypersensitivity to sulfonamides and similar drugs such as thiazide diuretics. Other contraindications include severe renal or hepatic impairment and adrenocortical insufficiency. Patients with preexisting electrolyte imbalances such as hyponatremia, hypokalemia, or hypochloremic acidosis should be treated with caution because acetazolamide may worsen these conditions.

Drug Interactions: The potential for hypokalemia is greatest early in the course of acetazolamide therapy and is accelerated by amphotericin B and corticosteroids. Because acetazolamide alkalinizes the urine, the renal excretion of many drugs may be decreased, including tricyclic antidepressants, procainamide, amphetamines, ephedrine, and quinidine. Renal excretion of lithium and phenobarbital may be increased. High-dose aspirin therapy can compete with tubular secretory mechanisms with acetazolamide, causing the Carbonic anhydrase inhibitor to accumulate to toxic levels. **Herbal/Food:** Unknown.

CONNECTIONS Complementary and Alternative Therapies

◖Dandelion

Description
The common dandelion, *Taraxacum officinale,* is found worldwide and is considered a weed by homeowners and gardeners; however, this plant has both culinary and medicinal uses.

History and Claims
Medicinal applications of dandelion have been recorded as early as the 10th century by Arab health care providers, and the plant was introduced by the Celts when Roman legions invaded Britain. Native Americans used the plant to treat heartburn and kidney disease. Leaves of the plant are rich in vitamin A, potassium, minerals, and fiber and have been eaten raw in salads or cooked like spinach as a major nutritional source. The dandelion root has been dried and used to treat a large variety of conditions, including constipation, liver ailments, bronchitis, gout, and arthritis, although there is insufficient evidence to suggest that it is effective for these conditions (National Center for Complementary and Alternative Medicine, 2012). The plant is also sold as a diuretic to ease premenstrual fluid retention.

Standardization
Dandelion is available in tea, liquid, or tablet form. Standardization is generally based on the amount of dandelion in grams (2–12 g/day).

Evidence
Research evidence to support most uses of dandelion is lacking, and data regarding the use of dandelion as a diuretic are conflicting. When taken in moderation, dandelion is safe and is a significant source of vitamins and minerals. High doses of dandelion should be discouraged due to potential interactions with prescription medications.

Pregnancy: Category C.

Treatment of Overdose: Overdose with acetazolamide results in metabolic acidosis, which may be treated by administering sodium bicarbonate. Electrolyte depletion and dehydration are treated with infusions of fluids containing electrolytes.

Nursing Responsibilities: Key nursing implications for patients receiving acetazolamide are included in the Nursing Practice Application for Patients Receiving Pharmacotherapy with Diuretics.

Drugs Similar to Acetazolamide (Diamox)
The other oral carbonic anhydrase inhibitor is methazolamide (Neptazane), which is used as a systemic antiglaucoma drug (see Chapter 74) rather than a diuretic.

CONNECTIONS: NURSING PRACTICE APPLICATION

Patients Receiving Pharmacotherapy with Diuretics

Assessment	Potential Nursing Diagnoses*
Baseline assessment prior to administration: • Obtain a complete health history including cardiovascular disease, diabetes, pregnancy, or breast-feeding. Obtain a drug history including allergies, current prescription and OTC drugs, herbal preparations, use of digoxin, lithium, or antihypertensive drugs, and alcohol use. Be alert to possible drug interactions. • Evaluate appropriate laboratory findings such as electrolytes, glucose, CBC, hepatic or renal function studies, uric acid levels, and lipid profiles. • Obtain baseline weight, vital signs (especially blood pressure and pulse), breath sounds, and cardiac monitoring (e.g., ECG, cardiac output) if appropriate. Assess for location, character, and amount of edema, if present. Assess baseline hearing and balance. • Assess the patient's ability to receive and understand instructions. Include the family and caregivers as needed.	• *Deficient Fluid Volume* • *Fatigue* • *Decreased Cardiac Output* • *Deficient Knowledge* (Drug Therapy) • *Risk for Falls*, related to hypotension and dizziness associated with adverse drug effects • *Risk for Injury*, related to hypotension and dizziness associated with adverse drug effects • *Risk for Urge Urinary Incontinence*
Assessment throughout administration: • Assess for desired therapeutic effects (e.g., adequate urine output, decreased edema or lowered blood pressure if given for HTN). • Continue periodic monitoring of electrolytes, glucose, CBC, lipid profiles, liver function studies, creatinine, and uric acid levels. • Assess for and promptly report adverse effects: hypotension, palpitations, dizziness or lightheadedness, musculoskeletal weakness or cramping, nausea, vomiting, abdominal cramping, diarrhea, or headache. Immediately report tinnitus or hearing loss, loss of balance or incoordination, severe hypotension accompanied by reflex tachycardia, dysrhythmias, decreased urine output, or weight gain or loss over 1 kg (2 lb) in a 24-h period.	

CONNECTIONS: NURSING PRACTICE APPLICATION (continued)

Implementation

Interventions and (Rationales)	Patient-Centered Care
Ensuring therapeutic effects: • Continue frequent assessments as above for therapeutic effects: urine output is increased, blood pressure and pulse are within normal limits or within the parameters set by the health care provider. (Diuresis may be moderate to extreme depending on the type of diuretic given. Blood pressure should be within normal limits without the presence of reflex tachycardia.) • Daily weights should remain at or close to baseline weight. (An increase in weight over 1 kg (2 lb) per day may indicate excessive fluid gain. A decrease of over 1 kg (2 lb) per day may indicate excessive diuresis and dehydration.)	• Teach the patient, family, or caregiver how to monitor the pulse and blood pressure. Ensure proper use and functioning of any home equipment obtained. • Have the patient weigh self daily and record weight along with blood pressure and pulse measurements.
Minimizing adverse effects: • Continue to monitor vital signs. Take blood pressure lying, sitting, and standing to detect orthostatic hypotension. **Lifespan:** Be particularly cautious with the older adult who is at increased risk for hypotension. (Diuretics reduce circulating blood volume, resulting in lowered blood pressure. Orthostatic hypotension may increase the risk of falls and injury.)	• Teach the patient to rise from lying or sitting to standing slowly to avoid dizziness or falls. If dizziness occurs, the patient should sit or lie down and not attempt to stand or walk, until the sensation passes. • Instruct the patient to stop taking the medication if blood pressure is 90/60 mmHg or below, or is below the parameters set by the health care provider, and promptly notify the provider.
• Continue to monitor electrolytes, glucose, CBC, lipid profiles, liver function studies, creatinine, and uric acid levels. (Most diuretics cause loss of Na^+ and K^+ and may increase lipid, glucose, and uric acid levels.)	• Instruct the patient on the need to return periodically for laboratory work and to inform laboratory personnel of diuretic therapy when providing blood or urine samples. • Advise the patient to carry a wallet identification card or wear medical identification jewelry indicating diuretic therapy.
• Continue to monitor hearing and balance, reporting persistent tinnitus or vertigo promptly. (Ototoxicity of cranial nerve VIII may occur, especially with loop diuretics. **Lifespan:** Because of pharmacokinetic differences, exercise additional caution when administering diuretics to infants and very young children. Audiology and additional monitoring may be ordered.)	• Have the patient report persistent tinnitus or balance or coordination problems immediately.
• Ensure patient safety, especially in the older adult. Observe for lightheadedness or dizziness. Monitor ambulation until the effects of the drug are known. (Dizziness from orthostatic hypotension may occur.)	• Instruct the patient to call for assistance prior to getting out of bed or attempting to walk alone, and to avoid driving or other activities requiring mental alertness or physical coordination until the effects of the drug are known.
• Weigh the patient daily and report weight gain or loss of 1 kg (2 lb) or more in a 24-h period. Measure intake and output in the hospitalized patient. (Daily weight is an accurate measure of fluid status and takes into account intake, output, and insensible losses. Diuresis is indicated by output significantly greater than intake.)	• Have the patient weigh self daily, ideally at the same time of day, and record weight along with blood pressure and pulse measurements. Have the patient report weight loss or gain of more than 1 kg (2 lb) in a 24-h period. • Advise the patient to continue to consume enough liquids to remain adequately, but not overly, hydrated. Drinking when thirsty, avoiding alcoholic beverages, and ensuring adequate but not excessive salt intake will assist in maintaining normal fluid balance. • Teach the patient that excessive heat conditions contribute to excessive sweating and fluid and electrolyte loss. Extra caution is warranted in these conditions.
• Monitor nutritional status and encourage appropriate intake to prevent electrolyte imbalances. (Electrolyte imbalances may occur dependent on the type of diuretic used. Most diuretics cause Na^+ and K^+ loss. Potassium-sparing diuretics may result in Na^+ loss but K^+ increase. **Lifespan:** Monitor electrolyte levels frequently in the older adult who is at greater risk for derangement related to age-related physiological changes.)	• Instruct patients taking potassium-wasting diuretics (e.g., thiazide, thiazide-like, and loop diuretics) to consume foods high in potassium: fresh fruits such as strawberries and bananas; dried fruits such as apricots and prunes; vegetables and legumes such as tomatoes, beets, and dried beans; juices such as orange, grapefruit, or prune; and fresh meats. • Instruct patients taking potassium-sparing diuretics to avoid foods high in potassium such as above, not to use salt substitutes (which often contain potassium salts), and to consult with a health care provider before taking vitamin and mineral supplements or specialized sports beverages. (Typical OTC sports beverages, e.g., Gatorade and Powerade, may have lesser amounts of potassium but have high carbohydrate amounts that may lead to increased diuresis, diarrhea, and the potential for dehydration from the hyperosmolarity.)
• Observe for signs of hypokalemia or hyperkalemia. Use with caution in patients taking corticosteroids, ACE inhibitors, ARBs, digoxin, or lithium. Report symptoms to the health care provider promptly. (Thiazide, thiazide-like, and loop diuretics can cause hypokalemia; potassium-sparing diuretics may cause hyperkalemia. Symptoms of *hypokalemia* include muscle weakness or cramping and palpitations. Symptoms of *hyperkalemia* include irritability or anxiety, fatigue, palpitations, nausea, and abdominal cramping. Concurrent use with corticosteroids may increase the risk of hypokalemia. Concurrent use with ACE inhibitors or ARBs may increase the risk of hyperkalemia. Concurrent use with digoxin increases the risk of potentially fatal dysrhythmias and with lithium may cause toxic levels of the drug.)	• Instruct the patient to report signs and symptoms of hypokalemia or hyperkalemia immediately to the health care provider. • Teach the patient to follow recommended dietary intake of high- or low-potassium foods as appropriate to the type of diuretic taken to avoid hypokalemia or hyperkalemia.

(continued)

CONNECTIONS: NURSING PRACTICE APPLICATION (continued)

• Observe for signs of hyperglycemia. Use with caution in patients with diabetes. (Thiazide, thiazide-like, and loop diuretics may cause hyperglycemia, especially in patients with diabetes.)	• Instruct the patient to report signs and symptoms of diabetes mellitus (e.g., polydipsia, polyphagia) or elevated blood glucose to the health care provider. Patients with diabetes may need to monitor their blood glucose levels more frequently until the effects of the diuretic are known.
• Observe for symptoms of gout. (Diuretics may cause hyperuricemia, which may result in gout-like symptoms including warmth, pain, tenderness, swelling, and redness around the joints, especially great toes, hand joints, elbows, and around ears; tophi (nodules); arthritis-like symptoms; and limited movement in affected joints.)	• Instruct the patient to report signs and symptoms of gout promptly to the health care provider. • Teach gout-prone patients to increase fluid intake and to avoid shellfish, organ meats (e.g., liver, kidneys), alcohol, and high-fructose beverages.
• Observe for sunburning if prolonged sun exposure has occurred. (Many diuretics cause photosensitivity and an increased risk of sunburning.)	• Instruct patients to wear sunscreen and protective clothing if prolonged sun exposure is anticipated.
• Observe for signs of infection. (Some diuretics may decrease white blood cell counts and the body's ability to fight infection. Agranulocytosis is a possible adverse effect of diuretic therapy.)	• Instruct the patient to report any flulike symptoms: shortness of breath, fever, sore throat, malaise, joint pain, or profound fatigue.
• **Lifespan:** Assess for the possibility of pregnancy or breast-feeding before beginning the drug. (Some diuretics are pregnancy category D drugs and should not be used during pregnancy.)	• Instruct female patients who may be considering pregnancy, or are pregnant or breast-feeding, to notify their provider before starting the drug.
Patient understanding of drug therapy: • Use opportunities during administration of medications and during assessments to discuss the rationale for the drug therapy, desired therapeutic outcomes, commonly observed adverse effects, parameters for when to call the health care provider, and any necessary monitoring or precautions. (Using time during nursing care helps to optimize and reinforce key teaching areas.)	• The patient, family, or caregiver should be able to state the reason for the drug, appropriate dose and scheduling, what adverse effects to observe for and when to report them, and the anticipated length of medication therapy.
Patient self-administration of drug therapy: • When administering the medication, instruct the patient, family, or caregiver in proper self-administration of the drug, e.g., early in the day to prevent disruption of sleep from nocturia. (Utilizing time during nurse-administration of these drugs helps to reinforce teaching.)	• The patient, family, or caregiver is able to discuss appropriate dosing and administration needs.

*Nursing Diagnoses—Definitions and Classification 2015–2017. Copyright © 2014, 1994–2014 by NANDA International. Used by arrangement with John Wiley & Sons Limited.

CHAPTER

32 Understanding the Chapter

Key Concepts Summary

32.1 The kidneys are major organs of excretion and body homeostasis.

32.2 The composition of filtrate changes dramatically as a result of the processes of reabsorption and secretion.

32.3 Renal failure may significantly impact the success of pharmacotherapy.

32.4 Diuretics are used to treat hypertension, heart failure, accumulation of edema fluid, and renal failure.

32.5 The most effective diuretics are the loop diuretics that block sodium reabsorption in the loop of Henle.

32.6 The thiazides are the most commonly prescribed class of diuretics.

32.7 Potassium-sparing diuretics have low effectiveness but can help prevent hypokalemia.

32.8 Osmotic diuretics cause diuresis by increasing the osmolality of the filtrate.

32.9 Carbonic anhydrase inhibitors are weak diuretics that have specific indications.

Case Study: Making the Patient Connection

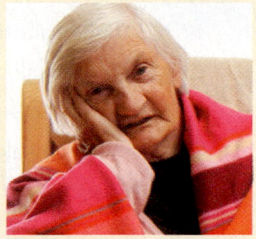

Remember the patient "Katherine Crosland" at the beginning of the chapter? Now read the remainder of the case study. Based on the information presented within this chapter, respond to the critical thinking questions that follow.

Katherine Crosland, a 79-year-old widow, has lived alone for the past 5 years. Although her son and daughters all reside in distant locations, they check on her at least weekly by telephoning. Katherine is fairly independent; however, she does not drive and is dependent on a neighbor to get her groceries and medications.

Three years ago, Katherine was hospitalized for an MI, which resulted in heart failure. She is adherent with her medications, which include digoxin (Lanoxin) 0.125 mg daily, furosemide (Lasix) 20 mg/day, and potassium supplements (K-Dur) 20 mEq daily.

Recently Katherine's neighbor went on an extended, out-of-town trip. Katherine was certain that she had enough of her medicine to last through that time. However, before the neighbor returned, Katherine discovered she had miscalculated her potassium supplement and only had enough for 10 days. Katherine figured that because the potassium was only a "supplement," she would be able to wait until her neighbor returned to get the medication refilled.

Today, she presents to the clinic with generalized weakness and fatigue. She has lost 3.6 kg (8 lb) since her last clinic visit 6 weeks ago. Her blood pressure is 104/62 mmHg, her heart rate is 98 beats/min, and she has a slightly irregular, respiratory rate of 20 breaths/min, and body temperature is 36.2°C (97.2°F). The blood specimen collected for diagnostic studies showed several outstanding findings such as a serum sodium level of 150 mEq/L and potassium level of 3.2 mEq/L. Katherine is diagnosed with dehydration and hypokalemia induced by diuretic therapy.

Critical Thinking Questions

1. Discuss fluid and electrolyte imbalances related to the following diuretic therapies:
   a. Loop diuretics
   b. Thiazide diuretics
   c. Potassium-sparing diuretics
   d. Osmotic diuretics

2. What relationship exists between this patient's diuretic therapy, digoxin therapy, and hypokalemia?

3. What patient education should the nurse provide about diuretic therapy?

See Answers to Critical Thinking Questions on student resource website.

Additional Case Study

During a recent visit to the clinic, Miles Davenport learned that his antihypertensive medication was not maintaining his blood pressure at the desired level. The nurse practitioner prescribed spironolactone (Aldactone) 50 mg twice daily in addition to his regular antihypertensive medications.

1. Discuss the mechanism of action for spironolactone.

2. Prepare a list of foods that should be eaten sparingly while taking spironolactone.

3. List the symptoms of hyperkalemia that Miles needs to know to manage his disease and medications.

See Answers to Additional Case Study on student resource website.

Chapter Review

1 The nurse is teaching a group of patients with cardiac conditions who are taking diuretic therapy. The nurse explains that individuals prescribed furosemide (Lasix) should:

1. Avoid consuming large amounts of cabbage, cauliflower, and kale.
2. Rise slowly from sitting or lying positions.
3. Count their pulse for 1 full minute before taking the medication.
4. Restrict fluid intake to no more than 1,000 mL in a 24-hour period.

2 The patient who is receiving bumetanide (Bumex) is instructed to watch for symptoms associated with electrolyte imbalances. Which condition would the patient most likely experience?

1. Hypernatremia
2. Hypokalemia
3. Hyperkalemia
4. Hypocalcemia

3 While preparing a patient for discharge, which of the following statements should the nurse include in the instructions regarding the patient's new prescription of hydrochlorothiazide (Microzide)?

1. "There are no limitations on the amount of salt and fluid intake."
2. "Ingest vitamin K-rich foods daily, such as green, leafy vegetables and broccoli."
3. "Report muscle cramps or weakness to the health care provider."
4. "Antihypertensive drugs taken concurrently may produce sleepiness."

4 Patients prescribed spironolactone (Aldactone) are often at risk for electrolyte imbalance. The nurse assesses for this adverse effect because this drug may cause the body to:

1. Retain potassium.
2. Release magnesium.
3. Excrete potassium.
4. Bind calcium.

5 Which nursing measures should be a nursing priority for a patient when first beginning mannitol (Osmitrol)?

1. Keep the urinal or bedpan available for patients with limited mobility.
2. Assess for hypokalemia and encourage foods high in potassium.
3. Monitor intake and output ratio, and weigh the patient daily.
4. Monitor blood pressure and assess for level of consciousness.

6 The nurse is monitoring a patient receiving acetazolamide (Diamox). Which acid–base imbalance is a potential risk for this patient?

1. Metabolic acidosis
2. Metabolic alkalosis
3. Respiratory acidosis
4. Respiratory alkalosis

See Answers to Chapter Review in Appendix A.

References

Axelrod, D. A., McCullough, K. P., Brewer, E. D., Becker, B. N., Segev, D. L., & Rao, P. S. (2010). Kidney and pancreas transplantation in the United States, 1999–2008: The changing face of living donation. *American Journal of Transplantation, 10*(4 Pt. 2), 987–1002. doi:10.1111/j.1600-6143.2010.03022.x

Cadwallader, A. B., De La Torre, X., Tieri, A., & Botrè, F. (2010). The abuse of diuretics as performance-enhancing drugs and masking agents in sports doping: Pharmacology, toxicology and analysis. *British Journal of Pharmacology, 161,* 1–16. doi:10.1111/j.1476-5381.2010.00789.x

Glover, M., & Clayton, J. (2012). Thiazide-induced hyponatraemia: Epidemiology and clues to pathogenesis. *Cardiovascular Therapeutics, 30*(5), e219–e226. doi:10.1111/j.1755-5922.2011.00286.x

Huang, A. R., Mallet, L., Rochefort, C. M., Eguale, T., Buckeridge, D. L., & Tamblyn, R. (2012). Medication-related falls in the elderly: Causative factors and preventive strategies. *Drugs & Aging, 29,* 359–376. doi:10.2165/11599460-000000000-00000

Mussi, C., Ungar, A., Salvioli, G., Menozzi, C., Bartoletti, A., Giada, F., . . . Brignole, M. (2009). Orthostatic hypotension as a cause of syncope in patients older than 65 years admitted to emergency departments for transient loss of consciousness. *The Journals of Gerontology, 64A,* 801–806. doi:10.1093/gerona/glp028

National Center for Complementary and Alternative Medicine. (2012). *Herbs at a glance: Dandelion.* Retrieved from http://nccam.nih.gov/health/dandelion

National Kidney and Urologic Diseases Information Clearinghouse. (2012). *Kidney disease statistics for the United States.* Retrieved from http://kidney.niddk.nih.gov/KUDiseases/pubs/kustats/index.aspx#5

Wehling, M. (2013). Morbus diureticus in the elderly: Epidemic overuse of a widely applied group of drugs. *JAMDA, 14,* 437–442. doi:10.1016/j.jamda.2013.02.002

World Anti-Doping Agency. (2014). *The World Anti-Doping Code: The 2014 prohibited list.* Retrieved from https://www.wada-ama.org/en/resources/science-medicine/prohibited-list#.VFAYf96XJUQ

Selected Bibliography

Alfie, J., Aparicio, L. S., & Waisman, G. D. (2011). Current strategies to achieve further cardiac and renal protection through enhanced renin-angiotensin-aldosterone system inhibition. *Reviews on Recent Clinical Trials, 6*(2), 134. doi:10.2174/157488711795177912

Armstrong, A. (2013). Practical tips for prescribing in renal impairment. *Nurse Prescribing, 11,* 222–227.

Brandimarte, F., Mureddu, G. F., Boccanelli, A., Cacciatore, G., Brandimarte, C., Fedele, F., & Gheorghiade, M. (2010). Diuretic therapy in heart failure: Current controversies and new approaches for fluid removal. *Journal of Cardiovascular Medicine, 11,* 563–570. doi:10.2459/JCM.0b013e3283376bfa

Daien, V., Duny, Y., Ribstein, J., Du Cailar, G., Mimran, A., Villain, M., . . . Fesler, P. (2012). Treatment of hypertension with renin–angiotensin system inhibitors and renal dysfunction: A systematic review and meta-analysis. *American Journal of Hypertension, 25,* 126–132. doi:10.1038/ajh.2011.180

Herdman, T. H., & Kamitsuru, S. (Eds.). (2014). *NANDA International nursing diagnoses: Definitions and classification, 2015–2017.* Oxford, United Kingdom: Wiley-Blackwell.

Khatib, R. (2011). Prescribing diuretics in the management of heart failure. *Nurse Prescribing, 9*(9), 436–441.

Martin, R. K. (2010). Acute kidney injury: Advances in definition, pathophysiology, and diagnosis. *AACN Advanced Critical Care, 21,* 350–356. doi:10.1097/NCI.0b013e3181f9574b

National Kidney Foundation. (2014). *Use of herbal supplements in chronic kidney disease.* Retrieved from http://www.kidney.org/atoz/content/herbalsupp.cfm

Reilly, R. F., & Jackson, E. K. (2011). Diuretics. In L. L. Brunton, B. A. Chabner, & B. C. Knollman (Eds.), *The pharmacological basis of therapeutics* (12th ed., pp. 671–720). New York, NY: McGraw-Hill.

St. Peter, W. L. (2010). Improving medication safety in chronic kidney disease patients on dialysis through medication reconciliation. *Advances in Chronic Kidney Disease, 17,* 413–419. doi:10.1053/j.ackd.2010.06.001

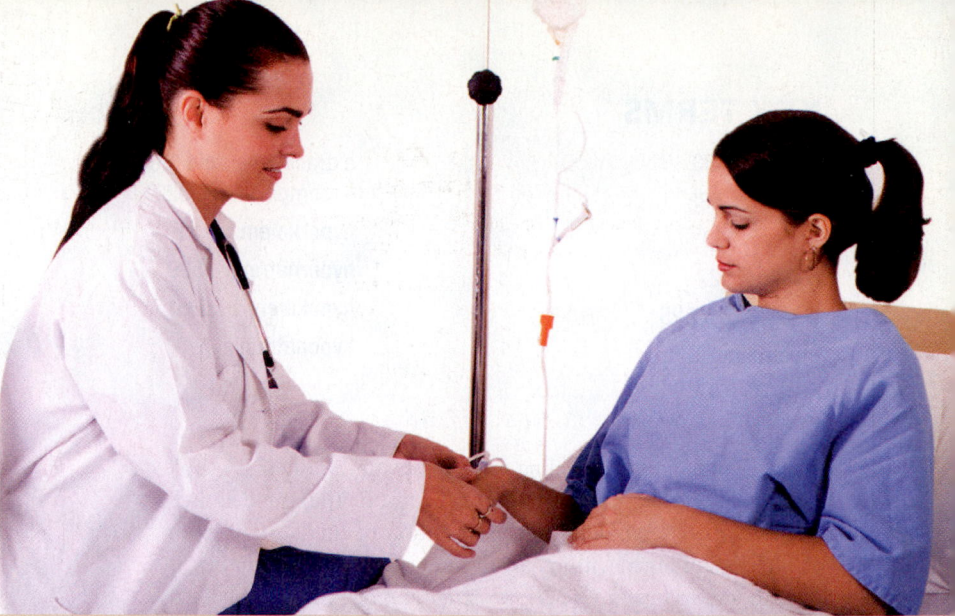

"I don't understand why I need an IV. I was told this was going to be a quick procedure."

Patient "Peggy Hover"

Pharmacotherapy of Fluid Imbalance, Electrolyte, and Acid–Base Disorders

LEARNING OUTCOMES

After reading this chapter, the student should be able to:

1. Describe the exchange of fluids that occurs among the different fluid compartments in the body.
2. Identify conditions for which intravenous fluid therapy may be indicated.
3. Explain how changes in the osmolality or tonicity of a fluid can cause water to move to a different compartment.
4. Compare and contrast the use of blood products, crystalloids, and colloids in intravenous therapy.
5. Explain the importance of electrolyte balance in the body.
6. Explain the pharmacotherapy of sodium and potassium imbalances.
7. Discuss medications used to treat acidosis and alkalosis.
8. Describe the nurse's role in the pharmacologic management of fluid imbalance, electrolyte, and acid–base disorders.
9. For each of the classes shown in the chapter outline, identify the prototype and representative drugs and explain the mechanism(s) of drug action, primary indications, contraindications, significant drug interactions, pregnancy category, and important adverse effects.
10. Apply the nursing process to care for patients receiving pharmacotherapy for fluid imbalance, electrolyte, and acid–base disorders.

CHAPTER OUTLINE

▸ **Principles of Fluid Balance**

▸ **Fluid Replacement Agents**
Blood Products
PROTOTYPE Normal Serum Albumin (Albuminar, Plasbumin, Others), *p. 525*
Crystalloids
PROTOTYPE 5% Dextrose in Water (D_5W), *p. 526*
Colloids
PROTOTYPE Dextran 40 (Gentran 40, Others), *p. 527*

▸ **Physiology of Electrolytes**

▸ **Pharmacotherapy of Electrolyte Imbalances**
PROTOTYPE Sodium Chloride (NaCl), *p. 530*
PROTOTYPE Potassium Chloride (KCl), *p. 531*
PROTOTYPE Magnesium Sulfate ($MgSO_4$), *p. 532*

▸ **Pharmacotherapy of Acid–Base Imbalances**
PROTOTYPE Sodium Bicarbonate, *p. 534*
PROTOTYPE Ammonium Chloride, *p. 535*

KEY TERMS

acidosis, 533

alkalosis, 535

buffers, 533

colloids, 527

crystalloids, 525

electrolyte, 528

extracellular fluid (ECF)
   compartment, 522

hyperkalemia, 531

hypernatremia, 529

hypokalemia, 531

hyponatremia, 529

intracellular fluid (ICF)
   compartment, 522

ion trapping, 534

osmolality, 522

osmosis, 523

tonicity, 522

Can too much pure, sparkling water hurt you? As often as people hear "drink plenty of fluids," too much (or too little) can definitely be harmful. The volume and composition of fluids in the body must be maintained within narrow limits. Excess fluid volume can lead to hypertension (HTN), heart failure, or peripheral edema, while depletion results in dehydration.

Body fluids must also contain specific amounts of essential ions or electrolytes and be maintained at particular pH values. Imbalances in electrolytes or changes in the pH of body fluids may have fatal consequences if left untreated. This chapter will examine drugs used to reverse fluid imbalance, electrolyte, or acid–base disorders.

Principles of Fluid Balance

33.1 Body fluids are exchanged between intracellular and extracellular compartments.

Body fluids travel between compartments separated by semipermeable membranes. Control of water balance in the various compartments is essential to homeostasis. Fluid imbalances are frequent indications for pharmacotherapy.

Not surprisingly, the greatest bulk of body fluid consists of water, which serves as the universal solvent in which electrolytes, minerals, and most nutrients are dissolved. Water alone is responsible for about 60% of the total body weight in a young adult. A newborn may contain 80% water, while an older adult may contain only 40%.

In a simple model, water in the body can be located in one of two places, or compartments. The **intracellular fluid (ICF) compartment**, which contains water that is inside cells, accounts for about two thirds of the total body water. The remaining one third of body fluid resides outside cells in the **extracellular fluid (ECF) compartment**. The ECF compartment is further divided into two parts: fluid in the plasma, or intravascular space, and fluid in the interstitial spaces between cells. The relationship between these fluid compartments is illustrated in Figure 33.1.

Once contained in a compartment, water and minerals do not stay there for very long. There is a continuous exchange, turnover, and mixing of fluids between compartments, as molecules travel across the membranes that separate them. For example, the plasma membranes of cells separate the ICF from the ECF. The capillary membranes separate plasma from the interstitial fluid. Although water travels freely among the compartments, processes of diffusion and active transport govern the movement of large molecules and those with electrical charges. Movement of ions and drugs across membranes is a primary topic of pharmacokinetics (see Chapter 3).

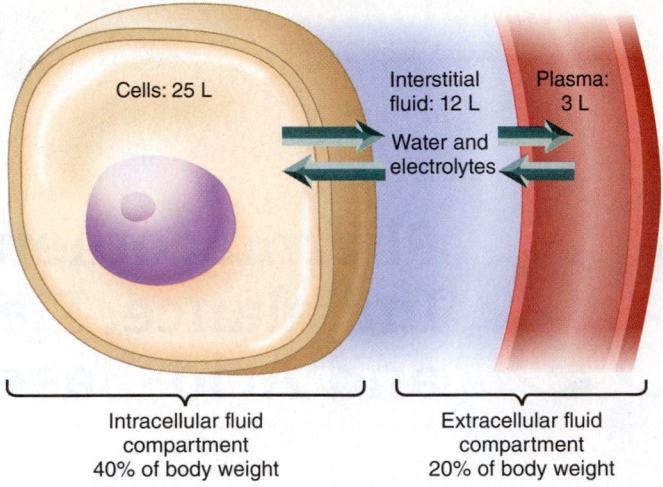

Figure 33.1 Major fluid compartments in the body.

CONNECTION Checkpoint 33.1

From what you learned in Chapter 3, what barriers does an oral drug face in moving from the gastrointestinal (GI) tract to the extracellular fluid compartment (plasma)? *See Answer to Connection Checkpoint 33.1 on student resource website.*

33.2 Osmolality or tonicity determines the movement of body fluids.

Osmolality and tonicity are two related terms central to understanding the pharmacotherapy of fluid imbalance disorders. Abnormalities in the osmolality or tonicity of a body fluid can cause significant shifts in water balance between compartments. The nurse will often administer intravenous (IV) fluids to compensate for these changes.

The **osmolality** is a measure of the number of dissolved particles, or solutes, in 1 kg (1 L) of water. In most body fluids, three solutes determine the osmolality: sodium, glucose, and urea. Sodium is the greatest contributor to osmolality due to its abundance in most body fluids. The normal osmolality of body fluids ranges from 275 to 295 milliosmoles per kilogram (mOsm/kg).

The term **tonicity** is sometimes used interchangeably with osmolality, although they are somewhat different. Tonicity is the ability of a solution to cause a change in water movement across a membrane due to osmotic forces. Whereas osmolality is a laboratory value that can be precisely measured, *tonicity* is a general term used to describe the *relative* concentration of IV fluids. The tonicity of normal plasma is considered isotonic and is used as the reference point when administering IV solutions. Solutions that are isotonic have the same concentration of solutes (same osmolality) as plasma. Hypertonic solutions contain a greater concentration of solutes than plasma, whereas hypotonic solutions have a lesser concentration of solutes than plasma.

Through **osmosis**, water moves from areas of low solute concentration (low osmolality) to areas of high solute concentration (high osmolality). If a hypertonic (hyperosmolar) IV solution is administered, water will move, by osmosis, from the cells, to the interstitial fluid compartment, to the plasma compartment. If a hypotonic solution is administered, water will move in the opposite direction, from plasma to the interstitial fluid, and eventually into cells. Isotonic solutions produce no net fluid shift. From a pharmacologic perspective, water movement between compartments following an IV infusion can be either a therapeutic effect or an adverse effect depending upon the patient's condition and the expected outcomes of the drug administration.

33.3 Overall fluid balance is regulated primarily by hormones acting upon the kidneys.

The average adult has a water intake of approximately 2,500 mL per day, most of which comes from ingested food and beverages. Water output occurs through the kidneys, lungs, skin, feces, and sweat. To maintain water balance, water intake must equal water output. Net gains or losses of water can be estimated by changes in total body weight.

The most important physiological mechanism regulating fluid intake is thirst. The sensation of thirst occurs when osmoreceptors in the hypothalamus sense that the ECF has become hypertonic. Saliva secretion diminishes and the mouth dries, motivating the person to drink fluids. As the ingested water is absorbed, the osmolality of the ECF falls and the thirst center in the hypothalamus is no longer stimulated.

In addition to triggering thirst, the hypothalamus also directs the pituitary gland to release antidiuretic hormone (ADH) when plasma osmolality rises. ADH acts directly on the distal tubules of the kidney to increase water reabsorption. This increased water in the intravascular space dilutes the plasma, thus lowering its osmolality. In high concentrations ADH, also called vasopressin, can cause vasoconstriction, which serves as an important compensatory mechanism during hypovolemic shock.

A second set of hormones assists in the maintenance of fluid balance. Through the renin-angiotensin-aldosterone system (RAAS) (see Chapter 31), the hormone aldosterone is secreted by the adrenal cortex. Aldosterone causes the kidneys to retain sodium and water in the body, thus increasing the osmolality of the ECF.

Failure to maintain adequate intake or output can lead to fluid imbalance disorders that are indications for pharmacologic intervention. Fluid *deficit* disorders can cause dehydration or shock, which are treated by administering oral (PO) or intravenous (IV) fluids. Fluid *excess* disorders are treated with diuretics (see Chapter 32). When treating fluid imbalances, the ultimate goal is to diagnose and correct the underlying cause of the disorder, while administering supporting fluids and medications to stabilize the patient.

CONNECTION Checkpoint 33.2

From what you learned in Chapter 31, name the two aldosterone antagonists and provide their indications. *See Answer to Connection Checkpoint 33.2 on student resource website.*

Fluid Replacement Agents

33.4 Dehydration may be treated with fluid volume expanders.

When fluid output exceeds fluid intake, volume deficits may result in shock, dehydration, or electrolyte loss. Left untreated, large-volume deficits may turn fatal. The following are common causes of fluid depletion:

- Loss of GI fluids due to vomiting, diarrhea, chronic laxative use, or GI suctioning
- Excessive sweating during hot weather, athletic activity, or prolonged fever
- Severe burns
- Hemorrhage
- Excessive diuresis due to diuretic therapy or uncontrolled diabetic ketoacidosis

The immediate goal in treating a volume deficit disorder is to replace the depleted fluid so that blood volume and blood pressure can be maintained. In nonacute circumstances, this may be achieved by drinking more liquids or by administering fluids via a feeding tube. In acute situations, IV fluid therapy is indicated.

Choice of IV fluid therapy depends upon the nature of the volume deficit. Careful attention must be paid to restoring normal levels of blood elements (erythrocytes, leukocytes, and thrombocytes) and electrolytes as well as fluid volume. If significant blood loss has occurred, blood products may be indicated. Loss of substantial sodium and other salts involves replacement therapy with hypertonic fluids. Excessive sweating can result in water loss that requires hypotonic IV fluids. Treating dehydration with an IV fluid with the incorrect tonicity may worsen the condition.

Fluid replacement should always be conducted in a controlled, stepwise manner. Rapid infusions can cause fluid overload, pulmonary edema, and cardiovascular stress. Vital signs and plasma electrolytes should be carefully monitored during therapy. Therapy for dehydration is summarized in Table 33.1. The three basic classes of fluid replacement agents are blood products, crystalloids, and colloids.

33.5 Transfusions of blood products are used to treat serious conditions that cannot be managed effectively by other means.

Blood products include whole blood, packed red cells, fresh frozen plasma, cryoprecipitate, immune globulins, and platelet infusions. A single unit of whole blood can be separated into its specific constituents (erythrocytes, leukocytes, platelets, plasma proteins, fresh frozen plasma, and globulins), which can be used to treat multiple patients. Indications for the various blood products are shown in Table 33.2.

TABLE 33.1	Types of Dehydration Disorders and Their Treatment		
Type	**Isotonic Contraction**	**Hypotonic Contraction**	**Hypertonic Contraction**
Fluid lost	Water and sodium in equal proportions	Loss of sodium, without a corresponding loss of water	Loss of water, without a corresponding loss of sodium
Pathophysiology	ECF remains isotonic; no net fluid shift	ECF becomes hypotonic; fluid shifts from ECF to ICF, lowering plasma fluid volume	ECF becomes hypertonic; fluid shifts from ICF to ECF, causing cellular dehydration
Causes	Vomiting, diarrhea, renal disease, diuretics	Diuretics, renal disease	Excessive sweating without replenishment, osmotic diuresis, burns
Treatment	Administer isotonic fluids; e.g., isotonic saline (0.9%)	Administer hypertonic fluids; e.g., hypertonic saline (3%)	Administer hypotonic fluids; e.g., hypotonic saline or 5% dextrose

PharmFACT

In the United States, over 9 million people donate almost 16 million pints of blood each year. More than 41,000 donations are needed every day (American Red Cross, n.d.).

Blood products may be administered to restore deficient numbers of blood cells or proteins, or to increase fluid volume depending on the clinical situation. Whole blood is indicated for the treatment of acute, massive blood loss (depletion of more than 30% of the total volume) when there is a need to replace plasma volume, as well as supply erythrocytes to increase the blood's oxygen-carrying capacity.

The administration of whole blood has been largely replaced by the use of blood components. Whole blood is rarely administered for several reasons. If the patient only needs one specific component

in blood, there is no need to expose the patient to unnecessary components that could potentially trigger an adverse effect. The supply of blood products depends on human donors and requires careful crossmatching to ensure compatibility between the donor and the recipient.

The most common complications of whole blood transfusion include febrile nonhemolytic and chill-rigor reactions. The patient experiences symptoms of an allergic reaction that include back pain and low-grade fever and chills. Dizziness, urticaria, and headache may occur during or immediately after the transfusion. Symptoms are generally mild and treated with acetaminophen (Tylenol) and diphenhydramine (Benadryl) as needed.

The most serious adverse effect from administration of whole blood is an acute hemolytic transfusion reaction. This occurs when the patient receiving the transfusion develops antibodies against

TABLE 33.2	Indications for Blood Products	
Product	**Description**	**Indication(s)**
Whole blood	Contains all blood components	Rapid, massive blood loss when safer agents are not available
Packed RBCs	One unit of packed RBCs increases hemoglobin by about 1 g/dL and hematocrit by about 3% Washed RBCs are nearly free of plasma, WBCs, and platelets and are reserved for patients who have severe reactions to plasma components	Product of choice to increase serum hemoglobin level
Fresh frozen plasma (FFP)	An unconcentrated source of all clotting factors, without platelets	Correction of bleeding secondary to factor deficiencies for which specific factor replacements are unavailable, multifactor deficiency states, and rapid warfarin reversal FFP should not be used for simple volume expansion
Cryoprecipitate	A concentrate prepared from FFP Each concentrate contains about 80 units each of Factor VIII and von Willebrand factor and about 250 mg of fibrinogen It also contains fibronectin and Factor XIII	Originally used for hemophilia and von Willebrand's disease, it is currently used as a source of fibrinogen in acute disseminated intravascular coagulation with bleeding, treatment of uremic bleeding, cardiothoracic surgery, and obstetric emergencies such as abruptio placentae
Immune globulins	Antibody preparations used to provide an immediate boost to the immune system	Rho [D] immune globulin (RhoGAM) prevents development of maternal Rh antibodies that can result from fetomaternal hemorrhage Other immune globulins are available for postexposure prophylaxis for patients exposed to certain infectious diseases, including cytomegalovirus, hepatitis A and B, measles, rabies, respiratory syncytial virus, rubella, tetanus, smallpox, and varicella
Platelets	One platelet concentrate increases the platelet count by about 10,000/mcL	Used to prevent bleeding in asymptomatic severe thrombocytopenia, for bleeding patients with less severe thrombocytopenia, for bleeding patients with platelet dysfunction due to antiplatelet drugs but with normal platelet count, for patients receiving a massive transfusion that causes dilutional thrombocytopenia, and before invasive surgery

donor red blood cell (RBC) antigens. ABO blood type incompatibility is the most common cause of this rare, though sometimes fatal, disorder. Another uncommon, though serious, adverse effect from whole blood is transfusion-related acute lung injury. This injury occurs when the patient receives donor antibodies that attack normal granulocytes in the lung. Acute respiratory symptoms develop and may be fatal.

Whole blood, despite being carefully screened, also has the potential to transmit serious infections such as hepatitis, cytomegalovirus, malaria, or HIV. In addition, platelet concentrates are stored at room temperature, which may promote the growth of bacteria in the sample. Although disease transmission from donor to recipient is possible, the risk is very low.

PROTOTYPE DRUG	Normal Serum Albumin (Albuminar, Plasbumin, Others)

Classification: Therapeutic: Fluid replacement agent
Pharmacologic: Blood product, colloid

Therapeutic Effects and Uses: Normal serum albumin is a protein extracted from whole human blood, plasma, or placental plasma that contains 96% albumin and 4% globulins and other proteins. After extraction from blood or plasma, the albumin is sterilized to remove possible contamination by hepatitis viruses or HIV. Plasma protein fraction (Plasmanate) is another albumin product that contains 83% albumin and 17% plasma globulins. Albumin is classified as both a blood product and a colloid.

The functions of endogenous albumin are to maintain plasma osmotic pressure and to bind certain substances traveling through the blood, including fatty acids, hormones, enzymes, and a substantial number of drug molecules. Binding to albumin renders these substances inactive until they become unbound.

Normal serum albumin may be administered to restore plasma volume and maintain cardiac output in patients with hypovolemic shock. It may also be administered to restore the level of blood proteins in patients with hypoproteinemia, which occurs with hepatic cirrhosis. Albumin is occasionally administered to bind and remove toxic bilirubin in hemolytic disease of the newborn. It may also offer protection against kernicterus, a toxic accumulation of bilirubin in infants that causes brain injury. It has an immediate onset of action and is available in concentrations of 5% and 25%.

Mechanism of Action: Administered IV, normal serum albumin rapidly increases the osmotic pressure of the blood and causes fluid to move from the tissues to the general circulation.

Pharmacokinetics: Because human albumin is a natural substance, it is not possible to obtain accurate pharmacokinetic values. Endogenous albumin has a half-life of 17 to 19 days.

Adverse Effects: Normal serum albumin is a natural blood product and the patient may have antibodies to the donor's albumin that cause allergic reactions. Because coagulation factors, antibodies, and most other blood proteins have been removed, such allergic reactions from albumin are rare. Signs of allergy include fever, chills, urticaria, rash, dyspnea, and, possibly, hypotension.

Contraindications/Precautions: The drug is contraindicated in patients with severe anemia or cardiac failure in the presence of normal or increased intravascular volume and in those with known allergy to albumin.

Drug Interactions: There are no clinically significant interactions. **Herbal/Food**: Unknown.

Pregnancy: Category C.

Treatment of Overdose: Protein overload may occur if excessive albumin is infused. There is no treatment for overdose.

Nursing Responsibilities: Key nursing implications for patients receiving normal serum albumin are included in the Nursing Practice Application for Patients Receiving Pharmacotherapy for Fluid and Electrolyte Imbalances.

Drugs Similar to Normal Serum Albumin (Albuminar, Plasbumin, Others)

Other blood products are described in Table 33.2 and include whole blood, packed red cells, fresh frozen plasma, cryoprecipitate, immune globulins, and platelet infusions.

33.6 Crystalloids are intravenous solutions that closely resemble the composition of extracellular fluid.

Crystalloids are IV solutions that contain electrolytes and other substances in concentrations that closely mimic the body's extracellular fluid. They are used to replace depleted fluids and to promote urine output. Crystalloid solutions are capable of quickly diffusing across membranes, leaving the plasma, and entering the interstitial fluid and ICF. Isotonic, hypotonic, and hypertonic solutions are available. Sodium is the most common crystalloid added to solutions, although some crystalloids contain dextrose, a form of glucose. Common crystalloids used to treat shock include normal saline, lactated Ringer's, Plasma-Lyte, and hypertonic saline. Selected crystalloids are listed in Table 33.3. Infusion of crystalloids will increase the total fluid volume in the body, but the compartment that is most expanded depends on the solute concentration of the fluid administered.

Isotonic crystalloids: Isotonic crystalloids expand the circulating intravascular (plasma) fluid volume, without causing major fluid shifts between compartments. This is because the osmotic pressures of the intravascular and extravascular compartments are equal. Isotonic crystalloids such as normal saline are often used to treat fluid loss due to vomiting, diarrhea, or surgical procedures, especially when blood pressure is low. The isotonic saline solutions may also be used to treat sodium deficiency (hyponatremia) because they contain sodium chloride. Because isotonic crystalloids can rapidly expand circulating blood volume, care must be taken not to cause fluid overload in the patient.

Hypertonic crystalloids: Infusion of hypertonic crystalloids raises the osmolality of the plasma and expands plasma volume by drawing water away from the cells and tissues. These drugs may be used to relieve cellular edema, especially cerebral edema. When patients are dehydrated and have hypertonic plasma, hypertonic solutions match the tonicity of the plasma as it is infused, but the dextrose in the IV solution is subsequently metabolized and the

TABLE 33.3   Selected Crystalloid IV Solutions

Drug	Tonicity
normal saline (0.9% NaCl)	Isotonic
hypertonic saline (3% NaCl)	Hypertonic
hypotonic saline (0.45% NaCl)	Hypotonic
lactated Ringer's	Isotonic
Plasma-Lyte 148	Isotonic
Plasma-Lyte 56	Hypotonic
Dextrose Solutions	
5% dextrose in water (D₅W)	Isotonic*
5% dextrose in normal saline	Hypertonic
5% dextrose in 0.2% saline	Isotonic
5% dextrose in lactated Ringer's	Hypertonic
5% dextrose in Plasma-Lyte 56	Hypertonic

*Because dextrose is metabolized quickly, the solution is sometimes considered hypotonic.

solution becomes hypotonic. This hypotonic solution then causes water to shift into the intracellular space, relieving the dehydration within the cells. Overtreatment with hypertonic crystalloids such as 3% normal saline can lead to excessive expansion of the intravascular (plasma) compartment, fluid overload, and HTN.

Hypotonic crystalloids: Hypotonic crystalloid infusions lower the serum osmolality. This causes water to move out of the plasma to the tissues and cells in the intracellular compartment; thus, these solutions are not plasma volume expanders. Hypotonic crystalloids are indicated for patients with hypernatremia and cellular dehydration. Care must be taken not to cause depletion of the intravascular compartment, which can result in hypotension, or too much expansion of the extracellular compartment, which can cause peripheral edema. Patients who are dehydrated with low blood pressure should be given normal saline; the isotonic saline will expand plasma volume and increase blood pressure while hydrating the patient. Patients who are dehydrated with normal blood pressure should be given a hypotonic solution; this infusion will hydrate cells without expanding plasma volume.

PROTOTYPE DRUG	5% Dextrose in Water (D₅W)

Classification: Therapeutic: Fluid expander
Pharmacologic: Crystalloid

Therapeutic Effects and Uses: Commonly found in concentrations of 2.5%, 5%, or 10%, dextrose solutions are infused to replace lost water and to enhance renal function. Being a form of glucose, dextrose provides nutritional value: 1 L of 5% dextrose supplies 170 calories. In addition, water is formed during the metabolism of dextrose, adding to the rehydration of the patient. D₅W is also used as a diluent for mixing other medications for IV delivery. Dextrose 50% is indicated for the emergency treatment of insulin hypoglycemia to restore blood glucose levels.

D₅W is isotonic in the container. When infused, however, the dextrose is quickly metabolized in the body, leaving only water, and

the solution becomes hypotonic. Water may then move from the plasma to the intracellular spaces, relieving cellular dehydration. Essentially, the infusion of D₅W has the same effect as administration of water. Because this may result in a lower plasma volume, patients needing fluid replacement for hypovolemia should receive lactated Ringer's or normal saline rather than D₅W.

Dextrose is added to other IV solutions, as shown in Table 33.3. It is also available in other concentrations. In all cases, the dextrose is simply added as a source of calories and nutrition.

Mechanism of Action: There are two forms of glucose in nature: L-glucose and D-glucose. Only D-glucose, also called dextrose, can be used by the human body for energy. If insulin is present, glucose (dextrose) enters cells and is converted into adenosine triphosphate (ATP), CO_2, and water.

Pharmacokinetics: Because dextrose and water are natural substances, it is not possible to obtain accurate pharmacokinetic values.

Adverse Effects: Infusion of too much D₅W may cause fluid overload, thus worsening peripheral edema, pulmonary edema, and heart failure. Hyperglycemia is possible, especially in patients with deficient insulin secretion. Pain may occur at the injection site. As D₅W dilutes the plasma, the concentration of sodium in the plasma may fall, resulting in hyponatremia. Hyponatremia in children is especially dangerous because it can lead to encephalopathy as the brain swells.

Contraindications/Precautions: Caution must be used when using D₅W in patients with heart failure or who are hyperglycemic. Patients with increased intracranial pressure should not receive hypotonic agents such as D₅W because they may worsen this condition. Dextrose is obtained from corn and patients allergic to this food may be hypersensitive to the drug.

Drug Interactions: There are no significant drug interactions with D₅W. **Herbal/Food**: Unknown.

Pregnancy: Category C.

Treatment of Overdose: Overdose is uncommon, but diuretics may be indicated in cases of fluid overload.

Nursing Responsibilities: Key nursing implications for patients receiving 5% dextrose in water are included in the Nursing Practice Application for Patients Receiving Pharmacotherapy for Fluid and Electrolyte Imbalances.

Drugs Similar to 5% Dextrose in Water (D₅W)

Other crystalloids include Ringer's solution and Plasma-Lyte.

Ringer's and Lactated Ringer's: Ringer's solution is named after the pharmacologist Sydney Ringer who created the drug in the mid-1800s. Ringer's solution is an isotonic fluid that contains sodium, chloride, potassium, and calcium ions in concentrations similar to those found in plasma. Lactated Ringer's solution also contains lactate, which serves as a chemical buffer in the blood to prevent acidosis. Lactated Ringer's is also available with 5% dextrose. Ringer's solutions are widely administered IV for fluid resuscitation following hemorrhage caused by trauma, surgery, or burns.

Plasma-Lyte: Plasma-Lyte solutions are electrolyte solutions used to correct volume and electrolyte deficiencies. The solutions also contain buffers such as lactate, acetate, or gluconate, which help to correct or prevent acidosis. Several formulations are available that differ in electrolyte composition and osmolarity. These include Plasma-Lyte-R, Plasma-Lyte-A, Plasma-Lyte 56, and Plasma-Lyte 148.

33.7 Colloids are intravenous solutions containing large molecules that remain in the blood.

Colloids are proteins, starches, or other large molecules that remain in the blood for a long time because they are too large to easily cross the capillary membranes. While circulating, they have the same effect as hypertonic solutions, drawing water molecules from the cells and tissues into the plasma through their ability to increase plasma osmolality and osmotic pressure. These drugs are sometimes called plasma volume expanders. Blood product colloids include normal serum albumin, plasma protein fraction, and serum globulins. The non–blood product colloids are dextran (40, 70, and high molecular weight) and hetastarch (Hespan). These medications are administered to provide life-sustaining support following massive hemorrhage and to treat shock as well as for the treatment of burns, acute liver failure, and neonatal hemolytic disease. Selected colloid solutions are given in Table 33.4.

PROTOTYPE DRUG	Dextran 40 (Gentran 40, Others)

Classification: Therapeutic: Plasma volume expander
Pharmacologic: Colloid

Therapeutic Effects and Uses: Dextran 40 is a synthetic polysaccharide that is too large to pass through capillary walls. It is similar to dextran 70, except dextran 40 has a lower molecular weight. Given as an IV infusion, it has the capability of doubling plasma volume within a few minutes after administration, although its effects last only about 12 hours. Cardiovascular responses include increased blood pressure, increased cardiac output, and improved venous return to the heart. Indications include fluid replacement for patients experiencing hypovolemic shock due to hemorrhage, surgery, or severe burns. When given for acute shock, it is infused as rapidly as possible until blood volume is restored.

Dextran 40 also reduces platelet adhesiveness and improves blood flow through capillaries by its ability to reduce blood

viscosity. These antithrombotic properties have led to its use in preventing deep vein thrombosis and postoperative pulmonary emboli. Dextran, however, is less effective than heparin or low-molecular-weight heparin (LMWH) in preventing thromboembolism (see Chapter 38).

Mechanism of Action: Dextran 40 acts by raising the osmotic pressure of the blood, thereby causing fluid to move from the interstitial spaces of the tissues to the blood. The larger blood volume increases cardiac output, stroke volume, blood pressure, and urinary output. Heart rate and blood viscosity decrease.

Pharmacokinetics:

Route(s)	IV
Absorption	Not absorbed
Distribution	Does not leave the vascular system
Primary metabolism	Unknown
Primary excretion	Renal
Onset of action	Several minutes
Duration of action	12–24 h

Adverse Effects: Vital signs should be monitored continuously during dextran 40 infusions to prevent HTN caused by the plasma volume expansion. Signs of fluid overload include tachycardia, peripheral edema, distended neck veins, dyspnea, or cough. A small percentage of patients are allergic to dextran 40, with urticaria being the most common sign. Anaphylaxis is possible.

Contraindications/Precautions: Dextran 40 is contraindicated in patients with renal failure because fluid overload may result. Adequate fluid intake should be ensured in patients with severe dehydration who receive dextran to prevent renal failure due to high urine viscosity. Other contraindications include severe heart failure and hypervolemic disorders.

Drug Interactions: There are no clinically significant interactions. **Herbal/Food**: Unknown.

Pregnancy: Category C.

Treatment of Overdose: For patients with normal renal function, discontinuing the infusion will reduce adverse effects. Patients with renal impairment may benefit from an osmotic diuretic.

Nursing Responsibilities: Key nursing implications for patients receiving dextran 40 are included in the Nursing Practice Application for Patients Receiving Pharmacotherapy for Fluid and Electrolyte Imbalances.

Drugs Similar to Dextran 40 (Gentran 40, Others)

The only solution similar to dextran is hetastarch.

Hetastarch: Hetastarch is a complex mixture of a nonprotein polymer of the starch amylopectin. It is a synthetic colloid with properties similar to those of 5% albumin, but with an extended duration of action. Hetastarch has a half-life of about 17 days and provides volume expansion for 24 to 36 hours. It is indicated for the treatment and prophylaxis of shock and acute edematous conditions. Hetastarch provides the same physiological actions as albumin. This drug is pregnancy category C.

TABLE 33.4 Selected Colloid IV Solutions

Drug	Tonicity
5% albumin	Isotonic
dextran 40 in normal saline	Isotonic
dextran 40 in D₅W	Isotonic
dextran 70 in normal saline	Isotonic
hetastarch 6% in normal saline	Isotonic
plasma protein fraction	Isotonic

◀ **Dehydration in the Older Adult**

Dehydration is one of the top reasons for hospitalization of the older adult. Older adults are more vulnerable to dehydration than the general population for multiple reasons including age-related changes in the body's ability to sense thirst, renal changes, and a decline in the percentage of total body water. Medications such as diuretics or laxatives may add to fluid and electrolyte depletion, and disease conditions such as a stroke may lead to the inability to seek or obtain water to drink or may impair swallowing. Dehydration may also lead to or worsen other conditions such as electrolyte imbalance, delirium, and susceptibility to infections. It is not exclusively a problem in nursing homes, and the hospitalized older adult and those living at home may also experience significant dehydration.

To prevent dehydration, simple strategies may be effective in increasing fluid intake: Leaving water within easy reach and around the house in easy-to-open bottles for the older adult living at home; providing occasional substitutes such as frozen ice pops or gelatin cups as an alternative to water; adding flavoring powders to water to make it more palatable; and encouraging the older adult to sip or drink small amounts throughout the day rather than trying to drink full cups at a time are all strategies that may prevent dehydration and the resultant need for IV hydration and hospitalization.

Electrolytes are essential to many body functions, including nerve conduction, membrane permeability, muscle contraction, water balance, and bone growth and remodeling. Levels of electrolytes in body fluids are maintained within very narrow ranges, primarily by the kidneys and gastrointestinal (GI) tract. Because electrolytes are lost due to normal excretory functions, they must be replaced by adequate intake; otherwise electrolyte imbalances will result, as shown in Table 33.5. Although imbalances can occur with any ion, sodium, potassium, and calcium are of greatest importance. The role of calcium in bone homeostasis is presented in Chapter 72.

When an electrolyte imbalance is identified, it is a sign of an underlying medical condition that needs attention. Imbalances are associated with a wide variety of acute and chronic disorders, with renal impairment being the most common cause. In some cases, drug therapy itself can cause the electrolyte imbalance. A classic example is the diuretic furosemide (Lasix), which can cause serious potassium depletion. In all cases, the therapeutic goal is to quickly correct the electrolyte imbalance while the underlying condition is being diagnosed and treated. Treatments for electrolyte imbalances depend on the severity of the problem and range from simple changes in dietary intake to rapid electrolyte infusions. In acute cases, serum electrolyte levels must be carefully monitored to prevent imbalances in the opposite direction; levels can change rapidly from hypoconcentrations to hyperconcentrations.

Physiology of Electrolytes

33.8 Electrolytes are charged substances that are essential to homeostasis.

Minerals are inorganic substances needed in very small amounts to maintain homeostasis (see Chapter 61). Minerals are held together by ionic bonds and dissociate or ionize when placed in water. The resulting ions have positive or negative charges and are able to conduct electricity, hence the name **electrolyte**. Positively charged electrolytes are called cations; those with a negative charge are anions. Electrolyte levels are measured in units of milliequivalents per liter (mEq/L).

Pharmacotherapy of Electrolyte Imbalances

33.9 Sodium balance is closely associated with water balance.

Sodium is the major electrolyte in extracellular fluid. Due to its central roles in neuromuscular physiology, acid–base balance, and overall fluid distribution, sodium imbalances can have serious consequences. Although definite sodium monitors or sensors have yet to be discovered in the body, the regulation of sodium balance

TABLE 33.5	**Electrolyte Imbalances**		
Ion	**Condition**	**Abnormal Serum Value (mEq/L)**	**Supportive Treatment***
calcium	Hypercalcemia	Greater than 11	Hypotonic fluid or calcitonin
	Hypocalcemia	Less than 4	Calcium supplements or vitamin D
chloride	Hyperchloremia	Greater than 112	Hypotonic fluid
	Hypochloremia	Less than 95	Hypertonic salt solution
magnesium	Hypermagnesemia	Greater than 4	Hypotonic fluid
	Hypomagnesemia	Less than 0.8	Magnesium supplements
phosphate	Hyperphosphatemia	Greater than 6	Dietary phosphate restriction
	Hypophosphatemia	Less than 1	Phosphate supplements
potassium	Hyperkalemia	Greater than 5	Hypotonic fluid, buffers, or dietary restriction
	Hypokalemia	Less than 3.5	Potassium supplements
sodium	Hypernatremia	Greater than 145	Hypotonic fluid or dietary restriction
	Hyponatremia	Less than 135	Hypertonic salt solution or sodium supplement

*For all electrolyte imbalances, the primary therapeutic goal is to identify and correct the cause of the imbalance.

is well understood. The normal range of serum sodium is 136 to 145 mEq/L of plasma.

Sodium balance and water balance are intimately connected. As sodium levels increase in a body fluid, solute particles accumulate and osmolality increases. Water will move toward this area of relatively high osmolality. In simplest terms, water travels toward or with sodium. The physiological consequences of this relationship cannot be overstated: As the sodium and water content of plasma increases, so does blood volume and blood pressure. Thus, sodium movement provides an important link between water retention, blood volume, and blood pressure.

In healthy individuals, sodium intake is equal to sodium output, which is regulated by the kidneys. High levels of aldosterone secreted by the adrenal cortex promote sodium and water retention by the kidneys as well as potassium excretion. Inhibition of aldosterone promotes sodium and water excretion. When a patient ingests high amounts of sodium, aldosterone secretion decreases, thus sending the excess sodium to the urine. This relationship is illustrated in Figure 33.2.

Hypernatremia: Sodium excess, or **hypernatremia**, occurs when the serum sodium level rises above 145 mEq/L. The most common cause of hypernatremia is decreased sodium excretion due to kidney pathology. Hypernatremia may also be caused by excessive intake of sodium, either through dietary consumption or by overtreatment with IV fluids containing sodium chloride or sodium bicarbonate. Overconsumption of table salt (NaCl) or processed foods with high sodium content will quickly exceed the daily amount needed by the body. Drinking too little water can cause hypernatremia due to the development of hypertonic plasma. Another cause of hypernatremia is high net water losses, such as that occurring from watery diarrhea, fever, or burns. High doses of glucocorticoids or estrogens also promote sodium retention.

A high serum sodium level increases the osmolality of the plasma, making the intravascular space hypertonic and drawing fluid from interstitial spaces and cells, thus causing cellular dehydration. Ordinarily, a small increase in serum sodium will trigger thirst. Other manifestations of hypernatremia include fatigue, weakness, muscle twitching, convulsions, altered mental status, and a decreased level of consciousness (LOC). For minor hypernatremia, a low-salt diet combined with adequate water intake may be effective in returning serum sodium to normal levels. In patients with acute hypernatremia, however, the treatment goal is to rapidly return the osmolality of the plasma to normal. If the patient is hypovolemic, infusing hypotonic fluids such as 5% dextrose or 0.45% NaCl will increase plasma volume and at the same time reduce osmolality by diluting the plasma. For the patient who is hypervolemic, diuretics may be used to remove sodium and excess water from the body.

Hyponatremia: **Hyponatremia** is the most common electrolyte abnormality in hospitalized patients and is defined as a serum sodium level of less than 135 mEq/L. Hyponatremia may occur through excessive dilution of the plasma caused by administration of hypotonic IV solutions or by high ADH secretion. Hyponatremia may also result from increased sodium loss due to disorders of the skin, GI tract, or kidneys. Significant loss of sodium by the skin may occur in burn patients and in those experiencing excessive sweating or prolonged fever. GI sodium losses may occur from vomiting,

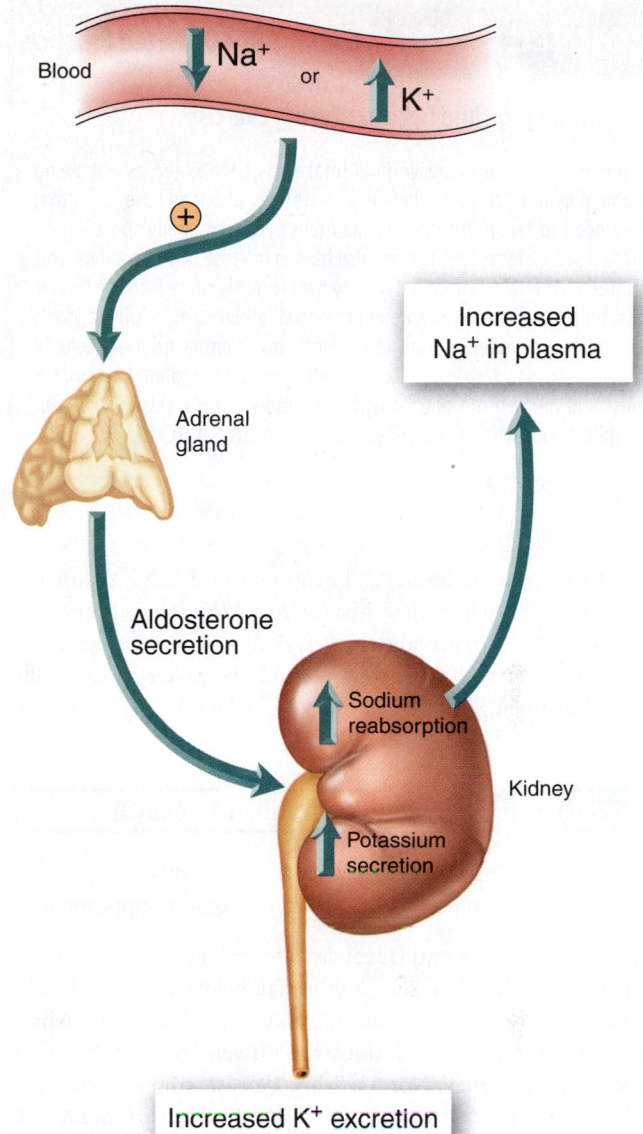

Figure 33.2 Renal regulation of sodium and potassium balance.

diarrhea, or GI suctioning, and renal sodium loss may occur with diuretic use and in certain advanced kidney disorders.

Early symptoms of hyponatremia include nausea, vomiting, anorexia, and abdominal cramping. Later signs include altered neurologic function such as confusion, lethargy, convulsions, coma, and muscle twitching or tremors. Hyponatremia caused by excessive dilution is treated with loop diuretics, which will remove the fluid overload that caused the hyponatremia (see Chapter 32). Hyponatremia caused by sodium loss may be treated with the administration of oral or parenteral sodium chloride, or with IV fluids containing salt, such as normal saline or lactated Ringer's solution.

In 2009, tolvaptan (Samsca) was approved to quickly raise serum sodium levels in hospitalized patients experiencing symptoms of hyponatremia. Tolvaptan is a vasopressin (antidiuretic hormone) antagonist that enhances water excretion. As the amount of water in the blood is reduced, the serum sodium concentration is increased. Tolvaptan carries several black box warnings. Therapy with the drug should only be conducted in a hospital

CONNECTIONS Community-Oriented Practice

◀ Maintaining Fluid Balance During Exercise

Hyponatremia from excessive fluid intake has been noted as a growing problem in athletes, particularly novice athletes who may have heard that they need to "keep drinking" to maintain hydration. Many sports drinks contain some electrolytes but are also high in fructose or other sugars. This creates a hypertonic solution that may paradoxically cause increased water loss. Unless exercise is extreme or prolonged, athletes, especially children, should be encouraged to drink when thirsty and maintain urine at a color of clear yellow, not dark yellow or colorless. Adequate fluid intake to match thirst will help ensure normal hydration and sodium levels and prevent complications such as exercise-associated hyponatremia (EAH).

where serum sodium levels can be monitored closely, because too rapid correction of hyponatremia can result in seizures, coma, and death. In patients with advanced liver disease, severe malnutrition, or alcoholism, hyponatremia should be corrected especially slowly. Treatment should be limited to 30 days due to the risk for liver injury.

PROTOTYPE DRUG   Sodium Chloride (NaCl)

Classification: Therapeutic: Drug for hyponatremia
Pharmacologic: Electrolyte, sodium supplement

Therapeutic Effects and Uses: Sodium chloride is administered for hyponatremia when serum levels fall below 130 mEq/L. The drug is available in several concentrations; the decision on which NaCl concentration to administer is driven by the severity of the sodium deficiency. Normal saline consists of 0.9% NaCl and is used to treat mild hyponatremia. When serum sodium falls below 115 mEq/L, a highly concentrated 3% NaCl solution may be infused. Other concentrations include 0.45% and 0.22%, and both hypotonic and isotonic solutions are available. For less severe hyponatremia, 1-g tablets are available.

Ophthalmic solutions of NaCl may be used to treat corneal edema, and an over-the-counter (OTC) nasal spray is available to relieve dry, inflamed nasal membranes. In conjunction with oxytocin, 20% NaCl may be used as an abortifacient late in pregnancy when instilled into the amniotic sac.

Mechanism of Action: Sodium chloride is a replacement solution for lost sodium.

Pharmacokinetics: Because sodium ions form natural electrolytes, it is not possible to obtain accurate pharmacokinetic values. The sodium ions in the drug are widely distributed and excreted by the kidneys in the same manner as endogenous sodium ions.

Adverse Effects: Patients receiving NaCl infusions must be monitored frequently to avoid symptoms of hypernatremia, which include lethargy, confusion, muscle tremor or rigidity, hypotension, and restlessness. Because some of these symptoms are also common to hyponatremia, periodic laboratory assessments must be taken to be certain that sodium values are moving toward

the normal range. When infusing 3% NaCl solutions, the nurse should continuously check for signs of pulmonary edema.

Contraindications/Precautions: This drug should not be administered to patients with hypernatremia, heart failure, or impaired renal function.

Drug Interactions: There are no clinically significant drug interactions. **Herbal/Food:** Unknown.

Pregnancy: Category C.

Treatment of Overdose: There is no specific treatment for overdose. If excess fluid accumulation has occurred, diuretics may be administered to remove excess sodium ion and water to reduce pulmonary or peripheral edema.

Nursing Responsibilities: Key nursing implications for patients receiving sodium chloride are included in the Nursing Practice Application for Patients Receiving Pharmacotherapy for Fluid and Electrolyte Imbalances.

Drugs Similar to Sodium Chloride (NaCl)

There is no other drug similar to sodium chloride.

33.10 Potassium imbalances must be quickly corrected to prevent serious cardiac consequences.

Potassium is the most abundant intracellular cation; 98% of the potassium present in the body is found inside cells, with the majority found in skeletal muscle. Potassium serves critical roles in muscular contraction and the conduction of nerve impulses.

To prevent imbalances, adequate dietary intake of potassium must be carefully balanced to potassium excretion. Patients with normal diets consume plenty of potassium for bodily functions because the mineral is abundant in fruits, vegetables, and meats.

Insulin is a key hormone for the regulation of potassium homeostasis. The uptake of potassium ion into cells is mediated by insulin. As serum potassium levels rise, the pancreas secretes additional insulin, which causes the ion to move out of the plasma and into cells, thus preventing hyperkalemia. In a typical feedback loop, as serum potassium levels fall, insulin secretion is diminished.

Acid–base imbalances may also affect potassium homeostasis. As the blood becomes acidic, the body attempts to raise plasma pH by pumping hydrogen ions (H^+) into cells. To maintain electrical neutrality, each H^+ entering the cell is exchanged for a K^+ leaving the cell. This can raise the serum potassium level, resulting in hyperkalemia. This is sometimes called a false hyperkalemia because the total body potassium is not actually increased; it has just shifted from intracellular to extracellular spaces.

Potassium ion is freely filtered at the glomerulus but is entirely reabsorbed as it travels along the kidney tubule. In the distal tubule, however, potassium is secreted back into the renal tubule and exits in the urine. Like sodium, potassium excretion is influenced by the actions of aldosterone on the kidney. In fact, the renal excretion of sodium and potassium ions is closely linked. For every sodium ion that is reabsorbed, one potassium ion is secreted into the renal tubules.

Potassium levels must be maintained within narrow limits. Both hyper- and hypokalemia are associated with fatal dysrhythmias and serious neuromuscular disorders. Because over 98% of potassium is intracellular, serum potassium may not be an accurate reflection of total body potassium. Normal adult values for serum potassium range from 3.5 to 5 mEq/L.

Hyperkalemia: **Hyperkalemia** occurs when the serum potassium level rises above 5 mEq/L. This condition may be caused by excessive consumption of potassium-rich foods or dietary supplements, particularly when patients are taking potassium-sparing diuretics such as spironolactone (see Chapter 32). In fact, overtreatment with potassium supplements is the most common cause of hyperkalemia. Excess potassium may also accumulate when renal excretion is diminished due to kidney pathology. The most serious consequences of hyperkalemia are related to cardiac function: dysrhythmias and heart block. Other symptoms are muscle twitching, fatigue, paresthesias, dyspnea, cramping, and diarrhea. Hyperkalemia is much less common than hypokalemia.

In mild cases of hyperkalemia, potassium levels may be returned to normal by restricting primary dietary sources of potassium such as bananas, citrus and dried fruits, peanut butter, broccoli, and green leafy vegetables. All potassium supplements and the use of salt substitutes containing potassium should be discontinued. If the patient is taking a potassium-sparing diuretic, the dose must be lowered, or a thiazide or loop diuretic substituted.

Several options are available for patients with severe hyperkalemia. Administration of the diuretic furosemide (Lasix) can significantly increase the urinary excretion of potassium within 5 to 15 minutes. Administering glucose or dextrose concurrently with insulin temporarily lowers serum potassium levels by causing potassium to leave the extracellular fluid and enter cells. In all patients who are symptomatic, calcium gluconate or calcium chloride is administered to prevent or treat potassium-induced cardiotoxicity. Sodium bicarbonate is sometimes infused to correct any acidosis that may be concurrent with the hyperkalemia.

Excess potassium may also be eliminated from the body by giving polystyrene sulfonate (Kayexalate) orally or rectally. This drug, which is not absorbed, exchanges Na^+ for K^+ as it travels through the intestine. The onset of action is 1 hour, and the dose may be repeated every 4 hours as needed. The drug is given concurrently with a laxative such as sorbitol to promote rapid evacuation of the potassium.

Hypokalemia: **Hypokalemia** is one of the most common electrolyte imbalances and occurs when the serum potassium level falls below 3.5 mEq/L. The most frequent cause of hypokalemia is pharmacotherapy with loop and thiazide diuretics. In addition, strenuous muscular activity and severe vomiting or diarrhea can lead to significant potassium loss. Because the body does not have large stores of potassium, adequate daily dietary intake is necessary. Neurons and muscle fibers are most sensitive to potassium loss, and muscle weakness, lethargy, anorexia, dysrhythmias, and cardiac arrest are possible consequences.

Mild hypokalemia is treated by increasing the dietary intake of potassium-rich foods. The foods highest in potassium content include dried fruit, nuts, molasses, avocados, lima beans, and bran cereals. If increasing dietary intake is not possible, a large number of potassium products are available for oral supplementation.

The most common supplements are the chloride salts, because these supply both potassium and chloride, which are lost during diuretic therapy. Liquid preparations are very effective, although many must be diluted with water or fruit juices prior to administration. Extended release (K-Dur 20, Slow-K, Micro-K) and powders (Klor-Con) are also available.

Severe hypokalemia may require parenteral potassium supplements. Caution must always be used when using IV potassium because rapid administration of the drug can be fatal, especially for patients with significant renal impairment. Cardiac function should be closely monitored during IV potassium therapy.

PROTOTYPE DRUG | **Potassium Chloride (KCl)**

Classification: **Therapeutic:** Drug for hypokalemia
Pharmacologic: Electrolyte, potassium supplement

Therapeutic Effects and Uses: Potassium chloride is a drug of choice for preventing or treating hypokalemia because potassium and chloride depletion usually occur concurrently. It is also used to treat mild forms of alkalosis. Oral formulations of potassium chloride include tablets, powders, and liquids, usually heavily flavored due to its unpleasant taste. Because potassium supplements can cause peptic ulcers, the drug should be diluted with plenty of water. When given IV, potassium must be administered slowly because bolus injections can overload the heart and cause cardiac arrest. Because pharmacotherapy with loop or thiazide diuretics is the most common cause of potassium depletion, patients taking these drugs are usually prescribed PO potassium supplements to prevent hypokalemia.

Mechanism of Action: Potassium chloride is a replacement solution for lost potassium.

Pharmacokinetics: Because potassium chloride is a natural electrolyte, it is not possible to obtain accurate pharmacokinetic values. The potassium ions in the drug are widely distributed and excreted by the kidneys in the same manner as endogenous potassium ions.

Adverse Effects: Nausea, vomiting, diarrhea, and abdominal pain are common, because potassium chloride irritates the GI mucosa. The drug may be taken with meals or antacids to lessen gastric distress. The most serious adverse effects of potassium chloride are related to the possible accumulation of excess potassium. Hyperkalemia may occur if the patient takes potassium supplements concurrently with potassium-sparing diuretics. Because the kidneys perform over 90% of the body's potassium excretion functions, reduced renal function can rapidly lead to hyperkalemia, particularly in patients taking potassium supplements.

Contraindications/Precautions: Potassium chloride is contraindicated in patients with hyperkalemia, systemic acidosis, severe dehydration, extensive tissue breakdown as in severe burns, or adrenal insufficiency. Oral potassium supplements are contraindicated in any condition for which transit through the GI tract is delayed because prolonged contact may damage the GI mucosa. The drug should be used with extreme caution in patients with chronic or acute renal failure because the drug may accumulate to high levels.

Drug Interactions: Potassium supplements should not be administered to patients who are taking potassium-sparing diuretics because hyperkalemia may result. Angiotensin-converting enzyme (ACE) inhibitors prevent aldosterone secretion and cause potassium retention, thus increasing the risk for hyperkalemia if administered with potassium supplements. Drugs that slow GI transit time, such as anticholinergics, may increase the GI toxicity of potassium supplements.

Herbal/Food: Unknown.

Pregnancy: Category C.

Treatment of Overdose: Potassium-sparing diuretics and all foods and medications containing potassium should be withheld. Treatment includes IV administration of 10% dextrose solution containing 10 to 20 units of crystalline insulin. Sodium bicarbonate may be infused to correct acidosis. Polystyrene sulfonate may be administered to enhance potassium elimination.

Nursing Responsibilities: Key nursing implications for patients receiving potassium chloride are included in the Nursing Practice Application for Patients Receiving Pharmacotherapy for Fluid and Electrolyte Imbalances.

Drugs Similar to Potassium Chloride (KCl)

Other potassium drugs include acetate, bicarbonate, citrate, and gluconate salts. Potassium acetate is used as an IV alternative to potassium chloride. Potassium bicarbonate supplies bicarbonate ion, which is alkaline and may be useful in treating acidosis. Potassium citrate makes the urine less acidic and is primarily used to reduce the formation of kidney stones. Potassium gluconate is commonly available in tablet form and dissociates to potassium ion and gluconate ion, a form of glucose.

33.11 Magnesium imbalances significantly affect cardiovascular and neuromuscular function.

Magnesium is the second most abundant intracellular cation and, like potassium, it is essential for proper neuromuscular function. Magnesium also serves a metabolic role in activating certain enzymes in the breakdown of carbohydrates and proteins; it is a cofactor in over 300 biochemical reactions. Patients with disorders of magnesium homeostasis generally present with cardiovascular and neuromuscular symptoms. Because the majority of magnesium is found in bone, serum magnesium levels are not accurate indicators of total body magnesium.

Magnesium levels are primarily controlled by the kidney. The ion is freely filtered and reabsorbed in the loop of Henle and loop diuretics such as furosemide can cause significant magnesium loss. Renal impairment is a major cause of magnesium imbalances. Magnesium is absorbed by the small intestine and small amounts are secreted in intestinal fluid.

Hypomagnesemia: Because it produces few symptoms until serum levels fall below 1 mEq/L, hypomagnesemia is sometimes called the most common undiagnosed electrolyte abnormality. Although the overall incidence for magnesium deficiency is 6% to 12%, the majority of critically ill patients present with this

condition. Renal causes of hypomagnesemia include kidney failure and therapy with loop diuretics. GI causes include malabsorption disorders and loss of significant amounts of body fluids due to diarrhea, chronic laxative abuse, or nasogastric suctioning. Hypomagnesemia may also present in alcoholics and in those receiving prolonged parenteral feeding with magnesium-free solutions. Patients may experience general weakness, dysrhythmias, HTN, loss of deep tendon reflexes, and respiratory depression—signs and symptoms that are sometimes mistaken for hypokalemia. Additional signs include muscle twitches, tetany, or seizures.

Magnesium supplements are available by both PO and parenteral routes. Oral formulations are used for minor hypomagnesemia. Because intramuscular (IM) preparations produce significant pain at the injection site, severe cases of hypomagnesemia are normally treated using the IV route. Pharmacotherapy with magnesium sulfate can quickly reverse symptoms of hypomagnesemia. Magnesium sulfate is a central nervous system (CNS) depressant and is sometimes given to prevent or terminate seizures associated with eclampsia.

Hypermagnesemia: Advanced renal failure is the only major cause of hypermagnesemia, although overtreatment with magnesium supplements may also lead to excessive serum magnesium levels. Clinical signs include CNS depression, respiratory depression, hypotension, dysrhythmias, bradycardia, complete heart block, and coma. Infusions of calcium salts will immediately reverse the neuromuscular and cardiovascular signs. If the magnesium elevation is minor, treatment with furosemide to increase urinary excretion may be sufficient to reverse the hypermagnesemia.

PROTOTYPE DRUG   **Magnesium Sulfate (MgSO₄)**

Classification: Therapeutic: Drug for hypomagnesemia
Pharmacologic: Electrolyte, magnesium supplement

Therapeutic Effects and Uses: Severe hypomagnesemia can be rapidly reversed by the administration of IM or IV magnesium sulfate. Parenteral formulations include 4%, 8%, 12.5%, and 50% solutions. After administration, magnesium sulfate is distributed throughout the body, and therapeutic effects are observed within 30 to 60 minutes. Plasma magnesium levels should be monitored frequently during therapy.

Oral forms of magnesium sulfate are used as cathartics, when complete evacuation of the colon is desired. Its action as a CNS depressant has led to its occasional use as an anticonvulsant in patients with preeclampsia or eclampsia (see Chapter 22). Magnesium sulfate has been used off-label to slow uterine contractions during preterm labor (see Chapter 69).

Mechanism of Action: Magnesium sulfate is a replacement solution for lost magnesium.

Pharmacokinetics:

Route(s)	PO, IM, IV
Absorption	Not absorbed
Distribution	Widely distributed; crosses the placenta; secreted in breast milk
Primary metabolism	Not metabolized
Primary excretion	Renal
Onset of action	PO: 1–2 h; IM: 1 h; IV: immediate
Duration of action	PO and IM: 3–4 h; IV: 30 min; half-life: unknown

Adverse Effects: Patients receiving IV infusions of magnesium sulfate require careful observation to prevent toxicity. Early signs of magnesium overdose include flushing of the skin, sedation, confusion, intense thirst, and muscle weakness. Extreme levels cause neuromuscular blockade with resultant respiratory paralysis, heart block, and circulatory collapse. Because of these potentially fatal adverse effects, the use of magnesium sulfate is restricted to patients with severe magnesium deficiency. Mild to moderate hypomagnesemia is treated with oral forms of magnesium such as magnesium gluconate or magnesium hydroxide. Oral magnesium sulfate, also known as Epsom salts, is a saline-type laxative and will cause diarrhea in patients. This may be a dose-limiting adverse effect for some patients.

Contraindications/Precautions: Magnesium is contraindicated in patients with serious cardiac disease. Oral administration is contraindicated in those with undiagnosed abdominal pain, intestinal obstruction, or fecal impaction. The drug should be used cautiously in patients with renal impairment because the drug may rapidly rise to toxic levels.

Drug Interactions: Use with neuromuscular blockers may increase respiratory depression and apnea. Because magnesium sulfate has CNS depression effects, patients receiving other CNS depressants may experience increased sedation. **Herbal/Food**: Magnesium salts may decrease the absorption of certain anti-infectives such as tetracycline.

Pregnancy: Category A.

Treatment of Overdose: Serious respiratory and cardiac suppression may result from overdose. Calcium gluconate or gluceptate may be administered IV as an antidote.

Nursing Responsibilities: Key nursing implications for patients receiving magnesium sulfate are included in the Nursing Practice Application for Patients Receiving Pharmacotherapy for Fluid and Electrolyte Imbalances.

Drugs Similar to Magnesium Sulfate (MgSO$_4$)

Several oral magnesium salts are available OTC. Magnesium citrate (citrate of magnesia) and magnesium hydroxide (milk of magnesia) are classified as laxatives or cathartics. Magnesium oxide (Mag-Ox) is an antacid, and magnesium salicylate (Doan's Pills) is used as an analgesic.

PharmFACT

Although the recommended dietary allowance for magnesium is 420 mg/day in men and 320 mg/day in women, certain patients need higher levels to maintain health. These include patients with Crohn's disease, poorly controlled diabetes, pregnant or lactating women, older adults, and patients with alcoholism (National Institutes of Health, Office of Dietary Supplements, 2013).

Pharmacotherapy of Acid–Base Imbalances

33.12 The pH of body fluids must be maintained between very narrow limits.

The degree of acidity or alkalinity of a solution is measured by its pH. A pH of 7.0 is defined as neutral, above 7.0 as basic or alkaline, and below 7.0 as acidic. To maintain homeostasis, the pH of plasma and most body fluids must be kept within the narrow range of 7.35 to 7.45 because nearly all proteins and enzymes in the body function optimally within this range. A few enzymes, most notably those in the digestive tract, require pH values outside the 7.35 to 7.45 range to function properly.

The body generates significant amounts of acids during normal metabolic processes. Without an effective means of neutralizing these metabolic acids, the overall pH of body fluids would quickly fall below the normal range. **Buffers** are chemicals that help maintain normal body pH by neutralizing strong acids and bases. The two primary buffers in the body are bicarbonate ions and phosphate ions.

The body uses two mechanisms to remove acid. The acidic carbon dioxide (CO_2) produced during body metabolism is efficiently removed by the lungs during exhalation. The kidneys remove excess acid in the form of hydrogen ion (H^+) by excreting it in the urine. If retained in the body, CO_2 and/or H^+ will lower body pH. Normal acid–base balance is maintained by the lungs and kidneys. Impairment of these organs commonly leads to change in pH.

Acidosis (excess acid) and alkalosis (excess base) are not diseases but are symptoms of an underlying medical disorder. Acidic drugs and basic drugs are administered to rapidly correct pH imbalances in body fluids, supporting the patient's vital functions while the underlying disease is being treated. The correction of acid–base imbalance is illustrated in Figure 33.3.

33.13 The pharmacotherapy of acidosis includes the administration of alkaline drugs.

Acidosis occurs when the pH of the plasma falls below 7.35, which is confirmed by measuring arterial pH, partial pressure of carbon dioxide (P_{CO_2}), and plasma bicarbonate levels. For proper pharmacotherapy, the diagnosis must differentiate between respiratory etiology and metabolic (renal) etiology. Occasionally, the cause has mixed respiratory and metabolic components.

The most profound symptoms of acidosis affect the CNS and include lethargy, confusion, and CNS depression leading to coma.

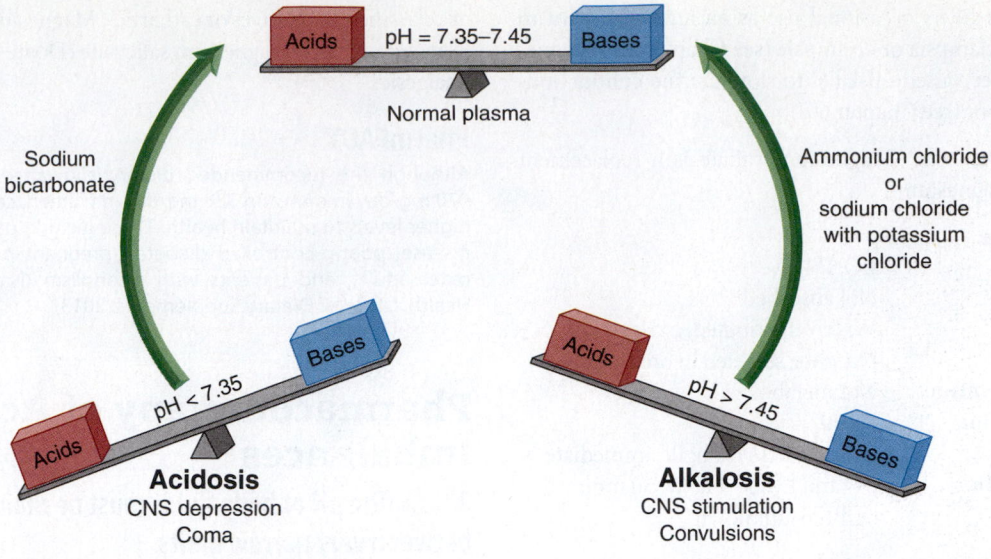

Figure 33.3 Acid–base imbalances.

A deep, rapid respiration rate indicates an attempt by the lungs to rid the body of excess acid. Common causes of acidosis are shown in Table 33.6.

In patients with acidosis, the therapeutic goal is to quickly reverse the adverse effects caused by excess acids in the blood. Mild acidosis may be treated with oral bicarbonate or citrate salts or other basic substances. For acute acidosis the treatment of choice is to administer infusions of sodium bicarbonate. Bicarbonate ion is a base that can quickly neutralize acids in the blood and other body fluids. The patient must be carefully monitored during infusions because this drug can "overcorrect" the acidosis, causing blood pH to turn alkaline. Sodium citrate, sodium lactate, and sodium acetate are alternative alkaline drugs that may be used in place of bicarbonate.

Alkalinizing drugs are also used to aid in the renal excretion of toxic substances through a phenomenon called **ion trapping**. Whenever a large pH gradient exists across a membrane, drug molecules will accumulate on the side where the opportunity for ionization is greatest. Recall from Chapter 3 that acids ionize in a basic environment; bases ionize in acidic solutions. The infusion of an alkalinizing drug will create an alkaline filtrate in the kidney tubule, a perfect environment for ionization of an acidic drug like aspirin. Rather than being absorbed back into the body, the ionized aspirin remains "trapped" in the filtrate and is excreted in the urine. Thus, through ion trapping, the alkalinizing drug was able to move aspirin from the blood to the urine.

PROTOTYPE DRUG	Sodium Bicarbonate

Classification: Therapeutic: Drug to treat acidosis or bicarbonate deficiency
Pharmacologic: Electrolyte, sodium, and bicarbonate supplement

Therapeutic Effects and Uses: Sodium bicarbonate is a drug of choice for correcting metabolic acidosis. After dissociation, the bicarbonate ion directly raises the pH of body fluids. Sodium bicarbonate may be given PO if acidosis is mild, or IV in cases of acute disease. IV concentrations range from 4.2% to 8.4%. Although sodium bicarbonate also neutralizes gastric acid, it is rarely used to treat peptic ulcers due to its tendency to cause uncomfortable gastric distention. The PO form of sodium bicarbonate is commonly known as baking soda.

Sodium bicarbonate may also be used to alkalinize the urine to speed the excretion of acidic medications such as aspirin and phenobarbital and as adjunctive therapy for certain chemotherapeutic drugs such as methotrexate. Sodium bicarbonate is also used in chronic renal failure to neutralize the metabolic acidosis that occurs when the kidneys cannot excrete hydrogen ion. When IV sodium bicarbonate is given, it causes the urine to become more

TABLE 33.6	Causes of Alkalosis and Acidosis
Acidosis	**Alkalosis**
Respiratory Origins of Acidosis	**Respiratory Origin of Alkalosis**
Hypoventilation or shallow breathing	Hyperventilation due to asthma, anxiety, or high altitude
Airway constriction	
Damage to respiratory center in medulla	
Metabolic Origins of Acidosis	**Metabolic Origins of Alkalosis**
Severe diarrhea	Constipation for prolonged periods
Kidney failure	Ingestion of excess sodium bicarbonate
Diabetes mellitus	Diuretics that cause potassium depletion
Excess alcohol ingestion	Severe vomiting
Starvation	

alkaline. Less acid is reabsorbed, so more acid and acidic medicine is excreted. This process is known as ion trapping.

Mechanism of Action: The bicarbonate ion in sodium bicarbonate buffers excess acid (H^+) to raise the pH of body fluids.

Pharmacokinetics:

Route(s)	IV, PO
Absorption	Rapidly absorbed
Distribution	Widely distributed in body fluids
Primary metabolism	Not metabolized
Primary excretion	Renal
Onset of action	PO: 15 min; IV: immediate
Duration of action	PO: 1–3 h; IV: 8–10 min

Adverse Effects: Most of the adverse effects of sodium bicarbonate therapy are the result of metabolic alkalosis created by receiving too much bicarbonate ion. Symptoms may include confusion, irritability, slow respiration rate, and vomiting. Discontinuing the sodium bicarbonate infusion often reverses these symptoms; however, potassium chloride or ammonium chloride may be administered to reverse acute alkalosis. During sodium bicarbonate infusions, serum electrolytes should be carefully monitored because sodium levels may lead to hypernatremia and fluid retention. In addition, high levels of bicarbonate ion passing through the kidney tubules increase potassium secretion, which could lead to hypokalemia.

Contraindications/Precautions: Patients who are vomiting, have severe diarrhea, or have continuous GI suctioning will lose acid and chloride and may be in a state of metabolic alkalosis; therefore, they should not receive sodium bicarbonate because it may worsen alkalosis. Due to the sodium content of this drug, it should be used cautiously in patients with cardiac disease, HTN, or renal impairment.

Drug Interactions: Sodium bicarbonate may decrease the absorption of ketoconazole and may decrease elimination of dextroamphetamine, ephedrine, pseudoephedrine, and quinidine. The elimination of lithium, salicylates, and tetracyclines may be increased. **Herbal/Food:** Chronic use with milk or calcium supplements may cause milk-alkali syndrome, a condition characterized by serious hypercalcemia and possible kidney failure.

Pregnancy: Category C.

Treatment of Overdose: Overdose results in metabolic alkalosis, which is treated by administering acidic drugs (see Section 33.10).

Nursing Responsibilities: Key nursing implications for patients receiving sodium bicarbonate are included in the Nursing Practice Application for Patients Receiving Pharmacotherapy for Fluid and Electrolyte Imbalances.

Drugs Similar to Sodium Bicarbonate

There are no drugs similar to sodium bicarbonate.

33.14 The pharmacotherapy of alkalosis includes the administration of acidic drugs.

At plasma pH values above 7.45, **alkalosis** develops. Mortality can reach as high as 80% if the pH rises above 7.65. Like acidosis,

alkalosis may have either respiratory or metabolic causes, as shown in Table 33.6. Also like acidosis, the CNS is greatly affected. Symptoms of CNS stimulation occur including nervousness, hyperactive reflexes, and convulsions. In metabolic alkalosis, slow, shallow breathing indicates that the body is attempting to compensate by retaining acid and lowering internal pH. Life-threatening dysrhythmias are the most serious adverse effects of alkalosis.

In mild cases, alkalosis may be corrected by administering sodium chloride combined with potassium chloride. This combination increases the renal excretion of bicarbonate ion, which indirectly increases the acidity of the blood. More severe alkalosis may be treated with infusions of an acidic drug such as ammonium chloride or hydrochloric acid.

PROTOTYPE DRUG	**Ammonium Chloride**

Classification: Therapeutic: Drug for lowering pH
Pharmacologic: Acidic drug

Therapeutic Effects and Uses: Ammonium chloride is an acidic substance that has been available as a drug for over 80 years. Severe metabolic alkalosis may be reversed by the administration of acidic drugs such as ammonium chloride. Ammonium chloride acidifies the urine, which is beneficial in treating certain urinary tract infections. Historically, it has been used as a mild diuretic, though safer and more effective agents have made its use obsolete. By acidifying the urine, ammonium chloride promotes the excretion of alkaline drugs such as amphetamines through ion trapping. Oral and IV forms are available; when given for alkalosis, the IV route is preferred. Because of the potential for causing acidosis, the drug is infused slowly.

Mechanism of Action: During the hepatic conversion of ammonium chloride to urea, Cl^- and H^+ are formed. The H^+ combines with bicarbonate to form the weak acid carbonic acid, which dissociates to water and carbon dioxide. By removing bicarbonate, ammonium chloride decreases the pH of body fluids. The chloride ion also combines with bases to reduce the alkalinity of extracellular fluids.

Pharmacokinetics:

Route(s)	IV, PO
Absorption	Rapidly absorbed
Distribution	Unknown
Primary metabolism	Hepatic
Primary excretion	Renal
Onset of action	Unknown
Duration of action	Unknown

Adverse Effects: Aggressive treatment with ammonium chloride can cause acidosis. Characteristic symptoms of acidosis include CNS depression, drowsiness, confusion, and coma. Periods of CNS excitement may alternate with coma. Oral forms of the drug are irritating to the gastric mucosa and may cause nausea and vomiting.

Contraindications/Precautions: Ammonium chloride should not be administered to patients with serious hepatic or renal impairment because the drug will accumulate to toxic levels. It should not be administered to patients with either metabolic or respiratory acidosis.

Drug Interactions: Ammonium chloride may cause crystalluria when taken with aminosalicylic acid. Antacids should not be administered concurrently because they are alkaline and will antagonize the acidifying effects of ammonium chloride. Ammonium chloride reduces levels of amphetamines, flecainide, mexiletine, methadone, ephedrine, and pseudoephedrine. Urinary excretion of sulfonylureas and salicylates is decreased. Serum magnesium values may decrease.

Herbal/Food: Unknown.

Pregnancy: Category B.

Treatment of Overdose: Overdose results in metabolic acidosis, which is treated by administering alkaline drugs (see Section 33.9).

Nursing Responsibilities: Key nursing implications for patients receiving ammonium chloride are included in the Nursing Practice Application for Patients Receiving Pharmacotherapy for Fluid and Electrolyte Imbalances.

Drugs Similar to Ammonium Chloride

The only similar drug is hydrochloric acid.

Hydrochloric acid: Hydrochloric acid may be administered IV in severe cases of metabolic acidosis. A central venous catheter must be used to administer the drug. Hydrochloric acid is only used when sodium or potassium chloride cannot be administered due to volume overload or advanced renal failure. This drug can cause severe tissue necrosis if it extravasates into the tissues.

CONNECTIONS: NURSING PRACTICE APPLICATION

Patients Receiving Pharmacotherapy for Fluid and Electrolyte Imbalances

Assessment	Potential Nursing Diagnoses*
Baseline assessment prior to administration: • Obtain a complete health history including cardiovascular (including HTN, myocardial infarction [MI]), neurologic (including stroke or head injury), burns, endocrine, hepatic, or renal disease. Obtain a drug history including allergies, current prescription and OTC drugs, and herbal preparations. Be alert to possible drug interactions. • Obtain baseline weight and vital signs, level of consciousness (LOC), breath sounds, and urinary output as appropriate. • Evaluate appropriate laboratory findings (e.g., electrolytes, CBC, urine specific gravity and urinalysis, blood urea nitrogen [BUN] and creatinine, total protein and albumin levels, activated partial thromboplastin time [aPTT], activated prothrombin time [aPT] or international normalized ratio [INR], renal and liver function studies). • Assess the patient's ability to receive and understand instructions. Include the family and caregiver as needed.	• *Deficient Fluid Volume* • *Decreased Cardiac Output* • *Fatigue* • *Activity Intolerance* • *Deficient Knowledge* (Drug Therapy) • *Risk for Falls*, related to hypotension and dizziness associated with adverse effects • *Risk for Injury*, related to hypotension and dizziness associated with adverse effects • *Risk for Deficient Fluid Volume* • *Risk for Imbalanced Fluid Volume*, related to drug therapy • *Risk for Electrolyte Imbalance* • *Risk for Ineffective Health Maintenance*, related to drug effects and dietary needs
Assessment throughout administration: • Assess for desired therapeutic effects dependent on the reason for the drug (e.g., electrolyte values return to within normal range, adequate urine output). • Continue monitoring vital signs, urinary output, and LOC as appropriate. • Assess for and promptly report adverse effects: tachycardia, HTN, dysrhythmias, decreasing LOC, increasing dyspnea, lung congestion, pink-tinged frothy sputum, decreased urinary output, muscle weakness or cramping, and allergic reactions.	

Implementation

Interventions and (Rationales)	Patient-Centered Care
Ensuring therapeutic effects: • Continue frequent assessments as above for therapeutic effects dependent on the reason the drug therapy is given. Assist the patient as needed with obtaining fluids and eating. (Urinary output is within normal limits. Electrolyte balance is restored or within the parameters set by the health care provider. **Lifespan:** Older adults, infants, and patients who cannot access fluids or eat by themselves [e.g., post-stroke] are at increased risk for fluid and electrolyte imbalance.)	• Teach the patient to continue to consume enough liquids to remain adequately, but not overly, hydrated. Drinking when thirsty, avoiding alcoholic beverages, maintaining a healthy diet, and ensuring adequate but not excessive salt intake will assist in maintaining normal fluid and electrolyte balance. • Have the patient weigh self daily, ideally at the same time of day, and record weight along with blood pressure and pulse measurements as appropriate. • Teach the patient, family, or caregiver how to monitor pulse and blood pressure if needed. Ensure proper use and functioning of any home equipment obtained.

CONNECTIONS: NURSING PRACTICE APPLICATION (continued)

Minimizing adverse effects:

- Monitor for signs of fluid volume excess or deficit, e.g., HTN (excess) or hypotension (deficit), tachycardia, or changes in the quality of pulse (bounding or thready). Notify the health care provider if blood pressure or pulse exceeds established parameters. Monitor for signs of potential electrolyte imbalance including nausea, vomiting, GI cramping, diarrhea, muscle weakness, cramping, twitching, paresthesia, and irritability. Immediately report any confusion, decreasing LOC, or increasing hypotension or HTN, especially if associated with tachycardia, decreased urine output, or seizures. (Many fluid and electrolyte imbalances have similar symptoms. When assessing the patient for adverse effects, consider past health history, drug history, and current condition and medications to correlate symptoms to possible causes.)

- Instruct the patient to report changes in muscle strength or function; numbness and tingling in the lips, fingers, arms, or legs; palpitations; dizziness; nausea or vomiting; GI cramping; or decreased urination.
- Instruct patients with hypokalemia to consume foods high in potassium: fresh fruits such as strawberries and bananas; dried fruits such as apricots and prunes; vegetables and legumes such as tomatoes, beets, and beans; juices such as orange, grapefruit, or prune; and fresh meats. Instruct patients with hyperkalemia to avoid the above as well as salt substitutes (which often contain potassium salts), and to consult with a health care provider before taking vitamin and mineral supplements or specialized sports beverages. Licorice should be avoided because it causes potassium loss and sodium retention.

- Frequently monitor CBC, electrolytes, aPTT, aPT, or INR levels. (Crystalloid solutions may cause electrolyte imbalances. Colloid solutions may reduce normal blood coagulation. Frequent monitoring of electrolyte levels while on replacement therapy may be needed to ensure therapeutic effects.)

- Instruct the patient on the need to return periodically for laboratory work.

- Continue to monitor vital signs. Take blood pressure lying, sitting, and standing to detect orthostatic hypotension. **Lifespan:** Be particularly cautious with the older adult who is at increased risk for hypotension. Ensure patient safety. (Dehydration and electrolyte imbalances may cause dizziness and hypotension. Orthostatic hypotension may increase the risk of falls and injury.)

- Teach the patient to rise from lying or sitting to standing slowly to avoid dizziness or falls. If dizziness occurs, the patient should sit or lie down and not attempt to stand or walk until the sensation passes.
- Instruct the patient to call for assistance prior to getting out of bed or attempting to walk alone and to avoid driving or other activities requiring mental alertness or physical coordination if dizziness or lightheadedness occurs.

- Weigh the patient daily and report a weight gain or loss of 1 kg (2 lb) or more in a 24-h period. (Daily weight is an accurate measure of fluid status and takes into account intake, output, and insensible losses. Weight gain or edema may signal excessive fluid volume or electrolyte imbalances.)

- Have the patient weigh self daily, ideally at the same time of day, and record weight along with blood pressure and pulse measurements. Have the patient report a weight loss or gain of more than 1 kg (2 lb) in a 24-h period.
- Teach the patient that excessive heat conditions contribute to excessive sweating and fluid and electrolyte loss, and extra caution is warranted in these conditions.

- Closely monitor for signs and symptoms of allergy if colloids are used. (Colloids such as plasma protein fraction, dextran, and hetastarch may cause allergic and anaphylactic reactions.)

- Instruct the patient to report dyspnea, itching, feelings of throat tightness, palpitations, chest pain or tightening, or headache immediately.

- Closely monitor IV sites when infusing potassium or ammonium. Double-check doses with another nurse before giving. (Potassium and ammonium are irritating to the vessel and phlebitis may result. Potassium is a "high-alert" medication and double-checking doses before giving prevents medication errors.)

- Instruct the patient to report any irritation, pain, redness, or swelling at the IV site or in the arm where the drug is infusing.

- Monitor LOC, deep tendon reflexes, urinary output, respiratory rate, and laboratory values frequently in patients receiving parenteral magnesium sulfate and newborns if the mother has received the drug. Keep calcium gluconate available as an antidote to magnesium toxicity. (Adverse effects from hypermagnesemia include respiratory and cardiac arrest and neuromuscular depression.)

- To allay anxiety, teach the patient and family the rationale for all equipment used and the need for frequent monitoring.
- Instruct patients with hypomagnesemia to consume foods high in magnesium: green leafy vegetables and legumes such as peas, beans, nuts, and whole grains, and to increase fluid intake.

Patient understanding of drug therapy:

- Use opportunities during administration of medications and during assessments to discuss the rationale for the drug therapy, desired therapeutic outcomes, and any necessary monitoring or precautions. (Using time during nursing care helps to optimize and reinforce supportive drug treatment and care.)

- The patient, family, or caregiver should be able to state the reason for the drug, appropriate dose and scheduling, what adverse effects to observe for and when to report them, and the anticipated length of medication therapy.

Patient self-administration of drug therapy:

- When administering the medication, instruct the patient, family, or caregiver in proper self-administration of the drug, e.g., early in the day to prevent disruption of sleep from nocturia. (Utilizing time during nurse-administration of these drugs helps to reinforce teaching.)

- The patient, family, or caregiver is able to discuss appropriate dosing and administration needs.
- **Lifespan:** Assess swallowing ability before giving or taking potassium chloride or ammonium chloride; they may cause mouth, esophageal, or gastric irritation. Liquid forms should always be diluted with water or fruit juice and tablets swallowed whole.

CHAPTER

33

Understanding the Chapter

Key Concepts Summary

33.1 Body fluids are exchanged between intracellular and extracellular compartments.

33.2 Osmolality or tonicity determines the movement of body fluids.

33.3 Overall fluid balance is regulated primarily by hormones acting upon the kidneys.

33.4 Dehydration may be treated with fluid volume expanders.

33.5 Transfusions of blood products are used to treat serious conditions that cannot be managed effectively by other means.

33.6 Crystalloids are intravenous solutions that closely resemble the composition of extracellular fluid.

33.7 Colloids are intravenous solutions containing large molecules that remain in the blood.

33.8 Electrolytes are charged substances that are essential to homeostasis.

33.9 Sodium balance is closely associated with water balance.

33.10 Potassium imbalances must be quickly corrected to prevent serious cardiac consequences.

33.11 Magnesium imbalances significantly affect cardiovascular and neuromuscular function.

33.12 The pH of body fluids must be maintained between very narrow limits.

33.13 The pharmacotherapy of acidosis includes the administration of alkaline drugs.

33.14 The pharmacotherapy of alkalosis includes the administration of acidic drugs.

Case Study: Making the Patient Connection

Remember the patient "Peggy Hover" at the beginning of the chapter? Now read the remainder of the case study. Based on the information presented within this chapter, respond to the critical thinking questions that follow.

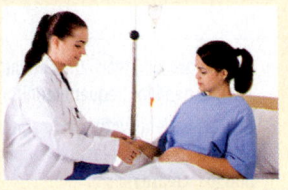

Peggy Hover is 26 years old and has been admitted to the short-stay surgical unit for an elective laparoscopic cholecystectomy. She has been in good health except for repeated bouts of gallbladder attacks and it is anticipated that she will be able to go home this afternoon after the surgery is completed.

As the nurse admitting Peggy, you have orders to start a D$_5$W infusion prior to surgery, to run at 15 mL/h. You have started the IV in her right hand. Peggy

asks you why she needs it, especially since she will be returning home that afternoon.

Critical Thinking Questions

1. Why do you think an IV was ordered for Peggy, and what will you explain to her?

2. What are the two main categories of IV solutions? Which category was ordered for Peggy?

3. Dextrose 5% in water (D$_5$W) is a common solution. What precautions should be taken with this fluid type?

See Answers to Critical Thinking Questions on student resource website.

Additional Case Study

Marvin Fields has been prescribed a loop diuretic, furosemide (Lasix), 40 mg daily, and a potassium supplement 40 mEq tablet daily. As you are preparing to discharge this patient, he states, "I understand why I need the diuretic, but why do I have to take this potassium?"

1. How would you respond to his question?

2. What adverse effect related to potassium supplementation would you advise him to watch for?

3. What advice would you give Marvin about his dietary consumption of potassium-rich foods?

See Answers to Additional Case Study on student resource website.

Chapter Review

1 The patient with a disorder causing metabolic acidosis is being treated with intravenous sodium bicarbonate. The nurse monitors for therapeutic effectiveness by noting which laboratory values?

1. Serum pH
2. Red blood cell count
3. Liver function test
4. Blood urea nitrogen

2 The nurse is teaching the patient about a liquid potassium chloride supplement. Which statement, if made by the patient, indicates that further teaching is necessary?

1. "I should avoid salt substitutes unless approved by my health care provider."
2. "Liquid preparations should not be diluted with other fluids."
3. "I should report signs of potassium deficit such as weakness and fatigue."
4. "Persistent vomiting will result in significant losses of potassium."

3 The nurse is administering dextran 40 (Gentran 40) to a patient with multiple traumatic injuries following a motor vehicle crash. The nurse knows that which adverse effect of this medication is toxic?

1. Dehydration
2. Increased urinary output
3. Hypovolemic shock
4. Bleeding

4 The patient will be receiving 5% dextrose in water (D_5W) intravenous infusion. Which statement is correct about this therapy?

1. D_5W can cause hypoglycemia in the patient who has diabetes.
2. D_5W may be used to dilute mixed intravenous drugs.
3. D_5W is considered a colloid solution.
4. D_5W has a sufficient number of calories to supply metabolic needs.

5 The health care provider orders intravenous magnesium sulfate for a pregnant patient with preeclampsia. The nurse should consult with the prescriber about which patient assessment finding that may affect the drug therapy?

1. Pupil constriction to direct light
2. Chest congestion and coughing
3. Elevated blood pressure
4. Decreased patellar deep tendon reflexes

6 Which of the following nursing actions should be included in the care plan for a patient receiving normal serum albumin (Albuminar)? Select all that apply.

1. Document past history of blood transfusion reactions.
2. Restrict dietary intake of food high in potassium.
3. Monitor blood pressure and pulse rate.
4. Measure urinary output hourly.
5. Observe for signs related to potassium deficit.

See Answers to Chapter Review in Appendix A.

References

American Red Cross. (n.d.). *Blood facts and statistics.* Retrieved from http://www.redcrossblood.org/learn-about-blood/blood-facts-and-statistics

National Institutes of Health, Office of Dietary Supplements. (2013). *Magnesium: Fact sheet for health professionals.* Retrieved from http://ods.od.nih.gov/factsheets/Magnesium-HealthProfessional/

Selected Bibliography

Bunn, F., & Trivedi, D. (2012). Colloid solutions for fluid resuscitation. *Cochrane Database of Systematic Reviews, 7.* doi:10.1002/14651858.CD001319.pub4

Coyle, J. D., Joy, M. S., & Hladik, G. A. (2011). Disorders of sodium and water homeostasis. In J. T. DiPiro, R. L. Talbert, C. Y. Yee, G. R. Matzke, B. G. Wells, & L. M. Posey (Eds.), *Pharmacotherapy: A pathophysiologic approach* (8th ed.). New York, NY: McGraw-Hill.

Herdman, T. H., & Kamitsuru, S. (Eds.). (2014). *NANDA International nursing diagnoses:* *Definitions and classification, 2015–2017.* Oxford, United Kingdom: Wiley-Blackwell.

Huang, L. H. (2012). *Dehydration.* Retrieved from http://emedicine.medscape.com/article/906999-overview

James, M. F. M. (2010). Magnesium in obstetrics. *Best Practice & Research Clinical Obstetrics & Gynaecology, 24,* 327–337. doi:10.1016/j.bpobgyn.2009.11.004

Lehnhardt, A., & Kemper, M. J. (2011). Pathogenesis, diagnosis and management of hyperkalemia. *Pediatric Nephrology, 26,* 377–384. doi:10.1007/s00467-010-1699-3

Matzke, G. R., Devlin, J. W., & Palevsky, P. M. (2011). Acid-base disorders. In J. T. DiPiro, R. L. Talbert, C. Y. Yee, G. R. Matzke, B. G. Wells, & L. M. Posey (Eds.), *Pharmacotherapy: A pathophysiologic approach* (8th ed.). New York, NY: McGraw-Hill.

Metheny, N. (2011). *Fluid and electrolyte balance: Nursing considerations.* Sudbury, MA: Jones & Bartlett.

Myburgh, J. A., & Mythen, M. G. (2013). Resuscitation fluids. *New England Journal of Medicine, 369,* 1243–1251. doi:10.1056/NEJMra1208627

Perel, P., Roberts, I., & Ker, K. (2013). Colloids versus crystalloids for fluid resuscitation in critically ill patients. *Cochrane Database of Systematic Reviews, 2.* doi:10.1002/14651858 .CD000567.pub6.

Rizoli, S. (2011). PlasmaLyte. *The Journal of Trauma and Acute Care Surgery, 70*

(Suppl. 5), S17–S18. doi:10.1097/TA.0b013e 31821a4d89

Rosanoff, A., Weaver, C. M., & Rude, R. K. (2012). Suboptimal magnesium status in the United States: Are the health consequences under-estimated? *Nutrition Reviews, 70,* 153–164. doi:10.1111/j.1753-4887.2011.00465.x

Sterns, R. H., Hix, J. K., & Silver, S. (2010). Treatment of hyponatremia. *Current Opinion in Nephrology and Hypertension, 19* (5), 493–498. doi:10.1097/MNH.0b013e 32833bfa64

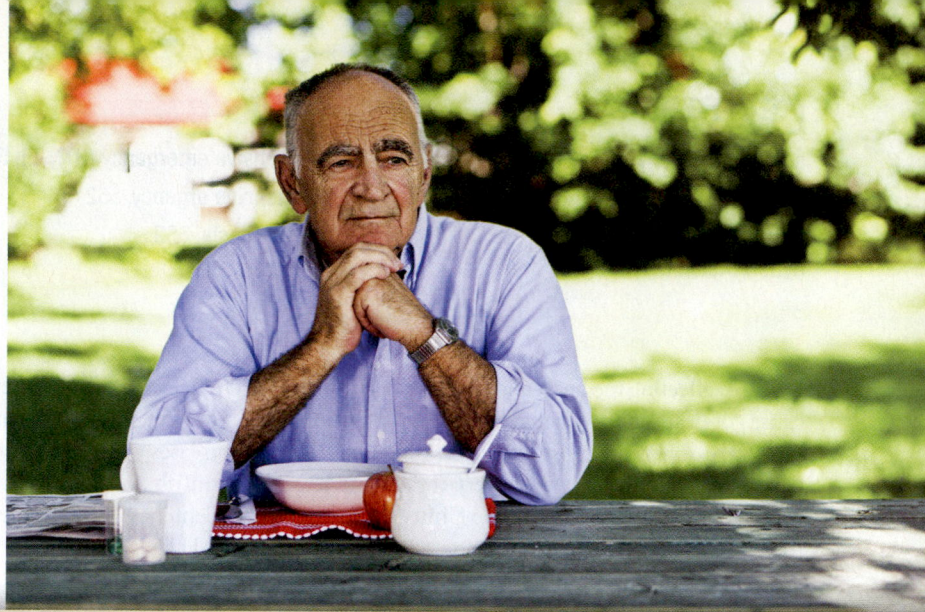

"I am doing everything my doctor has advised me to do to control my hypertension. My doctor has prescribed several different types of drugs over the last few months. My blood pressure is still elevated. What else can I do?"

Patient "Elmer Foley"

CHAPTER

34

Pharmacotherapy of Hypertension

LEARNING OUTCOMES

After reading this chapter, the student should be able to:

1. Summarize the long-term consequences of untreated hypertension.

2. Compare and contrast the roles of nonpharmacologic and pharmacologic methods in the management of hypertension.

3. Describe general principles guiding the pharmacotherapy of hypertension.

4. Identify drug classes used in the primary and alternate management of hypertension.

5. Describe the pharmacologic management of hypertensive emergencies.

6. For each of the classes shown in the chapter outline, identify the prototype and representative drugs and explain the mechanism(s) of drug action, primary indications, contraindications, significant drug interactions, pregnancy category, and important adverse effects.

7. Apply the nursing process to care for patients receiving antihypertensive drugs.

CHAPTER OUTLINE

▶ Etiology and Pathogenesis of Hypertension

▶ Nonpharmacologic Management of Hypertension

▶ Guidelines for the Management of Hypertension

▶ Pharmacotherapy of Hypertension

▶ Drug Classes for Hypertension

Diuretics

Calcium Channel Blockers

Drugs Affecting the Renin-Angiotensin-Aldosterone System

Angiotensin-Converting Enzyme Inhibitors

Angiotensin II Receptor Blockers

Adrenergic Antagonists

Beta-Adrenergic Antagonists

Alpha$_1$-Adrenergic Antagonists

Alpha$_2$-Adrenergic Agonists (Centrally Acting Drugs)

Adrenergic Neuron Blockers

Direct Vasodilators

PROTOTYPE Hydralazine (Apresoline) *p. 551*

▶ Management of Hypertensive Emergency

PROTOTYPE Nitroprusside Sodium (Nitropress) *p. 552*

KEY TERMS

angiotensin-converting enzyme
(ACE) inhibitors, 548

first-dose phenomenon, 549

hypertension (HTN), 543

hypertensive emergency (HTN-E), 552

hypertensive urgency, 552

hypertrichosis, 552

primary hypertension, 542

reflex tachycardia, 550

secondary hypertension, 542

Diseases affecting the heart and blood vessels are the most frequent causes of death in the United States. Hypertension (HTN) or high blood pressure is the most common of the cardiovascular diseases. Chronic HTN affects one in every three Americans and contributes to over 348,000 deaths in the United States each year (Centers for Disease Control and Prevention, 2014). Although mild HTN can be controlled with lifestyle modifications, moderate to severe HTN requires pharmacotherapy.

Because nurses encounter so many patients with this disease, it is critical for the nurse to understand the underlying principles of antihypertensive therapy. By improving public awareness of HTN and teaching the importance of early intervention, the nurse can contribute significantly to reducing cardiovascular mortality.

PharmFACT

Individuals whose blood pressure is higher than 140/90 mmHg (140 systolic or above or 90 diastolic or above) often become patients treated for serious cardiovascular problems. This includes:

- 75% of those who experience a first stroke
- 69% of those who have a first heart attack
- 74% of those with heart failure.

(American Heart Association, 2012).

Etiology and Pathogenesis of Hypertension

34.1 Failure to properly manage hypertension can lead to stroke, heart failure, or myocardial infarction.

Hypertension is a complex disease that is caused by a combination of genetic and environmental factors. Approximately 30% to 40% of HTN is thought to be due to genetic factors. Scientists have discovered specific genes that appear to predispose a patient to HTN. These genes control critical activities such as renal sodium and water transport and the renin-angiotensin-aldosterone system. Environmental factors related to diet and exercise also play an important role in the development of HTN.

For the large majority of patients with HTN, no specific cause can be identified. HTN having no identifiable cause is called idiopathic, essential, or **primary hypertension** and accounts for 90% of all cases. Although patients with primary HTN may not be cured, the disease can be managed such that the risk of serious, long-term consequences can be reduced.

In some cases, a specific cause of the HTN can be identified. This type, called **secondary hypertension**, accounts for 10% of all patients with HTN. Certain diseases, such as Cushing's syndrome, hyperthyroidism, chronic renal impairment, pheochromocytoma, and arteriosclerosis, are associated with elevated blood pressure. Certain drugs are also associated with HTN, including corticosteroids, oral contraceptives, estrogen, erythropoietin, and sibutramine. The therapeutic goal for secondary HTN is to treat or remove the underlying condition that is causing the blood pressure elevation. In many cases, correcting the comorbid condition will cure the associated HTN.

Research has clearly demonstrated that failure to control HTN can result in serious consequences. Prolonged or improperly controlled HTN damages blood vessels, particularly small arteries and arterioles. As it progresses, the walls of the arteries gradually thicken in an attempt to protect the vessels against injury from the increased pressure. The injured vessel walls become inflamed, increasing the permeability of the vessels and causing additional thickening of their walls. Eventually, the lumen of the artery permanently narrows, reducing blood flow to vital tissues. HTN accelerates atherosclerosis and will worsen conditions such as coronary artery disease (CAD).

Hypertension may exist for years, indeed decades, before becoming symptomatic. As the disease progresses, however, the risk of target-organ damage increases. Because sustained HTN may affect any artery in the body, damage may be widespread and symptoms vary greatly according to which vessels are affected.

The heart is a primary organ damaged by chronic HTN. Hypertension increases afterload, forcing the heart to work harder to pump blood to the tissues. The heart is subjected to chronic pressure overload, resulting in left ventricular hypertrophy. If untreated, this excessive workload eventually causes the heart to fail and the lungs to fill with fluid, a condition known as heart failure (HF). Drug therapy for HF is covered in Chapter 36.

Further damaging the heart is the effect of HTN on the coronary vessels. Hypertension accelerates the deposition of atherosclerotic plaque, creating or worsening CAD. This places the patient at greater risk of dysrhythmias, angina pectoris, and myocardial infarction (MI). Heart failure and MI are the most common causes of death in patients with HTN.

The brain is also a major target organ for hypertensive damage. Occlusion of the small vessels supplying blood and oxygen to the brain can cause transient ischemic attacks and stroke. These neurologic events are common in patients with HTN and are a major cause of disability.

Because a large percentage of blood pumped per minute circulates through the kidneys, chronic HTN creates major stress on these organs. As the small arteries supplying the kidney become injured, inflamed, and atherosclerotic, the patient's renal function gradually declines. Poorly managed HTN is an important contributor to kidney failure and end-stage kidney disease.

Hypertension is a major cause of visual impairment, which can occur when vessels in the eye become atherosclerotic. Although patients may remain asymptomatic for many years, small hemorrhages that affect vision may occur. Symptoms of retinal damage range from subtle vision changes to blindness. Retinopathy is particularly serious in patients who present with diabetes as a comorbid condition with HTN.

The importance of treating this disorder in the prehypertensive stage cannot be overstated. The long-term damage to target organs caused by HTN may become irreversible if the disease is allowed to progress unchecked. This is especially critical in people with diabetes and those with chronic kidney disease, as these patients are particularly susceptible to the long-term consequences of HTN.

Nonpharmacologic Management of Hypertension

34.2 Therapeutic lifestyle changes can reduce blood pressure and lessen the need for antihypertensive medications.

When a patient is first diagnosed with HTN, a comprehensive medical history is necessary to determine if the disease can be controlled by nonpharmacologic means. Therapeutic lifestyle changes should be recommended for all patients with HTN or at risk for the development of HTN. Of great importance is maintaining optimum weight, since obesity is closely associated with hyperlipidemia and HTN. A 5- to 9-kg (11- to 20-lb) weight loss often produces a measurable decrease in blood pressure, even in patients who are obese. Combining a medically supervised weight loss program with proper nutrition can delay the progression to HTN.

In some cases, implementing positive lifestyle changes may eliminate the need for pharmacotherapy altogether. Even if medication is required to manage the HTN, positive lifestyle changes may allow dosages to be minimized, thus lowering the potential for drug adverse effects. The nurse plays a vital role in educating patients about controlling their HTN. Because all blood pressure medications have potential adverse effects, it is important for patients to attempt to control their disease through nonpharmacologic means,

to the greatest extent possible. Nonpharmacologic methods for controlling HTN include the following:

- Limit intake of alcohol.
- Restrict sodium consumption.
- Reduce intake of saturated fat and cholesterol, and increase consumption of fruits and vegetables.
- Increase aerobic physical activity.
- Discontinue use of all tobacco products.
- Explore measures for dealing with excessive stress.
- Maintain optimum weight.

Guidelines for the Management of Hypertension

34.3 Research-based guidelines have been developed to aid the health care provider in providing optimum treatment for patients with hypertension.

Hypertension (HTN) is defined as the consistent elevation of systemic arterial blood pressure. When most people use the word *hypertension*, they are referring to systemic HTN, that which is measured routinely by a conventional blood pressure cuff on the upper arm over the brachial artery. Systemic HTN is a general measurement of arterial blood pressure in the body. Localized HTN may also occur. For example, patients with cirrhosis of the liver often develop portal HTN, which occurs in the portal vein and its branches serving the liver. Pulmonary HTN occurs in the pulmonary artery and its branches and is most often observed in patients with left-sided heart failure. These localized types of HTN respond to many of the same antihypertensive drugs used for systemic HTN.

To develop guidelines for treatment, many attempts have been made to define HTN and to determine when medical intervention

---

CONNECTIONS ❮ Complementary and Alternative Therapies

❮ Grape Seed Extract

Description
Grape seed extract is obtained from the seeds of grapes that are usually used in the process of winemaking.

History and Claims
Grapes and grape seeds have been used for medicinal purposes for thousands of years. The primary use of the extract has been to treat cardiovascular conditions such as HTN, high blood cholesterol, atherosclerosis, and to generally improve circulation. Some claim that it improves wound healing, prevents cancer, and lowers the risk for the long-term consequences of diabetes. The drug is being examined for its effects on Alzheimer's disease.

Standardization
The grape seeds are crushed and placed into tablet, capsule, or liquid forms. Typical doses are 50 to 300 mg/day. Standardization is based on percentage of polyphenols. The seeds also contain a high concentration of essential fatty acids and vitamin E.

Evidence
Thousands of studies have been conducted on the polyphenols contained in this supplement. Grape seed extract has antioxidant properties (University of Maryland Medical Center, 2013). In general, antioxidants improve wound healing and repair cellular injury. Preliminary evidence suggests it may have some benefit in repairing blood vessel damage that could lead to atherosclerosis and HTN (National Center for Complementary and Alternative Medicine, 2012). Controlled, long-term studies on the effects of grape seed extracts on HTN have not been conducted. It has few adverse effects. Caution should be used if taking anticoagulant drugs, because increased bleeding may result. Overall, the benefits of grape seed extract are no different than those of a diet balanced with natural antioxidants (and an occasional glass of red wine).

TABLE 34.1   Recommendations for Treating Hypertension

| Group | Blood Pressure Goal | FIRST-LINE DRUGS (ALONE OR IN COMBINATION) | |
		Nonblack	Black
Age 60 or greater without DM or CKD	Less than 150/90 mmHg	Thiazide diuretic, ACEI, ARB or CCB	Thiazide diuretic or CCB
Age 59 or lower without DM or CKD	Less than 140/90 mmHg	Thiazide diuretic, ACEI, ARB or CCB	Thiazide diuretic or CCB
All ages with DM present (no CKD)	Less than 140/90 mmHg	Thiazide diuretic, ACEI, ARB or CCB	Thiazide diuretic or CCB
All ages with CKD present (with or without DM)	Less than 140/90 mmHg	ACEI or ARB	ACEI or ARB

DM = diabetes mellitus; CKD = chronic kidney disease; ACEI = angiotensin-converting enzyme inhibitor; ARB = angiotensin receptor blocker; CCB = calcium channel blocker.

is beneficial in reducing mortality due to cardiovascular disease. In 2003, the National High Blood Pressure Education Program Coordinating Committee of the National Heart, Lung, and Blood Institute at the National Institutes of Health issued *The Seventh Report of the Joint National Committee on Prevention, Detection, Evaluation, and Treatment of High Blood Pressure* (JNC-7), which became the standard for treating HTN for the following decade. The JNC-7 defined HTN as a sustained systolic blood pressure of greater than 140 mmHg or diastolic pressure of greater than 90 to 99 mmHg.

Late in 2013, the Eighth Joint National Committee (JNC-8) significantly revised the HTN guidelines, based on newer research (James et al., 2014). The JNC-8 committee kept the same definition of hypertension as JNC-7: 140/90 mmHg. The primary difference is that research has shown that not all people with a blood pressure higher than 140/90 mmHg need pharmacotherapy. For example, patients over age 60 who do not have chronic kidney disease or diabetes do not need pharmacotherapy until the 150/90 mmHg threshold. Furthermore, the classes of medications recommended as first-line therapy have changed: Beta-adrenergic blockers are no longer considered first-line drugs.

In the past decade, research has determined that there are racial differences in response to antihypertensive medications. To account for these differences, the JNC-8 guidelines make a distinction between drugs used for black and nonblack patients. Nonblacks without chronic kidney disease (CKD) should be treated with thiazide diuretics, calcium channel blockers (CCBs), angiotensin-converting enzyme (ACE) inhibitors, or angiotensin receptor blockers (ARBs). Blacks without CKD are more effectively treated with thiazide diuretics either alone or in combination with CCBs. For patients with CKD, the therapy for blacks and nonblacks is the same. These recommendations are summarized in Table 34.1.

Pharmacotherapy of Hypertension

34.4 The choice of antihypertensive medication is determined by the degree of hypertension and the presence of other medical conditions.

The goal of antihypertensive therapy is to reduce the morbidity and mortality associated with chronic HTN. Research has confirmed that keeping blood pressure within normal limits reduces the risk of hypertension-related target-organ damage.

The pharmacologic management of HTN is individualized to the patient's risk factors, comorbid medical conditions, and degree

of blood pressure elevation. Patient responses to antihypertensive medications vary widely because of the many complex genetic and environmental factors affecting blood pressure.

Eleven different drug classes are used to treat HTN, as shown in Table 34.2. Each class has specific benefits and characteristic adverse effects. The mechanisms of action of the major classes of antihypertensive drugs are summarized in Pharmacotherapy Illustrated 34.1. Although many effective drugs are available, and the data supporting the benefits of therapy are strong, HTN remains a challenging disorder to treat successfully. Choice of therapy is often based on the clinician's experience. Although antihypertensive treatment varies, there are several principles that guide pharmacotherapy.

Initial Drug of Choice

The JNC-7 report recommended thiazide diuretics as initial drugs for the management of mild to moderate HTN. The JNC-8 expanded this recommendation to a choice of thiazide diuretics, ACE inhibitors, ARBs, or CCBs for most patients. Clinical research has clearly demonstrated that these four primary drug classes reduce HTN-related morbidity and mortality.

In most cases, low doses of the initial drug are prescribed and the patient is reevaluated after an appropriate time period. As therapy continues, dosage is adjusted to maintain optimum blood pressure.

Adding Drugs to the Antihypertensive Regimen

If the patient does not respond to the initial medication, a drug from a different antihypertensive class may be added to the

TABLE 34.2   Drug Classes for Hypertension

Type	Class
First-line drugs	Diuretics
	Angiotensin-converting enzyme (ACE) inhibitors
	Angiotensin receptor blockers (ARBs)
	Calcium channel blockers (CCBs)
Second-line drugs	Alpha$_2$-adrenergic agonists
	Alpha$_1$- adrenergic blockers
	Beta-adrenergic blockers
	Centrally acting alpha and beta blockers
	Direct-acting vasodilators
	Direct renin inhibitors
	Peripherally acting adrenergic neuron blockers

PHARMACOTHERAPY ILLUSTRATED 34.1

Mechanism of Action of Antihypertensive Drugs

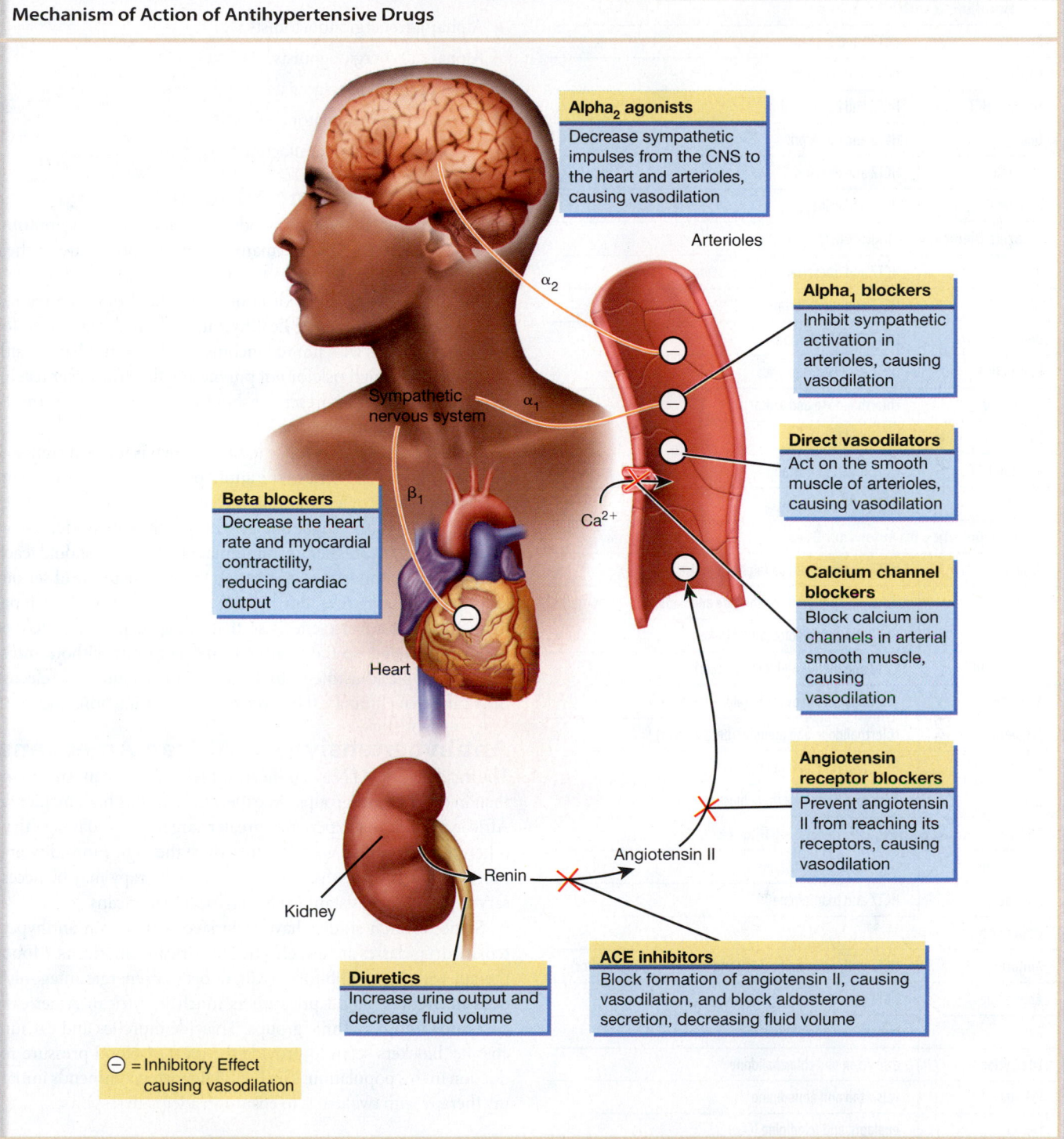

Alpha$_2$ agonists

Decrease sympathetic impulses from the CNS to the heart and arterioles, causing vasodilation

Arterioles

Alpha$_1$ blockers

Inhibit sympathetic activation in arterioles, causing vasodilation

Direct vasodilators

Act on the smooth muscle of arterioles, causing vasodilation

Calcium channel blockers

Block calcium ion channels in arterial smooth muscle, causing vasodilation

Angiotensin receptor blockers

Prevent angiotensin II from reaching its receptors, causing vasodilation

ACE inhibitors

Block formation of angiotensin II, causing vasodilation, and block aldosterone secretion, decreasing fluid volume

Beta blockers

Decrease the heart rate and myocardial contractility, reducing cardiac output

Sympathetic nervous system

Heart

Kidney

Diuretics

Increase urine output and decrease fluid volume

Renin

Angiotensin II

Ca^{2+}

⊖ = Inhibitory Effect causing vasodilation

regimen. Prescribing two antihypertensives concurrently results in additive or synergistic blood pressure reduction and is common practice when managing resistant HTN. The advantage of using two drugs is that lower doses of each may be used, resulting in fewer adverse effects and better patient adherence. Drug manufacturers sometimes combine two drugs into a single pill or capsule for dosing convenience and to improve patient adherence. The majority of these combinations include a thiazide diuretic, usually

hydrochlorothiazide, sometimes abbreviated as HCTZ combined with an ACE inhibitor or ARB. ACE inhibitors and ARBs are not used in combination with each other because they act by very similar mechanisms. Selected combination antihypertensives are shown in Table 34.3.

Certain antihypertensive classes cause a higher incidence of adverse effects and are generally prescribed when drugs from the four primary classes do not produce a satisfactory response. In some

TABLE 34.3 Selected Combination Medications for Hypertension

Thiazide Diuretic with ACE Inhibitor

Accuretic	HCTZ* and quinapril
Capozide	HCTZ and captopril
Lotensin HCT	HCTZ and benazepril
Uniretic	HCTZ and moexipril
Vaseretic	HCTZ and enalapril
Zestoretic	HCTZ and lisinopril

Thiazide Diuretic with Angiotensin II Blocker

Avalide	HCTZ and irbesartan
Atacand HCT	HCTZ and candesartan
Benicar HCT	HCTZ and olmesartan
Diovan HCT	HCTZ and valsartan
Edarbyclor	chlorthalidone and azilsartan
Hyzaar	HCTZ and losartan
Micardis HCT	HCTZ and telmisartan
Teveten HCT	HCTZ and eprosartan

Thiazide Diuretic with Autonomic Drug

Aldoril	HCTZ and methyldopa (alpha$_2$ agonist)
Corzide	HCTZ with bendroflumethiazide and nadolol (beta blocker)
Inderide	HCTZ and propranolol (beta blocker)
Lopressor HCT	HCTZ and metoprolol (beta blocker)
Minizide	polythiazide and prazosin (alpha blocker)
Tenoretic	chlorthalidone and atenolol (beta blocker)
Timolide	HCTZ and timolol (beta blocker)
Ziac	HCTZ and bisoprolol (beta blocker)

Thiazide Diuretic with Potassium-Sparing Diuretic

Aldactazide	HCTZ and spironolactone
Dyazide	HCTZ and triamterene

Other Combinations

Amturnide	HCTZ with amlodipine (CCB) and aliskirin (renin inhibitor)
Apresazide	HCTZ and hydralazine (direct vasodilator)
Azor	olmesartan and amlodipine
Edarbyclor	azilsartan and chlorthalidone
Exforge	valsartan and amlodipine
Lexxel	enalapril and felodipine (CCB)
Lotrel	benazepril and amlodipine
Tarka	trandolapril and verapamil (CCB)
Tekalmo	amlodipine and aliskiren (renin inhibitor)
Tekturna HCT	HCTZ and aliskiren
Tribenzor	HCTZ with olmesartan and amlodipine

*HCTZ = hydrochlorothiazide; CCB = calcium channel blocker.

cases, research studies have not demonstrated a firm link between drug use and lowered morbidity or mortality. The alternative antihypertensive drug classes include the following:

- Alpha$_1$-adrenergic antagonists
- Alpha$_2$-adrenergic agonists
- Beta-adrenergic antagonists
- Direct-acting vasodilators
- Peripheral adrenergic antagonists

Enhancing Patient Adherence

Because chronic HTN may produce no identifiable symptoms for as long as 10 to 20 years, many people are not aware of their condition. Convincing patients to change established lifestyle habits, spend money on medication, and take drugs on a regular basis when they are feeling healthy can be a challenging task for the nurse. Patients with limited income or who do not have health insurance are at high risk for not purchasing the drugs after receiving a prescription. The prescriber should consider generic forms of these drugs to reduce costs and increase adherence.

Further reducing adherence to the regimen is the occurrence of adverse drug effects. Some of the antihypertensive drugs cause embarrassing adverse effects such as impotence, which may go unreported. Others cause fatigue and generally make patients feel sicker than they were before therapy was initiated. The nurse should teach the patient the importance of treating the disease to avoid serious long-term consequences. Furthermore, the nurse should teach patients to report adverse effects so that dosage can be adjusted, or the drug changed, so the treatment may continue without interruption. Simple adjustments to the dosage or changing the selected drug can often eliminate the adverse effects causing nonadherence.

Antihypertensives in African Americans

The incidence of HTN is significantly higher in African Americans than in other ethnic groups. As expected from this high incidence, African Americans experience greater target-organ damage than other populations. In an effort to reduce the high morbidity and mortality risks, aggressive antihypertensive therapy may be necessary to overcome resistant HTN in African Americans.

Some research studies have suggested that certain antihypertensive drug classes are less effective in African Americans. Monotherapy with ACE inhibitors, ARBs, or beta-adrenergic antagonists does not reduce blood pressure as much in African Americans compared to other ethnic groups. Thiazide diuretics and calcium channel blockers seem to provide the greatest blood pressure reduction in this population. The JNC-8 Report recommends initiating therapy with two drugs to ensure an adequate response.

Drug Classes for Hypertension

34.5 Diuretics are often drugs of first choice for treating mild to moderate hypertension.

Diuretics were the first class of medications used to treat HTN in the 1950s. Despite the many advances in drug therapy, diuretics are still considered first-line drugs for this disease because they are very effective at controlling mild to moderate HTN with few serious adverse effects. Although sometimes used as monotherapy, they are

◀ **Sleep, Cardiovascular Disease, and Timing of Antihypertensives**

Sleep apnea has currently been linked to vascular events such as stroke. More recent clinical research suggests that not only sleep apnea, but the duration of sleep may play a role in cardiovascular conditions, including HTN and angina. Several recent studies have noted an increased occurrence of cardiovascular disease (CVD) in patients who slept 5 hours or less, or more than 9 hours (Magee, Iverson, & Caputi, 2009; Sabanayagam & Shankar, 2010). The lowest occurrence seemed to be associated with 7 hours of sleep. More research is needed to determine whether short- or long-duration sleep is a sign of CVD or whether it is a result of cardiovascular risk factors or disease. In the study by Sabanayagam and Shankar (2010), short- and long-duration sleep was associated with CVD risk factors such as HTN, obesity, and diabetes. It was postulated that sleep disturbances may be associated with endocrine or metabolic functions. In a related study, Hermida, Ayala, Mojón, and Fernández (2011) determined that patients with chronic kidney disease taking at least one antihypertensive drug at bedtime decreased the risk of cardiovascular events, including angina, MI, HF, and stroke. Patients taking their antihypertensive medications at bedtime also had lower sleep-time blood pressures and better daytime control of their blood pressure.

When taking the initial history and subsequent follow-up on a patient with known or suspected CVD, answers to questions about sleep duration or nighttime awakening may be important data to gather. Nurses often teach patients to take antihypertensive medication at night to reduce the risk for dizziness and falls related to orthostatic hypotension, and it may also be a strategy, even for once-daily medications, for reducing the occurrence of cardiovascular events.

frequently prescribed with other antihypertensive medications to enhance their effectiveness. Because this class of drugs was presented in detail in Chapter 32, the following section is a summary of their application to the treatment of HTN.

Although dozens of diuretics are available for the treatment of HTN, all produce a similar result: the reduction of blood volume through the urinary excretion of water and electrolytes. Reducing blood volume places less pressure on the arterial walls, thereby decreasing peripheral resistance and lowering systemic blood pressure. The mechanism by which diuretics increase the excretion of water and electrolytes, specifically where and how the kidney is affected, differs among the various classes of diuretics.

Whenever a medication changes urine flow or composition, dehydration and electrolyte depletion are possible. Dehydration may manifest as increased thirst or poor skin turgor. Excessive sodium loss (hyponatremia) is a concern for all diuretics. Potassium loss (hypokalemia) is of particular concern for loop and thiazide diuretics. The potassium-sparing diuretics such as triamterene (Dyrenium) have less tendency to cause hypokalemia.

Thiazide and thiazide-like diuretics: Thiazide and thiazide-like diuretics have been the mainstay for the pharmacotherapy of HTN for decades. The thiazide diuretics are inexpensive, and most are available in generic formulations. They are safe drugs, with excessive urinary potassium loss being the primary adverse effect. Because hypokalemia can induce serious dysrhythmias in susceptible patients, careful laboratory monitoring of serum

potassium is necessary. Patients should increase their amount of dietary potassium, and potassium supplements may be prescribed. These diuretics may also cause hyperglycemia; therefore, blood glucose levels should be monitored in patients with diabetes. Because thiazides may increase blood lipids, these drugs should be used cautiously in patients with existing hyperlipidemia. Hydrochlorothiazide, or HCTZ (Microzide), is featured as the prototype drug in this class in Chapter 32. In addition to HCTZ, thiazides indicated for HTN include chlorothiazide (Diuril), chlorthalidone (Hygroton), indapamide (Lozol), methyclothiazide (Enduron), and metolazone (Zaroxolyn).

Potassium-sparing diuretics: Although potassium-sparing diuretics such as spironolactone (Aldactone) and triamterene (Dyrenium) produce only a modest diuresis, their primary advantage is they do not cause potassium depletion. They are especially beneficial when the patient is at risk of developing hypokalemia due to a medical condition or the use of thiazide or loop diuretics. The primary concern when using potassium-sparing diuretics is the possibility of retaining too much potassium, which can cause serious dysrhythmias. Patients with diabetes and those with renal impairment are particularly susceptible to hyperkalemia. Patients should be instructed to avoid excess potassium in their diet, including salt substitutes containing KCl, and not to use potassium supplements during therapy. Concurrent use with an ACE inhibitor or ARB significantly increases the potential for development of hyperkalemia. Spironolactone is presented as a prototype drug for this class in Chapter 32. In addition to spironolactone and triamterene, other potassium-sparing diuretics indicated for HTN are amiloride (Midamor) and eplerenone (Inspra).

Loop (high-ceiling) diuretics: The loop diuretics such as furosemide (Lasix) cause greater diuresis and have the potential to produce a higher reduction in blood pressure than the thiazides or potassium-sparing diuretics. Although this makes them very effective at reducing blood pressure, they are not ideal drugs for maintenance therapy. The risk of adverse effects such as hypokalemia and dehydration is great because of their ability to remove large amounts of fluid from the body in a short time period. Loop diuretics are ototoxic, an effect more likely to occur in patients with renal insufficiency or when high doses are administered. Because of their greater toxicity, loop diuretics are sometimes reserved for patients with resistant HTN. Furosemide, the only loop diuretic in widespread use, is presented as a prototype drug in Chapter 32. In addition to furosemide, other loop diuretics indicated for HTN include bumetanide (Bumex), ethacrynic acid (Edecrin), and torsemide (Demadex).

CONNECTION Checkpoint 34.1

From what you learned in Chapter 32, why must the thiazide diuretics be used with great caution in patients taking digoxin (Lanoxin)? *See Answer to Connection Checkpoint 34.1 on student resource website.*

34.6 Calcium channel blockers have emerged as important drugs in the treatment of hypertension.

Calcium channel blockers (CCBs) are widely used in the treatment of HTN, angina pectoris, and dysrhythmias, as presented in Chapter 30. The following section summarizes their application to the treatment of HTN.

CCBs exert beneficial effects on the heart and blood vessels by blocking calcium ion channels in cardiac and arteriolar smooth muscle. The flow of calcium ions into muscle cells is inhibited, limiting the degree of muscular contraction. At low doses, CCBs relax arterial smooth muscle, thus decreasing peripheral resistance and lowering blood pressure. Some CCBs such as nifedipine (Adalat CC, Procardia XL) are selective for arterioles, whereas others such as verapamil (Calan, Isoptin, Verelan) affect channels in both arterioles and the myocardium. CCBs vary in potency and in the frequency and types of adverse effects produced. Nifedipine and verapamil are highlighted as drug prototypes in Chapter 30.

Due to their potent vasodilating effects, CCBs can cause reflex tachycardia, especially with those CCBs that are selective for arterioles. Because CCBs can slow myocardial conduction, they are contraindicated in patients with certain types of heart conditions such as sick sinus syndrome or third-degree AV block without the presence of a pacemaker. The CCBs that reduce myocardial contractility can worsen heart failure.

CCBs are usually not used as monotherapy for chronic HTN. They are, however, useful in combination therapy for treating certain populations such as older adults and African Americans who are sometimes less responsive to drugs in other antihypertensive classes. In addition to nifedipine and verapamil, other CCBs indicated for HTN include amlodipine (Norvasc), clevidipine (Cleviprex), diltiazem (Cardizem, Dilacor, others), felodipine, isradipine (DynaCirc), nicardipine (Cardene), and nisoldipine (Sular).

CONNECTION Checkpoint 34.2

Verapamil and nifedipine are both calcium channel blockers used for HTN. From what you learned in Chapter 30, why would a beta blocker be used concurrently with nifedipine but be contraindicated with verapamil? *See Answer to Connection Checkpoint 34.2 on student resource website.*

34.7 Blocking the renin-angiotensin-aldosterone system leads to a decrease in blood pressure and improved kidney function.

As discussed in Chapter 31, the renin-angiotensin-aldosterone system (RAAS) is one of the primary homeostatic mechanisms controlling blood pressure and fluid balance. Drugs inhibiting the RAAS are widely used in the treatment of cardiovascular disease. Clinical research suggests ACE inhibitors are as effective as the diuretics in reducing HTN-related morbidity and mortality. The following section summarizes their applications to HTN pharmacotherapy.

Angiotensin-converting enzyme (ACE) inhibitors block the formation of angiotensin II, decreasing blood pressure through two mechanisms. First, ACE inhibitors block the intense vasoconstriction of arterioles caused by angiotensin II, which decreases blood pressure due to diminished peripheral resistance. Second, these drugs block the effects of angiotensin II on the secretion of aldosterone, which lowers blood pressure by decreasing blood volume. Through their inhibition of aldosterone secretion, ACE inhibitors enhance the effects of the thiazide diuretics; thus drugs from these two classes may be used concurrently in the management of HTN. Lisinopril (Prinivil, Zestril) is the prototype drug for the ACE inhibitors in Chapter 31. Other ACE inhibitors indicated for HTN include benazepril (Lotensin), captopril (Capoten),

enalapril (Vasotec), fosinopril (Monopril), moexipril (Univasc), perindopril (Aceon), quinapril (Accupril), ramipril (Altace), and trandolapril (Mavik).

Adverse effects of ACE inhibitors are usually minor and include persistent cough and orthostatic hypotension, particularly following the first few doses of the drug. Hyperkalemia may occur and can be a major concern for patients with diabetes, those with renal impairment, and patients taking potassium-sparing diuretics. Though rare, the most serious adverse effect of ACE inhibitors is the development of angioedema. When it does occur, angioedema most often develops within days after beginning ACE inhibitor therapy. Cough and angioedema arise more frequently in African Americans than in other ethnic groups.

The ARBs afford a second method for altering the RAAS pathway. ARBs such as losartan (Cozaar) block receptors for angiotensin II in arteriolar smooth muscle and in the adrenal gland, thus causing blood pressure to fall. Their actions are similar to those of the ACE inhibitors.

Angiotensin II receptor blockers have the lowest incidence of serious adverse effects of any of the antihypertensive classes. Most ARB adverse effects are related to hypotension. Unlike the ACE inhibitors, they do not cause cough, and angioedema is rare. Medications in this class are often combined with drugs from other classes in the management of HTN. A drug prototype feature for losartan (Cozaar) is included in Chapter 31. Other ARBs indicated for HTN include candesartan (Atacand), eprosartan (Teveten), irbesartan (Avapro), olmesartan (Benicar), telmisartan (Micardis), and valsartan (Diovan).

Aliskiren (Tekturna) was the first in a new class of antihypertensives called "direct renin inhibitors" approved for HTN. They act by interfering with part of the RAAS system. The combination of aliskiren with HCTZ (Tekturna ACT) is also approved for treating HTN. The most common adverse effects of aliskiren are diarrhea, cough, flulike symptoms, and rash. The direct renin inhibitors are not considered first-line medications for HTN.

34.8 Adrenergic antagonists are commonly used to treat hypertension.

The adrenergic antagonists, or blockers, are used for a wide variety of cardiovascular disorders, including HTN, angina pectoris, dysrhythmias, and MI prophylaxis. Blocking adrenergic receptors in the sympathetic nervous system has a number of beneficial effects on the heart and vessels. For example, by blocking the "fight-or-flight" responses, heart rate slows, blood pressure declines, and the bronchi dilate.

Adrenergic blockers affect the sympathetic division through a number of distinct mechanisms, although all have in common the effect of lowering blood pressure. These mechanisms include the following:

- Blockade of $beta_1$-adrenergic receptors
- Blockade of $alpha_1$-adrenergic receptors
- Nonselective blockade of both $alpha_1$- and beta-adrenergic receptors
- Stimulation of centrally acting $alpha_2$-adrenergic receptors in the brainstem
- Blockade of peripheral adrenergic neurons

The earliest drugs for HTN were nonselective drugs that blocked nerve transmission at the ganglia or at both alpha- and beta-adrenergic receptors. Although the nonselective medications revolutionized the treatment of HTN, they caused a high incidence of adverse effects. These drugs are rarely used today because selective agents are more efficacious and better tolerated by patients. Of the five subclasses of adrenergic antagonists, the beta-adrenergic blockers are the most widely used group. All of the adrenergic inhibitors are considered second-line drugs for HTN.

Beta-adrenergic antagonists: In this section, the discussion of beta-adrenergic antagonists is limited to their use in treating HTN. The student should refer to Chapter 16 for a detailed discussion of the basic pharmacology of this drug class. Other important therapeutic applications of the beta blockers include angina pectoris and MI, dysrhythmias, heart failure, and migraines.

Beta-adrenergic antagonists may be cardioselective (beta$_1$) or nonspecific (beta$_1$ and beta$_2$). Cardioselective beta blockers decrease heart rate, myocardial contractility, and cardiac conduction velocity. Nonspecific beta blockers produce the same effects but also act on the respiratory system to cause bronchoconstriction. Decreasing the heart rate and contractility also reduces cardiac output and lowers systemic blood pressure. Some of their antihypertensive effect is also caused by the blockade of beta$_1$ receptors in the juxtaglomerular apparatus, which inhibits the secretion of renin and the formation of angiotensin II. Although they are not recommended by the JNC Report as first-line drugs for HTN, the beta-adrenergic antagonists are still widely used for this condition.

At low doses, beta blockers are well tolerated and serious adverse events are uncommon. As the dosage is increased, however, adverse effects can become numerous and potentially serious in certain patients. Because nonselective beta blockers will slow the heart rate and cause bronchoconstriction, they should be used with caution in patients with asthma or heart failure. Heart rate and rhythm should be regularly monitored during beta-blocker therapy. Many patients report fatigue and activity intolerance at higher doses because the reduction in heart rate causes the heart to become less responsive to exertion. When discontinuing a beta blocker, drug doses should be tapered over a several week period. Abrupt cessation of beta-blocker therapy can result in rebound HTN, angina, MI, and even death in patients with CAD.

Prototype features for beta-adrenergic antagonists can be found for propranolol (Inderal, InnoPran XL) and metoprolol (Lopressor, Toprol XL) in Chapter 16, atenolol (Tenormin) in Chapter 35, and timolol (Betimol, Istalol, Timoptic) in Chapter 74. In addition to atenolol, metoprolol, propranolol, and timolol, other beta-blockers approved for HTN include betaxolol (Kerlone), bisoprolol (Zebeta), and nadolol (Corgard).

CONNECTION Checkpoint 34.3

From what you learned in Chapter 16, should a hypertensive patient with asthma receive a selective beta$_1$ blocker or a nonselective beta blocker for HTN? *See Answer to Connection Checkpoint 34.3 on student resource website.*

Alpha$_1$-adrenergic antagonists: The alpha$_1$-adrenergic antagonists have several clinical applications, which were presented in Chapter 16. In addition to their use in HTN, they are prescribed for benign prostatic hyperplasia (BPH) because their ability to relax smooth muscle in the prostate and bladder neck reduces urethral resistance. A prototype drug feature for prazosin (Minipress) is included in Chapter 16, and the use of tamsulosin (Flomax) in treating BPH is discussed in Chapter 71. Terazosin is another alpha$_1$-adrenergic antagonist used for HTN.

The alpha$_1$-adrenergic antagonists lower blood pressure directly by blocking sympathetic receptors in arterioles, causing the vessels to dilate. They also dilate veins, which lowers blood pressure indirectly by decreasing venous return to the heart and reducing cardiac output. The alpha blockers are not first-line drugs for HTN because long-term clinical trials have shown them to be less effective at reducing the incidence of serious HTN-related cardiovascular events than diuretics. When used to treat HTN, the alpha blockers are used concurrently with other classes of antihypertensives, such as diuretics.

The alpha$_1$-adrenergic blockers may cause significant orthostatic hypotension. It is particularly serious with the initial doses of these medications and is referred to as the **first-dose phenomenon**, although orthostatic hypotension may persist throughout treatment. In severe cases, syncope can occur. Blood pressure should be assessed regularly during therapy to maintain patient safety. Other common adverse effects include weakness, dizziness, dry mouth, headache, and gastrointestinal (GI) complaints such as nausea and vomiting. Less common, though sometimes a major cause for nonadherence, are adverse effects on male sexual function that include decreased libido and erectile dysfunction.

Nonselective alpha$_1$- and beta-adrenergic antagonists: Carvedilol (Coreg) and labetalol (Trandate) are unique in that they block both alpha$_1$- and beta-adrenergic receptors. These drugs act by a combination of effects: reducing cardiac output, inhibiting renin secretion, and blocking vasoconstriction of arterioles and veins. As expected, their adverse effects are a combination of alpha and beta blockade and include orthostatic hypotension, bradycardia, and bronchoconstriction. The applications of carvedilol in treating heart failure are presented in Chapter 36.

Alpha$_2$-adrenergic agonists: If an alpha antagonist such as prazosin lowers blood pressure, it might be predicted that the administration of an alpha$_2$-adrenergic agonist would raise blood pressure. This is not the case. The answer to this contradiction lies in the different locations of the two subtypes of alpha receptors. The alpha$_1$ receptors blocked by prazosin lie in the peripheral nervous system (PNS) at arterioles. The alpha$_2$ receptors reside in the central nervous system (CNS).

When alpha$_2$ receptors are activated, the outflow of sympathetic nerve impulses from the CNS to the heart and arterioles is inhibited. In effect, this produces the same responses as inhibition of the alpha$_1$ receptor: slowing the heart rate and conduction velocity and dilating the arterioles. Thus, activating alpha$_2$ receptors (in the CNS) produces similar actions as inhibiting alpha$_1$ receptors (in the PNS).

The centrally acting alpha$_2$ agonists are used less frequently than the alpha$_1$ antagonists. The alpha$_2$ agonists have a tendency to cause excessive sedation, dizziness, and orthostatic hypotension, which can be especially troublesome in older adults. Extended use results in sodium and water retention, which increases blood volume and counteracts the antihypertensive action of these drugs. Alpha$_2$ agonists are usually reserved for treating resistant HTN that cannot be managed by safer medications. The two drugs in this class are methyldopa (Aldomet) and clonidine (Catapres, Duraclon, Kapvay, Nexiclon XR).

Methyldopa is an older drug approved in 1962. Its only indication is HTN that has not responded adequately to safer antihypertensives. The drug is normally administered by the oral (PO) route, although an intravenous (IV) form known as methyldopate is available for hypertensive crises. Compared to other antihypertensives given by the IV route, methyldopa has a relatively slow onset of action because it must first be metabolized inside neurons to an active metabolite, methyl norepinephrine. Methyldopa is sometimes used for treating HTN occurring during pregnancy because it maintains stable blood flow to the uterus, and its safety to the fetus has been demonstrated in long-term studies.

Because methyldopa is a centrally acting drug, CNS effects such as drowsiness, depression, headache, sedation, and bizarre dreams are relatively common. Orthostatic hypotension may occur, but it is less severe than that produced by the alpha$_1$ antagonists. Peripheral edema due to sodium retention may occur, which can be managed by administration of a thiazide diuretic. A significant number of patients develop a positive Coombs' test, which detects antibodies against the patient's own red blood cells. Because tolerance develops after 3 to 4 months of therapy, a dosage increase may be required to manage HTN. This drug is pregnancy category B.

Approved in 1974, clonidine (Catapres, Duraclon, Kapvay, Nexiclon XR) activates alpha$_2$-adrenergic receptors in the cardiovascular control centers in the brainstem. The reduced sympathetic outflow causes vasodilation and slows the heart rate. As an antihypertensive, it is available as regular oral tablets, extended release tablets or suspension (Nexiclon), or a transdermal patch (Catapres) that releases the drug at a constant rate over 7 days. A second approved indication for clonidine (Duraclon) is intractable pain in patients with cancer that is not relieved by opiates. Pain control is achieved by a continuous epidural infusion of the drug. To assist in pain management, transdermal clonidine may be used to provide some degree of analgesia so that the dose of opiate can be reduced. In 2010, an extended release form of clonidine (Kapvay) was approved to treat attention deficit/hyperactivity disorder.

Clonidine has many off-label indications. These include dysmenorrhea, menopausal flushing, migraine prophylaxis, smoking cessation, opiate and benzodiazepine withdrawal, and Tourette's syndrome.

The most common adverse effect of clonidine is dry mouth, which occurs in about 40% of the patients taking the drug. Like methyldopa, CNS adverse effects such as sedation, fatigue, drowsiness, and dizziness are common. Transdermal clonidine produces fewer serious adverse effects, although the patches can cause skin irritation and itching. The patient should be warned not to abruptly discontinue the drug, as severe rebound HTN, agitation, nervousness, and anxiety may result.

Adrenergic neuron blockers: The adrenergic neuron–blocker class consists of two drugs that inhibit the synthesis or release of norepinephrine (NE) in sympathetic neurons. With less NE available to cross the synapse, sympathetic activity is diminished at both alpha- and beta-adrenergic receptors. In effect, the actions of these drugs are the same as the nonselective

alpha$_1$- and beta-adrenergic antagonists: reduced heart rate and cardiac output (beta effects) combined with dilation of arterioles (alpha effect).

The adrenergic neuron blockers have mostly historical interest, as they are rarely prescribed today due to the availability of safer medications. Reserpine (Serpalan), approved in 1952, was one of the earliest drugs used for HTN. Reserpine lowers blood pressure by irreversibly binding to NE storage vesicles, causing depletion of NE and other neurotransmitters in both the central and peripheral nervous systems. The drug may take 2 to 6 weeks to deplete NE and produce an optimal antihypertensive effect. Unfortunately, reserpine can cause profound depression and sedation, and cardiovascular adverse effects such as bradycardia and orthostatic hypotension can be severe. Effects are often prolonged because once depleted of NE, neurons may take several weeks to synthesize adequate amounts of the neurotransmitter. Reserpine is only prescribed when patients are unable to tolerate safer antihypertensives.

Guanethidine (Ismelin) is also an adrenergic neuron–blocking drug. It acts by preventing the storage and release of NE in nerve terminals. As with reserpine, depletion of NE causes the heart rate to slow and blood pressure to fall. The limiting adverse effects of guanethidine are severe diarrhea and orthostatic hypotension, which occur frequently and can be serious enough to cause syncope. Guanethidine is rarely prescribed due to the potential for serious adverse effects. A third drug in this class, guanadrel (Hylorel), has similar actions and adverse effects to guanethidine, but its use has been discontinued in the United States.

34.9 Direct-acting vasodilators lower blood pressure by relaxing arteriolar smooth muscle.

The ability to cause vasodilation is a property shared by many different classes of drugs, as shown in Pharmacotherapy Illustrated 34.1. Most vasodilators are used to treat HTN, and some are also used for the pharmacotherapy of heart failure, angina pectoris, and MI. Some of the drugs presented in previous sections of this chapter produce vasodilation indirectly by affecting autonomic nerves or by influencing the renin-angiotensin-aldosterone pathway. The drugs presented in this section affect the vascular smooth muscle itself; thus, they are called direct vasodilators.

Direct relaxation of arteriolar smooth muscle is an effective way to reduce blood pressure. Indeed, sodium nitroprusside (Nitropress) and diazoxide (Hyperstat IV) are used in hypertensive emergencies and can lower blood pressure almost instantaneously. Unfortunately, the medications in this class have the potential to produce serious adverse effects. This limits their applications in the pharmacotherapy of HTN to hypertensive emergencies and for HTN unresponsive to medications from safer drug classes.

All direct vasodilators cause **reflex tachycardia**, a compensatory increase in heart rate due to the sudden decrease in blood pressure. The baroreceptor reflex is an essential component of the normal physiological control of blood pressure. However, when reflex tachycardia occurs as the result of vasodilator drugs, the heart is forced to work harder and the resultant blood pressure increase counteracts the effect of the antihypertensive drug. Patients with CAD may experience an acute angina attack due to the sudden increase in cardiac workload. Fortunately, reflex tachycardia can be prevented by administering a beta-adrenergic blocker, such as propranolol (Inderal). Beta blockers are often administered concurrently with direct vasodilators for this reason.

A second potentially serious adverse effect of direct vasodilator therapy is salt and water retention. The reduction in blood pressure from the vasodilator causes a compensatory increase in aldosterone secretion by the adrenal gland. The increased aldosterone level signals the kidney to retain more sodium and water. Blood volume increases, thus raising blood pressure and canceling the antihypertensive action of the vasodilator. A diuretic may be administered concurrently with a direct vasodilator in order to prevent fluid retention.

Other adverse effects are drug specific. Hydralazine can induce a lupus-like syndrome characterized by myalgia, arthralgia, fever, and the presence of antinuclear antibodies. Although rare, symptoms may persist for 6 months or longer and antinuclear antibodies may be present for 9 years. The occurrence of this lupus-like syndrome is more common in Caucasians who are slow acetylators (see Chapter 11). Antinuclear antibody titers should be determined prior to initiating therapy and periodically thereafter to identify the development of this syndrome.

PROTOTYPE DRUG | **Hydralazine (Apresoline)**

Classification: **Therapeutic:** Antihypertensive
Pharmacologic: Direct vasodilator

Therapeutic Effects and Uses: In 1952, hydralazine was one of the first oral antihypertensive medications marketed in the United States. It is most commonly administered in tablet form for moderate to severe HTN, usually in combination with other antihypertensives. Apresazide is a fixed-dose combination of hydralazine with HCTZ. When given PO, hydralazine is administered 2 to 4 times per day, usually with food because this increases its bioavailability. Therapy is generally begun with low doses, which are gradually increased until the desired therapeutic response is obtained. After several months of therapy, tolerance to the drug develops and a dosage increase may be necessary. Although it produces an effective reduction in blood pressure, drugs in other antihypertensive classes have largely replaced hydralazine.

Hydralazine is also available by the intramuscular (IM) and IV routes for hypertensive emergencies, especially those associated with preeclampsia, although it is not a drug of choice for this indication. It is sometimes administered to patients with acute heart failure because the drug reduces the workload on the heart due to its antihypertensive action. ACE inhibitors have largely replaced the drug for patients with heart failure. A fixed-dose combination therapy of isosorbide dinitrate and hydralazine (BiDil) is available for the treatment of HF in African American patients.

Mechanism of Action: By causing peripheral vasodilation, hydralazine acts directly to relax arterial smooth muscle. The decreased peripheral resistance is accompanied by an increase in heart rate and cardiac output. The overall result is a reduction in afterload. Because the drug is selective for arterioles and does not cause dilation of veins, orthostatic hypotension is not a major adverse effect.

Pharmacokinetics:

Route(s)	PO, IM, IV
Absorption	Rapidly absorbed PO and well absorbed IM
Distribution	Widely distributed; crosses the placenta and is secreted in breast milk; 87% bound to plasma protein
Primary metabolism	GI mucosa and liver; extensive first-pass metabolism
Primary excretion	90% renal, 10% feces
Onset of action	PO: 20–30 min; IM: 10–30 min; IV: 5–20 min
Duration of action	3–8 h (PO); 1–4 h (IV)

Adverse Effects: Hydralazine may cause several adverse events that have the potential to prompt discontinuation of therapy. Headache, tachycardia, palpitations, flushing, nausea, and diarrhea are common but may resolve as therapy progresses. Orthostatic hypotension, fluid retention, and peripheral edema may also occur. Patients who are slow acetylators and those with renal impairment or who are receiving high doses of hydralazine are susceptible to experiencing a lupus-like syndrome. Symptoms may include rash, urticaria, myalgia, fever, chills, and fatigue. Blood dyscrasias such as agranulocytosis and leukopenia are rare, though potentially serious, adverse effects.

Contraindications/Precautions: Patients with lupus should not receive hydralazine, as the drug can worsen symptoms. The drug is contraindicated in patients with cerebrovascular disease or rheumatic heart disease. Patients should discontinue hydralazine gradually because abrupt withdrawal may cause severe rebound HTN and anxiety. Because it is excreted primarily by the kidneys, the drug should be used with caution in patients with renal impairment. Caution must be used when administering hydralazine to patients who are known slow acetylators because plasma drug levels will be significantly higher in these patients. Caution should be used when treating patients with CAD, because hydralazine can precipitate angina attacks and an acute MI.

Drug Interactions: Administering hydralazine with other antihypertensives or monoamine oxidase inhibitors (MAOIs) may cause severe hypotension. This includes all drug classes used as antihypertensives. Nonsteroidal anti-inflammatory drugs (NSAIDs) may decrease the antihypertensive action of hydralazine. Beta blockers are usually used concurrently with hydralazine to block reflex tachycardia, and heart rate should be carefully monitored to avoid bradycardia. Hydralazine may produce false-positive Coombs' tests. **Herbal/Food:** Hawthorn should be avoided because it may cause additive hypotensive effects.

Pregnancy: Category C.

Treatment of Overdose: Treatment includes gastric lavage, activated charcoal, and administration of a plasma volume expander to raise blood pressure. Tachycardia may require treatment with a beta blocker.

Nursing Responsibilities: Key nursing implications for patients receiving hydralazine are included in the Nursing Practice Application for Patients Receiving Pharmacotherapy with Direct Vasodilators.

Drugs Similar to Hydralazine (Apresoline)

Other direct vasodilators used for HTN include diazoxide, minoxidil, and nitroprusside. Nitroprusside is a drug for hypertensive emergencies and is presented in Section 34.10. Diazoxide (Hyperstat IV) is a rapid-acting vasodilator that is no longer marketed for blood pressure control. An oral form of diazoxide (Proglycem) is available to treat various hypoglycemic states, usually caused by the presence of excessive insulin (hyperinsulinism).

Minoxidil (Loniten): Minoxidil is a direct vasodilator with profound vasodilation activity that is selective for arterioles: It does not dilate veins. It is administered PO for severe HTN that is unresponsive to drugs from other classes. Because of its efficacy and the potential for serious effects on the cardiovascular system, initial doses are very low, and the amount is increased gradually. It is a pregnancy category C drug.

Minoxidil is considerably more toxic than hydralazine. The most serious adverse effects are cardiovascular in nature, including reflex tachycardia and plasma volume expansion due to sodium and water retention. Beta blockers are usually administered concurrently to minimize tachycardia, and diuretics to prevent fluid retention. Although rare, pericardial effusion has been reported with minoxidil use. Minoxidil causes **hypertrichosis**: the elongation, thickening, and increased pigmentation of body hair. This is normal and will reverse when the drug is discontinued. The drug's effect on hair growth is used to the patient's advantage in Rogaine, a topical form of minoxidil used to stimulate hair growth in patients with male-pattern baldness. The topical form of the drug is not absorbed into the systemic circulation; thus Rogaine produces none of the serious cardiovascular effects observed with Loniten.

Management of Hypertensive Emergency

34.10 Hypertensive crisis is a medical emergency that is treated by the intravenous administration of antihypertensive medications.

A **hypertensive emergency (HTN-E)**, also called hypertensive crisis, is defined as a diastolic pressure of greater than 120 mmHg, with evidence of target-organ system damage. HTN-E requires aggressive treatment, usually within minutes to hours, to prevent further organ damage. A related condition, **hypertensive urgency**, is when a patient presents with severe HTN but has no evidence of target-organ damage.

Target-organ damage from extreme HTN most often occurs in the cardiovascular system, the kidneys, or the CNS. In the cardiovascular system, the increased workload on the heart leads to acute left heart failure with pulmonary edema, sometimes accompanied by myocardial ischemia or infarction. Chest pain and dyspnea are the most common symptoms in patients with HTN-E. Renal function is diminished, as evidenced by oliguria, hematuria, and proteinuria. Acute renal failure may occur, or preexisting chronic renal failure may worsen. In the brain, thrombotic or hemorrhagic stroke may occur. The capillaries in the brain become leaky, producing hypertensive encephalopathy, with resulting headache, paralysis, seizures, or coma. In addition, retinal hemorrhages and edema of the retina (papilledema) are signs of severe HTN.

The most common cause of HTN-E is untreated or poorly controlled essential HTN. In some cases, the patient has abruptly discontinued use of the antihypertensive medication. There are, however, a large number of possible secondary causes of HTN-E, including the following conditions:

- Renovascular hypertension
- Pheochromocytoma
- Cocaine use
- Eclampsia or preeclampsia
- Head injuries
- Primary hyperaldosteronism
- Coarctation of the aorta
- Hyperthyroidism or thyroid storm

In the management of HTN-E, the therapeutic goal is to lower blood pressure quickly. Care must be taken, however, to not decrease blood pressure too quickly because rapid and intense vasodilation can result in serious hypoperfusion of the cerebral, coronary, or renal vascular capillaries. This can cause ischemia or infarction, worsening target-organ damage to the brain, heart, kidneys, or retina. It is recommended that the pretreatment blood pressure be progressively reduced by 20% to 25%, over 30 to 60 minutes. Additional, gradual reductions are made over a 12- to 48-hour period until blood pressure is reduced to a value within the normal range. Parenteral antihypertensives are preferred over PO medications due to their rapid onset of action and because infusions offer more precise control during the gradual pressure reduction.

In patients with hypertensive urgencies, target-organ damage has not yet developed. These patients are treated more conservatively by increasing the dose of their current antihypertensive drug, or by adding a second drug to the regimen. Oral medications are used to lower blood pressure because these drugs are less toxic than parenteral antihypertensives. Oral drugs with a relatively rapid onset of action that may be used for hypertensive urgency include clonidine (Catapres), captopril (Capoten), or labetalol (Trandate). The patient should be monitored for several hours, and doses may be repeated at frequent intervals, as needed, to lower pressure to acceptable levels. All patients with hypertensive urgency should receive follow-up assessments after 1 to 3 days on the new regimen.

PROTOTYPE DRUG	Nitroprusside Sodium (Nitropress)

Classification: **Therapeutic:** Drug for hypertensive emergency
Pharmacologic: Direct vasodilator

Therapeutic Effects and Uses: Nitroprusside is a first-line drug for patients with aggressive, life-threatening HTN because it has the ability to lower blood pressure almost instantaneously upon IV administration. Indications include hypertensive crisis, acute HF, and promotion of controlled hypotension to reduce bleeding during surgery. The drug has a short half-life, and the hypotensive effects disappear approximately 3 minutes after the infusion is discontinued. Unlike most direct vasodilators, nitroprusside causes very little reflex tachycardia. Although discovered in 1850, the drug was not approved by the FDA until 1974.

Patients must be continuously monitored while receiving nitroprusside to prevent hypotension due to overtreatment. Therapy is limited to 72 hours because the drug is metabolized to toxic thiocyanate and cyanide compounds. This is of special concern to patients with renal impairment who are unable to excrete the cyanide. If serum thiocyanate exceeds 12 mg/dL, the nitroprusside infusion should be discontinued. As a general rule, patients are switched from nitroprusside to an oral antihypertensive as soon as blood pressure has stabilized.

Mechanism of Action: Nitroprusside dilates both arteries and veins; therefore, the hypotensive action of nitroprusside is due to direct relaxation of arteriolar smooth muscle and to blood pooling in the veins. In most patients, heart rate is mildly increased, while cardiac output is decreased. In patients with severe left ventricular hypertrophy, however, cardiac output may increase.

Pharmacokinetics:

Route(s)	IV
Absorption	N/A
Distribution	Unknown
Primary metabolism	Metabolized to thiocyanates in erythrocytes and other tissues
Primary excretion	Renal
Onset of action	1–2 min
Duration of action	1–10 min

Adverse Effects: Signs and symptoms of vasodilation such as hypotension, headache, dizziness, and flushing of the skin are expected adverse effects. With extended therapy, thiocyanate toxicity may manifest. Thiocyanate poisoning is characterized by hypotension, lethargy, blurred vision, metabolic acidosis, faint heart sounds, and loss of consciousness. Irritation may occur at the infusion site. **Black Box Warning**: Nitroprusside requires dilution prior to infusion and is not suitable for direct injection. The drug can cause irreversible ischemic injury and death due to significant drops in blood pressure. Accumulation of cyanide ion may occur.

Contraindications/Precautions: Patients with inadequate cerebral circulation or who have compensatory HTN should not receive nitroprusside. Because the kidneys excrete the toxic thiocyanate metabolite of the drug, patients with serious renal impairment should be treated cautiously. Nitroprusside is contraindicated in patients with high intracranial pressure because the drug may worsen this condition.

Drug Interactions: Antihypertensive drugs, ethanol, general anesthetics, and ganglionic blockers should be used with caution with nitroprusside because additive hypotension could result. Sympathomimetics such as epinephrine will block the antihypertensive actions of nitroprusside. Dobutamine (Dobutrex) and nitroprusside are sometimes administered concurrently because this interaction results in a beneficial synergistic increase in cardiac output and decrease in pulmonary capillary wedge pressure. **Herbal/Food**: Hawthorn may cause additive hypotensive effects.

Pregnancy: Category C.

Treatment of Overdose: Extreme hypotension may be treated with a vasopressor. Cyanide toxicity caused by the overdose may require the use of a cyanide antidote kit, which contains amyl nitrate, sodium nitrite, and sodium thiosulfate. The purpose of these drugs is to convert toxic cyanide into nontoxic thiocyanate.

Nursing Responsibilities: Key nursing implications for patients receiving nitroprusside are included in the Nursing Practice Application for Patients Receiving Pharmacotherapy with Direct Vasodilators.

Drugs Similar to Nitroprusside Sodium (Nitropress)

Other vasodilators for HTN-E are shown in Table 34.4, which summarizes their applications to the pharmacotherapy of hypertensive crisis.

PharmFACT

Hypertensive crisis is a common condition, affecting 1% of the patients with primary HTN. The most common presentation, occurring in 25% of patients, is stroke. The 1-year survival rate for a patient presenting with a HTN crisis has improved from only 20% prior to 1950 to more than 90% with current medical treatment (Hopkins, 2013).

TABLE 34.4 Drugs for Hypertensive Emergency

Drug	Class	Applications
clevidipine (Cleviprex)	Calcium channel blocker	Newer drug with an onset of action of 2–4 min and a short duration, allowing for rapid blood pressure reduction
enalaprilat (Enalapril IV)	ACE inhibitor	Onset of action is 15–30 min; useful in HTN-E associated with heart failure or high plasma levels of angiotensin II
esmolol (Brevibloc)	Beta-adrenergic antagonist	Onset of action is 1–5 min; useful for patients with severe left ventricular dysfunction or with peripheral vascular disease
fenoldopam (Corlopam)	Dopamine agonist	Onset of action is 5 min; useful for patients with renal impairment, as the drug increases renal blood flow
hydralazine (Apresoline)	Direct vasodilator	Onset of action is 5–20 min; useful in HTN-E due to eclampsia and preeclampsia because it increases uterine blood flow
labetalol (Trandate)	Alpha- and beta-adrenergic antagonist	Onset of action is 2–5 min; reduces incidences of MI and death
nicardipine (Cardene IV)	Calcium channel blocker	Onset of action is 1 min; rapid and effective for most HTN-E, with fewer adverse effects than some other HTN-E drugs
nitroprusside sodium (Nitropress)	Direct vasodilator	Onset of action is 1 min; preferred drug for many HTN-E
phentolamine (Regitine)	Alpha-adrenergic antagonist	Onset of action is 1–5 min; rarely used due to high incidence of reflex tachycardia and myocardial ischemia; useful for HTN-E due to pheochromocytoma

CONNECTIONS: NURSING PRACTICE APPLICATION

Patients Receiving Pharmacotherapy with Direct Vasodilators

Assessment	Potential Nursing Diagnoses*
Baseline assessment prior to administration: • Obtain a complete health history: cardiovascular (including MI, heart failure), cerebrovascular and neurologic (including level of consciousness [LOC], history of stroke, head injury, increased intracranial pressure), respiratory, and the possibility of autoimmune diseases, especially systemic lupus erythematosus. Obtain a drug history including allergies, current prescription and over-the-counter drugs, and herbal preparations. Be alert to possible drug interactions. • Evaluate appropriate laboratory findings: electrolytes, especially sodium and potassium levels, hepatic and renal function studies, and lipid profiles. • Obtain baseline weight, vital signs, pulse oximetry, breath and heart sounds, and cardiac monitoring (e.g., ECG, cardiac output). Assess location and character of peripheral edema if present. • Assess the patient's ability to receive and understand instructions. Include family and caregivers as needed.	• *Decreased Cardiac Output* • *Deficient Knowledge* (Drug Therapy) • *Risk for Decreased Cardiac Tissue Perfusion* • *Risk for Imbalanced Fluid Volume* • *Risk for Injury* • *Risk for Impaired Skin Integrity,* related to adverse effects from IV infusion of medication
Assessment throughout administration: • Assess for desired therapeutic effects (e.g., lowered blood pressure within established limits). • Continue frequent and careful monitoring of vital signs, pulse oximetry, urinary and cardiac output, and daily weight, especially if IV administration is used. Blood pressure and pulse must be monitored every 5 min or as ordered while on IV infusion of the drug. (Invasive monitoring, such as arterial lines, is often used for this purpose.) • Continue periodic monitoring of electrolytes, especially potassium. • Continue frequent physical assessments, particularly neurologic, cardiac, and respiratory systems. • Assess for and promptly report adverse effects: excessive hypotension, dysrhythmias, reflex tachycardia (from too rapid decrease in blood pressure or significant hypotension), headache, decreased urinary output, peripheral edema, and priapism (prolonged erection in the absence of sexual stimulation). Severe hypotension, seizures, dysrhythmias, or palpitations may signal drug toxicity and are immediately reported.	

Implementation

Interventions and (Rationales)	Patient-Centered Care
Ensuring therapeutic effects: • Continue frequent assessments as above for therapeutic effects. IV infusion of vasodilators may be titrated frequently to achieve desired effects. Vital signs, cardiac and urinary output, and daily weights should remain within the limits set by the health care provider. (Pulse, blood pressure, and respiratory rate should be within normal limits or acceptable parameters. An increase in weight of more than 1 kg [2 lb] per day may indicate excessive fluid gain, and may require judicious diuretic therapy.)	• To allay possible anxiety, teach the patient, family, or caregiver the rationale for all equipment used and the need for frequent monitoring. • Teach the patient, family, or caregiver how to monitor pulse and blood pressure as appropriate if the patient is on oral therapy at home. Ensure proper use and functioning of any home equipment obtained. • Have the patient weigh self daily along with blood pressure and pulse measurements. Report a weight gain or loss of more than 1 kg (2 lb) in a 24-h period.
Minimizing adverse effects: • Continue to monitor vital signs frequently. **Lifespan:** Be particularly cautious with older adults who are at increased risk for hypotension, patients with a preexisting history of cardiac or cerebrovascular ischemia, which may be worsened by decreased blood pressure, patients with dehydration, and patients with lupus erythematosus. Immediately notify the health care provider if the blood pressure or pulse decrease beyond established parameters or if hypotension is accompanied by reflex tachycardia. (Direct-acting vasodilators cause significant vasodilation, resulting in the potential for dramatically and rapidly lowered blood pressure accompanied by reflex tachycardia. Reflex tachycardia may require treatment with beta-blocking drugs.)	• Instruct the patient, family, or caregiver to report angina-like symptoms (e.g., chest, arm, back, or neck pain), palpitations, faintness, dizziness, drowsiness, or headache.
• Continue cardiac monitoring (e.g., ECG) and invasive monitoring (e.g., cardiac output, arterial line pressures) as ordered in the hospitalized patient. (Monitoring devices assist in detecting early signs of adverse effects as well as monitoring for therapeutic effects. **Diverse Patients:** Hydralazine is known to metabolize in patients who are slow acetylators, and because this cannot always be predicted, ensure that frequent monitoring continues, especially in the early stages of drug therapy.)	• To allay possible anxiety, teach the patient, family, or caregiver the rationale for all equipment used and the need for frequent monitoring.

CONNECTIONS: NURSING PRACTICE APPLICATION (continued)

- Continue frequent physical assessments, particularly neurologic, cardiac, and respiratory. Immediately report any changes in LOC, headache, or changes in heart or lung sounds. (Vasodilator therapy may worsen preexisting neurologic, cardiac, or respiratory conditions as blood pressure drops and perfusion to vital organs diminishes.)

- When on oral therapy at home, the patient, family, or caregiver should immediately report changes in mental status or LOC, palpitations, dizziness, dyspnea, increasing productive cough, especially if frothy sputum is present, and seek medical attention.

- Weigh the patient daily and report weight gain or loss of 1 kg (2 lb) or more in a 24-h period or significant peripheral edema. (Daily weight is an accurate measure of fluid status and takes into account intake, output, and insensible losses. Weight gain or edema may signal blood pressure has lowered too quickly, stimulating renin release, and may require judicious use of diuretic therapy to treat.)

- When on oral therapy at home, have the patient weigh self daily, ideally at the same time of day, and record weight along with blood pressure and pulse measurements. Have the patient report a weight gain or loss of more than 1 kg (2 lb) in a 24-h period, or peripheral edema, especially if increasing.

- Continue to monitor IV infusion sites frequently. (Direct-acting vasodilators may cause tissue damage if the drug extravasates.)

- Instruct the patient to report any burning or stinging pain, swelling, warmth, redness, or tenderness at the IV insertion site.

- Observe for signs and symptoms of lupus in patients taking vasodilators, particularly hydralazine. (Hydralazine has been linked to drug-induced/drug-related lupus. Other direct vasodilators are used with caution for this reason.)

- Instruct the patient to report symptoms such as a butterfly-shaped rash over the nose and cheeks, muscle aches, and fatigue when taking oral vasodilators, particularly hydralazine.

- Monitor for the development of priapism and notify the health care provider. (Priapism may result in tissue damage if unrelieved and is considered a medical emergency.)

- Instruct the patient to report a sustained erection that lasts more than 4 h if on vasodilator therapy at home and to seek immediate medical care.

- For oral drug therapy, give the first dose of the drug at bedtime. (A first-dose response may result in a greater initial drop in blood pressure than subsequent doses.)

- Instruct the patient to take the first dose of the medication at bedtime, immediately before going to bed, and to avoid driving or other substantial activities for 12 to 24 h after the first dose or when the dosage is increased until effects are known.

- Do not abruptly stop medication. (Rebound HTN and tachycardia may occur.)

- Teach the patient, family, or caregiver not to stop the medication abruptly and to call the health care provider if the patient is unable to take the medication for more than 1 day due to illness.

- Encourage appropriate lifestyle changes: lowered fat intake, gradual increase in exercise, limited alcohol intake, smoking cessation. Provide for dietitian consultation as needed. (Healthy lifestyle changes will support and minimize the need for drug therapy. Direct vasodilators decrease blood pressure substantially, and concurrent beta-blocker use may decrease heart rate. Given alone or together, this may lead to exercise intolerance. Activity levels should be increased gradually to patient tolerance. If dizziness or shortness of breath occurs, decrease exercise levels to a comfortable level. Alcohol consumption may increase the risk of blood pressure–related adverse effects.)

- Encourage the patient, family, or caregivers to adopt a healthy lifestyle of low-fat food choices, reduced sodium intake, increased exercise, decreased alcohol consumption, and smoking cessation.
- Caution the patient about sudden increases in activity level. Report dizziness, palpitations, or shortness of breath that occurs while exercising.

Patient understanding of drug therapy:
- Use opportunities during administration of medications and during assessments to discuss the rationale for drug therapy, desired therapeutic outcomes, commonly observed adverse effects, parameters for when to call the health care provider, and any necessary monitoring or precautions. (Using time during nursing care helps to optimize and reinforce key teaching areas.)

- The patient, family, or caregiver should be able to state the reason for the drug, appropriate dose and scheduling, what adverse effects to observe for and when to report them, and the anticipated length of medication therapy.

Patient self-administration of drug therapy:
- When administering medications, instruct the patient, family, or caregiver in proper self-administration techniques. (Utilizing time during nurse-administration of these drugs helps to reinforce teaching.)

- Instruct the patient in proper administration techniques, followed by return demonstration.
- The patient, family, or caregiver is able to discuss appropriate dosing and administration needs.

34 Understanding the Chapter

Key Concepts Summary

34.1 Failure to properly manage hypertension can lead to stroke, heart failure, or myocardial infarction.

34.2 Therapeutic lifestyle changes can reduce blood pressure and lessen the need for antihypertensive medications.

34.3 Research-based guidelines have been developed to aid the health care provider in providing optimum treatment for patients with hypertension.

34.4 The choice of antihypertensive medication is determined by the degree of hypertension and the presence of other medical conditions.

34.5 Diuretics are often drugs of first choice for treating mild to moderate hypertension.

34.6 Calcium channel blockers have emerged as important drugs in the treatment of hypertension.

34.7 Blocking the renin-angiotensin-aldosterone system leads to a decrease in blood pressure and improved kidney function.

34.8 Adrenergic antagonists are commonly used to treat hypertension.

34.9 Direct-acting vasodilators lower blood pressure by relaxing arteriolar smooth muscle.

34.10 Hypertensive crisis is a medical emergency that is treated by the intravenous administration of antihypertensive medications.

Case Study: Making the Patient Connection

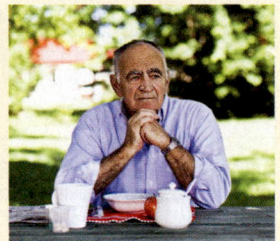

Remember the patient "Elmer Foley" at the beginning of the chapter? Now read the remainder of the case study. Based on the information presented within this chapter, respond to the critical thinking questions that follow.

Elmer Foley is a 72-year-old Caucasian male with a 10-month history of uncontrolled HTN. Initially, Elmer was prescribed the thiazide diuretic HCTZ (Microzide). However, after 1 week of therapy his blood pressure has remained at 168/102 mmHg. Next, Elmer's health care provider added an ACE inhibitor, captopril (Capoten), to the regimen. Still, Elmer's blood pressure remained above normal limits. Lastly, the health care provider discontinued the captopril and started Elmer on hydralazine (Apresoline). With this visit, his blood pressure is 146/90 mmHg.

When Elmer was first told he had HTN, he began many of the suggested lifestyle changes encouraged by his health care provider. He has lost a total of 15 kg (33 lb) since starting his diet 10 months ago. Elmer started walking daily for exercise and can now walk up to 1 mile without fatigue. He avoids all salty foods and diligently checks food labels for fat and salt content. Elmer occasionally drinks a glass of wine, although never more than 1 to 2 glasses per month. Although it was difficult for Elmer to stop smoking totally, he proudly claims he has been smokeless for 8 months.

Critical Thinking Questions

1. How would you respond to Elmer's question, "What else can I do?" Is there anything else he can do to reduce his blood pressure?

2. Elmer wants to know why the previous therapies were unsuccessful. What would you say as his nurse?

3. As the nurse, how can you support Elmer before he leaves the clinic?

See Answers to Critical Thinking Questions on student resource website.

Additional Case Study

Helen Edwards is a 44-year-old African American woman who presents to the ED with headache and shortness of breath. Helen has a long-standing history of HTN. She has never consistently adhered to any HTN management strategies and has been nonadherent with her medication regimen for the past 8 months. Upon arrival at the ED her blood pressure is 192/126 mmHg.

When you assess the patient, it is noted that she is approximately 1.7 m (5'6") in height and the self-reported weight is 107 kg (235 lb). She is slightly lethargic and reports having left arm numbness and tingling. Other physical assessment parameters are normal.

Helen is started on an infusion of nitroprusside (Nitropress) 50 mg in 250 mL in D_5W. The dose will be titrated between 0.5 and 10 mcg/kg/min to maintain the patient's diastolic pressure at less than 100 mmHg.

1. Describe the mechanism of action related to nitroprusside (Nitropress).
2. For what adverse effects should you monitor in patients receiving this drug therapy?
3. What factors does this patient have that predispose her to hypertensive crises?

See Answers to Additional Case Study on student resource website.

Chapter Review

1 Methyldopa (Aldomet) is being initiated for a patient with hypertension. Which health teaching would be most appropriate for this drug?

1. Avoid hot baths and showers and prolonged standing in one position.
2. This drug may discolor the urine a pinkish-brown color.
3. You may experience bloating and weight gain.
4. The tablet should be taken only with food or milk.

2 A patient is receiving hydralazine (Apresoline) for elevated blood pressure levels. The nurse would include in the care plan to monitor the patient for which adverse effects?

1. Atelectasis
2. Crystalluria
3. Photosensitivity
4. Orthostatic hypotension

3 The nurse determines that the patient understands an important principle in self-administration of hydralazine (Apresoline) when the patient makes which statement?

1. "I should not drive until the response to drug therapy is determined."
2. "I can stop taking this medication once I begin to feel better."
3. "If I experience dizziness, I should take only half the dose."
4. "I should avoid air travel while taking this medication."

4 A patient with hypertensive crisis is started on nitroprusside (Nitropress) therapy. The nurse would perform what priority intervention during the course of this treatment?

1. Monitor for the presence or absence of bowel sounds.
2. Obtain urine samples for specific gravity measurements and glucose levels.
3. Observe skin pressure points for turgor and integrity.
4. Titrate intravenous infusion rate according to the blood pressure response.

5 A 65-year-old Caucasian patient has been newly diagnosed with hypertension, with an average blood pressure of 164/92. Which of the following drug groups will potentially be ordered initially? Select all that apply.

1. Beta blockers
2. Calcium channel blockers
3. Thiazide diuretics
4. Angiotensin-converting enzyme (ACE) inhibitors or receptor blockers (ARBs)
5. Direct-acting vasodilators

6 A patient is receiving nitroprusside (Nitropress) and is being monitored in the intensive care unit. Because of toxic cyanide metabolites that develop, which of the following should the nurse evaluate in the patient? Select all that apply.

1. Cardiac status and cardiac output
2. Renal function and creatinine levels
3. Past history of alcohol use
4. Level of consciousness
5. Skin color and turgor

See Answers to Chapter Review in Appendix A.

References

American Heart Association. (2012). *Why blood pressure matters.* Retrieved from http://www.heart.org/HEARTORG/Conditions/HighBloodPressure/WhyBloodPressureMatters/Why-Blood-Pressure-Matters_UCM_002051_Article.jsp

Centers for Disease Control and Prevention. (2014). *High blood pressure facts.* Retrieved from http://www.cdc.gov/bloodpressure/facts.htm

Hermida, R. C., Ayala, D. E., Mojón, A., & Fernández, J. R. (2011). Bedtime dosing of antihypertensive medications reduces cardiovascular risk in CKD. *Journal of the American Society of Nephrology, 22,* 2313–2321. doi:10.1681/ASN.2011040361

Hopkins, C. (2013). *Hypertensive emergencies.* Retrieved from http://emedicine.medscape.com/article/1952052-overview

James, P. A., Oparil, S., Carter, B. L., Cushman, W. C., Dennison-Himmelfarb, C., Handler, J., . . . Ortiz, E. (2014). 2014 Evidence-based guideline for the management of high blood pressure in adults: Report from the panel members appointed to the Eighth Joint National Committee (JNC 8). *JAMA, 311,* 507–520. doi:10.1001/jama.2013.284427. Retrieved from http://jama.jamanetwork.com/article.aspx?articleid=1791497

Magee, C. A., Iverson, D. C., & Caputi, P. (2009). Factors associated with short and long sleep. *Preventive Medicine, 49,* 461–467. doi:10.1016/j.ypmed.2009.10.006

National Center for Complementary and Alternative Medicine. (2012). *Herbs at a glance: Grape seed extract.* Retrieved from http://nccam.nih.gov/health/grapeseed/ataglance.htm

National Institutes of Health, National Heart, Lung, and Blood Institute, National High Blood Pressure Education Program Coordinating Committee. (2003). *JNC-7 express: The seventh report of the Joint National Committee on Prevention, Detection, Evaluation, and Treatment of High Blood Pressure.* Bethesda, MD: Author. Retrieved from http://www.nhlbi.nih.gov/guidelines/hypertension/express.pdf

Sabanayagam, C., & Shankar, A. (2010). Sleep duration and cardiovascular disease: Results from the National Health Interview Survey. *Sleep, 33*(8), 1037–1042.

University of Maryland Medical Center. (2013). *Grape seed.* Retrieved from http://umm.edu/health/medical/altmed/herb/grape-seed

Selected Bibliography

Clark, C. E., Smith, L. F., Taylor, R. S., & Campbell, J. L. (2010). Nurse led interventions to improve control of blood pressure in people with hypertension: Systematic review and meta-analysis. *British Medical Journal, 341,* c3995. doi:10.1136/bmj.c3995

Colbert, B. J., & Mason, B. J. (2012). *Integrated cardiopulmonary pharmacology* (3rd ed.). Upper Saddle River, NJ: Pearson.

Herdman, T. H., & Kamitsuru, S. (Eds.). (2014). *NANDA International nursing diagnoses: Definitions and classification, 2015–2017.* Oxford, United Kingdom: Wiley-Blackwell.

Hill, M. N., Miller, N. H., & DeGeest, S. (2011). Adherence and persistence with taking medication to control high blood pressure. *Journal of the American Society of Hypertension, 5,* 56–63. doi:10.1016/j.jash.2011.01.001

Kotchen, T. A. (2010). The search for strategies to control hypertension. *Circulation, 122,* 1141–1143. doi:10.1161/CIRCULATIONAHA.110.978759

Michel, T., & Hoffman, B. B. (2011). Treatment of myocardial ischemia and hypertension. In L. L. Brunton, B. A. Chabner, & B. C. Knollman (Eds.), *The pharmacological basis of therapeutics* (12th ed., pp. 745–788). New York, NY: McGraw-Hill.

Touyz, R. M. (2011). Advancement in hypertension pathogenesis: Some new concepts. *Current Opinion in Nephrology and Hypertension, 20,* 105–106. doi:10.1097/MNH.0b013e328343f526

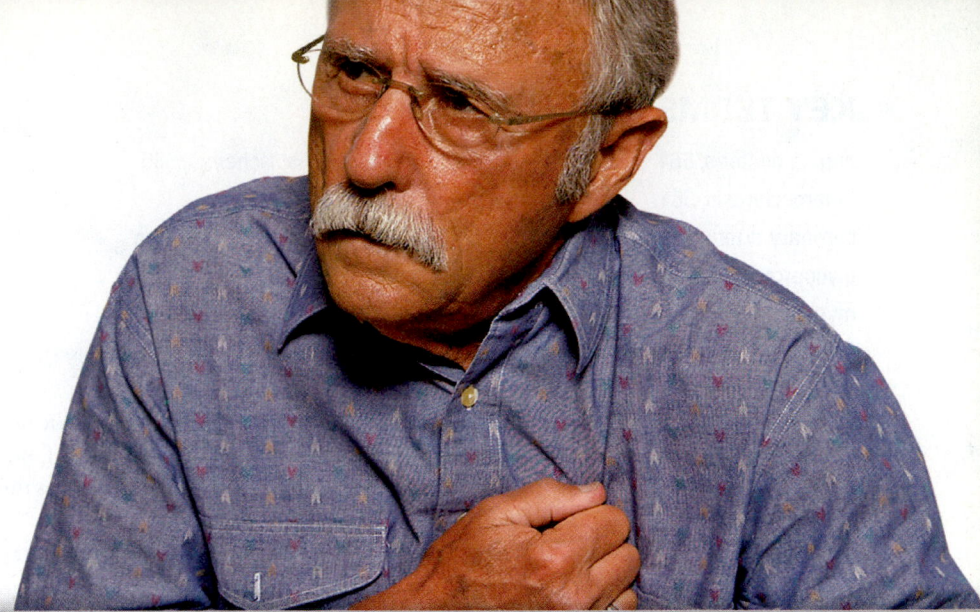

"I was simply sitting and reading the newspaper, when suddenly my chest felt tight, I felt weak, and I had difficulty breathing."

Patient "Michael Graff"

CHAPTER

35

Pharmacotherapy of Angina Pectoris and Myocardial Infarction

LEARNING OUTCOMES

After reading this chapter, the student should be able to:

1. Describe factors that affect myocardial oxygen supply and demand.

2. Explain the relationship between atherosclerosis and coronary artery disease.

3. Explain the pathophysiology of angina pectoris and myocardial infarction.

4. Discuss the role of therapeutic lifestyle changes in the management of coronary artery disease.

5. Describe the pharmacologic management of the different types of angina.

6. Describe the pharmacologic management of myocardial infarction.

7. For each of the classes shown in the chapter outline, identify the prototype and representative drugs and explain the mechanism(s) of drug action, primary indications, contraindications, significant drug interactions, pregnancy category, and important adverse effects.

8. Apply the nursing process to care for patients receiving pharmacotherapy for angina and myocardial infarction.

CHAPTER OUTLINE

▶ Pathophysiology of Myocardial Ischemia

▶ Etiology of Coronary Artery Disease

▶ Pathophysiology of Angina Pectoris

▶ Nonpharmacologic Therapy of Coronary Artery Disease

▶ Pharmacologic Management of Angina Pectoris

▶ Drug Classes for Angina Pectoris
  Organic Nitrates
  PROTOTYPE Nitroglycerin (Nitrostat, Nitro-Bid, Nitro-Dur, Others), *p. 565*
  Beta-Adrenergic Blockers
  PROTOTYPE Atenolol (Tenormin), *p. 566*
  Calcium Channel Blockers

▶ Pathophysiology of Myocardial Infarction

▶ Pharmacologic Management of Myocardial Infarction
  Thrombolytics and Adjunct Medications for Myocardial Infarction

KEY TERMS

angina pectoris, 561

atherosclerosis, 561

coronary artery disease (CAD), 560

glycoprotein IIb/IIIa, 571

myocardial infarctions (MIs), 567

myocardial ischemia, 560

nitric oxide, 564

partial fatty-acid oxidation
   inhibitors, 563

plaque, 561

silent angina, 561

stable angina, 561

unstable angina, 561

vasospastic (Prinzmetal's) angina, 561

The tissues of the body depend on a continuous supply of oxygen and vital nutrients to support life and health. The heart is particularly demanding of a steady source of oxygen. Insufficient arterial blood supply to cardiac muscle may result in angina pectoris, acute myocardial infarction (heart attack), and possibly death. This chapter focuses on the pharmacologic interventions related to angina pectoris and myocardial infarction (MI).

Pathophysiology of Myocardial Ischemia

35.1 Myocardial ischemia develops when there is inadequate blood supply to meet the metabolic demands of cardiac muscle.

Myocardial ischemia is a condition in which the heart is receiving an insufficient amount of oxygen to meet its metabolic demands. This occurs when there is an imbalance between oxygen supply and oxygen demand in myocardial cells. Knowledge of factors affecting myocardial oxygen supply and demand is necessary for understanding the pharmacotherapy of the diseases associated with myocardial ischemia.

Myocardial Oxygen Supply

The heart, from the moment it begins to function *in utero* until death, works to distribute oxygen and nutrients by means of its nonstop pumping action. It is the hardest working organ in the body, functioning continuously during both activity and rest. Because the heart is a muscle, it needs a steady supply of nourishment to sustain itself and maintain the systemic circulation in a balanced state of equilibrium. Any disturbance in blood flow to the myocardium—even for brief episodes—can result in life-threatening consequences. A review of the coronary circulation is provided in Section 28.5.

As with other arteries in the body, the amount of blood flow through the coronary arteries is dependent on a number of hemodynamic factors. Of these, blood pressure is the most important. When systolic blood pressure falls, the quantity of blood flowing to the coronary arteries is diminished. If this occurs suddenly, such as in acute shock, it could be life threatening. Immediate restoration of blood pressure is required to reestablish an adequate oxygen supply to the myocardium as well as to other vital tissues. Other hemodynamic factors contributing to the myocardial oxygen supply include changes in blood volume (e.g., hemorrhage) and disorders that reduce the oxygen content or carrying capacity of the blood (e.g., anemia).

The narrowing of a coronary artery resulting from atherosclerosis or coronary artery disease (CAD) deprives cells of needed oxygen and nutrients. If the narrowing develops over a long period

of time, the heart compensates for its inadequate blood supply and the patient may be asymptomatic. Indeed, coronary arteries may be occluded as much as 50% or more and cause no symptoms.

Myocardial Oxygen Demand

As CAD progresses, cardiac muscle does not receive enough oxygen to meet the body's metabolic demands. The physiological demands on the heart are highly variable and depend on a large number of hemodynamic and lifestyle factors.

Basically, anything that increases the workload of the heart will increase myocardial oxygen demand. It is not difficult to think of the many daily activities that increase cardiac workload. Exercise, for example, will cause the heart to beat faster in order to pump more blood to muscles. This physical activity need not be extreme: Simply walking at a normal pace will increase cardiac workload over resting levels.

In some patients, the increased cardiac workload can be the result of mental, rather than physical, stressors. Think of the first time (or last time) you had to give a speech in front of a group, or became angry with a child, spouse, or coworker. These activities resulted in your heart pumping harder or faster, even though there was no physical activity involved. What factors do physical exercise and mental stress have in common that produced the increased cardiac workload?

The answer is simple. Anything that increases heart rate, contractility, or tension on the ventricular walls causes the heart to work harder and affect cardiac oxygen consumption. For example, if heart rate increases due to exercise or hyperthyroidism, it is easy to understand why the heart needs more oxygen because it must beat more times per minute. Similarly, the heart will need more oxygen if it beats more forcefully (increased contractility). A patient with heart failure (HF) has a thickened myocardium (increased tension) that will require more work to contract. The heart of a patient with hypertension will have to work harder to overcome resistance and eject blood. It is important to remember that anything that makes the heart beat faster or contract with more force will increase myocardial oxygen demand. Drugs that diminish these factors are of value in the treatment of angina, MI, and HF.

Etiology of Coronary Artery Disease

35.2 Coronary artery disease is the major cause of myocardial ischemia.

Coronary artery disease (CAD) is one of the leading causes of mortality in the United States. The primary defining characteristic of CAD is narrowing or occlusion of one or more coronary arteries.

Narrowing can result in symptoms of angina pectoris, whereas occlusion results in MI. The two disorders are closely related, as most patients who experience an MI have narrowing of the coronary vessels.

The most common etiology of CAD in adults is **atherosclerosis**, the presence of **plaque**—a fatty, fibrous material—within the walls of the coronary arteries. Plaque develops progressively over time, producing varying degrees of intravascular narrowing that results in partial or total blockage of the vessel. During periods of rest, demands on the heart are less and a partially occluded artery may be able to provide adequate oxygen. During exercise (or a pharmacology test), however, workload on the heart increases, the cardiac muscle distal to the obstruction receives insufficient oxygen supply, and ischemia results.

A healthy heart responds to stress by changing the diameter of the coronary arteries. When the oxygen demands of the heart increase, the vessels will immediately dilate to bring more oxygen to the myocardium. Plaque impairs normal elasticity, and the coronary vessels are unable to dilate properly when the myocardium demands additional oxygen. Myocardial ischemia occurs when cardiac demands exceed the amount of oxygen that can be supplied through the narrowed, inelastic vessels characteristic of CAD.

Plaque accumulation occurs gradually, over periods of 40 to 50 years in some individuals, but actually begins to accrue very early in life. The development of atherosclerosis is illustrated in Figure 35.1.

CONNECTION Checkpoint 35.1

From what you learned in Chapter 28, predict what would happen to the cardiac workload when plasma volume is increased by an infusion of normal saline. What effect might this have on a patient with CAD? *See Answer to Connection Checkpoint 35.1 on student resource website.*

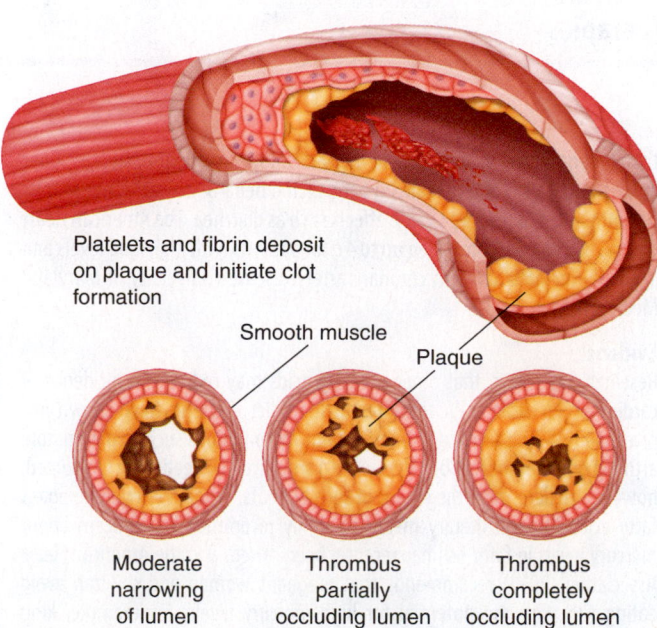

Platelets and fibrin deposit on plaque and initiate clot formation

Smooth muscle

Plaque

Moderate narrowing of lumen

Thrombus partially occluding lumen

Thrombus completely occluding lumen

Figure 35.1 Atherosclerosis in the coronary arteries.

Pathophysiology of Angina Pectoris

35.3 Angina pectoris is characterized by severe chest pain brought on by physical exertion or emotional stress.

Angina pectoris is acute chest pain caused by myocardial ischemia. The classic presentation of angina pectoris is steady, intense pain, sometimes with a crushing sensation in the anterior chest. Typically, the discomfort radiates to the left shoulder and proceeds down the left arm. It may also extend to the posterior thoracic region or move upward to the jaw, and in some patients the pain is experienced in the epigastrium or abdominal area. Accompanying the discomfort is severe emotional distress—a feeling of panic with fear of impending death. There is usually pallor, dyspnea with cyanosis, diaphoresis, tachycardia, and elevated blood pressure.

Anginal pain is usually precipitated by physical exertion or emotional excitement—events associated with increased myocardial oxygen demand. Angina pectoris episodes are of short duration. With physical rest and mental relaxation, the workload demands upon the heart diminish and the discomfort subsides within 5 to 10 minutes. Descriptions of the four basic types of angina follow.

When angina occurrences are fairly predictable in frequency, intensity, and duration, the condition is described as classic or **stable angina**. Rest usually relieves the pain associated with stable angina.

Vasospastic (Prinzmetal's) angina occurs when the decreased myocardial blood flow is caused by spasms of the coronary arteries. The vessels undergoing spasms may or may not contain atherosclerotic plaque. Thus, the primary cause of the narrowing and subsequent angina pain is vasoconstriction of the artery, rather than plaque buildup. Vasospastic angina pain occurs most often during periods of rest, although it may occur unpredictably, unrelated to rest or activity.

Although most people equate angina with chest pain, this is not always the case. When myocardial ischemia occurs in the absence of pain, it is called **silent angina**. Although one or more coronary arteries are partially occluded, the patient is asymptomatic. Some patients diagnosed with stable angina also experience silent angina. Although the mechanisms underlying silent angina are not completely understood, the condition is associated with a high risk for acute MI and sudden death.

Unstable angina occurs when episodes of angina occur suddenly, have added intensity, and occur during periods of rest. Unstable angina is a type of acute coronary syndrome in which an atherosclerotic plaque within a coronary artery ruptures. A thrombus quickly builds on the displaced plaque, and the artery becomes at serious risk of occlusion. This condition is a medical emergency requiring aggressive intervention because of the associated increased risk for MI.

Anginal pain often parallels the signs and symptomatology of MI. It is extremely important that the nurse be able to accurately identify the characteristics that differentiate the two conditions, since the pharmacologic interventions related to angina differ considerably from those of MI. Angina, while aggravating and uncomfortable, rarely leads to a fatal outcome and the chest pain is usually immediately relieved by nitroglycerin. MI, however, carries with it a high mortality rate if appropriate treatment is delayed (see Section 35.9). In the event of MI, pharmacologic intervention must be initiated immediately and systematically maintained. When a patient presents with chest pain, the foremost objective for the health care provider is to quickly determine the cause of the pain so that proper, effective interventions can be delivered.

PharmFACT

About 9.8 million Americans experience angina each year. The risk of angina increases with age and is more common in women. Only 18% of coronary attacks are preceded by angina (Alaeddini, 2014).

Nonpharmacologic Therapy of Coronary Artery Disease

35.4 Therapeutic lifestyle changes can decrease the frequency of anginal episodes and reduce the risk of coronary artery disease.

A combination of variables influences the development and progression of angina, including dietary patterns and lifestyle choices. The nurse is instrumental in teaching patients the means of preventing CAD as well as how to lower the rate of recurrence of anginal episodes. Such support includes the formulation of a comprehensive plan of care that incorporates psychosocial support and an individualized teaching plan. The patient needs to understand the causes of angina, identify the conditions and situations that trigger it, and develop the motivation to modify behaviors associated with their disease.

Listing therapeutic lifestyle changes that modify the development and progression of cardiovascular disease (CVD) may seem repetitious, as these same factors have been included in chapters on hypertension (HTN) and heart disease. However, the importance of prevention and management of CVD through nonpharmacologic means cannot be overemphasized. Making healthy lifestyle choices can prevent CAD and slow the progression of the disease in those who have existing plaque. The following interventions have been shown to reduce the incidence of CAD:

- Limit alcohol consumption to small or moderate amounts.
- Eliminate foods high in cholesterol or saturated fats.
- Keep blood cholesterol and other lipid indicators within the normal ranges.
- Keep blood pressure within the normal range.
- Maintain blood glucose levels within the normal range.
- Exercise regularly and maintain optimum weight.
- Do not use tobacco.

When the patient is unable or unwilling to adopt healthy lifestyle choices, preventive drug therapy may be used to lower CAD risk factors. For example, antihypertensives are often used to manage blood pressure, statins to lower blood lipids, and insulin or oral hypoglycemics to keep blood glucose within the normal range. The nurse should teach patients that therapeutic lifestyle changes should be incorporated into their daily routine, even if medications are necessary to control major risk factors.

Pharmacologic Management of Angina Pectoris

35.5 The pharmacologic management of angina includes organic nitrates, beta-adrenergic blockers, and calcium channel blockers.

There are several desired therapeutic goals for a patient receiving pharmacotherapy for angina. A primary goal is to reduce the frequency and intensity of angina episodes. Additionally, successful pharmacotherapy should improve exercise tolerance and allow the patient to actively participate in activities of daily living. Long-term goals include extending the patient's lifespan by preventing

---

CONNECTIONS | Complementary and Alternative Therapies

◖Omega-3 Fatty Acids

Description
Omega-3 fatty acids are unsaturated fats found in fatty fish such as salmon, mackerel, and tuna; vegetable oils such as canola and soybean; seeds such as flaxseed and flaxseed oil; and nuts, green leafy vegetables, and beans. Omega-3 fatty acids are essential to the body and necessary for regulating muscle function, blood clotting, digestion, cell growth, and other functions (National Center for Complementary and Alternative Medicine, 2013).

History and Claims
Omega-3 fatty acids have been claimed to reduce inflammation and prevent or treat conditions such as heart disease, high blood pressure, rheumatoid arthritis, lupus, asthma, inflammatory bowel disease, and cancer.

Standardization
There are different types of omega-3 fatty acids: alpha-linolenic acid (ALA), eicosapentaenoic acid (EPA), and docosahexaenoic acid (DHA). While a balance of omega-3 and omega-6 fatty acids in the diet is important, the average U.S. diet tends to contain as much as 10 to 25 times more omega-6

than omega-3, due in large part to the consumption of meats that are higher in omega-6. Doses of less than 3 g per day of omega-3 fatty acids are usually recommended to prevent GI side effects such as diarrhea. The American Heart Association has recommended up to 4 g for patients with high lipid levels and 1 g daily for patients with coronary artery disease (University of Maryland Medical Center, 2013).

Evidence
Research has shown that omega-3 fatty acids may reduce the incidence of cardiovascular disease. In some research studies, patients have shown improvement in lipid levels and in inflammatory conditions such as rheumatoid arthritis or inflammatory bowel disease. Larger studies need to be conducted, however, to determine the extent of such benefits. While obtaining omega-3 fatty acids through dietary means is highly recommended, concern about mercury levels in fatty fish has recently been raised, and the American Heart Association (2014) recommends that pregnant women and children avoid eating fish with the potential for high mercury levels, for example, king mackerel, shark, and swordfish.

the serious consequences of ischemic heart disease such as dysrhythmias, HF, and MI. Pharmacotherapy alone, however, cannot usually achieve these outcomes; the patient must be willing to implement therapeutic lifestyle changes that promote a healthy heart.

Medications for angina are sometimes placed into two categories: those that terminate an acute angina episode in progress, and those that decrease the frequency of angina episodes. The primary means by which antianginal medications act is by reducing the myocardial demand for oxygen. This may be accomplished by the following mechanisms:

- Slowing the heart rate
- Dilating veins so that the heart receives less blood (reduced preload)
- Causing the heart to contract with less force (reduced contractility)
- Lowering blood pressure (reduced afterload)

The pharmacotherapy of angina uses three primary classes of drugs: organic nitrates, beta-adrenergic blockers, and calcium channel blockers (CCBs). Rapid-acting organic nitrates are drugs of choice for *terminating* an acute angina episode. Beta-adrenergic blockers are first-line drugs for *prophylactic* treatment. CCBs are used when beta blockers are not tolerated well by a patient.

Long-acting nitrates, given by the oral (PO) or transdermal routes, are alternatives for prophylaxis. Persistent angina requires drugs from two or more classes, such as a beta blocker combined with a long-acting nitrate or a CCB. Pharmacotherapy Illustrated 35.1 illustrates the mechanisms of action of medications used to prevent and treat CAD.

Approved in 2006, ranolazine (Ranexa) belongs to a class of drugs called **partial fatty-acid oxidation inhibitors**. Although its exact mechanism is not known, ranolazine is believed to act by shifting the metabolism of cardiac muscle cells so that they utilize glucose as the primary energy source rather than fatty acids. This decreases the metabolic rate and oxygen demands of myocardial cells. Thus, this is the only antianginal that acts through its metabolic effects, rather than hemodynamic effects. Effects on heart rate and blood pressure are minimal. The drug is only approved for chronic angina that has not responded to other drugs.

CONNECTION Checkpoint 35.2

Many patients take HMG-CoA reductase inhibitors (statins) concurrently with antianginal medications. From what you learned in Chapter 29, what is the rationale for prescribing drugs from this class for a patient with CAD? *See Answer to Connection Checkpoint 35.2 on student resource website.*

PHARMACOTHERAPY ILLUSTRATED 35.1

Mechanisms of Action of Drugs Used to Treat Angina

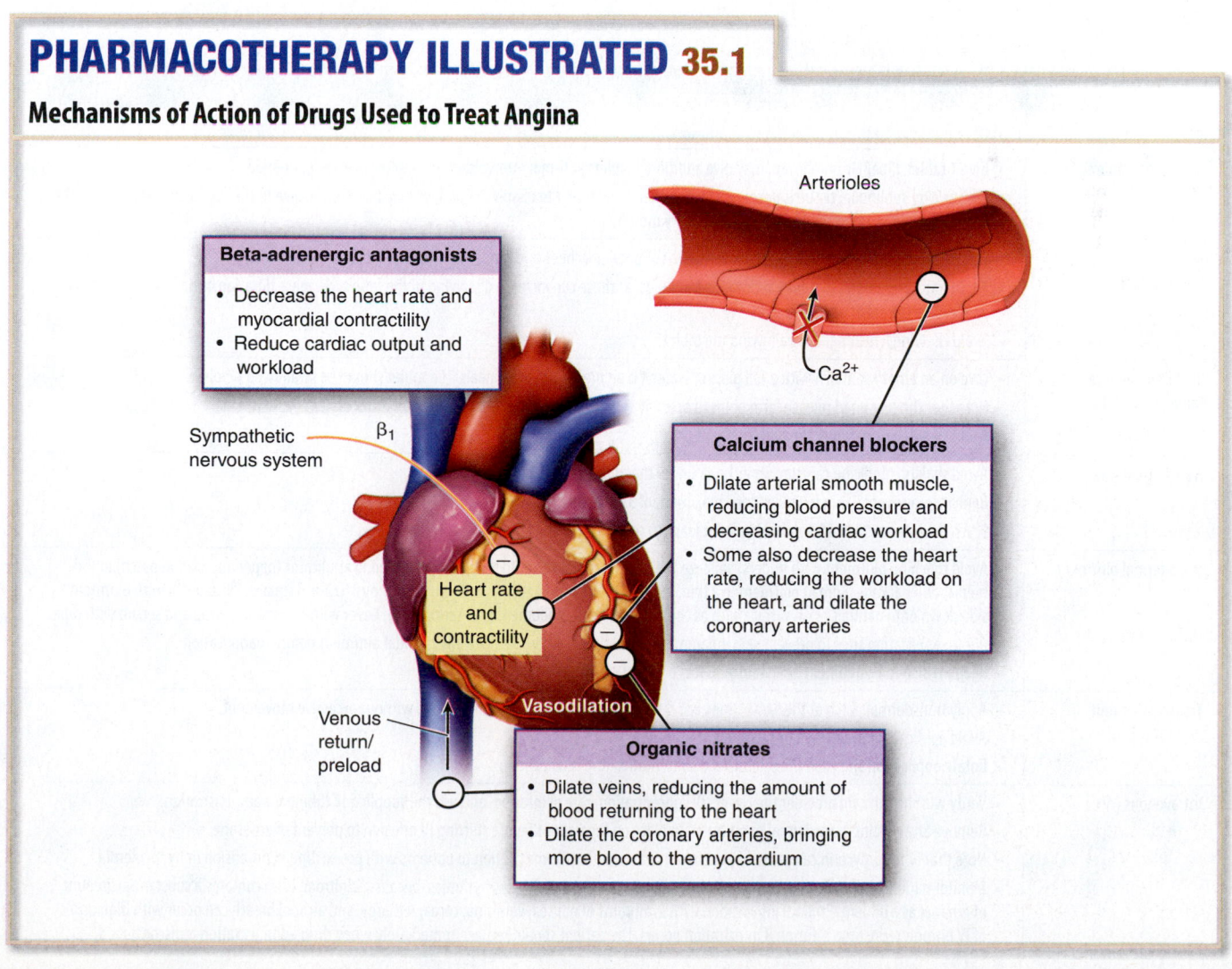

Drug Classes for Angina Pectoris

35.6 Organic nitrates may be used to terminate or prevent angina episodes.

After their medicinal properties were discovered in 1857, the organic nitrates became the mainstay for the treatment of angina for the next 100 years. The mechanism of action results from the formation of **nitric oxide** in vascular smooth muscle. Nitric oxide is an important cell-signaling molecule and a potent vasodilator, causing relaxation of both arterial and venous smooth muscle. Dilation of veins reduces the amount of blood returning to the heart (preload), and the chambers contain a smaller volume. With less blood for the ventricles to pump, cardiac output is reduced and the workload on the heart is decreased, thereby lowering myocardial oxygen demand. The therapeutic outcome is that chest pain is alleviated and episodes of angina become less frequent. The organic nitrates are listed in Table 35.1.

Organic nitrates also have the ability to dilate coronary arteries, which was once thought to be their primary mechanism of action. It seems logical that dilating a partially occluded coronary vessel would allow more oxygen to reach ischemic tissue. While this effect does indeed occur, it is no longer considered the primary mechanism of nitrate action in the treatment of stable angina. Coronary artery vasodilation, however, is crucial in treating vasospastic angina, in which the chest pain is caused by coronary artery spasm. The organic nitrates relax these spasms, allowing more oxygen to reach the myocardium, thereby terminating the pain.

Organic nitrates are classified by their onset and duration of action. The short-acting nitrates, such as nitroglycerin, may be taken sublingually or as an oral spray or buccal tablet to quickly terminate an acute anginal episode. Long-acting nitrates, such as isosorbide dinitrate (Isordil), are taken orally or are absorbed slowly through a transdermal patch to decrease the frequency and severity of angina episodes. Long-acting organic nitrates are occasionally used to treat symptoms of HF; their role in the treatment of that disease is presented in Chapter 36.

Tolerance is a common and potentially serious problem with the long-acting organic nitrates. The magnitude of the tolerance depends on the dosage and the frequency of drug administration. Although tolerance develops rapidly—as quickly as 24 hours after the initiation of therapy in some patients—it also disappears rapidly when the drug is withheld. Patients are often instructed to remove the transdermal patch for 6 to 12 hours each day or withhold a nighttime dose of the oral medications in order to delay the development of tolerance. Because the oxygen demands during sleep are diminished, the patient with stable angina experiences few angina episodes during this drug-free interval.

TABLE 35.1 Administration of Organic Nitrates	
Route	**Administration**
Sublingual tablet	• Give 1 tablet. If pain is unrelieved, may give additional tablets at 5-min intervals up to 3 tablets in a 15-min period. • Moisture on sublingual tissue is necessary for the sublingual tablet to dissolve. A patient may be unresponsive to sublingual nitroglycerin, as the anxiety caused by chest pain typically leads to dry mouth.
Sustained release buccal tablet	• Place 1 tablet between lip and gum above incisors or between cheek and gum. Allow to slowly dissolve over 3–5 h. • Avoid touching tongue to tablet or drinking hot fluids, as these can increase dissolving of the tablet, decrease duration of the medicinal effect, and lead to the onset of angina pain. • Avoid chewing, crushing, or swallowing the tablet.
Sustained release tablet or capsule	• Give on an empty stomach with a full glass of water 1 h before, or 2 h after, meals. The tablet should be swallowed whole. • Note that the sustained release form helps to prevent angina attacks but is not intended for immediate relief of angina. • Avoid chewing or crushing the tablet.
Translingual spray	• Avoid shaking medicine canister. Spray on or under the tongue. Never inhale spray. • Repeat spray every 5 min if needed for a maximum of 3 metered doses. • Teach the patient to avoid swallowing for at least 10 sec.
Transdermal ointment	• Avoid touching ointment with fingers. Squeeze the prescribed dosage onto the dose-determining applicator (paper application patch) in the medication package. Spread ointment in a thin, even layer to premarked 5.5- by 9-cm (2 1/4- by 3 1/2-in.) square. Place patch with ointment side down onto nonhairy skin surface such as the forearm, chest, abdomen, or anterior thigh. Cover with transparent wrap and secure with tape. • Rotate application sites to prevent skin inflammation and sensitization. Remove any residual ointment before reapplication. • Keep medication container closed and stored in a cool place.
Transdermal unit	• Apply transdermal patch at the same time each day to nonhairy or closely trimmed area without excessive movement. • Avoid application on irritated or scarred skin. • Rotate application site each time to prevent skin irritation and sensitization.
Intravenous (IV)	• Verify with health care provider the correct IV concentration, rate of infusion, and use the supplied IV tubing for administration. • Remove any existing transdermal or ointment in place on the patient before starting IV infusion to prevent overdosage. • Note that IV nitroglycerin can cause hypotension, so give with extreme caution to patients with preexisting hypotension or hypovolemia. • Monitor patient closely for any change in levels of consciousness and for dysrhythmias, because IV nitroglycerin contains a substantial amount of ethanol as a diluent. Ethanol intoxication with symptoms of nausea, vomiting, coma, lethargy, and alcohol breath can occur with high doses of IV nitroglycerin. Stop infusion if intoxication occurs. The patient should recover immediately when drug administration is discontinued.

Most adverse effects of organic nitrates are extensions of their hypotensive action. Flushing of the face and headache are common effects, related to vasodilation. Orthostatic hypotension is a frequent adverse effect of this drug class, and patients should be advised to change positions gradually to prevent lightheadedness. Blood pressure should be carefully monitored, and the nurse should hold nitrates and remove topical forms if serious hypotension is discovered. Taking organic nitrates concurrently with alcohol may cause severe hypotension and even cardiovascular collapse.

An additional adverse effect that can be limiting in some patients is reflex tachycardia. When the organic nitrates dilate vessels and blood pressure falls, the baroreceptor reflex is triggered. Sympathetic stimulation of the heart increases heart rate and contractility, which are undesirable effects in a patient with angina. This adverse effect is often transient and asymptomatic. Patients who report significant palpitations may be administered a beta blocker, which will prevent the reflex cardiac stimulation.

PROTOTYPE DRUG	Nitroglycerin (Nitrostat, Nitro-Bid, Nitro-Dur, Others)

Classification: Therapeutic: Antianginal drug
Pharmacologic: Organic nitrate, vasodilator

Therapeutic Effects and Uses: Nitroglycerin, the oldest and most widely used organic nitrate, can be delivered by a number of different routes: sublingual, lingual spray, PO, intravenous (IV), transmucosal, transdermal, topical, and extended release forms. The rapid-acting forms may be taken while an acute angina episode is in progress or just prior to physical activity. When given sublingually, it reaches peak plasma levels within minutes, thus quickly terminating angina pain. Chest pain that does not respond within 10 to 15 minutes after two or three doses of sublingual nitroglycerin may indicate MI, and emergency medical services (EMS) should be contacted. The transdermal and oral sustained release forms are for prophylaxis only, since they have a relatively slow onset of action. The long-acting forms should be discontinued gradually because vasospasm may result if they are abruptly withheld.

There are indications for nitroglycerin other than angina. When administered by the IV route, the drug is approved for controlled hypotension induction during anesthesia and the treatment of HF, acute pulmonary edema, acute MI, severe HTN, or hypertensive emergency. Off-label indications include use as a uterine relaxant to aid in the extraction of a retained placenta and for pain associated with anal fissures or hemorrhoids.

Mechanism of Action: Upon reaching vascular smooth muscle, nitroglycerin forms nitric oxide, which triggers a cascade resulting in the release of calcium ions in smooth muscle. Nitroglycerin relaxes both arterial and venous smooth muscle. The venous dilation decreases the amount of blood returning to the heart, reducing preload. With less blood for the ventricles to pump, myocardial oxygen demand is decreased. In addition, direct vasodilation of coronary arteries enhances the blood supply to the myocardium and is partially responsible for its therapeutic effects.

Pharmacokinetics:

Route(s)	PO: sublingual tablets, sublingual spray, buccal tablets; transdermal patch, topical ointment
Absorption	Rapid
Distribution	Widely distributed; 60% bound to plasma protein
Primary metabolism	Hepatic; extensive first-pass metabolism
Primary excretion	Renal
Onset of action	Sublingual: 1–3 min; buccal: 2–5 min; transdermal patch: 40–60 min; topical ointment: 20–60 min
Duration of action	Sublingual: 30–60 min; buccal: 2 h; transdermal patch: 18–24 h; topical ointment: 12 h

Adverse Effects: Most patients experience flushing of the face and a throbbing, transient headache, which result from the drug's vasodilation action. Orthostatic hypotension and syncope may occur. Stinging and rash may occur with ointments and transdermal patches. Methemoglobinemia is a rare adverse effect that can cause shock and coma. Anaphylaxis leading to circulatory collapse due to severe hypotension is rare. Tolerance develops with continuous therapy or large doses of the drug.

Contraindications/Precautions: Nitrates are contraindicated in patients with preexisting hypotension, shock, head injury with increased intracranial pressure, or head trauma because additive vasodilation would worsen these conditions. Drugs in this class are contraindicated in pericardial tamponade and constrictive pericarditis because the heart is unable to increase cardiac output to maintain blood pressure when the drug causes vasodilation. Sustained release forms of the medicine should not be given to patients with glaucoma because the drug may increase intraocular pressure. Nitroglycerin should be used cautiously in patients with severe liver or renal disease, as the drug could build to toxic levels. Dehydration or hypovolemia should be corrected before nitroglycerin is administered; otherwise serious hypotension may result.

Drug Interactions: Concurrent use with sildenafil (Viagra) or other phosphodiesterase-5 inhibitors may cause life-threatening hypotension and cardiovascular collapse. Nitrates should not be taken within 24 hours before or after taking these drugs. Concurrent use with ethanol, CCBs, antidepressants, phenothiazines, or antihypertensive drugs may cause additive hypotension. Sympathomimetics such as epinephrine will antagonize the vasodilation effects of nitroglycerin. **Herbal/Food**: Use with hawthorn may result in additive hypotension.

Pregnancy: Category C.

Treatment of Overdose: During overdose, hypotension may be reversed with the IV administration of normal saline. If methemoglobinemia is suspected, methylene blue may be administered.

Nursing Responsibilities: Key nursing implications for patients receiving nitroglycerin are included in the Nursing Practice Application for Patients Receiving Pharmacotherapy with Organic Nitrates for Angina and Myocardial Infarction.

Drugs Similar to Nitroglycerin (Nitrostat, Nitro-Bid, Nitro-Dur, Others)

Other organic nitrates include isosorbide dinitrate and isosorbide mononitrate. Another older drug in this class, amyl nitrite, is given by the inhalation route but is rarely used for angina.

Isosorbide dinitrate (Dilatrate SR, Isordil): Approved in 1961, isosorbide dinitrate is an organic nitrate used to terminate anginal attacks (sublingual) and for the prophylaxis of angina (extended release tablets). It is occasionally used to treat HF. The dosing schedule must allow for a drug-free period of at least 14 hours to prevent tolerance to the drug's effects. The PO forms of the drug should not be used to terminate angina attacks in progress because it takes as long as 60 minutes to reach therapeutic drug levels. The sublingual dosage forms may be taken 15 minutes prior to activities likely to precipitate angina. Adverse effects are similar to those of nitroglycerin. Like other nitrates, isosorbide dinitrate should not be administered within 24 hours of taking erectile dysfunction medications such as sildenafil. A fixed-dose combination of isosorbide dinitrate with hydralazine (BiDil) is available to reduce morbidity and mortality associated with HF. This drug is pregnancy category C.

Isosorbide mononitrate (Imdur, Ismo, Monoket): Approved in 1991, isosorbide mononitrate is an active, long-acting metabolite of isosorbide dinitrate. The mononitrate is only used for prophylaxis: Its 30- to 60-minute onset of action makes it unacceptable for termination of acute anginal pain. The dosing schedule must allow for a drug-free period of at least 7 hours to prevent the development of tolerance to the drug's effects. It is available as regular release or extended release tablets, which should be taken on an empty stomach at least 30 minutes before a meal. Imdur is an extended release form of the drug that permits once-daily dosing. Adverse effects are the same as the other organic nitrates. This drug is pregnancy category C.

35.7 Beta-adrenergic blockers are sometimes drugs of choice for stable angina.

Beta-adrenergic antagonists or blockers decrease cardiac workload by lowering blood pressure, slowing heart rate, and reducing contractility. These actions on the heart are particularly beneficial during exercise. Beta blockers are as effective as the organic nitrates in decreasing the frequency and severity of anginal episodes caused by exertion. For the pharmacotherapy of CAD, cardioselective beta$_1$ antagonists are preferred over nonselective beta antagonists because they are less likely to cause bronchoconstriction (a beta$_2$ response). Beta-adrenergic antagonists are not effective for treating vasospastic angina and may, in fact, worsen this condition.

Beta-adrenergic blockers offer several advantages over the organic nitrates. Tolerance does not develop to the antianginal effects of the beta blockers during prolonged therapy. They possess antidysrhythmic properties, which help prevent cardiac conduction abnormalities that are common complications of patients with ischemic heart disease. Beta blockers are ideal for patients who have both HTN and CAD due to their antihypertensive action. They have also been shown to reduce the incidence of MI. Because of these cardioprotective actions, beta blockers are considered drugs of choice for the prophylaxis of chronic angina. The beta blockers used for angina are listed in Table 35.1. Beta blockers have a variety of uses and additional details may be found in chapters

on adrenergic antagonists (see Chapter 16), HTN (see Chapter 34), HF (see Chapter 36), and dysrhythmias (see Chapter 37). A Nursing Practice Application for patients receiving beta blockers is included in Chapter 16.

Beta-adrenergic antagonists are well tolerated by most patients. In some patients, fatigue, lethargy, and depression are reasons for discontinuation of beta-blocker therapy. At high doses, drugs in this class can cause shortness of breath and respiratory distress due to bronchoconstriction, and they should be used cautiously in patients with asthma or chronic obstructive pulmonary disease (COPD). Because beta blockers slow the heart rate and myocardial conduction velocity, they are contraindicated in patients with bradycardia and greater than first-degree heart block. Heart rate should be closely monitored so that it does not fall below 50 to 60 beats/minute at rest or 100 beats/minute during exercise. Beta blockers are also contraindicated in cardiogenic shock and overt cardiac failure.

Patients with diabetes who are prescribed beta blockers should be aware that the actions of beta blockers can obscure the initial symptoms of hypoglycemia (palpitations, diaphoresis, and nervousness). Because of this, blood glucose levels should be monitored more frequently, and insulin doses may need to be adjusted accordingly.

Beta-adrenergic antagonists should never be abruptly discontinued. With long-term beta blocker use, the heart becomes more sensitive to catecholamines, which are blocked by these medications. When withdrawn abruptly, adrenergic receptors are activated and rebound excitation occurs. In patients with CAD, this can exacerbate angina, precipitate tachycardia, or cause an MI.

PROTOTYPE DRUG | Atenolol (Tenormin)

Classification: Therapeutic: Antianginal drug
Pharmacologic: Beta-adrenergic antagonist

Therapeutic Effects and Uses: Atenolol is one of the most frequently prescribed drugs in the United States, due to its relative safety and effectiveness in treating a number of chronic disorders, including HF, HTN, stable angina, and post-acute MI. Approved in 1981, it is given by the PO route and has a long duration of action that allows for once-daily dosing. Off-label indications for atenolol include ethanol withdrawal, migraine prophylaxis, and unstable angina.

Mechanism of Action: Atenolol selectively blocks beta$_1$-adrenergic receptors in the heart. Its effectiveness in angina is attributed to its ability to slow the heart rate and reduce contractility, both of which lower myocardial oxygen demand.

Pharmacokinetics:

Route(s)	PO, IV
Absorption	50% absorbed from the gastrointestinal (GI) tract
Distribution	Distributed to most tissues including the placenta; secreted in breast milk; does not readily cross the blood–brain barrier; 5–15% bound to protein
Primary metabolism	Not metabolized
Primary excretion	Renal (50%), feces (50%)
Onset of action	PO: 1 h; IV: immediate
Duration of action	PO/IV: 24 h; half-life: 6–7 h

Adverse Effects: Oral atenolol is well tolerated by most patients. Beta-blocking effects can result in bradycardia and hypotension. Fatigue, weakness, and dizziness are other potential adverse effects. Nausea and vomiting occur in some patients. **Black Box Warning**: Abrupt discontinuation should be avoided in patients with ischemic heart disease because this may worsen angina or cause an MI. Doses should be gradually reduced over a 1- to 2-week period if possible. If angina worsens during the withdrawal period, the drug should be reinstituted, at least temporarily.

Contraindications/Precautions: Because atenolol slows heart rate, it should not be used by patients with severe bradycardia, advanced atrioventricular (AV) heart block, cardiogenic shock, or decompensated HF. Due to its vasodilation effects, it is contraindicated in patients with severe hypotension. Patients with severe renal impairment should receive reduced doses or have longer time intervals between doses to prevent drug accumulation. Because atenolol reduces cardiac output, patients with stroke or low cerebrovascular blood flow should not receive this drug. Patients with major depression should not receive beta blockers because these drugs can worsen this condition.

Drug Interactions: Anticholinergics may decrease the absorption of atenolol from the GI tract. Use with digoxin or other antidysrhythmic drugs that depress myocardial conduction may cause AV heart block. Concurrent use of atenolol with other antihypertensives may result in additive hypotension. Although CCBs are often used concurrently with beta blockers for their additive therapeutic actions, patients must be monitored carefully due to the possibility of excessive cardiac suppression. **Herbal/Food**: Use with hawthorn may result in additive hypotension.

Pregnancy: Category D.

Treatment of Overdose: The most serious symptoms of atenolol overdose are hypotension and bradycardia. Atropine or isoproterenol may be used to reverse bradycardia, or a cardiac pacemaker may be used to stabilize cardiac rhythm. Atenolol can be removed from the systemic circulation by hemodialysis.

Nursing Responsibilities: Key nursing implications for patients receiving atenolol are included in the Nursing Practice Application for Patients Receiving Pharmacotherapy with Adrenergic Antagonists in Chapter 16.

Drugs Similar to Atenolol (Tenormin)

Atenolol, metoprolol, propranolol, and timolol are equally effective in treating chronic angina. Information on these beta-adrenergic antagonists is presented in other chapters. The student should review the general information on beta blockers in Chapter 16. Several are featured as prototype drugs: metoprolol (Lopressor, Toprol) and propranolol (Inderal, InnoPran XL) in Chapter 16 and timolol (Betimol, Istalol, Timoptic) is featured as an antiglaucoma medication in Chapter 74.

35.8 Calcium channel blockers are effective at reducing myocardial oxygen demand and treating stable and vasospastic angina.

Blockade of calcium channels has a number of effects on the heart, most of which are similar to those of beta blockers. Although the first approved indication for CCBs was for the treatment of angina, these medications are also used for HTN and dysrhythmias. The mechanisms of calcium channel blockade by drugs in this class are presented in detail in Chapter 30. The actions of CCBs relevant to ischemic heart disease are discussed in this section. The CCBs used for angina are listed in Table 35.2.

CCBs have several actions on the cardiovascular system that benefit the patient with angina. Most importantly, CCBs relax arteriolar smooth muscle, thus reducing blood pressure. This reduction in afterload decreases myocardial oxygen demand. Some of the CCBs also slow cardiac conduction velocity through the AV node, thereby decreasing heart rate and contributing to the reduced cardiac workload. An additional effect of the CCBs is their ability to dilate the coronary arteries, bringing more oxygen to the myocardium. This vasodilation is especially important in patients with vasospastic angina. CCBs are considered drugs of choice for that condition. For stable, exertional angina, they may be used as monotherapy in patients unable to tolerate beta blockers. In patients with persistent symptoms, CCBs may be administered concurrently with organic nitrates or beta blockers.

Adverse effects of CCBs are generally not serious and are related to vasodilation: headache, dizziness, and edema of the ankles and feet. CCBs should be used with caution in patients taking other cardiovascular medications that slow conduction through the AV node, particularly digoxin or beta-adrenergic blockers. The combined effects of these drugs may cause partial or complete AV heart block, HF, or dysrhythmias. Some CCBs worsen HF by reducing myocardial contractility.

CONNECTION Checkpoint 35.3

For patients with asthma, calcium channel blockers are generally the preferred antianginal agents, rather than beta-adrenergic antagonists. From what you learned in Chapter 16, why would calcium channel blockers be preferred for patients with this comorbid condition? *See Answer to Connection Checkpoint 35.3 on student resource website.*

Pathophysiology of Myocardial Infarction

35.9 Early diagnosis and pharmacotherapy of myocardial infarction increase chances of survival.

Myocardial infarctions (MIs), blood clots that block coronary arteries, are responsible for a substantial number of deaths each year. Many patients die before reaching a medical facility for treatment, or within 48 hours following the initial MI, due to complications of the disorder. Clearly, MI is a serious and frightening disease and one responsible for a large percentage of sudden deaths.

The primary cause of MI is advanced CAD: atherosclerotic plaque accumulation in the endothelial wall of one or more branches of the coronary arteries. Pieces of unstable plaque in a coronary artery can ulcerate or rupture and lodge in a small vessel serving a portion of the myocardium. Exposed plaque activates the clotting cascade, resulting in platelet aggregation. A new clot quickly builds on the existing plaque, making obstruction of the vessel imminent. A detailed discussion of coagulation and clot formation is included in Chapter 38.

Deprived of adequate oxygen supply, the obstructed region of the myocardium becomes ischemic. The myocytes shift to anaerobic

TABLE 35.2 Selected Drugs for Angina and Myocardial Infarction

Drug	Route and Adult Dose (Maximum Dose Where Indicated)	Adverse Effects
Organic Nitrates		
isosorbide dinitrate (Dilatrate SR, Isordil)	PO: 2.5–30 mg 4 times daily (max: 480 mg/day) Extended release: 40–80 mg daily (max: 160 mg/day) SL: 2.5–5 mg taken 15 min before exercise	*Headache, orthostatic hypotension, flushing of the face, dizziness, rash (transdermal patch), tolerance* <u>Anaphylaxis, circulatory collapse due to hypotension, syncope due to orthostatic hypotension</u>
isosorbide mononitrate (Imdur, Ismo, Monoket)	PO: 20 mg qid Ismo, Monoket: 20 mg bid (max: 40 mg/day) Imdur: 30–60 mg each morning (max: 240 mg/day)	
nitroglycerin (Nitrostat, Nitro-Dur, Nitro-Bid, Others)	SL: 1 tablet (0.3–0.6 mg) or 1 spray (0.4–0.8 mg) every 3–5 min (max: 3 doses in 15 min)	
Beta-Adrenergic Antagonists		
atenolol (Tenormin)	PO: 25–50 mg daily (max: 100 mg/day)	*Fatigue, insomnia, drowsiness, impotence or decreased libido, depression, bradycardia, and confusion* <u>Agranulocytosis, laryngospasm, Stevens–Johnson syndrome, anaphylaxis; if the drug is abruptly withdrawn, palpitations, rebound HTN, life-threatening dysrhythmias or myocardial ischemia may occur</u>
metoprolol (Lopressor, Toprol XL)	PO (for HTN or angina): 100 mg/day (max: 400 mg/day)	
propranolol (Inderal, Innopran XL, Inderal LA)	PO immediate release: 40–420 mg bid (max: 640 mg/day) PO extended release: 80–160 mg/day (max: 120 mg/day for Innopran; 640 mg/day for Inderal LA)	
timolol (Betimol)	PO: 15–45 mg tid (max: 60 mg/day)	
Calcium Channel Blockers		
amlodipine (Norvasc)	PO: 5–10 mg daily (max: 10 mg/day)	*Flushed skin, headache, dizziness, peripheral edema, lightheadedness, nausea, constipation* <u>Hepatotoxicity, MI, HF, confusion, mood changes</u>
diltiazem (Cardizem, Cartia XT, Dilacor XR, Others)	PO regular release: 30 mg tid–qid (max: 360 mg/day) Extended release: 120–240 mg bid (max: 540 mg/day)	
nicardipine (Cardene)	PO: 20–40 mg tid or 30–60 mg sustained release bid (max: 120 mg/day)	
nifedipine (Adalat, Procardia, Others)	PO: 10–20 mg tid (max: 180 mg/day) Extended release: 30–90 mg once daily	
verapamil (Calan, Covera-HS, Isoptin SR, Verelan)	PO immediate release: 80–120 mg 3–4 times daily (max: 480 mg/day) PO extended release: 180–540 mg/day	
Miscellaneous Drug		
ranolazine (Ranexa)	PO: 500–1,000 mg bid (max: 2,000 mg/day)	*Dizziness, constipation, headache, and nausea* <u>QT interval prolongation</u>

Note: Italics indicate common adverse effects. <u>Underline</u> indicates serious adverse effects.

metabolism after only 8 to 10 seconds of oxygen loss. Anaerobic metabolism, however, is inefficient and cannot produce enough ATP to keep the heart beating efficiently for prolonged periods. Lactic acid accumulates, causing acidosis, which affects contractility and suppresses normal conduction across the myocardium. As contractility diminishes, the patient may experience HF. Myocytes will begin to die in about 20 minutes unless the blood supply is quickly restored. The necrosis of myocardial tissue, which may be irreversible, releases certain "marker" enzymes, such as creatine phosphokinase (CK) or cardiac-specific troponin (cTn), which can be measured in the blood to confirm the patient has experienced an MI.

Extreme chest pain is often the first symptom of MI and the one that drives most patients to seek medical attention. An electrocardiogram (ECG) can give important clues as to the extent and location of the MI because the infarcted region of the myocardium is nonconducting, producing abnormalities of Q waves, T waves, and ST segments. Patients showing elevation of the ST segment on the ECG are at highest risk for death and require immediate treatment. Laboratory test results are used to aid in diagnosis and monitor progress after an MI. Table 35.3 describes some of these important laboratory values.

Early diagnosis and prompt pharmacotherapy of MI can significantly reduce the mortality and long-term disability associated with MI. The pharmacologic goals for treating a patient with an acute MI are as follows:

- If cardiac arrest has occurred, restart the heart and restore normal blood pressure with vasopressors.

- Restore blood supply (reperfusion) to the damaged myocardium as quickly as possible through the use of thrombolytics.

- Reduce myocardial oxygen demand with organic nitrates, beta blockers, or CCBs to lower the risk of additional infarctions.

TABLE 35.3 Changes in Blood Test Values with Acute Myocardial Infarction

Blood Test	Initial Elevation After MI	Peak Elevation After MI	Duration of Elevation	Normal Range
CK: Total creatine kinase (also called creatine phosphokinase)	3–8 h	12–24 h	2–4 days	Males: 5–35 mcg/L Females: 5–25 mcg/L
CK-MB	4–6 h	10–24 h	3–4 days	0–3% of CK
ESR (erythrocyte sedimentation rate)	2–3 days	4–5 days	Several weeks	Males: 15–20 mm/h Females: 20–30 mm/h
LDH: Total (lactate dehydrogenase)	12–24 h	2–5 days	6–12 days	70–250 units/L
Myoglobin	2–6 h	8–12 h	1–2 days	12–90 ng/mL
Troponin I	1–3 h	24–36 h	5–9 days	0.1–0.5 mcg/L
Troponin T	1–3 h	24–36 h	10–14 days	<0.2 mcg/L

- Control or prevent MI-associated dysrhythmias with amiodarone (Cordarone), beta blockers, or other antidysrhythmics.
- Reduce post-MI mortality with aspirin, beta blockers, and ACE inhibitors.
- Manage severe MI pain and associated anxiety with narcotic analgesics.

Pharmacologic Management of Myocardial Infarction

35.10 Thrombolytic drugs can restore perfusion to ischemic regions of the myocardium if administered soon after a myocardial infarction.

Thrombolytic therapy is administered to dissolve clots obstructing the coronary arteries in order to restore circulation to the ischemic region of the myocardium. Clinical research has confirmed that quick restoration of coronary circulation reduces mortality following an acute MI. After the clot is successfully dissolved, anticoagulant or antiplatelet therapy is initiated to prevent additional clot formation. Dosages and descriptions of the various thrombolytics are listed in Chapter 38 where alteplase (Activase) is presented as a drug prototype for this class. A Nursing Practice Application for thrombolytics is also included in Chapter 38.

Thrombolytics are most effective when administered from 20 minutes to 12 hours after the onset of MI symptoms. Ideally, the time from presentation in the emergency department to administration of the thrombolytic should be 30 minutes or less. Research has demonstrated little or no therapeutic benefit if the drugs are administered 24 hours or more after the MI onset. In addition, research suggests that patients over age 75 do not experience reduced mortality from these drugs. Because thrombolytic therapy is expensive and has the potential to produce serious adverse effects, it is important to identify circumstances that contribute to successful therapy. The development of clinical practice guidelines for thrombolytic therapy remains an area of active research. Pharmacotherapy Illustrated 35.2 illustrates this reperfusion process.

Thrombolytics exhibit a narrow margin of safety between dissolving clots and producing serious adverse effects. Although therapy is usually targeted to a single thrombus in a specific artery, once infused in the blood the drugs travel to all vessels and may cause adverse effects anywhere in the body. The primary risk of thrombolytics is excessive bleeding from interference with the clotting process. Vital signs must be monitored continuously and signs of bleeding call for discontinuation of therapy. Because these medications have a brief half-life and are rapidly destroyed in the blood, stopping the infusion normally results in the rapid termination of adverse effects. Physical and laboratory assessment for the possibility of abnormal bleeding should continue for 2 to 4 days after therapy is discontinued.

Thrombolytic therapy is contraindicated for many conditions, including recent trauma or surgery, internal bleeding (other than menses), active peptic ulcer, postpartum (within 10 days), history of intracranial hemorrhage, suspected ischemic stroke within the past 3 months, bleeding disorders, severe liver disease, or thrombocytopenia. Caution should be used when administering thrombolytics to patients taking anticoagulants or antiplatelet drugs.

35.11 Drugs are used to treat the symptoms and complications of acute myocardial infarction.

The most immediate needs of the patient with MI are to ensure that the heart continues to function adequately and that permanent damage from the infarction is minimized. In addition to restoring perfusion to the myocardium with thrombolytic therapy, drugs from several other classes are administered soon after the onset of symptoms to prevent reinfarction and to ultimately reduce mortality from the episode.

Aspirin

Unless contraindicated, 160 to 325 mg of aspirin is given as soon as an MI is suspected. Research has determined that aspirin use in the weeks following an acute MI dramatically reduces mortality. These effects from aspirin are believed to be due to several mechanisms. Clearly, aspirin has antiplatelet action that reduces platelet aggregation and thus the formation or enlargement of thrombi. Additionally, its anti-inflammatory properties decrease the formation of C-reactive protein, which is associated with an increased risk of MI.

The major concern over aspirin use is its tendency to promote GI bleeding in some patients. This could be a serious adverse effect, given that some post-MI patients receive anticoagulants.

PHARMACOTHERAPY ILLUSTRATED 35.2

Thrombolytic Pharmacotherapy

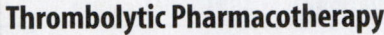

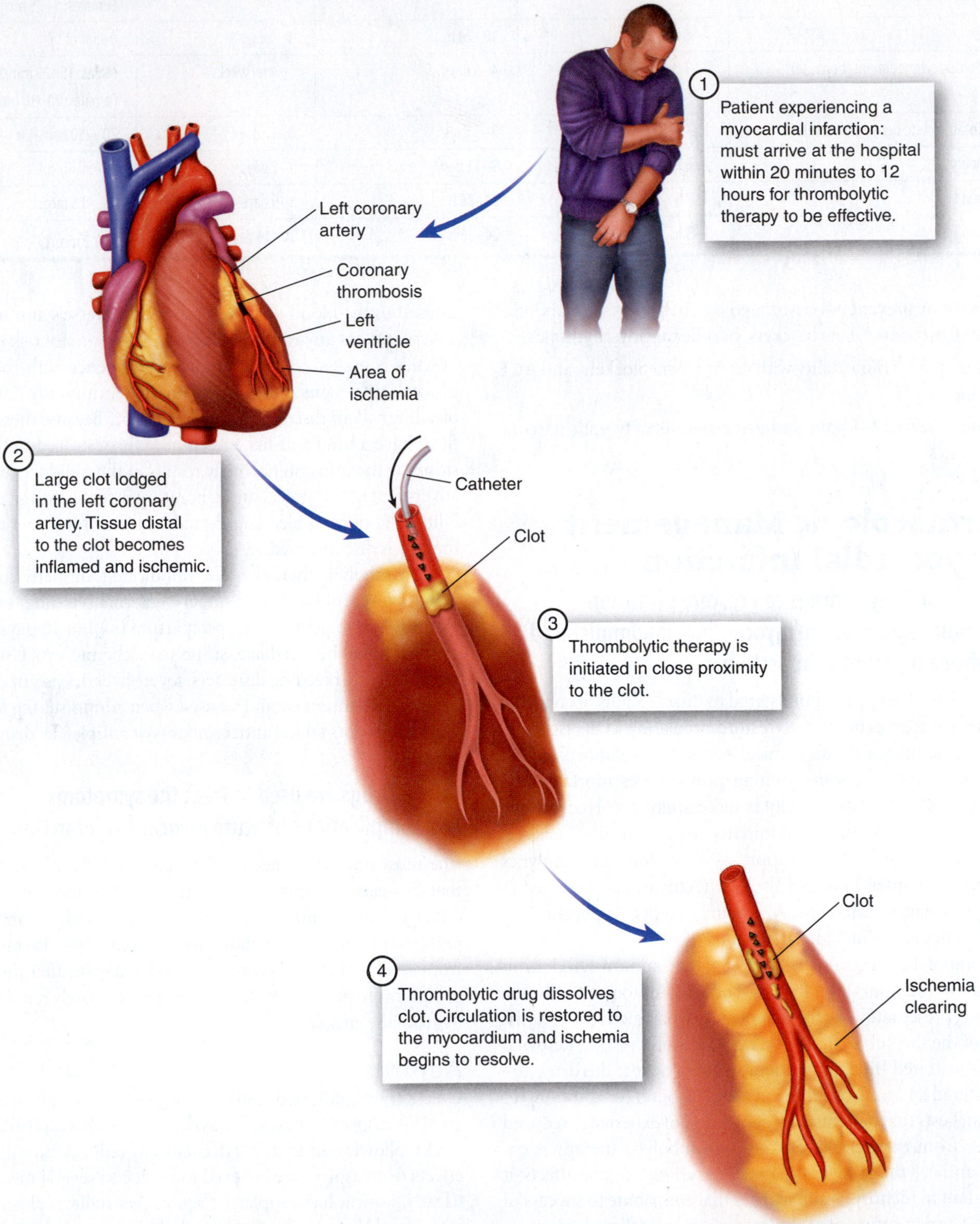

1 Patient experiencing a myocardial infarction: must arrive at the hospital within 20 minutes to 12 hours for thrombolytic therapy to be effective.

Left coronary artery

Coronary thrombosis

Left ventricle

Area of ischemia

2 Large clot lodged in the left coronary artery. Tissue distal to the clot becomes inflamed and ischemic.

Catheter

Clot

3 Thrombolytic therapy is initiated in close proximity to the clot.

Clot

Ischemia clearing

4 Thrombolytic drug dissolves clot. Circulation is restored to the myocardium and ischemia begins to resolve.

CONNECTIONS **Evidence-Based Practice**

Nitroglycerin and Chest Pain

Clinical Question
Does relief of chest pain by the administration of nitroglycerin indicate the presence of CAD with myocardial ischemia?

Evidence
Relief of chest pain following administration of nitroglycerin has been used as an indicator for CAD with myocardial ischemia since the late 1970s. More recent studies questioned the validity of that conclusion, and even complete relief of chest pain, experienced by only approximately 70% of patients, was not found to correlate directly with the presence or absence of CAD.

In a comprehensive review of clinical studies, the American Heart Association confirmed that relief of chest pain by nitroglycerin was not an adequate indicator of the presence or absence of CAD or cardiac pathologies and because it did not predict myocardial ischemia, it should not be used as the sole indicator (Amsterdam et al., 2010). Further diagnostic studies, including cardiac markers (e.g., troponin), ECG, and noninvasive or invasive studies such as echocardiography when appropriate, should be used to evaluate the presence of CAD with or without myocardial ischemia.

Implications
Nitroglycerin plays a key role in the treatment of myocardial ischemia and continues to be a part of the treatment plan. Health care providers should not rely on the presence or absence of chest pain following nitroglycerin use as an indicator of CAD, myocardial ischemia, or impending MI; other laboratory work and cardiac studies should also be used for an accurate diagnosis. The nurse can help patients understand that the provider should be notified if nitroglycerin is taken for chest pain, particularly if frequent or escalating use is required. The nurse can also teach the patient, family, or caregiver that the relief of chest pain after nitroglycerin use is not the only indicator that MI is not occurring or impending. Other symptoms such as fatigue, chest pressure, dizziness, sweating, or abdominal discomfort should be considered as possible symptoms of myocardial ischemia, and the patient should seek emergency assistance if the symptoms continue to exist after taking nitroglycerin for chest pain.

Critical Thinking Questions
In addition to angina, what are other signs and symptoms of myocardial ischemia? What should the nurse teach the patient if sublingual nitroglycerin is prescribed?

See Answers to Critical Thinking Questions on student resource website.

However, the benefits of taking aspirin following an acute MI generally outweigh the risks for most patients. Aspirin maintenance therapy can cut the risk of death due to a subsequent MI by as much as 50% in some populations. Furthermore, the low doses used in maintenance therapy (75–150 mg/day) rarely cause GI bleeding. Additional discussion of aspirin may be found in Chapter 41, where it is featured as a prototype drug.

Anticoagulants and Antiplatelet Drugs

Drugs from several classes are routinely used to prevent MIs by altering the coagulation properties of the blood. The primary goal for using these coagulation modifiers is to prevent new thrombi from being formed, or from enlarging.

Anticoagulants: Upon diagnosis of MI in the emergency department, patients may be placed on the anticoagulant heparin to prevent the formation of additional thrombi. Unfractionated heparin therapy is sometimes continued for 48 hours, or until percutaneous coronary intervention (PCI) is completed, at which time the patients are switched to warfarin (Coumadin) or an antiplatelet drug. An alternative is to administer a low-molecular-weight heparin, such as enoxaparin (Lovenox). A comparison of these different anticoagulants is presented in Chapter 38, along with prototype drug features for heparin and warfarin.

Some patients may remain on anticoagulant therapy after hospital discharge. These include patients at high risk for thromboembolic disease and those with chronic atrial fibrillation. Research has not shown that the use of warfarin lowers mortality in post-MI patients; however, it does increase the risk of bleeding. For most patients, anticoagulation with aspirin or antiplatelet drugs is sufficient for protection from thromboembolic events. The long-term use of heparin in post-MI patients is limited unless other conditions are present that warrant the use of the drug.

Adenosine diphosphate receptor blockers: Clopidogrel (Plavix) and ticlopidine (Ticlid) are antiplatelet drugs that are approved for the prevention of thrombotic stroke and MI. Research has demonstrated that these drugs reduce mortality associated with thromboembolic events. They are considered for antiplatelet therapy in patients who are allergic to aspirin or at high risk for GI bleeding from aspirin. Some protocols call for combination therapy with clopidogrel and aspirin. Clopidogrel is one of the most frequently used drugs for prevention of MI, and is featured as a prototype in Chapter 38.

Glycoprotein IIb/IIIa Inhibitors Glycoprotein IIb/IIIa is a receptor found on the surface of platelets. Glycoprotein IIb/IIIa inhibitors are sometimes indicated to prevent thrombi from forming in patients with unstable angina, MI, or for those undergoing PCI procedures such as angioplasty. The most common drug in this class, abciximab (ReoPro), is infused at the time of PCI and continued for 12 hours after the procedure is completed to prevent reinfarction. These drugs may be used in combination therapy with aspirin and heparin, thus increasing the need for careful monitoring for bleeding. Doses for the glycoprotein IIb/IIIa inhibitors and a prototype feature for abciximab are found in Chapter 38.

Other antiplatelet drugs: In 2014 the Food and Drug Administration (FDA) approved the first in a new class of antiplatelet drugs called the protease-activated receptor-1 antagonists. Vorapaxar (Zontivity) is administered to reduce the incidence of thrombotic events in patients with a history of MI or other clotting disorders. It is usually given in combination with aspirin or clopidogrel.

Nitrates

The value of nitrates in treating myocardial ischemia was presented in Section 35.6. Nitrates have additional uses in the patient with a suspected MI. At the initial onset of chest pain, sublingual nitroglycerin is administered to assist in the diagnosis, and three doses may be taken 5 minutes apart. Pain that persists 5 to 10 minutes after the initial dose may indicate an MI, and the patient should seek medical assistance. Thus, nitrates serve a diagnostic role for MI patients.

Patients with persistent pain, HF, or severe HTN may receive IV nitroglycerin for 24 hours following the onset of pain. The arterial and venous dilation produced by the drug reduces myocardial oxygen demand. Organic nitrates also relieve coronary artery vasospasm, which may be present during the acute stage of MI. Upon discharge from the hospital, organic nitrates are discontinued, unless the patient needs them for relief of stable anginal pain.

Beta-Adrenergic Blockers

Beta blockers have the ability to slow heart rate, decrease contractility, and reduce blood pressure. These three factors reduce myocardial oxygen demand, which is critical for patients experiencing a recent MI. In addition, they slow impulse conduction through the heart, suppressing dysrhythmias, which are serious and sometimes fatal complications following an MI. Research has clearly demonstrated that beta blockers can reduce MI-associated mortality if administered within 8 hours of MI onset. These drugs may be initially administered IV, and then switched to oral dosing for chronic therapy. Unless contraindicated, beta-blocker therapy continues for the remainder of the patient's life. For patients unable to tolerate beta blockers, CCBs are an alternative. The beta blockers most often used for MI are listed in Table 35.1.

Angiotensin-Converting Enzyme Inhibitors

Clinical research has demonstrated increased survival for patients administered the angiotensin-converting enzyme (ACE) inhibitors captopril (Capoten) or lisinopril (Prinivil, Zestoretic) following an acute MI. These drugs are most effective when therapy is started within 24 hours after the onset of symptoms. Oral doses are normally begun after thrombolytic therapy is completed and the patient's condition has stabilized. IV therapy may be used during the early stages of MI pharmacotherapy.

The benefit of ACE inhibitors is believed to be due to their ability to prevent cardiac remodeling and their ability to suppress dysrhythmias. Unless otherwise contraindicated, post-MI patients should receive an ACE inhibitor indefinitely to prevent HF and future ischemic development. The mechanisms of action and prototype features for several ACE inhibitors may be found in Chapter 31.

Pain Management

The pain associated with an MI can be debilitating and stressful, creating an increased workload for the myocardium. Pain control is essential in order to ensure patient comfort and to reduce stress. Narcotic analgesics such as morphine sulfate or meperidine (Demerol) are given to ease extreme pain, sedate the anxious patient, and decrease the workload of the heart. Pharmacology of the analgesics was presented in Chapter 25.

PharmFACT

About 1.5 million Americans experience a new or recurrent MI each year. About one third of the patients experiencing an MI will die within 24 hours of the onset of the attack (Zafari, 2014).

35.12 Vasopressors are used following cardiopulmonary arrest to reestablish coronary and cerebral blood flow.

Cardiopulmonary arrest is a complete stoppage of heart and lungs activity, usually resulting from a dysrhythmia such as ventricular fibrillation or pulseless ventricular tachycardia. Most patients who experience cardiopulmonary arrest have underlying CAD.

Cardiopulmonary resuscitation (CPR) must be initiated as quickly as possible to restore ventilation and blood circulation to avoid hypoxic injury to the tissues. Electrical defibrillation is used to restore normal cardiac rhythm.

Pharmacotherapy is an important component of CPR. The primary drugs used in the initial phase of resuscitation are sympathomimetics, and epinephrine is the drug of choice. Sympathomimetics cause vasoconstriction, immediately raising cerebral, coronary, and systemic blood pressure. Vasopressin, also called antidiuretic hormone, is an alternative therapy.

Following restoration of cardiac function and ventilation, it is critical that the heart maintain normal conduction in order to prevent the recurrence of ventricular fibrillation or the establishment of other serious dysrhythmias. Historically, lidocaine has been the preferred drug for ventricular dysrhythmias associated with MI. Clinical research, however, has shown that the administration of amiodarone (Cordarone) may result in improved patient survival. If the risk of dysrhythmia is high, a loading dose of amiodarone is given by infusion, and the patient is switched to oral forms after a therapeutic plasma level of the drug has been achieved. Amiodarone is featured as an antidysrhythmic drug prototype in Chapter 37.

CONNECTIONS: NURSING PRACTICE APPLICATION

Patients Receiving Pharmacotherapy with Organic Nitrates for Angina and Myocardial Infarction

Assessment	Potential Nursing Diagnoses*
Baseline assessment prior to administration: • Obtain a complete health history: cardiovascular (including previous MI, HF, valvular disease), cerebrovascular and neurologic (including level of consciousness, history of stroke, head injury, increased intracranial pressure), renal or hepatic dysfunction, dysrhythmias, pregnancy, or lactation. Obtain a drug history including allergies, current prescription and over-the-counter (OTC) drugs, herbal preparations, and alcohol use. Be aware that use of erectile dysfunction drugs (e.g., sildenafil [Viagra], vardenafil [Levitra], or tadalafil [Cialis]) within the past 24 to 48 h may cause profound and prolonged hypotension when nitrates are administered. Be alert to possible drug interactions. • Obtain baseline weight, vital signs (especially blood pressure and pulse), and ECG. Assess for location and character of angina if currently present. • Evaluate appropriate laboratory findings, electrolytes, renal function studies, and lipid profiles. Troponin and/or CK-MB laboratory values may be ordered to rule out MI. • Assess the patient's ability to receive and understand instructions. Include family and caregivers as needed.	• *Decreased Cardiac Output* • *Acute Pain* • *Fatigue* • *Activity Intolerance* • *Deficient Knowledge* (Drug Therapy) • *Risk for Decreased Cardiac Tissue Perfusion*, related to adverse effects of drug therapy • *Risk for Falls*, related to adverse effects of drug therapy • *Risk for Injury*, related to adverse effects of drug therapy
Assessment throughout administration: • Assess for desired therapeutic effects (e.g., chest pain has subsided or has significantly lessened), heart rate and blood pressure remain within normal limits, ECG remains within normal limits without signs of ischemia or infarction. • Continue periodic monitoring of ECG for ischemia or infarct. • Continue frequent monitoring of blood pressure and pulse whenever IV nitrates are used or when giving rapid-acting (e.g., sublingual) nitrates. With sublingual nitrates, take blood pressure before and 5 min after giving dose and hold the drug if blood pressure is less than 90/60 mmHg, pulse over 100 beats/min, or parameters as ordered, and check with the health care provider before continuing to give the drug. • Assess for and promptly report adverse effects: severe hypotension, dysrhythmias, reflex tachycardia (from too rapid decrease in blood pressure or severe hypotension), headache that does not subside within 15–20 min, or when accompanied by neurologic changes or decreased urinary output. Immediately report severe hypotension, seizures, dysrhythmias, or palpitations. Chest pain remaining present after three sublingual nitroglycerin tablets given 5 min apart should be reported immediately, even if pain has lessened, as this may be a sign of impending ischemia or infarction.	

Implementation

Interventions and (Rationales)	Patient-Centered Care
Ensuring therapeutic effects: • Continue frequent assessments as above for therapeutic effects. (Because nitrates cause vasodilation, preload and afterload diminish, decreasing myocardial oxygenation needs, and chest pain diminishes.)	• Ask the patient to briefly describe the location and character of pain (use a pain rating scale for rapid assessment) prior to and after giving nitrates to assess for extent of relief. Correlate with objective assessment findings. **Lifespan and Diverse Patients:** Due to differences in reporting pain, use subjective and objective data in evaluating pain relief in ethnically diverse and the older adult patient.
• Continue to monitor ECG, blood pressure, and pulse. (Nitrates cause vasodilation and possible hypotension. Blood pressure assessment aids in determining drug frequency and dose. ECG monitoring helps detect adverse effects such as reflex tachycardia, ischemia, or infarction.)	• Teach the patient, family, or caregiver how to monitor pulse and blood pressure. Ensure proper use and functioning of any home equipment obtained.
• Evaluate the need for adjunctive treatment with the health care provider for angina prevention and treatment (e.g., beta blockers, aspirin therapy) or further cardiac studies. (Patients with unstable angina may require adjunctive drug therapy or definitive cardiac studies to determine the need for other treatment options.)	• Encourage the patient to discuss any changes in character, severity, or frequency of angina episodes with the health care provider. Instruct the patient not to take routine (daily) aspirin without discussing with the provider first, because the drug may be contraindicated depending on other conditions or medications.
• For patients on transdermal nitroglycerin patches, remove patch for 6–12 h at night, or as directed by the health care provider. (Removing the transdermal patch at night helps prevent or delay the development of tolerance to nitrates.)	• Instruct the patient on proper use of nitroglycerin and the rationale for removing transdermal patches. Also instruct patients on transdermal patches to always remove the old patch, cleanse the skin underneath gently, and to rotate sites before applying a new patch.
• Encourage appropriate lifestyle changes: lowered fat intake, restricted sodium or fluid intake if ordered, gradually increased levels of exercise, limited alcohol intake, and smoking cessation. Provide for dietitian consultation as needed. (Healthy lifestyle changes will support the benefits of drug therapy.)	• Encourage the patient, family, and caregivers to adopt a healthy lifestyle of low-fat food choices, increased exercise, decreased alcohol consumption, and smoking cessation. Provide educational materials on low-fat, low-sodium food choices.

(continued)

CONNECTIONS: NURSING PRACTICE APPLICATION (continued)

Minimizing adverse effects:
- Continue to monitor vital signs frequently. **Lifespan:** Be particularly cautious with older adults who are at increased risk for hypotension, patients with a preexisting history of cardiac or cerebrovascular disease, or patients with a recent head injury, which may be worsened by vasodilation. Notify the health care provider immediately if angina remains unrelieved or if blood pressure or pulse decrease beyond established parameters, or if hypotension is accompanied by reflex tachycardia. (Nitrates may cause significant vasodilation, resulting in the potential for hypotension accompanied by reflex tachycardia. Reflex tachycardia increases myocardial oxygen demand, worsening angina.)

- Instruct the patient, family, or caregiver to report dizziness, faintness, palpitations, or headache unrelieved after taking nonnarcotic analgesics (e.g., acetaminophen).
- Instruct the patient on nitrates to rise from lying to sitting or standing slowly to avoid dizziness or falls, especially if taking sublingual nitrates, or until drug effects are known. If dizziness occurs, the patient should sit or lie down and not attempt to stand or walk, until the sensation passes.

- Continue cardiac monitoring (e.g., ECG) as ordered if IV nitrates are administered. (Monitoring devices assist in detecting early signs of adverse effects of drug therapy, myocardial ischemia or infarction, as well as monitoring for therapeutic effects.)

- To allay possible anxiety, teach the patient, family, or caregiver the rationale for all equipment used and the need for frequent monitoring.

- Continue frequent physical assessments, particularly neurologic, cardiac, and respiratory. Immediately report any changes in level of consciousness, headache, or changes in heart or lung sounds. (Nitrate therapy may worsen preexisting neurologic, cardiac, or respiratory conditions as blood pressure drops and perfusion to vital organs diminishes. Lung congestion may signal impending HF.)

- When on PO therapy at home, the patient, family, or caregiver should immediately report changes in mental status or level of consciousness, palpitations, dizziness, dyspnea, and increasing productive cough, especially if frothy sputum is present, and seek medical attention.

- Review the medications taken by the patient before sending the patient home, and review all prescription as well as OTC medications with the patient. Current use of erectile dysfunction drugs, as noted on medication history, is contraindicated with nitrates. (Erectile dysfunction drugs lower blood pressure and when combined with nitrates, can result in severe and prolonged hypotension.)

- Instruct the patient to not take sildenafil (Viagra), vardenafil (Levitra), or tadalafil (Cialis) while taking nitrates and to discuss treatment options for erectile dysfunction with the health care provider.

Patient understanding of drug therapy:
- Use opportunities during administration of medications and during assessments to discuss the rationale for the drug therapy, desired therapeutic outcomes, commonly observed adverse effects, parameters for when to call the health care provider, and any necessary monitoring or precautions. (Using time during nursing care helps to optimize and reinforce key teaching areas.)

- The patient, family, or caregiver should be able to state the reason for the drug; appropriate dose and scheduling; what adverse effects to observe for and when to report them; and the anticipated length of medication therapy.

Patient self-administration of drug therapy:
- When administering medications, instruct the patient, family, or caregiver in the proper self-administration of drugs and when to contact the provider. (Utilizing time during nurse-administration of these drugs helps to reinforce teaching.)

- The patient should be able to state how to use sublingual nitroglycerin at home:
  - Take one nitroglycerin tablet, under the tongue, for angina/chest pain. Remain seated or lie down to avoid dizziness or falls.
  - If chest pain continues, repeat one nitroglycerin tablet, under the tongue, in 5 min. Remain seated or lying down.
  - If chest pain continues, repeat nitroglycerin, under the tongue, in 5 min.
  - If chest pain continues, even if reduced, do not take further nitroglycerin unless specifically directed by the health care provider. Call EMS (e.g., 911) for assistance. Do *not* drive self, or have family drive the patient, to the emergency department.
- If blood pressure monitoring equipment is available at home, have the patient, family, or caregiver take blood pressure prior to the second and third nitroglycerin doses. Hold the drug and contact EMS if blood pressure is less than 90/60 mmHg.

---

*Nursing Diagnoses—Definitions and Classification 2015–2017. Copyright © 2014, 1994–2014 by NANDA International. Used by arrangement with John Wiley & Sons Limited.

CHAPTER
35

Understanding the Chapter

Key Concepts Summary

35.1 Myocardial ischemia develops when there is inadequate blood supply to meet the metabolic demands of cardiac muscle.

35.2 Coronary artery disease is the major cause of myocardial ischemia.

35.3 Angina pectoris is characterized by severe chest pain brought on by physical exertion or emotional stress.

35.4 Therapeutic lifestyle changes can decrease the frequency of anginal episodes and reduce the risk of coronary artery disease.

35.5 The pharmacologic management of angina includes organic nitrates, beta-adrenergic blockers, and calcium channel blockers.

35.6 Organic nitrates may be used to terminate or prevent angina episodes.

35.7 Beta-adrenergic blockers are sometimes drugs of choice for stable angina.

35.8 Calcium channel blockers are effective at reducing myocardial oxygen demand and treating stable and vasospastic angina.

35.9 Early diagnosis and pharmacotherapy of myocardial infarction increase chances of survival.

35.10 Thrombolytic drugs can restore perfusion to ischemic regions of the myocardium if administered soon after a myocardial infarction.

35.11 Drugs are used to treat the symptoms and complications of acute myocardial infarction.

35.12 Vasopressors are used following cardiopulmonary arrest to reestablish coronary and cerebral blood flow.

Making the Patient Connection

Remember the patient "Michael Graff" at the beginning of the chapter? Now read the remainder of the case study. Based on the information presented within this chapter, respond to the critical thinking questions that follow.

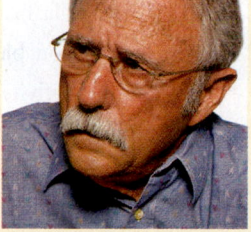

Early one morning, 60-year-old Michael Graff began to feel severe anterior crushing chest pain that lasted for 35 minutes. He experienced dizziness, cold sweats, and nausea. Although he considered driving to the local emergency department, his family insisted on calling an ambulance for emergency transport to the hospital.

Michael, a general contractor, is a 2-pack-per-day smoker and consumes alcohol (beer) two to three times per week. He has a family history of coronary artery disease, diabetes mellitus, and hyperlipidemia. It has been at least 10 years since his last physical examination.

Upon arrival at the emergency department, he presents with symptoms of anxiety, moderate chest pain, and cold extremities. Auscultation of the thorax revealed tachycardia and clear lung fields. Blood pressure was slightly above normal at 156/90 mmHg. He had no neck venous distention. His white

blood cell count was $7,600/mm^3$, hematocrit 43.8%, platelets $256,000/mm^3$, creatine phosphokinase (CPK) 87 international units/L, and troponin-I < 4.1 mcg/L. An ECG showed ST-segment elevation.

Once stabilized, Michael is transported to the coronary care unit with the admission diagnosis of unstable angina and to rule out MI. In the coronary care unit, he receives IV nitroglycerin 50 mg in D_5W 25 mL. The nurse begins the infusion at 10 mcg/min and titrates the rate based on his report of chest pain every 5 to 10 min (5–10 mcg/min).

Critical Thinking Questions

1. Michael and his family ask you to explain what is occurring with his heart. How would you describe the pathophysiology of Michael's condition to them?

2. Discuss the reason Michael is receiving nitroglycerin.

3. What adverse effects should the nurse monitor with patients receiving IV nitroglycerin?

4. How do nitroglycerin infusions differ from other IV infusions?

See Answers to Critical Thinking Questions on student resource website.

Additional Case Study

Bill Shackley, a 52-year-old man, is prescribed a daily nitroglycerin transdermal patch. While discussing his medications, Bill shares several of his concerns. How would you respond to the following questions?

1. "I heard that I can become 'tolerant' to this drug. What does this mean? How can it be avoided?"

2. "Sometimes, after applying the nitroglycerin patch, I get a throbbing headache. Is there anything I can do about this?"

3. "I was told to report episodes of dizziness when I stand up plus rapid heart rates. How does nitroglycerin cause these?"

See Answers to Additional Case Study on student resource website.

Chapter Review

1 Nitroglycerin topical ointment is being initiated for a patient with angina. Which health teaching would be most appropriate?

1. Keep the medication in the refrigerator.
2. Only take this medication when chest pain is severe.
3. Remove the old paste before applying the next dose.
4. Apply the ointment on the chest wall only.

2 A patient with chest pain is receiving sublingual nitroglycerin. The nurse would include in the care plan to monitor the patient for which adverse effect?

1. Photosensitivity
2. Elevated blood pressure
3. Vomiting and diarrhea
4. Decreased blood pressure

3 The patient states, "I always put my nitroglycerin patch in the same place so I do not forget to take it off." The nurse's response would be based on which of the following physiological concepts?

1. Patients are more likely to remember to apply the patch if the same site is used daily.
2. Repeated use of the same application site will enhance medication absorption.
3. Rebound phenomenon is likely to occur when the same site is used more than once.
4. Skin irritation due to the nitroglycerin ointment can occur if the same site is used repeatedly.

4 The nurse is caring for a patient with chronic angina pectoris. The patient is receiving isosorbide dinitrate (Isordil) oral tablets. Which patient manifestations would the nurse conclude are common adverse effects of this medication?

1. Flushing and headache
2. Tremors and anxiety
3. Lightheadedness and dizziness
4. Sleepiness and lethargy

5 The patient asks how atenolol (Tenormin) helps angina. The response provided by the nurse is based on which concept? This medication:

1. Slows the heart rate and reduces contractility.
2. Increases the heart rate and diminishes contractility.
3. Blocks sodium channels and elevates depolarization.
4. Decreases blood pressure and blocks the alpha$_2$ receptors.

6 Which of the following assessment findings, if discovered in a patient receiving verapamil (Calan) for angina, would be cause for the nurse to withhold the medication? Select all that apply.

1. Bradycardia: heart rate of 40 beats/minute
2. Tachycardia: heart rate of 126 beats/minute
3. Hypotension: blood pressure 76/46 mmHg
4. Tinnitus with hearing loss
5. Hypertension: blood pressure 156/92 mmHg

See Answers to Chapter Review in Appendix A.

References

Alaeddini, J. (2014). Angina pectoris. *Medscape Reference.* Retrieved from http://emedicine.medscape.com/article/150215-overview

American Heart Association. (2014). *Fish and omega-3 fatty acids.* Retrieved from http://www.heart.org/HEARTORG/GettingHealthy/NutritionCenter/HealthyDietGoals/Fish-and-Omega-3-Fatty-Acids_UCM_303248_Article.jsp

Amsterdam, E. A., Kirk, J. D., Bluemke, D. A., Diercks, D., Farkouh, M. E., Garvey, J. L., . . .

Thompson, P. D. (2010). Testing of low-risk patients presenting to the emergency department with chest pain: A scientific statement from the American Heart Association. *Circulation, 122*(17), 1756–1776. doi:10.1161/CIR.0b013e3181ec61df

National Center for Complementary and Alternative Medicine. (2013). *Omega-3 supplements: An introduction.* Retrieved from http://nccam.nih.gov/health/omega3/introduction.htm

University of Maryland Medical Center. (2013). *Omega-3 fatty acids.* Retrieved from http://umm.edu/health/medical/altmed/supplement/omega3-fatty-acids

Zafari, A. M. (2014). *Myocardial infarction.* Retrieved from http://emedicine.medscape.com/article/155919-overview

Selected Bibliography

Bhat, D. L. (2010). Acute coronary syndrome update for hospitalists. *Journal of Hospital Medicine, 5*(Suppl. 4), S15–S21. doi:10.1002/jhm.830

Gupta, A. K., Winchester, D., & Pepine, C. J. (2013). Antagonist molecules in the treatment of angina. *Expert Opinion on Pharmacotherapy, 14,* 2323–2342. doi:10.1517/14656566.2013.834329

Herdman, T. H., & Kamitsuru, S. (Eds.). (2014). *NANDA International nursing diagnoses: Definitions and classification, 2015–2017.* Oxford, United Kingdom: Wiley-Blackwell.

Jayasekara, R. (2010). Effect of early treatment with antihypertensive drugs on short- and long-term mortality in patients with an acute cardiovascular event. *International Journal of Evidence-Based Healthcare, 8,* 41. doi:10.1111/j.1744-1609.2010.00155.x

Jones, D. A., Timmis, A., & Wragg, A. (2013). Novel drugs for treating angina. *BMJ, 347.* doi:10.1136/bmj.f4726

Kee, J. L. (2014). *Laboratory and diagnostic tests with nursing implications* (9th ed.). Upper Saddle River, NJ: Pearson Education.

Maron, B. A., & Rocco, T. P. (2011). Pharmacotherapy of heart failure. In L. L. Brunton, B. A. Chabner, & B. C. Knollman (Eds.), *The pharmacological basis of therapeutics* (12th ed., pp. 789–814). New York, NY: McGraw-Hill.

Norton, C., Georgiopoulou, V., Kalogeropoulos, A., & Butler, J. (2011). Chronic stable angina: Pathophysiology and innovations in treatment. *Journal of Cardiovascular Medicine, 12,* 218–219. doi:10.2459/JCM.0b013e328343e974

Shah, A., & Fox, K. (2013). Stable angina: Current guidelines and advances in management. *Prescriber, 24*(17), 35–44. doi:10.1002/psb.1095

Sharma, V., Bell, R. M., & Yellon, D. M. (2012). Targeting reperfusion injury in acute myocardial infarction: A review of reperfusion injury pharmacotherapy. *Expert Opinion on Pharmacotherapy, 13,* 1153–1175. doi:10.1517/14656566.2012.685163

Wright, R. S., Anderson, J. L., Adams, C. D., Bridges, C. R., Casey, D. E., Ettinger, S. M., . . . Zidar, J. P. (2011). 2011 ACCF/AHA focused update of the guidelines for the management of patients with unstable angina/non–ST-elevation myocardial infarction (updating the 2007 guideline): A report of the American College of Cardiology Foundation/American Heart Association Task Force on Practice Guidelines. *Journal of the American College of Cardiology, 57,* 1929–1959. doi:10.1016/j.jacc.2011.02.009

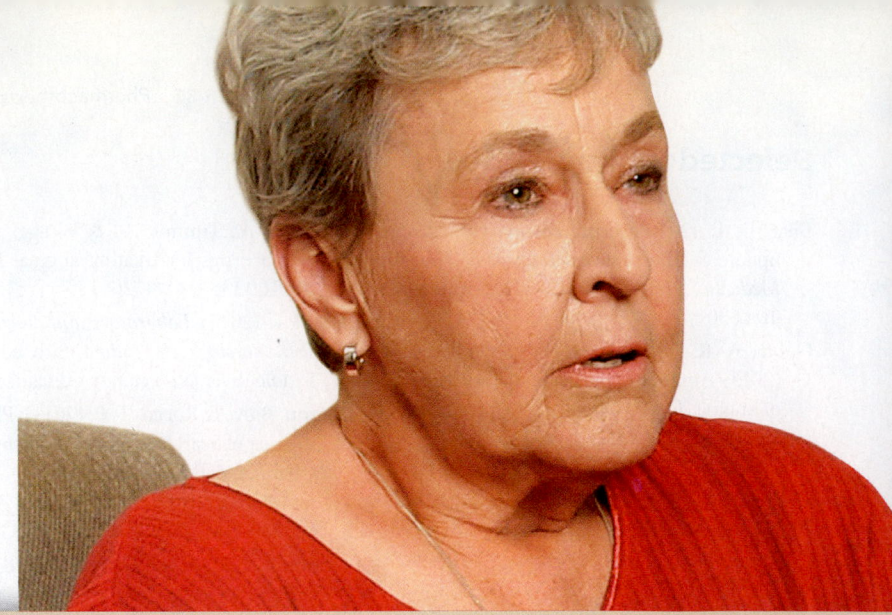

"It seems that over the past 2 weeks, I have become more short of breath just walking around my apartment. Walking up stairs and unloading my groceries have become impossible."

Patient "Thelma Walters"

LEARNING OUTCOMES

After reading this chapter, the student should be able to:

1. Identify the major diseases associated with heart failure.
2. Relate how the symptoms associated with heart failure may be caused by a weakened heart muscle and diminished cardiac output.
3. Identify compensatory mechanisms used by the body to maintain cardiac output in patients with heart failure.
4. Describe how heart failure is classified.
5. Describe the nurse's role in the pharmacologic management of heart failure.
6. For each of the classes shown in the chapter outline, identify the prototype and representative drugs and explain the mechanism(s) of drug action, primary indications, contraindications, significant drug interactions, pregnancy category, and important adverse effects.
7. Apply the nursing process to care for patients receiving pharmacotherapy for heart failure.

CHAPTER OUTLINE

▸ Etiology of Heart Failure

▸ Pathophysiology of Heart Failure
   Ventricular Hypertrophy

▸ Pharmacologic Management of Heart Failure

▸ Drugs for Heart Failure
   Angiotensin-Converting Enzyme Inhibitors and Angiotensin Receptor Blockers
   Diuretics
   Beta-Adrenergic Antagonists
   Vasodilators
   Cardiac Glycosides
   PROTOTYPE Digoxin (Lanoxin, Lanoxicaps), *p. 587*
   Beta-Adrenergic Agonists
   Phosphodiesterase III Inhibitors
   PROTOTYPE Milrinone (Primacor), *p. 589*

KEY TERMS

cardiac remodeling, 579	heart failure (HF), 579	phosphodiesterase III, 589
digitalization, 587	natriuretic peptides, 581	reverse remodeling, 586
diuretic resistance, 585		

Heart failure is one of the most common and fatal of the cardiovascular diseases, and its incidence is increasing as the population ages. Although improved treatment of myocardial infarction and hypertension has led to declines in mortality due to heart failure, approximately one in five patients still dies within a year of diagnosis of heart failure, and 50% die within 5 years. Historically, this condition was called *congestive heart failure*; however, because not all incidences of this disease are associated with congestion, the more appropriate name is *heart failure*.

PharmFACT

Each year, about 670,000 new cases of heart failure are diagnosed and about 277,000 deaths are attributed to HF in the United States. Although the incidence is equal in men and women, females develop HF later in life and survive longer with the disease (Dumitru, 2014).

Etiology of Heart Failure

36.1 Heart failure is closely associated with disorders such as chronic hypertension, coronary artery disease, and diabetes.

Heart failure (HF) is the inability of the heart to pump enough blood to meet the metabolic demands of the body. HF can be caused by any disorder that affects the heart's ability to receive or eject blood. While weakening of cardiac muscle is a natural consequence of aging, the process can be caused or accelerated by the following:

- Coronary artery disease (CAD)
- Mitral stenosis
- Myocardial infarction (MI)
- Chronic hypertension (HTN)
- Diabetes mellitus

The student should detect a common theme throughout the chapters on cardiovascular pharmacology. That theme is the ability to prevent major causes of morbidity and mortality through control of healthy lifestyle choices. Controlling lipid levels, implementing a regular exercise program, maintaining optimum body weight, and keeping blood pressure within recommended limits reduce the incidences of CAD and MI. Maintaining blood glucose within the normal range reduces the consequences of uncontrolled diabetes. Thus, for many patients, HF is a preventable condition; controlling associated diseases will greatly reduce the risk of development and progression of HF.

Since there is no cure for HF, the treatment goals are to prevent, treat, or remove the underlying causes whenever possible and treat its symptoms, so that the patient's quality of life can be improved. Advances in understanding the pathophysiology of HF during the past two decades have led to a change in pharmacotherapeutic goals. No longer is therapy of HF focused on end stages of the disorder.

Pharmacotherapy is now targeted at prevention and slowing the progression of HF. This change in emphasis has led to significant improvements in survival and quality of life in patients with HF.

Pathophysiology of Heart Failure

36.2 The body attempts to compensate for heart failure by increasing cardiac output.

HF is a general term used to describe several different types of cardiac dysfunction. The dysfunction may occur on the left side, the right side, or on both sides of the heart.

Left-sided HF is called congestive heart failure (CHF) because it is characterized by an accumulation of fluid causing congestion in the pulmonary capillary beds. Although left-sided HF is more common, the right side of the heart can also become weak, either simultaneously with the left side or independently from the left side. In right-sided HF, the blood pools in the veins, resulting in peripheral edema and engorgement of organs such as the liver.

Left-sided HF is further subdivided into two types. Systolic HF occurs when cardiac output (CO) is diminished due to decreased contractility of the myocardium. Approximately 60% to 80% of left-sided HF is the systolic type. Diastolic HF occurs when the lungs become congested even though cardiac output is normal. Diastolic HF is caused by a restriction in ventricular filling, resulting in higher-than-normal pressure in the ventricle. Although cardiac output is normal, the increased pressure in the ventricle creates higher pressure in the pulmonary capillaries, resulting in pulmonary edema. A patient may have both systolic and diastolic HF. Pharmacotherapy of the two types differs somewhat. For example, inotropic drugs that increase contractility are more successful with systolic HF than diastolic HF.

HF may progress slowly over many years, or it may have an acute onset. Once HF reaches the stage where cardiac output is affected, tissues receive inadequate perfusion and organ failure is possible. The body has developed a complex series of actions to compensate for HF. Knowledge of these compensatory mechanisms is important to understanding the pharmacotherapy of HF. Prior to continuing in this chapter, factors affecting cardiac output, stroke volume, afterload, and preload, discussed in Chapter 28, should be reviewed. The pathophysiology of HF is illustrated in Figure 36.1.

Ventricular Hypertrophy

In left HF, the left ventricle is forced to work harder due to the increased preload or afterload. Over time, the wall of the left ventricle thickens and enlarges (ventricular hypertrophy) in an attempt to compensate for the increased workload. Changes in the size, shape, and structure of the myocardial cells (myocytes) occur. These compensatory changes in structure benefit the heart by allowing it to better maintain adequate stroke volume and cardiac output. The term **cardiac remodeling** is sometimes used to describe these changes to myocyte structure and function.

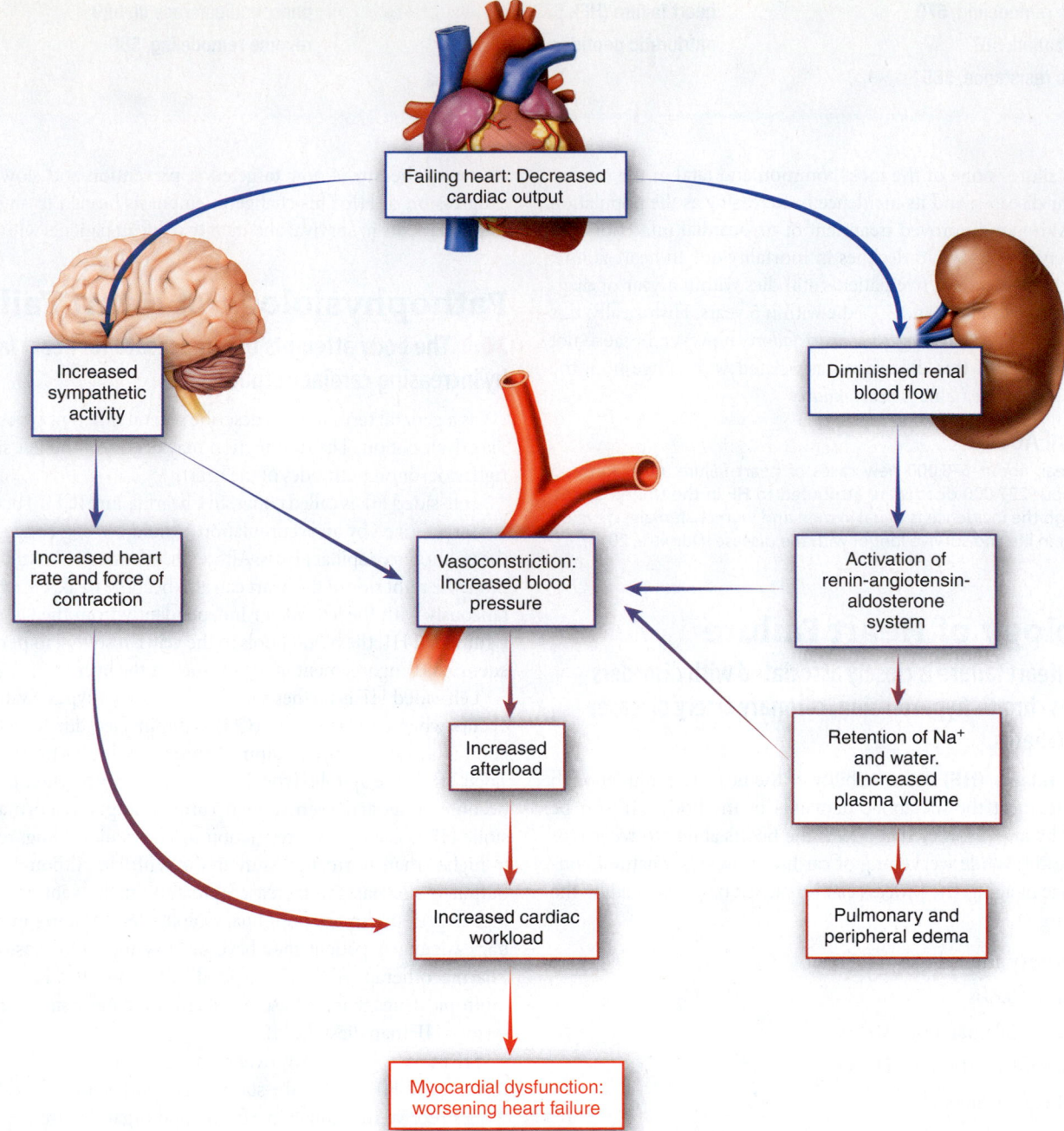

Figure 36.1 Pathophysiology of heart failure.

The benefits of cardiac remodeling as a compensatory mechanism, however, are limited. Myocytes continually die, likely due to workload injury, and fibrotic tissue fills the spaces between them. These tissue changes stiffen the myocardium, causing diminished contractility and reduced cardiac output. The heart responds with even more remodeling, continuing the destructive cycle. Without intervention, the abnormal structural changes can result in irreversible cardiac impairment.

Activation of the Sympathetic Nervous System

One of the fastest homeostatic responses to diminished cardiac output is activation of the sympathetic nervous system (SNS).

The increased heart rate resulting from sympathetic activation is a normal compensatory mechanism that serves to increase cardiac output.

The SNS, however, also constricts arteries and activates the renin-angiotensin-aldosterone system (RAAS). Higher angiotensin II levels raise blood pressure and afterload, causing the heart to work harder. The stressed myocardium, which already has reduced contractility and is having difficulty maintaining cardiac output, is faced with even greater challenges by this additional workload. The diminished cardiac output caused by the high afterload produces an ongoing activation of the SNS. Patients with preexisting CAD may experience an anginal attack from the increased SNS activity. Again, although there are certain compensatory benefits to activating the SNS to maintain cardiac output, a destructive cycle is created that can lead to or worsen HF.

CONNECTION Checkpoint 36.1

Propranolol (Inderal) is an example of a negative inotropic agent. From what you learned in Chapter 16, explain why this type of drug should be administered with caution to a patient with heart failure who also has asthma. *See Answer to Connection Checkpoint 36.1 on student resource website.*

Increased Plasma Volume and Preload

When cardiac output in a patient with HF is diminished, blood flow to the kidneys is reduced. The kidneys respond to the decreased perfusion by secreting renin and activating the RAAS. As a result of the action of angiotensin II, aldosterone secretion is increased, and the body retains sodium and water. This has the beneficial effects of increasing preload, stretching the myocardial fibers, and increasing contractility, thus returning cardiac output to normal levels. This is an important compensatory mechanism in normal hearts.

However, the heart has a limited ability to increase contractility. In a diseased heart, the increased preload leads to volume overload and pulmonary congestion. In addition, the increased plasma volume increases blood pressure, which further adds to afterload and to the burden of an already weak heart.

Research has discovered additional detrimental effects related to activation of the RAAS. Angiotensin II has been found to promote ventricular hypertrophy, myocyte death, and fibrosis formation in the myocardium. Aldosterone also has direct effects on the myocardium, promoting fibrosis and stiffening of the ventricular wall. Angiotensin-converting enzyme (ACE) inhibitors have become preferred drugs for HF, in part, because they are able to block these detrimental effects of angiotensin II and aldosterone on cardiac remodeling.

Natriuretic Peptides and Neurohumoral Factors

Natriuretic peptides are substances secreted in response to increased pressure in the heart. Three types have been identified:

1. Atrial natriuretic peptide (ANP) is secreted by the atria.
2. B-type natriuretic peptide (BNP) is secreted by the ventricles.
3. C-type natriuretic peptide (CNP) is secreted by the brain.

The physiological functions of ANP and BNP are to cause diuresis, vasodilation, and decreased aldosterone secretion, thus balancing the effects of the SNS and RAAS activation. Nesiritide (Natrecor), a drug structurally identical to BNP, has a limited role in the treatment of HF, as discussed in Section 36.8.

Research has identified several other substances as potential mediators in the progression of HF. Two proinflammatory substances, tumor necrosis factor (TNF) and interleukin, are found in high levels in patients with HF and are associated with a poor prognosis. The hormone endothelin is a vasoconstrictor that also is associated with a poor prognosis in HF patients. Vasopressin (antidiuretic hormone), which is elevated in HF patients, causes fluid retention and worsens this condition. It is likely that research will identify additional mediators of HF, along with potential novel therapies for the disease.

TABLE 36.1 Drugs That May Worsen Heart Failure

Mechanism	Example Drugs and Classes
Negative inotropic effect: slow heart rate or reduce contractility	Antidysrhythmics
	Beta-adrenergic blockers
	Calcium channel blockers
	Itraconazole (antifungal)
Cardiotoxicity: damage to the myocardium	Cyclophosphamide (antineoplastic)
	Daunomycin (antineoplastic)
	Doxorubicin (antineoplastic)
Increase blood volume: cause sodium and water retention and fluid overload	Androgens
	Estrogens
	Glucocorticoids
	NSAIDs
	Rosiglitazone and pioglitazone (antidiabetic)

36.3 Symptoms of heart failure occur when compensatory mechanisms fail to maintain adequate cardiac output.

The classic symptoms of HF are dyspnea on exertion, fatigue, pulmonary congestion, and peripheral edema. Lung congestion causes a cough and orthopnea (difficulty breathing when recumbent). If pulmonary edema occurs, the patient feels as if he or she is suffocating and extreme anxiety may result. The condition often worsens at night.

Through pharmacotherapy and lifestyle modifications, many patients with HF can be maintained in a symptom-free, compensated state for years. The most common reason patients experience decompensation is fluid overload due to nonadherence to sodium and water restrictions. The second most common reason is nonadherence to the pharmacotherapeutic regimen. The nurse must stress to patients the importance of sodium restriction and treatment adherence to maintain a properly functioning heart. Cardiac events such as myocardial ischemia, MI, or dysrhythmias can also precipitate acute HF. Certain medications can worsen HF, and the nurse should use these drugs with caution. A list of selected drugs that may worsen HF is shown in Table 36.1.

Pharmacologic Management of Heart Failure

36.4 The specific therapy for heart failure depends on the clinical stage of the disease.

Several models are available to guide the pharmacologic management of HF. The New York Heart Association (NYHA) classification has been widely used in clinical practice for the staging of HF. This model classifies symptomatic HF into four functional classes:

- I: Patients with cardiac disease but with no symptoms during physical activity
- II: Patients with cardiac disease who have slight limitations on physical activity, with symptoms such as fatigue, palpitations, dyspnea, or angina

TABLE 36.2   **Stages for Treating Heart Failure**

Stage	Description	Treatment Examples
A	Patients are at high risk of developing HF.	Make lifestyle modifications. Treat and control associated conditions: HTN, dyslipidemia, and diabetes. If hypertensive, use ACE inhibitor.
B	Patients have structural evidence of heart disease, such as a previous MI or valvular disease, but no symptoms of HF. (Includes NYHA Class I patients.)	Continue treatments for Stage A. Treat with ACE inhibitor (or ARB if patient is intolerant to ACE inhibitors). Beta blockers are added for those with prior HF symptoms or history of MI.
C	Patients have structural evidence of heart disease with symptoms of HF such as fatigue, fluid retention, or dyspnea. (Includes NYHA Class II and III patients.)	Continue lifestyle modifications. Treat with ACE inhibitor (or ARB) and beta blocker. If needed to control symptoms, add digoxin or diuretic or combination of isosorbide dinitrate with hydralazine (in African Americans). In patients with a history of atrial fibrillation or thromboembolic event, implement anticoagulation with drugs such as warfarin, dabigatran, apixaban, or rivaroxaban. Consider supplementation with omega-3 fatty acids.
D	Patients have symptoms at rest or minimal exertion despite optimal medical therapy; decompensated HF. (Includes NYHA Class IV patients.)	Continue lifestyle modifications. Treatment may include IV diuretics, dopamine, dobutamine, IV nitroglycerin, nitroprusside, nesiritide, or phosphodiesterase inhibitors.

From "2013 Focused Update: ACCF/AHA Guidelines for the Diagnosis and Management of Heart Failure in Adults. A Report of the American College of Cardiology Foundation/American Heart Association Task Force on Practice Guidelines Developed in Collaboration with the International Society for Heart and Lung Transplantation," 2013, *Journal of the American College of Cardiology, 53*, pp. 1343–1382; "ACCF/AHA Guideline for the Management of Heart Failure: A Report of the American College of Cardiology Foundation/American Heart Association Task Force on Practice Guidelines," by C. W. Yancy et al., 2013, *Circulation, 128*, e240. Published online before print June 5, 2013.

- III: Patients with cardiac disease who have marked limitations during physical activity
- IV: Patients with cardiac disease who are unable to perform physical activity, and who have symptoms at rest

A more recent model, proposed by the American College of Cardiology (ACC) and the American Heart Association (AHA), categorizes HF into four stages, as listed in Table 36.2. Although similar to the NYHA model, the ACC/AHA model better illustrates the progressive nature of the disease and the role of risk factor modification.

Drugs for Heart Failure

Pharmacotherapy of HF focuses on three primary goals:

1. Reduction of preload
2. Reduction of systemic vascular resistance (afterload reduction)
3. Inhibition of both the RAAS and vasoconstrictor mechanisms of the sympathetic nervous system.

The first two goals provide symptomatic relief but do not reverse the progression of the disease. In addition to reducing symptoms,

---

CONNECTIONS **Evidence-Based Practice**

◖ Diabetes and Heart Failure

Clinical Question
Does maintaining glucose control in diabetes decrease the incidence of heart failure?

Evidence
People with diabetes have a higher incidence of CAD and an increased risk of heart disease and HF. Studies of the incidence of HF often include multiple risk factors including smoking, physical inactivity, and lipid levels that make determining the impact of diabetes alone difficult to assess. Van Melle et al. (2010) analyzed data collected in the 2003 Heart and Soul Study of depression and quality-of-life indicators in patients with heart failure. Regression analyses demonstrated that for patients with diabetes, serum control as measured by the A1C level was an independent risk factor for the development of HF in patients with stable CAD. This finding was also noted by Dungan, Osei, Nagaraja, Schuster, & Binkley (2010), and further studies were suggested to support or refute the findings. When teaching patients, nurses can emphasize the need for stable glucose control (A1C levels) over time as an important means to decrease the risk of HF in patients with diabetes who also have CAD, even if no symptoms are present currently.

Implications
Maintaining glucose control is an important part of a diabetes regimen. People with diabetes have a higher incidence of CAD, which may progress to heart disease, MI, and HF. Recent studies suggest that poor glucose control is linked to the development of HF in people with diabetes. Nurses teaching the patient with diabetes should include a discussion of the risks for heart disease and HF, and emphasize the need to maintain stable glucose levels as measured by the A1C level.

Critical Thinking Questions
A patient is evaluated by a cardiologist for mild chest pain. The patient has type 2 diabetes managed with both oral medication and insulin therapy. What teaching would the nurse need to give this patient?

See Answers to Critical Thinking Questions on student resource website.

PHARMACOTHERAPY ILLUSTRATED 36.1

MECHANISMS OF ACTION OF DRUGS USED FOR HEART FAILURE

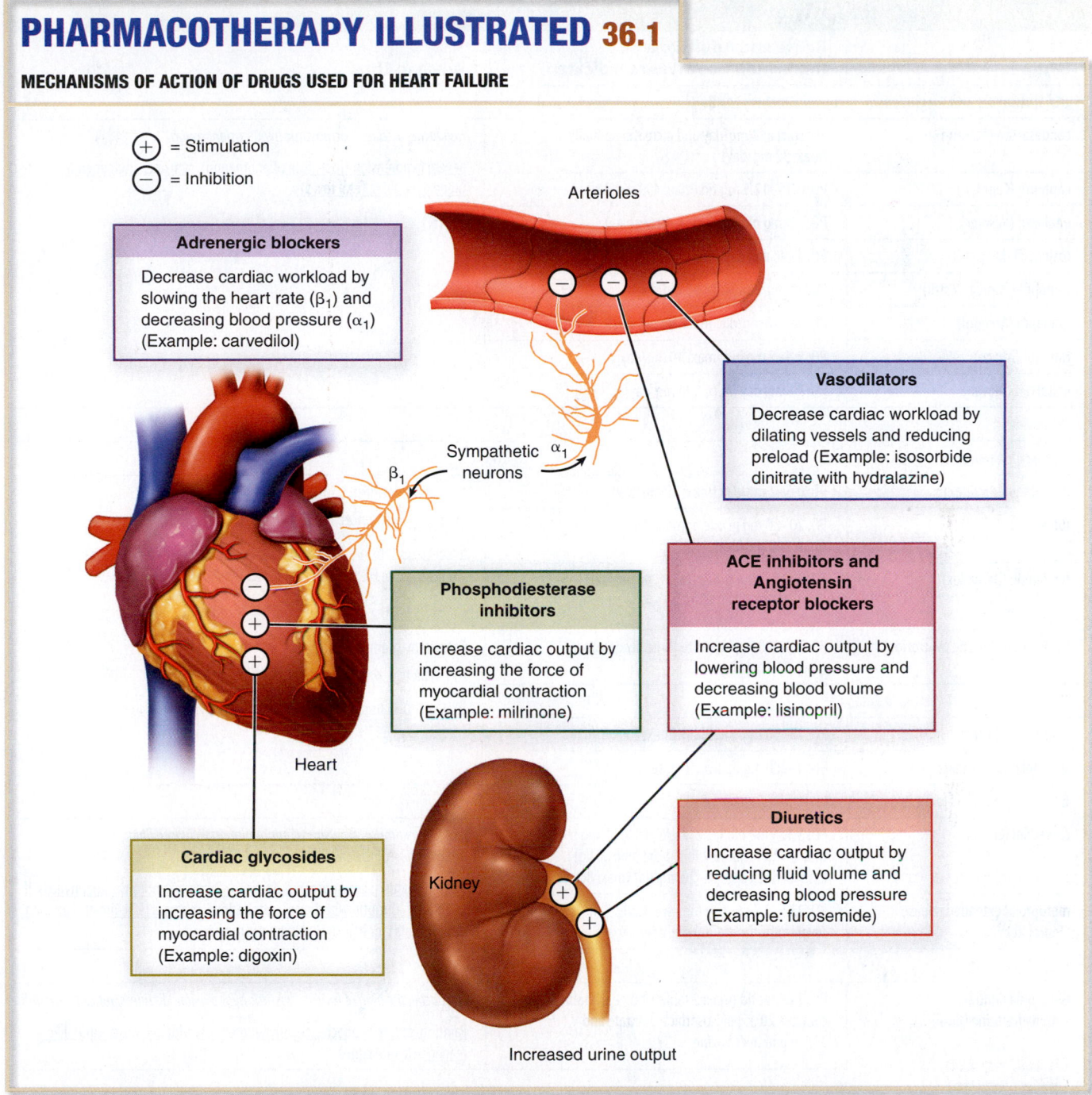

$\oplus$ = Stimulation
$\ominus$ = Inhibition

Adrenergic blockers
Decrease cardiac workload by slowing the heart rate (β_1) and decreasing blood pressure (α_1) (Example: carvedilol)

Arterioles

Vasodilators
Decrease cardiac workload by dilating vessels and reducing preload (Example: isosorbide dinitrate with hydralazine)

Sympathetic neurons α_1
β_1

Phosphodiesterase inhibitors
Increase cardiac output by increasing the force of myocardial contraction (Example: milrinone)

ACE inhibitors and Angiotensin receptor blockers
Increase cardiac output by lowering blood pressure and decreasing blood volume (Example: lisinopril)

Heart

Cardiac glycosides
Increase cardiac output by increasing the force of myocardial contraction (Example: digoxin)

Kidney

Diuretics
Increase cardiac output by reducing fluid volume and decreasing blood pressure (Example: furosemide)

Increased urine output

---

inhibition of the RAAS and vasoconstriction by the sympathetic nervous system also result in a significant reduction in morbidity and mortality from HF. These mechanisms are illustrated in Pharmacotherapy Illustrated 36.1.

36.5 Angiotensin-converting enzyme inhibitors are drugs of choice for heart failure.

Due to their effectiveness and relative safety, the ACE inhibitors have replaced digoxin as first-line drugs for the treatment of chronic HF. Indeed, unless specifically contraindicated, all patients with HF and many patients at high risk of HF should receive an ACE inhibitor. The student should refer to Chapter 31 for details on

the pharmacology of the drugs in this class. The following section focuses on the benefits of these drugs for patients with HF.

Clinical research has clearly demonstrated that ACE inhibitors slow the progression of HF and reduce mortality from this disease. Although this is probably true for all ACE inhibitors, the largest body of research has been conducted using captopril (Capoten) and lisinopril (Prinivil, Zestril). Doses for the ACE inhibitors indicated for HF are listed in Table 36.3.

The two primary actions of the ACE inhibitors are to lower peripheral resistance through the inhibition of angiotensin II formation, and to reduce blood volume through inhibition of aldosterone secretion. The resultant reduction of arterial blood pressure diminishes afterload and increases cardiac output. An additional effect of

TABLE 36.3	Drugs for Early and Moderate Heart Failure	

Drug	Route and Adult Dose (Maximum Dose Where Indicated)	Adverse Effects
ACE Inhibitors and Angiotensin Receptor Blockers (ARBs)		
candesartan (Atacand)	PO: start at 4 mg/day and increase gradually (max: 32 mg/day)	*Headache, dizziness, orthostatic hypotension, cough* Severe hypotension (first-dose phenomenon), syncope, angioedema, blood dyscrasias, fetal toxicity
captopril (Capoten)	PO: 6.25–12.5 mg tid (max: 450 mg/day)	
enalapril (Vasotec)	PO: 2.5 mg qid–bid (max: 40 mg/day)	
fosinopril (Monopril)	PO: 5–40 mg/day (max: 40 mg/day)	
lisinopril (Prinivil, Zestril)	PO: 10 mg/day (max: 80 mg/day)	
quinapril (Accupril)	PO: 10–20 mg/day (max: 40 mg/day)	
ramipril (Altace)	PO: 2.5–5 mg bid (max: 10 mg/day)	
valsartan (Diovan)	PO: 80 mg/day (max: 320 mg/day)	
Diuretics		
Loop or High Ceiling		
bumetanide (Bumex)	PO: 0.5–2 mg/day (max: 10 mg/day)	Loop and thiazides: *Electrolyte imbalances, fatigue, orthostatic hypotension* Severe hypotension, dehydration, serious hypokalemia, hyponatremia, hyperglycemia (thiazides), ototoxicity (loop diuretics)
furosemide (Lasix)	PO: 20–80 mg in one or more divided doses (max: 600 mg/day)	
torsemide (Demadex)	PO/IV: 10–20 mg/day (max: 200 mg/day)	
Thiazide and Thiazide-Like		
hydrochlorothiazide (Microzide)	PO: 25–200 mg in one to three divided doses (max: 200 mg/day)	Potassium-sparing: *Hyperkalemia, gynecomastia in males, fatigue* Dysrhythmias due to hyperkalemia
Potassium-Sparing (Aldosterone Antagonist)		
eplerenone (Inspra)	PO: 25–50 mg once daily (max: 100 mg/day)	
spironolactone (Aldactone)	PO: 5–200 mg in divided doses	
Beta-Adrenergic Blockers		
carvedilol (Coreg)	PO: 3.125 mg bid for 2 weeks (max: 25 mg bid if less than 85 kg or 50 mg bid if more than 85 kg) Extended release: 10–20 mg/day (max: 80 mg/day)	*Fatigue, insomnia, drowsiness, impotence or decreased libido, bradycardia, confusion* Agranulocytosis, laryngospasm, Stevens–Johnson syndrome, anaphylaxis; if the drug is abruptly withdrawn, palpitations, rebound HTN, life-threatening dysrhythmias, or myocardial ischemia may occur
metoprolol extended release (Toprol XL)	PO: 12.5–25 mg/day for 2 weeks; 12.5 mg/day for severe cases (max: 200 mg/day)	
Vasodilator		
isosorbide dinitrate with hydralazine (BiDil)	PO: 1 tablet tid (max: 2 tablets tid); each tablet contains 20 mg of isosorbide dinitrate and 37.5 mg of hydralazine	*Headache, flushing of face, orthostatic hypotension, dizziness, reflex tachycardia* Fainting, severe headache, severe hypotension with overdose, lupus-like reaction (hydralazine)
Cardiac Glycoside		
digoxin (Lanoxin, Lanoxicaps)	PO: 0.125–0.5 mg/day	*Nausea, vomiting, headache, and visual disturbances such as seeing halos, a yellow or green tinge, or blurring* Dysrhythmias, AV block

Note: Italics indicate common adverse effects. Underline indicates serious adverse effects.

the ACE inhibitors is dilation of veins. This action, which is probably not directly related to their inhibition of angiotensin, lowers preload and reduces pulmonary congestion and peripheral edema. The combined reductions in preload, afterload, and blood volume from the ACE inhibitors substantially decrease the workload on the heart and allow it to work more efficiently for patients with cardiac impairment. Patients taking ACE inhibitors experience fewer HF-related symptoms, hospitalizations, and treatment failures. Exercise tolerance is improved.

Research has also demonstrated that several ACE inhibitors are effective in preventing HF following an acute MI. Furthermore, post-MI therapy with ACE inhibitors reduces mortality and decreases reinfarction rates. Although these effects are most prominent when therapy is initiated within 36 hours after the onset of the MI, benefits are also obtained when therapy is begun later and continued for several years.

Therapy with ACE inhibitors is generally begun at low doses, and the amount is gradually increased until the desired therapeutic level is reached. Clinical research has not shown a significant difference in mortality between patients receiving low versus high doses. Because higher doses reduce HF symptoms more effectively, however, patients often receive doses in the higher range, as long as significant adverse effects do not interfere with therapy. Symptomatic relief from HF symptoms occurs within days of initiating therapy, but maximum benefits may take several weeks.

The ACE inhibitors are well tolerated by most patients with HF. Hypotension is the most common adverse effect, and the risk is increased when the patient is receiving other drugs that lower blood pressure such as diuretics and beta blockers. Hypotension is generally worse at the beginning of therapy or when dosage is increased. Multidrug therapy is common in these patients and the nurse serves a key role in teaching patients how to space drug administration times to minimize hypotensive adverse effects.

An additional concern during ACE inhibitor therapy is functional renal insufficiency. Patients with severe HF have high circulating levels of angiotensin II, which helps to maintain renal blood flow by constricting efferent arterioles in the kidney. When ACE inhibitors are administered, the level of angiotensin II declines rapidly, leading to reduced blood flow through the kidneys. During therapy with ACE inhibitors, renal insufficiency may also result from sodium depletion, often secondary to the concurrent use of diuretics. To avoid this potentially serious adverse effect, serum creatinine, serum electrolytes, and blood urea nitrogen (BUN) should be monitored during therapy. Should an assessment discover signs of renal impairment, the dose should be immediately decreased or the drug discontinued.

Other adverse effects of ACE inhibitors are angioedema, cough, and hyperkalemia. The student should refer to Chapter 31 for additional information on the adverse effects of ACE inhibitors and for a drug prototype feature for lisinopril (Prinivil, Zestril).

Another mechanism that blocks the effects of angiotensin II is the use of angiotensin receptor blockers (ARBs). Pharmacologically, the effects of the ARBs are very similar to those of the ACE inhibitors, as would be expected, because drugs from both classes inhibit the actions of angiotensin II. In patients with HF, ARBs show equivalent efficacy to the ACE inhibitors. Clinical research, however, has suggested that combining ARBs with ACE inhibitors does not improve patient survival but does increase the risk of adverse effects. Because they show no clear advantage over other HF medications, the use of ARBs in the treatment of HF is usually reserved for patients who are unable to tolerate the adverse effects of ACE inhibitors. Losartan (Cozaar) is an ARB featured as a prototype drug in Chapter 31.

36.6 Diuretics relieve symptoms of heart failure by reducing fluid overload and decreasing blood pressure.

Diuretics are common medications for the treatment of patients with HF, since they are effective at reducing peripheral edema and pulmonary congestion and produce few adverse effects. By reducing blood volume and lowering blood pressure, the workload on the heart is reduced, and cardiac output increases. Diuretics are rarely used alone for HF but are frequently prescribed in combination with ACE inhibitors, beta blockers, and other HF medications. Doses for selected diuretics are listed in Table 36.3.

Although diuretics are effective at relieving HF symptoms, clinical research has not demonstrated their effectiveness in slowing the progression of HF or in decreasing the mortality rate associated with the disease. Indeed, some of the actions of the diuretics, particularly effects on potassium balance, may increase the risk of adverse effects from other HF drugs. Because of this, diuretics are only indicated when there is evidence of fluid retention. In patients presenting with fluid retention, especially with symptoms of severe pulmonary congestion or peripheral edema, diuretics are essential medications.

Of the diuretic classes, the loop diuretics are most commonly prescribed for HF, due to their effectiveness in removing fluid from the body. Loop diuretics are also able to function in patients with renal impairment, an advantage for many patients with decompensated HF. Another major advantage in treating acute HF is that loop diuretics act quickly, within minutes for IV formulations. For chronic HF, therapy is begun with low doses of furosemide (Lasix), bumetanide (Bumex), or torsemide (Demadex) and gradually increased until the desired volume reduction is obtained.

As therapy continues with loop diuretics, some patients become less responsive, a phenomenon known as **diuretic resistance**. The loop diuretics exhibit a ceiling effect; once the "ceiling dose" is reached, increases in dosage will not produce additional diuresis. To obtain additional diuresis and volume reduction, the loop diuretic may be administered more frequently, or a diuretic from a different class may be added to the regimen.

Thiazide diuretics are also used in the pharmacotherapy of HF, sometimes combined with loop diuretics to achieve a more effective diuresis in patients with acute HF. Because they are less effective than the loop diuretics, thiazides are generally reserved for patients with mild-to-moderate HF.

In addition to being a potassium-sparing diuretic, spironolactone is also classified as an aldosterone antagonist. As a diuretic, spironolactone has a limited role in HF, due to its low efficacy. Clinical research, however, has demonstrated that the drug is able to block the deleterious effects of aldosterone on the heart. High levels of aldosterone promote cardiac remodeling and the deposition of fibrotic tissue in the myocardium of patients with HF. By blocking these cardiac effects, spironolactone decreases mortality due to sudden death as well as progression to advanced HF.

At the low doses used for HF patients (25 mg daily), spironolactone produces few adverse effects. The most common adverse effect at this dose is gynecomastia in male patients. More serious, however, is the risk of hyperkalemia. Caution must be used when administering spironolactone concurrently with ACE inhibitors due to the possibility of additive hyperkalemia. Care must be taken to educate patients to limit potassium-rich foods in the diet and eliminate potassium supplements.

Diuretic use in HF patients should be carefully monitored to avoid dehydration or electrolyte imbalances. These adverse effects are more likely to occur in HF patients who have comorbid renal impairment. During maintenance therapy, patients are urged to weigh themselves frequently and report significant changes to their health care provider. Frequent laboratory tests for blood electrolyte levels are obtained to prevent the development of hypokalemia during loop or thiazide diuretic therapy. This is especially important in patients who are also taking digoxin (Lanoxin), because hypokalemia may induce fatal dysrhythmias. Hydrochlorothiazide, furosemide, and spironolactone are featured as drug prototypes in Chapter 32.

CONNECTION Checkpoint 36.2

Conn's syndrome is characterized by excess secretion of aldosterone. From what you learned in Chapter 31, what effect would you predict this syndrome would have on the heart, and what medication might be a drug of choice? *See Answer to Connection Checkpoint 36.2 on student resource website.*

36.7 Beta-adrenergic antagonists can dramatically reduce hospitalizations and increase the survival of patients with heart failure.

Cardiac glycosides, beta-adrenergic agonists, and other medications that produce a positive inotropic effect serve important roles in reversing the diminished contractility that is the hallmark of HF. It may seem somewhat surprising, then, to find beta-adrenergic blockers—drugs that exhibit a *negative* inotropic effect—prescribed for this disease. Even though this class of drugs has the potential to worsen HF, beta-adrenergic blockers are standard therapy for many patients with this chronic disorder. Why is this the case?

In patients with HF, high levels of endogenous norepinephrine and other catecholamines cause excessive activation of the sympathetic nervous system and are associated with cardiac remodeling and progression of the disease. Beta-adrenergic antagonists block the actions of these catecholamines, slowing the heart rate and reducing blood pressure, thus decreasing the cardiac workload. After several months of therapy, heart size, shape, and function return to normal in some patients, in essence producing a **reverse remodeling** of the heart. Extensive clinical research has demonstrated that the careful use of beta-adrenergic antagonists can dramatically reduce the number of HF-associated hospitalizations and deaths. They are effective in all stages of symptomatic HF. Doses for selected beta-adrenergic antagonists are listed in Table 36.3.

To benefit patients with HF, however, beta-adrenergic antagonists must be administered in a very specific manner. Initial doses must be 1/10 to 1/20 of the target dose. Doses are doubled every 2 weeks until the target dose is reached. If therapy is begun with the target dose, or the dose is increased too rapidly, beta blockers can worsen HF. Carvedilol and metoprolol are the two beta-adrenergic antagonists approved for HF, although bisoprolol has also been shown to be effective. When treating HF, beta blockers are almost always combined with other agents, especially the ACE inhibitors.

Adherence to beta-blocker therapy can be a major clinical challenge for some patients. The patient may not report symptomatic improvement with the drug and, in fact, may feel worse at the initiation of therapy. To achieve maximum patient adherence, the nurse must teach the patient the important long-term benefits of beta blockers.

Beta-adrenergic antagonists are contraindicated in patients with chronic obstructive pulmonary disease (COPD), severe bradycardia, or heart block. These medications should be used with caution in patients with diabetes, peripheral vascular disease, and hepatic impairment. Caution is needed with older adults because these patients often require a reduced dose. Hepatic function tests should be performed periodically and the prescriber notified if signs or symptoms of liver toxicity become apparent.

The basic pharmacology of the beta-adrenergic antagonists is presented in Chapter 16, where metoprolol is featured as a prototype for this class. Other applications of the beta-adrenergic blockers are discussed elsewhere in this text: HTN is discussed in Chapter 34, angina and MI in Chapter 35, and dysrhythmias in Chapter 37.

36.8 Vasodilators reduce symptoms of heart failure by reducing preload or afterload.

Vasodilators relax blood vessels and lower blood pressure, creating less workload on the heart. They serve a limited role in the pharmacotherapy of HF.

Hydralazine with isosorbide dinitrate (BiDil): Hydralazine combined with isosorbide dinitrate (BiDil) is approved as an adjunct to standard therapy for HF. The combination appears to be particularly effective in treating African Americans, who are sometimes resistant to therapy for HTN and HF.

Hydralazine acts on arterioles to decrease peripheral resistance, reduce afterload, and increase cardiac output. It is an effective antihypertensive drug, although it is not a drug of first choice for this indication because hypotension and reflex tachycardia are common and may limit therapy. The drug must be taken three to four times daily, which places an extensive pill burden on patients with HF, who often are taking multiple drugs. Hydralazine is presented as a prototype vasodilator for HTN in Chapter 34.

Isosorbide dinitrate (Isordil) is a long-acting organic nitrate that reduces preload by directly dilating veins. The drug is not very effective as monotherapy, and tolerance develops to its actions with continued use. Isosorbide dinitrate is usually combined with hydralazine (BiDil) because the two drugs act synergistically when used in patients with HF. The high incidence of adverse effects in some patients such as reflex tachycardia and orthostatic hypotension limits their use. The use of isosorbide dinitrate in the pharmacotherapy of angina pectoris is presented in Chapter 35.

Nesiritide (Natrecor): A third vasodilator used for HF is very different from hydralazine or isosorbide dinitrate. Approved in 2001, nesiritide (Natrecor) is a small-peptide hormone, produced through recombinant DNA technology, that is structurally identical to human beta-type natriuretic peptide (hBNP). When heart failure occurs, the ventricles begin to secrete hBNP in response to the increased stretch on the ventricular walls. hBNP enhances diuresis and renal excretion of sodium.

In therapeutic doses, nesiritide causes vasodilation, which reduces preload. By lowering preload and afterload, the drug compensates for diminished cardiac function. The use of nesiritide is limited because it can rapidly cause severe hypotension, which can persist several hours after the infusion is discontinued. The drug is given by IV infusion, and patients require continuous monitoring. It is approved only for patients with acutely decompensated heart failure. The dosage for nesiritide is shown in Table 36.4. Nesiritide is pregnancy category C.

TABLE 36.4 Drugs for Advanced Heart Failure

Drug	Route and Adult Dose (Maximum Dose Where Indicated)	Adverse Effects
Beta-Adrenergic Agonists		
dobutamine (Dobutrex)	IV: Infused at a rate of 2.5–40 mcg/kg/min for a max of 72 h	*Headache, palpitations, nausea, vomiting, changes in blood pressure (hypo- or hypertension)* <u>Dysrhythmias, gangrene, severe HTN</u>
dopamine (Dopastat, Intropin)	IV: 2–5 mcg/kg/min initial dose; may be increased to 20–50 mcg/kg/min (max: 50 mcg/kg/min)	
epinephrine (Adrenalin)	Subcutaneous: 0.1–0.5 mL of 1:1,000 every 10–15 min prn IV: 0.1–0.25 mL of 1:1,000 every 10–15 min	
isoproterenol (Isuprel)	IV infusion: 0.5–5 mcg/min	
norepinephrine (Levophed)	IV: Initially, 0.5–1 mcg/min until pressure stabilizes, then 2–4 mcg/min for maintenance (max: 30 mcg/min)	
Phosphodiesterase Inhibitors		
inamrinone (Inocor)	IV: 0.75 mg/kg bolus given slowly over 2–3 min; then 5–10 mcg/kg/min (max: 10 mg/kg/day)	*Headache, hypotension* <u>Dysrhythmias</u>
milrinone (Primacor)	IV: 50 mcg/kg over 10 min; then 0.375–0.75 mcg/kg/min	
Vasodilator		
nesiritide (Natrecor)	IV: 2 mcg/kg bolus followed by continuous infusion at 0.1 mcg/kg/min	*Hypotension, increased serum creatinine* <u>Dysrhythmias</u>

Note: Italics indicate common adverse effects. <u>Underline</u> indicates serious adverse effects.

CONNECTION Checkpoint 36.3

Isosorbide dinitrate is also used for angina. From what you learned in Chapter 35, why is nitroglycerin a preferred drug for acute angina, rather than isosorbide dinitrate? *See Answer to Connection Checkpoint 36.3 on student resource website.*

36.9 Cardiac glycosides increase the force of myocardial contraction and were once drugs of choice for heart failure.

Once used as arrow poisons by African tribes and as medicines by the ancient Egyptians and Romans, the value of the cardiac glycosides in treating heart disorders has been known for over 2,000 years. Originally extracted from the beautiful flowering plants, *Digitalis purpura* (purple foxglove) and *Digitalis lanata* (white foxglove), the cardiac glycosides were the mainstay of HF treatment until the discovery of the ACE inhibitors. During the past 20 years, the role of the cardiac glycosides in the pharmacotherapy of HF has become more limited. The two primary cardiac glycosides, digoxin and digitoxin, are quite similar in efficacy; the primary difference is that the latter has a more prolonged half-life. Digitoxin is no longer available in the United States. The dose for digoxin is listed in Table 36.3.

Because of its long historical use, the effectiveness of digitalis in the pharmacotherapy of HF remained unquestioned until the late 1980s, when a controlled study of 6,800 patients with HF revealed no significant difference in mortality between patients who took digoxin and those who received a placebo. The drug did, however, produce symptomatic benefit in patients. Based on this study, and the development of safer and more effective drug classes, cardiac glycosides are now limited to late-stage HF, in combination with other agents. Digoxin remains an important therapy in HF patients with supraventricular tachyarrhythmias, because the drug has antidysrhythmic activity that can stabilize these types of cardiac conduction abnormalities.

The margin of safety between a therapeutic dose and a toxic dose of cardiac glycosides is very narrow, and severe adverse effects may result from poorly managed therapy. **Digitalization** refers to the procedure by which the dose of digoxin is gradually increased until tissues become saturated with the medication, and the symptoms of HF diminish. If the patient is critically ill, digitalization can be done rapidly with IV doses in a controlled clinical environment, where adverse effects may be carefully monitored. As an outpatient, digitalization may be completed over a period of 7 days, using oral (PO) dosing. In either case, the goal is to determine the proper dose of medication to be administered, without undue adverse effects.

PROTOTYPE DRUG	Digoxin (Lanoxin, Lanoxicaps)

Classification: Therapeutic: Drug for heart failure
Pharmacologic: Cardiac glycoside, inotropic agent

Therapeutic Effects and Uses: The primary benefit of digoxin is its ability to increase the strength of myocardial contraction, a positive inotropic action. By increasing myocardial contractility, digoxin directly increases cardiac output, which alleviates symptoms of HF and improves exercise tolerance. The higher cardiac output increases urine production and results in a desirable reduction in blood volume, relieving the distressing symptoms of pulmonary congestion and peripheral edema. In current clinical practice, digoxin use is usually limited to patients who are not responding adequately to ACE inhibitor therapy or to HF patients with atrial fibrillation.

In addition to its positive inotropic effect, digoxin also affects the speed of myocardial conduction. Through a mechanism not fully understood, digoxin decreases SNS activity and increases parasympathetic activity. This helps attenuate the excessive sympathetic activation that causes tachycardia and worsens HF (see Section 36.2). Digoxin has the ability to suppress the sinoatrial node and slow electrical conduction through the atrioventricular node. The heart rate decreases, allowing greater diastolic filling of the ventricles. Because the heart rate may decline too much, health care providers establish parameters for each patient. As a general rule, if the apical pulse falls below 60 beats per minute, the medication is withheld and the health care provider notified. Digoxin is sometimes used to treat dysrhythmias, as discussed in Chapter 37.

Digoxin is available by the PO or IV route. The capsule formulation (Lanoxicaps) has a more predictable bioavailability than the tablet form, but it is more expensive. Because differences in bioavailability of digoxin formulations can potentially affect drug action and the potential for adverse effects, it is advisable to continue with the same brand name, unless otherwise changed by the prescriber.

Mechanism of Action: Digoxin inhibits Na^+-K^+-ATPase, the critical enzyme responsible for pumping sodium ions out of the myocardial cells in exchange for potassium ions. As sodium ions accumulate in myocytes, calcium ions are released from their storage areas in the cell to activate contractile elements. The release of calcium ions produces a more forceful contraction of myocardial fibers.

Pharmacokinetics:

Route(s)	PO, IV
Absorption	70–90% absorbed from the gastrointestinal (GI) tract
Distribution	Widely distributed; crosses the placenta; secreted in breast milk; 20–25% bound to protein
Primary metabolism	Hepatic, 14%
Primary excretion	Renal
Onset of action	PO: 30–90 min; IV: 5–30 min
Duration of action	Half-life: 3–4 days

Adverse Effects: Adverse effects of digoxin involve multiple body systems and can be severe. The most dangerous adverse effect is its ability to cause ventricular dysrhythmias, which may result in sudden cardiac death. The most common cause of digoxin-induced dysrhythmias is hypokalemia due to diuretic use. Other factors placing patients at risk for digoxin-induced dysrhythmias include hypomagnesemia, hypercalcemia, and impaired renal function. Additional serious adverse cardiac effects include atrioventricular (AV) block, atrial dysrhythmias, and sinus bradycardia. Frequent electrocardiograms (ECGs) should be obtained to assess for cardiotoxicity.

Noncardiac adverse effects include general malaise, dizziness, headache, anorexia, nausea, and vomiting. The drug may produce unusual visual effects such as halos, changes in color perception, and photophobia.

Frequent serum digoxin levels should be obtained during therapy, and the dosage adjusted based on the laboratory results and the patient's clinical response. Clinical research suggests that digoxin levels from 0.5 to 2 ng/mL give the most therapeutic benefit, with an acceptable risk of adverse effects for most patients. Raising the dose does not increase the therapeutic effect, but it does increase the risk of serious digoxin toxicity. For each patient, the health care provider should establish acceptable parameters for serum digoxin levels, and the drug

should be discontinued should the level rise above the maximum. Digoxin levels greater than 2.0 ng/mL are considered toxic. However, the nurse should remember that toxicity should be based on patient symptoms rather than serum level. Levels should be taken 6 to 12 hours after a dose, because digoxin has a prolonged distribution time.

Contraindications/Precautions: Patients with AV block or ventricular dysrhythmias unrelated to HF should not receive digoxin, because the drug may worsen these conditions. Digoxin should be administered with caution to older adults because these patients experience a higher incidence of adverse effects. Patients with renal impairment should receive lower doses of digoxin, because the drug is excreted by this route. The drug should be used with caution in patients with MI, cor pulmonale, or hypothyroidism.

Drug Interactions: Digoxin interacts with many drugs. Concurrent use of digoxin with diuretics must be carefully monitored, since diuretics can cause hypokalemia and increase the risk of dysrhythmias. Use with ACE inhibitors, spironolactone, or potassium supplements can lead to hyperkalemia and reduce the therapeutic action of digoxin. Administration of digoxin with other positive inotropic agents can cause additive effects on myocardial contractility. Concurrent use with beta blockers may result in additive bradycardia. Antacids and cholesterol-lowering drugs can decrease the absorption of digoxin. If calcium is administered intravenously together with digoxin, it can increase the risk of dysrhythmias. Quinidine, verapamil, amiodarone, and alprazolam will decrease the distribution and excretion of digoxin, thus increasing the risk of digoxin toxicity. **Herbal/Food**: The drug should be used with caution with ginseng, which may increase the risk of digoxin toxicity.

Pregnancy: Category C.

Treatment of Overdose: Digoxin overdose can be fatal and the nurse should be prepared to administer digoxin immune Fab (Digibind). Digoxin immune Fab consists of digoxin-specific antibodies, which form a complex with digoxin that prevents the drug from reaching the tissues, and is removed through renal excretion. Reversal of adverse effects occurs quickly: 90% of patients respond within an hour after IV administration. As digoxin is removed from the body, the inotropic effects of the drug will diminish, and the patient may be at risk of HF. The patient must be monitored continuously during the infusion.

Nursing Responsibilities: Key nursing implications for patients receiving digoxin are included in the Nursing Practice Application for Patients Receiving Pharmacotherapy for Heart Failure.

Drugs Similar to Digoxin (Lanoxin, Lanoxicaps)

Digoxin is the only cardiac glycoside available in the United States.

CONNECTION Checkpoint 36.4

Cholestyramine reduces the bioavailability of digoxin, thus potentially decreasing the actions of the cardiac glycoside. From what you learned in Chapter 29, what is the primary indication for cholestyramine and what is the likely reason this drug causes a decrease in digoxin bioavailability? *See Answer to Connection Checkpoint 36.4 on student resource website.*

CONNECTIONS | Complementary and Alternative Therapies

◀ Carnitine (L-Carnitine)

Description

Carnitine is a natural substance that is structurally similar to amino acids. Its primary function in metabolism is to move fatty acids from the bloodstream into cells, where it assists in the breakdown of lipids in the mitochondria. This breakdown produces energy and increases the availability of oxygen, particularly in muscle cells. A congenital deficiency of carnitine leads to severe brain, liver, and heart damage. The best food sources of carnitine are organ meats, fish, muscle meats, and milk products.

History and Claims

Carnitine has been claimed to enhance energy and sports performance, heart health, memory, immune function, and male fertility. It is also being marketed as a "fat burner" for weight reduction.

Standardization

Carnitine is available as a supplement in several forms, including L-carnitine, D-carnitine, and L-acetylcarnitine. D-carnitine is associated with potential adverse effects and should be avoided. Doses range from 2 to 6 g/day.

Evidence

Carnitine has been well studied but large, controlled research trials are still needed to explore the effects for certain conditions. There is solid evidence to support supplementation in patients who are deficient in carnitine (Flanagan, Simmons, Vehige, Wilcox, & Garrett, 2010). Although a normal diet supplies 300 mg per day, certain patients may need additional amounts. Vegans are at risk for carnitine depletion, since plant protein supplies little or no carnitine.

Carnitine supplementation has been shown to improve exercise tolerance in patients with angina. The use of carnitine may prevent the occurrence of dysrhythmias in the early stages of heart disease. Carnitine has also been shown to decrease triglyceride levels while increasing HDL serum levels, thus helping to minimize one of the major risk factors associated with heart disease.

Research has not shown carnitine supplementation to be of significant benefit in enhancing sports performance, improving brain function in patients with Alzheimer's disease, or weight loss (University of Maryland Medical Center, 2011).

36.10 Phosphodiesterase III inhibitors and other positive inotropic agents are used for acute decompensated heart failure.

Advanced or decompensated HF can be a medical emergency, and prompt, effective treatment is necessary to avoid organ failure or death. In addition to high doses of loop diuretics, positive inotropic drugs are often necessary. The two primary classes of inotropic agents used for decompensated HF are beta-adrenergic agonists and phosphodiesterase inhibitors. Doses for these agents are listed in Table 36.4.

Beta-Adrenergic Agonists (Sympathomimetics): Beta-adrenergic agonists used for HF include isoproterenol (Isuprel), epinephrine, norepinephrine, dopamine (Dopastat, Intropin), and dobutamine (Dobutrex). Dobutamine has been a traditional drug of choice in this class because it has the ability to rapidly increase myocardial contractility, with minimal changes to heart rate or blood pressure. This is important because increases in heart rate or blood pressure will create greater oxygen demands on the heart and possibly worsen HF. Therapy with dobutamine is usually limited to 72 hours, as continuous infusion of the drug causes the heart to become tolerant to beta-adrenergic activation, making the drug less effective. The two most common adverse effects with beta agonists are tachycardia and dysrhythmias.

Patients who have both HF and hypotension benefit from dopamine, which not only increases myocardial contractility but also activates alpha-adrenergic receptors to increase blood pressure. However, tachycardia is more prominent with dopamine than with dobutamine. Patients who have been receiving a beta-adrenergic antagonist for their HF may require a higher initial dose of beta agonist. The basic pharmacology of the beta-adrenergic agonists was presented in Chapter 15, where epinephrine and isoproterenol were featured as prototypes for this drug class.

Phosphodiesterase III Inhibitors: In the 1980s, two medications became available that block the enzyme **phosphodiesterase III** in cardiac and smooth muscle, which leads to increases in the amount of calcium available for myocardial contraction. The enzyme inhibition results in two main actions that benefit patients with HF: a positive inotropic action and vasodilation. Cardiac output is increased due to the increase in contractility and the decrease in left ventricular afterload. There is little effect on heart rate. Arterial pressure is either decreased or, in some patients, it remains unchanged.

Although the actions of the phosphodiesterase III inhibitors are very similar to dobutamine, they have a much longer half-life. This makes it more difficult to make rapid changes in dose when controlling acute HF. In addition, if adverse effects do occur, they are more prolonged than with dobutamine.

Phosphodiesterase inhibitors have serious toxicity that limits their use to patients with resistant HF who have not responded to ACE inhibitors, digoxin, or other therapies. Therapy is limited to 2 to 3 days and the patient is continuously monitored for ventricular dysrhythmias, including ectopic beats, supraventricular dysrhythmias, premature ventricular contractions, ventricular tachycardia, and ventricular fibrillation. If the patient presents with hypokalemia, this should be corrected before administering phosphodiesterase III inhibitors because this can increase the likelihood of dysrhythmias. These medications can cause hypotension. When using inamrinone, frequent laboratory blood tests should be conducted to assess for thrombocytopenia.

PROTOTYPE DRUG | Milrinone (Primacor)

Classification: Therapeutic: Drug for heart failure
Pharmacologic: Phosphodiesterase inhibitor; inotropic agent

Therapeutic Effects and Uses: Approved in 1987, milrinone is indicated for the short-term treatment of patients with acute decompensated heart failure. Although inamrinone was the first drug in this class to be marketed, milrinone is generally preferred because it has a shorter half-life and fewer adverse effects. It is only given intravenously, and peak effects occur in 2 minutes. Immediate effects of milrinone include an increased force of contraction (positive inotropic effect) and a resulting increase in cardiac output. Research has not yet demonstrated any decrease in mortality or morbidity with the use of milrinone infusions. In patients with Class II or IV HF, drug therapy with milrinone is generally limited to 48 hours.

Mechanism of Action: Milrinone inhibits phosphodiesterase III, the enzyme responsible for the breakdown of cAMP to AMP, in cardiac and vascular smooth muscle. The rise in cAMP levels increases intracellular calcium, resulting in greater contractility. Cardiac output is increased and pulmonary capillary wedge pressure is decreased.

Pharmacokinetics:

Route(s)	IV
Absorption	N/A
Distribution	Unknown; 70% bound to plasma protein
Primary metabolism	83% is excreted unchanged; small amounts metabolized by liver
Primary excretion	Renal
Onset of action	2–10 min
Duration of action	Half-life: 3–6 h

Adverse Effects: The most serious adverse effect of milrinone is ventricular dysrhythmia, which can occur in more than 10% of patients taking the drug. The ECG is monitored continuously during infusion of the drug to prevent serious dysrhythmias. Blood pressure is also continuously monitored during the infusion to prevent hypotension. Patients with Class IV HF are at high risk for life-threatening cardiovascular reactions. Less serious adverse effects include headache, nausea, and vomiting.

Contraindications/Precautions: Milrinone is contraindicated in patients with severe obstructive valvular heart disease. The drug should be used with caution in patients with preexisting dysrhythmias. Hypovolemia or electrolyte imbalances should be corrected before starting the infusion, and the dose should be reduced in patients with renal impairment.

Drug Interactions: Caution should be used when administering milrinone with digoxin, dobutamine, or other inotropic drugs, since their cardiac effects may be additive. Use with antihypertensive agents may cause additive hypotension. **Food/Herbal**: Ginger may contribute to the cardiac actions of milrinone.

Pregnancy: Category C.

Treatment of Overdose: Overdose of milrinone causes hypotension, which may be treated with the administration of normal saline or a vasopressor.

Nursing Responsibilities: Key nursing implications for patients receiving milrinone are included in the Nursing Practice Application for Patients Receiving Pharmacotherapy for Heart Failure.

Drugs Similar to Milrinone (Primacor)

The only other drug in the phosphodiesterase inhibitor class is inamrinone.

Inamrinone (Inocor):   Approved in 1984, inamrinone has similar indications and inotropic actions as milrinone. Its only approved use is for the short-term therapy of serious or decompensated HF. Like milrinone, it is administered by IV infusion with continuous monitoring to detect the possibility of dysrhythmias and to avoid hypotension. One difference is that inamrinone causes a higher incidence of thrombocytopenia. The nurse should assess for signs and symptoms of bleeding during therapy. Because the liver metabolizes inamrinone, caution must be used when treating patients with hepatic impairment. Prior to 2000, inamrinone was called amrinone. The name was changed to avoid medication errors. The name amrinone looked and sounded too similar to amiodarone, an antidysrhythmic drug. This drug is pregnancy category C.

CONNECTIONS: NURSING PRACTICE APPLICATION

Patients Receiving Pharmacotherapy for Heart Failure

Assessment	Potential Nursing Diagnoses*
Baseline assessment prior to administration: • Obtain a complete health history: cardiovascular (including previous MI, HF, valvular disease, dysrhythmias [especially heart block]), renal dysfunction, pregnancy, or lactation. Obtain a drug history including allergies, current prescription and over-the-counter (OTC) drugs, herbal preparations, and alcohol use. Be alert to possible drug interactions. • Obtain baseline weight, vital signs (especially pulse and blood pressure), breath sounds, and ECG. Assess for location and character of edema if present. • Evaluate appropriate laboratory findings, electrolytes, especially potassium level, renal function studies, and lipid profiles. • Assess the patient's ability to receive and understand instructions. Include family and caregivers as needed.	• *Decreased Cardiac Output* • *Fatigue* • *Activity Intolerance* • *Excess Fluid Volume* • *Deficient Knowledge* (Drug Therapy) • *Risk for Reduced Cardiac Tissue Perfusion* • *Risk for Falls*, related to adverse drug effects • *Risk for Injury*, related to adverse drug effects
Assessment throughout administration: • Assess for desired therapeutic effects (e.g., heart rate and blood pressure return to, or remain within, normal limits; urine output returns to, or is within, normal limits; respiratory congestion [if present] is improved; peripheral edema [if present] is improved; level of consciousness, skin color, capillary refill, and other signs of adequate perfusion are within normal limits; fatigue lessens). • Continue periodic monitoring of electrolytes, especially potassium, renal function, and drug levels. • Assess for adverse effects: hypotension, fatigue, dizziness, or drowsiness. Bradycardia, nausea, vomiting, anorexia, visual changes (e.g., halos around lights, yellow or yellowish-green tint to colors) may also occur with digoxin. A pulse rate below 60 or above 100 beats/min, palpitations, significant dizziness or syncope, dyspnea, persistent anorexia or vomiting, or visual changes should be reported to the provider immediately. • **Lifespan:** Exercise extra caution when giving the drug to older adults, pediatric patients, or patients with renal insufficiency. Immature renal function or declines in renal function make these populations more susceptible to adverse effects.	

Implementation

Interventions and (Rationales)	Patient-Centered Care
Ensuring therapeutic effects: • Continue frequent assessments as above for therapeutic effects. (As the heart contracts more forcefully, blood pressure and pulse should return to within normal limits or within the parameters set by the health care provider; urine output returns to within normal limits, peripheral edema decreases, and lung sounds clear.)	• Teach the patient, family, or caregiver how to monitor the pulse and blood pressure. Ensure proper use and functioning of any home equipment obtained.
Encourage appropriate lifestyle changes: lowered fat intake, restricted sodium or fluid intake if ordered, gradually increased levels of exercise, limited alcohol intake, and smoking cessation. Provide for dietitian consultation as needed. (Healthy lifestyle changes will support the benefits of drug therapy.)	• Encourage the patient, family, or caregiver to adopt a healthy lifestyle of low-fat food choices, increased exercise, decreased alcohol consumption, and smoking cessation. Provide educational materials on low-fat, low-sodium food choices.
Minimizing adverse effects: • Continue to monitor vital signs. Take an apical pulse for 1 full minute before giving the drug. Hold the drug and notify the health care provider if heart rate is below 60 or above 100 beats/min and contact the provider. Monitor ECG during infusion of milrinone (Primacor) and during the digitalization period for dysrhythmias or bradycardia. (Drugs that are positive inotropes increase myocardial contractility but may affect cardiac conduction. Milrinone is associated with serious and potentially life-threatening dysrhythmias. Digoxin slows the heart rate and may cause bradycardia.)	• Teach the patient, family, or caregiver how to take a peripheral pulse for 1 full minute before taking the drug. Assist the patient to find the most convenient and easily felt pulse area. Record daily pulse rates and bring the record to each health care visit. Instruct the patient to not take the drug if pulse is below 60 or above 100 beats/min, and to contact the provider for further direction. If the patient, family, or caregiver chooses to buy a stethoscope to take pulse, ensure proper understanding of heart sounds (i.e., lub-dub of heartbeat is *ONE* heartbeat) and appropriate stethoscope placement. Have the patient, family, or caregiver return demonstrate. (With easier accessibility to OTC medical equipment such as stethoscopes, patients, family, or caregivers may try to emulate the health care provider. Ensure proper use before the patient goes home.) • Instruct patients receiving milrinone by infusion to immediately report any chest pain.
• Continue to monitor electrolyte levels periodically, especially potassium, renal function laboratory values, drug levels, and ECG. (Hypokalemia increases the risk of dysrhythmias from drugs used to treat HF.)	• Instruct the patient on the need to return periodically for laboratory work. • Advise the patient to carry a wallet identification card or wear medical identification jewelry indicating drug therapy for HF.

(continued)

• Weigh the patient daily and report a weight gain or loss of 1 kg (2 lb) or more in a 24-h period. (Daily weight is an accurate measure of fluid status and takes into account intake, output, and insensible losses. Weight gain or edema may signal impending HF with reduced organ perfusion, stimulating renin release.)	• Have the patient weigh self daily, ideally at the same time of day, and record weight along with pulse measurements. Instruct the patient to report a weight loss or gain of more than 1 kg (2 lb) in a 24-h period.
• Monitor for signs of worsening HF (e.g., increasing dyspnea or postural nocturnal dyspnea, rales or crackles in lungs, frothy pink-tinged sputum) and report immediately. (Positive inotropic drugs such as digoxin or phosphodiesterase inhibitors are usually reserved for patients with more advanced stages of HF. If signs and symptoms worsen, other treatment options may need to be considered.)	• Instruct the patient to immediately report any severe shortness of breath, frothy sputum, profound fatigue, or swelling of extremities as possible signs of HF.
• For patients taking digoxin, report signs of possible toxicity immediately to the provider and obtain a drug level. Digoxin levels should remain less than 1.8 mg/mL. Signs and symptoms such as bradycardia, nausea and vomiting, anorexia, visual changes, depression, changes in level of consciousness, fatigue, dizziness, or syncope should be reported. **Lifespan:** Digoxin is on the Beers List of potentially inappropriate drugs for the older adult and warrants careful monitoring. (Decreased excretion of digoxin and phosphodiesterase inhibitors due to age-related changes may increase the risk of adverse effects.)	• Instruct the patient, family, or caregiver on signs to report to the health care provider. Encourage the patient to report any significant change in overall health or mental activity promptly.
• **Lifespan:** Use extra caution when measuring the precise dose of medication ordered, and use extreme caution when measuring liquid doses, especially for pediatric patients. (For drugs such as digoxin with a long half-life and duration, toxic levels may result with only small amounts of additional drug.)	• Caution the patient on taking the precise dose of medication ordered, not doubling the dose if a dose is missed, and to use extreme caution when measuring liquid doses, especially for pediatric patients.
• **Lifespan**: Assess for the possibility of pregnancy before beginning the drug. (Many drugs for HF are pregnancy category C drugs and should be used with caution during pregnancy or breast-feeding.)	• Instruct female patients who may be considering pregnancy, or are pregnant or breast-feeding, to notify their provider before starting the drug.
Patient understanding of drug therapy: • Use opportunities during administration of medications and during assessments to discuss the rationale for the drug therapy, desired therapeutic outcomes, commonly observed adverse effects, parameters for when to call the health care provider, and any necessary monitoring or precautions. (Using time during nursing care helps to optimize and reinforce key teaching areas.)	• The patient, family, or caregiver should be able to state the reason for the drug, appropriate dose and scheduling, what adverse effects to observe for and when to report them, and the anticipated length of medication therapy.
Patient self-administration of drug therapy: • When administering medications, instruct the patient, family, or caregiver in the proper self-administration techniques. (Utilizing time during nurse-administration of these drugs helps to reinforce teaching.)	• The patient, family, or caregiver is able to discuss appropriate dosing and administration needs. • The drug should be taken at the same time each day, and doses should not be skipped or doubled. • The brand of the drug prescribed should not be switched without consultation with the provider to ensure consistent effects.

*Nursing Diagnoses—Definitions and Classification 2015–2017. Copyright © 2014, 1994–2014 by NANDA International. Used by arrangement with John Wiley & Sons Limited.

CHAPTER

36

Understanding the Chapter

Key Concepts Summary

36.1 Heart failure is closely associated with disorders such as chronic hypertension, coronary artery disease, and diabetes.

36.2 The body attempts to compensate for heart failure by increasing cardiac output.

36.3 Symptoms of heart failure occur when compensatory mechanisms fail to maintain adequate cardiac output.

36.4 The specific therapy for heart failure depends on the clinical stage of the disease.

36.5 Angiotensin-converting enzyme inhibitors are drugs of choice for heart failure.

36.6 Diuretics relieve symptoms of heart failure by reducing fluid overload and decreasing blood pressure.

36.7 Beta-adrenergic antagonists can dramatically reduce hospitalizations and increase the survival of patients with heart failure.

36.8 Vasodilators reduce symptoms of heart failure by reducing preload or afterload.

36.9 Cardiac glycosides increase the force of myocardial contraction and were once drugs of choice for heart failure.

36.10 Phosphodiesterase III inhibitors and other positive inotropic agents are used for acute decompensated heart failure.

Case Study: Making the Patient Connection

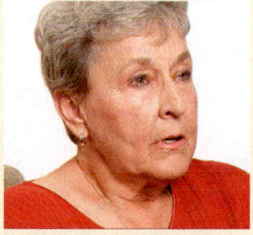

Remember the patient "Thelma Walters" at the beginning of the chapter? Now read the remainder of the case study. Based on the information presented within this chapter, respond to the critical thinking questions that follow.

Thelma Walters is a 77-year-old woman who arrives via EMS at the emergency department after experiencing increasing dyspnea for the past 2 days. She has also noticed swelling in her feet and ankles. Due to her onset of shortness of breath, she has had to sleep in a recliner and is unable to lie flat in bed at night. Her past medical history includes a myocardial infarction 3 years ago and an episode of heart failure 1 year ago. The heart failure was treated with captopril (Capoten) and furosemide (Lasix), which she has been taking since that time. Her surgical history includes a hysterectomy 20 years ago. She has never used tobacco or alcohol.

As the nurse performs the initial physical assessment the following relevant findings are discovered. The patient is 1.7 m (5'6") tall and weighs 82 kg (180 lb). The patient's blood pressure is 162/92 mmHg, her heart rate is 148 beats/min and irregular, and her respiratory rate is 38 breaths/min and labored. The neck veins of the patient are distended when she is placed at a 45-degree incline. She is orthopneic and cannot tolerate the head of the bed being lowered below 45 degrees. The nurse notes scattered crackles bilaterally throughout the lung fields. The patient has a productive cough with frothy,

pink-tinged sputum. 4+ pitting edema of both hands and legs is noted with the nail beds moderately cyanotic. Circumoral cyanosis is also noted.

Immediately upon arrival at the emergency department, the patient received oxygen therapy and an IV line was started. Blood is collected for initial laboratory data with the following results: serum sodium 136 mEq/L (normal 135–147 mEq/L), serum potassium 3.1 mEq/L (normal 3.5–5.2 mEq/L), and arterial blood gases on room air: pH 7.32, PaO_2 54, $PaCO_2$ 48, SpO_2 68%, indicating overall hypoxemia. Thelma is in acute distress and admitted to the intensive care unit (ICU) with a diagnosis of heart failure. She is given a dose of furosemide (Lasix) 20 mg intravenously and she will receive milrinone (Primacor) by IV infusion after admission to the ICU.

Critical Thinking Questions

1. Describe how milrinone (Primacor) aids in treating heart failure.

2. During the infusion of milrinone (Primacor), Thelma's ECG and blood pressure will be monitored closely. What adverse effects does milrinone have on the heart rhythm and blood pressure?

3. Because Thelma has been taking furosemide (Lasix) at home and has received another dose in the emergency department, what will the nurse assess prior to starting the milrinone (Primacor)? What electrolyte imbalance must be corrected before Thelma receives the milrinone (Primacor)?

See Answers to Critical Thinking Questions on student resource website.

Additional Case Study

Jim Mabry, a 77-year-old man, currently takes the following medications daily: digoxin (Lanoxin) 0.125 mg; furosemide (Lasix) 20 mg daily; and potassium supplementation (K-Dur) 20 mEq. As his nurse, you will be discussing Jim's medication regimen and his next health care provider office visit after discharge from the hospital.

1. Discuss the relationship among the three medications.

2. Jim will have a digoxin serum level collected during the health care provider office visit. What does he need to know about this procedure?

3. Jim asked you to compile a list of foods that are rich in potassium. Prepare the list.

See Answers to Additional Case Study on student resource website.

Chapter Review

1 A patient newly diagnosed with heart failure following an acute myocardial infarction has a prescription for enalapril (Vasotec). This drug class is frequently used in early heart failure because of what clinical improvement?

1. It strengthens the force of myocardial contraction to improve cardiac output.

2. It decreases peripheral resistance, increasing cardiac output.

3. It slows the heart rate, improving filling time and increasing cardiac output.

4. It has diuretic effects, decreasing peripheral edema and pulmonary congestion.

2 In providing the patient with heart failure information prior to discharge, the nurse will discuss digoxin (Lanoxin) therapy. Which point would the nurse include in the patient's teaching?

1. Take the drug in the morning before rising.

2. Monitor the pulse daily prior to taking the drug.

3. Discontinue the drug if the pulse rate is 70 beats per minute.

4. Eat a diet high in bran fiber and calcium.

3 The nurse is evaluating the therapeutic effects of milrinone (Primacor). The nurse knows that this drug is given to:

1. Increase the force of cardiac contractions and improve cardiac output.

2. Decrease the volume of the cardiac output to reduce hypertension.

3. Relax the myocardial muscle, decreasing myocardial oxygen requirements.

4. Inhibit cardiac irregularities, decreasing the sensation of palpitations.

4 The patient is receiving hydralazine with isosorbide (BiDil) for heart failure. The nurse should monitor this patient for:

1. Confusion and agitation.

2. Bleeding.

3. Tingling or cramping in the legs.

4. Dizziness and rapid heart rate.

5 A patient will begin taking carvedilol (Coreg) for heart failure. Before teaching the patient about this drug, the nurse will discuss the strategy for drug dosage with the health care provider because of which recommended routine for beta-adrenergic blockers in heart failure?

1. Significantly lower dosages are used first and gradually increased to a target dose.

2. A loading dose that is higher than the subsequent daily dose must be given.

3. The beta-adrenergic blocker dosage must be lowered if the patient is also on ACE inhibitors.

4. Beta-adrenergic blockers are almost never used in HF and the order must be confirmed.

6 When planning patient education, the nurse knows that patient adherence to beta-adrenergic blocker therapy in heart failure may be difficult to achieve despite the usefulness of these drugs. What will the nurse need to address in the teaching plan? Select all that apply.

1. The dosage must be gradually adjusted over time to a beneficial dose.

2. The patient may not notice significant improvement during early therapy.

3. The drug may require changes to many other medications the patient is taking.

4. The drug has significant benefit in reducing mortality from heart failure.

5. The drug will require extensive lifestyle changes.

See Answers to Chapter Review in Appendix A.

References

Dumitru, I. (2014). Heart failure. *Medscape Reference*. Retrieved from http://emedicine.medscape.com/article/163062-overview

Dungan, K. M., Osei, K., Nagaraja, H. N., Schuster, D. P., & Binkley, P. (2010). Relationship between glycemic control and readmission rates in patients hospitalized with congestive heart failure during implementation of hospital-wide initiatives. *Endocrine Practice, 16*(6), 945–951. doi:10.4158/EP10093.OR

Flanagan, J. L., Simmons, P. A., Vehige, J., Wilcox, M., & Garrett, Q. (2010). Role of carnitine in disease. *Nutrition and Metabolism, 7*, 30. doi:10.1186/1743-7075-7-30

University of Maryland Medical Center. (2011). *Carnitine (L-carnitine)*. Retrieved from http://www.umm.edu/altmed/articles/carnitine-l-000291.htm

van Melle, J. P., Bot, M., de Jonge, P., de Boer, R. A., van Veldhuisen, D. K., & Whooley, M. A. (2010). Diabetes, glycemic control, and new-onset heart failure in patients with stable coronary artery disease. *Diabetes Care, 33*(9), 2084–2089. doi:10.2337/dc10-0286

Yancy, C. W., Jessup, M., Bozkurt, B., Butler, J., Casey, D. E., Jr., Drazner, M. H., . . . Wilkoff, B. L. (2013). 2013 ACCF/AHA guideline for the management of heart failure: A report of the American College of Cardiology Foundation/American Heart Association Task Force on Practice Guidelines. *Circulation, 128*, e240–e327. Published online before print June 5, 2013. doi:10.1161/CIR.0b013e31829e8776

Selected Bibliography

Al-Mohammad, A., & Mant, J. T. (2011). The diagnosis and management of chronic heart failure: Review following the publication of the NICE guidelines. *Heart, 97*, 411–416. doi:10.1136/hrt.2010.214999

Case, R., Haynes, D., Holaday, B., & Parker, V. G. (2010). Evidence-based nursing: The role of the advanced practice registered nurse in the management of heart failure patients in the outpatient setting. *Dimensions of Critical Care Nursing, 29*, 57–62. doi:10.1097/DCC.0b013e3181c92efb

Corotto, P. S., McCarey, M. M., Adams, S., Khazanie, P., & Whellan, D. J. (2013). Heart failure patient adherence: Epidemiology, cause, and treatment. *Heart Failure Clinics, 9*(1), 49–58. doi:10.1016/j.hfc.2012.09.004

DeFelice, P., Masucci, M., McLoughlin, J., Salvatore, S., Shane, M., & Wong, D. (2010). Congestive heart failure: Redefining health care and nursing. *Journal of Continuing Education in Nursing, 41*(9), 390–391. doi:10.3928/00220124-20100825-03

Dupree, C. S. (2010). Primary prevention of heart failure: An update. *Current Opinion in Cardiology, 25*, 478–483. doi:10.1097/HCO.0b013e32833cd550

Herdman, T. H., & Kamitsuru, S. (Eds.). (2014). *NANDA International nursing diagnoses: Definitions and classification, 2015–2017*. Oxford, United Kingdom: Wiley-Blackwell.

Kee, J. L. (2014). *Laboratory and diagnostic tests with nursing implications* (9th ed.). Upper Saddle River, NJ: Pearson Education.

Krum, H., & Driscoll, A. (2013). Management of heart failure. *The Medical Journal of Australia, 199*, 334–339. doi:10.5694/mja12.10993

Lam, C., & Smeltzer, S. C. (2013). Patterns of symptom recognition, interpretation, and response in heart failure patients: An integrative review. *Journal of Cardiovascular Nursing, 28*, 348–359. doi:10.1097/JCN.0b013e3182531cf7

Maron, B. A., & Rocco, T. P. (2011). Pharmacotherapy of congestive heart failure. In L. L. Brunton, B. A. Chabner, & B. C. Knollman (Eds.), *The pharmacological basis of therapeutics* (12th ed., pp. 789–814). New York, NY: McGraw-Hill.

Rich, M. W. (2012). Pharmacotherapy of heart failure in the elderly: Adverse events. *Heart Failure Reviews, 17*, 589–595. doi:10.1007/s10741-011-9263-1

Stewart, S. (2013). What is the optimal place for heart failure treatment and care: Home or hospital? *Current Heart Failure Reports, 10*, 227–231. doi:10.1007/s11897-013-0144-x

Wakefield, B. J., Boren, S. A., Groves, P. S., & Conn, V. S. (2013). Heart failure care management programs: A review of study interventions and meta-analysis of outcomes. *Journal of Cardiovascular Nursing, 28*, 8–19. doi:10.1097/JCN.0b013e318239f9e1

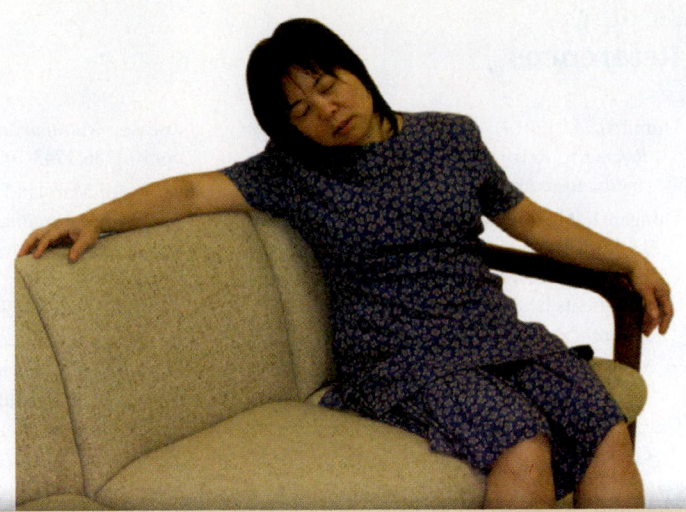

"I will never forget the fear that overwhelmed me as I woke up in the emergency department. I had no idea what had happened. I only remember a strange sensation in my chest. It was like my heart was fluttering. Then I must have passed out."

Patient "Jada Chinn Nguyen"

CHAPTER

37

Pharmacotherapy of Dysrhythmias

LEARNING OUTCOMES

After reading this chapter, the student should be able to:

1. Identify disorders associated with an increased risk of dysrhythmias.

2. Explain how rhythm abnormalities can affect cardiac function.

3. Sketch a typical cardiac action potential and label the flow of potassium, sodium, and calcium ions during each phase.

4. Design a table that indicates the classification of dysrhythmias and the types of drugs used to treat them.

5. Describe general principles guiding the management of dysrhythmias.

6. Identify the primary mechanisms of action of antidysrhythmic drugs.

7. For each of the classes shown in the chapter outline, identify the prototype and representative drugs and explain the mechanism(s) of drug action, primary indications, contraindications, significant drug interactions, pregnancy category, and important adverse effects.

8. Apply the nursing process to care for patients receiving pharmacotherapy for dysrhythmias.

CHAPTER OUTLINE

▸ Etiology of Dysrhythmias

▸ Phases and Measurement of the Cardiac Action Potential

▸ Classification of Dysrhythmias

▸ General Principles of Dysrhythmia Management

▸ Drugs for Dysrhythmias

Sodium Channel Blockers: Class I

PROTOTYPE Procainamide, *p. 604*

Beta-Adrenergic Antagonists: Class II

Potassium Channel Blockers: Class III

PROTOTYPE Amiodarone (Cordarone, Pacerone), *p. 607*

Calcium Channel Blockers: Class IV

Miscellaneous Antidysrhythmics

Dysrhythmias are disorders of cardiac rhythm characterized by abnormal heart rate or irregular contractions. Also called arrhythmias, they encompass a number of different disorders that range from harmless to life threatening. Diagnosis is difficult and patients often must be connected to an electrocardiogram (ECG) and must be experiencing symptoms in order to determine the exact type of rhythm disorder. Proper diagnosis and optimum pharmacotherapy can significantly affect the frequency of dysrhythmias and their consequences.

Etiology of Dysrhythmias

37.1 Some dysrhythmias produce no patient symptoms, while others may be life threatening.

Some dysrhythmias are asymptomatic and have no effect on cardiac function, while others require immediate treatment. Typical symptoms of dysrhythmias include dizziness, weakness, fatigue, decreased exercise tolerance, palpitations, dyspnea, and syncope. It is difficult to estimate the frequency of the disease, although it is likely that dysrhythmias are quite common in the population. Patients often wait until these symptoms occur more frequently or become acute before seeking medical intervention.

Dysrhythmias occur in all age groups and in both healthy and diseased hearts. While the actual cause of most dysrhythmias is elusive, the majority are closely associated with certain conditions, primarily heart disease and myocardial infarction (MI): 90% of patients experiencing an MI will develop a dysrhythmia. Persistent dysrhythmias are associated with increased risk of stroke and heart failure (HF), and severe dysrhythmias may result in sudden death. Conditions that promote the formation of cardiac rhythm abnormalities are called **prodysrhythmics**. Following are some of the diseases and conditions associated with dysrhythmias:

- Hypertension (HTN)
- Cardiac valve disease such as mitral stenosis
- Coronary artery disease (CAD)
- Low or high potassium levels in the blood
- Myocardial infarction (MI)
- Stroke
- Diabetes mellitus
- Heart failure

In addition to the preceding list, a number of medications have been found to cause new dysrhythmias or worsen existing ones. Caution must be used when administering prodysrhythmic drugs to patients with preexisting cardiac impairment or who may have any of the above conditions. Table 37.1 lists selected drugs known to have prodysrhythmic properties.

TABLE 37.1 Selected Prodysrhythmic Drugs

Class of Medication	Example Drugs
Antidysrhythmic drugs	amiodarone, disopyramide, dofetilide, flecainide, ibutilide, procainamide, propafenone, quinidine, sotalol
Autonomic drugs	atenolol, clonidine, methyldopa, nadolol, propranolol
Calcium channel blockers	diltiazem, nifedipine, verapamil
Cardiac glycosides	digoxin
Miscellaneous drugs	amitriptyline, chloroquine, cimetidine, haloperidol, lithium carbonate, phenothiazines

Phases and Measurement of the Cardiac Action Potential

37.2 The phases of cardiac action potential include rapid depolarization, a long plateau, and repolarization.

Dysrhythmias are alterations in the normal generation or conduction of electrical impulses, or action potentials, across the myocardium. Because antidysrhythmic drugs act by correcting or modifying impulse conduction, a firm grasp of cardiac electrical properties is essential to understanding drug mechanisms. Before proceeding, the student should review the normal pathway of impulse conduction in the heart presented in Chapter 28.

Action potentials occur in neurons and cardiac muscle cells (myocytes) due to the changes in the concentration of specific ions found inside and outside the cell. Under resting conditions, sodium ions (Na^+) and calcium ions (Ca^{2+}) are in higher concentrations *outside* of myocytes, whereas potassium ions (K^+) are found in higher concentration *inside* these cells. These imbalances are, in part, responsible for the inside of a myocyte plasma membrane having a slightly negative charge (80–90 mV), relative to the outside of the membrane. A cell having this negative membrane potential is **polarized**.

An action potential illustrating the steps in electrical conduction is shown in Figure 37.1. The changes in ions, or fluxes, occurring during an action potential may be grouped into five phases.

Phase 4: It is easiest to begin with phase 4 because this is the period during which the myocyte is "resting" and the action potential has not yet occurred. Note in Figure 37.1, however, that during phase 4 the membrane potential is slowly increasing toward a potential that will trigger an action potential: the **threshold potential**. Sodium is slowly "leaking" into the cell during this period, causing the change in potential, which gives certain regions such as the sinoatrial (SA) node the property of automaticity, the ability to depolarize spontaneously, without input from the nervous system.

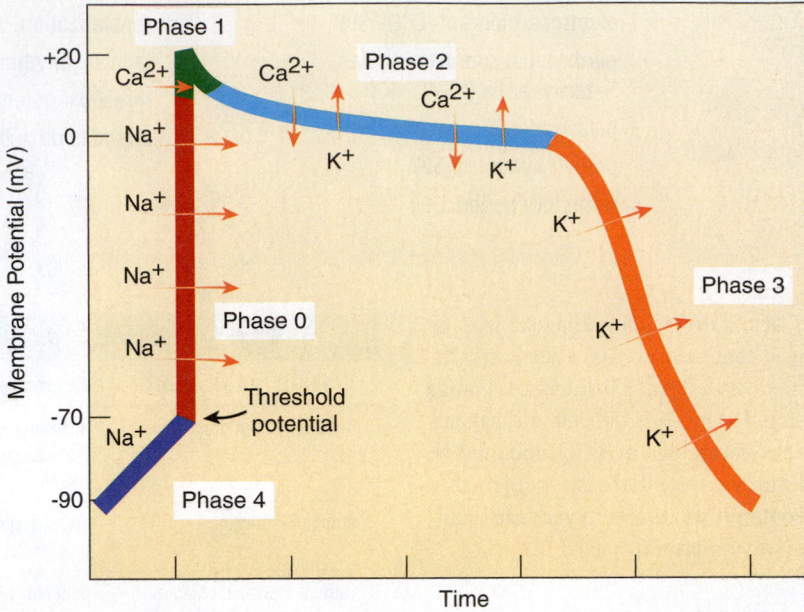

Figure 37.1 Phases of the myocardial action potential. Ion movements during each phase are shown.

Phase 0: An action potential begins when the threshold potential is reached and gated sodium ion channels located in the plasma membrane become activated and open. Sodium ions rush into the cell, producing a rapid **depolarization**, or loss of membrane potential. Because they open and close rapidly, these sodium channels are sometimes referred to as "fast" channels. During this period, Ca^{2+} also enters the cell through calcium ion channels, although the influx is slower than that of sodium. In myocytes located in the SA and atrioventricular (AV) nodes, it is the influx of Ca^{2+}, rather than Na^+, which generates the rapid depolarization of the membrane.

Phase 1: During depolarization, the inside of the plasma membrane temporarily reverses its charge, becoming positive. This is a brief, transient phase.

Phase 2: During phase 2, a plateau is reached in which depolarization is maintained. The entry of Ca^{2+} into the cells signals the release of additional calcium ions that had been held in storage inside the sarcoplasmic reticula. This large and sudden increase in intracellular Ca^{2+} is responsible for the contraction of cardiac muscle. Gated potassium ion channels open, causing an efflux of K^+ from the cells. The plateau is maintained as long as the positive calcium ions entering the myocytes are balanced by the positive potassium ions leaving the cell. Action potentials in skeletal muscle lack this plateau phase.

Phase 3: During phase 3, the calcium channels close and additional potassium channels open, thus causing a net loss of positive ions from the cell. This **repolarization** returns the negative resting membrane potential to the cell.

The synchronized pumping action of the heart requires alternating periods of contraction and relaxation. There is a brief period of time following depolarization and most of repolarization during which the cell cannot initiate a subsequent action potential. This **refractory period** ensures that the myocardial cell finishes contracting before a second action potential begins.

Although learning about the different ions involved in an action potential may seem complicated, they are very important to cardiac pharmacology. Blocking potassium, sodium, or calcium ion channels is a pharmacologic strategy used to terminate or prevent dysrhythmias. In addition, the therapeutic effect of some antidysrhythmic drugs is due to their prolongation of the refractory period. It is not possible to understand drug mechanisms without adequate knowledge of the normal electrical conduction properties of the heart. In general, most cardiac drugs:

- Increase impulse formation (or automaticity).
- Increase conduction velocity.
- Increase both impulse formation and conduction velocity.

  OR

- Decrease impulse formation or automaticity.
- Decrease conduction velocity.
- Decrease both impulse formation or automaticity and conduction.

CONNECTION Checkpoint 37.1

From what you learned in Chapter 30, what are the three types of calcium channels? Which type is blocked by calcium channel blocker medications? *See Answer to Connection Checkpoint 37.1 on student resource website.*

37.3 The electrocardiogram is used to measure electrical conduction across the myocardium.

The **electrocardiogram (ECG)** is a graphic recording of the wave of electrical conduction across the myocardium. The ECG is a primary tool in the diagnosis of dysrhythmias and other heart diseases. A normal ECG and its relationship to impulse conduction in the heart are shown in Figure 37.2.

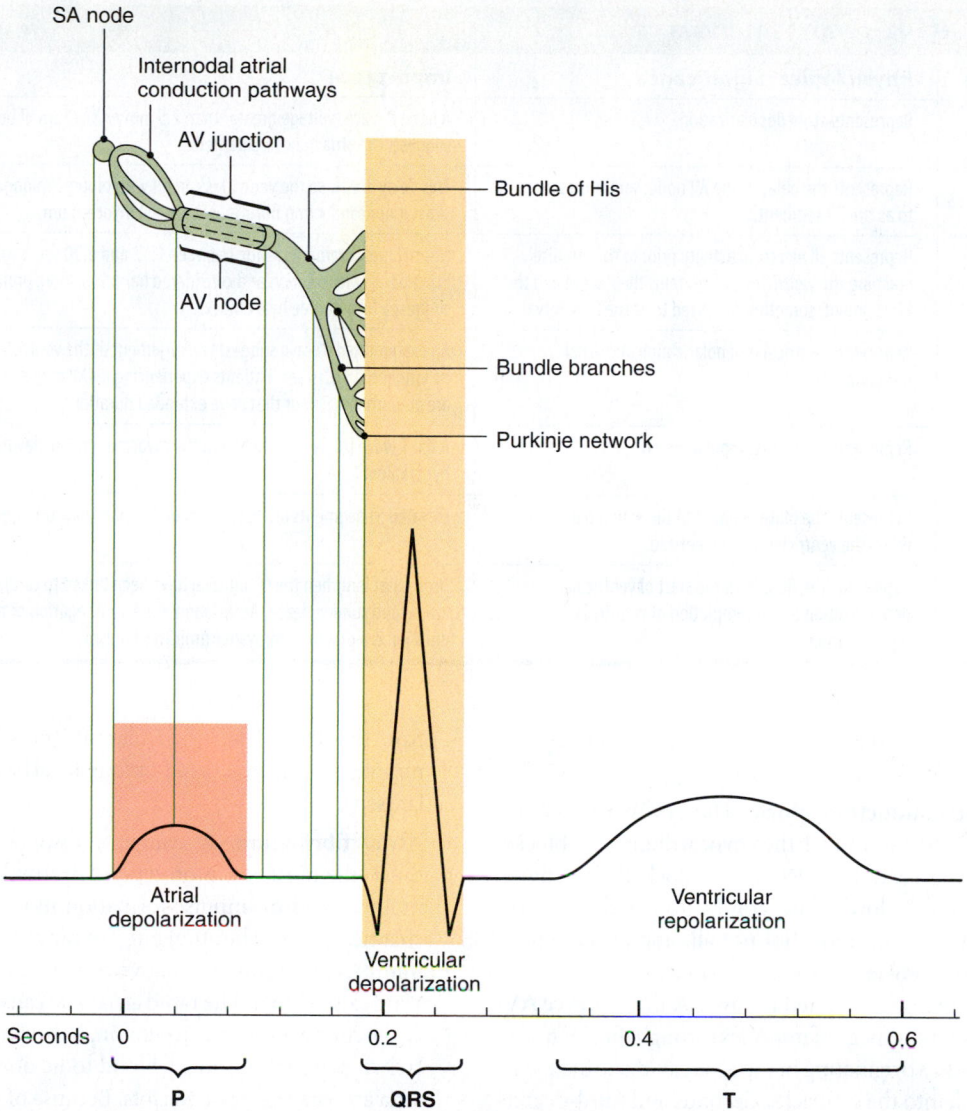

Figure 37.2 Relationship of the electrocardiogram to electrical conduction in the heart.

Three distinct waves are produced by a normal ECG: the P wave, the QRS complex, and the T wave. Changes to the wave patterns or in their timing are associated with certain pathologies. The different classes of antidysrhythmic drugs also affect the ECG in characteristic manners. A summary of the different waves, segments, and intervals, and their importance to cardiac physiology is given in Table 37.2.

PharmFACT

Inherited long QT syndrome (LQTS) is a dysrhythmia that causes about 3,000 to 4,000 sudden deaths in children and young adults each year. It is diagnosed during childhood and is more common in females than males. LQTS is usually treated with beta-adrenergic blockers (National Heart, Lung, and Blood Institute, 2011).

Classification of Dysrhythmias

37.4 Dysrhythmias are classified by the impulse origin and type of rhythm abnormality produced.

There are many types of dysrhythmias and they are classified by a number of different methods. The two broad categories of rhythm abnormalities are those that affect impulse formation and those that affect impulse conduction. Although a correct diagnosis of the type of dysrhythmia is sometimes difficult, it is essential for effective treatment.

Bradydysrhythmias are disorders characterized by a heart rate of less than 60 beats/minute. Bradydysrhythmias are very common in older adults because the number of cells in the SA node declines progressively such that by age 75 about 90% of the cells are nonfunctional. Similar age-related changes occur in the AV node, where normal cells progressively die and are replaced by fibrotic tissue. Bradydysrhythmias are the major indication for pacemaker implantation. Common bradydysrhythmias include the following:

- **Sinus bradycardia.** The most common slow heart rhythm. Sinus bradycardia generally does not require treatment unless the patient is experiencing syncope or dizziness due to lack of sufficient blood flow to the brain, or if the heart rate fails to increase during periods of exertion.

- **Sinoatrial node dysfunction (sick sinus syndrome).** The SA node fails to generate or transmit sufficient electrical impulses. Patients with this condition may experience severe bradycardia (less than 40 beats/minute resting), failure of the heart rate to increase with exercise, or significant sinus "pauses."

TABLE 37.2 ECG Waves and Intervals

Wave or Interval	Physiological Significance	Importance
P wave	Represents atrial depolarization.	A large P wave (voltage greater than 2.5 mm or 2 1/2 small boxes on the readout) suggests the atria may be enlarged.
PQ segment	Represents the delay at the AV node; sometimes referred to as the PR segment.	This delay is vital so the ventricles can fill with blood. Prolonged PQ segments suggest slow or nonconducting fibrotic areas in the myocardium.
PQ interval	Represents all electrical activity prior to the impulse reaching the ventricles and contains the P wave and the PQ segment; sometimes referred to as the PR interval.	Normal measurements range between 0.12 and 0.20 sec. Slightly prolonged PQ intervals are common and considered harmless. More prolonged PQ intervals suggest a first-degree heart block.
QRS complex	Represents ventricular depolarization and atrial repolarization.	An exaggerated R wave suggests enlargement of the ventricles. The QRS should not be longer than 0.10 sec. Patients experiencing an MI may show QRS complexes that are abnormally high or that have extended durations.
T wave	Represents ventricular repolarization.	A flat T wave suggests ischemia to the myocardium; an elevated T wave indicates hyperkalemia.
ST segment	Represents the plateau phase of the action potential when the ventricles are depolarized.	Elevated ST segments are used to guide the pharmacotherapy of MI.
QT interval	Represents the time from the start of ventricular depolarization to the completion of ventricular repolarization.	Drugs that lengthen the QT interval have been linked to cardiac dysrhythmias, cardiac arrest, and sudden death. At the same time, prolongation of the action potential duration is a primary antidysrhythmic mechanism.

Severe episodes of bradycardia may alternate with periods of abnormally rapid heart rates.

- **Atrioventricular conduction block.** The AV node fails to conduct impulses to the rest of the myocardium. AV blocks are classified by degree. In first-degree AV block, the AV node conducts the impulse slowly, and conduction is delayed. In second-degree AV block, some, but not all, impulses are prevented (blocked) from leaving the AV node. Second-degree AV block results in nonconducted P waves. A third-degree AV block results in total stoppage of impulses through the AV node. None of the impulses originating in the atria can make their way through the block into the ventricles. Second- and third-degree blocks require pharmacotherapy or the insertion of a temporary or permanent pacemaker. Some AV blocks are temporary in origin and can be due to cardiac drug toxicity. Any drug that slows AV conduction can cause a temporary form of AV block.

Tachydysrhythmias are disorders exhibiting a heart rate greater than 100 beats/minute. The incidence of tachydysrhythmias increases in older adults and in patients with preexisting cardiovascular disease. The simplest method for categorizing tachydysrhythmias is according to the type of rhythm abnormality produced and its location. Dysrhythmias that originate in the atria are sometimes referred to as supraventricular. Those that originate in the ventricles are generally more serious because they are more likely to interfere with the normal function of the heart.

- **Atrial tachycardia.** May be caused by a rapidly firing SA node or by an ectopic focus in the atria that suppresses the SA node and establishes a rapid heart rate, often between 160 and 200 beats/ minute. When these episodes alternate with periods of normal rhythm, it is called paroxysmal atrial tachycardia (PAT), or **paroxysmal supraventricular tachycardia (PSVT)**.
- **Atrial flutter.** A rapid, regular heartbeat in which the atria may beat 250 to 350 times per minute. During atrial flutter, the job of the AV node is to selectively block some of the impulses coming

from the atria, so the ventricular rate (pulse) is 125 to 175 beats/ minute (usually two, three, or four atrial beats for each ventricular beat).

- **Atrial fibrillation.** A complete disorganization of rhythm, this is the most common type of dysrhythmia. It is caused by multiple sites of impulse formation in the atria, all firing in a chaotic fashion. The atrial rate can range from 300 to 600 beats/ minute, causing an irregular ventricular rate ranging from 50 to 200 beats/minute. The rapid atrial rate causes a loss of organized atrial contraction and results in quivering (fibrillation). This lack of contraction causes blood to lie dormant in parts of the atria and may give rise to clots. Because of the potential for clot formation, atrial fibrillation is a leading risk factor for stroke.
- **Ventricular tachycardia.** Usually recognized by regular, rapid, wide beats with a ventricular rate of 100 to 200 beats/minute. Patients with sustained or symptomatic ventricular tachycardia must be treated immediately because this condition is associated with a high risk of sudden death. **Torsades de pointes** is a specific type of ventricular tachycardia that is characterized by rates between 200 and 250 beats/minute and "twisting of the points" of the QRS complex on the ECG.
- **Ventricular fibrillation.** A complete disorganization of rhythm in which the ventricles pump little or no blood, quickly starving the tissues of oxygen. Ventricular fibrillation is now considered cardiac arrest.

General Principles of Dysrhythmia Management

37.5 Antidysrhythmic drugs are only used when there is a clear benefit to the patient.

Most antidysrhythmic drugs have the potential to produce serious adverse effects. The very drugs used to treat dysrhythmias may actually worsen or create new dysrhythmias. Furthermore, research suggests that mortality may actually increase when some of these drugs are used to treat or prevent dysrhythmias. The following guidelines are used in the management of the patient with dysrhythmias.

Asymptomatic dysrhythmias: Research has shown little or no benefit to the patient in treating asymptomatic dysrhythmias with medications. Antidysrhythmic drugs are normally reserved for patients experiencing overt symptoms or for those whose condition cannot be controlled by other means.

Acute dysrhythmias: Some types of dysrhythmias are serious and may be life threatening. In these cases, pharmacotherapy or cardioversion is warranted. For example, ventricular dysrhythmias often interfere with cardiac output and have greater potential for harm than atrial dysrhythmias. Dysrhythmias that are sustained may worsen and affect cardiac function. Several antidysrhythmics available by the intravenous (IV) route have an immediate onset of action to terminate life-threatening dysrhythmias.

Prophylaxis of dysrhythmias: Patients who are afflicted with recurring dysrhythmias or who have a comorbid condition, such as preexisting heart disease, may benefit from prophylactic therapy with antidysrhythmics. These patients should be monitored regularly to assess for prodysrhythmic effects from the drugs. Drug combinations that have the potential to prolong the QT interval are avoided and doses are kept as low as possible to minimize risk. Prophylactic therapy should only be initiated for high-risk patients.

Nonpharmacologic treatment: Serious types of dysrhythmias are corrected through electrical stimulation of the heart, a treatment called **cardioversion** or **defibrillation**. The electrical shock momentarily stops all electrical impulses in the heart, both normal and abnormal. Under ideal conditions, the temporary cessation of electrical activity will allow the SA node to automatically return conduction to a normal sinus rhythm.

Other types of nonpharmacologic treatment include identification and destruction of the myocardial cells responsible for the abnormal conduction through a surgical procedure called catheter ablation. Cardiac pacemakers are sometimes inserted to correct the types of dysrhythmias that cause the heart to beat too slowly. Implantable cardioverter defibrillators (ICDs) are placed in a patient to restore normal rhythm by either pacing the heart or giving it an electric shock when dysrhythmias occur. In addition, the ICD is capable of storing information regarding the heart rhythm for the health care provider to evaluate.

Drugs for Dysrhythmias

37.6 Antidysrhythmic drugs are classified by their mechanism of action.

The therapeutic goals of antidysrhythmic pharmacotherapy are to terminate existing dysrhythmias or to prevent abnormal rhythms for the purpose of reducing the risks of sudden death, stroke, or other complications resulting from the disease. Antidysrhythmic drugs act by altering specific electrophysiologic properties of the heart. They do this through two basic mechanisms: blocking flow through ion channels (conduction) or altering autonomic activity (automaticity).

The most common method of classifying antidysrhythmic drugs is called the Vaughan Williams classification, which was begun in 1985. This classification scheme groups drugs as Classes I, II, III, and IV based on the stage at which they affect the action potential. A fifth group includes miscellaneous drugs not acting by one of the first four mechanisms. Although widely used, the Vaughan Williams classification method is simplistic because some of these drugs act by more than one mechanism and the drugs within each class have unique properties that distinguish them from each other. For example, the Class I drugs have three subclasses. The categories of antidysrhythmics and their mechanisms are shown in Table 37.3.

The use of antidysrhythmic drugs has significantly declined in recent years. The reason for this decline is that research studies determined that the use of antidysrhythmic medications for prophylaxis can actually increase patient mortality. Drugs affecting cardiac electrophysiology have a narrow margin of safety between a therapeutic effect and a toxic effect. While they have the ability to correct dysrhythmias, they can also worsen or even create new dysrhythmias. These prodysrhythmic effects have resulted in less use of these drugs, especially those medications in Class I.

Another reason for the decline in antidysrhythmic drug use is the success of nonpharmacologic techniques. Catheter ablation and implantable defibrillators are more successful in managing many types of dysrhythmias than is the prophylactic use of medications.

Sodium Channel Blockers: Class I

37.7 Class I antidysrhythmics act by blocking ion channels in myocardial cells.

Sodium channel blockers, the Class I drugs, are the largest group of antidysrhythmics. They are further divided into three subgroups (IA, IB, and IC) based on subtle differences in their mechanisms of action. Because initiation of the action potential is dependent on the opening of gated sodium ion channels, a blockade of these channels will prevent depolarization of the myocardium. The spread of the action potential will slow, and areas of ectopic pacemaker activity will be suppressed. The sodium channel blockers are shown in Table 37.4 and Figure 37.3.

CONNECTIONS | **Lifespan Considerations**

Dental Health and Dysrhythmias in the Older Adult

Studies have begun to link poor dental health with many diseases related to inflammation. Dental caries (tooth decay) has been shown to increase inflammatory chemicals in the body and some studies link the rise of these chemical mediators to coronary heart disease. Kaneko, Yoshihara, and Miyazaki (2011) studied adults age 70 or older for a period of 4 years. For nonsmokers, an increase in the number of oral sites with periodontal disease was associated with a statistically significant elevated risk of dysrhythmias. The same increase in risk was not found among those elders who smoked, although smoking is associated with the development of periodontal disease.

Aging is often associated with increasing dental concerns and tooth loss, and nurses should continue to encourage the older adult to maintain adequate dental hygiene. Hygiene is not only a method for preserving teeth and dental function, it is also a possible preventive measure against other more serious conditions such as coronary heart disease and dysrhythmias.

TABLE 37.3 Classification of Antidysrhythmics

Class	Actions	Primary Indications
I: Sodium Channel Blockers		
IA	Delays repolarization; slows conduction velocity; increases duration of the action potential	Atrial fibrillation, premature atrial contractions, premature ventricular contractions, tachycardia
IB	Accelerates repolarization; slows conduction velocity; decreases duration of action potential	Severe ventricular dysrhythmias
IC	No significant effect on repolarization; slows conduction velocity	Severe ventricular dysrhythmias
II: Beta-Adrenergic Blockers	Slows conduction velocity; decreases automaticity; prolongs refractory period	Atrial flutter and fibrillation, tachydysrhythmias, ventricular dysrhythmias
III: Drugs That Slow Repolarization	Slows repolarization; increases duration of action potential; prolongs refractory period	Severe atrial and ventricular dysrhythmias
IV: Calcium Channel Blockers	Slows conduction velocity; decreases contractility; prolongs refractory period	Paroxysmal supraventricular tachycardia, supraventricular tachydysrhythmias

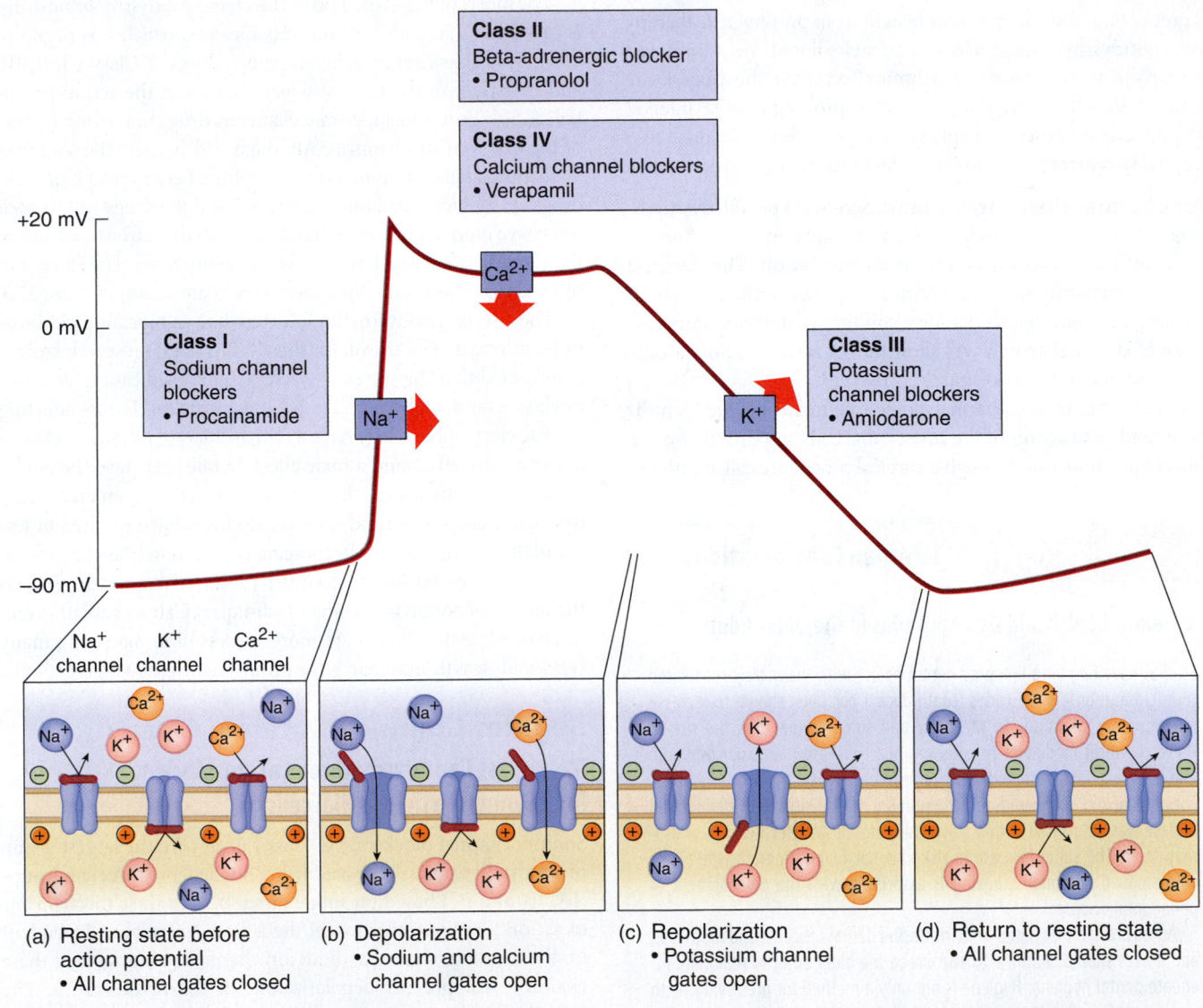

Figure 37.3 Ion channels in myocardial cells: (a) resting state before action potential (all channel gates closed); (b) depolarization (sodium and calcium channel gates open); (c) repolarization (potassium channel gates open); (d) return to resting state (all channel gates closed).

TABLE 37.4 Antidysrhythmic Drugs

Drug	Route and Adult Dose (Maximum Dose Where Indicated)	Adverse Effects
Class IA: Sodium Channel Blockers		
disopyramide (Norpace)	PO (Immediate release): 400–800 in divided doses PO (Controlled release): 300 mg bid	*Nausea, vomiting, diarrhea, dry mouth, urinary retention, cinchonism (quinidine), anorexia, rash, photosensitivity* May produce new dysrhythmias or worsen existing ones; hypotension, torsades de pointes, blood dyscrasias, hepatotoxicity (quinidine), lupus (procainamide)
procainamide	IV: 100 mg every 5 min at a rate of 25–50 mg/min (max: 1 g)	
quinidine gluconate	PO: 324–648 mg tid–qid (max: 3–4 g/day) IV: 0.25 mg/kg/min (max: 5–10 mg/kg)	
quinidine sulfate	PO: 200–400 mg tid–qid (max: 3–4 g/day); therapeutic serum drug level is 2–5 mcg/mL	
Class IB: Sodium Channel Blockers		
lidocaine (Xylocaine)	IV: 1–4 mg/min infusion (max: 3 mg/kg per 5–10 min)	*Nausea, vomiting, drowsiness, dizziness, lethargy, confusion (phenytoin)* May produce new dysrhythmias or worsen existing ones; hypotension, bradycardia, CNS toxicity (lidocaine), malignant hyperthermia (lidocaine), cardiac arrest (lidocaine), status epilepticus if abruptly withdrawn (phenytoin), blood dyscrasias (phenytoin)
mexiletine (Mexitil)	PO: 200–300 mg tid (max: 1,200 mg/day)	
phenytoin (Dilantin)	IV: 50–100 mg every 10–15 min until dysrhythmia is terminated (max: 1 g/day) PO: 100–200 mg tid (max: 625 mg/day)	
Class IC: Sodium Channel Blockers		
flecainide (Tambocor)	PO: 50 mg bid (max: 400 mg/day)	*Nausea, vomiting, fatigue, dizziness, headache, visual disturbances (flecainide)* May produce new dysrhythmias or worsen existing ones; hypotension, bradycardia, cardiac arrest (flecainide), blood dyscrasias, lupus (propafenone), HF (propafenone), acute liver injury (propafenone)
propafenone (Rythmol)	PO (Immediate release): 150–300 mg tid (max: 900 mg/day) PO (Extended release): 225 mg bid (max: 425 mg q12h)	
Class II: Beta-Adrenergic Antagonists		
acebutolol (Sectral)	PO: 200–600 mg bid–tid (max: 1,200 mg/day)	*Fatigue, insomnia, drowsiness, impotence, decreased libido, dizziness, bradycardia, confusion* Agranulocytosis, HF, bronchospasm, hypotension, Stevens–Johnson syndrome, anaphylaxis; if the drug is abruptly withdrawn, palpitations, rebound HTN, life-threatening dysrhythmias, or myocardial ischemia may occur
esmolol (Brevibloc)	IV: 500 mcg/kg/min loading dose; maintenance dose 50–300 mcg/kg/min (maintenance max: 200 mcg/kg/min)	
propranolol (Inderal, Innopran XL)	PO: 10–30 mg 3–4 times daily (max: 480 mg/day) IV: 0.5–3.1 mg every 4 h or prn	
Class III: Potassium Channel Blockers		
amiodarone (Cordarone, Pacerone)	PO: 400–600 mg/day in 1–2 divided doses (max: 1,600 mg/day as loading dose)	*Blurred vision (amiodarone), photosensitivity, nausea, vomiting, anorexia* May produce new dysrhythmias or worsen existing ones; hypotension, HF, heart block, bradycardia, pneumonia-like syndrome (amiodarone, dronedarone), angioedema (dofetilide), CNS toxicity (ibutilide)
dofetilide (Tikosyn)	PO: 125–500 mcg bid based on creatinine clearance	
dronedarone (Multaq)	PO: 400 mg bid	
ibutilide (Corvert)	IV: 1 mg infused over 10 min (for patients over 60 kg); 0.01 mg/kg (for patients under 60 kg); (max: 2 mg infused over at least 20 min)	
sotalol* (Betapace, Betapace AF, Sorine)	PO: 80 mg bid (max: 320 mg/day)	
Class IV: Calcium Channel Blockers		
diltiazem (Cardizem, Dilacor, Taztia XR, Tiazac)	IV: 5–10 mg/h continuous infusion for a maximum of 24 h (max: 15 mg/h)	*Flushed skin, headache, dizziness, peripheral edema, lightheadedness, nausea, diarrhea, syncope* Hepatotoxicity, MI, CHF, confusion, mood changes, hypotension
verapamil (Calan, Isoptin, Verelan)	PO: 240–480 mg/day in divided doses IV: 5–10 mg direct: may repeat in 15–30 min	
Miscellaneous Antidysrhythmics		
adenosine (Adenocard, Adenoscan)	IV: 6–12 mg given as a bolus injection every 1–2 min as needed (max: 12 mg/dose)	*Facial flushing, dyspnea, headache* May produce new dysrhythmias or worsen existing ones, AV block
digoxin (Lanoxin, Lanoxicaps)	PO: 0.125–0.5 mg 4 times daily Therapeutic serum drug level: 0.8–2 ng/mL	*Nausea, vomiting, headache, diarrhea, visual disturbances* May produce new dysrhythmias or worsen existing ones

Note: *Italics* indicate common adverse effects. <u>Underline</u> indicates serious adverse effects.

*Sotalol is a beta blocker, but because its cardiac effects are more similar to amiodarone, it is in Class III. Adverse effects are those of Class II and Class III.

The sodium channel blockers are similar in structure and action to local anesthetics. In fact, the Class I antidysrhythmic lidocaine is a prototype local anesthetic in Chapter 26. This anesthetic-like action slows impulse conduction across the heart. Some, such as quinidine and procainamide, are effective against many types of dysrhythmias. The remaining Class I drugs are more specific and indicated only for life-threatening ventricular dysrhythmias.

The adverse effects of the sodium blockers vary with each individual drug. All these agents can cause new dysrhythmias or worsen existing ones. The slowing of the heart rate can cause hypotension, dizziness, and fainting. During pharmacotherapy, the ECG should be monitored for signs of cardiotoxicity, such as increases in the PR and QT intervals and widening of the QRS complex. Some Class I drugs have significant anticholinergic adverse effects such as dry mouth, constipation, and urinary retention. Special precautions should be taken with older adults, because anticholinergic adverse effects may worsen urinary hesitancy in men with prostate enlargement.

Class IA: The Class IA antidysrhythmics include quinidine, disopyramide (Norpace), and procainamide. Although quinidine is the oldest and best known Class IA drug, procainamide is the prototype because it has been more widely used than quinidine in recent decades. All are available by the oral (PO) route and act by blocking sodium ion channels during phase 0 of the action potential.

The primary action responsible for the antidysrhythmic effects of the Class IA drugs is a slowing of conduction velocity. These drugs also inhibit potassium channels, which delays repolarization and increases the refractory period. Subsequent action potentials must wait slightly longer before triggering the next electrical impulse. These actions allow the Class IA drugs to inhibit the formation of ectopic foci in both the atria and ventricles.

The effects of the Class IA agents can be recognized on the ECG. The QRS complex widens, owing to the slowed depolarization of the ventricles. The QT interval is increased due to the delay in repolarization of the ventricles.

PROTOTYPE DRUG **Procainamide**

Classification: Therapeutic: Antidysrhythmic, Class IA
Pharmacologic: Sodium channel blocker

Therapeutic Effects and Uses: Approved in 1950, procainamide is a broad-spectrum antidysrhythmic chemically related to the local anesthetic procaine that has the ability to correct many different types of atrial and ventricular dysrhythmias. Indications include ventricular tachycardia during cardiopulmonary resuscitation (CPR); refractory ventricular fibrillation or pulseless ventricular tachycardia during CPR; conversion to sinus rhythm in patients with paroxysmal atrial tachycardia, atrial flutter, or atrial fibrillation; and treatment or prophylaxis of PSVT. Procainamide is now considered a drug of last choice for advanced cardiac life support due to its toxicity; it is used when other drugs have failed to reverse a severe dysrhythmia. The major hepatic metabolite of the drug, N-acetyl procainamide, also has antidysrhythmic activity. Because the rate of acetylation to the active metabolite is genetically determined, "slow acetylators" and "fast acetylators" will require adjustments in dosages to obtain optimum therapeutic results.

Procainamide is available in IV and intramuscular (IM) formulations: PO forms of procainamide have been discontinued. Dosage is guided by periodic serum drug levels, which are maintained between 4 and 8 mcg/mL. The supine position should be used during IV administration because severe hypotension may occur during the infusion. Use of procainamide must be terminated if the QRS widens more than 50% of its original width.

Mechanism of Action: Procainamide blocks sodium ion channels in myocardial cells, thus reducing automaticity and slowing the velocity of the action potential across the myocardium. This slight delay in conduction velocity prolongs the refractory period and can suppress dysrhythmias.

Pharmacokinetics:

Route(s)	IV, IM
Absorption	Readily absorbed
Distribution	Widely distributed; crosses the placenta; secreted in breast milk; 15% bound to plasma protein
Primary metabolism	Hepatic; metabolized to active metabolite
Primary excretion	Renal, 50–70% unchanged
Onset of action	IV: immediate; IM: 10–30 min
Duration of action	IM/IV: 3–4 h

Adverse Effects: Procainamide has a narrow therapeutic index and dosage must be monitored carefully to avoid serious adverse effects. Nausea, vomiting, abdominal pain, and headache are common during therapy. The drug can cause fever, accompanied by anorexia, weakness, nausea, and vomiting. High doses may produce central nervous system (CNS) effects such as confusion or psychosis. Rapid IV administration of procainamide can cause severe hypotension. **Black Box Warnings**: Chronic administration may result in an increased titer of antinuclear antibodies (ANAs). A lupus-like syndrome may occur in 30% to 50% of patients taking the drug for more than a year. Procainamide should be reserved for life-threatening dysrhythmias because it has the ability to produce new dysrhythmias or worsen existing ones. Agranulocytosis, bone marrow depression, neutropenia, hypoplastic anemia, and thrombocytopenia have been reported, usually within the first 3 months of therapy. Complete blood counts should be monitored carefully and the drug discontinued at the first sign of potential blood dyscrasia.

Contraindications/Precautions: Procainamide is contraindicated in patients with second- or third-degree AV block (unless controlled by a pacemaker), severe HF, peripheral neuropathy, and myasthenia gravis. Because procainamide may activate or worsen lupus, the drug is only used in these patients when there is no safer alternative. Doses must be lowered in patients with renal impairment due to possible accumulation of the drug. Patients in shock or with severe hypotension should not receive this drug due to additive hypotension. Procainamide may worsen blood dyscrasias; thus, it should be used with caution in patients with preexisting bone marrow suppression.

Drug Interactions: Additive cardiac depressant effects may occur if procainamide is administered with other antidysrhythmics. Additive anticholinergic adverse effects will occur if procainamide is used concurrently with anticholinergic drugs. Procainamide may increase plasma levels of amiodarone or quinidine. Use with antihypertensives may result in hypotension. **Herbal/Food**: Although no interactions have been well documented, the use of all herbal products or supplements should be avoided unless approved by the health care provider due to the toxicity of the drug.

Pregnancy: Category C.

Treatment of Overdose: No specific therapy is available for overdose. Supportive treatment is targeted to reversing hypotension with vasopressors and preventing or treating procainamide-induced dysrhythmias.

Nursing Responsibilities: Key nursing implications for patients receiving procainamide are included in the Nursing Practice Application for Patients Receiving Pharmacotherapy for Dysrhythmias.

Drugs Similar to Procainamide

There are similar Class IA, IB, and IC antidysrhythmics. Other Class IA antidysrhythmics include disopyramide and quinidine. Moricizine, a unique oral antidysrhythmic that possessed some properties attributed to all three Class I subclasses, was discontinued in 2007 due to lack of market demand.

Disopyramide (Norpace): Approved in 1977, disopyramide has actions and indications similar to those of other Class IA agents. Available only by the PO route, the drug is used infrequently due to a high incidence of anticholinergic effects such as xerostomia (dry mouth) and urinary retention in patients with benign prostatic hyperplasia. The anticholinergic effects cause an increase in heart rate, which may directly cancel out the therapeutic cardiac depressant effects of the drug. Off-label uses include maintenance of, or conversion to, sinus rhythm in patients with atrial flutter or atrial fibrillation. Disopyramide has a black box warning that the drug should be restricted to patients with life-threatening ventricular dysrhythmias. This drug is pregnancy category C.

Quinidine: Approved in 1938, quinidine is the oldest antidysrhythmic drug, originally obtained as a natural substance from the bark of the South American Cinchona tree. Like procainamide, quinidine is a broad-spectrum drug having the ability to correct many different types of atrial and ventricular dysrhythmias. The two salts of quinidine are sulfate, which is given PO, and gluconate, which is given PO and IV. Like other drugs in this class, quinidine blocks sodium ion channels in myocardial cells, thus reducing automaticity and slowing the velocity of the action potential across the myocardium. In addition to dysrhythmias, quinidine gluconate may be used to treat malaria and persistent hiccups. The most common adverse effect of quinidine is diarrhea, which occurs in about one third of patients and may be intense. The drug can induce various types of dysrhythmias when serum levels rise above normal. High doses result in a syndrome called **cinchonism** with symptoms such as tinnitus, headache, blurred vision, hearing loss, and dysrhythmias. These symptoms are reversible once the drug is discontinued. Quinidine is contraindicated in patients with incomplete AV block because it can induce total blockage of conduction. Quinidine carries a black box warning that the drug has resulted in increased mortality when used for non–life-threatening dysrhythmias. This drug is pregnancy category C.

Class IB: The Class IB antidysrhythmics include lidocaine, mexiletine, and phenytoin. Like other Class I drugs, these agents act by blocking gated sodium ion channels in cardiac muscle cells. Unlike the Class IA drugs, the Class IB agents shorten the refractory period and have little effect on conduction velocity. The Class IB drugs have minimal effects on the ECG and their primary indication is ventricular dysrhythmias. A fourth drug in this class, tocainide, was discontinued in 2003 due to a high incidence of adverse effects.

Lidocaine (Xylocaine): Lidocaine, the most frequently prescribed Class IB antidysrhythmic, was featured as a prototype local anesthetic in Chapter 30. It is an important treatment for life-threatening ventricular dysrhythmia, although amiodarone is considered a preferred drug for this indication. It is not effective in preventing or treating atrial dysrhythmias. Lidocaine decreases the refractory period of the action potential, especially in ischemic myocardial tissue. For acute conditions, lidocaine is administered by IV bolus or infusion; it is rarely given by the IM or subcutaneous routes. Serum lidocaine levels may be monitored and should be between 2 and 6 mcg/mL. The first signs of lidocaine toxicity usually involve the CNS and include confusion, anxiety, tremors, and paresthesias. As doses increase, the patient may become comatose and experience seizures or respiratory arrest. The correct lidocaine formulation must be used for IV infusions: Local anesthetic lidocaine preparations may contain preservatives and epinephrine and should not be given IV. This drug is pregnancy category B.

Mexiletine (Mexitil): Approved in 1985, mexiletine is chemically similar to lidocaine, has local anesthetic properties, and is used only for serious ventricular dysrhythmias. Mexiletine, however, is well absorbed orally. An off-label indication is for the treatment of neuropathic pain. The most common adverse effects are nausea and vomiting. CNS effects such as dizziness, tremor, and ataxia are common. Less common, though potentially serious, adverse effects include blood dyscrasias, pulmonary fibrosis, and worsening of HF. A black box warning has been issued regarding the possibility of acute liver damage in patients taking mexiletine. The target range for serum mexiletine concentration is 0.5 to 2 mcg/mL. This drug is pregnancy category C.

Phenytoin (Dilantin): The primary use for phenytoin is to treat seizures, and it was presented in Chapter 22 as a prototype antiseizure medication. As an antidysrhythmic, phenytoin may be administered by the oral or IV route. IV phenytoin must be pushed extremely slowly: 100 mg over 5 minutes. Phenytoin is rarely used for its antidysrhythmic properties and is not approved by the U.S. Food and Drug Administration (FDA) for this purpose. Historically, it has been used to treat dysrhythmias secondary to digoxin (Lanoxin) toxicity. If used for dysrhythmias, serum phenytoin levels should be carefully monitored to be 10 to 20 mcg/mL because the drug can have multiple serious adverse effects, including seizures, ataxia, coma, blood dyscrasias, and hepatotoxicity. This drug is pregnancy category D.

Class IC: The Class IC antidysrhythmics include two drugs: flecainide and propafenone. Like other Class I agents, these drugs block gated sodium ion channels in cardiac muscle cells. The Class IC antidysrhythmics profoundly decrease conduction velocity. Thus the PR, QRS, and QT intervals are often prolonged.

The refractory period may be shortened slightly but is mostly unchanged by the Class IC drugs. Their primary indication is for life-threatening atrial dysrhythmias, although they can also prevent ventricular dysrhythmias. Research has shown these drugs to have a pronounced prodysrhythmic effect that has the potential to increase mortality in patients who have experienced a recent MI.

Flecainide (Tambocor): Flecainide is an oral drug used primarily to treat or prevent paroxysmal atrial fibrillation or atrial flutter due to its ability to markedly decrease conduction velocity. It is indicated for the prophylaxis of life-threatening ventricular dysrhythmias, although it is rarely used for this purpose. The FDA has issued several black box warnings regarding flecainide. The prodysrhythmic effects of the drug may generate new ventricular dysrhythmias in about 10% of the patients. Due to an excessive mortality rate, the drug is contraindicated in patients with left ventricular dysfunction who have experienced a recent MI. Serum flecainide levels should be monitored, especially in patients with renal or hepatic impairment, and maintained between 0.2 and 1 mcg/mL. Pulmonary fibrosis and bone marrow suppression are potentially serious adverse effects. Other adverse effects include dizziness, headache, asthenia, tremor, and malaise. This drug is pregnancy category C.

Propafenone (Rythmol): Approved in 1989, propafenone is an oral drug similar to flecainide that is used primarily for atrial fibrillation and the prophylaxis of PSVT. Its prodysrhythmic activity limits its use in treating ventricular dysrhythmias. Unlike flecainide, propafenone exhibits clinically significant beta-adrenergic antagonist activity. This beta-blocker action may cause a negative inotropic effect that can worsen symptoms of CHF. Furthermore, the beta-blocking actions may cause bronchospasm in patients with asthma or chronic obstructive pulmonary disease (COPD). An extended release formulation (Rythmol SR) allows for twice-daily dosing. Propafenone is metabolized to active metabolites, which account for much of the drug's effects. In addition to exacerbating or creating new dysrhythmias, propafenone may cause dizziness and dysgeusia (altered sense of taste). Like some of the other antidysrhythmics, propafenone has a black box warning that the drug should be restricted to patients with life-threatening ventricular dysrhythmias. This drug is pregnancy category C.

Beta-Adrenergic Antagonists: Class II

37.8 Beta-adrenergic antagonists reduce automaticity as well as slow conduction velocity in the heart.

Beta-adrenergic antagonists, or blockers, are used to treat HTN, MI, HF, and dysrhythmias. The basic pharmacology of beta-adrenergic blockers was explained in Chapter 16; the student should refer to that chapter for nursing responsibilities and patient and family education related to this drug class. Only the actions of these drugs that relate to dysrhythmias are discussed in this section.

As expected from their effects on the autonomic nervous system, beta-adrenergic antagonists slow the heart rate (negative chronotropic effect) and decrease conduction velocity. These effects are primarily caused by the blockade of calcium ion channels in the SA and AV nodes, although these drugs also block gated sodium ion channels in the atria and ventricles. The reduction in myocardial automaticity stabilizes many types of dysrhythmias.

The main value of beta blockers as antidysrhythmic drugs is to treat atrial dysrhythmias associated with HF. When administered to post-MI patients, beta blockers decrease the likelihood of sudden death due to fatal dysrhythmias. Tachydysrhythmias respond well to beta blockers, including those that are induced by exercise.

Only a few beta blockers are approved for dysrhythmias, due to potential adverse effects, and these are listed in Table 37.4. Unless a functioning pacemaker is present, these drugs are contraindicated in patients with severe bradycardia, sick sinus syndrome, or advanced AV block because they depress conduction through the AV node. Blockade of beta-adrenergic receptors in the heart causes bradycardia, which may not be well tolerated in patients with preexisting cardiac disease, and hypotension may cause dizziness and possible fainting. Nonselective beta blockers may affect beta$_2$ receptors in the lung, causing bronchospasm in patients with asthma or COPD. Higher doses may produce depression, as well as hallucinations and psychosis, especially in older adults. Abrupt discontinuation of beta blockers can lead to dysrhythmias and HTN.

Acebutolol (Sectral): Approved in 1984, acebutolol is a cardioselective beta$_1$-adrenergic antagonist available only by the oral route. Like other beta blockers, acebutolol reduces sympathetic activity to the heart, thus lowering heart rate. It also has a negative inotropic effect. As an antidysrhythmic, it is used to treat premature ventricular contractions and reduce exercise-induced tachycardia. Other indications include chronic, stable angina, and HTN. Adverse effects such as hypotension and bradycardia are extensions of its beta-blocking action. At high doses, the selectivity for beta$_1$ receptors diminishes and the drug may cause bronchoconstriction (beta$_2$ receptors). Because the negative inotropic effects of the drug may worsen symptoms of HF, it is usually contraindicated in patients with HF. This drug is pregnancy category B.

Esmolol (Brevibloc): Approved in 1986, esmolol differs from the other antidysrhythmic beta blockers in that it has a very short half-life of 9 minutes and is only given by IV infusion. As an antidysrhythmic, esmolol is used for the immediate termination of atrial tachyarrhythmias and noncompensatory sinus tachycardia and to control ventricular rate in patients with atrial flutter or fibrillation. When a loading dose is administered, peak plasma levels can be reached after only 5 minutes. Off-label indications include treatment of hypertensive emergencies, acute MI, and unstable angina. Hypotension and bradycardia are common

---

CONNECTIONS   Treating the Diverse Patient

◀ **Asian Patients' Sensitivity to Propranolol**

Growing evidence from research studies has shown a differential drug response to propranolol among Asian Americans. These individuals typically lack a specific enzyme (mephenytoin hydroxylase) that is needed to metabolize propranolol. Because of this sensitivity, propranolol has a significantly greater effect on heart rate. In other words, individuals of Asian descent will develop signs of toxicity more quickly than non-Asians. The nurse should assess this population for signs and symptoms of early drug toxicity, possible overdosage, and adverse reactions due to high drug levels. Assessing for unique cultural sensitivity to drug therapies is necessary for safe drug administration of pharmacologic agents.

adverse effects but they quickly resolve once the infusion is discontinued. At therapeutic doses, the drug is selective for beta$_1$-adrenergic receptors. This drug is pregnancy category C.

Propranolol (Inderal, InnoPran XL): Propranolol is a nonselective beta-adrenergic antagonist. Because it slows automaticity, propranolol is indicated for many types of dysrhythmias including suppression of exercise-induced tachycardia, atrial dysrhythmias, ventricular dysrhythmias, premature ventricular contractions, and digoxin-induced tachydysrhythmias. Propranolol exhibits few serious adverse effects at therapeutic doses. At high doses, patients may experience bradycardia, hypotension, HF, and bronchospasm. Propranolol is featured as a prototype beta-adrenergic antagonist in Chapter 16. This drug is pregnancy category C.

CONNECTION Checkpoint 37.2

Both alpha$_1$ blockers and beta$_1$ blockers are used to treat HTN but only the beta$_1$ blockers are antidysrhythmics. From what you learned in Chapter 16, explain why the selective alpha$_1$ blockers are not used to treat dysrhythmias. *See Answer to Connection Checkpoint 37.2 on student resource website.*

Potassium Channel Blockers: Class III

37.9 Potassium channel blockers prolong the refractory period of the heart.

The potassium channel blockers are a small but diverse class of drugs that have very important applications to the treatment of dysrhythmias. After the action potential has passed and the myocardial cell is in a depolarized state, repolarization depends on removal of potassium from the cell. The drugs in Class III exert their actions by blocking potassium ion channels in myocardial cells. Although there are significant differences among the drugs, all have in common the ability to delay repolarization and prolong the refractory period. This action is reflected by an increase in the QT interval on the ECG. Automaticity is also reduced.

Most drugs in this class have multiple actions on the heart and also affect adrenergic receptors or sodium channels. For example, in addition to blocking potassium channels, sotalol (Betapace) is considered a beta-adrenergic blocker. The potassium channel blockers are listed in Table 37.4.

Drugs in this class have limited uses due to potentially serious toxicity. Like other antidysrhythmics, potassium channel blockers slow the heart rate, resulting in bradycardia and possible hypotension in a significant percentage of patients. These drugs can create or worsen dysrhythmias, especially during the first few doses. Older adults with preexisting HF must be carefully monitored because these patients are at higher risk for the cardiac adverse effects of potassium channel blockers.

PROTOTYPE DRUG	Amiodarone (Cordarone, Pacerone)

Classification: Therapeutic: Antidysrhythmic, Class III
Pharmacologic: Potassium channel blocker

Therapeutic Effects and Uses: Approved in 1985, amiodarone is the most frequently prescribed Class III antidysrhythmic. It is considered a broad-spectrum antidysrhythmic because it is effective in terminating both atrial and ventricular dysrhythmias. It is approved for the treatment of resistant ventricular tachycardia and recurrent fibrillation that may prove life threatening, and it has become a medication of choice for the treatment of atrial dysrhythmias in patients with HF.

Amiodarone is available as PO tablets and as an IV infusion. IV infusions are limited to short-term therapy (2 to 4 days). Although its onset of action may take several weeks when the medication is given PO, its effects can last 4 to 8 weeks after the drug is discontinued because it has an extended half-life that may exceed 100 days. Amiodarone is a structural analog of thyroid hormone. The therapeutic serum level for amiodarone is 1 to 2.5 mcg/mL.

Mechanism of Action: Amiodarone exerts multiple, complex actions on the heart, and its exact mechanism of action is not completely known. In addition to blocking potassium ion channels, some of this drug's actions relate to its blockade of sodium ion channels and inhibiting sympathetic activity to the heart. Repolarization is delayed, the refractory period prolonged, and automaticity reduced. In addition to prolonging the QT interval, amiodarone increases the PR interval and widens the QRS complex on the ECG.

Pharmacokinetics:

Route(s)	PO, IV
Absorption	Completely absorbed by the gastrointestinal (GI) tract
Distribution	Widely distributed; crosses the placenta; secreted in breast milk; concentrated in the lung, kidneys, spleen, and adipose tissue
Primary metabolism	Hepatic to active metabolites; some enterohepatic recirculation; inhibits some CYP enzymes
Primary excretion	Primarily biliary; some feces
Onset of action	PO: 2–3 days; IV: 2 h
Duration of action	PO/IV: 10–150 days

Adverse Effects: Potentially serious adverse effects limit the use of amiodarone. Amiodarone may cause nausea, vomiting, anorexia, fatigue, dizziness, and hypotension. Visual disturbances are common in patients taking this drug for extended periods and include blurred vision due to cornea deposits, photophobia, xerostomia, cataracts, and macular degeneration. Rashes, photosensitivity, and other skin reactions occur in 10% to 15% of patients taking the drug. Certain tissues concentrate this medication; thus, adverse effects may be slow to resolve, persisting long after the drug has been discontinued. **Black Box Warning (oral form only):** Amiodarone causes a pneumonia-like syndrome in the lungs. Because the pulmonary toxicity may be fatal, baseline and periodic assessment of lung function is essential. Amiodarone has prodysrhythmic action and may cause bradycardia, cardiogenic shock, or AV block. Mild liver injury is frequent with amiodarone.

Contraindications/Precautions: Amiodarone is contraindicated in patients with severe bradycardia, cardiogenic shock, sick sinus syndrome, severe sinus node dysfunction, or third-degree AV block. Because amiodarone contains iodine in its chemical structure, patients who have hypersensitivity to this element should not receive the drug. It should be used with caution in patients with HF because it has a negative inotropic effect that can worsen symptoms. Electrolyte imbalances, especially hypokalemia and hypomagnesemia, should be corrected before administering amiodarone because these conditions predispose the patient to the development of dysrhythmias. Due to the drug's pulmonary toxicity, it is contraindicated in patients with COPD or respiratory insufficiency. Breast-feeding during amiodarone therapy may cause infant hypothyroidism; thus, the drug is contraindicated during lactation.

Drug Interactions: Amiodarone is metabolized by the cytochrome P450 enzymes and markedly inhibits the metabolism of many other drugs. This can raise the serum levels of these drugs and cause toxicity. For example, amiodarone can increase serum digoxin levels by as much as 70%. Amiodarone greatly enhances the actions of anticoagulants; thus the dose of warfarin must be cut by as much as half. Use with beta-adrenergic blockers or calcium channel blockers (CCBs) may potentiate sinus bradycardia, sinus arrest, or AV block. Amiodarone may increase phenytoin levels two- to threefold. Caution must be used during therapy with loop diuretics because hypokalemia can enhance the prodysrhythmic properties of amiodarone. Because of the large number of potential drug interactions, the nurse should regularly check current reference sources when patients are taking amiodarone concurrently with other medications. **Herbal/Food**: Use with echinacea may increase the risk of hepatotoxicity. Aloe may cause an increased effect of amiodarone. When the drug is administered PO, grapefruit juice can increase serum amiodarone levels by over 80%.

Pregnancy: Category D.

Treatment of Overdose: Overdose will cause bradycardia, hypotension, and life-threatening dysrhythmias. Supportive treatment is targeted to reversing hypotension with vasopressors and bradycardia with atropine or isoproterenol.

Nursing Responsibilities: Key nursing implications for patients receiving amiodarone are included in the Nursing Practice Application for Patients Receiving Pharmacotherapy for Dysrhythmias.

Drugs Similar to Amiodarone (Cordarone, Pacerone)

Other Class III antidysrhythmics include dofetilide, dronedarone, ibutilide, and sotalol. A fifth drug in this class, bretylium, was discontinued in the United States due to the availability of safer and more effective antidysrhythmic drugs.

Dofetilide (Tikosyn): Approved in 1999, dofetilide is an oral drug indicated for conversion of symptomatic atrial flutter or fibrillation to normal sinus rhythm. Like other potassium channel blockers, dofetilide prolongs the refractory period and action potential duration, thus increasing the QT interval. Dofetilide does not exhibit a negative inotropic effect, as do amiodarone and sotalol. The drug has no effect on the PR interval and it does not widen the QRS complex. Dofetilide has many potentially serious adverse effects, and a black box warning states that therapy should begin in a clinical setting under continuous monitoring for a minimum of 3 days. The drug exhibits significant dose-related prodysrhythmic effects, including heart block, ventricular tachycardia, and torsades de pointes. The risk

for drug-induced dysrhythmias is increased when dofetilide is administered concurrently with other medications that prolong the QT interval, including Class I and Class III antidysrhythmics. Dofetilide may accumulate to toxic levels in patients with renal impairment. Therefore, serum creatinine levels are monitored frequently during therapy. Electrolyte imbalances, especially hypokalemia or hypomagnesemia, should be corrected before administering dofetilide because these conditions predispose the patient to developing dysrhythmias. This drug is pregnancy category C.

Dronedarone (Multaq): Approved in 2009, dronedarone is a newer antidysrhythmic. Given by the oral route, the drug is indicated to reduce the risk of hospitalization in patients with atrial dysrhythmias and associated cardiovascular risk factors such as HTN, diabetes, or previous stroke. The drug has a black box warning that it is contraindicated in patients with advanced HF with recent decompensation. It is also contraindicated in patients with bradycardia (less than 50 beats/minute), prolonged QT interval, and severe hepatic impairment. The most common adverse effects are diarrhea, nausea, abdominal pain, vomiting, and asthenia. Dronedarone inhibits CYP enzymes and can participate in multiple drug–drug interactions with other cardiovascular medications. Dronedarone is a category X drug and should not be taken during pregnancy or lactation.

Ibutilide (Corvert): Approved in 1995, ibutilide is only administered as an IV infusion. Continuous ECG monitoring should be conducted for at least 4 hours following the infusion to identify the potential development of new or worsening dysrhythmias. Administered over 10 minutes, ibutilide is a drug of choice for rapidly converting atrial flutter or fibrillation to normal sinus rhythm. The drug prolongs the duration of the cardiac action potential without affecting the PR interval or QRS complex. The infusion is stopped as soon as the dysrhythmia is terminated. Ibutilide is generally well tolerated, although it does have prodysrhythmic effects, including induction of ventricular tachycardia and torsades de pointes. Like other Class III drugs, precautions must be taken when administering this drug concurrently with other medications that prolong the QT interval or if given to patients with hypokalemia or hypomagnesemia, as these conditions increase the risk of dysrhythmias. This drug is pregnancy category C.

Sotalol (Betapace, Betapace AF, Sorine): Approved in 1992, sotalol is unique in that the drug has both Class II and Class III antidysrhythmic properties. As a Class II agent, it is a nonselective beta blocker that slows conduction through the AV node. Its Class III actions delay repolarization and prolong the refractory period, thus widening the QT interval. Its mixed mechanisms are reflected in the diversity of indications for the drug.

Betapace and its generic equivalents are indicated for sustained ventricular fibrillation that is deemed to be life threatening. Betapace AF converts atrial fibrillation to normal sinus rhythm and is indicated for highly symptomatic atrial dysrhythmias. The drugs contain a black box warning stating that they are not interchangeable.

Because of its prodysrhythmic activity, the first 3 days of therapy with sotalol are usually conducted in a controlled clinical setting with continuous monitoring. The drug should be used with caution when taken concurrently with other medications that prolong the QT interval or if given to patients with hypokalemia or hypomagnesemia, as these conditions increase the risk of dysrhythmias. Other adverse effects and contraindications for beta-adrenergic antagonists are given in Chapter 16. This drug is pregnancy category B.

Calcium Channel Blockers: Class IV

37.10 Calcium channel blockers are used to treat atrial dysrhythmias.

Although about 10 CCBs are available to treat cardiovascular disease, only a limited number are approved for dysrhythmias. Review Chapter 30 for details regarding the mechanism of actions, indications, and nursing responsibilities for this drug class. Only actions relevant to dysrhythmias are discussed in this section. The antidysrhythmic CCBs are listed in Table 37.4.

Blockade of calcium ion channels has a number of effects on the heart, which are very similar to those of beta-adrenergic blockers. Effects include reduced automaticity in the SA node and slowed impulse conduction through the AV node. These effects are predictable, because nodal tissues are more dependent on calcium channels than other areas of the myocardium. This slows the heart rate and prolongs the refractory period. On an ECG, the most prominent effect of CCBs is prolongation of the PR interval. Indications include the control of ventricular rate in cases of atrial flutter or fibrillation, and prophylaxis of PSVT. CCBs are only effective against atrial dysrhythmias.

CCBs are safe medications that are well tolerated by most patients. As with many other antidysrhythmics, patients should be carefully monitored for bradycardia and hypotension. Because their cardiac effects are almost identical to those of beta-adrenergic blockers, patients concurrently taking drugs from both classes are especially at risk for bradycardia and possible HF. Because older adults often have multiple cardiovascular disorders, such as HTN, HF, and dysrhythmias, it is not unusual to find elderly patients taking drugs from multiple classes.

CONNECTION Checkpoint 37.3

Nifedipine (Procardia) is a prototype CCB discussed in Chapter 30. From what you learned in Chapter 30, why is this drug (and other dihydropyridines) not effective in treating dysrhythmias? *See Answer to Connection Checkpoint 37.3 on student resource website.*

Diltiazem (Cardizem, Dilacor, Taztia XR, Tiazac): Like other CCBs, diltiazem inhibits the transport of calcium into myocardial cells. The actions and indications for diltiazem are the same as those of verapamil. The IV form of the drug is indicated for the management of acute atrial dysrhythmias, including paroxysmal supraventricular tachycardia. In addition to its use in treating and preventing atrial dysrhythmias, the oral forms are indicated for HTN as well as stable and vasospastic angina. Adverse effects of diltiazem are generally not serious and are related to vasodilation: headache, dizziness, and edema of the ankles and feet. Because of its profound depressant effects on nodal tissue, diltiazem is contraindicated in patients with severe bradycardia, AV block, or sick sinus syndrome. Concurrent use of diltiazem with digoxin or beta-adrenergic blockers may cause partial or complete heart block, HF, or dysrhythmias.

Verapamil (Calan, Isoptin SR, Verelan): Verapamil was the first CCB approved by the FDA. In the heart, verapamil slows conduction

velocity and stabilizes dysrhythmias. The IV form of the drug is indicated for the rapid control of acute atrial dysrhythmias. Because verapamil can cause bradycardia and AV block, patients with HF should be carefully monitored. Because the drug may produce profound bradycardia, patients should notify their health care provider if their heart rate falls below 60 beats/minute or if systolic blood pressure falls below 90 mmHg. The therapeutic serum level is 0.08 to 0.3 mcg/mL. A prototype drug feature that describes other indications for verapamil is presented in Chapter 30.

PharmFACT

Sudden cardiac arrest (SCA), also called sudden cardiac death, is usually caused by ventricular fibrillation (VF). VF is commonly the first expression of coronary artery disease and is responsible for about 50% of deaths from CAD, often within the first hour after the onset of an acute myocardial infarction. The mortality rate is as high as 95% (Goyal, 2014).

Miscellaneous Antidysrhythmics

37.11 Adenosine and digoxin are used for specific dysrhythmias.

Two other medications, adenosine and digoxin, are occasionally used to treat specific dysrhythmias, but they do not act by the mechanisms described above. Doses for these miscellaneous drugs are listed in Table 37.4.

Adenosine (Adenocard, Adenoscan): Adenosine is a naturally occurring nucleoside that activates potassium channels in the SA and AV nodes, causing the potassium to leave cardiac muscle cells. When given as a rapid 1- to 2-second IV bolus, adenosine blocks reentry pathways in the AV node and terminates the tachycardia. It is usually followed by a 1- to 5-second period of asystole. Patients should be laid supine prior to adenosine use, and warned that they may feel faint. The IV site used to give adenosine should be antecubital or above, and an 18-gauge angiocatheter or larger should be used. A rapid saline flush immediately after instillation of the medication is necessary due to its short half-life. Immediate medical assistance must be nearby during the procedure. If the tachycardia has not been eliminated in 1 to 2 minutes, a second rapid bolus may be given. The primary indication for adenosine is PSVT, for which it is a drug of choice. It is also used to assist in the diagnosis of coronary artery disease of dysrhythmias in patients who are unable to undergo a cardiac exercise stress test. It is not effective in treating ventricular dysrhythmias. Although the drug has prodysrhythmic effects and dyspnea is common, adverse effects are generally self-limiting because of its 10-second half-life. In 2013, the FDA issued a safety alert that the use of adenosine may be associated with an increased risk of heart attack and death. This drug is pregnancy category C.

Digoxin (Lanoxin, Lanoxicaps): Although digoxin is primarily used to treat HF, it is also prescribed for atrial flutter or fibrillation and PSVT because of its ability to decrease automaticity of the SA node and slow conduction through the AV node. The drug is not effective against ventricular dysrhythmias. Because excessive levels of digoxin can produce serious dysrhythmias, and interactions with other medications are common, patients must be carefully monitored during therapy. Additional information on the mechanism of action, adverse effects, and nursing responsibilities for digoxin may be found in Chapter 36, where the drug is featured as a prototype.

CONNECTIONS: NURSING PRACTICE APPLICATION

Patients Receiving Pharmacotherapy for Dysrhythmias

Assessment	Potential Nursing Diagnoses*
Baseline assessment prior to administration: • Obtain a complete health history including cardiovascular (including previous dysrhythmias, HTN, MI, HF), and the possibility of pregnancy. Obtain a drug history including allergies, current prescription and over-the-counter (OTC) drugs, herbal preparations, and alcohol use. Be alert to possible drug interactions. • Obtain baseline weight, vital signs (especially blood pressure and pulse), ECG (rate and rhythm), cardiac monitoring (such as cardiac output if appropriate), and breath sounds. Assess for location, character, and amount of edema, if present. • Evaluate appropriate laboratory findings: electrolytes, especially potassium, calcium and magnesium levels, renal and liver function studies, and lipid profiles. • Assess the patient's ability to receive and understand instructions. Include the family and caregivers as needed.	• *Decreased Cardiac Output* • *Anxiety* • *Fatigue* • *Activity Intolerance* • *Sexual Dysfunction* • *Deficient Knowledge* (Drug Therapy) • *Risk for Decreased Cardiac Tissue Perfusion* • *Risk for Injury, related to hypotension or dizziness associated with dysrhythmias or to adverse effects of drug therapy* • *Risk for Falls, related to hypotension or dizziness associated with dysrhythmias or to adverse effects of drug therapy*
Assessment throughout administration: • Assess for desired therapeutic effects (e.g., control or elimination of dysrhythmia, blood pressure and pulse within established limits). • Continue frequent monitoring of ECG (continuous if hospitalized). Check pulse quality, volume, and regularity, along with ECG. Assess for complaints of palpitations and correlate symptoms with ECG findings. Assess for changes in LOC. • Continue periodic monitoring of electrolytes, especially potassium and magnesium. • Assess for adverse effects: lightheadedness or dizziness, hypotension, nausea, vomiting, headache, fatigue or weakness, flushing, sexual dysfunction, or impotence. Immediately report bradycardia, tachycardia, or new or different dysrhythmias to the health care provider.	

Implementation

Interventions and (Rationales)	Patient-Centered Care
Ensuring therapeutic effects: • Continue frequent assessments as above for therapeutic effects. (Dysrhythmias have diminished or are eliminated. Blood pressure and pulse should be within normal limits or within parameters set by the health care provider.)	• To alleviate possible anxiety, teach the patient, family, or caregiver the rationale for all equipment used and the need for frequent monitoring.
• Encourage appropriate lifestyle changes: lowered fat intake, increased exercise, limited alcohol intake, limited caffeine intake, and smoking cessation. Provide for dietitian consultation as needed. (Healthy lifestyle changes will support and minimize the need for drug therapy.)	• Encourage the patient and family to adopt a healthy lifestyle of low-fat food choices, increased exercise, reduced caffeine intake, decreased alcohol consumption, and smoking cessation.
Minimizing adverse effects: • Continue to monitor ECG and pulse for quality and volume. Take the pulse for 1 full minute to assess for regularity. Continue to assess for complaints of palpitations and correlate palpitations or pulse irregularities with the ECG. (Not all dysrhythmias are symptomatic. Correlating symptoms with an ECG may help determine the need for further symptom management. **Diverse Patients:** Because of differences in acetylation and because some antidysrhythmics metabolize through the P450 pathways, monitor ethnically diverse patients more frequently to ensure optimal therapeutic effects and to minimize adverse effects.)	• Teach the patient, family, or caregiver how to take a peripheral pulse for 1 full minute before taking the drug. Assist the patient to find the pulse area most convenient and easily felt. Record daily pulse rates and regularity, and bring the record to each health care visit. Instruct the patient to notify the provider if the pulse is below 60 or above 100 beats/min, there is a noticeable change in regularity from previously felt pulse rate, or if palpitations develop or worsen.
• Take the blood pressure lying, sitting, and standing to detect orthostatic hypotension. **Lifespan:** Be particularly cautious with the first few doses of the drug and with the older adult who is at increased risk for hypotension. (Antidysrhythmic drugs may cause hypotension. A first-dose effect may occur with a significant drop in blood pressure with the first few doses. Orthostatic hypotension may increase the risk of falls and injury.)	• Teach the patient to rise from lying or sitting to standing slowly to avoid dizziness or falls. If dizziness occurs, the patient should sit or lie down and not attempt to stand or walk until the sensation passes. • Instruct the patient to take the first dose of the new prescription in the evening before bed if possible, and to be cautious during the next few doses until the drug effects are known. • Teach the patient, family, or caregiver how to monitor blood pressure if required. Ensure proper use and functioning of any home equipment obtained. • Instruct the patient to notify the health care provider if blood pressure is 90/60 mmHg or below, or below the parameters set by the health care provider.
• Continue to monitor periodic electrolyte levels, especially potassium, calcium, and magnesium, renal function laboratory values, and drug levels as needed. (Hypokalemia, hypocalcemia, and hypomagnesemia increase the risk of dysrhythmias. Inadequate or high levels of antidysrhythmic drugs may lead to increased or more lethal dysrhythmias.)	• Instruct the patient on the need to return periodically for laboratory work. • Advise the patient to carry a wallet identification card or wear medical identification jewelry indicating antidysrhythmic therapy.

CONNECTIONS: NURSING PRACTICE APPLICATION (continued)

• Weigh the patient daily and report weight gain or loss of 1 kg (2 lb) or more in a 24-h period. Continue to assess for edema, noting location and character. (Daily weight is an accurate measure of fluid status and takes into account intake, output, and insensible losses. Weight gain or edema may indicate adverse drug effects or worsening cardiovascular disease processes.)	• Have the patient weigh self daily, ideally at the same time of day, and record weight along with pulse measurements. Have the patient report weight loss or gain of more than 1 kg (2 lb) in a 24-h period.
• Monitor for breath sounds and heart sounds (e.g., increasing dyspnea or postural nocturnal dyspnea, rales or crackles in lungs, frothy pink-tinged sputum, murmurs, or extra heart sounds) and report immediately. (Increasing lung congestion or new or worsening heart murmurs may indicate impending HF. Potassium channel blockers are associated with pulmonary toxicity.)	• Instruct the patient to immediately report any severe shortness of breath, frothy sputum, profound fatigue, or swelling of extremities as possible signs of HF or pulmonary toxicity.
• Report any visual changes, skin rashes, or unusual sunburn to the health care provider. (Potassium channel blockers may cause photosensitivity, skin rashes, and blurred vision.)	• Teach the patient to report any visual changes promptly and to maintain regular eye examinations. • Teach the patient about the importance of wearing protective clothing and applying sunscreen regularly during periods of sun exposure.
• **Lifespan**: Assess for the possibility of pregnancy before beginning the drug. (Some antidysrhythmics such as amiodarone are pregnancy category D drugs and should not be used during pregnancy.)	• Instruct female patients who may be considering pregnancy, or are pregnant or breast-feeding, to notify their provider before starting the drug.
Patient understanding of drug therapy: • Use opportunities during administration of medications and during assessments to discuss the rationale for the drug therapy, desired therapeutic outcomes, commonly observed adverse effects, parameters for when to call the health care provider, and any necessary monitoring or precautions. (Using time during nursing care helps to optimize and reinforce key teaching areas.)	• The patient, family, or caregiver should be able to state the reason for the drug, appropriate dose and scheduling, what adverse effects to observe for and when to report them, equipment needed as appropriate and how to use that equipment, and the required length of medication therapy needed, with any special instructions regarding renewing or continuing the prescription as appropriate.
Patient self-administration of drug therapy: • When administering medications, instruct the patient, family, or caregiver in proper self-administration techniques. (Utilizing time during nurse-administration of these drugs helps to reinforce teaching.)	• Teach the patient to take drugs as evenly spaced apart as possible and not to double dose if a dose is missed. • Teach the patient, family, or caregiver not to stop the medication abruptly, and to call the health care provider if the patient is unable to take the medication for more than one day due to illness.

*Nursing Diagnoses—Definitions and Classification 2015–2017. Copyright © 2014, 1994–2014 by NANDA International. Used by arrangement with John Wiley & Sons Limited.

CHAPTER
37

Understanding the Chapter

Key Concepts Summary

37.1 Some dysrhythmias produce no patient symptoms, while others may be life threatening.

37.2 The phases of cardiac action potential include rapid depolarization, a long plateau, and repolarization.

37.3 The electrocardiogram is used to measure electrical conduction across the myocardium.

37.4 Dysrhythmias are classified by the impulse origin and type of rhythm abnormality produced.

37.5 Antidysrhythmic drugs are only used when there is a clear benefit to the patient.

37.6 Antidysrhythmic drugs are classified by their mechanism of action.

37.7 Class I antidysrhythmics act by blocking ion channels in myocardial cells.

37.8 Beta-adrenergic antagonists reduce automaticity as well as slow conduction velocity in the heart.

37.9 Potassium channel blockers prolong the refractory period of the heart.

37.10 Calcium channel blockers are used to treat atrial dysrhythmias.

37.11 Adenosine and digoxin are used for specific dysrhythmias.

Case Study: Making the Patient Connection

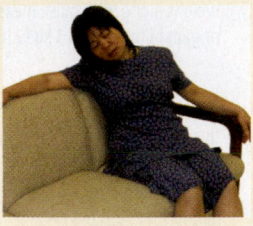

Remember the patient "Jada Chinn Nguyen" at the beginning of the chapter? Now read the remainder of the case study. Based on the information presented within this chapter, respond to the critical thinking questions that follow.

The day had been busy as Jada prepared for her daughter's upcoming wedding. There were so many arrangements to be made, and Jada felt overwhelmed. During the day she experienced heaviness in her chest, but she attributed it to the stress of the wedding and perhaps a touch of bronchitis. Nonetheless, she knew there was no time to stop and rest; there was too much to do.

Later that afternoon, she realized that she had to take it easy. Then she experienced that strange sensation once again. As she sat in a chair, Jada suddenly felt dizzy with extreme weakness and difficulty breathing. Her family members report that she became pale and unexpectedly collapsed. Emergency personnel were called to the scene, and Jada was taken to the nearest hospital.

In the emergency department, Jada's physical examination revealed the following findings: weak, middle-aged Asian female; vital signs: blood pressure 102/68 mmHg, heart rate 116 beats/min, respiratory rate 18 breaths/min, afebrile; weight 53 kg (116 lb). She has clear bilateral breath sounds and active bowel sounds heard in all four quadrants. Her ECG reveals atrial fibrillation with a ventricular rate of 116 beats/min. She is admitted to the coronary care unit for further testing and observation.

Critical Thinking Questions

1. Jada's ECG shows atrial fibrillation. Trace the electrical conduction system through the heart. What part of the ECG complex would be most affected with this patient's medical diagnosis?

2. While in the coronary care unit, Jada will receive amiodarone (Cordarone) IV infusion. She wants to know how long she will need to receive the IV medication and how it works. How would you respond to this patient's questions?

3. The patient is being discharged on amiodarone 400 mg twice daily. What instructions should this patient receive?

4. List any drug–food interaction concerns you should discuss with Jada.

See Answers to Critical Thinking Questions on student resource website.

Additional Case Study

Malcolm Hibbert is a 56-year-old man who was diagnosed with a rapid atrial dysrhythmia and placed on diltiazem (Cardizem) to control the condition. He has been surfing the Internet to find out more about his condition and drug therapy. When he returns to the clinic, he has multiple questions to ask you. How would you respond to each of the following?

1. "My neighbor had a fast heartbeat and now he's on something called digoxin. Why didn't they use that for me?"

2. "If I'm on a calcium channel blocker, does that mean my bones might get weak?"

3. "Might any of my medications cause an increase in dysrhythmias?"

See Answers to Additional Case Study on student resource website.

Chapter Review

1 A health care provider has ordered procainamide for each of four patients. A nurse should question the order for a patient with which condition?

1. Ventricular tachycardia
2. Paroxysmal atrial tachycardia
3. Atrial fibrillation
4. Severe heart failure

2 A patient is receiving intravenous lidocaine for ventricular dysrhythmias. Which nursing intervention is appropriate for this therapy?

1. Monitor the patient for decreased platelet levels.
2. Place the patient in a supine position during administration.
3. Monitor for paresthesias, drowsiness, or confusion.
4. Encourage coughing and deep breathing to remove secretions.

3 The patient with a rapid atrial dysrhythmia is being treated with verapamil (Calan). The nurse would monitor for therapeutic effectiveness by noting which of the following?

1. Change in the blood pressure
2. Increase in the serum potassium level
3. Changes in the cardiac rhythm
4. Reduction in the urine output

4 A patient is to receive adenosine (Adenocard) for rapid supraventricular tachycardia. This drug must be administered:

1. Over a 24-hour period by IV drip.
2. Along with potassium chloride to prevent electrolyte imbalance.
3. Over 20 to 30 minutes IV.
4. By a rapid IV bolus injection over 1 to 2 seconds.

5. The patient is prescribed propranolol (Inderal) for the treatment of atrial dysrhythmias associated with heart failure. The nurse knows this drug is used cautiously in patients with heart failure because of which effect?

   1. It causes sodium retention, worsening congestion.

   2. Its adverse effects include hypertension, worsening heart failure.

   3. It is a negative inotropic drug and will decrease myocardial contractility and cardiac output.

   4. It may cause bronchoconstriction.

6. A patient is being discharged with a diagnosis of dysrhythmias. The nurse is teaching the patient about amiodarone (Cordarone). What patient teaching is needed related to this medication?

   1. Avoid crowds while taking this medication.

   2. Avoid birth control pills and use an alternate form of birth control.

   3. Wear protective clothing and adequate sunscreen.

   4. Use an electric razor to shave.

See Answers to Chapter Review in Appendix A.

References

Goyal, S. K. (2014). *Ventricular fibrillation*. Retrieved from http://emedicine.medscape.com/article/158712-overview

Kaneko, M., Yoshihara, A., & Miyazaki, H. (2011). Relationship between root caries and cardiac dysrhythmia. *Gerodontology, 28,* 289–295. doi:10.1111/j.1741-2358.2010.00367.x

National Heart, Lung, and Blood Institute. (2011). *What is long QT syndrome?* Retrieved from http://www.nhlbi.nih.gov/health/dci/Diseases/qt/qt_whatis.html

Selected Bibliography

Antzelevitch, C., & Burashnikov, A. (2011). Overview of basic mechanisms of cardiac arrhythmia. *Cardiac Electrophysiology Clinics, 3*(1), 23–45. doi:10.1016/j.ccep.2010.10.012

Atwood, S., Stanton, C., & Storey-Davenport, J. (2011). *Introduction to basic cardiac dysrhythmias*. Burlington, MA: Jones & Bartlett.

Brenyo, A., & Aktas, M. K. (2013). Review of complementary and alternative medical treatment of arrhythmias. *The American Journal of Cardiology, 113,* 897–903. doi:10.1016/j.amjcard.2013.11.044

Dagres, N., Sommer, P., Anastasiou-Nana, M., & Hindricks, G. (2011). Treating arrhythmias: An expert opinion. *Expert Opinion on Pharmacotherapy, 12,* 1359–1367. doi:10.1517/14656566.2011.555397

Herdman, T. H., & Kamitsuru, S. (Eds.). (2014). *NANDA International nursing diagnoses: Definitions and classification, 2015–2017*. Oxford, United Kingdom: Wiley-Blackwell.

Ismail, H., & Lewin, R. J. (2013). The role of a new arrhythmia specialist nurse in providing support to patients and caregivers. *European Journal of Cardiovascular Nursing, 12,* 177–183. doi:10.1177/1474515112442446

Knapp, E., & Watson, K. (2011). Medication management of atrial fibrillation: Emerging therapies for rhythm control and stroke prevention. *Pharmacy and Therapeutics, 36,* 518–528.

National Heart, Lung, and Blood Institute. (2011). *What is sudden cardiac arrest?* Retrieved from http://www.nhlbi.nih.gov/health/health-topics/topics/scda/

Sampson, K. J., & Kaas, R. S. (2011). Antiarrhythmic drugs. In L. L. Brunton, B. A. Chabner, & B. C. Knollman (Eds.), *The pharmacological basis of therapeutics* (12th ed., pp. 815–848). New York, NY: McGraw-Hill.

Sullivan, S. D., Orme, M. E., Morais, E., & Mitchell, S. A. (2013). Interventions for the treatment of atrial fibrillation: A systematic literature review and meta-analysis. *International Journal of Cardiology, 165,* 229–236. doi:10.1016/j.ijcard.2012.03.070

Tsiperfall, A., Ottoboni, L. K., Beheiry, S., Al-Ahmad, A., Natale, A., & Wang, P. (2011). *Cardiac arrhythmia management: A practical guide for nurses and allied professionals*. Ames, IA: Wiley-Blackwell.

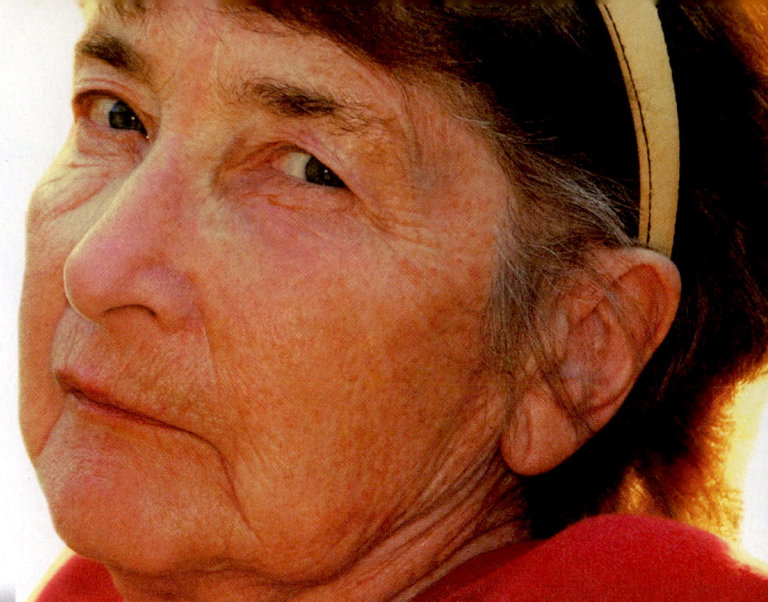

"Ever since I returned from my trip to Bangkok, my right calf has really hurt. I first thought my arthritis was flaring up again, especially after sitting on the plane for so long."

Patient "Ruby Dwyer"

38 Pharmacotherapy of Coagulation Disorders

LEARNING OUTCOMES

After reading this chapter, the student should be able to:

1. Describe primary risk factors for thromboembolic disorders.

2. Explain the etiology and symptoms of coagulation disorders.

3. Identify the primary mechanisms by which coagulation-modifying drugs act.

4. Explain how laboratory testing of coagulation parameters is used to monitor anticoagulant pharmacotherapy.

5. Describe the nurse's role in the pharmacologic management of patients with coagulation disorders.

6. For each of the classes shown in the chapter outline, identify the prototype and representative drugs and explain the mechanism(s) of drug action, primary indications, contraindications, significant drug interactions, pregnancy category, and important adverse effects.

7. Apply the nursing process to care for patients receiving pharmacotherapy for coagulation disorders.

CHAPTER OUTLINE

▶ **Disorders of Hemostasis**

▶ **Overview of Coagulation Modifiers**

▶ **Anticoagulants**
   PROTOTYPE Heparin, *p. 619*
   PROTOTYPE Warfarin (Coumadin), *p. 621*
   Direct Thrombin Inhibitors
   PROTOTYPE Dabigatran (Pradaxa), *p. 623*

▶ **Antiplatelet Drugs**
   Aspirin
   Adenosine Diphosphate Receptor Blockers
   PROTOTYPE Clopidogrel (Plavix), *p. 627*
   Glycoprotein IIb/IIIa Receptor Inhibitors
   PROTOTYPE Abciximab (ReoPro), *p. 629*

▶ **Drugs for Intermittent Claudication**

▶ **Thrombolytics**
   PROTOTYPE Alteplase (Activase), *p. 632*

▶ **Hemostatics**
   PROTOTYPE Aminocaproic Acid (Amicar), *p. 635*

▶ **Drugs for Hemophilia**

KEY TERMS

activated partial thromboplastin
time (aPTT), 617

anticoagulants, 615

antithrombin III (AT-III), 618

deep venous thrombosis (DVT), 615

fibrinolysis, 631

glycoprotein IIb/IIIa, 629

hemophilia, 616

hemostasis, 615

intermittent claudication (IC), 630

plasminogen, 631

procoagulants, 615

prothrombin time (PT), 617

pulmonary embolism, 615

thrombocytopenia, 616

thromboembolic disorder, 615

venous thromboembolism (VTE), 615

von Willebrand's disease (vWD), 638

Everyone is familiar with the bleeding associated with simple cuts and scrapes, and we take for granted that bleeding will stop in a few minutes. The stoppage of blood flow, or **hemostasis**, is complex and essential to our well-being. The underlying mechanisms of hemostasis promote blood clotting that protects us from injuries that could lead to shock and perhaps death. Too much clotting, however, can be just as dangerous. The physiological processes of hemostasis must maintain a delicate balance between blood fluidity and coagulation.

Many common diseases and conditions affect hemostasis, including myocardial infarction (MI), stroke, venous or arterial thrombosis, valvular heart disease, and indwelling catheters. Because these conditions are so prevalent in clinical practice, nurses will have frequent occasions to administer and monitor the effects of coagulation-modifying medications. Drugs may be used to enhance coagulation, inhibit coagulation, or dissolve existing clots to restore blood flow.

Disorders of Hemostasis

38.1 Thromboembolic disorders are abnormalities of hemostasis that include deep venous thrombosis and pulmonary embolism.

Coagulation is regulated by a large number of natural substances circulating in the blood. Some of these are **procoagulants**, which favor the formation of clots, while others are **anticoagulants**, which inhibit clot formation. Coagulation, then, can be thought of as a delicate balance between procoagulants and anticoagulants. For example, injuries to blood vessels release procoagulants that tip the balance in favor of initiating coagulation. The student should review the coagulation cascade presented in Chapter 28 before proceeding.

Once a stationary clot, or thrombus, forms in a vessel, it often grows larger as more fibrin is added. Pieces of the thrombus may break off and travel in the bloodstream to block other vessels. A traveling clot is called an *embolus*. Because these two conditions often occur concurrently in patients, the term **thromboembolic disorder** is used to describe conditions in which the body forms undesirable clots. Thromboembolic disorders may be classified as either venous or arterial.

Venous thromboembolism (VTE) is a common disease that occurs when blood flow through a vein is very slow (stasis). Venous stasis allows procoagulation factors to accumulate and overcome the natural anticoagulant substances in the blood. There are two manifestations of VTE: deep venous thrombosis and pulmonary embolism.

When thrombosis occurs in the legs it is called **deep venous thrombosis (DVT)**. Because blood flow is slowest in the deep veins of the lower limbs, these vessels are the most common sites for VTE. Conditions associated with venous stasis and DVT include the following:

- **Extended immobility.** During major illness or following surgery, patients may be supine or otherwise immobile for extended periods of time. Because the movement of blood through the deep veins is entirely dependent on the squeezing action from skeletal muscular contraction, blood in the deep veins of these patients has difficulty returning to the heart.

- **Major trauma.** Trauma often causes serious bleeding that activates procoagulation factors. In addition, stasis will likely occur surrounding the injured area, promoting the development of DVT. Trauma involving the lower extremities places the patient at high risk for DVT.

- **Major surgery.** Surgery of the lower extremities, especially knee and hip replacements, are common causes of DVT for the same reasons as trauma; bleeding activates procoagulation factors and stasis occurs around the surgical site.

- **Hypercoagulability states.** Malignancy, lupus, and pregnancy are examples of conditions associated with an increased risk of coagulation and DVT. Certain genetic disorders also produce hypercoagulability, the most common being a genetic deficiency of protein C, a natural anticoagulant.

- **Drug therapy.** High amounts of estrogen, prescribed as replacement therapy or as a component of oral contraceptives, have been associated with DVT in numerous studies. Selective estrogen receptor modulators (SERMs), such as raloxifene (Evista), are also associated with a higher risk of DVT.

The second primary thromboembolic disorder is **pulmonary embolism**, which occurs when a venous clot dislodges, migrates to the pulmonary vessels, and blocks arterial circulation to the lungs. Pulmonary emboli are the most serious consequence of VTE because death may occur within minutes after the onset of symptoms. The factors associated with an increased risk of pulmonary embolism are the same as those for patients with DVT: prolonged immobility, major trauma, lower extremity surgery, hypercoagulability states, and estrogen therapy. Prevention of pulmonary embolism is a primary goal for all patients with VTE and a major indication for pharmacotherapy.

Patients with DVT are sometimes asymptomatic, or report nonspecific symptoms such as pain, swelling, or warmth of the legs. The disorder may be present for years, causing progressive damage to venous valves, thus worsening blood flow in the region and increasing the risk of an acute episode. A pulmonary embolism, however, produces a sudden onset of cough, chest pain, tachypnea, dyspnea, tachycardia, and hemoptysis. Symptoms of pulmonary embolism resemble an MI, and rapid diagnosis and treatment are essential.

PharmFACT

Up to 30% of patients presenting with venous thrombosis have a malignancy. This is because about 90% of patients with cancer have some abnormal clotting factors (Patel, 2014).

Arterial thromboembolism may deprive an area of blood flow and is a medical emergency because tissue hypoxia and cellular death will result soon after blood stoppage. The most serious arterial thromboembolism disorders are MI and stroke.

Arterial thrombi and emboli commonly result from procedures involving arterial punctures such as angiography and stent placement. They may also originate from the heart. Emboli are common complications of mitral valve disease, prosthetic heart valves, and atrial dysrhythmias. Emboli originating from the left side of the heart may lodge in any organ in the body.

CONNECTION Checkpoint 38.1

Coagulation occurs by intrinsic and extrinsic pathways. From what you learned in Chapter 28, which pathway is activated when blood leaks from a vessel? Which is more complex and takes several minutes? Which results in the formation of fibrin? *See Answer to Connection Checkpoint 38.1 on student resource website.*

38.2 Coagulation disorders are caused by decreased numbers of platelets or by deficiencies in specific clotting factors.

Whereas thromboembolic disorders are caused by too much clotting, coagulation disorders result from too little clotting. Serious consequences result if the body does not form clots in a timely manner. The two most common etiologies of coagulation disorders are decreased numbers of platelets and deficiencies in one or more clotting factors.

Platelets are central to the process of coagulation. Recognizing a site of vessel injury, activated platelets release von Willebrand factor, which causes platelets to become "sticky" and adhere to the site. Following adhesion, platelets secrete substances such as adenosine diphosphate (ADP) and thromboxane A_2 that promote platelet aggregation and the formation of a platelet plug at the site. Procoagulation factors become activated on the platelets and a fibrin mesh clot results. Nearly every step of this pathway requires sufficient numbers of properly functioning platelets.

The most common coagulation disorder is a deficiency of platelets, or **thrombocytopenia**, which occurs when platelet counts fall below 150,000 mm^3. Thrombocytopenia is the result of either decreased platelet production or increased platelet destruction. Any condition or disease that suppresses bone marrow function has the potential to cause decreased platelet production. Other common causes of decreased platelet production are folic acid or vitamin B_{12} deficiencies and decreased production of thrombopoietin by the liver during hepatic failure. Increased destruction of platelets may occur in patients with thrombocytopenic purpura, disseminated intravascular coagulation (DIC), or lupus.

Of special concern is thrombocytopenia caused by drug therapy. A significant number of drugs have the potential to increase platelet destruction, either by direct toxic effects on bone marrow or by inducing the immune system to destroy them. When caring for patients receiving these drugs, the nurse must be vigilant in assessing the results of blood laboratory tests and observing for signs of thrombocytopenia such as bleeding gums, nosebleeds, and extensive bruising. Selected drugs that cause thrombocytopenia are listed in Table 38.1. Heparin-induced thrombocytopenia, a particularly serious form of this disorder, is discussed in Section 38.4.

Deficiencies in specific clotting factors may prolong coagulation and lead to excess bleeding. Deficiencies in multiple coagulation factors occur frequently in patients with serious hepatic impairment, because the liver synthesizes most clotting factors. Deficiency in a single coagulation factor suggests **hemophilia**: a series of coagulation disorders caused by genetic deficiencies in specific clotting factors. Hemophilia disorders are typified by prolonged coagulation times, resulting in persistent bleeding that can be acute or chronic. Patients may experience various forms of the disease, with symptoms ranging from mild to severe. Approximately two thirds of patients with hemophilia will report a family history of the disease. The pharmacotherapy of hemophilia is described in Section 38.14.

To diagnose coagulation and thromboembolic disorders, a thorough medical history and physical examination are necessary. Laboratory tests measuring coagulation must be obtained. These

TABLE 38.1   Selected Drugs That Cause Thrombocytopenia

Class	Examples
Analgesics	acetaminophen, aspirin, diclofenac, ibuprofen, indomethacin, morphine, naproxen
Anticoagulants and antiplatelets	heparin, clopidogrel, glycoprotein IIb/IIIa inhibitors
Anti-infectives	acyclovir, amphotericin B, ampicillin, clarithromycin, ethambutol, fluconazole, indinavir, isoniazid, itraconazole, linezolid, oxacillin, piperacillin, rifampin, sulfonamides, trimethoprim, vancomycin
Antineoplastic and immunotherapy drugs	carboplatin, interferon-alfa, methotrexate
Cardiovascular drugs	atorvastatin, captopril, digoxin, hydrochlorothiazide, inamrinone, nitroglycerin, procainamide, quinidine, simvastatin
Central nervous system drugs	carbamazepine, chlorpromazine, diazepam, haloperidol, lithium, phenobarbital, phenytoin, valproic acid
Other drug classes	cimetidine, isotretinoin, MMR vaccine, octreotide, ranitidine, sirolimus

usually include a whole-blood clotting time, **prothrombin time (PT)**, thrombin time, **activated partial thromboplastin time (aPTT)**, liver functions tests, platelet count, and, in some instances, a bleeding time. Additional tests, such as serum levels of specific clotting factors, may be indicated, based on the results of these laboratory analyses.

Overview of Coagulation Modifiers

38.3 The normal coagulation process can be modified by a number of different mechanisms.

Medications can be used to modify hemostasis in a number of ways. An overview of the basic mechanisms of coagulation-modifying drugs is presented in Table 38.2. These mechanisms are illustrated in Figure 38.1.

The most commonly prescribed coagulation modifiers are the anticoagulants, which are used to prevent clot formation. Patients usually call these drugs "blood thinners," which is an inaccurate description because they do not change the viscosity or thickness of the blood. Drugs may accomplish clot prevention by the following mechanisms:

- Inhibition of specific clotting factors in the coagulation cascade: examples include heparin and warfarin (Coumadin)
- Inhibition of the clotting action of platelets: examples include aspirin and clopidogrel (Plavix)

Regardless of the mechanism, all anticoagulant medications will increase the normal time the body takes to form clots. Anticoagulants are widely used for thromboembolic disease and are discussed in Sections 38.4 through 38.6.

Once an abnormal clot has formed, it may block blood vessels that serve critical tissues and it must be quickly removed to restore normal function. This is particularly important for vessels serving the heart, lungs, and brain. A specific class of drugs, the thrombolytics, has been developed to dissolve life-threatening clots. These drugs are presented in Section 38.12.

Coagulation modifiers are also used to promote the formation of clots. Drugs called hemostatics inhibit the normal removal of

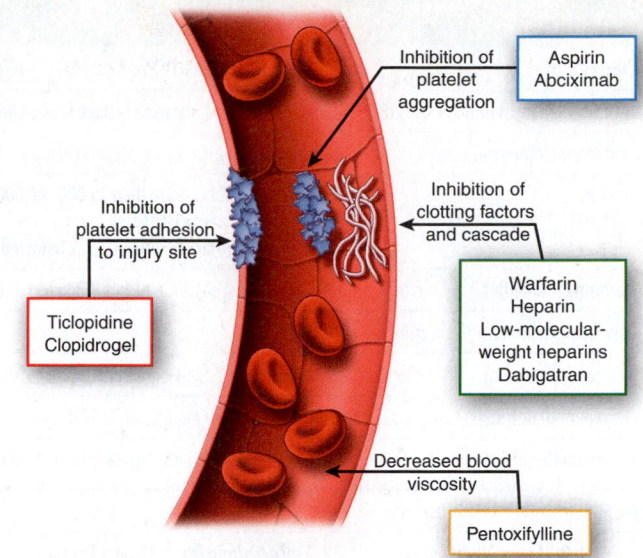

Figure 38.1 Mechanisms of action of coagulation modifiers.

fibrin, thus keeping the clot in place for a longer period of time. These drugs are primarily used to speed clot formation to limit bleeding from a surgical site, and are discussed in Section 38.12. For patients with hemophilia, clotting factors may be administered to promote clotting by providing a missing or deficient component in the coagulation cascade, as presented in Section 38.13.

Since hemostasis involves a fine balance of factors favoring clotting versus those inhibiting clotting, pharmacotherapy with coagulation modifiers is individualized to each patient. Serious adverse effects may occur if the drugs are not used properly; therefore, these patients will require frequent assessment and monitoring to ensure that the goal of normal coagulation is being achieved, without serious adverse events.

Anticoagulants

38.4 Heparin is the traditional drug of choice for rapid anticoagulation.

Extensively used in the treatment of thromboembolic disease, anticoagulants lengthen clotting time and prevent thrombi from forming or growing larger. Since thromboembolic disease can be life threatening, therapy is often begun by administering anticoagulants parenterally to achieve the most rapid onset of action. As the disease stabilizes and the desired degree of anticoagulation has been achieved, the patient is gradually switched to oral anticoagulants, with careful monitoring of appropriate coagulation laboratory values. Traditionally, the most frequently prescribed parenteral anticoagulant has been heparin; warfarin is the most common oral anticoagulant (see Section 38.5). The anticoagulants are listed in Table 38.3.

Heparin is a natural chemical found in the liver and the lining of blood vessels. As a drug, heparin has been used for many decades and is one of the few drugs still obtained from animal tissue, usually beef lung or pig intestine. Chemically, heparin is a special type of carbohydrate called a glycosaminoglycan that consists of repeated disaccharide units of differing lengths. Thus,

TABLE 38.2	Overview of Coagulation Modifiers	
Type of Modification	**Mechanism**	**Drug Classification**
Prevention of clot formation	Inhibition of specific clotting factors	Anticoagulants
	Inhibition of platelet actions	Antiplatelet drugs
Removal of an existing clot	Clot dissolved by the drug	Thrombolytics
Promotion of clot formation	Inhibition of fibrin destruction	Hemostatics
	Administration of missing clotting factors	Clotting factor concentrates

TABLE 38.3 Anticoagulants

Drug	Route and Adult Dose (Maximum Dose Where Indicated)	Adverse Effects
antithrombin, recombinant (ATryn)	IV infusion: Dose is individualized based on pretreatment antithrombin level and body weight	*Minor bleeding, nausea, vomiting, transient thrombocytopenia (heparin), anemia (fondaparinux)*
fondaparinux (Arixtra)	Subcutaneous: 2.5 mg/day starting at least 6 h postop for 5–9 days (max: 10 mg/day)	
heparin	IV: 5,000 unit bolus dose, then 20,000–40,000 units infused over 24 h (use agency-specific heparin nomogram) Subcutaneous: 10,000–20,000 units followed by 8,000–20,000 units every 8–12 h	Hemorrhage, anaphylaxis antithrombin, heparin
warfarin (Coumadin)	PO: Dose varies based on target INR, which is usually within the range of 2–3	
Low-Molecular-Weight Heparins (LMWHs)		
dalteparin (Fragmin)	Subcutaneous: 2,500–5,000 units/day for 5–10 days (max: 18,000 international units/day)	*Minor bleeding, nausea, vomiting, hematoma, local pain, fever*
enoxaparin (Lovenox)	Subcutaneous: 30 mg bid for 7–10 days	
tinzaparin (Innohep)	Subcutaneous: 175 units/kg daily for at least 6 days	Hemorrhage, thrombocytopenia, pancytopenia, anaphylaxis
Direct Thrombin Inhibitors		
argatroban (Acova, Novastan)	IV: 2 mcg/kg/min (max: 10 mcg/kg/min)	*Fever, nausea, allergic skin reactions, hepatic impairment, pneumonia, fever, minor bleeding, back pain (bivalirudin)*
bivalirudin (Angiomax)	IV: 0.75 mg/kg initial bolus followed by 1.75 mg/kg/h for 4 h; may continue at 0.2 mg/kg/h up to 20 h	
dabigatran (Pradaxa)	PO: 75–150 mg bid	Serious internal hemorrhage, hemoptysis, hematuria, sepsis, heart failure
desirudin (Iprivask)	Subcutaneous: 15 mg bid for 9–12 days (max: 80 mg/day)	
Factor Xa Inhibitors		
apixaban (Eliquis)	PO: 5 mg bid	*Minor bleeding*
rivaroxaban (Xarelto)	PO: 10–20 mg once daily	Major bleeding, including stroke; hypersensitivity reactions

Note: Italics indicate common adverse effects. Underline indicates serious adverse effects.

heparin is actually a mixture of different molecules, varying in size. This drug is also called unfractionated heparin because it contains a mixture of different molecular pieces or "fractions." This mixture affects protein binding and drug bioavailability and is partially responsible for the wide variation in patient responses to heparin.

Heparin produces its anticoagulant effects by binding to **antithrombin III (AT-III)**. As its name implies, antithrombin inactivates thrombin (as well as several other clotting factors). The binding to heparin produces a structural change in AT-III that makes it 1,000 times more active in inhibiting thrombin, Factor Xa, Factor IXa, and other substances involved in coagulation. Within minutes after intravenous (IV) administration, the loss of these activated clotting factors prevents the formation of fibrin clots.

Because responses to heparin anticoagulation vary considerably among patients, regular monitoring of laboratory values during heparin therapy is essential to patient safety. aPTT is the conventional measurement guiding heparin therapy, with normal values ranging from 25 to 40 seconds. For therapeutic anticoagulation, the aPTT should be between 1.5 and 2 times the patient's baseline, or 60 to 80 seconds. Elevated aPTT values indicate the patient is at high risk for bleeding and that a reduction in heparin dose is necessary. aPTT values of less than 60 seconds indicate the need for higher heparin doses. During continuous IV heparin therapy, the aPTT is measured daily and 6 to 8 hours after any changes in dosage.

Low-molecular-weight heparins: The heparin molecule has been shortened and modified to create a new class of drugs called low-molecular-weight heparins (LMWHs). Given subcutaneously, the mechanism of action of these drugs is very similar to that of heparin, except the shorter heparin molecules are unable to bind thrombin, making them more selective for Factor Xa inhibition. For some applications, the LMWHs have begun to replace traditional heparin anticoagulation.

LMWHs possess the same anticoagulant activity as heparin but have several advantages. They produce a more predictable anticoagulant response than heparin because there is less binding of the drug to proteins and macrophages; therefore, less frequent laboratory monitoring is required. They are about 10 times less likely to cause thrombocytopenia, a potentially serious adverse effect of heparin. They also exhibit a half-life that is two to four times longer than heparin that permits once-daily dosing, and family members or the patient can be trained to give the necessary subcutaneous injections at home. Like heparin, the LMWHs do not cross the placenta. LMWHs have become preferred drugs for a number of clotting disorders, including the prevention of DVT following surgery. One disadvantage is that LMWHs are considerably more expensive than heparin.

When using LMWHs, the aPTT laboratory value does not reflect the anticoagulant effects of the drugs because aPTT is insensitive to changes in Factor Xa. Instead, dosage calculations with LMWHs are fixed and based on the patient's weight. A given amount of subcutaneous LMWH results in a predictable plasma drug level. This is a major advantage over heparin, for which levels continually fluctuate and doses must be adjusted based on aPTT levels. In highly unstable patients or those with renal impairment, measurement of antifactor Xa activity may be used to gauge therapeutic response. Acceptable target values for antifactor Xa range from 0.5 to 1 unit/mL.

PROTOTYPE DRUG | **Heparin**

Classification: **Therapeutic:** Anticoagulant
Pharmacologic: Indirect thrombin inhibitor

Therapeutic Effects and Uses: Heparin is the traditional standard to which other parenteral anticoagulants are compared. Because it has an immediate onset of action when administered IV, heparin is a first-line drug for acute thromboembolic disorders where rapid anticoagulation is necessary. Subcutaneous heparin is injected into the deep fatty layers of the abdomen and may take up to 1 hour to achieve a therapeutic effect. A continuous IV infusion allows for better titration and finer management of aPTT values. Indications include DVT, pulmonary embolism, unstable angina, evolving MI, and prevention of thrombosis in high-risk patients. Heparin and LMWHs are preferred anticoagulants during pregnancy because heparin molecules are too large to cross the placenta. Heparin is also used to maintain the patency of peripheral catheters (heparin locks) and arterial lines.

Heparin prolongs coagulation time, thereby inhibiting excessive clotting within blood vessels. As a result, it prevents the enlargement of existing clots and the formation of new ones. It has no ability to dissolve existing clots. Clotting time is prolonged, although bleeding time is only affected at high doses.

Mechanism of Action: Heparin activates the enzyme antithrombin III, which in turn inhibits thrombin. To a lesser extent, and by a separate mechanism, heparin also inactivates Factor Xa. Other clotting factors are affected by heparin, but these have little clinical significance. High doses interfere with platelet aggregation.

Pharmacokinetics:

Route(s)	Subcutaneous, IV bolus injection, or continuous infusion
Absorption	Heparin is poorly absorbed by the gastrointestinal (GI) mucosa because of rapid metabolism by the hepatic enzyme, heparinase
Distribution	Unknown; does not cross the placenta and is not secreted in breast milk
Primary metabolism	Hepatic and by reticuloendothelial system
Primary excretion	Reticuloendothelial system
Onset of action	Subcutaneous: 30–60 min; IV: immediate
Duration of action	8–12 h; half-life: 90 min

Adverse Effects: Abnormal bleeding is common with heparin therapy, occurring in about 10% of patients, and is the most serious adverse effect. Bleeding may be major or minor and may involve

any system in the body. The risk of bleeding is dose dependent; the higher the dose, the higher the risk. Should the aPTT become excessively prolonged or bleeding be observed, discontinuation of the drug will result in loss of anticoagulant activity within hours. **Black Box Warning:** Epidural or spinal hematomas may occur when heparin or LMWHs are used in patients receiving spinal anesthesia or lumbar puncture. Because these can result in long-term or permanent paralysis, frequent monitoring for neurologic impairment is essential.

Heparin-induced thrombocytopenia (HIT) is a serious complication that occurs in up to 30% of patients taking the drug. Symptoms range from mild to severe. More severe symptoms usually appear after 5 to 10 days of therapy; thus, frequent blood laboratory testing should be conducted during this period. Although thrombocytopenia usually leads to excessive bleeding, HIT causes the opposite effect: an increase in adverse thrombotic events. HIT markedly increases platelet aggregation and the patient may experience serious and even life-threatening thrombosis. Although the half-life of heparin is brief, it may take a week after the drug is discontinued for platelets to recover. In addition, HIT may not even become evident until several weeks after the drug is discontinued.

Because heparin is derived from animal sources, hypersensitivity reactions are possible. Mild allergic symptoms include fever, chills, and urticaria. Anaphylaxis is rare. Osteoporosis has been reported in patients taking the drug longer than 30 days and may be severe enough to cause bone fractures. Skin lesions may develop, especially at the site of parenteral injections.

Contraindications/Precautions: Heparin should not be administered to patients with active internal bleeding, serious bleeding pathologies, severe hypertension (HTN), recent trauma, intracranial hemorrhage, or bacterial endocarditis. Some heparin products may contain sulfites and should not be administered to patients with sulfite sensitivity. Patients with severe thrombocytopenia or HIT should not be given heparin. Whenever possible, intramuscular (IM) injections of other medications should be avoided because they may cause serious bruising, bleeding, or hematomas. Although relatively safe during pregnancy, the drug should be used with caution during the peripartum period due to the risk of maternal hemorrhage. Caution must be used when administering heparin to patients with serious renal or hepatic impairment because the drug may rise to toxic levels.

Drug Interactions: Oral anticoagulants, including warfarin, potentiate heparin activity. Drugs that inhibit platelet aggregation (such as aspirin, indomethacin, and ibuprofen) may induce bleeding. Nicotine, digoxin, tetracyclines, or antihistamines may inhibit anticoagulation. **Herbal/Food:** Herbal supplements that may affect coagulation such as ginger, garlic, green tea, feverfew, or ginkgo should be avoided because they may increase the risk of bleeding.

Pregnancy: Category C.

Treatment of Overdose: If serious hemorrhage occurs, a specific antagonist, protamine sulfate, may be administered IV (1 mg for every 100 units of heparin) to neutralize the anticoagulant activity of heparin. Protamine sulfate has an onset of action of 5 minutes and a duration of 2 hours. Multiple doses may be necessary to control extensive hemorrhaging. Protamine is also an antagonist to the LMWHs.

Nursing Responsibilities: Key nursing implications for patients receiving heparin are included in the Nursing Practice Application for Patients Receiving Pharmacotherapy with Anticoagulants.

Drugs Similar to Heparin

The LMWHs include dalteparin, enoxaparin, and tinzaparin. Two drugs in this class, ardeparin (Normiflo) and danaparoid (Organ), have been discontinued in the United States. Antithrombin (recombinant) and fondaparinux are parenteral anticoagulants that act by unique mechanisms.

Antithrombin, recombinant (ATryn): ATryn is a unique coagulation modifier approved in 2009 to treat patients who have a congenital deficiency of antithrombin III. These patients have a high incidence of blood clots, especially DVT. The drug is indicated for the prevention of perioperative and peripartum thromboembolic events in hereditary antithrombin-deficient patients. Antithrombin (ATryn) is unusual because it is obtained from genetically engineered goats. The goats are engineered through recombinant DNA technology to secrete human antithrombin in their milk. The drug is then purified and powdered for reconstitution as an IV infusion.

Levels of antithrombin activity in the blood must be monitored before, during, and immediately following therapy. The initial and subsequent drug doses are based on the level of antithrombin activity. The most common adverse effects are hemorrhage and infusion site reaction. ATryn enhances the anticoagulant effect of heparin and LMWHs. This drug is pregnancy category C.

Dalteparin (Fragmin): As an LMWH, dalteparin has smaller glycosaminoglycan chains than unfractionated heparin. Approved in 1994, dalteparin is given by the subcutaneous route for the treatment and prophylaxis of DVT or pulmonary embolism. Other approved indications include thrombosis prophylaxis in patients at increased risk due to unstable angina, an acute MI, or cancer. It has a longer half-life than heparin, which allows for less frequent dosing. Like other LMWHs, bleeding is the most serious adverse effect and the drug should not be administered to patients with active bleeding. This drug is pregnancy category B.

Enoxaparin (Lovenox): Enoxaparin was the first LMWH approved by the U.S. Food and Drug Administration (FDA) in 1993. Indications include treatment and prophylaxis of DVT and pulmonary embolism. Following hip or lower extremity surgery, enoxaparin may be administered once daily for 7 to 10 days. Some orthopedic procedures such as repair of hip fractures require more prolonged therapy. Enoxaparin may also be administered for the prophylaxis of coronary artery thrombosis and the prevention of ischemic complications in patients with acute coronary syndrome, for patients with unstable angina, and patients having percutaneous coronary intervention (PCI). Bleeding is the most serious adverse effect and the drug should not be administered to patients with active bleeding. This drug is pregnancy category B.

Fondaparinux (Arixtra): Approved in 2001, fondaparinux is an anticoagulant used for many of the same indications as heparin and the LMWHs, but it has certain differences that make it unique. Fondaparinux is a synthetic agent that consists of only five saccharide units (a pentasaccharide) that is structurally identical to the region of the heparin molecule that binds AT-III.

The pentasaccharide unit is able to selectively inhibit Factor Xa without directly affecting thrombin. Fondaparinux is only given by the subcutaneous route and is approved for the prophylaxis of VTE following orthopedic surgery and the treatment of DVT or pulmonary embolism. Like the LMWHs, fondaparinux is administered as fixed doses based on the patient's weight, and routine laboratory monitoring is not required because aPTT and PT are not accurate measures of drug activity. Doses of fondaparinux are not interchangeable with heparin or the LMWHs. There is no specific antidote for overdose; administration of protamine is ineffective. This drug is pregnancy category B.

Tinzaparin (Innohep): Approved in 2000, tinzaparin is indicated for the therapy of acute, symptomatic DVT, with or without evidence of pulmonary embolism, when administered with warfarin. Therapy is continued for 6 days, or until the patient has been switched to oral anticoagulation with warfarin. Therapy may be prolonged for 3 to 6 months in patients with cancer at high risk for DVT or pulmonary embolism. Thrombosis prophylaxis is an off-label indication for tinzaparin. Bleeding is the most serious adverse effect and the drug should not be administered to patients with active bleeding. This drug is pregnancy category B.

38.5 Warfarin is the most widely used drug for oral anticoagulant therapy.

Although parenteral anticoagulants have the advantage of an almost immediate onset of action, drugs given by this route require close medical supervision because adverse effects such as bleeding can rapidly ensue. When the patient's condition allows, oral anticoagulants are used due to their convenience and greater safety.

Warfarin (Coumadin) has been available as an anticoagulant for over 50 years and is the most frequently used drug in this class. In acute situations, patients begin anticoagulation therapy with heparin and are switched to warfarin when their condition stabilizes. When transitioning, the two drugs must be administered concurrently for 2 to 3 days. This is because heparin has a brief half-life (90 minutes), and aPTT returns to normal within 2 to 3 hours following discontinuation of heparin. Warfarin, on the other hand, takes 1 to 3 days of therapy to achieve optimum anticoagulation. Thus, concomitant pharmacotherapy

CONNECTIONS | Patient Safety

◀ The Dangers of Similar Packaging

In the past several years, three premature infants received fatal overdoses of heparin, and almost 20 received overdoses but survived, including a highly publicized case of twins born to a celebrity couple. It was reported that in at least one case, 1-mL heparin vials with 10,000 units/mL were placed in an automated dispensing unit where 10-unit/mL vials were usually kept. In other cases, the packaging for the high-concentration heparin and the lower concentration vial used for IV flush used similar labeling, and a nurse gave the wrong concentration to flush the IV line of the infants. What errors were involved in these cases? What could the nurse do to avoid this error in the future?

See Answers to Patient Safety Questions on student resource website.

◀ Miscarriage Prevention with Anticoagulants

Miscarriage in pregnancy is devastating, and recurrent miscarriage even more so. Recent research suggests that undiagnosed thrombophilias (genetic hyper-coagulability disorders) such as antiphospholipid syndrome (APS) may play a role in some cases (Check, 2012), but clots have also been noted in the placenta after miscarriage in women without any confirmed genetic susceptibility for thrombophilia. Some studies and systematic reviews have noted that LMWH used for women who had experienced at least one miscarriage (early or late term) resulted in an increased rate of live births (Mantha, Bauer, & Zwicker, 2009; Monien et al., 2009). Other studies have not demonstrated the same results from LMWH, heparin, or aspirin, although it is recognized that there are many factors involved in recurrent miscarriage (Kaandorp et al., 2010; McNamee, Dawood, & Farquharson, 2012). Because there are insufficient studies to recommend that heparin, LMWH, or aspirin should be used routinely for women who have experienced a previous unexplained pregnancy loss, it is recommended that a woman experiencing such loss discuss the situation with her provider and whether genetic testing should be conducted. If genetic coagulation abnormalities are found, heparin or LMWH may be considered as an option.

is necessary to ensure continuous anticoagulation. During this transition, there is increased risk of bleeding, due to the additive anticoagulant action of the two drugs.

Unlike heparin, which is monitored with aPTT values, PT is the standard laboratory test used to monitor the effectiveness of warfarin. The normal PT range is 12 to 15 seconds. During therapeutic anticoagulation, PT should increase to 1.5 to 2 times the patient's baseline. Because laboratory testing methods for PT vary, however, PT time is also reported as an international normalized ratio (INR) value; INR values averaging 2.5 are considered therapeutic for most indications. PT is measured daily until the desired level of therapeutic anticoagulation is achieved. Then, the frequency of laboratory testing is decreased to weekly or monthly as the patient's condition stabilizes. Home monitoring devices are available to provide convenient and reliable INR values, which can guide the patients to adjust their own medication amounts. Self-monitoring has its limitations, however. The devices are expensive and the patient or their caregiver must be capable of understanding how to properly adjust the dosage.

Several newer drugs have emerged as significant alternatives to warfarin for stroke prevention. In 2011, rivaroxaban (Xarelto) became the first anticoagulant available by the oral (PO) route to directly inhibit Factor Xa, a component of the clotting cascade. Approval of a second Factor Xa inhibitor, apixaban (Eliquis), followed in 2012. A third option for oral stroke prevention is dabigatran (Pradaxa), a direct thrombin inhibitor. The three newer alternatives do not require INR monitoring and they do not exhibit extensive drug interactions compared to warfarin. Perhaps more important is that the three alternatives appear to be more effective than warfarin at preventing strokes. The alternatives are more expensive than warfarin and they have a much shorter half-life: Missing a single dose may increase stroke risk.

PROTOTYPE DRUG | **Warfarin (Coumadin)**

Classification: **Therapeutic:** Anticoagulant
Pharmacologic: Vitamin K antagonist

Therapeutic Effects and Uses: Indications for warfarin therapy include the long-term prophylaxis of arterial thromboembolism, including prevention of stroke and MI. Other uses include the prophylaxis and treatment of DVT or pulmonary embolism in patients undergoing hip or knee surgery, or in those with long-term indwelling central venous catheters or prosthetic heart valves. The drug may be given to prevent thromboembolic events in high-risk patients following an MI or an atrial fibrillation episode.

Warfarin is well absorbed after PO administration but takes several days to produce an optimum therapeutic effect. Ninety-nine percent of absorbed warfarin is bound to plasma proteins and is not immediately available to produce its effect. This high level of protein binding is also responsible for some of the many drug–drug interactions that occur with warfarin.

There is wide variation in response to warfarin therapy. Dosage levels must be determined individually for each patient and carefully monitored. Patients stabilized on warfarin should not switch brands of the drug unless recommended by the health care provider, due to differences in bioavailability. For most indications, the therapeutic range of serum warfarin levels varies from 1 to 10 mcg/mL to achieve a target INR value of 2 to 3.

Mechanism of Action: Warfarin inhibits two enzymes involved in the formation of activated vitamin K, which is required for the synthesis of clotting factors II, VII, IX, and X. Warfarin inhibits the synthesis of new clotting factors but does not affect clotting factors that are already circulating in the blood. It takes 3 to 4 days for the plasma levels of existing clotting factors to fall and for the anticoagulant effect of warfarin to appear. After discontinuing the drug, 3 to 4 days are needed for the body to make new clotting factors and return coagulation to baseline levels.

Pharmacokinetics:

Route(s)	PO
Absorption	Well absorbed
Distribution	Widely distributed; crosses the placenta but is not secreted in breast milk; 99% bound to plasma protein
Primary metabolism	Hepatic
Primary excretion	Renal, small amounts in bile
Onset of action	2–7 days
Duration of action	3–5 days; half-life: 0.5–3 days

Adverse Effects: Like all anticoagulants, the most serious adverse effect of warfarin is abnormal bleeding, which may occur in any body system. Warfarin may release pieces of atheromatous plaque from vessel walls, resulting in systemic cholesterol microembolization that may occlude small vessels. For example, "purple-toe syndrome" is caused by cholesterol microembolization and severe cases may lead to gangrene or amputation. Long-term use of warfarin may increase the risk of osteoporosis and bone fractures. **Black Box Warning**: Warfarin can cause major or fatal bleeding, and regular monitoring of INR is required. Patients should be instructed about prevention measures to minimize bleeding risk and to immediately notify health care providers of signs and symptoms of bleeding.

Contraindications/Precautions: Patients with recent trauma, active internal bleeding, serious bleeding disorders, intracranial hemorrhage, severe HTN, bacterial endocarditis, or severe hepatic or renal impairment should not take warfarin. When possible, warfarin should be discontinued or the dosage lowered before dental or elective surgical procedures. Patients with heart failure may exhibit excessive anticoagulation with warfarin, which requires lower doses. Whenever possible, IM injections of other medications should be avoided because they may cause bruising, bleeding, or hematomas. Warfarin should not be taken during pregnancy because the drug has been shown to produce numerous fetal abnormalities, induce fatal bleeding, and can cause fetal death. Warfarin is believed to be safe for lactating women who are at risk for postpartum venous thrombus because very little of the drug enters breast milk. Studies have shown no change in the INR values of lactating infants whose mothers are receiving warfarin.

Drug Interactions: Drug–drug interactions with warfarin are numerous. Because the therapeutic index of warfarin is very low, drugs that interact with warfarin have the potential to affect coagulation time and cause harm. Concurrent use with other drugs with anticoagulant activity, including aspirin, heparin, and antiplatelet drugs, may produce additive effects and excessive bleeding. Extensive protein binding is responsible for numerous drug–drug interactions, some of which include nonsteroidal anti-inflammatory drugs (NSAIDs), diuretics, selective serotonin reuptake inhibitors (SSRIs) and other antidepressants, steroids, antibiotics, vaccines, and vitamins (e.g., vitamin K). NSAIDs increase bleeding risk. During warfarin therapy, the patient should not take any other prescription or over-the-counter (OTC) drugs or herbal products unless approved by the health care provider. A listing of selected drugs and supplements affecting warfarin therapy is given in Table 38.4. **Herbal/Food**: Herbal supplements such as green tea, ginkgo, feverfew, garlic, cranberry, chamomile, and ginger may increase the risk of bleeding.

Pregnancy: Category X.

Treatment of Overdose: The specific treatment for warfarin overdose is PO or parenteral administration of vitamin K_1. When administered IV, vitamin K_1 can reverse the anticoagulant effects of warfarin within 6 hours.

Nursing Responsibilities: Key nursing implications for patients receiving warfarin are included in the Nursing Practice Application for Patients Receiving Pharmacotherapy with Anticoagulants.

TABLE 38.4 Drug–Drug Interactions with Warfarin

Interaction	Drug or Drug Class
Increased anticoagulant effect	acetaminophen, amiodarone, anabolic steroids, aspirin, azole antifungals, cephalosporins, cimetidine, clopidogrel, danazol, disulfiram, heparin, isoniazid, macrolides, metronidazole, nalidixic acid, NSAIDs, omeprazole, paroxetine, penicillin, propafenone, quinidine, tamoxifen, tetracyclines, thyroid hormone, ticlopidine, trimethoprim-sulfisoxazole, statins
Decreased anticoagulant effect	barbiturates, bile-acid sequestrants, carbamazepine, cyclosporine, dicloxacillin, oral contraceptives, rifampin
Mixed effect	allopurinol, corticosteroids, ethanol, phenytoin
Supplements and food	American ginseng, cranberry, feverfew, ginkgo, green tea, vitamin E, vitamin K

Drugs Similar to Warfarin (Coumadin)

Apixaban and rivaroxaban are oral anticoagulant alternatives to warfarin that inhibit steps in the clotting cascade.

Apixaban (Eliquis): Approved in 2012, apixaban is an oral anticoagulant approved to lower the risk of stroke and systemic embolism in patients with nonvalvular atrial fibrillation. Its effectiveness at preventing stroke appears to be greater than that of warfarin, and INR monitoring is not required during therapy. Apixaban acts by inhibitor clotting Factor Xa, resulting in prolonged clotting time. The most common adverse reactions are associated with excessive bleeding. There is no antidote for apixaban overdose. Apixaban carries a black box warning that abrupt discontinuation of the drug can increase the risk of thromboembolism. Unless discontinued for a pathologic reason (excessive bleeding), another drug should be immediately substituted so that continuous anticoagulation is obtained. This drug is pregnancy category B; however, its use during pregnancy is not recommended because it could increase the risk of hemorrhage during pregnancy or delivery.

Rivaroxaban (Xarelto): Rivaroxaban is a newer oral anticoagulant approved in 2011 to lower the risk of stroke and systemic embolism in patients with nonvalvular atrial fibrillation. It is also approved to treat DVT and pulmonary embolism and to prevent DVT and pulmonary embolism in patients undergoing knee or hip replacement surgery. Like apixaban, rivaroxaban selectively inhibits Factor Xa in the clotting cascade, does not require INR monitoring, and exhibits few drug interactions. Bleeding is the most common adverse effect. The drug carries a black box warning that spinal or epidural hematomas may occur in anticoagulated patients receiving epidural or spinal anesthesia or who are undergoing spinal puncture. A second black box warning mirrors that of apixaban: Abrupt discontinuation of the drug can increase the risk of thromboembolism. Unless discontinued for a pathologic reason (excessive bleeding), another drug should be immediately substituted so that continuous anticoagulation is obtained. These patients must be monitored frequently for signs of neurologic impairment. This drug is pregnancy category C.

38.6 The direct thrombin inhibitors are anticoagulants originally obtained from medical leeches that are used to treat or prevent venous thromboembolism.

The direct thrombin inhibitors have an interesting history; they were originally derived from chemicals found in leeches. Leeches are wormlike animals that survive by sucking and digesting blood from mammals. Medical leeches are an ancient treatment that dates back to early Egyptian and Greek civilizations. They were applied to the skin as a type of bloodletting, which was thought to remove harmful substances from the body. Known as hirudotherapy, the use of leeches was largely discontinued with the advent of modern medicine in the early 1900s. However, leeches are still an approved therapy for relieving venous congestion in transplanted or reattached fingers or limbs. While studying leeches, scientists isolated a potent chemical called hirudin, which prevented blood from coagulating in the leech.

The direct thrombin inhibitors bind reversibly to thrombin, preventing the formation of fibrin. They are highly specific for thrombin and do not require AT-III as an intermediate in promoting anticoagulation as does heparin. They bind to circulating thrombin as well as thrombin attached to fibrin clots. These drugs exhibit typical anticoagulant actions and are used for the same types of indications as heparin and the LMWHs.

Two drugs in the direct thrombin inhibitor class, bivalirudin and desirudin, were derived from the hirudin molecule found in leeches and are structurally very similar. They are administered by the parenteral route. Argatroban and dabigatran inhibit thrombin but are not chemically related to the hirudin molecule. Dabigatran is the only direct thrombin inhibitor that is given PO.

PROTOTYPE DRUG	Dabigatran (Pradaxa)

Classification: **Therapeutic:** Anticoagulant
Pharmacologic: Direct thrombin inhibitor

Therapeutic Effects and Uses: Dabigatran is a direct thrombin inhibitor that was approved in 2010 for stroke prophylaxis in patients with nonvalvular atrial fibrillation. In 2014 indications were extended to include treatment of DVT and pulmonary embolus in patients who have been treated with a parenteral anticoagulant for 5 to 10 days. Because it is administered PO, dabigatran is an alternative to both heparin and warfarin. Although considerably more expensive, dabigatran has equal efficacy to warfarin and does not require the same high degree of laboratory monitoring as does warfarin or heparin.

Mechanism of Action: Dabigatran directly inhibits the action of thrombin without requiring the intermediate step of antithrombin III inhibition.

Pharmacokinetics:

Route(s)	PO
Absorption	3–7% absorbed
Distribution	35% bound to plasma proteins; unknown if it crosses the placenta or is secreted in breast milk
Primary metabolism	Hepatic to active metabolites
Primary excretion	Renal 80%
Onset of action	30–90 min
Duration of action	Half-life: 12–17 h

Adverse Effects: Like other anticoagulants, the most serious adverse effect of dabigatran is bleeding. Symptoms may include bleeding from puncture or wound sites, epistaxis, hematuria, vaginal bleeding, or GI bleeding. Hypersensitivity reactions, including anaphylaxis, have been reported. Dyspepsia and gastritis are common during therapy. **Black Box Warnings**: Premature discontinuation of dabigatran increases the risk of thrombotic events. Epidural or spinal hematomas may occur when administering this drug to patients who are receiving neuraxial anesthesia or spinal puncture.

Contraindications/Precautions: Dabigatran should not be administered to patients with active bleeding or those with impaired hemostasis. Patients with mechanical heart valves should not receive this drug due to an increased risk of thrombotic events. Patients with severe renal impairment or on hemodialysis should not receive dabigatran. The drug should be used with caution in patients with recent hemorrhage, recent surgery, intracranial hemorrhage, and ulcerative GI disease or symptoms of gastritis.

Drug Interactions: Additive risk for bleeding may occur if dabigatran is administered concurrently with other coagulation modifiers, including warfarin, heparin, aspirin, and fibrinolytic drugs. **Herbal/Food**: Herbal supplements that affect coagulation such as ginger, garlic, green tea, feverfew, St. John's wort, or ginkgo should be avoided because they may increase the risk of bleeding.

Pregnancy: Category C.

Treatment of Overdose: There are no specific antidotes for dabigatran overdose. Administration of protamine and vitamin K are not effective. Hemodialysis may be used to remove some of the drug from the plasma.

Nursing Responsibilities: Key nursing implications for patients receiving dabigatran are included in the Nursing Practice Application for Patients Receiving Pharmacotherapy with Anticoagulants.

Drugs Similar to Dabigatran (Pradaxa)

Other direct thrombin inhibitors include argatroban, bivalirudin, and desirudin. Lepirudin (Refludan) was withdrawn from the market in 2012.

Argatroban (Acova, Novastan): Approved in 2000, argatroban is a synthetic thrombin inhibitor that is given by the IV route for HIT. It is also approved to treat or prevent thrombotic events associated with PCI. Unlike dabigatran, which is excreted by the kidneys, argatroban is metabolized and eliminated by the liver and therefore may be used in patients with renal impairment. Caution must be observed, however, when administering the drug to patients with hepatic impairment. Allergic reactions occur in up to 10% of patients receiving argatroban. Bleeding is the most serious adverse effect and the drug should not be administered to patients with active bleeding. This drug is pregnancy category C.

Bivalirudin (Angiomax): Approved in 2000, bivalirudin is a direct thrombin inhibitor that is only available by the IV route. Bivalirudin is given concurrently with aspirin to reduce the incidence of thromboembolic events associated with HIT and to provide anticoagulation in patients undergoing PCI. Back pain is

CONNECTIONS: NURSING PRACTICE APPLICATION

Patients Receiving Pharmacotherapy with Anticoagulants

Assessment	Potential Nursing Diagnoses*
Baseline assessment prior to administration: • Obtain a complete health history: cardiovascular (including HTN, MI, heart failure) and peripheral vascular disease (including thrombophlebitis), respiratory (including previous pulmonary embolism), neurologic (including recent head injury or stroke), hepatic or renal disease, diabetes, peptic ulcer disease, hypercholesterolemia, and the possibility of alcoholism or pregnancy. **Lifespan:** Ask women of menstrual age about length and heaviness of usual menstrual flow. Obtain a drug history including allergies, current prescription and OTC drugs, herbal preparations, and alcohol use. Be alert to possible drug interactions. • Obtain baseline weight, vital signs, ECG (if appropriate), and breath sounds. Assess for presence, quality, location of angina, and for presence of dyspnea or chest pain. Assess extremities for symptoms of thrombophlebitis (e.g., warmth, swelling, tenderness in calf, positive Homans' sign), and for location and character/amount of edema, if present. • Evaluate appropriate laboratory findings (e.g., aPTT, PT/INR), CBC, renal and liver function studies, arterial blood gases (ABGs) as appropriate, and lipid profiles. • Assess the patient's ability to receive and understand instructions. Include family and caregivers as needed.	• *Acute Pain* • *Ineffective Peripheral Tissue Perfusion* • *Impaired Skin Integrity* • *Anxiety* • *Deficient Knowledge* (Drug Therapy) • *Risk for Injury*, related to adverse effects of anticoagulant therapy
Assessment throughout administration: • Assess for desired therapeutic effects (e.g., existing area of phlebitis exhibits signs of improvement with no symptoms of thrombosis formation; signs and symptoms of existing thrombosis show gradual improvement: e.g., previous anginal or peripheral extremity pain has diminished or is eliminated; peripheral pulses are improving in quality and volume).	
• Continue periodic monitoring of appropriate laboratory values (e.g., aPTT, PT/INR). • Assess for adverse effects: bleeding at IV sites, wounds, excessive ecchymosis, petechiae, hematuria, black/tarry stools, rectal bleeding, coffee-ground emesis, epistaxis, bleeding from gums, hemoptysis, prolonged or heavy menstrual flow; and assess for occult bleeding: pallor, dizziness, hypotension, tachycardia, abdominal pain, areas of abdominal wall swelling or firmness, lumbar pain, or decreased level of consciousness.	

Implementation

Interventions and (Rationales)	Patient-Centered Care
Ensuring therapeutic effects: • Continue frequent assessments as above for therapeutic effects, e.g., existing area of phlebitis exhibits signs of improvement with no symptoms of thrombosis formation; signs and symptoms of existing thrombosis show gradual improvement: e.g., previous anginal or peripheral extremity pain has diminished or is eliminated; peripheral pulses are improving in quality and volume. (Anticoagulants help prevent the formation of thrombi or prevent existing thrombi from increasing in size. As the body's own thrombolysis factors activate, existing thrombi will gradually reduce in size.)	• To allay possible anxiety, teach the patient, family, or caregiver the rationale for all equipment used (e.g., antiembolic stockings, intermittent pneumatic sequential compression devices) and the need for frequent monitoring.
• Encourage early ambulation postoperatively in the hospitalized patient and active range of motion (ROM) if the patient is on bed rest or has limited mobility. Perform passive ROM for patients unable to perform active ROM. (Early ambulation and ROM prevent venous stasis and thrombosis formation, lessening the need for anticoagulant therapy.)	• Assist the patient with ambulation postoperatively, and teach active ROM. Teach the patient, family, or caregiver how to perform passive ROM exercises for patients unable to perform active ROM.
• Assess the patient's lifestyle and occasions of travel over extended lengths of time (e.g., air travel, lengthy driving trips) and the frequency of such trips. (Prolonged sitting during air or car travel may limit blood flow to lower extremities and venous return, promoting the formation of thrombi. Frequent stretching, ambulating when possible, and increasing fluids to maintain normal osmolarity/viscosity may decrease thrombosis formation and lessen the need for anticoagulant therapy.)	• Educate patients and consumers about thrombosis prevention during travel: periodic stretching, short periods of ambulation, avoid sitting for prolonged periods, increasing fluid intake.
• Encourage appropriate lifestyle changes: lowered fat intake, increased exercise, limited alcohol intake, limited caffeine intake, and smoking cessation. Provide for dietitian consultation as needed. (Smoking increases platelet aggregation and promotes the formation of thrombi. Healthy lifestyle changes will support and minimize the need for drug therapy.)	• Encourage the patient to adopt a healthy lifestyle of low-fat food choices, increased exercise, decreased alcohol consumption, and smoking cessation. Provide for appropriate consultation (e.g., dietitian) as needed.

CONNECTIONS: NURSING PRACTICE APPLICATION (continued)

Minimizing adverse effects:

- Monitor for signs and symptoms of excessive visible bleeding and for occult bleeding. (Bleeding is the most common adverse effect of anticoagulant therapy. Frequent assessment for both visible and occult bleeding is necessary to prevent hemorrhage and to start early corrective treatment as appropriate. **Diverse Patients:** Because some drugs such as clopidogrel [Plavix] metabolize through the P450 system pathways, monitor ethnically diverse patients to ensure optimal therapeutic effects and to minimize adverse effects.)

- Anticoagulant use is a high-risk safety concern and is included in The Joint Commission's National Patient Safety Goals.
- Teach the patient, family, or caregiver the signs and symptoms of excessive bleeding, including occult. If external bleeding occurs, pressure over the site should be held up to 15 min. If bleeding continues, is severe, or is accompanied by dizziness or syncope, immediate medical attention (e.g., 911) should be obtained.
- **Lifespan:** Women of menstrual age should report excessively heavy or prolonged menstrual bleeding and should keep a pad count and report to the health care provider.

- Continue to monitor frequent laboratory tests (aPTT, PT/INR), CBC, and platelets. (Therapeutic aPTT levels are usually 1.5–2.5 times the normal control value. INR is usually 2–3.5 or 4. Learn own laboratory provider's values. Values below the norm indicate less than optimal therapeutic levels of the drug; values above the norm indicate a high potential for bleeding and hemorrhage. CBC, especially RBC, hemoglobin [Hgb], and hematocrit [Hct], and platelet levels should remain within normal limits. Decreasing values on CBC may indicate excessive bleeding and the need to assess for location. **Lifespan:** Be especially cautious with the older adult as age-related hepatic changes may increase the risk of bleeding.)

- Instruct the patient on the need to return periodically for laboratory work and to alert laboratory personnel that anticoagulant therapy is being used.
- Instruct the patient to carry a wallet identification card or wear medical identification jewelry indicating anticoagulant therapy.

- Continue to monitor peripheral pulses for quality and volume, complaints of angina or chest pain, especially if new or of sudden onset or accompanied by dyspnea. (Anticoagulants prevent thrombus formation or extension; they do not prevent emboli from occurring. Monitoring for new or sudden onset of pain is necessary to ensure prompt treatment of possible emboli.)

- Teach the patient, family, or caregiver to report immediately any sudden pain in the chest, legs or calves, dyspnea, or new-onset anginal pain.

- Minimize opportunities for injury or bleeding where possible: Avoid IM injections, provide a soft toothbrush, and be cautious when providing care, especially with older adults who have more fragile skin. (Anticoagulants raise the risk of bleeding, and causes of even minor bleeding should be avoided when possible. If minor bleeding occurs, prolonged pressure, longer than expected, will be necessary to stop it, and the site should be assessed frequently for oozing. Warfarin and antiplatelet drugs may continue to have effects after the drug is stopped.)

- Instruct the patient on ways to minimize opportunities for injury or bleeding where possible:
  - Switch to a soft toothbrush and inspect gums after brushing.
  - Use an electric razor if possible, or be extra cautious with a safety razor, holding prolonged pressure over small nicks.
  - Be cautious with food preparation, especially when cutting food.
  - Avoid contact sports, amusement park rides, or other physical activities that may cause intense or violent bumping, jostling, or injury.
- **Lifespan:** Frequently assess older adult family members on anticoagulant therapy who have more fragile skin and may experience skin tears or ecchymosis more frequently.

- Closely evaluate all new prescriptions or use of OTC medications for drug interactions. (Many drugs interact with anticoagulants, enhancing the action and increasing the chance for bleeding. All OTC medications containing salicylates, e.g., aspirin, and NSAIDs are contraindicated.)

- Instruct the patient to consult the health care provider before taking any new prescription or OTC medication, including herbal preparations.

- Maintain a normal diet, avoiding increases or decreases in vitamin K–rich foods (e.g., asparagus, broccoli, cabbage, cauliflower, kale), and limit or eliminate alcohol intake. (Vitamin K is necessary for synthesis of clotting agents in the liver. Sudden increases or decreases in dietary intake of vitamin K–rich foods may increase or decrease the effectiveness of anticoagulants, particularly oral anticoagulant therapy. Excessive intake of alcohol, more than two drinks in men or one in women per day, may alter the effectiveness of oral anticoagulants.)

- Teach the patient to maintain a normal diet, avoiding increases or decreases in vitamin K–rich foods and limit or eliminate alcohol intake. Vitamin K supplements and protein supplement drinks (e.g., Ensure or Boost), which often have vitamin K added, should also be avoided.
- Advise patients to avoid excessive intake of alcohol while on oral anticoagulants.

- Assess for any symptoms of hepatitis (e.g., darkening urine, light or clay-colored stools, itchy skin, jaundice of sclera or skin, abdominal pain, especially in the RUQ) in patients receiving oral anticoagulant therapy. (Drug-induced hepatitis is a possible adverse effect of oral anticoagulant therapy.)

- Instruct the patient to report any signs of possible hepatitis immediately, especially abdominal discomfort that localizes in the RUQ.

- **Lifespan:** Assess for the possibility of pregnancy before beginning the drug. (Women on anticoagulant therapy will be monitored closely for labor and the possibility of excessive bleeding. Warfarin is a pregnancy category X drug.)

- Instruct female patients who may be considering pregnancy, or are pregnant, to notify their provider before starting the drug. Women taking warfarin should use extra precautions during sex, such as barrier contraceptive measures, to prevent pregnancy.

Patient understanding of drug therapy:

- Use opportunities during administration of medications and during assessments to discuss the rationale for drug therapy, desired therapeutic outcomes, commonly observed adverse effects, parameters for when to call the health care provider, and any necessary monitoring or precautions. (Using time during nursing care helps to optimize and reinforce key teaching areas.)

- The patient, family, or caregiver should be able to state the reason for the drug, appropriate dose and scheduling, what adverse effects to observe for and when to report them, equipment needed as appropriate and how to use that equipment, and the required length of medication therapy needed, with any special instructions regarding renewing or continuing the prescription as appropriate.

(continued)

CONNECTIONS: NURSING PRACTICE APPLICATION (continued)

Patient self-administration of drug therapy:

- When administering medications, instruct the patient, family, or caregiver in proper self-administration techniques followed by return demonstration. (Utilizing time during nurse-administration of these drugs helps to reinforce teaching.)

- Teach the patient, family, or caregiver in proper self-administration techniques:
  - Injections of heparin or LMWHs should be administered in the fatty layers of the abdomen or just above the iliac crest, avoiding the periumbilical area by 5 cm (2 in.).
  - Skin is drawn up (pinched), and the needle is inserted at a 90-degree angle.
  - Injection is given without aspirating for blood return.
  - Release the skin and hold slight pressure to the site, but do not massage the area.
- Have the patient, family, or caregiver return demonstrate until the proper technique is used and they are comfortable giving the injection.
- Teach the patient on oral anticoagulants to take the medication at the same time each day.

*Nursing Diagnoses—Definitions and Classification 2015–2017. Copyright © 2014, 1994–2014 by NANDA International. Used by arrangement with John Wiley & Sons Limited.

a common adverse effect of the drug, occurring in about 40% of patients. Nausea, vomiting, hypotension, and headache also occur in a significant number of patients. Bleeding is the most serious adverse effect and the drug should not be administered to patients with active bleeding. Bivalirudin is as effective as heparin and produces a lower incidence of serious bleeding, although it is very expensive. This drug is pregnancy category B.

Desirudin (Iprivask): Made through recombinant DNA technology, desirudin is nearly identical to hirudin and is the only direct thrombin inhibitor administered by the subcutaneous route. It acts by the same mechanism and has the same adverse effects and contraindications as bivalirudin. The drug was approved in 2003 for DVT prophylaxis in patients undergoing hip replacement surgery. Off-label uses include prevention of thromboembolic events in patients with unstable angina and those undergoing PCI. Allergic reactions, including anaphylaxis, are rare. Bleeding is the most serious adverse effect and the drug should not be administered to patients with active bleeding. This drug is pregnancy category C.

Antiplatelet Drugs

38.7 Antiplatelet drugs provide anticoagulation by reducing the aggregation properties of platelets.

Antiplatelet drugs modify coagulation primarily by interfering with platelet aggregation. Unlike the anticoagulants, which are used primarily to prevent thrombosis in veins, the primary indications for antiplatelet drugs are to prevent clot formation in arteries. The antiplatelet agents are listed in Table 38.5.

Because platelets are a central component of blood hemostasis, reducing the number of platelets or their function can profoundly

TABLE 38.5 Antiplatelet Drugs

Drug	Route and Adult Dose (Maximum Dose Where Indicated)	Adverse Effects
anagrelide (Agrylin)	PO: 0.5 mg qid or 1 mg bid (max: 10 mg/day)	*Nausea, vomiting, diarrhea, abdominal pain, dizziness, headache*
aspirin (ASA, acetylsalicylic acid)	PO: 80 mg daily to 650 mg bid	
dipyridamole (Persantine)	PO: 75–100 mg qid as adjunct to warfarin therapy	<u>Increased bleeding, central nervous system (CNS) effects (dipyridamole), anaphylaxis (aspirin), interstitial lung disease (anagrelide)</u>
vorapaxar (Zontivity)	PO: 2.08 mg/day	
ADP Receptor Blockers		
ticagrelor (Brilinta)	PO: 180 mg loading dose followed by 90 mg bid	*Minor bleeding, dyspepsia, abdominal pain, headache, rash, diarrhea*
clopidogrel (Plavix)	PO: 75 mg/day (max: 300 mg/day for life-threatening cases)	
prasugrel (Effient)	PO: 60 mg loading dose followed by 10 mg/day	<u>Increased clotting time, GI bleeding, blood dyscrasias, angina</u>
ticlopidine (Ticlid)	PO: 250 mg bid (max: 500 mg/day)	
Glycoprotein IIb/IIIa Receptor Antagonists		
abciximab (ReoPro)	IV: 0.25 mg/kg initial bolus over 5 min, then 0.125 mcg/kg/min for 12 h (max: 10 mcg/min)	*Dyspepsia, dizziness, pain at injection site, hypotension, bradycardia, minor bleeding*
eptifibatide (Integrilin)	IV: 180 mcg/kg initial bolus over 1–2 min, then 2 mcg/kg/min for 24–72 h (max: 180 mcg/kg bolus, 2 mcg/kg/min infusion)	<u>Major hemorrhage, thrombocytopenia</u>
tirofiban (Aggrastat)	IV: 0.4 mcg/kg/min for 30 min, then 0.1 mcg/kg/min for 12–24 h	
Drugs for Intermittent Claudication		
cilostazol (Pletal)	PO: 100 mg bid	*Dyspepsia, nausea, vomiting, dizziness, myalgia, headache*
pentoxifylline (Trental)	PO: 400 mg tid (max: 1,200 mg/day)	<u>Tachycardia and palpitations (cilostazol), CNS effects (pentoxifylline), heart failure, MI</u>

Note: *Italics* indicate common adverse effects. <u>Underline</u> indicates serious adverse effects.

increase bleeding time. Three groups of drugs are classified as antiplatelet drugs:

- Aspirin
- Adenosine diphosphate (ADP) receptor blockers
- Glycoprotein IIb/IIIa receptor blockers

Aspirin deserves special mention as an antiplatelet agent. Because it is available OTC, patients may not consider aspirin a potent medication; however, its anticoagulant activity is well documented. Aspirin acts by binding irreversibly to the enzyme cyclooxygenase (COX) in platelets. This binding inhibits the formation of thromboxane A_2, a powerful inducer of platelet aggregation. The anticoagulant effect of a single dose of aspirin may persist for as long as 1 week. Concurrent use of aspirin with other coagulation modifiers should be avoided, unless medically approved. Nursing responsibilities and a prototype feature for aspirin are given in Chapter 41.

38.8 The adenosine diphosphate receptor blockers are antiplatelet drugs prescribed for the prevention and treatment of arterial thrombosis.

Although platelets are simply fragments of cells that have no nucleus, they contain many receptors on their plasma membranes and their functions are complex. Chemicals such as epinephrine, thromboxane A_2, thrombin, serotonin, and fibrinogen can bind to these receptors and modify coagulation through their interaction with the platelets.

Following vessel injury, platelets become "sticky," bind to exposed collagen, and release substances that recruit additional platelets to the site. One of these chemicals is ADP, whose function is to promote platelet aggregation. The ADP receptor blockers comprise a small group of drugs that irreversibly alter the plasma membrane of platelets. For the remainder of their lifespan, the affected platelets are unable to recognize the chemical signals required for them to aggregate.

Ticlopidine (Ticlid), clopidogrel (Plavix), and prasugrel (Effient) are ADP receptor blockers given PO to prevent thrombi

formation in patients who have experienced a recent thromboembolic event such as stroke or MI. Ticlopidine can cause life-threatening neutropenia and agranulocytosis in a small percentage of patients. Clopidogrel is safer, having a lower incidence of adverse GI, hematologic, and cutaneous adverse effects. Prasugrel is a newer drug in this class that acts more rapidly than clopidogrel.

Drugs affecting platelet aggregation increase the risk of bleeding should the patient sustain trauma or undergo dental or surgical procedures. These drugs are sometimes given concurrently with anticoagulants, which can further increase bleeding risk. Prolonged direct pressure over injection or venipuncture sites may be required to control bleeding. Bleeding lasting more than 10 minutes may require special medical or nursing interventions, such as suturing or applying a sandbag to a venipuncture site that does not stop bleeding.

PROTOTYPE DRUG | Clopidogrel (Plavix)

Classification: **Therapeutic:** Antiplatelet drug
Pharmacologic: ADP receptor blocker

Therapeutic Effects and Uses: Approved in 1997, clopidogrel is used for the prophylaxis of arterial thromboembolism to reduce the risk of stroke and MI. The drug has been shown to be more effective than aspirin in reducing thromboembolic events in patients with recent stroke or MI. It may also be given to prevent thrombi formation in patients with unstable angina or coronary artery stents, and to prevent postoperative DVT. Clopidogrel has similar anticoagulant activity to aspirin but is much more expensive.

Clopidogrel is given PO and has the advantage of once-daily dosing. Inhibition of platelet function may persist for 7 to 10 days after the drug is discontinued. When possible, clopidogrel should be discontinued at least 5 days prior to surgery to avoid excessive bleeding.

Mechanism of Action: Clopidogrel inhibits ADP receptors on platelets and prolongs bleeding time by irreversibly inhibiting

---

CONNECTIONS | Complementary and Alternative Therapies

Garlic

Description:
Garlic (*Allium sativum*) is a perennial plant in the onion family that can be grown and cultivated worldwide.

History and Claims:
Garlic has been used for centuries by most cultures as a flavoring and as a medicine. Historical uses have included curing deafness and earaches, and treating leprosy and scurvy. Modern claims have focused on cardiovascular uses: treatment of high blood lipid levels, atherosclerosis, and HTN. Other modern claims are that garlic reduces blood glucose levels and has antibacterial and antineoplastic activity.

Standardization:
Substances called alliaceous oils have been isolated from garlic and shown to have pharmacologic activity. Dosage forms include eating prepared garlic oil or the fresh bulbs (cloves) from the plant. In tablet or capsule form, doses range from 1 to 4 g/day. Extracts may be standardized by percent allicin.

Evidence:
Garlic is one of the best-studied herbs. Like most other herbal products, garlic likely has some health benefits, but controlled, scientific studies are lacking and the results are mixed (National Center for Complementary and Alternative Medicine, 2012). It has been shown to decrease the aggregation or "stickiness" of platelets, thus producing an anticoagulant effect. There is some research to show that the herb has a small effect on lowering blood cholesterol, although the effects seem to be short term. Evidence on the effects of the herb on blood pressure and slowing the development of atherosclerosis is mixed (Drug Digest, n.d.). Although some studies have concluded that garlic may prevent certain types of cancer, this has not been supported by randomized controlled studies (Ernst & Posadzki, 2012).

Garlic is safe for consumption in small and moderate amounts. Patients taking anticoagulant medications should limit their intake of garlic to avoid bleeding complications. Patients with diabetes should monitor their blood glucose levels closely if taking high doses of garlic.

platelet aggregation. Clopidogrel itself has little activity; however, it is changed to a highly active metabolite in the liver through extensive first-pass metabolism.

Pharmacokinetics:

Route(s)	PO
Absorption	Rapidly absorbed
Distribution	Unknown; unknown if it crosses the placenta or is secreted in breast milk; 94–98% bound to plasma protein
Primary metabolism	Hepatic; metabolized to active metabolite
Primary excretion	Renal 50%; feces 50%
Onset of action	1–2 h
Duration of action	5 days

Adverse Effects: Clopidogrel has approximately the same tolerability as aspirin and adverse effects are rarely severe enough to cause discontinuation of therapy. Although excessive bleeding is a potential adverse effect, it only occurs in about 1% of patients. Older adults are more susceptible to bleeding during therapy and should be carefully monitored. The incidence of GI bleeding is less than that of aspirin. Common adverse effects are flulike syndrome, headache, diarrhea, dizziness, bruising, upper respiratory tract infection, and rash or pruritus. Clopidogrel does not exhibit the same degree of bone marrow toxicity as ticlopidine. **Black Box Warning**: Because the effectiveness of clopidogrel is dependent on its metabolic activation by CYP 450 enzymes, poor metabolizers will exhibit less therapeutic effect and more adverse cardiovascular events.

Contraindications/Precautions: Clopidogrel is contraindicated in patients with active bleeding and should be used with caution in patients at high risk for bleeding, including those with peptic ulcer disease. Severe hepatic disease may impair the ability of the liver to convert the drug to its active metabolite. The drug should be discontinued at least 5 days prior to elective surgery.

Drug Interactions: Use with anticoagulants, other antiplatelet drugs, thrombolytic agents, or NSAIDs, including aspirin, will increase the risk of bleeding. Drugs that inhibit hepatic metabolic enzymes—such as the azole antifungals, protease inhibitors, erythromycin, verapamil, or zafirlukast—may diminish the antiplatelet actions of clopidogrel. Drugs that increase hepatic metabolic enzyme activity, such as barbiturates, rifampin, or carbamazepine, may increase the anticoagulant activity of clopidogrel. **Herbal/Food**: Herbal supplements that affect coagulation such as feverfew, green tea, ginkgo, fish oil, ginger, or garlic may increase the risk of bleeding.

Treatment of Overdose: There is no specific therapy for clopidogrel overdose. Platelet transfusions may be beneficial in preventing hemorrhage.

Pregnancy: Category B.

Nursing Responsibilities: Key nursing implications for patients receiving clopidogrel are included in the Nursing Practice Application for Patients Receiving Pharmacotherapy with Anticoagulants. While nursing responsibilities are similar to those for the anticoagulant drugs, bleeding risk is lessened with the antiplatelet drugs.

Drugs Similar to Clopidogrel (Plavix)

Other antiplatelet drugs include dipyridamole, prasugrel, ticagrelor, ticlopidine, and vorapaxar. Aspirin also provides anticoagulation by this mechanism and is discussed in Section 38.7.

Dipyridamole (Persantine): Approved in 1961, the only approved use of dipyridamole is in combination with warfarin for postoperative prophylaxis of thromboembolic complications in patients with prosthetic heart valves. By itself, dipyridamole provides little antithrombotic protection, but it may be combined with aspirin or warfarin to produce an anticoagulant effect. Dipyridamole acts by a different mechanism than clopidogrel. Rather than blocking ADP receptors, dipyridamole elevates levels of cyclic AMP (cAMP), which is a potent inhibitor of platelet aggregation. Originally approved in 1961 for treating angina due to its vasodilation action on the coronary arteries, dipyridamole is no longer used for that indication. Dizziness, abdominal pain, and headache are the most common adverse effects. This drug is pregnancy category B.

Prasugrel (Effient): Prasugrel is an ADP receptor blocker that was approved in 2009 to reduce the risk for thrombotic events in patients with acute coronary syndrome who undergo PCI. Prasugrel is a prodrug that is rapidly metabolized to its active form as it crosses the intestinal mucosa. Antiplatelet effects begin to occur within 30 minutes, which is faster than other drugs in this class. Compared to clopidogrel, prasugrel is associated with a reduced risk of adverse cardiovascular events, such as stroke and MI, and it is less prone to interact with other medications. Prasugrel carries a black box warning that it can cause serious and life-threatening bleeding. It should not be used in patients with active bleeding or a history of transient ischemic attack or stroke. Prasugrel should be discontinued at least 7 days prior to expected surgery. This drug is pregnancy category B.

Ticagrelor (Brilinta): Approved in 2011, ticagrelor is a new coagulation modifier indicated to reduce the risk of thromboembolic events in patients with acute coronary syndrome. In patients with PCI, the drug reduces the risk of stent thrombosis. Like clopidogrel and pasugrel, ticagrelor acts by blocking the ADP receptor on platelets. The most frequent adverse effects are dyspnea and bleeding. Ticagrelor carries a black box warning that the drug can cause serious or fatal bleeding, that it is contraindicated in patients with a history of intracranial hemorrhage or pathologic bleeding, and that it should be discontinued at least 5 days prior to surgery. The black box warning also states that maintenance doses of aspirin should not exceed 100 mg/day because aspirin decreases the effectiveness of ticagrelor. This drug is pregnancy category C.

Ticlopidine (Ticlid): Approved in 1991, ticlopidine is an ADP receptor blocker with antiplatelet effects very similar to those of clopidogrel. Ticlopidine is approved to prevent thrombotic stroke and has been used to prevent thromboembolic events in those receiving coronary artery stents. The drug is administered PO and may take up to 5 to 6 days of therapy to achieve optimum effects. Anticoagulant action may persist 1 to 2 weeks after the drug is withdrawn, because new platelets must be synthesized to replace those bound to the drug. Common adverse effects include diarrhea, nausea, vomiting, and dyspepsia. Ticlopidine carries a black box warning that the drug may cause bone marrow toxicity, which may manifest as agranulocytosis, pancytopenia, thrombocytopenic purpura, or neutropenia. Although these cases are rare, they may be life threatening. Thus, ticlopidine is generally only used when other drugs such as aspirin and clopidogrel have failed to produce the desired therapeutic results. This drug is pregnancy category B.

Vorapaxar (Zontivity): In 2014 the FDA approved vorapaxar, a new type of antiplatelet drug, to reduce the risk for blood clots in patients with a history of MI or other thromboembolic disorders. Given PO, it is the first drug to cause anticoagulation by blocking the protease-activated receptor (PAR-1) on platelets. Like other anticoagulants, its primary adverse effect is increased bleeding risk. Vorapaxar carries a black box warning that it should not be administered to patients with a history of stroke, transient ischemic attack, or intracranial hemorrhage. This drug is pregnancy category B.

38.9 The glycoprotein IIb/IIIa receptor inhibitors are the most effective antiplatelet drugs for preventing coagulation.

Glycoprotein IIb/IIIa is a receptor found on the surface of platelets. The receptor contains two distinct protein chains: IIb and IIIa designate the two chains. Platelets contain a huge number of glycoprotein IIb/IIIa receptors: approximately 50,000 to 80,000 per cell. These receptors serve as docking stations, waiting for signals from chemical messengers that indicate injury may have occurred.

Substances that may bind to and activate glycoprotein IIb/IIIa receptors include thrombin, von Willebrand factor, ADP, and thromboxane A_2. Following activation of the surface glycoprotein, the platelets change shape, bind fibrinogen, and become sticky. Essentially, the platelets develop an enhanced ability to bind to each other, to fibrinogen, and to the exposed collagen of damaged vessels. This process is illustrated in Figure 38.2.

Glycoprotein IIb/IIIa receptor inhibitors are relatively new additions to the therapy of thromboembolic disease. Inhibition of the glycoprotein IIb/IIIa receptor prevents platelet activation and thrombus formation in patients with a recent MI, stroke, and PCI, with or without stent placement.

Although these medications are the most effective antiplatelet drugs, they are very expensive. Another major disadvantage is that they are given only by the IV route. PO forms of these drugs recently entered clinical trials but proved less effective than aspirin in reducing thromboembolic events.

PROTOTYPE DRUG	Abciximab (ReoPro)

Classification: Therapeutic: Antiplatelet drug
Pharmacologic: Glycoprotein IIb/IIIa inhibitor

Therapeutic Effects and Uses: Abciximab was the first glycoprotein IIb/IIIa inhibitor approved by the FDA in 1994. It is of value in decreasing the incidence of thromboembolic events in patients with acute coronary syndrome, and in conjunction with PCI, both before and after the procedure. Abciximab is only available by IV bolus injection and infusion. It is often given

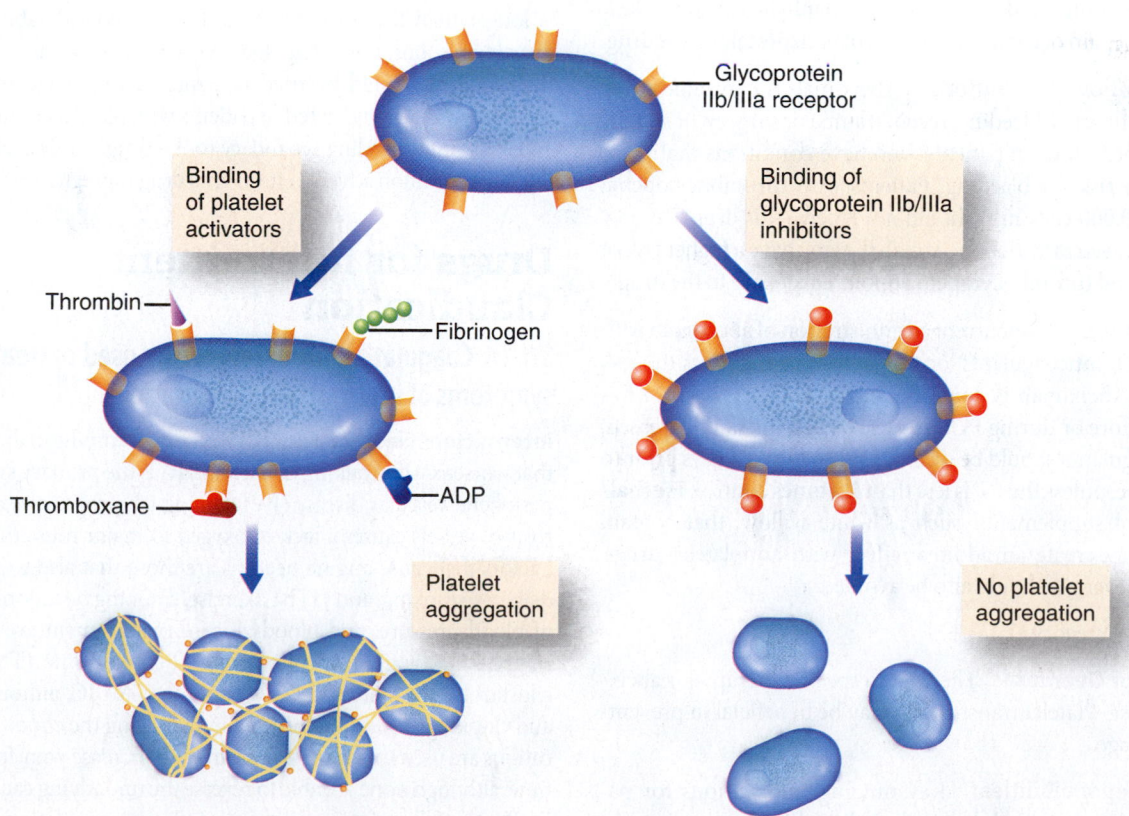

Figure 38.2 Glycoprotein IIb/IIIa receptor activation of platelet function.

concurrently with aspirin, clopidogrel, or heparin to achieve optimum therapeutic results.

Glycoprotein IIb/IIIa receptor inhibitors act very rapidly: Platelet function is reduced by as much as 90% in just 2 hours. Effects may persist for more than 10 days following discontinuation of the drug.

Mechanism of Action: Abciximab is an antibody fragment that binds to glycoprotein IIb/IIIa receptors on platelets, thus preventing fibrinogen, von Willebrand factor (vWF), and other procoagulants from activating platelets.

Pharmacokinetics:

Route(s)	IV
Absorption	NA
Distribution	Mostly bound to platelets, with very little circulating free; unknown if the drug crosses the placenta or is secreted in breast milk
Primary metabolism	Rapidly destroyed by proteases in plasma
Primary excretion	Unknown
Onset of action	10 min
Duration of action	72 h; half-life: 10–30 min

Adverse Effects: The most common adverse effect of abciximab is abnormal bleeding, which may occur in any body system. Major bleeding occurs in about 10% of patients, with the most common bleeding occurring at the arterial access site. Hypotension may occur secondary to loss of blood. Thrombocytopenia occurs in more than 5% of the patients; thus, blood counts must be periodically monitored during therapy. Anaphylaxis is rare. Back pain and chest pain occur in 11% to 18% of patients taking the drug.

Contraindications/Precautions: Abciximab is contraindicated in patients with active bleeding, recent trauma or surgery, or serious bleeding disorders, or in patients who have conditions that place them at high risk for bleeding. Patients with thrombocytopenia (less than 100,000 cells/mL) should not receive this drug. Patients who have received previous abciximab therapy have a higher risk of anaphylaxis and thrombocytopenia upon reexposure to the drug.

Drug Interactions: Concurrent administration of abciximab with heparin, other anticoagulants, or thrombolytics increases the risk of bleeding. Abciximab is contraindicated when IV dextran has been used before or during PCI because bleeding risk is increased. Oral anticoagulants should be discontinued at least 7 days prior to abciximab use, unless the PT is less than 1.2 times control. **Herbal/Food**: Herbal supplements, such as white willow, that contain salicylates may create an additive effect with antiplatelet drugs. Ginkgo and feverfew should also be avoided.

Pregnancy: Category C.

Treatment of Overdose: There is no specific therapy for abciximab overdose. Platelet transfusions may be beneficial in preventing hemorrhage.

Nursing Responsibilities: Key nursing implications for patients receiving abciximab are included in the Nursing Practice Application for Patients Receiving Pharmacotherapy with Anti-

coagulants. While nursing responsibilities are similar to those for the anticoagulant drugs, bleeding risk is lessened with the antiplatelet agents.

Drugs Similar to Abciximab (ReoPro)

The two other glycoprotein IIb/IIIa inhibitors are eptifibatide and tirofiban.

Eptifibatide (Integrilin): Approved in 1998, eptifibatide is a synthetic drug administered by the IV route that is highly specific to binding the glycoprotein IIa/IIIb receptor. Unlike abciximab, the binding of eptifibatide is rapidly reversible and a large amount of unbound drug may circulate in the plasma. In overdose situations, platelet infusions may be of little benefit because the unbound drug will quickly occupy glycoprotein IIb/IIIa receptors on the new platelets to prevent their activation by procoagulants. The drug is indicated for the prevention of thromboembolic events in patients with acute coronary syndrome and those undergoing PCI. Aspirin or heparin is usually administered concurrently with eptifibatide. Should platelet count decrease to less than $100,000/mm^3$, the aspirin or heparin is discontinued. The duration of action of eptifibatide is only 2 to 4 hours, compared to 24 to 48 hours for abciximab with eptifibatide. The kidneys primarily excrete the drug; thus, caution should be used in patients with renal impairment. Bleeding at the arterial access site is the most common adverse effect. This drug is pregnancy category B.

Tirofiban (Aggrastat): Like eptifibatide, tirofiban is an IV synthetic drug highly selective for binding the glycoprotein IIb/IIIa receptor in a rapid, reversible manner. The drug is indicated for the prevention of thromboembolic events in patients with acute coronary syndrome and those undergoing PCI. Aspirin or heparin is usually administered concurrently. Its duration of action (4 to 8 hours) is longer than that of eptifibatide but still considerably less than abciximab's duration. The kidneys primarily excrete the drug; thus, caution should be used in patients with renal impairment. Tirofiban is contraindicated in patients with platelet counts less than $100,000/mm^3$. Bleeding secondary to the drug's antiplatelet effect is the most common adverse effect. This drug is pregnancy category B.

Drugs for Intermittent Claudication

38.10 Coagulation modifiers can be used to treat symptoms of intermittent claudication.

Intermittent claudication (IC) is pain or cramping in the lower legs that worsens with walking or exercise. IC is the primary symptom of peripheral vascular disease (PVD), in which progressive atherosclerosis of vessels causes a lack of oxygen to major muscles of the leg. Factors that cause angina pectoris are those that also worsen PVD: diabetes, smoking, and HTN. Exercise, smoking cessation, reduction of blood pressure, and blood glucose management are important nonpharmacologic therapies for IC. Pentoxifylline (Trental) and cilostazol (Pletal) are specifically approved for IC, although aspirin and clopidogrel may also be used in managing the condition. Medications are used to reduce symptoms and increase pain-free walking time, although none are able to reverse the underlying cause of PVD.

Pentoxifylline is a unique drug with anticoagulation properties that acts on red blood cells to reduce their viscosity and increase

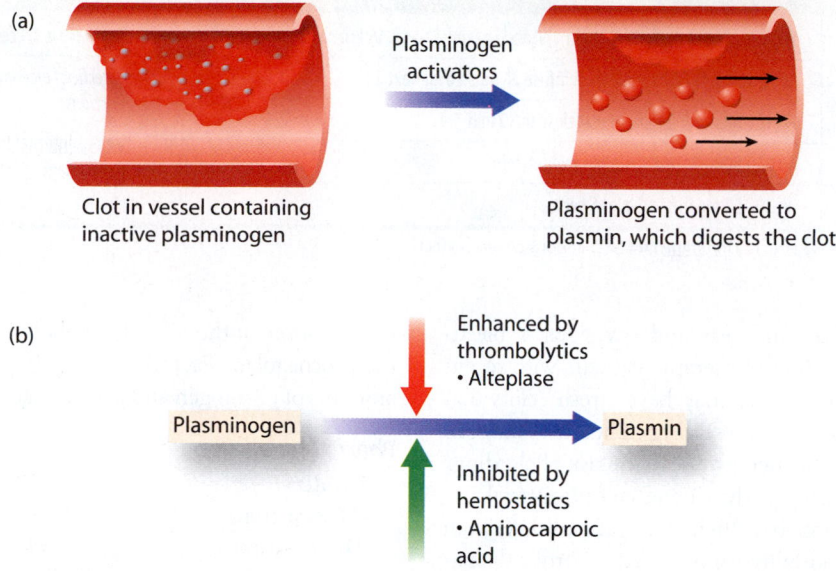

Figure 38.3 Steps in fibrinolysis: (a) clot dissolves when plasminogen is converted to plasmin. (b) thrombolytics enhance fibrinolysis; hemostatics inhibit fibrinolysis.

their flexibility, allowing them to enter vessels that are partially occluded and prevent thrombi formation. It also inhibits platelet aggregation. It is given PO to increase the microcirculation in patients with IC.

Cilostazol is indicated to reduce symptoms of IC and improve walking time. Given PO, the drug has antiplatelet and antithrombotic activity. Cilostazol should be used with care in patients with cardiac disease because it may cause palpitations and tachycardia.

38.11 Fibrinolysis is a process that removes thrombi.

The goal of hemostasis has been achieved once a blood clot is formed and the body is protected from excessive hemorrhage. The process of hemostasis, however, is a positive feedback mechanism in which small amounts of clotting lead to additional clotting. Without an effective means of controlling the process, clotting would spread far beyond the zone of injury and, indeed, occur throughout the vascular system until existing clotting factors were used up. Furthermore, fibrin clots can prevent blood flow to the surrounding area. Circulation must eventually be restored so that the tissue can resume normal activities.

Fibrinolysis is the physiological process that limits clot formation and removes existing clots. During the time a fibrin clot is forming, the surrounding damaged tissue secretes anticoagulant chemicals that limit the spread of the clot to the area of injury. Removal of the clot begins about 24 to 48 hours following clot formation and continues until it is dissolved.

Like hemostasis, fibrinolysis involves several cascading steps. The process is initiated by plasminogen activators. The two best studied plasminogen activators are tissue-plasminogen activator (tPA), which is secreted by the endothelium of blood vessels, and urokinase-plasminogen activator (uPA), secreted by the kidney. The function of tPA and uPA is to convert the inactive protein **plasminogen**, which is present in the fibrin clot, to its active form called plasmin. Plasmin is an enzyme that attacks the fibrin strands, breaking them into small fragments that are soluble and no longer able to hold the clot together. The procoagulation factors fibrinogen, prothrombin, and clotting Factors V and XII are also inactivated by plasmin. The body normally regulates fibrinolysis such that unwanted fibrin clots are removed, while fibrin present in wounds is left to maintain hemostasis. The steps of fibrinolysis are shown in Figure 38.3.

Thrombolytics

38.12 Thrombolytics are used to dissolve existing intravascular clots in patients with myocardial infarction and stroke.

It is often mistakenly believed that the purpose of anticoagulants such as heparin or warfarin is to digest clots. This is not the case. A totally different type of drug is needed for this goal. The thrombolytics, listed in Table 38.6, are administered very differently from the anticoagulants and antiplatelet drugs, and they produce their effects by different mechanisms. Thrombolytics are prescribed for disorders in which an intravascular clot has already formed, such as acute MI, pulmonary embolism, acute ischemic stroke, and DVT.

Thrombolytics promote fibrinolysis by converting plasminogen to plasmin. The enzyme plasmin then digests fibrin, breaking it into small soluble fragments. In essence, the thrombolytics simply accelerate the normal process of clot removal in the body. The thrombolytics are also called fibrinolytics, owing to their destructive effects on fibrin. The therapeutic outcomes of thrombolytic therapy are strongly dependent on the time frame in which they are administered. They are considerably more effective when given as soon as possible after the clot has formed—preferably within 4 hours. The mechanism of action of the thrombolytics is shown in a Pharmacotherapy Illustrated feature in Chapter 35.

Thrombolytics are nonspecific and have a very narrow margin of safety between dissolving "normal" and "abnormal" clots. Vital

TABLE 38.6 Thrombolytics

Drug	Route and Adult Dose (Maximum Dose Where Indicated)	Adverse Effects
alteplase (Activase, t-PA)	IV: Begin with 60 mg and then infuse 20 mg/h over next 2 h	*Superficial bleeding at injection sites, allergic reactions*
reteplase (Retavase)	IV: 10 units over 2 min; repeat dose in 30 min	
streptokinase (Streptase)	IV: 250,000–1.5 million units over 60 min	<u>Serious internal bleeding, intracranial hemorrhage, HTN</u>
tenecteplase (TNKase)	IV: 30–50 mg infused over 5 sec	

Note: *Italics* indicate common adverse effects. <u>Underline</u> indicates serious adverse effects.

signs must be monitored continuously and any signs of bleeding may call for discontinuation of therapy. Patients with recent trauma, active bleeding, or surgery may have "fresh" clots that could be disrupted by the action of these drugs. Thus, they may not be candidates for thrombolytic therapy due to the risk of bleeding.

The use of thrombolytics in elderly patients is controversial. Research has shown that thrombolytic therapy in patients older than age 75 does not decrease mortality from the MI or stroke the patient has experienced. The risks of serious bleeding following drug administration may outweigh the therapeutic benefits. Patients older than age 75 must be carefully screened for contraindicated conditions, such as uncontrolled HTN, recent ischemic stroke, or current use of anticoagulants.

Because these medications are rapidly destroyed in the bloodstream, discontinuing the infusion quickly terminates their thrombolytic activity. After the clot is successfully dissolved with the thrombolytic, anticoagulant therapy with an anticoagulant is initiated to prevent the reformation of clots.

Since the discovery of streptokinase, the first drug in this class, there have been several subsequent generations of thrombolytics. The newer drugs such as tenecteplase (TNK-tPA) are more fibrin specific and are reported to have fewer adverse effects than streptokinase. tPA, marketed as alteplase (Activase), has replaced urokinase as the preferred thrombolytic for clearing thrombosed central IV lines.

PROTOTYPE DRUG   Alteplase (Activase)

Classification: Therapeutic: None
Pharmacologic: Thrombolytic/fibrinolytic

Therapeutic Effects and Uses: Produced through recombinant DNA technology, alteplase is identical to human tPA. Alteplase is a drug of choice for the treatment of thrombotic stroke. An off-label use is to restore IV catheter patency (Cathflo Activase). Although not routinely indicated for treating venous clots, the drug may be used in cases where a limb is at risk of gangrene and possible amputation due to vessel occlusion. Like other drugs in this class, it is administered by the IV route.

To achieve maximum effect, alteplase therapy should begin within 6 hours of onset of MI symptoms and within 3 hours of thrombotic stroke. Therapy should be initiated only after intracranial hemorrhage has been ruled out. Alteplase does not exhibit the degree of allergic reactions seen with streptokinase.

Mechanism of Action: The primary action of alteplase is to convert plasminogen to plasmin, which then dissolves fibrin clots. Alteplase is more fibrin specific than streptokinase but less

so than some of the other thrombolytics. The drug also degrades the procoagulant Factors V and VIII and lowers the circulating amounts of fibrinogen and plasminogen.

Pharmacokinetics:

Route(s)	IV
Absorption	NA
Distribution	Unknown; unknown if the drug crosses the placenta or is secreted in breast milk
Primary metabolism	Hepatic
Primary excretion	Renal
Onset of action	Immediate
Duration of action	3 h; half-life: less than 10 min

Adverse Effects: The most common adverse effect of alteplase is bleeding, which may occur superficially at catheter access or needle puncture sites, or internally. Signs of bleeding such as spontaneous ecchymoses, hematomas, or epistaxis should be reported to the health care provider immediately. Fibrinolysis of clots in the coronary arteries may cause transient dysrhythmias. Angioedema and intracranial bleeding are rare, though serious, adverse effects.

Contraindications/Precautions: History of stroke within the past 3 months, recent trauma or surgery, active bleeding, severe uncontrolled HTN, intracranial neoplasm, or arteriovenous malformation are contraindications to the use of alteplase. Whenever possible, parenteral injections of other drugs should be avoided during alteplase therapy to avoid an increased risk of bleeding at the injection site. Alteplase should not be administered if the patient is on warfarin and INR is greater than 1.7 or PT is greater than 15 seconds.

Drug Interactions: Concurrent use with anticoagulants, antiplatelet drugs, or NSAIDs, including aspirin, will increase the risk of bleeding. Intravenous nitroglycerin enhances the hepatic degradation of alteplase, reducing its ability to dissolve clots. **Herbal/Food:** Use with supplements that affect coagulation such as feverfew, green tea, ginkgo, fish oil, ginger, or garlic should be avoided, because they may increase the risk of bleeding.

Pregnancy: Category C.

Treatment of Overdose: There is no specific treatment for overdose. Excessive bleeding may require the administration of blood, blood products, or hemostatics.

Nursing Responsibilities: Key nursing implications for patients receiving alteplase are included in the Nursing Practice Application for Patients Receiving Pharmacotherapy with Thrombolytics.

CONNECTIONS: NURSING PRACTICE APPLICATION

Patients Receiving Pharmacotherapy with Thrombolytics

Assessment	Potential Nursing Diagnoses*
Baseline assessment prior to administration: • Obtain a complete health history: cardiovascular, peripheral vascular disease, respiratory, neurologic (including recent head injury), recent surgeries or injuries, hepatic or renal disease, diabetes, peptic ulcer disease, recent childbirth (within 10 days), or the possibility of pregnancy. Obtain a drug history including allergies, current prescription and OTC drugs, herbal preparations, and alcohol use. Be alert to possible drug interactions. • Obtain baseline weight, vital signs, ECG, and breath sounds. Assess presence, quality, location of angina, and for presence of dyspnea or chest pain. Assess neurologic status. • Evaluate laboratory findings (aPTT, PT/INR, bleeding time), CBC and platelets, renal and liver function studies, ABGs as appropriate, and lipid profiles. Support the patient during other required tests (e.g., CT or MRI prior to thrombolytic therapy for stroke). • Establish all monitoring equipment and necessary lines, or arrange for their insertion (e.g., ECG monitoring, IV, Foley catheter, arterial line). • Assess the patient's ability to receive and understand instructions. Include family and caregivers as needed.	• *Pain* • *Ineffective Peripheral Tissue Perfusion* • *Impaired Gas Exchange* • *Impaired Skin Integrity* • *Anxiety* • *Deficient Knowledge* (Drug Therapy) • *Risk for Injury*, related to adverse effects of thrombolytic therapy
Assessment throughout administration: • Continue frequent assessments for therapeutic effects (e.g., angina has diminished significantly or is eliminated and ECG findings within normal limits, respiratory effort and ABGs significantly improved). • Continue frequent monitoring of appropriate laboratory values (e.g., Hgb, Hct, platelets, RBC, urinalysis, ABGs). • Monitor vital signs and ECG every 15 min during the first hour of infusion, and then every 30 min during the remainder of the infusion. Continue to monitor vital signs every 30 min to 1 h for the first 8 h following the infusion. • Assess for adverse effects: bleeding at IV sites, wounds, excessive ecchymosis, petechiae, hematuria, black/tarry stools, rectal bleeding, coffee-ground emesis, epistaxis, bleeding from gums, hemoptysis, dysrhythmias, and signs of occult bleeding: pallor, dizziness, hypotension, tachycardia, abdominal pain, areas of abdominal wall swelling or firmness, lumbar pain, or decreased level of consciousness. • Monitor neurologic status frequently, especially if thrombolytics are used for stroke.	

Implementation

Interventions and (Rationales)	Patient-Centered Care
Ensuring therapeutic effects: • Continue frequent assessments as above for therapeutic effects, e.g., previous angina has diminished significantly or is eliminated and ECG findings show decrease in ischemia. (Thrombolytics rapidly dissolve existing clots to allow reperfusion of the affected area.)	• Teach the patient about all procedures and their necessity prior to beginning thrombolytic therapy. • To allay anxiety, teach the patient, family, or caregiver the rationale for all equipment used.
• Post-therapy, encourage appropriate lifestyle changes: lowered fat intake, increased exercise, limited alcohol and caffeine intake, and smoking cessation. Provide for dietitian consultation as needed. (Smoking increases platelet aggregation and promotes the formation of thrombi. Healthy lifestyle changes will support and minimize the need for future drug therapy.)	• Encourage the patient to adopt a healthy lifestyle of low-fat food choices, increased exercise, decreased alcohol consumption, and smoking cessation. Provide for appropriate consultation (e.g., dietitian) as needed.
Minimizing adverse effects: • Monitor frequently for signs and symptoms of excessive visible bleeding: bleeding at IV sites, wounds, hematuria, rectal bleeding, coffee-ground emesis, bleeding from gums, hemoptysis, bleeding at previous recent incisional sites; and assess for occult bleeding: pallor, hypotension, tachycardia, dizziness, sudden severe headache, lumbar pain, and decreased level of consciousness. (Bleeding is the most common adverse effect of thrombolytic therapy. Frequent assessment for both visible and occult bleeding is necessary to prevent extensive hemorrhage and to start early corrective treatment as appropriate. Bleeding risk is elevated up to 2–4 days post-treatment and if the patient is maintained on anticoagulant or antiplatelet therapy post-thrombolytics.)	• Allay anxiety by reassuring the patient and explaining the rationale for frequent monitoring. Provide adequate pain relief as appropriate.

(continued)

• Monitor vital signs and ECG every 15 min during first hour of infusion, and then every 30 min during remainder of the infusion. Continue to monitor vital signs every 30 min to 1 h for the first 8 h following the infusion. Report any dysrhythmias immediately. (Frequent monitoring of vital signs assesses for adverse effects of the drug, including hypotension and tachycardia associated with bleeding, and for dysrhythmias. Dysrhythmias may occur postperfusion of the coronary arteries or may be associated with adverse effects. Further treatment may be necessary.)	• To allay possible anxiety, teach the patient, family, or caregiver the rationale for all equipment used and the need for frequent monitoring. • Teach the patient to report any palpitations, dyspnea, or angina postinfusion.
• Maintain the patient on bed rest and with limited activity during the infusion. (Limited physical activity and bed rest decrease the chance for bruising, injury, and bleeding.)	• Provide explanation and rationale that activity will be limited during the infusion and for up to 8 h post-treatment.
• Monitor neurologic status frequently, especially if thrombolytics are used for stroke. (A sudden change in neurologic status or sudden severe headache is a possible sign of an intracranial bleed with increased intracranial pressure.)	• To allay possible anxiety, teach the patient, family, or caregiver the rationale for the frequent assessments and provide reassurance. • Instruct the family to report immediately any change in the patient's mental status or level of consciousness during the postinfusion period.
• Avoid invasive procedures during infusion and up to 8 h postinfusion when possible. (Any puncture site or site of invasive procedure will create an additional site for bleeding. Whenever an invasive procedure must be used, e.g., ABGs, the site must be maintained under pressure for 30 min or longer to prevent hemorrhage.)	• Teach the patient that after any required procedures, pressure will be maintained on the site for a prolonged period of time.
• Continue to monitor laboratory work (Hgb, Hct, platelet counts, and bleeding time) frequently post-treatment. Periodic CBC and ABGs may also be monitored. Risk of bleeding remains high for 2–4 days postinfusion.	• Provide explanation for the need for activity restriction and frequent monitoring during this time.
Patient understanding of drug therapy: • Use opportunities during administration of thrombolytic therapy to explain the rationale for drug therapy, desired therapeutic outcomes, required monitoring for adverse effects, and precautions that will be taken during the infusion and during the immediate postinfusion time period. (Using time during nursing care helps to reassure the patient and allay anxiety.) • Provide support and reassurance to family and caregivers during the time of treatment. (Thrombolytics are used to treat potentially life-threatening conditions. Providing support, reassurance, and appropriate referrals, e.g., pastoral care or social service support, assists family members in a stressful situation.)	• The patient, family, or caregiver should have an understanding of the rationale behind thrombolytic therapy, equipment and monitoring that will be used, and the care required in the postinfusion period. • Allow family members time to discuss fears and concerns, and provide referral to support and ancillary providers as appropriate.
Patient self-administration of drug therapy: • Provide education during the postinfusion period about required medical care follow-up, postinfusion drug therapy (e.g., anticoagulants or antiplatelet drugs), and lifestyle changes. (Using time during nursing care helps to reinforce teaching and assess for any questions or concerns the patient or family may have.)	• Teach the patient, family, or caregiver in the proper self-administration techniques of anticoagulants or antiplatelet drugs as appropriate.

*Nursing Diagnoses—Definitions and Classification 2015–2017. Copyright © 2014, 1994–2014 by NANDA International. Used by arrangement with John Wiley & Sons Limited.

Drugs Similar to Alteplase (Activase)

Other thrombolytics include reteplase, streptokinase, and tenecteplase. Obtained from human blood donors, urokinase was removed from the market because of the possibility of viral contamination.

Reteplase (Retavase): Approved in 1996, reteplase is approved for the treatment of acute MI with ST elevation due to coronary artery thrombosis and for acute peripheral arterial thromboembolism. The drug is a modified form of human tPA produced through recombinant DNA technology. Reteplase has the same adverse effects and contraindications as alteplase. It has a more rapid onset of action than alteplase, perhaps because reteplase is better able to reach the inside of clots. Like alteplase, it is selective for lysing fibrin and the most serious adverse effect is bleeding. This drug is pregnancy category C.

Streptokinase (Streptase): Streptokinase, the first approved thrombolytic, is indicated for the treatment of acute MI with ST elevation due to coronary artery thrombosis, acute pulmonary embolism, DVT, or arterial thromboembolism. Streptokinase is obtained from beta-hemolytic streptococci and is less fibrin specific than the other drugs in this class; the drug also breaks down fibrinogen and other clotting factors. The drug may be administered by IV infusion into the general circulation or introduced via catheter directly at a site of occlusion.

Although it is much less expensive than other thrombolytics, streptokinase is considered a second-line drug because it is less effective at opening arteries. Allergic reactions such as urticaria, flushing, and headache occur in 1% to 4% of patients, although anaphylaxis is rare. The body develops antistreptokinase antibodies, which can cause resistance to the effects of the drug. Streptokinase shares the same contraindications and adverse effects with the other thrombolytics. The most common adverse effect is abnormal bleeding. Fever occurs in many patients and is managed by administering acetaminophen. This drug is pregnancy category C.

Tenecteplase (TNKase): Approved in 2000 for the treatment of acute MI with ST elevation with coronary artery thrombosis, tenecteplase is a modified form of human tPA. The drug has similar indications, contraindications, and adverse effects to alteplase but has greater fibrin specificity and a longer half-life. This may be responsible for a slightly lower incidence of noncerebral bleeding with tenecteplase. Another advantage is that it can be administered using a single, 5-second bolus injection. Allergic reactions are rare. This drug is pregnancy category C.

Hemostatics

38.13 Hemostatics are used to promote the formation of clots.

The hemostatics, or antifibrinolytics, have an action opposite to that of anticoagulants: to shorten bleeding time. Although their mechanisms differ, all drugs in this class prevent fibrin from dissolving, thus enhancing the stability of the clot and preventing excessive bleeding. The hemostatics, listed in Table 38.7, have very specific indications, and none are commonly prescribed.

Aminocaproic acid (Amicar) and tranexamic acid (Cyklokapron, Lysteda) are hemostatics that are administered IV. Injection sites should be monitored frequently for thrombophlebitis and extravasation. These drugs may affect muscles, causing wasting and weakness. High doses can promote the formation of abnormal clots. Chest pain and shortness of breath may indicate pulmonary thrombus or embolus. Use is contraindicated in patients with DIC or severe renal impairment.

PROTOTYPE DRUG	Aminocaproic Acid (Amicar)

Classification: Therapeutic: Hemostatic/antifibrinolytic
Pharmacologic: None

Therapeutic Effects and Uses: Aminocaproic acid is prescribed for conditions where there is excessive hemorrhage due to clots being dissolved rapidly or prematurely. Excessive fibrinolysis is associated with conditions such as aplastic anemia, hepatic cirrhosis, postoperative cardiac surgery, and in certain carcinomas. It is most commonly prescribed following surgery to reduce postoperative bleeding. Patients with hemophilia A (see Section 38.14) may receive aminocaproic acid immediately following dental procedures to control bleeding. The combination of aminocaproic acid with desmopressin (DDAVP) has been used to reduce postoperative bleeding in patients undergoing cardiopulmonary bypass.

During acute hemorrhage, aminocaproic acid can be given IV to reduce bleeding in 1 to 2 hours. It is also available in tablet form. The therapeutic serum level is 100 to 400 mcg/mL.

Mechanism of Action: Aminocaproic acid occupies binding sites on plasminogen and plasmin. This effectively prevents digestion of the fibrin clot by plasmin.

Pharmacokinetics:

Route(s)	PO, IV
Absorption	Rapidly absorbed from GI tract
Distribution	Widely distributed; unknown if it crosses the placenta or is secreted in breast milk
Primary metabolism	Unknown
Primary excretion	Renal
Onset of action	1–2 h
Duration of action	3–4 h

Adverse Effects: Aminocaproic acid is well tolerated and adverse effects are generally mild. By inhibiting fibrinolysis, the incidence of thrombosis may be increased. Myopathy is an uncommon adverse effect that requires monitoring because the drug may lead to rhabdomyolysis. Rapid IV administration may cause hypotension or bradycardia.

Contraindications/Precautions: Since aminocaproic acid tends to stabilize clots, it should be used cautiously in patients with a recent history of thromboembolic disease, including those with DIC. Aminocaproic acid is contraindicated in patients with urinary tract bleeding because the drug promotes the formation of clots in the renal pelvis or ureters that may cause obstruction. Caution must be used when administering the drug to patients with serious renal impairment because the drug may accumulate to toxic serum levels.

Drug Interactions: Aminocaproic acid antagonizes the action of thrombolytic drugs. Hypercoagulation may occur with concurrent use of estrogens and oral contraceptives. In hemophiliacs, concurrent administration of aminocaproic acid with Factor IX increases the risk of thrombosis and acute MI. **Herbal/Food**: Unknown.

Pregnancy: Category C.

Treatment of Overdose: Overdose may lead to hypotension and renal failure. No treatment for overdose is known, although hemodialysis or peritoneal dialysis may be used to remove the drug.

TABLE 38.7	Hemostatics	

Drug	Route and Adult Dose (Maximum Dose Where Indicated)	Adverse Effects
aminocaproic acid (Amicar)	IV: 4–5 g for 1 h, then 1–1.25 g/h until bleeding is controlled	*Allergic skin reactions, nausea, sinus and nasal symptoms, headache* <u>Anaphylaxis, thrombosis, bronchospasm, nephrotoxicity</u>
thrombin (Evithrom, Recothrom, Thrombinar)	Topical: Amount varies based on the size of the treated area	*Incision site complications, pruritus, nausea* <u>Antibody development, anaphylaxis, atrial fibrillation</u>
tranexamic acid (Cyklokapron, Lysteda)	PO: Two 650 mg tablets tid for a maximum of 5 days IV: 10 mg/kg, tid or qid, for 2–8 days	*Headache, nasal and sinus symptoms, back and abdominal pain* <u>Anaphylaxis, thromboembolic events</u>

Note: Italics indicate common adverse effects. <u>Underline</u> indicates serious adverse effects.

Nursing Responsibilities:

- Check IV site frequently for extravasation or thrombophlebitis and immediately change the site if this occurs.

- Monitor laboratory tests for creatine phosphokinase (CPK) activity, and obtain urinalyses for early detection of myopathy. Report fever, myalgia, reddish-brown urine, or decrease in urine output to the health care provider.

- Observe for signs of thrombophlebitis or embolism. If signs develop, immediately discontinue the drug and notify the provider.

- Monitor vital signs and urine output throughout therapy and for up to 24 hours post-therapy.

Lifespan and Diversity Considerations

- Monitor renal function labs more frequently with the older adult because normal changes related to aging or the development of myopathy or rhabdomyolysis may increase the risk of renal failure.

Patient and Family Education

- Immediately report any of the following to the health care provider: difficulty urinating, reddish-brown urine, arm or leg pain, chest pain, difficulty breathing, bleeding, clotting, dizziness, drowsiness, confusion, or convulsions.

- Make position changes slowly when moving from a lying to a standing position to prevent dizziness and possible fainting.

- Observe for increased toxicity with oral contraceptives and estrogen.

- Immediately notify the health care provider of any known or suspected pregnancy.

- Do not breast-feed while taking this drug without approval of the health care provider.

Drugs Similar to Aminocaproic Acid (Amicar)

Other hemostatics include desmopressin, thrombin (recombinant) (Recothrom), and tranexamic acid. Aprotinin (Trasylol) was voluntarily withdrawn from the market by the manufacturer in 2008 after several research studies determined that patients treated with this drug had a higher risk of renal failure, MI, heart failure, stroke, and death compared to patients who received aminocaproic acid or tranexamic acid.

Desmopressin (DDAVP, Stimate): Approved in 1978, DDAVP differs from other hemostatics in being a hormone similar to vasopressin (antidiuretic hormone [ADH]), a drug that promotes the renal conservation of water. As a hemostatic, it is approved for the treatment of spontaneous bleeding, trauma-induced hemorrhage or bleeding prophylaxis in patients with hemophilia A, or von Willebrand's disease type 1 with Factor VIII activity. The drug may be given parenterally in acute care scenarios, or by the nasal route (Stimate) for prophylaxis. Because desmopressin inhibits diuresis, caution must be used to prevent water intoxication. Headache and facial flushing are common adverse effects of the intranasal formulation. Tolerance rapidly develops to the actions of desmopressin, although this is usually not a problem when the drug is used to treat hemorrhage because only one to two doses are needed. Desmopressin has uses beyond hemostasis that include the control of excessive or nocturnal urination (enuresis) and polydipsia in patients with diabetes insipidus. This drug is pregnancy category B.

Thrombin, topical (Evithrom, Recothrom, Thrombinar): Topical thrombin is applied with a spray or gelatin sponge to areas that are oozing blood and for minor bleeding from capillaries. The drug is not to be used for serious arterial bleeding or bleeding over large areas. Care must be taken not to inject this drug or to allow systemic absorption due to the risk of thrombi formation.

Thrombin-JMI is an older form of thrombin prepared from cow blood. Allergic reactions may occur in patients hypersensitive to cow products. Approved by the FDA in 2007, human thrombin (Evithrom) is prepared from human plasma. Although screened and treated to inactivate viruses, products obtained from human plasma carry a small risk for transmission of infectious agents, such as viruses and the Creutzfeldt–Jakob disease agent. In 2008 the FDA approved thrombin (recombinant) (Recothrom), the first recombinant formulation of thrombin. The topical thrombins are pregnancy category C drugs.

Tranexamic acid (Cyklokapron, Lysteda): Like aminocaproic acid, tranexamic acid produces an antifibrinolytic effect by inhibiting plasminogen and plasmin activity. The drug was first approved in 1986 as an IV medication to reduce or prevent bleeding in patients with hemophilia who are undergoing dental procedures. In 2009, the PO form of the drug (Lysteda) was approved for the treatment of excessive menstrual bleeding. Because the drug inhibits clot removal, patients must be monitored carefully for signs and symptoms of thromboembolism. Taking Lysteda concurrently with hormonal contraceptives increases the risk of thromboembolic adverse effects. The drug is 8 to 10 times more potent and has a longer half-life than aminocaproic acid. Adverse effects are similar to those of aminocaproic acid. Tranexamic acid is pregnancy category B.

Drugs for Hemophilia

38.14 Hemophilia is treated by replacing the missing clotting factor(s) or by inhibiting coagulation.

Hereditary disorders of coagulation are relatively rare and may be caused by deficiency in any blood factor in the coagulation cascade. Symptoms of congenital coagulation disorders manifest as bleeding in muscles or weight-bearing joints, ecchymoses, epistaxis, gingival bleeding, and abnormally long bleeding times following trauma or surgery. Joint bleeding causes chronic inflammation and may result in permanent deformity and loss of mobility.

Some patients have mild forms of hemophilia, exhibiting no symptoms of excessive bleeding until they experience major trauma or surgery. The most severe forms of these disorders, however, are diagnosed shortly after birth and require a lifetime of lifestyle adjustment and pharmacotherapy. Because symptoms associated with the different clotting disorders are nonspecific, diagnosis requires laboratory assays for each of the clotting factors to determine which deficiency is causing the disorder.

The pharmacotherapy of hereditary coagulation disorders has resulted in a remarkable change in the lifespans of afflicted patients.

Prior to 1960, the average lifespan of a male with severe hemophilia A was 11 years; the lifespan is now 50 to 60 years.

PharmFACT

Hemophilia A: Lack of clotting Factor VIII results in hemophilia A, which accounts for approximately 80% of all hemophilia. Adequate amounts of Factor VIII are necessary to activate Factor X in the intrinsic coagulation pathway. Because the gene for Factor VIII is carried on the X chromosome, hemophilia A is a sex-linked disease with nearly all cases occurring in males. Females are asymptomatic carriers. Remarkably, patients may have a 75% reduction in the amount of Factor VIII in the blood and yet have no major symptoms. Those with 1% or less of Factor VIII have severe forms of the disease.

The traditional treatment for hemophilia A is administration of fresh frozen plasma. Plasma obtained from blood donors contains all the necessary components to replace the missing clotting factor(s). Unfortunately, contamination of blood products with the human immunodeficiency virus (HIV), hepatitis B, and hepatitis C in the early 1980s infected most patients with hemophilia and resulted in a significant percentage of deaths in transfusion recipients. Although all donated blood is screened for viral pathogens, fresh frozen plasma is now rarely used to treat hemophilia due to a small risk of viral contamination.

Hemophilia A is now treated with the administration of a concentrated solution of Factor VIII. A large number of products are available, and trade names include Advate, Alphanate, Bioclate, Helixate, Humate, Hyate, Koate, Kogenate, Monarc, Monoclate, NovoEight, Recombinate, ReFacto, and Xyntha. Factor VIII products differ in purity and whether they are derived from plasma or through recombinant DNA technology. Factor concentrates were once obtained by pooling the plasma from human donors, but this has been replaced by creating ultra-high-purity factors through recombinant DNA technology to lower the risk of viral contamination. There is still a very small risk of viral contamination and allergic reaction because human cells and albumin are used to prepare some of the recombinant DNA products. Most factor concentrates are subjected to dry heat, vapor heat, solvent detergent, or a monoclonal antibody to remove any viruses that may remain.

Factor VIII therapy in people with hemophilia is indicated for acute bleeding due to trauma and to prevent perioperative bleeding associated with medical and surgical procedures. Prompt and early therapy is required for acute bleeding events. A typical regimen for a bleeding episode includes an initial bolus dose followed 8 hours later by a second dose. Subsequent doses are administered every 12 hours until a target blood level of Factor VIII is reached: 30% to 50% of normal level for minor bleeding episodes and 100% for major bleeding. Some regimens substitute a continuous infusion of the drug, rather than bolus doses.

Patients with severe hemophilia A may receive prophylactic therapy with Factor VIII with the goal of preventing chronic joint damage and disability. For prophylaxis, a typical regimen is 10 to 20 international units/kg of Factor VIII given three times per week.

The target level for Factor VIII prophylaxis ranges from 1% to 5% of normal. To be most effective, therapy should begin before joint damage has occurred, usually prior to age 2. Prophylactic therapy is very expensive and must be continued throughout the patient's lifespan. A central venous access device may be installed to allow more convenient dosing.

Adverse reactions to Factor VIII administration are uncommon. Flushing, headache, dyspnea, and urticaria may signal an allergic reaction. Anaphylaxis is possible, though rare. About 30% of patients will develop antibodies (called inhibitors) to Factor VIII that can significantly decrease the therapeutic effect of the drug. Patients who experience this inhibition may receive higher doses of Factor VIII or they may receive activated Factor VIIIa. Factor VIIIa is very expensive and is only used when medically necessary.

Desmopressin is an alternative therapy for treating minor bleeding episodes in patients with mild hemophilia A. Available by infusion or intranasal spray, desmopressin causes the release of Factor VIII and vWF from storage sites within the body. The drug can cause a two- to fourfold increase in Factor VIII levels. Desmopressin therapy is usually limited to 2 to 3 days because repeated administration results in a diminished response. If desmopressin is used for a minor surgical procedure, a test dose is usually administered 1 week prior to surgery to determine if the patient is responsive to the drug. In adult hemophiliacs, 10% to 20% of patients will not respond to desmopressin therapy. Those with severe forms of the disease have no internal storage depots of Factor VIII or vWF; thus, the drug will be ineffective in these patients.

Other therapies for hemophilia A include the hemostatic drugs aminocaproic acid and tranexamic acid. These drugs are primarily used for short-term therapy to reduce bleeding related to dental procedures.

Hemophilia B: Hemophilia B, or Christmas disease, is caused by a deficiency of Factor IX, and comprises about 20% of those afflicted with hemophilia. Factor IX, in conjunction with activated Factor VIII, is required for the activation of Factor X in the coagulation cascade. Like Factor VIII, the gene for Factor IX is on the X chromosome. Thus symptomatic disease occurs predominantly in males. The disease is much less common than hemophilia A, but symptoms of excessive bleeding are the same. Laboratory testing is necessary to distinguish between the two diagnoses.

Treatment of hemophilia B is through replacement therapy with Factor IX. Like Factor VIII, fresh frozen plasma and pooled factor concentrates were historically used to supply the missing clotting factor. The development of a recombinant form of Factor IX in 1996, however, removed the risk of viral contamination and has become the therapy of choice for this disorder. The drug is administered for treating and preventing excessive bleeding events such as acute trauma or surgery. Products containing recombinant Factor IX include Alprolix, BeneFIX, and Rixubis. A typical regimen for acute bleeding includes an initial dose of 20 to 80 international units/kg, followed by repeat doses every 24 hours until the target level of Factor IX is obtained. Target levels can sometimes be achieved after a single dose and maintained with lower doses. Factor IX is also administered prophylactically to reduce the incidence of spontaneous bleeding. Hemostatic drugs such as aminocaproic acid and tranexamic acid may be used for short-term therapy to reduce bleeding related to dental procedures in patients with hemophilia B.

Hemophilia C: Factor XI deficiency, or hemophilia C, occurs in equal numbers of males and females and is a mild form of hemophilia. In the general population, hemophilia C occurs at a rate of 1 per million births, but it affects up to 13% of those with Ashkenazi Jewish heritage. No therapy is generally indicated unless the patient is undergoing a medical, surgical, or dental procedure. Administration of fresh frozen plasma supplies adequate amounts of Factor XI to prevent or slow bleeding during these procedures.

von Willebrand's Disease

The most common inherited coagulation disorder, **von Willebrand's disease (vWD)**, affects 1 in every 100 to 500 people. This disorder results in a decrease in quantity or quality of von Willebrand factor (vWF), which is required for platelet adhesion to injured blood vessel endothelium. vWF is also a carrier molecule for Factor VIII, protecting it from destruction as it circulates through the blood. Thus, a deficiency in vWF will decrease levels of Factor VIII and affect coagulation. Like hemophilia, the disease has mild and severe forms, both characterized by abnormal bleeding. The disease affects males and females equally, and life expectancy is usually normal.

This type of bleeding disorder is treated with Factor VIII concentrate as well as desmopressin, which promotes the release of stored vWF. For the most severely affected patients, plasma products containing vWF may be required.

CHAPTER
38

Understanding the Chapter

Key Concepts Summary

38.1 Thromboembolic disorders are abnormalities of hemostasis that include deep venous thrombosis and pulmonary embolism.

38.2 Coagulation disorders are caused by decreased numbers of platelets or by deficiencies in specific clotting factors.

38.3 The normal coagulation process can be modified by a number of different mechanisms.

38.4 Heparin is the traditional drug of choice for rapid anticoagulation.

38.5 Warfarin is the most widely used drug for oral anticoagulant therapy.

38.6 The direct thrombin inhibitors are anticoagulants originally obtained from medical leeches that are used to treat or prevent venous thromboembolism.

38.7 Antiplatelet drugs provide anticoagulation by reducing the aggregation properties of platelets.

38.8 The adenosine diphosphate receptor blockers are antiplatelet drugs prescribed for the prevention and treatment of arterial thrombosis.

38.9 The glycoprotein IIb/IIIa receptor inhibitors are the most effective antiplatelet drugs for preventing coagulation.

38.10 Coagulation modifiers can be used to treat symptoms of intermittent claudication.

38.11 Fibrinolysis is a process that removes thrombi.

38.12 Thrombolytics are used to dissolve existing intravascular clots in patients with myocardial infarction and stroke.

38.13 Hemostatics are used to promote the formation of clots.

38.14 Hemophilia is treated by replacing the missing clotting factor(s) or by inhibiting coagulation.

Case Study: Making the Patient Connection

Remember the patient "Ruby Dwyer" at the beginning of the chapter? Now read the remainder of the case study. Based on the information presented within this chapter, respond to the critical thinking questions that follow.

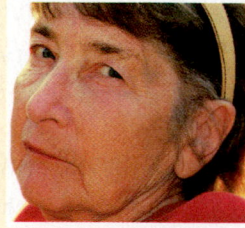

Ruby Dwyer had looked forward to the trip and was anxious to see her grandchildren. When her son accepted an executive position with his company, she had no idea that he would be relocated to Bangkok. The trip would be long but certainly worth the effort. She never dreamed in her 74 years that she would be flying out of the United States, much less to Thailand. When the opportunity came to see her son and his family, she jumped at the chance. After all, it had been 5 years since he had left their home in Chicago.

When she returned from her trip, she noticed some pain in her right leg. Although she sees herself as a healthy older woman, she does experience occasional arthritis pain. Considering that she was on a commercial airliner for more than 20 hours, she did not think much about the leg discomfort. However, after a few days, her leg became increasingly more painful and swollen. She could not imagine what was causing this problem. Finally, after 3 days, Ruby became worried about what seemed to be increasing leg swelling and pain. She is seen in her health care provider's office. The following health information is documented in her medical record:

> Ruby Dwyer, 74-year-old Caucasian woman. Her physical examination revealed the following findings: alert, oriented 74-year-old woman with chief complaint of swelling, painful right lower extremity × 3 days. Cardio: Heart rate regular without murmurs; blood pressure 118/74 mmHg; all pulses present equal and strong in all extremities; no respiratory distress—regular, clear, breath sounds; audible bowel sounds in all four quadrants. Her right mid-calf area has 3–4+ pitting edema, and is hot and painful to touch and she has a moderate amount of varicosities in lower extremities bilaterally.

Ruby had a hysterectomy 15 years ago, and does not drink alcohol or use tobacco. She takes occasional aspirin for muscle aches, and has no known allergies. Her family history indicates that her father died from a stroke and her mother died of "old age." She has one sister who has diabetes.

Ruby was diagnosed with deep venous thrombosis (DVT) in her right leg. The treatment plan was to admit her into the hospital for anticoagulant therapy and pain control. In the hospital setting, Ruby will receive heparin therapy. You are the nurse caring for this patient.

Critical Thinking Questions

1. Ruby asks, "How soon will the heparin dissolve my blood clot?" How would you respond to this question?
2. What patient education should you provide Ruby about anticoagulation therapy?
3. What is an activated partial thromboplastin time? How will this test be used to direct heparin therapy?
4. What factors predisposed this patient to deep venous thrombosis?
5. What should Ruby be taught about taking aspirin for arthritis pain?

See Answers to Critical Thinking Questions on student resource website.

Additional Case Study

You are attending your annual family reunion and begin talking to your favorite uncle Lewis about his recent hospitalization. Lewis Kinard, a 55-year-old man, was recently discharged from the hospital following an episode of atrial fibrillation. He returned home with instructions to take warfarin (Coumadin) 10 mg daily. He has many questions for you, his favorite relative.

1. Why would someone with atrial fibrillation be prescribed Coumadin?
2. What special precautions should Lewis take while on this drug?
3. Are there any foods that he should avoid or limit in his diet?
4. What laboratory testing will be done to determine this drug's effectiveness?

See Answers to Additional Case Study on student resource website.

Chapter Review

1 The patient with deep venous thrombosis is being treated with a heparin infusion. The nurse would monitor for therapeutic effectiveness by noting which of the following?
   1. Activated partial thromboplastin time (aPTT)
   2. Prothrombin time (PT)
   3. Platelet counts
   4. International normalized ratio (INR)

2 Which of the following should the nurse include in the teaching plan for a patient receiving subcutaneous heparin? Select all that apply.
   1. Inject medication in the deep fatty layer of the abdomen.
   2. When brushing your teeth, use a soft toothbrush.
   3. Hold direct pressure on any puncture sites for 15 minutes.
   4. Use dental floss daily after brushing.
   5. Take a daily aspirin tablet, 325 mg, to prevent inflammation at the injection site.

3 A patient who is taking warfarin (Coumadin) states, "I wake up every morning with arthritis pain and I always take aspirin or ibuprofen." The nurse's response would be based on which physiological concepts?

1. Aspirin and ibuprofen (Motrin) will counteract the therapeutic effects of many anticoagulants.

2. Anticoagulants will reduce the half-life of drugs such as aspirin and ibuprofen.

3. Many substances such as aspirin and ibuprofen will increase the risk of bleeding.

4. The combination of aspirin products with anticoagulants will worsen arthritis pain.

4 What should the nurse teach the patient who is to receive alteplase (Activase) as part of the treatment for myocardial infarction?

1. The drug will be given IV, and the patient should be able to go home later today.

2. The patient should remain quiet and lying down during drug administration and for up to 8 hours after infusion.

3. The risk of bleeding returns to normal within 24 hours after the drug has been infused.

4. An increase in vitamin K–rich foods or a supplement will be needed for the week following the treatment.

5 A patient who is taking clopidogrel (Plavix) to prevent another stroke asks the nurse how the medication works. The nurse's response should be based on an understanding that Plavix:

1. Inhibits platelet aggregation to prevent clot formation.

2. Activates antithrombin III and subsequently inhibits thrombin.

3. Inhibits enzymes involved in the formation of vitamin K.

4. Converts plasminogen to plasmin to dissolve fibrin clots.

6 A patient will be receiving dabigatran (Pradaxa). Which of the following is true concerning this drug therapy? Select all that apply.

1. Ginger, garlic, and green tea may increase the risk of bleeding.

2. Vitamin B_{12} is used to augment this drug's response.

3. Pradaxa is used for DVT.

4. Activated partial thromboplastin time may be monitored to determine effectiveness.

5. This drug is contraindicated for patients with gastritis.

See Answers to Chapter Review in Appendix A.

References

Check, J. H. (2012). The use of heparin for preventing miscarriage. *American Journal of Reproductive Immunology, 67,* 326–333. doi:10.1111/j.1600-0897.2012.01119.x

Drug Digest. (n.d.). *Drugs and herbs: Garlic.* Retrieved from http://www.drugdigest.org

Ernst, E., & Posadzki, P. (2012). Can garlic intake reduce the risk of cancer? A systematic review of randomised controlled trials. *Focus on Alternative and Complementary Therapies, 17,* 192–196. doi:10.1111/fct.12000

Kaandorp, S. P., Goddijn, M., van der Post, J. A., Hutten, B. A., Verhoeve, H. R., Hamulyák, K., . . . Middeldorp, S. (2010). Aspirin plus heparin or aspirin alone in women with recurrent miscarriage. *New England Journal of Medicine, 362,* 1586–1596. doi:10.1056/NEJMoa1000641

Mantha, S., Bauer, K. A., & Zwicker, J. I. (2009). Low molecular weight heparin to achieve live birth following unexplained pregnancy loss: A systematic review. *Journal of Thrombosis and Haemostasis, 8,* 263–268. doi:10.1111/j.1538-7836.2009.03687.x

McNamee, K., Dawood, F., & Farquharson, R. (2012). Recurrent miscarriage and thrombophilia: An update. *Current Opinions in Obstetrics and Gynecology, 24,* 229–234. doi:10.1097/GCO.0b013e32835585dc

Monien, S., Kadecki, O., Baumgarten, S., Salama, A., Dorner, T., & Kiesewetter, I. H. (2009). Use of heparin in women with early and late miscarriages with and without thrombophilia. *Clinical and Applied Thrombosis/Hemostasis, 15,* 636–644. doi:10.1177/1076029609335501

National Center for Complementary and Alternative Medicine. (2012). *Herbs at a glance: Garlic.* Retrieved from http://nccam.nih.gov/health/garlic/ataglance.htm

National Hemophilia Association. (n.d.). *HIV/AIDS.* Retrieved from http://www.hemophilia.org/NHFWeb/MainPgs/MainNHF.aspx?menuid=43&contentid=39&rptname=bloodsafety

Patel, K. (2014). Deep venous thrombosis. *Medscape Reference.* Retrieved from http://emedicine.medscape.com/article/1911303-overview

Selected Bibliography

Abad, R., Pitarch, J., & Rocha, E. (2010). Overview of venous thromboembolism. *Drugs, 70* (Suppl. 2), 3–10. doi:10.2165/1158583-S0-000000000-00000

Abraham, P., Rabinovich, M., Curzio, K., Patka, J., Chester, K., Holt, T., . . . Feliciano, D. V. (2013). A review of current agents for anticoagulation for the critical care practitioner. *Journal of Critical Care, 28,* 763–774. doi:10.1016/j.jcrc.2013.06.013

Franchini, M., & Mannucci, P. M. (2011). Inhibitors of propagation of coagulation (factors VIII, IX and XI): A review of current therapeutic practice. *British Journal of Clinical Pharmacology, 72,* 553–562. doi:10.1111/j.1365-2125.2010.03899.x

Gay, S. (2010). An inside view of venous thromboembolism. *Nurse Practitioner, 35*(9), 32–39. doi:10.1097/01.NPR.0000387141.02789.c5

Goldhaber, S. Z., & Bounameaux, H. (2012). Pulmonary embolism and deep vein thrombosis. *The Lancet, 379*(9828), 1835–1846. doi:10.1016/S0140-6736(11)61904-1

Herdman, T. H., & Kamitsuru, S. (Eds.). (2014). *NANDA international nursing diagnoses: Definitions and classification, 2015–2017.* Oxford, United Kingdom: Wiley-Blackwell.

Hughes, S. (2013). *Apixaban approved: Now which anticoagulant to use?* Retrieved from http://www.medscape.com/viewarticle/777887.

Lin, Y., Stanworth, S., Birchall, J., Doree, C., & Hyde, C. (2011). Use of recombinant factor VIIa for the prevention and treatment of bleeding in patients without hemophilia: A systematic review and meta-analysis. *Canadian Medical Association Journal, 183*(1), 223–247. doi:10.1503/cmaj.100408

Pernod, G., Albaladejo, P., Godier, A., Samama, C. M., Susen, S., Gruel, Y., . . . Sié, P. (2013). Management of major bleeding complications and emergency surgery in patients on long-term treatment with direct oral anticoagulants, thrombin or factor-Xa inhibitors: Proposals of the working group on perioperative haemostasis (GIHP). *Archives of Cardiovascular Diseases, 106*(6-7), 382–393. doi:10.1016/j.acvd.2013.04.009

Weltz, D. S., & Weltz, J. I. (2010). Update on heparin: What do we need to know? *Journal of Thrombosis and Thrombolysis, 29,* 199–207. doi:10.1007/s11239-009-0411-6

Wiltink, E. H. (2014). Anticoagulant therapy: We have to do better! A systematic review. *European Journal of Hospital Pharmacy, 21,* 108–112. doi:10.1136/ejhpharm-2013-000295

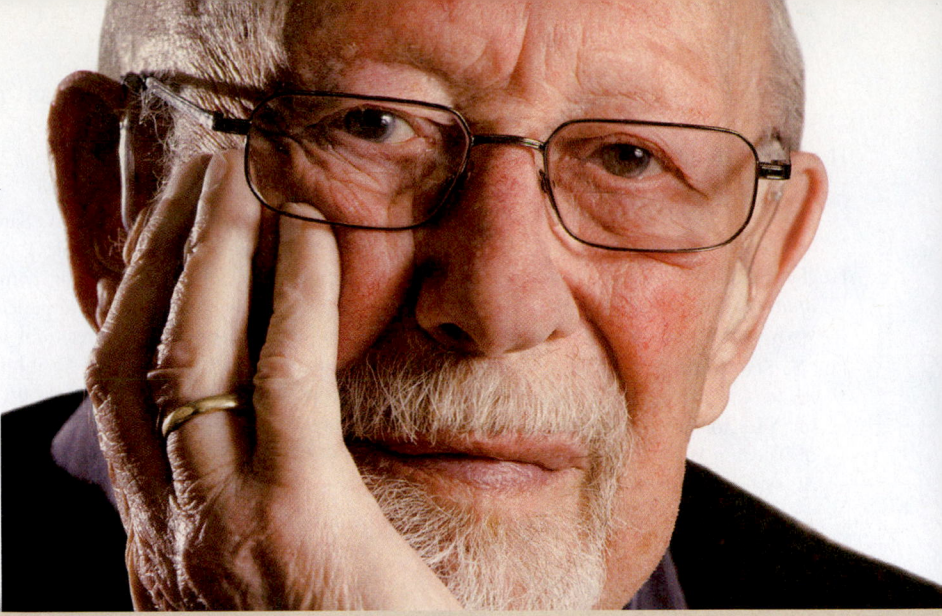

"For me, the worst part is the isolation from people. It's almost unbearable. I feel so lonely. If I could just be with people, I know I would feel better."

Patient "Carl Guenther"

CHAPTER

39 Pharmacotherapy of Hematopoietic Disorders

LEARNING OUTCOMES

After reading this chapter, the student should be able to:

1. Describe the physiology of hematopoiesis.
2. Describe how aspects of hematopoiesis can be modified by the administration of pharmacologic agents.
3. Explain the functions of erythropoietin.
4. Explain the functions of colony-stimulating factors.
5. Classify types of anemia based on their causes.
6. Illustrate the metabolism, storage, and transfer of iron in the body.
7. Identify the role of intrinsic factor in the absorption of vitamin B_{12}.
8. Compare and contrast anemias caused by vitamin B_{12} and folate deficiency.
9. Describe the nurse's role in the pharmacologic management of hematopoietic disorders.
10. For each of the classes shown in the chapter outline, identify the prototype and representative drugs and explain the mechanism(s) of drug action, primary indications, contraindications, significant drug interactions, pregnancy category, and important adverse effects.
11. Apply the nursing process to care for patients who are receiving pharmacotherapy for hematopoietic disorders.

CHAPTER OUTLINE

▸ **Physiology of Hematopoiesis**

▸ **Hematopoietic Growth Factors**
   Erythropoietin
   PROTOTYPE Epoetin Alfa (Epogen, Procrit), *p. 644*
   Colony-Stimulating Factors
   PROTOTYPE Filgrastim (Neupogen), *p. 646*
   Platelet Enhancers
   PROTOTYPE Oprelvekin (Neumega), *p. 651*

▸ **Classification of Anemias**

▸ **Antianemic Drugs**
   Iron Deficiency Anemia
   PROTOTYPE Ferrous Sulfate (Feosol, Feostat, Others), *p. 655*
   Pernicious Anemia
   PROTOTYPE Cyanocobalamin (Nascobal), *p. 658*

KEY TERMS

anemia, 652

colony-stimulating factors (CSFs), 646

erythropoietin, 643

ferritin, 654

folate, 657

folic acid, 657

hematopoiesis, 643

hemosiderin, 654

intrinsic factor, 657

multipotent stem cells, 643

pernicious anemia, 657

thrombopoietin, 649

transferrin, 654

The blood serves all other cells in the body and is the only fluid tissue. Because of its diverse functions, diseases affecting blood constituents have widespread effects on the body. This chapter examines medications used to enhance the functions of erythrocytes, leukocytes, and platelets. Pharmacology of the hematopoietic system is a small, though emerging, branch of medicine.

Physiology of Hematopoiesis

39.1 Hematopoiesis is a dynamic process that is responsive to the changing demands of the body.

Blood is a highly dynamic tissue; over 200 billion new blood cells are formed every day. The process of blood cell formation is called **hematopoiesis**, or hemopoiesis. In adults, hematopoiesis occurs primarily in red bone marrow and requires B vitamins, vitamin C, copper, iron, and other nutrients. Before proceeding, the student should read the brief review of blood found in Chapter 28.

Hematopoiesis responds to internal and external challenges faced by the body. For example, the production of white blood cells (WBCs) can increase tenfold in response to infection. The number of red blood cells (RBCs) can increase as much as fivefold in response to anemia or hypoxia. Homeostatic control of hematopoiesis is influenced by a number of hormones and growth factors, which allow for points for pharmacologic intervention. The process of hematopoiesis is illustrated in Figure 39.1.

The process of hematopoiesis begins with **multipotent stem cells**, which are capable of maturing (differentiating) into any blood cell type. What determines whether the stem cell produces RBCs, macrophages, lymphocytes, or perhaps platelets? The specific path taken by the multipotent stem cell depends on the internal needs of the body. These needs are transmitted to multipotent stem cells by regulatory substances that include various hormones and proteins. For example, high amounts of the hormone erythropoietin circulating through the blood signal the stem cells to differentiate into erythrocytes. Many types of cells secrete cytokines (interferons and interleukins) that signal the stem cells to increase or decrease the production of specific WBCs. Through recombinant deoxyribonucleic acid (DNA) technology some of these regulatory agents, shown in Figure 39.1, are now available in sufficient quantities to be used as medications.

PharmFACT

The recommended dietary allowance of iron for a woman is 10 to 15 mg. However, during pregnancy, a woman's body needs 1 g of iron daily: 300 mg for the fetus, 500 mg for expansion of the maternal RBCs, and 200 mg due to excretion (Office of Dietary Supplements, National Institutes of Health, 2014).

The pharmacologic management of hematopoietic disorders often involves simply replacing a deficient substance that is essential to hematopoiesis. In some cases, the drug is identical, or very closely resembles, the deficient endogenous factor. For example, the drug epoetin alfa (Epogen, Procrit) is identical to the natural hormone erythropoietin and stimulates the production of RBCs in the same manner. Administration of antianemic medications such as ferrous sulfate or vitamin B_{12} supplies the patient with essential factors that may be deficient.

Some of the hematopoietic drugs have become important adjunct medications in the pharmacotherapy of malignancies. Antineoplastic drugs often are toxic to bone marrow and cause neutropenia, a reduced number of WBCs. Neutropenia is a primary cause of patient morbidity and mortality in the treatment of cancer. Hematopoietic drugs can be used to boost the WBC counts in these patients.

Natural hormones that regulate some aspect of blood formation are called hematopoietic growth factors. These drugs and their doses are listed in Table 39.1.

CONNECTION Checkpoint 39.1

From what you learned in Chapter 28, name the three formed elements of blood. What percentage of whole blood do the formed elements comprise? *See Answer to Connection Checkpoint 39.1 on student resource website.*

Hematopoietic Growth Factors

39.2 Erythropoietin stimulates production of red blood cells and is used to treat anemia.

The process of RBC formation, or erythropoiesis, is regulated by the hormone **erythropoietin**. In adults, 90% of erythropoietin is secreted by the kidneys and 10% is secreted by the liver.

The primary signal to increase the renal secretion of erythropoietin is hypoxia: a reduction in oxygen reaching the proximal tubule cells in the kidney. Once secreted, erythropoietin travels to the bone marrow where it interacts with receptors on stem cells and delivers the message to increase erythrocyte production. Just as important, erythropoietin also stimulates the production of hemoglobin (Hgb), which is required for a functional erythrocyte. Hemorrhage, chronic obstructive pulmonary disease, anemia, or high altitudes may increase serum levels of erythropoietin as much as 1,000-fold in response to severe hypoxia. Erythropoietin is marketed as the drug epoetin alfa (Epogen, Procrit). Darbepoetin alfa (Aranesp) is closely related to epoetin alfa but has a duration of action that is two to three times longer. These drugs are sometimes called erythropoietic growth factors.

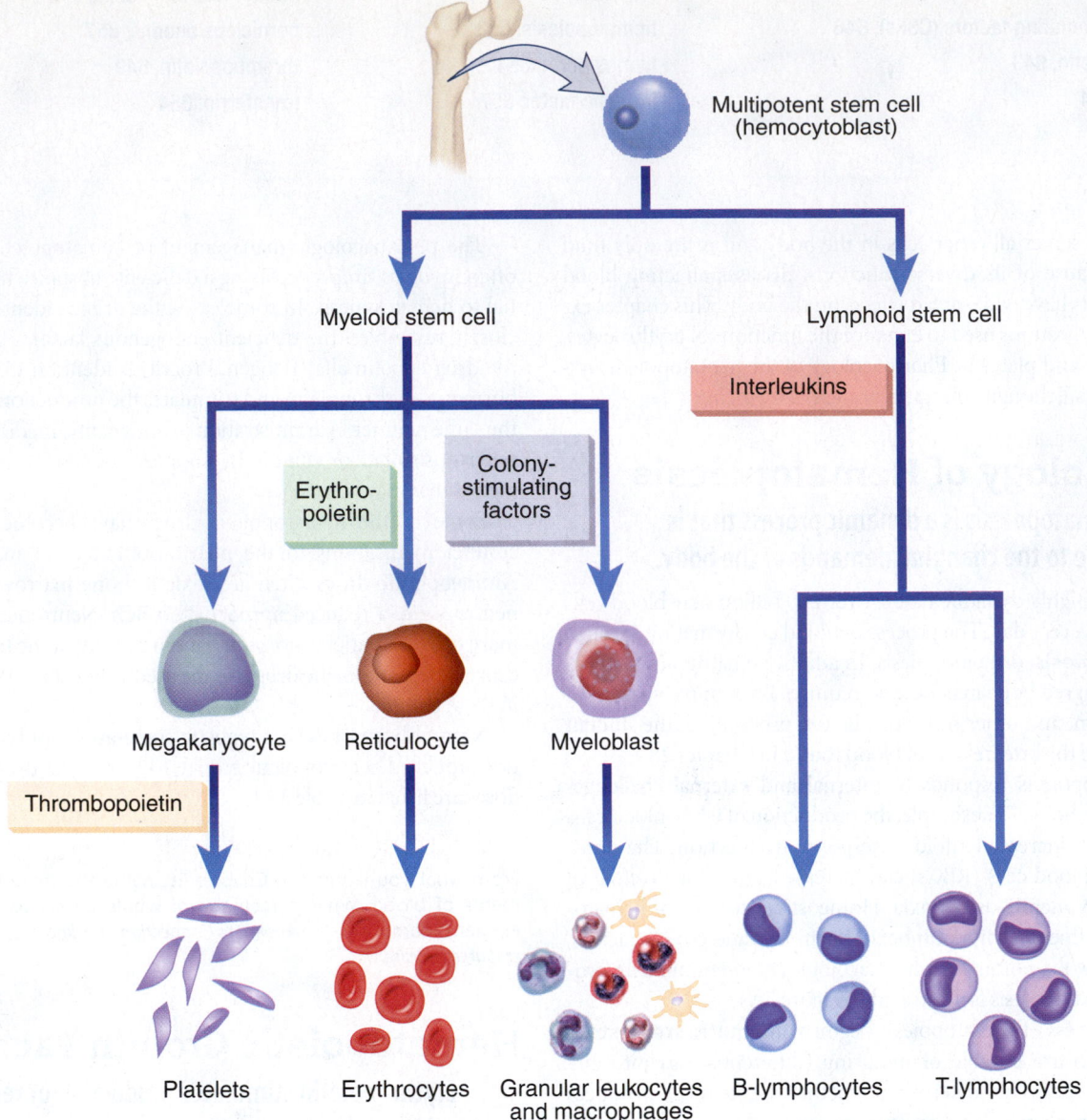

Figure 39.1 Hematopoiesis: Blood cells are formed from stem cells under the influence of hormones such as thrombopoietin, colony-stimulating factors, and erythropoietin.

PROTOTYPE DRUG | Epoetin Alfa (Epogen, Procrit)

Classification: Therapeutic: Hematopoietic growth factor, drug for anemia
Pharmacologic: Erythropoietin

Therapeutic Effects and Uses: Approved in 1989, epoetin alfa is made through recombinant DNA technology and is functionally identical to human erythropoietin. Although the drug may be administered intravenously (IV), the subcutaneous route is generally preferred because lower doses are needed, absorption is slower, and a more sustained response can be achieved. Epoetin is not used for the emergency correction of severe anemia or as a substitute for transfusion because it has a gradual onset of action. The hematocrit (Hct) increases 2% per week during the initial weeks of epoetin therapy and some patients require 2 to 6 weeks

for a change in Hct to occur. Most patients on epoetin therapy also receive iron supplements to meet the increased demands caused by the increased erythrocyte production. Although epoetin alfa does not cure any primary disease, it reduces anemia symptoms and dramatically improves the patient's ability to perform daily activities. A typical initial regimen for epoetin alfa requires 50 to 100 units/kg three times per week until a target Hgb level of 10 to 12 g/dL is achieved.

Epoetin is indicated for the treatment of anemia associated with chronic renal failure. Patients with chronic renal failure often experience anemia because they are unable to secrete sufficient endogenous erythropoietin. The drug is occasionally prescribed to reduce the need for transfusions in anemic patients prior to elective surgery, if a significant blood loss is expected. HIV-infected patients who are receiving zidovudine may receive epoetin alfa to treat anemia caused by antiretroviral drugs.

TABLE 39.1 Hematopoietic Growth Factors

Drug	Route and Adult Dose (Maximum Dose Where Indicated)	Adverse Effects
Erythropoietic Growth Factors		
darbepoetin alfa (Aranesp)	Subcutaneous/IV: 0.45 mcg/kg once per week (max: 74 mg/kg)	*Headache, fever, nausea, vomiting, diarrhea, insomnia, cough, upper respiratory infection, edema, pyrexia, rash* HTN, seizures, HF, MI
epoetin alfa (Epogen, Procrit): erythropoietin	Subcutaneous/IV: Start with 50–100 units/kg/dose and increase until target Hct range of 30–33% (max: 36%) is reached; Hct should not increase by more than 4 points in any 2-week period	
Colony-Stimulating Factors		
filgrastim (Neupogen): granulocyte-CSF	IV: 5 mcg/kg by 30-min infusion; may increase by 5 mcg/kg for each chemotherapy cycle Subcutaneous: 5 mcg/kg/day as single bolus dose; may increase by 5 mcg/kg for each chemotherapy cycle	*Flulike syndrome, fever, dyspnea, nausea, vomiting, bone pain (sargramostim)* Arthralgia, thrombocytopenia, cutaneous vasculitis, pericardial effusion (sargramostim), tachycardia (sargramostim)
pegfilgrastim (Neulasta)	Subcutaneous: 6 mg once per chemotherapy cycle at least 24 h after chemotherapy	
sargramostim (Leukine): GM-CSF	IV: 250 mcg/m^2/day infused over 2 h for 14 days, begin 2–4 h after bone marrow transfusion and not less than 24 h after last dose of chemotherapy or 12 h after last radiation therapy	
Platelet Enhancers		
eltrombopag (Promacta)	PO: 50 mg once daily (max: 75 mg/day)	*Arthralgia, myalgia, paresthesia, insomnia* Bone marrow fibrosis, thromboembolism, hematologic malignancy, hepatotoxicity
oprelvekin (Neumega)	Subcutaneous: 50 mcg/kg once daily starting 6–24 h after completing chemotherapy for 14–21 days or until platelet count is at least 50,000/mcL	*Edema, fever, headache, dizziness, dyspnea, fatigue, rash, nausea, vomiting* Tachycardia, febrile neutropenia, pleural effusion, anaphylaxis, dysrhythmias, candidiasis
romiplostim (Nplate)	Subcutaneous: 1 mcg/kg/week initial dose; may increase by increments of 1 mg/kg weekly until platelet count is at least 50,000/mcL	*Arthralgia, dizziness, insomnia, myalgia, abdominal pain, dyspepsia, paresthesia* Thromboembolism, bone marrow fibrosis

Note: Italics indicate common adverse effects. Underline indicates serious adverse effects.

Epoetin alfa is given to patients undergoing chemotherapy for nonmyeloid malignancies to counteract the anemia commonly caused by antineoplastic drugs. It should be carefully noted that the anemia must be secondary to the chemotherapy, not to the cancer itself. Research has shown that the administration of epoetin alfa does not benefit patients when the anemia is caused by the malignancy; in fact, mortality is increased in these patients by the administration of the drug. Care must be taken not to administer epoetin alfa to patients with myeloid malignancies such as myelogenous leukemia, because the drug may increase tumor growth.

Mechanism of Action: Epoetin alfa stimulates the division and differentiation of stem cells in the bone marrow to become erythrocytes. Erythropoietin also promotes the synthesis of Hgb and causes a shift of marrow reticulocytes into the circulation.

Pharmacokinetics:

Route(s)	IV, subcutaneous
Absorption	Readily absorbed (subcutaneous)
Distribution	Unknown if the drug crosses the placenta or is secreted in breast milk
Primary metabolism	Plasma
Primary excretion	Mostly feces; 10% renal
Onset of action	7–14 days
Duration of action	2 weeks; half-life: 4–13 h

Adverse Effects: The most serious adverse effect of epoetin alfa is hypertension (HTN), which occurs in 30% of patients receiving the drug. An antihypertensive drug may be indicated. Some patients with chronic renal failure develop neutralizing antibodies to subcutaneous epoetin alfa, which can lead to a rapidly developing severe anemia known as pure red cell aplasia. Seizures may occur during the first 90 days of therapy, especially if blood pressure and Hct rise rapidly. Common adverse effects include headache, fever, nausea, diarrhea, and edema. **Black Box Warning:** The risk of serious cardiovascular and thromboembolic events is increased with epoetin alfa therapy. Transient ischemic attacks (TIAs), myocardial infarctions (MIs), and strokes have occurred in patients with chronic renal failure who are on dialysis and being treated with epoetin alfa. Epoetin increased the rate of deep venous thrombosis (DVT) in patients not receiving concurrent anticoagulation. The lowest dose possible should be used in patients with cancer because the drug can promote tumor progression and shorten overall survival in some patients.

Contraindications/Precautions: The drug should not be given to patients with uncontrolled HTN because epoetin alfa may increase blood pressure. The risk of thromboembolic events, stroke, and MI greatly increases when Hgb rises above 12 g/dL. Patients with known hypersensitivity to products derived from mammal cells, such as albumin, should not receive this drug.

Drug Interactions: Androgens can increase blood viscosity, resulting in an increased response from epoetin alfa. The effectiveness of epoetin alfa will be greatly reduced in patients with iron deficiency or other vitamin-depleted states. Whenever possible, such deficiencies should be corrected prior to initiating epoetin alfa therapy. Hemodialysis patients with preexisting heart disease who are taking epoetin may require increased doses of heparin. **Herbal/Food**: Unknown.

Pregnancy: Category C.

Treatment of Overdose: Overdose may lead to polycythemia (too many erythrocytes), which can be corrected by phlebotomy.

Nursing Responsibilities: Key nursing implications for patients receiving epoetin alfa are included in the Nursing Practice Application for Patients Receiving Pharmacotherapy with Erythropoietin.

Drugs Similar to Epoetin Alfa (Epogen, Procrit)

The only other erythropoietic growth factor is darbepoetin alfa. A similar drug, peginesatide (Omontys), was approved in 2012 but recalled in 2013 due to serious safety concerns.

Darbepoetin alfa (Aranesp): Approved in 2001, darbepoetin alfa has a chemical structure that closely resembles epoetin alfa, differing only by two carbohydrate chains. It has the same mechanism of action, efficacy, and safety profile as epoetin alfa. It is administered by the subcutaneous or IV route and has an extended duration of action that allows it to be administered once weekly. Maximum response occurs in 2 to 4 weeks. Darbepoetin alfa is approved for the treatment of anemia associated with cancer chemotherapy or chronic renal failure. Like epoetin alfa, darbepoetin should only be administered to patients with anemia secondary to the chemotherapy and not caused by the malignancy itself. In addition, Hgb levels should be maintained below 12 g/dL to reduce the risks of serious cardiovascular adverse events. Darbepoetin has similar adverse effects and the same black box warning as epoetin alfa. This drug is pregnancy category C.

39.3 Colony-stimulating factors increase the production of leukocytes.

Regulation of WBC production, or leukopoiesis, is more complicated than erythropoiesis because there are different types of leukocytes in the blood. Adding to the complication is that a large number of substances modify the synthesis and activation of leukocytes and the processes of leukopoiesis regulation are incompletely understood. Pharmacologically, the most important substances are **colony-stimulating factors (CSFs)**. CSFs are hormones that stimulate the growth and differentiation of one or more types of leukocytes.

CSFs are produced by a diverse group of cells that include endothelial cells, fibroblasts, macrophages, and T lymphocytes. Normally present at minute levels in the blood, the production of CSFs rapidly increases when the body receives a bacterial challenge. The leukopoietic growth factors are active at very low concentrations; each stem cell stimulated by these growth factors is capable of producing as many as 1,000 mature leukocytes. The CSFs not only increase the production of new leukocytes, but they also activate existing white blood cells. Examples of enhanced functions include increased migration of leukocytes to antigens, increased antibody toxicity, and increased phagocytosis.

CSFs are named according to the types of blood cells that they stimulate. For example, granulocyte colony-stimulating factor (G-CSF) increases the production of neutrophils, the most common type of granulocyte. Granulocyte-macrophage colony-stimulating factor (GM-CSF) stimulates both neutrophil and macrophage production. The process of identifying the many endogenous CSFs, determining their normal functions, and discovering their potential value as therapeutic agents is an emerging area of pharmacology.

Through recombinant DNA technology, several CSFs are now available as medications (see Table 39.1). The goal of CSF therapy is to produce a rapid increase in the number of neutrophils in patients who have suppressed immune systems (neutropenia). CSF therapy shortens the length of time patients are neutropenic and susceptible to life-threatening infections. The degree of increase in circulating neutrophils is dose related. Indications include patients undergoing chemotherapy or radiation therapy, receiving transplants, or who have certain malignancies. Neutropenia is a limiting adverse effect with many antineoplastic drugs and may cause chemotherapy schedules to be delayed or abandoned. By raising neutrophil counts, CSFs can assist in keeping antineoplastic dosing regimens on schedule (and more effective).

It is often difficult to assess the adverse effects of CSF medications because the same types of patient symptoms may be caused by the condition or disease being treated. Nonspecific adverse effects include nausea, vomiting, fatigue, fever, and flushing. Therapy requires careful laboratory monitoring to avoid producing too many neutrophils. Several recent research studies have suggested that the risk of developing acute myeloid leukemia or myelodysplastic syndrome may be doubled when CSFs are administered to patients undergoing chemotherapy for breast cancer.

| PROTOTYPE DRUG | **Filgrastim (Neupogen)** |

Classification: Therapeutic: Drug for increasing neutrophil production
Pharmacologic: Colony-stimulating factor

Therapeutic Effects and Uses: Produced through recombinant DNA technology, filgrastim is nearly identical in structure to human G-CSF and has the same biologic activity. Its primary actions are to increase neutrophil production in the bone marrow and to enhance the phagocytic and cytotoxic functions of existing neutrophils. The subcutaneous route is preferred, although filgrastim may also be administered by slow IV infusion. A typical regimen is 5 to 10 mcg/kg given once or twice daily. Continued therapy is based on absolute neutrophil counts (ANCs): Therapy is usually discontinued once laboratory results indicate 10,000 cells/mm^3 or greater.

Filgrastim is indicated for various conditions associated with neutropenia, a condition that can lead to severe bacterial and

CONNECTIONS: NURSING PRACTICE APPLICATION

Patients Receiving Pharmacotherapy with Erythropoietin

Assessment	Potential Nursing Diagnoses*
Baseline assessment prior to administration: • Obtain a complete health history: cardiovascular (including HTN, MI) and peripheral vascular disease, respiratory (including previous pulmonary embolism), neurologic (including stroke), hepatic, or renal disease. Obtain a drug history including allergies, current prescription and OTC drugs, herbal preparations, and alcohol use. Be alert to possible drug interactions. • Obtain baseline weight and vital signs, especially blood pressure. • Evaluate appropriate laboratory findings (e.g., CBC, activated partial thromboplastin time [aPTT], international normalized ratio [INR], transferrin and serum ferritin levels, renal and liver function studies). • Assess the patient's ability to receive and understand instructions. Include the family and caregivers as needed.	• *Ineffective Peripheral Tissue Perfusion* • *Activity Intolerance* • *Fatigue* • *Deficient Knowledge* (Drug Therapy) • *Risk for Injury*, related to seizure activity secondary to drug
Assessment throughout administration: • Continue assessment for therapeutic effects (e.g., Hct, RBC count significantly improved), patient's activity level and ability to carry out ADLs has improved. • Continue frequent monitoring of appropriate laboratory values (e.g., CBC, aPTT, INR). • Monitor vital signs frequently, especially blood pressure, during the first 2 weeks of therapy. • Assess for adverse effects: HTN, headache, neurologic changes in level of consciousness, or premonitory signs and symptoms of seizure activity (e.g., aura), angina, signs of thrombosis development in peripheral extremities (e.g., leg pain, pale extremity, diminished peripheral pulses).	

Implementation

Interventions and (Rationales)	Patient-Centered Care
Ensuring therapeutic effects: • Continue frequent assessments as above for therapeutic effects. (RBC count increases rapidly in the first 2 weeks of therapy. CBC and platelet count should show continued improvement. Blood pressure and pulse should remain within normal limits or within the parameters set by the health care provider.)	• Instruct the patient on the need to return frequently for follow-up laboratory work.
• Encourage adequate rest periods and fluid intake. (The patient may be significantly fatigued due to low Hgb and Hct. Adequate fluid intake helps maintain adequate fluid balance as Hct levels rise.)	• Encourage the patient to rest when fatigued, and to space activities throughout the day to allow for adequate rest periods. • Encourage intake of water and nonhyperosmolar beverages.
Minimizing adverse effects: • Continue to monitor for adverse effects, especially HTN, peripheral thrombosis, or seizure activity. (Because Hct rapidly increases during the first 2 weeks of therapy, HTN or seizures may occur and should be reported immediately. Peripheral thrombosis, including coronary or cerebral, may also occur. **Lifespan:** Be especially cautious with the older adult who may be at greater risk for thromboembolic events due to age-related vascular changes.)	• Teach the patient, family, or caregiver how to monitor the pulse and blood pressure as appropriate. Ensure proper use and functioning of any home equipment obtained. • Instruct the patient, family, or caregiver to report headache (especially if sudden onset or severe), changes in level of consciousness, weakness or numbness in extremities, or premonitory signs and symptoms of seizure activity (e.g., aura), angina, or symptoms of peripheral thrombosis (e.g., leg pain, pale extremity, diminished peripheral pulses).
• Assess transportation needs of the patient and refer to appropriate resources as needed. (Driving may be restricted up to 90 days after initiation of drug therapy.)	• Advise the patient, family, or caregiver to consult with the health care provider about driving or other hazardous activities during the first several months of drug therapy.
• Continue to monitor aPTT prior to dialysis in patients with chronic renal failure. (Heparin dose during dialysis may need to be increased as Hct increases.)	• Explain any changes in the medication routine to the patient and provide rationale.
• **Lifespan:** Assess for the possibility of pregnancy or breast-feeding before beginning the drug. (Epoetin is a pregnancy category C drug and the effects during breast-feeding are not fully known.)	• Instruct female patients who may be considering pregnancy, or are pregnant or breast-feeding, to notify their provider before starting the drug.
• **Lifespan:** When administering epoetin alpha to premature infants, use preservative-free formulations. (Epoetin alfa may contain preservatives such as benzyl alcohol. Benzyl alcohol may cause fetal gasping syndrome.)	• To allay anxiety, offer parents rationales for all treatments provided for the infant.

(continued)

• Encourage adequate dietary intake of iron, folic acid, and vitamin B$_{12}$. Provide dietary consult as needed. Consider nutritional supplements of these nutrients if the diet is inadequate. (Response to epoetin alfa may be decreased if blood levels of iron, folic acid, and vitamin B$_{12}$ are deficient.)	• Teach the patient to maintain a healthy diet with adequate amounts of iron, folic acid, and vitamin B$_{12}$ (found in meats, dairy, eggs, fortified cereals and breads, leafy green vegetables, citrus fruits, dried beans and peas).
Patient understanding of drug therapy: • Use opportunities during administration of medications and during assessments to discuss the rationale for drug therapy, desired therapeutic outcomes, most commonly observed adverse effects, parameters for when to call the health care provider, and any necessary monitoring or precautions. (Using time during nursing care helps to optimize and reinforce key teaching areas.)	• The patient, family, or caregiver should be able to state the reason for the drug, appropriate dose and scheduling, what adverse effects to observe for and when to report them, and the anticipated length of medication therapy.
Patient self-administration of drug therapy: • When administering medications, instruct the patient, family, or caregiver in proper self-administration techniques followed by teach-back. (Utilizing time during nurse-administration of these drugs helps to reinforce teaching.) Proper technique includes: • The vial should be gently rotated to mix the content, never shaken. Vials are kept under refrigeration and should be gently warmed in the hand. • All vials are for one-time use only and any remaining amount should be discarded. • If an indwelling subcutaneous soft catheter (e.g., Insuflon soft catheter) is left in place, the patient, family, or caregiver should be taught appropriate site care, insertion technique as appropriate, and the schedule for rotating sites.	• Teach the patient, family, or caregiver proper self-administration techniques. If an indwelling subcutaneous soft catheter (e.g., Insuflon soft catheter) is left in place for injections, teach the patient, family, or caregiver proper care of the site and catheter, and any schedule for rotating sites. • Have the patient, family, or caregiver return demonstrate until the proper technique is used and the person is comfortable giving injections.

*Nursing Diagnoses—Definitions and Classification 2015–2017. Copyright © 2014, 1994–2014 by NANDA International. Used by arrangement with John Wiley & Sons Limited.

fungal infections. Administration of filgrastim shortens the length of time of neutropenia and is approved for the following patients:

- Patients with cancer whose bone marrow has been suppressed by antineoplastic drugs
- Patients with cancer who are receiving bone marrow transplants
- Patients with severe, chronic neutropenia (such as those with AIDS)
- Patients undergoing peripheral mobilization of hematopoietic progenitor cells for collection by leukapheresis

Mechanism of Action: Filgrastim acts by the same mechanism as endogenous G-CSF. The drug causes an increase in neutrophil production in the bone marrow, resulting in higher levels of circulating neutrophils.

Pharmacokinetics:

Route(s)	IV, subcutaneous
Absorption	Rapidly absorbed (subcutaneous)
Distribution	Unknown if the drug crosses the placenta or is secreted in breast milk
Primary metabolism	Unknown
Primary excretion	Renal
Onset of action	4 h
Duration of action	4 days

Adverse Effects: Although filgrastim is well tolerated, the drug is associated with potentially serious adverse effects and close monitoring is required. Nausea and vomiting occur in the majority of patients. Bone pain may occur in up to 33% of patients receiving filgrastim. The pain may be diffuse or localized to bones with the greatest amount of bone marrow: long bones, sternum, ribs, and pelvis. The degree of pain is dose dependent and can usually be managed with nonopioid analgesics. Frequent laboratory tests are conducted to ensure that excessive numbers of neutrophils (leukocytosis) do not occur. Leukocyte counts higher than 100,000 cells/mm^3 increase the risk of serious adverse effects

such as respiratory failure, intracranial hemorrhage or infarction, retinal hemorrhage, and MI. Hyperuricemia and elevated lactate dehydrogenase and alkaline phosphatase levels occur in a significant number of patients. Splenomegaly may occur in 30% of the patients receiving long-term therapy with filgrastim. Other common adverse effects include fatigue, rash, epistaxis, decreased platelet counts, neutropenic fever, alopecia, and diarrhea. Allergic reactions, including anaphylaxis, are rare.

Contraindications/Precautions: Patients with hypersensitivity to *Escherichia coli* (*E. coli*) proteins should not receive filgrastim because this microbe is used to produce the recombinant drug. Patients with sickle cell disease should be treated with caution because filgrastim may worsen this condition. Filgrastim should not be administered to patients with myeloid cancers.

Drug Interactions: Because antineoplastic drugs and CSFs produce opposite effects, filgrastim is not administered until at least 24 hours after a chemotherapy session. Lithium causes the release of neutrophils and may contribute to filgrastim-induced leukocytosis. **Herbal/Food**: Unknown.

Pregnancy: Category C.

Treatment of Overdose: Overdose can lead to leukocytosis and should be prevented by discontinuing the drug when ANC rises above 10,000 cells/mm^3. There is no specific therapy for overdose.

Nursing Responsibilities: Key nursing implications for patients receiving filgrastim are included in the Nursing Practice Application for Patients Receiving Pharmacotherapy with Colony-Stimulating Factors.

Drugs Similar to Filgrastim (Neupogen)

The two other CSFs are pegfilgrastim and sargramostim.

Pegfilgrastim (Neulasta): Approved in 2002, pegfilgrastim is a form of filgrastim bonded to a molecule of polyethylene glycol (PEG).

This delays the renal excretion of the molecule, allowing the drug to remain in the body with a sustained duration of action. Its only approved indication is prophylaxis of chemotherapy-induced neutropenia. The drug is given by the subcutaneous route, once per chemotherapy cycle. It should not be administered 14 days before or 24 hours after the administration of cytotoxic chemotherapy. Adverse effects, interactions, and contraindications are the same as those of filgrastim. This drug is pregnancy category C.

Sargramostim (Leukine): Sargramostim is structurally very similar to natural GM-CSF and has the same biologic activity. It may be administered IV, but subcutaneous is the preferred route. The drug has multiple effects that include increasing the number of circulating neutrophils, eosinophils, and monocytes; activating macrophages; increasing the cytotoxic activity of monocytes; and enhancing the bacteriocidal activity of other cells of the immune system. Indications include decreasing the period of neutropenia in patients treated for acute lymphocytic leukemia or Hodgkin's disease and those having autologous bone marrow transplantation. Typically, therapy with sargramostim is initiated when ANC is less than 500 cells/mm^3 and continues until an ANC of 1,500 cells/mm^3 for 3 consecutive days is achieved. To prevent leukocytosis, sargramostim should be discontinued if the ANC rises above 10,000 cells/mm^3.

Like filgrastim, bone pain is a common adverse effect. A serious adverse effect of sargramostim is respiratory distress that occurs during the IV infusion the first time the drug is administered, which appears to be related to the trapping of granulocytes in the pulmonary circulation. The patient develops difficulty breathing, tachycardia, low blood pressure, and lightheadedness. These symptoms usually call for discontinuing sargramostim therapy. This drug is pregnancy category C.

39.4 Platelet enhancers may be used to treat thrombocytopenia.

The production of platelets, or thrombocytopoiesis, begins when megakaryocytes in the bone marrow start shedding membrane-bound packets. These packets enter the bloodstream and become platelets. A single megakaryocyte can produce thousands of platelets.

Megakaryocyte activity is controlled by the hormone **thrombopoietin**, which is produced by the liver and bone marrow. Thrombopoietin is not available as a medication, although it has undergone clinical trials. The only hematopoietic growth factor available to enhance platelet production is oprelvekin (Neumega), which is functionally equivalent to endogenous interleukin-11 (IL-11). Interleukins are cytokines secreted by monocytes, lymphocytes, and other cell types that signal cells in the immune system to respond to an infection. Over 30 interleukins have been identified but only a few have been isolated and approved as drugs.

Romiplostim (Nplate) and eltrombopag (Promacta) are medications approved to improve platelet function in patients with chronic immune (idiopathic) thrombocytopenia purpura (ITP). Chronic ITP is a disorder characterized by inadequate platelet production and/or increased platelet destruction. Patients with ITP experience a high risk for bruising and bleeding, which may occur anywhere in the body. Both drugs increase the number of platelets by activating the natural receptor for thrombopoietin.

CONNECTIONS: NURSING PRACTICE APPLICATION

Patients Receiving Pharmacotherapy with Colony-Stimulating Factors

Assessment	Potential Nursing Diagnoses*
Baseline assessment prior to administration: • Obtain a complete health history including recent or current infections; recent surgeries, injuries, or wounds; yeast infections (e.g., thrush); vaccination history; cardiac conditions (e.g., dysrhythmias, HF); respiratory, renal, and hepatic conditions. Obtain a drug history including allergies, current prescription and OTC drugs, herbal preparations, and alcohol use. Be alert to possible drug interactions. • Obtain baseline weight and vital signs. Assess level of fatigue. • Evaluate appropriate laboratory findings (e.g., CBC, WBC, or ANC, renal and liver function studies, uric acid levels, and ECG). ANC = total WBC count multiplied by the total percentage of neutrophils (segmented plus bands); e.g., WBC 5,000 × (0.45 segs + 0.05 banded neutrophils) = 5,000 × 0.5 = ANC of 2,500. • Assess the patient's ability to receive and understand instructions. Include the family and caregiver as needed.	• *Anxiety* • *Activity Intolerance* • *Fatigue* • *Deficient Knowledge* (Drug Therapy) • *Risk for Infection* • *Risk for Caregiver Role Strain*
Assessment throughout administration: • Continue assessment for therapeutic effects (e.g., CBC, WBC, or ANC has increased, no signs or symptoms of infection). • Continue frequent monitoring of appropriate laboratory values (e.g., CBC, WBC, or ANC, Hct, platelet count, renal and hepatic labs, uric acid levels). • Monitor vital signs and level of fatigue. • Assess for adverse effects: bone pain (especially lower back, posterior iliac crests, and sternum), fever, nausea, anorexia, hyperuricemia, anemia, ST-segment depression on ECG, angina, respiratory distress, and allergic reaction. Continue to assess for infection and fatigue related to the drug treatment (e.g., chemotherapy).	

(continued)

CONNECTIONS: NURSING PRACTICE APPLICATION (continued)

Implementation

Interventions and (Rationales)	Patient-Centered Care
Ensuring therapeutic effects: • Continue frequent assessments as above for therapeutic effects. (Rise in WBC and/or ANC counts will depend on the condition treated, e.g., depth and length of nadir from cytotoxic chemotherapy. Counts are usually monitored twice per week or as ordered by the health care provider.)	• Instruct the patient on the need to return frequently for follow-up laboratory work.
• Encourage adequate rest periods and adequate fluid intake. (The patient may be significantly fatigued due to the drug therapy. Adequate fluid intake helps maintain adequate urinary output and prevent urinary tract infections.)	• Encourage the patient to rest when fatigued and to space activities throughout the day to allow for adequate rest periods. • Encourage intake of water and nonhyperosmolar beverages, and drinking whenever thirsty.
Minimizing adverse effects: • Continue to monitor for adverse effects: bone pain (especially lower back, posterior iliac crests, and sternum), fever, nausea, anorexia, hyperuricemia, anemia, ST-segment depression on ECG, angina, respiratory distress, and allergic reaction. Continue to assess for infection and fatigue related to drug treatment, e.g., chemotherapy. (Bone pain tends to occur 2–3 days prior to rise in circulating WBCs due to the production of WBCs in bone marrow. ST-segment depression on ECG may occur with potential for serious dysrhythmias. Respiratory distress may develop after administration of sargramostim and should be reported immediately. Hyperuricemia may cause gout-like conditions.)	• Instruct the patient to report any severe bone pain not relieved by nonnarcotic analgesics. • Teach the patient to report any palpitations, dizziness, angina, or dyspnea immediately. • Gout-prone patients should report signs and symptoms of gout and increase fluid intake to enhance renal elimination of uric acid.

• Maintain meticulous infection control measures. Immediately report any signs and symptoms of fever or infections, especially viral or fungal. (The patient will continue to be at risk for infections until WBC or ANC levels rise. Opportunistic infections, such as yeast, and viruses, such as herpes simplex, may occur. Parameters will be set by the health care provider for reporting fever, e.g., any temperature over 38°C [100.5°F], dependent on the underlying disease condition and drug therapy.)	• Instruct the patient in hygiene and infection control measures such as:
	  • Washing hands frequently.
	  • Avoiding crowded indoor places.
	  • Avoiding people with known infections or young children, because they have a higher risk of having an infection.
	  • Cooking food thoroughly and not consuming raw fruits or vegetables. Allow the family or caregiver to prepare raw meats or fish and to clean up.
	• Instruct the patient to report any fever per the parameters set by the health care provider, and symptoms of infection such as wounds with redness or drainage, increasing cough, increasing fatigue, white patches on oral mucous membranes, white and itchy vaginal discharge, or itchy blister-like vesicles on the skin.

• Monitor ECG periodically for ST-segment depression or dysrhythmias, and report immediately. (Sargramostim may cause significant ST-segment depression with potential for serious dysrhythmias, especially in patients with previous cardiac conditions.)	• Instruct the patient to report any palpitations, dizziness, or angina immediately.
• Monitor for signs of dyspnea or respiratory distress, especially when accompanied by tachycardia and hypotension, and report immediately. (Sargramostim may cause respiratory distress as granulocyte counts rise, especially in patients with preexisting respiratory disorders.)	• Instruct the patient to immediately report any dyspnea, respiratory distress, palpitations, or dizziness.
• Monitor for signs and symptoms of allergic-type reactions. (The patient may be hypersensitive to proteins used in the drug development process.)	• Instruct the patient to immediately report symptoms of allergic reaction such as rash, urticaria, wheezing, and dyspnea.
• Monitor hepatic status during drug administration period. (Filgrastim may cause an elevation in liver enzymes.)	• Instruct the patient to report any significant itching, yellowing of the sclera or skin, darkened urine, or light or clay-colored stools.
• Stop administration when WBC counts reach a level determined by the health care provider. (Filgrastim may be stopped when neutrophil counts reach 10,000/mm^3, sargramostim when neutrophil counts reach 20,000/mm^3, or as ordered by the provider.)	• Instruct the patient on the importance of returning regularly for laboratory work.
• Assess for spleen enlargement periodically and report. (Filgrastim has been associated with rare but potentially fatal cases of splenomegaly and rupture.)	• Instruct the patient, family, or caregiver to report any symptoms of left upper abdominal pain or left shoulder pain, which may indicate spleen enlargement or rupture.
• **Lifespan:** Monitor laboratory results for pediatric patients with forms of congenital neutropenia (e.g., congenital agranulocytosis) more frequently. (Patients with these disorders are at greater risk for developing acute myelogenous leukemia [AML] and myelodysplastic neutropenia [MDS] related to drug therapy.)	• Teach the patient, family, or caregivers that frequent laboratory studies may be needed.
• **Lifespan:** Assess for the possibility of pregnancy or breast-feeding before beginning the drug. (Colony-stimulating factors are pregnancy category C drugs and the effects during breast-feeding are not fully known.)	• Instruct female patients who may be considering pregnancy, or are pregnant or breast-feeding, to notify their provider before starting the drug.

CONNECTIONS: NURSING PRACTICE APPLICATION (continued)

Patient understanding of drug therapy:

- Use opportunities during administration of medications and assessments to discuss the rationale for drug therapy, desired therapeutic outcomes, commonly observed adverse effects, parameters for when to call the health care provider, and any necessary monitoring or precautions. (Using time during nursing care helps to optimize and reinforce key teaching areas.)

- The patient, family, or caregiver should be able to state the reason for the drug, appropriate dose and scheduling, what adverse effects to observe for and when to report them, and the anticipated length of medication therapy.

Patient self-administration of drug therapy:

- When administering medications, instruct the patient, family, or caregiver in proper self-administration techniques followed by teach-back. (Utilizing time during nurse-administration of these drugs helps to reinforce teaching.) Proper technique includes:
  - The vial should be gently rotated to mix the contents, never shaken. Vials are kept under refrigeration and should be gently warmed in the hand.
  - All vials are for one-time use only and any remaining amount should be discarded.
- If an indwelling subcutaneous soft catheter (e.g., Insuflon soft catheter) is left in place, the patient, family, or caregiver should be taught appropriate site care, insertion technique as appropriate, and schedule for rotating sites.

- Teach the patient, family, or caregiver in proper self-administration techniques. If indwelling subcutaneous soft catheter (e.g., Insuflon soft catheter) is left in place for injections, teach the patient, family, or caregiver proper care of the site, catheter, and any schedule for rotating sites.
- Have the patient, family, or caregiver return demonstrate until the proper technique is used and the person is comfortable giving the injection.

*Nursing Diagnoses—Definitions and Classification 2015–2017. Copyright © 2014, 1994–2014 by NANDA International. Used by arrangement with John Wiley & Sons Limited.

| PROTOTYPE DRUG | Oprelvekin (Neumega) |

Classification: Therapeutic: Platelet enhancer
Pharmacologic: Interleukin

Therapeutic Effects and Uses: Produced through recombinant DNA technology, oprelvekin is used to stimulate the production of platelets in patients who are at risk for severe thrombocytopenia caused by the chemotherapy of nonmyeloid cancers. The drug shortens the time that the patient is thrombocytopenic and most susceptible to adverse bleeding events. Dosing is initiated 6 to 24 hours after chemotherapy and continues daily until the platelet count is greater than 50,000/mm³. Dosing beyond 21 days is not recommended. Platelet counts will remain elevated for about 7 days after the last dose. Therapy with oprelvekin decreases the need for platelet infusion. Oprelvekin is only given by the subcutaneous route.

Mechanism of Action: Oprelvekin is equivalent to endogenous interleukin-11 and stimulates the synthesis and maturation of megakaryocytes into platelets.

Pharmacokinetics:

Route(s)	Subcutaneous
Absorption	80% absorbed
Distribution	Well distributed to highly perfused organs; unknown if the drug crosses the placenta or is secreted in breast milk
Primary metabolism	Not metabolized
Primary excretion	Renal
Onset of action	5–9 days
Duration of action	7 days; half-life: 6.9 h

Adverse Effects: Oprelvekin causes many adverse effects, although most are reversible upon discontinuation of therapy. The most common adverse effects include nausea, vomiting, edema, neutropenic fever, dyspnea, mucositis, and diarrhea. Fluid retention is a serious adverse effect that occurs in about 60% of patients and can be a concern for patients with preexisting cardiovascular or renal disease. Adverse effects related to fluid retention may be severe and include pulmonary edema, pericardial effusion, and ascites. Cardiovascular adverse effects include transient atrial dysrhythmias, sinus tachycardia, vasodilation, and peripheral edema. Papilledema (swelling of the optic nerve) can occur during therapy and result in blurred vision, loss of visual acuity, and blindness, in rare cases. **Black Box Warning**: Although not common, allergic reactions, including anaphylaxis, have been reported with oprelvekin. The drug should be permanently discontinued if a patient experiences a hypersensitivity reaction.

Contraindications/Precautions: Oprelvekin is contraindicated in patients who have shown hypersensitivity to the drug on a previous exposure. It should be used with caution in patients with cardiac disease, especially heart failure (HF), dysrhythmias, and left ventricular dysfunction, since fluid retention is a common adverse effect that can worsen these conditions. Oprelvekin should not be used following myeloablative therapy because the drug exhibits increased toxicity. The drug should be used with caution in patients with preexisting visual impairment; papilledema is a dose-limiting adverse effect in children receiving this drug.

Drug Interactions: Oprelvekin should not be administered within 24 hours of chemotherapy because the cytotoxic effects of the antineoplastic drugs decrease the effectiveness of the drug. Concurrent use with thiazide or loop diuretics may cause serious hypokalemia. **Herbal/Food**: Unknown.

Pregnancy: Category C.

Treatment of Overdose: Overdose may result in serious adverse effects and close monitoring of cardiovascular and renal function is necessary. No specific therapy is available.

Nursing Responsibilities:

- Notify the prescriber prior to administration if the patient has a history of leukemia, multiple myeloma, or other myeloid malignancies.
- Monitor for and immediately report signs and symptoms of fluid overload, hypokalemia, and cardiac dysrhythmias.

- Monitor patients with preexisting fluid retention conditions carefully, such as HF, pleural effusion, or ascites, for worsening of symptoms.

- This drug has a black box warning for possible anaphylaxis. Promptly report any signs and symptoms of allergic reaction to the provider and discontinue the drug.

Lifespan and Diversity Considerations:

- Tachycardia, cardiomegaly, papilledema, conjunctival redness, and bone changes may occur more frequently in children taking oprelvekin than in adults. Carefully monitor heart rate and heart sounds, changes in visual acuity or eye pain, and for complaints of bone pain or changes in gait. Further cardiac testing (e.g., echocardiography) and frequent eye exams may be warranted.

Patient and Family Education:

- Do not take any other prescription or nonprescription drugs, dietary supplements, or herbal products without the approval of the health care provider.

- Immediately report shortness of breath, swelling of feet or ankles, rapid weight gain, chest pain, unusual fatigue or weakness, irregular heartbeat, fever of 38°C (100.5°F) or higher, unusual bruising or bleeding, or blurred vision.

- For self-administration, follow the procedure demonstrated to prevent contamination of the vial, syringe, or medicine. Never touch the rubber stopper of the vial or the needle of the syringe with your fingers. Dispose of needles and syringes as directed by a health care provider.

- Do not drive or perform other hazardous activities until the effects of the drug are known because this drug may cause drowsiness or dizziness.

- Notify the health care provider of any difficulty walking or bone pain, changes in visual acuity or eye pain, or rapid heart rate.

- Immediately notify the health care provider of any known or suspected pregnancy.

- Do not breast-feed while using this drug without approval of the health care provider.

Drugs Similar to Oprelvekin (Neumega)

The two other platelet enhancers are eltrombopag and romiplostim.

Eltrombopag (Promacta): Approved in 2008, eltrombopag is an oral medication that increases the number of platelets in the blood by activating thrombopoietin receptors. Its only indication is for the treatment of thrombocytopenia in patients with chronic ITP who have not responded to corticosteroids, immunoglobulins, or splenectomy. The drug carries a black box warning that it may cause hepatotoxicity. Liver laboratory values (alanine aminotransferase [ALT], aspartate aminotransferase [ASP], and bilirubin) must be closely monitored and the drug discontinued if abnormal values persist. The most common adverse effects include nausea, diarrhea, upper respiratory tract infection, vomiting, increased ALT, myalgia, urinary tract infection, oropharyngeal pain, increased AST, pharyngitis, back pain, influenza, paresthesia, and rash. Because of the potential for serious adverse effects, the drug is available through a restricted distribution program. This drug is pregnancy category C.

Romiplostim (Nplate): Like eltrombopag, romiplostim was approved in 2008 and increases platelet count by activating the thrombopoietin receptor. Also like eltrombopag, the only indication is for the treatment of thrombocytopenia in patients with chronic ITP who have not responded to corticosteroids, immunoglobulins, or splenectomy. Romiplostim, however, does not exhibit hepatotoxicity. The most common adverse effects are arthralgia, dizziness, insomnia, myalgia, pain in extremity, abdominal pain, shoulder pain, dyspepsia, and paresthesia. It is only administered by subcutaneous injection and the drug has a restricted distribution program. This drug is pregnancy category C.

CONNECTION Checkpoint 39.2

Abciximab, eptifibatide, and tirofiban are drugs that can cause severe ITP. From what you learned in Chapter 38, to what class do these drugs belong and what is the primary indication for their use? *See Answer to Connection Checkpoint 39.2 on student resource website.*

Classification of Anemias

39.5 Anemias may be caused by hemorrhage or a change in red blood cell production or destruction.

Anemia is a condition in which RBCs have a diminished capacity to deliver oxygen to tissues. Anemia is a serious health problem that can have a major impact on the quality of life; it is estimated that over 3.4 million Americans have the disorder. Although there are dozens of possible causes of anemia, most fall into one of the following categories:

- Blood loss due to hemorrhage

- Increased erythrocyte destruction

- Decreased erythrocyte production

Anemia is considered a sign of an underlying disorder, rather than a distinct disease. For example, anemia is commonly associated with peptic ulcer, various malignancies, and chronic renal disease. For therapy to be successful, the underlying pathology must be identified and treated. Despite the fact it is often considered secondary to other diseases, proper treatment of anemia is necessary to improve the patient's ability to adequately perform activities of daily living.

Classification of anemia is generally based on a description of the erythrocyte's size and color. Sizes are described as normal (normocytic), small (microcytic), or large (macrocytic). Color is based on the amount of Hgb present and is described as normal red (normochromic) or light red (hypochromic). This classification is shown in Table 39.2. It is not unusual for patients to have more than one type of anemia concurrently.

Although each type of anemia has specific characteristics, all exhibit common signs and symptoms. Assessment includes sources and causes of potential bleeding, as well as a thorough dietary history to rule out deficiencies in the intake of nutrients essential to RBC production, such as vitamin B_{12}, folic acid, or iron. Some types of anemia, including sickle cell and thalassemia, are hereditary and discovered by family history. If the anemia occurs gradually, the patient may remain asymptomatic, except during periods of physical exercise. As the condition progresses, the patient often exhibits pallor, which is a paleness of the skin and mucous membranes due to Hgb deficiency. Decreased exercise tolerance, fatigue, and lethargy occur because of insufficient oxygen reaching muscles. Dizziness and fainting are common because the brain is not receiving enough

TABLE 39.2 Classification of Anemia

Morphology	Description	Examples
Macrocytic-normochromic	Large, abnormally shaped erythrocytes with normal Hgb concentration	Pernicious anemia, folate deficiency anemia
Microcytic-hypochromic	Small, abnormally shaped erythrocytes with decreased Hgb concentration	Iron deficiency anemia, thalassemia
Normocytic-normochromic	Destruction or depletion of normal erythroblasts or mature erythrocytes	Aplastic anemia, hemorrhagic anemia, sickle cell anemia, hemolytic anemia

CONNECTIONS Community-Oriented Practice

◀ Epoetin Alfa for Blood Doping

Blood doping, withdrawing blood from an athlete and then re-transfusing it before a competitive sporting event, has been used by some athletes in an attempt to gain a competitive edge. With increased RBCs and higher Hgb, oxygen-carrying capacity is thought to increase, boosting endurance. With the advent of epoetin alfa, blood doping took on new meaning and some athletes found that the use of epoetin well before an athletic meet achieved the same effects without the ability through testing to detect the dramatic increase that was apparent after a transfusion. Charges of blood doping with epoetin were initially difficult to prove, but as more sophisticated tests became available, detection of the presence of the drug was possible, and athletes were ejected from events or had their winnings disqualified. Newer drugs, without new tests to detect them initially, are on the horizon, and the race against cheating in sports continues.

Blood doping is not without a price, however. Increased blood volume and viscosity have led to hypertension, thrombosis, and death. Undeterred, some athletes, desperate for a competitive edge, continue to use it. Adolescents involved in competitive sports activities may have heard about epoetin and may question its advantages. The nurse plays a key role in providing accurate information about epoetin and related drugs and counseling adolescents about the risks and adverse effects of sports-enhancing drugs.

oxygen to function properly. The respiratory and cardiovascular systems compensate for the oxygen depletion by increasing respiration rate and heart rate. Chronic or severe disease can result in HF. Because symptoms are nonspecific, laboratory tests such as complete blood count, Hgb, Hct, and serum iron are essential to making a diagnosis so that appropriate pharmacotherapy can be initiated.

Depending on the type of anemia, several vitamins and minerals may be given to enhance the oxygen-carrying capacity of blood. The most common antianemic drugs are iron salts, cyanocobalamin (Nascobal), and folic acid. Doses of these drugs are listed in Table 39.3.

Antianemic Drugs

39.6 Administration of iron salts can rapidly reverse symptoms of iron deficiency anemia.

Iron is a mineral essential to the function of several mitochondrial enzymes involved in metabolism and energy production in the cell. It is also a component of certain antioxidant enzymes that assist in clearing the body of free radicals. Most iron in the body, 60% to 80%, is associated with Hgb inside erythrocytes. Knowledge of iron balance and homeostasis is necessary to understanding the pharmacotherapy of iron deficiency anemia. Factors affecting iron balance are illustrated in Figure 39.2.

The two basic forms of iron in biologic systems are ferrous (Fe^{2+}) and ferric (Fe^{3+}). Most food contains iron in the ferric state, which is not absorbed in the gastrointestinal (GI) tract. In the presence of stomach acid, however, the ferric form is converted to the ferrous form, which is readily absorbed in the duodenum. Iron absorption is dynamic; if the body senses a shortage of iron in the blood, GI absorption increases. When iron stores are plentiful, less iron is absorbed from food. Since adults only need about 8 mg of iron per day, a normal diet supplies sufficient amounts of the mineral for most people.

TABLE 39.3 Antianemic Drugs

Drug	Route and Adult Dose (Maximum Dose Where Indicated)	Adverse Effects
cyanocobalamin (Nascobal)	IM/deep subcutaneous: 30 mcg/day for 5–10 days, then 100–200 mcg/month Intranasal: one spray (500 mcg) in one nostril once weekly	*Diarrhea, hypokalemia, rash* <u>Anaphylaxis</u>
folic acid	PO/IM/subcutaneous/IV: less than 1 mg/day	No adverse effects
Iron Salts		
ferrous fumarate (Feostat, others)	PO: 200 mg tid or qid	*Nausea, heartburn, constipation, dark stools* <u>Cardiovascular collapse, aggravation of peptic ulcers or ulcerative colitis, hepatic necrosis, hypotension (Ferumoxytol), anaphylaxis (iron dextran), respiratory arrest (iron dextran), seizures (iron dextran)</u>
ferrous gluconate (Fergon, Ferralet)	PO: 325–600 mg qid, may be gradually increased to 650 mg qid as needed	
ferrous sulfate (Feosol, others)	PO: 750–1,500 mg/day in one to three divided doses	
ferumoxytol (Feraheme)	IV: single dose of 510 mg followed by a second 510-mg dose 3–8 days later	
iron dextran (Dexferrum)	IM/IV: Dose is individualized and determined from a table supplied by the drug manufacturer that correlates body weight to Hgb values (max: 100 mg within 24 h)	
iron sucrose (Venofer)	IV: 100–200 mg by slow IV injection or infusion	

Note: Italics indicate common adverse effects. <u>Underline</u> indicates serious adverse effects.

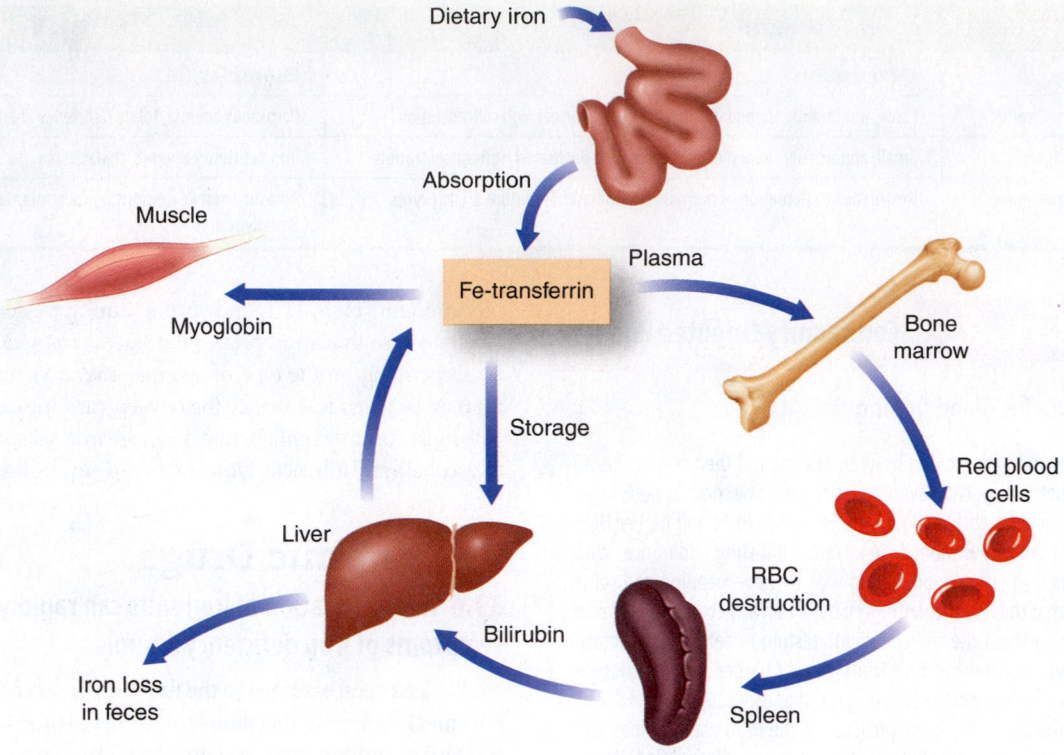

Figure 39.2 Iron metabolism.

Other factors affect the absorption of iron. Iron in heme, which is found in meat, fish, and poultry, is three times more absorbable than the nonheme iron found in vegetables and grains. Thus meats are considered the best natural source of absorbable iron. Calcium inhibits the absorption of iron; thus, those who drink milk with meals are at greater risk for iron deficiency. Vitamin C increases iron absorption about 30%, while black tea will diminish absorption.

Because free iron is toxic, the body binds the mineral to the protein complexes **ferritin**, **hemosiderin**, and **transferrin**. Ferritin and hemosiderin maintain iron stores inside cells, whereas transferrin transports iron to sites throughout the body where it is needed, such as to the bone marrow for incorporation into Hgb. Serum ferritin levels are a reliable indicator of how much iron is being stored by the body. Low serum ferritin levels (less than 12 ng/mL) are characteristic of iron deficiency anemia. In addition to Hgb, major storage depots for iron are the liver and myoglobin in skeletal muscle.

After erythrocytes die, nearly all of the iron in their Hgb is incorporated into transferrin and recycled for later use. Because of this efficient recycling, only about 1 mg of iron is excreted from the body per day, making daily dietary iron requirements in most individuals quite small. Vegetarians are at higher risk of iron deficiency anemia because of a lack of heme intake from meat and must take care to select foods rich in iron. Iron requirements may double during growth, pregnancy, and menses; thus, intake of iron must be increased to maintain proper iron balance.

Iron deficiency is the most common cause of anemia worldwide. More than 50% of patients diagnosed with iron deficiency anemia have GI bleeding, such as may occur from GI malignancies or chronic peptic ulcer disease (PUD). In the United States and Canada, iron deficiency most commonly occurs in women of childbearing age due to pregnancy, and blood losses during menses.

Low-dose iron supplements are recommended during pregnancy to prevent this condition. Certain individuals have an increased demand for iron, including those who are on meat-free diets or undergoing intensive athletic training. These conditions may require more than the recommended dietary allowance (RDA) of iron (see Chapter 61). In undeveloped countries, the primary cause of iron deficiency anemia is the lack of meat or fresh fruits and vegetables in the diet. The most significant effect of iron deficiency is a reduction in erythropoiesis, resulting in symptoms of anemia.

Iron therapy is initiated to alleviate symptoms of anemia caused by blood loss or dietary deficiency. Once diagnosed, a primary goal is to identify the etiology of the disorder and treat the underlying pathology. Choice of therapy depends on the etiology and severity of the deficiency:

- Mild anemia may be prevented or corrected in most patients by increasing the intake of iron-rich foods, such as fish, red meat, fortified cereal, and whole-grain breads.

CONNECTIONS   Patient Safety

◀ **Iron Poisoning in Children**

While talking with a group of young mothers, the nurse becomes concerned about the remarks made by one of the members. The mother states, "I insist that my children take iron-fortified vitamins every day. My children really enjoy taking the cute little cartoon vitamins. They call the vitamins their 'morning candy.'" Should the nurse be concerned? How should the nurse respond?

See Answers to Patient Safety Questions on student resource website.

- Moderate anemia is corrected by oral iron supplementation.
- Severe anemia, and that caused by iron malabsorption disorders, is corrected by parenteral iron therapy.

PROTOTYPE DRUG	Ferrous Sulfate (Feosol, Feostat, Others)

Classification: Therapeutic: Drug for anemia
Pharmacologic: Iron supplement

Therapeutic Effects and Uses: Ferrous sulfate is an iron supplement containing about 20% elemental iron. Desiccated (dried) ferrous sulfate contains 30% elemental iron. It is inexpensive and available in a wide variety of dosage forms to prevent or rapidly reverse symptoms of iron deficiency anemia. Enteric-coated and extended release forms are available. If tolerated, the drug should be taken on an empty stomach, at least 1 hour before or 2 hours after a meal.

In general, patients with iron deficiency respond rapidly to the administration of ferrous sulfate. Although a positive therapeutic response may be achieved in 48 hours, therapy may continue for several months to replenish the storage depots for iron. As the deficiency is corrected, the body will absorb a smaller percentage of elemental iron in each dose until iron intake balances iron loss. This is assuming, of course, that the source of the iron imbalance, such as bleeding or dietary insufficiency, has been corrected. Laboratory evaluation of Hgb, transferrin, and Hct levels is conducted regularly to assess the progress of pharmacotherapy. Dosage is decreased as therapy progresses and the deficiency is corrected.

If rapid, symptomatic improvement is not experienced, the reasons for the treatment failure must be carefully explored. The patient may be experiencing continued bleeding or may have a malabsorption disorder that prevents the iron from being absorbed. A common reason for treatment failure is lack of adherence to pharmacotherapy. Patients may stop taking the drug due to severe nausea and vomiting, or they may take the drug with food or other drugs that inhibit iron absorption. Excellent assessment and teaching skills of the nurse are key to achieving successful pharmacotherapeutic outcomes in these patients.

Mechanism of Action: After absorption, most iron is used by the body to make Hgb. Laboratory values of Hgb should increase 2 to 4 g/dL every 3 weeks until normal values are achieved. In addition, therapy is continued until serum ferritin levels return to normal, indicating that the iron storage depots are filled.

Pharmacokinetics:

Route(s)	PO
Absorption	5–30% absorbed
Distribution	Well distributed; crosses the placenta
Primary metabolism	Undergoes extensive enterohepatic recirculation
Primary excretion	Feces, urine, and skin
Onset of action	3 days to 4 weeks
Duration of action	Unknown

Adverse Effects: The most common adverse effects of ferrous sulfate are nausea and vomiting, which will occur to some degree in most patients. Taking the drug with food will diminish GI upset but can decrease the absorption of iron by 50% to 70%. The degree of nausea and vomiting is dose related and serious symptoms may require a dosage adjustment. Contact of liquid iron with teeth should be avoided because the drug can cause brown stains. Iron preparations will darken stools but this is a harmless adverse effect. Because constipation is common, especially in older adults, an increase in dietary fiber intake is indicated. **Black Box Warning:** Nonintentional overdoses of iron-containing products are a leading cause of fatal poisoning of children.

Contraindications/Precautions: Iron salts should not be administered for anemia other than that caused by iron deficiency, because iron will not correct these conditions and may build to toxic levels. The drug should not be administered to patients with hemochromatosis, a disease in which the patient has excess iron stores. Ferrous sulfate may irritate the stomach mucosa and increase bleeding in patients with PUD. The drug may cause diarrhea if administered to patients with regional enteritis or ulcerative colitis.

Drug Interactions: Absorption is reduced when oral iron salts are given concurrently with antacids, proton pump inhibitors, or calcium supplements. Iron decreases the absorption of tetracyclines, fluoroquinolones, levodopa, and etidronate. To prevent possible interactions, it is advisable to take iron supplements 1 to 2 hours before or after other medications. **Herbal/Food:** Food (especially dairy products), coffee, and tea will inhibit iron absorption. Vitamin C will increase absorption.

Pregnancy: Category A.

Treatment of Overdose: Iron is very toxic and most overdoses are accidental, occurring in children under the age of 6 years. The antidote for acute iron intoxication is the parenteral drug deferoxamine (Desferal). This chelating agent binds iron, which is removed by the kidneys, turning the urine a reddish-brown color.

Nursing Responsibilities:

- Give on an empty stomach if possible because oral iron preparations are best absorbed between meals. If GI adverse effects are prominent, give with or immediately after meals with adequate liquid.
- If the patient experiences difficulty swallowing tablets or capsules, recommend a liquid formulation or a less corrosive form, such as ferrous gluconate.
- Dilute liquid preparations well and give them through a straw or place them on the back of the tongue with a dropper to prevent staining of teeth and to mask the unpleasant taste.
- Mix Feosol elixir with water as it is not compatible with milk or fruit juice. Fer-In-Sol (drops) may be given in water or in fruit or vegetable juice, according to the manufacturer.
- Iron therapy may be continued for 2 to 3 months after the Hgb level has returned to normal (roughly twice the period required to normalize Hgb concentration).
- Monitor bowel movements because constipation is a common adverse effect. Increase the amount of fluids and soluble fiber in the diet.

Lifespan and Diversity Considerations

- Due to age-related changes in peristalsis and bowel function, monitor the older adult for constipation. Increase the amount of fluids and soluble fiber in the diet. A stool softener or laxative may be needed.

- Keep iron preparations in a secured location if there are young children in the household to prevent accidental poisoning.

Patient and Family Education

- Do not take tablets or capsules within 1 hour of bedtime.

- Do not crush tablets or empty the contents of capsules because this may cause GI distress.

- Take ferrous sulfate with a full glass of water. Rinse mouth with clear water immediately after ingestion.

- Consume citrus fruit or tomato juice with iron preparations (except the elixir form) because ascorbic acid (vitamin C) increases iron absorption.

- Avoid taking iron salts with milk, eggs, antacids, or caffeine beverages, because these inhibit drug absorption.

- Iron preparations cause dark green or black stools: This is a harmless side effect.

- Report constipation or diarrhea to the health care provider. Symptoms may be relieved by adjustments in dosage or diet, or by changing to another iron preparation.

Drugs Similar to Ferrous Sulfate (Feosol, Feostat, Others)

At least eight iron salts are available for administration to patients with iron deficiency anemia. Iron salts are often classified by their route of administration, either oral (PO) or parenteral.

Oral iron salts: Oral iron salts include ferrous fumarate, ferrous gluconate, polysaccharide-iron complex, and carbonyl iron. The choice of specific drug and dose are based on iron content and degree of GI tolerability. Table 39.4 lists the amount of elemental iron in these drugs.

A large number of brand-name iron products and formulations are available, including tablets, drops, elixirs, and suspensions. Nausea, vomiting, constipation, and diarrhea are common adverse effects with all oral iron preparations. Slow-release products, called carbonyl iron (Feosol-caps, Ferronyl), are more expensive but are

TABLE 39.4 Iron Content of Oral Iron Formulations

Preparation	Elemental Iron	Dose Needed to Provide 200 mg of Elemental Iron per Day
carbonyl iron	100%	200 mg
ferrous fumarate	33%	600 mg
ferrous gluconate	12%	720 mg
ferrous sulfate: desiccated	30%	660 mg
ferrous sulfate: regular	20%	1,000 mg
polysaccharide iron complex	100%	200 mg

less dangerous in children following accidental ingestion because there is a longer period for intervention before toxic effects materialize. Some products have an enteric coating so that the capsule or tablet dissolves in the intestine, thus causing less gastric irritation. Recall, however, that stomach acid is necessary to convert iron to its more absorbable form. In addition, enteric coatings are less reliable because they may dissolve after the drug has passed the duodenum, which is the primary site for iron absorption. Vitamin C is added to many oral iron supplements because it enhances iron absorption. Some products are formulated as multivitamins. For example, Niferex PN Forte, which is formulated specifically for pregnant or lactating women, contains a polysaccharide-iron complex and vitamins A, D, C, folic acid, B complex, calcium, iodine, magnesium, copper, and zinc. Adding extra enhancers such as additional vitamins, extended release properties, or an enteric coating increases the cost of the drug but not necessarily its effectiveness. The amount of elemental iron in the product and adverse effects should be the primary factors guiding therapy.

Parenteral iron salts: Iron dextran (Dexferrum), iron sucrose (Venofer), and ferric gluconate (Ferrlecit) are parenteral preparations reserved for patients who cannot tolerate oral iron preparations or who have a malabsorption disorder preventing iron absorption from the GI tract. Giving parenteral iron does not lead to a faster recovery for patients with iron deficiency anemia because the body is limited as to how quickly it can make Hgb and new RBCs. These drugs are clearly more toxic than the oral iron products and require careful monitoring during pharmacotherapy.

In 2009, the U.S. Food and Drug Administration (FDA) approved a new iron salt. Ferumoxytol (Feraheme) is approved to treat iron deficiency associated with chronic kidney disease (with or without dialysis). The drug consists of iron oxide protected by a carbohydrate shell. The shell remains intact until the drug enters macrophages, whereby the iron is released to its storage depots. The advantage of ferumoxytol over existing iron salts is that it can be administrated safely by the IV route and can raise iron levels more rapidly.

All parenteral agents are equally effective at raising iron levels. All are given IV. Iron dextran is also available by the IM route although this is rarely used due to pain at the injection site and unreliable absorption from the muscle. Iron sucrose and iron gluconate have more limited application. They are only approved for patients with iron deficiency anemia undergoing chronic hemodialysis who are also receiving erythropoietin.

Anaphylaxis has been reported with iron dextran and iron sucrose. Prior to administering an infusion of these drugs, the patient must receive a small IV test dose and be observed for 15 to 30 minutes to assess for possible allergic reactions, which may cause respiratory arrest and circulatory collapse. Vital signs should be monitored during the test dose infusion. Some health care providers order test doses conducted prior to every administration of IV iron salts, since anaphylaxis may occur on second and subsequent doses. Ferric gluconate produces a lower incidence of anaphylactic shock; although a test dose is not required, it is good clinical practice to conduct one prior to administration.

Common adverse reactions of iron dextran are hypotension, headache, muscle pain, and joint pain; these are more severe when given IV. Iron dextran appears to increase bone density in the joints, which is the probable cause of the muscle and joint pain.

Frequent adverse effects with ferric gluconate include cramping, nausea, vomiting, hypotension, and rash. Iron sucrose is well tolerated, with some patients experiencing leg cramps and hypotension.

CONNECTION Checkpoint 39.3

From what you learned in Chapter 8, explain why a patient who is pregnant has a substantially higher iron requirement compared to a nonpregnant woman. *See Answer to Connection Checkpoint 39.3 on student resource website.*

39.7 Pernicious anemia may be successfully treated with the administration of vitamin B$_{12}$.

Vitamin B$_{12}$ and folic acid are dietary nutrients essential for rapidly dividing cells. The continuous, high rate of erythropoiesis occurring throughout the lifespan demands a continuous supply of these vitamins. Without them, the normal production of RBCs is interrupted and large, immature erythrocytes that are unable to carry the same amount of oxygen as normal RBCs are released into the blood, and anemia results.

Vitamin B$_{12}$ is an essential component of two coenzymes required for normal cell growth and DNA replication. Neither plants nor animals synthesize vitamin B$_{12}$; only bacteria can make this vitamin. Because the body only requires miniscule amounts of vitamin B$_{12}$ (3 mcg/day), deficiency of this vitamin is usually not due to insufficient dietary intake. Instead, the most common cause of vitamin B$_{12}$ deficiency is absence of **intrinsic factor**, a protein secreted by stomach cells. Intrinsic factor forms a complex with vitamin B$_{12}$, which is then absorbed into the circulation. Without the formation of this complex, vitamin B$_{12}$ is not absorbed from the intestine. Figure 39.3 illustrates the metabolism of vitamin B$_{12}$.

Deficiency of intrinsic factor is caused by inflammatory diseases of the stomach or by gastric resection. Inflammatory diseases of the small intestine that affect food and nutrient absorption may also cause vitamin B$_{12}$ deficiency. Because vitamin B$_{12}$ is found primarily in foods of animal origin, strict vegetarians may require a vitamin supplement to avoid deficiency. The center portion of the vitamin B$_{12}$ molecule contains the metal ion cobalt, which is a micromineral essential to human nutrition.

The most profound consequence of vitamin B$_{12}$ deficiency is a megaloblastic anemia called **pernicious anemia**, which affects both the hematologic and nervous systems. In pernicious anemia, the hematopoietic stem cells produce abnormally large erythrocytes that do not fully mature. Although RBCs are most affected, lack of maturation of all blood cell types may occur in severe disease. Symptoms of pernicious anemia are often nonspecific and develop slowly, sometimes over several years. Profound nervous system symptoms distinguish this disease from most other anemias and include memory loss, confusion, unsteadiness, tingling or numbness in the limbs, delusions, mood disturbances, and even hallucinations in severe deficiencies. Permanent nervous system impairment may result if the disease remains untreated for 6 to 12 months. Pharmacotherapy includes the administration of cyanocobalamin, a form of vitamin B$_{12}$. Prior to administration of vitamin B$_{12}$, the nurse should assess for other causes of anemia including GI bleeding, GI surgery, tapeworm infestation, and gluten enteropathy.

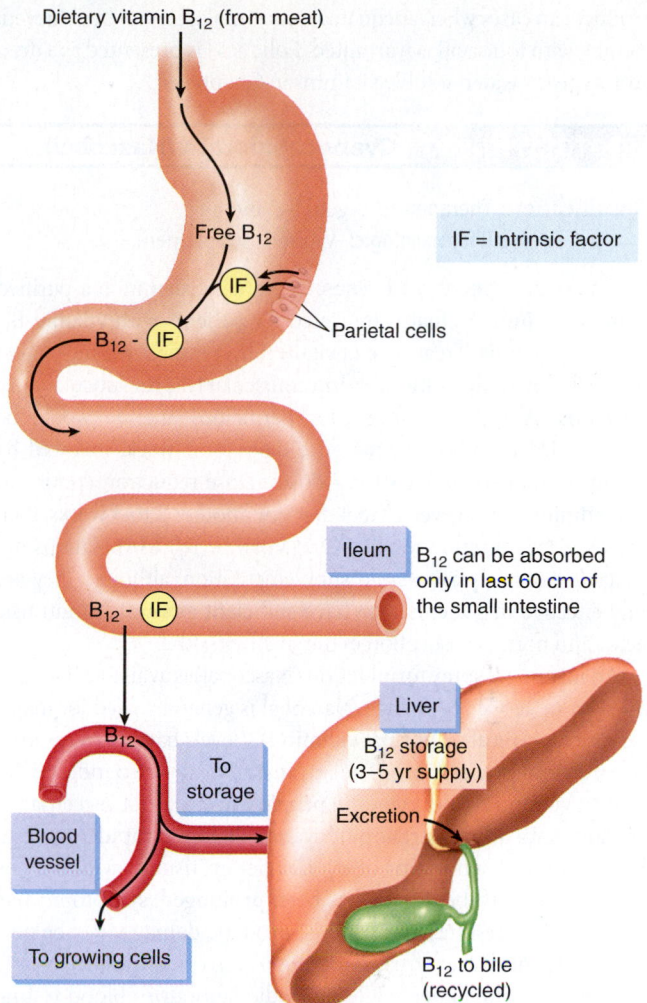

Figure 39.3 Metabolism of vitamin B$_{12}$.

Folic acid, or **folate**, is a B-complex vitamin that is essential for normal DNA and ribonucleic acid (RNA) synthesis. Like B$_{12}$ deficiency, insufficient folic acid levels can manifest as anemia. In fact, the metabolism of vitamin B$_{12}$ and folic acid are intricately linked; a B$_{12}$ deficiency will create a lack of activated folic acid. Folate deficiency is one of the most common types of anemias in the United States.

Folic acid does not require intrinsic factor for intestinal absorption, and the most common cause of deficiency is insufficient dietary intake. This is often observed in patients with chronic alcoholism because their diets are often deficient in this nutrient, and ethanol interferes with folate metabolism in the liver. Fad diets and absorption diseases of the small intestine can also lead to folate-deficiency anemia. Hematopoietic symptoms of folate deficiency are the same as those for B$_{12}$ deficiency; however, no neurologic signs are present. Folate deficiency during pregnancy has been linked to neural birth defects such as spina bifida. Mild deficiency or prophylaxis of folate deficiency is accomplished by increasing the dietary intake of folic acid through fresh green vegetables, dried beans, and wheat

PharmFACT

A deficiency of vitamin B$_{12}$, folate, or vitamin B$_6$ may increase the blood level of homocysteine, an amino acid normally found in the blood. An elevated blood level of homocysteine is a risk factor for heart disease and stroke (Office of Dietary Supplements, National Institutes of Health, 2011).

products. In cases when adequate dietary intake cannot be achieved, therapy with folic acid is warranted. Folic acid is presented as a drug prototype for water-soluble vitamins in Chapter 61.

PROTOTYPE DRUG | **Cyanocobalamin (Nascobal)**

Classification: Therapeutic: Agent for anemia
Pharmacologic: Vitamin supplement

Therapeutic Effects and Uses: Cyanocobalamin is a purified form of vitamin B_{12} that is indicated for patients with vitamin B_{12} deficiency anemia. Treatment of vitamin B_{12} deficiency is most often by weekly, biweekly, or monthly intramuscular (IM) or subcutaneous injections. A typical regimen for pernicious anemia would be 100 mcg IM or subcutaneous once daily for 1 week, followed by 100 mcg on alternate days for 7 doses. Dose reduction continues, with administration every 3 to 4 days for another 2 to 3 weeks, then 100 mcg IM monthly for life. Oral vitamin B_{12} formulations are available primarily as vitamin supplementation, although they are only effective in patients who have sufficient amounts of intrinsic factor and normal absorption in the small intestine.

An intranasal spray formulation (Nascobal) is available that provides for once-weekly dosage. Nascobal is generally used for maintenance therapy after normal vitamin B_{12} levels have been restored by parenteral preparations. The intranasal form is also indicated to prevent vitamin B_{12} deficiency in people who are strict vegetarians.

Parenteral administration of cyanocobalamin rapidly reverses most signs and symptoms of B_{12} deficiency, usually within a few days or weeks. If the disease has been prolonged, symptoms may take longer to resolve, and some neurologic damage may be permanent. In most cases, treatment must often be maintained for the remainder of the patient's life. Periodic laboratory blood testing and Hgb values are used to gauge the success of pharmacotherapy.

Mechanism of Action: Administration of cyanocobalamin reverses vitamin B_{12} deficiency and results in rapid improvement of anemia symptoms. Normal RBC production resumes, with laboratory evaluation of blood and bone marrow showing continuous improvement over about 7 days. Therapy may extend to several months to restore hepatic stores of the vitamin.

Pharmacokinetics:

Route(s)	PO, IM, deep subcutaneous, intranasal
Absorption	Well absorbed; PO absorption requires intrinsic factor
Distribution	Widely distributed; crosses the placenta; secreted in breast milk
Primary metabolism	Primarily converted in tissues to coenzyme B_{12} and stored in liver; extensive enterohepatic recirculation
Primary excretion	Renal
Onset of action	Peak serum level: 8–12 h (PO), 1–2 h (intranasal), and 1 h (IM/subcutaneous)
Duration of action	Half-life: 6 days

Adverse Effects: Adverse effects from cyanocobalamin are uncommon. Because hypokalemia may occur, serum potassium levels are monitored periodically. A small percentage of patients receiving

B_{12} exhibit rashes, itching, or other signs of allergy. Anaphylaxis is possible, though rare, with parenteral administration. Sodium retention occurs in some patients, with possible worsening of HF.

Contraindications/Precautions: Patients with suspected sensitivity to cobalt should receive an intradermal test dose because they may experience allergic reactions or anaphylaxis to the drug. Monotherapy with folic acid will not improve symptoms of vitamin B_{12} deficiency anemia. Cyanocobalamin is contraindicated in patients with severe pulmonary disease and should be used cautiously in patients with heart disease because of the potential for sodium retention caused by the drug.

Drug Interactions: Drug interactions with cyanocobalamin include a decrease in absorption when given concurrently with ethanol, aminosalicylic acid, omeprazole, neomycin, or colchicine. Chloramphenicol may interfere with the therapeutic response to cyanocobalamin. **Herbal/Food:** Unknown.

Pregnancy: Category A (C when used parenterally). Maternal requirements for vitamin B_{12} increase during pregnancy and lactation, although the drug should not be taken in higher than recommended amounts.

Treatment of Overdose: Overdosage has not been reported with this drug.

Nursing Responsibilities:

- Monitor serum potassium levels during the first 48 hours. Conversion to normal erythropoiesis increases the erythrocyte potassium requirement and can result in severe hypokalemia and sudden death.

- Monitor vital signs in patients with cardiac disease and in those receiving parenteral cyanocobalamin. Be alert to symptoms of pulmonary edema, which may occur early in therapy.

- Obtain a complete diet and drug history and inquire into alcohol drinking patterns for all patients receiving cyanocobalamin to identify and correct poor dietary habits.

Lifespan and Diversity Considerations:
- Evaluate the older adult's nutritional status and weight during each monthly visit for their injection and laboratory work.

- Due to undetected heart disease, monitor the older adult for edema or signs and symptoms of HF.

Patient and Family Education:
- Do not discontinue taking this drug without approval of the health care provider. The drug will be required lifelong.

- If using the spray form, prime the pump before the first use by pumping the spray a few times until a fine mist appears. If it has been longer than 5 days between uses, prime the pump again. Sniff gently while spraying.

- Eat foods that are rich sources of B_{12} (nonpernicious anemia) such as nutrient-fortified breakfast cereals, vitamin B_{12}-fortified soy milk, organ meats, clams, oysters, egg yolk, crab, salmon, sardines, muscle meat, milk, and dairy products.

Drugs Similar to Cyanocobalamin (Nascobal)

There are no drugs similar to cyanocobalamin.

CHAPTER

39

Understanding the Chapter

Key Concepts Summary

39.1 Hematopoiesis is a dynamic process that is responsive to the changing demands of the body.

39.2 Erythropoietin stimulates production of red blood cells and is used to treat anemia.

39.3 Colony-stimulating factors increase the production of leukocytes.

39.4 Platelet enhancers may be used to treat thrombocytopenia.

39.5 Anemias may be caused by hemorrhage or a change in red blood cell production or destruction.

39.6 Administration of iron salts can rapidly reverse symptoms of iron deficiency anemia.

39.7 Pernicious anemia may be successfully treated with the administration of vitamin B_{12}.

Case Study: Making the Patient Connection

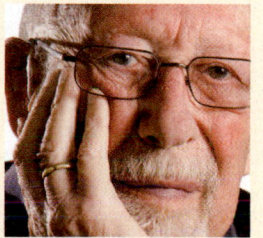

Remember the patient "Carl Guenther" at the beginning of the chapter? Now read the remainder of the case study. Based on the information presented within this chapter, respond to the critical thinking questions that follow.

"A real people-person who never met a stranger." That is how family and friends have always described Carl Guenther. His positive and outgoing personality is well known in the community. When Carl was informed about his prostate cancer, he handled the diagnosis well and with his usual optimism. He was confident that the chemotherapy would be successful. His mantra for years had been to "Live every day as if it were your last." However, the treatment for the cancer had adverse effects that he did not expect and his enthusiasm diminished.

Carl is a 72-year-old retired sales representative for a chain of department stores. His entire career was centered on interacting with all kinds of people. When he retired, his outgoing nature was an asset for the many community agencies at which he volunteered to help. He was active in the local Lions Club, his church's outreach ministry, and at the children's hospital. He had even considered working as a greeter at his neighborhood department store.

As he went through chemotherapy, the associated nausea and vomiting were well managed with antiemetic agents. His physical appearance did not change much since Carl had minimal hair loss due to the chemotherapy. Now he faces an exceedingly low white blood cell count and has been advised to avoid potential sources of infection, including people. By far this is the worst adverse effect of the chemotherapy for Carl. He feels socially isolated and depressed. Is this the end, he wonders? Am I to die lonely?

Critical Thinking Questions

1. The health care provider orders filgrastim (Neupogen) 10 mcg/kg daily for 4 days. Carl asks you, his nurse, "How does this drug work?" What is your response?

2. List interventions that should be followed during this period of chemotherapy-induced neutropenia to protect Carl from infection.

3. What adverse effects would you monitor in patients receiving Neupogen?

See Answers to Critical Thinking Questions on student resource website.

Additional Case Study

When the blood test returned from Betty Arnold's preemployment physical, the results indicated anemia. "No wonder I feel so exhausted all the time," she said. "I thought my fatigue was from taking care of my five children, my home, and my aging parents." When she saw her primary health care provider, she was diagnosed with iron deficiency anemia and prescribed ferrous sulfate (Feosol) 160-mg sustained release tablets daily.

1. As the nurse, you will provide teaching for this patient about dietary sources of iron. Create a list of foods high in iron.

2. What adverse effects should Betty watch for while taking Feosol?

3. Is there a best time of the day to take this medication? Why?

See Answers to Additional Case Study on student resource website.

Chapter Review

1 Which statement would the nurse include in the care plan for a patient receiving epoetin alfa?

1. Avoid fresh fruit and vegetables, or partially cooked meats.
2. Encourage frequent rest periods to minimize fatigue.
3. Limit exposure to direct sunlight and use sunscreen when outdoors.
4. Protect tissues and mucous membranes from traumatic injury.

2 Darbepoetin (Aranesp) is prescribed for each of the following patients. A nurse should question the order for which condition?

1. A patient with HIV who is receiving zidovudine
2. A patient with uncontrolled hypertension
3. A patient with chronic renal failure
4. A patient with chemotherapy-induced anemia

3 The patient is being treated with filgrastim (Neupogen). Which of the following would the nurse monitor to determine the effectiveness of this drug?

1. Red blood cell counts
2. Platelet counts
3. White blood cell counts
4. Reticulocyte count and mean cell volume (MCV)

4 The nurse is teaching the patient about oprelvekin (Neumega). Which statement, if made by the patient, indicates that additional health teaching is needed?

1. "This drug stimulates the production of platelets."
2. "I should weigh myself and watch for fluid retention."
3. "I will report vision changes to my health care provider."
4. "I will add more iron-rich foods to my diet."

5 A patient who regularly consumes significant amounts of alcohol is prescribed cyanocobalamin (Nascobal) and states, "I don't understand why my health care provider has prescribed B_{12} injections." The nurse's response would be based on which physiological concept?

1. Patients who regularly consume large amounts of alcohol are often deficient in this nutrient.
2. Alcohol facilitates folate metabolism in the liver, which destroys vitamin B_{12}.
3. Patients who regularly consume large amounts of alcohol are at high risk for neutropenia, a condition that develops from vitamin B_{12} loss.
4. Liver cirrhosis caused by large amounts of alcohol ingestion diminishes natural physiological deposits of B_{12}.

6 The nurse is teaching the patient about ferrous sulfate (Feosol). Which statement should be included in the teaching plan? Select all that apply.

1. This drug should be taken on an empty stomach at least 1 hour before or 2 hours after a meal.
2. Getting liquid iron on teeth should be avoided because the drug can cause brown stains.
3. Iron preparation may darken stools and cause constipation.
4. Vitamin E is added to many oral iron supplements because it enhances iron absorption.
5. This drug can be taken with caffeinated beverages.

See Answers to Chapter Review in Appendix A.

References

Office of Dietary Supplements, National Institutes of Health. (2011). *Dietary supplement fact sheet: Vitamin B_{12}.* Retrieved from http://ods.od.nih.gov/factsheets/VitaminB12-HealthProfessional/

Office of Dietary Supplements, National Institutes of Health. (2014). *Dietary supplement fact sheet: Iron.* Retrieved from http://ods.od.nih.gov/factsheets/Iron-HealthProfessional/#h2

Selected Bibliography

Fishbane, S., & Nissenson, A. R. (2010). Anemia management in chronic kidney disease. *Kidney International, 78*(S3–S9). doi:10.1038/ki.2010.188

Flores, I. Q., & Ershler, W. (2010). Managing neutropenia in older patients with cancer receiving chemotherapy in a community setting. *Clinical Journal of Oncology Nursing, 14,* 81–86. doi:10.1188/10.CJON.81-86

Freburger, J. K., Ng, L. J., Bradbury, B. D., Kshirsagar, A. V., & Brookhart, M. A. (2012). Changing patterns of anemia management in US hemodialysis patients. *The American Journal of Medicine, 125,* 906–914. doi:10.1016/j.amjmed.2012.03.011

Hamilton, J. A., & Achuthan, A. (2013). Colony stimulating factors and myeloid cell biology in health and disease. *Trends in Immunology, 34,* 81–89. doi:10.1016/j.it.2012.08.006

Herdman, T. H., & Kamitsuru, S. (Eds.). (2014). *NANDA International nursing diagnoses: Definitions and classification, 2015–2017.* Oxford, United Kingdom: Wiley-Blackwell.

Kaushansky, K., & Kipps, T. J. (2011). Hematopoietic agents: Growth factors, minerals and vitamins. In L. L. Brunton, B. A. Chabner, & B. C. Knollman (Eds.), *The pharmacological basis of therapeutics* (12th ed., pp. 1067–1100). New York, NY: McGraw-Hill.

Khan, M., & Mikhael, J. (2010). A review of immune thrombocytopenic purpura: Focus on the novel thrombopoietin agonists. *Journal of Blood Medicine, 1,* 21–31. doi: 10.2147/JBM.S6803

Sabol, V. K., Resnick, B., Galik, E., Gruber-Baldini, A., Morton, P. G., & Hicks, G. E. (2010). Anemia and its impact on function in nursing home residents: What do we know? *Journal of the American Academy of Nurse Practitioners, 22,* 3–16. doi:10.1111/j.1745-7599.2009.00471.x

Scialdone, L. (2012). Overview of supportive care in patients receiving chemotherapy antiemetics, pain management, anemia, and neutropenia. *Journal of Pharmacy Practice, 25,* 209–221. doi:10.1177/0897190011431631

Tucker, B. B., & Dauffenbach, V. (2011). *Nutrition and diet therapy for nurses.* Upper Saddle River, NJ: Pearson Education.

UNIT 6

Pharmacology of Body Defenses

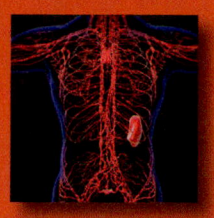 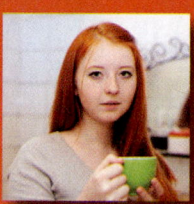 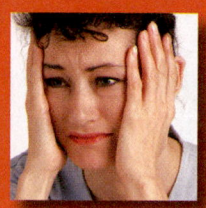 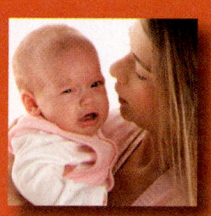

CHAPTER 40   Review of Body Defenses and the Immune System / 664

CHAPTER 41   Pharmacotherapy of Inflammation and Fever / 672

CHAPTER 42   Immunostimulants and Immunosuppressants / 689

CHAPTER 43   Immunizing Agents / 709

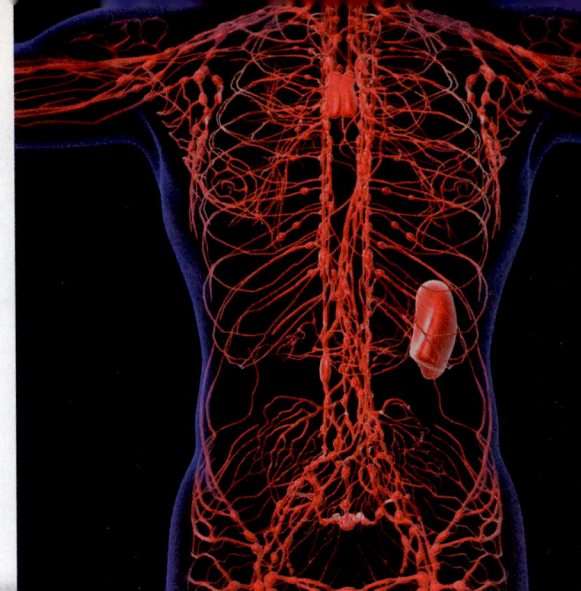

CHAPTER

40 Review of Body Defenses and the Immune System

LEARNING OUTCOMES

After reading this chapter, the student should be able to:

1. Identify the major components of the lymphatic system.
2. Describe the components of the nonspecific body defense system and their functions.
3. Compare and contrast specific and nonspecific body defenses.
4. Identify the signs and symptoms of inflammation.
5. Outline the basic steps in the acute inflammatory response.
6. Explain the role of histamine and other chemical mediators in the inflammatory response.
7. Compare and contrast the humoral and cell-mediated immune responses.

CHAPTER OUTLINE

▸ Organization of the Lymphatic System

▸ Innate (Nonspecific) Body Defenses
   Inflammation

▸ Specific (Adaptive) Body Defenses
   Humoral Immune Response
   Cell-Mediated Immune Response

The human body is under continuous attack from a host of foreign invaders, including viruses, bacteria, fungi, and even single-celled animals. Some of these pathogens intentionally seek out humans because it is an essential part of their life cycle, whereas others happen to be "at the right place and time" when a cut or scrape allows entrance into the body. Fortunately, the body's extensive defenses are capable of mounting a rapid and effective response against most of these pathogens. Drugs used to modify body defenses, which include anti-inflammatory agents, immunostimulants, immunosuppressants, and vaccines, are presented in Chapters 41 through 43. The purpose of this chapter is to review the fundamental concepts of body defenses that apply to the pharmacotherapy of the immune system and infectious disease. For a more thorough review of this topic, the student should consult an anatomy and physiology textbook.

Organization of the Lymphatic System

40.1 The lymphatic system is the primary organ system that protects the body from invasion by foreign agents.

The components of the lymphatic system provide the body with **immunity**, which is the ability to resist injury and infections. The **lymphatic system** comprises a network of cells, vessels, and tissues that provide immune surveillance. This monitoring function begins when fluid leaves the capillaries due to the osmotic forces and high pressure in the capillaries. This fluid, known as lymph, enters blind-ended lymphatic vessels and slowly travels on its journey through the lymphatic system. As much as 3 L of fluid per day travel through the highly branched lymphatic vessel network to eventually return to the cardiovascular circulation.

Lymphatic vessels carry more than escaped fluid. Viruses, bacteria, cellular debris, and even cancer cells can enter these vessels. Should these pathogens or cancer cells be permitted to return to the bloodstream, an infection (or cancer) could quickly spread throughout the body with potentially disastrous consequences. Fortunately, before these pathogens can return to the general circulation, they must pass through dozens of **lymph nodes**, which are the principal lymphoid organs in the body. Lymph nodes are solid, spherical bodies that are packed with macrophages and lymphocytes, which are cells specialized to recognize anything that is "nonself" or foreign to the body. Recognition of these foreign agents activates the immune response, which neutralizes or removes the pathogens before they can reach the general circulation. Each lymph node serves as a minifilter, removing up to 99% of the foreign agents entering the node. Should a pathogen be clever enough

to escape surveillance in a lymph node, it is then faced with passing through dozens, and sometimes hundreds, more lymph nodes in the lymphatic system.

In addition to lymph vessels and nodes, lymphoid tissues line connective tissue at every potential portal of entrance into the body, including the gastrointestinal (GI) tract, respiratory tract, and genitourinary tract. Lymphoid tissue contains lymphocytes, which "patrol" the region for potential injury or exposure to microbes. Other large collections of lymphoid tissue include the tonsils, spleen, and thymus. These are considered organs of the lymphatic system.

Although the lymphatic system can be divided into individual structures and components for ease of study, it is best to think of it as an integrated whole. The various components of this system are in continuous communication and work together as a single unit to accomplish effective immune surveillance. A malfunction in any one single component may affect the effectiveness of the entire lymphatic system. An overview of the primary divisions of immunity is shown in Figure 40.1.

PharmFACT

Lymphatic vessels are highly dynamic structures and are constantly being remodeled. This remodeling, called lymphangiogenesis, is involved in the pathophysiology of various inflammatory conditions (Kim, Kataru, & Koh, 2012).

Innate (Nonspecific) Body Defenses

40.2 Innate body defenses are the body's first line of defense against pathogens.

Innate body defenses are those that are present even before an infection has occurred and that provide the first line of protection from pathogens. These are sometimes referred to as nonspecific defenses because they are unable to distinguish one type of threat from another; the body's response is the same regardless of the particular pathogen. A summary of nonspecific body defenses is given in Table 40.1. A useful way of categorizing the innate defenses is to consider them as types of barriers:

- Physical barriers: skin and mucous membranes
- Cellular barriers: phagocytes, natural killer cells, and dendritic cells
- Process barriers: complement, fever, and inflammation

Physical barriers: The skin and mucous membranes are considered the first line of defense against pathogen invasion. The intact skin is a formidable physical barrier to pathogens. The cells

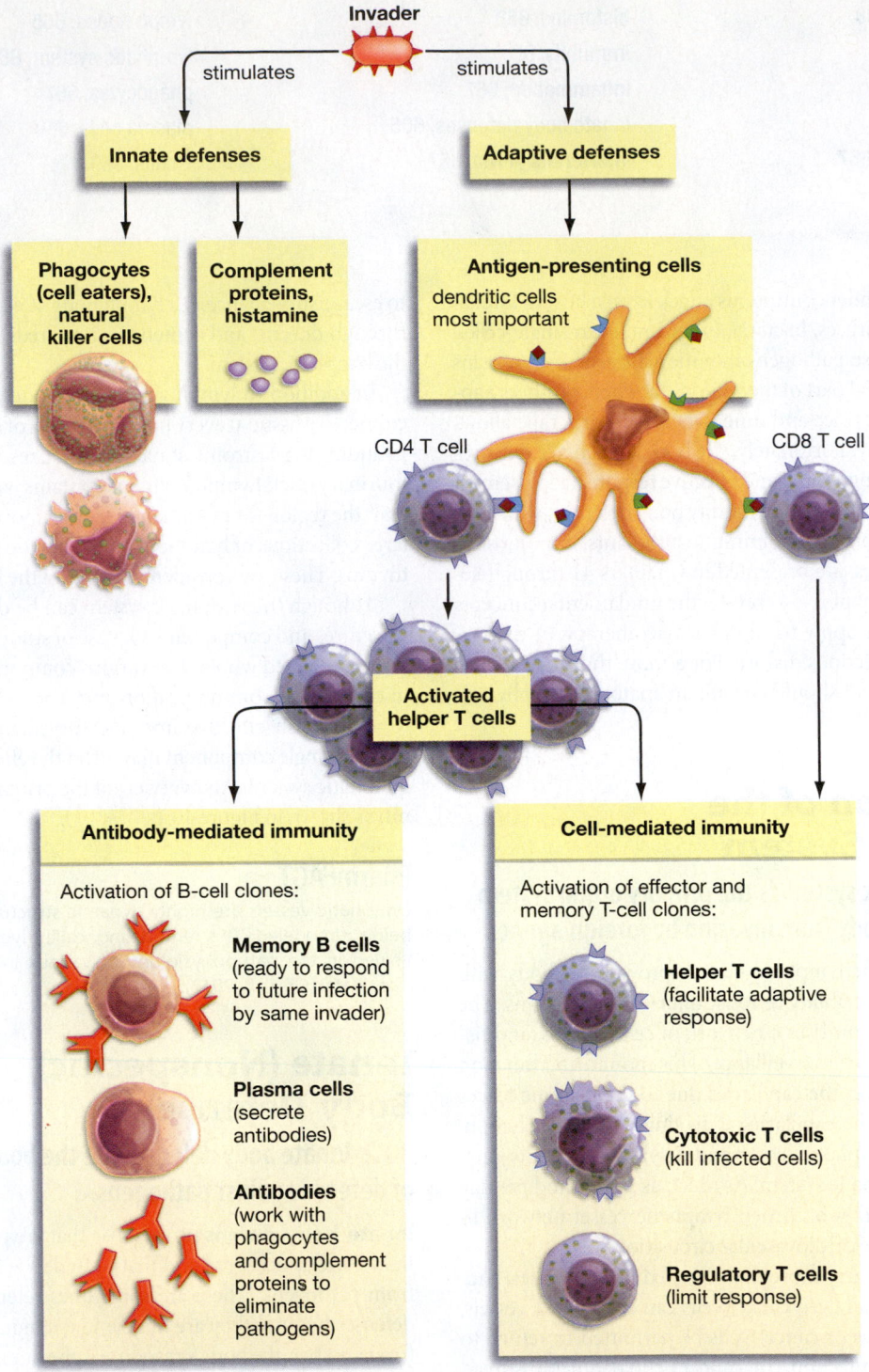

Figure 40.1 Overview of body defenses.

From *Biology: A Guide to the Natural World* (5th ed., p. 563), by D. Krogh, 2006. Printed and electronically reproduced by permission of Pearson Education, Inc., Upper Saddle River, NJ.

of the epidermis are packed tightly together, which discourages penetration by microbes. The outer layer of skin cells is continually shed, along with any microbes that may be clinging to them. The accessory structures of the skin secrete sebum (oil), sweat, and antimicrobial peptides that discourage microbial growth on the surface. The skin is also colonized with a variety of bacteria and fungi that are normally harmless to the host. This microbiota (flora) competes with pathogens for space and nutrients, thus creating an

unfavorable growth environment for harmful organisms. However, should the skin become broken or compromised by needlesticks or catheters, some species of normal flora may become pathogenic.

The body cavities that open to the outside environment are lined with a mucosal epithelium that not only provides a physical barrier, but also contains proteins, lysozymes, and other substances that discourage pathogen growth. The respiratory tract secretes a sticky mucus that traps microbes. The stomach and genitourinary

TABLE 40.1 Summary of Nonspecific Body Defenses

Component	Functions
Physical Barriers	
Skin	Forms a mechanical barrier to prevent pathogens and other harmful substances from entering the body. Surface contains keratin, which is resistant to water and acid.
Mucous membranes	Line the portals of entry to inhibit the entry of pathogens. Mucus inhibits microbial growth. Cilia in the respiratory tract and saliva in the mouth discourage pathogen entry.
Cellular Barriers	
Phagocytes	Ingest antigens. Specific types include neutrophils, eosinophils, and monocytes, which differentiate into macrophages. Also include dendritic cells that reside deep in the skin, in lymph nodes, and in the inner lining of the respiratory and digestive tracts.
Natural killer (NK) cells	Directly attack virus-infected and cancer cells by releasing substances that are toxic to the antigen.
Interferons	Proteins secreted by cells infected by viruses. They protect uninfected cells and also stimulate the activity of phagocytes and NK cells; used as medications to treat certain types of cancer.
Process Barriers	
Complement	Promotes inflammation and phagocytosis; lyses microbes.
Fever	Systemic response that increases body temperature to activate body defenses; inhibits the growth of some microbes.
Inflammation	Limits the spread of infection and releases substances that attract phagocytes; initiates repair of the injured area.

tracts provide an acidic environment that kills many microbes. Like the skin, the mucosa of the mouth, colon, and vagina have a normal population of flora, which discourages pathogen growth by competing for space and nutrients.

Cellular barriers: Once physical barriers are breached, **phagocytes** are the primary cells of innate immunity. The primary job of phagocytes is to engulf pathogens and other foreign substances that enter the body. Once engulfed, the phagocytes destroy the microbe in vesicles called lysosomes, which contain powerful destructive enzymes. As expected, phagocytes are found in large numbers in the blood, in lymphatic tissues, and in locations where pathogens have the highest likelihood of entering. For example, the deeper layers of the epidermis contain specialized phagocytes called dendritic cells, which are able to remove pathogens that penetrate the superficial layers. Phagocytes have the ability to migrate to distant sites when an infection is detected, a process called *chemotaxis*.

Phagocytes have proteins on their surface that allow them to recognize cells and cellular components that are "non-self." When recognized as "non-self," the pathogen is internalized and destroyed within the phagocyte. Pieces of the microbe are sometimes displayed on the plasma membrane of the phagocyte, which serves to activate other components of the immune response. Not all pathogens can be engulfed by phagocytosis. Some, such as *Mycobacterium tuberculosis*, are not only resistant to phagocytosis, but they can also multiply while residing inside macrophages.

Cancer cells or virus-infected cells attract a different type of innate cellular response: natural killer (NK) cells. Found in most lymphoid organs, NK cells are not phagocytic, but they do release toxins that kill cancer cells or virus-infected cells. NK cells also secrete chemicals that enhance inflammation and modulate the adaptive immune response.

Interferons (IFNs) are antimicrobial proteins that are crucial components of the innate body defense system. Released by infected macrophages and lymphocytes, IFNs protect uninfected cells from the pathogen. IFNs have been isolated and are now available as medications for the treatment of immune disorders (see Chapter 42), viral infections (see Chapter 54), and cancer (see Chapter 57).

Process barriers: Processes associated with innate defenses are complement activation, fever, and inflammation. The **complement system** is a cluster of 20 plasma proteins that combine in a specific sequence and order when an infection occurs. Activation of complement attracts phagocytes to the infection site, attacks and breaks down the cell walls of pathogens, and stimulates the inflammatory process.

Other key processes of the nonspecific defense system are fever and inflammation. Fever accelerates body defenses and associated repair processes by raising the temperature of the body. When excessive, however, fever can harm the body and must be treated with drugs known as antipyretics (see Chapter 41). From a pharmacologic perspective, one of the most important nonspecific defenses is inflammation. Because of its significance, inflammation is presented separately in Sections 40.3 and 40.4.

PharmFACT

The skin surface has a large population of resident bacteria, most of which are associated with sweat glands because these provide warm, humid places to grow. Common residents include *Staphylococcus, Propionibacterium, Acinetobacter*, and *Corynebacterium* (Madigan, Martinko, Stahl, & Clark, 2012).

Inflammation

40.3 Inflammation is a nonspecific defense mechanism that neutralizes or destroys foreign substances and microbes.

Inflammation occurs in response to many different stimuli, including physical injury, exposure to toxic chemicals, extreme heat, invading microorganisms, or death of cells. Inflammation is considered a nonspecific defense mechanism because it proceeds in the same manner regardless of the cause.

The central purposes of inflammation are to contain the injury, destroy the pathogen, and initiate repair of the area. The repair of the injured area can proceed at a faster pace by neutralizing the foreign agent and removing cellular debris and dead cells. Signs of inflammation include swelling, pain, warmth, and redness of the affected area.

Inflammation may be classified as acute or chronic. During acute inflammation, such as that caused by minor physical injury, 8 to 10 days are normally needed for the symptoms to resolve and for repair to begin. If the body cannot neutralize the damaging agent, inflammation may continue for long periods and become chronic. In chronic autoimmune disorders such as lupus and rheumatoid arthritis (RA), inflammation may persist for years, with symptoms becoming progressively worse over time. Other disorders such as seasonal allergy arise at predictable times during each year, and inflammation may produce only minor, annoying symptoms.

40.4 Inflammation proceeds with the release of chemical mediators.

During inflammation, pathogens, chemicals, or physical trauma cause the damaged tissue to release chemical mediators that act as alarms to notify the surrounding area of the injury. Chemical mediators of inflammation include histamine, leukotrienes, bradykinin, complement, and prostaglandins. These inflammatory mediators, which are listed in Table 40.2, are sometimes called proinflammatory substances. Some of the inflammatory mediators are important targets for anti-inflammatory drugs. For example, aspirin and ibuprofen are prostaglandin inhibitors that are effective at treating fever, pain, and inflammation.

The rapid release of the chemical mediators of inflammation on a large scale throughout the body is responsible for anaphylaxis, a life-threatening allergic response that may result in shock and death. A number of chemicals, insect stings, foods, and some therapeutic drugs can cause this widespread release of histamine from mast cells if the person has an allergy to these substances.

Histamine is a key chemical mediator of inflammation. It is stored primarily within mast cells located in tissue spaces under epithelial membranes such as the skin, bronchial tree, and digestive tract and along blood vessels. Mast cells detect foreign agents or injury and respond by releasing histamine, which initiates the inflammatory response within seconds. In addition to its role in inflammation, histamine also directly stimulates pain receptors and is a primary agent responsible for the symptoms of seasonal allergies.

When released at an injury site, histamine dilates nearby blood vessels, causing the capillaries to become more permeable. Plasma, complement proteins, and phagocytes can then enter the area to neutralize microbes or their toxins. The affected area may become congested with blood, which can lead to significant swelling and pain. Figure 40.2 illustrates the fundamental steps in acute inflammation.

Histamine interacts with two different receptors to elicit an inflammatory response. H_1 receptors are present in the smooth muscle of the vascular system, the respiratory passages, and the digestive tract. Stimulation of these receptors results in itching, pain, edema, vasodilation, bronchoconstriction, and the characteristic symptoms of inflammation and allergy. In contrast, H_2 receptors are present primarily in the stomach, and their stimulation results in the secretion of large amounts of hydrochloric acid.

Drugs that act as specific antagonists for H_1 and H_2 receptors are in widespread therapeutic use. H_1-receptor antagonists, which are used to treat allergies and inflammation, are discussed in Chapter 45. H_2-receptor antagonists are used to treat peptic ulcers and are discussed in Chapter 59.

CONNECTION Checkpoint 40.1

In addition to being a mediator of inflammation, bradykinin is responsible for one of the most common adverse effects of ACE inhibitors. From what you learned in Chapter 31, describe this adverse effect. *See Answer to Connection Checkpoint 40.1 on student resource website.*

Specific (Adaptive) Body Defenses

40.5 The specific body defenses include the humoral and cell-mediated immune systems.

The body also has the ability to mount a third line of defense that is specific to certain threats. For example, a specific defense may act against only a single species of bacteria and be ineffective against all others. These are known as **adaptive defenses** or, more commonly, the immune response. The primary cell of the immune response is the lymphocyte.

TABLE 40.2	Chemical Mediators of Inflammation
Mediator	**Description**
Bradykinin	Protein present in an inactive form in plasma and mast cells; increases vascular permeability and causes pain; effects are similar to those of histamine; broken down by angiotensin-converting enzyme (ACE).
Complement	Series of at least 20 proteins that combine in a cascade fashion to neutralize or destroy an antigen; stimulates histamine release by mast cells; causes cell lysis.
C-reactive protein	Occurs as an early response to acute inflammation; activates complement; used as a biomarker to gauge the extent of inflammation.
Histamine	Stored and released by mast cells; causes vasodilation, smooth muscle constriction, tissue swelling, and itching.
Leukotrienes	Lipids stored and released by mast cells; effects are similar to those of histamine; synthesized from arachidonic acid; responsible for some symptoms of asthma and allergies.
Prostaglandins	Lipid present in most tissues and stored and released by mast cells; increase capillary permeability, attract white blood cells to the site of inflammation, cause pain, and induce fever; aspirin inhibits their synthesis; some are available as medications.
Tumor necrosis factor (TNF)	A cytokine that promotes inflammation and the programmed death of cells (apoptosis).

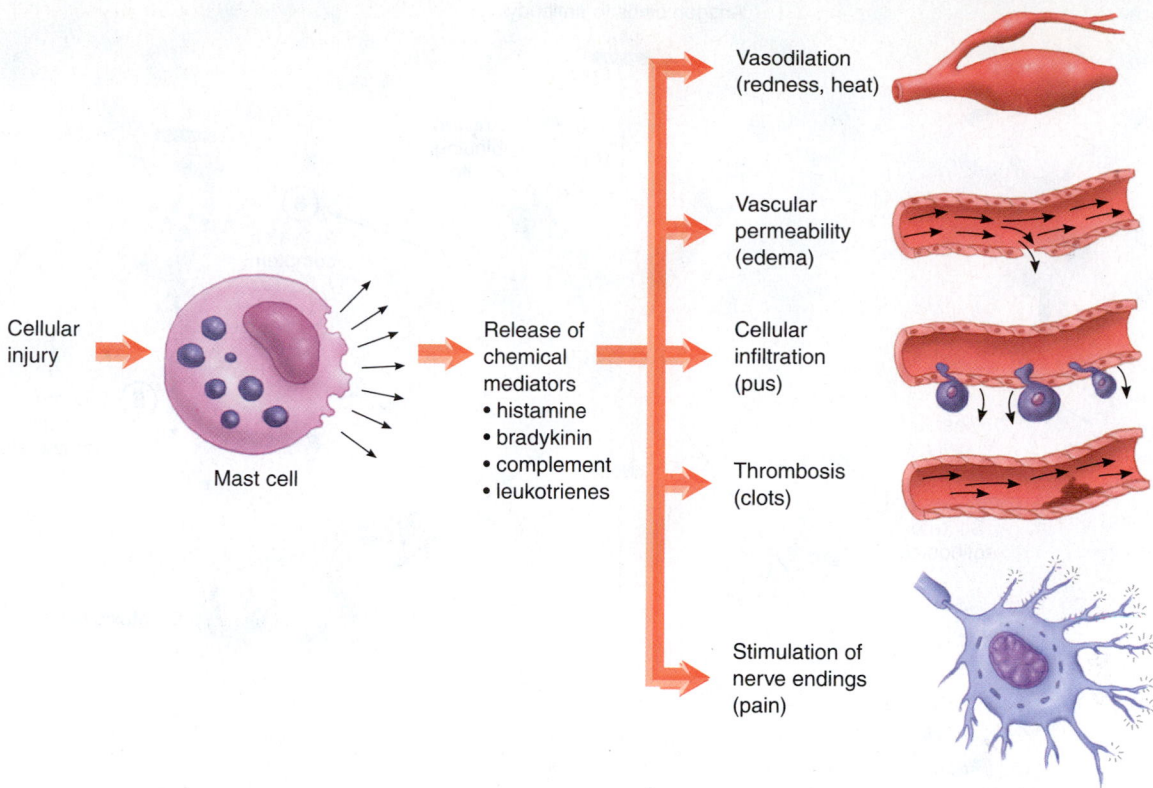

Figure 40.2 Steps in acute inflammation.

Microbes and foreign substances that elicit an immune response are called **antigens**. Foreign proteins, such as those present on the surfaces of pollen grains, bacteria, nonhuman cells, and viruses, are the strongest antigens. Typically, only a small fragment or piece of a foreign protein is required to activate the immune system. It is estimated that the immune system is able to recognize and react to over a billion different antigens.

The immune response is extremely complex. Following are several important aspects of the immune response.

Specificity: Each aspect of the immune response recognizes only particular pathogens and not others. Recognition of the antigen is dependent on the immune cells interacting with specific foreign proteins. Once an immune response is mounted, it generally only affects the one specific antigen that was recognized.

Systemic: Despite being specific to a particular antigen, the immune response is systemic. Thus antigens that exist in remote regions beyond the initial site of infection will be neutralized.

Memory: After an antigen interaction occurs, cells of the adaptive immune system remember the immune response. This is different from the components of nonspecific defenses, which have no memory. Upon subsequent exposures to the *same* antigen, the body is able to mount a stronger and more rapid response.

The basic steps of the immune response involve recognition of the antigen, communication and coordination with other defense cells, and destruction or suppression of the antigen. A large number of chemical messengers and complex interactions are involved in the immune response, many of which have yet to be discovered. The two primary divisions of the immune response are antibody-mediated (humoral) immunity and cell-mediated immunity.

Humoral Immune Response

40.6 The humoral immune response is mediated by B lymphocytes and includes the secretion of antibodies.

The humoral immune response is triggered when an antigen encounters a B lymphocyte, more simply known as a **B cell**. The activated B cell divides to form millions of identical copies of itself in a process known as clonal division. Most cells in this clone are called **plasma cells**, whose primary function is to secrete antibodies specific to the antigen that initiated the challenge. Each plasma cell is capable of manufacturing antibodies at an astounding rate, as many as 2,000 antibodies each second.

Circulating through body fluids are **antibodies**, also known as immunoglobulins (Ig), which physically interact with antigens to neutralize or mark them for destruction by other cells of the immune response. The activation of complement, with subsequent inflammation and enhanced phagocytosis, is a major defense mechanism resulting from the formation of antigen–antibody complexes. Peak production of antibodies occurs about 10 days after an initial antigen challenge. The important functions of antibodies are illustrated in Figure 40.3.

After the antigen challenge, memory B cells are formed that will remember the specific antigen–antibody interaction. Should the body be exposed to the same antigen in the future, the humoral immune system will manufacture even higher levels of antibodies in a shorter period, approximately 2 to 3 days. For some antigens, such as those for measles, mumps, or chickenpox, memory can be

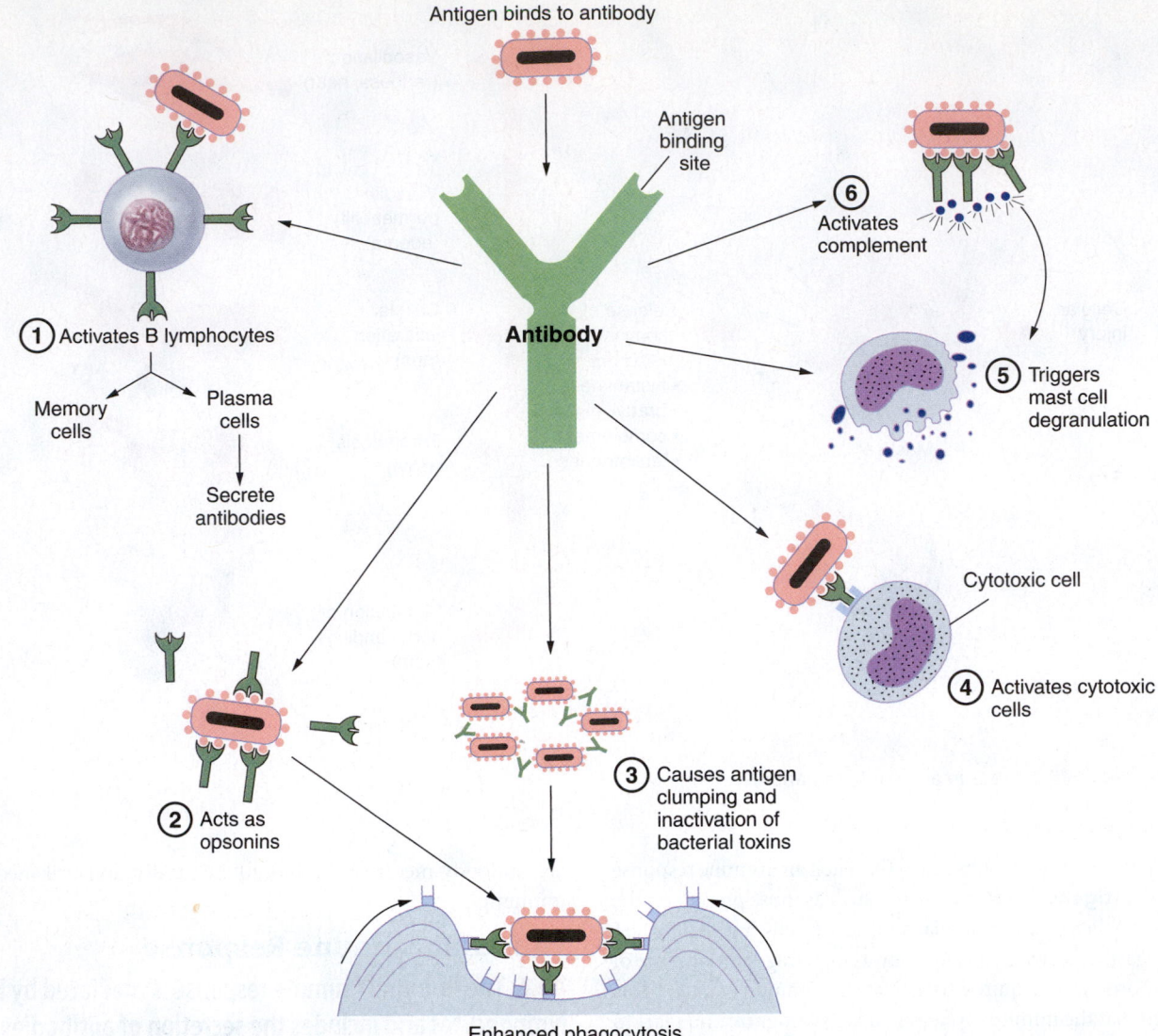

Figure 40.3 Functions of antibodies.

From *Human Physiology: An Integrated Approach* (5th ed.), by D. U. Silverthorn, 2013. Printed and Electronically reproduced by permission. Upper Saddle River, NJ: Pearson Education, Inc.

retained for an entire lifetime. Vaccines are sometimes administered to produce these memory cells in advance of exposure to the antigen, so that when the body is exposed to the actual organism it can mount a fast, effective response (see Chapter 43).

It is important to remember that the body contains millions of different B cells, each programmed to react to a specific antigen. These B cells, in turn, are able to construct millions of different types of antibodies, each specific to a particular antigen. The body is preprogrammed with the genetic information to defend against millions of different antigens. Although it is unlikely that an individual will ever be infected during a lifetime with all the different antigens, the body is waiting for the challenge.

Cell-Mediated Immune Response

40.7 The cell-mediated immune response is mediated by T lymphocytes and includes the secretion of cytokines.

A second branch of the immune response involves T lymphocytes, or **T cells**. Two major types of T cells are called helper T cells and cytotoxic T cells. These cells are named after a protein receptor on their

plasma membrane. The helper T cells have a CD4 receptor, and the cytotoxic T cells have a CD8 receptor. The helper (CD4) T cells are particularly important because they are responsible for activating most other immune cells, including B cells and other types of T cells. Cytotoxic (CD8) T cells travel throughout the body, directly killing certain bacteria, parasites, virus-infected cells, and cancer cells.

PharmFACT

T cells move quickly throughout the body. In a typical day, a T cell may spend 30 minutes in the blood, 5 to 6 hours in the spleen, and 15 to 20 hours in a lymph node (Martini, Nath, & Bartholomew, 2012).

T cells rapidly form clones after they are activated or sensitized following an encounter with their specific antigen. Unlike B cells, however, T cells do not produce antibodies. Instead, activated T cells produce huge amounts of **cytokines**, which are hormone-like proteins that regulate the intensity and duration of the immune response and mediate cell-to-cell communication. Some cytokines kill foreign organisms directly, whereas others induce inflammation or enhance the killing power of macrophages. Specific cytokines released by activated T cells include interleukins, gamma interferon, tumor necrosis factor (TNF), and perforin. Some cytokines are used therapeutically to stimulate the immune system (see Chapter 42). Small amounts of cytokines are also secreted by certain macrophages, B lymphocytes, mast cells, endothelial cells, and the stromal cells of the spleen, thymus, and bone marrow.

PharmFACT

T cells need help in recognizing intact antigens. Certain macrophages must phagocytize the antigen and present the foreign proteins on their surface to be recognized by T cells. These are called antigen-presenting cells (APCs) (Martini, Nath, & Bartholomew, 2012).

Like B cells, some sensitized T cells become memory cells. If the patient encounters the same antigen in the future, the memory T cells assist in mounting a more rapid immune response.

CONNECTION Checkpoint 40.2

Proinflammatory cytokines such as interleukin-1 and TNF have been associated with a higher risk of Alzheimer's disease and progression of this disorder. From what you learned in Chapter 21, describe the primary drug classes for treating Alzheimer's disease. *See Answer to Connection Checkpoint 40.2 on student resource website.*

CHAPTER 40

Understanding the Chapter

Key Concepts Summary

40.1 The lymphatic system is the primary organ system that protects the body from invasion by foreign agents.

40.2 Innate body defenses are the body's first line of defense against pathogens.

40.3 Inflammation is a nonspecific defense mechanism that neutralizes or destroys foreign substances and microbes.

40.4 Inflammation proceeds with the release of chemical mediators.

40.5 The specific body defenses include the humoral and cell-mediated immune systems.

40.6 The humoral immune response is mediated by B lymphocytes and includes the secretion of antibodies.

40.7 The cell-mediated immune response is mediated by T lymphocytes and includes the secretion of cytokines.

References

Kim, H., Kataru, R. P., & Koh, G. Y. (2012). Regulation and implications of inflammatory lymphangiogenesis. *Trends in Immunology, 33,* 350–356. doi:10.1016/j.it.2012.03.006

Krogh, D. (2011). *Biology: A guide to the natural world* (5th ed.). San Francisco, CA: Benjamin Cummings.

Madigan, M. T., Martinko, J. M., Stahl, D. A., & Clark, D. P. (2012). *Brock biology of microorganisms* (13th ed.). Upper Saddle River, NJ: Pearson Prentice Hall.

Martini, F. H., Nath, J. L., & Bartholomew, E. F. (2012). *Fundamentals of human anatomy and physiology* (9th ed.). San Francisco, CA: Benjamin Cummings.

Selected Bibliography

DiPiro, J. T., Talbert, R. L., Yee, G. C., Matzke, G. R., Wells, B. G., & Posey, L. M. (Eds.). (2012). *Pharmacotherapy: A pathophysiologic approach* (7th ed.). New York, NY: McGraw-Hill.

Silverthorn, D. U. (2013). *Human physiology: An integrated approach* (6th ed.). San Francisco, CA: Benjamin Cummings.

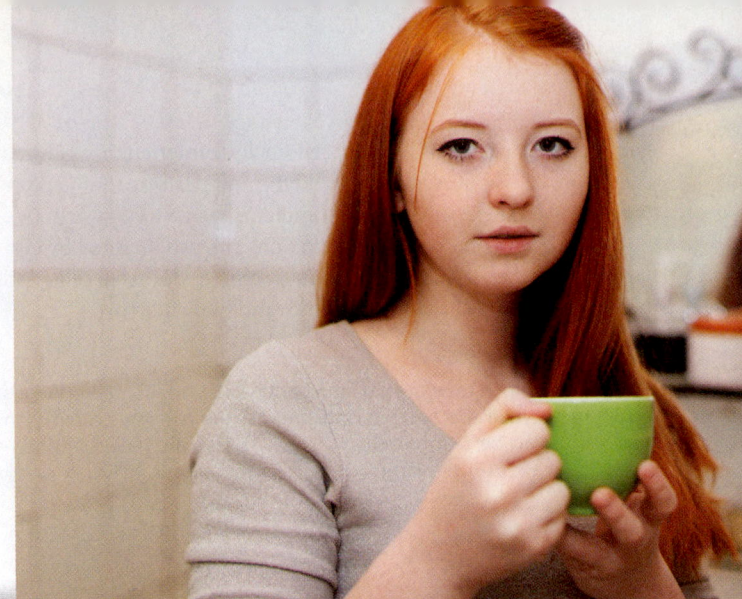

"I haven't been feeling good this week. It's probably just the flu like all my friends have. I'll just take some of the aspirin my mom uses for her arthritis so I don't miss school and I'll be fine."

Patient "Joycee Layne"

CHAPTER
41

Pharmacotherapy of Inflammation and Fever

LEARNING OUTCOMES

After reading this chapter, the student should be able to:

1. Explain the pathophysiology of inflammation and fever.
2. Identify drug classes used to treat inflammation and fever.
3. Explain how aspirin damages the gastrointestinal mucosa.
4. Describe the symptoms and treatment of salicylism.
5. Compare the actions and adverse effects of aspirin to ibuprofen and ibuprofen-like drugs.
6. Compare the actions and adverse effects of the cyclooxygenase-2 inhibitors to other nonsteroidal anti-inflammatory drugs.
7. Describe the nurse's role in the pharmacologic management of inflammation and fever.
8. For each of the classes shown in the chapter outline, identify the prototype and representative drugs and explain the mechanism(s) of drug action, primary indications, contraindications, significant drug interactions, pregnancy category, and important adverse effects.
9. Apply the nursing process to care for patients who are receiving pharmacotherapy for fever or inflammation.

CHAPTER OUTLINE

▶ Pathophysiology of Inflammation and Fever

▶ Pharmacotherapy of Inflammation

▶ Nonsteroidal Anti-Inflammatory Drugs
   Salicylates
   PROTOTYPE Aspirin (Acetylsalicylic Acid) *p. 676*
   Ibuprofen-Like Drugs
   PROTOTYPE Ibuprofen (Advil, Motrin, Others) *p. 679*
   Cyclooxygenase-2 Inhibitors
   PROTOTYPE Celecoxib (Celebrex) *p. 682*

▶ Antipyretic and Analgesic Drugs
   PROTOTYPE Acetaminophen (Tylenol) *p. 683*

KEY TERMS

anaphylaxis, 673
antipyretics, 674
cyclooxygenase (COX), 675

inflammation, 673
prostaglandins, 674

salicylates, 674
salicylism, 678

Inflammation is a response to injury that destroys agents that could damage human tissue. A large number of conditions can trigger inflammation, including physical trauma, burns, chemical injury, infections, hypersensitivity reactions, or tissue necrosis (death). Although it is a natural defense mechanism, excessive inflammation causes symptoms that range from minor discomfort to severe, disabling pain, fever, and limitation of mobility. This chapter examines drugs used to diminish the inflammatory response and reduce fever.

Pathophysiology of Inflammation and Fever

41.1 Inflammation is a nonspecific body response to antigens and tissue injury.

The basic process of inflammation and the proinflammatory chemical mediators involved are described in Chapter 40. The student should review that chapter before proceeding.

Acute inflammation: Acute inflammation has an immediate onset and lasts 1 to 2 weeks. The inflammatory process is initiated when the body is exposed to a foreign substance, or antigen. The antigen may be anything from ragweed pollen to a microorganism; it may even be a normal cell that has been damaged or changed. Once the inflammation process is initiated, nearby blood vessels become permeable, allowing phagocytic cells to reach and neutralize the antigen. The increased permeability causes edema of the surrounding tissue, which often leads to acute pain and, possibly, joint immobility. The greater the tissue damage from the antigen or the inflammation, the greater the edema and the greater the immobility at the site.

Occasionally, acute inflammation is initiated by a rapid, massive release of inflammatory chemical mediators throughout the entire body. This condition, known as **anaphylaxis**, is a life-threatening allergic response that may cause cardiovascular shock and death. A number of chemicals, insect stings, foods, and some therapeutic drugs can cause this widespread release of histamine from mast cells if the person has hypersensitivity to these substances.

The resolution of acute inflammation occurs when damaged tissue begins the process of regeneration and may conclude within a matter of weeks or continue throughout the individual's life with the regeneration of new tissue. Regeneration processes may replace normal cells with scar tissue, especially in nerve, cardiac, and muscle tissues. Replacement with fibrotic tissue can impair the function of the inflamed tissue.

Chronic inflammation: Chronic inflammation has a slow onset and may lack the distinct stages characteristic of acute inflammation. Whereas acute inflammation is the result of an influx of neutrophils, chronic inflammation is caused primarily by lymphocytes and macrophages. The chronic invasion of an area by macrophages and the resultant chemical reaction at the tissue site activates fibroblasts

and generates scar tissue, which may limit mobility or narrow vessel lumens. Lymphocytes sometimes surround macrophages, resulting in granulomas. For example, chronic inflammation from *Mycobacterium tuberculosis* in the lung may occur over many years and yield the development of granulomas. The granulomas serve as a means of protection, walling off the agent from the rest of the body. In the event that the host's immune response diminishes, the host is susceptible to the reemergence of inflammation and the possible onset of active infection.

When acute or chronic inflammation is caused by an infection, the patient is at risk for the development of a febrile episode, which is characterized by an increase in body temperature due to cytokine-induced changes in the hypothalamus. The systemic manifestations of inflammation associated with an infection are elevated temperature above 39°C (102°F), pulse rate greater than 90 beats/minute, respirations greater than 20 breaths/minute, and a white blood cell count greater than 12,000/mm³.

Pharmacotherapy of Inflammation

41.2 Treatment of inflammation includes nonpharmacologic therapies and the administration of anti-inflammatory drugs.

Because inflammation is a nonspecific process and may be caused by a variety of physical and infectious etiologies, it may occur in virtually any tissue or organ system. When treating the patient with inflammation, the following general principles apply:

- Inflammation is not a disease but a symptom of an underlying disorder. Whenever possible, the cause of the inflammation is identified and treated.

- Inflammation is a natural process for ridding the body of antigens, and it is usually self-limiting. Nonpharmacologic treatments such as ice packs and rest should be used for mild symptoms whenever applicable.

- Topical drugs should be used when applicable because they cause few adverse effects. Inflammation of the skin and mucous membranes of the mouth, nose, rectum, and vagina are best treated with topical drugs. These include creams, ointments, patches, suppositories, and intranasal sprays. Inhalation drugs may be used for pulmonary inflammation.

The goal of pharmacotherapy with anti-inflammatory drugs is to prevent or decrease the intensity of the inflammatory response and reduce fever, if present. Most anti-inflammatory agents are nonspecific; that is, whether the inflammation is caused by an injury, autoimmune disease, or allergy, the drug will exhibit the same inhibitory actions. Common diseases that benefit from anti-inflammatory medications include allergic rhinitis, anaphylaxis, ankylosing spondylitis, contact dermatitis, Crohn's disease, glomerulonephritis, Hashimoto's thyroiditis, peptic ulcer disease (PUD), rheumatoid arthritis (RA), systemic lupus erythematosus, and ulcerative colitis.

If fever is associated with the inflammation, medications used to reduce body temperature, or **antipyretics**, may be administered. The goal of antipyretic therapy is to lower body temperature while treating the underlying cause of the fever, which is usually an infection. Many of the drugs used for inflammation also reduce fever and relieve mild to moderate pain.

Two major drug classes are used for nonspecific inflammation: nonsteroidal anti-inflammatory drugs (NSAIDs) and the corticosteroids. For mild to moderate pain, inflammation, and fever, NSAIDs are the preferred class of drugs. Should inflammation become severe or disabling, corticosteroid therapy is begun. Due to the potential for serious long-term adverse effects, corticosteroids are usually used for only 1 to 3 weeks to bring inflammation under control. The patient is then switched to NSAIDs. Corticosteroids are used for a large number of conditions, and their pharmacotherapy is presented in Chapter 68.

A few anti-inflammatory drug classes are specific to certain disorders. For example, the 5-aminosalicylic acid drugs such as sulfasalazine (Azulfidine) are specific to treating inflammatory bowel disease (see Chapter 60). Colchicine and allopurinol (Zyloprim) are used for the inflammation specifically caused by gouty arthritis (see Chapter 72). These specific anti-inflammatory agents are less widely prescribed because they are more toxic than the NSAIDs.

PharmFACT

In the United States, approximately 70 million NSAID prescriptions are written and 30 billion OTC NSAID tablets are sold each year (Wiegand, 2012).

Nonsteroidal Anti-Inflammatory Drugs

The NSAIDs consist of three major classes: salicylates, ibuprofen (including ibuprofen-like agents), and the cyclooxygenase-2 (COX-2) inhibitors. These drug classes are sometimes grouped as first-generation NSAIDs (salicylates and ibuprofen-like drugs) and second-generation NSAIDs (cyclooxygenase-2 inhibitors). This is not a particularly useful means of grouping the drugs because there are over 20 first-generation NSAIDs and only one second-generation NSAID. The ibuprofen-like NSAIDs are described in Section 41.4 and the COX-2 inhibitors are presented in Section 41.5.

Salicylates

41.3 Aspirin is an inexpensive, effective, first-generation nonsteroidal anti-inflammatory drug commonly used by adults.

The first of the NSAIDs to be discovered was originally extracted from the bark of the common willow tree. The medical uses of willow bark, especially for pain relief and fever reduction, had been known for centuries but it was not until 1828 that the active ingredient, called salicin, was identified and converted to salicylic acid. Quite toxic in concentrated amounts, salicylic acid was converted into its most useful form, known as aspirin or acetylsalicylic acid, by a scientist at the Bayer Pharmaceutical Company in 1897. The chemical family to which aspirin belongs is known as the **salicylates**. Since its discovery, aspirin has become one of the most highly used therapeutic drugs in the world. Aspirin has the following indications for use:

- **Analgesic.** The ability to relieve mild to moderate pain
- **Anti-inflammatory.** The ability to decrease mild to moderate inflammation
- **Antipyretic.** The ability to lower body temperature
- **Suppression of platelet aggregation.** The ability to prevent and/or treat cardiovascular conditions such as acute myocardial infarction (MI) and stroke

Understanding the mechanism of action of aspirin is important because it explains both the therapeutic actions of the drug as well as its adverse effects. All NSAIDs act by inhibiting the synthesis of prostaglandins. **Prostaglandins** are local hormones found in virtually every tissue that have many diverse functions depending on

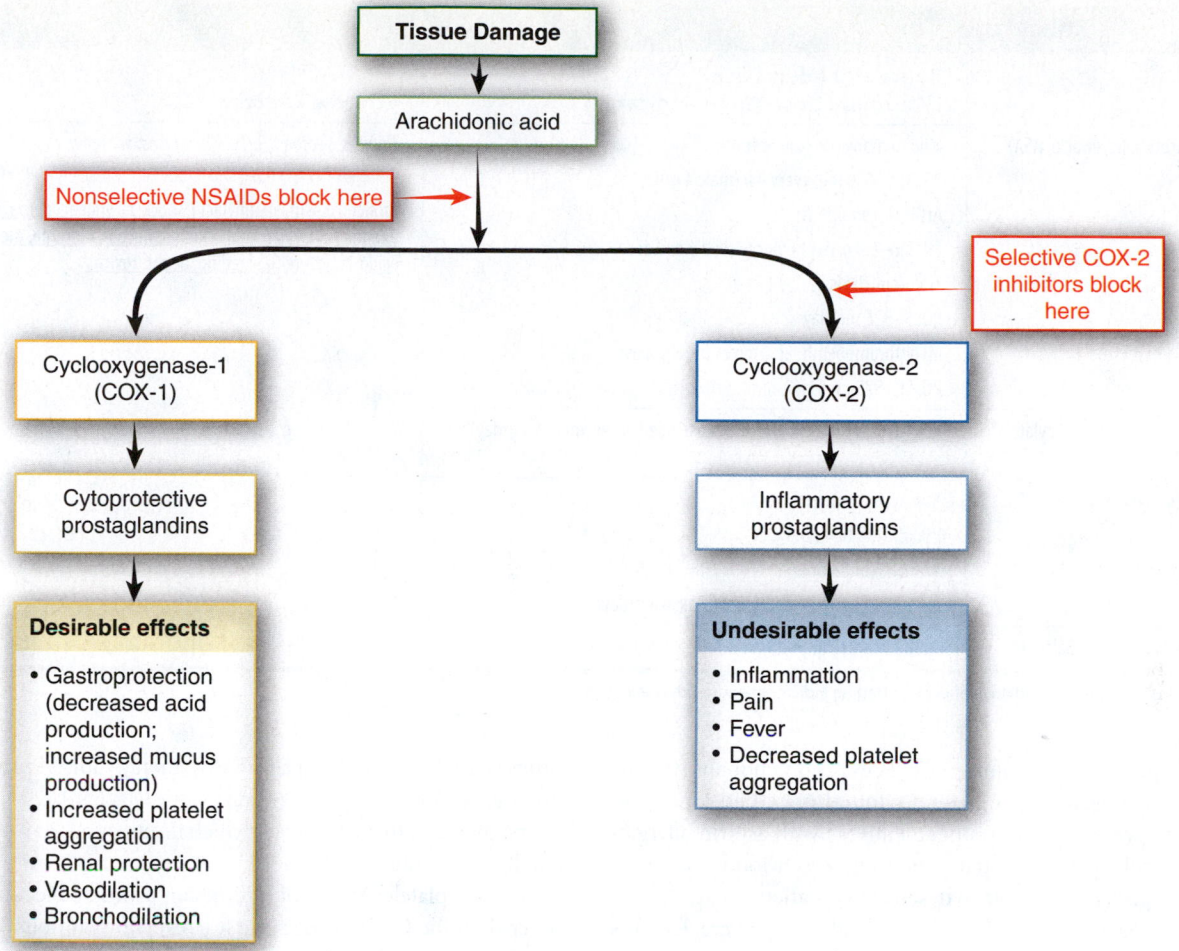

Figure 41.1 Inhibition of cyclooxygenase 1 and 2. Nonselective NSAIDs block the cytoprotective effects as well as inflammation. Selective COX-2 inhibitors block only the inflammation effects.

their location. Several prostaglandins are available as drugs, including carboprost (Hemabate, prostaglandin F_2 alpha), dinoprostone (Cervidil, prostaglandin E_2), and misoprostol (Cytotec prostaglandin E_1). The physiological properties of prostaglandins include the following:

- **Mediation of inflammation.** Cause vasodilation, increase capillary permeability, and cause pain

- **GI protection.** Increase bicarbonate and mucus production to protect the stomach mucosa from acid

- **Renal protection.** Help maintain blood flow through the kidneys

- **Smooth muscle.** Help regulate smooth muscle tone in blood vessels; increase smooth muscle tone in the uterus; may cause bronchodilation or bronchoconstriction

- **Blood clotting.** Increase platelet aggregation to promote clot formation

Aspirin blocks the synthesis of prostaglandins by inhibiting the enzyme **cyclooxygenase (COX)**. Aspirin and the ibuprofen-like NSAIDs block both forms of the enzyme, known as COX-1 and COX-2, by changing their structures and preventing the formation of prostaglandins. This inhibition of COX is responsible for their therapeutic and adverse effects, depending on the location and function of the prostaglandin that is being blocked. For example,

the inhibition of COX in peripheral tissues will reduce the pain and inflammation caused by prostaglandins. The inhibition of COX in the stomach, however, will remove the protective effect of prostaglandins and result in damage to the gastrointestinal (GI) mucosa. The mechanism by which aspirin produces its effects is illustrated in Figure 41.1.

The inhibition of the COX enzyme in platelets is especially prolonged and may last for the entire 8- to 11-day lifespan of the platelet. This antithrombotic action inhibits platelet aggregation and reduces the risk of adverse cardiovascular events, including MI and stroke. The antipyretic effect of aspirin results from a suppression of prostaglandin synthesis in the hypothalamus of the brain. It lowers temperature by indirectly causing centrally mediated peripheral vasodilation and sweating. The principal analgesic effect of aspirin occurs in the peripheral areas of the body and in the central nervous system (CNS). Doses for aspirin and the other salicylates are listed in Table 41.1.

Aspirin is sometimes combined with prescription and over-the-counter (OTC) medications, and its presence is not always obvious unless the label is carefully inspected. This is especially important for patients with aspirin allergy, which is present in about 1% of the population. Patients with asthma or food allergies are most likely to be allergic to aspirin. Aspirin allergy symptoms include rash, urticaria, dyspnea, wheezing, rhinorrhea, and cough. To prevent aspirin allergy, the patient should be instructed to read labels carefully

TABLE 41.1 Salicylates

Drug	Route and Adult Dose (Maximum Dose Where Indicated)	Adverse Effects
aspirin (acetylsalicylic acid, ASA)	Mild to moderate pain or fever: PO: 350–650 mg, every 4 h (max: 4 g/day) Arthritic conditions: PO: 3.6–5.4 g/day in four to six divided doses TIA prophylaxis: PO: 5–325 mg/day MI or thromboembolic disorder prophylaxis: PO: 80–325 mg/day	*Tinnitus, deafness, urticaria, nausea, vomiting, confusion, drowsiness, prolonged bleeding time, dyspepsia, stomach pain* <u>Bronchospasm, anaphylactic shock, laryngeal edema, hemolytic anemia, salicylism, angioedema, Reye's syndrome, metabolic acidosis, severe GI bleeding, hepatotoxicity</u>
choline magnesium trisalicylate (Trilisate)	PO: 1.0–2.5 g/day in one to three divided doses (max: 4.5 g/day)	
magnesium salicylate (Doan's Pills)	Analgesic/antipyretic: PO: 650 mg tid or qid Arthritic conditions: PO: 9.6 g/day in divided doses (max: 4.8 g/day)	
salsalate (Mono-gesic, Salsitab)	PO: 325–3,000 mg/day in divided doses (max: 4 g/day)	

Note: Italics indicate common adverse effects. <u>Underline</u> indicates serious adverse effects.

and avoid products containing salicylates. This is not always possible because salicylates are naturally found in certain foods and are used as preservatives in others. Patients with aspirin allergies should consult with a dietitian regarding which food sources to avoid. Allergists may be able to desensitize a patient if exposure to the drug is unavoidable or if the patient's allergy is severe. Patients who are hypersensitive to aspirin will likely be sensitive to other NSAIDs. For pain or fever relief, acetaminophen may be safely used in these patients.

The most significant adverse effect of aspirin and other NSAIDs is GI bleeding, which is shown in Pharmacotherapy Illustrated 41.1. Although the risk is dose related, even low doses of aspirin (75–325 mg/day) may double the risk of GI bleeding. Risk factors for aspirin-induced GI bleeding include history of peptic ulcers, age greater than 60, use of anticoagulants or corticosteroids, *Helicobacter pylori* infection, smoking, and use of alcohol. Aspirin has the following adverse effects on the GI mucosa:

- As aspirin is absorbed across the stomach mucosa, it causes direct cellular injury. This topical damage to the stomach may be lessened by the use of enteric-coated formulations.

- After aspirin is absorbed systemically, it inhibits COX-1 and depletes the GI mucosa of prostaglandins. Prostaglandins normally provide a protective function in the GI mucosa by directing the secretion of mucus and bicarbonate and promoting cellular repair of mucosal damage.

- If GI damage or active ulcers are already present, the antiplatelet effects of aspirin will prolong bleeding.

In addition to GI bleeding, aspirin can cause dyspepsia, nausea, and ulcer perforation. For patients who must take high doses of aspirin, proton pump inhibitors (PPIs), such as omeprazole, may provide some degree of protection against GI damage by reducing acid secretion in the stomach. PPIs are effective and relatively safe

drugs (see Chapter 59). An alternative therapy for GI protection is oral misoprostol (Cytotec), which is a prostaglandin. Misoprostol is a pregnancy category X drug, which limits its use in women with childbearing potential.

The antiplatelet effects of aspirin can promote bleeding at sites other than the GI tract. Because it irreversibly inhibits COX-1 in platelets, the antiplatelet action of aspirin can be prolonged. It may take longer for minor cuts and injuries to stop bleeding. Patients undergoing surgical or dental procedures should discontinue aspirin use a week prior to the procedure. Patients with known bleeding disorders should not take aspirin at all.

Children under age 19 should never be administered products that contain aspirin when they have flu symptoms, fever, or chickenpox due to the risk of Reye's syndrome, a potentially fatal disease. It is unclear how aspirin contributes to Reye's syndrome, because the condition can appear without aspirin use. The incidence of Reye's syndrome is now very rare due to public awareness of the risk associated with aspirin use.

PharmFACT

More than 20,000 salicylate poisonings occur each year of which about 50% are intentional overdoses. Approximately 60 deaths from acute salicylate overdose occur each year (Waseem, 2013).

PROTOTYPE DRUG	Aspirin (Acetylsalicylic Acid)

Classification: Therapeutic: Nonnarcotic analgesic, antipyretic, antiplatelet
Pharmacologic: Salicylate, NSAID

Therapeutic Effects and Uses: Approved by the U.S. Food and Drug Administration (FDA) in 1939, aspirin is one of the best known medications. The ability of aspirin to reduce pain, inflammation, and fever makes it an extremely versatile and widely

PHARMACOTHERAPY ILLUSTRATED 41.1

NSAID-INDUCED ULCER FORMATION

(a)

COX converts arachidonic acid to prostaglandins (○).
- Less acid
- More mucus protection

Digestive Acids

Mucosa

Submucosa

Muscularia

(b)

NSAIDs (▲) inhibit COX and prevent prostaglandin formation.
- More acid/less mucus
- Direct irritation of mucosa

Digestive Acids

Mucosa

Submucosa

Muscularia

used drug. It is used to reduce pain and inflammation that is mild to moderate in intensity. The doses of aspirin needed to control severe pain or inflammation often result in a high incidence of adverse effects.

Aspirin is approved by the FDA for the prevention of thromboembolic events. Aspirin is a first-line treatment for stroke prophylaxis in patients with a history of transient ischemic attacks (TIAs) or who have persistent or paroxysmal atrial fibrillation. It is approved for MI prophylaxis in patients who are at risk for a cardiac event and who are not already taking warfarin or an antiplatelet drug, including those with coronary artery disease who have already experienced an MI. To lower the risk of thromboembolic events, emergency medical services professionals administer aspirin to patients with a suspected coronary thrombosis prior to hospital arrival. Patients with a high risk for arterial thromboembolism may receive low-dose aspirin therapy.

An off-label use of aspirin is to prevent colorectal cancer. Regular, long-term aspirin use has been determined to reduce the risk of colorectal cancer (Rothwell et al., 2010). In some studies, high doses of aspirin were administered and it is unclear whether the reduction in the incidence of colorectal cancer from the drug is worth the increased risk of GI bleeding. The effectiveness of aspirin in preventing cancer is an area of active research.

Mechanism of Action: The anti-inflammatory action of aspirin is caused by the inhibition of COX-1 and COX-2 that leads to reduced prostaglandin synthesis. The analgesic action of aspirin occurs peripherally with limited action in the CNS on the hypothalamus. The suppression of prostaglandin synthesis in or near the hypothalamus results in the lowering of body temperature. Aspirin acts indirectly, causing centrally mediated peripheral vasodilation and sweating.

Pharmacokinetics:

Route(s)	Oral (PO), rectal
Absorption	80–100% absorbed
Distribution	Widely distributed; crosses the placenta; secreted in breast milk; 80–90% bound to plasma protein
Primary metabolism	Hepatic; metabolized to salicylic acid, an active metabolite, in the GI mucosa, plasma, and erythrocytes
Primary excretion	Renal
Onset of action	PO: 5–30 min; rectal: 1–2 h
Duration of action	PO: 1–4 h; rectal: 7 h

Adverse Effects: A major adverse effect of aspirin is the risk of a serious hypersensitivity reaction, which is noted with symptoms such as bronchospasm, laryngeal edema, and anaphylaxis. It also causes significant stomach irritation, heartburn, nausea, vomiting, diarrhea, and stomach pain in 10% to 30% of patients. The risk of GI bleeding increases with dose. The hematologic adverse effects of aspirin administration include thrombocytopenia, hemolytic anemia, and occult bleeding. Long-term administration of aspirin may produce nephrotoxic effects and hepatotoxicity. Tinnitus and hearing loss are common adverse effects with high doses.

Contraindications/Precautions: Patients who have a hypersensitivity to any salicylate (including that found in foods) should not be administered aspirin or other NSAIDs. Patients who have the "aspirin triad," which includes aspirin allergy, nasal polyps, and asthma, should not be administered aspirin. Aspirin is also contraindicated in chronic rhinitis, acute bronchospasm, agranulocytosis, head trauma, increased intracranial pressure, history of GI bleeding, hypoprothrombinemia, vitamin K deficiency, heart failure (HF), pregnancy, and lactation. Children and teenagers should not be administered aspirin or products containing aspirin if they have a fever or a flulike illness. Patients over age 60 are especially prone to GI ulceration and bleeding due to aspirin. It should be used cautiously in patients with hypothyroidism, immunosuppression, asthma, and gout. It should also be used cautiously in patients with renal and hepatic impairment, G6PD deficiency, anemia, preoperatively, and in the presence of Hodgkin's disease. Aspirin should not be taken during pregnancy, especially in the third trimester; it may prolong bleeding and inhibit natural contractions caused by prostaglandins in the uterus.

Drug Interactions: Concurrent administration of aspirin with other salicylates such as 5-aminosalicylic acid increases the risk of salicylate toxicity. The combined use of aspirin with acetaminophen may cause additive nephrotoxicity. Ammonium chloride and other acidifying agents decrease the renal elimination of aspirin, resulting in salicylate toxicity. The administration of aspirin with anticoagulants, thrombolytics, or antiplatelet agents increases the patient's risk for bleeding. When oral antidiabetic agents are administered concurrently with high doses of aspirin, hypoglycemic activity increases. Patients who consume three or more alcoholic drinks per day may experience additive GI ulceration. Corticosteroids increase the risk of gastric irritation and result in ulcerogenic effects when administered with aspirin. Methotrexate administered with aspirin results in methotrexate toxicity. Low doses of salicylates may antagonize the uricosuric effects of probenecid and sulfinpyrazone. The antihypertensive effects of beta blockers may decrease if administered concurrently

with aspirin. **Herbal/Food**: The administration of feverfew, garlic, ginger, horse chestnut, and red clover will increase the patient's risk for bleeding. Taking aspirin with caffeine will increase the rate of aspirin absorption. St. John's wort may increase sedation.

Pregnancy: Categories C (first and second trimester) and D (third trimester).

Treatment of Overdose: Acute or chronic overdose of aspirin is known as **salicylism**, which is defined as a serum salicylate level above 200 mcg/mL. The symptoms depend on the dose but include tinnitus, metabolic acidosis, hyperventilation, respiratory alkalosis (secondary to stimulation of the respiratory center), dehydration, agitation, CNS depression, nausea, and vomiting. Emesis, gastric lavage, and alkalinization of urine are indicated. Hemodialysis is of benefit in severe salicylate poisonings.

Nursing Responsibilities: Key nursing implications for patients receiving aspirin are included in the Nursing Practice Application for Patients Receiving Pharmacotherapy for Inflammation and Fever.

Drugs Similar to Aspirin (Acetylsalicylic Acid)

Agents that produce similar actions to aspirin include choline magnesium trisalicylate, magnesium salicylate, and salsalate.

Choline magnesium trisalicylate (Trilisate): Approved in 1938, this drug combines choline salicylate and magnesium salicylate. It is an oral drug approved for fever and mild to moderate pain and inflammation associated with osteoarthritis, RA, bursitis, and other muscle or joint conditions. This drug causes less GI irritation than aspirin, and it exhibits less antiplatelet activity. Choline magnesium trisalicylate should not be administered to patients with known hypersensitivity to other salicylates. Other contraindications and adverse effects are similar to those of aspirin. This drug is pregnancy category C; D if used for prolonged periods or near term.

Magnesium salicylate (Doan's Pills): Approved in 1938, magnesium salicylate is an oral drug approved for fever and mild to moderate pain and inflammation associated with osteoarthritis, RA, bursitis, and other muscle or joint conditions. It inhibits prostaglandin synthesis just as aspirin, but it is less potent, causes less GI irritation, and has less effect on platelet aggregation than aspirin. Magnesium salicylate should not be administered to patients with known hypersensitivity to other salicylates. Other contraindications and adverse effects are similar to those of aspirin. This drug is pregnancy category C for the first and second trimesters and D for the third trimester.

Salsalate (Mono-gesic, Salsitab): Approved in 1977, salsalate has analgesic properties similar to those of aspirin but it causes less gastric irritation. It is an oral drug approved to treat mild and moderate pain due to osteoarthritis and RA. Like other salicylates, salsalate produces its effects by inhibiting prostaglandin synthesis. It has little antipyretic activity and has less effect on platelet aggregation than aspirin. Salsalate

CONNECTION Checkpoint 41.1

Aspirin is classified as an antiplatelet drug in Chapter 38. Name the other two classes of drugs that are antiplatelet agents and state the prototype drug for each class. *See Answer to Connection Checkpoint 41.1 on student resource website.*

should not be administered to patients with known hypersensitivity to other salicylates. Other contraindications and adverse effects are similar to those of aspirin. This drug is pregnancy category C.

Ibuprofen-Like Drugs

41.4 Ibuprofen and similar nonsteroidal anti-inflammatory drugs are the most common drugs for treating mild to moderate pain and inflammation.

In the 1950s researchers began searching for safer alternatives to aspirin or corticosteroids for treating the severe inflammation of RA. An exhaustive search of over 600 potential compounds over a 15-year period resulted in the discovery of ibuprofen, one of the safest and most widely prescribed NSAIDs in the world. The drug was introduced in the United States in 1974, and it became one of the first prescription-only drugs to be changed to OTC status in 1984.

Since the discovery of ibuprofen, over 20 other nonaspirin NSAIDs have been approved by the FDA. Although their chemical structures vary, they are grouped as "ibuprofen-like" because they share very similar actions and adverse effects with the original drug. Doses for the NSAIDs are listed in Table 41.2. When used at recommended doses, NSAIDs have the following similarities:

- All have the same mechanism of action: They inhibit both COX-1 and COX-2.
- All have analgesic properties: They are widely prescribed to treat patients with mild to moderate pain.
- All have anti-inflammatory properties: Most are specifically approved for osteoarthritis and RA.
- All have antipyretic properties, although not all of them are approved for this indication.
- Most are weak acids that are readily absorbed in the GI tract.
- Most are strongly bound to albumin in the blood.
- Most are metabolized in the liver to inactive metabolites, which are excreted by the kidneys.
- All have the ability to damage the GI mucosa, including bleeding and ulcer formation.
- Many pose an increased risk of cardiac events, such as heart failure and MI.
- Many are nephrotoxic at high doses.

From the preceding list, it should be obvious that the available nonaspirin NSAIDs share many properties. There are, however, some differences in pharmacokinetic profiles. For example, some have longer half-lives or are available in sustained release formulations that permit once-daily dosing. Some are available by the parenteral route, and a few are formulated for children. Some are enteric coated, which may reduce stomach pain but does not appear to be protective against the formation of ulcers. Another consideration that is important to many consumers is cost. A month's supply of generic ibuprofen 200 mg or naproxen 220 mg costs less than $25 and is available OTC. At the opposite extreme are prescription-only celecoxib (Celebrex) 200 mg and flurbiprofen (Ansaid) 100 mg, which cost $150 to $240 for a monthly supply. Indications for each of the NSAIDs are listed in Table 41.3.

There are important differences between aspirin and the ibuprofen-like agents in their effects on the blood and heart. Although ibuprofen-like drugs affect blood coagulation, their action is short lived and they are relatively safe to use with anticoagulants. Because they have less antiplatelet effect, the ibuprofen-like agents are not used for the prophylaxis of adverse cardiovascular events. In fact, some of the nonaspirin NSAIDs such as indomethacin and sulindac significantly increase the risk of cardiovascular events. Caution should be used with all the nonaspirin NSAIDs when they are given for prolonged periods to patients with a history of cardiac disease.

NSAIDs are considered equivalent to aspirin in their effectiveness for treating pain, inflammation, and fever. For the occasional user who takes the medications at recommended doses and who has no risk factors, the drugs are very safe and rarely produce any significant adverse effects. For patients who must take high doses for a chronic illness, ibuprofen appears to cause less GI bleeding than aspirin, although both drugs place patients at high risk for GI adverse effects.

PROTOTYPE DRUG	**Ibuprofen (Advil, Motrin, Others)**

Classification: **Therapeutic:** Analgesic, anti-inflammatory drug, antipyretic
Pharmacologic: NSAID

Therapeutic Effects and Uses: Approved in 1974, ibuprofen was the first nonaspirin NSAID marketed in the United States. Like aspirin, it possesses analgesic, anti-inflammatory, and antipyretic properties. It is indicated for the relief of fever and mild to moderate pain associated with chronic symptomatic RA and osteoarthritis, myalgia, headache, dental pain, and dysmenorrhea. Chewable tablets, drops, and solutions are available in low doses for administration to children.

Unlike aspirin, ibuprofen is not indicated to treat or prevent any cardiovascular conditions. Ibuprofen inhibits platelet aggregation and prolongs the bleeding time without affecting the prothrombin time (PT) or whole-blood clotting times. Its effects on platelets are reversible within 24 hours after discontinuation of the drug.

Ibuprofen lysine (NeoProfen) is an intravenous (IV) form of the drug that was approved in 2006 to close patent ductus arteriosus in premature infants. The drug has a 75% success rate in infants who are no more than 32 weeks gestational age. Although the mechanism of action is not known, it is believed that prostaglandins delay closing of the ductus. By blocking prostaglandin synthesis with ibuprofen, the ductus closes.

Mechanism of Action: Ibuprofen inhibits COX-1 and COX-2, which block prostaglandin synthesis and modulate T-cell function. Ibuprofen inhibits inflammatory cell chemotaxis, decreases the release of superoxide radicals, and increases the scavenging of these products at the inflammatory sites.

Pharmacokinetics:

Route(s)	PO
Absorption	80% absorbed
Distribution	Crosses the placenta; unknown if secreted in breast milk; highly protein bound
Primary metabolism	Hepatic
Primary excretion	Renal; small amount biliary
Onset of action	1 h
Duration of action	6–8 h

TABLE 41.2   Nonaspirin NSAIDs and Acetaminophen

Drug	Route and Adult Dose (Maximum Dose Where Indicated)	Adverse Effects
acetaminophen (Tylenol, Others)	PO: 325–650 mg every 4–6 h (max: 4 g/day for all products containing this drug) Rectal: 650 mg every 4–6 h	*Epigastric pain, abdominal pain* <u>Hepatotoxicity, acute renal failure, GI bleeding</u>
celecoxib (Celebrex)	PO: 100–200 mg bid (max: 800 mg/day)	*Back pain, peripheral edema, abdominal pain, dyspepsia, flatulence, dizziness, headache, insomnia, HTN* <u>Increased risk of cardiovascular events, acute renal failure</u>
diclofenac (Cataflam, Voltaren, Others)	RA and osteoarthritis: PO: 150–200 mg/day in three to four divided doses Ankylosing spondylitis: PO: 25–50 mg qid	*Dyspepsia, dizziness, headache, drowsiness, tinnitus, rash, pruritus, increased liver enzymes, prolonged bleeding time, edema, nausea, vomiting, occult blood loss* <u>Peptic ulcer, GI bleeding, anaphylactic reactions with bronchospasm, blood dyscrasias, renal impairment, MI, HF, hepatotoxicity</u>
diflunisal	PO: 250–500 mg bid (max: 1,500 mg/day)	
etodolac	PO: 200–1,200 mg/day in two to four divided doses (max: 1,200 mg)	
fenoprofen (Nalfon)	PO: 200–600 mg tid or qid (max: 3,200 mg/day)	
flurbiprofen	PO: 200–300 mg in two to four divided doses (max: 300 mg/day and 100 mg/dose)	
ibuprofen (Advil, Motrin, Others)	Inflammatory disease: PO: 400–800 mg tid or qid (max: 3,200 mg/day) Pain, fever, dysmenorrhea: PO: 200–400 mg every 4–6 h (max: 1,200 mg/day)	
indomethacin (Indocin)	PO: 25–50 mg bid or tid (max: 200 mg/day and 100 mg/dose)	
ketoprofen	PO: 25–75 mg tid or qid (max: 300 mg/day) PO: 200 mg extended release once daily	
ketorolac (Acular, Sprix, Toradol)	IM/IV: 30–60 mg loading dose, then 15–30 mg qid (max: 150 mg/day then 120 mg for subsequent days) PO: 10 mg qid prn (max: 40 mg/day) Intranasal: one spray (15.75 mg) in each nostril every 4–6 h (max: 126 mg)	
meclofenamate	PO: 100–400 mg/day in three to four divided doses (max: 400 mg/day)	
mefenamic acid (Ponstel)	PO: 500-mg loading dose followed by 250-mg maintenance dose qid (max: 1,250 mg/day for no longer than 7 days)	
meloxicam (Mobic)	PO: 7.5–15 mg once daily (max: 15 mg/day)	
nabumetone (Relafen)	PO: 1,000 mg daily as a single dose (max: 2,000 mg/day)	
naproxen (Naprosyn) and naproxen sodium (Aleve, Anaprox, Others)	PO: 250–500 mg bid (naproxen/naproxen controlled release max: 1,500 mg/day; naproxen sodium max: 1,650 mg/day; nonprescription max: 660 mg/day)	
oxaprozin (Daypro)	PO: 600–1,200 mg daily (max: 1,800 mg/day or 26 mg/kg, whichever is lower)	
piroxicam (Feldene)	PO: 20 mg once daily (max: 20 mg/day)	
sulindac (Clinoril)	PO: 150–200 mg bid (max: 400 mg/day)	
tolmetin (Tolectin)	PO: 400 mg tid initially then maintenance dose of 600–1,800 mg/day in three to four divided doses (max: 1,800 mg/day)	

Note: Italics indicate common adverse effects. <u>Underline</u> indicates serious adverse effects.

Adverse Effects: In low to moderate doses, ibuprofen is well tolerated and serious adverse effects are uncommon. The most frequent adverse events are GI related and include bleeding, anorexia, heartburn, nausea, vomiting, and constipation or diarrhea. Adverse CNS effects include dizziness, headache, drowsiness, and lightheadedness. Other possible adverse effects include hypotension, HF, peripheral edema, occult blood loss, aplastic anemia, leukopenia, decreased hemoglobin and hematocrit, and increased aspartate transaminase (AST) and alanine transaminase (ALT). Chronic use of ibuprofen may lead to renal impairment, including acute renal failure, polyuria, azotemia, cystitis, hematuria, and increased creatinine and blood urea nitrogen (BUN) levels. **Black Box Warnings**: Ibuprofen may increase the risk of serious and potentially fatal cardiovascular thrombotic events, MI, and stroke. This risk may increase with duration of use and in patients with cardiovascular risk factors. Ibuprofen also increases the risk of

TABLE 41.3 Indications for Selected Nonsteroidal Anti-Inflammatory Drugs

NSAID	Arthritis	Mild to Moderate Pain	Fever	Dysmenorrhea	Other Approved Indications
celecoxib (Celebrex)	A	A		A	Ankylosing spondylitis; familial adenomatous polyposis
diclofenac (Cataflam, Voltaren, Others)	A	A		A	Ankylosing spondylitis; actinic keratosis (topical); ocular pain and inflammation (ophthalmic)
diflunisal	A	A			
etodolac	A	A			
fenoprofen (Nalfon)	A	A			
flurbiprofen	A				Miosis inhibition (ophthalmic)
ibuprofen (Advil, Motrin, Others)	A	A	A	A	Acute migraine
indomethacin (Indocin)	A	A			Ankylosing spondylitis; close patent ductus arteriosus (IV)
ketoprofen	A	A	A	A	
ketorolac (Acular, Sprix, Toradol)		A			Allergic conjunctivitis; reduce ocular pain and inflammation (ophthalmic)
meclofenamate	A	A		A	
mefenamic acid (Ponstel)		A		A	
meloxicam (Mobic)	A				
nabumetone (Relafen)	A				
naproxen/naproxen sodium (Aleve, Anaprox, Naprosyn, Others)	A	A	A	A	Ankylosing spondylitis
oxaprozin (Daypro)	A				
piroxicam (Feldene)	A				
sulindac (Clinoril)	A				Ankylosing spondylitis; acute painful shoulder
tolmetin (Tolectin)	A				

A = FDA approved.

serious GI adverse effects including bleeding, ulcer, and stomach or intestine perforation. These GI events may occur at any time during use and without prior warning. Older adults are at greater risk for serious GI events.

Contraindications/Precautions: Patients who have a known allergy to aspirin or other NSAIDs should not be administered ibuprofen. In addition, patients who have been diagnosed with PUD, bleeding abnormalities, and perioperative pain related to coronary artery bypass graft (CABG) should not receive ibuprofen. The drug should be used cautiously in patients with hypertension (HTN), history of GI bleeding, diabetes mellitus, and impaired renal or hepatic function. It should also be used cautiously in patients who have heart failure, serious HTN, or a history of stroke or MI. Children with asthma may experience diminished respiratory function when administered ibuprofen. Patients with severe hepatic impairment should not receive ibuprofen because the drug can accumulate to toxic levels.

Drug Interactions: Oral anticoagulants and antiplatelet drugs taken with ibuprofen increase the risk of bleeding. Ibuprofen may increase the toxicity of digoxin, lithium, or methotrexate if taken concurrently. Use with other NSAIDs, alcohol, or corticosteroids may cause serious adverse GI events. The antihypertensive action of diuretics, beta blockers, and angiotensin-converting enzyme (ACE) inhibitors may be reduced if taken with ibuprofen. **Herbal/Food**: Ibuprofen combined with feverfew, garlic, ginger, and ginkgo may result in an increased risk of bleeding.

Pregnancy: Categories B (first and second trimesters) and D (third trimester).

Treatment of Overdose: Overdose may lead to acute renal failure, apnea, cyanosis, drowsiness, GI bleeding, nausea, vomiting, and sweating. Treatment is supportive and includes the administration of activated charcoal and nasogastric suction.

Nursing Responsibilities: Key nursing implications for patients receiving ibuprofen are included in the Nursing Practice Application for Patients Receiving Pharmacotherapy for Inflammation and Fever.

Drugs Similar to Ibuprofen (Advil, Motrin, Others)

There are a number of subclasses of NSAIDs that are based on the chemical structures of the molecules. These subclasses include the propionic acids (e.g., ibuprofen), phenylacetic acids (e.g., diclofenac),

CONNECTIONS Evidence-Based Practice

◀ Treating Fevers with Ibuprofen, Acetaminophen, or Both

Clinical Question
When treating children with fevers, which is more effective: ibuprofen, acetaminophen, or both?

Evidence
Recent research suggests that alternating doses of ibuprofen and acetaminophen may provide better fever control than either drug alone. Paul et al. (2010) determined that when given either ibuprofen or acetaminophen for fever, both groups had reductions in temperature. Children receiving alternating or combined doses of ibuprofen and acetaminophen had significantly lower temperature readings than after using either ibuprofen or acetaminophen alone. Two other studies found both drugs to be effective in fever relief but that ibuprofen was slightly more effective than acetaminophen (Pierce & Voss, 2010; Wong et al., 2013).

Implications
For most children with fevers, alternating doses of acetaminophen and ibuprofen, or combining the two drugs, may provide enhanced fever relief, and control may be longer lasting than using either drug alone. Sullivan and Farrar (2011) supported the combination or alternating ibuprofen and acetaminophen. However, they raised a concern that combined treatment may be more complicated for parents to follow and could contribute to unsafe use of the drugs. Because the amount of each drug may vary, nurses must ensure that parents are appropriately measuring the correct dose of each drug and that adequate intervals are spaced between doses. This is particularly important if liquid preparations are used. Instructions on avoiding OTC cough and cold remedies, which often include acetaminophen, should also be included.

Critical Thinking Questions
How should a nurse respond to a parent's questioning about which drug is best to use for his or her child's fever: ibuprofen or acetaminophen?

See Answers to Critical Thinking Questions on student resource website.

indole acetic acids (e.g., indomethacin), fenamates (e.g., mefenamic acid), ketones (e.g., nabumetone), and oxicams (e.g., piroxicam). From a clinical perspective, the nonaspirin NSAIDs are remarkably similar to ibuprofen. Doses and indications for these drugs differ, as listed in Tables 41.2 and 41.3.

PharmFACT

It is estimated that NSAID use is associated with about 100,000 hospitalizations and 16,000 deaths annually in the United States, largely as a result of GI complications (Wiegand, 2012).

Cyclooxygenase-2 Inhibitors

41.5 Celecoxib is an effective second-generation nonsteroidal anti-inflammatory drug, but its use is limited due to an increased risk of myocardial infarction and stroke.

Celecoxib (Celebrex) is a second-generation NSAID that blocks COX-2 without inhibiting COX-1. The selective inhibition of COX-2 produces the analgesic, anti-inflammatory, and antipyretic effects typical of other NSAIDs, but without causing platelet aggregation or GI irritation. The primary advantage of celecoxib is that it causes less GI bleeding and ulcer formation than aspirin or ibuprofen. This medication is the newest and most controversial of the NSAIDs.

The ability to treat arthritis without adverse effects caused excitement throughout the medical field in the 1990s, and the three drugs originally in this class were widely prescribed. This elation quickly ended when postmarketing data revealed that rofecoxib (Vioxx) doubled the risk of MI and strokes in patients taking the drug for extended periods. At that time, more than 84 million people had used rofecoxib since its approval in 1999. Based on the research data, the drug manufacturer voluntarily removed rofecoxib from the market. Shortly afterward a second COX-2 inhibitor, valdecoxib (Bextra), was also voluntarily withdrawn, leaving celecoxib (Celebrex) the sole drug in this class. A large number of lawsuits were subsequently filed, and the marketing of new COX-2 inhibitors has ground to a halt in the United States. Other COX-2 inhibitors are still available outside the United States.

PROTOTYPE DRUG **Celecoxib (Celebrex)**

Classification: **Therapeutic:** Anti-inflammatory
Pharmacologic: COX-2 inhibitor, NSAID

Therapeutic Effects and Uses: Celecoxib is approved to treat mild to moderate pain and inflammation associated with RA, osteoarthritis, dysmenorrhea, dental procedures, headache, and ankylosing spondylitis. It is also an effective antipyretic agent. The effectiveness of celecoxib at reducing pain and inflammation is equivalent to that of other NSAIDs.

In addition to its anti-inflammatory indications, celecoxib also is used for the prophylaxis of adenomas or colorectal polyps in adults with familial adenomatous polyposis (FAP). Patients with this condition have an inherited mutation in a gene that results in hundreds of polyps and an almost 100% risk of colon cancer. Although celecoxib reduces the number of polyps in these patients, it has not been proven to reduce the risk of malignancies.

Mechanism of Action: Celecoxib selectively inhibits the enzyme COX-2. It inhibits prostaglandin synthesis to reduce inflammation. This action relieves pain and inflammation in the joints and smooth muscle tissue.

Pharmacokinetics:

Route(s)	PO
Absorption	Well absorbed
Distribution	Widely distributed; is likely secreted in breast milk; 97% protein bound
Primary metabolism	Hepatic by CYP2C9

Primary excretion	Primarily feces (57%), with some in urine (27%)
Onset of action	Peak: 3 h
Duration of action	Half-life: 11.2 h

Adverse Effects: The COX-2 inhibitors have been found to increase the risk of serious cardiovascular events, including fatal MI and stroke. Celecoxib produces the same GI-related adverse effects as other NSAIDs but at a lower rate. GI adverse effects include GI bleeding, ulcers, abdominal pain, diarrhea, dyspepsia, flatulence, and nausea. CNS adverse effects include headache, dizziness, and insomnia. Cardiovascular adverse effects include HTN, MI, and peripheral edema. Adverse effects of the integumentary system are generally rare and include erythema multiforme, exfoliative dermatitis, rash, Stevens–Johnson syndrome, and toxic epidermal necrolysis. Some patients have reported pharyngitis, rhinitis, sinusitis, and upper respiratory infection. The long-term use of celecoxib may cause renal and hepatic impairment.

Contraindications/Precautions: Celecoxib should not be administered to patients with hepatic insufficiency because the primary site of drug metabolism is the liver. It is also contraindicated in patients with advanced renal disease. Celecoxib is contraindicated in patients with anemia or in the postoperative phase of a CABG. Celecoxib is administered cautiously in patients who are poor CYP2C9 metabolizers. This drug is contraindicated in patients with a history of GI bleeding or PUD, and it should be administered with caution to patients receiving anticoagulants. Patients with a history of asthma, bone marrow suppression, stroke, peripheral vascular disease, elevated liver function tests, heart failure, kidney disease, and fluid retention should be administered celecoxib cautiously.

Drug Interactions: If taken with celecoxib, oral coagulation modifiers such as clopidogrel or warfarin may cause an increased risk of bleeding. Celecoxib may increase the toxicity of lithium if taken concurrently. Use with alcohol, corticosteroids, aspirin, or other NSAIDs may cause serious adverse GI events. The antihypertensive action of diuretics or ACE inhibitors may be reduced if taken with celecoxib. Concurrent use with fluconazole may increase serum celecoxib levels. **Herbal/Food:** Feverfew, garlic, ginger, ginkgo, horse chestnut, and red clover may increase the risk of bleeding if used during celecoxib therapy.

Pregnancy: Category C; category D in the third trimester.

Treatment of Overdose: Overdose may cause acute renal failure, apnea, cyanosis, drowsiness, GI bleeding, nausea, vomiting, and sweating. Treatment is supportive and includes the administration of activated charcoal and nasogastric suction.

Nursing Responsibilities: Key nursing implications for patients receiving celecoxib are included in the Nursing Practice Application for Patients Receiving Pharmacotherapy for Inflammation and Fever.

CONNECTION Checkpoint 41.2

Several NSAIDs are approved to treat mild migraines. From what you learned in Chapter 25, what non-NSAID drug classes are used to terminate severe migraine episodes? *See Answer to Connection Checkpoint 41.2 on student resource website.*

Drugs Similar to Celecoxib (Celebrex)

Celecoxib (Celebrex) is the sole medication in this class.

Antipyretic and Analgesic Drugs

41.6 Acetaminophen is administered for pain relief and to reduce fever, but it has no anti-inflammatory properties.

Acetaminophen (Tylenol) is administered for pain relief and to reduce fever. Unlike aspirin, ibuprofen, and celecoxib, acetaminophen has no anti-inflammatory properties, and therefore is not classified as an NSAID. Acetaminophen has equal effectiveness to the NSAIDs in reducing pain and fever, and it is often a preferred drug for treating noninflammatory pain. It is the primary alternative to NSAIDs when patients have a contraindication to taking aspirin or ibuprofen. Acetaminophen is frequently combined with other OTC drugs in treating severe flu symptoms. It is often combined with opioid analgesics; adding acetaminophen provides additive pain relief and allows for lower doses of the narcotic (see Chapter 25). In 2011, the FDA asked drug manufacturers to limit the strength of acetaminophen in prescription combination products to 325 mg per tablet, capsule, or dosing unit to lower the potential for acetaminophen-induced hepatotoxicity. All manufacturers have complied with this recommendation.

Acetaminophen has no effect on platelet aggregation and does not exhibit cardiotoxicity. Most importantly, it does not cause GI bleeding or ulcers, as do the NSAIDs.

| PROTOTYPE DRUG | Acetaminophen (Tylenol) |

Classification: Therapeutic: Nonopioid analgesic, antipyretic
Pharmacologic: Para-aminophenol derivative

Therapeutic Effects and Uses: Approved in 1950, acetaminophen relieves mild to moderate pain but has no effect on inflammation. Acetaminophen is approved to treat pain associated with osteoarthritis of the hip or knee, dysmenorrhea, dental procedures, headache, and myalgia. It is also an effective antipyretic agent. It is a preferred drug for reducing fever. Acetaminophen is administered as a substitute for aspirin when NSAIDs are contraindicated due to age, allergy, or gastric irritation. It is not linked with Reye's syndrome, as is aspirin; thus it is safe to administer to infants, children, and adolescents who have flulike symptoms or chickenpox.

Acetaminophen is available for the oral (suspension, tablets, chewable tablets, extended release tablets, and oral granules) or rectal route. Childhood and infant preparations are available.

Mechanism of Action: Acetaminophen acts centrally in the CNS by inhibiting COX. It has no effect on COX in peripheral tissues. It also may inhibit the chemical mediators of pain, but its mechanism is unclear. The reduction of fever occurs by its direct action on the heat-regulating center of the hypothalamus to produce peripheral vasodilation, sweating, and dissipation of heat.

CONNECTIONS ⟩ Treating the Diverse Patient

◀ Ethnic Differences in Acetaminophen Metabolism

Certain ethnic populations, including patients of Asian, African American, or Middle Eastern descent, may have higher rates of an enzyme deficiency that affects how they metabolize certain drugs. More than 200 million people worldwide are believed to have a hereditary deficiency of the enzyme glucose-6-phosphate dehydrogenase (G6PD). Patients with G6PD deficiency are at risk for developing hemolysis after ingesting certain drugs, including acetaminophen. In patients with the deficiency, therapeutic dosages of acetaminophen may cause hemolysis.

Because acetaminophen is one of the most common drugs used for fever, pain control, and in many OTC cough and cold medicines, and because patients may not know that they have the deficiency, health care providers should recommend that ethnically diverse patients exercise caution when using acetaminophen and report any signs or symptoms associated with anemia. Patients with known G6PD deficiency should avoid this drug. Patients receiving IV forms of acetaminophen should have frequent CBC laboratory monitoring.

Pharmacokinetics:

Route(s)	PO, rectal
Absorption	Rapid and complete absorption
Distribution	Distributed to all body fluids; crosses the placenta; secreted in breast milk; 25% bound to plasma protein
Primary metabolism	Hepatic
Primary excretion	Renal
Onset of action	30–60 min
Duration of action	3–8 h

Adverse Effects: At recommended doses, acetaminophen is well tolerated and serious adverse effects are rare. The risk for adverse effects is dose related and increases with the long-term use of this drug. Acute acetaminophen poisoning is very serious, and symptoms include anorexia, nausea, vomiting, dizziness, lethargy, diaphoresis, chills, epigastric or abdominal pain, and diarrhea. Excessive acetaminophen use is the number one cause of acute hepatic failure in the United States. The onset of hepatotoxicity is noted with elevated transaminases (ALT, AST) and bilirubin. The patient will also have hypoglycemia, hepatic coma, and acute renal failure. Chronic ingestion of acetaminophen results in neutropenia, pancytopenia, leukopenia, thrombocytopenic purpura, hepatotoxicity in alcoholics, and renal damage. In 2013, the FDA issued a safety alert that recommended the drug be immediately discontinued if skin reactions or blisters develop. These skin lesions may indicate the development of rare, though serious, disorders such as Stevens–Johnson syndrome. **Black Box Warning**: Acetaminophen has the potential to cause severe liver injury and may cause serious allergic reactions with symptoms of angioedema, difficulty breathing, itching, or rash.

Contraindications/Precautions: Patients who are allergic to acetaminophen should not be administered this medication. It should be used cautiously in patients with anemia, G6PD deficiency, or hepatic disease. Acetaminophen should be administered cautiously to patients with rheumatoid or osteoarthritis, malnutrition, bone marrow depression, and immunosuppression. Chronic administration of acetaminophen should be avoided in patients with renal impairment because this drug can worsen kidney function.

Drug Interactions: Acetaminophen should not be administered with alcohol or to patients who consume alcohol with regularity because this greatly increases the risk of hepatotoxicity. Alcohol-induced hepatotoxicity can occur at therapeutic doses of acetaminophen. Due to additive hepatotoxic effects, acetaminophen should not be administered with barbiturates, carbamazepine, diphenylhydantoin, isoniazid, rifampin, and sulfinpyrazone. Acetaminophen will decrease lamotrigine levels, if the drugs are administered concurrently. Long-term use of acetaminophen and warfarin will result in increased hypoprothrombinemic effects. Zidovudine administered with acetaminophen may increase the risk of bone marrow suppression. **Herbal/Food**: Caffeine will enhance the analgesic effects of acetaminophen. Hepatotoxicity has been reported with concurrent echinacea use.

Pregnancy: Category B.

Treatment of Overdose: Acetaminophen overdose is treated with oral or IV acetylcysteine (Acetadote). For maximum effectiveness, the antidote should be administered within 8 hours of acetaminophen ingestion. The IV form (Acetadote) is administered by the "three-bag method":

- **Loading dose.** Dilute 150 mg/kg in 200 mL of 5% dextrose and administer over 60 minutes.
- **Second dose.** Dilute 50 mg/kg in 500 mL of 5% dextrose and administer over 4 hours.
- **Third dose.** Dilute 100 mg/kg in 1,000 mL of 5% dextrose and administer over 16 hours.

Nursing Responsibilities: Key nursing implications for patients receiving acetaminophen are included in the Nursing Practice Application for Patients Receiving Pharmacotherapy for Inflammation and Fever.

Drugs Similar to Acetaminophen (Tylenol)

Acetaminophen is the only medication in this class.

CONNECTIONS: NURSING PRACTICE APPLICATION

Patients Receiving Pharmacotherapy for Inflammation and Fever

Assessment	Potential Nursing Diagnoses*
Baseline assessment prior to administration: • Obtain a complete health history including hepatic, renal, respiratory, cardiovascular or neurologic disease, pregnancy, or breast-feeding. Obtain a drug history including allergies, current prescription and OTC drugs, herbal preparations, caffeine, nicotine, and alcohol use. Be alert to possible drug interactions. • Obtain baseline vital signs and weight. • Evaluate appropriate laboratory findings (e.g., CBC, coagulation panels, bleeding time, electrolytes, glucose, lipid profile, and hepatic or renal function studies). • Assess the patient's ability to receive and understand instructions. Include the family and caregivers as needed.	• *Acute* or *Chronic Pain* • *Hyperthermia* • *Deficient Fluid Volume* • *Deficient Knowledge* (Drug Therapy) • *Risk for Injury*, related to adverse drug effects
Assessment throughout administration: • Assess for desired therapeutic effects (e.g., temperature returns to within normal range, pain is decreased or absent, signs and symptoms of inflammation such as redness or swelling are decreased). • Continue periodic monitoring of CBC, coagulation studies, bleeding time, electrolytes, glucose, lipids, hepatic, and renal function studies. • Assess vital signs and weight periodically or if symptoms warrant. Report any weight gain over 1 kg (2 lb) in a 24-h period or more than 2 kg (5 lb) in 1 week. • Assess for and promptly report adverse effects: symptoms of GI bleeding (dark or tarry stools, hematemesis, coffee-ground emesis, or blood in the stool), abdominal pain, severe tinnitus, dizziness, drowsiness, lightheadedness, palpitations, tachycardia, HTN, increased respiratory rate and depth, pulmonary congestion, or edema.	

Implementation

Interventions and (Rationales)	Patient-Centered Care
Ensuring therapeutic effects: • Continue assessments as above for therapeutic effects. (Diminished fever, pain, or signs and symptoms of infection should begin after taking the first dose and continue to improve. The provider should be notified if fever remains present after 3 days or if increasing signs of infection are present.)	• Teach the patient to supplement drug therapy with nonpharmacologic measures (e.g., RICE: rest, ice or cool compresses), compression bandage (e.g., ACE wrap), elevation of the inflamed joint or limb; increased fluid intake for fever; positioning for comfort, diversionary distractions (e.g., television or music), and rest for pain.
Minimizing adverse effects: • Continue to monitor vital signs, especially temperature if fever is present, and blood pressure and pulse for patients on ibuprofen and similar drugs. Immediately report undiminished fever, changes in level of consciousness, febrile seizures, tachycardia, blood pressure over 140/90, or per parameters as ordered to the health care provider. (Fever should begin to diminish within 1–3 h after taking the drug. Ibuprofen and similar drugs may increase the risk for cardiovascular thrombotic events such as MI and stroke.)	• Teach the patient to immediately report a fever that does not diminish below 37.8°C (100°F) or per parameters, febrile seizures, changes in behavior or level of consciousness, tachycardia, palpitations, or increased blood pressure to the health care provider. • Teach the patient on ibuprofen or similar drugs how to monitor the pulse and blood pressure. Ensure proper use and functioning of any home equipment obtained.
• Continue to monitor periodic laboratory work: hepatic and renal function tests, CBC, electrolytes, glucose, lipid levels, coagulation studies, or bleeding time. **Lifespan:** Monitor the older adult frequently because age-related physiological changes increase the risk of adverse renal and hepatic effects. (Aspirin and salicylates affect platelet aggregation and should be monitored if used long term or if excessive bleeding or bruising is noted. Acetaminophen can be hepatotoxic in large doses or if taken when hepatic dysfunction is present.)	• Instruct the patient on the need to return periodically for laboratory work. • Teach the patient to abstain from alcohol while taking acetaminophen. Men who consume more than two alcoholic beverages per day or women who consume more than one alcoholic beverage per day should consult their health care provider before taking acetaminophen.
• Monitor for abdominal pain, black or tarry stools, blood in the stool, hematemesis, coffee-ground emesis, dizziness, lightheadedness, and hypotension, especially if associated with tachycardia. **Lifespan:** Monitor the older adult frequently for GI irritation or bleeding because age-related physiological changes increase the risk of adverse effects. (NSAIDs may cause GI irritation and bleeding.)	• Instruct the patient to immediately report any signs or symptoms of GI bleeding. • Teach the patient to take the drug with food or milk to decrease GI irritation. Enteric-coated tablets should be swallowed whole without chewing, crushing, or breaking. Alcohol use should be avoided or eliminated.
• Monitor for tinnitus, difficulty hearing, lightheadedness, or difficulty with balance, and report promptly. (NSAIDs and salicylates may be ototoxic and cause hearing loss.)	• Instruct the patient to immediately report any signs or symptoms of ringing, humming, buzzing in ears, difficulty with balance, dizziness or vertigo, or nausea.

(continued)

CONNECTIONS: NURSING PRACTICE APPLICATION (continued)

• Monitor urine output and renal function studies periodically. Weigh patient on corticosteroids daily, and report weight gain of 1 kg (2 lb) or more in a 24-h period or more than 2 kg (5 lb) per week, or increasing peripheral edema. (NSAIDs and salicylates may be renal toxic and patients on long-term or high-dose therapy should monitor urine output and have periodic renal function studies. Daily weight is an accurate measure of fluid status and takes into account intake, output, and insensible losses.)	• Instruct the patient on NSAIDs and salicylates to report promptly any changes in the quantity of urine output, darkening of urine, or edema. • Teach the patient on NSAIDs and salicylates to increase fluid intake, especially if fever is present. • Instruct the patient to weigh self daily, ideally at the same time of day. The patient should report a weight gain of more than 1 kg (2 lb) in a 24-h period or more than 2 kg (5 lb) per week, or increasing peripheral edema.
• Periodically monitor vision in patients on NSAIDs. Immediately report unusual changes in visual acuity, blurred or diminished vision, reports of spots in vision, or changes in color sense to the provider. (NSAIDs may cause blurred or diminished vision, decreased color sense, diplopia, or scotomas.)	• Teach the patient on NSAIDs to obtain eye exams twice yearly or more frequently as instructed by the provider. Immediately report any eye pain, diminished or blurred vision, or changes in color sense.
• **Lifespan:** Avoid the use of aspirin or salicylates in children under age 19 unless explicitly ordered by the health care provider. (Aspirin has been associated with an increased risk of Reye's syndrome in children under age 19, particularly associated with the flu virus and varicella infections.)	• Instruct parents to use NSAIDs or acetaminophen in children under age 19 for fever or pain control, unless otherwise ordered by the provider. Do not use aspirin or salicylates in children under age 19 unless ordered by the provider or within 2–3 weeks after the varicella vaccination has been administered to these children. • Teach parents to read labels on all OTC medications and to avoid formulations with aspirin or salicylate on the label.
• **Lifespan:** Assess for the possibility of pregnancy before beginning the drug. (Many NSAIDs are pregnancy category C or D drugs.)	• Instruct female patients who may be considering pregnancy, or are pregnant, to notify their provider before starting the drug.
Patient understanding of drug therapy: • Use opportunities during administration of medications and during assessments to discuss the rationale for drug therapy, desired therapeutic outcomes, most commonly observed adverse effects, parameters for when to call the health care provider, and any necessary monitoring or precautions. (Using time during nursing care helps to optimize and reinforce key teaching areas.)	• The patient, family, or caregiver should be able to state the reason for the drug, appropriate dose and scheduling, what adverse effects to observe for and when to report them, and the anticipated length of medication therapy.
Patient self-administration of drug therapy: • When administering the medication, instruct the patient, family, or caregiver in proper self-administration, e.g., with food or milk. (Utilizing time during nurse-administration of these drugs helps to reinforce teaching. Household measuring devices such as teaspoons differ significantly in size and amount and should not be used for pediatric or liquid doses.)	• The patient, family, or caregiver is able to discuss appropriate dosing and administration needs, including: • NSAIDs should be taken with food or milk to decrease GI upset. • Liquid doses of acetaminophen or NSAIDs should be measured with the enclosed dosage cup, dropper, or spoon. If that measuring device is no longer available, do NOT use a household spoon. Obtain another calibrated measuring cup or dropper.

*Nursing Diagnoses—Definitions and Classification 2015–2017. Copyright © 2014, 1994–2014 by NANDA International. Used by arrangement with John Wiley & Sons Limited.

CHAPTER

41   Understanding the Chapter

Key Concepts Summary

41.1 Inflammation is a nonspecific body response to antigens and tissue injury.

41.2 Treatment of inflammation includes nonpharmacologic therapies and the administration of anti-inflammatory drugs.

41.3 Aspirin is an inexpensive, effective, first-generation nonsteroidal anti-inflammatory drug commonly used by adults.

41.4 Ibuprofen and similar nonsteroidal anti-inflammatory drugs are the most common drugs for treating mild to moderate pain and inflammation.

41.5 Celecoxib is an effective second-generation nonsteroidal anti-inflammatory drug, but its use is limited due to an increased risk of myocardial infarction and stroke.

41.6 Acetaminophen is administered for pain relief and to reduce fever, but it has no anti-inflammatory properties.

Case Study: Making the Patient Connection

Remember the patient "Joycee Layne" at the beginning of the chapter? Now read the remainder of the case study. Based on the information presented within this chapter, respond to the critical thinking questions that follow.

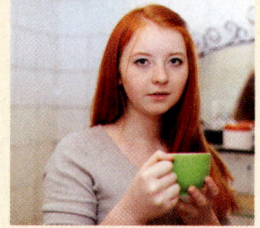

Joycee Layne is a 17-year-old high school student in her senior year. She is an honors student, works hard to get good grades, and hates to miss school. For the past 3 days, she has not been feeling well. This morning her temperature is 39°C (102.2°F), and she has chills and a headache. Several of her friends at school have the flu. She has taken ibuprofen for fevers and menstrual cramps in the past, but Joycee cannot find any in the house as she gets ready to head off to school. Her parents have already left for work, and they trust her to check with you, the nurse who lives next door, before taking any medication. Joycee calls you to ask "Is it OK to take the aspirin that my mom uses for her arthritis so I can go to school?" As the nurse, this presents an opportunity for you to teach Joycee about aspirin and her fever.

Critical Thinking Questions

1. Describe the pathophysiology of fever and inflammation.
2. Why is aspirin administered for fever?
3. Should Joycee take the aspirin? Why or why not?
4. What will you teach Joycee about aspirin and the flulike symptoms she is having? What additional patient teaching will she need?

See Answers to Critical Thinking Questions on student resource website.

Additional Case Study

Tameeka Jones has a postoperative infection following a vaginal hysterectomy. The infection is noted at the site of the laparoscopic incision of the lower abdomen. She has developed a fever of 38.8°C (102°F). The health care provider has ordered acetaminophen (Tylenol) 650 mg PO every 4 to 6 h as needed for the fever.

1. What is the action of acetaminophen (Tylenol)?
2. What pain medications should be avoided while the patient is receiving acetaminophen (Tylenol) for fever reduction?
3. What patient teaching is important for the patient who has a fever related to infection?

See Answers to Additional Case Study on student resource website.

Chapter Review

1 A 30-year-old patient with depression has attempted suicide by overdosing on acetaminophen (Tylenol). The nurse in the emergency department will anticipate that the patient's treatment will consist of:

1. An intravenous infusion with normal saline to infuse at 1,000 mL per hour.
2. The administration of acetylcysteine (Acetadote) by intravenous infusion.
3. Preparation for cardioversion due to the impending arrhythmia.
4. The assessment of liver hepatic enzymes to determine hepatotoxicity.

2 A patient has a fever and is allergic to aspirin. Which medication will the nurse anticipate administering to reduce the patient's fever?

1. Ibuprofen (Motrin, Advil)
2. Ketorolac (Toradol)
3. Acetaminophen (Tylenol)
4. Celecoxib (Celebrex)

3 An anti-inflammatory agent is ordered to be given intravenously to the patient for pain. Which anti-inflammatory agent is administered parenterally?

1. Ketorolac (Toradol, Acular)
2. Ketoprofen
3. Ibuprofen (Motrin, Advil)
4. Celecoxib (Celebrex)

4 An 80-year-old woman, who is scheduled for a total knee replacement next month, currently takes ibuprofen (Motrin, Advil) 600 mg three times per day. Which patient teaching intervention is most important?

1. Continue ibuprofen (Motrin, Advil) until surgery.
2. Stop ibuprofen (Motrin, Advil) today.
3. Decrease ibuprofen (Motrin, Advil) to two times per day.
4. Stop ibuprofen (Motrin, Advil) 7 to 14 days before surgery.

5 The nurse should question the order of acetaminophen (Tylenol) for which patient?

1. A patient with cirrhosis of the liver

2. A patient with chronic obstructive pulmonary disease

3. A patient with breast cancer

4. A patient who is taking warfarin (Coumadin)

6 A patient takes aspirin (acetylsalicylic acid) daily for pain in the right knee. Which toxic effects may be present with aspirin overdosage? Select all that apply.

1. Tinnitus

2. Hyperventilation

3. Gastrointestinal bleeding

4. Decreased urinary output

5. Peripheral neuropathy

See Answers to Chapter Review in Appendix A.

References

National Center for Complementary and Alternative Medicine. (2012). *Herbs at a glance: Goldenseal.* Retrieved from http://nccam.nih.gov/health/goldenseal

Paul, I. M., Sturgis, S. A., Yang, C., Engle, L., Watts, H., & Berlin, C. M. (2010). Efficacy of standard doses of ibuprofen alone, alternating, and combined with acetaminophen for treatment of febrile children. *Clinical Therapeutics, 32,* 2433–2440. doi:10.1016/j.clinthera.2011.01.006

Pierce, C. A., & Voss, B. (2010). Efficacy and safety of ibuprofen and acetaminophen in children and adults: A meta-analysis and qualitative review. *The Annals of Pharmacotherapy, 44,* 489–506. doi:10.1345/aph.1M332

Rothwell, P. M., Wilson, M., Elwin, C. E., Norrving, B., Algra, A., Warlow, C. P., & Meade, T. M. (2010). Long-term effect of aspirin on colorectal cancer incidence and mortality: 20-year follow-up of five randomised trials. *The Lancet, 376,* 1741–1750. doi:10.1016/S0140-6736(10)61543-7

Sullivan, J. E., & Farrar, H. C. (2011). Fever and antipyretic use in children. *Pediatrics, 127,* 580–587. doi:10.1542/peds.2010-3852

University of Maryland Medical Center. (2013). *Goldenseal.* Retrieved from http://umm.edu/health/medical/altmed/herb/goldenseal

Waseem, M. (2013). *Salicylate toxicity.* Retrieved from http://emedicine.medscape.com/article/1009987-overview#a0156

Wiegand, T. J. (2012). *Nonsteroidal anti-inflammatory agent toxicity.* Retrieved from http://emedicine.medscape.com/article/816117-overview

Wong, T., Stang, A. S., Ganshorn, H., Hartling, L., Maconochie, I. K., Thomsen, A. M., & Johnson, D. W. (2013). Combined and alternating paracetamol and ibuprofen therapy for febrile children. *Cochrane Database of Systematic Reviews, 10,* CD009572. doi:10.1002/14651858.CD009572.pub2

Selected Bibliography

Abramson, S. B. (2011). Clinical guidelines: Expert recommendations for NSAID use: A user-friendly model? *Nature Reviews Rheumatology, 7,* 133–134. doi:10.1038/nrrheum.2010.230

Barkin, R. L., Beckerman, M., Blum, S. L., Clark, F. M., Koh, E. K., & Wu, D. S. (2010). Should nonsteroidal anti-inflammatory drugs (NSAIDs) be prescribed to the older adult? *Drugs and Aging, 27*(10), 775–789. doi:10.2165/11539430-000000000-00000

Conaghan, P. G. (2012). A turbulent decade for NSAIDs: Update on current concepts of classification, epidemiology, comparative efficacy, and toxicity. *Rheumatology International, 32*(6), 1491–1502. doi:10.1007/s00296-011-2263-6

Farrell, S. E. (2013). *Acetaminophen toxicity.* Retrieved from http://emedicine.medscape.com/article/820200-overview#aw2aab6b2b4

Grosser, T., Smythe, E., & Fitzgerald, G. A. (2010). In L. L. Brunton, B. A. Chabner, & B. C. Knollman (Eds.), *The pharmacological basis of therapeutics* (12th ed., pp. 1067–1100). New York, NY: McGraw-Hill.

Herdman, T. H., & Kamitsuru, S. (Eds.). (2014). *NANDA International nursing diagnoses: Definitions and classification, 2015–2017.* Oxford, United Kingdom: Wiley-Blackwell.

Shah, S., & Mehta, V. (2012). Controversies and advances in non-steroidal anti-inflammatory drug (NSAID) analgesia in chronic pain management. *Postgraduate Medical Journal, 88,* 73–78. doi:10.1136/postgradmedj-2011-130291

Trepanier, C. H., & Milgram, N. W. (2010). Neuroinflammation in Alzheimer's disease: Are NSAIDs and selective COX-2 inhibitors the next line of therapy? *Journal of Alzheimer's Disease, 21*(4), 1089–1099. doi:10.3233/JAD-2010-090667

Venerito, M., Wex, T., & Malferthiner, P. (2010). Nonsteroidal anti-inflammatory drug-induced gastroduodenal bleeding: Risk factors and prevention strategies. *Pharmaceuticals, 3*(7), 2225–2237. doi:10.3390/ph3072225

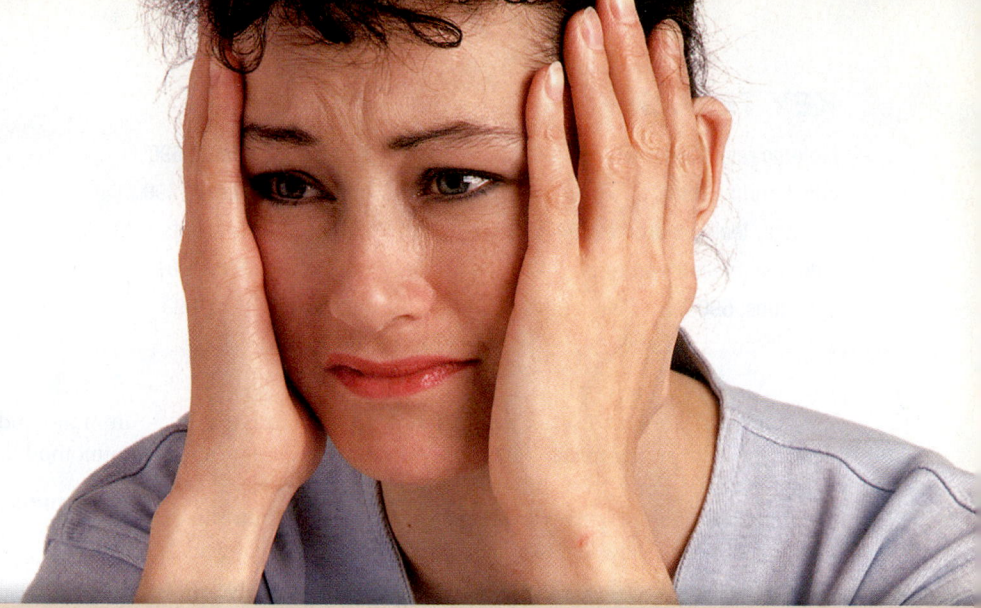

*"I don't know what's worse—
the symptoms or the treatment.
I feel terrible."*

Patient "Carol Banks"

CHAPTER

42

Immunostimulants and Immunosuppressants

LEARNING OUTCOMES

After reading this chapter, the student should be able to:

1. Compare and contrast the therapeutic applications of the immunostimulants and immunosuppressants.

2. Describe the roles of interferons, interleukins, and other cytokines in modulating the immune response.

3. Explain how pegylation of the interferon molecule allows for less frequent dosing.

4. Explain why therapy with immunosuppressant medications is necessary following organ transplants.

5. Identify the classes of drugs used as immunosuppressants.

6. Compare and contrast polyclonal and monoclonal antibodies.

7. For each of the classes shown in the chapter outline, identify the prototype and representative drugs and explain the mechanism(s) of drug action, primary indications, contraindications, significant drug interactions, pregnancy category, and important adverse effects.

8. Apply the nursing process to care for patients who are receiving immunostimulants and immunosuppressants.

CHAPTER OUTLINE

▸ **Immunostimulants**

Interferons

PROTOTYPE Interferon Alfa-2b (Intron A), *p. 691*

Interleukins

PROTOTYPE Aldesleukin (Proleukin), *p. 694*

▸ **Immunosuppressants**

Calcineurin Inhibitors

PROTOTYPE Cyclosporine (Gengraf, Neoral, Sandimmune), *p. 698*

Cytotoxic Drugs and Antimetabolites

PROTOTYPE Azathioprine (Azasan, Imuran), *p. 700*

Antibodies

PROTOTYPE Basiliximab (Simulect), *p. 703*

Corticosteroids

KEY TERMS

biologic response modifiers, 691

calcineurin, 698

capillary leak syndrome, 694

cytokine release syndrome, 703

cytokines, 690

immunomodulator, 690

immunostimulants, 690

immunosuppressants, 690

interferons (IFNs), 691

interleukins (ILs), 693

monoclonal antibody (MAB), 702

pegylation, 691

polyclonal antibodies, 702

transplant rejection, 695

The immune system and other body defenses are truly formidable deterrents to invading microorganisms. A healthy defense system can protect the body from life-threatening infections caused by thousands of different species of organisms often over an entire lifetime. In addition, body defenses can protect against internal invaders such as cancer cells. There are certain circumstances, however, when drugs may be necessary to modulate the body's defenses. This chapter examines pharmacotherapy with agents that either stimulate or suppress immune function.

42.1 Immunomodulators are substances that either enhance or suppress the ability of the body to fight infection and disease.

Body defenses are composed of a complex system of cells, tissues, and processes designed with a single goal: to protect the body from invasion by foreign substances, or antigens, that may cause harm. Some of these defenses are specific to a single species of microbe, whereas others are nonspecific and provide the same response or protection regardless of the invading pathogen. The student should review the components of body defenses in Chapter 43, before proceeding.

Immunomodulator is a general term referring to any drug or therapy that affects body defenses. An overview of the immunomodulators is given in Figure 42.1. Two basic types of immunomodulators are used for pharmacotherapy:

- **Immunostimulants** are drugs that increase the ability of the immune system to fight infection and disease. In most cases, these drugs are used to treat patients with cancer. The use of immunostimulants to treat cancer is called *immunotherapy*. Some immunostimulants are also used to treat hepatitis. The use of colony-stimulating factors to treat neutropenia was presented in Chapter 39 and the application of vaccines to boost the immune response is presented in Chapter 43.

- **Immunosuppressants** are drugs that diminish the ability of the immune system to fight infection and disease. Immunosuppressants are used to prevent transplant rejection and to dampen hyperactive immune responses, such as those that may occur during exacerbations of systemic lupus erythematosus (SLE) or rheumatoid arthritis (RA).

Immunostimulants

42.2 Interferons are biologic response modifiers that have antiviral and antineoplastic activity.

When challenged by antigens, certain cells of the immune system secrete **cytokines**, which are substances that help the body

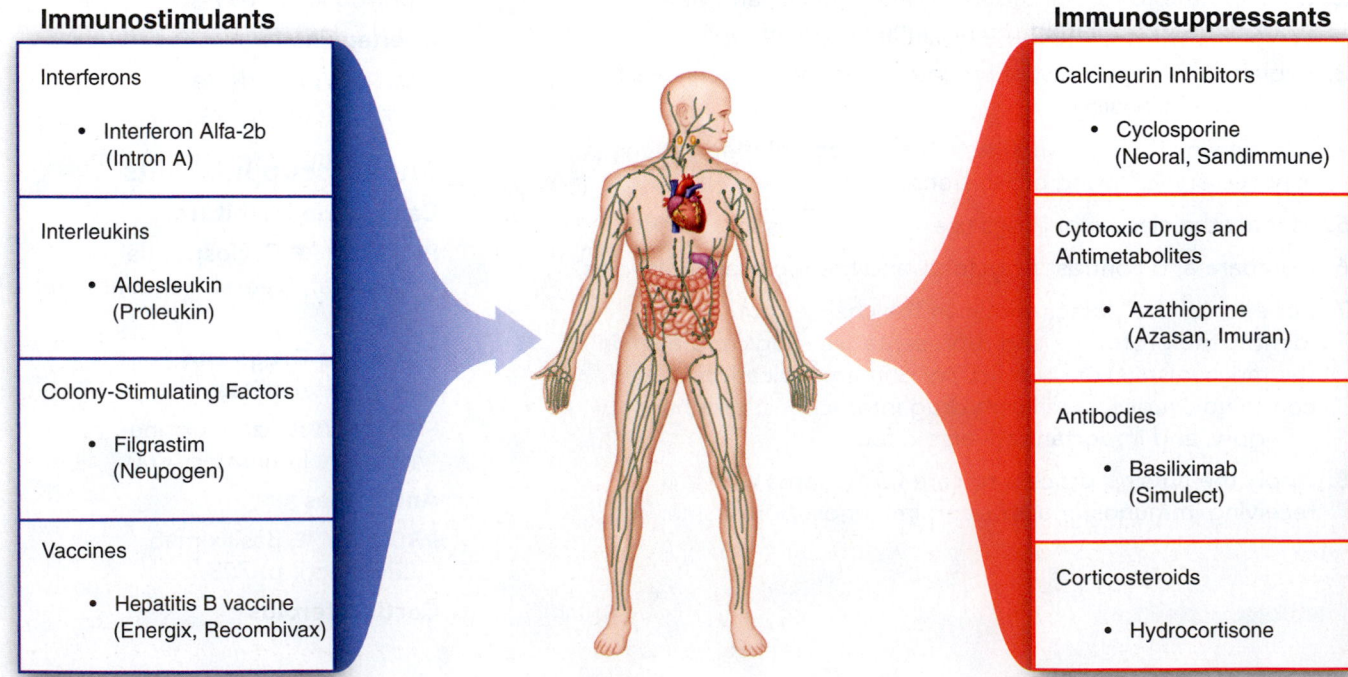

Immunostimulants

Interferons
- Interferon Alfa-2b (Intron A)

Interleukins
- Aldesleukin (Proleukin)

Colony-Stimulating Factors
- Filgrastim (Neupogen)

Vaccines
- Hepatitis B vaccine (Energix, Recombivax)

Immunosuppressants

Calcineurin Inhibitors
- Cyclosporine (Neoral, Sandimmune)

Cytotoxic Drugs and Antimetabolites
- Azathioprine (Azasan, Imuran)

Antibodies
- Basiliximab (Simulect)

Corticosteroids
- Hydrocortisone

Figure 42.1 Overview of immunomodulators.

mediate and intensify the immune response. Because cytokines have powerful actions on the immune system, the body generally only produces them when challenged by an antigen; their production is rapid though transient. Chronic, high levels of cytokines can contribute to diseases, such as psoriasis, Crohn's disease, or RA, and can greatly worsen symptoms of these disorders.

Cytokines exhibit multiple complex actions. A single cytokine can affect multiple target cells, each resulting in a different action. There is also considerable overlap or redundancy among the cytokines in that different cytokines can produce the same biologic actions. In addition to affecting their target cells, cytokines interact with each other by turning the synthesis of other cytokines on or off. The physiology of cytokines is complex and is an active research field.

Natural cytokines have been identified and, through recombinant deoxyribonucleic acid (DNA) technology, enough quantity has been made available to treat certain disorders. Also called **biologic response modifiers**, some of these agents have been approved to boost specific functions of the immune system.

Interferons (IFNs) are cytokines secreted by lymphocytes and activated macrophages that have been infected with a virus. IFNs are unable to protect the infected cell, but they warn surrounding cells that a viral infection has occurred. IFNs attach to nearby uninfected cells, inducing the production of protective antiviral proteins. When the virus attempts to attack the protected cell, the pathogen is inactivated.

IFNs are part of the nonspecific defense system. Their actions slow the spread of viral infections, stimulate the activity of existing leukocytes, increase phagocytosis, and enhance the cytotoxic ability of T cells. Interestingly, IFNs promote apoptosis in infected cells, which is a form of programmed cell death in which the infected cell kills itself to limit the replication and spread of the virus. In addition to their antiviral actions, IFNs have antineoplastic and antiinflammatory properties.

Many different cell types produce IFNs. Although their functions are nearly identical, each IFN has a slightly different structure, and some have different receptors. To distinguish among the different IFNs, each type is assigned numbers and a Greek letter. The most common types are IFN alfa-2b, IFN beta-1a, IFN beta-1b, and IFN gamma-1a. When the drug consists of a mixture of IFNs, the letter "n" is assigned. For example, IFN alfa-n3 is a mixture of IFN alfa subtypes.

The alfa IFNs have the greatest clinical utility. The formulations available include IFN alfa-2b, IFN alfacon-1, IFN alfa-n3, pegIFN alfa-2a, and pegIFN alfa-2b.

The two "peg" formulations have the molecule polyethylene glycol (PEG) bonded to the IFN. PEG is a polymer with low toxicity that can be found in skin creams, laxatives, lubricants, toothpastes, and many other products. The addition of PEG to another molecule, known as **pegylation**, increases the molecule's solubility and extends its stability. The addition of PEG to an IFN extends the half-life of the drug to allow for once-weekly dosing. Indications for IFN alfa therapy include hairy cell leukemia, non-Hodgkin's lymphoma, acquired immunodeficiency syndrome (AIDS)–related Kaposi's sarcoma, and chronic hepatitis B or C. The use of IFN alfa in the pharmacotherapy of hepatitis is presented in Chapter 54. Doses of the IFNs are listed in Table 42.1.

IFN beta consists of two different formulations, beta-1a and beta-1b, which are primarily reserved for the treatment of severe multiple sclerosis (MS) (see Chapter 21). A third drug in this class, called IFN gamma-1b, has limited clinical application in the treatment of chronic granulomatous disease and severe osteoporosis.

PROTOTYPE DRUG	Interferon Alfa-2b (Intron A)

Classification: Therapeutic: Immunostimulant
Pharmacologic: Interferon, biologic response modifier

Therapeutic Effects and Uses: Approved in 1986, IFN alfa-2b is a biologic response modifier prepared by recombinant DNA technology. Indications include neoplastic conditions such as hairy cell leukemia, malignant melanoma, non-Hodgkin's lymphoma, and AIDS-related Kaposi's sarcoma as well as viral infections (chronic hepatitis virus B and C). IFN alfa-2b is also indicated for the intralesional treatment of condylomata acuminata, which are genital warts caused by the human papillomavirus. Off-label indications include chronic myelogenous leukemia, bladder cancer, herpes simplex virus, multiple myeloma, renal cell cancer, human immunodeficiency virus (HIV), varicella-zoster virus (VZV), and West Nile virus. It is available for intravenous (IV), intramuscular (IM), and subcutaneous administration.

Rebetron is a combination drug containing IFN alfa-2b and ribavirin, an antiviral agent. Rebetron is indicated for the pharmacotherapy of hepatitis C infection.

Mechanism of Action: IFN alfa-2b has both antiviral and antineoplastic activities. It is a nonspecific inhibitor of viral replication. It affects cancer cells by two mechanisms. First, it enhances the general functions of the immune system: IFNs increase the phagocytic activity of macrophages and monocytes, resulting in enhanced cytotoxicity against tumor cells. Second, this drug suppresses the growth of cancer cells.

Pharmacokinetics:

Route(s)	IV, IM, subcutaneous
Absorption	80% absorbed
Distribution	Unknown if secreted in breast milk
Primary metabolism	Minimal hepatic metabolism
Primary excretion	Renal
Onset of action	Peak: 3–12 h
Duration of action	Half-life: 2–3 h

Adverse Effects: The most common adverse effect of IFN therapy is a flulike syndrome of fever, chills, dizziness, weight loss, and fatigue that occurs in about 50% of patients and that usually diminishes as therapy progresses. Fatigue may be severe at higher doses. Headache, nausea, vomiting, diarrhea, and anorexia are relatively common. Hair loss may occur with prolonged therapy. Depression and suicidal ideation have been reported and may be severe enough to require discontinuation of the drug. The depression may persist after the drug is discontinued. With prolonged therapy, serious adverse effects such as immunosuppression, hepatotoxicity, and neurotoxicity may be observed. **Black Box Warning**: IFNs may cause or aggravate fatal or life-threatening neuropsychiatric, autoimmune, ischemic, or infectious disorders. The drug should be discontinued if these symptoms are persistent or severe.

TABLE 42.1 Immunostimulants

Drug	Route and Adult Dose (Maximum Dose Where Indicated)	Adverse Effects
aldesleukin (Proleukin)	IV: 600,000 units/kg (0.037 mg/kg) every 8 h by a 15-min IV infusion for a total of 14 doses	*Flulike symptoms, rash, anemia, nausea, vomiting, diarrhea, confusion, dyspnea* <u>Cardiac arrest, hypotension, tachycardia, thrombocytopenia, oliguria, anuria, pulmonary edema, capillary leak syndrome</u>
bacillus Calmette-Guérin (BCG) vaccine (TheraCys, Tice)	Interdermal (Tice): 0.1 mL as vaccine Intravesical (TheraCys): bladder instillation for bladder carcinoma	*Flulike symptoms, dysuria, hematuria, anemia, lymphadenopathy* <u>Thrombocytopenia, cystitis, urinary tract infection, disseminated mycobacteria</u>
Interferons		
IFN alfa-2b (Intron A)	IM/subcutaneous: hairy cell leukemia: 2 million units/m^2 3 times/week for up to 6 months Kaposi's sarcoma: 30 million units/m^2 3 times/week for 16 weeks Chronic hepatitis B: 30–35 million units/week for 16 weeks	*Flulike symptoms, myalgia, fatigue, headache, anorexia, diarrhea* <u>Myelosuppression, thrombocytopenia, neutropenia, suicide ideation, seizures (IFN beta), MI (IFN gamma), anaphylaxis, hepatotoxicity</u>
IFN alfacon-1 (Infergen)	Subcutaneous: As monotherapy: 9 mcg 3 times/week for 24 weeks As combination therapy: 15 mcg daily with ribavirin for up to 48 weeks	
IFN alfa-n3 (Alferon N)	Intralesion: 0.05 mL (250,000 international units) per wart twice/week for up to 8 weeks	
IFN beta-1a (Avonex, Rebif)	IM (Avonex): 30 mcg/week Subcutaneous (Rebif): 44 mcg 3 times/week	
IFN beta-1b (Betaseron, Extavia)	Subcutaneous: 0.25 mg (8 million units) every other day	
IFN gamma-1b (Actimmune)	Subcutaneous: 50 mcg/m^2, 3 times weekly	
pegIFN alfa-2a (Pegasys)	Subcutaneous: 180 mcg once weekly for 48 weeks	
pegIFN alfa-2b (Pegintron, Sylatron)	Subcutaneous (Pegintron): 1.5 mcg/kg once weekly for 48 weeks Subcutaneous (Sylatron): 6 mg/kg/week for eight doses followed by 3 mg/kg/week for up to 5 years	

Note: Italics indicate common adverse effects. <u>Underline</u> indicates serious adverse effects.

Contraindications/Precautions: Contraindications include hypersensitivity to IFNs, autoimmune hepatitis, or hepatic decompensation. Neonates and infants should not receive this drug because it contains benzyl alcohol, which is associated with an increased incidence of neurologic and other serious complications in this age group. If infection occurs during therapy, antiinfectives should be started immediately. Hepatic enzymes may become elevated during IFN therapy and may require discontinuation of the drug. This effect is worse in patients with preexisting hepatic impairment. IFN alfa-2b should be used with caution in patients with cardiac disease, herpes zoster, and recent exposure to chickenpox. Triglycerides should be monitored during therapy because elevated levels have resulted in symptoms of pancreatitis in some patients.

Drug Interactions: IFN alfa-2b may increase theophylline levels. Zidovudine may increase hematologic toxicity and cause immunosuppression. **Herbal/Food:** Unknown.

Pregnancy: Category C. If used with ribavirin, the combination is category X.

Treatment of Overdose: Overdose with IFN may cause lethargy and coma. Treatment is by general supportive measures.

Nursing Responsibilities: Key nursing implications for patients receiving IFN alfa-2b are included in the Nursing Practice Application for Patients Receiving Pharmacotherapy with Immunomodulators.

Drugs Similar to Interferon alfa-2b (Intron A)

Other available IFNs include IFN alfacon-1, IFN alfa-n3, IFN beta-1a, IFN beta-1b, IFN gamma-1b, pegIFN alfa-2a, and pegIFN alfa-2b. IFN alfa-n1 (Wellferon) and IFN alfa-2a are no longer available in the United States.

IFN alfacon-1 (Infergen): Approved in 1997, IFN alfacon-1 is a drug that contains a mixture of all the IFN alfa subtypes. Given by the subcutaneous route, its only approved indication by the U.S. Food and Drug Administration (FDA) is for the treatment of chronic hepatitis C infection in patients at least 18 years old with compensated liver disease. The drug is nearly always used in combination with ribavirin because this increases the effectiveness of therapy. Contraindications, drug interactions, and adverse effects are the same as those for IFN alfa-2b. Mild flulike symptoms are common adverse effects. Patients should be monitored for depression and suicidal ideation. A black box warning for IFNs states that these drugs may cause or aggravate fatal or life-threatening neuropsychiatric, autoimmune, ischemic, or infectious disorders. This drug is pregnancy category C.

IFN alfa-n3 (Alferon N): Approved in 1989, IFN alfa-n3 is a mixture of IFN alfa subtypes purified from human leukocytes. Indications include genital warts and human papillomavirus. Two injections per week for 8 weeks are usually sufficient to cause warts to disappear. Unlike the other IFNs, this drug is injected directly into lesions (intralesionally). Its off-label indications include treatment of hepatitis C, herpes simplex, and other viral infections by the subcutaneous route. This product may contain egg protein and is contraindicated in patients with egg sensitivity. IFN alfa-n3 exhibits few adverse effects when administered intralesionally. This drug is pregnancy category C.

IFN beta-1a (Avonex, Rebif) and IFN beta-1b (Betaseron, Extavia): The beta interferons are first-line drugs for the pharmacotherapy of MS. These medications decrease the frequency of clinical exacerbations and slow the progression to physical disability, which is characteristic of MS. Both beta interferons are available by the subcutaneous route: beta-1b can also be administered. Adverse effects are similar to those of other IFNs, with flulike symptoms being observed in the majority of patients. Patients should be monitored for depression and suicidal ideation. Additional details on the pharmacotherapy of MS and a drug prototype feature for IFN beta-1b are presented in Chapter 21. The beta interferons are pregnancy category C.

IFN gamma-1b (Actimmune): Approved in 1999, IFN gamma-1b is produced by recombinant DNA technology and is very similar to natural IFN gamma. IFN gamma-1b has both direct and indirect antiviral activity. This drug activates macrophages to increase the production of interleukin-12 and tumor necrosis factor (TNF), which increases the killing ability of these cells. IFN gamma-1b also promotes the recruitment of leukocytes to the sites of infection or inflammation. IFN gamma-1b is the only IFN indicated for the treatment of chronic granulomatous disease (CGD). CGD is an inherited disorder of phagocytic cells that leads to recurrent life-threatening bacterial and fungal infections. A second characteristic of CGD is the development of nodular granulomas in the skin, gastrointestinal (GI) tract, and genitourinary (GU) tract due to chronic infections at these sites. IFN gamma-1b reduces the frequency and severity of infections in patients with CGD. Off-label indications include infections by *Mycobacterium avium* complex (MAC), pulmonary fibrosis, and ovarian cancer. The most common adverse effects include flulike symptoms, nausea, vomiting, diarrhea, rash, and elevated hepatic enzymes. Because of the potential for neutropenia and thrombocytopenia, periodic CBCs are required. This drug is pregnancy category C.

PegIFN alfa-2a (Pegasys): PegIFN alfa-2a is a biologic response modifier that has a molecule of PEG attached to IFN alfa-2a, which is identical to the natural IFN produced by human lymphocytes and macrophages. Approved in 2002, it is prepared through recombinant DNA technology and is available as single-use prefilled syringes and administered by the subcutaneous route. Approved indications for pegIFN alfa-2a include chronic hepatitis B and hepatitis C virus infections that show evidence that the virus is replicating. Off-label uses include renal cell carcinoma and chronic myelogenous leukemia. Patients should be monitored for depression and suicidal ideation. Neutropenia and thrombocytopenia are uncommon

but may be severe. Other potential adverse effects include colitis, pancreatitis, hyper- or hypothyroidism, hypertension (HTN), and dysrhythmias. A black box warning for IFNs states that these drugs may cause or aggravate fatal or life-threatening neuropsychiatric, autoimmune, ischemic, or infectious disorders. This drug is pregnancy category C.

PegIFN alfa-2b (Pegintron, Sylatron): Approved in 2001, pegIFN alfa-2b (Pegintron) is indicated for the treatment of chronic hepatitis C in patients age 3 years or older with compensated liver disease. It may be used off-label to treat chronic hepatitis B infections and neoplastic disease. Pegintron is usually given in combination with the antiviral ribavirin over a period of 24 to 48 weeks. It is important to note that ribavirin can cause fetal injury and death and is a possible carcinogen. Sylatron was approved in 2011 for the adjunctive treatment of melanoma that has lymph node involvement.

PegIFN alfa-2b has a molecule of PEG attached to the IFN molecule, which gives the drug an extended half-life. Peak concentrations can be sustained for 48 to 72 hours, which results in greater antiviral activity. The most frequently reported adverse effects with pegIFN alfa-2b are injection-site reactions, fatigue, headache, rigors, fever, nausea, myalgia, and emotional lability. A black box warning for IFNs states that these drugs may cause or aggravate fatal or life-threatening neuropsychiatric, autoimmune, ischemic, or infectious disorders. This drug is pregnancy category C (X if used with ribavirin).

42.3 Interleukins, vaccines, and colony-stimulating factors are used to boost the immune system.

Interleukins (ILs) are a class of cytokines synthesized by lymphocytes, monocytes, macrophages, and certain other cells in response to antigen exposure. Like IFNs, ILs are signaling molecules that enable cells of the immune system to communicate with each other. The ILs, however, work by different mechanisms than the IFNs. The ILs have widespread effects on immune function that include the following:

- Stimulation of cytotoxic T-cell activity against tumor cells
- Activation and increased production of natural killer (NK) cells
- Increased B-cell and plasma cell production
- Increased neutrophil chemotaxis
- Promotion of inflammation

More than 30 different ILs have been identified, though only a few are available as medications. IL-2, which is derived from helper T cells, promotes the proliferation of both T cells and activated B cells. It is available as aldesleukin (Proleukin), which is indicated for the treatment of metastatic renal carcinoma and metastatic melanoma. IL-11, which is derived from bone marrow cells, is a growth factor with multiple hematopoietic effects. It is marketed as oprelvekin (Neumega) for its ability to stimulate platelet production in patients with immunosuppression. Oprelvekin is featured as a prototype drug in Chapter 39. Some interleukins are used in the pharmacotherapy of RA.

Bacillus Calmette-Guérin (BCG) vaccine (TheraCys, Tice) is a biologic response modifier that is available to enhance the immune system. BCG is an attenuated strain of *Mycobacterium bovis* used for the pharmacotherapy of certain types of bladder cancer.

Vaccines are types of immunostimulants that have the ability to mobilize the body against specific antigens. A small amount of an inactivated antigen is administered and the patient develops an immune reaction. If reexposed to the antigen in future years, memory B or T cells will develop a rapid response, eliminating the antigen before it causes disease. Vaccines are presented in Chapter 43.

The final type of immunostimulant includes the colony-stimulating factors, which are drugs that promote the production of white blood cells (WBCs). For example, filgrastim (Neupogen) stimulates the production of granulocytes, and sargramostim (Leukine) activates multiple types of leukocytes. These drugs are used to shorten the length of neutropenia in patients with cancer and in those who have had a bone marrow transplant and whose bone marrow has been suppressed by drugs. Filgrastim, the prototype, and other colony-stimulating factors are presented in Chapter 39.

CONNECTION Checkpoint 42.1

From what you learned in Chapter 39, what is the primary indication of oprelvekin (Neumega) therapy, and what is its most important adverse effect? *See Answer to Connection Checkpoint 42.1 on student resource website.*

PROTOTYPE DRUG	Aldesleukin (Proleukin)

Classification: Therapeutic: Immunostimulant
Pharmacologic: Interleukin, biologic response modifier

Therapeutic Effects and Uses: Approved in 1992, aldesleukin has a structure very similar to natural IL-2, and it has identical actions in the body. It is FDA approved for the pharmacotherapy of metastatic renal cell carcinoma and metastatic malignant melanoma. It has been designated by the FDA as an orphan drug for the chemotherapy of non-Hodgkin's lymphoma and acute myelogenous leukemia. It is used off-label to treat leprosy.

CONNECTIONS | Community-Oriented Practice

◄ Fever in the Patient on Immunosuppressant Drugs

Immunosuppressant drugs are now given to treat a variety of conditions, and more uses are being discovered. Patients taking immunosuppressants are at great risk for infection but may not always experience symptoms to the same degree that patients with competent immune systems do. The patient must be assessed for subtle signs of infection including low-grade fevers (less than 37.8°C [100°F]), unusual skin lesions with or without drainage, excessive fatigue, malaise, arthralgias, cough, headache, diarrhea, or nausea. Any of these symptoms should be immediately reported to the health care provider so that appropriate follow-up examination can be conducted. Before going home with an immunosuppressant drug, the patient should receive explicit instructions on when to call the provider for a fever and how often the temperature should be taken when fever is present or symptoms such as those listed above are present. Antipyretics such as ibuprofen are usually not appropriate because they can mask the symptoms of a significant infection. Many patients on immunosuppressant drugs are able to live active, normal lives. However, they should be taught measures to reduce the exposure risk to infections, and should always receive appropriate instruction for fever management before they begin to take the medication.

Aldesleukin is a very toxic drug that should only be administered by personnel familiar with its use. It must be administered in multiple, brief IV infusions because of its short half-life.

Mechanism of Action: The mechanism of action of aldesleukin is identical to that of endogenous IL-2. It initiates a series of actions that activate IFNs, TNF, and other ILs. The drug promotes proliferation of both B cells and T cells, macrophages, and NK cells, which in turn increase the body's ability to fight cancer cells.

Pharmacokinetics:

Route(s)	IV
Absorption	N/A
Distribution	Widely distributed; unknown if secreted in breast milk
Primary metabolism	Renal
Primary excretion	Renal
Onset of action	Unknown
Duration of action	Half-life: 85 min

Adverse Effects: Aldesleukin is a toxic drug that has the potential to cause serious adverse effects in virtually any organ system. Many of the adverse effects are caused by **capillary leak syndrome**, a serious condition in which plasma proteins and other substances leave the blood and enter the interstitial spaces because of porous capillaries. If not monitored carefully, capillary leak syndrome can result in death. Over 70% of patients taking aldesleukin will experience hypotension, which can sometimes be severe enough to cause tissues and organs to receive an insufficient blood supply to function properly. Tachycardia and other dysrhythmias occur in a significant number of patients. Diarrhea, nausea, or vomiting may occur in as many as half the patients taking the drug. Other common adverse effects include confusion, drowsiness, oliguria, stomatitis, anorexia, hyperbilirubinemia, hypothyroidism, elevated hepatic enzymes, weight gain, dyspnea, and pulmonary congestion. Common changes in blood values include thrombocytopenia, anemia, and leukopenia. Flulike symptoms such as fever and malaise occur frequently. **Black Box Warnings**: Aldesleukin can cause capillary leak syndrome, which can be severe. Death may result from infection that can spread throughout the body because of impaired neutrophil function. If moderate to severe fatigue develops, the drug should be withheld. The drug should be used with extreme caution in patients with a history of cardiac or pulmonary disease.

Contraindications/Precautions: There are many contraindications to using aldesleukin, and a thorough baseline assessment of health status is required. If the assessment indicates a preexisting bacterial infection, this should be treated prior to initiating therapy with aldesleukin. Aldesleukin should not be administered to patients with developing moderate to severe lethargy because the drug may induce coma. Patients with significant cardiac, central nervous system (CNS), pulmonary, renal, or hepatic impairment should not receive this drug. Aldesleukin may cause seizures and should be used with caution in patients with epilepsy. This drug may worsen the condition of patients with autoimmune disease, including those with scleroderma, RA, diabetes mellitus, and thyroiditis.

Drug Interactions: Aldesleukin has the potential to interact with nearly any other drug. Given concurrently with aldesleukin, drugs that affect mental status such as many antianxiety agents, opioids, sedatives, or antipsychotic agents may cause mood disturbances and drowsiness. Concurrent administration with drugs that are hepatotoxic or nephrotoxic may cause additive organ damage. Caution should be used when using agents that modify coagulation such as aspirin, nonsteroidal anti-inflammatory agents (NSAIDs), or platelet inhibitors due to an increased risk of bleeding. Antihypertensive drugs may cause additive hypotension when used with aldesleukin. **Herbal/Food**: None known.

Pregnancy: Category C.

Treatment of Overdose: Dexamethasone may be used to reverse some of the toxicities observed from an overdose of aldesleukin.

Nursing Responsibilities: Key nursing implications for patients receiving aldesleukin are included in the Nursing Practice Application for Patients Receiving Pharmacotherapy with Immunomodulators.

Drugs Similar to Aldesleukin (Proleukin)

The only other IL approved by the FDA is IL-11, a platelet enhancer marketed as oprelvekin (Neumega), which is featured as a prototype in Chapter 39. BCG vaccine is a miscellaneous biologic response modifier. An additional immunostimulant, levamisole (Ergamisol), has been discontinued in the United States.

Bacillus Calmette-Guérin vaccine (TheraCys, Tice): BCG vaccine is a live, attenuated vaccine that is available in two distinct strains with different indications. Both forms are pregnancy category C.

TheraCys: TheraCys is approved for the prophylaxis and treatment of patients with superficial bladder cancer. This drug is instilled into the urinary bladder for 2 hours, after which the patient voids the medication. The treatment may be repeated at 3-month intervals. TheraCys produces a nonspecific immune reaction in the bladder that attracts lymphocytes, macrophages, and NK cells to the site of the cancer. Adverse effects include local reactions such as bladder irritability, hematuria, dysuria, cystitis, incontinence, and nocturia. A flulike syndrome may occur.

Tice: Tice is used to stimulate immunity against *Mycobacterium tuberculosis*. Vaccination with BCG simulates exposure to tuberculosis and induces an immune response against the organism. This drug is used to prevent tuberculosis and is not given to treat active infections. It is the only FDA-approved treatment for tuberculosis prophylaxis. The drug is not 100% effective and its length of protection is variable. Flulike symptoms often develop 1 to 2 days after administration. Minor skin papules appear at the site of percutaneous puncture.

Immunosuppressants

42.4 Immunosuppressants are used to prevent transplant rejection and for the treatment of autoimmune disorders.

Used to inhibit the immune response, immunosuppressants are prescribed for patients who are receiving transplanted tissues or organs and to treat autoimmune disorders. Doses for these agents are listed in Table 42.2.

Transplantation: Transplants may include specific cells, parts of tissues, or complete organs. They may originate from the patient's own body (autografts), genetically identical donors (isografts), or genetically dissimilar donors (allografts). Most transplantation procedures use allografts.

Typing for transplanted tissues attempts to match, as closely as possible, donor and recipient human leukocyte antigen (HLA) and ABO blood-type antigens. Despite accurate tissue matching, allografts always contain certain antigens that have the potential to trigger the patient's immune defenses. This response, called **transplant rejection**, is often acute; antibodies sometimes destroy the transplanted tissue within 48 hours after a transplant. The cell-mediated branch of the immune system responds more slowly to the transplant, attacking it about 2 weeks following surgery. Chronic rejection of the transplant may occur months or even years after surgery.

Successful transplantation requires the use of immunosuppressant drugs. One or more immunosuppressants are administered at the time of transplantation and are continued for several months following surgery. In some cases, they are continued indefinitely at low doses. Transplantation would be impossible without the use of effective immunosuppressant drugs. Although immunosuppressant therapies have proven very successful at preventing acute transplant rejection, they have been far less successful at preventing chronic rejection.

Prior to the initiation of immunosuppressant therapy, it is critical that the patient be carefully assessed to rule out active infections. This includes screening for viruses such as cytomegalovirus (CMV), hepatitis B and C viruses, Epstein-Barr virus (EBV), VZV, HIV, and herpes simplex virus (HSV). If an active infection is discovered, it should be treated prior to transplantation. In addition, patients should be screened for the presence of cancer prior to surgery because immunosuppressant drugs will allow preexisting cancers to grow rapidly.

During immunosuppressant therapy the patient is susceptible to infection from all types of pathogens: viral, bacterial, fungal, or protozoan. Infections in immunosuppressed patients are called opportunistic infections. Opportunistic pulmonary infections are the leading cause of morbidity and mortality in patients receiving a transplant. Many patients receive antibiotics for the prophylaxis of opportunistic infections for 4 to 12 months following surgery. Six months following the transplant, 80% of patients will return to their baseline risk of infection, but the remainder will remain at high risk indefinitely.

Long-term survivors of transplants are also at high risk of developing cancers. These include non-Hodgkin's lymphoma, squamous and basal cell skin cancer, cervical cancer, and Kaposi's sarcoma. Regular follow-up monitoring for cancer is required in these patients.

PharmFACT

More than 123,000 patients are waiting for organ transplants. About 82% of these are waiting for a kidney, 13% for a liver, and 3% for a heart (Organ Procurement and Transplantation Network, 2014).

Autoimmune disorders: Autoimmune disorders are those in which the body creates antibodies against normal tissues. The body attacks its own cells as if they were foreign, resulting in tissue injury. Examples of autoimmune disorders include RA, SLE, myasthenia gravis, and Hashimoto's thyroiditis.

TABLE 42.2 Immunosuppressants

Drug	Route and Adult Dose (Maximum Dose Where Indicated)	Adverse Effects
Antibodies		
antithymocyte globulin (Atgam, Thymoglobulin)	IV (Atgam): 10–30 mg/kg daily IV: (Thymoglobulin): 1.5 mg/kg daily infused over 4–6 h for 7–14 days	*Local reactions at the injection site (pain, erythema, myalgia), influenza-like symptoms (malaise, fever, chills), headache, dizziness* Anaphylaxis, HTN, infections (may occur in many different body systems), thrombocytopenia, leukopenia, renal impairment (basiliximab), antithymocyte globulin
basiliximab (Simulect)	IV: 20 mg times two doses (first dose 2 h before surgery; second dose 4 days after transplant)	
Cytotoxic Drugs and Antimetabolites		
anakinra (Kineret)	Subcutaneous: 100 mg (0.67 mL) once daily	*Injection-site reactions, urinary tract infection, headache, nausea, diarrhea, sinusitis, arthralgia, flulike symptoms* Leukopenia, infections, malignancy, anaphylaxis
azathioprine (Azasan, Imuran)	PO/IV: 3–5 mg/kg/day initially; may be able to reduce to 1–3 mg/kg/day	*Nausea, vomiting, anorexia* Severe nausea and vomiting, bone marrow suppression, thrombocytopenia, serious infections, malignancy, hepatotoxicity
belatacept (Nulojix)	IV: 5–10 mg/kg using enclosed silicone-free disposable syringe	*Anemia, diarrhea, urinary tract infection, peripheral edema, hypertension, pyrexia, cough, nausea, leukopenia* Post-transplant lymphproliferative disorder, progressive multifocal leukoencephalopathy, serious infections, malignancies
cyclophosphamide (Cytoxan)	PO: 2.5–3 mg/kg daily for a period of 60–90 days (higher doses are used for malignant disease)	*Nausea, vomiting, anorexia, neutropenia, alopecia* Anaphylaxis, leukopenia, pulmonary emboli, interstitial pulmonary fibrosis, toxic epidermal necrolysis, Stevens–Johnson syndrome, hemorrhagic cystitis, oligospermia
etanercept (Enbrel)	Subcutaneous: 50 mg once/week	*Injection-site reactions (pain, erythema, myalgia), abdominal pain, vomiting, headache* Infections, pancytopenia, leukopenia, anemia, myocardial infarction (MI), heart failure, malignancy
methotrexate (Rheumatrex, Trexall)	PO/IM/IV: 15–30 mg/day for 5 days; repeat every 12 weeks for three courses	*Headache, glossitis, gingivitis, mild leukopenia, nausea, alopecia* Ulcerative stomatitis, myelosuppression, aplastic anemia, hepatic cirrhosis, nephrotoxicity, sudden death, pulmonary fibrosis, or pneumonia
mycophenolate (CellCept, Myfortic)	PO/IV: 720 mg bid in combination with corticosteroids and cyclosporine; start within 24 h of transplant	*Peripheral edema, diarrhea, headache, tremor, dyspepsia, abdominal pain* Urinary tract infection, leukopenia, anemia, thrombocytopenia, sepsis, HTN
thalidomide (Thalomid)	PO: 100–300 mg/day (max: 400 mg/day) for at least 2 weeks	*Rash, mild leukopenia, fever, dizziness, diarrhea, malaise, drowsiness* Toxic epidermal necrolysis, birth defects (pregnancy category X), orthostatic hypotension, neutropenia, peripheral neuropathy
Calcineurin Inhibitors		
cyclosporine (Gengraf, Neoral, Sandimmune)	PO: Transplants: 5–10 mg/kg/day PO: Autoimmune disorders: 1.25–2.5 mg/kg/day (max: 4 mg/day)	*Hirsutism, tremor, nausea, vomiting* HTN, MI, nephrotoxicity, hyperkalemia, seizures, paresthesia, hepatotoxicity
tacrolimus (Prograf)	PO: 0.1–0.15 mg/kg/day in two divided doses every 12 h; give first PO dose 8–12 h after discontinuing IV therapy IV: 0.03–0.05 mg/kg/day as continuous infusion	*Oliguria, nausea, constipation, diarrhea, headache, abdominal pain, insomnia, peripheral edema, fever* Infections, HTN, nephrotoxicity, neurotoxicity (tremors, paresthesia, psychosis), hyperkalemia, anemia, hyperglycemia, malignancy, thrombocytopenia, seizures
Kinase Inhibitors (Rapamycins)		
everolimus (Afinitor, Zortress)	PO (Afinitor): 10 mg once daily PO (Zortress): Begin with 0.75 mg bid and adjust to achieve a trough concentration of 3–8 ng/mL	*Peripheral edema, hyperlipidemia, nausea, hypertension, UTI, asthenia, weight changes (loss or gain), elevated serum creatinine, hyperglycemia and fever* Leukopenia, anemia, thrombocytopenia, sepsis, secondary infections, malignancy, anaphylaxis, interstitial lung disease or pneumonia, birth defects
sirolimus (Rapamune)	PO: 6–15 mg loading dose immediately after the transplant, then 2–5 mg/day maintenance dose	
temsirolimus (Torisel)	IV: 25 mg once weekly infused over 30–60 min	

Note: Italics indicate common adverse effects. <u>Underline</u> indicates serious adverse effects.

Autoimmune diseases are characterized by symptomatic periods alternating with remissions. Although the remissions may last many months or even years, relapses are often progressive, with symptoms worsening as the disease progresses. During acute relapses, fever and signs of widespread inflammation may be present. Virtually any tissue or organ may be affected, depending on the specific autoimmune disease.

Unlike transplant recipients who may receive immunosuppressants indefinitely, patients with autoimmune disease are usually given these drugs for brief periods in high doses to control relapses. In some cases, however, these patients may receive low doses for longer periods for prophylaxis.

The immunosuppressant class includes drugs that block the immune response by several different mechanisms, as shown in Pharmacotherapy Illustrated 42.1. These include blocking the receptors and production of IL-2, inhibiting the proliferation of T cells, and using antibodies specific to certain receptors or cells of the immune response. The drugs may be classified into the following categories:

- Calcineurin inhibitors and similar drugs
- Cytotoxic drugs and antimetabolites
- Antibodies
- Corticosteroids (glucocorticoids)

PHARMACOTHERAPY ILLUSTRATED 42.1

Mechanism of Action of Immunosuppressants

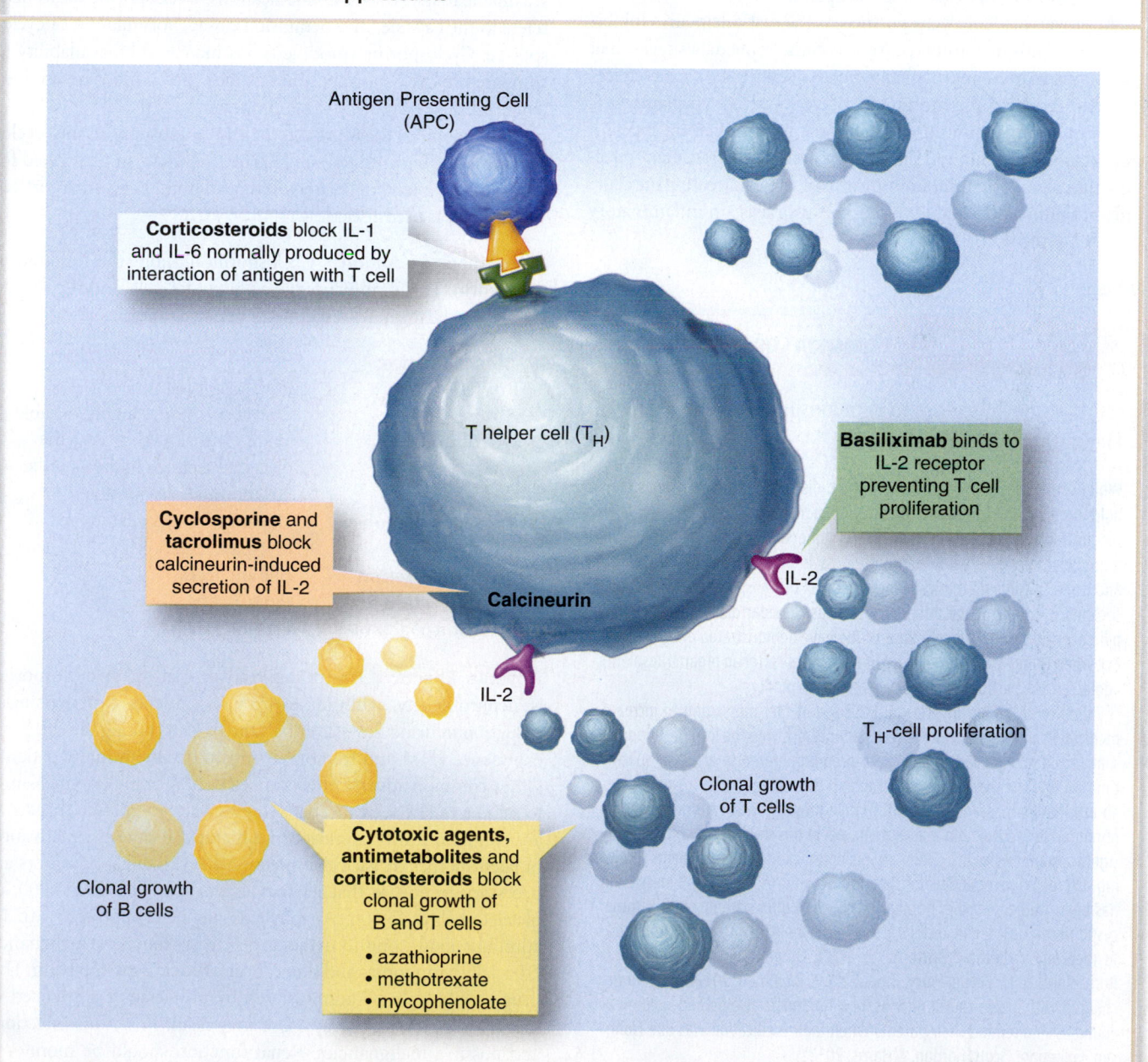

Antigen Presenting Cell (APC)

Corticosteroids block IL-1 and IL-6 normally produced by interaction of antigen with T cell

T helper cell (T$_H$)

Basiliximab binds to IL-2 receptor preventing T cell proliferation

Cyclosporine and **tacrolimus** block calcineurin-induced secretion of IL-2

Calcineurin

IL-2

IL-2

T$_H$-cell proliferation

Clonal growth of T cells

Cytotoxic agents, antimetabolites and **corticosteroids** block clonal growth of B and T cells
- azathioprine
- methotrexate
- mycophenolate

Clonal growth of B cells

42.5 Calcineurin inhibitors are preferred drugs for the prophylaxis of transplant rejection.

When a T cell encounters an antigen, calcineurin is activated. **Calcineurin** is an enzyme that acts as an intracellular messenger, telling the T cell to begin synthesizing IL-2. As described in Section 42.3, IL-2 is an important chemical mediator in promoting the proliferation of B cells, T cells, macrophages, and NK cells. Blocking IL-2 suppresses the immune response.

Two of the most important drugs in transplant medicine, cyclosporine (Sandimmune, Neoral) and tacrolimus (Prograf), are calcineurin inhibitors. These drugs revolutionized the pharmacotherapy of transplant rejection and have been the mainstay of transplant therapy since the 1980s. Although newer medications have been developed, the calcineurin inhibitors remain critical drugs for transplant recipients. The calcineurin inhibitors allow the doses of corticosteroids to be lowered, thereby reducing the incidence of opportunistic infections following transplants.

Approved in 1983, cyclosporine was the first calcineurin inhibitor and remains the prototype for this class. Some data suggest that tacrolimus may be more effective in preventing transplant rejection and reducing the mortality associated with transplants. It is the most common immunosuppressant used in certain types of transplants. In addition to their use in preventing transplant rejection, the calcineurin inhibitors are also of value in treating the acute inflammation associated with RA and psoriasis, an inflammatory disorder of the skin.

CONNECTIONS Lifespan Considerations

◀ Increasing Adherence to Immunosuppressive Medication in Pediatric Patients

While sometimes viewed as an unwanted distraction, text messages may hold promise for increasing medication adherence. Forgetting to take medication is a problem in maintaining adherence to any medication. In immunosuppressive therapy, forgetfulness is potentially life threatening and can result in a dramatically increased risk of transplant graft rejection. Techniques to encourage adherence such as calendar diaries or electronic pill boxes that signal when a dose is due have demonstrated effectiveness. But when trying to live as normal a life as possible after an organ transplant, adolescents may choose not to use standard reminders.

Miloh et al. (2009) investigated the use of text messaging to increase medication adherence in adolescent patients receiving the immunosuppressant tacrolimus. Text messages were preprogrammed to arrive at specific times before the medication was due and the patient had to respond with an affirmative message. If no affirmative message was returned, another reminder was sent within a set time frame. In this small study, a statistically significant difference in adherence was noted in adolescent patients receiving text message reminders for their medication. The use of text messaging has been studied in other populations including for patients with asthma, cystic fibrosis, HIV, and other chronic diseases with increased adherence to medication therapy (Britto et al., 2012; Horvath, Azman, Kennedy, & Rutherford, 2012; Petrie, Perry, Broadbent, & Weinman, 2012). For younger children with access to cell phones, text reminders also helped children as young as 7 to remind their parents when their medication was due (Johnson, Culpepper, Scott, Gordon, & Harris, 2011).

PROTOTYPE DRUG Cyclosporine (Gengraf, Neoral, Sandimmune)

Classification: **Therapeutic:** Immunosuppressant
Pharmacologic: Calcineurin inhibitor

Therapeutic Effects and Uses: Cyclosporine is a complex chemical obtained from a soil fungus. It is FDA approved for the prophylaxis of kidney, heart, and liver transplant rejection; psoriasis; severe RA; and xerophthalmia, an eye condition of diminished tear production caused by ocular inflammation. Off-label indications include a number of autoimmune and inflammatory conditions such as ulcerative colitis, SLE, myasthenia gravis, aplastic anemia, Crohn's disease, psoriatic arthritis, and graft-versus-host disease.

Cyclosporine may be administered as capsules, oral solution, or IV or as an ophthalmic solution (Restasis) for xerophthalmia. Due to the risk of anaphylaxis, the IV route is used only when patients are unable to take oral (PO) medications. Cyclosporine (modified) refers to the capsule, microemulsion dosage formulation of cyclosporine. Cyclosporine (modified) has increased bioavailability as compared to cyclosporine (nonmodified) and cannot be used interchangeably without close monitoring.

Unlike some of the more cytotoxic immunosuppressants, cyclosporine is less harmful to bone marrow cells. When prescribed for transplant recipients, it is often used in combination with a corticosteroid such as prednisone.

Mechanism of Action: Cyclosporine inhibits the function of calcineurin. This diminishes the activity of T cells and B cells and suppresses the immune response.

Pharmacokinetics:

Route(s)	PO, IV, ophthalmic
Absorption	Oral absorption is highly variable
Distribution	Widely distributed; crosses the placenta; secreted in breast milk; 90% bound to lipoproteins
Primary metabolism	Hepatic (CYP3A), extensive first-pass metabolism
Primary excretion	Bile and feces
Onset of action	Peak: 3–4 h
Duration of action	Half-life: 16–27 h

Adverse Effects: The primary adverse effect of cyclosporine is nephrotoxicity, with up to 75% of patients experiencing a reduction in urine flow. Over half the patients taking the drug will experience HTN and tremor. Hirsutism occurs in many patients. Other common adverse effects are elevated hepatic enzymes, mild to moderate HTN, headache, and gingival hyperplasia. Infections are common during cyclosporine therapy, including reactivation of latent herpes or varicella infections. Periodic blood counts are necessary to ensure that leukocytes do not fall below 4,000, or platelets below 75,000. Anaphylaxis has been reported with IV administration. Long-term therapy increases the risk of malignancy, especially lymphomas and skin cancers. **Black Box Warning**: This drug should only be administered by physicians experienced in immunosuppressive therapy. Use may result in serious infections and possible malignancies. Renal function should be monitored during therapy.

Contraindications/Precautions: Patients who are taking cyclosporine should avoid direct exposure to the sun due to an increased risk of skin cancer. Because cyclosporine is nephrotoxic, the drug is either contraindicated or should be used with extreme caution in patients with renal impairment: Renal laboratory function should be regularly evaluated. The drug should not be used during pregnancy or lactation. Because cyclosporine is primarily eliminated via the bile, its dose should be reduced in patients with hepatic or biliary impairment. Patients with active infections should be treated with anti-infectives prior to cyclosporine therapy. Caution should be used in patients with preexisting HTN because the drug may worsen this condition.

Drug Interactions: Cyclosporine is a major substrate of CYP3A4 and may interact with drugs that inhibit or induce this enzyme. Drugs that may decrease cyclosporine levels include phenytoin, phenobarbital, carbamazepine, and rifampin. Azole antifungal drugs, oral hypoglycemics, and macrolide antibiotics may increase cyclosporine levels. Because cyclosporine increases blood pressure, the doses of antihypertensives will require adjustment. Potassium-sparing diuretics should be avoided because their concurrent use with cyclosporine causes hyperkalemia. Cyclosporine should be given with caution with other nephrotoxic drugs due to the potential for additive kidney damage. Statins should not be used concurrently with cyclosporine due to the potential for myopathy or rhabdomyolysis. **Herbal/Food:** Food decreases the absorption of the drug. Grapefruit juice can raise cyclosporine levels by 50% to 200%. The immune-enhancing effects of astragalus and echinacea may interfere with the action of immunosuppressants.

Pregnancy: Category C.

Treatment of Overdose: An overdose of cyclosporine can result in significant nephrotoxicity and hepatotoxicity. General supportive measures are indicated.

Nursing Responsibilities: Key nursing implications for patients receiving cyclosporine are included in the Nursing Practice Application for Patients Receiving Pharmacotherapy with Immunomodulators.

Drugs Similar to Cyclosporine (Gengraf, Neoral, Sandimmune)

The only other calcineurin inhibitor is tacrolimus. Although not calcineurin inhibitors, everolimus, sirolimus, and temsirolimus are immunosuppressants similar to tacrolimus.

Everolimus (Afinitor, Zortress): Everolimus is a newer drug in this class initially approved in 2009 (Afinitor) to treat advanced renal cell carcinoma and astrocytoma. In 2010, the drug (Zortress) was approved for the prophylaxis of organ rejection in patients receiving a kidney transplant. The dose when used as an antineoplastic is much higher than that when used in transplant patients (see Table 42.2). In transplant medicine, the drug is given in combination with basiliximab and concurrently with reduced doses of cyclosporine and corticosteroids. To prevent potential toxicity, therapeutic drug monitoring is recommended.

Everolimus is functionally similar to sirolimus and temsirolimus and blocks a key kinase enzyme that activates B and T cells. Like most immunosuppressants, the drug carries a black box warning regarding its potent immunosuppressive actions and the possible development of serious infections and malignancies. In addition the black box warning includes an increased risk of kidney damage, including renal arterial and venous thrombosis. The drug is pregnancy category C.

Sirolimus (Rapamune): Approved in 1999, sirolimus is a PO drug isolated from a soil bacterium that shares a similar structure and potent immunosuppressant properties with tacrolimus. Sirolimus, however, acts by a unique mechanism; that is, it binds to a protein known as FKBP that prevents T-cell activation and proliferation and the production of antibodies by B cells. Sirolimus does not exhibit the serious organ toxicity characteristic of tacrolimus. This drug appears to be less effective than the calcineurin inhibitors, but it does exert synergistic immunosuppression when used with other immunosuppressive agents. Sirolimus is only approved for use in the prophylaxis of kidney transplant rejection in combination with cyclosporine and corticosteroids for the first year after transplantation. At 2 to 4 months post-transplantation, the cyclosporine may be gradually withdrawn over a 4- to 8-week period. The serum levels of sirolimus must be adjusted upward when cyclosporine is withdrawn. Adverse effects include hyperlipidemia, hypercholesterolemia, peripheral edema, tremor, azotemia, elevated serum creatinine, HTN, diarrhea, and anemia. Like most immunosuppressants, the drug carries a black box warning regarding its potent immunosuppressive actions and the possible development of serious infections and malignancies. In addition, the black box warning states that the use of this drug is not recommended in patients with liver transplants (excess mortality and graft loss) or lung transplants (bronchial rupture). This drug is pregnancy category C.

Tacrolimus (Prograf): Approved by the FDA in 1994, tacrolimus is available in PO capsule or IV forms for the prophylaxis of heart and liver transplant rejection. It is used off-label for other transplants as well as for graft-versus-host disease, nephritic syndrome, psoriasis, and uveitis. A topical form of tacrolimus (Protopic) is indicated for the short-term treatment of eczema and atopic dermatitis; the topical drug contains a black box warning of possible lymphoma and skin cancer. Tacrolimus is 100 times more potent than cyclosporine and appears to be more effective in some patients at preventing transplant rejection. Nephrotoxicity may occur in half the patients taking this drug. Neurotoxicity symptoms are common and include headache, tremor, paresthesias, insomnia, and dizziness. Hypertension, anemia, hyperglycemia, and GI complaints occur in a significant number of patients who are taking tacrolimus. Like cyclosporine, an increased incidence of infections and malignancies may occur with tacrolimus use. This drug is pregnancy category C.

Temsirolimus (Torisel): Approved in 2007, temsirolimus is structurally similar to sirolimus and acts by the same mechanism. In fact, temsirolimus is metabolized in the liver to sirolimus. It is approved to treat patients with advanced renal cell carcinoma that has not responded to other therapies. This drug is administered only by the IV route. Temsirolimus is toxic to the hematologic system; 94% of patients will experience anemia, 53% will experience lymphopenia, and 32% will experience leukopenia. Hyperglycemia occurs in most patients; thus patients with diabetes will require close monitoring. Most patients who are taking the drug will also experience hyperlipidemia that may be serious enough to require pharmacotherapy. Interstitial lung disease is a rare though potentially fatal adverse effect. This drug is pregnancy category D.

PharmFACT

Each day in the United States about 18 people die waiting for transplants. One organ donor can save up to eight lives (OrganDonor .Gov, n.d.).

42.6 Cytotoxic drugs and antimetabolites are used to suppress proliferating B cells and T cells.

Cytotoxic drugs are immunosuppressive agents used to kill B cells and T cells. Antimetabolites do not kill directly, but instead severely restrict the replication of B cells and T cells. Each of these medications acts by a different mechanism. Some of the drugs resemble essential chemical building blocks needed for the biosynthesis of DNA and block replication. Others inhibit protein synthesis. Most of the cytotoxic and antimetabolite immunosuppressants are nonspecific, affecting many different cells of the immune response. They have the same general indications and adverse effects as the calcineurin inhibitors.

PROTOTYPE DRUG	Azathioprine (Azasan, Imuran)

Classification: **Therapeutic:** Immunosuppressant
Pharmacologic: Cytotoxic agent

Therapeutic Effects and Uses: An older immunosuppressant approved in 1968, azathioprine is indicated for the prophylaxis of kidney transplant rejection and for the treatment of severe RA. Off-label indications include other inflammatory disorders such as Crohn's disease, autoimmune hepatitis, myasthenia gravis, SLE, and ulcerative colitis. When treating nontransplant conditions, it is generally prescribed only when standard treatments fail.

Azathioprine is usually given PO, but it may be given by the IV route to patients who are unable to take the drug by mouth. When used to prevent transplant rejection, it is usually administered in combination with other immunosuppressants.

Mechanism of Action: Azathioprine inhibits DNA synthesis, resulting in DNA damage and chromosome breakage. The drug is metabolized to mercaptopurine in the liver, an active substance marketed as an antineoplastic drug for leukemia.

Pharmacokinetics:

Route(s)	PO, IV
Absorption	Well absorbed
Distribution	Crosses the placenta; secreted in breast milk; 30% bound to plasma proteins
Primary metabolism	Hepatic; metabolized to mercaptopurine, an active metabolite
Primary excretion	Renal
Onset of action	7–14 days
Duration of action	Half-life: 3 h

Adverse Effects: Azathioprine causes bone marrow suppression that can result in pancytopenia, agranulocytosis, leukopenia, and thrombocytopenia. Serious infections may occur secondary to immunosuppression, and latent herpes or varicella infections may become reactivated during azathioprine therapy. Hepatotoxicity has been reported with this drug. Nausea and vomiting are common, especially during the first few weeks of therapy. Patients who have received a renal transplant and who are being treated with azathioprine have an increased risk of developing skin and lymphoid malignancies. The toxicities of azathioprine are dose related and occur more frequently in patients who have received a renal transplant compared

---

CONNECTIONS   Complementary and Alternative Therapies

◖Echinacea

Description
Nine species of echinacea have been identified, and all are native to the midwestern United States and central Canada. *Echinacea purpurea* (purple coneflower) and *Echinacea angustifolia* (narrow-leaf coneflower) are the two most commonly studied species. All portions of the plant contain chemicals that have potential pharmacologic activity.

History and Claims
Echinacea was used by Native Americans to treat various wounds and injuries. Until the widespread manufacture of antibiotics in the late 1940s, echinacea was commonly used as an anti-infective.

Standardization
The flowers, leaves, and stems of this plant are harvested and dried. Preparations include dried powder, tincture, fluid extracts, and teas. No single ingredient seems to be responsible for the herb's activity. A large number of potentially active chemicals have been identified from the extracts. Recommended doses include 300 mg dry powdered extract (standardized to 3.5% echinacoside) or 0.5 to 1 g dried root or tea.

Evidence
There has been wide variation in the quality and doses of echinacea used in research studies, which makes comparisons and conclusions extremely difficult. Echinacea is claimed to boost the immune system by increasing IFN levels, increasing phagocytosis, and inhibiting the bacterial enzyme hyaluronidase. Some substances in echinacea appear to have antiviral activity; thus the herb is sometimes taken to treat the common cold and influenza—indications for which it has received official approval in Germany. A recent study disputed this claim, however, and no significant difference was found between research participants taking echinacea and those taking a placebo (Barrett et al., 2010). In general, echinacea is used as a supportive treatment for any disease involving inflammation and to enhance the immune system. Adverse effects are rare, although it may cause allergic reactions in patients who are allergic to plants in the daisy family such as ragweed, marigolds, daisies, and chrysanthemums (National Center for Complementary and Alternative Medicine, 2012). It may also interfere with drugs that have immunosuppressant effects.

with those who are treated for RA. **Black Box Warning**: Use may result in serious or fatal infections and possible malignancies. Complete blood counts (CBCs) should be monitored during therapy.

Contraindications/Precautions: Azathioprine should be used with extreme caution in patients with preexisting hematologic disease or hepatic impairment. Blood counts and hepatic enzymes must be regularly monitored. Azathioprine is contraindicated during pregnancy and lactation.

Drug Interactions: Additive bone marrow suppression is expected if azathioprine is given concurrently with other immunosuppressants. Concurrent use of allopurinol with azathioprine can result in a large increase in azathioprine activity and hematologic toxicity. The use of angiotensin-converting enzyme (ACE) inhibitors with azathioprine may induce anemia and severe leukopenia. **Herbal/Food**: None known.

Pregnancy: Category D.

Treatment of Overdose: Hemodialysis may be of value in removing some azathioprine from the blood following an overdose. Other treatment measures are supportive.

Nursing Responsibilities: Key nursing implications for patients receiving azathioprine are included in the Nursing Practice Application for Patients Receiving Pharmacotherapy with Immunomodulators.

Drugs Similar to Azathioprine (Azasan, Imuran)

Other cytotoxic and antimetabolite drugs indicated for immunosuppression include anakinra, belatacept, cyclophosphamide, etanercept, methotrexate, mycophenolate, and thalidomide.

Anakinra (Kineret): Approved in 2001, anakinra is an IL-1 receptor antagonist that prevents the formation of certain inflammatory cytokines. This drug's only indication is for the treatment of moderate to severe RA that has not responded to first-line agents. It is administered only by the subcutaneous route and injection-site reaction is the most frequent adverse effect. Because the drug lowers WBC counts, secondary infections occur in almost 40% of patients taking anakinra. This drug is pregnancy category B.

Belatacept (Nulojix): Belatacept is a newer cytotoxic drug, approved in 2011 for the prophylaxis of organ rejection in patients receiving kidney transplants. The drug blocks specific receptors on T lymphocytes, inhibiting their proliferation and stopping the production of cytokines that could damage a newly transplanted organ. The drug acts by the same mechanism as abatacept (Orencia), which is approved to treat RA. Belatacept is always used in combination with basiliximab, mycophenolate mofetil, and corticosteroids. The drug carries a black box warning that it may increase the risk for developing post-transplant lymphoproliferative disorder (PTLD). PTLD is a condition in which B cells proliferate unchecked and may cause B-cell tumors. The warning also states that the drug may increase the risk for malignancies and that it should not be used for liver transplants due to possible graft rejection. Belatacept is pregnancy category C.

Cyclophosphamide (Cytoxan): Cyclophosphamide is one of the most commonly prescribed antineoplastic medications for patients with malignancies. It acts by forming cross-links in DNA, which

prevents cancer cell replication. It is a powerful immunosuppressant, affecting both B cells and T cells. It is used off-label for SLE, graft-versus-host disease, and RA, and for the transplant prophylaxis of solid organs. Hematologic toxicity (pancytopenia, leukopenia, anemia, and thrombocytopenia) is a major dose-limiting adverse effect. Cyclophosphamide is a prototype antineoplastic drug discussed in Chapter 57. This drug is pregnancy category D.

Etanercept (Enbrel): Approved in 1998, etanercept is a protein that mimics the natural receptor for TNF. Rather than binding to its receptors on T cells, TNF binds with the etanercept. This inhibition of TNF activity reduces the levels of damaging cytokines responsible for causing inflammation and joint destruction in patients with RA. The drug is FDA approved to treat RA, psoriatic arthritis, plaque psoriasis, and ankylosing spondylitis. It is used off-label to prevent transplant rejection. It is administered only by the subcutaneous route. The most common adverse effects are injection-site reactions and infections. Etanercept has a black box warning regarding the possibility of malignancy and serious infections during therapy, including tuberculosis and bacterial sepsis. This drug is pregnancy category B.

Methotrexate (Rheumatrex, Trexall): Methotrexate is an older antimetabolite approved in 1953 that acts by inhibiting the enzyme responsible for folic acid metabolism. Like cyclophosphamide, it is indicated for various cancers as well as serious inflammatory disorders such as RA, psoriasis, SLE, and ulcerative colitis. Methotrexate is used off-label to prevent transplant rejection. The most frequently reported adverse reactions include nausea, vomiting, stomatitis, esophagitis, oral ulceration, and abdominal distress. Hematologic adverse reactions are common. The drug carries a black box warning regarding the possibility of malignancy and serious hematologic, GI, hepatic, pulmonary, and dermatologic toxicity. Methotrexate is a prototype antineoplastic drug discussed in Chapter 57. This drug is pregnancy category X.

Mycophenolate (CellCept, Myfortic): Approved in 1995, mycophenolate is a potent immunosuppressant that acts by inhibiting the DNA synthesis of B cells and T cells. There are two forms of mycophenolate. Mycophenolate mofetil (CellCept) is a prodrug that is converted in the body to its active form, mycophenolic acid. It is given IV or PO, usually in combination with other immunosuppressants such as cyclosporine and corticosteroids. Mycophenolate sodium (Myfortic) is a delayed release tablet.

Indications for mycophenolate include the prophylaxis of heart, kidney, or liver transplant rejection. Mycophenolate appears to be more effective than azathioprine for the prophylaxis of transplant rejection. This drug was recently given orphan drug status for the treatment of patients with myasthenia gravis and pemphigus vulgaris. Off-label indications include SLE, graft-versus-host disease, and atopic dermatitis. GI adverse effects such as nausea, vomiting, constipation, diarrhea, dyspepsia, and abdominal pain are common. Other relatively frequent adverse effects include tachycardia, tremor, back pain, sinusitis, increased urinary frequency, and blood dyscrasias. Weekly CBCs should be obtained and the drug withheld if the absolute neutrophil count (ANC) falls below $1.3 \times (10)^3$ cells/mcL. Mycophenolate carries a black box warning regarding the possibility of malignancy and serious infections. This is a pregnancy category D drug.

Thalidomide (Thalomid): Thalidomide is an infamous drug that caused serious fetal malformations in patients who were pregnant and took the drug in the late 1950s. At that time the drug was not approved for use in the United States, but it was available in other countries as a sedative. Thalidomide has received orphan drug status for the treatment of a variety of neoplastic and immune-related disorders, including primary brain malignancies, graft-versus-host disease, Crohn's disease, Kaposi's sarcoma, HIV-wasting syndrome, leprosy, stomatitis, *Mycobacterium* infections, and multiple myeloma. Other off-label indications include SLE and renal cell cancer. The drug is highly regulated and is available only through a limited number of pharmacists and physicians. Because the drug is pregnancy category X, a negative pregnancy test is required prior to administration in women with childbearing potential. Adverse effects include teratogenesis, thromboembolic disease, drowsiness, and peripheral neuropathy. Thalidomide carries a black box warning regarding its teratogenic effects, as well as a high risk of thromboembolic events occurring during therapy.

42.7 Antibodies are used to prevent acute transplant rejection, autoimmune disorders, and malignancies.

Recall from Chapter 40 that antibodies are proteins that are produced following an antigen challenge. B cells become plasma cells, which subsequently produce massive amounts of antibodies that help rid the body of the antigen through several mechanisms. Antibodies that are produced by a plasma cell are very specific to the antigen. For example, exposure to *Streptococcus* would result in different antibodies than would *Escherichia coli*. In this example, antibodies *boost* the immune system. It may seem puzzling then to learn that certain antibodies may be administered to patients to *suppress* the immune response. How is this possible?

The answer is to create antibodies against human immune cells. A simple method is to inject animals (usually horses, rabbits, or mice) with human T cells, B cells, or thymocytes. The animal forms antibodies against the human immune cells, which can be collected and purified. When injected in humans, the animal's antibodies will attack the T cells (or T-cell receptors). These are called **polyclonal antibodies** because they contain a wide mixture of different antibodies. This polyclonal drug product, called

antithymocyte globulin (Atgam, Thymoglobulin), is a potent immunosuppressant and is available for the prophylaxis of kidney transplant rejection and aplastic anemia.

In the 1980s a technique was developed to harvest antibodies produced by a single B cell. Because a single B cell produces a single antibody, it is called a **monoclonal antibody (MAB)**. A MAB is very specific, targeting a single type of target cell or receptor. This allows greater effects on the target cell or receptor at lower doses and with fewer adverse effects than using polyclonal antibodies.

The first MABs were derived from mouse cells and had short half-lives. The human immune system quickly recognized them as foreign when they were injected in patients. Through genetic engineering, scientists have been able to replace the mouse portions of the antibody with human sequences, thus allowing it to escape detection by the immune system for longer periods and extending its half-life.

Scientists have created approximately 30 different MABs to attack a diverse number of targets. The majority of the MABs are designed to attack specific types of cancer cells. Others are used to treat autoimmune or inflammatory disorders such as RA or psoriasis by attacking specific cells of the immune system that secrete proinflammatory mediators. The FDA-approved MABs are listed in Table 42.3. Those used exclusively for cancer are found in Chapter 57.

Only one MAB is approved as an immunosuppressant in transplant medicine. Basiliximab (Simulect) is given concurrently with other drugs such as cyclosporine and azathioprine to prevent the acute rejection of kidney transplants. Two MABs previously approved for the prophylaxis of transplant rejection, daclizumab (Zenapax) and muromonab-3 (OKT-3), are no longer marketed in the United States.

The MABs are difficult to learn because many have similar names that end in -*mab* (for *m*onoclonal *a*nti*b*ody). There is, however, some consistency to the names—they reflect the origin of the antibody:

- MABs that have 75% human sequences are called chimeric and have -*xi* in the name (e.g., basiliximab).

- MABs that have 90% human sequences are called humanized and have -*zu* in their name (e.g., trastuzumab).

- MABs that are 100% human have -*mumab* in their name (e.g., golimumab).

TABLE 42.3	Selected Monoclonal Antibodies for Immunosuppression		
Drug/Antibody	**Approval Date**	**Target**	**Approved Treatment(s)**
adalimumab (Humira)	2002	Inhibition of TNF-α signaling	Inflammatory diseases (mostly autoimmune disorders)
basiliximab (Simulect)	1998	IL-2 receptor blocker	Transplant rejection
belimumab (Benlysta)	2011	B lymphocytes	Systemic lupus erythematosus
certolizumab pegol (Cimzia)	2008	TNF blocker	Crohn's disease and RA
eculizumab (Soliris)	2007	Complement system protein C5	Inflammatory diseases, including paroxysmal nocturnal hemoglobinuria
golimumab (Simponi)	2009	TNF blocker	Psoriatic arthritis, ankylosing spondylitis and RA
infliximab (Remicade)	1998	Inhibition of TNF-α signaling	Inflammatory diseases (mostly autoimmune disorders)
natalizumab (Tysabri)	2006	T-cell VLA4 receptor	Inflammatory diseases (mainly autoimmune-related MS therapy)
siltuximab (Sylvant)	2014	IL-6 receptor blocker	Castleman disease (rare blood disorder)
tofacitinib (Xeljanz)	2012	JAK enzyme inhibitor	RA
tocilizumab (Actemra)	2010	IL-2 receptor blocker	RA

| PROTOTYPE DRUG | Basiliximab (Simulect) |

Classification: Therapeutic: Immunosuppressant
Pharmacologic: Monoclonal antibody

Therapeutic Effects and Uses: Basiliximab is a monoclonal antibody approved in 1998 for the prophylaxis of transplant rejection. The drug dampens the immune response by inhibiting CD25, a receptor on the surface of activated T cells. By binding to CD25, basiliximab stops IL-2 from activating the T cell, and the immune response is prevented. This drug does not lower the total number of circulating T cells; it does, however, lower their ability to respond to an antigen challenge.

Administered by IV infusion, the standard regimen is two doses; one is given 2 hours prior to transplantation and the other is given 4 days later. Following the two infusions, the actions of basiliximab may last for 4 to 6 weeks. The only approved indication for basiliximab is for prophylaxis of kidney transplant rejection. It is administered in combination with other immunosuppressants, usually cyclosporine and corticosteroids.

Mechanism of Action: Basiliximab inhibits the binding of IL-2 to CD25 on the surface of activated T-cells. This prevents the rapid proliferation of T-cells that would normally release cytokines to attack transplanted tissue.

Pharmacokinetics:

Route(s)	IV
Absorption	N/A
Distribution	Unknown
Primary metabolism	Unknown
Primary excretion	Unknown
Onset of action	30 min
Duration of action	7.2 day half-life

Adverse Effects: Basiliximab causes few adverse effects compared to the calcineurin inhibitors or the cytotoxic immunosuppressants. The most common adverse effects are GI related such as nausea, vomiting, abdominal pain, and diarrhea. Anaphylaxis has been reported. **Black Box Warning**: Basiliximab should only be used by physicians experienced in immunosuppressive therapy.

Contraindications/Precautions: The only contraindication to the use of basiliximab is hypersensitivity to the drug. Because patients receiving this drug have suppressed immune systems, vaccinations are normally postponed until immune function returns.

Drug Interactions: Basiliximab does not interact significantly with the major drugs used in transplant medicine. However, caution must always be used when administering multiple drugs that suppress immune function. **Herbal/Food**: None known.

Pregnancy: Category B.

Treatment of Overdose: Overdose with this drug is very rare, since only 2 doses are administered.

Nursing Responsibilities: Key nursing implications for patients receiving basiliximab are included in the Nursing Practice Application for Patients Receiving Pharmacotherapy with Immunomodulators.

Drugs Similar to Basiliximab (Simulect)

The other antibody drug used in transplant medicine is antithymocyte globulin, although it is a polyclonal antibody rather than a MAB. The MABs used for RA such as adalimumab (Humira) and infliximab (Remicade) are discussed in Chapter 72.

Antithymocyte globulin (Atgam, Thymoglobulin): Approved in 1981, antithymocyte globulin consists of polyclonal antibodies obtained from the serum of horses (Atgam) or rabbits (Thymoglobulin) exposed to human T cells. Doses of the two are not interchangeable. The drug is a potent immunosuppressant used for the prophylaxis and management of transplant rejection and for the treatment of moderate to severe aplastic anemia in patients who are unable to have bone marrow transplantation. It is used off-label to treat graft-versus-host disease and myelodysplastic syndrome. Given by the IV route, a single infusion may lower the lymphocyte count by 85% to 90%. After discontinuation of therapy, T-cell counts take several months to return to baseline levels. The most common adverse effects are fever, chills, malaise, headache, diarrhea, itching, and other flulike symptoms. Corticosteroids, antihistamines, and acetaminophen may be administered 1 hour prior to antithymocyte globulin therapy to prevent **cytokine release syndrome**. Anaphylaxis has been reported. Like other immunosuppressants, an increased incidence of infections and malignancies is expected. A black box warning states that antithymocyte globulin should only be used by physicians experienced in immunosuppressive therapy. This drug is pregnancy category C.

CONNECTION Checkpoint 42.2

Basiliximab (Simulect) binds to CD25 and an immune response is prevented. From what you learned in Chapter 40, which type of immunity, humoral or cell-mediated, does this drug affect? *See Answer to Connection Checkpoint 42.2 on student resource website.*

42.8 Corticosteroids are widely used as immunosuppressants but have significant long-term adverse effects.

The corticosteroids, or glucocorticoids, are potent inhibitors of inflammation and are discussed in detail in Chapters 41 and 68. They are often the drugs of choice for the short-term therapy of severe inflammation.

In addition to their anti-inflammatory effects, corticosteroids affect nearly every aspect of the immune response. They intervene at multiple steps in the immune response, including antigen presentation, production of cytokines, and the proliferation of lymphocytes.

- **Lymphocyte effect.** A single dose of corticosteroid reduces circulating lymphocyte counts within a few hours. This inhibits the ability of the body to react to an antigen challenge.

- **Monocyte effect.** Corticosteroids quickly deplete the body of monocytes and macrophages. Macrophages are responsible for presenting antigens to lymphocytes.

- **Neutrophil effect.** Corticosteroids cause neutrophils to move from the bone marrow into the general circulation, resulting in increased numbers of circulating neutrophils. The drug then prevents the neutrophils from migrating out of the circulation to sites of inflammation.

CONNECTIONS: NURSING PRACTICE APPLICATION

Patients Receiving Pharmacotherapy with Immunomodulators

Assessment	Potential Nursing Diagnoses*
Baseline assessment prior to administration: • Obtain a complete health history including previous history or current case of cancer; fever; active infections (especially herpes, varicella, and CMV); hepatic, renal, cardiovascular, neurologic, or autoimmune disease; dermatologic conditions; HIV infection; pregnancy or breast-feeding. Obtain a drug history, especially the use of corticosteroids. • Obtain a dietary history, especially the intake of grapefruit or grapefruit juice. • Obtain baseline vital signs, especially blood pressure and temperature, height, and weight. • Assess oral and dental health. • Evaluate appropriate laboratory findings (e.g., CBC, platelets, electrolytes, glucose, hepatic and renal laboratory values, and lipid levels). • Assess the patient's ability to receive and understand instructions. Include the family and caregivers as needed.	• *Anxiety* or *Fear* • *Ineffective Family Therapeutic Regimen Management* • *Impaired Oral Mucous Membranes*, related to drug treatment • *Social Isolation* • *Deficient Knowledge* (Drug Therapy) • *Risk for Infection*, related to drug treatment • *Risk for Injury*, related to adverse drug effects
Assessment throughout administration: • Assess for desired therapeutic effects (e.g., no signs or symptoms of transplant rejection, no severe inflammatory response; suppression of autoimmune responses). • Continue monitoring CBC, platelets, electrolytes, glucose, liver and renal function studies, and lipid levels. • Assess vital signs, especially blood pressure and temperature. • Assess for and immediately report adverse effects: fever, chills, visible signs of infection, nausea, vomiting, dizziness, confusion, muscle weakness, tremors, tachycardia, HTN, angina, syncope, dyspnea, pulmonary congestion, skin rashes, bruising or bleeding, decreased urine output.	

Implementation

Interventions and (Rationales)	Patient-Centered Care
Ensuring therapeutic effects: • Continue assessments as above for therapeutic effects. (Monitoring will be specific to the transplant, e.g., maintenance of urine output, or specific patient condition. Severe inflammatory conditions and autoimmune disorders should show gradually lessening inflammation and pain.)	• Advise the patient on the treatment and condition-specific monitoring requirements (e.g., urine output, improvement of movement in joints with lessened swelling).
Minimizing adverse effects: • Continue to monitor vital signs, especially blood pressure and temperature. (Immunosuppressant drugs may cause HTN and increase the risk of infections. Immunostimulants may cause hypotension. **Lifespan:** Be particularly cautious with older adults who are at increased risk for hypotension and at greater risk for falls.)	• Teach the patient how to monitor blood pressure. Ensure proper use and functioning of any home equipment obtained. The patient should report blood pressure over 140/90 mmHg or parameters set by the health care provider. Chest pain or pressure should be reported immediately. • Teach the patient to report any fever over 38.3°C (101°F) or as instructed by the health care provider. • Instruct the patient taking immunostimulants to rise from lying to sitting or standing slowly to avoid dizziness or falls. If dizziness occurs, the patient should sit or lie down and not attempt to stand or walk until the sensation passes.

• Observe for signs and symptoms of infection: fever over 38.3°C (101°F) or parameters set by the health care provider, sore throat, diarrhea, malaise, white patches in the oral cavity, painful or vesicular rashes, reddened or warm areas at the site of injury, or lethargy. (Immunosuppressants increase the risk of infections, especially with opportunistic infections such as herpes, varicella, CMV, and fungal infections. **Diverse Patients**: Because some drugs such as cyclosporine (Gengraf, Neoral, Sandimmune) metabolize through the P450 system pathways, monitor ethnically diverse patients to ensure optimal therapeutic effects and to minimize adverse effects.)	• Teach the patient to immediately report signs and symptoms of infection such as wounds with redness or drainage, increasing cough, increasing fatigue, white patches on oral mucous membranes, white and itchy vaginal discharge, or itchy blister-like vesicles on the skin.
	• Instruct the patient, family, and caregivers on infection control measures, including:
	  • Washing hands frequently. Use lotion afterwards to prevent excessive drying and cracking of the skin.
	  • Avoiding large crowds, especially indoors.
	  • Avoiding people with known infection or young children because they have a higher risk of having an infection.
	  • Cooking food thoroughly, allowing the family or caregiver to prepare raw meat or fish and clean up, and not consuming raw fruits or vegetables.

CONNECTIONS: NURSING PRACTICE APPLICATION (continued)

• Assess for changes in level of consciousness, disorientation, confusion, or tremors. (Neurologic changes may indicate adverse drug effects.)	• Instruct the patient, family, or caregiver to immediately report increasing lethargy, disorientation, confusion, changes in behavior or mood, slurred speech, tremors, or ataxia.
• Continue to monitor CBC, platelets, electrolytes, glucose, liver and renal function studies, and lipid levels. (Immunosuppressants may cause leukopenia, anemia, thrombocytopenia, hyperglycemia, and hyperkalemia. **Lifespan:** Monitor the older adult frequently because age-related physiological changes increase the risk of adverse renal and hepatic effects.)	• Instruct the patient on the need to return frequently for follow-up laboratory work. • Advise the patient to carry a wallet identification card or wear medical identification jewelry indicating immunosuppressant therapy.
• Inspect oral mucous membranes, and schedule dental appointments prior to starting drug therapy and frequently thereafter. (Immunosuppression increases the risk of oral candidiasis and gingivitis. Oral antifungal rinses may be required.)	• Teach the patient to maintain excellent oral hygiene, inspecting the oral cavity daily. Keep regular dental visits, and consult the dentist about the required frequency.
• Assess diet and consumption of grapefruit or grapefruit juice. (Grapefruit juice significantly increases cyclosporine levels and should be avoided or eliminated while on immunosuppressant therapy.)	• Teach the patient to avoid or eliminate grapefruit and grapefruit juice while on cyclosporine. Flavored beverages without juice are permissible.
• **Lifespan:** Assess for pregnancy. (Pregnancy should be avoided during and for up to 4 months after discontinuing immunosuppressive therapy. Women who become pregnant while on the drug should consult with their health care provider.)	• Discuss pregnancy and family planning with women of childbearing age. Explain the effect of medications on pregnancy and breast-feeding and the need to discuss any pregnancy plans with the health care provider. Discuss the need for additional forms of contraception, including barrier methods, with patients taking immunosuppressants.
• Assess for development of hirsutism or alopecia. (Hirsutism is reversible when the drug is discontinued. Alopecia may indicate significant immunosuppression.)	• Advise the patient to notify the provider of changes to hair growth or texture.
• Continue to monitor neurologic and mental status in patients receiving IFN therapy. (Psychosis, depression, and suicidal ideations are potential adverse effects of IFN use.)	• Instruct the patient, family, or caregiver to immediately report increasing lethargy, disorientation, confusion, changes in behavior or mood, agitation or aggression, slurred speech, or ataxia.
Patient understanding of drug therapy: • Use opportunities during administration of medications and during assessments to discuss the rationale for drug therapy, desired therapeutic outcomes, commonly observed adverse effects, parameters for when to call the health care provider, and any necessary monitoring or precautions. (Using time during nursing care helps to optimize and reinforce key teaching areas.)	• The patient, family, or caregiver should be able to state the reason for the drug, appropriate dose and scheduling, what adverse effects to observe for and when to report them, and the anticipated length of medication therapy.
Patient self-administration of drug therapy: • When administering medications, instruct the patient, family, or caregiver in proper self-administration techniques followed by return demonstration. (Utilizing time during nurse-administration of these drugs helps to reinforce teaching.)	• Teach the patient to take the medication by: • Using the enclosed equipment to measure or mix the drug. • Using a glass, and not paper or plastic cups, unless the package directions indicate they are to be used. • Mixing the drug with milk, chocolate milk, or orange juice, and stirring well. After taking the drug, rinse the cup with additional liquid and drink it to ensure the entire dose is taken. • Taking the medication at the same time each day.

*Nursing Diagnoses—Definitions and Classification 2015–2017. Copyright © 2014, 1994–2014 by NANDA International. Used by arrangement with John Wiley & Sons Limited.

• **Other effects.** Corticosteroids block the production of prostaglandins and ILs. This results in T cells being unable to react to antigens and proliferate.

Two common drugs in this class, prednisone and methylprednisolone, have been widely used to prevent transplant rejection since the 1960s. When used for a few weeks, the corticosteroids are safe and effective immunosuppressants. The long-term adverse effects of corticosteroids, however, are serious and include osteoporosis, cataract formation, mental status changes, fluid and salt retention, HTN, hyperglycemia, obesity, and adrenal atrophy. Because of their long-term effects, health care providers have begun to look at the possibility of eliminating corticosteroids from the transplant regimen. Some regimens call for the initial use of corticosteroids, with their gradual withdrawal at some point, usually within 3 to 6 months following the transplant. The issue remains unresolved and an area of active research.

42 Understanding the Chapter

Key Concepts Summary

42.1 Immunomodulators are substances that either enhance or suppress the ability of the body to fight infection and disease.

42.2 Interferons are biologic response modifiers that have antiviral and antineoplastic activity.

42.3 Interleukins, vaccines, and colony-stimulating factors are used to boost the immune system.

42.4 Immunosuppressants are used to prevent transplant rejection and for the treatment of autoimmune disorders.

42.5 Calcineurin inhibitors are preferred drugs for the prophylaxis of transplant rejection.

42.6 Cytotoxic drugs and antimetabolites are used to suppress proliferating B cells and T cells.

42.7 Antibodies are used to prevent acute transplant rejection, autoimmune disorders, and malignancies.

42.8 Corticosteroids are widely used as immunosuppressants but have significant long-term adverse effects.

Case Study: Making the Patient Connection

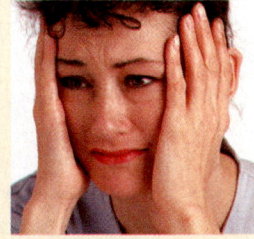

Remember the patient "Carol Banks" at the beginning of the chapter? Now read the remainder of the case study. Based on the information presented within this chapter, respond to the critical thinking questions that follow.

Carol Banks is a 42-year-old woman diagnosed with hepatitis C who was recently seen by her health care provider at an office visit. She reported having right upper quadrant pain, fatigue, anorexia, nausea, and vomiting. She has been feeling progressively worse for the past year but did not seek medical care for her problem. She has lost 5.4 kg (12 lb) over the past 6 months.

Carol was initially hospitalized to receive IV fluids for dehydration and to be further evaluated. Once in the hospital, a full hepatitis panel found that she was positive for hepatitis C virus (HCV).

During the initial interview with Carol, she discloses that she was addicted to illegal IV drugs for 15 years and was an alcohol abuser for 20 years.

However, Carol claims that she has abstained from substance abuse for the past 5 years. She resides with her husband and three children and is employed as a clerk in a local retail convenience store.

As part of the treatment for Carol's hepatitis she is prescribed IFN alfa-2b (Intron A). She is taught to self-administer (subcutaneously) the standard dose of IFN, 3 million units, given three times weekly.

Critical Thinking Questions

1. Discuss the rationale for the use of IFN alfa-2b (Intron A) in the treatment of hepatitis C.

2. What adverse effects is Carol experiencing with this drug therapy? How can the nurse assist Carol to cope with the related adverse effects?

3. Identify the patient education that Carol will need concerning her drug therapy.

See Answers to Critical Thinking Questions on student resource website.

Additional Case Study

Gordon Sharp had been on kidney dialysis since his car crash 2 years ago. He sustained severe traumatic injuries and subsequently developed renal failure. Gordon has recently received a kidney transplant and is currently on cyclosporine (Sandimmune).

1. How does cyclosporine work and why is Gordon receiving the drug?

2. Describe the patient teaching that the nurse should give to Gordon concerning this drug therapy.

3. What dietary precautions would be indicated for this patient?

See Answers to Additional Case Study on student resource website.

Chapter Review

1 The nurse is monitoring the laboratory findings of a patient who is taking interferon alfa-2b (Intron A). Which findings would indicate that the patient is experiencing common adverse effects?

1. Flulike symptoms of fever, chills, fatigue, and weight loss
2. Depression with thoughts of suicide
3. Edema, hypotension, and tachycardia
4. Fluid volume overload, hypertension, renal insufficiency

2 The patient is receiving basiliximab (Simulect) and cyclosporine (Sandimmune) after a kidney transplant to prevent transplant rejection. The patient develops a high fever and chills, with a temperature of 103°F (39.4°C). The nurse interprets that the patient is most likely experiencing:

1. Capillary leak syndrome.
2. A significant infection related to immunosuppression.
3. Graft-versus-host rejection.
4. Androgen-insensitivity syndrome.

3 The nurse who is caring for a patient receiving cyclosporine (Sandimmune) will discontinue the medication immediately and call the provider if which of the following occurs?

1. Red blood cell count above 8.5 million/mm³.
2. White blood cell count below 4,000/mm³.
3. Platelet count above 100,000/mm³.
4. Serum creatinine level less than 1.0 mg/100 mL.

4 Azathioprine (Imuran) is prescribed to a patient who had a renal transplant. A nurse reviews the patient's medical record and would question the medication order for the patient with a history of:

1. Benign prostatic hyperplasia.
2. Cataracts.
3. Varicella zoster.
4. Rheumatoid arthritis.

5 A nurse is instructing a patient who is receiving tacrolimus (Prograf) following a liver transplant. Which point should be included in the teaching plan?

1. Take a "baby" strength aspirin every day.
2. Increase physical activity to avoid weight gain.
3. Record radial pulse rate every morning in a journal.
4. Avoid raw fruits and vegetables and eat only fully cooked meats.

6 A nurse is particularly cautious in monitoring the patient who is prescribed aldesleukin (Proleukin). To monitor for the development of capillary leak syndrome, the nurse would frequently assess:

1. Skin condition and rashes.
2. Laboratory values for increasing amylase and lipase.
3. Blood pressure and urine output.
4. Vision and hearing.

See Answers to Chapter Review in Appendix A.

References

Barrett, B., Brown, R., Rakel, D., Mundt, M., Bone, K., Phyto, D., . . . Ewers, T. (2010). Echinacea for treating the common cold. *Annals of Internal Medicine, 153,* 769–777. doi:10.7326/0003-4819-153-12-201012210-00003

Britto, M. T., Munafo, J. K., Schoetker, P. J., Vockell, A. L., Wimberg, J. A., & Yi, M. S. (2012). Pilot and feasibility test of adolescent-controlled text messaging reminders. *Clinical Pediatrics, 51,* 114–121. doi:10.1177/0009922811412950

Horvath, T., Azman, H., Kennedy, G. E., & Rutherford, G. W. (2012). Mobile phone text messaging for promoting adherence to antiretroviral therapy in patients with HIV infection. *Cochrane Database of Systematic Reviews, 2012*(3), CD009756. doi:10.1002/14651858.CD009756

Johnson, K. B., Culpepper, D., Scott, P., Gordon, J. S., & Harris, C. (2011). The utility of providing automated medication dose reminders to young children on chronic medication. *Journal of Telemedicine and Telecare, 17,* 387–391. doi:10.1258/jtt.2011.110314

Miloh, T., Annunziato, R., Arnon, R., Warshaw, S. P., Suchy, F. J., Iyer, K., & Kerkar, N. (2009). Improved adherence and outcomes for pediatric liver transplant recipients by using text messaging. *Pediatrics, 124*(5), e844–850. doi:10.1542/peds.2009-0415

National Center for Complementary and Alternative Medicine. (2012). *Herbs at a glance: Echinacea.* Retrieved from http://nccam.nih.gov/health/echinacea/ataglance.htm

OrganDonor.Gov. (n.d.). *Becoming a donor: The need is real.* Retrieved from http://www.organdonor.gov/index.html

Organ Procurement and Transplantation Network. (2014). *Waiting list candidates.* Retrieved from http://optn.transplant.hrsa.gov/data/

Petrie, K. J., Perry, K., Broadbent, E., & Weinman, J. (2012). A text message programme designed to modify patients' illness and treatment beliefs improves self-reported adherence to asthma preventer medication. *British Journal of Health Psychology, 17,* 74–84. doi:10.1111/j.2044-8287.2011.02033.x

Selected Bibliography

Coelho, T., Tredger, M., & Dhawan, A. (2012). Current status of immunosuppressive agents for solid organ transplantation in children. *Pediatric Transplantation, 16,* 106–122. doi:10.1111/j.1399-3046.2012.01644.x

Gabardi, S., & Tichy, E. M. (2012). Overview of immunosuppressive therapies in renal transplantation. In A. Chandraker, M. H. Sayegh, & A. K. Singh (Eds.), *Core concepts in renal transplantation* (pp. 97–127). doi:10.1007/978-1-4614-0008-0_6

Herdman, T. H., & Kamitsuru, S. (Eds.). (2014). *NANDA International nursing diagnoses:* *Definitions and classification, 2015–2017.* Oxford, United Kingdom: Wiley-Blackwell.

Kaufman, C. (2011). The secret life of lymphocytes. *Nursing, 41*(6), 50–54. doi:10.1097/01.NURSE.0000396267.88998.f9

Krensky, A. M., Bennett, W. M., & Vincenti, E. (2011). Immunosuppressants, tolerogens, and immunostimulants. In L. L. Brunton, B. A. Chabner, & B. C. Knollman (Eds.), *The pharmacological basis of therapeutics* (12th ed., pp. 1005–1030). New York, NY: McGraw-Hill.

Linde, K., Barrett, B., Bauer, R., Melchart, D., & Woelkart, K. (2006). Echinacea for preventing and treating the common cold. *Cochrane Database of Systematic Reviews, 2006* (1), CD000530. doi:10.1002/14651858.CD000530.pub2

Maggi, E., Vultaggio, A., & Matucci, A. (2011). Acute infusion reactions induced by monoclonal antibody therapy. *Expert Review of Clinical Immunology, 7,* 55–63. doi:10.1586/eci.10.90

Pelligrino, B. (2013). Immunosuppression. *Medscape Reference.* Retrieved from http://emedicine.medscape.com/article/432316-overview#a1

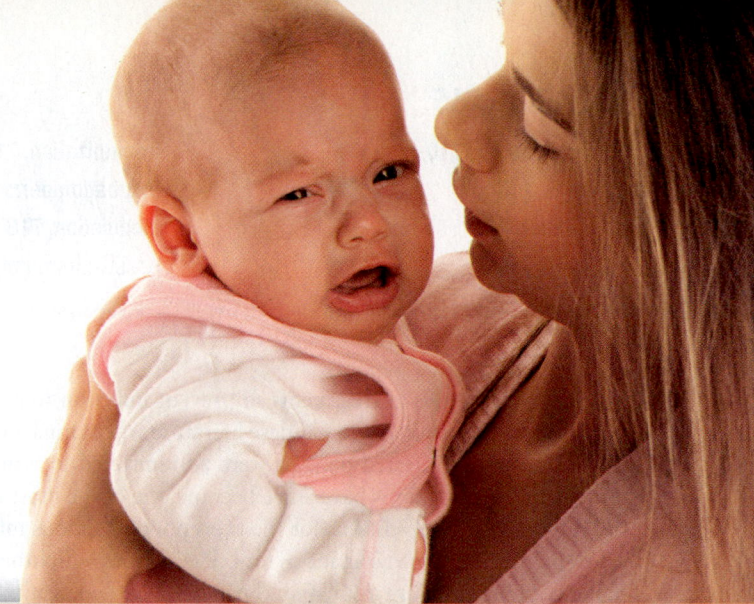

"I don't think these immunizations are necessary. They made her so sick last time!"

Mother of patient "Samantha Abbott"

CHAPTER

43

Immunizing Agents

LEARNING OUTCOMES

After reading this chapter, the student should be able to:

1. Explain why the development of vaccines was one of the most significant discoveries of modern medicine.

2. Compare and contrast active and passive immunity.

3. Explain the immune response that leads to the development of active immunity.

4. Prepare a table listing the types of vaccines, their indications, and potential adverse effects.

5. Explain why it is important to administer childhood vaccines at specific ages.

6. Identify contraindications for vaccine administration.

7. Describe the pathogenesis and immunization of bacterial infections, including diphtheria, pertussis, tetanus, pneumococcus, and meningococcus.

8. Describe the pathogenesis and immunization of viral infections, including hepatitis A and B, influenza, rabies, measles, mumps, rubella, polio, varicella zoster, human papillomavirus, and rotavirus.

9. Explain the rationale for administering antibodies to establish passive immunity.

10. For each of the major vaccines and patient age groups, identify the schedule for the recommended dosage sequence established by the Centers for Disease Control and Prevention.

11. Apply the nursing process to care for patients receiving immunizing agents.

CHAPTER OUTLINE

▸ Discovery of Vaccines

▸ Vaccines and the Immune System

▸ Types of Vaccines

▸ General Principles of Vaccine Administration

▸ Active Immunity: Bacterial Immunizations

▸ Active Immunity: Viral Immunizations

   PROTOTYPE Hepatitis B Vaccine (Engerix-B, Recombivax HB), *p. 716*

▸ Passive Immunity

   PROTOTYPE Rh$_o$ [D] Immune Globulin (RhoGAM), *p. 721*

KEY TERMS

active immunity, 710

antigens, 710

attenuated, 711

boosters, 710

immunization, 710

incubation period, 710

inoculation, 710

passive immunity, 710

postherpetic neuralgia, 719

shingles, 719

toxoids, 711

vaccination, 710

The earliest attempts at treatments to prevent infection were reported in ancient Indian and Chinese literature when dried, powdered scabs from infected persons were administered to healthy individuals. Vaccinations have since become one of the most important medical interventions for the prevention of serious infectious disease. Routine vaccinations for polio, pertussis, diphtheria, tetanus, and measles are estimated to prevent 3 million deaths annually. This chapter examines the role of vaccines in promoting the health of both children and adults and the potential adverse effects of these drugs.

Discovery of Vaccines

43.1 The eradication of smallpox was a great triumph in modern medicine.

In the 1790s, Dr. Edward Jenner was experimenting with the use of **inoculation**, the placement of a foreign substance on or in an individual for the purpose of disease prevention. Inoculation uses live virus particles obtained from an infected patient. Jenner used the cowpox virus, a benign pathogen in humans, because he predicted that exposure to that virus would provide immunity to smallpox, which was one of the most dreaded human diseases of that era. Case fatality rates of 30% or more were reported with smallpox infections. In the 18th century, the disease was a frequent cause of blindness and death for 400,000 people worldwide annually.

Jenner's inoculation of a single 8-year-old boy ultimately led to one of the greatest triumphs in disease prevention. On May 8, 1980, the World Health Assembly certified that global medical interventions had actually eradicated smallpox infections from the planet. Although this announcement was heralded by the scientific community as proof of the success of routine immunization, it also has presented new challenges. With the last known case of the disease, the need for smallpox immunization ceased, resulting in a growing, nonimmune population. The widespread release of a modified smallpox organism to an unvaccinated population could be a potential terrorist weapon (see Chapter 75).

Vaccines and the Immune System

43.2 Vaccines are used to activate the immune system for the purpose of disease prevention.

An immune response occurs when an antigen is recognized by the B or T lymphocytes. **Antigens** are microbes and foreign substances that elicit an immune response. Most microbes, nonhuman proteins, bacterial or plant toxins, and normal cells that become damaged or cancerous are considered antigens. Following the first exposure to an antigen, sufficient time is needed for the body to process the antigen and mount an effective response. It is during this time, known as the **incubation period**, that the symptoms of infection and tissue injury develop. During this first antigen exposure, memory B cells or T cells are formed. Should a second or subsequent exposure to the same antigen occur, the memory cells react quickly to produce a more rapid immune response with fewer (or no) symptoms of infection. The student should review Chapter 40 for a summary of the humoral and cell-mediated immune responses before proceeding.

Edward Jenner was the first to use the term *vaccination*. **Vaccination** is the process of introducing foreign proteins or inactive cells (vaccines) into the body to trigger immune activation *before* the patient is exposed to the real pathogen. As a result of the vaccination, memory B cells or T cells are formed. When later exposed to the real infectious organism, these cells will react quickly by producing large quantities of antibodies and cytokines that help to neutralize or destroy the antigen. Whereas some vaccinations are needed only once, most require follow-up doses, known as **boosters**, to provide prolonged protection. The type of response induced by the real pathogen, or its vaccine, is called **active immunity**. During this response the body produces its own antibodies in response to exposure. The active immunity induced by vaccines closely resembles that caused by natural exposure to the antigen, including the generation of memory cells. The term **immunization** is considered equivalent to the term *vaccination*, and either one may be used to describe this process of disease prevention.

The effectiveness of most vaccines can be assessed by measuring the amount of antibodies produced after the vaccine has been administered, a quantity called *titer*. If the titer falls below a specified, protective level over time, a booster dose is indicated. Antibodies are a product of the humoral immune system. The cell-mediated immune system is also important in producing immunity, but its cellular responses are less readily measured.

Passive immunity occurs when preformed antibodies are transferred or "donated" from one person to another. For example, maternal antibodies cross the placenta and provide protection for the fetus and newborn. Other examples of passive immunity include the administration of immune globulin following exposure to hepatitis, antivenins for snakebites, and sera to treat botulism, tetanus, and rabies. The drugs for passive immunity are administered when the patient has already been exposed to a virulent pathogen, or when the patient is at very high risk for exposure and there is not sufficient time to develop active immunity. Patients who are immunosuppressed may receive these agents to prevent infections. Because these drugs do not stimulate the patient's immune system, no memory cells are produced and protective effects last only 2 to 3 weeks. Passive immunity is presented in Section 43.7.

Most vaccines are administered with the goal of *preventing* illness. Common vaccines include those used to prevent patients from acquiring measles, influenza, diphtheria, polio, pertussis (whooping cough), tetanus, and hepatitis B. Anthrax vaccine has been used to immunize people who are at high risk for exposure to anthrax from a potential bioterrorism incident (see Chapter 75). In the case of infection by the human immunodeficiency virus (HIV), experimental HIV vaccines are given after infection has occurred for the purpose of enhancing the immune response, rather than preventing the disease. Unlike other vaccines, experimental vaccines for HIV have thus far been unable to prevent acquired immunodeficiency syndrome (AIDS).

CONNECTION Checkpoint 43.1

The humoral and cell-mediated immune responses are components of the specific (adaptive) body defenses. From what you learned in Chapter 40, compare and contrast the humoral and cell-mediated responses to an antigen. *See Answer to Connection Checkpoint 43.1 on student resource website.*

Types of Vaccines

43.3 There are four traditional methods of producing vaccines.

The goal of vaccine administration is to induce long-lasting immunity to a pathogen without producing an illness in an otherwise healthy person. Therefore, the microorganisms and other substances used as vaccines must be able to strongly activate the immune system but be modified to pose no significant risk of disease development. The vaccine must be economical to develop and be stable for storage and administration. For disease protection to be long standing, the vaccine must be able to stimulate the production of memory B cells and T cells. There are four traditional methods of producing safe and effective vaccines, as listed in Table 43.1. All four methods are capable of inducing active immunity.

Attenuated (live) vaccines: Live vaccine products contain microorganisms that are capable of replicating and causing disease. Live vaccines are very effective at inducing immunity but are not used for vaccination because of their risk. However, effective vaccines can be developed from organisms that are **attenuated** or rendered less able to cause disease through the application of heat or chemicals. Attenuated (live) vaccines cause the development of

a mild or subclinical case of the disease while still inducing lasting immunity. The type of immune response obtained from the administration of a live or attenuated organism is the same as if the patient had been exposed to the natural, nonattenuated organism. There must, however, be adequate immune functioning for the vaccine to work. The use of attenuated (live) vaccines is dangerous for individuals who are immunosuppressed because the organism may retain some residual ability to replicate and cause disease. In very rare cases, the attenuated virus may mutate to an infectious form in patients who received the vaccine. An example of a live or attenuated vaccine is the measles, mumps, and rubella (MMR) vaccine.

Inactivated (killed) vaccines: Inactivated or killed vaccines are of two types: whole agent and subunit. Whole-agent vaccines consist of microbes killed by heat or chemicals. Subunit vaccines consist of specific segments of a cell membrane, foreign proteins, or sequences of a chromosome rather than the whole microbe.

Inactivated or killed vaccines are safer than live vaccines because the organism is unable to replicate, mutate, or cause disease. Subsequent booster doses are required to maintain immunity if inactivated or killed vaccines are used. Examples of inactivated or killed vaccines include the influenza and hepatitis A vaccines. Examples of subunit vaccines are the human papillomavirus (HPV) vaccine and the acellular pertussis vaccine.

Toxoid vaccines: Some pathogens secrete toxins, which are responsible for the symptoms of the infection. **Toxoids** are bacterial toxins that have been chemically modified to be incapable of causing disease. When injected as a type of immunization, toxoids induce the formation of antibodies that are capable of neutralizing the real toxins. Toxoids attack the bacterial toxin, not the invading pathogen itself. Examples include the diphtheria and tetanus toxoids.

Recombinant technology vaccines: Modern biologic techniques have allowed the development of vaccines that include partial organisms or proteins that are generated in the laboratory. Perhaps the best example of the use of this form of biotechnology is for the development of the hepatitis B immunization. It was originally obtained from the serum of infected individuals but carried the risk of transmitting HIV when it was administered as a vaccine. Through advances in recombinant deoxyribonucleic acid (DNA) technology, yeast cells have been reengineered to produce proteins very similar to those found on the coating of the hepatitis B virus, allowing for the development of safe immune protection from this virus.

TABLE 43.1 Vaccine Types			
Type of Vaccine	**Immune System Response**	**Vaccine Examples**	**Remarks**
Attenuated (live) virus	B-cell response; T-cell response	Polio (oral), measles, mumps, rubella, varicella	Risk for disease in persons with reduced immune function
Inactivated (killed) virus	B-cell response	Salk polio (injectable), influenza, rabies, hepatitis A	Does not confer lifelong immunity
Toxoid	B-cell response	Tetanus toxoid, diphtheria toxoid	Large quantities of antigen needed
Recombinant technology vaccine	B-cell response	Hepatitis B	Area of current research interest

General Principles of Vaccine Administration

43.4 Vaccines should be administered by an established schedule with precautions taken for patients who are immunosuppressed or pregnant.

The effective use of vaccines requires that they be delivered according to a specified schedule at the proper dose. Childhood vaccines have a specific age range at which they should be administered. Should the child miss the recommended vaccination date, "catch-up" doses can sometimes be administered to provide adequate protection. In addition, comorbid health conditions sometimes cause the delay of vaccinations in certain patients. Although each vaccine has different indications, certain general principles apply to the administration of most immunizations.

In the United States, the Centers for Disease Control and Prevention (CDC) is the government agency that establishes immunization schedules. Immunization protocols are reviewed on a regular basis by the CDC's Advisory Committee on Immunization Practices, and revisions are frequently made based on current research. The practicing nurse should refer often to the CDC website for updates.

Many of vaccine-preventable diseases are rare in the United States, but endemic to specific regions of the world. The nurse should advise patients traveling to these regions to check that their vaccinations are current. The CDC provides updated country-specific health information for those traveling abroad.

Dose and timing: The total dose of a vaccine is important for the development of immunity. For some vaccinations, multiple doses are required to achieve immunity. Omitting subsequent doses could result in the lack of full disease protection.

To prevent childhood diseases, certain vaccinations should begin at birth and proceed with booster doses at specific ages according to the schedule recommended by the CDC. The timing established by the CDC allows the vaccine to be given prior to the expected exposure to the pathogen. For example, the pertussis vaccine is begun in the first few months of life because infection by *Bordetella pertussis* often occurs by age 1 or 2 years. On the other hand, vaccination for HPV is recommended at 11 to 12 years of age because this virus is spread by sexual contact, which often occurs during the teen years. Vaccination outside the guidelines of the vaccination schedule is permitted, but its effectiveness may be reduced.

Route of administration: Vaccines must be administered by the specific route indicated for each product. Failure to follow administration protocol may result in an insufficient immune response. For example, hepatitis B vaccine elicits a satisfactory response when administered into the deltoid muscle but not the gluteus muscle. Injection into the gluteus muscle also risks injury to the sciatic nerve. Attenuated (live) influenza vaccine is administered intranasally, whereas varicella vaccine is given subcutaneously.

Precautions and contraindications: There are few absolute contraindications for the use of vaccines. However, caution must be used in immunocompromised patients, such as those with cancer, recent tissue transplant recipients, or those infected with HIV. Patients receiving high-dose, systemic corticosteroid therapy may also have suppressed immune systems. Vaccinations in an immunocompromised patient should be avoided if the patient is having an exacerbation of his or her disorder. In some cases, only inactivated (killed) vaccines are indicated for these patients. Because it is suppressed, the patient's immune system may not be able to develop effective immunity in response to the vaccine, and subsequent laboratory results should be assessed to confirm that immunity has actually occurred.

Although most vaccines are pregnancy category C, vaccinations are sometimes delayed in pregnant patients until after delivery to avoid any potential harm to the fetus. Inactivated (killed) vaccines may be administered to pregnant patients if the benefits of disease prevention outweigh the possible risk to the mother and fetus. For example, exposure to hepatitis B, influenza, tetanus, or diphtheria can have serious or fatal results for the fetus, so the benefits of immunization of the mother may outweigh the vaccine risks for the fetus. The MMR vaccine should not be administered to pregnant women due to the theoretical risk of transmitting a live virus to the fetus.

Anaphylaxis and allergy: The most common adverse effects of vaccination are pain, swelling, and redness at the injection sites. Allergy or anaphylaxis following vaccination is extremely rare. Some preparations may contain preservatives such as gelatin or the mercury compound thimerosal, which could trigger an allergic response. Patients with confirmed vaccine anaphylaxis should not receive subsequent doses of that vaccine.

Adverse event reporting: Health care providers are required to report all vaccine-related adverse events requiring medical attention to the Vaccine Adverse Event Reporting System (VAERS). The VAERS is a postmarketing surveillance program conducted by the CDC and the U.S. Food and Drug Administration (FDA). Voluntary reports may be submitted to the VAERS by patients and parents as well as health care providers. Vaccine manufacturers are required to report any adverse effects of which they are aware.

VAERS has a number of limitations. VAERS merely collects data and reports incidences of adverse events; it does not attempt to confirm that the reported event was actually caused by the vaccine. Reports are not checked by the FDA or CDC for accuracy or completeness. Despite its limitations, VAERS serves as an important, central repository of information for identifying potential adverse effects to vaccines.

CONNECTION Checkpoint 43.2

Vaccines are sometimes contraindicated in patients who are receiving immunosuppressant drugs. From what you learned in Chapter 42, identify the following drugs as being either an immunosuppressant or an immunostimulant: aldesleukin (Proleukin), cyclosporine (Neoral, Sandimmune), basiliximab (Simulect), and hydrocortisone. *See Answer to Connection Checkpoint 43.2 on student resource website.*

Active Immunity: Bacterial Immunizations

43.5 Active immunity can be induced to prevent bacterial infections.

Vaccinations are performed to provide protection against both viral and bacterial pathogens. However, the role of vaccines is very different for each type of infectious agent. Table 43.2 gives a summary of

TABLE 43.2   Disease Epidemiology and Immunizations

Disease	Worldwide Incidence	U.S. Incidence	Immunization (Age)	Remarks
Cholera	Estimated 3–5 million cases annually	Very rare: fewer than 50 cases/year, usually in travelers to endemic countries	Not available in the United States; "boil it, cook it, peel it, or forget it"	Route: oral–fecal toxin from bacteria 80% can be successfully treated with rehydration salts
Diphtheria	Fewer than 1,000 cases, usually in developing countries	No reported cases since 1980	2, 4, 6, and 15–18 months; 4–6 years	Mucous membrane bacterial toxin infection
Hepatitis A	Estimated 1.4 million cases annually, usually in developing countries	Fewer than 2,700 new cases annually; has declined by 90% in the past 2 decades	Two-shot series: 12 months and 6–18 months later	Route: oral–fecal from carriers; immune globulin available
Hepatitis B	2 billion affected; 350 million chronic carriers worldwide	Fewer than 19,000 new cases annually; has declined by over 80% in the past 2 decades	Three-shot series: 0, 1, and 6–18 months	Vaccine recommended for all health care providers; immune globulin available
Influenza (*Haemophilus influenzae* type b [Hib])	Estimated 250,000–500,000 deaths annually; endemic during winter months	About 36,000 deaths annually (high risk to those older than 65 years of age and in general ill health)	Annual vaccine based on estimated exposure	Vaccine recommended for children, immunocompromised patients, older adults, and health care workers
Measles (rubeola)	About 1 million deaths annually, usually in developing countries (mostly children)	Fewer than 100 cases annually	MMR: 12–15 months; booster: 4–6 years	Highly contagious; airborne and droplet exposure
Meningococcus	About 1,600 deaths; major outbreaks every 8–12 years	Fewer than 1,000 cases; rates are highest for children under age 1	11–12 years, at high school entry, or college entry	Airborne droplet exposure; antibiotics if known exposure
Mumps	Endemic in many countries; rarely fatal	Large outbreak of mumps occurred in 2006 with over 3,500 cases	MMR: 12–15 months; booster: 4–6 years	Viral parotitis; respiratory droplet infection
Pertussis	Endemic worldwide; 30–50 million cases annually	About 17,000 cases annually	2, 4, 6, and 15–18 months; 4–6 years	Gram-negative bacterial infection, cough; increased incidence in adolescent age group
Poliomyelitis	Fewer than 34 deaths annually	Very rare	Inactivated virus: 2, 4, and 12 months; booster: 4–6 years	20% of children in Nigeria younger than 5 years are not vaccinated because of fear of AIDS and female infertility
Rabies	Canine rabies epidemic in Africa, Asia, and Central America; fewer than 200 deaths annually	Found in all continents	Preexposure vaccine for veterinarians; postexposure immune globulin	Viral infection; transmitted via contaminated saliva; from peripheral nervous system to central nervous system
Rubella	Common disease worldwide; rarely fatal	Almost no cases	MMR: 12–15 months; booster: 4–6 years	Mild disease but fetal cataracts, deafness, and cardiac malformations
Smallpox	Global eradication since 1980	Global eradication since 1980	No vaccine in use; concern for bioterrorism use	Live virus vaccine; contagious vesicle
Tetanus	Global health problem; incidence in unvaccinated persons; about 200 deaths annually	Less than 100 cases	2, 4, 6, and 15–18 months; 4–6 years	Spores in soil; illness follows inadequate or missed immunizations
Varicella (chickenpox)	Endemic worldwide; rarely fatal	90% decline in past 2 decades	One injection between 12 and 18 months old	Highly contagious; airborne spread; latent in nerve ganglia; reoccurs as herpes zoster (shingles)

the epidemiology and immunizations associated with these pathogens. Immunizations against viruses are presented in Section 43.6.

Many bacterial infections cause host cellular injury by releasing toxic substances. Vaccination for bacterial infections, therefore, may be achieved by exposing the immune system to inactive bacterial toxins. When later faced with the actual bacterial infection, the immune system will remember the protein-based toxin and respond rapidly by producing antibodies to neutralize it.

It is common practice to combine several childhood vaccines for a single administration. For example, DTaP combines diphtheria, tetanus, and pertussis into a single injection. Combining vaccines is less traumatic for the child and is more convenient and efficient for the caregiver and the health care provider.

Diphtheria

Pathophysiology: Diphtheria is an infection of the upper respiratory tract caused by the gram-positive bacterium *Corynebacterium diphtheriae*. The bacterium releases a potent toxin that causes a low-grade fever, malaise, and a painful oropharynx. The organism causes the formation of a thick, gray coating across the membranes of the soft palate, tonsillar areas, and uvula. The thickened membranes can partially occlude the airway and cause difficulty swallowing or a feeling of choking. Attempts to remove the membrane result in pain and bleeding. If untreated, the membrane softens and gradually disappears approximately 1 week following its appearance. A majority of deaths associated with diphtheria are related to toxin escape, leading to acute systemic toxicity or myocarditis. Because of effective immunization programs, the disease has almost been entirely eradicated from the United States.

Diphtheria toxoid: Diphtheria toxin is produced by organisms in culture that are rendered inactive by the addition of formalin. The diphtheria toxoid triggers immune memory without producing disease in the upper airways. Currently diphtheria toxin is available as a combination immunization with tetanus toxoid and acellular pertussis (DTaP) as well as in combination with other compatible immunizations. DTaP is part of the recommended routine immunization schedule for infants older than 6 months.

Pertussis (Whooping Cough)

Pathophysiology: Pertussis is a highly contagious infection by the gram-negative bacterium *Bordetella pertussis* that is transmitted via aerosolized droplets from an infected person. Once inhaled, the bacteria attach to the ciliated respiratory epithelial cells and release a toxin. Pertussis begins with a low-grade fever and irritated cough and progresses to spasmodic coughing episodes characterized by an inspiratory "whoop," leading to the common name "whooping cough." The coughing episodes are productive and may be induced by laughing, talking, or activity in children, and lead to gagging or vomiting. The cough will usually resolve at the termination of the infection in approximately 2 to 6 weeks. Exhaustion is common in patients experiencing pertussis, as are secondary respiratory infections. Active pertussis infection is treated with the antibiotic erythromycin, with the best results seen with early and aggressive treatment.

Immunization: Originally the pertussis vaccine was made from inactivated or killed whole cells and was highly effective in providing immunity. The whole-cell vaccines, however, were associated with adverse effects that prompted the development of an acellular form (aP). The aP vaccine remains highly effective in producing immunity but has a lower rate of adverse effects than the whole-cell vaccine. The acellular form of pertussis vaccine became available in 1996 and has replaced the original form.

Local injection-site reactions, drowsiness, persistent crying, and fever occur in 3% to 5% of patients receiving the vaccine. The vaccine is always administered concurrently with the diphtheria and tetanus toxoids. The childhood vaccine is called DTaP. Children receive five intramuscular (IM) doses of DTaP, one dose at each of the following ages: 2 months, 4 months, 6 months, 15 to 18 months, and 4 to 6 years. Because the severity of pertussis declines with age, vaccination for pertussis is not recommended for children after age 7 or for adults. Adults, however, may receive a booster vaccine (Tdap) if they are anticipating contact with patients with pertussis.

Tetanus

Pathophysiology: *Clostridium tetani* normally lives in soil as a spore but can infect humans when the gram-positive anaerobe enters an open wound. Symptoms of infection may present over a wide range of time, averaging from 3 days to 3 weeks after exposure. *C. tetani* produces a toxin that is one of the most toxic substances known; receiving 2.5 mg (one billionth of a gram) per kilogram of body weight can be lethal. The toxin enters the peripheral nervous system (PNS) and migrates to the central nervous system (CNS). The toxin causes continuous, painful muscular contractions. Symptoms range from local muscle spasm, including the muscles of the jaw (lockjaw), to neck stiffness and seizures that are sometimes unresponsive to drug therapy. Treatment includes the administration of antibiotics but is primarily supportive in advanced cases.

Immunization: Tetanus toxoid (TT) is available alone, combined with diphtheria (DT), or combined with both diphtheria and pertussis (DTaP). The initial series of recommended immunizations uses the DTaP and is given in five doses during the first 6 years of the child's life. A contaminated wound in an adult with an appropriate immunization history requires only the booster administration of TT. To retain immunity, the booster for tetanus prevention should be given to adults every 10 years. TT can be injected IM, subcutaneously, or via jet injector. In patients with symptomatic tetanus infection, the TT injection may be coupled with passive immunization of antibodies against the toxin. The vaccine is nearly 100% effective at preventing tetanus and its widespread use has nearly eradicated this disease in the United States.

Pneumococcus

Pathophysiology: Infection by *Streptococcus pneumoniae* is the most common cause of bacterial otitis media, meningitis, and pneumonia. Pneumococcal infection begins in the nasopharynx and may spread to the middle ear, sinuses, and lower respiratory tract. It occurs with a higher incidence in the winter months, when air pollution increases, or as a secondary infection following viral disease. The immune health of the patient greatly impacts the progress of *S. pneumoniae* infection and those with decreased immune function are at greater risk for the development of serious infections. Also at risk are patients with diminished cough and gag reflexes who have difficulty clearing secretions from the upper airways, such as in cases of neuromuscular diseases, or postanesthetic exposure. Smoking is a contributing factor in approximately half of the *S. pneumoniae* infections in nonelderly populations, probably due to the change in upper airway clearance of secretions in these patients. All strains of *S. pneumoniae* have a common polysaccharide in their cell wall that is used for vaccine development.

Immunization: The immunization for pneumococcal infection has changed over time and currently has two different formulations. The first to be approved by the FDA, called pneumococcal polysaccharide vaccine (PPV), is derived from the cell walls of 23 strains of *S. pneumoniae*. PPV is recommended for those who are age 65 or older and for patients from age 2 to 64 who have a chronic illness or who are living in environments where exposure risk is increased. The vaccine is also recommended in immunocompromised patients (ages 2–64) who have HIV infection, leukemia, lymphoma, Hodgkin's disease, or multiple myeloma; patients who receive dialysis; patients who are receiving high-dose corticosteroid therapy; and transplant recipients. A booster 5 or more years following the first vaccination is recommended.

Because the administration of PPV to young children with immature immune systems leads to a poor antibody response, this vaccine is not recommended in children under 2 years of age. A second vaccine, called pneumococcal conjugate vaccine (PCV), was specially developed for routine immunization in children under the age of 2. This immunization differs from PPV in that the *S. pneumoniae* polysaccharides are coupled with a protein that leads to improved immune activation in infants with immature immune function. The latest form of the pneumococcal conjugate vaccine, PCV13, was approved in 2010 and protects against 13 types of pneumococcal bacteria. PCV13 is used in a series of four IM injections at 2 months, 4 months, 6 months, and 12 to 15 months.

Both PPV and PCV vaccines are well tolerated and only contraindicated in individuals with prior severe reactions to immunizations. The most common symptoms following the administration of either PPV or PCV are mild fever, local redness, swelling, and pain at the injection site, which lasts from 1 to 3 days.

Meningococcus

Pathophysiology: Meningococcal infection (meningitis) is caused by *Neisseria meningitidis*, a highly virulent gram-negative, toxin-secreting organism. Although meningitis usually occurs sporadically in the United States, it sometimes causes epidemics in other nations. Early meningococcal infection is very difficult to discriminate from other viral or bacterial infections, because it initially presents with nonspecific fever and rash; frequently symptoms appear less than 24 hours before individuals are hospitalized. Neurologic symptoms rapidly develop, including nuchal rigidity, headache, photophobia, and seizures. Infants present with reduced feeding, irritability or lethargy, and bulging fontanels. A rash is seen in most cases, which appears as petechiae or larger purpuric eruptions on the arms, chest, or axilla. Early hospitalization and aggressive treatment with intravenous (IV) penicillin-based antibiotics have reduced the mortality and morbidity of meningococcal infection. About 10% of patients die from the infection and up to 20% experience some degree of permanent neurologic disability.

Immunization: Routine immunization for meningococcal infection is recommended at age 11 with a booster at 16 years of age. Special populations that should receive vaccination include individuals traveling to regions where meningococcal infection is endemic or those living in crowded conditions, such as college residence halls. Because college freshmen living in dormitories are at increased risk for infection, some colleges now require meningococcal vaccination for these students. This practice is required for all college students in the United Kingdom. Once an outbreak (three or more confirmed cases) is documented, immunization is recommended for all potentially exposed individuals, and antibiotic therapy is frequently offered to individuals having close contact with the infected persons.

There are two types of meningococcal vaccine. Meningococcal polysaccharide vaccine (MPSV-4) is administered by the subcutaneous route and is available for those ages 2 and older. Meningococcal conjugate vaccine (MCV, Menactra, Menveo) is a newer vaccine that contains *N. meningitidis* polysaccharides conjugated to diphtheria toxoid protein. Given by the IM route, MCV is believed to produce longer lasting immunity than MPSV-4. Neither vaccine contains live or attenuated organisms. MPSV-4 is recommended for patients age 2 to 10 and those over age 55; MCV is used for those age 11 to 55. In 2010, recommendations for MCV were changed to include a two-dose regimen at age 11 and 16 years; or two doses 2 months apart if the vaccine is given at other ages. Neither vaccine protects against meningococcus serogroup B, which is responsible for about one third of all cases of meningitis.

Active Immunity: Viral Immunizations

43.6 Effective vaccines that prevent viral infections have been developed.

Vaccinations for viral infections have a different form and function than those for bacterial infections. Viruses are nonliving and only contain a few strands of nucleic acid (DNA or ribonucleic acid [RNA]), an outer protein coat, and a few viral enzymes. Viruses require a host cell for replication and transmission. The signs and symptoms that follow viral invasion may be caused by either the effects of the viral infection itself or by the host's immune response.

Viral proteins are readily recognized as foreign by the immune system and will normally trigger an immune response. In some cases, immune cells are able to recognize that a virus has entered one of its own cells and has become infected. Recognition of infected cells takes place through the host secretion of special communication proteins called interferons (IFNs), which signal the surrounding noninfected cells of the approaching virus. The infected cells are programmed to undergo cell death, or apoptosis, when they are invaded, thus decreasing the viral spread to adjacent cells. Because viruses undergo rapid mutations that allow them to constantly change structure and evade the host's defense mechanisms, they present enormous challenges for effective vaccine development.

The term *live viral vaccine* is commonly used in clinical practice. The student should understand, however, that viruses are nonliving particles. In vaccine terminology, the term *live* refers to a virus's ability to infect the host and does not indicate that the virus is actually alive.

CONNECTION Checkpoint 43.3

From what you learned in Chapter 42, what are the indications for pharmacotherapy with interferons? *See Answer to Connection Checkpoint 43.3 on student resource website.*

Hepatitis B

Pathophysiology: Infection with hepatitis B virus (HBV) leads to a range of symptoms, from a self-limiting acute illness to life-threatening liver failure. Patients with HBV infection are at risk for developing a chronic carrier state, which is associated with the development of cirrhosis and hepatic cancer. Of the five viral infections known to cause hepatitis, HBV has the highest incidence worldwide.

Hepatitis B cannot be discriminated from the other forms of viral hepatitis by symptoms alone; serologic testing is required for diagnosis. The onset of symptoms ranges between 6 weeks and 6 months postexposure and includes low-grade fever, nausea, vomiting, malaise, fatigue, and anorexia. The patient may present with signs of hepatitis, including jaundice, dark urine, and clay-colored stools that appear 1 to 2 weeks following the onset of symptoms.

Approximately 30% of patients are hospitalized during the acute phase of hepatitis infection. End-stage hepatitis includes encephalopathy, confusion and disorientation, and coma, and carries a mortality rate of 60% to 70% without transplantation. Details on the pathophysiology and pharmacotherapy of HBV infections are presented in Chapter 54.

Immunization: The first HBV vaccine became available in 1982 and was derived from the blood of chronic carriers of the disease. Concerns regarding the possibility of transmitting HIV infection with the vaccine resulted in the development of a recombinant form of the vaccine in 1986. Current HBV vaccines contain highly antigenic proteins from the viral coat, which is known as hepatitis B surface antigen (HBsAg). Recombinant hepatitis vaccines contain no blood products and therefore do not represent a risk for HIV infection.

Because of the potential for occupational exposure, health care providers have a 10-fold increased risk of acquiring HBV. Dried HBV can remain infectious on an environmental surface for up to 1 week, and although needlestick injuries have the highest risk of infection (37–62%), the virus can gain entry via scratches, rashes, burns, or other disruptions of the mucosal surface. The CDC now recommends preexposure immunization against HBV infection for health care providers.

PROTOTYPE DRUG	**Hepatitis B Vaccine (Engerix-B, Recombivax HB)**

Classification: Therapeutic: Vaccine
Pharmacologic: Vaccine

Therapeutic Effects and Uses: The HBV vaccine is a noninfectious, highly immunogenic vaccine that provides immunity to HBV in 99% to 100% of patients when given in the recommended three-dose regimen. The effectiveness of the vaccine in producing immunity in adults declines with age. The vaccine is 98% effective in patients age 20 to 29, 94% in patients age 30 to 39, and 89% in those age 40 or older. The HBV vaccine may be administered in combination with hepatitis B immunoglobulin for postexposure prophylaxis or to prevent the perinatal transmission of the virus from mother to infant. The vaccine is indicated for immunity against all known subtypes of HBV. Indications for the HBV vaccine include the following:

- Routine infant immunization programs, including those born to hepatitis B–infected mothers
- Children born after November 21, 1991, and catch-up immunization of children 11 years old or younger at high risk for infection
- Sexually active adolescents
- Health care workers or caregivers who are at risk for contact with HBV-contaminated blood
- Subpopulations with known high rates of infection, including Alaskan natives, Pacific Islanders, refugees, or persons adopted from areas where HBV infection is endemic
- Persons with high-risk sexual practices, such as heterosexual activity with multiple partners, female prostitutes, homosexual or bisexual practices, or persons who repeatedly contract sexually transmitted infections

- Injecting drug abusers
- Prisoners in correctional facilities
- Dialysis patients
- Living or traveling for more than 6 months in countries where HBV is common

In adults 19 years of age or older, the HBV vaccine is administered 10 mcg IM, followed by repeat doses at 1 and 6 months. Travelers to high-risk areas or those who have been recently exposed to the virus may receive 20 mg IM, followed by subsequent doses at 1, 2, and 12 months.

Mechanism of Action: The HBV vaccine consists of HBsAg produced through recombinant DNA technology using yeast cells. Antibodies induced by the HBV vaccine decline over time and may require a booster dose for continued immunization.

Pharmacokinetics:

Route(s)	IM injection in the deltoid or anterolateral thigh in infants and small children
Absorption	Rapid, following IM injection
Distribution	Unknown
Primary metabolism	Unknown
Primary excretion	Unknown
Onset of action	Antibodies to HBV appear within 2 weeks
Duration of action	Immunity lasts 5–7 years

Adverse Effects: The most common adverse effects from HBV vaccination are pain at the injection site and mild to moderate fever. Approximately 15% of patients will experience systemic effects, usually fatigue, dizziness, fever, and headache. Children may experience irritability, fever, diarrhea, fatigue, weakness, diminished appetite, and rhinitis. Anaphylaxis is rare and is usually reported within a few hours after the vaccination. Guillain-Barré syndrome is a very rare adverse effect of the HBV vaccine.

Contraindications/Precautions: Known hypersensitivity to yeast or any component of the vaccine is an absolute contraindication. Patients who demonstrated severe hypersensitivity to the first dose should not receive subsequent doses. Although anaphylaxis is rare, proper emergency equipment or facilities should be available. Patients with active infections or unexplained fever should delay use of the vaccine unless the health of the patient is endangered by withholding the vaccine. Caution should be exercised when administering the vaccine to patients with severe cardiopulmonary impairment. The vaccine should be given to pregnant or lactating women only if clearly needed to protect the health of the mother or child.

Drug Interactions: Hepatitis B immunoglobulin should not be administered in the same syringe or at the same site as the vaccine because it can impair the development of immunity from the vaccine. Patients receiving immunosuppressant drugs may require a higher dose of vaccine. **Herbal/Food:** Unknown.

Pregnancy: Category C.

Treatment of Overdose: Overdose with this drug has not been reported.

Nursing Responsibilities: Key nursing implications for patients receiving hepatitis B vaccination are included in the Nursing Practice Application for Patients Receiving Immunizations.

Drugs Similar to Hepatitis B Vaccine (Engerix-B, Recombivax HB)

There are no other vaccines similar to the HBV vaccine.

Hepatitis A

Pathophysiology: Unlike HBV, which is mostly bloodborne, hepatitis A virus (HAV) is acquired by coming in contact with the stools of an infected person. At highest risk for HAV infection are household contacts or sexual partners of infected persons and travelers to regions of the world where HAV is endemic (Africa, South America, and most of Asia). Good personal hygiene and proper sanitation can prevent HAV infection. Children are at risk due to generally poor hygiene habits.

Approximately one third of the U.S. population has lifelong immunity to HAV based on a past infection. Symptoms associated with HAV infection are age dependent. In children less than 5 years old, 50% to 90% of infections are asymptomatic, whereas 70% to 95% of adults will exhibit symptoms. Signs and symptoms include elevation in the liver enzyme levels, jaundice, fatigue, anorexia, fever, dull abdominal pain, nausea, and vomiting. Symptoms are often mild, and most patients report the resolution of symptoms in several weeks. The disease is rarely fatal and normally produces no permanent hepatic impairment.

Immunization: When the HAV vaccine became available in 1995, the number of cases of HAV infection in the United States dropped dramatically. Current recommendations for hepatitis A vaccinations include all children at age 12 to 23 months; catch-up vaccination of older children in selected areas; and vaccination of persons at increased risk for hepatitis A, including travelers to endemic areas, illicit drug users, or men who have sex with men (CDC, 2013).

Given by the IM route, children should receive two doses: an initial vaccination at 12 months of age and a follow-up dose 6 to 12 months later. For individuals traveling to endemic regions, three doses may be given with 4 weeks between the three injections. This vaccine is highly immunogenic, with 95% to 100% of vaccinated individuals developing protective antibodies. Antibody coverage persists in both adults and children for 5 to 8 years following vaccination. Adverse effects of the HAV vaccine are mild and include soreness at the injection site, headache, anorexia, and fatigue.

Influenza

Pathophysiology: Influenza, or flu, is a respiratory disease spread by the three forms of the influenza virus: types A, B, and C. Influenza type A is the most dangerous and the primary focus for the annual development of a vaccine for the prevention of epidemic outbreaks. Influenza type A causes seasonal outbreaks during the winter months that are usually self-limiting but may lead to serious health consequences in patients who are debilitated, immunosuppressed, or who have chronic medical conditions. Influenza type A is also harbored in wild aquatic birds and is responsible for outbreaks of "bird flu." Influenza types B and C are less common and generally do not cause epidemics or result in serious symptoms. The influenza viruses mutate at a rapid rate and change their antigenic appearance; almost every time the viral RNA replicates, a new mutant is created. Once an outbreak of influenza occurs, immunization is no longer effective and pharmacotherapy of the active infection may be initiated. Because treatment of influenza infection is minimally effective, the best approach for dealing with this infection is through prevention. The pharmacotherapy of influenza infection is presented in Chapter 54.

Immunization: The first influenza immunization took place in 1945 following a worldwide outbreak during World War II. Throughout the history of influenza immunization, the viral particles used for the inoculation have been incubated in chicken eggs, leading to an increased risk of anaphylaxis in patients with egg allergies. With the development of recombinant human DNA preparations, the risk of allergy has decreased.

The development of the annual influenza vaccine begins with a prediction on the part of scientists as to what strains of the virus are most likely to appear that year. Each year one influenza vaccine is prepared that contains portions of the most likely strains of type A and type B. If their prediction is accurate, the vaccine will prevent 70% to 90% of the flu cases; however, the effectiveness of the vaccine is significantly lower in some years.

Two types of influenza vaccines are available. The trivalent inactivated influenza vaccine (TiIV) is a subcutaneous formulation that is approved for patients older than 6 months, including healthy people, women who anticipate being pregnant during the flu season, and those with chronic medical conditions. The live, attenuated intranasal vaccine (LAIV) is delivered as a nasal spray to healthy people 2 to 49 years of age who are not pregnant. Annual influenza vaccination is recommended for the following groups:

- Everyone over age 50
- Residents of nursing homes or long-term care facilities
- Adults and children who have chronic conditions such as asthma, diabetes, or heart disease
- Anyone whose immune system is compromised due to HIV or AIDS, high-dose corticosteroid therapy, or cancer chemotherapy
- Women who will be pregnant during the influenza season
- Health care providers
- Healthy household contacts (including children) and caregivers of persons at high risk of acquiring influenza

The most common adverse effects of the subcutaneous vaccine are soreness and redness at the injection site. Nasal congestion, headache, and sore throat are common adverse effects of the nasal spray vaccine. About 1% of patients may experience fever, chills, muscle aches, and other symptoms of influenza that last 1 to 2 days. Serious adverse effects are rare. Caution should be used in patients who are allergic to egg or mercury, which are sometimes used as preservatives.

Rabies

Pathophysiology: Rabies is caused by a virus that can invade the nervous system of most mammals. The rabies virus is carried in saliva and is passed to humans through animal bites from infected dogs, coyotes, wolves, foxes, raccoons, skunks, and bats. In unvaccinated individuals, the mortality rate is nearly 100%.

Following the bite of an infected animal, the incubation period for rabies infection is long, from 20 to 60 days. When possible, the biting animal is confined and examined for rabies infection. Because the infection is always fatal if untreated, therapy is immediately implemented while waiting for the results of animal testing.

Pain or paresthesia surrounding the bite is reported by most persons with rabies. Other symptoms include fever, headache, malaise, irritability, anxiety, and insomnia. Short periods of agitation, aggressiveness, hyperactivity, and disorientation are followed by normal behavior. Nuchal rigidity, seizures, bizarre behavior, and hydrophobia indicate a progression of the disease; if untreated, rabies will progress to cardiac or respiratory arrest or paralysis, requiring mechanical ventilation. Death usually occurs within 10 days of the onset of symptoms.

Immunization: preexposure and postexposure:

Prevention of rabies may be accomplished through vaccination. Although the vaccine is effective, few people are administered preexposure immunization because of the very small risk of coming into contact with a rabid animal during their lifetime. However, this immunization is offered to individuals with potential exposure to rabid animals, such as animal handlers or veterinarians, and to travelers to countries where rabies is prevalent. Cave explorers often receive prophylactic treatment because of their potential exposure to rabid bats. Preexposure immunization includes three inoculations.

Once a potential exposure to rabies is reported, the patient should immediately receive postexposure vaccination. The immune response to dead or attenuated organisms in a rabies vaccine takes approximately 2 weeks to develop, which is well within the incubation period of rabies. Patients receive one dose of rabies immune globulin, which offers immediate protection. Five doses of rabies vaccine are then administered over a 28-day period. If instituted promptly, postexposure vaccination is very successful. If the biting animal is shown not to have rabies, the sequence of vaccinations may be discontinued.

The most common adverse effects of the rabies vaccine are pain and redness at the injection site. Mild, transient flulike symptoms may occur. Pregnant women may receive the vaccine, if exposure to the rabies virus is suspected.

Measles, Mumps, and Rubella

Measles (rubeola) pathophysiology: The measles virus, *Morbillivirus*, is one of the most contagious viral pathogens, being readily transmitted by airborne particles and respiratory secretions. Because humans are the only known reservoir for the virus, routine immunization has eliminated measles as a common childhood disease in the United States. Measles is still widespread in other countries and occasional outbreaks across the United States emphasize the importance of continued MMR immunizations.

Symptoms of measles infection appear 10 to 12 days following airborne exposure and begin with nonspecific cough, malaise, and low-grade fever. The fever can subsequently spike to as high as 40.6°C (105°F). A rash appears first on the oral mucosa but then develops into a reddened, raised rash on the face, hairline, ears, and neck, spreading to the trunk and extremities. The rash lasts approximately 1 week and then fades and disappears. Individuals are considered to be infectious 4 days prior to and after rash appearance.

In developing countries, measles infection carries a mortality rate as high as 2% to 15%.

Mumps pathophysiology: Mumps is a viral infection in the parotid salivary glands that is transmitted by exposure to contaminated saliva. Symptoms develop 16 to 18 days after exposure, resulting in mild fever, headache, anorexia, and malaise. The fever usually lasts 1 to 6 days but the swelling in the parotid glands may continue for 10 days or more. The infection is usually self-limiting and mortality is rare. Complications of mumps include orchitis (swelling of the testes) in approximately 37% of infected, postpubescent males and deafness in children.

Rubella or German measles pathophysiology: Rubella, also called German measles, is a viral infection that produces mild symptoms in most people. The rubella virus is transmitted by infected aerosol droplets. Symptoms include enlarged cervical lymph nodes, mild fever, and malaise, followed by a raised rash 14 to 17 days later.

The major concerns with rubella are the consequences of maternal infection during pregnancy. Infection occurring during the first 12 weeks of pregnancy carries the greatest risk of fetal defects. Rubella infection rapidly spreads to all fetal organ systems and may cause a wide variety of consequences. The most frequently described are congenital cataracts and blindness from retinal destruction, heart disease, and deafness in infants. Since the initiation of routine rubella immunization and maternal antibody screening, the incidence of rubella infection of the fetus or newborn has declined to 0.01 per 10,000 pregnancies in the United States. A single, subcutaneous rubella vaccine made from attenuated (live) virus grown in human tissue cultures is available and usually very well tolerated.

Immunization: The MMR vaccine has incorporated live or attenuated viruses since its development in the 1960s, and widespread immunization has led to a 98% decrease in the incidences of these viral infections. Current recommendations include a two-dose subcutaneous immunization, with the first given at 12 to 15 months of age and the second at 4 to 6 years of age. The overall immunity rate for MMR vaccination is 92% to 95%. In 2005, the FDA approved the addition of varicella vaccine to the combination, which is known as MMRV (ProQuad).

A single dose of MMR vaccine is recommended for those individuals born after 1957 without contraindication or past history of measles infection or positive immunity. A second dose of MMR is recommended in the following situations: epidemic outbreak or exposure to measles infection, vaccination with an unknown vaccine between 1963 and 1967 or vaccination with killed organism, health care workers or those traveling internationally, or nonimmune students in postsecondary educational settings.

Although generally well tolerated, several groups are usually excluded from vaccination:

- Pregnant patients or women planning conception within 3 months of vaccination because the live or attenuated rubella virus poses a hypothetical risk of infection with subsequent congenital malformations.

- Patients who are immunosuppressed; however, MMR can be given to individuals living in the same setting with asymptomatic HIV disease and persons with mild immunosuppression.

- Persons reporting an allergy to neomycin or gelatin because the vaccine contains these substances. Persons reporting egg allergy have a very low risk of allergic reaction but it is recommended that these patients be observed for 90 minutes following immunization.

Adverse reactions to MMR vaccination are minimal and include fever and lymphadenopathy, rare encephalitis (1 occurrence per 1 million vaccinations), and arthralgia in adults. MMR is now available in an aerosolized formulation that has fewer associated adverse effects and an improved immunogenicity as compared to the injected forms.

Polio

Pathophysiology: Poliomyelitis was the leading cause of permanent disability in the era just prior to vaccines. Highly contagious, polio epidemics in the 1800s and early 1900s prompted the search for, and eventual discovery of, vaccines. The virus replicates in the gastrointestinal (GI) tract and is spread by the oral–fecal route via contaminated food and water.

Over 90% of those exposed to the poliovirus are asymptomatic. Rarely (less than 1%), the virus reaches the motor tracts of the spinal cord, where it leads to the development of flaccid muscle paralysis of the infected motor cells. On rare occasions the respiratory muscles are involved, leading to the need for artificial ventilation. Global immunization has made the disease extremely rare and global eradication is possible.

Immunization: Two forms of vaccination are currently used for the prevention of poliovirus infection. Developed by Dr. Jonas Salk, the inactivated polio vaccine (IPV) was first marketed in 1955. In 1978 it was reformulated to be more potent. The oral polio vaccine (OPV) was developed in the early 1960s and was used extensively until vaccine-associated paralytic polio (VAPP) was found to be a rare, though devastating, adverse effect. The OPV is still widely used in regions of the world where polio is endemic due to its ease of administration. The OPV also prevents the intestinal spread of the virus, which is of critical importance in areas of the world that have poor sanitation.

Since 2000, the IPV has been exclusively used in the United States for the immunization of infants. Children get four doses of IPV, at 2 months, 4 months, 6 to 18 months, and a booster dose at 4 to 6 years. IPV is available as a single suspension or in combination with DTaP, hepatitis B, or influenza vaccines. Routine IM administration of IPV results in redness, swelling, and tenderness at the administration site. Children receiving the complete IPV regimen are provided 99% to 100% lifelong immunity.

Varicella Zoster

Pathophysiology: Infection by the varicella zoster virus (VZV) leads to the development of two very different diseases. The initial outbreak of VZV, known as chickenpox (varicella), generally occurs during childhood. Following the initial infection, the virus becomes dormant for 30 to 40 years in nerve roots until it reactivates to cause herpes zoster (HZ) or shingles.

The initial VZV infection is transmitted through inhaled droplets or by direct contact with infectious skin lesions. The virus replicates in the local lymph nodes for several days and then becomes bloodborne. By day 10 to 14, a blistered rash appears, with new lesions opening, draining, and crusting within 24 hours. Intense itching may lead to secondary bacterial infections and permanent scarring. General illness is common in individuals for 5 to 7 days with fever, malaise, and anorexia. Adults with chickenpox have more intense symptoms than children and have a seven times greater risk of encephalitis. Furthermore, women who acquire VZV during pregnancy have a small risk of passing the infection to the fetus, resulting in birth defects.

Following the initial infection, the virus migrates to the spinal nerves, where it may remain dormant for the life of the individual. In about 20% of patients, however, the virus becomes reactivated and causes an HZ infection, or **shingles**, usually after age 50; this increases to approximately 50% for individuals over the age of 85. Shingles often begins with a burning or tingling pain, numbness, or itch in one particular location on the surface of the body. After several days or a week, fluid-filled blisters, similar to chickenpox, appear in one area of the body. Shingles lesions can be very painful and may require up to a month for resolution. In immunocompromised individuals the infection may be prolonged, taking 3 to 4 weeks for lesion scabbing and several months for complete resolution. Up to 30% of patients with shingles experience a serious form of the disease called **postherpetic neuralgia** in which the pain lasts for years. In about 15% of patients with shingles, the virus infects the eye and can cause blindness.

Antiviral drugs such as acyclovir (Zovirax) are sometimes administered to reduce the severity and duration of a shingles attack and postherpetic neuralgia. Other treatments for postherpetic neuralgia include corticosteroids and nonsteroidal anti-inflammatory drugs (NSAIDs).

Immunization: An attenuated or live VZV vaccine (Varivax) has been used in the United States since 1995, and it is estimated that widespread vaccination has reduced the incidence of varicella infection by more than 70%. In 2006, new standards were adopted with the following recommendations:

- Implementation of a routine two-dose varicella vaccination schedule for children. The first dose is administered at age 12 to 15 months and the second dose at age 4 to 6 years.

- Routine vaccination of all healthy persons over age 13, without evidence of immunity.

- Prenatal assessment and postpartum vaccination.

CONNECTIONS   Patient Safety

Adequate Patient History to Avoid Adverse Effects

A nurse new to working in the outpatient clinic is preparing an MMR injection for a patient who has just moved to the United States and was not vaccinated previously. The nurse-mentor assigned to the new nurse asks if the patient's history was taken and the nurse replies, "Yes, and there is no history of vaccination." What else should be assessed in the history before administering the MMR injection?

See Answer to the Patient Safety Question on student resource website.

- Expanding the use of the varicella vaccine for children infected with HIV.
- Establishing middle school, high school, and college entry vaccination requirements.

There is wide variation in the effectiveness of the vaccine, and 10% to 15% of immunized individuals will still acquire the infection, which is a condition known as breakthrough varicella. Breakthrough varicella infection produces milder symptoms as compared to those in nonimmunized patients.

Also in 2006, an advisory panel of the CDC recommended that all Americans receive the shingles vaccine (Zostavax) at age 60. The shingles vaccine contains a live or attenuated form of the virus and is 60% effective at preventing the reactivation of VZV. The shingles vaccine is essentially a booster of the VZV vaccine administered to prevent chickenpox. It is not effective at treating symptoms of shingles or postherpetic neuralgia once they develop.

Adverse effects associated with VZV vaccine include low-grade fever, tenderness at the injection site, and rash localized to the injection site. The vaccine should be used with caution in persons with a history of allergy to eggs or gelatin. Caution should be exercised with the use of this immunization in pregnant or breast-feeding women. Although there have been no documented problems with receiving the immunization while pregnant, VZV has been linked to the development of birth defects. Finally the administration of this vaccine in immunosuppressed patients may increase the incidence of adverse effects or cause a decrease in the developed immunity.

PharmFACT

Approximately 95% of adults in the United States have antibodies to the varicella zoster virus, indicating prior exposure to this pathogen. Incidence increases with advancing age due to declining immunity (Janniger, 2013).

CONNECTIONS | Lifespan Considerations

◀ The Shingles Vaccination

While most vaccinations are given in childhood, vaccination against varicella zoster virus (VZV), the virus that causes shingles (also known as herpes zoster), is recommended for adults age 60 or older. Like Varivax given in childhood to prevent varicella (chickenpox), Zostavax is given to boost immunity against shingles. An estimated 90% of older adults have had chickenpox or sufficient exposure, and an estimated 10–25% of the population will have shingles (Litchfield, 2010). The rash that develops in shingles is extremely painful, significantly impacts the patient's ability to work or carry on normal daily activities, and the blisters that occur with the rash represent an exposure risk to other people in the patient's environment, including pregnant women, people without immunity to varicella, and patients who are immunocompromised. Postherpetic neuralgia may develop, causing months or years of acute pain even after the shingles rash has resolved. Antiviral drugs such as acyclovir (Zovirax) may be used to reduce the overall period of active shingles, but they do not cure the disease and relapses may occur. Nurses working with the older adult population should review the patient's vaccination history and suggest booster vaccinations when needed. The VZV vaccine, Zostavax, should also be recommended for healthy older adults over the age of 60 and included as part of routine health care when the patient reaches age 60.

Human Papillomavirus

Pathogenesis: Genital human papillomavirus (HPV), the most common sexually transmitted disease in the United States, is associated with a higher risk of cervical cancer, which is a significant cause of cancer deaths in women. Although there are over 100 different forms of HPV, only 7 are associated with cervical cancer. HPV is also associated with a higher risk of other types of cancer, including vaginal, vulvar, and anal. Some types of HPV are responsible for causing genital warts. The virus may infect both males and females, and it may be transmitted from mother to child during vaginal delivery.

Spread through sexual contact, HPV infection may be asymptomatic or lead to the development of a low-grade infection that resolves spontaneously in individuals with a healthy immune system. A high-grade HPV infection may lead to the development of dysplasia, a precancerous change in the cervical cells that is directly related to the viral infection.

Immunization: The HPV vaccine has been created with virus-like particles using recombinant DNA technology. Great caution was necessary in the development of this vaccine because the HPV contains oncogenes, which are modified forms of a gene that are believed to lead to a cancerous transformation. Because of the potential cancer risk, the HPV vaccine is a noninfectious, virus-like particle (VLP) containing only proteins from the coat of the virus, rather than a complete attenuated virus. The HPV vaccine is intended to prevent cervical, vulvar, and vaginal cancer and certain precancerous lesions in women. In men and women, the HPV vaccine is indicated to prevent genital warts caused by HPV. It is not effective against existing cancers or genital diseases not caused by HPV.

The HPV vaccine (Gardasil, Cervarix) is administered through a series of three IM injections. The second and third doses should be given 2 and 6 months after the first dose. The vaccine has close to 100% effectiveness in preventing HPV infection and appears to offer long-lasting protection. The CDC recommends the routine vaccination of females 11 to 12 years old and of females age 13 to 26 years who were not vaccinated at an earlier age. Females who have already been infected with a strain of HPV experience less benefit from vaccination. However, it may still prevent infection from additional strains of the virus. Mild adverse effects include pain, swelling, and redness of the injection site. In 2011, the CDC recommended that Gardasil be administered to males age 9 through 26 years to prevent genital warts and anal cancer.

PharmFACT

Nearly all sexually active men and women will become infected with one type of HPV during their lives. About 79 million Americans are infected with HPV and 14 million new infections occur every year (CDC, 2014).

Rotavirus

Pathophysiology: Approximately 680,000 children die worldwide each year from rotavirus infection, mostly in developing countries. Although the virus rarely causes death in the United States, it is estimated that nearly every child is infected by age 5 and that most will experience gastroenteritis, resulting in severe diarrhea and dehydration. Viral replication of the rotavirus occurs only in mature red blood cells found in the tips of the intestinal villi, leading to a strictly oral–fecal means of viral transmission.

Immunization: The FDA approved the first rotavirus immunization (RotaShield) in August 1998. In the 10 months following FDA approval, over 1.5 million doses of the vaccine were administered and 15 cases of intussusception (a form of intestinal obstruction from a telescoping of the intestine into itself) were reported. In November 1999, RotaShield was removed from the market due to these safety concerns. Newer rotavirus vaccines received approval in 2006 (RotaTeq) and 2008 (Rotarix) for routine immunization in infants. The CDC recommends rotavirus vaccine in a three-dose oral series in infants 6 to 32 weeks of age for the prevention of gastroenteritis. The vaccine has been shown to reduce the overall incidence of gastroenteritis by 74% and of hospitalization due to the virus by 96%. There are no serious adverse effects associated with immunization with RotaTeq, but mild cases of diarrhea and vomiting occur in small numbers of patients receiving the drug.

Passive Immunity

43.7 Antibodies are administered to provide passive immunity.

Passive immunization is very different from active immunization. Whereas active immunity requires mobilization of the patient's immune response, which leads to the development of memory cells, passive immunity is the administration of preformed antibodies (immunoglobulins). During passive immunity the immune system is not activated and memory cells are not produced.

Passive immunization is typically used to provide immediate protection against a recent infection, a potential infection, or a disease in progress. Several examples serve to illustrate the benefits of passive immunization:

- A person has just been bitten by a potentially rabid dog. It will take several days to determine if the dog is infected with rabies.
- A person has been in a motorcycle crash and sustained serious trauma. He has never had a tetanus vaccination.
- A student nurse has learned that she has been exposed to blood from a patient with confirmed HBV. She has not been vaccinated for HBV.

What do these three scenarios have in common? First, immediate treatment is indicated because the consequences of infection can be serious or fatal. The use of a vaccine requires too much time for the activation of an immune response, and the disease would have the opportunity to create serious illness. In these cases, antibodies against the infection can be administered to provide immediate prevention against rabies, tetanus, or HBV infection. Antibodies are sometimes given concurrently with the vaccine series to provide complete immunity against the disease. For example, following an exposure to rabies the patient is given rabies immunoglobulin (RI) as well as the rabies vaccine.

The preceding scenarios illustrate a second message of importance to the nurse. If the patients had kept their tetanus and HBV vaccinations up to date, they would have developed active immunity to these pathogens and there would be no need to provide passive immunity.

A second indication for the use of passive immunity is for situations where the activation of the immune system and the development of memory are not desirable. In this case, the individual is given the antibodies against the foreign agent and the immune system does not mount a response. The administration of RhoGAM is an example of this type of indication.

Table 43.3 lists selected immune globulin preparations. Pharmacotherapy Illustrated 43.1 shows the development of immunity through vaccines or the administration of antibodies.

PROTOTYPE DRUG	Rh$_o$[D] Immune Globulin (RhoGAM)

Classification: Therapeutic: Immunizing agent (passive)
Pharmacologic: Antibody, immunoglobulin

Therapeutic Effects and Uses: Erythrocytes contain two types of surface antigens that are used to designate the blood type. The first identifier is ABO; the presence or absence of antigen A and antigen B will determine the blood type as A, B, AB, or O. A second identifier on the cell membrane of the red blood cell (RBC) is the Rhesus factor, or Rh antigen. If the antigen is present, the individual

TABLE 43.3 Immune Globulin Preparations

Drug	Route and Adult Dose (Maximum Dose Where Indicated)	Adverse Effects
cytomegalovirus immune globulin (CytoGam)	IV: 150 mg/kg within 72 h of transplantation; then 100 mg/kg for 2, 4, 6, and 8 weeks post-transplant; then 50 mg/kg for 12 and 16 weeks post-transplant	*Local reactions at the injection site (pain, erythema, myalgia), influenza-like symptoms (malaise, fever, chills), headache, joint stiffness* <u>Anaphylaxis</u>
hepatitis B immune globulin (HBIG)	IM: 0.06 mL/kg as soon as possible after exposure, preferably within 24 h, but no later than 7 days; repeat 28–30 days after exposure	
intravenous immune globulin (IVIG, Gammagard, Carimune, Octagam)	IV: 100–200 mg/kg per month IM: 1.2 mL/kg followed by 0.6 mL/kg every 2–4 weeks	
rabies immune globulin (BayRab, Imogam Rabies-HT, Hyperab)	IM (gluteal): 20 units/kg as a single dose with rabies vaccine	
Rh$_o$[D] immune globulin (RhoGAM)	IM/IV: one vial or 300 mcg at approximately 28 weeks; followed by one vial of minidose or 120 mcg within 72 h of delivery if infant is Rh$^+$	
tetanus immune globulin (BayTet, HyperTet, HyperTet S/D)	IM: 250 units for prophylaxis	
varicella zoster immune globulin (Varizig)	IM: 62.5–625 international units	

Note: *Italics* indicate common adverse effects. <u>Underline</u> indicates serious adverse effects.

PHARMACOTHERAPY ILLUSTRATED 43.1

Mechanisms of Active and Passive Immunity

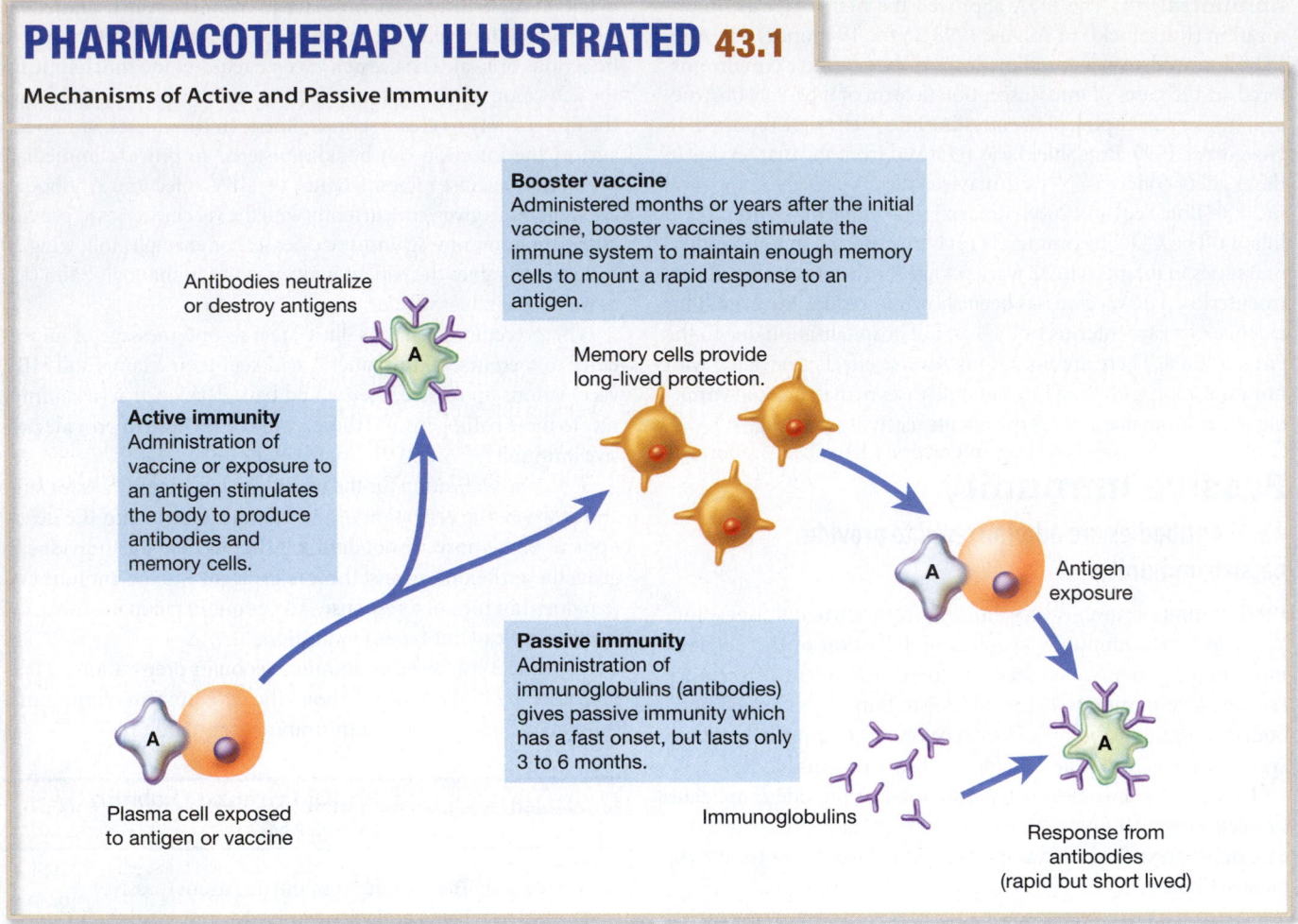

Active immunity
Administration of vaccine or exposure to an antigen stimulates the body to produce antibodies and memory cells.

Antibodies neutralize or destroy antigens

Booster vaccine
Administered months or years after the initial vaccine, booster vaccines stimulate the immune system to maintain enough memory cells to mount a rapid response to an antigen.

Memory cells provide long-lived protection.

Antigen exposure

Plasma cell exposed to antigen or vaccine

Passive immunity
Administration of immunoglobulins (antibodies) gives passive immunity which has a fast onset, but lasts only 3 to 6 months.

Immunoglobulins

Response from antibodies (rapid but short lived)

---

is said to be Rh positive (Rh^+) and if it is missing, Rh negative (Rh^-); 85% of individuals living in North America are Rh positive.

Erythroblastosis fetalis (EF), or hemolytic disease of the newborn, is a disorder that was first described in 1940 and is caused by an Rh incompatibility between the mother and her fetus. This condition can only occur if the mother is Rh negative.

EF does not occur with the first pregnancy because the two types of RBC (Rh^- mother and Rh^+ child) are separated by the placenta and the blood is not physically exchanged. At birth, however, their blood mixes and the mother's immune system reacts by producing antibodies against the foreign Rh^+ antigen. The presence of circulating antibodies against the Rh antigen creates a potential risk for an Rh incompatibility in future pregnancies. If in a subsequent pregnancy the fetus is Rh^+, the mother's antibodies against the Rh^+ antigen will cross the placenta and destroy erythrocytes in the fetus. This may lead to a severe anemia or brain damage in the developing fetus and even fetal death.

Rh_o immunoglobulins are obtained from filtered human serum for the prevention of Rh incompatibility in Rh^- women. This drug has been used to provide passive immunity since 1968 and has significantly reduced the incidence of EF. Administration of Rh_o immunoglobulins will prevent the mother from forming Rh antibodies, so that there will be no risk of incompatibility in subsequent pregnancies. Rh_o[D] immune globulin prophylaxis is not indicated if either the father or the fetus is Rh_o[D] negative.

The administration of RhoGAM is recommended:

- At 28 weeks' gestation
- Within 72 hours postpartum
- Within 3 hours of spontaneous or induced pregnancy termination
- Following any event that could lead to transplacental hemorrhage (such as amniocentesis, chorionic villi sampling, or abdominal trauma)

Mechanism of Action: Rh_o[D] antibodies act by suppressing the immune response of Rh^- mothers to Rh^+ fetuses or newborns. Sensitization to Rh_o[D]-positive blood in future pregnancies is therefore less likely to occur.

Pharmacokinetics:

Route(s)	IM, IV
Absorption	Unknown
Distribution	Unknown
Primary metabolism	Unknown
Primary excretion	Unknown
Onset of action	Peak antibody levels: 2 h (IV) or 5–10 days (IM)
Duration of action	Half-life: 24–30 days

Adverse Effects: The most commonly reported adverse reactions include local swelling, redness, and mild pain at the injection site.

A small number of patients experience low-grade fever. Hypersensitivity reactions are rare and may include hives, generalized urticaria, tightness of the chest, wheezing, hypotension, and anaphylaxis. Also rarely reported are anemia, anorexia, bruising, disseminated intravascular coagulation (DIC), dyspnea, dysuria, edema, hematuria, hemolysis, hypertension, increased risk of bleeding, lower back pain, malaise, nausea, polydipsia, vomiting, and weight gain.

Contraindications/Precautions: This drug is contraindicated in individuals with a history of hypersensitivity reaction to human immunoglobulin injection. $Rh_o[D]$ antibodies are also contraindicated in patients having immunoglobulin A (IgA) deficiencies or in patients with severe anemia and should be used with caution in patients who have DIC, hemolysis, renal disease, and splenectomy.

Drug Interactions: No drug interactions have been reported. **Herbal/Food:** Unknown.

Pregnancy: Category C.

Treatment of Overdose: Overdose with this drug has not been reported.

Nursing Responsibilities: Key nursing implications for patients receiving $Rh_o[D]$ immune globulin are included in the Nursing Practice Application for Patients Receiving Immunizations.

Drugs Similar to $Rh_o[D]$ Immune Globulin (RhoGAM)

Other immunoglobulins include cytomegalovirus immune globulin, hepatitis B immune globulin, and IV immune globulin.

Cytomegalovirus immune globulin (CytoGam): About half of the U.S. adult population has been exposed to cytomegalovirus (CMV). Few people, however, have experienced symptoms because healthy immune systems prevent symptomatic, active infections. When donating organs or tissues, CMV may be inadvertently transferred to a transplant recipient with a suppressed immune system. Cytomegalovirus immune globulin (CMV-IGIV) is recommended for the prevention of CMV infections in at-risk individuals receiving kidney, liver, pancreas, and heart transplants. The drug can lower the incidence of serious CMV-associated disease by 50%. Current dosage recommendations include the IV administration of seven doses, beginning within 72 hours of the receipt of the organ and ending 30 days later. The most common adverse effects are minor and include flushing, chills, muscle cramps, back pain, fever, nausea, vomiting, arthralgia, and wheezing.

Hepatitis B immune globulin (HBIG): The goal of HBIG administration is to prevent the transmission of HBV to those who have been exposed to the virus. The administration of HBIG is recommended for the following instances:

- Nonimmunized individuals who have had acute and significant exposure to hepatitis B–infected blood. This includes accidental needlestick, oral ingestion, or direct mucous membrane contact with infected blood or blood products. One dose is usually given immediately after exposure and another dose 1 month later. The administration of HBIG is effective in the prevention of clinical hepatitis B infection in approximately 75% of individuals who are treated.

- Infants born to women infected with HBV. These infants should receive HBIG and start the HBV vaccine series within 12 hours of birth. This regimen is 70% to 90% effective in preventing infection in the infant.

- Sexual partners of HBV-infected patients. A single dose of HBIG is 75% effective at preventing HBV infection if the drug is administered within 2 weeks of sexual contact.

- Household exposure of infants less than 12 months of age who are born to a mother or have a primary caregiver who is infected with HBV. These infants should receive HBIG and start the HBV vaccine series before 12 months of age.

The administration of HBIG is effective in the prevention of clinical hepatitis B infection in approximately 75% of individuals who are treated, but this immune protection is temporary, lasting approximately 2 to 3 months. HBIG is usually given concurrently (different IM site) with hepatitis immunization in infants born of hepatitis B–infected mothers. Adverse reactions to HBIG are rare and include local site reactions, such as tenderness, redness, and swelling. Hypersensitivity reactions have also been reported. HBIG is provided in a prefilled, single-dose syringe in either pediatric or adult preparations.

Intravenous immune globulin (IVIG, Gammagard, Carimune, Octagam): Immune globulin contains pooled antibodies obtained from human plasma that is used to provide passive immunity following exposure to an organism for which no active immunization exists, if there is inadequate time to develop active immunity, and as replacement therapy for those with antibody deficiencies. IVIG contains 95% or more immunoglobulin G (IgG). The passive immunity induced by IVIG is capable of attenuating or preventing a wide range of infectious diseases and adverse effects from toxins, mycoplasma, parasites, bacteria, and viruses. IVIG may be thought of as a "generic" treatment for balancing immune systems. It contains components that strengthen immune function as well as substances that can suppress overactive immune systems. Disease protection lasts for 3 weeks or longer. Because this drug contains antibodies to live viruses, active vaccinations should not be given until 3 to 5 months after IVIG has been administered.

CONNECTIONS: NURSING PRACTICE APPLICATION

Patients Receiving Immunizations

Assessment	Potential Nursing Diagnoses*
Baseline assessment prior to administration: • Obtain a complete health history including previous history of the actual disease (e.g., chickenpox), hepatic, renal, cardiovascular, neurologic, or autoimmune disease, HIV infection, fever or active infections, pregnancy or breast-feeding, previous allergic response to immunizations or to products contained within immunization (e.g., sensitivity to yeast, eggs, or albumin products). Obtain a drug history, especially the use of immunosuppressants or corticosteroids. • Obtain an immunization history and any unusual reactions or responses. • Obtain baseline vital signs, especially temperature. • Evaluate appropriate laboratory findings (e.g., CBC, platelets, electrolytes, titers, hepatic and renal tests). • Assess the patient's ability to receive and understand instructions. Include family and caregivers as needed.	• *Readiness for Enhanced Health management* • *Deficient Knowledge* (Vaccination Schedule, recommendations) • *Risk for Ineffective Health Maintenance, related to failure to complete immunization schedule* • *Risk for Injury, related to adverse drug effects*
Assessment throughout administration: • Assess for patient adherence to the recommended immunization schedule (e.g., need for repeated immunizations, boosters in adults). • Continue periodic monitoring of CBC, liver and renal function studies as appropriate to the type of immunizing agent. • Assess vital signs, especially temperature. • Assess for and immediately report adverse effects: fever, dizziness, confusion, muscle weakness, tachycardia, hypotension, syncope, dyspnea, pulmonary congestion, skin rashes, bruising or bleeding, anaphylactic reactions.	

Implementation

Interventions and (Rationales)	Patient-Centered Care
Ensuring therapeutic effects: • Continue assessments as above for therapeutic effects. (The patient should adhere to the recommended immunization schedule. Periodic titers may be needed to confirm immunity, especially in individuals who are over age 60 or those who are immunosuppressed.)	• Teach the patient, family, or caregivers to keep vaccination records, to copy records if needed for school or work situations but retain the originals, and to remain current with required immunizations. • Encourage older adults to consider having titers drawn to confirm immunity and to consult with the health care provider to arrange as appropriate.
• For patients considering overseas travel, obtain current immunization recommendations for the destination country. (Current recommendations may be found on the CDC Traveler's Health website.)	• Teach the patient to consult the CDC Traveler's Health website before planning overseas travel and to consult with the health care provider about risks and required immunizations.
Minimizing adverse effects: • Continue to monitor vital signs, especially temperature, and neurologic status. (Immunizations may cause dermatologic, cardiovascular, and neurologic adverse effects. Increase in temperature, localized ulcerations, signs of infection at the injection site, tachycardia, palpitations, dizziness, or changes in level of consciousness may indicate significant adverse effects.) • Report all significant adverse effects to the health care provider for reporting to VAERS.	• Teach the patient to immediately report any fever over 38°C (101°F) or as instructed by the health care provider, changes in consciousness such as drowsiness or disorientation, dyspnea, tachycardia, or palpitations.
• Treat minor adverse effects symptomatically. (Acetaminophen or the drug as ordered by the health care provider for low-grade fevers of less than 38°C [101°F], for localized tenderness, or for minor arthralgias and malaise, and cool compresses to the injection site may help alleviate malaise, fever, or injection-site soreness.)	• Teach the patient to treat minor symptoms as needed but to immediately report any adverse effects as noted above.
• **Lifespan and Diverse Patients:** Assess for the possibility of pregnancy, previous history of organ transplantation, and the home environment for any significantly immunocompromised patients at home, e.g., from chemotherapy, before giving live virus immunizations. (Some live vaccinations continue to be shed from the patient in the postvaccination period and may be transmitted to immunocompromised patients in the home environment. Pregnancy is a contraindication for vaccination with live viruses, and women who become pregnant within 3 months of immunization with a live vaccine should consult their health care provider. For religious or other reasons, some patients may refuse to accept administration of any component derived from human blood or serum, including Rh$_0$[D] immune globulin.)	• Teach the patient to alert the health care provider to any home situation that may require deferral of live vaccinations before the vaccination is given. Women who are pregnant or who may become pregnant within the first 3 months after vaccination should return to the health care provider for follow-up. • Encourage the patient with concerns about vaccination, including those with components derived from human blood or serum, to consult with the health care provider in order to make an educated choice about accepting or refusing the drug.

CONNECTIONS: NURSING PRACTICE APPLICATION (continued)

• Avoid or defer immunizations in any patient with a fever, autoimmune disease, or those taking corticosteroids. (Immune response to the vaccine may result in less than the desired immunity or an increased risk of adverse effects.)	• Explain to the patient the need to defer vaccinations under certain conditions. Ensure that follow-up appointments are made as appropriate to maintain currency with immunizations.
• Assess patients for previous use of Bacillus Calmette-Guérin (BCG) vaccine and consult with the health care provider before giving PPD skin testing for TB. (BCG stimulates immunity to the tuberculin, and recent vaccination may cause adverse reaction to PPD injection or result in a false-positive reaction. Other testing may be warranted.)	• Teach the patient that previous use of BCG may result in a false-positive TB test, or an unusual reaction to the PPD test, or that other testing may be required to confirm or refute current infection.
Patient understanding of drug therapy: • Use opportunities during administration of immunizations and during assessments to discuss the rationale for drug therapy, desired therapeutic outcomes, commonly observed adverse effects, parameters for when to call the health care provider, and any necessary monitoring or precautions. (Using time during nursing care helps to optimize and reinforce key teaching areas.)	• The patient should be able to state the reason for the drug, appropriate scheduling, what adverse effects to observe for, and when to report them.

*Nursing Diagnoses—Definitions and Classification 2015–2017. Copyright © 2014, 1994–2014 by NANDA International. Used by arrangement with John Wiley & Sons Limited.

CHAPTER
43

Understanding the Chapter

Key Concepts Summary

43.1 The eradication of smallpox was a great triumph in modern medicine.

43.2 Vaccines are used to activate the immune system for the purpose of disease prevention.

43.3 There are four traditional methods of producing vaccines.

43.4 Vaccines should be administered by an established schedule with precautions taken for patients who are immunosuppressed or pregnant.

43.5 Active immunity can be induced to prevent bacterial infections.

43.6 Effective vaccines that prevent viral infections have been developed.

43.7 Antibodies are administered to provide passive immunity.

Case Study: Making the Patient Connection

Remember the patient "Samantha Abbott" at the beginning of the chapter? Now read the remainder of the case study. Based on the information presented within this chapter, respond to the critical thinking questions that follow.

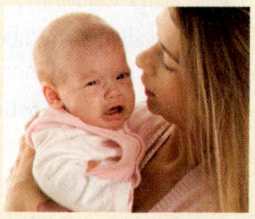

Mr. and Mrs. Abbott arrive in the office where you work with their 4-month-old infant, Samantha, for her checkup. She is scheduled to receive the following immunizations today: DTaP, Hib, PCV, and IPV. Samantha's mother states, "I don't think these immunizations are necessary. Don't these shots usually make children sick?"

As first-time parents, Mr. and Mrs. Abbott are new to the experience of childhood immunizations and require careful teaching. While obtaining her history, you find that 4-month-old Samantha has been doing well and is in the 90th percentile for height and 89th percentile for weight. She has achieved the developmental milestones for her age and is bright and interacts well with her environment.

Critical Thinking Questions

1. What information should be obtained from the Abbotts about Samantha's first response to immunization?
2. Why is it important to discuss the potential adverse effects of vaccines with Samantha's parents?
3. What educational information should be given to the Abbotts?

See Answers to Critical Thinking Questions on student resource website.

Additional Case Study

As a nurse working in the intensive care unit, your patient assignment today is to care for a critically ill patient who is known to be HIV positive and hepatitis B and C positive. You are cleaning up after assisting a first-year resident with the insertion of a central line and, as you are putting the disposable drapes into the trash, you feel a sharp pain in your right hand. As you pull your hands away you see a needle protruding through the glove into your hand. You report the incident to your supervisor and report to the emergency department (ED) per exposure protocol.

The ED physician orders you to have antibody testing for anti-HBsAg, to have baseline HIV testing, and to receive gamma globulin and antiviral prophylaxis.

1. What is the rationale for the hepatitis B testing?
2. What is the rationale for the HIV testing?
3. Why is gamma globulin ordered?
4. Why is antiviral prophylaxis appropriate?

See Answers to Additional Case Study on student resource website.

Chapter Review

1 Mary is a 4-month-old infant who is brought to the clinic for her first checkup. Her mother tells the nurse that the child has never been ill. Which factor would the nurse consider most significant in assessing the baby's likelihood of receiving immunizations?

1. Allergies to previously administered medications
2. Mother's preconceptions and reservations relating to vaccines
3. Maternal and paternal allergies or reactions to vaccine administration
4. The nurse's knowledge of the recommended pediatric immunization schedule

2 The nurse is preparing to administer an MMR vaccination to a 15-month-old child. What would cause the nurse to hold the injection and recheck this order with the provider?

1. The mother tells the nurse that the family will be going to the beach for the next few weeks.
2. The mother states that she was told that she had a reaction to the injection when she was a child.
3. The mother tells the nurse that her husband is having chemotherapy for Hodgkin's lymphoma.
4. The mother tells the nurse that the child's older brother is home with a cold virus.

3 A 7-year-old girl, who was bitten by a stray dog, is treated in the emergency department. The dog has not been tested to rule out rabies. The nurse will anticipate that this patient will receive which immunizations? Select all that apply.

1. Tetanus toxoid
2. DTaP vaccine
3. Rabies immunoglobulin
4. Rabies vaccine
5. Rabies toxoid

4 The nurse determines that the patient understands the teaching given for care required after receiving a tetanus toxoid injection when the patient states:

1. "I will keep my arm still for the next 24 hours to give the vaccine time to absorb."
2. "I will limit my fluid intake for the next 8 hours in case I have nausea."
3. "I will avoid crowds and people with viruses for the next 7 days."
4. "I will take some acetaminophen (Tylenol) or ibuprofen (Advil) if my arm is sore."

5 The occupational health nurse will be administering hepatitis B vaccine to a new employee. Which assessment finding discovered by the nurse would necessitate withholding the injection? The patient is:

1. A two-pack-per-day smoker.
2. Known to have transient hypertension.
3. Allergic to yeast and yeast products.
4. Frightened by needles and injections.

6 A postpartum patient received $Rh_o[D]$ immune globulin (RhoGAM) therapy after the delivery of an 8-lb baby boy. The nurse performs what important intervention during the course of this treatment?

1. Monitors the patient for 20 minutes following the administration for hypersensitivity reaction
2. Evaluates the laboratory results for thrombocytopenia, anemia, and increased liver enzymes
3. Provides the patient with the information needed to maintain a low-saturated fat, low-cholesterol diet
4. Instructs the patient to use nonmedicated sugar-free lozenges or hard candies to relieve cough

See Answers to Chapter Review in Appendix A.

References

Centers for Disease Control and Prevention. (2013). *Vaccine information statement: Hepatitis A*. Retrieved from http://www.cdc.gov/vaccines/hcp/vis/vis-statements/hep-a.html

Centers for Disease Control and Prevention. (2014). *Genital HPV infection fact sheet*. Retrieved from http://www.cdc.gov/std/HPV/STDFact-HPV.htm#a5

Janniger, C. K. (2013). *Herpes zoster*. Retrieved from http://emedicine.medscape.com/article/1132465-overview

Litchfield, S. M. (2010). Shingles. *AAOHN Journal, 58*(6), 228–231. doi:10.3928/08910162-20100526-05

Selected Bibliography

Ball, J. W., & Bindler, R. C. (2011). *Pediatric nursing: Caring for children* (5th ed.). Upper Saddle River, NJ: Pearson.

Centers for Disease Control and Prevention. (n.d.). *Smallpox*. Retrieved from http://www.bt.cdc.gov/agent/smallpox

Centers for Disease Control and Prevention. (n.d.). *Travelers' health*. Retrieved from http://wwwnc.cdc.gov/travel

Centers for Disease Control and Prevention. (2012). *Parent's guide to childhood immunizations* (2nd reprint). Retrieved from http://www.cdc.gov/vaccines/pubs/parents-guide/downloads/parents-guide-508.pdf

Centers for Disease Control and Prevention. (2012). *Vaccines and preventable diseases*. Retrieved from http://www.cdc.gov/vaccines/vpd-vac/default.htm

Centers for Disease Control and Prevention (2014). *ACIP vaccine recommendations*. Retrieved from http://www.cdc.gov/vaccines/hcp/acip-recs/index.html

Chatterjee, A., & O'Keefe, C. (2010). Current controversies in the USA regarding vaccine safety. *Expert Review of Vaccines, 9*, 497–502. doi:10.1586/erv.10.36

Herdman, T. H., & Kamitsuru, S. (Eds.). (2014). *NANDA International nursing diagnoses: Definitions and classification, 2015–2017*. Oxford, United Kingdom: Wiley-Blackwell.

Kessels, S. J., Marshall, H. S., Watson, M., Braunack-Mayer, A. J., Reuzel, R., & Tooher, R. L. (2012). Factors associated with HPV vaccine uptake in teenage girls: A systematic review. *Vaccine, 30*, 3546–3556. doi.10.1016/j.vaccine.2012.03.063

Luthy, K. E., Beckstrand, R. L., Callister, L. C., & Cahoon, S. (2012). Reasons parents exempt children from receiving immunizations. *The Journal of School Nursing, 28*, 153–160. doi:10.1177/1059840511426578

Markowitz, L. E., Tsu, V., Deeks, S. L., Cubie, H., Wang, S. A., Vicari, A. S., & Brotherton, J. M. (2012). Human papillomavirus vaccine introduction—the first five years. *Vaccine, 30*(Suppl. 5), F139–F148. doi:10.1016/j.vaccine.2012.05.039

Music, T. (2012). Protecting patients, protecting healthcare workers: A review of the role of influenza vaccination. *International Nursing Review, 59*, 161–167. doi:10.1111/j.1466-7657.2011.00961.x

Vaccine Adverse Event Reporting System (VAERS). (n.d.). *Vaccine event reporting system*. Retrieved from https://vaers.hhs.gov/index

Wharton, M. (2010). Vaccine safety: Current systems and recent findings. *Current Opinion in Pediatrics, 22*(1), 88–93. doi:10.1097/MOP.0b013e3283350425

Pharmacology of the Respiratory System and Allergy

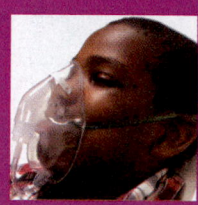
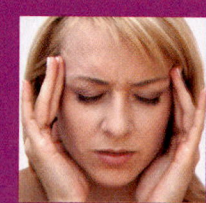

CHAPTER 44   Pharmacotherapy of Asthma and Other Pulmonary Disorders / 730

CHAPTER 45   Pharmacotherapy of Allergic Rhinitis and the Common Cold / 752

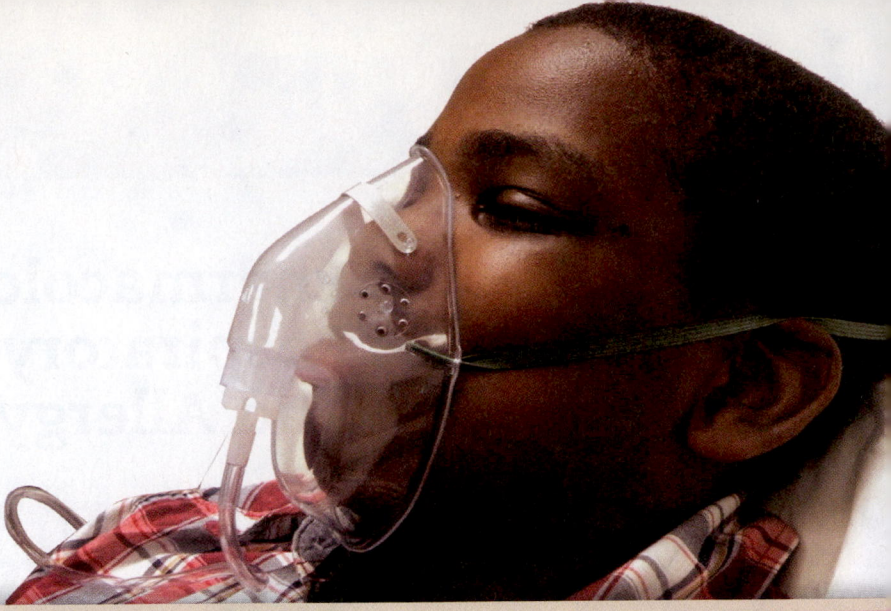

"I can't breathe! Help me!"

Patient "Nathan Almond"

44 Pharmacotherapy of Asthma and Other Pulmonary Disorders

LEARNING OUTCOMES

After reading this chapter, the student should be able to:

1. Identify the anatomic structures associated with the lower respiratory tract and their functions.

2. Explain how the autonomic nervous system regulates airway diameter.

3. Explain the role of inflammation and bronchospasm in the pathogenesis of asthma.

4. Compare the advantages and disadvantages of using the inhalation route of drug administration for pulmonary drugs.

5. Describe the types of devices used to deliver aerosol therapies via the inhalation route.

6. Explain the three basic principles of asthma management recommended by the National Asthma Education and Prevention Program.

7. Compare and contrast the indications for pharmacotherapy with the short- versus long-acting beta-adrenergic agonists.

8. Describe the nurse's role in the pharmacologic management of lower respiratory tract disorders.

9. For each of the classes shown in the chapter outline, identify the prototype and representative drugs and explain the mechanism(s) of drug action, primary indications, contraindications, significant drug interactions, pregnancy category, and important adverse effects.

10. Apply the nursing process to care for patients receiving pharmacotherapy for lower respiratory tract disorders.

CHAPTER OUTLINE

▶ **Physiology of the Lower Respiratory Tract**

▶ **Pathophysiology of Asthma**

▶ **Administration of Pulmonary Drugs via Inhalation**

▶ **Principles of Asthma Pharmacotherapy**

Beta₂-Adrenergic Agonists
PROTOTYPE Albuterol (Proventil, Ventolin, VoSpire), *p. 736*

Anticholinergics
PROTOTYPE Ipratropium (Atrovent), *p. 739*

Corticosteroids
PROTOTYPE Beclomethasone (Beconase AQ, Qvar), *p. 740*

Mast Cell Stabilizers
PROTOTYPE Cromolyn, *p. 742*

Leukotriene Modifiers
PROTOTYPE Zafirlukast (Accolate), *p. 743*

Methylxanthines
PROTOTYPE Theophylline (Theo-Dur, Others), *p. 744*

Monoclonal Antibodies

▶ **Chronic Obstructive Pulmonary Disea**

KEY TERMS

aerosol, 733	dry powder inhaler (DPI), 734	nebulizer, 734
asthma, 732	emphysema, 745	pulmonary perfusion, 731
bronchospasm, 732	leukotrienes, 743	small volume nebulizer, 734
chronic bronchitis, 745	metered-dose inhaler (MDI), 733	status asthmaticus, 733
chronic obstructive pulmonary disease (COPD), 745	methylxanthines, 744	ventilation, 731
	mucolytics, 746	

The flow of oxygen, carbon dioxide, and other gases in and out of the human body is in constant flux. Minute-by-minute control of the airways is necessary to bring an adequate supply of oxygen to the pulmonary capillaries and to rid the body of some of its most toxic waste products. Any restriction in this dynamic flow, even for brief periods, may result in serious consequences. This chapter examines drugs used in the pharmacotherapy of two primary pulmonary disorders: asthma and chronic obstructive pulmonary disease (COPD).

Physiology of the Lower Respiratory Tract

44.1 The physiology of the respiratory system involves two main processes: perfusion and ventilation.

The primary function of the respiratory system is to bring oxygen into the body and to remove carbon dioxide. The process by which these gases are exchanged is called respiration. The basic structures of the lower respiratory tract are shown in Figure 44.1.

Blood flow through the lung is called **pulmonary perfusion**. The bronchial tree ends in microscopic sacs called alveoli, which have no smooth muscle and inflate like balloons during inspiration. The alveoli are abundantly rich in capillaries. An extremely thin membrane in the alveoli separates the inspired air from the pulmonary capillaries, allowing gases to readily move between the internal environment of the blood and the inspired air. As oxygen crosses this membrane to enter the bloodstream, it is exchanged for carbon dioxide, which is a cellular waste product that leaves the bloodstream to enter the alveoli. The process of gas exchange is illustrated in Figure 44.1.

Ventilation is the process of moving air into and out of the lungs. As the diaphragm contracts and lowers in position, it creates a negative pressure that draws air into the lungs and inspiration occurs. During expiration the diaphragm relaxes and air leaves the lungs passively. Ventilation is a purely mechanical process that occurs approximately 12 to 18 times per minute in adults, which is a rate determined by neurons in the brainstem. This rate may be modified by a number of factors, including emotions, fever, stress, and the pH of the blood.

One of the most important factors that affect ventilation is the size of the thousands of tubes or passageways leading from the outside to the alveoli, collectively known as the airways. The nervous system controls ventilation by changing the diameter of the airways, specifically the very small and abundant bronchioles.

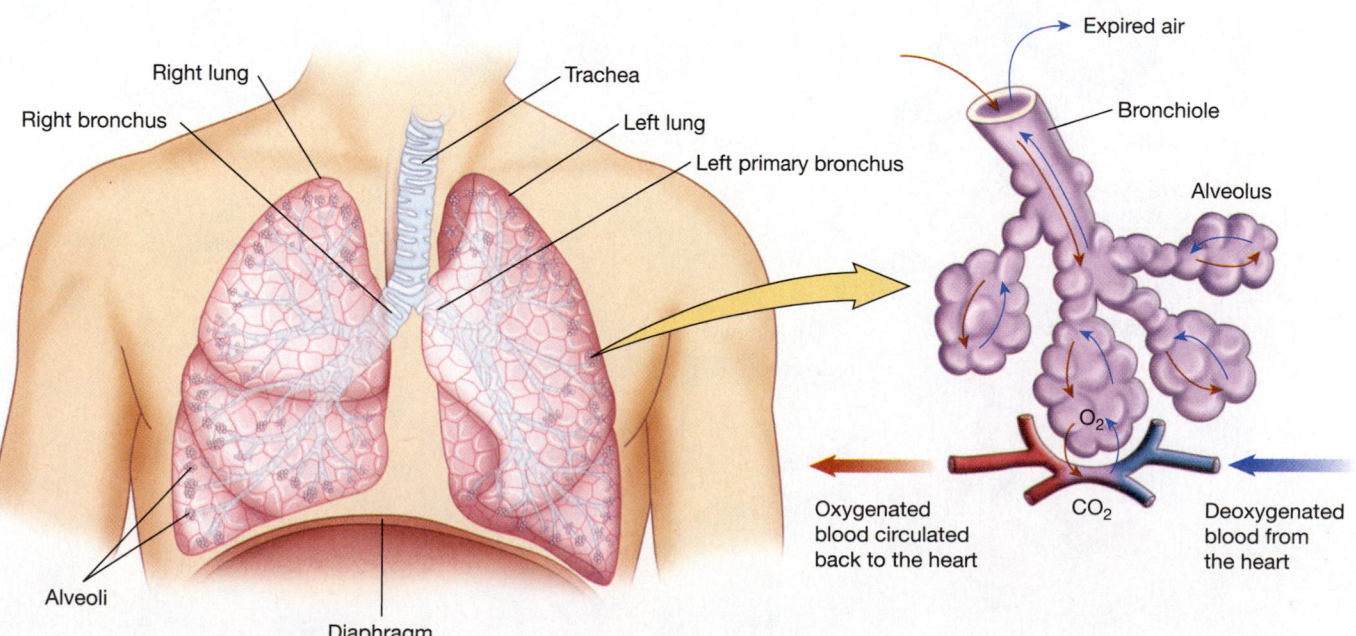

Figure 44.1 The lower respiratory tract and the process of gas exchange.

Bronchioles are muscular, elastic, tubular structures whose diameter, or lumen, varies with the contraction or relaxation of bronchiolar smooth muscle. Bronchodilation allows air to enter the alveoli more freely, thus increasing the supply of oxygen to the body's tissues during periods of exercise. Bronchoconstriction increases airway resistance, resulting in less airflow. Bronchodilation and bronchoconstriction are largely regulated by the two branches of the autonomic nervous system:

- The sympathetic branch activates beta$_2$-adrenergic receptors, causing bronchiolar smooth muscle to relax, the airway diameter to increase, and bronchodilation to occur.
- The parasympathetic branch causes bronchiolar smooth muscle to contract, the airway diameter to narrow, and bronchoconstriction to occur.

In practical terms, drugs that enhance bronchodilation enable the patient to breathe easier. On the other hand, drugs causing bronchoconstriction result in more labored breathing and the patient to become short of breath.

Bronchoconstriction is a common indication for pharmacotherapy. Bronchoconstriction may occur through several mechanisms, and the choice of pharmacotherapy will differ depending on the mechanism. The airways may narrow due to **bronchospasm**, a sudden contraction of the smooth muscle of the airways that causes acute dyspnea. Drug treatment for bronchospasm is targeted at immediately relaxing the smooth muscle spasm. A second mechanism of bronchoconstriction is the production of thick, viscous secretions that plug up the airways. Depending on the cause, treatment may involve antibiotics for an infection or drugs that break up viscous secretions (mucolytics). A third mechanism of bronchoconstriction is edema that is caused by engorgement of the pulmonary blood vessels. Treatment may include diuretics and drugs to enhance cardiac function.

Pathophysiology of Asthma

44.2 Asthma is a chronic disease that has both inflammatory and bronchospasm components.

Asthma is one of the most common chronic conditions in the United States, and it is increasing at an alarming rate. Asthma currently affects about 24 million Americans. The prevalence of asthma is three times greater among African Americans compared to European Americans, and women account for about 65% of all patients with asthma. Although often considered a condition of childhood, asthma can occur at any age.

Asthma is characterized by chronic inflammation that occurs when potent mediators of the immune and inflammatory responses are released by mast cells lining the bronchial passageways. These mediators include histamine, leukotrienes, prostaglandins, and interleukins. The result of inflammation is an increase in airway edema coupled with increased mucus secretion, which narrows the airways, compromises the process of respiration, and contributes to airway obstruction. This is illustrated in Figure 44.2.

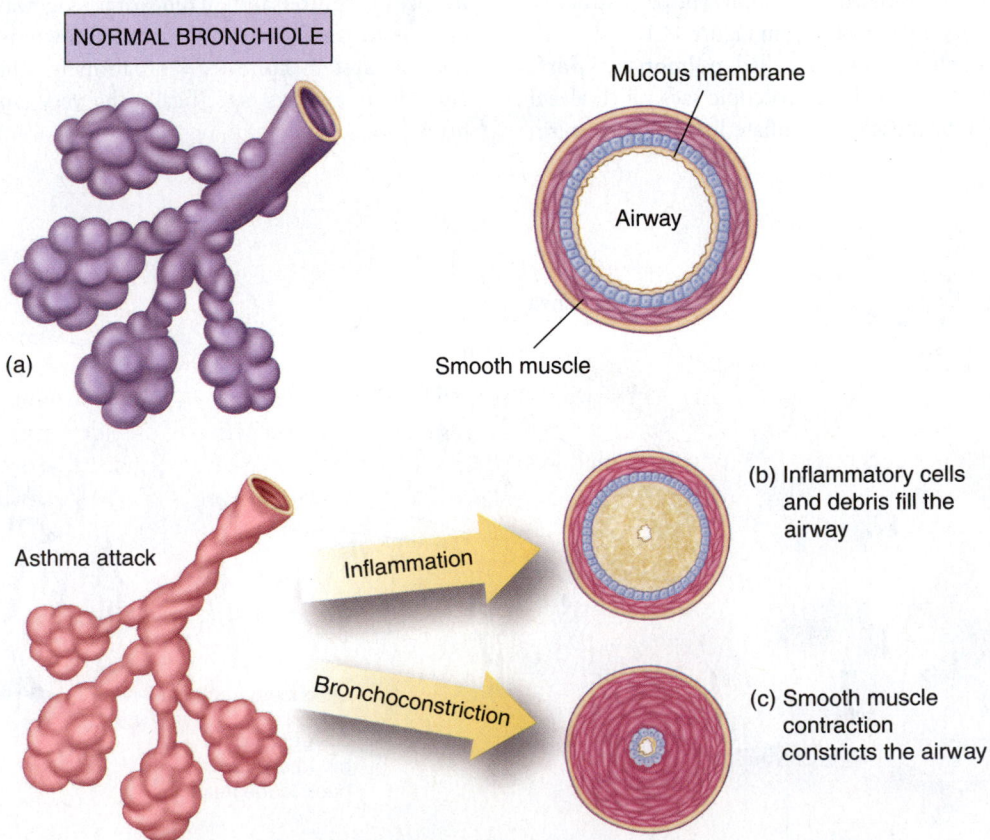

Figure 44.2 Changes in the bronchioles during an asthma attack: (a) Normal bronchiole. (b) The inflammatory component plugs the airway. (c) Bronchoconstriction narrows the airway.

TABLE 44.1	Common Triggers of Asthma
Cause	**Sources**
Air pollutants	Tobacco smoke
	Ozone
	Nitrous and sulfur oxides
	Fumes from cleaning fluids or solvents
	Burning leaves
Allergens	Pollen from trees, grasses, and weeds
	Animal dander
	Household dust
	Mold
Chemicals and food	Drugs, including aspirin, ibuprofen, and beta blockers
	Sulfite preservatives
	Food and condiments, including nuts, monosodium glutamate (MSG), shellfish, and dairy products
Respiratory infections	Bacterial, fungal, and viral
Stress	Emotional stress, anxiety, exercise in dry, cold climates

The second component in the pathogenesis of asthma is bronchospasm. The inflammatory conditions in the airway make the smooth muscle hyperresponsive to a variety of stimuli. Stimuli such as breathing smoke, pollutants, or cold air may trigger acute bronchospasm. Specific triggers are listed in Table 44.1. Some patients experience bronchospasm on exertion, a condition called exercise-induced asthma. Gastroesophageal reflux can trigger an asthma event when acid in the esophagus induces reflex bronchoconstriction.

PharmFACT

About 1 in every 12 Americans has asthma. Asthma is an associated cause of deaths for over 3,400 people each year (American Academy of Allergy, Asthma and Immunology, 2014).

The patient with asthma may present with a variety of symptoms, including evening cough, shortness of breath, chest tightness, and wheezing. Intervals between symptoms may vary from days to weeks to months. The severity of asthma is often graded by the frequency and intensity of acute episodes, as given in Table 44.2. **Status asthmaticus**, an emergency situation in which asthma is unresponsive to drug treatment, may lead to respiratory failure. Drugs may be given to prevent asthmatic attacks or to terminate attacks in progress.

Administration of Pulmonary Drugs via Inhalation

44.3 Inhalation is a common route of administration for pulmonary drugs because it delivers drugs directly to their sites of action.

Many drugs that are used to treat asthma are available for administration by the inhalation route. Inhalation offers a rapid and efficient mechanism for delivering drugs directly to their site of action in the lungs. The enormous surface area of the bronchioles and alveoli and the rich blood supply to these areas result in an almost instantaneous onset of action for inhaled substances.

Medications are delivered to the respiratory system by aerosol therapy. An **aerosol** is a suspension of minute liquid droplets or fine solid particles suspended in a gas. The major advantage of aerosol therapy is that it delivers the drugs directly to the site of action. Not only does this dramatically decrease the onset of action, but it also allows for much smaller doses of a drug. The small doses of drug given by the inhalation route minimize any systemic effects that might result from absorption across pulmonary capillaries when compared to PO medications. Several devices are used to deliver drugs via the inhalation route. The most common are metered-dose inhalers, dry powder inhalers, and nebulizers.

The **metered-dose inhaler (MDI)**, often simply called an inhaler, is the most common type of aerosol delivery device. It consists of a canister that holds the medicine and a mouthpiece. To use an MDI, the patient presses the canister toward the mouthpiece to deliver a measured dose or "puff" of medication. By inhaling during drug delivery, the patient helps to ensure that the drug reaches the site of action in the lungs. Even when MDIs are used properly, however, the majority of the aerosolized drug never reaches the lungs. There are two primary reasons for this problem. One is that heavier aerosolized particles fall out by gravity and are deposited in the oropharynx. The other reason is that proper coordination of drug delivery with inhalation can be difficult for some patients. To decrease oropharyngeal deposition and to enhance drug delivery to the lungs, many health

TABLE 44.2	Assessment of Asthma		
Level	**Frequency of Symptoms**	**Nocturnal Attacks**	**Activity**
Intermittent	Less than 2 times/week	Less than 2 times/month	Not limited
Mild persistent	3–6 days/week	More than 2 times/month	Attacks may limit activity
Moderate persistent	Daily	More than 1 time/week	Attacks affect activity
Severe persistent	Continual	Frequent	Attacks limit physical activity

From *Integrated Cardiopulmonary Pharmacology* (2nd ed.), by B. Colbert, L. S. Gonzales, and B. J. Kennedy, © 2008. Reprinted and electronically reproduced by permission of Pearson Education, Inc., Upper Saddle River, New Jersey.

care providers recommend that patients use a spacer with their MDI. A spacer is a special tube that attaches to the mouthpiece that is designed to hold the cloud of aerosolized medication. This serves two primary purposes. First, the spacer holds drops that fall out of the aerosol so that less medication is deposited on the oropharynx and in the mouth. Second, because the spacer holds the medication, the patient does not have to precisely coordinate inhalation with activation, so that more drug reaches the site of action.

A **dry powder inhaler (DPI)** delivers the medication as a fine dry powder. Whereas the MDI is activated by pressing the canister, the DPI is automatically activated when the patient inhales through the mouthpiece. Because the timing of drug delivery and inhalation does not have to be coordinated, more medication is delivered to the lung with a DPI. The DPI has no propellants in the canister (propellants can be harmful to some patients with lung problems).

A **nebulizer** (or **small volume nebulizer**) is a machine that delivers medication as a fine mist. When using a nebulizer, the medication to be delivered is poured into a receptacle. The machine then vaporizes the liquid medication into a mist that is inhaled by using a face mask or other handheld device. These "breathing treatments" may take up to 30 minutes to administer the drug so it may not work as quickly as a drug taken from an MDI or DPI; however, medication delivered in this fashion is often more effective because it is delivered over many inhalations that occur during the period of medication delivery.

Principles of Asthma Pharmacotherapy

44.4 The goals of asthma pharmacotherapy are to terminate acute bronchospasms and to reduce the frequency of asthma attacks.

The choice of medications for asthma is determined by evidence-based guidelines coupled with the patient's response to therapy and adjusted according to the patient's individual situation. Evidence-based guidelines have been developed by experts in asthma management and are based on research findings. In the United States, the National Asthma Education and Prevention Program (NAEPP) issued guidelines for asthma treatment in 1991, which were updated in 1997, 2002, and 2007. The NAEPP guidelines (2007) recommend a stepwise approach to asthma control based on the frequency and severity of symptoms, as shown in Figure 44.3. As patient symptoms worsen, the pharmacotherapy is adjusted accordingly by going to the next step. This provides for a rational, evidence-based approach to asthma management. The three general strategies for asthma management from the NAEPP are as follows:

- Incorporate four components of care: medications, patient education, environmental control measures, and management of comorbidities.

- Initiate therapy based on asthma severity. For patients not taking long-term control therapy, select the treatment step based

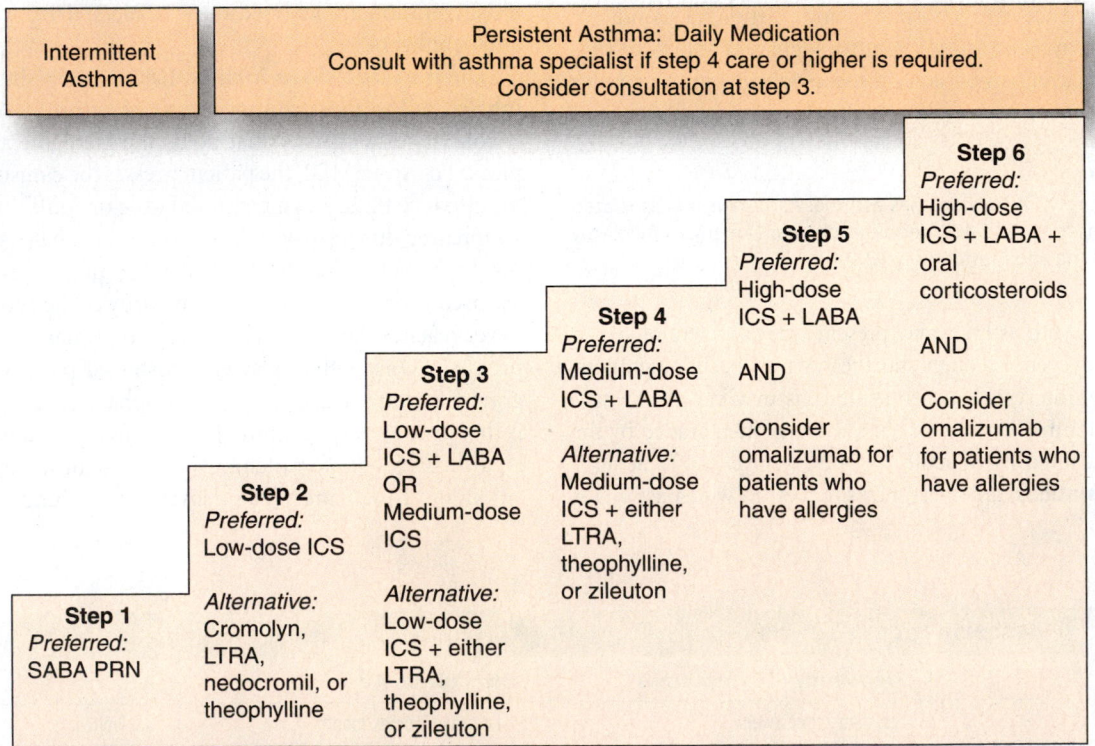

Key: ICS, inhaled corticosteroid; LABA, long-acting inhaled beta$_2$-agonist; LTRA, leukotriene receptor antagonist; SABA, inhaled short-acting beta$_2$ agonist

Figure 44.3 Stepwise approach for managing asthma in adults and patients 12 years and older.
Adapted from Figure 4.5 in *Expert Panel Report 3 (EPR3): Guidelines for the Diagnosis and Management of Asthma* by the National Asthma Education Prevention Program, coordinated by the National Heart, Lung, and Blood Institute of the National Institutes of Health, 2007. Retrieved from http://www.nhlbi.nih.gov/guidelines/asthma/asthgdln.htm.

TABLE 44.3	Overview of Drug Classes for Asthma Management	
Class	**Mechanism**	**Use**
Quick-Relief Medications		
Short-acting beta₂-adrenergic agonists (SABAs)	Bronchodilators	Preferred drugs for relief of acute symptoms.
Anticholinergics	Bronchodilators	Alternate drugs for those who cannot tolerate SABAs.
Corticosteroids: systemic	Anti-inflammatory	Although not rapid acting, these oral agents are used for short periods to reduce the frequency of acute exacerbations.
Long-Acting Medications		
Corticosteroids: inhaled	Anti-inflammatory	Preferred drugs for long-term asthma management. Oral doses may be required for severe, persistent asthma.
Mast cell stabilizers	Anti-inflammatory	Alternative drugs to control mild, persistent asthma or exercise-induced asthma.
Leukotriene modifiers	Anti-inflammatory	Alternative drugs to control mild, persistent asthma or as adjunctive therapy with inhaled corticosteroids.
Long-acting beta₂-adrenergic agonists (LABAs)	Bronchodilators	Used in combination with inhaled corticosteroids for prophylaxis of moderate to severe persistent asthma.
Methylxanthines	Bronchodilators	Used in combination with inhaled corticosteroids for prophylaxis of mild to moderate persistent asthma.
Immunomodulators	Monoclonal antibody	Used as adjunctive therapy for patients who have allergies and severe, persistent asthma.

Data from *Adults in Expert Panel Report 3 (EPR3): Guidelines for the Diagnosis and Management of Asthma* by the National Asthma Education Prevention Program, coordinated by the National Heart, Lung, and Blood Institute of the National Institutes of Health, 2007. Retrieved from http://www.nhlbi.nih.gov/guidelines/asthma/asthgdln.htm.

on severity. Patients who have persistent asthma require daily long-term control medication.

- Adjust the therapy based on asthma control. Once therapy is initiated, monitor the level of asthma control and adjust the therapy accordingly: step up if necessary and step down if possible to identify the minimum amount of medication required to maintain asthma control.

The goals of asthma pharmacotherapy are twofold: to terminate acute bronchospasms and to prevent or reduce the frequency of asthma attacks. Different medications are needed to achieve each of these goals. The NAEPP categorizes asthma drugs into two simple classes: quick-relief medications and long-term control medications. A summary of the different classes used for asthma management is given in Table 44.3.

PharmFACT

More than 10 million children have been diagnosed with asthma in the United States. Children from poor households are more likely to have asthma than those from nonpoor households (National Center for Health Statistics, 2012).

44.5 Beta₂-adrenergic agonists are the most effective drugs for relieving acute bronchospasm.

Beta-adrenergic agonists are some of the most frequently prescribed drugs for treating pulmonary disorders. Beta agonists are drugs that activate the sympathetic nervous system, which relaxes bronchial smooth muscle, resulting in bronchodilation. They are preferred drugs for the treatment of bronchoconstriction.

Beta-agonist medications may act on either beta₁ receptors, which are located primarily in the heart, or on beta₂ receptors, which are located in smooth muscle of the lung, uterus, and other organs. Beta agonists that activate both beta₁ and beta₂ receptors are called nonselective bronchodilators. Beta agonists that activate

only the beta₂ receptors are called selective agents. The selective beta₂-adrenergic agonists have largely replaced the older, nonselective agents such as epinephrine and isoproterenol (Isuprel) for asthma pharmacotherapy because they produce fewer adverse cardiac effects. For a review of the nonselective beta agonists and prototype features for epinephrine and isoproterenol, refer to Chapter 15.

Beta₂-adrenergic agonists are classified by their duration of action. Short-acting agents have a rapid onset of action, usually several minutes, so they are effective in terminating an acute asthma attack. Short-acting beta₂ agonists are the drugs currently recommended by the NAEPP to abort or terminate an acute asthma attack. For this reason, they are often referred to as rescue agents. Their effects, however, last only 2 to 6 hours, so the use of short-acting agents is generally limited to as-needed (prn) management of acute episodes. Doses of these drugs are listed in Table 44.4.

Intermediate-duration beta₂ agonists last approximately 8 hours, whereas long-acting agents last up to 12 hours. These agents have a relatively slow onset of action. In 2005, the U.S. Food and Drug Administration (FDA) issued a public health advisory regarding an increase in deaths among persons who take long-acting beta₂ agonists (LABAs). Because LABAs are not indicated to abort an asthma attack, taking a LABA instead of a short-acting beta agonist could result in unrelieved bronchospasm and subsequent death. The LABAs are also delivered via handheld inhalers and patients may assume that they have the same actions as the short-acting agents. Patients must be alerted to the dangers inherent in taking these during an acute episode. Although the risk of asthma-related death is small, LABAs should only be used as additional therapy for patients who are not adequately controlled on other asthma-controller medications, such as inhaled corticosteroids, or for patients with severe asthma who clearly require two medications for disease management (see Table 44.2). They are not to be used as monotherapy for this disease.

Asthma Management

Clinical Question
What role do elementary school teachers play in the management of asthma?

Evidence
Multiple risk factors for asthma have been determined including family history, low socioeconomic status, lack of insurance coverage, obesity, and environmental and allergen exposures. Research into best practices for drug management has recently suggested that the combination of a long-acting beta agonist (LABA) paired with an inhaled corticosteroid (ICS) works well in preventing and controlling asthma symptoms for many patients, especially for those whose asthma is not controlled by ICS alone (Lemanske & Busse, 2010; O'Connor, Patrick, Parasuraman, Martin, & Goldman, 2010). Despite current knowledge into the risks, etiology, and treatment of asthma, childhood asthmatic attacks still cause lost school days and learning, lost parent productivity as days off from work are required to care for the child, and increasing medical expenses.

Teachers are with children up to one third of their waking hours during the week and, as such, are in a key position to proactively assist the child and family to manage asthma. Bruzzese et al. (2010) found that despite experience with asthmatic children in the classroom, elementary school teachers were not always well prepared in asthma management. Overall, the majority of teachers had experience with children with asthma and could recognize common asthma triggers. While many could identify steps to prevent asthma attacks, such as trigger avoidance and activity limitation, few identified actually taking more than one step. Fewer teachers identified steps to manage asthma symptoms, with most identifying "contacting the nurse" as the usual step taken. And while the teachers communicated about the child's asthma with both the parents and the school nurse, more teachers discussed asthma-related information with the parents than with the nurse.

Implications
Teachers must manage multiple academic responsibilities as well as health-related concerns such as asthma. The school nurse may be the most important person in assisting elementary teachers to proactively manage childhood asthma rather than reactively seeking assistance when an attack occurs. Working together as a team, nurses can help teachers become more knowledgeable about asthma triggers, symptoms, and treatment, and teachers can become more skilled in symptom recognition and prevention measures.

Critical Thinking Questions
Discuss approaches that a school nurse could use to increase teachers' knowledge about asthma management. What are some strategies that could encourage students, parents, and their families to participate in a schoolwide effort to increase asthma knowledge?

See Answers to Critical Thinking Questions on student resource website.

Beta$_2$-adrenergic agonists are available in PO, inhaled, and parenteral formulations. When taken for asthma and other respiratory problems, inhalation is by far the most common route. Inhaled beta$_2$ agonists produce minimal systemic toxicity because only small amounts of the drugs are absorbed. When given PO a longer duration of action is achieved, but systemic adverse effects are more frequently experienced. Systemic effects may include some activation of beta$_1$ receptors in the heart, which could cause an angina attack or a dysrhythmia in patients with cardiac impairment. With chronic use tolerance may develop to the bronchodilation effect and the duration of action will become shorter. Should this occur, the dose of beta$_2$ agonist may need to be increased, or a second drug may be added to the therapeutic regimen.

PROTOTYPE DRUG	Albuterol (Proventil, Ventolin, VoSpire)

Classification: **Therapeutic:** Bronchodilator
Pharmacologic: Beta$_2$-adrenergic agonist

Therapeutic Effects and Uses: Approved in 1981, albuterol is a short-acting, beta$_2$-adrenergic agonist that is used to relieve and prevent the bronchospasm that is a characteristic pathophysiologic feature of asthma. Its rapid onset and excellent safety profile have made inhaled albuterol a drug of choice for the termination of acute bronchospasm. In addition to relieving bronchospasm, the drug facilitates mucus drainage and can inhibit the release of inflammatory chemicals from mast cells. When inhaled 15 to 30 minutes prior to physical activity, it can prevent exercise-induced bronchospasm for 2 to 3 hours. Inhaled albuterol is considered safe for use during pregnancy.

Oral forms of albuterol include immediate release and extended release tablets (VoSpire) and an oral solution. The PO forms have a longer onset of action and are not suitable for terminating acute asthma attacks. The NAEPP does not recommend the use of short-acting beta$_2$ agonists for the management of asthma prophylaxis.

Mechanism of Action: Albuterol acts by selectively binding to beta$_2$-adrenergic receptors in bronchial smooth muscle to cause bronchodilation.

Pharmacokinetics:

Route(s)	Inhalation, PO
Absorption	Slow by the inhalation route. Some of the inhaled drug is swallowed and absorbed by the gastrointestinal (GI) tract. Rapid when given PO
Distribution	Delivered directly to the lungs (site of action); crosses the blood–brain barrier; may cross the placenta; unknown if secreted in breast milk
Primary metabolism	Hepatic (CYP450)
Primary excretion	Renal (less than 10% feces)
Onset of action	Inhalation: 5–15 min; PO: 30 min; peak effect: 0.5–2 h
Duration of action	Inhalation: 2–6 h; PO, sustained release: 8–12 h

Adverse Effects: Serious adverse effects from inhaled albuterol are uncommon when taken as directed; PO forms cause more sympathomimetic adverse effects. Some patients experience palpitations, headaches, throat irritation, tremor, nervousness,

TABLE 44.4 Bronchodilators for Asthma

Drug	Route and Adult Dose (Maximum Dose Where Indicated)	Adverse Effects
Beta Agonists/Sympathomimetics		
albuterol (Proventil, Ventolin, VoSpire)	MDI: 2 inhalations every 4–6 h as needed (max: 12 inhalations/day) Nebulizer: 1.25–5 mg every 4–8 h as needed PO: 2–4 mg tid-qid (max: 32 mg/day); extended release tabs: 8 mg every 12 h (max: 32 mg/day divided)	*Headache, dizziness, tremor, nervousness, throat irritation, drug tolerance* <u>Tachycardia, dysrhythmia, hypokalemia, hyperglycemia, paradoxical bronchoconstriction, hypomagnesemia, maternal heart problems during pregnancy (terbutaline), increased risk for asthma-related death</u>
arformoterol (Brovana)	Nebulizer: 15 mcg twice daily (max: 30 mcg/day)	
formoterol (Foradil, Perforomist)	DPI: 12 mcg inhalation capsule every 12 h (max: 24 mcg/day) Nebulizer: 20 mcg bid (max: 40 mcg/day)	
indacaterol (Arcapta neohaler)	Inhalation: one 75 mcg capsule/day using the Neohaler	
levalbuterol HCl (Xopenex)	Nebulizer: 0.63 mg tid-qid MDI: 2 inhalations every 4–6 h	
metaproterenol	PO: 20 mg q6–8 h	
pirbuterol	MDI: 2 inhalations qid (max: 12 puffs/day)	
salmeterol (Serevent)	DPI: 2 aerosol inhalations bid or 1 powder diskus bid	
terbutaline sulfate (Brethine)	PO: 2.5–5 mg tid (max: 15 mg/day) Subcutaneous: 0.25 mg, followed by an additional 0.25 mg if no response is noted in 30 min	
Anticholinergics		
aclidinium (Tudorxa Pressair)	DPI: 2 inhalations (400 mcg) bid	*Headache, bad taste, cough, dry mouth, blurred vision, paradoxical bronchospasm, worsening of narrow-angle glaucoma* <u>Pharyngitis</u>
ipratropium (Atrovent)	MDI: 2 inhalations (50 mcg) qid (max: 12 inhalations/day) Nebulizer: 500 mcg every 6–8 h as needed	
tiotropium (Spiriva)	DPI: 1 capsule inhaled/day	
Methylxanthines		
aminophylline (Truphylline)	PO: 380 mg/day in divided doses every 6–8 h (max: 928 mg/day) IV: 0.1–0.5 mg/kg/h (rate dependent on certain patient parameters)	*Nervousness, tremors, dizziness, headache, nausea, vomiting, anorexia* <u>Tachycardia, dysrhythmias, hypotension, seizures, circulatory failure, respiratory arrest</u>
Dyphylline (Lufylline)	PO: 15 mg every 6 h	
theophylline (Theo-Dur, Others)	PO: 300–600 mg/day in divided doses (max: 900 mg/day) IV: 0.39–0.79 mg/kg/h (rate dependent on certain patient parameters)	

Note: *Italics* indicate common adverse effects. <u>Underline</u> indicates serious adverse effects.

restlessness, and tachycardia. Less common adverse reactions include insomnia and dry mouth. Uncommon adverse effects include chest pain, paradoxical bronchospasm, and allergic reactions.

Contraindications/Precautions: Albuterol use is contraindicated if the patient has hypersensitivity to the drug. Because albuterol may exhibit cardiovascular effects in some patients, caution is required when administering these agents to persons with a history of tachyarrhythmias, prolongation of the QT interval, coronary artery disease, or hypertension (HTN).

Drug Interactions: Concurrent use with beta blockers will inhibit the bronchodilation effect of albuterol and may induce bronchospasm in patients with asthma. To prevent hypertensive crisis, patients should also avoid monoamine oxidase inhibitors (MAOIs) within 14 days of beginning therapy. Concurrent use with thyroid hormone may produce additive stimulatory effects on the cardiovascular system. **Herbal/Food**: Products containing caffeine such as coffee and tea may cause nervousness, tremor, or palpitations.

Pregnancy: Category C.

Treatment of Overdose: Overdose results in an exaggerated sympathetic activation, causing dysrhythmias, hypokalemia, and hyperglycemia. Cardiac arrest and death have been reported. In severe cases, administration of a beta antagonist may be necessary.

Nursing Responsibilities: Key nursing implications for patients receiving albuterol are included in the Nursing Practice Application for Patients Receiving Pharmacotherapy for Asthma and COPD.

Drugs Similar to Albuterol (Proventil, Ventolin, VoSpire)

Other short-acting beta agonists include levalbuterol and pirbuterol. Long-acting beta agonists include arformoterol, formoterol, indacaterol, metaproterenol, salmeterol, and terbutaline. Bitolterol mesylate is a drug in this class that has been discontinued in the United States. Adverse effects are the same as those of other beta$_2$ agonists and include tachycardia, nervousness, angina, and headache.

Arformoterol (Brovana): Arformoterol was approved in 2007 for the treatment of COPD, including chronic bronchitis and emphysema. This drug is an isomer of formoterol and was the first LABA available by inhalation via nebulizer. Formoterol and salmeterol use DPIs. Arformoterol may be administered twice daily. Although it begins to relax bronchi within about 7 minutes, its maximum effects take 1 to 3 hours. Thus this drug is not suitable for terminating acute asthma attacks. Arformoterol is well tolerated and exhibits few serious adverse effects in most patients. The drug has a black box warning that it (and other LABAs) has been shown to increase the risk of asthma-related death; thus it should only be prescribed when short- and intermediate-acting drugs are unable to control symptoms. A combination drug (Dulera) containing arformoterol and mometasone was approved in 2010. Arformoterol is pregnancy category C.

Formoterol (Foradil, Perforomist): Approved in 2001, formoterol is a long-acting, selective beta$_2$ agonist that is administered using a DPI. Because the drug takes 1 to 3 hours for maximum effect, it is not suitable for terminating acute bronchospasm. Due to its long duration of action, formoterol is indicated for asthma prophylaxis, including the prevention of nocturnal symptoms and exercise-induced asthma. It is also approved by the FDA for the relief of bronchospasm due to COPD. This drug is well tolerated and has the same adverse effect profile as that of other drugs in this class. Formoterol has a black box warning that it (and other LABAs) has been shown to increase the risk of asthma-related death; thus it should only be prescribed when short- and intermediate-acting drugs are unable to control symptoms. This drug is pregnancy category C.

Indacaterol (Arcapta Neohaler): One of the newer drugs in this class, indacaterol was approved in 2011 as a maintenance bronchodilator for patients with COPD, including chronic bronchitis and emphysema. The drug comes as a capsule that is inserted into the neohaler device for inhalation. Its once-daily dosing schedule offers an advantage over other LABAs. Indacaterol is not indicated for the termination of acute bronchospasm. Like other LABAs, indacaterol carries a black box warning that it should not be used for long-term asthma control due to the possibility of an increased risk of asthma-related death. This drug is pregnancy category C.

Levalbuterol (Xopenex): Approved in 1999, levalbuterol is an isomer of albuterol and has almost identical indications, actions, and adverse effects. This drug is administered via nebulized or aerosolized oral inhalation. It is indicated for the relief of acute bronchospasm symptoms and can be administered three to four times daily. Regular, daily use of levalbuterol is not recommended by the NAEPP as a means to prevent bronchospasm. Like other drugs in this class, levalbuterol has few serious adverse effects, with nervousness and tremor being the most frequently reported. This drug is pregnancy category C.

Metaproterenol: Approved in 1981 to treat bronchospasm, metaproterenol is a short-acting beta agonist available by the oral route. It has a duration of 4 to 6 hours. The actions and adverse effects are similar to those of albuterol. This drug is pregnancy category C.

Pirbuterol: Approved in 1986, pirbuterol is a short-acting, selective beta$_2$ agonist that has a structure very similar to that of albuterol. Its rapid, 5-minute onset of action makes it suitable for the termination of acute bronchospasm symptoms. Doses may be repeated every 4 to 6 hours, as needed. Like the other short-acting beta$_2$ agonists, this drug must not be used on a regular, daily basis to prevent asthmatic attacks. It is also FDA approved for the relief of bronchospasm due to COPD and may be prescribed off-label to prevent exercise-induced bronchospasm. It is available only by the inhalation route. Adverse effects are uncommon and include tachycardia and palpitation. This drug is pregnancy category C.

Salmeterol (Serevent): Approved in 1994, salmeterol is a LABA that is prescribed for asthma prophylaxis and the long-term therapy of bronchospasm associated with COPD. The LABAs salmeterol and formoterol are considered less effective at preventing asthma attacks than the inhaled corticosteroids. Salmeterol has a slow onset of action and should not be used to terminate acute bronchospasm. The aerosol form of salmeterol has been discontinued in the United States, although the DPI route is still available. Overall, the drug is well tolerated, and few serious adverse effects are reported. Pharyngitis and upper respiratory tract infections occur in patients who are taking the drug, and headache is a common adverse effect. Salmeterol has a black box warning that it (and other LABAs) has been shown to increase the risk of asthma-related death; thus it should only be prescribed when short- and intermediate-acting drugs are unable to control symptoms. This drug is pregnancy category C.

Terbutaline (Brethine): An older drug approved in 1974, terbutaline is indicated for the treatment of bronchospasm. Terbutaline is given by the PO route and may take 30 minutes or longer to act; thus it is too slow to be used for acute conditions. A subcutaneous form of terbutaline can relieve bronchospasm within 15 minutes. PO terbutaline has a shorter duration of action than albuterol or salmeterol and it must be administered three times daily. An inhalation form of the drug (Brethaire) was removed from the U.S. market in 1999. Terbutaline is moderately selective for beta$_2$ receptors but may produce some activation of beta$_1$ receptors in the heart. Adverse effects are similar to those observed with other drugs in this class. Terbutaline has been used off-label to delay premature labor contractions due to its effects on beta$_2$ receptors in the uterus that cause smooth muscle relaxation (see Chapter 69). However, in 2011 the FDA issued a black box warning that *oral* terbutaline should not be used to prevent or treat preterm labor because it has not been shown to be effective and there is a potential for serious maternal heart problems and death. In very serious conditions, the *injectable* form of the drug may still be used but treatment is limited to no longer than 48 to 72 hours to delay preterm labor. This drug is pregnancy category B.

CONNECTION Checkpoint 44.1

The medications for asthma are selective for beta$_2$-adrenergic receptors. From what you learned in Chapter 15, what are the primary indications for the drugs selective for beta$_1$-adrenergic receptors? *See Answer to Connection Checkpoint 44.1 on student resource website.*

44.6 The inhaled anticholinergics are used for preventing bronchospasm.

Although short-acting beta agonists are the drugs of choice for treating acute bronchospasm, anticholinergics (cholinergic blockers or antagonists) are alternative bronchodilators. Although anticholinergics such as atropine have been available for many decades, the adverse effect profile of anticholinergics made them poorly suited for the management of asthma. With the delivery of the anticholinergics by inhalation, however, they have become important drugs in the arsenal of asthma pharmacotherapy. Three inhalation anticholinergics are available for the treatment of bronchospasm. The first to be developed was ipratropium (Atrovent), which is considered a short-acting agent. Aclidinium (Tudorza Pressair) and tiotropium (Spiriva) are newer, long-acting anticholinergics.

Anticholinergics block the parasympathetic nervous system. Blocking the parasympathetic nervous system results in actions similar to those of stimulating the sympathetic nervous system (see Chapter 14). It is predictable then that anticholinergic drugs would cause bronchodilation and have potential applications in the pharmacotherapy of asthma and COPD. Ipratropium is rapid acting and can be used to relieve acute bronchospasm, whereas tiotropium is better suited for maintenance therapy due to its longer onset of action.

Anticholinergics have actions that are similar to those of beta-adrenergic agonists and drugs from the two classes may be combined to produce a greater and more prolonged bronchodilation than either drug used separately. This additive effect is particularly useful for patients with persistent bronchospasm for whom either agent alone is inadequate to alleviate bronchoconstriction. Taking advantage of this increased effect, the pharmaceutical companies have developed inhalants that combine both an anticholinergic and a beta agonist into a single canister.

Anticholinergics are available in PO, inhaled, and injection formulations; however, when used for asthma and other respiratory conditions, the inhaled forms are typically prescribed. The inhaled anticholinergics are relatively safe medications. The wide range of anticholinergic adverse effects that is observed when drugs in this class are administered systemically rarely occurs when administered by inhalation.

| PROTOTYPE DRUG | Ipratropium (Atrovent) |

Classification: Therapeutic: Bronchodilator
Pharmacologic: Anticholinergic

Therapeutic Effects and Uses: Approved by the FDA in 1986, ipratropium is an anticholinergic medication that is delivered by the inhalation and intranasal routes. The inhalation form is approved to relieve and prevent the bronchospasm that is characteristic of asthma and COPD. It is a preferred drug for treating bronchospasms due to COPD (e.g., bronchitis and emphysema). Although it has not received FDA approval for the treatment of asthma, it is nevertheless prescribed off-label for the disorder. NAEPP guidelines state that the role of ipratropium in asthma management is as an alternative to short-acting beta agonists and for patients experiencing severe asthma exacerbations. It is sometimes combined with beta agonists or corticosteroids to provide additive bronchodilation. Ipratropium is much less effective than the beta$_2$ agonists at preventing exercise-induced bronchospasm.

When administered via inhalation, ipratropium can relieve acute bronchospasm within minutes of administration, although peak effects may take 1 to 2 hours. Bronchodilation action may continue for up to 6 hours.

The nasal spray formulation of ipratropium is indicated for the symptomatic relief of rhinorrhea associated with the common cold and perennial rhinitis. The drug inhibits nasal secretions but does not have decongestant action. Treatment is limited to 3 weeks.

Mechanism of Action: Ipratropium causes bronchodilation by blocking cholinergic receptors in bronchial smooth muscle. Intranasal administration blocks parasympathetic receptors, thus reducing nasal hypersecretion characteristic of the common cold.

Pharmacokinetics:

Route(s)	Inhalation, intranasal
Absorption	Minimal systemic absorption; some of the inhaled drug is swallowed but is not absorbed by the GI tract
Distribution	Small amount is secreted in breast milk; minimally bound to plasma protein
Primary metabolism	Hepatic (CYP450)
Primary excretion	Renal and feces
Onset of action	5–15 min; peak effect: 1.5–2 h
Duration of action	3–6 h; half-life: 1.5–2 h

Adverse Effects: Because it is not readily absorbed from the lungs, ipratropium produces few systemic adverse effects. Though rare it can worsen glaucoma with sufficient systemic absorption. Typical anticholinergic adverse effects such as dry mouth, nausea, and GI distress are among the most common adverse effects but occur in less than 3% of patients. Irritation of the upper respiratory tract may cause cough, drying of the nasal mucosa, or hoarseness. Paradoxical acute bronchospasm is a rare adverse effect that may be life threatening. This drug produces a bitter taste that some patients find problematic. Intranasal administration may cause epistaxis and excessive drying of the nasal mucosa.

Contraindications/Precautions: Ipratropium is contraindicated in patients with hypersensitivity to soya lecithin or related food products such as soybean and peanut. Soya lecithin is used as a propellant in the inhaler. Ipratropium is contraindicated in persons who have demonstrated a hypersensitivity to ipratropium. All anticholinergics should be used with caution in patients with closed-angle glaucoma or urinary tract obstruction because they may worsen these conditions.

Drug Interactions: Because it has little systemic absorption, ipratropium interacts with very few drugs. Use with other anticholinergics such as atropine may lead to additive anticholinergic adverse effects. Ipratropium should not be used concurrently with pramlintide (Symlin) because both slow GI peristalsis and can cause nausea, vomiting, or constipation. **Herbal/Food:** Unknown.

Pregnancy: Category B.

Treatment of Overdose: Overdose with ipratropium is unlikely because very little of the drug is absorbed.

Nursing Responsibilities: Key nursing implications for patients receiving ipratropium are included in the Nursing Practice Application for Patients Receiving Pharmacotherapy for Asthma and COPD.

Drugs Similar to Ipratropium (Atrovent)

The other anticholinergics currently approved for inhalation are aclidinium (Tudorza Pressair) and tiotropium.

Aclidinium (Tudorza Pressair): Aclidinium is the newest anticholinergic approved in 2012 for the long-term maintenance treatment of bronchospasm associated with COPD. It is administered twice daily by DPI and is used to prevent, not terminate, bronchospasm. It has very similar actions and adverse effects to those of the other two drugs in this class. Common side effects include headache, nasopharyngitis, and cough. This drug is pregnancy category C.

Tiotropium (Spiriva): Approved in 2004, tiotropium is closely related to ipratropium and is indicated for the long-term maintenance treatment and prophylaxis of bronchospasm in patients with COPD, including chronic bronchitis and emphysema. It is not to be used to terminate acute bronchospasm; short-acting adrenergic agonists are indicated for this condition. An advantage of tiotropium is its long duration of action. Unlike ipratropium, which must be taken four or more times a day, tiotropium only needs to be taken once a day so patients are less likely to miss doses. Another difference between the two agents is that ipratropium is administered by MDI, whereas tiotropium is administered by DPI (HandiHaler device). For patients with COPD who have difficulty using an MDI device, tiotropium can be a viable alternative. Adverse effects are the same as those of ipratropium. This drug is pregnancy category C.

44.7 Inhaled corticosteroids are the most effective drugs for the long-term control of asthma.

Corticosteroids are the most potent natural anti-inflammatory substances known. Because asthma has a major inflammatory component, it should not be surprising that drugs in this class play a major role in the management of this disorder. *Inhaled* corticosteroids are the drugs of choice for the prevention of asthmatic attacks and for the management of chronic asthma. *Oral* corticosteroids are used for the short-term management of acute asthma attacks. The therapeutic actions of the corticosteroids have resulted in their widespread use in the pharmacotherapy of allergic rhinitis (see Chapter 45) and other inflammatory disorders. Doses for the inhaled corticosteroids are given in Table 44.5.

Corticosteroids decrease inflammation of the airways by inhibiting the synthesis and release of inflammatory mediators, including histamine, leukotriene, cytokines, and prostaglandins. They also inhibit the number of circulating leukocytes and decrease vascular permeability. This results in diminished mucus production and edema, thus reducing airway obstruction. Although corticosteroids are not bronchodilators, they sensitize the bronchial smooth muscle to be more responsive to beta-agonist stimulation. In addition, they reduce the bronchial hyperresponsiveness to allergens, which is responsible for triggering many asthma attacks.

When inhaled on a daily schedule, corticosteroids suppress inflammation without producing major adverse effects. Although symptoms will improve in the first 1 to 2 weeks of therapy, 4 to 8 weeks may be required for maximum benefit. Because of the dangerous adverse effects of long-term therapy, systemic corticosteroids are generally reserved for short-term management of acute asthma exacerbations. For outpatient management in these instances, PO corticosteroids such as prednisone are given for the shortest length of time possible, usually 5 to 7 days. In the hospital setting, intravenous (IV) corticosteroids may be given. Regardless, at the end of the brief treatment period, patients are usually switched to inhaled corticosteroids for long-term management.

When taken long term, both PO and inhaled formulations of corticosteroids have the potential to affect bone physiology in adults and children. Adults who are at risk for osteoporosis should receive periodic bone mineral density tests and possibly pharmacotherapy with bisphosphonates to prevent fractures (see Chapter 72). In children, small decreases in linear bone growth have been documented. Although these effects are usually temporary, growth should be monitored and the prescriber should weigh the risks of growth suppression against the benefits of corticosteroid use. In all cases, effects on bone growth are dose and frequency dependent; thus patients should be administered the lowest doses possible to maintain adequate asthma control.

CONNECTIONS **Lifespan Considerations**

◀ Proper Inhaler Use by Older Adults

Inhaler use in the treatment of asthma and COPD is common. Correct use of the inhaler is necessary for adequate therapeutic outcomes and adherence to treatment. Proper inhaler use can be a challenge for all patients; however, the older adult is more likely to have one or more factors that impede appropriate use than does a younger patient (Lareau & Hodder, 2012). These factors include patient issues (e.g., cognitive ability, dexterity, presence of tremors, visual or hearing impairments); disease-based issues (e.g., ability to inhale adequately, decreased inspiratory volume); device issues (e.g., devices with differing instructions, use of multiple devices); and cost. Nurses working with respiratory patients should be familiar with the use and functioning of all types of inhalers and provide detailed instructions for appropriate use. Recognizing barriers that the older adult might experience helps nurses in planning teaching strategies to improve inhaler use by these patients, resulting in improved therapeutic outcomes.

PROTOTYPE DRUG **Beclomethasone (Beconase AQ, Qvar)**

Classification: Therapeutic: Anti-inflammatory
Pharmacologic: Corticosteroid

Therapeutic Effects and Uses: Approved in 1976, beclomethasone is a corticosteroid that is available for administration by aerosol inhalation for asthma (Qvar) or as a nasal spray (Beconase AQ) for allergic rhinitis. Guidelines from the NAEPP place beclomethasone and other drugs in this class as preferred drugs for the long-term management of persistent asthma in both children and adults. Two inhalations, two to three times per day, usually provide adequate prophylaxis, although 3 to 4 weeks of therapy may be necessary before optimum benefits are achieved. In 2000, a double strength formulation (Qvar) was developed with smaller drug particles. It is able to deliver half the usual dose and achieve the same therapeutic effect. Beclomethasone is not a bronchodilator and should not be used to terminate asthma attacks in progress.

TABLE 44.5 Anti-Inflammatory Drugs for Asthma and COPD

Drug	Route and Adult Dose (Maximum Dose Where Indicated)	Adverse Effects
Inhaled Corticosteroids*		
beclomethasone (Beconase AQ, Qvar)	MDI: 1–2 inhalations tid-qid (max: 20 inhalations/day)	*Hoarseness, dry mouth, cough, sore throat* Oropharyngeal candidiasis, hypercorticism, hypersensitivity reactions
budesonide (Pulmicort)	DPI: 1–2 inhalations (200 mcg/inhalation) qid (max: 800 mcg/day)	
ciclesonide (Alvesco)	Intranasal: 2 sprays per nostril (200 mcg) once daily Inhalation: 2 inhalations (160–320 mcg/inhalation) daily	
flunisolide	MDI: 2–3 inhalations bid-tid (max: 12 inhalations/day)	
fluticasone (Flovent)	MDI (44 mcg): 2 inhalations bid (max: 10 inhalations/day)	
mometasone (Asmanex)	DPI: 1 inhalation daily (max: 2 inhalations daily)	
triamcinolone	MDI: 2 inhalations tid-qid (max: 16 inhalations/day)	
Mast Cell Stabilizers		
cromolyn	MDI: 1 inhalation qid	*Nausea, sneezing, nasal stinging, throat irritation, unpleasant taste* Anaphylaxis, angioedema, bronchospasm
nedocromil	MDI: 2 inhalations qid	
Leukotriene Modifiers and Miscellaneous Drugs		
montelukast (Singulair)	PO: 10 mg/day in evening	*Headache, nausea, diarrhea, throat pain, weight loss (roflumilast)* Increased aspartate aminotransferase (AST), hepatotoxicity, psychiatric events including suicidality (roflumilast)
roflumilast (Daliresp)	PO: 500 mcg once daily	
zafirlukast (Accolate)	PO: 20 mg bid 1 h before or 2 h after meals	
zileuton (Zyflo CR)	PO: 1,200 mg bid (max: 2,400 mg/day)	

*For doses of systemic corticosteroids, refer to Chapter 68.

Note: Italics indicate common adverse effects. Underline indicates serious adverse effects.

The intranasal formulation is effective at reducing the symptoms of allergic rhinitis. Therapeutic effects may take as long as 2 weeks to be fully apparent. Intranasal beclomethasone is also approved to prevent recurrence of nasal polyps following surgical removal. Very little of this drug is absorbed in the systemic circulation when it is administered by this route.

Mechanism of Action: Beclomethasone acts by reducing inflammation and immune responses, thus decreasing the frequency of asthma attacks.

Pharmacokinetics:

Route(s)	Inhalation, intranasal
Absorption	Small amounts of systemic absorption
Distribution	Delivered directly to the lungs (site of action); small amount is secreted in breast milk
Primary metabolism	Liver (CYP450: 3A substrate) and lung
Primary excretion	Mostly feces with about 10% in urine
Onset of action	1–3 weeks
Duration of action	Half-life: 15 h

Adverse Effects: Inhaled beclomethasone produces few systemic adverse effects. Because small amounts may be swallowed with each dose, the patient should be observed for signs of corticosteroid toxicity (hypercorticism) when taking this drug for prolonged periods. Local effects may include hoarseness, dry mouth, and changes in taste. Inhaled corticosteroid use has been associated with the development of cataracts in adults. Some studies have shown that long-term intranasal or inhaled corticosteroids may cause growth inhibition in children.

Like all corticosteroids, the anti-inflammatory properties of beclomethasone can mask signs of infections and the drug is contraindicated if active infection is present. A large percentage of patients taking beclomethasone on a long-term basis will develop oropharyngeal candidiasis, a fungal infection in the throat, due to the constant deposits of drug in the oral cavity. Children who have not been vaccinated for varicella should receive the vaccine because of the potential for developing serious disseminated varicella infections during treatment with corticosteroids.

Contraindications/Precautions: The only contraindication to using beclomethasone is hypersensitivity to the drug.

Drug Interactions: Because very little of the drug is absorbed, no clinically significant drug interactions occur. **Herbal/Food**: None known.

Pregnancy: Category C.

Treatment of Overdose: Overdose does not occur when taken by the inhalation route.

Nursing Responsibilities: Key nursing implications for patients receiving beclomethasone are included in the Nursing Practice Application for Patients Receiving Pharmacotherapy for Asthma and COPD.

Drugs Similar to Beclomethasone (Beconase AQ, Qvar)

Other corticosteroids for inhalation include budesonide, ciclesonide, flunisolide, fluticasone, mometasone, and triamcinolone.

Budesonide (Pulmicort): Budesonide is a corticosteroid that is available by the intranasal route for allergic rhinitis (Rhinocort), oral inhalation, nebulizer for asthma prophylaxis (Pulmicort), or PO capsules for Crohn's disease (Entocort). The most common adverse effects with the inhaled use of budesonide include respiratory infections, rhinitis, cough, and otitis media. Visual impairment may occur. Growth effects should be monitored in pediatric patients. This drug is pregnancy category B.

Ciclesonide (Alvesco): Approved in 2006, ciclesonide is a corticosteroid available by the oral inhalation (Alvesco) route for asthma maintenance and prophylaxis in patients over 12 years of age or by the intranasal (Omnaris) route for allergic rhinitis. Ciclesonide is a prodrug that is converted to an active metabolite following administration. Like other drugs in this class, ciclesonide is not a bronchodilator and should not be used to treat acute bronchospasm. Actions and adverse effects are the same as those of other corticosteroids administered by inhalation. This drug is pregnancy category C.

Flunisolide: Flunisolide is a corticosteroid that is available by the intranasal route for allergic rhinitis (Nasarel) or by oral inhalation for asthma prophylaxis. The most common adverse effects with inhaled use include upper respiratory infections, dry mouth, hoarseness, nausea, vomiting, and taste changes. Like other drugs in this class, visual impairment may occur and growth effects should be monitored in pediatric patients. This drug is pregnancy category C.

Fluticasone (Flovent): Fluticasone is a corticosteroid that is available by the intranasal route for allergic rhinitis (Flonase); oral inhalation for asthma prophylaxis or COPD (Flovent); or topical cream or ointment for dermatitis, eczema, and other skin conditions (Cutivate). The most common adverse effects with the inhaled use of fluticasone include headache, throat irritation, and upper respiratory tract infections. Visual impairment may occur. Growth effects should be monitored in pediatric patients. Like other inhaled corticosteroids, fluticasone is not indicated for the relief of acute bronchospasm. This drug is pregnancy category C.

Mometasone (Asmanex): Mometasone is an inhaled corticosteroid that is available for the prevention of acute asthmatic attacks. When inhaled it may take an hour or longer to produce its effects; therefore, it is not indicated for the relief of acute bronchospasm. Actions and adverse effects are the same as those of other inhaled corticosteroids. An intranasal form is available for allergic rhinitis (Nasonex), and a topical preparation (Elocon) is used to treat various inflammatory skin conditions. This drug is pregnancy category C.

Triamcinolone: Triamcinolone is available in a wide variety of formulations: oral inhalation for asthma, intranasal for allergic rhinitis (Nasacort), ophthalmic for ocular inflammation (Triesence), and various topical formulations for inflammatory skin conditions. Parenteral formulations (Kenalog) are available for a large number of allergic and inflammatory disorders. When inhaled, the adverse effects are the same as those of other corticosteroids, such as throat irritation, dry mouth, hoarseness, visual changes, possible growth retardation in children, and upper respiratory tract infections. This drug is pregnancy category C.

CONNECTION Checkpoint 44.2

From what you learned in Chapter 42, describe strategies that could be used to limit the incidence of serious adverse effects when corticosteroids must be taken PO for prolonged periods. *See Answer to Connection Checkpoint 44.2 on student resource website.*

44.8 Mast cell stabilizers are used for the prophylaxis of asthma and act by preventing the release of histamine.

Mast cell stabilizers serve limited, though important, roles in the prophylaxis of asthma. Mast cells are large cells that contain inflammatory granules, such as histamine, that mediate inflammatory and allergic reactions. When these cells are sensitized, they degranulate and release the inflammatory substances into the body where they initiate an inflammatory response. Mast cell stabilizers are helpful in managing asthma and COPD because they prevent degranulation of the mast cell, preventing the release of histamine and other inflammatory mediators in the airways. There are two currently approved mast cell stabilizers: cromolyn and nedocromil. Doses of these agents are listed in Table 44.5. Mast cell stabilizers are administered by inhalation via an MDI or a nebulizer. An intranasal form is available for management of allergic rhinitis.

PROTOTYPE DRUG	Cromolyn

Classification: **Therapeutic:** Anti-inflammatory
Pharmacologic: Mast cell stabilizer

Therapeutic Effects and Uses: An older drug that was approved by the FDA in 1973, cromolyn prevents the inflammation that is a characteristic pathophysiologic feature of asthma and COPD. Because it has no effect on previously released inflammatory mediators from mast cell degranulation, the effects will not be noted immediately. The NAEPP guidelines place cromolyn as an alternate drug for the treatment of mild to moderate asthma when corticosteroids are contraindicated or have not proven effective. This drug should not be used to terminate acute asthma attacks.

For asthma therapy the drug is administered via oral inhalation. An intranasal over-the-counter (OTC) formulation (NasalCrom) is available for allergic rhinitis. An ophthalmic solution (Crolom) is used to treat various allergic disorders of the conjunctiva. Gastrocrom is a PO dosage form of cromolyn that is the only FDA-approved drug to treat systemic mastocytosis, which is a rare condition in which the patient has an excessive number of mast cells. Gastrocrom is also used off-label to treat ulcerative colitis and to prevent symptoms associated with food allergies.

Mechanism of Action: By stabilizing mast cells, cromolyn helps to prevent the inflammatory response that occurs when mast cells degranulate.

Pharmacokinetics:

Route(s)	Inhalation
Absorption	Minimal systemic absorption (less than 1%)
Distribution	Delivered directly to the lungs (site of action); small amount crosses the placenta; small amount is secreted in breast milk
Primary metabolism	Hepatic
Primary excretion	Bile (and, subsequently, feces) and renal
Onset of action	Adequate effect may not be noted until 2–4 weeks of use
Duration of action	Unknown

Adverse Effects: Adverse effects are uncommon when the drug is administered by oral inhalation. The most common effects are bronchospasm, cough, and pharyngeal irritation. Intranasal and ophthalmic administration may cause local burning and stinging.

Contraindications/Precautions: As with any drug, persons who have demonstrated a hypersensitivity to this drug should not take it. It should be discontinued if the patient develops pulmonary eosinophilia.

Drug Interactions: No significant interactions are known. **Herbal/Food**: Unknown.

Pregnancy: Category B.

Treatment of Overdose: There are no noted problems associated with overdosage. Toxicity is unlikely.

Nursing Responsibilities: Key nursing implications for patients receiving cromolyn are included in the Nursing Practice Application for Patients Receiving Pharmacotherapy for Asthma and COPD.

Drugs Similar to Cromolyn

Nedocromil is the only other mast cell stabilizer.

Nedocromil: Approved in 1992, the actions of this drug are similar to those of cromolyn with the exception of a very bitter taste that causes some people to discontinue it. This is a particularly important consideration for children who will be less willing to take distasteful medication. Like cromolyn, nedocromil is to be used only for asthma prophylaxis and not to terminate acute asthma attacks. The drug may require a week of therapy before benefits are obtained, and it must be taken on a continuous basis for asthma prophylaxis. An ophthalmic form (Alocril) is available to treat allergic conjunctivitis. This drug is pregnancy category B.

44.9 The leukotriene modifiers, which are primarily used for asthma prophylaxis, act by reducing the inflammatory component of asthma.

Leukotriene modifiers are one of the newest drug classes added to the arsenal of asthma management. They are able to ease bronchoconstriction by reducing inflammation. Because of their delayed onset, leukotriene modifiers are ineffective at terminating acute

asthma attacks. The NAEPP guidelines list the leukotriene modifiers as alternative drugs to be considered when inhaled corticosteroids and short-acting beta agonists are unable to control asthma symptoms. Doses for these drugs are listed in Table 44.5.

Leukotrienes are mediators of the immune and inflammatory responses that are involved in allergic and asthmatic reactions. Leukotrienes are synthesized by mast cells as well as neutrophils, basophils, and eosinophils. When released in the airway, they promote edema, inflammation, and bronchoconstriction. Leukotriene modifiers reduce inflammation by either blocking the enzyme that controls leukotriene synthesis or by blocking leukotriene receptors. They are not considered bronchodilators, although they do reduce bronchoconstriction indirectly. The leukotriene modifiers are only available by the PO route.

<table><tr><td>**PROTOTYPE DRUG**</td><td>**Zafirlukast (Accolate)**</td></tr></table>

Classification: **Therapeutic:** Agent for asthma prophylaxis, anti-inflammatory
Pharmacologic: Leukotriene modifier

Therapeutic Effects and Uses: Zafirlukast, the first leukotriene modifier, which was approved in 1996, is used for the prophylaxis of persistent, chronic asthma. This drug prevents the inflammation that is a characteristic pathophysiologic feature of asthma and COPD. It is less effective than inhaled corticosteroids. Off-label uses include allergic rhinitis and prevention of exercise-induced bronchospasm.

Zafirlukast is given by the PO route. Its relatively long onset of action makes it unsuitable for the termination of acute bronchospasm.

Mechanism of Action: Zafirlukast prevents airway edema and inflammation by blocking leukotriene receptors in the airways.

Pharmacokinetics:

Route(s)	PO
Absorption	Rapidly absorbed, but decreased in presence of food
Distribution	Secreted in breast milk; more than 99% bound to plasma protein
Primary metabolism	Extensive hepatic metabolism (CYP2C9, CYP3A4)
Primary excretion	Mostly bile; 10% renal
Onset of action	1 week
Duration of action	Unknown; half-life: 10 h

Adverse Effects: Zafirlukast produces few serious adverse effects. Headache is the most common complaint. Rhinitis, nausea, vomiting, and diarrhea are reported by some patients.

Contraindications/Precautions: The only absolute contraindication is hypersensitivity to this drug. Because a few rare cases of fatal hepatic failure have been reported, patients with preexisting hepatic impairment should be treated with caution. This drug should be avoided when breast-feeding.

Drug Interactions: Zafirlukast is metabolized by CYP450 enzymes and has the potential to interact with substrates of the inhibitors of this enzyme. Use with warfarin may significantly increase prothrombin time (PT). Erythromycin and theophylline may decrease the serum levels of zafirlukast. Concurrent use with aspirin can significantly increase zafirlukast levels. **Herbal/Food**: Food can reduce the bioavailability; thus the drug should be taken on an empty stomach.

Pregnancy: Category B.

Treatment of Overdose: Symptoms of overdose include headache, nausea, and vomiting. Treatment is supportive.

Nursing Responsibilities: Key nursing implications for patients receiving zafirlukast are included in the Nursing Practice Application for Patients Receiving Pharmacotherapy for Asthma and COPD.

Drugs Similar to Zafirlukast (Accolate)

Montelukast and zileuton are other leukotriene modifiers.

Montelukast (Singulair): Given by the PO route, montelukast acts by blocking leukotriene receptors in the airways. Montelukast is the only agent in this category that is approved for very young children, 12 months or older. For pediatric use it is available as chewable tablets and oral granules that may be sprinkled on soft food. The drug is approved for the prophylaxis of persistent, chronic asthma, allergic rhinitis, and exercise-induced bronchospasm. Like other drugs in this class, montelukast should not be used to treat acute asthma attacks. Adverse effects are generally mild. Headache is the most frequently reported adverse effect. This is a pregnancy category B drug.

Zileuton (Zyflo CR): Approved in 1996, zileuton is a PO drug that acts by inhibiting the lipoxygenase, which is the first enzyme in the pathway of leukotriene synthesis. Like other drugs in this class, zileuton is considered an alternate drug in the prophylaxis of persistent, chronic asthma. In 2007 an extended release formulation (Zyflo CR) was approved that allows for twice-daily dosing. Like other drugs in this class, zileuton should not be used to treat acute asthma attacks. This drug is generally well tolerated, with sinusitis, nausea, and throat pain being the most common adverse effects. The most serious concern with zileuton is the potential for liver damage. Zileuton raises liver enzymes (alanine aminotransferase), and cases of jaundice and severe hepatic injury have been reported. This drug is contraindicated in patients with hepatic impairment, and liver function tests should be conducted on a regular basis during therapy. Because zileuton can increase serum warfarin levels, PT should be regularly monitored. This is a pregnancy category C drug.

44.10 Methylxanthines were once the mainstay of asthma pharmacotherapy but are now rarely prescribed for that disorder.

The **methylxanthines** were considered the drugs of choice for treating asthma 30 years ago. Now they are primarily reserved for the long-term management of persistent asthma that is unresponsive to beta agonists or inhaled corticosteroids. One reason for the lessened use of methylxanthines is that their narrow therapeutic index increases the risk of toxicity, especially with prolonged use. These drugs also have significant interactions with numerous other drugs. Doses for these agents are listed in Table 44.4.

The methylxanthines are modest bronchodilators. They are chemically related to caffeine and share caffeine's stimulant effect. Methylxanthines are available in forms for PO, parenteral, and rectal administration. Because they are not available for inhalation, patients do not benefit from the smaller doses and direct effects that are provided by drugs that can be administered by the inhalation route. Interestingly, theobromine, an ingredient in chocolate, is also a methylxanthine.

PROTOTYPE DRUG	**Theophylline (Theo-Dur, Others)**

Classification: **Therapeutic:** Bronchodilator **Pharmacologic:** Methylxanthine

Therapeutic Effects and Uses: Approved by the FDA in 1940, theophylline is a natural substance found in small amounts in tea. Theophylline relaxes bronchial smooth muscle and may exert some anti-inflammatory action that is beneficial to patients with asthma. It is considered an alternate drug by the NAEPP guidelines to be considered for asthma prophylaxis when more effective drugs fail to bring symptomatic relief. It may be used in combination with a corticosteroid for persistent asthma. Although FDA approved for treating acute bronchospasm, theophylline is not recommended by the NAEPP guidelines because the short-acting beta$_2$-adrenergic agonists (SABAs) are more effective.

Theophylline has several off-label indications. As a respiratory stimulant, theophylline and caffeine may be used to treat sleep apnea in neonates and in adults with chronic heart failure. Given IV, theophylline has been found to reduce neurotoxicity resulting from the drug methotrexate.

Mechanism of Action: Theophylline works by two mechanisms. It relaxes bronchial smooth muscle, which promotes bronchodilation, and it suppresses airway responsiveness to stimuli that promote bronchospasm.

Pharmacokinetics:

Route(s)	PO, parenteral, suppository
Absorption	Rapid absorption
Distribution	About 40% protein bound; remainder is distributed well in fluids and less well in body lipids
Primary metabolism	Hepatic (CYP1A2, CYP2E1, CYP3A3)
Primary excretion	Renal
Onset of action	Peak: approximately 60 min (highly variable)
Duration of action	Half-life: 6–10 h (highly variable)

Adverse Effects: Theophylline has a very narrow therapeutic index. Therapeutic levels are 10 to 15 mcg/mL and the toxic level is anything above 20 mcg/mL. Serum theophylline levels should be obtained during therapy. Common adverse effects include nausea, vomiting, headache, irritability, and insomnia. More serious reactions include dysrhythmias, hypotension, and seizures.

Contraindications/Precautions: Theophylline should be used with great caution in patients who have seizure disorders, heart failure, or cardiac dysrhythmias. Theophylline has also been shown to increase the production of gastric acid so use in patients with active peptic ulcer disease is not recommended. Because of the extensive hepatic metabolism, theophylline should be closely monitored in patients with a history of liver disease. As with any drug, this drug is contraindicated in persons who have demonstrated a hypersensitivity to it.

Drug Interactions: Because theophylline is highly metabolized by the CYP450 enzyme system, there are numerous drug interactions, including many common antibiotics (ciprofloxacin, clarithromycin, erythromycin) and antianxiety agents (diazepam, flurazepam, lorazepam, midazolam). When treating a patient who is receiving multiple drugs concurrently with theophylline, the nurse should consult current sources for potential drug interactions. There are also a number of IV incompatibilities, including emergency medications such as epinephrine, norepinephrine, and isoproterenol. Compatibility of any medication should be checked prior to initiating infusions in the same line. **Herbal/Food**: Foods and beverages containing caffeine will cause additive central nervous system (CNS) stimulation. St. John's wort may decrease the effectiveness of theophylline.

Pregnancy: Category C.

Treatment of Overdose: There is no specific antidote to theophylline. Gastric lavage is indicated in the event of an overdose of PO medications. Seizures and other CNS effects may respond to barbiturates or benzodiazepines. Supportive measures need to be provided for hypotension, shock, dysrhythmias, and other toxic effects. Serum levels should be monitored periodically until they are within normal limits.

Nursing Responsibilities: Key nursing implications for patients receiving theophylline are included in the Nursing Practice Application for Patients Receiving Pharmacotherapy for Asthma and COPD.

Drugs Similar to Theophylline (Theo-Dur, Others)

Aminophylline and dyphylline are other methylxanthines. Oxtriphylline (Choledyl) is a drug in this class that has been discontinued in the United States.

Aminophylline: Approved in 1975, aminophylline is a theophylline salt that has enhanced water solubility. It is approved to treat symptoms of asthma and COPD. It has the same actions and adverse effects as theophylline. Aminophylline is shorter acting than theophylline and is available in PO, rectal, and IV forms. This drug is pregnancy category C.

Dyphylline (Lufyllin): Dyphylline is not a theophylline salt but it has similar actions. It is approved to treat acute bronchospasms associated with asthma and COPD. Approved in 1951, it is available in PO form and has a short half-life of only 2 hours, so it is usually given four times a day. It is 90% less potent than theophylline but exerts fewer adverse effects. The intramuscular (IM) form of the drug has been discontinued in the United States. Indications are the same as those of theophylline. This drug is pregnancy category C.

44.11 Monoclonal antibodies are a newer form of therapy for the prevention of asthma symptoms.

Approved in 2003, omalizumab (Xolair) was the first biologic therapy used to treat asthma, offering a new approach to the management of the disease. This drug is approved for treating allergic rhinitis and moderate to severe, persistent asthma that cannot be controlled satisfactorily with inhaled corticosteroids. To receive omalizumab, the patient must have tested positive for an airborne allergen such as mold, pollen, or animal dander. Although it is only available by the subcutaneous route, injections are scheduled every 2 to 4 weeks, depending on the patient's response to therapy. It is approved for asthma prophylaxis in patients 12 years of age or older.

Omalizumab is a monoclonal antibody. Monoclonal antibodies are designed to attach to a specific receptor on a target cell or molecule. Most monoclonal antibodies are designed to attack cancer cells. However, omalizumab is designed to attach to a receptor on immunoglobulin E (IgE). The normal function of IgE is to react to antigens and cause the release of inflammatory chemical mediators from mast cells and basophils. By binding to IgE, omalizumab prevents inflammation and dampens the body's response to allergens that sometimes trigger asthma. The student should refer to Chapter 42 for a complete discussion of monoclonal antibodies and a prototype feature for muromonab-CD3 (Orthoclone, OKT3).

Omalizumab is reserved for patients with persistent asthma because of its expense, potential adverse effects, and the need for regular parenteral injections. Although adverse effects are uncommon, they may be serious and include anaphylaxis, bleeding-related events, or severe dysmenorrhea. Less serious adverse effects include rash, headache, and viral infections.

CONNECTION Checkpoint 44.3

Most monoclonal antibodies are classified as immunosuppressants. From what you learned in Chapter 42, explain methods by which these drugs can be used to suppress the immune system. *See Answer to Connection Checkpoint 44.3 on student resource website.*

Chronic Obstructive Pulmonary Disease

44.12 Chronic obstructive pulmonary disease may be treated with bronchodilators, anti-inflammatory agents, and mucolytics.

Chronic obstructive pulmonary disease (COPD) is a progressive pulmonary disorder characterized by chronic and recurrent obstruction of airflow. The two most common examples of conditions that cause chronic pulmonary obstruction are **chronic bronchitis**, a condition in which excess mucus is produced in the lower respiratory tract, and **emphysema**, a condition in which there is loss of bronchiolar elasticity and destruction of alveolar walls.

The clinical distinction between chronic bronchitis and emphysema is sometimes unclear because patients may exhibit symptoms of both conditions concurrently. Both conditions are strongly associated with smoking tobacco products (cigarette smoking accounts for 85% to 90% of all cases of nonasthmatic COPD) and, secondarily, breathing air pollutants. In chronic bronchitis, excess mucus is produced in the lower respiratory tract due to the inflammation and irritation from cigarette smoke or pollutants. The airway becomes partially obstructed with mucus, resulting in the classic signs of dyspnea and coughing. An early sign of bronchitis is often a productive cough that occurs on awakening. Gas exchange may be impaired; thus wheezing and decreased exercise tolerance are additional clinical signs. Microbes thrive in the mucus-rich environment, and pulmonary infections are common.

Because most patients with COPD are lifelong tobacco users, they often have serious comorbid cardiovascular conditions such as heart failure and HTN. Emphysema is most often the result of years of chronic inflammation and is characterized by loss of elasticity of the bronchioles and damage and loss of alveolar wall structures. The loss of elasticity results in partial collapse of the airways on exhalation, leading to air trapping, and the destruction of alveolar walls leads to decreased perfusion and gas exchange at the alveolus. The patient with emphysema may experience extreme dyspnea from even the slightest physical activity.

Drugs may be used to bring symptomatic relief to patients with COPD, but they do not alter the progression of COPD or cure the disorder. The goals of pharmacotherapy of COPD are to relieve symptoms and avoid complications of the condition. Various classes of drugs are used to treat infections, control cough, and relieve bronchospasm. Most patients receive the same classes of bronchodilators and anti-inflammatory agents that are prescribed for asthma. A few of the newer agents and combination drugs are approved only for COPD. These include the following:

- Roflumilast (Daliresp), approved in 2011 is an oral drug for severe COPD that exhibits anti-inflammatory effects on the airways by inhibiting the enzyme phosphodiesterase-4.

- Incruse ellipta, approved in 2013, contains the anticholinergic umeclidinium that relaxes bronchial smooth muscle to cause bronchodilation. It is administered once daily by oral inhalation.

- Anora ellipta, approved in 2013, contains umeclidinium and vilanterol (a LABA). It is given by oral inhalation for the maintenance treatment of COPD.

- Breo ellipta, approved in 2013, is a fixed dose combination of vilanterol and fluticasone (a corticosteroid). Like anora ellipto, it is given once daily by oral inhalation for the maintenance treatment of COPD.

Mucolytics, which are agents given to loosen thick viscous bronchial secretions, and expectorants, which are agents given to aid in the removal of mucus, are sometimes prescribed (see Chapter 45). Long-term oxygen therapy is prescribed in later stages and it has been shown to decrease mortality in patients with advanced COPD. Antibiotics may be prescribed for patients who experience multiple bouts of pulmonary infections.

Patients with COPD should not receive drugs that have beta-adrenergic antagonist activity because these agents cause bronchoconstriction. Respiratory depressants such as opioids and barbiturates should also be avoided when possible. An important teaching point for the nurse is to strongly encourage smoking cessation in these patients. Smoking cessation has been shown to slow the progression of COPD and to result in fewer respiratory symptoms; however, it cannot undo damage that has already occurred.

CONNECTIONS: NURSING PRACTICE APPLICATION

Patients Receiving Pharmacotherapy for Asthma and COPD

Assessment	Potential Nursing Diagnoses*
Baseline assessment prior to administration: • Obtain a complete health history including previous history of symptoms and association with seasons, foods, or environmental exposures; existing cardiovascular, respiratory, hepatic, renal, or neurologic disease; glaucoma; prostatic hypertrophy; difficulty with urination; presence of fever or active infections; pregnancy or breast-feeding; alcohol use; or smoking. Obtain a drug history, noting the type of adverse reaction experienced to any medications. • If asthma symptoms are of new onset, particularly in infants and young children, assess for any recent changes in diet, soaps including laundry detergent, laundry softener, cosmetics, lotions, and environmental factors (e.g., pets, travel, or recent carpet-cleaning) that may correlate with the onset of symptoms. • Obtain baseline vital signs, noting respiratory rate and depth. • Assess pulmonary function with pulse oximeter, peak expiratory flow meter, and/or arterial blood gases to establish baseline levels. • Evaluate appropriate laboratory findings (e.g., CBC, hepatic, and renal tests). • Assess symptom-related effects on eating, sleep, and activity level. • Assess the patient's ability to receive and understand instructions. Include the family and caregivers as needed.	• *Impaired Gas Exchange* • *Anxiety* • *Disturbed Sleep Pattern*, related to adverse drug effects • *Activity Intolerance*, related to disease processes or ineffective drug therapy • *Deficient Knowledge* (Drug Therapy) • *Risk for Decreased Cardiac Tissue Perfusion*

CONNECTIONS: NURSING PRACTICE APPLICATION (continued)

Assessment throughout administration:
- Assess for desired therapeutic effects (e.g., increased ease of breathing, improvement in pulmonary function studies, improved signs of peripheral oxygenation and increased activity levels, maintenance of normal eating and sleep periods).
- Continue periodic monitoring of pulmonary function with pulse oximeter, peak expiratory flow meter, and/or arterial blood gases as appropriate.
- Assess vital signs, especially respiratory rate and depth. Assess breath sounds, noting the presence of adventitious sounds, and any mucus production.
- Assess for adverse effects: dizziness, tachycardia, palpitations, blurred vision, or headache. Immediately report fever, confusion, tachycardia, palpitations, hypotension, syncope, dyspnea, or increasing pulmonary congestion.

Implementation

Interventions and (Rationales)	Patient-Centered Care
Ensuring therapeutic effects:	
• Continue assessments as above for therapeutic effects. (Increased ease of breathing, lessened adventitious breath sounds, improved signs of tissue oxygenation, and normal appetite and eating and sleeping patterns should occur.)	• Teach the patient to supplement drug therapy with nonpharmacologic measures, such as increased fluid intake to liquefy and mobilize mucus, and to reduce exposure to allergens where possible. • Advise the patient to carry a wallet identification card or wear medical identification jewelry indicating the presence of asthma or a respiratory condition, any significant allergies or anaphylaxis, and use of inhaler therapy.
• Monitor pulmonary function periodically with pulse oximeter, peak expiratory flow meter, and/or arterial blood gases. (Periodic monitoring is necessary to assess drug effectiveness.)	• Teach the patient how to use the peak expiratory flow meter or other equipment ordered to monitor pulmonary function. • Instruct the patient to immediately report symptoms of deteriorating respiratory status such as increased dyspnea, breathlessness with speech, increased anxiety, or orthopnea.
• For treatment of acute asthmatic attacks, inhaler therapy should be started at first sign of respiratory difficulty to abort the attack. For preventive therapy, long-term bronchodilation by inhaler or orally will be used to maintain bronchodilation. *LABAs and long-acting bronchodilators are not to be used to abort an acute attack.* (Acute asthmatic attacks are managed with quick-acting bronchodilation such as beta₂ agonists. For maintaining bronchodilation and preventing attacks, LABAs, anticholinergics, mast cell stabilizers, and glucocorticoid or methylxanthine therapy may be used. It is crucial to know and recognize the difference between quick-acting and long-acting inhalers.)	• Provide explicit instructions on the use of quick-acting versus long-acting inhalers. Teach the patient to use quick-acting inhalers at the earliest possible appearance of symptoms. Long-acting inhalers or oral therapy may be used to maintain bronchodilation but *do not discard quick-acting inhalers if on long-term maintenance therapy.* They may still be needed for periodic acute attacks.
Minimizing adverse effects:	
• Continue to monitor respirations, rate, depth, breath sounds, mucus production, and for increasing dyspnea, adventitious breath sounds, and signs of tissue hypoxia (e.g., cyanosis), anxiety, confusion, or decreasing pulmonary function (e.g., pulse oximeter, peak expiratory flow). Immediately notify the provider if symptoms continue to increase, especially if respiratory involvement worsens or fever is present. (Increasing dyspnea, adventitious breath sounds, diminished oxygenation, or increasing anxiety or confusion may indicate inadequate drug therapy, worsening disease process, or respiratory infection and should be reported immediately. **Diverse Patients:** Because some drugs such as theophylline metabolize through the P450 system pathways, monitor ethnically diverse patients to ensure optimal therapeutic effects and to minimize adverse effects.)	• Instruct the patient to report immediately symptoms of deteriorating respiratory status such as increased dyspnea, breathlessness with speech, increased anxiety, or orthopnea.
• Provide explicit instruction on the use of quick-acting and long-acting inhalers. Ensure that the patient is able to identify the appropriate inhaler for the treatment of acute asthmatic attacks or for preventive therapy. (Acute asthmatic attacks are managed with quick-acting bronchodilation such as beta₂ agonists and the patient must be able to identify the appropriate inhaler to use. Provide written instructions, including drug name and when to use, if both quick-acting and long-acting inhalers are ordered.)	• Teach the patient to use the quick-acting inhaler at the earliest possible appearance of symptoms. Long-acting inhalers or oral therapy may be used to maintain bronchodilation but *do not discard quick-acting inhalers if on long-term maintenance therapy.* They may still be needed for periodic acute attacks. • Teach the patient not to rely on the color of the inhaler to indicate quick-acting versus long-acting inhalers. Depending on the manufacturer and trade versus generic drugs, the color may change. If the patient desires to color-code, suggest individual color stickers or tape be used per patient preference. Instruct the patient not to obscure the drug name with the sticker.

(continued)

CONNECTIONS: NURSING PRACTICE APPLICATION (continued)

• Monitor eating and sleep patterns and ability to maintain functional ADLs. Provide for calorie-rich, nutrient-dense foods, frequent rest periods between eating or activity, and a cool room for sleeping. (Respiratory difficulty and fatigue associated with hypoxia and the work of breathing may affect appetite, ability to eat during dyspnea, and maintenance of required ADLs. Adequate nutrition, fluids, rest, and sleep are essential to support optimal health.)	• Teach the patient to supplement drug therapy with nonpharmacologic measures including: • Increased fluid intake to liquefy and assist in mobilizing mucus • Small, frequent meals of calorie-rich, nutrient-dense foods to prevent fatigue and maintain normal nutrition • Adequate rest periods between eating and activities • Decreased room temperature for ease of breathing during sleep • Reduced exposure to allergens where possible. • Instruct the patient to immediately report any significant change in appetite, inability to maintain normal intake, inadequate sleep periods, or inability to carry out required ADLs.
• Eliminate smoking, limit exposure to secondhand smoke, and limit caffeine intake, especially if methylxanthines are prescribed. (Cigarette smoke irritates respiratory mucous membranes, increasing the risk of adverse effects and increasing bronchoconstriction. Caffeine may increase the risk of tachycardia in addition to the drugs' adverse effects, and both smoking and caffeine affect the metabolism of methylxanthines.)	• Teach the patient about smoking cessation programs, to avoid environments with secondhand smoke, and to limit or abstain from caffeine intake while taking bronchodilator therapy.
• Maintain consistent dosing of long-acting bronchodilators. LABAs, anticholinergics, mast cell stabilizers, and corticosteroids are used to prevent or limit acute bronchoconstrictive attacks. Regular, consistent dosing must be maintained for best results.	• Teach the patient the importance of continuing regular and consistent administration of all bronchodilation therapy to prevent acute attacks. Irregular use may increase the risk or severity of bronchoconstrictive events.
• Utilize the appropriate spacer between the inhaler and mouth and rinse mouth after using the inhaler, especially after corticosteroids. (Spacers between metered-dose inhalers may be ordered to assist in coordination and timing of inhalation and to prevent medication being delivered to the back of the pharynx. Rinsing the mouth after the use of inhalers prevents systemic absorption or localized reactions to the drug such as ulceration.)	• Instruct the patient in the proper use of spacers if ordered, followed by return demonstration. • Teach the patient to rinse the mouth after each use of the inhaler and not to swallow after rinsing.
• Continue to monitor cardiac status, hepatic function, and ophthalmology exam findings. (Beta-adrenergic drugs given for asthma and COPD may cause cardiac adverse effects. Corticosteroids may increase the risk of cataract formation. **Lifespan:** Monitor the older adult frequently because age-related physiological changes increase the risk of adverse effects.)	• Teach the patient about any follow-up laboratory or other testing needed, such as annual eye exams.
• Monitor for anticholinergic adverse effects in patients taking ipratropium (Atrovent) and other anticholinergic drugs. (**Lifespan:** Be aware that the male older adult is at higher risk for mechanical obstruction due to an enlarged prostate. The older adult is also at increased risk of constipation due to slowed peristalsis.)	• Teach the patient about the importance of drinking extra fluids and increasing fiber intake. Instruct the patient to notify the health care provider if difficulty with urination occurs or if constipation is severe.
Patient understanding of drug therapy: • Use opportunities during administration of medications and during assessments to discuss the rationale for drug therapy, desired therapeutic outcomes, commonly observed adverse effects, parameters for when to call the health care provider, and any necessary monitoring or precautions. (Using time during nursing care helps to optimize and reinforce key teaching areas.)	• The patient should be able to state the reason for the drug, appropriate dose and scheduling, what adverse effects to observe for, and when to report them.
Patient self-administration of drug therapy: • When administering the medication, instruct the patient, family, or caregiver in proper self-administration of the drug, e.g., take the drug at the first appearance of symptoms before they are severe. (Utilizing time during nurse-administration of these drugs helps to reinforce teaching.)	• The patient, family, or caregiver is able to discuss appropriate dosing and administration needs. • The patient recognizes the difference between quick-acting and long-acting inhalers and knows when each is to be used. • Instruct the patient in proper administration techniques for inhalers, followed by return demonstration, including: • Use a spacer if instructed between the metered-dose inhaler and the mouth. • Shake the inhaler or load it with a tablet or powder as instructed. • If using a bronchodilator and corticosteroid inhalers, use the bronchodilator first, wait 5 min, then use the corticosteroid to ensure the drug reaches deeply into the bronchial area. • Rinse mouth after using any inhaler. • Clean the inhaler at least weekly by running warm water through the plastic mouthpiece after removing the drug canister, shaking out excess water, and allowing to air dry. • **Lifespan:** Supervise children under the age of 5 to ensure proper inhaler use.

*Nursing Diagnoses—Definitions and Classification 2015–2017. Copyright © 2014, 1994–2014 by NANDA International. Used by arrangement with John Wiley & Sons Limited.

CHAPTER

44 Understanding the Chapter

Key Concepts Summary

44.1 The physiology of the respiratory system involves two main processes: perfusion and ventilation.

44.2 Asthma is a chronic disease that has both inflammatory and bronchospasm components.

44.3 Inhalation is a common route of administration for pulmonary drugs because it delivers drugs directly to their sites of action.

44.4 The goals of asthma pharmacotherapy are to terminate acute bronchospasms and to reduce the frequency of asthma attacks.

44.5 Beta$_2$-adrenergic agonists are the most effective drugs for relieving acute bronchospasm.

44.6 The inhaled anticholinergics are used for preventing bronchospasm.

44.7 Inhaled corticosteroids are the most effective drugs for the long-term control of asthma.

44.8 Mast cell stabilizers are used for the prophylaxis of asthma and act by preventing the release of histamine.

44.9 The leukotriene modifiers, which are primarily used for asthma prophylaxis, act by reducing the inflammatory component of asthma.

44.10 Methylxanthines were once the mainstay of asthma pharmacotherapy but are now rarely prescribed for that disorder.

44.11 Monoclonal antibodies are a newer form of therapy for the prevention of asthma symptoms.

44.12 Chronic obstructive pulmonary disease may be treated with bronchodilators, anti-inflammatory agents, and mucolytics.

Case Study: Making the Patient Connection

Remember the patient "Nathan Almond" at the beginning of the chapter? Now read the remainder of the case study. Based on the information presented within this chapter, respond to the critical thinking questions that follow.

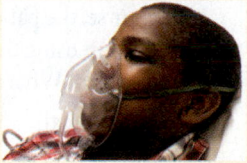

Nathan is a 12-year-old with a history of asthma, diagnosed 2 years ago. He is an outgoing, active boy and participates in a swim club and a basketball team, but he has had a difficult time adjusting to the limitations of his asthma. He has learned to control acute attacks by using an albuterol (Proventil) metered-dose inhaler, and because his asthma is often triggered by exercise, he has also been using a budesonide (Pulmicort) inhaler and taking montelukast (Singulair).

After competing in his swim meet at the local indoor pool, Nathan began experiencing respiratory distress. He alerted his coach, who retrieved the albuterol inhaler from Nathan's backpack. After two inhalations, Nathan was still in distress and the rescue squad was called.

On admission to the emergency department, Nathan is in obvious distress with pulse oximeter readings of 90% to 91%. He has nasal flaring and bilateral wheezing is heard in his lung fields, pulse rate is 122 beats/min, and he is orthopneic. While treatment is started, the nurse asks him questions that he can nod or shake his head to answer. He shakes his head "no" when asked if he used his budesonide inhaler today and shrugs when asked about his last dose of montelukast.

Critical Thinking Questions

1. Considering his history, medications, and the location where Nathan's asthma attack occurred, what might explain his acute attack?

2. What medications would you anticipate will be prescribed to treat Nathan's acute asthmatic attack and why?

3. What changes might be made to Nathan's medications? What teaching will Nathan and his family need prior to discharge?

See Answers to Critical Thinking Questions on student resource website.

Additional Case Study

As the home health nurse, you visit with Mr. Jonas Maxwell weekly to assess his pulmonary status and his adherence to his medication regimen. Jonas has end-stage COPD. He was diagnosed with the disease many years ago and his pulmonary status has deteriorated slowly during the past few years. Despite his health care provider's recommendation to change to another medication, Jonas insists that theophylline (Theo-Dur) is the only medication that helps him to breathe. He also uses several MDIs with spacers several times per day.

1. What symptoms would you expect to observe in Jonas if he is experiencing early signs of toxicity?

2. Create a list of things to avoid for an individual who is receiving theophylline therapy.

3. In your own words, how would you describe the function of the spacer used with Jonas's MDI?

See Answers to Additional Case Study on student resource website.

Chapter Review

1 A patient with asthma asks which of the prescribed medications should be used in the event of an acute episode of bronchospasm. The nurse will instruct the patient to use:

1. Albuterol, a beta-agonist bronchodilator, by inhalation.

2. Beclomethasone, a glucocorticoid anti-inflammatory drug, by inhalation.

3. Ipratropium, an anticholinergic bronchodilator, by inhalation.

4. Zafirlukast, a leukotriene modifier, by mouth.

2 A patient is prescribed beclomethasone (Qvar), a glucocorticoid inhaler. Education by the nurse will include:

1. "Check your heart rate because this may cause tachycardia."

2. "Limit your coffee intake while on this drug."

3. "Rinse your mouth out well after each use."

4. "You may feel shaky and nervous after using this drug."

3 The nurse should inform the patient who is prescribed a nebulizer treatment with albuterol (Proventil, VoSpire) that a common adverse effect is:

1. An increased heart rate with palpitations.

2. A predisposition to infection.

3. Sedation.

4. Temporary dyspnea.

4 The nurse should monitor the patient who is taking beclomethasone (Qvar) for evidence of (select all that apply):

1. Infection.

2. Hyperglycemia.

3. Urinary retention.

4. Tachycardia.

5. Photophobia.

5 A 4-year-old child with respiratory distress secondary to asthma has an order for a nebulizer treatment. The type of medication most likely to be given for asthma management is a:

1. Beta agonist.

2. Beta antagonist.

3. Corticosteroid.

4. Leukotriene modifier.

6 Despite repeated demonstrations of proper inhaler use by the nurse, the patient is unable to demonstrate proper technique in using the training inhaler. The patient is becoming frustrated. What is the best action for the nurse to take?

1. Encourage the patient to keep practicing just a little longer.

2. Notify the health care provider that the patient is incompetent.

3. Provide a spacer for use with the inhaler.

4. Switch to an oral form of a beta agonist.

See Answers to Chapter Review in Appendix A.

References

American Academy of Allergy, Asthma and Immunology. (2014). *Asthma statistics.* Retrieved from http://www.aaaai.org/about-the-aaaai/newsroom/asthma-statistics.aspx

Bruzzese, J. M., Unikel, L. H., Evans, D., Bornstein, L., Surrence, K., & Mellins, R. B. (2010). Asthma knowledge and asthma management behavior in urban elementary school teachers. *Journal of Asthma, 47,* 185–191. doi:10.3109/02770900903519908

Colbert, B. J., Gonzales, L. S., & Kennedy, B. J. (2012). *Integrated cardiopulmonary pharmacology* (3rd ed.). Upper Saddle River, NJ: Pearson Education.

Lareau, S. C., & Hodder, R. (2012). Teaching inhaler use in chronic obstructive pulmonary disease patients. *Journal of the American Academy of Nurse Practitioners, 24,* 113–120. doi:10.1111/j.1745-7599.2011.00681.x

Lemanske, R. F., & Busse, W. W. (2010). The U.S. Food and Drug Administration and long-acting β_2 agonists: The importance of striking the right balance between risks and benefits of therapy? *Journal of Allergy and Clinical Immunology, 126*(3), 449–452. doi:10.1016/j.jaci.2010.05.039

National Asthma Education and Prevention Program Coordinating Committee. (2007). *Expert panel report 3 (EPR3): Guidelines for the diagnosis and management of asthma.* Coordinated by the National Heart, Lung, and Blood Institute of the National Institutes of Health. Retrieved from http://www.nhlbi.nih.gov/guidelines/asthma/asthgdln.htm

National Center for Health Statistics. (2012). *Summary health statistics for U.S. children: National health interview survey, 2012.* Retrieved from http://www.cdc.gov/nchs/data/series/sr_10/sr10_258.pdf

O'Connor, R. D., Patrick, D. L., Parasuraman, B., Martin, P., & Goldman, M. (2010). Comparison of patient-reported outcomes during treatment with adjustable- and fixed-dose budesonide/formoterol pressurized metered-dose inhaler versus fixed-dose fluticasone propionate/salmeterol dry powder inhaler in patients with asthma. *Journal of Asthma, 47,* 217–223. doi:10.3109/02770900903497154

Selected Bibliography

Albertson, T. E., Schivo, M., Gidwani, N., Kenyon, N. J., Sutter, M. E., Chan, A. L., & Louie, S. (2013, November 2). Pharmacotherapy of critical asthma syndrome: Current and emerging therapies. *Clinical Reviews in Allergy & Immunology.* Advance online publication. doi:10.1007/s12016-013-8393-8

American Lung Association. (2012). *Trends in asthma morbidity and mortality.* Retrieved from http://www.lung.org/finding-cures/our-research/trend-reports/asthma-trend-report.pdf

American Lung Association. (2013). *Trends in COPD (chronic bronchitis and emphysema): Morbidity and mortality.* Retrieved from http://www.lung.org/finding-cures/our-research/trend-reports/copd-trend-report.pdf

Antus, B. (2013). Pharmacotherapy of chronic obstructive pulmonary disease: A clinical review. *ISRN Pulmonology,* Article ID 582807, 11 pp. doi:10.1155/2013/582807

Bjerg, A., Lundbäck, B., & Lötvall, J. (2012). The future of combining inhaled drugs for COPD. *Current Opinion in Pharmacology, 12,* 252–255. doi:10.1016/j.coph.2012.03.004

Centers for Disease Control and Prevention. (2014). *Asthma.* Retrieved from http://www.cdc.gov/nchs/fastats/asthma.htm

D'Amatol, G., Perticone, M., Bucchioni, E., Salzillo, A., D'Amato, M., & Liccardi, G. (2010). Treating moderate-to-severe allergic asthma with anti-IgE monoclonal antibody (omalizumab). An update. *European Annals of Allergy and Clinical Immunology, 42*(4), 135–140.

Ferry-Rooney, R. (2013). Asthma in primary care: A case-based review of pharmacotherapy. *Nursing clinics of North America, 48,* 25–34. doi:10.1016/j.cnur.2012.12.005

Herdman, T. H., & Kamitsuru, S. (Eds.). (2014). *NANDA International nursing diagnoses: Definitions and classification, 2015–2017.* Oxford, United Kingdom: Wiley-Blackwell.

Kaufman, G. (2012). Asthma: Assessment, diagnosis, and treatment adherence. *Nurse Prescribing, 10,* 331–338.

McIvor, A. R. (2011). Inhaler blues? *CMAJ, 183*(4), 464. doi:10.1503/cmaj.111-2025

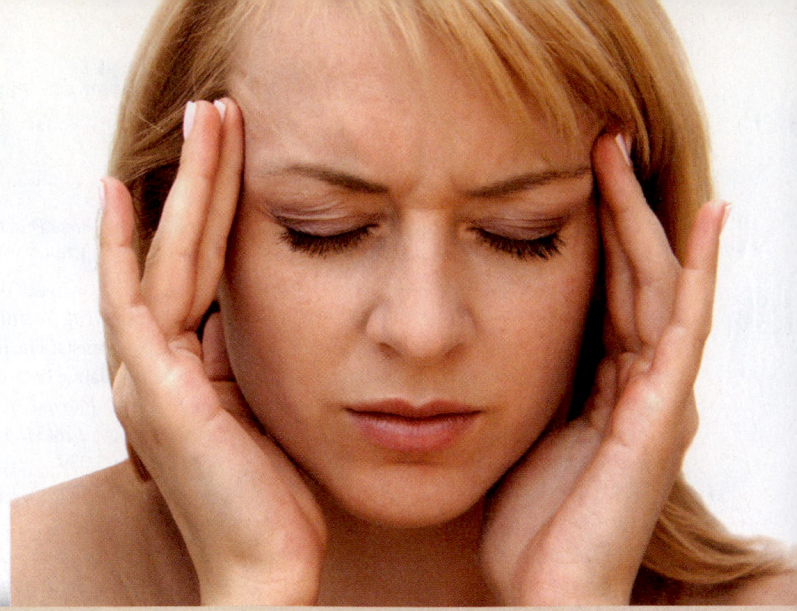

> "I can't stop coughing, I can't sleep, and my head hurts. I thought I had a summer cold but this is just dragging on. It's affecting my work!"
>
> Patient "Nancy Williams"

CHAPTER

45

Pharmacotherapy of Allergic Rhinitis and the Common Cold

LEARNING OUTCOMES

After reading this chapter, the student should be able to:

1. Identify structures of the upper respiratory tract that serve as body defenses against foreign substances.

2. Describe the common causes and symptoms of allergic rhinitis.

3. Differentiate between H_1 and H_2 histamine receptors.

4. Compare and contrast the first- and second-generation antihistamines.

5. Explain why intranasal corticosteroids are the drugs of choice for the treatment of allergic rhinitis.

6. Compare and contrast the oral and intranasal decongestants.

7. Explain why it is usually better to take individual drugs for the common cold, rather than a multisymptom combination product.

8. Describe the appropriate use of cough suppressants.

9. Describe the use of drugs prescribed to treat thick bronchial secretions.

10. For each of the classes shown in the chapter outline, identify the prototype and representative drugs and explain the mechanism(s) of drug action, primary indications, contraindications, significant drug interactions, pregnancy category, and important adverse effects.

11. Apply the nursing process to care for patients who are receiving pharmacotherapy for allergic rhinitis and the common cold.

CHAPTER OUTLINE

▶ **Physiology of the Upper Respiratory Tract**

▶ **Pathophysiology of Allergic Rhiniti**

▶ **Pharmacotherapy of Allergic Rhinitis**

H_1-Receptor Antagonists (Antihistamines)
PROTOTYPE Fexofenadine (Allegra), *p. 758*

Intranasal Corticosteroids
PROTOTYPE Fluticasone (Flonase, Veramyst), *p. 762*

Mast Cell Stabilizers

▶ **Decongestants**
PROTOTYPE Pseudoephedrine (Sudafed), *p. 763*

▶ **Drugs for the Common Cold**

▶ **Antitussives**
PROTOTYPE Dextromethorphan (Delsym Robitussin DM, Others), *p. 766*

▶ **Expectorants and Mucolytics**

KEY TERMS

allergen, 754

allergic rhinitis, 754

antitussives, 767

expectorants, 767

H₁ receptors, 755

mast cell stabilizers, 762

mucolytics, 767

rebound congestion, 765

The respiratory system begins at the nose and ends at the respiratory membrane: the dividing line between the alveoli and the pulmonary capillaries. The pharmacotherapy of asthma and chronic obstructive pulmonary disease (COPD), which are conditions of the lower respiratory tract, are discussed in Chapter 44. This chapter examines the drugs used for two conditions that are primarily associated with the upper respiratory tract: allergic rhinitis and the common cold. Because many of these medications are readily available over the counter (OTC), it is essential for the nurse to provide effective teaching for their use.

Physiology of the Upper Respiratory Tract

45.1 The upper respiratory tract acts as a defense in preventing systemic infection.

The upper respiratory tract (URT) consists of the nose, nasal cavity, pharynx, and paranasal sinuses. These passageways filter, warm, and humidify air during inhalation. The URT traps particulate matter and many pathogens, preventing them from being carried to the bronchioles and alveoli, where they would have access to the capillaries of the systemic circulation. The mucous membranes of the URT are lined with ciliated epithelium. The cilia projecting from the epithelium are found throughout the nasal passages and help to trap smaller particles. The cilia have a wavelike motion that sweeps the pathogens and particulate matter upward toward the oropharynx, where they are swallowed when a person coughs or clears the throat. A sneeze clears the nasal passages. The basic structures of the URT are shown in Figure 45.1.

The nasal mucosa is a dynamic structure richly supplied with vascular tissue that is controlled, in part, by the autonomic nervous system. Activation of the sympathetic nervous system constricts the arterioles in the nose, reducing the thickness of the mucosal layer. This serves to widen the airway and allow air to more freely enter the URT. Parasympathetic activation has the opposite effect: The arterioles dilate and more mucus is produced. This difference is important during therapy with drugs that affect the autonomic nervous system. For example, administration of a sympathomimetic will shrink the nasal mucosa, relieving nasal stuffiness associated with the common cold. These drugs are classified as decongestants. On the other hand, parasympathetic agents cause increased blood flow to the nose with increased nasal stuffiness and a runny nose as side effects.

The oral mucosa serves an important role in the body's defense against invasion by microbes. Saliva contains immunoglobulins (IgA) and lysozyme, which break down bacterial cell walls. Swallowed saliva or nasal mucus exposes microorganisms to the hostile environment of the stomach where they contact high gastric acidity and enzymes that kill them.

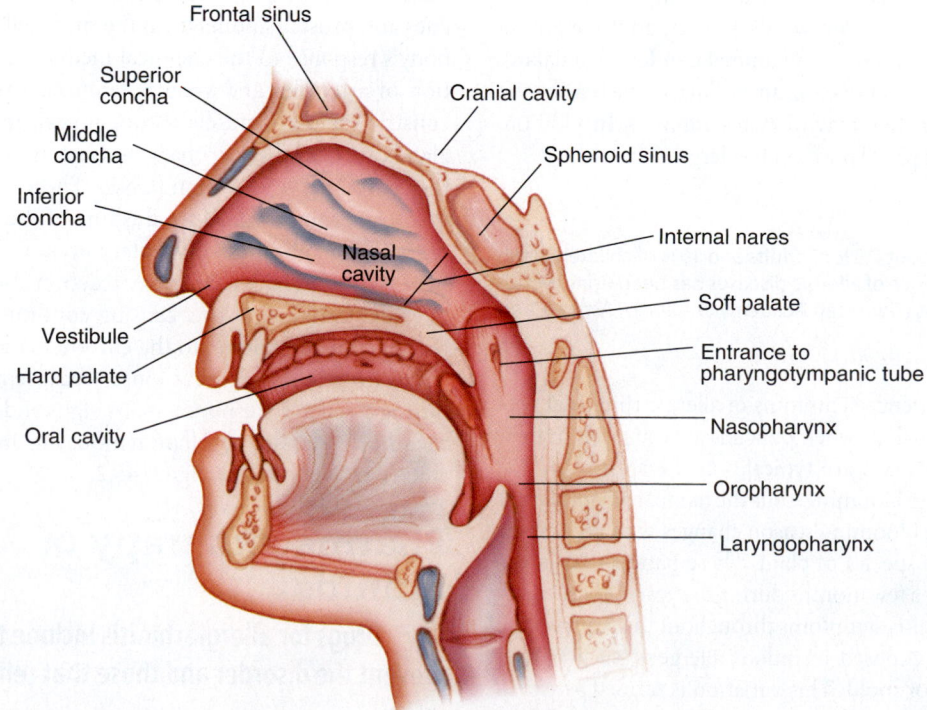

Figure 45.1 The respiratory system.

The nasal mucosa is also part of the first line of body defense, secreting up to a quart of mucus daily. This fluid is rich in immunoglobulins that are able to neutralize airborne pathogens. The nasal mucosa contains numerous nonspecific body defense cells that can activate complement or engulf microbes. Mast cells, which contain histamine, also line the nasal mucosa, and these play a major role in causing the symptoms of allergic rhinitis.

Pathophysiology of Allergic Rhinitis

45.2 Allergic rhinitis is caused by exposure to an environmental allergen, which leads to symptoms that resemble those of the common cold.

Allergic rhinitis is inflammation of the nasal mucosa due to exposure to allergens. Although not life threatening, allergic rhinitis is a condition that affects millions of people and one that is a common indication for pharmacotherapy.

Sometimes called hay fever, the symptoms of allergic rhinitis resemble those of the common cold and include tearing, burning, red, swollen, or itching eyes; sneezing; nasal itching or congestion; postnasal drip; cough; and scratchy throat. In addition to the acute symptoms, complications of allergic rhinitis may include loss of taste or smell, sinusitis, hoarseness, and plugged ears. Some people may not obtain restful sleep and awaken very fatigued. Symptoms can be severe enough to cause poor performance in or absence from school or work. Because of the smaller size of their anatomic structures, children are also at increased risk for middle ear infections.

As with other types of allergies, the cause of allergic rhinitis is exposure to an antigen. An antigen, also called an **allergen**, is anything that is recognized as foreign and provokes a response from the body's defense system. The specific allergen responsible for a patient's allergic rhinitis is often difficult to pinpoint; however, common agents are pollens from weeds, grasses, and trees; mold spores; dust mites; certain foods; and animal dander (skin flakes). Chemical fumes, tobacco smoke, or air pollutants such as ozone are nonallergenic factors that may worsen symptoms. In addition, there is a strong genetic predisposition to allergic rhinitis.

PharmFACT

Allergic rhinitis affects about 7.8% of adults and 10% of children in the United States. The incidence of allergic diseases has been rising worldwide for the past 50 years (American Academy of Allergy, Asthma, and Immunology, n.d.).

Some patients experience symptoms of allergic rhinitis at specific times of the year such as when pollen is at high levels in their environment. These periods are typically in the spring and fall when plants and trees are blooming; thus the name *seasonal* allergic rhinitis. Obviously, the blooming season changes with geographic location and with each species of plant. These patients may need symptom relief for only a few months during the year. Others are afflicted with allergic rhinitis symptoms throughout the year because they are continuously exposed to indoor allergens, such as dust mites, animal dander, or mold. This variation is termed *perennial* allergic rhinitis. These patients may require a treatment plan that includes continuous pharmacotherapy.

It is often not clear whether a patient is experiencing seasonal or perennial allergic rhinitis. Patients with seasonal allergies may also be sensitive to some of the perennial allergens. It is also common for one allergen to sensitize patients to another allergen. For example, during ragweed season, a patient may become hyperresponsive to other allergens such as mold spores or animal dander. The body's response and the symptoms of allergic rhinitis are the same, however, regardless of the specific allergen(s). Allergy testing can help pinpoint the particular allergens responsible for the symptoms and help direct a treatment plan that includes avoiding allergens that cause the symptoms and treating the symptoms.

The fundamental pathophysiology responsible for allergic rhinitis is inflammation of the mucous membranes in the nose, throat, and airways. The nasal mucosa is rich with mast cells (a type of connective tissue cell) and basophils (a type of leukocyte), both of which synthesize and store histamine. The release of histamine and other substances such as leukotrienes occurs after a patient has been exposed to specific allergens. The allergen stimulates the production of high amounts of immunoglobulin E (IgE). The IgE antibodies then bind to the outer surface of mast cells and basophils, thus sensitizing them. Sometime later when reexposed to an antigen such as pollen, the antigen attaches to the antibody and the antigen–antibody reaction begins. This reaction stimulates a process that begins by mobilizing intracellular calcium and, eventually, the sensitized cells release chemical mediators, including histamine. In certain cases, histamine can be released from mast cells without prior exposure to an antigen (allergen). These nonallergic releases of histamine can occur with cell damage, certain drugs, plasma expanders, or radiographic contrast media.

Patients with allergic rhinitis have greater numbers of mast cells. An immediate (or Type I) hypersensitivity response releases histamine and other chemical mediators such as leukotrienes and prostaglandins from the mast cells and basophils. The body's response to the chemical mediators is to cause vasodilation of arterioles and venules, increase capillary permeability, constrict smooth muscle (bronchioles), increase secretions of glands such as the lacrimals, and act as a neurotransmitter in the central nervous system (CNS). These responses, in the case of allergic rhinitis, produce flushing of the skin, sneezing, itching nasal membranes, and watery eyes, and may cause drowsiness. A delayed hypersensitivity reaction also occurs 4 to 8 hours after the initial exposure, causing continuous inflammation of the mucosa and adding to the chronic nasal congestion experienced from the allergic response. Because histamine is released during an allergic response, many signs and symptoms of allergy are similar to those of inflammation. The mechanism of allergic rhinitis is illustrated in Figure 45.2.

Pharmacotherapy of Allergic Rhinitis

45.3 Drugs for allergic rhinitis include those that prevent the disorder and those that relieve symptoms.

The therapeutic goals of treating allergic rhinitis are to prevent its occurrence and to relieve symptoms. Drugs that are used to treat

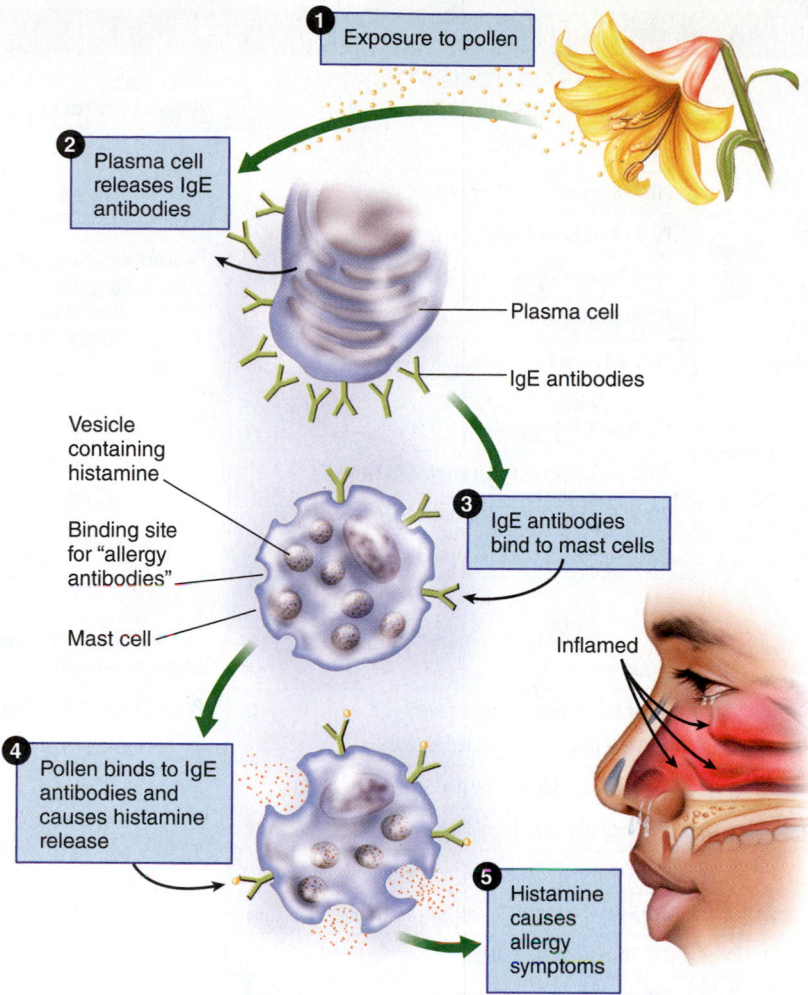

Figure 45.2 Pathophysiology of allergic rhinitis.

allergic rhinitis may thus be grouped into two simple categories—preventers and relievers:

- Preventers are used for prophylaxis. These include antihistamines, intranasal corticosteroids, and mast cell stabilizers.

- Relievers are used to provide immediate, though temporary, relief for acute allergy symptoms once they have occurred. Relievers include the oral and intranasal decongestants, which usually are drugs from the sympathomimetic class.

Nurses should help patients identify the sources of the allergy and recommend appropriate actions. These may include removing pets from the home environment or limiting their exposure (such as not allowing the pet on furniture); cleaning moldy surfaces; using and routinely cleaning or replacing microfilters on air-conditioning units; and frequent cleaning to remove dust mites from bedding, carpet, or furniture. Although dust mites can never be totally removed from mattresses, regularly decreasing their numbers can help lessen symptoms of allergic rhinitis. It may be interesting to know that dust mites feed primarily on naturally shedding human skin and that it is not the microscopic dust mite itself that a patient inhales and is allergic to, but rather its excrement.

45.4 Antihistamines are widely used to treat allergic rhinitis and other minor allergies.

There are two types of receptors for histamine: H_1 and H_2. Activation of **H_1 receptors** produces the typical symptoms of allergy. Drugs that block H_2 receptors such as ranitidine (Zantac) reduce gastric acid secretion and are used to treat peptic ulcer disease and gastroesophageal reflux disease. This histamine receptor activity is not related to allergic responses and is covered in Chapter 59.

H_1-receptor antagonists, also called *antihistamines*, are drugs that selectively block histamine from reaching its H_1 receptors, thus alleviating allergic symptoms. Because the term *antihistamine* is nonspecific and does not indicate which of the two histamine receptors is affected, H_1-receptor antagonist (or blocker) is a more accurate name. In clinical practice, as well as in this text, the two terms are used interchangeably. Antihistamines that selectively block H_1 receptors are widely used as OTC remedies for the relief of allergy symptoms, motion sickness, and insomnia. The antihistamines are listed in Table 45.1.

The most frequent therapeutic use of antihistamines is for the treatment of allergies. These medications provide symptomatic relief from the sneezing, runny nose, and itching of the eyes, nose, and throat of allergic rhinitis. Antihistamines are often combined

TABLE 45.1	H_1-Receptor Antagonists for Allergies	
Drug	**Route and Adult Dose (Maximum Dose Where Indicated)**	**Adverse Effects**
First-Generation Drugs		
brompheniramine (Dimetapp, Others)	PO: 4–8 mg every 4–6 h (max: 40 mg/day)	*Dry mouth, headache, dizziness, urinary retention, thickening of bronchial secretions, nausea, vomiting*
chlorpheniramine (Chlor-Trimeton, Others)	PO: 2–4 mg every 4–6 h (max: 24 mg/day)	Paradoxical excitation (usually in children), sedation, hypersensitivity reactions, hypotension, extrapyramidal symptoms (promethazine), agranulocytosis (brompheniramine, promethazine, clemastine)
clemastine (Tavist)	PO: 1.34–2.68 mg every 12 h (max: 8.04 mg/day)	
cyproheptadine	PO: 4–20 mg every 6–8 h (max: 0.5 mg/kg/day)	
dexchlorpheniramine (Dexchlor, Poladex, Polaramine)	PO: 2 mg every 4–6 h (max: 12 mg/day)	
dimenhydrinate (Dramamine)	PO: 50–100 mg every 4–6 h	
diphenhydramine (Benadryl, Others)	PO: 25–50 mg every 6–8 h (max: 300 mg/day)	
promethazine (Phenergan)	PO: 12.5–25 g every 6–24 h (max: 100 mg/day)	
triprolidine	PO: 2.5 mg every 4–6 h (max: 10 mg/day)	
Second-Generation Drugs		
acrivastine with pseudoephedrine (Semprex-D)	PO: One capsule daily (8 mg acrivastine/60 mg pseudoephedrine)	*Dry mouth, headache, dizziness, nausea, drowsiness (cetirizine), bitter taste (olopadine)*
azelastine (Astelin, Astepro, Optivar)	Intranasal: 2 sprays per nostril every 12 h Ocular: 1 drop in each affected eye bid	Paradoxical excitation, hypersensitivity reactions, hypotension
cetirizine (Zyrtec)	PO: 5–10 mg/day (max: 10 mg/day)	
desloratadine (Clarinex)	PO: 5 mg/day (max: 5 mg/day)	
fexofenadine (Allegra)	PO: 60 mg every 12 h or 180 mg once daily	
levocetirizine (Xyzal)	PO: 5 mg (1 tablet or 2 teaspoons) once daily	
loratadine (Claritin)	PO: 10 mg/day (max: 10 mg/day)	
olopatadine (Patanase, Patanol)	Intranasal: 2 sprays per nostril bid Ocular: 1 drop in each affected eye bid	

Note: *Italics* indicate common adverse effects. <u>Underline</u> indicates serious adverse effects.

with decongestants and antitussives in OTC cold and sinus medicines. Common OTC antihistamine combinations that are used to treat allergies are listed in Table 45.2.

Antihistamines are most effective when taken prophylactically to prevent allergic symptoms. Their effectiveness in reversing allergic symptoms that have already manifested is limited. This is because antihistamines block the effect of histamine at its receptor sites. They do not prevent the release of histamine from mast cells. Their effectiveness may diminish with long-term use.

In addition to producing antihistamine effects, these drugs also easily cross the blood–brain barrier and block cholinergic receptors to cause typical anticholinergic effects. Anticholinergic effects are responsible for certain beneficial effects of antihistamines, such as drying of mucous membranes, which results in less nasal congestion and tearing.

A large number of H_1-receptor antagonists are available as medications. They all have the same basic mechanism of action and are equally effective in treating allergic rhinitis and other mild allergies. Adverse effects are similar but differ in intensity among the various antihistamines. The older, first-generation antihistamines frequently cause significant drowsiness, which can be a limiting adverse effect in some patients. After a few doses tolerance generally

develops to sedation. The newer, second-generation antihistamines cause less sedation because they do not cross the blood–brain barrier. Alcohol and other CNS depressants should be used with caution when taking antihistamines, because their sedating effects may be additive, even for the second-generation agents. Some patients (especially young children) exhibit CNS stimulation, which can cause insomnia, nervousness, and tremors, or even convulsions. Other CNS adverse effects, such as dizziness, confusion, and even fatigue, more commonly affect the older adult.

The second major adverse effect of antihistamines relates to their anticholinergic effects. Excessive drying of mucous membranes can lead to dry mouth, and urinary hesitancy may be troublesome for patients, especially those with prostatic hyperplasia. Some antihistamines produce more pronounced anticholinergic effects than others. Diphenhydramine and clemastine exhibit a significant incidence of anticholinergic adverse effects, whereas the second-generation agents—loratadine, desloratadine, and fexofenadine—produce the least.

Although most antihistamines are given via the oral route (PO), azelastine (Astelin, Astepro) and olopatadine (Patanase) are available by the intranasal route. These drugs are as effective as the PO antihistamines, but because they are applied locally to the nasal

TABLE 45.2   Selected Over-the-Counter Antihistamine Combinations

Trade Name	Antihistamine	Decongestant	Analgesic
Actifed Cold and Allergy tablets	chlorpheniramine	phenylephrine	—
Actifed Plus	triprolidine	pseudoephedrine	acetaminophen
Benadryl Allergy/Cold caplets	diphenhydramine	phenylephrine	acetaminophen
Chlor-Trimeton Allergy/Decongestant tablets	chlorpheniramine	pseudoephedrine	—
Dimetapp Children's Cold and Allergy	brompheniramine	phenylephrine	—
Sudafed PE Nighttime Cold	diphenhydramine	phenylephrine	acetaminophen
Sudafed PE Sinus and Allergy tablets	chlorpheniramine	phenylephrine	—
Tavist Allergy tablets	clemastine	—	—
Triaminic Cold/Allergy	chlorpheniramine	phenylephrine	—
Tylenol Allergy Multi-Symptom Gels	chlorpheniramine	phenylephrine	acetaminophen
Tylenol PM Gelcaps	diphenhydramine	—	acetaminophen

mucosa, limited systemic absorption occurs. This may make the intranasal drugs slightly safer than PO antihistamines.

Antihistamines are used as adjuncts to the emergency treatment of anaphylaxis, which is the most severe form of allergic reaction. Although massive histamine release causes bronchoconstriction, edema, hypotension, and other symptoms of anaphylaxis, other inflammatory mediators, including leukotrienes and prostaglandins, contribute to the hypersensitivity response. Because antihistamines do not block these other mediators, antihistamines are only effective as adjunctive therapy in anaphylaxis. They are most effective if given as preventive medications before anaphylaxis for patients who are at high risk of having an allergic response. The major life-threatening symptoms of anaphylaxis are controlled with epinephrine and other vasoconstrictors.

H_1-receptor antagonists are effective in treating a number of other disorders, including the following:

- **Vertigo and motion sickness.** Nausea resulting from vertigo or motion sickness responds well to antihistamines. These drugs act by suppressing the vomiting center in the medulla and depressing the excitability of the neurons of the vestibular apparatus of the inner ear. To be effective, they must be taken prior to the onset of symptoms. Meclizine (Antivert) and dimenhydrinate (Dramamine) are the two most common antihistamines used for this purpose. Cyclizine (Marezine) is another older antihistamine that is occasionally used to reduce nausea and vertigo. The pharmacotherapy of nausea is discussed in Chapter 60.

- **Parkinson's disease.** Drugs with significant anticholinergic actions are used to treat mild forms of Parkinson's disease. They are also used to treat the tremor and extrapyramidal adverse effects from conventional antipsychotic drugs. Because diphenhydramine exerts great amounts of anticholinergic action, it is sometimes used to treat these conditions.

- **Insomnia.** Many patients become drowsy after taking first-generation antihistamines. OTC sleep aids usually include antihistamines such as diphenhydramine and doxylamine (Unisom SleepTabs). After a few days, patients will become tolerant to the drowsiness produced by these drugs; thus they should be used for 2 weeks or less.

- **Urticaria and other skin rashes.** Urticaria or hives is often caused by the release of histamine, and the condition responds well to H_1-receptor blockers. Symptomatic treatment may include any of the first- or second-generation agents, either using PO drugs or topical creams or lotions.

CONNECTION Checkpoint 45.1

Although drugs with anticholinergic action are used to treat Parkinson's disease, they are generally not drugs of first choice. From what you learned in Chapter 21, name the drug most commonly prescribed for Parkinson's disease and the neurotransmitter it replaces. *See Answer to Connection Checkpoint 45.1 on student resource website.*

CONNECTIONS   Lifespan Consideration

◀ Antihistamines and Drugs for Allergic Rhinitis for the Older Adult

While generally considered a condition of children and young and middle-aged adults, the older adult patient is also susceptible to allergic rhinitis. Changes to nasal structure and mucous membranes in older patients may increase symptoms of rhinitis. The older adult is also more sensitive to the effects of antihistamines, and drowsiness, dizziness, and fall risk are possible with the first-generation antihistamines. Second-generation antihistamines may require a dosage adjustment due to normal physiological changes as a person ages. For the older adult male, the anticholinergic effects of antihistamines may exacerbate symptoms of an enlarged prostate and worsen urinary symptoms.

Slavin (2010) determined that intranasal corticosteroid sprays were preferred for the older adult with symptoms of allergic rhinitis. They had limited systemic side effects due to the topical application; caused fewer adverse effects such as dizziness, drowsiness, or urinary problems; and were well tolerated. If an antihistamine was warranted, intranasal antihistamines or second-generation drugs were preferred over the traditional drugs. Leukotriene receptor antagonist drugs were also effective but were not considered superior to intranasal corticosteroids because of the potential for drug interactions.

Fexofenadine (Allegra)

Classification: **Therapeutic:** Drug for allergic rhinitis and minor allergies
Pharmacologic: H_1-receptor antagonist (second generation), antihistamine

Therapeutic Effects and Uses: Approved in 1996 for the treatment of allergic rhinitis, fexofenadine is a second-generation H_1-receptor antagonist with an effectiveness that is equivalent to that of diphenhydramine. Most effective when taken before symptoms develop, fexofenadine reduces the severity of nasal congestion, sneezing, and tearing of the eyes.

The long half-life of fexofenadine, over 14 hours, allows it to be administered once or twice daily. Fexofenadine is available in PO form as regular tablets, orally disintegrating tablets, and as a suspension. In addition to allergic rhinitis, it is also approved to treat chronic idiopathic urticaria. Allegra-D combines fexofenadine with pseudoephedrine, which is a decongestant.

Mechanism of Action: Fexofenadine acts by competing with histamine for binding to histamine (H_1) receptor sites. It does not prevent the release of histamine.

Pharmacokinetics:

Route(s)	PO (capsules, tablets, and suspension)
Absorption	Rapid
Distribution	Does not cross the blood–brain barrier; unknown if secreted in breast milk; 60–70% bound to plasma protein
Primary metabolism	Hepatic
Primary excretion	80% renal, 11% feces
Onset of action	Usually within 1 h
Duration of action	Half-life: 14.4 h; duration: 12–24 h

Adverse Effects: The major advantage of fexofenadine over first-generation antihistamines is that it does not readily cross the blood–brain barrier, so drowsiness is generally not a major adverse effect. Adverse effects are infrequent and usually minor and include headache, nausea, dyspepsia, and dysmenorrhea. Patients who are taking the drug have an increased incidence of viral infections. Anticholinergic effects such as dry mouth can occur in some patients.

Contraindications/Precautions: The only contraindication to fexofenadine is hypersensitivity to this drug. Patients with advanced renal disease should receive reduced doses.

Drug Interactions: Although considered nonsedating, fexofenadine can still cause drowsiness in certain patients at high doses and if combined with CNS depressants, including alcohol. Concurrent administration with ketoconazole or erythromycin increases the plasma concentrations of fexofenadine. Prolongation of the QT interval has occurred with other antihistamines but is infrequent with fexofenadine. Antacids that contain aluminum or magnesium may interfere with the absorption of fexofenadine. **Herbal/Food:** Absorption may be decreased when taken with grapefruit, orange, or apple juice, thereby reducing the bioavailability of fexofenadine.

Pregnancy: Category C.

Treatment of Overdose: Overdose may cause CNS depression, dry mouth, and dizziness. There is no specific antidote for overdose, and supportive treatment of symptoms is indicated.

Nursing Responsibilities: Key nursing implications for patients receiving fexofenadine are included in the Nursing Practice Application for Patients Receiving Pharmacotherapy with Antihistamines.

Drugs Similar to Fexofenadine (Allegra)

The second-generation H_1 antagonists include acrivastine with pseudoephedrine, azelastine, cetirizine, desloratadine, levocetirizine, loratadine, and olopatadine. Because the first-generation antihistamines are all very similar, a description of diphenhydramine is included in this section as an example of this group.

Acrivastine with pseudoephedrine (Semprex-D): Approved in 1994, Semprex-D is a fixed-dose combination product containing acrivastine (an antihistamine) and pseudoephedrine (a decongestant). Acrivastine is structurally similar to triprolidine, a first-generation antihistamine. The drug is approved for the treatment of seasonal allergic rhinitis with nasal congestion in adults and children age 12 and older. Adverse effects include headache, dry mouth, and somnolence. This drug is pregnancy category B.

Azelastine (Astelin, Astepro, Optivar): Originally approved in 2000, azelastine is a second-generation H_1 antagonist approved for relief of symptoms caused by seasonal allergic rhinitis. An intranasal formulation (Astepro) was subsequently approved to treat perennial allergic rhinitis and an ophthalmic formulation (Optivar) for allergic conjunctivitis. Dymista is a combination drug that combines azelastine with fluticasone, a corticosteroid. Adverse effects of intranasal azelastine include local effects on the nasal mucosa such as epistaxis (nosebleed), a bitter taste, and postnasal drip. The most common side effects of eyedrop therapy are headache, transient eye stinging, and a bitter taste. The drug can cause drowsiness, especially when combined with CNS depressants or alcohol. This drug is pregnancy category C.

Cetirizine (Zyrtec): Approved in 1995, cetirizine is a second-generation antihistamine that is commonly used for treating allergic rhinitis and itching due to hives. It is used off-label to treat atopic dermatitis and symptoms of allergy-induced asthma. Various PO formulations are available, including tablets to be swallowed, chewable tablets, and syrup. It is well tolerated and approved for children as young as 2 years of age. Adverse effects are uncommon. Cetirizine appears to be somewhat more sedating than other second-generation agents. Xerostomia and fatigue are additional adverse effects. The drug was moved from prescription to OTC status in 2007. Cetirizine is an active metabolite of hydroxyzine (Atarax, Vistaril), a first-generation antihistamine. This drug is pregnancy category B.

In 2007, an isomer of cetirizine was approved by the U.S. Food and Drug Administration (FDA). Levocetirizine (Xyzal) is a PO antihistamine that has the same indications and actions as those of cetirizine but is reported to cause less drowsiness.

Desloratadine (Clarinex): Desloratadine is a nonsedating, second-generation antihistamine that was approved in 2001 for the treatment of allergic rhinitis and itching due to hives. It is the active metabolite of loratadine (Claritin). Desloratadine is administered by the PO route and is approved to treat adults and children age 6 months and older. Like other second-generation drugs, sedation is minimal and adverse effects are uncommon. Headache, pharyngitis, and xerostomia are the most frequently reported adverse effects. This drug is pregnancy category C.

Diphenhydramine (Benadryl, Others): Diphenhydramine is a first-generation H_1-receptor antagonist that is commonly used to treat minor symptoms of allergy and the common cold such as sneezing, runny nose, and tearing of the eyes. It exhibits a strong anticholinergic drying action on mucous membranes. OTC diphenhydramine is often combined with an analgesic, decongestant, or expectorant when treating cold symptoms. Diphenhydramine is also used as a topical drug to treat rashes, and intramuscular (IM) and intravenous (IV) forms are available for severe allergic reactions. An elixir and syrup form is available for administration to young children. Other indications for diphenhydramine include Parkinson's disease, motion sickness, and insomnia. Diphenhydramine can cause significant drowsiness, although this usually diminishes with long-term use. Occasionally diphenhydramine is given to produce drowsiness as a treatment for insomnia. This drug may cause paradoxical excitement in some patients, which is an effect most commonly seen in children. This drug may cause anticholinergic adverse effects such as urinary retention, tachycardia, elevated blood pressure, xerostomia, thickening of bronchial secretions, and blurred vision. This drug is pregnancy category B.

Loratadine (Claritin): Loratadine was the first of the second-generation antihistamines, approved in 1993, to treat allergic rhinitis and itching due to hives. In 2002, the high safety record of loratadine led to the reclassification of the drug from prescription to OTC. Like other drugs in its class, loratadine causes very little drowsiness, and adverse effects are unusual. It is only available PO and may be administered to children age 2 and older. Drowsiness and headache may occur at higher doses. This drug is pregnancy category C.

Olopatadine (Patanase, Patanol): Olopatadine is a second-generation H_1 antagonist approved in 1996. The intranasal spray (Patanase) is approved for the treatment of seasonal allergic rhinitis in adults and children 6 years of age and older. Adverse effects of olopatadine include local effects on the nasal mucosa such as epistaxis, a bitter taste, and postnasal drip. Other adverse effects include headache, throat pain, and URT infection. Although uncommon, nasal ulceration and septal perforation are serious adverse effects. In some patients, the drug can cause drowsiness; thus it should be used with caution when combined with CNS depressants and alcohol. An ophthalmic formulation (Patanol) is approved for the treatment of allergic conjunctivitis. As eyedrops, the drug can cause local effects such as blurred vision, burning or stinging, and dry eyes. This drug is pregnancy category C.

CONNECTION Checkpoint 45.2

From what you learned in Chapter 44, what is the role of leukotriene antagonists in treating asthma? What drug classes are preferred for this condition? *See Answer to Connection Checkpoint 45.2 on student resource website.*

45.5 Intranasal corticosteroids are the drugs of choice for allergic rhinitis because of their effectiveness and safety.

Corticosteroids, also known as glucocorticoids, may be applied directly to the nasal mucosa to prevent symptoms of allergic rhinitis. These drugs are listed in Table 45.3.

Although corticosteroids are very effective at reducing allergy symptoms, their oral and parenteral uses are limited by potentially serious adverse effects. Intranasal formulations of these drugs, however, produce virtually no serious adverse effects. Because of their

TABLE 45.3 Intranasal Corticosteroids and Miscellaneous Drugs for Allergic Rhinitis

Drug	Route and Adult Dose (Maximum Dose Where Indicated)	Adverse Effects
Intranasal Corticosteroids		
beclomethasone (Beconase AQ, Qnasl, Qvar)	Intranasal: 1 spray bid–qid	*Transient nasal irritation, burning, sneezing, dryness*
budesonide (Rhinocort Aqua)	Intranasal: 2 sprays bid	
ciclesonide (Omnaris)	Intranasal: 2 sprays once daily (max: 200 mcg/day)	Hypercorticism (only if large amounts are swallowed), nasal ulceration, *Candida* infection
fluticasone (Flonase, Veramyst)	Intranasal: 1 spray in each nostril once (Veramyst) or twice (Flonase) daily	
mometasone (Nasonex)	Intranasal: 2 sprays/day	
triamcinolone (Nasacort AQ)	Intranasal: 2–4 sprays 4 times daily	
Miscellaneous Drugs		
cromolyn (NasalCrom)	Intranasal: 1 spray in each nostril tid–qid	*Nasal burning and irritation* Anaphylaxis
ipratropium (Atrovent)	Intranasal: 2 sprays per nostril 3 to 4 times daily	*Transient nasal irritation, burning, sneezing or dryness, cough* Urinary retention, worsening of glaucoma
montelukast (Singulair)	PO: 10 mg/day	*Headache, nausea, diarrhea* No serious adverse effects

Note: Italics indicate common adverse effects. Underline indicates serious adverse effects.

CONNECTIONS: NURSING PRACTICE APPLICATION

Patients Receiving Pharmacotherapy with Antihistamines

Assessment	Potential Nursing Diagnoses*
Baseline assessment prior to administration: • Obtain a complete health history including previous history of symptoms and association to seasons, foods, or environmental exposures; existing cardiovascular, respiratory, hepatic, renal, or neurologic disease; glaucoma; prostatic hypertrophy; difficulty with urination; presence of fever or active infections, pregnancy or breast-feeding, alcohol use, or smoking. Obtain a drug history, noting the type of adverse reaction or allergy experienced to any medications. • If allergy symptoms are of new onset, particularly for infants and young children, assess for any recent changes in diet, soaps including laundry detergent, laundry softener, cosmetics, lotions, environmental factors (e.g., pets, travel), or recent carpet cleaning. • Obtain baseline vital signs. An ECG may be ordered for patients with a history of cardiac conditions. • Evaluate appropriate laboratory findings (e.g., CBC, hepatic and renal laboratory tests). • Assess the patient's ability to receive and understand instructions. Include the family and caregiver as needed. **Assessment throughout administration:** • Assess for desired therapeutic effects (e.g., decreased nasal congestion and drainage, decreased eye watering or itching). • Continue periodic monitoring of CBC and liver and renal function studies as appropriate. • Assess vital signs, especially pulse rate and rhythm. • Assess for adverse effects: dizziness, drowsiness, dry mouth, blurred vision, or headache. Report immediately any increasing fever, confusion, muscle weakness, tachycardia, palpitations, hypotension, syncope, dyspnea, pulmonary congestion, urinary retention, sudden severe eye pain, or rainbow halos around lights.	• *Ineffective Airway Clearance* • *Ineffective Breathing Pattern* • *Disturbed Sleep Pattern* or *Insomnia*, related to adverse drug effects • *Fatigue*, related to adverse drug effects • *Deficient Knowledge* (Drug Therapy) • *Risk for Injury*, related to adverse drug effects • *Risk for Falls*, related to adverse drug effects

Implementation

Interventions and (Rationales)	Patient-Centered Care
Ensuring therapeutic effects: • Continue assessments as above for therapeutic effects. (Diminished nasal congestion and improvement in other signs and symptoms of allergy should begin after taking the first dose and continue to improve. Notify the provider if symptoms continue to increase, especially if respiratory involvement worsens.)	• Teach the patient to supplement drug therapy with nonpharmacologic measures, such as increased fluid intake to liquefy and mobilize mucus, and to reduce exposure to allergens where possible. • Advise the patient to carry a wallet identification card or wear medical identification jewelry indicating any significant allergies or anaphylaxis.
• For treatment of seasonal allergies, drug therapy should be started *before the beginning of the allergy season and the appearance of symptoms.* (Because antihistamines competitively bind to histamine receptors, beginning drug therapy before circulating histamine increases will result in better effects.)	• Teach the patient to begin taking the drug before allergy season begins or at the earliest possible appearance of symptoms for best effects, and to maintain consistent dosing. • **Lifespan:** Teach parents or caregivers that antihistamines are not recommended for use in children under 6 unless recommended by the health care provider.
Minimizing adverse effects: • Ensure patient safety, especially in the older adult. Observe for lightheadedness or dizziness. Monitor ambulation until the effects of the drug are known. (**Lifespan:** Drowsiness or dizziness from drug effects or orthostatic hypotension may occur and increases the risk of injury and falls, particularly in the older adult. Drowsiness tends to diminish over several doses as the patient becomes tolerant to the effects.)	• Instruct the patient to call for assistance prior to getting out of bed or attempting to walk alone, and to avoid driving or other activities requiring mental alertness or physical coordination until the effects of the drug are known. If dizziness occurs, the patient should sit or lie down and not attempt to stand or walk until the sensation passes.
• Continue to monitor vital signs, especially pulse rate and rhythm for patients with existing cardiac disease. ECGs may be ordered periodically for patients with a history of dysrhythmias. (Histamine plays a role in cardiac conduction and, when blocked by antihistamines, may cause dysrhythmias in patients with a history of dysrhythmias, cardiac disease, or in the sensitive patient. **Lifespan:** Undetected cardiac disease may place the older adult at greater risk for cardiovascular adverse effects.)	• Instruct the patient to immediately report dizziness, palpitations, or syncope. • Teach the patient, family, or caregiver how to monitor the pulse and blood pressure as appropriate. Ensure proper use and functioning of any home equipment obtained.

CONNECTIONS: NURSING PRACTICE APPLICATION (continued)

• Continue to monitor periodic hepatic and renal function laboratory values, especially in patients on long-term antihistamine use or those with previous history of hepatic or renal impairment. (Hepatic toxicity is a potential adverse effect of antihistamines. Impaired renal function will inhibit drug excretion and prolong drug effects with potentially increased adverse effects. **Lifespan:** Monitor the older adult more frequently because physiological changes related to aging may affect the drug's metabolism or excretion.)	• Instruct the patient on the need to return periodically for laboratory work.
• Monitor for persistent dry cough, increasing cough severity, increasing congestion, or dyspnea. (Antihistamines are used with extreme caution or are contraindicated in patients with existing respiratory disease, including COPD. Thickened mucus is a potential adverse drug effect. A change in the severity of the cough may indicate increasing allergic response, worsening disease process, or respiratory infection, and should be reported immediately.)	• Instruct the patient to promptly report any change in the severity or frequency of cough. Any cough accompanied by shortness of breath, increasing congestion, fever, or chest pain should be reported immediately. • Encourage the patient to increase fluid intake to assist in liquefying mucus secretions and to ease dry mouth effects.
• Assess for CNS effects including restlessness, nervousness, insomnia, headache, tremors, fatigue, or weakness. Frequently monitor for these symptoms in the patient with hyperthyroidism. Immediately report severe symptoms or any disorientation or confusion. (CNS depressant effects, such as drowsiness, fatigue, or mild weakness, are common. Paradoxical excitement, such as restlessness or nervousness, or insomnia may occur, especially in children. Patients with hyperthyroidism may experience pronounced CNS stimulatory effects. Immediately report any severe symptoms to the health care provider. Alcohol consumption increases the CNS depressant effects and should be avoided or eliminated.)	• Instruct the patient, family, or caregiver to immediately report increasing lethargy, disorientation, confusion, changes in behavior or mood, agitation or aggression, slurred speech, or ataxia. • Instruct the patient to avoid or eliminate alcohol consumption while on antihistamines.
• If an antihistamine is used for sleep (e.g., doxylamine), ensure patient safety, including on awakening. Avoid using antihistamines for sleep for more than 2 weeks and consult the health care provider if insomnia continues. (Morning or daytime grogginess, a hangover effect, may occur in some patients taking antihistamines for sleep and may impair normal activities. Patients may become tolerant to drowsiness-inducing effects within 2 weeks, and insomnia that continues beyond that time should be evaluated by a health care provider.)	• Caution the patient about possible morning or daytime sleepiness or grogginess, and to exercise caution with activities requiring mental alertness or physical coordination until daytime effects of the drug are known. Do not keep the medication at the bedside to prevent overdosage from occurring if additional doses are taken when drowsy. Do not take the medication concurrently with alcohol.
• Assess for changes in visual acuity, blurred vision, and immediately report any loss of peripheral vision, seeing rainbow halos around lights, acute eye pain, or pain accompanied by nausea and vomiting. (Increased intraoptic pressure in patients with narrow-angle glaucoma may occur in patients taking antihistamines.)	• Instruct the patient to immediately report any visual changes or eye pain.
• Assess for urinary retention. (Antihistamines may cause urinary retention as an adverse effect. **Lifespan:** Be aware that the male older adult is at higher risk for mechanical obstruction due to an enlarged prostate.)	• Instruct the patient to immediately report an inability to void, increasing bladder pressure, or pain.
• Monitor for gastrointestinal (GI) effects. Encourage the patient to take the drug with food to prevent adverse effects. (Nausea, vomiting, epigastric distress, anorexia, constipation, or diarrhea may occur and are treated symptomatically. Taking the drug with food or milk may decrease GI adverse effects.)	• Teach the patient to take the medication with food or milk. Report any significant GI symptoms (e.g., nausea with vomiting, diarrhea) to the health care provider for further treatment.
• Monitor for anticholinergic-related adverse effects including dry mouth, thickened mucus, nasal dryness, slightly blurred vision, or headache. (Mild anticholinergic adverse effects are common and are treated symptomatically. Significant symptoms as listed previously are reported immediately.)	• Teach the patient to increase fluid intake or suck on hard candy to relieve mouth and respiratory tract dryness. Exercise caution if blurred vision impairs normal activities and report significant visual disturbances as listed previously.
Patient understanding of drug therapy: • Use opportunities during administration of medications and during assessments to discuss the rationale for drug therapy, desired therapeutic outcomes, commonly observed adverse effects, parameters for when to call the health care provider, and any necessary monitoring or precautions. (Using time during nursing care helps to optimize and reinforce key teaching areas.)	• The patient should be able to state the reason for the drug, appropriate dose and scheduling, what adverse effects to observe for, and when to report them.
Patient self-administration of drug therapy: • When administering the medication, instruct the patient, family, or caregiver in the proper self-administration of the drug, e.g., take the drug before allergy season or before symptoms are severe. (Utilizing time during nurse-administration of these drugs helps to reinforce teaching.)	• The patient, family, or caregiver is able to discuss appropriate dosing and administration needs.

*Nursing Diagnoses—Definitions and Classification 2015–2017. Copyright © 2014, 1994–2014 by NANDA International. Used by arrangement with John Wiley & Sons Limited.

effectiveness and safety, the intranasal corticosteroids have joined antihistamines as first-line drugs in the therapy of allergic rhinitis. They are now considered the most effective drug treatment for seasonal and perennial allergic rhinitis. Intranasal corticosteroids are also used for patients undergoing nasal or sinus surgery for their anti-inflammatory action.

When sprayed onto the nasal mucosa, corticosteroids act by multiple mechanisms. They decrease the secretion of inflammatory mediators, reduce tissue edema, and cause a mild vasoconstriction. All corticosteroids are administered with a metered-spray device that delivers a consistent dose of drug per spray. All have equal effectiveness. Unlike sympathomimetics, however, the benefits of inhaled corticosteroids are not immediate. To achieve peak response, 1 to 3 weeks (often longer with perennial rhinitis than seasonal rhinitis) may be required. After the patient's symptoms are controlled, the dose of intranasal corticosteroids is reduced to the lowest amount required to control the symptoms. The intranasal corticosteroids must be taken daily to produce maximum benefit.

When administered appropriately, the actions of corticosteroids are limited to the nasal passages. The most frequently reported adverse effect is an intense burning sensation in the nose immediately after spraying. Excessive drying of the nasal mucosa may occur, leading to epistaxis.

PROTOTYPE DRUG	Fluticasone (Flonase, Veramyst)

Classification: Therapeutic: Drug for allergic rhinitis
Pharmacologic: Intranasal corticosteroid

Therapeutic Effects and Uses: Approved in 1990, fluticasone is an intranasal corticosteroid that is used for the management of nasal symptoms associated with seasonal and perennial rhinitis. Therapy usually begins with two sprays in each nostril, twice daily, and decreases to one dose per day. Prolonged use of corticosteroids can lead to tolerance to the drug's therapeutic effects.

Veramyst and Dymista are two newer formulations of this drug. Veramyst contains intranasal fluticasone that is approved for the treatment of both seasonal and perennial allergic rhinitis in patients 2 years and older. Veramyst offers the advantage of once-daily dosing along with improvement of both nasal and ocular symptoms associated with allergies. Dymista is a combination drug approved in 2012 that contains fluticasone and the antihistamine azelastine. Dymista nasal spray is taken twice daily to treat allergic rhinitis.

Fluticasone is also available in oral inhalation and topical formulations. The oral inhalation product (Flovent) is administered in a metered-dose inhaler (MDI) device for the treatment of asthma and COPD (see Chapter 44). Flovent reduces bronchial inflammation that is characteristic of asthma. In 2013 Breo Ellipta, a combination of fluticasone with vilanterol (a long-acting β_2 agonist), was approved to treat COPD. Topical ointments and creams are applied to the skin for various inflammatory conditions, including atopic dermatitis, eczema, exfoliative dermatitis, psoriasis, and contact dermatitis (see Chapter 73).

Mechanism of Action: Fluticasone acts to decrease local inflammation in the nasal passages through vasoconstrictor and anti-inflammatory mechanisms. It is thought to inhibit mast cells, macrophages, and inflammatory mediators such as prostaglandins, histamine, kinins, and leukotrienes.

Pharmacokinetics:

Route(s)	Intranasal spray, oral inhalation, topical
Absorption	Intranasal: drug is swallowed, with less than 2% absorbed systemically
	Oral inhalation: 30% reaches systemic circulation
	Topical: minimal absorption
Distribution	Widely distributed; 91–99% bound to plasma protein
Primary metabolism	Hepatic, extensive first-pass metabolism by CYP3A4
Primary excretion	Feces
Onset of action	12 h to several days
Duration of action	Several days

Adverse Effects: When administered by the intranasal route, adverse effects of fluticasone are uncommon and include headache, cough, nasal ulceration, epistaxis, and local burning. Swallowing large amounts increases the potential for systemic corticosteroid adverse effects (see Chapter 71).

Contraindications/Precautions: The only contraindication to fluticasone is prior hypersensitivity to the drug. Because corticosteroids can mask signs of infection, patients with known bacterial, viral, fungal, or parasitic infections (especially of the respiratory tract) should not receive these drugs until the infection has cleared. Safety has not been established in children under 4 years of age.

Drug Interactions: Concurrent use of fluticasone with an intranasal decongestant increases the risk of nasal irritation or bleeding. Use with ritonavir should be avoided, because this drug significantly increases plasma fluticasone levels. **Herbal/Food:** Use with caution with black licorice, which may potentiate the effects of corticosteroids.

Pregnancy: Category C.

Treatment of Overdose: Overdose with intranasal corticosteroids is unlikely. There is no specific treatment.

Nursing Responsibilities: Key nursing implications for patients receiving fluticasone are included in the Nursing Practice Application for Patients Receiving Pharmacotherapy for Symptomatic Cough and Cold Relief.

Drugs Similar to Fluticasone (Flonase, Veramyst)

All of the intranasal corticosteroids have the same indications, actions, and adverse effects. Due to individual variation, some patients experience more irritation or burning with one drug over another. All are equally effective when administered at their recommended doses. The other intranasal corticosteroids are listed in Table 45.3.

45.6 Cromolyn, ipratropium, and montelukast are alternatives to intranasal corticosteroids in the treatment of allergic rhinitis.

Although most patients with allergic rhinitis are successfully treated with intranasal corticosteroids or antihistamines, several alternatives exist. **Mast cell stabilizers** are drugs that inhibit the release of inflammatory mediators from mast cells. Mast cells contain granules that release histamine and leukotrienes during inflammatory and allergic reactions. Intranasal cromolyn (NasalCrom) is a mast cell stabilizer approved for the treatment of seasonal or perennial allergic rhinitis. Cromolyn is featured as a prototype in Chapter 44.

Most effective when given prior to allergen exposure, cromolyn has few adverse effects and is now designated as an OTC drug for the treatment of allergy and cold symptoms. It is just as effective as antihistamines but less effective than intranasal corticosteroids. This drug is very safe and adverse effects are uncommon. A major disadvantage is that cromolyn must be taken four times daily. If a patient is experiencing nasal congestion, a topical decongestant is used prior to administration of cromolyn. When administered by the oral inhalation route, cromolyn is approved for the treatment of asthma. A second mast cell stabilizer, nedocromil (Tilade), is approved only for asthma.

Ipratropium (Atrovent) nasal spray is an anticholinergic drug indicated for the symptomatic relief of runny nose (rhinorrhea) associated with seasonal allergic rhinitis or the common cold. Its actions are limited to decreasing nasal secretions; it does not stop the sneezing, postnasal drip, or itchy throat or eyes characteristic of allergic rhinitis or the common cold. The drug is well tolerated with epistaxis and nasal dryness experienced by a small percentage of patients. Like other anticholinergics, it should be used with caution in patients with narrow-angle glaucoma or with prostatic hyperplasia. The primary use of ipratropium is by the inhalation route as a bronchodilator in the treatment of chronic obstructive pulmonary disease. It is presented as a prototype drug for this disorder in Chapter 44.

Montelukast (Singulair) is an oral drug that acts by blocking leukotriene receptors. Leukotrienes are associated with inflammation and are responsible for some of the sneezing, nasal itching, and congestion characteristic of allergic rhinitis. Originally approved for the treatment of asthma in 1998, allergic rhinitis was subsequently added as an indication. It is approved for both the seasonal and perennial forms of the disease and can be used in children as young as 6 months of age. Like cromolyn, montelukast is not considered as effective as the intranasal corticosteroids. This drug is well tolerated and produces few serious adverse effects. This drug is pregnancy category B.

Decongestants

45.7 Intranasal and oral sympathomimetics are the most effective drugs for relieving nasal congestion.

Decongestants are drugs that relieve nasal congestion. They are administered by either the PO or intranasal route and are often combined with antihistamines in the pharmacotherapy of allergies or the common cold.

Sympathomimetics (also called adrenergic agonists) with alpha-adrenergic activity are effective at relieving the nasal congestion associated with the common cold and allergic rhinitis when given by either the PO or intranasal route. The intranasal preparations such as oxymetazoline (Afrin, Others) are available OTC as sprays or drops and produce a noticeable response within minutes. The nasal decongestants are listed in Table 45.4.

Intranasal sympathomimetics produce few systemic effects because only minimal amounts of these drugs are absorbed in the circulation. The most serious, limiting adverse effect of the intranasal preparations is **rebound congestion**. In almost all patients, prolonged use causes hypersecretion of mucus and worsening nasal congestion once the drug effects wear off. This leads to a cycle of increased drug use as the condition worsens to obtain the desired effect from these drugs. Because of this rebound congestion, intranasal sympathomimetics should be used for no longer than 3 to 5 days. Patients who develop dependence should be gradually switched to intranasal corticosteroids because they do not cause rebound congestion. The usual technique for switching to intranasal corticosteroids is by stopping the use of the decongestant in one nostril at a time.

When administered PO, sympathomimetics do not produce rebound congestion. Their onset of action by this route, however, is much slower than when administered intranasally, and they are less effective at relieving severe congestion. The possibility of systemic adverse effects is also greater with the PO drugs. Potential adverse effects include hypertension (HTN) and CNS stimulation that may lead to insomnia and anxiety. Pseudoephedrine and phenylephrine are common sympathomimetics found in oral OTC cold and allergy medicines.

The sympathomimetics relieve only nasal congestion and therefore are often combined with antihistamines to control sneezing and tearing. It is interesting to note that some OTC drugs having the same basic name (Neo-Synephrine, Afrin, and Vicks) may contain different sympathomimetics. For example, Neo-Synephrine decongestants with 12-hour duration contain the drug oxymetazoline; Neo-Synephrine preparations that last 4 to 6 hours contain phenylephrine.

PharmFACT

When legislation restricted the sale of products containing pseudoephedrine, the seizures of illegal methamphetamine (meth) laboratories by law enforcement agencies in the United States decreased 70% from 2003 to 2007. Since 2008, however, the number of illegal meth laboratories has been rapidly increasing, likely due to newer methods of synthesizing meth and by circumventing state laws on the purchase of pseudoephedrine (U.S. Government Accountability Office, 2013).

PROTOTYPE DRUG | Pseudoephedrine (Sudafed)

Classification: Therapeutic: Decongestant
Pharmacologic: Sympathomimetic

Therapeutic Effects and Uses: Approved in 1959, pseudoephedrine is available in tablet and elixir formulations. It is often combined with other medications in OTC preparations used to treat allergic rhinitis, sinus congestion, and the common cold symptoms. Pseudoephedrine promotes sinus drainage and can open obstructed Eustachian tubes in adults and children with chronic otic inflammation. It is also used off-label to prevent otitic barotraumas, pain or damage to the tympanic membrane caused by rapid pressure changes during air travel or diving.

Pseudoephedrine deserves special attention because of its potential for misuse. Pseudoephedrine is the starting chemical for the synthesis of illegal methamphetamine by drug traffickers. As of 2004, pseudoephedrine products must be kept in

TABLE 45.4   Nasal Decongestants

Drug	Route and Adult Dose (Maximum Dose Where Indicated)	Adverse Effects
naphazoline (Privine)	Intranasal: 2 drops every 3–6 h	*Intranasal: transient nasal irritation, burning, sneezing, or dryness, headache*
oxymetazoline (Afrin 12 Hour, Neo-Synephrine 12 Hour, Others)	Intranasal (0.05%): 2–3 sprays bid for up to 3 days	*Oral: CNS stimulation: nervousness, insomnia, headache, dry mouth*
phenylephrine (Afrin 4–6 Hour, Neo-Synephrine 4–6 Hour, Others)	Intranasal (0.1%): 1–2 sprays or drops every 4 h, as needed, up to 3 days	<u>Intranasal: rebound congestion</u>
pseudoephedrine (Sudafed)	PO: 30–60 mg 4–6 h (max: 240 mg/day) Sustained release: 120 mg every 12 h	<u>Oral: CNS excitation (in people with coronary artery disease or HTN), tremors, dysrhythmias, tachycardia, difficulty in voiding, HTN and peripheral and visceral vasoconstriction</u>
tetrahydrozoline (Tyzine)	Intranasal: 2–4 drops or sprays every 3 h	
xylometazoline (Otrivin)	Intranasal (0.1%): 1–2 sprays bid (max: 3 doses/day)	

Note: Italics indicate common adverse effects. <u>Underline</u> indicates serious adverse effects.

a locked box behind the pharmacy counter, so that pharmacists can monitor sales and distribution. Although still considered OTC drugs, pharmacists are required to keep a log of the names and addresses and check the photo identification of anyone who buys a pseudoephedrine product. At least two states have made pseudoephedrine a prescription drug. Note that these precautions are not being taken because pseudoephedrine itself is a dangerous drug, but instead to limit the availability of the drug to illicit makers of methamphetamine. Manufacturers have reformulated their OTC cold medicines to contain phenylephrine rather than pseudoephedrine.

Mechanism of Action: Pseudoephedrine activates $alpha_1$-adrenergic receptors, which causes vasoconstriction in the nasal mucosa, resulting in shrinking of mucosal swelling. It also stimulates $beta_2$-adrenergic receptors of the respiratory tract, which may result in some bronchodilation.

Pharmacokinetics:

Route(s)	PO (tablets, elixir)
Absorption	Well absorbed orally
Distribution	Widely distributed, including in cerebrospinal fluid (CSF); crosses the placenta; secreted in breast milk
Primary metabolism	Hepatic
Primary excretion	Renal
Onset of action	30 min; extended release: 60 min
Duration of action	4–8 h; extended release: 12 h

Adverse Effects: Pseudoephedrine is well tolerated at regular dosage levels. Some patients experience CNS stimulation with symptoms of insomnia, restlessness, anxiety, and dizziness. Excitability is especially a concern in infants and young children. At high doses, seizures and psychosis may occur. Other sympathomimetic effects include dysrhythmias, HTN, palpitations, tachycardia, dry mouth, and anorexia. Rebound congestion is not usually a concern with PO decongestants. Serious injury and deaths due to overdose have occurred in pediatric patients under 2 years of age who received high doses of cough and cold medicines.

Contraindications/Precautions: Pseudoephedrine should not be used by patients with severe HTN, severe coronary artery disease, or hypersensitivity to this drug or by those who take monoamine oxidase inhibitor (MAOI) drugs. Alpha-adrenergic agonists should be used with caution in patients with prostatic enlargement, because these drugs increase smooth muscle activity in the prostate gland and may diminish urinary outflow (see Chapter 71). The FDA has issued advisories that nonprescription cough and cold products (including those containing pseudoephedrine) not be used in children under 6 years of age, and that they be used with extreme caution in all children.

Drug Interactions: Pseudoephedrine interacts with MAOIs to cause a hypertensive crisis. Use with other sympathomimetic drugs, including caffeine, can lead to additive cardiovascular and CNS stimulation effects. Beta blockers and pseudoephedrine together can result in HTN or severe bradycardia. Concurrent use with tricyclic antidepressants may result in increased cardiovascular toxicity and severe headaches. Pseudoephedrine can antagonize the effects of antihypertensive drugs. Pseudoephedrine should be avoided in patients who are taking nitrates for angina due to the vasoconstriction caused by the stimulation of alpha-adrenergic receptors on systemic blood vessels. Use with digoxin may cause dysrhythmias. **Herbal/Food:** Bitter orange may increase the risk of HTN.

Pregnancy: Category C.

Treatment of Overdose: Overdose may cause coma, seizures, profuse sweating, and dysrhythmias. No specific treatment exists.

Nursing Responsibilities: Key nursing implications for patients receiving pseudoephedrine are included in the Nursing Practice Application for Patients Receiving Pharmacotherapy for Symptomatic Cough and Cold Relief.

Drugs Similar to Pseudoephedrine (Sudafed)

All the sympathomimetic intranasal decongestants have very similar actions and adverse effects. Additional details on this class of drugs are included in Chapter 15.

Drugs for the Common Cold

45.8 The common cold is caused by a virus and is treated with some of the same drugs as those used to treat allergic rhinitis.

The common cold is a viral infection of the upper respiratory tract that produces a characteristic array of annoying symptoms. It is fortunate that the disorder is self-limiting, because there is no cure or effective prevention for colds. Therapies used to relieve symptoms include some of the same drug classes used for allergic rhinitis, including antihistamines and decongestants. A few additional drugs, such as those that suppress cough and loosen bronchial secretions, are used for symptomatic cold treatment.

Many OTC preparations are available to treat cold symptoms. These OTC drugs are often made as combinations containing two or more drugs to treat a variety of symptoms. Some common OTC combination products are listed in Table 45.2. The most common ingredients of combination drugs for the common cold are antihistamines and decongestants; caffeine is sometimes added to combat the adverse effect of drowsiness from first-generation antihistamines. The caffeine is omitted from combination drugs if the medication is to be taken at night, for example, NyQuil. Almost all combination drugs contain some form of analgesic, such as acetaminophen, aspirin, or other nonsteroidal anti-inflammatory drug, to help with fever and muscular aches. Many combination products also contain a cough suppressant and an expectorant to help loosen congestion.

The wide variety of combination cold, flu, and sinus products that are available OTC can be confusing for consumers. Multi-symptom combination products should only be taken if the patient is experiencing the indicated symptoms. For example, if cough and fever are not present, products that contain cough suppressants, expectorants, or analgesics should not be taken. Consuming combination products without appropriate symptoms can increase the risk of unnecessary adverse effects. It is usually better to take only the drugs needed to treat specific symptoms rather than a combination product.

In 2011, the FDA issued an advisory that removed all unapproved *prescription* cough, cold, and allergy products from the market (U.S. FDA, 2011). Dozens of these prescription products contained ingredients that were also available OTC such as brompheniramine, chlorpheniramine, pseudoephedrine, guaifenesin, phenylephrine, and dextromethorphan. These products were never evaluated for safety, quality, or effectiveness by the FDA because they had initially been marketed before current laws were passed that require rigorous testing and approval. Furthermore, OTC alternatives existed for all the prescription medications.

PharmFACT

Adults average two to four colds per year, while children have six to eight per year. Colds account for more office visits per year than any other condition (American Lung Association, n.d.).

Antitussives

45.9 Antitussives are drugs used to suppress the cough reflex.

Cough is a natural reflex mechanism that serves to forcibly remove excess secretions and foreign material from the respiratory system. In diseases such as emphysema and bronchitis, or when liquids have been aspirated into the bronchi, it is not desirable to suppress the normal cough reflex. Dry, hacking, nonproductive coughing, however, can be irritating to the membranes of the throat and trigger inflammation, depriving patients of much needed rest. It is these types of conditions in which therapy with medications that control cough, known as **antitussives**, is warranted. Although there is clear evidence that antitussives are effective against chronic, nonproductive cough, there is less certainty about their value in treating acute coughs due to the common cold (Smith, Schroeder, & Fahey, 2012). Antitussives are classified as opioid or nonopioid and are listed in Table 45.5.

Opioids, the most effective antitussives, act by raising the cough threshold in the CNS. Codeine and hydrocodone are the most frequently prescribed opioid antitussives. Doses needed to suppress the cough reflex are very low; thus, there is minimal potential for

---

CONNECTIONS | Complementary and Alternative Therapies

◄ Ascorbic Acid (Vitamin C)

Description
Vitamin C is naturally occurring and found in a variety of foods. Citrus fruits are especially high in vitamin C, as is cranberry.

History and Claims
Vitamin C is well documented as a prevention and treatment for scurvy. In 1970, Linus Pauling, the only person to win two unshared Nobel prizes, published a book called *Vitamin C and the Common Cold* in which he asserted that the common cold could be almost completely controlled in the United States by improvement of nutrition through adequate intake of ascorbic acid. This book, more than anything else in recent times, helped the case of vitamin C as a treatment or preventive for the common cold.

Standardization
Vitamin C and the combination products can vary in the amount, strength, and quality of the vitamin found in them. The current recommended daily allowance (RDA) for vitamin C is 90 mg per day in adult males and 75 mg per day in adult females. An additional 35 mg is recommended if the adult also smokes. The upper limit of tolerance is about 2 g per day in an adult.

Evidence
Since the publication of Linus Pauling's book, many studies have been conducted to test the value of vitamin C in improving the immune system response to viruses that cause the common cold. Vitamin C has been found to be necessary for normal mental and physical growth in children as well as to enhance components of the immune system such as natural killer cell activities, lymphocyte growth, chemotaxis, and delayed-type hypersensitivity (Maggini, Wenzlaff, & Hornig, 2010). A recent analysis of 29 studies concluded that vitamin C does not reduce the incidence of colds in the general population, although there may be a slight reduction of the duration of cold symptoms (Hemilä & Chalker, 2013).

TABLE 45.5   Selected Antitussives and Expectorants

Drug	Route and Adult Dose (Maximum Dose Where Indicated)	Adverse Effects
Antitussives: Opioids		
codeine	PO: 10–20 mg every 4–6 h prn (max: 120 mg/24 h)	*Nausea, vomiting, constipation, confusion, dizziness, sedation*
hydrocodone combined with homatropine (Hycodan)	PO: 5 mL or 1 tablet every 4–6 h as needed (max: 30 mL/day or 6 tablets/day)	Hypotension, seizures, hallucinations, bradycardia, respiratory depression, severe somnolence
Antitussives: Nonopioids		
benzonatate (Tessalon)	PO: 100–200 mg tid prn up to 600 mg/day	*Drowsiness, constipation, GI upset, chest and tongue numbness (if capsules are opened or chewed)* Paradoxical excitation, tremors, euphoria, insomnia
dextromethorphan (Delsym, Robitussin-DM, Others)	PO: 10–20 mg every 4 h or 30 mg every 6–8 h (max: 120 mg/day)	*Drowsiness, headache, GI upset* CNS depression, paradoxical excitation, respiratory depression
Expectorant		
guaifenesin (Mucinex, Robitussin, Others)	PO: 200–400 mg every 4 h (max: 2.4 g/day) Extended release PO: 600–1,200 mg every 12 h (max: 2,400 mg/day)	*Drowsiness, headache, GI upset* No serious adverse effects
Mucolytics		
acetylcysteine (Mucomyst)	Inhalation: 1–10 mL of 20% solution every 4–6 h or 2–20 mL of 10% solution every 4–6 h	*Unpleasant odor, nausea, local irritation, stickiness on the face* Severe nausea and vomiting
dornase alfa (Pulmozyme)	Inhalation: 1–2 of 2.5 mg ampules once daily using nebulizer	*Voice alteration, laryngitis, rash* Dyspnea

Note: Italics indicate common adverse effects. Underline indicates serious adverse effects.

dependence. Most opioid cough mixtures are classified as Schedule III, IV, or V drugs and are reserved for more serious cough conditions. Though not common, overdose from opioid cough remedies may cause significant respiratory depression. Care must be taken when using these medications in patients with asthma because bronchoconstriction may occur. Codeine is usually not recommended for children. Opioids may be combined with other agents such as antihistamines, decongestants, and nonopioid antitussives in the therapy of severe cold or flu symptoms. Some of these combinations are listed in Table 45.6.

The three nonopioid antitussives are dextromethorphan, diphenhydramine (Benadryl), and benzonatate (Tessalon). Dextromethorphan is available OTC as a single drug but is usually found as a component of combination, multisymptom cold medications. Diphenhydramine is usually taken for its antihistamine effects, but it also has antitussive action. Benzonatate is a prescription drug.

PROTOTYPE DRUG   Dextromethorphan (Delsym, Robitussin DM, Others)

Classification: Therapeutic: Antitussive
Pharmacologic: Levorphanol derivative

Therapeutic Effects and Uses: Approved in 1954, dextromethorphan is the most frequently used and most effective nonopioid antitussive. Considered as effective as codeine, dextromethorphan carries no risk of dependence. Although used for over 50 years

TABLE 45.6   Opioid Combination Drugs for Severe Cold Symptoms

Trade Name	Opioid	Nonopioid Active Ingredients
Ambenyl Cough Syrup	codeine	bromodiphenhydramine
Calcidrine Syrup	codeine	calcium iodide
Codamine Syrup	hydrocodone	phenylpropanolamine
Codiclear DH Syrup	hydrocodone	guaifenesin
Codimal DH	hydrocodone	phenylephrine, pyrilamine
Hycodan	hydrocodone	homatropine
Hycomine Compound	hydrocodone	phenylephrine, chlorpheniramine, acetaminophen
Hycotuss Expectorant	hydrocodone	guaifenesin
Novahistine DH	codeine	pseudoephedrine, chlorpheniramine
Phenergan with Codeine	codeine	promethazine
Robitussin A-C	codeine	guaifenesin
Tega-Tussin Syrup	hydrocodone	phenylephrine, chlorpheniramine
Triaminic Expectorant DH	hydrocodone	phenylpropanolamine, pyrilamine, pheniramine, guaifenesin
Tussionex	hydrocodone	chlorpheniramine

to treat cough, controlled studies examining the effectiveness of dextromethorphan have given mixed results. Its present status is that the FDA considers it a safe and effective cough suppressant when used at recommended doses. It appears to be more effective at reducing nonproductive cough due to chronic throat irritation from tobacco use or emphysema rather than acute cough due to colds.

Reports of dextromethorphan abuse began to appear in the 1990s. Dextromethorphan has been reported to cause a mild stimulant effect at lower doses and altered sensory perceptions and complete dissociative effects (mind-out-of-body–like experiences) at very high doses. The effects typically last 6 to 8 hours. To produce these effects, 10 to 30 times the antitussive dose is used. Additional information on dextromethorphan abuse is presented in Chapter 27.

Mechanism of Action: Dextromethorphan is chemically similar to the opioids and acts directly on the cough center in the medulla to elevate the cough threshold. It has no effect on opioid receptors.

Pharmacokinetics:

Route(s)	PO
Absorption	Readily absorbed orally
Distribution	Unknown; may cross the placenta
Primary metabolism	Hepatic; metabolized by CYP2D6 and CYP3A to active metabolite
Primary excretion	Renal
Onset of action	15–30 min
Duration of action	3–8 h

Adverse Effects: There are almost no adverse effects at therapeutic doses. Sedation and dizziness have occurred at moderate doses. In abuse situations the drug can cause CNS toxicity with a wide variety of symptoms, including slurred speech, ataxia, hyperexcitability, stupor, respiratory depression, seizures, coma, and toxic psychosis.

Contraindications/Precautions: This medication is extensively metabolized by the liver and should be used cautiously in patients with hepatic impairment. The FDA has issued advisories that nonprescription cough and cold products (including those containing dextromethorphan) not be used in children under 6 years of age and that they be used with extreme caution in all children.

Drug Interactions: Patients who take MAOIs, triptans, or selective serotonin reuptake inhibitors (SSRIs) should not take dextromethorphan due to the risk of serotonin syndrome (nausea, changes in blood pressure, and confusion). Dextromethorphan has an additive CNS depressant effect with alcohol, antihistamines, antidepressants, and opioids. The analgesic effect of opioids can be almost doubled by giving them with dextromethorphan. **Herbal/Food**: Grapefruit juice can raise serum levels of dextromethorphan and cause toxicity.

Pregnancy: Category C.

Treatment of Overdose: Overdose may result in significant CNS toxicity. Treatment is symptomatic.

Nursing Responsibilities: Key nursing implications for patients receiving dextromethorphan are included in the Nursing Practice Application for Patients Receiving Pharmacotherapy for Symptomatic Cough and Cold Relief.

Drugs Similar to Dextromethorphan (Delsym, Robitussin DM, Others)

The only other nonopioid antitussive is benzonatate.

Benzonatate (Tessalon): Approved in 1958, benzonatate is an oral, nonopioid antitussive that acts by a unique mechanism. Chemically related to the local anesthetic tetracaine (Pontocaine), benzonatate suppresses the cough reflex by anesthetizing stretch receptors in the lungs. If chewed, this drug can cause numbing of the mouth and pharynx. Adverse effects are uncommon but may include sedation, nausea, headache, and dizziness. This drug should not be used in children under 10 years of age: Death has been reported from accidental ingestion in children. Like dextromethorphan the effectiveness of benzonatate in treating acute cough has not been clearly established. This drug is pregnancy category C.

Expectorants and Mucolytics

45.10 Expectorants and mucolytics are used to treat thick bronchial secretions.

Several drugs are available to control excess mucus production. **Expectorants** increase bronchial secretions, and **mucolytics** remove mucus by loosening thick bronchial secretions. These drugs are listed in Table 45.5.

Expectorants: Expectorants reduce the thickness or viscosity of bronchial secretions, thus increasing mucus flow that can then be removed more easily by coughing. The only commonly used OTC expectorant is guaifenesin (Mucinex). Like dextromethorphan, guaifenesin produces few adverse effects and is a common ingredient in many combination multisymptom OTC cold and flu preparations. It is most effective in treating dry, nonproductive cough but may also be of benefit for patients with productive cough. Like the antitussives the effectiveness of guaifenesin in reducing acute cold symptoms has been questioned. The dosage range used in cold remedies is usually too low to have much positive benefit for patients. Nonprescription cough and cold products (including those containing guaifenesin) should not be used in children under 6 years of age. High doses can induce nausea, vomiting, and abdominal pain. This drug is pregnancy category C.

Mucolytics: Acetylcysteine (Mucomyst) is one of the few drugs that directly loosen thick, viscous bronchial secretions. Drugs of this type, known as mucolytics, break down the chemical structure of mucus molecules. The mucus becomes thinner and can be removed more easily by coughing. Acetylcysteine is delivered by the PO and inhalation routes and is not available OTC. It is used in patients who have cystic fibrosis, chronic bronchitis, or other diseases that produce large amounts of thick bronchial secretions. Acetylcysteine is also administered by the IV route (Acetadote) to prevent the development of hepatotoxicity in patients who have received an overdose of acetaminophen. Its use in the pharmacotherapy of acetaminophen toxicity is presented in Chapter 41. Adverse effects include bronchospasm, nausea, vomiting, unpleasant odor, and fever. This drug is pregnancy category B.

CONNECTIONS: NURSING PRACTICE APPLICATION

Patients Receiving Pharmacotherapy for Symptomatic Cough and Cold Relief

Assessment	Potential Nursing Diagnoses*
Baseline assessment prior to administration: • Obtain a complete health history including previous history and length of symptoms; existing cardiovascular, respiratory, hepatic, or renal disease; presence of fever, pregnancy or breast-feeding, alcohol use, or smoking. Obtain a drug history, including allergies, current prescription and OTC drugs, herbal preparations, caffeine, nicotine, and alcohol use. Be alert to possible drug interactions. • Obtain baseline vital signs. • Evaluate appropriate laboratory findings (e.g., CBC, hepatic and renal laboratory tests). • Assess the patient's ability to receive and understand instructions. Include the family or caregiver as needed.	• *Ineffective Airway Clearance* • *Ineffective Breathing Pattern* • *Disturbed Sleep Pattern* or *Insomnia*, related to adverse drug effects • *Fatigue*, related to adverse drug effects • *Deficient Knowledge* (Drug Therapy) • *Risk for Injury*, related to adverse drug effects • *Risk for Falls*, related to adverse drug effects
Assessment throughout administration: • Assess for desired therapeutic effects (e.g., decreased cough, increased ease in expectorating mucus, clearer nasal passages). • Continue periodic monitoring of CBC, liver and renal function studies as needed. • Assess vital signs, especially pulse rate and rhythm in patients with existing cardiac disease. • Assess for adverse effects: dizziness, drowsiness, blurred vision, headache, epistaxis. Immediately report any increasing fever, tachycardia, palpitations, syncope, dyspnea, pulmonary congestion, or confusion.	

Implementation

Interventions and (Rationales)	Patient-Centered Care
Ensuring therapeutic effects: • Continue assessments as above for therapeutic effects. (Diminished cough, thinner secretions, increased ease of expectoration, and clearing nasal passages should begin after taking the first dose and continue to improve. Improvement in other signs and symptoms of the common cold should begin after taking the first dose and continue to improve.)	• Teach the patient to supplement drug therapy with nonpharmacologic measures, such as increased fluid intake, to liquefy and mobilize mucus and to moisten the respiratory tract. • Instruct the patient to contact the health care provider if symptoms worsen or if fever is present or increasing.
Minimizing adverse effects: • Ensure patient safety. Observe for lightheadedness or dizziness. (**Lifespan:** Drowsiness or dizziness from cough suppressant drug effects may occur, increasing the risk of falls, especially in the older adult.)	• Instruct the patient to call for assistance prior to getting out of bed or attempting to walk alone, and to avoid driving or other activities requiring mental alertness or physical coordination until the effects of the drug are known. If dizziness occurs, the patient should sit or lie down and not attempt to stand or walk until the sensation passes.
• Continue to monitor vital signs, especially pulse rate and rhythm for patients taking decongestants, including nasal decongestants. (Adrenergic decongestants may cause tachycardia and dysrhythmias in patients with a history of dysrhythmias or cardiac disease, or in the sensitive patient. **Lifespan:** Undetected cardiac disease may place the older adult at greater risk for cardiovascular adverse effects.)	• Instruct the patient to immediately report dizziness, palpitations, or syncope. • Teach the patient, family, or caregiver how to monitor the pulse and blood pressure as appropriate. Ensure proper use and functioning of any home equipment obtained.
• Monitor for persistent dry cough, increasing cough severity, increasing congestion, or dyspnea. The provider should be notified if symptoms continue to increase, especially if respiratory involvement worsens or if fever is present. (Drugs used for symptomatic relief of the common cold are used with extreme caution or are contraindicated in patients with existing respiratory disease, including COPD. A change in the severity of the cough may indicate a worsening disease process or a more serious respiratory infection and should be reported immediately.)	• Instruct the patient to promptly report any change in the severity or frequency of cough. Any cough accompanied by shortness of breath, increasing congestion, fever, or chest pain should be reported immediately. • Encourage the patient to increase fluid intake to assist in liquefying mucus secretions and to moisten the upper respiratory tract.
• Assess the color and consistency of any expectorated sputum. (Increasing thickness, color, hemoptysis, or increased quantity of sputum may indicate a serious respiratory infection and should be reported immediately.)	• Instruct the patient to report any significant change in the color, consistency, or quantity of the expectorated mucus to the health care provider.
• Monitor for GI effects. Encourage the patient to take tablets or capsules with a full glass of water. (Nausea, vomiting, or abdominal discomfort may occur with common cold preparations. Taking the drug with additional fluids or food may decrease GI adverse effects.)	• Teach the patient to take the medication with additional fluid or food. Report any significant GI symptoms (e.g., nausea with vomiting, diarrhea) to the health care provider for further treatment.

CONNECTIONS: NURSING PRACTICE APPLICATION *(continued)*

• Encourage use of single-symptom drug preparations when possible. (Many OTC formulations include a combination of drugs, increasing the risk of adverse drug effects. Drug therapy should be aimed at symptomatic relief and additional drugs that are not needed in multiuse preparations should be avoided when possible.)	• Teach the patient to consider symptoms when reading labels of OTC cold remedies and choose preparations based on current symptoms rather than multiuse remedies. • Instruct patients that multiuse cold remedies containing acetaminophen must be taken in prescribed doses, should not be taken if daily alcohol intake exceeds two glasses, and not increased to avoid acetaminophen overdose and potential liver damage.
• Do not use symptomatic cough or cold preparations in children under the age of 6 unless instructed to do so by the provider. (FDA guidelines recommend that cough and cold preparations should not be used in children under the age of 6.)	• Instruct the parents or caregivers of children under the age of 6 not to routinely give cold preparations to the child unless instructed to do so by the provider. • Recommend symptomatic relief measures for children under 6 years such as increased fluids and juice, ice pops, and cool or warm mist humidifiers. Frequently clean all humidifiers in use to avoid mold growth.
• Eliminate smoking and limit exposure to secondhand smoke. (Cigarette smoke irritates respiratory mucous membranes, increasing the risk of adverse effects.)	• Teach the patient about smoking cessation programs and to avoid environments with secondhand smoke.
Patient understanding of drug therapy: • Use opportunities during administration of medications and during assessments to discuss the rationale for drug therapy, desired therapeutic outcomes, commonly observed adverse effects, parameters for when to call the health care provider, and any necessary monitoring or precautions. (Using time during nursing care helps to optimize and reinforce key teaching areas.)	• The patient should be able to state the reason for the drug, appropriate dose and scheduling, what adverse effects to observe for, and when to report them.
Patient self-administration of drug therapy: • When administering the medication, instruct the patient, family, or caregiver in proper self-administration of the drug, e.g., take the drug before allergy season or before symptoms are severe. (Utilizing time during nurse-administration of these drugs helps to reinforce teaching.)	• The patient, family, or caregiver is able to discuss appropriate dosing and administration needs, including: • *Cough suppressants:* Cough syrups should be swallowed without water and allowed to coat the throat for soothing effects, followed by increased fluid intake 30–60 min later. The dose should not be increased beyond the recommended dose to avoid increased risk of adverse effects. • *Expectorants:* Syrups should be taken with a full glass of liquid with increased fluid intake throughout the day to assist in thinning mucus for ease of expectoration. • *Nasal decongestants:* Nasal passages should be cleared by blowing, followed by the nasal spray. If a second spray is ordered, administer 5 min after the first spray. If glucocorticoid or mast cell stabilizer sprays are ordered, the decongestant spray should be used first, followed by the additional drug 5–10 min later. Spit out any additional drug that drains into the mouth. Discontinue use of decongestant nasal sprays after 3–5 days to avoid rebound congestion, unless otherwise ordered by the provider. • *For all OTC cold preparations:* Single-symptom formulations should be used when possible to avoid additional drugs not needed for symptom relief or an increased risk of adverse effects.

*Nursing Diagnoses—Definitions and Classification 2015–2017. Copyright © 2014, 1994–2014 by NANDA International. Used by arrangement with John Wiley & Sons Limited.

A second mucolytic, dornase alfa (Pulmozyme), is an enzyme that was approved in 1993 for the management of thick bronchial secretions in patients with cystic fibrosis. Dornase alfa breaks down deoxyribonucleic acid (DNA) molecules in the mucus, causing it to become less viscous. It is administered by the oral inhalation route. Adverse effects include chest pain, conjunctivitis, hoarseness, and pharyngitis. This drug is pregnancy category B.

CHAPTER
45

Understanding the Chapter

Key Concepts Summary

45.1 The upper respiratory tract acts as a defense in preventing systemic infection.

45.2 Allergic rhinitis is caused by exposure to an environmental allergen, which leads to symptoms that resemble those of the common cold.

45.3 Drugs for allergic rhinitis include those that prevent the disorder and those that relieve symptoms.

45.4 Antihistamines are widely used to treat allergic rhinitis and other minor allergies.

45.5 Intranasal corticosteroids are the drugs of choice for allergic rhinitis because of their effectiveness and safety.

45.6 Cromolyn, ipratropium, and montelukast are alternatives to intranasal corticosteroids in the treatment of allergic rhinitis.

45.7 Intranasal and oral sympathomimetics are the most effective drugs for relieving nasal congestion.

45.8 The common cold is caused by a virus and is treated with some of the same drugs as those used to treat allergic rhinitis.

45.9 Antitussives are drugs used to suppress the cough reflex.

45.10 Expectorants and mucolytics are used to treat thick bronchial secretions.

Case Study: Making the Patient Connection

Remember the patient "Nancy Williams" at the beginning of the chapter? Now read the remainder of the case study. Based on the information presented within this chapter, respond to the critical thinking questions that follow.

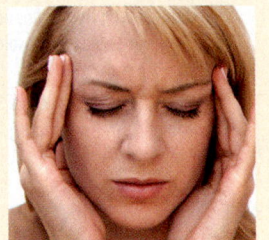

Nancy Williams is a 32-year-old female who is in good health except for her current problem. She has come to the urgent care center because of a stuffy nose; red, itchy eyes; and a slightly sore throat. She takes daily calcium supplements but no other medications. She is 1.68 m (5 ft 6 in.) tall and weighs 67 kg (148 lb).

Nancy is a fourth-grade teacher at a local elementary school and is worried about being able to finish her end of school term activities with the symptoms of a lingering "cold." Her vital signs are as follows: temperature, 37.4°C (99.4°F); pulse, 102 beats/min; respirations, 12 breaths/min; blood pressure, 148/88 mmHg; oxygen saturation, 98%.

After taking her vital signs, Nancy tells the nurse that her mother-in-law bought her a bottle of Neo-Synephrine nasal spray about 10 days ago. It helped, but she tells the nurse that it ran out yesterday and now her nose is even stuffier than before. She had been taking Tylenol but stopped using that, too, because she does not feel like she has a fever and it was not helping much anyway. Nancy says, "I went to the drug store after school and did not

stay. I felt so miserable that I couldn't even figure out what medicine does what and I just wanted to get home. I need some rest so I can take care of my girls, do a good job for my students, and get my report cards done." The nurse practitioner observes that Nancy has a cough, runny nose, and inflamed eyes, which she occasionally rubs during the conversation.

Critical Thinking Questions

1. Considering the history and the initial assessment that the nurse practitioner conducted, what further data would you as the nurse want to gather that are not listed in the scenario?

2. If Nancy has no history of heart disease or HTN and takes no medicines to treat those conditions, what do you think might be the cause of her elevated blood pressure and heart rate?

3. Nancy gave her two daughters a golden retriever puppy a few weeks ago. How does this information add to your assessment findings and patient teaching?

4. The nurse practitioner diagnoses Nancy with probable allergic rhinitis and prescribes intranasal fluticasone (Flonase). In addition, the nurse practitioner suggests getting two OTC cough suppressants, one with the main ingredient dextromethorphan and the other one with the main ingredient diphenhydramine. What do you tell Nancy is the reason she is being prescribed each one?

See Answers to Critical Thinking Questions on student resource website.

Additional Case Study

A 23-year-old woman arrives at the emergency department with her boyfriend. She is wheezing and short of breath. Her respiratory rate is 23 breaths/min, her heart rate is 104 beats/min, her blood pressure is 88/60 mmHg, and she has hives over most of her body. Her boyfriend says she was eating strawberries and suddenly started having trouble breathing. She has eaten strawberries for years and nothing like this has ever happened before. The health care provider prescribes epinephrine for her allergic response.

1. Why did the health care provider not prescribe an antihistamine for this allergic response?

2. A second dose of epinephrine is given and the nurse inserts an IV. With a reduction in her wheezing, the patient's respiratory rate is 18 breaths/min, heart rate is 100 beats/min, and blood pressure is 98/64 mmHg. The health care provider prescribes Benadryl, 10 mg IV. Describe why the health care provider is now prescribing an antihistamine for the patient.

See Answers to Additional Case Study on student resource website.

Chapter Review

1 The patient has been prescribed fluticasone (Flonase) for allergic rhinitis. Which points are appropriate to include in the teaching plan? Select all that apply.

1. Take with a full glass of water.
2. Prime the inhaler before the first use.
3. Take the drug only when symptoms are present.
4. Take for no more than 5 days to prevent rebound congestion.
5. Effects of the drug may not be noticeable for 2 to 3 weeks.

2 The nurse teaches the patient that which type of over-the-counter cough preparation is not effective on coughs associated with the common cold and allergic rhinitis?

1. Dextromethorphan
2. Diphenhydramine
3. Mucolytics
4. Pseudoephedrine

3 An older adult man informs the nurse that he is taking diphenhydramine (Benadryl) to reduce seasonal allergy symptoms. The nurse would be most concerned about an increased risk of _____ for this patient.

4 Fexofenadine (Allegra) is prescribed to treat the symptoms of allergic rhinitis for a patient with seasonal allergies. Before teaching the patient about this drug, what condition would the nurse assess for?

1. A history of osteoporosis
2. A history of peptic ulcer disease
3. A history of psoriasis
4. A history of cardiac disease

5 A patient has been prescribed fluticasone (Flonase). Place the instructions below in the order in which the nurse will instruct the patient to use the drug.

1. Instill one spray directed high into the nasal cavity.
2. Clear the nose by blowing.
3. Prime the inhaler prior to the first use.
4. Spit out any excess liquid that drains into the mouth.

6 The nurse is teaching the patient about the use of dextromethorphan with guaifenesin (Robitussin-DM) syrup for a cough accompanied by thick mucus. Which statement would be part of the patient's teaching?

1. "Lie supine for 30 minutes after taking the drug."
2. "Drink minimal fluids to avoid stimulating the cough reflex."
3. "Take the drug with food for best results."
4. "Avoid drinking fluids immediately following the syrup and then increase overall fluid intake."

See Answers to Chapter Review in Appendix A.

References

American Academy of Allergy, Asthma, & Immunology. (n.d). *Allergy statistics.* Retrieved from http://www.aaaai.org/about-the-aaaai/newsroom/allergy-statistics.aspx

American Lung Association. (n.d.). *Facts about the common cold.* Retrieved from http://www.lung.org/lung-disease/influenza/in-depth-resources/facts-about-the-common-cold.html

Hemilä, H., & Chalker, E. (2013). Vitamin C for preventing and treating the common cold. *Cochrane Database of Systematic Reviews, 1,* CD000980. doi:10.1002/14651858.CD000980.pub4

Maggini, S., Wenzlaff, S., & Hornig, D. (2010). Essential role of vitamin C and zinc in child immunity and health. *Journal of International Medical Research, 38,* 386–414. doi:10.1177/147323001003800203

Pauling, L. (1970). *Vitamin C and the common cold.* San Francisco, CA: W. H. Freeman.

Slavin, R. G. (2010). Special considerations in treatment of allergic rhinitis in the elderly: Role of intranasal corticosteroids. *Allergy and Asthma Proceedings, 31,* 179–184. doi:10.2500/aap.2010.31.3342

Smith, S. M., Schroeder, K., & Fahey, T. (2012). Over-the-counter medications for acute cough in children and adults in ambulatory settings. *Cochrane Database of Systematic Reviews, 8,* CD001831. doi:10.1002/14651858.CD001831.pub4

U.S. Food and Drug Administration. (2011). *Unapproved cough, cold and allergy products: FDA prompts removal from the market.* Retrieved from http://www.fda.gov/Safety/MedWatch/SafetyInformation/SafetyAlertsforHumanMedicalProducts/ucm245279.htm

U.S. Government Accountability Office. (2013). *Drug control: State approaches taken to control access to key methamphetamine ingredient show varied impact on domestic drug labs.* Retrieved from http://www.gao.gov/products/GAO-13-204

Selected Bibliography

Costa, D. J., Bosquet, P. J., Ryan, D., Price, D., Demoly, P., Brozek, J., … Bousquet, J. (2009). Guidelines for allergic rhinitis need to be used in primary care. *Primary Care Respiratory Journal, 18,* 250–257. doi:10.4104/pcrj.2009.00028

Greiner, A. N., Hellings, P. W., Rotiroti, G., & Scadding, G. K. (2011). Allergic rhinitis. *The Lancet, 378,* 2112–2122.

Herdman, T. H., & Kamitsuru, S. (Eds.). (2014). *NANDA International nursing diagnoses: Definitions and classification, 2015–2017.* Oxford, United Kingdom: Wiley-Blackwell.

Isbister, G. K., Prior, F., & Kilham, H. A. (2012). Restricting cough and cold medicines in children. *Journal of Paediatrics and Child Health, 48,* 91–98. doi:10.1111/j.1440-1754.2010.01780.x

Paul, I. M. (2012). Therapeutic options for acute cough due to upper respiratory infections in children. *Lung, 190*(1), 41–44. doi:10.1007/s00408-011-9319-y

Turner, P. J., & Kemp, A. S. (2012). Allergic rhinitis in children. *Journal of Paediatrics and Child Health, 48,* 302–310. doi:10.1111/j.1440-1754.2010.01779.x

Yanai, K., Rogala, B., Chugh, K., Paraskakis, E., Pampura, A. N., & Boev, R. (2012). Safety considerations in the management of allergic diseases: Focus on antihistamines. *Current Medical Research & Opinion, 28*(4), 623–642. doi:10.1185/03007995.2012.672405

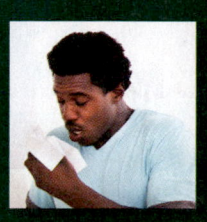
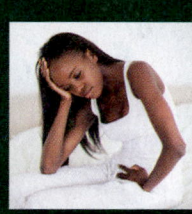
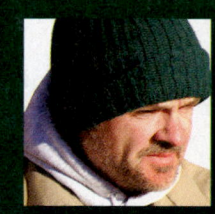
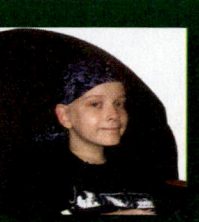

CHAPTER 46   Basic Principles of Anti-Infective Pharmacotherapy / 774

CHAPTER 47   Antibiotics Affecting the Bacterial Cell Wall / 786

CHAPTER 48   Antibiotics Affecting Bacterial Protein Synthesis / 804

CHAPTER 49   Fluoroquinolones and Miscellaneous Antibacterials / 821

CHAPTER 50   Sulfonamides and the Pharmacotherapy of Urinary Tract Infections / 833

CHAPTER 51   Pharmacotherapy of Mycobacterial Infections / 848

CHAPTER 52   Pharmacotherapy of Fungal Infections / 866

CHAPTER 53   Pharmacotherapy of Protozoan and Helminthic Infections / 884

CHAPTER 54   Pharmacotherapy of Non-HIV Viral Infections / 906

CHAPTER 55   Pharmacotherapy of HIV-AIDS / 926

CHAPTER 56   Basic Principles of Antineoplastic Therapy / 948

CHAPTER 57   Pharmacotherapy of Neoplasia / 962

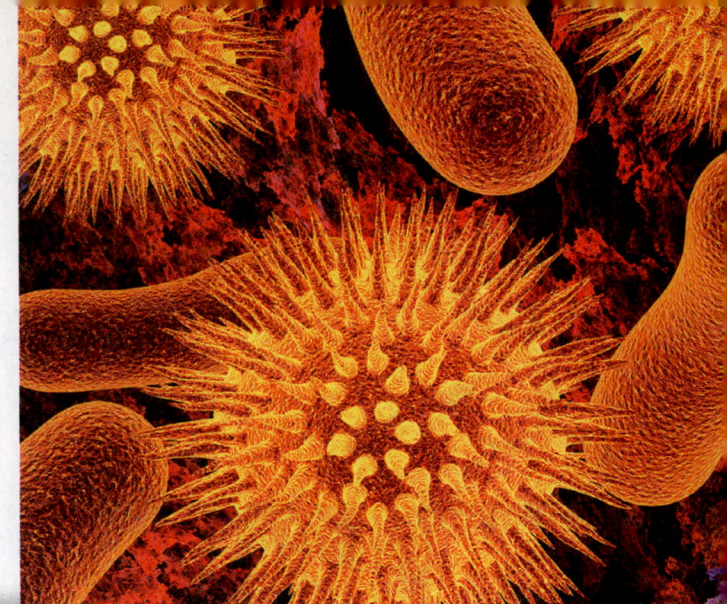

CHAPTER

46 Basic Principles of Anti-Infective Pharmacotherapy

LEARNING OUTCOMES

After reading this chapter, the student should be able to:

1. Explain the mechanisms by which pathogens infect the body.
2. Describe methods for classifying bacteria.
3. Explain the mechanisms by which anti-infective drugs act to kill pathogens or restrict their growth.
4. Describe the clinical significance of bacterial resistance.
5. Identify steps that the nurse can take to limit the development of resistance.
6. Describe the clinical rationale for selecting specific antibiotics.
7. Identify the role of the nurse in preventing, identifying, and treating adverse effects due to antibiotic therapy.
8. Explain how the patient's immune status, history of allergic reactions, age, pregnancy status, genetics, or local tissue conditions influence anti-infective pharmacotherapy.
9. Explain the clinical importance of selecting the correct antibiotic for the individual patient.
10. Describe the development of superinfections.

CHAPTER OUTLINE

▶ Pathogenicity and Virulence

▶ Describing and Classifying Bacteria

▶ Classification of Anti-Infectives

▶ Mechanisms of Action of Anti-Infectives

▶ Acquired Resistance

▶ Indications and Selection of Specific Anti-Infectives

▶ Host Factors Affecting Anti-Infective Selection

▶ Superinfections

acquired resistance, 779

aerobic, 776

anaerobic, 776

antibiotic, 776

anti-infective, 776

bacteriocidal, 776

bacteriostatic, 776

broad-spectrum antibiotic, 782

conjugation, 780

culture and sensitivity (C&S) testing, 782

endotoxins, 775

exotoxins, 775

gram negative, 776

gram positive, 776

health care–associated infections (HAIs), 780

host flora, 782

invasiveness, 775

microbial antagonism, 784

mutations, 780

narrow-spectrum antibiotic, 782

pathogenicity, 775

pathogens, 775

peptidoglycan, 778

superinfections, 784

virulence, 775

The human body has adapted quite well to living in a world teeming with microorganisms (microbes). In the air, water, food, and soil, microbes have been essential components of life on the planet for billions of years. In some cases, these microorganisms coexist in intimate contact with human beings. It is estimated that 10^{14} bacterial cells reside inside or on the surface of the body, which is more than the total number of human cells in an average person. Fortunately, of the millions of species of microbes, only a relative few are harmful to human health. The purpose of this chapter is to present the fundamental principles that apply to the pharmacotherapy of infectious diseases.

PharmFACT

In 1900, 5 of the 10 most frequent causes of death in the United States were infectious diseases. In 2010, only influenza or pneumonia and septicemia were in the top 10 causes of death (Madigan, Martinko, Stahl, & Clark, 2012).

Pathogenicity and Virulence

46.1 Pathogens cause disease due to their ability to invade tissues or secrete toxins.

The first challenge in studying the pharmacotherapy of infectious disease is to understand the terminology that is used to describe the organisms and drugs. Microbes that are capable of causing human disease, or **pathogens**, include viruses, bacteria, fungi, unicellular organisms (protozoans), and multicellular animals (e.g., fleas, mites, and worms).

Some pathogens are extremely infectious and life threatening to humans, whereas others simply cause annoying symptoms or none at all. **Pathogenicity**, the ability of an organism to cause disease, depends on an organism's speed of reproduction and its skill in bypassing or overcoming body defenses. Organisms that usually infect only when the body's immune system is suppressed are called *opportunistic* pathogens.

Virulence is a quantitative measure of an organism's pathogenicity. A highly virulent microbe is one that can produce disease when present in very small numbers. Virulent pathogens produce their devastating effects through two primary characteristics: invasiveness and toxicity.

Invasiveness is the ability of a pathogen to grow extremely rapidly and cause direct damage to surrounding tissues by their sheer numbers. Because a week or more may be needed to mount an immune response against the organism, this exponential growth can rapidly overwhelm body defenses and disrupt normal cellular function. Some streptococci, staphylococci, and clostridia secrete hyaluronidase, an enzyme that digests the matrix between human cells, allowing the bacteria to penetrate anatomic barriers more easily. *Staphylococcus aureus* secretes the enzyme coagulase, causing fibrin to be deposited on its cells, thereby protecting it from phagocytes.

The second characteristic of virulence is the production of toxins, or toxicity. **Exotoxins** are proteins released by bacteria into surrounding tissues that have the ability to inactivate or kill host cells. *Clostridium botulinum*, the organism responsible for botulism, produces one of the most potent toxins known that binds to presynaptic motor neurons to prevent the release of acetylcholine. Cholera toxin from *Vibrio cholerae* causes large amounts of fluid to be secreted into the intestinal lumen. Symptoms of exotoxin-producing bacteria are usually caused by the toxin itself, not the bacteria. For example, patients experience food poisoning by ingesting food containing the toxins produced by the organisms; growth of the bacteria in the body is not required. Most exotoxins are water soluble and can readily enter the blood to cause systemic toxemia.

Endotoxins are harmful nonprotein chemicals that are part of the outer layer of the normal cell wall of gram-negative bacteria. After the bacterial cell dies, endotoxins are liberated into the surrounding tissue and induce macrophages to release large amounts of cytokines, causing generalized inflammation, fever, and chills. Rapid decreases in the number of lymphocytes, leukocytes, and platelets may occur. The initial doses of antibiotic therapy may actually worsen symptoms by lysing bacteria and releasing larger amounts of endotoxins. Even very small amounts of some bacterial endotoxins may disrupt normal cellular activity and, in extreme cases, result in death. Examples of organisms producing endotoxins include *Proteus*, a common cause of urinary tract infections (UTIs), and *Neisseria meningitidis*, the agent that causes meningitis.

CONNECTION Checkpoint 46.1

From what you learned in Chapter 3, if your patient has a particularly virulent infection, which route of administration would likely be used during antibiotic therapy to most rapidly kill the organisms? *See Answer to Connection Checkpoint 46.1 on student resource website.*

Describing and Classifying Bacteria

46.2 Bacteria are described by their staining characteristics, shape, and ability to utilize oxygen.

Because of the enormous number of bacterial species, several descriptive systems have been developed to simplify their study. It is important for nurses to learn these classification schemes, because drugs that are effective against one organism in a class are likely to be effective against other pathogens in the same class. Common bacterial pathogens and their associated diseases are listed in Table 46.1.

One of the simplest methods of classifying microbes is to examine them microscopically after a crystal violet Gram stain has been applied to the microbes. Some bacteria contain a thick cell wall composed of peptidoglycan and retain the violet color after staining. These bacteria are called **gram positive** and include *Staphylococcus*, *Streptococcus*, and *Enterococcus*. Bacteria that have thinner cell walls will lose the violet stain and are called **gram negative**. Examples of gram-negative bacteria include *Bacteroides*, *Escherichia*, *Klebsiella*, *Pseudomonas*, and *Salmonella*. The distinction between gram-positive and gram-negative bacteria is a profound one that reflects important biochemical and physiological differences between the two groups. Many antibiotics are effective against only one of the two groups. For example, gram-negative bacteria are generally susceptible to the tetracycline class but are resistant to the sulfonamides. This generalization, however, quickly breaks down when resistant strains develop.

Bacteria are often described by their basic shape, which can be readily determined microscopically. Those with rod shapes are called bacilli, those that are spherical are called cocci, and those that are spiral are called spirilla. The shape, along with the Gram stain, helps pathologists to identify organisms that are isolated from infectious specimens.

A third factor used to categorize bacteria is their ability to use oxygen. Those that thrive in an oxygen-rich environment are called **aerobic**; those that grow optimally without oxygen are called **anaerobic**. Some organisms have the ability to change their metabolism and survive in either aerobic or anaerobic conditions, depending on their external environment. Antibiotics are often selective for either aerobes or anaerobes.

Classification of Anti-Infectives

46.3 Anti-infective drugs are classified by their susceptible organisms, chemical structures, and mechanisms of action.

Anti-infective is a general term that applies to any medication that is effective against pathogens. In its broadest sense, an anti-infective drug may be used to treat bacterial, fungal, viral, or parasitic infections. To distinguish among the various anti-infectives, these medications are classified as antibacterial, antifungal, antiviral, antiprotozoan, and antihelminthic based on the type of organism they treat.

The most frequent term used to describe an antibacterial drug is antibiotic. Technically, **antibiotic** refers to a natural substance produced by a microorganism that can kill other microorganisms. However, many of the newer drugs that are available to treat bacterial infections are now produced synthetically. In clinical practice, the terms *antibacterial* and *antibiotic* are used interchangeably to refer to any drug that is effective against bacteria. In this text, antibiotic and antibacterial are used interchangeably.

Classifying drugs only by their susceptible organism, such as an antibacterial, tells us nothing about the properties, actions, or adverse effects of a drug. With over 300 antibacterials available, it is helpful to group these drugs into subclasses that share similar therapeutic properties. Two means of grouping are widely used: chemical classes and pharmacologic classes.

Class names such as aminoglycoside, fluoroquinolone, and sulfonamide refer to the fundamental chemical structure shared by a group of anti-infectives. Anti-infectives that belong to the same chemical class have close structural similarities and usually share similar antibacterial properties and adverse effects. Although chemical names are sometimes long and difficult to pronounce, placing drugs into chemical classes will assist the student in mentally organizing these drugs into distinct therapeutic groups.

Pharmacologic classes are used to group anti-infectives by their mechanism of action. Like chemical classes, placing an antibiotic into a pharmacologic class allows the nurse to develop a mental framework on which to organize these medications and to predict similar actions and adverse effects. Examples of pharmacologic classes grouped by their mechanisms of action with representative drugs are listed in Table 46.2. It is important that the nurse learn both the chemical class and the pharmacologic class for each antibiotic because this will provide a deeper understanding of the drug's therapeutic action and potential adverse effects.

Mechanisms of Action of Anti-Infectives

46.4 Anti-infective drugs act by selectively targeting a pathogen's metabolism or life cycle.

Although the immune system provides elaborate defenses against microbial invaders, there are times when the body defenses become overwhelmed by an infection. Furthermore, there are times when acquiring an infection could be a serious health challenge for a patient, and it is best to prevent it. Whether it is used for treating or preventing disease, the primary goal of anti-infective therapy is to assist the body in eliminating a pathogen. Drugs that accomplish this goal by killing bacteria are called **bacteriocidal**. Some drugs do not kill pathogens but instead slow their growth, allowing natural body defenses to eliminate the microorganisms. These growth-slowing drugs are called **bacteriostatic**.

Bacterial cells have distinct anatomic and physiological differences compared to human cells. Bacteria incorporate different chemicals into their membranes and use unique biochemical pathways and enzymes to manage their rapid growth. Even the more complex pathogens such as fungi and protozoans have different cell structures and use certain metabolic pathways not found in human cells. Antibiotics exert selective toxicity by targeting these unique differences between human and bacterial, fungal, and protozoan cells. Through this selective action, these pathogens can be killed, or their growth severely hampered, without any major effects

TABLE 46.1	Common Bacterial Pathogens	
Name of Organism	**Disease(s)**	**Description**
Gram-Positive Bacilli		
Bacillus anthracis	Anthrax	Aerobe; appears in cutaneous and respiratory forms
Clostridium	Food poisoning, gas gangrene, tetanus	Anaerobe
Corynebacterium	Diphtheria	Aerobe or anaerobe
Gram-Positive Cocci		
Enterococci	Wounds, UTI, endocarditis, bacteremia	Aerobe; part of host flora of the genitourinary and intestinal tracts; common opportunistic pathogen
Staphylococcus aureus	Pneumonia, food poisoning, impetigo, wounds, bacteremia, endocarditis, toxic shock syndrome, osteomyelitis, UTI	Aerobe; some species are part of host flora on the skin and mucous membranes
Streptococci	Pharyngitis, pneumonia, skin infection, septicemia, endocarditis, otitis media, meningitis in children	Aerobe; some species are part of host flora of the respiratory, genital, and intestinal tracts
Gram-Negative Bacilli		
Bacteroides	Peritonitis, abdominal abscess	Anaerobe; part of host flora of the intestinal, respiratory, and genitourinary tracts
Campylobacter	Gastroenteritis, diarrhea	One of the most common causes of diarrheal illness in the United States
Enterobacter	UTI, blood or lung infections	Aerobe or anaerobe
Escherichia coli	Traveler's diarrhea, UTI, meningitis in children, bacteremia	Part of host flora of the intestinal tract
Haemophilus influenzae	Pneumonia, meningitis in children, bacteremia, otitis media, sinusitis	Some species are part of host flora of the upper respiratory tract
Klebsiella pneumoniae	Pneumonia, UTI	Common opportunistic pathogen; often fatal if not treated aggressively
Proteus mirabilis	UTI, skin infection	Part of host flora of the intestinal tract
Pseudomonas aeruginosa	UTI, skin infection, septicemia	Common opportunistic pathogen
Salmonella enteritides	Food poisoning	Acquired from infected animal products: raw eggs, undercooked meat or chicken
Salmonella typhi	Enteric (typhoid) fever	Acquired from contaminated food or water supplies
Serratia	Nosocomial infections of wounds and UTI	Aerobic or anaerobic
Shigella	Dysentery	Aerobic or anaerobic; part of host flora of the gastrointestinal (GI) tract
Vibrio cholerae	Cholera	Gram-negative aerobe; acquired from contaminated food or water
Gram-Negative Cocci		
Neisseria gonorrhoeae	Gonorrhea, urethritis, anorectal infection, pelvic inflammatory disease, neonatal eye infection	Gram-negative aerobe; some species are part of host flora of the upper respiratory tract
Neisseria meningitides	Meningitis, particularly in children	Gram-negative aerobe; may result in death within hours of onset of symptoms
Spirilla/Spirochetes		
Borrelia burgdorferi	Lyme disease	Acquired from tick bites
Treponema	Syphilis	Sexually transmitted infection (STI)
Other Organisms		
Chlamydia trachomatis	Venereal disease, eye infection	Gram-negative; most common cause of STIs in the United States
Mycobacterium leprae	Leprosy	Most cases in the United States occur in immigrants from Africa or Asia
Mycobacterium tuberculosis	Tuberculosis	Very high incidence in patients with human immunodeficiency virus (HIV) or acquired immunodeficiency syndrome (AIDS)
Mycoplasma pneumoniae	Pneumonia	Most common cause of pneumonia in patients age 5–35
Rickettsia rickettsii	Rocky mountain spotted fever	Gram-negative; acquired from tick bites

TABLE 46.2	**Classification of Anti-Infective Drugs**	
Mechanism of Action	**Chemical Class**	**Examples**
Inhibition of cell wall synthesis	Penicillins Cephalosporins Carbapenems	penicillin G cefotaxime (Claforan) imipenem (Primaxin) isoniazid (INH) vancomycin (Vancocin)
Inhibition of protein synthesis	Aminoglycosides Tetracyclines Macrolides Oxazolidinones	gentamicin (Garamycin) tetracycline (Achromycin) erythromycin (E-mycin) linezolid (Zyvox)
Disruption of plasma membrane	Azoles Polyenes	amphotericin B (Fungizone) fluconazole (Diflucan) nystatin (Fungizone)
Inhibition of nucleic acid synthesis	Fluoroquinolones	ciprofloxacin (Cipro)
Inhibition of metabolic pathways	Sulfonamides	dapsone (DDS) trimethoprim-sulfamethoxazole (Bactrim, Septra)

on human cells. Of course, there are limits to this selective toxicity, depending on the specific antibiotic and the dose employed. Adverse effects can be expected from all the anti-infectives. There are five major methods by which antibacterials exert their selective toxicity: inhibition of cell wall synthesis, inhibition of protein synthesis, disruption of the plasma cell membrane, inhibition of nucleic acid synthesis, and inhibition of metabolic pathways (antimetabolites). This is an oversimplification of antibacterial actions because some of these drugs act by multiple mechanisms and a few act by unknown mechanisms. Furthermore, as new drugs are developed they often act by new mechanisms and become the only medication in a class. Indeed although the five major classes encompass the majority of anti-infectives, the "miscellaneous" group of anti-infectives has expanded into a large class (see Chapter 49).

Inhibition of Cell Wall Synthesis

Unlike human cells, bacteria have rigid cell walls that create a high osmotic pressure within the cells. The cell wall primarily consists of **peptidoglycan**, a strong, repeating network of carbohydrate and protein chains found only in bacteria and that contains sugars bound to peptides. Disruption of this wall causes the cell to absorb water and eventually lyse. The presence of a unique cell wall gives several means by which antibiotics may act. Fungi also have a unique cell wall that contains lipids that are not used in human cells.

The penicillins and cephalosporins bind to specific proteins that are essential to building the bacterial cell wall. Vancomycin acts by preventing the formation of peptide chains that are used in the construction of the cell wall. Several drugs that are effective against *Mycobacterium tuberculosis*, including isoniazid, act by inhibiting the incorporation of mycolic acid, an important component of the cell wall of this mycobacterium. Uses of the cell wall inhibitors are presented in Chapter 47.

Inhibition of Protein Synthesis

Both bacterial and human cells conduct protein synthesis, so this may seem an unlikely target for antibiotics. However, proteins are constructed on the surface of ribosomes, and these organelles have different structures in humans and bacteria. This difference in ribosomal structure accounts for the selective toxicity of certain antibiotics for bacterial cells.

The fact that protein synthesis occurs in several steps affords different mechanisms by which antibiotics may act. For example, the tetracyclines interfere with the transfer of ribonucleic acid (RNA), which carries the amino acids to the ribosome. The aminoglycosides change the shape of the ribosome so that protein synthesis is impeded. Drugs that inhibit protein synthesis are discussed in Chapter 48.

Disruption of the Plasma Cell Membrane

A few antibacterial and antifungal medications act by interfering with the pathogen's plasma membrane. For example, when polymyxin B attaches to the phospholipids in bacterial plasma membranes, the permeability of the membrane changes and substances escape from the cell. The antifungal drug amphotericin B shuts down the synthesis of ergosterol, a lipid essential to the integrity of fungal plasma membranes.

Inhibition of Nucleic Acid Synthesis

Although deoxyribonucleic acid (DNA) and RNA synthesis are complex processes that occur in both human and bacterial cells, the molecular structures of the various enzymes required for these processes differ considerably. The largest group of antibiotics that inhibits DNA synthesis is the fluoroquinolones. These drugs affect bacterial DNA gyrase, an enzyme that uncoils DNA during the replication process. The fluoroquinolones are presented in Chapter 49.

Inhibition of Metabolic Pathways (Antimetabolites)

Because they divide rapidly, bacterial cells need a steady supply of nutrients and metabolites. A few drugs structurally resemble these building blocks and "fool" the bacterial cell into using them for growth. The sulfonamide antibiotics resemble para-amino benzoic acid (PABA), a precursor to folic acid. Folic acid, a B vitamin that is essential to human metabolism, is also essential to bacteria. When the bacteria attempt to use the sulfonamides, bacterial protein synthesis is blocked. The sulfonamides are presented in Chapter 50.

Other Mechanisms of Action

Anti-infectives act by a number of other miscellaneous mechanisms. The antifungal drug griseofulvin inhibits the formation of mitotic microtubules. Antiretrovirals such as zidovudine block the synthesis of viral DNA by inhibiting the enzyme reverse transcriptase. Mebendazole kills parasitic worms by preventing their absorption of nutrients.

Many other possible mechanisms exist. As the understanding of bacterial physiology increases, it is likely that pharmacologists will develop anti-infectives with entirely new mechanisms of action. The primary mechanisms of action of antibacterial drugs are shown in Pharmacotherapy Illustrated 46.1.

PHARMACOTHERAPY ILLUSTRATED 46.1

Mechanisms of Action of Antimicrobial Drugs

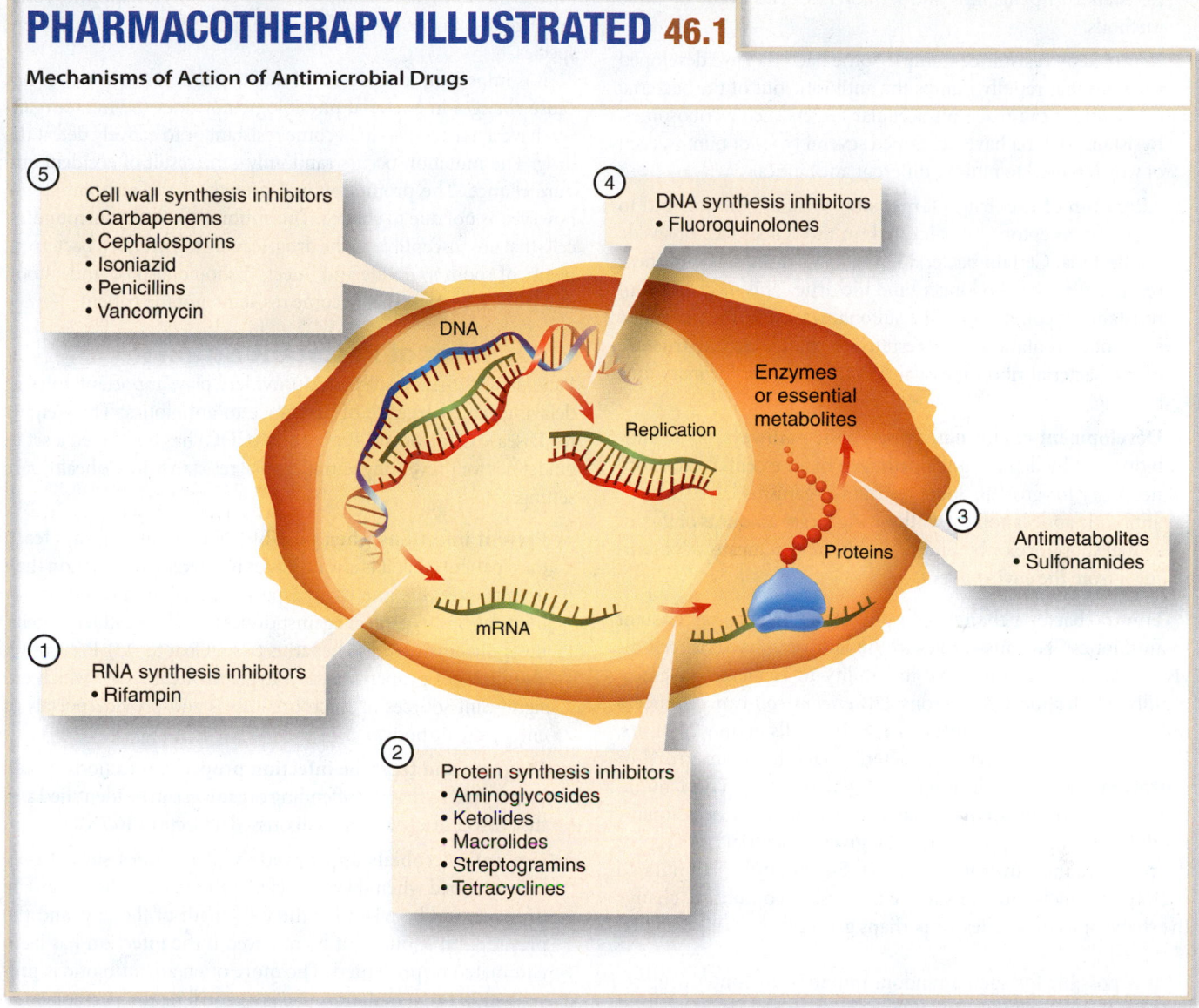

⑤ Cell wall synthesis inhibitors
- Carbapenems
- Cephalosporins
- Isoniazid
- Penicillins
- Vancomycin

④ DNA synthesis inhibitors
- Fluoroquinolones

③ Antimetabolites
- Sulfonamides

① RNA synthesis inhibitors
- Rifampin

② Protein synthesis inhibitors
- Aminoglycosides
- Ketolides
- Macrolides
- Streptogramins
- Tetracyclines

DNA · Replication · Enzymes or essential metabolites · Proteins · mRNA

PharmFACT

Antibiotic-resistant bacteria cause over 2 million illnesses and 23,000 deaths annually in the United States. Over half of these deaths are caused by antibiotic-resistant *Clostridium difficile* infections (Centers for Disease Control and Prevention, 2013).

Acquired Resistance

46.5 Acquired resistance is a major clinical problem that is worsened by the inappropriate use of anti-infectives.

In the 1950s, health care providers called antibiotics "miracle drugs" and predicted that all infectious disease would one day be eliminated. It did not take long, however, to discover that these miracle drugs were rapidly becoming ineffective. How could a drug that once killed nearly 100% of a species of bacteria soon prove to be ineffective? The answer is acquired resistance.

Acquired resistance is the ability of an organism to become unresponsive over time to the effects of an anti-infective. Resistance

can occur in bacteria, fungi, viruses, and protozoans. It is a major clinical problem that is growing in importance.

Mechanisms of Resistance

How can an organism become insensitive to a drug that kills other members of its species? Medicine has discovered a number of mechanisms by which pathogens acquire resistance:

- **Destruction of the drug.** Organisms can produce an enzyme that destroys or deactivates the drug. For example, some bacteria are able to produce beta lactamase, an enzyme that splits the active portion of the drug molecule. Organisms that produce beta lactamase are resistant to many of the penicillin and cephalosporin antibiotics.

- **Prevention of drug entry into the pathogen.** Some antibiotics must enter the pathogen to cause their action. Some bacteria have developed enzymes that inactivate the drug as it crosses the cell wall. Others have changed the structure of the channels or pores that the antibiotic normally uses to enter the cell.

Resistance to penicillins and tetracyclines can occur by these methods.

- **Removal by resistance pumps.** Some bacteria have developed a system that rapidly pumps the antibiotic out of the bacterial cell before it can reach intracellular targets such as ribosomes. Resistant bacteria have developed several types of pumps, each of which is used to remove different antibiotics.

- **Alteration of the drug's target site.** Most antibiotics bind to a specific receptor that is located on the cell surface or inside the bacteria. Certain bacteria have changed the shape of these receptors, so they no longer bind the drug. This mechanism of resistance is common for the sulfonamides. For the macrolide antibiotics, mutations have resulted in changes to the structure of the bacterial ribosome, which is the receptor for macrolide binding.

- **Development of alternative metabolic pathways.** Some antibiotics act by depleting the pathogen of an essential substance necessary for growth. Some resistant organisms have survived antibiotic application by synthesizing larger amounts of the essential substance or by finding an alternative means of obtaining it from the environment.

How do bacteria change their physiology to become resistant to antibiotics? The answer lies in the nature of bacterial cell division. Microorganisms have the ability to replicate extremely rapidly. Under ideal conditions *Escherichia coli* can produce a million cells every 20 minutes, or 1×10^{21} cells in only 24 hours. During exponential division, bacteria make frequent errors, or **mutations**, while duplicating their genetic code. These mutations, which occur spontaneously and randomly, occasionally result in a change in physiology that gives a bacterial cell a reproductive advantage over its neighbors. For example, the mutated bacterium may be able to survive in harsher conditions, change the shape of its organelles, or perhaps grow faster than other bacterial cells.

It is possible for such a random mutation to confer drug resistance for a microorganism. Once the mutation produces a resistant strain, the microbes permanently lose sensitivity to that specific drug and often to other drugs in the same pharmacologic and chemical class. Over several decades, these drug-resistant mutants may colonize a large segment of the human population, thus making the medication essentially useless as a first-line antibiotic.

Promotion of Resistance

The widespread and sometimes unwarranted use of antibiotics has promoted the development of drug-resistant bacterial strains. By killing strains of bacteria that are sensitive to the drug, the only bacteria remaining to replicate are those that acquired the mutations that made them insensitive to the effects of the antibiotic. These drug-resistant bacteria are then free to grow, unrestrained by their neighbors that are killed by the antibiotic. Soon the patient develops an infection that is resistant to conventional drug therapy. This concept is shown in Figure 46.1.

After acquiring resistance, the mutated bacterium may pass its resistance gene to other bacteria through **conjugation**, which is the direct transfer of small pieces of circular DNA called plasmids. Through conjugation, it is quite possible for a bacterium that has never been exposed to the antibiotic to become resistant.

Furthermore, because conjugation is not species specific, resistance genes may be passed from one species to a totally different species.

It is important to understand that the antibiotic itself does not cause changes in bacterial physiology, nor does the microorganism have a master plan to become resistant or to actively defeat the drug. The mutation occurs randomly—the result of accident and pure chance. The promotion and growth of the resistant strain, however, is not due to chance. The antibiotic kills the surrounding cells that are susceptible to the drug, leaving the mutated bacterium plenty of room to divide and infect. It should also be understood that it is the bacteria that become resistant, not the patient.

Prevention of Resistant Strains

Patients and their health care providers play important roles in delaying the emergence of resistance to antibiotics. The Centers for Disease Control and Prevention (CDC) has developed a set of guidelines for preventing antimicrobial resistance in the health care setting:

- **Prevent infections when possible.** Nurses must always teach their patients that it is always easier to prevent an infection than to treat one. One important aspect of prevention is getting immunizations to protect against diseases such as influenza, tetanus, polio, measles, and hepatitis B (see Chapter 43). Prevention also includes proper care and hygiene of catheters, which are significant sources of microorganisms and provide portals of entry into the body.

- **Diagnose and treat the infection properly.** Infections should be cultured so that the offending organism can be identified and the correct drug chosen, as discussed in Section 46.7.

- **Use antimicrobials appropriately.** Antibiotics should only be prescribed when there is a clear rationale for their use. The drugs should be taken for the full length of therapy, and the prescription should not be renewed if the infection has been eliminated or prevented. The more often an antibiotic is prescribed in the population, the larger will be the percentage of resistant strains.

- **Prevent transmission.** Nurses can contain infections and stop the spread of the disease in their work settings by using proper infection control procedures. Additionally, nurses should teach their patients the methods of proper hygiene to prevent the transmission of infectious disease in the home and community settings.

CONNECTION Checkpoint 46.2

From what you learned in Chapter 27, explain the difference between resistance and tolerance. *See Answer to Connection Checkpoint 46.2 on student resource website.*

46.6 Several resistant strains are major clinical challenges due to the lack of therapeutic options.

Infections that are acquired in a health care setting, called **health care–associated infections (HAIs)**, are often resistant to common antibiotics. The most common site of HAIs is the urinary tract, followed by surgical wounds, respiratory tract, and bacteremia. Table 46.3 lists the organisms that are frequently responsible for HAI infections.

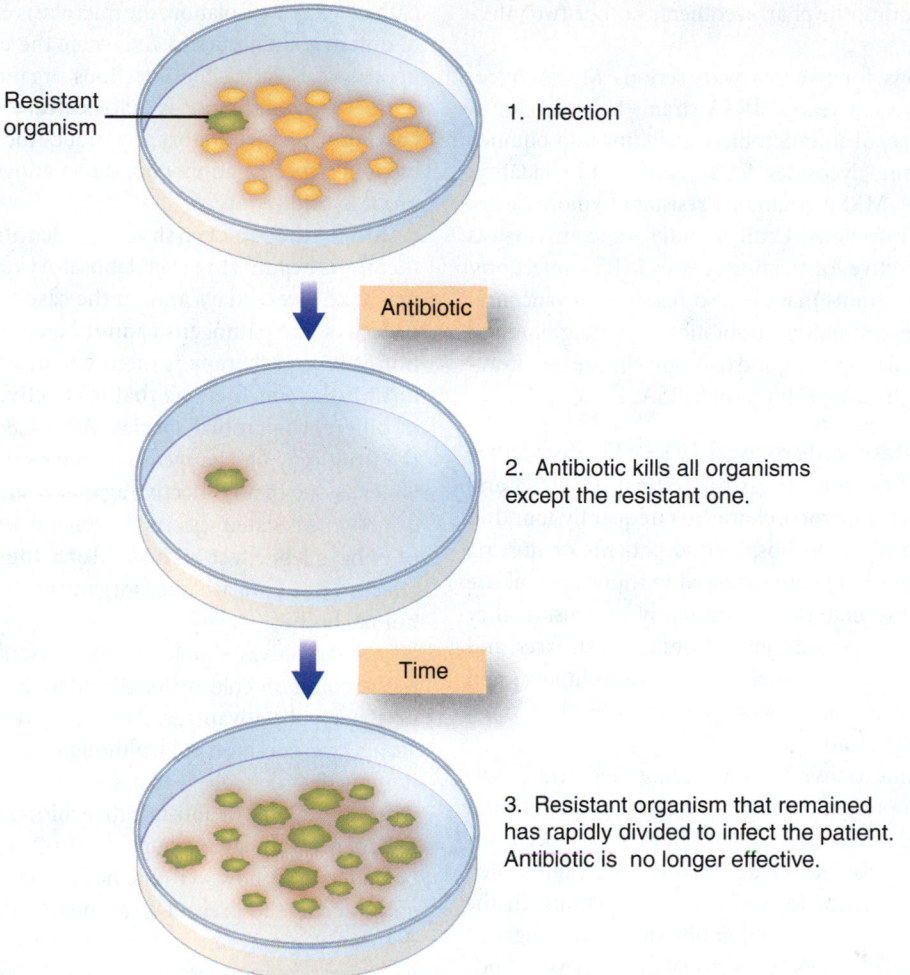

Figure 46.1 Acquired resistance.

1. Infection

Resistant organism

Antibiotic

2. Antibiotic kills all organisms except the resistant one.

Time

3. Resistant organism that remained has rapidly divided to infect the patient. Antibiotic is no longer effective.

TABLE 46.3   Common Pathogens Associated with Health Care–Associated Infections

Pathogen	Infection
Acinetobacter species (spp)	Bacteremia, pneumonia
Clostridium difficile	Colon
Enterobacter spp	Pneumonia
Enterococcus spp	Urinary tract
Escherichia coli	Urinary tract, primary bacteremia, pneumonia
Klebsiella pneumoniae	Pneumonia, urinary tract
Pseudomonas aeruginosa	Pneumonia, urinary tract
Staphylococcus aureus	Surgical wounds, pneumonia, bacteremia
Staphylococci (coagulase negative)	Bacteremia

There are four general sources of HAIs:

- **Patient flora.** Bacteria normally residing on the skin and in the lung or genitourinary tract
- **Invasive devices.** Urinary catheters, vascular catheters, endotracheal tubes, and endoscopes
- **Medical personnel.** Infected health care workers or noninfectious carriers
- **Medical environment.** Contaminated instruments, air, food, or fluids

Many times, patients are at risk for HAIs caused by resistant organisms. Two types of resistant strains are especially important to pharmacotherapy: methicillin-resistant *Staphylococcus aureus* and vancomycin-resistant enterococci.

Methicillin-resistant *Staphylococcus aureus* (MRSA): MRSA is a type of bacterium that is resistant to certain antibiotics such as methicillin, amoxicillin, and penicillin. At least 60% of *S. aureus* infections are now resistant to penicillin. The term *methicillin resistant* is still used for these infections despite the fact that methicillin was removed from the market many years ago.

MRSA infections are most frequently acquired in hospitals and long-term care facilities. These hospital-acquired infections (HA-MRSA) occur primarily in patients with weakened immune systems. MRSA infections that occur in nonhospitalized settings are called community-acquired infections. Community-acquired MRSA (CA-MRSA) infections occur in otherwise healthy people and are usually manifested as skin and soft tissue infections, such as pimples and boils. The strains that are responsible for HA-MRSA infections appear to be distinctly different from those that cause

CA-MRSA infections; thus the pharmacotherapy of the two infections differs somewhat.

Therapeutic options for patients with serious MRSA infections are limited. In recent years, MRSA strains have developed resistance to most classes of antimicrobials, including fluoroquinolones, macrolides, aminoglycosides, tetracyclines, and clindamycin. In general, the HA-MRSA strains are resistant to more classes than the CA-MRSA infections. Until recently, vancomycin was the only antibiotic effective for treating serious MRSA infections. Unfortunately, MRSA strains that are also resistant to vancomycin have appeared. Several newer antibiotics, including linezolid (Zyvox), quinupristin-dalfopristin, and daptomycin, are now available to treat multidrug-resistant strains of MRSA.

Vancomycin-resistant enterococci (VRE): Enterococci are normal inhabitants of the human gastrointestinal (GI) tract and the female genital tract. Enterococci are also frequently found in wounds and pressure ulcers in hospitalized patients or nursing home residents. Patients with compromised immune systems are at greatest risk. Because enterococci are hardy organisms, they can survive for prolonged periods on environmental surfaces, and health care workers using poor infection control techniques can easily spread them. More than 95% of VRE strains in the United States are *Enterococcus faecium*.

Like MRSA, VRE infections represent a major therapeutic challenge, and treatment options are limited. Strains that are resistant to the most commonly used classes of antibiotics have been isolated. Virtually all are resistant to high levels of ampicillin, which is the conventional treatment for enterococci infections. In the 1990s, vancomycin became the only antibiotic effective against multidrug-resistant VRE strains. Unfortunately, each year finds more VRE strains becoming resistant to vancomycin, and newer antibiotics must be used for these infections.

PharmFACT

Up to 90% of all *S. aureus* organisms isolated from individuals are now resistant to penicillin G. Over half of these are also methicillin resistant (Gumbo, 2011).

46.7 Careful selection of the correct antibiotic is essential for effective pharmacotherapy and to limit adverse effects.

It is essential for the health care provider to select an antibiotic that will be effective against the specific pathogen that is causing the patient's infection. Selecting an incorrect drug will delay proper treatment, giving the pathogens more time to invade or secrete toxins. For acute infections, treatment delays of just a few hours or days can lead to poorer patient prognosis and even death. Prescribing ineffective antibiotics also promotes the development of resistance and may cause unnecessary adverse effects in the patient.

For the correct antibiotic to be chosen, identification of the causative agent is necessary. Although gathering data on symptoms is important, many infections produce the same signs early in their course; thus more exact laboratory means of diagnosis are necessary.

Specimens such as urine, sputum, blood, or pus are examined in the laboratory for the purpose of isolating and identifying specific pathogens. After isolation, the microbe is exposed in the laboratory to different antibiotics to determine the most effective ones. This process of isolating the infectious organism and identifying the most effective antibiotic is called **culture and sensitivity (C&S) testing**. Other laboratory techniques include examination of the blood for specific antibodies, direct antigen detection, and DNA probe hybridization.

Ideally, the pathogen should be identified before anti-infective therapy is begun. However, laboratory testing and identification may take several days and, in the case of viruses, several weeks. Indeed, some pathogens cannot be cultured at all. If the infection is severe, therapy is often begun with a **broad-spectrum antibiotic**, which is one that is effective against a wide variety of different microbial species. After C&S testing is completed, the drug may be changed to a **narrow-spectrum antibiotic**, which is one that is effective against a smaller group of microbes or only the isolated species. In general, narrow-spectrum antibiotics have less effect on **host flora**, thus causing fewer adverse effects. Host flora are microorganisms that normally inhabit the human body.

Anti-infectives should not be prescribed for infections such as the common cold or for disorders for which antibiotics serve no therapeutic advantage. Antibiotics do not affect viral diseases such as the common cold, although many patients with this self-limiting disorder believe that these drugs will speed their recovery. Another example of anti-infective misuse is prescribing antibiotics to patients who have a cough due to chronic bronchitis. It should be understood, however, that health care providers may prescribe anti-infectives to prevent a secondary infection from developing. For example, an elderly patient with a severe cold may develop a weakened immune response. Thus the health care provider may order an antibiotic not for the viral infection, but to prevent a secondary bacterial infection from developing.

Indications and Selection of Specific Anti-Infectives

46.8 Depending on the pathogen, anti-infective therapy may be conducted with a single drug or a combination of drugs.

If C&S testing confirms that an infection is caused by only one species of microbe, antibiotic therapy is usually begun with a single drug. In some cases, combining two antibiotics may actually decrease each drug's effectiveness, a phenomenon known as *antagonism*. For example, giving a drug that slows bacterial growth may interfere with an antibiotic that depends on a high bacterial growth rate to produce its bacteriocidal effect. Use of multiple antibiotics can also promote the emergence of multidrug-resistant strains and produce unnecessary adverse effects.

In well-defined circumstances combination therapy with multiple antibiotics is warranted. For example, multiple anti-infective drugs are indicated if different species of pathogens are causing the infection. Patients may present with a life-threatening infection of unknown etiology and the health care provider may need to prescribe several antibiotics until the specific pathogens can be identified. In some cases, two antibiotics have been shown through clinical research to work synergistically, producing a greater kill rate than would be achieved by either antibiotic given alone. Examples of situations where multidrug therapy is clearly warranted are for the pharmacotherapy of tuberculosis (see Chapter 51) and HIV-AIDS (see Chapter 55).

CONNECTION Checkpoint 46.3

From what you learned in Chapter 5, why would there be potentially fewer adverse effects in a patient if two antibiotics are given at lower doses, rather than a single antibiotic given at a higher dose? *See Answer to Connection Checkpoint 46.3 on student resource website.*

46.9 Anti-infectives may be administered to prevent infections.

In most cases, anti-infectives are given when there is clear evidence of infection. This is because health care providers have developed clear rationales for prescribing these drugs to discourage the emergence of resistant strains.

However, anti-infectives are administered to prevent infections in certain high-risk patients. In these cases, research has demonstrated that the benefits of infection prophylaxis outweigh the increased risk of adverse effects or the potential for producing resistant strains. Prophylactic anti-infectives are indicated for the following clinical situations:

- Antibiotics for patients with suppressed immune systems, including those with HIV-AIDS or profound neutropenia
- Antibiotics for patients with deep puncture wounds such as from dog bites
- Antibiotics for patients with prosthetic heart valves, prior to receiving medical or dental surgery, to prevent bacterial endocarditis
- Antibiotics for patients who are undergoing specific types of surgery, such as cardiovascular surgery, orthopedic surgery, and surgery of the alimentary canal, where it has been shown that antibiotic use decreases the risk of postoperative infections
- Antimalarial drugs for patients who are entering areas of the world where malaria is endemic
- Antitubercular drugs for close personal contacts of patients who have confirmed or suspected active tuberculosis
- Antiretrovirals to prevent the transmission of HIV to newborns when the mother is HIV positive
- Antiretrovirals for health care workers who have a confirmed exposure to HIV-contaminated body fluids

Prophylactic therapy with anti-infectives is usually conducted using specific protocols that designate the duration of therapy. For example, chloroquine (Aralen) is given 1 week before expected exposure to malaria and continues for 4 weeks following exposure. Zidovudine (AZT) is given to the HIV-positive mother beginning by week 14 of pregnancy until birth, after which the drug is given to the neonate for 6 weeks. Only in rare cases are anti-infectives given prophylactically for indefinite time periods. Examples include the prevention of infections in patients with suppressed immune systems such as those with HIV infection, or those receiving immunosuppressants following an organ transplant.

Host Factors Affecting Anti-Infective Selection

46.10 Patient factors such as host defenses, local tissue conditions, history of allergic reactions, age, pregnancy status, and genetics influence the choice of anti-infective.

The most important factor in selecting an appropriate antibiotic is to be certain that the microbe is sensitive to the bacteriocidal or bacteriostatic effects of the drug. Once the appropriate drug has been chosen, the nurse must consider a number of host factors that have the potential to significantly influence the success of anti-infective therapy.

Host Defenses

Remember that the primary goal of antibiotic therapy is to kill enough of the pathogen or slow its growth such that natural body defenses can overcome the invading agents. An anti-infective is rarely able to eliminate a pathogen without help from a functioning immune system. Patients with weakened immune defenses often require the administration of prophylactic antibiotics. Should an infection occur in these patients, anti-infective therapy is more aggressive and prolonged. Examples of patients who may require this type of antibiotic therapy include those with AIDS and those with neutropenia caused by immunosuppressive or antineoplastic medications.

Local Tissue Conditions

Anti-infectives must be able to reach the area of infection in sufficient concentrations to be effective; thus local conditions at the infection site are important to the success of pharmacotherapy. Infections of the central nervous system (CNS) are particularly difficult to treat because many medications are unable to cross the blood–brain barrier to reach the brain and associated tissues. Injury or inflammation at an infection site can cause tissues to become acidic or anaerobic and have poor circulation. Excessive pus formation or large hematomas can impede drugs from reaching their targets. Pathogens such as mycobacteria, salmonella, toxoplasma, and listeria can reside intracellularly and thus be resistant to antibacterial action.

Factors that hinder the drug from reaching microbes will limit therapeutic success, and adjustments in treatment may be necessary. Increasing the dosage or switching to a different route of drug administration may be indicated. Occasionally, it is necessary to switch to a different antibiotic that is more effective for conditions specific to the infection site.

Allergy History

Although not common, serious hypersensitivity reactions to antibiotics may be fatal. The penicillins are the class of antibacterials that have the highest incidence of allergic reactions: Between 0.7% and 10% of all patients who receive these drugs exhibit some degree of hypersensitivity.

Patient assessment must always include a thorough medication history. A previous acute allergic incident with a drug is highly predictive of future hypersensitivity to the same medication. Because the patient may have been exposed to an antibiotic unknowingly, such as through food products or molds, allergic reactions can occur without any apparent previous exposure. If severe allergy to a drug is established, it is best to avoid all drugs in the same chemical class.

Other Host Factors

Age, pregnancy status, and genetics are additional factors that influence anti-infective pharmacotherapy. Infants and older adults are less able to metabolize and excrete antibiotics; thus doses are generally decreased. Because of polypharmacy in older patients, this group is more likely to be taking multiple drugs that could interact with antibiotics.

Some antibiotics are readily secreted in breast milk or cross the placenta. For example, tetracyclines taken by the mother can cause teeth discoloration in the newborn, and aminoglycosides can affect hearing. Some anti-infectives are pregnancy category D, such as minocycline, doxycycline, neomycin, and streptomycin. The benefits of antibiotic use in pregnant or lactating women must be carefully weighed against the potential risks to the fetus and neonate.

A genetic absence of certain enzymes can lead to an inability of a patient to metabolize antibiotics to their inactive forms. For example, patients with a deficiency of the enzyme glucose-6-phosphate dehydrogenase should not receive sulfonamides, chloramphenicol, or nalidixic acid due to the possibility of erythrocyte rupture.

CONNECTION Checkpoint 46.4

From what you learned in Chapter 42, what classes of drugs are administered to boost immune function so that the patient is less likely to experience an opportunistic infection? *See Answer to Connection Checkpoint 46.4 on student resource website.*

Superinfections

46.11 Superinfections can occur when an anti-infective antibiotic kills host flora.

Microorganisms that normally inhabit the human body, or host flora, are present on the surface of the skin and in the upper respiratory, genitourinary, and intestinal tracts. Some of these microbes serve useful purposes by producing natural antibacterial substances or by breaking down toxic agents. The various host flora are in competition with each other for physical space and nutrients. This **microbial antagonism** helps protect the host from being overrun by pathogenic organisms.

Antibiotics are unable to distinguish between host flora and pathogenic organisms. When an antibiotic kills the host's normal flora, additional nutrients and space are available for pathogenic microorganisms to grow unchecked. These new, secondary infections caused by antibiotic use are called **superinfections**, or suprainfections. The appearance of a new infection while receiving anti-infective therapy is highly suspicious of a superinfection. Signs and symptoms of superinfection commonly include diarrhea, bladder pain, painful urination, or abnormal vaginal discharges.

Broad-spectrum antibiotics are more likely to cause superinfections because they kill many microbial species, which sometimes includes host flora. Organisms that commonly cause superinfections are *Clostridium albicans* in the vagina, streptococci in the oral cavity, and *Clostridium difficile* in the colon.

CHAPTER

46 Understanding the Chapter

Key Concepts Summary

46.1 Pathogens cause disease due to their ability to invade tissues or secrete toxins.

46.2 Bacteria are described by their staining characteristics, shape, and ability to utilize oxygen.

46.3 Anti-infective drugs are classified by their susceptible organisms, chemical structures, and mechanisms of action.

46.4 Anti-infective drugs act by selectively targeting a pathogen's metabolism or life cycle.

46.5 Acquired resistance is a major clinical problem that is worsened by the inappropriate use of anti-infectives.

46.6 Several resistant strains are major clinical challenges due to the lack of therapeutic options.

46.7 Careful selection of the correct antibiotic is essential for effective pharmacotherapy and to limit adverse effects.

46.8 Depending on the pathogen, anti-infective therapy may be conducted with a single drug or a combination of drugs.

46.9 Anti-infectives may be administered to prevent infections.

46.10 Patient factors such as host defenses, local tissue conditions, history of allergic reactions, age, pregnancy status, and genetics influence the choice of anti-infective.

46.11 Superinfections can occur when an anti-infective antibiotic kills host flora.

References

Centers for Disease Control and Prevention. (2013). *Antibiotic resistance threats in the United States, 2013.* Retrieved from http://www.cdc.gov/drugresistance/threat-report-2013/

Gumbo, T. (2011). General principles of antimicrobial therapy. In L. L. Brunton, B. A. Chabner, & B. C. Knollman (Eds.), *The pharmacological basis of therapeutics* (12th ed., pp. 1365–1382). New York, NY: McGraw-Hill.

Madigan, M. T., Martinko, J. M., Stahl, A. A., & Clark, D. P. (2012). *Brock biology of microorganisms* (13th ed.). San Francisco, CA: Benjamin Cummings.

Selected Bibliography

Barnes, B. E., & Sampson, D. A. (2011). A literature review on community-acquired methicillin-resistant *Staphylococcus aureus* in the United States: Clinical information for primary care nurse practitioners. *Journal of the American Academy of Nurse Practitioners, 23,* 23–32. doi:10.1111/j.1745-7599.2010.00571.x

Bauman, R. W. (2012). *Microbiology with diseases by body system* (3rd ed.). San Francisco, CA: Benjamin Cummings.

Custodio, H. T. (2013). *Hospital-acquired infections.* Retrieved from http://emedicine.medscape.com/article/967022-overview#aw2aab6b2b5aa

Davey, P., Brown, E., Charani, E., Fenelon, L., Gould, I., Holmes, A., . . . Wilcox, M. (2013). Interventions to improve antibiotic prescribing practices for hospital inpatients. *Cochrane Database of Systematic Reviews, 4,* CD003543. doi:10.1002/14651858.CD003543.pub3

Gilbert, D. N., Moellering, R. C., & Sande, M. A. (2011). *The Sanford guide to antimicrobial therapy 2011* (41st ed.). Sperryville, VA: Antimicrobial Therapy.

Gurusamy, K. S., Koti, R., Toon, C. D., Wilson, P., & Davidson, B. R. (2013). Antibiotic therapy for the treatment of methicillin-resistant *Staphylococcus aureus* (MRSA) infections in surgical wounds. *Cochrane Database of Systematic Reviews, 8,* CD009726. doi:10.1002/14651858.CD009726

Kee, V. R. (2012). *Clostridium difficile* infection in older adults: A review and update on its management. *The American Journal of Geriatric Pharmacotherapy, 10*(1), 14–24. doi.org/10.1016/j.amjopharm.2011.12.004

Rice, L. B. (2012). Mechanisms of resistance and clinical relevance of resistance to β-lactams, glycopeptides, and fluoroquinolones. *Mayo Clinic Proceedings, 8,* 198–208. doi.org/10.1016/j.mayocp.2011.12.003

Spellberg, B., Bartlett, J. G., & Gilbert, D. N. (2013). The future of antibiotics and resistance. *New England Journal of Medicine, 368,* 299–302. doi:10.1056/NEJMp1215093

Tortora, G. J., Funke, B. R., & Case, C. L. (2012). *Microbiology: An introduction* (11th ed.). San Francisco, CA: Benjamin Cummings.

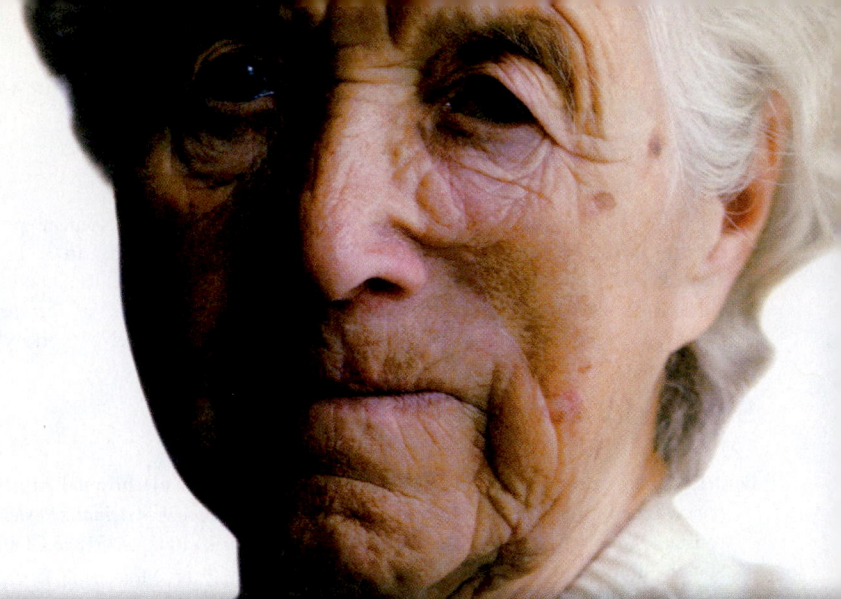

> *"Last month I underwent surgery for the removal of a skin lesion from my left arm. Unfortunately, I think the wound has become infected. The area is red, swollen, and painful and has a yellowish drainage."*
>
> Patient "Katie Dennison"

LEARNING OUTCOMES

After reading this chapter, the student should be able to:

1. Explain the structure of a bacterial cell wall and its importance to pharmacotherapy.
2. Identify the classes of antibiotics that act by affecting the synthesis of the bacterial cell wall.
3. Explain the mechanisms by which antibiotics affect the bacterial cell wall.
4. Compare and contrast the four classes of penicillins.
5. Compare and contrast the five generations of cephalosporins.
6. Identify similarities and differences among drugs in the carbapenem class.
7. For each of the classes shown in the chapter outline, identify the prototype and representative drugs and explain the mechanism(s) of drug action, primary indications, contraindications, significant drug interactions, pregnancy category, and important adverse effects.
8. Apply the nursing process to care for patients who are receiving pharmacotherapy with bacterial cell wall inhibitors.

CHAPTER OUTLINE

▶ Structure of Bacterial Cell Walls

▶ Penicillins

Natural Penicillins

PROTOTYPE Penicillin G, *p. 790*

Broad-Spectrum Penicillins (Aminopenicillins)

PROTOTYPE Ampicillin (Principen), *p. 792*

Extended-Spectrum (Antipseudomonal) Penicillins

Penicillinase-Resistant (Antistaphylococcal) Penicillins

▶ Cephalosporins

PROTOTYPE Cefazolin (Ancef, Kefzol), *p. 795*

▶ Carbapenems

PROTOTYPE Imipenem-Cilastatin (Primaxin), *p. 797*

▶ Miscellaneous Cell Wall Inhibitors

PROTOTYPE Vancomycin (Vancocin), *p. 7*

The discovery and development of the first anti-infective drugs in the mid-1900s was a milestone in the field of medicine. Humans no longer die in massive numbers from infectious organisms such as *Yersinia pestis*, which killed 25% of the known human population in the 14th century due to the bubonic plague. This chapter examines the penicillins, cephalosporins, and other antibiotic drugs that kill bacteria by disrupting their cell walls.

Structure of Bacterial Cell Walls

47.1 Bacterial cell walls consist of layers of carbohydrate and protein chains, which are constructed by enzymes called penicillin-binding proteins.

The cell wall is a structure that sets people apart from the bacterial world. Humans do not have them, but all bacteria do. The osmotic pressure is so high within a bacterial cell that the cell would rupture without the containment of this rigid structure. The cell wall also serves as a barrier to substances that try to enter the cell, including antibiotics. Simply, it protects the bacterial cell from a hostile environment. The cell walls of gram-positive bacteria are very thick, whereas the walls of gram-negative bacteria are thinner. The structure of a bacterial cell wall is illustrated in Figure 47.1.

The primary material in a bacterial cell wall is peptidoglycan, a strong, repeating network of carbohydrate and protein chains that contains sugars bound to peptides. In gram-positive bacteria, peptidoglycan is laid down in repeated layers that are cross-linked to each other to provide greater stability to the wall. The layers may be compared to a fort that is built to provide protection from invaders. A single wall could be easily destroyed, but five or six repeated walls would provide almost impenetrable protection to those inside.

Because of the critical importance of their cell walls, bacteria spend a lot of time and energy building them. At least 30 different bacterial enzymes participate in their construction. Some of these enzymes are targets for penicillins and related antibiotics and are called **penicillin-binding proteins (PBPs)**. Most penicillins affect transpeptidase, which is the final PBP enzyme in the construction of the cell wall that adds the cross-links to the peptidoglycan layers. Without the cross-linking, the cell wall becomes weakened and bulges due to the high osmotic pressure inside the cell. The bacterial cell eventually lyses (disintegrates). This process is illustrated in Figure 47.2. Because humans do not construct cell walls, they do not have PBPs. Therefore, antibiotics that affect the cell wall have selective toxicity to bacteria.

The PBPs are located on the outside of the plasma membrane of the bacterial cell. This location allows antibiotics to exert their bacteriocidal effect without actually entering the cell. Although all bacteria have a cell wall, the materials and PBPs used in their construction differ among species. Even slight structural changes to a PBP can cause lack of antibiotic binding to the enzyme. This

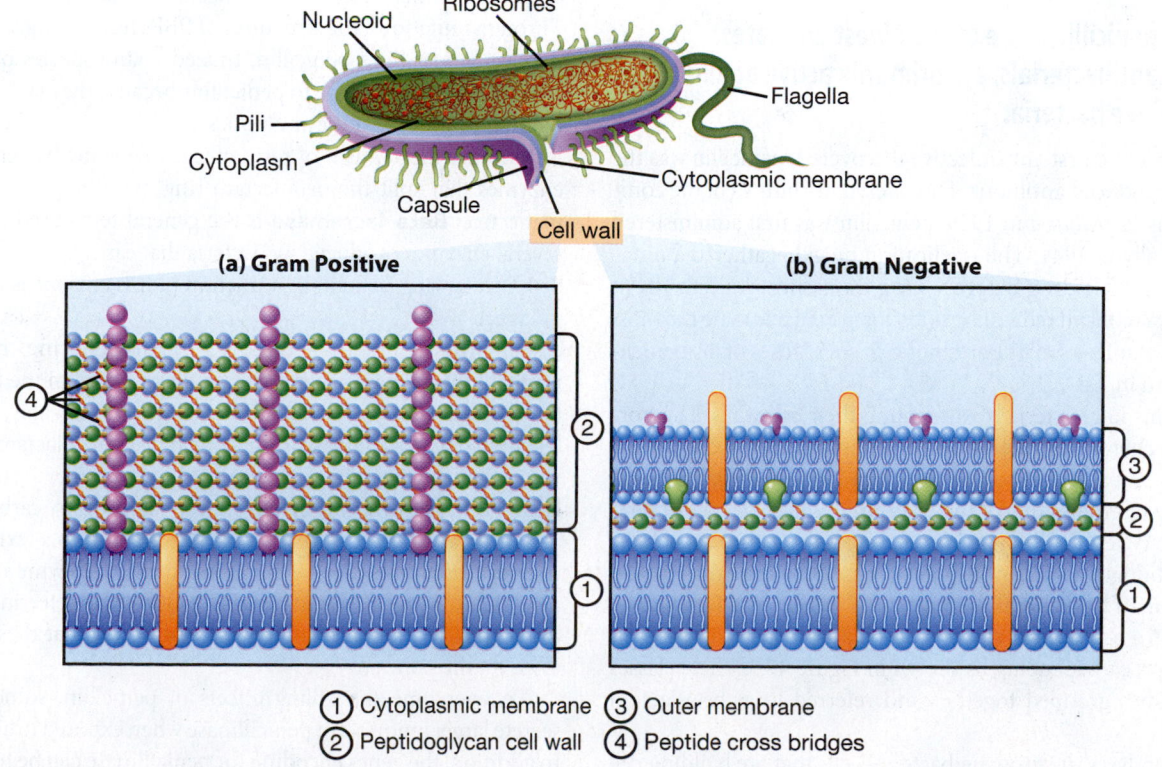

① Cytoplasmic membrane	③ Outer membrane
② Peptidoglycan cell wall	④ Peptide cross bridges

Figure 47.1 The bacterial cell wall: (a) gram-positive bacterium; (b) gram-negative bacterium.

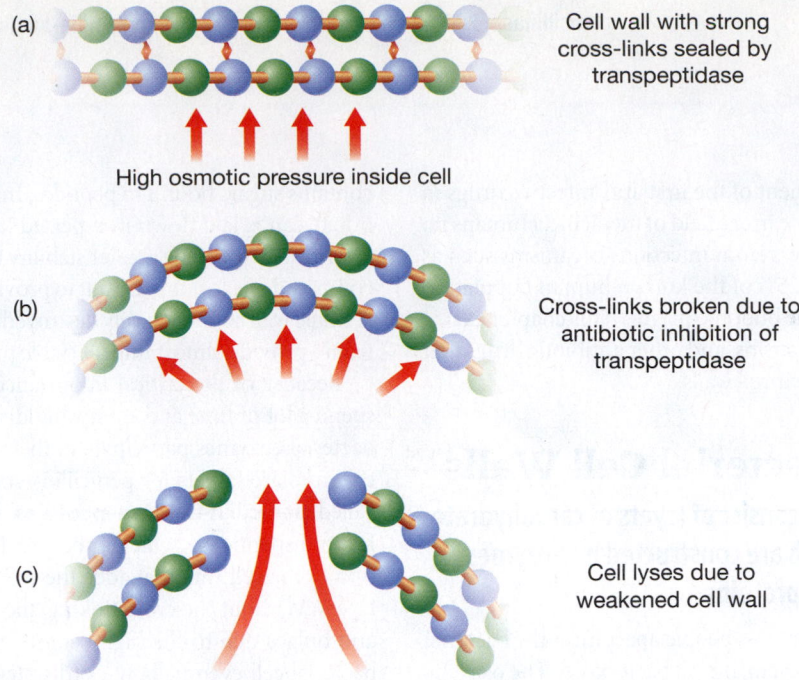

(a)   Cell wall with strong cross-links sealed by transpeptidase

High osmotic pressure inside cell

(b)   Cross-links broken due to antibiotic inhibition of transpeptidase

(c)   Cell lyses due to weakened cell wall

Figure 47.2   Mechanism of penicillin: (a) Bacterial cell wall strengthened by peptide cross-links. (b) Penicillin breaks cross-links. (c) Cell death due to weakened cell walls.

explains why penicillins are not effective against all species of microorganisms. This also provides an explanation as to how an organism develops resistance to the penicillins.

Penicillins

47.2 The penicillins, one of the oldest and safest groups of antibacterials, are primarily active against gram-positive bacteria.

Although not the first anti-infective discovered, penicillin was the first mass-produced antibiotic. Discovered in cultures of the common fungus *Penicillium* in 1929, penicillin was first administered therapeutically in 1941. The medication quickly gathered a reputation as a miracle drug by preventing thousands of deaths from what are now considered minor infections. Penicillins are the most extensively studied of all the antibiotic classes. Doses of the penicillins are listed in Table 47.1.

Penicillins kill bacteria by disrupting their cell walls. The portion of the chemical structure of penicillin that is responsible for its antibacterial activity is called the **beta-lactam ring**. The beta-lactam ring resembles one of the chemical building blocks of peptidoglycan. When the PBP enzyme attempts to add the next "link" in the peptidoglycan chain, it binds to the beta-lactam ring, and construction of the cell wall is terminated. Other antibiotic classes that contain a beta-lactam ring include the cephalosporins, monobactams, and carbapenems, as shown in Figure 47.3. These classes are sometimes grouped together and referred to as beta-lactam antibiotics.

Penicillin lyses the growing bacterial cells that are building cell walls; therefore, it is considered bacteriocidal. It has much less toxicity, however, on bacterial cells that have already constructed

their cell walls. Like all infections, the body's immune defenses are needed to eliminate stable, slow-growing bacterial cells.

Because of their extensive use during the past 70 years, large numbers of resistant bacterial strains have emerged to limit the therapeutic usefulness of the penicillins. There are several mechanisms by which bacteria may become resistant to penicillins. Through mutations, the structures of PBPs have changed such that they no longer bind penicillin. Indeed, many species of bacteria are inherently insensitive to penicillins because they lack the target binding protein for these antibiotics.

Another mechanism of resistance is that some bacteria secrete enzymes that split the beta-lactam ring, rendering the antibiotic ineffective. **Beta lactamase** is the general term used for any of several enzymes produced by bacteria that can split the four-atom beta-lactam ring structure. The action of this enzyme is illustrated in Figure 47.4.

Scientists who first discovered this enzyme named it **penicillinase**, a name that is still frequently used in medicine. Although the terms are sometimes used interchangeably, it should be noted that penicillinase is only one type of beta lactamase—that which splits the ring in penicillin antibiotics. Other forms of beta lactamase exist that can inactivate cephalosporins, carbapenems, and other antibiotics with this ring structure. In this textbook, the term *penicillinase* is used when referring to this enzyme's action on penicillins; the term *beta lactamase* is used when referring to other antibiotics. It should be understood, however, that these are two forms of the same enzyme.

To overcome the killing effects of penicillin, some bacteria secrete larger amounts of penicillinase when exposed to antibiotics. In addition, the genes encoding for penicillinase can be transferred to other bacteria through conjugation, thus spreading the development of resistance genes.

TABLE 47.1 Penicillins

Drug	Route and Adult Dose (Maximum Dose Where Indicated)	Adverse Effects
Natural Penicillins		
penicillin G benzathine (Bicillin)	IM: 1.2 million units as a single dose (max: 2.4 million units/day)	*Rash, pruritus, diarrhea, nausea, fever*
penicillin G potassium	IM/IV: 2–24 million units divided every 4–6 h (max: 80 million units/day)	Anaphylaxis symptoms, including angioedema, circulatory collapse, and cardiac arrest; nephrotoxicity
penicillin G procaine (Wycillin)	IM: 600,000–1.2 million units daily (max: 4.8 million units/day)	
penicillin V	PO: 125–250 mg qid (max: 7.2 g/day)	
Broad-Spectrum Penicillins (Aminopenicillins)		
amoxicillin (Amoxil, Trimox)	PO: 250–500 mg tid (max: 1,750 mg/day)	
amoxicillin-clavulanate (Augmentin)	PO: 250- or 500-mg tablet (each with 125 mg clavulanic acid) every 8–12 h	
ampicillin (Principen)	PO/IV/IM: 250–500 mg every 6 h (max: 4 g/day PO or 14 g/day IV/IM)	
ampicillin and sulbactam (Unasyn)	IV/IM: 1.5–3 g every 6 h	
Extended-Spectrum (Antipseudomonal) Penicillins		
piperacillin	IM/IV: 2–4 g tid–qid (max: 24 g/day)	
piperacillin-tazobactam (Zosyn)	IV: 3.375 g qid over 30 min	
ticarcillin-clavulanate (Timentin)	IV: 3.1 g every 4–6 h	
Penicillinase-Resistant (Antistaphylococcal) Penicillins		
dicloxacillin	PO: 125–500 mg qid (max: 4 g/day)	
nafcillin	IV/IM: 500 mg–1 g qid (max: 12 g/day)	
oxacillin	IV: 50–100 mg/kg/day divided every 4–6 h (max: 12 g/day)	

Note: *Italics* indicate common adverse effects. <u>Underline</u> indicates serious adverse effects.

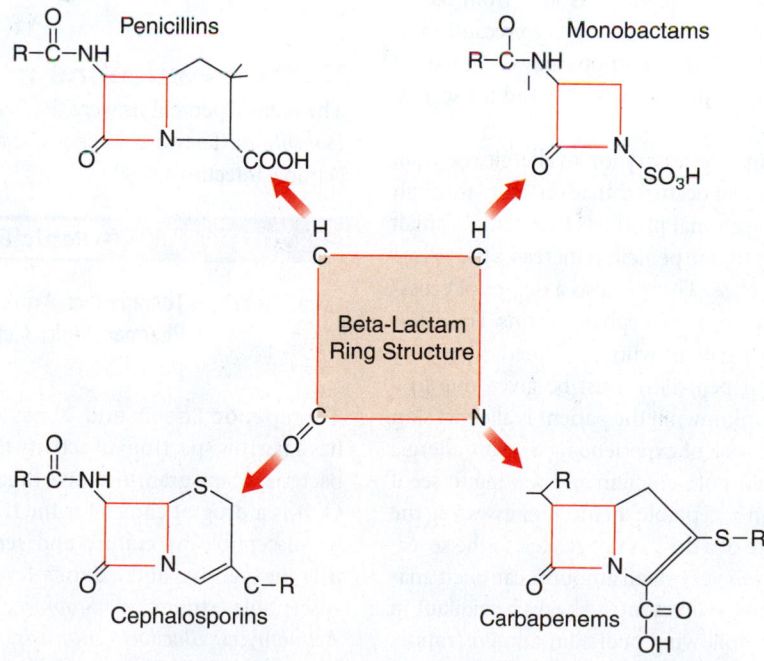

Figure 47.3 Beta-lactam antibiotics: The beta-lactam ring is common to many different classes of antibiotics.

Although each drug in this class has certain unique properties, some generalizations may be made about the penicillins:

- Most are more effective against gram-positive bacteria, although a few have activity against gram-negative bacteria.

- Most have a narrow spectrum of antimicrobial activity.

- They are widely distributed to most body tissues, although only small amounts reach the cerebrospinal fluid (CSF).

- Nearly all are rapidly excreted by the kidneys.

- Most have short half-lives.

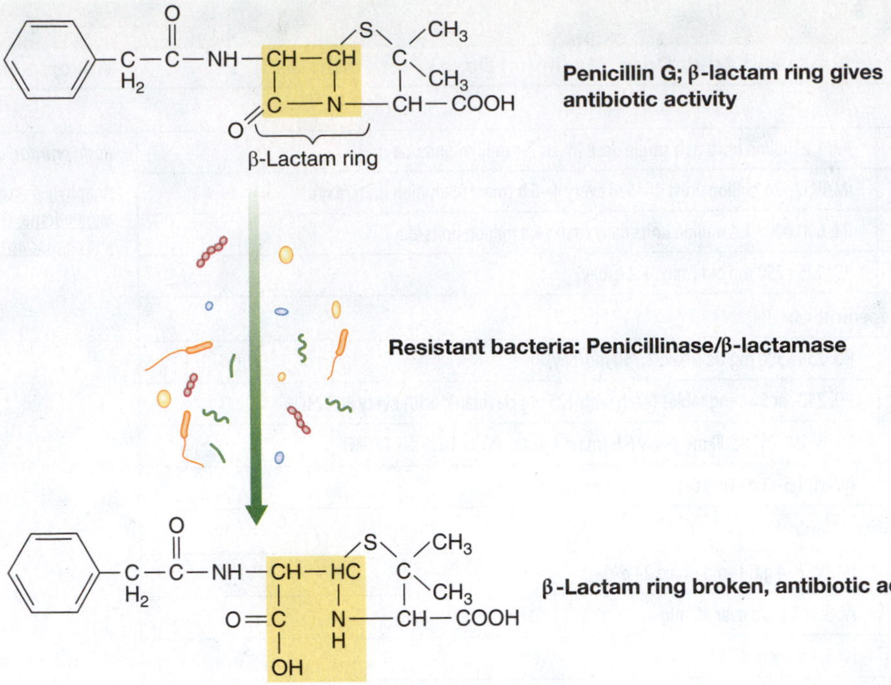

Figure 47.4 Action of penicillinase.

Allergic reactions are the most common adverse effects of the penicillins and ones that require careful attention by nurses. The overall incidence of penicillin allergy ranges from 0.7% to 10%. Symptoms range from mild rash and nausea to fever or anaphylaxis. Although the incidence of anaphylaxis is low, from 0.04% to 2%, mortality is high and nurses must take every precaution to identify patients at highest risk. Allergic reactions may occur within minutes after taking the drug, or they may be delayed for several days or weeks.

Prior exposure to penicillin is necessary for an allergic reaction, although this exposure may have occurred inadvertently through exposure to mold or by eating animal products that contain small amounts of penicillin. Allergy to one penicillin increases the risk of allergy to other drugs in this class. There is also a degree of cross-hypersensitivity between penicillins and cephalosporins. The nurse should not give penicillin to a patient who has a medical history of serious penicillin allergy. If penicillin must be given due to a patient's condition, and it is unknown if the patient is allergic, skin tests may be used to assess the risk of experiencing a severe allergic reaction. Giving a small amount of penicillin and waiting to see if anaphylaxis develops is not an acceptable method for assessing the probability of allergy. The size of a dose is not related to the severity of the response, because even very small amounts can elicit anaphylaxis in susceptible patients. Nurses must always be vigilant in observing for signs of allergy following penicillin administration, because there is no infallible method for predicting which patient will experience an allergy to the drug.

Chemical modifications to the original molecule have produced drugs that offer several advantages over the natural penicillins, including the following:

- Penicillinase resistance
- Broader antimicrobial spectrum
- Extended spectrum

PharmFACT

The U.S. Food and Drug Administration has determined that there is a lack of evidence to support the benefit of using consumer products, including hand washes, body washes, and others, that contain antibacterial additives (Centers for Disease Control and Prevention [CDC], 2013).

Natural Penicillins

The natural penicillins were the first to be isolated from the fungus *Penicillium*. They are inexpensive and the drugs of choice for susceptible infections.

PROTOTYPE DRUG	**Penicillin G**

Classification: Therapeutic: Antibacterial
Pharmacologic: Cell wall inhibitor, natural penicillin

Therapeutic Effects and Uses: Approved in 1943, penicillin G has a narrow spectrum of activity that includes most gram-positive bacteria. Many gram-negative organisms are resistant to penicillin G. It is a drug of choice for the treatment of infections shown to be susceptible by culture and sensitivity (C&S) testing because it is inexpensive and exhibits few adverse effects. These include susceptible strains of *Staphylococcus*, *Streptococcus*, *Neisseria*, *Actinomyces*, *Bacillus anthracis*, *Clostridium*, *Treponema*, and *Corynebacterium*. Penicillin is given for the prophylaxis of bacterial endocarditis in patients with prosthetic heart valves or congenital heart disease and for those at risk for recurrent bouts of rheumatic fever.

Penicillin G is available as a benzathine, potassium, or a procaine salt; each has slightly different pharmacokinetics. For example, while the intramuscular (IM) administration of penicillin G potassium is rapid, the benzathine and procaine salts are absorbed from an IM site very slowly, over a 24-hour period. However, there is no difference in effectiveness among the three salts because they all dissociate to penicillin G. Penicillin G benzathine and penicillin G procaine are administered IM; penicillin G potassium may be administered by either the IV or IM route. Penicillin G potassium was once available by the oral (PO) route, but the drug had low bioavailability due to destruction by gastric acid. Penicillin V and amoxicillin are more stable in acid and are used when oral penicillin therapy is desired.

Mechanism of Action: This drug inhibits bacterial wall synthesis by binding PBPs. Penicillin G is bacteriocidal and destroyed by penicillinase.

Pharmacokinetics:

Route(s)	IM, IV
Absorption	Rapid absorption (IM)
Distribution	Widely distributed; only small amounts cross the blood–brain barrier; secreted in breast milk; approximately 60% bound to plasma proteins
Primary metabolism	15–30% metabolized, primarily hepatic
Primary excretion	Renal
Onset of action	IM: 15–30 min; IV: immediate
Duration of action	4–6 h; half-life: 20–60 min

Adverse Effects: Penicillin G is well tolerated by most patients and adverse effects are uncommon. Urticaria and delayed skin reactions occasionally occur. The most serious adverse effect is severe hypersensitivity reaction. The anaphylactic response may include cardiovascular collapse; edema of the mouth, tongue, pharynx, and larynx; confusion; seizures; and hallucinations. While most allergic reactions to penicillin occur within minutes after administration, late hypersensitivity reactions may occur several weeks into the regimen.

Contraindications/Precautions: Penicillin G is contraindicated in patients who are allergic to any drug in the penicillin class and is used cautiously in those with hypersensitivity to cephalosporins. In cases where penicillin G is the only effective antibiotic in a patient with a known allergy to the drug, penicillin may be given via a desensitization procedure whereby the dose begins very small and gradually increases. Because 90% of a dose of penicillin G is excreted unchanged by the kidneys through tubular secretion, patients with significant renal impairment must be carefully monitored. Patients with heart failure should not receive the penicillin sodium salt. Hyperkalemia may result with high doses of the penicillin G potassium salt.

Drug Interactions: Penicillin G may decrease the effectiveness of oral contraceptives. Colestipol will decrease the absorption of penicillin. Probenecid decreases the excretion of penicillin G and can lead to antibiotic toxicity. Potassium-sparing diuretics such as spironolactone may cause hyperkalemia when administered with penicillin G potassium. Because penicillins can antagonize the actions of aminoglycoside antibiotics, drugs from these two classes are not administered concurrently. The bacteriostatic action of tetracyclines may inhibit the bacteriocidal action of penicillin G. **Herbal/Food**: Unknown.

Pregnancy: Category B.

Treatment of Overdose: No specific therapy is available. Patients are treated symptomatically.

Nursing Responsibilities: Key nursing implications for patients receiving penicillin G are included in the Nursing Practice Application for Patients Receiving Pharmacotherapy with a Penicillin, Cephalosporin, or Vancomycin Antibiotic.

Drugs Similar to Penicillin G

Other natural penicillins include penicillin G benzathine, penicillin G procaine, and penicillin V.

Penicillin G benzathine (Bicillin): Approved in 1943, penicillin G benzathine dissociates to form penicillin G; thus they share the same actions, indications, and adverse effects. Penicillin G benzathine is given only by the IM route and is absorbed very slowly, resulting in low peak serum levels with a prolonged duration of action that can last up to 26 days. Neurologic adverse effects have been reported with penicillin G benzathine, including severe agitation, confusion, hallucinations, and seizures. Injections of this drug are painful and injection-site reactions may occur. Permanent neurologic damage occurs if this drug is injected near a nerve. This drug is pregnancy category B.

Penicillin G procaine (Wycillin): Approved in 1943, penicillin G procaine is a repository form of penicillin given only by the IM route. Like the benzathine salt, it is absorbed slowly from its injection site and has a prolonged duration of action (15–20 hours). It shares the same actions, indications, and adverse effects as penicillin G. The procaine salt is less painful on administration than penicillin G administered by the IM route. Penicillin G procaine can cause neurotoxicity if the drug is accidentally injected near a nerve. Like the benzathine salt, neurologic adverse effects can occur with penicillin G procaine, including severe agitation, confusion, hallucinations, and seizures. Patients with allergies to the local anesthetic procaine (Novocain) should not receive this drug. This drug is pregnancy category B.

Penicillin V: Penicillin V is nearly identical to penicillin G, except that it is more acid stable, which allows it to be administered by the PO route. However, it should be taken on an empty stomach to maximize absorption. Approved in 1956, it shares the same actions, indications, and adverse effects as penicillin G. Some patients experience nausea, vomiting, and diarrhea. This drug is pregnancy category B.

CONNECTION Checkpoint 47.1

From what you learned in Chapter 5, explain how taking a good medical history can eliminate some allergic reactions to antibiotics. *See Answer to Connection Checkpoint 47.1 on student resource website.*

Broad-Spectrum Penicillins (Aminopenicillins)

A major limitation of the natural penicillins is their lack of activity against gram-negative organisms. The aminopenicillins, amoxicillin and ampicillin, are effective against gram-positive and certain gram-negative bacilli such as *Haemophilus influenzae, Escherichia coli, Salmonella,* and *Shigella*. This distinction is responsible for them being placed into a separate class called broad-spectrum penicillins.

Aminopenicillins are rapidly inactivated by penicillinase, which limits their therapeutic usefulness, particularly against

Staphylococcus aureus infections. Despite this limitation, the aminopenicillins are some of the most widely prescribed antibiotics for sinus and upper respiratory and genitourinary tract infections. Their widespread use over many decades has resulted in the emergence of a large number of resistant strains.

Combination drugs have been developed that offer certain advantages over single-drug therapy with aminopenicillins. The fixed-dose combination of Augmentin combines amoxicillin with clavulanate, a beta-lactamase (penicillinase) inhibitor. Another fixed-dose product, Unasyn, contains ampicillin and the beta-lactamase inhibitor sulbactam. By inhibiting penicillinase, these combined drugs allow a greater percentage of the aminopenicillin molecules to reach pathogens and affect cell wall synthesis. The beta-lactamase inhibitors are ineffective when used alone and therefore are always used in fixed combination formulations with other drugs.

PROTOTYPE DRUG | **Ampicillin (Principen)**

Classification: **Therapeutic:** Antibacterial
Pharmacologic: Cell wall inhibitor, aminopenicillin

Therapeutic Effects and Uses: Approved in 1963, the actions of ampicillin are similar to those of penicillin G except that ampicillin has a broader spectrum that includes enhanced activity over enterococci, *E. coli*, *Proteus mirabilis*, *Neisseria gonorrhoeae*, *H. influenzae*, *Salmonella*, *Shigella*, and *Bordetella pertussis*. Because a large percentage of resistant strains have developed, ampicillin is no longer a drug of choice for the treatment of gonococcal infections, childhood meningitis, or *Salmonella* or *Shigella* enteritis.

Mechanism of Action: Ampicillin inhibits bacterial wall synthesis by binding PBPs. This drug is bacteriocidal and inactivated by penicillinase.

Pharmacokinetics:

Route(s)	PO, IM, and IV
Absorption	50% absorbed PO
Distribution	Widely distributed; only small amounts cross the blood–brain barrier; secreted in breast milk; plasma protein binding is about 15–20%
Primary metabolism	Largely unmetabolized, 10% hepatic
Primary excretion	Renal
Onset of action	PO: 30–60 min; IM: 15–30 min
Duration of action	Half-life: 1–2 h

Adverse Effects: Ampicillin is a safe drug that rarely produces serious adverse effects. Rash and diarrhea are the most common adverse effects, and diarrhea occurs more frequently with ampicillin than with the other aminopenicillins. Pain at the injection site is common. Like all penicillins, anaphylaxis is rare, though potentially fatal. Anaphylactic response may include cardiovascular collapse; edema of the mouth, tongue, pharynx, and larynx; confusion; seizure; and hallucinations. Pseudomembranous colitis (PMC) is an additional rare, though serious, severe adverse effect. Very high doses may produce confusion and seizures.

Contraindications/Precautions: Ampicillin is contraindicated in patients who are allergic to any drug in the penicillin class and used cautiously in those with hypersensitivity to cephalosporins. Ampicillin is excreted primarily by the kidneys; therefore, drug therapy must be monitored carefully in patients with renal disease.

Drug Interactions: Ampicillin may decrease the effectiveness of oral contraceptives. Probenecid (Benemid) decreases the excretion of ampicillin and can lead to antibiotic toxicity. Penicillins can antagonize the actions of aminoglycoside antibiotics and must be administered at least 2 hours apart. The antibacterial actions of ampicillin are diminished when it is taken concurrently with chloramphenicol, erythromycin, or tetracyclines. **Herbal/Food**: Because food decreases its absorption, ampicillin should be taken on an empty stomach.

Pregnancy: Category B.

Treatment of Overdose: No specific therapy is available. Patients are treated symptomatically.

Nursing Responsibilities: Key nursing implications for patients receiving ampicillin are included in the Nursing Practice Application for Patients Receiving Pharmacotherapy with a Penicillin, Cephalosporin, or Vancomycin Antibiotic.

Drugs Similar to Ampicillin (Principen)

The only other aminopenicillin is amoxicillin.

Amoxicillin (Amoxil, Trimox): Approved in 1974, amoxicillin is closely related structurally to ampicillin and has many of the same characteristics. The drug is destroyed by penicillinase-producing organisms. It is more acid stable than ampicillin and offers greater gastrointestinal (GI) absorption with peak serum levels twice as high. It exhibits a lower incidence of diarrhea than ampicillin. Amoxicillin has largely replaced ampicillin, and it is one of the most frequently prescribed antibiotics. Amoxicillin should not be administered to patients with hypersensitivity to any penicillin. An extended release form of the drug (Moxatag) was approved in 2008 for treating *Streptococcus pyogenes* infections. This drug is pregnancy category B.

Extended-Spectrum (Antipseudomonal) Penicillins

Piperacillin and ticarcillin have broad spectrums of antimicrobial activity similar to those of the aminopenicillins. Their primary advantage is their additional activity against *Pseudomonas aeruginosa*; thus they are called extended-spectrum or antipseudomonal penicillins. A third drug in this class, carbenicillin, is no longer marketed in the United States.

P. aeruginosa is an opportunistic pathogen found in air, soil, and water. It can persist on environmental surfaces such as soap residues and hot tubs and can even survive in some antiseptic solutions. *P. aeruginosa* infections may occur anywhere in the body, primarily causing disease in patients whose health is already compromised in some manner. It is responsible for about 10% of all health care–associated infections (HAIs), including serious pneumonia in debilitated patients and a large number of infections in wounds and in patients with extensive burns.

P. aeruginosa has natural resistance to most antibiotics due in part to its ability to rapidly pump out antibiotic molecules that enter its cells. Because *Pseudomonas* infections are often persistent, aggressive combination anti-infective therapy is often indicated. A typical combination includes an aminoglycoside antibiotic with an antipseudomonal penicillin. Because penicillins inactivate aminoglycosides, they must be administered at least 2 hours apart. Other antibiotics such as ceftazidime (Ceptaz, Fortaz, Tazicef), ciprofloxacin (Cipro), or imipenem (Primaxin) may be needed.

As with the other penicillins, drugs in this class inhibit bacterial wall synthesis by binding PBPs. The antipseudomonal penicillins achieve their extended spectrum because they have greater penetration through the outer membrane of gram-negative bacteria and a higher affinity for penicillin-binding proteins. The two drugs in this class are similar, and there are few differences on which to distinguish them. Like most penicillins, the antipseudomonal penicillins are widely distributed to tissues and rapidly excreted mostly unchanged in the urine.

Because penicillinase-producing bacteria can inactivate the antipseudomonal penicillins, they are usually combined with a beta-lactamase inhibitor. Fixed-dose combinations with beta-lactamase inhibitors include piperacillin with tazobactam (Zosyn) and ticarcillin with clavulanate (Timentin).

Rash and diarrhea are the most common adverse effects of the antipseudomonal penicillins. These drugs prevent the aggregation of platelets, which can prolong bleeding time. Caution must therefore be used when using these drugs concurrently with agents that modify coagulation. Sodium salts of the antipseudomonal penicillins cause sodium overload in patients with heart failure. Like all penicillins, anaphylaxis is rare, though potentially fatal. PMC is an additional severe adverse effect. Very high doses may produce confusion and seizures. The antipseudomonal penicillins are pregnancy category B.

Piperacillin: Approved in 1981, piperacillin has one of the broadest spectrums of any of the penicillins and is effective against most gram-negative and many gram-positive anaerobic and aerobic microbes. It has been used to treat a variety of serious infections, including those of the skin, blood, sinuses, central nervous system (CNS), respiratory tract, and genitourinary tract. Available by the IM and IV routes, piperacillin is often used in combination with an aminoglycoside antibiotic because together they exert synergistic action on gram-negative microbes. High doses can lead to platelet dysfunction, although piperacillin seems to have less effect than other antipseudomonal penicillins. Electrolytes should be regularly monitored to prevent hypokalemia and hypernatremia. Piperacillin should not be administered to patients with hypersensitivity to any penicillin. Localized injection-site reactions include pain, inflammation, phlebitis, and hematomas. Zosyn is a fixed-dose combination of piperacillin and tazobactam.

Ticarcillin-clavulanate (Timentin): As with piperacillin, ticarcillin has one of the broadest spectrums of any penicillin. Approved in 1976, it has been used to treat moderate to severe gram-negative infections of the skin, blood, bone and joints, CNS, respiratory tract, and genitourinary tract. Available by the IV route, high doses can lead to hypernatremia, platelet dysfunction, and hypokalemia. Electrolytes should be regularly monitored to prevent hypokalemia and hypernatremia. Ticarcillin has a high sodium content that could affect patients with preexisting heart disease. Ticarcillin should not be administered to patients with hypersensitivity to any penicillin. Pain and phlebitis with thrombosis may occur at the injection site. To increase its effectiveness, it is combined with clavulanate.

Penicillinase-Resistant (Antistaphylococcal) Penicillins

This subclass of penicillins includes dicloxacillin, nafcillin, and oxacillin, which are drugs that are effective against penicillinase-producing bacteria. These medications are less effective than penicillin G against nonpenicillinase-producing strains and are ineffective against gram-negative bacteria. This narrow spectrum of activity has largely restricted their use to penicillinase-producing strains of *Staphylococcus*. Because they are often the preferred drugs for infections by this organism, they are referred to as antistaphylococcal penicillins. An older drug in this class, cloxacillin (Cloxapen), is no longer marketed in the United States.

The emergence of many methicillin-resistant *S. aureus* (MRSA) strains has limited the use of drugs in this class. As discussed in Chapter 46, the appearance of MRSA strains that are resistant to all penicillins is an emerging clinical problem. The first drug developed in the penicillinase-resistant class, called methicillin, was removed from the U.S. market for producing an unacceptable incidence of interstitial nephritis.

Drugs in the penicillinase-resistant class share similar actions and properties with penicillin G. Dicloxacillin is readily absorbed by the PO route, whereas nafcillin and oxacillin are given parenterally. They are rapidly excreted by the kidneys, having a half-life of 30 to 60 minutes. As with all penicillins, hypersensitivity reactions may occur. Some of these drugs are sodium salts, which may cause sodium overload in susceptible patients. PMC has been reported in a small number of patients taking these drugs. All are pregnancy category B drugs.

Dicloxacillin: Approved in 1968, dicloxacillin is a penicillinase-resistant penicillin available by the PO route. As with other drugs in this class, its use is primarily limited to the treatment of susceptible staphylococcal infections. It is not effective against MRSA. Nausea and vomiting are commonly reported adverse effects. It should be taken on an empty stomach to enhance absorption. Other adverse effects and contraindications are the same as those of other penicillins. This drug should not be given to a patient with hypersensitivity to any penicillin.

Nafcillin: Approved in 1964, nafcillin is used to treat susceptible infections of the blood, skin, upper and lower respiratory tract, bone and joints, and urinary tract. It is ineffective against MRSA infections. Unlike most penicillins, nafcillin is excreted primarily in the bile; thus dosage adjustments for patients with hepatic disease are necessary. It is available in both oral and parenteral formulations. Because only 10% to 20% of the drug is absorbed when given PO, it is normally given parenterally. The complete blood count (CBC) must be regularly monitored because nafcillin can cause neutropenia and other blood abnormalities in 10% to 20% of the patients taking it. This drug should not be given to a patient with hypersensitivity to any penicillin.

Oxacillin: Approved in 1962, oxacillin is used to treat a variety of staphylococcal infections of the blood, skin, upper and lower respiratory tract, bone and joints, and urinary tract. It is ineffective against MRSA infections. Because oxacillin causes fewer injection-site reactions than nafcillin, it is sometimes the parenteral drug of choice in its class. Indications and adverse effects are similar to those of other penicillinase-resistant penicillins. This drug should not be given to a patient with hypersensitivity to any penicillin.

CONNECTIONS | Lifespan Considerations

◀ Antibiotic Use and the Cost Burden for the Older Adult

Older adults may forego filling an expensive antibiotic prescription due to lack of adequate drug coverage on their insurance. Studies have noted that as the cost of the drug and the amount of cost sharing (copay) required increases, the number of prescriptions filled decreases. As with other drugs, newer antibiotics may be costly, and an older generic version may not be available to treat the infection. Because the older adult may not exhibit the same symptoms of an infection as a younger patient will, an untreated infection may quickly become more serious. Recent changes to Medicare and the implementation of the drug benefit (Part D) portion may increase the number of prescriptions filled. In a recent study, Zhang, Lee, and Donohue (2010) noted that as Medicare drug coverage improved, older adults increased their use of broad-spectrum, newer, and more expensive antibiotics. While this may be a double-edged sword with inappropriate use also occurring, it lessens the chance that an infection will remain untreated due to cost concerns.

Cephalosporins

47.3 The cephalosporins are similar in structure and function to the penicillins and are widely prescribed for gram-negative infections.

Isolated shortly after penicillin, the cephalosporins comprise the largest antibiotic class. Like the penicillins, many cephalosporins contain a beta-lactam ring that is responsible for their antimicrobial activity. In some cephalosporins, the structure of the beta-lactam ring is quite stable and resistant to enzyme destruction. The cephalosporins are bacteriocidal and inhibit cell wall synthesis by binding to PBPs. Growing bacterial cells are unable to build their cell walls properly, and lysis occurs in the same manner as penicillins. The cephalosporins are listed in Table 47.2.

The primary therapeutic use of the cephalosporins is for gram-negative infections and for patients who are allergic to penicillin or who have penicillin-resistant infections. Over 20 cephalosporins are available, all having similar sounding names that can challenge even the best memory. Selection of a specific cephalosporin is first

TABLE 47.2   Cephalosporins

Drug	Route and Adult Dose (Maximum Dose Where Indicated)	Adverse Effects
First Generation		
cefadroxil (Duricef)	PO: 500 mg–1 g once or twice a day (max: 2 g/day)	*Diarrhea, abdominal cramping, nausea, fatigue, rash, pruritus, pain at injection site, oral or vaginal candidiasis*
cefazolin (Ancef, Kefzol)	IM/IV: 250 mg–2 g tid (max: 12 g/day)	
cephalexin (Keflex)	PO: 250–500 mg qid (max: 4 g/day)	PMC, nephrotoxicity, anaphylaxis
Second Generation		
cefaclor (Ceclor)	PO: 250–500 mg tid (max: 2 g/day)	
cefotetan (Cefotan)	IV/IM: 1–2 g every 12 h (max: 6 g/day)	
cefoxitin (Mefoxin)	IV/IM: 1–2 g every 6–8 h (max: 12 g/day)	
cefprozil (Cefzil)	PO: 250–500 mg 1–2 times/day (max: 1 g/day)	
cefuroxime (Ceftin, Zinacef)	PO (Ceftin): 250–500 mg bid (max: 1 g/day) IM/IV (Zinacef): 750 mg–1.5 g every 8 h (max: 9 g/day)	
Third Generation		
cefdinir (Omnicef)	PO: 300 mg bid (max: 600 mg/day)	
cefditoren (Spectracef)	PO: 400 mg bid for 10 days (max: 800 mg/day)	
cefixime (Suprax)	PO: 400 mg/day or 200 mg bid (max: 800 mg/day)	
cefotaxime (Claforan)	IM: 1–2 g bid–tid (max: 12 g/day)	
cefpodoxime (Vantin)	PO: 200 mg every 12 h for 10 days (max: 800 mg/day)	
ceftazidime (Fortaz, Tazicef)	IV/IM: 1–2 mg every 8–12 h (max: 6 g/day)	
ceftibuten (Cedax)	PO: 400 mg/day for 10 days (max: 400 mg/day)	
ceftizoxime (Cefizox)	IV/IM: 1–2 g every 8–12 h, up to 2 g every 4 h (max: 12 g/day)	
ceftriaxone (Rocephin)	IV/IM: 1–2 g every 12–24 h (max: 4 g/day)	
Fourth Generation		
cefepime (Maxipime)	IV/IM: 0.5–1 g every 12 h for 7–10 days (max: 6 g/day)	
Fifth Generation		
ceftaroline (Teflaro)	IV: 600 mg every 12 h for 5–14 days	

Note: Italics indicate common adverse effects. Underline indicates serious adverse effects.

based on the sensitivity of the pathogen, and secondly on possible adverse effects.

The cephalosporins are classified chronologically by their generations, which are loosely based on differences in their spectrums of microbial activity. It is important to note that the placement of a drug in a particular generation is somewhat arbitrary and has little therapeutic usefulness. Drugs within each generation have different chemical structures, routes of administration, and spectrums of activity. Scientists do not always agree on placement. The following generalizations may be made regarding the generations:

- First-generation cephalosporins contain a beta-lactam ring; bacteria that produce beta lactamase are usually resistant to these drugs. They are the most effective cephalosporins against gram-positive bacteria, including staphylococci and streptococci and are sometimes the preferred drugs for these organisms. First-generation cephalosporins have only moderate activity against gram-negative bacteria. First-generation drugs do not cross the blood–brain barrier to any appreciable extent.

- Second-generation cephalosporins exhibit a broader spectrum against gram-negative organisms than do the first-generation drugs. They are more potent and less sensitive to beta lactamase than the first-generation drugs. Like the first-generation agents, however, they are unable to enter the CSF in sufficient concentration to treat infections of the CNS. In general, the second-generation drugs have largely been replaced by third-generation cephalosporins.

- Third-generation cephalosporins exhibit an even broader spectrum against gram-negative bacteria than the second-generation group. They generally have a longer duration of action and are resistant to beta lactamase. These cephalosporins are sometimes the preferred drugs against infections by *Pseudomonas, Klebsiella, Neisseria, Salmonella, Proteus,* and *H. influenzae.* Third-generation drugs are able to enter the CSF to treat CNS infections.

- Fourth-generation cephalosporins have a similar antimicrobial spectrum to third-generation agents but are more effective against organisms that have developed resistance to earlier cephalosporins. Fourth-generation drugs are capable of entering the CSF in sufficiently high concentrations to treat CNS infections.

- Fifth-generation cephalosporins are broad-spectrum drugs with extended gram-positive effectiveness. They are designed to be effective against MRSA infections. This generation is still in development and the first drug, ceftaroline, was approved in 2010.

CONNECTION Checkpoint 47.2

From what you learned in Chapter 46, what is the primary difference in physiology that distinguishes a gram-positive organism from a gram-negative organism? *See Answer to Connection Checkpoint 47.2 on student resource website.*

Over decades of use, many bacterial strains have developed resistance to the cephalosporins. Like the penicillins, the primary mechanism of resistance is the secretion of beta-lactamase enzymes (sometimes called cephalosporinases). Although third-generation agents were initially unaffected by beta lactamase, resistant strains that can inactivate drugs in this generation have been identified.

None of the cephalosporins has significant activity against MRSA or penicillin-resistant *Streptococcus pneumoniae.*

In general, the cephalosporins are safe drugs with adverse effects similar to those of the penicillins. Allergic reactions are the most common adverse effect. Although sometimes prescribed for patients who are allergic to penicillin, nurses must be aware that 5% to 10% of the patients who are allergic to penicillin will also exhibit hypersensitivity to cephalosporins. Despite this small incidence of cross-allergy, the cephalosporins offer a reasonable alternative for patients who are unable to take penicillin. Cephalosporins are contraindicated, however, for patients who have experienced anaphylaxis following penicillin exposure.

In addition to allergy, rash and GI complaints are common adverse effects of cephalosporins. Nurses should continually assess for the presence of superinfections. Because cephalosporins are secreted in small amounts in breast milk, they should be used with caution in nursing mothers.

Nearly all cephalosporins are eliminated by the kidneys. Earlier-generation cephalosporins exhibited kidney toxicity but this is diminished with the later-generation drugs in this class. Patients with preexisting renal impairment or those who are concurrently receiving nephrotoxic drugs should be monitored carefully during therapy with any cephalosporin. Kidney function tests should be evaluated on a regular basis.

Other adverse effects are specific to particular cephalosporins. For example, cefotetan interferes with vitamin K metabolism and increases the risk of bleeding due to hypoprothrombinemia. Nurses must carefully monitor prothrombin time (PT) in patients taking these drugs, particularly those who are concurrently taking anticoagulants. Cefotetan produces a disulfiram-like reaction when taken concurrently with alcohol. Cephalosporins cause pain at IM injection sites, and thrombophlebitis can occur when given IV. Over half of the cephalosporins are only administered parenterally.

PROTOTYPE DRUG	Cefazolin (Ancef, Kefzol)

Classification: Therapeutic: Antibacterial
Pharmacologic: Cell wall inhibitor, first-generation cephalosporin

Therapeutic Effects and Uses: Approved in 1973, cefazolin is a beta-lactam antibiotic used for the treatment and prophylaxis of bacterial infections, particularly those that are caused by susceptible gram-positive organisms. Its effectiveness extends to nonpenicillinase- and penicillinase-producing *S. aureus* and streptococci (except enterococci). Cefazolin is not effective against MRSA. Cefazolin has been used to treat infections of the respiratory tract, urinary tract, skin structures, biliary tract, bones, and joints. It has also been useful in the pharmacotherapy of genital infections, septicemia, and endocarditis. This drug is sometimes used for infection prophylaxis in patients who are undergoing surgical procedures. Cefazolin has a longer half-life than other first-generation cephalosporins, which allows for less frequent dosing. It is one of the most frequently prescribed parenteral antibiotics.

Mechanism of Action: Cefazolin inhibits bacterial wall synthesis by binding to specific PBPs. The drug is bacteriocidal, exhibits a broad spectrum, and is sensitive to beta lactamase.

Pharmacokinetics:

Route(s)	IM and IV
Absorption	Well absorbed when given IM
Distribution	Widely distributed; only small amounts cross the blood–brain barrier; crosses the placenta; secreted in breast milk; about 85% bound to plasma protein
Primary metabolism	Not metabolized
Primary excretion	Renal
Onset of action	Immediate
Duration of action	Half-life: 90–135 min

Adverse Effects: Like the penicillins, the cephalosporins are well tolerated by most patients. Rash and diarrhea are the most common adverse effects, and superinfections are likely when the antibiotic is used for prolonged periods. Approximately 1% to 4% of patients will experience some kind of an allergic reaction. Severe hypersensitivity reactions are rare, though potentially fatal. Anaphylactic response may include cardiovascular collapse; edema of the mouth, tongue, pharynx, and larynx; confusion; seizures; and hallucinations. Pain and phlebitis can occur at IM injection sites. However, cefazolin causes less pain than do other cephalosporins. Seizures are a rare, though potentially serious, adverse effect of cephalosporin therapy.

Contraindications/Precautions: Cefazolin is contraindicated in patients who are allergic to any drug in the cephalosporin class and is used cautiously in those with hypersensitivity to penicillins. Because most cefazolin is excreted unchanged by the kidneys, patients with significant renal impairment must be carefully monitored.

Drug Interactions: Probenecid decreases the excretion of cefazolin and can lead to antibiotic toxicity. Concurrent use of cefazolin with nephrotoxic drugs, such as aminoglycosides or vancomycin, increases the risk of nephrotoxicity. Cefazolin may have additive or synergistic antimicrobial action with other antibiotics such as aztreonam, carbapenems, and the penicillins. The anticoagulant effect of warfarin may be increased if given concurrently with cefazolin.

Herbal/Food: None known.

Pregnancy: Category B.

Treatment of Overdose: No specific therapy is available. Patients are treated symptomatically.

Nursing Responsibilities (includes all generations of cephalosporins): Key nursing implications for patients receiving cefazolin are included in the Nursing Practice Application for Patients Receiving Pharmacotherapy with a Penicillin, Cephalosporin, or Vancomycin Antibiotic.

Drugs Similar to Cefazolin (Ancef, Kefzol)

First generation: Other first-generation cephalosporins include cefadroxil (Duricef) and cephalexin (Keflex). These drugs are administered parenterally and have the same spectrum of microbial activity. They have the same basic indications (primarily gram-positive bacteria) and are eliminated by the kidneys. Cephradine (Velosef) is no longer available in the United States.

Second generation: Second-generation cephalosporins include cefaclor (Ceclor), cefotetan (Cefotan), cefoxitin (Mefoxin), cefprozil (Cefzil), and cefuroxime (Ceftin, Zinacef). All have the same spectrum of microbial activity and there is little difference among the drugs other than the route of administration (see Table 47.2). The kidneys eliminate all second-generation cephalosporins. Cefoxitin and cefotetan are the most active against *Bacteroides fragilis*.

Third generation: Third-generation cephalosporins are the largest group and include cefdinir (Omnicef), cefditoren (Spectracef), cefixime (Suprax), cefotaxime (Claforan), cefpodoxime (Vantin), ceftazidime (Fortaz, Tazicef), ceftibuten (Cedax), ceftizoxime (Cefizox), and ceftriaxone (Rocephin). The differences among third-generation cephalosporins are minor. Some are available by the PO route, whereas others are given only parenterally (see Table 47.2). Cefixime and ceftriaxone have longer durations that allow for once-daily dosing. Ceftazidime is one of the few third-generation drugs with significant activity against *P. aeruginosa*. Cefotaxime is a preferred drug for certain types of meningitis and for infection prophylaxis in patients who are undergoing surgical procedures. Cefoperazone (Cefobid) is no longer available in the United States.

Fourth generation: Cefepime (Maxipime) is the only drug in this generation. It is very similar to the third-generation drugs but appears to have a slightly broader spectrum of activity and is more stable against beta lactamase–producing organisms. It has been used for the treatment of serious infections in hospitalized patients with gram-positive microorganisms such as *Enterobacteriaceae* and *Pseudomonas*. It is not effective against MRSA.

Fifth generation: Ceftaroline (Teflaro), the first drug in this generation, was approved by the FDA in 2010 for acute bacterial

---

CONNECTIONS ‹ **Community-Oriented Practice**

‹ **Risk Factors for Pseudomembranous Colitis**

Clostridium difficile–associated diarrhea (CDAD) and pseudomembranous colitis (PMC), progressing from CDAD, are significant infections related to antibiotic use. They account for the majority of HAI diarrheal infections with an increase in mortality rate associated with these infections. PMC may be recurrent and the older adult is particularly at risk for CDAD and PMC. Symptoms include watery diarrhea with up to 5 to 10 or more occurrences per day, abdominal cramping, fever, blood and mucus in the stool, and dehydration. While it has long been recognized that the overuse of antibiotics, either prophylactically, at high doses, or beyond the time required to adequately treat the infection, contributes to CDAD and PMC, there are other risk factors. Proton pump inhibitors (PPIs), which lower gastric acidity, contribute to a favorable environment for *C. difficile*. Patients receiving tube feedings with elemental diets (i.e., without fiber, fructose, starches, or probiotics) are also at risk. O'Keefe (2010) recommends that the critically ill ICU patient be assessed for the need for prophylactic antibiotics, PPIs, or elemental tube feedings and that there be judicious use of broad-spectrum antibiotics as methods to reduce CDAD and PMC. When necessary, elemental tube feeding diets should be changed to those containing more healthful ingredients such as fiber, and PPIs should be limited to confirmed cases of hyperacidity. All patients on high-dose, broad-spectrum, or long-term antibiotics should be carefully monitored for the development of CDAD and PMC.

skin and skin structure infections and community-acquired bacterial pneumonia. It is effective against a broad spectrum of both gram-positive and gram-negative organisms, including MRSA. Available by the IV route, it is relatively safe, with the most common adverse effects being diarrhea, nausea, and rash.

Carbapenems

47.4 The carbapenems are resistant to beta lactamase and are broad-spectrum alternatives to penicillin.

Although the penicillins and cephalosporins comprise the largest groups of drugs affecting the bacterial cell wall, several other antibacterials also act by this mechanism. Doses of these drugs are listed in Table 47.3.

Imipenem (Primaxin), ertapenem (Invanz), doripenem (Doribax), and meropenem (Merrem IV) belong to a class of antibiotics called carbapenems. These drugs are bacteriocidal and have some of the broadest antimicrobial spectrums of any class of antibiotics. They contain a beta-lactam ring and kill bacteria by inhibiting construction of the cell wall. Though similar, the ring in carbapenems has a slightly different structure than other beta-lactam antibiotics that makes it very resistant to destruction by beta lactamase. These factors allow the carbapenems to provide better activity against serious gram-negative and multidrug-resistant infections than most cephalosporins or penicillins. A disadvantage is that they must be given parenterally. The primary role of the carbapenems is for the treatment of complicated bacterial infections. They are sometimes considered the antibiotics of "last resort" for treating multidrug-resistant infections.

All the carbapenems exhibit a low incidence of adverse effects. Diarrhea, nausea, rashes, and thrombophlebitis at injection sites are the most common adverse effects.

In recent years, bacteria have been isolated that are resistant to the carbapenems. These infections, called carbapenem-resistant *Enterobacteriaceae* (CRE), are usually health care associated and can be highly lethal.

PROTOTYPE DRUG | **Imipenem-Cilastatin (Primaxin)**

Classification: Therapeutic: Antibacterial
Pharmacologic: Cell wall inhibitor, carbapenem

Therapeutic Effects and Uses: Approved in 1985, imipenem is used for the treatment and prophylaxis of susceptible bacterial infections. Imipenem has a very broad antimicrobial spectrum and is the most widely used carbapenem. Because of its broad spectrum and beta-lactamase resistance, it is effective against most gram-positive and gram-negative microbes, including anaerobic bacteria. It is particularly useful for mixed infections containing both aerobic and anaerobic organisms, including those with *S. aureus. P. aeruginosa* and strains of MRSA are also susceptible to imipenem.

Although imipenem contains a beta-lactam ring, it is resistant to the actions of beta lactamase. This drug, however, is rapidly destroyed by dipeptidase, an enzyme found in the kidney tubules. Concurrent administration of the drug cilastatin, a renal dipeptidase inhibitor, with imipenem prevents the destruction of imipenem and allows for higher serum levels of the antibiotic. Cilastatin possesses no antimicrobial activity of its own. Imipenem is only marketed with cilastatin in a fixed-dose combination (Primaxin).

Primaxin is sometimes combined with antibiotics from other classes, such as the aminoglycosides or cephalosporins, when

---

TABLE 47.3 Carbapenems and Miscellaneous Cell Wall Inhibitors

Drug	Route and Adult Dose (Maximum Dose Where Indicated)	Adverse Effects
Carbapenems		
doripenem (Doribax)	IV: 500 mg every 8 h for 5–14 days (max: 500 mg every 8 h)	*Nausea, diarrhea, headache*
ertapenem (Invanz)	IV/IM: 1 g/day	Anaphylaxis, superinfections, PMC, confusion, seizures
imipenem-cilastatin (Primaxin)	IV: 250–500 mg tid–qid (max: 4 g/day)	
meropenem (Merrem)	IV: 1–2 g tid (max: 2 g tid)	
Miscellaneous Cell Wall Inhibitors		
aztreonam (Azactam, Cayston)	IM (Azactam): 0.5–2 g bid–qid (max: 8 g/day) Inhalation (Cayston): one vial in nebulizer tid for 28 days	*Nausea, vomiting, rash, thrombophlebitis (Azactam); cough, nasal congestion, wheezing (Cayston)* Anaphylaxis, superinfections, bronchospasm (Cayston)
fosfomycin (Monurol)	PO: 3 g sachet dissolved in 3–4 oz of water as a single dose	*Nausea, diarrhea, back pain, headache* Anaphylaxis, superinfections
telavancin (Vibativ)	IV: 10 mg administered over 60 min, once daily for 7–10 days	*Nausea, vomiting and foamy urine* Nephrotoxicity, QT interval prolongation, infusion-related reactions, birth defects
vancomycin (Vancocin)	IV: 500 mg qid; 1 g bid PO: 500 mg–2.0 g in three to four divided doses for 7–10 days	*Nausea, vomiting* Anaphylaxis, superinfections, nephrotoxicity, ototoxicity, red man syndrome

Note: Italics indicate common adverse effects. Underline indicates serious adverse effects.

treating *P. aeruginosa* infections. Primaxin has a short half-life that requires administration every 6 hours.

Mechanism of Action: Imipenem inhibits bacterial wall synthesis by binding to specific PBPs. Cilastatin blocks renal dipeptidase, which is the enzyme primarily responsible for the excretion of imipenem. The combination of imipenem-cilastatin is bacteriocidal.

Pharmacokinetics:

Route(s)	IM and IV
Absorption	Not absorbed PO
Distribution	Widely distributed, including in the CSF; secreted in breast milk; both imipenem and cilastatin cross the placenta
Primary metabolism	Hepatic
Primary excretion	Renal
Onset of action	IM: rapid; IV: immediate
Duration of action	Half-life: 1 h

Adverse Effects: The most frequent adverse effects of imipenem-cilastatin include nausea, vomiting, diarrhea, rash, and pain and phlebitis at the injection site. Rare, though serious, reactions include confusion, seizures, hallucinations, PMC, and anaphylaxis. Anaphylactic response may include cardiovascular collapse and edema of the mouth, tongue, pharynx, and larynx.

Contraindications/Precautions: Imipenem-cilastatin is contraindicated in patients who have experienced a severe allergic reaction to this drug, other carbapenems, cephalosporins, or penicillins. Because the kidneys excrete imipenem-cilastatin, patients with significant renal impairment must be carefully monitored and dosages lowered. This drug should be used cautiously in patients with brain lesions, head trauma, or a history of seizures due to an increased risk of seizures.

Drug Interactions: Certain other antibiotics, including penicillins, cephalosporins, and aztreonam antagonize the antimicrobial effects of imipenem-cilastatin; therefore, they should not be given concurrently. Concurrent use with cyclosporine, tramadol, theophylline, or ganciclovir may increase the risk of seizures and other CNS effects. Iminipenum-cilastatin decreases levels of valproic acid, resulting in seizures. **Herbal/Food**: None known.

Pregnancy: Category C.

Treatment of Overdose: Overdose may result in ataxia and seizures. Patients are treated symptomatically.

Nursing Responsibilities: Key nursing implications for patients receiving imipenem-cilastatin are included in the Nursing Practice Application for Patients Receiving Pharmacotherapy with a Penicillin, Cephalosporin, or Vancomycin Antibiotic.

Drugs Similar to Imipenem-Cilastatin (Primaxin)

Other carbapenems include doripenem, ertapenem, and meropenem.

Doripenem (Doribax): Doripenem (Doribax) is a newer drug in this class that was approved in 2007. It is similar to meropenem and has activity against both gram-positive and gram-negative organisms.

It is approved to treat complicated intra-abdominal infections and urinary tract infections (UTIs). It is administered by IV infusion over 60 minutes. Common adverse effects include headache, rash, nausea, vomiting, diarrhea, and phlebitis. Doripenem is contraindicated in patients who have experienced a severe allergic reaction to other carbapenems, cephalosporins, or penicillins. This drug is pregnancy category B.

Ertapenem (Invanz): A newer drug in this class, ertapenem, has a narrower spectrum than the other carbapenems, being active primarily against gram-negative aerobes. Its major advantage is its longer half-life, which allows for once-daily dosing. It is approved for the treatment of serious abdominopelvic and skin infections, community-acquired pneumonia, complicated UTIs, and diabetic foot infections without concomitant osteomyelitis. It is administered by the IV and IM routes. Adverse effects are similar to those of other carbapenems. Ertapenem is contraindicated in patients who have experienced a severe allergic reaction to other carbapenems, cephalosporins, or penicillins. This drug is pregnancy category B.

Meropenem (Merrem): Approved in 1996, meropenem has a similar spectrum of activity to imipenem, although it is only approved for peritonitis and skin and skin structure infections in adults and bacterial meningitis in children. The drug is used off-label for other indications. The antimicrobial spectrum of activity of meropenem is similar to that of imipenem. Meropenem may be more active against *Enterobacteriaceae*, gonococcus, *H. influenzae*, and *P. aeruginosa*. This drug is not destroyed by renal dipeptidase, so it is not administered with cilastatin. Adverse effects are similar to those of imipenem. Meropenem is contraindicated in patients who have experienced a severe allergic reaction to other carbapenems, cephalosporins, or penicillins. It is only available by the IV route. Bolus injections are given IV over 3 to 5 minutes, and infusions over 15 to 30 minutes. This drug is pregnancy category B.

PharmFACT

Central-line associated bloodstream infections are a deadly form of HAI with a mortality rate of 12% to 24%. The number of these infections declined from 43,000 in 2001 to 18,000 in 2009 (CDC, 2011).

Miscellaneous Cell Wall Inhibitors

47.5 Several miscellaneous cell wall inhibitors have activity against resistant microbes.

Several other cell wall inhibitors have important roles in the pharmacotherapy of infections. These agents are either new drugs or the only medication in a class.

PROTOTYPE DRUG	Vancomycin (Vancocin)

Classification: **Therapeutic:** Antibacterial
Pharmacologic: Cell wall inhibitor

Therapeutic Effects and Uses: Approved in 1964, vancomycin (Vancocin) is used for the treatment and prophylaxis of susceptible bacterial infections. It is effective against most gram-positive organisms, including *Streptococcus*, *Corynebacterium*, *Clostridium*, *Listeria*, and *Bacillus* species. Vancomycin is usually administered by slow IV infusion for systemic infections because it is not well absorbed from the GI tract. It has been administered off-label by the intrathecal or intraventricular route to treat meningitis. Oral vancomycin is approved for the treatment of antibiotic-induced PMC, which is caused by a toxin produced by *C. difficile*. When given orally, the drug acts locally in the intestine and very little is absorbed into the systemic circulation.

Current protocols restrict the use of vancomycin to severe infections that have become resistant to safer antibiotics. It is anticipated that this restriction will discourage or delay the appearance of resistant strains. Because vancomycin was used infrequently during the first 30 years following its discovery, the incidence of vancomycin-resistant organisms has been less than that of other antibiotics. Vancomycin is the most effective drug for treating MRSA infections. Vancomycin-resistant strains of *S. aureus*, however, have begun to appear in recent years. Vancomycin is often considered a "last resort" antibiotic. Therapeutic options for vancomycin-resistant infections are limited.

Mechanism of Action: Although vancomycin kills bacteria mainly by inhibiting bacterial cell wall synthesis, it also affects the plasma membrane and interferes with ribonucleic acid (RNA) synthesis. The fact that it has multiple mechanisms is probably responsible for the low rate of resistance from the drug. It is bacteriocidal and only effective against gram-positive organisms such as *S. aureus* and *S. pneumoniae*.

Pharmacokinetics:

Route(s)	IV, PO
Absorption	Poorly absorbed PO
Distribution	Oral form does not usually enter systemic circulation; IV form is widely distributed with small amounts in the CSF; secreted in breast milk; 55% bound to plasma proteins
Primary metabolism	Probably not metabolized
Primary excretion	Renal
Onset of action	IV: immediate
Duration of action	Half-life: 4–8 h

Adverse Effects: Vancomycin may cause a syndrome of flushing, hypotension, tachycardia, and rash on the upper body, a condition called the red man syndrome. This syndrome can be minimized by infusing the drug over at least 60 minutes. Other common adverse effects include nausea, rash, fever, and chills. Serious adverse effects include confusion, seizures, and hallucinations. If extravasation occurs, it may lead to tissue necrosis. Ototoxicity is associated with serum concentrations of vancomycin above 60 to 80 mcg/mL. Tinnitus and high-tone hearing loss precede deafness and may progress even after this drug is discontinued. The most susceptible are older adults and those on high doses. Nephrotoxicity can occur in patients with therapeutic concentrations but is more common if trough serum concentrations are kept above 10 mcg/mL. Anaphylactic response may include cardiovascular collapse or edema of the mouth, tongue, pharynx, and larynx.

Contraindications/Precautions: Vancomycin is contraindicated in patients who have experienced previous hypersensitivity to this drug. The nurse must monitor drug therapy carefully in patients with impaired renal function and those with a history of hearing loss.

Drug Interactions: Vancomycin adds to toxicity of aminoglycosides, amphotericin B, cisplatin, cyclosporine, polymyxin B, and other ototoxic and nephrotoxic medications. Vancomycin may increase the risk of lactic acidosis when administered with metformin, especially in patients with renal impairment. **Herbal/Food**: Unknown.

Pregnancy: Category C.

Treatment of Overdose: Because overdose may result in renal impairment, patients are treated supportively to maintain kidney function.

Nursing Responsibilities: Key nursing implications for patients receiving vancomycin are included in the Nursing Practice Application for Patients Receiving Pharmacotherapy with a Penicillin, Cephalosporin, or Vancomycin Antibiotic.

Drugs Similar to Vancomycin (Vancocin)

Other miscellaneous cell wall inhibitors include aztreonam, fosfomycin, and telavancin.

Aztreonam (Azactam, Cayston): Approved in 1986, aztreonam has a beta-lactam ring and belongs to a newer class of antibiotics known as monobactams. Like other cell wall inhibitors, aztreonam binds to specific penicillin-binding proteins to cause a bacteriocidal effect. Although considered narrow-spectrum antibiotics, monobactams are particularly useful against certain gram-negative aerobes, such as *P. aeruginosa*. Other organisms considered susceptible to aztreonam include *Citrobacter*, *Enterobacter*, *E. coli*, *H. influenzae*, *Neisseria*, *Proteus*, *Providencia rettgeri*, and *Shigella*. Monobactams have little or no activity against gram-positive bacteria or anaerobes. Although they have beta-lactam rings, they do not exhibit cross-hypersensitivity with penicillins or cephalosporins. Azactam is administered by the parenteral route and exhibits similar adverse effects as those of other cell wall inhibitors including nausea, vomiting, diarrhea, superinfections such as vaginal candidiasis, and local pain or phlebitis at the injection site. Anaphylaxis and PMC are rare. An inhalation form of the drug, Cayston, was approved in 2010 to improve respiratory symptoms in patients with cystic fibrosis who have *P. aeruginosa* infection. This drug is pregnancy category B.

Fosfomycin (Monurol): Approved in 1996, fosfomycin is a cell wall inhibitor that is currently approved for the treatment of uncomplicated UTI and bladder infections in women caused by *E. coli* and *Enterococcus faecalis*. It is given as an oral powder, which is mixed with water and taken PO as a single dose. Adverse effects are minor and include asthenia, nausea, vomiting, diarrhea, headache, and vaginitis. This drug is pregnancy category B.

Telavancin (Vibativ): Approved in 2009, telavancin is a synthetic derivative of vancomycin that acts by inhibiting the polymerization and cross-linking of peptidoglycan in bacterial cell walls. It is approved as a once-daily IV infusion for the treatment of complicated skin and skin structure infections caused by gram-negative bacteria, including MRSA. Common adverse effects include taste disturbances, nausea, vomiting, and foamy urine. Telavancin is nephrotoxic and kidney function should be monitored during therapy. Telavancin prolongs the QT interval and it should be used with caution with other medications that cause this effect. This drug is pregnancy category B.

CONNECTIONS: NURSING PRACTICE APPLICATION

Patients Receiving Pharmacotherapy with a Penicillin, Cephalosporin, or Vancomycin Antibiotic

Assessment	Potential Nursing Diagnoses*
Baseline assessment prior to administration: • Obtain a complete health history including neurologic, cardiovascular, respiratory, hepatic, or renal disease, and the possibility of pregnancy. Obtain a drug history including allergies, specific reactions to drugs, current prescription and over-the-counter (OTC) drugs, herbal preparations, and alcohol use. Be alert to possible drug interactions. • Assess signs and symptoms of the current infection, noting location, characteristics (what it looks like), presence or absence of drainage and the character of drainage, duration, and the presence or absence of fever or pain. • Evaluate appropriate laboratory findings (e.g., CBC, C&S, hepatic and renal function studies). • Assess the patient's ability to receive and understand instructions. Include family and caregivers as needed.	• *Acute Pain* • *Hyperthermia* • *Deficient Knowledge* (Drug Therapy) • *Risk for Injury*, related to adverse drug effects • *Risk for Deficient Fluid Volume*, related to fever and/or diarrhea caused by adverse drug effects
Assessment throughout administration: • Assess for desired therapeutic effects (e.g., diminished signs and symptoms of infection and fever). • Continue periodic monitoring of CBC, hepatic and renal function, urinalysis, and C&S as ordered. • Assess for adverse effects: nausea, vomiting, abdominal cramping, diarrhea, drowsiness, or dizziness. Severe diarrhea, especially containing mucus, blood, or pus; yellowing of the sclera or skin; decreased urine output; or darkened urine should be reported immediately.	

Implementation

Interventions and (Rationales)	Patient-Centered Care
Ensuring therapeutic effects: • Continue assessments as above for therapeutic effects. (Diminished fever, pain, or signs and symptoms of infection should begin after taking the first dose and continue to improve. The provider should be notified if fever and signs and symptoms of infection remain or increase after 3 days or if the entire course of antibacterial has been taken and signs of infection are still present.)	• Teach the patient to complete the entire course of antibacterial therapy; to not share doses with other family members with similar symptoms; and to return to the provider if symptoms have not resolved after an entire course of therapy.
Minimizing adverse effects: • Continue to monitor vital signs, especially temperature if fever is present. Immediately report undiminished fever, changes in level of consciousness (LOC), or febrile seizures to the health care provider. (Continued fever may be a sign of worsening infection, adverse drug effects, or antibiotic resistance.)	• Teach the patient to report fever that does not diminish below 37.8°C (100°F) or per parameters set by the health care provider within 3 days, increasing signs and symptoms of infection, or symptoms that remain after taking the entire course of antibacterial therapy. Immediately report febrile seizures, changes in behavior, or changes in LOC to the health care provider.
• Continue to monitor periodic laboratory work: renal function tests, CBC, urinalysis, and C&S as ordered. (Penicillins and cephalosporins may be renal toxic. Periodic C&S tests may be ordered if infections are severe or slow to resolve to confirm appropriate therapy.)	• Instruct the patient on the need for periodic laboratory work.
• Monitor for hypersensitivity and allergic reactions, especially with the first dose of the drug. Continue to monitor the patient for up to 2 weeks after completing antibacterial therapy. (Anaphylactic reactions are possible, particularly with the first dose of an antibacterial. Post-use, residual drug levels, dependent on length of half-life, may cause delayed reactions.)	• Teach the patient to immediately report any itching, rashes, swelling (particularly of tongue or face), urticaria, flushing, dizziness, syncope, wheezing, throat tightness, or difficulty breathing. • Instruct the patient with known antibacterial allergies to carry a wallet identification card or wear medical identification jewelry indicating allergy.
• Continue to monitor for renal toxicity; e.g., darkened urine, diminished urine output, or weight gain greater than 1 kg (2 lbs) in 24 hours. (Penicillins and cephalosporins may require frequent monitoring to prevent adverse effects. **Lifespan:** Age-related physiological differences may place the young child or older adult at greater-risk for renal toxicity.)	• Teach the patient to immediately report any diminished urine output, weight gain of more than 1 kg (2 lbs) in a 24 h period, darkening of urine. • Advise the patient to increase fluid intake to 2–3 L/day if permitted.
• Monitor for development of superinfections, e.g., CDAD or PMC, fungal or yeast infections. (Superinfections with opportunistic organisms may occur when normal host flora are diminished or killed by the antibacterial drug. Severe diarrhea may indicate the presence of CDAD or PMC, superinfections caused by *C. difficile*.)	• Instruct the patient to report any diarrhea that increases in frequency or amount, or contains mucus, blood, or pus. • Instruct the patient to consult the health care provider before taking any antidiarrheal drugs that slow gastric motility because these may cause the retention of harmful bacteria.

CONNECTIONS: NURSING PRACTICE APPLICATION (continued)

	• Teach the patient to observe for changes in stool, white patches in the mouth, whitish thick vaginal discharge, itching in the urogenital area, or blistering itchy rash, and to immediately report severe diarrhea. • Teach the patient infection control measures such as frequent hand washing, allowing for adequate drying after showering or bathing, and to increase intake of live-culture dairy foods.
• Monitor for signs and symptoms of neurotoxicity, e.g., dizziness, drowsiness, severe headache, changes in LOC, or seizures. (Penicillins and cephalosporins have an increased risk of neurotoxicity. **Lifespan**: Be particularly cautious with the older adult who is at greater risk for falls.)	• Instruct the patient to immediately report increasing headache, dizziness, drowsiness, changes in behavior or LOC, or seizures. • Caution the patient that drowsiness may occur and to be cautious with driving or other activities requiring mental alertness until the effects of the drug are known. If dizziness occurs, the patient should sit or lie down and not attempt to stand or walk, until the sensation passes.
• Monitor for development of "red man syndrome" in patients receiving vancomycin. Report any significantly large area of reddening such as trunk, head, neck, limbs, or gluteal area, especially if associated with decreased blood pressure or tachycardia. (Vancomycin hypersensitivity may cause the release of large amounts of histamine. If a significant area is involved, vasodilation from histamine may cause hypotension and reflex tachycardia. Prevancomycin antihistamines, e.g., diphenhydramine, may be ordered. IV infusions should be given slowly and monitored closely.)	• Instruct the patient to immediately report unusual flushing, especially involving a large body area, dizziness, dyspnea, or palpitations.
• Monitor for signs and symptoms of blood dyscrasias, e.g., low-grade fevers, bleeding, bruising, or significant fatigue. (Penicillins may cause blood dyscrasias with resulting decreases in RBCs, WBCs, and/or platelets.)	• Teach the patient to report any low-grade fevers, sore throat, rashes, bruising, nosebleeds, increased bleeding, unusual fatigue, or shortness of breath, especially after taking the antibiotic for a prolonged period.
• Monitor electrolytes, pulse, and ECG if indicated in patients on penicillin. (Some preparations of penicillin may be based in sodium or potassium salts and may cause hypernatremia and hyperkalemia.)	• Teach the patient to promptly report any palpitations, lightheadedness, dizziness, or swelling of feet or ankles.
• **Lifespan:** Women of childbearing age taking oral contraceptives and penicillin antibiotics should use an alternative form of birth control to prevent pregnancy. (Some penicillins may significantly reduce the effectiveness of oral contraceptives.)	• Teach women of childbearing age on oral contraceptives to consult their health care provider about birth control alternatives if penicillin antibiotics are ordered.
Patient understanding of drug therapy: • Use opportunities during administration of medications and during assessments to discuss the rationale for drug therapy, desired therapeutic outcomes, commonly observed adverse effects, parameters for when to call the health care provider, and any necessary monitoring or precautions. (Using time during nursing care helps to optimize and reinforce key teaching areas.)	• The patient, family, or caregiver should be able to state the reason for the drug, appropriate dose and scheduling, what adverse effects to observe for and when to report them, and the anticipated length of medication therapy.

Patient self-administration of drug therapy:
• When administering medications, instruct the patient, family, or caregiver in proper self-administration techniques followed by teach-back. (Utilizing time during nurse-administration of these drugs helps to reinforce teaching.)
	• Teach the patient to take the medication:
	  • Complete the entire course of therapy unless otherwise instructed. Do not share with other family members, and do not stop the medicine when starting to feel better.
	  • Avoid or eliminate alcohol. Cephalosporins may cause significant reactions when taken with alcohol, and alcohol increases adverse GI effects of the drug.
	  • Take the drug with food or milk, but avoid acidic or carbonated beverages to decrease adverse GI effects.
	  • Take the medication as evenly spaced throughout each day as feasible.
	  • Increase overall fluid intake while taking the antibacterial drug.
	  • Discard outdated medications or those no longer in use. Review medicine cabinet twice a year for old medications (e.g., at beginning and end of daylight saving time).

*Nursing Diagnoses—Definitions and Classification 2015–2017. Copyright © 2014, 1994–2014 by NANDA International. Used by arrangement with John Wiley & Sons Limited.

CHAPTER
47

Understanding the Chapter

Key Concepts Summary

47.1 Bacterial cell walls consist of layers of carbohydrate and protein chains, which are constructed by enzymes called penicillin-binding proteins.

47.2 The penicillins, one of the oldest and safest groups of antibacterials, are primarily active against gram-positive bacteria.

47.3 The cephalosporins are similar in structure and function to the penicillins and are widely prescribed for gram-negative infections.

47.4 The carbapenems are resistant to beta lactamase and are broad-spectrum alternatives to penicillin.

47.5 Several miscellaneous cell wall inhibitors have activity against resistant microbes.

Case Study: Making the Patient Connection

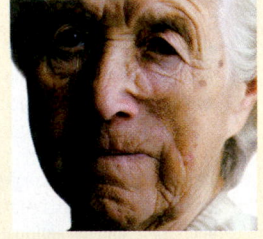

Remember the patient "Katie Dennison" at the beginning of the chapter? Now read the remainder of the case study. Based on the information presented within this chapter, respond to the critical thinking questions that follow.

Katie Dennison is an 83-year-old retired school teacher. She was recently seen by her health care provider for removal of a noncancerous skin lesion. Now she suspects that the wound on her arm has become infected. She has attempted to report this condition to her health care provider. However, due to the holidays she has been unable to reach him. Ms. Dennison presents to a local urgent care center for treatment.

The physical examination and diagnostic tests reveal the following findings. Vital signs are temperature, 38°C (100.9°F); pulse, 110 beats/min; respiratory rate, 20 breaths/min; and blood pressure, 108/68 mmHg. The large dressing on her left arm is saturated with dried yellow-green exudates. She states that it is painful to move her left arm and that the pain has limited her range of motion in the affected extremity. She is pale and has "paper thin" fragile skin.

Katie reports that she accidentally got the dressing wet while taking a shower. She did not change the dressing because she was not told to do so by her health care provider when the skin lesion was removed. A series of laboratory tests were completed. A sterile dressing was applied to the wound. Ms. Dennison was given an injection of cefazolin (Ancef) and a prescription for antibiotics. She was also instructed to follow up with her health care provider within the next 2 to 3 days.

Critical Thinking Questions

1. What factors possibly contributed to the wound infection in this patient?
2. What laboratory tests were probably obtained during this visit to the urgent care center?
3. What information should the nurse provide to the patient concerning the antibiotic?
4. Discuss the mechanism of action for cefazolin.

See Answers to Critical Thinking Questions on student resource website.

Additional Case Study

Mrs. Murphy is 80 years old and lives in a retirement community for lower income older adults. You are the community health nurse visiting with her. As part of your assessment, you ask Mrs. Murphy how she obtains her prescribed medications. The patient explains that most of the time, her neighbor will pick up prescriptions for her. She further explains that in some cases, however, she has "stockpiled" medicines she has been prescribed. When you investigate, you find that the patient has multiple bottles of various types of unused antibiotics. Some of the drugs were prescribed 5 or 6 years ago.

1. Describe how you should respond to this situation.
2. Identify the health teaching needs of this patient regarding "stockpiling" (saving) antibiotics.

See Answers to Additional Case Study on student resource website.

Chapter Review

1 Which instruction should the nurse give a 21-year-old female patient being treated with ampicillin (Principen)?

1. Stop taking oral contraceptives because serious adverse effects could occur.

2. Use oral contraceptives as prescribed because antibiotics do not react with birth control pills.

3. The antibiotic may decrease the effectiveness of oral contraceptives.

4. The antibiotic when taken with oral contraceptives causes toxicity.

2 The nurse is caring for a patient who is receiving intravenous vancomycin (Vancocin). Which symptom, if present, may indicate that the patient is experiencing drug-induced ototoxicity?

1. Erythema of the earlobes and ear canal

2. Inner ear pruritus after infusion is completed

3. Tinnitus and dizziness when remaining still

4. Ocular pain with purulent drainage

3 The patient reports abnormal vaginal discharge after completing a prescription of cefotaxime (Claforan). For which condition is the patient most likely exhibiting symptoms?

1. Hypersensitivity reaction

2. Superinfection

3. Pseudomembranous colitis

4. Antibiotic toxicity

4 The patient who has been taking cefixime (Suprax) for the past week and a half returns to the provider with reports of "explosive diarrhea, very watery, sometimes with a lot of mucus" up to eight times in the last 2 days. The patient reports significant weakness. For which condition is the patient describing symptoms?

1. Antibiotic-induced peptic ulcer disease

2. Antibiotic-associated malabsorption

3. GI-associated hypersensitivity

4. *Clostridium difficile*–associated diarrhea

5 The patient who is taking imipenem-cilastatin (Primaxin) reports shortness of breath, mouth and tongue swelling, and generalized itching. For which of the following does the nurse initially assess the patient?

1. Hypersensitivity reaction

2. Blood dyscrasias

3. Beta-lactamase induction

4. Drug toxicity

6 The nurse is teaching a patient who recently was diagnosed with an upper respiratory infection and is prescribed ampicillin (Principen). The nurse would evaluate the session as being successful if the patient states which of the following?

1. "I should take this medication on an empty stomach with a full glass of water."

2. "I can expect my tongue to become black and furry."

3. "Once I stop coughing, I should stop taking this medication."

4. "If I miss a dose, I should take two doses together to catch up."

See Answers to Chapter Review in Appendix A.

References

Centers for Disease Control and Prevention. (2011). Vital signs: Central line-associated blood stream infections—United States, 2001, 2008, and 2009. *Morbidity and Mortality Weekly Report, 60*(8), 243–248.

Centers for Disease Control and Prevention. (2013). *Get smart: Know when antibiotics work. Antibiotic resistance questions and answers.* Retrieved from http://www.cdc.gov/getsmart/antibiotic-use/antibiotic-resistance-faqs.html

O'Keefe, S. J. D. (2010). Tube feeding, microbiota, and *Clostridium difficile* infection. *World Journal of Gastroenterology, 16*, 139–142. doi:10.3748/wjg.v16.i2.139

Zhang, Y., Lee, B. Y., & Donohue, J. M. (2010). Ambulatory antibiotic use and prescription drug coverage in older adults. *Archives of Internal Medicine, 170*, 1308–1314. doi:10.1001/archinternmed.2010.235

Selected Bibliography

Centers for Disease Control and Prevention. (2013). *Healthcare-associated infections: Carbapenem-resistant enterobacteriaceae in healthcare settings.* Retrieved from http://www.cdc.gov/hai/organisms/cre/

Chang, C., Mahmood, M. M., Teuber, S. S., & Gershwin, M. E. (2012). Overview of penicillin allergy. *Clinical Reviews in Allergy & Immunology, 43*(1-2), 84–97. doi:10.1007/s12016-011-8279-6

Chen, L. F., Chopra, T., & Kaye, K. S. (2010). Pathogens resistant to antibacterial agents. *Medical Clinics of North America, 95*, 647–676. doi:10.1016/j.mcna.2011.03.005

Herdman, T. H., & Kamitsuru, S. (Eds.). (2014). *NANDA International nursing diagnoses: Definitions and classification, 2015–2017.* Oxford, United Kingdom: Wiley-Blackwell.

Karras, G., Giannakaki, V., Kotsis, V., & Miyakis, S. (2012). Novel antimicrobial agents against multi-drug-resistant gram-negative bacteria: An overview. *Recent Patents on Anti-Infective Drug Discovery, 7*(3), 175–181. doi:10.2174/157489112803521922

Matteo, B., Ginocchio, F., Giacobbe, D. R., & Malgorzata, M. (2011). Development of antibiotics for gram-negatives: Where now? *Clinical Investigation, 1*, 221–227. doi:10.4155/cli.10.31

Smith, S. M. (2010). Update on *Clostridium difficile* infection and its management. *Nursing for Women's Health, 14*, 391–397. doi:10.1111/j.1751-486X.2010.01578.x

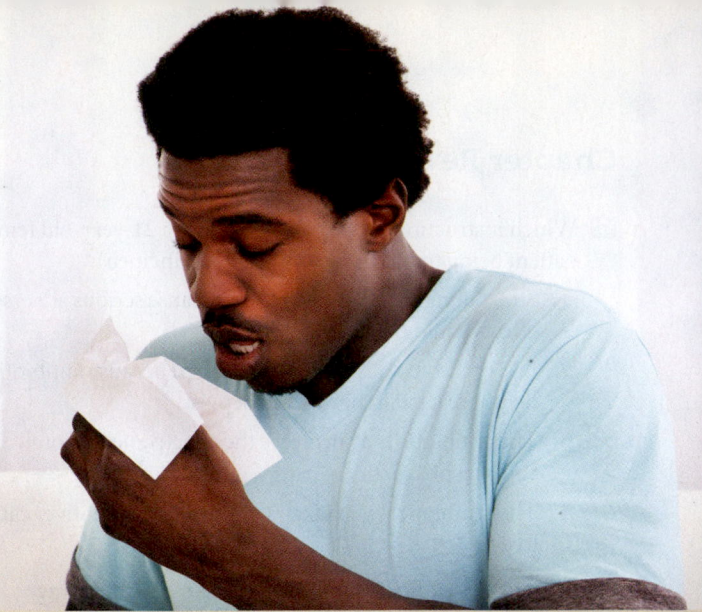

"Today is the fifth day since I started taking the medication and I'm still having chills and fever. I thought these antibiotics were supposed to get rid of this!"

Patient "John Travis"

48 Antibiotics Affecting Bacterial Protein Synthesis

LEARNING OUTCOMES

After reading this chapter, the student should be able to:

1. Explain the steps in the synthesis of bacterial proteins.
2. Identify the classes of antibiotics that act by inhibiting bacterial protein synthesis.
3. Explain mechanisms by which antibiotics inhibit bacterial protein synthesis.
4. Explain how protein synthesis inhibitors exert selective toxicity toward bacterial, rather than human, cells.
5. Describe means by which bacteria become resistant to protein synthesis inhibitors.
6. For each of the classes shown in the chapter outline, identify the prototype and representative drugs and explain the mechanism(s) of drug action, primary indications, contraindications, significant drug interactions, pregnancy category, and important adverse effects.
7. Apply the nursing process to care for patients who are receiving pharmacotherapy with bacterial protein synthesis inhibitors.

CHAPTER OUTLINE

▸ **Mechanisms of Antibiotic Inhibition of Bacterial Protein Synthesis**

▸ **Tetracyclines**
  PROTOTYPE Tetracycline (Sumycin, Others), *p. 808*

▸ **Macrolides**
  PROTOTYPE Erythromycin (EryC, Erythrocin, Others), *p. 810*

▸ **Aminoglycosides**
  PROTOTYPE Gentamicin (Garamycin, Others), *p. 813*

▸ **Miscellaneous Inhibitors of Bacterial Protein Synthesis**

KEY TERMS

cholestatic hepatitis, 811

gray baby syndrome, 815

oxazolidinones, 815

postantibiotic effect, 812

pseudomembranous colitis (PMC), 808

Svedberg unit, 806

translation, 805

To maintain the extreme metabolic rate required for exponential reproduction, bacteria must synthesize huge amounts of protein. Antibacterial drugs that inhibit this high rate of protein metabolism can either kill the bacterial cell or slow its replication rate. Tetracyclines, macrolides, and a few miscellaneous drugs are bacteriostatic inhibitors of protein synthesis. The aminoglycosides are bacteriocidal inhibitors.

Mechanisms of Antibiotic Inhibition of Bacterial Protein Synthesis

48.1 Antibiotics inhibit microbial protein synthesis by binding to the bacterial ribosome.

The importance of protein to a microbe is illustrated by the fact that up to 50% of the dry weight of a bacterial cell consists of protein. Bacterial proteins serve many of the same functions as human proteins. For example, the bacterial enzymes required for all biochemical reactions are proteins. Proteins are studded in the plasma membrane and serve as channels, pores, or transporters, assisting substances as they move into and out of cells. Like human proteins, bacterial proteins are composed of long chains of amino acids.

Several types of proteins, however, are unique to bacteria. Bacterial cells produce protein toxins, which kill other bacteria and can cause serious injury to human cells. The sticky gel-like substance that allows bacterial cells to cling to human epithelial cells on the skin surface, in bronchi, in the gastrointestinal (GI) tract, or in the genitourinary tract consists of proteins combined with carbohydrates. The structure of the bacterial cell wall (see Chapter 47) consists of peptidoglycan layers of protein and carbohydrates that protect the bacterium from its environment. From these examples, it is easy to understand why proteins are critical to bacterial cells.

Knowledge of how proteins are synthesized by bacterial cells is important to understanding how antibiotics act. The basic steps in protein synthesis, or **translation**, are the same in bacteria as they are in humans. Knowledge of translation, which is illustrated in Figure 48.1, is necessary to understand the mechanisms of action of antibiotics that inhibit protein synthesis.

Protein synthesis occurs in the cytoplasm and requires the following three components:

- Messenger ribonucleic acid (mRNA)
- Transfer ribonucleic acid (tRNA)
- Ribosomes, which consist of one large and one small subunit

The mRNA carries the encoded message for making a protein from the deoxyribonucleic acid (DNA) to the ribosome, which serves as the site for protein construction. The strand of mRNA squeezes between the two ribosomal subunits and begins to move through the subunits. As it does, a tRNA molecule arrives, carrying the specific amino acid that was encoded in the mRNA strand. As the mRNA proceeds through the ribosome, subsequent amino acids are added one at a time to the growing protein chain. This growing chain is known as a polypeptide. Eventually, a "stop signal" is reached on the mRNA strand, which tells the ribosome that the last amino acid has been added and the protein is ready to be released.

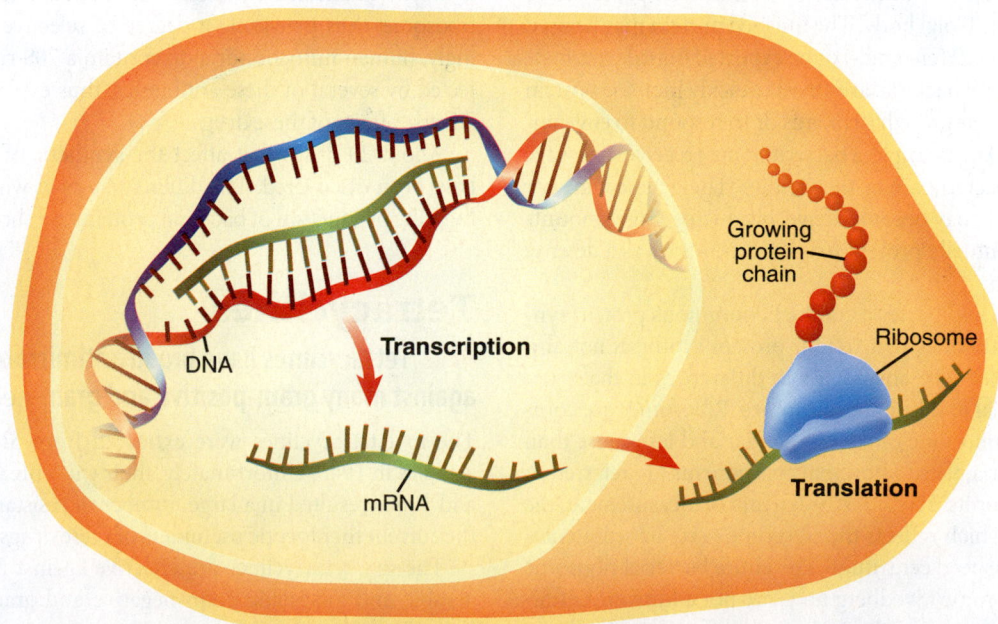

Figure 48.1 Steps in protein synthesis: The DNA is used as a template to make mRNA (transcription). The mRNA is sent to the ribosome to make the protein chain (translation).

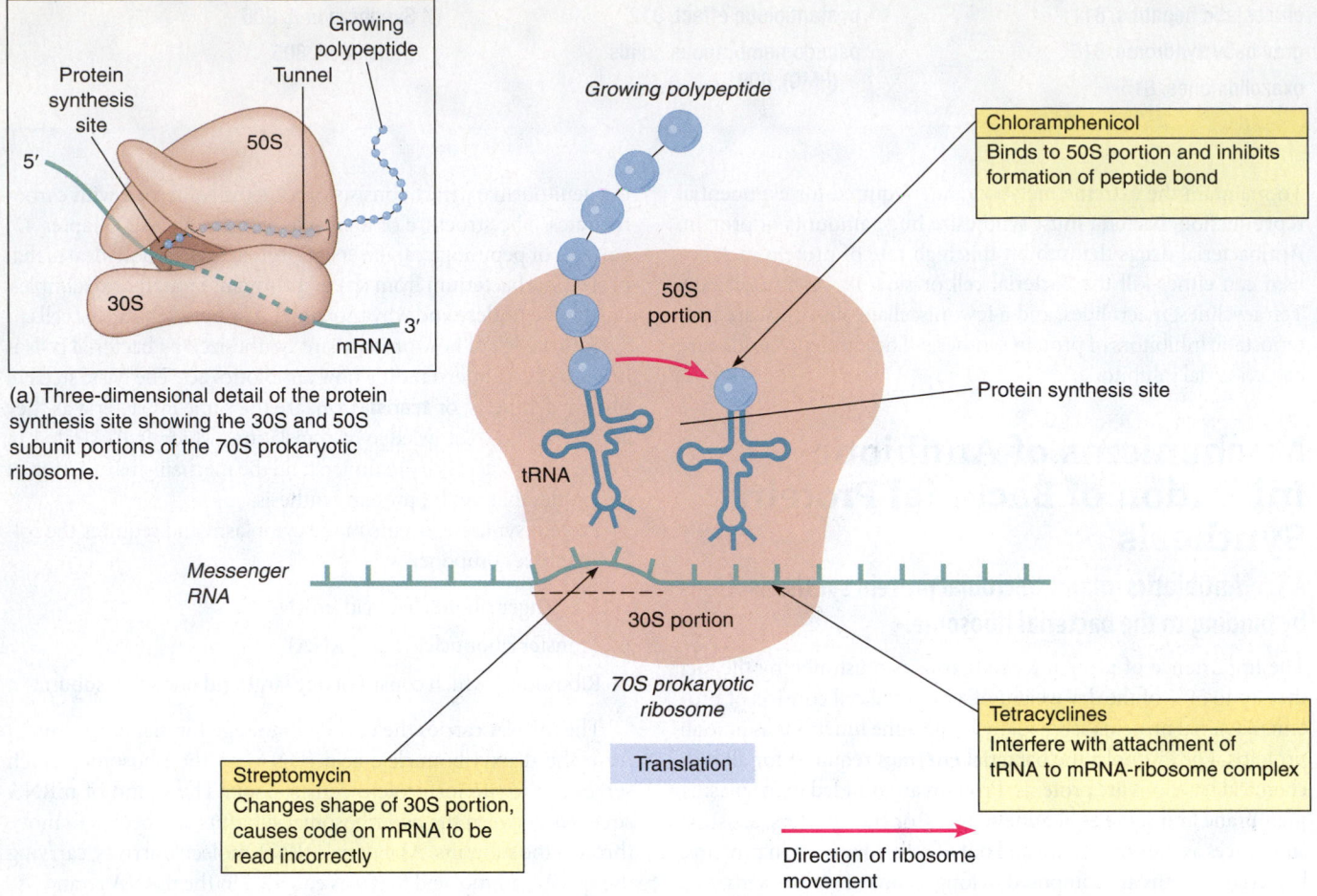

(a) Three-dimensional detail of the protein synthesis site showing the 30S and 50S subunit portions of the 70S prokaryotic ribosome.

Chloramphenicol
Binds to 50S portion and inhibits formation of peptide bond

Protein synthesis site

Tetracyclines
Interfere with attachment of tRNA to mRNA-ribosome complex

Translation

Streptomycin
Changes shape of 30S portion, causes code on mRNA to be read incorrectly

Direction of ribosome movement

(b) In the diagram the black arrows indicate the different points at which chloramphenicol, the tetracyclines, and streptomycin exert their activities.

Figure 48.2 Mechanisms of action of antibiotics inhibiting bacterial protein synthesis.

From *Microbiology: An Introduction* (10th ed., p. 558), by G. Tortora, B. Funke, & C. Case, 2010. Reprinted by permission of Pearson Education, Inc., Upper Saddle River, NJ.

The protein may be active immediately, or it may be processed to its active form in the Golgi body. The finished protein may be used within the bacterial cell (enzymes) or be exported outside (toxins).

All cells, including bacteria, are able to quickly increase protein synthesis to meet their growth demands or to respond to environmental challenges. For example, a bacterium may receive a message that competitive bacteria are in the vicinity. The gene coding for a toxin or antibiotic may become active, producing large amounts of mRNA and eventually protein toxin, which serves as a defense against the invaders.

If both humans and bacteria conduct continuous protein synthesis, why are antibiotics that inhibit protein synthesis not also toxic to human cells? The answer lies in differences in the structures of the bacterial and human ribosomes. Ribosomes are composed of two subunits, one of which is larger and less dense than the other. In bacteria, these ribosomal components are referred to as 30S and 50S subunits. The letter "S" is a unit of measurement, the **Svedberg unit**, which reflects the ribosome's size or sedimentation rate in a high-speed centrifuge. The entire bacterial ribosome is called a 70S ribosome (Svedberg units are not additive). Antibiotics that inhibit protein synthesis do so by affecting subunits of the bacterial ribosome. Humans have ribosomes that are larger and denser than the 70S bacterial ribosome. The 80S human ribosome

is mostly unaffected by antibiotics that bind to the bacterial 70S ribosome, thus providing a degree of selective toxicity. Interestingly, human mitochondria do contain a 70S ribosome that is affected by several of these antibiotics, thus explaining some of the adverse effects of these drugs.

About 20 drugs that affect the synthesis of bacterial proteins have been discovered. The different steps at which antibiotics inhibit the production of bacterial proteins are shown in Figure 48.2.

Tetracyclines

48.2 Tetracyclines have broad antimicrobial activity against many gram-positive and gram-negative bacteria.

The first tetracyclines were extracted from *Streptomyces* in soil samples in 1948. Unfortunately, their widespread use in the 1950s and 1960s resulted in a large number of resistant strains, limiting the current therapeutic usefulness of these drugs.

The five tetracyclines are effective against a large number of aerobic and anaerobic gram-negative and gram-positive organisms: They have one of the broadest antimicrobial spectrums of any class of antibiotics. They are effective against some species that are resistant to penicillins and other cell wall inhibitors. Because

❮ Traveler's Diarrhea

Clinical Question

What are the current recommendations for prevention or treatment of traveler's diarrhea?

Evidence

Traveler's diarrhea (TD) is an unpleasant but rarely fatal infection that affects travelers going to developing regions of the world, especially tropical or semitropical areas. *E. coli, Shigella, Campylobacter, Salmonella,* and the noroviruses are common causes of traveler's diarrhea. As many as 40% to 50% of travelers going abroad will develop TD (Kollaritsch, Paulke-Korinek, & Wiedermann, 2012). While mortality is low, the diarrhea may ruin a trip and result in long-term complications. Risk factors include age (toddler or adolescent), infrequent travel to developing regions, length of time in a region, mode of travel (e.g., backpacking), lack of infection control practices such as hand washing or care in eating or drinking, and daily use of a proton pump inhibitor (de la Cabada Bauche & DuPont, 2011; Kollaritsch et al., 2012). Chronic, postinfection inflammatory bowel syndrome (IBS) persisting for up to 5 years has been noted following TD infections.

Three antibiotics have shown the most promise in treating TD infections, dependent on the endemic pathogens in the area of travel: fluoroquinolones (ciprofloxacin [Cipro] or levofloxacin [Levaquin]), rifaximin (Xifaxan, Salix), and azithromycin (Zithromax, Zmax). While the time for initiation of treatment, after the first loose stool or after the classic TD definition of three loose stools, has not been determined, it is recommended that travelers visiting high-risk countries bring an antibiotic for self-treatment of TD.

Implications

More people are traveling to foreign countries than ever before. Nurses can be instrumental in teaching methods to avoid traveler's diarrhea. Travelers can decrease their risk by practicing frequent hand cleansing with hand sanitizers or antiseptic cloths; avoiding beverages with ice, not drinking water that has not been boiled, and not using tap water for teeth brushing; and not consuming raw fruits or vegetables that cannot be peeled because they may be contaminated. Over-the-counter (OTC) medications such as bismuth subsalicylate (Pepto-Bismol) or probiotics such as *Lactobacillus* and *Saccharomyces boulardii* may confer some protection against TD.

Depending on the area of the world that the traveler will be visiting and endemic pathogens most likely to be encountered there, an antibiotic may be prescribed to have on hand in case of TD. The nurse should assess for allergies and provide patient education on when the antibiotic should be used (e.g., after one or more loose stools). The nurse should teach that local health authorities should be contacted if the diarrhea worsens, is accompanied by severe abdominal pain or fever, or if blood is present in the stool. Upon returning home, the traveler should consult a health care provider, and any continued diarrhea or GI symptoms should be monitored for the development of postinfection IBS.

Critical Thinking Question

In what specific patient populations would TD be most serious? Why?

See Answers to Critical Thinking Questions on student resource website.

---

of widespread bacterial resistance, however, they are the drugs of choice for only a few diseases: Rocky Mountain spotted fever, typhus, cholera, Lyme disease, peptic ulcers caused by *Helicobacter pylori,* and chlamydial infections. In addition, *Treponema pallidum* (syphilis) responds well to tetracycline therapy for patients who are allergic to penicillin. Although traditionally used for gonorrhea, most strains of *Neisseria gonorrhoeae* are now resistant to tetracyclines. Drugs in this class are occasionally used for the treatment of acne vulgaris, for which they are given topically or orally (PO) at low doses. Almost all strains of *Pseudomonas aeruginosa* are resistant to tetracyclines. Once resistance develops to one tetracycline, it usually extends to all drugs in this class. Doses for the tetracyclines are listed in Table 48.1.

Tetracyclines exert a bacteriostatic effect by selectively inhibiting bacterial protein synthesis. As illustrated in Figure 48.2, the tetracyclines bind to the 30S bacterial ribosome, thereby preventing the addition of amino acids to the growing polypeptide chain. Resistance to tetracyclines develops when bacteria prevent tetracyclines from concentrating inside their cells, or when their ribosome shape is altered so the antibiotic can no longer bind. In addition to having ribosomes with different structures, human cells lack the active transport system required for tetracyclines to enter their cells. At high doses, however, tetracyclines begin to exert toxicity on human cells.

All tetracyclines have the same spectrum of antimicrobial activity and similar adverse effects. All except tigecycline may be given PO. Several have topical and parenteral formulations. They are sometimes classified by their duration of action as short acting, intermediate acting, or long acting.

Most PO tetracyclines should be taken on an empty stomach to maximize their absorption. Because gastric distress is relatively common with drugs in this class, patients will often take tetracyclines with food. However, these drugs bind metal ions such

TABLE 48.1 Tetracyclines		
Drug	**Route and Adult Dose (Maximum Dose Where Indicated)**	**Adverse Effects**
demeclocycline (Declomycin)	PO: 150 mg every 6 h or 300 mg every 12 h (max: 2.4 g/day)	*Nausea, vomiting, abdominal cramping, flatulence, diarrhea, mild phototoxicity, rash, dizziness, stinging or burning with topical applications*
doxycycline (Vibramycin, Others)	PO: 100 mg bid on day 1, then 100 mg daily (max: 200 mg/day)	
minocycline (Minocin, Others)	PO: 200 mg as one dose followed by 100 mg bid	Anaphylaxis, superinfections, hepatotoxicity, exfoliative dermatitis, permanent teeth discoloration in children
tetracycline (Sumycin, Others)	PO: 250–500 mg bid–qid (max: 2 g/day)	
tigecycline (Tygacil)	IV: 100 mg, followed by 50 mg every 12 h	

Note: Italics indicate common adverse effects. Underline indicates serious adverse effects.

CONNECTIONS Patient Safety

◀ Photosensitivity and Antibiotics

Having fun in the sun may be hazardous to some patients. Photosensitivity is a relatively common adverse reaction to some medications, especially antibiotics. Many pharmacologic therapies have photosensitivity as a possible adverse effect.

Any skin reaction to light is generally defined as photosensitivity. However, this medication-induced adverse effect can present in two categories: phototoxicity and photoallergic reactions. The more common of the two conditions is phototoxicity, which encompasses both sunburn and reactions caused by chemical photosensitizers such as medications. Both reactions are typically manifested by delayed redness and edema followed by hyperpigmentation. Phototoxicity may occur after first exposure to a drug.

Photoallergic reactions are less common. These reactions present as variations of contact dermatitis and are the result of hypersensitivity. In photoallergic reactions, the drug forms an immunogenic complex with cutaneous proteins due to the presence of light energy. Photoallergic reactions tend to become more pronounced with repeat exposures.

What role can nurses play to help patients prevent photosensitivity reactions from occurring?

See Answer to the Patient Safety Question on student resource website.

---

as calcium, magnesium, aluminum, and iron, and tetracyclines should not be taken with milk or iron supplements. Food, milk, or other dairy products can reduce drug absorption by 50% or more. Food does not interfere with absorption of the longer acting drugs doxycycline and minocycline.

Because most tetracyclines are incompletely absorbed, they remain in the GI tract in high concentrations, often killing normal flora in the colon. Tetracycline-induced diarrhea is common and could indicate toxic effects on normal flora or a bowel superinfection. The presence of diarrhea must be monitored carefully due to the possibility of **pseudomembranous colitis (PMC)**. Caused by *Clostridium difficile*, this is a rare though potentially severe disorder resulting from therapy with tetracyclines and other classes of antibiotics.

When administered parenterally or in high doses, certain tetracyclines can cause hepatotoxicity, especially in patients with preexisting liver disease. Some patients experience photosensitivity during therapy, making their skin especially susceptible to sunburn. Photosensitivity may appear as exaggerated sunburn within minutes to hours of exposure and is often accompanied by a tingling, burning sensation. Because of their broad spectrum, superinfections due to *Candida albicans* are relatively common. Women who are on oral contraceptives may be more susceptible to vaginal candidiasis. Tetracyclines are usually contraindicated in pregnant or lactating women and in children under the age of 8 because these drugs cause yellow-brown teeth discoloration and may slow the overall growth rate in fetuses or children.

PROTOTYPE DRUG	Tetracycline (Sumycin, Others)

Classification: Therapeutic: Antibacterial
Pharmacologic: Bacterial protein synthesis inhibitor, tetracycline

Therapeutic Effects and Uses: Approved in 1953, tetracycline is used for the treatment and prophylaxis of susceptible gram-positive and gram-negative bacteria as well as chlamydiae, rickettsiae, mycoplasmas, and certain protozoa. Tetracycline has one of the broadest spectrums of any antibiotic. Its use has increased during the past decade due to its effectiveness against *H. pylori* in the treatment of peptic ulcer disease. Oral and topical preparations are available for treating inflammatory acne vulgaris.

Mechanism of Action: Tetracycline inhibits bacterial protein synthesis by binding to the 30S ribosomal subunit, interfering with the attachment of the tRNA to the mRNA-ribosome complex. The growing amino acid chain is prematurely terminated and protein synthesis is inhibited. Tetracycline is usually considered bacteriostatic, although it can be bacteriocidal at high concentrations.

Pharmacokinetics:

Route(s)	PO, topical
Absorption	80% is absorbed PO
Distribution	Widely distributed; only small amounts cross the blood–brain barrier; crosses the placenta; secreted in breast milk
Primary metabolism	15–30% metabolized, primarily in the liver
Primary excretion	60% renal, small amounts excreted into bile
Onset of action	1–2 h
Duration of action	Half-life: 6–12 h

Adverse Effects: Being a broad-spectrum antibiotic, tetracycline has a tendency to affect vaginal, oral, and intestinal flora and cause superinfections. Other frequent adverse effects include nausea, vomiting, epigastric burning, diarrhea, discoloration of the teeth, and photosensitivity. Serious adverse reactions include anaphylaxis; fatty degeneration of the liver, producing jaundice; and exfoliative dermatitis. Although not nephrotoxic, tetracycline can worsen kidney impairment in patients with preexisting disease.

Contraindications/Precautions: Tetracycline is contraindicated in patients who are allergic to any drug in the tetracycline class. As a pregnancy category D agent, tetracycline should not be used during pregnancy. Drug therapy must be monitored carefully in patients with impaired hepatic or renal function, because this drug is excreted by these routes.

Drug Interactions: Oral supplements, laxatives, or antacids that contain metal ions such as calcium, iron, magnesium, or aluminum reduce the GI absorption and serum levels of oral tetracycline. Tetracycline binds with colestipol and cholestyramine, thereby decreasing the antibiotic's absorption. Tetracyclines decrease the effectiveness of oral contraceptives. **Herbal/Food**: Dairy products interfere with tetracycline absorption. Tetracycline eliminates vitamin K–producing bacteria in the intestines; patients taking warfarin may experience an increased anticoagulant effect.

Pregnancy: Category D.

Treatment of Overdose: No specific therapy is available. Patients are treated symptomatically.

Nursing Responsibilities: Key nursing implications for patients receiving tetracycline are included in the Nursing Practice Application for Patients Receiving Pharmacotherapy with a Tetracycline, Macrolide, or Aminoglycoside Antibiotic.

Drugs Similar to Tetracycline (Sumycin, Others)

Other tetracyclines include demeclocycline, doxycycline, minocycline, and tigecycline. The use of oxytetracycline (Terramycin) was discontinued in the United States.

Demeclocycline (Declomycin): Approved in 1960, demeclocycline has the same spectrum of antimicrobial action as other tetracyclines. Unrelated to its anti-infective properties, demeclocycline is the only drug in this class used off-label to treat syndrome of inappropriate antidiuretic hormone (SIADH). Because of its blocking action on antidiuretic hormone (ADH), demeclocycline is used to produce a diuresis in patients with excess ADH secretion (see Chapter 65). Photosensitivity is more severe with demeclocycline than with any other drug in this class. Demeclocycline undergoes extensive enterohepatic recirculation and is excreted in the bile; thus doses should be reduced for patients with hepatic impairment. This drug is pregnancy category D.

Doxycycline (Vibramycin, Others): Approved in 1967, doxycycline is the safest tetracycline for patients with impaired renal function because it is excreted primarily by nonrenal routes. Normally administered PO, an IV form is available for treating severe infections. It is absorbed well, with or without food, and offers the advantage of once- or twice-daily dosing. Doxycycline is included in the CDC "Sexually Transmitted Diseases: Treatment Guidelines" (2010) for treating syphilis, chlamydial infections, and pelvic inflammatory disease. Doxycycline is recommended as an alternative to ciprofloxacin for the prophylactic treatment of *Bacillus anthracis* (anthrax). Adverse effects and contraindications are the same as those of other tetracyclines.

Several newer formulations of doxycycline have been approved. Doryx is an extended release enteric-coated oral formulation. Oracea is a dual-release capsule, containing immediate and delayed release beads for the treatment of inflammatory lesions of the skin associated with rosacea. Oracea is not intended for the treatment or prevention of infections. Two doxycycline products are available for the treatment of chronic periodontitis in adults. Atridox is administered as a topical, subgingival controlled release product, and Periostat is given as an oral tablet. Doxycycline is pregnancy category D.

Minocycline (Minocin, Others): Approved in 1971, minocycline offers the advantage of once- or twice-a-day dosing and may be administered without regard to meals or dairy products. It is the only tetracycline that can cause reversible vestibular toxicity, resulting in dizziness, vertigo, and weakness that can limit therapy. Minocycline is active against some strains of bacteria that are resistant to other drugs in the tetracycline class. Hepatic function laboratory values should be monitored during therapy to assess for hepatotoxicity. Other adverse effects and contraindications are the same as those of other tetracyclines. A microsphere powder formulation, called Arestin, is introduced subgingivally to treat periodontitis. In 2006, Solodyn, an extended release tablet, was approved for the treatment of inflammatory lesions associated with moderate to severe acne vulgaris in patients over 12 years of age. This drug is pregnancy category D.

Tigecycline (Tygacil): Tigecycline is a tetracycline that was approved in 2005. Available only by the intravenous (IV) route, it has more limited indications than other drugs in this class: complicated skin and skin structure infections and complicated intra-abdominal infections in patients over age 18. Tigecycline is effective against certain bacterial strains resistant to other antibiotics, including methicillin-resistant *Staphylococcus aureus* (MRSA) and vancomycin-resistant enterococci (VRE). Nausea and vomiting are the most frequent adverse effects, and these may be severe enough to cause discontinuation of therapy. Life-threatening anaphylaxis and pancreatitis have been reported. Other adverse effects and contraindications are the same as those of other tetracyclines. Hepatic function laboratory values should be monitored during therapy to assess for hepatotoxicity. Tigecycline carries a black box warning that the drug is associated with an increased mortality risk and that its use should be reserved for infections not responsive to other anti-infectives. This drug is pregnancy category D.

PharmFACT

The bubonic plague caused by the bacterium *Yersinia pestis* was responsible for killing approximately 50% of the population during the 5th and 6th centuries AD, and 40% of the population between the 8th and 14th centuries. If antibiotics had been available back then, most of the estimated 200 million people who died would likely have survived after a 10-day treatment with tetracyclines or aminoglycosides (Dufel, 2013).

Macrolides

48.3 The macrolides are alternatives to penicillin for many gram-positive infections.

Erythromycin (EryC, Erythrocin, Others), the first macrolide antibiotic, was isolated from *Streptomyces* organisms in a soil sample in 1952. The name *macrolide* was chosen for this drug class because they all possess an unusually large 14- to 15-atom ring as part of their chemical structure. Doses for the macrolides are listed in Table 48.2.

Macrolides are considered alternative drugs for patients who are allergic to penicillin. They are widely prescribed although they are the drugs of first choice for relatively few diseases. Most effective against gram-positive bacteria, common indications for macrolides include the treatment of whooping cough, diphtheria, Legionnaire's disease, and infections by streptococci, *Haemophilus influenzae*, *Mycoplasma pneumoniae*, and chlamydia. Clarithromycin is one of several antibiotics used to treat peptic ulcer disease due to its activity against *H. pylori* (see Chapter 59). The macrolides are preferred drugs for the prophylaxis of recurring rheumatic fever in patients who are allergic to penicillins. One of the newest drugs in this class, fidaxomicin (Dificid), is approved for treatment of *C. difficile*–associated diarrhea.

The macrolides inhibit bacterial protein synthesis by binding to the 50S ribosomal subunit, thus preventing movement of the ribosome along the mRNA. Macrolides do not bind to human ribosomes, thus offering a degree of selective toxicity. These drugs are usually bacteriostatic, though they may be bacteriocidal depending on the dose and the target organism.

TABLE 48.2   Macrolides

Drug	Route and Adult Dose (Maximum Dose Where Indicated)	Adverse Effects
azithromycin (Zithromax, Zmax)	PO (Zithromax): 500 mg for one dose, then 250 mg/day for 4 days PO (Zmax): 2 g single dose	*Nausea, vomiting, diarrhea, abdominal cramping, dry skin or burning (topical route)* Anaphylaxis, ototoxicity, PMC, hepatotoxicity, superinfections, dysrhythmias
clarithromycin (Biaxin)	PO: 250–500 mg bid	
erythromycin (EryC, Erythrocin, Others)	PO: 250–500 mg bid or 333 mg tid	
fidaxomicin (Dificid)	PO: 200 mg bid for 10 days	*Nausea, vomiting, abdominal pain* GI bleeding, anemia, neutropenia, anaphylaxis

Note: Italics indicate common adverse effects. Underline indicates serious adverse effects.

The newer macrolides have longer half-lives and generally cause less GI irritation than erythromycin, which is the original drug from which macrolides were synthesized. Azithromycin (Zithromax) has an extended half-life such that it can be administered for only 5 days rather than the 10-day therapy required for most antibiotics. A single dose of azithromycin is effective against *N. gonorrhoeae*. The brief duration of therapy is thought to increase patient adherence and to offset the added cost of azithromycin.

Like most of the older antibiotics, macrolide-resistant strains are becoming more common. Many organisms develop resistance to macrolides by pumping it out of the cell before the antibiotic has a chance to reach an effective concentration. In some cases, bacteria have modified the shape of their 50S ribosomal subunit so that it no longer binds the drug.

The macrolides are well tolerated and considered to be one of the safest antibiotic classes. The most common adverse effects are GI related and include nausea, vomiting, abdominal cramping, and diarrhea. These GI symptoms occur whether the drug is administered PO or IV. Taking the drug with food can significantly inhibit the absorption of troleandomycin and azithromycin suspension. Thus these drugs should be taken on an empty stomach.

Many macrolides have an enteric coating, which serves two purposes. First, the coating allows the drug to dissolve in the small intestine rather than the stomach, causing less gastric irritation. Second, the macrolides are inactivated in gastric acid, and the enteric coating allows it to avoid destruction and reach the small intestine where they are readily absorbed in the alkaline environment.

Macrolides are metabolized and concentrated in the liver and excreted into bile. Because macrolides decrease the hepatic metabolism of other drugs, a number of drug–drug interactions are possible. When macrolides prevent the conversion of drugs to their less active form, the serum levels of these other drugs will increase and cause potential toxicity. For example, warfarin (Coumadin) is extensively metabolized to its inactive form in the liver. If given concurrently with erythromycin, the destruction of warfarin is diminished and greater amounts of "active" warfarin remain in the blood for longer periods. Because warfarin increases bleeding time, this could result in prolonged bleeding in a patient. In general, doses of drugs that are metabolized in the liver should be reduced, or at least carefully monitored, if they are given concurrently with macrolides.

CONNECTION Checkpoint 48.1

From what you learned in Chapter 38, what type of laboratory monitoring should be done for a patient who is taking warfarin concurrently with a macrolide? *See Answer to Connection Checkpoint 48.1 on student resource website.*

PROTOTYPE DRUG   Erythromycin (EryC, Erythrocin, Others)

Classification: Therapeutic: Antibacterial
Pharmacologic: Bacterial protein synthesis inhibitor, macrolide

Therapeutic Effects and Uses: Erythromycin (also called erythromycin base) is indicated for the treatment and prophylaxis of susceptible bacterial infections. The main application for erythromycin is for patients who are allergic to penicillins or who may have a penicillin-resistant infection. It has a spectrum similar to that of the penicillins and is effective against most gram-positive bacteria, including susceptible strains of *Staphylococcus* and *Streptococcus*. Susceptible gram-negative strains include *N. gonorrhoeae* and *H. influenzae*. It is a drug of choice for infections from *Bordetella pertussis* (whooping cough), *Legionella pneumophila* (Legionnaire's disease), *M. pneumoniae*, and *Corynebacterium diphtheriae*.

All oral forms of erythromycin are considered to have equal effectiveness. Topical and ophthalmic formulations are also available. Erythromycin is available in a number of salts:

- Erythromycin stearate (Erythrocin) and erythromycin ethylsuccinate (EryPed, Pediamycin) are acid stable and more readily absorbed in the stomach than erythromycin base. These forms are converted to the base form in the liver before they become bacteriostatic. The stearate salt should be taken on an empty stomach, whereas the ethylsuccinate salt may be taken without regard to food.

- Erythromycin lactobionate is given IV when the patient is unable to take oral medications, or when the infection is severe enough to warrant a faster onset of action.

Mechanism of Action: Erythromycin inhibits bacterial protein synthesis by binding to the 50S ribosomal subunit. Erythromycin is considered bacteriostatic but may be bacteriocidal in high doses.

Pharmacokinetics:

Route(s)	PO, topical, IV (gluceptate and lactobionate salts)
Absorption	Readily absorbed PO; enteric coated
Distribution	Widely distributed; only small amounts cross the blood–brain barrier; secreted in breast milk
Primary metabolism	Hepatic metabolism (CYP3A); concentrates in the liver and bile
Primary excretion	Bile
Onset of action	1 h
Duration of action	Half-life: 1.5–2 h

Adverse Effects: The most common adverse effects from erythromycin are nausea, vomiting, and abdominal cramping, although these are rarely serious enough to cause discontinuation of therapy. Concurrent administration with food reduces these adverse effects. When given by the IV route, phlebitis and intense pain at the injection site are common. Anaphylaxis is possible. Hearing loss, vertigo, and dizziness may be experienced when using high doses, particularly in older adults and in those with impaired hepatic or renal excretion. High doses of IV erythromycin may be cardiotoxic and pose a risk for torsades de pointes, which is a type of dysrhythmia that is potentially fatal. Like nearly all other antibiotics, PMC is possible with the use of erythromycin.

Contraindications/Precautions: Erythromycin is contraindicated in patients with hypersensitivity to drugs in the macrolide class and for those who are taking terfenadine, astemizole, or cisapride. Drug therapy must be monitored carefully in patients with impaired hepatic or biliary function, due to the possibility of **cholestatic hepatitis**, a type of liver inflammation caused by obstruction of the bile ducts. Because macrolides have been shown to prolong the QT interval, erythromycin should be used with caution in patients with known prolongation of the QT interval, a history of torsades de pointes, bradydysrhythmias, or uncompensated heart failure.

Drug Interactions: Erythromycin inhibits hepatic CYP 450 metabolic enzymes and can interact with many drugs. When used concurrently with erythromycin, the serum levels and toxicities of alfentanil, carbamazepine, cyclosporine, fentanyl, theophylline, and methadone may increase. Because erythromycin may increase the effects of digoxin or warfarin, leading to abnormal bleeding, the doses of these anticoagulants may need to be lowered. Erythromycin competes with clindamycin and chloramphenicol for binding sites on the 50S bacterial ribosomal subunit, causing an antagonistic effect. Thus these antibiotics should not be taken concurrently. The concurrent use of erythromycin with lovastatin or simvastatin is not recommended because it may increase the risk of myopathy and rhabdomyolysis. Because fluconazole also inhibits CYP3A4, especially at high dosages, its concurrent use with erythromycin should be avoided.

Herbal/Food: Grapefruit juice may increase the bioavailability of erythromycin.

Pregnancy: Category B.

Treatment of Overdose: No specific therapy is available. Patients are treated symptomatically.

Nursing Responsibilities: Key nursing implications for patients receiving erythromycin are included in the Nursing Practice Application for Patients Receiving Pharmacotherapy with a Tetracycline, Macrolide, or Aminoglycoside Antibiotic.

Drugs Similar to Erythromycin (EryC, Erythrocin, Others)

Other macrolides include azithromycin, clarithromycin, and fidaxomicin. The macrolide dirithromycin (Dynabac) is no longer available in the United States.

Azithromycin (Zithromax, Zmax): Approved in 1991, azithromycin has a long duration of action that allows for less frequent dosing. A "Tri-pak" consists of three 500 mg tablets (taken over 3 days) and a "Z-pak" contains six 250 mg tablets (taken over 5 days). For acute otitis media in children, a single dose has been found to be as effective as 3- or 5-day regimens. An IV form for infusions is available for the treatment of pelvic inflammatory disease and community-acquired pneumonia. An ophthalmic solution (AzaSite) was approved in 2007 for treating bacterial conjunctivitis. Azithromycin demonstrates greater activity over gram-negative organisms than erythromycin.

Azithromycin causes less nausea than erythromycin and may be taken with or without food. The extended release oral suspension should be administered on an empty stomach. Because azithromycin does not inhibit liver metabolism, it is safer for patients with hepatic impairment and causes fewer drug–drug interactions than erythromycin base. The most common adverse effects are diarrhea, nausea, and abdominal pain. Azithromycin has been shown to prolong the QT interval, which can increase the risk of cardiac dysrhythmia. The drug should be used with caution in patients with known prolongation of the QT interval, a history of torsades de pointes, bradydysrhythmias, or uncompensated heart failure. Patients with a known hypersensitivity to any macrolide should not receive azithromycin. This drug is pregnancy category B.

Clarithromycin (Biaxin): Approved in 1991, clarithromycin is similar to erythromycin but causes significantly less nausea, and the regular release tablets may be taken with or without food. The drug is commonly prescribed for infections of the respiratory tract, sexually transmitted infections, _H. pylori_–associated peptic ulcer disease, and otitis media. An extended release (XL) formulation is used to treat sinusitis, chronic bronchitis, and community-acquired pneumonia. The XL form should be administered with food because its absorption is increased. The most frequent adverse effects with clarithromycin are diarrhea, nausea, abnormal taste, dyspepsia, abdominal discomfort, and headache. Like erythromycin, clarithromycin is metabolized by CYP 450 enzymes and a significant number of drug–drug interactions may occur. Patients with a known hypersensitivity to any macrolide should not receive clarithromycin. This drug is pregnancy category C.

Fidaxomicin (Dificid): A newer macrolide, fidaxomicin was approved in 2011 specifically for infections proven or strongly suspected to be caused by _C. difficile_. The drug should only be prescribed for this indication because other uses could encourage the development of resistant strains. Taken as an oral tablet, the drug is not significantly absorbed and remains in the digestive tract where it produces its effects on _C. difficile_. Fidaxomicin appears to have equal efficacy to vancomycin, the primary antibiotic used to treat *C. difficile* diarrhea. Relapses are less frequent than with vancomycin. The drug is well tolerated with the most frequent adverse effects being nausea, vomiting, abdominal pain, and GI bleeding. This drug is pregnancy category B.

Aminoglycosides

48.4 The aminoglycosides are effective against aerobic gram-negative organisms but have the potential to cause ototoxicity and nephrotoxicity.

The first aminoglycoside, streptomycin, was named after *Streptomyces griseus*, the soil organism from which it was isolated in 1943. Once widely used, streptomycin is now usually reserved for the treatment of tuberculosis (TB) due to the development of safer alternatives and the appearance of a large number of resistant strains. Other aminoglycosides have since been isolated, and several have been produced semisynthetically. All have a common chemical structure of two or more amino sugars with a glycosidic, or sugar, link. The differences in spelling of some of these drugs, -*mycin* and -*micin,* reflects the different organisms from which the drugs were originally isolated. Doses for the aminoglycosides are listed in Table 48.3.

Aminoglycosides bind irreversibly to the 30S ribosomal subunit of bacteria, changing its shape and preventing the initiation stage of protein synthesis. Some drugs in this class also affect the 50S subunit. In addition, these antibiotics cause mRNA to be read incorrectly, resulting in abnormal proteins that are subsequently inserted into the bacterial plasma membrane, causing it to leak. Whereas most antibiotics that affect protein synthesis are bacteriostatic, aminoglycosides are bacteriocidal.

Although they have the ability to kill many different bacterial species, the aminoglycosides are considered narrow-spectrum drugs because they are normally reserved for serious systemic infections caused by aerobic gram-negative organisms, such as *Pseudomonas* and members of the Enterobacteriaceae family, which includes *E. coli, Serratia, Proteus,* and *Klebsiella.* Aminoglycosides are ineffective against most gram-positive bacteria. Because oxygen is required for aminoglycoside antibiotics to be transported inside bacterial cells, this class of drugs does not affect anaerobes.

Most aminoglycosides are polar compounds that are poorly absorbed from the GI tract. Less than 1% of an oral dose is absorbed; therefore they must be administered parenterally to treat systemic infections. Because aminoglycosides travel through the alimentary canal unchanged, they are occasionally given PO to sterilize the bowel prior to intestinal surgery. Neomycin is available for topical infections of the skin, eyes, and ears. Paromomycin (Humatin) is given orally for the treatment of parasitic infections.

Due to their polar nature, aminoglycosides cannot enter most human cells. Although distributed to most body fluids, not enough of the drugs enter the cerebrospinal fluid (CSF) for them to treat central nervous system infections. Aminoglycosides can, however, cross the placenta. If taken late in pregnancy, streptomycin can cause hearing loss in the child. In addition, aminoglycosides concentrate in renal tissue, which leads to potential nephrotoxicity.

Resistance develops quickly when aminoglycosides are administered as monotherapy. Resistance occurs when a species acquires an ability to degrade the antibiotic. Once degraded by the bacterial enzymes, these drugs are unable to bind with the bacterial ribosome. Some resistance also occurs when mutations change the shape of the bacterial ribosome so that it no longer binds the aminoglycoside. The emergence of aminoglycoside-resistant strains of *Enterococcus faecalis* and *Enterococcus faecium* has become a serious clinical problem because there are few therapeutic alternatives to treat these infections. Once resistance develops to an aminoglycoside, the mutant strain is usually resistant to the other drugs in this class. An exception is amikacin, which appears to have some activity against gentamicin-resistant strains.

Several techniques have been used to increase the effectiveness of the aminoglycosides. Administering these drugs in one large dose per day rather than smaller divided doses results in a greater bacteriocidal effect and fewer resistant microbes. A second technique is to administer aminoglycosides and penicillins concurrently (though not mixed in the same IV solution). The penicillin weakens the cell wall, allowing a greater amount of aminoglycoside to enter and reach its ribosomal targets.

Aminoglycosides are excreted almost exclusively by the kidneys. Because certain tissues bind the drugs very tightly, renal excretion may be prolonged up to 20 days after discontinuation of the drug. Although serum drug levels may fall below what is considered a minimally effective concentration, some antimicrobial activity continues during this time. This is known as a **postantibiotic effect**.

The clinical applications of the aminoglycosides are limited by their potential to cause serious adverse effects. The degree and types of toxicity are similar for all drugs in this class. For example,

TABLE 48.3	Aminoglycosides	
Drug	**Route and Adult Dose (Maximum Dose Where Indicated)**	**Adverse Effects**
amikacin	IV/IM: 5–7.5 mg/kg as a loading dose, then 7.5 mg/kg bid	*Pain or inflammation at the injection site, rash, fever, nausea, diarrhea, dizziness, tinnitus*
gentamicin (Garamycin, Others)	IV/IM: 1.5–2 mg/kg as a loading dose, then 1–2 mg/kg bid–tid	
kanamycin	IV/IM: 5–7.5 mg/kg bid–tid	Anaphylaxis, nephrotoxicity, irreversible ototoxicity, superinfections
neomycin	PO: 4–12 g/day in divided doses	
paromomycin (Humatin)	PO: 7.5–12.5 mg/kg tid	
streptomycin	IM: 15 mg/kg up to 1 g as a single dose	
tobramycin (Tobrex)	IV/IM: 1 mg/kg tid (max: 5 mg/kg/day)	

Note: Italics indicate common adverse effects. Underline indicates serious adverse effects.

all aminoglycosides can impair both hearing and balance. Damage to sensory cells in the cochlea causes hearing loss. Balance is affected by damage to sensory cells in the vestibular apparatus of the inner ear. As many as 25% of patients who are taking aminoglycoside antibiotics may experience some ototoxicity. This effect is more prominent when the medications are used for longer than 10 days, or when the patient has preexisting kidney impairment, causing high serum drug levels. The damage to sensory cells is cumulative; repeated doses of the drug can damage increasing numbers of cells. Because many older adults have some degree of preexisting hearing impairment, permanent deafness may occur in this group. Signs of impending inner ear damage include high-pitched tinnitus, headache, nausea, vomiting, and vertigo. Signs of ototoxicity may continue for several weeks after the drugs are discontinued. If hearing and balance functions are not carefully monitored during therapy and proper interventions are not implemented, the ototoxicity may become irreversible.

One of the most serious adverse effects of aminoglycosides is their potential to cause nephrotoxicity. Aminoglycosides directly injure renal tubule cells, and this nephrotoxicity may be severe, affecting up to 26% of patients receiving these antibiotics. As expected, patients who are receiving higher doses for longer periods are most affected. Those with preexisting renal impairment or who are receiving concurrent therapy with other nephrotoxic drugs must be monitored carefully: Regular evaluation of urinalysis, blood urea nitrogen (BUN), and serum creatinine results is essential. Serum drug concentrations should be obtained regularly and doses adjusted accordingly to prevent permanent damage. If recognized early, renal damage caused by aminoglycosides is reversible. Impaired kidney function may cause drug serum levels to rise, thus increasing the risk or worsening of ototoxicity.

A less common though serious adverse effect of aminoglycosides is neuromuscular blockade. Aminoglycosides inhibit the release of acetylcholine at synapses. Giving other drugs that affect acetylcholine release, such as anesthetics or neuromuscular blockers (see Chapter 26), can result in profound apnea and prolonged muscle paralysis. Because they have fewer acetylcholine receptors, patients with myasthenia gravis are especially at risk. To avoid the problem, aminoglycosides may be discontinued prior to surgery. IV calcium salts have been found to reverse aminoglycoside-induced neuromuscular blockade.

CONNECTION Checkpoint 48.2

From what you learned in Chapter 14, name the prototype drugs classified as neuromuscular blockers. Is muscle paralysis occurring at a nicotinic or muscarinic synapse? *See Answer to Connection Checkpoint 48.2 on student resource website.*

PROTOTYPE DRUG	Gentamicin (Garamycin, Others)

Classification: Therapeutic: Antibacterial
Pharmacologic: Bacterial protein synthesis inhibitor, aminoglycoside

Therapeutic Effects and Uses: Approved in 1966, gentamicin is used for the treatment and prophylaxis of susceptible bacterial infections. It is prescribed primarily for serious infections caused by

aerobic, gram-negative bacilli. Activity includes *Enterobacter, E. coli, Klebsiella, Citrobacter, Pseudomonas,* and *Serratia.* Gentamicin is effective against a few gram-positive bacteria, including some strains of MRSA. It has no activity against anaerobes. This drug is not absorbed by the PO route. A topical formulation (Genoptic) is available for infections of the external eye.

Therapy with gentamicin is generally limited to those cases in which a less toxic alternative is not available. Resistance to gentamicin is increasing, and some patients show cross-resistance to other aminoglycosides such as tobramycin. Gentamicin is sometimes given concurrently with a beta-lactam antibiotic such as a penicillin or cephalosporin to improve bacterial kill and to delay resistance.

Mechanism of Action: Gentamicin inhibits bacterial protein synthesis by binding to the 30S ribosomal subunit. Gentamicin is bacteriocidal in that it causes premature termination of the growing polypeptide chain.

Pharmacokinetics:

Route(s)	Intramuscular (IM), IV, topical (ophthalmic)
Absorption	Not absorbed PO; readily absorbed IM
Distribution	Distributed to most body tissues and fluids, except the CSF; concentrates in the kidney and inner ear; crosses the placenta; small amounts secreted in breast milk
Primary metabolism	Not metabolized
Primary excretion	Renal
Onset of action	Rapid
Duration of action	Half-life: 3–4 h

Adverse Effects: Resistance to gentamicin is increasing and some cross-resistance among aminoglycosides has been reported. Rash, nausea, vomiting, and fatigue are the most common adverse effects. **Black Box Warnings**: Adverse effects from parenteral gentamicin may be severe and include the following:

- Neurotoxicity may manifest as ototoxicity and produce a loss of hearing or balance, which may become permanent with continued use. Tinnitus, vertigo, and persistent headaches are early signs of ototoxicity. The risk of neurologic effects is higher in patients with impaired renal function. Other signs of neurotoxicity include paresthesias, muscle twitching, and seizures. Concurrent use with other neurotoxic drugs should be avoided.

- Neuromuscular blockade and respiratory paralysis are possible and the drug may cause severe neuromuscular weakness that lasts for several days.

- Nephrotoxicity is possible. Signs of reduced kidney function include oliguria, proteinuria, and elevated BUN and creatinine levels. Nephrotoxicity is of particular concern to patients with preexisting kidney disease and may limit pharmacotherapy. Concurrent use with other nephrotoxic drugs should be avoided.

Contraindications/Precautions: Gentamicin is contraindicated in patients who are hypersensitive to aminoglycosides. Drug therapy must be monitored carefully in patients with impaired renal function or in those with preexisting hearing loss. Gentamicin should not be used in pregnant or breast-feeding patients.

Drug Interactions: Concurrent use with other nephrotoxic drugs such as acyclovir, amphotericin B, capreomycin, cisplatin, cyclosporine, salicylates, polymyxin B, or vancomycin increases the risk of nephrotoxicity. Other drugs affecting the eighth cranial nerve such as ethacrynic acid and furosemide will increase the risk of ototoxicity if given concurrently with gentamicin. Penicillins can inactivate aminoglycosides if they are mixed together in the same solution. Antiemetics such as dimenhydrinate, meclizine, promethazine, and scopolamine may block the nausea characteristic of vestibular toxicity or motion sickness, thus masking the signs of aminoglycoside-induced ototoxicity. **Herbal/Food**: No significant interactions are known.

Pregnancy: Category D (parenteral).

Treatment of Overdose: Overdose can result in serious kidney damage and ototoxicity. No specific therapy is available. Patients are treated symptomatically.

Nursing Responsibilities: Key nursing implications for patients receiving gentamicin are included in the Nursing Practice Application for Patients Receiving Pharmacotherapy with a Tetracycline, Macrolide, or Aminoglycoside Antibiotic.

Drugs Similar to Gentamicin (Garamycin, Others)

Other aminoglycosides include amikacin, kanamycin, neomycin, paromomycin, streptomycin, and tobramycin. All aminoglycosides have similar spectrums of activity and adverse effects. They all carry the same black box warning as gentamicin.

Amikacin: Approved in 1976, amikacin has the broadest spectrum in this class and is sometimes effective against organisms that have developed resistance to other aminoglycosides. Amikacin has been used to treat multidrug-resistant TB. It is administered by the IV and IM routes. Indications, contraindications, and adverse effects (including the black box warning) are nearly the same as those for gentamicin. This is a pregnancy category D drug.

Kanamycin: Approved in 1958, kanamycin is the most toxic aminoglycoside, and resistant strains are common. Its use is limited to the adjunctive treatment of hepatic coma and for the short-term treatment of serious infections. Like amikacin, kanamycin may be used to treat multidrug-resistant TB after first-line drugs have failed. Kanamycin can be delivered IV, IM, by inhalation, or by intraperitoneal instillation. Contraindications and adverse effects (including the black box warning) are the same as those for gentamicin. This is a pregnancy category D drug. Concurrent therapy with other nephrotoxic and neurotoxic drugs should be avoided due to the potential for additive adverse effects.

Neomycin: Approved in 1952, neomycin is widely used for topical infections as an OTC ointment combined with polymyxin B and bacitracin (Neosporin). It is also combined in OTC creams with hydrocortisone for minor skin irritations and insect bites. Not available in parenteral form due to toxicity, neomycin may be used orally to sterilize the bowel. Oral neomycin can cause headache, lethargy, nausea, and vomiting. Oral neomycin carries a black box warning regarding neurotoxicity, nephrotoxicity, and ototoxicity. This is a pregnancy category C drug.

Paromomycin (Humatin): Approved in 1959, paromomycin is most active against gram-negative aerobic bacteria (with the exception of *Pseudomonas*). When administered orally, the drug is not absorbed and 100% is recovered in the feces. The primary use of this drug is for sterilizing the bowel and treating intestinal parasitic infections caused by protozoans and tapeworms. Because this drug is not absorbed systemically, it does not carry the same black box warnings as other aminoglycosides. This is a pregnancy category C drug.

Streptomycin: The use of streptomycin, the first aminoglycoside approved by the U.S. Food and Drug Administration (FDA) in 1945, was generally discontinued in 1993, but it is still available on a case-by-case basis. It is rarely used due to a large number of resistant strains and its high risk for ototoxicity. It is most often used in combination with other drugs in the pharmacotherapy of multidrug-resistant TB. Streptomycin carries a black box warning regarding neurotoxicity and nephrotoxicity. This is a pregnancy category D drug.

Tobramycin: Approved in 1975, tobramycin has a spectrum of activity similar to that of gentamicin, but it is more effective against *P. aeruginosa* than gentamicin. Most often administered parenterally, tobramycin is also available as an ophthalmic solution (Tobrex) and in nebulizer form for patients with cystic fibrosis who have *Pseudomonas* infections. Adverse effects (including the black box warning) and contraindications are similar to those of gentamicin. This is a pregnancy category D drug.

PharmFACT

This chapter discussed antibiotics selective for bacterial protein synthesis. However, bacteria can fight back. *Corynebacterium diphtheriae* produces a toxin that targets human protein synthesis (Madigan, Martinko, Stahl, & Clark, 2012).

Miscellaneous Inhibitors of Bacterial Protein Synthesis

48.5 Several inhibitors of protein synthesis are effective against resistant infections but may have significant adverse effects that limit their use.

Several bacterial protein synthesis inhibitors do not belong to the tetracycline, macrolide, or aminoglycoside classes. These miscellaneous drugs, listed in Table 48.4, have varying spectrums of activity and adverse effect profiles and thus must be considered individually. One of the medications in the miscellaneous class, spectinomycin (Trobicin), has been discontinued in the United States.

Chloramphenicol: Chloramphenicol is an older, broad-spectrum antibiotic that was approved in 1960 and has been available for nearly 60 years. It binds to the 50S subunit of the bacterial ribosome and may be bacteriostatic or bacteriocidal, depending on species and dose. Chloramphenicol is administered PO or IV as chloramphenicol succinate for serious infections. A topical form is available for ophthalmic and otic infections.

Effective in treating salmonellae, rickettsiae, streptococci, typhoid fever, and meningitis caused by *H. influenzae*, this drug was widely used before it was found to be associated with bone

TABLE 48.4 Miscellaneous Inhibitors of Bacterial Protein Synthesis

Drug	Route and Adult Dose (Maximum Dose Where Indicated)	Adverse Effects
chloramphenicol	PO: 12.5 mg/kg qid	*Nausea, vomiting, diarrhea* Anaphylaxis, superinfections, pancytopenia, bone marrow depression, aplastic anemia
clindamycin (Cleocin, Others)	PO: 150–450 mg qid IV: 600–1,200 mg/day in divided doses	*Nausea, vomiting, diarrhea, rash, burning, or pruritus (topical forms)* Anaphylaxis, superinfections, cardiac arrest, PMC, blood dyscrasias
lincomycin (Lincocin)	PO: 500 mg tid–qid (max: 8 g/day) IM: 600 mg every 12–24 h (max: 8 g/day)	*Nausea, vomiting, diarrhea* Anaphylaxis, superinfections, cardiac arrest, PMC, blood dyscrasias
linezolid (Zyvox)	PO/IV: 600 mg every 12 h (max: 1,200 mg/day)	*Nausea, diarrhea, headache* Anaphylaxis, superinfections, PMC, blood dyscrasias
quinupristin-dalfopristin (Synercid)	IV: 7.5 mg/kg infused over 60 min every 8 h	*Pain and inflammation at the injection site, myalgia, arthralgia, diarrhea* Superinfections, PMC
telithromycin (Ketek)	PO: 800 mg once a day	*Nausea, vomiting, diarrhea* Visual disturbances, hepatotoxicity, dysrhythmias

Note: Italics indicate common adverse effects. <u>Underline</u> indicates serious adverse effects.

marrow suppression and a very small, though fatal, incidence of aplastic anemia. Chloramphenicol carries a black box warning that serious and fatal blood dyscrasias have been reported with the drug. Peak and trough serum levels should be monitored regularly during therapy to avoid serious adverse effects. Chloramphenicol is now reserved for meningitis and other infections in which the benefits of the drug clearly outweigh the risks of serious drug toxicity.

Another serious toxicity from chloramphenicol is **gray baby syndrome**. Most often seen in premature or newborn infants, this syndrome occurs when the baby's liver is unable to metabolize or excrete this drug. Symptoms include failure to feed, abdominal distention, cyanosis, and cardiovascular collapse. The syndrome is rapidly fatal and can cause death in just a few hours. If done early, discontinuing chloramphenicol therapy can reverse the syndrome. This is a pregnancy category C drug.

Clindamycin (Cleocin, Others): Approved in 1970, clindamycin acts on the 50S bacterial ribosomal subunit in a manner similar to that of the macrolides. It is usually bacteriostatic. A drug of choice for abdominal infections caused by *Bacteroides fragilis*, it is also effective against *Fusobacterium*, *Actinomyces*, and *Clostridium*.

Three salts of clindamycin are available: clindamycin hydrochloride (PO), clindamycin palmitate (PO), and clindamycin phosphate (parenteral or topical). In 2004, an aerosol topical foam of 1% clindamycin (Evoclin) was approved for the treatment of acne vulgaris, and a single-dose suppository vaginal cream (Clindesse) was marketed for bacterial vaginosis.

Once widely prescribed as a penicillin alternative, the use of clindamycin has become limited due to the development of resistant strains, a high incidence of diarrhea, and a potential risk of drug-induced PMC caused by *C. difficile*, which can be fatal (black box warning). It is generally only used when safer alternatives are not effective. The nurse must advise patients to report incidences of diarrhea during clindamycin therapy. If PMC is suspected, clindamycin is discontinued and the patient is placed on a drug that

is effective against *C. difficile* such as vancomycin. This is a pregnancy category B drug.

Lincomycin (Lincocin): Approved in 1964, lincomycin is chemically similar to clindamycin. Lincomycin may be used for patients who cannot take penicillins or cephalosporins but it offers no therapeutic advantages over clindamycin. The drug is rarely prescribed due to a relatively high incidence of serious adverse effects, especially PMC (black box warning). It is available by both PO and parenteral routes. This is a pregnancy category B drug.

Linezolid (Zyvox): Approved in 2000, linezolid is in a class of antibiotics called **oxazolidinones** that act by binding to a part of the bacterial 50S ribosome known as the 23S portion. It is unique among antibiotics in that it prevents the first event in protein synthesis, which is the formation of an initiation complex. It is believed to be bacteriocidal. Linezolid is important because it is effective against infections that have become resistant to most other antibiotics, including MRSA and VRE. It is less effective against gram-negative organisms. Oral and IV formulations are available.

Adverse effects are usually minor and related to GI distress. Because this drug can cause transient dose-related myelosuppression, laboratory blood counts should be frequently monitored during therapy. Linezolid is a nonselective inhibitor of monoamine oxidase (MAO) and may cause hypertension in some patients. Risk for hypertension and palpitations is increased if the patient is taking sympathomimetics concurrently with linezolid; thus these medications should be avoided. Patients with diabetes should be cautioned of possible hypoglycemic events while taking linezolid. This is a pregnancy category C drug.

Quinupristin-dalfopristin (Synercid): Approved in 1999, quinupristin-dalfopristin is a fixed-dose bacteriocidal combination used for therapy of life-threatening *E. faecium* infections that are vancomycin resistant and for complicated infections caused by MRSA or *Streptococcus pyogenes*. It belongs to a class of antibiotics called *streptogramins* that act by binding the 50S bacterial ribosome

CONNECTIONS: NURSING PRACTICE APPLICATION

Patients Receiving Pharmacotherapy with a Tetracycline, Macrolide, or Aminoglycoside Antibiotic

Assessment	Potential Nursing Diagnoses*
Baseline assessment prior to administration: • Obtain a complete health history including neurologic, cardiovascular, respiratory, hepatic, or renal disease, and the possibility of pregnancy. Obtain a drug history including allergies, specific reactions to drugs, current prescription and OTC drugs, herbal preparations, and alcohol use. Be alert to possible drug interactions. • Assess signs and symptoms of the current infection, noting location, characteristics, presence or absence of drainage and the characteristics of drainage, duration, and presence or absence of fever or pain. • Evaluate appropriate laboratory findings (e.g., CBC, culture and sensitivity [C&S], hepatic and renal function studies). • Assess the patient's ability to receive and understand instructions. Include family and caregivers as needed.	• *Infection* (bacterial) • *Acute Pain* • *Hyperthermia* • *Deficient Knowledge* (Drug Therapy) • *Risk for Injury*, related to adverse drug effects • *Risk for Deficient Fluid Volume*, related to diarrhea caused by adverse drug effects
Assessment throughout administration: • Assess for desired therapeutic effects (e.g., diminished signs and symptoms of infection and fever). • Continue periodic monitoring of CBC, hepatic and renal function, urinalysis, and C&S as ordered. • Assess for adverse effects: nausea, vomiting, abdominal cramping, diarrhea, drowsiness, tinnitus, or dizziness. Severe diarrhea, especially that containing mucus, blood, or pus, yellowing of the sclera or skin, decreased urine output or darkened urine should be reported immediately.	

Implementation

Interventions and (Rationales)	Patient-Centered Care
Ensuring therapeutic effects: • Continue assessments as above for therapeutic effects. (Diminished fever, pain, or signs and symptoms of infection should begin after taking the first dose and continue to improve. The provider should be notified if fever and signs and symptoms of infection remain or increase after 3 days, or if the entire course of antibacterial has been taken and signs of infection are still present.)	• Teach the patient to complete the entire course of the antibacterial therapy; do not share doses with other family members with similar symptoms; and return to the provider if symptoms have not resolved after an entire course of therapy.
Minimizing adverse effects: • Continue to monitor vital signs, especially temperature if fever is present. Immediately report undiminished fever, changes in level of consciousness, or febrile seizures to the health care provider. (Fever should begin to diminish within 1–3 days after starting the drug. Continued fever may be a sign of worsening infection, adverse drug effects, or antibiotic resistance.)	• Teach the patient to report fever that does not diminish below 37.8°C (100°F) or per parameters set by the health care provider. Immediately report febrile seizures, changes in behavior, or changes in level of consciousness to the health care provider.
• Continue to monitor periodic laboratory work: hepatic and renal function tests, CBC, urinalysis, C&S, and peak and trough drug levels as ordered. (Tetracyclines and aminoglycosides may be renal toxic; macrolides may be hepatotoxic. Periodic C&S tests may be ordered if infections are severe or are slow to resolve to confirm appropriate therapy. Peak and trough drug levels will be monitored for aminoglycosides to prevent severe adverse effects.)	• Instruct the patient on the need for periodic laboratory work.
• Monitor for hypersensitivity and allergic reactions, especially with the first dose of the drug. Continue to monitor the patient for up to 2 weeks after completing antibacterial therapy. (Anaphylactic reactions are possible, particularly with the first dose of an antibacterial. Post-use, residual drug levels, dependent on the length of half-life, may cause delayed reactions.)	• Teach the patient to immediately report any itching, rashes, or swelling, particularly of the face or tongue, urticaria, flushing, dizziness, syncope, wheezing, throat tightness, or difficulty breathing. • Instruct the patient with known antibacterial allergies to carry a wallet identification card or wear medical identification jewelry indicating the allergy.
• Continue to monitor for nephrotoxicity; e.g., diminished urine output, or weight gain greater than 1 kg (2 lbs) in 24 h. (Tetracyclines and aminoglycosides may require frequent monitoring to prevent adverse effects. **Lifespan**: Age-related physiological differences may place the young child or older adult at greater risk for renal toxicity.)	• Teach the patient to immediately report any diminished urine output, visible swelling of feet or ankles, or weight gain greater than 1 kg (2 lbs) in 24 h. • Advise the patient to increase fluid intake to 2–3 L/day.

CONNECTIONS: NURSING PRACTICE APPLICATION (*continued*)

- Monitor for the development of superinfections, e.g., CDAD or PMC, fungal or yeast infections. (Superinfections with opportunistic organisms may occur when normal host flora are diminished or killed by the antibacterial drug and no longer hold pathogens in check. Severe diarrhea may indicate the presence of CDAD or PMC, superinfections caused by *C. difficile*.)

  - Instruct the patient to report any diarrhea that increases in frequency, amount, or contains mucus, blood, or pus.
  - Instruct the patient to consult the health care provider before taking any antidiarrheal drugs, which cause the retention of harmful bacteria.
  - Teach the patient to observe for changes in the color, consistency, or frequency of stool, white patches in the mouth, whitish thick vaginal discharge, itching in the genital area, or blistering itchy rash.
  - Teach the patient infection control measures such as frequent hand washing, adequate drying after showering or bathing, and to increase the intake of live-culture dairy foods.

- Monitor for significant throat irritation in patients taking tetracycline. (Esophagitis or esophageal ulceration may occur secondary to tetracycline use.)

  - Teach the patient taking tetracycline to immediately report any difficulty in swallowing or throat or epigastric pain.

- Monitor for signs and symptoms of neurotoxicity, e.g., dizziness, drowsiness, severe headache, tinnitus, increasing muscle weakness, paresthesias, twitching, or seizures. (Aminoglycosides have an increased risk of neurotoxicity. **Lifespan:** Be particularly cautious with the older adult who is at greater risk for falls.)

  - Instruct the patient to immediately report increasing headache, dizziness, twitching, or seizures. If dizziness occurs, the patient should sit or lie down and not attempt to stand or walk until the sensation passes.

- Monitor electrolytes, pulse, and ECG if indicated in patients taking erythromycin and related drugs. (Erythromycin and some related drugs may prolong the Q-T interval and increase the risk for potentially fatal dysrhythmias.)

  - Teach the patient to promptly report any palpitations, lightheadedness, or dizziness.

- Monitor for signs and symptoms of ototoxicity, e.g., dizziness, vertigo, tinnitus, or diminished hearing. (Erythromycin and aminoglycosides have an increased risk of ototoxicity.)

  - Instruct the patient to immediately report dizziness, vertigo, tinnitus, or diminished hearing.

- Monitor for the effects of other drugs if the patient is on erythromycin. (**Diverse Patients:** Because erythromycin metabolizes through the P450 system pathways, monitor ethnically diverse patients to ensure optimal therapeutic effects and to minimize adverse effects. Erythromycin also inhibits P450 enzymes and is known to increase the effects of some drugs such as anticoagulants and digoxin and decrease others. Grapefruit juice taken concurrently with erythromycin may increase drug levels.)

  - Teach the patient to report any unusual effects related to other drugs taken concurrently. If the patient is taking anticoagulants, an increase in bleeding should be immediately reported.
  - Teach the patient not to consume grapefruit or grapefruit juice while taking erythromycin.

- Continue to monitor for dermatologic effects including red or purplish skin rash, blisters, or sunburn. Immediately report severe rashes, especially when accompanied by blistering. (Tetracyclines may cause significant dermatologic effects including Stevens–Johnson syndrome.)

  - Teach the patient to wear sunscreen and protective clothing for sun exposure and to avoid tanning beds. Immediately report any severe sunburn or rashes.

- **Lifespan:** Assess for the possibility of pregnancy or breast-feeding in patients prescribed tetracycline or erythromycin antibiotics. (Tetracyclines affect fetal bone growth and teeth development, causing permanent yellowish-brown staining of teeth. Tetracycline use in children under age 8 or 9 should also be avoided. Erythromycin antibiotics may significantly reduce the effectiveness of oral contraceptives, and a secondary method to prevent conception should be used.)

  - Advise women who are pregnant, breast-feeding, or attempting to become pregnant to inform their health care provider before receiving any tetracycline antibiotic.
  - Teach women of childbearing age on oral contraceptives to consult their health care provider about birth control alternatives if erythromycin antibiotics are ordered.

Patient understanding of drug therapy:
- Use opportunities during administration of medications and during assessments to discuss the rationale for drug therapy, desired therapeutic outcomes, commonly observed adverse effects, parameters for when to call the health care provider, and any necessary monitoring or precautions. (Using time during nursing care helps to optimize and reinforce key teaching areas.)

  - The patient, family, or caregiver should be able to state the reason for the drug, appropriate dose and scheduling, what adverse effects to observe for and when to report them, and the anticipated length of medication therapy.

Patient self-administration of drug therapy:
- When administering the medications, instruct the patient, family, or caregiver in proper self-administration techniques followed by teach-back. (Utilizing time during nurse-administration of these drugs helps to reinforce teaching.)

  - Teach the patient to take the medication:
    - Complete the entire course of therapy unless otherwise instructed. Do not share with other family members and do not stop taking the medicine when starting to feel better.
    - Take the drug with food or milk and avoid acidic or carbonated beverages to decrease GI effects.
    - Do not take tetracycline with milk products, iron-containing preparations such as multivitamins, or with antacids. Take the tetracycline 1 h before or 2 h after consuming these products.
    - Take the medication as evenly spaced throughout each day as feasible.
    - Increase overall fluid intake while taking the antibacterial drug.
    - Discard outdated medications or those no longer in use. Review the medicine cabinet twice a year for old medications (e.g., at the beginning and end of daylight saving time).

in a manner similar to that of the macrolides. The combination of the two antibiotics is truly synergistic: The combination has 16 times more antimicrobial activity compared to either drug used alone. Synercid is bacteriocidal and only available by the IV route.

Joint and muscle pain, diarrhea, rash, and pain at the infusion site are common adverse effects. Venous irritation may be severe enough to cause the drug to be discontinued. Synercid inhibits hepatic drug metabolism enzymes, resulting in numerous drug–drug interactions. The nurse should use caution when administering drugs concurrently with Synercid, because those that rely on hepatic metabolism for detoxification may build to toxic levels in the blood. In addition, some cases of PMC have been reported. Quinupristin-dalfopristin carries a black box warning that it should be reserved for serious or life-threatening vancomycin-resistant *E. faecium* infections. Despite its potential for adverse effects, quinupristin-dalfopristin serves an important role in treating multidrug-resistant gram-positive pathogens, which have become a major clinical challenge. This is a pregnancy category B drug.

Telithromycin (Ketek): Approved in 2004, telithromycin is a broad-spectrum antibiotic structurally similar to the macrolides. Telithromycin is the sole member of a class called *ketolides*.

Ketolides inhibit bacterial protein synthesis by the same mechanism as the macrolides: by binding to the 50S ribosomal subunit. However, telithromycin binds more tightly to the ribosome than other protein synthesis inhibitors and is capable of causing greater bacterial kill. It also exhibits a significant postantibiotic effect in some organisms. Indications for telithromycin are similar to those of the macrolides except it has greater activity against *S. pneumoniae*. Because of this, its primary use is to treat bronchitis, sinusitis, and community-acquired pneumonia. It is effective against many other bacterial strains, including those that show macrolide resistance. This drug is available as oral tablets.

Although most adverse effects are minor and GI related, telithromycin has the potential to cause several serious adverse effects. Hepatotoxicity has occurred in a small number of patients. Telithromycin can cause blurred vision, double vision, and difficulty focusing, which can be severe enough to cause discontinuation of therapy. Telithromycin carries a black box warning that patients with myasthenia gravis should not take this drug because life-threatening respiratory failure may occur. As with some of the macrolides, telithromycin may increase the risk for ventricular dysrhythmias such as torsades de pointes and is contraindicated in patients with prolonged QT intervals. This is a pregnancy category C drug.

CHAPTER

48

Understanding the Chapter

Key Concepts Summary

48.1 Antibiotics inhibit microbial protein synthesis by binding to the bacterial ribosome.

48.2 Tetracyclines have broad antimicrobial activity against many gram-positive and gram-negative bacteria.

48.3 The macrolides are alternatives to penicillin for many gram-positive infections.

48.4 The aminoglycosides are effective against aerobic gram-negative organisms but have the potential to cause ototoxicity and nephrotoxicity.

48.5 Several inhibitors of protein synthesis are effective against resistant infections but may have significant adverse effects that limit their use.

Case Study: Making the Patient Connection

Remember the patient "John Travis" at the beginning of the chapter? Now read the remainder of the case study. Based on the information presented within this chapter, respond to the critical thinking questions that follow.

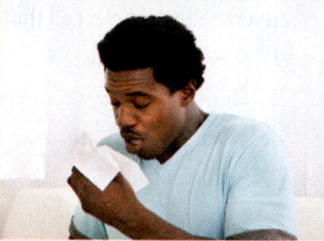

John Travis, a 31-year-old high school teacher, has had an upper respiratory infection for the past 2 weeks. Although he has seen his health care provider, he does not seem to be improving. He is convinced that if he takes the antibiotic just 1 more day, he will surely improve. However, after 5 days of drug therapy, John continues to experience chills, fever, and a productive cough. His wife insisted that he return to the clinic for further evaluation and treatment.

At the clinic the patient's physical examination and diagnostic tests reveal the following findings: Temperature is 39.2°C (102.6°F), pulse rate is 112 beats/min, respiratory rate is 30 breaths/min, and blood pressure is 134/88 mmHg. He is visibly short of breath and is experiencing intermittent coughing episodes. On auscultation of his lung fields, bilateral crackles and wheezes are discovered. His WBC count is 14,400 mm³. A chest x-ray is taken to confirm a diagnosis of pneumonia and reveals right lower lobe infiltrates (white areas in the lung that indicate infection).

The patient is diagnosed with bacterial pneumonia. He is hospitalized and prescribed IV antibiotic therapy. On the second hospital day you are assigned to care for John. He and his wife have multiple questions about the drug therapy prescribed.

Critical Thinking Questions

1. Why did the first antibiotic prescribed not cure the infection?
2. The patient has been told that a sputum specimen is needed for a "C and S" and asks what that is. What will the nurse teach him about this test and why it is needed?
3. John has been told that laboratory personnel will be collecting blood for a peak and trough level this afternoon and in the morning. How would the nurse explain this laboratory test to the patient?
4. What symptoms would indicate that the patient's condition is worsening?

See Answers to Critical Thinking Questions on student resource website.

Additional Case Study

Mr. Klein is an 85-year-old man seen in the outpatient clinic for an acute infection. He has informed the health care provider that he is allergic to a variety of antibiotics and is subsequently prescribed erythromycin estolate. The patient is a recovering alcoholic who has been abstinent for 10 years.

1. What is the significance of Mr. Klein's history of alcoholism?

2. What possible adverse effect should the nurse instruct the patient to watch for?
3. What laboratory diagnostic studies may be indicated in this patient?

See Answers to Additional Case Study on student resource website.

Chapter Review

1 While teaching the patient about taking oral tetracycline, which of the following does the nurse advise the patient to do?

1. Consume calcium-rich products to decrease the duration of the antibacterial effect.
2. Use a soft toothbrush and floss teeth gently to remove staining on teeth.
3. Report any ringing in the ears or dizziness.
4. Avoid direct exposure to sunlight and apply sun block when outdoors.

2 The nurse determines that the patient understands the use of azithromycin (Zithromax) when the patient makes which statement?

1. "It only needs to be taken once daily because it lasts longer."
2. "It causes more nausea than most other antibiotics in this classification."
3. "It must be taken on an empty stomach."
4. "It is ineffective if taken with calcium-rich foods."

3 The patient is receiving amikacin (Amikin) for a bacterial infection. Which adverse effects does the nurse include in the plan of care to monitor the patient's status?

1. Weight gain
2. Visual disturbances
3. Mental depression
4. Urinary frequency

4 The health care provider orders gentamicin (Garamycin) for a patient with a postoperative wound infection. Which laboratory result should prompt the nurse to consult with the prescriber about possible nephrotoxicity of this drug?

1. Elevated serum creatinine level
2. Decreased blood urea nitrogen (BUN) level
3. Increased white blood cell (WBC) count
4. Elevated serum iron level

5 The patient has received a prescription for tetracycline (Sumycin) for treatment of acne. The nurse will teach the patient to avoid taking the tetracycline concurrently with _____.

6 The patient is receiving gentamicin (Garamycin) IV for a significant infection. While the patient is receiving this drug, what assessment data will the nurse gather to monitor for adverse effects? Select all that apply.

1. Serum creatinine
2. Signs of muscle weakness
3. Liver function studies
4. Urine output
5. Hearing and balance assessments

See Answers to Chapter Review in Appendix A.

References

Centers for Disease Control and Prevention. (2010). Sexually transmitted diseases: Treatment guidelines 2010. *Morbidity and Mortality Weekly Report, 59*. Retrieved from http://www.uphs.upenn.edu/bugdrug/antibiotic_manual/cdcstdrx2010.pdf

de la Cabada Bauche, J., & DuPont, H. L. (2011). New developments in traveler's diarrhea. *Gastroenterology and Hepatology, 7*, 88–95.

Dufel, S. E. (2013). CBRNE—Plague. *Medscape Reference*. Retrieved from http://emedicine.medscape.com/article/829233-overview

Kollaritsch, H., Paulke-Korinek, M., & Wiedermann, U. (2012). Traveler's diarrhea. *Infectious Disease Clinics of North America, 26*, 691–706. doi:10.1016/j.idc.2012.06.002

Madigan, M. T., Martinko, J. M., Stahl, D. A., & Clark, D. P. (2012). *Brock biology of microorganisms* (13th ed.). San Francisco, CA: Benjamin Cummings.

Tortora, G. J., Funke, B. R., & Case, C. L. (2013). *Microbiology: An introduction* (11th ed.). San Francisco, CA: Benjamin Cummings.

Selected Bibliography

Anderson, R. J., Groundwater, P. W., Todd, A., & Worsley, A. J. (2012). *Antibacterial agents: Chemistry, mode of action, mechanisms of resistance and clinical applications* (pp. 173–196). Chichester, UK: John Wiley & Sons, Ltd. doi:10.1002/9781118325421.ch8

Barnes, B. E., & Sampson, D. A. (2011). A literature review on community-acquired methicillin-resistant *Staphylococcus aureus* in the United States: Clinical information for primary care nurse practitioners. *Journal of the American Academy of Nurse Practitioners, 23*, 23–32. doi:10.1111/j.1745-7599.2010.00571.x

Davey, P., Sneddon, K., & Nathwani, D. (2010). Overview of strategies for overcoming the challenge of antimicrobial resistance. *Expert Review of Clinical Pharmacology, 3*, 667–686. doi:10.1586/ecp.10.46

Guilbeau, J. R., & Fordham, P. N. (2010). Evidence-based management and treatment of outpatient community-associated MRSA. *Journal for Nurse Practitioners, 6*, 140–145. doi:10.1016/j.nurpra.2009.07.011

Herdman, T. H., & Kamitsuru, S. (Eds.). (2014). *NANDA International nursing diagnoses: Definitions and classification, 2015–2017.* Oxford, United Kingdom: Wiley-Blackwell.

Kee, V. R. (2012). *Clostridium difficile* infection in older adults: A review and update on its management. *The American Journal of Geriatric Pharmacotherapy, 10*(1), 14–24. doi.org/10.1016/j.amjopharm.2011.12.004

Kwok, C. S., Arthur, A. K., Anibueze, C. I., Singh, S., Cavallazzi, R., & Loke, Y. K. (2012). Risk of clostridium difficile infection with acid suppressing drugs and antibiotics: Meta-analysis. *The American Journal of Gastroenterology, 107*, 1011–1019. doi:10.1038/ajg.2012.108

Labby, K. J., & Garneau-Tsodikova, S. (2013). Strategies to overcome the action of aminoglycoside-modifying enzymes for treating resistant bacterial infections. *Future Medicinal Chemistry, 5*, 1285–1309. doi:10.4155/fmc.13.80

Paitan, Y., & Ron, E. Z. (2014). Gram-negative pathogens: Overview of novel and emerging resistant pathogens and drugs. In F. Marinelli & O. Genilloud (Eds.), *Antimicrobials* (pp. 29–56). Berlin, Heidelberg, Germany: Springer.

Rossolini, G. M., Mantengoli, E., Mantagnani, F., & Pollini, S. (2010). Epidemiology and clinical relevance of microbial resistance determinants versus anti-gram-positive agents. *Current Opinion in Microbiology, 13*, 582–588. doi:10.1016/j.mib.2010.08.006

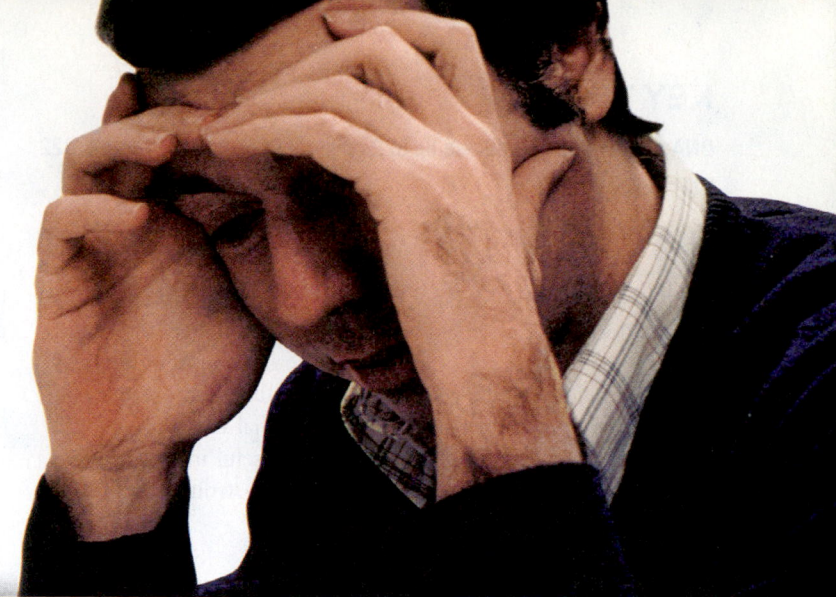

"Every morning for the last month I have had terrible headaches with pain directly on my forehead. Then my upper jaw and cheeks became tender to touch and my teeth ached."

Patient "Mike Springs"

LEARNING OUTCOMES

After reading this chapter, the student should be able to:

1. Explain the steps in bacterial DNA replication.

2. Identify the classes of drugs that act by affecting bacterial DNA replication.

3. Explain mechanisms by which fluoroquinolones inhibit bacterial DNA replication.

4. Describe means by which bacteria become resistant to fluoroquinolones.

5. For each of the classes shown in the chapter outline, identify the prototype and representative drugs and explain the mechanism(s) of drug action, primary indications, contraindications, significant drug interactions, pregnancy category, and important adverse effects.

6. Explain the nurse's role in the safe administration of fluoroquinolones.

7. Apply the nursing process to care for patients who are receiving pharmacotherapy with fluoroquinolones and miscellaneous antibacterials.

CHAPTER OUTLINE

▶ Bacterial DNA Replication

▶ Inhibition of DNA Replication

▶ Fluoroquinolones
  PROTOTYPE Ciprofloxacin (Cipro), *p. 825*

▶ Miscellaneous Antibacterials
  Bacitracin
  Daptomycin (Cubicin)
  Metronidazole (Flagyl)
  Polymyxin B
  Rifampin (Rifadin, Rimactane)
  Telithromycin (Ketek)

KEY TERMS

DNA gyrase (topoisomerase II), 822

DNA helicase, 822

DNA polymerase, 822

ketolides, 830

supercoil, 822

topoisomerase IV, 822

With resistance to other antibacterials developing rapidly, drugs in the fluoroquinolone class have become increasingly important in the pharmacotherapy of infectious diseases. Fluoroquinolones are bacteriocidal and are effective against many gram-positive and gram-negative microbes. They affect bacterial deoxyribonucleic acid (DNA) synthesis and are particularly useful in the management of respiratory, genitourinary, and gastrointestinal (GI) infections.

Bacterial DNA Replication

49.1 Bacterial DNA replication requires several different enzymes to uncoil, unwind, and duplicate the DNA.

Under optimal conditions, many pathogenic bacteria can divide every 1 to 3 hours. Under highly favorable conditions, *Escherichia coli* divides every 20 minutes, producing a billion cells in only 10 hours. The most critical step in bacterial reproduction is duplicating the DNA so that each daughter cell contains the same genetic material. Thus, bacteria are in the process of continuously replicating their DNA as well as constructing cell walls and synthesizing proteins.

Like human DNA, bacterial DNA uses the four bases, adenine, guanine, cytosine, and thymidine, and is arranged in a double-helical formation. Most bacteria, however, contain a single circular chromosome as illustrated in Figure 49.1. The helix is then twisted and coiled. This highly twisted arrangement is called a **supercoil**. This supercoiled arrangement is necessary for all the DNA to fit into the small bacterial cell. However, this supercoil must be relaxed and the two helices unwound immediately prior to replicating its DNA, so that duplication enzymes can reach the bases.

A large number of enzymes are needed for DNA replication, and some of these enzymes are targets for antibiotics. This is a complex process but may be simplified in four steps. The enzymes involved in this four-step process afford different sites at which drugs may act.

1. Relax: Supercoil is relaxed by the enzyme **DNA gyrase** (also called **topoisomerase II**).

2. Unwind: After the supercoil is relaxed, the enzyme **DNA helicase** unwinds the two strands.

3. Replicate: The enzyme **DNA polymerase** adds the precursor bases to replicate the original DNA and form new DNA strands.

4. Migrate: The two newly formed strands are interlocked until the enzyme **topoisomerase IV** frees them to migrate to opposite sides of the cell, where they are segregated into the two daughter cells.

Inhibition of DNA Replication

49.2 Drugs have been discovered that inhibit different steps in bacterial DNA replication.

Blocking the DNA replication of a pathogen is a common mechanism used by drugs across several different therapeutic classes. Drugs can block bacterial DNA replication in three basic ways:

- Drugs can inhibit the synthesis or availability of precursor bases or nucleotides.

- Drugs can bind to bacterial DNA, preventing the relaxation and uncoiling processes required for replication.

- Drugs can bind to enzymes of DNA replication, halting the formation of new DNA strands.

A number of drugs employed in cancer chemotherapy act by mimicking precursor molecules or by interacting with DNA. Cytarabine (Cytosar-U) and fluorouracil (5-FU) resemble nucleotides

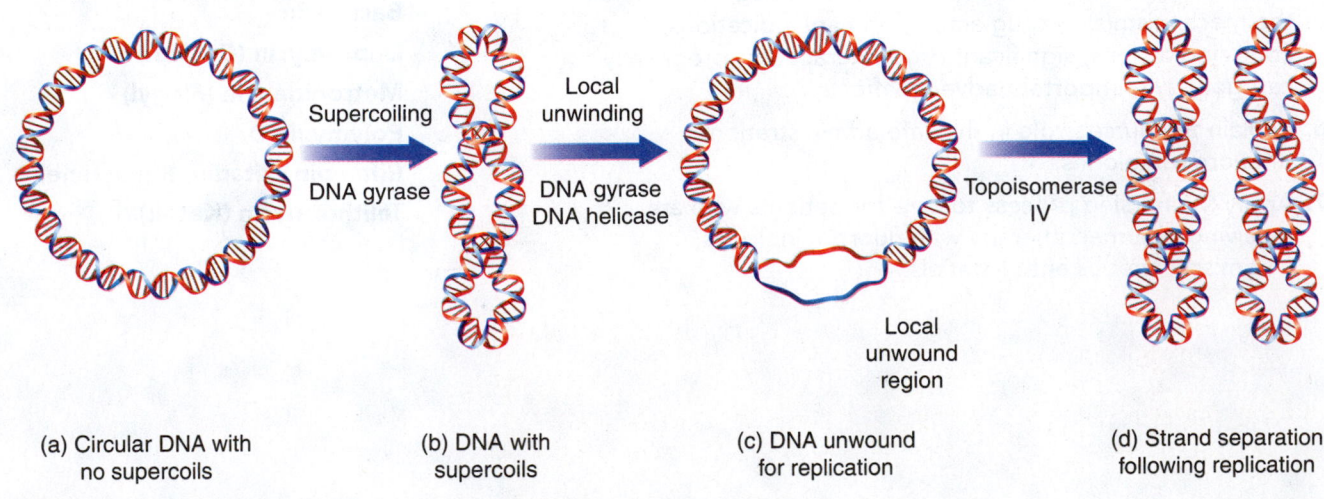

(a) Circular DNA with no supercoils

(b) DNA with supercoils

(c) DNA unwound for replication

(d) Strand separation following replication

Figure 49.1 The unwinding and replication of bacterial DNA.

and are mistakenly incorporated into newly formed DNA strands. Daunorubicin (Cerubidine) and bleomycin (Blenoxane) are highly toxic antibiotics that interact with DNA to physically block replication. Although classified as antibiotics, these drugs are too toxic to be used for infections but have therapeutic indications in the chemotherapy of specific types of cancer.

Several drugs act by inhibiting enzymes involved in DNA replication. Acyclovir (Zovirax) inhibits the DNA polymerase of herpesvirus and is a leading drug for treating this infection (see Chapter 54). Teniposide (Vumon) and etoposide (VePesid) are antineoplastic drugs that act by inhibiting topoisomerase I, an enzyme that helps repair DNA damage. By binding in a complex with topoisomerase and DNA, these antineoplastics cause strand breaks that accumulate and permanently damage the DNA.

The fluoroquinolone antibiotics act on two enzymes in the DNA replication process. First, they bind to DNA gyrase, inhibiting its ability to relax the supercoiling of the bacterial DNA. When the replication enzymes reach an area still in a supercoiled state, replication terminates. A second mechanism is binding to topoisomerase IV. When this occurs, the two daughter DNA strands cannot migrate to opposite sides of the cell, and division cannot be completed. It is thought that fluoroquinolones inhibit DNA gyrase in gram-negative organisms, and inhibit topoisomerase IV in gram-positive organisms. However, this is likely an oversimplification of their exact mechanism. These drugs have no effect on human enzymes involved in DNA replication because of significant differences in the chemical structures of the human and bacterial enzymes. These differences account for their selective toxicity on bacteria and their favorable safety profile.

Fluoroquinolones

49.3 Fluoroquinolones are antibiotics whose therapeutic applications have expanded in recent years to treat many gram-positive and gram-negative infections.

The first drug in this class, nalidixic acid (NegGram), was approved in 1962. Classified as a quinolone, the use of nalidixic acid was restricted to treating urinary tract infections (UTIs) due to its narrow spectrum of activity and a high incidence of bacterial resistance. Nalidixic acid is still used for the pharmacotherapy of UTIs, although it is not a drug of first choice. Nalidixic acid is important because it served as a building block for the synthesis of other drugs in this class.

In the late 1980s, the development of quinolones with a fluorine side chain resulted in drugs with wider spectrums of activity and longer durations of action. The fluoroquinolones, listed in Table 49.1, have become an increasingly important class of antibiotics in the past two decades. Fluoroquinolones are bacteriocidal and affect bacterial DNA synthesis by inhibiting both DNA gyrase and topoisomerase IV.

Four generations of fluoroquinolones are available, based on their antibacterial spectrums. All fluoroquinolones have activity against gram-negative pathogens, with the newer drugs being significantly more effective against gram-positive bacteria. The distinctions among the generations are listed in Table 49.2. The newer fluoroquinolones were developed and approved primarily for the treatment of respiratory infections.

Clinical applications of fluoroquinolones include infections of the respiratory, GI, and genitourinary tracts, and some skin and soft tissue infections. Their effectiveness against gram-negative

TABLE 49.1 Fluoroquinolones and Quinolones

Drug	Route and Adult Dose (Maximum Dose Where Indicated)	Adverse Effects
First Generation		*Nausea, headache, diarrhea, rash, insomnia, pain and inflammation at injection site, local burning, stinging, corneal irritation (ophthalmic)*
nalidixic acid (NegGram)	PO: Acute therapy: 1 g qid PO: Chronic therapy: 500 mg qid	
Second Generation		Anaphylaxis, tendon rupture, superinfections, photosensitivity, pseudomembranous colitis (PMC), seizure, peripheral neuropathy, hepatotoxicity
ciprofloxacin (Cipro)	PO: 250–750 mg bid (max: 1,500 mg/day)	
norfloxacin (Noroxin)	PO: 400 mg bid or 800 mg once daily	
ofloxacin (Floxin)	PO/IV: 200–400 mg bid (max: 800 mg/day)	
Third Generation		
gatifloxacin (Zymar, Zymaxid)	Drops (ophthalmic solution): 1 drop in each affected eye every 2–4 h	
levofloxacin (Levaquin)	PO/IV: 250–750 mg/day (max: 750 mg/day)	
Fourth Generation		
besifloxacin (Besivance)	Drops (ophthalmic solution): 1 drop in each affected eye every 8 h	
gemifloxacin (Factive)	PO: 320 mg/day (max: 320 mg/day)	
moxifloxacin (Avelox, Moxeza, Vigamox)	PO/IV (Avelox): 400 mg/day once daily (max: 400 mg/day) Ophthalmic solution: one drop in affected eye tid (Vigamox) or bid (Moxeza)	

Note: Italics indicate common adverse effects. Underline indicates serious adverse effects.

TABLE 49.2	Generations of Fluoroquinolones			
Generation	**Example**	**Route of Administration**	**Spectrum of Activity**	**Indications**
First generation	nalidixic acid	Oral	Enterobacteriaceae	Uncomplicated UTI
Second generation	ciprofloxacin	Oral and IV	Enterobacteriaceae, atypical pathogens, *P. aeruginosa*	Complicated UTI, gastroenteritis with severe diarrhea, sexually transmitted infections (STIs)
Third generation	levofloxacin	Oral and IV	Enterobacteriaceae, atypical pathogens, some streptococci	Complicated UTI, gastroenteritis with severe diarrhea, STIs, community-acquired pneumonia
Fourth generation	moxifloxacin	Oral	Enterobacteriaceae, atypical pathogens, some streptococci, MRSA, anaerobes	Bacterial conjunctivitis (ophthalmic drops), acute bacterial sinusitis, exacerbations of chronic bronchitis, community-acquired pneumonia, skin and skin structure infections

organisms makes them drugs of choice in the treatment of uncomplicated UTIs (see Chapter 53). A newer medication, moxifloxacin (Avelox), is effective against anaerobes, a group of bacteria that are often difficult to treat. Ciprofloxacin (Cipro) is the fluoroquinolone usually selected for infections by *Pseudomonas aeruginosa*. Recent studies have suggested that some fluoroquinolones may be effective against *Mycobacterium tuberculosis*, although the U.S. Food and Drug Administration (FDA) has not approved these drugs for this indication.

Along with doxycycline, streptomycin, and penicillin, several fluoroquinolones are indicated for pathogens that could potentially be of benefit following a bioterrorism incident. Ciprofloxacin (Cipro) is a drug of choice for postexposure prophylaxis to *Bacillus anthracis*, the causative agent of anthrax. Ciprofloxacin is also indicated for postexposure prophylaxis to other potential biologic warfare pathogens such as *Yersinia pestis* (plague), *Francisella tularensis* (tularemia), and *Brucella melitensis* (brucellosis). Details on the pharmacotherapy of bioterrorism agents are presented in Chapter 75.

Fluoroquinolones are well absorbed orally and may be administered either once or twice a day, making them ideal for outpatient therapy. The serum levels of these drugs after oral (PO) administration are nearly equivalent to the levels achieved during IV administration. This allows for a rapid, smooth transition from IV therapy to oral therapy, potentially decreasing the length of the hospital stay. Like aminoglycosides, fluoroquinolones exhibit a postantibiotic effect. Their bacteriocidal actions continue after serum levels fall to below minimum inhibitory concentrations. Once available by the PO route, gatifloxacin is now formulated as an ophthalmic solution.

Adverse Effects

In the 1990s, fluoroquinolones came into widespread use because they were well tolerated and few serious adverse effects were reported. Over time, several uncommon, although very serious, adverse effects were discovered. Since that time, almost half the fluoroquinolones approved by the FDA have been discontinued in the United States due to safety concerns.

Cartilage toxicity: Animal studies have suggested that fluoroquinolones can affect the extracellular matrix of cartilage during development, and tendon toxicity has been reported in children using these drugs. Although these abnormalities ceased upon termination of antibiotic therapy, fluoroquinolones are not approved for patients under age 18, and their use in children is restricted to instances where the benefits of pharmacotherapy clearly outweigh the potential risks.

Although rare, tendon abnormalities have also been reported in adults. Tendinitis and rupture of the shoulder, hand, and Achilles tendons have occurred several months after discontinuation of therapy. In 2007, the FDA approved safety labeling revisions that state patients older than 65 years are at increased risk for severe tendon disorders and that this risk is further increased by concurrent use of corticosteroids. Musculoskeletal complaints should be carefully monitored during therapy with fluoroquinolones, and patients should be advised to report unexplained joint or tendon pain.

GI toxicity: GI symptoms such as nausea, vomiting, and diarrhea occur in as many as 20% of patients taking fluoroquinolones. Although food does not affect their absorption, certain multivitamins or mineral supplements containing calcium, zinc, iron, aluminum, and magnesium can delay absorption of the antibiotic by as much as 90%. Substances containing these minerals should not be administered at the same time as fluoroquinolones.

In 2007, the FDA approved safety labeling revisions for certain antimicrobials to warn of the risk for *Clostridium difficile*–associated diarrhea (CDAD). This safety labeling applied to most fluoroquinolones as well as drugs from most other antibiotic classes.

Hypersensitivity reactions: Certainly not unique to fluoroquinolones, hypersensitivity may occur to any antibiotic. Although the FDA has always required label warnings on quinolones for the risk of hypersensitivity reactions that occur after the first dose, new labels warn of the rare risk for serious, and sometimes fatal, events after multiple doses.

Cardiotoxicity: Some of the most serious adverse effects of drugs in this class are dysrhythmias (moxifloxacin). Several of the drugs in this class were removed from the market due to the potential for fatal dysrhythmias. Nearly all fluoroquinolones prolong the QT interval.

Nervous system toxicity: Central nervous system (CNS) effects such as dizziness, headache, and sleep disturbances affect 1% to 8% of patients. Seizures, hallucinations, high intracranial pressure, confusion, and toxic psychoses have been reported in patients taking fluoroquinolones. These drugs should be used with caution in patients with preexisting seizure disorders. In 2013, the FDA issued a safety warning that serious nerve damage (peripheral neuropathy) caused by oral or parenteral fluoroquinolones may be permanent.

Phototoxicity: Moderate to severe phototoxicity may occur in patients exposed to direct or indirect sunlight, or to sunlamps during or following treatment with fluoroquinolones. Recovery may take several weeks.

Hepatotoxicity: Some of the fluoroquinolones elevate hepatic enzymes, which usually return to normal 1 to 2 months following completion of therapy. Trovafloxacin (Trovan) was discontinued due to an unacceptable incidence of liver damage, including fatal hepatic failure.

Resistance: Like other antibiotics, resistance of bacterial species to fluoroquinolones has been increasing and can occur by multiple mechanisms. Mutations to DNA gyrase can alter its ability to bind fluoroquinolones, thus rendering the drug less effective. Some bacteria have developed resistance pumps that remove fluoroquinolones from inside their cells, while others have developed a cell wall structure that is less permeable to the drugs. Fluoroquinolones were drugs of choice for treating *Neisseria gonorrhoeae* from 1993 to 2005. Because of the large number of resistant strains, however, the Centers for Disease Control and Prevention no longer recommends fluoroquinolones for the treatment of gonorrhea. Resistance to one fluoroquinolone sometimes confers resistance to all drugs in this class; therefore, resistance is becoming a limiting factor in the clinical utility of these drugs.

PharmFACT

Someone who is taking a fluoroquinolone antibiotic has a three times greater risk of tendon rupture than someone in the general population. If the person is over age 60 and also taking a corticosteroid, the risk is six times greater (Doyle, 2010).

PROTOTYPE DRUG	Ciprofloxacin (Cipro)

Classification: **Therapeutic:** Antibacterial
Pharmacologic: Bacterial DNA replication inhibitor, fluoroquinolone

Therapeutic Effects and Uses: Ciprofloxacin is a second-generation fluoroquinolone approved in 1987 that is the most widely used drug in this class. It is prescribed for UTI, sinusitis, pneumonia, skin infections, bone and joint infections, infectious diarrhea, and certain eye infections. It is a broad-spectrum antibiotic that is more effective against gram-negative organisms. It is active against *Enterobacter, Citrobacter, E. coli, Haemophilus, Klebsiella, Proteus, Staphylococcus, Shigella, Salmonella, Neisseria,* and *Serratia.* It is poorly effective against *Streptococcus pneumoniae* and is inactive against most anaerobic bacteria. Ciprofloxacin is a preferred drug for postexposure prophylaxis of inhalational *B. anthracis* spores.

Ciprofloxacin is available by multiple routes, including oral, IV, ophthalmic, and otic. As an ophthalmic solution (Ciloxan), it is used to treat corneal ulcers and conjunctivitis due to *Staphylococcus, Haemophilus,* and *Pseudomonas.* An otic suspension (Ciprodex otic) is a combination of ciprofloxacin and dexamethasone to treat acute otitis media and acute otitis externa in children age 6 months and older. Cipro HC otic combines ciprofloxacin with hydrocortisone to treat adults and children with acute otitis media.

Several extended release (XR) formulations are available that permit once-daily dosing, usually for treating UTI. Cipro XR contains two different ciprofloxacin salts: ciprofloxacin hydrochloride and ciprofloxacin betaine. Approved in 2005, Proquin XR contains only the hydrochloride salt and has been formulated to cause less nausea, vomiting, and diarrhea than other formulations. Proquin XR is administered for only 3 days and is only approved for uncomplicated UTI (acute cystitis).

Mechanism of Action: By inhibiting bacterial DNA gyrase and topoisomerase, ciprofloxacin affects bacterial replication and DNA repair. Ciprofloxacin is usually considered bacteriocidal and exhibits a prolonged postantibiotic effect.

Pharmacokinetics:

Route(s)	PO, IV, ophthalmic and otic drops
Absorption	60–80% absorbed
Distribution	Widely distributed to all body fluids; crosses the placenta; secreted in breast milk; small amounts in cerebrospinal fluid; 20–40% bound to plasma proteins
Primary metabolism	Mostly unchanged; small amounts of hepatic metabolism
Primary excretion	Primarily renal; 15% by biliary route
Onset of action	Rapid
Duration of action	12 h

Adverse Effects: Ciprofloxacin is well tolerated by most patients, and serious adverse effects are uncommon. GI adverse effects, such as nausea, vomiting, and diarrhea, may occur in patients taking high doses. Ciprofloxacin may be administered with food to diminish adverse GI effects. The patient should not, however, take this drug with antacids or mineral supplements, because drug absorption will be diminished. Some patients report phototoxicity, headache, and dizziness. Like most antibiotics, ciprofloxacin can cause serious pseudomembranous colitis (PMC). Although rare, seizures and toxic psychosis have been reported in patients receiving fluoroquinolones. **Black Box Warning**: Tendinitis and tendon rupture may occur in patients of all ages. Risk is especially high in patients over age 60; in kidney, heart, and lung transplant recipients; and in those receiving concurrent corticosteroid therapy. Fluoroquinolones may cause extreme muscle weakness in patients with myasthenia gravis.

Contraindications/Precautions: Ciprofloxacin is contraindicated in patients who are hypersensitive to fluoroquinolones and in pregnant patients. Drug therapy must be monitored carefully in patients with suspected CNS disorders, because this drug can be neurotoxic at high doses and can cause seizures when given by rapid IV infusion. Although prescribed for patients with UTIs, the drug should be used with caution in patients with serious renal impairment, because this drug is excreted by this route and may accumulate to toxic levels.

Drug Interactions: Concurrent administration with warfarin may increase anticoagulant effects and result in bleeding due to the decreased metabolism of warfarin. Antacids and vitamin supplements containing calcium or aluminum, iron or zinc sulfate, and sucralfate decrease the absorption of ciprofloxacin, thus causing decreased effectiveness of the antibiotic. Ciprofloxacin slows the hepatic metabolism of xanthines, including caffeine, theophylline, and theobromine. Theophylline levels may increase 15% to 30%. **Herbal/Food**: Patients ingesting large quantities of caffeinated products may experience excessive nervousness, anxiety, or tachycardia. Calcium-fortified juices may interfere with absorption of the antibiotic.

Pregnancy: Category C.

Treatment of Overdose: No specific therapy is available; patients are treated symptomatically.

Nursing Responsibilities: Key nursing implications for patients receiving ciprofloxacin are included in the Nursing Practice Application for Patients Receiving Pharmacotherapy with Fluoroquinolones.

Drugs Similar to Ciprofloxacin (Cipro)

Other fluoroquinolones include besifloxacin, gatifloxacin, gemifloxacin, levofloxacin, moxifloxacin, norfloxacin, and ofloxacin. With few exceptions, these drugs have very similar actions and adverse effects to ciprofloxacin. A black box warning regarding possible tendon rupture is included for all oral and parenteral drugs in this class. Cinoxacin (Cinobac), Enoxacin (Penetrex), lomefloxacin (Maxaquin), sparfloxacin (Zagam), and trovafloxacin (Trovan)/alatrofloxacin (Trovan IV) are drugs in this class that have been discontinued in the United States.

Besifloxacin (Besivance): Besifloxacin is one of the newer fluoroquinolones, approved in 2009 for the treatment of bacterial conjunctivitis. It is available as a 0.6% ophthalmic suspension. The most frequently reported adverse reaction is conjunctival redness. If used for a prolonged time period, the patient should be examined for the possibility of overgrowth of resistant microbes. Patients should be advised to discontinue use of contact lenses during therapy. This drug is pregnancy category C.

Gatifloxacin (Zymar, Zymaxid): Once available by the oral and parenteral routes, gatifloxacin is now only available as an ophthalmic solution for the treatment of bacterial conjunctivitis. The most frequently reported adverse reactions after ophthalmic administration include increased worsening of conjunctivitis, eye irritation, dysgeusia, and eye pain. Patients should be advised to discontinue use of contact lenses during therapy. This drug is pregnancy category C.

Gemifloxacin (Factive): Gemifloxacin was approved in 2003 for acute bacterial exacerbations of chronic bronchitis and community-acquired pneumonia. It is primarily effective against gram-positive bacteria, most importantly *S. pneumoniae* and *Staphylococcus aureus*, than many other drugs in this class. It is only available orally. The drug undergoes only minimal metabolism by the liver and is excreted almost equally by the kidneys and in the feces. Diarrhea, rash, and nausea are the most common adverse effects. It is contraindicated in patients with certain dysrhythmias, due to its effects on cardiac conduction. Other contraindications and adverse effects (including the black box warning) are similar to those of ciprofloxacin. This drug is pregnancy category C.

Levofloxacin (Levaquin): Approved in 1996, levofloxacin is prescribed for UTI, acute pyelonephritis, chronic bacterial prostatitis, pneumonia (nosocomial and community-acquired), acute bacterial sinusitis, acute bacterial exacerbations of chronic bronchitis, skin infections, and bacterial conjunctivitis. It is available for PO, IV, and ophthalmic (Iquix, Quixin) administration. Levofloxacin has a long half-life that allows for once-daily dosing. The most common adverse effects are nausea, headache, diarrhea, insomnia, constipation, and dizziness. Adverse effects of ophthalmic levofloxacin include transient blurred vision, foreign body sensation, headache, burning, pharyngitis, and photophobia. Caution should be used for patients with certain dysrhythmias, due to its effects on cardiac conduction. Although rare, hematologic toxicity, including agranulocytosis and thrombocytopenia, and renal toxicity may occur after multiple doses. Other contraindications and adverse effects for the oral and IV forms (including the black box warning) are similar to those of ciprofloxacin. This drug is pregnancy category C.

Moxifloxacin (Avelox, Moxeza, Vigamox): Approved in 1999, moxifloxacin is prescribed for skin infections, community-acquired pneumonia, acute sinusitis, and acute bacterial exacerbations of chronic bronchitis. It is available by the oral and IV routes and as an ophthalmic preparation (Moxeza, Vigamox) for bacterial conjunctivitis. The most common adverse effects are dizziness, diarrhea, nausea, and vomiting. For the ophthalmic drops, eye irritation, pyrexia, and conjunctivitis are the common adverse effects. Like gemifloxacin, it is contraindicated in patients with certain dysrhythmias, due to its effects on cardiac conduction. Other contraindications and adverse effects for the oral and IV forms (including the black box warning) are similar to those of ciprofloxacin. This drug is pregnancy category C.

Norfloxacin (Noroxin): Norfloxacin was approved in 1986 and is indicated for UTI and prostatitis. It has the shortest half-life of all fluoroquinolones and is available only by the PO route. The most common adverse effects are nausea, headache, asthenia, rash, and abdominal cramping. Other contraindications and adverse effects (including the black box warning) are similar to those of ciprofloxacin. An ophthalmic solution once used for bacterial conjunctivitis is no longer available in the United States. This drug is pregnancy category C.

Ofloxacin (Ocuflox, Floxin Otic): Approved in 1990, ofloxacin is indicated for acute bacterial exacerbations of chronic bronchitis, community-acquired pneumonia, chlamydial infections of the reproductive tract, cystitis, complicated UTI, prostatitis, superficial

---

CONNECTIONS   Patient Safety

◀ Levofloxacin (Levaquin)

Yesterday, Mrs. Rackey received the first dose of IV levofloxacin (Levaquin). While receiving the medication, she reported itching and a slight swelling of the tongue and lips (angioedema). However, later that day she had no discomfort or presence of the previous symptoms. She will receive the second dose of the medication again this morning. What should the nurse do?

See Answers to Patient Safety Questions on student resource website.

ocular infections (Ocuflox), and otitis media (Floxin Otic). The most common adverse effects are nausea, headache, insomnia, dizziness, and rash. The otic preparation can cause otic pruritus. Other contraindications and adverse effects for the oral and IV forms (including the black box warning) are similar to those of ciprofloxacin. It is available for the PO, IV, ophthalmic, and otic routes. This drug is pregnancy category C.

Miscellaneous Antibacterials

49.4 A number of miscellaneous antibacterials have specific clinical indications.

Several drugs act by miscellaneous mechanisms or are the only drugs in their class. Doses for the miscellaneous drugs are listed in Table 49.3.

Bacitracin: Bacitracin is an older antibiotic, approved in 1948, that acts by inhibiting cell wall synthesis. It is combined with polymyxin B in over-the-counter (OTC) first aid products (Neosporin, Polysporin) and is also available as monotherapy in OTC products such as Bacitracin First Aid. It is effective against a variety of gram-positive and a few gram-negative microbes. Although an intramuscular (IM) form is available, bacitracin is almost always used topically due to potential nephrotoxicity (black box warning). In addition to creams and ointments, bacitracin solutions may be used to soak compresses that can be applied to large areas of the skin. This drug is pregnancy category C.

Daptomycin (Cubicin): Approved in 2003, daptomycin belongs to a class of antibiotics known as the cyclic lipopeptides. The spectrum of activity of daptomycin includes a wide variety of gram-positive pathogens. It is indicated for the treatment of complicated skin infections caused by organisms such as *S. aureus*, including methicillin-resistant *S. aureus* (MRSA), *Streptococcus pyogenes*, and *Enterococcus faecalis* (vancomycin-susceptible strains only). Daptomycin is bacteriocidal and its mechanism of action is clearly distinct from that of any other antibiotic. When binding to bacterial membranes, daptomycin causes a rapid depolarization of membrane potential, leading to inhibition of protein, DNA, and ribonucleic acid (RNA) synthesis. It is given only by IV infusion. The most clinically significant adverse effects are abnormal liver function tests, elevated creatine phosphokinase (CPK), dyspnea, and pneumonia. Myopathy has been recorded in a small percentage of patients taking daptomycin; therefore, the nurse should carefully monitor for muscle pain or weakness. The drug should be withheld if the CPK becomes elevated above 1,000 units/L. This drug is pregnancy category B.

Metronidazole (Flagyl): Metronidazole is another older anti-infective, approved in 1963, that is effective against a large number of anaerobes. It acts by interfering with the DNA and RNA synthesis of pathogens. Metronidazole is one of only a few drugs that have dual activity against both bacteria and multicellular parasites. It is a preferred drug for trichomoniasis, giardiasis, and amebiasis. Unlike most antibiotics, resistance to metronidazole is uncommon. When given orally, adverse effects are generally minor and include nausea, dry mouth, and headache. High doses can produce neurotoxicity.

As an antibacterial, metronidazole has two indications: serious infections due to anaerobic bacteria, and peptic ulcer disease. Few antibacterials are effective against anaerobes because the organisms reside in sites that have tissue destruction and a poor blood supply. Anaerobic bacteria are common causes of abscesses, gangrene, diabetic skin ulcers, and deep wound infections. Serious

TABLE 49.3	Miscellaneous Antibacterials	
Drug	**Route and Adult Dose (Maximum Dose Where Indicated)**	**Adverse Effects**
bacitracin	Topical: Apply thin layer of ointment bid or tid or as solution of 250–1,000 units/mL in wet dressing	*Anorexia, nausea, vomiting* Nephrotoxicity, anaphylaxis
daptomycin (Cubicin)	IV: 4–6 mg/kg once every 24 h for 7–14 days	*Insomnia, diarrhea, headache, abnormal liver function tests, elevated CPK, edema* Anaphylaxis, superinfections, renal failure, myopathy, jaundice, PMC
metronidazole (Flagyl)	Anaerobic infections: PO: 7.5 mg/kg every 6 h (max: 4 g/day) IV loading dose: 15 mg/kg IV maintenance dose: 7.5 mg/kg every 6 h (max: 4 g/day)	*Dizziness, headache, anorexia, abdominal pain, metallic taste and nausea, Candida infections* Seizures, peripheral neuropathy, leukopenia
polymyxin B	IV: 15,000–25,000 units/kg/day divided every 12 h IM: 25,000–30,000 units/kg/day divided every 4–6 h	*Urticaria* Nephrotoxicity, neurotoxicity (confusion, blurred vision, paresthesias, paralysis), superinfections
rifampin (Rifadin, Rimactane)	PO/IV: 600 mg/day	*Nausea, vomiting, heartburn, anorexia, diarrhea, orange discoloration of the urine, sweat, and tears* PMC, acute renal failure, hepatotoxicity, blood dyscrasias
telithromycin (Ketek)	PO: 800 mg once daily	*Nausea, diarrhea, dizziness, headache, blurred vision* Superinfections, PMC, hepatotoxicity, dysrhythmias, respiratory failure, loss of consciousness

Note: *Italics* indicate common adverse effects. <u>Underline</u> indicates serious adverse effects.

CONNECTIONS: NURSING PRACTICE APPLICATION

Patients Receiving Pharmacotherapy with Fluoroquinolones

Assessment	Potential Nursing Diagnoses*
Baseline assessment prior to administration: • Obtain a complete health history including neurologic, cardiovascular, respiratory, hepatic, or renal disease, myasthenia gravis, and the possibility of pregnancy. Assess for previous organ transplantation surgery. Obtain a drug history including allergies, noting specific reactions to drugs, current prescriptions, particularly corticosteroids, and OTC drugs, herbal preparations, and alcohol use. Be alert to possible drug interactions. • Assess signs and symptoms of current infection noting location, characteristics, presence or absence of drainage and character of drainage, duration, and presence or absence of fever or pain. • Evaluate appropriate laboratory findings (e.g., CBC, culture and sensitivity [C&S], hepatic function studies). • Assess the patient's ability to receive and understand instructions. Include family and caregivers as needed.	• *Infection* (bacterial) • *Acute Pain* • *Hyperthermia* • *Impaired Physical Mobility*, related to adverse drug effects • *Deficient Knowledge* (Drug Therapy) • *Risk for Injury*, related to adverse drug effects • *Risk for Deficient Fluid Volume*, related to diarrhea caused by adverse drug effects
Assessment throughout administration: • Assess for desired therapeutic effects (e.g., diminished signs and symptoms of infection and fever). • Continue periodic monitoring of CBC, renal function, urinalysis, and C&S as ordered. • Assess for adverse effects: nausea, vomiting, abdominal cramping, diarrhea, headache, calf or ankle pain, weakness, numbness, or dizziness. Severe diarrhea, especially containing mucus, blood, or pus, or decreased urine output should be reported immediately.	

Implementation

Interventions and (Rationales)	Patient-Centered Care
Ensuring therapeutic effects: • Continue assessments as above for therapeutic effects. (Diminished fever, pain, or signs and symptoms of infection should begin after taking the first dose and continue to improve. The provider should be notified if fever and signs and symptoms of infection remain or increase after 3 days or if the entire course of antibacterial has been taken and signs of infection are still present.)	• Teach the patient to complete the entire course of the antibacterial therapy; do not share doses with other family members with similar symptoms; and return to the provider if symptoms have not resolved after an entire course of therapy.
Minimizing adverse effects: • Continue to monitor vital signs, especially temperature if fever is present. Immediately report undiminished fever, changes in level of consciousness, or febrile seizures to the health care provider. (Fever should begin to diminish within 1–3 days after starting drug. Continued fever may be a sign of worsening infection, adverse drug effects, or antibiotic resistance.)	• Teach the patient to report fever that does not diminish below 37.8°C (100°F) or per the health care provider parameters. Immediately report febrile seizures, changes in behavior, or changes in level of consciousness to the provider.
• Continue to monitor periodic laboratory work: renal function tests, CBC, urinalysis, and C&S as ordered. (Fluoroquinolones may be renal toxic. Periodic C&S tests may be ordered if infections are severe or are slow to resolve to confirm appropriate therapy.)	• Instruct the patient on the need for periodic laboratory work.
• Monitor for hypersensitivity and allergic reactions, especially with the first dose of the drug. Continue to monitor the patient for up to 2 weeks after completing antibacterial therapy. (Anaphylactic reactions are possible, particularly with the first dose of an antibacterial. Post-use, residual drug levels may cause delayed reactions, dependent on the length of half-life.)	• Teach the patient to immediately report any itching, rashes, or swelling, particularly of the tongue or face, urticaria, flushing, dizziness, syncope, wheezing, throat tightness, or difficulty breathing. • Instruct the patient with known antibacterial allergies to carry a wallet identification card or wear medical identification jewelry indicating allergy.
• Continue to monitor for renal toxicity, e.g., diminished urine output, or weight gain greater than 1 kg (2 lb) in 24 h. (Fluoroquinolones may require frequent monitoring to prevent adverse effects. Increasing fluid intake will help prevent drug accumulation in the kidneys. **Lifespan:** Age-related physiological differences may place the young child or older adult at greater risk for renal toxicity.)	• Teach the patient to immediately report any diminished urine output, visible swelling of feet or ankles, or weight gain greater than 1 kg (2 lb) in 24 h. • Advise the patient to increase fluid intake to 2–3 L/day.

CONNECTIONS: NURSING PRACTICE APPLICATION (continued)

• Monitor for development of superinfections, e.g., CDAD or PMC, fungal, or yeast infections. (Superinfections with opportunistic organisms may occur when normal host flora are diminished or killed by the antibacterial drug and no longer hold pathogens in check. Severe diarrhea may indicate the presence of CDAD or PMC, superinfections caused by *C. difficile*.)	• Instruct the patient to report any diarrhea that increases in frequency, amount, or contains mucus, blood, or pus. • Instruct the patient to consult the health care provider before taking any antidiarrheal drugs, which cause the retention of harmful bacteria. • Teach the patient to observe for changes in stool, white patches in the mouth, whitish thick vaginal discharge, itching in the genital area, blistering itchy rash, and to immediately report severe diarrhea. • Teach the patient infection control measures such as frequent hand washing, adequate drying after showering or bathing, and to increase the intake of live-culture dairy foods.
• Monitor for signs and symptoms of neurotoxicity, e.g., dizziness, severe headache, seizures, peripheral numbness, or paresthesia. (Fluoroquinolones have an increased risk of neurotoxicity. Previous seizure disorders or head injuries may increase this risk. Persistent or increasing headaches should be immediately reported. Peripheral neuropathies may be permanent. **Lifespan:** Be particularly cautious with the older adult who is a greater risk for falls.)	• Instruct the patient to immediately report persistent or increasing headache, dizziness, seizures, or numbness or tingling of the hands or feet. If dizziness occurs, the patient should sit or lie down and not attempt to stand or walk, until the sensation passes.
• Monitor for joint, tendon, leg, or heel pain, or difficulty with movement or walking in patients on fluoroquinolones. (Fluoroquinolones have been associated with tendinitis and tendon rupture, especially of the Achilles tendon. **Lifespan:** Be particularly cautious with the older adult, who is a greater risk for tendinitis and tendon rupture.)	• Instruct the patient to immediately report any significant or increasing joint, tendon, heel, lower leg or calf pain, or difficulty moving or walking to the health care provider.
• Monitor for the anticoagulation effects if the patient is on warfarin. (Fluoroquinolones decrease the metabolism of warfarin and may increase the anticoagulation effect and risk of bleeding.)	• Teach the patient to report any increase in bruising or bleeding while on warfarin. More frequent laboratory work may be needed.
• Continue to monitor for dermatologic effects including red or purplish skin rash, blisters, or sunburning. Immediately report severe rashes, especially associated with blistering. (Fluoroquinolones may cause significant dermatologic effects including Stevens–Johnson syndrome. Sunscreens and protective clothing should be used to prevent photosensitivity and photoallergic reactions.)	• Teach the patient to wear sunscreens and protective clothing for sun exposure and to avoid tanning beds. Immediately report any severe sunburn or rashes.
Patient understanding of drug therapy: • Use opportunities during administration of the medications and during assessments to discuss the rationale for drug therapy, desired therapeutic outcomes, commonly observed adverse effects, parameters for when to call the health care provider, and any necessary monitoring or precautions. (Using time during nursing care helps to optimize and reinforce key teaching areas.)	• The patient, family, or caregiver should be able to state the reason for the drug, appropriate dose and scheduling, what adverse effects to observe for and when to report them, and the anticipated length of medication therapy.
Patient self-administration of drug therapy: • When administering medications, instruct the patient, family, or caregiver in proper self-administration techniques followed by teach-back. (Utilizing time during nurse-administration of these drugs helps to reinforce teaching.)	• Teach the patient to take the medication: • Complete the entire course of therapy unless otherwise instructed. Do not share with other family members and do not stop the medicine when starting to feel better. • Take the drug with food but avoid taking the drug concurrently with dairy products or calcium-fortified juices, which may decrease absorption. Take the fluoroquinolone 1 h before or 2 h after consuming these products. • Do not take antacids or preparations containing iron or zinc at the same time as the fluoroquinolones dose. • Avoid excess consumption of beverages or foods containing caffeine, which may increase the chance of nervousness or anxiety. • Take the medication as evenly spaced throughout each day as feasible. • Increase overall fluid intake while taking the antibacterial drug. • Discard outdated medications or those no longer in use. Review the medicine cabinet twice a year for old medications (e.g., at beginning and end of daylight saving time).

*Nursing Diagnoses—Definitions and Classification 2015–2017. Copyright © 2014, 1994–2014 by NANDA International. Used by arrangement with John Wiley & Sons Limited.

intra-abdominal infections or septicemia due to *Bacteroides* and streptococci often respond well to IV infusions of the drug. It is a preferred drug for managing CDAD. Metronidazole has found a relatively new use in the treatment of *Helicobacter pylori* infections of the stomach associated with peptic ulcer disease. The drug carries a black box warning that it causes cancer in laboratory animals. Metronidazole is featured as a prototype drug in Chapter 53. This drug is pregnancy category B.

Polymyxin B: Approved in 1951, polymyxin B is an older, bacteriocidal drug that acts by disrupting the bacterial cell membrane. The drug is able to penetrate the phospholipid layer, make the membrane leaky, and cause the death of the bacterium. Although parenteral formulations are available, polymyxin B is rarely prescribed by these routes due to potential nephrotoxicity and neurotoxicity (black box warnings). Its primary application is in the treatment of topical infections of the skin, mucous membranes, or eye, caused by gram-negative organisms. It is not effective against gram-positive microbes. It is combined with bacitracin and neomycin in common OTC first aid products such as Neosporin Ointment, Bactine Antibiotic, and Polysporin. Topical application, including to denuded skin, results in negligible systemic absorption. Polymyxin B is combined with neomycin and hydrocortisone in prescription otic preparations. Topical polymyxin B is pregnancy category B.

Rifampin (Rifadin, Rimactane): Approved in 1958, rifampin is administered PO or IV and is usually associated with the pharmacotherapy of tuberculosis. The drug, however, is effective against a wide range of both gram-positive and gram-negative organisms. As an antibacterial, it is used for prophylaxis in contacts of patients with *Haemophilus influenzae* type B and for the prophylaxis of asymptomatic carriers of meningococcal disease. Occasionally, it is used for Legionnaire's disease, or when therapy with other antibiotics is unsuccessful. The reason its applications are limited is because of the rapid development of resistance, which can appear after only a few days of therapy. A flulike syndrome develops in about half the patients receiving the drug. Rifampin acts by inhibiting bacterial RNA polymerase, the enzyme that makes bacterial RNA. The use of rifampin in the pharmacotherapy of tuberculosis is presented in Chapter 51. This drug is pregnancy category C.

Telithromycin (Ketek): In 2004, the FDA approved telithromycin for respiratory infections, the first in a class of antibiotics known as the **ketolides**. Telithromycin blocks bacterial protein synthesis by binding to two different sites on the 50S ribosomal subunit. Telithromycin is an oral drug, with the most common adverse effects being diarrhea, nausea, and headache. The primary indication for this drug is community-acquired pneumonia due to *S. pneumoniae, H. influenzae, Moraxella catarrhalis,* or *Mycoplasma pneumoniae*. When post–market surveillance discovered several cases of hepatic failure in patients receiving this drug, the FDA withdrew its approval for the treatment of acute bacterial sinusitis and acute bacterial exacerbations of chronic bronchitis. Hepatic function tests must be monitored during therapy. Telithromycin has the potential to prolong the QT interval, which represents an increased risk for ventricular dysrhythmias. The drug may cause mild to moderate visual disturbances, including blurred vision, diplopia, and difficulty focusing. Telithromycin carries a black box warning that it should not be used in patients with myasthenia gravis because fatal respiratory depression may occur. This drug is pregnancy category C.

CHAPTER 49

Understanding the Chapter

Key Concepts Summary

49.1 Bacterial DNA replication requires several different enzymes to uncoil, unwind, and duplicate the DNA.

49.2 Drugs have been discovered that inhibit different steps in bacterial DNA replication.

49.3 Fluoroquinolones are antibiotics whose therapeutic applications have expanded in recent years to treat many gram-positive and gram-negative infections.

49.4 A number of miscellaneous antibacterials have specific clinical indications.

Case Study: Making the Patient Connection

Remember the patient "Mike Springs" at the beginning of the chapter? Now read the remainder of the case study. Based on the information presented within this chapter, respond to the critical thinking questions that follow.

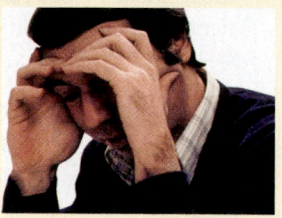

Mike Springs presents to the local health clinic. He is a 38-year-old male who has no history of chronic illness. His vital signs are normal with the exception of a slight increase in body temperature, 37.3°C (99.2°F). He denies shortness of breath. However, his nasal passages are congested, causing him to "mouth breathe." Mike is busy with work and family responsibilities. Until this most recent illness, he had started efforts toward a healthier lifestyle and weight reduction. Mike is now jogging for exercise and taking vitamin tablets. He is diagnosed with acute sinusitis, and the health care provider orders ciprofloxacin PO 500 mg twice daily for 10 days. Additional medications prescribed include a nasal decongestant and a mild analgesic.

As Mike is leaving the health clinic, he comments that he is responsible for multiple corporate offices and will soon be traveling. He is worried about remembering to take the medication and admits to a history of nonadherence with medication regimens because he sometimes forgets to take medications.

Critical Thinking Questions

1. Prepare a patient teaching handout for Mike that provides him with information about the antibiotics he is being prescribed.

2. Mike asks you, the nurse, if he should continue jogging and taking vitamins. What would you advise?

3. What tips can you provide someone who forgets to take scheduled medication?

See Answers to Critical Thinking Questions on student resource website.

Additional Case Study

Carolyn Ijams is doing her spring cleaning. As she is arranging the content of her medicine cabinet, she notices a tube of bacitracin antibiotic ointment that is about half-used. She wonders whether she should keep it or not and asks you, the nurse who lives next door, what she should do with the tube.

1. Should Carolyn keep the antibiotic ointment? What would you want to know before making a recommendation?

2. What would you teach Carolyn about the use of topical antibiotic ointments such as the bacitracin?

See Answers to Additional Case Study on student resource website.

Chapter Review

1 The patient is prescribed ciprofloxacin (Cipro) and is instructed to take each dose of medication as evenly spaced apart during the day as possible. The nurse recognizes that this instruction is essential because:

1. The medication can cause sleep pattern disturbances.
2. Pathogenic bacteria have extremely rapid growth and reproduction rates.
3. Superinfections may develop if a dose of the medication is missed.
4. Allergic reactions are more likely to occur if a dose is missed.

2 The patient is prescribed ofloxacin (Floxin) for treatment of acute bronchitis. The patient tells the nurse that he experienced an allergic reaction when he took ciprofloxacin (Cipro) previously. As reported by the patient, which of the following would be most indicative of an allergic reaction to this drug group? Select all that apply.

1. Headache
2. Nausea and vomiting
3. Itching without visible rash
4. Swelling of lips or tongue
5. Nervousness or anxiety

3 The nurse is instructing a patient on a new prescription for ciprofloxacin (Cipro) and will include which instructions? Select all that apply.

1. Increase fluid intake to 2–3 liters per day.

2. Avoid consuming dairy products or antacids when you take the antibiotic.

3. Limit vitamin C intake in both dietary and oral vitamin forms.

4. Take the pill with an antihistamine to avoid adverse effects.

5. Coffee or tea without milk, cream, or coffee-lightener is the preferred beverage for taking the antibiotic dose.

4 A patient has been receiving levofloxacin (Levaquin) IV for septicemia for 2 weeks and will be given the drug orally at home. Which discharge instruction would be most appropriate for the nurse to give this patient?

1. Report any unusual joint or tendon pain or difficulty with movement or walking.

2. Take a daily multivitamin supplement with the levofloxacin.

3. Exposure to direct sunlight will help increase absorption of vitamin D, which is impaired by this medication.

4. Limit fluid intake to less than 1,500 mL per day.

5 A patient has been given a prescription for ciprofloxacin (Cipro). The nurse checks the patient's history because this drug should be used cautiously, or is contraindicated, in patients with what condition?

1. A history of anxiety disorder and nervousness

2. Patients over the age of 65

3. A history of penicillin allergy

4. Patients with myasthenia gravis

6 Which is the most important goal of nursing care for a patient receiving polymyxin B ointment on a laceration?

1. Promote wound healing.

2. Sterilize the skin and mucous membranes.

3. Prevent allergic reaction.

4. Maximize pain relief.

See Answers to Chapter Review in Appendix A.

References

Doyle, H. E. (2010). Tendinopathy resulting from the use of fluoroquinolones: Managing risks. *Journal of the American Academy of Physician Assistants, 23*(12), 18–21.

Selected Bibliography

Albertson, T. E., Dean, N. C., El Solh, A. A., Gotfried, M. H., Kaplan, C., & Niederman, M. S. (2010). Fluoroquinolones in the management of community-acquired pneumonia. *International Journal of Clinical Practice, 64*, 378–388. doi:10.1111/j.1742-1241.2009.02239.x

Beauduy, C., & MacDougall, C. (2013). Update on management of *Clostridium difficile* infection. *Hospital Pharmacy, 48*(Suppl. 1), S7–S13. doi:10.1310/hpj4802-S7

Bouziana, D. G. (2010). Current and future medical approaches to combat the anthrax threat. *Journal of Medicinal Chemistry, 53*, 4505–4531. doi:10.1021/jm901024b

Dalhoff, A. (2012). Global fluoroquinolone resistance epidemiology and implications for clinical use. *Interdisciplinary Perspectives on Infectious Diseases, 2012*, Article ID 976273, 37 pages. doi:10.1155/2012/976273

Frei, C. R., Labreche, M. J., & Attridge, R. T. (2011). Fluoroquinolones in community-acquired pneumonia: Guide to selection and appropriate use. *Drugs, 71*, 757–770. doi:10.2165/11585430-000000000-00000

Herdman, T. H., & Kamitsuro, S. (Eds.). (2014). *NANDA International nursing diagnoses: Definitions and classification, 2015–2017.* Oxford, United Kingdom: Wiley-Blackwell.

Kaleagasioglu, F., & Olcay, E. (2012). Fluoroquinolone-induced tendinopathy: Etiology and preventive measures. *The Tohoku Journal of Experimental Medicine, 226*, 251–258. doi:10.1620/tjem.226.251

Madigan, M. T., Martinko, J. M., Stahl, D. A., & Clark, D. P. (2012). *Brock biology of microorganisms* (13th ed.). San Francisco, CA: Benjamin Cummings.

Parry, C. M. (2010). Fluoroquinolone resistance: Challenges for disease control. In T. J. Weber (Ed.), *Antimicrobial resistance: Beyond the breakpoint.* Basil, Switzerland: Karger.

Pugi, A., Longo, L., Bartoloni, A., Rossolini, G. M., Mugelli, A., Vannacci, A., & Lapi, F. (2012). Cardiovascular and metabolic safety profiles of the fluoroquinolones. *Expert Opinion on Drug Safety, 11*, 53–69. doi:10.1517/14740338.2011.624512

Redgrave, L. S., Sutton, S. B., Webber, M. A., & Piddock, L. J. (2014). Fluoroquinolone resistance: Mechanisms, impact on bacteria, and role in evolutionary success. *Trends in Microbiology, 22*, 438–445. doi:10.1016/j.tim.2014.04.007

Sousa, J., Alves, G., Fortuna, A., & Falcão, A. (2014). Third- and fourth-generation fluoroquinolone antibacterials: A systematic review of safety and toxicity profiles. *Current Drug Safety, 9*, 89–105. doi:10.2174/1574886308666140106154754

Somasundaram, S., & Manivannan, K. (2013). An overview of fluoroquinolones. *Annual Review & Research in Biology, 3*, 296–313.

Stahlman, R., & Hartmut, L. (2010). Safety considerations of fluoroquinolones in the elderly: An update. *Drugs and Aging, 27*, 193–209. doi:10.2165/11531490-000000000-00000

Stephenson, A. L., Wu, W., Cortes, D., & Rochon, P. A. (2013). Tendon injury and fluoroquinolone use: A systematic review. *Drug Safety, 36*, 709–721. doi:10.1007/s40264-013-0089-8

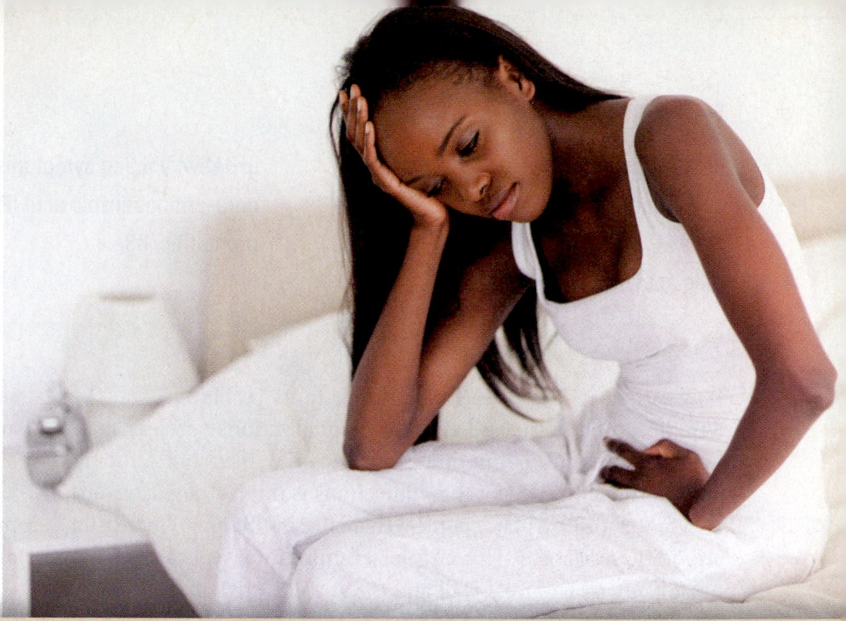

"It seems that I have been sick all winter. Yesterday, when I began having a fever, I took some antibiotic tablets that a doctor prescribed when I was sick last month. I'm sure glad I didn't take all of the prescription and had some of the pills left to take."

Patient "Sandra Phillipi"

CHAPTER 50 Sulfonamides and the Pharmacotherapy of Urinary Tract Infections

LEARNING OUTCOMES

After reading this chapter, the student should be able to:

1. Classify types of urinary tract infections based on their anatomic location.
2. Explain the epidemiology and pathogenesis of urinary tract infections.
3. Compare and contrast the pharmacotherapy of complicated versus uncomplicated urinary tract infections.
4. Identify the classes of antibiotics used to treat urinary tract infections.
5. Describe modifications in the pharmacotherapy of urinary tract infections for infants and children, pregnancy, older adults, and those with recurring infections.
6. Explain why folate inhibitors exert selective toxicity toward bacterial cells.
7. For each of the classes shown in the chapter outline, identify the prototype and representative drugs and explain the mechanism(s) of drug action, primary indications, contraindications, significant drug interactions, pregnancy category, and important adverse effects.
8. Apply the nursing process to care for patients receiving pharmacotherapy for urinary tract infections.

CHAPTER OUTLINE

- Pathophysiology of Urinary Tract Infections
- Pharmacotherapy of Urinary Tract Infections
- Sulfonamides
  - **PROTOTYPE** Trimethoprim-Sulfamethoxazole (Bactrim, Septra), *p. 839*
- Urinary Antiseptics
  - **PROTOTYPE** Nitrofurantoin (Furadantin) and Nitrofurantoin Macrocrystals (Macrobid, Macrodantin), *p. 841*

bacteriuria, 834

crystalluria, 839

cystitis, 834

folic acid, 837

irritative voiding symptoms, 834

para-aminobenzoic acid (PABA), 837

prostatitis, 834

pyelonephritis, 834

urethritis, 834

uropathogens, 834

It is estimated that urinary tract infections (UTIs) account for 8 million office visits and 100,000 hospitalizations per year, making them the most common type of bacterial infection. Although antimicrobial therapy of these infections is often straightforward, UTI is becoming a major clinical challenge in this era of increasing antibiotic resistance. This chapter examines the types of patients most likely to acquire a UTI and the anti-infective therapy that is most effective against this disease.

Pathophysiology of Urinary Tract Infections

50.1 Infections can occur in any portion of the urinary tract.

The urinary tract consists of the kidneys, ureters, urinary bladder, and urethra. The male and female urinary tracts are identical, with the exception of the urethra, which is shorter in the female and located closer to the anus. This anatomic difference results in the periurethral region of the female being populated by bacteria that are normally restricted to the gastrointestinal (GI) tract and could cause UTIs. In addition to the male having a longer urethra, the scrotum provides a physical barrier between the urethra and the anus. These anatomic differences result in a higher risk of UTI in females.

The continuous, peristaltic flow of urine from the kidneys, down the ureters, into the bladder, and voiding through the urethra provide formidable barriers to harmful microorganisms or **uropathogens** attempting to invade the urinary system. Although it is indeed difficult for uropathogens to go against the flow of urine and reach beyond the proximal portion of the urethra, this is the means by which the large majority of UTIs are acquired. Infections that travel from the urethra to the bladder or kidney are known as retrograde or ascending infections. The most successful uropathogens are those that secrete sticky adhesion proteins or that have structures called fimbriae that allow them to adhere to the epithelial lining of the urinary tract. Occasionally, pathogens traveling through the blood can infect the kidney. This mode of infection is called the hematogenous route and is responsible for only 5% of all UTIs.

Any portion of the urinary tract may be infected by uropathogens. Infection of the urethra, or **urethritis**, presents as discomfort during voiding and occurs in both men and women. It is usually distinguished from a bladder infection, or **cystitis**, because it causes less voiding urgency than cystitis and has a more gradual onset of symptoms. Urethritis is often a sign of a sexually transmitted infection.

A cluster of complaints known as **irritative voiding symptoms** accompanies cystitis. Occurring in both men and women, symptoms include dysuria and increased voiding urgency and frequency. Despite the increased urgency and frequency, only small volumes of urine are voided during each attempt. During and immediately following voiding, burning or aching may occur. The patient may have suprapubic tenderness upon palpation. Urinalysis usually identifies the presence of an offending uropathogen, or **bacteriuria**, as well as other signs of infection such as pyuria, hematuria, and changes in urine pH, nitrites, or proteins.

In females, symptoms of cystitis are frequently reported following intercourse with a new sexual partner. In males, cystitis is likely to occur following anal intercourse. Cystitis in males may be accompanied by acute **prostatitis**. Normally recognized by palpating the prostate, which will be tender during manual examination, prostatitis may include fever and has the potential to cause urinary obstruction as the prostate swells.

Bacteria that ascend the ureter and reach the kidney can cause **pyelonephritis**, an inflammation of the kidney, pelvis, and other renal cells. Irritative voiding symptoms occur, along with other signs similar to cystitis. More severe symptoms are manifested as nausea, vomiting, fever, chills, and acute costovertebral angle and flank tenderness. Because acute pyelonephritis may lead to shock, aggressive anti-infective therapy may be required.

Pharmacotherapy of Urinary Tract Infections

50.2 Choice of pharmacotherapy for acute urinary tract infection depends on the severity of the infection and the presence of comorbid conditions.

In addition to describing UTIs by their location, these infections are also classified as complicated or uncomplicated. The classification is an important clinical distinction because the pharmacotherapy for complicated UTI and uncomplicated UTI is quite different.

Acute Uncomplicated Cystitis

Acute uncomplicated cystitis (AUC) occurs in patients who have no serious or chronic health disorders that might impact the spread of the uropathogen or the treatment of the UTI. These infections occur mostly in women of reproductive age, with the highest incidence occurring from 18 to 24 years of age. Adult males rarely have AUC. Common risk factors for AUC include the following:

- Frequent sexual activity
- Use of spermicides for contraception
- Use of a diaphragm for contraception
- Estrogen deficiency

In many cases, a diagnosis of AUC is made by the health care provider based on symptoms and history alone, without additional serologic or urinary testing. Women who have experienced a prior AUC are often able to self-diagnose. Rapid dipstick tests are

CONNECTIONS | Evidence-Based Practice

◀ Urinary Tract Infection Symptoms and the Older Adult

Clinical Question

Are urinary tract symptoms a reliable indicator of UTI in the older adult?

Evidence

Woodford and George (2009) studied 265 hospitalized older adults over the age of 75 with a diagnosis of UTI upon discharge. Out of this population, 115 (43.4%) had a UTI confirmed by positive urine culture. Coliform bacteria (*E. coli*) was the most common pathogenic organism, but *Enterococcus*, *Pseudomonas*, *Staphylococcus aureus*, *Streptococcus*, and methicillin-resistant *S. aureus* were also cultured. Typical UTI symptoms were found to be an unreliable indicator of infection because less than one third (32.1%) of those patients with a positive urine culture had urinary tract symptoms. It was also noted that UTI symptoms were present in 13 patients (17%) with a negative urine culture. Costovertebral angle tenderness, fever, and discolored urine were more suggestive of the presence of a UTI than suprapubic tenderness, urine odor, or a smell of urine on the patient. Based on their study, the authors concluded that a UTI may be misdiagnosed up to 40% of the time, predominantly because of the reliance on the presence of urinary tract symptoms commonly used to diagnose a UTI in a group where those symptoms are not reliable indicators. Rowe and Juthani-Mehta (2014) also support these findings and note that while older adults may have acute symptoms similar to their younger counterparts, they may have more generalized symptoms. UTI in older adults may also be more difficult to diagnose in the presence of cognitive decline when these patients cannot accurately describe their symptoms.

Implications

UTIs are a frequent reason for hospitalization of the older adult, especially for those over the age of 75. They account for up to 70% of the causes for bacteremia (blood system infection) in the older adult (Lubart et al., 2011). Accurately identifying the presence of a UTI in these patients is difficult, and misdiagnosis may lead to unnecessary antibiotic use with an increased risk of adverse effects such as *Clostridium difficile*–associated diarrhea (CDAD). In younger patients, symptoms such as dysuria, urgency, suprapubic pain, hematuria, urine odor, and fever may signal the presence of a UTI. But in the older adult, these symptoms may not be present.

The presence of common symptoms such as dysuria, frequency, or suprapubic pain are unreliable indicators and a urine culture should be obtained when a UTI is suspected, even in patients without symptoms. Rapid-testing measures, such as urine dipstick, were found to be especially unreliable. The unnecessary use of antibiotics may increase the risk that older patients have of complications, such as CDAD. This may be avoided by accurate diagnosis on admission and the development of better criteria to aid in diagnosing a UTI in the older adult. This may hold especially true for patients with cognitive impairment who cannot accurately report symptoms.

Critical Thinking Question

Working on a unit with a high number of older adults, how could a nurse use these findings to change practice on the unit so that a misdiagnosis of UTI and resulting antibiotic treatment would be less likely?

See Answers to Critical Thinking Questions on student resource website.

---

available to examine for the presence of infection. *Escherichia coli* is the most common causative agent for AUC, being responsible for 80% to 90% of UTIs. *Staphylococcus saprophyticus* is isolated in about 10% to 15% of the cases. The most frequent uropathogens are listed in Table 50.1. Follow-up of AUC is usually by routine office visit; no additional testing or cultures are required if the symptoms promptly resolve.

Most patients with AUC begin pharmacotherapy immediately, prior to receiving the results of a urinalysis confirming the specific pathogen. The choice of initial antibiotic and duration of therapy vary widely among health care providers. The choice is often customized to an institution or community, based on local antibiotic resistance patterns and practitioner experience. Single-dose or short-course therapy is preferred for patient convenience and to maximize adherence.

Asymptomatic bacteriuria is frequently discovered on a routine urinalysis: Estimates range from 1% to 2% of young adult women to as high as 60% of women over age 60. In general, asymptomatic bacteriuria is not treated with medications because very few of these patients will progress to symptomatic UTI. Widespread therapy would be costly and increase the number of resistant strains in the community. Certain populations of patients, however, are treated when asymptomatic bacteriuria is discovered. These include pregnant women, those undergoing urologic procedures, and patients who are immunosuppressed or in otherwise poor health.

The traditional choice for AUC is trimethoprim-sulfamethoxazole (TMP-SMZ), a fixed-dose combination drug that is featured as a prototype in Section 50.4. Given as a 3-day regimen, TMP-SMZ is effective at eliminating most of the common species of uropathogens. The occurrence of many resistant strains, however, has begun to limit its use as a first-line drug.

An equally effective therapy for AUC is a 3-day regimen with a fluoroquinolone. An extended release form of ciprofloxacin (Cipro XR, Proquin XR) permits once-daily dosing. Other fluoroquinolones useful in treating AUC include norfloxacin (Noroxin), ofloxacin (Floxin), and levofloxacin (Levaquin). Fluoroquinolones have become preferred drugs for AUC in many communities because of their safety and the appearance of sulfonamide-resistant strains. Although prescribed for patients with UTIs, fluoroquinolones should be used with caution in patients with serious renal

---

TABLE 50.1 Most Common Uropathogens

Uncomplicated UTI	Complicated UTI
Escherichia coli	*E. coli*
Staphylococcus saprophyticus	Enterobacteriaceae
Klebsiella	*Klebsiella*
Proteus mirabilis	Group B streptococci
Enterobacter	*Enterococcus*
	Pseudomonas
	Proteus mirabilis

impairment, because they are excreted by the kidneys and may accumulate to toxic levels in these patients. Additional details about the fluoroquinolones are presented in Chapter 49.

An additional choice for AUC therapy in communities where TMP-SMZ resistance is high (over 20%) is urinary antiseptics such as nitrofurantoin, which is featured as a prototype in Section 50.5. If compliance is an issue, a single dose of fosfomycin (Monurol) has proven effective for many patients. Fosfomycin blocks cell wall synthesis, and its only indication is UTI.

CONNECTION Checkpoint 50.1

From what you learned in Chapter 49, what black box warning accompanies the oral and parenteral fluoroquinolones? *See Answer to Connection Checkpoint 50.1 on student resource website.*

Complicated Urinary Tract Infection

Complicated urinary tract infections (C-UTIs) are defined as infections that occur in a patient who has an underlying comorbid condition that increases the risk of treatment failure. C-UTIs may require aggressive pharmacotherapy, often involving more toxic drugs, higher doses, or prolonged therapy. Comorbid conditions include the following:

- Structural or functional abnormalities in the genitourinary tract such as neurogenic bladder, benign prostatic hyperplasia (BPH), renal tumor, or urinary stones
- Indwelling urinary catheters
- Older patients with generally ill health
- Recurring urinary infections
- Identification of resistant uropathogens
- Patients with poor toileting or periurethral hygiene
- All UTIs in men

While nearly all uncomplicated UTIs are caused by *E. coli* and *S. saprophyticus*, C-UTIs are caused by a wider variety of uropathogens (see Table 50.1). Hospital-acquired C-UTIs are sometimes caused by organisms such as *Klebsiella, Enterobacter, Proteus,* and *Pseudomonas.* When treating C-UTIs, a urine culture should be obtained to identify the specific microbe and the most effective antibiotic based on culture and sensitivity (C&S) testing. Therapy is sometimes begun with a broad-spectrum anti-infective, then adjusted based on C&S results. Patients who have mild or moderate C-UTIs can be treated with the same medications used for AUC: fluoroquinolones, TMP-SMZ, or nitrofurantoin (Furadantin, Macrobid, Macrodantin). Therapy is often continued for 14 days to be certain that all uropathogens have been eliminated. Severe disease requires hospitalization with parenteral administration of fluoroquinolones, aminoglycosides, cephalosporins, or ampicillin, depending on the sensitivity of the microbe. Follow-up urine cultures are performed several weeks after completion of therapy to ensure that the uropathogen has been eliminated.

PharmFACT

Although men have a much lower overall incidence of UTI than women, the presence of prostatic hypertrophy and catheterization in men over age 50 dramatically increases the risk of UTI (Brusch, 2014).

50.3 Infants, children, pregnant women, older adults, and those with recurring urinary tract infections require modifications to standard pharmacotherapy.

Certain populations require special consideration when selecting and initiating a course of pharmacotherapy to treat UTI. These include infants, children, pregnant women, older adults, and those with recurring infections.

Infants and Children

Although UTIs occur most frequently in sexually active adult women, they are also relatively common in infants and children. More than 2% of males have a UTI before 12 months of age, a higher percentage than girls of the same age. As many as 3% of all females and 1% of males experience a UTI during their school-age years. A concern with pediatric patients is that repeated UTIs may cause scarring of the kidneys, resulting in hypertension later in life. With this possibility in mind, health care providers have a goal of preventing recurring infections in children.

Like adults, *E. coli* causes most pediatric UTIs. Therapeutic options, however, are more limited in children. TMP-SMZ and nitrofurantoin are effective in children. However, fluoroquinolones are contraindicated in children under age 18 because these drugs have been found to affect cartilage development. The safety and efficacy of fosfomycin has not been established in children younger than 12 years old. Recurring UTIs in infants and children may require prolonged, prophylactic antibiotic therapy.

Pregnancy

During pregnancy, the enlarging uterus creates pressure on the urinary bladder, which increases the size of the ureters and promotes urinary stasis and reflux. UTIs in pregnant women are a risk factor for prematurity and newborn low birth weight. In addition, pyelonephritis is one of the most frequent reasons for hospitalization during pregnancy.

Urinary screening is routinely performed by the 16th week of pregnancy. Discovery of high levels of bacteria in the urine is an indication for antimicrobial therapy, even if the patient is asymptomatic at the time of testing. A follow-up culture is performed 1 to 2 weeks after therapy is completed. Continued asymptomatic bacteriuria is predictive of the development of symptomatic UTI later in pregnancy. Therapy for asymptomatic bacteriuria is continued until cultures are negative, or until delivery.

During pregnancy, C&S testing is generally conducted to identify the appropriate antibiotic. Pharmacotherapy, however, is limited to drugs that are pregnancy category B, unless the patient is gravely ill. Category B agents include cephalosporins, ampicillin, and nitrofurantoin. Ceftriaxone (Rocephin) is sometimes a preferred drug. Fluoroquinolones are contraindicated during pregnancy due to possible growth inhibition in the fetus, and TMP-SMZ is contraindicated during the first trimester. Asymptomatic patients are sometimes given a shorter treatment of 1 to 3 days, whereas those with clear symptoms of UTI receive a 7-day regimen.

CONNECTION Checkpoint 50.2

From what you learned in Chapter 47, if a pregnant patient has a history of allergy to ampicillin, should the nurse administer a cephalosporin such as ceftriaxone for UTI? *See Answer to Connection Checkpoint 50.2 on student resource website.*

Older Adults

UTIs are common in the geriatric population, especially for those in long-term care (LTC) facilities. Factors that predispose older adults to UTI are BPH, increased postvoid residual urine, and urinary incontinence. Residents of LTC facilities may have chronic diseases that require the use of indwelling catheters or IV lines. The large percentage of patients receiving antibiotics in these facilities promotes the emergence of multidrug-resistant strains, which can be difficult to eliminate in the LTC setting.

Pharmacotherapy in the geriatric population is conducted in the same manner as for younger adults, if the geriatric patient is otherwise healthy. Asymptomatic bacteriuria is generally not treated unless the patient has an underlying comorbid condition. Asymptomatic bacteriuria is present in 30% to 50% of older adults, and such widespread therapy would promote the emergence of resistant strains.

Older adults in generally poor health and those with a comorbid condition receive more aggressive pharmacotherapy. These patients may exhibit atypical symptoms, such as altered mental status, sudden incontinence, nausea, or vomiting. However, in as many as 60% of these patients, these symptoms are not indicative of a UTI but of other pathology (Woodford & George, 2009). If immunosuppressed, an antibiotic may be prescribed for prophylaxis against pneumonia, UTIs, and skin and soft tissue infections, which are the three most common infections in LTC facilities. Because of the prevalence of resistant strains, patients in an LTC setting with symptomatic UTI should undergo C&S testing to determine the most effective course of therapy. Pharmacotherapy may be prolonged and continue until urine cultures are negative.

By providing a direct route of entry to the bladder for uropathogens, catheter-associated UTI is one of the common hospital-acquired infections. Because the risk of infection increases over time, it is best to remove the catheter as soon as feasible. Patients with catheters should be carefully monitored for signs of UTI. Periodic urinalysis testing should be conducted to check for bacteriuria. A positive urine culture, with or without urinary tract symptoms, is an indication for removal of the catheter (if feasible) and initiation of pharmacotherapy.

Recurring Urinary Tract Infections

One in five patients with a UTI will experience a subsequent UTI within 6 months. Recurring UTIs are classified as either relapses or reinfections. A *relapse* occurs when the patient experiences a second UTI within 2 weeks after completing pharmacotherapy for the original infection. Normally, a relapse is caused by failure of the initial treatment to totally eliminate the uropathogen. A *reinfection* occurs when the patient recovers from the original infection but acquires another infection weeks or months later. Reinfections may be caused by the original microbe or by a different uropathogen.

Recurrent UTIs require extended antimicrobial therapy, either with the original antibiotic or with a different medication. It is necessary to identify the pathogen in order to examine for resistant strains.

Women who experience two or more UTIs within 6 months, or three or more UTIs over the course of a year, are candidates for prophylactic therapy. Choices for prophylaxis include administration of antibiotics at low doses either on a daily or three-times-per-week schedule. Another option is to allow the woman to initiate therapy herself. With this type of treatment, the patient is provided with a single dose or 3-day course of therapy, which is initiated by the woman after each act of coitus, or when symptoms first develop. Patients should be advised to see their health care provider if symptoms worsen, or if they do not resolve during prophylactic therapy, because this may be a sign of a more serious infection.

PharmFACT

Chronic UTIs in women have been associated with lack of the bacterium *Lactobacillus crispatus* in the vagina. Treatment with an intravaginal probiotic suppository containing *L. crispatus*, called LACTIN-V, has been found to reduce the recurrence of chronic UTI (Stapleton et al., 2011).

Sulfonamides

50.4 Sulfonamides are the traditional drugs of choice for urinary tract infections, but resistance limits their usefulness.

The discovery of the sulfonamides, also called sulfa drugs, in the 1930s heralded a new era in the treatment of infectious disease. Effective against both gram-positive and gram-negative bacteria, the sulfonamides significantly reduced mortality from susceptible microbes and earned its discoverer a Nobel Prize in medicine in 1938. Doses for the sulfonamides are listed in Table 50.2.

Sulfonamides are active against a broad spectrum of microorganisms including some staphylococci, many streptococci (except *Enterococcus faecalis*), *Haemophilus influenzae*, *Nocardia*, most Enterobacteriaceae, *Neisseria*, and *Chlamydia*. Sulfonamides have also been used to treat mycobacterial infections and some protozoans such as *Toxoplasma gondii*. Agents in this drug class are also given for treatment and prophylaxis of *Pneumocystis jiroveci* pneumonia and *Shigella* infections of the small bowel. The nurse should keep in mind that although these drugs appear to be effective against many species, the sensitivity of specific strains of these organisms to sulfonamides in a particular community setting must be confirmed, due to widespread resistance.

Sulfonamides suppress bacterial growth by inhibiting the synthesis of **folic acid**, or folate. In human physiology, folic acid is a water-soluble vitamin that serves a critical role as a coenzyme in the synthesis of ribonucleic acid (RNA) and deoxyribonucleic acid (DNA). But if folic acid is essential to both humans and bacteria, why are the sulfonamides not acutely toxic to humans? The answer lies in differences in the metabolic pathways in humans and bacteria.

Humans must obtain "premade" folic acid by eating foods rich in this vitamin. Humans are unable to synthesize this essential nutrient "from scratch." Bacteria, on the other hand, make their own folic acid using simpler precursor molecules. The basic steps in this pathway are shown in Figure 50.1. Sulfonamides inhibit the enzyme in step 1; the drug trimethoprim inhibits the enzyme in step 3. Note how closely the sulfonamides resemble the precursor molecule, **para-aminobenzoic acid (PABA)**, in Figure 50.2. It is easy to see how an enzyme could confuse the two similar molecules. Once the enzyme binds to the sulfonamide, however, folic acid synthesis stops, and bacterial growth slows. This explains why these agents are bacteriostatic; they slow bacterial growth rather than kill the cells.

TABLE 50.2 Drugs Used for Urinary Tract Infections

Drug	Adult Dose (Maximum Dose Where Indicated)	Adverse Effects
Sulfonamides		
silver sulfadiazine	Topical: Apply 1% cream 1–2 times per day to burn wounds to a thickness of 1.5 mm	*Nausea, vomiting, anorexia, rash, crystalluria* Anaphylaxis, Stevens–Johnson syndrome, blood dyscrasias, fulminant hepatic necrosis, hyperkalemia
sulfadiazine	PO: Loading dose: 2–4 g Maintenance dose: 2–4 g/day in four to six divided doses	
sulfadoxine-pyrimethamine (Fansidar)	PO: 1 tablet weekly (500 mg sulfadoxine, 25 mg pyrimethamine)	
sulfisoxazole (Gantrisin)	PO: Loading dose: 2–4 g Maintenance dose: 1–2 g qid (max: 12 g/day)	
trimethoprim-sulfamethoxazole (TMP-SMZ) (Bactrim, Septra)	PO: 160 mg TMP/800 mg SMZ bid IV: 8–10 mg/kg/day TMP, every 6–12 h infused over 60–90 min	
Urinary Antiseptics and Miscellaneous Drugs		
fosfomycin (Monurol)	PO: 3-g sachet dissolved in 3–4 oz of water as a single dose	*Nausea, diarrhea, back pain, headache* Anaphylaxis, superinfections
methenamine hippurate (Hiprex) or mandelate (Mandelamine)	PO: 1 g bid (hippurate) or 1 g qid (mandelate)	*Nausea, vomiting, diarrhea, increased urinary urgency* Anaphylaxis, crystalluria
nalidixic acid (NegGram)	PO: Acute infections: 1 g qid Chronic infections: 500 mg qid	*Nausea, vomiting, diarrhea, drowsiness, fatigue, headache, blurred vision* Anaphylaxis, hemolytic anemia
nitrofurantoin (Furadantin, Macrobid, Macrodantin)	PO: 50–100 mg qid (max: 7 mg/kg/day)	*Nausea, vomiting, anorexia, dark urine, rash* Anaphylaxis, superinfections, hepatic necrosis, interstitial pneumonitis, Stevens–Johnson syndrome, hemolytic anemia

Note: *Italics* indicate common adverse effects. <u>Underline</u> indicates serious adverse effects.

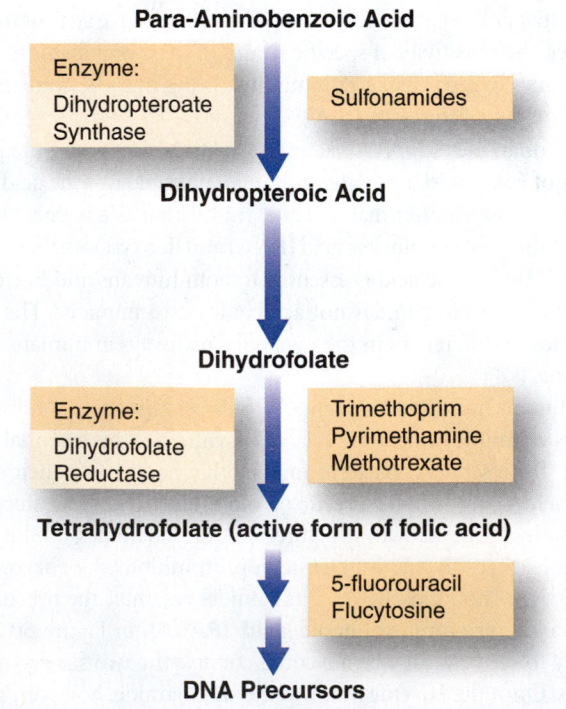

Figure 50.1 Drug inhibition of folic acid metabolism. Drugs inhibit multiple steps in the metabolic pathway leading to folic acid.

The widespread use of sulfonamides for over 60 years resulted in a substantial number of resistant strains. The mechanism of acquired resistance to sulfonamides is likely a mutation in the enzyme performing step 1 of folic acid synthesis. Mutant enzymes can still bind to PABA but can no longer bind to sulfonamides. Resistance to one sulfonamide often confers resistance to all members of this class.

In addition to resistance, several other factors have led to a significant decline in the use of sulfonamides. The development of the penicillins, cephalosporins, and macrolides gave practitioners larger choices of agents, some of which exhibited an improved safety profile over the sulfonamides. Approval of the combination antibiotic TMP-SMZ marked resurgence in the use of sulfonamides in treating UTIs. Decades of widespread use, however, have now resulted in a large number of strains resistant to TMP-SMZ. In communities with high resistance rates, TMP-SMZ is no longer a drug of first choice, unless C&S testing determines it to be the most effective drug for the specific uropathogen.

Sulfonamides are classified by their absorption and excretion characteristics. These subclasses include:

- Oral (PO) agents that are readily absorbed
- PO agents that are not absorbed
- Topical agents

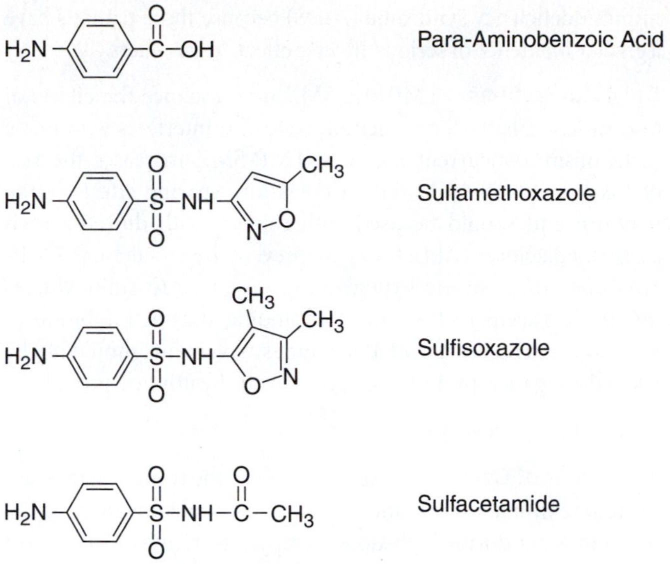

Figure 50.2 Chemical similarities between para-aminobenzoic acid and sulfonamides.

Drugs that are readily absorbed after a PO dose include sulfisoxazole (Gantrisin), sulfadiazine, and TMP-SMZ. These sulfonamides are distributed to most tissues in the body, and the amount of plasma protein binding may be significant. Once hepatic enzymes convert these drugs to inactive metabolites, the drugs are excreted rapidly by the kidney. Sulfadoxine is an exception, with an exceptionally long half-life of 7 to 9 days. For malarial prophylaxis, it is combined with pyrimethamine and marketed as Fansidar.

One sulfonamide comprises the second subclass: drugs that are given PO but undergo no significant absorption. Sulfasalazine (Azulfidine) remains unabsorbed in the alimentary canal, where it is used to treat intestinal infections and mild to moderate ulcerative colitis. Some systemic toxicity may be observed with this drug, because one of its metabolic products is absorbed from the intestine and enters the systemic circulation.

The third subclass includes topical sulfonamides. Silver sulfadiazine (Silvadene, Thermazene) is used for the prophylaxis and treatment of topical infections resulting from wounds or burns. Mafenide (Sulfamylon) is another drug in this class applied topically over burn wounds. Topical sulfonamides may be absorbed across denuded skin, resulting in significant plasma drug levels.

Sulfacetamide (Cetamide) is available as a solution or ointment to treat conjunctivitis and other external eye infections. Blephamide is a combination drug with sulfacetamide and prednisolone indicated for ocular infections that have inflammation as a significant component.

Adverse Effects

In general, the sulfonamides are safe drugs; however, some adverse effects may be serious. Of most concern are adverse effects on the urinary tract, hypersensitivity reactions, and blood abnormalities. Nausea, vomiting, and anorexia may also occur.

Agents in this class must be used with caution in patients with renal impairment. Sulfonamides have a low solubility, which may

CONNECTIONS Patient Safety

◀ **Trimethoprim-Sulfamethoxazole (Bactrim, Septra)**

The nurse will administer TMP-SMZ (Bactrim, Septra) to a patient with a UTI. Before giving the medication, the nurse reviews the patient's chart. The nurse notices that the patient is afebrile with a normal pulse, blood pressure, and respiratory rate. The most recent culture indicates a decline in the number of bacteria present in the urine. Other information found in the medical record indicates that the patient routinely takes medication for hypertension and arthritis. The patient has also reported allergies to chocolate and thiazide diuretics. Should the nurse give the medication as prescribed?

See Answer to Patient Safety Questions on student resource website.

cause **crystalluria**, crystals that form in the urine and potentially obstruct the kidneys or ureters. The risk is higher in dehydrated patients and when urine pH is abnormally low. To decrease the possibility of crystalluria, fluids in amounts up to 3,000 mL per day should be encouraged to achieve a urinary output of 1,500 mL in 24 hours.

Although not common, sulfonamides can cause potentially fatal blood abnormalities such as aplastic anemia, acute hemolytic anemia, and agranulocytosis. Baseline and periodic blood laboratory values should be assessed to prevent the development of anemia or other hematologic disorders. Patients with preexisting myelosuppression should be monitored carefully during therapy, because this increases the risks associated with drug-induced bone marrow depression.

Hypersensitivity to sulfa drugs is well documented. These drugs cause a number of dermal reactions ranging from urticaria to photosensitivity and exfoliative dermatitis. Patients may develop fever and malaise. Cross sensitivity exists with diuretics, such as acetazolamide (Diamox) and the thiazides, and with sulfonylurea antidiabetic drugs. These agents should be avoided in patients with a history of hypersensitivity to sulfonamides because this can induce Stevens–Johnson syndrome. At the first signs of rash, patients should be instructed to stop taking the drug and contact their health care provider.

Most sulfonamides readily cross the placenta and may reach sufficiently high levels to cause adverse effects in the fetus. Sulfonamides are contraindicated during lactation, because they enter breast milk. They are contraindicated for infants less than 2 months of age and for pregnant patients near term, because sulfonamides displace bilirubin from plasma proteins. The displaced, free bilirubin is toxic to the brain and causes kernicterus, a serious type of jaundice.

| PROTOTYPE DRUG | Trimethoprim-Sulfamethoxazole (Bactrim, Septra) |

Classification: Therapeutic: Antibacterial
Pharmacologic: Folic acid inhibitor, sulfonamide

Therapeutic Effects and Uses: Approved in 1973, TMP-SMZ is a folic acid inhibitor containing a fixed-dose combination of trimethoprim (TMP) and sulfamethoxazole (SMZ), a sulfonamide. The drug is commonly used for UTI prophylaxis and in the pharmacotherapy of complicated and uncomplicated UTI, depending on the sensitivity of the specific uropathogen. It is also approved for the treatment and prophylaxis of *P. jiroveci* pneumonia, *Shigella* infections of the small bowel, traveler's diarrhea due to *E. coli*, and for acute exacerbations of chronic bronchitis due to *Streptococcus pneumoniae* or *Haemophilus influenzae*. The drug is used off-label for many other indications, depending on the sensitivity of the microbe. PO and IV formulations are available.

Mechanism of Action: Both SMZ and TMP are inhibitors of the bacterial metabolism of folic acid. Each drug inhibits a separate enzyme in the metabolic pathway, creating a synergistic combination: A greater bacterial kill is achieved by the fixed combination than would be achieved with either drug used separately. Because humans obtain folate in their diets, these medications are selective toward bacterial folate metabolism.

Pharmacokinetics:

Route(s)	PO, IV
Absorption	Readily absorbed
Distribution	Widely distributed to all body fluids, including cerebrospinal fluid (CSF); crosses the placenta; secreted in breast milk; protein binding is 70% (SMZ) and 44% (TMP)
Primary metabolism	Hepatic
Primary excretion	Renal
Onset of action	PO: 1–4 h
Duration of action	Half-life: 8–10 h (TMP) and 10–13 h (SMZ)

Adverse Effects: Nausea and vomiting are the most common adverse effects of TMP-SMZ therapy. These normally diminish with time but may require treatment or cause discontinuation of therapy. Hypersensitivity is relatively common and usually manifests as skin rash, pruritus, and fever. Severe hypersensitivity reactions such as anaphylaxis, Stevens–Johnson syndrome, epidermal necrolysis, agranulocytosis, aplastic anemia, and allergic myocarditis have been reported. The drug should be discontinued at the first appearance of a skin rash. To prevent crystalluria and potential damage to tubular cells, it is important to maintain dilute urine during therapy to reduce the concentration of the drugs as they travel through the renal tubule. Due to the potential for photosensitivity, the patient should avoid direct sunlight during therapy.

Contraindications/Precautions: An allergy history should be taken prior to administration, because TMP-SMZ is contraindicated in patients with hypersensitivity to sulfites, sulfonamides, or chemically related agents such as thiazide diuretics. TMP-SMZ is contraindicated in patients with folate-deficiency anemia, since a folic acid inhibitor would worsen this condition. This medication is contraindicated in patients with severe renal impairment because this is the primary route of drug excretion and the drug may accumulate to toxic levels in these patients. It should be used with caution in patients with hepatic impairment because the liver metabolizes TMP-SMZ. Trimethoprim decreases potassium excretion and is contraindicated in patients with hyperkalemia. Caution must be used when treating patients with acquired immunodeficiency syndrome (AIDS) because these patients have a greater incidence of serious adverse effects than others.

Drug Interactions: TMP and SMZ may enhance the effects of oral anticoagulants. Since methotrexate also interferes with folate metabolism, concurrent use with TMP-SMZ increases the risk of toxicity. TMP-SMZ exerts a potassium-sparing effect on the nephron and should be used with caution with diuretics such as spironolactone (Aldactone) to prevent hyperkalemia. TMP-SMZ may increase the hypoglycemic response to sulfonylureas due to displacement from protein-binding sites or inhibition of metabolism. **Herbal/Food**: Potassium supplements should not be taken during therapy, unless directed by the health care provider.

Pregnancy: Category C.

Treatment of Overdose: Acidification of the urine will increase the renal elimination of trimethoprim. If signs of bone marrow depression occur during high-dose therapy, 5 to 15 mg of leucovorin should be given daily.

Nursing Responsibilities: Key nursing implications for patients receiving TMP-SMZ are included in the Nursing Practice Application for Patients Receiving Pharmacotherapy for Urinary Tract Infection.

Drugs Similar to Trimethoprim-Sulfamethoxazole (Bactrim, Septra)

Other orally absorbed sulfonamides include sulfadiazine and sulfisoxazole. Sulfadoxine-pyrimethamine (Fansidar) is used exclusively for treating malaria and is discussed in Chapter 53.

Sulfadiazine: Approved in 1941, sulfadiazine is a short-acting, oral sulfonamide that is given every 4 to 6 hours. It has a broad spectrum and is used for diverse infections, including UTI, nocardiosis, meningococcal meningitis, cerebral toxoplasmosis (in combination with pyrimethamine), and resistant malaria. Sulfadiazine is usually prescribed only when other, safer anti-infectives have failed to produce a therapeutic effect and C&S testing has determined the organism to be sensitive to the drug. Like other sulfonamides, hypersensitivity may be a major clinical limitation to therapy. Sulfadiazine is poorly soluble in urine and causes more crystalluria than other sulfonamides. Adequate fluid intake and frequent urinary testing are essential to avoid nephrotoxicity. Sulfadiazine carries a black box warning that it should be discontinued at the first sign of a skin rash due to the possibility for Stevens–Johnson syndrome. Sulfadiazine is pregnancy category C.

Silver sulfadiazine (Silvadene, Thermazene) is a topical cream indicated as an adjunct for the prevention and treatment of wound sepsis in patients with second- and third-degree burns. Adverse effects are rare when the cream is applied over small areas. However, when the drug is applied over large denuded areas some of the topical medication is absorbed and systemic adverse effects may occur. Silver sulfadiazine is pregnancy category B.

Sulfisoxazole (Gantrisin): Like sulfadiazine, this drug is short acting and must be taken PO every 4 to 6 hours. Approved in 1948, indications include UTI, acute otitis media due to *H. influenzae*, nocardiosis, and malaria, in combination with other antimalarial agents. It is sometimes preferred over other sulfonamides for UTI because it causes less crystalluria. Hypersensitivity is a common adverse effect. An ophthalmic formulation is available for the treatment of chlamydial conjunctivitis. A fixed-dose suspension of sulfisoxazole with erythromycin is available for the treatment of acute otitis media in penicillin-allergic patients. This drug is pregnancy category C.

Trimethoprim (Primsol): In addition to being part of the TMP-SMZ combination, trimethoprim is also available as monotherapy. Trimethoprim is approved to treat uncomplicated UTI and acute otitis media in children due to *S. pneumoniae* or *H. influenzae*. It has been used off-label for the treatment of traveler's diarrhea and for *Pneumocystis* pneumonia, in combination with either sulfamethoxazole or dapsone. Rash and pruritus are common adverse effects, and these may appear 1 to 2 weeks after therapy has begun. Some patients experience nausea, vomiting, and diarrhea. Trimethoprim is combined with polymyxin B in an ophthalmic solution for ocular infections. This drug is pregnancy category C.

Urinary Antiseptics

50.5 Urinary antiseptics are anti-infective drugs used exclusively for urinary tract infections.

As has been noted throughout this textbook, most medications are totally or partially excreted by the kidneys. The majority of drugs and their metabolites travel through the urinary system, producing little or no effect on the renal tubular cells or the other parts of the kidney. For the small class of drugs known as the urinary antiseptics, however, the urinary system is their target tissue. Being able to reach the urinary tract in high concentrations is essential to their therapeutic success.

Urinary antiseptics are given by the PO route for their antibacterial action in the urinary tract. While they do not reach high enough levels in the blood to be effective for systemic infections, the kidney concentrates the drugs; thus, their actions are specific to the urinary system. Urinary antiseptics reach therapeutic levels

in the kidney tubules, and their anti-infective action continues as they travel to the urinary bladder.

The advantage of the urinary antiseptics is that they are able to treat local infections in the urinary tract without reaching high levels in the blood that might produce systemic toxicity. Although not considered first-line drugs for UTI, they serve important roles as secondary medications, especially in patients who present with infections resistant to TMP-SMZ or the fluoroquinolones.

| PROTOTYPE DRUG | Nitrofurantoin (Furadantin) and Nitrofurantoin Macrocrystals (Macrobid, Macrodantin) |

Classification: Therapeutic: Antibacterial
Pharmacologic: Urinary tract antiseptic

Therapeutic Effects and Uses: Nitrofurantoin is an older drug that is indicated for the treatment of uncomplicated acute cystitis, most commonly for the prophylaxis of recurrent UTI. Nitrofurantoin is active against the *E. coli, S. saprophyticus,* and many other strains of gram-positive and gram-negative aerobes. It is not effective against the *Pseudomonas, Proteus,* or *Serratia* species. It is not indicated for the treatment of pyelonephritis.

Nitrofurantoin is available in three formulations: a microcrystalline form (Furadantin), a regular release macrocrystalline form (Macrodantin), and a sustained release macrocrystalline form (Macrobid). The macrocrystalline form is more slowly absorbed than the microcrystalline form and produces fewer GI-related adverse effects.

Despite being approved by the FDA in 1953, development of resistance has not been a significant problem. The broad-based mechanism of action may explain the relative lack of acquired bacterial resistance to nitrofurantoin. Multiple mutations at diverse locations of the bacterial chromosome would be necessary for a bacterium to acquire such resistance. Cross resistance with other antibiotics is very rare, if it occurs at all.

CONNECTIONS Complementary and Alternative Therapies

Cranberry

Description
Cranberry shrubs grow in diverse climates ranging from bogs to forests. The ripe berry is used for its potential medicinal effects.

History and Claims
Native Americans used the berries to treat wounds and to cure anorexia and other digestive complaints. In the early 1900s, it was noted that the acidity of urine increases after eating cranberries; thus began the belief that cranberry juice is a natural cure for UTIs.

Standardization
The herb is taken as juice or dried extract. Doses generally range from 120 to 4,000 mL of juice or 400 to 500 mg of the extract daily.

Evidence
Cranberry contains a significant amount of vitamin C and other antioxidants that can promote health. A meta-analysis of the clinical research involving

over 1,600 patients concluded that cranberry products are indeed effective for preventing UTIs (Wang et al., 2012). Previously, it was thought that this juice would change the pH of urine to become more acidic, discouraging bacteria growth. Recently, specific chemicals found in cranberry juice (e.g., proanthocyanidins) have demonstrated the ability to prevent the bacteria from sticking to the walls of the bladder. This makes it more difficult for the bacteria to colonize and reproduce. The juice should be 100% cranberry and not cocktail juice because that contains sugar, which enhances bacterial growth and may be contraindicated in patients with diabetes. Some individuals may prefer to take cranberry capsules, which are available at most drug stores. Cranberry should be used cautiously by people who take anticoagulants such as warfarin (National Center for Complementary and Alternative Medicine, 2012). GI intolerance and weight gain from extra caloric intake from the juice seem to be the dominant reasons for discontinuing the cranberry product.

Mechanism of Action: Nitrofurantoin acts by several unique mechanisms. When bacteria break down nitrofurantoin, the drug is converted to highly reactive intermediates. These intermediates attack bacterial ribosomal proteins. The drug inhibits bacterial protein synthesis, aerobic energy metabolism, DNA synthesis, RNA synthesis, and formation of the cell wall. Nitrofurantoin is bactericidal in the urine at therapeutic doses.

Pharmacokinetics:

Route(s)	PO
Absorption	Readily absorbed
Distribution	Widely distributed to body fluids; crosses the placenta; secreted in breast milk; 60% bound to plasma proteins
Primary metabolism	Hepatic
Primary excretion	Renal
Onset of action	30 min
Duration of action	Half-life: 20 min

Adverse Effects: Nitrofurantoin has the potential to produce many adverse effects. The most frequent include hypersensitivity reactions, anorexia, headache, rash, nausea, and vomiting. Acute and chronic pulmonary toxicity is a serious adverse effect and may include interstitial pneumonitis, persistent cough, and pulmonary fibrosis. Chronic pulmonary toxicity may not appear until months or years after therapy has been completed. Hepatotoxicity is rare, though potentially fatal, and may include cholestatic jaundice, hepatic necrosis, or hepatitis.

Contraindications/Precautions: Because nitrofurantoin is excreted by the kidneys, significant renal impairment (creatinine clearance under 60 mL/minute or significant elevated serum creatinine) is a contraindication. Successful treatment depends on achieving high amounts of drug in the urine, which will not occur in patients with oliguria or anuria. Because of the possibility of hemolytic anemia due to immature erythrocyte enzyme systems, the drug is contraindicated in pregnant patients or in neonates less than 1 month of age.

This drug should be used with caution in patients with preexisting pulmonary disease, and pulmonary function should be closely monitored throughout therapy. Although rare, reports have cited diffuse interstitial pneumonitis or pulmonary fibrosis as causes of death in patients receiving nitrofurantoin.

Nitrofurantoin should be used with caution in patients with preexisting hepatic disease. The drug should be discontinued immediately if changes are noted in liver function tests.

Drug Interactions: Nitrofurantoin should not be given with antacids containing magnesium because absorption will be decreased. Concurrent administration with nalidixic acid, and possibly fluoroquinolones, may result in antagonism and a decreased drug effect. **Herbal/Food**: Unknown.

Pregnancy: Category B.

Treatment of Overdose: Adequate fluid intake should be provided to ensure renal excretion of the drug. In extreme cases, dialysis may be of value in removing nitrofurantoin.

Nursing Responsibilities: Key nursing implications for patients receiving nitrofurantoin are included in the Nursing Practice Application for Patients Receiving Pharmacotherapy for Urinary Tract Infection.

Drugs Similar to Nitrofurantoin (Furadantin) and Nitrofurantoin Macrocrystals (Macrobid, Macrodantin)

Other urinary antiseptics include fosfomycin, methenamine, and nalidixic acid.

Fosfomycin (Monurol):   Approved in 1996, fosfomycin is approved for the treatment of uncomplicated UTI caused by susceptible strains of *E. coli* and *Enterococcus faecalis*. Technically classified as a cell wall inhibitor (see Chapter 47), it reaches high concentrations in the urine and bladder. Thus, it is sometimes called a bladder antiseptic. It is administered as a single PO dose. The most frequent adverse effects are diarrhea, headache, vaginitis, nausea, rhinitis, and pain. This drug is pregnancy category B.

Methenamine (Hiprex, Urex):   Methenamine is an older drug approved in 1939 that is available as hippurate salts. In the very acidic environment of urine, methenamine hippurate is metabolized to formaldehyde, a breakdown product toxic to microorganisms. The hippurate salt becomes an acid in the urine, thus providing an even greater environment (lower pH) for the generation of formaldehyde. At therapeutic doses, methenamine is a safe drug, although higher doses can result in dysuria, nausea, vomiting, and hematuria.

The only clinical application of methenamine is for prophylactic treatment of recurrent UTI, especially those with neurogenic bladder. Preventive therapy with methenamine is instituted after eradication of the infection by other appropriate anti-infectives. It is effective against most bacteria typically responsible for UTI. Urease-positive bacteria such as *Proteus* are resistant because they produce ammonia in the urine, which prevents the formation of formaldehyde. Concurrent therapy of methenamine with sulfamethoxazole is contraindicated because the combination promotes crystalluria. This drug is pregnancy category C.

Nalidixic acid (NegGram):   Approved in 1964, nalidixic acid was the first quinolone anti-infective marketed. Nalidixic acid and newer drugs in this class (fluoroquinolones) act by inhibiting DNA and RNA synthesis. While fluoroquinolones are prescribed for many diverse infections, the use of nalidixic acid is limited to UTI. Its spectrum of activity includes most bacteria responsible for UTI. Another first-generation quinolone, cinoxacin (Cinobac), was very similar to nalidixic acid but is no longer marketed in the United States.

Nalidixic acid is readily absorbed in the GI tract and is concentrated in the urine. GI distress is the most common adverse effect. At higher doses, patients may experience drowsiness, fatigue, headaches, and visual disturbances such as blurred vision.

Nalidixic acid is contraindicated in infants less than 3 months of age because it may create intracranial hypertension. The nurse should monitor laboratory blood counts, because nalidixic acid has been reported to cause hemolytic anemia and thrombocytopenia in some patients. This drug displaces warfarin from plasma protein-binding sites. Thus, a reduction in dose may be necessary for the anticoagulant. Resistance to nalidixic acid develops rapidly during therapy. This drug is pregnancy category C.

CONNECTIONS: NURSING PRACTICE APPLICATION

Patients Receiving Pharmacotherapy for Urinary Tract Infection

Assessment	Potential Nursing Diagnoses*
Baseline assessment prior to administration: • Obtain a complete health history including hepatic or renal disease, diabetes, AIDS, folate-deficiency anemia, and the possibility of pregnancy. Obtain a drug history including allergies (e.g., specific reactions to drugs), current prescription and over-the-counter (OTC) drugs, herbal preparations, and alcohol use. Be alert to possible drug interactions. • Assess signs and symptoms of current infection, noting location, characteristics, presence or absence of urinary tract symptoms or of fever. • Evaluate appropriate laboratory findings (e.g., complete blood count [CBC], C&S, hepatic, and renal function studies). • Assess the patient's ability to receive and understand instructions. Include family and caregivers as needed.	• *Infection* (bacterial) • *Acute Pain* • *Hyperthermia* • *Deficient Knowledge* (Drug Therapy) • *Risk for Injury*, related to adverse drug effects • *Risk for Deficient Fluid Volume*, related to diarrhea caused by adverse drug effects
Assessment throughout administration: • Assess for desired therapeutic effects (e.g., diminished signs and symptoms of infection and fever). • Continue periodic monitoring of CBC, renal function, urinalysis, and C&S as ordered. • Assess for adverse effects: nausea, vomiting, abdominal cramping, diarrhea, headache, or dizziness. Severe diarrhea, especially containing mucus, blood, or pus, or decreased urine output should be reported immediately.	

Implementation

Interventions and (Rationales)	Patient-Centered Care
Ensuring therapeutic effects: • Continue assessments as above for therapeutic effects. (Diminished fever, pain, or signs and symptoms of infection should begin after taking the first dose and continue to improve. The provider should be notified if fever and signs and symptoms of infection remain or increase after 3 days, or if the entire course of antibacterial has been taken and signs of infection are still present.)	• Teach the patient to complete the entire course of the antibacterial; do not share doses with other family members with similar symptoms; and return to the provider if symptoms have not resolved after an entire course of therapy.
Minimizing adverse effects: • Continue to monitor vital signs, especially temperature, if fever is present. Immediately report undiminished fever, changes in level of consciousness, or febrile seizures to the health care provider. (Fever should begin to diminish within 1–3 days after starting the drug. Continued fever may be a sign of worsening infection, adverse drug effects, or antibiotic resistance.)	• Teach the patient to report a fever that does not diminish below 37.8°C (100°F) or per the parameters set by the health care provider. Immediately report febrile seizures, changes in behavior, or changes in level of consciousness to the health care provider.
• Continue to monitor periodic laboratory work: renal function tests, CBC, urinalysis, and C&S as ordered. (Sulfonamides may be renal toxic. Periodic C&S tests may be ordered if infections are severe or are slow to resolve to confirm appropriate therapy.)	• Instruct the patient on the need for periodic laboratory work.
• Monitor for hypersensitivity and allergic reactions, especially with the first dose of the drug, and in patients with a history of allergy to thiazide diuretics. Continue to monitor the patient for up to 2 weeks after completing the antibacterial therapy. (Anaphylactic reactions are possible, particularly with the first dose of an antibacterial. Post-use, residual drug levels, dependent on the length of half-life, may cause delayed reactions.)	• Teach the patient to immediately report any itching, rashes, swelling, particularly of the face or tongue, urticaria, flushing, dizziness, syncope, wheezing, throat tightness, or difficulty breathing. • Instruct the patient with known antibacterial allergies to carry a wallet identification card or wear medical identification jewelry indicating the allergy.
• Continue to monitor for renal toxicity, e.g., diminished urine output, edema, or weight gain greater than 1 kg (2 lb) in 24 h. (Sulfonamides may require frequent monitoring to prevent adverse effects. Increasing fluid intake will help prevent drug accumulation in the kidneys and the development of urine crystals. **Lifespan:** Age-related physiological differences may place the young child or older adult at greater risk for renal toxicity.)	• Teach the patient to immediately report any diminished urine output, visible swelling of feet or ankles, or weight gain greater than 1 kg (2 lb) in 24 h. • Advise the patient to increase fluid intake to 2–3 L/day.

(continued)

CONNECTIONS: NURSING PRACTICE APPLICATION (continued)

• Monitor for development of superinfections, e.g., CDAD or PMC, fungal, or yeast infections. (Superinfections with opportunistic organisms may occur when normal host flora are diminished or killed by the antibacterial drug and no longer hold pathogens in check. Severe diarrhea may indicate the presence of CDAD or PMC, superinfections caused by *C. difficile*.)	• Instruct the patient to report any diarrhea that increases in frequency, amount, or contains mucus, blood, or pus. • Instruct the patient to consult the health care provider before taking any antidiarrheal drugs, which cause the retention of harmful bacteria. • Teach the patient to observe for changes in stool, white patches in mouth, whitish thick vaginal discharge, itching in the genital area, blistering itchy rash, and to immediately report severe diarrhea. • Teach the patient infection control measures such as frequent hand washing, adequate drying after showering or bathing, and to increase intake of live-culture dairy foods.
• Continue to monitor for dermatologic effects including red or purplish skin rash, blisters, or sunburn. Immediately report severe rashes, especially any associated with blistering. (Sulfonamides may cause significant dermatologic effects including Stevens–Johnson syndrome. Sunscreens and protective clothing should be used to prevent photosensitivity and photoallergic reactions.)	• Teach the patient to wear sunscreens and protective clothing for sun exposure and to avoid tanning beds. Immediately report any severe sunburn or rashes.
• Monitor for systemic effects in patients requiring topical sulfonamide creams for burns or infected wounds. (Large areas of treatment may result in excessive absorption of the drug, resulting in systemic effects. Stinging or burning may occur on application of the cream but does not indicate a systemic effect.)	• Teach the patient to report nausea, vomiting, abdominal cramping, diarrhea, headache, or dizziness while using the topical drug because these may indicate systemic absorption. • Instruct the patient in the appropriate application of the topical cream, applying a thin layer to the affected area, covered by a dry dressing.
• Monitor for anticoagulation effects if the patient is on warfarin. (Sulfonamides may increase the effects of warfarin, resulting in an increased risk of bleeding.)	• Teach the patient on warfarin to report any increase in bruising or bleeding. More frequent laboratory work may be needed.
• Monitor glucose levels more frequently in patients with diabetes on PO medication with sulfonylureas. Monitor potassium levels more frequently in the patient taking K-sparing diuretics or ACEIs. (Sulfonamides exert a K-sparing effect on the kidney and may cause hyperkalemia in patients taking K-sparing diuretics or ACEIs. The drugs also increase the hypoglycemic effect of sulfonylureas.)	• Instruct patients taking potassium-sparing diuretics (e.g., spironolactone [Aldactone]) or ACEIs (e.g., lisinopril [Prinivil, Zestril]) to avoid foods high in potassium, e.g., fresh fruits such as strawberries and bananas; dried fruits such as apricots and prunes; vegetables and legumes such as tomatoes, beets, and dried beans; juices such as orange, grapefruit, or prune; and fresh meats; to avoid the use of salt substitutes (which often contain potassium salts); and to consult with a health care provider before taking vitamin and mineral supplements or specialized sports beverages. • Instruct patients with diabetes who rely on PO medication with sulfonylureas (e.g., glyburide [DiaBeta, Micronase]) to monitor their blood sugar more frequently and to be aware of subtle signs of possible hypoglycemia (e.g., nervousness, irritability). Any consistent changes in their blood sugar levels while on a sulfonamide antibiotic should be reported to the health care provider.
Patient understanding of drug therapy: • Use opportunities during administration of medications and during assessments to discuss the rationale for drug therapy, desired therapeutic outcomes, commonly observed adverse effects, parameters for when to call the health care provider, and any necessary monitoring or precautions. (Using time during nursing care helps to optimize and reinforce key teaching areas.)	• The patient, family, or caregiver should be able to state the reason for the drug, appropriate dose and scheduling, what adverse effects to observe for and when to report them, and the anticipated length of medication therapy.
Patient self-administration of drug therapy: • When administering medications, instruct the patient, family, or caregiver in proper self-administration techniques followed by teach-back. (Utilizing time during nurse-administration of these drugs helps to reinforce teaching.)	• Teach the patient to: • Complete the entire course of therapy unless otherwise instructed. Do not share with other family members, and do not stop taking the medicine when starting to feel better. • Take the medication as evenly spaced throughout each day as feasible. • Increase overall fluid intake while taking the antibacterial drug. • Discard outdated medications or those no longer in use. Review the medicine cabinet twice a year for old medications (e.g., at the beginning and end of daylight saving time).

CHAPTER

50 Understanding the Chapter

Key Concepts Summary

50.1 Infections can occur in any portion of the urinary tract.

50.2 Choice of pharmacotherapy for acute urinary tract infection depends on the severity of the infection and the presence of comorbid conditions.

50.3 Infants, children, pregnant women, older adults, and those with recurring urinary tract infections require modifications to standard pharmacotherapy.

50.4 Sulfonamides are the traditional drugs of choice for urinary tract infections, but resistance limits their usefulness.

50.5 Urinary antiseptics are anti-infective drugs used exclusively for urinary tract infections.

Case Study: Making the Patient Connection

Remember the patient "Sandra Phillipi" at the beginning of the chapter? Now read the remainder of the case study. Based on the information presented within this chapter, respond to the critical thinking questions that follow.

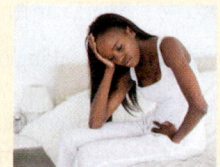

Sandra Phillipi is a 32-year-old woman who has experienced frequent UTIs. Sandra is married with two children and works as a branch manager in the local bank.

In the clinic, Sandra's physical examination reveals the following findings: temperature 38.4°C (101.2°F), pulse 106 beats/min, respiratory rate 18 breaths/min, and blood pressure 112/74 mmHg. She reports having a fever, chills, dysuria, frequency, urinary urgency, and suprapubic pain. Sandra also reports seeing a small amount of blood in the urine and the sensation of incomplete bladder emptying. She states that recently her urine has become cloudy and smells bad.

As you continue your interview with the patient, she states, "I can't believe I have another UTI. I had one just last month." The urinalysis reveals microscopic bacteriuria (greater than 10^5/mL). A urine culture is also collected during this visit, and the results will be reported within 48 h. The patient's preliminary diagnosis is recurrent UTI, and she receives a prescription for trimethoprim-sulfamethoxazole (TMP-SMZ) (Bactrim, Septra).

Critical Thinking Questions

1. How should you respond to the patient's statements about the recurrent infections?

2. What health teaching regarding antibiotic therapy should you stress to this patient?

3. What information should you give patients about saving medications?

See Answers to Critical Thinking Questions on student resource website.

Additional Case Study

Dorothy Janes is an 80-year-old female admitted to your unit for hypertension and a history of stroke with residual right-sided weakness. She is alert and oriented to person, time, and place but requires assistance with ambulation due to a history of falls. Her health care provider ordered Dorothy to be restricted to bed rest with bathroom privileges with assistance. When the patient's daughter comes to visit, she tells you that sometimes her mother has urinary incontinence due to her inability to walk to the bathroom by herself when the urge to urinate occurs. She wants to know if her mother can have a urinary catheter inserted to prevent accidents.

1. How would you respond to the daughter's request for her mother to have a urinary catheter inserted?

2. Brainstorm nursing actions that you could implement to avoid urinary incontinence for this patient.

See Answers to Additional Case Study on student resource website.

Chapter Review

1 An older patient is prescribed sulfisoxazole (Gantrisin). Knowing that one of the major adverse effects of this drug is crystalluria, what should the nurse instruct the patient to do?

1. Limit intake of foods high in calcium such as milk, cheese, and yogurt.
2. Avoid changing positions (lying down, sitting, or standing) rapidly.
3. Increase fluid intake to 2 to 3 L per day.
4. Avoid consuming alcoholic beverages while taking this medication.

2 The nurse understands that which of the following is the main purpose of nitrofurantoin (Furadantin)?

1. Prevent recurrent urinary tract infections.
2. Relieve the pain associated with urinary tract infections.
3. Promote effective urinary elimination and prevent stasis.
4. Reduce pathogenic microorganisms specific to pyelonephritis.

3 The nurse is collecting health data from a patient with diabetes who has a urinary tract infection before starting an order for trimethoprim-sulfamethoxazole (Bactrim, Septra). Which questions asked by the nurse would be most important? Select all that apply.

1. "Have you ever had migraine headaches?"
2. "Are you allergic to any sulfa drugs?"
3. "Do you empty your bladder before and after sexual intercourse?"
4. "When was your last menstrual period?"
5. "What drugs do you use to manage your diabetes?"

4 The nurse is providing the patient with discharge instructions concerning silver sulfadiazine (Silvadene) cream, which has been ordered to treat a significant skin infection. Which statement by the patient indicates to the nurse that the teaching session was effective?

1. "I should use this cream on noninfected surfaces surrounding the infection to prevent additional infection."
2. "If this medication causes stinging or burning, I should stop the drug and report that to my doctor immediately as a drug allergy."
3. "If I experience any nausea and it continues for more than 24 hours, I will contact my doctor."
4. "I must avoid foods high in potassium."

5 The patient is to receive nitrofurantoin (Furadantin) for a urinary tract infection. A nurse should question the order for the patient with which condition?

1. Pulmonary disease
2. Diabetes
3. Rheumatoid arthritis
4. Angina and hypertension

6 A patient taking trimethoprim-sulfamethoxazole (Bactrim, Septra) develops a reddish-purplish papular rash surrounded by areas of erythema. The rash should be evaluated by the provider because it may indicate which skin condition?

1. A fungal superinfection
2. Viral skin eruptions
3. Dermatologic toxicity including Stevens–Johnson syndrome
4. Nonadherence with drug therapy

See Answers to Chapter Review in Appendix A.

References

Brusch, J. L. (2014). *Urinary tract infections in males.* Retrieved from http://emedicine.medscape.com/article/231574-overview#a0156

Lubart, E., Segal, R., Haimov, E., Dan, M., Baumoehl, Y., & Leibovitz, A. (2011). Bacteremia in a multilevel geriatric hospital. *Journal of the American Medical Directors Association, 12,* 204–207. doi:10.1016/j.jamda.2010.02.017

National Center for Complementary and Alternative Medicine. (2012). *Herbs at a glance: Cranberry.* Retrieved from http://nccam.nih.gov/health/cranberry

Rowe, T. A., & Juthani-Mehta, M. (2014). Diagnosis and management of urinary tract infection in older adults. *Infectious Disease Clinics of North America, 28,* 75–89. doi:10.1016/j.idc.2013.10.004

Stapleton, A. E., Au-Yeung, M., Hooton, T. M., Fredericks, D. N., Roberts, P. L., Czaja, C. A., . . . Stamm, W. E. (2011). Randomized, placebo-controlled phase 2 trial of a *Lactobacillus crispatus* probiotic given intravaginally for prevention of recurrent urinary tract infection. *Clinical Infectious Diseases, 52,* 1212–1217. doi:10.1093/cid/cir183

Wang, C. H., Fang, C. C., Chen, N. C., Liu, S. S. H., Yu, P. H., Wu, T. Y., . . . Chen, S. C. (2012). Cranberry-containing products for prevention of urinary tract infections in susceptible populations: A systematic review and meta-analysis of randomized controlled trials. *Archives of Internal Medicine, 172,* 988–996. doi:10.1001/archinternmed.2012.3004

Woodford, H. J., & George, J. (2009). Diagnosis and management of urinary tract infection in hospitalized older people. *Journal of the American Geriatrics Society, 57,* 107–114. doi:10.1111/j.1532-5415.2008.02073.x

Selected Bibliography

Copp, H. L., Shapiro, D. J., & Hersh, A. L. (2011, May 9). National ambulatory antibiotic prescribing patterns for pediatric urinary tract infection, 1998–2007. *Pediatrics.* doi:10.1542/peds.2010-3465

Foxman, B., & Buxton, M. (2013). Alternative approaches to conventional treatment of acute uncomplicated urinary tract infection in women. *Current Infectious Disease Reports, 15,* 124–129. doi:10.1007/s11908-013-0317-5

Herdman, T. H., & Kamitsuro, S. (Eds.) (2014). *NANDA International nursing diagnoses: Definitions and classification, 2015–2017.* Oxford, United Kingdom: Wiley-Blackwell.

Hooton, T. M. (2012). Uncomplicated urinary tract infection. *New England Journal of Medicine, 366,* 1028–1037. doi:10.1056/NEJMcp1104429

Hooton, T. M., Bradley, S. F., Cardenas, D. D., Colgan, R., Geerlings, S. E., Rice, J. C., . . . Nicolle, L. E. (2010). Diagnosis, prevention, and treatment of catheter-associated urinary tract infection in adults: 2009 international clinical practice guidelines from the Infectious Diseases Society of America. *Clinical Infectious Diseases, 50,* 625–663. doi:10.1086/650482

Jepson, R. G., Williams, G., & Craig, J. C. (2012). Cranberries for preventing urinary tract infections. *Cochrane Database of Systematic Reviews, 10,* CD001321. doi:10.1002/14651858.CD001321.pub5

Lowe, N. K., & Ryan-Wenger, N. A. (2012). Uncomplicated UTIs in women. *The Nurse Practitioner, 37*(5), 41–48. doi:10.1097/01.NPR.0000413483.52003.f8

Mylonas, I. (2011). Antibiotic chemotherapy during pregnancy and lactation period: Aspects for consideration. *Archives of Gynecology and Obstetrics, 283,* 7–18. doi:10.1007/s00404-010-1646-3

Nosseir, S. B., Lind, L. R., & Winkler, H. A. (2012). Recurrent uncomplicated urinary tract infections in women: A review. *Journal of Women's Health, 21,* 347–354. doi:10.1089/jwh.2011.3056

O'Dell, K. K. (2011). Pharmacologic management of asymptomatic bacteriuria and urinary tract infections in women. *Journal of Midwifery and Women's Health, 56,* 248–265. doi:10.1111/j.1542-2011.2011.00063.x

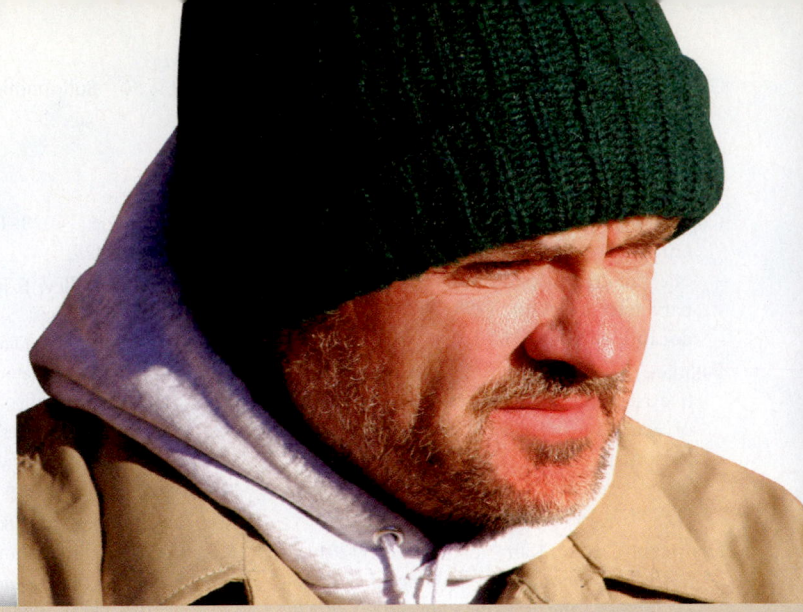

> *"A few years ago I lost my job and was unable to pay my rent. Since then, you could say that I'm homeless. I try to spend my nights at the shelter, but it is sometimes too crowded and I sleep on the street. About a month ago, I started feeling sick with a cough and fever. I'm exhausted and I have no energy."*

Patient "Sam Myers"

CHAPTER

51

Pharmacotherapy of Mycobacterial Infections

LEARNING OUTCOMES

After reading this chapter, the student should be able to:

1. Compare and contrast the types of infections caused by mycobacteria.
2. Explain the pathogenesis of tuberculosis.
3. Describe how the pharmacotherapy of tuberculosis differs from that of bacterial infections.
4. Identify the most common drug regimens for treating tuberculosis.
5. Describe the pathogenesis and treatment of leprosy.
6. Describe the pathogenesis and treatment of infections caused by *Mycobacterium avium* complex.
7. For each of the classes shown in the chapter outline, identify the prototype and representative drugs and explain the mechanism(s) of drug action, primary indications, contraindications, significant drug interactions, pregnancy category, and important adverse effects.
8. Explain significant patient variables that must be considered for effective pharmacotherapy with antimycobacterial drugs.
9. Apply the nursing process to care for patients receiving pharmacotherapy for mycobacterial infections.

CHAPTER OUTLINE

▶ **Types of Mycobacterial Infections**

▶ **Pathogenesis and Diagnosis of Tuberculosis**

▶ **Pharmacotherapy of Tuberculosis**

Antituberculosis Drugs

PROTOTYPE Isoniazid (INH), *p. 855*

▶ **Drugs for Leprosy**

PROTOTYPE Dapsone (DDS), *p. 859*

▶ **Drugs for *Mycobacterium avium* Complex Infections**

KEY TERMS

acetylation, 855

atypical mycobacterial infections (AMIs), 849

directly observed therapy (DOT), 851

leprosy, 859

Mycobacterium avium complex (MAC), 849

mycolic acid, 849

purified protein derivative (PPD), 851

rifamycin derivatives, 857

tubercles, 850

tuberculosis (TB), 849

Mycobacterial infections have been responsible for considerable human suffering and death throughout history. Mycobacterial disease was once called *consumption,* because of its ability to cause the body to waste away if left untreated. Although these infections usually respond to modern anti-infectives, therapy is prolonged, and resistant organisms have emerged as major clinical challenges. Despite the effective treatments available for the disease, tuberculosis (TB) still claims about 1.7 million lives each year worldwide. This chapter examines the pharmacotherapy of the three primary infections caused by mycobacteria.

PharmFACT

More than 11,000 new cases of tuberculosis are reported each year in the United States. From 1953 to 2010, the incidence decreased 87% (Centers for Disease Control and Prevention [CDC], 2013b).

Types of Mycobacterial Infections

51.1 Several species of mycobacteria are important human pathogens.

The genus *Mycobacterium* consists of about 100 species of aerobic organisms that have in common a unique and complex lipid, **mycolic acid**, which covers their cell surfaces. This waxy coating, comprising up to 40% of the cell's weight, protects the mycobacterium, making it resistant to many disinfectants, including chlorinated water. Although over 125 mycobacterial species have been identified in nature only about 10 are potential human pathogens, with *Mycobacterium tuberculosis* being the most common. Robert Koch, a pioneering microbiologist, identified *M. tuberculosis* as the causative agent of TB in 1882.

Nontuberculosis diseases caused by mycobacteria are known as **atypical mycobacterial infections (AMIs)**. These are considered opportunistic infections because they most often appear in people with compromised immune defenses. As the occurrences of human immunodeficiency virus (HIV) infection and acquired immunodeficiency syndrome (AIDS) rose during the 1980s and 1990s, the once-rare AMIs began to increase in frequency. In addition to HIV-AIDS, AMIs sometimes occur in patients with leukemia, or those who are undergoing antineoplastic or immunosuppressive therapy.

Mycobacterium leprae is an AMI that was identified as the causative agent of leprosy by G. A. Hansen in 1873. Leprosy is still sometimes called Hansen's disease, after its discoverer. The pharmacotherapy of leprosy is presented in Section 51.6.

Unlike *M. tuberculosis* and *M. leprae*, which have been described since antiquity, the characterization of **Mycobacterium avium complex (MAC)** infection is relatively recent. MAC usually arises as a secondary infection due to the immunosuppression caused by HIV-AIDS. MAC consists of two predominant species, *M. avium* and *Mycobacterium intracellulare*. Whereas *M. avium* is the cause of almost all infections in patients with HIV-AIDS, *M. intracellulare* is more common in immunocompetent patients. The pharmacotherapy of MAC is discussed in Section 51.7.

Several other species can cause AMIs in humans, but their incidence is rare. *Mycobacterium kansasii* is the second most common cause of AMI in patients with HIV-AIDS. *Mycobacterium bovis* is usually acquired from the ingestion of raw, unpasteurized milk. Infections by *M. kansasii* or *M. bovis* cause respiratory symptoms that are almost identical to those of TB.

Mycobacterium scrofulaceum usually affects children 1 to 3 years of age. The target for this pathogen is the lymph nodes, and infants have mild symptoms, such as low-grade fever. Infections by *Mycobacterium chelonae* and *Mycobacterium abscessus* can cause a variety of clinical syndromes including respiratory disease, local skin disease, osteomyelitis, joint infections, and ocular disease. Surgical-site infections due to *M. chelonae* are well documented.

PharmFACT

It is estimated that about a third of the world's population has latent TB. About 10% of the people with latent TB will develop symptoms during their lifetime (WHO, 2014).

Pathogenesis and Diagnosis of Tuberculosis

51.2 Tuberculosis is a respiratory infection that exhibits both active and latent stages.

Tuberculosis (TB) is a highly contagious infection caused by the organism *M. tuberculosis*. Although TB has been a major killer throughout human history, its incidence declined in the United States during most of the 20th century. With the appearance of HIV-AIDS, however, the incidence of TB greatly increased from 1985 to 1992. As many as 20% of all patients with AIDS may develop active TB. High immigration rates from areas of the world where TB is endemic also contributed to increases in this disease in the United States during this period. Since its peak in 1992, the incidence of TB in the United States has steadily declined, although the disease is still significant in racial/ethnic and foreign born minorities. Four states (California, Florida, New York, and Texas) account for almost half of the cases (CDC, 2013a).

Patients acquire *M. tuberculosis* by the respiratory route. During its infectious stages, the organism may be transmitted to others via airborne droplets by sneezing, coughing, and even talking. The organism can remain alive in these droplets for several hours outside the body. Unlike most species of mycobacteria, however, *M. tuberculosis* is not an environmental pathogen. It must reside in a living host to survive and reproduce. Left untreated, it is estimated that each person infected with this mycobacterium will spread the disease to 10 to 15 other people (World Health Organization [WHO], 2014).

TB infections may be classified as primary or postprimary. A *primary* TB infection occurs when the patient inhales mycobacteria from a person with an active TB infection. Because they are acquired via inhalation, most primary infections occur in the upper lobes of the lungs. The slow-growing mycobacteria activate cells of the immune response, which isolate the microorganisms by creating a wall of macrophages around them. In an attempt to neutralize the mycobacteria, the macrophages ingest them. The pathogens, however, can grow *inside* the macrophages, despite the presence of an ongoing immune response. An acute respiratory infection develops, with symptoms presenting as pneumonia. In those with healthy immune systems, the primary infection lasts a few weeks and then subsides.

Although the macrophages are eventually successful in isolating the pathogen, granulomatous lesions called **tubercles** are formed in the lung. Tissue within the tubercles undergoes necrosis, causing cavities within the lung, which can be identified on chest radiographs. The mycobacteria often become dormant, lying inside the tubercles for an extended time. Indeed, people can retain latent, inactive mycobacteria in tubercles for an entire lifetime.

If the immune system becomes suppressed later in life, the dormant mycobacteria may enter a *postprimary* or *reactivation* stage. Once reactivated, *M. tuberculosis* can be disseminated throughout the body via the blood or lymphatic system. Lymph nodes and organs of the genitourinary system are the most common nonrespiratory sites, although infections of the bone marrow and liver are possible. Reactivation frequently occurs in patients with HIV-AIDS, those with poor nutritional status, and those who have terminal or debilitating diseases. The pathogenesis of TB is illustrated in Pharmacotherapy Illustrated 51.1.

PHARMACOTHERAPY ILLUSTRATED 51.1

The Pathogenesis of Tuberculosis

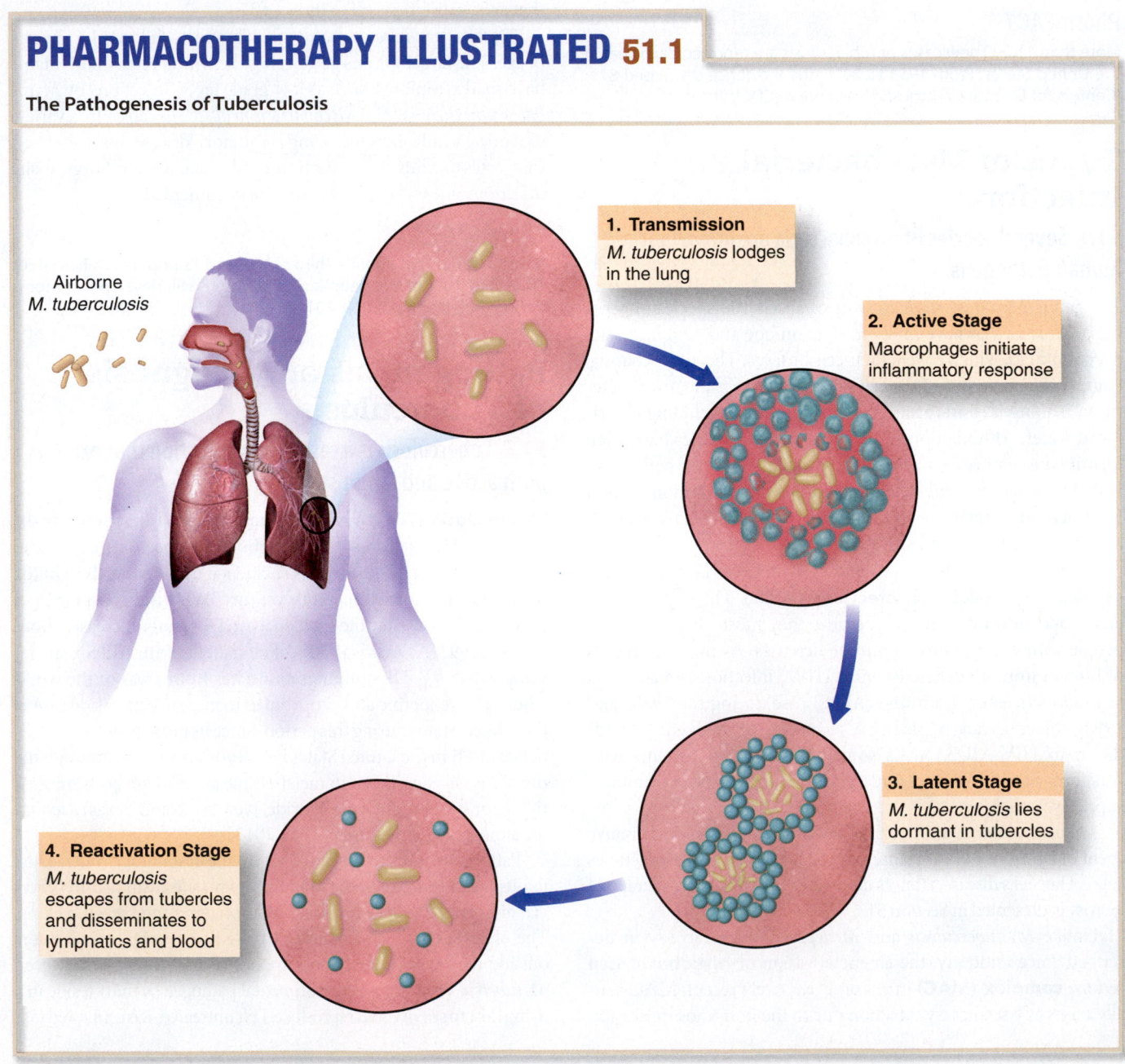

Airborne
M. tuberculosis

1. Transmission
M. tuberculosis lodges in the lung

2. Active Stage
Macrophages initiate inflammatory response

3. Latent Stage
M. tuberculosis lies dormant in tubercles

4. Reactivation Stage
M. tuberculosis escapes from tubercles and disseminates to lymphatics and blood

Some patients with TB remain asymptomatic throughout the infection. In others, the disease progresses so gradually that the individual may not seek medical interventions until the disease becomes advanced. Symptoms are nonspecific and include anorexia, weight loss, night sweats, fatigue, and low-grade fever. Cough becomes progressively worse, producing infectious sputum.

TB is diagnosed by several different means. Each of the following tests has advantages and drawbacks:

- **Tuberculin skin test (purified protein derivative [PPD]).** A positive PPD indicates the presence of memory T cells to *M. tuberculosis* but cannot determine whether the disease is active or latent. Once a positive PPD occurs, the test will always be positive due to the presence of these memory T cells, and the patient should never have subsequent PPDs because skin damage may result. Although inexpensive, the PPD test requires that the patient return to have the results examined.

- **Sputum culture.** Sputum is obtained to culture and identify *M. tuberculosis*. Unfortunately, samples may be negative even when the patient has confirmed TB. Because *M. tuberculosis* grows very slowly on cultured media, results may take 2 to 8 weeks to produce results.

- **Chest radiography.** Both active and chronic TB infections produce changes in the lung that can be identified on chest radiographs. X-ray evidence is not always specific to TB, however, and other diagnostic evidence is needed to confirm the disease. Annual chest x-rays are often used to exclude active TB in patients who exhibit positive PPDs.

- **Nucleic acid amplification test.** Diagnostic laboratory tests such as the Amplified *Mycobacterium Tuberculosis* Direct Test can identify the presence of *M. tuberculosis* RNA in a sample in 2 to 4 hours. Because these tests are rapid, they allow for earlier treatment of infected patients.

- **Interferon gamma release assay (IGRA).** The IGRA is a newer TB screening procedure that measures the response of the immune system to a sample of the patient's blood. Large amounts of interferon released by the immune cells during the IGRA test suggest a TB infection. Test results are ready in about 24 hours.

CONNECTION Checkpoint 51.1

From what you learned in Chapter 42, identify immunosuppressant drugs that may cause TB to enter the reactivation stage in a patient who is receiving pharmacotherapy with these drugs. *See Answer to Connection Checkpoint 51.1 on student resource website.*

Pharmacotherapy of Tuberculosis

51.3 The pharmacotherapy of tuberculosis requires special dosing regimens and schedules.

The primary goal of TB pharmacotherapy is to eliminate all tubercle mycobacteria, while avoiding the emergence of resistant strains. This involves an initial or induction phase of therapy during which the actively dividing mycobacterial cells are killed, and a continuation phase in which the remaining dormant mycobacteria are eliminated. Special pharmacotherapeutic strategies are required to successfully eradicate this persistent pathogen.

The pharmacotherapy of TB differs from that of other bacterial infections because the thick mycolic acid layer surrounding the mycobacterium is resistant to penetration by anti-infectives. For the drugs to reach the mycobacteria isolated in tubercles and inside macrophages, therapy must continue for 6 to 12 months. Although the patient is not infectious this entire time and, indeed, may have no symptoms, it is critical that therapy be continued for the entire period. Patients who develop multidrug-resistant infections may require therapy for as long as 2 years.

A second difference in the therapy of TB is that a minimum of two—and sometimes as many as seven—antimycobacterial drugs are administered concurrently. During the long treatment period, different combinations of drugs are used. Combination drug therapy is necessary because mycobacteria grow slowly and often develop resistance during the course of treatment. The incidence of multidrug-resistant TB is increasing. In some communities, as many as 10% of patients have infections resistant to at least one antituberculosis medication. The use of multiple drugs that kill mycobacteria by different mechanisms lowers the potential for resistance and increases pharmacotherapeutic success. Figure 51.1 illustrates the use of combination therapy during tuberculosis therapy. Doses for the antimycobacterial drugs are listed in Table 51.1.

A third difference in therapy is that antimycobacterial drugs are used extensively for preventing the disease, in addition to treating active infections. Because of the acute infectious nature of TB, prophylactic therapy is indicated for close contacts or family members of recently diagnosed patients. Therapy of infected patients and all close contacts begins immediately after a positive diagnosis has been established. Patients with compromised immune function, such as those with HIV-AIDS or those who are receiving immunosuppressant drugs, may also receive preventive treatment with antimycobacterials. A short-term therapy of 2 months, consisting of combination therapy with isoniazid (INH) and pyrazinamide, is approved for TB prophylaxis in patients who are HIV positive.

A major concern with TB pharmacotherapy is ensuring that patients fully comply with the prescribed regimen. Nonadherence to pharmacotherapy is the most common cause of treatment failure in TB patients. In high-risk patients, **directly observed therapy (DOT)** is necessary. DOT requires that a health care provider directly observe the patient swallowing the pills, whether it is in the hospital, office, or home care setting. Nurses serve essential roles in providing education about this disorder to their patients and stressing the importance of adherence.

CONNECTION Checkpoint 51.2

From what you learned in Chapter 6, identify at least three major factors that might explain why a patient may choose to stop taking antimycobacterials. *See Answer to Connection Checkpoint 51.2 on student resource website.*

51.4 First-line or primary antituberculosis drugs are the most efficacious and safest drugs for treating *M. tuberculosis* infections.

Medications for TB are placed into two categories. The safer and more effective agents are called *first-line drugs*. A second group of drugs, which exhibit greater toxicity, are less effective and prescribed

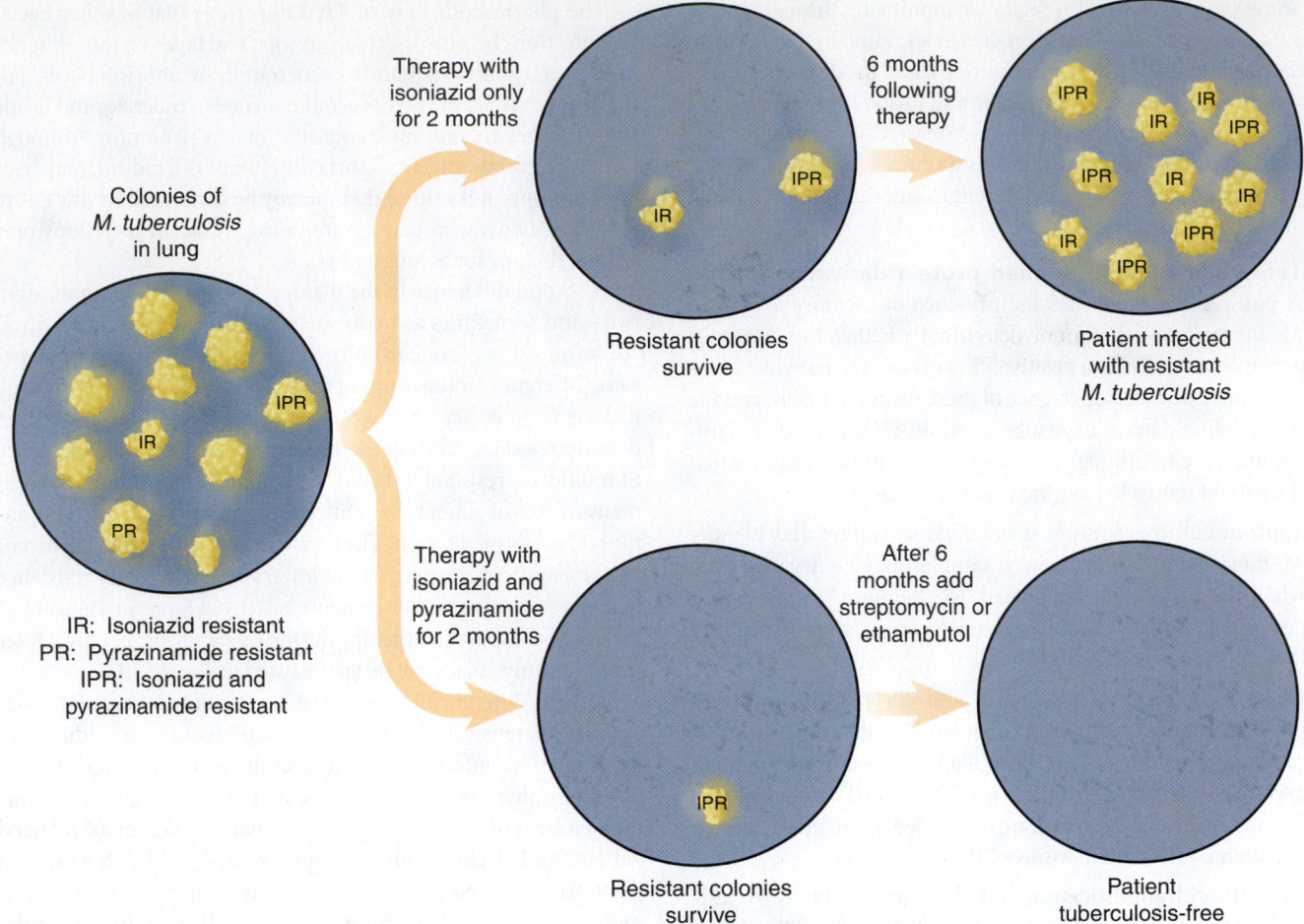

Figure 51.1 Use of combination therapy during tuberculosis therapy to avoid resistance.

when resistance develops to the first-line agents. The *second-line drugs* are discussed in Section 51.5.

The pharmacotherapy regimen for TB depends on drug sensitivity, disease stage, and the patient's immune status. Ideally, results of culture and sensitivity (C&S) testing should be obtained prior to treatment because of the possibility of drug-resistant strains. Definitive C&S results may take several weeks, however, and treatment must begin immediately. Therefore, the initial selection of pharmacotherapy is based on the experience of the prescriber and later adjusted when laboratory results become available.

Standard Regimen

The standard regimen is for patients who have a positive diagnosis of TB, or who have symptomology strongly suspicious of this infection. This therapy is recommended by the American Thoracic Society, the CDC, and the Infectious Diseases Society of America, and has remained unchanged since 2003. The regimen for patients with no complicating factors includes the following:

- **Initial phase.** Two months of daily therapy with isoniazid, rifampin (Rifadin, Rimactane), pyrazinamide (PZA), and ethambutol (Myambutol). If C&S results show that the strain is sensitive to the first three drugs, ethambutol is dropped from the regimen.

- **Continuation phase.** Four months of therapy with isoniazid and rifampin, two to three times per week.

The above regimen cures more than 95% of these patients. There are, however, many variations, based on patient variables. In regions where the incidence of isoniazid resistance is 4% or higher, ethambutol (Myambutol) or streptomycin is included as part of the initial therapeutic regimen. Three months of additional therapy may be indicated, depending on whether the sputum cultures have turned negative during therapy. Nine months of therapy is recommended for patients with evidence of nonrespiratory TB.

Patients Who Are HIV Positive

Coinfection with both TB and HIV can have mortal consequences: worldwide, about 25% of patients with HIV die of TB infection (WHO, 2014). Patients who are HIV positive often respond to the standard regimen. Because nonadherence has been frequently reported, DOT is recommended for patients who are HIV positive. In addition, patients taking numerous antiretroviral drugs are at greater risk for drug–drug interactions and must be monitored carefully. For example, rifampin and rifabutin are considered essential to TB elimination in this population, yet they can increase the metabolism of some antiretrovirals and decrease their effectiveness against HIV. Certain drug combinations, such as rifampin with single protease inhibitors, should be avoided to the extent possible or dosages adjusted accordingly. Nurses treating HIV-AIDS patients with TB should regularly consult recent pharmacology sources to identify the many drug–drug interactions because serious adverse effects can compromise the success of pharmacotherapy for both TB and HIV.

TABLE 51.1 Antimycobacterial Drugs

Drug	Route and Adult Dose (Maximum Dose Where Indicated)	Adverse Effects
First-Line Drugs		
ethambutol (Myambutol)	PO: 15–25 mg/kg/day (max: 1,600 mg for daily therapy)	*Nausea, vomiting, headache, dizziness* Anaphylaxis, optic neuritis (decreased acuity, color blindness or visual defects)
isoniazid (INH)	Latent TB PO: 300 mg/day or 900 mg twice weekly for 6–9 months Active TB PO: Daily therapy: 5 mg/kg/day or 300 mg/day; if given by DOT: 15 mg/kg or 900 mg twice weekly	*Nausea, vomiting, diarrhea, epigastric pain* Anaphylaxis, peripheral neuropathy, optic neuritis, hepatotoxicity, blood dyscrasias
pyrazinamide (PZA)	PO: 5–15 mg/kg tid–qid (max: 2 g/day)	*Nongouty polyarthralgia, increase in serum uric acid, rash* Anaphylaxis, hepatotoxicity, fatal hemoptysis, hemolytic anemia
rifabutin (Mycobutin)	TB Prophylaxis PO: 300 mg once daily Active TB 1st phase PO: 5 mg/kg/day 2nd phase PO: 5 mg/kg/day or twice weekly (max: 300 mg/day)	*Nausea, vomiting, epigastric pain, anorexia, diarrhea, orange discoloration of the urine, sweat, and tears, pyuria, hematuria, urinary tract infection, proteinuria, hypoglycemia* Pseudomembranous colitis (PMC), acute renal failure, hepatotoxicity, hyperuricemia, lymphopenia, neutropenia, anemia
rifampin (Rifadin, Rimactane)	Latent TB PO: 600 mg/day or 900 mg twice weekly for 4 months Active TB PO: 10 mg/kg/day or 600 mg/day IV and PO are same dose, but IV needs to be given over 30 min to 3 h and the final concentration should not exceed 6 mg/mL	
rifapentine (Priftin)	PO: 600 mg (four 150-mg tablets) given twice a week for 2 months with an interval of no less than 72 h between doses, then once a week for 4 months	
Second-Line Drugs		
amikacin (Amikin)	Intramuscular (IM): 10–15 mg/kg daily for 2 weeks in a large muscle	*Pain or inflammation at injection site, rash, fever, nausea, diarrhea, dizziness, tinnitus* Anaphylaxis, nephrotoxicity, PMC, ototoxicity
aminosalicylic acid (Paser)	PO: 150 mg/kg/day in three to four equally divided doses (max: 8g/day)	*GI intolerance, anorexia, diarrhea, fever, leukopenia* Hypersensitivity, inhibition of vitamin B_{12} absorption, hepatotoxicity
bedaquiline (Sirturo)	PO: 400 mg once daily for 2 weeks then 200 mg 3 times per week for 22 weeks	*Nausea, arthralgia, and headache* QT prolongation, increased risk of death, hepatotoxicity
capreomycin (Capastat)	IM: 1 g/day (not to exceed 20 mg/kg/day) for 60–120 days, then 1 g 2–3 times/week	*Rash, pain and inflammation at injection site, tinnitus* Blood dyscrasias, nephrotoxicity, ototoxicity, increase in urination, thirst
ciprofloxacin (Cipro)	PO: 250–750 mg bid	*Nausea, diarrhea, vomiting, rash, restlessness, pain and inflammation at injection site, local burning, stinging and corneal irritation (ophthalmic)* Anaphylaxis, tendon rupture, superinfections, photosensitivity, PMC, seizure, peripheral neuropathy, hepatotoxicity
cycloserine (Seromycin)	PO: 250 mg every 12 h for 2 weeks; may increase to 500 mg every 12 h (max: 1 g/day)	*Drowsiness, headache, lethargy* Convulsions, psychosis, confusion
ethionamide (Trecator-SC)	PO: 750 mg/day (max: 1 gram given in three to four divided doses)	*Nausea, vomiting, epigastric pain, diarrhea* Convulsions, hallucinations, mental depression, hepatotoxicity
kanamycin (Kantrex)	IM: 5–7.5 mg/kg bid–tid	(See amikacin)
ofloxacin (Floxin)	PO: 200–400 mg bid	(See ciprofloxacin)
streptomycin	IM: 15–30 mg/kg (max: 1–2 g/day) DOT: twice weekly IM: 25–30 mg/kg (max: 1.5 g) DOT: 3 times a week IM: 25–30 mg/kg	*Nausea, vomiting, pain at injection site, drowsiness, headache* Anaphylaxis, ototoxicity, profound CNS depression in infants, respiratory depression, exfoliative dermatitis, nephrotoxicity, teratogenicity

Note: *Italics* indicate common adverse effects. <u>Underline</u> indicates serious adverse effects.

Directly Observed Therapy and Multidrug-Resistant TB

Clinical Question

Multidrug-resistant TB (MDR-TB) is a growing public health concern. The length of drug therapy required to treat TB infections and lack of patient adherence to the regimen exacerbate the problem, allowing drug-resistant strains to develop. Many patients do not complete their course of treatment. DOT is a proven strategy to ensure that drug dosages are taken. Does DOT also reduce the incidence of MDR-TB?

Evidence

Moonan et al. (2011) used genotyping to identify specific strains of MDR-TB in order to study acquisition and transmission rates. They followed patients in counties that practiced a selective DOT program, that is, DOT for most patients with some patients self-administering medications without observation, and in counties with a universal DOT program where all patients suspected of having or proven to have TB received DOT. When comparing the two different populations, they found that the MDR-TB strain was more than 1.5 times more common in patients in the selective DOT program than in the universal DOT program. Based on the results of this study, the authors concluded that

MDR-TB may be better managed by using a universal DOT program in which all patients are observed taking their medications rather than a selective DOT in which some patients are not observed and adherence cannot be verified. The authors also suggested that essential components of a DOT program such as the location of and access to treatment, incentives, and cost still need to be defined.

Implications

Patient adherence to antituberculosis therapy is essential to reduce the acquisition and transmission of TB, including MDR-TB. In the past, high-risk patients were identified and followed with DOT. Based on the current study, lower acquisition and transmission rates occurred when all patients are followed with DOT.

Critical Thinking Question

1. As the nurse, how would you explain the need for DOT to a patient newly diagnosed with TB?

See Answers to Critical Thinking Questions on student resource website.

Pregnant Patients

Pregnant women with TB are at risk because drug choices are fewer. The safety of pyrazinamide during pregnancy has not been established; thus, it is usually avoided. Although ethambutol has been used successfully without adverse fetal effects, high doses in laboratory animals produced a low incidence of birth defects; therefore, it is used in pregnancy only if C&S testing shows it to be effective. Streptomycin is contraindicated during pregnancy because it can cause hearing impairment in the newborn. Fortunately, these drugs have not been shown to have adverse effects on the breast-feeding

neonate; thus, therapy can continue during lactation. Pregnant patients should receive isoniazid therapy supplemented with pyridoxine (vitamin B_6), which has been shown to prevent peripheral neuropathy.

Chemoprophylaxis Patients

Treatment of latent or dormant TB reduces the risk that the infection will progress to its active stage, thereby helping to prevent transmission of the disease. Although it would seem prudent to treat everyone suspected of having latent TB, pharmacotherapy is expensive

Travel and Tuberculosis Risk

The possibility of travel to all areas of the world increases the opportunity for acquisition, transmission, and spread of infectious diseases. A rare and exotic disease may be "only one plane flight away" from countries that have never encountered the disease before, but what about a disease such as TB, which is present throughout the world?

After a well-publicized case in the early 2000s of an air traveler with extensive drug-resistant TB (XDR-TB), WHO updated its guidelines for preventing or managing a potential TB exposure during air travel (Martinez, Thomas, & Figueroa, 2010). Per these guidelines, people with infectious or potentially infectious TB should postpone travel until they became noninfectious, with "noninfectious" being determined by negative sputum cultures. Health care providers, public health officials, and airlines should inform patients who are infectious or potentially infectious that they should not travel or should deny boarding to these patients. In addition, public health authorities should be alerted to any potential exposure to TB aboard a flight for follow-up screening and investigation. Airlines were given guidance for ventilation systems and the use of HEPA filters, disinfectant procedures, medical emergency

procedures, and national public health requirements for postexposure follow-up. While actual rates of exposure to and transmission of TB are difficult to assess, following WHO guidelines may limit the risk. Other authors have noted that merely being on antituberculosis medication does not prevent transmission. Kornylo-Duong et al. (2010) described the case of a highly infectious patient who had been started on antituberculosis drugs 12 days before a flight with several probable transmissions occurring during that flight. Even while on antituberculosis drugs, a negative sputum culture is needed.

Airline travel is not the only concern for TB transmission. Edelson and Phypers (2010) investigated the transmission of TB on public transportation by train, school bus, and commuter van. Lack of adequate ventilation, recirculation of air without HEPA filtering, and length of contact with and proximity to the infected individual were all identified as increasing the likelihood of transmission of TB. In addition, visitors to the United States who are classified as "nonimmigrant," including students who are admitted to study in the United States, may not be screened for either active or latent TB under current guidelines and may pose a small, but real risk (Aaron, Fotinas, West, Goodwin, & Mancuso, 2013).

and carries the risk of adverse drug reactions. Furthermore, not everyone with latent TB will progress to active disease. Patients with a possible latent TB infection are screened and only treated if they fall into a high-risk category. High-risk categories include patients who are HIV positive, those receiving immunosuppressive drugs, employees and residents of nursing homes, those living in residential facilities for patients with AIDS, those living in prisons, people born in countries where TB is endemic, and those who have been in close contact with patients with active TB. Pharmacotherapy of latent TB normally includes one of the following regimens:

- Nine months of therapy with isoniazid. This is considered the most effective treatment. Depending on anticipated patient adherence, the dose may be daily (300 mg) or twice weekly (15 mg/kg).

- Two months of therapy with both rifampin and pyrazinamide. This shorter duration therapy increases patient adherence, but serious liver injury has been reported and the patient must be monitored carefully for hepatotoxicity.

- Four months of therapy with rifampin. This monotherapy is used for patients who are unable to take isoniazid or pyrazinamide, or who have infections caused by organisms that are resistant to these drugs.

The pharmacotherapy of latent TB is modified for certain patients. Close contacts of HIV-AIDS patients with TB should be treated for at least 12 months. Contacts of patients with confirmed multidrug-resistant TB should receive at least two drugs known to be effective against the resistant *M. tuberculosis* strain. These patients usually require follow-up for 2 years to be certain the resistant strains have been killed.

PROTOTYPE DRUG	Isoniazid (INH)

Classification: Therapeutic: Antituberculosis drug, antimycobacterial
Pharmacologic: Mycolic acid inhibitor

Therapeutic Effects and Uses: Although a patient may take many different drugs during the long treatment period, isoniazid is considered the prototype antituberculosis drug. Approved by the U.S. Food and Drug Administration (FDA) in 1952, it remains a drug of choice for the treatment of *M. tuberculosis* infections because decades of experience have shown it to have a superior safety profile and to be the most effective, single drug for the disease. Isoniazid is used exclusively for the treatment and prophylaxis of mycobacterial infections. Isoniazid may be used alone for chemoprophylaxis, or in combination with other antituberculosis drugs for treating active disease. When used for prophylaxis, therapy may continue for as long as a year. While resistance to isoniazid can develop during therapy, the incidence is only about 10%. Treatment of active disease requires multidrug therapy.

The main route of metabolism of isoniazid is through enzymatic acetylation in the liver. **Acetylation** is a general biochemical process that adds a two-carbon chain to a drug molecule, which usually renders the medication less effective or allows it to be excreted more easily. Not all people are able to acetylate isoniazid at the same rate because of genetic differences in the activity of acetyltransferase, the hepatic enzyme that performs this action. Those of Japanese and Inuit descent often have increased enzyme activity and are known as *fast acetylators*. Those with decreased activity—*slow acetylators*—are most commonly of Scandinavian, North African Caucasian, or Jewish descent. The half-life of isoniazid ranges from 70 minutes in fast acetylators to 2 to 5 hours in slow acetylators. Fortunately, isoniazid is safe across a wide range of doses, and these variations do not generally result in toxicity. For optimal therapy, however, doses should be lowered in slow acetylators to avoid adverse effects, and increased in fast acetylators to keep plasma levels consistently in the therapeutic range. Dosage reductions should also occur in any patient with significant hepatic impairment because of diminished acetylation. The acetylation of isoniazid is illustrated in Figure 51.2.

Mechanism of Action: Isoniazid acts by inhibiting the synthesis of mycolic acid, an essential cell-wall component of mycobacteria. Because mycolic acids are unique to mycobacteria, isoniazid has no activity for other microbial species. It is bacteriocidal for rapidly dividing organisms but bacteriostatic for dormant mycobacteria.

Pharmacokinetics:

Route(s)	Oral (PO) and IM (only if PO is unavailable)
Absorption	Readily absorbed
Distribution	Widely distributed (can even enter the necrotic lung tubercles that are characteristic of TB); crosses the placenta, and enters the central nervous system (CNS); secreted in breast milk; about 15% bound to plasma protein
Primary metabolism	Metabolized by acetylation in the liver
Primary excretion	Renal (75%)
Onset of action	Rapid
Duration of action	Half-life: 1–4 h

Adverse Effects: Isoniazid exhibits few serious adverse effects, which is a major reason why it is a drug of choice for mycobacterial infections. Common adverse effects of isoniazid are rash and fever. Neurotoxicity is a concern during therapy, and patients may exhibit paresthesia of the feet and hands, convulsions, optic neuritis, dizziness, coma, memory loss, and various psychoses. A major factor responsible for the neurotoxicity of isoniazid is the ability of the drug to cause a deficiency of activated pyridoxine (vitamin B_6), which is required for synthesis of the neurotransmitter gamma-aminobutyric acid (GABA). Many practitioners routinely prescribe pyridoxine during isoniazid therapy to prevent the development of peripheral neuropathy. Pyridoxine is considered the antidote for reversing acute nervous system effects of isoniazid overdose. Blood dyscrasias such as agranulocytosis and aplastic anemia may occur, although they are uncommon. **Black Box Warning**: Although rare, hepatotoxicity is a potentially fatal adverse effect; thus, the patient should be monitored carefully for jaundice, fatigue, elevated hepatic enzymes, or loss of appetite. Liver enzyme tests are usually performed monthly during therapy to identify early hepatotoxicity. Hepatotoxicity usually appears in the first 1 to 3 months of therapy but may occur at any time during

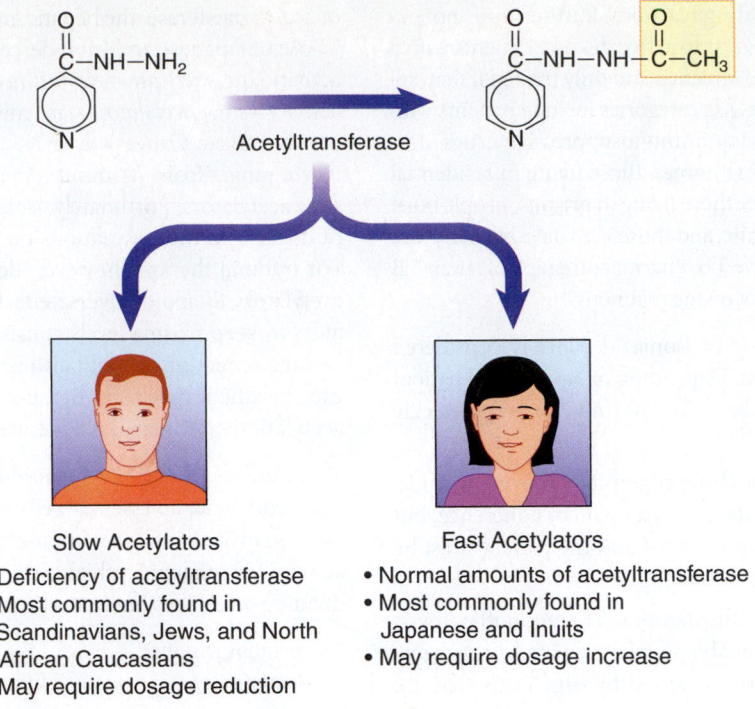

Acetyltransferase

Slow Acetylators
- Deficiency of acetyltransferase
- Most commonly found in Scandinavians, Jews, and North African Caucasians
- May require dosage reduction

Fast Acetylators
- Normal amounts of acetyltransferase
- Most commonly found in Japanese and Inuits
- May require dosage increase

Figure 51.2 Ethnic variation in the acetylation of isoniazid.

treatment. Older adults and those with daily alcohol consumption are at greater risk of developing hepatotoxicity.

Contraindications/Precautions: Isoniazid has no absolute contraindications other than previous allergy to the drug. Pharmacotherapy must be monitored carefully in patients with a history of chronic hepatic disease because the liver metabolizes the drug and fatal hepatitis has been reported. Serum aspartate transaminase (AST) levels should be monitored regularly during therapy in high-risk patients. If AST levels rise to three times baseline levels, liver damage is likely, and isoniazid should be discontinued. Patients with significant renal impairment usually require lower doses because the kidneys excrete the drug. Patients with seizure disorders should be carefully monitored because isoniazid can increase the incidence of seizures. Patients with a history of seizures often receive pyridoxine supplementation to prevent seizures during isoniazid therapy.

Drug Interactions: Isoniazid is a potent inhibitor of hepatic metabolic enzymes (CYP2C19 and CYP3A4) and is associated with numerous drug–drug interactions. Before adding a new drug to the regimen, the nurse should consult a drug guide for potential interactions. Aluminum-containing antacids should not be administered concurrently because they can decrease the absorption of isoniazid. Azole antifungals should not be used concurrently with isoniazid because this results in decreased levels of antifungals. Alcohol use should be avoided because it can increase the risk of hepatotoxicity. Isoniazid inhibits the metabolic breakdown of phenytoin, which may cause the anticonvulsant to build to toxic levels, an effect that occurs more often in slow acetylators. Isoniazid can increase serum levels of carbamazepine and cause carbamazepine toxicity. **Herbal/Food**: Food decreases the absorption of isoniazid.

Pregnancy: Category C.

Treatment of Overdose: Isoniazid overdose may be fatal and treatment is mostly symptomatic. Pyridoxine may be infused in a dose equal to that of the isoniazid overdose to prevent seizures and to correct metabolic acidosis. The dose may be repeated several times until the patient regains consciousness.

Nursing Responsibilities: Key nursing implications for patients receiving isoniazid are included in the Nursing Practice Application for Patients Receiving Pharmacotherapy for Tuberculosis.

Drugs Similar to Isoniazid (INH)

Other first-line antituberculosis drugs include ethambutol, pyrazinamide, rifampin, rifabutin, and rifapentine.

Ethambutol (Myambutol): Approved in 1967, ethambutol is included in multidrug regimens for TB because it is sometimes active against organisms that are resistant to other first-line drugs. It is also effective against atypical mycobacteria such as *M. kansasii*. The mechanism of action of ethambutol is not well understood, although its bacteriostatic effect is thought to be due to the inhibition of cell-wall synthesis and RNA synthesis. It is always given with other antimycobacterials because resistance develops rapidly if the drug is given as monotherapy. It is rapidly absorbed, distributed to most tissues, and excreted by both renal and fecal routes. Ethambutol has a short half-life of 1 to 4 hours; therefore, it must be taken daily.

Ethambutol has a unique adverse effect of optic neuritis that affects visual acuity and the ability to distinguish red from green. This effect is dose related, may be unilateral or bilateral, and is usually reversible when therapy is discontinued. A baseline ophthalmic exam should be conducted prior to therapy. Ethambutol may decrease the excretion of uric acid, causing hyperuricemia; patients with a history of gout should be closely monitored. This drug has few other significant adverse effects. Ethambutol is pregnancy category C.

Pyrazinamide (PZA): Pyrazinamide is an older drug approved in 1955 that is used for the initial therapy of active or advanced TB in combination with other antimycobacterials. It is usually taken in combination with rifampin, ethambutol, and INH for 8 weeks. If used alone, resistance develops rapidly. Like isoniazid, it acts by inhibiting the synthesis of mycolic acid in *M. tuberculosis*. Given PO, it is distributed to all body fluids and is excreted by the kidneys.

Pyrazinamide causes some degree of dose-related hepatotoxicity in as many as 15% of patients. Caution should be observed when giving pyrazinamide to patients with preexisting hepatic disease, and frequent laboratory monitoring of liver enzymes must be performed. Frequent use of ethanol increases the risk of hepatotoxicity. Hyperuricemia may occur because the drug slows the excretion of uric acid. Uric acid levels should be monitored and the nurse should assess for signs of gout or arthralgia, which can occur in up to 40% of the patients taking this drug. This drug is pregnancy category C.

Rifampin (Rifadin, Rimactane): Rifampin is widely used in combination with other drugs in the first-line treatment of TB: It is rarely given as monotherapy for the short-course therapy of latent *M. tuberculosis* infections. Rifampin exerts its bacteriocidal effects by inhibiting RNA synthesis. In addition to treating TB, rifampin is a broad-spectrum antibiotic approved for the short-term treatment of meningococci from the nasopharynx of asymptomatic carriers of *Neisseria meningitidis*. When given to meningococcal carriers, the length of therapy is only 2 days. Off-label uses include chemoprophylaxis of contacts of patients with *Haemophilus influenzae* type B and the treatment of Legionnaire's disease. It is also used to treat leprosy, in combination with dapsone. The drug should only be used when the infectious microbe has been demonstrated to be susceptible to the effects of the medication.

Rifampin is administered by either the PO or intravenous (IV) routes. Hypersensitivity reactions cause flulike symptoms in as many as 50% of the patients taking rifampin. Rash and urticaria are relatively common. Rifampin can be hepatotoxic and caution must be used when administering the drug to patients with preexisting liver disease or who are taking other hepatotoxic antituberculosis drugs such as isoniazid and pyrazinamide. Rifampin is a potent inducer of cytochrome P450 enzymes. Thus, it has the potential to increase the metabolism of other drugs metabolized by the liver, such as some antiretrovirals for HIV-AIDS, warfarin, and PO contraceptives. Because resistance develops rapidly, rifampin is almost always given in combination with other drugs. This drug is pregnancy category C.

Rifabutin (Mycobutin) and Rifapentine (Priftin): These two drugs are PO drugs closely related to rifampin that act by the same mechanism and cause the same adverse effects, including induction of P450 enzymes and potential hepatotoxicity. There is a high level of cross resistance among rifampin, rifabutin, and rifapentine, which, collectively, are called **rifamycin derivatives**. They are always used in combination with other antituberculosis medications.

Approved in 1998, rifapentine is approved only for the pharmacotherapy of TB and has a longer half-life than rifampin, thus offering the advantage of twice-a-week dosing. Rifabutin was approved in 1992 for the prophylaxis of MAC in patients infected with HIV. It offers little advantage over rifampin, other than it is thought to have less effect on hepatic enzymes. Rifapentine is pregnancy category C; rifabutin is category B.

Combination drugs: Rifamate and isonarif are capsules that contain both isoniazid and rifampin. Rifater is a tablet containing isoniazid, rifampin, and pyrazinamide. Combining multiple drugs into a single capsule or pill increases their ease of use and promotes patient adherence to therapy.

51.5 Second-line antituberculosis drugs are used when resistance develops to the first-line drugs.

If a patient develops multidrug-resistant strains of *M. tuberculosis* during the course of therapy, second-line antibiotics are added to the regimen. These drugs are either more toxic or less effective than the first-line agents. Some of them are occasionally included as part of the initial course of therapy if C&S testing demonstrates their effectiveness. As a general rule, a single antituberculosis drug should never be added to a regimen that has failed to control the mycobacterial infection. At least two, and preferably three, new medications to which the organism is likely to be susceptible should be added.

Aminoglycosides: Amikacin (Amikin), kanamycin (Kantrex), and streptomycin are aminoglycosides used as both antibacterials and antituberculosis agents. Like other second-line drugs, they are used for multidrug-resistant TB and always in combination with other antimycobacterials. They are administered parenterally because they are not absorbed when given by the PO route.

Approved in 1945, streptomycin has the distinction of being the first clinically effective drug used to treat TB. It was soon noticed, however, that resistance developed quickly when streptomycin was used as monotherapy. Streptomycin use has declined such that it is now a second-line TB drug. This is mostly because of the emergence of numerous streptomycin-resistant strains of *M. tuberculosis* and the need to administer the drug by the IM route. Other indications for streptomycin include tularemia, plague, brucellosis, and subacute bacterial endocarditis.

Streptomycin has a black box warning that renal function tests must be regularly assessed because the drug can accumulate to toxic levels in patients with kidney impairment. Additionally, the warning states that concurrent use with nephrotoxic or neurotoxic drugs should be avoided. IM injection of the drug is painful and can produce sterile abscesses at the site of injection. Also of serious concern is ototoxicity, which can cause tinnitus, deafness, and vertigo. This drug is pregnancy category D.

Amikacin and kanamycin are closely related structurally and have similar spectrums of activity, actions, and adverse effects. Like other aminoglycosides, these drugs are nephrotoxic, and kidney function must be monitored regularly during therapy. They are also ototoxic and can cause deafness and balance abnormalities. The risk of ototoxicity is greater in patients with impaired renal function. Amikacin appears to be less ototoxic than kanamycin and causes less pain when administered IM. Resistance of mycobacteria to either kanamycin or amikacin sometimes confers resistance to the other.

CONNECTION Checkpoint 51.3

From what you learned in Chapter 48, are aminoglycosides bacteriostatic or bacteriocidal? What is the mechanism of action of aminoglycosides? Are they most effective against gram-positive or gram-negative organisms? *See Answer to Connection Checkpoint 51.3 on student resource website.*

Aminosalicylic acid (Paser): Aminosalicylic acid (or para-aminosalicylic acid) was widely used to treat TB until more effective and safer drugs were discovered. It is structurally similar to para-aminobenzoic acid and is thought to have a similar mechanism of action as the sulfonamides. Aminosalicylic acid is given PO, but it has a half-life of only 1 hour. The drug is available as delayed-release granules that are taken several times a day.

The use of aminosalicylic acid is limited to the treatment of multidrug-resistant strains of *M. tuberculosis*. Higher doses can inhibit the acetylation of isoniazid, especially in patients who are rapid acetylators. Concurrent therapy of aminosalicylic acid with isoniazid, however, does not affect the serum level, half-life, or excretion of isoniazid.

Aminosalicylic acid has many adverse effects, the most common of which are gastrointestinal (GI) related and include nausea, vomiting, diarrhea, and abdominal pain. Taking the drug with food can diminish these types of adverse effects. Hypersensitivity is observed in 10% to 15% of patients and may begin with a rapid onset of high fever, lethargy, and joint pain. Aminosalicylic acid reduces the absorption of vitamin B_{12} by as much as 50%; thus, vitamin B_{12} supplements are indicated during long-term therapy. This is a pregnancy category C drug.

CONNECTION Checkpoint 51.4

From what you learned in Chapter 50, the synthesis of what essential vitamin is inhibited by the sulfonamides? What is the primary indication for sulfonamide pharmacotherapy? *See Answer to Connection Checkpoint 51.4 on student resource website.*

Bedaquiline (Sirturo): The newest antituberculosis drug, bedaquiline was approved in 2013 for the treatment of multidrug-resistant TB. Bedaquiline is always used in combination with at least three other antituberculosis drugs. It should not be used to treat TB strains that are sensitive to first-line drugs, for latent TB, or for nontuberculous mycobacterial infections. It is generally well tolerated, with nausea, headache, and joint pain being the most common side effects. However, the drug carries a black box warning because patients receiving the drug appear to have an increased risk of mortality. In addition, bedaquiline prolongs the QT interval, which is associated with dysrhythmias in some patients. This drug is pregnancy category B.

Capreomycin (Capastat): Approved in 1971, the only indication for capreomycin is the pharmacotherapy of multidrug-resistant strains of *M. tuberculosis*. Capreomycin is always given with other antimycobacterials because resistance quickly develops if it is administered alone. It is given only by IM injection. Because it is usually administered daily for the first 120 days of therapy, care must be taken to inject the drug deep into a large muscle mass and to rotate injection sites.

Capreomycin has a black box warning that the drug exhibits both neurotoxicity and nephrotoxicity. The drug is ototoxic, causing tinnitus and high-frequency hearing loss in up to 9% of patients. Auditory and vestibular function should be assessed prior to starting therapy and retested at least every other month during therapy. Renal toxicity is more common with capreomycin than with streptomycin. Older adults are generally more susceptible

to the nephrotoxic effects of capreomycin, and the maximal daily dosage should be reduced. Other nephrotoxic drugs such as aminoglycosides should be avoided during capreomycin pharmacotherapy. Renal function tests should be monitored regularly and the drug discontinued if blood urea nitrogen levels exceed 30 mg/dL. Because of these adverse effects, capreomycin is sometimes referred to as a last-line drug for TB. This is a pregnancy category C drug.

Cycloserine (Seromycin): Approved over 50 years ago, cycloserine is a PO drug used in the pharmacotherapy of multidrug-resistant strains of *M. tuberculosis*. The drug, which resembles the common amino acid D-alanine, acts by blocking mycobacterial cell-wall synthesis. In addition to being an antimycobacterial, cycloserine is also effective against certain gram-negative and gram-positive bacteria and may be used to treat urinary tract infections that are unresponsive to safer antibiotics. It is taken PO, usually twice daily.

Cycloserine use is limited because the difference between a toxic dose and an effective dose is small. Of most concern is neurotoxicity, which can manifest as different symptoms, including headache, lethargy, convulsions, psychotic states with suicidal ideation, depression, confusion, tremor, and paranoid reactions. Concurrent administration of isoniazid and ethionamide can increase the risk of neurotoxicity. The drug is contraindicated in patients with pre-existing psychoses or epilepsy because it may worsen these disorders. Because of its toxicity, serum levels of cycloserine are measured frequently during therapy, with normal levels ranging from 25 to 35 mcg/mL. Patients with renal impairment should not receive this drug because the primary route of excretion of this drug is via the kidneys. This is a pregnancy category C drug.

Ethionamide (Trecator-SC): Approved in 1962, ethionamide is a PO drug used as a second-line drug in the pharmacotherapy of multidrug-resistant TB or when patients are unable to tolerate first-line drugs. Ethionamide is always used in combination with other antituberculosis drugs because resistance develops rapidly if given alone. It is thought to act by inhibiting mycobacterial protein synthesis. The drug has only a 3-hour half-life and therefore must be administered several times daily.

The most common and limiting adverse effects of ethionamide are GI-related and include nausea, vomiting, diarrhea, abdominal pain, excessive salivation, metallic taste, anorexia, and weight loss. GI effects may be diminished by decreasing dosage, by taking the drug with food, or by the concurrent administration of an antiemetic. Concomitant administration of pyridoxine is recommended to decrease the incidence of peripheral neuropathy. Depression and drowsiness are common, and seizures have been reported with ethionamide. Hepatic function should be monitored regularly because hepatitis occurs in about 5% of the patients taking the drug. Alcohol use should be discouraged during ethionamide therapy because of additive harmful effects on the liver. Ethionamide is a pregnancy category C drug.

Fluoroquinolones: Ciprofloxacin (Cipro) and ofloxacin (Floxin) have undergone considerable testing for use as antituberculosis drugs. Many multidrug-resistant strains of *M. tuberculosis* are sensitive to the actions of the fluoroquinolones. Because this class of antibiotics is widely used in the pharmacotherapy of bacterial infections, there is concern in the medical community that use of these drugs for TB could produce resistant strains of

◀ **Accidental Overdose of Isoniazid**

Isoniazid (INH) and ethambutol (Myambutol) were prescribed for Mr. Abdullah for his TB treatment. He is used to taking multiple pills and uses a pill box with divisions for days of the week and morning, noon, evening, and night-time doses. He takes 300 mg of isoniazid and 1,200 mg of ethambutol daily. He usually takes one 300-mg tablet of isoniazid and three 400-mg tablets of ethambutol each day, but the outpatient clinic pharmacy has run out of ethambutol 400-mg tablets and has dispensed 100-mg tablets instead. He will need to take 12 tablets of ethambutol instead of 3 and the nurse goes over the change in pills with Mr. Abdullah before he leaves the clinic.

Two days later, Mr. Abdullah is taken to the emergency department with palpitations, nausea, vomiting, vertigo, and progressive confusion. He is admitted and his serum isoniazid level is found to be in toxic range. His wife brings in his pill dispenser for the pharmacist to check. Mr. Abdullah has accidentally overdosed by taking 12 isoniazid tablets instead of ethambutol tablets. Both isoniazid and ethambutol came as round, white, scored tablets. How could this overdose have been prevented? What could the nurse recommend to prevent this from recurring?

See Answers to Patient Safety Questions on student resource website.

other pathogens in addition to *M. tuberculosis*. Although they are sometimes given for multidrug-resistant TB, they have not been approved by the FDA for this indication. They are the safest of the second-line drugs available for this infection.

Drugs for Leprosy

51.6 Leprosy is caused by a mycobacterium and is treated by a multidrug regimen.

Leprosy is a chronic infection caused by *M. leprae*. Leprosy has been known for thousands of years but the term *leper* has been used by different cultures to designate someone sinful or unclean, not necessarily someone with the disease we now call leprosy.

Although rare in the United States, it is estimated that 6 million people worldwide have leprosy. Patients with leprosy present with macular skin lesions that can become quite large. The organism invades peripheral nervous tissue, causing nerve thickening that results in loss of sensation or paresthesia. If left untreated, the infection causes extreme disfigurement and bone resorption, resulting in loss of digits. The disease is diagnosed through identification of the pathogen from a skin biopsy.

Leprosy may be infectious or noninfectious, depending on the stage of the disease and the progress of pharmacotherapy. Although the mode of transmission is not clear, *M. leprae* is likely spread by the respiratory route. The disease may have a very long incubation period extending from several months to years.

PharmFACT

About 200 to 300 cases of leprosy are reported in the United States each year. Nearly all cases are diagnosed in immigrants from countries where leprosy is endemic (Lewis, 2014).

There are two presentations of leprosy, and pharmacotherapy differs for the different types. *Lepromatous* leprosy occurs in patients with defective cell-mediated immunity and is characterized by a slow, progressive development of nodular skin lesions and nerve involvement. Because the patient has an impaired immune system, the mycobacteria may disseminate throughout the body and cause death. *Tuberculoid* leprosy is less progressive and may have long periods of remission followed by reactivation with more severe nerve involvement. These patients have an intact cell-mediated immune response; thus, the disease is more benign and less often fatal.

Like tuberculosis, leprosy is treated with prolonged combination pharmacotherapy because monotherapy causes rapid development of resistant strains. Although improvement in skin lesions may occur within a few months, therapy must continue during the entire treatment period to eliminate all the mycobacteria. A typical regimen includes the following:

- **Lepromatous leprosy.** Initial three-drug regimen that includes dapsone, clofazimine (Lamprene), and rifampin (Rifadin) given for 2 to 5 years.
- **Tuberculoid leprosy.** Initial two-drug regimen with dapsone and rifampin for 6 to 12 months, followed by dapsone alone for 2 to 3 years.

Other drugs may be substituted when the patient cannot tolerate the standard regimen. Ofloxacin (Floxin), clarithromycin (Biaxin), and minocycline (Minocin) are antibacterials that have activity against *M. leprae* and may be used during the long course of leprosy pharmacotherapy.

During the first year of pharmacotherapy, skin lesions may actually worsen because of activation of the cell-mediated immune response. Skin edema may occur and new lesions may appear on normal skin. Most of these reactions occur because immune cells are attacking antigens released by the mycobacteria. If this occurs, corticosteroids such as prednisone are added to the regimen to reduce the severe inflammation.

Patients with leprosy are examined monthly throughout the initial course of treatment and less frequently as therapy progresses. Follow-up may continue for 3 years or longer after the completion of pharmacotherapy. Close contacts of patients with leprosy normally do not receive chemoprophylaxis as do those of patients with TB, although follow-up examinations are conducted to ensure that they have not acquired the infection.

PROTOTYPE DRUG | **Dapsone (DDS)**

Classification: **Therapeutic:** Antileprosy drug, antimycobacterial, antiacne drug
Pharmacologic: Folic acid inhibitor

Therapeutic Effects and Uses: Approved in 1955, dapsone is a drug of choice for the treatment of *M. leprae* infections, usually in combination with other antileprosy drugs. It has several off-label uses that include the chemoprophylaxis of malaria in combination with pyrimethamine. In combination with trimethoprim, dapsone is used for the prophylaxis and treatment of *Pneumocystis jiroveci* pneumonia in patients with AIDS. It may take 3 to 6 months of

CONNECTIONS: NURSING PRACTICE APPLICATION

Patients Receiving Pharmacotherapy for Tuberculosis

Assessment	Potential Nursing Diagnoses*
Baseline assessment prior to administration: • Obtain a complete health history including neurologic, cardiovascular, respiratory, GI, hepatic, or renal disease, and the possibility of pregnancy. Obtain a drug history including allergies (e.g., specific reactions to drugs), current prescription and over-the-counter drugs, herbal preparations, and alcohol use. Be alert to possible drug interactions. • Assess for signs and symptoms of current infection, noting symptoms, duration, or any recent changes. Assess for concurrent infections, particularly HIV. • Evaluate appropriate laboratory and diagnostic findings (e.g., CBC, acid-fast bacillus [AFB], C&S, hepatic and renal function studies, uric acid levels, visual acuity, and red-green color vision tests). • Assess the patient's ability to receive and understand instructions. Include the family or caregivers as needed.	• *Infection* • *Fatigue* • *Imbalanced Nutrition: Less than Body Requirements*, related to fatigue, adverse drug effects • *Noncompliance*, related to adverse drug effects, deficient knowledge, length of treatment required, or cost of medication • *Social Isolation* • *Deficient Knowledge* (Drug Therapy)
Assessment throughout administration: • Assess for desired therapeutic effects (e.g., diminished signs and symptoms of infection, fever, night sweating, increasing ease of breathing, decreased sputum production, improved radiographic evidence of improving infection). • Continue periodic monitoring of CBC, hepatic, and renal function. • Assess for adverse effects: nausea, vomiting, abdominal cramping, diarrhea, drowsiness, dizziness, paresthesias, tinnitus, vertigo, blurred vision, changes in visual color sense, increasing fatigue. Eye pain, acute blurring of vision or loss of color sense, sudden or increasing numbness or tingling in extremities, decreased hearing or significant tinnitus, or increase in bruising or bleeding should be reported immediately.	

Implementation

Interventions and (Rationales)	Patient-Centered Care
Ensuring therapeutic effects: • Continue assessments as above for therapeutic effects. (Diminished fever, cough, sputum, and other signs and symptoms of infection should be noted.) • Recognize that TB treatment requires long-term adherence and many reasons exist for nonadherence, e.g., cost, adverse effects, concerns for family members with similar symptoms. (Nonadherence may increase risk to the patient's health and family and community health and lead to development of resistant organisms.)	• Teach the patient to *complete* the prescribed course of therapy; do not share doses with other family members with similar symptoms; and return to the provider if adverse effects develop to ensure that drug therapy is maintained. • Discuss concerns about cost, family members who have similar symptoms or may need prophylactic treatment, and how to manage adverse effects with the patient to help encourage adherence. In cases of significant nonadherence, DOT may be required.
Minimizing adverse effects: • Continue to monitor vital signs, especially temperature if fever is present, breath sounds, and sputum production and quality. Immediately report undiminished fever, increases in sputum production, hemoptysis, or increase in adventitious breath sounds to the health care provider. (Increasing signs of infection may signify drug resistance or significant nonadherence to the drug regimen.)	• Teach the patient to report fever that does not diminish below 37.8°C (100°F) or per the parameters set by the health care provider, continued symptoms of disease (e.g., night sweating, fatigue), or increased sputum production to the health care provider promptly.
• Continue to monitor periodic laboratory work: hepatic and renal function tests, CBCs, sputum culture for AFB. (Antituberculosis drugs are hepatic and renal toxic. **Lifespan:** Monitor the older adult more frequently because age-related physiological changes may affect the drug's metabolism or excretion. Periodic C&S tests may be ordered if infections are severe or are slow to resolve to confirm appropriate therapy. Drug levels will be monitored on drugs with known severe adverse effects. **Diverse Patients:** Because some drugs such as isoniazid [INH] metabolize through the P450 system pathway, monitor ethnically diverse patients to ensure optimal therapeutic effects and to minimize adverse effects.)	• Instruct the patient on the need for periodic laboratory work.
• Continue to monitor for hepatic, renal, and/or ototoxicity, e.g., jaundice, right upper quadrant pain, darkened urine, diminished urine output, tinnitus, or vertigo. (Antituberculosis drugs that are hepatic, renal, or ototoxic require frequent monitoring to prevent adverse effects. Increasing fluid intake will help to prevent drug accumulation in the kidneys.)	• Teach the patient to report any nausea, vomiting, yellowing of the skin or sclera, abdominal pain, light or clay-colored stools, diminished urine output, darkening of urine, ringing, humming, or buzzing in ears, dizziness, or vertigo immediately. • Advise the patient to increase fluid intake to 2–3 L/day and to eliminate all alcohol use.

CONNECTIONS: NURSING PRACTICE APPLICATION (continued)

• Monitor for signs and symptoms of neurotoxicity, particularly peripheral and optic neuropathy, e.g., dizziness, drowsiness, headache, changes in visual acuity, blurred vision, loss of color sense, or paresthesia. (Neurotoxicity and peripheral and optic neuritis are adverse effects of antituberculosis drugs. **Lifespan:** Be particularly cautious with the older adult who is a greater risk for falls. Vitamin B$_6$ may be ordered to decrease the risk of peripheral neuropathy, especially that associated with isoniazid use. Monitor visual acuity and color vision sense in patients taking ethambutol.)	• Instruct the patient to report drowsiness, dizziness, numbness or tingling in peripheral extremities, blurred vision, changes in visual color sense, or changes in visual acuity. Eye pain, acute blurring of vision or loss of color sense, sudden or increasing numbness or tingling in extremities should be reported immediately. If dizziness occurs, the patient should sit or lie down and not attempt to stand or walk until the sensation passes. • Encourage the patient to increase intake of vitamin B$_6$–rich foods (e.g., fortified cereals, baked potato with skin on, bananas, lean meats, garbanzo beans) and discuss vitamin B$_6$ supplements with the health care provider.
• Monitor blood glucose levels in patients taking isoniazid. (Isoniazid may increase glucose levels. Patients with diabetes may require a change in their antidiabetic drug routine.)	• Teach patients with diabetes to test their glucose levels more frequently, reporting any consistent elevations to the health care provider.
• Monitor uric acid levels and for signs and symptoms of gout in patients taking ethambutol and pyrazinamide. (These drugs decrease the renal excretion of uric acid and hyperuricemia may result.)	• Teach the patient to report signs and symptoms of gout such as inflammation and pain around joints, redness, or swelling, particularly of toes or fingers. • Teach the patient to increase fluid intake to 2–4 L/day, taken throughout the day. • Teach the patient to avoid foods high in purine, eliminate alcohol consumption, and avoid increased vitamin C intake or supplementation. Provide dietitian consult as needed.
• Monitor dietary routine in patients taking isoniazid. (Foods high in tyramine can interact with the drug and cause palpitations, flushing, and hypertension.)	• Advise patients taking isoniazid to avoid foods containing tyramine, such as aged cheese, smoked and pickled fish, beer, red wine, bananas, and chocolate, and to immediately report headache, palpitations, tachycardia, or fever.
• Patients taking rifampin should be cautioned that the drug may turn body fluids (tears, sweat, saliva, urine) reddish-orange. (The effect is harmless but may stain soft, hydrophilic contact lenses or clothing.)	• Teach the patient to consult with an eye provider before using hydrophilic contact lenses. Consider wearing nonwhite clothing or use undergarments if sweating is excessive.
Patient understanding of drug therapy: • Use opportunities during administration of medications and during assessments to discuss the rationale for drug therapy, desired therapeutic outcomes, commonly observed adverse effects, parameters for when to call the health care provider, and any necessary monitoring or precautions. (Using time during nursing care helps to optimize and reinforce key teaching areas.)	• The patient, family, or caregiver should be able to state the reason for the drug, appropriate dose and scheduling, what adverse effects to observe for and when to report them, and the anticipated length of medication therapy.
Patient self-administration of drug therapy: • When administering medications, instruct the patient, family, or caregiver in proper self-administration techniques followed by teach-back. (Utilizing time during nurse-administration of these drugs helps to reinforce teaching.)	• Teach the patient to take the medication: • Complete the entire course of therapy unless otherwise instructed. The duration of the required therapy may be quite lengthy but it is necessary to prevent active infection. Do not stop taking the medicine when starting to feel better. • Do not share the medicine with other family members. If there is reason to believe they need medication, they should be assessed by a health care provider. • Eliminate alcohol while on these medications. These drugs cause significant reactions when taken with alcohol. • Take the drug with food or milk but avoid acidic beverages. If instructed to take the drug on an empty stomach, take with a full glass of water. • Take the medication as evenly spaced throughout each day as feasible. • Increase overall fluid intake while taking these drugs.

dapsone therapy before symptoms begin to improve. Pharmacotherapy for the prophylaxis of toxoplasmosis combines dapsone, pyrimethamine, and leucovorin. In 2005 dapsone 5% gel (Aczone) was approved as topical therapy for acne vulgaris.

Dapsone is the primary therapy for dermatitis herpetiformis and for autoimmune disease characterized by severe blistering skin lesions. Although its name implies herpes virus as a causative agent, the etiology of the disorder is sensitivity to gluten in the diet. Gluten is a protein found in wheat products.

Mechanism of Action: The mechanism of action of dapsone is incompletely understood but is thought to be the same as that of the sulfonamides: It inhibits folic acid metabolism.

Pharmacokinetics:

Route(s)	PO
Absorption	Readily absorbed
Distribution	Widely distributed; crosses the placenta; secreted in breast milk; up to 90% protein bound
Primary metabolism	Hepatic, through acetylation by CYP2E1 and CYP3A4
Primary excretion	Renal, with small amounts in the feces
Onset of action	4–8 h
Duration of action	Half-life: 20–30 h

Adverse Effects: The most frequent adverse effects of oral dapsone relate to the hematologic system: dose-related hemolysis and methemoglobinemia with cyanosis. Aplastic anemia and agranulocytosis are rare, though potentially severe, adverse effects. Toxic hepatitis has been reported. The drug concentrates in the skin, causing dermatologic reactions that include photosensitivity and toxic epidermal necrolysis. When administered topically, the most frequent side effects are erythema and skin dryness..

Contraindications/Precautions: Contraindications include hypersensitivity to dapsone or related drugs, such as sulfonamides. Because of its adverse effects on the hematologic system, caution should be used in treating patients with preexisting blood disorders. Frequent blood assessments are conducted during therapy to avoid serious adverse effects. Frequent liver enzyme testing should be conducted to monitor for hepatotoxicity, especially in patients with preexisting liver impairment.

Drug Interactions: Some patients receiving pyrimethamine and dapsone concurrently developed agranulocytosis during the second and third month of therapy; therefore, concurrent administration of these drugs must be carefully monitored. Increased dapsone levels have been reported in patients receiving trimethoprim, and patients receiving this combination may be at increased risk for dapsone toxicity. Rifampin may significantly reduce serum levels of dapsone. The H_2 receptor blockers such as ranitidine will decrease gastric pH and lower the effectiveness of dapsone. **Herbal/Food**: Dapsone levels may be decreased by St. John's wort.

Pregnancy: Category C.

Treatment of Overdose: Acute overdose may result in cyanosis, which may be treated by the slow IV administration of 1–2 mg/kg of methylene blue.

Nursing Responsibilities:
- Monitor periodic laboratory tests including white blood cell (WBC) count with differential, serum electrolytes, serum albumin, and liver function.
- Monitor for serious adverse effects such as GI bleeding, bone and joint pain, or diminished vision. Although reactions are usually reversible, they may require months or years to diminish. Other symptoms include colicky abdominal pain, nausea, and vomiting.
- Assess for any reddish-brown discoloration of the skin, cornea, conjunctiva, and body fluids. This adverse effect occurs in 75% to 90% of patients within a few weeks of treatment.
- Assess for tender, erythematous nodules with lymphadenopathy, joint swelling, epistaxis, and iritis, which can suggest a type 2 leprosy reactional state.

Lifespan and Diversity Considerations:
- Monitor hepatic function laboratory values more frequently in the older adult because normal physiological changes related to aging may affect the drug's metabolism and excretion.
- Because dapsone is metabolized through acetylation, monitor ethnically diverse populations more frequently to ensure optimal therapeutic effects and minimize adverse effects.

Patient and Family Education:
- Maintain strict adherence to the established drug regimen and do not change the drug dosage without the approval of the health care provider.
- Do not drive or perform other hazardous activities until the effects of the drug are known because this drug may cause drowsiness or dizziness.
- Minimize the use of soap and rinse thoroughly, especially if the skin is dry.
- Keep all appointments for follow-up care because drug resistance and relapse may occur.
- Immediately report any of the following to the health care provider: changes in vision or hearing, dark urine, unusual fatigue, unusual bruising or bleeding, bluish fingernails, or yellowing of the eyes or skin.

Drugs Similar to Dapsone (DDS)

Other primary antimycobacterial drugs for leprosy include clofazimine and rifampin. Rifampin is also used for TB and is discussed in Section 51.4.

Clofazimine (Lamprene): Clofazimine is a drug that exhibits selective activity toward mycobacteria. Although its only approved indication is leprosy, clofazimine is sometimes used in the pharmacotherapy of MAC. Given only by the PO route, the drug has a 70-day half-life—one of the longest of any drug. It may take up to 50 days before it exerts a bacteriocidal effect. The drug has anti-inflammatory and immunosuppressive properties. Clofazimine, a bright-red dye, can cause a reddish-brown discoloration of the skin, conjunctiva, and body fluids that may take years to disappear after discontinuing therapy. Therapy of dapsone-resistant infections may require daily administration of clofazimine for several years. This drug is pregnancy category C.

Drugs for Mycobacterium Avium Complex Infections

51.7 *Mycobacterium avium* complex infections are common in patients with impaired immune function.

MAC is the most common cause of lung disease due to atypical mycobacterial infections. Although rare in healthy people, MAC is a frequent cause of infection among those with impaired immune systems and is an expected complication in many patients with AIDS. It is also found in higher incidence in patients with chronic obstructive pulmonary disease. The infection is caused by *M. avium*, *M. intracellulare*, or a combination of atypical mycobacteria.

Unlike TB, MAC infections are not believed to be contagious or spread by human-to-human contact. The mode of transmission is not understood, although the organisms are widely distributed in soil and water and these may be the primary sources of infection. Once inside the body, MAC resides in the lungs like *M. tuberculosis*, and the initial respiratory symptoms are identical. The pathogen may travel through the lymphatics and bloodstream to infect any organ. The frequency of disseminated MAC disease has been markedly reduced in patients with AIDS because of successes in the pharmacotherapy of HIV-AIDS.

Treatment of MAC should include at least two drugs (and often three or four) because monotherapy has been shown to promote the emergence of resistant strains. Treatment is prolonged, and relapse rates for treating pulmonary MAC approach 20%. Drugs for this infection include the following:

- **Macrolide antibiotics.** Clarithromycin (Biaxin) and azithromycin (Zithromax) are relatively safe and effective against MAC and are included in most regimens. High doses of clarithromycin (1,000 mg bid) are associated with increased mortality rates.

- **Ethambutol (Myambutol).** Usually used for TB, this drug may be combined with clarithromycin in the pharmacotherapy of MAC.

- **Rifabutin (Mycobutin).** If a third drug is needed, rifabutin is often effective. Rifabutin, however, can cause many drug interactions, and high doses (600 mg/day) are associated with greater risk of serious uveitis with eye pain. Rifabutin is approved only for the prophylaxis of MAC in patients with HIV infection, although it is also used off-label to treat active infections.

Pharmacotherapy for AIDS patients with MAC infections involves antimicrobial drugs with activity against MAC, including clarithromycin, azithromycin, rifabutin, ethambutol, levofloxacin, and amikacin. MAC infections in patients with AIDS may be fatal; therefore, chemoprophylaxis is indicated when the CD4 lymphocyte count falls to less than 50 cells/mL. Clarithromycin and azithromycin are preferred drugs for prophylaxis. Rifabutin and ethambutol are alternatives to the macrolides. Many health care providers will discontinue chemoprophylaxis if a patient who is HIV positive regains normal immunologic status.

CHAPTER
51 Understanding the Chapter

Key Concepts Summary

51.1 Several species of mycobacteria are important human pathogens.

51.2 Tuberculosis is a respiratory infection that exhibits both active and latent stages.

51.3 The pharmacotherapy of tuberculosis requires special dosing regimens and schedules.

51.4 First-line or primary antituberculosis drugs are the most efficacious and safest drugs for treating *M. tuberculosis* infections.

51.5 Second-line antituberculosis drugs are used when resistance develops to the first-line drugs.

51.6 Leprosy is caused by a mycobacterium and is treated by a multidrug regimen.

51.7 *Mycobacterium avium* complex infections are common in patients with impaired immune function.

Case Study: Making the Patient Connection

Remember the patient "Sam Myers" at the beginning of the chapter? Now read the remainder of the case study. Based on the information presented within this chapter, respond to the critical thinking questions that follow.

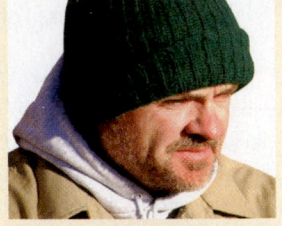

Sam Myers is a 58-year-old man who is homeless and spends some nights in shelters and some nights on the street. For the past 6 weeks, he has experienced anorexia, weight loss, and low-grade fever. He comes to the local church health center and presents with a productive cough that has progressively worsened.

A history and physical examination is completed with an evaluation for TB. The physical examination reveals the following findings: the patient's height is 1.9 meters (6'1") and his weight is 56.2 kg (124 lb). He is emaciated and obviously malnourished. His vital signs are blood pressure, 112/82 mmHg;

heart rate, 102 beats/min; respiratory rate, 26 breaths/min; and body temperature, 38.2°C (100.9°F). On auscultation, crackles are heard in the upper lung fields. The patient is experiencing moderate dyspnea. Sam's chest x-ray reveals multiple calcifications and two cavitary masses in the apical posterior segments of the upper lobes with lymphadenopathy also present. Sam admits to drinking alcohol almost every day and smoking at least one pack of cigarettes per day. He is admitted to a local acute care hospital for treatment of pulmonary TB.

Critical Thinking Questions

1. Describe the mechanism of transmission for *M. tuberculosis*.
2. Discuss how Sam's living conditions predispose him to pulmonary TB.
3. Why is Sam at high risk for hepatic-related adverse drug effects?

See Answers to Critical Thinking Questions on student resource website.

Additional Case Study

Georgia Sully has been diagnosed with an active TB infection after several months of increasing fevers, night sweats, productive cough, and weight loss. She is prescribed isoniazid (INH), ethambutol (Myambutol), rifampin (Rifadin), and pyrazinamide (PZA) for 6 months. She is also given instructions to take a daily dose of pyridoxine (vitamin B₆). She lives in a state that requires DOT for all patients receiving treatment for active TB.

1. Georgia is worried and questions the nurse about why she is receiving four different drugs for her tuberculosis. How would you respond?
2. Discuss why Georgia is receiving vitamin B₆ supplements.
3. Georgia asks what "directly observed therapy" is and why she needs it. What would you explain about DOT?

See Answers to Additional Case Study on student resource website.

Chapter Review

1 A patient who is receiving isoniazid (INH) reports tingling and numbness of the fingers and toes. The nurse knows that these symptoms are most likely due to the drug's ability to:

1. Increase the sensitivity of nerve endings.
2. Decrease the activity of pyridoxine (vitamin B₆).
3. Accelerate the excretion of neurotransmitters.
4. Enhance skin receptors for ascorbic acid (vitamin C).

2 Ethambutol (Myambutol) has been included as part of a multidrug regimen to treat a patient with active tuberculosis. Prior to starting this drug, which screening tests should the patient have? Select all that apply.

1. Coagulation studies
2. Sputum cultures
3. Uric acid level
4. Hepatic function tests
5. Vision acuity and vision color sense screening

3 A patient is identified by ethnic background as a possible slow acetylator and will be closely followed after beginning isoniazid therapy for latent tuberculosis. To ensure that this patient does not experience adverse effects related to the acetylation process, both _____ and _____ will be monitored frequently.

4 A patient with HIV infection who also has a *Mycobacterium avium* complex infection is started on clarithromycin (Biaxin) and ethambutol (Myambutol). What appropriate teaching should the nurse give this patient?

1. You will remain contagious until drug treatment is completed.
2. These drugs will only be required for a short period of time, approximately 2 to 3 weeks.
3. Drug therapy will be stopped if CD4 counts drop below 50 cells/mL.
4. It will be necessary to continue these drugs for a prolonged period of time to adequately treat the infection.

5 The patient is diagnosed with *Mycobacterium leprae* (leprosy) and is being treated with dapsone (DDS). Which nursing assessment findings would indicate that the patient is experiencing adverse effects from this therapy?

1. Discoloration of skin, cornea, and conjunctiva

2. Chronic constipation, chills, and dehydration

3. Hypoglycemia, impaired memory, and impotence

4. Memory loss, nervousness, and pruritus

6 Patients with diabetes who take isoniazid (INH) may require more frequent monitoring of blood glucose levels. What effect does isoniazid have on glucose levels?

1. It may decrease glucose levels.

2. It has no known effects on glucose levels.

3. It may increase glucose levels.

4. It causes rapid rises and falls of glucose levels.

See Answers to Chapter Review in Appendix A.

References

Aaron, C. L., Fotinas, M. J., West, K. B., Goodwin, D. J., & Mancuso, J. D. (2013). Tuberculosis among nonimmigrant visitors to US military installations. *Military Medicine, 178*(3), 346–352. doi:10.7205/MILMED-D-12-00297

Centers for Disease Control and Prevention. (2013a). *Reported tuberculosis in the United States, 2012: Executive summary.* Retrieved from http://www.cdc.gov/tb/statistics/reports/2012/executivecommentary.htm

Centers for Disease Control and Prevention. (2013b). Tuberculosis: United States 1993–2010. *Morbidity and Mortality Weekly Report, 62*(03), 149–154. Retrieved from http://www.cdc.gov/mmwr/preview/mmwrhtml/su6203a25.htm?s_cid=su6203a25_w

Edelson, P. J., & Phypers, M. (2010). TB transmission on public transportation: A review of published studies and recommendations for contact tracing. *Travel Medicine and Infectious Disease, 9*, 27–31. doi:10.1016/j.tmaid.2010.11.001

Kornylo-Duong, K., Kim, C., Cramer, E. H., Buff, A. M., Rodriguez-Howell, D., Doyle, J., . . . Marienau, K. J. (2010). Three air travel-related contact investigations associated with infectious tuberculosis, 2007–2008. *Travel Medicine and Infectious Disease, 8*, 120–128. doi:10.1016/j.tmaid.2009.08.001

Lewis, F. S. (2014). *Dermatologic manifestations of leprosy.* Retrieved from http://emedicine.medscape.com/article/1104977-overview#a0101

Martinez, L., Thomas, K., & Figueroa, J. (2010). Guidance from WHO on the prevention and control of TB during air travel. *Travel Medicine and Infectious Disease, 8*, 84–89. doi:10.1016/j.tmaid.2009.02.005

Moonan, P. K., Quituguo, T. N., Pogoda, J. M., Woo, G., Drewyer, G., Sahbazian, B., . . . Weis, S. E. (2011). Does directly observed therapy (DOT) reduce drug resistant tuberculosis? *BMC Public Health, 11*, 19. doi:10.1186/1471-2458-11-19

World Health Organization. (2014). *Tuberculosis factsheet N104.* Retrieved from http://www.who.int/mediacentre/factsheets/fs104/en

Selected Bibliography

American Thoracic Society, CDC, and Infectious Diseases Society of America. (2003). Treatment of tuberculosis. *Morbidity and Mortality Weekly Report, 52*(RR11), 1–77. Retrieved from http://www.cdc.gov/mmwr/preview/mmwrhtml/rr5211a1.htm

Centers for Disease Control and Prevention. (2013). *Tuberculosis (TB).* Retrieved from http://www.cdc.gov/tb/?404;http://www.cdc.gov:80/tb/pubs/mmwr/maj_guide.htm

Field, S. K., Fisher, D., Jarand, J. M., & Cowie, R. L. (2012). New treatment options for multidrug-resistant tuberculosis. *Therapeutic Advances in Respiratory Disease, 6*, 255–268. doi:10.1177/1753465812452193

Gumbo, T. (2011). Chemotherapy of tuberculosis, *Mycobacterium avium* complex disease, and leprosy. In L. L. Brunton, B. A. Chabner, & B. C. Knollman (Eds.), *The pharmacological basis of therapeutics* (11th ed., pp. 1549–1570). New York, NY: McGraw-Hill.

Herdman, T. H., & Kamitsuru, S. (Eds.). (2014). *NANDA International nursing diagnoses: Definitions and classification, 2015–2017.* Oxford, United Kingdom: Wiley-Blackwell.

Koirala, J. (2014). *Mycobacterium avium-intracellulare.* Retrieved from http://emedicine.medscape.com/article/222664-overview

Lienhardt, C., Raviglione, M., Spigelman, M., Hafner, R., Jaramillo, E., Hoelscher, M., . . . Gheuens, J. (2012). New drugs for the treatment of tuberculosis: Needs, challenges, promise, and prospects for the future. *Journal of Infectious Diseases, 205*(Suppl. 2), S241–S249. doi:10.1093/infdis/jis034

Nahid, P., & Menzies, D. (2012). Update in tuberculosis and nontuberculous mycobacterial disease 2011. *American Journal of Respiratory and Critical Care Medicine, 185*, 1266–1270. doi:10.1164/rccm.201203-0494UP

Pontali, E., Matteelli, A., & Migliori, G. B. (2013). Drug-resistant tuberculosis. *Current Opinion in Pulmonary Medicine, 19*, 266–272. doi:10.1097/MCP.0b013e32835f1bf3

Sterling, T. R., Pham, P. A., & Chaisson, R. E. (2010). HIV infection-related tuberculosis: Clinical manifestations and treatment. *Clinical Infectious Diseases, 50*(Suppl. 3), S223–S230. doi:10.1086/651495

Swaminathan, S., Padmapriyadarsini, C., & Narendran, G. (2010). HIV-associated tuberculosis: Clinical update. *Clinical Infectious Diseases, 50*, 1377–1386. doi:10.1086/652147

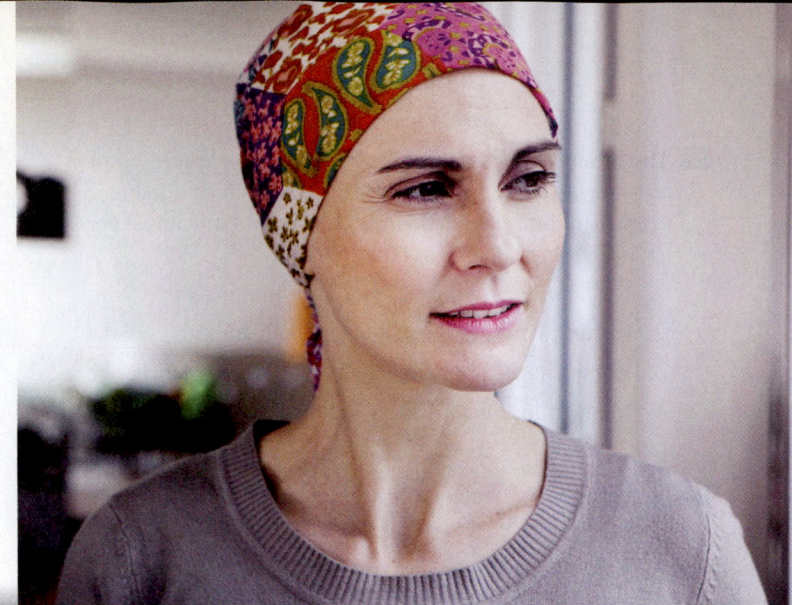

"*Since I started chemotherapy, these white patches have appeared on my tongue and sometimes my throat burns when I swallow. So I decided to come to the clinic to find out what's going on with me.*"

Patient "Sarah Williams"

52 Pharmacotherapy of Fungal Infections

LEARNING OUTCOMES

After reading this chapter, the student should be able to:

1. Compare and contrast the pharmacotherapy of fungal and bacterial infections.
2. Classify mycoses based on the location of the infection and the causative organism.
3. Compare and contrast the pharmacotherapy of superficial and systemic fungal infections.
4. Identify the types of patients at greatest risk of acquiring serious fungal infections.
5. Describe the nurse's role in the pharmacologic management of fungal infections.
6. For each of the classes shown in the chapter outline, identify the prototype and representative drugs and explain the mechanism(s) of drug action, primary indications, contraindications, significant drug interactions, pregnancy category, and important adverse effects.
7. Apply the nursing process to care for patients receiving pharmacotherapy for fungal infections.

CHAPTER OUTLINE

▶ **Characteristics of Fungi and Fungal Infections**

▶ **Drugs for Systemic Fungal Infections**

   PROTOTYPE Amphotericin B Deoxycholate (Fungizone), *p. 870*

▶ **Drugs for Both Systemic and Superficial Fungal Infections**

   PROTOTYPE Fluconazole (Diflucan), *p. 873*

▶ **Drugs for Superficial Fungal Infections**

   PROTOTYPE Nystatin (Mycostatin, Nystop, Others), *p. 877*

KEY TERMS

azole, 872

β-glucan, 868

dermatomycoses, 874

ergosterol, 868

fungi, 867

mycoses, 868

onychomycosis, 876

The past few decades have seen a dramatic rise in the incidence of fungal infections due to acquired immunodeficiency syndrome (AIDS), aggressive cancer chemotherapy, the widespread use of indwelling intravenous (IV) catheters, and the use of broad-spectrum antibiotics. Fungi are much more complex than bacteria and require a different approach to pharmacotherapy. Because of these structural and functional differences, most antibacterial drugs are ineffective against fungi. Although there are fewer drugs to treat fungal infections, the available medications are usually effective.

Characteristics of Fungi and Fungal Infections

52.1 Serious fungal infections are uncommon in people with healthy immune defenses.

Fungi are single-celled or multicellular organisms that serve essential roles on the planet as decomposers of dead plants and animals, returning their elements to the soil for recycling. Fungi include mushrooms, yeasts, and molds. Although 100,000 to 200,000 species of fungi exist in soil, air, and water, only about 50 species are associated with disease in humans. A few species of fungi survive as part of the normal host flora on the skin, mouth, and urogenital tract.

Unlike bacteria, which produce toxins or grow rapidly to overwhelm hosts' defenses, some fungi grow slowly and infections may progress for many months before symptoms develop. With a few exceptions (such as athlete's foot), fungal infections are not easily transmitted through casual contact. In addition to causing infections, fungal antigens may trigger hypersensitivity responses in susceptible patients, resulting in allergies to mold or mildew. A few fungi, such as *Aspergillus flavus*, secrete toxins that can cause illness in humans through ingestion of contaminated grains or other foods.

The human body is remarkably resistant to infection by these organisms and patients with healthy immune defenses experience few serious fungal diseases. However, patients with a suppressed immune system (immunocompromised), especially those infected with HIV, may experience frequent fungal infections and require aggressive pharmacotherapy. A systemic fungal infection in an immunocompromised patient may be rapidly fatal.

The species of pathogenic fungi that attack hosts with healthy immune defenses are often distinct from those that infect immunocompromised patients. Patients with intact immune defenses are afflicted with community-acquired infections such as sporotrichosis, blastomycosis, histoplasmosis, and coccidioidomycosis. Opportunistic fungal infections acquired in a hospital setting are more likely to be candidiasis, aspergillosis, cryptococcosis, and mucormycosis. Thus, assessing the immune status of a patient may help in diagnosing the specific infection and in determining the course of pharmacotherapy. Table 52.1 lists the species of fungi that most commonly cause disease in humans.

TABLE 52.1 Fungal Pathogens

Name of Fungus	Description
Systemic	
Aspergillus fumigatus and other species	Aspergillosis: Opportunistic; most commonly affects the lungs but can spread to other organs
Blastomyces dermatitides	Blastomycosis: Begins in the lungs and spreads to other organs
Candida albicans and other species	Candidiasis: Most common opportunistic fungal infection; may affect nearly any organ
Coccidioides immitis	Coccidioidomycosis: Begins in the lungs and spreads to other organs
Cryptococcus neoformans	Cryptococcosis: Opportunistic; begins in the lungs but is the most common cause of meningitis in patients with AIDS
Histoplasma capsulatum	Histoplasmosis: Begins in the lungs and spreads to other organs
Mucorales species	Mucormycosis: Opportunistic; affects blood vessels, causes sinus infections, stomach ulcers, and other disorders
Pneumocystis jirovecii	*Pneumocystis* pneumonia: Opportunistic; primarily pneumonia of the lung but can spread to other organs
Superficial	
Candida albicans and other species	Candidiasis: Affects the skin, nails, oral cavity (thrush), vagina
Epidermophyton floccosum	Athlete's foot (tinea pedis), jock itch (tinea cruris), and other skin infections
Microsporum species	Ringworm of the scalp (tinea capitis)
Trichophyton species	Affects the scalp, skin, and nails
Cutaneous and Subcutaneous	
Sporothrix schenckii	Sporotrichosis: Primarily affects the skin and superficial lymph nodes
Mixed species	Chromoblastomycosis: Chronic skin mycosis found in tropical and subtropical climates

52.2 Mycoses are classified as superficial, subcutaneous, or systemic.

Fungal infections are called **mycoses** (singular, mycosis). A simple and useful method of classifying fungal infections is to consider them as superficial, subcutaneous, or systemic.

Superficial mycoses affect the scalp, skin, nails, and mucous membranes such as the oral cavity and vagina. Only the surface layers of these regions are affected. Mycoses of this type are often treated with topical agents, because these drugs can penetrate into the keratin layer of the skin while producing few systemic adverse effects.

Subcutaneous and cutaneous mycoses are infections that affect deeper skin layers, including the dermis and subcutaneous layers. Often, the organisms that cause subcutaneous and cutaneous infections are different from those that cause superficial infections, as listed in Table 52.1. Because these fungal species often reside in soil, gardeners or people working in occupations involving exposure to soil can acquire these infections through cuts or abrasions on their skin. In addition, these infections occur in greater incidence in regions where the population travels barefoot. Topical antifungal preparations may not penetrate deep enough to reach the pathogen, thus oral (PO) antifungal therapy may be indicated. Some textbooks consider subcutaneous mycoses as subtypes of superficial mycoses.

Systemic mycoses are those that affect internal organs, typically the lungs, brain, and digestive organs. These infections often originate in the lungs, through inhalation of fungal spores. Although less common than superficial or subcutaneous mycoses, systemic fungal infections affect multiple body systems and may be fatal to patients with severely suppressed immune systems. Invasive systemic mycoses require aggressive oral or parenteral medications that produce more adverse effects than the topical agents.

Historically, antifungal drugs used for superficial infections were clearly distinct from those prescribed for systemic infections. In recent years, this distinction has blurred. Some of the newer antifungals may be used for superficial, subcutaneous, or systemic infections. Furthermore, some superficial infections may be treated with parenteral, oral, or topical drugs. This therapeutic division, however, is still useful because it separates the pharmacotherapy of relatively benign infections (superficial) from those that may be life threatening (systemic).

52.3 Antifungal drugs act by disrupting the fungal cell membrane or wall, affecting fungal enzymes, or disrupting replication.

Biologically, fungi are classified as eukaryotes: Their cellular organelles and metabolic pathways are more similar to those of humans, than to bacteria. Antibiotics that are efficacious against bacteria are ineffective in treating mycoses due to these differences in physiology; thus, an entirely different set of agents is needed to eliminate fungal pathogens.

Like antibacterials, the antifungal drugs may either slow the growth of the organisms (fungistatic) or kill them (fungicidal). The five mechanisms of action of the antifungal drugs are illustrated in Figure 52.1.

One important difference between fungal cells and human cells is the specific steroid used in constructing plasma membranes. While cholesterol is essential for animal cell membranes, **ergosterol** is present in fungi. The largest class of antifungals, the azoles, inhibits ergosterol biosynthesis, causing the fungal plasma membrane to become porous or leaky. Amphotericin B (Fungizone), terbinafine (Lamisil), and nystatin (Mycostatin) also act by this mechanism.

Caspofungin (Cancidas) disrupts fungal cell walls by inhibiting the synthesis of **β-glucan**, an essential component that shapes and strengthens the cell wall. Without sufficient β-glucan, the wall weakens and becomes porous, causing the death of the cell.

Some antifungals act by mechanisms that take advantage of enzymatic differences between fungi and humans. In fungi, flucytosine (Ancobon) is converted to the potent antimetabolite 5-fluorouracil, which inhibits both deoxyribonucleic acid (DNA) and ribonucleic acid (RNA) synthesis. Humans do not have the

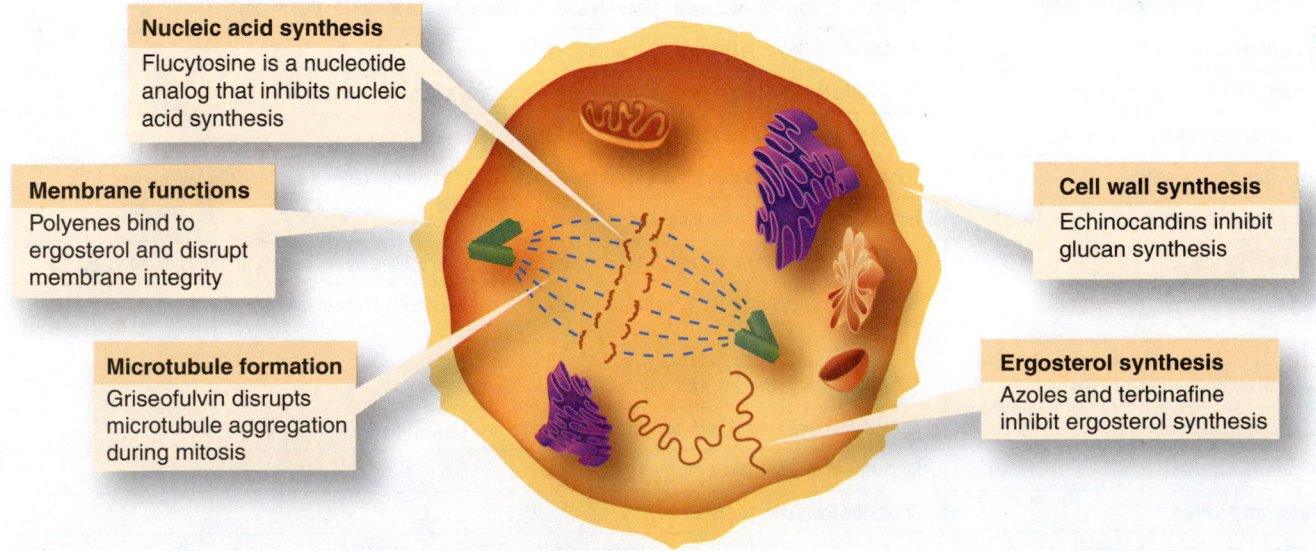

Figure 52.1 Mechanisms of action of antifungal drugs.

From *Brock Biology of Microorganisms* (11th ed., p. 691), by M. Madigan and J. Martinko, 2006. Reprinted and Electronically reproduced by permission of Pearson Education, Inc., Upper Saddle River, NJ.

◖ **Reducing Exposure of Patients with Neutropenia to Fungal Pathogens**

Clinical Question

What factors reduce the exposure of a patient with neutropenia to fungal pathogens?

Fungal infections are a major factor associated with mortality and morbidity in patients with cancer who develop neutropenia. Quality of life is severely affected by the symptoms and stress associated with cancer-related fungal invasions. Preventing fungal infection is a priority in the care of both hospitalized and ambulatory cancer patients.

Lessening the exposure to fungal pathogens is one method for decreasing the occurrence of infection in patients both in the hospital and in the community. Nursing professionals must examine environmental factors that may place these patients at risk for infections.

Evidence

Although the overall incidence of invasive fungal infections may be relatively low, the cost in terms of treatment, length of stay, and mortality rates is high (des Champs-Bro et al., 2011). Treatment with antifungal drugs has been effective, but with antifungals used prophylactically, there has been a rise in unusual and drug-resistant strains such as non-*albicans* types of *Candida* and non-*Aspergillus* species. Early diagnosis and treatment of fungal infections is crucial, but the prophylactic or empiric use of antifungals is still controversial with concerns about the rise of resistant strains, especially as broad-spectrum antifungal drugs such as posaconazole are used (Auberger et al., 2012). Empiric therapy is recommended for patients with neutropenia who have continued fevers not relieved by other drug treatment because the symptoms are often due to occult fungal infection. In these cases empiric antifungal drug therapy may be lifesaving.

Implications

Preventing an infection before it begins is the ideal clinical strategy. Infection control measures such as frequent and thorough hand washing, the use of disposable gowns and supplies, and thorough decontamination of the patient

environment help to reduce the chance of transmission of fungi, molds, and spores (Gould, 2011). In addition, other factors that may reduce the patient's exposure to fungal pathogens include:

- Utilize strict aseptic technique when performing all invasive procedures, especially when inserting a urinary catheter or performing endotracheal suctioning, because these procedures are done in areas where fungal infections are common.
- Modify the environment to minimize airborne contamination. Negative airflow with HEPA filtration significantly reduces the risk of airborne spores, and appropriate housekeeping measures keep down dust.
- Eliminate potentially contaminated reservoirs such as soil, damp or moist fabrics, dried or fresh flowers, and standing water when possible.
- Keep patients who are neutropenic away from construction areas in the health care agency. This prevents transmission of airborne spores released during the construction process. Areas of construction should be sealed off with appropriate impermeable barriers.
- Provide high-filtration masks if patients must leave their rooms for procedures to minimize inhalation risk.

Because invasive fungal infections often occur in the lungs (Auberger et al., 2012), thorough assessment of the respiratory system should occur during each physical assessment of the patient. Patients who are neutropenic may exhibit subtle signs of infection, such as low-grade fever and fatigue, even when an infection is present. Frequent respiratory assessments will assist the nurse in noting these subtle changes over time.

Critical Thinking Question

Why are patients with neutropenia more susceptible to opportunistic infections such as fungal infections?

See Answers to Critical Thinking Questions on student resource website.

---

enzyme necessary for this conversion. 5-Fluorouracil itself is a common antineoplastic medication (see Chapter 57).

A final mechanism is used by the drug griseofulvin. This drug is incorporated into newly formed keratin where it provides a protective effect against fungal invasion. Once it has entered the fungal cell, it disrupts the mitotic spindle, preventing replication.

CONNECTION Checkpoint 52.1

From what you learned in Chapter 47, what major classes of antibacterials act by disrupting cell walls? Why are these drugs not effective against fungi? *See Answer to Connection Checkpoint 52.1 on student resource website.*

Drugs for Systemic Fungal Infections

52.4 Systemic or invasive fungal disease may require intensive pharmacotherapy for extended periods.

Because human body defenses provide a formidable barrier to fungi, systemic mycoses are rarely encountered in persons with healthy immune systems. The AIDS epidemic, however, resulted

in the frequent clinical occurrence of previously rare mycoses, such as cryptococcosis and coccidioidomycosis. The opportunistic disease in patients with AIDS spurred the development of several new drugs for systemic fungal infections. In addition to occurring in patients with AIDS, others who may experience systemic mycoses include those receiving prolonged therapy with corticosteroids, having extensive burns, receiving antineoplastic drugs, having indwelling vascular catheters, or receiving organ transplants. Prophylactic antifungal therapy is sometimes indicated for these high-risk patients.

Pharmacotherapy of systemic mycoses is often continued for many months to ensure that the fungus is eliminated. Unlike the superficial antifungal drugs, systemic agents have the potential to cause serious adverse effects and therapy must be carefully monitored. The systemic antifungal drugs are listed in Table 52.2.

Pharmacologic options for serious systemic mycoses are limited. Amphotericin B (Fungizone) has been the traditional drug of choice for systemic fungal infections since the 1960s. Azole drugs such as itraconazole, however, are considerably safer and have become preferred drugs for less severe infections. Although rarely used as a monotherapy, flucytosine (Ancobon) is sometimes used in combination with amphotericin B in the pharmacotherapy of

TABLE 52.2   Drugs for Systemic Mycoses

Drug	Route and Adult Dose (Maximum Dose Where Indicated)	Adverse Effects
amphotericin B (Abelcet, AmBisome, Amphotec, Fungizone)	IV: 0.3–1.5 mg/kg/day, infused over 2–4 h (max: 1.5 mg/kg/day)	*Hypokalemia, hypomagnesemia, rash, fever and chills, nausea, vomiting, anorexia, headache* Nephrotoxicity, liver failure, anaphylaxis, cardiac arrest, thrombocytopenia, leukopenia, agranulocytosis, anemia
anidulafungin (Eraxis)	Candidemia IV: 200 mg on day 1, then 100 mg/day for 14 days Esophageal candidiasis IV: 100 mg on day 1, then 50 mg/day for 7–14 days Infusion rate should not exceed 1.1 mg/min	*Diarrhea, nausea, vomiting, mild allergic reactions, hypokalemia* Neutropenia, dysrhythmias, hepatic impairment, anaphylaxis
caspofungin (Cancidas)	IV: 70 mg on day 1, then 50 mg/day infused over 1 h for 14 days	*Fever, chills, diarrhea, increased serum alkaline phosphatase, hypokalemia* Anaphylaxis, hepatic impairment
flucytosine (Ancobon)	PO: 25 mg/kg every 6 h to reach a peak concentration of 50–100 mcg/mL	*Nausea, vomiting, headache* Blood dyscrasias, cardiac toxicity, renal failure, psychosis
micafungin (Mycamine)	IV: 150 mg/kg/day over 1 h for active *Candida* infection; 50 mg/kg/day over 1 h for *Candida* prophylaxis	*Headache, fever, nausea, vomiting, diarrhea, rash* Thrombocytopenia, hemolytic anemia, anaphylaxis, hepatic and renal impairment
Azoles		
fluconazole (Diflucan)	PO/IV: 200–400 mg on day 1, then 100–200 mg/day for 2–4 weeks PO (for vaginal candidiasis): 150 mg single dose	*Fever, chills, rash, dizziness, drowsiness, nausea, vomiting, diarrhea* Hepatotoxicity, anaphylaxis, blood dyscrasias, visual disturbances (voriconazole), dysrhythmias (posaconazole, voriconazole)
itraconazole (Sporanox)	PO: 200 mg/day (max: 400 mg/day)	
ketoconazole (Nizoral)	PO: 200–400 mg/day	
posaconazole (Noxafil)	PO (delayed release tablet): 100–300 mg daily (max: 400 mg/day)	
voriconazole (Vfend)	IV: 6 mg/kg on day 1, then 4 mg/kg every 12 h PO (maintenance dose): 200 mg q12h	

Note: Italics indicate common adverse effects. <u>Underline</u> indicates serious adverse effects.

severe *Candida* infections. Caspofungin (Cancidas) is becoming an important alternative to amphotericin B in the treatment of aspergillosis. Typical protocols for systemic mycoses are listed in Table 52.2.

PROTOTYPE DRUG Amphotericin B Deoxycholate (Fungizone)

Classification: **Therapeutic:** Antifungal (systemic type)
Pharmacologic: Polyene

Therapeutic Effects and Uses: Approved in 1957, amphotericin B has a broad spectrum of activity that includes most fungi that are pathogenic to humans. It is a drug of choice for treating severe systemic mycoses and may also be indicated as prophylactic antifungal therapy for patients with severe immunosuppression. Because it is not absorbed from the gastrointestinal (GI) tract, it is normally given by IV infusion. Topical preparations are available for superficial mycoses that have not responded favorably to other antifungals. Several months of pharmacotherapy may be required for a complete cure. Fungal resistance to amphotericin B is not common but is increasing in incidence.

To reduce the toxicity of amphotericin B, the original molecule has been formulated with several different types of lipid molecules:

- **Liposomal amphotericin B (AmBisome).** Consists of closed spherical vesicles. Amphotericin B is integrated into the membrane, as illustrated in Figure 52.2.
- **Amphotericin B lipid complex (Abelcet).** Contains amphotericin B complexed with two phospholipids in a 1:1 ratio.
- **Amphotericin B cholesteryl sulfate complex (Amphotec).** Consists of a colloidal suspension of amphotericin B in a 1:1 ratio with the lipid cholesteryl sulfate in microscopic disk-shaped particles.

The principal advantage of the lipid formulations is reduced nephrotoxicity and less infusion-related fever and chills. The reduced toxicity is believed to be due to the decreased plasma levels of the drug. Macrophages ingest the lipid formulations and deliver the medication to its fungal targets before it can accumulate to high serum levels that cause toxicity. Because of their expense, however, the lipid preparations are not considered first-line drugs and are generally used only after therapy with other antifungals has failed. A single treatment with the lipid formulations of amphotericin B can cost several thousand dollars.

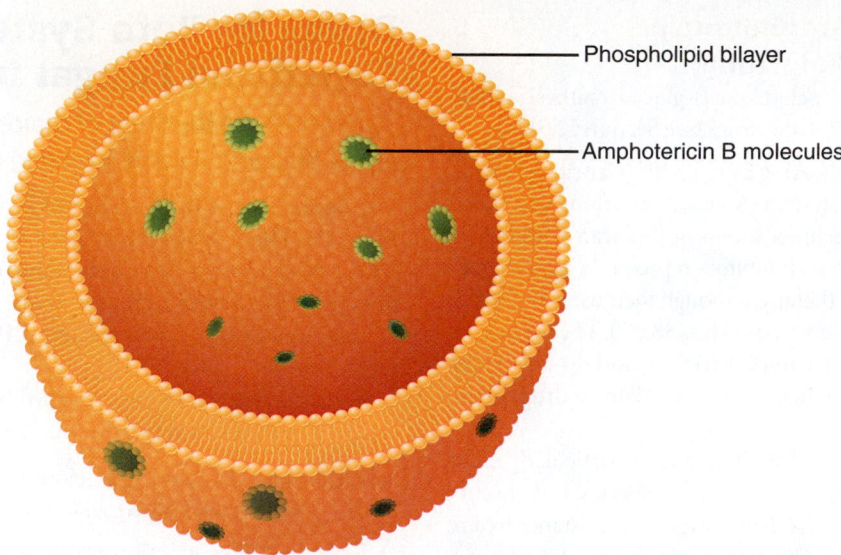

Phospholipid bilayer

Amphotericin B molecules

Figure 52.2 Liposomal amphotericin B: Drug molecules are embedded in the lipid bilayer.

Mechanism of Action: Amphotericin B acts by binding to ergosterol in fungal cell membranes, causing them to become permeable.

Pharmacokinetics:

Route(s)	IV, topical
Absorption	Not absorbed topically
Distribution	Widely distributed; very little enters the cerebrospinal fluid (CSF) or amniotic fluid; about 90% bound to plasma protein
Primary metabolism	Hepatic
Primary excretion	Renal
Onset of action	IV: immediate
Duration of action	Half-life: 24–48 h; drug may persist several weeks after therapy is discontinued

Adverse Effects: Amphotericin B can produce frequent and sometimes serious adverse effects. At the onset of therapy, as many as 50% of patients experience acute, infusion-related fever and chills, vomiting, anorexia, and headache. These symptoms usually subside as treatment continues. Phlebitis is also common during IV therapy, and alternate-day dosing is sometimes needed to reduce this adverse effect. Amphotericin B can cause ototoxicity, potentially affecting both branches, cochlear and vestibular, of cranial nerve VIII.

The most toxic effects of amphotericin B are related to its effects on the kidney. Some degree of nephrotoxicity is observed in 80% of the patients taking amphotericin B; thus laboratory tests of kidney function are regularly performed throughout the treatment period. Electrolyte imbalance, especially hypokalemia and hypomagnesemia, may develop as a result of renal damage, and place the patient at greater risk of developing life-threatening dysrhythmias and cardiac arrest. Concurrent therapy with other medications that reduce liver or renal function, such as aminoglycosides, is not recommended.

Amphotericin B is occasionally hepatotoxic. Anaphylaxis is possible, and cardiac arrest has been reported. Blood abnormalities, including thrombocytopenia, leukopenia, agranulocytosis, and anemia, are potentially serious adverse effects. **Black Box Warning**: The nonliposomal form of this drug should only be used for patients with a progressive and potentially life-threatening fungal infection. Caution should be exercised to prevent inadvertent overdosage.

Contraindications/Precautions: Amphotericin B should be infused slowly, over 2 to 6 hours, because hypotension, hypokalemia, and shock may result if the medication is administered too rapidly. The drug should be withheld if blood urea nitrogen exceeds 40 mg/dL or if serum creatinine rises above 3 mg/dL.

Drug Interactions: Drug interactions with amphotericin B focus on worsening two of its potentially serious adverse effects: nephrotoxicity and hypokalemia. For example, concurrent therapy with aminoglycosides, cyclosporine, vancomycin, carboplatin, and furosemide is not recommended. Corticosteroids, skeletal muscle relaxants, and thiazole may potentiate hypokalemia caused by amphotericin B. Drug-induced hypokalemia will also increase the risk of digoxin toxicity. Because animal studies have indicated an antagonistic effect between amphotericin B and certain azoles (imidazoles), concurrent therapy with this class of antifungals is usually avoided. **Herbal/Food**: Unknown.

Pregnancy: Category B.

Treatment of Overdose: Overdose may result in cardiorespiratory arrest. No specific therapy is available. Patients are treated symptomatically.

Nursing Responsibilities: Key nursing implications for patients receiving amphotericin B are included in the Nursing Practice Application for Patients Receiving Pharmacotherapy with Antifungals.

Drugs Similar to Amphotericin B Deoxycholate (Fungizone)

Other systemic antifungals include the β-glucan synthesis inhibitors, flucytosine, and certain azole drugs (see Section 52.5).

β-Glucan synthesis inhibitors: Caspofungin (Cancidas), anidulafungin (Eraxis), and micafungin (Mycamine) belong to a newer class of antifungals called echinocandins or β-glucan synthesis inhibitors. The glucan synthesis inhibitors represent a major development in antifungal drug therapy, although their use is limited by cost. A single treatment can cost as much as $8,000. The echinocandins are better tolerated than amphotericin B and do not exhibit significant nephrotoxicity or hepatotoxicity. All three drugs in this class are pregnancy category C.

Caspofungin was approved in 2001 and is particularly effective against invasive *Candida* and *Aspergillus* species. It is effective against some fungal species that have developed resistance to amphotericin B and the azoles. The drug is not absorbed if administered PO and must be given by slow IV infusion. Adverse effects with caspofungin include fever and rash and infusion-related reactions such as phlebitis, diarrhea, headache, and nausea. Caution should be used when administering caspofungin to patients with hepatic impairment.

Micafungin, approved in 2005, is used to treat acute disseminated candidiasis, esophageal candidiasis, and *Candida* infections in patients undergoing bone marrow transplants. It is available by slow IV infusion. Micafungin causes transient increases in hepatic enzymes, headache, nausea, and vomiting. Although rare, serious cases of renal and hepatic impairment and hematologic toxicity have occurred with micafungin.

Anidulafungin, the newest drug in this class, was approved in 2006 for candidemia and other systemic *Candida* infections. Like other drugs in this class, anidulafungin is only administered by slow IV infusion. The drug is generally well tolerated with adverse reactions occurring in 2% or less of patients. These adverse effects are generally not severe and include fever, diarrhea, hypokalemia, and increases in liver function test values.

Flucytosine (5-fluorocytosine, Ancobon): Unlike amphotericin B and caspofungin, which must be given parenterally, flucytosine is well absorbed from the GI tract. Approved in 1990, flucytosine is structurally similar to cytosine, a nucleotide used in DNA synthesis. When the fungus attempts to use flucytosine to construct its DNA, cell division is inhibited. It is approved to treat septicemia and pulmonary and urinary tract infections due to *Candida* and *Cryptococcus* species. Unfortunately, resistance to flucytosine is becoming a major clinical problem. The drug is usually used in combination with amphotericin B to reduce the potential for treatment failure due to resistance. Combination therapy also permits the use of lower doses of amphotericin B, thus reducing the risk of nephrotoxicity.

Although adverse GI effects are common with flucytosine, they are usually not severe. The drug carries a black box warning that extreme caution should be used in patients with renal impairment. The warning urges close monitoring of hematologic, renal, and hepatic status during therapy. Flucytosine can cause bone marrow toxicity, leukopenia, agranulocytosis, and thrombocytopenia. Serum concentrations of flucytosine should be less than 100 g/mL to avoid bone marrow suppression. Flucytosine may cause hepatitis and elevate serum levels of hepatic enzymes. This drug is pregnancy category C.

Drugs for Both Systemic and Superficial Fungal Infections

52.5 Azoles are the drugs of choice for many mycoses due to their efficacy and favorable safety profile.

The **azole** class is the largest and most versatile group of antifungals. These drugs have broad spectrums and are used to treat nearly any systemic, subcutaneous, or superficial fungal infection. They have replaced many of the older antifungals because they can be administered PO and have a superior safety profile.

The azoles are sometimes grouped by chemical or therapeutic classes. The azoles form two distinct chemical classes, as follows:

- **Imidazoles.** Butoconazole, clotrimazole, econazole, ketoconazole, miconazole, oxiconazole, sulconazole, and ticonazole

- **Triazoles.** Fluconazole, itraconazole, posaconazole, terconazole, and voriconazole

The triazoles are more slowly metabolized and appear to elicit fewer adverse effects than the imidazoles. Most of the newer azoles under development are in the triazole class. In clinical practice, imidazoles and azoles exhibit the same spectrum of activity and act by the same mechanism.

A second method of classifying azoles is by their therapeutic utility as either systemic or topical agents. Fluconazole (Diflucan), itraconazole (Sporanox), ketoconazole (Nizoral), posaconazole (Noxafil), and voriconazole (Vfend) are used for both systemic and topical infections. The remainder of the azoles are prescribed for superficial infections (see Section 52.6).

Azoles interfere with the biosynthesis of ergosterol, which is essential for the construction of fungal cell membranes. By depleting fungal cells of ergosterol, fungal growth is impaired.

The systemic azoles have a spectrum of activity similar to that of amphotericin B, are considerably less toxic, and have the major advantage that they can be administered PO. Because of these characteristics, azoles have replaced amphotericin B in the pharmacotherapy of less serious systemic fungal infections.

The most common adverse effects of the systemic azoles are nausea and vomiting, which occur in 10% to 20% of patients. Giving the drugs with food or in divided doses may relieve minor GI distress. Severe nausea may require dose reduction or the concurrent administration of an antiemetic. Asymptomatic elevations of serum aminotransferase levels are common during therapy. Anaphylaxis and rash have been reported. Fatal drug-induced hepatitis has occurred with ketoconazole, though the incidence is rare and has not been reported with the other systemic azoles. Because of this, itraconazole has largely replaced ketoconazole in the therapy of systemic mycoses. With all the systemic azoles, liver function tests should be obtained before therapy begins and throughout the course of treatment. Azoles may affect glycemic control, so blood glucose should be monitored regularly in patients with diabetes and those with metabolic syndrome.

Various reproductive abnormalities have been reported with systemic azoles, including menstrual irregularities, gynecomastia in males, and drops in plasma testosterone levels. Decreased libido and temporary sterility in males are other potential adverse effects. Fluconazole is teratogenic in laboratory animals and the safety of the azoles during pregnancy has not been established. The risk–benefit ratio should be carefully weighed before initiating azole therapy in a pregnant patient.

PROTOTYPE DRUG	Fluconazole (Diflucan)

Classification: Therapeutic: Antifungal
Pharmacologic: Inhibitor of fungal cell membrane synthesis, triazole (azole)

Therapeutic Effects and Uses: Approved in 1990, fluconazole is available as tablets, oral suspension, and IV injection. It is particularly effective against *Candida albicans* and is used to treat oropharyngeal candidiasis, esophageal candidiasis, vulvovaginal candidiasis, and various systemic infections by this species. It is also effective against cryptococcal meningitis and may be used for mycoses that are resistant to other antifungals. Fluconazole is less effective against non-*albicans Candida* species, which account for a significant percentage of opportunistic fungal infections. The drug is approved for prophylaxis of fungal infections in patients with AIDS, those undergoing bone marrow transplants, or those receiving antineoplastic drugs.

Fluconazole offers several advantages over other systemic antifungals. It is rapidly and completely absorbed when given PO and is also available by the IV route. Compared to itraconazole and ketoconazole, it more easily penetrates body membranes to reach infections in the central nervous system (CNS), bone, eye, urinary tract, and respiratory tract.

Mechanism of Action: Like other azoles, fluconazole acts by interfering with the synthesis of ergosterol.

Pharmacokinetics:

Route(s)	IV, PO
Absorption	Readily absorbed PO
Distribution	Widely distributed, including the CSF; secreted in breast milk; 12% bound to plasma protein
Primary metabolism	Hepatic
Primary excretion	Renal
Onset of action	Peak effect: 1–2 h
Duration of action	Half-life: 20–50 h

Adverse Effects: Fluconazole causes few serious adverse effects. Nausea, vomiting, and diarrhea are reported at high doses. Because the kidneys excrete most of the drug, it should be used cautiously in patients with preexisting renal impairment. Hepatotoxicity with fluconazole is less common than with ketoconazole. Stevens–Johnson syndrome has been reported in patients with immunosuppression.

Contraindications/Precautions: The only contraindication to fluconazole is hypersensitivity to the drug or another azole. Fluconazole should be used with caution in patients with hepatic impairment because the drug is metabolized in the liver: Hepatic injury has occurred with this drug. When given by the IV route, fluconazole is usually prepared without added medications because it is incompatible with a number of drugs. Patients with hypokalemia should be treated with caution because fluconazole may worsen this electrolyte imbalance.

Drug Interactions: Fluconazole is a strong inhibitor of CYP2C9, CYP2C19, and CYP3A4; therefore, it has the potential to interact with several drugs. Use with warfarin (Coumadin) may increase prothrombin time and cause increased risk for bleeding. Hypoglycemia may result if fluconazole is administered concurrently with certain oral hypoglycemics, including glyburide. Fluconazole levels may be decreased with concurrent rifampin or cimetidine use. The effects of fentanyl, alfentanil, benzodiazepines, tricyclic antidepressants, zidovudine, or methadone may be prolonged with concurrent administration of fluconazole. Fluconazole increases the serum level of phenytoin; careful monitoring of phenytoin concentrations is recommended to avoid CNS toxicity. Rifampin increases the metabolism of fluconazole; thus, the dose of fluconazole may need to be increased to maintain therapeutic plasma levels. Concurrent use of fluconazole and erythromycin increases the risk of cardiotoxicity and possibly sudden heart death. **Herbal/Food**: Unknown.

Pregnancy: Category C.

Treatment of Overdose: No specific therapy is available; patients are treated symptomatically. Dialysis can be used to lower serum drug level.

Nursing Responsibilities: Key nursing implications for patients receiving fluconazole are included in the Nursing Practice Application for Patients Receiving Pharmacotherapy with Antifungals.

Drugs Similar to Fluconazole (Diflucan)

Other systemic azoles include itraconazole, ketoconazole, posaconazole, and voriconazole.

Itraconazole (Sporanox): Approved in 1992, itraconazole is available as capsules, PO solution, and IV injection. Its spectrum is similar to that of other azoles, except it may have greater activity against *Aspergillus*. It is metabolized in the liver to hydroxyitraconazole, which also has antifungal activity. Because the drug may take 2 or more weeks to reach therapeutic levels, a loading dose is infused when treating invasive mycoses. The PO capsules should be taken with food to enhance absorption; however, the PO solution should be taken on an empty stomach. Both PO formulations require an acidic stomach environment for absorption and thus should not be taken concurrently with drugs or foods that decrease stomach acidity.

The most common adverse effects of itraconazole are GI related, especially nausea, which occurs in about 10% of patients. Hepatotoxicity is a rare, though potentially serious, adverse effect, which warrants periodic monitoring of liver laboratory tests. Itraconazole carries a black box warning that the drug should be discontinued if any signs of cardiotoxicity or heart failure arise during therapy. The warning also states that care should be taken when administering itraconazole with other medications, since numerous drug–drug interactions have been reported. Concurrent administration of itraconazole with benzodiazepines or statins is contraindicated. This drug is pregnancy category C.

Ketoconazole (Nizoral): Approved in 1981, ketoconazole is available as tablets for systemic mycoses and as a topical preparation for superficial mycoses. The topical drugs are used to treat dandruff and various tinea infections (see Section 52.6). PO ketoconazole requires an acidic stomach environment for absorption and thus should not be taken concurrently with drugs or foods that decrease stomach acidity. As a systemic drug, it is reserved for invasive mycoses, because it is the most hepatotoxic of the azoles. The most common adverse effects are nausea and vomiting, which can affect over 50% of patients taking high doses of the drug.

Ketoconazole carries several black box warnings, and in 2013 the FDA issued a safety alert that the oral form of the drug should only be used when alternative antifungal therapies have not proven successful. Ketoconazole has been associated with serious hepatotoxicity that can result in death or the need for liver transplantation. Hepatic function must be monitored regularly during therapy and it should not be used in patients with acute or chronic liver disease. Ketoconazole reduces the amount of corticosteroids secreted by the adrenal glands, which can cause symptoms of adrenal insufficiency. Ketoconazole may interact with other medications to cause serious drug–drug interactions; all drugs taken while undergoing ketoconazole must be monitored for potential interactions. Ketoconazole tablets are no longer indicated for fungal infections of the skin and nails. The above safety warnings do not apply to the topical forms of the drug. This drug is pregnancy category C.

Posaconazole (Noxafil): Posaconazole is the newest azole, approved in 2013. It is approved in two formulations for different indications. As delayed release tablets, the drug is approved for *prophylaxis* of invasive *Aspergillus* and *Candida* infections, which can be life threatening in patients with severely compromised immune systems. An oral suspension is approved for the treatment of oropharyngeal candidiasis. Caution must be used when treating patients taking calcineurin inhibitors such as tacrolimus or cyclosporine because posaconazole can increase the serum concentrations of these drugs and cause calcineurin toxicity. Posaconazole should also be used with caution in patients with dysrhythmias because the drug can prolong the QT interval. Its use is contraindicated in patients taking sirolimus, statins, and ergot alkaloids. Common adverse effects include fever, diarrhea, and nausea. This drug is pregnancy category C.

Voriconazole (Vfend): Approved in 2002, voriconazole is a second-generation triazole synthesized from fluconazole that is approved to treat invasive *Aspergillus* infections and serious *Candida* infections. It is believed to be safer and more effective than amphotericin B for these indications. It is available by PO and slow IV infusion. Extreme caution should be used when administering voriconazole to patients with severe renal or hepatic impairment, because this can result in toxic accumulation of the drug. The most frequent adverse events affect vision: enhanced brightness, changes in color vision, and blurred vision. Headache, nausea, vomiting, and rash are also common adverse effects. Although visual impairment occurs in 35% to 45% of patients, it is reversible following discontinuation of therapy. Dermatologic toxicity includes photosensitivity and the potential for Stevens–Johnson syndrome. Because it participates in many drug interactions, the nurse should seek information from a current drug guide when administering voriconazole concurrently with other medications. This drug causes teratogenicity in laboratory animals and is rated as pregnancy category D.

CONNECTION Checkpoint 52.2

Antifungal medications are sometimes administered to patients taking calcineurin inhibitors such as tacrolimus. From what you learned in Chapter 42, what is the primary indication for the calcineurin inhibitors? *See Answer to Connection Checkpoint 52.2 on student resource website.*

Drugs for Superficial Fungal Infections

52.6 Drugs for superficial mycoses are safe and effective at eliminating fungi on the skin, nails, or mucous membranes.

Superficial fungal infections of the hair, scalp, nails, and the mucous membranes of the mouth and vagina are rarely medical emergencies. Infections of the nails may be ongoing for months or even years before a patient seeks treatment. Unlike systemic fungal infections, superficial infections may occur in any patient, not just those who have suppressed immune systems. Drugs used to treat superficial mycoses are listed in Table 52.3.

Superficial antifungal drugs are much safer than their systemic counterparts because penetration into the deeper layers of the skin is limited, and only small amounts are absorbed into the circulation. Many are available as over-the-counter (OTC) creams, gels, and ointments. If the infection has grown into the deeper skin layers, PO antifungal drugs are indicated. Extensive superficial or subcutaneous mycoses are sometimes treated with both PO and topical antifungal agents to ensure that the infection is eliminated from deeper skin layers.

Dermatomycoses: Fungal infections of the skin and hair are called **dermatomycoses**. These infections are named by their Latin terms, beginning with tinea. For example, tinea capitis is an infection of the scalp, and tinea pedis is an infection of the feet.

Fungi that cause dermatomycoses grow in the keratin layer of the skin. Because fungi multiply more rapidly in warm, moist areas, dermatomycoses occur more frequently during the summer months and in warmer climates. They tend to favor skin creases that stay moist due to sweat or following bathing. Because relapse rates following pharmacotherapy are high, the patient should be taught proper personal hygiene measures to help eliminate the pathogen. These include frequent bathing with thorough drying of the infected area, the use of separate towels for the groin area, and wearing loose clothing.

Tinea corporis is an infection in which the fungus invades relatively hairless skin. The fungus typically appears as a ring pattern, thus resulting in the name ringworm. Transmission may occur through direct contact with infected animals (especially cats and dogs), infected humans, or contaminated furniture or clothing. The most common pathogens are *Trichophyton* and *Microsporum* species. Topical therapies are usually successful in controlling tinea corporis. In cases of inflammatory lesions, oral therapy with griseofulvin (Fulvicin), terbinafine (Lamisil), itraconazole (Sporanox), or fluconazole (Diflucan) is recommended.

Tinea cruris, commonly called jock itch, is a form of tinea corporis that occurs in the groin, perineum, and perianal region. Topical powders and creams are usually sufficient to cure tinea cruris.

TABLE 52.3 Selected Drugs for Superficial Mycoses

Drug	Route and Adult Dose (Maximum Dose Where Indicated)	Adverse Effects
butenafine (Mentax)	Topical: Apply daily for 2–4 weeks for tineas	*Drying of skin, stinging sensation at application site, pruritus, urticaria, contact dermatitis*
ciclopirox cream, gel, shampoo (Loprox), or nail lacquer (Penlac)	Topical: Apply cream bid for 4 weeks for tineas Topical: Apply lacquer to nail for 48 weeks for onychomycosis	
griseofulvin (Fulvicin)	PO: 500 mg microsize or 330–375 mg ultra microsize daily for tineas and onychomycosis	Granulocytopenia (griseofulvin), cholestatic hepatitis (oral terbinafine), neutropenia (oral terbinafine)
naftifine (Naftin)	Topical: Apply cream daily or gel bid for 4 weeks for tineas	
nystatin: topical powder (Mycostatin, Nystop); oral suspension (Nilstat) capsule (Bio-Statin); cream, ointment (Mycostatin, Nystex)	Suspension PO: 400,000–600,000 units 4 times/day Topical: Apply 2–3 times/day to the affected area Capsule: PO: 500,000 to 1 million units every 6 h Vaginal tablets: Insert 1 tablet daily for 2 weeks	
tavaborole (Kerydin)	Topical: Apply 5% solution once daily for 48 weeks	
terbinafine (Lamisil)	Topical: Apply once daily or bid for 7 weeks for tineas PO: 250 mg/day for 6–12 weeks for onychomycosis	
tolnaftate (Aftate, Tinactin)	Topical: Apply to the affected area twice daily for 2 weeks for tinea cruris and 4 weeks for tinea pedis or corporis	
undecylenic acid (Fungi-Nail, Gordochom, Others)	Topical: Apply once or twice daily for tineas for up to 4 weeks	

Azoles

Drug	Route and Adult Dose (Maximum Dose Where Indicated)	Adverse Effects
butoconazole (Femstat, Gynazole)	Intravaginal: Femstat: 1 applicator for 3 days Gynazole: 1 applicator as a single dose	*Drying of the skin, stinging sensation at application site, pruritus, urticaria, contact dermatitis*
clotrimazole: topical cream (Lotrimin AF); intravaginal (Gyne-Lotrimin, Mycelex, Others); troche (Mycelex)	Topical: Apply 1% cream bid for 4 weeks Intravaginal: 1 applicator for 7 days; one 100-mg tablet vaginally for 7 days or one 500-mg tablet once Troche: Dissolve one in the mouth over 15–30 min	Topical drugs exhibit few serious adverse effects except hypersensitivity
econazole (Spectazole)	Topical: Apply 1% cream bid for 4 weeks for tineas or cutaneous candidiasis	
fluconazole (Diflucan)	PO: 150 mg once, for vulvovaginal candidiasis (VVC)	
itraconazole (Sporanox)	PO: 200 mg daily for 1–2 weeks for OPC PO: 200 mg daily for 3 days for VVC PO: 200 mg daily for 3 months for onychomycosis	
ketoconazole (Nizoral)	Topical: Apply 2% cream or shampoo 1–2 times/day to affected area for tineas	
luliconazole (Luzu)	Topical: Apply 1% cream once daily for 2 weeks for tineas	
miconazole (Micatin, Monistat-3, Oravig)	Topical (Micatin): Apply 2% cream bid for 2–4 weeks Intravaginal (Monistat-3): Insert one suppository daily for 3 days for VVC Buccal (Oravig): Apply one tablet to the gum region daily for 2 weeks for oral candidiasis	
oxiconazole (Oxistat)	Topical: Apply 1% cream daily for 2 months for tineas and cutaneous candidiasis	
sulconazole (Exelderm)	Topical: Apply 1% cream daily or bid for 2–6 weeks for tineas	
terconazole (Terazol)	Intravaginal: 1 applicator for 3–7 weeks for VVC	
tioconazole (Monistat-1, Vagistat-1)	Intravaginal: 1 applicator as a single dose	

Note: Italics indicate common adverse effects. Underline indicates serious adverse effects.

PO antifungal drugs such as griseofulvin (Fulvicin), terbinafine (Lamisil), itraconazole (Sporanox), or fluconazole (Diflucan) may be necessary for severe cases.

Tinea pedis, commonly called athlete's foot, is a type of tinea corporis occurring on the feet, principally occurring between the toes and on the sole. It is associated with the wearing of shoes and contact with infected bath or pool floors. Tinea pedis is the most common dermatomycosis, affecting about 70% of adults at some time during their life. Topical antifungals are effective for noninflammatory tinea pedis. PO therapy is sometimes used to treat more severe infections and areas such as the soles. Typical therapy includes terbinafine (Lamisil) or itraconazole (Sporanox) for 2 to 4 weeks.

Tinea capitis involves the hair of the head, eyebrows, or eyelashes, and primarily affects children between 4 and 14 years of age. *Trichophyton* is responsible for more than 90% of cases. In contrast with other dermatomycoses, tinea capitis is routinely treated with PO agents. Typical regimens include the following:

- Griseofulvin (Fulvicin): 10 mg/kg/day for 8 to 10 weeks
- Itraconazole (Sporanox): 5 mg/kg/day for 1 to 4 weeks
- Terbinafine (Lamisil): 62.5 to 250 mg/day for 4 weeks

Onychomycosis: **Onychomycosis**, or tinea unguium, is the invasion of the nail plate by a fungus. It is a relatively common infection, affecting 2% to 3% of Americans. Rates among men are twice that of women, and infections increase with age. The higher incidence in elderly patients is believed to be due to reduced peripheral circulation, general inactivity, increased nail trauma, and difficulty (or inability) in maintaining proper nail hygiene. One in four patients with diabetes will acquire onychomycosis, likely due to reduced circulation to the area.

The most common fungal pathogens responsible for onychomycosis are *Trichophyton* and *Epidermophyton* species. Although any part of the nail may be affected, most commonly the infection begins with invasion of the hyponychium, the place where the nail separates from the nail bed. Toenails are more often affected than fingernails. The nail becomes markedly disfigured and distorted.

Although certainly not a life-threatening infection, onychomycosis is one of the most difficult superficial fungal infections to treat. Nails grow slowly and the nail plate is hard, preventing antifungal agents from penetrating. The traditional drug for onychomycosis has been griseofulvin (Fulvicin), but this drug has a narrow spectrum of activity. In addition, cure rates are low and recurrence is common. In recent years, terbinafine (Lamisil) and itraconazole (Sporanox) have become drugs of choice for onychomycosis. Both of these drugs are absorbed into the nail matrix and remain active for several months. Itraconazole can be detected in nail clippings for up to a year after administration and terbinafine for up to 3 months. This long duration is important, because nails may take 9 to 12 months to be totally replaced. Typical therapies have an 80% cure rate and include the following:

- Terbinafine (Lamisil): 250 mg daily for 3 months
- Itraconazole (Sporanox): 200 mg twice daily for 1 week/month. This cycle is repeated twice for fingernails and three to four times for toenails
- Ciclopirox Nail Lacquer (Penlac): Daily application to the affected nails for 48 weeks
- Fluconazole (Diflucan): 150 to 450 mg weekly for 6 to 9 months. This drug is used for persistent infections

Until recently, topical therapy alone was not successful for the treatment of onychomycosis because the available drugs could not penetrate deeply enough to eradicate the fungus. Ciclopirox solution (Penlac) is a newer drug applied as a topical nail lacquer for the treatment of mild to moderate onychomycosis. The drug is applied daily, covering the entire nail plate and surrounding skin for 12 months. Ciclopirox has a relatively high relapse rate and does not appear to be as effective as terbinafine or itraconazole.

Superficial candidiasis: Although there are at least 10 species of *Candida* that cause disease in humans, *C. albicans* is responsible for nearly 100% of cases of oropharyngeal fungal infections and at least 90% of cases of vulvovaginal candidiasis. A small yeast, *Candida* is often found as part of normal host flora on body surfaces. *Candida* species are the most common pathogens causing fungal disease in patients with compromised immune defenses.

Oropharyngeal candidiasis (OPC) is an oral mycosis, sometimes called thrush. About 50% of people carry *Candida* in the mouth as part of their host flora. Infection occurs when the patient's defenses are weakened; thus the highest incidence of OPC is seen in patients with AIDS, diabetes, or cancer, and in hospitalized patients. Patients taking inhaled corticosteroids are also at greater risk because these drugs cause a local immunosuppression in the oral cavity. Although not life threatening, OPC may predispose a patient to esophageal candidiasis, which is a serious, invasive mycosis.

Several options are available for the pharmacotherapy of OPC. Topical therapy is generally preferred and is often successful for milder, uncomplicated infections. Troches and PO suspensions are the most common formulations for topical therapy. Symptoms generally subside in 2 to 3 days but the nurse should encourage the patient to complete the full 1- to 2-week course of therapy. Typical treatments for OPC are as follows:

- Nystatin: lozenges, 200,000 units, or PO suspension, 500,000 units, by swish and swallow, four times daily for 7 to 14 days

---

CONNECTIONS | **Lifespan Considerations**

Oropharyngeal Candidiasis in Infants

Oropharyngeal candidiasis (OPC) (thrush) is commonly seen in infants. It is often difficult to distinguish from milk and appears as white patches on the tongue, palate, and inner aspects of the cheeks. Frequently, the infant with thrush may refuse to suck or feed because of mouth irritation. Transmission of this fungal infection may occur during a vaginal birth when the infant comes in contact with the mother's normal flora, or during feedings, including breast-feeding. In most cases, thrush is self-limiting and resolves spontaneously. However, it may take as long as 2 months to resolve, during which time it may spread to the larynx, trachea, bronchi, lungs, and GI tract.

The condition is treated with good hygiene, application of a fungicide, and correction of any underlying causes. Because the mother is often the source of the infection, she should also be treated to prevent reinfections. Fluconazole (Diflucan) and nystatin (Mycostatin) are commonly used, including for topical treatment of the nipple area of the mother if continued thrush is present.

Antifungal medications should be administered to the infant after feedings. When possible, sips of water may be useful to rinse away milk sugars and proteins after the feeding. Using an applicator or syringe, the medication should be distributed over the entire surface of the oral mucosa and tongue. After swabbing the area, the remainder of the dose is then deposited in the infant's mouth to be swallowed to treat any more extensive infection.

- Clotrimazole (Mycelex): 10-mg troche, slowly dissolved in the mouth five times a day for 7 to 14 days
- Fluconazole (Diflucan): 100 to 200 mg/day for 7 to 14 days
- Itraconazole (Sporanox): suspension, 200 mg (20 mL) daily by swish and swallow for 7 to 14 days; or capsules, 200 mg/day for 2 to 4 weeks

Extensive OPC, especially in immunosuppressed patients and in those with esophageal involvement, is treated with systemic therapy. Prolonged therapy with regular follow-up may be required in these patients. Prophylactic therapy of OPC using azole antifungals may be warranted in patients with AIDS. Prolonged prophylactic therapy, however, leads to azole-resistant *Candida* species. The practice is generally discouraged because OPC has a low mortality rate, and empirical treatment of the infection in these patients is generally successful.

PharmFACT
Oropharyngeal candidiasis in the neonate is most commonly acquired from the infected mucosa of the mother during passage of the infant through the birth canal. Neonatal candidiasis presents 3 to 7 days after birth with oral thrush and diaper dermatitis (Scheinfeld, 2014).

Candida species are part of the normal vaginal flora in about 50% of healthy women. Because vulvovaginal candidiasis (VVC) occurs in both healthy and immunosuppressed women, it is not considered an opportunistic infection. The biggest risk factors for VVC are sexual activity, pregnancy, diabetes mellitus, the use of oral contraceptives with high estrogen content, or broad-spectrum antibiotics. *Candida* may be transmitted to male sexual partners. Its highest incidence occurs between the ages of 30 and 40. *C. albicans* is by far the most common species, although *Candida glabrata* is an emerging pathogen for VVC.

Several effective topical agents for VVC are available without a prescription. The various topical regimens have equal effectiveness in treating VVC, with response rates of 80% to 90%. Many women prefer PO therapies because of their convenience. Oral therapy has the same efficacy as topical treatment.

Regimens for VVC are classified by their duration of therapy. The most popular therapies are 1-day PO regimens, due to their ease of use. Although 1-day treatments are effective for most women with VVC, there are limitations to this brief therapy. Because 1-day treatments may take up to 48 hours to produce relief, faster acting topical agents may be more beneficial for patients with severe symptoms. In addition, patients with complicated, persistent, or severe infections require 10 to 14 days of therapy for successful elimination of the pathogen, regardless of the route of administration. Typical therapies for VVC include the following:

- Single topical application: ticonazole (Vagistat-1, Monistat-1), 6.5% ointment; butoconazole (Gynazole), 2% cream (sustained release formulation); miconazole, 2% cream
- Single PO dose: fluconazole, one 150-mg tablet; itraconazole, 200 mg bid for 1 day; clotrimazole, one 500-mg tablet for 1 day
- Multiday regimens: butoconazole (Femstat), 2% cream, for 1 to 7 days; clotrimazole (Lotrimin AF), 1% cream or 100-mg tablets for 1 to 7 days; miconazole, 2% cream or 100- to 200-mg suppositories for 1 to 7 days; or nystatin, 100,000-unit vaginal tablet daily for 7 to 14 days

Because recurrent VVC may occur in 5% of patients treated for this infection, cultures may be necessary to identify the specific pathogen. Treatment begins with a 14-day induction phase that uses the same drugs as for nonrecurring infections. A maintenance phase follows, typically with azole antifungals taken once weekly (fluconazole) or once monthly (itraconazole) for 6 months.

PharmFACT
Three of every four women will experience vulvovaginal candidiasis at least once during their lifetime (Hidalgo, 2014).

CONNECTION Checkpoint 52.3
From what you learned in Chapter 46, why might broad-spectrum antibacterial therapy cause a *Candida* infection of the vagina? *See Answer to Connection Checkpoint 52.3 on student resource website.*

PROTOTYPE DRUG	Nystatin (Mycostatin, Nystop, Others)

Classification: Therapeutic: Antifungal, superficial type
Pharmacologic: Polyene

Therapeutic Effects and Uses: Approved in 1954, nystatin belongs to the same chemical class as amphotericin B, the polyenes. Although it acts by the same mechanism as the polyenes, nystatin has very different indications and is available in a wider variety of formulations, including cream, ointment, powder, tablets, and lozenges. Too toxic for parenteral administration, it is usually used topically to treat *Candida* infections of the vagina, skin, and mouth because it is not absorbed in these areas. Although available as vaginal tablets, the azoles have largely replaced nystatin due to their higher efficacy. PO suspensions are available to treat OPC, using a swish-and-swallow technique. Some formulations, such as Mytrex and Mycolog II cream, combine nystatin with triamcinolone (a corticosteroid) for treating inflamed subcutaneous lesions. It is available as tablets to treat candidiasis of the intestine, since it travels through the GI tract without being absorbed. It is not effective for treating onychomycosis.

Mechanism of Action: Nystatin binds to sterols in the fungal cell membrane, allowing leakage of intracellular contents across the weakened membrane.

Pharmacokinetics:

Route(s)	PO suspensions, troches, topical creams, and vaginal tablets; PO tablets for intestinal infections
Absorption	Poorly absorbed
Distribution	Not distributed
Primary metabolism	Not metabolized
Primary excretion	Excreted unchanged in the feces
Onset of action	Rapid
Duration of action	Half-life: 6–12 h

Adverse Effects: When given topically, nystatin produces few adverse effects other than minor skin irritation and burning at the site of application. There is a high incidence of contact dermatitis, related to the preservatives found in some of the formulations. When given PO, it may cause diarrhea, nausea, and vomiting.

Contraindications/Precautions: The only contraindication to nystatin therapy is hypersensitivity to the drug. Although no teratogenic effects have been reported, safety during pregnancy and lactation has not been established.

Drug Interactions: Unknown.

Pregnancy: Category B.

Treatment of Overdose: No specific therapy is available; patients are treated symptomatically.

Nursing Responsibilities: Key nursing implications for patients receiving nystatin are included in the Nursing Practice Application for Patients Receiving Pharmacotherapy with Antifungals.

Drugs Similar to Nystatin (Mycostatin, Nystop, Others)

Other superficial antifungals include griseofulvin, terbinafine, topical azoles, and several miscellaneous drugs.

Griseofulvin (Grifulvin V, Gris-PEG): Approved in 1959, griseofulvin is an inexpensive antifungal that is indicated for the PO therapy of mycoses of the hair, skin, and nails that have not responded to conventional topical preparations. It is not given topically because the drug is unable to penetrate into the deeper skin layers when given by this route. In an attempt to reduce adverse GI effects and increase its bioavailability, griseofulvin is available as microsize particles (Grifulvin V) and ultramicrosize particles (Gris-PEG). Grifulvin V is 25% to 70% absorbed and Gris-PEG is almost 100% absorbed.

The length of treatment for tinea pedis is 4 to 8 weeks and for tinea unguium, 3 to 6 months. Griseofulvin is deposited in keratin, where it accumulates and inhibits mitosis of the fungal cells. It exhibits few adverse effects, other than headache. Although rare, hepatitis and neutropenia have been reported with prolonged therapy.

Griseofulvin has a higher incidence of long-term adverse effects and has a greater relapse rate than some other superficial antifungal agents. This drug is pregnancy category C.

Terbinafine (Lamisil): Approved in 1993, terbinafine may be administered by the PO or topical route. Terbinafine acts by inhibiting ergosterol biosynthesis. The PO form of the drug is available by prescription to treat onychomycosis. The drug rapidly accumulates in nails, although therapy of persistent onychomycosis may require 6 to 12 weeks. The cure rate for onychomycosis is 50% to 70%, which is higher than that for griseofulvin. Oral preparations are well tolerated, with nausea, vomiting, abdominal pain, and diarrhea being the most common adverse effects. Rare, though serious, adverse effects include Stevens–Johnson syndrome, blood dyscrasias, and hepatic failure.

Nonprescription formulations such as Lamisil AT include topical creams and sprays for treating tinea corporis, tinea pedis, and tinea cruris. Adverse effects are rare with topical terbinafine; irritation or urticaria occurs in less than 1% of patients. The drug is not absorbed when administered topically. Both PO and topical forms of terbinafine are pregnancy category B.

Topical Azoles: Eleven azoles are used to treat superficial mycoses. Itraconazole, voriconazole, posaconazole, and fluconazole may be used PO to treat superficial mycoses, whereas the others are for topical use only. Among the topical drugs, all have equal effectiveness and similar adverse effects. Miconazole and clotrimazole are preferred drugs available OTC for vulvovaginal *Candida* infections, although a number of other azoles are available that are equally effective. Transient burning and irritation at the application sites are the most common adverse effects of the topical azoles.

Miscellaneous Topical Antifungals: Several agents are less commonly used for superficial fungal infections. These drugs are applied topically, for tineas, or intravaginally, for VVC. The doses and indications for these drugs are shown in Table 52.3.

CONNECTIONS: NURSING PRACTICE APPLICATION

Patients Receiving Pharmacotherapy with Antifungals

Assessment	Potential Nursing Diagnoses*
Baseline assessment prior to administration: • Obtain a complete health history including neurologic, cardiovascular, respiratory, hepatic, or renal disease, and the possibility of pregnancy. Obtain a drug history including allergies (e.g., specific reactions to drugs), current prescription and OTC drugs, herbal preparations, and alcohol use. Be alert to possible drug interactions. • Assess for signs and symptoms of current infection, noting location, characteristics, presence or absence of drainage, and character of drainage, duration, presence or absence of fever or pain. • Evaluate appropriate laboratory findings (e.g., complete blood count [CBC], electrolytes, urinalysis, culture and sensitivity [C&S], hepatic and renal function studies). • Obtain baseline weight and vital signs, especially blood pressure and pulse. • Assess the patient's ability to receive and understand instructions. Include family and caregivers as needed.	• *Infection* • *Acute Pain* • *Hyperthermia* • *Decreased Cardiac Output*, related to adverse drug effects • *Deficient Knowledge* (Drug Therapy) • *Risk for Injury*, related to adverse drug effects • *Risk for Deficient Fluid Volume*, related to adverse drug effects
Assessment throughout administration: • Assess for desired therapeutic effects (e.g., diminished signs and symptoms of infection and fever, surface lesions are improving or cleared). • Continue periodic monitoring of CBC, electrolytes, hepatic and renal function, C&S. • Continue to monitor vital signs, especially blood pressure and pulse, in patients on IV antifungal drugs. • Assess for adverse effects: nausea, vomiting, abdominal cramping, diarrhea, malaise, muscle cramping or pain, chills, drowsiness, dizziness, headache, tinnitus, vertigo, flushing, skin rash, urticaria, seizures, hypotension, electrolyte imbalances (e.g., hypokalemia, hypomagnesemia). Immediately report hypotension, tachycardia, dysrhythmia, changes in level of consciousness, diminished urine output, or seizures.	

Implementation

Interventions and (Rationales)	Patient-Centered Care
Ensuring therapeutic effects: • Continue assessments as above for therapeutic effects. (Diminished fever, pain, or signs and symptoms of infection should be noted.)	• Teach the patient on oral antifungals that several months of treatment may be required. The entire course of therapy should be completed and the patient should return to the provider if symptoms have not resolved.
Minimizing adverse effects: • Continue frequent monitoring of vital signs, especially blood pressure and pulse, and respiratory rate and depth in patients on IV antifungal drugs. Immediately report dysrhythmias, increasing pulmonary congestion, hypotension, or tachycardia. (Hypotension, tachycardia, dysrhythmias, cardiac collapse, and cardiac arrest are possible adverse effects of antifungal drugs given IV. **Lifespan:** Be particularly cautious with older adults who are at increased risk for hypotension and falls.)	• Instruct the patient on the need for frequent monitoring. Explain the rationale for all monitoring equipment used. • Teach the patient to rise from lying to sitting or standing slowly to avoid dizziness or falls if hypotension is noted. If dizziness occurs, the patient should sit or lie down and not attempt to stand or walk until the sensation passes.
• Continue to monitor periodic laboratory work: hepatic and renal function tests, CBC, urinalysis, C&S, electrolyte levels. (Antifungals are hepatic and renal toxic. Antifungals, particularly when given IV, may cause electrolyte imbalances, especially hypokalemia and hypomagnesemia, and electrolyte replacement may be needed.)	• Teach the patient the need for frequent laboratory testing. If prescribed oral antifungals for home use, instruct the patient on the need for periodic laboratory work, depending on the type of drug and the length of therapy.
• Ensure adequate hydration in patients on oral or IV antifungal drugs. Weigh the patient daily and report weight gain of 1 kg (2 lb) or more in a 24-h period. Measure intake or output in a 24-h period and monitor intake and output in the hospitalized patient. (Systemic antifungal drugs may be renal toxic. Adequate hydration helps to prevent adverse renal effects. Daily weight is an accurate measure of fluid status and takes into account intake, output, and insensible losses. Excessive weight gain or edema may indicate renal dysfunction.)	• Teach the patient to increase fluid intake to 2 L/day if on oral antifungal drugs. • Have the patient taking oral antifungal drugs at home weigh self daily, ideally at the same time of day, and record the weight. Have the patient report weight gain of more than 1 kg (2 lb) in a 24-h period.

(continued)

- Monitor for hypersensitivity and allergic reactions, especially with the first dose of an antifungal given IV. Continue to monitor the patient throughout therapy. (Anaphylactic reactions are possible and most common with the first IV infusion. Fever, chills, nausea, and headache are common reactions. A test dose of a small amount given slowly may be given before the main infusion. Premedication, including antipyretics, antihistamines or corticosteroids, and antiemetics, may be required to prevent reactions.)

  - Instruct the patient to promptly report any chills, nausea, tremors, palpitations, or headache.

- Continue to monitor for signs of ototoxicity; e.g., tinnitus, dizziness, or vertigo, and report promptly. (Antifungals given systemically may cause ototoxicity and require frequent monitoring to prevent adverse effects.)

  - Teach the patient to immediately report any ringing, humming, or buzzing in the ears, dizziness, or vertigo.

- Continue to monitor for hepatic toxicity; e.g., jaundice, right upper quadrant pain, darkened urine, diminished urine output, tinnitus, or vertigo in patients on systemic antifungal therapy. (Antifungals may cause hepatic toxicity. **Diverse Patients:** Because fluconazole is metabolized through the P450 system pathways, monitor ethnically diverse patients frequently to ensure optimal therapeutic effects and minimize adverse effects.)

  - Teach the patient to immediately report any nausea, vomiting, yellowing of the skin or sclera, abdominal pain, light or clay-colored stools, or darkening of urine.

- Monitor the IV site frequently for any signs of extravasation or thrombophlebitis. (IV antifungal medication is irritating to the vein and the IV site should be monitored frequently. A central line may be used when possible.)

  - Instruct the patient to immediately report any pain, burning, or redness at the site of peripheral IV. Explain the rationale for all equipment used.

- Monitor blood glucose levels in patients taking azole antifungal drugs such as fluconazole or ketoconazole. (Azole antifungals may increase glucose levels. Patients with diabetes may require a change in their antidiabetic drug routine.)

  - Teach patients with diabetes to test their glucose more frequently, reporting any consistent elevations to the health care provider.

- Monitor for significant GI effects, including nausea, vomiting, abdominal pain, or cramping. Give the drug with food or milk to decrease adverse GI effects. (Food or milk may decrease GI effects but an antiemetic may also be required if nausea is severe.)

  - Teach the patient to take the drug with food or milk but to avoid acidic foods and beverages or carbonated drinks.

Patient understanding of drug therapy:

- Use opportunities during administration of medications and during assessments to discuss the rationale for drug therapy, desired therapeutic outcomes, commonly observed adverse effects, parameters for when to call the health care provider, and any necessary monitoring or precautions. (Using time during nursing care helps to optimize and reinforce key teaching areas.)

  - The patient, family, or caregiver should be able to state the reason for the drug, appropriate dose and scheduling, what adverse effects to observe for and when to report them, and the anticipated length of the medication therapy.

Patient self-administration of drug therapy:

- When administering medications, instruct the patient, family, or caregiver in proper self-administration techniques. (Utilizing time during nurse-administration of these drugs helps to reinforce teaching.)

  - Teach the patient to take oral or topical antifungal medication:
    - Complete the entire course of therapy unless otherwise instructed. Several months of oral therapy may be required to adequately treat the infection.
    - Avoid or eliminate alcohol while on oral antifungals to avoid hepatic complications.
    - Dissolve oral antifungal lozenges (troches) in the mouth, or rinse with liquids after meals and at bedtime. If dentures are worn, remove them before using the drug and leave them out overnight. Swish the liquid drug around the mouth and hold in the mouth at least 2 min before expectorating. Do not swallow unless instructed to do so by the provider and do not rinse the mouth with water afterward.
    - Do not use occlusive dressings when topical antifungals are used. Apply a thin even layer to the affected area.
    - Allow affected skin areas to air dry when possible, and wear loose-fitting and breathable fabric clothes to allow adequate ventilation. Gently cleanse areas with mild soap and water. Avoid vigorous scrubbing.

CHAPTER

52   Understanding the Chapter

Key Concepts Summary

52.1 Serious fungal infections are uncommon in people with healthy immune defenses.

52.2 Mycoses are classified as superficial, subcutaneous, or systemic.

52.3 Antifungal drugs act by disrupting the fungal cell membrane or wall, affecting fungal enzymes, or disrupting replication.

52.4 Systemic or invasive fungal disease may require intensive pharmacotherapy for extended periods.

52.5 Azoles are the drugs of choice for many mycoses due to their efficacy and favorable safety profile.

52.6 Drugs for superficial mycoses are safe and effective at eliminating fungi on the skin, nails, or mucous membranes.

Case Study: Making the Patient Connection

Remember the patient "Sarah Williams" at the beginning of the chapter? Now read the remainder of the case study. Based on the information presented within this chapter, respond to the critical thinking questions that follow.

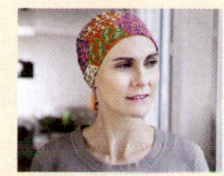

Sarah Williams is a 54-year-old female with lung cancer who recently finished her second round of chemotherapy. She comes to her appointment at the oncology clinic with concerns about white patches on her tongue and mouth. She states that her mouth is not sore but her throat burns when she swallows. This has made it very difficult for her to eat and drink.

A history and physical exam are completed. She is 5'3" tall and weighs 52.7 kg (116 lb). The health care provider evaluates Sarah for oropharyngeal

candidiasis. Sarah was diagnosed with lung cancer several months prior and is taking chemotherapy and corticosteroids. Upon initial assessment, her vital signs are normal, and she has no complaints except her expressed concerns about her mouth and throat. She has worn dentures for about 5 years.

Critical Thinking Questions

1. What are the signs and symptoms that you, as the nurse, look for to determine if Sarah is experiencing oropharyngeal candidiasis?

2. Why do you think that Sarah is at risk for this type of infection?

3. What treatment do you anticipate that Sarah will receive? What patient teaching will she need regarding this treatment?

See Answers to Critical Thinking Questions on student resource website.

Additional Case Study

Sean Seales is a 23-year-old patient with Hodgkin's lymphoma who is undergoing chemotherapy. He has experienced chills and fever with increasing fatigue for the past several days. Sean was assessed by his oncologist and was hospitalized for possible early sepsis. He is neutropenic and will be started on IV antibiotics and fluconazole (Diflucan) IV.

1. Why was Sean started on both IV antibiotics and antifungal medication?

2. What possible adverse effects might Sean experience from the fluconazole (Diflucan)? As his nurse, what will you monitor?

See Answers to Additional Case Study on student resource website.

Chapter Review

1 A patient is admitted to the intensive care unit for systemic fungal infections. Amphotericin B has been ordered and the nurse will administer this drug slowly IV. When administered too rapidly, amphotericin B may cause what significant adverse effects? Select all that apply.

1. Laryngeal spasms
2. Hypotension
3. Hypokalemia
4. Shock
5. Hypoglycemia

2 A patient with AIDS has been given a prescription for oral fluconazole (Diflucan) to prevent *Candida* infection. Considering the patient's primary diagnosis and the order for fluconazole, what essential teaching will the nurse provide?

1. Keep a food diary and request antinausea medication if eating becomes problematic.
2. Maintain regular low-impact exercise daily to avoid loss of muscle mass.
3. Wear a high-filtration mask if going out in public.
4. Avoid all fat-based soaps and allow the body to air-dry after bathing.

3 Nystatin (Mycostatin) suspension has been ordered for treatment of thrush (oropharyngeal *Candida*) in a 6-week-old infant. What instructions should the caregiver receive? Select all that apply.

1. Give the infant a small amount of water after feedings and before the drug to rinse the mouth.
2. Using an applicator or syringe, distribute the solution around the mouth and tongue, allowing the infant to swallow the remainder.
3. Chill the suspension in the refrigerator before giving for better taste.
4. Give the suspension before feeding the infant to prevent adverse GI effects.
5. Add the suspension to a bottle of formula for easier administration.

4 The nurse is caring for a patient with onychomycosis (nail fungus) who is receiving oral terbinafine (Lamisil) for treatment. The patient questions the need for 3 months' worth of pills. What is the nurse's best response?

1. "The health care provider will evaluate the nails monthly and stop treatment earlier if warranted."
2. "It is cheaper to buy more pills at one time than on a monthly schedule."
3. "The extensive prescription avoids the need for shorter term, potentially toxic doses."
4. "Nails grow slowly and the nail beds must receive adequate length of treatment to eliminate the infection."

5 The nurse knows that pretreatment with corticosteroids, antihistamines, and antipyretics prior to the administration of amphotericin B is given for what effect?

1. They enhance the effectiveness of amphotericin B.
2. They eliminate toxic by-products of amphotericin B.
3. They reduce the severity of adverse effects associated with amphotericin B.
4. They increase the half-life of amphotericin B.

6 A patient with diabetes treated with oral antidiabetic medications is receiving oral fluconazole (Diflucan) for treatment of long-standing tinea cruris (jock itch). The nurse will instruct the patient to monitor blood sugar more frequently while on this drug because of what potential drug effects?

1. Fluconazole (Diflucan) antagonizes the effects of antidiabetic drugs.
2. Fluconazole (Diflucan) may increase blood sugar levels.
3. Fluconazole (Diflucan) may decrease blood sugar levels.
4. Fluconazole (Diflucan) may enhance the effects of antidiabetic drugs.

See Answers to Chapter Review in Appendix A.

References

Auberger, J., Lass-Flörl, C., Aigner, M., Clausen, J., Gastl, G., & Nachbaur, D. (2012). Invasive fungal breakthrough infections, fungal colonization and emergence of resistant strains in high-risk patients receiving antifungal prophylaxis with posaconazole: Real-life data from a single-centre institutional retrospective observational study. *Journal of Antimicrobial Chemotherapy, 67,* 2268–2273. doi:10.1093/jac/dks189

des Champs-Bro, B., Leroy-Cotteau, A., Mazingue, F., Pasquier, F., Francois, N., Corm, S., ... Sendid,

B. (2011). Invasive fungal infections: Epidemiology and analysis of antifungal prescriptions in onco-haematology. *Journal of Clinical Pharmacy and Therapeutics, 36,* 152–160. doi:10.1111/j.1365-2710.2010.01166.x

Gould, D. (2011). Diagnosis, prevention and treatment of fungal infections. *Nursing Standard, 25*(33), 38–48. doi:10.7748/ns2011.04.25.33.38.c8464

Hidalgo, J. A. (2014). *Candidiasis.* Retrieved from http://emedicine.medscape.com/article/213853-overview

Madigan, M., & Martinko, J. (2006). *Brock biology of microorganisms* (11th ed., p. 691). Upper Saddle River, NJ: Pearson.

Scheinfeld, N. S. (2014). *Cutaneous candidiasis.* Retrieved from http://emedicine.medscape.com/article/1090632-overview#a0101

Tosti, A. (2014). *Onychomycosis.* Retrieved from http://emedicine.medscape.com/article/1105828-overview

Selected Bibliography

Alangaden, G. J. (2011). Nosocomial fungal infections: Epidemiology, infection control, and prevention. *Infectious Disease Clinics of North America, 25,* 201–225. doi:10.1016/j.idc.2010.11.003

Anderson-Berry, A. L. (2010). Health care–associated infections in the neonatal intensive care unit, a review of impact, risk factors, and prevention strategies. *Newborn and Infant Nursing Reviews, 10,* 187–194. doi:10.1053/j.nainr.2010.09.007

Bennet, J. E. (2011). Antifungal agents. In L. L. Brunton, B. A. Chabner, & B. C. Knollman (Eds.), *The pharmacological basis of therapeutics* (12th ed.). New York, NY: McGraw-Hill.

Carver, P. L. (2011). Invasive fungal infections. In J. T. De Piro (Ed.), *Pharmacotherapy: A pathophysiologic approach* (6th ed.). New York, NY: McGraw-Hill.

Chen, S. C., Playford, E. G., & Sorrell, T. C. (2010). Antifungal therapy in invasive fungal infections. *Current Opinion in Pharmacology, 10,* 522–530. doi:10.1016/j.coph.2010.06.002

de Sá, D. C., Lamas, A. P. B., & Tosti, A. (2014). Oral therapy for onychomycosis: An evidence-based review. *American Journal of Clinical Dermatology, 15*(1), 17–36. doi:10.1007/s40257-013-0056-2

Donders, G. G., Bellen, G., & Mendling, W. (2010). Management of recurrent vulvo-vaginal candidosis as a chronic illness. *Gynecologic and Obstetric Investigation, 70,* 306–321. doi:10.1159/000314022

Herdman, T. H., & Kamitsuru, S. (Eds.). (2014). *NANDA International nursing diagnoses: Definitions and classification, 2015–2017.* Oxford, United Kingdom: Wiley-Blackwell.

Kontoyiannis, D. P. (2012). Invasive mycoses: Strategies for effective management. *The American Journal of Medicine, 125*(Suppl. 1), S25–S38. doi:10.1016/j.amjmed.2011.10.009

Madigan, M. T., Martinko, J. M., Stahl, A. A., & Clark, D. P. (2012). *Brock biology of microorganisms* (13th ed.). San Francisco, CA: Benjamin Cummings.

Pfaller, M. A. (2012). Antifungal drug resistance: Mechanisms, epidemiology, and consequences for treatment. *The American Journal of Medicine, 125*(Suppl. 1), S3–S13. doi:10.1016/j.amjmed.2011.11.001

Rotta, I., Sanchez, A., Gonçalves, P. R., Otuki, M. F., & Correr, C. J. (2012). Efficacy and safety of topical antifungals in the treatment of dermatomycosis: A systematic review. *British Journal of Dermatology, 166,* 927–933. doi:10.1111/j.1365-2133.2012.10815.x

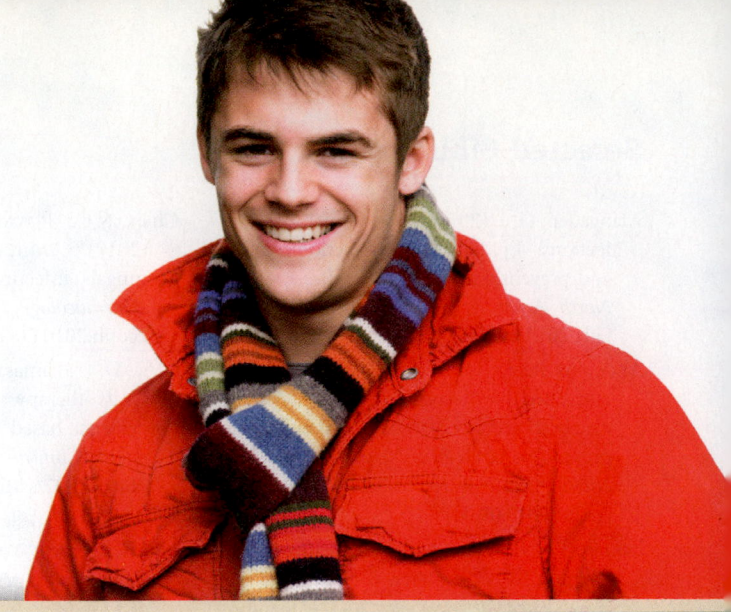

> *"Sure, I've thought about the possibility I may catch something on this trip. But it's the chance of a lifetime!"*
>
> Patient "Trevor Skales"

53 Pharmacotherapy of Protozoan and Helminthic Infections

LEARNING OUTCOMES

After reading this chapter, the student should be able to:

1. Identify features of protozoa and helminths that distinguish them from bacteria.
2. Identify protozoan and helminthic infections that may benefit from pharmacotherapy.
3. Explain why an understanding of *Plasmodium's* life cycle is important to the successful pharmacotherapy of malaria.
4. Explain the etiology, pathogenesis, and pharmacotherapy of amebiasis, giardiasis, cryptosporidiosis, toxoplasmosis, trichomoniasis, trypanosomiasis, and leishmaniasis.
5. Explain the etiology, pathogenesis, and pharmacotherapy of ascariasis, enterobiasis, hookworm, and tapeworm infections.
6. Describe the nurse's role in the pharmacologic management of protozoan and helminthic infections.
7. For each of the classes shown in the chapter outline, identify the prototype and representative drugs and explain the mechanism(s) of drug action, primary indications, contraindications, significant drug interactions, pregnancy category, and important adverse effects.
8. Apply the nursing process to care for patients receiving pharmacotherapy for protozoan and helminthic infections.

CHAPTER OUTLINE

▶ Classification and Pathogenesis of Protozoan Infections

▶ Drugs for Malaria
  PROTOTYPE Chloroquine (Aralen), *p. 887*

▶ Drugs for Nonmalarial Protozoan Infections
  PROTOTYPE Metronidazole (Flagyl), *p. 891*
  PROTOTYPE Pyrimethamine (Daraprim), *p. 895*

▶ Classification and Pathogenesis of Helminthic Infections

▶ Drugs for Helminthic Infections
  PROTOTYPE Mebendazole (Vermox), *p. 899*

KEY TERMS

cinchonism, 889	malaria, 886	sporozoite, 886
cysts, 885	merozoites, 886	trophozoite, 885
erythrocytic stage, 886	protozoan, 885	vectors, 885
helminths, 897		

Protozoa and parasitic worms, or helminths, are more complex than bacteria and cause significant morbidity and mortality worldwide. Pharmacotherapy is complicated by the life cycles of the organisms, during which they may change form and travel to infect distant organs. Some may remain infectious in contaminated soil or water for months or years. With few exceptions, the anti-infective drugs used to treat these disorders are different from those for bacterial or fungal infections.

Classification and Pathogenesis of Protozoan Infections

53.1 Protozoa are diverse, single-celled organisms that can cause widespread disease.

A **protozoan** is a single-celled organism that inhabits water, soil, and animal hosts. Although only a few of the more than 20,000 species are pathogenic in humans, they cause significant morbidity and mortality in Africa, South America, Central America, and Asia. These parasites thrive in conditions where sanitation and personal hygiene are poor and population density is high. The nurse needs to be familiar with these infections because travelers may acquire protozoan diseases overseas and bring them back to the United States and Canada. In addition, some of the protozoan infections frequently occur in patients with immunosuppression, such as those in the advanced stages of acquired immunodeficiency syndrome (AIDS) or those receiving chemotherapy or immunosuppressants. Selected protozoan infections important to human health are listed in Table 53.1.

Protozoa are an extremely diverse group of organisms, with each class having very different physiologies and survival strategies. Drugs that are effective against one species of protozoan are often not effective against others.

Some pathogenic protozoa have complex life cycles. The active, growing stage during which the organism feeds, often at the expense of its host, is the **trophozoite** stage. When faced with adverse conditions, some protozoa can form protective capsules called **cysts** that allow the organism to survive in harsh environments in a dormant state for prolonged time periods. Both trophozoite and cyst forms may reside within the human body simultaneously; however, some protozoa enter the cyst stage after they exit from the human body through coughing, sneezing, or fecal excretion. Protozoa remain in the cyst form until the organism is able to reinfect another host. When cysts occur inside the host, the parasite is often resistant to drug therapy.

Several of the major protozoan infections are spread by **vectors**, organisms that harbor the pathogen and carry it from one host to another. Some vectors, such as house flies, simply pick

TABLE 53.1 Selected Protozoan Infections		
Name of Disease and Protozoan Species	**Description**	**Source of Infection**
Amebiasis *Entamoeba histolytica*	Primarily infects the large intestine, causing severe diarrhea; commonly travels to the liver to form liver abscesses; rarely travels to other organs such as the brain, lungs, or kidney	Fecal-contaminated water
Cryptosporidiosis *Cryptosporidium parvum*	Infects the intestines, causing diarrhea; often seen in immunocompromised patients	Fecal-contaminated water; humans and other animals
Giardiasis *Giardia lamblia*	Infects the intestines, causing malabsorption, fatigue, and abdominal pain	Fecal-contaminated water
Leishmaniasis *Leishmania* (various species)	Affects many body systems including the skin, liver, spleen, or blood depending on the species	Bite of sand fly
Malaria *Plasmodium* (various species)	Infects red blood cells to cause fever, chills, and fatigue; some *Plasmodia* invade the liver and other tissues	Bite of female *Anopheles* mosquito
Toxoplasmosis *Toxoplasma gondii*	Can invade any organ; causes a fatal encephalitis in immunocompromised patients	Congenital transmission; cat feces
Trichomoniasis *Trichomonas vaginalis*	Common sexually transmitted infection (STI) that causes vaginitis in females and urethritis in males	Transmission through sexual contact with infected fluids
Trypanosomiasis *Trypanosoma cruzi* (American) *Trypanosoma brucei* (African)	The American form (Chagas' disease) invades cardiac tissue and autonomic ganglia; the African form (sleeping sickness) causes fatigue and central nervous system (CNS) depression	Bite of the kissing bug (American) or the tsetse fly (African)

up pathogens on their feet and transport them to human food or water. In other cases, the protozoan lives and multiplies inside the insect, which serves as an intermediate host. The protozoan *Plasmodium*, for example, reproduces in the gut of a mosquito and is transmitted to humans during a mosquito bite, causing malaria. The discovery that mites, ticks, or insects could spread infections was a major advance in medicine because researchers then realized that disease outbreaks could be prevented or controlled by eliminating the vectors.

53.2 The female *Anopheles* mosquito is the carrier of several species of *Plasmodium*, the parasite responsible for malaria.

Although rare in the United States and Canada, 300 to 500 million cases of malaria occur annually worldwide. Approximately 1,300 cases are diagnosed in the United States each year, almost all of which occur in immigrants or travelers returning from regions where the disease is endemic.

PharmFACT
Since 2000 efforts to control malaria have saved about 3.3 million lives worldwide, reducing malaria rates by 45% (World Health Organization, 2013).

Malaria is caused by four species of the protozoan *Plasmodium*. Each species has a characteristic geographical distribution and pattern of infection, although several species may coexist in the same location. *Plasmodium vivax*, the most common malarial species, occurs predominantly in India, Pakistan, and Central America. *Plasmodium falciparum* occurs with greater incidence in Africa, South America, Haiti, and the Dominican Republic. Although less common, *P. falciparum* causes the most severe symptoms, including a significant number of deaths in endemic areas, and is often more resistant to antimalarial drugs than the other *Plasmodium* species. The fatality rate for *P. falciparum* malaria approaches 10% of the patients infected with the parasite. The other two species, *Plasmodium malariae* and *Plasmodium ovale*, are less common, and current medical sources should be consulted for information on these species.

The carrier of *Plasmodium* is a mosquito. *Plasmodium* resides in the gut of the female *Anopheles* mosquito where it matures to its infective form, called a **sporozoite**. When the mosquito bites a human, some of the sporozoites, contained in mosquito saliva, are injected.

Once inside the human host, the blood carries the sporozoites to the liver, where they multiply and transform into millions of progeny called **merozoites**. There is an incubation period of 1 to 6 weeks following the mosquito bite, during which the patient experiences no ill effects.

After the incubation period, merozoites are released into the blood, where they enter red blood cells (RBCs) and multiply. The infected erythrocytes eventually rupture, releasing more merozoites and causing acute symptoms. This is the **erythrocytic stage** of the infection. Diagnosis is usually confirmed by the identification of *Plasmodium* on a blood smear. The bite of another *Anopheles* mosquito can pick up the merozoites from infected human blood, and the cycle begins anew. *P. vivax* can remain in body tissues for extended periods to cause relapses months, or even years, after the

initial infection. Unlike the human host, which can experience severe illness, the mosquito is unaffected by the presence of *Plasmodium*. The life cycle of *Plasmodium* is shown in Figure 53.1.

Symptoms of *P. vivax* malaria occur in a predictable, cyclic manner every 48 hours. This is because the merozoites grow and rupture erythrocytes on a regular time schedule. The uncomplicated or classic malaria attack lasts 6 to 10 hours and occurs in the following stages:

- **Cold stage.** Intense chills and shivering
- **Hot stage.** Fever, headache, vomiting; possible seizures in young children
- **Sweating stage.** Profuse diaphoresis, followed by return to normal body temperature, and fatigue

Complicated malaria may involve multiple organ failures and can be fatal. Nervous system involvement, called cerebral malaria, leads to abnormal behaviors, impairment of consciousness, seizures, or coma. Loss of large numbers of erythrocytes can cause severe anemia. Pulmonary edema and renal failure can occur. Complicated symptoms are nearly always indicative of infection by *P. falciparum*; the other three species rarely cause severe manifestations or death.

Drugs for Malaria

53.3 The three goals of malaria pharmacotherapy are chemoprophylaxis, treatment of acute attacks, and prevention of relapses.

Pharmacotherapy of malaria attempts to interrupt the complex life cycle of *Plasmodium*. Treatment becomes increasingly difficult as the parasite enters different phases of its life cycle. The goals of antimalarial therapy depend on the stage of the infection. These goals include chemoprophylaxis, treatment of acute attacks, and prevention of relapse. Drugs for malaria are listed in Table 53.2.

Chemoprophylaxis: A rule of thumb to remember about malaria (and many other diseases) is that it is much easier to prevent than to treat. The Centers for Disease Control and Prevention (CDC) recommends that travelers to infested areas receive prophylactic antimalarial drugs prior to travel, during their visit, and for at least 1 week after leaving. Chloroquine (Aralen) is the traditional drug of choice, unless travel is to a region known to have a high incidence of chloroquine-resistant strains of *Plasmodium*. Chloroquine therapy begins 1 to 2 weeks before travel and continues once a week during travel and for 4 weeks after returning.

Several options are available for patients unable to take chloroquine or for those who are traveling to areas where chloroquine-resistant species are prevalent. These include the combination drugs atovaquone-proguanil (Malarone), doxycycline, mefloquine, or primaquine. Of these medications, mefloquine is the only one recommended for prophylaxis during pregnancy.

Treatment of acute attacks: Once a *Plasmodium* infection has occurred, pharmacotherapy of malaria is more successful if it is begun immediately. Treatment is sometimes delayed, however, because the initial symptoms are nonspecific and may resemble the common cold or flu. The patient often does not seek medical

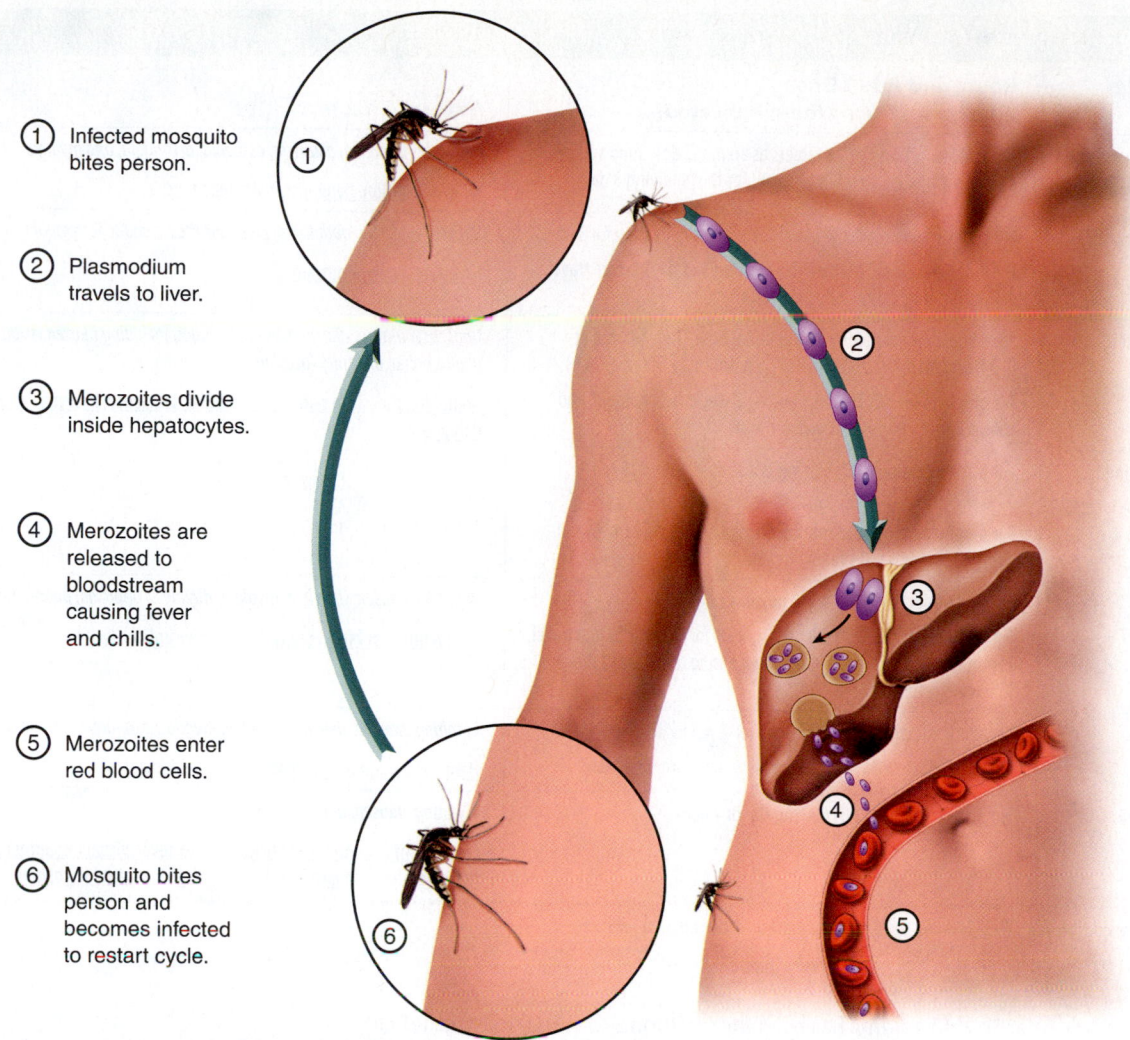

① Infected mosquito bites person.

② Plasmodium travels to liver.

③ Merozoites divide inside hepatocytes.

④ Merozoites are released to bloodstream causing fever and chills.

⑤ Merozoites enter red blood cells.

⑥ Mosquito bites person and becomes infected to restart cycle.

Figure 53.1 Life cycle of *Plasmodium*.

attention immediately. Classic malaria symptoms in a patient with a history of recent travel to an endemic region are sufficient evidence to begin antimalarial therapy, without waiting for laboratory confirmation.

Medications are used to interrupt the erythrocytic stage and eliminate the merozoites from RBCs. Elimination will break the life cycle of the protozoan and stop the acute symptoms. Chloroquine is the traditional antimalarial for treating the acute stage of the disease. It is the preferred drug for all species of *Plasmodia* causing uncomplicated malarial symptoms.

Several alternatives are available for treating chloroquine-resistant infections. These include primaquine, mefloquine, artemether-lumefantrine, atovaquone-proguanil, or quinine sulfate. In addition, several antibiotics are effective when used in combination with an antimalarial. Antibiotics used in the pharmacotherapy of malaria include tetracycline, doxycycline, and clindamycin. Tetracycline antibiotics are avoided in pregnant patients because they have the potential to cause birth defects (see Chapter 48).

Patients with complicated malaria are treated aggressively with high doses of parenteral antimalarials. Quinidine gluconate infusions are indicated, along with intravenous (IV) tetracycline, doxycycline, or clindamycin.

Prevention of relapse: Patients who acquire an acute malaria infection will almost always experience subsequent attacks unless drugs are given to eliminate dormant *P. vivax* residing in the liver. Primaquine is one of the few drugs able to eliminate hepatic cysts. To achieve a total cure, primaquine therapy is started near the conclusion of chloroquine therapy. Because *P. falciparum* does not invade the liver, relapses are not a problem with this species; thus, prophylactic drug therapy is unnecessary.

CONNECTION Checkpoint 53.1

From what you learned in Chapter 48, what adverse effects of tetracyclines, such as doxycycline, cause these drugs to be used with caution during pregnancy? *See Answer to Connection Checkpoint 53.1 on student resource website.*

PROTOTYPE DRUG | **Chloroquine (Aralen)**

Classification: Therapeutic: Antimalarial drug
Pharmacologic: Heme complexing agent

Therapeutic Effects and Uses: Developed in response to the high incidence of malaria among American soldiers in the Pacific

TABLE 53.2   Drugs for Malaria

Drug	Route and Adult Dose (Maximum Dose Where Indicated)	Adverse Effects
artemether-lumefantrine (Coartem)	For acute infections: PO: 4 tablets as an initial dose followed by 4 tablets 8 h later, then 4 tablets bid for the following 3 days	*Headache, anorexia, dizziness, asthenia, arthralgia, and myalgia* QT prolongation, hypersensitivity reactions
atovaquone-proguanil (Malarone)	For acute infections: PO: 4 tablets as a single daily dose for 3 days For prophylaxis: PO: 1 tablet/day starting 1–2 days before travel and continuing 7 days following return	*Nausea, vomiting, abdominal pain, diarrhea, headache, myalgia* Neutropenia, hypotension
chloroquine (Aralen)	For acute infections: PO: 600 mg initial dose, then 300 mg at 6, 24, and 48 h; IM: 200 mg every 6 h prn (max: 800 mg/24 h) For prophylaxis: PO: 300 mg starting 2 weeks before travel and continuing 7–14 days following return	*Nausea, vomiting, diarrhea, visual changes, including blurred vision, photophobia, difficulty focusing* Hemolytic anemia in patients with G6PD deficiency; irreversible retinal damage
hydroxychloroquine (Plaquenil)	For acute infections: PO: 620 mg initial dose, then 310 mg at 6, 18, and 28 h For prophylaxis: PO: 310 mg starting 2 weeks before travel and continuing 4–6 weeks following return	
mefloquine	For acute infections: PO: 1,250 mg as a single dose For prophylaxis: PO: 250 mg once a week for 4 weeks before travel; continuing 250 mg every other week during travel and 2 doses following return	*Vomiting, nausea, diarrhea, myalgia, dizziness, anorexia, abdominal pain* Atrioventricular block, bradycardia, tachycardia, psychosis
primaquine	For acute infection: PO: 15 mg/day for 2 weeks For prophylaxis: PO: 15 mg/day following return for 14 days	*Vomiting, nausea, diarrhea, myalgia, headache, anorexia, abdominal pain* Hemolytic anemia in patients with G6PD deficiency
quinine (Qualaquin)	For acute infections: PO: 650 mg tid for 7 days	*Vomiting, nausea, diarrhea* Cinchonism (tinnitus, ototoxicity, vertigo, fever, visual impairment), hypothermia, coma, cardiovascular collapse, agranulocytosis

Note: Italics indicate common adverse effects. <u>Underline</u> indicates serious adverse effects.

islands during World War II, chloroquine has been the traditional prototype medication for malarial prophylaxis and treatment for over 60 years. Chloroquine is very effective in treating acute symptoms of the erythrocytic stage but has no activity against dormant *P. vivax* or *P. ovale*. It can reduce the high fever of patients in the acute stage in less than 48 hours. It is also effective for the chemoprophylaxis of malaria caused by *P. malariae* and sensitive strains of *P. falciparum*, when taken 2 weeks before entering an endemic area and continuing 4 to 6 weeks after leaving. Although chloroquine is a drug of choice, many other antimalarials are available because resistance to chloroquine has become a major clinical challenge in certain regions of the world.

Both chloroquine and the closely related drug hydroxychloroquine (Plaquenil) are also used in the treatment of rheumatic and inflammatory disorders, including systemic lupus erythematosus and rheumatoid arthritis. When used for these disorders, doses are higher than those needed for malaria. Because hydroxychloroquine is less toxic at higher doses, this drug is preferred over chloroquine for treating inflammatory diseases.

Mechanism of Action: Chloroquine concentrates in the food vacuoles of *Plasmodia* residing in human red blood cells. Once in the vacuole, the drug likely prevents the destruction of heme and other proteins, which then build to toxic levels within the parasite. The anti-inflammatory effects of chloroquine occur because the drug inhibits the actions of histamine and serotonin and inhibits prostaglandin synthesis.

Pharmacokinetics:

Route(s)	Oral (PO), intramuscular (IM)
Absorption	Rapid and completely absorbed
Distribution	Widely distributed; crosses the placenta; secreted in breast milk
Primary metabolism	Hepatic; two active metabolites
Primary excretion	Renal
Onset of action	Peak effect: 1–2 h
Duration of action	Half-life: 70–120 h

Adverse Effects: Chloroquine exhibits few serious adverse effects at low to moderate doses. Nausea and diarrhea may occur. At higher doses, central nervous system (CNS) and cardiovascular toxicity may be observed. Symptoms include confusion, delirium, convulsions, reduced reflexes, hypotension, and dysrhythmias. Blood dyscrasias are possible. Chloroquine can cause retinal toxicity, including blurred vision, photophobia, and difficulty focusing.

Contraindications/Precautions: Patients with preexisting retinal field changes should not receive chloroquine, because the drug concentrates in this tissue and high doses can cause irreversible retinal damage. Baseline and periodic vision screening should be conducted during therapy. Because this drug can affect heme metabolism, it is contraindicated in patients with porphyria. Patients with known glucose-6-phosphate dehydrogenase (G6PD) deficiency should be treated cautiously, if at all, because chloroquine may cause hemolysis in these patients. Because chloroquine is metabolized in the liver, patients with chronic alcoholism or hepatic impairment should be monitored regularly. The drug should be used with caution in patients with eczema or psoriasis, because rare cases of exfoliative dermatitis have been reported. It is also contraindicated in patients with renal impairment and in those with hypersensitivity to the drug. Patients with preexisting hematologic disease should be treated with caution because chloroquine may cause blood dyscrasias.

Drug Interactions: Antacids and laxatives containing aluminum and magnesium can decrease absorption and must not be given within 4 hours of oral chloroquine administration. Cimetidine may also decrease the absorption of chloroquine. Chloroquine may interfere with the antibody response to rabies vaccine. Because chloroquine is associated with an increased risk for QT prolongation and torsades de pointes, it should not be administered concurrently with other drugs known to prolong the QT interval, such as many antidysrhythmics, phenothiazines, and beta-adrenergic agonists. **Herbal/Food**: Unknown.

Pregnancy: Category C.

Treatment of Overdose: Chloroquine overdose may be fatal. Symptomatic treatment includes anticonvulsants and vasopressors for shock. Ammonium chloride may be used to acidify the urine to hasten excretion of chloroquine.

Nursing Responsibilities: Key nursing implications for patients receiving chloroquine are included in the Nursing Practice Application for Patients Receiving Pharmacotherapy for Protozoan and Helminthic Infections.

Drugs Similar to Chloroquine (Aralen)

Other antimalarials include artemether-lumefantrine, atovaquone, halofantrine, hydroxychloroquine, mefloquine, primaquine, proguanil, and quinine. Halofantrine, approved by the U.S. Food and Drug Administration (FDA) in 1992, has not been marketed in the United States but is widely available in other countries. The combination drug pyrimethamine-sulfadoxine (Fansidar), once used for malaria, was discontinued due to the development of a large number of resistant strains.

Artemether-lumefantrine (Coartem): In 2009, the FDA approved the use of a fixed-dose combination of artemether and lumefantrine to treat acute, uncomplicated malaria. Artemether is prepared from substances obtained from the Chinese herb *Artemisia annua*, which has been known to have antimalarial properties for over a thousand years. Lumefantrine extends the half-life of the combination drug. Coartem is significant because it is very effective and offers an additional option for treating chloroquine-resistant infections. This drug is approved for treatment, not prevention, of malaria. Side effects are generally mild. Because this drug prolongs the QT interval, it should be used with caution in patients with cardiac impairment. This drug is pregnancy category C.

Atovaquone-proguanil (Malarone): The fixed-dose combination drug Malarone was approved in 2000 for the prevention and treatment of malaria. The two drugs have synergistic antimalarial activity and the combination results in less protozoan resistance than when either drug is used as monotherapy. Malarone may be given for prophylaxis or to lessen the severity of acute

symptoms. For acute attacks, a 3-day regimen is usually sufficient. For prevention, the drug is begun 1 to 2 days before entering an endemic region and continued for 7 days after returning. The drug combination rarely produces serious adverse effects; rash and gastrointestinal (GI) upset are the two most common complaints. Atovaquone (Mepron) is approved as monotherapy to treat *Pneumocystis jiroveci* pneumonia in patients who are intolerant to trimethoprim-sulfamethoxazole (TMP-SMZ). This drug is pregnancy category C.

Hydroxychloroquine (Plaquenil): As its name implies, hydroxychloroquine is closely related to chloroquine and has essentially the same actions. Approved in 1955, it is indicated for the prevention and treatment of malaria. Like chloroquine, retinal toxicity is a concern. Hydroxychloroquine is also prescribed to treat patients with cutaneous and systemic forms of systemic lupus erythematosus and for rheumatoid arthritis. Hydroxychloroquine is a prototype drug in Chapter 72. It is administered by the oral route and is pregnancy category C.

Mefloquine: Approved in 1989, mefloquine was developed during the Vietnam War to protect American soldiers from multidrug-resistant *P. falciparum* malaria. It is approved for both treatment and prophylaxis. It is a drug of choice for the prophylaxis of malaria caused by chloroquine-resistant strains of *Plasmodium*. Prophylactic dosing begins 1 week before entering an endemic area and continues for 4 weeks after leaving. Because of the rapid emergence of resistant strains, it is reserved for multidrug-resistant strains of *Plasmodium*. Nausea and vomiting are the most common adverse effects. The primary limitation of mefloquine is nervous system toxicity, including dizziness, nightmares, aggression, and psychoses, which can appear at high doses. Patients with preexisting psychiatric disorders should not take mefloquine. This is a pregnancy category C drug.

Primaquine: Approved in 1951, primaquine is a preferred drug for preventing relapses due to dormant *P. vivax* in the liver. Because it has no activity against the blood forms of *Plasmodium*, it must always be used in combination with other antimalarials. Standard therapy is for 14 days, although 5-day regimens have proved successful. The drug is well tolerated, even at high doses. The most serious adverse effect is hemolytic anemia in patients who are deficient in G6PD. Unlike some of the other drugs in this class, resistance is not a major clinical problem with primaquine. It is also used to treat *P. jiroveci* pneumonia in combination with clindamycin. This is a pregnancy category C drug.

Quinine (Qualaquin): First described in the 1600s, quinine is the oldest drug used to treat malaria, and it is still obtained from the bark of the South American cinchona tree. Although safer alternatives have since been discovered, quinine is still used for chloroquine-resistant *Plasmodia*, in combination with other antimalarials. It is only approved for the treatment (not prophylaxis) of uncomplicated malaria caused by *P. falciparum*. For many years, the majority of quinine use in the United States was to treat nighttime leg cramps, an off-label indication. However, in 2010, the FDA issued a black box warning against the off-label use of this drug for leg cramps because of the potential for developing severe and sometimes fatal thrombocytopenia. **Cinchonism**, a syndrome characterized by tinnitus, deafness, headache, vision abnormalities, and diarrhea, can occur at therapeutic doses.

A major limiting factor is cardiotoxicity, which produces quinidine-like dysrhythmias at high doses. This drug is pregnancy category X and should not be taken by pregnant patients.

Quinidine gluconate is closely related chemically to quinine. Given by infusion, the drug is used to treat severe, life-threatening malaria. Rarely, it may be used to treat symptomatic atrial dysrhythmias and life-threatening ventricular dysrhythmias when safer and more effective drugs have proven ineffective. Adverse effects are the same as for quinine.

Drugs for Nonmalarial Protozoan Infections

53.4 Amebiasis, giardiasis, and cryptosporidiosis are caused by intestinal parasites and are usually acquired through contaminated water or food.

Although infection by *Plasmodium* is the most significant protozoan disease worldwide, infections caused by other protozoa affect significant numbers of people in endemic areas. Each of the organisms has unique differences in its distribution pattern and physiology.

Many areas of the world do not enjoy the high level of sanitation found in the United States and Canada. In developing countries, drinking water may not be disinfected before consumption and may be contaminated with pathogens from human waste. In regions with poor sanitation, infectious diseases are endemic and contribute significantly to mortality, especially in children, who are often more susceptible to the pathogens. Amebiasis, giardiasis, and cryptosporidiosis are protozoan infections of the intestines, spread primarily by poor sanitation.

PharmFACT

It is estimated that 50 million cases of amebiasis occur each year worldwide, resulting in 100,000 deaths annually. Worldwide, it is the third leading cause of death due to parasites (Lacasse, 2013).

Amebiasis: Although not endemic to the United States, as much as 10% of the world's population is infected with this protozoan disease. The infection may be carried to the United States by travelers from regions where the disease is endemic, such as Mexico, India, Western and Southern Africa, and portions of Central and South America. The parasite is spread by drinking contaminated water, or by food handlers who transfer the cysts to raw vegetables or other consumables. Less commonly, amebiasis is transmitted through anal sex. Amebiasis also occurs with higher incidence in patients with AIDS, due to their inability to mount an effective immune response to the pathogen. The infection is asymptomatic in about 90% of patients.

Amebiasis begins when a person ingests cysts of *Entamoeba histolytica*. The trophozoite form of the protozoan invades the colon mucosa, causing ulcerations and considerable abdominal pain, distention, cramping, and bloody diarrhea. Diagnosis of amebiasis is generally through identification of the trophozoites in the stool; however, serum and stool antigen detection tests specific for *E. histolytica* are available. The life cycle of *E. histolytica* is illustrated in Figure 53.2.

Amebiasis is not restricted to the intestine. The trophozoite may gain access to the general circulation through colon ulcers and travel to other organs, particularly the liver, where it produces hepatic abscesses. Liver involvement causes high fever and right

upper quadrant (RUQ) pain. Other possible sites of infection include the brain, genitalia, and lung.

Regimens for amebiasis include combination therapy with two to three drugs to eliminate the parasites from their many potential sites. The drug of choice for both intestinal and hepatic amebiasis is metronidazole, due to its safety and efficacy. In cases of acute disease, IV metronidazole may be administered concurrently with an opioid to control severe diarrhea. Tinidazole (Tindamax) is an option for patients unable to take metronidazole.

If the infection is limited to the intestine, paromomycin (Humatin) and iodoquinol (Yodoxin) are preferred drugs because these agents are able to reach high concentrations in the intestinal lumen without producing significant systemic toxicity. These drugs are sometimes prescribed to eliminate the protozoan in patients who are asymptomatic carriers of the infection.

Pharmacotherapy for amebiasis is continued until multiple negative stool specimens are obtained. Drugs for amebiasis and other nonmalarial protozoan infections are listed in Table 53.3.

Giardiasis: Giardiasis is an infection caused by the protozoan *Giardia lamblia* that has much in common with amebiasis. They are both endemic to regions with poor sanitation, where the water supply is contaminated with human fecal matter. Both affect the intestine, causing acute cramping pain, severe diarrhea, fatigue, and marked weight loss. Both have a trophozoite and cyst stage, with no intermediate host or vector. Identification of *Giardia* trophozoites or cysts in the stool can help distinguish between the two diseases. Another potential cause of giardiasis in the United States is the unsanitary handling of soiled diapers in day care centers. It is interesting to note that *Giardia* was the very first protozoan discovered, originally identified by the inventor of the microscope, von Leeuwenhoek, in the 1600s.

Giardiasis is more common than amebiasis. It is the most common intestinal parasite responsible for diarrhea symptoms throughout the world. When contaminated food or water is ingested, the acidic environment of the stomach causes the parasite to transform from the cyst to the trophozoite stage. The incubation period is 1 to 3 weeks, and symptoms last 2 to 6 weeks. As many as 50% of the patients acquiring *Giardia* are asymptomatic.

Unlike *E. histolytica*, infections of *G. lamblia* remain localized to the intestine and are often self-limiting. A chronic form of giardiasis, however, can last for months and lead to malabsorption, steatorrhea, weakness, and chronic diarrhea. Although giardiasis is not fatal, it can weaken patients and make them susceptible to infection by opportunistic pathogens. Family members of infected patients, food handlers, and day care workers who are asymptomatic carriers should receive treatment.

Pharmacotherapy of giardiasis includes metronidazole (Flagyl), tinidazole (Tindamax), nitazoxanide (Alinia), or paromomycin (Humatin). Diarrhea generally stops within 48 hours after pharmacotherapy is initiated and a typical regimen continues for 3 to 5 days. Follow-up stool specimens are analyzed to confirm that the pharmacotherapy has been successful. For persistent cases, therapy may last 3 to 4 weeks.

PharmFACT

Someone infected with giardiasis may shed as many as 10 billion *Giardia* cysts each day for several months. It is believed that swallowing as few as 10 cysts might cause a person to develop symptoms of giardiasis (CDC, 2012).

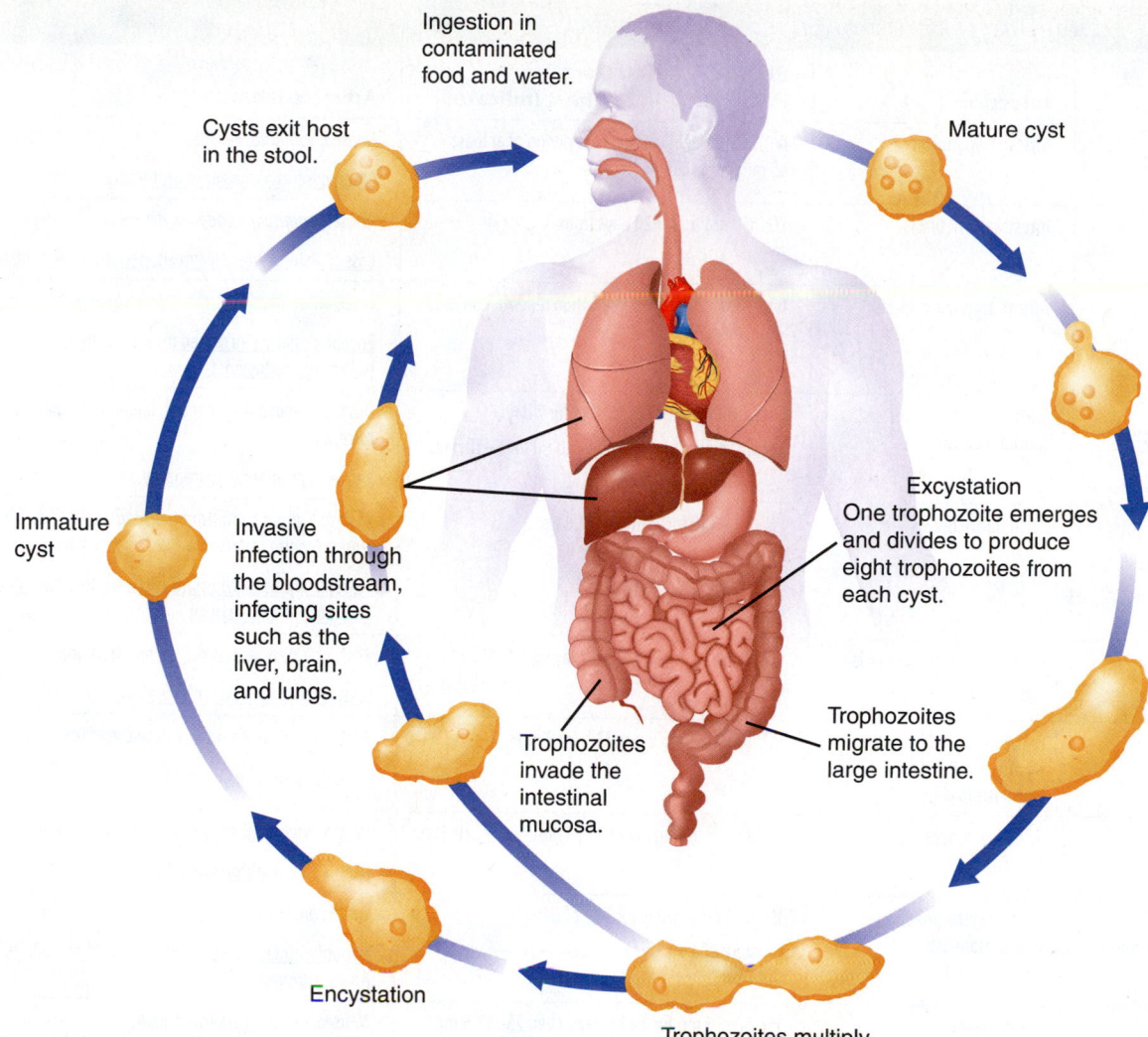

Figure 53.2 Life cycle of *Entamoeba histolytica*.

Cryptosporidiosis: Cryptosporidiosis is an infection caused by the protozoan *Cryptosporidium parvum* that causes severe diarrhea. Like *E. histolytica* and *G. lamblia*, *C. parvum* is primarily an intestinal parasite, acquired through the consumption of fecal-contaminated food or water. It has also been isolated from recreational water. A waterborne outbreak of cryptosporidiosis led to 400,000 cases in Milwaukee, Wisconsin, in 1993, and resulted in at least 100 deaths. This was the largest outbreak of waterborne illness in American history. Cysts of *C. parvum* survive harsh conditions, including chlorination of water: The Milwaukee outbreak occurred despite the fact that the water quality met all existing government standards. Although only about 3,000 cases of cryptosporidiosis are reported in the United States each year, it is responsible for a significant proportion of infectious diarrhea worldwide.

Pharmacotherapy of cryptosporidiosis is targeted at stopping the severe diarrhea through the symptomatic use of antidiarrheal drugs. In patients with healthy immune systems, the disease is self-limiting and no antiprotozoan drugs are necessary.

In immunosuppressed patients, cryptosporidiosis has a high mortality rate. Patients with AIDS can develop diarrhea that may cause the loss of as much as 17 L of fluid per day.

In addition, the disease can spread to other tissues, especially the gallbladder and biliary tree. Antiprotozoan drug therapy is necessary for these patients, with paromomycin (Humatin) being a preferred drug. Other agents that may be of benefit include azithromycin and nitazoxanide (Alinia). Combination therapy with these drugs may continue for 14 to 28 days, depending on patient response. Fortunately, the rate of cryptosporidiosis in patients with AIDS has declined because antiretroviral therapy has lessened the degree of immunosuppression in many patients with HIV infection.

PROTOTYPE DRUG	Metronidazole (Flagyl)

Classification: Therapeutic: Anti-infective, antiprotozoan
Pharmacologic: Nitroimidazole drug

Therapeutic Effects and Uses: Approved in 1963, metronidazole is the prototype medication for amebiasis, being effective against both the intestinal and hepatic phases of the disease. Resistant forms of *E. histolytica* have not yet emerged as a clinical problem with metronidazole. Metronidazole is also a preferred drug for giardiasis (off-label) and trichomoniasis.

		TABLE 53.3	Drugs for Nonmalarial Protozoan Infections

Drug	Infection	Route and Adult Dose (Maximum Dose Where Indicated)	Adverse Effects
eflornithine (Ornidyl)	African trypanosomiasis	IV: 100 mg/kg injected over a period of at least 45 min every 6 h for 14 days	*Nausea, vomiting, diarrhea* <u>Blood dyscrasias, seizures, ototoxicity</u>
iodoquinol (Yodoxin)	Intestinal amebiasis	PO: 650 mg tid for 20 days (max: 2 g/day)	*Nausea, vomiting, headache, dizziness* <u>Loss of vision, agranulocytosis, peripheral neuropathy</u>
melarsoprol (Arsobal)	African trypanosomiasis	IV: 2–3.6 mg/kg for 3 days, then repeated on day 7 and days 10–21	*Fever, albuminuria, transient arthralgias, dermatitis* <u>Encephalopathy, increased mental excitement, twitching, confusion, tremor, seizures</u>
metronidazole (Flagyl)	Trichomoniasis, giardiasis, Gardnerella vaginitis	For giardiasis: PO: 500 mg bid for 7 days For amebiasis: PO: 500–750 mg tid for 5–10 days	*Dizziness, headache, anorexia, abdominal pain, metallic taste, nausea* <u>Seizures, peripheral neuropathy</u>
miltefosine (Impavido)	Leishmaniasis	PO: 100–150 mg daily for 28 days	*Skin rash, elevated transaminases and creatinine levels, reduced sperm counts* <u>Stevens–Johnson syndrome, melena, thrombocytopenia, embryo and fetal toxicity</u>
nifurtimox (Lampit)	American trypanosomiasis	PO: 8–10 mg/kg 3–4 times/day for 90–120 days	*Rash, dizziness, headache, nausea, vomiting* <u>Seizures, paresthesia with myalgia, pneumonia</u>
nitazoxanide (Alinia)	Diarrhea caused by cryptosporidiosis or giardiasis in children	PO: 100–200 mg every 12 h for 3 days	*Abdominal pain, diarrhea, nausea, vomiting, headache* <u>No serious adverse effects</u>
paromomycin (Humatin)	Intestinal amebiasis	PO: 25–35 mg/kg divided in 3 doses for 5–10 days	*Nausea, vomiting, headache, diarrhea, abdominal cramps* <u>Ototoxicity, nephrotoxicity</u>
pentamidine (NebuPent, Pentam)	*Pneumocystis* pneumonia, trypanosomiasis, leishmaniasis	IM/IV: 4 mg/kg/day for 14–21 days Inhaled: 300 mg per nebulizer every 3–4 weeks	*Cough, bronchospasm* <u>Hypoglycemia, severe hypotension, kidney failure, pneumothorax</u>
pyrimethamine (Daraprim)	Toxoplasmosis	PO: 50–75 mg for 1–3 weeks, then 25–37.5 mg for 4–5 weeks	*Nausea, vomiting, diarrhea, rash* <u>Folic acid deficiency, blood dyscrasias</u>
sodium stibogluconate (Pentostam)	Leishmaniasis	IV or IM: 20 mg/kg/day for 20 days	*Nausea, vomiting, diarrhea, anorexia, cough, substernal pain* <u>ECG changes, pneumonia, blood dyscrasias</u>
suramin (Germanin)	African trypanosomiasis	IV: 1 g on days 1, 3, 7, 14, and 21	*Nausea, vomiting, malaise, fatigue, fever, diarrhea, rash* <u>Loss of consciousness, seizures, nephrotoxicity, adrenal insufficiency, blood dyscrasias, hepatotoxicity, severe hypersensitivity reactions</u>
tinidazole (Tindamax)	Amebiasis Giardiasis Trichomoniasis Bacterial vaginosis	For amebiasis: PO: 2 g/day for 3 days For giardiasis or trichomoniasis: PO: 2 g as single dose For vaginosis: PO: 2 g/day for 3 days	*Anorexia, constipation, dyspepsia, dizziness, bitter or metallic taste, nausea, vomiting* <u>Seizures, peripheral neuropathy, angioedema</u>

Note: *Italics* indicate common adverse effects. <u>Underline</u> indicates serious adverse effects.

In addition to its classification as an antiprotozoan agent, the drug has strong activity against anaerobic bacteria and may be given PO or IV to treat a number of serious respiratory, bone, skin, and CNS infections.

Topical forms of metronidazole (MetroGel, MetroCream, MetroLotion) are used to treat rosacea, a chronic, inflammatory condition characterized by skin reddening and hyperplasia of the sebaceous glands, particularly around the nose and face. MetroGel-vaginal is approved to treat susceptible vaginal infections. Helidac (metronidazole, bismuth, and tetracycline) is approved to eradicate *Helicobacter pylori*, an infection associated with peptic ulcer disease. Flagyl-ER is an extended duration form of the drug for treating bacterial vaginosis.

Off-label uses of metronidazole include the pharmacotherapy of pseudomembranous colitis, Crohn's disease, and colitis. When used for intestinal pathogens, metronidazole therapy is sometimes followed by administration of iodoquinol to more effectively eliminate residual parasites harbored in the colon.

Mechanism of Action: Metronidazole enters pathogens and binds to deoxyribonucleic acid (DNA), ribonucleic acid (RNA), and intracellular proteins. Cell death is likely the result of an absence of DNA repair and abnormalities in RNA synthesis.

Pharmacokinetics:

Route(s)	PO, IV, topical
Absorption	Well-absorbed PO (80%)
Distribution	Widely distributed, including the CSF and abscesses; crosses the placenta; secreted in breast milk
Primary metabolism	Hepatic (30–60%)
Primary excretion	Renal (77%), feces (6–15%)
Onset of action	PO/IV: Rapid; topical: 3 weeks
Duration of action	PO/IV: 6–8 h; topical: 12 h

Adverse Effects: Although adverse effects occur frequently during metronidazole therapy, most are not serious enough to cause discontinuation of the drug. The most common adverse effects are anorexia, nausea, vomiting, diarrhea, abdominal pain, dizziness, and headache. Dryness of the mouth and an unpleasant metallic taste may be experienced. Seizures and peripheral neuropathy have been reported. Patients receiving the drug by the IV route should be monitored for injection-site reactions. Use of the vaginal gel may lead to vaginal candidiasis in more than 10% of patients. **Black Box Warning**: Metronidazole (oral and injection) is carcinogenic in laboratory animals and should only be used for approved indications.

Contraindications/Precautions: Although rare, metronidazole can cause bone marrow suppression. Thus, it is contraindicated for patients with blood dyscrasias. Complete blood counts (CBCs) should be monitored during therapy to rule out any developing leukopenia. Metronidazole crosses the blood–brain barrier and is contraindicated in patients with active CNS pathology. Metronidazole should be discontinued if signs of CNS toxicity appear. Liver function tests should be carefully monitored in patients with alcoholism or hepatic impairment, because metronidazole is extensively metabolized in the liver. Doses of metronidazole should be lowered in these patients. The injectable form of metronidazole contains significant amounts of sodium, which can lead to edema in patients with heart failure.

Drug Interactions: Concurrent administration with PO anticoagulants can potentiate hypoprothrombinemia; thus, warfarin doses may require adjustment. Alcohol use may elicit a disulfiram-like reaction. Concurrent use with disulfiram can induce acute psychosis. This includes medications such as cough remedies that contain alcohol. Because metronidazole may elevate lithium levels, doses of lithium may need to be decreased to avoid toxicity. **Herbal/Food**: The extended release form of the drug should be taken on an empty stomach.

Pregnancy: Category B.

Treatment of Overdose: No specific therapy for overdose is available. Patients are treated symptomatically.

Nursing Responsibilities: Key nursing implications for patients receiving metronidazole are included in the Nursing Practice Application for Patients Receiving Pharmacotherapy for Protozoan and Helminthic Infections.

Drugs Similar to Metronidazole (Flagyl)

Other selected antiprotozoan drugs for amebiasis, giardiasis, or cryptosporidiosis include furazolidone, iodoquinol, nitazoxanide, paromomycin, and tinidazole. Furazolidone (Furoxone) is not available in the United States but is available in other countries.

Iodoquinol (Yodoxin): Approved in 1953, iodoquinol is prescribed for amebiasis to treat the trophozoite and cyst forms of *E. histolytica*. The usual regimen lasts for 20 days. Iodoquinol contains iodine; therefore, it should be used with caution in patients with thyroid disease and can influence thyroid function tests for as long as 6 months after discontinuation of therapy. Common adverse effects include diarrhea, nausea, vomiting, and stomach pain. Less common, although more serious, adverse effects include optic neuritis, loss of vision, anaphylaxis, and agranulocytosis. Iodoquinol also has activity against *Trichomonas vaginalis* and certain bacteria and fungi. This drug is pregnancy category C.

Nitazoxanide (Alinia): Approved in 1996, nitazoxanide is approved for the treatment of infectious diarrhea caused by cryptosporidiosis and giardiasis in adults and children. For children, it is formulated as a PO suspension. Off-label uses include diarrhea caused by other agents such as *E. histolytica* and *Clostridium difficile*. Clinical trials are examining its efficacy in patients with AIDS and cryptosporidiosis, because this infection can be fatal in immunosuppressed patients. A typical regimen is 500 mg bid for 3 days. The drug is well tolerated, with abdominal pain and GI distress being the most common adverse effects. This drug is pregnancy category B.

Paromomycin (Humatin): Approved in 1959, paromomycin is a broad-spectrum aminoglycoside antibiotic with antiprotozoan activity. The drug has activity against most gram-negative bacteria (except *Pseudomonas aeruginosa*), many gram-positive bacteria, some protozoa, and many parasitic worms. Because it is poorly absorbed from the GI tract, PO dosing is used to kill intestinal bacteria, protozoa, and helminths. It is approved for the treatment of intestinal *E. histolytica* infections, with a typical regimen consisting of 10 to 14 days of therapy. The drug has an orphan drug designation for treating multidrug-resistant tuberculosis and *Mycobacterium avium* complex infections. Although only the oral form is approved for use in the United States, an injectable form of paromomycin is available for the treatment of visceral leishmaniasis in other countries. The most common adverse effects are GI related: nausea, vomiting, cramping, and diarrhea. Like other aminoglycosides, the drug may exhibit ototoxicity and nephrotoxicity. This drug is pregnancy category C.

Tinidazole (Tindamax): Approved in 2004, tinidazole is in the same chemical class as metronidazole but has a longer half-life that allows for less frequent dosing intervals. Like metronidazole, tinidazole exhibits both antibacterial and antiprotozoan activity. It is highly active against *E. histolytica*, *T. vaginalis*, *G. lamblia*, and certain anaerobic bacteria. Typical regimens include single PO doses for giardiasis and trichomoniasis and 3-day therapy for amebiasis. In 2007, Tindamax was approved to treat bacterial vaginosis, the most common vaginal infection in the United States. Tinidazole interacts with anticoagulants to increase the risk of bleeding. When taken concurrently with alcohol, a disulfiram-like reaction occurs. Adverse effects are mild and include a bitter or metallic taste and GI distress. Tinidazole carries a black box warning that the drug is carcinogenic in laboratory animals and should only be used for approved indications. Tinidazole is contraindicated during the first trimester of pregnancy (category D) and should be used with caution in the second and third trimesters (category C).

53.5 Other protozoan infections that can cause significant disease include toxoplasmosis, trichomoniasis, trypanosomiasis, and leishmaniasis.

Protozoa can invade nearly any tissue in the body. As has been discussed earlier in this chapter, *Plasmodia* prefer erythrocytes, *Giardia* the colon, and *Entamoeba* travel to the liver. This section presents less common protozoa that invade additional sites. These infections include toxoplasmosis, trichomoniasis, trypanosomiasis, and leishmaniasis.

Toxoplasmosis: Toxoplasmosis is an infection caused by the protozoan *Toxoplasma gondii*. The domestic cat is an intermediate host to the parasite and serves as a primary means of transmission to humans. The only method of direct human-to-human transmission is from an infected mother to her fetus.

The cycle of *Toxoplasma* infection begins when a cat ingests cysts of *T. gondii*, either through fecal contaminated food or in the flesh of their prey. Once inside the cat, the cysts become trophozoites and invade the small intestine. The cysts are excreted and become infectious after they leave the cat's body. *Toxoplasma* cysts can remain infectious in the environment for up to a year, given ideal conditions such as warm, moist soil.

Toxoplasmosis can occur if humans are exposed to contaminated cat feces, or if they eat raw or undercooked meat containing the cysts. In otherwise healthy persons, toxoplasmosis is usually asymptomatic or presents with mononucleosis-like symptoms such as sore throat, fever, and malaise that rarely require medical intervention. Those who are pregnant or immunosuppressed, however, require pharmacotherapy because the disease can cause significant morbidity in these populations.

Once *T. gondii* enters the body, it can invade nearly any organ. The most common symptom is nonspecific lymphadenopathy. In patients with AIDS the brain is sometimes affected, resulting in a variety of CNS symptoms from headache to seizures. The cysts can form necrotic regions in the brain, resulting in focal neurologic abnormalities and changes in mental status. Fatal encephalitis from *Toxoplasma* infection was common in the early years of the AIDS epidemic. Lung infections were also frequent in these patients.

A pregnant woman acquiring *Toxoplasma* during the first two trimesters of pregnancy is at high risk of transmitting the infection to her fetus. The protozoan may cause stillbirth or abortion. Babies may present with ocular toxoplasmosis, a form of the infection that occurs when the cysts are deposited near the retina. Approximately 85% of the newborns who appear normal will develop brain or eye infections from *T. gondii*, sometimes years after birth.

The most effective regimen for acute toxoplasmosis is pyrimethamine (Daraprim) for 4 to 5 weeks. Clarithromycin, azithromycin, or a sulfonamide may be added to the regimen in combination with pyrimethamine or as alternatives. Leucovorin (Folinic acid), a form of folic acid, added to the regimen reduces the potential for pyrimethamine-induced bone marrow suppression. Because

relapse rates for toxoplasmosis in patients with AIDS approach 100%, lifelong prophylaxis may be necessary.

Trichomoniasis: Trichomoniasis is a parasitic infection caused by the protozoan *T. vaginalis*. It is a common sexually transmitted infection (STI), affecting approximately 15% of women visiting STI clinics in the United States (2.5 to 3 million women). Coinfection with other STIs is common.

Because *T. vaginalis* can survive on moist surfaces for several hours, the infection may also be spread by nonsexual means, although this mode of transmission is believed to be uncommon. In addition, there is a small risk of transmission of the infection from mother to baby during childbirth. Thus, trichomoniasis in pregnant patients is usually treated.

Trichomoniasis most commonly presents with malodorous vaginal discharge, accompanied by vulvar pruritus. Intense scratching may cause erythema and secondary infections in surrounding areas. Dysuria and discomfort during intercourse are common. Fifty percent of *Trichomonas* infections are asymptomatic or subclinical. Most infections in men are asymptomatic, or small amounts of urethral discharge may be noted. Because of the nonspecific nature of the symptoms, diagnosis may be difficult. Culturing of the vaginal discharge is conducted in patients who do not respond to standard therapy, and a specific monoclonal antibody test is available, but expense limits its use.

With pharmacotherapy, cure rates for trichomoniasis are high. A single PO dose of metronidazole (Flagyl) has been demonstrated to be as effective as prolonged therapy, and more effective than topical agents. The single dose also enhances patient adherence to therapy. However, the higher amount administered as a single dose causes a greater incidence of adverse effects, particularly GI upset. For these patients, 7 days of metronidazole therapy at a lower daily dose is equally effective and produces less GI upset. Therapy should also include the patient's sexual partners, even if they are asymptomatic, to break the cycle of reinfection.

Trypanosomiasis: Trypanosomiasis is actually two distinct parasitic infections: American and African trypanosomiasis. The two infections are caused by different organisms and have different vectors, clinical manifestations, and treatments.

American trypanosomiasis, or Chagas' disease, is caused by *Trypanosoma cruzi*, a parasite found throughout central and northern South America, Central America, and Mexico. The disease is rare in the United States. The vector for Chagas' disease is the "kissing" bug that ingests *T. cruzi* when it feeds on an infected human. The protozoan reproduces in the bug and is transmitted when the vector defecates on the host's skin at the same time that it feeds. *T. cruzi* usually enters the human host by being rubbed into the vector's bite, an open cut, or the mucous membranes of the eye, nose, or mouth. Other carriers are suspected for *T. cruzi*, including dogs, cats, and rodents. It is estimated that 50,000 die each year from the infection.

Acute Chagas' disease occurs more commonly in children and presents as a granuloma at the entry site, lymphadenopathy, and hepatomegaly. The acute form is not common and is often self-limiting. If pharmacotherapy is initiated, the drug of choice is benzimidazole, a medication that is only available in Brazil. Nifurtimox, available from the CDC, has been shown to benefit some patients. Pharmacotherapy for the acute phase is prolonged, at 90 to 100 days.

The chronic stage of Chagas' disease may appear decades after the initial infection and primarily affects the nervous system and heart. Signs and symptoms include cardiomyopathy and degeneration of autonomic ganglia that can result in megacolon, megaesophagus, and uncoordinated peristalsis. Unfortunately, treating the chronic phase with antiprotozoan drugs has not been shown to slow the progression of the disease. The chronic disease is treated symptomatically. Untreated, Chagas' disease is often fatal.

African trypanosomiasis, commonly known as sleeping sickness, is caused by the protozoan *Trypanosoma brucei*. The infection is transmitted to humans by the bite of a tsetse fly carrying *T. brucei*. African trypanosomiasis is restricted to sub-Saharan Africa, and its incidence ranges from 20,000 to 300,000 new infections annually, with about 50,000 deaths a year due to the infection.

Symptoms of *T. brucei* infection include a chancre at the site of the insect bite, extreme malaise (thus the name "sleeping sickness"), intermittent fever, muscle aching, weight loss, and body rash. The parasitic invasion may reach the CNS, causing personality changes, confusion, encephalitis, coma, and possibly death. The infection also affects the liver, heart, and other organs.

Pharmacotherapy of *T. brucei* infection depends on the stage of the disease. Early stages may be treated with suramin (Germanin) or pentamidine (Pentam). These drugs have been available for many decades, and resistance has become a problem. The standard drug for treating the late CNS manifestations is melarsoprol (Arsobal), a medication that has several toxic adverse effects. Eflornithine (Ornidyl), the first new drug for *T. brucei* in over 50 years, also causes serious adverse effects. There is a need for new, effective drugs for this infection.

Leishmaniasis: Most prevalent in Brazil, Peru, Afghanistan, Bolivia, Bangladesh, India, Sudan, Iran, Syria, and Saudi Arabia, leishmaniasis is an infection caused by about 20 different species of the protozoan *Leishmania*. Worldwide, 350 million are believed to be afflicted with the disease. Carriers for *Leishmania* include dogs, foxes, squirrels, and rodents. The disease is transmitted to humans by the bite of the sand fly. Three distinct forms of leishmaniasis have been identified, based on clinical signs and symptoms:

- **Visceral leishmaniasis.** Begins as a skin lesion but progresses to infect the spleen, liver, bone marrow, and lymph nodes. Visceral leishmaniasis is transmitted by contaminated blood or needlesticks and may occur in patients with advanced AIDS. It is usually fatal if untreated. This type most commonly occurs in India, Bangladesh, and Nepal.

- **Cutaneous leishmaniasis.** Characterized by skin lesions that spontaneously heal in 2 to 10 months. Occurs mostly in Mideastern countries such as Afghanistan, Iran, and Saudi Arabia but also is found in southern Texas, Central America, and South America.

- **Mucocutaneous leishmaniasis.** Characterized by ulcers of the mucous membranes of the nose, pharynx, or oral cavity. Found primarily in South America, these lesions cause severe disfigurement.

The CDC recommends sodium stibogluconate (Pentostam) as the standard treatment for visceral leishmaniasis. This drug is available only through the CDC. Stibogluconate must be administered by the IV or IM routes for 4 to 6 weeks, which makes the treatment of visceral leishmaniasis procedurally difficult in underdeveloped countries where the disease is most prevalent. In addition, resistance is common, particularly in India, the country with the highest rate of the disease. Relapse may occur as long as 10 years after the initial exposure. Alternative pharmacotherapy for visceral leishmaniasis includes amphotericin B for 20 doses, pentamidine (Pentam) for 15 days, or IM paromomycin (aminosidine) for 30 days.

Cutaneous leishmaniasis heals spontaneously in 5 to 12 months in immunocompetent patients and does not require pharmacotherapy. Mucocutaneous leishmaniasis is a much more serious condition, and secondary bacterial infections are common. Pharmacotherapy of these types of leishmaniasis includes many of the same drugs used for the visceral form. A topical therapy is paromomycin (aminosidine) with methyl benzalkonium chloride that is given for 10 days. In 2014, the FDA approved miltefosine (Impavido). This is the first FDA-approved drug to treat cutaneous or mucocutaneous leishmaniasis.

CONNECTIONS Community-Oriented Practice

◀ Risk of Disease from Consuming Sushi and Sashimi

Eating raw fish and other marine life is common in many areas of the world and has become popular in the United States. Raw fish, squid, and other animals may carry parasites that infect humans after consuming an infected meal. Tapeworms such as *Diphyllobothriasis nihonkaiense*, nematodes such as *Anisakis simplex* and *Pseudoterranova decipiens*, and more common infections such as *Escherichia coli* and *Salmonella* may be ingested during a meal of sushi or sashimi (Hochberg & Hammer, 2010; Jones, Anderson, Schulkin, Parise, & Eberhard, 2011). Because these parasites are microscopic, there is no method to tell good sushi from bad sushi when purchasing.

Ideally, fish and marine life should be cooked before consuming to kill parasites and bacteria. Freezing the flesh until solid at −35°C (−31°F) for 15 hours or at −20°C (−4°F) for 7 days will kill many parasites (FDA, 2012), including *Anisakis simplex*. However, freezing noticeably alters the taste and texture. Purchasing sushi and sashimi from trained sushi chefs and reputable restaurants may decrease the risk of infection, but it does not eliminate the risk. Pregnant women, young children, and immunocompromised patients should not consume any raw fish or meat.

PROTOTYPE DRUG | Pyrimethamine (Daraprim)

Classification: Therapeutic: Antiprotozoan
Pharmacologic: Folic acid antagonist

Therapeutic Effects and Uses: Available for over 30 years, pyrimethamine is a PO drug of choice for treating toxoplasmosis. Acute toxoplasmosis is treated for 2 to 4 weeks, whereas chronic stages that exhibit organ involvement may require months of therapy. Treatment of pneumonia caused by *Pneumocystis jiroveci* is an off-label indication for pyrimethamine.

Pyrimethamine is primarily effective against the acute phase of *T. gondii* infection and is less effective once the protozoan has entered the cystic phase of its life cycle. To boost its efficacy, pyrimethamine is sometimes combined with other anti-infectives such as clarithromycin, clindamycin, or azithromycin.

Fansidar, a fixed dose combination drug containing pyrimethamine and sulfadoxine, was once used for the treatment of malaria caused by *P. falciparum* in regions of the world showing high chloroquine resistance. The drug has been discontinued in the United States due to the large number of malarial strains that are resistant to the drug.

Mechanism of Action: Pyrimethamine inhibits the synthesis of folic acid in protozoa, thus inhibiting cell division.

Pharmacokinetics:

Route(s)	PO
Absorption	Pyrimethamine is well absorbed
Distribution	Widely distributed; crosses the placenta; secreted in breast milk; over 80% bound to plasma protein
Primary metabolism	Hepatic
Primary excretion	Kidneys
Onset of action	1 h
Duration of action	Half-life: 100 h

Adverse Effects: Common adverse effects of pyrimethamine include nausea, vomiting, anorexia, abdominal cramping, and rash. Serious adverse effects such as folic acid deficiency, megaloblastic anemia, pancytopenia, thrombocytopenia, and leukopenia may occur.

Contraindications/Precautions: Because pyrimethamine is a folic acid inhibitor, it is contraindicated in patients with preexisting megaloblastic anemia caused by folate deficiency. To prevent the development of anemia during therapy, leucovorin (Folinic acid) is administered concurrently. Pyrimethamine can stimulate the CNS and cause seizures. Therefore, it is used with caution in patients with seizure disorders. It should be used with caution in patients with significant renal or hepatic impairment and in those with G6PD deficiency.

Drug Interactions: Few significant drug interactions occur with pyrimethamine. Other folic acid antagonists such as TMP-SMZ should not be used concurrently because this will increase the possibility of severe folic acid depletion in the patient. Folic acid supplements should not be given because they will reduce the effectiveness of pyrimethamine. Pyrimethamine increases the half-life of phenytoin and may cause phenytoin toxicity. **Herbal/Food**: Unknown.

Pregnancy: Category C.

Treatment of Overdose: Overdose can cause seizures and serious blood dyscrasias. Parenteral diazepam may be used to control seizures and leucovorin may be administered to prevent folic acid deficiency.

Nursing Responsibilities: Key nursing implications for patients receiving pyrimethamine are included in the Nursing Practice Application for Patients Receiving Pharmacotherapy for Protozoan and Helminthic Infections.

Drugs Similar to Pyrimethamine (Daraprim)

Other selected antiprotozoan drugs for toxoplasmosis, trichomoniasis, trypanosomiasis, or leishmaniasis include eflornithine, melarsoprol, nifurtimox, sodium stibogluconate, and suramin.

Eflornithine (Ornidyl): Eflornithine is prescribed for African trypanosomiasis, especially late occurring CNS disease. It is less toxic than melarsoprol, but it is more expensive and is thus considered for therapy when melarsoprol fails to provide relief. Given by the IV route, therapy is continued for 7 to 14 days. Close medical supervision is required to monitor for the many serious adverse reactions, such as anemia, diarrhea, seizures, and vomiting. The parenteral form of eflornithine is only available from the World Health Organization. Unrelated to its antiprotozoan action, eflornithine cream (Vaniqa) was approved by the FDA in 2000 as the first topical prescription treatment for women with unwanted facial hair. Adverse effects from the topical formulation are mild and transient. Both IV and topical forms are pregnancy category C.

Melarsoprol (Arsobal): Melarsoprol is an older antiprotozoan, approved in 1949, that is used for the late CNS stages of African trypanosomiasis. It is one of only a few antiprotozoan drugs that can cross the blood–brain barrier to reach the parasite in the CNS. Melarsoprol contains arsenic, an element acutely toxic to life-forms. The most common regimen is a series of three IV injections administered with a rest period of 8 to 10 days between each series. Melarsoprol is a toxic drug and severe adverse effects are possible, including fatal encephalopathy convulsions, coma, thrombophlebitis, and necrosis at the injection site, if the drug is extravasated. Significant drug resistance, up to 30% in some regions, has occurred. Melarsoprol is only available from the CDC. This drug is pregnancy category C.

Nifurtimox (Lampit): Nifurtimox is used for the treatment of American trypanosomiasis. It is given PO for 14 to 21 days. Adverse effects include nausea, vomiting, anorexia, and neurologic disturbances. Only 50% to 70% of patients will respond favorably to nifurtimox therapy, indicating a need for additional drugs for this infection. Nifurtimox is only available through the CDC. This drug is pregnancy category D.

Sodium stibogluconate (Pentostam): Sodium stibogluconate is the traditional drug for treating leishmaniasis; however, decades of use have led to near-total resistance in certain strains of *Leishmania*. The drug must be given parenterally for 2 to 3 weeks. The most common adverse effects are pain at the injection site, pancreatitis, muscle and joint pain, and decreases in white and red blood cell counts. Treatment failures and relapses are common, indicating a need for more effective drugs for this infection. Sodium stibogluconate is only available through the CDC. This drug is pregnancy category C.

Suramin: Suramin is one of the oldest drugs for African trypanosomiasis, discovered in 1921. It is used exclusively for pharmacotherapy of the initial phase of the infection, since it is unable to cross the blood–brain barrier to treat the CNS symptoms characteristic of late disease. The usual regimen is one IV injection per week for 5 weeks. Nausea and malaise are common during infusions. Renal toxicity is common, though reversible with continued therapy. Suramin is only available through the CDC.

CONNECTION Checkpoint 53.2

Sulfonamides have been common antibiotics for many decades. From what you learned in Chapter 50, what are the primary indications for sulfonamide pharmacotherapy? *See Answer to Connection Checkpoint 53.2 on student resource website.*

Classification and Pathogenesis of Helminthic Infections

53.6 Helminthic infections cause significant intestinal disease, particularly in areas with poor sanitation.

Helminths consist of various species of parasitic worms. Unlike the single-celled protozoa, helminths have many cells, and thus their anatomy, physiology, and life cycles are more complex. Diseases caused by these pathogens affect more than 2 billion people worldwide and are quite common in areas of the world lacking high standards of sanitation. Helminth infections in the United States and Canada are neither common nor fatal, although drug therapy may be indicated.

Like protozoa, helminths have different stages in their life cycles, which include both immature and mature forms. Typically, the immature forms enter the body through the skin or the digestive tract. Most attach to the intestinal tract, although some form cysts in skeletal muscle or in organs such as the liver. Helminths are classified as roundworms (nematodes), flukes (trematodes), or tapeworms (cestodes).

Ascariasis: Ascariasis, caused by the roundworm *Ascaris lumbricoides,* is the most common helminth disease worldwide, affecting more than 1.4 billion people. This parasite is endemic to Latin America and Asia and afflicts 4 million Americans, generally in the warm climates of the southeast, and in areas where hygiene and sanitation are poor. This infection occurs most commonly in children between the ages of 3 and 8 years, because this group is most likely to be exposed to contaminated soil without proper hand washing. Although fatalities are rare in the United States, severe infections can lead to complete intestinal obstruction if left untreated. Worldwide, it is estimated that ascariasis causes approximately 60,000 deaths annually, mostly in children.

Transmission of *A. lumbricoides* occurs when a person accidentally ingests eggs from the parasite. Once in the stomach, immature worms hatch from the eggs, and larvae attach to the intestinal wall. The larvae can travel through veins and lymphatics and be carried to the lungs, where they burrow through alveolar walls and migrate up the bronchi. Once reaching the throat, the larvae are swallowed and the cycle begins again.

A. lumbricoides develops into adult worms in the intestines. The female adult worm, which can grow to over 40 cm in length, lays as many as 240,000 eggs daily, which enter the feces. Under unsanitary conditions, *Ascaris* eggs reach soil where they may remain infective for years. The life cycle of *Ascaris* is shown in Figure 53.3.

Ascariasis presents with both pulmonary and intestinal symptoms. As the larvae reach the lungs, the patient experiences cough, dyspnea, and low-grade fever. The intestinal phase is asymptomatic until large masses of worms are present. Vague upper abdominal pain, distention, and occasional vomiting may be present. Diagnosis is through identification of *Ascaris* eggs or worms in the feces. Occasionally, a worm is observed passing through the anus, mouth, or nose.

Pharmacotherapy for ascariasis is generally successful in eliminating the helminth from the body, without causing significant adverse effects. Oral mebendazole (Vermox) for 3 days is the standard treatment, with albendazole (Albenza) and pyrantel pamoate (Antiminth) as alternative medications. Stools are rechecked 2 weeks after therapy is completed to confirm elimination of the roundworms. When possible, pregnant patients are treated after the first trimester to minimize risks to the fetus.

Enterobiasis: Infection by the pinworm *Enterobius vermicularis* is the most common helminth infection in the United States, afflicting as many as 40 million people, mostly children. The disease causes intense perineal itching due to the presence of deposited *Enterobius* eggs or migrating female worms. The itching is worse at night and may cause restlessness, enuresis, and insomnia. Diagnosis is by identification of eggs on the perianal skin or worms in the stool.

Transmission of *Enterobius* is by diapers, toys, hands, or food contaminated with the eggs. After ingestion, eggs hatch in the duodenum within 6 hours and worms mature in 2 weeks. Only 1 cm in size, adult worms infest the terminal ileum and colon. The female worm is either expelled during defecation or migrates to the perineum where 11,000 eggs per day may be released. After leaving the body, *Enterobius* eggs can remain infectious in the environment for up to 3 weeks. If proper hygiene is not observed, eggs deposited under the fingernails during scratching may be placed in the mouth, renewing the infectious cycle. Like ascariasis, enterobiasis is more common in children, due to the inattention to hand washing. Enterobiasis, however, does not cause mortality.

Pharmacotherapy of enterobiasis includes mebendazole (Vermox), albendazole (Albenza), or pyrantel (Antiminth). A single dose is usually sufficient to eradicate the pinworms, although the dose may be repeated in 2 weeks to maximize therapeutic success. Antipruritic ointments are available for topical application to the perianal region for symptomatic relief of pruritus. Asymptomatic infestation of other household members is frequent; therefore, it is prudent for all close contacts to receive antihelminthic treatment.

Hookworms: Two human hookworms, *Ancylostoma duodenale* and *Necator americanus,* infect 900,000,000 people each year worldwide, usually in warm subtropical and tropical regions. Only about 1 cm in length, the adult hookworms live in the small intestine of the host. The female produces about 10,000 to 25,000 eggs per day, which are passed in the feces. Five days after exiting the body, hookworm eggs hatch and develop into an infective stage. The parasite is transmitted when an infective larva penetrates the skin, often to a child walking barefoot through contaminated soil. Diagnosis of infestation is confirmed by identification of hookworm eggs in the feces.

The initial symptom of hookworm infection is an itchy rash called "ground itch" at the site of skin penetration. As larvae migrate through the host's blood, they travel to the lung and up the throat, where they are swallowed and eventually end up in the small intestine. Pulmonary symptoms include cough, blood-tinged sputum, and low-grade fever. Later symptoms include vague abdominal pain, anorexia, and diarrhea.

The mouthparts of hookworms are modified cutting plates that cause hemorrhage when the worms attach to the intestinal mucosa to suck blood from the host. Children are particularly affected by the loss of blood. Although not directly fatal, hookworm infections can weaken the body by causing anemia and may cause death from infection by opportunistic pathogens.

The larvae of dog and cat hookworms can also infect humans, although they will not mature into adult worms in the human host. Transmitted to humans through contaminated soil or cat litter, these larvae remain in the skin where they migrate for many

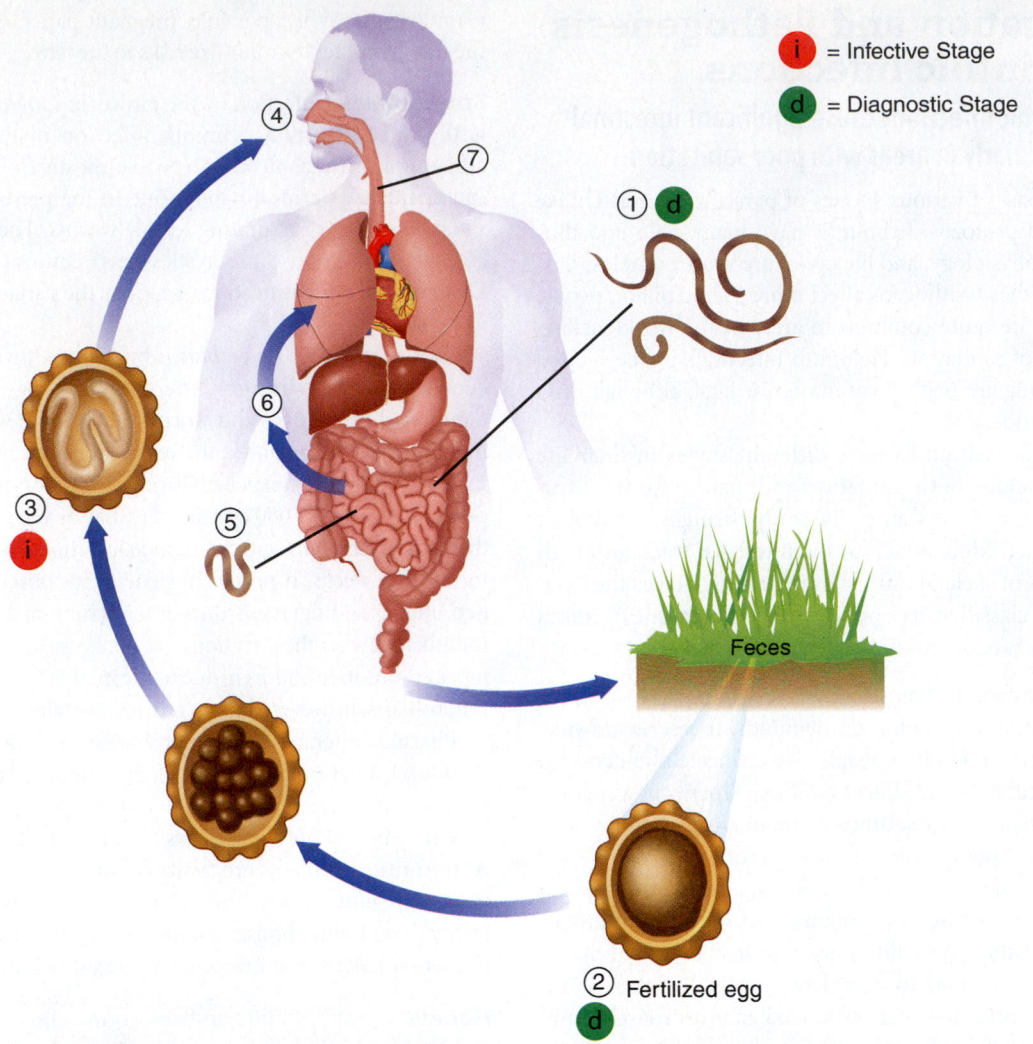

i = Infective Stage

d = Diagnostic Stage

Feces

② Fertilized egg

Figure 53.3 Life cycle of *Ascaris*: Adult worms (1) live in the lumen of the small intestine. A female may produce approximately 200,000 eggs per day, which are passed with the feces (2). Fertile eggs become infective after 18 days to several weeks (3), depending on the environmental conditions (optimum: moist, warm, shaded soil). After infective eggs are swallowed (4), the larvae hatch (5), invade the intestinal mucosa, and are carried via circulation to the lungs (6). The larvae mature further in the lungs (10 to 14 days), ascend the bronchial tree to the throat, and are swallowed (7). Upon reaching the small intestine, they develop into adult worms.

weeks and cause intense itching. This results in a condition known as *cutaneous larva migrans* or "creeping eruption." Thiabendazole (Mintezol) is a treatment of choice, although therapy with albendazole or ivermectin (Stromectol) may be necessary to eliminate persistent infections.

Mebendazole (Vermox), pyrantel (Antiminth), and albendazole (Albenza) are preferred drugs for hookworm infections. Albendazole and pyrantel are given as a single dose; mebendazole therapy is generally for 3 days. Iron supplements and antianemic drugs may be necessary for patients who have lost an extensive amount of blood.

Tapeworms: Several species of tapeworms infect humans. Beef and pork tapeworms are acquired when raw or undercooked meat is eaten that contains cysts or larvae of the parasites. Similarly, fish tapeworms may be acquired through ingestion of raw or poorly cooked fish containing the parasites. Some of the tapeworms reach enormous lengths; the beef tapeworm, *Taenia*

saginata, grows to 25 meters and the pork tapeworm, *Taenia solum*, is 7 meters.

Tapeworm infections may be asymptomatic or produce nonspecific symptoms such as nausea, diarrhea, hunger, fatigue, or abdominal pain. Diagnosis is through identification of perianal eggs or by finding tapeworm eggs in a stool specimen.

The treatment of choice for most tapeworm infections is a single dose of praziquantel (Biltricide). For some infections, a laxative is given 2 hours after treatment to remove all parts of the worm and its eggs.

Other helminthic infections: Several other helminths cause significant disease worldwide in areas where sanitation is inadequate and food-handling techniques are poor. Drugs used to treat these infections are either the same as those described above or are only available in other countries. Nurses traveling to these regions should consult medical sources for the most up-to-date pharmacotherapeutic information.

Drugs for Helminthic Infections

53.7 Antihelminthic drugs are usually successful in rapidly eliminating the parasites and have few serious adverse effects.

Drugs used to treat worm infections are called *antihelminthics*. Pharmacotherapy is not indicated for all helminthic infections because some are self-limiting and the adult parasites die without reinfecting the host. When the infestation is severe or if complications occur, however, drug therapy is initiated. Complications caused by extensive infestations may include physical obstruction in the intestine, malabsorption, extensive loss of blood, increased risk for opportunistic bacterial infections, and severe fatigue. Pharmacotherapy is targeted at killing the parasites locally in the intestine, and systemically in the tissues and organs they have invaded. Some antihelminthics have a broad spectrum and are effective against multiple species of worms, while others are indicated for a single species. Resistance is not a clinical problem with antihelminthics. Drugs for helminthic infections are listed in Table 53.4.

Because helminthic infections are often the result of poor sanitation or unhealthy hygiene habits, assessment of the patient's living conditions should be conducted. Often, all family members and close contacts of the patient should be treated in order to prevent reinfestation. Family teaching about ways to prevent reinfestation is essential to break the life cycle of the parasite.

PROTOTYPE DRUG	Mebendazole (Vermox)

Classification: Therapeutic: Antihelminthic
Pharmacologic: Microtubule inhibitor

Therapeutic Effects and Uses: Mebendazole, albendazole, and thiabendazole belong to the same chemical family, known as the benzimidazoles. Although the three benzimidazoles have similar properties and spectrums of action, mebendazole is the most widely prescribed in the United States.

Approved in 1974, mebendazole is used in the treatment of a wide range of helminthic infections, including those caused by roundworm (ascariasis), pinworm (enterobiasis), and hookworm species. As a broad-spectrum drug it is particularly valuable in mixed helminthic infections, which are common in areas with poor sanitation. It is effective against both the adult and larval stages of these parasites. For pinworm infections, a single dose is taken, followed by a second dose in 2 weeks. Other helminthic infections require 3 consecutive days of therapy. Although not approved by the FDA for tapeworm infections, it is sometimes prescribed for these parasites.

Mebendazole is poorly absorbed after PO administration, which allows it to maintain high concentrations in the intestine without causing systemic adverse effects.

Mechanism of Action: Mebendazole kills helminths by several biochemical mechanisms, including inhibition of glucose transport and uncoupling energy metabolism in the parasite's mitochondria. The drug binds to β-tubulin and is thought to disrupt the microtubular network in parasitic cells.

Pharmacokinetics:

Route(s)	PO
Absorption	Poorly absorbed
Distribution	Very little reaches the systemic circulation; 95% bound to plasma proteins
Primary metabolism	Hepatic
Primary excretion	Feces
Onset of action	Rapid
Duration of action	Half-life: 3–9 h

Adverse Effects: Because so little of the drug is absorbed, mebendazole does not cause serious systemic adverse effects. As the worms die, some abdominal pain, distention, and diarrhea may be experienced. Rare cases of seizures, agranulocytosis, neutropenia, and angioedema have been reported.

TABLE 53.4 Drugs for Helminthic Infections

Drug	Route and Adult Dose (Maximum Dose Where Indicated)	Adverse Effects
albendazole (Albenza)	PO: 400 mg bid with meals (max: 800 mg/day)	*Abnormal liver function tests, abdominal pain, nausea, vomiting* <u>Agranulocytosis, leukopenia</u>
ivermectin (Stromectol)	PO: 150–200 mcg/kg as a single dose	*Fever, pruritus, dizziness, arthralgia, lymphadenopathy* <u>Acute allergic or inflammatory response</u>
mebendazole (Vermox)	PO: 100 mg as a single dose or 100 mg bid for 3 days	*Abdominal pain, diarrhea, rash* <u>Angioedema, convulsions, agranulocytosis, neutropenia</u>
praziquantel (Biltricide)	PO: 5 mg/kg as a single dose or 25 mg/kg tid	*Headache, dizziness, malaise, fever, abdominal pain* <u>Cerebrospinal reaction syndrome</u>
pyrantel (Antiminth, Ascarel, Pin-X, Pinworm Caplets)	PO: 11 mg/kg as a single dose (max: 1 g)	*Nausea, tenesmus, anorexia, diarrhea, fever* <u>No serious adverse effects</u>
thiabendazole (Mintezol)	PO: 1.5 g bid for 2 days (max: 3 g/day)	*Dizziness, anorexia, nausea, vomiting* <u>Nephrotoxicity, jaundice, leukopenia</u>

Note: Italics indicate common adverse effects. <u>Underline</u> indicates serious adverse effects.

Contraindications/Precautions: Other than hypersensitivity, there are no contraindications for mebendazole. Because it is metabolized by the liver, patients with serious hepatic impairment should be monitored carefully. The drug is a potent teratogen in laboratory animals and should be avoided during pregnancy, especially the first trimester. Use in children under 2 years of age is not advised.

Drug Interactions: Carbamazepine and phenytoin can increase the metabolism of mebendazole, although dosage adjustment is not required because so little mebendazole is absorbed.

Pregnancy: Category C.

Treatment of Overdose: No specific therapy is available; patients are treated symptomatically.

Nursing Responsibilities: Key nursing implications for patients receiving mebendazole are included in the Nursing Practice Application for Patients Receiving Pharmacotherapy for Protozoan and Helminthic Infections.

Drugs Similar to Mebendazole (Vermox)

Other selected drugs for helminthic infections include albendazole, ivermectin, praziquantel, pyrantel, and thiabendazole. Bithionol (Bitin) is an antihelminthic available from the CDC for treating *Fasciola hepatica* (a liver fluke). Also available only through the CDC, diethylcarbamazine (Hetrazan) is only used to treat helminthic infections known as lymphatic filariasis, which are caused by various species of threadlike worms found in tropical climates.

Albendazole (Albenza): Approved in 1996, albendazole belongs to the same chemical class as mebendazole. It is incompletely absorbed when given PO, although enough of the drug is distributed to kill parasitic cysts in some tissues. It is a drug of choice for larval forms of the beef tapeworm *T. solium* and for hydatid cysts in the liver that form following infection by the dog tapeworm *Echinococcus granulosus*. Although only approved for these two indications, it is often prescribed off-label for other helminthic infections. Albendazole is well tolerated and exhibits few adverse effects. The most common adverse effect is a transient increase in serum aminotransferase activity caused by its effects on liver function. This is a pregnancy category C drug.

Ivermectin (Stromectol): Approved in 1996, ivermectin has become a mainstay in the pharmacotherapy of several helminthic infections due to its superior safety profile and single-dose efficacy. It is a preferred drug for treating onchocerciasis or "river blindness," an especially debilitating filarial infection in Africa, the Middle East, and Latin America. Annual doses have caused a significant reduction of this disease in endemic areas. It is a drug of choice (off-label) for the cutaneous therapy of larva migrans, or "creeping eruption." Because of its wide spectrum of action, it is of great importance in treating mixed helminthic infections, which are so common in underdeveloped countries. Adverse effects are minor and include fever, rash, and pruritus resulting from allergic and inflammatory reactions to the death of the parasites. This is a pregnancy category C drug.

Praziquantel (Biltricide): Approved in 1982, praziquantel is a broad-spectrum antihelminthic drug of choice for schistosomiasis, a helminthic infection caused by blood flukes that affects 200 million people worldwide. People acquire the parasite by bathing or swimming in feces-contaminated water. Although not found in the United States, the parasite is endemic to tropical regions across the globe, causing chronic ill health. Praziquantel is also approved for Chinese liver fluke infections and is prescribed worldwide for other helminthic infections. It is a safe medication, with dizziness, headache, and abdominal pain being the most common adverse effects. This is a pregnancy category B drug.

Pyrantel (Antiminth, Pin-Rid): Approved in 1971, pyrantel is poorly absorbed when given PO; thus, it is only effective against intestinal helminths. As a single dose, it has been a traditional drug of choice for treating enterobiasis, ascariasis, and hookworm infections. It is available over the counter (OTC). Adverse effects are usually minor and include nausea, vomiting, headache, dizziness, and rash. Pyrantel is usually considered an alternative to mebendazole. This is a pregnancy category C drug.

Thiabendazole (Mintezol): Although it is an effective, broad-spectrum drug, thiabendazole use is limited by a high incidence of adverse effects such as anorexia, nausea, vomiting, and dizziness. Approved in 1967, it is used for various worm infestations, although it has largely been replaced by albendazole and mebendazole for most indications. Topical formulations of thiabendazole cream for "creeping eruption" have been replaced by treatment with PO ivermectin. This is a pregnancy category C drug.

CONNECTIONS: NURSING PRACTICE APPLICATION

Patients Receiving Pharmacotherapy for Protozoan and Helminthic Infections

Assessment	Potential Nursing Diagnoses*
Baseline assessment prior to administration: • Obtain a complete health history including neurologic, cardiovascular, respiratory, hepatic, or renal disease, hematologic disorders, and the possibility of pregnancy. Obtain a drug history including allergies (e.g., specific reactions to drugs), current prescription and OTC drugs, herbal preparations, and alcohol use. Be alert to possible drug interactions. • Assess signs and symptoms of current infection and assess family members or others living in the home. • Obtain a travel history, noting dates of travel and when current symptoms started in relation to travel (i.e., before, during, or after travel). • Evaluate appropriate laboratory and diagnostic test findings (e.g., CBC, culture and sensitivity [C&S], fecal ova and parasites, hepatic and renal function studies, vision screening and retinal examination, ECG as appropriate). • Assess the patient's ability to receive and understand instructions. Include family and caregivers as needed.	• *Diarrhea* • *Nausea* • *Deficient Fluid Volume* • *Fatigue* • *Imbalanced Nutrition: Less Than Body Requirements* • *Acute Pain* • *Impaired Skin Integrity* • *Deficient Knowledge* (Drug Therapy)
Assessment throughout administration: • Assess for desired therapeutic effects (e.g., diminished diarrhea, chills, fever, muscle pain). • Continue periodic monitoring of CBC, hepatic and renal function, C&S, fecal ova and parasites, vision and retinal examination, ECG as appropriate. • Assess for adverse effects: nausea, vomiting, abdominal cramping, increasing diarrhea, drowsiness, dizziness, paresthesia, metallic taste, darkened urine, dysrhythmias, palpitations. Immediately report severe diarrhea, especially that containing mucus, blood, or pus; yellowing of the sclera or skin; decreased urine output; numbness of extremities; blurring of vision or difficulty with vision clarity; photophobia; seizures; dysrhythmias; hypotension; and tachycardia.	

Implementation

Interventions and (Rationales)	Patient-Centered Care
Ensuring therapeutic effects: • Continue assessments as above for therapeutic effects. (Diminished fever, pain, diarrhea, or signs and symptoms of infection should begin soon after taking the first dose and continue to improve. Notify the provider if signs and symptoms of infection remain or increase after 3 days or if the entire course of treatment has been taken and signs of infection are still present.)	• Teach the patient to report a fever that does not diminish below 37.8°C (100°F) or per parameters set by the health care provider within 3 days, increasing signs and symptoms of infection, or symptoms that remain present after taking the entire course of the drug. • Teach the patient to *complete* the entire course of medication; to not share doses with other family members with similar symptoms; and to return to the provider if symptoms have not resolved after the entire course of therapy.
Minimizing adverse effects: • Continue to monitor vital signs, especially temperature if fever is present. Immediately report undiminished fever or changes in level of consciousness (LOC) to the health care provider. (Fever should begin to diminish within 1–3 days after starting the drug. Continued fever may be a sign of worsening infection, adverse drug effects, or drug resistance.)	• Teach the patient to report fever that does not diminish below 37.8°C (100°F) or per parameters set by the health care provider. Immediately report changes in behavior or LOC to the health care provider.
• Continue to monitor periodic laboratory work: hepatic and renal function tests, CBC, ECG, C&S, fecal ova and parasites, and results of vision and retinal screening. (Hepatic and renal laboratory studies, particularly with IV therapy, should be monitored to prevent adverse effects. Periodic C&S or fecal ova and parasite tests may be ordered if infections are severe or are slow to resolve to confirm appropriate therapy. Periodic vision and retinal screening will be required with chloroquine therapy because the drug can cause irreversible damage to the retina. ECG monitoring may be required with some antimalarial drugs.)	• Instruct the patient on the need for periodic laboratory work. Provide a kit and instructions for home use if fecal specimens are required. • Cultures should be collected *before* the drug therapy is started or if started in an emergency (e.g., overwhelming infection with significant body-wide symptoms), as soon as feasibly possible, and thereafter as ordered by the provider. • Instruct the patient to immediately contact the provider if blurring, difficulty focusing, or photophobia is severe, continues, or worsens.
• Monitor for hypersensitivity and allergic reactions, especially with the first few doses of any drug treatment. (Anaphylactic reactions are possible, particularly with the first dose. As parasites die, increasing diarrhea, abdominal pain, or chills may occur.)	• Teach the patient to immediately report any itching, rashes, swelling, particularly of the face or tongue, urticaria, flushing, dizziness, syncope, wheezing, throat tightness, or difficulty breathing. Report significant increases in abdominal pain, diarrhea, chills, or fever to the health care provider.

(continued)

CONNECTIONS: NURSING PRACTICE APPLICATION (continued)

• Continue to monitor for hepatic or renal toxicity; e.g., jaundice, RUQ pain, darkened urine, or diminished urine output. (Increasing fluid intake will prevent drug accumulation in the kidneys. **Lifespan**: Age-related physiological differences may place older adults at greater risk for hepatic or renal toxicity.)	• Teach the patient to report immediately any nausea, vomiting, yellowing of the skin or sclera, abdominal pain, light- or clay-colored stools, diminished urine output, or darkening of urine. • Advise the patient to increase fluid intake to 2–3 L/day. Alcohol use should be avoided or eliminated.
• Monitor for significant GI effects, including nausea, vomiting, abdominal pain, or cramping. Give the drug with food or milk to decrease adverse GI effects. (Food or milk may decrease GI effects, but an antiemetic may be considered if nausea is severe. Alcohol use, especially in patients on metronidazole, may cause a disulfiram-like reaction with excessive nausea, vomiting, and possible hypotension.)	• Teach the patient to take the drug with food or milk but to avoid acidic foods, beverages or carbonated drinks, and alcohol, especially in patients on metronidazole.
• Monitor for signs and symptoms of neurologic effects, e.g., dizziness, drowsiness, or headache, and ensure patient safety. **Lifespan**: Be particularly cautious with the older adult who may be at increased risk for dizziness and falls. (Dizziness or drowsiness increases the risk for falls.)	• Teach the patient to rise from lying or sitting to standing slowly to avoid dizziness or falls, and to avoid driving or other activities requiring mental alertness or physical coordination until the effects of the drug are known. If dizziness occurs, the patient should sit or lie down and not attempt to stand or walk until the sensation passes. • Instruct the hospitalized patient to call for assistance prior to getting out of bed or attempting to walk alone.
• Monitor pulse and ECG as indicated in patients on antimalarial treatment. (Some antimalarials may cause dysrhythmias and hypotension.)	• Teach the patient to report any palpitations, lightheadedness, or dizziness promptly.
• Monitor for signs and symptoms of bone marrow suppression and blood dyscrasias, e.g., low-grade fevers, bleeding, bruising, significant fatigue. (Bone marrow suppression is an adverse effect and may cause blood dyscrasias with resulting decreases in RBCs, white blood cells [WBCs], and/or platelets. Periodic monitoring of CBC may be required.)	• Teach the patient to report any low-grade fevers, sore throat, rashes, bruising or increased bleeding, unusual fatigue or shortness of breath, especially after taking drug therapy for a prolonged period.
• Assess the patient's sexual partners for infection and treat current partners to avoid reinfection. (Infection may be reintroduced by an untreated sexual partner.)	• Have the patient notify sexual partners for assessment and treatment.
• Teach general hygiene measures to prevent reinfestation with parasites. (Families with young children should practice scrupulous hand washing and proper disposal of diapers, and notify day care or child care providers of the infection. Assess family pets that may carry infection and also require treatment. International travelers should practice scrupulous hygiene, especially in developing countries.)	• Teach the patient, family, and caregivers appropriate hygiene measures. Encourage veterinary assessment of family pets, even if asymptomatic. • Encourage international travelers to consult the CDC's website on "Traveler's Health" to learn the latest information about potential disease risk, preventive and treatment measures, and other valuable travel-related health information before embarking on their trip.
Patient understanding of drug therapy: • Use opportunities during administration of medications and during assessments to discuss the rationale for drug therapy, desired therapeutic outcomes, commonly observed adverse effects, parameters for when to call the health care provider, and any necessary monitoring or precautions. (Using time during nursing care helps to optimize and reinforce key teaching areas.)	• The patient, family, or caregiver should be able to state the reason for the drug, appropriate dose and scheduling, what adverse effects to observe for and when to report them, and the anticipated length of medication therapy.
Patient self-administration of drug therapy: • When administering medications, instruct the patient, family, or caregiver in proper self-administration techniques followed by teach-back. (Utilizing time during nurse-administration of these drugs helps to reinforce teaching.)	• Teach the patient to take the medication: • Complete the entire course of therapy unless otherwise instructed. Do not share with other family members and do not stop the medicine when starting to feel better. • Avoid or eliminate alcohol. Some medications (e.g., metronidazole) cause significant reactions when taken with alcohol, and alcohol increases the adverse GI effects of many drugs. • Take the drug with food or milk, but avoid acidic beverages. If instructed to take the drug on an empty stomach, take it with a full glass of water. • Take the medication as evenly spaced throughout each day as feasible. • Increase overall fluid intake while taking the drug. • Discard outdated medications or those no longer in use. Review the medicine cabinet twice a year for old medications (e.g., at beginning and end of daylight saving time).

*Nursing Diagnoses—Definitions and Classification 2015–2017. Copyright © 2014, 1994–2014 by NANDA International. Used by arrangement with John Wiley & Sons Limited.

CHAPTER 53

Understanding the Chapter

Key Concepts Summary

53.1 Protozoa are diverse, single-celled organisms that can cause widespread disease.

53.2 The female *Anopheles* mosquito is the carrier of several species of *Plasmodium*, the parasite responsible for malaria.

53.3 The three goals of malaria pharmacotherapy are chemoprophylaxis, treatment of acute attacks, and prevention of relapses.

53.4 Amebiasis, giardiasis, and cryptosporidiosis are caused by intestinal parasites and are usually acquired through contaminated water or food.

53.5 Other protozoan infections that can cause significant disease include toxoplasmosis, trichomoniasis, trypanosomiasis, and leishmaniasis.

53.6 Helminthic infections cause significant intestinal disease, particularly in areas with poor sanitation.

53.7 Antihelminthic drugs are usually successful in rapidly eliminating the parasites and have few serious adverse effects.

Case Study: Making the Patient Connection

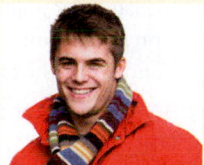

Remember the patient "Trevor Skales" at the beginning of the chapter? Now read the remainder of the case study. Based on the information presented within this chapter, respond to the critical thinking questions that follow.

Trevor Skales is a 23-year-old with an upcoming month-long eco-tour vacation planned to a rain forest in South America. He has been planning this trip since he graduated from college and will be leaving in 3 weeks with two college friends. He has researched the trip and knows about the possible endemic diseases in the area including tuberculosis, dengue fever, leishmaniasis, leprosy, and malaria. After discussing the trip with his health care provider, malaria carries the biggest threat for transmission during Trevor's trip.

He has had a complete physical exam and is up to date on all required vaccinations. His provider has also screened for the possibility of a G6PD

deficiency, and Trevor has had a thorough eye examination. The provider has ordered chloroquine (Aralen) for Trevor. He is to begin taking it 2 weeks before his trip, every week throughout his trip, and for 1 month after returning home.

Critical Thinking Questions

1. Why was chloroquine (Aralen) ordered for Trevor before he has started his trip?

2. Why are special screening for G6PD deficiency and an eye examination important?

3. Trevor asks why he needs to continue to take the chloroquine (Aralen) after he returns home. As his nurse, what would you teach him about the drug dosing schedule and about symptoms to watch for?

4. What adverse effects are associated with chloroquine (Aralen) therapy?

See Answers to Critical Thinking Questions on student resource website.

Additional Case Study

Mary Porter is a 19-year-old woman who visits the local clinic with malodorous vaginal discharge, accompanied by vulvar pruritus. She also reports dysuria and discomfort during sexual intercourse. Mary is diagnosed with trichomoniasis and started on metronidazole (Flagyl).

1. Why are female patients more likely to contract trichomoniasis?

2. What health teaching would you provide to the patient who is being treated for trichomoniasis?

3. Develop a list of adverse effects this patient may experience while taking metronidazole.

See Answers to Additional Case Study on student resource website.

Chapter Review

1 The patient is taking chloroquine (Aralen) prophylactically before traveling to a developing country and asks the nurse how long the drug will need to be taken after returning from the trip. Which response from the nurse would be correct? Chloroquine (Aralen) is:

1. Recommended for 4 weeks after returning from the malaria-infested location.
2. Not necessary after leaving the location.
3. Suggested for 3 days after returning from the trip.
4. Optional unless the patient reports symptoms of malaria.

2 A patient has been started on hydroxychloroquine (Plaquenil) for prevention of malaria on an overseas trip. In addition to the prevention and treatment of malaria, hydroxychloroquine is also indicated for what other conditions? Select all that apply.

1. Systemic lupus erythematosus
2. Roundworm infections
3. Urinary tract infections
4. Rheumatoid arthritis
5. Leishmaniasis infections

3 A patient is being treated with metronidazole (Flagyl) for *Giardia lamblia* infection. When instructing the patient about this drug, the nurse should caution about the possibility of which adverse reaction?

1. Flatus and intestinal bloating
2. Halitosis
3. Unpleasant metallic taste
4. Alopecia

4 The patient is diagnosed with toxoplasmosis and will be treated with pyrimethamine (Daraprim). Because of significant adverse effects, what teaching should the nurse give this patient?

1. Increase intake of fiber-rich foods to prevent constipation.
2. Report unusual bruising, fatigue, sores that do not heal, or low-grade fever.
3. Increase fluid intake to 3 L per day.
4. Schedule eye examinations every 6 months for 2 years after taking this drug.

5 A 6-year-old boy is diagnosed with an *Enterobius vermicularis* (pinworm) infection and has been prescribed mebendazole (Vermox). What appropriate instructions should the nurse give the boy's caregiver?

1. The drug will be continued for 2 weeks and then a stool sample will be retested.
2. Because the infection is not easily transmitted, it is not necessary to test or treat family members.
3. Eliminate all citrus and dairy products while this medication is taken.
4. Wash all bedding and undergarments thoroughly after the medication is given.

6 A nurse is monitoring a patient receiving metronidazole (Flagyl) for potential adverse effects. Which symptom, if present, would cause the nurse to discontinue the medication and notify the prescriber?

1. Ataxia and confusion
2. Nausea and diarrhea
3. Anorexia and thirst
4. Weight gain and irritability

See Answers to Chapter Review in Appendix A.

References

Centers for Disease Control and Prevention. (2012). *Parasites—Giardia: Epidemiology and risk factors.* Retrieved from http://www.cdc.gov/parasites/giardia/epi.html

Hochberg, N. S., & Hammer, D. H. (2010). Anisakidosis: Perils of the deep. *Clinical Infectious Diseases, 51,* 806–812. doi:10.1086/656238

Jones, J. L., Anderson, B., Schulkin, J., Parise, E., & Eberhard, M. L. (2011). Sushi in pregnancy, parasitic diseases—obstetrician survey. *Zoonoses and Public Health, 58,* 119–125. doi:10.1111/j.1863-2378.2009.01310.x

Lacasse, A. (2013). *Amebiasis.* Retrieved from http://emedicine.medscape.com/article/212029-overview#a0101

U.S. Food and Drug Administration (FDA). (2012). *Bad bug book: Handbook of foodborne pathogenic microorganisms and natural toxins: Anisakis simplex and related worms.* Retrieved from http://www.fda.gov/downloads/Food/FoodborneIllnessContaminants/UCM297627.pdf

World Health Organization. (2013). *World malaria report 2013 shows major progress in fight against malaria, calls for sustained financing.* Retrieved from http://www.who.int/mediacentre/news/releases/2013/world-malaria-report-20131211/en/

Selected Bibliography

Baird, J. K. (2012). Elimination therapy for the endemic malarias. *Current Infectious Disease Reports, 14,* 227–237. doi:10.1007/s11908-012-0250-z

Carmona, E. M., & Limper, A. H. (2011). Update on the diagnosis and treatment of *Pneumocystis* pneumonia. *Therapeutic Advances in Respiratory Disease, 5,* 41–59. doi:10.1177/1753465810380102

Fleckenstein, J. M., Bartels, S. R., Drevets, P. D., Bronze, M. S., & Drevets, D. A. (2010). Infectious agents of food- and water-borne illnesses. *The American Journal of the Medical Sciences, 340,* 238–246. doi:10.1097/MAJ.0b013e3181e99893

Gülmezoglu, A. M., & Azhar, M. (2011). Interventions for trichomoniasis in pregnancy. *Cochrane Database of Systematic Reviews, 5,* CD000220. doi:10.1002/14651858. CD000220.pub2

Herdman, T. H., & Kamitsuru, S. (Eds.). (2014). *NANDA International nursing diagnoses:* *Definitions and classification, 2015–2017.* Oxford, United Kingdom: Wiley-Blackwell.

Huang, Y. C., Su, C. C., & Wang, H. P. (2013). Hookworm infestation, an old but not vanished disease. *Journal of Acute Medicine.* doi:10.1016/j.jacme.2013.01.002

Mittal, V., & Ichhpujani, R. L. (2011). Toxoplasmosis—an update. *Tropical Parasitology 1,* 9–14. doi:10.4103/0000-0205 .72109

Nilles, E. J., & Arguin, P. M. (2012). Imported malaria: An update. *American Journal of Emergency Medicine, 30,* 972–980. doi.10.1016/j. ajem.2011.06.016

Phillips, M. A., & Stanley, S. L. (2011). Chemotherapy of protozoal infections: Amebiasis, giardiasis, trichomoniasis, trypanosomiasis, leishmaniasis and other protozoal infections. In L. L. Brunton, B. A. Chabner, & B. C. Knollman (Eds.), *The pharmacological basis of therapeutics* (12th ed., pp. 1419–1442). New York, NY: McGraw-Hill.

Sevene, E., Gonzalez, R., & Menendez, C. (2010). Current knowledge and challenges of antimalarial drugs for treatment and prevention in pregnancy. *Expert Opinion in Pharmacotherapy, 11,* 1277–1293. doi:10.1517/14656561003733599

Slavin, M. A., Croft, S., & Pillay, D. (2010). Drug combinations for visceral leishmaniasis. *Current Opinion in Infectious Diseases, 23,* 595–602. doi:10.1097/QCO.0b013e32833fca9d

van Lieshout, L., & Jaco, J. (2010). Newer diagnostic approaches to intestinal protozoa. *Current Opinion in Infectious Diseases, 23,* 488–493. doi:10.1097/QCO.0b013e32833de0eb

Vinetz, J. M., Clain, J., Bounkeua, V., Eastman, R. T., & Fidock, D. T. (2011). Chemotherapy of malaria. In L. L. Brunton, B. A. Chabner, & B. C. Knollman (Eds.), *The pharmacological basis of therapeutics* (11th ed., pp. 1383–1418). New York, NY: McGraw-Hill.

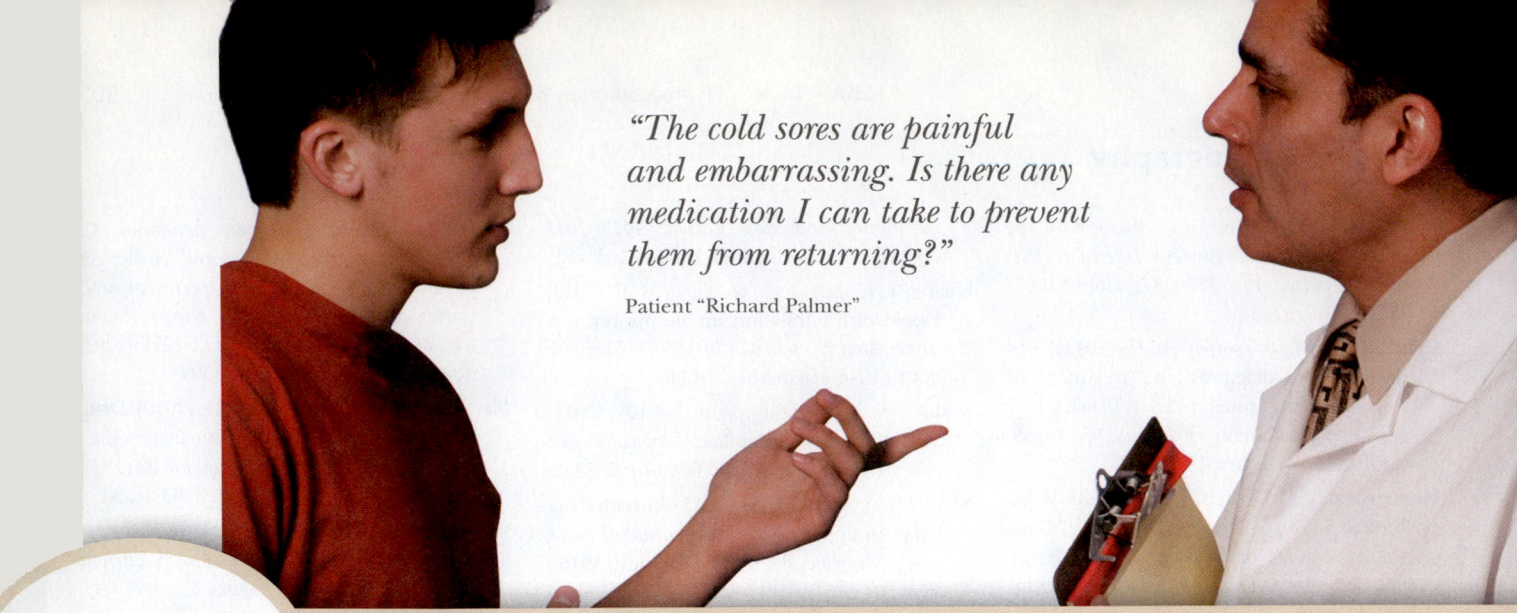

"The cold sores are painful and embarrassing. Is there any medication I can take to prevent them from returning?"

Patient "Richard Palmer"

CHAPTER

54 Pharmacotherapy of Non-HIV Viral Infections

LEARNING OUTCOMES

After reading this chapter, the student should be able to:

1. Describe the major structural components of viruses.
2. Identify viral infections that benefit from pharmacotherapy.
3. Explain the five principal stages in the pathogenesis of a viral infection.
4. Explain general principles related to the pharmacotherapy of viral infections.
5. Describe the nurse's role in the pharmacologic management of patients receiving medications for herpesviruses, influenza viruses, and hepatitis viruses.
6. For each of the classes shown in the chapter outline, identify the prototype and representative drugs and explain the mechanism(s) of drug action, primary indications, contraindications, significant drug interactions, pregnancy category, and important adverse effects.
7. Apply the nursing process to care for patients receiving pharmacotherapy for viral infections.

CHAPTER OUTLINE

▸ Characteristics of Viruses

▸ Pharmacotherapy of Non-HIV Viral Infections

▸ Drugs for Herpesviruses
Antivirals for Herpesviruses
PROTOTYPE Acyclovir (Zovirax), *p. 911*

▸ Drugs for Influenza Viruses
Antivirals for Influenza Viruses
Neuraminidase Inhibitors
PROTOTYPE Amantadine (Symmetrel), *p. 914*

▸ Drugs for Hepatitis Viruses
Antivirals for Hepatitis
PROTOTYPE Tenofovir (Viread), *p. 919*
Interferons

KEY TERMS

capsid, 907

hemagglutinin, 913

hepatitis, 915

influenza, 913

intracellular parasites, 907

neuraminidase, 913

provirus, 909

virion, 907

viruses, 907

Viruses are tiny infectious agents capable of causing disease in humans and other organisms. Because they possess only a few simple molecules, viruses use host enzymes and cellular mechanisms to replicate. Although the number of antiviral drugs has increased dramatically in recent years due to research into the acquired immunodeficiency syndrome (AIDS) epidemic, antiviral drugs remain the least effective of all the anti-infective classes. This chapter examines the pharmacotherapy of non-HIV viral infections, including herpesviruses, influenza viruses, and hepatitis viruses. Drugs for human immunodeficiency virus (HIV) infection are presented in Chapter 55.

Characteristics of Viruses

54.1 Viruses are infectious agents with simple structures.

Viruses are nonliving agents that do not contain any of the cellular organelles necessary for self-survival that are present in living organisms. Viruses infect bacteria, plants, and animals by entering a host cell and then using the enzymes inside that cell to replicate. Thus, viruses are **intracellular parasites**: They must be inside a host cell to cause infection. A mature infective virus particle is called a **virion**. Figure 54.1 shows the basic structure of a virus.

The structure of viruses is quite primitive, compared to even the simplest bacterial cell. The virus is surrounded by a protein coat or **capsid**, which helps to protect it from the surrounding environment. The structural proteins or glycoproteins that comprise the capsid are arranged in distinct, repeating subunits. These proteins help the virus attach to the cell membrane of its host.

All viruses contain genes, which carry the genetic information needed for viral replication, either in the form of ribonucleic acid (RNA) or deoxyribonucleic acid (DNA). Most possess only a few dozen genes.

Some viruses have an envelope surrounding the capsid and genetic material. The viral envelope consists of phospholipids, glycoprotein, and protein "spikes." The phospholipids actually are derived from the host cell membrane as the virus buds off the host cell. The protein spikes are entirely viral in nature. Recognized as foreign by the host's immune system, viral proteins trigger body defenses that attempt to remove the invader.

Although the host cell supplies most of the metabolic machinery needed by the virus, virions contain a few enzymes that serve key roles in the infection process. These enzymes are virus specific and assist the pathogen in entering the host cell, duplicating its genetic material, inserting its genes into the host's chromosome, or assembling newly formed virions. These unique viral enzymes serve as important targets for antiviral drug action.

54.2 The replication cycle of a virus occurs in five stages.

Despite their simple structures viruses are diverse, each having a distinct spectrum of infection. While some viruses are lethal, others can coexist with their host and produce no detectable symptoms. Only a handful of viruses cause significant disease in humans. Selected human pathogenic viruses are listed in Table 54.1. Not all viral infections warrant pharmacotherapy. Viruses that may be treated with antiviral medications include herpes simplex, cytomegalovirus, Epstein-Barr, varicella zoster, respiratory syncytial virus, and hepatitis.

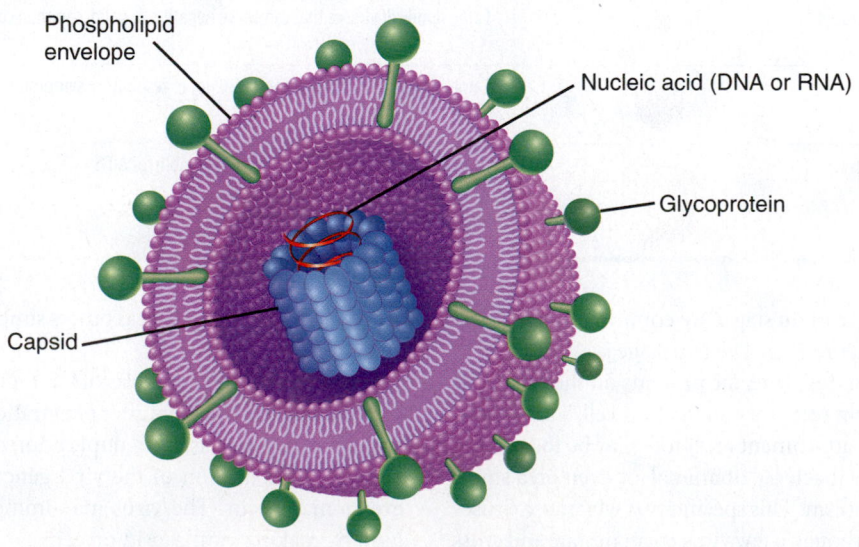

Figure 54.1 General structure of a virus.

	Virus		Description
DNA viruses	Adenoviruses		More than 40 species that primarily infect the human upper respiratory tract but can also cause conjunctivitis, GI infections, hemorrhagic cystitis, and serious infections in neonates
	Hepadnaviruses		Causes hepatitis B by invading hepatocytes; primarily transmitted by injection of infected blood or by use of contaminated needles
	Herpesviruses		Family of viruses that causes cold sores, genital herpes, infectious mononucleosis, chickenpox, and shingles
	Papovaviruses		Family of viruses that can cause tumors or warts
	Poxvirus		Responsible for smallpox, monkeypox, and molluscum contagiosum (a sexually transmitted infection)
RNA viruses	Arenaviruses		Family of 15 viruses, one of which causes Lassa fever, a severe form of epidemic hemorrhagic fever that is highly fatal
	Coronaviruses		Family of viruses, some of which cause upper respiratory tract infections with symptoms similar to the common cold
	Myxoviruses and paramyxoviruses		Family of viruses that includes the influenza virus, respiratory syncytial virus, measles virus, and mumps virus
	Orthomyxoviruses		Responsible for human influenza and avian (bird) flu
	Picornaviruses		Large family of viruses that can cause hepatitis A, polio, common cold, meningitis, and myocarditis
	Reoviruses		Large family of viruses that can cause upper respiratory symptoms and gastroenteritis in infants
	Retroviruses		Family that includes HIV, the virus responsible for AIDS

TABLE 54.1 Selected Human Viral Diseases

Despite their diversity, certain stages are common to most viral infections, as shown in Figure 54.2. The first stage is attachment of the virus to its host cell. In this stage, the proteins on the surface of the virion fuse with protein receptors on the host cell. This attachment is very specific; the "attachment receptor" may be found only in a single species of plant, bacteria, or animal, or even on a single type of cell within an organism. This specificity is why most viruses infect only one species, although a few viruses can mutate and cross species, as is likely the case for HIV.

The second stage of viral infection is penetration of the viral genes and enzymes into the host cell. For some viruses, the entire virion enters the cell, whereas others simply "inject" their genes and enzymes into the host cell.

The third stage is synthesis of viral nucleic acid and proteins by the host cell. Immediately after penetration, a few viral proteins are constructed, which assist in duplication of the viral DNA or RNA. Following duplication of the viral genetic material, two possible events may occur. The virus may immediately begin replicating itself by making viral capsid proteins and viral enzymes and then assembling more virions. In some cases, however, the viral DNA enters the nucleus of the host cell, where it inserts into the chromosome and remains for a period of time ranging from weeks to years

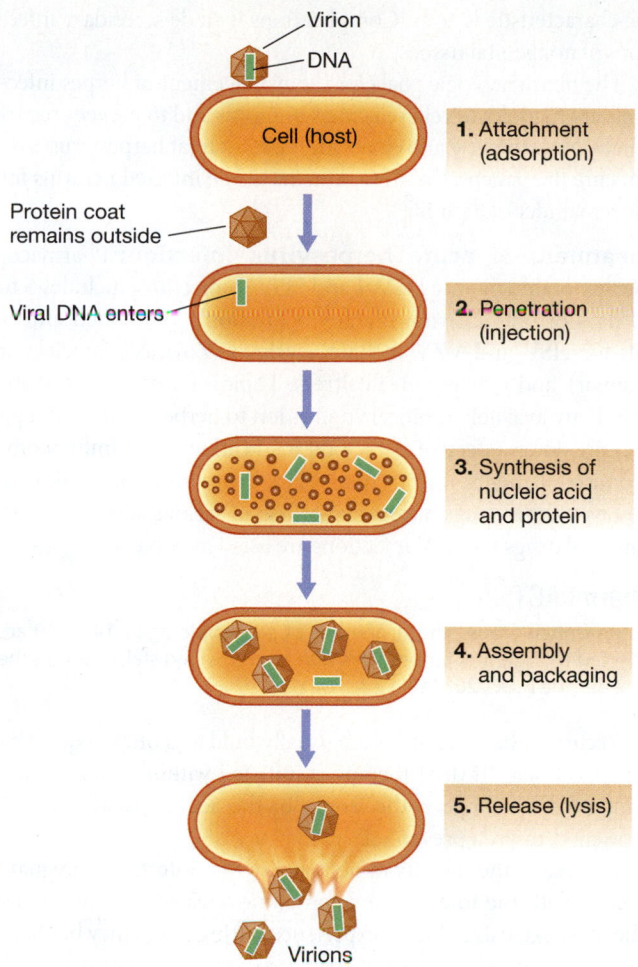

Figure 54.2 The five stages of viral infection.
From *Brock Biology of Microorganisms* (11th ed.), by M. Madigan and J. Martinko, 2006. Reprinted and Electronically reproduced by permission of Pearson Education, Inc., Upper Saddle River, NJ.

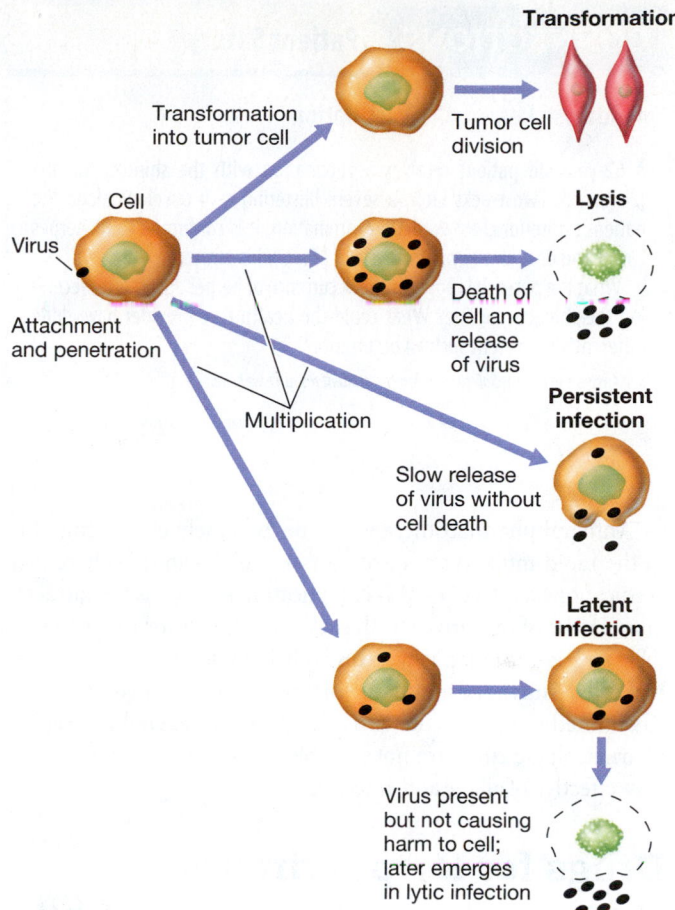

Figure 54.3 Effects of viruses on their host cells.
From *Brock Biology of Microorganisms* (11th ed., p. 251), by M. Madigan and J. Martinko, 2006. Reprinted and Electronically reproduced by permission of Pearson Education, Inc., Upper Saddle River, NJ.

before it proceeds to the replication stage. Once the viral DNA integrates into the host chromosome, it is called a **provirus**.

Assembly is the fourth stage of viral infection. All the viral components, structural proteins, enzymes, and nucleic acids are packaged and made ready for leaving the cell.

The final stage is the release of virions from the host cell. The number of virions may be so large that the cell bursts, releasing all the infectious particles at one time, killing the cell. In other cases, the virions bud off the host's plasma membrane in a slower, continuous process that does not result in death of the host cell.

Pharmacotherapy of Non-HIV Viral Infections

54.3 Antiviral drugs target a specific viral structure or stage of its replication cycle.

Viruses can produce significant effects on their host cells, as illustrated in Figure 54.3. Some viral infections, such as the common cold, cause acute symptoms but they are self-limiting. While symptoms may be annoying, they resolve in 7 to 10 days and the virus causes no permanent effects if the patient is otherwise healthy. For

these viral infections, drug therapy is not warranted due to the expense and the possibility of producing adverse effects that may be worse than the symptoms of the viral infection itself.

Some viral infections are not self-limiting, and drug therapy can be used to prevent the infection or alleviate symptoms. For example, HIV is uniformly fatal if left untreated. Certain hepatitis viruses can result in permanent liver damage and increase a patient's risk of hepatocellular carcinoma. Although not life threatening in most patients, herpesviruses can cause significant pain and, in the case of ocular herpes, permanent disability. Some viruses may even transform normal cells into tumor cells.

Antiviral therapy is targeted to a specific structure of the virus or an aspect of its replication cycle. For example, antiviral drugs are available that inhibit specific viral enzymes or change the shape of proteins that can prevent attachment to the host cell. Many of these drugs have only become available recently, due to research prompted by the AIDS epidemic.

Another approach to treating viral infections is to boost the immune system's response to viral antigens. Prevention of some viral infections can be accomplished through vaccines, which prepare body defenses in advance of the infection (see Chapter 43). Treatment of acute disease may utilize immunomodulators such as interferons (IFNs) that enhance aspects of the immune response. These are of particular value in treating hepatitis (see Section 54.6).

CONNECTIONS   Patient Safety

◀ Adverse Reaction to Vaccination

A 62-year-old patient receives a vaccination with the shingles vaccine (Zostavax). Two weeks later, a severe blistering rash develops along the patient's anterior chest wall. On examination, it is confirmed to be herpes zoster and drug therapy with acyclovir (Zovirax) is initiated.

What is a potential cause for the occurrence of herpes zoster after receiving the shingles vaccine? What could the health care provider have done differently to prevent such an occurrence?

See Answers to Patient Safety Questions on student resource website.

Antiviral pharmacotherapy can be extremely challenging due to the rapid mutation rates of viruses, which can quickly render medications ineffective. Also complicating therapy is the intracellular nature of the virus, which makes it difficult for drugs to find their targets without giving excessively high doses that injure normal cells. Antiviral drugs have narrow spectrums of activity, usually limited to one specific virus. For most of the viral pathogens, pharmacologic cures are not possible; thus, antivirals remain the least effective of all the anti-infective classes.

Drugs for Herpesviruses

54.4 Pharmacotherapy can lessen the severity of acute herpes simplex infections and prolong latency.

Herpes simplex viruses (HSVs) are a family of DNA viruses that cause blister-like lesions on the skin, genitals, and mucous membranes. Herpesviruses are usually acquired through direct physical contact with an infected person, but they can also be transmitted from infected mothers to their newborns, sometimes resulting in severe central nervous system (CNS) disease. Neonatal herpes infection is estimated to have a mortality rate of 50%. The herpesvirus family includes the following:

- **HSV type 1.** Primarily infections of the eye, mouth, and lips, although the incidence of genital infections is increasing
- **HSV type 2.** Primarily genital infections
- **Cytomegalovirus (CMV).** Affects multiple body systems in immunosuppressed patients
- **Varicella-zoster virus (VZV).** Shingles (zoster) and chickenpox (varicella)
- **Epstein-Barr virus (EBV).** Infectious mononucleosis and a form of cancer known as Burkitt's lymphoma
- **Herpesvirus-type 6.** Roseola in children and hepatitis or encephalitis in immunosuppressed patients

Humans are believed to be the only reservoir for HSV. Following its initial entrance into the human host, HSV may remain in a latent, asymptomatic, nonreplicating state in sensory or autonomic nerve root ganglia for many years. Infection is lifelong. Immunosuppression, physical challenge, or emotional stress can promote active replication of the virus and the reappearance of the characteristic lesions. Complications include secondary infections of nongenital tissues.

The pharmacologic goals for the management of herpes infections are twofold: to relieve acute symptoms and to prevent recurrences. Note that the antiviral drugs used to treat herpesviruses do not cure the patient; the virus remains inside infected neurons for the remainder of their life.

Treatment of acute herpesvirus infection: Pharmacotherapy of initial acute HSV-1 and HSV-2 infections includes 5 to 10 days of oral antiviral therapy. Commonly prescribed antivirals for HSV and VZV include acyclovir (Zovirax), famciclovir (Famvir), and valacyclovir (Valtrex). Topical forms of several antivirals are available for local application to herpes lesions, though they are not as effective as the oral medications. In immunocompromised patients, intravenous (IV) drugs may be indicated; however, these drugs have a higher risk of serious adverse effects. Antiviral drugs for HSV infections are listed in Table 54.2.

PharmFACT

In the United States about one out of six people aged 14 to 49 are infected with genital herpes. This rate has remained stable during the past decade (CDC, 2014a).

Recurrent herpes lesions are usually mild and often require no drug treatment. If drug therapy is initiated within 24 hours after symptoms first appear, the length of the acute episode may be shortened, or even prevented.

Because of the severity of neonatal herpes infections, pregnant women with the infection are sometimes treated with antivirals. The most extensive clinical experience during pregnancy has been with acyclovir, which has not been associated with teratogenic effects. The safety and effectiveness of these drugs during pregnancy, however, have not been clearly established. The greatest risk for transmission of HSV occurs when the mother acquires the infection late in the pregnancy.

Herpes of the eye is the most common infectious cause of corneal blindness in the United States. Ocular herpes causes a painful, inflamed lesion on the eyelid or surface of the eye. Prompt treatment with antiviral drugs can stop the herpesvirus from multiplying and destroying epithelial cells. Like genital herpes, once patients acquire ocular herpes they often experience recurrences, which may occur years after the initial symptoms. Use of the antiglaucoma medication latanoprost (Xalatan) (see Chapter 74) has been associated with reactivation of latent ocular HSV.

Pharmacotherapy of ocular herpes is through the local application of drops or ointment. The goal of therapy is to prevent permanent visual disability by limiting corneal involvement of the infection. Trifluridine (Viroptic) and idoxuridine (Dendrid, Herplex) are available in ophthalmic formulations. Oral acyclovir is used in situations where topical drops or ointments are contraindicated. Uncomplicated ocular herpes resolves after 1 to 2 weeks of pharmacotherapy.

Prophylaxis of herpesvirus infection: Due to the expense and potential adverse effects, antiviral drugs are not routinely prescribed for prophylaxis. However, patients who experience particularly severe or frequent recurrences (more than six episodes per year) may benefit from low doses of prophylactic antivirals. Suppressive therapy may also benefit immunocompromised

TABLE 54.2 Drugs for Herpesvirus Infections

Drug	Route and Adult Dose (Maximum Dose Where Indicated)	Adverse Effects
Systemic Drugs		
acyclovir (Zovirax)	Initial episode: PO: 200 mg every 4 h while awake for 10 days or 400 tid for 5–10 days Mild HSV labialis (cold sore or fever blister): 400 mg tid for 7 days Mild genital or perirectal HSV: 400 tid for 7 days Severe genital or perirectal HSV: IV 5–10 mg/kg every 8 h for 7–14 days	*Nausea, vomiting, diarrhea, headache, pain, inflammation at injection sites (parenteral drugs)* Thrombocytopenic purpura or hemolytic uremic syndrome, nephrotoxicity, seizures (foscarnet), electrolyte imbalances (foscarnet), hematologic toxicity or bone marrow suppression (ganciclovir, valganciclovir), neutropenia (cidofovir)
cidofovir (Vistide)	IV: 5 mg/kg once weekly for 2 weeks	
famciclovir (Famvir)	PO: 500 mg tid for 7 days (max: 1,500 mg/day)	
foscarnet (Foscavir)	IV: 40–60 mg/kg infused over 1–2 h tid (max: 180 mg/kg/day)	
ganciclovir (Cytovene, Zirgan)	IV: 5 mg/kg infused over 1 h bid (max: 6 mg/kg/dose) PO: 1,000 mg tid with food (max: 3,000 mg/day) Topical (Zirgan): 1 drop in the affected eye 3–5 times/day	
valacyclovir (Valtrex)	PO: 1 g tid (max: 3 g/day)	
valganciclovir (Valcyte)	PO: 900 mg once daily (max: 900 mg/day; 1,800 mg/day during CMV retinitis induction therapy)	
Topical Drugs		
docosanol (Abreva)	Topical: 10% cream applied to cold sore up to 5 times/day for 10 days	*Burning, irritation, or stinging at site of application, headache* Photophobia, keratopathy, edema of eyelids (ocular drugs)
idoxuridine (Dendrid, Herplex)	Topical: 1 drop in each eye every 1 h during waking hours and every 2 h during the night	
penciclovir (Denavir)	Topical: Apply every 2 h while awake for 4 days	
trifluridine (Viroptic)	Topical: 1 drop in each eye every 2 h during waking hours (max: 9 drops/day)	

Note: Italics indicate common adverse effects. <u>Underline</u> indicates serious adverse effects.

patients, such as those undergoing antineoplastic therapy or those with AIDS.

CONNECTION Checkpoint 54.1

From what you learned in Chapter 3 about the pharmacokinetics of topical drugs, why are topical drugs not as effective as oral agents in the case of herpes infections? *See Answer to Connection Checkpoint 54.1 on student resource website.*

PROTOTYPE DRUG	Acyclovir (Zovirax)

Classification: Therapeutic: Antiviral for herpesviruses
Pharmacologic: Nucleoside (deoxyguanosine) analog

Therapeutic Effects and Uses: Approved in 1982 as one of the first antiviral medications, the activity of acyclovir is limited to the herpesviruses, for which it is a drug of choice. It is most effective against HSV-1 and HSV-2 and effective only at high doses against CMV and varicella-zoster. Acyclovir has no activity against HIV. Resistance has developed to the drug, particularly in patients with HIV-AIDS.

Acyclovir decreases the duration and severity of acute herpes symptoms. When given for prophylaxis, it decreases the frequency of herpes recurrences, but it does not cure the patient. It is available in topical form for placing directly on active lesions, in oral (PO) form for prophylaxis, and in an IV form for severe conditions such

as herpes simplex encephalitis. Because of its 2.5- to 5-hour half-life, acyclovir is sometimes administered PO up to five times a day. PO formulations include capsule, tablet, and oral suspension. A 5% ointment is available for application to cold sores.

Mechanism of Action: Acyclovir is a nucleoside analog that inhibits viral replication by affecting two viral enzymes. First, it enters the host cell where it is activated by a viral enzyme known as thymidine kinase. The activated drug molecule resembles dGTP, one of the building blocks for DNA. As the virus begins to construct its DNA, it uses acyclovir, rather than dGTP. Once the acyclovir is inserted into the growing DNA chain, viral DNA synthesis is terminated, thus stopping the replication cycle of the virus. Simply stated, acyclovir acts by preventing viral DNA synthesis.

Pharmacokinetics:

Route(s)	PO, IV, topical
Absorption	15–30% is absorbed PO, minimal topical absorption
Distribution	Widely distributed, including the cerebrospinal fluid (CSF); crosses the placenta; secreted in breast milk; 9–33% bound to plasma protein
Primary metabolism	Not metabolized
Primary excretion	Renal excretion, unchanged
Onset of action	Peak effect: 1.5–2 h
Duration of action	4–8 h

Adverse Effects: Acyclovir has few adverse effects when it is administered topically or PO. Nausea, vomiting, anorexia, and elevated hepatic enzymes have been reported. Minor skin irritation, rash, and localized pruritus may occur with the dermatologic formulations.

When given by the IV route, acyclovir is associated with nephrotoxicity, and frequent laboratory tests should be performed to monitor renal function. Ensuring that the infusion is administered slowly and that the patient is properly hydrated can lessen the potential for IV toxicity. Neurotoxicity has also been reported at high doses when acyclovir is given IV, including dizziness, confusion, delirium, and coma.

Contraindications/Precautions: Acyclovir should be used with caution in patients with renal impairment because the antiviral is excreted entirely by the kidneys. Doses should be lowered in these patients and proper hydration should be implemented to prevent crystalluria.

Drug Interactions: Acyclovir interacts with only a few drugs. Probenecid decreases acyclovir elimination and can lead to toxic levels of the antiviral. Zidovudine may increase drowsiness and lethargy. Systemic acyclovir may result in additive nephrotoxicity if used with other drugs affecting renal function such as aminoglycosides. **Herbal/Food**: Unknown.

Pregnancy: Category B.

Treatment of Overdose: Overdose may result in coma, seizures, and renal failure. No specific therapy is available; hemodialysis may be initiated.

Nursing Responsibilities: Key nursing implications for patients receiving acyclovir are included in the Nursing Practice Application for Patients Receiving Pharmacotherapy with Antivirals for Non-HIV Viral Infections.

Drugs Similar to Acyclovir (Zovirax)

Other antivirals effective for treating herpesvirus infections include cidofovir, docosanol, famciclovir, foscarnet, ganciclovir, penciclovir, trifluridine, valacyclovir, and valganciclovir.

Cidofovir (Vistide): Once activated, cidofovir resembles a natural nucleoside (dCTP) and is incorporated into the viral DNA chain, causing premature termination. Approved in 1996, its use is restricted to the prevention or treatment of cytomegalovirus retinitis in patients with AIDS, although it has been used off-label to treat HSV, Epstein-Barr, and other viruses. Cidofovir is only available by the IV route. It has an extended intracellular half-life that permits once-weekly dosing, versus foscarnet or ganciclovir, which must be infused daily. Common adverse effects include rash, headache, alopecia, chills, anorexia, and anemia. Cidofovir carries a black box warning that the primary dose-limiting adverse effect is nephrotoxicity. This occurs in a large percentage of patients receiving the drug. Other drugs that cause nephrotoxicity should be avoided during therapy and serum creatinine and urine protein should be monitored within 48 hours of each dose. The black box warning also states that the patient should be monitored for neutropenia during therapy. This is a pregnancy category C drug.

Docosanol (Abreva): Approved in 2000, docosanol is one of the few nonprescription drugs for cold sores and fever blisters. Available as a 10% cream, the drug shortens the healing time and duration of symptoms of the lesions. It acts by blocking the fusion of HSV with its target cells, which is a very different mechanism than other drugs in this class. Docosanol is not absorbed from the skin; thus, no significant adverse effects occur. This is a pregnancy category C drug.

Famciclovir (Famvir): Famciclovir is a nucleoside analog that inhibits viral DNA synthesis in a manner similar to acyclovir, although it has a longer half-life that permits less frequent dosing. Approved in 1994, it is a prodrug, being activated to penciclovir after gastrointestinal (GI) absorption. When used PO for treating acute genital herpes, it reduces the severity of symptoms and shortens the healing time of the lesions. It is also used for prophylaxis of genital herpes and for treatment of acute herpes zoster (shingles). In herpes zoster management, famciclovir shortens healing time from 7 to 5 days and reduces pain. It is well tolerated, with headache, nausea, vomiting, and diarrhea being the most common adverse effects. This is a pregnancy category B drug.

Foscarnet (Foscavir): Approved in 1991, foscarnet is an IV medication that is effective against CMV and herpesviruses. It is indicated for CMV retinitis, acyclovir-resistant infections, and HSV infections in patients with AIDS. Off-label uses include nonocular CMV infections and VZV infections in patients with AIDS. Foscarnet is an expensive drug that exhibits greater toxicity than ganciclovir. Foscarnet has a short half-life that requires daily infusions throughout the therapy period. Headache, nausea, vomiting, and diarrhea are common during therapy. Foscarnet carries a black box warning that nephrotoxicity is a dose-limiting adverse effect that occurs in about 30% of the patients receiving the drug. Serum creatinine must be monitored carefully during therapy. Foscarnet is highly ionized in body fluids and may interfere with mineral and electrolyte metabolism, including serum calcium, phosphate, potassium, and magnesium levels. Electrolyte abnormalities with foscarnet use have been associated with seizures and cardiac abnormalities; thus, regular monitoring of serum electrolytes is essential. This is a pregnancy category C drug.

Ganciclovir (Cytovene, Zirgan): Approved in 1989, ganciclovir is structurally similar to acyclovir and has the same mechanism of action. It is indicated for acute treatment of CMV retinitis and for prophylaxis of CMV infection in immunosuppressed patients. Initial therapy is conducted by IV infusion. Thereafter the patient is switched to PO doses for continued therapy. Ganciclovir has a short half-life and must be administered daily by slow IV infusion during the treatment period. An intraocular implant containing ganciclovir (Vitrasert) is available that releases the drug slowly over 5 to 8 months. Diarrhea, nausea, vomiting, anorexia, abnormal dreams, anxiety, and confusion are frequent adverse effects. A black box warning for ganciclovir states that the principal dose-limiting adverse effect is bone marrow suppression, which can manifest as anemia, neutropenia, thrombocytopenia, or pancytopenia. Complete blood counts (CBCs) and platelet counts must be carefully monitored to assess for leukopenia and thrombocytopenia, because these adverse effects occur in up to 40% of patients taking ganciclovir. Ganciclovir is a known teratogen in laboratory animals. Women of childbearing potential should use effective contraception during treatment. Similarly, men should use barrier contraception for at least 90 days following treatment with ganciclovir. This is a pregnancy category C drug.

Penciclovir (Denavir): Approved in 1996, penciclovir is the active metabolite of famciclovir and acts by the same mechanism. Unlike famciclovir, which is taken PO, penciclovir is available by prescription only as a 1% cream to apply to recurrent cold sores on the lips or face. It should not be applied to lesions on mucous membranes of the nose or mouth. Penciclovir is not absorbed from the skin; thus, no systemic adverse effects occur. To be effective, it should be applied to lesions every 2 hours while awake. This is a pregnancy category B drug.

Trifluridine (Viroptic): Approved in 1980, trifluridine is a 1% ophthalmic solution indicated for primary keratoconjunctivitis and recurrent epithelial keratitis due to HSV types 1 and 2. The drug has no systemic adverse effects and causes only minor eye irritation. This is a pregnancy category C drug.

Valacyclovir (Valtrex): Approved in 1995, valacyclovir is a prodrug that is rapidly transformed into acyclovir after oral absorption. It offers the advantage of greater absorption and higher plasma levels than acyclovir. It has the same mechanism of action, indications, and adverse effects as acyclovir. It was originally approved to treat herpes zoster (shingles), but its indications have since been expanded to include initial and recurrent episodes and prophylaxis of herpes genitalis and herpes labialis. This is a pregnancy category B drug.

Valganciclovir (Valcyte): Approved in 2001, valganciclovir is a prodrug that is rapidly converted to ganciclovir after absorption. Given PO, it has the same mechanism of action, indications (cytomegalovirus), and adverse effects as ganciclovir. Patients must be monitored carefully for neutropenia and anemia during therapy. Patients may exhibit cross resistance between the two drugs. The black box warnings given for ganciclovir also apply for valganciclovir. This is a pregnancy category C drug.

Drugs for Influenza Viruses

54.5 Pharmacotherapy of influenza viruses includes drugs to prevent infection as well as agents to treat active infections.

Influenza, or flu, is a viral infection characterized by acute symptoms that include sore throat, sneezing, coughing, fever, and chills. The infectious viral particles are easily transmitted via airborne droplets or by hand-to-hand contact. In immunosuppressed patients, an influenza infection may be fatal, and flu outbreaks in long-term care facilities can be devastating. In 1919, a worldwide outbreak of influenza killed approximately 20 million people.

Influenza viruses are designated with the letters A, B, or C. Type A is the most common, causes the most severe symptoms, and has been responsible for serious pandemics throughout history. Due to its rapid mutation rate, there are multiple subtypes of influenza A, and each "flu season" is usually caused by a new subtype. Influenza B is much less common, produces milder symptoms, and has no major subtypes. Type C is even less common and produces symptoms similar to those of the common cold. The influenza viruses should not be confused with *Haemophilus influenzae*, a bacterium that causes respiratory symptoms.

PharmFACT

Each year in the United States over 50,000 people die from pneumonia resulting from influenza infection. This is the ninth leading cause of death in the United States (Heron, 2013).

The influenza viruses contain single-stranded RNA genetic material and have an envelope that contains two types of protein spikes important for pharmacotherapy. One spike contains **hemagglutinin**, an enzyme that facilitates the attachment of the virus to host cells. The other protein spike is composed of an enzyme called **neuraminidase**, which assists the virus in exiting the host cell. Continual mutations to the chemical structures of these spikes create new influenza strains that are able to evade the immune system. New strains are named by the hemagglutinin (H) and neuraminidase (N) proteins. For example, the Spanish flu subtype is H1N1, whereas the avian (bird) flu subtype is H5N1. Attempts to develop vaccines for influenza strains been challenging because of these many variants.

The best approach to influenza infection is prevention through annual vaccination. Both inactivated (killed) and live (attenuated) influenza vaccine are available. Those who benefit the most from vaccinations include healthy adults age 65 or older, residents of long-term care facilities, those with chronic diseases, and women who will be in their second or third trimester during the peak flu season. Patients with HIV-AIDS are at increased risk of influenza complications and should be immunized using the inactivated vaccine. Influenza vaccination is also recommended for health care workers who deliver direct care to patients at high risk for acquiring influenza, including patients with HIV infection. Adequate immunity is achieved about 2 weeks after vaccination and lasts for several months up to a year.

CONNECTION Checkpoint 54.2

From what you learned in Chapter 43, explain the difference between a live and an attenuated vaccine. *See Answer to Connection Checkpoint 54.2 on student resource website.*

Only a few antiviral drugs are available to treat influenza. Although these antiviral medications may be useful in preventing influenza or decreasing the severity of influenza symptoms, they should not be considered substitutes for vaccination. The drug amantadine (Symmetrel) has been available to prevent and treat influenza A since 1966. Chemoprophylaxis with amantadine, or the closely related drug rimantadine, is indicated for unvaccinated individuals after a confirmed outbreak of influenza A. Therapy with these antivirals is sometimes begun concurrently with vaccination and continued for 2 weeks. The antiviral offers protection during the period before proper antibody titers are achieved from the vaccine. These drugs are only prescribed for patients who are at greatest risk for the severe complications of influenza due to their expense and the possibility of adverse effects. It is estimated that the antivirals are 70% to 90% effective at preventing influenza A infections. Antivirals for influenza are listed in Table 54.3.

A class of drugs called neuraminidase inhibitors was introduced in 1999 to treat active influenza infections. Neuraminidase is a viral enzyme that allows newly formed, mature virions to bud from infected cells and disperse throughout the respiratory system. Neuraminidase also promotes the penetration of the virus into respiratory epithelial cells and prevents viral inactivation by

TABLE 54.3 Drugs for Influenza Infections

Drug	Route and Adult Dose (Maximum Dose Where Indicated)	Adverse Effects
Influenza Prophylaxis		
amantadine (Symmetrel)	PO: 100 mg every 12 h continued for at least 10 days after exposure or 2–4 weeks after vaccination (max: 400 mg/day)	*Nausea, dizziness, nervousness, difficulty concentrating, insomnia*
rimantadine (Flumadine)	PO: 100 mg bid (max: 200 mg/day)	<u>Leukopenia, hallucinations, orthostatic hypotension, urinary retention, seizures</u>
Influenza Treatment: Neuraminidase Inhibitors		
oseltamivir (Tamiflu)	Treatment: PO: 75 mg every 12 h for 5 days (must be started within 48 h of symptoms for documented efficacy) Prophylaxis: PO: 75 mg once daily for at least 7 days following close contact, or up to 6 weeks during a community outbreak	*Nausea, vomiting, diarrhea, dizziness* <u>Bronchitis, bronchospasm, serious skin hypersensitivity reactions</u>
zanamivir (Relenza)	Treatment: Two 5-mg inhalations bid for 5 days (must be administered within 2 days of symptom onset) Prophylaxis: One 5-mg inhalation every 24 h	

Note: Italics indicate common adverse effects. <u>Underline</u> indicates serious adverse effects.

respiratory mucus. When viral neuraminidase is inhibited, the virions will cling to the surface of the host cell and be noninfectious.

Given within 48 hours of the onset of symptoms, the two neuraminidase inhibitors, oseltamivir (Tamiflu) and zanamivir (Relenza), will shorten the normal 7-day duration of influenza symptoms to 5 days. Oseltamivir is given PO, whereas zanamivir is inhaled. Oseltamivir is the only antiviral approved to treat both A and B influenza viruses in patients 12 months of age or older. Cross resistance has been reported between the two drugs in this class. Because these drugs are expensive and produce only modest results, prevention through vaccination remains the best alternative.

It is important to remember that these antivirals are not effective against the common cold virus. About 200 different viruses, including rhinoviruses, cause symptoms characteristic of the common cold. Despite considerable attempts to develop a vaccine to prevent this annoying infection, success has not yet been achieved. Some drugs, however, may relieve symptoms of the common cold, and these were presented in Chapter 45.

| PROTOTYPE DRUG | Amantadine (Symmetrel) |

Classification: Therapeutic: Antiviral for influenza
Pharmacologic: Viral replication inhibitor

Therapeutic Effects and Uses: Amantadine has both therapeutic and prophylactic applications for influenza infections. When given during an active infection, amantadine significantly reduces the duration of influenza symptoms. When given for prevention, it is estimated that 70% of the patients taking the drug develop protection against influenza A. Amantadine is sometimes used immediately following influenza vaccination to give the patient protection during the 2 weeks it takes for protective antibodies to the vaccine to develop.

Use of amantadine is reserved for patients at high risk for influenza exposure. This includes immunocompromised patients, long-term care residents, health care workers, and close personal contacts of high-risk patients. Furthermore, the Centers for Disease

Control and Prevention (CDC) has recommended that the distribution of the drug be further restricted due to the large number of influenza strains becoming resistant to amantadine. This drug should not be used as a substitute for influenza virus vaccination.

Quite by accident, amantadine was found to have anticholinergic effects that can benefit patients with Parkinson's disease. Although approved for this disorder, the effectiveness of amantadine in relieving symptoms of Parkinson's disease is modest and it is not a major drug for this disorder (see Chapter 21).

Mechanism of Action: The precise mechanism of action of amantadine is not known. It is thought to inhibit viral replication by preventing uncoating, although it may also affect assembly of new virions. The antiparkinsonism effects are likely due to the drug's ability to release dopamine and norepinephrine from neuronal storage sites and possibly prevent their reuptake.

Pharmacokinetics:

Route(s)	PO
Absorption	Completely absorbed
Distribution	Widely distributed, including the CSF; crosses the placenta; secreted in breast milk
Primary metabolism	Not metabolized
Primary excretion	Renal
Onset of action	48 h
Duration of action	Half-life: 20–50 h

Adverse Effects: Up to 33% of patients taking amantadine experience CNS effects that may include insomnia, dizziness, light-headedness, nervousness, loss of concentration, and mental confusion. These symptoms quickly resolve when treatment is stopped. Amantadine can worsen mental problems in patients with a history of psychiatric disorders or substance abuse and cause or increase suicidal ideation. In patients with renal impairment, the drug can build to toxic levels, resulting in symptoms such as visual or auditory hallucinations, seizures, coma, or dysrhythmias. Dosage adjustment in these patients is necessary to avoid toxicity.

Older adults exhibit a higher incidence of adverse effects and often require reduced dosages.

Contraindications/Precautions: Amantadine should be used cautiously in patients with CNS disease, suicidal ideation, or psychiatric disorders, including seizures or psychoses, because the antiviral may worsen these conditions. Because the drug is excreted almost entirely by the kidneys, patients with preexisting renal disease must be monitored regularly. Although rare, amantadine has caused peripheral edema and heart failure and therefore should be used with caution in patients with preexisting cardiac disease. The drug should not be abruptly withdrawn in patients with Parkinson's disease because symptoms of parkinsonism may dramatically worsen.

Drug Interactions: Patients should avoid alcohol use while taking amantadine, because the combination can lead to increased CNS toxicity, including dizziness, confusion, and orthostatic hypotension. Anticholinergic drugs will exhibit additive effects with amantadine. Dopamine antagonists such as haloperidol will reduce the antiparkinson effects of amantadine. Coadministration with trimethoprim-sulfamethoxazole may impair renal clearance of amantadine, resulting in higher plasma concentrations of the antiviral. **Herbal/Food**: Unknown.

Pregnancy: Category C.

Treatment of Overdose: Overdose of amantadine can result in serious CNS toxicity and death. Physostigmine may be administered by the IV route to control some of the CNS symptoms and anticonvulsants may be necessary. Administration of acidic drugs enhances the renal excretion of the drug. Antidysrhythmics and antihypertensives may be administered to manage cardiovascular toxicity.

Nursing Responsibilities: Key nursing implications for patients receiving amantadine are included in the Nursing Practice Application for Patients Receiving Pharmacotherapy with Antivirals for Non-HIV Viral Infections.

Drugs Similar to Amantadine (Symmetrel)

Other drugs for treating influenza include oseltamivir, rimantadine, and zanamivir.

Oseltamivir (Tamiflu): Oseltamivir is a neuraminidase inhibitor available as a PO suspension or capsule that is indicated for the treatment of influenza A or B in patients over 12 months of age. It is also approved for influenza chemoprophylaxis in patients age 12 months or older. Approved in 1999, the drug must be started within 48 hours of the onset of flu symptoms to be effective. Symptoms in patients infected with influenza resolve 1.3 days (30%) faster if oseltamivir is administered. The drug is well tolerated, with nausea, vomiting, and diarrhea being the most common adverse effects. Oseltamivir should not be administered until 2 weeks after administration of the live attenuated influenza vaccine. This drug is pregnancy category C.

Rimantadine (Flumadine): Approved in 1993, rimantadine is chemically similar to amantadine and acts by a similar mechanism. It is approved for the treatment of influenza A infections in adults and for prophylaxis in children. Formulations include tablets as well as syrup for pediatric use. Like amantadine, it is not effective against influenza B. Rimantadine is less toxic than amantadine, with GI complaints such as nausea, vomiting, and abdominal pain being most commonly reported. Older adults experience more adverse effects to rimantadine; thus, doses in this population should be reduced. Like amantadine, the CDC has recommended that use of rimantadine be restricted due to the appearance of resistant viral strains. This drug is pregnancy category C.

Zanamivir (Relenza): Zanamivir is a neuraminidase inhibitor available as an inhaled, powdered formulation. It was approved in 1999 for the treatment of active influenza infections in patients age 7 or older. In 2006, the drug was approved for influenza chemoprophylaxis. Like oseltamivir, the drug must be started within 48 hours of the onset of flu symptoms to be effective. Symptoms in patients infected with influenza resolve 1 to 2 days faster if zanamivir is administered. Zanamivir is well tolerated and devoid of significant adverse effects in most patients. Those with preexisting respiratory disease should use zanamivir with caution, because the drug may initiate bronchospasm in these patients and the use of a bronchodilator may be indicated. Zanamivir should not be administered until 2 weeks after administration of the live attenuated influenza vaccine. This drug is pregnancy category C.

Drugs for Hepatitis Viruses

54.6 The most effective therapies for hepatitis infections are antivirals and drugs that boost the immune system to rid the body of the virus.

Hepatitis, or inflammation of the liver, may be caused by drugs, alcohol, autoimmune disorders, metabolic diseases, or infections. Viral hepatitis is a common infection caused by a number of different viruses. Although each virus has its own unique clinical features, they all invade hepatocytes, producing the same symptoms.

Hepatitis may be acute or chronic. Symptoms of acute hepatitis include fever, chills, fatigue, anorexia, nausea, and vomiting. Chronic hepatitis may result in prolonged fatigue, jaundice, liver cirrhosis, and, ultimately, hepatic failure. Neonates and immunocompromised patients are at higher risk for developing chronic hepatitis. Some patients infected with hepatitis viruses, especially children, are asymptomatic.

The three primary types of viral hepatitis are hepatitis A (HAV), hepatitis B (HBV), and hepatitis C (HCV). These are summarized in Table 54.4. Drugs used to manage viral hepatitis infections are listed in Table 54.5.

Hepatitis A: Hepatitis A, an RNA virus, is spread by the oral–fecal route and causes epidemics in regions of the world having poor sanitation. Outbreaks in the United States, however, are most often sporadic events caused by contaminated food.

HAV has an incubation period of 4 weeks. During this period, and for 1 to 10 days after symptoms appear, the virus is excreted in the stool and the patient is infectious. Clinical presentation includes an abrupt onset of nausea, anorexia, fatigue, and right upper quadrant (RUQ) pain. Hyperbilirubinemia and very high transaminase values are usually observed.

HAV is the most common cause of acute hepatitis in the United States. Although approximately 20% of patients require some hospitalization for symptoms related to the infection, most recover

TABLE 54.4 Summary of Viral Hepatitis Types

Type	Transmission	People at Risk	Prevention	Treatment
Hepatitis A	Primarily through food or water contaminated by feces from an infected person. Rarely, it spreads through contact with infected blood	International travelers; people living in areas where hepatitis A outbreaks are common; people who live with or have sex with an infected person; and, during outbreaks, day care children and employees, men who have sex with men, and injection drug users	Hepatitis A vaccine; also, avoiding tap water when traveling internationally, and practicing good hygiene and sanitation	Hepatitis A usually resolves on its own over several weeks
Hepatitis B	Through contact with infected blood, through sex with an infected person, and from mother to child during childbirth	People who have sex with an infected person, men who have sex with men, injection drug users, children of immigrants from disease-endemic areas, infants born to infected mothers, people who live with an infected person, health care workers, hemodialysis patients, people who received a transfusion of blood or blood products before July 1992 or clotting factors made before 1987, and international travelers	Hepatitis B vaccine	Chronic hepatitis B: drug treatment with alpha IFN, peginterferon (pegIFN), lamivudine, or adefovir dipivoxil Acute hepatitis B usually resolves on its own; severe cases can be treated with lamivudine
Hepatitis C	Primarily through contact with infected blood; less commonly, through sexual contact and childbirth	Injection drug users, people who have sex with an infected person, people who have multiple sex partners, health care workers, infants born to infected women, hemodialysis patients, and people who received a transfusion of blood or blood products before July 1992 or clotting factors made before 1987	There is no vaccine for hepatitis C; the only way to prevent the disease is to reduce the risk of exposure to the virus. This means avoiding behaviors like sharing drug needles or sharing personal items like toothbrushes, razors, and nail clippers with an infected person	Chronic hepatitis C: Drug treatment with pegIFN alone or combination treatment with pegIFN and the drug ribavirin or boceprevir Acute hepatitis C: Treatment is recommended if it does not resolve within 2 to 3 months
Hepatitis D	Through contact with infected blood; this disease occurs only in people who are already infected with hepatitis B	Anyone infected with hepatitis B; injection drug users who have hepatitis B have the highest risk. People who have hepatitis B are also at risk if they have sex with a person infected with hepatitis D or if they live with an infected person. Also at risk are people who received a transfusion of blood or blood products before July 1992 or clotting factors made before 1987	Immunization against hepatitis B for those not already infected; also, avoiding exposure to infected blood, contaminated needles, and an infected person's personal items	Chronic hepatitis D: Drug treatment with alpha IFN
Hepatitis E	Through food or water contaminated by feces from an infected person; uncommon in the United States	International travelers, people living in areas where hepatitis E outbreaks are common, and people who live or have sex with an infected person	There is no vaccine for hepatitis E; the only way to prevent the disease is to reduce the risk of exposure to the virus. This means avoiding tap water when traveling internationally and practicing good hygiene and sanitation	Hepatitis E usually resolves on its own over several weeks to months

without treatment and develop lifelong immunity to HAV. Fatalities due to chronic disease are rare, with only a small number of patients developing liver failure. Thus, HAV is normally considered an acute disease, having no significant chronic form. This makes HAV very different from hepatitis B or C.

Like all forms of hepatitis, the best approach for HAV is prevention: No antiviral drugs are available to treat acute HAV infection. Thorough hand washing after toileting is the most effective method for preventing the transmission of HAV. When visiting endemic regions, travelers should drink bottled or boiled water and not eat raw food.

HAV vaccine (Havrix, VAQTA) has been available since 1995 and consists of inactivated HAV. It is indicated for all children age 2 to 18, travelers to countries with high endemic HAV infection rates, men who have sex with men, and illegal drug users. When a booster is given 6 to 12 months after the initial dose, close to 100%

immunity is obtained. The length of protection has been shown to be 5 to 8 years, although it is predicted that antibody levels may provide protection for 20 years or longer. Adverse effects are mild and include pain or swelling at the injection site, headache, fatigue, and anorexia. The availability of the HAV vaccine has led to a dramatic drop in the rate of this infection in the United States.

For someone who has been recently exposed to the HAV, hepatitis A immunoglobulin (HAIg), a concentrated solution of antibodies, may provide some degree of passive immunity. HAV immunoglobulin is administered as prophylaxis for people traveling to endemic areas and to close personal contacts of infected patients to prevent transmission of the virus. A single IM dose of HAIg can provide prophylaxis for about 3 months. It is estimated that the immunoglobulins are 85% effective at preventing HAV in patients exposed to the virus. Serious adverse effects to HAV immunoglobulins are rare.

TABLE 54.5 Drugs for Viral Hepatitis

Drug	Route and Adult Dose (Maximum Dose Where Indicated)	Adverse Effects
Antivirals		
adefovir dipivoxil (Hepsera)	PO: 10 mg once daily	*Headache, nausea, dizziness, fatigue, nasal disturbances (lamivudine), phototoxicity (simeprevir)* Nephrotoxicity, lactic acidosis (adefovir, tenofovir), pancreatitis (lamivudine), hepatomegaly with steatorrhea (lamivudine, entecavir, tenofovir), cardiac arrest (ribavirin), hemolytic anemia (ribavirin), apnea (ribavirin), myopathy (telbivudine), peripheral neuropathy (telbivudine)
boceprevir (Victrelis)	PO: 800 mg tid	
entecavir (Baraclude)	PO: 0.5 mg once daily; 1 mg once daily for patients with history of lamivudine resistance	
lamivudine (Epivir)	PO: 150 mg bid	
ribavirin (Copegus, Rebetol, Others)	PO: 3,200-mg capsules in the a.m. and 3,200-mg capsules in the p.m.	
simeprevir (Olysio)	PO: 150 mg once daily	
sofosbuvir (Sovaldi)	PO: 400 mg once daily	
telaprevir (Incivek)	PO: Two 375 mg tablets/day	
telbivudine (Tyzeka)	PO: 600 mg/day	
tenofovir (Viread)	PO: 300 mg once daily	
Interferons		
IFN alfa-2b (Intron A)	IM/subcutaneous: 2 million units/m^2 3 times/week	*Flulike symptoms, myalgia, fatigue, headache, anorexia, diarrhea* Myelosuppression, thrombocytopenia, suicide ideation, anaphylaxis, hepatotoxicity
IFN alfacon-1 (Infergen)	Subcutaneous: As monotherapy: 9 mcg 3 times/week for 24 weeks As combination therapy: 15 mcg daily with ribavirin for up to 48 weeks	
pegIFN alfa-2a (Pegasys)	Subcutaneous: 180 mcg once weekly for 48 weeks	
pegIFN alfa-2b (PEG-Intron)	Subcutaneous: 1.5 mcg/kg once weekly for 48 weeks	

Note: *Italics* indicate common adverse effects. <u>Underline</u> indicates serious adverse effects.

CONNECTION Checkpoint 54.3

From what you learned in Chapter 43, what is an immunoglobulin? Name some other disease or conditions treated with immunoglobulins. *See Answer to Connection Checkpoint 54.3 on student resource website.*

Hepatitis B: Hepatitis B (HBV) is caused by a DNA virus. Although transmission in the United States is primarily through exposure to contaminated blood and body fluids, in endemic regions of the world the infection is widely transmitted by the perinatal route and from child to child.

The incubation period in adults is approximately 4 weeks, while in children the asymptomatic period may last decades. Symptoms of HBV infection are indistinguishable from those of other hepatitis viruses and include anorexia, nausea, vomiting, fatigue, and abdominal pain. The acute stage can cause severe jaundice. Treatment of acute HBV infection is symptomatic, because no specific antiviral therapy is available. Although infectious, infants are almost always asymptomatic, which is partly responsible for the spread of the virus from child to child. Ninety percent of acute HBV infections in adults resolve with complete recovery and do not progress to chronic disease. Lifelong immunity to HBV is usually acquired following resolution of the infection.

Chronic HBV infection may be asymptomatic, and it may take as long as 10 years before the chronic stage develops. HBV has a much greater incidence of chronic hepatitis and a greater mortality rate than does HAV. Although adults rarely progress from acute to chronic hepatitis, infants who acquire the infection have a 90% probability of progressing to chronic hepatitis later in life. The final stage of the infection is hepatic cirrhosis. In addition, chronic HBV infections are associated with an increased risk of hepatocellular carcinoma.

Like HAV, the best treatment for HBV infection is prevention through immunization. HBV vaccine (Engerix-B, Recombivax HB) consists of preparations of hepatitis B surface antigen (HBsAg), rather than inactivated virus. In recent years, the recommendations regarding populations who should receive the HBV vaccine have expanded to include many diverse groups, as listed in Table 54.6. Hepatitis B vaccine is very safe, with mild reactions such as pain at the injection site and low-grade fever being the most frequent adverse effects. Three doses of the vaccine provide up to 90% of the patients with protection against HBV following exposure to the virus. Combination vaccines that contain HBV vaccine include Comvax (hepatitis B-*Haemophilus influenzae* type b conjugate vaccine), Pediatrix (hepatitis B, diphtheria, tetanus, acellular pertussis [DTaP], and inactivated poliovirus vaccine), and Twinrix (HAV and HBV vaccine).

For someone who has been recently exposed to the HBV, therapy with hepatitis B immunoglobulins (HBIg) may be initiated. Indications for HBIg therapy include probable exposure to HBV through the perinatal, sexual, or parenteral routes, or known exposure of an infant to a caregiver with HBV. To be effective, HBIg should be administered within 48 hours after parenteral exposure to HBV, within 2 weeks of sexual contact, or to newborns of HBV-positive mothers 12 hours postpartum.

TABLE 54.6   Individuals Who Should Be Vaccinated Against Hepatitis B

- All children, with the first dose beginning at birth
- All children less than 19 years of age who have not been vaccinated previously
- Susceptible sex partners of hepatitis B surface antigen (HBsAg)-positive persons
- Sexually active persons who are not in a long-term, mutually monogamous relationship (e.g., more than one sex partner during the previous 6 months)
- Persons seeking evaluation or treatment for a sexually transmitted disease or HIV
- Men who have sex with men
- Injection drug users
- Susceptible household contacts of HBsAg-positive persons
- Health care and public safety personnel at risk for exposure to blood or blood-contaminated body fluids
- Persons with end-stage renal disease, including predialysis, hemodialysis, peritoneal dialysis, and home dialysis patients
- Residents and staff of facilities for people with developmental disabilities
- Travelers to regions with intermediate or high rates of HBV infection
- Persons with chronic liver disease
- Persons with HIV infection
- Unvaccinated adults with diabetes mellitus age 19 to 59
- All other persons seeking protection from HBV infection—acknowledgment of a specific risk factor is not a requirement for vaccination

From *Hepatitis B FAQs for Health Professionals*, CDC, 2010. Retrieved from http://www.cdc.gov/hepatitis/HBV/HBVfaq.htm

Once chronic hepatitis B becomes symptomatic, pharmacotherapy is indicated with the drugs listed in Table 54.5. The two basic strategies to eliminate HBV are to stop viral replication (i.e., suppress viral load) with antivirals or to boost body defenses with immunomodulators. Three drugs have demonstrated the greatest effectiveness at reducing viral load and are thus considered first-line drugs for chronic HBV infection.

- **IFN alfa or pegIFN.** Thirty to forty percent of patients respond to 4 months of therapy. Five to ten percent of these patients relapse after completing therapy.

- **Tenofovir disoproxil (Viread).** Following 48 weeks of therapy, about 78% of patients respond to tenofovir. Long-term studies show that resistance to tenofovir is very low.

- **Entecavir (Baraclude).** About 70% of patients respond after 48 weeks of therapy. Long-term studies show that resistance to entecavir is very low.

The remaining medications for HBV infection are considered second-line agents because they exhibit lower effectiveness, increased adverse effects, or greater resistance than the first-line agents. The second-line drugs such as lamivudine (Epivir) and adefovir (Hepsara) may be useful when resistance to the first-line drugs develops, or when used in combination with those agents. Clinical guidelines for the treatment of chronic HBV infection continue to evolve as long-term research becomes available.

Because patient symptoms do not reliably indicate the extent of infection, pharmacotherapy is guided by laboratory markers. Hepatic enzymes such as serum alanine transferase (ALT) and aspartate transaminase are used as indicators of liver damage. Hepatitis B DNA, hepatitis B surface antigen (HBsAg), and hepatitis Be antigen (HBeAg) confirm the presence of the virus. Pharmacotherapy is considered successful when hepatic transaminases return to normal values, HBV DNA disappears, and HBeAg is eliminated.

PharmFACT

The rate of new hepatitis B infections in the United States has decreased 82% since 1991. The number of new cases in the United States is estimated to be 38,000 new infections annually (CDC, 2014b).

Hepatitis C and other hepatitis viruses: The hepatitis C, D, E, and G viruses are sometimes referred to as non A–non B viruses. Research is continuing to identify additional hepatitis viruses. Of the non A–non B viruses, hepatitis C has the greatest clinical importance.

Transmitted primarily through exposure to infected blood or body fluids, hepatitis C (HCV) is more common than HBV. About 40% to 50% of all patients with HIV-AIDS are coinfected with HCV. Perinatal transmission rates are very low.

The incubation period for HCV is 50 days. Like other hepatitis infections, HCV symptoms include nausea, vomiting, anorexia, and jaundice. Although acute symptoms occasionally accompany an HCV infection, the majority of patients are asymptomatic. About 70% of patients infected with HCV proceed to chronic hepatitis, and up to 30% may develop end-stage cirrhosis. HCV is the most common cause of chronic hepatitis and is the most frequent indication for liver transplants.

Unlike HAV and HBV, no vaccine is available for hepatitis C due to the very high mutation rate of the virus. In addition, postexposure prophylaxis of HCV with immunoglobulins following exposure to the virus is not recommended because its effectiveness has not been demonstrated.

Current pharmacotherapy for chronic HCV infection includes combination therapy with IFN and the antiviral ribavirin. Combination therapy has been found to produce a more sustained viral suppression than monotherapy with either agent used alone. The sustained success rate for treating hepatitis C is about 50%.

Interferons (IFNs) are immunomodulatory proteins secreted by macrophages, B lymphocytes, and other body defense cells in response to viral infection. Actions of IFNs include suppression of cell division, inhibition of viral replication, and enhancement of macrophage and T-lymphocyte activity. Only the alpha family of IFNs is used in hepatitis therapy, and each IFN has slightly different applications and indications. Information on IFNs used for other indications may be found in Chapter 42.

Boceprivir (Victelis) or telaprivir (Incivek) have emerged as important drugs in the pharmacotherapy of chronic HCV infections. These drugs inhibit HCV protease, an enzyme that is essential to viral replication in infected host cells. Addition of a protease inhibitor to the PEG-IFN–ribavirin regimen is becoming the standard of care for treating this infection. The three-drug combination produces a more sustained viral inhibition, especially in patients with cirrhosis.

In 2013 two new protease inhibitors were approved by the FDA. Simeprevir (Olysia) and sofosbuvir (Sovaldi) are recommended as combination therapy with PEG-IFN and ribavirin. Both are administered PO once daily and exhibit few serious adverse effects. Sofosbuvir may be used with ribavirin alone (without PEG-IFN). The role of these new drugs in the treatment of HCV infection will be determined as more research becomes available.

| PROTOTYPE DRUG | Tenofovir (Viread) |

Classification: Therapeutic: Antiviral
Pharmacologic: Reverse transcriptase inhibitor

Therapeutic Effects and Uses: Originally approved for the treatment of HIV in 2001, tenofovir was approved in 2008 to treat chronic HBV in adults and in children 12 years and older. Tenofovir is given PO, usually in combination with other drugs. When used to treat HIV infection, tenofovir is always combined with at least two other drugs to delay the development of HIV resistance (see Chapter 55). Tenofovir is a preferred drug for treating combined HIV-HBV infections due to its dual effectiveness.

Tenofovir is one of the most effective medications for chronic HBV infection and is considered a first-line therapy. A major advantage of tenofovir over other drugs for chronic HBV infection is that resistance is extremely low during long-term therapy.

Mechanism of Action: Resembling a natural nucleoside, tenofovir inhibits viral DNA synthesis by inhibiting the reverse transcriptase enzyme.

Pharmacokinetics:

Route(s)	PO
Absorption	25% absorbed; taking the drug with high-fat meals increases absorption to 40%
Distribution	Distribution to milk and cerebral spinal fluid is unknown; minimal protein binding
Primary metabolism	Not metabolized by hepatic CYP enzymes
Primary excretion	Renal
Onset of action	Unknown; peak plasma levels reached in 1 h
Duration of action	12 h

Adverse Effects: The most frequent adverse effects include abdominal pain, nausea, insomnia, pruritus, vomiting, dizziness, and pyrexia. Because the drug may cause or worsen acute renal failure, renal function should be monitored prior to initiating therapy and periodically during treatment. Decreases in bone mineral density have been recorded, which may cause fractures in patients with osteoporosis. **Black Box Warning**: Tenofovir can cause a type of liver abnormality called lactic acidosis and severe hepatomegaly with steatosis. Although rare, this type of hepatotoxicity has resulted in several deaths. Also part of the warning, tenofovir may cause acute exacerbations of hepatitis B in patients who are coinfected with HBV and HIV and discontinue this drug abruptly.

Contraindications/Precautions: There are no contraindications to the use of tenofovir. However, patients with renal impairment should receive a lower dose and be monitored frequently for changes in urinary laboratory values. Hepatic enzyme values should be monitored regularly during therapy. If any signs of lactic acidosis or hepatotoxicity are noted, the drug should be immediately discontinued.

Drug Interactions: Tenofovir should not be used concurrently with Atripla, Complera, Stribild, or Truvada; these are combination drugs for HIV that contain tenofovir as one of their components.

Herbal/Food: May be taken with or without food, although food increases the rate of drug absorption.

Pregnancy: Category B.

Treatment of Overdose: There is no antidote for tenofovir overdose. Patients are treated symptomatically.

Nursing Responsibilities: Key nursing implications for patients receiving tenofovir are included in the Nursing Practice Application for Patients Receiving Pharmacotherapy with Antivirals for Non-HIV Viral Infections.

Drugs Similar to Tenofovir

Other antivirals for chronic hepatitis include adefovir dipivoxil, boceprevir, entecavir, lamivudine, ribavirin, telaprevir, and telbivudine. Although structurally different, the IFNs are discussed with this group because they are used to treat hepatitis.

Adefovir Dipivoxil (Hepsera): Approved in 2002, adefovir structurally resembles a natural nucleotide and inhibits viral DNA synthesis of HBV. It is active against several species of viruses, although it is only approved for the oral therapy of chronic HBV infection that shows evidence of active viral replication. Adefovir is an antiviral alternative for patients who have developed resistance to first-line antivirals. Other than headache and abdominal pain, the drug is well tolerated at the doses used to treat HBV. Resistance has not been a clinical problem. This drug has a black box warning that in patients with preexisting renal impairment, urinary laboratory values should be monitored regularly because nephrotoxicity has been reported. Severe exacerbation of hepatitis has been reported in patients who have discontinued therapy with adefovir and some other antivirals. Lactic acidosis and hepatomegaly with steatosis have resulted in several deaths in patients taking adefovir. This drug is pregnancy category C.

Boceprevir (Victrelis): One of the newest antivirals, boceprevir was approved in 2011 for the treatment of chronic HCV infections. Boceprevir acts by inhibiting HCV protease, an enzyme essential for viral replication. Boceprevir is only approved for combination therapy with pegIFN alfa and ribavirin in adults with compensated liver disease, including cirrhosis, who are previously untreated or who have failed previous IFN and ribavirin therapy. Therapy is initiated for 4 weeks with pegIFN alfa and ribavirin before boceprevir is added to the regimen. The most frequent adverse effects of combination therapy with boceprevir are fatigue, anemia, nausea, headache, and dysgeusia. Boceprevir may worsen neutropenia caused by pegIFN alfa and ribavirin. This drug combination is contraindicated during pregnancy (category X) because ribavirin is highly teratogenic.

Entecavir (Baraclude): Entecavir was approved in 2005 for the treatment of chronic HBV that exhibits evidence of active viral replication. Indications for entecavir were expanded in 2010 to include its use as a pretreatment for chronic HBV in patients with decompensated liver disease. Like lamivudine, entecavir is a reverse transcriptase inhibitor that inhibits viral DNA synthesis. Given PO, the drug is well tolerated and the most common adverse effects include nausea, headache, fatigue, and dizziness. A major advantage of this drug is that viral resistance is very low. Because of its effectiveness and relatively high safety profile, entecavir has become a first-line drug in the pharmacotherapy of HBV infection. A black box warning indicates that fatal lactic acidosis and severe hepatomegaly with steatosis have been reported. Exacerbation of hepatitis may occur following discontinuation of therapy with antivirals. Entecavir is not recommended for patients coinfected with HIV who are not receiving pharmacotherapy for HIV. This drug is pregnancy category C.

Lamivudine (Epivir): Originally approved for HIV infection in combination with other antiviral drugs in 1995, lamivudine was later approved for chronic hepatitis B infections that have evidence of viral replication and active liver inflammation. Lamivudine is given PO, often in combination with other drugs. Compared to tenofovir, patients on lamivudine are more likely to develop resistant strains during long-term therapy. The dose recommended for treating HBV (100 mg/day) is much less than that recommended for treating HIV (300 mg/day). Its use in treating HIV is discussed in Chapter 55.

Most patients tolerate lamivudine well, with the most frequent side effects being nausea, vomiting, abdominal pain, and diarrhea. Ear, nose, and throat infections and fatigue may occur in as many as 25% of the patients taking the drug. Lamivudine carries the same black box warning as tenofovir. Both can cause lactic acidosis and severe hepatomegaly with steatosis. In addition, both of these drugs cause severe exacerbations of hepatitis B in patients who are coinfected with HBV and HIV who discontinue this drug abruptly. Hepatic enzyme values should be monitored regularly during therapy. If any signs of lactic acidosis or hepatotoxicity are noted, the drug should be immediately discontinued. This drug is pregnancy category C.

Ribavirin (Copegus, Rebetol, Others): Ribavirin resembles a natural nucleoside and inhibits the viral synthesis of both DNA and RNA. Unlike many antivirals, it has a broad spectrum of activity against both RNA and DNA viruses. Ribavirin is given PO as a tablet (Rebetol) or capsule (Copegus) when treating HCV, always in combination with alfa IFNs. The inhalation form (Virazole) is approved to treat severe infections from the respiratory syncytial virus. Off-label uses include treatment of influenza, herpes, and other viruses. The drug can affect the heart and should be used with caution in patients with preexisting cardiac disease. Resistance has not been a clinical problem with ribavirin. According to the black box warning issued for this drug, the most serious adverse effect of ribavirin is hemolytic anemia, and patients must be assessed regularly for changes in laboratory blood values. In addition, ribavirin has produced embryotoxicity and fetal defects in every animal studied; it is pregnancy category X. Indeed, pregnant health care workers should not care for patients receiving aerosolized ribavirin due to the risk of incidental exposure.

Simeprevir (Olysio): Simeprevir is one of the newest drugs for the treatment of chronic HCV infection, approved in 2013. It is approved as combination therapy with PEG-IFN alfa and ribavirin in patients with compensated liver disease, including cirrhosis. It is given once daily by the PO route. The most frequent adverse effects, when used in combination with PEG-IFN and ribavirin, included rash, photosensitivity, pruritus, and nausea. Sun protection measures should be used when taking this drug. Patients of East Asian descent will exhibit increased risk of adverse effects. The drug is pregnancy category X (due to its combination with ribavirin).

Sofosbuvir (Solvadi): Sofosbuvir is an oral protease inhibitor approved in 2013 for the treatment of chronic HCV infection. It is recommended as combination therapy with PEG-IFN alfa and ribavirin. It may be used with ribavirin alone in patients for whom PEG-IFN is contraindicated. Fatigue and headaches are the most common side effects when used in combination with ribavirin. The drug is pregnancy category X (due to its combination with ribavirin).

Telaprevir (Incivek): Approved in 2011 for chronic HCV infections, telaprevir was approved the same month as boceprevir, and it acts by the same mechanism. Like boceprevir, telaprevir must be used in combination therapy along with ribavirin and pegIFN alfa. Rash, fatigue, nausea, vomiting, anemia, and pruritus are common adverse effects. Cases of Stevens–Johnson syndrome have been reported. This drug combination is contraindicated during pregnancy (category X) because ribavirin is highly teratogenic.

Telbivudine (Tyzeka): Telbivudine was approved in 2006 for the treatment of chronic HBV in patients with evidence of active disease. Like lamivudine, it is an oral drug that inhibits viral DNA synthesis by inhibiting the reverse transcriptase enzyme. Viruses may develop cross resistance between lamivudine and telbivudine. Long-term use of telbivudine with incomplete viral suppression can increase the risk for development of viral resistance. A baseline HBV DNA level should be obtained and subsequent levels determined every 24 weeks to determine if treatment is effective. The most frequent adverse effects include flulike symptoms, upper respiratory tract infection, fatigue, abdominal pain, and diarrhea. According to the black box warning for this drug, fatal lactic acidosis and severe hepatomegaly with steatosis have been reported. Exacerbation of hepatitis may occur following discontinuation of therapy with antivirals. This drug is pregnancy category B.

Interferons: Several IFNs are commercially available as drugs through recombinant DNA technology. Additional information on these drugs is presented in Chapter 42.

- **IFN alfa-2b (Intron A).** This drug is approved for chronic HBV infection. After 4 months of pharmacotherapy, approximately one third of patients will experience long-term loss of HBV DNA and HBsAg. In the second or third month of therapy, patients may experience an exacerbation of symptoms, probably due to removal of infected hepatocytes by the immune system. Patients most likely to respond to IFN therapy include those with a low viral load (HBV less than 20 copies/mL) and ALT greater than 100. Although the majority of patients respond to IFN monotherapy with normalization of transaminases and a reduction in liver degeneration, relapse rates are high. Permanent resolution of chronic HCV occurs in only about 10% to 25% of patients. Combination therapy with ribavirin increases the therapeutic success rate. Interferon alfa-2b is also used to treat hairy cell leukemia and Kaposi's sarcoma (see Chapter 42).

- **IFN alfacon-1 (Infergen).** This drug is approved only for chronic HCV infections. Its antiviral activity is estimated to be five times greater than IFN alfa-2a or 2b. Like IFN alfa-2b, it is administered subcutaneously three times per week. Actions and adverse effects are the same as those for IFN alfa-2b.

- **PegIFN alfa-2a (Pegasys) and PegIFN alfa-2b (PEG-Intron).** These drugs are pegylated formulations of IFNs that produce a more sustained serum drug level over a longer period of time. Pegylation permits the IFN to maintain a consistently high serum level and to be administered less frequently. Whereas standard IFN formulations must be administered three times per week, pegylated versions require only one dose per week. The PEG molecule is inert and does not influence antiviral activity. Pegasys and PEG-Intron are thought to be equivalent in terms of efficacy.

Approved indications for pegIFN alfa-2a include chronic HBV and HCV infections that show evidence that the virus is replicating. PegIFN alfa-2b is indicated for the treatment of chronic hepatitis C in patients 3 years or older with compensated liver disease. PegIFN alfa-2b is usually given in combination with the antiviral ribavirin (Rebetol) over a period of 24 to 48 weeks. Actions and adverse effects are the same as those for IFN alfa-2b.

CONNECTIONS: NURSING PRACTICE APPLICATION

Patients Receiving Pharmacotherapy with Antivirals for Non-HIV Viral Infections

Assessment	Potential Nursing Diagnoses*
Baseline assessment prior to administration: • Obtain a complete health history including immunizations; respiratory, neurologic, hepatic or renal disease; and the possibility of pregnancy. Obtain a drug history including allergies (e.g., specific reactions to drugs), current prescription and over-the-counter drugs, herbal preparations, and alcohol use. Be alert to possible drug interactions. • Assess signs and symptoms of the current infection, noting onset, duration, characteristics, presence or absence of fever, or pain. • Evaluate appropriate laboratory findings (e.g., CBC, hepatic and renal function studies, and viral cultures). • Assess the patient's ability to receive and understand instructions. Include the family and caregivers as needed.	• *Infection* • *Impaired Skin Integrity* • *Fatigue* • *Activity Intolerance* • *Social Isolation* • *Deficient Knowledge* (Drug Therapy) • *Risk for Deficient Fluid Volume*, related to adverse drug reactions • *Risk for Imbalanced Nutrition: Less than Body Requirements*, related to adverse drug reactions
Assessment throughout administration: • Assess for desired therapeutic effects (e.g., diminished or absence of signs and symptoms of concurrent infections). • Continue periodic monitoring of CBC and hepatic and renal function. • Assess for adverse effects: nausea, vomiting, diarrhea, anorexia, fatigue, drowsiness, dizziness, and headache. Decreased urine output or darkened urine, increased bruising or bleeding, increasing fever, or symptoms of infections should be reported immediately.	

Implementation

Interventions and (Rationales)	Patient-Centered Care
Ensuring therapeutic effects: • Continue assessments for therapeutic effects: diminishing signs of original infection, maintenance of normal appetite and fluid intake, and increasing energy level. (Drug therapy effects may not be immediately observable. Gradual improvement should be noted, and the patient should be encouraged to continue taking the medication.)	• Teach the patient to complete the full course of medication. • Encourage adequate nutrition, rest, and activity levels as improvement is noted.
Minimizing adverse effects: • Continue to monitor vital signs, especially temperature if fever is present. Report increasing fever, dizziness, headache, or diminished urine output to the health care provider immediately. (Increasing fever, especially when accompanied by worsening symptoms, may be a sign of worsening infection or adverse drug effects.)	• Teach the patient, family, or caregiver to promptly report a fever that exceeds 38.3°C (101°F) or per parameters set by the health care provider, an inability to maintain hydration or nutrition, or dizziness to the health care provider.
• Continue to monitor periodic laboratory work: CBC, hepatic and renal function tests, viral cultures. (Antiviral drugs may be hepatic and renal toxic. Bone marrow suppression and resulting blood dyscrasias, particularly thrombocytopenia, are also adverse effects.)	• Instruct the patient on the need for periodic laboratory work, correlating any symptoms with the need for possible laboratory tests (e.g., increased bruising or bleeding).
• Continue to monitor for hepatic and renal toxicities; e.g., jaundice, RUQ pain, darkened urine, and diminished urine output. (Hepatic and renal toxicities may occur. **Lifespan:** Age-related physiological differences may place older adults at greater risk for hepatic or renal toxicity. Increasing fluid intake will prevent drug accumulation in the kidneys.)	• Teach the patient to immediately report any nausea, vomiting, yellowing of the skin or sclera, abdominal pain, light- or clay-colored stools, diminished urine output, or darkening of urine. • Advise the patient to increase fluid intake to 2–3 L/day.
• Monitor for signs and symptoms of neurotoxicity, particularly in patients on IV acyclovir, e.g., drowsiness, dizziness, tremors, headache, confusion, changes in level of consciousness, or seizures. Ensure patient safety and have the patient rise slowly from lying or sitting to standing. (Acyclovir, especially when given IV, may be neurotoxic. **Lifespan:** The older adult patient should be monitored closely to prevent falls.)	• Instruct the patient, family, or caregiver to report increasing headache, dizziness, drowsiness, tremors, confusion, or changes in level of consciousness immediately. If dizziness occurs, the patient should sit or lie down and not attempt to stand or walk until the sensation passes. • Caution the patient that drowsiness may occur and to be cautious with driving or other activities requiring mental alertness until the effects of the drug are known.

(continued)

CONNECTIONS: NURSING PRACTICE APPLICATION (continued)

• Monitor patients on amantadine for changes in behavior, psychiatric symptoms, or suicidal thoughts. (An increased risk of CNS or psychiatric symptoms such as suicidal thoughts have been known to occur with amantadine, especially in patients with preexisting CNS or psychiatric disorders.)	• Have the patient, family, or caregiver immediately report any changes in behavior, confusion, delusion, or expressed thoughts of suicide.
• Monitor for signs and symptoms of blood dyscrasias, e.g., bleeding, bruising, significant fatigue, or increasing signs of infection. (Bone marrow suppression may occur and may cause blood dyscrasias with resulting decreases in red blood cells, white blood cells, and/or platelets.)	• Teach the patient to report any low-grade fevers, sore throat, rashes, bruising or increased bleeding, unusual fatigue, or shortness of breath, especially if on drug therapy for a prolonged period.
• Monitor for, and immediately report, signs and symptoms of lactic acidosis in patients taking lamivudine (Epivir) or several other drugs similar to lamivudine. (Lactic acidosis is a possible life-threatening adverse effect of lamivudine and similar drugs.)	• Teach the patient to immediately report symptoms such as abdominal pain, anxiety, fatigue, palpitations, lethargy, rapid breathing and heart rate, weakness, chest pain or tightness, fever, or shortness of breath to the health care provider.
• Monitor for significant GI effects, including nausea, vomiting, and diarrhea. Ensure adequate nutrition and caloric intake. Immediately report any severe or increasing abdominal pain. (Adverse GI effects are common and the patient may also have disease-related effects, e.g., mouth sores. Maintaining adequate nutrition and fluids is essential to healing. Lamivudine [Epivir] is known to cause or worsen pancreatitis, particularly in children with a history of pancreatitis.)	• Instruct the patient to immediately report any severe or increasing abdominal pain to the health care provider. • Teach the patient to avoid acidic foods and beverages, carbonated drinks, or excessively hot or cold foods and beverages that may cause mouth irritation. • Encourage the patient to try small, frequent meals, which may be better tolerated than fewer, larger meals. High-caloric foods and supplemental beverages (e.g., UnJury™, Boost™, or Ensure™) may help add additional calories and supply additional fluids. Assist the patient in obtaining a dietary consultation as needed if nausea or diarrhea makes maintaining intake difficult.
• Encourage infection control and good hygiene measures based on the disease condition, and follow established protocol in hospitalized patients. (Antiviral drugs decrease the level of infection but do not cure the disease. Excellent hygiene measures will limit the chance for secondary infections in the immunocompromised patient.)	• Teach the patient about adequate infection control and hygiene measures such as frequent hand washing, appropriate disposal of dressing material, and adequate nutrition and rest, especially if currently immunocompromised. • The patient may need to be isolated in the hospital or stay at home during peak transmission periods, leading to social isolation. Ascertain if the patient has assistance available if a prolonged period of homebound status is anticipated. • Teach the patient to practice abstinence or always use barrier protection during sexual activity even if genital lesions are not present. Genital HSV infections may be transmitted even in the asymptomatic period. Have the patient consult with the health care provider about suppressive therapy.
• Maintain hydration during antiviral therapy, providing preadministration hydration if the drug is given IV. Hydration may be ordered in the immediate pre- and postadministration periods. Monitor intake and output in the hospitalized patient. (Acyclovir and other antiviral drugs may be renal toxic and adequate hydration is essential to prevent adverse renal effects.)	• Teach the patient on oral antiviral drugs to increase fluids to 2 L/day throughout therapy.
Patient understanding of drug therapy: • Use opportunities during administration of medications and during assessments to discuss the rationale for drug therapy, desired therapeutic outcomes, commonly observed adverse effects, parameters for when to call the health care provider, and any necessary monitoring or precautions. (Using time during nursing care helps to optimize and reinforce key teaching areas.)	• The patient, family, or caregiver should be able to state the reason for the drug, appropriate dose and scheduling, what adverse effects to observe for and when to report them, and the anticipated length of medication therapy.
Patient self-administration of drug therapy: • When administering medications, instruct the patient, family, or caregiver in proper self-administration techniques followed by teach-back. (Utilizing time during nurse-administration of these drugs helps to reinforce teaching.)	• Teach the patient to take the medication: • Complete the entire course of therapy unless otherwise instructed. Suppressive therapy may be used to maintain a symptom-free period. Do not stop the medicine when starting to feel better. • Do not share the medicine with other family members. If there is reason to believe they need medication, they should be assessed by a health care provider. • Take the medication as evenly spaced throughout each day as feasible. • Increase overall fluid intake while taking these drugs. • If using ointments or creams, wash hands well before applying and again after application. If family or caregivers administer the medicine, gloves should be worn.

*Nursing Diagnoses—Definitions and Classification 2015–2017. Copyright © 2014, 1994–2014 by NANDA International. Used by arrangement with John Wiley & Sons Limited.

CHAPTER
54

Understanding the Chapter

Key Concepts Summary

54.1 Viruses are infectious agents with simple structures.

54.2 The replication cycle of a virus occurs in five stages.

54.3 Antiviral drugs target a specific viral structure or stage of its replication cycle.

54.4 Pharmacotherapy can lessen the severity of acute herpes simplex infections and prolong latency.

54.5 Pharmacotherapy of influenza viruses includes drugs to prevent infection as well as agents to treat active infections.

54.6 The most effective therapies for hepatitis infections are antivirals and drugs that boost the immune system to rid the body of the virus.

Case Study: Making the Patient Connection

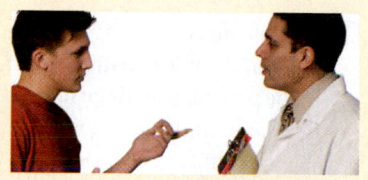

Remember the patient "Richard Palmer" at the beginning of the chapter? Now read the remainder of the case study. Based on the information presented within this chapter, respond to the critical thinking questions that follow.

Richard Palmer, a 19-year-old university student, has come to the health clinic. He states that he gets cold sores at least six to eight times per year. He informs the nurse that the cold sores usually start with lip pain or tingling, often followed by small, painful, fluid-filled blisters on a raised, red, painful area of his lip. The blisters usually last 2 to 3 days in duration then form yellowish crusts that slough off to reveal pinkish skin.

With his final exams coming up, Richard admits to feeling stressed. He also works part time serving at a local restaurant to help meet the expenses

of college. Like other college students his age, Richard eats on the run and seldom sleeps more than 4 to 5 hours per night. His weekends are even more hectic with the job, school, and social activities. Richard requests something to help rid him of the existing cold sore immediately.

Critical Thinking Questions

1. How would you explain the mode of transmission and onset of symptoms for herpes simplex viruses (HSV) to Richard?

2. How would you respond when Richard asked, "Is there any medication that I can take to prevent the cold sores from returning?"

3. Topical acyclovir is prescribed for this patient. What patient education would you provide?

See Answers to Critical Thinking Questions on student resource website.

Additional Case Study

Jeanie Schinkle is a 43-year-old factory worker who has just started a new job. Today, she presents to the employee health services with a fever (temperature: 38.3°C [101.1°F]), headache, myalgia, and cough that developed less than 24 hours ago.

As she is talking to the nurse, she expresses concern that she will lose her job if she is absent from work. "If only I had taken the flu shot, maybe I wouldn't have gotten sick," says Jeanie.

1. Is Jeanie a possible candidate for oseltamivir (Tamiflu)? Why or why not?

2. What health teaching should the nurse provide Jeanie about the flu?

See Answers to Additional Case Study on student resource website.

Chapter Review

1 Acyclovir (Zovirax) has been ordered IV for a patient with a herpes zoster infection to the upper torso and face. Which nursing intervention will help prevent a common adverse effect?

1. Administer the drug slowly IV over an hour, and encourage fluid intake throughout the day.

2. Keep skin areas dry to prevent fungal overgrowth.

3. Administer antihistamines 1 hour before giving the infusion to prevent itching.

4. Assess visual acuity periodically and provide for eye comfort such as lubricating eye drops.

2 The patient is receiving acyclovir (Zovirax) for genital herpes. Which statement, made by the patient, would indicate that patient teaching for this condition has been successful?

1. "Neither the topical nor the oral drug will prevent me from giving herpes to someone else."

2. "I will clean the affected areas with soap and water every other day."

3. "I should wear tight-fitting clothes over affected areas to prevent the spread of the infection."

4. "I should start the antiviral therapy after the lesion forms a crust."

3 Which assessment data would be most important for the nurse to monitor frequently in the patient receiving amantadine (Symmetrel)? Select all that apply.

1. White blood cell and platelet counts

2. Serum creatinine and urine output

3. Mental status and level of consciousness

4. Sodium and potassium levels

5. Lung sounds and signs of peripheral edema

4 The patient has received a prescription for zanamivir (Relenza) for flu symptoms but tells the nurse, "I think I can hold off on starting this, I don't feel that bad yet." What would be the nurse's best response?

1. "That should be fine and the drug has a stable shelf-life so it can be saved for later infections."

2. "It can be saved for later but you will also require an additional antibiotic to treat the symptoms at that point."

3. "It can be started within 2 weeks after the onset of symptoms."

4. "To be effective, it must be started within 48 hours after the onset of symptoms."

5 A patient with chronic hepatitis B has been prescribed tenofovir (Viread). The nurse will teach the patient to immediately report symptoms of what adverse and potentially life-threatening drug effect?

1. Systemic yeast infection

2. Lactic acidosis

3. Heart failure

4. Ventricular dysrhythmias

6 The patient is receiving ribavirin (Copegus, Rebetol) for treatment of chronic hepatitis B. Which manifestation, if present in the patient, would the nurse conclude is an adverse effect of this medication?

1. Neurologic symptoms such as headaches and dizziness

2. Respiratory symptoms such as dyspnea and congestion

3. Skin disruptions such as acne and ulcerations

4. Hematologic symptoms such as excessive fatigue or dizziness

See Answers to Chapter Review in Appendix A.

References

Centers for Disease Control and Prevention. (2010). *Hepatitis B FAQs for health professionals.* Retrieved from http://www.cdc.gov/hepatitis/HBV/HBVfaq.htm

Centers for Disease Control and Prevention. (2014a). *Genital herpes—CDC fact sheet.*

Retrieved from http://www.cdc.gov/std/herpes/stdfact-herpes.htm

Centers for Disease Control and Prevention. (2014b). *Surveillance for viral hepatitis—United States, 2011.* Retrieved from http://www.cdc.gov/hepatitis/Statistics/2011Surveillance/Commentary.htm#hepB

Heron, M. (2013). Deaths: Leading causes for 2010. *National Vital Statistics Report, 62*(6), 20 pp. Retrieved from http://www.cdc.gov/nchs/data/nvsr/nvsr62/nvsr62_06.pdf

Selected Bibliography

Acosta, E. P., & Flexner, C. (2011). Antiviral agents (nonretroviral). In L. L. Brunton, B. A. Chabner, & B. C. Knollman (Eds.), *The pharmacological basis of therapeutics* (12th ed., pp. 1593–1622). New York, NY: McGraw-Hill.

Buggs, A. M. (2012). *Viral hepatitis.* Retrieved from http://emedicine.medscape.com/article/775507-overview

Chou, R., Hartung, D., Rahman, B., Wasson, N., Cottrell, E. B., & Fu, R. (2013). Comparative effectiveness of antiviral treatment for hepatitis C virus infection in adults: A systematic review. *Annals of Internal Medicine, 158,* 114–123. doi:10.7326/0003-4819-158-2-201301150-00576

Derlet, R. W. (2014). *Influenza.* Retrieved from http://emedicine.medscape.com/article/219557-overview

Fiore, A. E., Fry, A., Shay, D., Gubareva, L., Bresee, J. S., & Uyeki, T. M. (2011). Antiviral agents for the treatment and chemoprophylaxis of influenza. *Morbidity and Mortality Weekly Report, 60*(RR1), 1–24.

Herdman, T. H., & Kamitsuru, S. (Eds.). (2014). *NANDA International nursing diagnoses: Definitions and classification, 2015–2017.* Oxford, United Kingdom: Wiley-Blackwell.

Kiser, J. J., & Flexner, C. (2013). Direct-acting antiviral agents for hepatitis C virus infection. *Annual Review of Pharmacology and Toxicology, 53,* 427–449. doi:10.1146/annurev-pharmtox-011112-140254

Kroger, A. T., Sumaya, C. V., Pickering, L. K., & Atkinson, W. L. (2011). General Recommendations on Immunization, Recommendations of the Advisory Committee on Immunization Practices (ACIP). *Morbidity and Mortality Weekly Report, 60*(RR2), 1–24.

Kuehn, B. M. (2011). Antiviral drugs underused in U.S. patients for 2009 influenza A (H1N1) pandemic. *The Journal of the American Medical Association, 305,* 1080–1083. doi:10.1001/jama.2011.284

Lee, H., Park, W., & You, K. S. (2010). Management of hepatitis B infection. *Gastroenterology Nursing, 33*(2), 120–126. doi:10.1097/SGA.0b013e3181d72c59

Muir, P. (2014). Management of herpes simplex and varicella-zoster infections. *Prescriber, 25*(3), 14–23. doi:10.1002/psb.1156

Pearlman, B. L. (2012). Protease inhibitors for the treatment of chronic hepatitis C genotype-1 infection: The new standard of care. *The Lancet Infectious Diseases, 12,* 717–728. doi:10.1016/S1473-3099(12)70060-9

Pyrsopoulos, N. T. (2013). *Hepatitis B.* Retrieved from http://emedicine.medscape.com/article/177632-overview

Salvaggio, M. R. (2012). *Herpes simplex.* Retrieved from http://emedicine.medscape.com/article/218580-overview

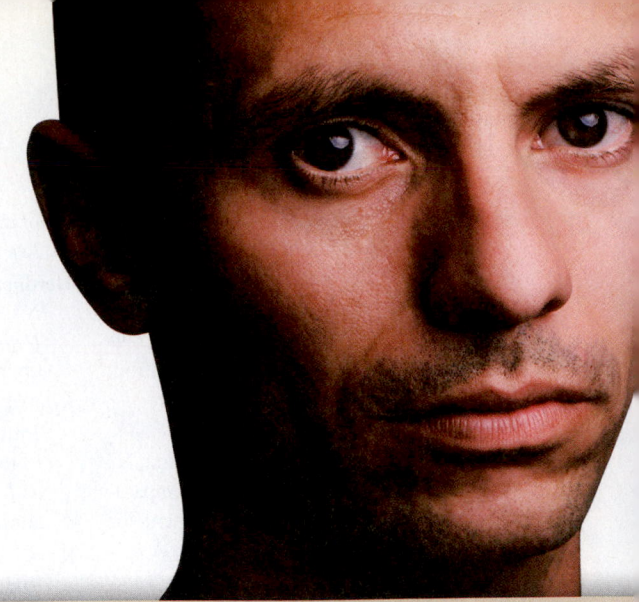

> *"Yeah, I admit it. I'm scared and practically out of my mind with worry. I've known several people who have died because of AIDS. What if this happens to me?"*
>
> Patient "Ryan Orre"

Pharmacotherapy of HIV-AIDS

LEARNING OUTCOMES

After reading this chapter, the student should be able to:

1. Describe the primary steps in the pathogenesis of HIV infection.
2. Explain the therapeutic goals for HIV-AIDS pharmacotherapy.
3. Identify reasons for treatment failure during HIV-AIDS pharmacotherapy.
4. Describe the advantages of highly active antiretroviral therapy in the pharmacotherapy of HIV infection.
5. Compare and contrast the classes of antiretroviral medications.
6. Describe the difficulties in developing a vaccine to prevent HIV-AIDS.
7. Explain the protocol and rationale for postexposure prophylaxis following occupational exposure to HIV.
8. Explain recent advances in the preexposure prophylaxis of HIV infection.
9. Describe the antiretroviral protocols used for reducing the risk of perinatal transmission and for treating pediatric patients with HIV-AIDS.
10. Identify opportunistic infections commonly acquired by patients with AIDS and the drugs used to treat them.
11. Describe the nurse's role in the pharmacologic management of patients receiving antiretroviral medications.
12. For each of the classes shown in the chapter outline, identify the prototype and representative drugs and explain the mechanism(s) of drug action, primary indications, contraindications, significant drug interactions, pregnancy category, and important adverse effects.
13. Apply the nursing process to care for patients receiving pharmacotherapy for HIV-AIDS.

CHAPTER OUTLINE

▶ Pathogenesis of HIV Infection

▶ General Principles of HIV Pharmacotherapy

▶ Classification of Antiretroviral Drugs

▶ Antiretroviral Drugs

  Nucleoside and Nucleotide Reverse Transcriptase Inhibitors

  PROTOTYPE Zidovudine (Retrovir, AZT), *p. 93*

  Nonnucleoside Reverse Transcriptase Inhibitors

  PROTOTYPE Efavirenz (Sustiva), *p. 935*

  Protease Inhibitors

  PROTOTYPE Lopinavir with Ritonavir (Kaletra), *p. 937*

  Entry Inhibitors and Integrase Inhibitors

▶ Prophylaxis of HIV Infections

  Vaccines

  Occupational Exposure to HIV

  Perinatal Transmission of HIV

▶ Pharmacotherapy of Opportunistic Infections Associated with HIV-AIDS

KEY TERMS

acquired immunodeficiency
  syndrome (AIDS), 927
acute retroviral syndrome, 928
antiretrovirals, 927
CD4 receptor, 927

highly active antiretroviral therapy
  (HAART), 931
human immunodeficiency virus (HIV), 927
integrase, 927
lipodystrophy, 933

mitochondrial toxicity, 933
protease, 928
reverse transcriptase, 927
viral load, 929

Recognized by the medical community as a distinct disease in 1981, the first documented case of **acquired immunodeficiency syndrome (AIDS)** has since been traced back to 1959. The syndrome is characterized by profound immunosuppression, leading to opportunistic infections (OIs) and malignancies not commonly acquired by people with intact immune defenses. The **human immunodeficiency virus (HIV)** was quickly identified as the causative agent for AIDS. HIV-AIDS has resulted in a tragic, worldwide epidemic, causing the deaths of millions of people. The infection continues to be a major public health challenge.

PharmFACT

More than 1 million Americans are living with HIV; 20% do not know they are infected (Lowes, 2011).

Pathogenesis of HIV Infection

55.1 HIV causes a profound loss of immune function.

The two primary types of HIV are HIV-1 and HIV-2. Because more than 99% of the global AIDS cases are caused by HIV-1, the discussion in this text will apply only to HIV-1. HIV uses the same stages of viral infection described in Chapter 54. There are, however, additional details that are important to understanding the pharmacotherapy of HIV infection.

Transmission: HIV infection occurs by exposure to contaminated body fluids, most commonly blood or semen, because these fluids have the highest concentration of the virus. Transmission may also occur through sexual activity or through contact of infected fluids with broken skin, mucous membranes, or needlesticks. Newborns of a mother infected with HIV may acquire the virus during birth or breast-feeding. Although in industrialized nations the majority of patients with HIV-AIDS are men who have sex with other men, heterosexual transmission is significant and is the predominant means of acquiring the infection in developing countries.

PharmFACT

About 32,000 new cases of AIDS are diagnosed each year in the United States. Approximately half of these involve male-to-male sexual contact. However, about one in every four people who acquire this disease is a woman who acquired the infection through heterosexual contact (Centers for Disease Control and Prevention [CDC], 2013a).

Replication cycle: Like other viruses, HIV must infect a host cell to duplicate its genetic material and assemble more virus particles (virions). Knowledge of the replication cycle of HIV is critical to understanding the pharmacotherapy of HIV-AIDS and is shown in Pharmacotherapy Illustrated 55.1.

The first stage of HIV pathogenesis is the attachment of the virus to its preferred target: the **CD4 receptor** on the surface of T4 lymphocytes. (Note that the terms *CD4 cells*, *T4 cells*, and *T4 lymphocytes* are used interchangeably in this text.) During this initial stage, structural proteins on the surface of HIV fuse with the CD4 receptor. Because these receptors are also present on monocytes, macrophages, and dendritic cells, multiple cell types become infected. In addition to the CD4 receptor, coreceptors known as CCR5 and CXCR4 have been discovered that assist HIV in binding to the T4 lymphocyte.

The second stage of pathogenesis is the penetration of HIV into the T4 lymphocyte. The virus uncoats and the single-stranded ribonucleic acid (RNA) genetic material enters the host cell. HIV converts its RNA strands to double-stranded deoxyribonucleic acid (DNA), using the viral enzyme **reverse transcriptase**. Only a few viruses are able to construct DNA from RNA; no bacteria, plants, or animals are able to perform this unique metabolic function. All living organisms make RNA from DNA. Because of their "backward" or reverse DNA synthesis, these viruses are called *retroviruses* and drugs used to treat HIV infections are called **antiretrovirals**. Although unique to HIV, reverse transcriptase is an inefficient enzyme that makes many errors when converting the viral RNA to double-stranded DNA. The enzyme has no "proofreading" ability, which allows errors in the viral genetic code to accumulate. This produces a high mutation rate, making it difficult to develop effective vaccines.

The viral DNA eventually enters the nucleus of the T4 lymphocyte where it becomes incorporated into the host's chromosomes. This action is performed by HIV **integrase**, another enzyme unique to HIV. Once incorporated into human chromosomes, the HIV is called a provirus, and it remains for the lifetime of the cell. It is impossible to recognize the HIV provirus or remove it. Indeed, despite the fact that the T4 lymphocyte is infected with a deadly virus, the host's immune system is unable to effectively remove the defective cells.

This *latent phase* of the infection may last only a few weeks, or it may continue for decades. During this phase, patients are asymptomatic and do not realize they are infected. It was once thought that the virus was truly "silent" during the latent phase but research has demonstrated that continuous HIV replication and immune system damage are occurring.

At some point, the latent provirus becomes activated and produces large amounts of viral messenger RNA, with the first strands producing viral proteins that amplify the replication process. All structural components of HIV are subsequently synthesized, and the cell is ready to assemble more virions.

The individual structural components of HIV migrate to the plasma membrane of the host cell, where they are packaged, and eventually bud from the host cell. The new virions, however, are not

PHARMACOTHERAPY ILLUSTRATED 55.1

Replication of HIV

yet infectious. As a final step, the viral enzyme **protease** cleaves some of the larger proteins to smaller, functional forms. Once budding occurs, the immune system recognizes that the cell is infected and kills the T4 lymphocyte. Unfortunately, it is too late; it is estimated that a patient infected with HIV may produce as many as 10 billion new virions every day, and the immune system becomes overwhelmed by the infection.

Symptoms: Many people incorrectly assume that because the body cannot rid itself of HIV, the immune system does not recognize invasion by the virus. Indeed, the immune system mounts an immediate, massive defense to the entry of HIV, producing an acute inflammatory response that rids the body of many of the infectious virions. It is estimated that a billion HIV virions are destroyed each day during this early stage. Patients experience sore throat, fever, rash, malaise, and weight loss that may last several weeks. However, because patients often mistake these vague symptoms for the common cold or flu, they do not realize that HIV infection has occurred and rarely seek medical intervention. Symptoms during this initial phase are known as

the **acute retroviral syndrome**. Although body defenses may suppress the viral invasion, tragically they are unable to eliminate the virus.

Progression to AIDS is characterized by gradual destruction of the immune system, as measured by the steady decline in the number of CD4 lymphocytes. Unfortunately, the CD4 lymphocyte is the primary cell coordinating the immune response for both the humoral and cell-mediated branches of the immune system. When the CD4 cell count falls below a critical level, the patient begins to experience opportunistic bacterial, fungal, and viral diseases and certain malignancies. Left untreated, the patient eventually is unable to mount any immune defense, and death occurs.

CONNECTION Checkpoint 55.1

Patients who are receiving immunosuppressant drugs have low white blood cell counts and, like patients with AIDS, are at risk for contracting OIs. From what you learned in Chapter 42, what are the major indications for immunosuppressant therapy? *See Answer to Connection Checkpoint 55.1 on student resource website.*

General Principles of HIV Pharmacotherapy

55.2 Treatment of HIV infection is difficult due to the latent nature of the virus and the development of resistant strains.

The widespread appearance of HIV infection in 1981 created enormous challenges for public health and an unprecedented need for the development of new antiviral drugs. HIV-AIDS is unlike any other infectious disease because it is sexually transmitted, uniformly fatal, and demands a continuous supply of new drugs for patient survival. Over 20 new antiretroviral drugs were developed over the past 30 years, but the disease remains incurable. Although the infection can be managed, stopping antiretroviral therapy always results in a rapid rebound in HIV replication. With HIV mutating extremely rapidly and resistant strains developing so quickly, the creation of new, novel approaches to antiretroviral drug therapy must remain a high priority in treating HIV infection.

While pharmacotherapy for HIV-AIDS has not produced a cure, it has resulted in a number of therapeutic successes. For example, many patients with HIV infection are able to live symptom free with their disease for a longer time period due to medications. Furthermore, the transmission of the virus from a mother infected with HIV to her newborn has been reduced dramatically due to intensive drug therapy of the mother prior to delivery and of the baby immediately following birth. Along with better patient education and prevention, successes in pharmacotherapy have produced a steep and steady decline in the death rate due to HIV-AIDS in the United States from a high of almost 41,000 in 1985 to around 15,000 now. Unfortunately, this decline has not been observed in African countries, where antiretroviral drugs are not as readily available, largely due to their high cost.

The therapeutic goals for the pharmacotherapy of HIV-AIDS include the following:

- Reduce HIV-related morbidity and prolong survival
- Improve quality of life
- Restore and preserve immunologic function
- Suppress viral load
- Prevent transmission from mother to child in pregnant patients who have HIV infection

Initiation of antiretroviral therapy: Should pharmacotherapy of HIV infection start as soon as the disease is diagnosed, or should it be postponed until symptoms develop? The optimum time to begin antiretroviral therapy remains controversial and has been a subject of much debate and research. In current clinical practice, the following serve as guidelines for initiating antiretroviral therapy:

- Antiretroviral therapy should be initiated in patients with a history of an AIDS-defining illness or with a CD4 cell count below 350 cells/mm^3.
- Antiretroviral therapy should also be initiated in the following groups of infected patients regardless of CD4 cell count: pregnant women, patients with HIV-associated nephropathy, and patients coinfected with hepatitis B virus (HBV) when HBV treatment is indicated.

- Antiretroviral therapy may be considered in some patients with CD4 cell counts above 350 cells/mm^3. This includes those patients with HIV who also have tuberculosis (TB), Kaposi's sarcoma, non-Hodgkin's lymphoma, and other malignancies.

The primary advantage of initiating therapy during the asymptomatic stage of HIV infection is that the number of replicating virions can be reduced. Early antiretroviral therapy has been shown to delay the onset of acute symptoms and the progression to AIDS. OIs can be prevented. Pharmacotherapy is beneficial even when started late in the course of an infection. However, organ damage to the kidneys and heart caused by ongoing viral replication may not be repairable if pharmacotherapy is initiated in the later stages of the disease.

The decision to begin treatment during the asymptomatic stage has certain negative consequences. Medications for HIV-AIDS treatment are expensive, ranging from $24,000 to $60,000 per year. Antiretrovirals can produce serious adverse effects and may interact with other drugs the patient is taking. Continuous pharmacotherapy over many years promotes viral resistance so that when the acute stage eventually develops, the medications may no longer be effective. These serious consequences must be weighed against the risk of deferring therapy; postponing treatment may cause the disease to reach a critical point at which antiretroviral rescue is not possible.

The decision to begin therapy in patients with *symptomatic* HIV disease is much easier, since the severe symptoms of AIDS can rapidly progress to death. Thus, pharmacotherapy nearly always occurs during this phase.

Patients receiving their first treatment for HIV infection are called antiretroviral *naïve*. Therapy for antiretroviral naïve patients is often different from that for antiretroviral experienced patients because drug-resistant strains of HIV develop during therapy.

Monitoring the progress of antiretroviral therapy: Two laboratory tests used to guide pharmacotherapy are absolute CD4 cell count and measurement of HIV RNA in the plasma. Figure 55.1 illustrates the value of using these two tests in predicting the prognosis of patients with this infection.

The number of CD4 lymphocytes is an important indicator of immune function that indicates the actual degree of immune system damage caused by the virus. It is a good predictor of the likelihood of the patient acquiring an OI. Normal values range from 500 to 1,600 cells/mcL. Patients with HIV infection whose CD4 lymphocyte count falls below 250 cells/mcL are said to have AIDS. Once treatment has succeeded in raising the CD4 cell count above the level for OI risk, this laboratory test is conducted every 6 to 12 months.

The **viral load** is determined by measuring the amount of HIV RNA in the blood, which provides an estimate of how rapidly the virus is replicating in the body. Plasma viral load is considered the most reliable indicator of response to drug treatment. HIV RNA levels are determined every 3 to 6 months to monitor progression of the disease and to assess the degree of success of antiretroviral therapy. The goal of antiretroviral therapy is to reduce plasma HIV

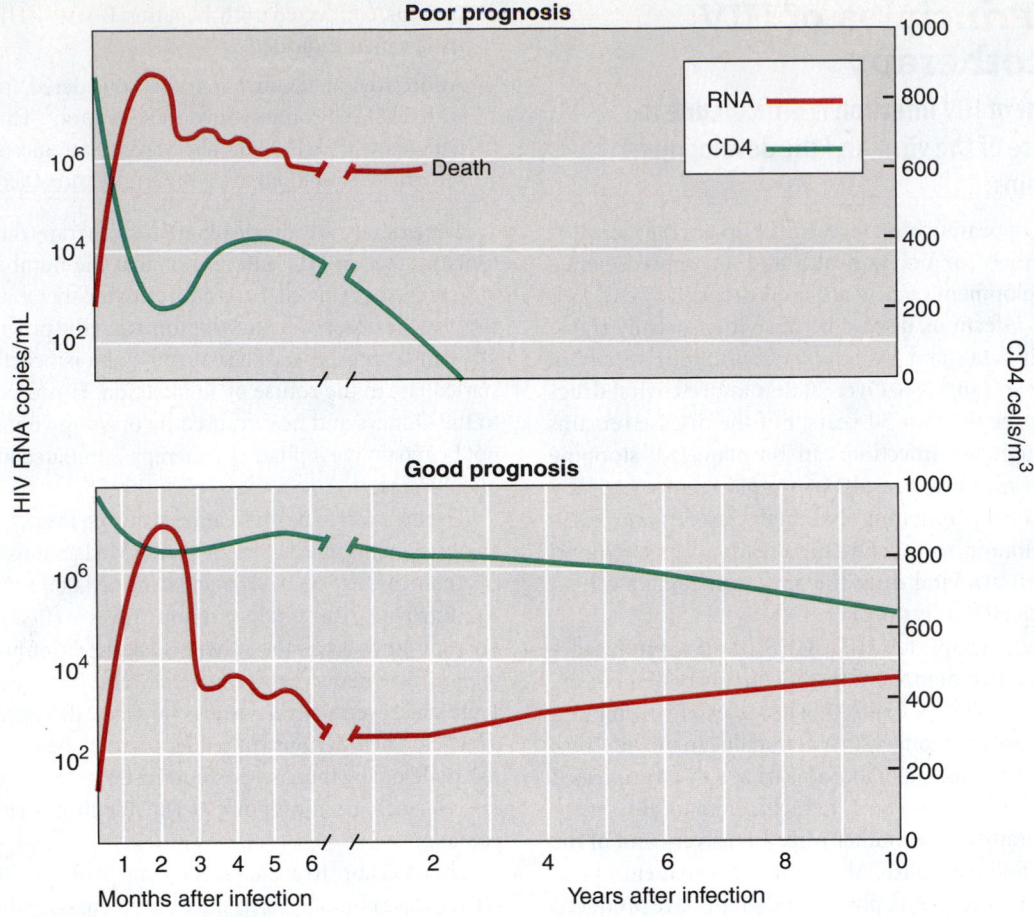

Figure 55.1 Use of CD4 lymphocyte and HIV RNA counts to predict therapeutic outcomes.

From *Brock Biology of Microorganisms* (11th ed.), by M. Madigan, J. Martinko, D. Stahl, and D. Clark, 2006. Reprinted by permission of Pearson Education, Inc., Upper Saddle River, NJ.

RNA to less than 48 copies/mL. For most patients, 12 to 24 weeks of HIV pharmacotherapy is required to achieve this level.

Treatment failures: Antiretroviral therapy does not totally eliminate the virus from the body and treatment must continue for the lifetime of the patient infected with HIV. Given the high mutation rate of the virus and decades of therapy, it is easy to understand why treatment failures are so common. Therapeutic failures are extremely challenging for nurses, other health care providers, and patients. The primary factors responsible for treatment failure are adverse effects of the medications, lack of adherence to drug therapy, emergence of resistant HIV strains, and the genetic variability among patients.

Should treatment failure occur, laboratory drug resistance testing is conducted to determine which drug(s) are affected. Higher doses are generally not indicated, because they lead to an increased incidence of serious adverse effects. Ideally, the patient is switched to at least two (preferably three) drugs from chemical classes that will yield full antiviral activity. Unless the treatment failure is severe, adding only a single new drug to the regimen is discouraged because it often leads to the rapid development of resistance.

Antiretroviral drugs cause many adverse effects, including nausea, diarrhea, rash, lipid abnormalities, hepatotoxicity, neuropathy, and increased risk of cardiovascular events. Patients always take at least two of these drugs (and usually more), which often interact with other medications to cause additional adverse effects. Identifying the specific drug interaction causing a toxic effect is challenging for the clinician. Serious adverse effects often require an immediate change in pharmacotherapy. Once the offending drug is identified, it is normally replaced with another drug from the same class. Other times, a simple adjustment, such as changing the amount per dose or spacing doses further apart, may prevent or eliminate the adverse effect. Adding antinausea drugs or antidiarrheal drugs to the regimen can diminish some of the more common adverse effects.

To be successful, antiretroviral therapy requires strict patient adherence to a complex regimen. Unfortunately, many factors deter patients from adhering to the regimen. Some antiretroviral drugs have inconvenient schedules and must be taken three to four times per day or be given parenterally. Some are expensive or simply not available to patients in developing countries. Others make the patients feel quite ill; patients may actually feel much better without taking the drugs. Given these complicating factors, and the prospect of a lifetime of drug therapy, it is easy to understand why adherence to the medication regimen is difficult, even for a motivated patient. The nurse is the key to helping develop a rational daily plan of treatment that best fits the lifestyle of the patient and family.

Drug resistance has become a serious barrier to pharmacotherapeutic success in treating HIV-AIDS. When standard therapies fail, viral resistance must always be considered as a potential source of the failure. Baseline HIV drug resistance testing is now recommended when patients enter care. Follow-up drug resistance testing is performed following a failed regimen to determine the future direction of therapy.

For some drugs such as nevirapine and lamivudine, a single mutation in HIV can produce a strain that will be resistant to all drugs in the same class. Indeed, resistance has been demonstrated after only a single dose of nevirapine. For others, such as the protease inhibitors, several mutations are necessary to confer resistance. Resistant strains may be transmitted between patients through sexual activity or injectable drug abuse. Some patients have developed HIV strains resistant to all four primary classes of antiretrovirals. This situation produces a critical need for the development of new antiretrovirals that act by novel mechanisms. Considerable research is ongoing to determine the optimal therapeutic regimens that delay the emergence of resistant strains.

Why do some patients succumb to HIV infections within months after diagnosis while others survive for decades? Considerable research over three decades has focused on genetic factors that have allowed some individuals to live with HIV for a long time without progressing to AIDS. These patients are known as long-term nonprogressors (LTNPs). Scientists have looked for specific antibodies, cytokines, and protective immune responses in these patients with the hope of developing therapies to help other infected patients. While some progress has been made in this area, researchers are far from understanding the protective genetic makeup of these LTNPs. Until knowledge advances, HIV infection will continue to be potentially fatal in every patient who acquires the infection.

Structured treatment interruptions: Health care providers once recommended the use of structured treatment interruptions: periods of time where all antiretroviral drugs were withdrawn. It was thought that treatment interruptions reduced levels of adverse effects, gave patients a welcome drug-free holiday, and diminished the potential for resistant HIV strains. Research has now clearly demonstrated that treatment interruptions and total discontinuation of medication is not effective and will result in an immediate increase in viral load.

Sexual lifestyle adjustments: Patients with HIV infection often face serious mental health challenges because of their illness. Most patients are young and sexually active. Knowing that they will likely die prematurely of the infection and that they could kill others through unsafe sexual practices is difficult to accept. Many patients benefit from psychotherapy, and all benefit from compassionate, nonjudgmental nursing care. Teaching patients with HIV-AIDS how to care for themselves and how to protect others from their disease is a major task of the nurse.

Studies have shown that antiretroviral therapy can markedly reduce the amount of HIV viral load in blood and body secretions. This should not be interpreted to mean that the patient is noninfectious. Patients who are asymptomatic, whether they are receiving antiretroviral therapy or not, are still infectious. Patients must observe abstinence or safe sexual practices for the remainder of their lifetimes to protect others from this lethal viral infection.

Classification of Antiretroviral Drugs

55.3 Six classes of antiretroviral drugs are available to treat HIV infection.

Antiretroviral drugs target specific phases of the HIV replication cycle. The standard pharmacotherapy for HIV-AIDS includes aggressive treatment with multiple drugs concurrently, a regimen called **highly active antiretroviral therapy (HAART)**. The goal of HAART is to reduce the replication of HIV as much as possible, as measured by a reduction in plasma HIV RNA to its lowest possible (or undetectable) level. The simultaneous use of medications from several classes reduces the probability that HIV will become resistant to treatment.

It is important to understand that eliminating the virus from the blood is not a cure because HIV is harbored in locations other than the blood, such as lymph nodes. In fact, only a small percentage of the total CD4 lymphocytes in the body is circulating in the blood at any given time. Should a patient reach a stage where HIV RNA levels are undetectable, it is important for the nurse to stress that the disease has not been cured and that antiretroviral therapy must be continued for the lifetime of the patient.

Antiretroviral drugs, listed in Table 55.1, are classified into the following groups, based on their mechanism of action:

- Nucleoside/nucleotide reverse transcriptase inhibitors (NRTIs/NtRTIs)
- Nonnucleoside reverse transcriptase inhibitors (NNRTIs)
- Protease inhibitors (PIs)
- Entry inhibitors (includes fusion inhibitors and CCR5 antagonists)
- Integrase inhibitors

Throughout the AIDS epidemic, pharmacotherapeutic regimens for treating the infection have continuously evolved based on ongoing research. Recommendations vary based on comorbid conditions such as hepatitis, TB, liver disease, or kidney disease. In current clinical practice, the following regimens have been shown to be the most successful choices for the *initial* therapy of HIV infection (Panel on Antiretroviral Guidelines for Adults and Adolescents, 2013):

- **NNRTI-based regimen:** efavirenz + tenofovir + emtricitabine (available as a fixed-dose combination: Atripla)
- **PI-based regimens:**
  - atazanavir (ritonavir-boosted) + tenofovir + emtricitabine
  - darunavir (ritonavir-boosted) + tenofovir + emtricitabine
- **Integrase inhibitor–based regimen:** raltegravir + tenofovir + emtricitabine

Although the preceding drug combinations are recommended, divergence to other regimens is necessary, especially as resistant strains develop. The pharmacotherapy of HIV-AIDS is rapidly evolving, and health care providers are still learning what drug combinations are most effective. The nurse should always review the latest medical literature before treating patients with HIV-AIDS.

TABLE 55.1 Antiretroviral Drugs for HIV-AIDS

Drug	Route and Adult Dose (Maximum Dose Where Indicated)	Adverse Effects
Nonnucleoside Reverse Transcriptase Inhibitors		
delavirdine (Rescriptor)	PO: 400 mg tid (max: 1,200 mg/day)	*Rash, fever, nausea, diarrhea, headache, stomatitis*
efavirenz (Sustiva)	PO: 600 mg/day (max: 600 mg/day)	Paresthesia, hepatotoxicity (nevirapine), Stevens–Johnson syndrome (SJS), CNS toxicity (efavirenz), severe depression (rilpivirine)
etravirine (Intelence)	PO: 200 mg bid following a meal (max: 400 mg/day)	
nevirapine (Viramune)	PO: 200 mg/day for 14 days, then increase to bid	
rilpivirine (Edurant)	PO: 25 mg once daily	
Nucleoside and Nucleotide Reverse Transcriptase Inhibitors		
abacavir (Ziagen)	PO: 300 mg bid (max: 600 mg/day)	*Fatigue, generalized weakness, myalgia, nausea, headache, abdominal pain, vomiting, anorexia, rash, sleep disorders*
didanosine (ddI, Videx EC)	PO: 125–300 mg bid 30 min before a meal	Bone marrow suppression, neutropenia, anemia, granulocytopenia, lactic acidosis with steatorrhea, neurotoxicity, peripheral neuropathy (stavudine), pancreatitis (lamivudine)
emtricitabine (Emtriva)	PO: 200 mg once daily (max: 200 mg/day)	
lamivudine (Epivir, 3TC)	PO: 150 mg bid (max: 300 mg/day)	
stavudine (d4T, Zerit)	PO: 40 mg bid (max: 80 mg/day)	
tenofovir (Viread)	PO: 300 mg once daily with a meal	
zidovudine (Retrovir, AZT)	PO: 200 mg every 4 h (1,200 mg/day), after 1 month may reduce to 100 mg every 4 h (600 mg/day) IV: 1–2 mg/kg every 4 h (1,200 mg/day)	
Protease Inhibitors		
atazanavir (Reyataz)	PO: 400 mg daily with food	*Nausea, vomiting, diarrhea, abdominal pain, headache*
darunavir (Prezista)	PO: 600 mg taken with 100 mg ritonavir bid with food	Anemia, leukopenia, deep venous thrombosis, pancreatitis, lymphadenopathy, hemorrhagic colitis, nephrolithiasis (indinavir), cardiac arrest (atazanavir), thrombocytopenia (saquinavir), pancytopenia (saquinavir)
fosamprenavir (Lexiva)	PO: 700–1,400 mg bid in combination with 100–200 mg ritonavir bid (max: 2,800 mg/day)	
indinavir (Crixivan)	PO: 800 mg tid 60 min before a meal	
lopinavir-ritonavir (Kaletra)	PO: 400/100 mg (3 capsules or 5 mL of suspension) bid, increase dose to 533/133 mg (4 capsules or 6.5 mL) bid, with concurrent efavirenz or nevirapine	
nelfinavir (Viracept)	PO: 750 mg tid with a meal	
ritonavir (Norvir)	PO: 600 mg bid (max: 1,200 mg/day)	
saquinavir (Invirase)	PO: 1,000 mg bid (max: 2,000 mg/day)	
tipranavir (Aptivus)	PO: 500 mg taken with 200 mg ritonavir bid with food (max: 2,000 mg/day)	
Miscellaneous Antiretrovirals		
dolutegravir (Tivicay)	PO: 50 mg once daily	*Insomnia and headache* Severe hypersensitivity reactions, hepatotoxicity
elvitegravir (only administered concurrently with cobicistat, tenofovir, and emtricitabine)	PO: 150 mg	*Nausea and diarrhea* Acute renal failure, Fanconi syndrome, decrease in bone mineral density, lactic acidosis, severe hepatomegaly with steatosis
enfuvirtide (Fuzeon)	Subcutaneous: 90 mg bid	*Local injection-site reactions, nausea, diarrhea, fatigue* Hypersensitivity, neutropenia, thrombocytopenia, nephrotoxicity, pneumonia
maraviroc (Selzentry)	PO: 150–600 mg bid (max: 1,200 mg/day)	*Respiratory tract infections, cough, pyrexia, rash, and dizziness* Hepatotoxicity, myocardial infarction
raltegravir (Isentress)	PO: 400 mg bid (max: 800 mg/day)	*Headache, diarrhea, nausea, fatigue, insomnia* Hypersensitivity reaction, myopathy, rhabdomyolysis

Note: Italics indicate common adverse effects. Underline indicates serious adverse effects.

Pharmacokinetic considerations: Pharmacokinetic variables become very important when treating patients with HIV-AIDS and can, in fact, contribute in a major way to the success or failure of pharmacotherapy. The bioavailability of some antiretrovirals is greatly affected by food in the stomach. The absorption of certain antiretrovirals (e.g., indinavir) is decreased in the presence of food. Some (e.g., lopinavir) have a significantly increased absorption with high-fat meals and others (e.g., nevirapine) are not affected by the presence of food.

In addition to changes in absorption, most antiretrovirals are metabolized by the liver. Several can significantly increase or decrease the hepatic metabolism of other drugs, resulting in large numbers of potential drug–drug interactions. These effects differ, even within the same drug class. For example, nevirapine induces the hepatic P450 enzyme system, thus decreasing the levels of other drugs. Delavirdine, an antiretroviral in the same class, inhibits the P450 system, thus increasing the levels of other drugs. Predicting and avoiding complex drug interactions in patients with HIV requires truly skilled and dedicated nurses and other health care providers who are current on the most recent medical literature.

Antiretroviral Drugs

55.4 Reverse transcriptase inhibitors block the synthesis of viral DNA.

Following penetration into a T4 lymphocyte, the single-stranded viral RNA is used as a template to synthesize double-stranded proviral DNA. HIV virions come "prepackaged" with reverse transcriptase, the enzyme necessary to perform this critical step. Because reverse transcriptase is a viral enzyme not found in human cells, it has been possible to design drugs with the ability to selectively inhibit viral replication.

As proviral DNA is synthesized, biochemical building blocks known as nucleosides and nucleotides are required. Nucleosides/nucleotides form the backbone of the DNA molecule and are composed of the four bases, adenine, guanine, thymine, and cytosine. These same nucleosides/nucleotides are used to make human DNA.

Drugs in the nucleoside and nucleotide reverse transcriptase inhibitor classes (NRTIs and NtRTIs) chemically resemble the natural building blocks of DNA. In essence, reverse transcriptase is fooled by these drugs and inserts them into the proviral DNA strand. As the "fake" nucleosides and nucleotides are used to build DNA, however, the proviral DNA chain is prevented from lengthening. Because the growing DNA strand is prematurely terminated, the viral DNA chain is unable to insert into the host chromosome. Reverse transcriptase inhibitors (NRTIs and NtRTIs) have less effect on the progression of the infection if the proviral DNA has already been integrated into the host chromosome.

There are differences in pharmacokinetic and toxicity profiles and choice of drug depends on patient response and the experience of the clinician. Tenofovir and emtricitabine are considered the most effective drugs for reducing viral load and are included in all treatment guidelines for the initial therapy of HIV infection. With the exception of zidovudine, which may be used as monotherapy to prevent the perinatal transmission of HIV, the NRTIs and NtRTIs are always used in multidrug combinations with drugs from other classes.

The NRTIs are prodrugs. They must first be metabolized to their active, triphosphate form inside their target cells before they become effective. Unlike many other antiretrovirals, the NRTIs do not interact extensively with other drugs undergoing hepatic metabolism. The NtRTIs are nucleotide inhibitors that are already in their active, triphosphate forms; thus, no metabolic activation is necessary. Tenofovir is the only NtRTI approved for HIV therapy although a second drug in this class, adefovir, is available for treating hepatitis B infection.

Zidovudine was the first antiretroviral used in HIV-AIDS pharmacotherapy. Because zidovudine and some other NRTIs have been used consistently for over 25 years, drug resistance must be considered when selecting the specific agent. There is a high degree of cross resistance among the NRTIs.

As a class, the NRTIs are well tolerated, although nausea, vomiting, diarrhea, headache, and fatigue are common during the first few weeks of therapy. Some of the serious adverse effects of NRTIs are caused by **mitochondrial toxicity**. NRTIs inhibit a human enzyme called gamma-polymerase, which is responsible for the replication of DNA in mitochondria. This small, obscure DNA molecule encodes subunits for mitochondrial enzymes in the respiratory chain, which generates ATP. All the NRTIs have been associated with a low incidence of an unusual form of mitochondrial toxicity known as lactic acidosis–severe hepatomegaly with steatosis. This syndrome, which occurs more commonly in women and in those with preexisting hepatic impairment, includes lipid deposits in the liver, elevated transaminase values, and possible hepatic failure. Symptoms are often vague and include nausea, right upper quadrant (RUQ) pain, and myalgia. The nurse must carefully monitor liver function tests and assess for hepatic disease, because some fatalities have resulted from this adverse effect.

Another manifestation of mitochondrial toxicity from NRTIs is **lipodystrophy**, a disorder in which fat is redistributed in specific areas in the body. Areas such as the face, arms, and legs tend to lose fat, while the abdomen, breasts, and base of the neck (buffalo hump) develop excess fat. The fat redistribution may be associated with hyperlipidemia and hyperglycemia. In 2010, the FDA approved tesamorelin (Egrifta), a drug similar to growth hormone that is prescribed to reduce the excess abdominal fat in patients with lipodystrophy who are infected with HIV.

PROTOTYPE DRUG | **Zidovudine (Retrovir, AZT)**

Classification: Therapeutic: Antiretroviral
Pharmacologic: Nucleoside reverse transcriptase inhibitor

Therapeutic Effects and Uses: Zidovudine was first discovered in the 1960s and its antiviral activity was demonstrated prior to the AIDS epidemic. It was approved by the U.S. Food and Drug Administration (FDA) in 1987 for both symptomatic and asymptomatic patients with HIV infection, as well as for postexposure prophylaxis in HIV-exposed health care workers (see Section 55.9). An important indication is to reduce the transmission rate of HIV from an HIV-positive mother to her fetus (see Section 55.10).

Because of its widespread use since the beginning of the AIDS epidemic, HIV strains resistant to zidovudine are common.

Because of the potential for resistant strains, zidovudine is usually prescribed in combination with other antiretrovirals to slow the development of resistance. Current treatment guidelines for nonpregnant patients do not include zidovudine as a drug of first choice due to the potential for resistance. Combination products containing zidovudine include Combivir (zidovudine and lamivudine) and Trizivir (zidovudine, lamivudine, and abacavir).

Mechanism of Action: Structurally, zidovudine resembles thymidine, one of four nucleoside building blocks of DNA. As the reverse transcriptase enzyme begins to synthesize viral DNA, it mistakenly uses zidovudine instead of thymidine, thus terminating the growing chain and creating a defective proviral DNA strand.

Pharmacokinetics:

Route(s)	Intravenous (IV), oral (PO)
Absorption	Readily absorbed
Distribution	Widely distributed, including the cerebrospinal fluid (CSF); secreted in breast milk
Primary metabolism	Hepatic
Primary excretion	Renal
Onset of action	Peak effect: 1–2 h
Duration of action	Half-life: 1 h

Adverse Effects: Many patients experience headache, anorexia, nausea, and diarrhea. Patients may report fatigue, myalgia, and generalized weakness. It is often difficult to determine if adverse effects are due to zidovudine, other drugs the patient is taking concurrently, or the progression of the HIV-AIDS illness. **Black Box Warnings**: Rare cases of fatal lactic acidosis with severe hepatomegaly and steatosis have been reported with zidovudine and other drugs in this class. Bone marrow suppression may result in neutropenia or severe anemia. Myopathy may occur with long-term use.

Contraindications/Precautions: Because zidovudine can suppress bone marrow function after 4 to 6 weeks of therapy, it should be used with caution in patients with preexisting anemia or neutropenia. Blood counts and other laboratory blood tests should be monitored frequently during therapy to prevent hematologic toxicity. Patients with significant renal or hepatic impairment require a reduction in dosage, because zidovudine may accumulate to toxic levels in these patients. Breast-feeding should be suspended because both the virus and the drug may be transmitted through breast milk. Discontinuation of therapy should always be conducted under the guidance of a health care provider.

Drug Interactions: Zidovudine interacts with many drugs. Concurrent administration with other drugs that depress bone marrow function, such as ganciclovir, interferon-alfa, dapsone, flucytosine, or vincristine should be avoided due to cumulative immunosuppression. Stavudine, ribavirin, and doxorubicin compete for intracellular activation sites and will diminish the effects of zidovudine. Probenecid, fluconazole, atovaquone, valproic acid, amphotericin B, and aspirin increase the blood levels of zidovudine and may increase adverse effects from the antiretroviral. Other antiretroviral drugs may contribute to the lactic acidosis and hepatomegaly caused by zidovudine. **Herbal/Food**: Zidovudine should be used with caution with herbal supplements such as St. John's wort, which may cause a decrease in antiretroviral activity.

Pregnancy: Category C.

Treatment of Overdose: No specific therapy is available; patients are treated symptomatically.

Nursing Responsibilities: Key nursing implications for patients receiving zidovudine are included in the Nursing Practice Application for Patients Receiving Pharmacotherapy with Antiretrovirals.

Drugs Similar to Zidovudine (Retrovir, AZT)

Other NRTIs/NtRTIs include abacavir, didanosine, emtricitabine, lamivudine, stavudine, and tenofovir. All of the NRTIs/NtRTIs are used in combination with other antiretrovirals. Fixed-dose combinations with NRTIs/NtRTIs include Combivir (zidovudine and lamivudine), Trizivir (zidovudine, lamivudine, and abacavir), Truvada (tenofovir and emtricitabine), Atripla (emtricitabine, tenofovir, and efavirenz), and Epzicom (abacavir and lamivudine). Zalcitabine (ddC, Hivid) has been discontinued in the United States.

All drugs in this class carry a black box warning for lactic acidosis and severe hepatomegaly with steatosis. Some carry additional warnings.

Abacavir (Ziagen): Abacavir chemically resembles the natural nucleoside guanosine and is indicated for the treatment of HIV infection as part of a multidrug regimen. Approved in 1998, it is given orally once daily and is widely distributed throughout the body, including the CSF.

The most common adverse effects are gastrointestinal (GI) related and include nausea, vomiting, anorexia, and diarrhea. Alcohol use during abacavir therapy should be avoided, because blood levels of the antiretroviral can increase as much as 40%. Cross resistance is common among the NRTIs. Abacavir carries a black box warning regarding the potential for hypersensitivity reactions. This unique hypersensitivity syndrome occurs in 4% to 6% of patients taking the drug. Symptoms, which include fever, rash, dyspnea, cough, or GI distress, occur within the first 6 weeks of treatment. It is essential that these symptoms be monitored and the medication immediately discontinued should allergy be suspected, because deaths have been recorded from this syndrome. This drug is pregnancy category C.

Didanosine (ddI, Videx EC): Approved in 1991, didanosine chemically resembles the naturally occurring nucleoside inosine and is indicated for the treatment of HIV infection as part of a multidrug regimen. An off-label indication is for HIV prophylaxis following suspected occupational exposure to HIV. Given orally once daily, it should be administered on an empty stomach to enhance absorption. Didanosine is not a preferred drug for treating HIV.

Diarrhea and peripheral neuropathy involving numbness and tingling in the hands and feet are common adverse effects occurring in over 20% of patients taking the drug. There are black box warnings for this drug. Of greatest concern is pancreatitis, which is a serious adverse effect that occurs in up to 10% of the patients taking the drug. Patients should be carefully monitored for signs and symptoms that may suggest pancreatitis, such as nausea, vomiting, elevated serum amylase, and increased serum triglycerides, because deaths have occurred due to this disorder. This drug is pregnancy category B.

Emtricitabine (Emtriva): Approved in 2003, emtricitabine is a cytosine analog, also known as FTC, which is approved for the treatment of HIV infection as part of a multidrug regimen. Although chemically similar to lamivudine, it has the advantages of once-daily dosing and fewer adverse effects. The most frequently reported adverse effects are nausea, headache, dizziness, depression, rhinitis, skin rash, and skin discoloration on the palms and soles. Of the NRTIs, emtricitabine is believed to have the least mitochondrial toxicity. Emtricitabine carries a black box warning that it should not be administered to patients coinfected with HBV because severe exacerbations of HBV symptoms may occur after discontinuation of emtricitabine. Emtricitabine is one of the preferred drugs for initial HIV therapy. This drug is pregnancy category B.

Lamivudine (Epivir, 3TC): Also known as 3TC, lamivudine is a chemical analog of cytosine, a naturally occurring nucleoside. Approved in 1995, lamivudine is rapidly absorbed orally and better tolerated than most NRTIs. Minor adverse effects include transient insomnia and headache. Because significant adverse effects from lamivudine are uncommon, it is one of the most widely used components of HAART regimens. This drug is also approved for treatment of hepatitis B (Epivir HBV) (see Chapter 54). An off-label indication is for HIV prophylaxis following perinatal or suspected occupational exposure to HIV. Its primary disadvantage is rapid emergence of resistance. A black box warning states that severe exacerbations of HBV illness may occur when the drug is withdrawn from patients infected with HIV. This drug is pregnancy category C.

Stavudine (d4T, Zerit): Approved in 1994, stavudine is a chemical analog of thymidine, a naturally occurring nucleoside that is approved for the treatment of HIV infection as part of a multidrug regimen. An off-label indication is for HIV prophylaxis following suspected occupational exposure to HIV. Given orally, the use of stavudine has declined because the drug exhibits greater mitochondrial toxicity than others in this class. Of special concern is a high degree of lipodystrophy, evidenced by excessive loss of fat tissue, which persists long after the drug is discontinued. Headache and peripheral neuropathy occur in 50% or more of patients taking the drug. Black box warnings include serious pancreatitis that may occur if this drug is given concurrently with didanosine. This drug is pregnancy category C.

Tenofovir (Viread): Approved in 2001, tenofovir is an NtRTI that is indicated in combination with other antiretrovirals for the treatment of HIV infection in adults and children 2 years of age and older. Other than having an extra phosphate group, nucleotides are the same as nucleosides, and tenofovir has the same actions on reverse transcriptase as the NRTIs. Tenofovir is administered PO on an empty stomach to increase absorption. Tenofovir is a preferred drug for the initial treatment of HIV infection and chronic HBV infections, for which it is a prototype drug in Chapter 54.

The most frequently reported adverse effects of tenofovir are nausea, vomiting, depression, and diarrhea. Because tenofovir has less effect on mitochondrial enzymes than other drugs in this class, it is better tolerated. The drug can lower bone mineral density, placing the patient at risk for osteopenia or bone fractures. Due to nephrotoxicity, the use of tenofovir in patients with renal impairment should be carefully monitored, and it should be used cautiously in patients receiving other nephrotoxic drugs. A black box warning states that severe exacerbations of HBV illness may occur when tenofovir is withdrawn from patients with HIV infection. This drug is pregnancy category B.

55.5 The nonnucleoside reverse transcriptase inhibitors inhibit viral DNA replication by binding to reverse transcriptase.

The nonnucleoside reverse transcriptase inhibitors (NNRTIs) act by a mechanism distinct from the NRTIs. Drugs in this class bind in proximity to the active site of reverse transcriptase, causing a change in shape of the enzyme molecule. Because of this structural change, reverse transcriptase is unable to add more nucleotides to the proviral DNA chain, resulting in a direct inhibition of enzyme function.

Because resistance develops rapidly to NNRTIs, they are always used in combination with other antiretrovirals. Resistance to one NNRTI usually confers resistance to all drugs in this class. However, cross resistance between NNRTIs and drugs from other antiretroviral classes is not common.

The NNRTIs are generally well tolerated and exhibit few serious adverse effects. The adverse effects are different than the NRTIs. Rash is common with NNRTIs and rare cases of Stevens–Johnson syndrome (SJS) have been reported. They all affect hepatic metabolism, increasing the risk of drug–drug interactions. Liver function should be regularly assessed, especially in patients with preexisting liver disease.

PROTOTYPE DRUG	Efavirenz (Sustiva)

Classification: **Therapeutic:** Antiretroviral
Pharmacologic: Nonnucleoside reverse transcriptase inhibitor

Therapeutic Effects and Uses: Approved in 1998, efavirenz is given PO in combination with other antiretrovirals in the treatment of HIV infection. Efavirenz has the advantage of once-daily dosing and penetration into the CSF. Efavirenz is a preferred drug for the initial therapy of HIV infection. In 2013, the indications for efavirenz were extended to include pediatric patients who are 3 months or older and weigh at least 3.5 kg.

Resistance to NNRTIs can develop rapidly and cross resistance among drugs in this class can occur. High-fat meals increase the absorption by over 20%, which may result in toxicity. Because of this, efavirenz should be taken on an empty stomach. Atripla is a fixed-dose combination of efavirenz, emtricitabine, and tenofovir that offers the convenience of once-daily dosing.

Mechanism of Action: Efavirenz binds directly to reverse transcriptase, disrupting the shape of the enzyme's active site. This inhibition prevents viral DNA from being synthesized from HIV RNA.

Pharmacokinetics:

Route(s)	PO
Absorption	Readily absorbed
Distribution	Widely distributed, including the CSF; unknown if secreted in breast milk; 99% bound to plasma protein
Primary metabolism	Hepatic (CYP3A4 and CYP2B6)
Primary excretion	Renal
Onset of action	Peak effect: 3–5 h
Duration of action	Half-life: 52–76 h

Adverse Effects: CNS adverse effects are observed in at least 50% of patients when first initiating therapy, including sleep disorders, nightmares, dizziness, reduced ability to concentrate, and delusions. The CNS adverse effects usually diminish after 3 to 4 weeks of therapy. Like other drugs in this class, rash is common and must be monitored carefully.

Contraindications/Precautions: Efavirenz causes birth defects and should not be given to pregnant patients unless the benefits outweigh the risk to the fetus. Patients in the childbearing years should be advised to use reliable methods of birth control to avoid pregnancy. Contraceptive measures should continue for 12 weeks after the drug is discontinued. Liver function should be monitored during therapy due to the risk for hepatotoxicity. Efavirenz should be used cautiously in patients with a history of seizures.

Drug Interactions: Efavirenz induces CYP3A4 and can interact with drugs that are substrates for, or antagonists of, this isozyme. Patients who are receiving antiepileptic medications metabolized by the liver, such as carbamazepine, phenytoin, and phenobarbital, may require periodic monitoring of plasma levels because efavirenz may increase the incidence of seizures. Efavirenz can decrease serum levels of the following: statins, methadone, sertraline, and calcium channel blockers. The CNS adverse effects of efavirenz are worsened if the patient takes psychotropic drugs or consumes alcohol. Levels of warfarin may either increase or decrease. **Herbal/Food:** Efavirenz should be used with caution with herbal supplements, such as St. John's wort, which may cause a decrease in antiretroviral activity.

Pregnancy: Category D.

Treatment of Overdose: No specific therapy is available; patients are treated symptomatically.

Nursing Responsibilities: Key nursing implications for patients receiving efavirenz are included in the Nursing Practice Application for Patients Receiving Pharmacotherapy with Antiretrovirals.

Drugs Similar to Efavirenz (Sustiva)

Other NNRTIs include delavirdine, etravirine, nevirapine, and rilpivirine.

Delavirdine (Rescriptor): Approved in 1997, delavirdine is given orally and is very similar to other NNRTIs in actions and adverse effects. It may be administered with or without food. Delavirdine is the least commonly prescribed NNRTI because it must be administered three times per day and does not appear to be as effective as nevirapine or efavirenz. Many patients taking this drug develop a skin rash. In most cases, this rash disappears after several weeks of therapy, but it must be monitored carefully because cases of SJS have been reported in patients receiving this drug. GI distress, headache, and fatigue are also common adverse effects. Because delavirdine can decrease hepatic metabolism, many drug–drug interactions are possible, including those listed for efavirenz. This drug is pregnancy category C.

Etravirine (Intelence): Approved in 2008, etravirine is used in combination with other oral drugs in the pharmacotherapy of HIV infection. It is only approved for treatment-experienced adults. Because the fasting state can increase absorption of the

drug significantly and cause potential toxicity, it should always be taken with food. It is excreted primarily in the feces; therefore, no dose adjustment is necessary in patients with renal impairment. Because etravirine can decrease hepatic metabolism, many drug–drug interactions are possible, including those listed for efavirenz. The drug does not exhibit the hepatotoxicity of nevirapine or the CNS toxicity of efavirenz. The drug is generally well tolerated, with the most frequently reported adverse effect being rash. This drug is pregnancy category B.

Nevirapine (Viramune): Nevirapine was the first drug in this class, approved in 1996, for the treatment of HIV infection in combination with other antiretroviral agents. By inducing P450 enzymes, nevirapine increases its own breakdown; thus, dosage may need to be increased after several weeks of therapy to maintain its effectiveness. In addition, because the metabolism of protease inhibitors is decreased, dosage adjustments in these antiretrovirals may be necessary. Unlike some other antiretrovirals that negatively impact lipid metabolism, nevirapine may improve the lipid profile by increasing HDL. Common adverse effects include nausea, diarrhea, fever, fatigue, and rash, which is occasionally severe enough to require discontinuation of therapy. A black box warning states that during the first 18 weeks of therapy, the patient should be carefully monitored for hepatic function because potentially life-threatening hepatotoxicity has occurred with nevirapine. Patients with a history of hepatitis or other liver disease are at greater risk for nevirapine-induced hepatotoxicity. In addition, severe dermal reactions, including SJS, have been reported. Serum transaminase levels should be checked for all patients developing a rash in the first 18 weeks. This drug is pregnancy category C.

Rilpivirine (Edurant): One of the newer NNRTIs, rilpivirine was approved in 2011 for the treatment of HIV infection in treatment-naïve patients with HIV RNA levels of 100,000 copies/mL or less at the start of therapy. It is a PO drug that offers the convenience of once-daily dosing. The most common adverse effects are depression, insomnia, headache, and rash. Patients should be monitored for possible suicide ideation during therapy. Liver function should be monitored during therapy due to the risk for hepatotoxicity. Because rilpivirine can decrease hepatic CYP metabolism, many drug–drug interactions are possible. Complera is a combination drug for HIV infections that contains rilpivirine, emtricitabine, and tenofovir. This drug is pregnancy category B.

55.6 Protease inhibitors prevent HIV protease from completing the final step in HIV maturation.

Near the end of its replication cycle, HIV has assembled all the necessary components to create new virions. As the newly formed virions bud from the host cell and are released into the surrounding extracellular fluid, one final step remains before the HIV matures and becomes infectious: A long polypeptide chain must be cleaved to produce the final HIV proteins. The enzyme performing this step is HIV protease.

Drugs in the protease inhibitor (PI) class attach to the active site of HIV protease, thus preventing the final synthesis of HIV proteins. Without this final step in HIV maturation, the virions are noninfectious. When combined with other antiretroviral drug classes in a HAART regimen, the PIs are capable of lowering plasma

HIV RNA levels to an undetectable range. The PIs are included in most treatment guidelines for the treatment of HIV-AIDS.

PIs are metabolized in the liver and induce hepatic enzymes; thus, they have the potential to interact with numerous medications. In general, they are well tolerated, with GI complaints being the most common adverse effects. Lipodystrophies have been reported, including elevated cholesterol and triglyceride levels, and abdominal obesity. Some of the PIs are associated with hyperglycemia and can cause diabetes or worsen existing diabetes. Blood glucose levels should be monitored regularly in patients taking PIs.

The available PIs are very similar but there are some noticeable differences in pharmacokinetic properties and adverse effect profiles. Atazanavir and darunavir (both combined with ritonavir) are preferred drugs for the initial therapy of HIV. Cross resistance among the PIs may occur.

The initial choice of a primary PI most often includes low doses of ritonavir. Addition of small amounts of ritonavir allows longer dosing intervals and increases the plasma concentration of the primary PI. This is known as ritonavir boosting.

PROTOTYPE DRUG	Lopinavir with Ritonavir (Kaletra)

Classification: Therapeutic: Antiretroviral
Pharmacologic: Protease inhibitor

Therapeutic Effects and Uses: Approved in 2000, Kaletra is a combination drug containing the protease inhibitors lopinavir and ritonavir. Lopinavir is the active component of the combination. Ritonavir inhibits the hepatic breakdown of lopinavir, thus permitting serum levels of lopinavir to increase by more than 100-fold. Kaletra tablets may be taken with or without food, but the oral solution form must be taken with a meal to enhance absorption. It has an extended half-life that allows for once- or twice-daily dosing. Resistance to lopinavir-ritonavir has been reported in patients treated with other protease inhibitors prior to Kaletra therapy.

Mechanism of Action: By effectively inhibiting HIV protease, the final step in the assembly of an infectious HIV virion is prevented.

Pharmacokinetics:

Route(s)	PO
Absorption	Readily absorbed (but quickly destroyed through hepatic first-pass metabolism)
Distribution	Widely distributed; 98% bound to plasma proteins
Primary metabolism	Hepatic (lopinavir is metabolized by CYP3A; ritonavir inhibits CYP3A)
Primary excretion	Renal (10%); feces (83%)
Onset of action	Peak effect: 3–4 h
Duration of action	Half-life: 5–6 h

Adverse Effects: Kaletra is well tolerated, with the most frequently reported problem being diarrhea. Headache and GI-related effects are common, including nausea, vomiting, dyspepsia, and abdominal pain. Kaletra may cause or worsen symptoms of diabetes mellitus, and hyperglycemia has been reported. Lipodystrophy syndrome occurs in many patients receiving long-term therapy with PIs and large increases in total cholesterol and triglycerides may occur during therapy. This syndrome is associated with hyperglycemia and fat redistribution. Kaletra should be used with caution in patients with cardiac disease because the drug can prolong the PR interval and cause third-degree heart block. Pancreatitis is a rare, though potentially fatal, adverse event.

Contraindications/Precautions: Because of its extensive hepatic metabolism, patients with liver impairment, especially those with preexisting viral hepatitis, should be carefully monitored. Hepatic enzyme levels should be regularly evaluated in these patients to prevent hepatic failure. Patients with diabetes should be monitored regularly because Kaletra may exacerbate this condition.

Drug Interactions: Lopinavir is extensively metabolized by hepatic CYP3A, and drugs that undergo hepatic metabolism may interact with Kaletra. Drugs that increase hepatic P450 enzymes will reduce the effectiveness of the antiretroviral. These include nevirapine, efavirenz, barbiturates, rifampin, rifabutin, phenytoin, and carbamazepine. Conversely, drugs that inhibit the P450 enzymes will increase levels of lopinavir, including aldesleukin, ketoconazole, delavirdine, indinavir, and ritonavir. Statins should not be administered with Kaletra due to an increased risk for myopathy. Concurrent use of rifampin may lower the effectiveness of Kaletra. Potentially life-threatening dysrhythmias may occur if Kaletra is used concurrently with cisapride, pimozide, and certain other antidysrhythmic drugs. Kaletra may increase adverse effects associated with selective serotonin reuptake inhibitors (SSRIs), tricyclic antidepressants, and phenothiazines. **Herbal/Food**: St. John's wort should be used with caution, because it may decrease antiretroviral activity.

Pregnancy: Category C.

Treatment of Overdose: No specific therapy is available; patients are treated symptomatically.

Nursing Responsibilities: Key nursing implications for patients receiving lopinavir with ritonavir are included in the Nursing Practice Application for Patients Receiving Pharmacotherapy with Antiretrovirals.

Drugs Similar to Lopinavir with Ritonavir (Kaletra)

Other PIs include atazanavir, darunavir, fosamprenavir, indinavir, nelfinavir, ritonavir, saquinavir, and tipranavir. Amprenavir (Agenerase) has been discontinued in the United States.

Atazanavir (Reyataz): Approved in 2003, atazanavir offers the advantages of once- or twice-daily dosing and fewer adverse effects on lipid levels than other PIs. Atazanavir boosted with ritonavir is a preferred drug in the initial pharmacotherapy of HIV infection. Headache, insomnia, dizziness, myalgia, depression, fever, and nausea are common adverse effects. Atazanavir increases bilirubin levels and cholelithiasis is possible. Liver function should be regularly monitored during therapy. Atazanavir has been shown to prolong the PR interval of the electrocardiogram (ECG) and produce first-degree atrioventricular block and other conduction abnormalities. The drug should be discontinued if rash occurs due to the risk for SJS. Atazanavir may cause hyperglycemia and worsen the symptoms of diabetes. Other adverse effects, contraindications, and drug interactions are similar to those of lopinavir. This drug is pregnancy category B.

Darunavir (Prezista): Approved in 2006, darunavir is a second-generation PI that is indicated for the treatment of HIV infection in adults and in pediatric patients age 6 years and older. When concurrently administered with ritonavir, darunavir is a preferred drug for this infection. Although cross resistance has been reported, darunavir retains some activity against viral strains resistant to other PIs. Because both darunavir and ritonavir decrease hepatic metabolism, numerous drug–drug interactions are possible. Darunavir should be administered with food to increase its absorption. Diarrhea, nausea, vomiting, rash, and headache are the most common adverse effects. Because drug-induced hepatitis has been reported with this drug, hepatic enzymes should be monitored regularly. Severe rashes are possible, and these call for discontinuation of therapy. Other adverse effects, contraindications, and drug interactions are similar to those of lopinavir. This drug is pregnancy category B.

Fosamprenavir (Lexiva): Approved in 2003, fosamprenavir is a PI that is administered with low doses of ritonavir as a booster. Both tablet and oral solution formulations are available and fosamprenavir may be taken with or without food. Like other PIs, fosamprenavir affects the hepatic metabolism of many drugs, making interactions likely. The drug can cause hyperglycemia and thus should be used cautiously in patients with diabetes. Other adverse effects, contraindications, and drug interactions are similar to those of lopinavir. This drug is pregnancy category C.

Indinavir (Crixivan): Approved in 1996, indinavir is a PI used to treat HIV infection and for HIV postexposure prophylaxis. It is administered PO, usually with a high-fat meal to increase drug absorption. It has a short half-life that requires three doses per day. Boosting with low doses of ritonavir is recommended. Like other PIs, indinavir should be used cautiously in patients with diabetes due to the risk of hyperglycemia. The most serious potential adverse effect is the formation of crystals in the urine, causing nephrolithiasis, which is unique among the protease inhibitors. Renal function should be monitored regularly and the patient should be encouraged to consume adequate amounts of fluid to dilute the urine in order to prevent crystalluria. Because indinavir can decrease the hepatic metabolism of drugs, numerous drug–drug interactions are possible. This drug is pregnancy category C.

Nelfinavir (Viracept): Approved in 1997, nelfinavir was one of the most frequently used PIs for many years. Its use has declined because newer PIs offer a lower pill burden and fewer adverse effects. Nelfinavir is given orally, usually with meals, in order to increase drug absorption. Unlike some other antiretrovirals, nelfinavir is 98% bound to plasma proteins and excreted almost entirely in the feces. Because large amounts of the drug and its metabolites reach the colon, severe diarrhea is frequent and antidiarrheal medications may be indicated. Patients taking oral contraceptives should be advised to use a second method of birth control, because nelfinavir decreases plasma levels of ethinyl estradiol. Patients with diabetes should be monitored carefully due to the hyperglycemic effect of the antiretroviral. This drug is pregnancy category B.

Ritonavir (Norvir): Approved in 1995, ritonavir is well absorbed orally and is available in both capsule and solution formulations. Because of low tolerability, the use of ritonavir is now almost entirely limited to boosting the function of other PIs. The drug undergoes extensive hepatic metabolism and is excreted primarily in the feces. Like other PIs, ritonavir inhibits P450 hepatic metabolizing enzymes, which reduces the elimination of many drugs. This is used to advantage in dual PI regimens. Giving low doses of ritonavir to boost serum levels of other PIs permits lower doses of the second PI. Ritonavir increases several other drug metabolizing enzymes in the liver; therefore, drug–drug interactions are common.

Most adverse effects of ritonavir are GI related and may limit therapy. Peripheral and perioral paresthesias are possible. Because ritonavir induces enzymes that increase its own metabolism, its effectiveness will diminish unless doses are increased. This drug is pregnancy category B.

Saquinavir (Invirase): Saquinavir was the original protease inhibitor approved by the FDA in 1995. When combined with ritonavir, saquinavir serum levels increase, making the drug more effective. Resistance to saquinavir develops with continued use and may include cross resistance with other PIs. Saquinavir is well tolerated, with the most frequently reported problems being GI related, such as nausea, vomiting, dyspepsia, and diarrhea. Other adverse effects are similar to those of lopinavir. Because of its extensive hepatic metabolism, patients with liver impairment should be carefully monitored. This drug is pregnancy category B.

Tipranavir (Aptivus): Approved in 2005, tipranavir is indicated for the management of HIV infection in treatment-experienced patients and those with strains of HIV that are resistant to more than one PI. To optimize antiviral activity, it should always be administered with ritonavir. Tipranavir capsules and solution can be taken without regard to food but the tablets should be taken with a high-fat meal to enhance absorption. The most common adverse effects are diarrhea, nausea, pyrexia, vomiting, fatigue, headache, and abdominal pain. Tipranavir contains sulfur and should be used with caution in patients with allergies to sulfa drugs. Like other PIs, tipranavir may be associated with the development or worsening of diabetes, elevations in cholesterol and triglycerides, and lipodystrophies. Tipranavir inhibits platelet aggregation and should be used with caution in patients who may be at risk of increased bleeding from trauma, surgery, or other medical conditions or who are receiving anticoagulants or antiplatelet drugs. The drug should be discontinued if a severe skin rash occurs. Black box warnings state that tipranavir has been associated with intracranial hemorrhage. Caution should be used when prescribing tipranavir to patients with elevated transaminases or preexisting hepatic impairment. Patients coinfected with hepatitis B or hepatitis C have a higher risk for hepatotoxicity. This drug is pregnancy category C.

55.7 Entry inhibitors and integrase inhibitors are newer strategies for managing HIV infections.

Because HIV develops resistance to most of the frequently prescribed antiretrovirals, scientists have been looking intensively for unique mechanisms of drug action. In recent years, several such mechanisms have been discovered. The role of these drugs in treating HIV infection is evolving.

Entry inhibitors: Entry inhibitors prevent the entry of the viral nucleic acid into the T4 lymphocyte. The two drugs in this class block the entry of HIV by different mechanisms.

In 2003, enfuvirtide (Fuzeon) was welcomed by the medical community as a novel way to attack a key component of the HIV replication cycle. This drug blocks the fusion of the viral membrane with the bilipid layer of the host's plasma membrane, a step required for entry of the virus. Because this mechanism is so different from other antiretrovirals, many patients resistant to other drug classes are still sensitive to the effects of enfuvirtide. However, the use of enfuvirtide is limited because it is expensive to manufacture and it is given by subcutaneous injection twice daily. Its current use is for treating HIV infections in treatment-experienced patients with strains resistant to other antiretrovirals. Almost every patient taking enfuvirtide will experience an injection-site reaction, usually during the first week of therapy. These reactions may involve severe pain, pruritus, erythema, cysts, abscesses, and cellulitis. Nausea, diarrhea, and fatigue are other common adverse effects. Patients should be carefully monitored for lung infections because an increased incidence of pneumonia has been reported in patients taking enfuvirtide. A major advantage is that no significant drug interactions have been found with enfuvirtide. This drug is pregnancy category B.

The second entry inhibitor, maraviroc (Selzentry), was developed in 2007 after scientists discovered that HIV needs coreceptors (in addition to the CD4 receptor) to enter into human cells. CCR5 is the name of one of the coreceptors required for entry. Maraviroc is the first of a new class of HIV drugs called CCR5 inhibitors or chemokine receptor antagonists. This drug blocks CCR5 and has the ability to significantly reduce viral load and increase T-cell production. Before treatment is initiated the patient must receive a tropism assay, which is used to determine if the strain of HIV has the CCR5 receptor (CCR5-tropic HIV). It may be administered with or without food. Maraviroc is approved for combination therapy with other antiretrovirals in treatment-naïve patients. The drug is well tolerated, with the most frequently reported adverse effects being upper respiratory tract infections, cough, pyrexia, rash, and dizziness. Caution should be used when administering this drug to patients with preexisting cardiac disease because the drug may increase the risk for myocardial ischemia or infarction. Maraviroc carries a black box warning regarding the possibility of hepatoxicity, which may be preceded by signs of a systemic allergic reaction. This drug is pregnancy category B.

Integrase inhibitors: In 2007, the FDA approved the first drug in a class of antiretrovirals called the integrase inhibitors. HIV requires the integrase enzyme to insert its viral DNA strand into the human chromosome. These drugs are sometimes called integrase strand transfer inhibitors (ISTIs). Like entry inhibitors, the integrase inhibitors offer a new mechanism for managing patients with HIV infections that have developed resistance to older antiretrovirals.

Raltegravir (Isentress), the first integrase inhibitor, is indicated for combination therapy with other antiretroviral drugs for the treatment of HIV infection in adult patients. It may be administered with or without food. Insomnia, fatigue, headache, and GI-related symptoms such as diarrhea and nausea are the most frequently reported adverse effects. Caution should be used when administering this drug to patients with myopathy or rhabdomyolysis because raltegravir may worsen these conditions. This drug is pregnancy category C. In 2014, a second oral integrase inhibitor, dolutegravir, was approved in a three drug combination (Triumeq) with abacavir and lamuvidine.

Prophylaxis of HIV Infections

55.8 The development of vaccines to prevent HIV has produced disappointing results.

Early in the history of the AIDS epidemic, scientists were optimistic that vaccines could be quickly developed that would prevent the spread of HIV infection. After all, scientists had totally eradicated the smallpox virus as a human threat and essentially controlled major viral infections such as measles and mumps. Such a vaccine could be given in childhood, offering lifetime protection against the fatal disease.

After decades of research, the FDA has not approved a single vaccine. Only a few HIV vaccines are currently in clinical trials, and none is expected to cause a major impact on the HIV epidemic. At best, the HIV vaccines produced thus far only boost the immune response; they are unable to prevent the infection. While this may help a patient already infected with the virus to better control the disease, it does not prevent new infections. Why is this the case?

HIV has an extremely rapid replication rate, combined with a high "error" or mutation rate. While creating new viral DNA at a breakneck pace, reverse transcriptase frequently inserts an incorrect nucleotide. It is estimated that, given the size of the HIV genome at 10,000 base pairs, every possible mutation probably occurs at every nucleotide daily in an untreated patient. These errors create huge numbers of genetic variants, or mutant strains, with new and different characteristics from the original. It is not unusual to find dozens of genetic variants of HIV replicating within the same patient. Thus, vaccine development, and indeed antiretroviral therapy, is trying to hit a "moving target" that is changing its genetic makeup literally every minute.

Also challenging is determining the most effective type of vaccine for HIV. The classic type of vaccine uses live, attenuated viruses because this mimics a natural exposure and produces the greatest immunologic response (see Chapter 43). However, given the extreme rate of HIV mutation, scientists are concerned that an attenuated form of HIV could mutate back to a live form and infect the patient. Thus, the approach with HIV has been to take various fragments of the virus, such as envelope protein subunits and portions of HIV genes, and produce a vaccine "cocktail" to administer to the patient. Unfortunately, these mixes have so far proven ineffective at preventing infection.

An additional challenge is to produce a vaccine-mediated immune response that will reach viruses lying latent inside T cells. HIV-infected cells reside in virtually every compartment in the body and serve as reservoirs for the latent virus, protecting it from the immune response produced by the vaccine. How do scientists coax the immune system to recognize these infected cells and dispose of them? Perhaps a better question is: Can a vaccine be designed to prevent the entry of the virus into cells to begin with? And how can this vaccine be ethically tested, since no animals have the same immune system as humans to serve as an experimental model?

Vaccine research has not been a total failure. Scientists have learned an enormous amount about the immune system's response to HIV infection. This has promoted the development of new drugs and advanced our understanding of how to treat and control the infection. It is likely that a preventive vaccine will become available in the future, but not soon enough for the millions already infected.

CONNECTIONS: NURSING PRACTICE APPLICATION

Patients Receiving Pharmacotherapy with Antiretrovirals

Assessment	Potential Nursing Diagnoses*
Baseline assessment prior to administration: • Obtain a complete health history including neurologic, cardiovascular, respiratory, hepatic, or renal disease, and the possibility of pregnancy. Obtain a drug history including allergies (e.g., specific reactions to drugs), current prescription and over-the-counter (OTC) drugs, herbal preparations, and alcohol use. Obtain a vaccination history, especially a history of recent vaccinations with live agents. Be alert to possible drug interactions. • Assess signs and symptoms of current infection, noting onset, duration, characteristics, and presence or absence of fever or pain. • Evaluate appropriate laboratory findings (e.g., complete blood count [CBC], CD4 count, HIV viral load, culture and sensitivity [C&S] for any concurrent infections, hepatic and renal function studies, lipid levels, serum amylase, and glucose). • Assess the patient's ability to receive and understand instructions. Include the family and caregivers as needed.	• *Infection* • *Activity Intolerance* • *Fatigue* • *Anxiety* • *Imbalanced Nutrition: Less Than Body Requirements* • *Deficient Fluid Volume* • *Diarrhea* • *Impaired Oral Mucous Membrane* • *Impaired Skin Integrity* • *Insomnia* • *Social Isolation* • *Disturbed Body Image* • *Confusion (Acute or Chronic)* • *Ineffective Health Management* • *Hopelessness*
Assessment throughout administration: • Assess for desired therapeutic effects (e.g., CD4 counts and HIV viral load remain within acceptable limits, able to attend to normal activities of daily living [ADLs], absence of signs and symptoms of concurrent infections). • Continue periodic monitoring of CBC, hepatic and renal function, CD4 and HIV viral load, lipid levels, serum amylase, glucose. • Assess for adverse effects: nausea, vomiting, anorexia, abdominal cramping, diarrhea, fatigue, drowsiness, dizziness, mental changes, insomnia, delusions, chills, fever, muscle or joint pain, paresthesia, hypotension, syncope, hyperglycemia. Severe diarrhea, jaundice, decreased urine output or darkened urine, purplish-red blistering rash on body or oral mucous membranes, acute abdominal pain, increasing mental or behavioral changes, or decreased level of consciousness (LOC) should be reported immediately.	• *Spiritual Distress* • *Deficient Knowledge (Drug Therapy)* • *Risk for Infection* • *Risk for Injury*, related to adverse drug effects • *Risk for Falls*, related to adverse drug effects • *Risk for Caregiver Role Strain*

Implementation

Interventions and (Rationales)	Patient-Centered Care
Ensuring therapeutic effects: • Continue assessments as above for therapeutic effects: maintenance of normal or increasing appetite, increasing energy level and ability to maintain ADLs, CD4 counts and HIV viral load within acceptable limits and stabilized, and maintenance of therapeutic regimen. (Drugs will be required long term and have many potential adverse effects, making adherence to the medication regimen difficult. The provider should be notified if fever and signs and symptoms of concurrent infections increase, excessive fatigue is present, or adverse effects place adherence to drug therapy at risk.)	• Teach the patient to continue taking the course of medications, to not share doses with others, and to return to the health care provider if adverse effects make adherence to the therapeutic regimen difficult to continue.
Minimizing adverse effects: • Continue to monitor vital signs, especially temperature if fever is present. Immediately report increasing fever, diarrhea or vomiting, dyspnea, tachycardia, dizziness, syncope, changes in behavior or LOC, or lethargy to the health care provider. (Increasing fever, especially when accompanied by worsening symptoms, may be a sign of worsening infection, adverse drug effects, or drug resistance.)	• Teach the patient, family, or caregiver to immediately report a fever that exceeds 33.8°C (101°F) or per parameters set by the health care provider, changes in behavior or LOC, shortness of breath, inability to maintain hydration or nutrition, or dizziness and fainting to the health care provider.
• Continue to monitor periodic laboratory work: hepatic and renal function tests, CBC, CD4 counts, HIV viral load, lipid levels, serum amylase, glucose, and C&S if concurrent infections are present. (Drugs used for the treatment of HIV are hepatic and renal toxic. Bone marrow suppression and blood dyscrasia, particularly anemia and leukopenia, are also adverse effects and will be monitored by CBC. Lipid levels and serum amylase will be monitored to assess for pancreatitis, and glucose levels checked for hyperglycemia.)	• Instruct the patient on the need for periodic laboratory work, correlating any symptoms with the need for possible laboratory tests (e.g., serum amylase if the patient is having upper abdominal pain). Advise laboratory personnel of HIV status.
• Monitor for hypersensitivity and allergic reactions, especially with the first dose of any antiretroviral or protease inhibitor. Continue to monitor the patient as needed based on drug used or patient condition. (Anaphylactic reactions are possible and reactions may not always be predictable.)	• Teach the patient to immediately report any itching, rashes, swelling, particularly of face or tongue, urticaria, flushing, dizziness, syncope, wheezing, throat tightness, or difficulty breathing.

CONNECTIONS: NURSING PRACTICE APPLICATION (continued)

- Continue to monitor for hepatic and renal toxicities; e.g., jaundice, RUQ pain, darkened urine, or diminished urine output. (Antiretrovirals and protease inhibitors may be hepatic and renal toxic. **Lifespan:** Age-related physiological differences may place older adults at greater risk for hepatic or renal toxicity. **Diverse Patients:** Because zidovudine is metabolized through the P450 system pathways, monitor ethnically diverse patients frequently to ensure optimal therapeutic effects and minimize adverse effects. Increasing fluid intake will prevent drug accumulation in the kidneys.)

- Teach the patient to immediately report any nausea, vomiting, yellowing of the skin or sclera, abdominal pain, light- or clay-colored stools, diminished urine output, or darkening of urine.
- Advise the patient to increase fluid intake to 2–3 L/day if permitted.

- Continue to monitor for dermatologic effects such as red or purplish skin rash, blisters, or peeling skin, including oral mucous membranes. Assess oral mucous membranes for signs of stomatitis because drug effects or immunosuppression may result in overgrowth of oral flora. Immediately report severe rashes, especially those associated with blistering. (These drugs may cause significant dermatologic effects including stomatitis, and SJS, a potentially fatal condition.)

- Teach the patient to inspect the oral cavity at least once a day and obtain regular dental exams. Maintain good oral hygiene and rinse mouth with plain water or solution as prescribed by the health care provider after eating. Use protective clothing for sun exposure and immediately report any significant rashes or sunburned appearance.

- Monitor for signs and symptoms of neurotoxicity, e.g., drowsiness, dizziness, mental changes, insomnia, delusions, paresthesia, headache, changes in LOC, or seizures. (Many HIV-AIDS drugs cause peripheral neuropathy and have neurologic adverse effects. Frequent monitoring is needed to prevent or minimize adverse effects.)

- Instruct the patient, family, or caregiver to immediately report increasing headache, dizziness, drowsiness, worsening insomnia, numbness of hands, feet, or extremities, or changes in behavior or LOC.
- Caution the patient that drowsiness may occur and to be cautious with driving or other activities requiring mental alertness until the effects of the drug are known.
- Instruct the patient to be cautious when in contact with heat or cold, because numbness from peripheral neuropathy may make sensing accurate temperatures more difficult.
- Encourage sleep hygiene measures, e.g., restful routines before bed, and avoiding large meals within 1–2 h of sleep. Have the patient consult with the health care provider if insomnia causes daytime sleepiness or continues.

- Monitor for signs and symptoms of blood dyscrasias, e.g., low-grade fevers, bleeding, bruising, or significant fatigue. (Bone marrow suppression may occur and may cause blood dyscrasias with resulting decreases in red and white blood cells and/or platelets. Periodic monitoring of CBC will be required.)

- Teach the patient to report any low-grade fevers, sore throat, rashes, bruising or increased bleeding, unusual fatigue or shortness of breath, especially after taking drug therapy for a prolonged period.

- Monitor for, and immediately report, signs and symptoms of lactic acidosis. (Some antiretroviral drugs may cause lactic acidosis with hepatomegaly and steatosis. Lactic acidosis is a possible life-threatening adverse effect.)

- Teach the patient to immediately report symptoms such as abdominal pain, anxiety, fatigue, palpitations, lethargy, rapid breathing and heart rate, weakness, chest pain or tightness, fever, or shortness of breath to the provider.

- Monitor for significant GI effects, including nausea, vomiting, abdominal pain or cramping, and diarrhea. Administer drugs as per guidelines. Additional pharmacologic treatment may be necessary to limit adverse GI effects. Ensure adequate nutrition and caloric intake. (Adverse GI effects are a common adverse effect of most antiretrovirals and protease inhibitors.)

- Teach the patient to take the drug with food or milk if appropriate, or to take the drug on an empty stomach with a full glass of water. Avoid acidic foods and beverages or carbonated drinks that may cause stomach upset.
- Assist the patient in obtaining a dietary consultation as needed if nausea or diarrhea makes maintaining intake difficult.

- Monitor for symptoms of pancreatitis including severe abdominal pain, nausea, vomiting, and abdominal distention. (Some antiretroviral drugs may cause pancreatitis. Serum amylase and lipid levels should be monitored periodically.)

- Instruct the patient to immediately report fever, severe abdominal pain, nausea, vomiting, and abdominal distention.

- Monitor blood glucose in patients taking antiretrovirals. (Many antiretroviral drugs may cause hyperglycemia. Patients with diabetes may require a change in their antidiabetic drug routine.)

- Teach the patient with diabetes to test blood glucose level more frequently, reporting any consistent elevations to the health care provider.

- Monitor cholesterol and triglyceride levels. For patients on long-term antiretroviral therapy, assess for fat distribution and effects on patient body image. Provide for counseling and support for body image concerns. (Lipodystrophy syndrome occurs in many patients receiving long-term therapy with many antiretroviral drugs, and large increases in total cholesterol and triglycerides may occur during therapy.)

- Instruct the patient on the need for periodic laboratory work.
- Provide emotional empathy and referral to support services as needed (e.g., counseling services, nutritional support) if the patient expresses concerns about body image or overall health while on long-term antiretroviral therapy.

- Women of childbearing age should use an alternative form of birth control to prevent pregnancy. (Some antiretroviral drugs may significantly reduce the effectiveness of oral contraceptives.)

- Teach women of childbearing age on oral contraceptives to consult their health care provider about birth control alternatives.

- Provide resources for medical and emotional support. (Treatment requires a multidisciplinary approach.)

- Advise the patient about community resources and support groups. Assist the family or caregiver with respite care as needed.

(continued)

CONNECTIONS: NURSING PRACTICE APPLICATION *(continued)*

Patient understanding of drug therapy: • Use opportunities during administration of medications and during assessments to discuss the rationale for drug therapy, desired therapeutic outcomes, commonly observed adverse effects, parameters for when to call the health care provider, and any necessary monitoring or precautions. (Using time during nursing care helps to optimize and reinforce key teaching areas.)	• The patient, family, or caregiver should be able to state the reason for the drug, appropriate dose and scheduling, what adverse effects to observe for and when to report them, and the anticipated length of medication therapy.

Patient self-administration of drug therapy:
• When administering medications, instruct the patient and/or family in proper self-administration techniques followed by teach-back. (Utilizing time during nurse-administration of these drugs helps to reinforce teaching.)
	• Teach the patient to take the medication:
	  • Complete the entire course of therapy unless otherwise instructed. The duration of the required therapy may be quite lengthy but it is necessary to prevent active infection. Do not stop taking the medicine when starting to feel better.
	  • Do not share the medicine with other family members. If there is reason to believe that family members need medication, they should be assessed by a health care provider.
	  • Eliminate alcohol while on these medications. These drugs cause significant reactions when taken with alcohol.
	  • Take the drug with food or milk if instructed to take with food, but avoid acidic beverages. If instructed to take the drug on an empty stomach, take with a full glass of water.
	  • Take the medication as evenly spaced throughout each day as feasible.
	  • Increase overall fluid intake while taking these drugs.

Nursing Diagnoses—Definitions and Classification 2015–2017. Copyright © 2014, 1994–2014 by NANDA International. Used by arrangement with John Wiley & Sons Limited.

CONNECTION Checkpoint 55.2

From what you learned in Chapter 43, explain the difference between active immunity and passive immunity. Which type of immunity would an HIV vaccine produce? *See Answer to Connection Checkpoint 55.2 on student resource website.*

55.9 Postexposure prophylaxis of HIV infection is designed to prevent transmission to health care workers.

Since the start of the AIDS epidemic, nurses and other health care workers caring for patients with HIV-AIDS have been concerned about acquiring the disease from their patients. Fortunately, if proper precautions are observed, the disease is rarely transmitted from patient to health care worker. Accidents have occurred, however, in which the health care provider has acquired the infection by exposure to the blood or body fluids of patients infected with HIV. Although the risk is small, the question remains: Can HIV transmission be prevented following accidental occupational exposure to HIV? The answer is a qualified yes.

The success of postexposure prophylaxis (PEP) for occupational HIV exposure is difficult to assess due to the lack of controlled studies and the small numbers of cases. Enough data have accumulated, however, to demonstrate that PEP is successful in certain circumstances. For prevention to be most successful, PEP should be started within 24 to 36 hours after exposure to a source person who is known to be HIV positive. Although the exact interval remains undefined, longer periods allow the infection to progress to stages where prophylaxis would not be successful. The health care worker should receive a baseline HIV viral load level as soon as possible after exposure.

If the HIV status of the source person is unknown, PEP is decided case by case, based on the type of exposure (percutaneous or mucous membrane) and the likelihood the blood contained HIV. In some cases, PEP is initiated for a few days, until the source person can be tested. PEP should only be initiated if the exposure was sufficiently severe and the source fluid is known, or strongly suspected, to contain HIV. Using PEP outside established guidelines is both expensive and dangerous; the antiretrovirals used for PEP produce adverse effects in most recipients.

Low-risk PEP is initiated when the source person is asymptomatic for HIV or is known to have a low viral load (below 1,500 HIV RNA copies/mL). The basic PEP treatment includes one of the following regimens, conducted over a 4-week period:

- Zidovudine and lamivudine, or
- Zidovudine and emtricitabine, or
- Lamivudine and tenofovir, or
- Tenofovir and emtricitabine

If the accidental HIV exposure was severe, and the source is a symptomatic HIV-infected person with a high viral load, a third drug may be added to the regimen. If available, the medical records of the source person should be consulted to determine the possibility of resistance to specific antiretrovirals. The enhanced PEP treatment includes one of the basic regimens listed previously, plus lopinavir-ritonavir.

Guidelines have also been established for the nonoccupational postexposure prophylaxis (nPEP) of HIV. These guidelines are largely based on animal studies and analysis of the existing data for occupational exposure. Because nPEP is expensive and may result in adverse drug effects, it is only recommended for specific nonoccupational exposures. First, the person should have been exposed to the blood or body fluids of a person known to be infected with HIV. Second, the nature of the exposure must be such that there is a substantial risk for transmission. Third, the exposure must have occurred no later than 72 hours before antiretroviral therapy is initiated. The sooner nPEP is initiated, the more successful the outcome. The health care provider considers nPEP for exposures outside these guidelines on a case-by-case basis. Recommended therapy is a 28-day regimen with one of the following:

- Efavirenz plus lamivudine, or
- Emtricitabine plus zidovudine or tenofovir, or
- Lopinavir/ritonavir plus lamivudine or emtricitabine, plus zidovudine

55.10 Preexposure prophylaxis has been shown to be partially effective in certain groups.

Significant research has been conducted to determine if HIV infection can be prevented by medications. The goal of preventing infection is an important one to consider because prevention of HIV infection is always preferable to treatment. This type of therapy is called preexposure prophylaxis (PrEP).

Research has demonstrated that, if taken continuously on a daily basis, the two-drug combination of emtricitabine and tenofovir can prevent HIV infection in men (and transgendered women) who have sex with men. Based on this research, the Centers for Disease Control and Prevention (CDC) also recommends this regimen for heterosexually active men and women and for intravenous drug users (CDC, 2013b). PrEP is only 40% successful in preventing HIV infection, so it is clear that other means should be taken to prevent this lethal infection.

55.11 The risk of perinatal transmission of HIV can be markedly reduced by specialized drug protocols.

Treatment regimens for HIV infection do not differ between men and women. Because some antiretrovirals have pharmacokinetic interactions with oral contraceptives, a second method of birth control is recommended.

Should pregnancy occur, the therapeutic outcomes focus on keeping the viral load low in the mother while aggressively protecting the transmission of HIV to the unborn child. Efavirenz has been shown to cause fetal malformations; therefore, its use is not recommended during pregnancy.

In 1994, clinical trials determined that perinatal transmission of HIV could be markedly reduced through pharmacotherapy. A reduction of approximately 70% in transmission from mother to infant was achieved using antepartum pharmacotherapy in the mother followed by aggressive treatment of the newborn child.

In pregnant women with HIV, antiretroviral therapy is recommended regardless of the viral level or CD4 count. Reducing the viral load in the mother has been shown to reduce the risk of HIV transmission to the fetus. Recommended protocols for the pregnant woman include two NRTIs (zidovudine and lamivudine) with either an NNRTI (nevirapine) or a PI (lopinavir boosted with ritonavir). The specific regimen is adjusted based on resistance testing.

Regardless of the antepartum therapy, it is recommended that the woman receive a continuous infusion of zidovudine during labor. Zidovudine rapidly crosses the placenta. This may provide some protection for the fetus because most perinatal transmission of HIV occurs near to or during labor and delivery.

> ### CONNECTIONS Community-Oriented Practice
>
> #### ◄ "Test and Treat" Prevention Strategy
>
> With recent data confirming that early antiretroviral therapy after diagnosis of HIV significantly lessens the chance for transmission to others (Grinsztejn et al., 2014), the earlier a patient can be identified as having HIV infection, the earlier treatment can be started. Early symptoms of HIV infection such as fever, chills, sore throat, and malaise are often mistaken for flu or other routine infections, and the patient may not seek treatment until the viral load has significantly increased. The fear and stigma associated with a diagnosis of HIV may also prevent some patients from seeking care. Routine testing for HIV infection and the immediate initiation of antiretroviral therapy (HAART) would significantly reduce the chance for transmission by substantially reducing the viral load as well as improving patient quality of life. With 100% testing coverage, early antiretroviral treatment could substantially reduce rates of transmission and the epidemic of HIV could feasibly be stopped completely, at least theoretically. Unfortunately, 100% testing coverage of the population is probably not possible at this time due to many factors including cost and the manpower required to maintain testing services. Other concerns include the long-term risk of adverse drug effects when antiretroviral therapy is started early, balanced against therapeutic benefits, ethical concerns, and motivation and adherence questions (Kulkarni, Shah, Sarma, & Mahjan, 2013). Nurses can advocate for testing regardless of HIV risk factors to help increase the numbers of patients having testing, while also being aware of the ongoing debate as to the effectiveness and feasibility of test-and-treat strategies.

Therapy of neonates born to mothers infected with HIV should begin immediately after delivery, no later than 6 to 12 hours postpartum. HIV infection is established in infants by age 1 to 2 weeks and beginning antiretroviral therapy more than 48 hours after birth has been shown to be ineffective in preventing the infection. It is recommended that zidovudine be given orally to the newborn for 6 weeks. In addition, three doses of nevirapine are given during the first week of life. In addition, mothers must be advised not to breast-feed their infants, because this is a possible route of HIV transmission, and many antiretrovirals are secreted in breast milk.

Although initial HIV antibody tests on the newborn may be positive, these antibodies may be due to maternal infection and not HIV infection in the child. Definitive diagnosis on infants less than 18 months of age requires virologic testing. If diagnostic testing reveals that the infant is not infected before the 6-week prophylactic treatment period is completed, zidovudine therapy is discontinued. On the other hand, if HIV diagnosis is confirmed during this period, the infant is switched to combination HAART therapy. In addition to antiretrovirals, all infants born to women with HIV infection should receive trimethoprim-sulfamethoxazole to prevent *Pneumocystis jiroveci* pneumonia (PJP) at age 4 to 6 weeks.

Approximately 12 antiretrovirals are approved for pediatric indications. The other antiretrovirals are too toxic for pediatric use, not available in convenient formulations, or the doses remain to be established. Like adults, the specific regimen is chosen based on the experience of the prescriber and resistance patterns of the HIV strain. The possibility that the child may have inherited a strain already resistant to some of the antiretrovirals must be considered when developing the regimen.

Pharmacotherapy of Opportunistic Infections Associated with HIV-AIDS

55.12 Loss of immune function due to HIV often results in opportunistic infections that require anti-infective therapy.

In the early 1980s, all patients with AIDS acquired serious OIs from pathogenic bacteria, viruses, fungi, and protozoans. Profound loss of immune function allowed dormant pathogens to flourish and also lowered the defense barriers for infection by newly acquired organisms. Often, the presentation of an acute OI was the reason the patient first sought medical attention for HIV disease. For example, in the early years of the epidemic,

70% to 80% of all patients with AIDS developed *Pneumocystis* pneumonia, which carried a mortality rate of up to 40% in these patients. Since the advent of HAART, *Pneumocystis* pneumonia is now rare.

OIs still occur in patients with HIV-AIDS; however, they are less common and mortality is diminished. This is because HAART increases the numbers of CD4 lymphocytes, allowing patients with HIV infection to maintain a higher level of immunologic defense. In addition, the anti-infective pharmacotherapy of OIs has evolved due to a better understanding of these diseases. Patients with CD4 counts below 200 cells/mcL are placed on prophylactic antibiotics because the risk of an OI in these patients is very high. Most other patients with HIV-AIDS are monitored carefully for signs of infectious disease and treated as symptoms indicate.

Drugs used for treating OIs have been presented in previous anti-infective chapters, and the student should refer to those chapters for specific drug information. A selected list of preferred drugs for selected OIs is given in Table 55.2.

TABLE 55.2	**Pharmacotherapy of Selected Opportunistic Infections in Patients with HIV-AIDS**	
Disease	**Preferred Drug(s) for Prevention**	**Comments**
Bacterial enteric infections	PO: fluoroquinolone (ciprofloxacin preferred) or TMP-SMZ	Most common pathogens are *Salmonella*, *Campylobacter*, and *Shigella*
Bacterial respiratory infections	Pneumococcal vaccine (PPV); inactivated influenza vaccine	Most common pathogens are *S. pneumoniae* and *H. influenzae*
Candidiasis (mucocutaneous)	PO: fluconazole	Topical azoles may be used for vulvovaginal or oropharyngeal disease
Cryptococcosis	No prevention recommended; treatment is with amphotericin B with flucytosine for 2 weeks, followed by fluconazole for 8 weeks	Lifelong prophylaxis with fluconazole is indicated in certain patients
Cryptosporidiosis	No specific anti-infective is indicated; clarithromycin or rifabutin may be effective	Therapy includes symptomatic treatment of diarrhea
Herpes simplex	PO: famciclovir or acyclovir for 7–14 days	IV therapy is indicated in severe infections
Histoplasmosis (disseminated)	PO: itraconazole daily	Lifelong prophylaxis with itraconazole is indicated in certain patients
Mycobacterial tuberculosis	PO: isoniazid plus pyridoxine for 9 months	Serious drug interactions can occur between rifamycin and the NNRTIs and protease inhibitors
Pneumocystis pneumonia (PJP)	PO: TMP-SMZ for 21 days	Lifelong prophylaxis is indicated in certain patients; pentamidine may be used for severe cases
Syphilis	IM: benzathine penicillin	If allergic to penicillin, penicillin desensitization is attempted or an alternate drug such as doxycycline is substituted
Toxoplasma gondii encephalitis	PO: TMP-SMZ	Clindamycin may be used instead of sulfadiazine

CHAPTER

55

Understanding the Chapter

Key Concepts Summary

55.1 HIV causes a profound loss of immune function.

55.2 Treatment of HIV infection is difficult due to the latent nature of the virus and the development of resistant strains.

55.3 Six classes of antiretroviral drugs are available to treat HIV infection.

55.4 Reverse transcriptase inhibitors block the synthesis of viral DNA.

55.5 The nonnucleoside reverse transcriptase inhibitors inhibit viral DNA replication by binding to reverse transcriptase.

55.6 Protease inhibitors prevent HIV protease from completing the final step in HIV maturation.

55.7 Entry inhibitors and integrase inhibitors are newer strategies for managing HIV infections.

55.8 The development of vaccines to prevent HIV has produced disappointing results.

55.9 Postexposure prophylaxis of HIV infection is designed to prevent transmission to health care workers.

55.10 Preexposure prophylaxis has been shown to be partially effective in certain groups.

55.11 The risk of perinatal transmission of HIV can be markedly reduced by specialized drug protocols.

55.12 Loss of immune function due to HIV often results in opportunistic infections that require anti-infective therapy.

Case Study: Making the Patient Connection

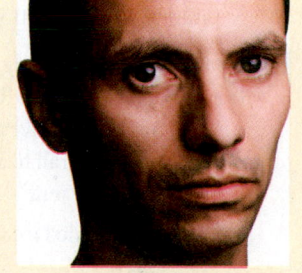

Remember the patient "Ryan Orre" at the beginning of the chapter? Now read the remainder of the case study. Based on the information presented within this chapter, respond to the critical thinking questions that follow.

Ryan Orre is a 37-year-old single male who has come to his health care provider because of the recent onset of a chronic sore throat and flulike symptoms, including swollen lymph nodes in the neck and armpits, tiredness, fever, and night sweats. During this office visit, Ryan appears extremely anxious and troubled.

When questioned about his apparent nervousness, Ryan states, "You don't understand; I'm gay. But I've always been very careful and practice safe sex. What if I have AIDS? What will I do? I don't want to die." The health care provider acknowledges Ryan's fears and spends additional time allowing Ryan to express his concerns. The process of diagnosing HIV infection is discussed with the patient and initiated.

Ryan's medical history reveals that he is allergic to penicillin, which results in rash and pruritus. Although Ryan does not currently take any prescribed medications, he recently started multivitamin and nutritional supplements due to a recent loss of weight. The patient denies any current recreational drug use but admits that he occasionally used IV drugs during his college years. He has not used them in the past 8 years. No past history of medical or psychiatric illness exists. He has never had surgery.

Ryan does not use tobacco products. He reports drinking alcoholic beverages several times weekly but never to excess. Ryan explains that he has had several male sexual partners over the past 10 years but feels that he has been consistent in his use of condoms. He currently lives alone and works as a sales representative with a local computer firm. A series of laboratory diagnostic tests found the following abnormal results: white blood cell (WBC) count of 2,950/mm^3 and CD4 count of 550/mm^3. Ryan is hospitalized with the preliminary diagnosis of sepsis and to rule out HIV. A test for HIV viral load is ordered.

Critical Thinking Questions

1. You are the nurse caring for Ryan in the hospital. On the first evening he is hospitalized, Ryan asks if you think his provider will be prescribing antiretroviral therapy. Given this situation, how would you explain the factors that determine when antiretroviral therapy should be initiated?

2. Ryan's CD4 count is still within low-normal range but his HIV viral load comes back significantly increased, indicating HIV infection. After talking with the provider, Ryan asks you to explain again the difference between HIV infection and AIDS. How would you explain this?

3. Ryan's provider has decided to start him on antiretroviral therapy and Ryan will begin taking efavirenz (Sustiva), tenofovir (Viread), and emtricitabine (Emtriva). What will be the best method of teaching Ryan about these drugs? What other factors should be considered when talking with Ryan?

See Answers to Critical Thinking Questions on student resource website.

Additional Case Study

Alexa Trihan is referred to an HIV clinic after she is diagnosed as having the HIV infection at the free clinic she goes to for medical care, most likely acquired by IV drug use. She is prescribed antiretroviral therapy using a HAART regimen. Although the health care provider has explained the therapy, Alexa's anxiety results in her inability to comprehend the entire explanation provided. Alexa begins asking you, her nurse, questions about HAART.

1. Using simple language, how would you, as Alexa's nurse, explain HIV and HAART therapy?

2. Alexa tells you that she may be pregnant. How will this potentially affect her treatment?

See Answers to Additional Case Study on student resource website.

Chapter Review

1 Zidovudine (Retrovir, AZT) is prescribed for a patient. Which statement by the patient would indicate that further medication-related teaching is needed?

1. "Antiretroviral therapy must be continued for the remainder of my life."
2. "The human immunodeficiency virus vaccine only creates temporary immunity against the disease."
3. "The medication schedule can be adjusted daily depending on my activities."
4. "Many individuals infected with the human immunodeficiency virus are able to live symptom free due to the medication."

2 A patient has been taking lopinavir with ritonavir (Kaletra) for the past 8 years and has noticed a redistribution of body fat in the arms, legs, and abdomen (lipodystrophy). In addition to this effect, the nurse knows that this drug may be associated with which additional adverse effects? Select all that apply.

1. Renal failure
2. Hyperglycemia
3. Pancreatitis
4. Bone marrow suppression
5. Hepatic failure

3 Emtricitabine (Emtriva) is included as part of a HAART regimen for a patient newly diagnosed with HIV. While lower in toxicity than other NRTIs, a potentially fatal adverse effect known to occur is:

1. Ventricular cardiac dysrhythmias.
2. Pulmonary fibrosis.
3. Necrotic bowel syndrome.
4. Lactic acidosis.

4 The nurse is aware that myelosuppression may be a problem for some patients receiving zidovudine (Retrovir). Which finding would indicate that this adverse effect is present?

1. Increase in serum blood urea nitrogen levels
2. Increase in white blood cell count
3. Decrease in platelet count
4. Decrease in blood pressure

5 The nurse is planning a teaching session with a patient who will be receiving highly active antiretroviral therapy (HAART). Which of the following should be included in the teaching plan? Select all that apply.

1. Avoid crowds and other people with colds, flu, and other infections.
2. Notify the health care provider at the first sign of any rash.
3. The medications will reduce transmission of the disease.
4. The drugs will be stopped periodically to give the immune system a chance to respond.
5. Herbal supplements will not interfere with this therapy.

6 A patient has been taking tenofovir (Viread) for the past 5 years as part of a HAART regimen. The patient would like to include some alternative and complementary health activities to improve his overall health. Which activity may be contraindicated for this patient?

1. Yoga and guided imagery
2. Massage therapy
3. Meditation and journaling
4. Weekly visits to a chiropractor

See Answers to Chapter Review in Appendix A.

References

Centers for Disease Control and Prevention. (2013a). Diagnoses of HIV infection and AIDS in the United States and dependent areas, 2011. *HIV Surveillance Report, Volume 23*. Retrieved from http://www.cdc.gov/hiv/library/reports/surveillance/2011/surveillance_Report_vol_23.html

Centers for Disease Control and Prevention. (2013b). Update to interim guidance for preexposure prophylaxis (PrEP) for the prevention of HIV infection: PrEP for injecting drug users. *Morbidity and Mortality Weekly Report, 62*(23), 463–465.

Grinsztejn, B., Hosseinipour, M. C., Ribaudo, H. J., Swindells, S., Eron, J., Chen, Y. Q., . . . Cohen, M. S. (2014). Effects of early versus delayed initiation of antiretroviral treatment on clinical outcomes of HIV-1 infection: Results from the phase 3 HPTN 052 randomised clinical trial. *The Lancet Infectious Diseases, 14*, 281–290. doi:10.1016/S1473-3099(13)70692-3

Kulkarni, S. P., Shah, K. R., Sarma, K. V., & Mahjan, A. P. (2013). Clinical uncertainties, health service challenges, and ethical complexities of HIV "test-and-treat": A systematic review. *American Journal of*

Public Health, 103(6), e14–23. doi:10.2105/AJPH.2013.301273

Lowes, R. (2011). Peril, progress and promise: 30 years of HIV/AIDS. *Medscape Medical News.* Retrieved from http://www.medscape.com/viewarticle/743927

Madigan, M. T., Martinko, J. M., Stahl, D. A., & Clark, D. P. (2012). *Brock biology of microorganisms* (13th ed.). Upper Saddle River, NJ: Prentice Hall.

Panel on Antiretroviral Guidelines for Adults and Adolescents. (2013). *Guidelines for the use of antiretroviral agents in HIV-1-infected adults and adolescents.* Washington, DC: U.S. Department of Health and Human Services. Retrieved from http://aidsinfo.nih.gov/contentfiles/lvguidelines/adultandadolescentgl.pdf

Selected Bibliography

Eisenhut, M. (2013). An update on HIV in children. *Paediatrics and Child Health, 23*(3), 109–114. doi:10.1016/j.paed.2012.06.003

Hankins, C. (2013). Overview of the current state of the epidemic. *Current HIV/AIDS Reports, 10,* 113–123. doi:10.1007/s11904-013-0156-x

Herdman, T. H., & Kamitsuru, S. (Eds.). (2014). *NANDA International nursing diagnoses: Definitions and classification, 2015–2017.* Oxford, United Kingdom: Wiley-Blackwell.

Hoyle, B. (2011). *2- or 3-drug regimen lessens intrapartum HIV transmission.* Retrieved from http://www.medscape.com/viewarticle/738814

Kuhar, D. T., Henderson, D. K., Struble, K. A., Heneine, W., Thomas, V., Cheever, L. W., . . . Panlilio, A. L. (2013). Updated U.S. Public Health Service guidelines for the management of occupational exposures to human immunodeficiency virus and recommendations for postexposure prophylaxis. *Infection Control and Hospital Epidemiology, 34*(9), 875–892. doi: 10.1086/672271

National Institute of Allergy and Infectious Diseases. (2011). *NIH news: Treating HIV-infected people with antiretrovirals protects partners from infections: Findings result from NIH-funded international study.* Retrieved from http://www.niaid.nih.gov/news/newsreleases/2011/Pages/HPTN052.aspx

Panel on Antiretroviral Therapy and Medical Management of HIV-Infected Children. (2014). *Guidelines for the use of antiretroviral agents in pediatric HIV infection.* Retrieved from http://aidsinfo.nih.gov/contentfiles/PediatricGuidelines.pdf

Panel on Treatment of HIV-Infected Pregnant Women and Prevention of Perinatal Transmission. (2014). *Recommendations for use of antiretroviral drugs in pregnant HIV-1-infected women for maternal health and interventions to reduce perinatal HIV transmission in the United States.* Retrieved from http://aidsinfo.nih.gov/contentfiles/lvguidelines/perinatalgl.pdf

Rathburn, R. C. (2013). *Antiretroviral therapy for HIV infection.* Retrieved from http://emedicine.medscape.com/article/1533218-overview

Smith, D. K., Grohskopf, L. A., Black, R. J., Auerbach, J. D., Veronese, F., Struble, K. A., . . . Greenberg, A. E. (2005). Antiretroviral postexposure prophylaxis after sexual, injection-drug use, or other nonoccupational exposure to HIV in the United States: Recommendations from the U.S. Department of Health and Human Services. *Morbidity and Mortality Weekly Report, 54*(RR-2), 1–20.

Tissot, F., Erard, V., Dang, T., & Cavassini, M. (2010). Nonoccupational HIV post-exposure prophylaxis: A 10-year retrospective analysis. *HIV Medicine, 11,* 584–592. doi:10.1111/j.1468-1293.2010.00826.x

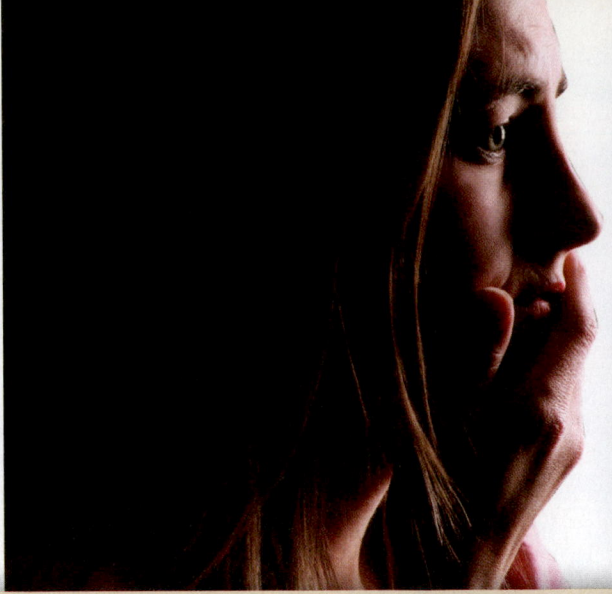

"When the doctor first told me that I had cancer, I was scared. Now after hearing all of the things that the chemotherapy can do to my body, I'm petrified."

Patient "Cheryl Ogen"

CHAPTER

56

Basic Principles of Antineoplastic Therapy

LEARNING OUTCOMES

After reading this chapter, the student should be able to:

1. Compare and contrast the differences between normal cells and cancer cells.
2. Identify etiologic factors associated with an increased incidence of cancer.
3. Construct a table categorizing the major primary and secondary means of cancer prevention.
4. Compare and contrast the following goals of chemotherapy: cure, control, palliation, prophylaxis, adjuvant therapy, and neoadjuvant therapy.
5. Explain the purposes of staging and grading cancers.
6. Explain the significance of growth fraction and the cell cycle to the success of chemotherapy.
7. Assess the ability of antineoplastic drugs to achieve a total cancer cure based on the cell kill hypothesis.
8. Explain how special chemotherapy protocols increase the effectiveness of therapy.
9. Discuss the types of toxicity and adverse effects of chemotherapeutic agents on the various organ systems.

CHAPTER OUTLINE

▸ Characteristics of Cancer

▸ Etiology of Cancer

▸ Detection and Prevention of Cancer

▸ Goals of Chemotherapy

▸ Staging and Grading of Cancer

▸ The Cell Cycle and Growth Fraction

▸ Cell Kill Hypothesis

▸ Improving the Success of Chemotherapy

▸ Toxicity of Antineoplastic Agents

adjuvant chemotherapy, 951

alopecia, 958

angiogenesis, 950

cachexia, 958

cancer, 949

carcinogens, 950

cell kill hypothesis, 954

chemotherapy, 951

emetic potential, 957

grading, 952

growth fraction, 954

metastasis, 950

mucositis, 957

nadir, 957

neoadjuvant chemotherapy, 951

neoplasm, 949

palliation, 951

peripherally inserted central catheter
 (PICC) line, 956

sclerosing, 956

staging, 952

telomerase, 950

telomeres, 950

tumor, 949

vesicants, 958

Cancer is one of the most feared diseases in society for a number of valid reasons. In the United States, cancer accounts for one out of every four deaths. It is often silent, producing no symptoms until it reaches an advanced stage. It sometimes requires painful and disfiguring treatments such as surgery or radiation. Cancer may strike at an early age, even during infancy, to deprive patients of a normal life span. Perhaps worst of all, the medical treatment of cancer often cannot offer a cure, and progression to death is sometimes slow, painful, and psychologically difficult for patients and their loved ones.

Despite its feared status, many successes have been made in the diagnosis and treatment of cancer. Modern treatment methods result in a cure for nearly two of every three people and the 5-year survival rate has steadily increased for most types of cancer. This chapter examines the basic principles of cancer therapy. Chapter 57 examines the medications used to treat cancer.

PharmFACT

The American Cancer Society (2013) estimates that more than 1,665,500 new cancer cases occur each year in the United States, with more than 581,700 deaths (about 1,600 people each day).

Characteristics of Cancer

56.1 Cancer is characterized by rapid, uncontrolled growth of cells that eventually invade normal tissues and metastasize.

A **tumor** is a swelling, an abnormal enlargement, or a mass. The word **neoplasm** is often used interchangeably with *tumor*. Tumors may be benign or malignant. Whereas benign tumors are usually slow growing, remain localized, and rarely cause death, malignant tumors are rapidly growing, invasive, and will kill the host if left untreated. Malignant tumors are classified as carcinomas or sarcomas. Examples of various types of benign and malignant tumors are listed in Table 56.1.

Cancer or carcinoma is a disease characterized by abnormal, uncontrolled cell division. Cell division is a normal process that occurs extensively in most body tissues from conception to late childhood. At some point in time, whether it occurs during fetal life, childhood, or adulthood, the degree of cell division in every tissue must be controlled.

Each cell in the body has the ability to regulate its growth (proliferation) by turning specific genes on and off. For example, growth-promoting genes can be turned on when it is necessary to replace worn-out cells, as in the case of blood stem cells, skin epithelial cells, and the lining of the digestive tract. Growth suppressor genes are responsible for slowing the duplication rate and can completely shut down replication, as in the case of muscle cells and most neuron cells. If the suppressor genes become damaged or mutated and do not slow down or stop cell growth, the cells will undergo abnormal proliferation. Because of the critical importance of cell growth to life, it is likely that each cell has multiple genes that regulate division, all of which are responsive to various chemical signals or messages originating from both inside and outside the cell.

Cancer is thought to result from damage to the genes controlling cell growth. Once damaged, cells may become unresponsive to the chemical signals that normally check growth. The cancer cells lose their normal functions, dividing rapidly and invading surrounding tissues. Unlike most normal cells, cancerous cells are able to move to other places in the body. The abnormal cells often travel to distant

TABLE 56.1 Classification and Naming of Tumors

Name	Description	Examples
Benign tumor	Slow growing; does not metastasize and rarely requires drug treatment	Adenoma, papilloma, lipoma, osteoma, meningioma
Carcinoma	Cancer of epithelial tissue; most common type of malignant neoplasm; grows rapidly and metastasizes	Malignant melanoma, renal cell carcinoma, adenocarcinoma, hepatocellular carcinoma
Glioma	Cancer of glial (interstitial) cells in the brain, spinal cord, and pineal gland	Telangiectatic glioma, brainstem glioma, posterior pituitary gland, or retina
Leukemia	Cancer of the blood-forming cells in bone marrow; may be acute or chronic	Myelocytic leukemia, lymphocytic leukemia
Lymphoma	Cancer of lymphoid tissue	Hodgkin's disease, lymphoblastic lymphoma
Sarcoma	Cancer of connective tissue; grows extremely rapidly and metastasizes early in the progression of the disease	Osteogenic sarcoma, fibrosarcoma, Kaposi's sarcoma, angiosarcoma

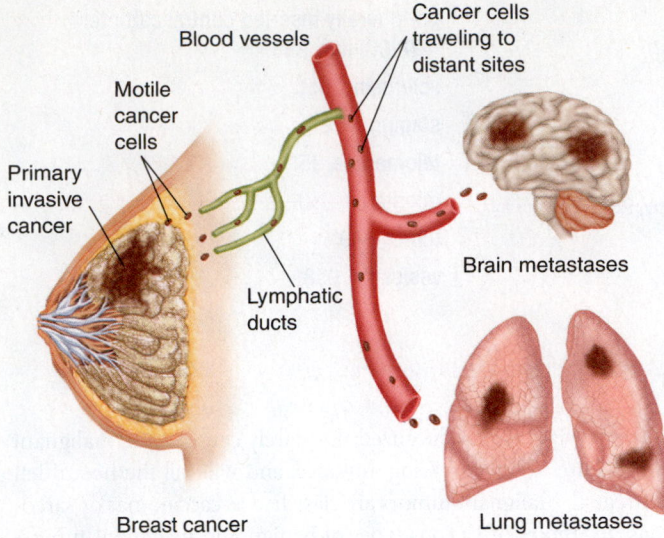

Figure 56.1 Invasion and metastasis by cancer cells.

sites where they populate new tumors, a process called **metastasis**. Figure 56.1 illustrates some characteristics of cancer cells.

Each time a cell divides, it loses a small amount of deoxyribonucleic acid (DNA) at the end of each chromosome. These regions of "extra" repetitive DNA, called **telomeres**, serve to protect the vital sequences of DNA from being destroyed. Normal cells are able to undergo mitosis 50 to 60 times before the cell loses the protective telomeres. Certain human stem cells contain the enzyme **telomerase**, which can lengthen the DNA chains and allow continued replication. Interestingly, this enzyme is not produced in mature cells, which dooms the cells to eventual death.

Cancer cells are different from normal cells in that they do not die as quickly and can divide and form new cancer cells indefinitely. One explanation for this difference is that most cancer cells produce large amounts of telomerase, which continues to add pieces to the telomeres so that the cell can continue to divide. It is believed that the cancer cell begins to produce telomerase soon after it has mutated and that this may be an important factor in the progression to cancer.

To divide rapidly (and indefinitely) tumor cells need an adequate supply of nutrients. Solid tumors need to create a new capillary network to "feed" themselves. The process of **angiogenesis**, which is the formation of new blood vessels, is controlled by a cascade of events similar to blood coagulation. Some factors that are secreted by cells promote angiogenesis, whereas others inhibit it. Cancer cells appear to have the ability to control angiogenesis and to establish their own blood supply, which not only brings in nutrients, but also provides an "escape route" during metastasis.

Etiology of Cancer

56.2 The etiology of cancer may be chemical, physical, or biologic.

Numerous factors have been found that cause cancer or are associated with a higher risk for acquiring the disease. Agents that cause cancer are called **carcinogens**.

Many chemical carcinogens have been identified. For example, chemicals in tobacco smoke are responsible for about one third of

all cancers in the United States. Alcohol ingestion has also been linked to certain cancers, including esophageal, oral, breast, and liver cancers. Chemicals such as asbestos and benzene have been associated with a higher incidence of cancer in the workplace. In some cases, the site of the cancer may be distant from the entry location, as is the case with bladder cancer, which is caused by the inhalation of certain industrial chemicals.

A number of physical factors are also associated with cancer. For example, exposure to large amounts of x-rays is associated with a higher risk of leukemia. Ultraviolet (UV) light from the sun is a common cause of skin cancer.

It is estimated that viruses and bacteria contribute to 15% to 20% of all human cancers. The common bacterium *Helicobacter pylori*, is associated with a higher incidence of gastric cancer. Examples of viruses include hepatitis B and C, Epstein–Barr, human papillomavirus (HPV), and human T-lymphotrophic viruses. If patients remain free from infection with these viruses, their chances of developing certain types of cancer diminish greatly. For example, a vaccine against HPV is available to prevent infection from the two major types of HPV that cause cervical cancer and genital warts. On the other hand, factors that depress immune function, such as the human immunodeficiency virus (HIV) or immunosuppressant drugs given after transplant surgery, may promote the growth of cancer cells.

Some cancers have a strong genetic component. The fact that twins or close relatives may acquire the same type of cancer suggests that certain genes may confer a predisposition to the condition. These abnormal genes interact with chemical, physical, and biologic agents to promote the formation of cancer. Gender can also be considered a risk factor for certain types of cancer. For instance, breast cancer is more commonly associated with women, whereas bladder cancer is more frequent in men.

Although the development of cancer has a genetic component, it is also greatly influenced by factors in the environment. Maintaining or adopting healthy lifestyle habits may reduce the risk of acquiring cancer. Following proper nutrition, avoiding chemical and physical risks (especially tobacco), and maintaining a regular schedule of health checkups can help prevent cancer from developing into a fatal disease.

Detection and Prevention of Cancer

56.3 The keys to successful cancer treatment are prevention and early detection.

If allowed to grow unchecked and untreated, cancer is fatal in nearly 100% of those who acquire it. The keys to successful cancer treatment are prevention and early detection. Prevention of cancer falls into two categories: primary prevention and secondary prevention.

Primary prevention of cancer includes interventions that keep cancer from ever developing. Interventions for primary prevention are targeted at avoiding known carcinogens and promoting a healthy lifestyle. Examples of primary prevention include the following:

- Health counseling and education delivered by the nurse
- Elimination of tobacco use to prevent lung, oral, and other cancers

- Receiving the HPV vaccination to prevent cervical cancer
- Maintaining a healthy diet low in fat and high in fresh vegetables and fruits
- Maintaining weight within recommended levels
- Decreasing excess stress
- Avoiding chronic or prolonged exposure to direct sunlight or wearing protective clothing or sunscreen

Secondary prevention includes interventions leading to the discovery and control of cancerous or precancerous lesions while they are small and localized. Examples of secondary prevention include the following:

- Receiving a Papanicolaou (Pap) smear every 3 years, for females between 21 and 29; every 5 years between the ages of 30 and 65; and testing can be stopped at age 65 if previous tests have been negative
- Receiving a screening colonoscopy, according to the schedule recommended by the health care provider
- Receiving mammograms, according to the schedule recommended by the health care provider
- Receiving prostate screening, as recommended by the health care provider
- Performing regular skin self-examinations to check for abnormal lesions

The American Cancer Society recommends using the following acronym to help people remember what to look for when self-assessing for cancer:

Caution

C: Change in bowel or bladder habits
A: A sore that does not heal
U: Unusual bleeding or discharge
T: Thickening or lump in the breast or elsewhere
I: Indigestion or difficulty swallowing
O: Obvious change in a wart or mole
N: Nagging cough or hoarseness

CONNECTION Checkpoint 56.1

From what you learned in Chapter 43, describe the immunization schedule for receiving the HPV vaccine. *See Answer to Connection Checkpoint 56.1 on student resource website.*

Goals of Chemotherapy

56.4 The three primary goals of chemotherapy are cure, control, and palliation.

Pharmacotherapy of cancer is sometimes simply referred to as **chemotherapy**. Transported through the blood, drugs have the potential to reach cancer cells in virtually any location. Certain chemotherapeutic drugs are specifically designed to be able to cross the blood–brain barrier to reach brain tumors. Others are instilled directly into body cavities such as the urinary bladder to bring the highest dose possible to the cancer cells without producing systemic adverse effects. Chemotherapy has three general goals: cure, control, and palliation.

When diagnosed with cancer, the primary goal desired by most patients is to achieve a complete cure; that is, permanent removal of all cancer cells from the body. The possibility for cure is much greater if a cancer is identified and treated when the tumor is small and localized to a well-defined region. The 5-year survival rates for nearly all types of cancers have increased in the past two decades due to improved detection and more effective therapies. Examples in which chemotherapy has been used successfully as curative treatment include Hodgkin's lymphoma, certain leukemias, and choriocarcinoma.

PharmFACT
The highest 5-year survival rates are for cancers of the prostate, testis, and thyroid. The lowest survival rates are for pancreatic, liver, and lung cancers (American Cancer Society, 2014).

When cancer has progressed and cure is not possible, a second goal of chemotherapy is to control or manage the disease. Although the cancer is not eliminated, preventing the growth and spread of the tumor may extend a patient's life. Essentially, the cancer is managed as a chronic disease, such as hypertension or diabetes.

In its advanced stages, cure or control of the cancer may not be achievable. For these patients, chemotherapy is used as **palliation**. Chemotherapy drugs are administered to reduce the size of the tumor, easing the severity of pain and other tumor symptoms and thus improving the quality of life. Examples of advanced cancers for which palliation is frequently used include osteosarcoma, pancreatic cancer, and Kaposi's sarcoma.

Chemotherapy may be used alone or in combination with other treatment modalities such as surgery or radiation therapy. Surgery is especially useful for removing solid tumors that are localized. Surgery lowers the number of cancer cells in the body so that radiation therapy and pharmacotherapy can be more successful. When only a portion of the tumor is removed, it is referred to as *debulking*. Surgery is not an option for tumors of blood cells or when it would not be expected to extend a patient's life span or improve the quality of life.

Approximately 50% of patients with cancer receive radiation therapy as part of their treatment. Radiation therapy is most successful and produces the fewest adverse effects for cancers that are localized when high doses of ionizing radiation can be aimed directly at the tumor and be confined to a small area. Radiation treatments are frequently prescribed postoperatively to kill cancer cells that may remain following an operation. Radiation is sometimes given as palliation for inoperable cancers to shrink the size of a tumor that may be pressing on vital organs and to relieve pain, difficulty breathing, or difficulty swallowing.

Adjuvant chemotherapy is the administration of antineoplastic drugs after surgery or radiation therapy. The purpose of adjuvant chemotherapy is to rid the body of any cancerous cells that were not removed during the surgery or to treat any micrometastases that may be developing.

Neoadjuvant chemotherapy is the administration of antineoplastic drugs before surgery or radiation therapy with the goal of shrinking a large tumor to a more manageable size. This may also be done if the tumor has invaded vital tissue around it, such as may happen with brain tumors. Shrinking the tumor preoperatively results in less surgical invasion when removing the tumor.

In a few cases, drugs are given as chemoprophylaxis with the goal of preventing cancer from occurring in patients at high risk for developing tumors. For example, patients with a close family history of breast cancer who have had a primary breast cancer removed may receive tamoxifen, even if there is no evidence of metastases. Tamoxifen has been shown to prevent the recurrence of breast cancer in these patients. Chemoprophylaxis of cancer is uncommon because most of these drugs have potentially serious adverse effects.

CONNECTION Checkpoint 56.2

Corticosteroids are administered to most patients who are receiving tissue or organ transplants. From what you learned in Chapter 42, what is the rationale for administering corticosteroids to these patients? *See Answer to Connection Checkpoint 56.2 on student resource website.*

Staging and Grading of Cancer

56.5 Cancers are described by their stage and grade.

Staging and grading must be done to determine the extent to which a cancer has invaded the body. These processes are performed on the initial diagnosis of cancer to determine the best course of therapy and predict patient outcomes.

Staging is the process of determining where the cancer is located and the extent of its invasion. Staging helps the health care provider to more accurately communicate the prognosis of the disease with the patient and helps to determine the best course of treatment.

During the staging of solid tumors, diagnostic testing determines the size of the tumor, whether the tumor has invaded surrounding tissue, the involvement of lymph nodes, and the presence or absence of metastasis (Table 56.2). The patient's disease is assigned numerical values for the tumor (T), node (N), and metastasis (M). Once these are determined, an overall stage is assigned: I, II, III or IV. Stage I is assigned to cancers that are the least invasive and which have the best prognosis. Stage IV is given for the cancer that is the most aggressive and has the poorest prognosis.

TABLE 56.2	Staging of Cancer*
T Category: Describes the Primary Tumor	
TX	Primary tumor cannot be assessed
T0	No evidence of primary tumor
T$_{is}$	Tumor is confined to the primary area
T1–T4	Tumor has invaded areas surrounding the primary tumor (number based on extent and size of the tumor)
N Category: Describes Whether or Not the Cancer Has Spread to Lymph Nodes	
NX	Nearby lymph nodes cannot be assessed
N0	No regional lymph nodes metastasis
N1–N3	Primary tumor has spread to regional lymph nodes
M Category: Describes Whether or Not Distant Metastases Are Present	
MX	Distant metastases cannot be assessed
M0	No distant metastases were found
M1	Distant metastases are present

*The exact staging of a tumor varies somewhat with each specific type of cancer. Most have multiple subcategories to better define the tumor.

TABLE 56.3	Grading of Cancer Cells
Grade	**Description**
GX	Grade cannot be determined
G1	Well differentiated: The cancer cells look like normal cells and are replicating slowly
G2	Moderately differentiated: The cancer cells look somewhat like normal cells and are replicating moderately fast
G3	Poorly differentiated: The cancer cells look clearly different from normal cells and are replicating rapidly
G4	Undifferentiated: The cancer cells do not look anything like normal cells and are replicating aggressively

Once a cancer is staged, the level does not change even if the cancer progresses. For example, if a cancer is staged as level II on diagnosis, the cancer will always be referred to as a Stage II even if it spreads to other sites. At this point, it may receive a qualifier, such as Stage II *with metastasis* or Stage II *recurrent*. Statistics regarding cancer survival and treatment are based on the initial stage at which the cancer was diagnosed.

Grading is a process that examines potential cancer cells under a microscope and compares their appearance to normal parent cells. Normal cells are highly differentiated: They have developed, become fully mature, look like the parent cell, and carry on the functions of the parent cell. For example, it is very easy to distinguish a liver cell from a muscle cell or a nerve cell microscopically. When a normal cell becomes cancerous, however, it gradually changes and becomes less differentiated in both structure and function. Once fully undifferentiated, the cancer cell will look very different from the parent cell from which it came and will not carry on the functions of the parent cell.

In the grading process, if the biopsy cells appear differentiated and very similar to the parent cells, the tumor is classified as a Grade 1 (G1) and has the best prognosis. G4 cells are grossly abnormal and clearly different from normal cells. Patients with these malignant and aggressive cells have the worst prognosis. The different grades are described in Table 56.3.

Grading has certain limitations. For instance, solid tumors often contain many different types of cells that vary in appearance from near normal to grossly abnormal. One part of the tumor may have cells consistent with G2, whereas other parts of the same tumor may have cells consistent with G4. Unlike staging, grading may change over time as the tumor evolves.

The Cell Cycle and Growth Fraction

56.6 Many antineoplastic drugs are more effective when given at specific stages of the cell cycle and in tumors with a high growth fraction.

Both normal and cancerous cells go through a sequence of events known as the cell cycle, which is illustrated in Figure 56.2. Knowledge of the cell cycle is important to understanding the effectiveness of anticancer drugs.

In simplest terms, a cell is either performing its daily functions or it is undergoing cell division. There are certain cellular activities

CONNECTIONS | Complementary and Alternative Therapies

◀ Acupuncture

Description

Acupuncture involves stimulating anatomic points on the body to treat pain and other health conditions. Based on traditional Chinese medicine, the body is viewed as having a delicate balance between two opposing forces, yin and yang, that when out of balance, results in symptoms or disease. Acupuncture is an attempt to correct the balance of energy between the two. There are at least 2,000 acupuncture points along pathways known as meridians or channels. It is these meridians or channels that acupuncture seeks to unblock and rebalance so that energy can flow. There are more than 12 primary meridians consisting of many interconnected acupuncture points (American Academy of Medical Acupuncture, n.d.).

History and Claims

Acupuncture has been used as a component of traditional Chinese medicine for thousands of years. Early needles were made of wood, bone, or stone. Metal needles the approximate width of a human hair are currently used. The World Health Organization and the National Institutes of Health recognize acupuncture as a legitimate health option for treating disorders such as asthma, bronchitis, carpal tunnel syndrome, constipation, diarrhea,

menopausal symptoms, and fibromyalgia, among many others (University of Maryland Medical Center, 2011).

Evidence

There is growing evidence that acupuncture has a physiological basis for its efficacy. While not fully understood, it appears to stimulate cholinergic nerves to increase the release of neurotransmitters and change brain function (Cassileth & Keefe, 2010). A recent meta-analysis of 29 clinical trials determined that acupuncture was beneficial in treating chronic pain such as osteoarthritis, back pain, shoulder pain, and chronic headache (Vickers & Linde, 2014). Other studies have shown that it may be beneficial to treat xerostomia induced by radiation (O'Sullivan & Higginson, 2010) and hot flashes and night sweats caused by hormonal-based chemotherapy such as tamoxifen (de Valois, Young, Robinson, McCourt, & Maher, 2010). Controlled studies of acupuncture often yield mixed results. For example, based on large systematic reviews of randomized controlled trials, there is still insufficient evidence to suggest effectiveness in treating cancer pain (Paley, Johnson, Tashani, & Bagnall, 2011). A meta-analysis of 38 studies did not find acupuncture to be beneficial in promoting smoking cessation (White, Rampes, Liu, Stead, & Campbell, 2014).

---

that occur in between these two basic functions of the cell that allow its life cycle to be divided into five stages or phases.

Stage G$_0$: Although sometimes called the resting stage, G$_0$ is the phase during which cells conduct their everyday activities such as metabolism, impulse conduction, contraction, or secretion. A cell may enter its G$_0$ phase at any point in the cycle and remain there for

extended periods, depending on the specific tissue and surrounding cellular signals. Cells spend most of their lifetime in the G$_0$ phase.

Stage G$_1$ (Gap 1): If a cell receives a signal to divide, it leaves the G$_0$ phase and enters the G$_1$ phase, during which it synthesizes the ribonucleic acid (RNA), proteins, and other components needed to duplicate its DNA.

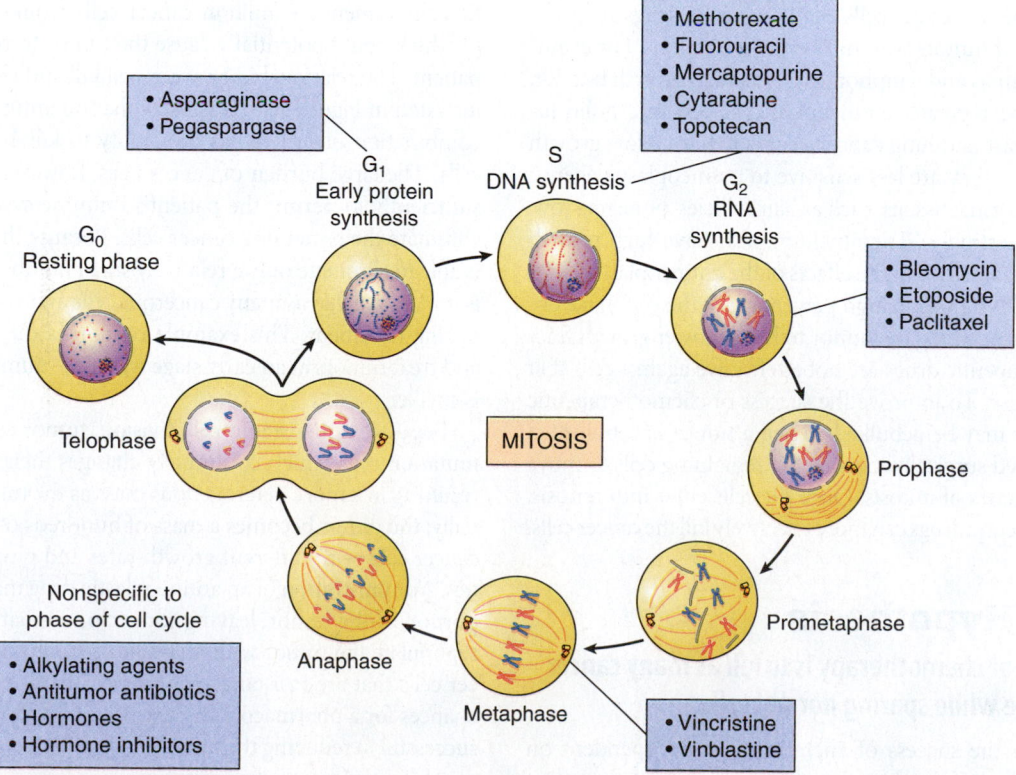

Figure 56.2 Antineoplastic agents and the cell cycle.

Stage S (Synthesis): During the S phase the cell duplicates its DNA.

Stage G₂ (Gap 2): During the G_2 or premitotic phase the cell makes additional proteins and the spindle apparatus that are necessary for cell division or mitosis.

Stage M (Mitosis): The cell undergoes mitosis, which includes prophase, metaphase, anaphase, and telophase. Following mitosis in the M phase, the cell has split into two identical cells that will either start the process over at the G_1 phase or enter the G_0 phase depending on the needs of the body. This is the briefest stage of the cell cycle.

The actions of some antineoplastics are specific to certain phases of the cell cycle, whereas others are mostly independent of the cell cycle. Cell cycle specific drugs kill the most cancer cells when they are administered in divided but frequent doses. Cell cycle specific drugs are most effective in treating hematologic malignancies and other cancers that have a relatively large proportion of cells proliferating at any given point in time. Examples include mitotic inhibitors such as vincristine (Oncovin), which affect cells in the M phase, and antimetabolites such as fluorouracil (Adrucil), which are most effective against cells during the S phase. In general, cell cycle specific drugs are not effective against tumors that have a large percentage of resting cells.

Cell cycle nonspecific drugs can kill cancer cells in any stage of the cell cycle, including the G_0 resting phase. Often, these drugs are incorporated into resting cancer cells and have no effects until the cells attempt to divide. These drugs act relatively slowly and are given intermittently to give normal cells an opportunity to recover. The effects of alkylating agents such as cyclophosphamide (Cytoxan), antitumor antibiotics, and hormonal therapies are generally independent of the phases of the cell cycle.

The **growth fraction** is a measure of the number of cells undergoing mitosis in a tissue. It is a ratio of the number of replicating cells to the number of resting cells. Antineoplastic drugs are more toxic to tissues and tumors with high growth fractions. For example, certain leukemias and lymphomas have a high growth fraction and therefore have a greater antineoplastic success rate. Solid tumors such as breast and lung cancer generally have a low growth fraction; therefore, they are less sensitive to antineoplastic agents. Because certain normal tissues, such as hair follicles, bone marrow, and the gastrointestinal (GI) epithelium, also have high growth fractions, they are sensitive to the effects of the antineoplastics.

With large solid tumors, a high percentage of the cells have entered the G_0 phase, causing the tumor to have a lower growth fraction. Chemotherapeutic drugs are not as effective against cells that are in the G_0 phase. To improve the success of chemotherapeutic drugs, the tumor may be debulked. When a tumor is debulked, a portion is removed surgically, causing the remaining cells to move into the active phases of mitosis. Once the cells enter into mitosis, the chemotherapeutic drugs can more effectively kill the cancer cells.

Cell Kill Hypothesis

56.7 The goal of chemotherapy is to kill as many cancer cells as possible while sparing normal cells.

Measurement of the success of chemotherapy is dependent on the therapeutic goal. If the desirable outcome is a total cure, then success is measured by how long the patient remains cancer free following treatment. If the goal is palliation, success is measured by the degree to which the patient's quality of life is improved. Because chemotherapy is often prolonged and physically challenging, it is crucial that the patient understand the goals of treatment and how they will be measured. In cases of palliation, the patient must weigh whether the adverse effects associated with treatment are worth the anticipated increase in the quality of life.

Patients who are undergoing chemotherapy usually receive several rounds of treatment spaced over a designated time, usually several weeks or months. This is because each round of chemotherapy kills a set percentage of cancer cells, usually those that are rapidly dividing at the time of treatment. Subsequent rounds kill additional cells. Another reason is that the chemotherapy always damages normal cells and can cause serious adverse effects. Patients need time to recover between treatments. For example, neutrophils are especially sensitive to chemotherapy and the patients' absolute neutrophil count (ANC) will usually plummet after a therapy session. Intervals between treatments allow the body to make more neutrophils so that body defenses are able to fight infections.

The **cell kill hypothesis** is a theoretical model that predicts the ability of antineoplastic drugs to eliminate cancer cells. This hypothesis predicts that a drug will kill a certain percentage, rather than a constant number, of cancer cells. Why is this important?

Theoretically, every single cell in a malignant tumor must be eliminated from the body to cure a patient. Leaving even a single malignant cell could result in regrowth of the tumor. Eliminating every cancer cell, however, is a very difficult task. As an example, consider that a small, 1-cm breast tumor may already contain 1 billion cancer cells before it can be detected during a manual examination. A drug that is able to kill 99% of these cells would be considered a very effective drug indeed. Yet even with this fantastic achievement, 10 million cancer cells would remain, any one of which could potentially cause the tumor to return and kill the patient. The relationship between cell kill and chemotherapy is illustrated in Figure 56.3. It is likely that no antineoplastic drug (or combination of drugs) has the ability to kill 100% of the tumor cells. The large burden of cancer cells, however, may be lowered sufficiently to permit the patient's immune system to control or eliminate the remaining cancer cells. Because the immune system is able to eliminate only a relatively small number of cancer cells, it is imperative that as many cancerous cells as possible be eliminated during treatment. This example reinforces the need to diagnose and treat tumors at an early stage when the number of cancer cells is smaller.

Because of their rapid cell division, tumor cells express a high mutation rate, which continually changes their genetic structure, resulting in a more heterogenous mass as the tumor grows. Essentially, the tumor becomes a mass of hundreds of different types of cancer cells with different growth rates and physiological properties. Administration of an antineoplastic drug may kill only a small portion of the tumor, leaving some clones unaffected and able to repopulate the tumor with resistant cells. The appearance of cancer cells that are resistant to antineoplastic drugs complicates the chances for a pharmacologic cure because a therapy that was very successful in reducing the tumor mass at the start of chemotherapy may become less effective over time.

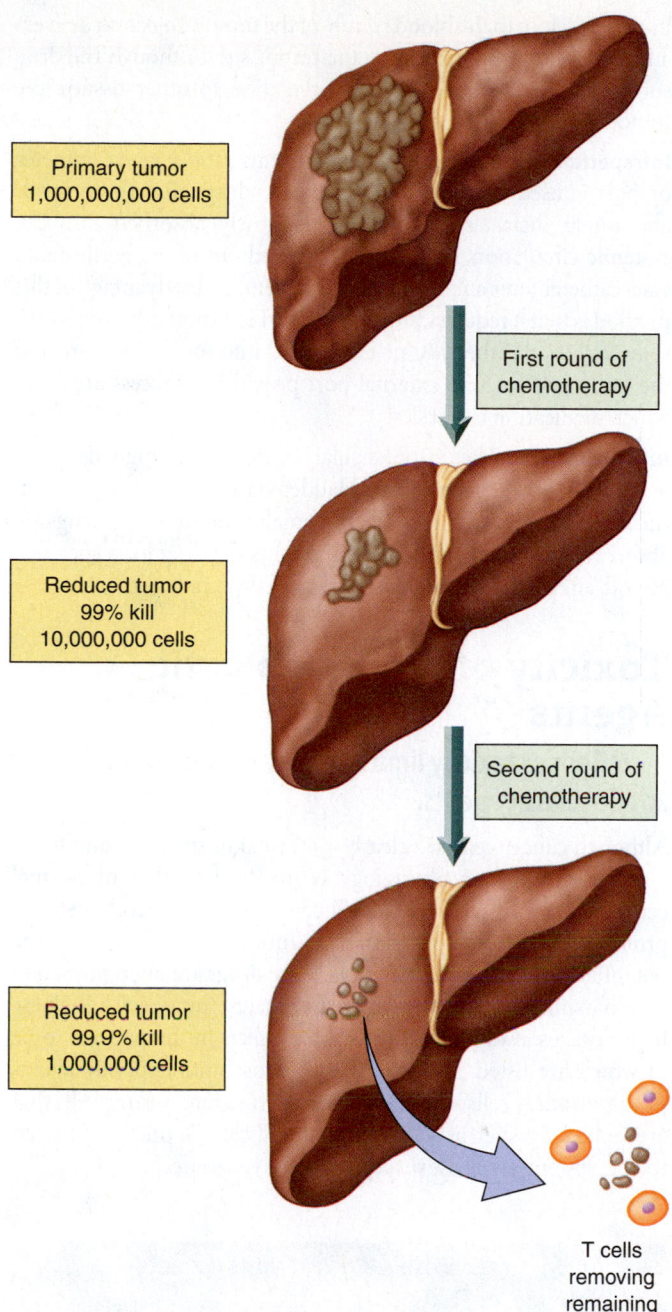

| Primary tumor |
| 1,000,000,000 cells |

First round of chemotherapy

| Reduced tumor |
| 99% kill |
| 10,000,000 cells |

Second round of chemotherapy

| Reduced tumor |
| 99.9% kill |
| 1,000,000 cells |

T cells removing remaining cancer cells

Figure 56.3 Cell kill and chemotherapy.

Improving the Success of Chemotherapy

56.8 Use of multiple drugs and intermittent dosing are strategies that allow for greater success of chemotherapy.

As has been seen throughout this text, the majority of pharmacotherapy is conducted with a single drug given in a constant amount over a specified time period. For most indications, the use of multiple drugs increases the expense of treatment and can cause additional adverse effects. Cancer chemotherapy is an important

exception: The concurrent use of multiple drugs, combined with intermittent dosing, results in improved patient outcomes.

Combination Chemotherapy

Chemotherapy is conducted using established protocols that are specific to the type of cancer and its stage. A cancer treatment protocol describes the specific combination of antineoplastics that will be given, their doses, and the cycles in which they will be administered. Using multiple drugs affects the different stages of the cancer cell's life cycle and attacks the various clones within the tumor via several mechanisms of action, thus increasing the percentage of cell kill. Combination chemotherapy also allows for lower dosages of each individual agent, thereby reducing toxicity and slowing the development of resistance. Examples of established protocols using combination therapy include cyclophosphamide-methotrexate-fluorouracil (CMF) for breast cancer and cyclophosphamide-adriamycin-vincristine (CAV) for lung cancer. Each type of cancer has its own individual protocol, which was established through clinical trials. These protocols are being refined and revised continually based on current research.

CONNECTION Checkpoint 56.3

From what you learned in Chapters 46 through 55, name two infectious diseases that require several years' therapy with anti-infectives, using multiple drugs. *See Answer to Connection Checkpoint 56.3 on student resource website.*

Dosing Schedules

Most chemotherapeutic medications are administered intermittently using specific dosing schedules that have been determined through research to increase the effectiveness of the antineoplastic agents. For example, some of the anticancer drugs are given as a single dose or perhaps several doses over a few days. A few weeks may pass before the next series of doses begins. This gives normal cells time to recover from the adverse effects of the drugs and allows tumor cells that may not have been replicating at the time of the first dose to begin dividing and become more sensitive to the next round of chemotherapy. Sometimes the optimum dosing schedule must be delayed until the patient sufficiently recovers from the drug toxicities, especially bone marrow suppression. Delays or reductions in the planned dosages are likely to negatively affect treatment outcomes. The specific dosing schedule chosen depends on the type of tumor, stage of the disease, and overall condition of the patient.

Route of Administration

Antineoplastic agents are available for administration by virtually any route. Whenever possible, the oral (PO) route is used because it is most acceptable to the patient and eliminates risks associated with intravenous (IV) administration, such as phlebitis or tissue necrosis. Antineoplastics may be given locally by topical application to the lesion or through direct instillation into the tumor region. Regional administration causes less systemic toxicity. The most common route for delivering antineoplastics is via the venous system.

Oral: The PO route is the easiest, most convenient, and least expensive route for chemotherapy administration. Patients can self-administer their PO chemotherapy medications at home. One problem associated with PO administration is the inconsistency of absorption. Chemotherapeutic agents that are administered PO produce many of the same adverse reactions as the injectable agents, and the patient and caregivers must be aware of these. They must also be taught safe handling and disposal of these drugs. Examples of antineoplastics available as PO preparations include methotrexate, mercaptopurine, cyclophosphamide, and melphalan.

Intravenous: IV is the most common route for delivery of chemotherapy agents. One advantage to the IV route is that a constant and consistent serum level of the drug can be obtained by fine adjustments to the infusion rate. A disadvantage is that **sclerosing**, or abnormal tissue hardening of the veins, may occur during prolonged administration. Another disadvantage to the patient is that chemotherapy administration is done in a cancer center, health care provider's office, or some other place away from the patient's home. This may require many miles of commuting and present a hardship to the patient and family. In addition, traveling out of the home may expose the patient to viruses and other infectious agents, which can be hazardous to those with diminished immune function. In some geographic areas, an oncology nurse will come to the patient's home and administer the chemotherapy.

Administration of chemotherapeutic agents can be done through a centrally located access device such as a Groshong catheter, which is inserted by being tunneled under the skin on the chest into a major vein for long-term medication instillation, or through a peripheral vein via a **peripherally inserted central catheter (PICC) line**. A PICC line is a central catheter that is threaded into the vena cava for administration of chemotherapy. The advantages of a central line are that it is less likely to infiltrate and it is inserted in a large vein, which is less likely to become irritated during chemotherapy. A disadvantage of a central line is that it increases the patient's risk of acquiring an infection.

Because IV administration requires a free-flowing IV in a large vein, it is imperative that the nurse constantly assesses the insertion site of the IV for signs of infiltration or phlebitis. Some antineoplastics can cause extreme cellular damage if the solution is allowed to enter surrounding tissues. Because of the potential for tissue damage, most antineoplastics are not administered by the intramuscular (IM) or subcutaneous routes. Examples of IV antineoplastics are carmustine, cisplatin, doxorubicin, and mitomycin.

Intrathecal: Some antineoplastic medications may be delivered intrathecally into the subarachnoid space of the spinal cord. In intrathecal administration, the drug bypasses the blood–brain barrier and circulates with the cerebrospinal fluid (CSF) to expose central nervous system (CNS) tumors to high concentrations of the drug. A specially trained individual must conduct the procedure because it requires a lumbar puncture or surgical placement of a reservoir or implanted pump for drug delivery. An advantage to intrathecal administration is that it provides a consistent drug level in the CSF. Potential adverse effects include headaches, confusion, lethargy, seizures, nausea, or vomiting, all of which are signs of increased intracranial pressure.

Intra-arterial: Occasionally the health care provider may choose to administer chemotherapeutic medications through an artery. Intra-arterial administration requires a surgical procedure for catheter placement and, often, special x-ray techniques. In most cases, a catheter is passed via the femoral or brachial artery so that its end lies close to the blood supply of the tumor. Injection delivers a high dose of drug directly to the tumor site. Although the drug subsequently distributes via the circulation to other tissues, the tumor area receives the highest dose.

Intraperitoneal: Intraperitoneal administration via a catheter or port is used to deliver antineoplastic drugs directly to intra-abdominal metastases. The drug is slowly absorbed into the systemic circulation, or it may be drained out of the peritoneum via a catheter after a few hours of treatment. A disadvantage of this method is that it requires the placing of a Tenckhoff catheter, which is a specialized catheter. One end placed into the peritoneum and the other end with an external port provides an access area into which medication is instilled.

Intravesicular: The intravesicular route instills high doses of antineoplastics into the urinary bladder via a Foley catheter to treat tumors of the bladder mucosa. Only small amounts of the drugs are absorbed systemically. The patient retains the drug for a specified period, after which it is voided or removed via catheter.

Toxicity of Antineoplastic Agents

56.9 Serious toxicity limits therapy with most antineoplastic agents.

Although cancer cells are clearly abnormal in structure and function, much of their physiology is identical to that of normal cells. Because it is difficult to kill cancer cells selectively without profoundly affecting normal cells, all antineoplastic drugs have the potential to cause serious toxicity. These drugs are often pushed to their maximum dosages to obtain the greatest tumor cell kill. These high dosages always result in adverse effects in the patient, some of which are listed in Table 56.4. Because antineoplastic agents primarily affect cells with a high growth fraction, normal cells that are replicating, such as cells in the hair follicles, GI tract, and hematologic system, are most susceptible to adverse effects.

TABLE 56.4 Examples of Adverse Effects of Anticancer Drugs

Common Expected Adverse Effects	Drug-Specific Adverse Effects	Dose-Limiting Adverse Effects
Nausea and vomiting	Fetal malformations (pemetrexed, methotrexate, mercaptopurine)	Bone marrow suppression
Stomatitis	Peripheral-sensory neuropathy (cisplatin)	Acute renal failure
Anorexia	Sterility (mechlorethamine)	Pulmonary fibrosis
Alopecia	Cardiotoxicity (doxorubicin, daunorubicin)	Diarrhea
Immunosuppression		
Fatigue		

Hematologic System

Erythrocytes, leukocytes, and platelets have relatively short life spans and must be continually replaced by hematopoietic stem cells residing in the bone marrow. Stem cells may be destroyed by antineoplastic agents, resulting in bone marrow suppression (myelosuppression). Myelosuppression is the most common dose-limiting adverse effect of chemotherapy and the one that most often causes discontinuation or delays of chemotherapy. Severe bone marrow suppression is a contraindication to therapy with most antineoplastic drugs.

Chemotherapy causes erythrocyte, leukocyte, and platelet counts to decrease until they reach their lowest value, known as the **nadir**. Patients are most susceptible to the symptoms, such as anemia, infections, or bleeding, during the nadir. Following the nadir, blood counts begin their recovery back to normal values. The nadir is specific for each chemotherapeutic agent and for each type of blood cell. For example, antimetabolites produce rapid nadirs for neutrophils in 7 to 14 days after the initiation of chemotherapy, with recovery within 7 to 21 days following the nadir. Other agents such as the nitrosoureas produce a delayed nadir for neutrophils at 26 to 63 days, with recovery at 35 to 89 days after the nadir.

Neutrophils are the type of white blood cells (WBCs) most affected by chemotherapy. This is primarily because the normal life span of a neutrophil is only 7 to 12 hours, and without continual replacement by stem cells the number of circulating neutrophils quickly falls. A patient is diagnosed with neutropenia when the neutrophil count is less than 1,500 cells/mL. Patients are very susceptible to infections while they are neutropenic. Many times patients who are neutropenic are placed in reverse isolation to protect them from exposure to any infections from family members or health care providers. Even an infection from a mild cold could be fatal to patients with extremely low neutrophil counts. If a patient who is neutropenic and receiving chemotherapy acquires an infection, an increase in WBCs may not be evident. If a patient who is neutropenic does develop a fever, this may be an indication of sepsis, and antibiotics are indicated.

Medications such as colony-stimulating factors (filgrastim [Neupogen] and sargramostim [Leukine]) are sometimes administered to accelerate recovery of suppressed bone marrow cells and to increase the WBC count. The administration of these drugs shortens the time of neutropenia, thus lowering the risk of opportunistic infections and allowing the patient to maintain an optimum chemotherapy dosing schedule. Filgrastim is presented as a prototype drug in Chapter 39.

Because the life span of a platelet is only 7 to 8 days, these blood elements require constant replenishment by bone marrow stem cells. A patient is diagnosed with thrombocytopenia when the platelet count is less than 100,000 per milliliter of blood. Chemotherapy is often delayed if this occurs. In patients who are receiving chemotherapy, thrombocytopenia usually occurs concurrently with neutropenia. Thrombocytopenia can cause the patient to exhibit abnormal bleeding, with symptoms ranging from bruising to petechiae to serious hemorrhage. Bleeding precautions must be implemented if the platelet count falls below 50,000 per milliliter of blood. To prevent the platelet count from decreasing to a harmful level, platelet infusions may be necessary. Oprelvekin (Neumega) is a thrombopoietic growth factor that may be administered to increase platelet production. This drug is presented as a prototype hematopoietic agent in Chapter 39.

Because erythrocytes have a longer life span (90–120 days) than neutrophils or platelets, reductions in red blood cells (RBCs), or anemia, occur later in the course of chemotherapy. Hemoglobin carries oxygen to all tissues in the body; thus anemia may affect every system in the body. An infusion of RBCs may be required to increase a patient's RBC count and hemoglobin value. A medication that the nurse may administer to help increase the number of RBCs is epoetin alfa (Epogen), which is presented as a prototype in Chapter 39. When assessing for anemia, it should be remembered that the etiology may be the result of nonchemotherapy-related causes, such as bleeding, iron deficiency, or kidney damage.

Gastrointestinal Tract

The vomiting center in the medulla is triggered by many antineoplastics. Acute nausea and vomiting often begin within minutes of chemotherapy administration and may last for 24 hours. Delayed nausea and vomiting begin 24 hours after chemotherapy and may continue for up to 6 days. Anticipatory nausea and vomiting may occur before chemotherapy because the patient may be expecting an unpleasant experience. Antineoplastics are sometimes classified by their **emetic potential**. Before starting therapy with the highest emetic potential agents, patients may be pretreated with antiemetic drugs such as ondansetron (Zofran), prochlorperazine (Compazine), or lorazepam (Ativan). It is not uncommon to administer several different antiemetic medications that have several modes of action. Antiemetic medications are presented in detail in Chapter 60.

The epithelial lining of the GI tract is very sensitive to the effects of chemotherapeutic agents. The GI mucosa commonly becomes inflamed, a condition known as **mucositis**. Consequences of mucositis include painful ulcerations in the mouth and esophagus, difficulty eating or swallowing, GI bleeding, intestinal infections, or severe diarrhea. Some research has shown that eating popsicles during chemotherapy infusions can decrease the severity of mucositis. The nurse may also instruct the patient to eat a bland diet and to use a soft toothbrush for oral care. Some health care providers may order a "medical cocktail," which may include lidocaine viscous, liquid diphenhydramine, and Carafate to decrease the pain associated with the mucositis. The patient should also be instructed to report any signs of thrush, which is an oral yeast infection.

Most patients receiving antineoplastics experience anorexia, usually due to a combination of nausea, vomiting, and mucositis. At times the patient's appetite is decreased such that tube feedings or parenteral feedings may be indicated. The body needs sufficient nutrients and calories for normal cells to repopulate and for repair of body tissues. When assessing for anorexia, it should be remembered that this symptom may be the result of direct effects from the tumor itself or from associated psychological changes such as depression or anxiety.

The patient may experience constipation or diarrhea depending on the specific drugs administered. Some chemotherapeutic medications damage the intestinal lining, inhibiting the reabsorption of fluids and producing loose stools. Replacement of fluids and electrolytes as well as treatment with an antidiarrheal drug may be indicated. Some chemotherapeutic medications decrease the motility of the GI tract, resulting in greater reabsorption of fluids, which leads to constipation. When assessing for constipation, it should be remembered that other common reasons for this symptom include therapy with opioid analgesics and inadequate water and fiber intake.

Many patients with cancer experience a general wasting of muscle and other tissues referred to as **cachexia**. Cachexia may be caused by toxic effects from the cancer itself or from its treatment. Symptoms from the chemotherapy such as anorexia, mucositis, nausea, and vomiting may contribute to cachexia, but other non-GI factors also contribute such as serious chronic pain, depression, and fatigue.

Cardiopulmonary System

Some of the chemotherapeutic medications can be toxic to the heart and lungs. For example, doxorubicin (Adriamycin) is specifically known for its cardiotoxicity and the nurse should monitor the patient for any changes in the electrocardiogram (ECG) and assess for any signs of heart failure. This adverse effect can be serious enough to later cause the patient to need cardiac monitoring or a heart transplant. A cardioprotective drug such as dexrazoxane (Zinecard) is administered just prior to a doxorubicin infusion to prevent permanent heart damage.

Bleomycin (Blenoxane) is specifically known for causing pneumonitis in patients. Nursing care of the patient who is receiving bleomycin should include monitoring the patient's pulse oximeter and respiratory status. Auscultating crackles in the lung fields may be a sign of a developing pneumonitis. Chest x-rays may be necessary two to three times per week to assess for lung changes.

Urinary System

Some of the chemotherapeutic medications can exhibit considerable nephrotoxicity. For example, cisplatin (Platinol) can lead to kidney failure if the dosage limit is exceeded. When administering chemotherapeutic agents that are nephrotoxic, the nurse should closely monitor intake and output and urine dipstick results for red cells. The patient should remain well hydrated during the treatment to help prevent renal damage. Diuretics may be administered to help balance the intake and output of the patient. In addition, the drug mesna (Mesnex) is administered to prevent hemorrhagic cystitis during chemotherapy with cyclophosphamide or ifosfamide.

Reproductive System

Some antineoplastics, particularly the alkylating agents, affect the gonads and have been associated with infertility in both males and females. If a woman is pregnant while receiving treatment, the fetus may be severely damaged due to the high growth fraction of the fetus's cells or it may be killed during the treatment. Sexually active male and female patients should be instructed to use reliable contraception while receiving chemotherapy and for 3 to 6 months following treatment.

Antineoplastic medications are more likely to cause permanent sterility in men than in women. Some patients choose to have their sperm or eggs harvested prior to treatment in case the chemotherapy does affect their fertility.

Many hospitals have protocols specifying that female nurses and pharmacists not handle chemotherapeutic agents if they are pregnant or are trying to become pregnant due to the toxic effects that the chemotherapy may have on the fetus.

Nervous System

Several chemotherapeutic agents are toxic to the nervous system. For instance, vincristine (Oncovin) may cause muscle weakness and peripheral neuritis. It is important for the nurse to assess the patient's neurologic status frequently when administering this medication. Patients should also be informed of the potential adverse effects so that they may inform the nurse of any tingling or pain in their extremities or if changes occur in muscle strength.

Cisplatin (Platinol) has been known to cause hearing loss and deafness in some patients. The nurse should assess the patient's hearing throughout the course of treatment and document any changes noted in the patient's ability to hear.

Skin and Soft Tissue

Many antineoplastics are classified as **vesicants**, agents that can cause serious tissue injury if they escape from an artery or vein during an infusion or injection. Extravasation or infiltration from an injection site can produce severe tissue and nerve damage, local infection, and even loss of a limb. If a nurse is concerned that a peripheral IV is no longer working properly, the IV should not be used for chemotherapy administration. Although rare, extravasation can still occur with a central line so the nurse should continue to frequently assess the insertion site of a central line while administering chemotherapy. Rapid treatment of extravasation is necessary to limit tissue damage, and certain antineoplastics have specific antidotes. For example, extravasation of carmustine (BiCNU, Gliadel) is treated with injections of equal parts of sodium bicarbonate and normal saline into the extravasation site. Before administering IV antineoplastic agents, the nurse should know the emergency treatment for extravasation. Antineoplastics with the strongest vesicant activity include busulfan, carmustine, dacarbazine, dactinomycin, daunorubicin, idarubicin, mechlorethamine, mitomycin, plicamycin, streptozocin, vinblastine, vincristine, and vinorelbine.

Other Effects

Fatigue is a common complaint during chemotherapy. The precise etiology of the fatigue is often difficult to determine. If the patient has anemia, the lack of hemoglobin to carry oxygen to the tissue can cause the patient to feel fatigued. The patient may be experiencing anxiety or depression due to the diagnosis of cancer, which may lead to sleep deprivation. The process of cellular regeneration after chemotherapy treatments may also cause feelings of fatigue. A nutritional consultation may be helpful in determining if the fatigue has a nutritional origin. Coping strategies for dealing with stress and scheduled periods of rest may benefit the patient.

Hair follicles are damaged by many chemotherapeutic agents, resulting in hair loss or **alopecia**. Hair loss usually begins within 1 to 2 weeks of the first treatment, and regrowth may take 3 to 5 months after the last chemotherapeutic treatment. The potential for alopecia should be discussed with patients before treatment begins so that they may choose to wear a hat, bandana, wig, or other accessory.

One of the ironies of chemotherapy is that the medications that are given to kill the cancer may cause a secondary cancer to develop elsewhere in the body. This is not a common adverse effect but it has been clearly demonstrated in patients. The secondary malignancy usually occurs many years after the initial cancer; thus this adverse effect is of most concern to children being treated with chemotherapy. It is estimated that pediatric cancer survivors have a 10 to 20 times greater risk than other children for developing a secondary malignancy. The most common secondary malignancy is nonlymphocytic leukemia.

Hyperuricemia is most frequently associated with chemotherapy for lymphomas and leukemias due to the rapid cell kill. A patient is diagnosed with hyperuricemia when uric acid levels in the blood are elevated, which can lead to renal failure if the uric crystals deposit in the renal tubules. Signs of hyperuricemia are nausea, vomiting, and oliguria. Keeping the patient well hydrated helps to preserve renal function by flushing microscopic crystals out of the kidney before they have a chance to form larger crystals. The nurse who is caring for a patient who is suspected of developing or has been diagnosed with hyperuricemia should monitor the patient's intake and output closely.

PharmFACT

The morbidity and mortality rates for most types of cancer remain higher in the African American population than in Caucasians. However, the overall disparity has narrowed over the past 20 years, especially in males (American Cancer Society, 2013).

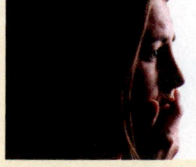

CHAPTER 56

Understanding the Chapter

Key Concepts Summary

56.1 Cancer is characterized by rapid, uncontrolled growth of cells that eventually invade normal tissues and metastasize.

56.2 The etiology of cancer may be chemical, physical, or biologic.

56.3 The keys to successful cancer treatment are prevention and early detection.

56.4 The three primary goals of chemotherapy are cure, control, and palliation.

56.5 Cancers are described by their stage and grade.

56.6 Many antineoplastic drugs are more effective when given at specific stages of the cell cycle and in tumors with a high growth fraction.

56.7 The goal of chemotherapy is to kill as many cancer cells as possible while sparing normal cells.

56.8 Use of multiple drugs and intermittent dosing are strategies that allow for greater success of chemotherapy.

56.9 Serious toxicity limits therapy with most antineoplastic agents.

Case Study: Making the Patient Connection

Remember the patient "Cheryl Ogen" at the beginning of the chapter? Now read the rest of the case study. Based on the information presented within this chapter, respond to the critical thinking questions that follow.

Cheryl Ogen is a 39-year-old patient who is employed as a kindergarten teacher. She has been married for 15 years and has never had any children. Her medical history confirms that both her mother and maternal grandmother died from breast cancer. Now Cheryl has been diagnosed with breast cancer. She is admitted to the hospital for tumor resection and chemotherapy. Cheryl's breast cancer is Stage T1, N0, M0, and G2. Cheryl has undergone the lumpectomy with regional lymph node biopsy and is now about to begin chemotherapy.

Critical Thinking Questions

1. Cheryl would like to know why she is receiving chemotherapy after the surgeon has removed the cancerous tumor. What would you tell her?

2. Why is it important to understand the staging and grading system used with cancer? How would you interpret the staging and grading of Cheryl's cancer?

3. Identify some of the hematologic changes that Cheryl may experience while receiving chemotherapy.

See Answers to Critical Thinking Questions on student resource website.

Additional Case Study

Jonah Cooper is a patient who is newly diagnosed with acute lymphocytic leukemia. He is 28 years old and is the father of two children age 9 months and 2 years. Jonah is admitted to the hospital for his initial round of chemotherapy.

1. Will Jonah's children be allowed to visit him during his hospital admission?

2. Why is Jonah receiving more than one type of chemotherapy?

3. Why was Jonah's cancer not staged on diagnosis?

See Answers to Additional Case Study on student resource website.

Chapter Review

1 The health care provider has written in the patient's chart that the cancer is at Stage I. The nurse knows that the implications for this staging are that the:

1. Cancer is advanced and the patient has a poor prognosis.
2. Cancerous cells are only moderately differentiated from the parent cells.
3. Cancer has been detected at an early stage.
4. Tumor is large and is invading surrounding tissue.

2 Which of the following statements by a patient who is undergoing chemotherapy would be of concern to the nurse? Select all that apply.

1. "I attended a meeting of a cancer support group this week."
2. "My husband and I are planning a short trip next week."
3. "I try to eat six small meals plus two protein shakes each day."
4. "I am taking my 15-month-old granddaughter to the pediatrician next week for her baby shots."
5. "I am going to go shopping at the mall next week."

3 The nurse determines that the patient understands an important principle of chemotherapy when the patient makes which statement?

1. "The use of multiple chemotherapy drugs affects different stages of the cancer cell's life cycle."
2. "Staging describes the process of determining how responsive the cancer is to the prescribed chemotherapy."
3. "Antineoplastic drugs kill the entire tumor, including the clones, and prevent repopulation."
4. "Combination chemotherapy requires higher dosages of each individual agent and increases toxicity."

4 Chemotherapy is being initiated for a patient with prostate cancer who is experiencing mucositis. Which health teaching would be most appropriate for this condition?

1. Use an over-the-counter mouthwash to eliminate bacteria.
2. Increase intake of citrus-containing foods and beverages.
3. Eat a bland diet with low roughage and use a soft toothbrush or plain water rinses for oral care.
4. This adverse effect is expected and will disappear within a few days.

5 The nurse is collaborating with the interdisciplinary team regarding the care of a patient with a brain tumor. The nurse knows that the most common reason that subsequent rounds of chemotherapy may be delayed is due to what condition?

1. Myelosuppression
2. Alopecia
3. Mucositis
4. Cachexia

6 A patient with cancer is started on a chemotherapeutic agent that is a known vesicant. The nurse performs which priority activity related to this drug? Monitor the patient's:

1. Response to antinausea drugs.
2. Intake of calcium-rich foods.
3. Respiratory status for cough.
4. IV port site for redness, swelling, and pain.

See Answers to Chapter Review in Appendix A.

References

American Academy of Medical Acupuncture. (n.d.). *NCCAM acupuncture information*. Retrieved from http://www.medicalacupuncture.org/ForPatients/ArticlesByPhysiciansAboutAcupuncture/NCCAMAcupunctureInformation.aspx

American Cancer Society. (2013). *Cancer facts and figures for African Americans 2013–2014*. Retrieved from http://www.cancer.org/acs/groups/content/@epidemiologysurveilance/documents/document/acspc-036921.pdf

American Cancer Society. (2014). *Cancer facts and figures 2014*. Retrieved from http://www.cancer.org/acs/groups/content/@research/documents/webcontent/acspc-042151.pdf

Cassileth, B. R., & Keefe, F. J. (2010). Integrative and behavioral approaches to the treatment of cancer-related neuropathic pain. *The Oncologist, 15*(Suppl. 2), 19–23. doi:10.1634/theoncologist.2009-S504

de Valois, B. A., Young, T., Robinson, N., McCourt, C., & Maher, E. J. (2010). Using traditional acupuncture for breast cancer-related hot flashes and night sweats. *Journal of Alternative and Complementary Medicine, 16*, 1047–1057. doi:10.1089/acm.2009.0472

O'Sullivan, E. M., & Higginson, I. J. (2010). Clinical effectiveness and safety of acupuncture in the treatment of irradiation-induced xerostomia in patients with head and neck cancer: A systematic review. *Acupuncture in Medicine, 28,* 191–199. doi:10.1136/aim.2010.002733

Paley, C. A., Johnson, M. I., Tashani, O. A., & Bagnall, A. M. (2011). Acupuncture for cancer pain in adults. *Cochrane Database of Systematic Reviews, 1,* CD007753. doi:10.1002/14651858.CD007753.pub2

University of Maryland Medical Center. (2011). *Acupuncture.* Retrieved from https://umm.edu/health/medical/altmed/treatment/acupuncture

Vickers, A. J., & Linde, K. (2014). Acupuncture for chronic pain. *The Journal of the American Medical Association, 311,* 955–956. doi:10.1001/jama.2013.285478.

White, A. R., Rampes, H., Liu, J. P., Stead, L. F., & Campbell, J. (2014). Acupuncture and related interventions for smoking cessation. *Cochrane Database of Systematic Reviews, 1,* CD000009. doi:10.1002/14651858.CD000009.pub4.

Selected Bibliography

American Cancer Society. (2012). *Find support and treatment: Staging.* Retrieved from http://www.cancer.org/treatment/%20understandingyourdiagnosis/staging

American Cancer Society. (2013). *Guidelines for the early detection of cancer.* Retrieved from http://www.cancer.org/healthy/findcancerearly/cancerscreeningguidelines/american-cancer-society-guidelines-for-the-early-detection-of-cancer

Bruce, S. D. (2013). Before you press that button: A look at chemotherapy errors. *Clinical Journal of Oncology Nursing, 17*(1), 31–32. doi:10.1188/13.CJON.31-32

Chen, R. (2011). Cochrane review summary for cancer nursing: Drug therapy for the management of cancer-related fatigue. *Cancer Nursing, 34,* 250–251. doi:10.1097/NCC.0b013e31820aeb72

Esper, P. (2013). Identifying strategies to optimize care with oral cancer therapy. *Clinical Journal of Oncology Nursing, 17*(6), 629–636. doi:10.1188/13.CJON.629-636

Given, B. A., Spoelstra, S. L., & Grant, M. (2011). The challenges of oral agents as antineoplastic treatments. *Seminars in Oncology Nursing, 27,* 93–103. doi:10.1016/j.soncn.2011.02.003

Kee, J. L. (2013). *Laboratory and diagnostic tests with nursing implications* (9th ed.). Upper Saddle River, NJ: Pearson.

Lemone, P., Burke, K., & Bauldoff, G. (2011). *Medical-surgical nursing: Critical thinking in client care* (5th ed.). Upper Saddle River, NJ: Pearson.

Neuss, M. N., Polovich, M., McNiff, K., Esper, P., Gilmore, T. R., LeFebvre, K. B., . . . Jacobson, J. O. (2013). 2013 Updated American Society of Clinical Oncology/Oncology Nursing Society chemotherapy administration safety standards including standards for the safe administration and management of oral chemotherapy. *Oncology Nursing Forum, 40,* 225–233. doi:10.1188/13.ONF.40-03AP2

Simmons, C. (2010). Oral chemotherapeutic drugs: Handle with care. *Nursing, 40*(7), 44–47. doi:10.1097/01.NURSE.0000383452.55906.e7

Yarbro, C. H., Wujcik, D., & Gobel, B. H. (2011). *Cancer nursing: Principles and practice* (7th ed.). Sudbury, MA: Jones-Bartlett.

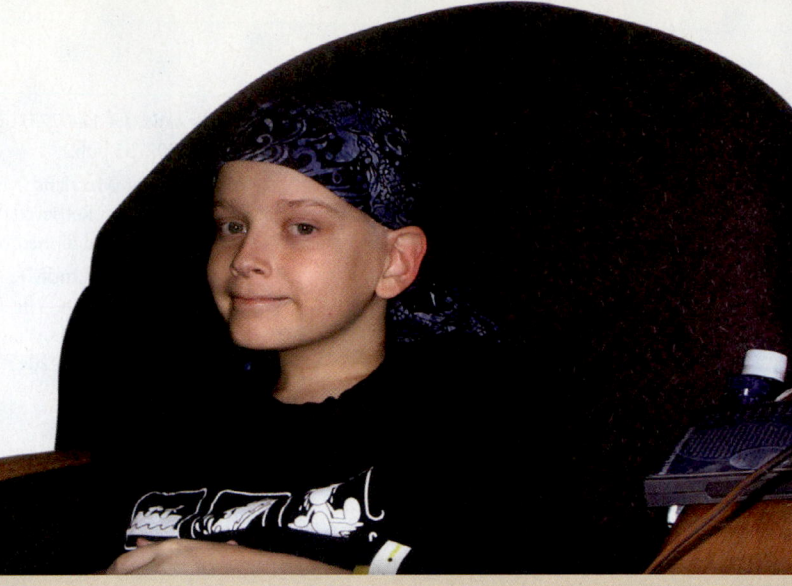

"Being tired all the time isn't so bad; I get to play a lot of video games. And I'm used to wearing my bandana. I just wish people would stop staring at me."

Patient "Zack Amos"

CHAPTER

57

Pharmacotherapy of Neoplasia

LEARNING OUTCOMES

After reading this chapter, the student should be able to:

1. Explain why it is difficult to accurately classify antineoplastic drugs.
2. Describe the common and dose-limiting toxicities of antineoplastics.
3. Describe how the process of alkylation kills rapidly growing cells.
4. Describe how antimetabolites kill cancer cells.
5. Describe mechanisms by which antitumor antibiotics kill cancer cells.
6. Explain applications of hormones and hormone antagonists to cancer chemotherapy.
7. Identify natural products that have the ability to kill tumor cells.
8. Explain the use of biologic response modifiers and targeted therapies in cancer chemotherapy.
9. For each of the classes shown in the chapter outline, identify the prototype and representative drugs and explain the mechanism(s) of drug action, primary indications, contraindications, significant drug interactions, pregnancy category, and important adverse effects.
10. Describe the types of drugs prescribed to reduce or prevent the adverse effects of antineoplastic drugs.
11. Discuss ways nurses can protect themselves from exposure to antineoplastics.
12. Apply the nursing process to care for patients receiving cancer chemotherapy.

CHAPTER OUTLINE

▶ Classification of Antineoplastic Drugs

▶ Antineoplastic Medications

Alkylating Agents

PROTOTYPE Cyclophosphamide (Cytoxan), *p. 964*

Antimetabolites

PROTOTYPE Methotrexate (MTX, Rheumatrex, Trexall), *p. 969*

Antitumor Antibiotics

PROTOTYPE Doxorubicin (Adriamycin), *p. 973*

Hormones and Hormone Antagonists

PROTOTYPE Tamoxifen, *p. 976*

Natural Products

PROTOTYPE Vincristine (Oncovin), *p. 981*

Biologic Response Modifiers and Targeted Therapies

Miscellaneous Antineoplastics

▶ Drugs for Reducing Adverse Effects

▶ Preparing and Administering Antineoplastics

KEY TERMS

alkylating agents, 963

hematopoietic growth factors, 988

oncology nurse, 992

biologic response modifier, 983

leucovorin rescue therapy, 969

targeted therapy, 988

The decision to begin cancer chemotherapy is a collaborative one made by the patient, the family, and the health care provider. Although there have been some remarkable successes in treating cancer, patients will experience adverse effects that can challenge their resolve to complete the chemotherapy regimen. Nurses must be prepared to assist patients and their families in dealing with the common adverse effects of the antineoplastics, the more serious adverse reactions, and the psychological impact of the decision to continue or discontinue treatment. This chapter examines the types of medications used in cancer chemotherapy and their applications to clinical practice.

Classification of Antineoplastic Drugs

57.1 Antineoplastic drugs kill or stop the growth of cancer cells and may be classified in multiple ways.

Drugs that are used in cancer chemotherapy come from diverse pharmacologic and chemical classes. Antineoplastics have been extracted from plants and bacteria as well as created entirely in the laboratory. Some of the drug classes attack cellular macromolecules in cancer cells, such as deoxyribonucleic acid (DNA) and proteins, whereas others poison vital metabolic pathways of rapidly growing cells. The common theme among all the antineoplastic drugs is their toxicity. They have the ability to kill or stop the growth of cancer cells.

Classification of the antineoplastics is difficult because some of these drugs kill cancer cells by multiple mechanisms and have characteristics from more than one class. For example, paclitaxel (Taxol) can be classified as a natural product (it was derived from a plant), a taxane (its chemical structure), a mitotic inhibitor (its mechanism of action), or a cell cycle inhibitor. Furthermore, the mechanisms by which some antineoplastics act are incompletely understood. A simple method of classifying this complex group of drugs includes the following categories:

- Alkylating agents
- Antimetabolites
- Antitumor antibiotics
- Hormones and hormone antagonists
- Natural products
- Biologic response modifiers and targeted therapies
- Miscellaneous antineoplastic drugs

PharmFACT

Prostate cancer is the most common non-skin cancer in America, affecting one in six men. One new case occurs every 2.3 minutes, and one man dies from prostate cancer every 16 minutes (Prostate Cancer Foundation, 2014).

Antineoplastic Medications

The antineoplastic medications include alkylating agents, antimetabolites, antitumor antibiotics, hormones and hormone antagonists, natural products, biologic response modifiers, targeted therapies, and miscellaneous antineoplastics.

Alkylating Agents

57.2 Alkylating agents change the shape of the deoxyribonucleic acid double helix and prevent cancer cells from dividing normally.

Alkylation, which is the transfer of a carbon group (alkyl group) from one molecule to another, is a common biochemical reaction. In the specific case of chemotherapy, alkylation involves covalent bonding of the antineoplastic drug to the DNA of the cancer cell. The drug may form a "bridge" or cross-link between the two DNA strands and markedly affect the function of the DNA.

Alkylating agents kill cancer cells by altering the shape of the DNA double helix and preventing the DNA from duplicating during cell division. Each alkylating agent attaches to DNA in a different manner; however, they all have the effect of inducing cell death or at least slowing the replication of tumor cells. Although the process of alkylation may occur at any time during the cell cycle, the killing action occurs when the affected cell attempts to duplicate the defective DNA strands. The alkylating agents have a broad spectrum and are used against many types of malignancies, including certain types of lymphomas, myelomas, leukemias, and pancreatic cancers, and some testicular, ovarian, and breast cancers. They are the oldest classification of antineoplastics, having been available since the 1940s, and are the most widely used antineoplastic drugs. Alkylating agents are sometimes subdivided into chemical classes, which include the nitrogen mustards, nitrosoureas, and platinum compounds, as listed in Table 57.1. Figure 57.1 illustrates the process of alkylation.

Because blood cells are particularly sensitive to the actions of alkylating agents, myelosuppression (bone marrow suppression) is the primary dose-limiting toxicity of these drugs. Within days after administration, the numbers of erythrocytes, leukocytes, and platelets begin to decline, reaching a nadir at 9 to 14 days. These drugs are withheld if red blood cell (RBC), white blood cell (WBC), and platelet counts fall below a predetermined limit during therapy. Epithelial cells lining the gastrointestinal (GI) tract are also damaged with alkylating agents, causing nausea, vomiting, and diarrhea. Alopecia may be expected from most of the alkylating agents. The nitrosoureas and mechlorethamine are also strong vesicants, and great care must be taken to avoid skin contact or extravasation. Like many other antineoplastics, secondary malignancies may occur with the alkylating agents. A small percentage of the patients treated with alkylating agents develop acute myelogenous leukemia 4 years or more after chemotherapy has been completed.

TABLE 57.1 Alkylating Agents

Drug	Route and Adult Dose (Maximum Dose Where Indicated)	Adverse Effects
Nitrogen Mustards		*Headache, alopecia, nausea, vomiting, stomatitis, anorexia, rash, fluid retention*
bendamustine (Treanda)	IV: 100 mg/m^2 on days 1 and 2 of a 28-day cycle (max: 6 cycles)	
chlorambucil (Leukeran)	PO: 0.1–0.2 mg/kg/day for 3–6 weeks	Myelosuppression, severe nausea, vomiting, diarrhea, Stevens–Johnson syndrome (SJS), hemorrhagic cystitis (ifosfamide), neurotoxicity, ototoxicity (platinum agents), pulmonary toxicity, nephrotoxicity (platinum agents), hepatic necrosis (dacarbazine), anaphylaxis and other hypersensitivity reactions, tissue necrosis (due to extravasation)
cyclophosphamide (Cytoxan)	PO: 1–5 mg/kg/day	
estramustine (Emcyt)	PO: 14 mg/kg/day in three to four divided doses	
ifosfamide (Ifex)	IV: 1.2 g/m^2/day for 5 consecutive days, repeated in 3 weeks	
mechlorethamine (Mustargen)	IV: 0.4 mg/kg as a single or divided dose	
melphalan (Alkeran)	PO: 6 mg/day for 2–3 weeks	
Nitrosoureas		
carmustine (BiCNU, Gliadel)	IV: 150–200 mg/m^2 once every 6 weeks	
lomustine (CeeNU, CCNU)	PO: 130 mg/m^2 as a single dose, once every 6 weeks	
streptozocin (Zanosar)	IV: 500 mg/m^2 for 5 consecutive days, every 6 weeks	
Platinum Compounds		
carboplatin (Paraplatin)	IV: 360 mg/m^2 once every 4 weeks	
cisplatin (Platinol)	IV: 20 mg/m^2/day for 5 days	
oxaliplatin (Eloxatin)	IV: 85 mg/m^2 for 2 h	
Miscellaneous Alkylating Agents		
busulfan (Busulfex, Myleran)	PO: 4–8 mg/day IV: 0.8 mg/kg qid for 4 days	
dacarbazine (DTIC-Dome)	IV: 2–4.5 mg/kg/day for 10 days, repeated every 4 weeks	
procarbazine (Matulane)	PO: 2–4 mg/kg/day in single or divided dose for 1 week, then 4–6 mg/kg/day until WBCs are less than 4,000/mm^3 or platelets are less than 100,000/mm^3, or when maximum response is obtained	
temozolomide (Temodar)	PO/IV: 75–150 mg/m^2/day	
thiotepa	IV: 0.3–0.4 mg/kg every 1–4 weeks	

Note: *Italics* indicate common adverse effects. <u>Underline</u> indicates serious adverse effects.

When alkylating agents are taken for prolonged periods, cancer cells can develop resistance to them. The mechanism of resistance is incompletely understood. However, possible mechanisms include decreased drug uptake by cancer cells, increased cellular inactivation of the drug, and increased production of DNA repair enzymes.

CONNECTION Checkpoint 57.1

From what you learned in Chapter 43, explain why vaccinations are usually contraindicated in patients who are receiving antineoplastic drugs. *See Answer to Connection Checkpoint 57.1 on student resource website.*

PROTOTYPE DRUG | **Cyclophosphamide (Cytoxan)**

Classification: Therapeutic: Antineoplastic
Pharmacologic: Alkylating agent, nitrogen mustard, disease-modifying antirheumatic drug, immunosuppressant

Therapeutic Effects and Uses: Approved in 1959 by the U.S. Food and Drug Administration (FDA), cyclophosphamide is available as an oral (PO) or injectable preparation. It has a very broad spectrum of action and is approved in combination with other antineoplastics in the chemotherapy of Hodgkin's and non-Hodgkin's lymphoma, acute lymphocytic and myelogenous leukemia, ovarian cancer, breast cancer, multiple myeloma, chronic lymphocytic and myelogenous leukemia, mycosis fungoides, neuroblastoma, sarcomas, and retinoblastoma. It may be used off-label to treat lung cancer, endometrial cancer, Ewing's sarcoma, osteogenic sarcoma, prostate cancer, rhabdomyosarcoma, and other neoplastic conditions. It is used in both children and adults.

Cyclophosphamide is an effective immunosuppressant. Although it is considered an adverse effect during cancer chemotherapy, this drug is used to intentionally cause immunosuppression, often in combination therapy with corticosteroids. Off-label immunosuppressive indications include prophylaxis of organ transplant rejection, nephrotic syndrome, severe progressive rheumatoid arthritis (RA), systemic lupus erythematosus (SLE), and scleroderma.

Mechanism of Action: Cyclophosphamide is a prodrug that is converted to its active form (phosphoramide mustard) in the liver. Cyclophosphamide binds to DNA and forms cross-links, which prevent the synthesis of DNA, ribonucleic acid (RNA), and protein. It is a cell cycle nonspecific drug.

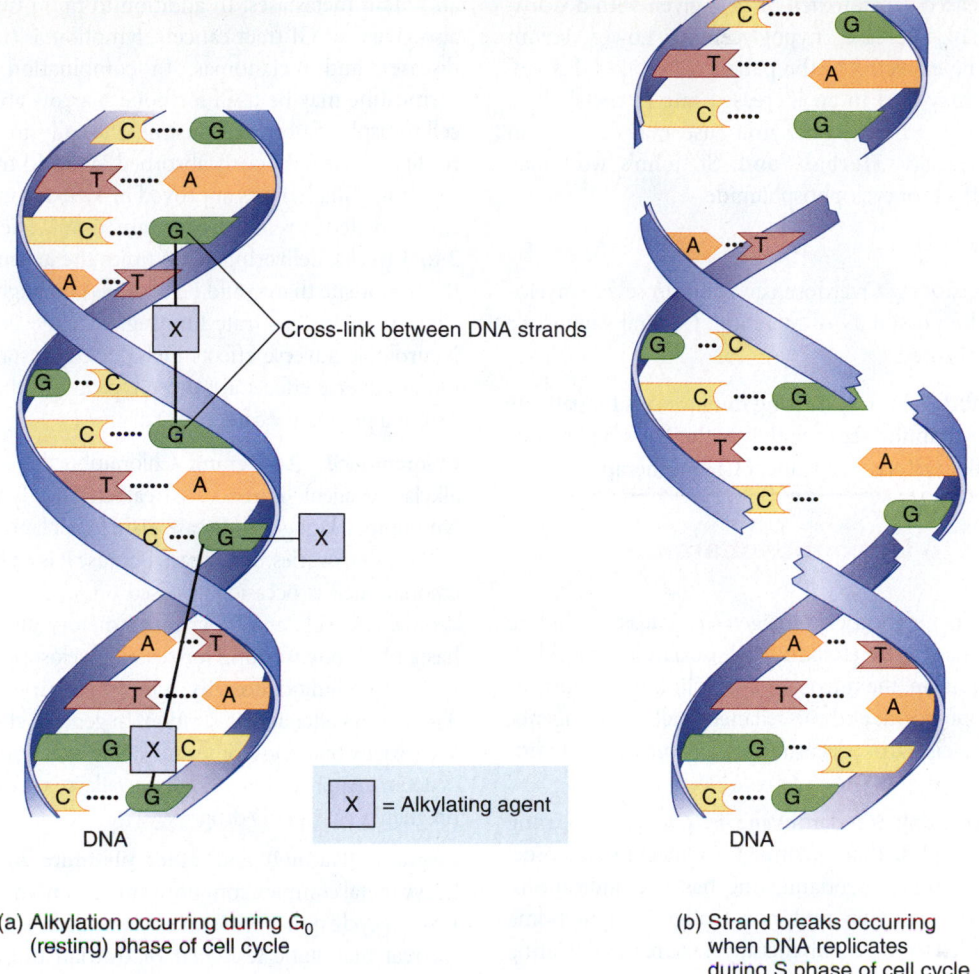

Cross-link between DNA strands

X = Alkylating agent

(a) Alkylation occurring during G_0
(resting) phase of cell cycle

(b) Strand breaks occurring
when DNA replicates
during S phase of cell cycle

Figure 57.1 Mechanism of action of the alkylating agents.

Pharmacokinetics:

Route(s)	PO, IV
Absorption	Well absorbed from the GI tract
Distribution	Widely distributed; crosses the placenta; secreted in breast milk; also found in brain tissue
Primary metabolism	Extensive hepatic metabolism by CYP2B6 and other CYP isozymes
Primary excretion	Renal
Onset of action	7 days
Duration of action	Half-life: 3–12 h; metabolites can still be identified in serum after 21 days

Adverse Effects: Adverse effects include those common to other antineoplastic drugs, such as anorexia, nausea, vomiting, weight loss, diarrhea, and mouth sores. Alopecia occurs more frequently with cyclophosphamide than with other antineoplastics; 50% of patients will develop total baldness. Other common adverse effects are jaundice, acne, blistered skin, and darkened or thickened skin. Bone marrow suppression is a potentially life-threatening adverse reaction that occurs between days 9 and 14 of therapy; the patient is at dangerous risk for severe infection and sepsis during this period. Bone marrow recovery occurs by days 18 through 25.

Other life-threatening adverse effects include secondary cancers, cardiotoxicity, and pulmonary fibrosis. Hematuria may signal hemorrhagic cystitis, which can be severe and even fatal. Interference with the ability to reproduce may occur in both males and females, and this may be irreversible. Cyclophosphamide can cause sterility in both males and females and can cause fetal harm. This drug is associated with increased risk of secondary malignancies, including bladder cancer, lymphoma, and leukemia, that may take several years after completion of chemotherapy to become apparent.

Contraindications/Precautions: The only contraindications to the use of cyclophosphamide are pregnancy, lactation, and severe myelosuppression. The drug must be used cautiously in persons with leukopenia, thrombocytopenia, previous radiation therapy, bone marrow infiltration of tumor cells, impaired renal or hepatic function, recent history of steroid use, or previous therapy that caused cytotoxicity.

Drug Interactions: Many drug interactions are possible with cyclophosphamide due to its extensive hepatic metabolism. This drug has additive immunosuppressive effects if administered with other agents that cause bone marrow toxicity. There may be an increased anticoagulant effect if it is given with anticoagulants.

There may be increased cardiotoxicity if it is given with doxoru-bicin. Insulin may increase hypoglycemia. Lower serum digoxin levels can be expected in the patient who takes digoxin. Phenobarbital use may lead to an increased rate of metabolism of cyclophosphamide, whereas phenytoin use may lead to an increased risk of toxicity. **Herbal/Food:** St. John's wort may increase the toxic effects of cyclophosphamide.

Pregnancy: Category D.

Treatment of Overdose: Overdose can result in severe myelo-suppression with the possibility of infection. General supportive measures are administered.

Nursing Responsibilities: Key nursing implications for patients receiving cyclophosphamide are included in the Nursing Practice Application for Patients Receiving Cancer Chemotherapy.

Drugs Similar to Cyclophosphamide (Cytoxan)

Alkylating agents include other nitrogen mustards, including bendamustine, chlorambucil, estramustine, ifosfamide, mechlor-ethamine, and melphalan; the nitrosoureas, including carmustine, lomustine, and streptozocin; and miscellaneous alkylating agents, including busulfan, cisplatin, dacarbazine, procarbazine, temo-zolomide, and thiotepa.

Bendamustine (Treanda): Bendamustine is a newer alkylating agent, approved in 2008, that is similar to mechlorethamine. Available by the IV route, bendamustine has two indications: chronic lymphocytic leukemia and non-Hodgkin's lymphoma that has not responded to rituximab therapy. Like many alkylating agents, the dose-limiting toxicity is myelosuppression. The most common nonhematologic adverse effects are pyrexia, nausea, and vomiting. Rare, though serious, toxicity includes anaphylaxis, Stevens–Johnson syndrome (SJS), and tumor lysis syndrome. It is a pregnancy category D drug.

Busulfan (Busulfex, Myleran): Approved in 1954, busulfan is a potent alkylating agent that is used for palliative treatment of chronic myelogenous leukemia for those patients who are no longer responsive to radiation therapy or other chemotherapeutic agents. It does not appreciably extend survival times. In combination with cyclophosphamide, busulfan is given for bone marrow ablation prior to stem cell transplantation. Busulfan is available as a PO preparation for cancer treatment and as an IV preparation (Busulfex) when used for patients who are undergoing stem cell transplant. Busulfan has a black box warning that myelosuppression is a serious adverse effect, and blood counts must be closely monitored. Pancytopenia occurs in 100% of patients who are taking high doses of this drug, and this condition may last as long as 2 years. Nausea, vomiting, stomatitis, and anorexia are common adverse effects. Because of the potential for infertility, men and women within childbearing years should be counseled regarding the drug's adverse reproductive effects. It is a pregnancy category D drug.

Carmustine (BiCNU, Gliadel): Carmustine, a nitrosourea, is an alkylating agent and is one of the few drugs in its class that can penetrate the blood–brain barrier. Thus it is used to treat brain tumors such as malignant glioma, astrocytoma, ependymoma, and brain metastases. In addition to brain tumors, carmustine is also given for GI tract cancers, lymphomas (including Hodgkin's disease), and melanomas. In combination with other drugs, carmustine may be used for bone marrow ablation prior to stem cell transplantation. Carmustine is usually administered by the IV route because it is poorly absorbed in the GI tract. A wafer form of the drug (Gliadel) was approved in 1996 for implantation into the cavity created by removal of a brain tumor. The wafer dissolves over 2 to 3 weeks, delivering 1,000 times the amount of carmustine to the tumor site than could be obtained through IV administration. The most serious rate-limiting toxicity is myelosuppression. Neurologic adverse effects include seizures and encephalopathy. Other adverse effects are those typical of other alkylating agents. This is a pregnancy category D drug.

Chlorambucil (Leukeran): Chlorambucil, a nitrogen mustard alkylating agent, is used to treat chronic lymphocytic leukemia, lymphomas, Hodgkin's disease, giant follicular lymphoma, and cancer of the testes, ovaries, and breast. Because it is an immunosuppressant, chlorambucil is occasionally used off-label to treat nephrotic syn-drome, RA, SLE, and other inflammatory disorders. Chlorambucil has a black box warning for severe myelosuppression, which is the major dose-limiting toxicity. Blood values usually return to baseline 3 to 4 weeks after administration. In general, chlorambucil produces less toxicity than most other alkylating agents and has a slower onset of action. Approved in 1957, it is available via the PO route. This is a pregnancy category D drug.

Cisplatin (Platinol) and other platinum agents: Cisplatin is a heavy metal complex containing platinum, chloride, and ammonia. It is cell cycle nonspecific and usually used as combination therapy to treat metastatic testicular or ovarian tumors, bladder cancer, osteosarcoma, and soft tissue sarcomas and as adjuvant therapy in head, neck, esophageal, prostate, lung, and cervical cancers. It is available only as an injectable preparation. Cisplatin carries black box warnings for myelosuppression, ototoxicity, anaphylaxis, nausea and vomiting, and nephrotoxicity, the major dose-limiting toxicity. Acute renal failure may occur within 24 hours after administration, and permanent damage to renal tubular cells may eventually cause chronic renal failure. Renal function must be closely monitored during therapy. Peripheral neuropathy is another potentially serious adverse effect with symptoms that include numbness that begins in the fingers and toes and proceeds up the limbs toward the trunk. Ototoxicity is common and can result in permanent impairment. The nurse should be prepared for anaphylactic-like reactions that may occur within minutes of cisplatin administration. Cisplatin is a pregnancy category D drug.

Carboplatin (Paraplatin): Approved for the first-line palliative treatment of advanced ovarian cancer, carboplatin is used off-label to treat acute lymphocytic leukemia, acute myelogenous leukemia, bladder cancer, breast cancer, and other tumors. Approved in 1989, carboplatin is administered by the IV route, is structurally similar to cisplatin, and works by the same mechanism but is estimated to be 45 times less toxic. The drug carries a black box warning for anaphylaxis and severe myelosuppression, the dose-limiting toxicity. Neurotoxicity and nephrotoxicity occur less often than with cisplatin. The nurse should be prepared for anaphylactic-like reactions that may occur within minutes of carboplatin administration. This is a pregnancy category D drug.

Oxaliplatin (Eloxatin): Approved in 2002, oxaliplatin is a platinum compound that is approved only to treat advanced colorectal cancer in combination with 5-fluorouracil, although it may be used off-label for other solid tumors. It acts by a different mechanism than cisplatin and exhibits little ototoxicity or nephrotoxicity. It does, however, cause significant levels of peripheral neuropathy, which can be dose limiting. An acute form of peripheral neuropathy begins within days of chemotherapy and resolves in 1 to 2 weeks. A more persistent form has a delayed onset and can cause functional impairment and discontinuation of therapy. The drug carries a black box warning for anaphylactic-like reactions that may occur within minutes of oxaliplatin administration. This is a pregnancy category D drug.

Dacarbazine (DTIC-Dome): Approved in 1998, dacarbazine is an alkylating agent that is available only for IV administration. It is approved to treat metastatic malignant melanoma, refractory Hodgkin's disease, and off-label for sarcomas and neuroblastomas. Adverse GI effects occur in most patients, but tolerance to these adverse effects may develop over subsequent administrations. Myelosuppression occurs during therapy, although to a lesser extent than many other drugs in this class. Dacarbazine carries a black box warning that hepatic necrosis has occurred with the use of this drug. Unlike other alkylating agents, dacarbazine is a pregnancy category C drug, although use during the first trimester of pregnancy is contraindicated.

Temozolomide (Temodar): Temozolomide is a prodrug that is metabolized to the same active compound as dacarbazine. Unlike dacarbazine, however, temozolomide can be administered by either the IV or PO route. Approved in 1999, it is indicated to treat malignant glioma (glioblastoma multiforme) concomitantly with radiotherapy and for refractory astrocytoma. It may also be used off-label to treat advanced metastatic melanoma. Adverse effects are similar to those of dacarbazine and include myelosuppression and nausea or vomiting. This is a pregnancy category D drug.

Estramustine (Emcyt): Estramustine is unusual because it is a dual molecule. One portion is a nitrogen mustard alkylating agent and the other is a molecule of estradiol. Thus, the drug may be classified as either an alkylating agent or a hormone. It is administered by the PO route for the palliative therapy of metastatic or advanced prostate cancer and may be used off-label to treat metastatic renal carcinoma. Unlike other alkylating agents, however, myelosuppression is infrequent. Nausea and vomiting are the dose-limiting toxicities. The estrogen component of the drug can cause gynecomastia, mastalgia, thromboembolic disease, and fluid retention. This is a pregnancy category D drug.

Ifosfamide (Ifex): Ifosfamide is a nitrogen mustard alkylating agent approved in 1988 for the treatment of testicular cancer. Off-label indications include breast, lung, pancreatic, bladder, and cervical cancers, sarcomas, and non-Hodgkin's lymphoma. The drug has black box warnings for urotoxicity, central nervous system (CNS) toxicity, and myelosuppression. Myelosuppression is the primary dose-limiting toxicity, with blood count nadirs occurring after 5 days and recovering by 4 weeks. Nephrotoxicity also limits its use and hematuria, hemorrhagic cystitis, and renal insufficiency occur in many patients. Signs of CNS toxicity such as confusion, drowsiness, hallucinations, and depression occur in about 12% of patients who are taking the drug. Cardiac toxicity occurs in as many

as 15% of patients and may include dysrhythmias, heart failure, and myocarditis. This is a pregnancy category D drug.

To prevent hemorrhagic cystitis in patients who are taking ifosfamide, the drug mesna (Mesnex) is administered at the time of chemotherapy by the IV route and 2 to 6 hours later by the IV or PO route. Mesna binds the toxic metabolites in the urinary bladder, reducing the incidence of hematuria by 70% to 100%, depending on the dose of ifosfamide. Mesna may be used off-label for patients taking cyclophosphamide.

Lomustine (CeeNU, CCNU): Approved in 1976, lomustine is an oral nitrosourea alkylating agent that has actions similar to those of carmustine. It is used as palliative therapy in combination with other chemotherapeutic agents or other treatment modalities in primary and metastatic brain tumors and as secondary therapy in Hodgkin's disease. The drug carries a black box warning for myelosuppression, which is its most serious dose-limiting toxicity. Delayed myelosuppression may occur up to 6 weeks following administration of the drug. Severe nausea and vomiting occur in most patients and require antiemetic therapy. This is a pregnancy category D drug.

Mechlorethamine (Mustargen): Mechlorethamine is one of the oldest antineoplastics, approved in 1949. It is available by the IV, intrathecal, or topical routes. It is usually used to provide palliation in patients with Hodgkin's disease (Stages 3 and 4), lymphosarcoma, polycythemia vera, bronchogenic carcinoma, and chronic myelocytic or chronic lymphocytic leukemia. It may also be used for palliative treatment of metastatic cancer in intrapleural, intrapericardial, and intraperitoneal spaces when effusion has occurred as a result of the tumor. Nausea and vomiting are acute and require antiemetic therapy. Myelosuppression occurs in 8 to 14 days after drug administration and can be severe. Like cyclophosphamide, infertility is a potential adverse effect. This drug carries a black box warning to use extreme care in handling the drug because exposure to mucous membranes or inhaling the dust can cause toxicity. This drug is a vesicant; extravasation requires the administration of sodium thiosulfate to the injection site. This is a pregnancy category D drug.

Melphalan (Alkeran): Melphalan is a nitrogen mustard approved for the palliative treatment of ovarian cancer and multiple myeloma. It may also be used off-label to treat breast or testicular cancer, osteogenic sarcoma, and non-Hodgkin's lymphoma. Because it has strong immunosuppressive and myelosuppressive effects, it has been used off-label for bone marrow ablation prior to stem cell transplantation in combination with other drugs. It is available as both a PO and an IV preparation. Melphalan carries black box warnings regarding myelosuppression, hypersensitivity reactions, and the possibility of secondary leukemia. Hematologic toxicity is the primary dose-limiting toxicity. Blood count nadirs usually occur in 2 to 3 weeks after therapy starts, and recovery is seen 4 to 5 weeks after treatment. Unlike some of the other alkylating agents, melphalan is not highly emetogenic. The nurse should use extra caution to prevent skin exposure (to both nurse and patient) to the drug because it can cause skin necrosis. Because of the potential for infertility, men and women in childbearing years should be counseled regarding the drug's adverse reproductive effects. This is a pregnancy category D drug.

Procarbazine (Matulane): Procarbazine is an oral alkylating agent that was approved in 1969 for the treatment of Hodgkin's disease.

It may be used off-label for treating non-Hodgkin's lymphomas and CNS tumors such as medulloblastoma, malignant glioma, and astrocytoma. It is also used as an adjunct in the palliative treatment of Hodgkin's disease. Because it has strong immunosuppressive effects, it may be used off-label for bone marrow ablation prior to stem cell transplantation in combination with other drugs. Myelosuppression is the primary dose-limiting toxicity. Blood count nadirs usually occur in week 4 after therapy starts, and recovery is seen 6 weeks after treatment. Nausea and vomiting are also common adverse effects that may be severe. CNS adverse effects are common and may include paresthesias, peripheral neuropathy, seizures, depression, and psychosis. When given by the IV route, neurotoxicity can be dose limiting. This is a pregnancy category D drug.

Streptozocin (Zanosar): Approved in 1982, streptozocin is a nitrosourea alkylating agent that is more toxic and has a lower therapeutic index than many other alkylating agents. It is available IV to treat metastatic islet cell cancers of the pancreas either as monotherapy or in combination with fluorouracil. It may be used off-label to treat colorectal cancer and other solid tumors. A clinically effective response most likely will be accompanied by some evidence of serious toxicity. Streptozocin carries black box warnings regarding nephrotoxicity, nausea, vomiting, diarrhea, hepatotoxicity, and hematologic toxicity. The most serious dose-limiting toxicity is nephrotoxicity, which occurs in more than half of the patients taking the drug and can cause permanent impairment and death. Nausea and vomiting are also severe adverse effects of streptozocin. This is a pregnancy category D drug.

Thiotepa: Thiotepa is an alkylating agent approved in 1994 to treat bladder, ovarian, and breast cancers and both Hodgkin's and non-Hodgkin's lymphomas. It is administered IV or by the intravesical route for bladder tumors. Myelosuppression is the primary dose-limiting toxicity, although neurotoxicity may also cause delay or discontinuation of therapy. Nausea and vomiting are uncommon. Injections and instillations of thiotepa can cause intense local pain. Intravesical administration causes bladder irritation, dysuria, and increased urgency. It should be noted that the drug may be absorbed during intravesical administration and cause serious myelosuppression. This is a pregnancy category D drug.

Antimetabolites

57.3 Antimetabolites disrupt the critical cellular pathways of cancer cells.

Rapidly growing cancer cells require large quantities of nutrients to construct proteins and nucleic acids. Antimetabolite drugs are structurally similar to these nutrients, but they do not perform the same functions as their natural counterparts. When cancer cells attempt to synthesize proteins, RNA, or DNA using the antimetabolites, metabolic pathways are disrupted, and the cancer cells die or their growth is slowed. Some of these structural similarities are illustrated in Figure 57.2.

Some antimetabolites become incorporated into the DNA of cancer cells and interfere with DNA replication and function. Others inhibit the enzymes that synthesize the vital components of the cell. All antimetabolites are cell cycle specific, with most of them affecting the S phase, although some can act during any of the active phases of the cell cycle. The three classes of antimetabolites are the folic acid analogs, the purine analogs, and the pyrimidine analogs. These drugs are listed in Table 57.2.

Folic acid analogs: Folic acid, or folate, is vitamin B9, which is essential for the growth and maintenance of cells. It is especially important during periods of rapid cell growth because this vitamin is needed to replicate DNA. Lack of this vitamin during pregnancy can cause neural tube defects in the fetus. Additional details on folic acid are presented in Chapter 61.

Three folic acid analogs are used as antineoplastic drugs. Methotrexate, approved in 1953, is the oldest and is prescribed for several autoimmune disorders in addition to cancer. Pemetrexed (Alimta) and pralatrexate (Folotyn) have very limited therapeutic applications. Some folic acid analogs are used as anti-infectives. These include trimethoprim (Primsol), pyrimethamine (Daraprim), and trimetrexate (Neutrexin).

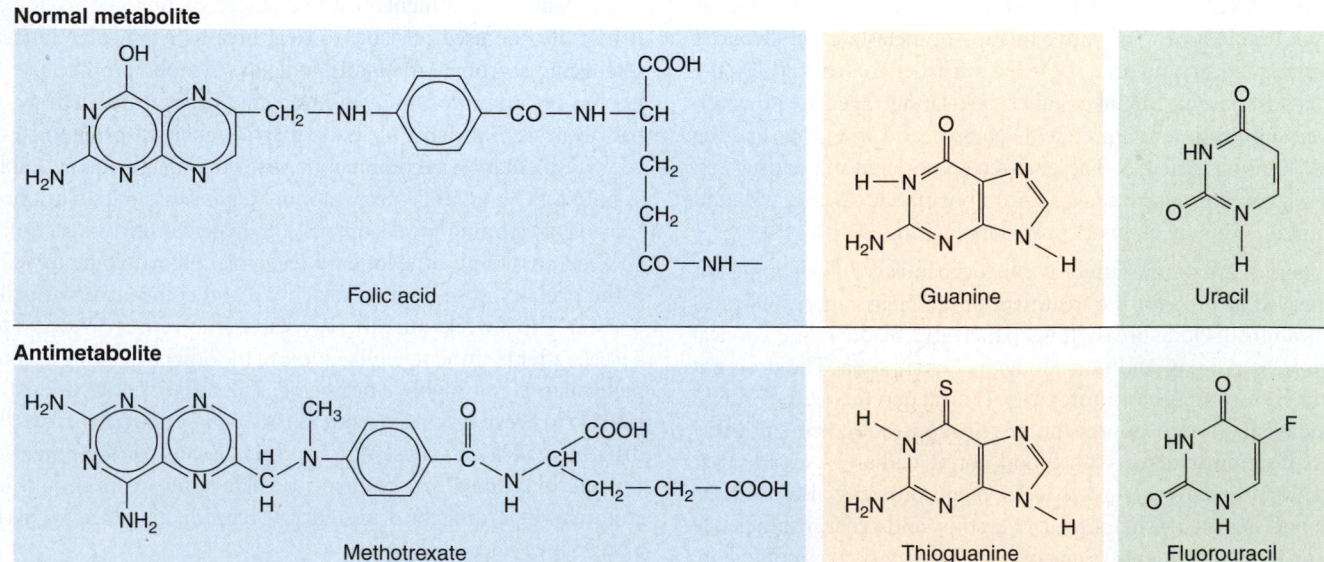

Figure 57.2 Structural similarities between antimetabolites and their natural counterparts.

TABLE 57.2   Antimetabolites

Drug	Route and Adult Dose (Maximum Dose Where Indicated)	Adverse Effects
Folic Acid Analogs		*Nausea, vomiting, stomatitis, anorexia, rash, fatigue, alopecia, headache*
methotrexate (MTX, Rheumatrex, Trexall)	PO: 10–30 mg/day for 5 days	Myelosuppression, severe nausea, vomiting, diarrhea, mucositis, hepatotoxicity, pulmonary toxicity, cytarabine syndrome, neurotoxicity (nelarabine), anaphylaxis and other hypersensitivity reactions
pemetrexed (Alimta)	IV: 500 mg/m^2 on day 1 of each 21-day cycle	
pralatrexate (Folotyn)	IV: 30 mg/m^2 once weekly for 6 weeks in 7-week cycles	
Purine Analogs		
cladribine (Leustatin)	IV: 0.09 mg/kg/day as a continuous infusion for 7 days	
clofarabine (Clolar)	IV: 52 mg/m^2/day over 2 h for 5 days	
fludarabine (Fludara)	IV: 25 mg/m^2/day for 5 consecutive days	
mercaptopurine (Purinethol)	PO: 1.5–2.5 mg/kg/day	
nelarabine (Arranon)	IV: 1,500 mg/m^2 on days 1, 3, and 5; repeat every 21 days	
pentostatin (Nipent)	IV: 4 mg/m^2 every other week	
thioguanine (Tabloid)	PO: 2 mg/kg/day	
Pyrimidine Analogs		
capecitabine (Xeloda)	PO: 1,250 mg/m^2/day twice daily for 2 weeks	
cytarabine (Cytosar-U, Depot-Cyt)	IV: 100 mg/m^2 as a continuous infusion over 24 h	
floxuridine (FUDR)	Intra-arterial: 0.1–0.6 mg/kg/day as an intra-arterial infusion	
fluorouracil (5-FU, Adrucil, Carac, Efudex)	IV: 12 mg/kg/day for 4 consecutive days	
gemcitabine (Gemzar)	IV: 1,000–1,250 mg/m^2 once weekly for 7 weeks	

Note: *Italics* indicate common adverse effects. <u>Underline</u> indicates serious adverse effects.

As antineoplastics, folic acid analogs are given at high doses, which can be toxic to normal cells as well as cancer cells. To "rescue" normal cells, the drug leucovorin is administered following chemotherapy with methotrexate. Leucovorin, or folinic acid, is a reduced form of folic acid that is able to enter normal cells but not cancer cells. The normal cells can thus continue metabolism and replication using leucovorin. Available by both the IV and PO routes, **leucovorin rescue therapy** must be initiated at very specific times following the methotrexate dose. Leucovorin is also used to treat overdose or prevent toxicity with other folic acid analogs such as pyrimethamine and trimethoprim. When used with fluorouracil (5-FU) in the treatment of colorectal cancer, leucovorin has been found to enhance cell killing. A new form of leucovorin, levoleucovorin (Fusilev), was approved in 2008. Given by IV infusion, levoleucovorin is an isomer of leucovorin that is reported to have fewer adverse effects.

Purine and pyrimidine analogs: Purines and pyrimidines are bases used in the biosynthesis of DNA and RNA. The purine and pyrimidine analogs are drugs structurally similar to their naturally occurring counterparts that can act in several ways. They can inhibit the synthesis of purine or pyrimidine bases, thus limiting the precursors needed for DNA and RNA biosynthesis. The analogs can also become incorporated into the structures of DNA and RNA, resulting in a disruption of nucleic acid function.

Most of the purine and pyrimidine analogs used as antineoplastics are prodrugs that are converted to their active forms on entering the body. A few purine analogs are used for immunosuppression, gout, and antiviral therapy.

CONNECTION Checkpoint 57.2

Trimethoprim is a folic acid analog that is nearly always combined with another antibiotic medication. From what you learned in Chapter 50, name the antibiotic combination that contains trimethoprim and give its primary indications. *See Answer to Connection Checkpoint 57.2 on student resource website.*

PROTOTYPE DRUG	**Methotrexate (MTX, Rheumatrex, Trexall)**

Classification: **Therapeutic:** Antineoplastic
Pharmacologic: Antimetabolite, folic acid analog, immunosuppressant, disease-modifying antirheumatic drug (DMARD)

Therapeutic Effects and Uses: Approved in 1953, methotrexate is an antimetabolite available by the PO, parenteral, and intrathecal routes. The PO route is preferred for low-dose therapy. It is approved for a large number of neoplasms, including osteosarcoma, acute lymphocytic and lymphoblastic leukemias, and lymphosarcomas in children; certain inoperable head, neck, and pelvic cancers; breast cancers; lung cancers; and advanced stage non-Hodgkin's lymphoma. Its primary use as an antineoplastic is in combination therapy to maintain induced remissions in those persons who have had surgical resection or amputation for a primary tumor.

Because of its powerful immunosuppressant properties, methotrexate is used with success in patients with severe RA who have had inadequate response to nonsteroidal anti-inflammatory drugs (NSAIDs) and at least one or more antirheumatic drugs. It also is used to treat severe psoriasis that is unresponsive to other forms of therapy. Off-label uses include other autoimmune disorders such as active Crohn's disease, ulcerative colitis, psoriasis, and SLE. Methotrexate may be used to terminate pregnancy, usually in combination with misoprostol.

Mechanism of Action: Methotrexate is specific for the S phase of the cell cycle. It blocks an enzyme that is responsible for converting folic acid to reduced folate, which interferes with DNA synthesis, repair, and cellular replication mainly in actively proliferating tissues. This action is what enables it to be effective in treating psoriasis and arthritis in addition to treating cancer.

Pharmacokinetics:

Route(s)	PO, intramuscular (IM), IV, subcutaneous, intrathecal
Absorption	Variable absorption from the GI tract; well absorbed by the subcutaneous or IM routes
Distribution	Widely distributed; crosses the placenta and blood–brain barrier; secreted in breast milk; 60% bound to plasma protein
Primary metabolism	Hepatic, extensive first-pass metabolism
Primary excretion	Renal
Onset of action	Peak: 1–4 h PO, and 0.5–2 h IM, IV
Duration of action	Half-life: 2–4 h

Adverse Effects: Methotrexate has many adverse effects, some of which can be serious. Nausea and vomiting are severe at high doses. **Black Box Warnings:** Methotrexate combined with NSAIDs may cause severe and sometimes fatal myelosuppression, which is the primary dose-limiting toxicity of this drug. The drug is hepatotoxic and may cause liver cirrhosis with prolonged use. Ulcerative stomatitis and diarrhea require suspension of therapy because they may lead to hemorrhagic enteritis and death from intestinal perforation. Potentially fatal opportunistic infections, including *Pneumocystis* pneumonia, may occur during therapy. Pulmonary toxicity may result in acute or chronic interstitial pneumonitis at any dose level. Severe, sometimes fatal, dermatologic reactions such as toxic epidermal necrolysis and SJS have been reported.

Contraindications/Precautions: The use of methotrexate as an antineoplastic is contraindicated in thrombocytopenia, anemia, leukopenia, concurrent administration of hepatotoxic drugs and hematopoietic suppressants, alcoholism, or lactation. Precautions must be taken in patients with impaired renal or hepatic function, active infections, ulcerative colitis, and peptic ulcers; in patients with cancer who have preexisting bone marrow impairment; in the very young or old or debilitated; and in those with poor nutritional status. This drug is a confirmed teratogen and precautions must be taken to avoid pregnancy during therapy. Caution should be used in handling this drug because it can cause severe skin reactions.

Drug Interactions: Methotrexate interacts with many drugs. Increased serum methotrexate levels can occur with the penicillins, vancomycin, cyclosporine, and para-amino benzoic acid (PABA). Chloramphenicol may decrease the intestinal absorption of methotrexate. An increased methotrexate effect can occur with probenecid, ibuprofen, aspirin, and tetracyclines. Folic acid may alter the body's response to methotrexate. Methotrexate may cause increased theophylline levels. Sulfonamides can lead to an increased risk of methotrexate-induced immunosuppression. Methotrexate can cause decreased phenytoin effects, leading to increased seizure activity. Immunization during methotrexate therapy is not effective and any live vaccine use may lead to a severe reaction that is secondary to the immunosuppressant activity of methotrexate. **Herbal/Food**: Food delays the oral absorption of methotrexate. Echinacea may increase the risk of hepatotoxicity. More than 180 mg per day of caffeine (3 to 4 cups of coffee) may decrease the effectiveness of methotrexate when taken for arthritis.

Pregnancy: Category X.

Treatment of Overdose: Leucovorin or levoleucovorin (Fusilev) is given as soon as possible after overdose to decrease the toxic effects of methotrexate. In some cases, leucovorin is given 24 to 36 hours after methotrexate chemotherapy to "rescue" normal cells from the adverse effects of the antineoplastic.

Nursing Responsibilities: Key nursing implications for patients receiving methotrexate are included in the Nursing Practice Application for Patients Receiving Cancer Chemotherapy.

Drugs Similar to Methotrexate (MTX, Rheumatrex, Trexall)

Pemetrexed and pralatrexate are other folic acid analogs used in cancer chemotherapy. The purine analogs used for cancer chemotherapy include cladribine, clofarabine, fludarabine, mercaptopurine, nelarabine, pentostatin, and thioguanine. The pyrimidine analogs include capecitabine, cytarabine, floxuridine (FUDR), fluorouracil, and gemcitabine.

Capecitabine (Xeloda): Capecitabine is a pyrimidine analog that is converted into 5-fluorouracil, another antimetabolite, by a series of three enzymatic steps. One of these enzymes, thymidine phosphorylase, is found in especially high amounts in cancer cells; thus the drug is converted to a toxic form inside the cancer cell. Capecitabine blocks the synthesis of pyrimidines and can also be incorporated into nucleic acid molecules. It is available PO to treat metastatic breast cancer refractory to other treatments, colorectal cancer, or as adjuvant therapy for colon cancer following resection. Capecitabine causes less immunosuppression than many antineoplastics. Diarrhea is the dose-limiting toxicity; antidiarrheal therapy with loperamide is often indicated during chemotherapy. Nausea, vomiting, stomatitis, and abdominal pain are common adverse effects. An unusual adverse effect with this drug is palmar-plantar erythrodysesthesia (hand and foot syndrome), which can occur in over half the patients receiving the drug. Hand and foot syndrome is characterized by numbness, tingling, swelling, erythema, blistering, and severe pain. Capecitabine carries a black box warning that patients receiving warfarin (Coumadin) must be closely monitored to prevent serious or fatal bleeding. It is a pregnancy category D drug.

Cladribine (Leustatin): Cladribine is an IV purine analog that is a preferred drug for active hairy cell leukemia. It may be used off-label to treat chronic lymphocytic leukemia, non-Hodgkin's lymphoma, acute and chronic myelogenous leukemia, and mycosis fungoides. Approved in 1993, cladribine differs from other purine analogs in that it is effective against both dividing (S phase) and nondividing cancer cells. Cladribine carries black box warnings regarding myelosuppression, neurotoxicity, and nephrotoxicity. Myelosuppression is the primary dose-limiting toxicity, with a nadir occurring in 14 days and recovery at 5 weeks. Lymphocyte counts may take up to a year to return to normal values, resulting in a high number of opportunistic infections in patients treated with cladribine. Fever and chills, which are often associated with infections, are common. Rash occurs in most patients but is not usually serious. Nausea and vomiting are mild compared to other antineoplastics. This is a pregnancy category D drug.

Clofarabine (Clolar): Clofarabine is an IV purine analog that was approved in 2004. It only has one indication: the treatment of relapsed or refractory acute lymphocytic leukemia after at least two prior regimens have proven unsuccessful. It is also only approved for patients age 1 to 21 years. Common adverse events include myelosuppression, opportunistic infections, nausea, vomiting, diarrhea, anorexia, fever, fatigue, abdominal pain, and edema. This is a pregnancy category D drug.

Cytarabine (Cytosar-U, Depot-Cyt): Approved in 1969, cytarabine is a pyrimidine antimetabolite available for IV, subcutaneous, or intrathecal administration. It is approved for remission induction in acute myelogenous leukemia. It may be used off-label for other hematologic malignancies, including acute lymphatic leukemia, chronic myelogenous leukemia, Hodgkin's and non-Hodgkin's lymphoma, and lymphomatous meningitis. Cytarabine is specific for the S phase of the cell cycle. It is converted to its active form, Ara-CTP, and then becomes incorporated into DNA, where it suppresses further DNA synthesis. Cytarabine carries a black box warning regarding myelosuppression. The myelosuppression has a nadir occurring at week 1 and resolution by week 3 or 4. High-dose therapy can cause severe nausea, vomiting, and other GI toxicities. A cluster of symptoms, called the cytarabine syndrome, can occur within 6 to 12 hours of treatment. Symptoms include bone pain, fever, myalgia, rash, and fatigue. Other serious adverse effects include peripheral neuropathy, respiratory distress, encephalopathy, palmar-plantar erythrodysesthesia, and hepatotoxicity. This is a pregnancy category D drug.

Depot-Cyt, a newer formulation of cytarabine, is a liposomal delivery system that requires less frequent dosing than conventional cytarabine. It is only administered by the intrathecal route for carcinomatous meningitis due to solid tumors. Liposomal cytarabine has been associated with potentially fatal chemical arachnoiditis that occurs within 48 hours of administration. Nervous system symptoms such as confusion, ataxia, dizziness, and impaired cognition are common. This is a pregnancy category D drug.

Floxuridine (FUDR): Floxuridine is a pyrimidine analog antimetabolite that was approved in 1970. Because it is nearly entirely removed by hepatic first-pass metabolism, it has very limited applications. Its only approved indication is as a continuous intra-arterial infusion via a hepatic artery catheter for the palliative treatment of metastatic liver cancer. Due to its high concentration in the liver, floxuridine can cause elevated liver function enzymes and serious hepatotoxicity. This drug carries a black box warning regarding myelosuppression. Other adverse effects, such as nausea,

vomiting, anorexia, diarrhea, rash, and alopecia, are common to other antineoplastics. This is a pregnancy category D drug.

Fludarabine (Fludara): Approved in 1991, fludarabine is an IV purine analog with a similar action to cladribine. It is approved only to treat chronic lymphocytic leukemia that has not responded to treatment with alkylating agents, but it may be used off-label to treat other leukemias and non-Hodgkin lymphomas. It is believed to be cell cycle specific for the S phase, where it inhibits DNA replication. Fludarabine carries black box warnings regarding myelosuppression, neurotoxicity, autoimmune complications, and pulmonary toxicity. Severe myelosuppression is the most common dose-limiting toxicity. Like cladribine, lymphocyte levels may take up to a year to return to normal levels. Rare instances of life-threatening autoimmune hemolytic anemia have been reported with this drug. High doses of fludarabine are neurotoxic and can result in blindness, coma, and death. Fever and infections are common, including serious interstitial pneumonitis. Nausea and vomiting are mild compared to other antineoplastics but may be severe at high doses. This is a pregnancy category D drug.

Fluorouracil (5-FU, Adrucil, Carac, Efudex): Approved in 1962, fluorouracil is an antimetabolite that inhibits DNA and RNA synthesis in the S phase of the cell cycle. It is available as an injection, a topical solution, and a topical cream. The IV form is used to treat solid tumors, including inoperable breast, ovarian, cervical, urinary bladder, liver, colon, rectal, stomach, and pancreatic cancers. As a topical preparation it is used to treat superficial basal cell carcinomas and multiple actinic keratoses. A formulation of fluorouracil cream using a microsponge delivery system (Carac) was approved in 2000 that allows for once-daily dosing and a sustained release of the drug. Fluorouracil carries a black box warning regarding myelosuppression, which may be dose limiting with a nadir at 9 to 14 days and recovery by 30 days. Palmar-plantar erythrodysesthesia occurs in up to 40% of patients receiving a prolonged IV infusion of this drug. Serious GI toxicity, including ulceration, stomatitis, diarrhea, anorexia, and vomiting, is common. Topical applications may cause local photosensitivity, burning, erythema, swelling, and desquamation. Fluorouracil is a pregnancy category D drug.

Gemcitabine (Gemzar): Gemcitabine is an IV pyrimidine analog approved in 1996 that kills cancer cells during the S phase of the cell cycle. Indications include locally advanced or metastatic solid tumors of the pancreas, breast, ovary, or lung. Gemcitabine is the most effective drug for treating advanced pancreatic cancer, which has a very poor 5-year survival rate. The dose-limiting toxicity for gemcitabine is myelosuppression, which occurs in nearly all patients taking the drug. Serious pulmonary, renal, and hepatic toxicity has been reported. Fever, nausea, vomiting, and infection are common adverse effects. This is a pregnancy category D drug.

Mercaptopurine (6-MP, Purinethol): Mercaptopurine is an older purine analog, approved in 1953, that is cell cycle specific to the S phase. It is a prodrug that has very similar actions, indications, and adverse effects to thioguanine. Mercaptopurine is indicated for acute lymphocytic and myelogenous leukemia in both adults and children. It is less effective in treating adults than children but remains a preferred drug. It can produce a temporary remission in patients with chronic granulocytic leukemia. Due to its powerful immunosuppressant activity, it may be used off-label to produce temporary remissions in patients with ulcerative colitis and Crohn's disease. The most frequent dose-limiting toxicity of mercaptopurine is myelosuppression, which results in leukopenia, thrombocytopenia, and anemia in nearly every patient. Nausea and vomiting are not severe, but diarrhea may require fluid replacement therapy. This is a pregnancy category D drug.

Nelarabine (Arranon): Approved in 2005, nelarabine is an IV purine analog approved to treat T-cell acute lymphoblastic leukemia and T-cell lymphoblastic lymphoma in both adults and children. Its use is limited to patients who have not responded to or have relapsed during treatment with at least two chemotherapy regimens. The drug carries a black box warning for neurotoxicity, which is the major dose-limiting adverse effect with nelarabine. Neurologic signs and symptoms may include impaired cognition, severe somnolence, seizures, peripheral neuropathies, ataxia, tremor, dizziness, and cerebral hemorrhage. Myelosuppression occurs in most patients; fatigue, fever, and infection occur frequently. Nausea, vomiting, and other GI complaints are usually not a major cause of discontinuation. This is a pregnancy category D drug.

Pemetrexed (Alimta) and pralatrexate (Folotyn): Pemetrexed and pralatrexate are folic acid inhibitors given by IV injection that have very specific therapeutic applications. Approved in 2004, pemetrexed is approved to treat malignant pleural mesothelioma that is unresectable or for patients who are not candidates for surgery. It is administered along with cisplatin in these patients. It is also used to treat locally advanced or metastatic non–small cell lung cancer after prior chemotherapy. Pralatrexate was approved in 2009 for the treatment of refractory T-cell lymphoma.

Myelosuppression is the primary dose-limiting toxicity for these drugs. GI adverse effects may be serious and include nausea, vomiting, anorexia, and mucositis. Patients may experience serious and even fatal skin reactions. With pemetrexed, caution must be used to ensure adequate kidney function because impairment may cause pemetrexed to accumulate to fatal levels in the blood. To reduce toxicity from pemetrexed and pralatrexate, patients usually receive folic acid and vitamin B12 supplements preceding therapy. These are pregnancy category D drugs.

Pentostatin (Nipent): Pentostatin is an IV purine analog approved in 1991 to treat active hairy cell leukemia that has not responded to interferon (INF) alfa. It may be used off-label to treat other leukemias and lymphomas. It is cell cycle specific in the S phase. Pentostatin has black box warnings regarding renal, liver, and pulmonary toxicities. Hematologic toxicity is dose limiting and patients experience a high rate of fever, chills, and infections. Rash and other skin reactions occur in most patients and may be severe. Neurologic toxicity is a serious problem with high doses. This is a pregnancy category D drug.

Thioguanine (Tabloid): Approved in 1966, thioguanine is very similar to mercaptopurine in its actions and adverse effects. Like other antimetabolites, it is active in the S phase of the cell cycle. It is available in a PO formulation, and it is used mainly to treat acute nonlymphocytic leukemia. Off-label indications include chronic myelogenous leukemia, psoriasis, refractory ulcerative colitis, and Crohn's disease. Myelosuppression is the most common dose-limiting toxicity. Long-term, continuous use of thioguanine is not recommended due to the risk for serious hepatotoxicity. Adverse GI effects are generally not severe at normal doses. This is a pregnancy category D drug.

PharmFACT

Although breast cancer is the second leading cause of cancer death in women, death rates have been declining since 1989. This is likely due to earlier detection and increased awareness of the disease (American Cancer Society, 2014b).

Antitumor Antibiotics

57.4 The antibiotic antineoplastics contain substances obtained from bacteria that have the ability to kill cancer cells.

Antitumor properties have been identified in a number of chemicals isolated from microorganisms. These substances are more cytotoxic than traditional antibiotics, and their use is restricted to treating a few specific types of cancer. For example, the only indication for idarubicin (Idamycin) is acute myelogenous leukemia. Testicular carcinoma is the only indication for plicamycin (Mithramycin). The antitumor antibiotics are listed in Table 57.3.

TABLE 57.3 Antitumor Antibiotics

Drug	Route and Adult Dose (Maximum Dose Where Indicated)	Adverse Effects
bleomycin (Blenoxane)	IV: 0.25–0.5 units/kg every 4–7 days	*Nausea, vomiting, stomatitis, anorexia, headache, rash, alopecia*
dactinomycin (Actinomycin-D, Cosmegen)	IV: 400–600 mcg/m^2/day for a maximum of 5 days	
daunorubicin (Cerubidine)	IV: 30–45 mg/m^2/day for 3–5 days	Myelosuppression, severe nausea, vomiting, diarrhea, mucositis, pulmonary or cardiac toxicity, anaphylaxis and other hypersensitivity reactions, tissue necrosis (due to extravasation), hemolytic uremic syndrome (mitomycin), hepatotoxicity (dactinomycin)
daunorubicin liposomal (DaunoXome)	IV: 40 mg/m^2 every 2 weeks	
doxorubicin (Adriamycin)	IV: 40–60 mg/m^2 as a single injection every 21–28 days when used in combination with other antineoplastics	
doxorubicin liposomal (Doxil, Evacet)	IV: 20 mg/m^2 every 3 weeks	
epirubicin (Ellence)	IV: 100–120 mg/m^2 as a single dose	
idarubicin (Idamycin)	IV: 8–12 mg/m^2/day for 3 days	
mitomycin (Mutamycin)	IV: 20 mg/m^2 as a single dose	
mitoxantrone (Novantrone)	IV: 12 mg/m^2 every 3 days	

Note: Italics indicate common adverse effects. <u>Underline</u> indicates serious adverse effects.

The antitumor antibiotics bind to DNA and affect its function by a mechanism similar to that of the alkylating agents; therefore, their general actions and adverse effects are like those of the alkylating agents. Unlike the alkylating agents, however, all the antitumor antibiotics must be administered IV or through direct instillation via a catheter into a body cavity or organ. As with many other antineoplastics, the primary dose-limiting toxicity of drugs in this class is myelosuppression. These drugs can cause major damage to the skin, subcutaneous tissue, and nerves should extravasation occur.

The antitumor antibiotics are divided into two groups, the anthracyclines and nonanthracyclines. The anthracyclines include doxorubicin, daunorubicin, epirubicin, idarubicin, and mitoxantrone. The anthracyclines are closely related in structure, and all exhibit cardiotoxicity, a major limiting adverse effect. Cardiotoxicity may occur within minutes of administration, or it may be delayed for months or years after chemotherapy has been completed. The nonanthracyclines, which include bleomycin, dactinomycin, and mitomycin, tend to cause less cardiotoxicity than the anthracyclines.

In 1995, the cardioprotective drug dexrazoxane (Totec, Zinecard) was approved to specifically treat doxorubicin cardiotoxicity. Started by slow IV infusion 30 minutes before doxorubicin, dexrazoxane reduces the incidence and severity of cardiomyopathy from the antitumor antibiotic. In 2007, a second form of dexrazoxane (Totect) was approved to treat the pain, inflammation, and tissue necrosis associated with extravasation of anthracyclines. For this indication, IV dexrazoxane is administered as soon as possible after confirmation of anthracycline extravasation, with subsequent doses at 24 and 48 hours. Dexrazoxane may add to the myelosuppression caused by anthracyclines.

PROTOTYPE DRUG	Doxorubicin (Adriamycin)

Classification: **Therapeutic:** Antineoplastic
Pharmacologic: Antitumor antibiotic, anthracycline

Therapeutic Effects and Uses: Approved in 1975, doxorubicin is a cytotoxic antibiotic obtained from *Streptomyces* that has a wide spectrum of antitumor activity and is considered one of the most effective single drugs against solid tumors. Doxorubicin is highly toxic to rapidly proliferating cells as well as slowly developing tumors. It is approved to treat neuroblastoma and solid tumors of the bone, bladder, breast, ovary, GI tract, lung, and thyroid. It is also part of many chemotherapy regimens for other tumors, such as acute lymphoblastic and myeloblastic leukemias, Wilms' tumor, soft tissue sarcomas, and multiple myeloma. Given by the IV route, it may also be instilled into the bladder for bladder cancer. It is also effective as a preradiation therapy to sensitize superficial tumors.

Doxorubicin liposomal (Doxil, Evacet) is a form of the drug incorporated into liposomes, closed, spherical molecules that encase the drug. Administered IV the liposomes have a long half-life and produce a prolonged duration of action. In addition, the liposomes tend to stay in the circulation until they reach tumors, which often have leakier capillaries than normal tissues. Once inside the tumor, the drug is released from its carrier. Doxorubicin liposomal

is approved for use in patients with acquired immunodeficiency syndrome (AIDS)–related Kaposi's sarcoma, refractory ovarian tumors, and relapsed multiple myeloma.

Mechanism of Action: Doxorubicin binds to DNA, causing strand splitting and inhibition of DNA synthesis. It is cell cycle nonspecific.

Pharmacokinetics:

Route(s)	IV
Absorption	N/A
Distribution	Widely distributed, crosses the placenta but does not cross the blood–brain barrier; secreted in breast milk; 75% bound to plasma protein
Primary metabolism	Hepatic
Primary excretion	Bile
Onset of action	Peak: 1/2–2 h
Duration of action	Triphasic half-life: 12 min, 3.3 h, and 30–40 h

Adverse Effects: Doxorubicin has many adverse effects, some of which are serious. These include severe nausea, vomiting, mucositis, rash, excessive lacrimation, hepatotoxicity, anaphylaxis, complete alopecia, and radiation recall phenomenon (a skin reaction due to prior radiation therapy). Doxorubicin turns urine and tears a red color, which is harmless but anxiety provoking. Temporary decreased fertility is likely in both men and women. **Black Box Warnings:** Severe myelosuppression may occur, which is the major dose-limiting toxicity. It may manifest as thrombocytopenia, leukopenia (especially granulocytes), and anemia. The neutropenia nadir occurs at 7 days and recovers by 14 days. Doxorubicin exhibits significant cardiotoxicity, which may be either acute or chronic. Cardiac adverse effects can be life threatening and may include sinus tachycardia, bradycardia, delayed heart failure, acute left ventricular failure, and myocarditis. Heart failure may occur months or years after the termination of chemotherapy. Acute, infusion-related reactions may occur, including anaphylaxis. Severe local necrosis may result if extravasation occurs. Secondary malignancies, especially acute myelogenous leukemia, may occur 1 to 3 years following therapy.

Contraindications/Precautions: Contraindications to the use of doxorubicin include pregnancy, lactation, myelosuppression, thrombocytopenia, preexisting cardiac disease, obstructive jaundice, lactation, or previous treatment with complete cumulative doses of doxorubicin or daunorubicin. Precautions include impaired hepatic or renal function, history of atopic dermatitis, and patients who have received cyclophosphamide or pelvic radiation therapy to areas surrounding the heart. Doxorubicin is a severe vesicant and precautions must be taken to avoid contact with the skin or soft tissue. Skin contact or extravasation should be treated immediately with local ice packs to reduce absorption of the drug.

Drug Interactions: Increased toxicity may occur with other antineoplastics, radiation therapy, or mercaptopurine. Cyclophosphamide may increase the risk of hemorrhagic cystitis or cardiac toxicity. Paclitaxel may decrease the clearance of doxorubicin, leading to more profound neutropenia and stomatitis. Phenobarbital and other barbiturates increase the elimination of doxorubicin. Possible decreased phenytoin levels may occur. Concurrent use with verapamil can raise the serum levels of doxorubicin, thus increasing the risk for cardiotoxicity. Use with paclitaxel will result in an increased incidence of stomatitis, neutropenia, and heart failure. Because doxorubicin causes thrombocytopenia, concurrent use with NSAIDs, anticoagulants, or platelet inhibitors may cause excessive bleeding. **Herbal/Food**: Unknown.

Pregnancy: Category D.

Treatment of Overdose: If myelosuppression occurs, administration of antibiotics, platelets, and granulocytes may be necessary. Symptoms of mucositis and heart failure must be treated symptomatically.

Nursing Responsibilities: Key nursing implications for patients receiving doxorubicin are included in the Nursing Practice Application for Patients Receiving Cancer Chemotherapy.

Drugs Similar to Doxorubicin (Adriamycin)

The anthracyclines include doxorubicin, doxorubicin liposomal, daunorubicin, epirubicin, idarubicin, and mitoxantrone. The nonanthracyclines are bleomycin, dactinomycin, and mitomycin. One nonanthracycline, valrubicin (Valstar), was withdrawn from the market in 2004.

Anthracyclines:

Daunorubicin (Cerubidine): Approved in 1979, daunorubicin is an IV antitumor antibiotic obtained from *Streptomyces*. Cell cycle specific for the S phase, daunorubicin binds to DNA, causing strand splitting and inhibition of DNA synthesis. Closely related structurally to doxorubicin, daunorubicin is approved to induce remission in acute myelogenous leukemia in adults and acute lymphocytic leukemia in children and adults. It is less effective than doxorubicin in treating solid tumors. Daunorubicin carries black box warnings regarding tissue necrosis following extravasation, cardiotoxicity, and myelosuppression. Myelosuppression is the major dose-limiting toxicity, and the drug exhibits the same types of cardiotoxicity as doxorubicin although to a lesser extent. Other adverse effects, such as nausea, vomiting, alopecia, urine discoloration, and vesicant properties, are the same as those of doxorubicin. This drug is pregnancy category D.

Daunorubicin liposomal (DaunoXome) is an IV formulation of daunorubicin in a liposomal vehicle that increases the amount of the drug delivered to tumor cells while decreasing the amount in normal cells. The only approved use for this drug is AIDS-related Kaposi's sarcoma, but it may be administered off-label to treat acute myelogenous leukemia, breast cancer, multiple myeloma, and non-Hodgkin's lymphoma. Adverse effects are the same as those of daunorubicin.

Epirubicin (Ellence): Approved in 1999, epirubicin is an IV antitumor antibiotic closely related to doxorubicin in both structure and function. Epirubicin is approved only for adjuvant therapy for axillary node–positive breast cancer but may be used off-label for bladder, gastric, lung, head, neck, and liver cancers. Carrying black box warnings for extravasation, cardiotoxicity, myelosuppression, and secondary malignancies, epirubicin exhibits the same types

of adverse effects as doxorubicin. Myelosuppression is the major dose-limiting toxicity, with a nadir occurring at 10 to 14 days and recovery at 21 days. Cardiotoxicity, including fatal heart failure, has been reported. Moderate to severe nausea, vomiting, and alopecia occur in many patients. Severe local tissue necrosis can occur with extravasation. Secondary acute myelogenous leukemia has been reported in patients treated with epirubicin. This is a pregnancy category D drug.

Idarubicin (Idamycin): Approved in 1990, idarubicin is an IV antitumor antibiotic structurally similar to daunorubicin. Its only approved indication is for acute myelogenous leukemia, although it may be used off-label for other leukemias, advanced metastatic breast cancer, and refractory non-Hodgkin's lymphoma. Idarubicin carries black box warnings regarding tissue necrosis following extravasation, cardiotoxicity, and myelosuppression. Like other drugs in this class, myelosuppression is the primary dose limitation, with a nadir by day 15 and recovery by day 25. Idarubicin is a vesicant, and care must be taken to not allow extravasation or exposure to skin. Other common adverse effects include alopecia, cardiotoxicity, and moderate nausea and vomiting. This is a pregnancy category D drug.

Mitoxantrone (Novantrone): Although not an anthracycline, mitoxantrone is structurally similar to the anthracyclines and shares some common properties. Approved in 1987, it is approved to treat acute myelogenous leukemia and for the palliation of severe pain associated with advanced prostate cancer. Off-label antineoplastic indications include other leukemias, breast cancer, metastatic ovarian cancer, liver cancer, and non-Hodgkin's lymphoma. It is one of the few drugs approved to treat symptoms of chronic multiple sclerosis. It is administered by IV infusion. Mitoxantrone carries black box warnings regarding extravasation, cardiotoxicity, myelosuppression, and secondary malignancies. The dose-limiting toxicity is myelosuppression, with a nadir at 10 to 14 days and recovery by 2 to 3 weeks. It is less cardiotoxic than the anthracyclines, but this is still a significant adverse effect of mitoxantrone. Other adverse effects include stomatitis, moderate nausea, vomiting, alopecia, injection-site reactions, and secondary malignancy (leukemia). This is a pregnancy category D drug.

Nonanthracyclines:

Bleomycin (Blenoxane): Approved in 1973, bleomycin is an antitumor antibiotic obtained from *Streptomyces* that is cell cycle specific to the G2 phase. Bleomycin is used for palliative therapy for many different cancers, including Hodgkin's and non-Hodgkin's lymphomas, testicular cancer, vulvar cancer, cervical cancer, and squamous cell carcinoma. It can be administered by the IM, IV, subcutaneous, and intrapleural routes. Bleomycin causes less myelosuppression than other drugs in this class. A black box warning states that the drug can cause severe and potentially fatal lung injury, with signs such as pulmonary fibrosis, or pleural effusions. Patients who have received radiation treatment to the chest or cumulative doses of bleomycin are at increased risk for lung injury. The warning also states that bleomycin can cause a severe idiosyncratic reaction, similar to anaphylaxis, consisting of hypotension, mental confusion, fever, chills, and wheezing. Serious dermatologic reactions may require lower doses or discontinuation of the drug. Nausea and vomiting are generally mild; however, anorexia and weight loss are common. This is a pregnancy category D drug.

Dactinomycin (Actinomycin-D, Cosmegen): Approved in 1973, dactinomycin is an IV antitumor antibiotic obtained from *Streptomyces* that binds to DNA to inhibit RNA synthesis and is cell cycle nonspecific. Its primary indication is to treat Wilms' tumor and rhabdomyosarcoma, but it is also approved for choriocarcinoma, Ewing's sarcoma, and testicular carcinoma. Off-label indications include Kaposi's sarcoma, malignant melanoma, and osteogenic sarcoma. Dactinomycin has several dose-limiting toxicities. Myelosuppression can be severe and lead to serious infections with a nadir at 7 to 21 days. Nausea and vomiting are severe and require antiemetic therapy. Other GI effects include oral or esophageal ulceration, anorexia, and diarrhea. Hepatotoxicity, including hepatomegaly, ascites, hepatitis, and hyperbilirubinemia, can be serious, especially at high doses. Alopecia and dermatologic skin reactions are common. This drug carries a black box warning that special handling is required because the powder, dust, and solution are extremely irritating to soft tissue and mucous membranes. This is a pregnancy category D drug.

Mitomycin (Mutamycin): Mitomycin is an IV antitumor antibiotic extracted from *Streptomyces* that was approved in 1974. It is very effective against both slowly developing and rapidly proliferating cells in solid tumors, including some tumors unresponsive to radiation and other chemotherapeutic drugs. Mitomycin is approved only for gastric and pancreatic cancers but may be used off-label for bladder cancer, colorectal cancer, breast cancer, and squamous cell carcinoma of the head, neck, lung, or cervix. Mitomycin carries black box warnings regarding myelosuppression and hemolytic uremic syndrome. The primary dose-limiting toxicity is bone marrow suppression with a nadir at 3 weeks. Recovery may take 4 to 8 weeks. Hemolytic uremic syndrome is a serious complication involving hemolytic anemia, thrombocytopenia, and irreversible renal failure. Severe skin reactions such as ulceration and cellulitis can occur, especially following extravasation. Lung toxicity is rare, but occurrences of interstitial pneumonitis can be fatal. Nausea, vomiting, anorexia, and fatigue may be delayed and persistent during therapy. This is a pregnancy category X drug.

Hormones and Hormone Antagonists

57.5 Hormones and hormone antagonists block the substances necessary for continued growth of tumors.

A number of hormones are used in cancer chemotherapy, including corticosteroids, progestins, estrogens, and androgens. In addition, several hormone antagonists have been found to exhibit antitumor activity. Endocrine, or hormonal therapy, is limited to treating hormone-sensitive tumors of the breast or prostate.

The mechanism of hormone antineoplastic activity is largely unknown. It is likely, however, that these antitumor properties are independent of their normal hormone mechanisms because the doses utilized in cancer chemotherapy are magnitudes larger than the amount normally present in the body. The student should refer to other chapters in this text for a complete discussion of hormone therapy. The antitumor hormones and hormone antagonists are listed in Table 57.4.

In general, the hormones and hormone antagonists act by blocking the substances essential for tumor growth. Because these drugs are not cytotoxic, they produce few of the life-threatening toxic effects of antineoplastics from other classes. They can, however, produce significant adverse effects when given at high doses for prolonged periods. Because they rarely produce cancer cures when used singly, these drugs are normally given for palliation. There are four general classes of hormone antagonists:

- Selective estrogen receptor modifiers
- Aromatase inhibitors
- Gonadotropin-releasing hormone analogs
- Androgen receptor blockers

Selective estrogen receptor modifiers: Estrogen is a hormone produced by the ovary and the adrenal gland that has profound metabolic actions on many organs. Estrogen produces its actions throughout the body by activating estrogen receptors (ERs). Estrogen receptors are overexpressed in many breast cancers, which are known as ER-positive tumors. Estrogen promotes the growth of ER-positive breast tumors.

Selective estrogen receptor modifiers (SERMs) are drugs that act to either activate or inhibit the ER. SERMs have the ability to activate ERs in some tissues (such as bone), while blocking ERs in other tissues (such as breast). SERMs that block ERs have an antiestrogen effect that slows tumor growth of ER-positive breast cancer. Tamoxifen is the most widely prescribed SERM and serves as the prototype for antineoplastic hormones.

Aromatase inhibitors: Aromatase is the enzyme that catalyzes the last step in the synthesis of estrogen. During this step, aromatase converts androgens (testosterone and androstenedione) to estrogens (estradiol) in the peripheral tissues such as fat and muscle. Blocking this step will reduce the levels of estrogen in the blood, starving ER-dependent tumors of a major growth stimulus.

The aromatase inhibitors cannot prevent estradiol formation in the ovary, which is the primary site of estrogen synthesis in premenopausal women. Because of this, the drug is only effective in postmenopausal women, who secrete almost no estrogen from their ovaries.

The American Society of Clinical Oncology (ASCO) recommends aromatase inhibitor therapy with exemestane (Aromasin) as an option for all postmenopausal women with ER-positive breast cancer (Visvanathan et al., 2013). Aromatase inhibitors can be started as primary therapy, or instituted after the completion of 2 to 3 years of tamoxifen therapy. For most patients, the total length of endocrine therapy (tamoxifen plus aromatase inhibitor) is 5 years.

Gonadotropin-releasing hormone analogs: Gonadotropin-releasing hormone (GnRH) analogs mimic the actions of endogenous GnRH and provide feedback to the pituitary gland. Initially, the effect is to increase the production of interstitial cell-stimulating hormone (ICSH), which increases the secretion of testosterone by the testes. ICSH is also known as follicle-stimulating hormone (FSH). With continued therapy, the pituitary becomes insensitive to the effects of GnRH, and the production of testosterone falls. In fact, testosterone secretion declines to near zero levels such that treatment with a GnRH analog is considered a type of chemical or pharmacologic castration. All are approved for the management of prostate cancer. The loss of testosterone "starves" prostate cancer cells of the hormone essential for their growth. Some drugs in this

TABLE 57.4   **Hormone and Hormone Antagonists Used for Neoplasia**

Drug	Route and Adult Dose (Maximum Dose Where Indicated)	Adverse Effects
Hormones		
dexamethasone (Decadron, others)	PO: 2 mg bid–qid	*Weight gain, insomnia, abdominal distention, sweating, flushing, diarrhea, nervousness, gynecomastia, hirsutism (testosterone)*
diethylstilbestrol (DES, Stilbestrol)	PO: For treatment of prostate cancer, 500 mg tid; for palliation, 1–15 mg/day	
ethinyl estradiol (Estinyl, others)	PO: For treatment of breast cancer, 1 mg tid for 2–3 months; for palliation of prostate cancer, 0.15–3 mg/day	Thrombophlebitis, muscle wasting (prednisone, dexamethasone), osteoporosis, hepatotoxicity
fluoxymesterone	PO: 10 mg tid	
medroxyprogesterone (Provera, Depo-Provera)	IM: 400–1,000 mg every week	
megestrol (Megace)	PO: 40–160 mg bid–qid	
prednisone (Deltasone, others)	PO: 20–100 mg/day	
testosterone (Androgel, Delatestryl, Testred, others)	IM: 200–400 mg every 2–4 weeks	
Hormone Antagonists		
abiraterone (Zytiga)	PO: 1 g once daily in combination with prednisone	*Hot flashes, insomnia, breast enlargement or pain, headache, diarrhea, asthenia, nausea, joint swelling (abiraterone)*
anastrozole (Arimidex)	PO: 1 mg/day	
bicalutamide (Casodex)	PO: 50 mg/day	Hypersensitivity reactions (including anaphylaxis), thrombophlebitis, heart failure (bicalutamide, goserelin), hepatotoxicity (flutamide, abiraterone), sexual dysfunction (goserelin, nilutamide, tamoxifen), ocular toxicity (toremifene), adrenocortical deficiency (abiraterone)
degarelix (Firmagon)	Subcutaneous: 240 mg loading dose followed by 80 mg every 28 days	
enzalutamide (Xtandi)	PO: 160 mg once daily	
exemestane (Aromasin)	PO: 25 mg/day after a meal	
flutamide (Eulexin)	PO: 250 mg tid	
fulvestrant (Faslodex)	IM: 500 mg once monthly	
goserelin (Zoladex)	Subcutaneous implant: 3.6 mg every 28 days	
histrelin (Supprelin LA, Vantas)	Subcutaneous implant: 1 implant every 12 months (50 mg)	
letrozole (Femara)	PO: 2.5 mg/day	
leuprolide (Eligard, Lupron, Viadur)	Subcutaneous implant: 1 implant every 12 months (65 mg) IM depot: 22.5–45 mg every 3–6 months	
nilutamide (Nilandron)	PO: 300 mg/day for 30 days; then 150 mg/day	
raloxifene (Evista)	PO: 60 mg once daily	
tamoxifen	PO: 10–20 mg 1–2 times/day	
toremifene (Fareston)	PO: 60 mg/day	
triptorelin (Trelstar)	IM: 3.75 mg once monthly	

Note: Italics indicate common adverse effects. Underline indicates serious adverse effects.

class are also approved to treat endometriosis and uterine leiomyomata and for the palliative treatment of advanced breast cancer. The GnRH analogs are administered by the IM route or subcutaneous implants. All GnRH analogs are pregnancy category X drugs and contraindicated during pregnancy.

Androgen receptor blockers: Growth of prostatic carcinoma is usually androgen dependent. The androgen receptor blockers prevent testosterone and other androgens from reaching their receptors on cancer cells, thus depriving the cells of an important growth promoter. Drugs in this group are all administered PO and are used only to treat prostate cancer. They have an additive or synergistic effect when used in combination with GnRH analogs.

PROTOTYPE DRUG   **Tamoxifen**

Classification: **Therapeutic:** Antineoplastic
Pharmacologic: Hormonal agent, estrogen receptor blocker

Therapeutic Effects and Uses: Approved in 1985, tamoxifen is an oral SERM that has an antiestrogen effect on ER-positive tumors. It has no effect on ER-negative cancers. Tamoxifen is approved for the palliative treatment of advanced, metastatic, ER-positive breast cancer in men and postmenopausal women. Off-label indications include astrocytoma, malignant glioma, malignant melanoma, and ovarian cancer.

CONNECTIONS | Lifespan Considerations

Neurotoxicity and Mobility Effects of Chemotherapy for the Older Adult

Many chemotherapy drugs used in the treatment of cancer have neurotoxic effects, some of which persist for years after treatment or cause permanent dysfunction. Peripheral neuropathy caused by chemotherapy may be severe and unpredictable and often causes sensory effects such as decreased touch, temperature, and other sensations, including muscle cramping. Neuropathic pain is also common and may be severe enough to result in the need to slow or stop treatment. Reduced deep tendon reflexes (DTRs) may be an early sign of peripheral neuropathy, and autonomic dysfunction may also occur, resulting in symptoms such as orthostatic hypotension and constipation (Cavaletti, Alberti, Frigeni, Piatti, & Susani, 2011).

While adults over the age of 65 account for a significant number of cancer patients and survivors, they are not well represented in research. There are few studies of the effects of chemotherapy on the older adult's mobility and balance. It is known that indicators of frailty such as grip strength, and functional dependence, i.e., requiring assistance for activities of daily living (ADLs), are associated with a poorer prognosis and tolerance to cancer therapy (Versteeg, Konings, Lagaay, van de Loosdrecht, & Verheul, 2014). Whereas positive therapeutic responses to chemotherapy may be similar to those of younger colleagues (Hung & Mullins, 2013), older adults often experience adverse effects of chemotherapy at more severe levels and for longer periods. With the increased risk of chemotherapy-related peripheral neuropathy and other neurotoxic effects associated with many drugs, the older adult is at extreme risk for falls and injury, especially when there are preexisting visual or hearing conditions.

Nurses can be proactive in helping the older adult to plan for and manage potential adverse effects from chemotherapy. Prior to beginning the drug regimen, a physical therapy consultation may be beneficial to establish baseline function. Periodic consultations thereafter can assist in the detection of developing neuropathies and other adverse effects so that they can be managed appropriately or the drug regimen reevaluated if needed. Because weakness or mobility problems related to chemotherapy may have a profound impact on the older adult, the nurse is a valuable member of the collaborative oncology team and is often the member who will have the most frequent contact with the patient. Early intervention may help reduce the impact of chemotherapy on mobility for the older adult.

A unique feature of tamoxifen is that it is the only antineoplastic that is approved for the *prophylaxis* of breast cancer in women who have a high risk of developing the disease. In addition, it is approved as adjunctive therapy in women following a mastectomy to decrease the potential for cancer in the contralateral breast. It is not to be used for prophylaxis in women at low risk of acquiring breast cancer because the risks may outweigh the benefits in this population. Risk factors that may qualify a woman for tamoxifen prophylactic therapy depend on age and also include the following:

- One first-degree relative with a history of breast cancer
- Two or more benign biopsies and a history of a breast biopsy showing atypical hyperplasia
- At least two first-degree relatives with a history of breast cancer and a personal history of at least one breast biopsy
- Lobular carcinoma *in situ*
- Age at first live birth less than or equal to 25 years of age and age at menarche less than or equal to 11 years

- At least two first-degree relatives with a history of breast cancer and age at first live birth of less than or equal to 19 years
- One first-degree relative with a history of breast cancer and a personal history of a breast biopsy showing atypical hyperplasia

Tamoxifen has several nonneoplastic indications, all of which are off-label. For the treatment of infertility, it may be used to induce ovulation in women who do not ovulate but desire to become pregnant. It may be used to reduce the pain associated with gynecomastia in both women and men. The drug is being examined for its potential use in patients with osteoporosis.

Mechanism of Action: Tamoxifen binds to ERs, producing agonist effects in some tissues (bone) and antagonist effects in other tissues (breast). The binding in breast tissue inhibits DNA replication and affects other growth factors in cancer cells.

Pharmacokinetics:

Route(s)	PO
Absorption	Slowly from the GI tract
Distribution	Widely distributed; crosses the placenta; unknown if secreted in breast milk
Primary metabolism	Hepatic by CYP3A, CYP2C9, and CYP2D6
Primary excretion	Feces
Onset of action	Peak serum concentration: 5 h
Duration of action	Half-life: 5–7 days

Adverse Effects: Tamoxifen has few serious adverse effects other than nausea and vomiting, which occurs in 12% to 25% of patients who are taking the drug. This can be controlled with antiemetics as necessary. Other common adverse effects include hot flashes, vaginal discharge, irregular menses, vaginal bleeding, fluid retention, headaches, light-headedness, and rash. **Black Box Warnings:** The most serious problem associated with tamoxifen use is the increased risk of endometrial cancer. The benefits of tamoxifen outweigh the risks in women taking tamoxifen to *treat* breast cancer. The benefit versus risk is not as clear in women who are taking tamoxifen to *prevent* breast cancer. There is also a slightly increased risk of thromboembolic disease, including stroke, pulmonary embolism, and deep venous thrombosis (DVT) with the use of tamoxifen. The risk of a thromboembolic event is believed to be about the same as for oral contraceptives.

Contraindications/Precautions: Contraindications to the use of tamoxifen include anticoagulant therapy, preexisting endometrial hyperplasia, history of thromboembolic disease, pregnancy, and lactation. Precautions should be observed in patients with leukopenia, thrombocytopenia, visual disturbances, cataracts, bone marrow suppression, hypercalcemia, and hypercholesterolemia.

Drug Interactions: Tamoxifen is extensively metabolized by hepatic CYP enzymes and may interact with inducers or inhibitors of these enzymes. Use with warfarin increases the risks of bleeding. Cytotoxic antineoplastics may increase the risk of thromboembolism. Bromocriptine may increase tamoxifen levels, whereas aminoglutethimide, medroxyprogesterone, or rifamycin may decrease tamoxifen levels. Selective serotonin reuptake inhibitors (SSRIs) may decrease the effectiveness of tamoxifen. This drug should not be used concurrently with oral contraceptives. **Herbal/Food:**

Black cohosh should not be taken unless approved by the health care provider.

Pregnancy: Category D.

Treatment of Overdose: Seizures, neurotoxicity, and QT-interval changes may occur with overdose. The patient is treated symptomatically.

Nursing Responsibilities: Key nursing implications for patients receiving tamoxifen are included in the Nursing Practice Application for Patients Receiving Cancer Chemotherapy.

Drugs Similar to Tamoxifen

The drugs in this broad category of antineoplastics are divided into SERMs, aromatase inhibitors, gonadotropin-releasing hormone analogs, and androgen receptor blockers. Dexamethasone, diethylstilbestrol, medroxyprogesterone, prednisone, and testosterone are hormones used for nonneoplastic indications. Information on these drugs may be found in other chapters of this text. Abarelix (Plenaxis) is a hormone antagonist that has been discontinued in the United States.

Selective estrogen receptor modifiers:

Fulvestrant (Faslodex): Approved in 2002, fulvestrant selectively binds to the ERs of breast cancer cells and inhibits cell division. It is used to treat advanced breast cancer in ER-positive, postmenopausal women with disease progression following antiestrogen therapy. Fulvestrant is a pure estrogen antagonist and, unlike tamoxifen, it has no estrogen agonist activity. Administered by IM injection once a month, it appears to be as effective as the aromatase inhibitors. It is well tolerated, with the most common adverse effects being nausea, vomiting, constipation, diarrhea, headache, abdominal pain, hot flashes, back pain, and pharyngitis. Temporary injection-site pain and inflammation are possible. Fulvestrant is a pregnancy category D drug.

Raloxifene (Evista): Raloxifene is an oral SERM that has antagonist effects on the ERs in the breast. It activates ERs in bone, which decreases bone resorption and increases bone mineral density. Unlike tamoxifen, it does not have agonist actions on the ERs in the uterus. Originally approved in 1997 for osteoporosis, its indications were expanded in 2007 to include prophylaxis of breast cancer in postmenopausal women who are at high risk for developing the disease. It is used off-label to treat uterine leiomyomata in postmenopausal women. Raloxifene is associated with an increased risk of thromboembolic disorders such as DVT, pulmonary embolism, and retinal thrombosis. Hot flashes and leg cramps are common adverse effects. It is classified as pregnancy category X. A prototype feature for raloxifene is presented in Chapter 72.

Toremifene (Fareston): Approved in 1997, toremifene is a PO medication closely related to tamoxifen that exerts antiestrogenic effects at ERs in the breast. Toremifene is indicated for the treatment of metastatic breast cancer in postmenopausal women with ER-positive or unknown tumors. Common adverse effects include hot flashes, vaginal discharge, diaphoresis, and fluid retention. Serious adverse effects are uncommon but may include stroke, angina, and increased intraocular pressure. Toremifene carries a black box warning that the drug prolongs the QT interval, resulting in dysrhythmias. It should not be given to patients with preexisting QT prolongation or uncorrected hypokalemia or hypomagnesemia. This is a pregnancy category D drug.

Aromatase inhibitors:

Anastrozole (Arimidex): Anastrozole is an oral hormone antagonist highly specific for the aromatase enzyme. Anastrozole restricts tumor growth by inhibiting the biosynthesis of estrogens, thus depriving the tumor of necessary estrogen. Although first approved in 1995 for the treatment of advanced breast cancer, indications were expanded in 2008 to include the adjuvant treatment of early breast cancer in postmenopausal women with ER-positive disease. An off-label indication of anastrozole is for the treatment of uterine leiomyomata. It is contraindicated in premenopausal women. Serious adverse effects are uncommon during anastrozole therapy. The most common adverse effects are hot flashes, asthenia, arthritis, pharyngitis, bone pain, nausea, vomiting, and depression. Osteoporosis during therapy may lead to an increased incidence of spinal fractures. Women with preexisting ischemic heart disease have an increased incidence of ischemic cardiovascular events. As an antiestrogen, anastrozole will block the effects of estrogen-containing products. Anastrozole is a pregnancy category D drug.

Exemestane (Aromasin): Exemestane is an oral aromatase inhibitor that reduces serum estradiol concentrations by binding irreversibly to the aromatase enzyme. Exemestane has greater antiestrogen actions than tamoxifen or anastrozole and is effective when tumors develop resistance to other drugs in this class. First approved in 1999 for the treatment of advanced breast cancer, indications were expanded in 2005 to include the adjuvant treatment of early breast cancer in postmenopausal women with ER-positive disease. It is contraindicated in premenopausal women. Adverse effects are the same as those of other aromatase inhibitors and include hot flashes, nausea, vomiting, arthralgia, and fatigue. Bone mineral density often decreases during exemestane use. An increase in ischemic heart disease has been reported during therapy. Exemestane is a pregnancy category D drug.

Letrozole (Femara): Letrozole is an oral aromatase inhibitor that reduces serum estrogen levels. First approved in 1997, its indications include the adjuvant treatment of early breast cancer in patients who have received 5 years of adjuvant tamoxifen therapy; first-line treatment of patients with ER-positive or unknown, locally advanced, or metastatic cancer; advanced breast cancer with disease progression following antiestrogen therapy; and the adjuvant treatment of patients with hormone receptor-positive early breast cancer. Off-label indications include the treatment of infertility in anovulatory women who wish to become pregnant and to increase the height of boys with idiopathic short stature or delayed puberty. It is contraindicated in premenopausal women. This drug is generally well tolerated, with the most common adverse effects being nausea, vomiting, asthenia, fatigue, headache, and bone and other musculoskeletal pain. Like other drugs in this class, bone mineral density decreases during therapy. Letrozole is a pregnancy category D drug.

Gonadotropin-releasing hormone analogs and related drugs:

Degarelix (Firmagon): Approved in 2008, degarelix acts by a different mechanism than other drugs in this class. Rather than being an analog of GnRH, it is an antagonist, blocking the receptors for GnRH in the pituitary. Although its mechanism differs, the pharmacologic indications, actions, and adverse effects are similar to those of the GnRH agonists. It is given by the IM route for the treatment of patients with advanced prostate cancer. The most common adverse effects are pain and swelling at the injection site, hot flashes, increased weight, and increases in serum levels of transaminases and gamma-glutamyltransferase. Long-term use can prolong the QT interval. This drug is pregnancy category X.

Goserelin (Zoladex): Approved in 1989, goserelin is a GnRH analog that is administered as a depot implant into the abdominal wall every 28 days. By inhibiting pituitary GnRH secretion, goserelin reduces testosterone levels in men to castration levels and lowers estrogen levels in women to postmenopausal levels. In men, the drug is approved for the treatment of early prostate cancer in combination with flutamide and radiotherapy and for the palliative management of advanced prostate cancer. In women, indications for goserelin include endometriosis and the palliative treatment of advanced breast cancer. It may be used off-label to treat uterine leiomyomata or benign prostatic hyperplasia. Hot flashes occur in most patients. Men experience sexual dysfunction and gynecomastia, whereas women experience amenorrhea, decreased libido, and breast atrophy. Bone pain and irritation at the injection site are common. Tumor flare phenomenon may occur, which includes a transient worsening of tumor symptoms during the first few weeks of treatment. Men have an increased risk of sudden cardiac death when using GnRH analogs. Goserelin is classified as a pregnancy category X drug.

Histrelin (Supprelin LA, Vantas): Approved in 2004, histrelin is a GnRH analog that is given subcutaneously as an implant, usually in the inner aspect of the upper arm. This drug is slowly released over a period of 12 months, at which time the implant is removed. Histrelin (Vantas) is approved for the palliation of advanced prostate cancer. Hot flashes occur in the majority of patients and inflammation may occur at the site of implantation. Men may experience impotence, gynecomastia, and testicular atrophy. Tumor flare phenomenon may occur during the first few weeks of treatment. Men have an increased risk of sudden cardiac death when using GnRH analogs. Histrelin is classified as a pregnancy category X drug.

Histrelin (Supprelin LA) uses the same implant technology to treat central precocious puberty in children. This condition is defined by the premature development of pubertal body characteristics earlier than age 8 in males or age 9 in females. Children with this disorder may have reduced adult height and psychosocial problems. Supprelin LA reduces estradiol levels (in girls) and testosterone levels (in boys) and stabilizes the condition. The most common adverse effect in these children is implant-site soreness and pain.

Leuprolide (Eligard, Lupron, Viadur): Leuprolide is a GnRH analog that is an effective androgen antagonist for treating hormone-dependent tumors. It reduces testosterone levels in men to castration levels and lowers estrogen levels in women to postmenopausal levels. It is used as a palliative treatment for advanced prostate cancer as an alternative to orchiectomy or estrogen therapy. It may be used off-label to induce ovarian ablation in premenopausal women with ER-positive breast cancer. Nonneoplastic indications include the treatment of endometriosis, uterine leiomyomata (fibroids), and central precocious puberty. It is occasionally used to treat female infertility by hyperstimulating the ovary (see

Chapter 70). Viadur and Eligard are subcutaneous implants for prostate cancer that release the drug over a period of 1 to 12 months, depending on the formulation. Lupron Depot is an IM formulation that releases the drug over 1 to 6 months, depending on the dose. Leuprolide causes nausea, vomiting, hot flashes, and diaphoresis in both men and women. Women develop amenorrhea and men experience testicular atrophy due to reduced testosterone levels. CNS effects such as migraines, depression, insomnia, asthenia, and dizziness may occur. Injection-site reactions are frequent. This is a pregnancy category X drug.

Triptorelin (Trelstar): Triptorelin is a GnRH analog that was approved in 2000 for the palliative management of advanced prostate cancer. This drug is administered once monthly by the IM route, and most patients achieve the castration levels of androgens in less than a month. Off-label uses include advanced breast cancer, uterine leiomyomata, and precocious puberty. Adverse effects are similar to those of other GnRH analogs. This is a pregnancy category X drug.

Androgen blockers:

Bicalutamide (Casodex), flutamide (Eulexin), and nilutamide (Nilandron): Bicalutamide, flutamide, and nilutamide are antiandrogen agents that are all closely related in structure and function. All have only one indication: the chemotherapy of metastatic prostate cancer. Because androgens promote the growth of prostate cancer, blocking androgen receptors can slow tumor growth. Bicalutamide and flutamide are used in combination with a GnRH analog such as goserelin or leuprolide. Bicalutamide and flutamide block androgen receptors, whereas the added GnRH analog decreases the secretion of testosterone. Nilutamide is given following an orchiectomy. The androgen receptor blockers are administered by the PO route. Adverse effects are mild to moderate and are those expected of blocking androgen secretion such as hot flashes, mastalgia, impotence, decreased libido, and gynecomastia. They are only indicated for prostate cancer and thus should not be administered to women. Flutamide carries a black box warning regarding the potential for serious hepatotoxicity. A black box warning for nilutamide states that 2% of patients receiving the drug develop pulmonary fibrosis. Bicalutamide and flutamide are pregnancy category X drugs, whereas nilutamide is a pregnancy category C drug.

Abiraterone (Zytiga) and enzalutamide (Xtandi): Abiraterone (approved in 2011) and enzalutamide (approved in 2012) are oral medications for the treatment of castration-resistant prostate cancer in patients who have received prior therapy with docetaxel. Both drugs lower testosterone levels by inhibiting enzymes required for the biosynthesis of androgens. Abiraterone must be taken on an empty stomach because the presence of food results in increased risk of toxicity. Common adverse effects for abiraterone include joint swelling, peripheral edema, hypokalemia, hypertension, and urinary tract infection. Abiraterone carries a black box warning that serious depression and suicidal ideation may occur during therapy. The most common adverse effects with enzalutamide are fatigue, back pain, diarrhea, arthralgia, hot flashes, peripheral edema, headache, respiratory infection, dizziness, insomnia, spinal cord compression, hematuria, paresthesia, anxiety, and hypertension. This drug is pregnancy category C.

Natural Products

57.6 Natural products that are derived from plants include the vinca alkaloids, taxanes, and topoisomerase inhibitors.

Agents with antineoplastic activity have been isolated from a number of plants, including the common periwinkle (*Vinca rosea*), Pacific yew (*Taxus baccata*), mandrake (May apple), and the shrub *Camptotheca acuminata*. Although structurally very different, medications in this class have the common ability to arrest cell division; thus, some of them are called mitotic inhibitors. The plant extracts, or natural products, are listed in Table 57.5. There are three subdivisions of natural products used as antineoplastics:

- Vinca alkaloids
- Taxanes
- Topoisomerase inhibitors

Vinca alkaloids: The vinca alkaloids vincristine (Oncovin) and vinblastine (Velban) are two older drugs derived from more than 100 alkaloids isolated from the periwinkle plant. The medicinal properties of this plant were described in folklore in several regions of the world long before their antineoplastic properties were discovered. Despite being derived from the same plant, vincristine, vinblastine, and the semisynthetic vinorelbine (Navelbine) exhibit different effects and toxicity profiles.

Taxanes: The taxanes, which include cabazitaxel (Jevtana), paclitaxel (Taxol), and docetaxel (Taxotere), were originally isolated from the bark of the Pacific yew, an evergreen found in forests throughout the western United States. More than 19 different taxane alkaloids have been isolated from the tree, and several have potential antineoplastic activity. Although the taxanes are mitotic inhibitors like the vinca alkaloids, they act by a different mechanism. Myelosuppression is usually the dose-limiting factor for the taxanes.

Topoisomerase inhibitors: DNA exists in a double-stranded supercoiled state. The two strands must be separated if the macromolecule is to replicate or serve as a template for RNA synthesis (see Chapter 56). Topoisomerase is an enzyme that cuts the DNA strand, thus changing it to a more relaxed structure that can be used for DNA and RNA synthesis. The topoisomerase enzyme exists in two closely related forms: Topoisomerase I causes breaks in one strand of the DNA molecule, and topoisomerase II causes breaks in both DNA strands.

Topoisomerase inhibitors bind to the enzyme, preventing it from causing the strand breaks necessary for DNA to perform its functions. The cancer cell is unable to properly uncoil its DNA, and DNA replication prematurely terminates. Topoisomerase inhibitors are natural products, and they are available for IV administration only.

American Indians described uses of the May apple or wild mandrake (*Podophyllum peltatum*) long before pharmacologists isolated podophyllotoxin, which is the primary active ingredient in the plant. As a botanical, podophyllum has been used as an antidote for snakebites, as a cathartic, and as a topical treatment for warts. Teniposide (Vumon) and etoposide (VePesid) are semisynthetic products of podophyllotoxin that inhibit topoisomerase II.

The topoisomerase I inhibitors include topotecan (Hycamtin) and irinotecan (Camptosar). These agents are sometimes called camptothecins because they were first isolated from *Camptotheca*

TABLE 57.5	Natural Products Used as Antineoplastic Therapy	
Drug	**Route and Adult Dose (Maximum Dose Where Indicated)**	**Adverse Effects**
Vinca Alkaloids		*Nausea, vomiting, stomatitis, anorexia, rash, alopecia, fatigue*
vinblastine (Velban)	IV: 3.7–18.5 mg/m^2 every 7–10 days	<u>Myelosuppression, severe nausea, vomiting, diarrhea, mucositis, pulmonary or cardiac toxicity, nephrotoxicity (vincristine), neurotoxicity (vincristine, docetaxel), anaphylaxis and other hypersensitivity reactions, severe fluid retention (docetaxel), severe diarrhea with electrolyte imbalances (topoisomerase inhibitors), hemorrhage (omacetaxine)</u>
vincristine (Marquibo, Oncovin)	IV: 1.4 mg/m^2 every week (max: 2 mg/m^2) IV (Marquibo): 2.25 mg/m^2 once every week	
vinorelbine (Navelbine)	IV: 30 mg/m^2 every week	
Taxanes		
cabazitaxel (Jevtana)	IV: 25 mg/m^2 every 3 weeks	
docetaxel (Taxotere)	IV: 60–100 mg/m^2 every 3 weeks	
paclitaxel (Abraxane, Taxol)	IV: 100–260 mg/m^2 every 3 weeks	
Topoisomerase Inhibitors		
etoposide (VePesid)	IV: 35–100 mg/m^2 daily for 5 days	
irinotecan (Camptosar)	IV: 125 mg/m^2 once every week for 4 weeks	
teniposide (Vumon)	IV: 165 mg/m^2 every 3–4 days for 4 weeks	
topotecan (Hycamtin)	IV: 1.5 mg/m^2 daily for 5 days	
Miscellaneous Natural Products		
eribulin (Halaven)	IV: 1.4 mg/m^2 on days 1 and 8 of a 21-day cycle	
omacetaxine (Synribo)	Subcutaneous: 1.25 mg/m^2 for 14 consecutive days	

Note: *Italics* indicate common adverse effects. <u>Underline</u> indicates serious adverse effects.

acuminata, a tree native to China. The camptothecins are administered IV, and their indications are limited. As with many other cytotoxic natural products, myelosuppression is the dose-limiting toxicity for the camptothecins.

PROTOTYPE DRUG	Vincristine (Oncovin)

Classification: **Therapeutic:** Antineoplastic
Pharmacologic: Vinca alkaloid, mitotic inhibitor, natural product

Therapeutic Effects and Uses: Vincristine is an antineoplastic obtained from the periwinkle plant that is specific for the M phase of the cell cycle where it inhibits cell division. It is approved to treat acute lymphocytic leukemia, Hodgkin's and non-Hodgkin's lymphomas, lymphosarcoma, malignant glioma, neuroblastoma, rhabdomyosarcoma, soft tissue sarcoma, and Wilms' tumor. It may be used off-label for breast, colorectal, and lung cancers. It is only administered by the IV route. A newer form of vincristine (Marquibo) encased in a liposomal carrier was approved in 2012 for acute lymphoblastic leukemia.

Mechanism of Action: Vincristine binds to tubulin, which is a protein that makes up the microtubules of the cell that are necessary for cell division. This disrupts the process whereby chromosomes are distributed to the daughter cells during mitosis, resulting in cell death. Paclitaxel and colchicine also produce pharmacologic actions by binding to tubulin, but they bind at a different location than vincristine.

Pharmacokinetics:

Route(s)	IV
Absorption	N/A
Distribution	Widely distributed; does not cross the blood–brain barrier; crosses the placenta; unknown if secreted in breast milk
Primary metabolism	Hepatic
Primary excretion	Bile and feces (80%); renal (20%)
Onset of action	15–20 min
Duration of action	Triphasic half-life: 0.85 min, 7.4 min, and 164 min

Adverse Effects: Vincristine is a toxic medication, and even therapeutic doses may result in serious adverse effects. The major dose-limiting toxicity of vincristine is neurotoxicity. This manifests as motor difficulties, peripheral neuropathy, paresthesias (especially of the hands and feet), weakness, cranial nerve palsies (diplopia, hoarseness, deafness, trigeminal neuralgia, vocal cord paralysis), and decreased reflexes. Neurotoxicity may take several months to resolve. CNS effects may include seizures, depression, hallucinations, and coma. GI-related adverse effects include nausea, vomiting, anorexia, stomatitis, severe constipation, and abdominal pain. Other adverse reactions include hepatotoxicity, rash, paralytic ileus (especially in children), and alopecia. **Black Box Warnings:** Myelosuppression may be severe and predispose to opportunistic infections. Extravasation can cause intense pain, inflammation, and tissue necrosis. If extravasation occurs, treatment with warm compresses and hyaluronidase is implemented; cold compresses will significantly increase the toxicity of vinca alkaloids.

Contraindications/Precautions: Contraindications to the use of vincristine include obstructive jaundice, men and women of childbearing age, active infection, adynamic ileus, radiation of the liver, infants, pregnancy, and lactation. Cautions must be taken when administering vincristine to patients with leukopenia, preexisting neuromuscular or neurologic disease, hypertension, or hepatic or renal disease; those who are taking drugs with neurotoxic properties; and the elderly. Doses should be reduced in patients with hepatic or biliary disease. Vincristine is a vesicant and caution must be used to avoid exposure of the skin to this drug.

Drug Interactions: Vincristine is a substrate for CYP3A4, and agents that induce CYP3A4 (such as carbamazepine or phenytoin) may increase the metabolism of vincristine and decrease the effects of the drug. Vincristine will increase the action of methotrexate, bleomycin, and anticoagulants. Decreased digoxin and phenytoin levels will occur. Administration of L-asparaginase just prior to vincristine will cause additive neurotoxicity. Concurrent administration with mitomycin may cause acute dyspnea and severe bronchospasm. Neurotoxicity may occur with peripheral nervous system drugs. **Herbal/Food**: Unknown.

Pregnancy: Category D.

Treatment of Overdose: Overdose may cause life-threatening symptoms or death. Symptoms are extensions of the adverse effects of vincristine. There is no antidote and patients are treated symptomatically.

Nursing Responsibilities: Key nursing implications for patients receiving vincristine are included in the Nursing Practice Application for Patients Receiving Cancer Chemotherapy.

Drugs Similar to Vincristine (Oncovin)

The two additional vinca alkaloids include vinblastine and vinorelbine. Other classes of natural products include the taxanes (cabazitaxel, docetaxel, and paclitaxel) and the topoisomerase inhibitors (irinotecan, topotecan, etoposide, and teniposide).

Vinblastine (Velban): Vinblastine is obtained from the periwinkle plant and has a chemical structure and mechanism of action very similar to those of vincristine. However, the toxicities and spectrum of actions of the two drugs differ. The use of vinblastine has declined because of the development of newer effective drugs, but it has traditionally been used to treat Hodgkin's disease and testicular tumors. Off-label uses include treatment of prostate, bladder, and lung cancers and metastatic malignant melanoma. It is only administered by the IV route. Unlike vincristine, neurotoxicity with vinblastine is infrequent. Instead, myelosuppression is the dose-limiting toxicity (especially neutropenia) with a nadir at 4 to 10 days and recovery between days 7 and 21. Extravasation can cause intense pain, inflammation, and tissue necrosis. This drug carries the same black box warnings as vincristine. Nausea and vomiting are generally mild. Other potential adverse effects include hypertension, stroke, dyspnea, and Raynaud's phenomenon. This is a pregnancy category D drug.

Vinorelbine (Navelbine): Vinorelbine is a semisynthetic drug derived from vinblastine to which it shares structural and functional similarities. In addition to having the same mechanism of action as the vinca alkaloids, vinorelbine also inhibits RNA synthesis and blocks the cellular use of glutamic acid that is needed for purine synthesis. Its only approved use is to treat non–small cell lung cancer but it may be used off-label to treat metastatic breast cancer, head and neck cancers, ovarian cancer, and Hodgkin's disease. The primary dose-limiting toxicity is myelosuppression (especially neutropenia) with a nadir at 7 to 14 days and recovery between days 14 and 24. Like vinblastine neurotoxicity is infrequent. Extravasation can cause intense pain, inflammation, and tissue necrosis. This drug carries the same black box warnings as vincristine and vinblastine. Other adverse effects include mild nausea, vomiting, thromboembolic events, asthenia, fatigue, and pulmonary hypersensitivity. Vinorelbine is a pregnancy category D drug.

Taxanes:

Cabazitaxel (Jevtana):   The newest of the taxanes, approved in 2010, cabazitaxel is indicated for hormone-refractory metastatic prostate cancer that has not responded to a docetaxel-containing regimen. Cabazitaxel carries black box warnings regarding severe hypersensitivity reactions and low neutrophil counts. Deaths due to severe neutropenia have been reported and the drug is contraindicated in patients with neutrophil counts of less than 1,500 cells/mm³. To reduce the incidence of severe hypersensitivity reactions, patients should be premedicated with dexamethasone, diphenhydramine, and ranitidine at least 30 minutes prior to cabazitaxel administration. Diarrhea may be extreme and requires premedication with antidiarrheals. Nonhematologic adverse effects include fatigue, nausea, vomiting, constipation, asthenia, abdominal pain, hematuria, and peripheral neuropathy. This is a pregnancy category D drug.

Docetaxel (Taxotere):   Approved in 1996, docetaxel is a semisynthetic taxane that is administered only by the IV route. It disrupts normal microtubule function and is a mitotic inhibitor. Docetaxel is approved to treat solid tumors, including advanced gastric cancer, head and neck cancers, metastatic breast or refractory prostate cancer, and non–small cell lung cancer that has failed to respond to therapy with platinum antineoplastics. Off-label indications include metastatic malignant melanoma and advanced ovarian cancer. Docetaxel is a toxic drug that carries multiple black box warnings regarding increased mortality in patients with hepatic impairment, myelosuppression, skin toxicity, severe hypersensitivity reactions, and fluid retention. To reduce the incidence and severity of fluid retention and hypersensitivity reactions, patients receiving docetaxel are administered dexamethasone for 3 days prior to chemotherapy. Without premedication, a hypersensitivity reaction occurs in about 20% of patients within minutes of the injection. Severe fluid retention occurs in some patients and may include peripheral or generalized edema, dyspnea, pleural effusion, cardiac tamponade, and ascites. The major dose-limiting toxicity is myelosuppression, especially neutropenia, which occurs in nearly all patients. The nadir occurs at 7 days with recovery at 14 days. This drug is contraindicated in patients with neutrophil counts of less than 1,500 cells/mm³. Skin reactions, primarily erythema, rash, and pruritus on the feet and hands, occur in the majority of patients. Severe skin toxicity occurs in about 5% of patients. Neurologic toxicity such as paresthesias and peripheral neuropathy occur in half the patients taking this drug. Mild to moderate nausea, vomiting, diarrhea, stomatitis, and esophagitis are common. Docetaxel is a pregnancy category D drug.

Paclitaxel (Abraxane, Taxol):   Approved in 1992, paclitaxel is a semisynthetic taxane that is administered by the IV route and approved to treat solid tumors, including metastatic breast cancer, ovarian cancer, Kaposi's sarcoma, and non–small cell lung cancer in combination with cisplatin. Off-label indications include the chemotherapy of bladder, head, and neck cancers. Paclitaxel carries black box warnings regarding severe hypersensitivity reactions and low neutrophil counts. The major dose-limiting toxicity is myelosuppression, which occurs in nearly all patients. The nadir occurs at 11 days. This drug is contraindicated in patients with neutrophil counts of less than 1,500 cells/mm³. Anaphylaxis and severe hypersensitivity reaction may occur, usually within an hour after the start of the infusion. To reduce the incidence of severe hypersensitivity reactions, patients should be premedicated with dexamethasone and diphenhydramine prior to paclitaxel administration. A protein-bound form of this drug (Abraxane) approved in 2013 does not require premedication. Abraxane is approved to treat late-stage pancreatic cancer (in combination with gemcitabine), non–small cell lung cancer (in combination with carboplatin), and metastatic breast cancer. Extravasation of paclitaxel can result in an acute and delayed injection-site reaction. A local hyaluronidase injection may be beneficial in treating severe extravasation symptoms. Other common adverse events include musculoskeletal pain, asthenia, hypotension, rash, peripheral neuropathy, mild to moderate nausea, vomiting, diarrhea, and stomatitis. Alopecia occurs in nearly every patient. Paclitaxel is a pregnancy category D drug.

Topoisomerase inhibitors:

Irinotecan (Camptosar):   Approved in 1996, irinotecan is a cytotoxic alkaloid obtained from *Camptotheca acuminata*. Like topotecan, it acts by inhibiting topoisomerase I, which interferes with DNA replication during the S phase of the cell cycle. Irinotecan is indicated for the treatment of metastatic colorectal cancer that has progressed despite treatment with fluorouracil. Off-label uses include advanced breast, cervical, ovarian, gastric, and lung cancers. Hematologic toxicity is dose limiting, with anemia, leukopenia, and neutropenia occurring in most patients. Irinotecan carries a black box warning about diarrhea, which can be severe and dose limiting. Early diarrhea occurs during or immediately after the infusion and may be accompanied by cholinergic symptoms such as rhinitis, increased salivation, miosis, lacrimation, diaphoresis, and abdominal cramping. Late diarrhea occurs more than 24 hours after the infusion and may be life threatening due to prolonged dehydration and electrolyte imbalances. Nausea and vomiting are common and severe enough to require pretreatment with antiemetics. Other adverse events that occur at a high rate include asthenia, fever, dyspnea, abdominal pain, anorexia, and dizziness. This drug is pregnancy category D.

Topotecan (Hycamtin):   Approved in 1996, this drug is an IV camptothecin, topoisomerase I inhibitor very similar to irinotecan, although its indications are different. Topotecan is approved to treat small cell lung cancer after failure of traditional chemotherapy and inoperable cervical cancer. It may be used off-label to treat rhabdomyosarcoma in children. Topotecan carries a black box warning regarding myelosuppression, which is a dose-limiting toxicity. The drug is contraindicated in patients with neutrophil counts of less than 1,500 cells/mm³. Nausea and vomiting are usually mild. Topotecan can cause infertility in both males and females. Other common adverse events include alopecia, fatigue, asthenia, fever, musculoskeletal pain, dyspnea, interstitial lung disease, and headache. This drug is pregnancy category D.

Etoposide (VePesid): Approved in 1983, etoposide is a derivative of podophyllotoxin that inhibits topoisomerase II. It is one of the few antineoplastic natural products that are administered by both PO and IV routes. It is approved for patients with small cell lung cancer and for testicular tumors in patients who have already received surgery, chemotherapy, and radiation without success. Off-label indications may include acute leukemia, Hodgkin's and non-Hodgkin's lymphoma, refractory ovarian cancer, gastric cancer, neuroblastoma, and malignant glioma. Etoposide carries a black box warning for severe, dose-limiting myelosuppression that has a nadir at day 16 and recovery by days 20 through 22. Alopecia occurs in a majority of patients. Anaphylaxis has been reported in up to 2% of patients who are receiving this drug. Secondary malignancies, especially acute nonlymphocytic leukemia, may occur in children who are treated with this drug. Etoposide is a pregnancy category D drug.

Teniposide (Vumon): Approved in 1992, teniposide is an IV derivative of podophyllotoxin that inhibits topoisomerase II. It is only approved to treat refractory childhood acute lymphoblastic leukemia but may be used off-label for neuroblastoma, bladder cancer, lung cancer, and non-Hodgkin's lymphoma. Teniposide carries black box warnings regarding myelosuppression and hypersensitivity reactions. Bone marrow toxicity (especially neutropenia) is its most common dose-limiting toxicity. Hypersensitivity reactions occur in about 5% of patients. GI adverse reactions occur in most patients and include severe stomatitis, diarrhea, mild nausea, and vomiting. Alopecia occurs in about 9% of patients. Secondary malignancies, especially acute nonlymphocytic leukemia, may occur

in children who receive this drug for prolonged periods. This drug is pregnancy category D.

PharmFACT

Lung cancer is the most common type of cancer, but it has one of the lowest survival rates because it is rarely discovered in its early stages. The 5-year survival rate from Stage I non–small cell lung cancer is 49%, but at Stage IV it is only 1% (American Cancer Society, 2014a).

Biologic Response Modifiers and Targeted Therapies

57.7 Biologic response modifiers and targeted therapies enhance the body's ability to kill tumor cells.

A **biologic response modifier** is a substance that enhances the ability of body defenses to remove cancer cells. Biologic response modifiers may produce their effects directly, by binding to cancer cells and destroying them, or indirectly, by activating general aspects of the immune response. Biologic response modifiers may be grouped into two general classes: cytokines and monoclonal antibodies. These drugs are listed in Table 57.6.

Cytokines that act as biologic response modifiers include the following:

- Interferons are natural proteins produced by T cells in response to viral infection and other antigens. They bind to specific receptors on cancer cell membranes and suppress cell division, enhance the phagocytic activity of macrophages, and promote the cytotoxic activity of T lymphocytes. PegINF alfa-2a (Pegasys, Sylatron) and IFN alfa-2b (Intron-A) are approved to treat hairy cell leukemia, chronic myelogenous leukemia, Kaposi's sarcoma, and chronic hepatitis B and C. In 2011, the

---

CONNECTIONS: NURSING PRACTICE APPLICATION

Patients Receiving Cancer Chemotherapy

Assessment	Potential Nursing Diagnoses*
Baseline assessment prior to administration: • Understand the reason the drug has been prescribed in order to assess for therapeutic effects. • Obtain a complete health history including neurologic, cardiovascular, respiratory, hepatic or renal disease, and the possibility of pregnancy. Obtain a drug history including allergies (e.g., specific reactions to drugs), current prescription and OTC drugs, herbal preparations, and alcohol use. Be alert to possible drug interactions. • Assess signs and symptoms of current infections and for history of herpes zoster or chickenpox. • Obtain an immunization history, especially recent vaccinations with live vaccines, particularly varicella. • Evaluate appropriate laboratory findings (e.g., complete blood count [CBC], platelet count, urinalysis, hepatic and renal function studies, uric acid, electrolytes, glucose). • Assess findings from other diagnostic tests specific to type of antineoplastic therapy regimen planned (e.g., audiology or cardiac testing, ECG, electromyography [EMG]). • Obtain baseline height, weight, and vital signs. Assess level of fatigue and presence of pain. Assess DTRs. • Assess the patient's ability to receive and understand instructions. Include the family and caregiver as needed.	• *Infection* • *Activity Intolerance* • *Fatigue* • *Anxiety* • *Imbalanced Nutrition: Less Than Body Requirements* • *Deficient Fluid Volume* • *Diarrhea* • *Impaired Oral Mucous Membrane* • *Impaired Skin Integrity* • *Pain (Acute or Chronic)* • *Social Isolation* • *Ineffective Health Management* • *Hopelessness* • *Spiritual Distress* • *Deficient Knowledge (Drug Therapy)* • *Risk for Decreased Cardiac Output*, related to adverse drug effects • *Risk for Injury*, related to adverse drug effects • *Risk for Falls*, related to adverse drug effects • *Risk for Caregiver Role Strain*

(continued)

CONNECTIONS: NURSING PRACTICE APPLICATION (continued)

Assessment throughout administration:

- Assess for desired therapeutic effects (e.g., indicators of treatment success or palliation specific to the type of cancer: slowed growth in solid tumors, able to attend to normal ADLs, absence of signs and symptoms of concurrent infections).
- Continue frequent monitoring of laboratory work (e.g., CBC, absolute neutrophil count [ANC], platelet count, urinalysis, hepatic and renal function studies, uric acid, electrolytes, glucose). ANC = WBC count multiplied by the total percentage of neutrophils (segmented plus banded): e.g., WBC 5,000 × (0.45 segs 1 0.5 bands) = 5,000 × 0.5 = ANC of 2,500. An ANC of less than 500 indicates that the patient is at great risk for infection.
- Continue to monitor findings from other diagnostic tests specific to the type of antineoplastic therapy regimen planned (e.g., audiology or cardiac testing, ECG, EMG).
- Assess for the presence of nausea or pain.
- Assess DTRs and ECG as specific to the type of antineoplastic drugs given.
- Continue to record daily weights and report any weight gain or loss of more than 1 kg (2 lb) in 24 hours.
- Assess for adverse effects: nausea, vomiting, anorexia, abdominal cramping, diarrhea, constipation, chills, fever, fatigue, dizziness, dysrhythmia, angina, dyspnea, muscle or joint pain, paresthesia, diminished or absent DTRs, hypotension, hyperglycemia, bruising, or bleeding. Fever exceeding parameters established by the oncology provider, severe diarrhea, jaundice, decreased urine output or hematuria, excessive bruising or bleeding, respiratory distress, or angina should be reported immediately.

Implementation

Interventions and (Rationales)	Patient-Centered Care
Ensuring therapeutic effects: • Continue assessments as above for therapeutic effects: radiographic evidence of diminished tumor mass, decreased production of abnormal cell growth, absence of signs and symptoms of infection, maintenance of appetite, food and fluid intake, nausea and vomiting are decreased or absent, able to perform acceptable levels of ADLs. (Antineoplastic drugs do not have immediately observable results. Results will be measured over time. These drugs have many potential adverse effects affecting many body systems.)	• Provide explanations for all testing and treatments used. Provide general information on the expected course of chemotherapy: requirements for invasive lines (e.g., peripheral and central access ports), initial infusion or dosing, frequency of expected treatments, nausea control, hydration and nutrition needs, frequent laboratory testing, onset of alopecia, techniques for managing fatigue, nutrition and fluid needs, follow-up appointments, in-hospital versus outpatient clinic locations, and how to reach the oncology team, especially during off-hours. Involve the family and caregivers in information sessions and provide written materials whenever possible.
Minimizing adverse effects: General Care • Continue to monitor vital signs, especially temperature. Report increasing temperature that exceeds parameters (e.g., three temperatures taken every 4 h over 38.1°C [100.5°F] or any single temperature over 38.3°C [101°F]) to the oncology provider. Avoid taking rectal temperatures. (Increasing fever, even low-grade temperatures less than 38.3°C, may be a sign of infection. Significant myelosuppression may allow infections to occur and disseminate rapidly. GI endothelial cells are affected by chemotherapy, and rectal mucosa may be damaged if rectal temperatures are used.)	• Teach the patient to take their temperature every 4 h if behavior or symptoms indicate the need (e.g., increased body warmth, general malaise, lethargy) or as ordered by the oncology provider. Include instructions on when to call the oncology team if parameters are exceeded. • Instruct the patient that antipyretics are not to be used unless explicitly approved by the oncology provider. Antipyretics may mask the symptoms of an infection, allowing rapid dissemination.
• Continue to monitor frequent laboratory work: CBC, ANC, platelet count, hepatic and renal function tests, electrolytes, glucose, and urinalysis. (Myelosuppression and resulting blood dyscrasias are expected adverse effects and will be monitored by ANC, CBC, and platelet counts.)	• Teach the patient the need for frequent laboratory work. Provide instructions for outpatient laboratory tests, and have the patient alert laboratory personnel of chemotherapy use. • If peripheral veins are used for phlebotomy, scrupulous cleansing of the site prior to the needlestick and prolonged pressure may be required during periods around the nadir. If central line access is used, scrupulous cleansing of the port is required and appropriate flush solution(s) used afterward to maintain catheter patency.
• Continue to monitor nutritional and fluid intake. (Nausea and vomiting are common adverse effects and usually require antiemetic therapy to manage. Dietary consultation may be required to maintain optimal nutrition.)	• Provide antiemetic therapy routinely during administration of drugs with high and moderate emetic potential. If the patient has had previous treatment with the chemotherapy regimen, assess the extent of nausea and vomiting and which antiemetics or routines had the most success in preventing nausea. • Encourage increased fluid intake, up to 2 L/day, taken in frequent small amounts as allowed. • Encourage small, high-calorie, nutrient-dense meals rather than large infrequent meals. Nutritional supplements, such as Boost or Ensure, may help boost caloric intake.

CONNECTIONS: NURSING PRACTICE APPLICATION (continued)

	• Avoid spicy, highly scented foods and excessively hot or cold foods during periods of nausea. Small sips of carbonated beverages, especially ginger ale, may provide nonmedicinal relief. If GI effects predominate (e.g., diarrhea), avoid high-roughage foods. • Encourage frequent oral hygiene: rinsing the mouth, especially after eating, applying lip balm, and avoiding alcohol-based mouthwash, which can be drying to the mucosa. • Provide referral to a dietary consultation as needed.
• Continue to assess for presence of pain and provide for adequate pain medication. (Pain may result from advanced disease or adverse drug effects. In advanced disease, pain medication is not withheld. Assess possible drug-related causes for pain, and treat the cause when possible.)	• Encourage the patient to seek pain relief when needed. Teach the patient, family, and caregiver that the absence of pain is a goal in the treatment of advanced disease, and pain medication should not be withheld.
• Provide for adequate rest. Schedule daily routines, diagnostic studies, and meals throughout the day if fatigue is profound. (Fatigue related to anemia and adverse drug effects is common, especially around the nadir and immediately after. Fatigue may continue after cell counts return to normal and may persist for several years after chemotherapy.)	• Teach the patient the importance of spacing daily routines throughout the day. Encourage rest whenever fatigue occurs. • Assess transportation needs if fatigue affects the ability to drive. Provide referral to social services as needed.

• Protect the patient from infection: e.g., frequent hand washing before patient care, maintaining scrupulous infection control measures for all IV lines or venous punctures, and encouraging the patient to maintain daily hygiene measures to limit skin flora. Assess for symptoms of opportunistic infections such as yeast, and acquire early treatment or prophylaxis. (Myelosuppression places patients at high risk for infection. Prophylactic therapy with antifungal and antibacterial mouth rinses or protective isolation may be required dependent on the level of neutropenia.)	• Teach the patient, family, and caregiver infection control measures:
	  • Avoiding crowded indoor places.
	  • Avoiding people with known infections or young children, who have a higher risk of having an infection.
	  • Cook food thoroughly, allowing the family or caregiver to prepare raw foods and perform cleanup; avoid consuming raw fruits or vegetables, which may carry bacteria on the surface.
	  • Report any fever per the parameters set by the health care provider, and report symptoms of infection such as wounds with redness or drainage, increasing cough, increasing fatigue, white patches on oral mucous membranes, white and itchy vaginal discharge, or itchy blister-like vesicles on the skin.

• Provide for emotional support for the patient, family, and caregiver. (Cancer results in profound emotional reactions from all involved. Encourage discussion of concerns, appropriate referrals for social support or spiritual assistance, and assess the patient or family for distress that may require a mental health referral. Cost issues may be a concern, and financial assistance may be required.)	• Encourage the patient, family, and caregiver to discuss concerns or questions and to seek appropriate spiritual or social support as desired. • Assess financial concerns and provide appropriate social service referral as needed.
Minimizing adverse effects: Care Specific to Drug Therapy • Monitor DTRs, neurologic status, and level of consciousness. (*Alkylating agents* such as cyclophosphamide and *natural product* antineoplastics such as vincristine have neurologic adverse effects. Changes may occur in DTRs that are not noticeable to the patient in early stages but may affect dexterity or steadiness when walking. **Lifespan:** Be particularly cautious with older adults who are at increased risk for falls. Monitor infants and children for growth or developmental delays.)	• Teach the patient to be cautious when walking or performing manual tasks requiring extra dexterity or when carrying hot or heavy objects. Promptly report any significant difficulty with dexterity or clumsiness when carrying out ADLs or when walking. • Encourage increased intake of fluids and moderate fiber in the diet if constipation is experienced related to decreased peristalsis. Drug therapy such as MiraLAX may be required if constipation is severe or to prevent straining during defecation.
• Monitor cardiovascular status including ECG, heart and breath sounds, presence of edema, angina, or chest wall pain. (*Alkylating agents* such as cyclophosphamide, *antitumor antibodies* such as doxorubicin, *natural product* antineoplastics such as vincristine, and *hormone and hormone antagonists* such as tamoxifen have cardiovascular adverse effects such as pericarditis and effects on the cardiac conduction system.)	• Teach the patient about the need for frequent monitoring of cardiac status. Report any chest wall pain, angina, palpitations, dyspnea, lung congestion, or dizziness immediately.
• Monitor respiratory status including breath sounds and pulmonary function tests. (*Alkylating agents* such as cyclophosphamide, *antimetabolites* such as methotrexate, *antitumor antibodies* such as doxorubicin, *natural product* antineoplastics such as vincristine, and *biologic response modifiers* such as INF alpha-2 have respiratory adverse effects such as interstitial pneumonitis.)	• Teach the patient about the need for frequent monitoring of respiratory status. Report any chest wall pain, dyspnea, lung congestion, or dizziness immediately. • Teach the patient pulmonary hygiene measures such as increasing fluid intake to moisten the respiratory tract, avoiding crowded indoor places and people with known respiratory disease, and avoiding the use of room or body sprays that may irritate the respiratory tract.

(continued)

CONNECTIONS: NURSING PRACTICE APPLICATION (continued)

• Monitor hepatic and renal status and for urinary tract dysfunction, including hepatic and renal function tests, urinalysis, and signs and symptoms such as jaundice, decreased urine output, or hematuria. (Antineoplastic drugs may cause significant hepatic and renal toxicity. *Alkylating agents* such as cyclophosphamide may cause hemorrhagic cystitis. **Diverse Patients:** Because some antineoplastics [e.g., tamoxifen, vincristine] are metabolized through the P450 system, monitor ethnically diverse patients frequently to ensure optimal therapeutic effects and minimize adverse effects. **Lifespan:** Age-related physiological differences place older adults at greater risk for hepatic or renal toxicity.)	• Teach the patient to immediately report any nausea, vomiting, yellowing of the skin or sclera, abdominal pain, light- or clay-colored stools, diminished urine output, darkening of urine, suprapubic pain, or blood in the urine. • Advise the patient to increase fluid intake to 2 to 3 L/day as allowed.
• Monitor for ototoxicity. Periodic audiology testing may be ordered. (Alkylating agents such as cyclophosphamide and *antimetabolites* such as methotrexate may cause ototoxicity, affecting hearing or balance, or both.)	• Teach the patient about the need for periodic monitoring of hearing. Immediately report any dizziness, vertigo, or nausea related to motion, buzzing, ringing, or humming in ears.
• Monitor for ocular toxicity. Periodic ophthalmology exams may be ordered. (*Hormone and hormone antagonists* such as tamoxifen may cause ocular toxicity. Frequent monitoring is necessary to prevent or limit toxicity.)	• Teach the patient about the need for periodic eye exams. Immediately report any blurred vision, eye pain, halos, or other visual disturbances. • Encourage the patient to wear eye protection (sunglasses) when in sunlight.
• Monitor for dermatologic toxicity. (*Alkylating agents* such as cyclophosphamide may cause significant skin reactions including SJS.)	• Teach the patient to promptly report any unusual changes to skin, rashes, or sunburn-like appearance. Immediately report any purplish-red, blistering rash, or peeling skin.
• Monitor for mucositis. (Antineoplastic drugs may cause significant mucositis related to the effects of rapidly dividing GI endothelial cells.)	• Teach the patient to inspect the oral cavity at least once daily and maintain regular dental exams. Maintain good oral hygiene and rinse the mouth with plain water or solution as prescribed by the health care provider after eating. Use antibacterial and antifungal mouth rinses as ordered, and do not rinse the mouth with water after using; swallow mouth rinse if directed to do so by the health care provider. Avoid excessively hot or cold foods. • Teach the patient to avoid high-roughage foods, spicy foods, carbonated and acidic beverages, alcohol, and caffeine. If diarrhea is severe, drug therapy may be required. Immediately report any excessive diarrhea, especially if it contains mucus or blood.
• Monitor for hypersensitivity and allergic reactions. (Antineoplastic drugs may cause significant hypersensitivity and allergic responses, including anaphylaxis. Because reactions may not always be predictable, caution and frequent monitoring are essential to ensure prompt treatment.)	• Teach the patient to immediately report any itching, rashes, swelling, particularly of the face or tongue, urticaria, flushing, dizziness, syncope, wheezing, throat tightness, or difficulty breathing.
• Follow agency-specific policies and procedures related to antineoplastic administration, and spill management, before working with or giving chemotherapy. All IV infusions with antineoplastics will be given via monitored pump. IV push drugs may utilize a push-pull technique, i.e., aspirate for blood return, administer dose, aspirate, administer. All spills will be managed via OSHA and agency protocols. Larger spills may require HAZMAT intervention. (Intensive education programs are required prior to administering vesicants and other chemotherapy. Protection of the nurse, pharmacy personnel, and others involved in the preparation and administration of chemotherapy is essential.)	• Provide the patient, family, and caregiver education and support when giving chemotherapy. • Instruct the patient, family, or caregiver on the specific procedures of handling and administering the drugs if any drug solutions are to be used in the home. Gloves will be required when working with oral solutions. Specific instructions should be obtained from the oncology provider or pharmacist if a spill occurs at home.
Patient understanding of drug therapy: • Use opportunities during administration of medications and during assessments to discuss the rationale for drug therapy, desired therapeutic outcomes, commonly observed adverse effects, parameters for when to call the health care provider, and any necessary monitoring or precautions. (Using time during nursing care helps to optimize and reinforce key teaching areas.)	• The patient, family, and caregiver should be able to state the reason for the drug, appropriate dose and scheduling, what adverse effects to observe for and when to report them, and the anticipated length of medication therapy.
Patient self-administration of drug therapy: • When administering medications, instruct the patient, family, and caregiver in proper self-administration techniques followed by teach-back as needed. (Utilizing time during nurse-administration of these drugs helps to reinforce teaching.)	• Provide explicit instructions for the patient, family, and caregiver on the routine to follow for any antineoplastic drugs used at home. Encourage the use of calendars for recording drugs and doses used; provide information on handling a liquid spill and on proper disposal of any unused drug. (Consult local pharmacies; many will accept unused drugs for proper disposal. Chemotherapy should *never* be flushed down the toilet, poured in a drain, or thrown away in the trash.)

TABLE 57.6 Selected Monoclonal Antibodies and Targeted Therapies

Drug	Route and Adult Dose (Maximum Dose Where Indicated)	Adverse Effects
alemtuzumab (Campath)	IV: 3–30 mg/day	*Nausea, vomiting, diarrhea, asthenia, stomatitis anorexia, rash, alopecia, tremors (alemtuzumab), fever, chills*
axitinib (Inlyta)	PO: 5 mg bid	Myelosuppression (neutropenia, anemia, thrombocytopenia), severe nausea, vomiting, diarrhea, pulmonary toxicity, severe hypersensitivity reactions, pancreatitis (gefitinib), severe fluid retention (imatinib), heart failure (bevacizumab, trastuzumab, pertuzumab), dysrhythmias (rituximab), GI perforation (bevacizumab, ziv-aflibercept, cabozantinib), tumor cell mobilization (plerixafor), sudden cardiac death (vandetanib), cutaneous squamous cell carcinoma (vemurafenib), fetal toxicity and death (vismodegib), severe hepatotoxicity (pazopanib, regorafenib, ceritinib), progressive multifocal leukoencephalopathy (obinutuzumab), severe hemorrhage (ramucirumab)
bevacizumab (Avastin)	IV: 5 mg/kg every 14 days	
bortezomib (Velcade)	IV: 1.3 mg/m^2 as bolus twice weekly for 2 weeks	
bosutinib (Bosulif)	PO: 500 mg once daily	
brentuximab (Adcetris)	IV: 1.8 mg/kg infused over 30 min every 3 weeks	
carfilzomib (Kyprolis)	IV: 20–27 mg/m^2/day on 2 consecutive days each week for 3 weeks	
cabozantinib (Cometriq)	PO: 140 mg once daily	
ceritinib (Zykadia)	PO: 750 mg once daily	
cetuximab (Erbitux)	IV: 400 mg/m^2 over 2 h; then continue with 250 mg/m^2 over 1 h weekly	
crizotinib (Xalkori)	PO: 250 mg bid	
dasatinib (Sprycel)	PO: 70 mg bid	
erlotinib (Tarceva)	PO: 150 mg/day	
gefitinib (Iressa)	PO: 250–500 mg/day	
gemtuzumab (Mylotarg)	IV: 9 mg/m^2 for 2 h	
ibritumomab (Zevalin)	IV: 250 mg/m^2 of rituximab is infused followed by 0.3–0.4 mCi/kg of Zevalin in a 10-min IV push	
ibrutinib ((Imbruvica)	PO: 420–560 once daily	
imatinib (Gleevec)	PO: 400–600 mg/day	
ipilimumab (Yervoy)	IV: 3 mg/kg once every 3 weeks	
lapatinib (Tykerb)	PO: 1,250 mg (5 tablets) once daily on days 1 to 21 continuously in combination with capecitabine	
nilotinib (Tasigna)	PO: 400 mg bid	
obinutuzumab (Gazyva)	IV: 100–1,000 mg depending on cycle	
ofatumumab (Arzerra)	IV: 300 mg initial dose followed 7 days later by 2 g weekly for 7 doses, followed 4 weeks later by 2 g every 4 weeks for 4 doses	
panitumumab (Vectibix)	IV: 6 mg/kg administered over 60 min every 14 days	
pazopanib (Votrient)	PO: 800 mg once daily	
pertuzumab (Parjeta)	IV: 840 mg, followed every 3 weeks by 420 mg	
plerixafor (Mozobil)	Subcutaneous: 0.24 mg/kg for up to 4 consecutive days	
ramucirumab (Cyramza)	IV: 8 mg/kg every 2 weeks	
regorafenib (Stivarga)	PO: 160 mg once daily for the first 21 days of each 28-day cycle	
rituximab (Rituxan)	IV: 375 mg/m^2/day as a continuous infusion	
sorafenib (Nexavar)	PO: 400 mg bid	
sunitinib (Sutent)	PO: 50 mg once daily for 4 weeks followed by 2 weeks off	
tositumomab (Bexxar)	IV: 450 mg over 60 min	
trastuzumab (Herceptin) and ado-trastuzumab (Kadcycla)	IV (Herceptin): 4 mg/kg as a single dose; then 2 mg/kg every week IV (Kadcycla): 3.6 mg/kg given every 3 weeks (21-day cycle)	
vandetanib (Caprelsa)	PO: 300 mg once daily	
vemurafenib (Zelboraf)	PO: 960 mg bid	
vismodegib (Erivedge)	PO: 150 mg once daily	
ziv-aflibercept (Zaltrap)	IV: 4 mg/kg every 2 weeks	

Note: *Italics* indicate common adverse effects. <u>Underline</u> indicates serious adverse effects.

indications for pegINF alfa-2a were extended to include melanoma with nodal involvement. Doses of the interferons and a prototype feature for INF alfa-2b are included in Chapter 42.

- Interleukin-2 activates cytotoxic T lymphocytes and promotes other actions of the immune response. Marketed as aldesleukin (Proleukin), this drug is indicated only for metastatic renal cell carcinoma. A prototype feature for aldesleukin is included in Chapter 42.

- **Hematopoietic growth factors** promote the formation of specific blood cells. These drugs enhance the ability of the immune system to respond and reduce some of the myelosuppression caused by antineoplastic medications. Hematopoietic growth factors include epoetin alfa (Epogen, Procrit), filgrastim (Neupogen), and sargramostim (Leukine). The doses and prototype features for epoetin alfa and filgrastim are given in Chapter 39.

Research into the mechanisms of cancer formation has allowed scientists to identify specific proteins (antigens) on the surface of cancer cells that are not present in normal cells. Different types of cancer cells exhibit different antigens. For example, cells in a brain tumor would have different antigens than those of a pancreatic tumor. Indeed, a single type of tumor in a patient may contain cancer cells with varied surface antigens. A **targeted therapy** is an antineoplastic drug that has been specially engineered to attack these cancer antigens.

Monoclonal antibodies (MABs) are biologic response modifiers that are a type of targeted therapy. Once the MAB binds to its specific antigen, the cancer cell is either killed directly by the drug or is marked for destruction by other cells of the immune response. For example, rituximab (Rituxan) is an MAB that binds to CD20, a surface protein present on premature B lymphocytes involved in certain leukemias and lymphomas. Once bound, rituximab lyses the tumor cells. As is typical of MABs, the action of rituximab is very specific: It was designed to only affect cells with the CD20 protein, in this case tumor B cells. The key point about MABs is that the tumor cells must possess the specific protein receptor; otherwise, the MAB will be ineffective. The general mechanism of action of MABs is shown in Pharmacotherapy Illustrated 57.1.

A few MABs carry a toxin that directly kills the tumor cell once it is bound. For example, gemtuzumab ozogamicin (Mylotarg) carries a cytotoxic antitumor antibiotic. The MAB reaches its target antigen and enters the cancer cell, where the toxic antibiotic is released to cause cell death. Tositumomab (Bexxar) carries radioactive iodine, ^{131}I, to its specific antigen, whereby the tumor cell receives a dose of ionizing radiation.

Other types of targeted therapies are available that affect key metabolic pathways in tumor cells. While these are not MABs they still have highly specific targets. Examples include the following:

- Tyrosine kinase (TK) is an enzyme that activates certain proteins in internal signaling pathways that regulate cell growth. In normal cells, the TK enzyme is turned on and off, depending on the cell's need for growth. Certain types of cancer cells turn on the TK enzyme permanently, leading to uncontrolled cell growth. Imatinib (Gleevec), dasatinib (Sprycel), and crizotinib (Xalkori) are examples of drugs that are able to inhibit TKs, thus stopping this unchecked cell growth. Everolimus (Afinitor, Zortress) inhibits a different type of kinase and is approved as an

antineoplastic drug as well as for the prophylaxis of transplant rejection (see Chapter 42). Approved in 2011, vemurafenib (Zelboraf) was designed to specifically inhibit multiple types of kinases and is indicated for malignant melanoma.

- The epidermal growth factor receptor (EGFR) is a cell-surface receptor that, when activated, results in cell growth. Mutations of the EGFR can result in uncontrolled cell growth and cancer. Antineoplastic drugs known as EGFR inhibitors are targeted to shut down this activation and slow the growth of certain neoplasms. Cetuximab (Erbitux), erlotinib (Tarceva), and trastuzumab (Herceptin) are examples of drugs that target the EGFR.

- Vascular endothelial growth factor (VEGF) is a protein that signals the formation of new blood vessels during embryonic development or following injury or blockage to tissues. VEGF, also called "angiogenesis inhibitors," prevents the formation of new blood vessels that are vital to the formation of new tumors. These drugs do not kill cancer cells, but they are able to slow tumor growth. Bevacizumab (Avastin) was the first drug to specifically target angiogenesis. An additional VEGF inhibitor, ramucirumab (Cyramza) was approved in 2014 to treat advanced gastric cancer. Thalidomide (Thalomid) and lenalidomide (Revlimid) are miscellaneous drugs, shown in Table 57.7, that possess antiangiogenic properties.

- CD20 is a protein located on the surface of B lymphocytes. While the normal function of CD20 is not completely understood, it has been found in high concentrations in certain lymphomas and leukemias. Monoclonal antibody drugs have been developed that target CD20 and kill the cancer cells expressing this protein. Examples of CD20 antibody medications include rituximab (Rituxan), ofatumumab (Azerra), tositumumab (Bexxar), and ibritumomab (Zevalin).

CONNECTION Checkpoint 57.3

PegIFN alfa-2a and -2b are used as antineoplastics. From what you learned in Chapter 42, what are the indications for INF alfacon-1 (Infergen), INF alfa-n3 (Alferon N), and INF beta-1a (Avonex, Rebif)? *See Answer to Connection Checkpoint 57.3 on student resource website.*

Miscellaneous Antineoplastics

57.8 Several miscellaneous antineoplastics act by unique mechanisms.

Some antineoplastics are classified as miscellaneous because they are structurally dissimilar to any of the previously discussed groups. Because these medications are unique, their adverse reactions vary. Doses for the miscellaneous antineoplastics are listed in Table 57.7.

Altretamine (Hexalen): Altretamine is an oral antineoplastic that has effects similar to those of alkylating agents. When metabolized it forms toxic metabolites that bind to cellular macromolecules, resulting in a cytotoxic effect. Its only indication is for refractory ovarian cancer that has not responded well to other therapies. Severe myelosuppression is observed in 15% of patients with a nadir at 3 to 4 weeks and recovery at 6 weeks. The most frequent adverse effects are mild to moderate nausea and vomiting. Altretamine causes mild to moderate neurotoxicity, including peripheral neuropathy,

PHARMACOTHERAPY ILLUSTRATED 57.1

Monoclonal Antibodies and Cancer Cells

1 Normal cells have no tumor-specific antigens On their surfaces.

2 Tumor cells with tumor-specific antigens. The antigen present is different for each type of cancer.

Administer MAB

3 Monoclonal antibodies (MABs) are created for each specific type of tumor antigen.

Administer MAB

4 Tumor cells die due to phagocytosis, complement fixation, or induction of apoptosis.
Examples:
   Rituximab (Rituxan)
   Alemtuzumab (Campath)

5 Tumor cells stop growing due to inhibition of growth factor receptors.
Examples:
   Cetuximab (Erbitux)
   Trastuzumab (Herceptin)

mood disorders, disorders of consciousness, ataxia, dizziness, and vertigo. This is a pregnancy category D drug.

Arsenic trioxide (Trisenox): Approved in 2000, arsenic trioxide is a toxic metal that has only one indication: acute promyelocytic leukemia. Its mechanism of action is incompletely understood but it appears to cause DNA fragmentation that is characteristic of apoptosis. It is administered by IV infusion. Leukocytosis, thrombocytopenia, anemia, nausea, vomiting, abdominal pain, diarrhea, constipation, and anorexia are common adverse effects. Skin reactions include injection-site inflammation, dermatitis, and pruritus. Neurotoxicity is relatively common and manifests as headache, insomnia, paresthesias, anxiety, dizziness, and tremors. Because arsenic trioxide can cause QT-interval prolongation and complete atrioventricular block, other drugs that prolong the QT interval should be discontinued during therapy. This is a pregnancy category D drug.

Asparaginase (Elspar): Asparaginase is an enzyme that deprives cancer cells of asparagine, an essential amino acid, causing a marked reduction in protein, RNA, and DNA synthesis. It is only approved to treat acute lymphocytic leukemia in combination with other antineoplastics. It is administered by the IM, IV, or subcutaneous routes. Hypersensitivity reactions occur in 40% of patients with symptoms ranging from urticaria to anaphylactic shock. Pretreatment with corticosteroids reduces the incidence of hypersensitivity reactions. This drug is hepatotoxic and may cause hypoalbuminemia and decreased synthesis of coagulation factors. Asparaginase may cause fatal pancreatitis. Lethargy, confusion, impaired cognition, and drowsiness are common neurotoxic effects. This is a pregnancy category C drug.

Pegaspargase (Oncaspar) is asparaginase with a molecule of PEG bonded to it. Pegylation increases the half-life of the drug and allows for less frequent dosing: 3 injections of pegaspargase versus

TABLE 57.7	Miscellaneous Antineoplastics	
Drug	**Route and Adult Dose (Maximum Dose Where Indicated)**	**Adverse Effects**
altretamine (Hexalen)	PO: 260 mg/m^2/day in divided doses for 14–21 days	*Hyporeflexia, paresthesias, nausea, vomiting, muscle weakness, peripheral numbness* Leukopenia, thrombocytopenia, Parkinson-like tremors
arsenic trioxide (Trisenox)	IV: 0.15 mg/kg/day (max: 60 doses)	*Fever, leukocytosis, nausea, vomiting, diarrhea, abdominal pain, anorexia, rash, pruritus, fatigue, edema, headache, insomnia* Thrombocytopenia, anemia, ecchymosis, epistaxis, bleeding, dysrhythmias
asparaginase (Elspar)	IV, IM: 200 international units/kg/day for 28 days, or 5,000–10,000 units/m^2/day every 3 weeks, or 10,000–40,000 units every 2–3 weeks	*Skin rash, urticaria, severe vomiting, nausea, decreased circulating platelets and fibrinogen, reduced clotting factors* Anaphylaxis, fatal hyperthermia, renal failure
belinostat (Beleodaq)	IV: 1000 mg/m^2 on days 1–5 of 21 day cycle	*Nausea, fatigue, pyrexia, anemia, vomiting* Blood dyscrasias, hepatotoxicity, tumor lysis syndrome, embryotoxicity
bexarotene (Targretin)	PO: 100–400 mg/m^2/day Topical: 1% gel applied to lesion 1–4 times/day	*Hyperlipidemia, leukopenia, rash, pruritus, headache, asthenia, nausea, vomiting* Acute pancreatitis, elevated hepatic enzymes, hypothyroidism
hydroxyurea (Droxia, Hydrea, Mylocel)	PO: 80 mg/kg every 3 days or 30 mg/kg/day	*Nausea, vomiting, diarrhea, stomatitis, rash* Myelosuppression
ixabepilone (Ixempra)	IV: 40 mg/m^2 infused over 3 h every 3 weeks	*Alopecia, diarrhea, fatigue, asthenia, musculoskeletal pain, peripheral sensory neuropathy, stomatitis, mucositis, nausea, and vomiting* Anemia, neutropenia, thrombocytopenia
lenalidomide (Revlimid)	PO: 25 mg/day	Same as thalidomide
mitotane (Lysodren)	PO: 9–10 g/day in divided doses tid or qid	*Anorexia, nausea, vomiting, diarrhea, rash, lethargy, drowsiness* Hemorrhagic cystitis
pegaspargase (Oncaspar)	IV: 2,500 international units/m^2 every 14 days	Same as asparaginase
pomalidomide (Pomalyst)	PO: 4 mg per day taken orally on days 1–21 of repeated 28-day cycles	Same as thalidomide
romidepsin (Istodax)	IV: 14 mg/m^2 on days 1, 8, and 15 of a 28-day cycle	*Nausea, fatigue, infections, vomiting, anorexia* Blood dyscrasias, anemia, ECG T-wave changes
sipuleucel-T (Provenge)	IV: 3 doses at 2-week intervals: Each dose contains 50 million autologous CD54 cells	*Chills, fatigue, fever, back pain, nausea, joint ache, headache* Acute infusion-related reactions
thalidomide (Thalomid)	PO: 200–400 mg/day	*Fatigue, constipation, nausea, diarrhea, dyspnea, respiratory infections, back pain, pyrexia* Neutropenia, venous thromboembolism
vorinostat (Zolinza)	PO: 400 mg once daily	*Diarrhea, nausea, vomiting, anorexia, fatigue, chills, taste disorders* Blood dyscrasias, pulmonary embolism
zoledronic acid (Zometa)	IV: 4 mg over at least 15 min	*Flulike symptoms, bone, muscle pain* Dysrhythmias, electrolyte imbalances, osteonecrosis of jaw

Note: Italics indicate common adverse effects. Underline indicates serious adverse effects.

21 injections of asparaginase. The two drugs share the same adverse effects and indications.

Belinostat (Beleodaq), romidepsin (Istodax) and vorinostat (Zolinza): These three drugs induce apoptosis in cancer cells by inhibiting the activity of the enzyme histone deacetylase. They are both approved for the treatment of cutaneous or peripheral T-cell lymphoma in patients who have progressive, persistent, or recurrent disease. Fatigue, diarrhea, nausea, anorexia, and blood dyscrasias are common adverse effects. Pulmonary embolism is a rare, though serious, adverse effect of vorinostat. These drugs are pregnancy category D.

Bexarotene (Targretin): Approved in 1999, bexarotene is a retinoid, a group of drugs related to vitamin A that are usually used for skin conditions such as psoriasis and acne (see Chapter 76). This drug is approved by the PO and topical routes to treat cutaneous T-cell lymphoma that has not responded to other therapies. Off-label indications include lung cancer, Kaposi's sarcoma, metastatic breast cancer, and severe psoriasis. Adverse effects of the oral formulation include hyperlipidemia, hypothyroidism, acute pancreatitis, leukopenia, headache, asthenia, anemia, anorexia, and photosensitivity. Topical bexarotene can cause rash, erythema, and pruritus. This is a pregnancy category X drug.

Hydroxyurea (Droxia, Hydrea, Mylocel): Hydroxyurea is an oral antineoplastic approved in 1967 for chemotherapy of chronic myelogenous leukemia, head and neck cancers, malignant melanoma, and ovarian cancer. It may be used off-label for acute myelogenous leukemia, astrocytoma, lung cancer, and malignant glioma. Sickle cell anemia is a nonneoplastic indication for the drug. Hydroxyurea causes myelosuppression, especially neutropenia. This drug carries a black box warning that long-term use may cause secondary leukemias. Nausea, vomiting, stomatitis, and diarrhea are common. Skin ulcers and gangrene have been reported. This is a pregnancy category C drug.

Ixabepilone (Ixempra): Approved in 2007, ixabepilone acts by the same mechanism as the taxanes but it has different pharmacokinetic properties. It is used in combination with capecitabine to treat metastatic or advanced breast cancer resistant to treatment with first-line medications such as the taxanes. At least 20% of patients experience alopecia, diarrhea, fatigue, asthenia, musculoskeletal pain, peripheral sensory neuropathy, stomatitis, mucositis, nausea, and vomiting. More than 40% of patients experience anemia, neutropenia, and thrombocytopenia. Ixabepilone carries a black box warning that it must not be given to patients with elevated serum aspartate alanine aminotransferase (AST), alanine aminotransferase, or bilirubin levels due to increased risk of toxicity and neutropenia-related death. This is a pregnancy category D drug.

Mitotane (Lysodren): Mitotane, which is similar to the insecticide DDT, poisons cancer cells by forming links to proteins. Given by the PO route, its only indication is for the chemotherapy of advanced, inoperable adrenocortical cancer. Because the drug is cytotoxic to the adrenal gland, symptoms of acute adrenal insufficiency may emerge. Mitotane carries a black box warning that the drug should be temporarily stopped after shock or severe trauma due to its adrenal suppression effects. Most patients experience adverse GI effects such as nausea, vomiting, and diarrhea. CNS effects such as lethargy, drowsiness, and vertigo are observed in up to 40% of patients who are taking the drug. Mitotane is a pregnancy category C drug.

Sipuleucel-T (Provenge): Approved in 2010, sipuleucel-T is very different from other antineoplastic medications. Three days prior to sipuleucel-T administration, the patient undergoes leukapheresis during which antigen-presenting cells (APCs) are collected. The APCs are then incubated with granulocyte-macrophage colony-stimulating factor (GM-CSF) and a prostate cancer antigen, which activates the collected cells. The product, consisting of GM-CSF mature and activated APCs, is reinfused into the patient to cause an immune response against prostate cancer cells. The product can only be used for the patient from whom the APCs were collected. Because acute infusion-related effects such as chills and fever have been reported, the patient is usually premedicated with acetaminophen and an antihistamine. The drug is not indicated for women so it carries no pregnancy rating.

Zoledronic acid (Reclast, Zometa): Approved in 2001, zoledronic acid is a bisphosphonate, a drug class commonly used to treat osteoporosis. The primary action of the drug is to inhibit bone resorption by osteoclasts. In addition to its use in managing osteoporosis, this drug is approved to treat multiple myeloma in patients with osteolytic metastases, severe hypercalcemia caused by malignancy, and Paget's disease. It is given by IV infusion. Adverse effects include flulike symptoms, fever, fatigue, headache, anemia, anorexia, bone pain, arthralgia, and osteonecrosis of the jaw. Reclast and Zometa are different strengths and may not be used interchangeably. This is a pregnancy category D drug.

Drugs for Reducing Adverse Effects

57.9 Medications are used to relieve the adverse effects experienced by patients undergoing chemotherapy.

Most patients who are undergoing chemotherapy will require drugs to treat the severe adverse effects of antineoplastic medications. In many cases, medications are given to prevent adverse effects from occurring. Some of these are well-established drugs with usefulness that has been proven over the years. Others are drugs that were developed specially to deal with the adverse effects of chemotherapy.

Antiemetics are given to nearly all patients who are undergoing chemotherapy to decrease or prevent nausea and vomiting. Examples include ondansetron (Zofran), lorazepam (Ativan), dronabinol (Marinol), and prochlorperazine (Compazine). The type and dose of the antiemetic is based on the known emetogenic potential of the specific antineoplastic drugs employed. Chapter 60 provides complete information on the antiemetics.

Drugs for bowel disorders may be ordered to decrease either constipation or diarrhea. Laxatives or stool softeners may be indicated, such as polyethylene glycol 3350 (MiraLAX), Milk of Magnesia, psyllium (Metamucil), or docusate (Surfak, Colace). Patients may require a medication such as diphenoxylate with atropine (Lomotil), loperamide (Imodium), or bismuth salts (Pepto Bismol) to stop or decrease diarrhea. The student should refer to Chapter 60 for information on drugs for bowel disorders.

Myelosuppression is a disabling adverse effect of many chemotherapy drugs. Three types of drugs are commonly used to prevent serious complications of myelosuppression:

- Epoetin alfa (Epogen, Procrit) is a hematopoietic growth factor that stimulates the production of RBCs, which may prevent the development of anemia. A prototype feature for epoetin alfa is included in Chapter 39.

- Colony-stimulating factors such as filgrastim (Neupogen) increase neutrophil production in the bone marrow and enhance the phagocytic and cytotoxic functions of existing neutrophils. Administration of filgrastim shortens the duration of neutropenia in patients with cancer. A prototype feature for filgrastim is included in Chapter 39.

- Oprelvekin (Neumega) is used to stimulate the production of platelets in patients who are at risk for severe thrombocytopenia caused by chemotherapy. A prototype feature for oprelvekin is included in Chapter 39.

Denosumab (Xgeva), approved in 2010, is a newer drug given to patients with bone metastases. This drug inhibits osteoclasts, which cause excessive bone resorption, pain, and possible fractures in these patients. Given by the subcutaneous route once every 4 weeks, denosumab is being investigated as a treatment for osteoporosis.

Other medications are ordered as the patient's condition warrants, including analgesics, antibiotics, appetite stimulants, and antidepressants. The pharmacotherapy of neoplasia may include a dozen or more drugs, which makes patient care extremely challenging.

Preparing and Administering Antineoplastics

57.10 Nurses who are preparing and delivering antineoplastics must exercise extreme caution to protect themselves from medication exposure.

Many health care agencies only allow an **oncology nurse** who has received special training to care for patients with cancer and to administer chemotherapy. A large number of antineoplastic medications are absorbed through the skin and mucous membranes, so the person preparing and administering them is at risk for absorbing them. The nurse and other health care professionals engaged in the preparation or administration of antineoplastics must be extremely diligent about always wearing protective clothing, including gloves, whenever handling them. Both the Oncology Nursing Society and the Occupational Safety and Health Administration (OSHA) have established and publicized guidelines for safe handling of antineoplastic medications. The guidelines include information on safe storage and disposal as well as safe handling.

CHAPTER
57

Understanding the Chapter

Key Concepts Summary

57.1 Antineoplastic drugs kill or stop the growth of cancer cells and may be classified in multiple ways.

57.2 Alkylating agents change the shape of the deoxyribonucleic acid double helix and prevent cancer cells from dividing normally.

57.3 Antimetabolites disrupt the critical cellular pathways of cancer cells.

57.4 The antibiotic antineoplastics contain substances obtained from bacteria that have the ability to kill cancer cells.

57.5 Hormones and hormone antagonists block the substances necessary for continued growth of tumors.

57.6 Natural products that are derived from plants include the vinca alkaloids, taxanes, and topoisomerase inhibitors.

57.7 Biologic response modifiers and targeted therapies enhance the body's ability to kill tumor cells.

57.8 Several miscellaneous antineoplastics act by unique mechanisms.

57.9 Medications are used to relieve the adverse effects experienced by patients undergoing chemotherapy.

57.10 Nurses who are preparing and delivering antineoplastics must exercise extreme caution to protect themselves from medication exposure.

Case Study: Making the Patient Connection

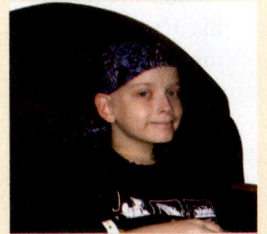

Remember the patient "Zack Amos" at the beginning of the chapter? Now read the remainder of the case study. Based on the information presented within this chapter, respond to the critical thinking questions that follow.

Zack is a 12-year-old boy who had been in good health with no significant medical history until 6 months ago. At that time he began to experience episodic migraine-like headaches, and with a paternal family history of migraines, Zack was evaluated for possible antimigraine therapy if the headaches continued. After 3 months of increasing severity of the headaches, he was diagnosed by CT scan with a brain tumor. Zack underwent craniotomy for evacuation of a malignant tumor and began chemotherapy 1 month after surgery, prior to planned radiation therapy treatments. He has completed one cycle of chemotherapy over 2 months and will have a second cycle prior to radiation. He visits the oncology clinic today for evaluation prior to his second round of chemotherapy.

Physical examination on this clinic visit reveals a pleasant young male in no obvious distress. Zack weighs 43.6 kg (96 lb) and is 157.5 cm (62 in.) in height. BP is 92/40 mmHg, pulse rate is 92 beats/min, respirations of 24 breaths/min, and temperature of 37.1°C (98.8°F). Zack denies having any pain and his neurologic exam is unremarkable except for diminished patellar DTRs, graded at 1 (decreased but present; normal of 2). His WBC count is 3,420/mm³; ANC, 1,800; hemoglobin (Hgb), 13 g/dL; hematocrit (Hct), 36.5%; and his platelet count is 225,000. CBC is within the range expected postchemotherapy. Zack will be hospitalized for approximately 2 days for administration of cyclophosphamide (Cytoxan), carboplatin (Paraplatin), and vincristine (Oncovin) and will continue to receive doses of vincristine as an outpatient and start etoposide (VePesid) in several weeks. Because he experienced significant nausea and vomiting with the last round of chemotherapy, he will also be given ondansetron (Zofran) regularly with supplemental corticosteroids IV as needed.

Critical Thinking Questions

1. Why are four antineoplastic drugs used for Zack? What is the pharmacologic classification of each of the drugs used?

2. What overlapping toxicities might Zack experience with these drugs? Considering his physical assessment findings from today, what system toxicities would be of most concern?

3. Fifteen days after the start of the second cycle of chemotherapy, Zack experiences his nadir. At this time his WBC count is 340/mm^3; ANC, 98; Hgb, 9.3 g/dL; Hct, 25.7%; and the platelet count is 55,000. Zack has been receiving filgrastim (Neupogen) subcutaneously since discharge and will continue until the WBC count begins to rise. Considering these laboratory values, what would be of most concern to the oncology team? What teaching should Zack and his family receive?

See Answers to Critical Thinking Questions on student resource website.

Additional Case Study

Ansen Rosenthal is a 25-year-old male who has recently begun chemotherapy at the local oncology center for treatment of Hodgkin's lymphoma. He has tolerated the chemotherapy fairly well but has experienced mild, daily nausea with occasional vomiting, usually controlled by granisetron (Kytril). His main concern is the fatigue he experiences and the impact it has on his work as a computer science engineer. He also admits that he has been experiencing anorexia and "just doesn't feel like eating much," something which

may be contributing to his fatigue. He has lost 2 kg (more than 4 lb) since his last clinic visit two weeks ago.

1. If you were Ansen's nurse, how might you manage his chemotherapy-related nausea and anorexia?

2. What suggestions might assist Ansen in managing his fatigue?

See Answers to Additional Case Study on student resource website.

Chapter Review

1 The nurse is preparing to administer cyclophosphamide (Cytoxan) and knows that the patient will experience a nadir in approximately 9 to 14 days. Which laboratory value(s) will indicate to the nurse that the patient has reached the nadir?

1. Blood urea nitrogen and creatinine
2. White blood cell count and absolute neutrophil count
3. Ionized calcium
4. Serum albumin

2 A patient has been receiving vincristine (Oncovin) as one of the drugs in a chemotherapy regimen. What important findings will the nurse monitor to prevent or limit the main dose-related toxicity for this patient? Select all that apply.

1. Numbness of the hands or feet
2. Angina and dysrhythmias
3. Constipation
4. Diminished reflexes
5. Dyspnea and pleuritis

3 A nurse is caring for a patient who is receiving tamoxifen for treatment of breast cancer. The nurse will teach the patient that postchemotherapy monitoring will be necessary to detect or treat which drug-associated adverse effect?

1. Paralytic ileus
2. Alopecia
3. Pulmonary fibrosis
4. Endometrial cancer

4 A patient with acute lymphoblastic leukemia has started therapy with doxorubicin (Adriamycin). The nurse will assist the patient with what important intervention during the course of this treatment?

1. Perform active or assisted range-of-motion (ROM) exercises to maintain strength.
2. Participate in relaxation therapy to control pain.
3. Use daily mouth rinses as prescribed.
4. Maintain bed rest during treatment.

5 The patient will continue to take methotrexate (MTX, Rheumatrex, Trexall) for treatment of osteosarcoma. When teaching the patient prior to discharge, what over-the-counter (OTC) drugs must not be taken concurrently with methotrexate?

1. Nonsteroidal anti-inflammatory drug pain relievers
2. Antihistamines
3. Laxatives
4. Cough suppressants

6 A patient receiving carboplatin (Paraplatin) is also receiving filgrastim (Neupogen). The nurse will explain to the patient that the filgrastim is used for what effect?

1. It boosts the effects of the carboplatin so a decreased dosage is needed.
2. It prevents the development of secondary cancers related to the carboplatin.
3. It shortens the duration of neutropenia and associated infection risk related to the carboplatin.
4. It prevents bone loss and osteoporosis.

See Answers to Chapter Review in Appendix A.

References

American Cancer Society. (2014a). *Non-small cell lung cancer survival rates by stage*. Retrieved from http://www.cancer.org/cancer/lungcancer-non-smallcell/detailedguide/non-small-cell-lung-cancer-survival-rates

American Cancer Society. (2014b). *What are the key statistics about breast cancer?* Retrieved from http://www.cancer.org/cancer/breastcancer/detailedguide/breast-cancer-key-statistics

Cavaletti, G., Alberti, P., Frigeni, B., Piatti, M., & Susani, E. (2011). Chemotherapy-induced neuropathy. *Current Treatment Options in Neurology, 13,* 180–190. doi:10.1007/s11940-010-0108-3

Hung, A., & Mullins, C. D. (2013). Relative effectiveness and safety of chemotherapy in elderly and nonelderly patients with stage III colon cancer: A systematic review. *The Oncologist, 18,* 54–63. doi:10.1634/theoncologist.2012-0050

Prostate Cancer Foundation. (2014). *Prostate cancer FAQs*. Retrieved from http://www.pcf.org/site/c.leJRIROrEpH/b.5800851/k.645A/Prostate_Cancer_FAQs.htm

Versteeg, K. S., Konings, I. R., Lagaay, A. M., van de Loosdrecht, A. A., & Verheul, H. M. (2014). Prediction of treatment related toxicity and outcome with geriatric assessment in elderly patients with solid malignancies treated with chemotherapy: A systematic review. *Annals of Oncology*. Advance online publication. doi:10.1093/annonc/mdu052

Visvanathan, K., Hurley, P., Bantug, E., Brown, P., Col, N. F., Cuzick, J., . . . Lippman, S. M. (2013). Use of pharmacologic interventions for breast cancer risk reduction: American Society of Clinical Oncology clinical practice guideline. *Journal of Clinical Oncology, 31,* 2942–2962. doi:10.1200/JCO.2013.49.3122

Selected Bibliography

American Cancer Society. (2014). *Cancer facts and figures 2014*. Retrieved from http://www.cancer.org/research/cancerfactsstatistics/cancerfactsfigures2014/index

Bruce, S. D. (2013). Before you press that button: A look at chemotherapy errors. *Clinical Journal of Oncology Nursing, 17*(1), 31–32. doi:10.1188/13.CJON.31-32

Chabner, B. A., Barnes, J., Neal, J., Olson, E., Mujagic, H., Sequist, L., . . . Richardson, P. (2011). Targeted therapies: Tyrosine kinase inhibitors, monoclonal antibodies and cytokines. In L. L. Brunton, B. A. Chabner, & B. C. Knollman (Eds.), *The pharmacological basis of therapeutics* (12th ed., pp. 1731–1754). New York, NY: McGraw-Hill.

Chabner, B. A., Bertino, J., Cleary, J., Ortiz, T., Lane, A., Supko, J. G., & Ryan, D. (2011). Cytotoxic agents. In L. L. Brunton, B. A. Chabner, & B. C. Knollman (Eds.), *The pharmacological basis of therapeutics* (12th ed., pp. 1677–1730). New York, NY: McGraw-Hill.

Halfdanarson, T. R., & Jatoi, A. (2010). Oral cancer chemotherapy: The critical interplay between patient education and patient safety. *Current Oncology Reports, 12,* 247–252. doi:10.1007/s11912-010-0103-6

Herdman, T. H., & Kamisuru, S. (Eds.). (2014). *NANDA International nursing diagnoses: Definitions and classification, 2015–2017*. Oxford, United Kingdom: Wiley-Blackwell.

Lizée, G., Overwijk, W. W., Radvanyi, L., Gao, J., Sharma, P., & Hwu, P. (2013). Harnessing the power of the immune system to target cancer. *Annual Review of Medicine, 64,* 71–90. doi:10.1146/annurev-med-112311-083918

Mendelsohn, J. (2013). Personalizing oncology: Perspectives and prospects. *Journal of Clinical Oncology, 31,* 1904–1911. doi:10.1200/JCO.2012.45.3605

Montagna, E., Cancello, G., & Colleoni, M. (2013). The aromatase inhibitors (plus ovarian function suppression) in premenopausal breast cancer patients: Ready for prime time? *Cancer Treatment Reviews, 39,* 886–890. doi:10.1016/j.ctrv.2013.04.007

Moy, B., Lee, R. J., & Smith, M. (2011). Natural products in cancer chemotherapy: Hormones and related agents. In L. L. Brunton, B. A. Chabner, & B. C. Knollman (Eds.), *The pharmacological basis of therapeutics* (12th ed., pp. 1755–1770). New York, NY: McGraw-Hill.

Watts, R. G., & Parsons, K. (2013). Chemotherapy medication errors in a pediatric cancer treatment center: Prospective characterization of error types and frequency and development of a quality improvement initiative to lower the error rate. *Pediatric Blood & Cancer, 60,* 1320–1324. doi:10.1002/pbc.24514

Yarbro, C. H., Wujcik, D., & Gobel, B. H. (2011). *Cancer nursing: Principles and practice* (7th ed.). Sudbury, MA: Jones-Bartlett.

UNIT

9

Pharmacology of the Gastrointestinal System

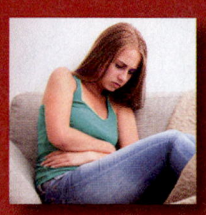 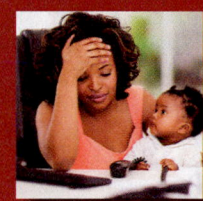 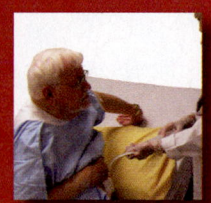 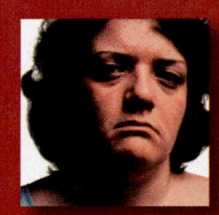

CHAPTER 58   Review of the Gastrointestinal System / 996

CHAPTER 59   Pharmacotherapy of Peptic Ulcer Disease / 1004

CHAPTER 60   Pharmacotherapy of Bowel Disorders and Other Gastrointestinal Conditions / 1023

CHAPTER 61   Vitamins and Minerals / 1047

CHAPTER 62   Enteral and Parenteral Nutrition / 1062

CHAPTER 63   Weight Reduction Strategies and the Pharmacotherapy of Obesity / 1078

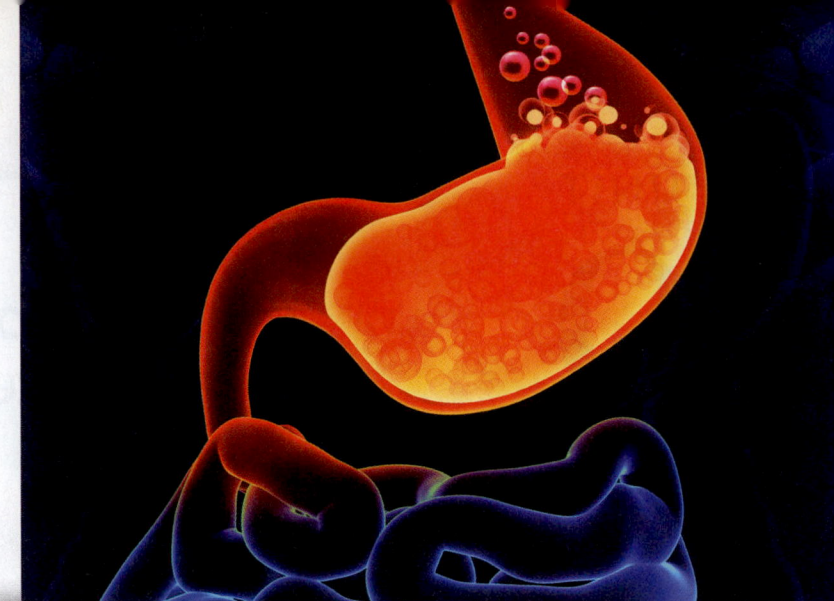

Review of the Gastrointestinal System

LEARNING OUTCOMES

After reading this chapter, the student should be able to:

1. Describe the major anatomic structures of the digestive system.
2. Outline the steps in the process of digestion.
3. Describe the primary functions of the stomach.
4. Analyze how the anatomic structures of the small intestine promote the absorption of nutrients and drugs.
5. Describe the primary structures and functions of the large intestine.
6. Describe the functions of the liver and their relevance to drug therapy.
7. Explain the hepatic portal system and its importance to drug therapy.
8. Explain the nervous control of digestion.
9. Explain the enzymatic breakdown of nutrients by the digestive system.

CHAPTER OUTLINE

▶ Overview of the Digestive System

▶ Physiology of the Upper Gastrointestinal Tract

▶ Physiology of the Lower Gastrointestinal Tract

▶ Physiology of the Accessory Organs of Digestion

▶ Regulation of Digestive Processes

▶ Nutrient Categories and Metabolism

Very little of the food we eat is directly available to body cells. Food must be broken down, absorbed, and chemically modified before it is in a form that is useful to cells. The digestive system performs these functions and many more. This chapter focuses on the aspects of digestion and physiology that are applicable to pharmacotherapy. For a complete review of the digestive system, the student should refer to an anatomy and physiology textbook.

Overview of the Digestive System

58.1 The function of the digestive system is to extract nutrients from food to fuel metabolic processes in the body.

The **digestive system** consists of two basic anatomic divisions: the alimentary canal and the accessory organs. The **alimentary canal**, or gastrointestinal (GI) tract, is a long, continuous, hollow tube that extends from the mouth to the anus. The **accessory organs of digestion** include the salivary glands, liver, gallbladder, and pancreas. The major structures of the digestive system are illustrated in Figure 58.1.

The overall function of the digestive system is to extract nutrients from food so that they may be used to fuel the metabolic processes in the body. Because food is a complex substance, multiple steps are necessary before cells can use its components. These steps are ingestion, propulsion, digestion, absorption, and defecation.

Ingestion is taking food into the body by mouth. In some patients, ingestion bypasses the mouth and delivers nutrients directly into the stomach or small intestine via a feeding tube.

Substances are propelled along the GI tract by **peristalsis**, which is the rhythmic contractions of layers of smooth muscle. The speed at which substances move through the GI tract is critical to the absorption of drugs, nutrients, and water and for the removal of wastes. If peristalsis is too fast, substances will not have sufficient contact with the GI mucosa to be absorbed. In addition, the large intestine will not have enough time to absorb water, and diarrhea may result. Abnormally slow transit may result in constipation or even obstructions in the small or large intestine.

Digestion is the mechanical and chemical breakdown of food into a form that may be absorbed into the systemic circulation. To chemically break down ingested food, a large number of enzymes and other substances are required. Digestive enzymes are secreted by the salivary glands, stomach, small intestine, and pancreas. The liver makes bile, which is stored in the gallbladder until it is needed for lipid digestion.

Absorption is the movement of nutrients and other substances from the alimentary canal to the circulation. The inner lining of the alimentary canal, called the mucosa layer, provides a surface area

for the various acids, bases, and enzymes to break down food. In many parts of the alimentary canal, the mucosa is folded and contains deep grooves and pits. The small intestine is lined with tiny projections called villi and microvilli that provide a huge surface area for the absorption of nutrients and medications.

Not all components of ingested food are useful to the human body or can be digested. The elimination of indigestible substances from the body is called **defecation**.

Physiology of the Upper Gastrointestinal Tract

58.2 The upper gastrointestinal tract is responsible for mechanical and chemical digestion.

The upper GI tract consists of the mouth, pharynx, esophagus, and stomach. From a pharmacologic perspective, the most important regions of the upper GI tract are the buccal and sublingual areas of the mouth and the stomach.

PharmFACT

Most people believe that obese people have larger stomachs. However, people who are naturally thin have the same size as or even larger stomachs than people who have problems with weight control. Weight has nothing to do with the size of the stomach (Bouchez, n.d.).

The epithelial mucosa of the buccal and sublingual regions is very thin, being only 40 to 50 cells in thickness. The mucosal layer, along with the salivary glands, secretes mucus, which lubricates and moistens the oral cavity. The mucus also serves as a liquid medium for drug administration inside the mouth. The oral mucosa in the sublingual region is relatively permeable, and drugs are rapidly absorbed. The buccal region is less permeable, and drug absorption is slower. The buccal region, however, has less salivary flow and drugs can be retained longer, making it better suited for sustained release delivery systems. For example, Striant is a buccal form of testosterone that is designed to release the drug over an 8- to 12-hour period.

The pharynx and esophagus serve as passageways for ingested food and liquids. Obstruction of these areas, or a loss of the swallowing reflex, precludes the administration of oral drugs. Little absorption occurs across the pharyngeal or esophageal mucosa because drugs travel quickly through these regions of the alimentary canal.

Food passes from the esophagus to the stomach by traveling through the lower esophageal (cardiac) sphincter. This ring of smooth muscle usually prevents the stomach contents from moving backward, a condition known as gastroesophageal reflux. The stomach has both mechanical and chemical functions. The muscular squeezing of the stomach churns and mixes the food, breaking it down mechanically to a semisolid known as **chyme**. Strong

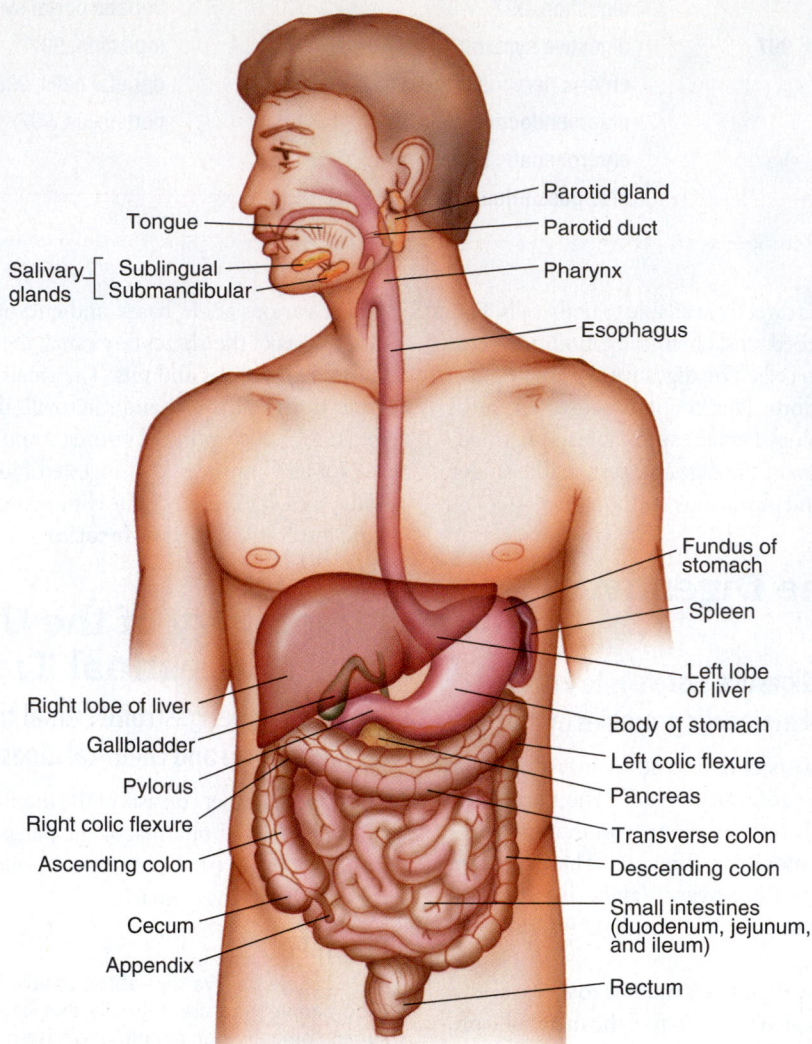

Figure 58.1 The digestive system.

peristaltic contractions push the chyme toward the pylorus, where it encounters a second ring of smooth muscle called the pyloric sphincter. Located at the entrance to the small intestine, this sphincter regulates the flow of substances leaving the stomach. Chyme moves in "spurts" through the sphincter into the small intestine. Large pieces of food are refluxed back into the body of the stomach, where they are subjected to more churning to reduce them in size to about 2 mm so that they may pass through the sphincter.

The stomach also secretes substances that promote the processes of chemical digestion. Gastric glands extending deep into the mucosa of the stomach contain several cell types that are critical to digestion and that are important to the pharmacotherapy of digestive disorders:

- **Chief cells** secrete pepsinogen, an inactive form of the enzyme pepsin that chemically breaks down proteins.
- **Parietal cells** secrete 1 to 3 liters of hydrochloric acid each day. This strong acid helps to break down food, activates pepsinogen, and kills microbes that may have been ingested. Parietal cells also secrete intrinsic factor, which is essential for the absorption of vitamin B_{12}.

- **Enteroendocrine cells** secrete hormones that modify the digestive processes. In the stomach, the most important secretion is gastrin, which stimulates acid production by the parietal cells.

The combined secretion of the chief and parietal cells, known as gastric juice, is the most acidic fluid in the body, having a pH of 1.5 to 3.5. A number of natural defenses protect the stomach mucosa against this extremely acidic fluid. Certain cells that line the surface of the stomach secrete a thick, mucous layer and bicarbonate ion to neutralize the acid. These form such an effective protective layer that the pH at the mucosal surface is nearly neutral. On reaching the duodenum, the stomach contents are further neutralized by bicarbonate from pancreatic and biliary secretions.

The pharmacologic importance of the stomach lies in its capacity to absorb drugs. For most oral drugs, the stomach is not the primary site of absorption because the drug does not stay long in the organ. Stomach acidity (pH 1 to 2) can either assist in the absorption process or destroy the drug entirely. Drugs that are weak acids tend to be absorbed in the stomach. Protein drugs are destroyed by pepsin in the stomach before they are absorbed or have a chance to reach the small intestine.

CONNECTION Checkpoint 58.1

Nitroglycerin is the most frequently prescribed sublingual medication. From what you learned in Chapter 35, what is the primary indication for nitroglycerin and what is the onset of action time of the drug when it is given by the sublingual route? *See Answer to Connection Checkpoint 58.1 on student resource website.*

Physiology of the Lower Gastrointestinal Tract

58.3 The small intestine is the longest portion of the alimentary canal and is the primary organ for absorption.

The lower GI tract consists of the small and large intestines. With its many folds and finger-like projections of villi and microvilli, the small intestine is highly specialized for absorption. The lining of each villus is composed of a single layer of epithelial cells and contains blood capillaries, as illustrated in Figure 58.2. Essentially, only a single cell separates a nutrient or drug molecule from the intestinal lumen of the body's circulatory system.

The first 10 inches of the small intestine, known as the duodenum, is the site where chyme mixes with bile from the gallbladder and digestive enzymes from the pancreas. Bile and pancreatic juice enter through an opening in the duodenum known as the duodenal papilla. The duodenum is sometimes considered part of the upper GI tract because of its proximity to the stomach. Peptic ulcer, the most common disorder of the duodenum, is discussed in Chapter 59.

PharmFACT

Energy drinks are consumed by 30% to 50% of children, adolescents, and young adults (Seifert, Schaechter, Hershorin, & Lipshultz, 2011). Because these drinks are classified as nutritional supplements, they avoid the limit of 71 mg of caffeine per 12 fluid ounces that the U.S. Food and Drug Administration has set for soda. Energy drinks contain as much as 75 to 400 mg of caffeine per container and sometimes contain even more caffeine (not included on the label) coming from additives such as guarana, kola nut, yerba mate, and cocoa.

The remainder of the small intestine consists of the jejunum and ileum. Because of its length and enormous absorptive surface, the first 1 to 2 meters of the jejunum is the site of the majority of nutrient and drug absorption. As the jejunum becomes the ileum, the diameter of the intestinal lumen diminishes and the villi become fewer in number. The terminal ileum is a primary site for the absorption of vitamin B$_{12}$, long-chain fatty acids, and fat-soluble vitamins. The ileum empties its contents into the large intestine

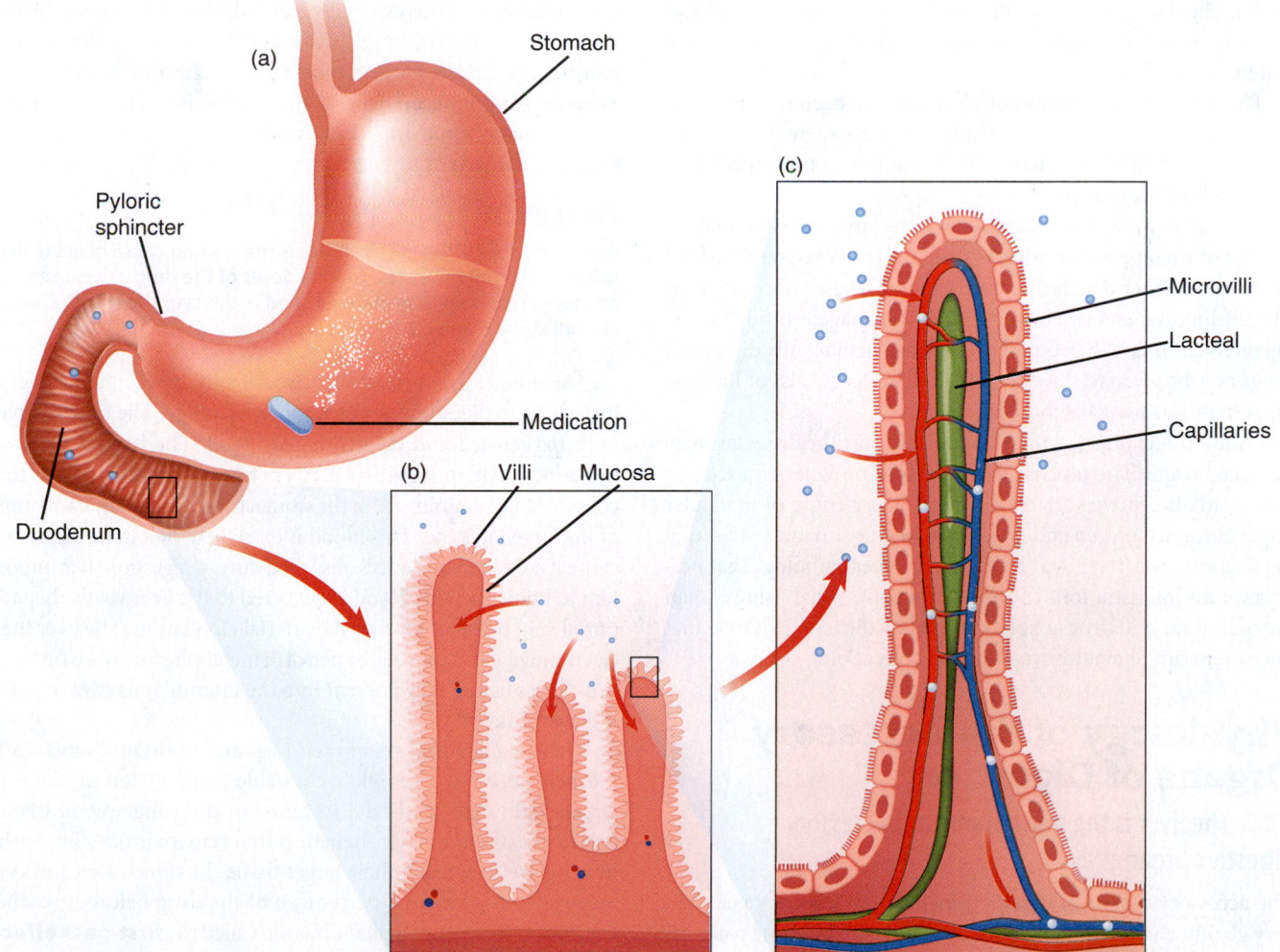

Figure 58.2 Villi and microvilli of the small intestine: (a) Tablet dissolves in the stomach. (b) Medication reaches the villi of the duodenum. (c) Drug molecules are absorbed into the microvilli capillaries.

through the ileocecal valve. Travel time for chyme through the entire small intestine varies from 3 to 6 hours.

The mucosa of the small intestine secretes intestinal juice, which is a mixture of mucus and digestive enzymes. The mucus has an alkaline pH, which neutralizes the acidity from the stomach. The small intestine also secretes cholecystokinin, a hormone that promotes pancreatic enzyme secretion and secretin, which stimulates bicarbonate production to make the small intestine more alkaline.

CONNECTION Checkpoint 58.2

Many oral drugs have enteric coatings. From what you learned in Chapter 3, what is the purpose of the enteric coating and why are these drugs not to be split or crushed? *See Answer to Connection Checkpoint 58.2 on student resource website.*

58.4 The large intestine contains host flora and is a major site of water reabsorption.

The large intestine, or colon, receives chyme from the ileum in a fluid state. The large intestine does not secrete digestive enzymes nor does it have enteroendocrine cells to secrete hormones. With few exceptions, little reabsorption of nutrients occurs during the 12- to 24-hour journey through the colon. The large intestine does secrete a large amount of mucus, which helps lubricate the fecal matter. The major functions of the colon are to reabsorb water and electrolytes from the waste material and excrete the remaining fecal material from the body.

The colon harbors a substantial amount of bacteria and fungi, called the host flora, which serve a useful purpose by synthesizing B-complex vitamins and vitamin K. Disruption of the normal host flora can lead to diarrhea.

From a pharmacologic perspective, the large intestine may be the site of therapeutic or adverse drug effects. A large number of drugs cause either diarrhea or constipation. These effects are usually self-limiting and can be prevented or managed through nursing interventions. When bowel patterns are significantly disrupted, drugs may be given to slow the activity (antidiarrheals) or increase the activity (laxatives) of the large intestine.

Of additional pharmacologic importance are the drugs given by the rectal route. The mucosa of the rectum provides an excellent and rapid absorptive surface for drugs. It is a route of particular importance in children and in patients who are unable to take oral medications due to nausea, vomiting, or other pathology that prevents oral administration. The onset of action is usually slower than the oral route, and drug action is limited by the length of time that the patient can retain the drug without defecation.

Physiology of the Accessory Organs of Digestion

58.5 The liver is the most important accessory digestive organ.

The accessory organs of digestion include the teeth, tongue, salivary glands, pancreas, gallbladder, and liver. Of these, the pancreas and liver have the most pharmacologic importance. The endocrine functions of the pancreas, which include the secretion of insulin and glucagon, are presented in Chapter 66.

The liver is one of the most important organs in pharmacology. Along with the kidneys, any drug that reaches the circulation, regardless of its route of administration, will pass through the liver. The overall function of the liver is to filter and process the nutrients and drugs delivered to it. Substances may be stored, chemically altered, or removed from the blood before they reach the general circulation. The following are some of the primary functions of the liver:

- **Regulation.** Stabilizes the serum levels of glucose, triglycerides, and cholesterol
- **Protection.** Removes toxic substances and waste products such as ammonia
- **Synthesis.** Synthesizes bile, plasma proteins, and certain clotting factors
- **Storage.** Stores iron and fat-soluble vitamins

When most drugs reach the liver, they are metabolized to less toxic substances that are more easily excreted by the kidney. The cytochrome P450 enzyme system in liver cells is especially active at metabolizing drugs; the various isozymes of CYP450 are discussed in Chapter 3. In a few cases, the liver changes the drug to a more active form. It is important to note that the handling of drugs and toxic substances by the liver can damage hepatocytes and impair their functions. This is especially true if the hepatocytes are chronically exposed to harmful substances such as alcohol. Hepatic impairment is a relatively common adverse effect of certain drugs. Whereas drug-induced hepatic impairment is often transient and asymptomatic, some drugs can cause severe, permanent, and even fatal liver damage.

PharmFACT

Acetaminophen (Tylenol) overdose is the leading cause of acute liver failure in the United States. Normal doses of the drug can cause acetaminophen poisoning in malnourished patients or those with chronic alcohol abuse (Farrell, 2014).

The unique structure of the vascular system serving the liver is important to digestion as well as pharmacology. The liver receives both oxygenated and deoxygenated blood. The **hepatic portal system**, shown in Figure 58.3, is a network of venous vessels that collects blood draining from the stomach, small intestine, and most of the large intestine. This blood is extremely rich in nutrients because it contains substances absorbed during digestion. It is important to know that this blood is delivered to the liver via the hepatic portal vein before it reaches the arterial circulation. The liver then can remove, store, excrete, or perform metabolic functions on these substances before they are sent into the inferior vena cava to reach other organs.

The hepatic portal system serves as an important homeostatic mechanism, allowing a relatively stable composition of blood to circulate through the body. In terms of drug therapy, nearly all oral medications enter the hepatic portal vein for processing by the liver before they reach their target tissue. In some cases, the liver inactivates a substantial percentage of the drug before it reaches the inferior vena cava, a phenomenon called the **first-pass effect**. Drugs that have a significant first-pass effect may be given by other routes, such as intramuscular, intravenous, subcutaneous, or topical. Although a drug will still eventually reach the liver by

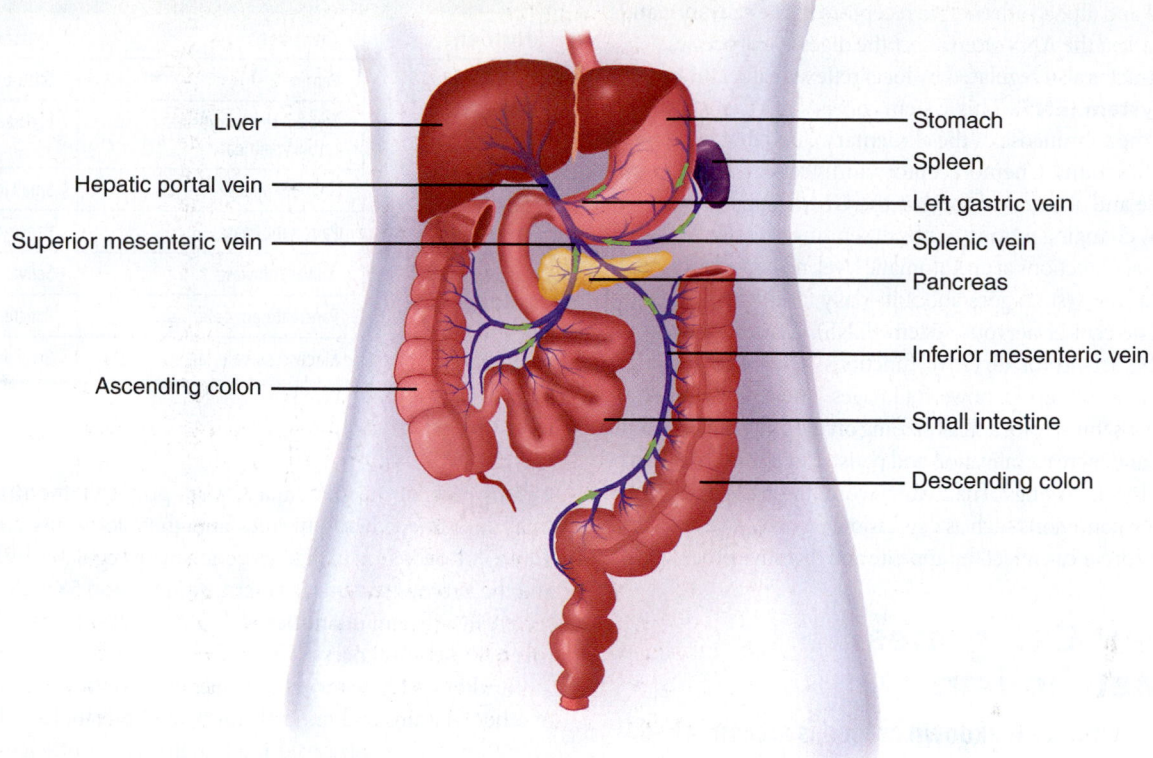

Figure 58.3 Hepatic portal circulation.

these routes, it will have an opportunity to also reach its target tissue. Note that the venous systems serving the head and the lower rectum are not parts of the hepatic portal system. Thus, drugs that are given by the buccal, sublingual, or rectal routes bypass the first-pass effect of the liver.

As the liver makes bile, the bile is sent to the gallbladder where it is stored. When lipids enter the small intestine, the gallbladder contracts and sends its contents into the duodenum. The bile salts emulsify the lipids, making them easier to digest enzymatically. When bile salts reach the terminal portion of the ileum, 95% are reabsorbed back into the hepatic portal circulation by a process called **enterohepatic recirculation**. This process has direct implications to pharmacotherapy. Certain drugs, including digoxin (Lanoxin), morphine, and estrogens, are eliminated in the bile and are reabsorbed by enterohepatic recirculation. Enterohepatic recirculation recycles the drug multiple times and can significantly extend a drug's half-life. Interactions can occur if one drug interferes with the enterohepatic recycling of another drug. Preventing this recycling can speed the elimination of a drug and reduce its therapeutic effectiveness. An example of such an interaction is when cholestyramine (Questran) interferes with the recycling of lorazepam (Ativan) and increases the clearance of lorazepam from the body.

The pancreas is an essential accessory digestive organ, secreting about a quart of pancreatic fluid into the duodenum each day. This fluid is alkaline (pH 7.5 to 8.8) and contains digestive enzymes to chemically break down carbohydrates, lipids, proteins, and nucleic acids. From a pharmacologic perspective, the pancreas is relatively protected from drugs and there are only a few therapies for pancreatic digestive disorders.

CONNECTION Checkpoint 58.3

The tricyclic antidepressant imipramine is a substrate for the CYP2D6 enzyme, and the selective serotonin reuptake inhibitor (SSRI) fluoxetine is a potent inhibitor of this enzyme. From what you learned in Chapter 5, predict the type of drug interaction that will occur to a patient stabilized on imipramine therapy when fluoxetine is added to the regimen. *See Answer to Connection Checkpoint 58.3 on student resource website.*

Regulation of Digestive Processes

58.6 Digestion is regulated by numerous hormonal and nervous factors.

Digestion is controlled through a large number of hormonal and nervous factors that influence the speed of peristalsis and the amount of saliva, mucus, acid, and enzyme secretions. Various negative feedback loops help to regulate these activities so that digestion is a smooth, continuous process. Disruption of normal homeostatic mechanisms can cause cramping, due to excessive peristalsis, or peptic ulcers, due to the overproduction of gastric acid.

The nervous control of digestion is provided at several levels. Chapter 12 discusses the role of the autonomic nervous system (ANS) in controlling the contraction of smooth muscle and glandular secretion. Activation of the parasympathetic nervous system stimulates the digestive processes by increasing peristalsis, salivation, and digestive gland secretion. The sympathetic nervous system has the opposite effects, with beta$_2$-adrenergic receptors in the intestinal wall and alpha$_1$-adrenergic receptors in the salivary glands. Drugs that affect the ANS often affect the digestive processes.

The GI tract is also regulated by local reflexes called the **enteric nervous system (ENS)**. This system consists of a vast network of neurons in the submucosa of the alimentary canal that has sensory and motor functions. Chemoreceptors and stretch receptors sense the presence and amount of food in the GI tract and respond accordingly by changing motility without sending signals to the ANS.

The GI tract functions at an automatic level; no conscious thought is required as the system goes about its daily tasks of secretion and digestion. The central nervous system (CNS), however, can greatly influence the activity of digestive functions. For example, merely thinking of food can evoke powerful images. These may be positive, such as perhaps thinking of a steak sizzling on the grill or bread baking in the oven, and increase salivation and peristalsis. Images may also be negative and evoke feelings of nausea and vomiting at the sight of food. Mental health conditions such as depression, anxiety, excessive stress, or bipolar disorder can affect the appetite and digestive processes.

Nutrient Categories and Metabolism

58.7 The chemical breakdown of food is accomplished by digestive enzymes.

The three basic nutrients are carbohydrates, lipids, and proteins. In food these nutrients are large molecules that cannot be absorbed across the mucosa of the alimentary canal. Chemical digestion must break down these complex food molecules into simpler substances so that they can be absorbed and used by the body for metabolic processes.

The breakdown of complex carbohydrates, lipids, and proteins requires digestive enzymes to be delivered when food is present at

TABLE 58.1	Major Digestive Enzymes	
Nutrient	**Enzyme**	**Source**
Proteins and polypeptides	Pepsin	Gastric glands
	Trypsin, chymotrypsin, carboxypeptidase	Pancreatic juice
	Aminopeptidase	Small intestine
Lipids	Pancreatic lipase	Pancreatic juice
Carbohydrates and starches	Salivary amylase	Saliva
	Pancreatic amylase	Pancreatic juice
	Maltase, sucrase, lactase	Small intestine

various parts of the alimentary canal, primarily the stomach and small intestine. These enzymes and their locations are listed in Table 58.1. Secretion of digestive enzymes is regulated by hormones and the nervous system, as described in Section 58.6. Patients who secrete insufficient quantities of digestive enzymes may be administered these substances as drugs.

In addition to the three basic nutrients, the body requires a host of other vitamins and minerals for proper metabolism. Deficiency symptoms will be observed if a patient has insufficient intake of these substances. The pharmacotherapy of vitamins and minerals is presented in Chapter 61.

The intake of various nutrients in sufficient amounts is necessary to maintain good health and to allow the body to heal during periods of illness or injury. The intake of sufficient amounts of proteins, carbohydrates, fats, vitamins, and minerals can often be achieved by eating a well-balanced diet of foods and fluids. When this does not occur, enteral or parenteral therapy may be indicated, as presented in Chapter 62.

CHAPTER

58 Understanding the Chapter

Key Concepts Summary

58.1 The function of the digestive system is to extract nutrients from food to fuel metabolic processes in the body.

58.2 The upper gastrointestinal tract is responsible for mechanical and chemical digestion.

58.3 The small intestine is the longest portion of the alimentary canal and is the primary organ for absorption.

58.4 The large intestine contains host flora and is a major site of water reabsorption.

58.5 The liver is the most important accessory digestive organ.

58.6 Digestion is regulated by numerous hormonal and nervous factors.

58.7 The chemical breakdown of food is accomplished by digestive enzymes.

References

Bouchez, C. (n.d.). *9 surprising facts about your stomach*. Retrieved from http://www.webmd.com/women/features/stomach-problems

Farrell, S. E. (2014). *Acetaminophen toxicity*. Retrieved from http://emedicine.medscape.com/article/820200-overview

Seifert, S. M., Schaechter, J. L., Hershorin, E. R., & Lipshultz, S. E. (2011). Health effects of energy drinks on children, adolescents, and young adults. *Pediatrics, 127*, 511–528. doi:10.1542/peds.2009-3592

Selected Bibliography

Krogh, D. (2011). *Biology: A guide to the natural world* (5th ed.). San Francisco, CA: Benjamin Cummings.

Martini, F. H., Nath, J. L., & Bartholomew, E. F. (2012). *Fundamentals of human anatomy and physiology* (9th ed.). San Francisco, CA: Benjamin Cummings.

Silverthorn, D. U. (2012). *Human physiology: An integrated approach* (5th ed.). San Francisco, CA: Benjamin Cummings.

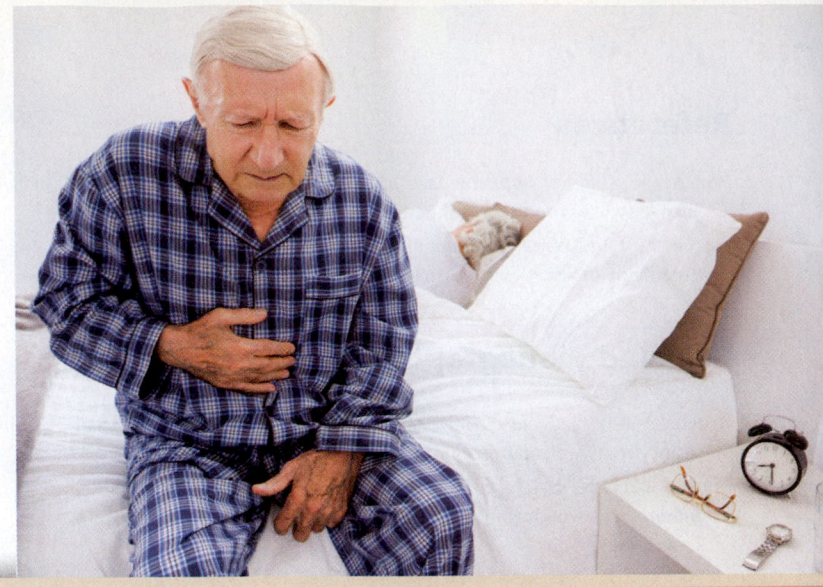

"I was diagnosed with a duodenal ulcer yesterday. Why do I need to take these antibiotics if I don't have an infection?"

Patient "Hugh Marshall"

59 Pharmacotherapy of Peptic Ulcer Disease

LEARNING OUTCOMES

After reading this chapter, the student should be able to:

1. Explain the physiological regulation of gastric acid secretion.
2. Describe factors that suppress and those that promote the formation of peptic ulcers.
3. Compare and contrast duodenal ulcers and gastric ulcers.
4. Identify the etiology, signs, and symptoms of peptic ulcer disease and gastroesophageal reflux disease.
5. Outline the treatment goals for the pharmacotherapy of peptic ulcer disease and gastroesophageal reflux disease.
6. Identify the classification of drugs used to treat peptic ulcer disease and gastroesophageal reflux disease.
7. Explain the pharmacologic strategies for eradicating *Helicobacter pylori*.
8. Describe the nurse's role in the pharmacologic management of patients with peptic ulcer disease and gastroesophageal reflux disease.
9. For each of the classes shown in the chapter outline, identify the prototype and representative drugs and explain the mechanism(s) of drug action, primary indications, contraindications, significant drug interactions, pregnancy category, and important adverse effects.
10. Apply the nursing process to care for patients who are receiving pharmacotherapy for peptic ulcer disease and gastroesophageal reflux disease.

CHAPTER OUTLINE

▸ Physiology of the Upper Gastrointestinal Tract

▸ Etiology and Pathogenesis of Peptic Ulcer Disease

▸ Etiology and Pathogenesis of Gastroesophageal Reflux Disease

▸ Pharmacotherapy of Peptic Ulcer Disease and Gastroesophageal Reflux Disease

Pharmacotherapy with Proton Pump Inhibitors
PROTOTYPE Omeprazole (Prilosec), *p. 101*

Pharmacotherapy with H₂-Receptor Antagonists
PROTOTYPE Ranitidine (Zantac), *p. 1014*

Pharmacotherapy with Antacids
PROTOTYPE Aluminum Hydroxide (AlternaGEL, Others), *p. 1016*

Pharmacotherapy of *Helicobacter pylori* Infection

Miscellaneous Drugs Used for Peptic Ulcer Disease and Gastroesophageal Reflux Disease

adhesins, 1017

antacids, 1015

Barrett's esophagus, 1008

gastroesophageal reflux disease (GERD), 1008

H^+, K^+-ATPase, 1010

H_2-receptor antagonists, 1013

milk-alkali syndrome, 1016

pepsin, 1005

peptic ulcer, 1005

prostaglandin E_2, 1005

proton pump inhibitors (PPIs), 1010

somatostatin, 1005

Zollinger-Ellison syndrome (ZES), 1007

Acid-related diseases of the upper gastrointestinal (GI) tract are some of the most common medical conditions. Drugs for these disorders are available over the counter (OTC), and many patients attempt self-treatment before seeking assistance from their health care provider. Signs and symptoms of acid-related conditions of the upper GI tract, however, may indicate more serious disease. This chapter examines the pharmacotherapy of two common disorders of the upper digestive system: peptic ulcer disease (PUD) and gastroesophageal reflux disease (GERD).

Physiology of the Upper Gastrointestinal Tract

59.1 The stomach secretes acid, enzymes, and hormones that are essential to digestive physiology.

The upper GI tract consists of the mouth, pharynx, esophagus, and stomach. The duodenum, the first 10 inches of the small intestine, is sometimes considered part of the upper GI tract because of its proximity to the stomach. The structures and functions of the upper GI tract are reviewed in Chapter 58.

Gastric glands in the stomach contain several cell types that are critical to digestion and important to the pharmacotherapy of digestive disorders. Chief cells secrete the enzyme pepsinogen, which is then activated to become **pepsin**, which is the digestive enzyme that breaks down proteins from food. Parietal cells secrete gastric (hydrochloric) acid in the stomach, which provides a strongly acidic environment that promotes the conversion of pepsinogen to pepsin, helps to break down food, and kills microbes that may have been ingested. Parietal cells also secrete intrinsic factor, which is essential for the absorption of vitamin B_{12} (see Chapter 58). Parietal cells are targets for the classes of drugs that reduce acid secretion. The cell types present in gastric glands are shown in Figure 59.1.

Parietal cells receive messages from several sources, which signal them to increase or decrease acid production. These cells contain receptors for the hormone gastrin, histamine (H_2), and the neurotransmitter acetylcholine, which are the three principal physiological stimuli that regulate acid secretion from the proton pump, or H^+, K^+-ATPase, located on the surface of parietal cells.

Ingestion of food and distention of the stomach stimulate the secretion of the hormone gastrin into the bloodstream. The target cells for gastrin are enteroendocrine cells in the gastric glands. When gastrin binds to their cell surface, the enteroendocrine cells produce and secrete histamine. Histamine then binds to the H_2 receptor on the parietal cell to stimulate acid secretion. In addition to promoting acid secretion, gastrin signals the chief cells to secrete pepsin, promotes the production of pancreatic enzymes, and increases gastric blood flow.

Like most hormones, gastrin is regulated by a negative feedback loop. As the stomach contents reach pH 3 or lower, the hormone **somatostatin** is released by cells in the stomach, small intestine, and pancreas. This hormone suppresses the secretion of gastrin, thus lowering acid secretion. Interestingly, somatostatin is also released by the anterior pituitary gland and is known as growth hormone-inhibiting hormone. However, the nervous system secretion and actions are independent of its digestive actions.

Cells lining the surface of the stomach mucosa secrete a thick mucous layer that provides a continuous, protective physical barrier against acid and pepsin. Bicarbonate ion is also secreted by the epithelial cells in the stomach and serves to neutralize gastric acid on the mucosal surface. The mucus and bicarbonate ion form such an effective protective layer that the pH at the mucosal surface is nearly neutral. Once the stomach contents reach the duodenum, they are further neutralized by the bicarbonate ion from pancreatic and biliary secretions.

Another protective substance is the hormone **prostaglandin E_2**. This hormone stimulates the secretion of mucus and bicarbonate, promotes repair of damaged gastric mucosal cells, and increases blood flow to the mucosa to help maintain optimal mucosal conditions. Several frequently prescribed drugs, including corticosteroids and nonsteroidal anti-inflammatory drugs (NSAIDs), cause peptic ulcers because they are prostaglandin antagonists. The natural defenses of the stomach are shown in Figure 59.2.

Etiology and Pathogenesis of Peptic Ulcer Disease

59.2 Peptic ulcer disease is associated with a number of etiologic risk factors.

A **peptic ulcer** is a lesion or erosion located in either the stomach (gastric) or small intestine (duodenal) mucosa that is usually associated with acute inflammation. PUD was an uncommon condition until the 19th century. Thus it is considered to be a "disease of civilization." Although PUD occurs most often in middle age, it may occur at any time, including infancy and childhood. A significant family history is present in at least half of children with PUD.

PUD occurs when there is an imbalance of protective factors versus aggravating factors: The levels of protective mucus and bicarbonate ion secretions are unable to protect against the aggravating factors of pepsin and gastric acid. Complications of PUD include bleeding, perforation, penetration, and GI obstruction due to scarring. The incidence of PUD is associated with the following risk factors:

- Infection with the bacterium *Helicobacter pylori* (*H. pylori*)
- Close family history of PUD
- Use of drugs, particularly corticosteroids, NSAIDs, and platelet inhibitors such as aspirin and clopidogrel

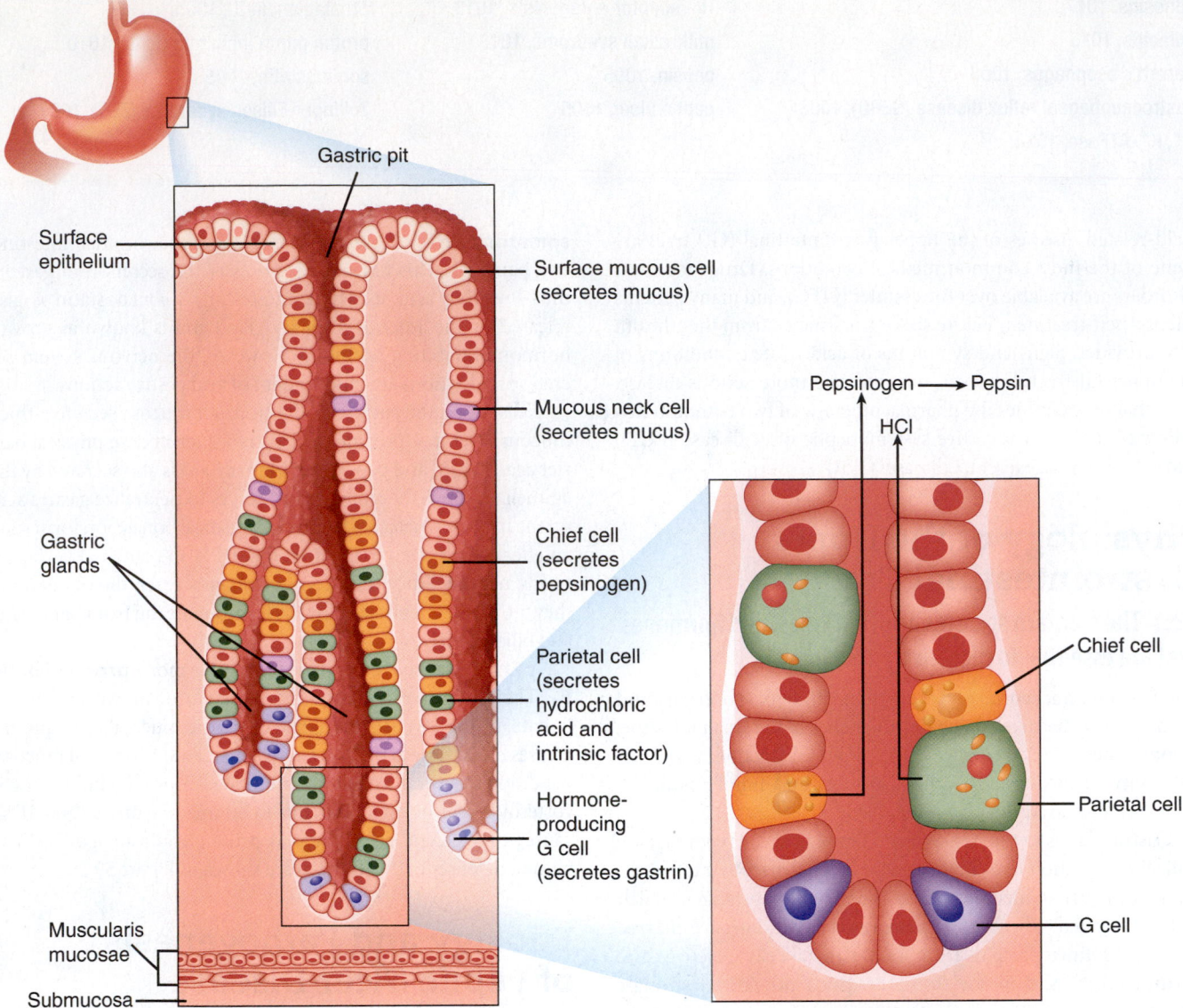

Figure 59.1   The stomach lining: gastric glands and the secretion of hydrochloric acid.

- Blood group O (the antigen may be a target of *H. pylori* attachment)
- Smoking tobacco (increases gastric acid secretion and reduces bicarbonate production)
- Consumption of beverages and foods that contain excessive caffeine
- Excessive psychological stress

PharmFACT

Approximately 4.5 million Americans are affected by PUD, and about 10% of Americans will experience an ulcer in their lifetime (Anand, 2012).

For many decades, it was thought that mental and physiological stress, smoking, and spicy foods were the primary causes of PUD. It was theorized that bacteria could not survive the acidic environment of the stomach; thus the hypothesis that an infectious agent could be the cause of PUD was not accepted. In the 1980s, however, researchers discovered an association between the gram-negative bacterium *H. pylori* and PUD. Over time, the hypothesis was accepted, and treatment of PUD as an infectious disease was aggressively promoted by the Centers for Disease Control and Prevention (CDC). The pharmacotherapy of *H. pylori* is described in Section 59.8.

Many causes of PUD are not related to *H. pylori* infection. For example, drug therapy with NSAIDs is likely responsible for almost half of peptic ulcer cases. Gastric and duodenal ulcers occur in about 20% of patients using NSAIDs on a regular basis, with 4% experiencing serious bleeding.

NSAIDs promote ulcer formation and inflammation both topically and systemically. Topically, NSAIDs cause direct cellular damage to GI mucosal cells. Systemically NSAIDs interfere with prostaglandin synthesis via the enzyme cyclooxygenase (COX) in the stomach, which normally aids in the production of mucus and bicarbonate. NSAIDs decrease gastric blood flow and slow cellular repair. NSAIDs are also weak acids that are nonionized in gastric acid and able to diffuse across the mucous barrier into the gastric epithelial cells, which leads to further cellular damage.

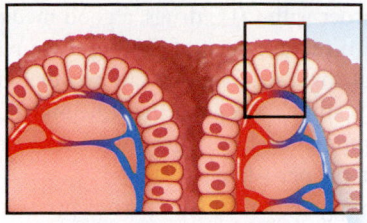

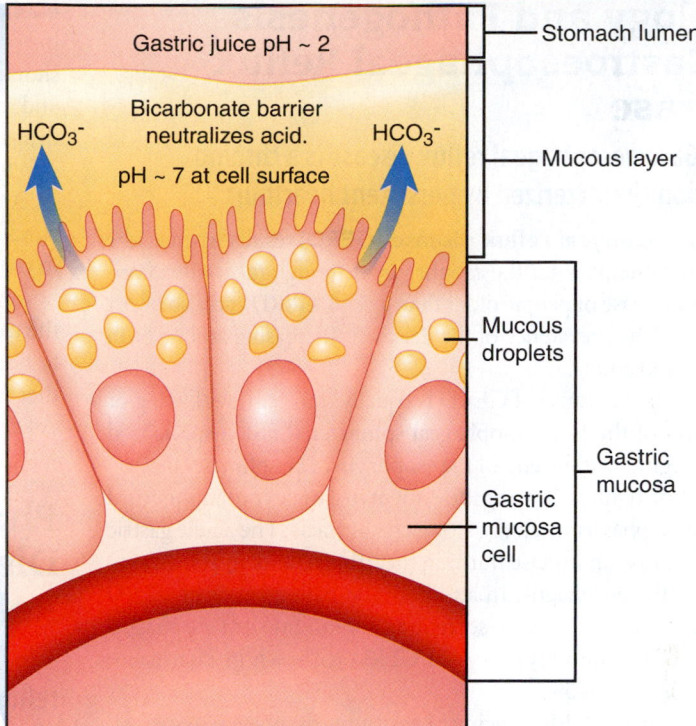

Stomach lumen

Gastric juice pH ~ 2

Bicarbonate barrier neutralizes acid.
pH ~ 7 at cell surface

HCO₃⁻   HCO₃⁻

Mucous layer

Mucous droplets

Gastric mucosa cell

Gastric mucosa

Figure 59.2 Natural defenses against stomach acid.

Risk factors for NSAID-induced PUD include long-term use of NSAIDs, advanced age, history of ulcers, concomitant use of corticosteroids or anticoagulants, or alcohol and cigarette smoking. In addition, *H. pylori* infection and NSAIDs act synergistically to promote ulcers. The combination poses a 3.5-fold greater risk of ulcers than either factor alone.

The characteristic symptom of duodenal ulcer is a gnawing or burning, upper abdominal pain that occurs 1 to 3 hours after a meal. The pain is usually worse when the stomach is empty and often disappears with ingestion of food. This is because the presence of food closes the pyloric sphincter and allows the acid to remain in the stomach, rather than to come into contact with the duodenal ulcer. Night-time pain may awaken the patient. If the erosion progresses deeper into the mucosa, bleeding occurs and may be evident as either bright red blood in vomit or black, tarry stools. Many duodenal ulcers heal spontaneously, although scar tissue remains, predisposing the mucosa to future ulceration, and they frequently recur after months of remission. Perforation and hemorrhage are sometimes the first signs of a duodenal ulcer in infants. Many patients with PUD are asymptomatic.

Gastric ulcers are less common than the duodenal type and have different symptoms. Pain is often relieved with food; however, in some patients the pain is exacerbated with eating. Anorexia, weight loss, and vomiting are more common with gastric ulcers. Remissions may be infrequent or absent. Medical follow-up of gastric ulcers should continue for several years because a small percentage of the erosions become cancerous. The most severe ulcers may penetrate the wall of the stomach and cause death. Whereas duodenal ulcers most frequently occur in males in the 30- to 50-year age group, gastric ulcers are more common in women over age 60. NSAID-related ulcers are more likely to produce gastric ulcers, whereas *H. pylori*–associated ulcers are more likely to be duodenal.

Patients who are experiencing physiological stress resulting from severe trauma, surgery, burns, illness, or shock may experience stress ulcers. Stress ulcers are typically asymptomatic initially, and about 25% of patients present with painless upper GI bleeding. Vasoconstriction secondary to sympathetic nervous system involvement causes decreased blood flow to the small intestine, which may play a role in the development of stress ulcers. Patients who are placed on mechanical ventilation and other seriously ill patients are sometimes administered prophylactic antiulcer drugs to prevent complications due to PUD.

Zollinger-Ellison syndrome (ZES) is a less common cause of PUD. It is caused by a gastrinoma, a tumor of the pancreas or duodenum that secretes large amounts of the hormone gastrin. Because gastrin is the hormonal signal for increasing hydrochloric acid secretion, the huge amounts of acid easily overcome the protective defenses, leading to multiple gastric and duodenal ulcers. Peptic ulcers are persistent, difficult to treat, and slow to heal. Symptoms of ZES are the same as those of PUD. The acid also irritates the GI tract, resulting in diarrhea. Treatment involves aggressive acid suppression with drugs.

Ulceration in the distal small intestine is known as Crohn's disease, and erosions in the large intestine are called ulcerative colitis. These diseases, together categorized as inflammatory bowel disease (IBD), are discussed in Chapter 60.

CONNECTION Checkpoint 59.1

Although surgery is often indicated for ZES, chemotherapy with doxorubicin (Adriamycin) plus streptozocin (Zanosar) is a common combination. From what you learned in Chapter 57, what are the drug classes for these two antineoplastics? *See Answer to Connection Checkpoint 59.1 on student resource website.*

Etiology and Pathogenesis of Gastroesophageal Reflux Disease

59.3 Gastroesophageal reflux disease is a chronic condition characterized by persistent heartburn.

Gastroesophageal reflux disease (GERD) results when acidic stomach contents enter the esophagus. Although most often considered a disease of people older than age 40, GERD can also occur in infants. The prevalence of the disease is increasing among both children and adults.

In adults, the cause of GERD is usually transient weakening or relaxation of the lower esophageal sphincter (LES), a specialized muscle segment at the end of the esophagus. The sphincter may no longer close tightly, allowing movement of gastric contents upward into the esophagus when the stomach contracts. The acidic gastric contents cause an intense burning (heartburn) and, in some cases, injury to the esophagus. In addition, the pathogenesis of GERD involves decreased salivary secretions and diminished esophageal motility. The pathophysiology of GERD is shown in Pharmaco-therapy Illustrated 59.1.

Symptoms of GERD include heartburn, dysphagia, dyspepsia, chest pain, nausea, and belching. Symptoms worsen following large meals, exercise, or when in a reclining or recumbent position. There is growing evidence that patients with GERD may also present with symptoms such as chronic cough, wheezing, bronchitis, sore throat, or hoarseness. GERD is a chronic condition with alternating periods of exacerbation and remission.

A large number of substances and conditions can worsen GERD symptoms. These include caffeine, alcohol, citrus fruits, tomato-based products, onions, carbonated beverages, spicy food, chocolate, smoking, pregnancy, and obesity. Certain medications may also contribute to or worsen GERD. They include nitrates, benzodiazepines, anticholinergics, beta blockers, alpha blockers, estrogen, progesterone, iron, calcium channel blockers, NSAIDs, tricyclic antidepressants, opioids, levodopa, bisphosphonates, and some chemotherapy drugs.

Left untreated, GERD can lead to complications such as esophagitis, esophageal ulcers, or strictures. Approximately 10% of patients diagnosed with GERD will develop **Barrett's esophagus**, a condition that is associated with an increased risk of esophageal cancer. Warning signs and symptoms of GERD that suggest a more complicated disease may include unexplained weight loss, early satiety, anemia, vomiting, initial onset of symptoms after age 50, and prolonged anorexia or dysphagia. Patients who are experiencing these symptoms should notify their health care provider.

PharmFACT

Twenty-five to forty percent of adults in the United States have GERD. Males are two to three times more likely to have the condition than females (Patti, 2014).

If a patient's GERD is associated with obesity, losing weight may eliminate the symptoms. Other lifestyle changes that can improve GERD symptoms include elevating the head of the bed, avoiding fatty or acidic foods, eating smaller meals at least 3 hours before sleep, and eliminating tobacco and alcohol use. Because patients often self-treat this disorder with OTC drugs, a good medication history may give clues to the presence of GERD. Also, patients should be informed that some medications can provoke GERD, and reviewing their medication history may prove helpful. Because drugs provide only symptomatic relief, surgery may become necessary to eliminate the cause of persistent GERD.

An emerging theory suggests that GERD may be a premalignant condition and that chronic acid suppression leads to an increase in esophageal malignancy. This theory is not universally accepted, however, and acid suppression currently remains the mainstay in the treatment of GERD. The presence of GERD does not warrant testing for *H. pylori* infection. Large studies have shown that neither the presence nor absence of *H. pylori* has any influence on the development of GERD.

Pharmacotherapy of Peptic Ulcer Disease and Gastroesophageal Reflux Disease

59.4 Peptic ulcer disease and gastroesophageal reflux disease are best treated with a combination of pharmacotherapy and lifestyle changes.

Before initiating pharmacotherapy, patients are usually advised to change lifestyle factors that may be contributing to the severity of PUD or GERD. For example, eliminating tobacco and alcohol use and reducing stress often allow healing of the ulcer and cause it to go into remission. Avoiding certain foods and beverages can lessen the severity of symptoms. For patients with GERD, losing weight may alleviate symptoms of the disorder.

The goals of PUD pharmacotherapy are to provide immediate relief from symptoms, promote healing of the ulcer, prevent complications, and prevent future recurrence of the disease. Eradication of *H. pylori* and discontinuing NSAIDs or other ulcer-promoting medications when possible are key factors.

For patients who are taking NSAIDs, the initial approach to PUD is to switch to an alternative medication, such as acetaminophen or another analgesic. This is not always possible, however, because NSAIDs are the drugs of choice for treating chronic arthritis and other disorders associated with pain and inflammation. Those with a history of PUD should be advised to avoid NSAIDs in the future to prevent ulcer recurrences. If discontinuation of the NSAID is not possible, concurrent antiulcer drugs are indicated. Platelet inhibitors such as aspirin or clopidogrel should be used cautiously in patients at risk for ulcer complications.

For patients with PUD with *H. pylori* infection, elimination of the bacteria using anti-infective therapy is the primary goal of pharmacotherapy. If the treatment includes only antiulcer drugs without eradicating *H. pylori*, a very high recurrence rate of PUD is observed. It has also been found that eradicating *H. pylori* infection prophylactically decreases the incidence of peptic ulcers in patients who subsequently take NSAIDs.

Once NSAIDs and *H. pylori* have been addressed, suppressing or neutralizing gastric acid is the aim of the pharmacologic treatment of both PUD and GERD. A wide variety of both prescription and OTC drugs are available to suppress acid secretion. The mechanisms of action of the major drug classes for PUD are shown

PHARMACOTHERAPY ILLUSTRATED 59.1

Treatment of Gastroesophageal Reflux Disease (GERD)

Symptoms
- Heartburn
- Nausea
- Chest pain
- Belching

Pathogenesis
- Gastric acid reflux to the esophagus
- Esophageal injury

Esophagus

Stomach

Esophageal sphincter

Stomach acid

H^+

H^+ H^+

Proton pump

H_2-receptor

Treatment
- Remove acid-causing food and drugs
- Administer proton pump inhibitors
- Administer H_2 receptor antagonists

in Pharmacotherapy Illustrated 59.2. These drugs fall into three primary classes and one miscellaneous group:

- Proton pump inhibitors
- H_2-receptor antagonists
- Antacids
- Miscellaneous drugs

Because medications used in treating GERD and PUD suppress acid, it should be kept in mind that certain nutrients and drugs need an acidic environment for complete absorption. For example, long-term acid suppression could lead to a deficiency in folic acid, iron, and vitamin B_{12}. Also, the effects of certain drugs such as fluconazole, tetracyclines, and indomethacin may be decreased because these drugs require an acidic environment for complete absorption.

PHARMACOTHERAPY ILLUSTRATED 59.2

Mechanisms of Action of Antiulcer Drugs

Proton pump inhibitors

Proton pump

H₂-receptor blockers

H₂-receptor

Proton pump inhibitors bind to the enzyme H⁺, K⁺-ATPase and prevent acid from being secreted.

H₂-receptor antagonists occupy the histamine receptors and prevent acid secretion.

Acid secretion

Parietal cell with proton pump

K⁺

Parietal cell with H₂-receptor

Ulcer with *H. pylori*

Antibiotic

Antacid

+ HCL ⟶ water + salt

Antibiotics eradicate *H. pylori*, the primary cause of peptic ulcers.

Alkaline antacids chemically combine with acids to increase stomach pH.

Pharmacotherapy with Proton Pump Inhibitors

59.5 Proton pump inhibitors block gastric acid secretion and are the drugs of choice in the therapy of peptic ulcer disease and gastroesophageal reflux disease.

The **proton pump inhibitors (PPIs)** act by blocking **H⁺, K⁺-ATPase**, the enzyme that is responsible for secreting hydrochloric acid in the stomach. PPIs are indicated for treatment of gastric

and duodenal ulcers for 4 to 8 weeks, treatment of GERD, maintenance therapy to prevent recurrence, and treatment of ZES. Omeprazole and lansoprazole are available OTC. These drugs are listed in Table 59.1.

PPIs reduce acid secretion in the stomach by binding irreversibly to the H⁺, K⁺-ATPase enzyme at the surface of the parietal cell, thereby blocking the final step in acid production. This enzyme acts as a pump to release acid (also called H⁺, or protons) onto the surface of the GI mucosa. The PPIs reduce acid secretion to a greater extent than the H₂-receptor antagonists and have a longer duration

CONNECTIONS Complementary and Alternative Therapies

◀ Ginger's Effect on the Gastrointestinal Tract

Description
Originally from Asia, ginger (*Zingiber officinalis*) is now cultivated in most tropical regions of the world. The active ingredients of ginger, and those that create its spicy flavor and pungent odor, are located in its roots or rhizomes. It has both culinary and medicinal uses.

History and Claims
The use of ginger for medicinal purposes dates to antiquity in India and China, and it is found in many ancient pharmacopeias. Its claimed uses are many and diverse, including antiemetic, antithrombotic, diuretic, anti-inflammatory, promotion of gastric secretions, promotion of blood glucose, and stimulation of peripheral circulation.

Standardization
Like most herbs, ginger contains multiple substances that may contribute to its pharmacologic activity. It is sometimes standardized according to its active substances, known as gingerols and shogaols. It is sold in pharmacies as dried ginger root powder and is readily available at most grocery stores for home cooking. A typical dose is 250 mg of dried root two to four times per day.

Evidence
Ginger is one of the best studied herbs, and it appears to be useful for a number of digestive-related conditions. Perhaps its widest use is for treating nausea, including that caused by motion sickness, pregnancy morning sickness, chemotherapy, and postoperative procedures. It has been shown to stimulate appetite, promote gastric secretions, and increase peristalsis. Newer research has shown that ginger may inhibit the effects of *H. pylori* and may help heal peptic ulcers. Its effects appear to stem from direct action on the GI tract, rather than on the CNS. Ginger has no toxicity when used at recommended doses. Adverse effects include abdominal discomfort and diarrhea. Overdoses may lead to CNS depression, inhibition of platelet aggregation, and cardiotonic effects.

TABLE 59.1 Proton Pump Inhibitors

Drug	Route and Adult Dose (Maximum Dose Where Indicated)	Adverse Effects
esomeprazole (Nexium)	PO: 20–40 mg daily or bid for up to 8 weeks IV: 20–40 mg daily for up to 10 days	*Diarrhea, nausea, rash, abdominal pain* <u>Increased risk for osteoporosis-related fractures of the hip, wrist, or spine</u>
lansoprazole (Prevacid)	PO: 15–30 mg daily for 4–8 weeks IV: 30 mg over 30 min daily for up to 7 days	
omeprazole (Prilosec)	PO: 20–60 mg daily or bid	
pantoprazole (Protonix)	PO: 40 mg daily or bid IV: 40 mg IV daily for up to 7 days	
rabeprazole (AcipHex)	PO: 20–60 mg once daily	

Note: Italics indicate common adverse effects. Underline indicates serious adverse effects.

of action. About 95% of the acid production is blocked, making the PPIs the most efficient drugs available for treating acid-related disease.

Because the proton pump is activated by food intake, the PPI should be taken 20 to 30 minutes before the first major meal of the day. This allows the peak serum drug levels to coincide with the time at which the proton pumps are activated. PPIs are formulated in a delayed release formation because the drug would be destroyed in the acidic environment of the stomach.

Although the PPIs have a short serum half-life (about 1.5 hours), they continue to suppress acid for about 24 hours because the inactivation of the proton pump is irreversible. Because not all of the proton pumps are inactivated with the first dose, several days of PPI therapy are needed to achieve maximal acid inhibition. Beneficial effects continue for 3 to 5 days after the drugs have been discontinued.

The PPIs are highly protein bound, metabolized in the liver, and excreted in the urine (80%) and feces (20%). Doses do not need to be adjusted for patients with renal insufficiency because there is negligible renal clearance.

All drugs in this class have similar effectiveness and adverse effects. The incidence of adverse effects with PPIs is very low, with headache, abdominal pain, diarrhea (including that associated with *Clostridium difficile*), nausea, and vomiting being the most commonly reported ones. Rashes and blood dyscrasias are rare. Rebound hypersecretion of acid does not appear to occur after the drugs are discontinued. PPIs can mask an *H. pylori* infection because of the marked reduction in the bacterial load that they initiate. Long-term therapy with PPIs increases the risk for osteoporosis-related fractures, perhaps due to their interference with calcium absorption. Some health care providers recommend calcium supplements during therapy to prevent these types of fractures.

PPIs heal more than 90% of duodenal ulcers within 4 weeks and about 90% of gastric ulcers in 6 to 8 weeks. GERD may require 8 to 12 weeks of therapy for symptoms to diminish, and long-term maintenance therapy may be needed. PPIs are best suited for the long-term prevention of heartburn rather than the treatment of acute symptoms. In patients with PUD who must take NSAIDs for a chronic pain or inflammatory condition, PPIs taken once daily are effective in reducing the incidence of ulcers.

PROTOTYPE DRUG Omeprazole (Prilosec)

Classification: Therapeutic: Antiulcer drug
Pharmacologic: Proton pump inhibitor

Therapeutic Effects and Uses: Omeprazole was the first PPI to be approved in 1989 for PUD and is available by prescription and OTC. By prescription it is approved for the short-term, 4- to 8-week therapy of active duodenal and gastric ulcers, GERD, and maintenance of erosive esophagitis. OTC, it is indicated for the relief of heartburn. Most patients are symptom free after 2 weeks of

◀ **Use of Proton Pump Inhibitors and Increased Risk of Infections**

Clinical Question
The acidic environment of the stomach is known to be a natural barrier to infection caused by ingested bacteria and it plays a role in the destruction of respiratory pathogens. The long-term effects of decreasing the acidity of the gastric fluid are uncertain. Because PPIs decrease the acidity, is there an association between PPI use and GI or respiratory infections?

Evidence
An increased risk of enteric bacterial infection (such as salmonella) has been demonstrated to exist in patients taking PPIs (Bavishi & Dupont, 2011). Evidence also suggests a link between PPI use and an increased risk of respiratory infections, including pneumonia (Ramsay, Pratt, Ryan, & Roughead, 2013). These effects may be related to the decrease in gastric acidity and the protective mechanism against respiratory bacteria that it provides. Bacterial overgrowth may be of concern in patients who take PPIs and subsequently develop *Clostridium difficile*–associated diarrhea (CDAD). This infection has been associated previously with prior antibiotic use or immunosuppression. Recently, an increased risk for the development of hospital-acquired *C. difficile* colitis in hospitalized patients who are receiving PPIs has been noted, especially with long-term use (Barletta, El-Ibiary, Davis, Nguyen, & Raney, 2013). The use of PPIs, as well as other gastric acid inhibitors such as H_2-antagonists, has also been shown to increase the risk of pneumonia, sepsis, and GI infections in infants and children (Chung & Yardley, 2013).

Implications
In patients who are receiving PPIs, the nurse should frequently assess for the development of severe diarrhea, especially that which is watery and contains mucus, blood, or pus. Respiratory symptoms such as cough, congestion, adventitious breath sounds, and dyspnea, especially when associated with fever, should also be assessed and reported.

Critical Thinking Question
What categories of patients may be at increased risk for developing infections associated with PPI use?

See Answers to Critical Thinking Questions on student resource website.

---

therapy. It is used for longer periods and in higher doses in patients who have ZES. It is combined with antibiotics in regimens for eliminating *H. pylori*. Omeprazole may be prescribed off-label to prevent PUD in patients taking NSAIDs.

Although omeprazole can take 2 hours to reach therapeutic levels, its effects last up to 72 hours. Omeprazole is available only in oral (PO) form in the United States and is approved for pediatric use in children age 2 years and older. Zegerid is a combination drug that contains omeprazole and the antacid sodium bicarbonate.

Mechanism of Action: Omeprazole reduces acid secretion in the stomach by binding irreversibly to the enzyme H^+, K^+-ATPase. It inhibits the final pathway involved in acid secretion and effectively inhibits the active proton pumps.

Pharmacokinetics:

Route(s)	PO
Absorption	Rapidly absorbed; food does not influence bioavailability
Distribution	Bioavailability after oral dosing: 50–60%; crosses the placenta; secreted in breast milk; 95% bound to plasma protein
Primary metabolism	Hepatic; significant first-pass effect due to metabolism by CYP2C19
Primary excretion	Renal with small amounts in bile
Onset of action	0.5–3.5 h
Duration of action	3–4 days; half-life: 0.5–1.5 h

Adverse Effects: PPIs are generally well-tolerated drugs. The most common adverse effects are minor and include headache, nausea, diarrhea, rash, and abdominal pain. Although rare, blood disorders may occur, causing unusual fatigue and weakness. Long-term studies have been conducted on the possible effects of omeprazole on cardiovascular events and gastric tumors. None of the studies has shown any significant increase in cardiovascular adverse effects or gastric cancer. Delayed release omeprazole has been associated with an increased risk of *Clostridium difficile*–associated diarrhea in hospitalized patients.

Contraindications/Precautions: The only contraindication is hypersensitivity to the drug. It is not recommended for children under 2 years of age. Patients with hepatic impairment should be treated with caution. The drug should be avoided or used with caution in pregnant or lactating patients.

Drug Interactions: Clinically significant interactions with PPIs are uncommon. Omeprazole has been shown to both inhibit and induce certain hepatic P450 enzyme systems. Therefore, concurrent use with other drugs using the P450 system, including warfarin, carbamazepine, diazepam, and phenytoin, may inhibit or delay metabolism and cause increased blood levels of these drugs. Concurrent use of omeprazole and clopidogrel (Plavix) reduces the conversion of clopidogrel to its active metabolite, thus reducing its effectiveness. Thus concurrent use with warfarin may increase the likelihood of bleeding. Coadministration of omeprazole and clarithromycin has been shown to increase plasma levels of both omeprazole and clarithromycin.

PPIs increase gastric pH and have the potential to affect the bioavailability of medications that depend on a lower pH for absorption (e.g., iron salts, digoxin, ampicillin, ketoconazole, atazanavir). Because an acidic environment promotes mineral absorption, mineral deficiencies could occur with long-term PPI use. Decreased vitamin B_{12} absorption may occur because an acid is optimal for vitamin B_{12} absorption. **Herbal/Food:** Ginkgo and St. John's wort may decrease the plasma concentration of omeprazole.

Pregnancy: Category C.

Treatment for Overdose: Overdose is uncommon and is treated symptomatically.

Nursing Responsibilities: Key nursing implications for patients receiving omeprazole are included in the Nursing Practice Application for Patients Receiving Pharmacotherapy for Peptic Ulcer Disease.

Drugs Similar to Omeprazole (Prilosec)

The other PPIs include esomeprazole, lansoprazole, pantoprazole, and rabeprazole.

Esomeprazole (Nexium): Approved in 2001, this drug is very similar in structure, effectiveness, and safety to omeprazole. Its effects may last longer than those of omeprazole. It is available by the PO and intravenous (IV) routes. Adverse effects include headache, diarrhea, and nausea. Similar to other PPIs, esomeprazole is available as once-daily dosing for uncomplicated PUD and GERD and twice-daily dosing for complicated conditions such as ZES. It is approved by the U.S. Food and Drug Administration (FDA) for the prophylaxis of ulcers in patients who are taking NSAIDs. Esomeprazole capsules can be opened and the pellets mixed with soft foods and swallowed without chewing. With all PPIs there is a risk of pneumonia due to the elevation in gastric pH. Esomeprazole is pregnancy category B.

Lansoprazole (Prevacid) and dexlansoprazole (Dexilant): Approved in 1995, lansoprazole has a similar effectiveness and safety profile to omeprazole and is available by both the PO and IV routes. Its antisecretory effects can last up to 24 hours. Similar to other PPIs, its adverse effects include headache, diarrhea, and nausea. As with other PPIs, lansoprazole offers once-daily dosing for uncomplicated PUD and GERD and twice-daily dosing for ZES. With lansoprazole, as with other PPIs, there is a risk of pneumonia due to the elevation in gastric pH. This drug is eliminated from the body by the biliary system. It is available by prescription as well as OTC.

For patients who have difficulty swallowing capsules, lansoprazole is available in an oral liquid suspension or as a PO disintegrating tablet (Prevacid SoluTab) that is placed under the tongue and disintegrates within 1 minute. Capsules of lansoprazole should be swallowed whole and not crushed or split. Dexlansoprazole (Dexilant) is a stereoisomer of lansoprazole that has identical effects to its parent drug. Lansoprazole is pregnancy category B.

Pantoprazole (Protonix): Approved in 2000, pantoprazole has a similar efficacy and safety profile to omeprazole and is available intravenously. Adverse effects include headache, diarrhea, and nausea. Because pantoprazole does not inhibit CYP450 enzymes, it is not likely to affect the metabolism of other drugs.

As with the other PPIs, pantoprazole offers once-daily dosing for uncomplicated PUD and GERD and twice-daily dosing for ZES. With all PPIs, there is a risk of pneumonia due to the elevation in gastric pH. Pantoprazole may be prescribed off-label to prevent ulcers in patients taking NSAIDs. Pantoprazole is pregnancy category B.

Rabeprazole (AcipHex): Although rabeprazole is similar to omeprazole, it causes reversible inhibition of the proton pump; thus its effects are of shorter duration. Approved in 1999, rabeprazole is available by the PO route. The tablets should be swallowed whole and not crushed or chewed. Like other PPIs rabeprazole accentuates the eradication of *H. pylori* when used with appropriate

antibiotics. Although rabeprazole is metabolized by the hepatic CYP450 drug-metabolizing system, it exhibits few significant drug interactions. Adverse effects are mild and transient and include headache, diarrhea, nausea, malaise, dizziness, and rash. Rabeprazole is pregnancy category B.

Pharmacotherapy with H₂-Receptor Antagonists

59.6 The H$_2$-receptor antagonists suppress gastric acid secretion and are widely prescribed for treating peptic ulcer disease and gastroesophageal reflux disease.

The discovery of the **H$_2$-receptor antagonists**, or H$_2$ blockers, in the 1970s marked a major breakthrough in the treatment of PUD. Since then they have become available OTC and are used extensively in the treatment of mild to moderate hyperacidity disorders of the GI tract. H$_2$-receptor antagonists are indicated for treatment of PUD and GERD to promote healing and prevent recurrence. Duodenal ulcers usually heal in 6 to 8 weeks, and gastric ulcers may require up to 12 weeks of therapy. All of the H$_2$-receptor antagonists are available OTC for the short-term (2 weeks) treatment of heartburn. These drugs are listed in Table 59.2.

Histamine has two types of receptors: H$_1$ and H$_2$. Activation of the H$_1$ receptors produces the classic symptoms of inflammation and allergy, whereas the H$_2$ receptors, which are located on the parietal cells in the stomach, promote gastric acid secretion when activated. The H$_2$-receptor antagonists effectively reduce both fasting and food-stimulated secretion and are also helpful in decreasing nocturnal acid secretion, which is largely dependent on histamine.

Pharmacokinetic properties of drugs in this class include rapid absorption from the small intestine, which is not affected by food, and a 30-minute onset of action. These drugs undergo hepatic metabolism and renal excretion and their half-lives range from 1 to 4 hours. Although there are no known harmful effects on the

---

TABLE 59.2 H₂-Receptor Antagonists

Drug	Route and Adult Dose (Maximum Dose Where Indicated)	Adverse Effects
cimetidine (Tagamet)	Active ulcers: PO: 300 mg every 6 h or 800 mg at bedtime or 400 mg bid with food; IV: 300 mg every 6 h (over a minimum of 5 min) or 37.5 mg/h by continuous infusion GERD: 400 mg every 6 h or 800 mg bid for 12 weeks	*Diarrhea, constipation, headache, fatigue, nausea, gynecomastia* Rare: <u>hepatitis, blood dyscrasias, anaphylaxis, dysrhythmias, skin reactions, galactorrhea, confusion, or psychoses</u>
famotidine (Pepcid)	Active ulcers: PO: 40 mg/day for 4–8 weeks, then 20 mg at bedtime GERD: PO: 20 mg bid for 6 weeks IV: 20 mg every 12 h	*Headache, nausea, dry mouth* Rare: <u>musculoskeletal pain, tachycardia, blood dyscrasias, blurred vision</u>
nizatidine (Axid)	Active ulcers: PO: 150 mg bid or 300 mg at bedtime GERD: PO: 150 mg bid IV: 20 mg every 12 h	
ranitidine (Zantac)	PO: 150 mg bid or 300 mg once daily after the evening meal IV/IM: 50 mg every 6–8 h by intermittent bolus or infusion	

Note: Italics indicate common adverse effects. <u>Underline</u> indicates serious adverse effects.

fetus, these drugs cross the placenta and are secreted in breast milk. All drugs in this class have similar safety profiles: Their adverse effects are minor and rarely cause discontinuation of therapy. Patients who are receiving higher doses, those with renal or hepatic disease, or older adults may experience confusion, restlessness, hallucinations, or depression. With moderate to severe kidney disease, doses of H₂-receptor antagonists should be cut in half to avoid toxicity. Antacids should not be taken at the same time as H₂-receptor antagonists because absorption is diminished.

PROTOTYPE DRUG | Ranitidine (Zantac)

Classification: Therapeutic: Antiulcer drug
Pharmacologic: H₂-receptor antagonist

Therapeutic Effects and Uses: Approved in 1983, ranitidine has a higher potency than cimetidine, which allows it to be administered PO, once daily, usually at bedtime. Adequate healing of the ulcer takes 4 to 8 weeks, although those at high risk for PUD may continue on drug maintenance for prolonged periods to prevent recurrence. Gastric ulcers heal more slowly than duodenal ulcers and thus require longer therapy. IV and intramuscular (IM) forms are available for the treatment of acute stress-induced bleeding ulcers or hypersecretory conditions in hospitalized patients. Tritec is a combination drug with ranitidine and bismuth citrate. An OTC preparation of ranitidine is also available.

Ranitidine is indicated for duodenal ulcers, gastric ulcers, hypersecretory conditions, heartburn, and GERD. In some cases, it is used off-label to prevent PUD in those who are taking medications known to cause peptic ulcers. It is not effective as monotherapy for the elimination of *H. pylori*. Ranitidine is available in a dissolving tablet form (EFFERdose) for treating GERD in children and infants older than 1 month of age.

Mechanism of Action: Ranitidine acts by blocking H₂ receptors on the parietal cells in the stomach to decrease acid production. Both daytime and nocturnal basal gastric acids are suppressed.

Pharmacokinetics:

Route(s)	PO, IV, IM (rare)
Absorption	Rapid absorption following PO administration; all three routes achieve comparable blood levels
Distribution	PO bioavailability is approximately 50%; very little enters the central nervous system (CNS); crosses the placenta; secreted in breast milk; 15% bound to plasma protein
Primary metabolism	Hepatic
Primary excretion	Renal (mostly unchanged)
Onset of action	30–60 min; peak effect: 1–3 h
Duration of action	6–12 h; half-life: 2–3 h

Adverse Effects: Adverse effects are uncommon and transient. Although rare, blood dyscrasias, especially neutropenia and thrombocytopenia, have been reported; thus, periodic blood counts should be performed. Confusion may occur rarely and is usually in the elderly or with IV dosing. High doses may result in gynecomastia, impotence, or loss of libido in men, although these effects are more common with cimetidine.

Contraindications/Precautions: Contraindications include hypersensitivity to H₂-receptor antagonists, acute porphyria, and OTC administration in children younger than 12 years of age. The drug should be used with caution in patients with renal impairment; dosages should be reduced.

Drug Interactions: Because ranitidine has much less affinity for CYP450 enzymes, it is less likely to participate in drug–drug interactions than cimetidine. Ranitidine may reduce the absorption of cefpodoxime, ketoconazole, and itraconazole because of the increase in gastric pH induced by H₂-receptor antagonists. Concurrent use can increase the effects of alcohol, sulfonylureas, salicylates, and warfarin. Antacids should not be given within 1 hour of H₂-receptor antagonists because their effectiveness may be decreased due to reduced absorption. Smoking decreases the effectiveness of ranitidine. **Herbal/Food:** Absorption of vitamin B_{12} depends on an acidic environment, so deficiency may occur. Iron is also better absorbed in an acidic environment.

Pregnancy: Category B.

Treatment of Overdose: Overdose is uncommon and is treated symptomatically.

Nursing Responsibilities: Key nursing implications for patients receiving ranitidine are included in the Nursing Practice Application for Patients Receiving Pharmacotherapy for Peptic Ulcer Disease.

Drugs Similar to Ranitidine (Zantac)

Other H_2-receptor antagonists include cimetidine, famotidine, and nizatidine.

Cimetidine (Tagamet): The first of the H_2 blockers that was approved in 1977, cimetidine is used less frequently than other drugs in this class because (1) it inhibits hepatic drug-metabolizing enzymes and exhibits numerous drug–drug interactions; (2) it has a high incidence of adverse effects; and (3) it must be taken up to four times a day. Because cimetidine interacts with CYP450 enzymes, it may delay the metabolism of other drugs metabolized in the liver, including warfarin, phenytoin, diazepam, and theophylline. Cimetidine also may cause gynecomastia or impotence, because it binds to androgen receptors, causing antiandrogenic effects. Cimetidine crosses the blood–brain barrier and therefore is more likely to cause CNS depression and confusion than the other H_2-receptor antagonists. A low-dose OTC preparation is available. Routes of administration include PO, IM, and IV. This drug is pregnancy category B.

Famotidine (Pepcid): Approved by the FDA in 1986, famotidine has indications, actions, and adverse effects that are almost identical to those of ranitidine. Famotidine does not inhibit CYP450 enzymes; therefore, it exhibits fewer drug–drug interactions than cimetidine. Famotidine is the most potent of the H_2-receptor

antagonists. It is available OTC and may be given by the PO or IV route. This drug is pregnancy category B.

Nizatidine (Axid): Although thought to have a similar safety and adverse effect profile to ranitidine and famotidine, nizatidine is not metabolized by the liver CYP450 enzyme system and therefore causes fewer drug interactions. Adverse effects are infrequent and transient. Nizatidine is indicated for up to 8 weeks of PUD therapy (12 weeks for GERD) and is available as PO capsules or a PO solution. Prescription nizatidine was approved in 1988. An OTC preparation is also available. This drug is pregnancy category B.

CONNECTION Checkpoint 59.2

From what you learned in Chapter 3, how is the excretion of drugs affected when they are metabolized through the hepatic CYP450 system? *See Answer to Connection Checkpoint 59.2 on student resource website.*

Pharmacotherapy with Antacids

59.7 Antacids are alkaline substances that neutralize stomach acid to treat symptoms of heartburn.

Prior to the development of H_2-receptor antagonists and PPIs, antacids were the mainstay of peptic ulcer and GERD pharmacotherapy. Indeed, many patients still use these inexpensive and readily available OTC drugs. Antacids may provide temporary relief from heartburn or indigestion, but they are no longer recommended as the primary drug class for acid-related disorders. Although antacids relieve symptoms of heartburn, they do not promote ulcer healing or help to eliminate *H. pylori*. These drugs are listed in Table 59.3.

Antacids are inorganic compounds containing aluminum, magnesium, sodium, or calcium that neutralize gastric acid and inactivate pepsin. They are also thought to stimulate prostaglandin production in the mucosa and increase LES tone, which reduces

TABLE 59.3 Antacids

Drug	Route and Adult Dose (Maximum Dose Where Indicated)	Adverse Effects
aluminum hydroxide (AlternaGEL, Others)	PO: 600 mg tid–qid	*Constipation, nausea* Fecal impaction, hypophosphatemia with chronic use
calcium carbonate (Titralac, Tums)	PO: 1–2 g bid–tid	*Constipation, flatulence*
calcium carbonate with magnesium hydroxide (Mylanta Supreme, Rolaids)	PO: 2–4 capsules or tablets prn (max: 12 tablets/day)	Fecal impaction, metabolic alkalosis, hypercalcemia, renal calculi
magaldrate (Riopan)	PO: 540–1,080 mg/day (5–10 mL suspension or 1–2 tablets) (max: 20 tablets or 100 mL/day)	*Diarrhea, nausea, vomiting, abdominal cramping*
magnesium hydroxide (Milk of Magnesia)	PO: 5–15 mL or 2–4 tablets as needed up to 4 times daily	Hypermagnesemia (in patients with renal disease), dysrhythmias (when given parenterally)
magnesium trisilicate and aluminum hydroxide (Gaviscon)	PO: 2–4 tablets prn (max: 16 tablets/day)	
magnesium hydroxide and aluminum hydroxide with simethicone (Mylanta, Maalox Plus, Others)	PO: 10–20 mL prn (max: 120 mL/day) or 2–4 tablets prn (max: 24 tablets/day)	
sodium bicarbonate (Alka-Seltzer, baking soda)	PO: 325 mg–2 g 1 to 4 times/day	*Abdominal distention, belching* Metabolic alkalosis, fluid retention, edema, hypernatremia

Note: Italics indicate common adverse effects. Underline indicates serious adverse effects.

gastroesophageal reflux. These drugs do not protect the stomach by coating the stomach wall. To be considered therapeutic, the dose of antacids should increase the gastric pH to a minimum of 3.5.

Self-medication with antacids is safe when taken in doses as directed on the labels. Although antacids act within 10 to 15 minutes, their duration of action is only 2 hours; thus, they must be taken often during the day. Combinations of aluminum hydroxide and magnesium hydroxide, the most common types, are capable of rapidly neutralizing stomach acid.

All the antacids are equally effective at neutralizing acid and reducing symptoms of heartburn when given in therapeutic doses. Each type has certain disadvantages that may preclude their use:

- **Sodium.** Antacids that contain sodium should not be taken by patients on sodium-restricted diets or by those with hypertension (HTN), heart failure, or renal impairment because they may promote fluid retention.

- **Magnesium.** Absorption of magnesium from high doses of magnesium-containing antacids can cause symptoms of hypermagnesemia (fatigue, hypotension, and dysrhythmias). Magnesium also acts as a laxative when it reaches the large intestine.

- **Calcium.** Antacids that contain calcium can cause constipation and may cause or aggravate kidney stones. When absorbed, hypercalcemia is possible, and renal failure may occur at very high doses. Administering calcium carbonate antacids with milk or any items with vitamin D can cause **milk-alkali syndrome** to occur. Early symptoms are the same as those of hypercalcemia and include headache, urinary frequency, anorexia, nausea, and fatigue. Milk-alkali syndrome may result in permanent renal damage if the drug is continued at high doses.

- **Aluminum.** Aluminum antacids are not absorbed to any great extent but they can cause constipation. The constipation effect is balanced when aluminum is combined with magnesium salts. Aluminum carbonate and aluminum hydroxide may interfere with dietary phosphate absorption to cause hypophosphatemia.

- **Bicarbonate.** Being a base, antacids that contain bicarbonate may provoke metabolic alkalosis (e.g., fatigue, mental status changes, muscle twitching, depressed respiratory rate) in patients at risk. Bicarbonate combines with gastric acid to form carbon dioxide, which causes bloating and belching.

Drug interactions with antacids occur by several mechanisms. Because antacids increase stomach pH, they affect the solubility and absorption of many oral drugs. Drugs that are weak acids are nonionized in the acidic environment of the stomach and are thus readily absorbed. If an antacid is given concurrently with a weak acid, the pH of the stomach will rise and result in a more ionized drug that is less readily absorbed. On the other hand, a drug that is a weak base is absorbed in a more alkaline medium. In other words, when taken with antacids, acidic drugs may have less therapeutic effect, and basic drugs may exhibit a greater effect. Examples of acidic drugs include NSAIDs, sulfonylureas, salicylates, warfarin, barbiturates, isoniazid, and digoxin. Basic drugs include morphine sulfate, antihistamines, tricyclic antidepressants, amphetamines, and quinidine.

Enteric-coated or delayed release drugs are designed to dissolve when they reach the alkaline environment in the small intestine. By raising the pH of the stomach, antacids may "fool" enteric-coated tablets into dissolving early and releasing their contents into the stomach. The drug may either irritate the stomach lining, causing nausea or vomiting, or be inactivated.

Drug interactions may also occur if the antacid physically binds to other drugs. For example, certain antacids form chemical complexes with tetracyclines, preventing the antibiotic from being absorbed. Digoxin is another drug whose absorption is affected by binding to antacids.

A third mechanism of drug interaction is due to the effects of antacids on urine pH. Making the urine pH more alkaline increases the excretion of acidic drugs such as aspirin and inhibits the excretion of basic drugs such as amphetamines.

Because antacids are widely used OTC by patients for self-treatment, nurses must emphasize that these drugs be used only as directed on the label due to the potential for adverse effects. To decrease the potential for antacid–drug interactions, nurses should advise that other medications be taken at least 1 hour before or 2 hours after giving an antacid.

PROTOTYPE DRUG | **Aluminum Hydroxide (AlternaGEL, Others)**

Classification: Therapeutic: Antiheartburn drug
Pharmacologic: Antacid

Therapeutic Effects and Uses: Aluminum hydroxide is an inorganic drug used alone or in combination with other antacids such as magnesium hydroxide. Combining aluminum compounds with magnesium (Gaviscon, Maalox, Mylanta) increases their effectiveness and reduces the potential for constipation. Unlike calcium-based antacids that can be absorbed and cause systemic effects, aluminum compounds are minimally absorbed. Their primary action is to neutralize stomach acid by raising the pH of the stomach contents. Unlike H_2-receptor antagonists and PPIs, aluminum antacids do not reduce the volume of acid secretion. They are most effectively used in combination with other antiulcer drugs for the symptomatic relief of heartburn due to PUD or GERD. A second aluminum salt, aluminum carbonate (Basaljel), is also available to treat heartburn.

CONNECTIONS | **Treating the Diverse Patient**

Global Health Implications of *H. Pylori* Infection

H. pylori occurs worldwide and has a noted association with an increased risk of gastric cancer, particularly in genetically susceptible subgroups. *H. pylori* is also associated with gastritis and PUD. Infection with the bacteria usually occurs in infancy or childhood, years before symptoms of gastric effects may appear, and close contact between family members in crowded housing may be associated with a higher incidence of the infection (Melius et al., 2013). Because gastric cancer is a significant cause of death worldwide, public health measures such as adequate sanitation, drinking water, and nutrition may decrease the risk of transmission and improve the general health of those infected with the disease. The need for these measures takes on special importance in light of the global increase in antibiotic-resistant strains of *H. pylori*, including in the United States (Gatta, Vakil, Vaira, & Scarpignato, 2013).

Mechanism of Action: Aluminum hydroxide combines with gastric (hydrochloric) acid to produce aluminum chloride and water. This raises the pH of the stomach contents and inactivates pepsin.

Pharmacokinetics:

Route(s)	PO
Absorption	17–30% absorbed
Distribution	Widely distributed
Primary metabolism	Hepatic
Primary excretion	Renal
Onset of action	20–40 min
Duration of action	2 h when taken with food; 3 h when taken 1 h after meals

Adverse Effects: Aluminum antacids frequently cause constipation. At high doses aluminum products bind with phosphate in the GI tract and long-term use can result in phosphate depletion. Those at risk include people who are malnourished, those who have alcoholism, and those with renal disease. The antacids are often combined with magnesium compounds, which counteract the constipation commonly experienced with aluminum antacids.

Contraindications/Precautions: Prolonged use in patients with low serum phosphate levels should be avoided. This drug should not be used in patients with suspected bowel obstruction.

Drug Interactions: Aluminum compounds should not be taken with other medications because they may interfere with their absorption. Concurrent use decreases the absorption of cimetidine, ciprofloxacin and other fluoroquinolones, digoxin, isoniazid, chloroquine, NSAIDs, iron salts, phenytoin, tetracycline, and thyroxine. Use with sodium polystyrene sulfonate may cause systemic alkalosis. Use of anticholinergic drugs can increase the effects of antacids. **Herbal/Food:** Aluminum antacids may inhibit the absorption of dietary iron.

Pregnancy: Category C.

Treatment of Overdose: There is no specific treatment for overdose.

Nursing Responsibilities: Key nursing implications for patients receiving aluminum hydroxide are included in the Nursing Practice Application for Patients Receiving Pharmacotherapy for Peptic Ulcer Disease.

Drugs Similar to Aluminum Hydroxide (AlternaGEL, Others)

All aluminum salts have similar effects to those of aluminum hydroxide.

Pharmacotherapy of *Helicobacter pylori* Infection

59.8 The gram-negative bacterium *H. pylori* is associated with approximately 70% of patients with peptic ulcer disease.

It is estimated that 60% to 80% of patients with duodenal ulcers are infected with *H. pylori* and that the majority of patients with gastric ulcers have the bacterium. Research has shown that the eradication of *H. pylori* decreases the recurrence of PUD. Risk factors for *H. pylori* include residing in a developing country, domestic crowding, unclean water, and exposure to the gastric contents of an infected individual. It is the only known microorganism that has been found to survive the hostile conditions in the stomach.

H. pylori has adapted well to the acidic environment in the stomach. It has devised ways to neutralize the high acidity surrounding it and make chemicals called **adhesins** that allow the organism to penetrate the GI mucosa and alter the epithelial cell structure, which initiates inflammation. The inflammatory and immune responses lead to the chronic production of inflammatory cells, including lymphocytes, plasma cells, and macrophages. This response then leads to the formation of immunoglobulin G antibodies and increased production of cytokines, including interleukins and tumor necrosis factor, all of which contribute to the inflammation of the gastric mucosa. Increased gastrin secretion and decreased bicarbonate production also play a role in ulcer formation caused by *H. pylori*.

Another mechanism involves ammonia. *H. pylori* produces large amounts of urease, an enzyme that breaks down urea to ammonia and carbon monoxide. Ammonia neutralizes the acid around the bacterium and allows *H. pylori* to survive in the acidic environment of the stomach. Unfortunately, the ammonia is toxic to mucosal cells and erodes the mucous barrier. *H. pylori* then finds its home in the submucosal layer of the stomach, producing damage to the gastric and duodenal mucosae, which allows pepsin and gastric acid to further damage the mucosae. There may also be a genetic predisposition that determines one's susceptibility to *H. pylori* infection.

Perforated, bleeding, or refractory ulcers are usually tested for the presence of *H. pylori*. The most reliable means of diagnosis is by obtaining a culture during endoscopy. Less invasive means include checking for antibodies to *H. pylori* in a blood sample or by using a breath test to check for urease, which is given off by the bacterium.

Prior to the identification of the link between *H. pylori* and ulcers, PUD was treated with acid-reducing drugs. Although this therapy was successful at treating symptoms, the majority of patients experienced relapses. This is because the acid-reducing drugs have little effect on *H. pylori*, which can remain active for life if not treated appropriately. Thus for infected patients, elimination of this bacterium is the prime pharmacologic objective. Eradication of the organism allows ulcers to heal more rapidly and remain in remission longer, often permanently.

A combination of antibiotics is used concurrently to eradicate *H. pylori* and help decrease antibiotic resistance. A PPI or bismuth compound is usually included in the regimen. Once eliminated from the stomach, reinfection with *H. pylori* is uncommon. Those with peptic ulcer who are not infected with *H. pylori* should not receive antibiotics because it has been shown that these patients have a worse outcome if they receive *H. pylori* treatment. Thus, patients should be tested for *H. pylori* before initiating treatment for infection. Example regimens used to eradicate *H. pylori* include the following:

- **Initial regimen.** Omeprazole, clarithromycin (Biaxin), and amoxicillin (Amoxil, Others)
- **Alternative regimens.**
  - Omeprazole (or other PPI), clarithromycin (Biaxin), and metronidazole (Flagyl), or
  - Omeprazole (or other PPI), bismuth subsalicylate (Pepto-Bismol), metronidazole (Flagyl), and tetracycline

Although technically not antibiotics, bismuth compounds inhibit bacterial growth by disrupting their cell wall and preventing *H. pylori* from adhering to the gastric mucosa. The PPI further suppresses *H. pylori*, and the increased pH that results from PPI administration creates a hostile environment for *H. pylori*, thus enhancing the effectiveness of the antibiotics.

H. pylori therapy generally continues for 7 to 14 days. Should resistance occur, rifabutin (Mycobutin) and fluoroquinolones have been and can be used as part of the regimen. Drug regimens continue to evolve as antibiotic resistance patterns change. The American College of Gastroenterology publishes periodic guidelines offering different pharmacologic strategies.

Indiscriminate use of antibiotics can lead to antibiotic resistance; thus treatment should be reserved for patients who would benefit from the regimen. Patient adherence is vital to successful eradication of *H. pylori*. Patients should be instructed on the importance of completing the drug regimen, because discontinuing the anti-infectives too soon may result in reinfection. Interestingly, following treatment for eradication of *H. pylori* infection, certain other conditions such as idiopathic thrombocytopenic purpura (ITP), a blood disorder, have been alleviated.

CONNECTION Checkpoint 59.3

From what you learned in Chapter 46, explain why antibiotic resistance has become a major public health problem throughout the world. *See Answer to Connection Checkpoint 59.3 on student resource website.*

Miscellaneous Drugs Used for Peptic Ulcer Disease and Gastroesophageal Reflux Disease

59.9 Several miscellaneous drugs, including sucralfate, bismuth subsalicylate, and misoprostol, are beneficial in treating peptic ulcer disease.

A few additional drugs are used in the pharmacotherapy of PUD and GERD. These drugs act by mechanisms other than the ones described for PPIs, H_2-receptor blockers, or antacids.

Sucralfate: Sucralfate (Carafate) is a PO medication that consists of sucrose (a sugar) plus aluminum hydroxide (an antacid). This drug stimulates mucus, bicarbonate, and prostaglandin secretion, all of which enhance mucosal defenses. Sucralfate also acts locally to produce a thick protective barrier that coats and binds to the ulcer, protecting it against further erosion from acid and pepsin to promote healing. It does not affect the secretion of gastric acid. It is intended for short-term therapy (up to 8 weeks). It is sometimes used in critically ill patients to prevent bleeding from stress-related gastritis. Sucralfate is not effective in preventing NSAID-related ulcers.

Other than constipation, the adverse effects of sucralfate are minimal because little of the drug is absorbed from the GI tract. Because sucralfate requires an acid medium to work effectively, concurrent use of antacids, H_2-receptor antagonists, and PPIs will reduce its effectiveness. Sucralfate may bind to other drugs and decrease their absorption, especially digoxin, warfarin, the quinolones and tetracyclines, and phenytoin. Antacids and other medications should be taken 2 hours before or after a dose of sucralfate. A major disadvantage of sucralfate is that it must be taken four times daily.

Bismuth compounds: In the United States the only bismuth compound available is bismuth subsalicylate (Kaopectate, Pepto-Bismol), a nonprescription formula containing both bismuth and salicylate. Bismuth subsalicylate stimulates mucosal bicarbonate and prostaglandin production and inhibits *H. pylori* from adhering to the ulcerated tissue. It has been shown to have local antimicrobial actions to *H. pylori* by causing cell wall death to the bacterium. Bismuth is often included as a component of a multidrug regimen containing tetracycline and metronidazole (Pylera, Helidac) to eradicate *H. pylori* infection. As monotherapy, it is approved to treat dyspepsia, heartburn, and diarrhea.

Therapeutic doses of bismuth produce no significant adverse effects. This drug can cause stools to turn black, which is a normal side effect. In stomach acid bismuth subsalicylate is converted to salicylic acid, which is absorbed. Patients who are taking other salicylates, such as aspirin, may experience adverse effects such as tinnitus, headache, nausea, vomiting, or dizziness. In addition, it is not recommended for use in pediatric patients under the age of 19 because of the increased risk of Reye's syndrome associated with salicylate use. A "Children's Pepto" is available that contains the antacid calcium carbonate but no salicylates.

Misoprostol: Misoprostol (Cytotec) is a synthetic form of prostaglandin E_2 that stimulates the production of protective mucus and inhibits gastric acid secretion. Normally, the stomach synthesizes a number of prostaglandins, which suppress acid, promote bicarbonate secretion, and maintain blood flow to the gastric mucosa. The primary use of misoprostol is for the prevention of gastric ulcers in patients who are taking high doses of NSAIDs or corticosteroids. It has a serum half-life of less than 30 minutes and is administered three to four times per day.

Diarrhea and abdominal cramping are relatively common with misoprostol. The drug carries a black box warning that it is contraindicated during pregnancy (pregnancy category X) and it should only be prescribed for patients with gastric ulcers following a negative pregnancy test. Patients must be advised that the drug may induce abortions if taken during pregnancy. This drug is combined with mifepristone for pregnancy termination (see Chapter 70). The use of misoprostol as an antiulcer drug is rare because of the availability of safer, more effective drugs.

Metoclopramide: Approved in 1985, metoclopramide (Reglan) is occasionally used for the short-term (4 to 12 weeks) therapy of symptomatic GERD or PUD in patients who fail to respond to first-line agents. It is more commonly prescribed to treat nausea and vomiting associated with surgery or cancer chemotherapy. Metoclopramide is available by the PO, IM, or IV routes. It causes muscles in the upper intestine to contract, resulting in faster emptying of the stomach. It also decreases esophageal relaxation and blocks food from entering the esophagus, which is of benefit in patients with GERD.

CNS adverse effects such as drowsiness, fatigue, confusion, and insomnia may occur in a significant number of patients. Metoclopramide carries a black box warning that it can cause tardive dyskinesia. Because the risk of this serious condition increases with duration of treatment, therapy should be limited to a maximum of 12 weeks. Due to the availability of safer, more effective drugs metoclopramide is rarely prescribed to treat peptic ulcer. This drug is pregnancy category B.

CONNECTIONS: NURSING PRACTICE APPLICATION

Patients Receiving Pharmacotherapy for Peptic Ulcer Disease

Assessment	Potential Nursing Diagnoses*
Baseline assessment prior to administration: • Obtain a complete health history including GI, hepatic, renal, respiratory, or cardiovascular disease, pregnancy, or breast-feeding. Obtain a drug history including allergies, current prescription and OTC drugs, herbal preparations, caffeine, nicotine, and alcohol use. Be alert to possible drug interactions. • Obtain a history of past and current symptoms, noting any correlations between onset and presence of any pain related to meals, sleep, positioning, or other medications. Also note what measures have been successful to relieve the pain (e.g., eating). • Obtain baseline vital signs and weight. • Evaluate appropriate laboratory findings (e.g., CBC, platelets, electrolytes, hepatic or renal function studies). • Assess the patient's ability to receive and understand instructions. Include family and caregivers as needed.	• *Acute Pain* • *Imbalanced Nutrition: Less Than Body Requirements* • *Constipation* or *Diarrhea, related to adverse drug effects* • *Deficient Knowledge (Drug Therapy)* • *Risk for Ineffective Health Maintenance*
Assessment throughout administration: • Assess for desired therapeutic effects (e.g., diminishing gastric area pain, lessened bloating or belching). • Continue periodic monitoring of CBC, electrolytes, hepatic and renal function laboratory values. Testing for *H. pylori* may be needed if symptoms fail to resolve. • Assess for adverse effects: nausea, vomiting, diarrhea, headache, drowsiness, or dizziness. Immediately report severe abdominal pain, vomiting, coffee-ground emesis, hematemesis, blood in stool, or tarry stools.	

Implementation

Interventions and (Rationales)	Patient-Centered Care
Ensuring therapeutic effects: • Follow appropriate administration guidelines. (For best results, follow administration guidelines regarding timing of the drug around meals. See "Patient Self-Administration" below.)	• Teach the patient to take the drug, following appropriate guidelines, and not to crush, open, or chew tablets unless directed to do so by the health care provider or label directions.
• Encourage appropriate lifestyle changes: lowered fat intake, eliminating alcohol intake, smoking cessation, increasing intake of yogurt and acidophilus-containing foods. (Smoking and alcohol use are known to increase gastric acid and irritation and should be eliminated. Correlating symptoms with dietary intake or activities may help to eliminate a triggering factor. Overall healthy lifestyle changes will support and minimize the need for drug therapy.)	• Encourage the patient to adopt a healthy lifestyle of low-fat food choices, increased exercise, and elimination of alcohol consumption and smoking. Provide for dietitian consultation or information on smoking cessation programs as needed. • Teach the patient to keep a food diary, noting correlations between discomfort or pain and meals or activities.
Minimizing adverse effects: • Continue to monitor for the presence of gastric area pain. Continued discomfort or pain should be reported. (Continued symptoms may indicate ineffectiveness of the current drug therapy, or the need to test for *H. pylori.*)	• Teach the patient that while some easing of discomfort may be noticed after beginning drug therapy, full effects may take several days to weeks or longer. Consistent drug therapy will provide the best results. If gastric discomfort or pain continue or worsen after several weeks of therapy, the health care provider should be notified.
• Monitor for any severe abdominal pain, vomiting, coffee-ground emesis or hematemesis, blood in stool, or tarry stools, and report immediately. (The drugs decrease gastric acidity, making the gastric environment less favorable for ulcer development, but they do not heal existing ulcers. Severe abdominal pain or blood in emesis or stools may indicate a worsening of the disease or a more serious condition and should be reported immediately.)	• Teach the patient that severe abdominal pain or any blood in emesis or stools should be reported immediately to the health care provider.
• Continue to monitor periodic electrolyte levels. (PPIs have been associated with a possible increase in osteopenia and osteoporosis. Calcium and magnesium supplements or other preventive drug therapy may be needed.)	• Instruct the patient on the need to return periodically for laboratory work.
• Monitor respiratory status and for fever, congestion, adventitious breath sounds such as crackles or wheezing, and dyspnea. Immediately report adventitious sounds or dyspnea accompanied by fever to the provider. (The drugs raise the gastric pH and impact the body's normal defense mechanisms against respiratory pathogens. Antibacterial therapy may be needed if respiratory infections develop.)	• Teach the patient to report symptoms of respiratory infection and report lung congestion or dyspnea accompanied by fever to the health care provider.

(continued)

CONNECTIONS: NURSING PRACTICE APPLICATION (continued)

• Monitor for severe diarrhea, especially if mucus, blood, or pus is present. (Severe diarrhea may indicate the presence of CDAD, or PMC. Drugs that raise gastric pH have been associated with an increased risk for CDAD.)	• Instruct the patient to immediately report any diarrhea that increases in frequency or amount or that contains mucus, blood, or pus. • Instruct the patient to consult the health care provider before taking any antidiarrheal drugs, which cause the retention of harmful bacteria. • Teach the patient to increase intake of dairy products containing live active cultures, such as yogurt, kefir, or buttermilk, to help restore normal intestinal flora.
• Continue to monitor periodic hepatic and renal function tests and CBC, platelets, and electrolyte levels. (Abnormal liver function tests may indicate drug-induced adverse hepatic effects. **Diverse Patients:** Because some drugs used in PUD therapy [e.g., omeprazole, cimetidine] are metabolized through the P450 system, monitor ethnically diverse patients frequently to ensure optimal therapeutic effects and minimize adverse effects. **Lifespan:** Age-related physiological differences may place older adults at greater risk for hepatic or renal toxicity. (Decreased RBC, WBC, or platelets have been noted with long-term H_2-receptor antagonist therapy, and decreases should be reported to the health care provider. Excessive use of antacids may affect electrolyte levels.)	• Instruct the patient on the need to return periodically for laboratory work.
• Monitor the effectiveness of other drugs taken along with PUD therapy. (PPIs, H_2 blockers, and antacids may significantly impair the effects of other drugs [e.g., clopidogrel].)	• Instruct the patient to immediately report any unusual symptoms related to other drugs used (e.g., increased risk of GI bleeding or bruising, or increased angina if clopidogrel is taken concurrently).
Patient understanding of drug therapy: • Use opportunities during administration of medications and during assessments to discuss the rationale for drug therapy, desired therapeutic outcomes, commonly observed adverse effects, parameters for when to call the health care provider, and any necessary monitoring or precautions. (Using time during nursing care helps to optimize and reinforce key teaching areas.)	• The patient, family, or caregiver should be able to state the reason for the drug, appropriate dose and scheduling, what adverse effects to observe for and when to report them, and the anticipated length of medication therapy.
Patient self-administration of drug therapy: • When administering the medication, instruct the patient, family, or caregiver in proper self-administration of the drug, e.g., during the evening meal. (Utilizing time during nurse-administration of these drugs helps to reinforce teaching.)	• Teach the patient to take the drug following appropriate guidelines as follows: • **PPIs:** Take 30 min before meals. If once-daily dosing is ordered, take the drug in the morning before breakfast. Antacids may be used concurrently. Do not continue taking beyond 3 to 4 months unless directed by the health care provider. • **H_2-receptor blockers:** Take the drug with or immediately after meals unless otherwise instructed. Do not take concurrently with antacids unless using a combination product (e.g., famotidine with calcium and magnesium-based antacids such as Pepcid-Complete). Exceeding the recommended dose increases the risk of adverse effects such as dizziness or drowsiness. • **Antacids:** Take 2 h before or after meals with a full glass of water. Do not take other medications concurrently unless available as a combination product or directed to do so by the health care provider. If relief is not achieved after several weeks of therapy, consult the health care provider for additional treatment recommendations.

*Nursing Diagnoses—Definitions and Classification 2015–2017. Copyright © 2014, 1994–2014 by NANDA International. Used by arrangement with John Wiley & Sons Limited.

CHAPTER
59

Understanding the Chapter

Key Concepts Summary

59.1 The stomach secretes acid, enzymes, and hormones that are essential to digestive physiology.

59.2 Peptic ulcer disease is associated with a number of etiologic risk factors.

59.3 Gastroesophageal reflux disease is a chronic condition characterized by persistent heartburn.

59.4 Peptic ulcer disease and gastroesophageal reflux disease are best treated with a combination of pharmacotherapy and lifestyle changes.

59.5 Proton pump inhibitors block gastric acid secretion and are the drugs of choice in the therapy of peptic ulcer disease and gastroesophageal reflux disease.

59.6 The H_2-receptor antagonists suppress gastric acid secretion and are widely prescribed for treating peptic ulcer disease and gastroesophageal reflux disease.

59.7 Antacids are alkaline substances that neutralize stomach acid to treat symptoms of heartburn.

59.8 The gram-negative bacterium *H. pylori* is associated with approximately 70% of patients with peptic ulcer disease.

59.9 Several miscellaneous drugs, including sucralfate, bismuth subsalicylate, and misoprostol, are beneficial in treating peptic ulcer disease.

Case Study: Making the Patient Connection

Remember the patient "Hugh Marshall" at the beginning of the chapter? Now read the remainder of the case study. Based on the information presented within this chapter, respond to the critical thinking questions that follow.

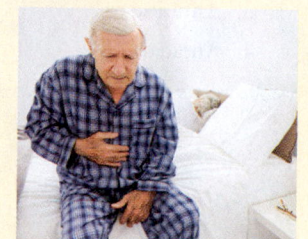

Hugh Marshall is a 71-year-old man who has been taking ibuprofen (Motrin) for a shoulder injury and assumed that this was the cause of his stomach pain. He is a one-pack-per-day smoker and drinks one glass of wine every night with dinner. His medical history includes HTN for which he takes a combination diuretic and ACE inhibitor. He stopped taking his ibuprofen, but the stomach pain did not subside. Because

of worsening symptoms, an endoscopy was performed, which confirmed the presence of *H. pylori*. He is worried about taking antibiotics because he has been allergic to penicillin in the past.

Critical Thinking Questions

1. Based on the scenario above, what risk factors for PUD does Hugh have?

2. How would you as the nurse describe the recommended treatment for *H. pylori*–induced PUD to him?

3. Why would you be concerned about this patient with a history of HTN using NSAIDs?

See Answers to Critical Thinking Questions on student resource website.

Additional Case Study

Sara Gaggi is a 51-year-old overweight white female with HTN who presents for an evaluation of heartburn that has been increasing in both intensity and frequency during the past 18 months. She reports epigastric burning after eating. It is worse after eating spicy foods or drinking red wine. She is occasionally awakened at night with symptoms. OTC antacids and H_2-receptor antagonists relieved her symptoms initially, but lately they have provided only minimal relief. Her only routine medication is amlodipine, a calcium channel blocker for her high blood pressure. Because the symptoms are increasing and her current therapy is not relieving her symptoms, an endoscopy was performed, which revealed the presence of GERD.

1. How would you describe to Sara the dangers of self-medicating GERD symptoms with OTC medications?

2. What three risk factors in this case predispose Sara for the development of GERD?

3. What medications will her health care provider likely prescribe?

See Answers to Additional Case Study on student resource website.

Chapter Review

1 The patient has developed severe diarrhea following 4 days of self-administered antacid preparation. The nurse suspects that the diarrhea may be caused by which type of antacid?

1. Aluminum compounds
2. Magnesium compounds
3. Calcium compounds
4. Sodium compounds

2 Omeprazole (Prilosec) is prescribed for a patient with gastroesophageal reflux disease. The nurse would monitor a reduction in which symptom to determine if the drug therapy is effective? Select all that apply.

1. Dysphagia
2. Dyspepsia
3. Appetite
4. Nausea
5. Belching

3 The nurse is scheduling the patient's daily medication. When would be the most appropriate time for the patient to receive proton pump inhibitors?

1. At night
2. After fasting at least 2 hours
3. About 1/2 hour before a meal
4. About 2 to 3 hours after eating

4 A patient who has duodenal ulcers is receiving long-term therapy with ranitidine (Zantac). The nurse includes in the care plan that the patient should be monitored for which adverse effects?

1. Photophobia and skin irritations
2. Neutropenia and thrombocytopenia
3. Dyspnea and productive coughing
4. Urinary hesitation and fluid retention

5 The prescriber orders sucralfate (Carafate) for a patient with peptic ulcer disease. The nurse should question the order if the patient is concurrently taking:

1. Proton pump inhibitors.
2. Calcium salt antacids.
3. H_2-receptor antagonists.
4. Aluminum salt antacids.

6 The nurse who is caring for a patient with gastroesophageal reflux disease should question the order for which drug?

1. H_2-receptor antagonists
2. Proton pump inhibitors
3. Antibiotics
4. Antacids

See Answers to Chapter Review in Appendix A.

References

Anand, B. S. (2012). *Peptic ulcer disease.* Retrieved from http://emedicine.medscape.com/article/181753-overview#a0101

Barletta, J. F., El-Ibiary, S. Y., Davis, L. E., Nguyen, B., & Raney, C. R. (2013). Proton pump inhibitors and the risk for *Clostridium dificile* infection. *Mayo Clinic Proceedings, 88,* 1085–1090. doi:10.1016/j.mayocp.2013.07.004

Bavishi, C., & Dupont, H. L. (2011). Systematic review: The use of proton pump inhibitors and increased susceptibility to enteric infection. *Alimentary Pharmacology & Therapeutics, 34,* 1269–1281. doi:10.1111/j.1365-2036.2011.04874.x

Chung, E. Y., & Yardley, J. (2013). Are there risks associated with empiric acid suppression treatment in infants and children suspected of having gastroesophageal reflux disease? *Hospital Pediatrics, 3*(1), 16–23. doi:10.1542/peds.2012-0077

Fraser, L. A., Leslie, W. D., Targownik, L. E., Papaioannou, A., & Adachi, J. D. (2013). The effect of proton pump inhibitors on fracture risk: Report from the Canadian multicentre osteoporosis study. *Osteoporosis International, 24,* 1161–1168. doi:10.1007/s00198-012-2112-9

Gatta, L., Vakil, N., Vaira, D., & Scarpignato, C. (2013). Global eradication rates for *Helicobacter pylori* infection: Systematic review and meta-analysis of sequential therapy. *BMJ (Clinical Research Ed.), 347,* f4587. doi:10.1136/bmj.f4587

Gill, J. M., Player, M. S., & Metz, D. C. (2011). Balancing the risks and benefits of proton pump inhibitors. *Annals of Family Medicine, 9,* 200–202. doi:10.1370/afm.1269

Melius, E. J., Davis, S. I., Retid, J. T., Lewin, M., Herlihy, R., Henderson, A., . . . Cheek, J. E. (2013). Estimating the prevalence of active *Helicobacter pylori* infection in a rural community with global positioning system technology-assisted sampling. *Epidemiology and Infection, 141,* 472–480. doi:10.1017/S0950268812000714

Patti, M. G. (2014). *Gastroesophageal reflux disease.* Retrieved from http://emedicine.medscape.com/article/176595-overview

Ramsay, E. N., Pratt, N. L., Ryan, P., & Roughead, E. E. (2013). Proton pump inhibitors and the risk of pneumonia: A comparison of cohort and self-controlled case series designs. *BMC Research Methodology, 13,* 82. doi:10.1186/1471-2288-13-82

Selected Bibliography

Ahn, J. S., Eom, C. S., Jeon, C. Y., & Park, S. M. (2013). Acid suppressive drugs and gastric cancer: A meta-analysis of observational studies. *World Journal of Gastroenterology: WJG, 19,* 2560. doi:10.3748/wjg.v19.i16.2560

Gurney, S., Carvalho, L., Gonzalez, C., Galaviz, E., & Sonstein, F. (2014). An efficacious and cost-effective pharmacologic treatment for *Helicobacter pylori. The Journal for Nurse Practitioners, 10,* 22–29. doi:10.1016/j.nurpra.2013.09.013

Hart, A. M. (2013). Evidence-based recommendations for GERD treatment. *The Nurse Practitioner, 38*(8), 26–34. doi:10.1097/01.NPR.0000431881.25363.84

Herdman, T. H., & Kamitsuru, S. (Eds.). (2014). *NANDA International nursing diagnoses: Definitions and classification, 2015–2017.* Oxford, United Kingdom: Wiley-Blackwell.

Hernández-Díaz, S., Martín-Merino, E., & Rodríguez, L. A. G. (2013). Risk of complications after a peptic ulcer diagnosis: Effectiveness of proton pump inhibitors. *Digestive Diseases and Sciences, 58,* 1653–1662. doi:10.1007/s10620-013-2561-9

Marmo, R., Bucci, C., Rea, M., & Rotondano, G. (2013). Treat the patient, not just the source of bleeding. *The American Journal of Gastroenterology, 108*(9), 1533–1534. doi:10.1038/ajg.2013.190

National Center for Complementary and Alternative Medicine. (2012). *Herbs at a glance: Ginger.* Retrieved from http://nccam.nih.gov/health/ginger

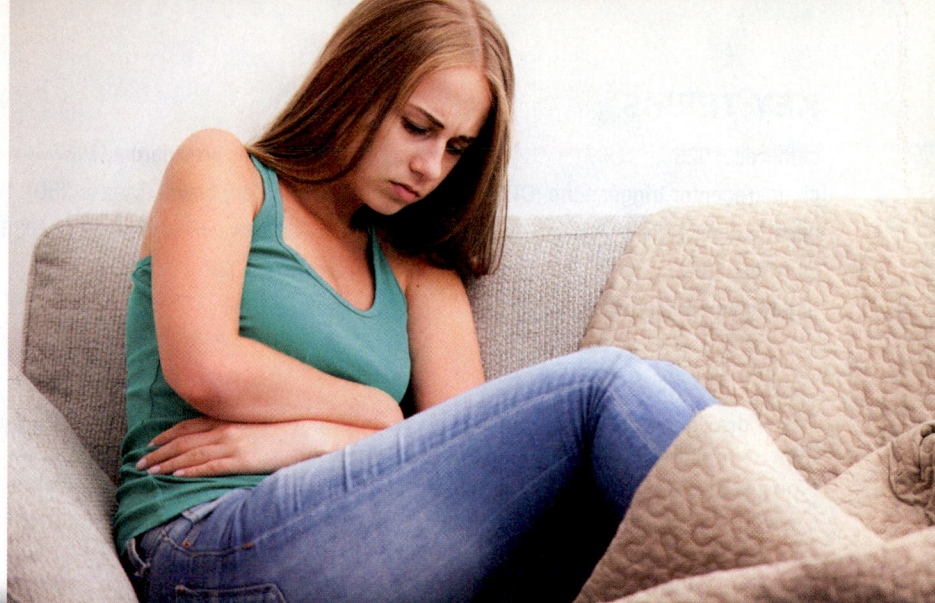

"This is ruining my life! I can't go to class; I can't go out with friends! I wish I'd never heard the term 'irritable bowel syndrome'!"

Patient "Kerry O'Grady"

CHAPTER 60

Pharmacotherapy of Bowel Disorders and Other Gastrointestinal Conditions

LEARNING OUTCOMES

After reading this chapter, the student should be able to:

1. Compare and contrast the definition of constipation used by patients to that used for diagnosis by health care providers.

2. Compare and contrast the different mechanisms of action of laxatives.

3. Explain the pathogenesis of constipation and diarrhea.

4. Compare and contrast the types of drugs used to treat inflammatory bowel disease and irritable bowel syndrome.

5. Explain conditions in which the pharmacotherapy of nausea and vomiting is indicated.

6. Identify drugs that are used to treat acute and chronic pancreatitis.

7. Describe the nurse's role in the pharmacologic management of bowel disorders, nausea and vomiting, and other gastrointestinal conditions.

8. For each of the classes shown in the chapter outline, identify the prototype and representative drugs and explain the mechanism(s) of drug action, primary indications, contraindications, significant drug interactions, pregnancy category, and important adverse effects.

9. Apply the nursing process to care for patients who are receiving pharmacotherapy for bowel disorders, nausea and vomiting, and other gastrointestinal conditions.

CHAPTER OUTLINE

▸ Pathophysiology of Constipation
▸ Pharmacotherapy with Laxatives
   PROTOTYPE Psyllium Mucilloid (Metamucil, Others), *p. 1026*
▸ Pathophysiology of Diarrhea
▸ Pharmacotherapy of Diarrhea
   PROTOTYPE Diphenoxylate with Atropine (Lomotil), *p. 1029*
▸ Pharmacotherapy of Inflammatory Bowel Disease
   PROTOTYPE Sulfasalazine (Azulfidine), *p. 1033*
▸ Pharmacotherapy of Irritable Bowel Syndrome
▸ Pathophysiology of Nausea and Vomiting
▸ Pharmacotherapy of Nausea and Vomiting
   PROTOTYPE Ondansetron (Zofran, Zuplenz), *p. 1040*
▸ Pharmacotherapy of Pancreatitis
   PROTOTYPE Pancrelipase (Creon, Pancreaze, Zenpep), *p. 1041*

KEY TERMS

cathartic, 1025

chemoreceptor trigger zone (CTZ), 1036

constipation, 1024

diarrhea, 1027

emetogenic potential, 1037

hyperemesis gravidarum, 1037

inflammatory bowel disease (IBD), 1030

irritable bowel syndrome (IBS), 1035

laxatives, 1025

nausea, 1036

pancreatitis, 1041

steatorrhea, 1041

vomiting, 1036

vomiting center, 1036

Bowel disorders, nausea, and vomiting are among the most common complaints for which patients seek medical consultation. Nonspecific symptoms of gastrointestinal (GI) distress may be caused by a large number of infectious, metabolic, inflammatory, neoplastic, or neuropsychological disorders. In addition, nausea, vomiting, constipation, and diarrhea are the most common adverse effects of oral (PO) medications. Although symptoms often resolve without the need for pharmacotherapy, when severe or prolonged, these conditions may lead to serious consequences unless drug therapy is initiated. This chapter examines the pharmacotherapy of these and other conditions associated with the GI tract. The anatomy and physiology of the lower GI tract are reviewed in Chapter 58.

Pathophysiology of Constipation

60.1 Constipation is characterized by infrequent or difficult bowel movements.

A large percentage of the water we drink is reabsorbed as it travels through the large intestine. Reabsorption of the proper amount of water results in stools of a normal, soft-formed consistency. If feces remain in the colon for an extended period too much water will be reabsorbed, leading to small, hard stools that are difficult to evacuate from the rectum without straining. Abdominal distention, discomfort, and flatulence may result.

Patients often define **constipation** as the infrequent passage of abnormally hard and dry stools. This definition, however, is not entirely satisfactory for diagnosis because the normal frequency of bowel movements varies widely among individuals, from two to three per day to as few as one per week. Constipation occurs more frequently in older adults because fecal transit time through the colon slows with aging. This population also exercises less, has diminished food intake, and is more likely to take certain drugs that cause constipation at a higher rate than in younger adults. Variations in frequency are normal and a daily bowel movement is not a requirement for good health.

Constipation is not a disease but a symptom of an underlying disorder or condition, some of which are shown in Table 60.1. A diagnosis of chronic constipation includes at least two of the following symptoms without the use of laxatives over the course of a year:

- Two or fewer bowel movements per week
- Lumpy or hard stools at least 25% of the time
- Straining to pass stools at least 25% of the time
- A feeling of incomplete evacuation at least 25% of the time

Occasional constipation is self-limiting and does not require drug therapy. Lifestyle modifications that incorporate increased dietary fiber, fluid intake, and physical activity should be considered before drugs are utilized for constipation. Chronic, infrequent, and painful bowel movements that are accompanied by severe straining may justify initiation of treatment. Excessive straining may lead to anorectal pathology such as anal fissures, hemorrhoids, or rectal prolapse. In its most severe form, constipation can lead to a fecal impaction and complete obstruction of the bowel.

Constipation that is accompanied by acute pain and abdominal distention are signs of a potential bowel obstruction or paralytic

TABLE 60.1 Etiology of Constipation

Condition	Causes
Dietary	Inadequate fiber intake
	Inadequate fluid intake
	Inadequate food intake
	Specific foods: alcoholic beverages, products with a high content of refined white flour, dairy products, and chocolate
GI disorders	Bowel obstruction
	Diverticulitis
	Irritable bowel syndrome
	Tumors
Lifestyle	Lack of exercise
Medications	Antacids containing bismuth, calcium, or aluminum
	Barium sulfate
	Calcium channel blockers
	Drugs with anticholinergic action: antihistamines, phenothiazines, tricyclic antidepressants, some antiparkinsonism agents
	Iron supplements
	Nonsteroidal anti-inflammatory drugs (NSAIDs)
	Opioids
Metabolic disorders	Diabetes
	Hypercalcemia or hypocalcemia
	Hypothyroidism
Neurogenic/Central nervous system (CNS) disorders	Clinical depression
	Diminished peristalsis
	Head or spinal trauma
	Parkinson's disease
	Strokes
Pregnancy	Diminished exercise, change in diet, pressure of fetus on the colon

ileus. These conditions are medical emergencies, and laxatives, enemas, and other therapies are absolutely contraindicated until the patient receives a full medical evaluation.

Pharmacotherapy with Laxatives

60.2 Laxatives are drugs that increase the frequency and quality of bowel movements.

Laxatives, drugs that promote defecation (evacuation of the bowel), are commonly used to prevent and treat constipation. **Cathartic** is a related term that implies an accelerated, stronger, and more complete bowel emptying. A variety of prescription and over-the-counter (OTC) laxatives, including tablet and liquid formulations, are available. Suppositories are used for infants or patients who are unable to take PO drugs. Laxatives and their doses are listed in Table 60.2.

Laxatives have several important indications. These may be divided into prophylaxis of constipation and treatment of constipation:

Prophylaxis

- Patients who have had a myocardial infarction (MI) or those with rectal pathology who should not be straining
- Patients receiving drug therapies who have constipation as a known adverse effect
- Patients who are bedridden or otherwise unable to exercise
- Patients who are pregnant
- Elderly patients with weak abdominal or perineal muscles

Treatment

- Relieve simple, chronic constipation
- Accelerate the removal of ingested toxic substances following overdose or poisoning
- Accelerate the removal of dead parasites following antihelminthic drug therapy
- Cleanse the bowel prior to diagnostic or surgical procedures of the colon or genitourinary tract, including colonoscopy or barium enema

TABLE 60.2 Laxatives and Cathartics

Drug	Route and Adult Dose (Maximum Dose Where Indicated)	Adverse Effects
Bulk Forming		
calcium polycarbophil (Equalactin, FiberCon, Others)	PO: 1 g daily	*Abdominal fullness or cramping, fainting*
methylcellulose (Citrucel)	PO: 5–20 mL tid in 8–10 oz liquid	Esophageal or GI obstruction if taken with insufficient fluid
psyllium mucilloid (Metamucil, Naturacil)	PO: 1–2 tablespoons in 8 oz liquid daily prn	
Saline and Osmotic		
magnesium hydroxide (Milk of Magnesia)	PO: 20–60 mL or 6–8 tablets daily prn	*Diarrhea, abdominal cramping*
polyethylene glycol (MiraLAX)	PO: 17 g/day in 8 oz of liquid daily for 2–4 days	Hypermagnesemia with magnesium hydroxide (dysrhythmias, respiratory failure)
sodium biphosphate (Fleet Phospho-Soda)	PO: 15–30 mL mixed in liquid daily prn	
Stimulant		
bisacodyl (Correctol, Dulcolax, Others)	PO: 10–15 mg daily prn	*Abdominal cramping, nausea, fainting, diarrhea*
castor oil (Emulsoil, Neoloid)	PO: 15–60 mL daily prn	Fluid and electrolyte loss
Stool Softener/Surfactant		
docusate (Colace, Dulcolax Stool Softener)	PO: 50–500 mg daily	*Abdominal cramping, diarrhea* No serious adverse effects
Herbal Agents		
castor oil	PO: 15–60 mL daily	*Abdominal cramping, diarrhea* No serious adverse effects
senna (Ex-Lax, Senokot, Others)	PO: 8.6–17.2 mg daily	
Miscellaneous Laxatives		
lubiprostone (Amitiza)	PO (idiopathic constipation): 24 mcg bid; PO (IBS with constipation): 8 mcg bid	*Diarrhea, nausea, headache, abdominal pain* Allergic reaction, dyspnea
methylnaltrexone (Relistor)	Subcutaneous: 8 or 12 mg every other day	*Diarrhea, nausea, abdominal pain, flatulence, hyperhidrosis* GI perforation
mineral oil	PO: 15–30 mL bid	*Diarrhea, nausea* Nutritional deficiencies, pneumonia (with aspiration)
naloxegol (Movantik)	PO: 25 mg in the morning	*Abdominal pain, nausea, vomiting, diarrhea, flatulance* GI perforation, opioid withdrawal

Note: *Italics* indicate common adverse effects. <u>Underline</u> indicates serious adverse effects.

The most common adverse effects of laxatives include abdominal distention and cramping. Diarrhea may result from excessive use. When cleansing the bowel prior to a colonoscopy or purging the bowel of toxic substances or parasites, forceful, frequent bowel movements are expected outcomes. Care must be taken to rule out acute abdominal pathology such as bowel obstruction prior to administration, because the drugs will increase colon pressure and possibly cause bowel perforation.

Laxatives may be classified into five primary groups and a miscellaneous category. The choice of a particular drug depends on the reason for use (treatment or prophylaxis), the onset of action desired (rapid or slow), and the completeness of evacuation needed (cathartic or laxative).

Bulk-forming laxatives: Bulk-forming agents absorb water, thus adding size to the fecal mass. Because fiber absorbs water and expands to provide bulk, these drugs must be taken with plenty of water. Bulk-forming laxatives are first-line drugs for the treatment and prevention of chronic constipation and may be taken on a regular basis without ill effects. Because of their slow onset of action, they are not used when a rapid and complete bowel evacuation is necessary. Bulk-forming laxatives are pregnancy category C and their onset of action is 24 to 48 hours.

Stimulant laxatives: Stimulant laxatives promote peristalsis by irritating the bowel. They are rapid acting and are more likely to cause diarrhea and cramping than the bulk-forming type of laxatives. They should not be used routinely, because they may cause laxative dependence, abdominal cramping, and depletion of fluid and electrolytes. These products are often used to prepare the bowel prior to colon examination or surgery, sometimes in combination with other laxatives and enemas. Stimulant laxatives are pregnancy category C and their onset of action is 6 to 12 hours (PO) or 1 to 6 hours (rectal).

Surfactant laxatives: Surfactants, commonly called stool softeners, cause more water and fat to be absorbed into the stools. They are ineffective at treating constipation but are most often used to prevent the condition. Stool softeners are generally prescribed for patients who have a condition that puts them at risk for constipation, such as a surgery, an injury, or an MI where straining during defecation should be avoided. Stimulant laxatives are pregnancy category C and their onset of action is 24 to 48 hours.

Saline/osmotic cathartics: Saline cathartics, also called osmotic laxatives, are poorly absorbed in the intestine. They pull water into the fecal mass to create a more watery stool. These drugs can produce a bowel movement very quickly but should not be used on a regular basis due to the possibility of dehydration and fluid and electrolyte depletion. Saline laxatives are highly effective and are an important component of colonoscopy prep and for purging toxins from the body. Most saline cathartics are pregnancy category B. Their onset of action is 1 to 6 hours in high doses.

Herbal laxatives: Herbal agents are natural products that are available OTC and that are widely used for self-treatment of constipation. The most commonly used herbal laxative is senna, a potent herb that stimulates the bowel and increases peristalsis. Other natural laxatives include rhubarb, cascara sagrada, aloe, flaxseed, and dandelion. Patients should be advised to exercise caution when using herbal products because many have not been evaluated through controlled studies for safety or effectiveness.

The pregnancy category for natural products has not been determined and their onset of action is variable.

Miscellaneous agents: Mineral oil is a miscellaneous drug that acts by lubricating the stool and the colon mucosa. The use of mineral oil should be discouraged because it interferes with the absorption of fat-soluble vitamins and can cause other potentially serious adverse effects. Its onset of action is 24 to 48 hours. Approved in 2006, lubiprostone is used to treat chronic idiopathic constipation as well as the constipation form of irritable bowel syndrome (IBS) in women. Approved in 2008, methylnaltrexone (Relistor) is specifically used to treat chronic constipation in patients with advanced illness who are receiving opioids for palliative care. Methylnaltrexone blocks the effects of the opioids in the colon without affecting analgesia. The newest of the miscellaneous drugs is naloxegol (Movantik) which was approved in 2014 specifically for constipation induced by opioid medications. When taken for prolonged periods or at high doses, opioids cause constipation in most patients.

PROTOTYPE DRUG	**Psyllium Mucilloid (Metamucil, Others)**

Classification: Therapeutic: Agent for constipation
Pharmacologic: Bulk-type laxative

Therapeutic Effects and Uses: Psyllium is derived from a natural product—the seeds of the plantain plant. Like other bulk-forming laxatives, psyllium is an insoluble fiber that is indigestible and not absorbed from the GI tract. When taken with a sufficient quantity of water, psyllium swells and increases the size of the fecal mass. The larger the size of the fecal mass, the greater will be the neural stimulus for defecation.

Several doses of psyllium may be needed over 1 to 3 days to produce an optimum therapeutic effect. Several 2.4-g doses may be taken each day. Frequent use of psyllium (7 g/day) may effect a small reduction in blood cholesterol level. This drug is available as granules, powder, and wafers.

Mechanism of Action: Psyllium expands the size of the stool and promotes colon peristalsis that closely resembles a natural bowel movement.

Pharmacokinetics:

Route(s)	PO
Absorption	Not absorbed; remains in the GI tract
Distribution	Not distributed
Primary metabolism	Not metabolized
Primary excretion	Feces
Onset of action	12–24 h
Duration of action	Unknown

Adverse Effects: Psyllium is the safest laxative and rarely produces adverse effects. It generally causes less cramping than the stimulant-type laxatives and results in a more natural bowel movement. If taken with insufficient water, psyllium may swell in the esophagus and cause obstruction.

Contraindications/Precautions: Psyllium should not be administered to patients with undiagnosed abdominal pain, suspected intestinal obstruction, or fecal impaction.

Drug Interactions: Psyllium may decrease the absorption and effects of warfarin, digoxin, nitrofurantoin, antibiotics, and salicylates. **Herbal/Food:** Unknown.

Pregnancy: Category C.

Treatment of Overdose: Overdose from psyllium is unlikely.

Nursing Responsibilities: Key nursing implications for patients receiving psyllium are included in the Nursing Practice Application for Patients Receiving Pharmacotherapy with Laxatives or Antidiarrheals.

Drugs Similar to Psyllium Mucilloid (Metamucil, Others)

Other popular laxatives include bisacodyl, castor oil, docusate, and magnesium salts.

Bisacodyl (Correctol, Dulcolax, Others): Bisacodyl is the most frequently used stimulant-type laxative. It acts by irritating the mucosa in the colon and by altering intestinal and electrolyte absorption. Only 15% of the drug is absorbed after oral administration. Onset of action is 8 to 12 hours (PO) if taken at bedtime or 15 to 60 minutes per rectal suppository. Bisacodyl should not be taken with milk or other dairy products because these can dissolve the enteric coating and cause dyspepsia. The enteric-coated tablets should not be crushed or chewed. Minor adverse effects include abdominal pain and cramping. Prolonged use may lead to laxative dependence and fluid and electrolyte loss. Bisacodyl is pregnancy category C.

Castor oil (Emulsoil, Neoloid): Castor oil is one of the oldest and worst-tasting laxatives. It was approved by the U.S. Food and Drug Administration (FDA) in 1939. A stimulant-type laxative, castor oil acts on the small intestine and produces a bowel movement in 2 to 6 hours. It causes more adverse effects than other laxatives, including diarrhea, cramping, nausea, vomiting, and dizziness. This drug is pregnancy category X and must not be used during pregnancy.

Docusate (Colace): Docusate is the most frequently prescribed surfactant-type laxative or stool softener. This drug permits additional water and lipids to penetrate the stool, making it softer. Docusate takes several days to act and therefore is not effective when a rapid and complete bowel evacuation is necessary. Only small amounts are absorbed systemically. Adverse effects are rare. Docusate sodium (Colace) should not be given to patients on sodium restriction. Docusate potassium (Dialose) should not be given to patients with renal impairment. Docusate increases the systemic absorption of mineral oil, so these two medications should not be given concurrently. Docusate should not be taken with certain herbal products such as senna, cascara, rhubarb, or aloe, because it will increase their absorption and the risk of liver toxicity. Docusate is pregnancy category C.

Magnesium hydroxide (Milk of Magnesia, MOM): Magnesium hydroxide has two effects on the GI tract. Taken PO it exerts an antacid effect because this drug neutralizes gastric hydrochloric acid to form magnesium chloride. About 30% of the magnesium chloride is absorbed systemically. The remainder continues along the GI tract and reaches the colon, where it exerts a laxative effect by drawing water and electrolytes to form a larger and softer fecal mass. This drug has a chalky taste and has a small incidence of nausea, vomiting, and abdominal cramping. Patients with impaired renal function should be monitored for hypermagnesemia. Magnesium hydroxide can bind to other drugs, delaying their absorption; thus it should be taken at least 2 hours apart from other medications. Drugs that may result in decreased absorption include H_2-receptor antagonists, iron salts, phenytoin, digoxin, and tetracyclines. Magnesium citrate and magnesium sulfate are other saline-type laxatives with rapid onsets of action (30 minutes to 4 hours).

CONNECTION Checkpoint 60.1

From what you learned in Chapter 22, describe the indications for using magnesium to treat seizure disorders. *See Answer to Connection Checkpoint 60.1 on student resource website.*

Pathophysiology of Diarrhea

60.3 Diarrhea is an abnormal increase in the frequency and fluidity of bowel movements.

The small intestine receives about 9 L of fluid, or chyme, daily. Most is reabsorbed, such that only about 1 L reaches the colon. Travel through the colon results in even more reabsorption, and only about 100 mL remains to form stools. Should the small or large intestines fail to reabsorb sufficient fluids, diarrhea may occur. **Diarrhea** is an increase in the frequency and fluidity of bowel movements.

Like constipation, occasional diarrhea is a self-limiting disorder that does not warrant drug therapy. In some cases, diarrhea is a type of body defense, rapidly and completely eliminating the body of toxins and pathogens. When prolonged or severe, especially in children, diarrhea can result in a significant loss of body fluids, and pharmacotherapy is indicated. In underdeveloped countries, diarrhea is

---

CONNECTIONS | Community-Oriented Practice

◀ Laxative Abuse

Laxatives are one of the most frequently abused OTC medication classes. Abuse occurs when patients overuse laxatives due to a false belief that daily bowel movements are necessary. Laxative abuse is also seen in patients who do not include sufficient fiber or water in their diets. Patients may also abuse laxatives to lose weight. Some have eating disorders, such as binge eaters who may want to get rid of large meals.

Nurses should monitor for laxative abuse and provide patients with the appropriate education about the use of these drugs. Laxative abuse can have serious effects, such as damage to the muscular function of the bowel and removal of the body's water, vitamins, and minerals. Loss of minerals and salts can cause electrolyte imbalances. Older adults are most vulnerable to these types of changes. Laxatives can also affect the effectiveness of other medications.

The nurse should instruct the older adult who expresses concern about overuse of laxatives to see a health care provider to determine the cause of the chronic constipation. Also, the nurse should instruct the patient that tapering off laxative overuse may be better than stopping abruptly. Changing to products containing psyllium may help. Additional alternatives to prevent constipation include the following:

- Drink plenty of water with each meal and throughout the day.
- Eat more fresh fruits, vegetables, and whole grains to increase dietary fiber.
- Go to the bathroom when you feel the urge. (This may occur right after a meal.)
- Exercise regularly to promote bowel movements.

a major cause of illness and death in young children. Prolonged diarrhea may lead to fluid, acid–base, or electrolyte imbalances.

Because diarrhea is a nonspecific symptom of an underlying condition or disease, a primary treatment goal is to identify and treat the cause. Assessing the patient's recent travels, dietary habits, immune system competence, and drug history may provide important clues about the etiology. Because such a large number of conditions can cause diarrhea, pinpointing an exact cause may be difficult. Therefore, symptomatic therapy is provided for the diarrhea while identifying its cause. Common etiologies include the following:

- **Infection.** Viral and bacterial infections are the most common cause of diarrhea. Intestinal protozoans and helminths are less common causes. The most frequently encountered diarrhea-producing organisms are *Campylobacter, Salmonella, Cryptosporidium, Giardia, Shigella, Escherichia coli* (traveler's diarrhea), and *Staphylococcus*.

- **Drugs.** Antibiotics often cause diarrhea by killing normal intestinal flora, thereby allowing an overgrowth of opportunistic pathogenic organisms. Laxatives, magnesium antacids, digoxin, orlistat, and NSAIDs are also common causes.

- **Inflammation.** Ulcerative colitis, Crohn's disease, and IBS cause inflammation of the bowel mucosa, leading to periods of intense diarrhea.

- **Foods.** Various foods can cause diarrhea, such as dairy products in lactose-intolerant patients, foods with capsaicin (hot pepper), and chronic alcohol ingestion.

- **Malabsorption.** Diseases of the small intestine and pancreas can cause insufficient absorption of foods and fluid.

Pharmacotherapy of Diarrhea

60.4 Opioids are the most effective drugs for controlling severe diarrhea.

Pharmacotherapy related to diarrhea depends on the severity of the condition and any identifiable etiologic factors. If the cause is an infectious disease, then an antibiotic or antiparasitic drug is indicated. Should the etiology be inflammatory, then anti-inflammatory drugs are warranted. When the cause appears to be due to an adverse effect of pharmacotherapy, the health care provider should discontinue the offending medication, lower the dose, or substitute an alternative drug.

The most effective drugs for the symptomatic treatment of diarrhea are the opioids, which can dramatically slow peristalsis in the colon. The most common opioid antidiarrheals are codeine and diphenoxylate with atropine (Lomotil). Diphenoxylate is a Schedule V agent that acts directly on the intestine to slow peristalsis, thereby allowing for more fluid and electrolyte absorption in the large intestine. The opioids cause central nervous system (CNS) depression at high doses and are generally reserved for the short-term therapy of acute diarrhea due to potential adverse effects and the potential for dependence. Details on the indications and adverse effects of opioids are found in Chapter 25.

OTC drugs for diarrhea act by a number of different mechanisms. Loperamide (Imodium) is an analog of meperidine (Demerol), although it has no narcotic effects and is not classified as a controlled substance. Low-dose loperamide is available OTC; higher doses are available by prescription. Other OTC treatments include bismuth subsalicylate (Pepto-Bismol), which acts by binding and absorbing toxins. Psyllium preparations may also slow diarrhea because they absorb large amounts of fluid, which helps to form bulkier stools. Probiotic supplements containing *Lactobacillus*, a normal inhabitant of the human gut and vagina, are sometimes taken to correct the altered GI flora following a serious diarrhea episode. A good source of healthy *Lactobacillus* is yogurt with active cultures, although a freeze-dried form of the bacteria is available in tablets. The antidiarrheals are listed in Table 60.3.

Antidiarrheal medications should never be used to treat diarrhea caused by poisoning or infection by toxin-producing organisms. For these patients, it is important that the toxic substances and organisms be expelled from the body. Use of antidiarrheals will retain these harmful substances. Antidiarrheal use is contraindicated in cases of diarrhea caused by pseudomembranous colitis that is caused by *Clostridium difficile*. This infection can cause fatal toxic megacolon.

TABLE 60.3 Antidiarrheals

Drug	Route and Adult Dose (Maximum Dose Where Indicated)	Adverse Effects
Opioids		
camphorated opium tincture (Paregoric)	PO: 5–10 mL 1–4 times daily	*Drowsiness, lightheadedness, nausea, dizziness, dry mouth (from atropine), constipation*
difenoxin with atropine (Motofen)	PO: 1–2 mg after each diarrhea episode (max: 8 mg/day)	
diphenoxylate with atropine (Lomotil)	PO: 5 mg 4 times daily (max: 20 mg/day)	Paralytic ileus with toxic megacolon, respiratory depression, CNS depression
loperamide (Imodium)	PO: 4 mg as a single dose, then 2 mg after each diarrhea episode (max: 16 mg/day)	
Miscellaneous Antidiarrheals		
bismuth subsalicylate (Kaopectate, Pepto-Bismol)	PO: 2 tablets or 30 mL prn	*Constipation, nausea, tinnitus* Impaction, Reye's syndrome
octreotide (Sandostatin)	Subcutaneous/intravenous (IV): 100–600 mcg/day in 2–4 divided doses	*Nausea, diarrhea, abdominal pain* Hypo- or hyperglycemia, gallstones, cholestatic hepatitis

Note: *Italics* indicate common adverse effects. Underline indicates serious adverse effects.

PROTOTYPE DRUG	**Diphenoxylate with Atropine (Lomotil)**

Classification: Therapeutic: Antidiarrheal
Pharmacologic: Opioid

Therapeutic Effects and Uses: Approved in 1960, diphenoxylate is an oral opioid available by liquid or tablet that is a Schedule V controlled substance. Like other opioids, diphenoxylate slows peristalsis, allowing time for additional water reabsorption from the intestine and the formation of solid stools. It acts within 45 to 60 minutes. It is effective for moderate to severe diarrhea, but it is not recommended for infants. The atropine in Lomotil is not added for its anticholinergic effect but to discourage patients from taking too much of the drug. At recommended doses the effects of atropine are negligible.

Diphenoxylate is discontinued as soon as the diarrhea symptoms resolve. A low-maintenance dose may be continued for up to 10 days if additional diarrhea is anticipated. Lomotil is approved for use in children 2 years and older.

Mechanism of Action: Diphenoxylate acts on the smooth muscle of the intestine to slow peristalsis.

Pharmacokinetics:

Route(s)	PO
Absorption	90% absorbed
Distribution	Small amounts are secreted in breast milk
Primary metabolism	Hepatic; metabolized to active metabolite
Primary excretion	Bile and feces
Onset of action	45–60 min
Duration of action	3–4 h

Adverse Effects: Unlike most opioids, diphenoxylate has no analgesic properties and has an extremely low potential for abuse. The drug is well tolerated at normal doses. Some patients experience dizziness, lethargy, or drowsiness, and care should be taken not to drive or operate machinery until the effects of the drug are known. At higher doses the anticholinergic effects of atropine, which include drowsiness, flushing, dry mouth, and tachycardia, may be observed.

Contraindications/Precautions: Contraindications to diphenoxylate include hypersensitivity to the drug, severe hepatic impairment, obstructive jaundice, and diarrhea associated with pseudomembranous colitis. Dehydration or electrolyte imbalances should be corrected before diphenoxylate therapy is initiated.

Drug Interactions: Other CNS depressants, including alcohol, will cause additive sedative effects. Opiate antagonists such as naloxone will reduce the effectiveness of diphenoxylate. When taken with monoamine oxidase inhibitors (MAOIs), diphenoxylate may cause hypertensive crisis. **Herbal/Food:** Unknown.

Pregnancy: Category C.

Treatment of Overdose: Overdose with Lomotil may be serious. Narcotic antagonists such as naloxone may be administered parenterally to reverse respiratory depression within minutes.

Nursing Responsibilities: Key nursing implications for patients receiving diphenoxylate with atropine are included in the Nursing Practice Application for Patients Receiving Pharmacotherapy with Laxatives or Antidiarrheals.

Drugs Similar to Diphenoxylate with Atropine (Lomotil)

Other antidiarrheal agents include bismuth subsalicylate, difenoxin with atropine, loperamide, octreotide, and paregoric.

Bismuth subsalicylate (Kaopectate, Pepto-Bismol): Bismuth subsalicylate is an oral OTC drug approved for indigestion, heartburn, and diarrhea. Its more recent use is in the treatment of *Helicobacter* infections in patients with peptic ulcer disease. Doses may be taken every 30 to 60 minutes (max: 4 doses/day) until the diarrhea resolves. Adverse effects do not occur at recommended doses. Stools may become discolored, but this is not harmful. In stomach acid, bismuth subsalicylate forms salicylic acid, which is absorbed systemically. Thus this drug should be used with caution by patients using aspirin; otherwise salicylate toxicity may result. In addition, this drug should not be used in children with chickenpox or flu symptoms due to the possibility of Reye's syndrome. A "Children's Pepto" is available that contains calcium carbonate without salicylates. This drug is pregnancy category C.

Difenoxin with atropine (Motofen): Difenoxin is an opioid that is an active metabolite of diphenoxylate; thus the two drugs have the same actions, contraindications, and adverse effects. Like Lomotil, atropine is added to Motofen to discourage substance abusers from using the drug. It is a Schedule IV controlled substance and is pregnancy category C.

Loperamide (Imodium): Approved in 1976, loperamide is an oral drug that is a drug of choice for the symptomatic treatment of acute diarrhea and the maintenance therapy of chronic diarrhea. Chemically related to the opioids, it shares the antidiarrheal properties of the opioids but has no analgesic action and does not produce dependence. This drug slows peristalsis, increasing the transit time, thus allowing for better formed stools. If diarrhea is not controlled after 48 hours of loperamide therapy, the patient should seek medical attention. Adverse effects are rare. A dose may last up to 24 hours. Safety has been established in children less than 2 years of age. This drug is pregnancy category C.

Octreotide (Sandostatin): Approved in 1988, octreotide is closely related to somatostatin (growth hormone–inhibiting hormone). It is approved to treat acromegaly and severe diarrhea associated with cancer. Octreotide is used off-label to treat a wide variety of other conditions including acquired immunodeficiency syndrome (AIDS)–related diarrhea, ileostomy-related diarrhea, and childhood diarrhea. Octreotide prevents the release of serotonin and other active peptides that promote diarrhea. It also directly inhibits intestinal secretions and enhances absorption. It is only given by the intramuscular (IM) or intravenous (IV) route. A long-acting depot form (Sandostatin LAR) is available for long-term use. The most frequent adverse effects are GI related, such as nausea, diarrhea, and abdominal pain. During long-term therapy, more than half of the patients who are taking octreotide experience gallbladder pathology, including gallstones, or cholestatic hepatitis. This drug is pregnancy category B.

Paregoric (camphorated opium): Paregoric contains opium, which has morphine and codeine as the active ingredients. Although once widely used in the treatment of severe diarrhea, it can cause opioid-related adverse effects and is a Schedule III controlled substance. This drug may also be used to prevent withdrawal symptoms in newborns born to opioid-dependent mothers. Safer agents have replaced paregoric. For short-term use, paregoric is pregnancy category C.

Pharmacotherapy of Inflammatory Bowel Disease

60.5 Inflammatory bowel disease is treated with immunosuppressants and anti-inflammatory drugs.

Inflammatory bowel disease (IBD) is characterized by the presence of ulcers in the intestinal tract. Crohn's disease or Crohn's lesions typically appear in the distal region of the small intestine (terminal ileum), although they can affect any region of the GI tract from the mouth to the anus. Crohn's lesions usually are discontinuous: Affected areas of the intestinal mucosa alternate with normal areas. The mucosal erosions characteristic of ulcerative colitis begin in the rectum and progress in an uninterrupted manner throughout the rest of the large intestine. It is estimated that 1 to 2 million Americans have IBD.

The etiology of IBD remains largely unknown. Several genes involved with immune responses are associated with the disorder. It is hypothesized that these defective genes cause hyperactivity of T-cell responses to normal flora in the terminal ileum and colon. These hyperactive responses result in chronic intestinal inflammation.

In addition to genetic susceptibility, certain environmental triggers exacerbate symptoms of IBD. The best studied trigger for Crohn's disease is smoking. Infections, the use of NSAIDs, and a high level of stress are additional environmental factors that have been identified. Less well known are triggers for ulcerative colitis; in many patients, triggers cannot be identified. It is known that symptoms of ulcerative colitis tend to peak between age 15 and 30 and again between 50 and 70.

Symptoms of IBD range from mild to acute, and the condition is characterized by alternating periods of remission and exacerbation. The most common clinical presentation of ulcerative colitis is abdominal cramping with frequent bowel movements. Severe

---

CONNECTIONS: NURSING PRACTICE APPLICATION

Patients Receiving Pharmacotherapy with Laxatives or Antidiarrheals

Assessment	Potential Nursing Diagnoses*
Baseline assessment prior to administration: • Obtain a complete health history including GI, cardiovascular, hepatic or renal disease, pregnancy, or breast-feeding. Obtain a drug history including allergies, current prescription and OTC drugs, herbal preparations, caffeine, nicotine, and alcohol use. Be alert to possible drug interactions. • Obtain a history of past and current symptoms, noting what measures have been successful to relieve the symptoms (e.g., increased fluids, fiber, dietary changes). • Obtain baseline weight and vital signs. • Evaluate appropriate laboratory findings (e.g., CBC, electrolytes, hepatic or renal function studies). • Obtain an abdominal assessment (e.g., bowel sounds, softness or firmness, distention, presence of tenderness). • Assess the patient's ability to receive and understand instructions. Include the family and caregivers as needed.	• *Constipation* • *Diarrhea* • *Deficient Knowledge* (Drug Therapy) • *Risk for Deficient Fluid Volume*
Assessment throughout administration: • Assess for desired therapeutic effects (e.g., adequate pattern of elimination, normal stool consistency and volume). • Continue periodic monitoring of abdominal assessment findings, especially bowel sounds. • Continue periodic monitoring of CBC, electrolytes, and hepatic and renal function laboratory values as appropriate. • Assess for adverse effects: nausea, vomiting, diarrhea, constipation, headache, drowsiness, and dizziness. Severe abdominal pain, vomiting, coffee-ground emesis, hematemesis, blood in the stool, or tarry stools should be reported **immediately.**	

Implementation

Interventions and (Rationales)	Patient-Centered Care
Ensuring therapeutic effects: • Treat the cause: If a definitive cause for the current symptoms can be identified (e.g., infection, food poisoning, inadequate fluid intake), correct the cause where possible. (Constipation and diarrhea are usually symptoms of other underlying conditions such as infections, inadequate fluid or fiber intake, stress, or sedentary lifestyle. The nursing history can assist in determining the cause of the symptoms.)	• For recurrent constipation or diarrhea, encourage the patient to maintain a diary of correlations between symptoms, foods, beverages, stress, or medications to help identify causative factors. • Review medications or possibility of illness with the patient or family to help identify factors that may require treatment or alterations in medication.

CONNECTIONS: NURSING PRACTICE APPLICATION (continued)

- Encourage appropriate lifestyle changes. (Ensuring adequate daily amounts of fluids and dietary fiber and increasing activity levels assist in encouraging normal peristaltic activity. Smoking and alcohol use are known to alter normal peristalsis and should be limited or eliminated. Correlating symptoms with medications or stress may help to identify a triggering factor.)

- Encourage the patient to adopt a healthy lifestyle of increased dietary fiber and fluid intake, increased exercise, increasing yogurt and *acidophilus*-containing foods, managing stress as needed, and limiting or eliminating alcohol consumption and smoking. Provide for dietitian consultation or information on smoking cessation programs as needed.
- Encourage the patient to keep a diary, noting correlations between symptoms and foods, beverages, stress, or medications.

- Follow appropriate administration guidelines for best results. Do not administer laxatives if bowel obstruction is possible. Do not administer antidiarrheal drugs if infection is possible. (Bowel obstruction must be ruled out in the presence of hypoactive or absent bowel sounds. If infection is a possible cause of diarrhea, giving antidiarrheal drugs may decrease peristalsis, giving the infection an opportunity to increase and spread.)

- Teach the patient to take the drug following appropriate guidelines or label directions, particularly for any additional fluid intake required, for best results.
- Instruct the patient that diarrhea or constipation associated with increasing nausea or vomiting, especially if accompanied by abdominal pain or fever, should be reported to the health care provider before taking the drug.

Minimizing adverse effects:
- Continue to monitor abdominal assessment findings. Any significant increase or decrease in bowel sounds, new onset, or increased discomfort or pain should be reported promptly. (Any significant change in bowel sound activity or increased discomfort or pain may signal the development of worsening bowel disease or adverse drug effects.)

- Teach the patient that some easing of discomfort related to constipation or diarrhea may be noticed soon after beginning drug therapy, but full effects may take several days or longer. If gastric discomfort or pain continues or worsens, the health care provider should be notified.

- Monitor for any severe abdominal pain, vomiting, coffee-ground emesis or hematemesis, blood in stool, or tarry stools, and report immediately. (Severe abdominal pain or blood in emesis or stools may indicate a worsening of disease or more serious conditions and should be reported immediately.)

- Teach the patient that severe abdominal pain or any blood in emesis or stools should be reported immediately to the health care provider.

- Ensure patient safety. Observe for lightheadedness or dizziness. Monitor ambulation until the effects of the drug are known. Obtain electrolyte levels if dizziness continues. (Drowsiness or dizziness from opioid-based or related antidiarrheals may occur. **Lifespan:** The older adult is at increased risk of injury and falls. Diphenoxylate with atropine may cause agitation, confusion, or hallucinations in the older adult, particularly if dementia is a preexisting condition. Continued dizziness may indicate electrolyte imbalance, and electrolyte levels should be assessed.)

- Instruct the patient to call for assistance prior to getting out of bed or attempting to walk alone if dizziness or drowsiness occurs. Provide for a commode or bedpan nearby. For home use, avoid driving or other activities requiring mental alertness or physical coordination until the effects of the drug are known. Immediately report any agitation, confusion, or hallucinations to the health care provider.

- Continue to monitor periodic hepatic and renal function tests and electrolyte levels as needed. (Abnormal liver function tests may indicate adverse hepatic effects from drugs such as diphenoxylate with atropine or octreotide. Excessive use of laxatives or continued diarrhea may affect electrolyte levels.)

- Instruct the patient on the need to return periodically for laboratory work.

- Monitor vital signs, particularly respiratory rate and depth, in patients taking opioid or opioid-related drugs. (Drugs such as diphenoxylate with atropine may depress CNS activity and decrease respiratory rate and depth. Intervention with narcotic antagonists may be needed if overdose occurs.)

- Teach the patient to take the drug as ordered and not to increase dose or frequency unless instructed to do so by the health care provider. Any drowsiness, dizziness, or disorientation should be reported to the provider promptly.

Patient understanding of drug therapy:
- Use opportunities during administration of medications and during assessments to discuss the rationale for drug therapy, desired therapeutic outcomes, commonly observed adverse effects, parameters for when to call the health care provider, and any necessary monitoring or precautions. (Using time during nursing care helps to optimize and reinforce key teaching areas.)

- The patient, family, or caregiver should be able to state the reason for the drug, appropriate dose and scheduling, what adverse effects to observe for and when to report them, and the anticipated length of medication therapy.

Patient self-administration of drug therapy:
- When administering the medication, instruct the patient, family, or caregiver in proper self-administration of the drug, e.g., taken with additional fluids. (Utilizing time during nurse-administration of these drugs helps to reinforce teaching.)

- Teach the patient on laxatives to take the drug following appropriate guidelines as follows:
  - **All laxative drugs:** Take the drug with additional fluids and increase fluid intake throughout the day. Increase the intake of dietary fiber, especially whole grains, fruits, and vegetables. Exceeding the recommended dose or frequent laxative use increases the risk of adverse effects and decreases normal peristalsis over time, resulting in laxative dependence.
  - **Bulk-forming laxatives:** Take other medications 1 h before or 2 h after the laxative. Powdered formulations should be mixed with a full glass of liquid and immediately taken, followed by an additional full glass of liquid. Powders should never be swallowed dry or esophageal obstruction may result.
  - **Mineral oil laxatives:** Should not be taken if nausea is present and should not be taken at bedtime to avoid the possibility of aspiration.

---

*Nursing Diagnoses—Definitions and Classification 2015–2017. Copyright © 2014, 1994–2014 by NANDA International. Used by arrangement with John Wiley & Sons Limited.

disease may lead to weight loss, bloody diarrhea, high fever, and dehydration. The patient with Crohn's disease also presents with abdominal pain, cramping, and diarrhea, which may have been present for years before seeking treatment. Symptoms of Crohn's disease are often similar to those of ulcerative colitis. Patients with IBD have an increased risk of acquiring GI cancer.

The expected outcomes for the pharmacotherapy of IBD are as follows:

- Reduce the acute symptoms of active disease by induction therapy and place the disease in remission.
- Keep the disease in remission with maintenance therapy.
- Change the natural course or progression of the disease.

Multiple medications are utilized to treat IBD, and pharmacotherapy is conducted in a stepwise manner, starting with the safest and best established medications for the disorder, as shown in Pharmacotherapy Illustrated 60.1. The first step of IBD treatment is usually with 5-aminosalicylic acid (5-ASA) agents that include sulfasalazine (Azulfidine), olsalazine (Dipentum), balsalazide (Colazal), and mesalamine (Asacol, Canasa, Lialda, others). These drugs act rapidly and exhibit a higher safety profile than the second-line agents. While effective at initially reducing symptoms, the 5-ASA medications are not as effective in maintaining remission. Doses

for the 5-ASA drugs are listed in Table 60.4. In some cases, a short course of antibiotics may benefit the patient experiencing mild symptoms.

When IBD symptoms are more intense or when patients have not responded well to the 5-ASA drugs, oral corticosteroids such as prednisone are used. Because of their potentially serious long-term adverse effects, however, they are prescribed for the shortest length of time needed to send the disease into remission. In hospitalized patients, IV corticosteroids may be used to put IBD into remission. For a detailed discussion of corticosteroid therapy, refer to Chapter 68.

Budesonide (Entocort-EC) is a corticosteroid with interesting properties that allow it to be used as a first-line therapy for IBD. Entocort-EC is encapsulated to avoid significant absorption in the stomach or duodenum. This drug is released slowly and reaches a high concentration in the terminal ileum and proximal colon—the two most frequently affected sites for IBD. Thus budesonide is in direct contact with the GI mucosa and produces a topical anti-inflammatory effect. In addition, when budesonide is absorbed, it is almost entirely removed by first-pass metabolism in the liver. Thus this drug shows few of the adverse effects seen with the long-term use of the other corticosteroids. It is approved for mild to moderate Crohn's disease. In 2012, a delayed release form of budesonide (Uceris), administered once daily, was approved to treat ulcerative colitis.

PHARMACOTHERAPY ILLUSTRATED 60.1

Inflammatory Bowel Disease

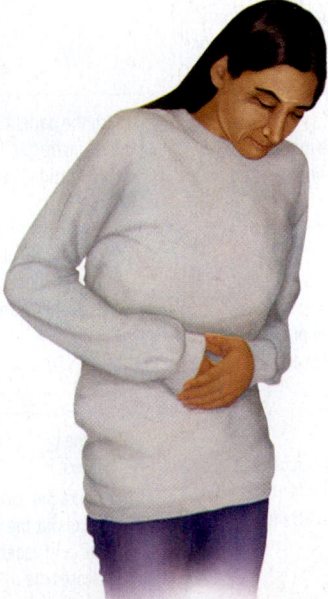

Mild Symptoms

Aminosalicylates
- Balsalazide
- Mesalamine
- Olsalazine
- Sulfasalazine

Antibiotics
- Ciprofloxacin
- Metronidazole

Moderate Symptoms

Oral corticosteroids
- Budesonide
- Dexamethasone
- Prednisolone
- Prednisone

IV corticosteroids
- Hydrocortisone
- Methylprednisolone

Severe Symptoms

Immunomodulators
- Azathioprine
- Cyclosporine
- 6-mercaptopurine
- Methotrexate
- Tacrolimus

Biologic therapies
- Adalimumab
- Certolizumab
- Infliximab
- Natalizumab

TABLE 60.4	Selected Drugs for Inflammatory Bowel Disease and Irritable Bowel Syndrome	
Drug	**Route and Adult Dose (Maximum Dose Where Indicated)**	**Adverse Effects**
First-Line Drugs for Inflammatory Bowel Disease		
balsalazide (Colazal, Giazo)	PO (Colazal): 2.25 g tid for 8–12 weeks PO (Giazo): 3.3 g bid for up to 8 weeks	*Headache, abdominal pain, diarrhea, nausea, vomiting, rash, flulike illness, allergic reactions*
mesalamine (Asacol, Canasa, Lialda, Others)	PO (delayed release tablets): 800 mg tid for 6 weeks PO (delayed release capsules): 1 g qid for 8 weeks	<u>Hepatotoxicity, blood dyscrasias, renal impairment, salicylate hypersensitivity, crystalluria (sulfasalazine)</u>
olsalazine (Dipentum)	PO: 500 mg bid (max: 3 g/day)	
sulfasalazine (Azulfidine)	PO: 1–2 g/day in four divided doses (max: 8 g/day)	
Drugs for Irritable Bowel Syndrome		
alosetron (Lotronex)	PO: Begin with 1 mg daily for 4 weeks; may increase to 1 mg bid (max: 2 mg/day)	*Constipation, abdominal discomfort, nausea, and rash* <u>Ischemic colitis, ileus</u>
dicyclomine (Bentyl)	PO/IM: 20–40 mg qid (max: 160 mg/day PO; 80 mg/day IM)	*Dry mouth, blurred vision, drowsiness, constipation, urinary hesitancy, and tachycardia*
hyoscyamine (Anaspaz, Gastrosed, Levsin)	PO: 0.15–0.3 mg 1–4 times/day	<u>Confusion, paralytic ileus</u>
linaclotide (Linzess)	PO: 145–290 mcg once daily	*Abdominal pain and distention, flatulence* <u>Severe diarrhea</u>
lubiprostone (Amitiza)	Chronic idiopathic constipation: PO: 24 mcg taken twice daily IBS with constipation: PO: 8 mcg taken twice daily (max: 48 mcg/day)	*Nausea, diarrhea, headache, dyspnea* <u>Allergic reactions</u>

Note: Italics indicate common adverse effects. <u>Underline</u> indicates serious adverse effects.

Should therapy with corticosteroids fail, step 3 of IBD therapy includes immunosuppressive drugs, such as azathioprine (Imuran), mercaptopurine (Purinethol), or methotrexate (MTX, Rheumatrex, Trexall). These medications are not used for induction therapy because they have a 3-month onset of action. They are, however, effective at extending the time between relapses. For a detailed discussion of immunosuppressant therapy, refer to Chapter 42.

The introduction of biologic therapies in the late 1990s gave clinicians another valuable tool in the pharmacotherapy of IBD. The biologic therapies for IBD comprise two classes.

- Tumor necrosis factor (TNF) inhibitors, such as infliximab (Remicade), have been shown to effectively reduce the acute symptoms of and provide maintenance therapy for both Crohn's disease and ulcerative colitis. Newer anti-TNF drugs include adalimumab (Humira), certolizumab pegol (Cimzia), and golimumab (Simponi).

- Integrin inhibitors: The two drugs in this class are monoclonal antibodies that bind integrins, which are receptors that mediate cell to cell communication. This binding impedes the ability of T-lymphocytes to migrate to inflamed lymphoid tissue in the intestinal tract. Natalizumab (Tysabri) was approved in 2008 to treat severe Crohn's disease. This drug was previously approved for multiple sclerosis (see Chapter 21). Natalizumab has adverse effects that limit its use, the most serious of which is an increased risk for progressive multifocal leukoencephalopathy (PML), an often-fatal opportunistic viral infection of the brain. In 2014, a second integrin inhibitor, vedolizumab (Entyvio),

was approved to treat IBD. No cases of PML have been recorded with vedolizumab. Both natalizumab and vedolizumab are administered by the IV route for patients who have not responded to immunomodulators or TNF inhibitors.

The biologic therapies are expensive, costing thousands of dollars per injection, and some patients experience a high rate of serious infections due to their immunosuppressive actions. Biologic therapies are usually recommended only when therapy with first-line drugs is unable to control symptoms. Because they cause healing of the GI mucosa, it is possible that early use of these drugs could change the progressive course of IBD. This is an area of active research. For a detailed discussion of biologic therapies and doses of these drugs, refer to Chapter 42.

PROTOTYPE DRUG | **Sulfasalazine (Azulfidine)**

Classification: Therapeutic: Drug for inflammatory bowel disease, DMARD
Pharmacologic: 5-aminosalicylate, anti-inflammatory, sulfonamide

Therapeutic Effects and Uses: Approved in 1950, sulfasalazine is a PO drug with anti-inflammatory properties that is approved to treat mild to moderate symptoms of ulcerative colitis for adults and children age 6 years and older. It is approved as an alternate drug in the pharmacotherapy of rheumatoid arthritis and is classified as a disease-modifying antirheumatic drug (DMARD) (see Chapter 72). Sulfasalazine is used off-label to treat Crohn's disease.

Colon bacteria metabolize sulfasalazine to two active metabolites: sulfapyridine and 5-ASA. These metabolites are responsible for its anti-inflammatory properties.

Mechanism of Action: Sulfasalazine and its metabolites inhibit the mediators of inflammation in the colon such as prostaglandins and leukotrienes.

Pharmacokinetics:

Route(s)	PO
Absorption	Sulfasalazine is only 10–15% absorbed but its metabolites in the colon produce the therapeutic effects
Distribution	Crosses the placenta; secreted in breast milk; 93% bound to plasma protein
Primary metabolism	Hepatic; intestinal metabolism to the active metabolites sulfapyridine and 5-ASA
Primary excretion	Renal; active metabolites excreted in the feces
Onset of action	Peak: 1.5–6 h
Duration of action	Half-life: 5–10 h

Adverse Effects: The most common adverse effects of sulfasalazine are GI related and include nausea, vomiting, diarrhea, dyspepsia, and abdominal pain. Dividing the total daily dose evenly throughout the day and using the enteric-coated tablets may improve adherence. Headache is common. Blood dyscrasias occur infrequently during therapy. Skin rashes are relatively common and may be a sign of a more serious adverse effect such as Stevens–Johnson syndrome. This drug may impair male fertility, which reverses when the drug is discontinued. Sulfasalazine can cause photosensitivity.

Contraindications/Precautions: Sulfasalazine is contraindicated in patients with sulfonamide or salicylate (aspirin or 5-ASA) hypersensitivity. Patients with preexisting anemia, folate, or other hematologic disorders should use this drug with caution because it may worsen blood dyscrasias. Sulfasalazine should be used with caution in patients with hepatic impairment because this drug can cause hepatotoxicity. This drug is contraindicated in patients with urinary obstruction and should be used with caution in dehydrated patients because it may cause crystalluria. Patients with diabetes or hypoglycemia should use sulfasalazine with caution because the drug can increase insulin secretion and worsen hypoglycemia.

Drug Interactions: Sulfasalazine may worsen bone marrow suppression caused by methotrexate and also result in additive hepatotoxicity. Absorption of digoxin may be decreased. Sulfasalazine is a folic acid antagonist and will inhibit absorption of this vitamin. Sulfasalazine can displace warfarin from its protein-binding sites, causing increased anticoagulant effects.

Herbal/Food: Unknown.

Pregnancy: Categories B and D (near term).

Treatment of Overdose: Overdose will cause abdominal pain, anuria, drowsiness, gastric distress, nausea, seizures, and vomiting. Treatment is mostly supportive with gastric lavage, emesis, and alkalinization of urine.

Nursing Responsibilities:
- Obtain a complete health history, including allergies, drug history, and possible drug interactions.
- Perform a complete assessment of GI functioning and symptoms of IBD, which include abdominal cramping with frequent bowel movements, weight loss, bloody diarrhea, fever, and dehydration.
- Monitor for GI distress, including nausea, vomiting, diarrhea, dyspepsia, and abdominal pain. If symptoms persist, the prescriber may withhold the drug for 5 to 7 days and restart it at a lower dosage level.
- Be aware that adverse reactions generally occur within a few days to 12 weeks after the start of therapy. They are most likely to occur in patients who are receiving high doses.
- Monitor laboratory tests for red blood cell counts and folate levels in patients on high doses (more than 2 g/day); a daily supplement may be prescribed. Patients with preexisting anemia, folate, or other hematologic disorders should use the drug with caution because it may worsen blood dyscrasias.
- Response to therapy and duration of treatment are determined by endoscopic examinations.

Lifespan and Diversity Considerations:
- Because of normal physiological changes in bowel tone related to aging, monitor bowel sounds in the older adult and for the development of constipation, particularly from prolonged use of the drug.
- Monitor hepatic and renal function laboratory values more frequently in the older adult because normal changes related to aging may affect the drug's metabolism and excretion.
- Monitor electrolyte levels frequently in the older adult who is at greater risk for the development of electrolyte imbalances secondary to the diarrhea.

Patient and Family Education:
- Examine stools and report to the health care provider if enteric-coated tablets have passed intact in feces. If this occurs, a conventional tablet form can be ordered.
- Increase fluid intake to 2 to 3 L/day because this drug may cause crystals in the urine. Be aware that this drug may color urine and skin orange-yellow.
- Attend all follow-up examinations. Relapses occur in about 40% of patients after an initial satisfactory response.
- It is recommended that the interval between doses not exceed 8 hours (even if administered at night).
- Men may experience a decreased production of sperm and infertility, which is reversed with the discontinuation of this drug.
- Avoid prolonged sun exposure because the skin may be more sensitive. Wear sunscreen, protective clothing, and sunglasses if exposed to direct sunlight. Report any sunburn or other skin rashes to the provider.

Drugs Similar to Sulfasalazine (Azulfidine)

Other 5-aminosalicylates include balsalazide, mesalamine, and olsalazine.

Balsalazide (Colazal, Giazo): Approved in 2000, balsalazide is a PO anti-inflammatory agent approved for the symptomatic treatment of ulcerative colitis in patients age 5 and above. In 2013, a newer formulation of the drug (Giazo) was approved for male patients age 18 and above. Like sulfasalazine, balsalazide is metabolized in the intestinal mucosa to 5-ASA, which is responsible for its therapeutic effects. Almost 100% of this drug reaches the colon without being absorbed; thus the primary action of the drug is topical rather than systemic. The drug is well tolerated, with headache, abdominal pain, diarrhea, nausea, and vomiting being the most common adverse effects. Patients with salicylate hypersensitivity should not take this drug. Rare cases of hepatotoxicity have occurred. This drug is pregnancy category B.

Mesalamine (Asacol, Canasa, Lialda, Others): Approved in 1987, mesalamine is sometimes referred to by its chemical name, 5-ASA. It is FDA approved for the treatment of active ulcerative colitis and used off-label for Crohn's disease. A delayed release formulation (Asacol) was developed for maintenance therapy, and a rectal suppository (Canasa) is available to treat ulcerative proctitis. Like other drugs in this class, mesalamine tablets and capsules are designed to release the drug in the terminal ileum and colon to produce its effects topically in the intestinal mucosa. Headache, abdominal pain, diarrhea, nausea, and vomiting are the most common adverse effects. Rectal irritation may be caused by the suppository forms of the drug. Patients with salicylate hypersensitivity should not take this drug. This drug is pregnancy category B.

Olsalazine (Dipentum): Like other drugs in this class, olsalazine is an oral agent that is metabolized in the intestinal mucosa to 5-ASA, which produces a topical anti-inflammatory effect. Nearly 100% of this drug reaches the colon without being absorbed systemically. Approved in 1990, the only indication for this drug is for the maintenance of remission of ulcerative colitis in patients who are unable to tolerate sulfasalazine. The most commonly reported adverse effects are diarrhea, abdominal pain, and rash. Rare cases of hepatotoxicity have occurred. This drug is pregnancy category C.

Pharmacotherapy of Irritable Bowel Syndrome

60.6 Irritable bowel syndrome is treated with dietary management, symptomatic therapy, and drugs that regulate intestinal motility.

Irritable bowel syndrome (IBS), also known as spastic colon or mucous colitis, is a common disorder of the lower GI tract characterized by symptoms that include abdominal pain, visible bloating, excessive gas, and colicky cramping. Bowel habits are altered, with diarrhea alternating with constipation, and there may be mucus in the stool. Pain is usually relieved by defecation, although the patient usually feels as if the evacuation is incomplete. Symptoms of IBS are likely caused by altered GI motility, increased peristalsis, and increased pain sensitivity of the GI tract.

CONNECTIONS | **Patient Safety**

◀ **Infusion Calculations**

A nurse is starting an infusion of infliximab (Remicade) on a patient with Crohn's disease. To save time, the nurse prepares the infusion based on the patient's body weight from the last infusion 6 weeks ago. What error has occurred? How could it have been avoided?

See Answers to Patient Safety Questions on student resource website.

PharmFACT

Irritable bowel syndrome affects 10% to 20% of adults. Women are two to three times more likely than men to have the disorder (Lehrer, 2014).

The diagnosis of IBS is sometimes one of exclusion, ruling out other diseases such as colon cancer, ulcerative colitis, intestinal infections, Crohn's disease, and diverticulitis. It is not a precursor of more serious disease, and symptoms such as bleeding, anorexia, weight loss, or fever are not usually experienced by patients with IBS. IBS is considered a functional bowel disorder, meaning that the normal operation of the digestive tract is impaired without the presence of detectable organic disease. A diagnosis of IBS requires that the patient has experienced recurrent abdominal pain or discomfort for at least 3 days per month during the previous 3 months that is associated with two or more of the following:

- Relieved by defecation
- Onset associated with a change in stool frequency
- Onset associated with a change in stool form or appearance

Treatment of IBS is supportive, with drug therapy targeted at symptomatic treatment depending on whether constipation or diarrhea is the predominant symptom. There is no single treatment that is effective for all, or even most, patients.

Lifestyle changes, diet, and aggravating medications: Stress is not a cause of IBS, but it can influence the condition. Attempts should be made to identify stressors and develop positive coping strategies. Psychotherapy, relaxation techniques, and hypnosis may benefit some patients. Food-specific triggers are not always apparent. However, the patient should keep a food diary in an attempt to recognize and avoid foods that appear to worsen the condition. Dietary restriction of caffeine, wheat, or lactose-based products may be attempted. Foods that cause bloating and flatulence such as beans, cabbage, and peas should be avoided.

Part of a medical history for IBS should include drugs that may be contributing to the symptoms of IBS. Common drugs that may cause constipation include NSAIDs, calcium channel blockers, anticholinergics, and opioids. Diarrhea may result from the use of laxatives, magnesium-containing antacids, or antibiotics. Sometimes a change in medication can help reduce IBS symptoms.

Dietary fiber and laxatives: Constipation, diarrhea, cramping, painful bowel movements, and rectal urgency occur frequently in patients with IBS. Because constipation and diarrhea often alternate, pharmacotherapy can be challenging. Fiber supplementation with nonprescription bulk laxatives such as psyllium has long been recommended as a treatment for IBS and can help regulate bowel movements to bring relief to some patients. Unfortunately, increased fiber intake will worsen the symptoms in some patients. Loperamide (Imodium), an antidiarrheal, is effective at relieving symptoms of diarrhea in patients with IBS.

Antidepressant therapy: For many years the tricyclic antidepressants such as amitriptyline, desipramine (Norpramin), and doxepin (Sinequan) have been used to treat patients with IBS who have pain as a major symptom. Studies on the effectiveness of these drugs in reducing pain and diarrhea in patients with IBS are conflicting, but they may be indicated for those who have depression as a comorbid condition. Selective serotonin reuptake inhibitors (SSRIs) such as paroxetine (Paxil) have also been studied but results suggest that their effectiveness at treating IBS is mild at best. While antidepressants may relieve pain for some patients, they are not first-line drugs for IBS.

Drug-specific therapies: Alosetron (Lotronex) is a serotonin ($5-HT_3$) antagonist approved for diarrhea-predominant IBS in women. Doses for the antispasmodics are listed in Table 60.4.

Drugs that are used to treat IBS do not alter the course of the disease and, in some cases, may actually worsen the symptoms. Research has not demonstrated that these drugs are any more effective than nonpharmacologic treatments such as IBS support groups, relaxation therapy, or dietary changes. There is no prototype drug for this condition. Drugs that provide symptomatic relief for some patients include alosetron, antispasmodic drugs (dicyclomine and hyoscyamine), linaclotide (Linzess), and lubiprostone.

Alosetron (Lotronex): By inhibiting serotonin ($5-HT_3$) receptors, alosetron reduces GI-related sensitivity and slows peristalsis in patients with diarrhea-predominant IBS. Alosetron was approved in 2000 but was withdrawn later that same year due to several deaths from ischemic colitis. This drug was allowed to return to the market in 2002 but with severe restrictions on its use. It is approved only for severe diarrhea-predominant IBS in women who have not responded to conventional therapy. The starting dose was lowered from 1 mg bid to 1 mg daily. No refills are allowed without a follow-up exam by the prescribing health care provider. A risk–benefit statement must be signed by the patient and health care provider that they agree to adhere to therapy plans. A black box warning states that alosetron can cause serious adverse GI reactions, including ischemic colitis and serious complications of constipation that can cause death. The warning also states that health care providers who wish to prescribe alosetron must receive special training and testing to learn to appropriately diagnose and treat IBS. Furthermore, other therapies must have been attempted (and failed) prior to alosetron use. Other adverse effects include abdominal discomfort, nausea, and rash. This drug is pregnancy category B.

Antispasmodic drugs: Antispasmodic drugs are those that relax smooth muscle and slow peristalsis. Dicyclomine (Bentyl) and hyoscyamine (Anaspaz, Gastrosed, Levsin) are older anticholinergic drugs that are used to reduce bowel spasms in patients with IBS (see Chapter 14). Dicyclomine was approved in 1950 for diarrhea-predominant IBS and other functional disorders of GI motility. Dicyclomine may be administered PO or by IM injection.

Frequent adverse effects include typical anticholinergic effects such as dry mouth, blurred vision, drowsiness, urinary hesitancy, and tachycardia. This drug is pregnancy category B.

Available since the FDA was established in 1938, hyoscyamine is an anticholinergic drug that is usually administered PO, but parenteral forms are available. It is approved to treat peptic ulcer disease and diarrhea-predominant IBS because the drug decreases acid secretion of the stomach and slows peristalsis. It has also been used to reverse bradycardia, to relieve symptoms of allergic rhinitis, and to dry respiratory and salivary secretions prior to surgery. Whereas in 1938 hyoscyamine may have been a drug of choice for these conditions, it has been replaced by safer and more effective drugs for nearly every indication. This drug is pregnancy category C.

Linaclotide (Linzess): One of the newest drugs for IBS, linaclotide was approved in 2012 for chronic idiopathic constipation and for constipation-dominant IBS. It is an oral drug that acts by a unique mechanism: activating the enzyme guanylate cyclase in the intestine. This causes increased secretion of chloride and bicarbonate ion into the intestinal lumen, resulting in increased amounts of intestinal fluid and accelerated fecal transport. The most common adverse effects are diarrhea, abdominal pain, flatulence, and abdominal distention. The drug carries a black box warning that it is contraindicated in children up to age 6 and should be avoided in children age 6 through 17. This drug is pregnancy category C.

Lubiprostone (Amitiza): Lubiprostone was approved in 2006 for the treatment of chronic idiopathic constipation. In 2008, approval was granted for the use of this drug in treating constipation-predominant IBS in women over age 18. Lubiprostone increases fluid secretion by activating chloride channels in the intestinal luminal cells, thereby altering stool consistency and promoting regular bowel movements. The most common adverse effect is nausea, which can be reduced by taking the drug with food. Lubiprostone should not be administered to patients with diarrhea or suspected GI obstruction. This drug is pregnancy category C.

CONNECTION Checkpoint 60.2

Anticholinergic drugs can inhibit muscarinic or nicotinic receptors. From what you learned in Chapter 14, which type do dicyclomine and hyoscyamine inhibit? What drug is the prototype for this class? *See Answer to Connection Checkpoint 60.2 on student resource website.*

Pathophysiology of Nausea and Vomiting

60.7 Nausea and vomiting occur when the vomiting center in the medulla is stimulated.

Nausea is an unpleasant feeling of the need to vomit that is accompanied by weakness, diaphoresis, dizziness, and hyperproduction of saliva. Intense nausea often leads to **vomiting**, or emesis, in which the stomach contents are forced upward into the esophagus and out of the mouth. Vomiting is a defense mechanism used by the body to rid itself of toxic substances.

Vomiting is a reflex primarily controlled by a portion of the medulla of the brain known as the **vomiting center**, which receives sensory signals from the digestive tract, the inner ear, and the **chemoreceptor trigger zone (CTZ)** in the cerebral cortex.

Interestingly, the CTZ is not protected by the blood–brain barrier, as is the vast majority of the brain; thus these neurons can directly sense the presence of toxic substances in the blood. Once the vomiting reflex is triggered, wavelike contractions of the stomach quickly propel its contents upward and out of the body.

The treatment outcomes for nausea or vomiting should focus on removal of the cause whenever feasible. Nausea and vomiting are common symptoms associated with a wide variety of conditions. Some conditions originate in the GI tract itself, such as peptic ulcer disease, GI obstruction, gallbladder disease, food poisoning, or ingestion of a toxic substance that irritates the mucosa. The nausea and vomiting may originate from systemic sources such as those caused by cancer, pregnancy, radiation sickness, migraine headache, trauma to the head or abdominal organs, inner ear disorders, extreme pain, diabetes, or systemic drug use. In addition to the CTZ, other parts of the nervous system may promote nausea and vomiting in response to nervousness, emotional imbalances, changes in body position (motion sickness), extreme stress, or when confronted with unpleasant sights, smells, or sounds.

The nausea and vomiting experienced by many women during the first trimester of pregnancy is referred to as morning sickness. The cause of nausea and vomiting during pregnancy is not completely understood but is probably due to hormonal changes, especially in levels of estrogen and human chorionic gonadotropin (hCG). All women of childbearing years who present with nausea or vomiting should receive a pregnancy test because this is a common explanation for these symptoms. Should this condition become acute, such as continual vomiting, it may lead to **hyperemesis gravidarum**, a situation in which the health and safety of the mother and developing baby can become severely compromised. Complications may include dehydration, electrolyte imbalances, and significant weight loss. Pharmacotherapy with fluid and electrolyte solutions and antiemetics is initiated after other antinausea measures have proven ineffective.

PharmFACT

Morning sickness occurs in 70% to 85% of pregnancies. Morning sickness has a peak incidence at 8 to 12 weeks of pregnancy but usually ends by week 20 (Wilcox, 2013).

Nausea and vomiting are the most frequently listed adverse effects for oral medications. The nurse should remember that because the vomiting center lies in the brain, nausea and vomiting occur just as frequently with parenteral formulations as with oral drugs. The most extreme example of this occurs with the antineoplastic drugs, most of which cause intense nausea and vomiting regardless of the route by which they are administered. The capacity of a chemotherapeutic drug to cause vomiting is called its **emetogenic potential**. Nausea and vomiting are common reasons for patient lack of adherence to the therapeutic regimen and for discontinuation of drug therapy.

When large amounts of fluids are vomited, dehydration and significant weight loss may occur. Because the contents lost from the stomach are strongly acidic, vomiting may cause a change in the pH of the blood, resulting in metabolic alkalosis. With excessive loss, severe acid–base disturbances can lead to vascular collapse, resulting in death if medical intervention is not initiated. Electrolytes such as sodium, potassium, and chloride are also lost during vomiting and may need to be replaced, especially in the infant, child, and older adult. Dehydration is especially dangerous for infants, small children, and the older adult and is evidenced by dry mouth, sticky saliva, and reduced urine output that is dark yellow-orange to brown in color.

Pharmacotherapy of Nausea and Vomiting

60.8 Antiemetics are prescribed to treat nausea, vomiting, and motion sickness.

Drugs from at least eight different classes are used to prevent or treat nausea and vomiting. Most of these drugs were originally developed for other indications, and their antiemetic characteristics were discovered later. Selection of a specific drug depends on the cause of the nausea and vomiting and its severity.

Patients who are seeking self-treatment can find several available OTC options. For example, simple nausea and vomiting are sometimes relieved by antacids or diphenhydramine (Benadryl). Peppermint and ginger are the most popular herbal therapies for nausea and vomiting.

Relief of serious nausea or vomiting requires prescription medications. Patients who are receiving antineoplastic drugs may receive three or more antiemetics concurrently to reduce the nausea and vomiting from chemotherapy. In fact, therapy with antineoplastic drugs is one of the most common reasons for prescribing antiemetic drugs. Many antiemetic agents are available through the IM, IV, or suppository route to prevent loss of the medication due to vomiting. Pharmacotherapy Illustrated 60.2 shows the mechanisms of action of antiemetic medications. Doses for selected antiemetics are listed in Table 60.5.

Anticholinergics and antihistamines: These medications are effective for treating simple nausea, with some being available OTC. For example, nausea due to motion sickness is effectively treated with anticholinergics or antihistamines. Motion sickness is a disorder that affects a portion of the inner ear that is associated with significant nausea. The most common drug used for motion sickness is scopolamine (Hyoscine, Transderm-Scop), an anticholinergic drug that is usually administered as a transdermal patch. Antihistamines such as dimenhydrinate (Dramamine), doxylamine, and meclizine (Antivert) are also effective but may cause significant drowsiness in some patients. Drugs that are used to treat motion sickness are most effective when taken 20 to 60 minutes before travel is expected.

Serotonin (5-HT3) receptor antagonists: The serotonin antagonists include dolasetron (Anzemet), granisetron (Kytril), ondansetron (Zofran, Zuplenz), and palonosetron (Aloxi). There are no major differences in effectiveness or toxicity of the serotonin receptor antagonists in treating acute nausea and vomiting. They are available by the PO or parenteral route. Since the 1990s these drugs have become the most widely prescribed drugs for chemotherapy-induced nausea and vomiting. For severe symptoms, the serotonin receptor antagonists are combined with a corticosteroid such as dexamethasone. The serotonin antagonists are most effective in the management of acute nausea and vomiting but are less effective at treating delayed symptoms. The few adverse effects they cause include headache, constipation or diarrhea, and dizziness.

PHARMACOTHERAPY ILLUSTRATED 60.2

Mechanisms of Action of Antiemetic Medications

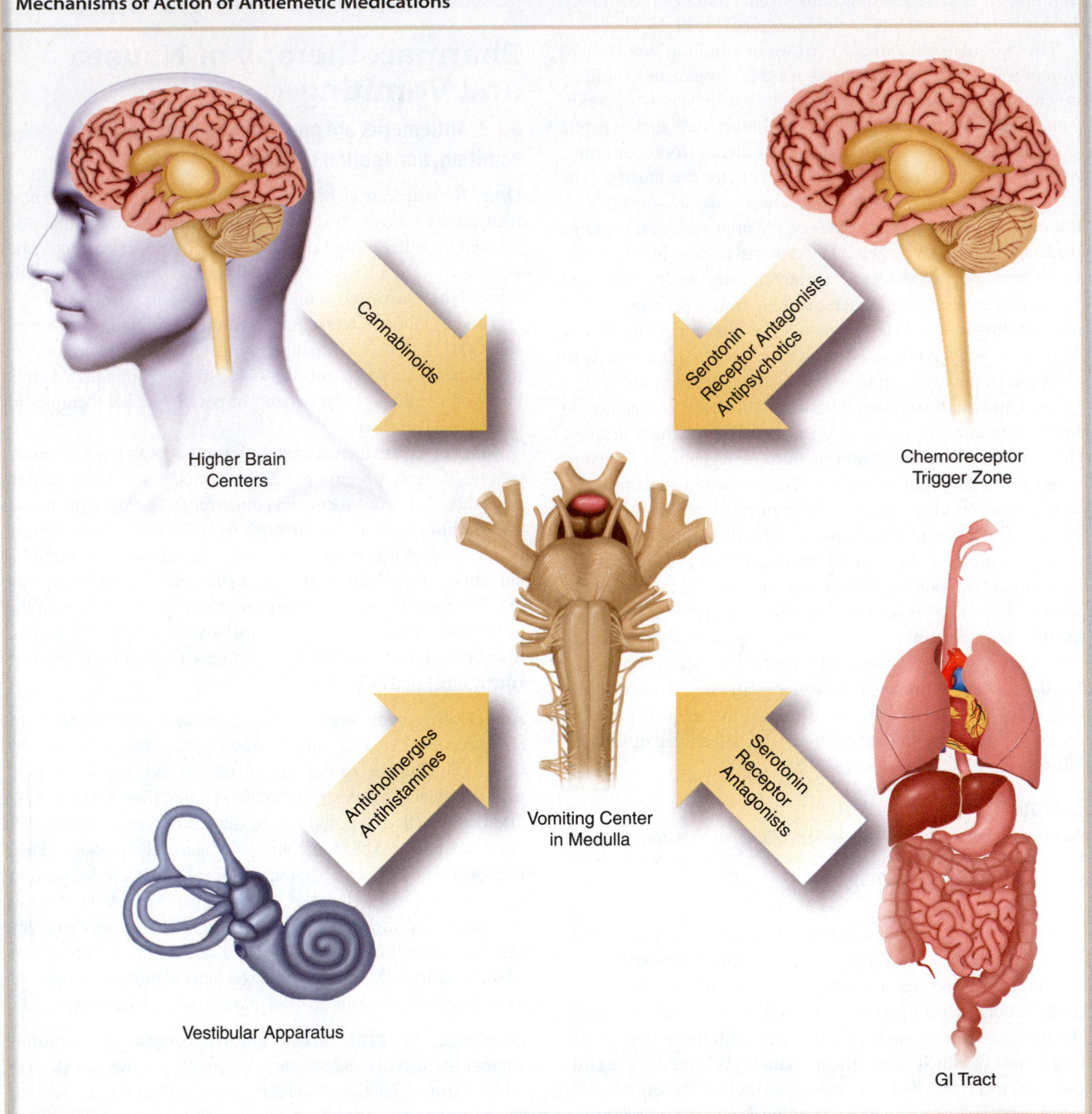

Higher Brain Centers

Cannabinoids

Serotonin Receptor Antagonists Antipsychotics

Chemoreceptor Trigger Zone

Anticholinergics Antihistamines

Vomiting Center in Medulla

Serotonin Receptor Antagonists

Vestibular Apparatus

GI Tract

Phenothiazines and related drugs (dopamine antagonists): The primary indication for phenothiazines is the treatment of psychoses (see Chapter 20), but they are also very effective antiemetics. Phenothiazines inhibit dopaminergic receptors in the CTZ, and the severe nausea and vomiting associated with antineoplastic therapy are often treated with these agents. Some of the phenothiazines may cause sedation, and extrapyramidal symptoms (EPS) are a concern with long-term therapy. Promethazine (Phenergan) is an older phenothiazine that is available by the PO, rectal, and parenteral routes that also has significant anticholinergic properties.

Benzodiazepines: The primary indication for benzodiazepines is anxiety. Benzodiazepines are ineffective as antiemetics when used as monotherapy. However, they relax the patient and decrease the anxiety associated with chemotherapy and the anticipation of severe nausea and vomiting. Lorazepam (Ativan) is the drug in this class that is most frequently used as an off-label antiemetic adjunct.

Cannabinoids: Cannabinoids are drugs that contain the same active ingredient as marijuana. Dronabinol (Marinol) and nabilone (Cesamet) are given PO to produce antiemetic effects and relaxation

TABLE 60.5 Selected Antiemetics

Drug	Route and Adult Dose (Maximum Dose Where Indicated)	Adverse Effects
Anticholinergics-Antihistamines		
cyclizine (Marezine)	PO: 50 mg every 4–6 h (max: 200 mg/day)	*Drowsiness, dry mouth, blurred vision (scopolamine), hypotension (cyclizine)*
dimenhydrinate (Dramamine, Others)	PO: 50–100 mg every 4–6 h (max: 400 mg/day)	Hypersensitivity reaction, sedation, tremors, seizures, hallucinations, paradoxical excitation (more common in children), hypotension
diphenhydramine (Benadryl, Others)	PO: 25–50 mg tid–qid (max: 300 mg/day)	
doxylamine and pyridoxine (Diclegis)	PO: 20–40 mg daily	
hydroxyzine (Atarax, Vistaril)	PO: 25–100 mg tid or qid (max: 400 mg/day)	
meclizine (Antivert, Bonine, Others)	PO: 25–50 mg daily, take 1 h before travel (max: 50 mg/day)	
scopolamine (Hyoscine, Transderm-Scop)	Transdermal: 0.5 mg (patch) every 72 h	
Benzodiazepines		
lorazepam (Ativan)	PO: 0.5–2 mg every 4–6 h (max: 10 mg/day)	*Dizziness, drowsiness, ataxia, fatigue, slurred speech*
		Paradoxical excitation (more common in children), seizures (if abruptly discontinued), coma
Cannabinoids		
dronabinol (Marinol)	PO: 5 mg/m^2 1–3 h before administration of chemotherapy, then every 2–4 h after chemotherapy for a total of 4–6 doses	*Dizziness, drowsiness, euphoria, confusion, ataxia, asthenia, increased sensory awareness*
nabilone (Cesamet)	PO: 1–2 mg bid	Paranoia, decreased motor coordination, hypotension
Corticosteroids		
dexamethasone (Decadron)	PO: 0.25–4 mg bid–qid	*Mood swings, weight gain, acne, facial flushing, nausea, insomnia, sodium and fluid retention, impaired wound healing, menstrual abnormalities, insomnia*
methylprednisolone (Medrol, Solu-Medrol, Others)	PO: 4–48 mg/day in divided doses	
		Peptic ulcer, hypocalcemia, osteoporosis with possible bone fractures, loss of muscle mass, decreased growth in children, possible masking of infections
Neurokinin Receptor Antagonist		
aprepitant (Emend)	PO: 125 mg 1 h prior to chemotherapy	*Fatigue, constipation, diarrhea, anorexia, hiccups*
	IV: 115–150 mg 30 min prior to chemotherapy	Dehydration, peripheral neuropathy, blood dyscrasias, pneumonia
Phenothiazine and Phenothiazine-Like Drugs		
metoclopramide (Reglan)	PO: 1–2 mg/kg 1 h prior to chemotherapy	*Dry eyes, blurred vision, dry mouth, constipation, drowsiness, photosensitivity*
perphenazine (Phenazine, Trilafon)	PO: 8–16 mg bid–qid	EPS, neuroleptic malignant syndrome, agranulocytosis, orthostatic hypotension
prochlorperazine (Compazine, Others)	PO: 5–10 mg tid or qid Rectal: 25 mg bid IM: 5–10 mg tid or qid IV: 2.5–10 mg tid or qid (max: 10 mg/dose or 40 mg/day)	
promethazine (Phenergan, Others)	PO: 12.5–25 mg every 4 h or qid	
trimethobenzamide (Tigan)	PO: 300 mg once daily IM: 200 mg 3–4 times/day	
Serotonin (5-HT$_3$) Receptor Antagonists		
dolasetron (Anzemet)	PO: 100 mg 1 h prior to chemotherapy	*Headache, drowsiness, fatigue, constipation, diarrhea, flulike symptoms*
granisetron (Kytril, Sancuso)	PO: 2 mg/day 1 h prior to chemotherapy IV: 10 mcg/kg 30 min prior to chemotherapy Transdermal patch: 1 patch 24–48 h prior to chemotherapy	Dysrhythmias, EPS, hepatic failure
ondansetron (Zofran, Zuplenz)	PO: 8 mg bid or tid IV: 32 mg 30 min prior to chemotherapy	
palonosetron (Aloxi)	PO: 0.5 mg single dose 1 h prior to chemotherapy IV: 0.25 mg 30 min prior to chemotherapy	

Note: Italics indicate common adverse effects. Underline indicates serious adverse effects.

CONNECTIONS Complementary and Alternative Therapies

◀ Lactobacillus Acidophilus

Description

Lactobacillus acidophilus is a probiotic bacterium that is normally found in the human alimentary canal and vagina.

History and Claims

Lactobacillus acidophilus is considered to be protective flora, inhibiting the growth of potentially pathogenic species such as *E. coli*, *Candida albicans*, *Helicobacter pylori*, and *Gardnerella vaginalis*. The primary use of *L. acidophilus* is to restore the normal flora of the intestine following diarrhea, particularly from antibiotic therapy.

Standardization

Supplements include capsules, tablets, and granules. Doses are not standardized, and tablet doses range from 50 to 500 mg. *L. acidophilus* may be obtained by drinking acidophilus milk or by eating yogurt or kefir containing live (or active) cultures. Those wishing to obtain *L. acidophilus* from yogurt should read the labels carefully, because not all products contain active cultures.

Evidence

One mechanism used by *L. acidophilus* to limit the growth of other bacterial species is the generation of hydrogen peroxide, which is toxic to most cells. It has also been shown to be effective at shortening episodes of acute infectious diarrhea. These supplements should probably not be used in severely immunosuppressed patients because they may cause infection. Some patients with IBS may benefit from the use of *Lactobacillus* supplements.

---

with less euphoria compared to marijuana. Cannabinoids are not as effective as other antiemetics.

Corticosteroids: Dexamethasone (Decadron) and methylprednisolone (Solu-Medrol) are used to prevent chemotherapy-induced and postsurgical nausea and vomiting. They are reserved for acute cases due to the possibility of serious adverse effects and are most often used in combination with other antiemetics. Dexamethasone is used for the treatment of delayed nausea and vomiting, which are common problems with certain antineoplastic drugs.

Other drugs: Aprepitant (Emend) belongs to a class of antiemetics called the neurokinin (NK) receptor antagonists that reduce the level of substance P, which is involved in the emesis reflex. Aprepitant was FDA approved in 2003 as part of a 3-day antiemetic regimen for antineoplastic chemotherapy in conjunction with a corticosteroid (dexamethasone) and a $5\text{-}HT_3$ antagonist (ondansetron). It is also approved to treat postoperative nausea and vomiting. The IV form of this drug, fosaprepitant, was approved in 2008. Aprepitant is pregnancy category B. Tricyclic antidepressants such as amitriptyline (Elavil) have also been used to reduce chronic idiopathic nausea.

On some occasions, it is desirable to stimulate the vomiting reflex with drugs called emetics. Indications for emetics include ingestion of poisons and overdoses of oral drugs. Ipecac syrup, given PO, or apomorphine, given subcutaneously, will induce vomiting in about 15 minutes.

CONNECTION Checkpoint 60.3

From what you learned in Chapter 20, define extrapyramidal adverse effects and provide examples of symptoms that a patient with EPS might exhibit. *See Answer to Connection Checkpoint 60.3 on student resource website.*

PROTOTYPE DRUG	Ondansetron (Zofran, Zuplenz)

Classification: **Therapeutic:** Antiemetic
Pharmacologic: Serotonin ($5\text{-}HT_3$) receptor antagonist

Therapeutic Effects and Uses: Ondansetron and other drugs in the serotonin receptor antagonist class have replaced older drugs for the treatment of serious nausea and vomiting due to their superior effectiveness and relative safety. To prevent chemotherapy-induced nausea and vomiting the medication is started at least 30 minutes prior to chemotherapy and continued for several days after. For radiation-induced nausea and vomiting the drug is administered 1 to 2 hours before therapy and continued for 1 to 2 days. It is available by the PO, IV, IM, oral disintegrating tablet, and oral soluble film routes. The drug may be used off-label to treat cholestatic pruritus or opioid-induced pruritus.

Mechanism of Action: Ondansetron acts by blocking serotonin receptors in the chemoreceptor trigger zone, an area of the brain responsible for nausea and vomiting.

Pharmacokinetics:

Route(s)	PO, IV
Absorption	Rapidly absorbed
Distribution	Widely distributed; secreted in breast milk; over 70% bound to plasma proteins
Primary metabolism	Extensive hepatic metabolism by various CYP enzymes
Primary excretion	Renal (44–60%) and feces (25%)
Onset of action	PO: 1–1.5 h
Duration of action	Unknown

Adverse Effects: Ondansetron is well tolerated, with the most common adverse effects being headache, dizziness, drowsiness, and constipation or diarrhea.

Contraindications/Precautions: This drug should not be used in patients with hypersensitivity to other serotonin receptor antagonists. Caution should be used when treating patients with cardiac abnormalities because ondansetron can prolong the QT interval and cause dysrhythmias.

Drug Interactions: Ondansetron exhibits few clinically significant drug interactions. Because the drug is extensively metabolized by hepatic CYP450 enzymes, inhibitors or inducers of these enzymes may affect the availability of ondansetron. **Herbal/Food**: Unknown.

Pregnancy: Category B.

Treatment of Overdose: There is no specific therapy for ondansetron overdose and general supportive measures should be used.

Nursing Responsibilities: Key nursing implications for patients receiving ondansetron are included in the Nursing Practice Application for Patients Receiving Pharmacotherapy with Antiemetics.

Drugs Similar to Ondansetron (Zofran, Zuplenz)

Other serotonin receptor antagonists include dolasetron (Anzemet), granisetron (Kytril), and palonosetron (Aloxi). All drugs in this class have similar effectiveness and safety profiles.

Pharmacotherapy of Pancreatitis

60.9 Pancreatic enzymes are administered as replacement therapy for patients with chronic pancreatitis.

The pancreas secretes insulin as well as essential digestive enzymes. The enzymatic portion of pancreatic juice contains carboxypeptidase, chymotrypsin, and trypsin, which are converted to their active forms once they enter the small intestine. Three other pancreatic enzymes—lipase, amylase, and nuclease—are secreted in their active form but require the presence of bile for optimum activity. When lack of pancreatic enzyme secretion results in malabsorption disorders, replacement therapy is warranted.

PharmFACT

Drugs are the cause of 0.1% to 2% of all cases of acute pancreatitis. The most frequently reported drugs associated with the disorder are mesalazine, azathioprine, and simvastatin (Nitsche, Jamieson, Lerch, & Mayerle, 2010).

Pancreatitis results when digestive enzymes remain in the pancreas rather than being released into the duodenum. Upon becoming activated and escaping into the surrounding tissue, the enzymes cause inflammation in the pancreas, which can lead to hemorrhage and necrosis. The backed-up enzymes and enteric bacteria may leak into the peritoneum, causing a severe systemic reaction and, possibly, death. Pancreatitis can be either acute or chronic. The two types of pancreatitis have different symptoms, mortality rates, and treatments.

Acute pancreatitis: Acute pancreatitis occurs most frequently in middle-aged adults and is often associated with gallstones in women and alcoholism in men. Symptoms of acute pancreatitis present suddenly, often after eating a fatty meal or consuming excessive amounts of alcohol. The most common symptom is a continuous severe pain in the epigastric area often radiating to the back. Fever, tachycardia, abdominal tenderness, and muscular guarding (involuntary spasm of the abdominal muscles when palpated) are common. Although most patients recover from the illness and regain normal pancreatic functions, a small percentage of patients experience recurring attacks and progress to chronic pancreatitis.

Many patients with acute pancreatitis require only bed rest, fasting, and adequate fluid and electrolyte therapy for a few days for the symptoms to subside. For patients with acute pain, an opioid such as hydromorphone (Dilaudid) brings effective relief. To reduce gastric and pancreatic juice secretions, H_2-receptor blockers, such as cimetidine (Tagamet), or proton pump inhibitors, such as omeprazole (Prilosec), may be prescribed. To decrease the amount of pancreatic enzymes secreted, carbonic anhydrase inhibitors, such as acetazolamide (Diamox), or antispasmodics, such as dicyclomine (Bentyl), may be used. In severe cases where enteral nutrition is not tolerated, total parenteral nutrition (TPN) may be necessary.

Cases of pancreatitis accompanied by a high fever and infection have a very high mortality rate. Pharmacotherapy with an antibiotic from the imipenem class is usually begun immediately.

Chronic pancreatitis: Seventy to eighty percent of chronic pancreatitis cases are associated with alcoholism. Other causes include pancreatic cancer and stones. Alcohol is thought to promote the formation of insoluble proteins that occlude the pancreatic duct. Pancreatic juice is prevented from flowing into the duodenum and remains in the pancreas, damaging cells and causing inflammation. Symptoms include chronic epigastric or left upper quadrant pain, anorexia, nausea, vomiting, and weight loss. **Steatorrhea**, the passing of bulky, foul-smelling fatty stools, occurs late in the course of the disease. Chronic pancreatitis causes permanent structural damage to the organ and may cause scarring of the pancreatic duct system. Chronic pancreatitis is a risk factor for the development of pancreatic cancer. The disease eventually leads to pancreatic insufficiency that may necessitate insulin therapy as well as replacement of pancreatic enzymes.

Drugs that are prescribed for the treatment of acute pancreatitis may also be used for patients with chronic pancreatitis. Fasting, IV fluids, and opioid analgesics may be necessary. The chronic, severe pain may lead to high doses of opioids and a possibility of drug dependence. In addition, the patient with chronic pancreatitis may require insulin and antiemetics.

Pancreatic enzyme supplementation is often used in patients with chronic pancreatitis. Supplementation sends a negative feedback message to stop secreting endogenous pancreatic enzymes, which can reduce pain. These supplements are given orally. Pancrelipase (Creon, Pancreaze, Zenpep) is a pancreatic enzyme supplement that helps to digest fats and prevent steatorrhea.

PROTOTYPE DRUG	Pancrelipase (Creon, Pancreaze, Zenpep)

Classification: Therapeutic: Pancreatic enzymes
Pharmacologic: None

Therapeutic Effects and Uses: Pancrelipase contains lipase, protease, and amylase of pork origin and is used as replacement therapy for patients with insufficient pancreatic exocrine secretions, including those with pancreatitis and cystic fibrosis. Given PO the capsule dissolves in the alkaline environment of the duodenum and releases its enzymes. The enzymes act locally in the GI tract and are not absorbed. Pancrelipase is available in powder, tablet, and delayed release capsule formulations.

Patients Receiving Pharmacotherapy with Antiemetics

Assessment	Potential Nursing Diagnoses*
Baseline assessment prior to administration: • Obtain a complete health history including GI, cardiovascular, hepatic or renal disease, pregnancy, or breast-feeding. Obtain a drug history including allergies, current prescription and OTC drugs, herbal preparations, caffeine, nicotine, and alcohol use. Be alert to possible drug interactions. • Obtain baseline weight and vital signs, especially blood pressure and pulse. • Evaluate appropriate laboratory findings (e.g., electrolytes, glucose, CBC, hepatic or renal function studies). • Obtain an abdominal assessment (e.g., bowel sounds, softness or firmness, distention, presence of tenderness). • Assess emesis for amount, color, and presence of blood. • Assess the patient's ability to receive and understand instructions. Include the family and caregiver as needed.	• *Deficient Fluid Volume* • *Deficient Knowledge* (Drug Therapy) • *Risk for Injury,* related to adverse drug effects • *Risk for Falls,* related to adverse drug effects
Assessment throughout administration: • Assess for desired therapeutic effects (e.g., nausea is decreased, no vomiting present, able to tolerate fluids and increasing solids). • Continue to monitor and measure any emesis. Assess urine output and maintain intake and output measurements in the hospitalized patient. • Monitor vital signs, especially blood pressure and pulse, and report any hypotension or tachycardia to the health care provider. • Continue periodic monitoring of abdominal assessment findings, especially bowel sounds. • Continue periodic monitoring of electrolytes, glucose, CBC, and hepatic and renal function laboratory values as appropriate. • Assess for adverse effects: headache, drowsiness, dizziness, dry mouth, blurred vision, or fatigue. Immediately report any continued vomiting, severe nausea, emesis with coffee-ground appearance or hematemesis, hypotension, tachycardia, or confusion.	

Implementation

Interventions and (Rationales)	Patient-Centered Care
Ensuring therapeutic effects: • Treat the cause: If a definitive cause for the current symptoms can be identified (e.g., infection, adverse drug effects), correct the cause where possible. (Nausea and vomiting are often symptoms of other underlying conditions such as adverse drug effects or infections.)	• Review medications, foods, or possibility of illness with the patient or family to help identify causative factors. • Decrease noxious stimuli (e.g., strong odors, rapid changes in position) that may increase nausea or vomiting.
• Encourage a small amount of fluids or ice chips and decreased activity level while nauseated, and abstinence from alcohol, smoking cessation, and increased intake of yogurt and *acidophilus*-containing foods after nausea has ceased. (Limiting amounts of fluids and solids during periods of nausea or vomiting and limiting physical activity or movement may help ease symptoms during the acute phase. Ensuring adequate amounts of fluids, including IV if necessary, will help maintain normal fluid balance. Smoking and alcohol use are known to cause gastric irritation.)	• Encourage the patient to limit physical movement or activity during periods of acute nausea or vomiting. Encourage increasing fluid intake gradually, with ice chips or small sips of water. Ginger ale may act as a natural antinausea beverage and may be palatable for some patients.
• Administer antiemetics 30–60 min before anticipated nausea-inducing travel or drug administration (e.g., chemotherapy). Ensure adequate hydration prior to the onset of anticipated nausea. (Antiemetics are most effective when taken before nausea occurs. Ensuring adequate prehydration decreases the risk of dehydration should vomiting occur.)	• Teach the patient to take the antiemetic 30–60 min before travel if nausea is anticipated. If drowsiness or dizziness may occur, encourage the patient to consider a trial run with the medication taken in the evening before bedtime to ascertain the effects prior to taking if driving is required. • Teach patients on at-home chemotherapy to take antiemetics prior to chemotherapy doses or routinely as ordered by the provider.
Minimizing adverse effects: • Monitor vital signs, particularly blood pressure and pulse. Take the blood pressure lying, sitting, and standing to detect orthostatic hypotension. **Lifespan:** Be particularly cautious with the older adult who is at increased risk for hypotension. Report any hypotension, especially associated with tachycardia, immediately. (Excessive vomiting may cause dehydration and decreased blood pressure or hypotension. Antiemetics such as anticholinergics, antihistamines, and phenothiazine or phenothiazine-like drugs may also cause a decrease in blood pressure.)	• Teach the patient to rise slowly from lying or sitting to standing to avoid dizziness or falls. If dizziness occurs, the patient should sit or lie down and not attempt to stand or walk until the sensation passes.

CONNECTIONS: NURSING PRACTICE APPLICATION (continued)

• Continue to monitor abdominal assessment findings. Any significant increase or decrease in bowel sounds, distention, new onset or increase in discomfort or pain, any severe abdominal pain, coffee-ground emesis, or hematemesis should be reported immediately. (Increasing or severe abdominal pain or hematemesis may indicate a worsening of disease and should be reported immediately.)	• Teach the patient to report any increasing gastric discomfort or pain. • Instruct the patient that severe abdominal pain or any blood in emesis should be reported immediately to the health care provider.
• Continue to monitor periodic electrolyte, glucose levels, and hepatic and renal function tests as needed. (Loss of electrolytes may occur with severe vomiting. Abnormal liver function tests may indicate drug-induced adverse hepatic effects.)	• Instruct the patient on the need for laboratory work.
• Monitor intake and output in the hospitalized patient. Initiate IV fluid replacement as ordered when indicated. Hold oral fluids until acute vomiting has ceased and then gradually increase fluid intake, beginning with small sips of water or ice chips. (Continuing oral intake may perpetuate or increase nausea and vomiting. Gradually resuming fluids will allow for hydration without stimulating nausea. IV fluid replacement may be required if fluid loss has been severe and if dehydration is present.)	• Instruct the patient on the need to withhold fluids and food until vomiting has ceased. Initiate incremental increases in intake beginning with small sips of water and clear fluids. • Explain the rationale for any IV hydration required and any equipment used.
• **Lifespan:** If pregnancy is suspected or confirmed, hold the antiemetic until the health care provider has been consulted. (Alternative antinausea measures should be used to control or ease nausea when possible. Drug pregnancy class and pregnancy trimester will be considered by the health care provider before prescribing the drug to avoid detrimental effects.)	• Teach pregnant patients, or if pregnancy is suspected, to consult with the health care provider before taking any antiemetic drug for morning sickness. • Encourage the use of nondrug measures such as dry and unsweetened cereals or crackers taken in small amounts, ginger ale to aid in diminishing nausea, and avoidance of noxious stimuli (e.g., strong odors) during periods of nausea.
Patient understanding of drug therapy: • Use opportunities during administration of medications and during assessments to discuss the rationale for drug therapy, desired therapeutic outcomes, the most commonly observed adverse effects, parameters for when to call the health care provider, and any necessary monitoring or precautions. (Using time during nursing care helps to optimize and reinforce key teaching areas.)	• The patient, family, or caregiver should be able to state the reason for the drug, appropriate dose and scheduling, what adverse effects to observe for and when to report them, and the anticipated length of medication therapy.
Patient self-administration of drug therapy: • When administering the medication, instruct the patient, family, or caregiver in proper self-administration of the drug, e.g., taken with small sips of fluid. (Utilizing time during nurse-administration of these drugs helps to reinforce teaching.)	• The patient, family, or caregiver is able to discuss appropriate dosing and administration needs.

*Nursing Diagnoses—Definitions and Classification 2015–2017. Copyright © 2014, 1994–2014 by NANDA International. Used by arrangement with John Wiley & Sons Limited.

The different brand names of pancrelipase are not interchangeable because the amounts of pancreatic enzymes in each product may vary. Dose is based on the amount of fat in the diet. Doses are taken just prior to meals or with meals.

Mechanism of Action: This agent facilitates the breakdown and conversion of lipids into glycerol and fatty acids, starches into dextrin and sugars, and proteins into peptides.

Pharmacokinetics:

Route(s)	PO
Absorption	Not absorbed
Distribution	Not distributed
Primary metabolism	Metabolized in the small bowel
Primary excretion	Feces
Onset of action	Immediate
Duration of action	Unknown

Adverse Effects: Adverse effects of pancrelipase are uncommon because the enzymes are not absorbed. The most common adverse effects are GI symptoms of nausea, vomiting, and diarrhea. Very high doses are associated with a risk for hyperuricemia. A rare condition known as fibrosing colonopathy may occur when very high doses of pancreatic enzyme replacements are given to patients with cystic fibrosis.

Contraindications/Precautions: Pancrelipase is contraindicated in patients who are allergic to this drug or to pork products. The delayed release products should not be given to patients with acute pancreatitis.

Drug Interactions: Pancrelipase interacts with iron, which may result in decreased absorption of iron. Calcium and magnesium antacids may diminish the effectiveness of pancrelipase. **Herbal/Food**: Unknown.

Pregnancy: Category C.

Treatment of Overdose: High levels of uric acid may occur with overdose. Patients are treated symptomatically.

Nursing Responsibilities:

- Assess for abdominal pain. Determine the type, intensity, and location of pain.

- Assess the patient for pork allergy because the enzymes in pancrelipase come from pork.

- Monitor intake and output ratio and weight. Note the patient's appetite and quality of stools, weight loss, abdominal bloating, polyuria, thirst, hunger, and itching. Pancreatic insufficiency is frequently associated with steatorrhea, bulky stools, and insulin-dependent diabetes. Dose may need to be regulated based on fat intake in the diet.

Lifespan and Diversity Considerations:

- Evaluate the child's or older adult's nutritional status and weigh weekly to ensure that adequate nutritional requirements are being met.

Patient and Family Education:

- Take this drug just before, during, or immediately after meals.

- Capsules may be opened and sprinkled over food, but avoid chewing or crushing the microspheres inside the capsules.
- Do not switch to a different brand of pancrelipase without consulting the prescriber.
- Continue to take pancrelipase even if feeling well. Pancrelipase may control symptoms but will not cure the condition.
- Do not take this drug with iron supplements or with calcium or magnesium antacids unless directed by the provider because they may diminish the effectiveness of this drug.

Drugs Similar to Pancrelipase (Creon, Pancreaze, Zenpep)

There are no drugs similar to pancrelipase. Several unapproved forms of pancreatic enzyme products were removed from the market in 2010, per a directive from the FDA.

CHAPTER

60   Understanding the Chapter

Key Concepts Summary

60.1   Constipation is characterized by infrequent or difficult bowel movements.

60.2   Laxatives are drugs that increase the frequency and quality of bowel movements.

60.3   Diarrhea is an abnormal increase in the frequency and fluidity of bowel movements.

60.4   Opioids are the most effective drugs for controlling severe diarrhea.

60.5   Inflammatory bowel disease is treated with immunosuppressants and anti-inflammatory drugs.

60.6   Irritable bowel syndrome is treated with dietary management, symptomatic therapy, and drugs that regulate intestinal motility.

60.7   Nausea and vomiting occur when the vomiting center in the medulla is stimulated.

60.8   Antiemetics are prescribed to treat nausea, vomiting, and motion sickness.

60.9   Pancreatic enzymes are administered as replacement therapy for patients with chronic pancreatitis.

Case Study: Making the Patient Connection

Remember the patient "Kerry O'Grady" at the beginning of the chapter? Now read the remainder of the case study. Based on the information presented within this chapter, respond to the critical thinking questions that follow.

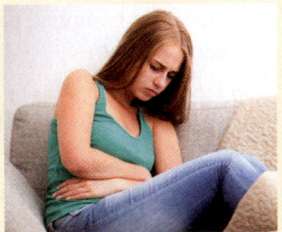

Kerry O'Grady is a 20-year-old college sophomore studying to be a middle-school teacher. She was diagnosed with IBS at the end of her freshman year after enduring multiple bouts of abdominal cramping, diarrhea, constipation, gas, and bloating. She thought it was just the stress of her first year of college because her symptoms eased over the summer break. Now it has returned and the diarrhea occurs more often than constipation. Some days she finds that she is unable to sit through an entire class without having to leave for

the restroom. She is increasingly worried about her grades and she is sure that the stress is not helping her condition either.

The nurse practitioner in the Student Health Services office has prescribed several weeks of dicyclomine (Bentyl) to be followed by loperamide (Imodium) after the diarrhea has slowed from the dicyclomine.

Critical Thinking Questions

1. How will the dicyclomine (Bentyl) and loperamide (Imodium) help treat Kerry's symptoms?

2. Considering the adverse effects of dicyclomine and loperamide, what should you as the nurse teach Kerry about her college course schedule?

3. What other nondrug measures might Kerry try to ease her symptoms?

See Answers to Critical Thinking Questions on student resource website.

Additional Case Study

Scott Mobley is a 25-year-old male with a diagnosis of ulcerative colitis. He currently reports having three to five loose bowel movements per day, associated with gas, cramps, and urgency of evacuation. He was diagnosed with ulcerative colitis 2 years earlier. Once he is stabilized, he will be placed on sulfasalazine.

1. Scott has asked you, his nurse, how this medication works. What is your response?

2. What adverse effects of this medication should you share with Scott?
3. What contraindications would you teach Scott about the drug sulfasalazine?

See Answers to Additional Case Study on student resource website.

Chapter Review

1 The patient is taking diphenoxylate with atropine (Lomotil). What does the nurse assess when monitoring for therapeutic effects?
   1. Reduction of abdominal cramping
   2. Minimal passage of flatus
   3. Decrease in loose, watery stools
   4. Increased bowel sounds

2 The patient who is taking sulfasalazine (Azulfidine) develops a sore throat, bruising, and severe fatigue. The nurse determines that the patient is most likely experiencing drug-induced:
   1. Stevens–Johnson syndrome.
   2. Blood dyscrasias.
   3. Idiosyncratic reaction.
   4. Hypersensitivity response.

3 Ondansetron (Zofran) has been ordered prior to chemotherapy for a patient receiving treatment for lymphoma. Prior to administering this drug, the nurse will review the patient's past medical history for what condition?
   1. Allergy to soy or soy products
   2. History of chronic constipation
   3. Glaucoma
   4. Cardiac dysrhythmias

4 A nurse should question the order for pancrelipase (Pancreaze) for which patient?
   1. The patient with allergy to pork products
   2. The patient with hypertension
   3. The patient with coronary artery disease
   4. The patient with hypersensitivity to iodine products

5 A health care provider orders magnesium hydroxide (Milk of Magnesia) for a patient with constipation, secondary to postoperative opioid use. Before administering the drug, the nurse would assess:
   1. Blood pressure.
   2. Dosage of the opioid drug prescribed.
   3. The patient's ability to ambulate to the bathroom.
   4. Bowel sounds.

6 A patient asks the nurse about giving an over-the-counter drug, bismuth subsalicylate (Pepto-Bismol), to treat a daughter's diarrhea. On which of the following will the nurse base the recommendation? Select all that apply.
   1. Cause of diarrhea
   2. Normal activity level
   3. Age
   4. Weight
   5. School schedule

See Answers to Chapter Review in Appendix A.

References

Lehrer, J. K. (2014). *Irritable bowel syndrome.* Retrieved from http://emedicine.medscape.com/article/180389-overview

Nitsche, C. J., Jamieson, N., Lerch, M. M., & Mayerle, J. V. (2010). Drug-induced pancreatitis. *Best Practice and Research in Clinical Gastroenterology, 24,* 143–155. doi:10.1016/j.bpg.2010.02.002

Wilcox, S. R. (2013). *Hyperemesis gravidarum in emergency medicine.* Retrieved from http://emedicine.medscape.com/article/796564-overview

Selected Bibliography

Bharucha, A. E., Pemberton, J. H., & Locke, G. R., III. (2013). American Gastroenterological Association technical review on constipation. *Gastroenterology, 144*(1), 218–238. doi:10.1053/j.gastro.2012.10.028

Ford, A. C., Brenner, D. M., & Schoenfeld, P. S. (2013). Efficacy of pharmacological therapies for the treatment of opioid-induced constipation: Systematic review and meta-analysis. *The American Journal of Gastroenterology, 108*, 1566–1574. doi:10.1038/ajg.2013.169

Grundmann, O., & Yoon, S. L. (2014). Complementary and alternative medicines in irritable bowel syndrome: An integrative view. *World Journal of Gastroenterology, 20*, 346–362. doi:10.3748/wjg.v20.i2.346

Haniadka, R., Popouri, S., Palatty, P. L., Arora, R., & Baliga, M. S. (2012). Medicinal plants as antiemetics in the treatment of cancer: A review. *Integrative Cancer Therapies, 11*, 18–28. doi:10.1177/1534735411413266

Herdman, T. H., & Kamitsuru, S. (Eds.). (2014). *NANDA International nursing diagnoses: Definitions and classification, 2015–2017.* Oxford, United Kingdom: Wiley-Blackwell.

Herrstedt, J., Rapoport, B., Warr, D., Roila, F., Bria, E., Rittennberg, C., & Hesketh, P. J. (2011). Acute emesis: Moderately emetogenic chemotherapy. *Supportive Care in Cancer, 19*(Suppl. 1), S15–23. doi:10.1007/s00520-010-0951-5

Kumar, A., & Kumar, A. (2013). Antiemetics: A review. *International Journal of Pharmaceutical Sciences & Research, 4*(1), 113–123.

Peyrin-Biroulet, L., Fiorino, G., Buisson, A., & Danese, S. (2013). First-line therapy in adult Crohn's disease: Who should receive anti-TNF agents? *Nature Reviews Gastroenterology and Hepatology, 10*, 345–351. doi:10.1038/nrgastro.2013.31

Rowe, W. A. (2014). *Inflammatory bowel disease.* Retrieved from http://emedicine.medscape.com/article/179037-overview#a0156

Salari, P., Nikfar, S., & Abdollahi, M. (2012). A meta-analysis and systematic review on the effect of probiotics in acute diarrhea. *Inflammation & Allergy-Drug Targets, 11*(1), 3–14. doi:10.2174/187152812798889394

Sharkey, K. A., & Wallace, J. L. (2011). Treatment of disorders of bowel motility and water flux; antiemetics; agents used in biliary and pancreatic disease. In L. L. Brunton, B. A. Chabner, & B. C. Knollman (Eds.), *The pharmacological basis of therapeutics* (12th ed., pp. 1323–1350). New York, NY: McGraw-Hill.

Wallace, J. L., & Sharkey, K. A. (2011). Pharmacotherapy of inflammatory bowel disease. In L. L. Brunton, B. A. Chabner, & B. C. Knollman (Eds.), *The pharmacological basis of therapeutics* (12th ed., pp. 1351–1362). New York, NY: McGraw-Hill.

Whelan, K., & Quigley, E. M. (2013). Probiotics in the management of irritable bowel syndrome and inflammatory bowel disease. *Current Opinion in Gastroenterology, 29*, 184–189. doi:10.1097/MOG.0b013e32835d7bba

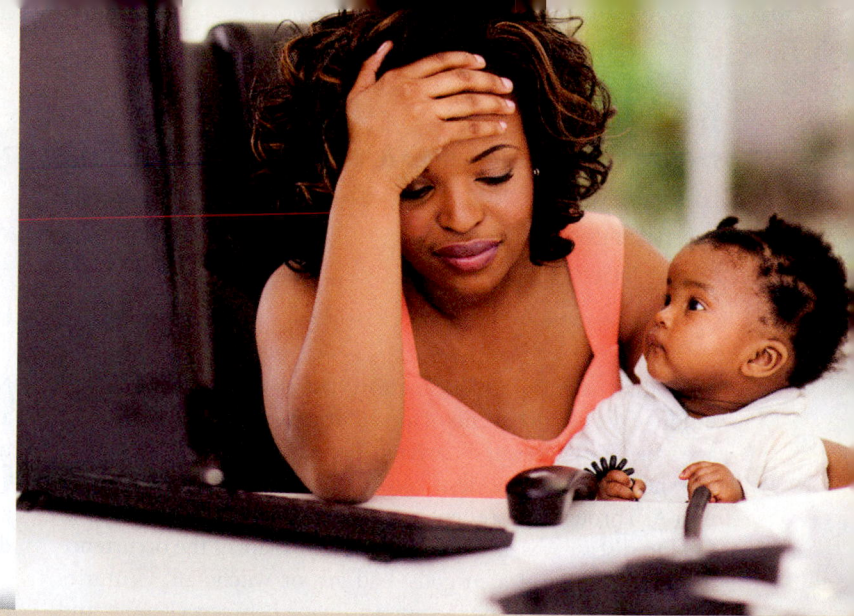

"I still have some prenatal vitamins left over. I've been feeling pretty stressed and tired lately. Maybe they'll give me more energy."

Patient "Charlene Garrett"

CHAPTER 61

Vitamins and Minerals

LEARNING OUTCOMES

After reading this chapter, the student should be able to:

1. Describe the role of vitamins in maintaining wellness.
2. Identify conditions for which vitamin and mineral therapy may be indicated.
3. Explain the governmental regulation of vitamins and minerals.
4. Discuss the role of the recommended dietary allowance in determining the standardized requirement of various vitamins and minerals.
5. Compare and contrast fat-soluble and water-soluble vitamins.
6. For each of the major vitamins, identify the mechanism(s) of action, primary indications, contraindications, significant drug interactions, pregnancy category, and important adverse effects.
7. Identify the major functions of macrominerals and microminerals.
8. Apply the nursing process to care for patients who are receiving vitamin and mineral supplementation therapy.

CHAPTER OUTLINE

▶ Role of Vitamins in Health and Disease

▶ Regulation of Vitamins

▶ Recommended Dietary Allowance

▶ Fat-Soluble Vitamins

▶ Water-Soluble Vitamins

▶ Minerals
   Macrominerals
   Microminerals

KEY TERMS

Council for Responsible Nutrition (CRN), 1049

fat-soluble vitamins, 1048

hypervitaminosis, 1049

macrominerals, 1056

microminerals, 1057

minerals, 1056

recommended dietary allowances (RDAs), 1050

supplements, 1048

vitamins, 1048

water-soluble vitamins, 1048

More than half of all Americans take vitamin supplements. Recognition of the health benefits of food nutrients dates back 3,500 years ago when the Egyptians discovered that eating certain foods such as liver helped night blindness. Today, this nutrient is known as vitamin A. Through subsequent years the relationship of nutrients in food to disease was largely ignored. Many blamed the occurrence of disease on displeased gods, bad air, or witchcraft. Centuries would pass before a connection was made between vitamins and health. This chapter examines the rationales for vitamin and mineral pharmacotherapy.

Role of Vitamins in Health and Disease

61.1 Although the importance of nutrition has been known for centuries, the specific vitamins were discovered in the 1900s.

When ocean voyages became a preferred way of travel in the Renaissance, extended periods onboard a ship often meant limited access to fresh fruits and vegetables. People began to develop scurvy, a disease that causes bleeding of the gums, loss of teeth, ulcers on the lower legs, loss of hair, aching joints, fatigue, depression, hallucinations, blindness, and open wounds with decreased ability to heal. In 1774, James Lind, a Scottish surgeon in the Royal Navy, made a major discovery that saved the lives of many sailors. In fact, Lind surmised that more men died from scurvy than from war injuries. Although he was not the first person to suspect that citrus fruit was important to health, he was the one who performed clinical experiments to address this illness. He divided the affected sailors into groups and added different substances, such as cider, vinegar, barley water, oranges, or lemons, to their diets. Those who ate citrus fruit recovered from scurvy. Lind was ahead of his time because about 40 years passed before authorities accepted the connection between disease and nutrition.

Even in the early 1900s, most people believed that diseases like beriberi and pellagra were infectious processes. Beriberi is now known as a nutritional disease characterized by progressive neuropathy and accompanying dysfunction of the sensory process and an unsteady gait. In the late 1880s, Christian Eijkman studied beriberi in the West Indies and determined the cure for beriberi to be rice. He did not understand that it was a specific substance within the rice that caused the cure. In 1905, Dr. William Fletcher observed inmates who had beriberi at a mental asylum and found that ingesting unpolished rice could prevent the disease. This English physician determined that the rice husks contained some substance (thiamine) that treated beriberi. In 1907, Sir Frederick Gowland, an English biochemist, confirmed the positive relationship of food to health. He later joined with Eijkman to win the 1929

Nobel Prize for his work with food nutrients and vitamins. In 1911, a Polish chemist named Casimir Funk coined the term *vitamines*, meaning nutrients vital for life.

In the 1920s and 1930s, scientists determined that small amounts of specific food substances (vitamins) prevented certain diseases. More than 160 years after Lind's discovery to prevent scurvy, Dr. Albert Szent-Györgi, a Hungarian researcher, received the Nobel Prize in medicine by isolating and naming vitamin C.

61.2 Vitamins are essential for optimal health.

Today **vitamins** are defined as substances that are required in small amounts for normal growth and nutrition. These naturally occurring organic substances are critical for metabolism as well as regulation of cell function and human growth and development. They contain carbon, are found in living organisms such as plants and animals, and function primarily as catalysts that speed up biochemical processes. Vitamins must be taken into the body from the external environment, usually through the diet, and are not manufactured by the body with the exception of vitamin D. Lack of sufficient amounts of vitamins results in symptoms of deficiency. People must consume vitamin supplements when their diet is lacking in these necessary nutrients or when they have health conditions that cause vitamin deficiencies. The vitamins and their functions are summarized in Table 61.1.

Vitamins are divided into two basic groups: those that dissolve in water (water soluble) and those that dissolve in lipids (fat soluble). Vitamin C and the B-complex vitamins are the primary **water-soluble vitamins**. This group of vitamins is stored briefly in the body and then excreted in the urine. The body's supply of water-soluble vitamins must be replenished on a daily basis. One exception is B_{12}, which is stored in the liver. In contrast, **fat-soluble vitamins** are stored in the liver and fatty tissue of the human body and only need intermittent renewal. Because they are stored and not readily excreted, the possibility of toxicity from overdosing is greater with the fat-soluble group, which includes vitamins A, D, E, and K.

Most people have no need for vitamins as long as they eat a well-balanced diet. However, many Americans rely on nutrient-poor fast foods and processed edibles as their main diet. Also, vitamins can be destroyed by heat, sunlight, exposure to moisture and air, mold, and oxidation. Although a healthy diet is the best way to maintain adequate vitamin and mineral intake, individual **supplements** are available as an additional way to meet the minimum daily requirements for some people. However, it is important to remember that vitamin and mineral products should supplement a healthy balanced diet; they are not substitutes for good nutrition. Doses for the fat-soluble vitamin supplements are listed in Table 61.2. The water-soluble vitamin doses are listed in Table 61.3.

TABLE 61.1 Essential Vitamins

Vitamin	Function(s)	Common Cause(s) of Deficiency
A	Visual pigments, epithelial cells	Prolonged dietary deprivation, particularly when rice is the main food source; pancreatic disease; cirrhosis
B vitamins		
Vitamin B_1: thiamine	Coenzyme in metabolic reactions, RBC formation	Prolonged dietary deprivation, particularly when rice is the main food source; hyperthyroidism, pregnancy, liver disease, alcoholism
Vitamin B_2: riboflavin	Coenzyme in oxidation–reduction reactions	Inadequate consumption of milk or animal products, chronic diarrhea, liver disease, alcoholism
Vitamin B_3: niacin	Coenzyme in oxidation–reduction reactions	Prolonged dietary deprivation, particularly when Indian corn (maize) or millet is the main food source; chronic diarrhea; liver disease; alcoholism
Vitamin B_6: pyridoxine	Coenzyme in amino acid metabolism and red blood cell (RBC) production	Alcoholism, oral contraceptive use, malabsorption diseases
Vitamin B_9: folic acid/folate	Coenzyme in amino acid and nucleic acid metabolism	Pregnancy, alcoholism, cancer, oral contraceptive use
Vitamin B_{12}: cyanocobalamin	Coenzyme in nucleic acid metabolism	Lack of intrinsic factor, inadequate intake of foods with animal origin
C (ascorbic acid)	Coenzyme and antioxidant	Inadequate intake of fruits and vegetables, pregnancy, chronic inflammatory disease, burns, diarrhea, alcoholism
D	Calcium and phosphate metabolism	Low dietary intake, inadequate exposure to sunlight
E	Antioxidant	Prematurity, malabsorption diseases
K	Cofactor in blood clotting	Newborns, liver disease, long-term parenteral nutrition, certain drugs such as cephalosporins and salicylates

Regulation of Vitamins

61.3 Government regulations and consumer knowledge about vitamins are limited.

A 2007 survey by the **Council for Responsible Nutrition (CRN)**, a Washington-based trade association representing ingredient suppliers and manufacturers in the dietary supplement industry, reported that 68% of adults in America take vitamin supplements. Those considered "regular users" increased from 46% in 2006 to 52% in 2007, with 84% believing that these supplements are safe. Most patients are unaware that taking too much of a vitamin or mineral can cause serious adverse effects. **Hypervitaminosis**, or toxic levels of vitamins, has been reported for vitamins A, C, D, E, B_6, niacin, and folic acid. In the United States, it is actually more common to observe syndromes of vitamin *excess* than of vitamin *deficiency*.

Consumers may assume that the U.S. Food and Drug Administration (FDA) regulates and approves nutritional supplements, as it does prescription and over-the-counter (OTC) drugs. However, the legislative regulation of supplements is much more limited as compared to drugs. The FDA regulates herbal, vitamin, and mineral products as "dietary supplements." In 1994, the Dietary Supplement Health and Education Act required labeling of supplements. In 2007, the FDA passed the "current Good Manufacturing

TABLE 61.2 Fat-Soluble Vitamins for Treating Nutritional Disorders

Drug	Route and Adult Dose (Maximum Dose Where Indicated)	Adverse Effects
Vitamin A (Aquasol A)	PO: 100,000 units/day for 3 days, followed by 50,000 units/day for 2 weeks; then 10,000–20,000 units/day for 2 months IM: 100,000 units/day for 3 days followed by 50,000 units/day for 2 weeks	*Uncommon at recommended doses* High doses: nausea, vomiting, fatigue, irritability, night sweats, alopecia, dry skin
Vitamin D (Calcijex, Rocaltrol)	PO: 0.25 mcg/day; may be increased by 0.25 mcg/day every 4–8 weeks for patients receiving dialysis or every 2–4 weeks for patients with hypoparathyroidism	*Uncommon at recommended doses, metallic taste* High doses: nausea, vomiting, fatigue, headache, polyuria, weight loss, hallucinations, dysrhythmias, muscle, and bone pain
Vitamin E (Aquasol E, Vita-Plus E, Others)	PO/IM: 60–75 units/day	*Uncommon at recommended doses* High doses: nausea, vomiting, fatigue, headache, blurred vision
Vitamin K (AquaMEPHYTON)	PO/IM/subcutaneous: 2.5–10 mg (up to 25 mcg); may be repeated after 6–8 h if needed	*Facial flushing, pain at the injection site* IV route may result in dyspnea, hypotension, shock, cardiac arrest

Note: Italics indicate common adverse effects. Underline indicates serious adverse effects.

TABLE 61.3 Water-Soluble Vitamins for Treating Nutritional Disorders

Drug	Route and Adult Dose (Maximum Dose Where Indicated)	Adverse Effects
Vitamin B₁: thiamine	IV/IM: 50–100 mg tid PO: 5–30 mg/day	*Pain at the injection site* IV route may result in angioedema, cyanosis, pulmonary edema, GI bleeding, and cardiovascular collapse
Vitamin B₂: riboflavin	PO: 5–10 mg/day	*Adverse effects have not been reported*
Vitamin B₃: niacin (Nicobid, Niospan, Others)	PO: 10–20 mg/day IV/IM/subcutaneous: 25–100 mg 2–5 times/day	*Uncommon at doses recommended for vitamin therapy* High doses: flushing, rash, diarrhea, hepatotoxicity
Vitamin B₆: pyridoxine (Hexa-Betalin, Nestrex)	PO/IM/IV: 2.5–10 mg/day for 3 weeks; then may reduce to 2.5–5 mg/day	*Pain at the injection site* High doses: neuropathy, ataxia, seizures
Vitamin B₉: folic acid (Folvite)	PO/IM/IV/subcutaneous: 0.4–1 mg/day	*Uncommon at recommended doses* Parenteral routes: allergic hypersensitivity
Vitamin B₁₂: cyanocobalamin (Betalin 12, Cobex, Cynapin, Others)	IM/deep subcutaneous: 30 mcg/day for 5–10 days; then 100–200 mcg/month	*Rash, diarrhea* High doses: thrombosis, hypokalemia, pulmonary edema, heart failure
Vitamin C: ascorbic acid (Ascorbicap, Cebid, Vita-C, Others)	PO/IV/IM/subcutaneous: 150–500 mg/day in one to two doses	*Uncommon at recommended doses* High doses: deep venous thrombosis (IV route), crystalluria

Note: *Italics* indicate common adverse effects. <u>Underline</u> indicates serious adverse effects.

Practice" (cGMP) regulations, which mandated manufacturers to evaluate supplements for purity, strength, and composition (see Chapter 7).

The FDA's Division of Dietary Supplement Programs offers guidelines and tips for consumer safety. The best advice is to be knowledgeable about the purchase and use of supplements. This agency encourages consumers to consult with their health care providers before using supplements and to be leery of false claims. Supplements can be expensive, and choosing foods with needed vitamins and minerals is a more natural way to reach nutritional health goals.

PharmFACT

Vitamin toxicity is responsible for over 60,000 calls to poison control centers each year in the United States (Rosenbloom, 2013).

Recommended Dietary Allowance

61.4 The recommended dietary allowance is the dietary intake level that is sufficient to meet the nutrient requirements for most people.

The Food and Nutrition Board of the National Academy of Sciences has established the **recommended dietary allowances (RDAs)** for healthy adults. These values represent the minimum amount of vitamins and minerals needed to prevent disease and are based on scientific nutritional research. A newer value, the dietary reference intake (DRI), is based on four parameters: the estimated average requirement, RDA, adequate intake, and tolerable upper intake level.

Although a well-balanced diet provides the necessary vitamins and minerals for most people, the amount of vitamins and minerals needed varies based on certain factors. For example,

infants, pregnant women, nursing mothers, older adults, those eating a vegan or vegetarian diet, and those with chronic diseases often require larger amounts of vitamins and minerals to maintain optimal health. Men and women can have different vitamin and mineral needs as do persons who participate in vigorous exercise. With normal aging, the absorption of food diminishes and the quantity of ingested food is often reduced, leading to a higher risk of vitamin deficiencies in older adults. Vitamin deficiencies in patients with chronic liver and kidney disease are well documented. In cases where dietary needs are increased, the RDAs will need adjustment and supplements are indicated to achieve optimum wellness.

Certain drugs have the potential to affect vitamin metabolism. Alcohol is known for its ability to inhibit the absorption of thiamine and folic acid: Alcohol abuse is the most common cause of thiamine deficiency in the United States. Folic acid levels may be reduced in patients who are taking phenothiazines, oral contraceptives, phenytoin (Dilantin), or barbiturates. Vitamin D deficiency can be caused by therapy with certain anticonvulsants. Inhibition of vitamin B₁₂ absorption has been reported with a number of drugs, including omeprazole (Prilosec) and metformin (Glucophage), alcohol, and oral contraceptives. Nurses must be aware of these drug interactions and recommend vitamin supplements when appropriate.

Vitamin deficiencies follow certain patterns. The following are general characteristics of vitamin deficiency disorders:

- Patients more commonly present with multiple vitamin deficiencies than with a single vitamin deficiency.
- Symptoms of deficiency are nonspecific and often do not appear until the deficiency has been present for a long period.
- Deficiencies in the United States are most often the result of poverty, fad diets, chronic alcohol or drug abuse, or prolonged parenteral feeding.

◀ **Vitamins During Pregnancy**

Pregnancy is a time when vitamin supplements are necessary to provide additional nutritional support. Essentially, the mother is eating for two, because the fetus demands nutritional support as much as the woman's body does. Supplementation with vitamins can support the mother's diet and ensure that both she and her baby get the nutrients they need. However, vitamins should be seen as a *supplement* to a healthy diet during pregnancy.

A common practice in prenatal care is for pregnant women to take prenatal vitamin supplements. These vitamins contain numerous nutrients, and folic acid, calcium, and iron are especially important. Each of these substances is necessary for a healthy mother and baby.

Folic acid (vitamin B_9) is often highlighted as a need in pregnancy because it prevents birth defects such as spina bifida, other neural tube problems, and congenital heart conditions. Because birth defects can take place early in pregnancy, taking prenatal vitamins is recommended if a woman is trying to get pregnant.

Calcium is another mineral that is needed in adequate amounts during pregnancy. Supplementation can stop the loss of bone density from the mother as the fetus absorbs calcium for bone growth. This is especially important during the second and third trimesters.

Iron is a mineral that is often supplemented in pregnancy because it is the central component in hemoglobin that carries oxygen for both mother and baby. Anemia can occur with insufficient iron intake. Women who experience morning sickness and vomiting are at risk for dietary iron deficiency. Also, women with poor diets or heavy menstrual periods before pregnancy can start their pregnancy with a mineral deficiency. Iron supplements should be taken separately from calcium-rich food and caffeine because these interfere with iron absorption. Vitamin C enhances the absorption of iron so the two can be taken concurrently. Because high amounts are extremely toxic, iron supplements should be kept away from children to avoid accidental poisoning.

Fat-Soluble Vitamins

61.5 Fat-soluble vitamins include vitamins A, D, E, and K.

The fat-soluble vitamins A, D, E, and K are found in fatty foods and oils. Because they are stored in lipid tissue, the body may go several weeks or months with insufficient dietary intake before signs of deficiency are noted. Excessive intake of these vitamins may be harmful.

Vitamin A (Aquasol A)

Therapeutic Effects and Uses: Vitamin A is essential for the normal growth and development of bones and teeth, natural immunity, integrity of epithelial and mucosal surfaces, and vision with the synthesis of visual purple necessary for adaptation to the dark (treats night blindness). Vitamin A replacement therapy is used when metabolic needs are increased such as in pregnancy, during lactation, or with infections. Vitamin A can be used in replacement therapy for conditions affecting the absorption, mobilization, or storage of vitamin A such as steatorrhea, severe biliary obstruction, liver cirrhosis, or total gastrectomy. Some skin conditions such as folliculosis keratosis or psoriasis respond favorably to topical preparations of vitamin A. Vitamin A has antioxidant properties and can be used as a screening test for fat malabsorption.

Mechanism of Action: As a fat-soluble vitamin, vitamin A acts as a cofactor in the synthesis of mucopolysaccharides, synthesis of cholesterol, and the metabolism of steroids. It is easily absorbed through the gastrointestinal (GI) tract with bile salts, pancreatic lipase, and dietary fat, and it is stored in the liver. Small amounts may also be stored in the kidney and body fat. Vitamin A can pass to the newborn through breast milk. Vitamin A is metabolized in the liver and excreted in feces and urine.

Adverse Effects: Adverse effects with vitamin A are rare but the health care provider should be notified of difficulty breathing; hives; swelling of the lips, face, or tongue; or closing of the throat. Overdose may result in hypervitaminosis syndrome symptoms such as fatigue, nausea, vomiting, decreased appetite, headache, gingivitis, dryness or cracking of the lips or skin, irritability, or loss of hair. Rare adverse effects include increased intracranial pressure, jaundice, leukopenia, anemia, and elevated prothrombin time (PT).

Contraindications/Precautions: Contraindications to vitamin A therapy include a history of sensitivity to vitamin A or to any ingredient in the formulation or hypervitaminosis. Oral (PO) administration to patients with malabsorption syndrome is also contraindicated. Its safe use in amounts exceeding 6,000 international units during pregnancy is not established. Vitamin A may falsely increase serum cholesterol determinations or falsely elevate bilirubin determination.

Drug Interactions: Caution should be used if the patient is taking vitamin A analogs such as isotretinoin because their actions are additive. The patient should consult with the health care provider if using mineral oil because this can deplete fat-soluble vitamins. Cholestyramine may decrease the absorption of vitamin A. Oral contraceptives can increase serum levels of vitamin A.

Pregnancy: Category A (at RDA value).

Recommended Intake: RDA: 2,500 international units for children, 4,000 international units for women, and 5,000 international units for men. DRI: 300–400 mcg/day for children, 700 mcg/day for women, and 900 mcg/day for men.

Nursing Responsibilities: Key nursing implications for patients receiving vitamin A are included in the Nursing Practice Application for Patients Receiving Pharmacotherapy with Vitamin or Mineral Supplements.

Vitamin D (Calcijex, Rocaltrol)

Therapeutic Effects and Uses: Vitamin D plays a major regulatory role in serum calcium levels. It maintains normal blood calcium and phosphate electrolyte levels by enhancing their intestinal absorption and by promoting mobilization of calcium from bone and the renal reabsorption of phosphate. This fat-soluble vitamin is necessary to develop and maintain strong bones. Vitamin D is used to treat skeletal diseases that weaken the bones such as familial hypophosphatemia (vitamin D–resistant rickets), osteomalacia (adult rickets), osteoporosis, renal osteodystrophy, and hypocalcemia associated with hypoparathyroidism. Vitamin D is used as prophylaxis for and treatment of nutritional rickets, and hypophosphatemia in Fanconi's syndrome. Sometimes vitamin D is helpful in treating psoriasis, rheumatoid arthritis, and lupus vulgaris. A drug prototype feature for calcitriol, the active form of vitamin D, is included in Chapter 72.

Mechanism of Action: Vitamin D is a fat-soluble vitamin that is found in food and that is also made by the body after exposure to ultraviolet (UV) rays from the sun. Sunlight is a significant source of vitamin D because UV rays trigger vitamin D synthesis in the skin. Vitamin D is readily absorbed from the GI tract and distributed in the lymph. The body stores vitamin D in the liver, skin, brain, spleen, and bones. About half of each vitamin D dose is excreted in bile but it may be stored in tissues for months.

Adverse Effects: Adverse effects of vitamin D therapy are uncommon at therapeutic doses. At higher doses possible adverse effects include fatigue, weakness, dizziness, ataxia, muscle and joint pain, hypotonia (infants), pruritus, headache, drowsiness, photophobia, or convulsions. GI symptoms include anorexia, nausea, vomiting, diarrhea, metallic taste, dry mouth, constipation, and abdominal cramps. Some patients present with anemia. Musculoskeletal symptoms include calcification of soft tissues in the kidneys, myocardium, lungs, or skin. Nephrotoxicity could occur with symptoms such as polyuria, polydipsia, nocturia, albuminuria, hematuria, and kidney failure. Vitamin D is rarely but possibly implicated in hypertension and some cardiac dysrhythmias. Chronic hypervitaminosis with vitamin D can occur in children, resulting in mental and physical retardation or suppression of linear growth.

Contraindications/Precautions: Precaution should be taken in patients with a known hypersensitivity to vitamin D, hypervitaminosis, hypercalcemia, hyperphosphatemia, renal osteodystrophy with hyperphosphatemia, malabsorption syndrome, or decreased kidney function. Use cautiously in patients with coronary disease, arteriosclerosis (especially in older adults), history of kidney stones, biliary tract disease, or during lactation.

Drug Interactions: Consult with the health care provider if using mineral oil because it can deplete the supply of fat-soluble vitamins in the body. Cholestyramine may decrease the absorption of vitamin D. Vitamin D can cause a false increase in serum cholesterol measurements. Prescribers should avoid calcitriol and its analogs because they may increase the incidence of hypercalcemia.

Pregnancy: Category C. The safe use of vitamin D in amounts exceeding 400 international units (10 mcg) daily during pregnancy has not been established.

Recommended Intake: **RDA:** Children, men, and women until age 50 need 200 international units of vitamin D per day. For individuals ages 51 to 70, the minimum dose increases to 400 international units per day. Those age 71 and older need 600 international units per day. **DRI:** 15 mg/day for children, and 15 mg/day for adults (20 mg/day over age 70).

Nursing Responsibilities: Key nursing implications for patients receiving vitamin D are included in the Nursing Practice Application for Patients Receiving Pharmacotherapy with Vitamin or Mineral Supplements.

PharmFACT

Indoor tanning has become increasingly popular with claims that it increases the level of vitamin D. However, most indoor tanning devices use UVA radiation, which is very inefficient at producing vitamin D in the skin (Woo & Elde, 2010).

Vitamin E (Aquasol E, Vita-Plus E, Others)

Therapeutic Effects and Uses: Vitamin E has many therapeutic uses. It prevents cell membrane and protein damage, protects against blood clot formation by decreasing platelet aggregation, enhances vitamin A utilization, and promotes the normal growth and development and tone of muscles. As an antioxidant, vitamin E prevents preoxidation, which releases free radicals or highly reactive chemical structures that damage cell membranes and alter nuclear proteins. Free radicals are associated with various conditions such as aging and disease.

Deficiencies of vitamin E often result in hemolytic anemia. Vitamin E therapy can reverse or prevent hemolytic anemia in premature neonates that is caused by vitamin E deficiency. It is also used to prevent retinopathy associated with vitamin E deficiency in neonates and to treat diseases with secondary erythrocyte membrane abnormalities (e.g., sickle cell anemia and G6PD deficiency). Vitamin E is used as a supplement in malabsorption syndromes. Topical vitamin E is used for dry or chapped skin and minor skin disorders.

Some people report improvement in muscular dystrophy symptoms and a number of other conditions although there is no conclusive evidence of its value. Vitamin E is included in most multivitamin formulations and may appear in deodorant preparations as an antioxidant.

Mechanism of Action: When fat absorption is adequate, 20% to 60% of vitamin E is absorbed across the GI tract. It enters blood through the lymph and is stored in adipose (fat) tissue. Vitamin E is metabolized in the liver and is eliminated primarily in bile. Vitamin E crosses the placenta.

Adverse Effects: Adverse reactions to vitamin E are rare. With excessive doses symptoms may include fatigue, headache, skeletal muscle weakness, nausea, diarrhea, intestinal cramps, thrombophlebitis, contact dermatitis, blurred vision, or abnormal bleeding. With toxic levels laboratory tests may reveal increased serum creatine kinase, cholesterol, and triglycerides; decreased serum thyroxine and triiodothyronine; increased urinary estrogens and androgens; and creatinuria.

Contraindications/Precautions: Vitamin E should be used with caution in bleeding disorders and thrombocytopenia or during pregnancy. Vitamin E can prolong the PT by inhibition of vitamin K–dependent carboxylase in someone with abnormally low vitamin K levels. Large doses may worsen iron deficiency anemia because it may impair the hematologic response to iron.

Drug Interactions: Mineral oil should be avoided because it can deplete fat-soluble vitamins. Cholestyramine may decrease absorption of vitamin E. Vitamin E may enhance the anticoagulant activity of warfarin.

Pregnancy: Category A (at RDA levels).

Recommended Intake: **RDA:** Ranges from 4 mg (6 international units) to 11 mg (16.5 international units) in children under 13 years, depending on the age, and 15 mg (22.5 international units) for persons age 14 through adult. Pregnant women need a minimum of 19 mg (28.5 international units) per day. **DRI:** 6–7 mg/day for children and 15 mg/day for adults.

Nursing Responsibilities: Key nursing implications for patients receiving vitamin E are included in the Nursing Practice Application for Patients Receiving Pharmacotherapy with Vitamin or Mineral Supplements.

Vitamin K (AquaMEPHYTON)

Therapeutic Effects and Uses: Vitamin K promotes the liver synthesis of clotting factors and is used in the production of red blood cells (RBCs). It helps maintain healthy bones, assists in healing fractures, and minimizes osteoporosis. It is the drug of choice as an antidote for the overdosage of warfarin and indandione PO anticoagulants. Vitamin K reverses hypoprothrombinemia secondary to the administration of PO antibiotics, quinidine, salicylates, sulfonamides, and excessive vitamin A, and secondary to inadequate absorption and synthesis of vitamin K (as in obstructive jaundice, biliary fistula, ulcerative colitis, intestinal resection, or prolonged hyperalimentation). Vitamin K is used as prophylaxis of and therapy for neonatal hemorrhagic disease.

Mechanism of Action: The body makes most of its needed vitamin K through bacteria in the GI tract. Phytonadione is a fat-soluble substance that is chemically identical to and has similar activity as naturally occurring vitamin K. It is absorbed readily in the intestinal lymph if bile is present. Vitamin K is essential for the hepatic biosynthesis of blood-clotting Factors II, VII, IX, and X. Hemorrhage is usually controlled within 3 to 8 hours, with normal PT obtained in 12 to 14 hours after vitamin K administration. Phytonadione is concentrated briefly in the liver after absorption, crosses the placenta, and is secreted in the breast milk of nursing mothers. It is metabolized quickly in the liver and eliminated in the urine and bile.

Adverse Effects: Reported effects after PO dosing include headache, GI upset, paradoxical hypoprothrombinemia (in patients with severe liver disease), severe hemolytic anemia, hyperbilirubinemia, kernicterus, bronchospasm, and dyspnea. Possible pain at the injection site, hematoma and nodule formation, erythematous skin eruptions (with repeated injections), and peculiar taste sensations may occur. **Black Box Warning**: Severe reactions such as shock, anaphylaxis, and cardiac arrest have occurred when vitamin K is given by the IV or IM route. These routes should only be used when subcutaneous or oral routes are not feasible.

Contraindications/Precautions: Caution should be used in patients with biliary tract disease, obstructive jaundice, or severe liver disease. Patients should be monitored for hypersensitivity to phytonadione, benzyl alcohol, or castor oil. Some interference may occur with diagnostic tests such as falsely elevated urine steroids.

Drug Interactions: Vitamin K decreases the anticoagulant effects of warfarin. Patients may have decreased absorption with the use of cholestyramine, colestipol, or mineral oil.

Pregnancy: Category C.

Recommended Intake: **RDA:** 80 mcg/day. **DRI:** 30–55 mcg/day for children, 90 mcg/day for women, and 120 mcg/day for men.

Nursing Responsibilities: Key nursing implications for patients receiving vitamin K are included in the Nursing Practice Application for Patients Receiving Pharmacotherapy with Vitamin or Mineral Supplements.

CONNECTION Checkpoint 61.1

From what you learned in Chapter 38, describe how vitamin K reverses the therapeutic effects of warfarin (Coumadin). *See Answer to Connection Checkpoint 61.1 on student resource website.*

Water-Soluble Vitamins

61.6 Water-soluble vitamins include the B-complex vitamins and vitamin C.

The water-soluble vitamins are found in rich abundance in fresh fruits and vegetables. Unlike the fat-soluble vitamins, vitamin C and most B-complex vitamins are not stored to any great extent, and signs of deficiency may be noted quickly if they are omitted from the diet. Excessive intake of these vitamins is usually not harmful because they are rapidly excreted.

Thiamine: Vitamin B₁

Therapeutic Effects and Uses: Thiamine, also known as vitamin B_1, functions as an essential coenzyme in the metabolism of carbohydrates and has a role in converting tryptophan to nicotinamide. This vitamin is used in the treatment and prophylaxis of beriberi, to correct anorexia due to thiamine deficiency, and in the treatment of neuritis associated with pregnancy, pellagra, and alcoholism. Severe deficiency is characterized by paralysis of the eye muscle (ophthalmoplegia), neuropathy, muscle wasting, edema, serous effusions, and heart failure. Its effectiveness is evidenced by improvement of the clinical manifestations of thiamine deficiency, such as anorexia, gastric distress, depression, irritability, insomnia, palpitations, tachycardia, loss of memory, paresthesias, muscle weakness and pain, elevated blood pyruvic acid level (diagnostic test for thiamine deficiency), and elevated lactic acid level.

Because of its abundance in food, thiamine deficiency in the United States is not common, except in people with chronic alcoholism or chronic liver disease and in patients following bariatric surgery. Therapy generally includes other members of the B-complex vitamins because thiamine deficiency rarely occurs alone. Thiamine is sometimes used in combination with other B vitamins to reduce depression and anxiety as well as to prevent motion sickness. Some believe that in certain amounts, this vitamin causes a chemical change on the skin that repels biting insects like mosquitoes.

Mechanism of Action: Thiamine is necessary for the conversion of carbohydrates to energy and is essential in maintaining the proper functioning of the heart, nervous system, and muscles. Thiamine is absorbed from the GI tract and widely distributed, and it is secreted in breast milk. This vitamin is eliminated in the urine.

Adverse Effects: Thiamine has few adverse effects. Excessive doses may cause a feeling of warmth, weakness, sweating, restlessness, tightness of the throat, angioneurotic edema, cyanosis, pulmonary edema, cardiovascular collapse, or hypotension after rapid IV administration. Other adverse effects may include GI hemorrhage, nausea, urticaria, and pruritus.

Contraindications/Precautions: There are no contraindications if the dosage is within the RDA.

Drug Interactions: Antibiotics such as erythromycin and azithromycin may decrease thiamine levels by altering intestinal flora.

Pregnancy: Category A; category C if doses are greater than the RDA.

Recommended Intake: **RDA:** 1.5 mg/day. **DRI:** 0.5–0.6 mg/day for children and 1.1–1.2 mg/day for adults.

Nursing Responsibilities: Key nursing implications for patients receiving vitamin B_1 (thiamine) are included in the Nursing Practice Application for Patients Receiving Pharmacotherapy with Vitamin or Mineral Supplements.

Riboflavin: Vitamin B₂

Therapeutic Effects and Uses: Vitamin B_2, or riboflavin, is a component of coenzymes that participate in a number of different oxidation–reduction reactions. As with thiamine, a deficiency of riboflavin is most commonly observed in people with chronic alcoholism. Clinical symptoms of deficiency include digestive disturbances, headache, burning sensation of the skin (especially "burning" feet), cracking at the corners of the mouth (cheilosis), glossitis, seborrheic dermatitis (and other skin lesions), mental depression, corneal vascularization (with photophobia, burning and itchy eyes, lacrimation, roughness of eyelids), anemia, and neuropathy. Riboflavin therapy is used to prevent riboflavin deficiency and microcytic anemia and to supplement other B vitamins in the treatment of pellagra and beriberi.

Mechanism of Action: As a component of the flavoprotein enzymes, riboflavin works together with a wide variety of proteins to catalyze many cellular respiratory reactions by which the body derives its energy. The vitamin is readily absorbed from the GI tract. Little riboflavin is stored and excess amounts are excreted in urine.

Adverse Effects: Riboflavin is nontoxic. It may discolor urine bright yellow. In large doses, riboflavin may produce yellow-green fluorescence in urine, which can cause false elevations in certain fluorometric determinations of urinary catecholamines.

Contraindications/Precautions: Unknown.

Drug Interactions: Unknown.

Pregnancy: Category A; category C if doses exceed the RDA.

Recommended Intake: **RDA:** 1.7 mg/day. **DRI:** 0.5–0.6 mg/day for children and 1.1–1.3 mg/day for adults.

Nursing Responsibilities: Key nursing implications for patients receiving vitamin B_2 (riboflavin) are included in the Nursing Practice Application for Patients Receiving Pharmacotherapy with Vitamin or Mineral Supplements.

Niacin: Vitamin B₃

The primary use for niacin is for the medical management of elevated cholesterol levels in patients at risk for atherosclerotic disease. It may be used as monotherapy or in combination with other antihyperlipidemic drugs. Additional details about niacin are included in Chapter 29.

Pyridoxine: Vitamin B₆

Therapeutic Effects and Uses: Pyridoxine deficiency occurs with inadequate dietary intake due to alcoholism, drug-induced deficiency (e.g., isoniazid, oral contraceptives), and inborn errors of metabolism (vitamin B_6–dependent convulsions or anemia). Pyridoxine is used to improve symptoms of vitamin deficiency such as nausea, vomiting, and skin lesions. Other symptoms that resemble those of riboflavin and niacin deficiency include edema, central nervous system (CNS) symptoms, and hypochromic microcytic anemia. Pyridoxine is administered to prevent chloramphenicol-induced optic neuritis. It is used to treat acute toxicity caused by overdosage of cycloserine, hydralazine, or isoniazid (INH); alcoholic polyneuritis; and sideroblastic anemia associated with high serum iron concentration. Pyridoxine has been used to manage many other conditions, including nausea and vomiting in radiation sickness and pregnancy, suppression of postpartum lactation, and diabetes; to decrease the symptoms of premenstrual syndrome (PMS); to minimize joint pain caused by some types of arthritis; and to treat carpal tunnel syndrome.

Mechanism of Action: Pyridoxine is usually available as part of a water-soluble complex of three closely related compounds with vitamin B_6 activity. Pyridoxine is essential to human nutrition, although a deficiency syndrome is not well defined. It is converted in the body to pyridoxal, a coenzyme that functions in protein, fat, and carbohydrate metabolism and in facilitating the release of glycogen from the liver and muscle. In protein metabolism, pyridoxine participates in many enzymatic transformations of amino acids and in the conversion of tryptophan to niacin and serotonin. It aids in energy transformation in the brain and nerve cells and is thought to stimulate heme production. Pyridoxine is readily absorbed from the GI tract. It is distributed and stored in the liver and crosses the placenta. Metabolism of this vitamin takes place in the liver. Pyridoxine is eliminated in urine.

Adverse Effects: Adverse events are few but the patient could experience paresthesias, slight flushing or feeling of warmth, temporary burning or stinging pain at the injection site, somnolence seizures (particularly following large parenteral doses), low folic acid levels, insomnia, or anxiety.

Contraindications/Precautions: Pyridoxine should be used with caution in patients with renal impairment, neonatal prematurity with renal impairment, or cardiac disease.

Drug Interactions: Use of isoniazid, cycloserine, penicillamine, hydralazine, and oral contraceptives may increase pyridoxine requirements. This vitamin may reverse or antagonize the therapeutic effects of the antiparkinsonism drug levodopa because it reduces the amount of dopamine entering the brain by facilitating the breakdown of levodopa in peripheral circulation.

Recommended Intake: **RDA:** 2 mg/day. **DRI:** 0.5–0.6 mg/day for children and 1.3–1.7 mg/day for adults.

Pregnancy: Category A; category C if doses exceed the RDA.

Nursing Responsibilities: Key nursing implications for patients receiving vitamin B_6 (pyridoxine) are included in the Nursing Practice Application for Patients Receiving Pharmacotherapy with Vitamin or Mineral Supplements.

CONNECTION Checkpoint 61.2

From what you learned in Chapter 51, how does the antitubercular drug isoniazid affect levels of pyridoxine (vitamin B_6)? *See Answer to Connection Checkpoint 61.2 on student resource website.*

Folic Acid: Vitamin B_9

Therapeutic Effects and Uses: Folic acid is used to treat folate deficiency, macrocytic anemia, and megaloblastic anemias, which are associated with inadequate dietary intake, alcoholism, primary liver disease, malabsorption syndromes, pregnancy, infancy, and childhood. Studies have shown that up to 80% of neural tube defects in newborns can be prevented with supplementation of folic acid prior to pregnancy.

Mechanism of Action: Vitamin B_9 is essential for the synthesis of nucleoproteins and the maintenance of RBCs, neurons, and proteins. It stimulates production of RBCs, white blood cells (WBCs), and platelets in patients with megaloblastic anemias. Folic acid counters folic acid deficiency, which can result in the production of defective deoxyribonucleic acid (DNA), leading to megaloblast formation and arrest of bone marrow maturation. Folic acid is readily absorbed in the proximal small intestine, is distributed to all body tissues, crosses the placenta in pregnancy, and is secreted in breast milk in lactating women. It is metabolized in the liver and excreted in urine.

Adverse Effects: The patient may feel warmth or flushing with IV doses. Although rare, the possible adverse effects include irritability, depression, loss of appetite, rash, itching, nausea, or dyspnea.

Contraindications/Precautions: Folic acid should not be used in patients with allergic sensitivity to B vitamins. It should be administered with caution if using folic acid alone to correct pernicious anemia or other vitamin B_{12} deficiency states as well as normocytic, refractory, aplastic, or undiagnosed anemia. Caution should be used with neonates. Folic acid can cause false low serum folate levels in patients who are receiving antibiotics such as tetracyclines.

Drug Interactions: Folic acid inhibitors such as methotrexate can antagonize the effects of folate therapy. Folic acid therapy increases the metabolism of phenytoin (Dilantin), possibly causing increased seizure activity.

Pregnancy: Category A.

Recommended Intake: **RDA:** 180–200 mcg/day. **DRI:** 150–200 mcg for children and 400 mcg/day for adults.

Nursing Responsibilities: Key nursing implications for patients receiving vitamin B_9 (folic acid) are included in the Nursing Practice Application for Patients Receiving Pharmacotherapy with Vitamin or Mineral Supplements.

Cyanocobalamin: Vitamin B_{12}

Therapeutic Effects and Uses: Cyanocobalamin is used to treat vitamin B_{12} deficiency and anemia due to malabsorption syndrome, such as in pernicious anemia; sprue; GI pathology, dysfunction, or surgery; fish tapeworm infestation; and gluten enteropathy. This drug is also used in vitamin B_{12} deficiency caused by increased physiological requirements or inadequate dietary intake and in the vitamin B_{12} absorption (Schilling) test. It may be used to prevent and treat toxicity associated with sodium nitroprusside, to treat asthma, and possibly to aid in healing following surgery. A prototype drug feature for this vitamin is presented in Chapter 39.

Mechanism of Action: Vitamin B_{12} is a cobalt-containing B-complex vitamin that is essential for normal growth, cell reproduction, maturation of RBCs, synthesis of nucleoproteins, and maintenance of the nervous system (myelin synthesis). It is believed to be involved in protein and carbohydrate metabolism as well. Vitamin B_{12} deficiency results in megaloblastic anemia, dysfunction of the spinal cord with paralysis, and GI lesions. Intestinal absorption requires the presence of intrinsic factor in the terminal ileum. It is widely distributed and is principally stored in the liver, kidneys, and adrenals. It crosses the placenta and is excreted in breast milk. In metabolism this vitamin is converted in the tissues to active coenzymes and is enterohepatically cycled. Vitamin B_{12} is eliminated in urine in 48 hours.

Adverse Effects: Adverse effects are rare but may include the feeling of a swelling body, anaphylactic shock, peripheral vascular thrombosis, pulmonary edema, heart failure, mild transient diarrhea, unmasking of polycythemia vera (with correction of vitamin B_{12} deficiency), hypokalemia, itching, rash, flushing, severe optic nerve atrophy, and sudden death.

Contraindications/Precautions: Contraindications include a history of sensitivity to vitamin B_{12}, other cobalamins, or cobalt; early Leber's disease (hereditary optic nerve atrophy); and indiscriminate use in folic acid deficiency. Caution should be used in patients with heart disease, anemia, or pulmonary disease.

Drug Interactions: Alcohol, aminosalicylic acid, neomycin, and colchicine may decrease the absorption of PO cyanocobalamin. Chloramphenicol may interfere with the therapeutic response to cyanocobalamin.

Pregnancy: Category A; category C (parenteral).

Recommended Intake: **RDA:** 2.4 mcg/day for age 19 and older, 2.6 mcg/day during pregnancy, and 2.8 mcg/day during lactation. **DRI:** 0.9–1.2 mcg/day for children and 2.4 mcg/day for adults.

Nursing Responsibilities: Key nursing implications for patients receiving vitamin B_{12} (cyanocobalamin) are included in the Nursing Practice Application for Patients Receiving Pharmacotherapy with Vitamin or Mineral Supplements.

Vitamin C: Ascorbic Acid

Therapeutic Effects and Uses: Vitamin C is essential for the synthesis and maintenance of collagen and intercellular ground substance of body tissues, blood vessels, cartilage, bones, teeth, skin, and tendons. It helps maintain the functions of the immune system for improved wound healing and increased resistance to infection. Vitamin C is used for both prophylaxis and treatment of scurvy and as a dietary supplement. Off-label uses include acidification of urine, prevention and treatment of cancer, treatment of idiopathic methemoglobinemia, and use as an adjuvant during deferoxamine therapy for iron toxicity. In megadoses vitamin C may possibly reduce the severity and duration of the common cold. It is used as an antioxidant in formulations of parenteral tetracycline and other drugs.

Mechanism of Action: Vitamin C is readily absorbed and widely distributed to body tissues. It crosses the placenta and is secreted in breast milk. Vitamin C is metabolized in the liver and eliminated rapidly in urine when the plasma level exceeds the renal threshold of 1.4 mg/dL. Unlike most mammals, humans are unable to synthesize ascorbic acid in the body; thus it must be consumed daily.

Adverse Effects: Possible adverse effects from large doses include nausea, vomiting, heartburn, diarrhea or abdominal cramps, acute hemolytic anemia, sickle cell crisis, headache, insomnia, urethritis, dysuria, crystalluria, hyperoxaluria, or hyperuricemia. With rapid IV administration temporary dizziness and soreness at the injection site may occur. Vitamin C may produce false-negative tests for occult blood in stools if taken within 48 to 72 hours of testing.

Contraindications/Precautions: Sodium ascorbate should not be used in patients on sodium restriction; calcium ascorbate is contraindicated in patients who are receiving digoxin (Lanoxin). Excessive doses should be avoided in patients with G6PD deficiency, hemochromatosis, thalassemia, sideroblastic anemia, or sickle cell anemia, or in patients prone to gout or renal calculi.

Drug Interactions: Large doses may attenuate the hypoprothrombinemic effects of PO anticoagulants. Aspirin and other salicylates may inhibit ascorbic acid uptake by leukocytes and tissues, and ascorbic acid may decrease elimination of salicylates. Chronic high doses of ascorbic acid may diminish the effects of disulfiram.

Pregnancy: Category C.

Recommended Intake: **RDA:** 60 mg/day. **DRI:** 15–25 mg/day for children and 75–90 mg/day for adults.

Nursing Responsibilities: Key nursing implications for patients receiving vitamin C (ascorbic acid) are included in the Nursing Practice Application for Patients Receiving Pharmacotherapy with Vitamin or Mineral Supplements.

Minerals

Minerals are essential substances that constitute about 4% of the body weight and serve many diverse functions. Some are essential ions or electrolytes in body fluids; others are bound to organic molecules such as hemoglobin, phospholipids, or metabolic enzymes. Those minerals that function as critical electrolytes in the body, most notably sodium and potassium, are covered in detail in Chapter 33.

Because minerals are needed in very small amounts for human metabolism, a balanced diet will supply the necessary quantities for most patients. Like vitamins, excess amounts of minerals can lead to toxicity, and patients should be advised not to exceed the recommended doses. Mineral supplements are, however, indicated for certain disorders. Iron deficiency anemia is the most common nutritional deficiency in the world and is a common indication for iron supplements. Women at high risk for osteoporosis are advised to consume extra calcium, either in their diet or as a dietary supplement.

61.7 Macrominerals are inorganic substances needed in amounts of at least 100 mg per day for normal body functioning.

Macrominerals are major inorganic substances that must be consumed daily in amounts of 100 mg or higher. Included in this group are calcium, chloride, magnesium, phosphorus, potassium, sodium, and sulfur. Two of the body's most important minerals affecting fluid and electrolyte balance, sodium and potassium, are presented in Chapter 33, with prototype features for sodium bicarbonate, sodium chloride, and potassium chloride. Each macromineral is listed in Table 61.4 along with the recommended daily allowance and function. Brief descriptions of some of the common macrominerals and their therapeutic uses are given next.

Calcium: Calcium is primarily stored in the teeth and bones to provide strength. Calcium may also be found in blood, muscle, and in the body fluid between cells. A consistent level of calcium is needed for vital body processes and functions such as bone matrix construction, muscle contraction, hormone and enzyme secretion, hemostasis, and nerve conduction. When a calcium deficiency occurs, the patient may become irritable and restless, with muscular cramps, spasms, and cardiac abnormalities. Fractures may result from continued hypocalcemia. Calcium compounds are available for pharmacotherapy in many PO salts such as calcium carbonate, calcium citrate, calcium gluconate, or calcium lactate. IV preparations are administered in severe cases. Calcium salts are featured as a prototype drug for hypocalcemia and osteoporosis in Chapter 72.

Chloride: Chloride is a chemical that the human body needs for metabolism and to maintain acid–base balance. In the CNS the inhibitory actions of certain neurotransmitters rely on the entry of chloride into specific neurons. The amount of chloride in the blood is carefully controlled by the kidneys. Isolated imbalances of chloride are due to imbalances in fluid, electrolytes, or acid base. Chloride imbalances are corrected by treating the underlying pathology.

Magnesium: Magnesium is required for more than 300 biochemical reactions in the body. This mineral helps maintain

TABLE 61.4 Minerals: Functions and RDAs

Mineral	RDA (adults)	Function
Macrominerals		
Calcium	1.0–1.2 g	Forms bony matrix; regulates nerve conduction and muscle contraction
Chloride	1.8–2.3 g	Major anion in body fluids; part of gastric acid secretion
Magnesium	Men: 400–420 mg Women: 310–320 mg	Cofactor for many enzymes; necessary for normal nerve conduction and muscle contraction
Phosphorus	700 mg	Forms bone matrix; part of ATP and nucleic acids
Potassium	4.7 g	Necessary for normal nerve conduction and muscle contraction; principal cation in intracellular fluid; essential for acid–base and electrolyte balance
Sodium	1.2–1.5 g	Necessary for normal nerve conduction and muscle contraction; principal cation in extracellular fluid; essential for acid–base and electrolyte balance
Sulfur	Not established	Component of proteins, B vitamins, and other critical molecules
Microminerals		
Chromium	20–35 mcg	Potentiates insulin; necessary for proper glucose metabolism
Cobalt	0.1 mcg	Cofactor for vitamin B_{12} and several oxidative enzymes
Copper	900 mcg	Cofactor for hemoglobin synthesis
Fluoride	3–4 mg	Influences tooth structure and possibly affects growth
Iodide	150 mcg	Component of thyroid hormones
Iron	Men: 8 mg Women: 8–18 mg	Component of hemoglobin and some enzymes of oxidative phosphorylation
Manganese	1.8–2.3 mg	Cofactor in some enzymes of lipid, carbohydrate, and protein metabolism
Molybdenum	45 mg	Cofactor for certain enzymes
Selenium	55 mcg	Antioxidant cofactor for certain enzymes
Zinc	8–11 mg	Cofactor for certain enzymes, including carbonic anhydrase; needed for proper protein structure, normal growth, and wound healing

normal muscle and nerve function, keeps cardiac rhythm steady, supports a healthy immune system, and maintains bone strength. The pharmacologic use of magnesium includes multiple pathologic conditions. For example, magnesium citrate is used for bowel evacuation, as is magnesium hydroxide, which can also be used as an antacid. Magnesium salicylate is used for the relief of pain and inflammation in rheumatoid arthritis. Lastly, the mineral can also be used as a CNS depressant because magnesium sulfate is frequently used as an anticonvulsant in labor and delivery. Magnesium sulfate is featured as a drug prototype in Chapter 33.

Most recently, magnesium has been used to help regulate blood sugar levels, promote normal blood pressure, and assist in energy metabolism and protein synthesis. The metabolism of magnesium is important to insulin sensitivity and blood pressure regulation. Magnesium deficiency is common in people with diabetes. Several epidemiologic studies indicate that magnesium may play an important role in regulating blood pressure. Furthermore, magnesium assists in the metabolism of carbohydrates and may influence the release and activity of insulin, which is the hormone that helps control blood glucose (sugar) levels.

Phosphorus: Phosphorus, another essential macromineral, binds to calcium to form calcium phosphate in bones. In addition to playing a role in bone structure, phosphorus is a component of

protein, adenosine triphosphate (ATP), and nucleic acids. Dietary sources of phosphorus are widely available; thus hypophosphatemia is most often seen in patients with severe malnutrition, intestinal malabsorption disorders, or kidney impairment that results in excess phosphorus loss in the urine. When serum phosphorus levels fall below 1.5 mEq/L, phosphate supplements are usually administered. Sodium phosphate and potassium phosphate are available for treating phosphorus deficiencies.

61.8 Microminerals are inorganic substances needed in amounts of at least 20 mg per day for normal body functioning.

Commonly called trace minerals, the **microminerals** are required daily in amounts of 20 mg or less. Although they are needed in minute amounts, their functions should not be underestimated. Profound illness may result with deficits of some of the microminerals. Each micromineral is listed in Table 61.4 along with the RDA and function. Brief descriptions of some of the common microminerals and their therapeutic uses are given next.

Fluoride: Fluoride, a trace mineral, is best known as the mineral that is helpful for bone and teeth health. Dental professionals may apply concentrated fluoride topically to the teeth to prevent cavities, especially in children. Many cities have added fluoride to the municipal water supply to improve dental health. Because high amounts of fluoride can be quite toxic to children, the use of fluoride-containing products should be closely monitored.

Iodide: Iodide is a micromineral needed to synthesize thyroid hormone. The most common source of dietary iodide is iodized salt. When dietary intake of iodide is low, hypothyroidism occurs and enlargement of the thyroid gland results. At high concentrations iodide suppresses thyroid function. Lugol's solution, a mixture containing 5% elemental iodine and 10% potassium iodide, is given to patients with hyperthyroid prior to thyroidectomy or during a thyrotoxic crisis. Sodium iodide is a drug that acts by rapidly suppressing the secretion of thyroid hormone and is indicated for patients who are having an acute thyroid crisis. Radioactive iodine (I-131) is given to destroy overactive thyroid glands (see Chapter 67). As an expectorant, the iodine ion increases mucous secretion formation in the bronchi and decreases viscosity of the mucus. Iodine salts such as iothalamate and diatrizoate are very dense and serve as diagnostic contrast agents in radiologic procedures of the urinary and cardiovascular systems.

Iron: Iron is essential to normal human physiology as an integral part of many proteins and enzymes that maintain good health. Iron is an essential component of proteins involved in oxygen transport; a deficiency limits oxygen delivery to cells, resulting in fatigue, poor work performance, and decreased immune function. It is also essential for the regulation of cell growth and differentiation. Dietary sources include meat, shellfish, nuts, and legumes.

Iron can be supplemented using various pharmacologic preparations, which often have ascorbic acid added to improve the absorption of PO iron. Generally, iron supplementation therapy is a PO therapy, and parenteral IV or intramuscular (IM) iron therapy is only given when absorption is seriously compromised by illnesses or when the patient cannot swallow. A prototype drug feature for ferrous sulfate is presented in Chapter 39.

CONNECTION Checkpoint 61.3

From what you learned in Chapter 39, what are the most common adverse effects experienced by patients taking iron salts such as ferrous sulfate by the oral route? *See Answer to Connection Checkpoint 61.3 on student resource website.*

Zinc: Zinc is found in at least 100 enzymes and has a role in regulating nucleic acid synthesis as well as wound healing, bone formation, cell-mediated immunity, and male fertility. Sources of zinc include protein foods, beans, lentils, nuts, seeds, and whole-grain cereals. Zinc sulfate, zinc acetate, and zinc gluconate are available to prevent and treat deficiency states at doses of 60 to 120 mg per day. Lozenges that contain zinc can be purchased OTC for treating sore throats and cold symptoms.

CONNECTIONS: NURSING PRACTICE APPLICATION

Patients Receiving Pharmacotherapy with Vitamin or Mineral Supplements

Assessment	Potential Nursing Diagnoses*
Baseline assessment prior to administration: • Obtain a complete health history including cardiovascular, neurologic, endocrine, hepatic, or renal disease. Obtain a drug history including allergies, current prescription and OTC drugs, and herbal preparations, alcohol use, or smoking. Be alert to possible drug interactions. • Obtain a history of any current symptoms that may indicate vitamin deficiencies or hypervitaminosis (e.g., dry itchy skin, alopecia, sore and reddened gums or tongue, tendency to bleed easily or excessive bruising, nausea or vomiting, or excessive fatigue). • Obtain a dietary history, noting adequacy of essential vitamins, minerals, and nutrients obtained from food sources. • Note sunscreen use and amount of sun exposure. • Obtain baseline weight and vital signs. • Evaluate appropriate laboratory findings (e.g., CBC, electrolytes, hepatic and renal function studies, and ferritin and iron levels). • Assess the patient's ability to receive and understand instructions. Include family or caregivers as needed.	• *Imbalanced Nutrition: Less Than Body Requirements* • *Ineffective Health Maintenance* • *Deficient Knowledge* (Drug Therapy) • *Risk for Injury*, related to adverse drug effects
Assessment throughout administration: • Assess for desired therapeutic effects dependent on the reason for the drug (e.g., symptoms of deficiency are diminished or absent). • Continue monitoring vital signs and periodic laboratory values as appropriate. • Assess for and promptly report adverse effects: nausea, vomiting, excessive fatigue, tachycardia, palpitations, hypotension, constipation, drowsiness, dizziness, disorientation, hyperreflexia, and electrolyte imbalances.	

CONNECTIONS: NURSING PRACTICE APPLICATION (continued)

Implementation

Interventions and (Rationales)	Patient-Centered Care
Ensuring therapeutic effects: • Treat the cause: If a definitive cause of vitamin or mineral deficiency is identified, correct the deficiency using natural sources of the nutrient where possible. Encourage an adequate diet to ensure sufficient intake of essential nutrients is enhanced. (The dietary history can assist in determining the cause of the symptoms and the adequacy of the patient's current diet to correct the deficiency. Natural food sources provide additional nutrients, fiber, and essential requirements not found in vitamin and mineral supplementation.)	• Review the dietary history with the patient and discuss food source options for correcting any deficiencies. Encourage the patient to adopt a healthy lifestyle of increased variety in the diet and limited or eliminated alcohol consumption. Provide for dietitian consultation as needed. • Assist the patient, family, or caregiver to become educated consumers, aware of the marketing of supplements that may not be required if diet is adequate. Provide educational pamphlets or web-based references to reputable sources as needed (e.g., NIH Office of Dietary Supplements).
Minimizing adverse effects: • Review the dietary and supplement history to correct any existing possibility for hypervitaminosis and adverse drug effects. (In the United States, hypervitaminosis from excessive vitamin and mineral intake is more common than deficiencies for most nutrients. Excessive intake of vitamins A, C, D, E, B_6, niacin, and folic acid may cause toxic effects.)	• Discuss the need for nutritional supplements if a normal diet is unable to supply these or if disease conditions (e.g., pernicious anemia) prevent absorption or utilization. • Discourage the overuse of supplementation and provide information on adverse effects and symptoms related to hypervitaminosis to watch for and report.
• Continue to monitor periodic laboratory work as needed. (Laboratory tests appropriate to the condition, e.g., pernicious anemia and Hgb and Hct levels, will help to ensure that therapeutic effects are met. With mineral replacement, electrolytes should return to, and maintain, normal levels.)	• Instruct the patient on the need to return periodically for laboratory work.
• Monitor the use of fat-soluble vitamins (A, D, E, and K). Excessive intake may lead to toxic effects. (Fat-soluble vitamins are stored in the body and may accumulate and result in toxic levels. Monitor liver function studies and for symptoms such as nausea, vomiting, headache, fatigue, dry and itchy skin, blurred vision, or palpitations. Report any symptoms immediately.)	• Instruct the patient not to take additional or large amounts of fat-soluble vitamins unless instructed by the health care provider. • Encourage the patient to obtain fat-soluble vitamins from natural sources through a balanced diet whenever possible.
• Assess for pregnancy or the possibility of pregnancy. Assess storage availability for any prenatal vitamins kept in the house. (Folic acid supplementation has been demonstrated to reduce the incidence of neurologic birth defects, and adequate folic acid intake should begin ideally before conception. Excessive vitamin intake may have deleterious effects on the developing fetus and prenatal vitamin use should be monitored by the health care provider. Poisonings with vitamins and iron are common in children.)	• Provide education to women of childbearing age pertaining to folic acid and its potential usefulness in preventing neurologic-related birth defects. Encourage adequate intake of vitamin and folic acid–rich foods (e.g., fortified and enriched grains, cereals and bread, spinach, and liver) *prior* to conception. • Instruct the patient to keep prenatal vitamins in a secure location if young children are in the household to prevent accidental ingestion and poisonings.
• Ensure adequate hydration if large doses of water-soluble vitamins are taken. (Water-soluble vitamins are not stored in the body but are excreted. Large doses of vitamins, particularly vitamin C, may cause adverse effects such as renal calculi.)	• Encourage the patient to increase fluid intake to 2 L/day, divided throughout the day.
• Monitor the use of mineral supplements. Excessive intake may lead to toxic effects. (Mineral toxicity is rare but may occur with excessive intake or underexcretion. Symptoms similar to Parkinson's disease, anemia, cirrhosis, dermatologic effects, hyper- or hypothyroidism, hair loss, or peripheral neuritis may signal mineral toxicity and should be reported to the provider for further testing.)	• Encourage the patient to obtain trace minerals from natural sources such as are found in a well-balanced, mixed diet containing both locally grown and other produce when possible. • Instruct the patient to consult the provider before taking large doses of any trace mineral and to report any unusual symptoms for further follow-up testing.
Patient understanding of drug therapy: • Use opportunities during administration of medications and during assessments to discuss the rationale for drug therapy, desired therapeutic outcomes, commonly observed adverse effects, parameters for when to call the health care provider, and any necessary monitoring or precautions. (Using time during nursing care helps to optimize and reinforce key teaching areas.)	• The patient should be able to state the reason for the drug, appropriate dose and scheduling, adverse effects to observe for and when to report them, and the anticipated length of medication therapy.
Patient self-administration of drug therapy: • When administering the medication, instruct the patient, family, or caregiver in proper self-administration of the drug, e.g., taken with additional fluids. (Utilizing time during nurse-administration of these drugs helps to reinforce teaching.)	• The patient, family, or caregiver is able to discuss appropriate dosing and administration needs.

CHAPTER

61 Understanding the Chapter

Key Concepts Summary

61.1 Although the importance of nutrition has been known for centuries, the specific vitamins were discovered in the 1900s.

61.2 Vitamins are essential for optimal health.

61.3 Government regulations and consumer knowledge about vitamins are limited.

61.4 The recommended dietary allowance is the dietary intake level that is sufficient to meet the nutrient requirements for most people.

61.5 Fat-soluble vitamins include vitamins A, D, E, and K.

61.6 Water-soluble vitamins include the B-complex vitamins and vitamin C.

61.7 Macrominerals are inorganic substances needed in amounts of at least 100 mg per day for normal body functioning.

61.8 Microminerals are inorganic substances needed in amounts of at least 20 mg per day for normal body functioning.

Case Study: Making the Patient Connection

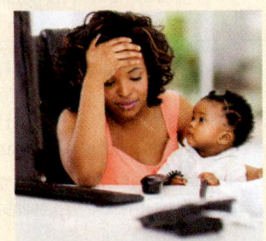

Remember the patient "Charlene Garrett" at the beginning of the chapter? Now read the remainder of the case study. Based on the information presented within this chapter, respond to the critical thinking questions that follow.

Charlene Garrett is a 32-year-old mother of a 1-year-old baby girl. She returned to work part time 3 months ago as a special-education instructor working with a group of preschoolers with special needs. Her husband watches their daughter two evenings a week so that Charlene can resume work toward a master's degree in special education at the local university.

Lately Charlene has begun feeling more stressed and tired. It is almost the end of the semester and papers are due; the holidays arrive in another month and both sides of the family will be coming to visit; and they've delayed celebrating the baby's birthday this month so that the families can enjoy the celebration when they visit.

Charlene lives next door and asks you, a nurse and the "reference for the neighborhood," about vitamin therapy to help her through this stressful period and to increase her energy level. She tells you that she still has some prenatal vitamins and wonders if she should take them.

Critical Thinking Questions

1. What other assessment data might you want to gather from Charlene before recommending vitamin therapy?

2. Should Charlene take the prenatal vitamins? Why or why not?

3. What other recommendations would you give to Charlene regarding vitamin therapy?

See Answers to Critical Thinking Questions on student resource website.

Additional Case Study

Jerrod is a 16-year-old Hispanic youth with moderate to severe developmental disabilities and mental retardation. He is cared for by his mother in their home. Jerrod has been admitted for possible seizure activity after his mother reported that he began atypical twitching and jerking of the extremities. The mother reports that Jerrod was unresponsive to her commands throughout the episode, which lasted approximately 4 to 5 minutes.

On further questioning, Jerrod's mother discloses that until approximately 6 months ago he attended a day care center for individuals with disabilities. However, due to his increased unpredictable irritability and combative behavior, his mother feared Jerrod venturing outside of the home. Typically, Jerrod spends his days watching television in a dark room or staring endlessly at a fish tank. Additionally, Jerrod is extremely selective about food intake and refuses to consume any dairy products, eggs, fish, or cereals. His daily intake consists mostly of chicken tenders and French fries.

1. One notable laboratory finding is Jerrod's elevated serum calcium and phosphate levels. What vitamin deficiency is most likely present given these findings and the patient's previous history?

2. What adverse effects should you monitor Jerrod for once the vitamin supplement therapy is initiated?

3. What environmental changes would you recommend to Jerrod's caregivers?

See Answers to Additional Case Study on student resource website.

Chapter Review

1 A health care provider has ordered oral vitamin A (Aquasol A) supplements for a patient. The serum level of vitamin A may be increased if the patient is also taking:

1. Vitamins D and E.
2. Oral contraceptives.
3. Mineral oil.
4. Antibiotics.

2 Vitamin C (ascorbic acid) may cause a false-negative result in _____ if taken within 48 to 72 hours of testing.

3 Pyridoxine (vitamin B$_6$) may cause antagonistic drug effects for the patient taking:

1. Isoniazid (INH).
2. Oral contraceptives.
3. Hydralazine (Apresoline).
4. Antiparkinsonism drugs.

4 The nurse is teaching the patient about the need for adequate intake of zinc in the diet. The nurse will teach the patient to increase consumption of:

1. Protein foods such as beans, lentils, and nuts.
2. Vegetables such as leafy greens, carrots, and squash.
3. Citrus such as grapefruit, oranges, and lemons.
4. Cruciferous vegetables such as broccoli, cauliflower, and Brussels sprouts.

5 A nurse should anticipate the administration of vitamin K (AquaMEPHYTON) for which of the following patients? Select all that apply.

1. A newborn infant
2. The patient with visual disturbances
3. The patient who received an overdose of certain oral anticoagulants
4. The patient with hypothyroidism
5. A teenager with chronic acne

6 The nurse would suspect a calcium deficiency in the patient exhibiting:

1. Night blindness.
2. Anemia.
3. Muscle cramping and spasms.
4. Bleeding abnormalities.

See Answers to Chapter Review in Appendix A.

References

Rosenbloom, M. (2013). *Vitamin toxicity*. Retrieved from http://emedicine.medscape.com/article/819426-overview

Woo, D. K., & Elde, M. J. (2010). Tanning beds, skin cancer and vitamin D: An examination of the scientific evidence and public health implications. *Dermatologic Therapy, 23,* 61–71. doi:10.1111/j.1529-8019.2009.01291.x

Selected Bibliography

Hark, L., Ashton, K., & Deen, D. (Eds.). (2012). *The nurse practitioner's guide to nutrition* (2nd ed.). Oxford, United Kingdom: Wiley-Blackwell.

Herdman, T. H., & Kamitsuru, S. (Eds.). (2014). *NANDA International nursing diagnoses: Definitions and classification, 2015–2017.* Oxford, United Kingdom: Wiley-Blackwell.

Hitt, E., & Barclay, L. (2011). *Updated USDA dietary guidelines released.* Retrieved from http://www.medscape.org/viewarticle/736605

Hughes, P. J., Kutner, A., & Brown, G. (2013). The physiology and pharmacology of vitamin D. *Nurse Prescribing, 11*(7), 344–352.

Howes, R. M. (2011). Mythology of antioxidant vitamins? *Journal of Evidence-Based Complementary and Alternative Medicine, 16,* 149–159. doi:10.1177/1533210110392955

Kapsak, W. R., Smith Edge, M., White, C., Childs, N. M., & Geiger, C. J. (2013). Putting the dietary guidelines for Americans into action: Behavior-directed messages to motivate parents—phase I and II observational and focus group findings. *Journal of the Academy of Nutrition and Dietetics, 113,* 196–204. doi:10.1016/j.jand.2012.10.019

McDaniel, J. C., & Belury, M. A. (2012). Are young adults following the dietary guidelines for Americans? *The Nurse Practitioner, 37*(5), 1–9. doi:10.1097/01.NPR.0000413484.90121.d8

Soni, M. G., Thurmond, T. S., Miller, E. R., Spriggs, T., Bendich, A., & Omaye, S. T. (2010). Safety of vitamins and minerals: Controversies and perspective. *Toxicology Sciences, 118,* 348–355. doi:10.1093/toxsci/kfq293

Tucker, S., & Dauffenbach, V. (2011). *Nutrition and diet therapy.* Upper Saddle River, NJ: Pearson.

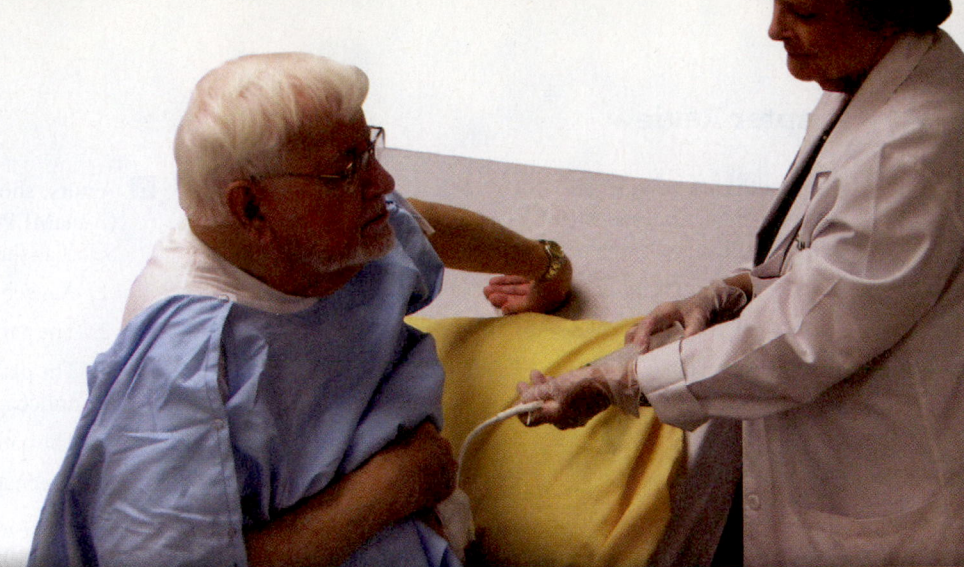

"They say this might just be temporary and I sure hope so. Being fed through a tube is no way to live."

Patient "Christopher Jones"

CHAPTER

62

Enteral and Parenteral Nutrition

LEARNING OUTCOMES

After reading this chapter, the student should be able to:

1. Identify conditions that may benefit from parenteral or enteral nutrition.
2. Compare and contrast enteral and parenteral methods of nutrition.
3. Compare and contrast methods by which enteral feedings are administered.
4. Distinguish among polymeric, elemental, semielemental, and modular formulas for enteral nutrition.
5. Identify the basic classes of nutrients contained in enteral formulas and their functions.
6. Identify the possible complications and adverse effects of enteral nutrition administration.
7. Describe the types of drug interactions that can occur when enteral nutrition formulas are given.
8. Explain the differences between delivering parenteral nutrition through a peripheral line versus a central line.
9. Describe the components of total parenteral nutrition solutions and the function of each element in attaining the body's daily requirements.
10. Describe the possible complications of parenteral nutrition therapy.
11. Identify drugs that may be incompatible with parenteral nutrition solutions.
12. Apply the nursing process to care for patients who are receiving enteral or parenteral nutrition.

CHAPTER OUTLINE

▶ **Enteral Nutrition**
  Methods of Administration
  Enteral Formulations
  Elements of Enteral Nutrition
  Complications of Enteral Therapy
  Drug and Food Interactions

▶ **Parenteral Nutrition**
  Components of Total Parenteral Nutrition Solutions
  Complications of Parenteral Therapy
  Drug and Food Interactions

KEY TERMS

bolus feedings, 1064

central vein total parenteral nutrition, 1069

continuous infusion feedings, 1064

cyclic feedings, 1064

dumping syndrome, 1064

elemental (monomeric) formulas, 1064

enteral nutrition (EN), 1063

intermittent feedings, 1064

modular formulas, 1065

parenteral nutrition, 1063

partial parenteral nutrition, 1069

peripheral vein parenteral nutrition, 1069

polymeric formulas, 1064

refeeding syndrome, 1068

semielemental (oligomeric) formulas, 1064

total parenteral nutrition (TPN), 1069

The intake of various nutrients in predetermined amounts or in combinations is necessary to maintain good health and to allow the body to heal during periods of illness. The intake of sufficient amounts of amino acids (proteins), carbohydrates, fats, vitamins, and minerals can often be achieved by eating a well-balanced diet of foods and fluids. In some circumstances, however, the daily nutritional needs of the body may require supplementation. Furthermore, certain diseases and conditions prevent feeding by the normal oral (PO) route. This chapter examines the methods and types of products available for providing enteral and parenteral nutrition.

62.1 Nutritional supplementation is required for patients with certain medical conditions.

Ensuring that patients have the necessary nutritional intake for proper health and wellness is a primary responsibility of the nurse. This responsibility extends to all patients, regardless of age, condition, or disease status. Although healthy patients can maintain their required caloric and nutritional requirements by eating a balanced diet, certain disease states, such as the following, may require nutritional intervention:

- Severe infections, such as human immunodeficiency virus–acquired immunodeficiency syndrome (HIV-AIDS)
- States of malnutrition
- Bowel rest for inflammatory bowel disease and disorders of the gastrointestinal (GI) tract
- Coma
- Postsurgical complications
- Major burns and trauma
- Neuromuscular and central nervous system disorders
- Advanced age or prematurity
- Eating disorders
- Cancer-related chemotherapy or radiation therapy

Although mechanical causes such as the inability to chew or swallow properly may limit caloric or nutritional intake, psychological and social reasons also play a role in inadequate nutrition. For example, stress related to a hospitalization may alter a patient's normal eating habits or regimen. Unfamiliar foods and generalized malaise or fear associated with a patient's medical condition may also result in a decreased appetite. For the older patient, ill-fitting dentures or issues with dysphagia may lead to nutritional deficits. Younger patients may be on a fad diet with limited intake of specific nutrients or may engage in activities related to bulimia or anorexia.

Clinical nutritional support is utilized in all settings, including hospitals and extended or long-term care facilities, as well as in the individual patient's home. Pediatric patients are now provided various forms of nutritional support by specially trained providers at day care facilities and schools.

Malnutrition in hospitalized persons or residents of nursing homes may present as dry, flaky skin and hair loss as a result of their poor nutritional state. More serious complications of malnutrition may include delayed wound healing, muscle atrophy, impaired immune function, infection, and even death. Secondary complications may include peripheral edema caused by a reduction in plasma proteins and a decreased oncotic pressure.

62.2 Supplemental nutrition may be provided by the oral or parenteral route.

Two basic routes are used to administer nutritional support: enteral and parenteral. **Enteral nutrition (EN)** is used for patients who have a functioning GI tract but are unable to orally ingest an adequate amount of nutrients to meet their metabolic needs. **Parenteral nutrition** involves the administration of high-caloric nutrients via a central vein, such as the subclavian vein.

Before initiating any form of nutritional support therapy, the medical team of health care providers, dietitians, and nurses must thoroughly evaluate the patient and determine which is the best method of treatment. It is also important to examine which route of nutritional support will achieve the desired optimum result. Areas that must be addressed include the amount of weight lost by the individual patient, the percentage of meals consumed, the patient's albumin level, and the patient's overall health and appearance. Other factors to consider when planning nutritional support are the patient's primary diagnosis, the patient's ability to swallow, any anticipated diagnostic testing and treatments (e.g., nothing by mouth [NPO] for more than 3 days), and the patient's overall prognosis. Socioeconomic factors of convenience, feasibility, and cost play a role in the decision-making process as well.

Enteral Nutrition

62.3 Various methods are utilized to administer enteral feedings to the patient.

EN includes products that are administered via the GI tract, either PO or through a feeding tube. When the patient's condition permits, EN is best administered by the PO route. Administering nutrition this way allows the natural digestive process to occur and requires less direct nursing supervision. Oral administration does require patient adherence to the planned feeding regimen and the ability to safely swallow the substance.

If the patient is unable to swallow properly, a feeding tube is passed either through the nose to the GI tract or surgically inserted directly into the stomach or small intestine. A nasogastric (nose to stomach) tube is more commonly used for short-term therapy and is often inserted by the nurse. If the patient displays symptoms of decreased gastric motility, a nasoduodenal or nasojejunal tube is usually inserted by the health care provider. Placement of this tube is confirmed by x-ray, and initiation of its use requires approval from the health care provider. If therapy is expected to last longer than 4 weeks, surgical or percutaneous endoscopic insertion of a gastrostomy or jejunostomy tube by the health care provider may be appropriate. A percutaneous endoscopic gastrostomy (PEG) tube remains the preferred route for long-term therapy and is usually better tolerated than a nasogastric tube.

An advantage of providing nutritional support via a feeding tube is that the amount of enteral solution can be precisely controlled and measured, and calories can be recorded. Contraindications to total enteral nutrition include peritonitis, intestinal obstruction, intractable vomiting, paralytic ileus, intractable diarrhea, and GI ischemia.

Methods of Administration

62.4 Enteral feedings can be delivered by bolus, intermittent drip or infusion, continuous infusion, or cyclic intermittent infusion.

Bolus feedings were the first method introduced and typically deliver 250 to 400 mL of formula every 4 to 6 hours via a syringe or funnel. This method takes about 15 minutes to complete and may not be well tolerated due to the large volume of solution introduced in such a short period. The bolus method can cause nausea, vomiting, abdominal cramping, and diarrhea, and there is a greater risk of aspiration. It is used with medically stable or ambulatory patients who have adequate absorptive capacity to tolerate the larger volume of fluid.

Intermittent feedings are administered every 3 to 6 hours and take about 30 to 60 minutes to infuse. They can be delivered either by gravity drip or by feeding pump infusion, with 300 to 400 mL of solution administered at each feeding. These feedings commonly use a feeding bag and are considered an inexpensive method of administering EN to the patient.

Continuous infusion feedings are often prescribed for critically ill patients or those with duodenal or jejunal entry feeding tubes. This type of feeding is often delivered by an infusion pump at a slow rate over a 16- to 24-hour period. Continual enteral feeding methods result in the patient meeting his or her nutritional goals much quicker. Furthermore, the continuous method of delivery is more successful because it helps to prevent complications such as the dumping syndrome and avoids the need for frequent irrigation of the tube. **Dumping syndrome** is the result of a sudden influx of feeding into the GI tract and the creation of a high osmotic gradient within the small intestine. This in turn causes a sudden shift of fluid from the vascular compartment to the intestinal lumen. Plasma volume decreases, causing vasomotor responses such as an increased pulse rate, decreased blood pressure, pallor, sweating, weakness, and dizziness. The increased intestinal fluid results in distention and produces a feeling of fullness, abdominal cramping, nausea, vomiting, and diarrhea.

Cyclic feedings are commonly infused over 8 to 16 hours daily (day or night). Infusions during the daytime hours are recommended for patients who are restless during sleep or have a greater risk of aspiration. Nighttime infusion allows patients more freedom during the day and is frequently used for ambulatory patients.

Enteral Formulations

62.5 Several types of liquid nutrition formulas are commercially available for enteral feedings.

Enteral solutions differ according to the various nutrients, the caloric values, and the osmolality of the solutions. There are four basic groups of solutions for EN: polymeric, elemental, semielemental, and modular:

- **Polymeric formulas** contain various mixtures of protein, lipids, and carbohydrates in high molecular weight form and are considered the most common type of enteral preparation. Typical composition includes 30% fat, 50% to 55% carbohydrate, and 15% to 20% protein. These formulas are used for patients who are generally undernourished but have a fully functioning GI tract. Polymeric formulas include blenderized diets and meal replacement formulas. Blenderized diets are generally high-residue, highly viscous products. Meal replacement formulas are either milk based or lactose free. These preparations are nutritionally complete, generally meet the recommended dietary allowance (RDA) for vitamins and minerals (see Chapter 61), and are palatable for oral ingestion. Examples include Osmolite and Promote.

- **Elemental (monomeric) formulas** include products that are usually lactose free and contain only a small percentage (1–3%) of calories from fats. Individual amino acids are provided, which are able to be absorbed without the aid of digestive enzymes. These formulas are used for patients who have malabsorption disorders. Examples include Precision HN, Criticare HN, and Vivonex T.E.N.

- **Semielemental (oligomeric) formulas** contain slightly larger molecules than elemental products such as free amino acids and small peptides that require little or no digestion and are easily absorbed into the body. They contain a higher percentage of fats than elemental products but they are in the form of medium-chain triglycerides (MCTs) that can be directly absorbed by the intestine without digestive enzymes or bile salts. They are used in patients with digestive disorders such as malabsorption syndrome, partial bowel obstruction, inflammatory bowel disease, short bowel syndrome, bowel fistulas, and antibiotic- or radiation-induced intestinal damage. Because there is little stimulation of digestive secretions, these products are also useful for patients with chronic pancreatitis. Oligomeric formulas are more expensive than polymeric preparations, with the main caloric source coming from carbohydrates. They are usually low in fat, which allows for rapid gastric emptying, and many of these preparations are designed for administration directly into the intestines. Flavor packets are available to improve the taste, but they are generally unpalatable and best suited for tube feedings. Examples of oligomeric products include Pepti-2000, Vital HN, Peptamen, and Subdue.

- **Modular formulas** or disease-specific supplements contain nutrients that are designed to meet a specific nutrient deficiency or disease state. For example, protein modules can be utilized to meet the extra nitrogen needs of patients with burns or severe trauma. Other conditions include renal failure, hepatic failure, pulmonary disease, or a specific genetic enzyme deficiency.

Elements of Enteral Nutrition

62.6 Most enteral nutrition formulas contain four basic classes of nutrients.

There are many different enteral products, each containing various amounts of nutritional substances. The four basic nutrient classes and their functions are as follows.

Carbohydrates: Carbohydrates are the major source of energy in the diet and function to spare body protein, prevent ketosis, and regulate blood glucose levels. Carbohydrate sources in enteral formulas must be soluble, digestible, and have a low osmolality. Commonly used sources of carbohydrates include corn syrup solids, hydrolyzed corn starch, maltodextrin, and other glucose polymers. Some special formulas include various types of fiber, fructose, and fructo-oligosaccharides. Simple sugars, such as sucrose, glucose, dextrose, and lactose, enhance the palatability of the oral preparations but increase the product's osmolality. These simple sugars retain water in the intestinal tract and can therefore promote diarrhea in the patient. The percentage of total calories derived from carbohydrates varies from 30% to 90%, depending on the particular preparation and the specific condition for which it was designed to treat. Most available EN products do not contain lactose and thus should not pose a problem for patients experiencing lactose intolerance.

Proteins: Proteins are essential to the diet because they support cellular growth as well as maintain and repair body tissues. They may be delivered as intact proteins, partially digested (hydrolyzed) proteins, or free amino acids. The selection of a particular protein product is based on the patient's medical condition and his or her ability to absorb the protein. Soy protein and caseinates are common sources of intact proteins and are found in polymeric formulas. Oligomeric formulas contain enzymatically hydrolyzed casein or whey. Elemental formulas contain free amino acids. Proteins may make up approximately 4% to 32% of the total calories of enteral formulas, depending on the specific product. Products that are designed for patients with renal impairment may contain no protein, whereas patients who are receiving immune-enhancing formulas may receive as much as 80 g of protein per 1,000 kcal.

Lipids: Lipids provide an isotonic, high-caloric source of energy for the body. Soybean and corn oil are common lipid sources, and canola and safflower oils are also available. Long-chain triglycerides provide essential fatty acids, limit the osmolality, and enhance the palatability of the product. The fat content of the enteral product can vary from 1% to 55% of the total calories. Products that are designed for patients with glucose intolerance or pulmonary disease are generally high in fat, whereas products that are designed for patients with intestinal malabsorption contain lower amounts of total fat.

Other nutrients: Most commercially prepared enteral formulas are fortified with vitamins and minerals. When given in adequate volume, they provide most of the elements needed to maintain body functioning. However, the volume required to provide the RDA varies greatly among the numerous products available to the consumer. Fiber such as cellulose and pectin is added to enteral formulas to improve stool consistency but can create complications in patients who are fluid restricted or have delayed GI motility. Because most enteral formulas do not provide enough water in solution to maintain adequate hydration, additional free water is needed to meet the minimum fluid requirements.

Complications of Enteral Therapy

62.7 Although considered physiological in nature, total enteral nutrition can predispose the patient to various complications.

Total enteral nutrition therapy poses a risk of mechanical complications such as aspiration, gastroesophageal reflux, diarrhea, metabolic and electrolyte disturbances, and procedural-related problems, such as tube clogging, tube migration, and dislodgment. Localized infections and sepsis are also potential problems during treatment. Table 62.1 summarizes the various complications of EN therapy.

Aspiration: The most serious potential complication for patients receiving enteral feedings is tracheobronchial aspiration of gastric contents. Symptoms of aspiration may include dyspnea, tachypnea, wheezing, rales, tachycardia, agitation, and cyanosis. Aspiration of a small amount of enteral formula may not produce immediate symptoms, but a subsequent fever may suggest the development of aspiration pneumonia. The risk for aspiration is increased if the patient is fed while lying flat or if the patient is unconscious. The head of the bed should be elevated at least 30 degrees during the administration of the feeding and should remain elevated for at least 30 minutes after the feeding. The nurse should check for gastric residual volume by gently aspirating the stomach contents before administering the next feeding, or every 4 to 6 hours if the patient is on a continuous infusion. Other risk factors for aspiration include a diminished gag reflex, neurologic injury, gastroesophageal reflux, and the use of large-bore feeding tubes.

Nausea and vomiting: A small percentage of patients who receive enteral tube feedings experience nausea and vomiting, which increase the risk of aspiration. The most common cause for this problem is delayed gastric emptying. If this cause is suspected, the following steps should be considered:

- Reduce the doses of opioid or other medications that slow GI motility.
- Switch to a low-fat preparation.
- Administer the feeding at room temperature.
- Reduce the rate of administration.
- Administer a promotility agent such as metoclopramide (Reglan).
- Consider antiemetic medications if gastric residues are low yet nausea persists.

Diarrhea: One of the major problems in patients who require tube feeding is diarrhea, which is commonly due to the rapid

TABLE 62.1	Complications of Enteral Nutrition	
Complication	**Possible Cause**	**Intervention**
Gastrointestinal		
Diarrhea (more than four bowel movements per day or large loose stool)	Medications	• Eliminate antibiotics or antacids if possible.
	Fat intolerance	• Eliminate feedings containing sorbitol. • Change to low-fat formula.
	Bacterial overgrowth	• Culture stool for pathogens. • Administer lactobacillus (acidophilus, Lactinex) if the patient is receiving antibiotics.
	Contaminated formula	• Stop administration of the current formula. • Replace the bag and tubing using aseptic technique. • Adhere to clean standards when changing or manipulating the feeding.
	Osmotic overload	• Decrease the concentration of the formula. • Change to an isotonic formula. • Further dilute hypertonic medications.
	Decreased bulk	• Administer medications by an alternate route. • Change to a high-fiber formula. • Administer bulking agents.
	Patient positioning	• Position the patient on the right side to facilitate passage of gastric contents through the pylorus.
	Volume overload	• Decrease the total volume. • Decrease the delivery rate to one previously tolerated. • Advance the delivery rate slowly over 12–24 h. • Stop feeding for 2 h and check for residuals.
Nausea or vomiting	Delayed gastric emptying	• Change to a low-fat formula. • Administer a medication that stimulates GI tract motility (cisapride, metoclopramide).
	Specific nutrient intolerances	• Change to a lactose-free or low-fat formula.
Constipation (no stool for 3 days)	GI tract obstruction; dehydration and impaction; decreased fiber	• Change to a high-fiber formula. • Administer a bulking agent. • Stop the feeding. • Provide free water. • Remove impaction.
	GI tract obstruction	• Stop the feeding.
Mechanical		
Pulmonary aspiration	Patient lying flat	• Elevate the head of the bed 30–45 deg during continuous feedings or for 30–60 min after bolus feedings.
	Absent or depressed gag reflex	• Infuse feedings into the duodenum or jejunum. • Change to a smaller bore tube.
	Esophageal reflux	• Infuse feedings into the duodenum or jejunum.
	Improper tube placement	• Confirm proper placement of the tube by x-ray after insertion after episodes of severe coughing, vomiting, or a seizure. • Reconfirm placement prior to each feeding by checking for residuals. • Tape the tube in place and mark the tube at the exit point for reference. • Restrain the patient if necessary to prevent the tube from being pulled or dislodged.
Tube obstruction	Acid precipitation of formula	• Flush the tube with water before and after checking for gastric residuals. • Infuse feedings into the duodenum or jejunum. • Do not mix medications with the enteral formula.
	Insufficient tube irrigation	• Flush the tube with warm water before and after each bolus feeding and every 8 h during continuous feedings or whenever feeding is stopped. • Adequately crush medications and mix powder with water.
	Medications	• Use liquid medications whenever possible. • Flush the tube before and after medication administration with at least 30 mL of warm water.

TABLE 62.1	Complications of Enteral Nutrition *(continued)*	
Complication	**Possible Cause**	**Intervention**
Nasal mucosal damage	Extended use of large-bore tubes	• Avoid administering bulk-forming agents via a small-bore tube. • Alternate nares. • Change to a smaller bore tube. • Change to a permanent gastrostomy or jejunostomy tube for extended enteral support. • Tape the tube in place to minimize rubbing.
Metabolic		
Overhydration	Refeeding syndrome; fluid overload	• Decrease the delivery rate. • Restrict free water. • Change to a concentrated formula. • Administer diuretics. • Change formula.
Dehydration	High osmolality formula; diarrhea; excessive protein intake with inadequate fluid intake	• Change formula. • Manage diarrhea. • Change to a decreased protein content formula. • Provide additional water.
Hyperglycemia	Too many calories; lack of adequate insulin	• Adjust insulin dose. • Change formula to higher fat or lower carbohydrate content. • Taper feedings.
Hypoglycemia	Holding or discontinuing feedings abruptly	• Monitor blood glucose if feedings are interrupted. • Taper feedings.
Hyperkalemia	Renal insufficiency; anabolic metabolism	• Reduce potassium intake or use a reduced potassium formula. • Administer polystyrene sulfonate (Kayexalate). • Reduce potassium intake or use a reduced potassium formula.
Hypokalemia	Refeeding syndrome; insulin administration; diuretics; diarrhea	• Monitor serum potassium daily and repeat until the levels stabilize. • Lower dose or discontinue.
Hyperphosphatemia	Renal insufficiency	• Discontinue if possible. • Use a reduced phosphate formula. • Administer a phosphate binder.
Hypophosphatemia	Refeeding syndrome, insulin administration	• Monitor serum phosphate daily and repeat until stable.
Hypomagnesemia	Refeeding syndrome, alcoholism	• Monitor serum magnesium daily and repeat until stable.
Hyponatremia	Fluid overload	• Restrict free water. • Use normal saline to flush the tube and provide hydration instead of water. • Reassess medications. • Increase free water.
Elevated BUN	Renal failure, excess protein intake, dehydration, medications (diuretics and steroids)	• Reassess renal function. • Reassess protein needs.
Rapid and excessive weight gain	Excess calories, excess fluid, electrolyte imbalance	• Change the formula. • Evaluate electrolytes.
Insufficient weight gain	Inadequate calories; malabsorption; catabolic state	• Change the formula or increase the delivery rate. • Change to a semielemental formula. • Provide nutrition support for weight maintenance while addressing medical issues.
Depression, withdrawal, nonadherence	Altered body image; loss of oral gratification	• Encourage socialization at mealtimes. • Provide emotional support. • Provide ice chips, sugar-free gum, or hard candy. • Provide oral care during every shift.

TABLE 62.2	Drug Administration Guidelines with Enteral Feedings

The following are guidelines for administering medications to patients who are receiving enteral nutrition:

- If the patient is able to take medications by mouth, the PO route is preferred over administration through the tube.
- Alternate routes of administration (IV, intramuscular [IM], rectal, sublingual, or transdermal) should be considered for certain medications that cannot be crushed, are not available in liquid form, or which repeatedly clog or block the tubing.
- Sterile technique is usually not required when administering enteral feedings or medications. Sterile technique may be required for severely immunocompromised patients.
- Check the compatibility of the medication with the tube feeding formula first before administering it through the tube.
- If a tablet is to be administered through the feeding tube, check with the pharmacist first to make sure that crushing the medication will not alter its effectiveness. Then crush the tablet into a fine powder and mix the powder with warm water before administering the drug.
- For individual doses of most medications, the tube should be flushed with at least 30 mL of water before and after administration. This will clear the tube for the drug delivery, facilitate the transport of the drug to the intestine, and indicate if the tube is patent.
- When several medications are to be administered, all medications should be given separately and the feeding tube flushed with at least 5 mL of water after each one.
- Most drugs in elixir form are hypertonic. Highly concentrated drug solutions or suspensions should be diluted with at least 60 mL of water before administration in order to decrease gastric mucosal irritation and to prevent osmotic diarrhea.
- Medications should never be added directly to the feeding formula. This may result in a decrease in the potency of the medication as well as a decrease in the stability of the feeding formula.
- For most medications enteral feedings should be stopped for at least 15 min before and after the administration of a drug.

administration of the feeding, high-caloric solutions, or bacterial contamination of the feeding formula or equipment. A patient who develops diarrhea while receiving EN should be evaluated for *Clostridium difficile*, which usually results secondary to antibiotic therapy. Drugs that contain magnesium, such as antacids, may contribute to the problem of diarrhea, as well as drugs containing sorbitol, liquid cimetidine (Tagamet), and various multivitamin preparations. Diarrhea frequently coincides with the initiation of the enteral treatments because many of the medications that had been given by the intravenous (IV) route are changed to the PO route when enteral feeding is begun. If diarrhea develops during enteral therapy, the following should be considered:

- Add fiber, such as psyllium (see Chapter 60).
- Consider switching to a formula containing fiber.
- Decrease the rate of infusion.
- Dilute the solution.
- Administer an antidiarrheal drug.
- If *C. difficile* is confirmed, administer an appropriate antibiotic.

Metabolic complications: Refeeding syndrome can occur when nutritional support, including EN therapy, is introduced to severely malnourished patients. This syndrome consists of metabolic complications, such as dehydration, electrolyte imbalances, and hyperglycemia. In severe cases, nervous system complications such as confusion, seizures, and coma may occur.

Careful monitoring can minimize or prevent metabolic complications. To prevent refeeding syndrome, those at high risk should first be identified, including patients with anorexia nervosa, kwashiorkor, chronic alcohol abuse, prolonged fasting, and prolonged IV hydration. Any electrolyte abnormalities should be corrected before starting nutritional support therapy, and vital signs, intake and output (I&O), and laboratory values should all be carefully monitored.

Clogged feeding tube: Tube clogging is more likely to occur with the use of intact protein and highly viscous products. Routine flushing of the feeding tube with 20 to 30 mL of warm water every 4 hours during continuous feedings and before and after each

intermittent feeding and drug administration can prevent most clogs. Aseptic technique should be utilized in order to minimize formula contamination, and extreme care should be maintained when administering medications via the feeding tube (Table 62.2).

Various methods are used to unclog a blocked feeding tube. The first is to instill warm water via a syringe, using slight manual pressure. If this fails, a sodium bicarbonate solution may be instilled in order to break down the clog. Pancrelipase (Creon, Pancreaze, Zenpep) crushed and instilled along with the sodium bicarbonate solution and left in place up to an hour may also break down the clog. These techniques may be repeated two to three times. If the tube remains clogged, the health care provider should be contacted.

Interrupted infusions: In the hospitalized patient, EN is sometimes interrupted for various diagnostic tests and procedures. These may include feedings held due to drug–food incompatibilities, hemodialysis treatment, "NPO after midnight" for surgery or procedures, physical or occupational therapy sessions, transportation from the unit, or GI intolerance (diarrhea, nausea, vomiting). When frequent interruptions are expected, recalculating the goal flow rate on a 22- or 23-hour basis instead of 24 hours may be more practical.

Drug and Food Interactions

62.8 Most medications that are administered orally can also be delivered to the patient via an enteral tube.

Medications that are delivered via an enteral tube must be in a liquid form (elixir or suspension), or finely crushed and dissolved in a liquid vehicle. Drugs that must not be crushed or dissolved are enteric-coated pills, time release forms, sublingual medications, and bulk-forming laxatives. If a tablet must be administered through the feeding tube, the nurse should check with the pharmacist to make sure that crushing the medication will not alter its effectiveness.

When liquid forms of drugs are mixed with enteral preparations, physical incompatibilities can cause the mixture to thicken and clog the feeding tube. Hyperosmolar liquid medications can also be poorly tolerated by the GI tract, resulting in abdominal

TABLE 62.3 Interaction of Drugs with Enteral Formulas

Interaction with Enteral Formula	Drugs
Physically incompatible	Antacids, cimetidine (Tagamet), dicyclomine (Bentyl), Dimetapp elixir, iron preparations, KCl liquid, MCT oil, Robitussin, thioridazine (Mellaril)
Increased osmolality	digoxin (Lanoxin), furosemide (Lasix), methyldopa (Aldomet), phenytoin (Dilantin), theophylline
Decreased drug effect	carbamazepine (Tegretol), ciprofloxacin (Cipro), digoxin, lithium, levodopa (L-dopa), phenytoin, theophylline, warfarin (Coumadin)

distention and cramping, vomiting, and diarrhea. Both of these problems can be avoided by simply flushing the feeding tube with water and by diluting the medication first with warm water before instilling it into the feeding tube.

Enteral feeding products are usually delivered as a constant infusion and contain high concentrations of proteins and certain metals such as calcium, magnesium, and iron. These important nutrients can bind with certain medications, hindering the bioavailability of the drug and, in turn, reducing the total delivered dose of the medication. The fluoroquinolone antibiotics such as ciprofloxacin (Cipro) are a frequently prescribed class of drugs that can interact with these metals. The effectiveness of liquid phenytoin (Dilantin) is often reduced by the drug's ability to bind with proteins in the enteral formula, resulting in subtherapeutic levels of the medication. Likewise, therapeutic levels of warfarin (Coumadin) may also be affected due to protein binding and the presence of vitamin K in the feeding preparation. Holding the enteral feeding for 1 hour before and after an antibiotic dose and 2 hours before and after giving phenytoin or warfarin will help minimize the drug's interaction with the enteral feeding. Table 62.3 lists the various drugs that interact with enteral formulas.

CONNECTION Checkpoint 62.1

From what you learned in Chapter 3, explain why drugs that have an enteric coating and those that are extended release should not be crushed and used in enteral feeding. *See Answer to Connection Checkpoint 62.1 on student resource website.*

Parenteral Nutrition

62.9 Parenteral nutrition is used when patients are unable to tolerate enteral feedings.

Parenteral nutrition is utilized for patients who are unable to eat or tolerate any form of EN. It is frequently given to patients with severe GI disorders such as diseases of the small bowel (Crohn's disease, fistulas, adhesions, postoperative ileus), necrotizing pancreatitis, hyperemesis gravidarum (maternity patients), and pediatric patients with congenital anomalies or prolonged diarrhea. It is also used for patients with demonstrated undernutrition (less than 50% of the metabolic needs met for more than 7 days) as well as patients with AIDs, cancer chemotherapy or radiation-induced enteritis, burns, severe trauma, or anorexia.

Parenteral nutrition is also referred to as **total parenteral nutrition (TPN)** or hyperalimentation and is administered solely by the IV route. It can be delivered via a peripheral line or a central line, depending on the hypertonicity of the solution. TPN can provide all the calories, glucose, protein, fats, minerals, and trace elements needed by the body to sustain growth and to promote weight gain as well as wound healing. A **partial parenteral nutrition** solution is one that lacks an essential element, usually fats or lipids.

Peripheral vein parenteral nutrition is used when a central venous line cannot be accessed or when it is not appropriate for the patient. These situations may include patients in whom the subclavian vein is inaccessible due to scar tissue from repeated IV line punctures or in patients with extensive trauma, severe burns, or cancer in the region of the upper torso or chest. These patients may be relatively healthy with only a slight nutritional deficit that cannot be met with enteral therapy. Peripheral parenteral nutrition (PPN) is considered a temporary measure until a central line can be placed, and the solution administered is usually lower in osmolality than the solution delivered through a central line. PPN is advantageous because there are fewer risks associated with the catheter placement, care of the infusion site is simpler, and the complications associated with hyperosmolar solutions can be avoided.

Problems associated with PPN include the need for several large peripheral veins, because the catheter site is routinely rotated to prevent infection. The vein must also be able to accommodate the larger sized venous catheter. PPN is associated with a high risk of phlebitis and is therefore reserved for patients with robust veins. Peripherally inserted central catheters (PICC lines) are often inserted in patients for home therapy with peripheral vein total parenteral nutrition.

Central vein total parenteral nutrition is the administration of the solution through a central vein such as the subclavian or the internal jugular vein. Because of the hypertonicity of the parenteral solution, the catheter tip must always be positioned in the superior vena cava so that the solution can be immediately diluted to a more tolerable concentration. The central vein total parenteral nutrition solution usually consists of crystalline amino acids, dextrose, and lipid emulsions with the addition of vitamins, minerals, trace elements, essential electrolytes, and water.

Central vein total parenteral nutrition is used in patients with limited peripheral access or in those patients whose nutritional needs cannot be met by peripheral vein total parenteral nutrition formulas. It is usually considered the access of choice for long-term parenteral therapy and is always administered using an infusion pump in order to precisely monitor the amount of solution given. Figure 62.1 shows the location of a central venous catheter for TPN therapy.

PharmFACT

When assessing undernourished patients for potential enteral therapy, the nurse should consider that the lack of dietary intake may be caused by drugs that cause bleeding gums (anticoagulants), altered taste (captopril), candidiasis (broad-spectrum antibiotics), or nausea and vomiting (antineoplastic drugs and many others) (Dawodu, 2013).

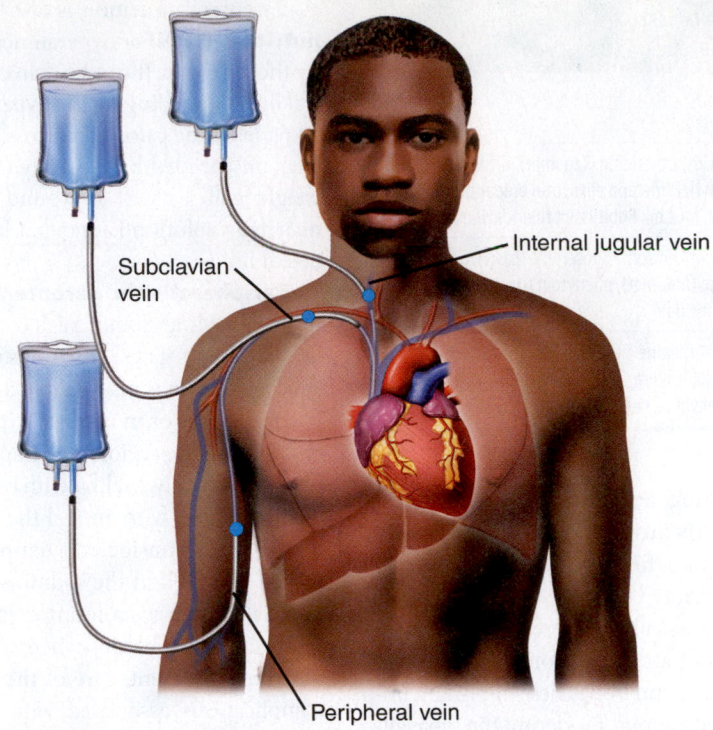

Subclavian vein

Internal jugular vein

Peripheral vein

Figure 62.1 Routes of administration for parenteral nutrition.

Components of Total Parenteral Nutrition Solutions

62.10 The basic total parenteral nutrition solution consists of carbohydrates, lipids, amino acids, electrolytes, minerals, and vitamins.

TPN solutions may be modified daily based on the patient's laboratory results, the underlying disorder, the rate of metabolism, and other factors. Like the enteral products, the basic components include carbohydrates, lipids, amino acids (proteins), electrolytes, minerals, and vitamins.

Carbohydrates: Carbohydrates and lipids are the primary sources of calories for the patient on TPN. Dextrose is the most common carbohydrate source because it is inexpensive and readily available from cornstarch, beet, or cane sugar. The RDA of carbohydrates for adult patients ranges from 25 to 35 kcal/kg. When administered through a central line, the concentration of dextrose in the TPN solution usually comprises 25% to 35% of the overall solution.

When dextrose is administered as the primary calorie source (without lipids added), hyperglycemia can occur. Because insulin is required for dextrose utilization, a combination of dextrose and lipids may help reduce the risk of hyperglycemia and the patient's need for supplemental insulin injections. Dextrose increases the metabolic rate and the production of carbon dioxide, which may increase the demands placed on the patient's respiratory system. The addition of lipids will also decrease this risk. Abruptly stopping the TPN solution can result in hypoglycemia due to the

continued release of endogenous insulin. This problem can be avoided by substituting a dextrose 10% solution until the new TPN solution bag is available, or by gradually tapering the solution over a 24-hour period when discontinuing parenteral therapy.

CONNECTION Checkpoint 62.2

From what you learned in Chapter 36, what are the primary indications for an infusion of dextrose in water (D_5W)? Why should a patient with severe heart failure not receive D_5W? *See Answer to Connection Checkpoint 62.2 on student resource website.*

Lipids: Unlike amino acids and concentrated dextrose solutions, fat emulsions are isotonic, which means that they can be infused through either a peripheral or central line. They are often a requirement for patients who are receiving TPN therapy for longer than 5 days. Lipid preparations that are currently available are produced from either safflower oil (Liposyn) or soybean oil (Intralipid). The principal fatty acids used in these preparations are linoleic, linolenic, oleic, palmitic, and stearic acids.

Fat emulsions can be hazardous for patients with liver disease, pulmonary disease, anemia, or blood coagulation disorders, with the most common adverse effect being hyperlipidemia. Fat emboli and death can occur when lipids are administered to premature, preterm, or low-birth-weight infants.

Amino acids: Amino acids are needed by the body to synthesize proteins, to conserve lean body mass, and to help promote wound healing. The RDA for infants and children ranges from 1.4 to 2.5 g/kg per day, whereas adults require 0.8 to 1 g/kg daily. Essential amino acids cannot be produced by the body, whereas nonessential amino acids can be synthesized from a nitrogen source, such as ammonium salts or urea. Amino acids must be closely monitored in patients with renal failure, because the BUN level can become elevated. For the patient with liver failure, the administration of amino acids may result in hepatic coma due to the liver's inability to process nitrogen.

Electrolytes and minerals: Electrolytes, including sodium, potassium, magnesium, calcium, phosphorus, chloride, and acetate, can be added to the TPN formula as salts. Specific electrolyte amounts are ordered daily by the health care provider, based on preexisting deficiencies and the patient's current medical condition. To prevent interactions between specific elements and crystallization of the solution, the pharmacist should add the electrolytes.

Trace mineral mixtures typically contain copper, chromium, manganese, selenium, and zinc and are commercially available to meet the specific nutritional needs of the patient. Trace minerals are metabolic cofactors that are essential for the proper functioning of several enzyme systems.

Although it is routine to monitor serum electrolyte levels, serum levels of the trace minerals are generally not monitored. Trace mineral administration should be decreased or withheld in patients with a limited capacity to excrete them. For example, selenium and chromium should not be used in patients with renal impairment, whereas copper and manganese should be withheld in patients with severe hepatic disease.

Vitamins: Vitamins are essential components of the TPN regimen. Most commercially prepared vitamin formulas can be given on alternate days in order to meet the patient's need for both fat-soluble vitamins as well as the water-soluble vitamins, and they can be added to the existing TPN solution. Vitamin K is usually administered weekly by subcutaneous or IM injection.

CONNECTION Checkpoint 62.3

Vitamin K is used as an antidote for overdose from a coagulation modifier. From what you learned in Chapter 38, what is the specific coagulation modifier and what would be the symptoms of an overdose from that drug? *See Answer to Connection Checkpoint 62.3 on student resource website.*

Complications of Parenteral Therapy

Despite improvements made in the delivery of parenteral nutrition over the past decade, patients may encounter certain problems during TPN therapy. These are classified as mechanical, metabolic, or infectious in nature. Selected complications of TPN therapy are summarized in Table 62.4.

62.11 As with enteral therapy, patients who are receiving parenteral nutrition therapy can experience various complications.

Regular monitoring is important during TPN therapy. The patient's individual nutritional requirements should be reviewed regularly, taking into account the patient's current condition, drug therapy, nutritional status, concurrent treatments (e.g., hemodialysis), response to TPN, and supporting laboratory data.

Mechanical complications: Improper or incorrect placement of the catheter can result in subclavian artery puncture, pneumothorax, hemothorax, carotid artery injury, thromboembolism,

TABLE 62.4 Selected Complications of Total Parenteral Nutrition

Complication	Cause	Symptom
Mechanical		
Pneumothorax	Accidental puncture of the pleural cavity by the catheter during insertion.	Sharp chest pain, decreased breath sounds
Hemothorax	Catheter damages a vein with blood entering the chest cavity.	Same as above
Hydrothorax	Catheter perforates a vein, releasing TPN solution into the chest. Clot in the subclavian vein.	Same as above
Venous thrombus	IV tubing is disconnected. Catheter is not clamped. Infusion cap fell off.	Distended neck veins, swelling of the face and arm
Air embolism		Cough, shortness of breath, chest pain, and cyanosis
Metabolic		
Hyperglycemia	Fluid is infused too quickly. Insufficient insulin coverage.	Nausea, headache, weakness, thirst, increased blood glucose level
Hypoglycemia	Fluid stopped abruptly. Too much insulin administered.	Pallor, cold clammy skin, increased pulse, headache, tremors, blurred vision
Fluid overload	Increased IV rate. Fluid shifts from the cellular to the vascular space due to hyperosmolar solution.	Cough, dyspnea, distended neck veins, rales, weight gain
Infection		
Sepsis	Poor aseptic technique when the catheter is inserted. Contamination of the catheter when changing tubing or when the TPN solution is mixed. Contamination when dressing is changed.	Fever, chills, tachycardia, drainage from the insertion site, lethargy, increased white blood cells (WBCs), positive blood cultures

catheter malposition, brachial plexus injury, subcutaneous emphysema, endocarditis, cardiac arrhythmias and tamponade, and phrenic nerve paralysis. Venous thrombosis is the most common problem and is associated with significant morbidity rates. Signs of venous thrombosis include distended neck veins as well as swelling of the face and arm on the side of the IV catheter.

Metabolic complications: Metabolic complications of parenteral nutrition therapy fall into two broad categories: early or late complications. Early complications can usually be anticipated and include fluid volume overload, refeeding syndrome, and various electrolyte and mineral imbalances. Hypertriglyceridemia can lead to pancreatitis and altered pulmonary function if left untreated. The early complications can be prevented by carefully monitoring the patient and adjusting the composition of the TPN formula or the rate of infusion.

Late metabolic complications are less predictable and may be caused by the exacerbation of preexisting conditions, inadequate solution composition, or failure to monitor the patient adequately. Late complications can include fatty acid, mineral, and vitamin deficiencies and metabolic bone disease or bone demineralization, which may develop in patients who receive TPN for periods extending beyond 3 months. Although the exact mechanism is not known, metabolic bone disease can cause severe pain in the lower extremities and the back. The only known treatment is to temporarily or permanently discontinue the TPN infusion. Hepatic steatosis (fatty liver) and gallbladder complications (cholelithiasis and cholecystitis) are also late complications of TPN therapy.

Infectious complications: Parenteral nutrition therapy creates a chronic breach in the patient's physiological line of defense. The IV infusion system from the solution container to the tip of the catheter may serve as a source for the introduction of bacterial or fungal organisms into the patient's bloodstream. The health care provider inserting the venous catheter, the pharmacist mixing the TPN solution, or the nurse hanging the IV bag or changing the central venous catheter dressing may inadvertently contaminate the patient's "lifeline."

Peripheral IV lines are at high risk for infection and infiltration, and the site of the peripheral line should be changed, if possible, every 48 hours in order to eliminate that risk. Unfortunately, severely debilitated patients often have few robust veins available for selection, necessitating the eventual placement of a central line.

Strict asepsis should be maintained when changing the IV tubing and dressings at the IV insertion site. TPN is an excellent medium for the growth of organisms; thus most TPN solutions are prepared by the pharmacist with the use of a laminar airflow hood. Whenever possible, the central line should be used exclusively for the infusion of the TPN solution. Other preventive measures to reduce the patient's risk for infection include:

- Changing the dressing routinely (every 48 to 72 hours, per institutional policy) or when it becomes soiled, wet, or loose. The caregiver should wear a mask and gloves while changing the dressing.

- Extending the application of antimicrobial solution (e.g., iodine) at least 1 inch beyond the edges of the final dressing.

- Placing a sterile sponge over the catheter, then covering with an occlusive, waterproof dressing.

- Inspecting the site for signs of tenderness, redness, edema, loose sutures, or any bleeding or drainage.

- Changing the TPN tubing every 24 hours with the first bag of the day. A 0.22-micron inline filter should be used to reduce the introduction of bacteria from the TPN solution.

- Avoiding the use of the TPN catheter for central venous pressure (CVP) monitoring or the administration of IV medications or blood products.

Drug and Food Interactions

62.12 Certain drugs are incompatible and should not be added to parenteral nutrition solutions.

The major issue associated with the addition of medications to the parenteral formula is the potential for drug incompatibilities. A significant risk is that of a precipitate forming in the solution but being obscured by the opaque fat emulsion. Therefore, drug additions to the TPN solution should never be undertaken unless sufficient data exist to ensure the stability of the solution. Medications that are routinely added to parenteral preparations and are physiologically stable in solution are the H_2-receptor antagonists, such as ranitidine (Zantac) and insulin.

When there is no other option but to administer a medication through the same access site as the TPN, it is best to use a separate lumen in a multilumen catheter to avoid the potential for incompatibility. The use of a Y site or piggyback drug delivery has helped to decrease the risk of drug compatibility problems. Flushing the IV line prior to and after the medication administration, along with temporarily turning off the TPN infusion during the drug administration for 15 to 30 minutes, will help lower the possibility of interactions.

Drugs with demonstrated physical incompatibilities with TPN include ampicillin, tetracycline, and amphotericin B. For administration of these medications, a second IV line should be sought. Medications that have a decreased therapeutic drug effect when given to patients who are receiving TPN with lipids include kanamycin and warfarin. It is important for the nurse to always check with the pharmacist to confirm compatibility and drug effectiveness when administering TPN with any medication.

CONNECTION Checkpoint 62.4

From what you learned in Chapter 59, to what drug class does ranitidine belong? Why would it be added to TPN solutions? *See Answer to Connection Checkpoint 62.3 on student resource website.*

CONNECTIONS Community-Oriented Practice

◀ Home Care of Patients on Total Parenteral Nutrition Therapy

Patients may be sent home on TPN. The patient and the patient's family should have the opportunity to practice the procedure for delivering TPN therapy while they are in the hospital setting under the supervision of the nurse.

Review the procedure for the storage of the solution. Instruct the patient to keep the containers refrigerated and to allow the container to come to room temperature before administering the solution. Instruct the patient never to warm the TPN in the microwave or the oven. Advise the patient to check the expiration date, label of contents, and the appearance of the solution. The patient should not use the solution if the TPN is cloudy, discolored, or has solid pieces floating in it. The solution should not be used if any separation (oil and water) is visible. The patient should check the integrity of the bag by gently squeezing it in order to detect any leakage.

The dressing should be changed at least every 2 days. Teach the patient, family, or caregiver how to use aseptic technique when changing the dressing. The supplies for the dressing and the infusion should be kept in a clean, dry place when not in use. The IV site should be inspected for any signs of swelling, redness, or drainage, which should be reported to the health care provider immediately. Demonstrate to the family how to irrigate the catheter and how to change the bags and the tubing. Instruct the patient in the various settings of the infusion pump, paying particular attention to reviewing what to do if the alarm goes off during the infusion. Review the local Environmental Protection Agency (EPA) policy regarding the proper disposal of used syringes and IV equipment.

Explain that the patient should be weighed daily, and that the patient's I&O should be closely monitored. Ask the family to observe the patient for signs of edema. Demonstrate to the family how to check the glucose level and ensure that all supplies needed are available. Review the potential complications of TPN, such as chills, fever, dyspnea, chest pain, coughing, reaction to lipid infusion, air embolism, nausea, vomiting, and hypo- or hyperglycemia. Instruct the patient never to stop the TPN infusion without conferring first with the health care provider. Recommend that the family keep the telephone number of the health care provider, the nursing service, and the community emergency services readily available in case an emergency or other need should arise. Whenever possible, provide written instructions for the patient and family to use as a reference before the patient is discharged.

CONNECTIONS: NURSING PRACTICE APPLICATION

Patients Receiving Pharmacotherapy with Enteral and Parenteral Nutrition

Assessment	Potential Nursing Diagnoses*
Baseline assessment prior to administration: • Obtain a complete health history including cardiovascular, neurologic, endocrine, hepatic, or renal disease. Obtain a drug history including allergies, current prescription and over-the-counter (OTC) drugs, and herbal preparations, alcohol use, and smoking. Be alert to possible drug interactions. • Obtain a dietary history, noting the ability to swallow, eat, and take adequate fluids. • Obtain baseline height, weight, and vital signs. • Evaluate appropriate laboratory findings (e.g., CBC, electrolytes, glucose, blood urea nitrogen [BUN], hepatic and renal function studies, total protein, serum albumin, lipid profile, serum iron levels). • Assess the patient's ability to receive and understand instructions. Include the family or caregiver as needed.	• *Imbalanced Nutrition: Less Than Body Requirements* • *Deficient Knowledge* (Drug Therapy) • *Risk for Imbalanced Fluid Volume* • *Risk for Infection*
Assessment throughout administration: • Assess for desired therapeutic effects (e.g., weight is maintained, electrolytes, glucose, proteins, and lipid levels remain within normal limits). • Continue monitoring vital signs and periodic laboratory values as appropriate. • Weigh daily at the same time each day and record. • Assess for and promptly report adverse effects: fever, nausea, vomiting, tachycardia, palpitations, hypotension, dyspnea, drowsiness, dizziness, disorientation, hypo- or hyperglycemia, and electrolyte imbalances.	

Implementation

Interventions and (Rationales)	Patient-Centered Care
Ensuring therapeutic effects: • Assess the patient's ability to take oral nutrition during replacement nutrition and encourage small PO feedings if allowed. (Supplementation with PO feedings may be allowed if enteral or parenteral nutrition will be used short term. Encouraging small amounts of PO intake will help the patient maintain normal salivation and ability to perform activities of daily living [ADLs] during the time of replacement nutrition.)	• If allowed, encourage the patient to maintain small, frequent PO intake, or have the family or caregiver assist the patient with PO nutrition and hydration.

(continued)

- Provide water between bolus feedings or each time a new enteral feeding amount is added with continuous feedings. If the patient is unable to take fluids PO, provide additional water through the enteral tube in addition to amounts used to flush the tube. Monitor skin turgor and oral mucous membranes. (Additional water will assist in maintaining adequate dilution of concentrated feedings and replenish body water. Decreased skin turgor and dry mucous membranes may indicate dehydration and the need for additional water.)

- Encourage the patient to consume small amounts of water if allowed, assisted by the family or caregiver as needed.
- Teach the patient, family, or caregiver to monitor for dry mouth or lips, dry skin, or tenting of the skin as signs that insufficient water is being given.

Minimizing adverse effects:
- Monitor vital signs, particularly temperature, throughout nutrition replacement. Assess all access sites (e.g., gastric tube insertion site, IV cannula, tubing, or port sites) frequently for redness, streaking, swelling, or drainage. Report any fever, chills, malaise, or changes in mental status immediately. (Nutritional replacement solutions contain high glucose, protein, and lipid sources that may serve as a reservoir for infection. Tube insertion and access sites may also serve as points of entry for infection.)

- Instruct the patient, family, or caregiver to immediately report any fever, chills, unusual changes to the insertion site, or changes in level of consciousness to the health care provider.

- Use aseptic technique with all insertion-site dressing changes, and refrigerate opened enteral solutions until approximately 30 min before using or as per agency protocol. Follow agency guidelines on the length of time solutions and equipment are allowed to remain in use and change accordingly. (Insertion sites are at high risk for development of infection and must be monitored frequently. Solutions must be refrigerated to inhibit bacterial growth.)

- Explain the rationale for all dressing and equipment monitoring and changes.
- Teach appropriate technique (aseptic or clean) to the family or caregiver if the nutrition is to be continued at home. Follow with demonstration and then teach-back until the family or caregiver is comfortable with the routine.
- Provide written instructions on the frequency of bag/tubing changes and how often the solution should be changed.

- Monitor blood glucose levels. Observe for signs of hyperglycemia or hypoglycemia and obtain capillary glucose levels as ordered. (Blood glucose levels may be affected if the nutrition feeding is stopped or the rate is reduced, or dependent on other medications the patient is on. Supplemental insulin may be required.)

- Instruct the patient on the need for frequent glucose monitoring. Teach the patient, family, or caregiver to promptly report signs of hyperglycemia (excessive thirst, copious urination, insatiable hunger) or hypoglycemia (nervousness, irritability, and dizziness).
- Instruct the patient, family, or caregiver in the technique to monitor capillary glucose, followed by teach-back, if the patient is to continue nutrition replacement at home.

- Monitor for signs of fluid overload. (Solutions are hypertonic and can create fluid shifting with resulting decreased intravascular fluid. Monitoring for a noticeable increase in the pulse rate and quality, changes in blood pressure from the baseline, dyspnea, or edema will assist in noting adverse effects quickly.)

- Instruct the patient, family, or caregiver to immediately report shortness of breath, heart palpitations, swelling, decreased urine output, dizziness, disorientation, or confusion.

- Monitor renal status. (I&O ratio, daily weight, and laboratory studies such as serum creatinine and BUN should be monitored to assess renal function.)

- Instruct the patient on home therapy to weigh self daily at the same time each day and record. An increase or loss in weight of over 1 kg (2 lb) per 24 h should be reported to the health care provider. Immediately report any edema or dyspnea.

- Monitor for signs of venous thrombosis on the same side as the IV catheter. (Venous thrombosis may occur in or around the catheter tubing. Signs and symptoms include the inability to obtain blood on aspiration from the catheter, inability to run fluids through the catheter, neck vein distention, and facial and neck edema on the side of the catheter. The infusion should be stopped and the provider immediately contacted).

- Instruct the patient, family, or caregiver to immediately report a stoppage in the infusion, neck vein distention, or swelling of the face or neck on the side of the IV placement.

- Assess for appropriate enteral tube placement before administering any feeding. Assess for residual amount by aspiration prior to beginning a new enteral feeding if continuous or by bolus. Hold the feeding if the amount returned is 50% or greater of the last bolus feeding or two times the hourly amount given by continuous feeding and contact the health care provider. Flush the tube with adequate amounts of warm water before and after each bolus feeding or every 2–4 h with continuous feedings or as per agency protocol. (Proper tube insertion should be confirmed radiographically before any feeding is initiated. Dependent on agency policy, confirmation of placement by observing the characteristics of the gastric aspirate or pH may be used to confirm placement. If any doubt exists about placement, hold the feeding and alert the health care provider to obtain an x-ray to confirm the placement site. Excessive residual amounts may indicate decreased absorption of the feeding or other conditions and increase the risk of aspiration. Return aspirated amounts unless agency policy requires otherwise.)

- Explain the rationale for checking tube placement prior to each feeding to the patient, family, or caregiver. If home enteral therapy is ordered, teach the patient, family, or caregiver the appropriate methods for checking placement prior to feeding, tube flushing, and aspiration technique for residual amounts. Follow with demonstration and then teach-back until the family or caregiver feels comfortable with the technique.

- Assess lung sounds every 4 h or per agency protocol. Immediately report any dyspnea, lung congestion, or changes in sputum to the health care provider. Maintain the head of the bed at a 30-degree angle or greater per agency policy for patients on enteral feedings. (Keeping the head of the bed elevated may help prevent regurgitation and aspiration.)

- Teach the patient, family, or caregiver to keep the patient in a semi-upright position and to immediately report dyspnea or lung congestion.

CONNECTIONS: NURSING PRACTICE APPLICATION (continued)

• Assess bowel sounds every 4 h, whenever a new amount of feeding is added to continuous feedings, before each bolus feeding, or per agency protocol. Assess for and report diarrhea, especially if profuse, watery, or containing blood or mucus. (Diarrhea or constipation may occur with enteral feedings. Patients on enteral feeding, particularly with elemental formulas, are at increased risk of *Clostridium difficile*–associated diarrhea [CDAD] or from other pathogens.)	• Teach the patient, family, or caregiver to report diarrhea or constipation to the health care provider. Immediately report any diarrhea that is profuse, watery, or contains blood or mucus.
• Review all oral medications the patient is to receive for appropriateness to be given via enteral tube. Contact the health care provider for alternative forms when necessary. (Oral medications may be crushed for administration via enteral tube in most cases. Enteric-coated, sustained release, gel capsules, and others may not be crushed and an alternative form or drug may be required.)	• Instruct the patient, family, or caregiver to review any new medication ordered with the provider who has ordered the enteral feeding to ensure appropriateness for administration via the enteral tube.
Patient understanding of drug therapy: • Use opportunities during administration of medications and during assessments to discuss the rationale for drug therapy, desired therapeutic outcomes, commonly observed adverse effects, parameters for when to call the health care provider, and any necessary monitoring or precautions. (Using time during nursing care helps to optimize and reinforce key teaching areas.)	• The patient, family, or caregiver should be able to state the reason for the enteral feedings, appropriate amount and scheduling, what adverse effects to observe for and when to report them, and the anticipated length of enteral therapy.
Patient self-administration of drug therapy: • When administering the feeding, instruct the patient, family, or caregiver in the proper administration of feeding, e.g., that it is taken with additional fluids. (Utilizing time during nurse-administration of feedings helps to reinforce teaching.)	• The patient, family, or caregiver is able to discuss appropriate administration needs. • The patient, family, or caregiver is able to provide teach-back on appropriate administration of the nutritional feeding and the care of access and insertion sites and tubes prior to home use.

*Nursing Diagnoses—Definitions and Classification 2015–2017. Copyright © 2014, 1994–2014 by NANDA International. Used by arrangement with John Wiley & Sons Limited.

CHAPTER

62 Understanding the Chapter

Key Concepts Summary

62.1 Nutritional supplementation is required for patients with certain medical conditions.

62.2 Supplemental nutrition may be provided by the oral or parenteral route.

62.3 Various methods are utilized to administer enteral feedings to the patient.

62.4 Enteral feedings can be delivered by bolus, intermittent drip or infusion, continuous infusion, or cyclic intermittent infusion.

62.5 Several types of liquid nutrition formulas are commercially available for enteral feedings.

62.6 Most enteral nutrition formulas contain four basic classes of nutrients.

62.7 Although considered physiological in nature, total enteral nutrition can predispose the patient to various complications.

62.8 Most medications that are administered orally can also be delivered to the patient via an enteral tube.

62.9 Parenteral nutrition is used when patients are unable to tolerate enteral feedings.

62.10 The basic total parenteral nutrition solution consists of carbohydrates, lipids, amino acids, electrolytes, minerals, and vitamins.

62.11 As with enteral therapy, patients who are receiving parenteral nutrition therapy can experience various complications.

62.12 Certain drugs are incompatible and should not be added to parenteral nutrition solutions.

Case Study: Making the Patient Connection

Remember the patient "Christopher Jones" at the beginning of the chapter? Now read the remainder of the case study. Based on the information presented within this chapter, respond to the critical thinking questions that follow.

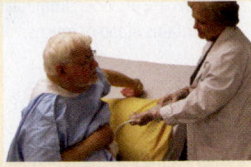

Christopher Jones is a 62-year-old man with a long-standing history of diabetes, the past 20 years as an insulin-dependent diabetic. During the past few months, Christopher has been having increasing difficulty with eating. At first he noticed that he felt full almost immediately and then nausea began in waves, eventually resulting in vomiting. He began to lose weight and have trouble controlling his blood glucose levels, experiencing more frequent bouts of hypoglycemia. He visited his health care provider, and after an upper GI series, esophagogastroduodenoscopy, and a gastric emptying study, Christopher was diagnosed with gastroparesis diabeticorum. His provider has told him that it is most likely due to his diabetes and may be temporary. He has been started on a prokinetic drug (metoclopramide [Reglan]) and erythromycin in an attempt to increase gastric emptying.

The provider inserted a jejunostomy tube for feedings until the outcomes of drug therapy can be determined. Christopher has returned on his first postoperative visit to the provider's office and will need teaching about his feeding tube.

Critical Thinking Questions

1. Christopher wants to know if he can still eat foods "normally." Give a rationale for your answer.

2. Christopher does not know how to take care of his tube and wants to know if any special care is required. What would you teach him?

3. Create a list of potential complications to which Christopher and his family should be alerted.

See Answers to Critical Thinking Questions on student resource website.

Additional Case Study

Misty Moore is a 36-year-old woman who was admitted to the hospital with a complete bowel obstruction, multiple abdominal adhesions, and a flare-up of Crohn's disease. She stands 5 ft 5 in. and weighs 65 kg (143 lb). Her usual weight is 75 kg (165 lb). Her past medical condition includes Crohn's disease since age 16, as well as a 10-year history of type 2 diabetes. Exploratory surgery is scheduled to remove the diseased portion of her small bowel as well as to perform lysis of the adhesions, which occurred as a result of her previous bowel operations. Because of her depleted nutritional state and the 10% drop in her weight, nutritional support is indicated. Her GI tract is not expected to be accessible for at least 10 to 14 days.

1. What type of nutritional support do you think will be ordered for Misty? Why?

2. Considering the patient's condition, what metabolic problem would you suspect she is at risk for developing?

3. How can the risk of developing this problem be reduced?

See Answers to Additional Case Study on student resource website.

Chapter Review

1 To meet his nutritional goals, the patient is placed on enteral feedings via a nasogastric (NG) tube. Which intervention should the nurse perform in order to ensure that the patient is maintaining a proper fluid balance?

1. Weigh the patient every other day.

2. Maintain a strict record of intake and output, and flush the nasogastric tube once a day.

3. Provide additional free water in addition to that used for irrigating the tube.

4. Assess the skin around the tube insertion site for any drainage or irritation.

2 Before hanging a bag of total parenteral nutrition, the nurse checks the various components of the solution. Which elements would the nurse expect to see on the solution label? Select all that apply.

1. Electrolytes

2. Diuretic

3. Trace minerals

4. Isophane (NPH) insulin

5. Multivitamins

3 The nurse is making rounds at the beginning of the shift and notes that the patient's total parenteral nutrition bag is empty. Which solution should the nurse hang until the total parenteral nutrition solution can be properly prepared and delivered to the nursing unit?

1. 5% dextrose in water (D_5W)
2. 5% dextrose in Ringer's lactate (D_5RL)
3. 5% dextrose in 0.9% sodium chloride (D_5NS)
4. 10% dextrose in water ($D_{10}W$)

4 The patient has been discharged home on total parenteral nutrition therapy. When making the home visits, which assessments should the home care nurse closely monitor?

1. Temperature and blood pressure
2. Temperature and weight
3. Pulse and blood pressure
4. Pulse and weight

5 The nurse is preparing to hang a lipid (fat) solution and notes that fat globules are visible at the top of the bag. Which action should be taken?

1. Roll the solution container gently.
2. Shake the solution container vigorously.
3. Run the solution container under warm water.
4. Obtain a different container of solution.

6 The patient who is receiving enteral nutrition via a PEG tube suddenly spikes a fever of 38.6°C (101.5°F). The nurse notifies the health care provider, who orders that the solution and tubing be changed immediately. Preventive measures to limit the risk of infection from enteral feedings include which of the following? Select all that apply.

1. Refrigerate unused portions of feeding.
2. Hang a feeding solution no longer than 4 hours.
3. Wash out tube feeding bags and tubings before reusing.
4. Use plain water to irrigate the tube between feedings.
5. Maintain sterile technique whenever initiating a new feeding solution.

See Answers to Chapter Review in Appendix A.

References

Dawodu, S. T. (2013). *Nutritional management in the rehabilitation setting.* Retrieved from http://emedicine.medscape.com/article/318180-overview#a1

Selected Bibliography

Abu-Hilal, M., Hemandas, A. K., McPhail, M., Jain, G., Panagiotopoulou, I., Scibelli, T., . . . Pearce, N. (2010). A comparative analysis of safety and efficacy of different methods of tube placement for enteral feedings following major pancreatic resection. A non-randomized study. *Journal of the Pancreas, 11*(1), 8–13. Retrieved from http://www.joplink.net/prev/201001/06.html

Bistrian, B. R. (2012). The who, what, where, when, why, and how of early enteral feeding. *The American Journal of Clinical Nutrition, 95*, 1303–1304. doi:10.3945/ ajcn.112.039826

Dibb, M., Teubner, A., Theis, V., Shaffer, J., & Lal, S. (2013). Review article: The management of long-term parenteral nutrition. *Alimentary Pharmacology & Therapeutics, 37*, 587–603. doi:10.1111/apt.12209

Herdman, T. H., & Kamitsuru, S. (Eds.). (2014). *NANDA International nursing diagnoses: Definitions and classification, 2015-2017.* Oxford, United Kingdom: Wiley-Blackwell.

Kelly, D., Bremner, R., Hartley, J., & Flynn, D. (Eds.). (2014). Parenteral nutrition: Initiating and monitoring. In *Practical approach to paediatric gastroenterology, hepatology and nutrition.* Oxford, United Kingdom: John Wiley & Sons. doi:10.1002/9781118898536.ch45

Martínez, R. A., Ortega, E. R., Munuera, C. C., Medina, J. M. F., Vinuesa, M. D. S., & Barrado-Narvión, M. J. (2014). Effectiveness of continuous enteral nutrition versus intermittent enteral nutrition in intensive care patients: A systematic review. *JBI Database of Systematic Reviews and Implementation Reports, 12*(1), 281–317. doi:10.11124%2Fjbisrir-2014-1129

Munroe, C., Frantz, D., Martindale, R. G., & McClave, S. A. (2011). The optimal lipid formulation in enteral feeding in critical illness: Clinical update and review of the literature. *Current Gastroenterology Reports, 13*, 368–375. doi:10.1007/s11894-011-0203-y

Rollins, C. J. (2010). Drug–nutrient interactions in patients receiving enteral nutrition. In J. I. Boullata & V. T. Armenti (Eds.), *Handbook of drug–nutrient interactions.* New York, NY: Humana.

Seres, D. S., Valcarcel, M., & Guillaume, A. (2013). Advantages of enteral nutrition over parenteral nutrition. *Therapeutic Advances in Gastroenterology, 6*, 157–167. doi:10.1177/1756283X12467564

Walmsley, R. S. (2013). Refeeding syndrome: Screening, incidence, and treatment during parenteral nutrition. *Journal of Gastroenterology and Hepatology, 28*(S4), 113–117. doi:10.1111/jgh.12345

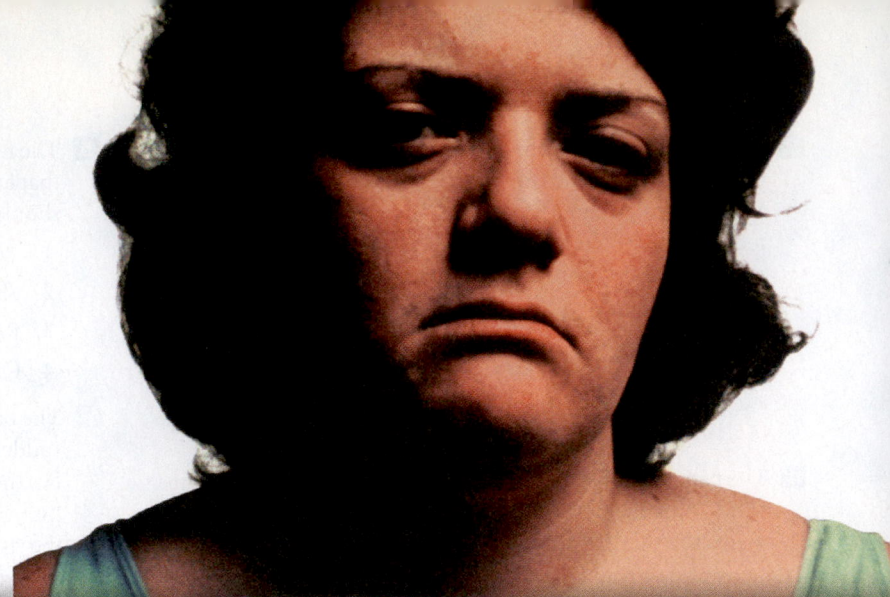

"I was shocked when the nurse weighed me in the office today: 30 pounds more! I didn't think I'd changed my habits all that much. Where did all that weight come from? I need to do something about this."

Patient "Rosemary Goodman"

CHAPTER

63

Weight Reduction Strategies and the Pharmacotherapy of Obesity

LEARNING OUTCOMES

After reading this chapter, the student should be able to:

1. Identify genetic and lifestyle factors that contribute to obesity.
2. Explain how energy imbalances can cause weight gain or loss.
3. Describe the role of the hypothalamus in regulating appetite.
4. Explain how leptin and brain neurotransmitters regulate appetite.
5. Describe how obesity is measured.
6. Outline the major components of a successful weight management program.
7. Identify several weight loss agents that were removed from the market due to their adverse effects.
8. Describe the nurse's role in the pharmacologic management of obesity.
9. For each class shown in the chapter outline, identify the prototype and representative drugs and explain the mechanism(s) of drug action, primary indications, contraindications, significant drug interactions, pregnancy category, and important adverse effects.
10. Apply the nursing process to care for patients receiving antiobesity therapy.

CHAPTER OUTLINE

▶ Etiology of Obesity

▶ Pathogenesis of Obesity

▶ Measurement of Obesity

▶ Nonpharmacologic Therapies for Obesity

▶ Pharmacotherapy of Obesity
   Lipase Inhibitors
   PROTOTYPE Orlistat (Alli, Xenical), *p. 1082*
   Anorexiants

▶ Adjuncts to Obesity Therapy

KEY TERMS

adipocytes, 1080
anorexiants, 1082
appetite, 1079

body mass index (BMI), 1080
leptin, 1080

satiety, 1079
satiety center, 1079

Americans spend $30 to $50 billion each year in attempts to lose weight. In the majority of cases, people experience little long-term success in sustaining weight loss. Obesity is closely associated with increased health risks that include premature death, hypertension (HTN), hyperlipidemia, diabetes mellitus, heart disease, sleep apnea, osteoarthritis, and some cancers. This chapter examines the etiology, pathogenesis, and treatment of obesity.

Etiology of Obesity

63.1 Genetic and lifestyle factors contribute to the etiology of obesity.

Obesity is a growing epidemic in the United States: It is estimated that 78 million adults are overweight or obese. This represents 35% of the adult population over age 20. Along with the increase in adult obesity, infant and childhood obesity has also increased. About 14% of children age 2 to 5 are now considered obese. All of these percentages have doubled or tripled since the mid-1970s. The trend is expected to continue, because studies have shown that those who were obese as children are more likely to be obese as adults.

Despite considerable research, the specific causes of obesity have not been identified. The etiology is likely a complex combination of genetic, lifestyle, and physiological factors. In a few cases, weight gain can be attributed to medical conditions, the most common being hypothyroidism. Certain rare disorders of the hypothalamus can also cause overeating. Drugs such as corticosteroids are clearly causes of weight gain.

PharmFACT

Although obesity is increasing in the total population, the incidence is not uniform. The highest incidences (more than 30%) in adults are in Louisiana, Mississippi, and West Virginia. The lowest incidences (less than 24%) are in Colorado, Massachusetts, and Hawaii (Centers for Disease Control and Prevention, 2013).

Studies of family histories and twins support a strong genetic component to obesity. Researchers have identified a few genetic mutations that lead to obesity, although these are rare and do not contribute significantly to the extent of obesity currently observed in the population. While a family history does not cause a person to be obese, it predisposes them to weight gain. The predisposition is best overcome by preventing weight gain. This is particularly important in identifying children at risk of adult obesity and implementing interventions aimed at prevention.

Lifestyle factors play a key role in the development of obesity, the two most obvious factors being diet and physical activity. The fundamental shift in obesity levels in the past three decades has likely been due to high-fat, calorie-dense diets combined with sedentary lifestyles.

There are many theories on the relationship between specific dietary practices and obesity. Often, these are fueled by fad diets rather than research. While it is certainly true that the body metabolizes and stores carbohydrates, lipids, and proteins differently, no specific dietary nutrient limitation has been clearly demonstrated to prevent obesity or to result in more sustainable weight loss.

Despite the ongoing debate on the "best" diet, the fact remains that body weight is most likely determined by energy (calorie) balance. Simply stated, if the number of calories consumed equals the number of calories expended, the person will maintain (balance) body weight at the current level. Changes in weight occur when there is an energy imbalance. For example, an imbalance of as little as 10 surplus calories per day can lead to a 1-lb weight gain each year. While this seems insignificant, if the imbalance persists over several decades it can lead to obesity in older adults. Of course, this calculation holds true for losing weight, but few are patient enough to wait an entire year to lose a single pound.

Therefore, to lose weight one has to expend more calories than one consumes. In terms of weight loss or gain, the source of the calories, carbohydrates, proteins, or lipids, probably does not matter. Of course, the source is indeed important in terms of overall health and wellness. Indeed, there remains considerable debate in the medical community as to which of the energy sources (carbohydrate, protein, or lipid) contributes the most to adult obesity.

The second half of the energy equation is energy expenditure. Physical activity expends calories and can result in either prevention of weight gain or a faster loss of weight. The most successful diet plans always combine a reduction in calories with an increase in physical activity.

Pathogenesis of Obesity

63.2 Appetite is regulated by the satiety center in the hypothalamus and is influenced by various hormones.

Hunger occurs when the hypothalamus recognizes the levels of certain chemicals (glucose) or hormones (insulin) in the blood. Hunger is a normal physiological response that drives people to seek nourishment. Appetite is somewhat different than hunger. **Appetite** is a psychological response that drives food intake based on associations and memory. For example, people often eat, not because they are experiencing hunger, but because it is a particular time of day or because they find the act of eating pleasurable or social. The psychological feeling of fullness or satisfaction following a meal is called **satiety**. The degree of satiety is directly recognized by a region of the hypothalamus known as the **satiety center**.

CONNECTION Checkpoint 63.1

The hypothalamus is part of the limbic system of the brain. From what you learned in Chapter 17, what are the primary functions of the limbic system? *See Answer to Connection Checkpoint 63.1 on student resource website.*

Another hormone that regulates hunger and weight balance is **leptin**, a protein secreted by **adipocytes** (fat cells). When a certain amount of fat has been stored, adipocytes increase their secretion of leptin. Receptors for leptin are located in the satiety center in the hypothalamus. Binding of leptin to its receptors signals the hypothalamus that the body has ingested enough food and tells the brain how much adipose tissue is present. Leptin suppresses appetite and increases body temperature (thermogenic) and energy expenditure. Leptin thus serves as a natural appetite suppressant.

Scientists have intensively searched for a means of reducing appetite by intervening in the leptin pathway. It would seem that administering leptin would be a natural method for suppressing appetite and promoting weight loss. However, patients who are obese already have high levels of leptin circulating in the blood. Leptin receptors in these patients appear to have become desensitized and developed resistance to the satiety effects of leptin. The result is an increase in appetite. At this time, the experimental administration of leptin does not have any effect on obesity.

Binding of the leptin receptors in the hypothalamus creates a signal cascade that leads to the secretion of a number of different hormones. Of primary interest is the action of neuropeptide Y (NPY), a hormone concentrated in the hypothalamus that has been associated with increased appetite and food consumption. If the body has too much adipose tissue, adipocytes will secrete more leptin, which signals the hypothalamus to inhibit NPY release, thus decreasing appetite. Unfortunately, experimental drugs that block NPY receptors have not been found to promote weight loss in patients with obesity.

Another important finding in the pathogenesis of obesity is the role of neurotransmitters in appetite suppression. Activation of certain subreceptors of the neurotransmitter serotonin (5-HT_{1B} and 5-HT_{2C}) reduces appetite and the consumption of calories at meals. In addition, activation of alpha$_1$- or beta$_2$-adrenergic receptors and the release of norepinephrine seem to decrease appetite. Antiobesity drugs are currently available that promote the release of these neurotransmitters.

Lipids are the most energy-dense nutrients for fueling metabolic processes; more calories can be obtained from lipids than from any other molecule. While the body can store only small amounts of protein and carbohydrate, fat stores are nearly unlimited. The ability of adipocytes to increase in size and store a nearly unlimited quantity of fat is likely a consequence of evolutionary adaptation. For most of human history, starvation has been a major cause of death, and hard physical activity was necessary to survive. Those who had more efficient lipid-storage capacity survived the times of famine. Although starvation is still a problem in parts of the world, it is no longer a major cause of death in developed countries. Unfortunately, human metabolic systems are still programmed for low-fat diets, combined with lots of physical exercise. What was once a survival mechanism has become a liability when a person consumes a high-fat diet and chooses a sedentary lifestyle.

Measurement of Obesity

63.3 Obesity is measured by using the body mass index and waist circumference.

Obesity is defined by several different measures. In simple terms, obesity is being more than 20% above the ideal weight. The ideal weight fluctuates depending on the person's gender, height, and general build.

The most commonly accepted measurement of obesity is the **body mass index (BMI)**. BMI is determined by dividing body weight (in kilograms) by the square of height (in meters). In adults, a BMI of 25 kg/m^2 indicates the person is overweight. Obesity is defined by a BMI of 30 kg/m^2. Figure 63.1 illustrates a simple graph of BMI for estimating obesity. BMI measurement is not accurate in athletes due to the higher proportion of muscle to fat in these persons.

Another clinical measure of obesity is waist circumference, as measured by a simple tape measure. Waist circumference values of 80 cm (32 in.) for women and 94 cm (37 in.) for men are associated with increased health risk. Waist measurements greater than 88 cm (35 in.) for women and 102 cm (40 in.) for men have the greatest health risks. Waist circumference correlates well with BMI and also provides an estimate of abdominal (visceral) fat, which is more strongly associated with health risk than fat stored in other regions of the body. Table 63.1 combines the waist circumference and BMI measurements in assessing the health risks for obesity.

PharmFACT

Obesity rates vary considerably by race, ethnic group, and gender. In 2009 to 2010, 59% of non-Hispanic black women and 45% of Mexican American women over age 20 were obese compared with 32% of non-Hispanic white women (National Center for Health Statistics, 2012).

Nonpharmacologic Therapies for Obesity

63.4 Nonpharmacologic treatment of obesity should be attempted prior to initiating pharmacotherapy.

Prior to initiation of drug therapy, the health care provider and patient must first attempt to achieve weight management through nonpharmacologic means. This involves making three major lifestyle changes: diet, exercise, and behavior modification. To obtain successful, sustained weight loss, lifestyle changes can be physically and emotionally demanding for a patient who is obese.

Choosing a sustainable diet is often the biggest hurdle for patients. Although it may have taken decades or longer to become obese, no one wants to take decades to lose weight. Weight loss schemes and fad diets that claim rapid weight loss while making few changes in dietary habits provide strong attractions to patients with obesity who are desperate to lose weight. The nurse should assist patients in setting realistic goals and steer them away from fad diets that may be unhealthy as well as unsuccessful. Severe restriction of any of the food groups—proteins, carbohydrates, or lipids—is not necessary or recommended by nutritionists. Examining the patient's diet and reducing the normal intake to 1,000 to 1,200 kcal/day for women and 1,200 to 1,600 kcal/day for men is

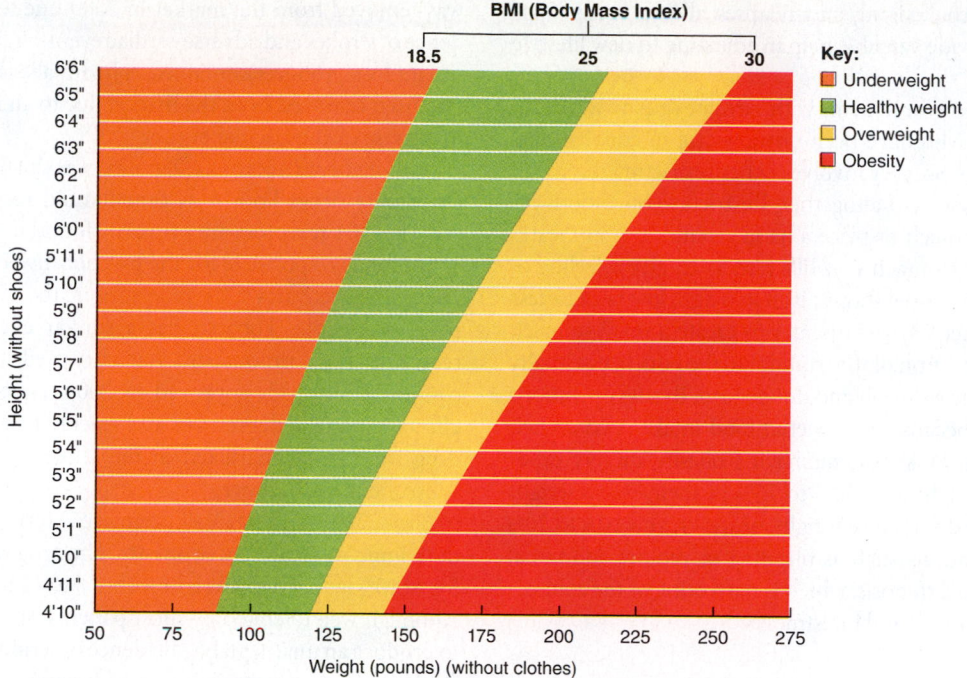

Figure 63.1 Calculation of body mass index. To determine your BMI, find the value for your height on the left and follow this line to the right until it intersects with the value for your weight on the bottom axis. The area in the graph where the two points intersect is your BMI.
From *Nutrition: An Applied Approach* (4th ed., p. 391), by Thompson and Manore, 2015. Upper Saddle River, NJ: Pearson Education, Inc.

usually sufficient, although small, progressive steps will be needed to achieve these values in patients who are accustomed to consuming two to six times the recommended daily calorie values. Weight loss of 0.5 to 1 kg (1 to 2 lb) per week is usually a realistic goal and is physically safe.

Exercise is an essential component of any weight management program. Many patients with obesity, however, have other chronic health problems that could impact an exercise program, the most common being diabetes, HTN, and heart disease. The patient should receive a thorough medical work-up to be certain there are no physical contraindications to starting an exercise program. The patient who is obese should begin with very modest exercise goals and proceed to more challenging physical activity under the guidance of a health care provider. Exercise should be combined with calorie restriction because increased physical activity, by itself, is not an efficient method for losing weight.

Behavior modification is another essential component of successful weight management programs. The patient likely became obese due to poor eating habits and behaviors, which must be changed for the remainder of the person's life. For extremely obese patients, the weight loss program will extend a year or longer; therefore, support groups should be encouraged. Breaking learned

TABLE 63.1	Classification of Overweight and Obesity by BMI, Waist Circumference, and Associated Disease Risks			
			DISEASE RISK* RELATIVE TO NORMAL WEIGHT AND WAIST CIRCUMFERENCE	
	BMI (kg/m²)	**Obesity Class**	**Men 102 cm (40 in.) or Less** **Women 88 cm (35 in.) or Less**	**Men > 102 cm (40 in.)** **Women > 88 cm (35 in.)**
Underweight	<18.5		—	—
Normal[+]	18.5–24.9		—	—
Overweight	25.0–29.9		Increased	High
Obesity	30.0–34.9	I	High	Very high
	35.0–39.9	II	Very high	Very high
Extreme obesity	40.0[+]	III	Extremely high	Extremely high

*Disease risk for type 2 diabetes, HTN, and cardiovascular disease.
[+]Increased waist circumference can also be a marker for increased risk even in persons of normal weight.
From *Clinical Guidelines on the Identification, Evaluation, and Treatment of Overweight and Obesity in Adults: The Evidence Report*, by the National Institutes of Health, National Heart, Lung, and Blood Institute, 1998, p. xvii, Washington, DC: Department of Health & Human Services. Retrieved from http://www.nhlbi.nih.gov/guidelines/obesity/ob_gdlns.htm

habits of eating is challenging and relapses always occur. Support groups can provide valuable help in adjusting to new lifestyle patterns.

Surgery is an option for patients with extreme obesity who have a BMI over 40 and who have been unsuccessful in conventional weight loss programs. Surgery involves either restricting the size of the stomach or bypassing it altogether. Restriction operations remove part of the stomach or place a band around it. This creates a smaller, pouchlike stomach that fills rapidly to give a feeling of fullness. The restriction operations result in weight loss because less food can be consumed. Bypass operations create a small stomach pouch and attach a portion of the jejunum to the pouch, essentially bypassing most of the stomach and duodenum. Bypass operations lead to weight loss because the lowered food intake is combined with malabsorption. Most patients having obesity surgery experience significant weight loss: 50% to 75% of their excess weight within 1 year. Some do not lose weight, however, and 10% to 20% experience complications such as bleeding or require additional surgery due to stromal stenosis, which is narrowing of the connection between the stomach and intestines.

Pharmacotherapy of Obesity

63.5 Drugs used for weight management affect appetite or the absorption of fats.

Because of the prevalence of obesity in society and the difficulty most patients experience when following weight reduction plans for extended periods, drug manufacturers have long sought to develop safe drugs that induce and sustain weight loss. The quest for the "magic weight loss pill," however, has been disappointing. Indeed, many of the popular weight loss products have been discontinued due to health concerns. A brief history of these discontinued products is included because the nurse may still receive questions from patients regarding their use.

In the 1970s, amphetamine and dextroamphetamine (Dexedrine) were widely prescribed to reduce appetite. Although these drugs have strong appetite-suppressant actions, their effects are short lived due to the development of tolerance, which leads to higher and higher doses. Although amphetamine, methamphetamine, and dextroamphetamine are still available, they have high abuse potential, and the therapy of obesity is no longer an acceptable indication for these drugs. Amphetamine is featured as a prototype central nervous system (CNS) stimulant in Chapter 24.

CONNECTION Checkpoint 63.2

Methylphenidate (Ritalin) is an amphetamine-like drug. From what you learned in Chapter 24, what are the primary indications for amphetamine and methylphenidate? *See Answer to Connection Checkpoint 63.2 on student resource website.*

In the 1990s, the combination of fenfluramine and phentermine (Fen-Phen) was found to be effective at promoting weight loss. However, fenfluramine was subsequently removed from the market for causing heart valve defects. Phentermine is still used as an adjunct to weight loss (see Section 63.7).

Two over-the-counter (OTC) appetite suppressants were widely used to promote weight loss in the 1980s and 1990s. Phenylpropanolamine, which was also used as a decongestant in cold remedies,

was removed from the market in 2000 due to an increased incidence of strokes and adverse cardiac events. Until 2004, alternative weight loss products contained ephedra alkaloids, but these have also been removed from the market due to an increased incidence of adverse cardiovascular events.

Rimonabant (Acomplia, Zimulti) was the first of a new class of antiobesity drugs known as cannabinoid receptor (CB1) blockers. The CB1 receptors are primarily found in the brain, and their activation is responsible for the psychoactive effects of marijuana. Overeating activates CB1 receptors in the CNS; blocking them reduces appetite. Tobacco has a similar effect on cannabinoid receptors; thus, rimonabant was also used to promote tobacco cessation. Although approved in 2006, concerns about adverse effects, especially depression and suicide ideation, prevented the drug from being marketed in the United States. Approval was subsequently withdrawn.

From 2007 until 2010, sibutramine (Meridia) was approved for the adjunctive treatment of obesity. The drug was able to produce a 5% to 10% loss of body weight within 6 to 12 months of treatment. Although well tolerated by most patients, sibutramine was found to produce an unacceptable incidence of serious cardiac events and stroke and was voluntarily removed from the market.

Given all these pharmacologic disappointments, current pharmacologic strategies for weight management focus on two sites of action. The lipase inhibitors act by reducing the absorption of fats in the small intestine. The approved antiobesity drugs produce only modest effects, and pharmacotherapy must be combined with a calorie-restricted diet. The appetite suppressants (also called **anorexiants** or anorectics) act centrally by increasing the amounts of norepinephrine, serotonin, and dopamine in the regions of the brain that affect appetite. Current drugs used as adjuncts in the treatment of obesity are shown in Table 63.2.

63.6 Lipase inhibitors cause weight loss by interfering with the absorption of fats.

One strategy to reduce weight is to block the absorption of dietary fats. Lipids are a very dense energy source and most of the accumulated fat in patients is derived from dietary sources.

Chemical digestion of lipids occurs through the enzymatic action of pancreatic lipase, which splits dietary triglycerides into glycerol and free fatty acids. Once absorbed, the fatty acids can be recombined with glycerol and stored in adipocytes. Attempts to produce antiobesity drugs that block lipid absorption have resulted in one approved drug: orlistat (Xenical).

PROTOTYPE DRUG	Orlistat (Alli, Xenical)

Classification: **Therapeutic:** Antiobesity drug
Pharmacologic: Lipase inhibitor

Therapeutic Effects and Uses: Approved in 1999, orlistat is indicated for the treatment of obesity in combination with a reduced-calorie diet and exercise. Orlistat is indicated for patients with a BMI of 30 or greater, or a BMI of 27 or greater if the patient has other risk factors such as HTN, hyperlipidemia, or diabetes. This drug produces only a modest weight reduction compared to placebos.

TABLE 63.2 Drugs for Treating Obesity

Drug	Route and Adult Dose (Maximum Dose Where Indicated)	Adverse Effects
bupropion and naltrexone (Contrave)	PO: Begin with 1 tablet in week 1 (90 mg bupropion/8 mg naltrexone); increase by 1 tablet/day each subsequent week until daily maintenance dose of 2 tablets twice daily is achieved at the start of week 4	*Nausea, constipation, headache, vomiting* Suicidal behavior, seizures, HTN, liver impairment, hypoglycemia
diethylpropion (Tepanil)	PO (immediate release): 25 mg tid PO (extended release): 75 mg once daily	*Vomiting, diarrhea, dry mouth, changes in libido, nervousness, dizziness* Dysrhythmia, hypertension, psychotic episodes, euphoria
lorcaserin (Belviq)	PO: 10 mg bid	*Headache, dizziness, fatigue, nausea, dry mouth, constipation, and hypoglycemia (in patients with diabetes)* Serotonin syndrome, valvular heart disease, euphoria, suicidal thoughts, priapism
orlistat (Alli, Xenical)	PO: 60–120 mg with each meal containing fat	*Flatus with discharge, fatty/oily stool, increased defecation, and fecal urgency or incontinence* Hepatic toxicity, increased renal oxalate
phentermine (Adipex-P, Suprenza)	PO (capsule): 37.5 mg daily PO (orally disintegrating tablet): 15–37.5 mg daily	*Paresthesia, dizziness, dysgeusia, insomnia, constipation, and dry mouth* Fetal toxicity, increased heart rate, suicidal behavior, acute myopia and glaucoma, mood and sleep disorders, cognitive impairment, metabolic acidosis
phentermine and topiramate (Qsymia)	PO: 3.75–15 mg phentermine and 23–92 mg topiramate once daily in the morning	*Paraesthesia, dizziness, dysgeusia, insomnia, constipation, dry mouth* Suicidal behavior, fetal toxicity, increased heart rate, metabolic acidosis, cognitive impairment

Note: *Italics* indicate common adverse effects. Underline indicates serious adverse effects.

CONNECTIONS | **Complementary and Alternative Therapies**

◀ **Green Tea and Weight Loss**

Description

Green tea is a natural substance made from the leaves of the plant *Camellia sinensis*, which is native to mainland China but is cultivated worldwide. There are many varieties and types of green teas.

History and Claims

In China, green tea has been used for thousands of years for ceremonial functions as well as to treat a diverse variety of ailments. In modern times, the health effects of green teas have focused on improving cardiovascular function, preventing cancer, and weight loss. There is some research examining the role of green tea for improving symptoms or treatment of neurodegenerative diseases such as multiple sclerosis, Parkinson's disease, and Alzheimer's disease.

Standardization

Green tea extracts contain large amounts of catechins (also called polyphenols), a group of chemicals that have strong antioxidant properties that are the most active compounds used medicinally and found in green tea. Green tea itself contains caffeine, although this is sometimes removed during processing. Extracts are sometimes standardized to percent polyphenols, which varies widely from 14% to 98%, depending on the product. Some products report the amount of epigallocatechin gallate (EGCG), which is the most abundant catechin in green tea extracts.

Evidence

The administration of green tea extract has been shown to decrease body weight in laboratory animals (Grove & Lambert, 2010). Epidemiologic studies suggest that those who consume green tea have a lower percentage of body fat and lower BMIs than non–tea drinkers. Interventions designed to increase weight loss in patients who are obese have shown mixed results. A meta-analysis of 15 studies concluded that green tea does induce a small amount of weight loss, but that the amount of loss is not large enough to be clinically significant (Jurgens et al., 2012). To conclude, consumption of green tea extract likely has a small positive effect on weight loss when consistently taken in moderate amounts over long periods.

The prescription form of orlistat (Xenical) is available at 120 mg and is given three times daily, during or up to 1 hour after a meal containing fat. In 2007, an OTC dosage form (Alli) was approved at 60 mg. The drug is only effective if taken with meals containing lipids; the dose may be omitted if the meal contains no fat. Orlistat is not approved for children under age 12.

Mechanism of Action: Orlistat inhibits pancreatic lipase and acts by blocking lipid absorption in the gastrointestinal (GI) tract. It primarily lowers the absorption of free fatty acids but also has an effect on cholesterol absorption. The decreased lipid absorption lowers calories and promotes weight loss. Orlistat inhibits fat absorption by approximately 30%.

Pharmacokinetics:

Route(s)	PO
Absorption	Minimal absorption
Distribution	Not distributed; remains in the GI tract; does not cross the placenta; is not secreted in breast milk
Primary metabolism	Wall of the GI tract
Primary excretion	Feces
Onset of action	24–48 h
Duration of action	Half-life: 1–2 h

CONNECTIONS · Treating the Diverse Patient

◀ Weight Loss from a Diabetes Treatment?

Can it be possible that a diagnosis of diabetes ever results in something positive? While a diagnosis of diabetes can mean a lifelong need to monitor, treat, and worry about complications, newer treatments for diabetes have resulted in significant gains, especially in the decrease in serious adverse effects normally associated with the disease, such as acute myocardial infarction (MI), stroke, and amputations (Gregg et al., 2014). Now one of the treatments might hold promise as a treatment for obesity.

Glucagon-like peptides-1 (GLP-1) are one of the newer classes of drugs used in the treatment of diabetes. They belong to a group known as incretin enhancers (see Chapter 66) and act as the natural hormones, incretins, do in the body. Activation of incretins results in increased pancreatic insulin secretion, decreased glucagon secretion, delayed gastric emptying, and increased feelings of satiety, resulting in decreased food intake. It had been noted that patients treated with GLP-1 drugs such as exenatide (Byetta) and liraglutide (Victoza) experienced weight loss along with their glucose control. New studies suggest that this class of drugs may be used in patients who do not have diabetes to achieve weight loss as well (Katout et al., 2014; Ottney, 2013; Torekov, Madsbad, & Holst, 2011). Additional benefits to GLP-1 drugs have been noted in research and include lowering of systolic blood pressure not related to weight loss or improvement in HbA1C levels (Katout et al., 2014) and decreases in the incidence of prediabetes conditions (Ottney, 2013). Future research may focus on combinations of drugs to achieve both weight loss and improvement in cardiovascular and metabolic outcomes.

Adverse Effects: Some of the adverse effects of orlistat are directly related to its inhibition of lipid absorption. As more lipids reach the large intestine, flatus with discharge, oily stool, and fecal urgency are common, especially during the first 4 weeks of therapy. To avoid serious adverse GI effects, patients should restrict their fat intake. Rare cases of liver toxicity have been reported with this drug.

Contraindications/Precautions: Orlistat should be used with caution in patients with cholestasis because the drug inhibits gallbladder contractions. Orlistat is contraindicated for patients who have a known cause of obesity, such as hypothyroidism, and in patients with severe malabsorption disorders. The drug is contraindicated in patients with anorexia nervosa or bulimia because it may worsen these disorders. Orlistat is contraindicated during pregnancy because the benefits of weight loss do not outweigh the potential risks to the fetus.

Drug Interactions: Because orlistat inhibits the absorption of the lipid-soluble vitamins A, D, and E, a supplement containing these vitamins should be taken at least 2 hours before or after a dose of orlistat. Vitamin K levels may decrease in patients taking orlistat, which can affect anticoagulation produced by warfarin. Orlistat decreases the absorption of cyclosporine and the two drugs should not be used concurrently. Orlistat may also decrease the absorption of warfarin (Coumadin); therefore, coagulation values in these patients should be monitored closely. **Herbal/Food**: Unknown.

Pregnancy: Category X.

Treatment of Overdose: Overdose with orlistat is not a clinical problem because the effects of the drug are rapidly reversible.

Nursing Responsibilities:

- Obtain a complete health history including allergies, drug history, and possible drug interactions.
- Perform a physical assessment including vital signs and apometric measurements such as BMI and body weight.
- Assess laboratory values as indicated to determine hepatic and renal function.
- Consult a dietitian to prepare and educate the patient on the recommended nutritional intake.

- Administer the drug during or up to 1 hour after a meal containing fat. Omit the dose if eating a meal that does not contain fat or if a meal is skipped.
- Monitor weight and BMI; closely monitor people with diabetes for hypoglycemia.
- Monitor prothrombin time (PT) and international normalized ratio (INR) if the patient is taking warfarin. Assess for signs of vitamin K deficiency such as bruising or prolonged oozing from minor cuts.
- Monitor blood pressure frequently, especially in patients with preexisting HTN.
- Assess for medications that can interact with orlistat such as warfarin, cyclosporine, pravastatin, diabetes drugs, and fat-soluble vitamin supplements such as A, D, E, and K. Vitamin deficiencies can occur, causing changes in eyesight, hair, and skin.

Lifespan and Diversity Considerations:

- Assess the older adult's diet, medication history, and alcohol intake. Vitamin deficiency may occur as a result of normal physiological changes related to aging and nutrient absorption, alcohol use, or medication. Medication interactions may be impaired further with the use of orlistat. Supplementation may be required.

Patient and Family Education:

- Take a daily multivitamin containing fat-soluble vitamins at least 2 hours before or after orlistat.
- Adverse GI effects are common but typically resolve after 4 weeks of therapy.
- Avoid high-fat meals to minimize adverse GI effects. Distribute fat calories over three main meals daily. Do not skip meals.
- Monitor weight several times weekly. If diabetic, monitor blood glucose carefully following any weight loss.
- Expect that certain adverse effects can occur such as stomach discomfort, an increased number of stools, loss of control of defecation, gas released with bowel movements, oily stools, or the urgent desire to defecate.
- Increase physical activity as tolerated and approved by the health care provider.

- Provide the health care provider with a list of all drugs and supplements currently taken because orlistat can interact with other drugs and vitamins.
- Immediately notify the health care provider of any known or suspected pregnancy.

Drugs Similar to Orlistat (Alli, Xenical)

Orlistat is the only lipase inhibitor indicated for obesity.

63.7 Anorexiants are drugs used to induce weight loss by suppressing appetite and hunger.

A second strategy to reduce weight is to block parts of the nervous system responsible for recognizing and reacting to hunger. Currently, only four anorexiant products are approved as adjuncts for treating obesity. All of the anorexiants have the potential to produce serious adverse effects; thus their use is limited to short-term therapy. Like the lipase inhibitors, anorexiants are prescribed for patients with a BMI of at least 30 or greater, or a BMI of 27 or greater if the patient has other risk factors such as HTN, hyperlipidemia, or diabetes.

Lorcaserin (Belviq) is one of the newer anorexiants, approved in 2012, for weight loss when combined with a reduced-calorie diet and increased exercise. It is believed to act by activating serotonin receptors in the hypothalamus, causing increased satiety. If a 5% weight loss has not occurred after 12 weeks of therapy, it is recommended that the drug be discontinued. Safety and effectiveness in patients younger than 18 has not been established. Lorcaserin does produce euphoria in some patients; thus it has some potential for abuse. This drug is contraindicated during pregnancy because the benefits of weight loss do not outweigh the potential risks to the fetus.

In 2014, the FDA approved Contrave, a combination of bupropion and naltrexone for the short-term pharmacotherapy of obesity. Bupropion was previously approved as an atypical antidepressant and naltrexone as an opioid agonist. The combination reduces appetite by increasing dopamine activity and blocking opioid receptors in the brain. Contrave should be discontinued in four months if a weight loss of less than 5% is observed. The drug carries a black box warning that it may cause suicidal behavior. It is pregnancy category X.

Although phentermine was initially approved in 1959 and was part of the now-discontinued Fen-Phen combination, it is still available as monotherapy and in combination with topiramate.

Phentermine (Adipex-P, Suprenza) and phentermine with topiramate (Qsymia) are PO drugs approved only for the short-term treatment of obesity. Topiramate is a drug previously approved to treat epilepsy (see Chapter 22). These drugs should be used with a reduced-calorie diet and increased physical activity. Phentermine is structurally similar to amphetamine and is a Schedule IV controlled substance. Nervous system adverse effects include nervousness, insomnia, and tremors. Caution should be used in treating patients with HTN or diabetes. Abuse of phentermine can cause dependence and psychoses. Both phentermine products are pregnancy category X.

The final FDA-approved appetite suppressant is diethylpropion (Tepanil), which is structurally similar to amphetamine and has similar pharmacologic effects. It acts by increasing the levels of norepinephrine in regions of the brain regulating appetite. Given orally, its use is limited to 12 weeks of therapy because tolerance develops rapidly to the anorexiant effects of the drug. If the patient has not lost at least 4 lb after the first month of therapy, treatment should be discontinued. Nervous system adverse effects include confusion, agitation, nervousness, insomnia, and tremors. Pulmonary HTN is a rare, though potentially fatal adverse effect. The drug may worsen HTN or cause dysrhythmias. Diethylpropion is a Schedule IV drug and is pregnancy category B.

CONNECTION Checkpoint 63.3

Orlistat may decrease the absorption of fat-soluble vitamins. From what you learned in Chapter 61, describe the types of effects that could result from deficiencies in the fat-soluble vitamins A and D. *See Answer to Connection Checkpoint 63.3 on student resource website.*

Adjuncts to Obesity Therapy

63.8 Artificial sweeteners and fat substitutes are sometimes used as adjuncts to weight management programs.

A primary component of any weight management program is reduction of caloric intake. In an attempt to reduce total calories, many people have turned to artificial sweeteners and fat substitutes.

Artificial sweeteners include saccharin (Sweet'N Low®, Sugar-Twin®), aspartame (NutraSweet®, Equal®), acesulfame (ACK, Sweet One®, Sunett®), and sucralose (Splenda®). These agents are 200 to 600 times sweeter than table sugar, or sucrose, and thus less quantity is needed for sweetening food and beverages. Artificial sweeteners are regulated by the FDA because they are classified as food additives. Safety studies suggest that these substances are safe when used in usual amounts. Consumers should be aware that "sugar-free" foods that contain artificial sweeteners may have just as many calories and have a higher fat content than regular foods. Patients who have diabetes or are pregnant should consult with their health care providers before consuming artificial sweeteners.

Stevia (Truvia) is a genus of a plant in the sunflower family from which natural sweeteners are extracted. More than 30 times sweeter than sucrose, stevia is recognized by the FDA as a dietary supplement, not as a food additive. It has gained wide acceptance as an artificial sweetener in the United States. Stevia has a bitter taste when used in large amounts. Safety concerns have caused it to be banned in several countries.

Fats give food a smooth texture as well as calories. It is easy to identify fat-free or low-fat foods because they generally lack the taste and feel of normal fat. Fat substitutes attempt to simulate the feel of normal fat without the calories or effects of raising lipid levels in the blood. Olestra is a popular fat substitute that consists of a sucrose molecule surrounded by fatty acids. It has the appeal of fat but passes through the digestive tract undigested. It offers zero calories and zero fat but has the unpleasant adverse effects of loose stools and anal leakage. It is primarily restricted to use in snack foods. Simplesse® is a second fat substitute. It is derived from natural whey protein and is used in baked goods and dairy products. Many other products are under development.

Do artificial sweeteners and fat substitutes actually help patients who are obese lose weight? The answer depends on the dietary habits of the consumer. Certainly, drinking a liter of a regular soft drink gives one many more calories than drinking the same amount of a diet soft drink. Likewise, eating 8 ounces of potato chips using olestra gives fewer calories and fat than eating 8 ounces of regular chips. However, patients with serious weight problems should probably make better food choices than soft drinks and chips. A few studies have suggested that the body compensates by craving sucrose and high-fat meals. It should be remembered that the FDA has only evaluated these food additives for safety, not for their effectiveness in maintaining or losing body weight. Just as there are no miracle pills for weight loss, there are no miracle foods that will promote weight loss. The answer lies in the simple rules of limiting calorie intake, proper nutrition, and exercise.

CHAPTER 63

Understanding the Chapter

Key Concepts Summary

63.1 Genetic and lifestyle factors contribute to the etiology of obesity.

63.2 Appetite is regulated by the satiety center in the hypothalamus and is influenced by various hormones.

63.3 Obesity is measured by using the body mass index and waist circumference.

63.4 Nonpharmacologic treatment of obesity should be attempted prior to initiating pharmacotherapy.

63.5 Drugs used for weight management affect appetite or the absorption of fats.

63.6 Lipase inhibitors cause weight loss by interfering with the absorption of fats.

63.7 Anorexiants are drugs used to induce weight loss by suppressing appetite and hunger.

63.8 Artificial sweeteners and fat substitutes are sometimes used as adjuncts to weight management programs.

Case Study: Making the Patient Connection

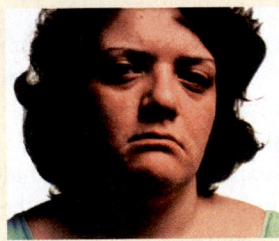

Remember the patient "Rosemary Goodman" at the beginning of this chapter? Now read the remainder of the case study. Based on the information presented within this chapter, respond to the critical thinking questions that follow.

Rosemary, a 55-year-old female, has just had her annual physical examination with the nurse practitioner. She was shocked to learn that she has gained just under 13.6 kg (30 lb) since her office visit 2 years ago, 7.7 kg (17 lb) in the last year alone. She went through menopause 2 years ago and thought that some of the mild edema and resulting weight gain she used to experience around the time of her menses was over. Rosemary has always been under or at normal weight except for the last office visit. At the time she was going through a personally stressful time and was not concerned about the weight gain. She works in an office as a financial manager, spending most of her day at her desk. Although she tries to get out for a lunchtime walk, most days, there is just too much to do in the office.

The rest of her physical was unremarkable except for a borderline hypertensive reading on her blood pressure of 138/82 mmHg. Her height is 1.6 meters (5 ft 6 in.), and she now weighs 79.5 kg (175 lb). She states that she "watches what she eats" and normally eats three meals per day: a hurried breakfast of "something from the local fast-food place" on the drive to work, a sandwich at her desk or "whatever the rest of the office is ordering for take-out" for lunch, and a "regular dinner" at home at night with her husband. On the evenings when her husband is not home for dinner, Rosemary picks up something at the local supermarket from the prepared food aisle. She also enjoys a glass of wine with dinner. When the nurse and Rosemary add up the approximate number of calories she consumes, the average total is over 2,000 per day. Rosemary is upset and asks the nurse about weight loss strategies.

Critical Thinking Questions

1. Rosemary asks about diet pills because her mother used to take them on occasion. What would you tell her about the availability of these drugs today?

2. Rosemary would like to try orlistat (Alli), which she has noticed on the shelf in the supermarket. What does Rosemary need to know about orlistat before deciding to take it? What teaching does she need about taking orlistat?

3. What factors have contributed to Rosemary's weight gain over the past 2 years? What general health teaching would be appropriate for Rosemary to aid her in her weight reduction?

See Answers to Critical Thinking Questions on student resource website.

Additional Case Study

Kathryn is a 52-year-old woman who has been grossly overweight for more than 15 years. In that time she has tried many diets, exercise regimens, diet clubs, and drug therapies but all to no avail. She weighs 143 kg (315 lb) and has a BMI of 48. Her health care provider has prescribed orlistat (Xenical). She informs you that she has tried diet pills in the past. She has heard that amphetamines cause people terrible problems and is fearful that she will become dependent on orlistat or experience serious complications.

1. How would you address Kathryn's fears about diet drugs and the use of orlistat (Xenical)?

2. How is prescription strength orlistat different from the OTC dosage? What adverse effects may occur at the higher dosage?

3. What effect does orlistat have on vitamin absorption? If Kathryn's provider prescribes a multivitamin, what should Kathryn know about taking it?

See Answers to Additional Case Study on student resource website.

Chapter Review

1 A patient is prescribed lorcaserin (Belviq) for the treatment of obesity and is concerned about the risks involved with the drug. Which of the following should the nurse include when teaching this patient?

1. If less than a 5% weight loss has been achieved after 3 months, a different weight loss regimen may be needed.

2. There is no need to worry about any long-term effects if they do not occur when the drug is taken.

3. Begin to see a cardiologist monthly until any cardiovascular risk has been ruled out.

4. Contact the drug company about follow-up programs.

2 A patient asks the provider about a prescription for phentermine (Adipex-P) for obesity. Which of the following would be considered a contraindication for the use of this drug?

1. Extreme obesity

2. A history of type 2 diabetes managed with oral antidiabetic drugs

3. A history of hypertension managed with beta blockers

4. Pregnancy

3 The patient has been started on orlistat (Xenical). The nurse would teach this patient to take this medication:

1. Once in the morning.

2. When a feeling of hunger is noticed.

3. Before daily exercise.

4. Just prior to each meal containing fats.

4 While taking orlistat (Alli), the nurse would instruct the patient to do which of the following?

1. Drink at least 2 to 3 liters of diet soda per day.

2. Always wear sunscreen when outdoors or when exposed to direct sunlight.

3. Rise slowly from a sitting or supine position.

4. Take a daily vitamin supplement containing fat-soluble vitamins.

5 A nurse is instructing a patient taking orlistat (Xenical) about adverse effects of the medication. Which symptoms indicate the presence of an expected adverse effect?

1. Flatus with discharge and oily stool

2. Heartburn and dyspepsia

3. Constipation with fecal impaction

4. Nausea with projectile vomiting

6 Which of the following measures is used to assess the presence of obesity? Select all that apply.

1. Body weight

2. Body mass index

3. Waist circumference

4. Treadmill test

5. Buoyancy analysis

See Answers to Chapter Review in Appendix A.

References

Centers for Disease Control and Prevention. (2013). *Overweight and obesity*. Retrieved from http://www.cdc.gov/obesity/data/adult .html

Gregg, E. W., Li, Y., Wang, J., Burrows, N. R., Ali, M. K., Rolka, D.,... Geiss, L. (2014). Changes in diabetes-related complications in the United States, 1990–2010. *The New England Journal of Medicine, 370*, 1514–1523. doi:10.1056/NEJMoa1310799

Grove, K. A., & Lambert, J. D. (2010). Laboratory, epidemiological, and human intervention studies show that tea (*Camellia sinensis*) may be useful in the prevention of obesity. *The Journal of Nutrition, 140*, 446–453. doi:10.3945/ jn.109.115972

Jurgens, T. M., Whelan, A. M., Killian, L., Doucette, S., Kirk, S., & Foy, E. (2012). Green tea for weight loss and weight maintenance in overweight or obese adults. *Cochrane Database of Systematic Reviews, 12*, CD008650. doi:10.1002/14651858.CD008650.pub2

Katout, M., Zhu, H., Rutsky, J., Shah, P., Brook, R. D., Zhong, J., & Rajagopalan, S. (2014). Effects of GLP-1 mimetics on blood pressure and relationship to weight loss and glycemic lowering: Results of a systematic meta-analysis and meta-regression. *American Journal of Hypertension, 27*, 130–139. doi:10.1093/ajh/hpt196

National Center for Health Statistics. (2012). *Prevalence of overweight, obesity, and extreme obesity among adults: United States, trends 1960–1962 through 2009–2010*. Retrieved from http:// www.cdc.gov/nchs/data/hestat/obesity_ adult_09_10/obesity_adult_09_10.pdf

National Institutes of Health, National Heart, Lung, and Blood Institute. (1998). *Clinical guidelines on the identification, evaluation, and treatment of overweight and obesity in adults: The evidence report* (p. xvii). Washington, DC: Author. Retrieved from http://www .nhlbi.nih.gov/guidelines/obesity/ob_gdlns .htm

Ottney, A. (2013). Glucagon-like peptide-1 receptor agonists for weight loss in adult patients without diabetes. *American Journal of Health-System Pharmacy, 70*, 2097–2103. doi:10.2146/ajhp130081

Torekov, S. S., Madsbad, S., & Holst, J. J. (2011). Obesity—an indication for GLP-1 treatment? Obesity pathophysiology and GLP-1 treatment potential. *Obesity Reviews, 12*(8), 593–601. doi:10.1111/j.1467-789X.2011.00860.x

Selected Bibliography

Clark, A., Franklin, J., Pratt, I., & McGrice, M. (2010). Overweight and obesity: Use of portion control in management. *Australian Family Physician, 39*(6), 407–411. Retrieved from http://www.racgp.org.au/afp/201006/ 37655

Derosa, G., & Maffioli, P. (2012). Anti-obesity drugs: A review about their effects and their safety. *Expert Opinion on Drug Safety, 11*, 459–471. doi:10.1517/14740338.2012.675326

Greenway, F. L., & Bray, G. A. (2010). Combination drugs for treating obesity. *Current Diabetes Reports, 10*, 108–115. doi:10.1007/ s11892-010-0096-4

Halford, J. C., Boyland, E. J., Blundell, J. E., Kirkham, T. C., & Harrold, A. (2010). Pharmacological management of appetite expression in obesity. *Nature Reviews Endocrinology, 6*, 255–269. doi:10.1038/nrendo.2010.19

Jensen, M. D., Ryan, D. H., Hu, F. B., Stevens, F. J., Hubbard, V. S., Stevens, V. J., . . . Yanovski, S. Z. (2013). *2013 AHA/ACC/TOS guideline for the management of overweight and obesity in adults*. Retrieved from http://circ .ahajournals.org/content/early/2013/11/11/01 .cir.0000437739.71477.ee.full.pdf+html

Kang, J. G., & Park, C. Y. (2012). Anti-obesity drugs: A review about their effects and safety. *Diabetes & Metabolism Journal, 36*, 13–25. doi:10.4093/dmj.2012.36.1.13

Kaplan, L. M. (2010). Pharmacologic therapies for obesity. *Gastroenterology Clinics of North America, 39*, 69–79. doi:10.1016/ j.gtc.2010.01.001

Powell, A. G., Apovian, C. M., & Aronne, L. J. (2011). New drug targets for the treatment of obesity. *Clinical Pharmacology & Therapeutics, 90*, 40–51. doi:10.1038/clpt.2011.82

Schwarz, S. (2011). *Obesity in children*. Retrieved from http://emedicine.medscape.com/article/ 985333-overview

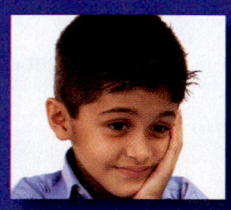
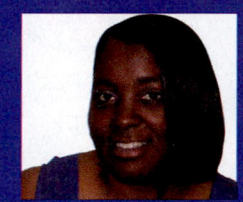
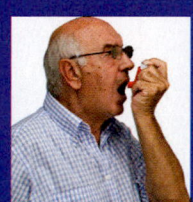
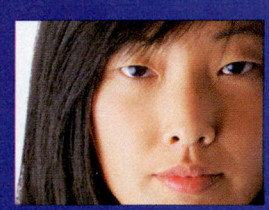

CHAPTER 64   Review of the Endocrine System / 1090

CHAPTER 65   Hypothalamic and Pituitary Drugs / 1096

CHAPTER 66   Pharmacotherapy of Diabetes Mellitus / 1111

CHAPTER 67   Pharmacotherapy of Thyroid Disorders / 1137

CHAPTER 68   Corticosteroids and Drugs Affecting the Adrenal Cortex / 1151

CHAPTER 69   Estrogens, Progestins, and Drugs Modifying Uterine Function / 1166

CHAPTER 70   Drugs for Modifying Conception / 1189

CHAPTER 71   Drugs for Disorders and Conditions of the Male Reproductive System / 1208

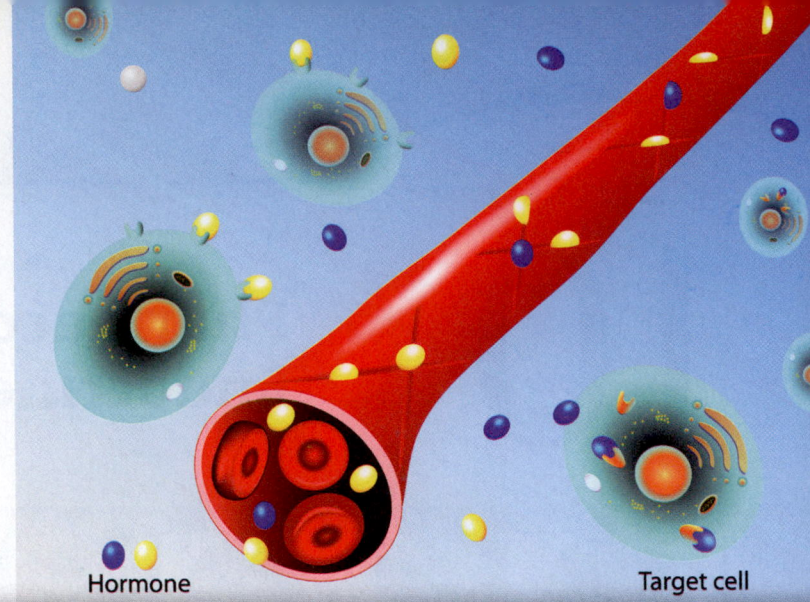

Hormone

Target cell

CHAPTER

64

Review of the Endocrine System

LEARNING OUTCOMES

After reading this chapter, the student should be able to:

1. Describe the general structure and functions of the endocrine system.

2. Compare and contrast the nervous and endocrine systems in the control of homeostasis.

3. Explain circumstances in which hormone receptors may be up-regulated or down-regulated.

4. Through the use of a specific example, explain the concept of negative feedback in the endocrine system.

5. Explain the three primary types of stimuli that regulate hormone secretion.

6. Identify indications for hormone pharmacotherapy.

CHAPTER OUTLINE

▸ Overview of the Endocrine System

▸ Hormone Receptors

▸ Negative Feedback Mechanisms

▸ Hormone Pharmacotherapy

KEY TERMS

down-regulation, 1091

endocrine system, 1091

hormones, 1091

negative feedback, 1091

replacement therapy, 1093

target cells, 1091

up-regulation, 1091

Like the nervous system, the endocrine system is a major controller of homeostasis. Whereas a nerve exerts instantaneous control over a single muscle fiber or gland, a hormone from the endocrine system may affect all body cells and take as long as several days to produce an optimum response. Hormonal balance is kept within a narrow range: Too little or too much of a hormone may produce profound physiological changes. This chapter reviews endocrine anatomy and physiology and its relevance to pharmacotherapy. For a more detailed review of the endocrine system, the student should refer to an anatomy and physiology textbook.

Overview of the Endocrine System

64.1 The endocrine system controls homeostasis through the secretion of hormones.

The **endocrine system** consists of various glands that secrete **hormones**, chemical messengers that the body releases in response to a change in the body's internal environment. The role of hormones is to maintain homeostasis in the body. For example, when the level of glucose in the blood rises above normal, the pancreas secretes insulin to return glucose levels to normal. The various endocrine glands and their hormones are illustrated in Figure 64.1.

After secretion from an endocrine gland, hormones enter the blood and are transported throughout the body. Compared to the nervous system, which reacts to body changes within milliseconds, the endocrine system responds relatively slowly. A few hormones, such as epinephrine, act within seconds, whereas others, such as testosterone, may take several days or even months to produce noticeable changes. Although slower in onset, the effects of hormones have a longer duration than those of the nervous system.

Hormone Receptors

64.2 Hormones must bind to specific receptors to cause physiological changes.

The cells affected by a hormone are called its target cells. **Target cells** have specific protein receptors on their plasma membrane that bind to the hormone. For some hormones, the receptors are in the cytoplasm or nucleus of the target cell. Once binding occurs, a change is produced in the cell, resulting in an action that is characteristic for the hormone. For example, when epinephrine binds to receptors on smooth muscle cells, they contract. When prolactin binds to secretory cells in the breast, milk production occurs.

Although a hormone travels throughout the body via the circulation, it only affects cells that have receptors for that specific hormone. Epinephrine does not affect breast secretory cells, because these cells have no epinephrine receptors. Prolactin does not cause muscular contraction because smooth muscle cells do not have prolactin receptors. This concept is illustrated in Figure 64.2.

In some cases, the target cells for a hormone are limited and specific. For example, the only receptors for thyroid-stimulating hormone are in the thyroid gland. However, some hormones, such as insulin and cortisol, have receptors on nearly every cell in the body; thus, these hormones have widespread effects.

The number of protein receptors for a hormone is dynamic and changes with the needs of the body. Cells can create more receptors on their plasma membrane to capture hormone molecules as they pass by, a process called **up-regulation**. This may occur if the cell is receiving signals that a hormone action is needed, such as the need for production of more breast milk or additional secretion of thyroid hormone. Once the hormone is up-regulated (secreted in large quantities), the cell no longer needs to capture every hormone molecule so it makes fewer receptors on its surface, a process called **down-regulation**. Receptors are very efficient at capturing hormone molecules; although most hormones are secreted only in small amounts, they produce profound changes.

Down-regulation has important implications for pharmacotherapy. When a hormone is administered as pharmacotherapy for long periods, the body recognizes an abundance of the hormone, and cells will down-regulate the number of receptors for that hormone. This causes a desensitization of the target cells; that is, they are less responsive to the effects of the hormone. When therapy is discontinued, the cells will need time, usually several days, to synthesize more protein receptors and adjust to the new hormone level.

It is important to understand that the amount of hormone secreted by an endocrine gland is only partially responsible for the therapeutic response. Other critical components include the number of receptors and their sensitivity. During pharmacotherapy, increasing the dose of a hormone will produce little additional pharmacologic effect if all the receptors are already occupied, or if they are no longer sensitive to the hormone.

Negative Feedback Mechanisms

64.3 Most hormone action is regulated through negative feedback.

Because hormones can produce profound effects on the body, their secretion and release is carefully regulated by several levels of control. The most important mechanism is **negative feedback**, which is illustrated in Figure 64.3. A hormone causes an output or action in its target cell or tissue. As the levels of hormone rise, so does its action. The increased output or action is monitored by sensors. Once homeostasis is restored, the sensor signals the endocrine tissue to stop secreting the hormone; that is, the target tissue provides negative feedback.

Depending on the specific hormone, the negative feedback mechanism may be based on three primary types of stimuli: neuronal, humoral, and hormonal. In some cases, regulation involves multiple stimuli. The various hormones and their regulation are summarized in Table 64.1.

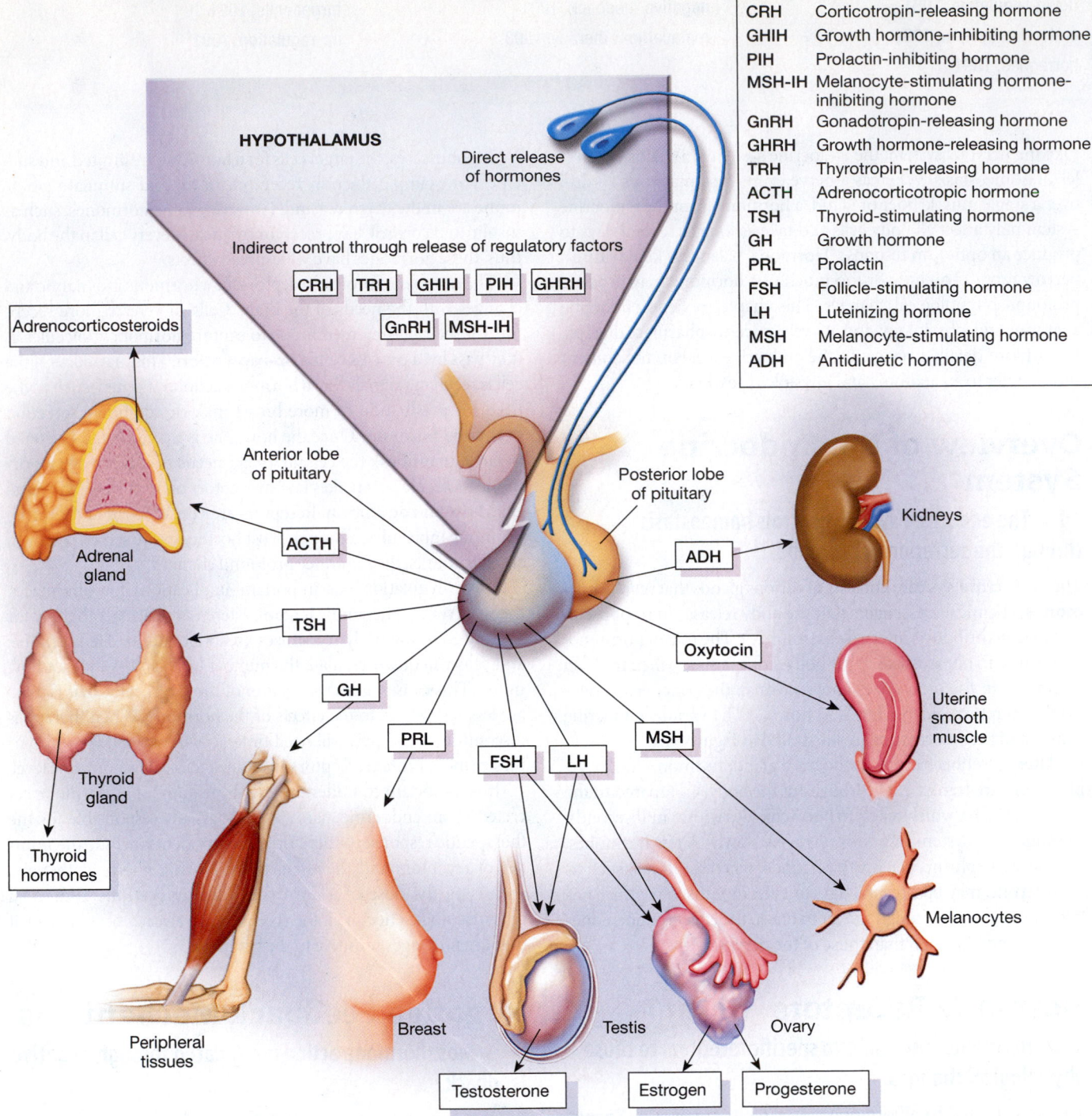

CRH	Corticotropin-releasing hormone
GHIH	Growth hormone-inhibiting hormone
PIH	Prolactin-inhibiting hormone
MSH-IH	Melanocyte-stimulating hormone-inhibiting hormone
GnRH	Gonadotropin-releasing hormone
GHRH	Growth hormone-releasing hormone
TRH	Thyrotropin-releasing hormone
ACTH	Adrenocorticotropic hormone
TSH	Thyroid-stimulating hormone
GH	Growth hormone
PRL	Prolactin
FSH	Follicle-stimulating hormone
LH	Luteinizing hormone
MSH	Melanocyte-stimulating hormone
ADH	Antidiuretic hormone

Figure 64.1 Hormones and the endocrine system.

Neuronal stimuli: A few hormones are regulated by nerve impulses. The best example is epinephrine, which is released when a neuronal impulse from the sympathetic nervous system reaches the adrenal medulla. Another example is the release of oxytocin from the pituitary gland.

Humoral stimuli: Some endocrine glands sense the levels of specific substances in the blood and release the hormone when the substance rises above or falls below the normal range. For example, pancreatic islet cells can sense the level of glucose in the blood. If glucose levels become too high, insulin is secreted. Another example is the release of parathyroid hormone when blood calcium levels fall.

Hormonal stimuli: In the endocrine system, it is common for one hormone to control the secretion of another hormone. In some cases, the sequence involves three hormones. For example, thyrotropin-releasing hormone (TRH, from the hypothalamus) stimulates thyroid-stimulating hormone (TSH, from the pituitary), which causes the release of thyroid hormone (TH, from the thyroid gland). In a loop typical of the endocrine system, the

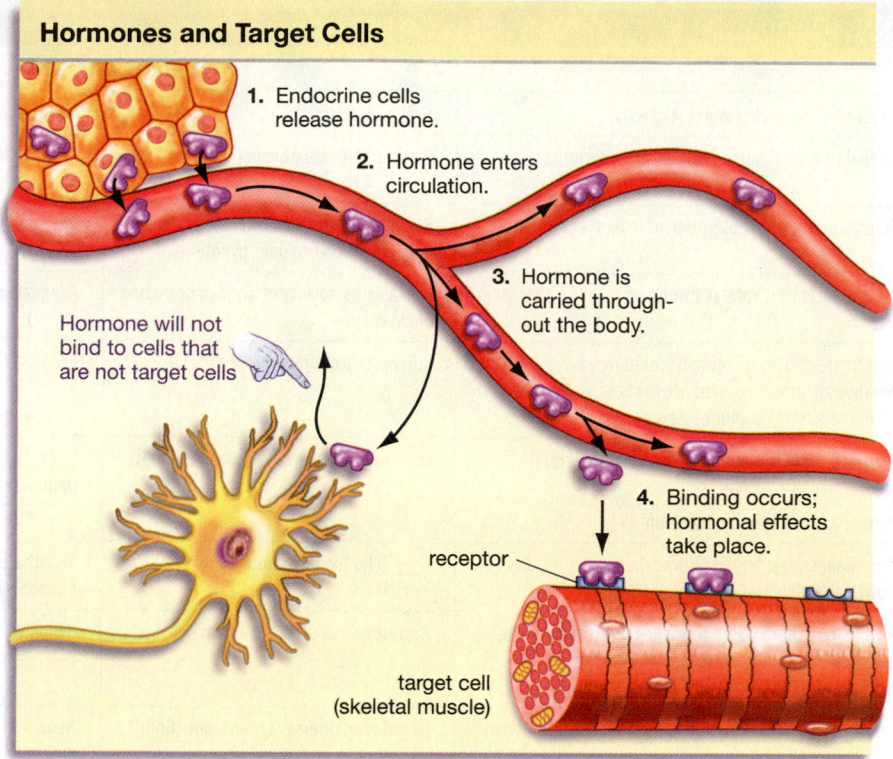

Hormones and Target Cells

1. Endocrine cells release hormone.

2. Hormone enters circulation.

3. Hormone is carried throughout the body.

Hormone will not bind to cells that are not target cells

4. Binding occurs; hormonal effects take place.

receptor

target cell (skeletal muscle)

Figure 64.2 Hormones and their target cells.

From *Biology: A Guide to the Natural World,* 5th ed., by D. Krogh, 2011. Reprinted and electronically reproduced by permission of Pearson Education, Inc., Upper Saddle River, New Jersey.

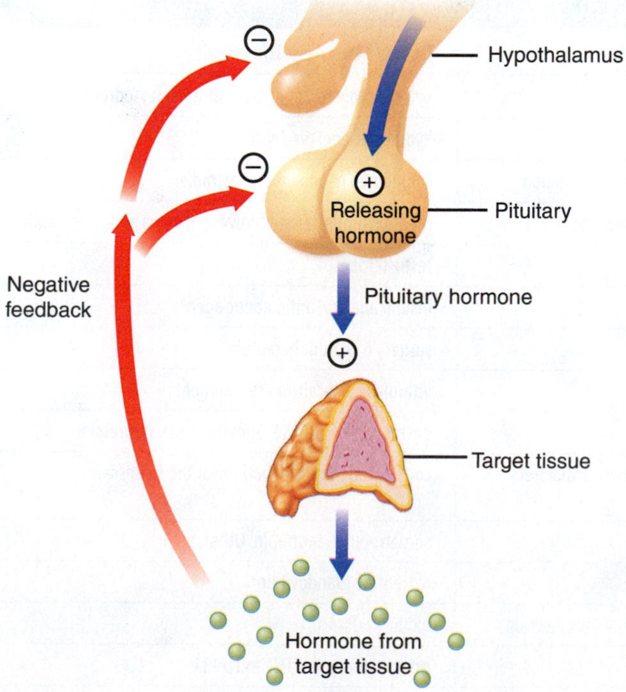

Hypothalamus

Releasing hormone — Pituitary

Pituitary hormone

Negative feedback

Target tissue

Hormone from target tissue

Figure 64.3 Negative feedback mechanism.

last hormone in the pathway (TH) provides negative feedback to shut off secretion of the initial hormone (TRH).

CONNECTION Checkpoint 64.1

From what you learned in Chapter 15, identify indications for epinephrine pharmacotherapy. *See Answer to Connection Checkpoint 64.1 on student resource website.*

Hormone Pharmacotherapy

64.4 Hormone pharmacotherapy is indicated for a diverse variety of conditions.

The goals of hormone pharmacotherapy vary widely. In many cases, a hormone is administered as **replacement therapy** for patients who are unable to secrete sufficient quantities of their own endogenous hormones. Examples of replacement therapy include the administration of thyroid hormone after the thyroid gland has been surgically removed, supplying insulin to patients whose pancreas is not functioning, or administering growth hormone to children with short-stature disorder. The pharmacologic goal of replacement therapy is to supply the same physiological, low-level amounts of the hormone that would normally be present in the body. Selected endocrine disorders and their drug therapy are summarized in Table 64.2.

Some hormones are used in cancer chemotherapy to shrink the size of hormone-sensitive tumors. For example, certain breast cancers are strongly dependent on estrogen for their growth. Giving the "opposite" hormone, testosterone, will shrink the

TABLE 64.1   Selected Hormones and Their Regulation

Hormone	Target Organ(s) and Action	REGULATION Stimulation	REGULATION Inhibition
Adrenocorticotropic hormone (ACTH)	Adrenal cortex: stimulates release of glucocorticoids	Corticotropin-releasing hormone	Negative feedback from corticosteroids
Aldosterone	Kidneys: promotes reabsorption of sodium and water	Renin-angiotensin-aldosterone pathway, decreased blood volume, hypotension	Increased blood volume or hypertension
Antidiuretic hormone (ADH)	Kidneys: increases water reabsorption	Increased osmolarity of blood or decreased blood volume	Adequate hydration
Corticosteroids (glucocorticoids)	Most tissues: increases protein breakdown and glucose metabolism, provides resistance to stress, suppresses inflammation and immune response	Adrenocorticotropic hormone (ACTH)	Negative feedback from corticosteroids
Follicle-stimulating hormone (FSH)	Ovaries: promotes maturation of ovarian follicles and estrogen production Testes: increases sperm production	Gonadotropin-releasing hormone (GnRH)	Negative feedback from estrogen (females) or testosterone (males)
Growth hormone (GH)	Most tissues: including bone, muscle, liver: stimulates growth and mobilizes lipids	Growth hormone-releasing hormone (GHRH)	Negative feedback from GH or growth hormone-inhibiting hormone (GHIH)
Insulin	Most tissues: promotes movement of glucose into cells, lowers blood glucose, decreases glycogen synthesis, and increases lipogenesis and protein synthesis	Hyperglycemia	Hypoglycemia
Luteinizing hormone (LH)	Ovaries: stimulates ovulation and production of estrogen Testes: produces testosterone	Gonadotropin-releasing hormone (GnRH)	Negative feedback from estrogen and progesterone (females) or testosterone (males)
Oxytocin	Uterus: stimulates contractions Breasts: ejects milk	Stretching of uterus or infant suckling	Lack of stretching of the uterus or discontinuation of breast-feeding
Parathyroid hormone	Kidneys, gastrointestinal tract, bone: increases calcium levels in blood	Hypocalcemia	Hypercalcemia
Prolactin	Breasts: promotes lactation	Prolactin-releasing hormone	Prolactin-inhibiting hormone
Thyroid hormone	Most tissues: increases basal metabolic rate and growth	Thyroid-stimulating hormone	Negative feedback from thyroid hormone

TABLE 64.2   Selected Endocrine Disorders and Their Pharmacotherapy

Gland	Hormone(s)	Disorder	Drug Therapy Examples
Adrenal cortex	Corticosteroids	Hypersecretion: Cushing's syndrome	ketoconazole (Nizoral) and mitotane (Lysodren)
		Hyposecretion: Addison's disease	hydrocortisone, prednisone
Gonads	Ovaries: estrogen	Hyposecretion: menstrual and metabolic dysfunction	conjugated estrogens and estradiol
	Ovaries: progesterone	Hyposecretion: dysfunctional uterine bleeding	medroxyprogesterone (Provera, Others) and norethindrone
	Testes: testosterone	Hyposecretion: hypogonadism	testosterone
Pancreatic islets	Insulin	Hyposecretion: diabetes mellitus	insulin and oral antidiabetic agents
Parathyroid	Parathyroid hormone	Hypersecretion: hyperparathyroidism	surgery (no drug therapy)
		Hyposecretion: hypoparathyroidism	vitamin D and calcium supplements
Pituitary	Antidiuretic hormone	Hyposecretion: diabetes insipidus	desmopressin (DDAVP, Stimate) and vasopressin
		Hypersecretion: syndrome of inappropriate antidiuretic hormone (SIADH)	conivaptan (Vaprisol) and tolvaptan (Samsca)
	Growth hormone	Hyposecretion: small stature	somatropin (Genotropin, Others)
		Hypersecretion: acromegaly (adults)	octreotide (Sandostatin)
	Oxytocin	Hyposecretion: delayed delivery or lack of milk ejection	oxytocin (Pitocin)
Thyroid	Thyroid hormone (T_3 and T_4)	Hypersecretion: Graves' disease	propylthiouracil (PTU) and I-131
		Hyposecretion: myxedema (adults), cretinism (children)	thyroid hormone and levothyroxine (T4)

tumor. In a similar manner, estrogen is used to shrink the size of testicular cancer, which is dependent on testosterone for its growth. Exactly how these hormones produce their antineoplastic action is largely unknown. When hormones are used as antineoplastics, their doses far exceed physiological levels normally present in the body. Hormones are nearly always used in combination with other antineoplastic medications.

Another goal of hormonal pharmacotherapy may be to produce an exaggerated response that is part of the normal action of the hormone. Administering hydrocortisone to suppress inflammation takes advantage of the normal action of the corticosteroids but at higher amounts than would normally be present in the body. Hydrocortisone is indicated for acute inflammatory disorders such as lupus or rheumatoid arthritis. As another example, supplying estrogen or progesterone at specific times during the uterine cycle can prevent ovulation and pregnancy. In this example, the patient is given natural hormones; however, they are taken at a time when levels in the body are normally low.

Endocrine pharmacotherapy also involves the use of "antihormones." These hormone antagonists block the actions of endogenous hormones. For example, propylthiouracil (PTU) is given to block the effects of an overactive thyroid gland. Tamoxifen is given to block the actions of estrogen in estrogen receptor–dependent breast cancers (see Chapter 57).

CONNECTION Checkpoint 64.2

Glucocorticoids, or corticosteroids, are important drugs in treating inflammation. From what you learned in Chapter 42, explain their role in treating autoimmune disease. *See Answer to Connection Checkpoint 64.2 on student resource website.*

CHAPTER 64

Understanding the Chapter

Key Concepts Summary

64.1 The endocrine system controls homeostasis through the secretion of hormones.

64.2 Hormones must bind to specific receptors to cause physiological changes.

64.3 Most hormone action is regulated through negative feedback.

64.4 Hormone pharmacotherapy is indicated for a diverse variety of conditions.

References

Krogh, D. (2011). *Biology: A guide to the natural world* (5th ed.). San Francisco, CA: Benjamin Cummings.

Selected Bibliography

Colbert, J. B., Ankney, J., & Lee, K. T. (2011). *Anatomy and physiology for health professionals: An interactive journey* (2nd ed.). Upper Saddle River, NJ: Pearson Education.

Greenstein, B., & Wood, D. (2011). *The endocrine system at a glance* (3rd ed.). Malden, MA: Wiley-Blackwell.

Marieb, E. N., & Hoehn, K. (2014). *Human anatomy and physiology* (9th ed.). San Francisco, CA: Benjamin Cummings.

Martini, F. H., Nath, J. L., & Bartholomew, E. F. (2014). *Fundamentals of human anatomy and physiology* (10th ed.). San Francisco, CA: Benjamin Cummings.

Molina, P. (2013). *Endocrine physiology,* (4th ed.). McGraw Hill Medical: Blacklick, OH.

Silverthorn, D. U. (2012). *Human physiology: An integrated approach* (6th ed.). San Francisco, CA: Benjamin Cummings.

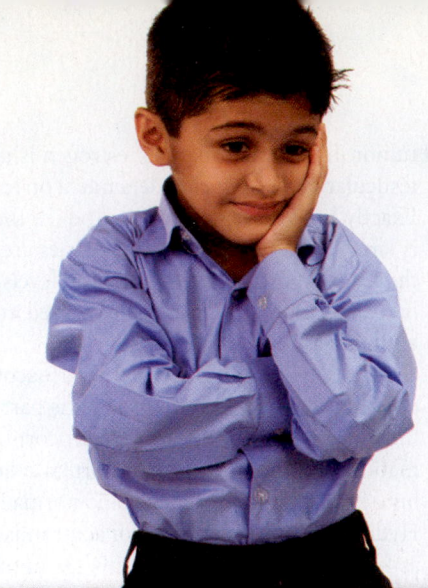

"I'm really worried about Raj. He's always been small for his age, and today the pediatrician told me he is only at the 5th percentile for height and weight for his age. The doctor is referring us to a pediatric endocrinologist. Could it be something serious?"

"Jasdeep Singh," mother of 8-year-old patient "Raj"

65 Hypothalamic and Pituitary Drugs

LEARNING OUTCOMES

After reading this chapter, the student should be able to:

1. Explain the principal actions of the hormones secreted by the hypothalamus and pituitary gland.

2. Identify indications for hypothalamic hormone therapy.

3. Explain the pharmacotherapy of growth hormone disorders in children and adults.

4. Explain the pharmacotherapy of antidiuretic hormone disorders.

5. For each of the classes shown in the chapter outline, identify the prototype and representative drugs and explain the mechanism(s) of drug action, primary indications, contraindications, significant drug interactions, pregnancy category, and important adverse effects.

6. Apply the nursing process to the care of patients receiving pharmacotherapy for disorders of the hypothalamus and pituitary gland.

CHAPTER OUTLINE

▶ **Functions of the Hypothalamus**

▶ **Functions of the Pituitary Gland**

▶ **Pharmacotherapy of Growth Hormone Disorders**

Growth Hormone Analogs

PROTOTYPE Somatropin (Genotropin, Humatrope, Norditropin, Nutropin, Saizen, Serostim, Zorbtive), *p. 1099*

Growth Hormone Antagonists

PROTOTYPE Octreotide (Sandostatin), *p. 1102*

▶ **Pharmacotherapy of Antidiuretic Hormone Disorders**

PROTOTYPE Desmopressin (DDAVP), *p. 1106*

KEY TERMS

acromegaly, 1102

anterior pituitary gland, 1098

antidiuretic hormone (ADH), 1103

diabetes insipidus (DI), 1105

dwarfism, 1098

gigantism, 1102

growth hormone (GH), 1098

insulin-like growth factor (IGF), 1098

posterior pituitary gland, 1098

short stature, 1099

syndrome of inappropriate antidiuretic hormone (SIADH), 1105

tropic hormones, 1098

In the specialty of endocrinology, understanding the complex relationship between the hypothalamus and pituitary gland is important because these organs regulate so many homeostatic functions. The two collaborate to secrete hormones that control functions of the gonads, adrenal glands, thyroid gland, kidneys, and the milk-producing tissues of the breast. The functioning of these two glands serves as the control center that provides integration between the nervous and endocrine systems. This chapter examines drugs that directly affect the functions of the pituitary and hypothalamus.

Functions of the Hypothalamus

65.1 The hypothalamus controls many diverse body processes and secretes hormones that influence pituitary function.

Roughly the size of an almond, the hypothalamus lies in the center of the diencephalon of the brain, just superior to the brainstem. The general purpose of the hypothalamus is to maintain homeostasis. To achieve this, the hypothalamus receives input from numerous vital regions of the nervous system, recognizes imbalances, and makes adjustments to bring the body back to homeostasis. Examples of the multiple and diverse functions of this organ include control of body temperature, thirst, appetite, fatigue, circadian rhythms, anger, and the rate of overall body metabolism. The hypothalamus also controls vital functions of the autonomic nervous system such as heart rate, vasoconstriction, digestion, and sweating. For the purposes of this chapter, only the endocrine functions of the hypothalamus are presented.

Every hormone has target cells that possess receptors for that specific hormone. For the hormones secreted by the hypothalamus, there is only one target organ: the pituitary gland. All hypothalamic hormones travel by the blood a short distance to the pituitary, which lies immediately below the hypothalamus. Upon reaching their receptors, the hypothalamic hormones simply increase or decrease the release of hormones by the pituitary gland. Because of this, hormones from the hypothalamus are called releasing hormones or inhibiting hormones. The major hypothalamic hormones and their actions on the pituitary gland are given in Table 65.1.

There are very few indications for the administration of hypothalamic hormones. Rather than give hypothalamic hormones, it is more effective (and less expensive) to administer pituitary hormones or the secretions of a target endocrine organ such as thyroid hormone, estrogen, testosterone, or corticosteroids.

The hypothalamic hormones that do have clinical applications are analogs or antagonists of gonadotropin-releasing hormone (GnRH). Initially the effect of the GnRH analogs is to increase the production of interstitial cell-stimulating hormone (in males) or follicle-stimulating hormone (in females), which increases the secretion of sex hormones. With continued therapy, however, the pituitary becomes insensitive to the effects of GnRH, and the production of sex hormones falls to near castration levels. Indications for these drugs include the following:

- Endometriosis, a common cause of female infertility (see Chapter 69)
- Central precocious puberty, the premature onset of puberty in children

TABLE 65.1	Hormones Secreted by the Hypothalamus and Pituitary Glands		
Hypothalamic Hormone	**Pituitary Hormone**	**Target Organ**	**Principal Actions**
Corticotropin-releasing hormone (CRH)	Adrenocorticotropic hormone (ACTH)	Adrenal cortex	Stimulates release of corticosteroids
Gonadotropin-releasing hormone (GnRH)	Follicle-stimulating hormone (FSH)	Ovaries, testes	Stimulates release of estrogen and ovarian follicle development in females, and sperm production in males
	Luteinizing hormone (LH)	Ovaries, testes	Triggers ovulation and secretion of estrogen and progesterone in females, increases testosterone secretion in males
Growth hormone-inhibiting hormone (GHIH) Growth hormone-releasing hormone (GHRH)	Growth hormone (GH)	Most body cells	Regulates growth and development of bones, muscles, cartilage, organs; general body metabolism
None	Melanocyte-stimulating hormone (MSH)	Skin	Stimulates pigmentation
Prolactin-inhibiting hormone (PIH) Prolactin-releasing hormone (PRH)	Prolactin	Mammary glands	Regulates lactation
Thyrotropin-releasing hormone (TRH)	Thyroid-stimulating hormone (TSH)	Thyroid gland	Stimulates release of thyroid hormone

- Palliative treatment of advanced prostate cancer
- Uterine leiomyomata, a benign tissue of smooth muscle sometimes called fibroids

GnRH analogs include goserelin (Zoladex), histrelin (Supprelin LA, Vantas), leuprolide (Eligard, Lupron, Viadur), nafarelin (Synarel), and triptorelin (Trelstar). GnRH antagonists include cetrorelix (Cetrotide), degarelix (Firmagon), and ganirelix. The effects of these drugs on the reproductive system are discussed in Chapter 69.

CONNECTION Checkpoint 65.1

Target tissues can up-regulate or down-regulate the number of receptors for a specific hormone. From what you learned in Chapter 64, which of the two occurs when a hormone is administered as pharmacotherapy for long periods? *See Answer to Connection Checkpoint 65.1 on student resource website.*

Functions of the Pituitary Gland

65.2 The pituitary gland secretes hormones that control many diverse body functions.

Although the pituitary gland is often referred to as the "master gland," its function is largely controlled by releasing or inhibiting hormones from the hypothalamus. The pituitary gland is divided into anterior and posterior lobes, which have very different structures and functions.

The **anterior pituitary gland** (adenohypophysis) comprises glandular tissue that manufactures and secretes hormones that control major body functions and systems. Four of these are called **tropic hormones**, a term that refers to the ability of these hormones to regulate the secretory actions of other endocrine glands. The anterior pituitary hormones are synthesized and stored in the pituitary until they receive a message from the hypothalamus. The message from the hypothalamus is usually to *enhance* the release of hormones, as is the case for growth hormone-releasing hormone (GHRH), thyrotropin-releasing hormone (TRH), prolactin-releasing hormone (PRH), corticotropin-releasing hormone (CRH), and gonadotropin-releasing hormone (GnRH). Two of the hypothalamic secretions, growth hormone-inhibiting hormone (GHIH) and prolactin-inhibiting hormone (PIH), *prevent* the release of pituitary hormones.

The **posterior pituitary gland** (neurohypophysis), by contrast, consists of nervous tissue and is basically an extension of the hypothalamus. It secretes two hormones: antidiuretic hormone (ADH) and oxytocin. These hormones are manufactured in the hypothalamus and travel down neurons to the posterior pituitary where they are stored until factors stimulate their release. The primary stimulus causing ADH secretion is an increased serum osmolality, or a high concentration of solutes in the blood. Oxytocin release is stimulated by touch receptors in the nipples of lactating women. Pharmacotherapy with oxytocin is presented in Chapter 69.

Regulation of hormone levels is an essential function because too little or too much of any of these endocrine secretions can cause profound symptoms. Many are controlled by negative feedback loops. As circulating levels of a hormone rise above normal, a message is sent to the hypothalamus, pituitary, or other endocrine gland to shut down the manufacture and secretion of the hormone. This prevents excess hormone levels. When hormones are administered as drug therapy, they can influence this normal negative feedback mechanism. One of the most important examples of this phenomenon is the negative feedback suppression of the adrenal glands caused by administration of corticosteroid medications. The student should review the information on negative feedback in Chapter 64 before proceeding.

Because of the widespread effects of the hormones secreted and controlled by the hypothalamus and pituitary glands, disorders of these glands are quite complex. In general, the pathologies of endocrine glands can be categorized as causing hypofunction or hyperfunction of the particular gland. Pituitary disorders can be the result of tumors, surgery, radiation therapy, infection, injury, infarction (loss of blood supply), or bleeding (hemorrhage) in the area. Congenital defects may also result in absent or impaired function of a hormone, or the lack of an enzyme necessary for hormone production.

Pharmacotherapy of Growth Hormone Disorders

65.3 Growth hormone deficiency in adults and children can be treated by administering recombinant growth hormone.

Growth hormone (GH), also called somatotropin or somatropin, is produced and secreted by the anterior pituitary gland. This hormone was once believed to be of importance only during periods of active growth, but it is now recognized that adults produce nearly as much GH as children. Although its major targets are bone and skeletal muscle, GH stimulates many types of body cells to increase in size and replicate. It is considered an anabolic (tissue-building) hormone. The primary effects of GH, illustrated in Figure 65.1, are as follows:

- Increases length and width of bone
- Stimulates cartilage growth
- Stimulates the growth and development of most visceral and endocrine organs, skeletal and cardiac muscle, and skin and connective tissue
- Enhances cellular uptake of amino acids and increased protein synthesis
- Breaks down adipose tissue to release fatty acids for use as fuel
- Decreases use of glucose; impairs glucose tolerance and induces insulin resistance in peripheral tissues

Many of the effects of GH are dependent on **insulin-like growth factor (IGF)**, a family of peptides that promote cartilage and bone growth. IGFs are produced in the liver and are released when hepatic cells become activated by GH. Secretion of GH fluctuates during the day, peaking 1 to 4 hours following the onset of sleep. These nighttime bursts in GH are greater in children than in adults.

The overall regulation of serum GH levels resides in the hypothalamus, with the secretion of GHRH and GHIH. A large number of secondary factors, such as exercise and sleep, influence the release of GH, and these are listed in Table 65.2.

In children, GH deficiency results in dwarfism. **Dwarfism** is associated with normal birth length followed by a slowing of the growth rate. These children have normal intelligence, short stature,

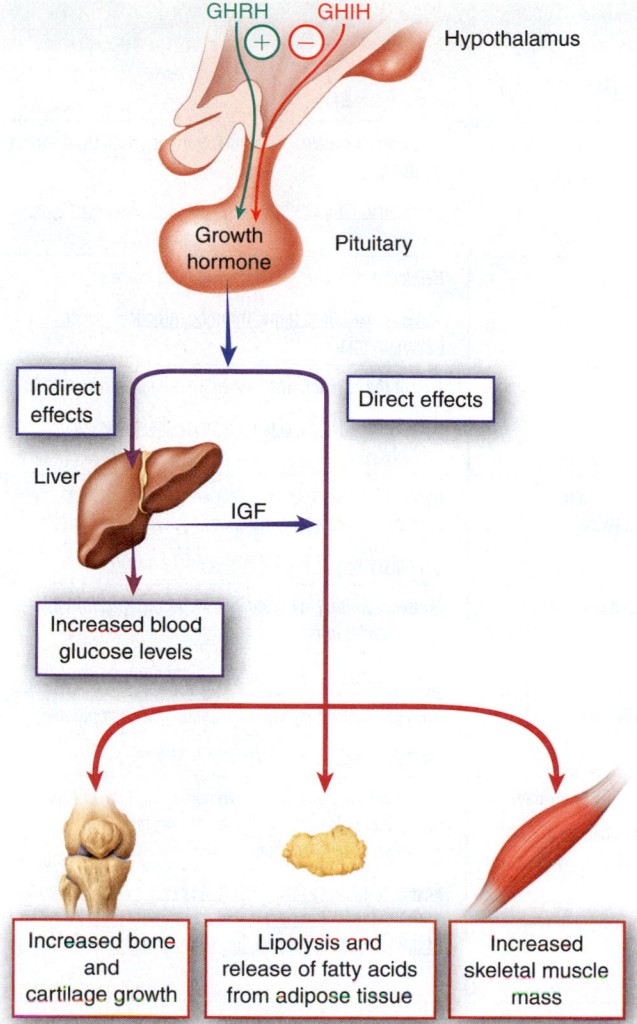

Figure 65.1 Physiological and pharmacologic effects of growth hormone.

GHRH GHIH
Hypothalamus
+ −
Growth hormone   Pituitary
Indirect effects
Direct effects
Liver
IGF
Increased blood glucose levels
Increased bone and cartilage growth
Lipolysis and release of fatty acids from adipose tissue
Increased skeletal muscle mass

TABLE 65.2 Selected Factors Affecting the Release of Growth Hormone	
Factors Increasing Release of GH	**Factors Decreasing Release of GH**
Amino acids: leucine, arginine	Beta-adrenergic agonists
Androgens and estrogens	Carbohydrate-rich diet
Clonidine	Cortisol
Elevated body temperature	Free fatty acids
Gamma-hydroxybutyrate	Increased serum glucose level
Growth hormone-releasing hormone (GHRH)	Obesity
Hypoglycemia, fasting, starvation	Somatostatin
L-dopa	
Stress, trauma	
Vigorous exercise	

immature facial features, obesity, and delayed skeletal maturation. In this context, **short stature** is defined as well below the fifth percentile for age and gender, or more than two standard deviations below the mean (average) height for age and gender. Acquired GH deficiency develops later in childhood and can be caused by a hypothalamic-pituitary tumor or an infection. Children who have been severely neglected or emotionally deprived can develop a psychosocial dwarfism, with poor growth, a potbelly, and poor nutritional habits. GH levels often return to normal once the child is removed from the dysfunctional environment.

When GH deficiency is the cause of short stature, replacement therapy is the treatment of choice. Until 1985, GH was obtained from the pituitary glands of human cadavers, a practice that was halted following the deaths of several recipients who developed Creutzfeldt–Jakob disease. GH is now obtained using recombinant DNA technology. GH obtained through recombinant technology is called somatropin. Doses for the GH analogs are listed in Table 65.3.

Therapy with recombinant GH is expensive, with an annual cost of approximately $30,000 to $50,000. The hormone is administered subcutaneously, several times a week during the period of active growth, and therapy may continue until adulthood. Females with Turner's syndrome and children with chronic renal insufficiency may also be treated with GH. Often, treatment with GH produces only modest gains in final adult height, but these gains are considered beneficial to the psychological well-being of the patient.

Adult GH deficiency is associated with reduced muscle mass, increased cardiovascular mortality, central adiposity and increased visceral fat, insulin resistance, and dyslipidemia. This hormonal deficiency may develop during adulthood, or it may be a continuation of childhood deficiency. Several forms of recombinant human GH formulations (Humatrope and Genotropin) have been approved for use in adults with body-wasting–type disorders. Treatment can result in increased lean body mass, decreased fat mass, increased bone mineral density, and decreased lipid levels.

Human GH has been abused for its anabolic effects. Athletes have used the drug to build muscle, increase strength, and maintain less body fat. It has also been called an antiaging drug because it promotes younger looking skin, improved memory, and reduced wrinkles. The administration of GH for these purposes is illegal, and prolonged use may lead to long-term adverse effects in patients. Despite potential adverse health effects, products advertised as "human growth hormone supplements" are readily marketed without a prescription. These do not contain any GH (which must be administered parenterally) but instead contain a mixture of oral (PO) supplements that are claimed to stimulate the pituitary gland. The safety and effectiveness of these products have not been evaluated adequately.

PROTOTYPE DRUG	**Somatropin (Genotropin, Humatrope, Norditropin, Nutropin, Saizen, Serostim, Zorbtive)**

Classification: Therapeutic: Human growth hormone
Pharmacologic: Pituitary hormone

Therapeutic Effects and Uses: Approved in 1987, somatropin is prepared through recombinant DNA technology and is identical to endogenous human GH. It is available in several different

TABLE 65.3	Hypothalamic and Pituitary Drugs	

Drug	Route and Adult Dose (Maximum Dose Where Indicated)	Adverse Effects
bromocriptine (Cycloset, Parlodel)	PO (Cycloset): 0.8 mg daily, increased weekly to achieve 1.6–4.8 mg daily PO: 1.25–2.5 mg/day for 3 days, then increase dose every 3–7 days to 30–60 mg/day	*Orthostatic hypotension, nausea, vomiting, fatigue, dizziness, headache* Shock, acute MI, cerebral ischemia, confusion, agitation, psychosis
desmopressin (DDAVP)	IV/subcutaneous: 2–4 mcg in two divided doses PO: 0.2–0.4 mg/day	*Headache, nasal congestion or irritation, nausea* Water intoxication, coma, thromboembolic disorder, hyponatremia
lanreotide (Somatuline Depot)	Subcutaneous: 60–120 mg every 4 weeks	*Pain at the injection site, nausea, vomiting, diarrhea, itching* Gallstones, abdominal pain, bradycardia, hyper- or hypoglycemia
mecasermin (Increlex)	Subcutaneous: 0.04–0.08 mg/kg twice daily. Must be administered within 20 min of a meal or snack (max: 0.12 mg/kg given twice daily)	*Injection-site reaction, iron deficiency anemia, goiter, antibody development, headache, hypertrophy of tonsils* Hypoglycemia, increased intracranial pressure
octreotide (Sandostatin)	Subcutaneous/IV: 100–600 mcg/day in two to four divided doses; after 2 weeks may switch to IM depot, 20 mg every 4 weeks	*Nausea, vomiting, diarrhea, headache, flushing, injection-site pain, cholelithiasis* Dysrhythmia, worsening heart failure, sinus bradycardia
pegvisomant (Somavert)	Subcutaneous: 40 mg loading dose, then 10 mg/day (max: 30 mg/day)	*Nausea, diarrhea, injection-site pain, flulike symptoms* Liver damage, elevated transaminase levels
somatropin (Genotropin, Humatrope, Norditropin, Nutropin, Saizen, Serostim, Zorbtive)	Humatrope: Subcutaneous: 0.006 mg/kg daily (max: 0.0125 mg/kg/day) Serostim: Subcutaneous: Weight more than 55 kg: 6 mg at bedtime; 45–55 kg: 5 mg at bedtime; 35–45 kg: 4 mg at bedtime; less than 35 kg: 0.1 mg/kg at bedtime Child: Genotropin: Subcutaneous: 0.16–0.24 mg/kg/week in six to seven divided doses Norditropin: 0.024–0.034 mg/kg 6–7 times/week	*Pain at injection site, hyperglycemia, arthralgia, myalgia, abdominal pain, otitis media, headache, bronchitis, hypothyroidism, HTN, flulike symptoms* Severe respiratory impairment in severely obese patients with Prader-Willi syndrome, diabetes, pancreatitis, scoliosis of the spine, papilledema, intracranial tumor
vasopressin	IM/subcutaneous: 5–10 units aqueous solution 2–4 times/day IV: 0.2–0.4 units/min up to 1 unit/min	*Tremor, pallor, nausea, vomiting, water retention, intoxication* Angina, acute MI, gangrene, anaphylaxis, cardiac arrest

Note: Italics indicate common adverse effects. Underline indicates serious adverse effects.

Self-Administration of Growth Hormone by Pen Device

Treatment of GH deficiencies is useful; however, to achieve the best outcome, it must be continued without interruptions, often for many years. Because recombinant human growth hormone (rhGH) is given by daily injection, adherence can be difficult, even for the most motivated patients.

Because pen devices have been used successfully for administering insulin and for auto-injection of epinephrine for acute allergic reactions, Rapaport et al. (2013) studied the outcomes of using a similar pen device for self-administration of rhGH. Participants were trained how to prepare, use, and disassemble the device. Overall, 86% of participants successfully used the device, and nearly 100% were satisfied with it.

GH treatment is lengthy and may be costly. Ensuring that a patient is able to take his or her medication consistently and safely ensures adherence. Pen devices for self-administration may result in better adherence with better outcomes of therapy.

formulations that vary by dose and regimen. The preferred route of administration is subcutaneous, although some forms may be given via the intramuscular (IM) route. GH produces growth of long bones in children prior to epiphyseal closure. The gain in growth is very rapid at the initiation of therapy but slows over time. Treatment may continue until the desired height is achieved, epiphyseal closure occurs, or the patient fails to respond to treatment. If treatment does not result in growth, it is stopped, and the diagnosis is reevaluated. The metabolic effects of the drug include increased protein synthesis, reduced carbohydrate utilization, and increased use of fatty acids for energy.

GH is used in the management of a number of growth-related disorders, including the following:

- Growth failure in children due to GH deficiency or Prader-Willi syndrome (Genotropin)

- Growth failure in children due to chronic renal insufficiency (Nutropin)

- Short stature associated with Turner's syndrome (Genotropin, Humatrope, Norditropin, Nutropin)

- Adult GH deficiency (Genotropin, Humatrope, Norditropin, Nutropin, Saizen)
- Acquired immunodeficiency syndrome (AIDS) wasting, cachexia, and severe thermal injuries (Serostim)
- Short bowel syndrome in patients receiving specialized nutrition support (Zorbtive)

Although the various brand-name products of GH have the same effectiveness, they differ in potency and are not interchangeable. Some are available in prefilled syringes, whereas others are longer acting. The nurse should check the package insert for specific dosing instructions.

Mechanism of Action: Somatropin has the same amino acid sequence as endogenous human GH and produces the same effects as the naturally occurring form of the hormone. The effects of GH are mediated by IGF.

Pharmacokinetics:

Route(s)	Subcutaneous; IM
Absorption	Well absorbed following injection
Distribution	Distributed to highly perfused organs (liver, kidneys); circulates bound to GH binding protein
Primary metabolism	Hepatic; some metabolism in kidneys
Primary excretion	Renal
Onset of action	Peak action variable: days to weeks
Duration of action	Half-life: 3.8–5 h

Adverse Effects: Adverse effects of somatropin include hyperglycemia and insulin resistance, which is made worse in patients with preexisting diabetes mellitus. It can also cause hypothyroidism. Edema of the hands and feet, headache, and hypertension (HTN) often occur initially but may resolve with continued therapy. Joint pain, muscle aches, and pain at the injection site are common. Carpal tunnel syndrome may occur with use of Serostim. Development of antibodies to GH may rarely occur. Hypercalciuria, possibly asymptomatic, may occur in the first few months of therapy.

Contraindications/Precautions: Somatropin is contraindicated for use in patients with closed epiphyses. It is also contraindicated in patients with severe obesity, respiratory impairment, or sleep apnea due to potentially fatal respiratory impairment. Somatropin is contraindicated in patients with intracranial tumor due to the risk for increased growth or recurrence of tumor. The drug is contraindicated in patients who are sensitive to glycerin. Somatropin should be used with caution in patients with severe renal or hepatic disease due to reduced clearance, and in patients with diabetes mellitus due to hyperglycemia and insulin resistance. It should be used with caution in pregnant or lactating patients because safety has not been established.

Drug Interactions: Corticosteroids interfere with the bone growth–promoting action of GH; thus, the two should not be given concurrently. Concurrent use with anabolic steroids, androgens, estrogens, or thyroid hormone may increase the rate of epiphyseal closure. Patients receiving insulin should be monitored carefully because somatropin decreases the actions of insulin. **Herbal/Food**: Unknown.

Pregnancy: Category B or C, depending on the specific formulation.

Treatment of Overdose: Overdose with somatropin has not been reported.

Nursing Responsibilities: Key nursing implications for patients receiving somatropin are included in the Nursing Practice Application for Patients Receiving Pharmacotherapy with Growth Hormone.

Drugs Similar to Somatropin (Genotropin, Humatrope, Norditropin, Nutropin, Saizen, Serostim, Zorbtive)

Mecasermin is the only other drug that has actions similar to GH.

Mecasermin (Increlex): Approved in 2005, mecasermin is a solution of insulin-like growth factor (IGF) produced through recombinant DNA technology. This drug is identical to endogenous IGF and therefore has the same actions as GH. Mecasermin is indicated for only two specific indications: the long-term treatment of growth failure in children with severe primary IGF deficiency, or for those who have developed neutralizing antibodies to GH. It is not intended to be used for any other forms of GH deficiency. It should not be used in adults after the epiphyses have closed. Adverse effects include hypoglycemia, local and systemic hypersensitivity, and tonsillar hypertrophy. Rare adverse effects include intracranial HTN, slipped capital epiphysis, and progression of scoliosis. Mecasermin use should be monitored carefully in patients taking insulin or oral antidiabetic drugs because mecasermin can increase the actions of these medications. This drug is pregnancy category C.

CONNECTIONS **Treating the Diverse Patient**

◀ Use of Growth Hormone in HIV Infected Patients on HAART

For untreated human immunodeficiency virus (HIV) infection, GH deficiency leads to AIDS wasting syndrome with loss of fat and lean muscle mass. For patients on highly active antiretroviral therapy (HAART), conditions such as cardiovascular disease and metabolic disorders with dyslipidemias, truncal obesity, and glucose changes have been noted. These conditions are usually noted in older adults and associated with normal aging. Although the causes of these changes are many, deficiency or relative deficiency of GH has been implicated as a cause. Using GH therapy in these patients has been found to increase lean muscle mass, decrease visceral adipose tissue and truncal obesity, and improve hyperlipidemias (Falutz, 2011). Impaired glucose metabolism may occur, although this may be managed with antidiabetic drugs if needed. Research is ongoing as to what form of GH and what dosages are needed for optimum therapy. The use of GH to improve the quality of life for patients with HIV infection who are on HAART is promising.

65.4 Overproduction of growth hormone in adults can be treated by administering growth hormone antagonists.

Excessive GH secretion that occurs prior to puberty and the sealing of epiphyseal plates of the long bones results in **gigantism**, or unusual tallness. Gigantism is rare due to early recognition of the cause of the oversecretion: a benign pituitary adenoma. GH excess in children is usually treated with surgery as soon as the disorder is diagnosed.

Excessive GH secretion in adults causes a condition known as **acromegaly**. Excess levels of GH stimulate the secretion of insulin-like growth factors from the liver, which then produce the clinical manifestations of the disorder. Because the epiphyseal plates are closed in adults, bones become deformed rather than elongated with this disorder. The onset is gradual, with enlargement of the bones of the hands, feet, face, and skull, a broad nose, protruding lower jaw, and slanting forehead. The cartilage of the larynx enlarges, deepening the voice. Spinal changes can lead to kyphosis. Arthralgias and degenerative arthritis may occur, and enlargement of organs, including the heart, can result in an early death due to atherosclerosis. Metabolic changes lead to insulin resistance and impaired glucose tolerance. Treatment may consist of a combination of surgery, radiation therapy, and pharmacotherapy to suppress GH secretion and correct metabolic abnormalities. Doses of the GH antagonists are listed in Table 65.3.

PROTOTYPE DRUG	Octreotide (Sandostatin)

Classification: Therapeutic: Growth hormone antagonist; antidiarrheal
Pharmacologic: Somatostatin

Therapeutic Effects and Uses: Approved in 1988, octreotide, which is also called somatostatin, is a long-acting peptide that mimics the actions of GHIH. Octreotide is effective in both children and adults with GH excess. To treat acromegaly, the drug is initially given three times daily by the subcutaneous route. A long-acting IM form (Sandostatin LAR Depot) is available that reduces dosing to every 4 weeks.

Although GHIH is primarily secreted by the hypothalamus, small amounts are also secreted by the stomach, intestine, and pancreas. Thus, in addition to its effect of blocking GH secretion in the anterior pituitary, octreotide suppresses the release of multiple gastrointestinal (GI) hormones, including gastrin, cholecystokinin (CCK), secretin, vasoactive intestinal peptide, insulin, and glucagon. This has resulted in its use in treating multiple secretory and bleeding conditions of the intestinal tract. Because it stimulates the absorption of fluid and electrolytes from the GI tract and prolongs intestinal transit time, it is approved to treat severe diarrhea and flushing episodes associated with metastatic carcinoid tumors, or vasoactive intestinal peptide tumors. Octreotide inhibits enzymes that cause vasodilation, decreases hepatic and GI blood flow, and reduces hepatic-portal venous pressure. These properties make the drug useful in treating portal HTN and upper GI bleeding caused by esophageal varices. It is also used off-label to reduce the output from pancreatic and other GI fistulas.

Mechanism of Action: Octreotide produces the same effects as the natural hormone somatostatin to suppress secretion of GH.

It also suppresses secretion of serotonin, pancreatic peptides, gastrin, vasoactive intestinal peptides, secretin, motilin, insulin, and glucagon.

Pharmacokinetics:

Route(s)	Subcutaneous or IM (depot formulation)
Absorption	Absorbed rapidly following subcutaneous injection
Distribution	May cross the placenta; may be secreted in breast milk; 65% bound to lipoproteins
Primary metabolism	Liver
Primary excretion	Renal
Onset of action	15–30 min (subcutaneous); 60 min (IM)
Duration of action	12 h; half-life: 1.5 h

Adverse Effects: The most common adverse effects of octreotide are related to the GI system: nausea, vomiting, diarrhea, abdominal discomfort, development of gallstones, and elevated liver enzymes. The nausea, vomiting, and abdominal pain diminish with continued therapy. It can also cause headache, fatigue, flushing, and edema. Because hypoglycemia or hyperglycemia can develop with long-term use, an adjustment in insulin doses in patients with diabetes may be necessary. It can also cause cardiac dysrhythmias, heart failure, and chest pain. Pain at the injection site is very common.

Contraindications/Precautions: Octreotide is contraindicated in patients who are sensitive to it. It is used with caution in patients with renal impairment or failure, liver disease, cardiac disease, diabetes, and hypothyroidism. Because the drug can cause cholelithiasis, biliary obstruction, or cholecystitis, it should be used cautiously in patients with preexisting gallbladder disease. In addition, it is used with caution in older adult patients due to a significantly longer half-life and delayed clearance; dose adjustments are necessary for these patients.

Drug Interactions: Octreotide may decrease cyclosporine levels and may alter the absorption of other drugs and nutrients because it slows intestinal motility. Concurrent administration of octreotide with PO antidiabetic drugs or insulin can produce hypoglycemia. Additive bradycardia may occur when administered with cardiac drugs such as beta blockers and calcium channel blockers. Concurrent use of octreotide with antidiarrheals and opioids can lead to severe constipation, intestinal obstruction, or paralytic ileus. **Herbal/Food**: Octreotide decreases the absorption of dietary fat and vitamin B_{12}.

Pregnancy: Category B.

Treatment of Overdose: Overdose with octreotide has not been reported.

Nursing Responsibilities:
- Assess baseline height and weight and monitor regularly to determine drug effectiveness.
- Assess baseline and periodic electrocardiograms (ECGs) because the drug may cause bradycardia and other dysrhythmias.

- Assess baseline and periodic vitamin B_{12} levels because the drug can reduce the absorption of this vitamin. Recommend supplementation as needed.

- Assess baseline and periodic hepatic and biliary function tests because this drug may cause or aggravate existing gallbladder disease.

- Administer octreotide by subcutaneous injection as the preferred route, alternating among the recommended sites between the abdomen, thigh, and buttock. Allow the solution to reach room temperature before administering.

- Monitor serum glucose levels frequently because this drug can cause hypoglycemia and may require adjustments in insulin dose.

- Monitor the patient's cardiac status, thyroid function, and electrolyte balance.

Lifespan and Diversity Considerations:

- Monitor all laboratory studies and other diagnostic testing more frequently in the older adult because normal physiological changes related to aging may increase the risk of adverse effects.

- Because genetic, individual variations may affect the results of drug therapy, monitor ethnically diverse populations more frequently to ensure optimal therapeutic effects and minimize adverse effects.

Patient and Family Education:

- Administer the drug between meals and at bedtime to minimize adverse GI effects. Rotate injection sites, and use the preferred sites for injections: the abdomen, thigh, or buttock.

- Reconstitute the drug gently, and avoid shaking the vial to prevent damaging the drug. Allow the solution to come to room temperature prior to injecting and refrigerate any unused solution. Discard any discolored solution or if particulate matter is present.

- Immediately report to the health care provider any yellowing of skin or the whites of the eyes, sharp right upper abdomen pain, nausea, or vomiting, because these may indicate the development of liver or gallbladder disease.

- Report abdominal pain or changes in bowel habits, either diarrhea or constipation, that is severe or that lasts more than 2 days.

- Be aware that treatment is expensive, and therapy may be prolonged.

- Immediately notify the health care provider of any known or suspected pregnancy.

- Do not breast-feed during drug therapy without approval of the health care provider.

Drugs Similar to Octreotide (Sandostatin)

Drugs with similar actions to octreotide include bromocriptine, lanreotide, and pegvisomant.

Bromocriptine (Cycloset, Parlodel): Approved in 1978, bromocriptine is a PO drug that is classified as a dopamine agonist. Dopamine itself is not used for acromegaly due to an unacceptable incidence of adverse effects. Bromocriptine inhibits the secretion of GH as well as prolactin from the pituitary. It is primarily indicated for Parkinson's disease and infertility caused by prolactin excess, but it has been used in combination with octreotide in children with GH excess. In 2009, the FDA approved bromocriptine (Cycloset) as an adjunct to diet and exercise to improve glycemic control in adults with type 2 diabetes mellitus.

The most common dose-limiting adverse effects are psychological reactions including confusion, agitation, hallucinations, paranoid delusions, or nightmares. Other adverse effects include orthostatic hypotension, headache, nausea, vomiting, anorexia, or rash on the face and arms. Bromocriptine interferes with lactation and should not be used during breast-feeding. It is a pregnancy category B drug.

Lanreotide (Somatuline Depot): Approved in 2007, lanreotide is a somatostatin analog indicated for the treatment of patients with acromegaly who have not responded to radiation therapy or who are unable to undergo surgical treatment. The drug lowers levels of GH, thus improving symptoms related to acromegaly. Lanreotide is a depot formulation that requires dosing only once per month. It is available in prefilled syringes and is delivered by deep subcutaneous injection. Adverse effects associated with lanreotide include pain at the injection site, nausea and vomiting, diarrhea, gallstones, skin reactions such as itching, bradycardia, and changes in blood glucose levels (either hyper- or hypoglycemia). This drug is pregnancy category C.

Pegvisomant (Somavert): Approved in 1997, pegvisomant is a specific GH receptor antagonist, making it very effective for acromegaly. The drug is structurally very similar to GH, although when it binds to GH receptors, it causes no cellular response. The multiple polyethylene glycol (PEG) molecules attached to the drug prolong its half-life and allow for once-daily dosing. It is administered subcutaneously once daily and is supplied as a powder for reconstitution. Adverse effects include nausea, vomiting, elevated liver enzymes, angina, chest pain and myocardial infarction (MI), HTN, flulike syndrome, and injection-site pain. Patients with diabetes should be monitored regularly to avoid hypoglycemia. Therapy for this drug is expensive and is continued indefinitely. It is a pregnancy category B drug.

Pharmacotherapy of Antidiuretic Hormone Disorders

65.5 Pharmacotherapy is used to treat deficient or excess secretion of antidiuretic hormone.

It is essential that the amount of fluid in the body be maintained within narrow limits. Loss of large amounts of water leads to dehydration, a serious condition that can lead to shock and death. Too much body fluid leads to congestion, edema, and water intoxication. **Antidiuretic hormone (ADH)** is one of the most important means the body uses to maintain fluid homeostasis. For a complete discussion of fluid balance and the drugs used as fluid replacement agents, see Chapter 33.

The hypothalamus senses fluid balance by recognizing the osmolarity of the blood. Osmolarity is the number of dissolved particles, or solutes, in a fluid. As water is lost, the osmolality, or

CONNECTIONS: NURSING PRACTICE APPLICATION

Patients Receiving Pharmacotherapy with Growth Hormone

Assessment	Potential Nursing Diagnoses*
Baseline assessment prior to administration: • Obtain a complete health history including cardiovascular, GI, hepatic, or renal disease, diabetes, pregnancy, or breast-feeding. Obtain a growth and development related history including congenital conditions such as Prader-Willi syndrome. Obtain a drug history including allergies, current prescription and OTC drugs, herbal preparations, alcohol use, or smoking. Be alert to possible drug interactions. • Evaluate appropriate laboratory findings (e.g., CBC, electrolytes, glucose, hepatic and renal function studies, thyroid hormone panels, insulin-like growth factor-1 [IGF-1], IGF binding protein [IGFBP]). • Obtain baseline height, weight, and vital signs. Obtain radiologic assessment of epiphyseal plates if ordered. • Assess the patient's ability to receive and understand instructions. Include the family or caregiver as needed.	• *Acute* or *Chronic Pain*, related to adverse drug effects • *Disturbed Body Image* • *Imbalanced Nutrition: Less Than Body Requirements* • *Deficient Knowledge* (Drug Therapy) • *Risk for Disproportionate Growth* • *Risk for Situational Low Self-Esteem* • *Risk for Impaired Social Interaction* • *Risk for Loneliness* • *Risk for Unstable Blood Glucose Level*, related to adverse drug effects
Assessment throughout administration: • Assess for desired therapeutic effects dependent on the reason the drug is given (e.g., measurable increase in height, improved nutritional intake, weight). • Continue periodic monitoring of CBC, electrolytes, glucose, hepatic and renal function studies, and thyroid and GH panels. • Continue monitoring vital signs, height, and weight. • Assess for adverse effects: nausea, vomiting, diarrhea, headache, peripheral edema, elevated serum glucose, joint pain or muscle aches. Patients with diabetes should promptly report consistent elevations in glucose.	

Implementation

Interventions and (Rationales)	Patient-Centered Care
Ensuring therapeutic effects: • Monitor height and weight at each clinical visit. Report lack of growth to the provider. (Lack of growth after a period of consistent growth may indicate the development of antibodies against GH or closure of the epiphyseal plates.)	• Teach the patient, family, or caregiver to measure and record height and weight weekly and bring the record to each clinical visit. • Instruct the patient on the need to return periodically for laboratory work. • Advise the patient, family, or caregiver of the cost of the drug before beginning therapy. Explore the ability to maintain drug therapy for the duration of the treatment prescribed. Assess financial concerns, and provide appropriate social service referrals as needed.
Minimizing adverse effects: • Monitor for any reports of muscle, joint, or bone pain, particularly in the knee or hip, or any changes in gait. (Carpal tunnel syndrome may occur, especially with Serostim. Avascular necrosis is an adverse drug effect of GH. Increasing or severe pain in joints or changes in gait should be reported promptly for follow-up evaluation.)	• Instruct the patient, family, or caregiver to report any changes in walking, discomfort or pain in knee or hip joints, bone pain, or consistent muscle pain over joint areas to the health care provider.
• Monitor serum glucose levels, particularly in patients with diabetes. Report consistent elevations to the health care provider. (GH may cause increases in glucose level. Patients with diabetes may need alterations in their normal medication routines if hyperglycemia occurs.)	• Instruct the patient on the need to return periodically for laboratory work. • Teach patients with diabetes to monitor capillary glucose levels more frequently during therapy. Report any consistent elevations in blood glucose to the health care provider.
• Continue to monitor vital signs, especially pulse and blood pressure for patients with existing cardiac disease. Monitor daily weight, output, lung sounds, and for peripheral edema. (Fluid retention with an increased intravascular volume, HTN, and peripheral edema may occur in early therapy but should resolve over time. Immediately report any continuing or worsening symptoms to the health care provider.)	• Instruct the patient to immediately report pounding headache, dizziness, palpitations, or syncope. • Teach the patient, family, or caregiver how to monitor pulse and blood pressure as appropriate. Ensure the proper use and functioning of any home equipment obtained. • Instruct the patient on how to monitor urine output if ordered, and provide measuring equipment as needed. Have the patient keep a record of daily weight and output and bring the record to each clinical visit.
• Periodically monitor urine calcium levels, especially in the first few months of therapy. Report any flank pain, GI symptoms, or dysuria to the health care provider. (Hypercalciuria may occur in early therapy, sometimes without symptoms. Renal calculi are a possible adverse effect.)	• Instruct the patient on the need to return periodically for laboratory work. • Encourage increased fluid intake, up to 2 L/day if allowed.

CONNECTIONS: NURSING PRACTICE APPLICATION (continued)

• Continue to monitor nutritional and fluid intake. (Wasting syndromes caused by conditions such as AIDS or chronic kidney disease may result in nutritional deficits and dehydration until the drug therapy is effective. Dietary consultation may be required to reach and maintain optimum nutrition.)	• Encourage increased fluid intake, up to 2 L/day if allowed, taken in frequent small amounts. • Encourage small, high-calorie, nutrient-dense meals rather than large infrequent meals. • Obtain a dietary consult if the patient requests or if malnutrition is severe.
Patient understanding of drug therapy: • Use opportunities during administration of medications and during assessments to discuss the rationale for drug therapy, desired therapeutic outcomes, commonly observed adverse effects, parameters for when to call the health care provider, and any necessary monitoring or precautions. (Using time during nursing care helps to optimize and reinforce key teaching areas.)	• The patient, family, or caregiver should be able to state the reason for the drug, appropriate dose and scheduling, what adverse effects to observe for, and when to report them.

Patient self-administration of drug therapy:
• When administering the medication, instruct the patient, family, or caregiver in proper self-administration of the drug, e.g., during the evening meal, followed by teach-back. (Utilizing time during nurse-administration of these drugs helps to reinforce teaching.)
	• Teach the patient to take the drug following appropriate guidelines:
	  • Reconstitute the parenteral drug exactly per package directions and do not shake the vial; gently rotate it to avoid breaking down the drug. Follow the manufacturer's instruction if the automated pen injector (e.g., Nutropin) is used.
	  • Store any unused reconstituted solutions in the refrigerator; do not freeze the solution. Discard any discolored solution or if particulate matter is present.
	  • Administer GH drugs in the evening to mimic the body's natural rhythms.
	  • Administer subcutaneous injections in the abdomen, buttock, or thigh areas, rotating injection sites. Do not use gluteal sites for children under the age of 2; these muscles are not well developed until the child has been walking for a year or more.

*Nursing Diagnoses—Definitions and Classification 2015–2017. Copyright © 2014, 1994–2014 by NANDA International. Used by arrangement with John Wiley & Sons Limited.

concentration of the blood, increases and the hypothalamus directs the posterior pituitary gland to release ADH. This hormone acts on the renal tubules to enhance water reabsorption. The increased amount of water in the body reduces serum osmolality to normal levels and ADH secretion stops. Other factors stimulating release of ADH include hypotension, decreased fluid volume, dehydration, pain, nausea, and vomiting. Factors inhibiting ADH release include decreased serum osmolality and increased fluid volume. Many drugs also affect ADH release, as listed in Table 65.4. ADH is also called vasopressin because it has the ability to cause vasoconstriction at high doses.

CONNECTION Checkpoint 65.2

In addition to ADH, the renin-angiotensin-aldosterone system (RAAS) is essential for maintaining fluid balance. From what you learned in Chapter 31, how does the RAAS affect sodium and water balance? *See Answer to Connection Checkpoint 65.2 on student resource website.*

TABLE 65.4 Drugs Interacting with Antidiuretic Hormone

Drugs Stimulating ADH Secretion	Drugs Inhibiting ADH Secretion
acetaminophen	alcohol
anesthetics	beta-adrenergic agonists
barbiturates	chlorpromazine
carbamazepine	demeclocycline
chlorpropamide	heparin
corticosteroids	lithium
diuretics	norepinephrine
tricyclic antidepressants	opioids
	phenytoin

A deficiency in ADH results in **diabetes insipidus (DI)**, a condition characterized by the production of large volumes of very dilute urine, usually accompanied by increased thirst. DI may be either nephrogenic or neurogenic. Nephrogenic DI is caused by the inability of the kidneys to respond to ADH. Drugs, such as lithium (Eskalith), or electrolyte disturbances can cause nephrogenic DI. Because nephrogenic DI results from an inability to respond to ADH, replacement therapy is not effective.

Neurogenic or central DI results from a lack of adequate production or secretion of ADH in the brain. The etiology of neurogenic DI can be genetic or acquired following head injury, surgery, tumors, infections, or vascular lesions of the region. Pharmacologic preparations of ADH can be used for replacement therapy for neurogenic DI. The preferred drug for treating chronic neurogenic DI is desmopressin (DDAVP). A PO hypoglycemic drug, chlorpropamide, can be used to stimulate ADH release in partial neurogenic DI. Paradoxically, both forms of DI respond in part to thiazide diuretics such as hydrochlorothiazide.

The primary symptoms of DI are polyuria and polydipsia (excessive thirst). Extremely large volumes of fluid (up to 30 L/day) may be ingested and the urine will be very dilute. The intense thirst and frequent urination usually keeps patients awake during the night. Failure to ensure adequate fluid intake will result in hypovolemia and dehydration due to the large renal water loss.

PharmFACT

Diabetes insipidus is uncommon with a prevalence of 3 cases per 100,000 people. Thirty percent of the cases are idiopathic with no identifiable cause (Khardori, 2014).

Excess secretion of ADH is the cause of the **syndrome of inappropriate antidiuretic hormone (SIADH)**, a condition characterized by marked fluid retention, elevated urine osmolality, low serum osmolality, and sodium loss in the urine. SIADH may occur as a transient or chronic condition. The resulting hyponatremia and water retention cause muscle cramps, weakness, headache, apprehension, nausea, vomiting, and lethargy, progressing to stupor and coma. Treatment involves fluid restriction and diuretics such as mannitol or furosemide (Lasix) to remove excess fluid. Conivaptan (Viprostol) and tolvaptan (Samsca) are vasopressin receptor antagonists that promote renal water excretion and increased serum sodium levels in patients with SIADH. The antibiotic demeclocycline (Declomycin) is a tetracycline used off-label to treat SIADH due to its ability to cause diuresis through the inhibition of ADH-induced water reabsorption in the tubules and collecting ducts of the kidneys. In severe cases, IV infusion of a hypertonic sodium chloride solution may be necessary to raise serum osmolality.

PROTOTYPE DRUG	Desmopressin (DDAVP)

Classification: Therapeutic: Antidiuretic hormone replacement **Pharmacologic:** Pituitary hormone

Therapeutic Effects and Uses: Approved in 1978, desmopressin is a synthetic analog of human ADH that has a longer duration of action than the natural hormone. It controls the acute symptoms of polyuria and polydipsia in patients with neurogenic DI but not nephrogenic diabetes insipidus. For DI, the PO route is preferred, although IV and subcutaneous forms are available for SIADH.

Desmopressin has vasoconstrictor activity that causes contraction of smooth muscle in the vascular system, uterus, and GI tract. It produces fewer vasoconstrictive effects than natural vasopressin. Desmopressin also produces an increase in plasma Factor VIII and von Willebrand's factor and is thus indicated for the management of bleeding in patients with hemophilia A and von Willebrand's disease (type I). An intranasal form of desmopressin (Stimate) is available for these indications. The use of desmopressin in treating coagulation disorders is presented in Chapter 38. This drug is the most effective pharmacologic intervention for controlling enuresis (bed-wetting) in children. For enuresis, desmopressin is administered 1 hour before bedtime in children age 6 or older, for up to 6 months.

Mechanism of Action: Desmopressin increases the permeability of renal collecting tubules to water, thereby increasing the reabsorption of water. It produces vasoconstriction of blood vessels at higher doses. The vasoconstriction produced is greatest in portal vessels and less in cerebral, coronary, pulmonary, and peripheral vessels. Desmopressin enhances GI motility and tone through contraction of smooth muscle in the GI tract.

Pharmacokinetics:

Route(s)	Subcutaneous, IV, PO
Absorption	5% through GI mucosa
Distribution	Small amount may cross the blood–brain barrier; secreted in breast milk
Primary metabolism	Metabolized rapidly by the liver
Primary excretion	Renal
Onset of action	PO: 1 h, with a peak at 4–7 h; IV: 1 min with a peak at 30 min
Duration of action	PO: 8–20 h; IV: 3 h

Adverse Effects: Desmopressin can cause water intoxication. Early signs include drowsiness, headache, and listlessness, progressing to convulsions and coma. Other adverse effects include transient headache, nasal congestion, rhinitis, nausea, mild abdominal pain and cramping, facial flushing, HTN, or pain or swelling at the injection site. A rare adverse effect of desmopressin is a severe allergic reaction or anaphylaxis (IV administration). Tolerance to the effects of desmopressin develops when it is administered more frequently than every 48 hours or by the IV route.

Contraindications/Precautions: Desmopressin is contraindicated in patients with nephrogenic DI. It is used with caution in patients with coronary artery disease, HTN, and in patients at risk for hyponatremia or thrombi. The drug is contraindicated in patients with moderate or severe renal impairment because the drug can worsen fluid retention and overload. Young children and the older adult should be treated with caution because these patients are more prone to water intoxication and hyponatremia.

Drug Interactions: Increased antidiuretic action can occur with carbamazepine, chlorpropamide, clofibrate, and nonsteroidal anti-inflammatory drugs (NSAIDs). Decreased antidiuretic action can occur with lithium, alcohol, heparin, and epinephrine. **Herbal/Food:** Unknown.

Pregnancy: Category B.

Treatment of Overdose: In case of overdose, or if water intoxication develops, symptomatic treatment with diuretics is recommended.

Nursing Responsibilities: Key nursing implications for patients receiving desmopressin are included in the Nursing Practice Application for Patients Receiving Pharmacotherapy with Antidiuretic Hormone.

Drugs Similar to Desmopressin (DDAVP)

The only drug that is similar to desmopressin is vasopressin.

Vasopressin: A synthetic analog of antidiuretic hormone, vasopressin is given IM or subcutaneously for central or neurogenic DI. Approved in 1941, it has a shorter duration of action than desmopressin and a more pronounced vasoconstrictor action, which can result in serious adverse effects.

Because vasopressin is a potent vasoconstrictor, it is given IV as an alternative to epinephrine for many off-label indications. These include bleeding from esophageal varices or the upper GI tract, cardiac arrest, and the treatment of severe hypotension or shock. Vasopressin may precipitate MI or angina. It may cause water intoxication. When used for its vasopressor effects, possible adverse effects include tissue necrosis and gangrene. Vasopressin is a pregnancy category C drug.

CONNECTION Checkpoint 65.3

Desmopressin is used to treat von Willebrand's disease, the most common inherited coagulation disorder. From what you learned in Chapter 38, what is the function of von Willebrand's factor? *See Answer to Connection Checkpoint 65.3 on student resource website.*

CONNECTIONS Treating the Diverse Patient

◀ Gender Differences in Desmopressin Dose for Nocturia in Adults

Although nocturnal enuresis is commonly considered a childhood condition, it occurs in the adult population as well. Excessive fluid intake and alcohol use are known causative factors. Increasing age and female gender have also been noted to be risk factors for desmopressin-induced hyponatremia, secondary to fluid retention. Juul, Klein, Sandström, Erichsen, and Nørgaard (2011) sought to determine whether gender indicated differences in desmopressin dosage. Appropriate dosage would assist in the prevention of desmopressin-induced hyponatremia and fluid retention. The authors found that women were significantly more sensitive to desmopressin and required approximately half to one quarter of the dose required by men. Juul, Klein, and Nørgaard (2013) also found that women had greater responses to lower doses of desmopressin and that these effects persisted up to a year later. While it is still not clear why women seem to have a greater response to the drug, large-scale clinical trials are recommended to determine appropriate doses for men and women.

CONNECTIONS: NURSING PRACTICE APPLICATION

Patients Receiving Pharmacotherapy with Antidiuretic Hormone

Assessment	Potential Nursing Diagnoses*
Baseline assessment prior to administration: • Obtain a complete health history including cardiovascular, GI, hepatic or renal disease, pregnancy, or breast-feeding. Obtain a drug history including allergies, current prescription and OTC drugs, herbal preparations, alcohol use, or smoking. Be alert to possible drug interactions. • Evaluate appropriate laboratory findings (e.g., urine and serum osmolality, urine specific gravity, serum protein, CBC, electrolytes, hepatic and renal function studies). • Obtain baseline height, weight, and vital signs. • Assess the patient's ability to receive and understand instructions. Include the family or caregiver as needed.	• *Deficient Fluid Volume* • *Impaired Urinary Elimination* • *Deficient Knowledge* (Drug Therapy) • *Excess Fluid Volume*, related to adverse drug effects • *Risk for Bleeding*
Assessment throughout administration: • Assess for desired therapeutic effects dependent on the reason the drug is being given (e.g., diuresis slows and urine output and serum osmolality return to normal, bleeding stops or slows). • Continue periodic monitoring of urine and serum osmolality, urine specific gravity, CBC, electrolytes, glucose, hepatic and renal function studies. • Continue monitoring vital signs and weight. • Assess for adverse effects: nausea, vomiting, diarrhea, headache, nasal congestion, or rhinitis. Immediately report drowsiness, dizziness, lethargy, hypotension or HTN, tachycardia, dysrhythmias, or angina to the health care provider.	

Implementation

Interventions and (Rationales)	Patient-Centered Care
Ensuring therapeutic effects: • For patients with DI, monitor urine output, urine and serum osmolality, and urine specific gravity for return to normal limits. If given for nocturnal enuresis, have the patient or family keep a diary of sleep patterns, noting any bed-wetting. (Urine output, osmolality, and specific gravity should return to normal limits. Bed-wetting should decrease or stop.)	• Teach the patient, family, or caregiver to measure and record height and weight weekly and bring the record to each clinical visit. • Instruct the patient on the need to return periodically for laboratory work. • Instruct the patient to monitor output (provide measuring equipment as needed) and to keep a record of daily weight and output. • Teach the patient, family, or caregiver to keep a diary of nighttime sleep habits and any bed-wetting. Limit oral fluids within 4 h of bedtime. Bring the record to each clinical visit. • Advise the patient of the cost of the drug before beginning therapy. Explore the ability to maintain drug therapy for the duration of the treatment prescribed. Assess financial concerns and provide appropriate social service referral as needed.
Minimizing adverse effects: • Continue to monitor vital signs, especially pulse and blood pressure for patients with existing cardiac disease. ECGs may be ordered periodically for patients with a history of dysrhythmias. Monitor daily weight, urine output, level of consciousness, lung sounds, and for peripheral edema. (Fluid retention secondary to antidiuretic hormone treatment may lead to increased intravascular volume, HTN, and water intoxication.)	• Instruct the patient to immediately report pounding headache, dizziness, palpitations, or syncope. • Teach the patient, family, or caregiver how to monitor pulse and blood pressure as appropriate. Ensure proper use and functioning of any home equipment obtained. • Instruct the patient to monitor urine output (provide measuring equipment as needed) and to keep a record of daily weight and urine output. • Instruct the patient, family, or caregiver to immediately report any drowsiness, dizziness, lethargy, or decreased level of consciousness to the health care provider.

(continued)

CONNECTIONS: NURSING PRACTICE APPLICATION (continued)

• Continue to monitor laboratory studies, especially serum sodium levels and osmolality. (DI or water retention triggered by the use of ADH replacement may result in alterations in serum sodium and osmolality. **Lifespan:** Normal physiological changes may place the older adult at greater risk for adverse effects related to electrolyte or fluid changes.)	• Instruct the patient on the need to return periodically for laboratory work.
• Monitor for and immediately report signs of peripheral ischemia, HTN, or angina. (Vasoconstriction caused by vasopressin may cause cardiac or peripheral ischemia, angina, or infarction.)	• Instruct the patient to immediately report any chest pain, pain or numbness in toes or fingers, or cramping when walking to the health care provider.
• Monitor nasal passages. Report any excoriation or bleeding. (Long-term intranasal ADH therapy may cause nasal irritation and ulceration.)	• Teach the patient to report nasal congestion, irritation, increase in nasal discharge, or bleeding to the health care provider.
Patient understanding of drug therapy: • Use opportunities during administration of medications and during assessments to discuss the rationale for drug therapy, desired therapeutic outcomes, commonly observed adverse effects, parameters for when to call the health care provider, and any necessary monitoring or precautions. (Using time during nursing care helps to optimize and reinforce key teaching areas.)	• The patient should be able to state the reason for the drug, the appropriate dose and scheduling, what adverse effects to observe for, and when to report them.

Patient self-administration of drug therapy:
• When administering the medication, instruct the patient or caregiver in proper self-administration of the drug, e.g., during the evening meal, followed by teach-back. (Utilizing time during nurse-administration of these drugs helps to reinforce teaching.)
	• Teach the patient to take the drug following appropriate guidelines:
	  • Direct nasal sprays high into the nasal cavity rather than back to the nasopharynx. Do not shake a nasal spray before using; gently rotate it.
	  • Store any unused solutions in the refrigerator. Nasal sprays may be kept at room temperature but avoid excessive heat over 26.7°C (80°F). Discard any discolored solution or if particulate matter is present.

*Nursing Diagnoses—Definitions and Classification 2015–2017. Copyright © 2014, 1994–2014 by NANDA International. Used by arrangement with John Wiley & Sons Limited.

CHAPTER

65

Understanding the Chapter

Key Concepts Summary

65.1 The hypothalamus controls many diverse body processes and secretes hormones that influence pituitary function.

65.2 The pituitary gland secretes hormones that control many diverse body functions.

65.3 Growth hormone deficiency in adults and children can be treated by administering recombinant growth hormone.

65.4 Overproduction of growth hormone in adults can be treated by administering growth hormone antagonists.

65.5 Pharmacotherapy is used to treat deficient or excess secretion of antidiuretic hormone.

Case Study: Making the Patient Connection

Remember the patient "Raj" at the beginning of the chapter? Now read the remainder of the case study. Based on the information presented in this chapter, answer the critical thinking questions that follow.

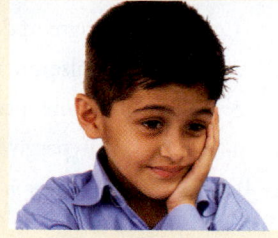

Raj, an 8-year-old boy, was referred to the pediatric endocrinology clinic for evaluation of his short stature. He had been healthy and developmentally normal until 3 years ago. Since that time, his growth has been extremely slow and almost imperceptible. On his initial exam, Raj's weight and height were 17 kg (37.4 lb) and 108 cm (42.5 in.), respectively. His height standard deviation score was −4.0 with a body mass index of 14.6. The remainder of his physical examination was normal.

When the pediatrician reviewed the results of hormonal assay tests with Raj's parents, everyone was relieved to find out that, although there is a problem, it is not due to a tumor or other life-threatening disorder. Raj has a congenital deficiency in GH, and the pediatrician begins to discuss replacement therapy with the parents. They agree that Raj should have this therapy and want to start it as soon as possible. Somatropin (Humatrope) has been ordered. As the nurse working with Raj and his family, address each of the following questions.

Critical Thinking Questions

1. What teaching will you need to provide to Raj's parents regarding drug therapy for his disorder?
2. Raj's father states, "I hope my health insurance will cover this medication." What would you say in response to this comment?
3. The parents ask about the adverse effects that might occur with this therapy. How would you respond?

See Answers to Critical Thinking Questions on student resource website.

Additional Case Study

Edward Keithy, a 10-year-old boy, and his parents visit the pediatrician's office where you are a nurse. The parents are concerned with Edward's continuing nocturnal enuresis, or nighttime bed-wetting. Increasingly, they see this condition as adversely affecting his self-image, self-esteem, and psychosocial well-being. Edward tells you that he is reluctant to take part in sleepovers at his friends' houses or to attend camping trips with his scouting troop.

1. What type of pharmacotherapy do you anticipate for Edward?
2. What information will Edward and his parents need as part of patient drug teaching?

See Answers to Additional Case Study on student resource website.

Chapter Review

1 A teaching plan for a parent whose child is receiving somatropin (Nutropin) should include what important information?
1. The patient must adhere to therapy to prevent mental retardation.
2. The medication cannot be given orally; it can be given only parenterally.
3. If growth hormone is begun in adolescence, it can add up to 6 inches in height.
4. Growth hormone therapy requires frequent blood work.

2 Which of the following findings would the nurse consider to be effects of somatropin? Select all that apply.
1. Increase in the length and width of long bones
2. Organ, muscle, and connective tissue growth
3. Increased synthesis of proteins
4. Lowering of serum glucose levels
5. Increase in fat deposits around the abdomen

3 The patient with neurogenic diabetes insipidus is being started on an oral dose of desmopressin (DDAVP). Which instruction should the nurse include in the teaching plan?
1. Use the drug only if urine output is excessive.
2. Use twice the prescribed dose if you miss a dose.
3. Obtain and record your weight each morning.
4. Use an NSAID such as ibuprofen if leg cramping occurs during walking.

4 A patient with metastatic colon cancer is experiencing bowel-related complications of the cancer and treatment. Octreotide (Sandostatin) has been ordered. The nurse will anticipate which therapeutic effect from this drug?
1. Decrease in the number of diarrheal stools per day
2. Slowing of the metastatic spread of the cancer
3. Increase in lean body mass and fat deposits
4. Episodes of hypo- or hyperglycemia

5 Prior to starting a patient on vasopressin for control of esophageal varices, the nurse will obtain the patient's past health history. If present, what condition might indicate the need to verify the order with the prescriber?

1. Glaucoma

2. Alcoholism

3. Chronic obstructive pulmonary disease (COPD)

4. Angina

6 Which of the following assessment findings would indicate that therapeutic goals have been achieved for a patient with diabetes insipidus being treated with desmopressin (DDAVP)?

1. Decreasing signs of dehydration

2. Increasing pulse and urine output

3. Decreasing urine specific gravity

4. Decreasing hyperglycemia

See Answers to Chapter Review in Appendix A.

References

Falutz, J. (2011). Growth hormone and HIV infection: Contribution to disease manifestations and clinical implications. *Best Practices and Research in Clinical Endocrinology and Metabolism, 25*, 517–529. doi:10.1016/j.beem.2010.11.001

Juul, K. V., Klein, B. M., & Nørgaard, J. P. (2013). Long-term durability of the response to desmopressin in female and male nocturia patients. *Neurourology and Urodynamics, 32*, 363–370. doi:10.1002/nau.22306

Juul, K. V., Klein, B. M., Sandström, R., Erichsen, L., & Nørgaard, J. P. (2011). Gender difference in antidiuretic response to desmopressin. *American Journal of Physiology, Renal Physiology, 300*, F1116–1122. doi:10.1152/ajprenal.00741.2010

Khardori, R. (2014). *Diabetes insipidus.* Retrieved from http://emedicine.medscape.com/article/117648-overview

Rapaport, R., Saenger, P., Schmidt, H., Hasegawa, Y., Colle, M., Loche, S., . . .

Litshitz, F. (2013). Validation and ease of use of a new pen device for self-administration of recombinant human growth hormone: Results from a two-center usability study. *Medical Devices, 6*, 141–146. doi:10.2147/MDER.S50088

Selected Bibliography

Chernausek, S. D. (2010). Growth and development: How safe is growth hormone therapy for children? *Nature Reviews Endocrinology, 6*, 251–253. doi:10.1038/nrendo.2010.43

Ferguson, L. A. (2011). Growth hormone use in children: Necessary or designer therapy? *Journal or Pediatric Health Care, 25*(1), 24–30. doi:10.1016/j.pedhc.2010.03.005

Herdman, T. H., & Kamitsuru, S. (Eds.). (2014). *NANDA International nursing diagnoses: Definitions and classification, 2015-2017.* Oxford, United Kingdom: Wiley-Blackwell.

Molitch, M. E., Clemmons, D. R., Malozowski, S., Merriam, G. R., & Vance, M. L. (2011).

Evaluation and treatment of adult growth hormone deficiency: An Endocrine Society clinical practice guideline. *The Journal of Clinical Endocrinology & Metabolism, 96*, 1587–1609. doi:10.1210/jc.2011-0179

Robson, L. M. (2014). *Enuresis.* Retrieved from http://emedicine.medscape.com/article/1014762-overview

Rosenfeld, R. G., Cohen, P., Robison, L. L., Bercu, B. B., Clayton, P., Hoffman, A. R., . . . Wit, J. M. (2011). Long-term surveillance of growth hormone therapy. *The Journal of Clinical Endocrinology & Metabolism, 97*, 68–72. doi:10.1210/jc.2011-2294

Sherlock, M., Woods, C., & Sheppard, M. C. (2011). Medical therapy in acromegaly. *Nature Reviews Endocrinology, 7*, 291–300. doi:10.1038/nrendo.2011.42

Simmons, S. (2010). Flushing out the truth about diabetes insipidus. *Nursing Critical Care, 5*(1), 35–39. doi:10.1097/01.CCN.0000365701.89988.69

Vallette, S., Ezzat, S., Chik, C., Ur, E., Imran, S. A., Uum, S., . . . Serri, O. (2013). Emerging trends in the diagnosis and treatment of acromegaly in Canada. *Clinical Endocrinology, 79*(1), 79–85. doi:10.1111/cen.12112

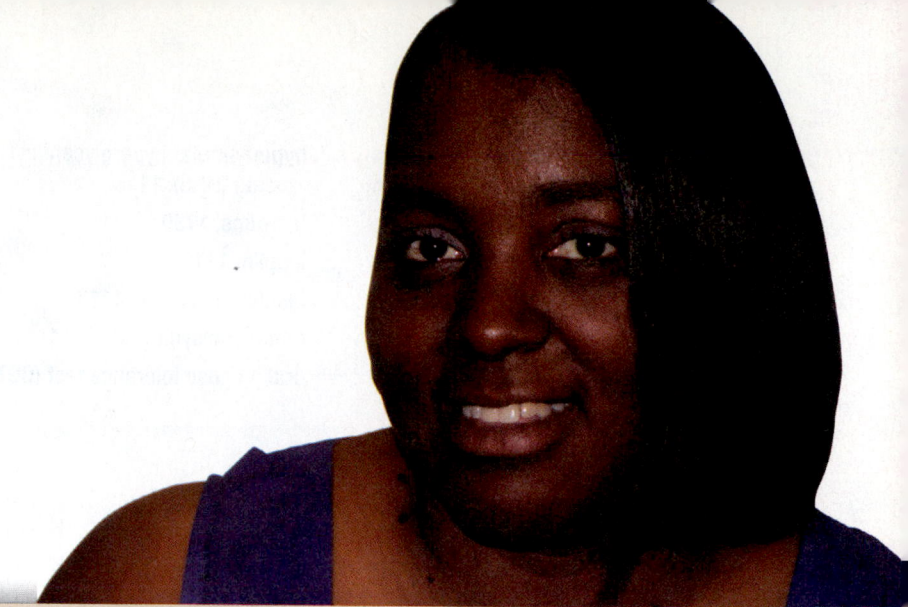

CHAPTER 66

Pharmacotherapy of Diabetes Mellitus

LEARNING OUTCOMES

After reading this chapter, the student should be able to:

1. Explain how blood glucose levels are maintained within narrow limits by insulin and glucagon.
2. Compare and contrast the etiology and pathogenesis of type 1, type 2, and gestational diabetes.
3. Describe the signs and diagnosis of diabetes.
4. Describe the acute complications of diabetes.
5. Identify the chronic complications of diabetes.
6. Compare and contrast the pharmacotherapy of the different types of diabetes.
7. For each type of insulin, identify the onset of action, peak action and duration of action, administration routes, when it is given related to meals, compatibility with other insulins, and adverse effects.
8. For each of the classes shown in the chapter outline, identify the prototype and representative drugs and explain the mechanism(s) of drug action, primary indications, contraindications, significant drug interactions, pregnancy category, and important adverse effects.
9. Apply the nursing process to the care of patients receiving pharmacotherapy for diabetes.

CHAPTER OUTLINE

▶ **Physiology of Serum Glucose Control**
▶ **Pathophysiology of Diabetes Mellitus: Types of Diabetes**
▶ **Symptoms and Diagnosis of Diabetes**
▶ **Complications of Diabetes Mellitus**
   PROTOTYPE Glucagon (GlucaGen), *p. 1115*
▶ **Insulin Therapy**
   PROTOTYPE Human Regular Insulin (Humulin R, Novolin R), *p. 1119*
▶ **Antidiabetic Drugs for Type 2 Diabetes**
   Sulfonylureas
   PROTOTYPE Glyburide (DiaBeta, Glynase, Micronase), *p. 1125*
   Biguanides
   PROTOTYPE Metformin (Glucophage, Glumetza, Others), *p. 1126*
   Meglitinides
   PROTOTYPE Repaglinide (Prandin), *p. 1127*
   Thiazolidinediones
   PROTOTYPE Rosiglitazone (Avandia), *p. 1128*
   Alpha-Glucosidase Inhibitors
   PROTOTYPE Acarbose (Precose), *p. 1129*
   Incretin Enhancers
   PROTOTYPE Sitagliptin (Januvia), *p. 1130*
▶ **Miscellaneous Antidiabetic Drugs**

KEY TERMS

diabetes mellitus, 1113

diabetic ketoacidosis (DKA), 1114

fasting plasma glucose (FPG) test, 1114

gestational diabetes, 1114

gluconeogenesis, 1112

glycogenolysis, 1112

hemoglobin A1C (HbA1C), 1114

hyperosmolar hyperglycemic
state (HHS), 1115

incretins, 1130

insulin, 1112

insulin resistance, 1113

metabolic syndrome, 1114

oral glucose tolerance test (OGTT), 1114

polydipsia, 1114

polyphagia, 1114

polyuria, 1114

prediabetes, 1114

type 1 diabetes, 1113

type 2 diabetes, 1113

It is estimated that over 29 million people in the United States have diabetes mellitus, with more than 8 million of those being undiagnosed. Diabetes is one of the leading causes of death in the United States. Mortality has risen in recent years, causing some public health officials to refer to it as an epidemic. Diabetes can lead to serious acute and chronic complications, including heart disease, stroke, blindness, kidney failure, and amputations. Because nurses frequently care for patients with diabetes, it is imperative that they thoroughly understand the disorder, its treatment, and possible complications. There is an unrelated disorder, diabetes insipidus, which results from a deficiency of antidiuretic hormone (see Chapter 65). When the term *diabetes* is used in this chapter, it is referring to diabetes mellitus.

Physiology of Serum Glucose Control

66.1 Serum glucose is maintained within a narrow range by the hormones insulin and glucagon.

Because diabetes is essentially a disorder of carbohydrate metabolism, it is important to understand the way the body obtains, metabolizes, and stores glucose. Of all the different molecules available, the body prefers to use glucose as its primary energy source. The brain relies almost exclusively on glucose for its energy needs because it is unable to synthesize glucose and it will exhaust its supply after just a few minutes of activity. Most other tissues can use fatty acids and proteins for energy production, if necessary, but they too prefer to use glucose. One of the most important roles of the liver and pancreas is to regulate the body's carbohydrate fuel supply so that all tissues of the body have sufficient energy to perform their functions.

Although the normal range for serum glucose is considered to be 60 to 100 mg/dL, it is usually tightly regulated by the body to remain between 80 and 90 mg/dL. Two pancreatic hormones contribute to maintaining a stable serum glucose level: **insulin**, which acts to decrease blood glucose levels, and glucagon, which acts to increase blood glucose levels.

Following a meal, glucose is rapidly absorbed from the gastrointestinal (GI) tract, and serum levels rise. Some of the glucose is taken up by cells and used for immediate energy needs, but about two thirds is stored in liver and muscle cells as glycogen, the storage form of glucose. When glucose levels fall between meals, glycogen is broken down in a process called **glycogenolysis**, and glucose is released into the bloodstream. Maintaining a stable serum glucose level is simply a matter of storing glucose during times of excess, and returning it to the bloodstream in times of deficiency. The importance of maintaining this delicate balance, however, cannot be overstated. Too much glucose or too little glucose can have lethal consequences.

Following a meal, the pancreas recognizes the rising serum glucose levels and releases insulin. Without insulin, glucose is not able to enter cells of the body. The cells may be surrounded by high amounts of glucose but they are unable to use it until insulin arrives. It may be helpful to visualize insulin as a transporter or "gatekeeper." When present, insulin swings open the gate, transporting glucose inside cells—if there is no insulin, there is no entry. The physiological actions of insulin are summarized as follows:

- Promotes the entry of glucose into cells
- Provides for the storage of glucose, as glycogen
- Inhibits the breakdown of fat and glycogen
- Increases protein synthesis and inhibits **gluconeogenesis**, which is the production of new glucose from noncarbohydrate molecules

Insulin is produced in beta cells of the pancreas known as islets of Langerhans, whereas alpha cells in the pancreas secrete glucagon. Glucagon maintains stable blood glucose levels between meals and during periods of fasting and has actions that are opposite to those of insulin. It removes glucose from its storage in the liver and sends it to the blood (glycogenolysis), raising serum glucose within minutes.

The level of glucose in the blood regulates the release of both insulin and glucagon. A hypoglycemic state (low serum glucose) stimulates the release of glucagon and inhibits the release of insulin, whereas a hyperglycemic state (high serum glucose) has the opposite effect: It stimulates the release of insulin and inhibits the release of glucagon. The physiological dynamics of insulin and glucagon release are shown in Figure 66.1.

Additional factors that decrease blood glucose levels are fasting, exercise, and alcohol. Factors that increase blood glucose levels include stress from infection, injury, or surgery, which triggers release of the epinephrine and norepinephrine; large meals or overconsumption of carbohydrates; growth hormone; and corticosteroids.

PharmFACT

According to the American Diabetes Association (ADA, 2014b), the incidence of diabetes mellitus in the United States is as follows:

- 1 in every 400 children and adolescents has diabetes.
- 11.3% of all people 20 years or older have diabetes.
- 26.9% of all people 65 years or older have diabetes.
- 1.9 million new cases of adult diabetes are diagnosed each year.

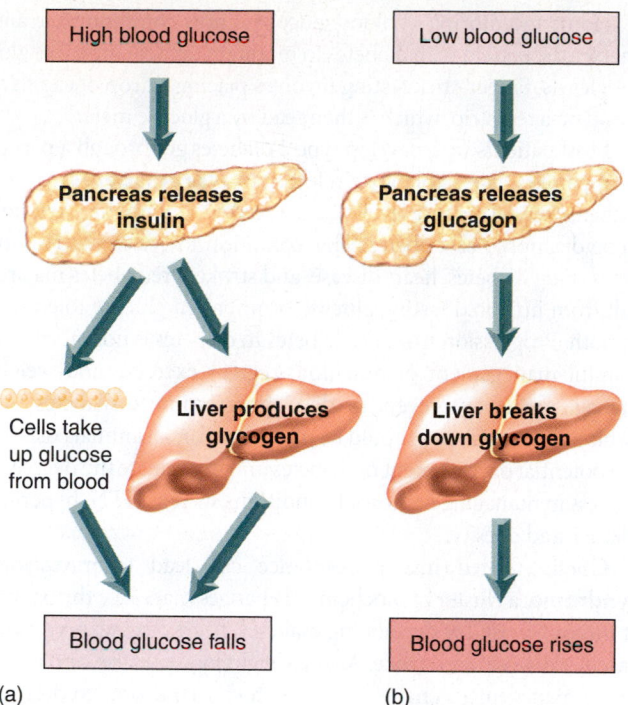

Figure 66.1 Insulin, glucagon, and blood glucose.

Pathophysiology of Diabetes Mellitus: Types of Diabetes

66.2 Type 1 diabetes is characterized by insufficient insulin synthesis by the pancreas, whereas type 2 diabetes is characterized by insulin resistance in the target cells.

Diabetes mellitus is a metabolic disorder characterized by an imbalance between insulin availability and insulin need. The two primary forms of diabetes are called type 1 and type 2. There are significant differences between the two types in terms of pathophysiology and disease management. A third form of the disease occurs during pregnancy and is known as gestational diabetes.

Type 1 diabetes results from an absolute lack of insulin secretion due to destruction of pancreatic beta cells. The destruction of beta cells is believed to result from a combination of autoimmune, genetic, and environmental factors. Type 1 is the less common form of diabetes, accounting for only 5% to 10% of all patients with the disorder. It is seen most frequently among children and young adults, but it may occur at any age.

Because of the lack of sufficient insulin in patients with type 1 diabetes, glucose cannot enter cells and fatty acids are used as the primary energy source. Metabolic by-products of lipid metabolism known as ketones accumulate in the blood, producing diabetic ketoacidosis (DKA), a dangerous and potentially life-threatening condition (see Section 66.4).

Patients with type 1 diabetes must receive insulin therapy to survive. In the past, type 1 was called juvenile or insulin-dependent diabetes. While these terms are still in use, they do not accurately reflect the nature of the disease.

Type 2 diabetes is the more common form of the disorder, representing 90% to 95% of people with diabetes. The primary physiological

characteristic of type 2 diabetes is hyperglycemia, caused by a relative deficiency of insulin. The disorder is characterized by **insulin resistance**, a condition in which cells become unresponsive to insulin due to a defect in insulin receptor function. The pancreas may be producing sufficient amounts of insulin but target cells do not recognize it.

As cells become more resistant to insulin, blood glucose levels rise and the pancreas responds by secreting even more insulin. Eventually, the hypersecretion of insulin leads to beta cell exhaustion, and, ultimately, to beta cell death. As type 2 diabetes progresses, it becomes a disorder characterized by insufficient insulin levels as well as insulin resistance. The activity of insulin receptors can be increased by exercise, which lowers the level of circulating insulin. In fact, adhering to a healthy diet and regular exercise have been shown to reverse insulin resistance and to delay or prevent the development of type 2 diabetes.

Eighty percent of persons with type 2 diabetes are overweight, and the degree of obesity directly affects the degree of insulin resistance. In particular, persons with upper body obesity (central or visceral obesity) are at increased risk for developing insulin resistance and type 2 diabetes. Although most patients with type 2 diabetes are older, this disease is increasingly being diagnosed in obese adolescents. Risk factors for type 2 diabetes are a family history of diabetes, obesity, and race and ethnicity. African Americans, Native Americans, Hispanic Americans, Asian Americans, and Pacific Islanders are at increased risk for type 2 diabetes (ADA, 2014b). Other risk factors are age older than 45 years; a history of elevated fasting serum glucose levels or impaired glucose tolerance; hypertension (HTN); low levels of high-density lipoproteins; triglycerides above 250 mg/dL; and a history of gestational diabetes or delivery of a baby over 9 pounds, or both. Table 66.1 compares and contrasts type 1 and type 2 diabetes.

Most patients with type 2 diabetes do not require insulin administration, at least initially; their condition can be managed with oral antidiabetic drugs. Type 2 diabetes was formerly called adult-onset diabetes and non–insulin-dependent diabetes, but these are not accurate descriptions of the disorder because it occurs in children and may require insulin administration.

TABLE 66.1	Comparison of Type 1 and Type 2 Diabetes Mellitus	
Diabetes Mellitus	**Type 1**	**Type 2**
Cause	Destruction of beta cells with lack of insulin	Insulin resistance; insulin deficiency may develop
Incidence	5–10%	90–95%
Age at onset	Children, young adults, usually younger than 35 years	Usually older than 35 years
Symptom onset	Rapid	Gradual
Body weight	Usually underweight	Usually overweight or obese
Symptoms	Polyuria, polydipsia, polyphagia, weight loss	Same as type 1, plus blurred vision, fatigue, recurrent infections
Ketosis	Often present with poor control	Infrequent
Pharmacologic treatment	Insulin replacement	Oral antidiabetes drugs with or without insulin

Gestational diabetes is a condition resulting from glucose intolerance with an onset, or first recognition, during pregnancy. This is a serious disorder that puts both the woman and fetus at risk for complications and so requires careful management during pregnancy. In addition, women who develop gestational diabetes are at increased risk for developing diabetes 5 to 10 years after delivery. It occurs most frequently in women with a family history of diabetes, a history of stillbirth or spontaneous abortion, a previous large-for-gestational-age baby, women who are obese or of advanced maternal age, women who have had five or more pregnancies, or women who are members of a high-risk population (Hispanic, Native American, Asian, or African American). If careful nutritional management combined with an approved exercise plan is unable to normalize serum glucose levels, insulin therapy is initiated. Traditionally, oral antidiabetic drugs have not been used for gestational diabetes due to concerns regarding potential teratogenicity; however, the results of research may change that practice in the future.

Symptoms and Diagnosis of Diabetes

66.3 The classic signs and symptoms of diabetes include polyuria, polydipsia, and polyphagia.

The classic triad of signs and symptoms for either type of diabetes is known as the three "polys": **polyuria**, excessive urine production; **polydipsia**, excessive thirst; and **polyphagia**, excessive appetite.

Glucose is one of the body's most valuable energy molecules, and nondiabetic patients excrete very little. As glucose levels rise in the blood in patients with diabetes, however, the kidneys are unable to reabsorb the large amounts passing through the renal tubules, so glucose is eliminated in the urine (glucosuria). Glucose molecules create increased osmotic pressure in body fluids, pulling water along with it; thus, osmotic diuresis (polyuria) occurs. The glucose increases osmotic pressure in the bloodstream, pulling water out of tissue cells and causing cellular dehydration. This triggers thirst and causes the person to increase fluid intake (polydipsia). The excess hunger (polyphagia) occurs primarily with type 1 diabetes, when nutrient stores become too depleted to meet the body's energy needs and weight is lost. Other signs and symptoms include blurred vision, fatigue, paresthesias, and skin infections. Nocturia, secondary to the polyuria, may occur.

Although symptomology is important for recognizing the possibility of diabetes, many patients with the disease have no symptoms. Laboratory tests are required for proper diagnosis. The primary blood tests for diagnosing diabetes are the **fasting plasma glucose (FPG) test**, **oral glucose tolerance test (OGTT)**, and **hemoglobin A1C (HbA1C)**.

- FPG: obtained following a fast of at least 8 hours. A value of 126 mg/dL or higher indicates diabetes.
- OGTT: A loading dose of 75 g of glucose is ingested and the plasma glucose level is obtained 2 hours later. A value of 200 mg/dL or higher indicates diabetes.
- HbA1C: As serum glucose increases, more glucose becomes bound to hemoglobin. A value of 6.5% or higher indicates diabetes. The advantage of HbA1C is that it does not require fasting and it provides an average measure of glucose control over the 8 to 12 weeks prior to the test.

Home monitoring of blood glucose is now commonplace and enables the patient with diabetes to maintain tighter control of glucose levels. Finger-stick testing involves placing a drop of capillary blood on a test strip, which is then read by a glucose meter.

Most patients who develop type 2 diabetes go through a period of impaired glucose tolerance referred to as **prediabetes**. In prediabetes, serum glucose levels are elevated but are not high enough to be diagnosed as diabetes. This condition increases the risk for developing diabetes, heart disease, and stroke. Prediabetes may result from impaired fasting glucose or impaired glucose tolerance, or both. Progression from prediabetes to diabetes is not inevitable. Careful management of nutrition, regular exercise, and weight management may prevent or delay progression to diabetes. Patients with prediabetes should be monitored on an annual basis for the potential development of diabetes and to evaluate the degree of success in managing comorbid conditions such as HTN, hyperlipidemia, and obesity.

Obesity-related insulin resistance can lead to **metabolic syndrome**, a cluster of biochemical changes that place the patient at increased risk for developing diabetes, heart disease, peripheral vascular disease, and stroke. Again, weight loss, exercise, and nutritional management enable people with this syndrome to delay or prevent the progression to type 2 diabetes. The metabolic syndrome is diagnosed by the presence of three or more of the following:

- Central (visceral) obesity, with waist circumference more than 35 in. for women or more than 40 in. for men
- Serum triglycerides equal to or greater than 150 mg/dL
- High-density lipoprotein (HDL) cholesterol less than 50 mg/dL in women or less than 40 mg/dL in men
- Blood pressure more than 130/85 mmHg
- Fasting plasma glucose more than 100 mg/dL (Porth, 2011)

Complications of Diabetes Mellitus

66.4 Acute complications of diabetes include diabetic ketoacidosis, hyperosmolar hyperglycemic state, and hypoglycemia.

Although most patients experience chronic diabetes, which develops over many years, acute episodes may occur suddenly in those with uncontrolled or poorly controlled diabetes. Diabetic ketoacidosis, hyperosmolar hyperglycemic state (HHS), and hypoglycemia are the three primary acute conditions. The chronic complications are discussed in Section 66.5.

Diabetic ketoacidosis (DKA) is an acute condition that occurs primarily in patients with type 1 diabetes. The three major disturbances that occur with DKA are hyperglycemia, metabolic acidosis, and osmotic diuresis. DKA typically develops over several days with symptoms such as polyuria, polydipsia, nausea, vomiting, and severe fatigue, progressing to stupor and eventual coma. The patient may report having abdominal pain or tenderness, and the breath has a typical fruity smell as the lungs attempt to remove volatile ketoacids. As the acidosis worsens, Kussmaul's respirations may develop, with an increased rate and depth of respirations. Tachycardia and hypotension occur in response to dehydration and fluid depletion.

DKA may be the first presenting symptoms of a person previously undiagnosed with diabetes. Treatment includes fluid replacement to improve circulating blood volume and tissue perfusion, normalization of blood glucose levels, and correction of electrolyte imbalances and metabolic acidosis. Insulin therapy is begun, usually with an IV loading dose, followed by a continuous low-dose infusion. Serum glucose levels must be lowered gradually because too rapid a drop can cause a fluid shift back into the cells that can lead to cerebral edema. Although DKA is a very serious disorder, the mortality rate for this complication has been reduced to less than 5% with proper treatment.

CONNECTION Checkpoint 66.1

From what you learned in Chapter 33, what is the clinical definition of acidosis? What is the drug of choice for reversing metabolic acidosis? *See Answer to Connection Checkpoint 66.1 on student resource website.*

Hyperosmolar hyperglycemic state (HHS) is a serious, acute complication of diabetes that carries a mortality rate of 20% to 40%. HHS is generally seen in persons with type 2 diabetes and is characterized by extreme hyperglycemia (above 600 mg/dL), hyperosmolarity (above 310 mOsm/L) with dehydration, the absence of ketoacidosis, and central nervous system (CNS) dysfunction. The typical patient is elderly, obese, and has comorbid medical problems, such as heart failure or renal impairment. The elevated serum glucose levels and increased osmolarity produce a large osmotic diuresis with marked dehydration, confusion, and lethargy. Other possible neurologic symptoms are seizures, hemiparesis, abnormal reflexes, aphasia, and visual disturbances. Symptoms can progress to stupor and coma. Tachycardia and hypotension result from fluid depletion and poor tissue perfusion. Acidosis may develop, caused by an accumulation of lactic acid rather than ketoacids.

The onset of HHS is gradual and, because of the neurologic manifestations, may be mistaken for a stroke in older adults. Treatment consists of careful fluid replacement while avoiding cerebral and pulmonary edema and correction of electrolyte imbalances, particularly potassium. Low-dose insulin is given by continuous IV infusion to slowly lower glucose levels to 250 to 300 mg/dL. Seizure precautions should be instituted, and hemodynamic monitoring should be used in these critically ill patients. The nurse should closely monitor intake and output, blood pressure, heart rate, lung sounds, weight, peripheral pulses, and neurologic status. Finally, the underlying cause of the episode should be investigated and treated as needed.

Hypoglycemia, or abnormally low serum glucose, occurs most often in patients improperly treated with insulin and may occur during therapy with some oral antidiabetic drugs. The manifestations of hypoglycemia result from changes in mental status and by the activation of the sympathetic nervous system. Because the brain relies on a continuous supply of glucose, falling glucose levels may lead to headache, difficulty concentrating, confusion, and behavioral changes, progressing to seizures and coma. The sympathetic nervous system activation results from the body's attempt to increase serum glucose by the release of catecholamines (epinephrine and norepinephrine). These catecholamines cause symptoms that include tachycardia, anxiety, sweating, and the constriction of surface vessels, leading to cool, clammy skin. Acute hypoglycemia is considered a medical emergency, and if prolonged or severe, can lead to brain damage or death.

The symptoms of hypoglycemia may have a very rapid onset. Patients who have had diabetes for an extended time may develop hypoglycemic unawareness, which is the inability to recognize symptoms. Some drugs, such as beta-adrenergic blockers, interfere with the sympathetic symptoms of hypoglycemia, making it more difficult for the patient to recognize the condition and for the body to correct the low glucose levels.

Factors that cause hypoglycemia in patients with diabetes include errors in insulin dosage, failure to eat at regular intervals, increased exercise, medication adjustments, or changes in the insulin injection site. Alcohol consumption can lead to hypoglycemia by decreasing gluconeogenesis. The treatment for hypoglycemia is always glucose, given in a concentrated source of 15 to 20 g. This can be repeated as necessary, while taking care not to overtreat the patient and cause hyperglycemia. If the person is unconscious, or unable to swallow safely, a small amount of glucose gel or spray can be administered to the buccal mucosa. Intravenous (IV) glucose is immediately effective in treating hypoglycemia and glucagon may be administered.

PROTOTYPE DRUG	Glucagon (GlucaGen)

Classification: **Therapeutic:** Antihypoglycemic drug
Pharmacologic: Pancreatic hormone

Therapeutic Effects and Uses: Glucagon is used for the emergency treatment of severe hypoglycemia in patients with diabetes who are unconscious or unable to eat sugar or drink a sweetened beverage. It is also used for radiographic studies to relax the smooth muscle of the GI tract. GlucaGen is obtained through recombinant DNA technology and is identical in structure to human glucagon.

Glucagon can be given intramuscularly (IM), subcutaneously, or IV. Glucagon will raise serum glucose levels in 10 to 20 minutes. Because glucagon raises glucose levels by stimulating breakdown of stored glycogen, it is not effective in patients who experience hypoglycemia due to starvation, because their glycogen stores are depleted.

From 1930 to 1950, massive doses of insulin were administered to agitated psychiatric patients with serious mental illnesses to induce seizures and coma, a procedure called insulin shock therapy. Upon administration of glucose or glucagon, the patient awakened in a more sedated state. Although glucagon is still approved for this purpose, this inhumane practice was discontinued when antipsychotic drugs were discovered in the 1950s.

Mechanism of Action: Glucagon increases glucose levels by increasing glycogenolysis; therefore, its actions are dependent on the presence of adequate liver glycogen stores. Glucagon stimulates the uptake of amino acids, increases their conversion to glucose (gluconeogenesis), and promotes lipolysis in the liver, with the release of fatty acids and glycerol.

Pharmacokinetics:

Route(s)	IM, IV, subcutaneous
Absorption	Easily absorbed IM or subcutaneous
Distribution	Throughout plasma
Primary metabolism	Liver, plasma, and kidneys
Primary excretion	Renal and through the bile
Onset of action	IV: 5–20 min; IM: 30 min; subcutaneous: 30–45 min
Duration of action	1–1.5 h

Adverse Effects: Glucagon is well tolerated. Adverse effects include nausea, vomiting, hypersensitivity reactions, transient changes in blood pressure (either hypotension or HTN), tachycardia, hyperglycemia, and hypokalemia.

Contraindications/Precautions: Glucagon is contraindicated in patients sensitive to protein compounds, in patients with depleted glycogen stores, or in patients with insulinoma or pheochromocytoma. It is used with caution in persons with coronary artery disease because it may affect blood pressure, heart rate, and myocardial oxygen demand.

Drug Interactions: Glucagon increases serum glucose and will antagonize the effects of antidiabetic drugs. Beta-adrenergic blockers will inhibit the glucose-elevating effect of glucagon and will also increase the risk of blood pressure or heart rate adverse effects associated with glucagon. **Herbal/Food:** None known.

Pregnancy: Category B.

Treatment of Overdose: An overdose can cause hyperglycemia, which may be treated with insulin, IV fluids, and monitoring of electrolytes.

Nursing Responsibilities:

- Assess the patient's blood glucose level before, during, and after glucagon administration.
- Reconstitute the dry powder of glucagon with the diluent supplied by the manufacturer. Gently roll the vial to mix the drug but do not shake the vial. If glucagon fails to cause a response, IV glucose must be given.
- Administer supplemental oral carbohydrates once consciousness has been achieved to restore glycogen levels and prevent secondary hypoglycemia.
- Instruct the patient on the proper use of the GlucaGen emergency kit.

Lifespan and Diversity Considerations:

- Calculate pediatric dosages carefully. In general, children under the age of 6 require one half the adult dose.

Patient and Family Education:

- Immediately report signs of impending hypoglycemia such as headache, difficulty concentrating, confusion, seizures, palpitations, nervousness, sweating, and cool, clammy skin to the health care provider.
- At the first signs of hypoglycemia, eat sugar or other carbohydrate because this may eliminate the need to administer glucagon. Follow any carbohydrate with a protein source for longer lasting effects.
- Do not mix the GlucaGen solution with the powder until it is ready to be used. Discard any unused portion.
- Wear a medical alert bracelet or jewelry that identifies your medical condition and its treatment.

Drugs Similar to Glucagon (GlucaGen)

There are no drugs similar to glucagon.

66.5 Serious complications of chronic diabetes include neuropathy, nephropathy, retinopathy, and vascular disease.

Most patients with type 2 diabetes experience no symptoms of their illness for many years, perhaps even decades. There may be no acute symptoms to motivate the patient to seek medical care. However, while years may pass without symptoms, the effects of uncontrolled blood glucose levels are progressively producing major, irreversible changes on body systems, especially the nervous and circulatory systems.

Teaching patients about the long-term consequences of untreated diabetes can be a major challenge for the nurse. When diagnosed at an asymptomatic stage, it is difficult to convince patients to make radical changes to their lifestyle and to spend money on prescriptions when they do not feel ill. Patients must clearly understand that if they delay treatment until symptoms appear, it will likely be too late to prevent serious, chronic complications. Intensive management of blood glucose levels has been found to dramatically reduce the incidence of long-term complications of diabetes.

Neuropathies are common, affecting an estimated 60% to 70% of persons with diabetes. Diabetic neuropathies affect both the somatic and autonomic nervous systems. Somatic neuropathies include paresthesias, numbness, tingling and pain, motor weakness, and muscle wasting. Autonomic neuropathies include postural hypotension, altered GI functioning including gastroparesis, or gastric atony, diarrhea, altered genitourinary functioning with difficulty voiding or erectile dysfunction, and possible cranial nerve impairment. Intensive management of blood glucose has been shown to reduce the occurrence of neuropathies.

Diabetic nephropathy is the leading cause of end-stage renal disease, which affects patients with both type 1 and type 2 diabetes. Most commonly, the renal glomeruli are damaged, and progressive loss of kidney function leads to eventual renal failure. Comorbid conditions that put the patient at high risk for nephropathy include HTN, poor glucose control, smoking, and hyperlipidemia.

Diabetic retinopathy is the leading cause of acquired blindness in the United States. Twenty years after the onset of diabetes, almost all persons with type 1 diabetes, and over 60% of those with type 2 diabetes, show some degree of retinopathy (Porth, 2011). Regular eye exams are important for everyone who has diabetes.

Diabetes is a major risk factor for the development of vascular disease, including premature atherosclerosis, which leads to coronary artery disease, cerebrovascular disease, and peripheral vascular disease. Heart disease and stroke account for about 65% of deaths in persons with diabetes. Preventive measures are directed toward reducing risk factors: control of blood pressure, smoking cessation, lowering lipid levels, and optimal glucose control. In addition, antiplatelet drugs are often indicated.

Foot ulcers occur in patients with diabetes due to peripheral neuropathies and poor circulation. Neuropathies may impair sensation, so a small area of irritation may go unnoticed. Vascular insufficiency and elevated glucose levels inhibit healing of the ulcer. If the ulcer becomes infected, it is often resistant to treatment and can ultimately result in the need for amputation. Diabetes is the leading cause of nontraumatic amputations.

Insulin Therapy

66.6 Insulin is the cornerstone of therapy for patients with type 1 and gestational diabetes.

Because patients with type 1 diabetes are severely deficient in insulin production, insulin replacement therapy is required to survive. Insulin is also required for those with type 2 diabetes who are unable to manage their blood glucose levels with diet, exercise, and oral antidiabetic drugs. Among adults with diabetes in the United States, 12% take only insulin, 14% take insulin with oral antidiabetic drugs, 58% take oral antidiabetic drugs only, and 16% take neither insulin nor antidiabetic drugs (Centers for Disease Control and Prevention, 2011).

The therapeutic goal for patients with type 1 diabetes is to administer insulin as replacement therapy in normal physiological amounts. Because insulin secretion varies greatly in response to daily activities, pharmacotherapy must be carefully planned in conjunction with proper meal planning and lifestyle habits. The desired outcome of insulin therapy is to prevent the long-term consequences of diabetes by maintaining blood glucose levels strictly within the normal range.

The fundamental principle to remember about insulin therapy is that the right amount of insulin must be available to cells when glucose is present in the blood. Administering insulin when glucose is not available can lead to hypoglycemia and, possibly, coma. This situation occurs when a patient administers insulin correctly but skips a meal. The insulin is available to cells, but glucose is not. In another example, the patient participates in strenuous exercise. The insulin may have been administered on schedule, and food eaten, but the active muscles quickly use up all the glucose in the blood, and the patient becomes hypoglycemic. Patients with diabetes who engage in competitive sports need to consume food or sports drinks just prior to and during the activity to maintain their blood glucose at normal levels. The nurse plays a key role in helping patients plan their meals, activities, and insulin dosages correctly. Figure 66.2 illustrates the management of type 1 diabetes and correct timing of the insulin dose with meals.

Many types of insulin are available, differing in their source, time of onset, and peak effect and duration of action. Until the 1980s, the primary source of insulin was beef or pork pancreas. Almost all insulin today, however, is human insulin obtained through recombinant DNA technology because it is more effective, causes fewer allergies, and has a lower incidence of resistance. Pharmacologists have modified human insulin to create certain pharmacokinetic advantages, such as a more rapid onset of action (Humalog) or a more prolonged duration of action (Lantus). These modified forms are called insulin *analogs*. The different types of insulins available are listed in Table 66.2.

Doses of insulin are highly individualized for the precise control of blood glucose levels in each patient. Because the GI tract destroys insulin, it must be given by injection. Some patients require two or more injections daily for proper diabetes management. For ease of administration, two different compatible types of insulin may be mixed, using a standard method, to obtain the desired therapeutic effects. Some of these combinations are marketed in cartridges containing premixed solutions. A long-acting insulin may be taken daily to provide a basal blood level, with a supplemental

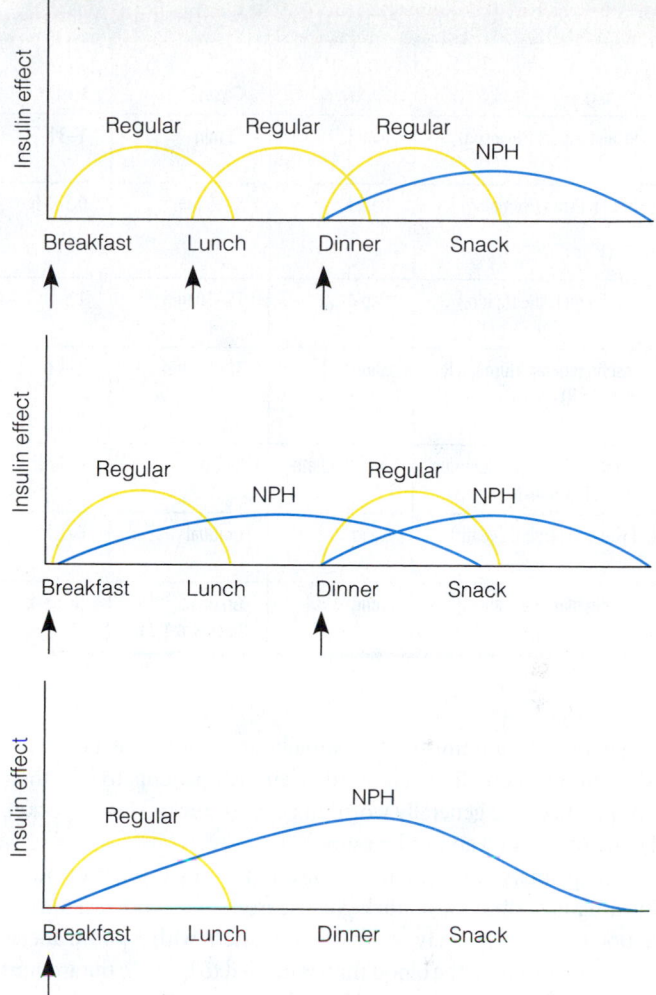

Figure 66.2 Insulin regimens.

rapid-acting insulin given shortly before a meal. It is important for nurses and patients to know the time of peak action of any insulin, because that is when the risk for hypoglycemic adverse effects is greatest.

All insulin products used clinically are U-100, meaning 1 mL contains 100 units of insulin, and are administered using U-100 syringes. One type of human regular insulin has been formulated in the U-500 strength, but this is available from the manufacturer only and is reserved for patients who require very large doses of insulin (more than 200 units/day). Insulin preparations are either clear or cloudy. Those that are cloudy require mixing the solution by rolling the vial prior to drawing out the desired dose. Insulins that are clear do not require mixing. Regular insulin is the only type that can be administered by IV injection.

Rapid- or regular-acting insulin can be used in continuous subcutaneous infusion devices, often called insulin pumps. An infusion set, which holds a syringe of the drug, delivers insulin from the pump to a needle anchored in the subcutaneous tissue of the abdomen. The infusion set is replaced every 3 days, at which time the injection site should be moved, preferably to 1 inch away from the old site. The pump is programmed to release small subcutaneous doses of insulin into the abdomen at predetermined intervals, with

TABLE 66.2	Types of Insulin: Actions and Administration					
Drug	**Action**	**Onset**	**Peak**	**Duration**	**Administration and Timing**	**Compatibility**
Insulin aspart (NovoLog)	Rapid	15 min	1–3 h	3–5 h	Subcutaneous: 5–10 min before meal	Can give with NPH; draw aspart up first, give immediately
Insulin lispro (Humalog)	Rapid	5–15 min	0.5–1 h	3–4 h	Subcutaneous: 15 min before or immediately after a meal	Can give with NPH; draw lispro up first, give immediately
Insulin glulisine (Apidra)	Rapid	15–30 min	1 h	3–4 h	Subcutaneous: 15 min before meal	Can give with NPH; draw glulisine up first, give immediately
Insulin regular (Humulin R, Novolin R)	Short	30–60 min	2–4 h	5–7 h	Subcutaneous: 30–60 min before meal; IV	Can mix with NPH, sterile water, normal saline; do not mix with glargine
Isophane insulin suspension (NPH, Humulin N)	Intermediate	1–2 h	4–12 h	18–24 h	Subcutaneous: Mix (cloudy)	Can mix with aspart, lispro, reg; do not mix with glargine
Insulin detemir (Levemir)	Long	Gradual	6–8 h	To 24 h	Subcutaneous: 1/day or 2/day	Do not mix with any other insulin
Insulin glargine (Lantus)	Long	Gradual: begins at 1.1 h	No peak	To 24 h	Subcutaneous: 1/day, same time each day	Do not mix with any other insulin

larger boluses administered manually at mealtime if necessary. Most pumps contain an alarm that reminds patients to take their insulin. They are generally worn on a belt or tucked into a pocket. Figure 66.3 shows an insulin pump.

The primary adverse effect of insulin therapy is overtreatment; insulin may remove too much glucose from the blood, resulting in hypoglycemia. This may occur when a patient with type 1 diabetes has more insulin in the blood than is needed to balance the amount of circulating blood glucose. Hypoglycemia may occur when the insulin level peaks, during exercise, when the patient receives too much insulin due to a medication error, or if the patient skips

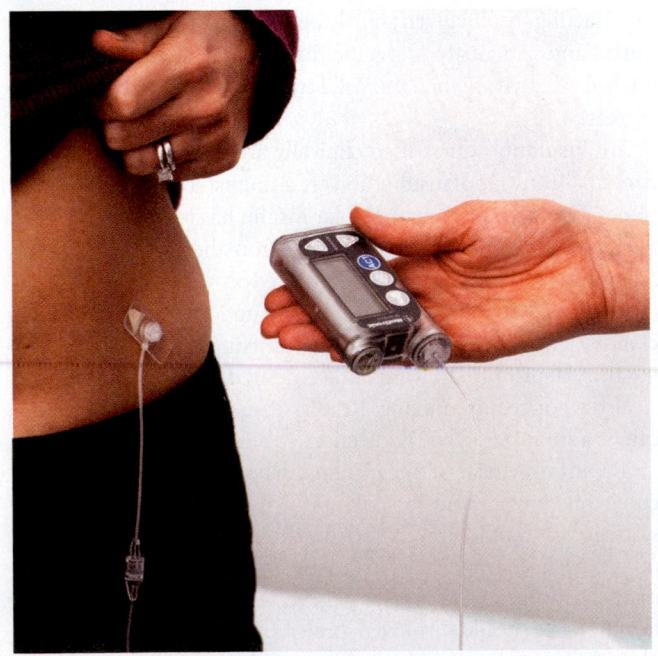

Figure 66.3 Insulin pump.
© ACE Stock Limited/Alamy

a meal. Some of the symptoms of hypoglycemia are the same as those of DKA. Those that differ and help to determine that a patient is hypoglycemic include pale, cool, and moist skin, with blood glucose less than 50 mg/dL and a sudden onset of symptoms. Left untreated, severe hypoglycemia may result in death.

Other adverse effects of insulin include injection-site reactions, generalized urticaria, and swollen lymph glands. Some patients will experience Somogyi phenomenon, a rapid decrease in blood glucose, usually during the night, which stimulates the release of hormones that elevate blood glucose (epinephrine, cortisol, and glucagon), resulting in an elevated morning blood glucose level. Administration of insulin above the patient's normal dose may produce a rapid rebound hypoglycemia. The hormone glucagon is administered as a replacement therapy for some patients with diabetes when they are in a hypoglycemic state and have impaired glucagon secretion.

Patients with diabetes who forget their insulin dose face equally serious consequences. Again, remember the fundamental principle of insulin pharmacotherapy: The right amount of insulin must be available to cells when glucose is present in the blood. Without insulin present, glucose from a meal can build up to high levels in the blood, causing hyperglycemia and possible coma. Proper planning and teaching by the nurse is essential to achieve successful outcomes and maximize patient adherence with therapy.

Insulin Adjunct

Pramlintide (Symlin) is an antihyperglycemic drug approved in 2005 that is used along with insulin in persons with type 1 or type 2 diabetes who are not able to achieve glucose control by the use of insulin alone. The drug is a synthetic analog of amylin, a natural hormone released by the beta cells of the pancreas at the same time as insulin. Its natural function is to act synergistically with insulin in glycemic control. The therapeutic actions of pramlintide are to slow gastric emptying time, reduce postprandial glucagon secretion, and increase satiety, thereby leading to reduced calorie intake.

Pramlintide is administered subcutaneously immediately prior to each meal, using U-100 insulin syringes. It cannot be mixed with insulin, and it must be injected into a different site than insulin. When initiating treatment, rapid- or short-acting insulin doses are usually reduced by 50%. Adverse effects include nausea, vomiting, abdominal pain, headache, dizziness, fatigue, coughing, allergic reaction, or arthralgia. The drug carries a black box warning that severe hypoglycemia may occur during therapy. Hypoglycemia may be prolonged and severe, usually occurring within 3 hours following an injection.

PROTOTYPE DRUG	**Human Regular Insulin (Humulin R, Novolin R)**

Classification: **Therapeutic:** Antidiabetic drug, pancreatic hormone
Pharmacologic: Short-acting hypoglycemic drug

Therapeutic Effects and Uses: Human regular insulin is used to maintain blood glucose levels within normal limits. The primary effects of human regular insulin are promotion of cellular uptake of glucose, amino acids, and potassium; promotion of protein synthesis, glycogen formation and storage, and fatty acid storage as triglycerides; and conservation of energy stores by promoting the utilization of glucose for energy needs and inhibiting gluconeogenesis. Indications for insulin include the following:

- As monotherapy to lower blood glucose levels in patients with type 1 diabetes
- In combination with oral antidiabetic drugs in patients with type 2 diabetes
- For the emergency treatment of DKA or hyperosmolar hyperglycemic state
- For gestational diabetes

Because regular insulin is short acting, it is most often used in combination with intermediate- or long-acting insulin to achieve 24-hour glucose control. Nondiabetic indications for insulin include stimulation of growth hormone secretion in the evaluation of growth hormone deficiency and the treatment of hyperkalemia to promote a shift of potassium into cells.

Mechanism of Action: Regular insulin is identical to endogenous insulin. Insulin decreases blood glucose levels by increasing cellular uptake of glucose and stimulating storage of glucose as glycogen; it also inhibits the release of glucagon.

Pharmacokinetics:

Route(s)	Subcutaneous; IV (only regular insulin can be given IV); inhalation
Absorption	Rapidly absorbed following subcutaneous injection; absorption time can vary by site of injection
Distribution	Throughout extracellular fluids
Primary metabolism	Hepatic
Primary excretion	Liver and kidneys
Onset of action	Subcutaneous: 30–60 min; IV: 15 min
Duration of action	6–10 h

Adverse Effects: The most common adverse effect of insulin therapy is hypoglycemia. Rebound hyperglycemia (Somogyi phenomenon) may occur. Irritation at injection sites may occur, including lipohypertrophy, the accumulation of fat in the area of injection. This effect is lessened with rotation of injection sites. Weight gain is a possible adverse effect. Because insulin facilitates the intracellular uptake of potassium, hypokalemia is possible.

Contraindications/Precautions: Beef or pork insulins (which are now rarely used) are contraindicated in persons with hypersensitivity to these animal proteins. Insulin is used with caution in pregnancy, renal impairment or failure, fever, thyroid disease, among the elderly, or in children or infants. Insulin should not be administered to patients with hypoglycemia. Patients with hypokalemia should be monitored carefully because insulin may worsen this condition.

Drug Interactions: Insulin must be used cautiously in conjunction with drugs that can produce hypoglycemia, including sulfonylureas, meglitinides, beta-adrenergic blockers, salicylates, anabolic steroids, monamine oxidase inhibitors (MAOIs), and alcohol. Several drugs can antagonize the glucose-lowering effects of insulin including dextrothyroxine, corticosteroids, epinephrine or norepinephrine, furosemide, and thiazide diuretics. Angiotensin-converting enzyme (ACE) inhibitors increase insulin sensitivity and may enhance the hypoglycemic effects of insulin. Many other drugs can influence blood glucose and the nurse should consult current drug references when treating patients who take high insulin doses or who have unstable diabetes.

Herbal/Food: Garlic, chromium, black cohosh, bitter melon, bilberry, and ginseng may potentiate the hypoglycemic effects of insulin. Cocoa and rosemary may have a hyperglycemic effect.

Pregnancy: Insulin glargine is pregnancy category C; other forms of insulin are category B.

Treatment of Overdose: An overdose of insulin can cause profound hypoglycemia, which is treated with a concentrated source of glucose (dextrose), such as D_5W or glucagon, by the parenteral route.

Nursing Responsibilities: Key nursing implications for patients receiving regular insulin are included in the Nursing Practice Application for Patients Receiving Pharmacotherapy with Insulin.

Drugs Similar to Human Regular Insulin (Humulin R, Novolin R)

Many types of insulin are available. They are categorized by their onset of action and duration of action, as given in Table 66.2. There are also premixed formulations of insulin available, such as human insulin Humulin 70/30. This type contains 70% NPH insulin and 30% regular insulin, so it can be given before a meal to help control postprandial glucose while also providing longer coverage of insulin needs. Other combination insulins include Humalog 75/25, Humulin 50/50, Novolin 70/30, and NovoLog 70/30. The characteristics of selected insulin combinations are shown in Table 66.3.

Insulin aspart (NovoLog): Insulin aspart is a rapid-onset drug, with a structure very similar to that of endogenous insulin. Insulin

TABLE 66.3	Premixed Insulin Combinations						
Drug	**Description**	**Route and Adult Dose (Maximum Dose Where Indicated)**	**Onset (min)**	**Peak (h)**	**Duration (h)**	**Adverse Effects**
Humulin 70/30	70% NPH insulin/ 30% regular insulin	Subcutaneous: individualized doses	30–60	1.5–16	Up to 36	*Pain and swelling at injection site* Hypoglycemia, DKA
Novolin 70/30	70% NPH insulin/ 30% regular insulin	Subcutaneous: individualized doses	30–60	2–12	Up to 36	
Humulin 50/50	50% NPH insulin/ 50% regular insulin	Subcutaneous: individualized doses	30–60	2–5.5	Up to 24	
NovoLog Mix 70/30	70% insulin aspart protamine/ 30% insulin aspart	Subcutaneous: individualized doses	15–60	1–4	Up to 24	
Humalog Mix 75/25	75% insulin lispro protamine/ 25% insulin lispro	Subcutaneous: individualized doses	15–60	1–6.5	Up to 24	

Note: Italics indicate common adverse effects. Underline indicates serious adverse effects.

aspart has a more rapid onset of action than regular insulin, acting within about 15 minutes when given subcutaneously. Because insulin aspart acts rapidly, injections should be made 5 to 10 minutes before meals. It also has a short duration of action, 3 to 5 hours when compared to regular insulin. Because of its short duration, insulin aspart is usually given in combination with an intermediate- or long-acting form of insulin. Insulin aspart is available in 10-mL vials and 3-mL prefilled cartridges.

Insulin detemir (Levemir): Insulin detemir is a long-acting insulin with a slow onset and dose-dependent duration of action. Detemir may be given once or twice a day, depending on the dose; low doses provide shorter durations of action than larger doses, and so dosing is individualized to the patient. At low doses (0.2 unit/kg), effects persist about 12 hours. At higher doses (0.4 unit/kg), effects last 20 to 24 hours. Because of its slow onset and prolonged duration, insulin detemir is used to provide basal glycemic control. It is not injected before meals to control postprandial hyperglycemia. It cannot be mixed with any other type of insulin and is only given by subcutaneous injection. Insulin detemir is supplied in 10-mL vials, 3-mL cartridges, a 3-mL pen, and a 3-mL InnoLet dosing device. The InnoLet dosing injection device is disposable and has an easy-to-read dial, large push button for injection, and audible clicks that indicate each unit injected.

Insulin glargine (Lantus): Insulin glargine is a newer recombinant insulin analog that exhibits constant, long-duration insulin activity. It has no defined peak effect and provides for the maintenance of steady blood levels; therefore, there is less risk of hypoglycemia with this type of insulin. Insulin glargine allows for once-daily dosing as basal insulin coverage. Although it can be given without regard to meals, it should be given at the same time each day to provide steady blood levels. It cannot be mixed with any other type of insulin and is only given by subcutaneous injection. Insulin glargine may also help improve the lipid profiles and A1C levels of type 2 diabetes when added to therapy. Insulin glargine is supplied in 10-mL vials and in 3-mL cartridges.

Insulin glulisine (Apidra): Insulin glulisine has a 10- to 15-minute onset and a short duration of 3 to 5 hours. Because of its rapid onset, the drug should be administered no sooner than 15 minutes before eating and no later than 20 minutes after starting a meal. Apidra is only given by subcutaneous injection.

Insulin lispro (Humalog): Insulin lispro is a rapid-acting analog of regular insulin, with effects beginning within 15 to 30 minutes of subcutaneous injection. Insulin lispro acts faster than regular insulin but has a shorter duration of action, 5 hours or less. Because of its rapid onset, insulin lispro should be administered immediately before eating, or even after eating. It is meant to help control the rise in blood glucose brought on by a meal and is normally given concurrently with an intermediate- or long-acting drug that provides a basal coverage of insulin. It is a clear insulin and does not require mixing prior to injecting. Lispro cannot be given IV. It is often used with insulin infusion pumps.

Isophane insulin (NPH, Humulin N): Isophane insulin is the only intermediate-acting insulin. It has a slower onset of action (1 to 4 hours) than regular insulin and a duration of action of up to 18 to 24 hours. It is used to provide a basal level of insulin coverage for between meals and at night. NPH insulin is normally administered 30 minutes before the first meal of the day, but in some instances a second, smaller dose is taken before the evening meal or at bedtime. Many patients are prescribed insulin that is premixed, such as 70% NPH with 30% regular or rapid acting. If the patient is prescribed a premixed insulin solution, it is important that proper instructions be given, especially if the patient will be using additional regular or rapid-acting insulin on a sliding scale. NPH is a cloudy suspension and requires mixing prior to drawing up a dose. NPH can be given with aspart, lispro, or regular insulin, but it cannot be mixed with glargine insulin. When mixed with another type of insulin, NPH should be drawn up after the other insulin, and the mixture should be administered immediately. The term *NPH* stands for Neutral Protamine Hagedorn. Hans Christian Hagedorn was a scientist who developed the drug in the 1920s.

◖ **Diabetes in the School Setting**

Caring for the school-age child with diabetes in a school setting requires teamwork between the parents or caregiver, school nurse, school staff, the child's health care provider, and, most often, the child. For each child, an individual diabetes medical management plan (DMMP) should be established that addresses all aspects of the diabetes care. The ADA (2014a) recommends the following specific instructions be included in each child's DMMP:

- Blood glucose monitoring instructions, including the frequency and circumstances for requiring monitoring. Provision should be made for privacy during testing or insulin administration if the child, parents, or caregiver desires.
- Information on insulin injections, if used, to include type(s) of insulin, dose, times for administration, storage, and provider permission for adjustments in insulin dosage if needed.
- Information on meals and snacks, including scheduling, the need for the child to be able to eat prn (as needed) to prevent hypoglycemia, and content and calories of a school lunch.
- Symptoms and treatment for hypoglycemia and hyperglycemia. Specific levels of training should be provided to school personnel based on whether they will administer basic, intermediate, or advanced treatment in caring for the child.
- Information on participation in physical activity.
- Emergency plans for emergency evacuation, shelter-in-place, or school lockdowns.

By establishing a DMMP, routine daily care as well as emergency contingencies can be addressed. When all participants work as a team, a child with diabetes can participate fully and safely in the school setting.

◖ **Incorrect Insulin Dose**

A patient with diabetes has 30 units of Humulin R (regular) insulin ordered for the morning dose. There are several patients with diabetes on the unit and the nurse has given many doses of insulin that morning. The nurse prepares the insulin but draws up Humalog 30 units instead. The patient begins experiencing symptoms of hypoglycemia within 15 minutes and is treated successfully.

What errors occurred and how could they be prevented in the future?

See Answers to Patient Safety Question on student resource website.

type 2 diabetes include alpha-glucosidase inhibitors, biguanides, incretin enhancers, meglitinides, sulfonylureas, and thiazolidinediones. An additional group includes miscellaneous drugs from other classes. All the medications used to treat type 2 diabetes require some degree of pancreatic insulin secretion. These antidiabetic medications are not effective in treating type 1 diabetes because these patients have a total lack of insulin secretion.

Treatment goals recommended by the American Association of Clinical Endocrinologists (AACE, 2011) are designed to target an HbA1C level of 6.5% or less with an FPG of less than 110 g/dL. In general, all of the antidiabetic drugs are similar in their ability to lower HbA1C levels in the short term. There are some differences, however, in long-term control. For example, drugs in the thiazolidinedione class appear to maintain glycemic control for 5 to 6 years, while the sulfonylureas peak at 6 months and slowly decline in efficacy. The adverse effects observed for each class differ: Some cause hypoglycemia, whereas others cause weight gain or GI complaints such as diarrhea. Because there is no perfect drug for type 2 diabetes, choice of therapy is guided by the experiences of the prescriber and the results achieved by the individual patient. A comparison of the antidiabetic drug classes is presented in Table 66.4. Doses of the individual medications are listed in Table 66.5.

Therapy for type 2 diabetes is usually initiated with a single drug. If glycemic control is not achieved with monotherapy, a second medication is added to the therapeutic regimen. Failure to achieve glycemic control with two oral hypoglycemic agents indicates the need for insulin to be added to the regimen.

Antidiabetic Drugs for Type 2 Diabetes

66.7 Antidiabetic drugs from multiple classes are used to treat type 2 diabetes.

The six primary classes of antidiabetic drugs used to treat type 2 diabetes are differentiated by their chemical structures and their mechanisms of action. Drug classes prescribed for patients with

TABLE 66.4 Summary of Antidiabetic Drug Classes		
Drug	**Action(s)**	**Nursing Considerations**
Alpha-Glucosidase Inhibitors	Interferes with carbohydrate breakdown and absorption; acts locally in GI tract with little systemic absorption	Common GI effects; hypoglycemia can occur if combined with another oral drug; if this occurs, treat with glucose, not sucrose; take with meals
Biguanides	Decreases production and release of glucose from the liver; increases cellular uptake of glucose; lowers lipid levels; promotes weight loss	Common GI adverse effects; risk for lactic acidosis (rare); avoid alcohol; low risk for hypoglycemia
Incretin Enhancers	Slows the breakdown of insulin, keeping it circulating in the blood longer; slows the rate of digestion, which increases satiety	Well tolerated; minor nausea, vomiting, and diarrhea; some weight loss is likely; low risk for hypoglycemia
Meglitinides	Stimulates insulin release	Can cause hypoglycemia, GI effects; well tolerated; administer shortly before meals
Sulfonylureas	Stimulates insulin release; decreases insulin resistance	Can cause hypoglycemia, GI disturbances, rash; cross sensitivity with sulfa drugs and thiazide diuretics; possible disulfiram response with alcohol
Thiazolidinediones	Decreases production and release of glucose from the liver; increases insulin sensitivity in fat and muscle tissue	Can cause fluid retention and worsening of heart failure; therapeutic effects take several weeks to develop

TABLE 66.5 Antidiabetic Drugs for Type 2 Diabetes

Drug	Route and Adult Dose (Maximum Dose Where Indicated)	Adverse Effects
Alpha-Glucosidase Inhibitors		
acarbose (Precose)	PO: 25–100 mg tid (max: 300 mg/day)	*Flatulence, diarrhea, abdominal distention*
miglitol (Glyset)	PO: 25–100 mg tid (max: 300 mg/day)	<u>Hypoglycemia (tremors, palpitations, sweating)</u>
Biguanides		
metformin immediate release (Glucophage, Riomet)	PO: 500 mg 2 times/day or 850 mg once daily; increase to 1,000–2,550 mg in two to three divided doses/day (max: 2.55 g/day)	*Flatulence, diarrhea, nausea, anorexia, abdominal pain, bitter or metallic taste, decreased vitamin B$_{12}$ levels*
extended release (Fortamet, Glucophage XR, Glumetza)	Glumetza: 1,000–2,000 mg once daily (max: 2 g/day) Glucophage XR: 500 mg once daily (max 2 g/day) Fortamet: 1,000 mg once daily (max: 2.5 g/day)	<u>Lactic acidosis</u>
Incretin Enhancers (GLP-1 Agonists)		
albiglutide (Tanzeum)	Subcutaneous: 30–50 mg once weekly	*Nausea, vomiting, diarrhea, headache, nervousness*
exenatide (Byetta)	Subcutaneous: 5–10 mcg 2 times/day 60 min prior to morning and evening meals	<u>Hypoglycemia (tremors, palpitations, sweating), antibody formation, pancreatitis (exenatide), renal impairment (exenatide), thyroid tumors (liraglutide, albiglutide)</u>
dulaglutide (Trulicity)	Subcutaneous: 0.75–1.5 mg once weekly	
liraglutide (Victoza)	Subcutaneous: 0.6–1.8 mg once daily, any time of day	
Incretin Enhancers (DPP-4 Inhibitors)		
alogliptin (Nesina)	PO: 25 mg once daily	*Headache, upper respiratory and urinary tract infections*
linagliptin (Tradjenta)	PO: 5 mg once daily	<u>Hypoglycemia (tremors, palpitations, sweating), anaphylaxis, peripheral edema, exfoliative dermatitis, Stevens–Johnson syndrome</u>
saxagliptin (Onglyza)	PO: 2.5–5 mg once daily	
sitagliptin (Januvia)	PO: 100 mg once daily	
Meglitinides		
nateglinide (Starlix)	PO: 60–120 mg tid, 1–30 min prior to meals	*Flulike symptoms, upper respiratory infection, back pain*
repaglinide (Prandin)	PO: 0.5–4 mg bid–qid, 1–30 min prior to meals (max: 16 mg/day)	<u>Hypoglycemia (tremors, palpitations, sweating), anaphylaxis, pancreatitis</u>
Sulfonylureas, First Generation		
chlorpropamide (Diabinese)	PO: 100–500 mg/day (max: 750 mg/day)	*Nausea, heartburn, dizziness, headache, drowsiness*
tolazamide (Tolinase)	PO: 100–500 mg 1–2 times/day (max: 1 g/day)	<u>Hypoglycemia (tremors, palpitations, sweating), cholestatic jaundice, blood dyscrasias</u>
tolbutamide (Orinase)	PO: 250–1,500 mg 1–2 times/day (max: 3 g/day)	
Sulfonylureas, Second Generation		
glimepiride (Amaryl)	PO: 1–4 mg/day (max: 8 mg/day)	*Nausea, heartburn, dizziness, headache, drowsiness*
glipizide (Glucotrol)	PO: 2.5–20 mg 1–2 times/day (max: 40 mg/day)	<u>Hypoglycemia (tremors, palpitations, sweating), cholestatic jaundice, blood dyscrasias</u>
glyburide (DiaBeta, Micronase) glyburide micronized (Glynase)	PO: 1.25–10 mg 1–2 times/day (max: 20 mg/day) PO: 0.75–12 mg 1–2 times/day (max: 12 mg/day)	
Thiazolidinediones		
pioglitazone (Actos)	PO: 15–30 mg/day (max: 45 mg/day)	*Upper respiratory infection, myalgia, headache, edema, weight gain*
rosiglitazone (Avandia)	PO: 4–8 mg 1–2 times/day (max: 8 mg/day)	<u>Hypoglycemia (tremors, palpitations, sweating), hepatotoxicity, bone fractures, heart failure, MI</u>
Miscellaneous Drugs		
bromocriptine (Cycloset)	PO: 0.8–4.8 mg/day upon awakening	*Nausea, fatigue, dizziness, vomiting, and headache* <u>Hypotension, psychosis, drowsiness</u>
canagliflozin (Invokana)	PO: 100 mg once daily (max: 300 mg/day) taken before first meal	*Female genital mycotic infections, urinary tract infection, and nasopharyngitis*
dapagliflozin (Farxiga)	PO: 5–10 mg once daily in the morning, with or without food	<u>Hypotension, renal impairment, hyperkalemia, hypoglycemia</u>
empagliflozin (Jardiance)	PO: 10–25 mg once daily in the morning, with or without food	

Note: Italics indicate common adverse effects. <u>Underline</u> indicates serious adverse effects.

CONNECTIONS: NURSING PRACTICE APPLICATION

Patients Receiving Pharmacotherapy with Insulin

Assessment	Potential Nursing Diagnoses*
Baseline assessment prior to administration: • Obtain a complete health history including endocrine, cardiovascular, hepatic, or renal disease; pregnancy; or breast-feeding. Obtain a drug history including allergies, current prescription and over-the-counter (OTC) drugs, herbal preparations, caffeine, nicotine, and alcohol use. Be alert to possible drug interactions. • Obtain a history of current symptoms, duration and severity, and other related signs or symptoms (e.g., paresthesias of hands or feet). Assess feet and lower extremities for possible injury, infection, or ulcerations. • Obtain a dietary history including caloric intake if on an ADA diet, number of meals and snacks per day. Assess fluid intake and type of fluids consumed. • Obtain baseline vital signs, height, and weight. • Evaluate appropriate laboratory findings (e.g., CBC, electrolytes, glucose, HbA1C level, lipid profile, osmolality, and hepatic and renal function studies). • Assess the patient's ability to receive and understand instructions. Include family and caregivers as needed.	• *Imbalanced Nutrition: Less Than Body Requirements* (type 1 diabetes) • *Obesity* (type 2 diabetes) • *Ineffective Health Management* • *Deficient Knowledge* (Drug Therapy) • *Risk for Unstable Blood Glucose Level* • *Risk for Deficient Fluid Volume* • *Risk for Injury*, related to adverse drug effects • *Risk for Infection*
Assessment throughout administration: • Assess for desired therapeutic effects (e.g., glucose levels remain within normal limits, electrolytes and osmolality remain normal, HbA1C levels demonstrate adequate control of glucose). • Assess for and report promptly any adverse effects: signs of hypoglycemia (e.g., nausea, paleness, sweating, diaphoresis, tremors, irritability, headache, light-headedness, anxiety, decreased level of consciousness) and hyperglycemia (e.g., flushed, dry skin, polyuria, polyphagia, polydipsia, drowsiness, glycosuria, ketonuria, acetone-breath), lipodystrophy, infection.	

Implementation

Interventions and (Rationales)	Patient-Centered Care
Ensuring therapeutic effects: • Continue assessments as above for therapeutic effects. (Dependent on the severity of hyperglycemia, blood glucose levels should return gradually to normal.)	• Teach the patient to report any return of original symptoms. • Teach the patient the symptoms of hyper- and hypoglycemia to observe for and instruct the patient to check the capillary glucose level routinely and if symptoms are present. Promptly report any noticeable symptoms and concurrent capillary glucose level to the health care provider.
• Administer insulin correctly and per the schedule ordered (e.g., routine dosing with or without additional sliding-scale coverage), plan insulin administration and peak times around mealtimes. Maintaining a steady level of insulin with mealtimes arranged to match peak insulin activity will assist in maintaining a steady blood glucose level.	• Teach the patient or caregiver appropriate administration techniques for all types of insulin used, followed by return demonstration until the patient or caregiver is comfortable with the technique and able to perform correctly. • Teach the patient or caregiver the importance of peak insulin levels and the need to ensure that adequate food sources are consumed to avoid hypoglycemia. Provide written materials for future reference whenever possible.
• Ensure that dietary needs are met based on the need to lose, gain, or maintain current weight and glucose levels. Consult with the dietitian as needed. Limit or eliminate alcohol use. (Adequate caloric, protein, carbohydrate, and fat amounts support an insulin regimen for glucose control. Activity and lifestyle will also be factored into dietary management. As alcohol is metabolized, it can raise and then precipitously lower blood sugar, raising the risk of hypoglycemia.)	• Review current diet, lifestyle, and activity level with the patient. Arrange a dietitian consult based on the need to alter diet or food choices. Teach the patient to limit or eliminate alcohol use. If alcoholic beverages are consumed, limit to one per day, and consume along with a complete meal to ensure that food intake balances alcohol metabolism.
Minimizing adverse effects: • Continue to monitor capillary glucose levels. Hold insulin dose if blood sugar is less than 70 mg/dL or per parameters as ordered, and contact the health care provider for further orders. (Daily glucose levels, especially before meals, will assist in maintaining adequate control of blood glucose and aid in assessing the appropriateness of current insulin types and dosages.)	• Instruct the patient on blood glucose monitoring the appropriate techniques to obtain capillary blood glucose levels, followed by return demonstration, and when to contact the health care provider (e.g., glucose less than 70 mg/dL). Monitor use and ensure proper functioning of all equipment to be used at home.
• Continue to monitor periodic laboratory work: CBC, electrolytes, glucose, HbA1C level, lipid profile, osmolality, hepatic and renal function studies. (Periodic monitoring of laboratory work assists in determining glucose control and the need for any change in insulin amounts and assesses for complications. HbA1C levels provide a measure of glucose control over several months' time.)	• Instruct the patient on the need to return periodically for laboratory work.

(continued)

CONNECTIONS: NURSING PRACTICE APPLICATION (continued)

- Assess for symptoms of hypoglycemia, especially around the time of insulin peak activity. If symptoms of hypoglycemia are noted, provide a quick-acting carbohydrate source (e.g., juice or other simple sugar), and then check capillary glucose level. Report to the health care provider if glucose is less than 70 mg/dL or as ordered. If mealtime is not immediate, provide a longer acting protein source to ensure that hypoglycemia does not recur. (Hypoglycemia is especially likely to occur around peak insulin activity, especially if food sources are inadequate. **Lifespan:** Age-related physiological differences may place the older adult at greater risk for hypoglycemia. Providing a quick-acting carbohydrate source and then checking the capillary glucose level will ensure that glucose does not decrease further while locating the glucose testing equipment. When in doubt, treating symptoms for suspected hypoglycemia is safer than allowing further decreases in glucose and possible loss of consciousness with adverse effects. Small additional amounts of carbohydrates will not dramatically increase blood sugar if testing shows a hyperglycemic episode.)

- Teach the patient to always carry a quick-acting carbohydrate source in case symptoms of hypoglycemia occur. If unsure whether symptoms indicate hypo- or hyperglycemia, treat as hypoglycemia and then check capillary glucose. If symptoms are not relieved in 10–15 min, or if blood sugar is below 70 mg/dL (or parameters as ordered), immediately notify the health care provider.

- Monitor blood glucose more frequently during periods of illness or stress. (Insulin needs may increase or decrease during periods of illness or stress. Frequent monitoring during these times helps to prevent hypoglycemia and ensures adequate glucose control.)

- Instruct the patient to check glucose levels more frequently when ill or under stress. Stress may increase insulin needs because the stress response can cause glycogenolysis. Illness, especially associated with anorexia, nausea, or vomiting, may decrease insulin needs. Notify the health care provider if unable to eat normal meals during periods of illness or stress for possible change in insulin dose.

- Encourage increased activity and exercise, but monitor blood glucose before and after exercise and begin any new or increased exercise routine gradually. Continue to monitor for hypoglycemia for up to 48 h after exercise. (Exercise assists muscles to use glucose more efficiently and increases insulin receptor sites in the tissues, lowering the blood sugar. Benefits of exercise and lowered blood sugar may continue for up to 48 h, increasing the risk of hypoglycemia during this time. Frequent monitoring helps to prevent hypoglycemia and ensures adequate glucose control.)

- Teach the patient the benefits of increased activity and exercise and to begin any new routine or increase in exercise gradually. Exercise should occur an hour after a meal or after a 10- or 15-g carbohydrate snack to prevent hypoglycemia. If exercise is prolonged, small frequent carbohydrate snacks can be consumed every 30 min during exercise to maintain blood sugar.
- Instruct the patient to check glucose levels more frequently before, during, and after exercise.

- Rotate insulin administration sites weekly. If the patient is hospitalized, use sites that have been less used or are difficult for the patient to reach. Insulin pump subcutaneous catheters should be changed every 2 to 3 days or as recommended by the health care provider. (Rotating injection sites weekly helps to prevent lipodystrophy. Use caution if using a new site, especially if the previous site used by the patient exhibits signs of lipodystrophy. Insulin in an unused site may absorb more quickly than a site with lipodystrophy or tissue changes, resulting in hypoglycemia. Insulin pump subcutaneous catheters should be changed every 2 to 3 days to prevent infections at the site of insertion.)

- Instruct the patient on the need to rotate insulin injection sites on a weekly basis to prevent tissue damage or to rotate subcutaneous catheter sites (insulin pumps) every 2 to 3 days.

- Ensure proper storage of insulin to maintain maximum potency. (Unopened insulin may be stored at room temperature, but avoid direct sunlight and excessive heat. Opened insulin vials may be stored at room temperature for up to 1 month. If noticeable change in solution occurs or if precipitate forms, discard the vial.)

- Teach the patient methods for proper storage of insulin and for storage during travel.

Patient understanding of drug therapy:
- Use opportunities during administration of medications and during assessments to discuss the rationale for drug therapy, desired therapeutic outcomes, commonly observed adverse effects, parameters for when to call the health care provider, and any necessary monitoring or precautions. (Using time during nursing care helps to optimize and reinforce key teaching areas.)

- The patient, family, or caregiver should be able to state the reason for the drug, appropriate dose and scheduling, what adverse effects to observe for and when to report them, and any special requirements of the medication therapy (e.g., insulin needs during exercise or illness).
- Instruct the patient to carry a wallet identification card and wear medical identification jewelry indicating diabetes.

Patient self-administration of drug therapy:
- When administering the medication, instruct the patient, family, or caregiver in the proper self-administration of the drug followed by teach-back. (Utilizing time during nurse-administration of these drugs helps to reinforce teaching.)

- The patient, family, or caregiver is able to discuss appropriate dosing and administration needs including:
- Proper preparation of insulin: Rotate vials gently between the palms and do not shake; if insulins are mixed, draw up the quickest acting insulin and then the longer acting one if insulins are compatible; insulin glargine or insulin detemir should not be mixed with any other type of insulin; use the appropriate syringe (100 unit) unless small amounts of insulin are ordered, then obtain syringes with smaller volumes to ensure accurate dosing.
- Proper subcutaneous injection techniques: selection and cleansing of the site with rotation every week, injecting at 90-degree angle, and applying a pad to the site after injection but not massaging the site.
- Proper use of all equipment: blood glucose monitoring equipment, insulin pump.

*Nursing Diagnoses—Definitions and Classification 2015–2017. Copyright © 2014, 1994–2014 by NANDA International. Used by arrangement with John Wiley & Sons Limited.

TABLE 66.6 Selected Combination Oral Antidiabetic Drugs

Brand Name Drug	Generic Drug Combination	Route and Adult Dose (Maximum Dose Where Indicated)
Actoplus Met	pioglitazone/metformin	PO: 15 mg/500–850 mg once or twice daily. Starting dose depends if patient was previously treated with metformin or pioglitazone combination or had an inadequate response with either drug alone (max: 45 mg/2,550 mg daily)
Avandamet	rosiglitazone/metformin	Patients with no prior treatment: PO: 2 mg/500 mg once or twice daily Previously treated patients: PO: 2–4 mg/500–1,000 mg twice daily (max: 8 mg/2,000 mg daily)
Avandaryl	rosiglitazone/glimepiride	PO: Start with 4 mg/2 mg once daily with the first meal of the day (max: 8 mg/4 mg daily)
Duetact	pioglitazone/glimepiride	PO: Start with 30 mg/2 mg once daily (max: 45 mg/8 mg daily)
Glucovance	glyburide/metformin	Patients with no prior treatment: PO: 1.25 mg/250 mg once or twice daily Previously treated patients: PO: 2.5 mg/500 mg to 5 mg/500 mg twice daily (max: 20 mg/2,000 mg daily)
Janumet	sitagliptin/metformin	PO: Starting dose 50 mg/500 mg twice daily with meals (max: 100 mg/2,000 mg/day)
Jentadueto	linagliptin/metformin	PO: 2.5 mg/1,000 mg bid with meals
Juvisync	sitagliptin/simvastatin	PO: Start with 100 mg/40 mg once daily in the evening
Kazano	alogliptin/metformin	PO: 12.5 mg/500 mg bid with food
Metaglip	glipizide/metformin	PO: 2.5 mg/500 mg or 5 mg/500 mg twice daily (max: 20 mg/2,000 mg daily)
Oseni	alogliptin/pioglitazone	PO: 25 mg/15 mg once daily
PrandiMet	repaglinide/metformin	PO: Start with 1 mg/500 mg given twice daily, 15 min before meals (max: 10 mg/2,500 mg daily)

Many fixed-dose combination products are available for the treatment of people with type 2 diabetes. The main advantage of taking a combination drug is that it is more convenient than taking two separate drugs and may improve adherence to the therapeutic regimen. Combination products are indicated for patients who fail to adequately control glucose levels with the use of a single drug. Doses for selected combination products are listed in Table 66.6.

Sulfonylureas

The first oral antidiabetic drug class available, sulfonylureas are divided into first- and second-generation categories. Although drugs from both generations are equally effective at lowering blood glucose, the second-generation drugs exhibit fewer drug–drug interactions.

The sulfonylureas act by stimulating the release of insulin from pancreatic islet cells and by increasing the sensitivity of insulin receptors on target cells. The most common adverse effect is hypoglycemia, which is usually caused by taking too much medication or not eating enough food. Hypoglycemia from these drugs may be prolonged and require administration of dextrose to return serum glucose to normal levels. Other adverse effects include weight gain, hypersensitivity reactions, GI distress, and hepatotoxicity. When alcohol is taken with sulfonylureas, some patients experience an uncomfortable disulfiram-like reaction, with flushing, palpitations, and nausea.

PROTOTYPE DRUG | **Glyburide (DiaBeta, Glynase, Micronase)**

Classification: Therapeutic: Antidiabetic drug
Pharmacologic: Sulfonylurea

Therapeutic Effects and Uses: Approved in 1984, glyburide is a second-generation sulfonylurea used to lower blood glucose levels in patients with type 2 diabetes. Glyburide can be used alone or in combination with another oral hypoglycemic drug. It should be used only if diet and exercise have proven ineffective in controlling the elevated blood glucose levels.

Two types of glyburide are available: the conventional form (DiaBeta, Micronase) and a micronized form (Glynase). Glynase allows for lower doses, compared to the conventional forms. Glucovance is a combination product that contains glyburide and metformin.

Mechanism of Action: Glyburide stimulates the release of insulin from pancreatic beta cells and increases the sensitivity of peripheral tissues to insulin. The stimulation of insulin release relies on some residual beta cell functioning; therefore, the drug is not effective for type 1 diabetes.

Pharmacokinetics:

Route(s)	Oral (PO)
Absorption	Readily absorbed following PO administration
Distribution	Distributed widely to body tissues, with greatest concentrations in liver, kidneys, and intestines; crosses the placenta
Primary metabolism	Extensive hepatic metabolism
Primary excretion	Equal in urine and feces
Onset of action	15–60 min
Duration of action	Up to 24 h

Adverse Effects: The primary adverse effect of glyburide is hypoglycemia. Patients at increased risk for hypoglycemia include those with renal or hepatic insufficiency, those consuming an improper diet, and patients who are elderly or malnourished. Excessive exercise or alcohol consumption also increases the risk for hypoglycemia. Other adverse effects of therapy include heartburn, nausea, vomiting, diarrhea, pruritus, erythema, urticaria, photosensitivity, and blurred vision. Rare, though serious, adverse effects include hepatotoxicity, cholestatic jaundice, aplastic anemia, leukopenia, thrombocytopenia, and agranulocytosis.

Contraindications/Precautions: Glyburide is contraindicated in patients with a known sensitivity to sulfa drugs or thiazide diuretics because sulfonylureas are chemically similar to sulfa drugs. It is contraindicated as the primary treatment for type 1 diabetes, diabetic coma, or DKA. The drug is used with caution in patients with renal or hepatic disease because the drug may accumulate to toxic levels. If used during pregnancy, glyburide should be discontinued at least 1 month before delivery because newborns exposed to sulfonylureas may develop severe hypoglycemia lasting several days.

Drug Interactions: Using alcohol with glyburide can cause hypoglycemia or hyperglycemia and has resulted in a disulfiram-type response, with severe nausea, vomiting, flushing, and palpitations. Drugs that can increase hypoglycemia when taken with glyburide are oral anticoagulants, MAOIs, probenecid, sulfonamides, chloramphenicol, oxyphenbutazone, phenylbutazone, salicylates, and clofibrate. Increased risk of hyperglycemia can occur with use of rifampin and thiazides. **Herbal/Food**: Ginseng, garlic, black cohosh, juniper berries, fenugreek, coriander, or dandelion root can cause hypoglycemia.

Pregnancy: Category C.

Treatment of Overdose: Treatment is the same as for acute hypoglycemia: A concentrated source of glucose is administered.

Nursing Responsibilities: Key nursing implications for patients receiving glyburide are included in the Nursing Practice Application for Patients Receiving Pharmacotherapy for Type 2 Diabetes.

Drugs Similar to Glyburide (DiaBeta, Glynase, Micronase)

First-generation sulfonylureas are typically less potent, require larger doses, have a shorter duration of action, and require more frequent dosing than the second-generation sulfonylureas. Thus, the second-generation drugs are more widely prescribed.

First-generation sulfonylureas:

Chlorpropamide (Diabinese):   Approved in 1958, chlorpropamide is the longest acting of the first-generation sulfonylureas, with a duration of action of 24 to 72 hours. In addition to treating type 2 diabetes, an unlabeled use is the treatment of neurogenic diabetes insipidus. Rarely, it can produce an antidiuretic effect, with resulting hyponatremia, water intoxication, and edema. Due to the long half-life of the drug (36 hours), hypoglycemia can be severe and prolonged. It is a pregnancy category C drug.

Tolazamide (Tolinase):   Approved in 1965, tolazamide is structurally related to tolbutamide but is five times more potent. It is taken once daily with breakfast. It can also be used in patients who fail to respond to other sulfonylureas. It is a pregnancy category C drug.

Tolbutamide (Orinase):   Tolbutamide is a short-acting sulfonylurea, with a duration of 6 to 12 hours, given once or twice daily after meals. Approved in 1957, it has been used in patients being treated with insulin who have failed to respond to other sulfonylureas. It is a pregnancy category C drug.

Second-generation sulfonylureas:

Glimepiride (Amaryl):   Approved in 1995, glimepiride can be used alone or in combination with insulin for patients with type 2 diabetes. It is most often given once a day with the first meal of the day. More recently, glimepiride has been included in fixed-dose combinations with pioglitazone (Duetact) and rosiglitazone (Avandaryl). Because of the increased risk for myocardial infarction (from rosiglitazone and pioglitazone), the fixed-dose combinations contain a black box warning regarding the increased risk for heart failure and myocardial infarction.

Glipizide (Glucotrol):   Approved in 1984, glipizide is available in a standard tablet form and an extended release (XL) tablet, which should not be crushed or chewed. In addition to treating patients with type 2 diabetes who are unable to achieve glucose control with diet alone, it can be used for short-term therapy for those who normally can control their glucose levels by diet. Once-a-day dosing is given 30 minutes before the first meal of the day. Metaglip is a combination product approved in 2002 that contains glipizide and metformin.

CONNECTION Checkpoint 66.2

Glyburide combined with alcohol can cause a disulfiram reaction. From what you learned in Chapter 27, what causes the symptoms of the disulfiram reaction and what are common symptoms of this reaction? *See Answer to Connection Checkpoint 66.2 on student resource website.*

Biguanides

Metformin (Glucophage) is the only drug in this class. It is a preferred drug for managing type 2 diabetes because of its effectiveness and safety.

PROTOTYPE DRUG	Metformin (Glucophage, Glumetza, Others)

Classification: **Therapeutic:** Antidiabetic drug
Pharmacologic: Biguanide

Therapeutic Effects and Uses: Approved in 1994, metformin lowers blood glucose levels in patients with type 2 diabetes who are unable to control glucose levels by diet and exercise. It can be used alone or in combination with sulfonylureas, alpha-glucosidase inhibitors, or insulin. It is approved for use in children age 10 and older. Several formulations of metformin are available:

- **Regular release tablets.** Administered once or twice daily, absorption is decreased with food, and the peak plasma level is 2.5 hours.
- **Solution (Riomet).** Administered once or twice daily, absorption is slightly increased with food, and the peak plasma level is 2.3 hours.
- **Sustained release (Fortamet, Glucophage XR, and Glumetza).** These are extended duration systems where the drug is slowly released from a semipermeable membrane

(Fortamet), gel (Glucophage XR), or gastric-retentive technology (Glumetza). Administered once daily, absorption is significantly increased with food, and the peak plasma level is 6 to 8 hours.

Metformin reduces fasting and postprandial glucose levels. Because it does not promote insulin release, it does not cause hypoglycemia, which is a major advantage of the drug. The drug actions do not depend on stimulating insulin release, so it is able to lower glucose levels in patients who no longer secrete insulin. In addition to lowering blood glucose levels, it lowers triglyceride levels, lowers total and low-density lipoprotein (LDL) cholesterol levels, and promotes weight loss.

Metformin is used off-label to treat women with polycystic ovary syndrome. Women with this syndrome have insulin resistance and high serum insulin levels. Metformin reduces insulin resistance, which in turn lowers insulin and androgen levels, thus restoring normal menstrual cycles and ovulation.

Mechanism of Action: Metformin reduces blood glucose levels by multiple mechanisms. The drug reduces gluconeogenesis, thereby suppressing hepatic production of glucose. In addition, the drug decreases the intestinal reabsorption of glucose and increases the cellular uptake of glucose.

Pharmacokinetics:

Route(s)	PO (regular release tablets, solution, and extended release preparations)
Absorption	Approximately 50–60% of a dose reaches systemic circulation; extended release forms are absorbed very slowly
Distribution	Distributed to most tissues; crosses the placenta; secreted in breast milk; not protein bound
Primary metabolism	Not metabolized
Primary excretion	Kidneys
Onset of action	Less than 1 h; peak action: 1–3 h
Duration of action	12 h (regular release); 24 h (extended release)

Adverse Effects: The most common adverse effects that occur in 30% of patients taking metformin are GI related and include nausea, vomiting, abdominal discomfort, metallic taste, diarrhea, anorexia, and moderate weight loss. It may also cause headache, dizziness, agitation, and fatigue. Unlike the sulfonylureas, metformin rarely causes hypoglycemia or weight gain. **Black Box Warning**: Lactic acidosis is a rare, though potentially fatal, adverse effect of metformin therapy. The risk for lactic acidosis is increased in patients with renal insufficiency or any condition that puts them at risk for increased lactic acid production, such as liver disease, severe infection, excessive alcohol intake, shock, or hypoxemia. Another drug in this class, phenformin, was withdrawn from the market in 1977 due to fatal cases of lactic acidosis.

Contraindications/Precautions: Metformin is contraindicated in patients with impaired renal function, because the drug can rise to toxic levels. It is also contraindicated in patients with heart failure, liver failure, history of lactic acidosis, concurrent serious infection, or with any condition that predisposes the patient to hypoxemia. It is contraindicated for 2 days prior to, and 2 days

after, receiving IV radiographic contrast. Metformin is used with caution in patients with anemia, diarrhea, vomiting, dehydration, fever, gastroparesis, or GI obstruction; in older adults; and in those with hyperthyroidism, pituitary insufficiency, trauma, or during pregnancy and lactation. Safety in children under age 10 has not been established.

Drug Interactions: Alcohol increases the risk for lactic acidosis and should be avoided. Captopril, furosemide, and nifedipine may increase the risk for hypoglycemia. Use with IV radiographic contrast may cause lactic acidosis and acute renal failure. The following drugs may decrease renal excretion of metformin: amiloride, cimetidine, digoxin, dofetilide, midodrine, morphine, procainamide, quinidine, ranitidine, triamterene, trimethoprim, and vancomycin. Acarbose may decrease blood levels of metformin. Use with other antidiabetic drugs potentiates hypoglycemic effects. **Herbal/Food**: Metformin decreases the absorption of vitamin B_{12} and folic acid. Garlic and ginseng may increase hypoglycemic effects.

Pregnancy: Category B.

Treatment of Overdose: For overdose or development of lactic acidosis, hemodialysis can be used to correct the acidosis and remove excess metformin.

Nursing Responsibilities: Key nursing implications for patients receiving metformin are included in the Nursing Practice Application for Patients Receiving Pharmacotherapy for Type 2 Diabetes.

Drugs Similar to Metformin (Glucophage, Glumetza, Others)

Metformin is the only biguanide available.

Meglitinides

The meglitinides act by stimulating the release of insulin from pancreatic islet cells in a manner similar to that of the sulfonylureas. Both drugs in this class have short durations of action of 2 to 4 hours. Their efficacy is equal to that of the sulfonylureas, and they are well tolerated. Hypoglycemia is the most common adverse effect.

PROTOTYPE DRUG	Repaglinide (Prandin)

Classification: Therapeutic: Antidiabetic drug
Pharmacologic: Meglitinide

Therapeutic Effects and Uses: Approved in 1997, repaglinide is used to lower blood glucose levels in patients with type 2 diabetes as an adjunct to diet and exercise. It may be used alone or in combination with metformin or a thiazolidinedione.

Because repaglinide is rapidly absorbed, it should be taken shortly before each meal. It is effective in lowering postprandial glucose levels and in reducing hemoglobin A1C levels but has little effect on fasting glucose levels. It undergoes almost no renal excretion, and so it can be used in patients with renal insufficiency.

Mechanism of Action: Repaglinide lowers glucose levels by stimulating insulin release from pancreatic beta cells. Patients must have some ability to secrete insulin for the drug to be effective.

Pharmacokinetics:

Route(s)	PO
Absorption	Rapidly absorbed following PO administration
Distribution	98% protein bound
Primary metabolism	Hepatic (CYP3A4)
Primary excretion	90% in feces
Onset of action	15–30 min; peak: 1 h
Duration of action	4 h

Adverse Effects: Repaglinide is generally well tolerated; the most common adverse effect is hypoglycemia. Other adverse effects include nausea, vomiting, diarrhea, and dyspepsia. Headache, paresthesias, upper respiratory infections, sinusitis, rhinitis, or bronchitis may also occur.

Contraindications/Precautions: Repaglinide is contraindicated in persons with type 1 diabetes or DKA. It should be used with caution in patients with hepatic impairment, during pregnancy or lactation, in elderly patients, or in those with systemic infection, surgery, or trauma. Its safety in children has not been established.

Drug Interactions: Drugs that induce hepatic CYP3A4 enzyme such as barbiturates, carbamazepine, rifampin, and pioglitazone may increase repaglinide metabolism and cause hyperglycemia. Drugs that inhibit CYP3A4 such as erythromycin, ketoconazole, and miconazole inhibit repaglinide metabolism and may potentiate hypoglycemia. Gemfibrozil may increase risk for hypoglycemia. Use with isophane insulin may cause myocardial ischemia. **Herbal/Food**: The concurrent intake of grapefruit juice inhibits metabolism and may result in increased repaglinide levels and hypoglycemia. Garlic and ginseng may increase hypoglycemic effects.

Pregnancy: Category C.

Treatment of Overdose: During overdose, provide symptomatic therapy and a concentrated source of glucose for hypoglycemia, preferably by the IV route.

Nursing Responsibilities: Key nursing implications for patients receiving repaglinide are included in the Nursing Practice Application for Patients Receiving Pharmacotherapy for Type 2 Diabetes.

Drugs Similar to Repaglinide (Prandin)

The only other meglitinide is nateglinide.

Nateglinide (Starlix):   Approved in 2000, nateglinide has actions and uses similar to those of repaglinide. It is used alone or in combination with metformin for managing glucose levels in persons with type 2 diabetes who have not achieved glycemic control through diet and exercise. It is not effective for type 1 diabetes. Like repaglinide, it is given 5 to 20 minutes before meals. An important difference between these drugs is that nateglinide is primarily renally excreted, and so it should be used with caution in patients with renal impairment. Like repaglinide, nateglinide is well tolerated and hypoglycemia is usually mild. The drug is pregnancy category C.

Thiazolidinediones

The thiazolidinediones (TZDs), or glitazones, reduce blood glucose by decreasing insulin resistance and inhibiting hepatic gluconeogenesis. Optimal lowering of blood glucose may require 3 to 4 months of therapy. The most common adverse effects are fluid retention, headache, and weight gain. Hypoglycemia does not occur with drugs in this class. Because of their tendency to promote fluid retention, thiazolidinediones are contraindicated in patients with serious heart failure or pulmonary edema.

PROTOTYPE DRUG   **Rosiglitazone (Avandia)**

Classification: Therapeutic: Antidiabetic drug
Pharmacologic: Thiazolidinedione

Therapeutic Effects and Uses: Rosiglitazone is used to lower blood glucose levels in persons with type 2 diabetes as an adjunct to diet and exercise. It can be used as monotherapy or in combination with metformin, a sulfonylurea, or insulin. It is effective in lowering fasting glucose levels and hemoglobin A1C levels. Optimum therapeutic effects take several weeks to occur.

Mechanism of Action: Rosiglitazone lowers blood glucose levels by increasing cellular sensitivity to insulin, thereby reducing insulin resistance. In addition, it decreases gluconeogenesis by the liver.

Pharmacokinetics:

Route(s)	PO
Absorption	Rapidly absorbed
Distribution	Greater than 99% protein bound
Primary metabolism	Hepatic (CYP2C8)
Primary excretion	Primarily renal, with approximately 25% in feces
Onset of action	Within 1 h; peak: 1 h
Duration of action	12–24 h

Adverse Effects: Rosiglitazone is generally well tolerated. The most prominent adverse effect is edema, including macular edema. Anemia, headache, back pain, fatigue, diarrhea, upper respiratory infection, or sinusitis may occur. The drug can also raise serum lipid levels, including HDL cholesterol, triglycerides, and LDL cholesterol. It is recommended that baseline liver function tests be obtained prior to initiating treatment, and then assessed every 3 to 6 months while on this drug. Patients should be informed of the signs of liver damage (nausea, fatigue, dark urine, jaundice) as well as the signs of heart failure (dyspnea, weight gain, edema, fatigue) while taking rosiglitazone. Research has also raised the concern of increased fracture risk among women taking drugs in this class. **Black Box Warning**: Drugs in this class can cause or worsen heart failure due to increased fluid retention. In addition, rosiglitazone may increase the risk of myocardial infarction (MI).

Contraindications/Precautions: Rosiglitazone is contraindicated in persons with severe heart failure, liver disease, or elevated liver enzymes, pregnancy, and lactation. Its safety in children has not been established. Rosiglitazone is contraindicated in persons with type 1 diabetes or DKA.

Drug Interactions: Inducers of hepatic CYP2C8 such as rifampin may decrease the effects of rosiglitazone. Inhibitors of CYP2C8 such as azole antifungals, fluvoxamine, gemfibrozil, and trimethoprim may elevate rosiglitazone plasma levels and increase the risk for adverse reactions. Concurrent use of rosiglitazone with insulin can increase edema and the risk for heart failure and myocardial ischemia. Other antidiabetic agents, angiotensin II receptor antagonists, and gemfibrozil can increase the hypoglycemic effects. Use of rosiglitazone with nitrates is not recommended due to the potential for myocardial ischemia. Thiazide diuretics, phenothiazines, and atypical antipsychotic drugs can decrease the hypoglycemic effects of rosiglitazone by increasing blood glucose levels. **Herbal/Food**: Garlic and ginseng can increase the risk for hypoglycemia if used with rosiglitazone. Cocoa and rosemary may decrease the therapeutic effect and have a hyperglycemic effect.

Pregnancy: Category C.

Treatment of Overdose: Standard treatment for hypoglycemia is initiated during overdose, along with symptomatic treatment of edema or fluid overload.

Nursing Responsibilities: Key nursing implications for patients receiving rosiglitazone are included in the Nursing Practice Application for Patients Receiving Pharmacotherapy for Type 2 Diabetes.

Drugs Similar to Rosiglitazone (Avandia)

The only other drug in this class is pioglitazone. Troglitazone (Rezulin) was withdrawn from the market in 2000 because of drug-related deaths due to hepatic failure.

Pioglitazone (Actos): Approved in 1999, pioglitazone has actions and uses similar to those of rosiglitazone. It is rapidly absorbed following PO administration, with peak effects occurring within 7 days of beginning therapy. Pioglitazone has shown more favorable effects on triglyceride and HDL-cholesterol levels than rosiglitazone, with more benefits seen among women than men (ADA, 2007). Pioglitazone can decrease serum levels of oral contraceptives and can cause nonovulating premenopausal women to resume ovulation; therefore, a reliable form of contraception is recommended. There is no evidence of liver damage from this drug, but hepatic function should be assessed for a baseline and periodically thereafter as with rosiglitazone. The drug carries the same black box warnings regarding heart failure and myocardial ischemia as rosiglitazone. The drug is pregnancy category C.

Alpha-Glucosidase Inhibitors

The alpha-glucosidase inhibitors act by blocking enzymes in the small intestine responsible for breaking down complex carbohydrates into monosaccharides. Because carbohydrates must be in the monosaccharide form to be absorbed, digestion of glucose is delayed. These drugs have minimal adverse effects, with the most common being GI related, such as abdominal cramping, diarrhea, and flatulence. Although alpha-glucosidase inhibitors do not produce hypoglycemia when used alone, hypoglycemia may occur when these drugs are combined with insulin or a sulfonylurea.

PROTOTYPE DRUG	Acarbose (Precose)

Classification: Therapeutic: Antidiabetic drug
Pharmacologic: Alpha-glucosidase inhibitor

Therapeutic Effects and Uses: Approved in 1995, acarbose lowers blood glucose levels in persons with type 2 diabetes who cannot adequately manage glucose levels by diet and exercise alone. It may be used alone or in combination with a sulfonylurea, metformin, or insulin. By slowing the breakdown and absorption of carbohydrates, the rise in postprandial glucose level is reduced. Hemoglobin A1C level is lowered as well.

Mechanism of Action: Acarbose lowers glucose levels by interfering with carbohydrate absorption from the GI tract. It acts locally in the GI tract to inhibit the enzyme responsible for carbohydrate breakdown.

Pharmacokinetics:

Route(s)	PO
Absorption	Only 2% absorbed (low absorption is desired because the drug acts locally in the GI tract); some metabolites are absorbed
Distribution	Acts locally in the digestive tract
Primary metabolism	Metabolized in the GI tract by intestinal bacteria and digestive enzymes
Primary excretion	Primarily in feces, 30% in urine
Onset of action	Peak: 1 h
Duration of action	2–4 h

Adverse Effects: The most common adverse effects of acarbose are diarrhea, flatulence, abdominal distention, borborygmi, anemia (iron deficiency), urticaria, and erythema. The GI-related effects may diminish as therapy progresses; however, they will worsen if the patient does not adhere to the prescribed diabetic diet. Hypoglycemia may occur if acarbose is combined with other hypoglycemic agents. If hypoglycemia does develop, it must be treated with glucose and not sucrose (table sugar), because the drug inhibits the absorption of sucrose. Acarbose may cause elevation of liver enzymes (plasma transaminases), although liver damage has not been reported, but levels return to normal following drug withdrawal.

Contraindications/Precautions: Acarbose is contraindicated in patients with inflammatory bowel disease, bowel obstruction, colon ulcers, or in those predisposed to bowel obstructions. It is used with caution in patients with GI distress or liver disorders and in pregnancy or lactation. Safety in children has not been established.

Drug Interactions: Use with sulfonylureas may increase the risk for hypoglycemia. Drugs that cause hyperglycemia such as thiazide diuretics, corticosteroids, phenothiazines, estrogens, phenytoin, or isoniazid may decrease the effectiveness of acarbose. **Herbal/Food**: Ginseng, garlic, black cohosh, juniper berries, aloe, or dandelion root can cause hypoglycemia. Cocoa and rosemary have a hyperglycemic effect and may decrease the therapeutic effect of acarbose.

Pregnancy: Category B.

Treatment of Overdose: Unlike the sulfonylureas, overdose with acarbose will not cause hypoglycemia. Abdominal pain, flatulence, and diarrhea are treated symptomatically.

Nursing Responsibilities: Key nursing implications for patients receiving acarbose are included in the Nursing Practice Application for Patients Receiving Pharmacotherapy for Type 2 Diabetes.

Drugs Similar to Acarbose (Precose)

The only other drug in this class is miglitol.

Miglitol (Glyset): Approved in 1996, miglitol is an alpha-glucosidase inhibitor used as monotherapy or in combination with other antidiabetic drugs for the pharmacotherapy of type 2 diabetes. It acts by delaying the conversion of complex carbohydrates to monosaccharides (glucose), thereby lessening the rise in postprandial serum glucose levels. Like acarbose, the drug must be present in the intestine at the same time the carbohydrates are being digested; thus, the drug must be taken with a meal. The adverse effects are similar with the notable exception of not causing increased liver enzymes. Acarbose and miglitol both act locally in the intestine, although miglitol is completely absorbed and has the potential to produce systemic effects. Overdose does not cause hypoglycemia. The drug is pregnancy category B.

Incretin Enhancers

66.8 Incretin therapies offer a different approach to treating type 2 diabetes.

Incretins are hormones released by the mucosa of the small intestine in response to meals. The most important incretin is glucagon-like peptide (GLP-1), which acts rapidly to produce the following effects:

- Increase the amount of insulin secreted by the pancreas.
- Decrease the amount of glucagon secreted by the pancreas.
- Delay gastric emptying (slow glucose absorption).
- Decrease food intake by increasing the level of satiety.

Two groups of drugs have been developed that can influence incretin release. The first activates the GLP-1 receptor, causing essentially the same glucose-lowering actions as the natural hormone. Exenatide (Byetta), albiglutide (Tanzeum), and liraglutide (Victoza) are synthetic drugs that mimic the action of incretin. They are all administered by the subcutaneous route, although albiglutide offers the advantage of once-weekly dosing.

The second class of drugs that enhance incretin actions are the dipeptidyl peptidase 4 (DPP-4) inhibitors. Alogliptin (Nesina), linagliptin (Tradjenta), saxagliptin (Onglyza), and sitagliptin (Januvia) prevent the breakdown of incretins, allowing the hormone levels to rise and produce a greater response. These drugs are given orally and are effective at lowering blood glucose with few adverse effects. They work well with other antidiabetic drugs and do not cause hypoglycemia.

PROTOTYPE DRUG	**Sitagliptin (Januvia)**

Classification: Therapeutic: Antidiabetic drug
Pharmacologic: DPP-4 inhibitor, incretin enhancer

Therapeutic Effects and Uses: Approved in 2006, sitagliptin is an oral incretin enhancer that is used to help lower glucose levels in patients with type 2 diabetes who are unable to achieve normal glucose levels with diet and exercise. The drug is used as adjunct therapy along with diet and exercise and can be administered as monotherapy or in combination with other oral antidiabetic drugs. In 2011, the FDA approved Juvisync, a fixed-dose combination of sitagliptin with simvastatin. The combination is indicated for patients with type 2 diabetes who also have high serum cholesterol levels.

The actions of sitagliptin are glucose dependent: They occur only in the presence of elevated serum glucose, and so the risk for hypoglycemia is reduced. Sitagliptin has the added benefit of increasing satiety, or the feeling of fullness following a meal, resulting in a lower calorie intake and improved weight control. Sitagliptin lowers both fasting and postprandial glucose levels. Janumet is a fixed-dose combination drug containing sitagliptin and metformin.

Mechanism of Action: Sitagliptin inhibits DPP-4, the enzyme responsible for breaking down incretins. Inhibition of DPP-4 reduces the destruction of incretins. Levels of incretin hormones increase, thus decreasing blood glucose levels in patients with type 2 diabetes.

Pharmacokinetics:

Route(s)	PO
Absorption	Rapidly absorbed
Distribution	Approximately 38% protein bound
Primary metabolism	20% metabolized in the liver by CYP3A4 and CYP2CB
Primary excretion	Renal
Onset of action	30–60 min; peak: 1–4 h
Duration of action	Half-life: 12 h

Adverse Effects: Sitagliptin is well tolerated by most patients and adverse effects are generally not serious. Possible adverse effects include headache, diarrhea, nasopharyngitis, and upper respiratory infection. Allergic skin reactions and anaphylaxis have been reported. As monotherapy, sitagliptin does not cause hypoglycemia; however, when used concurrently with a sulfonylurea or insulin, hypoglycemia may occur.

Contraindications/Precautions: Sitagliptin is contraindicated in type 1 diabetes and DKA. It is used with caution in persons with renal disorders or renal failure, among older adults, or during pregnancy and lactation. Safety for children under age 18 has not been established.

Drug Interactions: Sitagliptin may increase digoxin levels. **Herbal/Food**: Cocoa and rosemary may decrease the therapeutic effect and have a hyperglycemic effect.

Pregnancy: Category C.

Treatment of Overdose: Overdose is treated symptomatically. If used in combination with other glucose-lowering agents and hypoglycemia occurs, a concentrated source of glucose should be administered by the IV route.

Nursing Responsibilities: Key nursing implications for patients receiving sitagliptin are included in the Nursing Practice Application for Patients Receiving Pharmacotherapy for Type 2 Diabetes.

Drugs Similar to Sitagliptin (Januvia)

Other incretin enhancers include the GLP-1 agonists albiglutide, exenatide, dulaglutide, and liraglutide, and the DPP-4 inhibitors alogliptin, linagliptin, and saxagliptin.

Albiglutide (Tanzeum): Albiglutide is a newer GLP-1 inhibitor, approved in 2014 to improve glycemic control in adults with type 2 diabetes mellitus. It is not for patients with type 1 diabetes mellitus or as first-line therapy for those unable to control blood glucose through diet and exercise. Although it must be administered by the subcutaneous route, it has the advantage of once-weekly dosing and may be given without regard to meals or time of day. It is packaged as a single-dose pen for ease of administration. The drug carries a black box warning that it may increase the risk for thyroid gland tumors. It is contraindicated in patients with a health or family history of thyroid tumors or multiple endocrine neoplasia syndrome type 2. Acute pancreatitis has occurred in some patients taking this medication. This drug is pregnancy category C.

Alogliptin (Nesina): One of the newest of the DPP-4 inhibitors, alogliptin was approved in 2013 for patients who are unable to control their blood glucose through exercise and diet. The drug works by the same mechanism and has the same effectiveness and side effects as the other DPP-4 inhibitors. When approving alogliptin, the FDA simultaneously approved two fixed-dose combinations of alogliptin with metformin (Kazano) and pioglitazone (Oseni). Kazano carries a black box warning due to the possibility of lactic acidosis (from metformin), and Oseni due to the possibility of heart failure (from pioglitazone). Alogliptin is pregnancy category B.

Dulaglutide (Trulicity): One of the newest drugs in this class, dulaglutide was approved in 2014 as an adjunct to diet and exercise in improving glycemic control in patients with type 2 diabetes. Given by the subcutaneous route once weekly, dulaglutide is a GLP-1 agonist that causes increased insulin release by the pancreas. The drug may be used alone or in combination with metformin. Actions and side effects are the same as other GLP-1 agonists such as albiglutide. Like albiglutide, dulaglutide carries a black box warning that it may increase the risk for thyroid gland tumors and thus is contraindicated in patients with a history of thyroid tumors or multiple endocrine neoplasia syndrome type 2. This drug is pregnancy category C.

Exenatide (Byetta): Exenatide was approved in 2005 for patients with type 2 diabetes who are unable to achieve adequate glycemic control following metformin or sulfonylurea monotherapy. The drug is a synthetic peptide that stimulates the release of insulin from pancreatic beta cells. It mimics the actions of the incretin hormones normally secreted by the intestines, which slow the absorption of glucose. It is effective in lowering fasting and postprandial glucose levels and causes a consistent, slow weight loss. A major disadvantage of exenatide is that it must be given twice daily by the subcutaneous route, within 60 minutes before the morning and evening meals. It is available as a pen injector. Adverse effects include nausea, vomiting, diarrhea, dyspepsia, anorexia, and gastroesophageal reflux. It can also cause nervousness, dizziness, and diaphoresis. Like sitagliptin, it does not cause hypoglycemia. The drug is pregnancy category C.

Linagliptin (Tradjenta): Approved in 2011, linagliptin is one of the newer DPP-4 inhibitors. The drug is well tolerated and has the same actions and adverse effects as sitagliptin. One potential advantage over the other DPP-4 inhibitors is that linagliptin is excreted through the liver rather than the kidneys. This allows the drug to be used in patients with significant renal impairment. In 2012 a fixed-dose combination of linagliptin with metformin (Jentadueto) was approved. Jentadueto carries a black box warning that patients may be at risk for lactic acidosis from accumulation of metformin. The drug is pregnancy category B.

Liraglutide (Victoza): Approved in 2010, liraglutide is an incretin enhancer that acts by the same mechanism as exenatide. Like exenatide, liraglutide is effective at reducing HbA1C levels as well as decreasing appetite and producing a desirable weight loss. An advantage over exenatide is that it can be given once daily. Both drugs are given by the subcutaneous route. Liraglutide is well tolerated, with the most common adverse effects being headache, nausea, diarrhea, and anti-liraglutide antibody formation. Hypoglycemia is not a problem with monotherapy but it may occur if used in combination with other antidiabetic drugs. Pancreatitis has been reported with other incretin enhancers and may also occur in patients taking liraglutide. Like albiglutide, the drug carries a black box warning about the possibility of thyroid tumors. Patients with a personal or family history of thyroid cancer should not take this drug. This drug is pregnancy category C.

Saxagliptin (Onglyza): Saxagliptin is a DPP-4 inhibitor approved in 2009 to improve glycemic control in patients with type 2 diabetes. The drug is well tolerated and has the same actions and adverse effects as sitagliptin. Kombiglyze XR is a fixed-dose combination of saxagliptin and metformin. This drug is pregnancy category B.

Miscellaneous Antidiabetic Drugs

A few miscellaneous drugs play minor roles in treating type 2 diabetes. Bromocriptine (Cycloset) is an older drug that was approved for a new indication, treating type 2 diabetes, in 2009. Bromocriptine is a dopamine receptor agonist but its mechanism for improving glycemic control is not known. The drug is also approved for acromegaly, Parkinson's disease, and hyperprolactinemia. Common adverse effects include nausea, fatigue, dizziness, vomiting, and headache.

In 2013, the FDA approved canagliflozin (Invokana), the first in a new class of drugs called the sodium-glucose co-transporter (SGLT) inhibitors. Inhibiting the SGLT in the kidney allows more glucose to leave the blood and be excreted via the urine. This drug has the advantage of promoting weight loss. It is contraindicated in patients with severe renal impairment. The added glucose in the urine serves as a substrate for bacterial and fungal growth, thus increasing the frequency of mycotic infections of the urinary tract and genitalia. Canagliflozin is pregnancy category C. Two additional drugs in this class, dapagliflozin (Farxiga) and empagliflozin, were approved in 2014 and have very similar actions and adverse effects.

CONNECTIONS: Complementary and Alternative Therapies

◀ Chromium for Hyperglycemia

Description
Chromium is a trace mineral naturally found in various foods, including whole-grain cereals, prunes, nuts, and seafood.

History and Claims
The relationship between chromium intake and glucose metabolism was first reported in the 1950s, when chromium-containing brewer's yeast was reported to prevent diabetes in laboratory animals. Since that time, the use of chromium supplements among persons with diabetes has become more common practice. Chromium is thought to increase the number of insulin receptors and improve insulin's ability to bind to receptors, therefore lowering blood glucose levels. This, in theory, would lower insulin requirements in persons with type 1 diabetes.

Standardization
The recommended dietary intake for chromium is 25 to 35 mcg/day. Most over-the-counter chromium picolinate supplements range from 250 to 500 mg/day. The long-term effects of high-dose nutritional supplementation are unknown.

Evidence
The evidence for the effects of chromium is inconclusive, with some reporting positive and some negative benefits. Nahas and Moher (2009) conducted a meta-analysis of 41 clinical trials and determined that evidence existed for the efficacy of chromium in lowering finger-stick blood glucose and A1C levels at doses of 200 to 1,000 mcg over periods of up to 26 weeks. But the authors cite the need for definitive clinical trials. The ADA has concluded that there is no evidence that supplemental chromium enhances glycemic control in patients with diabetes (Evert et al., 2014). More rigorous, well-controlled studies are needed to fully assess the efficacy and mechanism of action of chromium supplementation as an adjuvant therapy for type 2 diabetes and impaired glucose tolerance.

CONNECTIONS: NURSING PRACTICE APPLICATION

Patients Receiving Pharmacotherapy for Type 2 Diabetes

Assessment Data	Potential Nursing Diagnoses*
Baseline assessment prior to administration: • Obtain a complete health history including endocrine, cardiovascular, hepatic, or renal disease; pregnancy; or breast-feeding. Obtain a drug history including allergies, current prescription and OTC drugs, herbal preparations, caffeine, nicotine, and alcohol use. Be alert to possible drug interactions. • Obtain a history of current symptoms, duration and severity, and other related signs or symptoms (e.g., paresthesias of hands or feet). Assess feet and lower extremities for possible ulcerations. • Obtain a dietary history including caloric intake and number of meals and snacks per day. Assess fluid intake and type of fluids consumed. • Obtain baseline vital signs, height, and weight. • Evaluate appropriate laboratory findings (e.g., CBC, electrolytes, glucose, HbA1C level, lipid profile, hepatic and renal function studies). • Assess the patient's ability to receive and understand instructions. Include family and caregivers as needed.	• *Obesity* • *Ineffective Health Management* • *Deficient Knowledge* (Drug Therapy) • *Risk for Unstable Blood Glucose Level* • *Risk for Injury*, related to adverse drug effects • *Risk for Infection*
Assessment throughout administration: • Assess for desired therapeutic effects (e.g., glucose levels remain within normal limits, HbA1C levels demonstrate adequate control of glucose). • Continue periodic monitoring of hepatic function studies. • Assess for and report promptly any adverse effects appropriate to the type of oral drug: signs of hypoglycemia (e.g., nausea, paleness, sweating, diaphoresis, tremors, irritability, headache, light-headedness, anxiety, or decreased level of consciousness) most commonly associated with sulfonylureas and meglitinides, and hyperglycemia (e.g., flushed or dry skin, polyuria, polyphagia, polydipsia, drowsiness, glycosuria, ketonuria, or acetone breath), gastric upset, diarrhea, infection, edema.	

Implementation

Interventions and (Rationales)	Patient-Centered Care
Ensuring therapeutic effects: • Continue assessments as above for therapeutic effects. (Dependent on the severity of hyperglycemia, supplemental insulin may be needed for blood glucose levels to return gradually to normal.)	• Teach the patient to report any return of original symptoms. • Teach the patient the symptoms of hyper- and hypoglycemia to observe for and to check capillary glucose level routinely and if symptoms are present. Promptly report any noticeable symptoms and concurrent capillary glucose level to the health care provider.

CONNECTIONS: NURSING PRACTICE APPLICATION (continued)

- Ensure that dietary needs are met based on the need to lose, gain, or maintain current weight and glucose levels. Consult with the dietitian as needed. Limit or eliminate alcohol use. (Adequate caloric protein, carbohydrate, and fat amounts support the oral hypoglycemic regimen for glucose control. Activity and lifestyle will also be factored into dietary management. As alcohol is metabolized, it can raise and then precipitously lower blood glucose, raising the risk of hypoglycemia. Patients on sulfonylureas should avoid or eliminate alcohol entirely because a disulfiram-like reaction with severe nausea, vomiting, and potential hypotension may result.)

- Review current diet, lifestyle, and activity level with the patient. Arrange a dietitian consult based on the need to alter diet or food choices. Teach the patient to limit or eliminate alcohol use. If alcoholic beverages are consumed, limit to one per day and consume along with a complete meal to ensure food intake balances alcohol metabolism.
- Instruct patients on sulfonylureas (e.g., glyburide) to avoid or eliminate alcohol use.

Minimizing adverse effects:
- Continue to monitor capillary glucose levels. Check with the health care provider before giving an oral hypoglycemic if blood sugar is less than 70 mg/dL or per the parameters as ordered by the health care provider. (Daily glucose levels, especially before meals, will assist in maintaining adequate control of blood glucose and aid in assessing the appropriateness of current drug therapy.)

- Instruct the patient on appropriate blood glucose monitoring techniques to obtain capillary blood glucose levels, followed by return demonstration, and when to contact the health care provider (e.g., glucose less than 70 mg/dL). Monitor use and ensure proper functioning of all equipment to be used at home.

- Continue to monitor periodic laboratory work: CBC, electrolytes, glucose, A1C level, lipid profile, hepatic and renal function studies. (Periodic monitoring of laboratory work assists in determining glucose control and the need for any change in medication and assesses for complications. HbA1C levels provide a measure of glucose control over several months' time. Sulfonylureas may cause hepatic toxicity. Biguanides may cause lactic acidosis. **Lifespan:** Age-related physiological differences may place the older adult at greater risk for hepatic toxicity.)

- Instruct the patient on the need to return periodically for laboratory work.
- Teach patients on sulfonylureas to immediately report any nausea, vomiting, yellowing of the skin or sclera, abdominal pain, light or clay-colored stools, or darkening of urine to the health care provider.
- Teach patients on biguanides to immediately report any drowsiness, malaise, decreased respiratory rate, or general body aches to the health care provider.

- Assess for symptoms of hypoglycemia. If symptoms are noted, provide a quick-acting carbohydrate source (e.g., juice or other simple sugar), and then check capillary glucose level. Report to the health care provider if glucose is less than 70 mg/dL or as ordered. If mealtime is not immediate, provide a longer acting protein source to ensure that hypoglycemia does not recur. (Hypoglycemia is especially likely to occur if the patient is taking sulfonylureas or meglitinides, although it may occur with other types of oral antidiabetic drugs, especially if food sources are inadequate. **Lifespan:** Age-related physiological differences may place the older adult at greater risk for hypoglycemia. Providing a quick-acting carbohydrate source and then checking the capillary glucose level will ensure glucose does not decrease further while locating the glucose testing equipment. When in doubt, treating symptoms for suspected hypoglycemia is safer than allowing further decreases in glucose and possible loss of consciousness with adverse effects. Small additional amounts of carbohydrates will not dramatically increase blood sugar if testing shows a hyperglycemic episode.)

- Teach the patient to always carry a quick-acting carbohydrate source in case symptoms of hypoglycemia occur. If unsure whether symptoms indicate hypo- or hyperglycemia, treat as hypoglycemia and then check capillary glucose. If symptoms are not relieved in 10–15 min, or if blood sugar is below 70 mg/dL (or the parameters as ordered), immediately notify the health care provider.

- Monitor blood glucose more frequently during periods of illness or stress. (Blood glucose levels may increase or decrease during periods of illness or stress. Frequent monitoring during these times helps to prevent hypoglycemia and ensures adequate glucose control.)

- Instruct the patient to check glucose levels more frequently when ill or under stress. Stress may increase blood glucose because the stress response can cause glycogenolysis and supplemental insulin may be required if oral antidiabetic drugs do not adequately control the blood sugar. Illness, especially associated with anorexia, nausea, or vomiting, may decrease the need for an oral hypoglycemic drug. Notify the health care provider if unable to eat normal meals during periods of illness or stress for possible change in drug regimen.

- Encourage increased activity and exercise, but monitor blood glucose before and after exercise and begin any new or increased exercise routine gradually. Continue to monitor for hypoglycemia for up to 48 h after exercise. (Exercise assists muscles to use glucose more efficiently and increases insulin receptor sites in the tissues, lowering the blood sugar and assisting with weight control. Benefits of exercise and lowered blood sugar may continue for up to 48 h, increasing the risk of hypoglycemia during this time. Frequent monitoring helps to prevent hypoglycemia and ensures adequate glucose control.)

- Teach the patient the benefits of increased activity and exercise and to begin any new routine or increase in exercise gradually.
- Instruct the patient to check glucose levels more frequently before and after exercise.

- Monitor for hypersensitivity and allergic reactions. Continue to monitor the patient throughout therapy. (Anaphylactic reactions are possible although rare. As sensitivity occurs, reactions may continue to develop.)

- Teach the patient to immediately report any itching, rashes, swelling, particularly of the face or tongue, urticaria, flushing, dizziness, syncope, wheezing, throat tightness, or difficulty breathing.

- Assess for pregnancy or the possibility of pregnancy. (Some oral antidiabetic drugs are category C and must be stopped during pregnancy. Due to the increasing metabolic needs of pregnancy, supplemental insulin or switching to insulin coverage may be required for the duration of the pregnancy.)

- Teach female patients of childbearing age to monitor for pregnancy and alert the health care provider if pregnant or if pregnancy is suspected to discuss medication needs.

(continued)

CONNECTIONS: NURSING PRACTICE APPLICATION (continued)

• Continue to monitor for edema, blood pressure, and lung sounds in patients taking thiazolidinediones. (Drugs such as rosiglitazone may cause edema and worsening of heart failure.)	• Instruct the patient to immediately report any edema of the hands or feet, dyspnea, or excessive fatigue to the health care provider.
• Monitor for hypoglycemia more frequently in patients on concurrent beta-blocker therapy. (Beta blockers antagonize the action of some oral antidiabetic drugs and may mask the symptoms of a hypoglycemic episode, allowing the blood sugar to drop lower before it is perceived.)	• Teach patients on concurrent beta-blocker therapy to monitor capillary blood glucose more frequently and to check blood glucose if minor changes in overall feeling are perceived (e.g., minor agitation or anxiety, slight tremors).
Patient understanding of drug therapy: • Use opportunities during administration of medications and during assessments to discuss the rationale for drug therapy, desired therapeutic outcomes, commonly observed adverse effects, parameters for when to call the health care provider, and any necessary monitoring or precautions. (Using time during nursing care helps to optimize and reinforce key teaching areas.)	• The patient, family, or caregiver should be able to state the reason for the drug, appropriate dose and scheduling, what adverse effects to observe for and when to report them, and any special requirements of medication therapy (e.g., drug needs during exercise or illness). • Instruct the patient to carry a wallet identification card and wear medical identification jewelry indicating diabetes.

Patient self-administration of drug therapy:
• When administering the medication, instruct the patient, family, or caregiver in the proper self-administration of drug. (Utilizing time during nurse-administration of these drugs helps to reinforce teaching.)
	• The patient, family, or caregiver is able to discuss appropriate dosing and administration needs, including:
	  • Timing of doses: Most oral antidiabetic drugs are taken once or twice a day. For drugs given once a day, take approximately 30 min before the first meal of the day. Alpha-glucosidase inhibitors (e.g., acarbose) should be taken with meals.
	  • Insulin requirements: While patients with type 2 diabetes produce some insulin, insulin injections may be required in addition to the oral antidiabetic drug on occasion. This does not necessarily signal a worsening of the disease condition but may be a temporary need.

*Nursing Diagnoses—Definitions and Classification 2015–2017. Copyright © 2014, 1994–2014 by NANDA International. Used by arrangement with John Wiley & Sons Limited.

CHAPTER

66 Understanding the Chapter

Key Concepts Summary

66.1 Serum glucose is maintained within a narrow range by the hormones insulin and glucagon.

66.2 Type 1 diabetes is characterized by insufficient insulin synthesis by the pancreas, whereas type 2 diabetes is characterized by insulin resistance in the target cells.

66.3 The classic signs and symptoms of diabetes include polyuria, polydipsia, and polyphagia.

66.4 Acute complications of diabetes include diabetic ketoacidosis, hyperosmolar hyperglycemic state, and hypoglycemia.

66.5 Serious complications of chronic diabetes include neuropathy, nephropathy, retinopathy, and vascular disease.

66.6 Insulin is the cornerstone of therapy for patients with type 1 and gestational diabetes.

66.7 Antidiabetic drugs from multiple classes are used to treat type 2 diabetes.

66.8 Incretin therapies offer a different approach to treating type 2 diabetes.

Case Study: Making the Patient Connection

Remember the patient "Ellen McIntosh" at the beginning of the chapter? Now read the remainder of the case study. Based on the information presented within this chapter, respond to the critical thinking questions that follow.

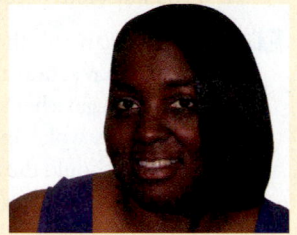

Ellen is a 44-year-old woman who works full time as an art teacher in a local high school. She also teaches art courses on the weekends at the local senior center. She visited her health care provider last week for her annual physical exam and to update her TB screening (PPD) for the coming school year. The office called her back this morning with her laboratory reports and requested that she make an appointment to return tomorrow to discuss the results. Her serum glucose level was elevated at 224 mg/dL and she will need further testing to rule out type 2 diabetes.

Ellen has follow-up testing with the results of a fasting serum glucose level returning at 131 mg/dL and a 2-hour 75-g oral glucose test of 242 mg/dL. A diagnosis of new-onset type 2 diabetes is confirmed. Ellen expresses disbelief and tells you, the nurse, "I can't believe it! I watch what I eat; I don't eat a lot of sugar, cookies, or candy. I drink only diet soda. I don't have any of the symptoms you hear about. And no one in my family has ever had diabetes." A health history and the results of Ellen's recent physical examination confirm

overall good health. Her height is 167.6 cm (66 in.) and weight 79.5 kg (175 lb) with a BMI of 28.2 kg/m², placing her in the "overweight" category. Vital signs, physical exam, and all other laboratory work are within acceptable limits. Ellen admits that she has been thirstier lately, "But it's summertime and I always drink more when it's hot." She has also been urinating more frequently but attributes that to her increased fluid intake.

Ellen's provider will start her on glyburide (Micronase) and metformin (Glucophage) and will recheck her serum glucose in 1 month. In the meantime, she is to begin capillary blood glucose testing before meals and at bedtime, and to bring her log to the next visit. She is given dietary instructions and you will be providing instruction on her medications.

Critical Thinking Questions

1. Why are two oral antidiabetic drugs prescribed for Ellen?
2. What essential teaching does Ellen need about her glyburide (Micronase) and metformin (Glucophage)?
3. Ellen asks why she is not being started on insulin. Why is insulin not being used at this time?
4. Ellen tells you that she occasionally enjoys a glass of wine with her dinner and wants to know if this is allowed. How will you answer?

See Answers to Critical Thinking Questions on student resource website.

Additional Case Study

Nicholas Jefferson is 8 years old and has just been diagnosed with type 1 diabetes. After increasing symptoms during the past month, he was hospitalized for continuous nausea, vomiting, and gradually increasing lethargy. His parents report that over the past month or two, Nicholas has had blurry vision and has been thirsty and hungry constantly. He has been eating frequently but does not seem to be gaining any weight. They also tell you that on several occasions, Nicholas has wet the bed, which is very unusual for him. On admission, his serum glucose level is 420 mg/dL with a urine sample positive for glucose and ketones. Nicholas is to remain NPO and will be started on an IV with 0.45 normal saline for fluid replacement, given an IV bolus of insulin, and then started on an insulin drip at 0.5 unit per hour.

Finger-stick glucose levels are to be checked every hour with serum blood glucose levels drawn every 4 hours. The IV insulin drip is to be discontinued when Nicholas's blood glucose level is 240 mg/dL and subcutaneous insulin will be started at that time.

1. What type of insulin do you anticipate using for the IV bolus dose and IV drip?
2. Why do you think the insulin IV will be stopped when the blood glucose level is 240 mg/dL and not at the normal level of 70 to 100 mg/dL?
3. What essential teaching will Nicholas and his family need at this time?

See Answers to Additional Case Study on student resource website.

Chapter Review

1 A patient with type 1 diabetes will use a combination insulin that includes NPH and regular insulins. The nurse is explaining the importance of knowing the peak times for both insulins. Why is this important information for the patient to know?

1. The patient will be able to estimate the time for the next injection of insulin based on these peaks.

2. The risk of a hypoglycemic reaction is greatest around the peak of insulin activity.

3. It is best to plan activities or exercise around peak insulin times for the best utilization of glucose.

4. Additional insulin may be required at the peak periods to prevent hyperglycemia.

2 Before administering a morning lispro insulin (Humalog) injection, which activity should the nurse perform? Select all that apply.

1. Obtain a morning urine sample for glucose and ketones.
2. Check the patient's finger-stick glucose level.
3. Ensure that breakfast trays are present on the unit and the patient may eat.
4. Obtain the patient's pulse and blood pressure.
5. Assess for symptoms of hypoglycemia.

3 The nurse would consider which of the following assessment findings as adverse effects to metformin therapy?

1. Hypoglycemia
2. Gastrointestinal distress
3. Lactic acidosis
4. Weight loss

4 A patient was started on rosiglitazone for type 2 diabetes. He tells the nurse that he has been taking it for 5 days, but his glucose levels are unchanged. What is the nurse's best response?

1. "You should double the dose. That should help."
2. "You need to give the drug more time. It can take several weeks before it becomes fully effective."

3. "You will need to add a second drug since this one has not been effective."
4. "You most likely require insulin now."

5 A young woman calls the clinic and reports that her mother had an insulin reaction and was found unconscious. The young woman gave her a glucagon injection 20 minutes ago, and her mother woke up but is still groggy and "does not make sense." What should the nurse tell the daughter?

1. "Let her wake up on her own, then give her something to eat."
2. "Place some hard candies in her mouth."
3. "Just let her sleep. People are sleepy after hypoglycemic episodes."
4. "Give her another injection and call the paramedics."

6 The nurse explains the benefit of using the long-acting insulin glargine (Lantus) over other insulins. What will the nurse tell the patient about this insulin?

1. It does not need to be administered by injection.
2. It can be given by intramuscular or subcutaneous injection.
3. It does not require blood glucose monitoring.
4. It has no definite peak but maintains a steady state of insulin in the body.

See Answers to Chapter Review in Appendix A.

References

American Association of Clinical Endocrinologists. (2011). Medical guidelines for clinical practice for developing a diabetes mellitus comprehensive care plan. *Endocrine Practice, 17*(Suppl. 2), 1–53. Retrieved from https://www.aace.com/files/dm-guidelines-ccp.pdf

American Diabetes Association. (2007). *From insulin to incretins: A report from the 67th scientific session of the American Diabetes Association.* Chicago, IL: Author.

American Diabetes Association. (2014a). Diabetes care in the school and day care setting. *Diabetes*

Care, 37(Suppl. 1), S91–S96. doi:10.2337/dc14-S091

American Diabetes Association. (2014b). *Statistics about diabetes.* Retrieved from http://www.diabetes.org/diabetes-basics/statistics/?loc=db-slabnav

Centers for Disease Control and Prevention. (2011). *National diabetes fact sheet.* Retrieved from http://www.cdc.gov/diabetes/pubs/pdf/ndfs_2011.pdf

Evert, A. B., Boucher, J. L., Cypress, M., Dunbar, S. A., Franz, M. J., Mayer-Davis, E. J., . . .

Yancy, W. S. (2014). Nutrition therapy recommendations for the management of adults with diabetes. *Diabetes Care, 37*(Suppl. 1), S120–S143. doi:10.2337/dc14-S120

Nahas, R., & Moher, M. (2009). Complementary and alternative medicine for the treatment of type 2 diabetes. *Canadian Family Physician, 55,* 591–596.

Porth, C. M. (2011). *Essentials of pathophysiology* (3rd ed.). Philadelphia, PA: Lippincott Williams & Wilkins.

Selected Bibliography

Anguita, M. (2013). Next generation of diabetes drugs arriving, but approach with caution. *Nurse Prescribing, 11,* 59.

Bennett, W. L., Maruthur, N. M., Singh, S., Segal, J. B., Wilson, L. M., Chatterjee, R., . . . Bolen, S. (2011). Comparative effectiveness and safety of medications for type 2 diabetes: An update including new drugs and 2-drug combinations. *Annals of Internal Medicine, 154,* 602–613. doi:10.7326/0003-4819-154-9-201105030-00336

Gates, B. J., & Walker, K. M. (2014). Physiological changes in older adults and their effect on diabetes treatment. *Diabetes Spectrum, 27,* 20–29. doi:10.2337/diaspect.27.1.20

Herdman, T. H., & Kamitsuru, S. (Eds.). (2014). *NANDA International nursing diagnoses: Definitions and classification, 2015-2017.* Oxford, United Kingdom: Wiley-Blackwell.

LeMone, P., Burke, K., & Bauldoff, G. (2011). *Medical-surgical nursing: Critical thinking in client care* (5th ed.). Upper Saddle River, NJ: Pearson Prentice-Hall.

Nathan, D. M. (2014). The diabetes control and complications trial/epidemiology of diabetes interventions and complications study at 30 years: Overview. *Diabetes Care, 37,* 9–16. doi:10.2337/dc13-2112

National Diabetes Information Clearinghouse. (2012). *Complementary and alternative*

medical therapies for diabetes. Retrieved from http://diabetes.niddk.nih.gov/dm/pubs/alternativetherapies

Powers, A. C., & D'Alessio, D. (2011). Endocrine pancreas and pharmacotherapy of diabetes mellitus and hypoglycemia. In L. L. Brunton, B. A. Chabner, & B. C. Knollman (Eds.), *The pharmacological basis of therapeutics* (12th ed., pp. 1237–1274). New York, NY: McGraw-Hill.

Wang, S. S. (2014). *Metabolic syndrome.* Retrieved from http://emedicine.medscape.com/article/165124-overview

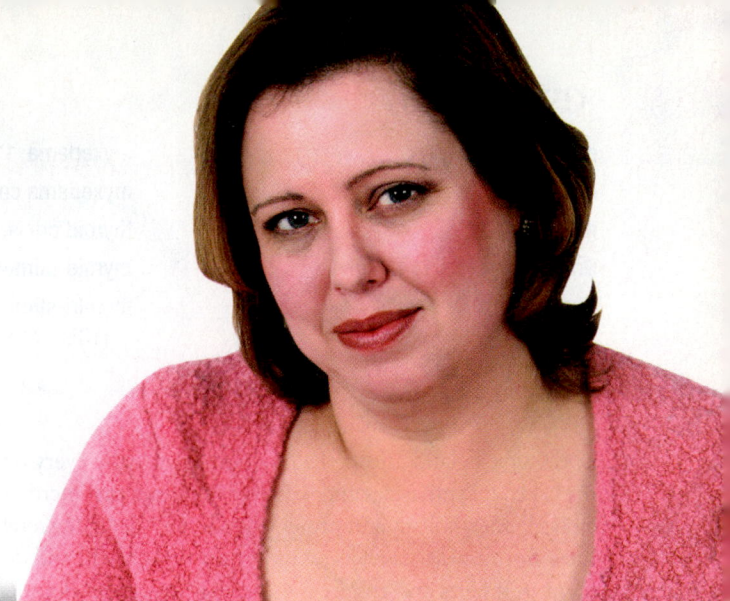

"I don't know why I've been so tired lately. Maybe it's just hormones, or my age catching up with me. I've also been gaining weight and it seems like I'm cold all the time. Maybe I should have it checked out."

Patient "Helen Mercado"

CHAPTER

67

Pharmacotherapy of Thyroid Disorders

LEARNING OUTCOMES

After reading this chapter, the student should be able to:

1. Explain the functions of thyroid hormone.
2. Explain the negative feedback control of thyroid function.
3. Explain how thyroid disorders are diagnosed.
4. Describe the pathophysiology of thyroid disorders.
5. Describe the pharmacotherapy of thyroid disorders.
6. For each of the classes shown in the chapter outline, identify the prototype and representative drugs and explain the mechanism(s) of drug action, primary indications, contraindications, significant drug interactions, pregnancy category, and important adverse effects.
7. Apply the nursing process to the care of patients receiving pharmacotherapy for thyroid disorders.

CHAPTER OUTLINE

▶ **Physiology of the Thyroid Gland**

▶ **Diagnosis of Thyroid Disorders**

▶ **Pathophysiology of Hypothyroid Disorders**

▶ **Pharmacotherapy of Hypothyroid Disorders**
   PROTOTYPE Levothyroxine (Levothroid, Levoxyl, Synthroid, Unithroid), *p. 1141*

▶ **Pathophysiology of Hyperthyroid Disorders**

▶ **Pharmacotherapy of Hyperthyroid Disorders**
   PROTOTYPE Propylthiouracil (PTU), *p. 1145*

KEY TERMS

cretinism, 1140

exophthalmos, 1142

goiter, 1138

Graves' disease, 1142

Hashimoto's thyroiditis, 1140

iodism, 1146

myxedema, 1140

myxedema coma, 1140

thyroid crisis, 1144

thyroid-stimulating hormone (TSH), 1138

thyroid-stimulating immunoglobulins (TSIs), 1144

thyroid storm, 1144

thyrotoxicosis, 1144

thyrotropin-releasing hormone (TRH), 1138

thyroxine (T$_4$), 1138

thyroxine-binding globulin (TBG), 1138

tri-iodothyronine (T$_3$), 1138

The thyroid gland affects the function of virtually every organ of the body. It synthesizes and secretes hormones that increase overall body metabolism and protein synthesis. Adequate secretion of these hormones is also necessary for normal growth and development in infants and children, including mental development and attainment of sexual maturity. The thyroid strongly affects functions of the cardiovascular, respiratory, gastrointestinal (GI), and neuromuscular systems. Thyroid disorders are common, affecting women 5 to 10 times more often than men. This chapter presents the pharmacotherapy of thyroid imbalances.

Physiology of the Thyroid Gland

67.1 Thyroid hormones contain iodine and stimulate the basal metabolic rate of nearly all tissues.

The thyroid gland lies on both sides of the trachea just below the larynx. The gland contains two distinct types of endocrine cell types: follicular cells and parafollicular cells. Follicular cells produce, store, and secrete thyroid hormone. Parafollicular cells produce calcitonin, a hormone totally unrelated to the structure or function of thyroid hormone. Calcitonin regulates calcium metabolism and is used as a drug in the pharmacotherapy of osteoporosis (see Chapter 72).

Thyroid hormone actually consists of two distinct hormones: **tri-iodothyronine (T$_3$)** and **thyroxine (T$_4$)**. Both T$_3$ and T$_4$ are synthesized from the amino acid tyrosine and iodine; the subscript numeral refers to the number of iodine molecules each hormone contains. Because the two have very similar actions, they are usually considered a single hormone.

When secreted into the bloodstream, more than 99% of T$_3$ and T$_4$ are bound to **thyroxine-binding globulin (TBG)**, a plasma protein manufactured by the liver. Any condition that causes decreased amounts of plasma proteins, such as protein malnutrition or liver impairment, can lead to a larger percentage of free thyroid hormone, with subsequent symptoms of hyperthyroidism.

Most circulating thyroid hormone is in the form of T$_4$. Upon entering target cells, however, T$_4$ is converted in peripheral tissues to T$_3$, which is three to five times more biologically active. This offers an additional level of control (tissue level) of thyroid hormone function.

The two thyroid hormones are metabolized by the liver and excreted by the kidneys, with small amounts excreted in the stool. Iodine is conserved in the process and returned to the thyroid gland for the production of more hormone molecules. Therefore, only a small daily intake of iodine is needed to meet the demands of the thyroid gland. High amounts of iodine are found in shellfish, but the main dietary source is the use of iodized salt. Thyroid hormones are the only known use for iodine in the body.

Thyroid hormone stimulates the basal metabolic rate of all tissues except the brain, anterior pituitary, spleen, lymph nodes, testes, and lungs. In the presence of large amounts of thyroid hormone, the basal metabolic rate of cells can increase by 60% to 100%. This increases the oxidation of energy sources (glucose, fats, and proteins), which in turn increases oxygen consumption and generates large amounts of heat. The rapid metabolic rate increases the body's demands for vitamins. Thyroid hormone affects GI function and motility, appetite, and body weight. Thyroid hormone increases the number of beta$_1$- and beta$_2$-adrenergic receptors and enhances their affinity to catecholamines (norepinephrine, epinephrine, and dopamine). The increase in sympathetic activity leads to increased heart rate and force of contraction, cardiac output, and cardiac demands for oxygen. Thyroid hormones also stimulate the secretion of growth hormone and are therefore essential for the normal growth and development of the skeletal and nervous systems. Thyroid hormone affects reflexes, thought processes, and overall level of consciousness (LOC). Signs and symptoms of thyroid hormone deficiency and excess are presented in Sections 67.3 and 67.5, respectively.

The secretion of thyroid hormone is regulated by the hypothalamus and anterior pituitary gland through a negative feedback loop, as shown in Figure 67.1. When blood levels of thyroid hormone are low, the hypothalamus secretes **thyrotropin-releasing hormone (TRH)**. Secretion of TRH stimulates the anterior pituitary to secrete **thyroid-stimulating hormone (TSH)**. TSH then stimulates the thyroid to produce and secrete T$_3$ and T$_4$. As blood levels of free, unbound thyroid hormone increase, negative feedback suppresses the secretion of TSH and TRH. High levels of iodine can also cause a temporary decrease in thyroid activity that can last for several weeks. One of the strongest stimuli for increased thyroid hormone production is exposure to cold.

Disorders of the thyroid result from a hypofunction or hyperfunction of the thyroid gland. Hormonal imbalances may occur due to disease within the thyroid gland itself or be caused by abnormalities of the pituitary or hypothalamus.

Thyroid disorders can be due to a congenital defect, or they may develop later in life. They may have an insidious or sudden onset. An increase in the size of the thyroid gland is referred to as a **goiter**. This can occur with normal, high, or low levels of thyroid hormone. Goiters may be diffuse, involving the entire gland, or nodular. When they become considerably enlarged, the goiter can compress the trachea and esophagus, causing difficulty swallowing, a choking sensation, and possibly inspiratory stridor (abnormal high-pitched sounds when breathing). They may also compress the superior vena cava, causing distention of the neck veins and facial edema.

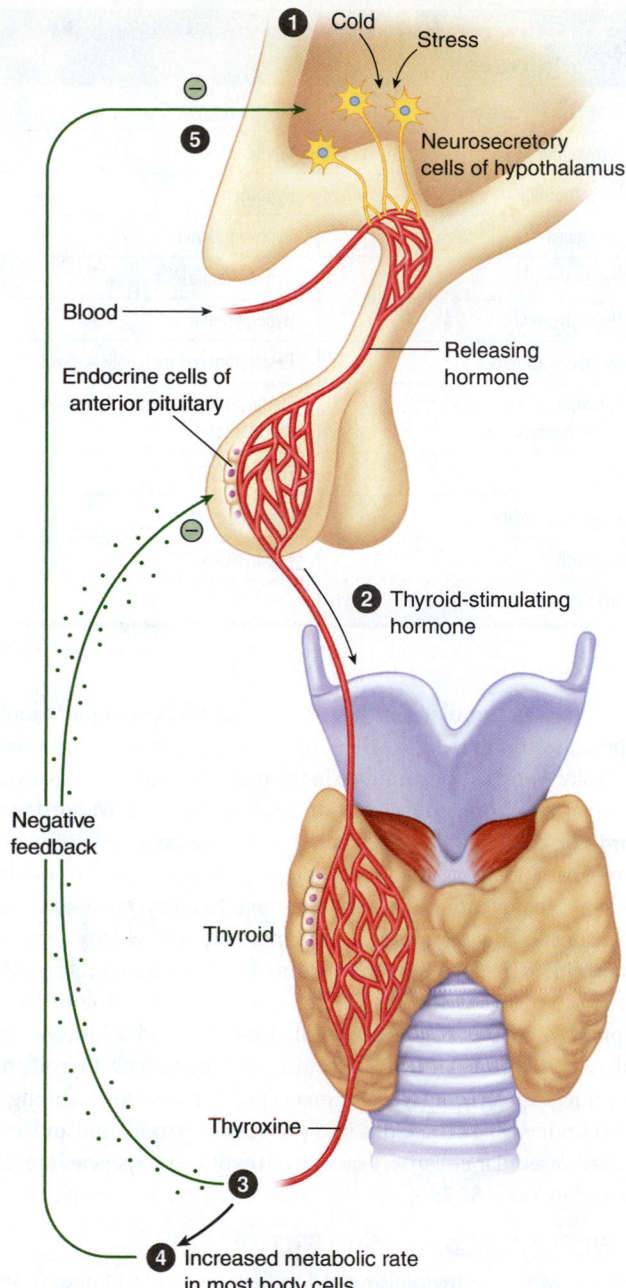

Figure 67.1 Feedback mechanisms of the thyroid gland.

Diagnosis of Thyroid Disorders

67.2 An accurate diagnosis of thyroid hormone dysfunction is based on the patient's symptoms and the results of diagnostic tests.

Because the thyroid gland is located close to the skin surface, palpation of the thyroid gland is conducted for routine screening of enlargements and nodules. Serum laboratory tests for T_3, T_4, and TSH are commonly used for diagnosis, as listed in Table 67.1. TSH is the preferred laboratory value for diagnosing and monitoring the progression of thyroid disease. Primary hypothyroidism is characterized by a low serum T_4 level and an elevated TSH level.

Abnormal laboratory values must be carefully evaluated because a number of conditions, including stress in critically ill adults, can affect TSH and T_4 levels. In addition, these laboratory values are influenced by abnormalities in serum protein levels because both T_3 and T_4 are heavily protein bound. Any condition that affects protein levels requires careful analysis of these test results. Another laboratory test useful in the diagnosis of thyroid pathology is antithyroid antibody titer. Patients with Hashimoto's thyroiditis, an autoimmune type of thyroid disease, will show abnormal levels of antithyroid antibody titer.

The diagnostic tool of choice for detecting malignancy of a thyroid nodule is the fine needle biopsy. Ultrasonography can be used to assess masses, cysts, and enlargement of the thyroid gland. The radioactive iodine uptake test measures the rate of iodine uptake by the thyroid gland after administration of ^{123}I tracer. This test can detect areas of increased and decreased function. Computed tomography (CT) and magnetic resonance imaging (MRI) scans can be used to determine tracheal compression or pressure on neighboring structures caused by thyroid gland enlargement.

An accurate diagnosis of thyroid hormone dysfunction is essential. Proper treatment of the disorder will depend on whether the abnormality lies within the thyroid gland itself or is the result of a defect in the negative feedback control by the hypothalamus or pituitary.

PharmFACT

The demands on the mother's thyroid gland increase by 50% or more early in pregnancy. Until week 20 of gestation, the fetus is entirely dependent on maternal thyroid hormones. Because even mild to moderate iodine deficiency can have adverse effects on neonatal outcomes, iodine supplementation during pregnancy is recommended (Yarrington & Pearce, 2011).

TABLE 67.1	Serum Values for Thyroid Function Tests		
Thyroid Test	**Normal Value**	**Hypothyroid**	**Hyperthyroid**
T_3 (serum)	80–200 ng/dL	Decreased	Increased
T_3 uptake	25–35% relative percentage uptake	No change	Increased
Free T_4	1–2.3 ng/dL	Decreased	Increased
Total T_4 (radioimmunoassay)	5–12 mcg/dL	Decreased	Increased
TSH (serum)	0.35–5.5 microinternational units/mL	Increased	Decreased

Pathophysiology of Hypothyroid Disorders

67.3 Hypothyroidism, or thyroid deficiency, can occur as a congenital or acquired disorder.

Hypothyroidism may occur as a congenital disorder, or it may be acquired in adulthood. Congenital hypothyroidism is a common, preventable cause of mental retardation. The infant appears normal at birth due to hormones supplied by the mother while *in utero*. If untreated, congenital hypothyroidism results in a condition known as **cretinism**, marked by profound mental retardation and impaired growth. Almost half of normal brain development occurs during the first 6 months of life, and thyroid hormone is essential for this to occur. Studies show that if thyroid replacement therapy is begun in the first 6 weeks of life, normal growth and development takes place and cretinism can be prevented. In the United States and Canada, screening for hypothyroidism is conducted for all neonates.

Hypothyroidism in older children and adults results in a general slowing of metabolic processes and **myxedema**, a mucous type of edema caused by an accumulation of hydrophilic substances in connective tissues. Primary hypothyroidism, the most common type in children and adults, results from dysfunction of the thyroid gland. Secondary hypothyroidism is due to pathology of the pituitary gland. Tertiary hypothyroidism is a result of a disorder of the hypothalamus. Causes of hypothyroidism include thyroidectomy or ablation of the thyroid gland with radiation, the use of lithium (in the treatment of bipolar disorder), or treatment with antithyroid drugs. Large amounts of iodine or substances that contain iodine, such as kelp tablets, certain cough syrups, the cardiac drug amiodarone, or iodine-containing radiographic contrast media, can block thyroid hormone production and cause goiter and hypothyroidism. Iodine deficiency is rarely a cause of hypothyroidism in the United States due to the widespread use of iodized salt.

The most common cause of hypothyroidism is an autoimmune disorder known as **Hashimoto's thyroiditis**. This is predominantly a disease of women, striking women 5 to 10 times more often than men. Because hypothyroidism during the first trimester of pregnancy has been shown to cause mental and developmental problems in the fetus, it is recommended that all women receive screening for hypothyroidism early in a pregnancy. By the second trimester, when the fetus is able to synthesize thyroid hormone, this threat disappears. Women also experience a high incidence of postpartum thyroiditis, which occurs following approximately 10% of pregnancies.

Hypothyroidism affects nearly all major organ systems, with manifestations arising from two factors: a hypometabolic state and myxedematous changes in body tissues. The hypometabolic state is marked by a gradual onset of weakness and fatigue, a tendency to gain weight despite a decreased appetite, and cold intolerance. Hypotension, bradycardia, hypoventilation, and subnormal temperature may occur. In time, the skin becomes rough and dry and may have a yellowish cast; the hair becomes coarse and brittle; and GI motility slows, causing chronic constipation, flatulence, and abdominal distention. Mental dullness, lethargy, slowed reflexes, and memory problems may occur.

TABLE 67.2 Signs and Symptoms of Thyroid Emergencies

Thyroid Storm	Myxedema Coma
Tachycardia	Bradycardia
Hyperthermia	Hypothermia
Tachypnea	Hypoventilation
Hypercalcemia	Hyponatremia
Hyperglycemia	Hypoglycemia
Metabolic acidosis	Respiratory and metabolic acidosis
Cardiovascular collapse: cardiogenic shock, hypovolemia, arrhythmias	Cardiovascular collapse: decreased vascular tone
Depressed LOC	Depressed LOC
Emotional lability	Seizures, coma
Psychosis	Hyporeflexia
Tremors, restlessness	

As fluid accumulates in tissues, the face takes on a puffy look, especially around the eyes; the tongue enlarges; and the voice may be husky. Fluid can accumulate in the pericardial or pleural spaces, causing effusions, cardiac dilation, and bradycardia. **Myxedema coma** or crisis is a life-threatening end-stage condition of hypothyroidism, characterized by coma, hypothermia, cardiovascular collapse, hypoventilation, hyponatremia, hypoglycemia, and lactic acidosis. This condition occurs most often in elderly women. Even with early detection and treatment, the mortality rate is 30% for those who develop myxedema coma. Treatment consists of supportive measures, correction of electrolyte and acid–base imbalances, treatment of hypotension, and immediate thyroid replacement therapy. If hypothermia is present, active rewarming is contraindicated, because this may precipitate vasodilation and lead to cardiovascular collapse. Features of thyroid emergencies are described in Table 67.2.

CONNECTION Checkpoint 67.1

Patients with hypothyroidism tend to have low rates of angina and myocardial infarction. From what you learned in Chapter 35, explain this link. *See Answer to Connection Checkpoint 67.1 on student resource website.*

Pharmacotherapy of Hypothyroid Disorders

67.4 Hypothyroidism is treated by replacement therapy with thyroid hormone.

Hypothyroidism is treated by replacement therapy with T_3 or T_4. The standard replacement regimen consists of levothyroxine (T_4), although combined therapy with levothyroxine plus liothyronine (T_3) is an option. Although T_4 is less biologically active than T_3, it is readily converted to T_3 in peripheral tissues. In most cases, thyroid replacement therapy is lifelong.

◀ The Effects of Soy Intake on Drug Treatment for Hypothyroidism

Soy and soy products are known to interact with, and inhibit absorption of, thyroid replacement drugs such as levothyroxine. Fruzza, Demeterco-Berggren, and Jones (2012) reported on the impact of soy formula and soy milk on infants and toddlers who had been diagnosed with congenital hypothyroidism. Signs of clinical hypothyroidism were observed until the soy formula (infant) or soy milk (toddler) was switched to a non-soy alternative. Because the implications of hypothyroidism in infants and young children during crucial periods of brain growth are significant and may result in developmental and growth delays, parents of children with congenital hypothyroidism should be cautioned about the use of soy products, and appropriate substitutions explored. This study also has implications for adult patients on thyroid replacement therapy. Depending on the amount of soy intake, hypothyroidism may result if the intake interferes with thyroid replacement absorption. Because some patients may switch to soy as a supplement or substitute for animal proteins in the diet, nurses should include a dietary assessment for adult patients on replacement therapy, especially for those who are experiencing hypothyroidism after a period of a euthyroid state.

In children with cretinism, therapy should continue for 3 years, after which it should be stopped for 1 month. During this time, thyroid hormone levels are monitored to assess the status of the deficiency and to determine if further treatment is needed.

In adults, serum TSH levels are used to evaluate the progress of therapy. When initiating therapy in older adults, the precaution is to "go low and go slow," because there is a risk for inducing acute coronary syndromes in susceptible individuals. Table 67.3 lists the doses of the drugs used to treat hypothyroidism.

PROTOTYPE DRUG	Levothyroxine (Levothroid, Levoxyl, Synthroid, Unithroid)

Classification: Therapeutic: Thyroid hormone
Pharmacologic: Thyroid hormone replacement

Therapeutic Effects and Uses: Levothyroxine is a synthetic form of T_4, with actions identical to endogenous thyroid hormone. It is used for primary or secondary hypothyroidism, congenital hypothyroidism, hypothyroid state resulting from the surgical removal of the thyroid gland, radiation or antithyroid drugs, management of thyroid cancer, or treatment of myxedema coma. The drug is given by the oral (PO) route for routine replacement therapy and intravenously (IV) for myxedema coma.

To avoid adverse effects, doses of thyroid hormone are highly individualized for each patient. When given by the PO route, 1 to 3 weeks may be required to obtain full therapeutic benefits. Doses for patients with preexisting cardiac disease are usually increased at 4- to 6-week intervals to avoid the possibility of dysrhythmias or angina attacks.

TABLE 67.3 Drugs for Hypothyroidism

Drug Name	Dose for Adults (Maximum Dose Where Indicated)	Adverse Effects
levothyroxine (Levothroid, Levoxyl, Synthroid, Others)	PO: 100–400 mcg/day IV: initial loading dose of 300–500 mcg followed by maintenance doses of 50–100 mcg	*Weight loss, headache, tremors, nervousness, heat intolerance, irritability, sweating, insomnia, menstrual irregularities*
liothyronine (Cytomel, Triostat)	PO: 25–75 mcg/day IV: 25–100 mcg/day	<u>Dysrhythmias, hypertension, palpitations, angina</u>
liotrix (Thyrolar)	PO: 12.5–30 mcg/day	
thyroid, desiccated (Armour thyroid, Thyroid USP)	PO: 60–180 mg/day	

Note: Italics indicate common adverse effects. <u>Underline</u> indicates severe adverse effects.

Mechanism of Action: The actions of levothyroxine are identical to endogenous thyroid hormone. The drug increases the metabolic rate, thereby increasing oxygen consumption, respiration, and heart rate; increases the rate of fat, protein, and carbohydrate metabolism; and promotes growth and maturation. Because levothyroxine is converted to T_3, it is not necessary to also give T_3.

Pharmacokinetics:

Route(s)	PO, IV
Absorption	Variable; partial absorption from the GI tract (50% to 80%)
Distribution	Gradually released to peripheral tissues; crosses the placenta; secreted in breast milk; more than 99% bound to protein
Primary metabolism	Hepatic
Primary excretion	Kidneys, with some secreted in bile and excreted in feces
Onset of action	PO: Slow; IV: 6–8 h
Duration of action	1–3 weeks; half-life: 6–7 days

Adverse Effects: At therapeutic doses, adverse effects of levothyroxine therapy are rare. At high doses, treatment may cause central nervous system (CNS) excitability such as tremors, headache, nervousness, or insomnia. Cardiovascular adverse effects include palpitations, tachycardia, angina, and cardiac arrest. Other possible adverse events include allergic skin reactions, diarrhea, nausea, and vomiting. Synthroid 100-mcg and 300-mcg tablets contain tartrazine, which may cause an allergic reaction in some patients, especially those sensitive to aspirin. **Black Box Warning**: Use of thyroid hormone for weight loss or the treatment of obesity is contraindicated.

Contraindications/Precautions: The use of levothyroxine is contraindicated if the patient is hypersensitive to the drug, is experiencing thyrotoxicosis, or has severe cardiovascular conditions or acute myocardial infarction (MI). If thyroid hormone is given to patients with adrenal insufficiency, it may cause a serious adrenal crisis; thus, the insufficiency should be corrected prior to administration of levothyroxine. It should be used with caution in patients with cardiac disease, angina pectoris, cardiac dysrhythmias, hypertension, and impaired kidney function, and in older adults. Symptoms of diabetes mellitus may be worsened with administration of thyroid hormone and doses of antidiabetic drugs may require adjustment.

Drug Interactions: A large number of medications can interact with thyroid hormone and result in either increased or decreased effects. Drugs that decrease the absorption of levothyroxine include cholestyramine, colestipol, calcium- or aluminum-containing antacids, sucralfate, and iron supplements. Several drugs are known to accelerate the metabolism of levothyroxine, including phenytoin, carbamazepine, rifampin, phenobarbital, and sertraline. Levothyroxine increases the effects of warfarin, resulting in an increased risk of bleeding. Digoxin decreases the effectiveness of levothyroxine. Thyroid hormone sensitizes cardiac responsiveness to catecholamines; therefore, administration of epinephrine or norepinephrine must be carefully monitored in these patients to prevent dysrhythmias. **Herbal/Food**: Soybean flour (infant formula), cottonseed meal, walnuts, and dietary fiber may bind and decrease the absorption of levothyroxine sodium from the GI tract. Calcium or iron supplements should be taken at least 4 hours after taking levothyroxine to prevent interference with drug absorption. The patient should also avoid consuming large amounts of foods that can inhibit thyroid secretion, such as strawberries, peaches, pears, cabbage, turnips, spinach, kale, Brussels sprouts, cauliflower, radishes, and peas.

Pregnancy: Category A.

Treatment of Overdose: The treatment of levothyroxine overdose is the same as the treatment of thyroid crisis or thyroid storm, as discussed in Section 67.6. Treatment is directed at reducing the level of circulating thyroid hormone with antithyroid drugs and decreasing sympathetic stimulation with corticosteroids and beta-adrenergic blockers.

Nursing Responsibilities: Key nursing implications for patients receiving levothyroxine are included in the Nursing Practice Application for Patients Receiving Pharmacotherapy with Thyroid Hormone Replacements.

Drugs Similar to Levothyroxine (Levothroid, Levoxyl, Synthroid, Others)

Other thyroid replacement medications include liothyronine, liotrix, and desiccated thyroid. All thyroid drugs carry a black box warning stating they should not be used for weight loss or to treat obesity.

Liothyronine (Cytomel, Triostat): Approved in 1954, liothyronine is a synthetic form of T_3 used in replacement therapy for hypothyroidism. Its actions, adverse effects, and contraindications are similar to those for endogenous thyroid hormone. It has a shorter onset, half-life, and duration of action than levothyroxine

---

CONNECTIONS | Treating the Diverse Patient

◀ Improved Kidney Function from Thyroid Hormone Replacement

Because thyroid hormones affect nearly all body systems, even slight changes in the amount of circulating hormones may have profound effects. Recent research suggests that subclinical hypothyroidism may have significant effects on chronic kidney disease (CKD), or the development of the disease (Hataya, Igarashi, Yamashita, & Komatsu, 2013; Shin et al., 2012). Correcting even subclinical hypothyroidism to a euthyroid state appears to improve and preserve kidney function as measured by glomerular filtration rate (GFR). Several theories exist as to why thyroid replacement improves renal function, including improvement in cardiac status, improvement in dyslipidemias, or the effect on vascular endothelium (Shin et al., 2012). It is recommended that patients with CKD be assessed for hypothyroidism and that thyroid replacement therapy should be started as needed, if appropriate (Hataya et al., 2013).

---

and is more expensive. Liothyronine is readily converted to T_3 in the bloodstream. The injectable form of liothyronine is a preferred drug for the treatment of myxedema coma. It is available in oral and IV formulations. This drug is pregnancy category A.

Liotrix (Thyrolar): Liotrix is a synthetic mixture of T_4 and T_3, in a 4:1 ratio, available in PO form only for the treatment of hypothyroidism. Because levothyroxine is readily converted to T_3, there is no apparent advantage in using liotrix over levothyroxine. Its actions, adverse effects, and contraindications are similar to those for endogenous thyroid hormone. This drug is pregnancy category A.

Thyroid, desiccated (Armour, Thyroid USP): Desiccated thyroid is an older formulation, approved in 1939, obtained from the dried thyroid glands of pigs. The drug contains T_3 and T_4 in their natural proportions. Desiccated thyroid is less pure and has less reliable content than synthetic formulations and has been replaced by levothyroxine. It is only used for patients who have taken it for years—newly diagnosed cases of hypothyroidism are treated with synthetic thyroid hormone.

Pathophysiology of Hyperthyroid Disorders

67.5 Hyperthyroidism, or Graves' disease, is an autoimmune disorder accompanied by ophthalmopathy and goiter.

Symptoms of hyperthyroidism have been recorded in medical documents dating back to the 12th century. The most common cause of hyperthyroidism is **Graves' disease**, named after the Irish doctor Robert Graves who described the disorder in 1835. The condition is characterized by the excessive secretion of thyroid hormone.

The two most visible signs of Graves' disease are goiter and **exophthalmos**, an outward bulging of the eyes. Up to one third

CONNECTIONS: NURSING PRACTICE APPLICATION

Patients Receiving Pharmacotherapy with Thyroid Hormone Replacements

Assessment	Potential Nursing Diagnoses*
Baseline assessment prior to administration: • Obtain a complete health history including cardiovascular, GI, hepatic, and renal disease; pregnancy; or breast-feeding. Obtain a drug history including allergies, current prescription and over-the-counter (OTC) drugs, herbal preparations, alcohol use, or smoking. Be alert to possible drug interactions. • Evaluate appropriate laboratory findings (e.g., T_3, T_4, and TSH levels; CBC; platelets, electrolytes, glucose, and lipid levels). • Obtain baseline height, weight, and vital signs. Obtain an ECG as needed. • Assess the patient's ability to receive and understand instructions. Include the family or caregiver as needed.	• *Activity Intolerance* • *Fatigue* • *Constipation* • *Deficient Knowledge* (Drug Therapy) • *Risk for Infection*, related to adverse drug effects • *Risk for Imbalanced Body Temperature*
Assessment throughout administration: • Assess for desired therapeutic effects, dependent on the reason the drug is given (e.g., T_3, T_4, and TSH levels return to normal, associated symptoms ease). • Continue periodic monitoring of T_3, T_4, and TSH levels and glucose levels. • Continue monitoring vital signs, height, and weight. Monitor ECG as needed. • Assess for adverse effects: nausea, vomiting, diarrhea, epigastric distress, skin rash, itching, headache, tachycardia, palpitations, dysrhythmia, sweating, nervousness, paresthesia, tremors, insomnia, heat intolerance, and angina. Hypo- or hypertension, tachycardia, especially associated with dysrhythmia, or angina should be immediately reported to the health care provider.	

Implementation

Interventions and (Rationales)	Patient-Centered Care
Ensuring therapeutic effects: • Monitor vital signs, appetite, weight, sensitivity to heat or cold, sleep patterns, and ability to perform activities of daily living (ADLs). (As metabolic activity controlled by thyroid hormones stabilizes, the patient should return to normal weight, ADLs, and feelings of wellness.)	• Advise the patient that the drug will help to stabilize thyroid hormone levels quickly, but full effects may take a week or longer to occur. • Instruct the patient to maintain consistent dosing to allow the drug to reach therapeutic levels. • Instruct the patient to weigh self two to three times per week and record the findings. Bring the record to each clinic visit.
• Avoid iodine-containing foods (e.g., iodized salt, soy sauce, tofu, yogurt, milk, strawberries, eggs) unless approved by the health care provider. (Iodine is necessary for the synthesis of thyroid hormone. Increasing or decreasing normal intake may result in adverse drug effects.)	• Provide dietary instruction on foods to avoid. Provide for a dietitian consultation as needed.
• Monitor thyroid function tests. (Results help determine the effectiveness of the drug therapy and the need for dosage changes.)	• Instruct the patient on the need to return periodically for laboratory work.
Minimizing adverse effects: • Monitor for return of original symptoms and report consistent occurrence. (Daily fluctuations in symptoms may occur because hormone replacement therapy does not precisely approximate the body's own levels. Significant increases in original symptoms may signal less-than-optimal therapeutic results. Dramatic "opposite" effect and hypo- or hyperthyroid symptoms may signal drug toxicity.)	• Teach the patient that small daily fluctuations may occur, especially during periods of stress or illness. Any significant or increasing changes in pulse rate, weight, nervousness or fatigue, intolerance to heat or cold, and diarrhea or constipation should be reported to the health care provider.
• **Lifespan:** Monitor symptoms in older adults more frequently. (Older patients are more sensitive to thyroid replacement therapy. Minor changes in daily thyroid levels may cause a significant change in symptoms.)	• Teach the patient, family, or caregiver that the lowest dose will be started and gradually increased to find the optimal level. Any significant change in symptoms should be promptly reported to the health care provider.
• **Lifespan:** Monitor height, weight, and developmental growth in infants and young children. (Infants and children receiving thyroid replacement therapy should continue to display normal growth and development curves.)	• Teach the parents or caregivers to weigh the child weekly and record. Bring the record to each health care visit. • Encourage the parents or caregivers to discuss concerns or any unusual findings that would suggest developmental or growth delays with the health care provider if they are noted in the child between health care visits.
• Monitor serum glucose levels, especially in patients with diabetes. Patients with diabetes should monitor capillary levels more frequently. (Thyroid replacement therapy may cause changes in glucose levels and an adjustment in antidiabetic medications may be needed.)	• Teach patients with diabetes to monitor capillary glucose levels more frequently during therapy. Report any consistent changes to the health care provider.

(continued)

CONNECTIONS: NURSING PRACTICE APPLICATION (continued)

• Ensure patient safety. Observe for lightheadedness or dizziness. Monitor ambulation until the effects of the drug are known. (Dizziness may be secondary to changes in pulse or blood pressure and should be assessed by the health care provider. **Lifespan:** The older adult is especially at risk for falls related to dizziness. Effects of thyroid hormone on bone remodeling may place the patient at risk for fractures.)	• Instruct the patient to call for assistance prior to getting out of bed or attempting to walk alone if dizziness occurs. If dizziness occurs, the patient should sit or lie down and not attempt to stand or walk until the sensation passes. • Assess the safety of the home environment and discuss modifications that may be needed with the family or caregiver.
• Continue to monitor the effectiveness of all other medications the patient is taking. Teach patients to take thyroid replacement 1 h before or 4 h after foods high in fiber or medications such as cholestyramine, calcium or aluminum antacids, or iron supplements. (Thyroid replacement drugs interact with many drugs and may cause suboptimal or excessive responses. Drugs such as calcium and aluminum antacids decrease absorption of thyroid hormone.)	• Teach the patient to report any unusual symptoms of concern to the health care provider.
Patient understanding of drug therapy: • Use opportunities during administration of medications and during assessments to discuss the rationale for drug therapy, desired therapeutic outcomes, commonly observed adverse effects, parameters for when to call the health care provider, and any necessary monitoring or precautions. (Using time during nursing care helps to optimize and reinforce key teaching areas.)	• The patient should be able to state the reason for the drug, appropriate dose and scheduling, what adverse effects to observe for, and when to report them.

Patient self-administration of drug therapy:
• When administering the medication, instruct the patient, family, or caregiver in proper self-administration of the drug, e.g., take the drug in the morning at the same time each day. (Utilizing time during nurse-administration of these drugs helps to reinforce teaching.)
	• Teach the patient to take the drug following appropriate guidelines:
	  • Take the drug at the same time each morning to approximate normal body hormone levels. If night shift hours are worked, consult with the health care provider about scheduling appropriate time of drug administration.
	  • Avoid foods high in iodine unless approved by the health care provider.
	  • To ensure optimal therapeutic response, take the same brand of drug and request the same manufacturer each time the prescription is filled. If the same drug is unavailable, consult with the health care provider about dosage or observe for adverse drug effects. Do not switch brand names until the provider has been consulted.

*Nursing Diagnoses—Definitions and Classification 2015–2017. Copyright © 2014, 1994–2014 by NANDA International. Used by arrangement with John Wiley & Sons Limited.

of those with Graves' disease develop ophthalmopathy, leading to severe eye problems. These include paralysis of the ocular muscles, damage to the optic nerve with some vision loss, and corneal ulceration due to the inability of the eyelids to close. These eye problems are aggravated by smoking, which should be strongly discouraged in persons with Graves' disease. The ophthalmopathy usually stabilizes with treatment but not all eye changes are reversible with therapy. A rare skin disorder, pretibial myxedema, may also occur, with thickening of the skin, plaques, and nodules over the shins and dorsal surface of the feet. Like the ophthalmic changes, these skin changes may persist despite effective treatment of the disease.

Causes of Graves' disease include adenoma and excessive intake of thyroid hormone. The onset is usually between the ages of 20 and 40 years, and it occurs five times more often in women than in men. Graves' disease is an autoimmune disorder in which the thyroid gland is stimulated by **thyroid-stimulating immunoglobulins (TSIs)**. It may occur concurrently with other autoimmune disorders, and there is a familial tendency to the condition.

The manifestations of hyperthyroidism are caused by the hypermetabolic state and the increase in sympathetic nervous system activity. The symptoms include nervousness, irritability and fatigability, insomnia, weight loss despite a large appetite, tachycardia, palpitations, hypertension, shortness of breath, increased sweating, muscle cramps, hyperthermia, and heat intolerance. A fine muscle tremor may occur. Approximately 15% of older adults with new-onset atrial fibrillation, a common cardiac dysrhythmia, have thyrotoxicosis.

Very high levels of circulating thyroid hormone may cause **thyrotoxicosis**. **Thyroid crisis**, or **thyroid storm**, is a rare, life-threatening form of thyrotoxicosis. If untreated, it is associated with mortality rates of 80% to 90%. Even with treatment, mortality from thyroid storm exceeds 20%. It occurs most often in teenage and young adult women with undiagnosed or untreated cases of hyperthyroidism and can be precipitated by the stress of an acute infection, diabetic ketoacidosis, trauma, or manipulation of the thyroid gland during surgery. Manifestations include high fever, cardiovascular effects (tachycardia, heart failure, angina, and MI), and CNS effects (agitation, restlessness, delirium, progressing to coma). It is treated with supportive measures, efforts to reduce body temperature without causing shivering, fluid, glucose and electrolyte replacement, and beta-adrenergic blockers. Aspirin should not be used to lower the body temperature of a person in thyroid storm because it displaces thyroid hormone from its protein-binding sites in the serum, increasing the level of free, or active, thyroid hormone, which worsens the condition. Antithyroid drugs may be used to decrease thyroid hormone production.

PharmFACT

Although Graves' disease most commonly occurs in adults, it also occurs in children. About 10% of infants born to women with Graves' disease have hyperthyroidism, but most are asymptomatic. Concordance for Graves' disease is 30% to 50% in identical twins (Levitsky, 2013).

Pharmacotherapy of Hyperthyroid Disorders

67.6 Hyperthyroidism is treated with surgery or drugs that reduce the production of thyroid hormone.

Treatment of hyperthyroidism often requires surgical removal of all or part of the thyroid gland. In less serious cases of the disorder, pharmacotherapy can be used to diminish the secretion of thyroid hormone.

One strategy to lower thyroid hormone secretion is to destroy part of the gland (ablation) by administering radioactive iodide (^{131}I). The goal of thyroid ablation is to use the ionizing radiation from the drug to destroy just enough of the thyroid gland to return the patient to a normal thyroid state. This therapy is preferred by many endocrinologists because it results in a permanent, long-term solution to hyperthyroidism. This therapy is contraindicated during pregnancy due to the risk of exposing the fetus to ionizing radiation.

Antithyroid drugs may be administered to manage hyperthyroidism. Propylthiouracil (PTU) and methimazole (Tapazole) prevent the incorporation of iodine into the thyroid hormone molecule and block the conversion of T_4 to T_3 in peripheral tissues. Doses of the antithyroid drugs are listed in Table 67.4.

Treatment of thyroid storm is a medical emergency. Methimazole is preferred by some health care providers because it can be given by either the oral route or the IV route and the risk for serious adverse effects is lower than with propylthiouracil. Propylthiouracil has equal effectiveness and is preferred for pregnant patients. Potassium iodide solution can be given to immediately block the release of thyroid hormone but should not be given until 1 hour after the administration of antithyroid medications.

Several drugs are used as adjuncts in the therapy of thyroid storm. During hyperthyroid states, beta-adrenergic blocking drugs such as propranolol (Inderal), esmolol (Brevibloc), or metoprolol (Toprol) are given to block the effects of the thyroid hormones on sympathetic receptors in the heart. The actions include a decrease in heart rate and strength of contraction, thereby decreasing myocardial oxygen demands. These effects occur quickly, while the actions of antithyroid drugs take longer to occur. Refer to Chapter 16 for the specific pharmacology of beta-adrenergic blockers.

IV corticosteroids such as hydrocortisone (Solu-Cortef) or dexamethasone (Decadron) may be ordered to treat acute hyperthyroid states. Corticosteroids block the conversion of T_4 to T_3 in peripheral tissues. In addition, severe hyperthyroid states create high levels of stress that deplete adrenal corticosteroids in the body, and administration of replacement doses is necessary. The pharmacology of the corticosteroids is presented in Chapter 68.

CONNECTION Checkpoint 67.2

Patients with Graves' disease have increased hepatic gluconeogenesis, rapid glucose absorption, and increased insulin resistance. From what you learned in Chapter 66, what insulin dosage adjustment is necessary for these patients who also have diabetes mellitus? *See Answer to Connection Checkpoint 67.2 on student resource website.*

PROTOTYPE DRUG	Propylthiouracil (PTU)

Classification: **Therapeutic:** Antithyroid drug
Pharmacologic: Thyroid hormone inhibitor

Therapeutic Effects and Uses: Approved in 1947, propylthiouracil decreases thyroid hormone levels in hyperthyroid states that are caused by the overproduction of thyroid hormone. It is also used to establish the normal thyroid state prior to surgery or radioactive iodine treatment and for palliative control of toxic nodular goiter. Propylthiouracil is not effective in treating thyroiditis because this condition is due to overrelease, not overproduction, of thyroid hormone.

Mechanism of Action: Propylthiouracil inhibits the first step in the synthesis of thyroid hormone and suppresses the peripheral conversion of T_4 to T_3. It does not affect thyroid hormone that has already been synthesized, so therapeutic response may be delayed by 3 to 12 weeks, until existing supplies of thyroid hormone have been depleted.

TABLE 67.4 Antithyroid Drugs

Drug Name	Dose for Adults (Maximum Dose Where Indicated)	Adverse Effects
methimazole (Tapazole)	PO: 5–15 mg tid (max: 60 mg/day)	*Nausea, rash, pruritus, urticaria, fever, numbness in fingers, peripheral neuropathy, leukopenia, hypothyroidism* <u>Agranulocytosis, bradycardia, hepatotoxicity</u>
potassium iodide and iodine (Lugol's solution, Thyro-Block)	PO: 125 mg daily	*Diarrhea, nausea, vomiting, stomach pain, fever, weakness, irregular heartbeat, hypothyroidism* <u>Angioneurotic edema, iodine poisoning</u>
propylthiouracil (PTU)	PO: 300–450 mg tid	*Nausea, rash, pruritus, headache, fever, numbness in fingers, diarrhea, myelosuppression, hypothyroidism* <u>Agranulocytosis</u>
radioactive iodide (^{131}I)	PO: 0.8–150 millicurie (a curie is a unit of radioactivity)	*Adverse effects are uncommon* <u>Thyroiditis, hypothyroidism, hypersensitivity</u>

Note: Italics indicate common adverse effects. <u>Underline</u> indicates severe adverse effects.

Pharmacokinetics:

Route(s)	PO
Absorption	Rapidly absorbed
Distribution	Concentrated by the thyroid gland; crosses the placenta; secreted in breast milk; 60–80% bound to plasma protein
Primary metabolism	Hepatic
Primary excretion	Kidneys
Onset of action	Absorbed within 30 min, but therapeutic effects may take up to 3 weeks
Duration of action	Half-life: 1–2 h; peak: 1–1.5 h

Adverse Effects: Approximately 15% to 20% of patients taking this drug will experience leukopenia, which is normally asymptomatic. Serious hypersensitivity reactions are rare but may be serious and include agranulocytosis, aplastic anemia, thrombocytopenia, rash, urticaria, and glomerulonephritis. Arthralgias and joint swelling occur in 5% of patients. CNS effects include headache, vertigo, neuritis, and paresthesias. Propylthiouracil can also cause hypothyroidism and goiter at high doses. **Black Box Warning**: Severe liver injury and acute hepatic failure have been reported in patients taking propylthiouracil. This drug should be reserved for those unable to tolerate methimazole and in whom radioactive iodine therapy or surgery are not appropriate treatments for hyperthyroidism.

Contraindications/Precautions: The use of propylthiouracil is contraindicated if the patient has a hypersensitivity to the drug. Although contraindicated during pregnancy, the drug occasionally must be administered to women who experience a thyrotoxic crisis during pregnancy, and it is preferred over methimazole because less of the drug crosses the placenta. It should be used with caution during active infection, lactation, and bone marrow depression. Because propylthiouracil can cause liver impairment, caution should be used when treating patients with preexisting hepatic disease.

Drug Interactions: Propylthiouracil increases the actions of anticoagulants, which creates an increased risk of bleeding. Iodine-containing drugs (amiodarone, potassium iodide, sodium iodide, radioactive iodine) and thyroid hormones can antagonize the effectiveness of this drug. Altered serum levels of metoprolol, propranolol, and digoxin can occur as the patient moves from a hyperthyroid to a normal thyroid state. Cross hypersensitivity occurs in about 50% of patients who have experienced a hypersensitivity reaction to methimazole, the other major antithyroid medication. Propylthiouracil should not be used with carbamazepine or clozapine because this may increase the risk of agranulocytosis. **Herbal/Food**: Unknown.

Pregnancy: Category D.

Treatment of Overdose: When propylthiouracil is taken in high doses, it can induce hypothyroidism; the administration of thyroid hormone may be necessary.

Nursing Responsibilities: Key nursing implications for patients receiving propylthiouracil are included in the Nursing Practice Application for Patients Receiving Pharmacotherapy with Antithyroid Drugs.

Drugs Similar to Propylthiouracil (PTU)

Drugs similar to propylthiouracil include Lugol's solution, methimazole, potassium iodide, and radioactive iodide.

Lugol's solution (5% elemental iodine and 10% potassium iodide):   This strong iodine solution is given orally to treat hyperthyroidism, as adjunctive therapy 10 to 14 days prior to thyroid surgery, or for the treatment of thyrotoxicosis. It has been used as a topical antiseptic. Although iodine is necessary for the synthesis of thyroid hormone, high levels inhibit both the synthesis and release of thyroid hormone. Chronic use can result in toxicity known as **iodism**, which is characterized by burning in the mouth and throat, a metallic taste, sore teeth and gums, increased salivation and nasal discharge, swollen eyelids, gastric irritation, and diarrhea. The distribution of Lugol's solution is now regulated by the U.S. Drug Enforcement Administration because strong iodine solutions are used in the manufacture of crystal methamphetamine. Potassium iodide is pregnancy category D.

Methimazole (Tapazole):   Approved in 1950, methimazole is given by the oral route to correct hyperthyroidism by inhibiting the synthesis of thyroid hormone. Like PTU, it does not affect existing stores of thyroid hormone; thus it may take many weeks before a normal thyroid state is achieved. Its uses, contraindications, and adverse effects are similar to those for PTU, except that methimazole does not induce hypothyroidism or cause serious liver injury. Other important differences are that methimazole does not inhibit conversion of T_4 to T_3; therefore, its effects may take longer to occur. Methimazole has a longer half-life, allowing for once-a-day dosing, while PTU must be taken three times a day. Methimazole is usually administered for 12 to 18 months, then tapered or discontinued if TSH levels are normal. This drug is pregnancy category D.

Potassium iodide (Thyro-Block):   Potassium iodide is given orally prior to thyroid surgery to reduce the vascularity (risk of bleeding), fragility, and size of the thyroid gland. It may also be used alone for hyperthyroidism or in combination with antithyroid drugs and beta-adrenergic blockers in the treatment of thyroid storm. Like other forms of iodide, it suppresses the synthesis and release of thyroid hormone. It is also used to protect the thyroid gland in instances of radiation exposure secondary to a nuclear accident. It is taken up by the thyroid gland, thereby blocking the uptake of radioactive iodide in the thyroid gland, reducing the risk for developing thyroid cancer. As a protective agent, it must be given immediately prior to, or within 3 hours following, radiation exposure. This drug is pregnancy category D.

Radioactive iodide (^{131}I):   Radioactive iodide is an isotope of iodine used for hyperthyroidism. Like all iodine, ^{131}I is taken up by the thyroid gland, where its radioactivity destroys thyroid tissue. The goal is to destroy part of the gland, thereby decreasing the amount of thyroid hormone produced and secreted. In some patients, too much thyroid gland is destroyed and hypothyroidism results, which is then treated with levothyroxine. Approximately two thirds of patients treated with ^{131}I respond to a single treatment, while the rest require two or more treatments. Therapeutic effects develop slowly over 2 to 3 months, and the tissue damage is limited to the thyroid gland with no surrounding structures affected. While it is contraindicated during pregnancy and breast-feeding, and usually not used in children, ^{131}I has not been known to cause cancer or other serious adverse effects to the thyroid gland or elsewhere in the body. It is used in patients wishing to avoid surgery or those who do not tolerate antithyroid drugs. It is administered PO and is also used to treat thyroid cancer (in high doses) and for the diagnosis of thyroid disorders. This drug is pregnancy category X.

CONNECTIONS: NURSING PRACTICE APPLICATION

Patients Receiving Pharmacotherapy with Antithyroid Drugs

Assessment	Potential Nursing Diagnoses*
Baseline assessment prior to administration: • Obtain a complete health history including cardiovascular, GI, hepatic, or renal disease; pregnancy; or breast-feeding. Obtain a drug history including allergies, current prescription and OTC drugs, herbal preparations, alcohol use, and smoking. Be alert to possible drug interactions. • Evaluate appropriate laboratory findings (e.g., T_3, T_4, and TSH levels; CBC; and platelets). • Obtain baseline height, weight, and vital signs. Obtain ECG as needed. • Assess the patient's ability to receive and understand instructions. Include the family or caregiver as needed.	• *Activity Intolerance* • *Fatigue* • *Constipation* • *Deficient Knowledge* (Drug Therapy) • *Risk for Infection*, related to adverse drug effects • *Risk for Imbalanced Body Temperature*
Assessment throughout administration: • Assess for desired therapeutic effects, dependent on the reason the drug is given (e.g., T_3, T_4, and TSH levels return to normal, associated symptoms of hyperthyroidism ease). • Continue periodic monitoring of T_3, T_4, and TSH levels; CBC; platelets; and glucose. • Continue monitoring vital signs, height, and weight. Monitor ECG as needed. • Assess for adverse effects: nausea, vomiting, diarrhea, epigastric distress, skin rash, itching, headache, vertigo, and paresthesias.	

Implementation

Interventions and (Rationales)	Patient-Centered Care
Ensuring therapeutic effects: • Monitor vital signs, appetite, weight, sensitivity to heat or cold, sleep patterns, and ability to perform ADLs. (As metabolic activity controlled by thyroid hormones stabilizes, the patient should return to more normal weight, ADLs, and feelings of wellness. Weight and pulse rate are measured to assist in the assessment of the therapeutic response to drug therapy.)	• Advise the patient that the drug will help to stabilize thyroid hormone levels quickly, but other methods (e.g., surgery, radioactive iodine) may be required for long-term management. • Instruct the patient to maintain consistent dosing to allow the drug to reach therapeutic levels. • Instruct the patient to weigh self two to three times per week and record the findings along with the pulse rate. Bring the record of weight and pulse to each health care provider visit.
• Avoid iodine-containing foods (e.g., iodized salt, soy sauce, tofu, yogurt, milk, strawberries, eggs) unless approved by the health care provider. (Iodine is necessary for the synthesis of thyroid hormone. Increasing or decreasing normal intake may result in adverse drug effects.)	• Provide dietary instruction on which foods to avoid to reduce excessive intake of foods with high iodine content. Provide for dietitian consultation as needed.
• Monitor thyroid function tests. (Results help determine the effectiveness of the drug therapy and need for dosage changes.)	• Instruct the patient on the need to return periodically for laboratory work.
Minimizing adverse effects: • Monitor for the return of original symptoms and report consistent occurrence. (Significant return of hyperthyroid symptoms may indicate that inadequate therapeutic levels are being maintained; symptoms of hypothyroidism may signal drug toxicity.)	• Teach the patient that small daily fluctuations in symptoms may occur, especially during periods of stress or illness. Any significant changes in pulse rate, weight, nervousness, or fatigue, intolerance to heat or cold, and diarrhea or constipation should be reported to the health care provider.
• Monitor for signs of infection: fever, rashes, sore throat, malaise, fatigue, or weakness. Monitor CBC and platelet counts. (Antithyroid drugs may cause agranulocytosis.)	• Instruct the patient to report fever, rashes, sore throat, chills, malaise, or weakness to the health care provider.
• Continue to monitor the effectiveness of all other medications the patient is taking. (Antithyroid replacement drugs interact with many drugs, particularly those containing iodine such as amiodarone. As a more normal thyroid state is reached, doses of cardiac drugs may need to be adjusted.)	• Review the patient's medication list at each health visit. Instruct the patient to report any unusual symptoms of concern to the health care provider.
• **Lifespan:** Monitor symptoms in older adults more frequently. (Older patients are more sensitive to thyroid hormone levels and minor changes in daily thyroid levels may cause a significant change in symptoms.)	• Teach the patient, family, or caregiver that the lowest dose will be started and gradually increased to find the optimal level. Any significant change in symptoms should be promptly reported to the health care provider.
• Monitor serum glucose levels, especially in patients with diabetes. Patients with diabetes should monitor capillary levels more frequently. (Antithyroid drugs may cause changes in glucose levels.)	• Teach patients with diabetes to monitor capillary glucose levels more frequently during therapy. Report any consistent changes to the health care provider.

(continued)

CONNECTIONS: NURSING PRACTICE APPLICATION (continued)

• Ensure patient safety. Observe for lightheadedness or dizziness. Monitor ambulation until the effects of the drug are known. (Dizziness may be secondary to changes in pulse or blood pressure or related to adverse drug effects and should be assessed by the health care provider. **Lifespan:** The older adult is especially at risk for falls related to dizziness.)	• Instruct the patient to call for assistance prior to getting out of bed or attempting to walk alone if dizziness occurs. If dizziness occurs, the patient should sit or lie down and not attempt to stand or walk until the sensation passes. • Assess the safety of the home environment and discuss modifications that may be needed with the family or caregiver.
• Ensure the patient and caregiver safety if radioactive iodine is used. (Even though radioactive iodine provides just low-dose radiation, prolonged contact by care providers or visitors should be avoided.)	• Teach the patient to limit contact with family to 1 h per day per person until the treatment period is over. Young children and pregnant women should avoid contact with the patient. • Advise the patient to increase fluid intake up to 2 L/day as allowed and to void frequently to avoid irradiation to gonads from radioactivity in urine excretion. • Instruct the patient not to expectorate and to cover the mouth when coughing. Any contaminated tissues should be disposed of per the protocol of the agency or health care provider.
Patient understanding of drug therapy: • Use opportunities during administration of medications and during assessments to discuss the rationale for drug therapy, desired therapeutic outcomes, commonly observed adverse effects, parameters for when to call the health care provider, and any necessary monitoring or precautions. (Using time during nursing care helps to optimize and reinforce key teaching areas.)	• The patient should be able to state the reason for the drug, appropriate dose and scheduling, what adverse effects to observe for, and when to report them.

Patient self-administration of drug therapy:
• When administering the medication, instruct the patient, family, or caregiver in proper self-administration of the drug, e.g., take the drug in the morning at the same time each day. (Utilizing time during nurse-administration of these drugs helps to reinforce teaching.)
	• Teach the patient to take the drug following appropriate guidelines:
	  • Take the drug at the same time each day.
	  • Take the drug with food or a meal.
	  • Avoid foods high in iodine unless approved by the health care provider.

*Nursing Diagnoses—Definitions and Classification 2015–2017. Copyright © 2014, 1994–2014 by NANDA International. Used by arrangement with John Wiley & Sons Limited.

CHAPTER 67

Understanding the Chapter

Key Concepts Summary

67.1 Thyroid hormones contain iodine and stimulate the basal metabolic rate of nearly all tissues.

67.2 An accurate diagnosis of thyroid hormone dysfunction is based on the patient's symptoms and the results of diagnostic tests.

67.3 Hypothyroidism, or thyroid deficiency, can occur as a congenital or acquired disorder.

67.4 Hypothyroidism is treated by replacement therapy with thyroid hormone.

67.5 Hyperthyroidism, or Graves' disease, is an autoimmune disorder accompanied by ophthalmopathy and goiter.

67.6 Hyperthyroidism is treated with surgery or drugs that reduce the production of thyroid hormone.

Case Study: Making the Patient Connection

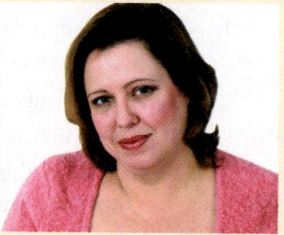

Remember the patient "Helen Mercado" at the beginning of the chapter? Now read the remainder of the case study. Based on the information presented within this chapter, respond to the critical thinking questions that follow.

Helen is a 42-year-old mother of three children, who works full time in a department store. She has been feeling extremely tired, has been gaining weight, and she says she feels cold all the time. Acting on her feelings that something might be wrong, she goes to her health care provider. Her vital signs at that time are as follows: blood pressure 94/60 mmHg, heart rate 58 beats/min, temperature 36.3°C (97.4°F). Her weight has increased 13.6 kg (30 lb) from when she was last seen 6 months ago. She confirms that her appetite has decreased. After completing a physical examination, the health care provider orders some laboratory tests including T_3, T_4, and TSH.

Critical Thinking Questions

1. Based on the patient's symptoms, what test results would you anticipate?

2. The health care provider orders levothyroxine (Synthroid) 200 mcg PO daily for Helen. What will you teach Helen about this drug and when to take it?

3. Helen asks you if she will need to be on the medication for very long. How will you answer her?

4. What symptoms should Helen report to the provider while she is taking the Synthroid?

See Answers to Critical Thinking Questions on student resource website.

Additional Case Study

The nurse receives a new patient admission onto a cardiac unit: Carolyn James, a 72-year-old female, with new-onset atrial fibrillation with rapid ventricular response. The nurse connects the patient to a cardiac monitor and obtains the following vital signs: blood pressure 168/96 mmHg, respirations 28 breaths/min, heart rate 162 beats/min, temperature 38.7°C (101.6°F). The nurse learns from the patient's daughter that the patient was recently diagnosed with Graves' disease, but she has not been taking her medications.

1. What diagnostic tests do you expect to see ordered for this patient?

2. What drug therapy do you anticipate for this patient?

3. What long-term therapy do you believe is appropriate for this patient?

See Answers to Additional Case Study on student resource website.

Chapter Review

1 The patient on replacement therapy with levothyroxine (Synthroid) reports feeling nervous and is having occasional palpitations and tremors. The nurse recognizes that these symptoms may indicate what effect is occurring?

1. The patient is still experiencing hypothyroidism and the dose may need to be increased.

2. The patient now has normal thyroid function and the levothyroxine (Synthroid) is no longer needed.

3. The patient has developed diabetes and needs further evaluation.

4. The patient is experiencing symptoms of hyperthyroidism and the drug dosage may need to be decreased.

2 Which of the following assessment findings would the nurse expect to observe in an adult patient experiencing therapeutic effects from levothyroxine (Synthroid)? Select all that apply.

1. Constipation and weight gain

2. Decreased blinking and exophthalmos

3. Decreased reports of fatigue

4. Decreased blood cholesterol levels

5. Pulse rate between 60 and 100 beats/minute

3 A patient will be treated with propylthiouracil (PTU) for hyperthyroidism. While the patient is taking this drug, which symptoms will the nurse teach the patient to report to the health care provider?

1. Sore throat, low-grade fever, chills

2. Increase in appetite and caloric intake

3. Tinnitus, altered taste, thickened saliva

4. Insomnia, nightmares, and night sweats

4 Which assessment finding would cause the nurse to withhold the regularly scheduled dose of levothyroxine?

1. A 2-lb weight gain

2. A blood pressure reading of 100/70 mmHg

3. A heart rate of 110 beats/minute

4. A temperature of 37.9°C (100.2°F)

5 A patient is taking a solution of 5% iodine and 10% potassium iodide (Lugol's solution) prior to a thyroidectomy. The patient asks why iodine solution is used since iodine is needed to make thyroid hormone. What is the nurse's best answer?

1. "The symptoms you were having indicate you were not receiving enough iodine."

2. "High levels of iodine can temporarily reduce the amount of thyroid hormone your body makes and secretes."

3. "High levels of iodine are always used prior to thyroidectomy to make up for the loss of iodine when the thyroid is removed."

4. "The high levels of iodine help prevent diabetes from developing."

6 What should the nurse teach the patient who is newly diagnosed with hypothyroidism and will take levothyroxine (Synthroid)?

1. Take the pill in the afternoon with a high-fiber snack to prevent stomach upset.

2. Eat plenty of fruits and vegetables such as strawberries, spinach, and kale to replace vital nutrients.

3. Take the dose in the morning before breakfast, as close to the same time each day as possible.

4. The drug may be taken every other day if diarrhea occurs.

See Answers to Chapter Review in Appendix A.

References

Fruzza, A. G., Demeterco-Berggren, C., & Jones, K. L. (2012). Unawareness of the effects of soy intake on the management of congenital hypothyroidism. *Pediatrics, 130,* e699–702. doi:10.1542/peds.2011-3350

Hataya, Y., Igarashi, S., Yamashita, T., & Komatsu, Y. (2013). Thyroid hormone replacement therapy for primary hypothyroidism leads to significant improvement of renal function in chronic kidney disease patients. *Clinical and Experimental Nephrology, 17,* 525–531. doi:10.1007/s10157-012-0727-y

Levitsky, L. L. (2013). *Pediatric Graves' disease.* Retrieved from http://emedicine.medscape.com/article/920283-overview

Shin, D. H., Lee, M. J., Kim, S. J., Oh, H. J., Kim, H. R., Han, J. H., . . . Kang, S. W. (2012). Preservation of renal function by thyroid hormone replacement therapy in chronic kidney disease patients with subclinical hypothyroidism. *Journal of Clinical Endocrinology and Metabolism, 97,* 2732–2740. doi:10.1210/jc.2012-1663

Yarrington, C., & Pearce, E. N. (2011). Iodine and pregnancy. *Journal of Thyroid Research, 2011,* Article ID 934104, 8 pages. doi:10.4061/2011/934104

Selected Bibliography

Bahn, R. S., Burch, H. B., Cooper, D. S., Garber, J. R., Greenlee, M. C., Klein, I., . . . Stan, N. M. (2011). Hyperthyroidism and other causes of thyrotoxicosis: Management guidelines of the American Thyroid Association and American Association of Clinical Endocrinologists. *Thyroid, 21,* 593–646. doi:10.1089/thy.2010.0417

Brent, G. A., & Koenig, R. J. (2011). Thyroid and antithyroid drugs. In L. L. Brunton, B. A. Chabner, & B. C. Knollman (Eds.), *The pharmacological basis of therapeutics* (12th ed., pp. 1129–1162). New York, NY: McGraw-Hill.

Citkowitz, E. (2013). *Myxedema coma or crisis.* Retrieved from http://emedicine.medscape.com/article/123577-overview

Crawford, A., & Harris, H. (2013). Tipping the scales: Understanding thyroid imbalances. *Nursing2013 Critical Care, 8*(1), 23–28. doi:10.1097/01.CCN.0000418818.21604.22

Donangelo, I., & Braunstein, G. D. (2011). Update on subclinical hyperthyroidism. *American Family Physician, 83,* 933–938.

Fatourechi, V. (2014). Hyperthyroidism and thyrotoxicosis. In *Endocrinology and diabetes* (pp. 9–21). New York, NY: Springer.

Figaro, M. K., Fassler, C. A., Jagasia, S., & Lakhani, V. T. (2013). Thyroid disease: Monitoring and management guidelines. In B. N. Savini (Ed.), *Blood and marrow transplantation long-term management: Prevention and complications* (pp. 225–232). doi:10.1002/9781118473306.ch22

Hampton, J. (2013). Thyroid gland disorder emergencies: Thyroid storm and myxedema coma. *AACN Advanced Critical Care, 24,* 325–332. doi:10.1097/NCI.0b013e31829bb8c3

Herdman, T. H., & Kamitsuru, S. (Eds.). (2014). *NANDA International nursing diagnoses: Definitions and classification, 2015-2017.* Oxford, United Kingdom: Wiley-Blackwell.

Misra, M. (2013). *Thyroid storm.* Retrieved from http://emedicine.medscape.com/article/925147-overview

Pearson, T. (2013). Hypothyroidism: Challenges when treating older adults. *Journal of Gerontological Nursing, 39*(1), 10–14. doi:10.3928/00989134-20121204-02

Simmons, S. (2010). A delicate balance: Detecting thyroid disease. *Nursing, 40*(7), 22–29. doi:10.1097/01.NURSE.0000383445.23626.82

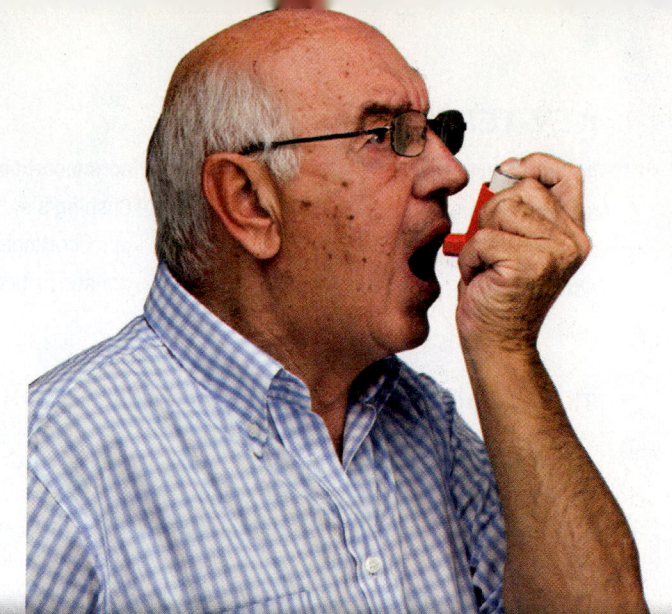

"After reading information on the Internet about the effects my steroid inhaler might have, I'm really worried. But with my lungs flaring up, I can't breathe without it."

Patient "Charlie Harness"

CHAPTER 68

Corticosteroids and Drugs Affecting the Adrenal Cortex

LEARNING OUTCOMES

After reading this chapter, the student should be able to:

1. Identify the functions of the three classes of hormones secreted by the adrenal gland.
2. Diagram the negative feedback regulation of corticosteroid secretion.
3. Identify common properties of the corticosteroid medications.
4. Describe the potential adverse effects of long-term corticosteroid therapy.
5. Compare and contrast the pharmacotherapy of acute and chronic adrenocortical insufficiency.
6. Explain how corticosteroids affect the inflammatory and immune responses.
7. Recognize nonendocrine disorders that respond to corticosteroid therapy.
8. Describe indications for pharmacotherapy with mineralocorticoids.
9. Explain the pharmacotherapy of Cushing's syndrome.
10. Describe the nurse's role in the pharmacologic management of adrenal disorders.
11. For each of the classes shown in the chapter outline, identify the prototype and representative drugs and explain the mechanism(s) of drug action, primary indications, contraindications, significant drug interactions, pregnancy category, and important adverse effects.
12. Apply the nursing process to the care of patients who are receiving pharmacotherapy with corticosteroids and mineralocorticoids.

CHAPTER OUTLINE

▶ **Physiology of the Adrenal Gland**

▶ **Overview of Corticosteroid Pharmacotherapy**

▶ **Adverse Effects of Corticosteroids**

▶ **Replacement Therapy with Corticosteroids**
  PROTOTYPE Hydrocortisone (Cortef, Solu-Cortef, Others), *p. 1157*

▶ **Corticosteroids for Nonendocrine Conditions**

▶ **Mineralocorticoids**
  PROTOTYPE Fludrocortisone, *p. 1162*

▶ **Antiadrenal Drugs**

KEY TERMS

Addison's disease, 1155

adrenal atrophy, 1156

adrenal crisis, 1156

adrenocortical insufficiency, 1155

adrenocorticotropic hormone (ACTH), 1153

Cushing's syndrome, 1163

glucocorticoids, 1153

gonadocorticoids, 1153

hyperaldosteronism, 1162

hypoaldosteronism, 1162

mineralocorticoids, 1152

Though small, the adrenal glands secrete hormones that affect every body tissue. The primary secretions of the adrenal glands, the corticosteroids, are some of the most widely used drugs in medicine. They can be delivered by any route to treat conditions as diverse as dermatitis, lymphoma, ulcerative colitis, allergic rhinitis, and arthritis. This chapter examines the pharmacologic properties of corticosteroids that make them so important to pharmacotherapy.

Physiology of the Adrenal Gland

68.1 The adrenal glands secrete gonadocorticoids, mineralocorticoids, and corticosteroids.

Weighing only two tenths of an ounce, each pyramid-shaped adrenal gland sitting atop each kidney is divided into two major portions: an inner medulla and an outer cortex. The secretions from these two portions have very different functions.

The adrenal medulla secretes 75% to 80% epinephrine, with the remainder of the secretion being norepinephrine. Adrenal release of epinephrine is triggered by activation of the sympathetic division of the autonomic nervous system. Symptoms of the fight-or-flight response resulting from the secretion of these hormones are described in Chapters 16 through 20.

The adrenal cortex secretes three essential classes of steroid hormones: mineralocorticoids, glucocorticoids, and gonadocorticoids. Collectively, the mineralocorticoids and glucocorticoids are called corticosteroids or adrenocortical hormones. Although the terms *corticosteroid* and *glucocorticoid* are sometimes used interchangeably in clinical practice, the term *corticosteroid* technically refers to a hormone or drug that has both glucocorticoid and mineralocorticoid activity. The hormones secreted by the adrenal gland are illustrated in Figure 68.1.

Mineralocorticoids: Aldosterone accounts for more than 95% of the **mineralocorticoids** secreted by the adrenal glands.

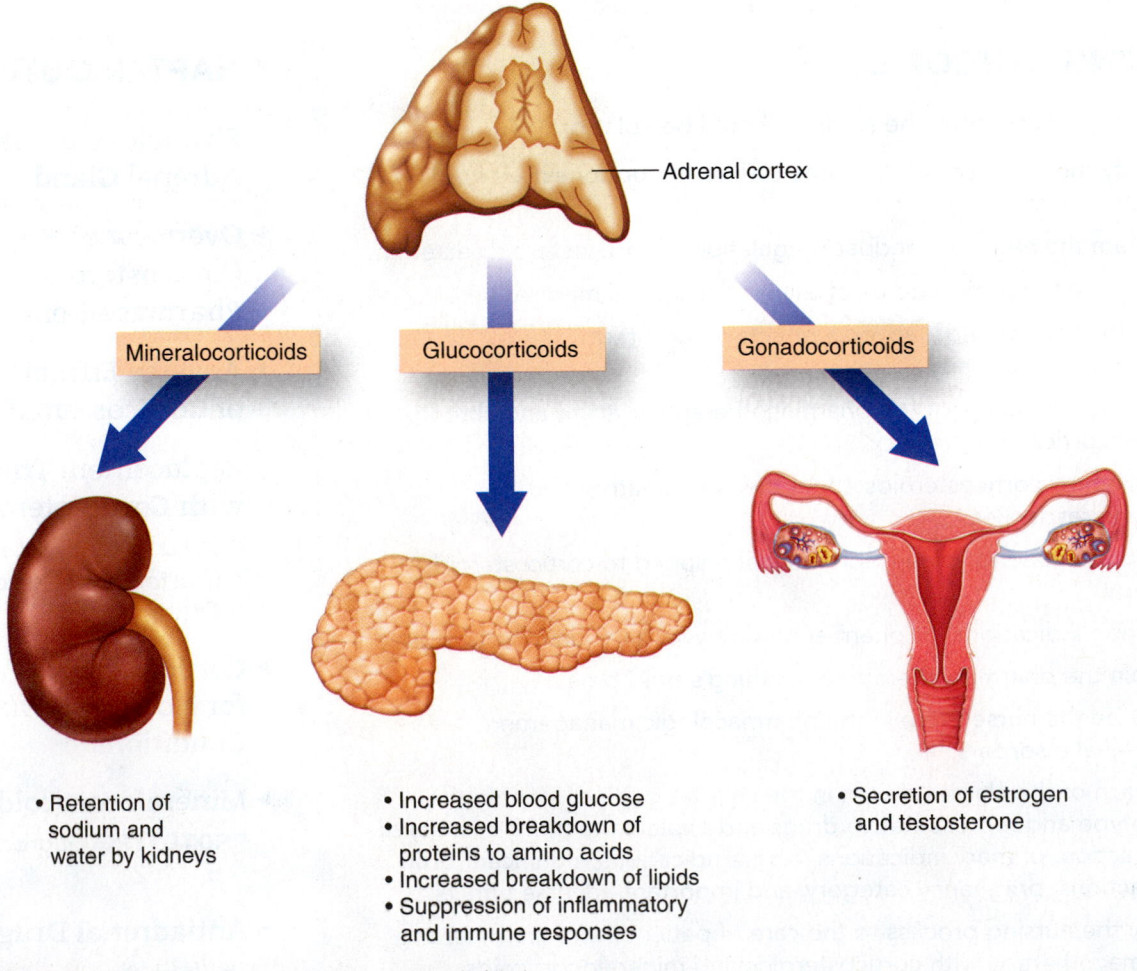

• Retention of sodium and water by kidneys

• Increased blood glucose
• Increased breakdown of proteins to amino acids
• Increased breakdown of lipids
• Suppression of inflammatory and immune responses

• Secretion of estrogen and testosterone

Adrenal cortex

Mineralocorticoids   Glucocorticoids   Gonadocorticoids

Figure 68.1 Hormonal secretions of the adrenal gland.

The primary function of aldosterone is to conserve sodium and water and promote the excretion of potassium by the renal tubule, thus regulating plasma volume. Pharmacotherapy with mineralocorticoids is presented in Section 68.6.

Glucocorticoids: More than 30 different **glucocorticoids** are secreted from the adrenal cortex. Cortisol, also called hydrocortisone, is secreted in the highest amount and is the most important pharmacologically. The liver converts hydrocortisone into cortisone, an active metabolite that is also available as a drug. Corticosterone is an additional steroid secreted by the adrenal cortex.

Glucocorticoids prepare the body for long-term stress and affect the metabolism of nearly every cell. The effects of glucocorticoids are diverse, and include the following:

- Increase the level of blood glucose (hyperglycemic effect) by inhibiting insulin secretion and promoting gluconeogenesis, which is the synthesis of carbohydrates from lipid and protein sources. This decreases glucose utilization by tissues and promotes the storage of glycogen in the liver.

- Increase the breakdown of proteins to amino acids. Amino acids are then converted to glucose and glycogen in the liver, resulting in protein depletion.

- Increase the breakdown of lipids (lipolysis). The fatty acids are then utilized as energy sources.

- Suppress the inflammatory and immune responses.

- Increase the sensitivity of vascular smooth muscle to the actions of norepinephrine and angiotensin II, thus modifying smooth muscle tone.

- Influence the central nervous system (CNS) by affecting mood and maintaining normal nerve excitability.

- Increase the breakdown of bony matrix, resulting in bone demineralization.

- Promote bronchodilation by making bronchial smooth muscle more responsive to sympathetic nervous system activation.

- Stabilize mast cells, inhibiting the release of inflammatory mediators.

As this list confirms, the glucocorticoids are essential hormones for maintaining homeostasis. When given as medications, some of the physiological actions of glucocorticoids are considered therapeutic effects, while others are adverse effects. Unfortunately, it is impossible to totally separate therapeutic effects from adverse effects when drugs with such widespread actions are used in pharmacotherapy.

The physiological levels of glucocorticoids vary based on a circadian rhythm. The lowest serum levels occur during early sleep. Secretion rises during the night, with levels peaking at awakening and declining during the day, depending on the needs of the body. Stress can cause a rapid increase in glucocorticoid levels; when faced with internal inflammatory or stressful conditions, the secretion of glucocorticoids can increase to 10 times their baseline level.

Regulation of glucocorticoid levels begins with corticotropin-releasing factor (CRF), secreted by the hypothalamus. CRF travels to the pituitary where it causes the release of **adrenocorticotropic hormone (ACTH)**. ACTH then travels via the blood to reach the adrenal cortex, causing it to release glucocorticoids. When the serum level of cortisol rises, it provides negative feedback to the

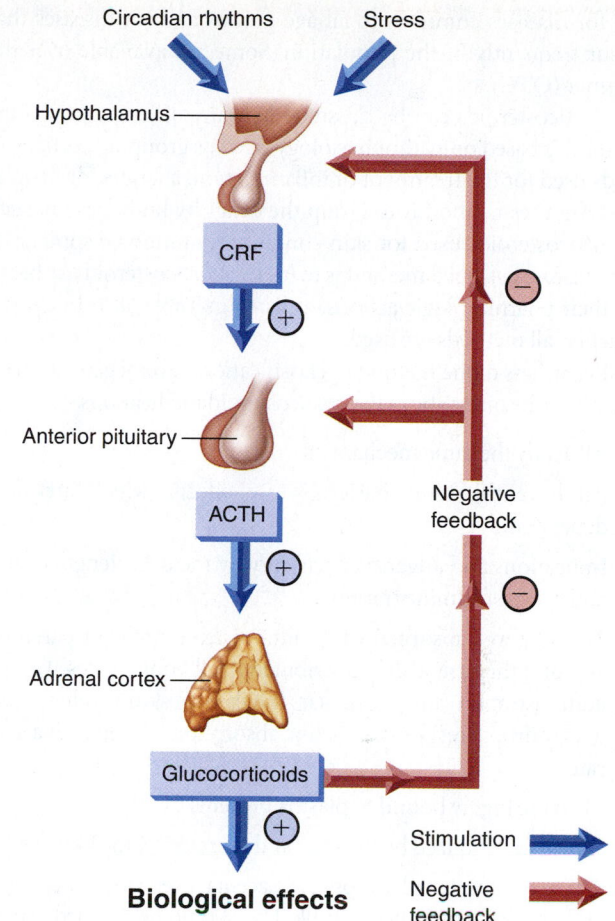

Figure 68.2 Feedback control of the adrenal cortex.

hypothalamus and pituitary to shut off further release of glucocorticoids. This negative feedback mechanism is illustrated in Figure 68.2.

Gonadocorticoids: The **gonadocorticoids** or sex hormones secreted by the adrenal cortex are mostly androgens, though small amounts of estrogens are also produced. The amounts of adrenal sex hormones are far less than the levels secreted by the testes or ovaries during the reproductive years. Though their amount is small, the adrenal gonadocorticoids contribute to the onset of puberty and are the primary source of endogenous estrogen in postmenopausal women (see Chapter 69). Tumors of the adrenal cortex can cause hypersecretion of gonadocorticoids, resulting in hirsutism and masculinization, signs that are more noticeable in women than men. The physiological effects of androgens are discussed in Chapter 71.

Overview of Corticosteroid Pharmacotherapy

68.2 Corticosteroids are widely used, and all drugs in the class have very similar indications, actions, and adverse effects.

Corticosteroids are some of the most widely prescribed medications because they are useful in treating conditions affecting nearly every body system. Furthermore, some of their indications are for diseases common to all age groups and for diseases that occur frequently in the population. Some are available over the counter (OTC).

Corticosteroids can be classified in many different ways. One method is based on pathophysiology, such as grouping corticosteroids used for the treatment of inflammation, allergies, or neoplasias. Another method is to group the drugs by body system, such as corticosteroids used for skin conditions, immune disorders, or lung diseases. A third method is to look at corticosteroid use based on their pharmacologic actions, as listed in Table 68.1. In clinical practice, all methods are used.

Regardless of the method of classification, several general statements can be made about the corticosteroid medications:

- All act by the same mechanism.
- All have the same basic adverse effects, which are dose dependent.
- Indications and adverse effects vary by the dose, length of use, and route of administration.
- They are well absorbed when administered orally or parenterally, and they are widely distributed to all body tissues. Topical administration (intra-articular, inhalation, skin products, and ocular drops) results in systemic absorption, although at a slow rate.
- Most are highly bound to plasma proteins.
- All are metabolized by the liver and excreted by the kidneys.
- All have the potential to cross the placenta (pregnancy category C) and are secreted in breast milk. Use should be avoided during pregnancy and lactation.

More than 20 corticosteroids are available as medications, and the choice of a particular drug depends primarily on the pharmacokinetic properties of the drug. The duration of action, which is sometimes used to classify these drugs, ranges from short to long acting. Some, such as hydrocortisone, also have mineralocorticoid activity and may cause sodium and fluid retention; others, such as prednisone, have no such effect. Some corticosteroids are available by only one route, such as topical for dermal conditions or

TABLE 68.1   Actions and Indications for Corticosteroids

Pharmacologic Action	Indications
Reduce cell reproduction	Lymphomas and other neoplasms
Reduce joint inflammation	Rheumatoid arthritis, osteoarthritis, bursitis, tendonitis
Reduce lung inflammation	Asthma, chronic obstructive pulmonary disease (COPD)
Reduce skin inflammation	Dermatitis, psoriasis
Supply exogenous corticosteroids	Replacement therapy
Suppress allergic response	Allergic rhinitis; anaphylaxis
Suppress gastrointestinal (GI) inflammation	Inflammatory bowel disease
Suppress general inflammatory response	Systemic lupus erythematosus
Suppress immune response	Prophylaxis of transplant rejection Autoimmune hemolytic anemia
Suppress ocular inflammation	Conjunctivitis

intranasal for allergic rhinitis. An overview of the indications for corticosteroid therapy is given in Table 68.1.

Adverse Effects of Corticosteroids

68.3 Long-term therapy with corticosteroids has the potential to cause serious adverse effects in multiple body systems.

Low-dose or brief-duration regimens of corticosteroids produce few adverse effects. On the other hand, high doses taken for prolonged periods offer a significant risk for serious adverse effects. These adverse effects of corticosteroid therapy are well documented and can impact nearly any body system. The following list

---

CONNECTIONS | **Complementary and Alternative Therapies**

◀ Fish Oils for Inflammation

Description
Fish oils, also known as marine oils, are lipids found primarily in coldwater fish such as salmon, mackerel, tuna, and herring, as well as in algae oils, green leafy vegetables, beans, and nuts. These oils are rich sources of long-chain polyunsaturated fatty acids of the omega-3 type. The two most studied fatty acids found in fish oils are eicosapentaenoic acid (EPA) and docosahexaenoic acid (DHA).

History and Claims
Fish oils are sometimes used for their anti-inflammatory, antithrombotic, antidysrhythmic, and antihyperlipidemic properties.

Standardization
Fish oils are standardized by the amount of omega-3 fatty acids they contain. There is no standard dose; capsules may range from 300 to 2,000 mg.

Evidence
Omega-3 fatty acids are known for their triglyceride-lowering activity and their anti-inflammatory actions (National Center for Complementary and Alternative Medicine, 2013). Several mechanisms are believed to account for the anti-inflammatory activity of EPA and DHA. The two competitively inhibit the conversion of arachidonic acid to the proinflammatory prostaglandins, thus reducing their synthesis.

Many studies have examined a proposed relationship between cognitive ability and high intake of omega-3 fatty acids. A recent meta-analysis confirmed that omega-3 fatty acids benefit attention and processing speed in people with mild cognitive impairment (Mazereeuw, Lanctôt, Chau, Swardfager, & Herrmann, 2012). No benefits, however, were shown in patients with Alzheimer's disease.

includes the most significant adverse events from long-term corticosteroid therapy:

- **Immune response.** Suppression of inflammation and immune responses increases patients' susceptibility to infections. Latent infections, such as herpesvirus or tuberculosis, may be reactivated during corticosteroid therapy. In addition, the anti-inflammatory actions of the corticosteroids may mask the signs of an existing infection.

- **Peptic ulcers.** Prolonged corticosteroid use is associated with the development of peptic ulcers, especially when these drugs are combined with nonsteroidal anti-inflammatory drugs (NSAIDs). Both classes of drugs reduce prostaglandin synthesis in the gastric mucosa, which normally provides protection from the high acidity in the stomach. Use of proton pump inhibitors may reduce the incidence of peptic ulcers in patients who are taking corticosteroids (see Chapter 59).

- **Osteoporosis.** Corticosteroids inhibit calcium absorption, suppress bone formation, and accelerate bone resorption—all actions that weaken the bony matrix. Up to 50% of patients on long-term corticosteroid therapy will sustain a fracture due to osteoporosis. Treatment with a bisphosphonate may reduce the incidence of fractures in these patients (see Chapter 72).

- **Behavioral changes.** By an unknown mechanism, corticosteroids can induce psychological changes. These may be minor, such as nervousness or moodiness, or may involve hallucinations and increased suicidal tendencies.

- **Eye changes.** Cataracts and open-angle glaucoma are frequent adverse events of long-term corticosteroid therapy.

- **Metabolic changes.** Corticosteroids have a hyperglycemic action that raises serum glucose and can cause glucose intolerance, especially in patients with diabetes. Mobilization of lipids may cause hyperlipidemia and abnormal fat deposits. Electrolyte changes include hypocalcemia, hypokalemia, and hypernatremia. Fluid retention, weight gain, hypertension (HTN), and edema are other possible effects.

- **Myopathy.** Muscle wasting induced by corticosteroids may cause weakness and fatigue. The myopathy may involve ocular or respiratory muscles.

CONNECTION Checkpoint 68.1

From what you learned in Chapter 41, what drug class includes drugs of choice for treating mild to moderate inflammation? *See Answer to Connection Checkpoint 68.1 on student resource website.*

Corticosteroids interact with many drugs. Their hyperglycemic effects may decrease the effectiveness of antidiabetic medications. Combining glucocorticoids with other ulcerogenic drugs such as aspirin and other NSAIDs markedly increases the risk of peptic ulcer disease. Administration with certain diuretics may lead to hypocalcemia and hypokalemia.

An important goal during long-term corticosteroid therapy is to prevent the development of serious adverse effects. The following strategies are often used to minimize the incidence of serious adverse effects:

- Doses are kept to the lowest amount that will achieve the therapeutic goal. In some cases, concurrent drug therapy with

CONNECTIONS | Lifespan Considerations

◀ Advances in Treating Acute Asthma in Pediatric Patients

Systemic corticosteroids have been recommended for children experiencing an acute asthma attack who failed to respond promptly and completely to a short-acting beta agonist (SABA) for bronchodilation. Inhaled corticosteroids (ICSs) alone, or with a long-acting beta agonist (LABA) if the ICS is insufficient, have been used for prevention therapy. With genetic analysis available to detect differences in the phenotypes of asthma, individualized treatment options may be targeted to specific types (Szefler, 2014). For example, low maternal vitamin D levels during pregnancy and low vitamin D levels in some children have been linked to an increase in the occurrence of allergies and asthma (Muehleisen & Gallo, 2013). One-day supplementation with vitamin D may be used to decrease the incidence or prevent asthma in children with specific phenotypes of asthma. Research has also found that exposure to a greater diversity of foods in the first year of life, including eggs, fish, wheat, and other grains, seems to decrease the occurrence of allergic disorders and asthma (Nwaru et al., 2014), although the mechanism behind this is still unclear. Until newer prevention and treatment strategies are found, current recommendations for the use of a stepped-care approach to asthma treatment and prevention through the use of SABAs, ICS, and LABAs remain. The overuse of LABAs is not recommended, and consideration of the antileukotriene drugs as a safer alternative to ICS or in combination with ICS when needed remain viable options (Robinson & Van Asperen, 2013).

a noncorticosteroid may be implemented to produce additive therapeutic effects, while keeping the corticosteroid dose low. Careful monitoring of the effectiveness of the drug is necessary.

- Corticosteroids are sometimes administered every other day (alternate-day dosing) to minimize adrenal atrophy (see Section 68.4). This prevents constant, negative feedback on the pituitary and forces the patient's adrenal glands to secrete endogenous corticosteroids every other day.

- For acute conditions, patients are administered large doses of corticosteroids for a few days and then the drug dose is gradually decreased until discontinued. This prevents the severe symptoms of adrenal atrophy from developing.

- Whenever possible, corticosteroids should be administered locally by inhalation, intra-articular injections, or topical applications to the skin, eyes, or ears to diminish the extent of systemic effects. Local administration rarely produces systemic adverse effects.

Replacement Therapy with Corticosteroids

68.4 Adrenocortical insufficiency is treated by administering physiological levels of corticosteroids.

Lack of adequate secretion by the adrenal cortex, or **adrenocortical insufficiency**, involves a lack of both glucocorticoids and mineralocorticoids. When pathology of the adrenal glands is the cause of the hyposecretion, it is called primary adrenocortical insufficiency, or **Addison's disease**. The most common etiology of primary adrenocortical insufficiency is the autoimmune destruction of both adrenal glands. Hemorrhage, infections, or metastases in the adrenal glands are other potential causes. Addison's disease is rare and includes a deficiency of both glucocorticoids and mineralocorticoids.

PharmFACT

One of the earliest symptoms of Addison's disease is hyperpigmentation of the oral and vaginal mucosas and the sun-exposed areas of the skin. This occurs because high ACTH levels stimulate melanocytes to produce excessive amounts of melanin (Griffing, 2014).

Secondary adrenocortical insufficiency occurs when the adrenal glands are normal, but they are not receiving adequate stimulation due to lack of sufficient ACTH from the pituitary. Low serum levels of both ACTH and cortisol are diagnostic of secondary adrenocortical insufficiency because this indicates that the adrenal gland is not receiving ACTH stimulation. Secondary adrenocortical insufficiency is much more common than primary and can occur when corticosteroids are suddenly withdrawn during pharmacotherapy. Symptoms of primary and secondary adrenocortical insufficiency are the same because both are characterized by inadequate corticosteroid secretion.

The onset of chronic adrenocortical insufficiency may take several months or even years before an accurate diagnosis is made. Symptoms include hypoglycemia, fatigue, muscle weakness, hypotension, increased skin pigmentation, and GI disturbances such as anorexia, vomiting, and diarrhea. Replacement therapy with corticosteroids is indicated. The goal of replacement therapy is to achieve the same physiological level of hormones in the blood that would be present if the adrenal glands were functioning properly. Patients requiring replacement therapy usually must take corticosteroids their entire lifetime, and concurrent therapy with a mineralocorticoid such as fludrocortisone is necessary.

Acute adrenocortical insufficiency has a sudden onset and usually occurs when corticosteroids are abruptly withdrawn from a patient who has been on long-term therapy. This is because constant, high amounts of corticosteroid medications provide continuous negative feedback to the hypothalamus and pituitary, shutting down

the secretion of ACTH. Without stimulation by ACTH, the adrenal cortex shrinks and stops secreting endogenous corticosteroids, a condition known as **adrenal atrophy**. If the corticosteroid medication is abruptly withdrawn, the shrunken adrenal glands will not be able to secrete sufficient corticosteroids, and symptoms of **adrenal crisis** will appear. Symptoms of this condition include nausea, vomiting, lethargy, confusion, myalgia, arthralgia, fever, asthenia, acute abdominal pain, hypotension, seizures, renal failure, and coma. Immediate administration of IV hydrocortisone is essential because shock may quickly result if symptoms remain untreated. To prevent adrenal crisis, corticosteroids should be discontinued gradually. The mechanism by which adrenal atrophy is induced by corticosteroid use is illustrated in Pharmacotherapy Illustrated 68.1.

The most frequently prescribed corticosteroids for treating adrenal insufficiency are hydrocortisone, prednisone, and dexamethasone. Doses of these drugs are individualized to the specific amount of replacement therapy needed by the patient, and doses will need to be increased during periods of high stress. Hydrocortisone and dexamethasone can be administered by the intramuscular (IM) or intravenous (IV) routes for acute disease, or orally for maintenance doses. Prednisone is administered by the oral (PO) route. Because dexamethasone and prednisone have little or no mineralocorticoid activity, concurrent fludrocortisone therapy is necessary. Hydrocortisone has some intrinsic mineralocorticoid activity; therefore, concurrent administration of fludrocortisone may not be necessary. Doses for selected corticosteroids are listed in Table 68.2.

Cosyntropin (Cortrosyn) is a drug structurally similar to ACTH that is used as a simple diagnostic test for adrenocortical deficiency. For this test, cosyntropin is injected IV and the plasma levels of cortisol are measured 30 to 60 minutes later. If the adrenal gland responds by secreting corticosteroids after the cosyntropin injection, the pathology lies at the level of the pituitary or hypothalamus (secondary adrenocortical insufficiency). If plasma cortisol levels fail to rise after the injection, the pathology is at the level of the adrenal gland (primary adrenocortical insufficiency).

TABLE 68.2 Selected Corticosteroids

Drug	Route and Adult Dose (Maximum Dose Where Indicated)	Adverse Effects
betamethasone (Celestone, Diprolene)	PO: 0.6–7.2 mg/day IM: 0.5–9 mg/day	*Mood swings, weight gain, acne, facial flushing, nausea, insomnia, sodium and fluid retention, impaired wound healing, menstrual abnormalities* Peptic ulcer, hypocalcemia, osteoporosis with possible bone fractures, loss of muscle mass, decreased growth in children, possible masking of infections
budesonide (Entocort EC, Pulmicort, Rhinocort)	Intranasal: 1–2 sprays in each nostril/day (each spray: 32 mcg) PO: 9 mg/day	
cortisone	PO: 20–300 mg/day in divided doses	
dexamethasone	PO: 0.25–9 mg/day in divided doses	
hydrocortisone (Cortef, Solu-Cortef)	PO: 10–320 mg/day in three to four divided doses IV/IM: 15–800 mg/day in three to four divided doses (max: 2 g/day)	
methylprednisolone (Depo-Medrol, Medrol, Others)	PO: 4–48 mg/day in divided doses	
prednisolone	PO: 5–60 mg one to four times/day	
prednisone	PO: 5–60 mg one to four times/day	
triamcinolone (Aristospan, Kenalog, Others)	PO: 4–48 mg one to four times/day	

Note: Italics indicate common adverse effects. Underline indicates serious adverse effects.

PHARMACOTHERAPY ILLUSTRATED 68.1

Corticosteroids and Adrenal Atrophy

1. Normal adrenal glands
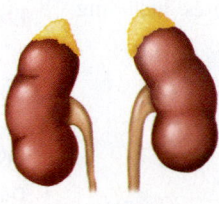

Corticosteroid Therapy

2. Adrenal gland atrophy following corticosteroid therapy
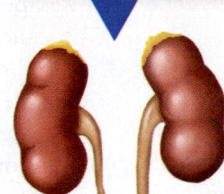

Gradual Discontinuation

Sudden Discontinuation

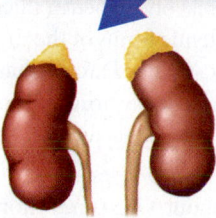
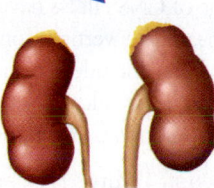

3. Gradual withdrawal of corticosteroids allows adrenal glands to resume normal function

4. Sudden withdrawal of corticosteroids leads to acute
- adrenal insufficiency
- hypotension
- lethargy
- renal failure
- asthenia
- nausea/vomiting

CONNECTION Checkpoint 68.2

From what you learned in Chapter 43, explain why immunizations are sometimes contraindicated in patients receiving high-dose corticosteroid therapy. *See Answer to Connection Checkpoint 68.2 on student resource website.*

PROTOTYPE DRUG | **Hydrocortisone (Cortef, Solu-Cortef, Others)**

Classification: **Therapeutic:** Adrenal hormone
Pharmacologic: Corticosteroid

Therapeutic Effects and Uses: Structurally identical to the natural hormone cortisol, hydrocortisone is a synthetic corticosteroid that is the drug of choice for treating adrenocortical insufficiency. When used for replacement therapy, it is given at physiological doses. Once proper dosing has been achieved, its therapeutic effects should mimic those of endogenous corticosteroids. Hydrocortisone is also available for the treatment of inflammation, allergic disorders, and many other conditions. Intra-articular injections may be given to decrease severe inflammation in affected joints.

Hydrocortisone is available in six different salts: base, acetate, cypionate, sodium phosphate, sodium succinate, and valerate. Some of the salts, such as hydrocortisone acetate, are designed for topical use, whereas others such as hydrocortisone sodium succinate are for parenteral use only. When administering hydrocortisone, care should be taken to use the correct route for the prescribed formulation of this drug.

Mechanism of Action: The actions of hydrocortisone are complex and the drug is thought to act by multiple mechanisms in different tissues. As a replacement drug, it restores deficient levels of glucocorticoids and, to a lesser extent, mineralocorticoids. As an anti-inflammatory drug, it blocks the actions of various chemical mediators in the inflammatory and allergic responses, including histamine, prostaglandins, and kinins.

Pharmacokinetics:

Route(s)	PO, IV, IM, subcutaneous, rectal, intra-articular, topical
Absorption	Rapid
Distribution	Widely distributed when given PO or parenterally; crosses the placenta; secreted in breast milk; extensively bound to plasma protein
Primary metabolism	Hepatic
Primary excretion	Renal
Onset of action	PO: 1–2 h; IM: 20 min
Duration of action	1–1.5 days (PO or IM)

Adverse Effects: When used at low doses for replacement therapy, or by the topical or intranasal routes, adverse effects of hydrocortisone are uncommon. However, signs of Cushing's syndrome can develop with high doses or with prolonged use. Hydrocortisone possesses some mineralocorticoid activity, so sodium and fluid retention may be observed. A wide range of CNS effects have been reported, including insomnia, anxiety, headache, vertigo, confusion, and depression. Cardiovascular effects may include HTN and tachycardia. Long-term therapy may result in peptic ulcer disease, osteoporosis, hyperglycemia, cataracts, HTN, and impaired wound healing.

Contraindications/Precautions: Hydrocortisone is contraindicated in patients who are hypersensitive to the drug or who have known infections, unless the patient is being treated concurrently with anti-infectives. Patients with diabetes, osteoporosis, psychosis, liver disease, or hypothyroidism should be treated with caution. Patients with heart failure (HF) or HTN should be treated with caution due to the possibility of fluid retention with hydrocortisone. If taken for longer than 2 weeks, hydrocortisone should be discontinued gradually. Caution should be used in treating children because the drug may delay normal growth and development. PO corticosteroids must be used with caution in patients with pre-existing GI disease such as peptic ulcers or ulcerative colitis because it may worsen these conditions. Use with potassium-wasting drugs such as thiazide or loop diuretics may increase the risk of hypokalemia. Anticholinesterase drugs may produce severe weakness. Hydrocortisone may cause a decrease in immune response to vaccines and toxoids. Patients on high doses of hydrocortisone should not receive live vaccines due to the possibility of infection. Because hydrocortisone can cause hyperglycemia, doses of insulin and oral hypoglycemic drugs may require adjustment. Vitamin D supplements are recommended to prevent corticosteroid-induced osteoporosis. **Herbal/Food**: Use with aloe, senna, cascara, or buckthorn may cause potassium deficiency with chronic use.

Pregnancy: Category C.

Treatment of Overdose: Hydrocortisone has no acute toxicity and deaths are rare. No specific therapy is available and patients are treated symptomatically.

Nursing Responsibilities: Key nursing implications for patients receiving hydrocortisone are included in the Nursing Practice Application for Patients Receiving Pharmacotherapy with Systemic Corticosteroids.

Drugs Similar to Hydrocortisone (Cortef, Solu-Cortef, Others)

There are many other corticosteroids, all having the same actions. In addition to hydrocortisone, dexamethasone and prednisone are most frequently used for adrenocortical insufficiency.

Dexamethasone: Dexamethasone is a synthetic corticosteroid that has almost no mineralocorticoid activity. It is 20 to 30 times more potent than hydrocortisone and is available by PO, IV, IM, topical, aerosol, and ophthalmic routes. The parenteral formulations (dexamethasone sodium phosphate) are used for serious disorders such as anaphylaxis, reduction of cerebral edema, or acute adrenocortical insufficiency, or when oral therapy is not possible. Dexamethasone may be injected intra-articularly for the short-term therapy of inflamed joints, or intralesionally into acute inflamed lesions associated with discoid lupus, psoriatic plaques, and granulomatous disorders. It is also indicated for the palliative management of leukemias and lymphomas. Dexamethasone is sometimes found in fixed-dose combinations with antibiotics such as ciprofloxacin to treat otic or ocular infections that have significant inflammation. Systemic forms of the drug are metabolized by the liver to inactive metabolites. Dexamethasone has one of the longest durations of action of any drug in its class. This drug is pregnancy category C.

Prednisone: Prednisone is rapidly absorbed and is the most frequently prescribed corticosteroid for oral administration. It is about four times more potent than hydrocortisone and has a longer duration of action. It has little mineralocorticoid activity. Prednisone is a synthetic corticosteroid whose actions are the result of being metabolized to an active form, which is also available as the drug prednisolone. Although prednisone is only available by the PO route, prednisolone may be administered PO, parenterally, or topically and may be of value in patients with liver impairment because it does not require hepatic activation. Oral solutions (Oraped, Prelone) and an oral disintegrating tablet (Oraped ODT) are primarily prescribed for treating childhood asthma. When used for inflammation, duration of prednisone therapy is commonly 4 to 10 days. For long-term therapy, alternate-day dosing is used. Prednisone is occasionally used to terminate acute bronchospasm in patients with asthma and as an antineoplastic drug for cancers such as Hodgkin's disease, acute childhood leukemias, and lymphomas. Prednisone has the same adverse effects and contraindications as hydrocortisone. This drug is pregnancy category C.

Corticosteroids for Nonendocrine Conditions

68.5 Corticosteroids are frequently used to suppress the inflammatory and immune responses.

One of the most important physiological effects of corticosteroids is their natural ability to dampen the immune response and inhibit the synthesis of inflammatory mediators. When used to treat conditions characterized by hyperactive body defenses, the

CONNECTIONS   Treating the Diverse Patient

◖ Corticosteroid Use by Mothers at Risk for Preterm Labor

Giving corticosteroids to mothers at risk for preterm labor helps to develop the baby's lungs and reduces the chance for serious complications such as infant respiratory distress syndrome if the baby is born preterm. However, the benefit does not last long, approximately 7 days. Due to concerns about effects on birth weight and later childhood disabilities related to repeated corticosteroid use, repeated doses may not be ordered. Crowther, McKinlay, Middleton, and Harding (2011) conducted an analysis of 10 randomized controlled trials found in the Cochrane Pregnancy and Childbirth Group's Trials Register to assess the effect of repeated corticosteroid use prior to preterm labor. Repeated dosages were found to have positive effects in reducing the risk for respiratory distress syndrome in the newborn. Although slight reductions in mean birth weight were noted in these babies, when adjusted for gestational age, these differences were insignificant. And no statistically significant differences in disability outcomes were noted at early childhood follow-up assessments between children whose mothers had received repeated corticosteroids and those who had not received the drug. The authors conclude that the research supports the use of repeated corticosteroids for women at risk for preterm birth to reduce the incidence of respiratory distress and serious health problems in the infant. Recently, research seems to suggest that the maximum benefit of antenatal corticosteroid therapy may be between 26 and 29 weeks' gestation, with the risk of neonatal complications equalling the risk of adverse effects of the corticosteroids on/after 29 weeks' gestation (Zephyrin et al., 2013).

---

anti-inflammatory effects of the corticosteroids are therapeutic. When the drugs are administered as replacement therapy, however, suppression of the immune response can result in an increased incidence of infections.

Part of the reason for the effectiveness of the corticosteroids in reducing inflammation and the immune response is that they act by multiple mechanisms. These mechanisms include the following:

- Decreased numbers of circulating lymphocytes, eosinophils, monocytes, and basophils
- Inhibited movement of macrophages and leukocytes to areas of inflammation
- Decreased production of inflammatory cytokines, including histamine, bradykinin, interferons, interleukins, and granulocyte-macrophage colony-stimulating factor
- Decreased formation of prostaglandins

It is important to note that the doses necessary to treat inflammatory and other nonendocrine diseases are much higher than those used to treat adrenocortical insufficiency. For example, a daily maintenance dose of prednisone for a patient with Addison's disease is 7.5 mg/day. This amount approximates what would normally be secreted by the adrenal glands. Daily doses of prednisone for nonendocrine disorders range from 5 to 30 mg for transplant prophylaxis; 80 mg for chronic lymphocytic leukemia; 40 to 60 mg for Crohn's disease; and 20 to 300 mg for systemic lupus erythematosus. At these high doses, the adverse effects of corticosteroids will quickly manifest and the adrenal gland will begin to atrophy in only 2 to 4 weeks. Interventions should be planned to prevent anticipated adverse effects.

Arthritis: Arthritis is one of the most common diseases affecting older adults. Rheumatoid arthritis (RA) is a chronic autoimmune disease that causes inflammation of joints and is characterized by disfigurement and inflammation of multiple joints. Osteoarthritis is also a progressive joint disease but it occurs with more advanced age and is characterized by less inflammation than RA. Both types of arthritis are treated with NSAIDs early in the course of the disease. Corticosteroids are administered when inflammation becomes severe, with therapy being limited to 1 to 2 weeks, or until the pain and inflammation subside. If the pain and inflammation are localized to one or two joints, intra-articular injections may be used. Corticosteroids offer only symptomatic treatment and do not alter the course of either type of arthritis. Arthritis pharmacotherapy is presented in Chapter 72.

Inflammatory bowel disease: Inflammatory bowel disease (IBD) is characterized by ulceration in the distal portion of the small intestine (Crohn's disease) or in the large intestine (ulcerative colitis). Various drugs, including the 5-aminosalicylic acid drugs, are used to control inflammation, cramping, and diarrhea. Exacerbations are treated with corticosteroids for brief time periods. Budesonide (Entocort-EC, Ulceris) is a corticosteroid that has a delayed release and remains in the intestine to treat the inflammation locally, without causing significant systemic effects. IBD pharmacotherapy is presented in Chapter 60.

Asthma: Asthma is characterized by chronic inflammation that causes bronchoconstriction in the respiratory passages. Inhaled corticosteroids are preferred drugs for the prevention of asthmatic attacks and the management of chronic asthma. The inhaled agents produce few systemic adverse effects. Oral corticosteroids are used for the short-term management of acute asthma exacerbations. Asthma pharmacotherapy is presented in Chapter 44.

Allergies: Allergic rhinitis is inflammation of the nasal mucosa caused by exposure to allergens. Corticosteroids are applied directly to the nasal mucosa to prevent symptoms of allergic rhinitis. They have largely replaced antihistamines as drugs of choice for this condition. When administered intranasally, the corticosteroids do not exhibit systemic adverse effects. For acute allergies, corticosteroids may be administered parenterally. Because their onset of action is slow, however, they are always administered concurrently with other drugs, such as epinephrine, for this indication. The pharmacotherapy of allergic rhinitis is presented in Chapter 45.

Transplant rejection prophylaxis: Successful tissue transplantation requires the use of immunosuppressant drugs; otherwise, the patient's immune system would reject the transplant. One or more immunosuppressants are administered at the time of transplantation and are continued for several months following surgery. Corticosteroids are part of most therapeutic regimens to prevent transplant rejection. They may be used for several weeks or maintained for 3 to 6 months following surgery. The prophylaxis of transplant rejection is presented in Chapter 42.

Dermatologic conditions: Topical corticosteroids are the most effective therapy for treating the inflammation and itching of dermatitis. These corticosteroids are specially formulated to penetrate deep into the skin layers. Topical corticosteroids such as betamethasone and hydrocortisone acetate are also the primary, initial treatment for psoriasis. High-potency corticosteroids are used for 1 to 2 weeks, followed by moderate- to low-potency corticosteroids for maintenance therapy. The pharmacotherapy of dermatologic diseases is presented in Chapter 73.

Neoplasms: Corticosteroids such as prednisone and dexamethasone are used as adjuncts in the treatment of certain neoplasms, especially acute childhood leukemias and Hodgkin's disease. They are always used in combination with other antineoplastics. The pharmacotherapy of cancer is presented in Chapter 57.

Edema: Corticosteroids are occasionally used to treat disorders characterized by edema. They have been used for many years to reduce intracranial edema associated with trauma, tumors, and cerebral ischemia. These hormones tend to stabilize capillary membranes. Their effectiveness in treating edema is controversial.

CONNECTIONS: NURSING PRACTICE APPLICATION

Patients Receiving Pharmacotherapy with Systemic Corticosteroids

Assessment	Potential Nursing Diagnoses*
Baseline assessment prior to administration: • Obtain a complete health history including cardiovascular, respiratory, neurologic, hepatic, or renal disease; pregnancy; or breast-feeding. Obtain a drug history including allergies, current prescription and OTC drugs, herbal preparations, caffeine, nicotine, and alcohol use. Be alert to possible drug interactions. • Obtain baseline vital signs and weight. • Evaluate appropriate laboratory findings (e.g., CBC, platelets, electrolytes, glucose, lipid profile, hepatic or renal function studies). • Assess the patient's ability to receive and understand instructions. Include the family and caregivers as needed.	• *Deficient Knowledge* (Drug Therapy) • *Risk for Imbalanced Fluid Volume*, related to fluid retention properties of corticosteroids • *Risk for Electrolyte Imbalance*, related to adverse drug effects • *Risk for Unstable Blood Glucose Level*, related to adverse drug effects • *Risk for Injury*, related to adverse drug effects • *Risk for Infection*, related to adverse drug effects • *Risk for Impaired Skin Integrity*, related to adverse drug effects
Assessment throughout administration: • Assess for desired therapeutic effects (e.g., signs and symptoms of inflammation such as redness or swelling are decreased). • Continue periodic monitoring of CBC, platelets, electrolytes, glucose, lipid profile, hepatic or renal function studies. • Assess vital signs and weight periodically or if symptoms warrant. Obtain weight daily and report any gain over 1 kg (2 lb) in a 24-h period or more than 2 kg (5 lb) in 1 week. Obtain height and weight of children on long-term corticosteroid therapy. • Assess for and promptly report adverse effects: nausea, vomiting, symptoms of GI bleeding (dark or tarry stools, hematemesis, coffee-grounds emesis, blood in the stool), abdominal pain, dizziness, light-headedness, confusion, agitation, euphoria or depression, palpitations, tachycardia, HTN, increased respiratory rate and depth, pulmonary congestion, significant weight gain, edema, blurred vision, fever, or infections.	

Implementation

Interventions and (Rationales)	Patient-Centered Care
Ensuring therapeutic effects: • Continue assessments as above for therapeutic effects. (Diminished inflammation, allergic response, and increased feelings of wellness should begin after taking the first dose and continue to improve.)	• Teach the patient to report any return of original symptoms or an increase in inflammation, allergic response, or generalized malaise to the health care provider.
Minimizing adverse effects: • Continue to monitor vital signs, especially blood pressure (BP) and pulse. Immediately report tachycardia or BP over 140/90 mmHg, or per parameters as ordered, to the health care provider. (Corticosteroids may cause increased BP, HTN, and tachycardia due to increased retention of fluids.)	• Teach the patient how to monitor pulse and BP. Ensure proper use and functioning of any home equipment obtained. Immediately report tachycardia, palpitations, or increased BP to the health care provider.
• Continue to monitor periodic laboratory work: CBC, electrolytes, glucose, lipid levels, and hepatic and renal function tests. (Corticosteroids have effects on the CBC and may cause hyperglycemia, hypernatremia, hyperlipidemia, and hypokalemia. Patients with diabetes may require a change in antidiabetic medication if the glucose remains elevated.)	• Instruct the patient on the need to return periodically for laboratory work. • Advise the patient taking corticosteroids long term to carry a wallet identification card and wear medical identification jewelry indicating corticosteroid therapy. • Teach the patient with diabetes to test for blood glucose more frequently, notifying the health care provider if a consistent elevation is noted.

CONNECTIONS: NURSING PRACTICE APPLICATION (continued)

• **Lifespan:** Monitor symptoms in older adults more frequently. (Older patients are at increased risk of adverse effects in all body systems due to normal physiological changes related to aging.)	• Teach the patient, family, or caregiver to follow administration guidelines. Any significant change in symptoms should be promptly reported to the health care provider.
• Monitor for and report abdominal pain, black or tarry stools, blood in the stool, hematemesis, coffee-ground emesis, dizziness, light-headedness, and hypotension, especially if associated with tachycardia. (GI bleeding is an adverse drug effect.)	• Instruct the patient to immediately report any signs or symptoms of GI bleeding. • Teach the patient to take the drug with food or milk to decrease GI irritation. Alcohol use should be avoided or eliminated.
• Monitor for signs and symptoms of infection in patients taking corticosteroids. (Corticosteroids suppress the body's normal immune and inflammatory response and may mask the signs and symptoms of infection.)	• Instruct the patient to report any signs or symptoms of infection (e.g., increasing temperature or fever, sore throat, redness or swelling at the site of injury, white patches in the mouth, vesicular rash).
• Monitor for osteoporosis (e.g., bone density testing) periodically in patients on long-term corticosteroids. Encourage adequate calcium intake, weight-bearing exercise, and avoidance of carbonated sodas. (Corticosteroids affect bone metabolism and may cause osteoporosis and fractures. Weight-bearing exercise stresses bone and encourages normal bone remodeling. Excessive or long-term consumption of carbonated sodas has been linked to an increased risk of osteoporosis.)	• Teach the patient to maintain adequate calcium in the diet, avoid carbonated sodas, and do weight-bearing exercises at least three to four times per week. • Teach postmenopausal women and patients on prolonged corticosteroid therapy to consult with their provider about the need for vitamin D or additional drug therapy (e.g., bisphosphonates) for osteoporosis prevention.
• Monitor for unusual changes in mood or affect. (Corticosteroids may cause increased or decreased mood, euphoria, depression, or severe mental instability.)	• Teach the patient, family, or caregiver to promptly report excessive mood swings or unusual changes in mood.
• Weigh the patient daily and report a gain of 1 kg (2 lb) or more in a 24-h period, or more than 2 kg (5 lb) per week, or increasing peripheral edema. Measure intake and output in the hospitalized patient. (Daily weight is an accurate measure of fluid status and takes into account intake, output, and insensible losses. Patients will experience some fluid retention but should report weight gain, as above, or edema to the health care provider.)	• Instruct the patient to weigh self daily, ideally at the same time of day. The patient should report weight gain of more than 1 kg (2 lb) in a 24-h period, or more than 2 kg (5 lb) per week, or increasing peripheral edema to the health care provider.
• **Lifespan:** Monitor height and weight in children. (Children receiving long-term corticosteroid therapy should continue to display normal growth and development curves.)	• Teach the parents or caregivers to weigh the child periodically at home and record. Bring the record to each health care visit. • Encourage the parents or caregivers to discuss concerns or any unusual findings that would suggest developmental or growth delays with the health care provider if they are noted in the child between health care visits.
• Monitor vision periodically in patients taking corticosteroids. (Corticosteroids may cause increased intraocular pressure and an increased risk for glaucoma, and may cause cataracts.)	• Teach the patient to have eye exams twice yearly or more frequently as instructed by the health care provider. Immediately report any eye pain, rainbow halos around lights, diminished vision, blurring, and inability to focus.
• Do not stop the drug abruptly. Drug dosages must be tapered off if used for longer than 1 or 2 weeks. (Adrenal insufficiency and crisis may occur with profound hypotension, tachycardia, and other adverse effects if the drug is stopped abruptly.)	• Teach patients to not stop corticosteroids abruptly and to notify the health care provider if unable to take medication for more than 1 day due to illness.
• Patients taking corticosteroids for replacement therapy for adrenal insufficiency should obtain and carry PO and injectable medication forms, especially when traveling. (In an emergency, replacement medication may not be readily available, and the patient may be unable to take an oral dose. Having doses readily available ensures that the drug can be taken or given if another replacement is not available.)	• Instruct patients on replacement therapy to obtain and carry replacement doses in both PO and parenteral forms for emergency use.
Patient understanding of drug therapy: • Use opportunities during administration of medications and during assessments to discuss the rationale for drug therapy, desired therapeutic outcomes, commonly observed adverse effects, parameters for when to call the health care provider, and any necessary monitoring or precautions. (Using time during nursing care helps to optimize and reinforce key teaching areas.)	• The patient, family, or caregiver should be able to state the reason for the drug, appropriate dose and scheduling, what adverse effects to observe for and when to report them, and the anticipated length of medication therapy.
Patient self-administration of drug therapy: • When administering the medication, instruct the patient, family, or caregiver in proper self-administration of the drug, e.g., with food or milk, followed by teach-back. (Utilizing time during nurse-administration of these drugs helps to reinforce teaching. Household measuring devices such as teaspoons differ significantly in size and amount and should not be used for pediatric or liquid doses.)	• The patient, family, or caregiver is able to discuss appropriate dosing and administration needs, including: • Take the drug in the morning at the same time each day. • Take the drug with food, milk, or a meal to prevent GI upset. • Do not use household measuring spoons to measure liquid or pediatric doses. Use the measuring device included with the drug or obtain a dose syringe or other device from a pharmacy or the health care provider.

*Nursing Diagnoses—Definitions and Classification 2015–2017. Copyright © 2014, 1994–2014 by NANDA International. Used by arrangement with John Wiley & Sons Limited.

Mineralocorticoids

68.6 Patients with adrenal insufficiency often require replacement therapy with mineralocorticoids.

Aldosterone is the primary hormone regulating sodium and potassium balance in the body. Regulation of aldosterone secretion is through activation of the renin-angiotensin-aldosterone system. When plasma volume falls, the kidney secretes renin, which results in the production of angiotensin II. Angiotensin II then promotes aldosterone secretion, which in turn acts on the renal tubules to promote sodium and water retention and increased excretion of potassium.

Lack of adequate aldosterone secretion, or **hypoaldosteronism**, may be caused by a number of disorders. The three broad categories of hypoaldosteronism are as follows:

- **Decreased stimulation of the adrenal cortex.** Beta blockers, NSAIDs, and calcium channel blockers may reduce renin serum levels and suppress the stimulation of aldosterone secretion. Angiotensin-converting enzyme (ACE) inhibitors block the formation of angiotensin II, which is the normal signal for aldosterone secretion.

- **Hyposecretion of aldosterone.** Low aldosterone secretion may result from primary adrenal insufficiency (Addison's disease), which is usually a deficiency in the secretion of both glucocorticoids and mineralocorticoids. Heparin can also suppress aldosterone synthesis and secretion.

- **Aldosterone resistance.** The renal tubules may become resistant to the actions of aldosterone. Aldosterone resistance occurs during diseases of the renal tubules and may also result from therapy with spironolactone (Aldactone) or progestins.

Whenever possible, the cause of hypoaldosteronism is identified and treated. In some cases, replacement therapy with fludrocortisone is necessary.

Excessive secretion of aldosterone, or **hyperaldosteronism**, is usually caused by a benign tumor of the adrenal gland. Also known as Conn's syndrome, symptoms include HTN caused by fluid retention and muscle weakness due to hypokalemia. Surgical excision of the adrenal tumor is the treatment of choice for most patients; however, pharmacotherapy with spironolactone (Aldactone) may benefit patients who are at high surgical risk. Spironolactone is a potassium-sparing diuretic that blocks the actions of aldosterone in the renal tubule. Spironolactone is featured as a drug prototype in Chapter 32.

CONNECTION Checkpoint 68.3

From what you learned in Chapter 31, name the two drugs classified as aldosterone antagonists and give their indications. *See Answer to Connection Checkpoint 68.3 on student resource website.*

PROTOTYPE DRUG	Fludrocortisone

Classification: Therapeutic: Drug for hypoaldosteronism
Pharmacologic: Mineralocorticoid

Therapeutic Effects and Uses: Approved in 1954, fludrocortisone is an oral corticosteroid that possesses a high degree of mineralocorticoid activity that mimics aldosterone. Although it has some glucocorticoid activity, this action is minimal at therapeutic doses. It is approved for the treatment of Addison's disease and for salt-losing forms of adrenogenital syndrome, a life-threatening congenital disorder that occurs during the first few weeks of life. It has been used off-label to treat neurogenic orthostatic hypotension.

Mechanism of Action: Fludrocortisone has the same pharmacologic actions as aldosterone. It acts on the distal renal tubule to promote sodium and water reabsorption and increased urinary potassium excretion.

Pharmacokinetics:

Route(s)	PO
Absorption	Rapidly absorbed
Distribution	Distributed to most tissues; crosses the placenta; secreted in breast milk; highly bound to plasma protein
Primary metabolism	Hepatic to inactive metabolites
Primary excretion	Renal
Onset of action	Peak plasma level: 1.5 h
Duration of action	Half-life: 3.5 h

Adverse Effects: Most adverse effects of fludrocortisone are the result of excessive mineralocorticoid activity: sodium and fluid retention, edema, cardiomegaly, HTN, and HF. Excessive urinary loss of potassium may result in symptoms of hypokalemia: nausea, vomiting, prolongation of the QT interval, muscle cramps, and fatigue.

Contraindications/Precautions: Fludrocortisone must be used with caution if the patient has any disorders in which fluid accumulation could be hazardous, such as HF, HTN, and renal or hepatic impairment. Because the drug has glucocorticoid properties that could lead to immunosuppression, it should not be administered to patients with a known systemic fungal infection.

Drug Interactions: If used with drugs that cause potassium loss, fludrocortisone use will result in additive hypokalemia. Potassium-wasting drugs include thiazide and loop diuretics and amphotericin B. Fludrocortisone should be used with caution in patients taking digoxin due to the potential for hypokalemia-induced digoxin toxicity. Concurrent use with androgens may cause additive sodium retention and edema. Fludrocortisone may affect glycemic control in patients with diabetes; doses of antidiabetic drugs may need to be increased. **Herbal/Food**: Sodium intake should be monitored because high levels may lead to sodium retention.

Pregnancy: Category C.

Treatment of Overdose: Overdosage results in HTN, edema, and hypokalemia. Treatment is symptomatic. Potassium supplements may be beneficial.

Nursing Responsibilities: Key nursing implications for patients receiving fludrocortisone are included in the Nursing Practice Application for Patients Receiving Pharmacotherapy with Systemic Corticosteroids.

Drugs Similar to Fludrocortisone

Fludrocortisone is the only drug in its class.

Antiadrenal Drugs

68.7 Antiadrenal drugs may be administered to lower serum corticosteroid levels in patients with Cushing's syndrome.

Cushing's syndrome occurs when high levels of corticosteroids are present in the body over a prolonged time period. Although hypersecretion of these hormones can occur due to pituitary or adrenal tumors, the most common cause of Cushing's syndrome is long-term therapy with high doses of systemic corticosteroids. Signs and symptoms include adrenal atrophy, osteoporosis, HTN, increased risk of infections, delayed wound healing, acne, peptic ulcers, general obesity, and a redistribution of fat around the face (moon face), shoulders, and neck (buffalo hump). Mood and personality changes are common, and the patient may become psychologically dependent on the drug. Some corticosteroids, including hydrocortisone, also have mineralocorticoid activity and can cause retention of sodium and water. Because of their anti-inflammatory and immunosuppressant properties, corticosteroids may mask signs of infection. It is important to note that corticosteroids do not have anti-infective properties. Even though the patient may not exhibit signs and symptoms of infections, the microorganisms continue duplicating and spreading. This could result in a delay in the initiation of antibiotic therapy.

PharmFACT

Cushing's syndrome caused by adrenal or pituitary tumors has a peak incidence between the ages of 25 and 40 years and afflicts five times as many women as men (Adler, 2014).

Because Cushing's syndrome has a high mortality rate, medical intervention is necessary. The primary therapeutic goal is to identify and treat the cause of the excess corticosteroids. If the patient is receiving high doses of a corticosteroid medication, gradual discontinuation of the drug is often sufficient to reverse the syndrome. When the cause of the hypersecretion is an adrenal tumor or an ectopic tumor secreting ACTH, surgical removal is indicated.

The antifungal drug ketoconazole (Nizoral) has become a preferred drug for long-term therapy of Cushing's syndrome. This drug rapidly blocks the synthesis of glucocorticoids, lowering serum levels. Unfortunately, the falling glucocorticoid level signals the pituitary to release more ACTH. Eventually, the very high levels of ACTH may overcome ketoconazole's inhibition of glucocorticoid synthesis. Ketoconazole should not be used during pregnancy because it has been shown to be teratogenic and embryotoxic at high doses in animals. It also causes hepatotoxicity in some patients; liver function should be carefully monitored.

A newer approach to treating Cushing's disease is the drug pasireotide (Signifor), which was approved in 2012. Pasireotide is closely related to somatostatin: growth hormone-inhibiting hormone. Binding of pasireotide to somatostatin receptors causes inhibition of ACTH secretion by the pituitary and subsequently corticosteroid secretion from the adrenals. Given by the subcutaneous route, several weeks or months of therapy may be needed for optimal suppression of corticosteroid secretion. The drug is pregnancy category C.

Mitotane (Lysodren) is an antineoplastic drug, specific for cells of the adrenal cortex, that is approved to treat inoperable tumors of the adrenal gland. Although not specifically approved for Cushing's syndrome, it will reduce symptoms of this disorder if they were caused by an adrenal cancer. Gastrointestinal symptoms such as anorexia, nausea, and vomiting will occur in 80% of patients. CNS adverse effects, including depression, lethargy, and dizziness, occur in 40% of patients. The drug is pregnancy category C.

Metyrapone (Metopirone) is an antiadrenal drug used for diagnostic purposes. A single dose is administered orally at midnight, and blood samples are taken 8 hours later. Levels of ACTH, glucocorticoids, and their metabolites are measured to see whether the adrenal glands responded to the inhibiting action of metyrapone. The drug inhibits glucocorticoid synthesis and it may be used off-label to treat Cushing's syndrome. Approved in 1961, metyrapone is pregnancy category C.

CHAPTER

68 Understanding the Chapter

Key Concepts Summary

68.1 The adrenal glands secrete gonadocorticoids, mineralocorticoids, and corticosteroids.

68.2 Corticosteroids are widely used, and all drugs in the class have very similar indications, actions, and adverse effects.

68.3 Long-term therapy with corticosteroids has the potential to cause serious adverse effects in multiple body systems.

68.4 Adrenocortical insufficiency is treated by administering physiological levels of corticosteroids.

68.5 Corticosteroids are frequently used to suppress the inflammatory and immune responses.

68.6 Patients with adrenal insufficiency often require replacement therapy with mineralocorticoids.

68.7 Antiadrenal drugs may be administered to lower serum corticosteroid levels in patients with Cushing's syndrome.

Case Study: Making the Patient Connection

Remember the patient "Charlie Harness" from the beginning of the chapter? Now read the remainder of the story. Based on the information presented within this chapter, answer the critical thinking questions that follow.

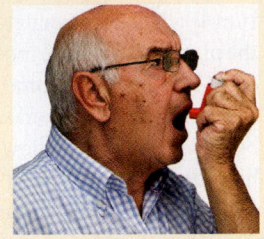

Charlie Harness is a 61-year-old man, newly diagnosed this year with early COPD secondary to bouts of chronic bronchitis. Charlie had been a cigarette smoker since age 15 but proudly tells everyone that he "quit cold turkey 5 years ago and hasn't touched one since!" He was surprised by the diagnosis of COPD even though he had been having increasingly long bouts of bronchitis and had noticed that he seemed more out of breath after each one. Charlie's father died at age 52 "from some kind of lung problem," which Charlie thinks might have been caused by smoking. Charlie still works as a service technician in the local tire and battery store and hopes to work until he is 70. His daughter just had a baby last year and he tells you, his nurse, "I want to be around to see my grandson graduate from high school!" Charlie has come to his health care provider today because of increasing shortness of breath. He relates this to "allergy season" when he feels his bronchitis flare and with it, increasing dyspnea. His physical exam reveals that Charlie is experiencing mild to moderate shortness of breath with him pausing for a breath after two or three sentences. His pulse is 108 beats/min, respiratory rate 28 breaths/

min, blood pressure 150/80 mmHg, and he is afebrile. A pulse oximeter reading is 94% and you note that Charlie's past readings have averaged between 94% and 97%. His breath sounds reveal a prolonged expiratory phase and are distant. He has inspiratory wheezing and he tells you that he frequently coughs up small amounts of beige-white mucus. He denies abdominal distention or tenderness. His provider gives him a prescription for an antibiotic and refill prescriptions for his bronchodilator and budesonide (Pulmicort) inhalers. Charlie is to return in 2 days for reassessment but tells you, "This should do the trick, it always does if I stay ahead of it." In the evenings, Charlie spends much of his time on the Internet, video-chatting with his daughter and son-in-law, viewing photos of his grandson, and reading articles on various websites. He has recently discovered information about steroids and expresses some concern about the information he has read. He is considering not taking his budesonide inhaler anymore and asks you what he should do.

Critical Thinking Questions

1. Create a list of questions you would ask Charlie to determine if he is experiencing any adverse effects from the corticosteroids.

2. What would you tell this patient related to abruptly discontinuing this medication? Why?

3. Charlie asks you if there are any precautions that he should take related to his budesonide (Pulmicort). How would you respond?

See Answers to Critical Thinking Questions on student resource website.

Additional Case Study

Monica Hamric, a 53-year-old woman, is referred to the endocrinologist for evaluation after being seen by the advanced practice nurse. She has a history of systemic lupus erythematosus, managed with corticosteroids, and has begun to experience weight gain, facial hirsutism with thinning of the hair on her head, spontaneous bruising, muscle weakness, and a recent diagnosis of diabetes. She has been taking prednisone (Deltasone) for the past 3 months. The physical examination reveals that Monica has developed a "buffalo hump" on her shoulder and red striae on her abdominal

and underarm areas. Her BP is also elevated, measuring 162/100 mmHg. The health care provider has diagnosed Monica with Cushing's syndrome related to her prednisone use. Monica will be withdrawn from the prednisone and started on immunosuppressant therapy. Because Monica has taken the prednisone for some time, how do you anticipate the drug will be stopped and why?

See Answers to Additional Case Study on student resource website.

Chapter Review

1 A patient has been ordered methylprednisolone (Medrol Dosepak) for treatment of a significant poison ivy rash. The nurse will teach the patient to report which adverse effects to the health care provider? Select all that apply.

1. Edema
2. Tinnitus
3. Eye pain or vision changes
4. Dizziness upon standing
5. Abdominal pain

2 A patient has been taking a thiazide diuretic for treatment of hypertension and has been prescribed hydrocortisone (Cortef) for a significant allergic reaction to shellfish. Which symptom should be immediately reported to the provider?

1. Irregular heart rate and rhythm
2. Delayed wound healing
3. Weight gain of 2 to 3 pounds in 1 week
4. Elevated serum lipid levels

3 An older adult patient with chronic bronchitis has been receiving low-dose therapy with dexamethasone for several months to reduce the inflammation occurring secondary to the bronchitis. What teaching should this patient receive to reduce the risk of osteoporosis related to dexamethasone use? Select all that apply.

1. Perform weight-bearing exercises at least three to four times weekly.
2. Increase dietary intake of calcium and vitamin D–rich foods.
3. Remain sedentary except during periods of exercise.
4. Increase fluid intake, including carbonated sodas, but avoid alcohol.
5. Request a prescription for a bisphosphonate drug from the provider.

4 A patient with adrenocortical insufficiency has started therapy with fludrocortisone (Florinef). What important intervention related to this drug therapy should the nurse teach the patient?

1. "Report any abdominal pain or changes in your stool color."
2. "Return monthly for laboratory work to assess blood lipid levels."
3. "Report any unusual changes in your mood."
4. "Weigh yourself daily, ideally at the same time each day."

5 A patient who has been taking dexamethasone for rheumatoid arthritis was unable to take the drug for several days due to an intestinal virus. The patient seeks treatment in the emergency department for complaints of severe nausea, vomiting, lethargy, fever, and hypotension. What drug does the nurse anticipate will be given to this patient?

1. Fludrocortisone
2. Ketoconazole (Nizoral)
3. Hydrocortisone (Solu-Cortef)
4. Metyrapone (Metopirone)

6 A patient with chronic adrenal insufficiency taking hydrocortisone (Cortef) and fludrocortisone is planning a family vacation. What essential teaching does this patient need prior to taking this trip?

1. "Take your blood pressure once or twice while you're gone."
2. "Avoid crowded indoor areas to avoid infections."
3. "Have your vision checked before you leave."
4. "Carry an oral and injectable form of both drugs with you on your trip."

See Answers to Chapter Review in Appendix A.

References

Adler, G. K. (2014). *Cushing syndrome*. Retrieved from http://emedicine.medscape.com/article/117365-overview

Crowther, C. A., McKinlay, C. J. D., Middleton, P., & Harding, J. E. (2011). Intervention review: Repeat doses of prenatal corticosteroids for women at risk of preterm birth for improving neonatal health outcomes. *Cochrane Database of Systematic Reviews, 6*, CD003935. doi:10.1002/14651858.CD003935.pub3

Griffing, G. T. (2014). *Addison disease clinical presentation*. Retrieved from http://emedicine.medscape.com/article/116467-clinical

Mazereeuw, G., Lanctôt, K. L., Chau, S. A., Swardfager, W., & Herrmann, N. (2012). Effects of omega-3 fatty acids on cognitive performance: A meta-analysis. *Neurobiology of Aging, 33*, 1482.e17-29. doi:10.1016/j.neurobiolaging.2011.12.014

Muehleisen, B., & Gallo, R. L. (2013). Vitamin D in allergic disease: Shedding light on a complex problem. *Journal of Allergy and Clinical Immunology, 131*(2), 324–239. doi:10.1016/j.jaci.2012.12.1562

National Center for Complementary and Alternative Medicine. (2013). *Omega-3 supplements: An introduction*. Retrieved from http://nccam.nih.gov/health/omega3/introduction.htm

Nwaru, B. I., Takkinen, H. M., Kaila, M., Erkkola, M., Pekkanen, J., Simell, O., … Virtanen, S. M. (2014). Food diversity in infancy and the risk of childhood asthma and allergies. *Journal of Allergy and Clinical Immunology, 133*(4), 1084–1091. doi:10.1016/j.jaci.2013.12.1069

Robinson, P. D., & Van Asperen, P. (2013). Update in paediatric asthma management: Where is evidence challenging current practice? *Journal of Paediatrics and Child Health, 49*, 346–352. doi:10.1111/j.1440-1754.2010.01975.x

Szefler, S. J. (2014). Advances in pediatric asthma in 2013: Coordinating asthma care. *Journal of Asthma and Clinical Immunology, 133*(3), 654–661. doi:10.1016/j.jaci.2014.01.012

Zephyrin, L. C., Hong, K. N., Wapner, R. J., Peaceman, A. M., Sorokin, Y., Dudley, D. J., … Sibai, B. (2013). Gestational age-specific risks vs benefits of multicourse antenatal corticosteroids for preterm labor. *American Journal of Obstetrics and Gynecology, 209*(4), 330.e1–7. doi:10.1016/j.ajog.2013.06.009

Selected Bibliography

Biddie, S. C., Conway-Campbell, B. L., & Lightman, S. L. (2012). Dynamic regulation of glucocorticoid signalling in health and disease. *Rheumatology, 51*, 403–412. doi:10.1093/rheumatology/ker215

Falorni, A., Minarelli, V., & Morelli, S. (2013). Therapy of adrenal insufficiency: An update. *Endocrine, 43*, 514–528. doi:10.1007/s12020-012-9835-4

Feelders, R. A., & Hofland, L. J. (2013). Medical treatment of Cushing's disease. *The Journal of Clinical Endocrinology & Metabolism, 98*, 425–438. doi:10.1210/jc.2012-3126

Fleseriu, M., & Petersenn, S. (2012). Medical management of Cushing's disease: What is the future? *Pituitary, 15*, 330–341. doi:10.1007/s11102-012-0397-5

Gardner, D. G., & Shoback, D. (Eds.). (2011). *Greenspan's basic and clinical endocrinology* (9th ed.). New York, NY: McGraw-Hill.

Herdman, T. H., & Kamitsuru, S. (Eds.). (2014). *NANDA International nursing diagnoses: Definitions and classification, 2015-2017*. Oxford, United Kingdom: Wiley-Blackwell.

Quinkler, M., & Hahner, S. (2012). What is the best long-term management strategy for patients with primary adrenal insufficiency? *Clinical Endocrinology, 76*, 21–25. doi:10.1111/j.1365-2265.2011.04103.x

Tritos, N. A., & Biller, B. M. (2012). Advances in medical therapies for Cushing's syndrome. *Discovery Medicine, 13*(69), 171–179.

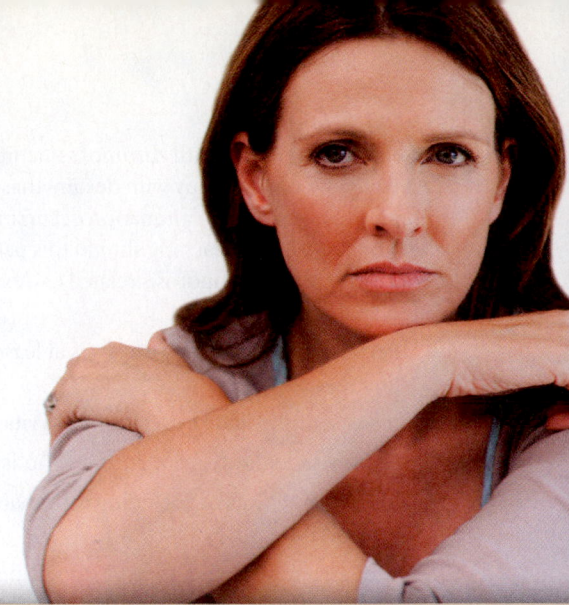

"I get fatigued so easily. I'm having mood swings, headaches, bouts of depression, and irritability; but my main concern is that I have absolutely no desire to have sexual intercourse. What's happening to me, and what can I do about it?"

Patient "Eileen John"

CHAPTER

69 Estrogens, Progestins, and Drugs Modifying Uterine Function

LEARNING OUTCOMES

After reading this chapter, the student should be able to:

1. Describe the roles of the hypothalamus, pituitary, and ovaries in maintaining female reproductive function.

2. Identify indications for estrogen pharmacotherapy.

3. Identify indications for progestin pharmacotherapy.

4. Compare and contrast the advantages and disadvantages of hormone replacement therapy during menopause.

5. Explain the use of uterine stimulants to promote labor and delivery.

6. Discuss the use of uterine relaxants in suppressing preterm labor.

7. Explain how drug therapy may be used to treat female infertility.

8. Describe the nurse's role in the pharmacologic management of disorders and conditions of the female reproductive system.

9. For each of the classes shown in the chapter outline, identify the prototype and representative drugs and explain the mechanism(s) of drug action, primary indications, contraindications, significant drug interactions, pregnancy category, and important adverse effects.

10. Apply the nursing process to the care of patients who are receiving pharmacotherapy for disorders and conditions of the female reproductive system.

CHAPTER OUTLINE

▶ **Hormonal Regulation of Female Reproductive Function**

▶ **Estrogens**
   PROTOTYPE Conjugated Estrogens (Cenestin, Enjuvia, Premarin), *p. 1168*

▶ **Progestins**
   PROTOTYPE Medroxyprogesterone (Depo-Provera, Depo-SubQ-Provera, Provera), *p. 1171*

▶ **Hormone Replacement Therapy**

▶ **Uterine Stimulants: Oxytocics**
   Ergot Alkaloids
   Prostaglandins
   PROTOTYPE Oxytocin (Pitocin), *p. 1177*

▶ **Uterine Relaxants: Tocolytics**
   Magnesium Sulfate
   Calcium Channel Blockers
   Beta$_2$-Adrenergic Agonists

▶ **Pharmacotherapy of Female Infertility**
   PROTOTYPE Clomiphene (Clomid, Serophene), *p. 1183*

KEY TERMS

anovulatory cycles, 1171

climacteric, 1174

corpus luteum, 1167

dysfunctional uterine
bleeding, 1171

endometriosis, 1183

hormone replacement therapy (HRT), 1174

infertility, 1181

menopause, 1174

ovarian hyperstimulation syndrome
(OHS), 1183

ovulation, 1167

ovulatory dysfunction, 1181

oxytocics, 1176

polycystic ovary syndrome, 1181

preterm labor, 1179

progestins, 1171

tocolytics, 1179

The steroid hormones estrogen and progesterone are responsible for the growth, development, and reproductive health of females throughout the lifespan. Deficiencies or excesses of these hormones can result in profound changes that extend beyond the reproductive system. These hormones impact virtually every body system including effects on coagulation, blood vessels, bone, muscles, overall body metabolism, and behavior. Stimulating hormones from the pituitary also affect reproductive function, including fertility, labor, delivery, and the production and ejection of breast milk. This chapter examines hormones and drugs used to treat conditions associated with the female reproductive system.

Hormonal Regulation of Female Reproductive Function

69.1 Regulation of the female reproductive system is achieved by hormones from the hypothalamus, pituitary gland, and ovary.

The two primary hormones of the female reproductive system are estrogen and progesterone. During a woman's childbearing years, nearly all estrogen and progesterone is secreted by the ovaries. Small amounts of estrogen are secreted by nonreproductive organs, including the adrenal glands, liver, kidney, skeletal muscle, and adipose tissue. In postmenopausal females, nearly all estrogen and progesterone is secreted by these nonreproductive tissues. In males, estrogen and progesterone are also secreted in small amounts by the testes.

Unlike males, who secrete steady and continuous levels of testosterone throughout adult life, secretion of the female sex hormones is variable and complex. Knowledge of these complexities is essential to understanding the pharmacotherapy of the female reproductive system. Although this section reviews physiology that is relevant to drug therapy, the student should refer to an anatomy and physiology textbook for more detailed information.

Secretion of female reproductive hormones varies on a 28-day menstrual cycle. The menstrual cycle is described by changes that occur in the ovaries (ovarian cycle) and in the lining of the uterus (uterine cycle). Both cycles are controlled by hormones from the hypothalamus and pituitary. The first day of menstruation is considered day 1 of the cycle. The hormonal changes that occur during the ovarian and uterine cycles are illustrated in Figure 69.1.

The hypothalamus secretes gonadotropin-releasing hormone (GnRH), which travels a short distance to the pituitary to stimulate the secretion of the gonadotropins: follicle-stimulating hormone (FSH) and luteinizing hormone (LH). Both of these anterior pituitary hormones act on the ovary and promote the development of immature ovarian follicles. Under the influence of FSH and LH, several ovarian follicles begin the maturation process each month during the reproductive lifespan. As ovarian follicles mature, they secrete increasing amounts of estrogen. On approximately day 14 of the ovarian cycle, a surge of LH (and to a lesser extent FSH) secretion causes one follicle to expel its oocyte (egg), a process called **ovulation**. The LH surge is an absolute requirement for ovulation, and thus conception. The oocyte begins its journey through the uterine tube and eventually reaches the uterus.

The ruptured follicle, minus the oocyte, remains in the ovary and is transformed into the **corpus luteum**, an endocrine tissue that secretes steadily increasing amounts of progesterone for the next 12 days. Progesterone thickens the uterine mucosa, readying this organ for implantation and potential pregnancy.

High progesterone and estrogen levels in the final third of the uterine cycle provide negative feedback to shut off GnRH, FSH, and LH secretion, as illustrated in Figure 69.2. Without stimulation from FSH and LH, estrogen and progesterone levels fall sharply, the endometrium is shed, and menstrual bleeding begins a new monthly cycle.

Estrogens

69.2 Estrogens are administered as replacement therapy, to prevent conception, and for certain neoplasms.

Estrogen is actually a general term for three different steroid hormones: estradiol, estrone, and estriol. Estradiol is present in the largest amount. Estrogens are responsible for the maturation of the reproductive organs and for the appearance of the secondary sex characteristics of the female during puberty. When women enter menopause at approximately age 50 to 55, the secretion of estrogen by the ovaries diminishes and eventually stops.

Apart from its reproductive functions, estrogen also affects the heart, liver, blood vessels, and bones. Estrogen decreases the levels of low-density lipoprotein (LDL) and increases the amount of high-density lipoprotein (HDL) in the blood. These effects are cardioprotective and help lower the risk of myocardial infarction (MI) in premenopausal women. By blocking resorption of the bony matrix, estrogen causes bones to grow longer and stronger in younger women. As estrogen levels decrease in postmenopausal women, the risk of osteoporosis and bone fractures dramatically increases.

Estrogens are used as contraception and to treat menopausal symptoms, female hypogonadism, and primary ovarian failure.

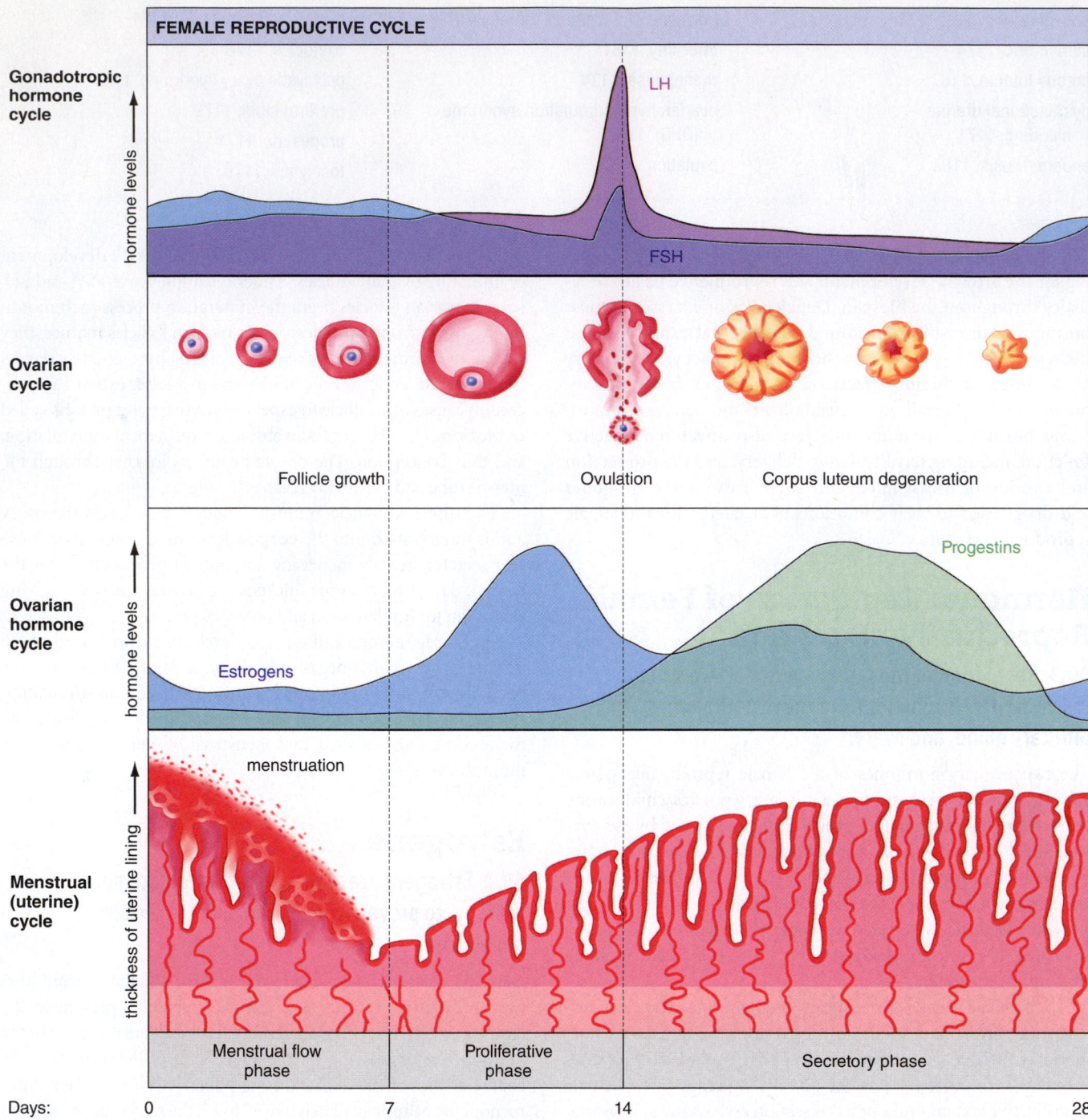

FEMALE REPRODUCTIVE CYCLE

Gonadotropic hormone cycle

LH

FSH

Ovarian cycle

Follicle growth   Ovulation   Corpus luteum degeneration

Ovarian hormone cycle

Progestins

Estrogens

Menstrual (uterine) cycle

menstruation

Menstrual flow phase   Proliferative phase   Secretory phase

Days: 0   7   14   28

Figure 69.1 Hormonal changes during the ovarian and uterine cycles.

When used as replacement therapy following surgical removal of the ovaries, estrogen is usually combined with a progestin. The purpose of the progestin is to counteract some of the adverse effects of estrogen on the uterus. Estrogen drugs are listed in Table 69.1. The contraceptive uses of estrogen are presented in Chapter 70.

High doses of estrogens are sometimes used to treat advanced prostate and breast cancer. Prostate cancer is usually dependent on androgens for growth, and administration of estrogens will suppress androgen secretion. In the treatment of cancer, estrogen is nearly always used in combination with other antineoplastics.

PROTOTYPE DRUG   **Conjugated Estrogens (Cenestin, Enjuvia, Premarin)**

Classification: Therapeutic: Hormone
Pharmacologic: Estrogen

Therapeutic Effects and Uses: Conjugated estrogen, equine (Premarin) was approved in 1938 and contains a mixture of different natural estrogens, traditionally obtained from pregnant mares' urine. Conjugated estrogen A (Cenestin) and conjugated

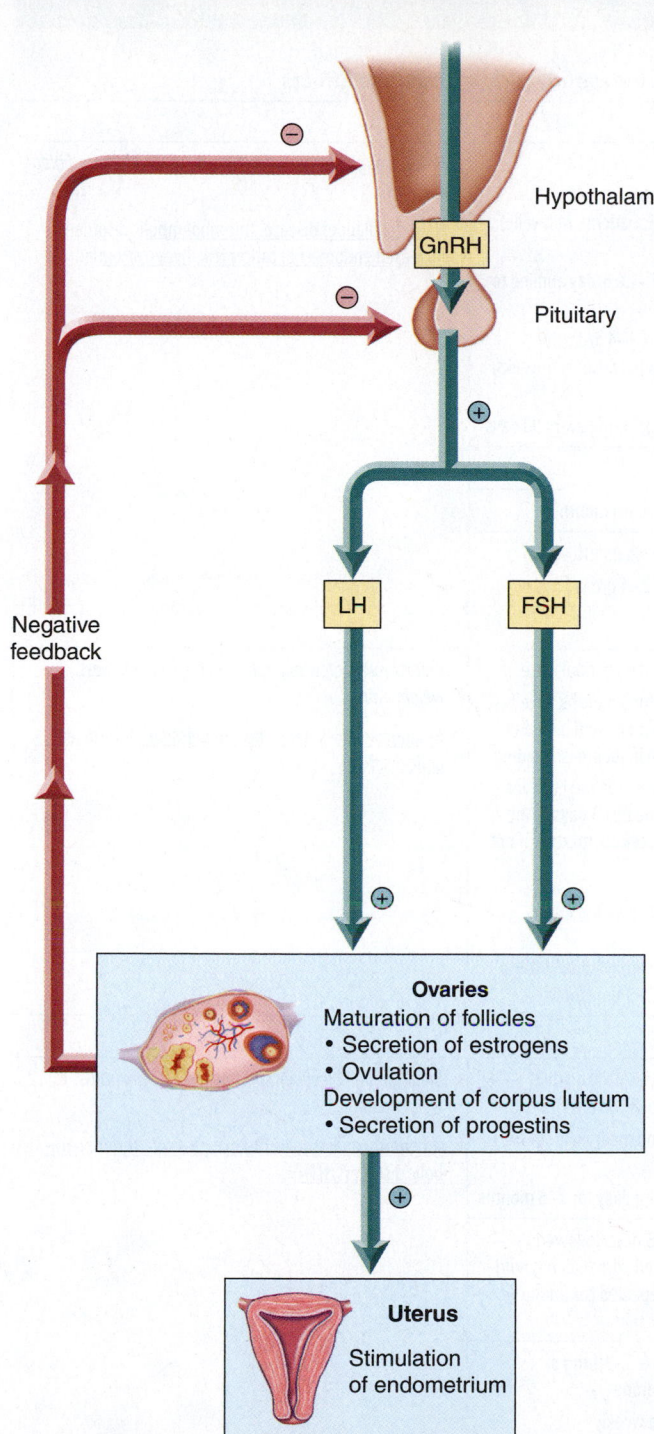

Figure 69.2 Negative feedback control of the female reproductive hormones.

estrogen B (Enjuvia) contain a mixture of 9 to 10 different synthetic plant estrogens.

The primary indication for conjugated estrogens has been to treat moderate to severe vasomotor symptoms of menopause, such as hot flashes and night sweats, caused by diminished estrogen secretion by the ovaries. Topical preparations may be used to treat symptoms of vulvar and vaginal atrophy, such as pain during

intercourse, associated with menopause. Replacement therapies include treatment of female hypogonadism and use following oophorectomy. Premarin is approved for the palliative treatment of prostate cancer and certain types of breast cancer. Conjugated estrogens have been used in the past for osteoporosis prophylaxis in postmenopausal women but safer therapies have replaced these drugs for this indication.

Conjugated estrogens are usually administered by the oral (PO) route. For dysfunctional uterine bleeding, they may be administered by the intramuscular (IM) or intravenous (IV) routes.

Mechanism of Action: Conjugated estrogens bind to intracellular estrogen receptors that stimulate deoxyribonucleic acid (DNA) and ribonucleic acid (RNA) to synthesize proteins responsible for the biologic effects of estrogens.

Pharmacokinetics:

Route(s)	PO, IM, IV, intravaginal
Absorption	Rapid absorption from the gastrointestinal (GI) tract, readily absorbed through the skin and mucous membranes, slow absorption through IM injections
Distribution	Widely distributed; crosses the placenta; secreted in breast milk; bound primarily to albumin
Primary metabolism	Hepatic metabolism by CYP3A4 to estrone, estradiol, and estriol
Primary excretion	Renal
Onset of action	PO: 30–60 min; IM: 15–30 min
Duration of action	Half-life: 4–18 h

Adverse Effects: The most frequently reported adverse effects of conjugated estrogens include headache, infections, abdominal cramps and bloating, breast tenderness, and vaginal bleeding. Other less common adverse effects may include thromboembolic events, fluid retention, edema, acute pancreatitis, appetite changes, skin eruptions, mental depression, decreased or increased libido, fatigue, nervousness, and weight gain. The risks of adverse effects increase in patients over age 35. Effects are dose dependent. **Black Box Warnings**: Estrogens, when used alone, have been associated with a higher risk of endometrial cancer in postmenopausal women (see Section 69.4). Although adding a progestin may exert a protective effect by lowering the risk of uterine cancer, studies suggest that progestin may increase the risk of breast cancer following long-term use. Estrogens when used alone increase the risk of stroke, deep venous thrombosis (DVT), MI, and pulmonary emboli. Estrogens should not be used to prevent cardiovascular disease or to treat dementia.

Contraindications/Precautions: Estrogens should be avoided in patients who have a history of breast cancer, cervical cancer, endometrial cancer, endometrial hyperplasia, prostate cancer, and hepatic diseases or cancer. Additionally, because estrogens have been associated with thromboembolic disorders, hypercalcemia, and lupus, they should not be prescribed without a thorough investigation of these conditions. Estrogens should be used with caution in patients with lipid disorders because they may increase HDL cholesterol and triglycerides. They are contraindicated in

TABLE 69.1 Selected Estrogens and Progestins

Drug	Route and Adult Dose (Maximum Dose Where Indicated)	Adverse Effects
Estrogens		
estradiol (Alora, Climara, Divigel, Elestrin, Estraderm, Estrace, Others)	PO (Estrace): 0.5–2 mg daily Transdermal patch: 1 patch either once weekly (Climara) or twice weekly (Alora, Estraderm, Minivelle) (0.025–0.1 mg/day) Topical gel (Divigel, Elestrin): 0.25–1.0 g/day applied to skin of upper thigh or arm Intravaginal cream (Estrace): Insert 2–4 g/day for 2 weeks, then reduce to 1/2 the initial dose for 2 weeks, then use 1 g 1–3 times/week Intravaginal ring (Estring, Femring): 1 ring every 90 days	*Breakthrough bleeding, spotting, breast tenderness, libido changes* HTN, gallbladder disease, thromboembolic disorders, increased endometrial cancer risk, hypercalcemia
estradiol valerate (Delestrogen)	IM: 10–20 mg every 4 weeks	
estrogen, conjugated (Cenestin, Enjuvia, Premarin)	PO: 0.3–1.25 mg daily for 21 days each month	
stropipate (Ogen)	PO: 0.75–6 mg daily for 21 days each month Intravaginal cream (Ogen): Insert 2–4 g/day	
Progestins		
medroxyprogesterone (Depo-Provera, depo-subQ-Provera, Provera)	PO: 5–10 mg daily on days 1–12 of menstrual cycle IM (Depo-Provera): 150 mg daily for 3 months. Give first dose during the first 5 days of the menstrual period or within the first 5 days postpartum if not breast-feeding Subcutaneous (depo-subQ-Provera): 104 mg daily for 3 months. Give first dose during the first 5 days of the menstrual period or at the sixth week postpartum if not breast-feeding	*Breakthrough bleeding, spotting, breast tenderness, weight gain* Amenorrhea, dysmenorrhea, depression, thromboembolic disorders
progesterone (Crinone, Endometrin, Prochieve, Prometrium)	Amenorrhea or functional uterine bleeding: IM: 5–10 mg/day Assisted reproductive technology: intravaginal: 90-mg gel once daily or 100-mg tablets 2–3 times/day	
Estrogen–Progestin Combinations		
conjugated estrogens with medroxyprogesterone (Premphase, Prempro)	PO (Premphase): estrogen 0.625 mg/daily on days 1–28; add 5 mg medroxyprogesterone daily on days 15–28 PO (Prempro): estrogen 0.3 mg and medroxyprogesterone 1.5 mg daily Intravaginal cream: insert 1/2 to 2 g daily for 3–6 months	*Breakthrough bleeding, spotting, breast tenderness, weight gain* Amenorrhea, dysmenorrhea, depression, thromboembolic disorders, HTN
estradiol with norgestimate (Prefest)	PO: 1 tablet of 1 mg estradiol for 3 days, followed by 1 tablet of 1 mg estradiol combined with 0.09 mg norgestimate for 3 days. Regimen is repeated continuously without interruption	
ethinyl estradiol with norethindrone acetate (Activella)	PO: 1 tablet daily, which contains 0.5–0.1 mg of estradiol and 0.5–1 mg norethindrone Transdermal patch: 1 patch, twice weekly	

Note: Italics indicate common adverse effects. <u>Underline</u> indicates serious adverse effects.

patients with undiagnosed vaginal bleeding. Because estrogens are classified as category X, pregnancy and lactation are contraindications for this drug.

Drug Interactions: Estrogen is metabolized by CYP450 enzymes and may interact with other drugs metabolized in the liver. Interactions include a decreased effect of tamoxifen, enhanced corticosteroid effects, and decreased effects of anticoagulants, especially warfarin. The effects of estrogen may be decreased if taken with barbiturates or rifampin and there is a possible increased

effect of tricyclic antidepressants if taken with estrogens. **Herbal/Food**: St. John's wort, red clover, and black cohosh have weak estrogenic effects and may interfere with estrogen therapy. Effects of estrogen may be enhanced if combined with ginseng. Estrogen may decrease the absorption of folic acid. If allergic to soy products, patients should not take Cenestin because it contains soy estrogens.

Pregnancy: Category X.

Treatment of Overdose: Overdose will cause nausea, vomiting, and breakthrough bleeding, which are treated symptomatically.

Nursing Responsibilities: Key nursing implications for patients receiving conjugated estrogens are included in the Nursing Practice Application for Patients Receiving Pharmacotherapy with Estrogen.

Drugs Similar to Conjugated Estrogens (Cenestin, Enjuvia, Premarin)

Other estrogens are listed in Table 69.1. These drugs have the same actions, adverse effects, and contraindications as those of conjugated estrogens.

CONNECTION Checkpoint 69.1

The majority of drugs in this chapter are pregnancy category X. From what you learned in Chapter 2, what is the difference between a category D drug and a category X drug? *See Answer to Connection Checkpoint 69.1 on student resource website.*

Progestins

69.3 Progestins are administered to treat dysfunctional uterine bleeding, to prevent conception, and for certain neoplasms.

Progestins are synthetic hormones that have actions identical to natural, endogenous progesterone. In combination with estrogen, progesterone promotes breast development and regulates the monthly changes of the uterine cycle. Under the influence of estrogen and progesterone, the uterine endometrium becomes vascular and thickens in preparation for receiving a fertilized egg. If implantation does not occur, levels of progesterone fall dramatically and menses begins. If pregnancy does occur, the ovary will continue to secrete progesterone, maintaining a healthy endometrium until the placenta develops sufficiently to begin producing the hormone.

Whereas the function of estrogen is to cause proliferation of the endometrium, progesterone limits and stabilizes endometrial growth. Progestins are drugs of choice for treating many uterine abnormalities. They are also a component of HRT and are used as contraceptives (see Chapter 70).

The primary noncontraception indication for progestins is **dysfunctional uterine bleeding**, a condition in which hemorrhage occurs on a noncyclic basis or in abnormal amounts. Dysfunctional uterine bleeding is common in adolescents and menopausal women and is often associated with anovulatory menstrual cycles. **Anovulatory cycles** are those that occur without ovulation. Dysfunctional uterine bleeding is the health problem most frequently reported by women and a common reason for a hysterectomy.

PharmFACT

Dysfunctional uterine bleeding most commonly occurs at the extreme ages of the reproductive years. The most severe cases occur in adolescents during the first 2 years after the onset of menstruation. Abnormal bleeding also occurs in 50% of perimenopausal women (Estephan, 2012).

Ninety percent of the cases of dysfunctional uterine bleeding result from anovulation. Possible causes of uterine bleeding include early abortion, pelvic neoplasms, thyroid disorders, pregnancy, and infection. Types of dysfunctional uterine bleeding include the following:

- **Amenorrhea.** Absence of menstruation
- **Endometriosis.** Abnormal location of endometrial tissues

- **Oligomenorrhea.** Infrequent menstruation
- **Menorrhagia.** Prolonged or excessive menstruation
- **Breakthrough (intermenstrual) bleeding.** Hemorrhage between menstrual periods
- **Premenstrual syndrome (PMS).** Symptoms developed during the luteal phase
- **Postmenopausal bleeding.** Hemorrhage following menopause
- **Endometrial carcinoma.** Cancer of the endometrium

Dysfunctional uterine bleeding is often due to a hormonal imbalance between estrogen and progesterone. Although estrogen increases the thickness of the endometrium, bleeding occurs sporadically unless it is balanced by adequate progesterone secretion. Administration of a progestin in a regimen starting 5 days after the onset of menses and continuing for the next 20 days can sometimes help to reestablish a normal, monthly cyclic pattern. Oral contraceptives may also be prescribed for this disorder.

In patients experiencing heavy bleeding, high doses of conjugated estrogens may be administered for 3 weeks prior to adding medroxyprogesterone for the last 10 days of therapy. Treatment with nonsteroidal anti-inflammatory drugs (NSAIDs) helps to ease painful menstrual flow. If aggressive hormonal therapy fails to stop the heavy bleeding, dilation and curettage (D&C) may be necessary.

Progestins are occasionally prescribed for the treatment of metastatic endometrial carcinoma. In these cases, they are used for palliation, in combination with other antineoplastics. Selected progestins and their dosages are shown in Table 69.1.

PROTOTYPE DRUG	Medroxyprogesterone (Depo-Provera, Depo-SubQ-Provera, Provera)

Classification: Therapeutic: Hormone, drug for dysfunctional uterine bleeding
Pharmacologic: Progestin

Therapeutic Effects and Uses: Approved in 1959, medroxyprogesterone is a synthetic progestin with a prolonged duration of action. Like progesterone, the primary target tissue for medroxyprogesterone is the uterine endometrium. It antagonizes the effects of estrogen on the uterus, thus restoring normal hormonal balance. It also inhibits the midcycle LH surge, which prevents ovulation, and causes a thick cervical mucus that is resistant to the passage of sperm. Approved indications include dysfunctional uterine bleeding, secondary amenorrhea, and contraception.

Medroxyprogesterone may also be given by sustained release IM (Depo-Provera) or subcutaneous (depo-subQ-Provera) depot injection. This is available in two doses: a lower dose for contraception, and a higher dose for the palliation of inoperable metastatic uterine or renal carcinoma. The use of medroxyprogesterone in contraception is presented in Chapter 70. The drug has been used off-label to treat symptoms of menopause.

Mechanism of Action: This drug is a synthetic derivative of progesterone with prolonged, variable duration of action and androgenic and antiestrogenic activity. The drug inhibits GnRH, thus preventing the LH surge and ovulation.

Patients Receiving Pharmacotherapy with Estrogen

Assessment	Potential Nursing Diagnoses*
Baseline assessment prior to administration: • Obtain a complete health history including cardiovascular, peripheral vascular, thyroid, hepatic, or renal disease; migraine headaches; diabetes; pregnancy; or breast-feeding. Note personal or family history of thromboembolic disorders (e.g., MI, stroke, peripheral vascular disease) and of reproductive cancers (e.g., breast, uterine, or ovarian cancer). • Obtain a drug history including allergies, current prescription and over-the-counter (OTC) drugs, herbal preparations, alcohol use, and smoking. Be alert to possible drug interactions. • Evaluate appropriate laboratory findings (e.g., CBC, platelets, electrolytes, glucose, lipid, and thyroid function levels), Pap test, HPV screening, and pregnancy test. • Obtain baseline height, weight, and vital signs. • Assess the patient's ability to receive and understand instructions. Include the family or caregiver as needed.	• *Decisional Conflict* • *Disturbed Body Image* • *Deficient Knowledge* (Drug Therapy) • *Risk for Imbalanced Fluid Volume*, related to adverse drug effects • *Risk for Ineffective Tissue Perfusion: Peripheral, Cerebral*, related to adverse drug effects • *Risk for Decreased Cardiac Tissue Perfusion*
Assessment throughout administration: • Assess for desired therapeutic effects dependent on the reason the drug is given (e.g., symptoms of menopause or ease of dysfunctional uterine bleeding). • Continue periodic monitoring of CBC, platelets, and hepatic function studies. • Monitor vital signs and weight at each health care visit. • Assess for adverse effects: nausea, vomiting, headache, weight gain, breast tenderness, skin rash, acne, fluid retention, changes in mood, and midcycle breakthrough bleeding. Immediately report tachycardia, palpitations, HTN, especially associated with angina, severe headache, cramping in calves, chest pain, or dyspnea.	

Implementation

Interventions and (Rationales)	Patient-Centered Care
Ensuring therapeutic effects: • Monitor appropriate medication administration for optimum results. (Maintaining consistent daily doses for treatment of menopausal symptoms or dysfunctional uterine bleeding will ensure that hormone levels stay stable and symptoms ease.)	• Instruct the patient to take the drug at the same time daily to help with remembering to take the pill. Do not omit doses or increase or decrease the dose without consulting the health care provider. Omitting doses increases the chance of breakthrough bleeding.
Minimizing adverse effects: • Monitor for symptoms of cardiopulmonary, cerebrovascular, and peripheral vascular thromboembolism. Monitor blood pressure at each clinical visit. (Thromboembolic events are a possible adverse effect of estrogen drugs. The risk increases with age over 35, in women with a previous history of cardiovascular disease, and in women who smoke. Monitor for symptoms of peripheral thrombophlebitis, pulmonary embolism, MI, stroke, or other complications related to blood clots.)	• Instruct the patient to immediately report: • Dyspnea, chest pain, or blood in sputum (possible pulmonary embolism). • Heaviness, chest pain, or overwhelming feeling of fatigue and weakness accompanied by nausea and diaphoresis (possible MI). • Sudden, severe headache, especially if associated with a preheadache aura, dizziness, difficulty with speech, numbness in arm or leg, and difficulty with vision (possible stroke). • Warmth, redness, swelling, or tenderness in calf or pain on walking (possible thrombophlebitis). • Teach the patient to monitor blood pressure periodically and report any blood pressure above 140/90 mmHg or per parameters set by the health care provider.
• Encourage smoking cessation and provide information about smoking cessation programs. (Smoking greatly increases the risk of adverse effects of hormone therapy.)	• Advise the patient of the risk of smoking while using estrogens and discuss smoking cessation programs, providing referrals to appropriate support groups and literature on smoking cessation programs.
• Monitor Pap tests, HPV screening, and breast exams as ordered. (Pap tests and breast exams, including mammography as appropriate, will monitor for the development of breast tumors or of cervical cancer.)	• Teach the patient how to perform breast self-exams, noting that monthly exams may not be recommended by the health care provider except for women at high risk for breast cancer. For women over age 40, advise the patient on the need for follow-up mammography per health care provider recommendations. • Advise the patient on the need for routine gynecologic exams appropriate to age to ensure continued health. Exam frequency may be decreased after age 65 after consultation with the health care provider.
• Monitor for the occurrence of any breakthrough bleeding. Report any continuous, unusual, or heavy bleeding. (Small amounts of spotting may occur, especially with low-dose hormone therapy, at midcycle. Any continuous, unusual, or heavy bleeding may indicate adverse effects or disease and should be reported because an increased risk of endometrial cancer has been noted with estrogen use.)	• Teach the patient that slight spotting may occur midcycle while on estrogens but to report any unusual changes in the amount or if the bleeding continues.

CONNECTIONS: NURSING PRACTICE APPLICATION (continued)

• Monitor hepatic function tests and symptoms of liver dysfunction, lipid profile studies, and thyroid levels periodically. (Estrogens are associated with increased risk of gallbladder disease and a rare risk of hepatotoxicity. **Diverse Patients**: Because estrogens metabolize through the P450 system pathways, monitor ethnically diverse patients to ensure optimal therapeutic effects and to minimize adverse effects.)	• Instruct the patient to return periodically for laboratory tests. • Teach the patient to report any symptoms of abdominal or right upper quadrant discomfort or pain, yellowing of the skin or sclera, fatigue, anorexia, darkened urine, or clay-colored stools immediately.
• Monitor concurrent drug therapy and any new prescriptions received. (Many drugs decrease or alter the effectiveness of estrogens including drugs in the penicillin, barbiturate, antiseizure, antidepressant, and benzodiazepine classifications. Check for drug interactions that may affect hormone effectiveness before any new prescription is started.)	• Teach the patient to advise all health care providers of the use of estrogens before beginning any new prescription.
Patient understanding of drug therapy: • Use opportunities during administration of medications and during assessments to discuss the rationale for drug therapy, desired therapeutic outcomes, commonly observed adverse effects, parameters for when to call the health care provider, and any necessary monitoring or precautions. (Using time during nursing care helps to optimize and reinforce key teaching areas.)	• The patient should be able to state the reason for the drug, appropriate dose and scheduling, what adverse effects to observe for, and when to report them.

Patient self-administration of drug therapy:
• When administering the medication, instruct the patient in proper self-administration of the drug, e.g., consistently at the same time each day to help remember the dose, followed by teach-back. (Utilizing time during nurse-administration of these drugs helps reinforce teaching.)
	• Teach the patient to take the drug following appropriate guidelines:
	  • Oral drugs should be taken at the same time each day to help remember the dose. Follow instructions if a dose is missed.
	  • Transdermal patches (e.g., Climara) are changed weekly or every other week per the health care provider's directions.
	  • Apply topical gels or creams only to the area to be treated. Do not wear tampons after intravaginal application.

*Nursing Diagnoses—Definitions and Classification 2015–2017. Copyright © 2014, 1994–2014 by NANDA International. Used by arrangement with John Wiley & Sons Limited.

Pharmacokinetics:

Route(s)	PO, IM, subcutaneous, IV
Absorption	Readily absorbed from the GI tract or IM
Distribution	Crosses the placenta; secreted in breast milk; 90% bound to protein
Primary metabolism	Hepatic
Primary excretion	Feces
Onset of action	PO: 30–60 min; IM: 15–30 min
Duration of action	Half-life: 30 days (PO) and 50 days (IM)

Adverse Effects: The most common adverse effects of medroxyprogesterone are breast tenderness and breakthrough bleeding and other menstrual irregularities. Weight gain, depression, hypertension (HTN), nausea, vomiting, fluid retention, and vaginal candidiasis may also occur. **Black Box Warning**: Progestins combined with conjugated estrogens may increase the risk of stroke, DVT, myocardial infarction, pulmonary emboli, and invasive breast cancer. Women age 65 or older have an increased risk of dementia when treated with progestins. Women receiving injectable medroxyprogesterone are at significant risk for loss of bone mineral density.

Contraindications/Precautions: Patients with a history of thromboembolic disorders, or who are pregnant or lactating, should not take progestins. Doses should be reduced in patients with hepatic impairment. Patients with preexisting breast, uterine, or vaginal cancer should not receive medroxyprogesterone unless it is for palliation of advanced cancer. The drug should be used cautiously in patients with a history of psychic depression, and the drug should be discontinued at the first sign of recurring depression. The drug is absolutely contraindicated in patients with known or suspected pregnancy (category X) or in those with undiagnosed vaginal bleeding.

Drug Interactions: Serum levels of medroxyprogesterone are decreased by aminoglutethimide, barbiturates, primidone, rifampin, rifabutin, and topiramate. **Herbal/Food**: St. John's wort may cause intermenstrual bleeding and loss of efficacy.

Pregnancy: Category X.

Treatment of Overdose: Overdose is treated symptomatically.

Nursing Responsibilities: Key nursing implications for patients receiving medroxyprogesterone are included in the Nursing Practice Application for Patients Receiving Pharmacotherapy with Progestin.

Drugs Similar to Medroxyprogesterone (Depo-Provera, Depo-SubQ-Provera, Provera)

Progestins used as contraceptives include desogestrel, dienogest, levonorgestrel, norgestrel, and norethindrone. These are presented in Chapter 70.

Progesterone (Crinone, Endometrin, Prochieve, Prometrium): Approved in 1978, progesterone is available in a variety of formulations. As a vaginal suppository (Endometrin) or vaginal gel (Crinone, Prochieve), progesterone is used to treat infertile women with progesterone deficiency as part of an assisted reproductive technology system. The vaginal formulations may also be used as progesterone supplements to support embryo implantation and early pregnancy. When used intravaginally, the drug may be absorbed and cause systemic adverse effects such as breast tenderness, bloating, drowsiness, headaches, irritability, and mood swings.

Oral capsules (Prometrium) are approved to treat secondary amenorrhea and may be used off-label to ease symptoms of PMS. Prometrium is also indicated for the prevention of endometrial hyperplasia in postmenopausal women who are receiving conjugated estrogens.

Progesterone IM injections are indicated for amenorrhea and to stop abnormal uterine bleeding. Adverse effects and contraindications are the same as those for medroxyprogesterone. The PO and IM progesterone formulations are pregnancy category X. The vaginal gel is category B.

Hormone Replacement Therapy

69.4 Hormone replacement therapy provides relief from menopause symptoms but may have serious long-term negative effects.

Menopause is characterized by a progressive decrease in estrogen secretion by the ovaries resulting in the permanent cessation of menses. The **climacteric** is the period of endocrine, somatic, and psychological changes occurring in the transition to menopause. There are over 30 million menopausal women in North America and each decade millions more reach the climacteric. Menopause is neither a disease nor a disorder, but is a natural consequence of aging that is often accompanied by unpleasant symptoms that include hot flashes, night sweats, irregular menstrual cycles, vaginal dryness, and bone mass loss.

PharmFACT

When a women enters early menopause (age less than 45 years) her risk of future stroke and cardiovascular disease doubles. Smokers reach menopause about 2 years earlier than nonsmokers (Wellons, Ouyang, Schreiner, Herrington, & Vaidya, 2012).

During the past 40 years, health care providers have commonly prescribed **hormone replacement therapy (HRT)** during menopause. HRT supplies physiological doses of estrogen, sometimes combined with a progestin, to treat unpleasant symptoms of menopause and to prevent the long-term consequences of estrogen loss listed in Table 69.2.

Beginning in the mid-1960s, large numbers of perimenopausal and menopausal women received conjugated estrogen (Premarin). Premarin was widely prescribed, despite a lack of research on its effectiveness and long-term effects. The drug's popularity extended several more decades, making Premarin one of the most frequently prescribed medications in the United States. In addition, a significant number of women were prescribed conjugated estrogens combined with medroxyprogesterone (Prempro).

In the mid-1970s, however, studies showed that women who had used estrogen (without progestin) for 7 years or longer were more likely to develop uterine (endometrial) cancer. Progestins were then added to the HRT regimen to lower the risk of endometrial cancer.

Two large, randomized, double-blind, placebo-controlled studies have challenged the safety of using HRT during menopause. The Women's Health Initiative (WHI) and the Heart and Estrogen/Progestin Replacement Study (HERS) helped disprove

TABLE 69.2 Potential Consequences of Estrogen Loss Related to Menopause	
Stage	**Symptoms and Conditions**
Early menopause	Headaches
	Hot flashes
	Insomnia
	Irregular menstrual cycles
	Mood disturbances, depression, irritability
Midmenopause	Sexual disinterest
	Skin atrophy
	Stress urinary incontinence
	Vaginal atrophy, increased infections, painful intercourse
Postmenopause	Alzheimer's-like dementia
	Cardiovascular disease
	Colon cancer
	Osteoporosis

some of the benefits of HRT for postmenopausal women. More than 26,000 women were enrolled in these studies, which were discontinued early when it became clear that the potential benefits of long-term HRT were not being realized. The results of the study depended on whether the HRT consisted of estrogen alone or an estrogen–progestin combination. Researchers reached the following conclusions:

- Women taking estrogen–progestin combination HRT experienced a statistically significant increased risk of MI, stroke, breast cancer, dementia, and venous thromboembolism. The risks were higher in women older than age 60; women age 50 to 59 actually experienced a slight decrease in adverse cardiovascular events.

- Women taking estrogen–progestin combination HRT experienced a decreased risk of hip fractures and colorectal cancer.

- Women taking estrogen alone experienced an increased risk of stroke and other thromboembolic disorders.

- Women taking estrogen alone did not experience an increased risk of breast cancer or MI.

The adverse effects documented in the WHI study and others were significant enough to suggest that the potential benefits of long-term HRT may not outweigh the risks for many women.

To be clear, HRT does offer relief from the immediate, distressing vasomotor menopausal symptoms, prevents osteoporosis-related fractures, and may offer some degree of protection from colorectal cancer. These are certainly significant and important benefits from HRT. The risks of HRT include increased incidence of MI, thromboembolic events, breast cancer (estrogen–progestin combinations), ovarian cancer (estrogen alone), and possibly dementia, urinary incontinence, and gallbladder disease. Until research provides more definitive answers, the choice of HRT to treat menopausal symptoms remains a highly individualized one, between the patient and her health care provider.

In recent years, several drugs have been marketed to treat symptoms of menopause while lowering the potential adverse effects of estrogen–progestin combinations. Duavee is a combination drug that contains conjugated estrogens with bazedoxifene, which belongs to a class of drugs called selective estrogen receptor modifiers (SERMs). Duavee offers the advantages of preventing intense hot flashes (the estrogen component) while reducing the risk of osteoporosis-related fractures that are common in postmenopausal women (the SERM component). Approved in 2013, Duavee is the first HRT that includes a SERM instead of a progestin. This drug carries the same black box warning as that for conjugated estrogens regarding an increased risk of endometrial cancer and DVT. Duavee is given by the oral route and is pregnancy category X.

Another SERM, ospemiphene (Osphema), was approved in 2013 to treat dyspareunia, a type of acute pain in postmenopausal women that may occur during intercourse. Ospemiphene acts as an estrogen agonist on the vagina, increasing the thickness of the vaginal epithelium. This drug carries the same black box warning as conjugated estrogens regarding an increased risk of endometrial cancer and DVT. Ospemiphene is given by the oral route and is pregnancy category X.

CONNECTIONS: NURSING PRACTICE APPLICATION

Patients Receiving Pharmacotherapy with Progestin

Assessment	Potential Nursing Diagnoses*
Baseline assessment prior to administration: • Obtain a complete health history including cardiovascular, peripheral vascular, thyroid, hepatic, or renal disease; migraine headaches; diabetes; pregnancy; or breast-feeding. Note personal or family history of thromboembolic disorders (e.g., MI, stroke, peripheral vascular disease) and of reproductive cancers (e.g., breast, uterine, or ovarian cancer). • Obtain a drug history including allergies, current prescription and OTC drugs, herbal preparations, alcohol use, and smoking. Be alert to possible drug interactions. • Evaluate appropriate laboratory findings (e.g., CBC, platelets, electrolytes, glucose, lipid, and thyroid function levels), Pap test, HPV screening, pregnancy test. • Obtain baseline height, weight, and vital signs. • Assess the patient's ability to receive and understand instructions. Include the family or caregiver as needed.	• *Decisional Conflict* • *Disturbed Body Image* • *Deficient Knowledge* (Drug Therapy) • *Risk for Nausea*, related to adverse drug effects • *Risk for Injury*, related to adverse drug effects
Assessment throughout administration: • Assess for desired therapeutic effects dependent on the reason the drug is given (e.g., symptoms of menopause or ease of dysfunctional uterine bleeding). • Continue periodic monitoring of CBC, platelets, and hepatic function studies. • Monitor vital signs and weight at each health care visit. • Assess for adverse effects: nausea, vomiting, headache, weight gain, breast tenderness, skin rash, acne, fluid retention, changes in mood, midcycle breakthrough bleeding. Immediately report tachycardia, palpitations, HTN, especially associated with angina, severe headache, cramping in calves, chest pain, or dyspnea.	

Implementation

Interventions and (Rationales)	Patient-Centered Care
Ensuring therapeutic effects: • Monitor appropriate medication administration for optimal results. (Maintaining consistent daily doses for treatment of menopausal symptoms or dysfunctional uterine bleeding will ensure that hormone levels stay stable and symptoms ease.)	• Instruct the patient to take the drug at the same time daily to help with remembering to take the pill. Do not omit doses or increase or decrease dose without consulting the health care provider. Omitting doses increases the risk of breakthrough bleeding.
Minimizing adverse effects: • Monitor for symptoms of cardiopulmonary, cerebrovascular, and peripheral vascular thromboembolism. Monitor blood pressure at each clinical visit. (Thromboembolic events are a possible adverse effect of progestin drugs. The risk increases with age over 35, in women with a previous history of cardiovascular disease, and in women who smoke. Monitor for symptoms of peripheral thrombophlebitis, pulmonary embolism, MI, stroke, or other complications related to blood clots.)	• Instruct the patient to immediately report: • Dyspnea, chest pain, or blood in sputum (possible pulmonary embolism). • Heaviness, chest pain, or an overwhelming feeling of fatigue and weakness accompanied by nausea and diaphoresis (possible MI). • Sudden, severe headache, especially if associated with a preheadache aura, dizziness, difficulty with speech, numbness in arm or leg, difficulty with vision (possible stroke). • Warmth, redness, swelling, or tenderness in calf or pain on walking (possible thrombophlebitis). • Teach the patient to monitor blood pressure periodically and report any blood pressure above 140/90 mmHg or per parameters set by the health care provider.

(continued)

CONNECTIONS: NURSING PRACTICE APPLICATION (continued)

• Encourage smoking cessation and provide information about smoking cessation programs. (Smoking greatly increases the risk of adverse effects of hormone therapy.)	• Advise the patient of the risk of smoking while using progestins and discuss smoking cessation programs, providing referral to appropriate support groups and literature on smoking cessation programs.
• Assess for the presence of bone or musculoskeletal pain on each health care visit, especially in patients taking injectable progestins. (Progestins are associated with an increased risk of loss of bone density. Bone density monitoring, e.g., DEXA scan, may be ordered periodically. Immediately report any sudden, severe pain or difficulty with ambulation or movement.)	• Instruct the patient to immediately report any sudden and severe pain, or continuous moderate pain, in joints or muscles, loss of motion, or difficulty with ambulation or movement to the health care provider.
• **Lifespan:** Monitor mental status in patients age 65 or older or patients with a history of depression or psychiatric illness. (Progestins are associated with increased risk of dementia in women age 65 or older.)	• Instruct the patient, family, or caregiver to promptly report any changes in behavior, depression, or mental status to the health care provider.
• Monitor concurrent drug therapy and any new prescriptions received. (Many drugs decrease or alter the effectiveness of progestins including drugs in the penicillin, barbiturate, antiseizure, antidepressant, and benzodiazepine classifications. Check for drug interactions that may affect hormone effectiveness before any new prescription is started.)	• Teach the patient to advise all health care providers of the use of progestins before beginning any new prescription.
• Monitor Pap tests, HPV screening, and breast exams as ordered. (Pap tests and breast exams, including mammography as appropriate, will monitor for the development of breast tumors or of cervical cancer.)	• Teach the patient how to perform breast self-exams, noting that monthly exams may not be recommended by the health care provider except for women at high risk for breast cancer. For women over age 40, advise the patient on the need for follow-up mammography per health care provider recommendations. • Advise the patient on the need for annual gynecologic exams to ensure continued health. Exam frequency may be decreased after age 65 after consultation with the health care provider.
• Monitor for the occurrence of any breakthrough bleeding. Report any continuous, unusual, or heavy bleeding. (Small amounts of spotting may occur, especially with low-dose hormone therapy, at midcycle. Any continuous, unusual, or heavy bleeding may indicate adverse effects or disease and should be reported.)	• Teach the patient that slight spotting may occur midcycle while on progestin but to report any unusual changes in the amount or if the bleeding continues.
Patient understanding of drug therapy: • Use opportunities during administration of medications and during assessments to discuss the rationale for drug therapy, desired therapeutic outcomes, commonly observed adverse effects, parameters for when to call the health care provider, and any necessary monitoring or precautions. (Using time during nursing care helps to optimize and reinforce key teaching areas.)	• The patient should be able to state the reason for the drug, appropriate dose and scheduling, what adverse effects to observe for, and when to report them.

Patient self-administration of drug therapy:
• When administering the medication, instruct the patient or caregiver in proper self-administration of the drug, e.g., consistently at the same time each day to help remember the dose, followed by teach-back. (Utilizing time during nurse-administration of these drugs helps to reinforce teaching.)
	• Teach the patient to take the drug following appropriate guidelines:
	  • Oral drugs should be taken at the same time each day to help remember the dose. Follow instructions if dose is missed.
	  • Take the drug with food or milk to decrease the possibility of nausea.

*Nursing Diagnoses—Definitions and Classification 2015–2017. Copyright © 2014, 1994–2014 by NANDA International. Used by arrangement with John Wiley & Sons Limited.

Uterine Stimulants: Oxytocics

69.5 Oxytocics are drugs used to stimulate the uterus and promote labor and delivery.

Oxytocics are drugs that stimulate uterine contractions and promote the induction of labor. The most widely used oxytocic is the natural hormone oxytocin, which is secreted by the posterior pituitary gland. The target organs for oxytocin are the uterus and the breast. Increasing amounts of oxytocin are secreted as the uterus is distended by the growing fetus. As blood levels of oxytocin rise, uterine smooth muscle is stimulated to contract, thus promoting labor and the delivery of the baby and the placenta. As pregnancy progresses, the number of oxytocin receptors in the uterus increases, making it even more sensitive to the effects of the hormone.

Oxytocin and other uterine stimulants are only indicated when there are demonstrated risks to the mother or fetus in continuing the pregnancy. Parenteral oxytocin (Pitocin) may be given to induce labor. Doses in an IV infusion are increased gradually, every 15 to 60 minutes, until a normal labor pattern is established. After delivery, IV oxytocin is administered to control postpartum uterine bleeding by temporarily restricting blood flow to this organ. Doses of these agents are listed in Table 69.3.

In postpartum women, oxytocin is released in response to suckling, whereby it promotes the ejection (letdown) of milk from the mammary glands. Oxytocin does not increase the volume of milk production: This function is provided by the pituitary hormone prolactin, which increases the synthesis of milk. Although rare, deficiencies of prolactin can result in insufficient milk to conduct breast-feeding. The actions of oxytocin during breast-feeding are illustrated in Figure 69.3.

Ergot alkaloids are drugs obtained from a fungus that grows on rye plants that are used as alternatives to oxytocin to control postpartum hemorrhage. The primary drug in this class, methylergonovine

TABLE 69.3 Uterine Stimulants and Relaxants

Drug	Route and Adult Dose (Maximum Dose Where Indicated)	Adverse Effects
Stimulants (Oxytocics)		
oxytocin (Pitocin)	To control postpartum bleeding: 10–40 units per infusion pump in 1,000 mL of IV fluid at a rate to prevent uterine atony To induce labor: IV: 0.5–2 milliunits/min, gradually increasing the dose no greater than 1–2 milliunits/min at 30- to 60-min intervals until contraction pattern is established	*Nausea, vomiting, maternal dysrhythmias* <u>Fetal bradycardia, uterine rupture, fetal intracranial hemorrhage, water intoxication, fetal brain hemorrhage</u>
Ergot Alkaloid		
methylergonovine (Methergine)	PO: 0.2–0.4 mg bid–qid	*Nausea, vomiting, uterine cramping* <u>Shock, severe HTN, severe dysrhythmias</u>
Prostaglandins		
carboprost (Hemabate)	IM: initial: 250 mcg (1 mL) repeated at 1½- to 3½-h intervals if indicated by uterine response	*Nausea, vomiting, cramping, diarrhea, fever* <u>Uterine laceration, rupture, or hemorrhage</u>
dinoprostone (Cervidil, Prepidil, Prostin E$_2$)	Intravaginal insert (Cervidil): 10 mg (1 insert) Intravaginal gel (Prepidil): 0.5 mg Intravaginal suppository: 20 mg (1 suppository)	
Relaxants (Tocolytics)		
magnesium sulfate	IV: 1–4 g in 5% dextrose by slow infusion (initial max dose: 10–14 g/day, then no more than 30–40 g/day at a max rate of 1–2 g/h)	*Flushing, sweating, muscle weakness* <u>Complete heart block, circulatory collapse, respiratory paralysis</u>
nifedipine (Adalat, Procardia)	PO: initial dosage of 20 mg, followed by 20 mg after 30 min. If contractions persist, therapy can be continued with 20 mg every 3–8 h for 48–72 h with a maximum dose of 160 mg/day After 72 h, if maintenance is still required, long-acting nifedipine 30–60 mg daily can be used	*Flushing, sweating, muscle weakness* <u>Complete heart block, circulatory collapse, respiratory paralysis</u>
terbutaline (Brethine)	IV: 2.5–10 mcg/min; increase every 10–20 min; duration of infusion: 12 h (max: 17.5–30 mcg/min) PO: maintenance dose: 2.5–10 mg every 4–6 h as long as necessary to prevent pregnancy	*Nervousness, tremor, drowsiness* <u>Bronchoconstrictions, dysrhythmias, altered maternal and fetal heart rates</u>

Note: Italics indicate common adverse effects. Underline indicates serious adverse effects.

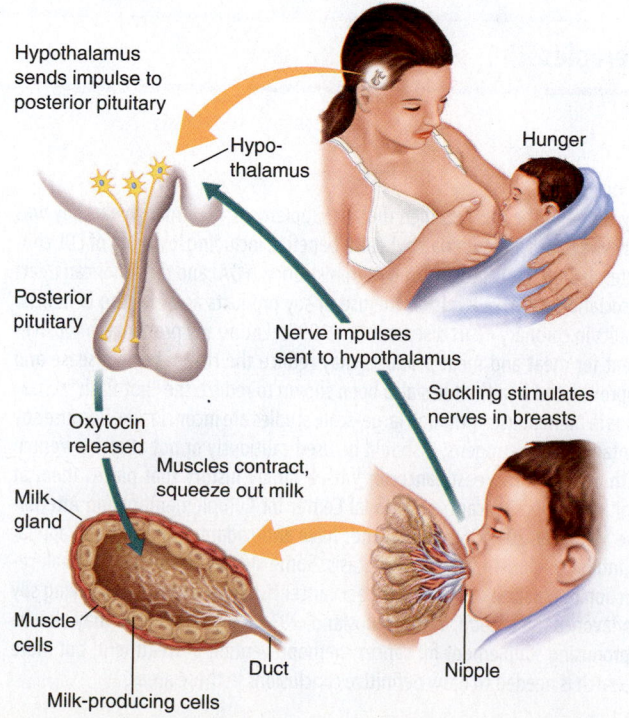

Figure 69.3 Oxytocin and breast-feeding.

(Methergine), is quite effective at promoting uterine contractions but is rarely prescribed due to the risk of serious HTN. Ergot alkaloids are also second-line drugs in the pharmacotherapy of migraines.

Several prostaglandins are also used as uterine stimulants. Unlike most hormones that travel through the blood to affect distant tissues, prostaglandins act directly at the site where they are secreted. In the uterus, prostaglandins cause intense smooth muscle contractions. Carboprost (Hemabate) may be used to control postpartum hemorrhage. Dinoprostone (Cervidil, Prepidil, Prostin E$_2$) is used intravaginally to promote cervical ripening, a softening and dilation of the cervix that must occur prior to vaginal delivery. Misoprostol (Cytotec) is another prostaglandin that has been used off-label to promote cervical ripening. When used in high doses, the prostaglandins can induce pharmacologic abortion (see Chapter 70).

PROTOTYPE DRUG Oxytocin (Pitocin)

Classification: Therapeutic: Drug to induce labor, uterine stimulant
Pharmacologic: Hormone, oxytocic

Therapeutic Effects and Uses: Oxytocin (Pitocin), identical to the natural hormone secreted by the posterior pituitary gland, is the drug of choice for inducing labor. Given by IV infusion

Pharmacokinetics:

Route(s)	IV or IM
Absorption	Destroyed in the GI tract
Distribution	Widely distributed in the extracellular fluid; small amounts may cross the placenta; secreted in breast milk
Primary metabolism	Rapidly destroyed in the kidney and the liver
Primary excretion	Small amounts via renal
Onset of action	IV: immediate; IM: 3–5 min
Duration of action	Half-life: 3–5 min

Adverse Effects: The most common adverse effects of oxytocin are rapid, painful uterine contractions and fetal tachycardia. Uterine rupture or fetal trauma from too-rapid expulsion through the pelvis, seizure, and coma are regarded as the most serious adverse effects. There is an increased risk of uterine rupture in women who have delivered five or more children. When given IV, vital signs of the fetus and mother must be monitored continuously to prevent fetal complications, such as dysrhythmias or intracranial hemorrhage. **Black Box Warning**: Oxytocin is not indicated for the elective induction of labor. Elective induction is the initiation of labor in a pregnant patient who has no medical indications for induction.

antepartum, oxytocin induces labor almost immediately by increasing the frequency and force of contractions of uterine smooth muscle. It is administered during the final stages of labor, after the cervix is dilated, membranes have ruptured, and presentation of the fetus has occurred. It is also used to induce labor in cases of maternal diabetes, pre-eclampsia, eclampsia, and erythroblastosis fetalis. It should not be used for elective induction of labor, due to potential adverse effects to the mother or baby.

Oxytocin is also approved to reduce postpartum hemorrhage following expulsion of the placenta and to aid in returning normal muscular tone to the uterus. This drug is approved at higher doses for the adjunct management of incomplete or inevitable abortion. Intranasal forms once used to promote milk letdown are no longer available in the United States.

Contraindications/Precautions: Oxytocin has an antidiuretic effect and care must be taken to avoid water intoxication. Oxytocin is contraindicated when there is evidence of fetal distress, placenta previa, uterine prolapse, active herpes infection, abnormal fetal position, and cervical cancer. Breast-feeding should be delayed for at least 24 hours after the drug is discontinued.

Mechanism of Action: Oxytocin increases the intensity and frequency of uterine smooth muscle contractions. When stimulated by sucking, oxytocin causes smooth muscle in alveolar ducts to contract, thus ejecting milk from the breast.

Drug Interactions: Vasoconstrictors used concurrently with oxytocin may cause severe HTN. Oxytocin may cause adverse cardiovascular effects when administered with fibrinolysin,

CONNECTIONS Complementary and Alternative Therapies

Soy as a Phytoestrogen

Description:
Soy, or soybean, is a nutritional food that is a major source of protein for many cultures, especially those in China and Japan. In the United States, soy has become increasingly popular and is one of the top 10 most utilized supplements. In addition to its nutritional value, soy contains estrogen-like (phytoestrogen) substances known as isoflavones. Soy milk is made by grinding soybeans into a fine powder, which is then mixed with water. Other products include soy sauce, soy flour, tofu, nutritional snack bars, and soy protein drinks.

History and Claims:
Soy has been used as a nutritional source for thousands of years. Claims for soy's benefits include anticancer effects, treatment of osteoarthritis, cholesterol-lowering effects, and reduction of menopausal symptoms. Soy isoflavones have been identified as dietary components that have an important role in reducing the incidence of breast and prostate cancers.

Standardization:
Standardization of soy is either to the amount of bean extract or to the amount of isoflavones in the product. The standard dose has not been established.

Evidence:
Soy is one of the most studied dietary supplements. For many years soy was believed to provide superlative health benefits, including lowering of LDL cholesterol. Both the Food and Drug Administration (FDA) and the American Heart Association (AHA) recognized the use of soy products as providing beneficial results in coronary heart disease in the 1990s. Eating soy protein as a replacement for meat and meat products may reduce the risk of heart disease and improve heart health. It has also been shown to reduce the "hot flash" sensations in menopause, although large-scale studies are inconclusive. Because soy contains phytoestrogens, it should be used cautiously or not at all by women with a history of breast cancer or with a family history that places them at high risk for breast cancer (National Center for Complementary and Alternative Medicine, 2012). Soy isoflavones have antioxidant properties and appear to inhibit angiogenesis and metastasis. Some studies have found a small reduction in prostate cancer and breast cancer risk for those who are taking soy isoflavones (Mahmoud, Yang, & Bosland, 2014). Soy isoflavones may also be a promising supplement for cancer chemoprevention or treatment, but more research is needed to draw definitive conclusions in these areas.

warfarin, and cyclopropane anesthesia. **Herbal/Food**: Ephedra used with oxytocin may lead to HTN.

Pregnancy: Category X.

Treatment of Overdose: Overdose will cause severe cramping and possible damage to the uterus. Discontinuation of the infusion will result in a rapid resolution of symptoms due to the short half-life of the drug.

Nursing Responsibilities: Key nursing implications for patients receiving oxytocin are included in the Nursing Practice Application for Patients Receiving Pharmacotherapy with Oxytocin (Pitocin).

Drugs Similar to Oxytocin (Pitocin)

Uterine stimulants also include prostaglandins (carboprost and dinoprostone) and the ergot alkaloid methylergonovine.

Carboprost (Hemabate): Carboprost, equivalent to endogenous prostaglandin F$_2$ alpha, is approved for controlling postpartum bleeding that has not responded to oxytocin and for inducing pharmacologic abortion between weeks 13 and 20 of gestation. For postpartum bleeding, it is administered by the IM route every 15 to 90 minutes until hemorrhage is controlled. Nausea, vomiting, diarrhea, and fever are common adverse effects. This drug is pregnancy category C.

Dinoprostone (Cervidil, Prepidil, Prostin E$_2$): Dinoprostone, or prostaglandin E$_2$, is approved to prepare the cervix for labor or to abort a fetus that has died. To promote cervical ripening, it is administered intravaginally. The gel form of the drug is placed into the cervical canal using prefilled syringes and doses may be repeated every 6 hours, as needed. The vaginal insert releases the drug slowly, over 12 hours. The insert may be quickly and easily removed once labor begins. Both the gel and the insert may stimulate the uterus to begin contracting. Like carboprost, GI effects and fever are very common adverse effects. This drug is pregnancy category C.

Methylergonovine (Methergine): Ergonovine is an older drug, approved in 1946. It may be administered by the PO, IM, or IV routes to control postpartum hemorrhage and restore uterine tone. The IV route is only used in emergency situations because it may produce serious HTN or stroke in the mother. Uterine contractions begin in 3 to 5 minutes after an IM dose. Cramping and GI-related adverse effects are common with this drug. The drug is contraindicated during pregnancy because it can cause immediate uterine contractions that could injure the fetus. This drug is pregnancy category C.

Uterine Relaxants: Tocolytics

69.6 Uterine relaxants are used to suppress preterm labor.

Preterm labor is the initiation of labor prior to week 37 of gestation. The most common cause of preterm labor is premature rupturing of membranes or infections of the chorion or uterus. If the organ systems of the fetus are determined to be immature, attempts may be made to delay labor because preterm infants have a high morbidity and mortality rate. Suppressing labor allows additional time for the fetal organs to develop and may permit the pregnancy to reach normal term. Bed rest is mandatory and corticosteroids may be administered to accelerate fetal lung maturity and reduce the incidence of neonatal respiratory distress syndrome.

Antibiotics such as ampicillin or erythromycin are indicated if the preterm labor is due to a uterine or chorionic infection. Preterm labor can be stopped and delivery delayed in about 50% of women, if the membranes have not yet ruptured. The success rate is only 25% in patients with membrane rupture.

Tocolytics are uterine relaxants prescribed to suppress preterm labor contractions. Typically, the mother is given a monitor with a sensor that records uterine contractions and this information is used to determine the doses and timing of tocolytic medications. Tocolytics can generally delay labor by only 24 to 72 hours, but this is often enough time for the fetus to develop normal lung function. The benefits of these drugs must be carefully weighed against their potential adverse effects, which include tachycardia in both the mother and the fetus. There is no clear evidence that tocolytics reduce perinatal or neonatal mortality.

Only a few drugs are available as tocolytics, and none can be realistically considered a prototype. For over 30 years, magnesium sulfate was the preferred drug for delaying preterm labor, but some evidence suggests that it may be ineffective and that it poses undue risks to the fetus and mother. The only drug that is FDA approved for this indication is ritodrine (Yutopar), but it is no longer available in the United States. Calcium channel blockers and beta-adrenergic agonists appear to be effective and are used off-label for this indication. Doses for these drugs are listed in Table 69.3.

Magnesium sulfate: A traditional tocolytic of choice, magnesium sulfate is administered by continuous IV infusion via a controlled pump device until preterm contractions diminish, usually in about 30 minutes. It is used off-label for this indication. During therapy, careful monitoring of deep tendon reflexes, blood pressure, respirations, urinary output, and serum magnesium concentrations are necessary. Early signs of magnesium overdose include flushing of the skin, sedation, confusion, intense thirst, and muscle weakness. Extreme levels cause neuromuscular blockade with resultant respiratory paralysis, heart block, and circulatory collapse. This drug is featured as a prototype electrolyte in Chapter 33 for the treatment of magnesium deficiency. Magnesium sulfate is pregnancy category A.

Nifedipine (Adalat, Procardia): Nifedipine is a calcium channel blocker widely prescribed for the treatment of HTN and angina. The drug has been used off-label as a tocolytic as an option to magnesium sulfate. Nifedipine is given either by the PO or sublingual route. A typical regimen includes a loading dose followed by additional PO doses every 15 to 20 minutes until contractions diminish. Nifedipine appears to be as effective as magnesium sulfate and the beta-adrenergic agonists but exhibits fewer adverse effects. Adverse effects include acute pulmonary edema, dysrhythmias, and hypotension. A prototype feature for nifedipine is presented in Chapter 30. This drug is pregnancy category C.

Terbutaline (Brethine): Terbutaline is a beta$_2$-adrenergic agonist that is FDA approved to treat acute bronchospasm due to asthma. It has been used off-label to suppress preterm contractions due to its ability to relax smooth muscle. It is given by the subcutaneous route either by injection every 20 minutes or by using a continuous infusion device; it may also be administered orally. Serious adverse reactions may occur. The mother may experience increased heart rate, dysrhythmias, myocardial ischemia, transient hyperglycemia, hypokalemia, and pulmonary edema. The fetus may experience increased heart rate and neonatal hypoglycemia. This drug is pregnancy category B.

CONNECTIONS: NURSING PRACTICE APPLICATION

Patients Receiving Pharmacotherapy with Oxytocin (Pitocin)

Assessment	Potential Nursing Diagnoses*
Baseline assessment prior to administration: • Obtain a complete health history including current length of pregnancy duration; presence of pre-eclampsia or eclampsia; recent labor; type of delivery; history of labors or cesarean sections; cardiovascular, neurologic, hepatic, or renal disease; diabetes; or breast-feeding. • Obtain a drug history including allergies, current prescription and OTC drugs, herbal preparations, alcohol use, and smoking. Be alert to possible drug interactions. • Evaluate appropriate laboratory findings (e.g., CBC, platelets, coagulation studies, electrolytes, glucose, magnesium level, and hepatic and renal function studies). • Obtain baseline height, weight, and vital signs. • Obtain fetal heart rate, intrauterine positioning. • Check for presence of cervical dilation and effacement. Monitor quality and duration of any existing contractions. Monitor fetal response to contractions, noting any sign of fetal distress. • Check for postpartum bleeding and note the number of pads saturated. • Assess the patient's ability to receive and understand instructions. Include the family or caregiver as needed.	• *Acute Pain* • *Deficient Knowledge* (Drug Therapy) • *Risk for Injury* (Patient or Fetus), related to adverse drug effects • *Risk for Excess Fluid Volume,* related to adverse drug effects
Assessment throughout administration: • Assess for desired therapeutic effects dependent on the reason the drug is given (e.g., strong, regular contractions supportive of labor, control of postpartum bleeding). • Continuously monitor timing, quality, and duration of contractions. Immediately report sustained uterine contractions to the health care provider. • Continuously monitor fetal heart rate and response to contractions. Immediately report signs of fetal distress to the health care provider. • Continue periodic monitoring of CBC, platelets, electrolytes, glucose, and magnesium levels. • Monitor vital signs frequently and immediately report any blood pressure above 140/90 mmHg or less than 90/60 mmHg, especially if accompanied by tachycardia, or per set parameters to the health care provider. • Continue to monitor postpartum bleeding and pad count. Notify health care provider if more than two full-size pads are saturated in 2-h time. • Assess for adverse effects: nausea, vomiting, or headache. Immediately report tachycardia, palpitations, HTN, especially associated with angina, severe headache, or dyspnea. Immediately report any severe abdominal pain, sustained uterine contraction, diminished urine output, dizziness, drowsiness, confusion, changes in level of consciousness, or seizures.	

Implementation

Interventions and (Rationales)	Patient-Centered Care
Ensuring therapeutic effects: • Monitor appropriate medication administration for optimal results. IV oxytocin must be given via infusion pump to allow for precise dosing. (Infusion pumps allow for rapid dosage adjustments to maintain uterine contractions supportive of labor until cervical dilation has reached approximately 5 to 6 cm.)	• Teach the patient about the rationale for all IV and monitoring equipment and the need for frequent monitoring to allay anxiety. • Teach the patient that labor contractions will gradually increase and that the drug will be decreased or stopped once contractions reach an optimal level. • Encourage laboring patients to use pain control measures (e.g., therapeutic breathing), or use pain control drugs as needed and as ordered.
Minimizing adverse effects: • Monitor timing, quality, and duration of contractions continuously. Immediately report any sustained uterine contractions to the health care provider. Stop the drug infusion, infuse normal saline or solution as ordered, and place the patient on her side until follow-up orders are obtained if contractions continue sustained. (Oxytocin may cause sustained uterine muscle contractions with potential uterine rupture. Uterine contractions must be monitored and any continuous, sustained contractions reported immediately.)	• Teach the patient that labor contractions will increase in strength and duration and will be monitored throughout. Instruct the patient to immediately report any sustained contraction or severe abdominal pain.

CONNECTIONS: NURSING PRACTICE APPLICATION (continued)

• Continuously monitor the fetal heart rate and response to contractions. Immediately report any signs of fetal distress to the health care provider. (Uterine contractions can affect the amount of blood flow through the placenta with diminished oxygenation to the fetus. Changes in fetal heart rate may signal fetal distress, and the patient should be placed on her side, oxygen administered unless otherwise ordered, the infusion stopped, and the health care provider notified.)	• Teach the patient that the fetal heart rate will also be monitored along with uterine contractions. Explain the purpose of all monitoring equipment to allay anxiety.
• Monitor vital signs and urine output frequently, and immediately report any blood pressure above 140/90 mmHg or less than 90/60 mmHg, especially if accompanied by tachycardia or diminished urine output, to the health care provider. (Oxytocin has vasoconstrictive and water-retention properties. Blood pressure and heart rate may increase and water intoxication is a possible adverse effect. Blood pressure or pulse rate exceeding parameters, increasing disorientation or confusion, and diminished urine output may signify adverse drug effects or possible complications.)	• Instruct the patient to immediately report any headache, dizziness, disorientation or confusion, palpitations, chest pressure, or pain.
• Monitor fundal firmness and location, postpartum bleeding, and pad count. Notify the health care provider if more than two full-size pads are saturated in 2-h time. (Oxytocin may be given to control postpartum bleeding. Lochia that increases, or if two or more pads are saturated over a 2-h period, should be immediately reported to the health care provider.)	• Instruct the patient to report any sudden increase in lochia, dizziness, light-headedness, or if more than two pads are saturated after 2 h.
Patient understanding of drug therapy: • Use opportunities during administration of medications and during assessments to discuss the rationale for drug therapy, desired therapeutic outcomes, commonly observed adverse effects, parameters for when to call the health care provider, and any necessary monitoring or precautions. (Using time during nursing care helps to optimize and reinforce key teaching areas.)	• The patient should be able to state the reason for the drug, monitoring needs, what adverse effects to observe for, and when to report them.

*Nursing Diagnoses—Definitions and Classification 2015–2017. Copyright © 2014, 1994–2014 by NANDA International. Used by arrangement with John Wiley & Sons Limited.

CONNECTION Checkpoint 69.2

Calcium channel blockers, including nifedipine, are widely used to treat cardiovascular disorders. From what you learned in Chapter 30, what effects would you expect nifedipine to have on vascular smooth muscle, myocardial oxygen demand, and myocardial conduction? *See Answer to Connection Checkpoint 69.2 on student resource website.*

Pharmacotherapy of Female Infertility

69.7 Female infertility may be treated with drugs that promote oocyte maturation and ovulation.

Infertility is defined as the inability to become pregnant after at least 1 year of frequent, unprotected intercourse. Infertility is a common disorder: 25% of couples experience difficulty in conceiving children at some point during their reproductive lifetimes. It is estimated that female reproductive tract conditions contribute to approximately 60% of the infertility disorders. Drugs used to treat female infertility are listed in Table 69.4. Treatment of male infertility is presented in Chapter 71.

PharmFACT

The most important preventable causes of infertility are chlamydia and gonorrhea infections. These infections can cause pelvic inflammatory disease, which can lead to infertility and ectopic pregnancies (Centers for Disease Control and Prevention, 2013).

The three primary causes of female infertility are pelvic infections, physical obstruction of the uterine tubes, and lack of ovulation. Extensive testing is often necessary to determine the exact cause, and it is not uncommon to find multiple etiologies for the infertility.

For women whose infertility is due to inadequate ovulation, pharmacotherapy may be of value. **Ovulatory dysfunction** is defined as the presence of abnormal, irregular, or absent ovulation. Signs and symptoms of ovulatory dysfunction include irregular or absent menses, excessive abdominal bloating, and mood lability. Confirmation of the disorder is made by measuring hormone levels.

Ovulatory dysfunction may occur at the level of the hypothalamus, pituitary, or ovary, and pharmacotherapy is targeted to the specific cause of the dysfunction. The most common etiology of ovulatory dysfunction is **polycystic ovary syndrome**, a condition in which the ovaries are filled with follicular cysts and the patient has elevated levels of androgens and estrogen. Hirsutism is commonly observed in these women due to the excessive androgen levels. Another cause of ovulatory dysfunction is hyperprolactinemia, excessive levels of the hormone prolactin, which is most frequently caused by a tumor of the pituitary gland.

Many women with ovulatory dysfunction can be successfully treated with drug therapy; restoring regular, monthly ovulation is an essential goal of fertility management. Ovulation induction protocols are sometimes divided into the following three medication groups, which are shown in Pharmacotherapy Illustrated 69.1:

• Drugs used to promote maturation of ovarian follicles

• Drugs used to trigger ovulation at the end of follicular maturation

• Drugs that promote ovulation to occur on a regular, monthly basis, at the midpoint of the menstrual cycle

Promotion of follicle maturation: Ovulation cannot occur unless the ovarian follicles receive a hormonal signal to mature each month. This signal is normally supplied by LH and FSH during the first few weeks of the menstrual cycle. Clomiphene

TABLE 69.4   Drugs for Female Infertility

Drug	Route and Adult Dose (Maximum Dose Where Indicated)	Adverse Effects
bromocriptine (Parlodel)	PO: 1.25–2.5 mg/daily (max: 2.5 mg 2–3 times/day)	*Nausea, vomiting, cramping, constipation, drowsiness, headache, orthostatic hypotension, anorexia* GI bleeding, psychosis, seizures, syncope
clomiphene (Clomid, Serophene)	PO first course: 50 mg/day for 5 days; start on fifth day of cycle following start of spontaneous or induced bleeding (with progestin) Second course if ovulation: Repeat first course until conception or for 3 cycles Second course if no ovulation: 100 mg/day for 5 days as above (max: 100 mg/day)	*Weight gain, symptoms of PMS, hot flashes, dermatitis* Blurred vision, ovarian hyperstimulation, cataracts, thrombosis of temporal arteries
danazol (Danocrine)	PO: 200–400 mg bid for 3–6 months, start during menstruation or if pregnancy test is negative, may extend to 9 months if necessary	*Hirsutism, alopecia, voice deepening, weight gain, vaginal dryness, reduction in breast size, edema, emotional lability, hot flashes* Thromboembolic events, hepatotoxicity, intracranial HTN
FSH- and LH-Enhancing Drugs		
chorionic gonadotropin-HCG (Novarel, Ovidrel, Pregnyl)	IM: 5,000–10,000 units 1 day following last dose of menotropins	Females: *Pelvic pain, depression, fatigue* Ovarian hyperstimulation syndrome Males: *Gynecomastia, acne* Aggressive behavior, depression
follitropin alfa (Gonal-F)	Subcutaneous: 75 international units/day initially, then increased by 37.5 international units at the end of 14 days. Further 37.5-unit dose increases may be made every 7 days if needed (max: 300 international units/day)	*Headache, nausea, abdominal pain, diarrhea, increased infections* Ovarian hyperstimulation syndrome, thromboembolic disorders
follitropin beta (Follistim)	Subcutaneous: 50–75 international units/day initially, then increased by 25–50 international units at the end of 14 days (max: 300 international units/day)	
menotropins (Menopur, Repronex)	Subcutaneous: 225 international units initially with 125 international unit dosage increases not more often than every 2 days	*Abdominal cramps, fullness, or pain, injection-site reaction, nausea* Ovarian hyperstimulation syndrome, thromboembolic disorders, respiratory disorders
urofollitropin (Bravelle)	For ovulatory females: subcutaneous: 150 international units once daily until sufficient follicular development is attained For anovulatory females: subcutaneous: 75 international units once daily. The dose should not be increased more than twice in any cycle or by more than 75 international units per adjustment	*Headache, nausea, abdominal pain, diarrhea, increased infections* Ovarian hyperstimulation syndrome, thromboembolic disorders
GnRH Antagonists		
cetrorelix (Cetrotide)	Subcutaneous: 0.25 mg/day during the early to midfollicular phase of the cycle following the initiation of FSH	*Hot flashes, headache, menstrual irregularities* Fetal death, ovarian hyperstimulation syndrome
ganirelix	Subcutaneous: 250 mcg once daily during the early to midfollicular phase of the cycle following the initiation of FSH	
GnRH Analogs/Agonists		
goserelin (Zoladex)	Subcutaneous implant for endometriosis: 3.6 mg every 28 days Subcutaneous implant for advanced carcinoma: 10.8 mg every 3 months	Females: *Headache, depression, sweating, acne, vaginitis, vaginal dryness, menstrual irregularities, bone density loss, emotional lability* Tumor flare (goserelin and leuprolide) Males: *Erectile dysfunction, lethargy, gynecomastia* Heart failure All patients: *Pain at injection site, hot flashes, loss of libido* Bone density loss, fractures
leuprolide (Eligard, Lupron, Viadur)	IM for endometriosis: 3.75 mg every month or 11.25 mg every 3 months Subcutaneous for infertility: 0.5–1 mg/day. By day 3 of the menstrual cycle, the dosage is typically decreased by 50%	
nafarelin (Synarel)	Intranasal: 2 inhalations/day (200 mcg/inhalation), one in each nostril; begin between days 2 and 4 of menstrual cycle (may increase to 800 mcg/day as 2 inhalations)	

Note: Italics indicate common adverse effects. Underline indicates serious adverse effects.

(Clomid, Serophene) is a drug of choice for treating female infertility because it stimulates the release of LH, resulting in the maturation of more ovarian follicles than would normally occur. The rise in LH level induced by clomiphene is sufficient to induce ovulation in about 80% of treated patients. The use of clomiphene assumes that the pituitary gland is able to respond by secreting LH, and that the ovaries are responsive to LH. If either of these assumptions is false, other treatment options must be considered.

If the infertility is a result of endocrine disruption at the pituitary level, therapy with human menopausal gonadotropin (HMG) or GnRH may be indicated. These therapies are generally indicated only after clomiphene has failed to induce ovulation. Also known as menotropins (Menopur, Repronex), HMG acts on the ovaries to increase follicle maturation and results in a 25% incidence of multiple pregnancies. Successful therapy with HMG assumes that the ovaries are responsive to LH and FSH. Newer formulations use recombinant DNA technology to synthesize gonadotropins containing nearly pure FSH, rather than extracting the FSH-LH mixture from urine.

Promotion of ovulation: Unless maturing follicles receive the final "burst" of LH, ovulation will not occur. HMG is similar in structure to natural LH and produces the same effect: ovulation.

Restoration of a normal monthly pattern of ovulation: The success of conception will be improved if a regular, monthly pattern of ovulation is established. Premature ovulation, the expulsion of the oocyte from the ovary before it has fully matured, is prevented by the use of two antagonists of GnRH: ganirelix and cetrorelix (Cetrotide).

Stimulation of the ovary by certain fertility drugs causes the ovaries to enlarge. Mild enlargement may cause pelvic pain but is generally benign and disappears when therapy is discontinued. One serious complication of certain fertility drugs is **ovarian hyperstimulation syndrome (OHS).** The onset of OHS is characterized by rapid, massive enlargement of the ovaries accompanied by nausea, vomiting, rapid weight gain, ascites, respiratory difficulties, increased risk of thromboembolism, and progressive kidney impairment. Progressive symptoms call for discontinuation of drug therapy, fluid restriction, bed rest, and symptomatic treatment of nausea, vomiting, and pain. Although OHS can be fatal, most cases resolve in 1 to 2 weeks.

Endometriosis, a cause of infertility, is characterized by the presence of endometrial tissue that has implanted outside the uterus in locations such as the surface of pelvic organs or the ovaries. Approximately 25% to 50% of infertile women have endometriosis. Being responsive to hormonal stimuli, this abnormal tissue can cause pain, dysfunctional uterine bleeding, and dysmenorrhea. The pain, discomfort, and infertility brought on by endometriosis may be treated by danazol, nafarelin, and leuprolide. These drugs suppress the production of estrogen and progesterone, resulting in a decrease in growth potential of endometrial tissues. Surgical removal, ablation, or laser vaporization of the abnormal endometrial lesions may be necessary. Women who have completed their childbearing or who are postmenopausal may consider a hysterectomy with oophorectomy.

Leuprolide (Lupron) and nafarelin (Synarel) are GnRH agonists that produce an initial release of LH and FSH, followed by suppression due to the negative feedback effect on the pituitary. Many women experience relief from the symptoms of endometriosis after 3 to 6 months of leuprolide therapy, and the benefits may extend well beyond the treatment period. As an alternative choice, danazol (Danocrine) is an anabolic steroid that suppresses FSH production, which in turn shuts down both ectopic and normal endometrial activity. While leuprolide is given only by the parenteral route, danazol is given orally. Estrogen–progestin oral contraceptives are also useful in treating endometriosis.

PROTOTYPE DRUG | **Clomiphene (Clomid, Serophene)**

Classification: **Therapeutic:** Infertility drug **Pharmacologic:** Ovarian stimulant

Therapeutic Effects and Uses: Approved in 1967, clomiphene is a drug of choice for female infertility caused by ovulatory dysfunction. It acts by inducing ovulation in anovulatory women. The pregnancy rate of patients taking clomiphene is high, and twins occur in about 3% to 5% of treated patients. Therapy is usually begun with a low dose for 5 days following menses because this is the time of greatest follicle maturation. If ovulation does not occur, the dose is increased. If ovulation still is not induced, HCG is added to the regimen. If pregnancy has not occurred following six cycles of successful ovulation, the drug is usually discontinued and other means of restoring fertility are explored. The use of clomiphene does not permanently restore normal follicle maturation. Its effects diminish once the drug is discontinued.

Clomiphene is used off-label to treat low sperm counts (oligospermia) in men. Just as in females, the drug increases the secretion of LH. In men, LH stimulates the testes to produce testosterone and additional sperm.

Mechanism of Action: Clomiphene is a SERM that has both estrogen agonist and antagonist effects, depending on the tissue. In the pituitary and hypothalamus, clomiphene acts as an "antiestrogen," shutting off LH secretion, which is required for ovulation. Clomiphene competes for estrogen receptors in the hypothalamus, sending a message that estrogen levels are low; thus, LH is secreted, leading to ovarian stimulation.

Pharmacokinetics:

Route(s)	PO
Absorption	Readily absorbed
Distribution	Crosses the placenta; unknown if secreted in breast milk; 90% bound to protein
Primary metabolism	Hepatic
Primary excretion	Feces; small amounts in urine
Onset of action	30–60 min
Duration of action	Half-life: 5–7 days; peak effects: 4–10 days

Adverse Effects: Few serious adverse effects occur during clomiphene therapy. The most common are weight gain, symptoms of PMS, hot flashes, allergic dermatitis, and urticaria. The most serious adverse effects are blurred vision, ovarian hyperstimulation, cataracts and other visual impairments, and thrombosis of temporal arteries. The drug may cause ovarian enlargement with subsequent pelvic pain in about 14% of women taking the drug.

Contraindications/Precautions: Clomiphene should be avoided in patients with lactation, gynecomastia, fibrocystic breast disease, liver disease, ovarian cysts not due to polycystic ovary syndrome, and hepatic, thyroid, or adrenal dysfunction. The drug is contraindicated in patients with dysfunctional uterine bleeding until the cause can be determined. Pregnant patients must not take this drug.

Drug Interactions: Androgens will reduce the success of clomiphene therapy. **Herbal/Food:** Black cohosh and chasteberry have estrogen effects that may reduce the effectiveness of clomiphene.

PHARMACOTHERAPY ILLUSTRATED 69.1

Mechanisms of Action of Drugs Used to Treat Female Infertility

(5) Antiestrogens shut off negative feedback to the hypothalamus, allowing more secretion of LH and a greater chance of ovulation
• Clomiphene

Hypothalamus

GnRH

(1) GnRH analogs desensitize pituitary GnRH receptors, resulting in sharply reduced levels of estrogen
• Goserelin, leuprolide, nafarelin

Pituitary

(2) GnRH antagonists block GnRH receptors in the pituitary to inhibit premature LH surge and allow follicles to finish maturing and normal ovulation to occur
• Cetrorelix, ganirelix

−

+

LH

FSH

Negative feedback

(3) Similar to LH, this drug induces ovulation
• Chorionic gonadotropin

(4) Similar to FSH, these drugs stimulate maturation of ovarian follicles
• Follitropins, menotropins

−

−

Ovary

Pregnancy: Category X.

Treatment of Overdose: Symptoms of overdose include nausea or vomiting, visual blurring, hot flashes, and pelvic pain. The patient is treated symptomatically.

Nursing Responsibilities:
• Prior to beginning therapy, obtain a pregnancy test to confirm that the patient is not pregnant. This is a category X drug that could cause fetal abnormalities.
• Assess for abnormal vaginal bleeding. If present, ensure that neoplastic lesions are not present prior to initiating therapy.

• Prior to initiating therapy, exclude other causes of infertility, such as thyroid disorders, adrenal disorders, hyperprolactinemia, and male factor infertility.
• Monitor laboratory results for increased levels of FSH and LH, and pregnancy.
• Counsel patients regarding the timing of drug therapy and intercourse to achieve pregnancy.
• Monitor for signs of ovarian hyperstimulation syndrome such as rapid weight gain, increased abdominal girth, nausea, vomiting, dyspnea, and chest pain. Report symptoms immediately to the prescriber.

Patient and Family Education:

- Record basal temperature at the same time each day on a graph to determine if ovulation has occurred. Ovulation occurs on days 4 through 10 in women who respond to treatment. There is an increased possibility of a multiple pregnancy.

- Take the medication at the same time each day to maintain consistent drug levels.

- Discontinue the drug and notify the health care provider if pelvic pain or abdominal distention occurs. This may indicate ovarian enlargement or presence of a ruptured ovarian cyst.

- Immediately report blurred vision, spots or flashes in the eyes, severe hot flashes, uterine bleeding, headache, and nausea to the health care provider.

- Report signs of jaundice such as yellowing of the skin or eyes, light-colored stool, and fever.

- Immediately notify the health care provider of any known or suspected pregnancy.

Drugs Similar to Clomiphene (Clomid, Serophene)

Other drugs for female infertility include bromocriptine, cetrorelix, chorionic gonadotropin-HCG, danazol, follitropins, ganirelix, goserelin, leuprolide, menotropins, and nafarelin.

Bromocriptine (Parlodel): Approved in 1978, bromocriptine is chemically related to the ergot alkaloids and is indicated for a large number of diverse conditions. The drug is a dopamine agonist, activating dopaminergic receptors in the hypothalamus. For infertility, its primary use is to treat prolactin-secreting tumors of the pituitary, which often cause amenorrhea and female infertility. Normal menses is usually restored after 6 to 8 weeks of therapy. This reduces elevated serum prolactin levels and restores ovulation and ovarian function in amenorrheic women. It is used as a short-term treatment of amenorrhea in the absence of pituitary tumors. It is also FDA approved to treat acromegaly and Parkinson's disease and to improve glycemic control in patients with type 2 diabetes. Off-label indications include mastalgia associated with PMS, alcoholism, cocaine withdrawal, and neuroleptic malignant syndrome. Bromocriptine causes frequent adverse effects that include nausea, vomiting, cramping, constipation, drowsiness, headache, orthostatic hypotension, and anorexia. This drug is pregnancy category C.

Cetrorelix (Cetrotide): Approved in 2000, cetrorelix is a GnRH antagonist given by the subcutaneous route that blocks GnRH receptors in the pituitary. Women undergoing ovarian stimulation with FSH or menotropin therapy experience a sharp rise in estrogen levels due to the maturing follicles, which can trigger an early surge of LH and premature ovulation. Cetrorelix inhibits this premature LH surge in women who are undergoing controlled ovarian stimulation for assisted reproduction, thus allowing follicles to finish maturing and normal ovulation to occur. The only indication for cetrorelix is infertility. Adverse effects are minor and include hot flashes and headache. It is contraindicated for use in primary ovarian failure, renal failure, and pregnancy. This drug is pregnancy category X.

Chorionic gonadotropin-HCG (Novarel, Ovidrel, Pregnyl): This drug has two forms. HCG is secreted by the placenta and obtained and purified from the urine of pregnant women. Choriogonadotropin alfa (r-HCG, Ovidrel) is a recombinant form with actions identical to those of HCG. The chorionic gonadotropin drugs have the same actions as LH and can mimic the LH surge that normally causes ovulation. As part of an assisted reproductive program, chorionic gonadotropin is administered at midcycle, after clomiphene or FSH has been used to mature sufficient numbers of ovarian follicles. A single IM dose is sufficient to induce ovulation. The drug has few adverse effects when administered as a single dose in females. This drug is pregnancy category X.

In males, HCG is approved to treat prepubertal cryptorchidism, hypogonadism, and oligospermia. Therapy in males may continue for several months. In males, gynecomastia, acne, and behavioral changes may occur.

Danazol (Danocrine): Danocrine is a PO drug used to treat endometriosis. Approved in 1976, the drug exerts antiestrogenic and weak androgenic properties, which causes ectopic endometrial tissue to atrophy. After 6 weeks of therapy, danazol causes anovulation and amenorrhea, which are its therapeutic effects. When the drug is discontinued, normal ovulation and menstrual cycles return in about 2 to 3 months. Danazol is also FDA approved to treat fibrocystic breast disease and for the prophylaxis of hereditary angioedema. The drug has androgenic actions that may cause permanent masculinization effects such as hirsutism, alopecia, voice deepening, and weight gain. Females may experience effects of estrogen deficiency such as vaginal dryness, reduction in breast size, emotional lability, and hot flashes. Serious adverse effects include thromboembolism, hepatic adenoma, and intracranial HTN. This drug is pregnancy category X.

Follitropins: The follitropins are three different drugs with the same actions. All are versions of human FSH. Urofollitropin (Bravelle) is FSH purified from the urine of postmenopausal females. Follitropin alfa (Gonal-F) and follitropin beta (Follistim) are FSH obtained through recombinant DNA technology. All three FSH products are given by the parenteral route. The function of FSH (and the follitropins) is to stimulate the maturation of ovarian follicles. The drugs are given early in the menstrual cycle, followed by a dose of chorionic gonadotropin, which provides the boost for ovulation. Multiple births, including triplets, quadruplets, and quintuplets, are common during therapy with follitropins. Care must be taken not to overtreat with follitropins because this can cause OHS. In males, follitropins are used to stimulate spermatogenesis in patients with hypogonadism and oligospermia. Minor adverse effects include headache, nausea, abdominal pain, diarrhea, and increased infections. The most serious potential adverse effects are OHS, thromboembolism, acute respiratory distress syndrome, and exacerbation of asthma. The follitropins are pregnancy category X.

Ganirelix: Like cetrorelix, ganirelix is a GnRH antagonist given by the subcutaneous route that blocks GnRH receptors in the pituitary. Approved in 1999, its only indication is for female infertility. Ganirelix inhibits the premature LH surge in patients undergoing controlled ovarian stimulation for assisted reproduction. Adverse effects are minor and include hot flashes, menstrual irregularities, and headache. It is contraindicated for use in primary ovarian failure, renal failure, and pregnancy. This drug is pregnancy category X.

Goserelin (Zoladex): Goserelin is a GnRH hormone analog or agonist. It has the same physiological actions as endogenous GnRH; however, the way it is administered causes the opposite effect. Natural GnRH is released by the hypothalamus in an "on–off" pulsatile manner, which stimulates the release of LH and FSH (and eventually estrogen). Like GnRH, goserelin first stimulates LH and FSH secretion. With continuous administration, however, the pituitary receptors become insensitive to the effects of GnRH and the gland stops releasing LH and FSH. Without FSH or LH, the levels of estrogen in females and testosterone in males fall dramatically. This hypoestrogenic state relieves the symptoms of endometriosis. It is also approved for palliative treatment of estrogen-dependent breast cancer and for advanced prostatic cancer. Goserelin is available subcutaneously as a once-monthly implant (for males or females) and a 3-month implant for males with prostate cancer. Females may experience hypoestrogenic effects such as vaginal dryness, depression, menstrual irregularities, bone density loss, emotional lability, and hot flashes. Males may experience erectile dysfunction, gynecomastia, and loss of libido. Pain at the injection site is common. This drug is pregnancy category X.

Leuprolide (Eligard, Lupron, Viadur): Like goserelin, leuprolide is a GnRH agonist/analog. The two drugs act by the same mechanism: desensitizing pituitary GnRH receptors, resulting in sharply reduced levels of estrogen and testosterone. For relief of endometriosis symptoms, a depot IM injection is given once monthly or once every 3 months, depending on the dose. Treatment of endometriosis is limited to 6 months. Like goserelin, it is also approved for the palliative treatment of advanced prostatic cancer and used off-label for breast cancer. Leuprolide is an orphan drug for treating precocious (early) puberty in children less than 9 years old. The drug was once widely used to treat infertility by inhibiting premature LH surges but the GnRH antagonists are now used for this indication.

The adverse effects are the same as those for goserelin. This drug is pregnancy category X.

Menotropins (Menopur, Repronex): Approved in 1975, menotropins is sometimes referred to as HMG. Menotropins is a product containing a combination of FSH and LH purified from the urine of postmenopausal women. The FSH activity of menotropins is significantly higher than its LH activity. Like the follitropins, menotropins is given by the parenteral route during the first half of the menstrual cycle to promote follicle maturation. At the end of therapy, HCG is often administered to supply the LH surge necessary for ovulation. Menotropins therapy is associated with a 20% to 35% possibility of multiple births. In males, menotropins is FDA approved to stimulate spermatogenesis in patients with hypogonadism and oligospermia. In males, gynecomastia, acne, and behavioral changes may occur. In females, the drug often causes ovarian enlargement and OHS is possible. Serious pulmonary conditions such as acute respiratory distress syndrome and exacerbation of asthma have been reported. This drug is pregnancy category X.

Nafarelin (Synarel): Like goserelin and leuprolide, nafarelin is a GnRH agonist/analog. The three drugs act by the same mechanism: desensitizing pituitary GnRH receptors, resulting in sharply reduced levels of estrogen and testosterone. Unlike the other GnRH analogs, nafarelin is applied topically to the nasal mucosa, where the drug is rapidly absorbed. When used to treat endometriosis, the typical dose is one spray in each nostril daily. It is also approved to treat precocious puberty and used off-label for hirsutism. Nafarelin may be used off-label to prevent premature LH surges in women with infertility; however, ganirelix and cetrorelix are more frequently prescribed for this indication. Adverse effects are the same as those of the other GnRH agonists goserelin and leuprolide. This drug was approved in 1990 and is pregnancy category X.

CHAPTER

69 Understanding the Chapter

Key Concepts Summary

69.1 Regulation of the female reproductive system is achieved by hormones from the hypothalamus, pituitary gland, and ovary.

69.2 Estrogens are administered as replacement therapy, to prevent conception, and for certain neoplasms.

69.3 Progestins are administered to treat dysfunctional uterine bleeding, to prevent conception, and for certain neoplasms.

69.4 Hormone replacement therapy provides relief from menopause symptoms but may have serious long-term negative effects.

69.5 Oxytocics are drugs used to stimulate the uterus and promote labor and delivery.

69.6 Uterine relaxants are used to suppress preterm labor.

69.7 Female infertility may be treated with drugs that promote oocyte maturation and ovulation.

Case Study: Making the Patient Connection

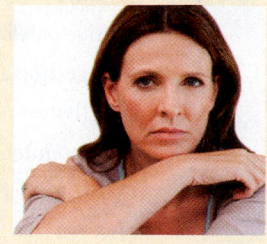

Remember the patient "Eileen John" at the beginning of the chapter? Now read the remainder of the case study. Based on the information presented within this chapter, respond to the critical thinking questions that follow the case study.

Eileen John is 46 years old and exhibiting signs of menopause. She reports a change in her menstrual cycle regularity. For the past year, her periods have occurred between 6 and 8 weeks apart and have lasted only 2 to 3 days. Previously, she experienced her periods approximately every 28 days and they lasted from 4 to 5 days. She reports to the nurse that she is now feeling easily fatigued, has more mood swings, occasional headaches, hot flashes, insomnia, bouts of depression, and irritability. She is also concerned about her loss of libido. She admits to smoking half a pack of cigarettes a day and drinking several cups of coffee during work hours. She has a family history of HTN, cardiac disease, and diabetes, but she has never been diagnosed with any of those disorders.

A complete history and physical examination, along with a vaginal examination and a Pap smear were performed.

Critical Thinking Questions

1. Do you think that Eileen is a candidate for hormone replacement therapy? Why or why not?
2. Create a list of some treatment options for Eileen.
3. Eileen asks about the precautions related to suggested treatment options. How would you respond?

See Answers to Critical Thinking Questions on student resource website.

Additional Case Study

Prithi Kaur, a 23-year-old woman, and her 25-year-old husband attend the infertility clinic for evaluation. Efforts at becoming pregnant naturally for the past 2 years have failed. They inform the nurse that the husband has a 3-year-old son from an earlier relationship. The wife has never conceived. Both denied any sexually transmitted infections. The patient is started on clomiphene (Clomid) 50 mg for 5 days.

1. Prithi asks you, the nurse, "What are some causes of infertility?" How would you respond?
2. What instructions would you give to the patient regarding the administration of this drug?

See Answers to Additional Case Study on student resource website.

Chapter Review

1 A 52-year-old patient experiencing symptoms of menopause is interested in taking hormone replacement therapy (HRT) with conjugated estrogen (Premarin). Which conditions may be a contraindication for HRT for this patient? Select all that apply.

1. History of type 2 diabetes mellitus
2. History of deep venous thrombosis
3. History of breast cancer with "lumpectomy" treatment
4. History of hyperlipidemia, controlled by drug therapy
5. History of two cesarean sections

2 The nurse is evaluating the effect of an oxytocin infusion in a laboring woman. Which of the following indicates that the drug is exerting therapeutic effects?

1. Hemorrhage is controlled.
2. Contractions are sustained at 60 seconds long.
3. Contractions are occurring every 4 minutes and lasting 20 seconds.
4. Milk letdown has begun in preparation of breast-feeding.

3 Which instruction about clomiphene (Clomid) will the nurse provide to a woman with infertility?

1. "The drug will be taken for a year and then reevaluated for an increased dose."
2. "After you are pregnant, the drug will be continued for the first 3 months of pregnancy to guard against miscarriage."
3. "You may stay on this indefinitely until pregnancy occurs. There are few adverse effects."
4. "If pregnancy does not occur within six cycles, other options for treatment will be explored."

4 A 48-year-old patient has received a prescription for medroxyprogesterone (Provera) for treatment of dysfunctional uterine bleeding. Because of related adverse effects, the nurse will teach the patient to monitor and report which symptoms?

1. Insomnia or difficulty falling asleep
2. Excessive mouth, eye, or vaginal dryness
3. Joint pain or pain on ambulation
4. Breakthrough spotting between menstrual periods

5 The patient informs the health care provider that she has been trying to become pregnant for more than 2 years and has not used any form of contraception. The health care provider prescribed clomiphene (Clomid) 50 mg/day for 5 days. The nurse should instruct the patient to begin taking the drug on the:

1. First day of the menstrual cycle.
2. Fifth day of the menstrual cycle.
3. Fifth day after ovulation.
4. Last day of the menstrual cycle.

6 A patient in preterm labor is receiving magnesium sulfate by IV infusion. Which early sign of magnesium toxicity would prompt the nurse to stop the infusion and notify the provider?

1. Hyperactive patellar reflexes
2. Chest congestion and coughing
3. Seizure activity
4. Sedation and intense thirst

See Answers to Chapter Review in Appendix A.

References

Centers for Disease Control and Prevention. (2013). *STDs and infertility*. Retrieved from http://www.cdc.gov/std/infertility/default.htm

Estephan, A. (2012). *Dysfunctional uterine bleeding in emergency medicine*. Retrieved from http://emedicine.medscape.com/article/795587-overview

Mahmoud, A. M., Yang, W., & Bosland, M. C. (2014). Soy isoflavones and prostate cancer: A review of molecular mechanisms. *The Journal of Steroid Biochemistry and Molecular Biology, 140*, 116–132. doi:10.1016/j.jsbmb.2013.12.010

National Center for Complementary and Alternative Medicine. (2012). *Herbs at a glance: Soy*. Retrieved from http://nccam.nih.gov/health/soy/ataglance.htm

Wellons, M., Ouyang, P., Schreiner, P. J., Herrington, D. M., & Vaidya, D. (2012). Early menopause predicts future coronary heart disease and stroke: The multi-ethnic study of atherosclerosis. *Menopause, 19*, 1081. doi:10.1097/gme.0b013e3182517bd0

Selected Bibliography

Bennington, L. (2010). Can complementary/alternative medicine be used to treat infertility? *American Journal of Maternal Child Nursing, 35*, 140–147. doi:10.1097/NMC.0b013e3181d76594

Bhagavath, B., & Carson, S. A. (2012). Ovulation induction in women with polycystic ovary syndrome: An update. *American Journal of Obstetrics and Gynecology, 206*(3), 195–198. doi.org/10.1016/j.ajog.2011.06.007

Davidson, M. R., London, M. L., & Ladewig, P. L. (2012). *Maternal newborn nursing and women's health across the lifespan* (9th ed.). Upper Saddle River, NJ: Pearson Prentice Hall.

deVilliers, T. J., Gass, M. L., Haines, C. J., Hall, J. E., Lobo, R. A., Pierroz, D. D., & Rees, M. (2013). Global consensus statement on menopausal hormone therapy. *Climacteric, 16*, 203–204. doi:10.3109/13697137.2013.771520

Herdman, T. H., & Kamitsuru, S. (Eds.). (2014). *NANDA International nursing diagnoses: Definitions and classification, 2015-2017*. Oxford, United Kingdom: Wiley-Blackwell.

Howles, C. M., Ezcurra, D., & Homburg, R. (2012). Ovarian stimulation protocols in assisted reproductive technology: An update. *Expert Review of Endocrinology & Metabolism, 7*, 319–330. doi:10.1586/eem.12.18

Levin, E. R., & Hammes, S. R. (2011). Estrogens and progestins. In L. L. Brunton, B. A. Chabner, & B. C. Knollman (Eds.), *The pharmacological basis of therapeutics* (12th ed., pp. 1163–1194). New York, NY: McGraw-Hill.

Mao, A. J., & Anastasi, J. K. (2010). Diagnosis and management of endometriosis: The role of the advanced practice nurse in primary care. *Journal of the American Academy of Nurse Practitioners, 22*, 109–116. doi:10.1111/j.1745-7599.2009.00475.x

National Heart, Lung and Blood Institute. (2010). *Women's health initiative*. Retrieved from http://www.nhlbi.nih.gov/whi

Ray, A., Shah, A., Gudi, A., & Homburg, R. (2012). Unexplained infertility: An update and review of practice. *Reproductive Biomedicine Online, 24*, 591–602. doi.10.1016/j.rbmo.2012.02.021

Schimmer, B. P., & Parker, K. L. (2011). Contraception and the pharmacotherapy of obstetrical and gynecological disorders. In L. L. Brunton, B. A. Chabner, & B. C. Knollman (Eds.), *The pharmacological basis of therapeutics* (12th ed., pp. 1833–1852). New York, NY: McGraw-Hill.

Taylor, H. S., & Manson, J. E. (2011). Update in hormone therapy use in menopause. *Journal of Clinical Endocrinology and Metabolism, 96*, 255–264. doi:10.1210/jc.2010-0536

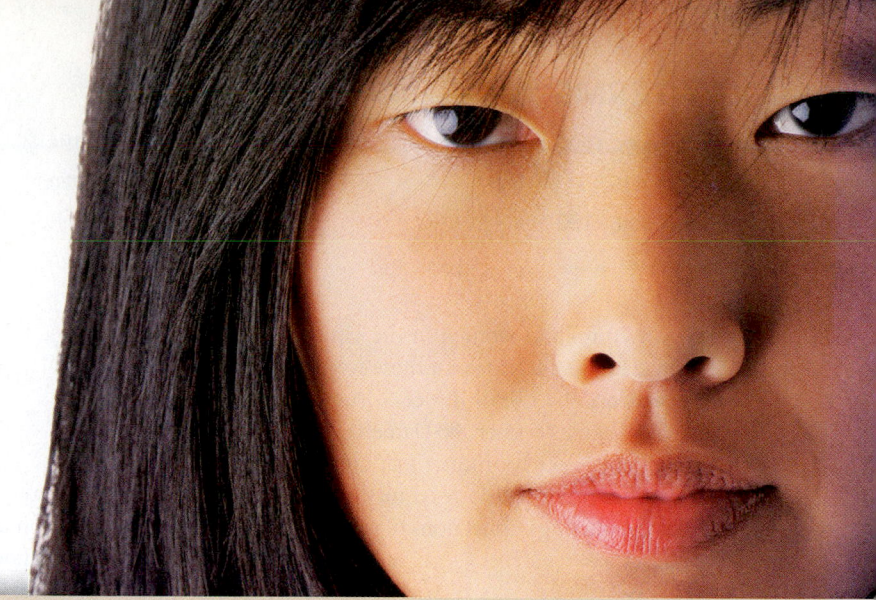

"I really don't want to ruin my chances of going to college by becoming pregnant right now in my life. What can I do?"

Patient "Lila Bastian," 19 years old

LEARNING OUTCOMES

After reading this chapter, the student should be able to:

1. Identify the choices available for birth control.
2. Delineate advantages and disadvantages of the different contraceptive options.
3. Explain the mechanisms by which estrogens and progestins prevent conception.
4. Compare the safety and effectiveness of different birth control methods.
5. Explain how drugs may be used to provide emergency contraception and to terminate pregnancy.
6. Describe the nurse's role in the pharmacologic management of patients who are taking oral contraceptives.
7. Compare and contrast the options available for long-term contraception.
8. Explain the use of drugs for emergency contraception and inducing pharmacologic abortion.
9. For each of the classes shown in the chapter outline, identify the prototype and representative drugs and explain the mechanism(s) of drug action, primary indications, contraindications, significant drug interactions, pregnancy category, and important adverse effects.
10. Apply the nursing process to the care of patients who are receiving pharmacotherapy for contraception.

CHAPTER OUTLINE

▶ **Options and Choices for Birth Control**

▶ **Combination Oral Contraceptives**
Estrogen/Progestin Combinations
PROTOTYPE Estradiol and Norethindrone (Ortho-Novum, Others), *p. 1194*

▶ **Progestin-Only Oral Contraceptives**

▶ **Adverse Effects of Combined Oral Contraceptives**

▶ **Drugs for Long-Term Contraception and Newer Contraceptive Delivery Methods**

▶ **Spermicides**
PROTOTYPE Nonoxynol-9, *p. 1200*

▶ **Emergency Contraception**

▶ **Drugs for Pharmacologic Abortion**
PROTOTYPE Mifepristone (Mifeprex), *p. 1203*

KEY TERMS

abortifacients, 1202

chloasma, 1197

contraception, 1190

ectopic pregnancy, 1194

emergency contraception
(EC), 1200

estrogen, 1190

progesterone, 1190

spermicides, 1199

More than 70 million women in the United States are of child-bearing age (15 to 44 years). Of these women about 62% practice **contraception**, the use of devices, drugs, or surgery to prevent pregnancy (Jones, Mosher, & Daniels, 2012). This chapter discusses the female sex hormones that are used to modify conception, describes other widely used methods of contraception, and identifies the nursing connections to patient and family education.

PharmFACT

Four out of five sexually active women have used oral contraceptives during their lifetime. This number has remained essentially unchanged since 1995. Use of 3-month duration contraceptives and transdermal patches has significantly increased during this time period (Daniels, Mosher, & Jones, 2013).

Options and Choices for Birth Control

70.1 Selection of a contraceptive is based on effectiveness, safety, and personal choice.

The decision to engage in sexual activity is one of the most important decisions in life; the choice affects not just the partners, but may impact generations to follow. A couple who is engaging in intercourse on a regular basis without contraceptive protection has a 90% probability of conceiving a child over the course of a year. Thus, the voluntary choice to use contraceptive measures is a critical decision faced by most women in the childbearing years.

Prior to the 1960s, the three primary methods of avoiding pregnancy were total abstinence, abstinence during periods of greatest fertility (rhythm or calendar method), and withdrawal prior to ejaculation (coitus interruptus). The discovery of oral contraceptives and the development of novel long-term contraceptives have given couples more effective choices for birth control. Many options are now available, each having specific advantages and disadvantages. The primary options, their effectiveness, and advantages and disadvantages are listed in Table 70.1.

Women make personal birth control decisions based on several factors. The effectiveness for preventing pregnancy and the safety of the medication or device are the highest priorities. Other factors, however, may be of personal concern. Women who engage in intercourse frequently or who are likely to forget to take their medication may prefer the convenience of the long-acting contraceptives. For patients who have a history of thromboembolic disorders, barrier protection or the use of progestin-only types of contraceptives are safer options. Factors that influence their decisions include the following:

- Effectiveness of the chosen method
- Adverse effects and safety
- Age
- Frequency of intercourse
- Ease of use and the ability to adhere to the required regimen
- Preexisting medical conditions
- Cultural beliefs and practices

Women seeking to prevent conception need to discuss the available options with their health care provider. Final decisions on choosing a contraceptive should be made voluntarily with full knowledge of its advantages and disadvantages, effectiveness, adverse effects, contraindications, and potential long-term risks. When the desire to have children in the future no longer exists, sterilization of either the male or female is the most common and effective option for birth control. Whatever the choice of birth control, personal motivation must be taken into consideration because it is important that the woman be consistent in using the chosen method if pregnancy is to be prevented.

Contraceptives act in different regions of the female reproductive tract. The student should refer to Pharmacotherapy Illustrated 70.1 often while reading this chapter to obtain an overall perspective on the sites and mechanisms of contraceptive action.

Combination Oral Contraceptives

70.2 The most effective oral contraceptives include combinations of low-dose estrogens and progestins.

The physiology and pharmacologic indications for the female sex hormones estrogen and progesterone are presented in Chapter 69. Because estrogen and progesterone are the two classes of drugs used most frequently for contraception, the student should review that chapter before proceeding.

The most widespread pharmacologic use of estrogen and progesterone is to prevent pregnancy. **Estrogen** is a general term that refers to several female sex hormones. The ones used in oral contraceptives are the synthetic estrogens ethinyl estradiol and, rarely, mestranol. All estrogens have the same pharmacologic actions.

Progestin is a general term that refers to synthetic hormones that have actions identical to progesterone. Although **progesterone** is the natural progestin secreted by the corpus luteum, it is rarely used for contraception. Instead, synthetic progestins including norethindrone, norgestrel, desogestrel, and levonorgestrel are used. The synthetic progestins have a much longer half-life than progesterone, which allows for the convenience of once-daily dosing. All progestins have the same pharmacologic activity.

The majority of oral contraceptives (OCs), known as "the pill," contain combinations of estrogen and progestin. Approximately 30% of the women who choose contraceptive methods select OCs. These inexpensive, readily available drugs are nearly 100% effective at preventing pregnancy when taken daily. They are excellent methods of contraception for women who are healthy and have no

TABLE 70.1   Effectiveness of Conception Modifiers

Type	Description	Pregnancy Rate (%/Year)* With Perfect Use	With Typical Use	Selected Advantages	Selected Disadvantages
Hormonal Methods					
Combination oral contraceptives (OCs)	Daily tablets	0.3%	9%	Very effective, decreased risk of ovarian and endometrial cancer	Fluid retention, venous thromboembolism, amenorrhea, nausea, vomiting, irregular bleeding, headache; must be taken daily
Progestin-only OCs	Daily tablets	0.5%	9%	No estrogen adverse effects; may be used in women with history of thromboembolic disease	Less effective than combination OCs; frequent spotting, amenorrhea, ectopic pregnancy
Progestin injections	Every 3 months	0.2%	6%	Do not have to take daily pills; long-term protection	Amenorrhea, irregular bleeding, headache, loss of bone density, may delay return of fertility when discontinued
Transdermal patches	Weekly patch	0.3%	5%	Do not have to take daily pills; easy to apply	Similar to OCs; higher risk of thromboembolic disease compared to OCs, irritation at application site
Subdermal progestin implants	Every 3 years	0.05%	1%	Do not have to take daily pills; long-term protection	Amenorrhea, irregular bleeding, headache
Barrier and Miscellaneous Methods					
Condoms (male), diaphragms	Coitus based	2–6%	12–18%	Inexpensive; some protection against sexually transmitted infections, no hormonal adverse effects; few significant adverse effects	Less convenient than hormonal methods
Spermicides	Coitus based	18	28	Inexpensive, no hormonal adverse effects	Ineffective if used without barrier protection; requires reapplication if intercourse lasts longer than 1 h; inconvenient; vaginal irritation
Contraceptive sponge	Coitus based	9–20%	12–24%	Inexpensive; no hormonal adverse effects; protection lasts 24 h	Allergic reactions, vaginal dryness or irritation; less convenient
Intrauterine devices/systems	Mirena, Skyla, Copper T380A; every few years	0.2–0.6%	0.2–0.8%	Effective, long-term contraception; decreased menstrual flow and cramping; inexpensive; no hormonal adverse effects (Copper T380A), quick return of fertility	Irregular bleeding, pelvic pain, spontaneous expulsion, uterine perforation
Withdrawal method	Coitus based	4%	22%	Free; no adverse effects	Requires cooperation of partner, inconvenient and ineffective
Biologic	Calendar/rhythm	3–5%	24%	Free; no adverse effects	Requires cooperation of partner, inconvenient and ineffective

*Pregnancy rates from using the various methods listed vary considerably in the scientific literature.

contraindications. One advantage of OCs is that they can be discontinued at any time without long-lasting adverse effects. In addition, one of the OCs, Nataxia, has an additional indication: heavy menstrual bleeding.

A large number of combination OC preparations are available, differing in dose and by type of estrogen and progestin, as listed in Table 70.2. Selection of a specific drug is individualized for each patient and determined by which product gives the best contraceptive protection with the fewest adverse effects. Treatment is generally initiated with the lowest dose that effectively provides

contraceptive protection. Daily doses of estrogen in OCs have declined from 150 mcg 40 years ago to about 20 mcg in modern formulations. This reduction has resulted in a significant decrease in estrogen-related adverse effects.

Typically, administration of an OC begins on day 5 of the menstrual cycle and continues for 21 days. During the other 7 days of the month, the patient takes a placebo. Although the placebo serves no pharmacologic purpose, it does encourage the patient to take the pills on a daily basis. Some of these placebos contain iron, which replaces iron lost due to menstrual bleeding.

PHARMACOTHERAPY ILLUSTRATED 70.1

Mechanisms of Action of Contraceptives

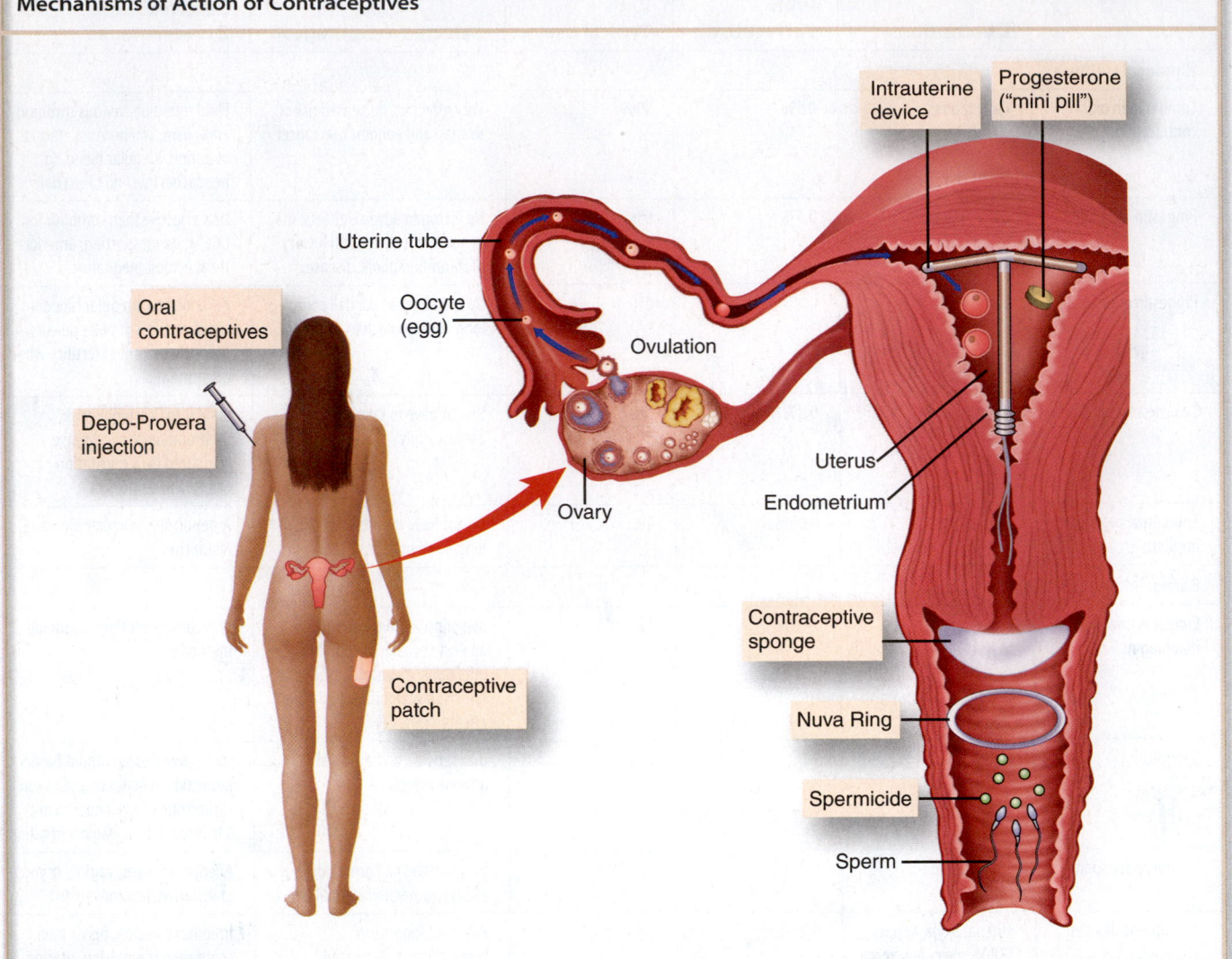

CONNECTIONS | Complementary and Alternative Therapies

◀ Black Cohosh

Description
Black cohosh (*Cimicifuga racemosa*) is a perennial that grows in open woods in the eastern United States and parts of Canada. "Black" refers to the color of its roots.

History and Claims
Use of this herb by Native Americans for more than 100 years has been recorded. These peoples used the herb for a variety of conditions, including sore throat, kidney ailments, fatigue, menstrual cramps, and to ease the pain of labor. Modern use of this herb has focused on its actions on the female reproductive system.

Standardization
Doses of black cohosh are sometimes standardized by the amount of the chemical 27-deoxyactein, which is an active ingredient. A typical dose of black cohosh ranges from 40 to 80 mg of dried herb per day. (Approximately 1 mg of 27-deoxyactein is present in each 20-mg tablet or in 20 drops of the liquid formulation.)

Evidence
Studies on the use of black cohosh in the management of menopausal symptoms have shown mixed results (National Center for Complementary and Alternative Medicine, 2012). A meta-analysis of 16 research studies found insufficient evidence to conclude that the herb has any effect on hot flashes, vaginal dryness, or night sweats (Leach & Moore, 2012). Although black cohosh was once thought to have phytoestrogenic effects, new research questions this fact and suggests that the supplement may act by reducing pain (Johnson & Fahey, 2012). Its actual mechanism of action is still unknown. Adverse effects include hypotension, uterine stimulation, and gastrointestinal (GI) complaints such as nausea. A number of research studies have reported that the herb is hepatotoxic (Abdualmjid & Sergi, 2013). Patients with a history of liver impairment should not take this herb.

TABLE 70.2 Selected Oral Contraceptives

Trade Name	Estrogen	Progestin
Monophasic		
Desogen	ethinyl estradiol, 30 mcg	desogestrel, 0.15 mg
Loestrin 1.5/30 Fe	ethinyl estradiol, 30 mcg	norethindrone, 1.5 mg
Ortho-Cyclen-28	ethinyl estradiol, 35 mcg	norgestimate, 0.25 mg
Yasmin	ethinyl estradiol, 30 mcg	drospirenone, 3 mg
Zovia 1/50E-28	ethinyl estradiol, 50 mcg	ethynodiol diacetate, 1 mg
Biphasic		
Mircette	ethinyl estradiol, 20 mcg for 21 days; 10 mcg for 5 days	desogestrel, 0.15 mg for 21 days
Triphasic		
Ortho-Novum 7/7/7-28	ethinyl estradiol, 35 mcg	norethindrone, 0.5 mg
	ethinyl estradiol, 35 mcg	norethindrone, 0.75 mg
	ethinyl estradiol, 35 mcg	norethindrone, 1 mg
Ortho Tri-Cyclen	ethinyl estradiol, 35 mcg	norgestimate, 0.18 mg
	ethinyl estradiol, 35 mcg	norgestimate, 0.215 mg
	ethinyl estradiol, 35 mcg	norgestimate, 0.25 mg
Tri-Norinyl-28	ethinyl estradiol, 35 mcg	norethindrone, 0.05 mg
	ethinyl estradiol, 35 mcg	norethindrone, 0.1 mg
	ethinyl estradiol, 35 mcg	norethindrone, 0.5 mg
Trivora-28	ethinyl estradiol, 30 mcg	levonorgestrel, 0.05 mg
	ethinyl estradiol, 40 mcg	levonorgestrel, 0.075 mg
	ethinyl estradiol, 30 mcg	levonorgestrel, 1.25 mg
Four-phasic		
Natazia	ethinyl valerate, 3 mg	—
	ethinyl valerate, 2 mg	dienogest, 2 mg
	ethinyl valerate, 2 mg	dienogest, 2 mg
	ethinyl valerate, 1 mg	—
Progestin Only		
Micronor	None	norethindrone, 0.35 mg
Nor-QD	None	norethindrone, 0.35 mg
Emergency Contraceptive		
Plan B and Plan B One Step	None	levonorgestrel, 1.5 mg

PharmFACT

The percentage of teens age 13 to 18 taking OCs increased from 12% in 2002 to 18% in 2009. At least part of this increase was likely due to expanded coverage for OCs in health insurance plans (Ehrlich, Gibson, & Mark, 2011).

A common problem with OCs, and likely the most frequent reason for treatment failure (pregnancy), is forgetting to take the medication daily. If one dose is missed, taking two pills the following day usually provides for continuous contraception. If two consecutive doses are missed, two tablets should be taken on both the day the missed doses are remembered and the following day. The regular schedule should then be continued, but a second method of contraception should be used for at least 7 days after restarting the pills. If 3 or more consecutive days are missed, the patient should implement other contraceptive precautions until the regimen can be restarted in the next monthly cycle. Figure 70.1 shows a typical monthly OC packet with the 28 pills.

Estrogen-progestin combination OCs act by preventing ovulation. They accomplish this by providing negative feedback to the pituitary, which suppresses the secretion of luteinizing hormone (LH) and follicle-stimulating hormone (FSH). Without the influence of LH and FSH, the ovarian follicles cannot mature and ovulation is prevented. The estrogen-progestin combination drugs also make the uterine

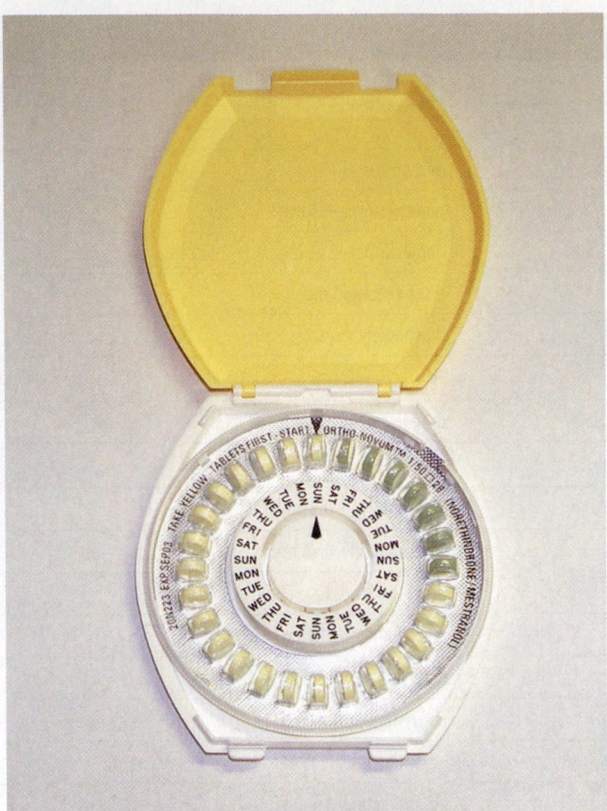

Figure 70.1 An oral contraceptive showing the daily doses and the different formulation taken in the last 7 days of the 28-day cycle.

endometrium less favorable to receiving an embryo, thus reducing the likelihood of implantation. In addition, the hormones promote the formation of a thick cervical mucus that slows sperm transport and inhibits the process that allows sperm to penetrate the ovum. The student should refer to Figure 69.2 in Chapter 69 for a review of the negative feedback control of female reproductive hormones.

CONNECTION Checkpoint 70.1

Certain drugs that are used to treat infertility block the negative feedback cycle by occupying the estrogen receptors in the hypothalamus. From what you learned in Chapter 69, name this class of drugs and explain how they are used to increase fertility. *See Answer to Connection Checkpoint 70.1 on student resource website.*

The four types of estrogen-progestin OC formulations are monophasic, biphasic, triphasic, and a four-phase version. The monophasic OC delivers a constant dose of estrogen and progestin throughout the 21-day treatment cycle. In biphasic drugs, the amount of estrogen in each pill remains constant, but the amount of progestin is increased toward the end of the treatment cycle to better nourish the uterine lining. In triphasic formulations, the amounts of both estrogen and progestin vary in three distinct phases during the treatment cycle. In 2010 the first four-phase OC, called Natazia, was introduced. Natazia contains a synthetic estrogen called estradiol valerate and a progestin called dienogest; this is the first time this specific combination has been used. The manufacturer claims that this four-phase combination more closely resembles the natural monthly hormonal variation. In 2012, Natazia was also the first OC approved to treat heavy menstrual bleeding.

When discontinuing OCs it may take several months for ovulation to return to normal and for monthly menstrual periods to become regular. Some women can conceive in the first month, whereas others experience a delay for up to a year before fertility is restored. The length of contraceptive use does not appear to affect fertility. The incidence of miscarriage is not increased in women who conceive after having taken OCs.

Although the main purpose for taking combination OCs is to prevent pregnancy, there are several other benefits. Women who are taking OCs report less painful menstruation and may have reduced incidences of the following disorders: **ectopic pregnancy**, which is the development of the fetus elsewhere rather than in the uterus; pelvic inflammatory disease (PID); ovarian and endometrial cancer; colorectal cancer; iron deficiency anemia; and benign breast diseases. Women on OCs also experience a better regulated menstrual flow and fewer outbreaks of acne.

Seasonale is an "extended regimen" OC that consists of tablets containing levonorgestrel and ethinyl estradiol that are taken for 84 consecutive days, followed by seven placebo tablets (without hormones). This allows for continuous contraceptive protection while extending the time between menses; only four periods are experienced per year. Seasonique is similar, but instead of inert tablets for 7 days, the patient takes low-dose estrogen tablets. Seasonique, which was approved in 2006, is claimed by the manufacturer to have a lower incidence of bloating and breakthrough bleeding. In 2008, a lower dose formulation of Seasonique, called LoSeasonique, was marketed.

PROTOTYPE DRUG	**Estradiol and Norethindrone (Ortho-Novum, Others)**

Classification: Therapeutic: Combination oral contraceptive
Pharmacologic: Estrogen-progestin

Therapeutic Effects and Uses: The primary use of Ortho-Novum is to prevent conception, for which it is nearly 100% effective. Ortho-Novum is available in monophasic, biphasic, and triphasic formulations. Off-label indications for the drug include acne vulgaris (in females who have achieved menarche), endometriosis, hypermenorrhea, dysfunctional uterine bleeding, and hirsutism related to hyposecretion of estrogen or oversecretion of androgens. Noncontraceptive benefits of Ortho-Novum include improvement in menstrual cycle regularity and decreased incidence of dysmenorrhea.

Mechanism of Action: Ortho-Novum decreases the potential for conception by inhibiting ovulation. When the right combination of estrogens and progestins is present in the bloodstream, the release of FSH and LH is inhibited, thus preventing ovulation.

Pharmacokinetics:

Route(s)	Oral (PO)
Absorption	83% (norethindrone) and 47–73% (ethinyl estradiol)
Distribution	Widely distributed; secreted in breast milk
Primary metabolism	Hepatic and GI mucosa; extensively metabolized
Primary excretion	Renal and feces
Onset of action	30–60 min
Duration of action	Half-life: 3–27 h

Adverse Effects: The most common adverse effects of Ortho-Novum are nausea, breast tenderness, weight gain, and breakthrough bleeding. Less common serious adverse effects include edema, unexplained loss of vision, diplopia, intolerance to contact lenses, gallbladder disease, nausea, abdominal cramps, changes in urinary function, dysmenorrhea, breast fullness, fatigue, skin rash, acne, headache, vaginal candidiasis, photosensitivity, and changes in urinary patterns. Cardiovascular adverse effects, the most serious of all, may include hypertension (HTN) and thromboembolic disorders. The estrogen component of the pill can lead to venous and arterial thrombosis, which results in pulmonary, myocardial, and thrombotic strokes.

Other conditions that are associated with OCs are abnormal uterine bleeding; benign hepatic adenoma; multiple births; elevated plasma glucose; retinal disorder; and melanoderma, a patchy or generalized skin discoloration caused by increased production of melanin. These conditions, though rare, have been reported, and tend to disappear immediately after discontinuing the use of OCs. **Black Box Warning**: Cigarette smoking increases the risk of serious cardiovascular adverse effects in women taking OCs containing estrogen. This risk increases markedly with age (over age 35) and with heavy smoking (more than 15 cigarettes per day).

Contraindications/Precautions: There are many contraindications and precautions regarding the use of OCs. The risk of cancer following long-term OC use has been extensively studied. Because some studies have shown a small increase in the incidence of breast cancer, OCs are contraindicated in patients with known or suspected breast cancer. The incidences of endometrial and ovarian cancers, however, are significantly reduced after long-term OC administration. It is likely that the relationship between the long-term use of these drugs and cancer will continue to be a controversial and frequently researched topic. Obesity is a risk factor for treatment failure and for increased possibilities of thromboembolic events. OCs may significantly worsen symptoms of lupus. Mood disorders, including depression, may be worsened in patients taking OCs. All combination OCs are pregnancy category X and are contraindicated in pregnancy.

Drug Interactions: A number of anticonvulsants (phenobarbital, phenytoin, carbamazepine, and primidone) and antibiotics (tetracyclines, rifampin, and ampicillin) can reduce the effectiveness of OCs, thus increasing a woman's risk of pregnancy. Women who are taking these drugs should be advised to use additional means of birth control or to have their OC dosages revised. Because OCs can reduce the effectiveness of warfarin (Coumadin), insulin, and certain oral hypoglycemic drugs, dosage adjustment may be necessary. Tranquilizers are known to cause false-positive pregnancy test results. Patients who are taking theophylline for asthma or imipramine as an antidepressant in conjunction with OCs should be evaluated often because these drugs may accumulate to toxic levels in these individuals. **Herbal/Food**: OCs have been shown to cause breakthrough bleeding when used concurrently with St. John's wort.

Pregnancy: Category X.

Treatment of Overdose: There is no specific treatment for overdose. The patient is treated symptomatically.

Nursing Responsibilities: Key nursing implications for patients receiving conjugated estrogens are included in the Nursing Practice Application for Patients Receiving Hormonal Contraceptives.

Drugs Similar to Estradiol and Norethindrone (Ortho-Novum, Others)

Dozens of different estrogen-progestin combinations are available as OCs. All have the same types of adverse effects. Those with higher doses may be expected to produce more adverse effects.

Progestin-Only Oral Contraceptives

70.3 Oral contraceptives that contain only progestin are often used when estrogen is contraindicated.

Although most OCs use a combination of estrogen and progestin, a few products contain only progestin. The progestin-only OCs, sometimes called minipills, are less effective at preventing ovulation. They prevent pregnancy primarily by causing a thick, viscous cervical mucus at the entrance to the uterus that discourages sperm penetration. They also tend to inhibit implantation of a fertilized egg.

Progestin-only oral contraceptives are taken daily throughout the month without the use of placebo tablets. Minipills are somewhat less effective than estrogen-progestin combinations, having a failure rate of 1% to 4%. Their use also results in a higher incidence of irregular menstrual cycles, including amenorrhea, prolonged bleeding, or breakthrough spotting. Menstrual irregularity is the most frequently reported adverse effect. The risk of ectopic pregnancy is higher with progestin-only products. Progestin-only PO drugs are generally reserved for patients who are at high risk for estrogen-related adverse effects or who are lactating. Unlike estrogens, progestins are not associated with a higher risk of thromboembolic events, and they do not have any

---

CONNECTIONS | **Treating the Diverse Patient**

◀ **The Possibility of a Male Birth Control Pill**

The search for a male equivalent to women's OCs continues. As for existing OCs, any drug would need to be safe, reliable, reversible, and affordable. One of the difficulties with modeling a male contraceptive pill after female OCs is similar: Potential systemic effects that are unwanted and potentially detrimental may occur. Several approaches to finding a male birth control pill are feasible, including suppressing or halting sperm production or blocking or inhibiting sperm function. Two of the more promising lines of research have been into the use of a form of retinoic acid (Vitamin A) and a new class of cancer drugs currently under study (Kean, 2012). Both drug groups disrupt spermatogenesis and have been shown to cause a reversible disruption of male fertility in mice. Human trials, large-scale clinical trials, and comparative studies among different ethnic groups will be needed for these drugs and the possibility of a male birth control pill is still many years away.

effect on breast cancer. The progestin-only products are pregnancy category X.

Products that contain norethindrone only include Aygestin, Camila, Errin, Jolivette, Nora-BE, and Ortho Micronor. In addition to contraception, norethindrone therapy is approved to treat amenorrhea, dysfunctional uterine bleeding, and endometriosis. The doses used for contraception are only 0.35 mg per day, whereas those for uterine conditions are 2.5 to 10 mg per day. Detailed information on the contraindications, drug interactions, and adverse effects of progestins are included in Chapter 69, along with a prototype feature for medroxyprogesterone (Provera).

Adverse Effects of Combined Oral Contraceptives

70.4 The adverse effects of combined oral contraceptives are uncommon but may be serious in some women.

The adverse effects of combination OCs have been extensively studied, and various risk factors have been identified. These are summarized in Table 70.3. For the large majority of patients, OCs are safe and serious adverse effects are uncommon. A few of the adverse effects, however, may be serious. Because OCs are so widely prescribed, nurses should become familiar with the adverse effects and incorporate them into the teaching component of the treatment plan.

Much of the early research on OCs was performed on women who were taking high doses of estrogens and progestins. Most, and perhaps all, of the serious adverse effects of OCs are dose dependent. The newer low-dose formulations result in far less risk than the original OCs. Furthermore, much less research has been conducted on the newer delivery methods for contraception (see Section 70.5), which may have a different spectrum of adverse effects.

The Centers for Disease Control and Prevention and the World Health Organization have developed a comprehensive list of preexisting medical conditions as absolute contraindications for the use of hormonal contraceptives (Division of Reproductive Health, N. C., 2013). These include current breast cancer, severe hepatic cirrhosis, major surgery with prolonged immobilization, migraines (with aura), impaired cardiac function, complicated valvular heart disease, HTN (systolic ≥ 160 or diastolic ≥ 100), smoking (age ≥ 35, ≥15 cigarettes/day), history of stroke, systemic lupus erythematosus (positive or unknown antiphospholipid antibodies), and high risk for thromboembolic disorders. Relative contraindications exist when there are preexisting disorders such as depression, migraines (without aura), epilepsy, epilepsy therapy (with certain anticonvulsants), and controlled HTN. The nurse should discuss nonhormonal contraceptive choices for women who have serious medical conditions for which OCs are contraindicated.

CONNECTION Checkpoint 70.2

Thromboembolic events are a serious concern for many patients who are taking OCs. From what you learned in Chapter 38, identify the classes of drugs that may be used to reduce the risk of thromboembolic events in high-risk patients. *See Answer to Connection Checkpoint 70.2 on student resource website.*

About 5% of women who are taking OCs will develop HTN because the drugs elevate angiotensin and aldosterone levels. Angiotensin is a vasopressor substance produced by the kidney, and aldosterone is a hormone secreted by the adrenal cortex of the

---

TABLE 70.3 Adverse Effects Associated with Oral Contraceptives

Adverse Effect	Prevention
Breast milk reduction	Some studies suggest that OCs may reduce the quantity of breast milk. They should not be taken until 6 weeks postpartum.
Cancer	Women who test positive for the HPV have an increased risk of cervical cancer. These patients should have regular checkups. Because estrogens promote the growth of certain types of breast cancer, patients with a history of this cancer should not take OCs.
Glucose elevation	OCs may cause slight increases in blood glucose. Patients with diabetes should monitor their serum glucose carefully during OC therapy.
Hypertension	Risk is increased with age, dose, and length of therapy. Blood pressure should be monitored periodically and antihypertensives prescribed as needed.
Increased appetite, weight gain, fatigue, depression, acne, hirsutism	These are common effects that are often caused by high amounts of progestin. The dose of progestin may need to be lowered.
Lupus exacerbation	Symptoms of systemic lupus erythematosus may worsen in some patients. A progestin-only OC may be an option for these patients.
Menstrual irregularities	Amenorrhea or hypermenorrhea is often caused by low amounts of progestin. The dose of progestin may need to be increased. Breakthrough bleeding and spotting are common with the low-dose OCs. The patient may need a higher dose product.
Migraines	Estrogen may decrease or increase the incidence of migraines. Because migraines are a risk factor for stroke, patients with migraines should seek advice from their health care provider.
Nausea, edema, breast tenderness	These are common effects that are often caused by high amounts of estrogen. The dose of estrogen may need to be lowered.
Teratogenicity	Estrogens are pregnancy category X. Patients should be advised to discontinue OCs if pregnancy is confirmed.
Thromboembolic disorders	Estrogens promote blood clotting. OCs should not be prescribed for patients with a history of thromboembolic disorders, strokes, coronary artery disease, or who are heavy smokers.

kidney (see Chapter 31). The action of both substances can result in HTN. The mean elevation from high doses of OCs is about 3 to 6 mmHg systolic and 2 to 5 mmHg diastolic. Low-dose formulations do not pose a major risk for HTN.

OCs can mimic certain symptoms of pregnancy, including breast tenderness, nausea, bloating, and **chloasma**, which is a darkened pigmentation found on the forehead, temples, cheeks, and upper lips. If a woman suspects pregnancy while taking an OC, the drug should be discontinued immediately because estrogen and progestin can cause fetal harm.

Because estrogen and progesterone can stimulate the growth of some types of cancers, the incidence of cancer in women taking OCs has been studied for several decades in large numbers of women. Some studies have demonstrated that long-term use may pose a slightly higher risk of breast cancer, whereas others have shown no relationship. Cervical cancer is also slightly increased, and this has been closely associated with human papillomavirus (HPV) infections. The risk of liver cancer may be increased. However, OCs appear to have protective effects for ovarian and endometrial cancers that continue for many years after the drugs are discontinued. A protective effect has also been observed for colorectal cancer. Conclusions of these studies are that women who have a personal or very close family history of breast cancer should explore nonhormonal means of contraception. All women who are taking OCs should be instructed to perform breast self-examinations, as recommended by their health care provider, and be aware of the importance of routine scheduling of mammograms that are appropriate for their age range.

Other conditions associated with OCs are abnormal uterine bleeding, benign hepatic adenoma, multiple births, retinal disorders, and melanoderma. These conditions, though rare, have been reported and they normally resolve after discontinuing the use of OCs. OCs may accelerate the formation of gallstones in patients who have preexisting gallbladder disease. The drugs may increase glucose levels and suppress insulin responsiveness, although this can be prevented by adjustments in the insulin dose of patients with diabetes.

Although not an adverse effect, health care providers and their patients should be aware that some studies have indicated an increased risk for pregnancy in overweight or obese women (Lopez et al., 2013). Among the various methods of birth control, transdermal patches appear to be least effective in obese women. The correlation between effectiveness and weight (or BMI) is an ongoing area of research.

When discussing the risks and benefits of hormonal contraception with patients, the nurse should place the drug in context with the health risks associated with pregnancy and delivery. Many patients do not understand that pregnancy itself may cause many challenging health conditions for the mother. Pregnancy-related deaths in the United States are approximately 14.5 per 100,000 live births, with African American women having the highest incidence of death (Berg, Callaghan, Syverson, & Henderson, 2010). Maternal morbidity includes conditions such as hemorrhages, preeclampsia or eclampsia, obstetric trauma, infections, gestational diabetes, and HTN. Placed in the proper context, the risks of pregnancy for most patients (those without absolute contraindications for OC use) are likely as great, or greater, than hormonal contraception.

Drugs for Long-Term Contraception and Newer Contraceptive Delivery Methods

70.5 Long-acting contraceptives and novel delivery methods offer women additional birth control choices.

Delivery methods have been developed that are able to provide effective contraceptive protection for periods lasting from weeks to years. The long-acting drugs and novel delivery systems were developed to offer ease of use and improve adherence. They vary in efficacy, reversibility, and discreteness of use. It is important for nurses and patients to understand that the long-acting methods are not more effective than the daily OCs and that they have the same types of contraindications and adverse effects. These long-acting contraceptives deliver medications by patches, vaginal inserts, injections, subdermal implants, and intrauterine devices.

Transdermal delivery method: Transdermal hormonal contraception is a safe, effective, and easy-to-use birth control method. Approved in 2001, Ortho-Evra is a topical patch worn on the skin of the buttock, arms, or trunk that contains ethinyl estradiol and norelgestromin. The patch slowly releases the hormones, which penetrate the skin and are distributed throughout the body. The patch is changed every 7 days for the first 3 weeks, followed by a patch-free week 4 (days 22–28). The patch may be worn during bathing, exercise, and other daily activities. Should the patch fall off, which occurs in about 5% of the applications, it should be replaced as soon as possible. Forgetting to replace or change the patch will result in a rapid loss of contraceptive protection. After the patch is removed, hormone levels return to normal within 3 days. The serum estrogen levels of patients who use the patch are 60% higher compared to those of patients who take combination OCs.

The most frequently reported adverse effects of the Ortho-Evra patch include headache, vomiting, nausea, breast discomfort, breakthrough bleeding, and dysmenorrhea. Long-term effects and contraindications are the same as those of OCs. Some research suggests that patients using the patch have an increased risk of venous thromboembolism (VTE) compared to women taking OCs. In 2008, the U.S. Food and Drug Administration (FDA) added a statement to the label of Ortho-Evra that women with a history of serious blood clots should discuss other means of contraception with their health care provider. To reduce postpartum risk for VTE, 3 to 6 weeks should elapse between delivery and use of the transdermal patch. Used patches still contain significant levels of hormones and must be discarded in a waste container away from children and pets. They should not be flushed down the toilet because residual estrogen can pollute wastewater, lakes, and streams.

Vaginal delivery method: The NuvaRing, illustrated in Figure 70.2, is a flexible, soft vaginal ring impregnated with a low-dose, sustained release, combined hormonal contraceptive. It is approximately 2 to 3 inches in diameter and contains ethinyl estradiol and etonogestrel. The ring is inserted into the vagina once a month to provide 3 weeks of contraceptive protection. The ring slowly releases the hormones, which are absorbed across the vaginal mucosa into the blood and distributed throughout the body. The contraceptive action is systemic in nature and not

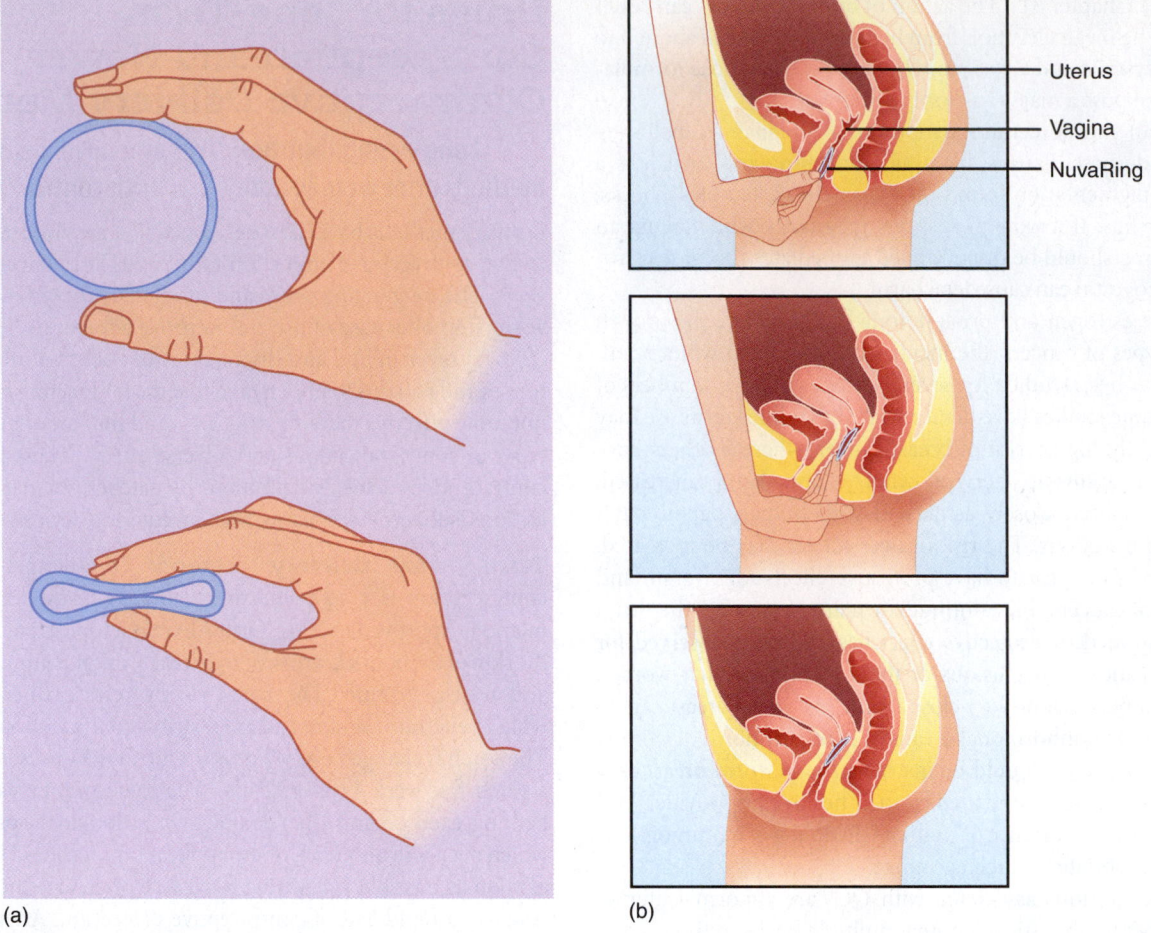

Figure 70.2 Vaginal medication administration: (a) The NuvaRing® contraceptive; (b) proper insertion of the NuvaRing.

localized to the vagina. The ring is removed at the end of week 3, and a new ring is inserted a week later during the first week of the next menstrual cycle. If forgotten and left in place for more than 3 weeks, contraceptive action will be lost.

The main adverse effects of NuvaRing are similar to those of combination OCs. Women sometimes discontinue using the vaginal delivery method due to discomfort of the device during intercourse. Women who are experiencing uterine prolapse must monitor the ring frequently because it may fall out. Adverse effects include nausea, bloating, headaches, breast tenderness, and break-through bleeding. If the ring is expelled from the vagina, it may be rinsed with water and replaced. Local effects may include vaginal irritation, sensation of a foreign body, and vaginitis. The NuvaRing should be discarded in a waste container away from children and not flushed down the toilet.

Depot injection methods: Intramuscular medroxyprogesterone acetate (Depo-Provera, depo-subQ-Provera) was approved for contraceptive use in the United States in 2004. A single deep intramuscular (IM) injection of 100 mg of Depo-Provera provides 3 months of contraceptive protection. The same drug may be injected subcutaneously (depo-subQ-Provera) with the same duration of action and effectiveness. Medroxyprogesterone suppresses ovulation, inhibits sperm from reaching the egg by thickening the cervical mucus, and prevents a fertilized egg from implanting in the uterus. Neither of the depot delivery methods contains estrogen. The drug is usually given on days 1 through 5 of the menstrual cycle to postpartum women who are not breast-feeding. Breast-feeding women should wait until week 6 postpartum to take the drug. The dose is repeated every 3 months as long as contraception is desired. The depot injection methods are very effective at preventing pregnancy.

Once injected the actions of the drug cannot be reversed and fertility may not be restored for up to 12 months after discontinuation. The most common adverse effects are menstrual disturbances, headache, acne, injection-site reactions, weight gain, and decreased libido. This drug carries a black box warning that long-term use causes significant loss of bone mineral density. This drug is pregnancy category X. Medroxyprogesterone is also approved to treat inoperable endometrial and renal carcinomas and menstrual disturbances. A prototype feature for medroxyprogesterone may be found in Chapter 69.

Subdermal implant delivery: Although several contraceptive subdermal implants have been approved since 1996, only Implanon is available. A single plastic tube about the size of a matchstick, Implanon contains 68 mg of the progestin etonogestrel. Inserted on the inner side of the upper arm, the device releases the progestin slowly, for up to 3 years. Although the device can be readily removed, some women may experience pain, inflammation, or hematoma at the removal site. Other side effects are the same as those of other progestins.

Intrauterine devices: Three intrauterine devices (IUDs) are available. These devices, ParaGard, Mirena, and Skyla, are all designed in a T shape and have been in use for many years. They are safe, inexpensive, and reliable methods of contraception. They offer a major advantage for women who are likely to forget a daily pill or who prefer greater ease of use. The IUD is not felt by the woman or her partner during intercourse and it can be removed at any time. Fertility returns quickly after removal of the device. Despite these advantages, only 2% of women who use birth control use IUDs.

The oldest product, ParaGard, also known as Copper T380A, is a plastic device that is partially covered with copper. It is inserted into the uterus, where the copper triggers a spermicidal-like reaction in the body that slows sperm motility and prevents the sperm from reaching the ovum. If fertilization does occur, implantation is not likely to happen because the copper causes endometrial changes to make the lining less favorable. Unlike the hormonal methods, ParaGard has no effect on ovulation. It can be left in place for up to 10 years, and the main adverse effects are bleeding between menses, dysmenorrhea, and expulsion of the device. ParaGard is an important nonhormonal option for patients who have contraindications to using estrogen or progesterone.

Mirena is an intrauterine system consisting of a polyethylene reservoir containing levonorgestrel that is slowly released. Contraception results from a thickening of the endometrium and increased cervical mucus that slows down sperm motility. Mirena decreases menstrual pain and lowers blood loss. This drug acts locally to prevent conception for up to 5 years. The effectiveness of Mirena is similar to that of OCs. This device may be removed at any time, and fertility returns quickly. The most common adverse effects of this IUD are uterine/vaginal bleeding alterations, amenorrhea, intermenstrual bleeding and spotting, abdominal/pelvic pain, and ovarian cysts.

Skyla is a newer IUD, approved in 2013. It contains the same progestin as Mirena, but it is smaller and is approved for up to 3 years of contraceptive use. While Mirena is recommended for women who have had at least one child, Skyla may be inserted into women who have not had children.

Spermicides

70.6 Spermicides are safe but should be combined with barrier protection for maximum effectiveness.

Spermicides are drugs that kill sperm. They come in a variety of creams, foams, jellies, and suppositories that immobilize or destroy sperm when inserted into the vagina prior to intercourse. Two spermicides used in contraceptive products are nonoxynol-9 and octoxynol-9. Spermicides are available over the counter (OTC).

To be effective spermicides must be applied high into the vagina, as close to the cervix as possible, approximately 20 minutes before intercourse. Most spermicides have a duration of action of only 1 hour and must be reapplied if coitus extends beyond this time.

The contraceptive sponge (Today Sponge), which is illustrated in Figure 70.3, is a soft absorbent sponge impregnated with nonoxynol-9. The sponge is moistened with water to activate the spermicides and inserted into the vagina to cover the cervix. The sponge releases the drug slowly and may provide up to 24 hours of contraceptive protection. It is left in place for 6 hours after intercourse but must be removed by 30 hours after insertion. The sponge delivery system has the same effectiveness as spermicidal gels, creams, and suppositories. Adverse effects include local irritation and vaginal dryness.

Patients should be informed that spermicides have low levels of effectiveness when used alone and should therefore be used in conjunction with barrier methods such as condoms and diaphragms. Research has also determined that nonoxynol-9 does not offer any protection against chlamydia, gonorrhea, or the human immunodeficiency virus (HIV) as previously thought. In fact, frequent use of spermicides disrupts the vaginal epithelium and may actually increase the risk of HIV transmission from an infected partner. This drug also disrupts the anal mucosa, possibly increasing the risk of HIV transmission and should not be used for anal intercourse. Patients must be instructed to take added precautions to prevent such transmissions.

CONNECTIONS Community-Oriented Practice

◀ Macular Edema in Women on Oral Contraceptives

A higher risk of thromboembolic conditions is associated with OC use. Women are advised to immediately report any signs or symptoms such as calf redness and swelling, chest pain, dyspnea, or severe headache to their provider. Macular edema, secondary to retinal vascular occlusion, is also possible. If untreated, it may lead to progressive vision loss and blindness (Aggarwal, Gujarant, Mishra, & Aggarwal, 2013). Because vision loss from macular edema may be insidious or sudden, with or without pain, *any* decrease in visual acuity while a woman is on OCs should be evaluated by an ophthalmologist and retinal vascular occlusion ruled out as a causative factor.

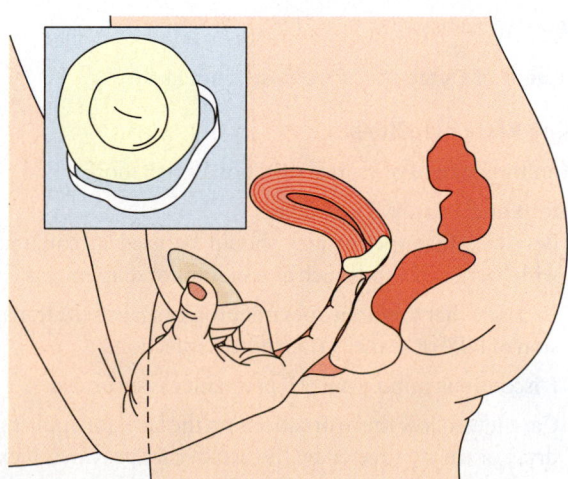

Figure 70.3 The contraceptive sponge is moistened well with water and inserted into the vagina with the concave portion positioned over the cervix.

PROTOTYPE DRUG	**Nonoxynol-9**

Classification: Therapeutic: Intravaginal contraceptive
Pharmacologic: Spermicide

Therapeutic Effects and Uses: Originally approved in 1963, nonoxynol-9 is a topical contraceptive that acts by inhibiting the ability of sperm to reach the ovum. Most products have a duration of spermicidal action of 60 minutes; the contraceptive sponge provides 24 hours of protection.

Pharmacokinetics: Nonoxynol-9 disrupts the cell membrane of sperm, causing it to lose motility and function. The carrier (foam, sponge, cream, etc.) may also act as a physical barrier to sperm motility.

Route(s)	Apply or insert vaginally
Absorption	Minimal absorption
Distribution	Acts locally, killing the sperm on contact
Primary metabolism	Not metabolized
Primary excretion	Small amounts by the kidneys and in feces
Onset of action	Immediate for creams, foams, gels, and sponge; 5–15 min for suppositories
Duration of action	Up to 24 h after intercourse (sponge)

Adverse Effects: Adverse effects are uncommon. Vaginal irritation and dryness, increase in vaginal infections, irritation of the genitalia of the sexual partner, and toxic shock syndrome have been reported.

Contraindications/Precautions: Women with cystocele, prolapsed uterus, sensitivity or allergy to nonoxynol-9, vaginitis, or toxic shock syndrome, or those who are pregnant, postabortion, or postpregnancy should avoid this drug.

Drug Interactions: Intravaginal azole antifungals may inactivate the spermicides.

Pregnancy: Category C.

Treatment of Overdose: Overdose is not likely.

Nursing Responsibilities:
- Monitor for signs of vaginal infection or irritation.

  Patient and Family Education:
  - Be aware that spermicides should be used in conjunction with barrier methods such as condoms or diaphragms.
  - Be aware that this drug does not protect against the transmission of HIV or sexually transmitted infections.
  - Discontinue nonoxynol-9 if pregnancy is suspected.
  - Carefully follow the instructions on the label for applying the drug, or use as directed by the health care provider. If excessive burning, stinging, or irritation occurs, try a product with a lower strength of nonoxynol-9.
  - If using a diaphragm, place 1 to 3 tsp of the spermicide in the dome prior to insertion.
  - Leave the spermicide and diaphragm in place 6 hours after intercourse.
  - Use the spermicide before the first and every subsequent act of intercourse.
  - Report burning; inflammation; intense vaginal and vulvar itching; cheesy, curd-like discharge; painful intercourse; and dysuria to the health care provider.

Drugs Similar to Nonoxynol-9
There are no drugs that are similar to nonoxynol-9.

Emergency Contraception
70.7 Emergency contraception provides a reproductive option for women who have unprotected sex or contraceptive failure.

Emergency contraception (EC) is the prevention of implantation following unprotected intercourse or contraceptive failure. Statistics suggest that almost half the pregnancies in the United States are unplanned and some of these occur due to the inconsistent use or failure of contraceptive devices. EC, commonly referred to as the "morning after pill," offers a means of protecting against unwanted pregnancies.

The treatment goal for these patients is to provide effective and immediate contraception. These medications must be taken as soon as possible after unprotected intercourse or contraceptive failure. When used accordingly, these drugs act by preventing ovulation; they do not cause abortion. If implantation of an embryo has already occurred, the drugs used for EC will have no effect on the established pregnancy. Two different medications are approved for EC: Plan B and ulipristal (Ella). Table 70.4 lists drugs, routes, and dosages for EC. These drugs are not intended to replace regular methods of contraception.

Plan B is approved for OTC purchase by women 17 years of age or older. Females younger than age 17 require a prescription to obtain the drug. Plan B has largely been replaced by Plan B One Step, which offers the convenience of a single 1.5-mg dose.

The active drug in Plan B is levonorgestrel, which is the same progestin used for contraception in the intrauterine system Mirena (see Section 70.5). There is, however, a large difference in doses. Whereas the long-acting Mirena releases 20 mcg per day of levonorgestrel over a 5-year period, Plan B delivers a total of 1,500 mcg of levonorgestrel in a single day. The drug is most effective when taken either within 72 hours (Plan B) or 120 hours (Plan B One Step) after unprotected intercourse.

Plan B is not 100% effective. The normal rate of pregnancy from a single unprotected sex act is 8%; Plan B is estimated to lower this risk to 1% to 2%. Serious adverse effects with Plan B are uncommon. Nausea and vomiting are the most common adverse effects, and abdominal pain, fatigue, headache, irregular (increased or decreased) menstrual bleeding, and dizziness are reported by a number of patients. Plan B is not intended to be a primary method of birth control because the long-term effects of multiple doses have not been established. Fertility returns quickly after taking Plan B; therefore, the patient should be encouraged to implement routine contraception measures as soon as possible.

CONNECTIONS: NURSING PRACTICE APPLICATION

Patients Receiving Hormonal Contraceptives

Assessment	Potential Nursing Diagnoses*
Baseline assessment prior to administration: • Obtain a complete health history including cardiovascular, peripheral vascular, migraine headaches, thyroid, hepatic, or renal disease; diabetes; pregnancy; or breast-feeding. Note personal or family history of thromboembolic disorders (e.g., MI, stroke, peripheral vascular disease) and of reproductive cancers (e.g., breast, uterine, or ovarian cancer). • Obtain a drug history including allergies, current prescription and OTC drugs, herbal preparations, alcohol use, and smoking. Be alert to possible drug interactions. • Evaluate appropriate laboratory findings (e.g., CBC, platelets, electrolytes, glucose, lipid, and thyroid function levels), Pap test, HPV screening, and pregnancy test. • Obtain baseline height, weight, and vital signs. • Assess the patient's ability to receive and understand instructions. Include the family or caregiver as needed.	• *Decisional Conflict* • *Disturbed Body Image* • *Deficient Knowledge* (Drug Therapy) • *Risk of Excess Fluid Volume*, related to adverse drug effects • *Risk for Ineffective Peripheral Tissue Perfusion*, related to adverse drug effects • *Risk for Ineffective Cerebral Tissue Perfusion*, related to adverse drug effects • *Risk for Decreased Cardiac Tissue Perfusion*, related to adverse drug effects
Assessment throughout administration: • Assess for desired therapeutic effects dependent on the reason the drug is given (e.g., pregnancy prevention). • Continue periodic monitoring of CBC, platelets, and glucose. • Monitor vital signs and weight at each health care visit. • Assess for adverse effects: nausea, vomiting, headache, weight gain, breast tenderness, skin rash, acne, fluid retention, changes in mood, or midcycle breakthrough bleeding. Immediately report tachycardia, palpitations, HTN, especially associated with angina, severe headache, cramping in calves, chest pain, or dyspnea.	

Implementation

Interventions and (Rationales)	Patient-Centered Care
Ensuring therapeutic effects: • Monitor appropriate medication administration for optimum results. (OCs are nearly 100% effective when taken as required. Skipping doses increases the risk of pregnancy. Newer types of contraception such as transdermal patches or depot injections may be desirable for women who experience difficulty adhering to OCs or for those who choose not to take daily medication.)	• Instruct the patient to take the pill at the same time daily to help with remembering to take it. Do not omit, increase, or decrease doses without consulting the health care provider. Omitting or decreasing doses increases the chance of pregnancy; increasing doses may increase the risk of adverse effects. • Encourage women to discuss other available options (e.g., transdermal patches, depot injections, subdermal implants) with their health care provider as appropriate.

Minimizing adverse effects:
• Monitor for symptoms of cardiopulmonary, cerebrovascular, and peripheral vascular thromboembolism. Monitor blood pressure at each clinical visit. (Thromboembolic events are a possible adverse effect of OC drugs. The risk increases in women with a previous history of cardiovascular disease, women classified as obese, and in women who smoke. Monitor for symptoms of peripheral thrombophlebitis, pulmonary embolism, MI, stroke, or other complications related to blood clots.)
	• Instruct the patient to immediately report:
	  • Dyspnea, chest pain, or blood in sputum (possible pulmonary embolism)
	  • Heaviness, chest pain, or overwhelming feeling of fatigue and weakness accompanied by nausea and diaphoresis (possible MI)
	  • Sudden, severe headache, especially if associated with a preheadache aura, dizziness, difficulty with speech, numbness in an arm or leg, or difficulty with vision (possible stroke)
	  • Eye problems such as blurred vision or loss of vision (possible stroke, retinal hemorrhage or thrombus)
	  • Warmth, redness, swelling, or tenderness in calf, or pain on walking (possible thrombophlebitis).
	• Teach the patient to monitor blood pressure periodically and report any blood pressure above 140/90 mmHg or per parameters as ordered by the health care provider.

• Encourage smoking cessation and provide information about smoking cessation programs. (Smoking greatly increases the risk of experiencing the adverse effects of hormone therapy.)	• Advise the patient of the risk of smoking while using OCs; discuss and provide literature on smoking cessation programs, providing referral to appropriate support groups.
• Monitor Pap tests, HPV screening, and breast exams as ordered. (Pap tests and breast exams, including mammography as appropriate, will monitor for the development of breast tumors or cervical cancer.)	• Teach the patient how to perform breast self-exams, but monthly exams may not be recommended by the health care provider except for women at high risk for breast cancer. For women over age 40, advise the patient on the need for follow-up mammography as per the health care provider recommendations. • Advise the patient on the need for regularly scheduled gynecologic exams to ensure continued health.

(continued)

• Monitor the occurrence of any breakthrough bleeding. Report any continuous, unusual, or heavy bleeding. (Spotting may occur, especially with low-dose hormone therapy, at midcycle. Any continuous, unusual, or heavy bleeding may indicate adverse effects, pregnancy loss, or disease and should be reported.)	• Teach the patient that spotting may occur midcycle while on OCs but to report any unusual changes in the amount or if the bleeding continues.
• Monitor hepatic function tests and symptoms of liver dysfunction, lipid profile studies, and thyroid levels periodically. (OCs are associated with an increased risk of gallbladder disease and a rare risk of hepatotoxicity.)	• Instruct the patient to return periodically for laboratory tests. • Teach the patient to report any symptoms of abdominal or right upper quadrant discomfort or pain, yellowing of the skin or sclera, fatigue, anorexia, darkened urine, or clay-colored stools. Report any severe abdominal pain immediately.
• Monitor concurrent drug therapy and any new prescriptions received. (Many drugs decrease or alter the effectiveness of OCs including drugs in the penicillin, tetracycline, barbiturate, antiseizure, antidepressant, and benzodiazepine classifications.)	• Teach the patient to advise all health care providers of the use of OCs before beginning any new prescription.
Patient understanding of drug therapy: • Use opportunities during administration of medications and during assessments to discuss the rationale for drug therapy, desired therapeutic outcomes, commonly observed adverse effects, parameters for when to call the health care provider, and any necessary monitoring or precautions. (Using time during nursing care helps to optimize and reinforce key teaching areas.)	• The patient should be able to state the reason for the drug, appropriate dose and scheduling, what adverse effects to observe for, and when to report them.
Patient self-administration of drug therapy: • When administering the medication, instruct the patient in proper self-administration of the drug, e.g., consistently at the same time each day to help with remembering to take the dose, followed by teach-back. (Utilizing time during nurse-administration of these drugs helps to reinforce teaching.)	• Teach the patient to take the pill at the same time daily to help with remembering to take it. If a dose is missed, take the drug as follows: • *For estrogen-progestin combination OCs:* If a dose is missed, take it as soon as it is remembered, and take the next pill at its normally scheduled time. If two consecutive doses are missed, take 2 tablets on both the day the missed doses are remembered and on the following day. Follow the remaining schedule of pills, but a second method of contraception (e.g., a barrier method) should be used for at least 7 days after restarting the pills. If 3 or more consecutive days are missed, use another form of contraception until the pills can be restarted in the next monthly cycle. • *For progestin-only OCs:* If a dose is missed, take the pill as soon as remembered, but use an additional form of contraception until the next cycle of pills is started. • *Transdermal patches (e.g., Ortho-Evra) and vaginal rings (e.g., NuvaRing):* Patches and rings are changed weekly for 3 weeks, followed by 1 week of being patch- or ring-free. If the patch falls off or the ring falls out, it should be replaced with a new patch or ring. Safely discard used patches or rings in the trash.

*Nursing Diagnoses—Definitions and Classification 2015–2017. Copyright © 2014, 1994–2014 by NANDA International. Used by arrangement with John Wiley & Sons Limited.

In 2010, ulipristal (Ella) was approved as a single-dose product for EC. This drug is a mixed progesterone agonist/antagonist that acts by preventing ovulation. Unlike Plan B, which is available OTC, ulipristal requires a prescription. One advantage of ulipristal is that it retains its effectiveness for 5 days following unprotected sex.

Drugs for Pharmacologic Abortion

70.8 Abortifacients are drugs that are used to terminate pregnancy.

A woman who is in early pregnancy may decide that she is no longer able to carry the child to term. The nurse should use his or her knowledge of the stages of fetal growth and development to counsel the patient regarding the available options. The risks and benefits of the different options should be provided to the patient. One option for the patient if the pregnancy is 9 weeks or less is a medical abortion. Pharmacologic (medical) abortion is the removal of an embryo by the use of drugs after implantation has occurred. Drugs used to induce abortion are called **abortifacients**.

Once the ovum has been fertilized, several pharmacologic choices are available to terminate the pregnancy, as listed in Table 70.4.

A single dose of mifepristone (Mifeprex) followed 36 to 48 hours later by a single dose of misoprostol (Cytotec) is a frequently used regimen. Although mifepristone-misoprostol should never be used as a substitute for an effective means of contraception such as abstinence or OCs, these medications do offer women a safer alternative than surgical abortion. The actions of the two drugs are as follows:

• Mifepristone is a synthetic steroid that blocks progesterone receptors in the uterus. If given within 3 days of intercourse, mifepristone alone is almost 100% effective at preventing pregnancy. Given up to 9 weeks after conception, mifepristone aborts the implanted embryo.

• Misoprostol is a prostaglandin that causes uterine contractions, thus increasing the effectiveness of the pharmacologic abortion.

Pharmacologic abortion must be conducted under the close supervision of a health care provider. The patient is required to sign detailed consent forms after it has been determined that the pregnancy is under 49 days. The patient receives an assessment by the health care provider 2 days after dosing. If abortion has not occurred, additional misoprostol is taken and the patient returns to the health care provider in 14 days to confirm that abortion is complete. Occasionally pharmacologic abortion does not occur and the patient is referred for surgical abortion. The primary adverse effect

TABLE 70.4 Drugs for Emergency Contraception and Pharmacologic Abortion

Drug	Route and Adult Dose (Maximum Dose Where Indicated)	Adverse Effects
Drugs for Emergency Contraception		
levonorgestrel (Plan B, Plan B One Step)	PO (Plan B): 1 tablet within 72 h of unprotected intercourse followed by 1 tablet 12 h later (0.75 mg in each pill) PO (Plan B One Step): 1 tablet (1.5 mg) within 120 h of unprotected sex	*Nausea, heavy menstrual bleeding, lower abdominal pain, headache, fatigue, and dizziness* Serious adverse effects are rare when only one or two doses are administered
ulipristal (Ella)	PO: 1 tablet (30 mg) within 5 days of unprotected intercourse or contraceptive failure	*Headache, abdominal pain, nausea, dysmenorrhea, fatigue, dizziness* Serious adverse effects are rare when only one dose is administered
Drugs for Pharmacologic Abortion		
carboprost (Hemabate)	IM: Initial: 250 mcg (1 mL) repeated at 1/2- to 3 1/2-h intervals if indicated by uterine response. Dosage may be increased to 500 mcg (2 mL) if uterine contractility is inadequate after several doses of 250 mcg (1 mL), not to exceed a total dose of 12 mg or continuous administration for 1 month	*Nausea, vomiting, cramping, diarrhea, fever* Uterine laceration, rupture, or hemorrhage
dinoprostone (Cervidil, Prepidil, Prostin E$_2$)	Intravaginal: Insert 20-mg suppository high in the vagina; repeat every 2–5 h until abortion occurs or membranes rupture (max: total dose 240 mg)	*Nausea, vomiting, cramping, diarrhea, fever* Uterine laceration, rupture, or hemorrhage
methotrexate with misoprostol	IM methotrexate (50 mg/m^2) followed 5 days later by intravaginal 800 mcg of misoprostol	*Nausea, vomiting, diarrhea* Abdominal pain, headache, uterine hemorrhage, respiratory arrest
mifepristone (Mifeprex) with misoprostol	PO: Day 1: 600 mg of mifepristone; day 3 (if abortion has not occurred): 400 mcg of misoprostol	*Nausea, vomiting, diarrhea* Abdominal pain, headache, uterine hemorrhage

Note: Italics indicate common adverse effects. <u>Underline</u> indicates serious adverse effects.

of mifepristone-misoprostol is cramping that occurs soon after taking misoprostol. Nausea is common. The most serious adverse effect is prolonged bleeding, which may continue for 1 to 2 weeks after dosing.

Methotrexate, an antineoplastic drug, is sometimes combined with intravaginal misoprostol (Cytotec). Methotrexate 50 mg/m^2 is given IM, followed in 5 days by 800 mcg of intravaginal misoprostol. If abortion does not occur within 24 hours, the misoprostol is repeated. The treatment is 96% effective at causing abortion. Most patients experience adverse effects such as nausea, vomiting, diarrhea, headache, dizziness, abdominal cramping, and hot flashes.

Prostaglandins may also be used to induce abortion. Prostaglandins are natural hormones that produce a diverse number of local actions in virtually every body system. In the uterus, the normal function of prostaglandins is to cause contraction of smooth muscle. They serve a valuable function in inducing contractions at the beginning of labor and in promoting cervical ripening.

The three approved prostaglandins include dinoprostone (Cervidil, Prepidil, Prostin E$_2$), carboprost (Hemabate), and misoprostol (Cytotec). All three may be used to induce uterine contractions that can expel an implanted embryo and result in abortion up to the second trimester. Dinoprostone is used early in pregnancy and comes in preparations of vaginal suppositories (Prostin E), vaginal inserts (Cervidil), and gel, which are inserted high into the vaginal canal. Carboprost is administered by deep IM injection and misoprostol by tablet. When used for abortion, misoprostol is administered with either mifepristone or methotrexate. Nausea, vomiting, and diarrhea are common adverse effects of prostaglandins and uterine cramping is expected. Drug-induced fever occurs in the majority of

patients and may last up to 6 hours. Because rare instances of uterine laceration and rupture have been reported, the patient is monitored closely for uterine activity, excessive pain, and vaginal bleeding. Indications for the prostaglandins are given in Table 70.5.

PROTOTYPE DRUG | **Mifepristone (Mifeprex)**

Classification: **Therapeutic:** Drug for abortion
Pharmacologic: Abortifacient, progesterone antagonist

Therapeutic Effects and Uses: The only FDA-approved indication for mifepristone is to terminate pregnancies that are less than 49 days of gestation. Due to the controversial nature of this drug, distribution is restricted and tightly controlled. This drug is only available via restricted access to registered prescribers in the United States. This drug is not available in pharmacies but is sold directly to approved, registered prescribers. Surgical intervention must be readily available in case of incomplete abortion or severe bleeding or other serious complications. Pharmacotherapy with mifepristone requires three office visits by the patient:

- Day 1: Three 200-mg tablets of mifepristone are taken as a single dose.
- Day 3: If abortion is not confirmed, 400 mcg of misoprostol are administered as a single dose. The patient is usually observed for at least 4 hours to determine potential adverse effects. Complete termination usually occurs in 4 to 24 hours.
- Day 14: Confirmation of abortion.

TABLE 70.5	Indications for Prostaglandins				
	INDICATIONS				
Drug	**Abortifacient**	**Control of Postpartum Bleeding**	**Cervical Ripening Induction**	**Labor Induction**	**Other**
carboprost (Hemabate) prostaglandin F$_2$	A	A	O	O	Hemorrhagic cystitis (O); hydatidform mole (O)
dinoprostone (Cervidil, Prepidil, Prostin E$_2$) prostaglandin E$_2$	A	—	A	—	Hydatidform mole (A)
misoprostol (Cytotec) prostaglandin E$_1$	O	O	O	O	Nonsteroidal anti-inflammatory drug–induced ulcer prophylaxis (A); kidney transplant rejection prophylaxis (O)

Note: A = FDA-approved indication; O = off-label indication.

Mifepristone may be used off-label as a means of EC. Given as a single 600-mg dose, it has the same effectiveness and safety profile as Plan B. Other off-label indications include breast cancer, endometriosis, uterine leiomyomata, Cushing's syndrome, and termination of ectopic pregnancy (in combination with methotrexate).

Mechanism of Action: Mifepristone is a strong antagonist of progesterone and corticosteroids. This drug blocks the supportive effects of progesterone on the uterine lining. If given within 72 hours of unprotected intercourse, a fertilized ovum will not be able to implant in the uterus. During early pregnancy, mifepristone acts by increasing the synthesis of prostaglandins and sensitizing the uterus to the effects of prostaglandins. When misoprostol (a prostaglandin) is given on day 3 of treatment, the large amount of prostaglandin promotes increased uterine contractions, which expel the embryo from the uterus.

Pharmacokinetics:

Route(s)	PO
Absorption	Rapidly absorbed
Distribution	Crosses the placenta; it is unknown if secreted in breast milk; 98% bound to plasma protein
Primary metabolism	Hepatic (CYP3A4)
Primary excretion	Mostly feces, small amounts in urine
Onset of action	Rapid
Duration of action	Half-life: 18 h

Adverse Effects: Nearly all patients who take the mifepristone-misoprostol combination experience adverse effects, especially after misoprostol is given on day 3. The most frequent adverse effects of mifepristone are headache, dizziness, nausea, vomiting, fatigue, and abdominal pain or cramping. Vaginal bleeding and spotting will occur for about 16 days. **Black Box Warning:** Serious and sometimes fatal infections and prolonged heavy bleeding have occurred. Excessive or continued bleeding may require medical intervention with vasoconstrictor medications or curettage. Rare cases of septic shock have been reported.

Contraindications/Precautions: Because mifepristone is a corticosteroid antagonist, its use in patients who are taking long-term corticosteroid therapy or who have chronic adrenal failure is contraindicated. The mifepristone-misoprostol combination is contraindicated in patients with ectopic pregnancy because the therapy will be ineffective. Those on anticoagulant therapy or who otherwise have an increased risk for bleeding should not receive mifepristone. Patients with an IUD in place should have the device removed before mifepristone is administered. The drug is contraindicated for use in patients who are unable to understand the implications of abortion or who may not comply with the established regimen. Safety in patients under age 18 has not been established. When administered for nonabortion indications, this drug is contraindicated in pregnancy (category X).

Drug Interactions: Because mifepristone is only taken in one or two doses, serious drug interactions are unlikely. This drug does, however, have an extended half-life that may cause interactions after it is discontinued. Mifepristone is metabolized by hepatic CYP450 enzymes and may interact with drugs that induce or inhibit this enzyme system. For example, phenytoin, phenobarbital, and carbamazepine induce CYP3A4, increasing the metabolism of mifepristone and lowering its serum levels. **Herbal/Food:** St. John's wort and grapefruit juice may decrease serum levels of mifepristone.

Pregnancy: Category X.

Treatment of Overdose: Overdose has rarely occurred with mifepristone. Treatment is supportive.

Nursing Responsibilities:
- Conduct a comprehensive health assessment, including the patient's ability to understand the consequences of drug therapy and her ability to comply with the regimen.
- Confirm a positive pregnancy test and that the length of gestation is less than 9 weeks.

- Ensure that the proper emergency medical support is available in case of partial abortion or excessive bleeding.

- Assess the patient's medical history for the presence of an IUD, use of anticoagulants, presence of bleeding disorders, or corticosteroid therapy.

- Instruct the patient on the expected adverse effects, especially cramping, and that vaginal bleeding may continue for several weeks to a month.

- Instruct the patient on steps to take in case of emergency, including the phone number and address of the nearest emergency center.

Lifespan and Diversity Considerations:
- Because mifepristone is metabolized through the P450 system pathways, monitor ethnically diverse populations more frequently to ensure optimal therapeutic effects and minimize adverse effects.

Patient and Family Education:
- Follow the therapeutic regimen exactly as prescribed by the health care provider.

- Attend all follow-up appointments because these are essential for safe and effective drug therapy.

- Immediately report heavy vaginal bleeding (use of more than two thick sanitary pads per hour for 2 consecutive hours), persistent vomiting, severe abdominal cramps, fever of 38°C (100.4°F) or higher, or weakness to the health care provider.

- Do not take any other prescription or nonprescription drugs, dietary supplements, or herbal products without approval of the health care provider.

- Resume or initiate birth control immediately after the treatment ends or as directed by the health care provider.

Drugs Similar to Mifepristone (Mifeprex)

There are no drugs that are similar to mifepristone.

CHAPTER

70

Understanding the Chapter

Key Concepts Summary

70.1 Selection of a contraceptive is based on effectiveness, safety, and personal choice.

70.2 The most effective oral contraceptives include combinations of low-dose estrogens and progestins.

70.3 Oral contraceptives that contain only progestin are often used when estrogen is contraindicated.

70.4 The adverse effects of combined oral contraceptives are uncommon but may be serious in some women.

70.5 Long-acting contraceptives and novel delivery methods offer women additional birth control choices.

70.6 Spermicides are safe but should be combined with barrier protection for maximum effectiveness.

70.7 Emergency contraception provides a reproductive option for women who have unprotected sex or contraceptive failure

70.8 Abortifacients are drugs that are used to terminate pregnancy.

Case Study: Making the Patient Connection

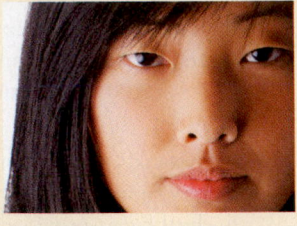

Remember the patient "Lila Bastian" from the beginning of the chapter? Now read the remainder of the case study. Based on the information presented within this chapter, respond to the critical thinking questions that follow.

Lila, a 19-year-old college student, comes to the clinic for renewal of her prescription for oral contraceptive pills. She finished her last pack of pills (Ortho-Novum) 10 days ago. She has been unable to get to the clinic to have her prescription renewed before today. She remembers having unprotected intercourse 2 days ago, and now she is concerned that she will become pregnant. Lila asks the nurse, "How can you help me?"

A complete history and physical finds Lila in very good health. Her vital signs are temperature, 36.7°C (98°F); pulse, 68 beats/min; respiratory rate, 18 breaths/min; and blood pressure, 118/71 mmHg. Her weight is 62.6 kg (138 lb) and her height is 1.7 m (5 ft 7 in.). Her skin is dry and warm to the touch, mucous membranes are pink and moist, and there are no outward signs of distress. Her abdomen is soft and not tender, and there are no signs of bloating or distention. She has no vaginal bleeding at this time. Lila emphasizes that she only had sex once, 2 days ago. A urine pregnancy test is negative. Lila is prescribed the emergency contraceptive, Plan B.

Critical Thinking Questions

1. Lila asks you, the nurse, if it is too late to prevent pregnancy. How would you respond to her question?

2. How does Plan B work to prevent pregnancy? What is another emergency contraceptive option that Lila could use?

3. What instructions would you give Lila regarding pregnancy and Plan B for emergency contraception?

See Answers to Critical Thinking Questions on student resource website.

Additional Case Study

Gina Martin, age 22, has been taking combined OCs for the past 2 years. Her health care provider orders antibiotics for a recurrent throat infection. As she is leaving the clinic, she asks you, the nurse, if she should temporarily discontinue her OC.

1. Explain the relationship between antibiotics and oral contraceptives.

2. What advice would you give Gina with regard to continuing the oral contraceptives?

See Answers to Additional Case Study on student resource website.

Chapter Review

1 Estradiol and norethindrone (Ortho-Novum) is prescribed for each of the following patients. Which patients would the nurse consider at highest risk for an adverse response to this therapy? Select all that apply.

1. A 38-year-old with a BMI classified as overweight
2. A 16-year-old athlete with asthma
3. A 22-year-old who smokes two packs of cigarettes per day
4. An 18-year-old with a history of chronic clinical depression
5. A 42-year-old who has delivered four healthy children

2 The patient who is taking estradiol and drospirenone (Yasmin) informs the nurse that she forgot to take her pills for the past 2 days. Which response by the nurse would be best when addressing this concern?

1. "Take two pills today and tomorrow then resume your normal dosage."
2. "Take one pill now and resume your normal dosage time tomorrow."
3. "Skip another day and then resume the normal medication schedule."
4. "Stop taking the pills and have a pregnancy test performed as soon as possible."

3 The patient is interested in taking levonorgestrel and estradiol (Seasonique) and asks how to take it. Which would be the correct response provided by the nurse?

1. "Seasonique is taken one pill per day for 3 weeks, then 1 week of 'dummy pills' with inert ingredients."
2. "Seasonique is taken year-round without a break and without a period."
3. "Seasonique is taken for 2 months then off for 1 month using regular oral contraceptives."
4. "Seasonique is taken for 84 days followed by 7 days of a lower dose that comes with the pack."

4 The nurse is teaching the patient who has received a prescription for mifepristone (Mifeprex) and misoprostol (Cytotec) to terminate a pregnancy. When should the patient be instructed to take the misoprostol (Cytotec)?

1. Take it after taking one additional dose of mifepristone (Mifeprex).
2. Take it the day after taking the mifepristone (Mifeprex).
3. Take it only after reassessment by her health care provider in 2 days.
4. Take it only if she is still bleeding in 3 days.

5 The nurse is providing health education about contraceptive methods to a group of young adults. Which of the following statements is correct about the use of spermicides?

1. They are extremely effective in preventing pregnancy.

2. They have relatively low levels of effectiveness when used alone.

3. They are the main causes of HIV and pelvic inflammatory disease.

4. They can prevent ectopic pregnancy.

6 Rank the following contraceptive methods in order of effectiveness from most to least effective:

1. Depo-Provera

2. Spermicides

3. Calendar rhythm

4. Oral contraceptives

5. Transdermal (Ortho-Evra)

See Answers to Chapter Review in Appendix A.

References

Abdualmjid, R. J., & Sergi, C. (2013). Hepatotoxic botanicals—an evidence-based systematic review. *Journal of Pharmacy & Pharmaceutical Sciences, 16,* 376–404.

Aggarwal, R. S., Gujarant, I., Mishra, V. V., & Aggarwal, S. V. (2013). Oral contraceptive pills: A risk factor for retinal vascular occlusion in in-vitro fertilization patients. *Journal of Human Reproductive Sciences, 6,* 79–81. doi:10.4103/0974-1208.112389

Berg, C. J., Callaghan, W. M., Syverson, C., & Henderson, Z. (2010). Pregnancy-related mortality in the United States, 1998–2005. *Obstetrics and Gynecology, 116,* 1302–1309. doi:10.1097/AOG.0b013e3181fdfb11

Daniels, K., Mosher, W. D., & Jones, J. (2013). Contraceptive methods women have ever used: United States, 1982–2010. *National Health Statistics Reports* (62). Retrieved from http://www.cdc.gov/nchs/products/nhsr.htm

Division of Reproductive Health, N. C. (2013). U.S. selected practice recommendations for contraceptive use, 2013: Adapted from the World Health Organization selected practice recommendations for contraceptive use (2nd ed.). *Morbidity and Mortality Weekly Report Recommendations and Reports, 62*(RR05), 1–46.

Ehrlich, E., Gibson, T. B., & Mark, T. L. (2011). Trends in prescriptions for oral contraceptives among U.S. teenagers. *Truven Health Analytics.* Retrieved from http://truvenhealth.com/portals/0/assets/ACRS_11225_0712_OralContraceptives_RB_Web.pdf

Johnson, T. L., & Fahey, J. W. (2012). Black cohosh: Coming full circle? *Journal of Ethnopharmacology, 141,* 775–779. doi:10.1016/j.jep.2012.03.050

Jones, J., Mosher, W., & Daniels, K. (2012). Current contraceptive use in the United States, 2006–2010, and changes in patterns of use since 1995. *National Health Statistics Reports, 60,* 1–25.

Kean, S. (2012). Contraception research. Reinventing the pill: Male birth control. *Science, 338,* 318–320. doi:10.1126/science.338.6105.318

Leach, M. J., & Moore, V. (2012). Black cohosh (Cimicifuga spp.) for menopausal symptoms. *Cochrane Database of Systematic Reviews, 9,* CD007244. doi:10.1002/14651858.CD007244.pub2

Lopez, L. M., Grimes, D. A., Chen, M., Otterness, C., Westhoff, C., Edelman, A., & Helmerhorst, F. M. (2013). Hormonal contraceptives for contraception in overweight or obese women. *Cochrane Database of Systematic Reviews, 4,* CD008452. doi:10.1002/14651858.CD008452.pub3

National Center for Complementary and Alternative Medicine. (2012). *Herbs at a glance: Black cohosh.* Retrieved from http://nccam.nih.gov/health/blackcohosh/ataglance.htm

Selected Bibliography

Dorflinger, L. J. (2013). New developments in contraception for US women. *Contraception, 87,* 343–346. doi:10.1016/j.contraception.2012.12.013

Freeman, S., & Schulman, L. P. (2010). Considerations for the use of progestin-only contraceptives. *Journal of the American Academy of Nurse Practitioners, 22,* 81–91. doi:10.1111/j.1745-7599.2009.00473.x

Herdman, T. H., & Kamitsuru, S. (Eds.). (2014). *NANDA International nursing diagnoses: Definitions and classification, 2015–2017.* Oxford, United Kingdom: Wiley-Blackwell.

Kavanaugh, M. L., Williams, S. L., & Schwarz, E. B. (2011). Emergency contraception use and counseling after changes in United States prescription status. *Fertility and Sterility, 95*(8), 2578–2581. doi:10.1016/j.fertnstert.2011.03.011

Koyama, A., Hagopian, L., & Linden, J. (2013). Emerging options for emergency contraception. *Clinical Medicine Insights. Reproductive Health, 7,* 23–35. doi:10.4137/CMRH.S8145

Mansour, D., Gemzell-Danielsson, K., & Jensen, J. T. (2011). Fertility after discontinuation of contraception: A comprehensive review of the literature. *Contraception, 84,* 465–477. doi:10.1016/j.contraception.2011.04.002

Marchbanks, P. A., Curtis, K. M., Mandel, M. G., Wilson, H. G., Jeng, G., Folger, S. G., . . . Spirtas, R. (2012). Oral contraceptive formulation and risk of breast cancer. *Contraception, 85,* 342–350. doi:10.1016/j.contraception.2011.08.007

Salcedo, J., Rodriguez, M. I., Curtis, K. M., & Kapp, N. (2013). When can a woman resume or initiate contraception after taking emergency contraceptive pills? A systematic review. *Contraception, 87,* 602–604. doi:10.1016/j.contraception.2012.08.013

Shaw, K. A., & Edelman, A. B. (2013). Obesity and oral contraceptives: A clinician's guide. *Best Practice & Research Clinical Endocrinology & Metabolism, 27*(1), 55–65. doi:10.1016/j.beem.2012.09.001

Upadhya, K. K., Breuner, C. C., Trent, M. E., Blythe, M. J., Adelman, W. P., Levine, D. A., . . . Seigel, W. M. (2012). Emergency contraception. *Pediatrics, 130*(6), 1174–1182. doi:10.1542/peds.2012-2962

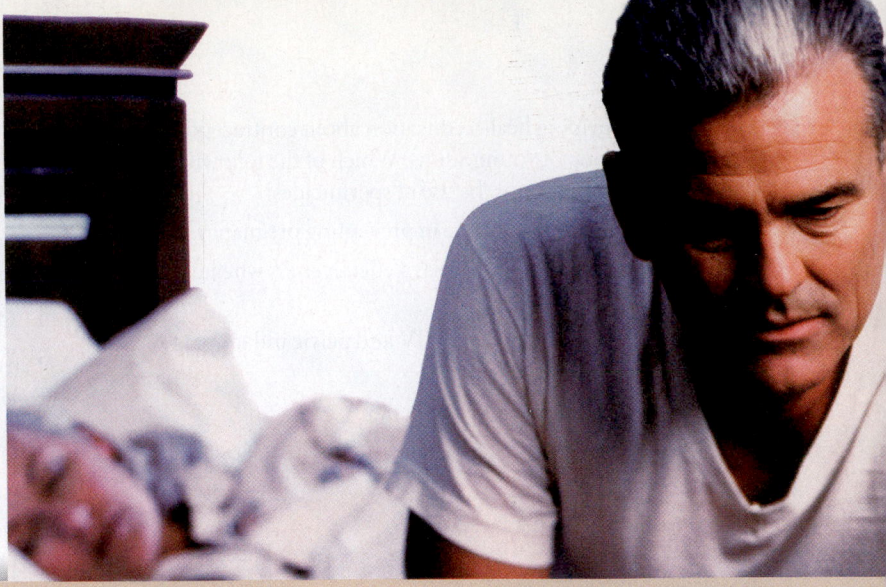

"What's wrong with me? Dana excites me so much, but when we get into bed I just can't please her sexually."

Patient "Mike Mayhew"

CHAPTER

71

Drugs for Disorders and Conditions of the Male Reproductive System

LEARNING OUTCOMES

After reading this chapter, the student should be able to:

1. Explain the physiological effects of androgens.
2. Describe the roles of the hypothalamus, pituitary, and testes in regulating male reproductive function.
3. Explain the role of androgens in the treatment of male hypogonadism, delayed puberty, and breast cancer.
4. Describe the potential consequences associated with the use of anabolic steroids to enhance athletic performance.
5. Identify the types and causes of male sexual dysfunction disorders.
6. Explain the role of drugs in the management of male infertility.
7. Describe the etiology, pathogenesis, and pharmacotherapy of erectile dysfunction.
8. Describe the pathogenesis and pharmacotherapy of benign prostatic hyperplasia.
9. Compare and contrast the nonpharmacologic and pharmacologic management of disorders and conditions of the male reproductive system.
10. For each of the classes shown in the chapter outline, identify the prototype and representative drugs and explain the mechanism(s) of drug action, primary indications, contraindications, significant drug interactions, pregnancy category, and important adverse effects.
11. Apply the nursing process to the care of patients who are receiving pharmacotherapy for disorders and conditions of the male reproductive system.

CHAPTER OUTLINE

▶ **Regulation of Male Reproductive Function**

▶ **Pharmacotherapy with Androgens**
   PROTOTYPE Testosterone, *p. 1211*

▶ **Anabolic Steroids**

▶ **Etiology of Male Sexual Dysfunction**

▶ **Pharmacotherapy of Male Infertility**

▶ **Pharmacotherapy of Erectile Dysfunction**
   PROTOTYPE Sildenafil (Viagra), *p. 1218*

▶ **Pathophysiology of Benign Prostatic Hyperplasia**

▶ **Pharmacotherapy of Benign Prostatic Hyperplasia**
   Alpha₁-Adrenergic Blockers
   5-Alpha Reductase Inhibitors
   PROTOTYPE Finasteride (Proscar), *p. 1221*

As in women, reproductive function in men is regulated by a small number of hormones from the hypothalamus, pituitary, and gonads. Because hormonal secretion in men is relatively constant throughout the adult lifespan, the pharmacologic treatment of reproductive disorders in men is less complex and more limited than in women. This chapter examines the drugs used to treat the disorders and conditions of the male reproductive system.

Regulation of Male Reproductive Function

71.1 Male reproductive function is controlled through the secretion of androgens.

Male reproduction function is controlled by **androgens**, which are hormones secreted by **Leydig cells** in the testes. Testosterone, the primary androgen, is responsible for maturation of the male reproductive system and the secondary sex characteristics of men. Other important androgens include androstenedione and dehydroepiandrosterone (DHEA). Androgens are sometimes referred to as anabolic steroids.

Androgens are responsible for the development of the male urogenital system in the fetus. After birth the Leydig cells are quiet until activated by the gonadotropins, which are hormones secreted by the pituitary gland. The resulting increased production of testosterone by the testes begins the cascade of changes that accompany the onset of puberty in the male adolescent. The increased testosterone levels are responsible for the process of **virilization**, or the development of the male sexual characteristics. During the next several years, the testes, scrotum, and penis enlarge until they reach adult proportions. Pubic and axillary hair grows and other body hair becomes more adult-like in nature. The production of sperm that are capable of fertilizing an ovum begins in the seminiferous tubules of the testes. The cartilage of the larynx grows, causing the deeper toned male voice. Sebaceous gland activity is stimulated, resulting in an increase in the level of acne. The final change is the growth of facial hair.

Testosterone also has profound metabolic effects in nonreproductive tissues. Of particular importance is its ability to build skeletal muscle mass and to stimulate bone growth, which contributes to the differences in muscle strength and body composition between men and women. Testosterone promotes the synthesis of erythropoietin, resulting in an increased production of red blood cells (RBCs) and accounting for the higher hemoglobin and hematocrit levels found in males.

Androgen secretion is regulated by the same pituitary hormones that control reproductive function in women. Although the name follicle-stimulating hormone (FSH) applies to its target in the female ovary, this same hormone influences testosterone secretion in men. Luteinizing hormone (LH), more accurately called interstitial cell–stimulating hormone (ICSH) in the male reproductive system, regulates the production of testosterone by the Leydig cells of the testes. Unlike the 28-day cyclic secretion of estrogen and progesterone in women, testosterone secretion is relatively constant in adult men. Beginning in puberty, testosterone production increases rapidly and continues to maintain a high level of production until later adulthood, after which it slowly declines. Normal plasma concentrations of testosterone are 250 to 1,000 mg/dL. If the level of testosterone in the blood rises above normal, negative feedback to the pituitary shuts off the secretion of LH and FSH. The relationship among the hypothalamus, pituitary, and the male reproductive hormones is illustrated in Figure 71.1.

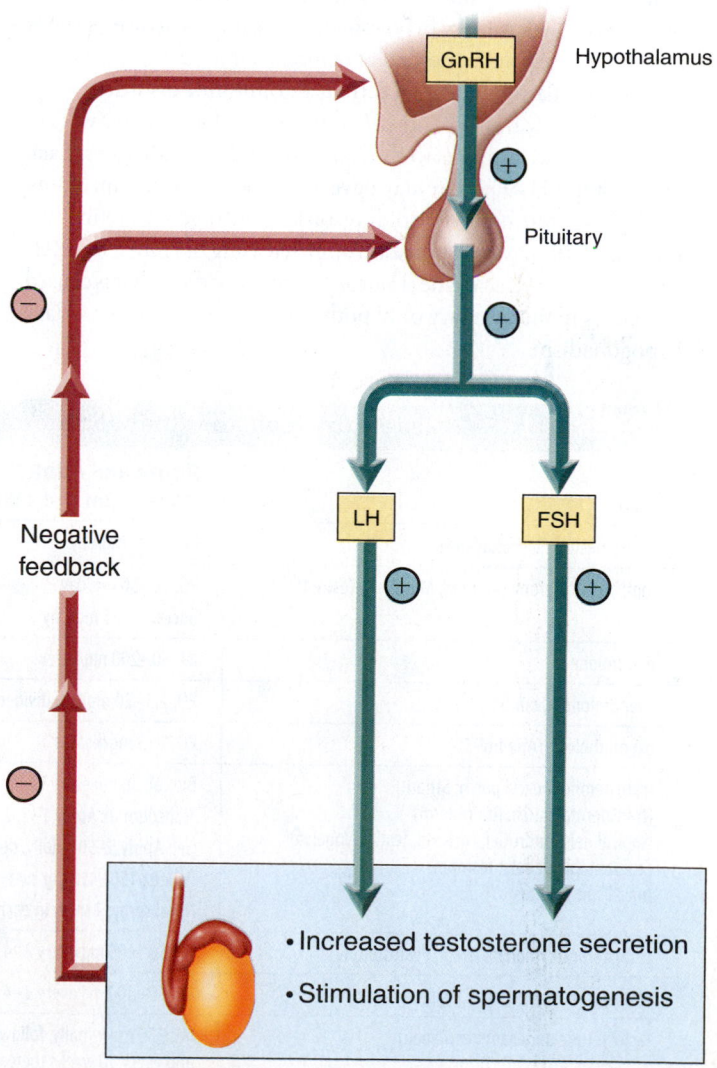

Figure 71.1 Hormonal control of the male reproductive hormones.

Precursor molecules of testosterone, androstenedione and DHEA, are secreted in small amounts by the adrenal glands. Their production in the adrenal gland is controlled by the secretion of adrenocorticotropic hormone (ACTH). These weaker androgens are converted to testosterone once they reach peripheral tissues. Adrenal androgens have a role in the growth of pubic hair and are thought to influence the skeletal growth spurt in adolescents. In adult males, the adrenal androgens have minimal effects due to the comparatively larger amount of testosterone secreted by the testes.

Pharmacotherapy with Androgens

71.2 Androgens are used to treat hypogonadism and delayed puberty in males and breast cancer in females.

Androgens are used to treat testosterone deficiency in men, delayed puberty, oligospermia, hypogonadism, anemia, muscle-wasting disorders, and certain cancers. These hormones are listed in Table 71.1.

Lack of sufficient testosterone secretion by the testes can result in male **hypogonadism**. Hypogonadism may be congenital or acquired later in life. When the condition is caused by a testicular disorder, it is called primary hypogonadism. Examples of disease states that may cause primary testicular failure include mumps, testicular trauma or inflammation, and certain autoimmune disorders.

A deficiency in FSH and LH secretion by the pituitary will result in a lack of stimulus to the testes to produce androgens. Lack of FSH and LH secretion may have a number of causes, including Cushing's syndrome, thyroid disorders, estrogen-secreting tumors, and therapy with gonadotropin-releasing hormone (GnRH) agonists such as leuprolide (Lupron). Hypogonadism that is caused by defects in the pituitary or hypothalamus is known as secondary hypogonadism.

Insufficient testosterone secretion may delay the onset of puberty. If total lack of testosterone secretion occurs, puberty will not occur at all. In the adult male symptoms of hypogonadism include diminished secondary sex characteristics such as sparse axillary, facial, and pubic hair; increased subcutaneous fat; reduced muscle mass; and smaller testes. The lack of testosterone can lead to erectile dysfunction (ED); low sperm counts (oligospermia); a decrease in the amount of ejaculate; and decreased **libido**, or a lack of interest in sexual intercourse. Nonspecific complaints may include behavioral and mood changes such as irritability, fatigue, depression, and a general loss of motivation.

Hypogonadism can be easily confirmed by obtaining serum testosterone levels. Assessment of LH and FSH levels, as well as prolactin, estradiol, and thyroid hormone levels, may be useful in determining causation. Low serum levels of testosterone concurrent with normal or elevated levels of FSH and LH suggest that the testes are unresponsive to hormonal activation; thus the patient has primary hypogonadism. If testosterone, FSH, and LH levels are all low, this would indicate secondary hypogonadism.

Pharmacotherapy of hypogonadism includes replacement therapy with testosterone or other androgens. For young males experiencing delayed puberty, puberty is generally induced when the boy reaches 15 to 17 years of age using a long-acting testosterone preparation. A 6-month period of androgen therapy is given, followed by 6 months without the drug. If further therapy is needed, then testosterone cypionate (Depo-Testosterone) may be administered every 2 to 4 weeks. Therapy may be continued for up to 4 years. Once appropriate physiological hormonal levels have been attained, the normal progression of pubertal changes typically occurs.

In the adult patient a variety of testosterone replacement preparations are available. The patient should experience improved libido, increased amount of ejaculate, and correction of ED within days or weeks of initiating therapy. Male sex characteristics become better defined, depression resolves, and muscle strength rapidly

TABLE 71.1 Selected Androgens and Anabolic Steroids

Drug	Route and Adult Dose (Maximum Dose Where Indicated)	Adverse Effects
fluoxymesterone (Halotestin)	PO: 5–20 mg/day	*Acne, gynecomastia, hirsutism and male sex characteristics (in women), sodium and water retention, emotional lability, amenorrhea, decreased libido, hypercholesterolemia*
methyltestosterone (Android, Methitest, Testred)	PO: 10–50 mg/day Buccal: 5–25 mg/day	
nandrolone	IM: 50–200 mg/week	<u>Anaphylaxis, testicular atrophy and oligospermia at high doses, priapism, peliosis hepatis, benign intracranial hypertension (HTN), thromboembolism</u>
oxandrolone (Oxandrin)	PO: 2.5–20 mg/day divided 2–4 times/day for 2–4 weeks	
oxymetholone (Anadrol-50)	PO: 1–5 mg/kg/day	
testosterone (buccal patch: Striant) (transdermal patch: Androderm) (topical gels: AndroGel, Fortesta, Testim, Vogelxo) (implantable pellets: Testopel) (nasal spray: Natesto)	Buccal: 30 mg every 12 h Transdermal: Apply 1–2, 2.5 mg patches daily (max: 5 mg/day) Gel: Apply 5–50 g daily, depending upon product Pellets: 150–450 mg every 6 months (each pellet is 75 mg) Nasal spray: 1 spray in each nostril tid	
testosterone cypionate (Depo-Testosterone)	IM: 50–400 mg every 2–4 weeks	
testosterone enanthate (Delatestryl)	IM: 50–400 mg every 2–4 weeks	
testosterone undecanoate (Aveed)	IM: 750 mg initially, followed by the same dose at 4 weeks and every 10 weeks thereafter	

Note: *Italics* indicate common adverse effects. <u>Underline</u> indicates serious adverse effects.

improves. Therapy with androgens is targeted to return serum testosterone to normal physiological levels. Above-normal levels serve no therapeutic purpose and increase the risk of adverse effects.

Nonreproductive uses: Because androgens have widespread physiological effects, they have been used to treat certain nonreproductive disorders. Testosterone promotes the synthesis of erythropoietin, which is essential for RBC production, and the drug may be used to correct anemia unresponsive to other treatments. These indications include aplastic anemia and anemias associated with chronic renal disease and chemotherapy. Taking advantage of the anabolic effects of testosterone on bone and skeletal muscle, the drug is sometimes given to debilitated patients who have muscle-wasting disease, such as that seen in patients with acquired immunodeficiency syndrome (AIDS).

High doses of androgens are occasionally used for the palliative management of certain types of breast cancer in combination with other antineoplastics. The high doses required for breast cancer treatment will cause virilization in women. Androgen therapy is contraindicated in males with breast cancer because it promotes the growth of the cancer. Similarly, because the growth of most prostate carcinomas is testosterone dependent, androgens should not be prescribed for older men unless the possibility of prostate cancer has been ruled out. Patients with prostate carcinoma are sometimes given a GnRH agonist such as leuprolide (Lupron) to reduce circulating testosterone levels.

Testosterone formulations: Testosterone is available in a number of different preparations. All formulations are equally effective and the choice is based on health care provider experience, ease of use, and the personal preference of the patient. Common to all dosage forms is the need for regular follow-up health care visits to ensure that the serum testosterone level is maintained within the designated range.

Intramuscular (IM) testosterone: Testosterone cypionate (Depo-Testosterone), testosterone undecanoate (Aveed), and testosterone enanthate (Delatestryl) are IM forms of testosterone. These drugs are slowly absorbed, metabolized to free testosterone, and result in blood levels that will vary widely after administration. This variation in serum levels may cause patients to experience fluctuations in their libido and energy and experience mood swings. Patients tend to report soreness at the site of injection. IM injections are given deep in the gluteal muscle every 2 to 4 weeks.

Implantable testosterone pellets: Testopel is a long-acting form of testosterone that is implanted subcutaneously, usually on the anterior abdominal wall. One to six pellets are implanted depending on the dose required. Testosterone levels are obtained regularly during therapy and the number of pellets adjusted accordingly. To induce puberty, low doses are usually used for 4 to 6 months. For adult replacement therapy higher doses are administered, with the effectiveness of the pellets lasting 3 to 4 months.

Transdermal testosterone patch: The Androderm patch is applied to the upper arm, thigh, back, or abdomen, rotating application sites. The patch is not to be applied to the scrotum or to damaged skin. A rash at the site of the application tends to be the only adverse effect noted. The patches are applied in the evening and changed daily. Because the used patches contain some testosterone, they should be disposed of safely, away from children and pets.

Transdermal testosterone gel: AndroGel, Fortesta, Testim, and Vogelxo are testosterone gels that are indicated for the treatment of hypogonadism. The drug is applied once daily in the morning to clean and dry skin of the upper arms, shoulders, or abdomen (not the genitals). Showering or swimming should be avoided for several hours after application to avoid washing off the drug. The alcohol-based gels dry quickly: The testosterone is absorbed in the skin in about 30 minutes and released slowly to the blood. Many patients prefer the use of gels because they cause less local irritation, the gel does not fall off like the patches, and a more consistent level of testosterone is delivered. A disadvantage is that the gel can be transferred to another person by skin-to-skin contact, causing virilization of female contacts and potential fetal harm. Testosterone levels should be measured after a few weeks of therapy and at regular intervals thereafter to ensure that physiological levels have been achieved.

Approved in 2014, Natesto delivers testosterone gel via intranasal spray. Absorption is rapid across the nasal mucosa but the drug needs to be applied three times daily. The most common side effects are nasal-related and include nasopharyngitis, rhinorrhea, and epistaxis.

Testosterone buccal tablets: Striant is a form of testosterone that produces a continuous supply of testosterone in the blood. Patients are instructed to place a tablet in the gum area just above the incisor, holding it in place for 30 seconds. Usual doses are one tablet every 12 hours, alternating sides of the cheek. Patients may eat, drink, and chew gum with the buccal tablet in place. There have been only minor adverse effects to this route such as local irritation to the area, bad taste, and altered taste perceptions.

PROTOTYPE DRUG | **Testosterone**

Classification: Therapeutic: Male sex hormone
Pharmacologic: Androgen, anabolic steroid, antineoplastic

Therapeutic Effects and Uses: The primary therapeutic use of testosterone is to treat delayed puberty and hypogonadism in males by promoting virilization, including maturation of the sexual organs, growth of facial hair, and a deepening of the voice. In adult males testosterone administration will increase libido and restore masculine characteristics that may be deficient. Testosterone is approved to treat ED when the cause is associated with low androgen levels. The drug is also approved by the U.S. Food and Drug Administration (FDA) for the palliative treatment of inoperable breast cancer in women. Off-label indications for testosterone include treatment of postpubertal cryptorchidism, microphallus, anemia in patients with chronic renal failure, female-to-male gender change, and AIDS-associated wasting syndrome.

Testosterone base is administered by the IM route, although other salts are available for the transdermal, implantable pellets, and buccal routes. Testosterone was classified as a Schedule III controlled substance in 1991 because it was being widely abused by weight lifters and other athletes.

Mechanism of Action: Testosterone binds to specific receptors located in the cell cytoplasm. The hormone-receptor complex then migrates to the nucleus where it acts on the deoxyribonucleic acid (DNA) to promote the synthesis of specific messenger ribonucleic acid (RNA) molecules. These form templates for the production of specific proteins that mediate testosterone effects.

Pharmacokinetics:

Route(s)	Buccal, transdermal, IM, implantable pellets
Absorption	Cypionate and enanthate are slowly absorbed from IM sites
Distribution	98% bound to sex hormone–binding globulin; unknown if secreted in breast milk
Primary metabolism	Hepatic
Primary excretion	90% renal, 6% feces
Onset of action	Steady-state levels are reached in 3–4 weeks
Duration of action	2–4 weeks cypionate and enanthate; half-life: 10–100 min

Adverse Effects: Androgens may cause either decreased or increased libido. Salt and water are often retained, causing edema, and a diuretic may be indicated. Liver damage and hepatic cancer are potentially serious adverse effects and are of special concern when high doses are taken for prolonged periods. Acne and skin irritation are common during therapy. High doses may suppress spermatogenesis, reduce ejaculatory volume, and cause oligospermia. **Black Box Warning**: Virilization in children and women may occur following secondary exposure. Children and women should avoid the application sites in men using testosterone gel. Signs of virilization in women include suppression of ovulation, lactation, or menstruation; hoarseness or deepening of their voice, which is often irreversible; hirsutism; oily skin; clitoral enlargement; regression of breasts; and male-pattern baldness.

Contraindications/Precautions: Testosterone is contraindicated in men with known or suspected breast or prostatic carcinomas because it can promote the growth of these tumors. It is contraindicated in women who are or may become pregnant (category X). The drug may worsen prostatic hyperplasia. Testosterone should be used with caution in patients with preexisting renal or hepatic impairment. Caution must be used if testosterone is administered to patients with diabetes mellitus, history of myocardial infarction (MI), coronary artery disease (CAD), benign prostatic hyperplasia (BPH), and acute intermittent porphyria and in geriatric patients. Monitoring of serum cholesterol and serum electrolytes, as well as liver function tests, is needed throughout therapy because testosterone may increase these values.

Drug Interactions: Testosterone may potentiate the effects of oral (PO) anticoagulants and increase the risk of severe bleeding. Concurrent use of testosterone with corticosteroids may cause additive edema, which can be a serious concern for those with heart failure. Hepatotoxic drugs should be avoided because their use with testosterone can cause additive liver damage. The 5-alpha reductase drugs (finasteride) used to treat prostatic hyperplasia are antiandrogenic and their use with testosterone will inhibit the therapeutic effects of both drugs. **Herbal/Food**: Insulin requirements may decrease, and the risk of hepatotoxicity may increase when used with echinacea. Evaluation of calcium levels is necessary because hypercalcemia may result.

Pregnancy: Category X.

Treatment of Overdose: There is no specific treatment for overdose.

Nursing Responsibilities: Key nursing implications for patients receiving testosterone are included in the Nursing Practice Application for Patients Receiving Pharmacotherapy with Androgens.

Drugs Similar to Testosterone

The two other androgens are fluoxymesterone and methyltestosterone.

Fluoxymesterone (Halotestin): Approved in 1983, fluoxymesterone is a PO androgen that is indicated for male hypogonadism and the palliative therapy of inoperable breast cancer in women. This drug has the same adverse effects, contraindications, and actions as those of testosterone. Like other androgens, hepatitis and hepatic neoplasms may occur with long-term use. Fluoxymesterone should be used with caution in patients with preexisting cardiac or renal disease because the edema caused by the drug can worsen these disorders. Older men have an increased risk for prostate cancer when taking this androgen. This drug is pregnancy category X.

Methyltestosterone (Android, Methitest, Testred): Methyltestosterone is available as PO tablets, capsules, or buccal tablets. It is indicated for male hypogonadism, delayed male puberty, and inoperable breast cancer in women. This drug has the same adverse effects, contraindications, and actions as those of testosterone. Caution must be used during long-term use because of the potential for hepatotoxicity and for the development of prostate cancer in older men. This drug is pregnancy category X.

Anabolic Steroids

71.3 Often abused by athletes, anabolic steroids can cause serious adverse effects.

Testosterone has both androgenic and anabolic effects. Its androgenic effects are responsible for creating and maintaining the male sexual characteristics. The hormone's **anabolic effects** relate to its ability to accelerate the growth of RBCs, muscle, bone, and neural tissues.

Anabolic steroids are testosterone-like substances that were originally developed to produce the anabolic effects of androgens while minimizing the androgenic effects. They are rarely prescribed but are often taken inappropriately by athletes who hope to build muscle mass and strength, thereby obtaining a competitive edge. The use of anabolic steroids to improve athletic performance is illegal and strongly discouraged by health care providers. All major athletic organizations prohibit the use of anabolic steroids by their participants.

Interestingly, despite their regulation, many formulations of anabolic steroids can be purchased over the counter (OTC) or on Internet websites. They are promoted as natural steroid alternatives

CONNECTIONS: NURSING PRACTICE APPLICATION

Patients Receiving Pharmacotherapy with Androgens

Assessment	Potential Nursing Diagnoses*
Baseline assessment prior to administration: • Obtain a complete health history including cardiovascular, peripheral vascular, thyroid, hepatic, or renal disease; diabetes; prostatic hyperplasia; or breast cancer. • Obtain a drug history including allergies, current prescription and OTC drugs, herbal preparations, alcohol use, and smoking. Be alert to possible drug interactions. • Evaluate appropriate laboratory findings (e.g., CBC, electrolytes, glucose, lipid levels). • Obtain baseline height, weight, and vital signs. • Assess the patient's ability to receive and understand instructions. Include the family or caregiver as needed.	• *Disturbed Body Image*, related to adverse drug effects • *Sexual Dysfunction*, related to adverse drug effects • *Excess Fluid Volume*, related to adverse drug effects • *Deficient Knowledge* (Drug Therapy)
Assessment throughout administration: • Assess for desired therapeutic effects dependent on the reason the drug is given (e.g., hormone levels normalize, normal signs of masculinization are present). • Continue periodic monitoring of CBC, electrolytes, glucose, lipid levels, hepatic and renal function laboratory values. • Monitor vital signs, height, and weight at each health care visit. • Assess for adverse effects: nausea, vomiting, headache, weight gain, fluid retention, edema, increased blood pressure (BP), changes in mood, irritability, or agitation. Immediately report tachycardia, palpitations, HTN, especially associated with angina or dyspnea, or abdominal pain, especially right upper quadrant and associated with yellowed skin or sclera, darkened urine, or clay-colored stools.	

Implementation

Interventions and (Rationales)	Patient-Centered Care
Ensuring therapeutic effects: • Monitor appropriate medication administration for optimal results. (Appropriate administration, especially of gels or transdermal forms, will optimize drug absorption and therapeutic effects.)	• Teach the patient the appropriate administration techniques.
Minimizing adverse effects: • Monitor BP at each clinical visit. Check weight and for the presence of edema. (Androgens cause sodium and water retention with resulting increases in weight, BP, and possible edema. Immediately report any BP over 140/90 mmHg, peripheral edema, or weight gain.)	• Teach the patient to monitor BP on a weekly basis. Report any BP over 140/90 mmHg, or as directed, to the health care provider. Report any weight gain of 1 kg (2 lb) in 24 h or 2 kg (5 lb) in 1 week to the health care provider. Report any peripheral edema. Ensure proper functioning of any equipment used at home.
• Continue to monitor electrolytes, lipid levels, and hepatic function laboratory values periodically. (Androgens may cause increases in cholesterol and calcium levels. Hepatotoxicity and hepatic neoplasms are rare but potential adverse effects. **Lifespan:** Age-related physiological differences may place the older adult at greater risk for hepatic toxicity.)	• Instruct the patient to return periodically for laboratory tests. • Teach the patient to immediately report any symptoms of abdominal or right upper quadrant discomfort or pain, yellowing of the skin or sclera, fatigue, anorexia, darkened urine, clay-colored stools, weakness, lethargy, nausea, or vomiting.
• Monitor blood glucose levels in patients with diabetes more frequently. Report consistent elevations to the health care provider. (Androgens may affect carbohydrate metabolism, leading to increased glucose levels.)	• Teach men with diabetes to monitor capillary blood sugar more frequently while on the drug and report consistent elevations to the health care provider.
• Monitor height and growth in children and adolescents. (Androgen administration may result in premature closure of epiphyseal bone endings and loss of normal growth patterns.)	• Teach the patient, family, or caregiver to measure height once per month or as directed. Return for clinical assessments as needed, approximately every 6 months, to monitor bone growth.
• Monitor drug use in adolescent patients. (Abuse of androgens and anabolic steroids may occur, along with resulting adverse effects.)	• Teach the adolescent patient, family, or caregiver to maintain daily dosing as instructed and not to increase the dosage unless instructed to do so by the health care provider. The drug should never be shared with others.
Patient understanding of drug therapy: • Use opportunities during administration of medications and during assessments to discuss the rationale for drug therapy, desired therapeutic outcomes, commonly observed adverse effects, parameters for when to call the health care provider, and any necessary monitoring or precautions. (Using time during nursing care helps to optimize and reinforce key teaching areas.)	• The patient, family, or caregiver should be able to state the reason for the drug, appropriate dose and scheduling, what adverse effects to observe for, and when to report them.

(continued)

CONNECTIONS: NURSING PRACTICE APPLICATION *(continued)*

Patient self-administration of drug therapy:

- When administering the medication, instruct the patient or caregiver in proper self-administration of the drug, e.g., consistently at the same time each day to help with remembering to take the dose, followed by teach-back. (Utilizing time during nurse-administration of these drugs helps to reinforce teaching.)

- Teach the patient to take the drug following appropriate guidelines:
  - *Oral drugs* should be taken at the same time each day to help with remembering the dose.
  - *Transdermal patches* (e.g., Testoderm, Androderm) should be applied to the upper arm, thigh, back, or abdomen. Change the patch and rotate sites daily, and report any skin irritation. Discard used patches safely in the trash. Do not apply the patch to the scrotal area or on broken or irritated skin.
  - *Buccal tablets* (e.g., Striant) should be placed between the cheek and upper gum near the incisor and held in place for 30 sec. Eating, drinking, and chewing gum may continue while the tablet is in place. Rotate from side to side, avoiding areas of irritation.
  - *Gels and creams* (e.g., AndroGel and Testim) should be applied to the upper arms, shoulders, or abdomen. Do not apply the gel or cream to the scrotal area or to broken or irritated skin. Swimming and showering should be avoided for several hours following administration. Do not allow women or children to come in contact with the drug or application sites, because the drug may rub off and cause adverse effects.
  - *Transdermal pellets* (e.g., Testopel) are implanted in the abdominal wall every 3–6 months.
  - *Injections* should be given into deep gluteal muscle. If the patient is to administer his own injections, teach the appropriate technique, followed by teach-back until the patient is comfortable and demonstrates proper technique.

*Nursing Diagnoses—Definitions and Classification 2015–2017. Copyright © 2014, 1994–2014 by NANDA International. Used by arrangement with John Wiley & Sons Limited.

---

for building muscle mass. Many anabolic steroid products, including oxymetholone (Anadrol-50) and nandrolone, are potent anabolic steroids that are classified as Schedule III drugs under the Anabolic Steroid Control Act of 2004 because of their abuse potential.

PharmFACT

Approximately 3% of high school boys take anabolic steroids annually. The number of high school students trying the drugs peaked in 2000 to 2001 at 8% to 12% and has been declining since then (Fronczak, Kim, & Barqawi, 2012).

One of the few FDA-approved anabolic steroids, oxandrolone (Oxandrin), is used in the treatment of constitutional growth delay, promotion of weight gain in the severely ill, and delayed puberty in boys. Those who are receiving oxandrolone for growth delay should have bone growth assessed every 6 months. Other steroids are used for the treatment of advanced estrogen-dependent breast cancer and anemia that is unresponsive to other treatment. The anabolic steroids are listed in Table 71.1.

When taken in large doses for prolonged periods, anabolic steroids can produce significant adverse effects, some of which may persist for months after discontinuation of the drugs. When given in higher doses, androgen administration suppresses the release of LH and FSH, resulting in oligospermia, testicular atrophy, and impotence in men. In female athletes menstrual irregularities are likely with an obvious increase in masculine appearance, such as hair growth and reduction in breast size. In teen or preteen males and females, androgens can promote premature epiphyseal plate closure, thereby reducing adult height. Anabolic steroids are hepatotoxic, and permanent liver damage or hepatic carcinoma may result with prolonged use. Accompanying salt and water retention can result in HTN. These drugs tend to raise low-density lipoprotein (LDL) and lower high-density lipoprotein (HDL) cholesterol levels, possibly accelerating atherosclerosis. Acne is common.

Behavioral changes include an increase in aggressive behavior and psychological dependence. Another unusual adverse effect is peliosis hepatis, which is a condition in which liver, and sometimes splenic, tissue is replaced with blood-filled cysts. These cysts are sometimes asymptomatic and may not be recognized until life-threatening hepatic failure or intra-abdominal hemorrhage occurs. Anabolic steroids are pregnancy category X medications and their use is contraindicated during pregnancy.

CONNECTION Checkpoint 71.1

Anabolic steroids are often taken illegally by "stacking" or "pyramiding." From what you learned in Chapter 27, define the use of these terms in the abuse of these drugs. *See Answer to Connection Checkpoint 71.1 on student resource website.*

Etiology of Male Sexual Dysfunction

71.4 Male sexual dysfunction may have both medical and psychological etiologies.

Approximately 50% of males will experience some form of sexual dysfunction during their adult life. The primary types of male dysfunction disorders may be classified as the following:

- Diminished libido: lack of interest in sexual activity
- Erectile dysfunction (ED): inability to obtain or maintain an erection
- Ejaculation disorder: premature, delayed, or retrograde ejaculation
- Infertility: inability to conceive a child

Certain causes of male sexual dysfunction are treatable, either medically or surgically, or can be improved to the degree that a couple can achieve successful conception or maintain a satisfactory sexual lifestyle. For example, therapy with testosterone can rapidly increase libido in patients who have insufficient serum testosterone levels or hypogonadism. Many men with ED can now be successfully treated with medications.

A large number of drugs can cause or worsen male sexual dysfunction, as listed in Table 71.2. In most cases, the dysfunction is dose related and is much less evident when a single drug is taken at low doses. However, taking multiple drugs that have the potential to cause sexual adverse effects may result in additive sexual dysfunction. The two most common drug classes that cause sexual dysfunction are antihypertensives and antidepressants. Because sexual adverse effects are a potential cause of nonadherence, nurses should ask specific questions regarding changes in sexual function when their patients are taking these drugs.

Many comorbid medical conditions are associated with sexual dysfunction. Conditions that result in general debility, such as pain, muscle weakness, shortness of breath, or stroke, may cause dysfunction. Diabetes and HTN are the two chronic medical conditions most frequently associated with male sexual dysfunction. Patients who present with psychological conditions such as anxiety and depression have a high incidence of sexual dysfunction. Other factors associated with ED include obesity and cigarette smoking. Combining multiple risk factors, for example, a man who has diabetes, is obese, takes antihypertensive drugs, and smokes, will result in a high risk for sexual dysfunction.

Nurses play a key role in treating male sexual dysfunction by obtaining a thorough medical history and by recognizing factors that contribute to the disorder. Should patients experience unacceptable sexual adverse effects from their medications, alternative drugs can usually be substituted. Encouraging patients to receive treatment for anxiety, depression, and other comorbid conditions sometimes helps improve the sexual dysfunction. All men at risk for ED should be encouraged to maintain optimum weight, stop smoking, and limit their alcohol use.

TABLE 71.2 Drugs That May Cause or Worsen Male Sexual Dysfunction

Drug/Drug Class	Sexual Adverse Effect(s)
Antihypertensives	
alpha-adrenergic blockers (e.g., prazosin)	Retrograde ejaculation, priapism
angiotensin-converting enzyme (ACE) inhibitors (e.g., lisinopril)	ED
beta-adrenergic blockers (e.g., propranolol)	Diminished libido, ED
methyldopa	Diminished libido, ED
spironolactone	Diminished libido, ED
thiazide diuretics	ED
Nervous System Drugs	
carbamazepine	ED
haloperidol	Inhibited ejaculation, priapism
lithium carbonate	ED
phenothiazines (e.g., chlorpromazine)	Diminished libido, ED, inhibited ejaculation, priapism
selective serotonin reuptake inhibitors (e.g., fluoxetine)	Anorgasmy, inhibited ejaculation, diminished libido
trazodone	Priapism
tricyclic antidepressants (e.g., imipramine)	Diminished libido, ED, inhibited ejaculation
Other Drugs	
alcohol	ED
anabolic steroids	Infertility
antineoplastics (e.g., cyclophosphamide)	Infertility
cimetidine	Diminished libido, ED, gynecomastia
digoxin	ED
finasteride	ED
methotrexate	Infertility

Pharmacotherapy of Male Infertility

71.5 Male infertility is treated with endocrine drugs that boost sperm production.

Infertility affects approximately 6.1 million persons in the United States, or roughly 10% of the reproductive age population. It is estimated that 30% to 40% of infertility among couples is due to difficulties with the male reproductive system.

Like female infertility, male infertility may have a number of complex causes. The most common congenital cause is Klinefelter's syndrome, which is the presence of an extra X chromosome. Acquired infertility may result from testicular trauma; pituitary or hypothalamus disorders; and infections such as mumps, chronic tuberculosis, and sexually transmitted infections. Infertility may occur with or without signs of hypogonadism. Rarely, life-threatening conditions such as testicular cancer and pituitary tumors may be the cause. In addition, the lack of ability to conceive may be caused by factors such as ED or ejaculation disorders. Identifying the etiology of infertility is important because not all causes can be successfully treated with pharmacotherapy.

The most obvious etiology of male infertility is lack of sufficient sperm production. **Oligospermia** is the presence of less than 20 million sperm per milliliter of ejaculate. **Azoospermia**, which occurs in 15% of men with infertility, is the complete absence of sperm in ejaculate. Azoospermia can be caused by severely reduced or absent sperm production, or it may indicate an obstruction of the vas deferens or ejaculatory duct that can be corrected surgically. Drug therapy with calcium channel blockers, colchicine, spironolactone, and cimetidine can lower sperm production.

Depending on the cause of the condition, one goal of pharmacotherapy for male infertility may be to increase sperm production. If the cause of the infertility is decreased testosterone secretion due to hypogonadism, administration of this hormone can increase sperm production and cure the condition.

Another method of increasing sperm production is to stimulate the testes with pituitary hormones. Pharmacotherapy often begins with IM injections of human chorionic gonadotropin (HCG) three times per week over 1 year. Although HCG is secreted by the placenta, its effects in men are identical to those of LH: increased testosterone secretion and spermatogenesis. Sperm counts are conducted periodically to assess therapeutic progress. If HCG is unsuccessful, therapy with menotropins (Menopur, Repronex) or newer recombinant forms of FSH may be attempted. Menotropins consist of a mixture of purified FSH and LH, which increases testosterone and sperm production.

Once testosterone levels rise, either through the administration of testosterone or HCG, the natural feedback mechanism of the body will signal the pituitary to shut down testosterone secretion in the testes. To boost testosterone levels, antiestrogen drugs such as tamoxifen (Nolvadex) and clomiphene (Clomid) have been used to block the negative feedback of adrenal estrogen to the pituitary and hypothalamus, thus increasing the levels of FSH and LH. Unfortunately, these drugs produce only a small increase in sperm count and can produce such adverse effects as gynecomastia, decreased libido, and weight gain. Clomiphene is presented as a prototype drug for female infertility in Chapter 69.

Other pharmacologic approaches to treating male infertility have been attempted. If retrograde ejaculation has been identified as a probable cause, sympathomimetics may be used to convert to normal, antegrade ejaculation. Various nutritional supplements, such as zinc to improve sperm production, L-carnitine to improve sperm motility and sperm count, and vitamins C and E as antioxidants to reduce reactive intermediates, have been tested. Unfortunately these and other therapies have not conclusively been shown to have any positive effect on male infertility.

Drug therapy of male infertility is not as successful as pharmacotherapy in women because only about 5% of infertile males have an endocrine etiology for their disorder. Many years of therapy may be required. Because of the expense of pharmacotherapy, the large number of injections needed, and the relative lack of success, other means of conception for the infertile man should be explored. A wide range of assistive reproduction procedures, including *in vitro* fertilization or intrauterine insemination, may be pursued.

CONNECTION Checkpoint 71.2

Clomiphene is used for both male and female infertility. From what you learned in Chapter 69, how does this drug act to improve female fertility? *See Answer to Connection Checkpoint 71.2 on student resource website.*

Pharmacotherapy of Erectile Dysfunction

71.6 Erectile dysfunction is a common disorder that may be successfully treated with inhibitors of the enzyme phosphodiesterase-5.

Erectile dysfunction (ED) is defined as the consistent inability to either attain an erection or to sustain an erection long enough to achieve satisfactory sexual intercourse. **Impotence**, a term often used interchangeably with ED, is the total inability to achieve an erection, an inconsistent ability to achieve an erection, or the ability to have only brief erections. An estimated 15 to 30 million men in the United States have ED. The incidence of ED increases with age, although it may occur in men of any age.

Penile erection is a complex event that has psychological, neuromuscular, and vascular components. Sexual arousal results in the release of neurotransmitters, primarily nitric oxide and epinephrine, from the hypothalamus. This stimulation along the autonomic nerves results in the release of an enzyme that makes cyclic guanosine monophosphate (cGMP). cGMP causes dilation of the arterioles leading to the major erectile tissues of the penis, called the **corpora cavernosa**. Rigidity of the penis results when the increased local blood flow and pressure fill the vascular spaces within the corpora. This engorgement causes occlusion of the veins that drain blood from the corpora, allowing the penis to remain rigid long enough for successful coitus. When stimulation ends or after ejaculation, cGMP is removed by the enzyme phosphodiesterase-5 (PDE-5). At this point, the pressure in the penis decreases, the veins dilate, blood leaves the corpora, and the penis quickly loses its rigidity. The anatomy of the penis is illustrated in Figure 71.2.

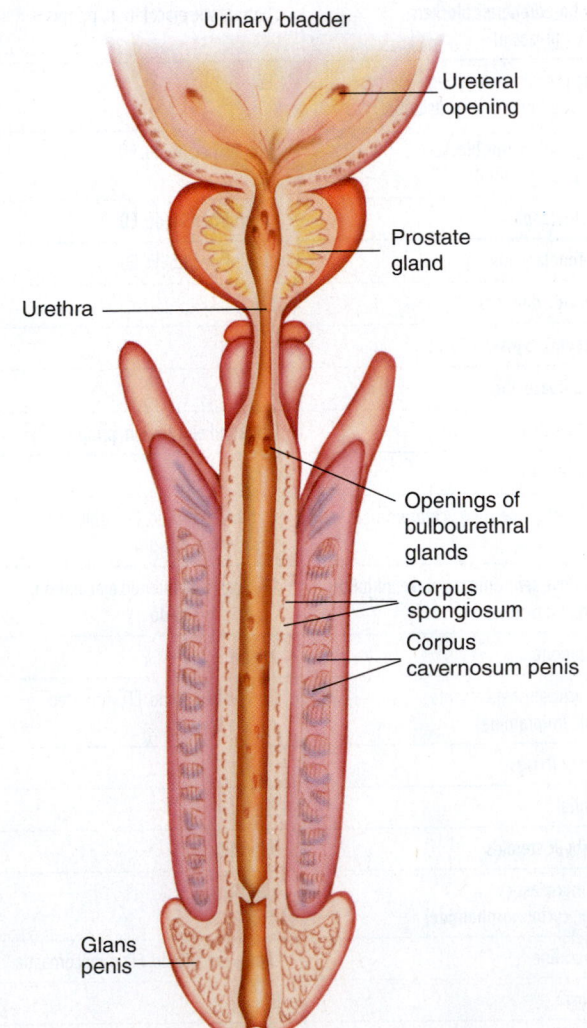

Figure 71.2 Anatomy of the penis.

Urinary bladder

Ureteral opening

Prostate gland

Urethra

Openings of bulbourethral glands

Corpus spongiosum

Corpus cavernosum penis

Glans penis

Organic causes of ED may include damage to the nerves serving the penis or a decrease in blood flow through the blood vessels involved in the erection reflex. Many chronic illnesses have the potential to damage the arteries, smooth muscle, and fibrous tissues of the penis, most notably atherosclerosis, diabetes, stroke, kidney disease, and HTN. Psychogenic causes may include depression, fatigue, stress, or fear of sexual failure. In some men, a number of common drugs cause impotence as an adverse effect, including thiazide diuretics, phenothiazines, selective serotonin reuptake inhibitors (SSRIs), tricyclic antidepressants (TCAs), propranolol (Inderal), and diazepam (Valium). Another potential cause of ED is hypogonadism, which can cause an inability to develop an erection, owing to the loss of libido. Nerve innervation and blood flow to the penis may be damaged by surgery, particularly during procedures involving the prostate gland.

A thorough health history of male patients should include questions regarding sexual function. Laboratory tests to check for possible metabolic or hormonal causes of ED include serum testosterone, prostate-specific antigen (PSA), blood chemistries, prolactin, and thyroxin levels. A nocturnal penile tumescence and rigidity (NPTR) test may be ordered. This test monitors the number of erections during sleep and is used to differentiate between the psychological and physiological causes of ED. A penile blood flow test is also used to determine whether there is sufficient arterial and venous flow through the penis. Patients who have diminished or abnormal blood flow may find that the drugs used to treat ED are not effective. These patients may have more success with penile implants.

The treatment of ED is becoming more prevalent as the population ages because more men are becoming affected by the disorder. If hormones are the cause of the dysfunction, treatment is aimed at correcting the abnormality. In some, testosterone replacement therapy by IM injection or transdermal patches may assist with ED, particularly if associated with hypogonadism or low libido. If the cause is found to be psychological, treatment will usually consist of a combination of psychotherapy and pharmacotherapy.

The development of sildenafil (Viagra), the first PDE-5 inhibitor, revolutionized the treatment of ED. When sildenafil was approved in 1998, it set a record for pharmaceutical sales of any new drug in U.S. history. Three other PDE-5 inhibitors have been approved by the FDA: avanafil (Stendra), vardenafil (Levitra, Staxyn), and tadalafil (Cialis). Drugs for ED are listed in Table 71.3.

The PDE-5 inhibitors do not cause an erection. They merely enhance the erection resulting from physical contact or other sexual stimuli by maintaining relaxation of the smooth muscle in the penis and increasing blood flow. These drugs are not as effective in promoting erections in men who do not have ED. Despite considerable research interest, PDE-5 inhibitors have no effects on female sexual function. These drugs are not approved for use by women.

The three PDE-5 inhibitors are equally effective at promoting erections in 60% to 80% of male patients, and the adverse effects are similar. The most common adverse effects are nasal congestion, headache, facial flushing, and dizziness. These drugs produce a 5- to 10-mm fall in blood pressure, but this drop is usually not clinically important. In patients who are taking nitrates or multiple antihypertensive medications, however, this blood pressure change may produce symptoms of hypotension. Therefore, PDE-5 inhibitors are contraindicated in patients who are taking organic nitrates in any form. Organic nitrates include nitroglycerin and isosorbide mononitrate.

Prior to the discovery of sildenafil, the treatment of ED consisted of rigid or inflatable penile prostheses being implanted into the corpora. As an alternative to prostheses, drugs such as alprostadil (Caverject) or the combination of papaverine plus phentolamine (Pavabid, Genabid, Cerespan) were injected directly into the corpora cavernosa just prior to intercourse. Penile injections cause pain and reduce the spontaneity associated with pleasurable intercourse. Intracavernous injections may cause fibrous tissue within the penis, hypotension, dizziness, pain, and priapism. These alternative therapies are rare today, though they may be used for patients in whom PDE-5 inhibitors are contraindicated.

Alprostadil (Caverject) can be used as a minisuppository that can be administered into the urethra as a medicated urethral system for erection (MUSE) or by direct injection into the cavernosa. As with papaverine, erection results from a relaxation of smooth muscle, increasing blood flow into the corpora. MUSE is available in four dosage strengths: 125, 250, 500, and 1,000 mcg. Alprostadil by either method should not be used more than three times per week and not more than once in 24 hours. Penile pain, burning sensations, and priapism are common adverse effects and, more rarely, penile fibrosis. The effectiveness of alprostadil is less than that of the PDE-5 inhibitors or intracavernosal therapy, and the strength of the erection can be improved by using a constriction ring.

TABLE 71.3 Drugs for Erectile Dysfunction

Drug	Route and Adult Dose (Maximum Dose Where Indicated)	Adverse Effects
avanafil (Stendra)	PO: 100 mg approximately 30 min before intercourse (max: 200 mg once/day)	*Nasal congestion, headache, facial flushing, dizziness, vision abnormalities, myalgia*
sildenafil (Viagra)	PO: 25–50 mg approximately 30–60 min before intercourse (max: 100 mg once/day)	
tadalafil (Cialis)	PO: 10 mg approximately 30 min before intercourse (max: 20 mg/day); Once-daily dosing: 2.5–5 mg daily	<u>Hypotension when taken with nitrates, priapism, hearing loss, nonarteritic anterior ischemic optic neuropathy</u>
vardenafil (Levitra, Staxyn)	PO: 10 mg approximately 1 h before intercourse (max: 20 mg once/day)	

Note: Italics indicate common adverse effects. <u>Underline</u> indicates serious adverse effects.

PROTOTYPE DRUG | Sildenafil (Viagra)

Classification: Therapeutic: Drug for treating impotence
Pharmacologic: Phosphodiesterase-5 inhibitor

Therapeutic Effects and Uses: Approved in 1998, sildenafil is a PO drug and was the first PDE-5 inhibitor approved for ED. The onset of action is relatively rapid (less than 1 hour), and its effects last up to 4 hours.

In 2005, sildenafil (Revatio) was approved for the treatment of pulmonary arterial HTN. For this indication, blocking PDE-5 in pulmonary vascular smooth muscle causes vasodilation and reduction in arterial HTN. The drug improves exercise capacity in these patients. The dosing for Revatio is 5 to 20 mg three times daily. Off-label indications include prevention of pulmonary HTN induced by altitude sickness and treatment of Raynaud's phenomena resistant to vasodilator therapy.

Mechanism of Action: Sildenafil inhibits PDE-5 and increases and preserves cGMP levels in the penis. This relaxes smooth muscle in the corpus cavernosa, allowing increased blood flow into the penis and allowing a harder and longer lasting erection in about 70% of men taking the drug.

Pharmacokinetics:

Route(s)	PO
Absorption	Rapid; bioavailability: 40%
Distribution	96% protein bound
Primary metabolism	Hepatic (CYP3A4 and 2C9)
Primary excretion	80% feces, 12% renal
Onset of action	20–60 min
Duration of action	24 h; half-life: 4 h

Adverse Effects: Sildenafil is well tolerated and adverse effects are usually transient and mild. Common adverse effects include headache, dizziness, flushing, rash, and nasal congestion. The most serious adverse effect, hypotension, occurs in patients who are concurrently taking organic nitrates for angina and can result in MI and sudden cardiac death. Sildenafil can produce blurred vision, increased sensitivity to light, or changes in color perception in 10% of patients using it. Priapism, a sustained erection lasting longer than 6 hours, has been reported with sildenafil use and may lead to permanent damage of penile tissue.

Contraindications/Precautions: Sildenafil is contraindicated in patients who are taking nitrates and in those with hypersensitivity to this drug. It is contraindicated in patients with severe cardiovascular disease, recent MI, stroke, heart failure, or dysrhythmias, and in the presence of anatomic deformities of the penis. This drug should be used with caution in patients with renal or hepatic impairment. Patients with preexisting visual disturbances should not use sildenafil.

Drug Interactions: Cimetidine, erythromycin, and ketoconazole will increase serum levels of sildenafil and necessitate lower drug doses. Concurrent use with nitrates is contraindicated and will result in hypotension and possibly death. Protease inhibitors (ritonavir, amprenavir, others) will cause increased sildenafil levels, which may lead to toxicity. Rifampin may decrease sildenafil levels, leading to decreased effectiveness. Concurrent use of sildenafil with drugs that lower blood pressure, including alpha-adrenergic blockers, should be avoided due to the potential for additive hypotension. **Herbal/Food:** Administration of sildenafil with high-fat meals should be avoided because absorption is decreased. Grapefruit juice increases the plasma concentrations of sildenafil and may cause adverse effects.

Pregnancy: Category B (not approved for women).

Treatment of Overdose: There is no specific treatment for overdose.

Nursing Responsibilities:

- Obtain a complete physical examination, including a history of sexual dysfunction; cardiovascular or peripheral vascular disease; thyroid, hepatic, or renal disease; diabetes; or prostatic hyperplasia.
- Obtain a complete drug history including prescription, OTC, and recreational or illicit drug use.
- Obtain baseline vital signs and notify the health care provider of blood pressure below 90/60 mmHg.
- Notify the prescriber if the patient takes a drug for angina or HTN such as nitroglycerin because these drugs may cause a sudden, unsafe drop in blood pressure.
- Monitor liver function tests. Patients with cirrhosis or severe decreased liver function may start with lower doses to prevent hepatotoxicity.
- Monitor for visual adverse effects such as blurred vision, the inability to differentiate between green and blue, perception of a blue tinge to objects, or photophobia. Observe safety precautions until it is known whether sensory-perceptual alterations occur to prevent falls and other injuries.
- Monitor for presence of headache, dizziness, flushing, rash, and nasal congestion.

Lifespan and Diversity Considerations:

- Monitor hepatic and renal function laboratory values and cardiac status more frequently in the older adult because normal physiological changes related to aging may increase the risk of adverse effects.

Patient and Family Education:

- Keep all laboratory visits to evaluate liver function.
- Take this drug 30 to 60 minutes before anticipated sexual activity. Do not take more than one dose in a 24-hour period.
- Alert all health care providers to the use of sildenafil before starting any new medication.
- Avoid high-fat meals before taking this drug because it may cause a delay in drug action.
- Immediately report any chest pain, unrelieved visual changes, eye pain, lights or flashes in the eyes, or an erection that lasts longer than 4 hours or is painful to the health care provider.

Drugs Similar to Sildenafil (Viagra)

The other PDE-5 inhibitors are avanafil, tadalafil, and vardenafil.

Avanafil (Stendra): The newest ED drug, avanafil, was approved in 2012 and acts by the same mechanism as the other three

PDE-5 inhibitors. It acts in 15 to 30 minutes, which is the fastest of the drugs in this class. It has a duration of about 6 hours, which is short compared to 36 hours for tadalafil. Avanafil may be taken twice daily. This drug's absorption is not affected by food. The adverse effects and contraindications are the same as those of other drugs in this class. This drug is pregnancy category C (not approved for women).

Tadalafil (Cialis):   Initially approved in 2003, tadalafil acts by the same mechanism as sildenafil, which is relaxation of penile arterial and trabecular smooth muscle. This drug's absorption is not affected by food. It acts within about 60 minutes and has a longer duration of action than sildenafil: up to 36 hours. The longer duration allows for more spontaneity of sexual activity. Contraindications include patients who take nitrates, and dosing can be prescribed every 72 hours. Tadalafil produces less blood pressure decrease than the other drugs in this class, making it safer for patients with heart failure or a history of MI. It also results in a lower incidence of visual disturbances. Other adverse effects are similar to those of sildenafil. A daily dosing of 2.5-mg tadalafil for erectile dysfunction was approved in 2008. This drug is pregnancy category B (not approved for women).

Like sildenafil, tadalafil (Adcirca) is also approved to treat pulmonary arterial HTN. The dose for this indication is higher, at 40 mg/day. In 2011, tadalafil (Cialis) was approved for the symptomatic treatment of BPH. Although its exact mechanism is still being investigated, tadalafil is believed to reduce BPH symptoms by relaxing urinary smooth muscles and increasing blood perfusion and oxygenation of the bladder and prostatic tissue.

Vardenafil (Levitra, Staxyn ODT):   Like other drugs in this class, vardenafil allows for relaxation of arterial and trabecular smooth muscle in the penis. Approved in 2003, vardenafil acts within 30 to 60 minutes and its effects continue for 4 to 5 hours. In 2010, an orally disintegrating tablet (ODT) form of this drug (Syaxyn) was approved. Headache, flushing, rhinitis, and dyspepsia are the common adverse effects. Vardenafil may prolong the QT interval and is to be used with caution in patients who are taking nitrates. Administration with high-fat meals should be avoided because absorption is decreased. This drug is pregnancy category B (not approved for women).

Pathophysiology of Benign Prostatic Hyperplasia

71.7 Benign prostatic hyperplasia is an enlargement of the prostate that occurs in older men.

The prostate is a gland the size of a walnut that surrounds the male urethra. Its primary function is to contribute fluids to the ejaculate. The prostate contains two major types of tissues:

- **Epithelial tissue.** This is the glandular portion of the prostate that secretes fluids for the ejaculate. The growth of prostatic epithelial tissue is controlled by the presence of androgens. Testosterone is converted to its active metabolite, dihydrotestosterone (DHT), in the epithelial cells of the prostate by the enzyme 5-alpha reductase.

- **Stomal tissue.** This is smooth muscle tissue, which is controlled by alpha$_1$-adrenergic receptors. When activated these receptors cause the smooth muscle to contract around the urethra.

Benign prostatic hyperplasia (BPH), an abnormal enlargement of the prostate, is the most common benign neoplasm in men. The exact cause of BPH is unknown, but it exists to some degree in all older men. It is present in 70% of men by age 60 and 90% by age 80. Other than age, the risk factors for BPH include a family history of the disorder, smoking, heavy alcohol consumption, HTN, diabetes, a diet high in meats and fats, and African American ancestry. BPH is not considered to be a precursor to prostate carcinoma, though it is well known that many men with BPH eventually experience prostate cancer.

PharmFACT

Until recently, the PSA test was the gold standard for screening men over age 50 for prostate cancer. This test is no longer recommended for routine screening because it results in very small or no reduction in prostate cancer mortality and is associated with unnecessary medical treatments (Chou et al., 2011).

The characteristic feature of BPH is an enlargement of the prostate gland that decreases the outflow of urine by obstructing the urethra, causing difficult urination. The pathogenesis of BPH involves two components: static and dynamic. The static factors are caused by the physical enlargement of the prostate gland due to the overgrowth of the epithelial cells. The gland can double or triple in size with aging, creating a blockage of urine outflow at the neck of the bladder. The dynamic factors are due to excessive numbers of alpha$_1$-adrenergic receptors located in stromal tissue in the neck of the urinary bladder and in the prostate gland. When activated, these receptors compress the urethra and provide resistance to urine outflow from the bladder. The two mechanisms of disease, static and dynamic, have led to two different classes of drugs for treating the symptoms of BPH. These mechanisms are shown in Pharmacotherapy Illustrated 71.1.

Certain frequently used medications may worsen symptoms of BPH. Alpha-adrenergic drugs, which include decongestants such as pseudoephedrine and phenylephrine, activate alpha$_1$-adrenergic receptors in the bladder neck, restricting urine flow. Drugs with anticholinergic effects such as antihistamines, TCAs, or phenothiazines may worsen the associated urinary retention. Testosterone and other anabolic steroids may increase prostate enlargement,

CONNECTIONS   Patient Safety

◀ Increased Plasma Drug Concentrations

A 53-year-old male is prescribed sildenafil (Viagra) for treatment of erectile dysfunction. His medical history reveals no cardiovascular disease and no other medication use, and his blood pressure is within normal range. Later that evening, he is admitted to the emergency department complaining of chest pain and dizziness and has a blood pressure of 80/48 mmHg. The triage nurse notes in the EHR that the patient took two acetaminophen (Tylenol) tablets 4 hours before taking the sildenafil. A dietary history reveals that he follows a gluten-free diet and drinks three glasses of grapefruit juice daily. What is a potential cause of this patient's symptoms, and what should the nurse teach this patient?

See Answers to Patient Safety Questions on student resource website.

PHARMACOTHERAPY ILLUSTRATED 71.1

Mechanism of Action of Antiprostatic Drugs

Bladder

Prostate gland

Urethra

Static factors:
- Gland enlarges under the influence of testosterone
- Enlarged gland creates physical obstruction of urethra

Dynamic factors:
- Alpha$_1$-adrenergic receptors are activated in smooth muscle in urethra and neck of bladder
- Smooth muscle contracts to narrow the lumen of the urethra

Shrunken gland

Open lumen

Relaxed smooth muscle

Open lumen

Alpha-reductase inhibitors interfere with testosterone metabolism.

Alpha$_1$-adrenergic blockers prevent the activation of alpha receptors.

which contributes to the physical obstruction of the urethra. Drugs that worsen symptoms of BPH should be avoided in older men.

There is no clear correlation between the symptoms experienced by patients and the size of the prostate. Some men may have minimal enlargement and experience moderate symptoms, whereas others may have extremely enlarged glands and be asymptomatic. This is because the smooth muscle in the urinary bladder has the ability to compensate for the obstruction by contracting with greater force to eject the urine stream. Over time, the bladder is no longer able to compensate and symptoms of BPH manifest, such as increased urinary frequency (usually with small amounts of urine), increased urgency to urinate, postvoid leakage, excessive nighttime urination (nocturia), decreased force of the urine stream, and a sensation that the bladder did not completely empty.

Some patients do not seek medical attention until complications caused by the long-standing obstruction at the neck of the urinary bladder arise. Serious complications include recurrent urinary infections, incontinence, gross hematuria, bladder stones, and chronic renal failure.

Pharmacotherapy of Benign Prostatic Hyperplasia

71.8 In its early stages, benign prostatic hyperplasia may be treated successfully with drug therapy.

The goal of treatment for patients with BPH focuses on minimizing the urinary obstruction and preventing complications. Drug therapy can only treat symptoms; it cannot reverse or cure BPH. Patients who are asymptomatic or who present with mild symptoms generally do not receive pharmacotherapy. Not all BPH is progressive, and many patients never experience moderate or advanced symptoms. Patient education such as avoiding caffeine or alcohol intake, eliminating drugs that worsen BPH, and restricting fluids close to bedtime may be sufficient to achieve symptomatic improvement. Morning diuretic therapy may be used to reduce nighttime diuresis. The patient is reevaluated at 6- to 12-month intervals to assess for worsening symptoms.

When symptoms of BPH worsen, pharmacotherapy is indicated. Only a few drugs are available for the pharmacotherapy of

TABLE 71.4 Drugs for Benign Prostatic Hyperplasia

Drug	Route and Adult Dose (Maximum Dose Where Indicated)	Adverse Effects
Alpha₁-Adrenergic Blockers		
alfuzosin (Uroxatral)	PO: 10 mg/day (max: 10 mg/day)	*Orthostatic hypotension, headache, dizziness, decreased libido, decreased ejaculate volume*
doxazosin (Cardura)	PO: 1–8 mg/day (max: 8 mg/day)	
doxazosin XL (Cardura XL)	Extended release: 4–8 mg/day (max: 8 mg/day)	First-dose phenomenon (severe hypotension and syncope), tachycardia
silodosin (Rapafo)	PO: 8 mg once daily with a meal	
tamsulosin (Flomax)	PO: 0.4 mg 30 min after a meal (max: 0.8 mg/day)	
terazosin (Hytrin)	PO: Start with 1 mg at bedtime, then 1–5 mg/day (max: 20 mg/day)	
5-Alpha Reductase Inhibitors		
dutasteride (Avodart)	PO: 0.5 mg/day	*Sexual dysfunction, decreased libido, decreased ejaculate volume, gynecomastia*
finasteride (Proscar)	PO: 5 mg/day (max: 5 mg/day)	Possible increased risk for prostate cancer
Phosphodiesterase-5 Inhibitors		
tadalafil (Cialis)	PO: 5 mg once daily	See Table 71.3

Note: Italics indicate common adverse effects. Underline indicates serious adverse effects.

BPH, and these are listed in Table 71.4. Drugs that are used to treat BPH have limited effectiveness and have value only in treating mild to moderate disease as an alternative to surgery. Because pharmacotherapy does not cure the disease, these medications must be taken for the remainder of the patient's life or until surgery is indicated. If the drugs are discontinued, the prostate returns back to its enlarged state and symptoms of BPH return. In advanced cases, transurethral resection of the prostate or a laser prostatectomy is needed to restore the patency of the urethra.

The two major drug classes for treating BPH are the alpha₁-adrenergic blockers and the 5-alpha reductase inhibitors. Research has shown that combination therapy with an alpha₁ blocker and a 5-alpha reductase inhibitor is more effective than therapy with either drug alone. This is the treatment of choice for patients with moderate symptoms of BPH. Recently, tadalafil (Cialis), a PDE-5 inhibitor, joined the list of approved drugs for BPH.

The alpha₁-adrenergic blockers act on the stromal tissue of the prostate to relax smooth muscle in the prostate gland, bladder neck, and urethra, thus easing the urinary obstruction. Doxazosin (Cardura) and terazosin (Hytrin) are of particular value to patients who have both HTN and BPH; these two disorders occur concurrently in about 25% of men older than 60. Three alpha₁ blockers, silodosin (Rapaflo), tamsulosin (Flomax), and alfuzosin (Uroxatral), are selective for the prostate and have no effect on blood pressure at normal doses. Drugs in this class improve urine flow and reduce other symptoms of BPH after 1 to 2 weeks of therapy. Common adverse effects include headache, fatigue, and dizziness. Doxazosin and terazosin are not associated with an increased risk of sexual dysfunction, but ejaculatory disorders have been reported with silodosin, tamsulosin, and alfuzosin. Reflex tachycardia due to stimulation of baroreceptors is common with alpha₁ blockers. Additional information on the alpha₁ blockers is presented in Chapter 16.

Some patients are unable to tolerate the cardiovascular adverse effects of the alpha₁-adrenergic blockers. For these patients, the 5-alpha reductase inhibitors are used as monotherapy. These drugs act by blocking 5-alpha reductase, the enzyme responsible for converting testosterone to DHT, which is its active metabolite. Without DHT the hormonal signal for prostatic epithelial tissue growth is eliminated, thus causing the enlarged prostate to shrink in size. The most commonly prescribed drug in this class is finasteride (Proscar), which is featured below as a prototype for BPH. These drugs may take several months to shrink the size of the prostate; thus, they are not appropriate for severe disease. The 5-alpha reductase inhibitors produce few adverse effects, although they can cause sexual dysfunction and gynecomastia in some patients. Because they are pregnancy category X, patients who are taking these drugs should not donate blood because of the possibility that the donated blood would be given to a pregnant woman.

CONNECTION Checkpoint 71.3

Alpha₁-adrenergic blockers are very susceptible to causing the "first-dose phenomenon." From what you learned in Chapter 16, define this phenomenon and describe what should be done to minimize its effects. *See Answer to Connection Checkpoint 71.3 on student resource website.*

PROTOTYPE DRUG	Finasteride (Proscar)

Classification: Therapeutic: Drug for BPH
Pharmacologic: Antiandrogen, 5-alpha reductase inhibitor

Therapeutic Effects and Uses: Approved in 1992, finasteride is a PO drug that inhibits the metabolism of testosterone. The drug is sometimes called an antiandrogen. Finasteride shrinks enlarged prostates, helping to restore urinary function. It is most effective in patients with larger prostates. It is sometimes prescribed in combination with doxazosin to reduce the risk of symptomatic progression of BPH. This drug is also marketed as Propecia, which is prescribed to promote hair regrowth in patients with male-pattern baldness. Doses of finasteride are five times higher when prescribed for BPH than when prescribed for baldness.

CONNECTIONS   Complementary and Alternative Therapies

◖ Saw Palmetto

Description

Saw palmetto (*Serenoa repens*) is a dwarf palm tree that grows in the coastal regions of the southern United States. The berries of the saw palmetto are used in supplements. More than 2 million men in the United States use saw palmetto each year in the hopes that it will treat their symptoms of BPH.

History and Claims

Like finasteride, saw palmetto is thought to help stop a cascade of prostate-damaging enzymes that may create BPH. In theory, it occupies binding sites on the prostate that are typically occupied by DHT, an enzyme that may trigger BPH, inhibiting growth of the prostate gland.

Standardization

Saw palmetto is available in capsule, tablet, and liquid dosage forms. PO saw palmetto products should be standardized to contain 80% or more of the active ingredients, which are fatty acids.

Evidence

Although several clinical studies have suggested that saw palmetto may be beneficial in treating BPH symptoms, there is insufficient evidence to conclude that it is as effective as finasteride in treating mild to moderate BPH (National Center for Complementary and Alternative Medicine [NCCAM], 2012). A meta-analysis of 17 randomized clinical trials found that therapy with saw palmetto had no effect over the placebo in improving lower urinary tract symptoms (MacDonald, Tacklind, Rutks, & Wilt, 2012). Although considered a safe supplement, saw palmetto may cause damage to the liver and pancreas, and it is vital that the nurse obtain a thorough health and supplement use history and advise the patient of its potential adverse effects.

Off-label indications for finasteride take advantage of its anti-androgen effects. It may be used to treat mild to moderate hirsutism in females. Although some clinical trials suggested the drug exerted a protective effect against prostate cancer, the drug insert from the manufacturer clearly states it is not to be prescribed for this purpose.

Mechanism of Action: Finasteride acts by inhibiting 5-alpha reductase, which is the enzyme responsible for converting testosterone to one of its metabolites, 5-alpha dihydrotestosterone. This active metabolite causes proliferation of prostate cells and promotes enlargement of the gland. Finasteride promotes regression of prostate epithelial tissue and decreases mechanical obstruction of the urethra.

Pharmacokinetics:

Route(s)	PO
Absorption	Well absorbed
Distribution	Crosses the blood–brain barrier; found in semen; 90% bound to plasma protein
Primary metabolism	Hepatic (CYP3A4)
Primary excretion	39% renal, 57% feces
Onset of action	Maximum effects take 3–6 months
Duration of action	2 weeks

Adverse Effects: Finasteride is well tolerated and adverse effects are generally mild and transient. Finasteride causes various types of sexual dysfunction in up to 16% of patients, including gynecomastia, impotence, diminished libido, and ejaculatory disorders such as decreased volume of ejaculate. The drug reduces sperm production and may impair fertility. The actual incidence of drug-induced sexual dysfunction is difficult to estimate because a large percentage of older males develop these symptoms as a consequence of aging or comorbid conditions. Other minor adverse effects include headache, nausea, rash, dizziness, and asthenia. Men over age 55 may have a slightly increased risk of developing high-grade prostate cancer.

Contraindications/Precautions: Contraindications to finasteride include hypersensitivity to the drug, pregnancy (category X), lactation, females, and children. The pregnant nurse or pharmacist should avoid handling crushed medication because it may be absorbed through the skin and cause harm to a male fetus. Caution must be used when administering the drug to patients with hepatic or renal impairment.

Drug Interactions: Use with anticholinergics may decrease the effects of finasteride. Use of finasteride with testosterone will result in a reduction in the effects of both drugs. **Herbal/Food**: Saw palmetto may potentiate the effects of finasteride.

Pregnancy: Category X.

Treatment of Overdose: There is no specific treatment for overdose.

Nursing Responsibilities: Key nursing implications for patients receiving finasteride are included in the Nursing Practice Application for Patients Receiving Pharmacotherapy for Benign Prostatic Hyperplasia.

Drugs Similar to Finasteride (Proscar)

The only other 5-alpha reductase inhibitor is dutasteride.

Dutasteride (Avodart): Approved in 2001, dutasteride is a PO drug approved only for the treatment of BPH. Compared to finasteride, dutasteride causes a greater inhibition of 5-alpha reductase and thus is able to more effectively lower DHT levels. It is estimated that serum DHT levels are lowered 90% to 93% with dutasteride and 70% by finasteride. Dutasteride has a half-life of 5 weeks and it remains in the body for several months after the drug is stopped. Like finasteride, sexual adverse effects such as reduced ejaculate volume, diminished libido, and ED occur in some patients. Other warnings, contraindications, and actions are the same as those of finasteride. Jalyn is a fixed-dose combination drug that contains dutasteride with tamsulosin. The drug is pregnancy category X.

CONNECTIONS: NURSING PRACTICE APPLICATION

Patients Receiving Pharmacotherapy for Benign Prostatic Hyperplasia

Assessment	Potential Nursing Diagnoses*
Baseline assessment prior to administration: • Obtain a complete health history including cardiovascular, peripheral vascular, thyroid, hepatic, or renal disease; diabetes; prostatic hyperplasia; or prostatic cancer. • Obtain a drug history including allergies, current prescription and OTC drugs, herbal preparations, alcohol use, and smoking. Be alert to possible drug interactions. • Evaluate appropriate laboratory findings (e.g., CBC, hepatic and renal function). • Obtain baseline vital signs. • Assess the patient's ability to receive and understand instructions. Include the family or caregiver as needed.	• *Sexual Dysfunction,* related to adverse drug effects • *Deficient Knowledge* (Drug Therapy) • *Risk for Falls,* related to adverse effects of alpha-adrenergic drug therapy
Assessment throughout administration: • Assess for desired therapeutic effects dependent on the reason the drug is given (e.g., urinary stream increases, lessened urinary retention). • Continue periodic monitoring of CBC, hepatic and renal function laboratory values, and PSA levels. • Monitor vital signs at each health care visit. • Assess for adverse effects: nausea, headache, rash, dizziness, or sexual dysfunction.	

Implementation

Interventions and (Rationales)	Patient-Centered Care
Ensuring therapeutic effects: • Monitor appropriate medication administration for optimal results. (Full therapeutic effects from 5-alpha reductase inhibitors may take 3–6 months to be achieved.)	• Teach the patient to continue taking the medication consistently during the early months of therapy and that the drug may take several months to achieve its full effects.
Minimizing adverse effects: • Continue to monitor hepatic function laboratory values periodically. (Hepatotoxicity is a potential adverse effect. **Lifespan:** Age-related physiological differences may place the older adult at greater risk for hepatic toxicity. **Diverse Patients:** Because erythromycin metabolizes through the P450 system pathways, monitor ethnically diverse patients to ensure optimal therapeutic effects and to minimize adverse effects.)	• Teach the patient to immediately report any increasing symptoms of urinary retention or slowing of the urinary stream. A prostate exam may be indicated. • Teach the patient to immediately report any symptoms of abdominal or right upper quadrant discomfort or pain, yellowing of the skin or sclera, fatigue, anorexia, darkened urine, clay-colored stools, weakness, lethargy, nausea, or vomiting.
• Monitor BP at each clinical visit. Check weight and for presence of edema. (Alpha-adrenergic blockers may trigger sodium and water retention with resulting increases in weight, BP, and possible edema. Immediately report any BP over 140/90 mmHg, peripheral edema, or weight gain.)	• Teach the patient taking alpha-adrenergic blockers to monitor BP on a weekly basis. Report any BP over 140/90 mmHg, or as directed, to the health care provider. Report any weight gain of 1 kg (2 lb) in 24 h or 2 kg (5 lb) in 1 week to the health care provider. Report any peripheral edema. Ensure proper functioning of any equipment used at home.
• Monitor urine output and symptoms of dysuria such as hesitancy or nocturia. (5-Alpha reductase inhibitors may cause urinary frequency, nocturia, or hesitancy.)	• Have the patient promptly report urinary hesitancy, frequency, or an increase in nocturia.
• Give the first dose of any alpha-adrenergic blocker at bedtime. (A first-dose response may result in a greater initial drop in BP than subsequent doses. This may also occur if the dose is increased. **Lifespan:** Be cautious with the older adult who is a greater risk for falls.)	• Instruct the patient to take the first dose of medication at bedtime, immediately before going to bed, and to avoid driving for 12–24 h after the first dose, or when the dosage is increased, until the effects are known. If dizziness occurs, the patient should sit or lie down and not attempt to stand or walk until the sensation passes.
• Do not abruptly stop alpha-adrenergic blockers used for BPH. (Rebound HTN and tachycardia may occur.)	• Teach the patient not to stop the medication abruptly and to call the health care provider for instructions if the patient is unable to take the medication for more than 2 days due to illness.
• Protect against accidental exposure to 5-alpha reductase inhibitors by women of childbearing age and children, including through handling of crushed or broken drugs. (The drug has teratogenic effects and handling by women of childbearing age should be avoided. Men should wear condoms during sexual activity and should not donate blood while taking the drug and up to 1 month after stopping the drug.)	• Teach the patient to keep the drug in a secure location to guard against accidental exposure to women of childbearing age or children. • Teach the patient to use condoms consistently for sexual activity to avoid exposing women of childbearing age to semen, which may also contain the drug. • Instruct the patient not to donate blood during the time the drug is taken and up to 1 month after the drug is stopped.

(continued)

Patient understanding of drug therapy: • Use opportunities during administration of medications and during assessments to discuss the rationale for drug therapy, desired therapeutic outcomes, commonly observed adverse effects, parameters for when to call the health care provider, and any necessary monitoring or precautions. (Using time during nursing care helps to optimize and reinforce key teaching areas.)	• The patient, family, or caregiver should be able to state the reason for the drug, the appropriate dose and scheduling, what adverse effects to observe for, and when to report them.
Patient self-administration of drug therapy: • When administering the medication, instruct the patient or caregiver in proper self-administration of the drug, e.g., consistently over several months of therapy, followed by teach-back. (Utilizing time during nurse-administration of these drugs helps to reinforce teaching.)	• The patient is able to discuss the appropriate dosing and administration needs.

*Nursing Diagnoses—Definitions and Classification 2015–2017. Copyright © 2014, 1994–2014 by NANDA International. Used by arrangement with John Wiley & Sons Limited.

CHAPTER

71

Understanding the Chapter

Key Concepts Summary

71.1 Male reproductive function is controlled through the secretion of androgens.

71.2 Androgens are used to treat hypogonadism and delayed puberty in males and breast cancer in females.

71.3 Often abused by athletes, anabolic steroids can cause serious adverse effects.

71.4 Male sexual dysfunction may have both medical and psychological etiologies.

71.5 Male infertility is treated with endocrine drugs that boost sperm production.

71.6 Erectile dysfunction is a common disorder that may be successfully treated with inhibitors of the enzyme phosphodiesterase-5.

71.7 Benign prostatic hyperplasia is an enlargement of the prostate that occurs in older men.

71.8 In its early stages, benign prostatic hyperplasia may be treated successfully with drug therapy.

Case Study: Making the Patient Connection

Remember the patient "Mike Mayhew" at the beginning of the chapter? Now read the remainder of the case study. Based on the information presented within this chapter, respond to the critical thinking questions that follow.

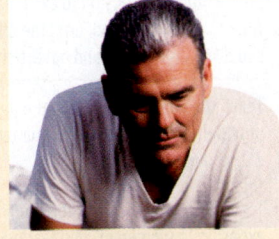

One year after his divorce, Mike, a 54-year-old white male, began dating and soon met Dana. The couple found that they had a lot in common and enjoyed each other's company. As the relationship grew, the couple became more intimate and sexually involved. However, the emotional scars from his previous marriage were painful and deeply affected him.

After the divorce, Mike was depressed and had low self-esteem. The condition required short-term hospitalization, and he now follows up on an outpatient basis with a psychiatrist. He has been taking antidepressants and was recently prescribed tadalafil (Cialis) for a diagnosis of ED. Mike also has a past history of HTN and is taking nifedipine (Procardia).

Critical Thinking Questions

1. What factors in Mike's life and health history do you think are contributing to the diagnosis of ED?

2. If you were the nurse, what patient education instructions would you provide to Mike regarding administration of tadalafil (Cialis) along with nifedipine (Procardia)?

3. After considering both options, Mike would rather be prescribed sildenafil (Viagra) instead of tadalafil (Cialis). What should the health care provider discuss with Mike about this request?

See Answers to Critical Thinking Questions on student resource website.

Additional Case Study

Morrie Jones, a 72-year-old white male, has been having difficulty with urinary frequency and excessive nighttime urination. He scheduled an appointment with his health care provider and is diagnosed with BPH. He is prescribed finasteride (Proscar) and needs to see his health care provider again in 6 months.

1. How would you explain the purpose of finasteride (Proscar) in treating BPH?

2. What education would you provide Mr. Jones that he may find helpful in dealing with BPH?

3. What additional health history and physical assessment findings would be considered in diagnosing this condition?

See Answers to Additional Case Study on student resource website.

Chapter Review

1 An adult patient has been receiving testosterone (Testoderm) for the treatment of primary hypogonadism. Which laboratory test would the nurse monitor to determine that this drug therapy is effective?

1. Red blood cell count
2. Sperm count
3. FSH
4. LH

2 The patient with erectile dysfunction is being evaluated for pharmacotherapy. Which question should the nurse ask prior to initiating therapy with sildenafil (Viagra)?

1. "Are you currently taking medications for angina?"
2. "Do you have a history of diabetes?"
3. "Have you ever had an allergic reaction to penicillin products?"
4. "Have you ever been treated for gastric ulcers?"

3 The nurse is teaching a patient who has received a prescription testosterone gel (AndroGel) for treatment of symptoms related to low androgen levels. What instructions should the nurse give the patient? Select all that apply.

1. "Apply the gel to the scrotal and perineal area daily."
2. "Avoid exposing women to the gel or to areas of skin where gel has been applied."
3. "Report any weight gain over 2 kilograms (5 pounds) in 1 week's time."
4. "Avoid showering or swimming for at least 12 to 14 hours after applying the gel."
5. "Maintain a low-fat diet and return periodically for blood lipid laboratory studies."

4 The nurse is counseling a patient about the goal of therapy with sildenafil (Viagra). What will the nurse teach the patient about the drug's effects?

1. It should always result in a penile erection within 10 minutes.
2. It is not effective if sexual dysfunction is psychological in nature.
3. It will result in less intense feelings with prolonged use.
4. It may heighten sexual response in female partners.

5 The nurse is teaching the patient about the use of finasteride (Proscar). What patient teaching related to this medication is needed? Select all that apply.

1. Finasteride promotes shrinkage of an enlarged prostate and helps restore urinary function.
2. The drug should not be handled by women who may be pregnant.
3. Finasteride affects both near and far vision in older adult males.
4. Six to 12 months may be required before the benefits of finasteride are achieved.
5. The drug may cause significant dizziness, which can be avoided by making position changes slowly.

6 A patient who has taken finasteride (Proscar) for the past 8 months reports a sudden increase in urinary hesitancy, urinary retention, and slowing of the urinary stream. What will the nurse teach this patient to do?

1. Continue to take the drug to achieve full effects.
2. Decrease the intake of coffee, tea, and alcohol.
3. Discuss the use of a low-dose diuretic with the health care provider.
4. Return to the health care provider for a prostate exam.

See Answers to Chapter Review in Appendix A.

References

Chou, R., Croswell, J. M., Dana, T., Bougatsos, C., Blazina, I., Fu, R., … Lin, K. (2011). Screening for prostate cancer: A review of the evidence for the U.S. Preventive Services Task Force. *Annals of Internal Medicine, 155,* 762–771. doi:10.7326/0003-4819-155-11-201112060-00375

Fronczak, C. M., Kim, E. D., & Barqawi, A. B. (2012). The insults of illicit drug use on male fertility. *Journal of Andrology, 33,* 515–528. doi:10.2164/jandrol.110.011874

MacDonald, R., Tacklind, J. W., Rutks, I., & Wilt, T. J. (2012). Serenoa repens monotherapy for benign prostatic hyperplasia (BPH): An updated Cochrane systematic review. *BJU International, 109*(12), 1756–1761. doi:10.1111/j.1464-410X.2012.11172.x

National Center for Complementary and Alternative Medicine (NCCAM). (2012). *Herbs at a glance: Saw palmetto.* Retrieved from http://nccam.nih.gov/health/palmetto/ataglance.htm

Selected Bibliography

Bruzziches, R., Francomano, D., Gareri, P., Lenzi, A., & Aversa, A. (2013). An update on pharmacological treatment of erectile dysfunction with phosphodiesterase type 5 inhibitors. *Expert Opinion on Pharmacotherapy, 14,* 1333–1344. doi:10.1517/14656566.2013.799665

Centers for Disease Control and Prevention. (2014). *Prostate cancer.* Retrieved from http://www.cdc.gov/cancer/prostate/

Filson, C. P., Wei, J. T., & Hollingsworth, J. M. (2013). Trends in medical management of men with lower urinary tract symptoms suggestive of benign prostatic hyperplasia. *Urology, 82*(6), 1386–1392. doi:10.1016/j.urology.2013.07.062

Hellstrom, W. J., Douglass, L. M., & Powers, M. K. (2012). *How does avanafil compare for erectile dysfunction?* Retrieved from http://www.medscape.com/viewarticle/768904

Herdman, T. H., & Kamitsuru, S. (Eds.). (2014). *NANDA International nursing diagnoses: Definitions and classification, 2015–2017.* Oxford, United Kingdom: Wiley-Blackwell.

Kim, E. D. (2014). *Erectile dysfunction.* Retrieved from http://emedicine.medscape.com/article/444220-overview

Lunenfeld, B., Mskhalaya, G., Kalinchenko, S., & Tishova, Y. (2013). Recommendations on the diagnosis, treatment and monitoring of late-onset hypogonadism in men—a suggested update. *The Aging Male, 16,* 143–150. doi:10.3109/13685538.2013.853731

Roehrborn, C. G. (2011). Male lower urinary tract symptoms (LUTS) and benign prostatic hyperplasia (BPH). *Medical Clinics of North America, 95,* 87–100. doi:10.1016/j.mcna.2010.08.013

Samplaski, M. K., Loai, Y., Wong, K., Lo, K. C., Grober, E. D., & Jarvi, K. A. (2014). Testosterone use in the male infertility population: Prescribing patterns and effects on semen and hormonal parameters. *Fertility and Sterility, 101,* 64–69. doi:10.1016/j.fertnstert.2013.09.003

Ullah, M. I., Riche, D. M., & Koch, C. A. (2014). Transdermal testosterone replacement therapy in men. *Drug Design, Development and Therapy, 8,* 101. doi:10.2147/DDDT.S43475

Winters, B. R., & Walsh, T. J. (2014). The epidemiology of male infertility. *Urologic Clinics of North America, 41,* 195–204. doi:10.1016/j.ucl.2013.08.006

Additional Drug Classes

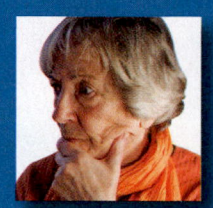
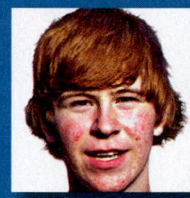
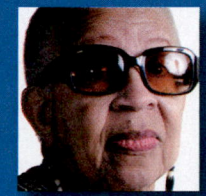
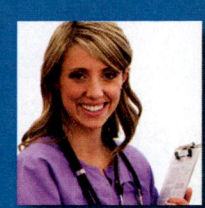

CHAPTER 72   Pharmacotherapy of Bone and Joint Disorders / 1228

CHAPTER 73   Pharmacotherapy of Dermatologic Disorders / 1261

CHAPTER 74   Pharmacotherapy of Eye and Ear Disorders / 1283

CHAPTER 75   Emergency Preparedness: Bioterrorism and Management of Poisoning / 1302

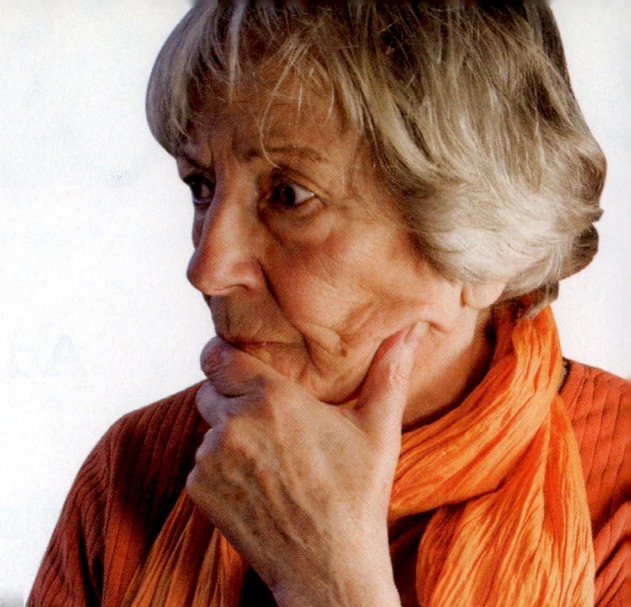

"My clothes just don't seem to fit right anymore. My pant legs are dragging on the ground. Is it possible that I'm getting shorter?"

Patient "Darlene Coleman"

Pharmacotherapy of Bone and Joint Disorders

LEARNING OUTCOMES

After reading this chapter, the student should be able to:

1. Describe the role of calcium in maintaining homeostasis in the nervous, muscular, skeletal, and cardiovascular systems.

2. Identify the recommended dietary allowance and the normal serum levels of calcium.

3. Explain the roles of parathyroid hormone, calcitonin, and vitamin D in maintaining calcium balance.

4. Explain the etiology, pathogenesis, and pharmacotherapy for hypocalcemia, osteomalacia, osteoporosis, rickets, osteoarthritis, rheumatoid arthritis, and gout.

5. Describe the nurse's role in the pharmacologic management of bone and joint disorders.

6. For each of the classes shown in the chapter outline, identify the prototype and representative drugs and explain the mechanism(s) of drug action, primary indications, contraindications, significant drug interactions, pregnancy category, and important adverse effects.

7. Apply the nursing process to the care of patients who are receiving pharmacotherapy for bone and joint disorders.

CHAPTER OUTLINE

▸ **Role of Calcium in Body Homeostasis**

▸ **Regulation of Calcium Balance**

▸ **Pharmacotherapy of Hypocalcemia**
   Calcium Supplements
   PROTOTYPE Calcium Salts, *p. 1232*

▸ **Pathophysiology of Metabolic Bone Disease**

▸ **Pharmacotherapy of Metabolic Bone Disease**
   Vitamin D Therapy
   PROTOTYPE Calcitriol (Calcijet, Rocaltrol), *p. 1237*
   Bisphosphonates
   PROTOTYPE Alendronate (Fosamax), *p. 1240*
   Selective Estrogen Receptor Modulators
   PROTOTYPE Raloxifene (Evista), *p. 1242*
   Calcitonin and Miscellaneous Drugs

▸ **Pathophysiology and Pharmacotherapy of Joint Disorders**
   Osteoarthritis
   Rheumatoid Arthritis
   PROTOTYPE Hydroxychloroquine (Plaquenil), *p. 1249*

▸ **Pharmacotherapy of Gout and Hyperuricemia**
   PROTOTYPE Colchicine (Colcrys), *p. 1253*
   PROTOTYPE Allopurinol (Lopurin, Zyloprim), *p. 1255*

KEY TERMS

acute gouty arthritis, 1253

bisphosphonates, 1239

bone deposition, 1231

bone resorption, 1231

calcitonin, 1231

calcitriol, 1232

cholecalciferol, 1232

disease-modifying antirheumatic drugs (DMARDs), 1247

gout, 1253

hyperuricemia, 1253

metabolic bone disease (MBD), 1233

osteoarthritis (OA), 1244

osteomalacia, 1236

osteoporosis, 1236

Paget's disease, 1237

rheumatoid arthritis (RA), 1246

selective estrogen receptor modulators (SERMs), 1242

uricosurics, 1255

xanthine oxidase, 1255

The bones and joints are at the core of body movement. Disorders that are associated with the skeletal system can lead to immobility and affect a patient's ability to fulfill activities of daily living (ADLs). In addition, the skeletal system serves as the primary repository for calcium, which is one of the body's most important minerals.

This chapter focuses on the pharmacotherapy of important skeletal and joint disorders such as osteomalacia, osteoporosis, arthritis, and gout. The importance of calcium balance and the action of vitamin D are stressed because they are critical to the proper structure and function of bones.

Role of Calcium in Body Homeostasis

72.1 Adequate levels of calcium in the body are necessary to transmit nerve impulses, to prevent muscle spasms, and for proper bone health.

Calcium balance is critical to the proper functioning of the nervous, muscular, skeletal, and cardiovascular systems. In the nervous system calcium ions influence the release of neurotransmitters and the excitability of all neurons. Contraction is dependent on calcium ion movement in skeletal, smooth, and cardiac muscle cells. Calcium is important for the normal functioning of other body processes such as blood coagulation by converting prothrombin into thrombin and in activating enzymes that catalyze many essential chemical reactions.

Calcium is the major cation for the structure of the bones and teeth. Total body content of calcium is about 1,200 g or approximately 2% of the total body weight. More than 99% of that calcium is in the skeletal system and is bound as a hard matrix known as hydroxyapatite crystals. Only about 1% of the calcium in bone is rapidly exchangeable with blood calcium; the remaining calcium is more stable and slowly exchanged.

Much of the calcium found outside of bone circulates in the blood. Calcium exists in plasma in three forms: ionized, bound, and complexed. About 50% of the serum calcium is in an active, ionized form that participates in intracellular functions, including neuromuscular activity and blood coagulation. This is the only physiologically and clinically significant form of calcium. An adequate amount of free or ionized calcium is required for normal body functions. Most of the remaining 50% of calcium in plasma is bound to plasma proteins, primarily albumin, and other substances and is unavailable for general use by the body.

To maintain homeostasis, the body must obtain sufficient amounts of calcium through proper nutrition and dietary supplements. Unfortunately, only 30% to 50% of dietary calcium is absorbed from the small intestine. The amount absorbed, however, is dynamic and changes with body conditions. Absorption is increased by moderate amounts of fat or high protein intake, high gastric acidity, and when certain hormones are secreted in response to low blood calcium. Decreased absorption occurs with vitamin D deficiency, high-fat diet, decreased gastric acidity, certain hormones secreted in response to high blood calcium, and conditions that increase gastrointestinal (GI) motility such as diarrhea. Dietary calcium that remains unabsorbed is excreted in feces. Calcium can also be lost through the nails, hair, sweat, and other body fluids. In lactating women, large amounts are lost through breast milk.

The recommended dietary allowance (RDA) of calcium for healthy adults is 1,000 to 1,200 mg per day. Higher amounts are needed by pregnant and lactating females, growing children, and postmenopausal women, as given in Table 72.1. The best dietary sources of calcium are dairy products. The calcium found in milk is the most readily available form because milk contains sufficient amounts of vitamin D, which is necessary for calcium absorption. Other rich sources of calcium include seafood, such as salmon, oysters, and clams, and green leafy vegetables, such as kale, broccoli, spinach, and mustard greens. If the body does not obtain enough dietary calcium, it will remove calcium from the bones, resulting in bones that become soft and weakened and that eventually develop osteoporosis. The importance of meeting the daily RDA for

TABLE 72.1 Normal Recommended Daily Intakes for Calcium

Age/Condition	U.S. RDA (mg)
0–6 months	200
7–12 months	260
1–3 years	700
4–8 years	1,000
9–18 years	1,300
19–70 years	1,000*
71+	1,200
Pregnant and lactating women (14–18 years)	1,300
Pregnant and lactating women (19–50 years)	1,000

*1,200 for women 51–70 years

calcium is vital to both women and men. Although not as prevalent, men may develop bone conditions such as osteoporosis, and adequate calcium intake should be added to their list of preventive health care interventions.

The normal serum calcium range is 4.5 to 5.5 mEq/L or 8.5 to 10.5 mg/dL. Serum calcium concentrations that exceed 5.5 mEq/L result in hypercalcemia, which causes a decrease in sodium permeability across cell membranes. This is a dangerous state because nerve conduction depends on the proper influx of sodium into cells. When calcium levels in the bloodstream are below 4.5 mEq/L, a state of hypocalcemia develops and the cell membranes become hyperexcitable. If this situation becomes severe, convulsions or muscle spasms may result.

PharmFACT

In the United States, 1.5 million osteoporotic fractures occur each year. Of these, 700,000 are spinal fractures; 300,000 are hip fractures; and 200,000 are wrist fractures (Jacobs-Kosmin, 2013).

Regulation of Calcium Balance

72.2 Calcium balance is regulated by parathyroid hormone, calcitonin, and vitamin D.

Calcium balance is controlled by parathyroid hormone, calcitonin, and vitamin D. Acting together, these three substances regulate the rate of absorption of calcium from the small intestine, the excretion of calcium from the kidney, and the movement of calcium into and out of bone. Calcium balance is illustrated in Figure 72.1.

Parathyroid hormone: Parathyroid hormone (PTH) is secreted from the parathyroid gland, as illustrated in Figure 72.1. The parathyroid glands contain calcium receptors that are able to sense very small changes in serum calcium concentration. When the serum levels of ionized calcium decrease, the parathyroid glands secrete PTH. PTH directly increases calcium reabsorption in the renal tubule and releases calcium from bone (resorption). PTH indirectly increases serum calcium by promoting the formation of activated vitamin D,

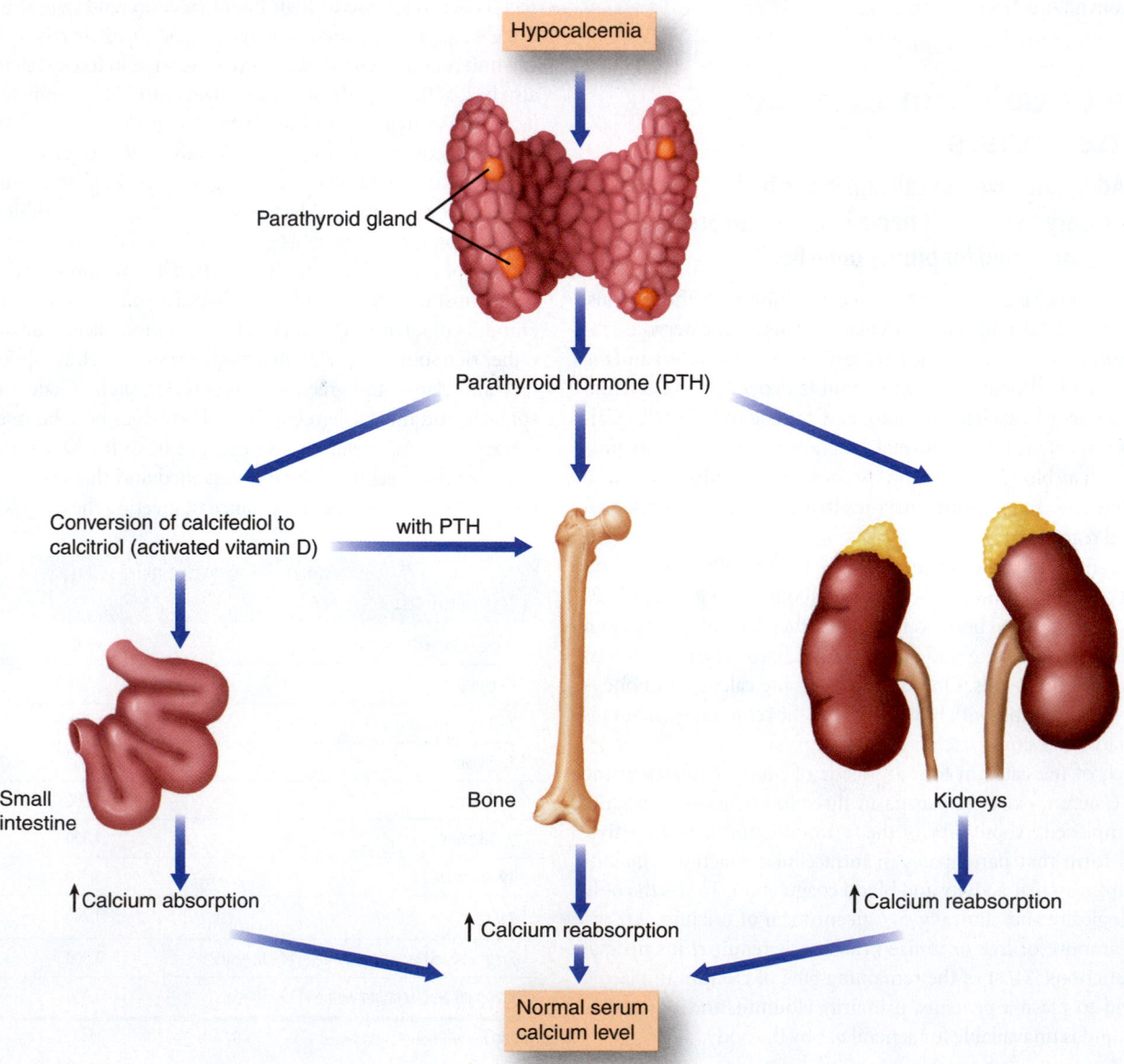

Figure 72.1 Calcium balance.

which then increases calcium absorption from the GI tract. The overall effect of these physiological changes is to rapidly (within minutes) increase serum calcium, returning it to normal levels.

The parathyroid glands are regulated by a typical negative feedback loop. An increase in the ionized serum calcium is recognized by calcium receptors in the parathyroid gland, which suppress PTH secretion. A second piece of the negative feedback loop is that activated vitamin D also shuts down PTH secretion. Without PTH present, the absorption of calcium from the GI tract is diminished, the reabsorption in the kidney tubule decreases, and calcium remains deposited in bone.

The exchange of calcium between the serum and bones is influenced by PTH and calcitonin. PTH stimulates bone cells called osteoclasts. These cells accelerate the process of **bone resorption**, or demineralization, which breaks down bone into its mineral components. Once bone is broken down (resorbed), calcium becomes available to be transported and used elsewhere in the body. The opposite of this process is **bone deposition**, or bone building, which is accomplished by cells called osteoblasts. This process, which removes calcium from the blood to be placed in bone, is stimulated by the hormone calcitonin. It is important to note that maintaining normal serum calcium levels takes precedence over the calcium requirements of the bone. If serum calcium levels are low, bone resorption will occur even if it compromises the structural integrity of the bone matrix.

Calcitonin: When serum calcium levels become elevated, the hormone **calcitonin** is released by the thyroid gland. Calcitonin acts in opposition to PTH and vitamin D to decrease the plasma levels of calcium by inhibiting the resorption of calcium from bone and increasing the excretion of calcium by the kidney, thus decreasing the concentration of serum calcium. It is important to note that calcitonin does not affect the rates of calcium absorption from the small intestine. Calcitonin is available as a medication for the treatment of osteoporosis.

Vitamin D: The regulation of the rate of absorption of calcium from the small intestine is influenced primarily by PTH, but vitamin D is a required component. Vitamin D and calcium metabolism are intimately related: Absorption of calcium is increased in the presence of vitamin D, and absorption is inhibited by vitamin D deficiency. Thus, calcium disorders are often associated with vitamin D disorders.

Vitamin D is unique among vitamins because it is the only vitamin that the body is able to synthesize from precursor molecules. Several steps, however, are required before vitamin D can act on target tissues. Figure 72.2 illustrates the metabolism of vitamin D.

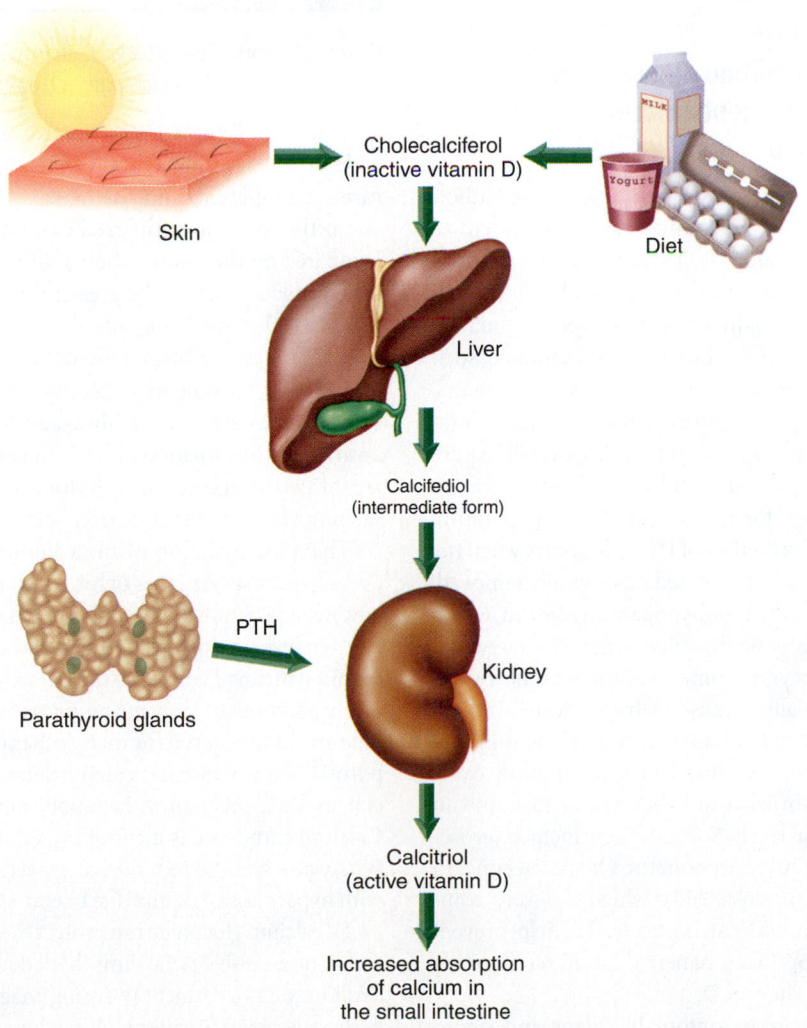

Figure 72.2 Pathway for vitamin D activation.

In the skin, **cholecalciferol**, the inactive form of vitamin D, is synthesized from cholesterol. Exposure of the skin to sunlight or ultraviolet light increases the level of cholecalciferol in the blood. Cholecalciferol can also be obtained from dietary products such as milk or other foods fortified with vitamin D.

Following its absorption from dietary sources or formation in the skin, cholecalciferol is converted to an intermediate vitamin form called calcifediol. Enzymes in the kidneys then metabolize calcifediol to **calcitriol**, the active form of vitamin D. PTH stimulates the formation of calcitriol at the level of the kidneys. Patients with extensive kidney disease are unable to adequately synthesize calcitriol and thus frequently experience calcium and vitamin D abnormalities. The primary function of calcitriol is to increase calcium absorption from the GI tract. Dietary calcium is absorbed more efficiently in the presence of active vitamin D and PTH, resulting in higher serum levels of calcium, which is then transported to bone, muscle, and other tissues.

CONNECTION Checkpoint 72.1

Inhibition of calcium transport into cells can have important physiological effects. From what you learned in Chapter 30, what are the primary indications for pharmacotherapy with calcium channel blockers? *See Answer to Connection Checkpoint 72.1 on student resource website.*

Pharmacotherapy of Hypocalcemia

72.3 Hypocalcemia is a condition that requires therapy with calcium supplements, often concurrently with vitamin D.

Hypocalcemia is not a disease but is a sign of underlying pathology. Therefore, diagnosis of the cause of hypocalcemia is essential. Many factors can cause hypocalcemia. Lack of sufficient dietary calcium or vitamin D intake is a common cause and one that can be easily reversed by nutritional adjustments. If hypocalcemia occurs with normal dietary intake, GI causes must be examined, such as excessive vomiting or the presence of malabsorption disorders. Damage to renal tubular cells may cause excessive loss of calcium in the urine. Most patients with chronic kidney disease will require calcium and vitamin D therapy to prevent hypocalcemia.

Another common etiology for hypocalcemia is hypoparathyroidism leading to decreased secretion of PTH, as occurs when the thyroid and parathyroid glands are diseased or surgically removed. A rare cause of hypocalcemia is pseudohypoparathyroidism, which is an uncommon group of genetic disorders where the target organs for PTH (bone and kidneys) become resistant to the hormone.

Drug therapy is occasionally a cause of hypocalcemia. Blood transfusions and certain anticonvulsants such as phenytoin and phenobarbital can lower serum calcium levels. In addition, overtreatment with drugs that are used to lower serum calcium can result in overshooting normal levels. Some of these include furosemide, phosphate therapy, or bisphosphonates. Of special concern is long-term therapy with corticosteroids, which is a very common cause of hypocalcemia and osteoporosis. To help prevent corticosteroid-induced osteoporosis, patients should receive daily supplements of calcium and vitamin D.

Hypocalcemia is frequently asymptomatic. Signs and symptoms of hypocalcemia are those of nerve and muscle excitability.

The symptoms include confusion, paresthesias around the mouth and in the digits, carpopedal spasms, and hyperreflexia. Muscle twitching, tremors, or cramping may be evident. Two clinical signs are Chvostek's sign and Trousseau's sign. Chvostek's sign is elicited by tapping on the facial nerve just below the temple. A positive sign is a twitch of the nose or lip. Trousseau's sign is the contraction of the hand and fingers when the arterial blood flow in the arm is occluded for 5 minutes.

Intestinal cramping and hyperactive bowel sounds may be present because the low calcium levels affect the smooth muscle of the GI tract. Severe symptoms include convulsions, laryngeal spasms, and tetany. Tetany is a continuous muscle spasm that can interfere with breathing and even cause death. The characteristic electrocardiogram (ECG) change is a prolonged QT interval, indicating prolonged ventricular depolarization with characteristically weak cardiac muscle contractions.

Unless the hypocalcemia is especially severe or life threatening, adjustments in diet should be attempted prior to initiating therapy with calcium supplements. Increasing the consumption of calcium-rich foods, especially dairy products, fortified orange juice, cereals, and green leafy vegetables, is often sufficient to restore calcium balance.

PROTOTYPE DRUG	Calcium Salts

Classification: Therapeutic: Calcium supplement
Pharmacologic: Drugs for hypocalcemia

Therapeutic Effects and Uses: Calcium salts are available in a wide variety of products and formulations. Calcium has two major forms: complexed and elemental. Most calcium supplements are in the form of complexed calcium. These products are often compared on the basis of their ability to release elemental calcium into the bloodstream. The greater the ability of complexed calcium to release elemental calcium, the more potent is the supplement. Table 72.2 lists the doses for selected calcium supplements.

For mild, chronic hypocalcemia, effective and inexpensive calcium supplements are readily available over the counter (OTC) in a variety of formulations. Calcium carbonate and calcium citrate are the two most common salts for routine supplementation. Many calcium supplements also contain vitamin D.

The administration of intravenous (IV) calcium salts may be necessary for severe cases of hypocalcemia or if the patient is in tetany. Repeated infusions are sometimes required to return the serum calcium level to normal. Constant monitoring of serum calcium is required during IV administration to prevent hypercalcemia.

In addition to preventing or treating hypocalcemia, calcium salts are administered for many other conditions, including osteoporosis, Paget's disease, osteomalacia, chronic hypoparathyroidism, rickets, pregnancy, lactation, and rapid childhood growth. Calcium carbonate is a common antacid used to treat heartburn. It may also be used to bind excessive dietary phosphate in patients with hyperphosphatemia due to end-stage renal disease.

IV calcium gluconate can protect the heart against the hyperexcitability of excessive potassium (hyperkalemia) and help to maintain cardiorespiratory function during magnesium sulfate toxicity (hypermagnesemia) situations. IV calcium salts have been administered during cardiac arrest due to their ability to increase cardiac muscle

TABLE 72.2 Selected Calcium Salts

Drug	Calcium Content	Route and Adult Dose (Maximum Dose Where Indicated)	Adverse Effects
Calcium Supplements (All doses are in terms of elemental calcium.)			*Constipation, nausea, vomiting, metallic taste*
calcium acetate (PhosLo)	25%	Oral (PO): 2–4 tablets with each meal (each tablet contains 169 mg calcium)	
calcium carbonate (Rolaids, Tums, OsCal, Others)	40%	PO: 1–2 g bid–tid	<u>Hypercalcemia (drowsiness, lethargy, headache, anorexia, nausea, vomiting, increased urination, and thirst), dysrhythmias, cardiac arrest, confusion, delirium, stupor, coma</u>
calcium chloride	27 mg Ca/mL	IV: 0.5–4 g by slow infusion (1 mL/min)	
calcium citrate (Citracal)	21%	PO: 1–2 g bid–tid	
calcium gluconate (Kalcinate)	9% (PO); 9 mg Ca/mL (IV)	PO: 0.5–2 g bid–tid IV: 0.5–4 g by slow infusions (1 g/h)	
calcium lactate (Cal-Lac)	13%	PO: 100–200 mg tid with meals	
calcium phosphate tribasic (Posture)	39%	PO: 1–2 g bid–tid	

Note: Italics indicate common adverse effects. <u>Underline</u> indicates serious adverse effects.

tone and the force of systolic contraction (positive inotropic effect). However, the use of calcium salts in cardiac resuscitation has declined and is limited to patients with cardiac disease who have hypocalcemia because calcium salts may cause dysrhythmias at high doses.

Mechanism of Action: Calcium salts restore the normal serum levels of calcium, which promotes deposition of the mineral in bone. This helps to restore bone strength and prevent fractures. Calcium also restores normal neuromuscular function and muscular contraction.

Pharmacokinetics: The pharmacokinetics of calcium salts varies by the route of administration and the specific formulation. They are widely distributed and excreted primarily in the feces, with about 20% in the urine. The duration of action of calcium salts is generally only a few hours.

Adverse Effects: Oral calcium products are safe and produce few adverse effects when used as directed. The most common adverse effect of calcium supplements is hypercalcemia, which is caused by taking too much of this supplement. This can be especially serious in the IV formulations. Symptoms of hypercalcemia include drowsiness, lethargy, weakness, headache, anorexia, constipation, increased gastric acid secretion, nausea, vomiting, a tingling sensation, increased urination, and thirst. IV administration of calcium may cause pain and burning at the IV site, severe venous thrombosis, necrosis, sloughing of the skin (with extravasation), hypotension, sensations of heat waves (peripheral vasodilation), fainting, bradycardia, cardiac dysrhythmias, and cardiac arrest. Large doses of supplemental calcium may lead to the formation of symptomatic kidney stones.

Contraindications/Precautions: Calcium salts are contraindicated in patients with ventricular fibrillation, metastatic bone disease, renal calculi, hypercalcemia, predisposition to hypercalcemia, hyperparathyroidism, certain malignancies, and digoxin toxicity. Calcium salts should not be injected into the myocardium or administered by the subcutaneous or intramuscular (IM) route. Caution must be used with patients who have renal or cardiac insufficiency, dysrhythmias, dehydration, diarrhea, hyperphosphatemia, sarcoidosis, or history of kidney stones. Immobilized patients are at high risk for the development of hypercalcemia.

Drug Interactions: Concurrent use with digoxin increases the risk of dysrhythmias and enhances the inotropic effects of digoxin. Magnesium may compete for GI absorption. Calcium decreases the absorption of tetracyclines and fluoroquinolones, such as ciprofloxacin. Their use may antagonize the effects of verapamil and possibly other calcium channel blockers. **Herbal/Food:** Zinc-rich foods such as shellfish, dried beans, sesame seeds, pumpkin seeds, and many meats may decrease the absorption of calcium. Alcohol, caffeine, and carbonated beverages affect the absorption of calcium. Oxalic acid in spinach, rhubarb, Swiss chard, and beets can suppress calcium absorption. Phytic acid, which is present in bran and whole-grain cereals, depresses calcium absorption.

Pregnancy: Category B or C.

Treatment of Overdose: Measures may be taken to treat cardiac abnormalities caused by the hypercalcemia that results from overdose.

Nursing Responsibilities: Key nursing implications for patients receiving calcium supplementation are included in the Nursing Practice Application for Patients Receiving Pharmacotherapy for Osteoporosis.

Drugs Similar to Calcium Salts

A large number of calcium salts are available. A summary of their indications is shown in Table 72.3.

Pathophysiology of Metabolic Bone Disease

72.4 Metabolic bone disease is characterized by abnormal bone structure.

Metabolic bone disease (MBD) is a general term that refers to a cluster of disorders that have in common defects in the structure of bone. MBDs are caused by abnormal amounts of the minerals or hormones responsible for bone homeostasis, such as calcium, phosphate, vitamin D, or PTH. Some MBDs have a genetic etiology, whereas others are iatrogenic and caused by certain drugs and therapies.

TABLE 72.3 Indications for Selected Calcium Salts

Salt	Antacid	Management of Hyperkalemia	Management of Hypermagnesemia	Management of Hyperphosphatemia	Prevention and Treatment of Hypocalcemia	Cardiotonic	Mineral Supplement	Electrolyte Replenishment
calcium acetate				X				
calcium carbonate	X			X	X		X	
calcium chloride	X	X	X			X		X
calcium citrate				X	X		X	
calcium glubionate					X		X	
calcium gluconate injection		X	X		X	X		X
calcium lactate					X		X	
calcium phosphate, dibasic					X		X	

CONNECTIONS: NURSING PRACTICE APPLICATION

Patients Receiving Pharmacotherapy for Osteoporosis

Assessment	Potential Nursing Diagnoses*
Baseline assessment prior to administration: • Obtain a complete health history including musculoskeletal, GI, cardiovascular, neurologic, endocrine, hepatic, or renal disease. Obtain a drug history including allergies, current prescription and OTC drugs, and herbal preparations, alcohol use, or smoking. Be alert to possible drug interactions. • Obtain a history of any current symptoms and their effect on ADLs. Assess muscle strength and gait and note any pain or discomfort on movement or at rest. Obtain bone density studies if ordered. • Obtain a dietary history, noting adequacy of essential vitamins, minerals, and nutrients obtained through food sources, particularly calcium, vitamin D, and magnesium. Note amount of soda or other nondairy fluids intake daily. • Note sunscreen use and amount of sun exposure. • Obtain baseline height, weight, and vital signs. • Evaluate appropriate laboratory findings (e.g., CBC, electrolytes, calcium, phosphorus, and magnesium levels, hepatic and renal function studies). • Assess the patient's ability to receive and understand instructions. Include the family or caregiver as needed.	• *Acute* or *Chronic Pain*, bone or joints; related to disease condition • *Deficient Knowledge* (Drug Therapy) • *Risk for Injury*, related to adverse drug effects • *Risk for Falls*, related to adverse drug effects
Assessment throughout administration: • Assess for desired therapeutic effects dependent on the reason for the drug (e.g., calcium, phosphate, and magnesium levels are within normal limits, bone density studies show improvement). • Continue monitoring laboratory values as appropriate, especially calcium, phosphorus, and magnesium. • Assess for and promptly report adverse effects: nausea, vomiting, abdominal pain, esophageal irritation, constipation, diarrhea, or symptoms of electrolyte imbalances. Severe GI irritation or pain should be reported immediately.	

CONNECTIONS: NURSING PRACTICE APPLICATION (continued)

Implementation

Interventions and (Rationales)	Patient-Centered Care
Ensuring therapeutic effects: • Review the dietary history with the patient and discuss food source options for correcting any deficiencies, particularly calcium and vitamin D intake. Encourage the patient to adopt a healthy lifestyle of increased activity or exercise, adequate sun exposure, limited caffeine and soda intake, and limited or eliminated alcohol consumption. (Adequate amounts of calcium, vitamin D, and magnesium are needed for bone health. Any deficiencies should be corrected before bisphosphonates are started. Adequate sun exposure, approximately 15–20 min/day without sunscreens, may assist in vitamin D formation. Excessive soda, caffeine, or other nondairy intake may increase the risk of osteoporosis due to lessened calcium consumption and decreased calcium absorption from caffeine effects.)	• Encourage adequate amounts of calcium, vitamin D, and magnesium from food sources. Provide educational pamphlets or web-based references to reputable sources as needed (e.g., NIH Office of Dietary Supplements). Provide dietitian referral as needed. • Encourage limited amounts of sun exposure daily without sunscreens, approximately 15–20 min. Discourage prolonged sun exposure beyond that time. • Teach the patient that excessive soda intake may take the place of beverages with milk or dairy. Excessive soda, caffeine, and other nondairy consumption may diminish absorption of dietary calcium. • Encourage adequate activity and exercise, especially weight-bearing exercise, three to five times per week.
• Follow administration guidelines for optimal results. (Calcium supplements and vitamin D should be taken with meals or within 1 h after meals for best absorption. Bisphosphonates should be taken on an empty stomach with a full glass of water and the patient should remain upright for 30 min to 1 h. Bisphosphonates and calcium preparations should be taken 2 h apart.)	• Teach the patient the appropriate administration guidelines for best results. Ensure that the patient is able to remain upright if bisphosphonates are used.
Minimizing adverse effects: • Monitor for GI irritation or abdominal pain. (Bisphosphonates may cause esophageal irritation and erosion. Increasing nausea, gastric, or abdominal pain should be reported immediately.)	• Instruct the patient to immediately report any new onset of nausea or any increasing or severe chest or abdominal discomfort or pain.
• Continue to monitor periodic laboratory work, especially calcium, magnesium, phosphorus, vitamin D, and creatinine as needed. Assess for signs or symptoms of hypo- or hypercalcemia. (Calcium, magnesium, phosphorus, and vitamin D levels should return to, and remain within, normal limits. Increased creatinine levels may indicate renal effects and may require discontinuation of medications.)	• Instruct the patient on the need to return periodically for laboratory work. • Instruct the patient to immediately report symptoms of hypocalcemia (muscle spasms, facial grimacing, irritability, hyperreflexes) or hypercalcemia (increased bone pain, anorexia, nausea, vomiting, constipation, thirst, lethargy, or fatigue).
• Monitor the use of vitamin D. Excessive intake may lead to toxic effects. (Fat-soluble vitamins are stored in the body and may accumulate and result in toxic levels. Monitor liver function studies and for symptoms such as nausea, vomiting, headache, fatigue, dry and itchy skin, blurred vision, or palpitations. Report any symptoms immediately.)	• Instruct the patient not to take additional or large amounts of vitamin D unless instructed by the provider. • Encourage the patient to obtain fat-soluble vitamins from natural sources through a balanced diet whenever possible.
• Increase fluid intake, avoiding caffeine or soda. (Increased fluid intake decreases the risk of renal calculi formation.)	• Encourage the patient to increase fluid intake to 2 L/day, divided throughout the day, but avoid highly caffeinated beverages and excessive soda intake.
• Monitor adherence to the recommended regimen. (Bone remodeling occurs over several months and effects may not be noted immediately. The patient may discontinue drug therapy because of a perceived lack of response.)	• Teach the patient to continue taking the drug therapy regularly to ensure full effects. Therapeutic response may take 1–3 months and effects continue after the drug has been discontinued.
• Note and promptly report any new-onset thigh or groin pain, unilaterally or bilaterally. (An increased incidence of atypical fractures has been noted in some patients taking bisphosphonates, particularly with long-term use or with concurrent corticosteroid use. Thigh or groin pain has been noted to occur prior to fracture and should be reported to the provider for assessment.)	• Teach the patient to promptly report any new onset of groin or thigh pain, either unilaterally or bilaterally. • Advise the patient to review the need for continued bisphosphonate use with the health care provider based on bone density studies on a regular basis.
Patient understanding of drug therapy: • Use opportunities during administration of medications and during assessments to discuss the rationale for drug therapy, desired therapeutic outcomes, commonly observed adverse effects, parameters for when to call the health care provider, and any necessary monitoring or precautions. (Using time during nursing care helps to optimize and reinforce key teaching areas.)	• The patient should be able to state the reason for the drug, appropriate dose and scheduling, what adverse effects to observe for and when to report them, and the anticipated length of the medication therapy.
Patient self-administration of drug therapy: • When administering the medication, instruct the patient, family, or caregiver in proper self-administration of the drug, e.g., taken with additional fluids, followed by teach-back. (Utilizing time during nurse-administration of these drugs helps to reinforce teaching.)	• The patient, family, or caregiver is able to discuss appropriate dosing and administration needs including: • *Calcium supplements:* Take with meals or immediately after meals. • *Bisphosphonates:* Take with a full glass of plain water and remain in an upright position for 30 min to 1 h after taking.

Osteoporosis: Osteoporosis is an MBD characterized by bone demineralization, decreased bone density, and subsequent fractures. Osteoporosis is the most prevalent MBD in the United States and is responsible for as many as 1.5 million fractures annually. This disorder is usually asymptomatic until the bones become brittle enough to fracture or for vertebrae to collapse.

Normal bone remodeling requires a balance between bone deposition (gain) and bone resorption (loss). The exact pathophysiology of osteoporosis is unknown, but there are two major theories. In the first, osteoporosis may be caused by defective osteoblasts that have an abnormally short lifespan or work less efficiently, resulting in slow bone deposition. The second and more popular theory suggests that the osteoclasts have increased activity, resorbing bone at an increased rate. The common factor between the two theories is that normal bone turnover is altered, with the rate of resorption greater than bone formation, resulting in a decrease in total bone density and an altered bone structure.

Although the exact cause of osteoporosis is unknown, numerous risk factors have been identified. Women are four times as likely as men to develop osteoporosis, and the most common risk factor associated with the development of osteoporosis is the onset of menopause. When women reach menopause, estrogen secretion declines, and bones become weak and fragile. In women with osteoporosis, fractures often occur in the hips, wrists, forearms, or spine. In some cases, a lack of dietary calcium and vitamin D contributes to bone deterioration. The metabolism of calcium in osteoporosis is illustrated in Figure 72.3.

Major risk factors for osteoporosis include the following:

- Menopause
- Age over 60 years
- Family history of osteoporosis
- Caucasian or Asian race
- High alcohol intake
- Estrogen deficiency
- Smoking history
- Androgen deficiency
- Anorexia nervosa
- Low calcium or vitamin D intake
- Physical inactivity
- Thin, lean body build

Several methods are available for measuring bone mineral density (BMD) but the "gold standard" for the diagnosis of osteoporosis is dual-energy x-ray absorptiometry (DEXA). BMD at the spine and hip is measured and data are reported as T-scores. Positive T-scores represent the BMD values of a young adult between the ages of 30 and 35, which is the period of peak bone strength. Negative T-scores indicate some loss in BMD. Osteopenia, or a low bone mass, is present when the T-score is between –1 and –2.5. Osteoporosis is defined as a T-score of less than –2.5. Nutritional adjustments and/or drug therapy are initiated when T-scores fall into the osteopenic or osteoporosis ranges.

Drug therapies for osteoporosis include calcium and vitamin D therapy, estrogen replacement therapy (ERT), estrogen receptor modulators, statins, slow release sodium fluoride, bisphosphonates,

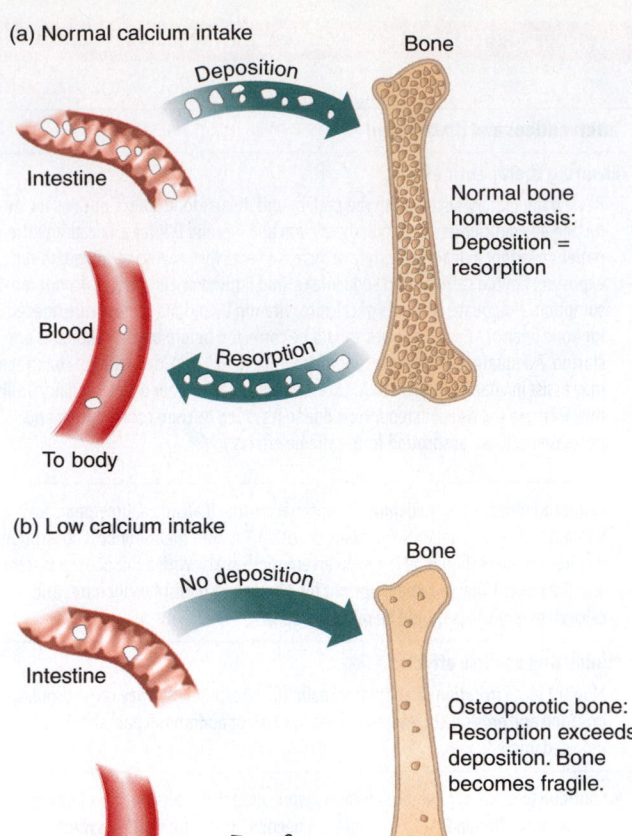

(a) Normal calcium intake

Deposition

Intestine

Blood

Resorption

To body

Bone

Normal bone homeostasis: Deposition = resorption

(b) Low calcium intake

No deposition

Intestine

Blood

Excess resorption

To body

Bone

Osteoporotic bone: Resorption exceeds deposition. Bone becomes fragile.

Figure 72.3 Calcium metabolism in osteoporosis.

and calcitonin. Teriparatide (Forteo) is a new drug for osteoporosis that is a structural analog of PTH produced through recombinant deoxyribonucleic acid (DNA) technology.

Osteomalacia: Osteomalacia, referred to as rickets in children, is a disorder characterized by softening of bones without alteration of basic bone structure. Weight-bearing stress on the softened bones causes skeletal deformities. Many factors contribute to the development of osteomalacia and rickets, but the most important is a deficiency of vitamin D and calcium. This risk factor for the disease is extremely rare in the United States, being most prevalent in the elderly, in premature infants, and in individuals on strict vegetarian diets. Other factors that may result in the development of osteomalacia include malabsorption disorders of the small bowel, damage to the renal tubules, adverse effects of anticonvulsant therapy, hepatic impairment, or a limited exposure to sunlight.

Recent research has documented a global resurgence of rickets. The promotion of breast-feeding over vitamin D–fortified formulas is thought to be responsible for part of the increase, particularly in mothers who are vitamin D deficient. In addition, the increased use of sunscreens to prevent skin cancer inhibits the formation of adequate vitamin D by sunlight. The replacement of vitamin D–fortified milk with carbonated beverages by children and teens also contributes to the possibility of rickets. Nurses need to emphasize the importance of getting enough extra dietary vitamin D to children and pregnant women. Drug therapy for children and adults consists of calcium salts and vitamin D.

Symptoms of osteomalacia include hypocalcemia, muscle weakness, muscle spasms, and diffuse bone pain, especially in the hip area. Patients may also experience pain in the arms, legs, and spine. Classic signs of rickets in children include bowlegs and a pigeon breast. Children may also develop a slight fever and become restless at night.

Tests that are performed to verify osteomalacia include bone biopsy; bone radiographs; computed tomography (CT) scan of the vertebral column; and determination of serum calcium, phosphate, and vitamin D levels. Many of these tests are routine for bone disorders and are performed as needed to determine the extent of bone health.

Paget's disease: **Paget's disease**, or osteitis deformans, is a chronic, progressive condition characterized by accelerated remodeling of the bone, producing enlarged and softened bones. With this disorder, the processes of bone resorption and bone formation occur simultaneously but at a very high rate. The rapid turnover causes new bone to be weak and brittle, resulting in deformities and fractures. Paget's disease can occur in any bone, but it most often affects the vertebrae, skull, sternum, pelvis, femur, and tibia. Paget's disease occurs with equal frequency in men and women over 40 years of age. The cause of Paget's disease is unknown.

Although many patients with Paget's disease are asymptomatic, approximately 10% experience vague, nonspecific complaints for many years. Symptoms include pain of the hips and femurs, joint inflammation, headaches, facial pain, and hearing loss if bones around the ear are affected. Nerves along the spinal column may be pinched because of the abnormal vertebral bone growth.

The evaluation of Paget's disease is based on radiographic and laboratory findings. The enzyme alkaline phosphatase (ALP) is elevated in the blood because of the extensive bone turnover. The disease is usually confirmed by early detection of this enzyme in the blood. Calcium is also liberated because of its close association with phosphate. If diagnosed early enough, symptoms can be treated successfully. If the diagnosis is made late in the progression of the disease, permanent skeletal abnormalities develop and other disorders may appear, including arthritis, kidney stones, and heart disease.

The pharmacotherapy of patients with Paget's disease includes bisphosphonates and calcitonin. Patients with Paget's disease should consume adequate amounts of calcium and vitamin D on a daily basis.

Pharmacotherapy of Metabolic Bone Disease

72.5 Vitamin D therapy is indicated for treating osteomalacia, hypoparathyroidism, and osteoporosis.

Inactive, intermediate, and active forms of vitamin D are available as medications. Patients' vitamin D needs vary depending on how much sunlight they receive. After age 70, the RDA of vitamin D increases from 400 units per day to 600 units per day. In severe cases of malabsorption disorders, patients may receive 50,000 to 100,000 units per day. Because vitamin D is needed to absorb calcium from the GI tract, many supplements combine vitamin D and calcium into a single tablet.

Several forms of vitamin D are available for therapy. Three of those products—ergocalciferol, cholecalciferol, and calcitriol—are identical to the forms of vitamin D that occur in nature. Each vitamin D product has a slightly different potency and pharmacokinetics. Indications for vitamin D products include the following:

- Hypocalcemia
- Hypophosphatemia
- Osteomalacia or rickets
- Osteoporosis prophylaxis
- Parathyroid dysfunction
- Vitamin D deficiency

Vitamin D is a fat-soluble vitamin that is stored by the body. It is possible to consume too much of this vitamin or to show signs of overdose from prescription medications. Excess vitamin D will cause calcium to leave bones and enter the blood. The signs and symptoms of hypercalcemia, such as anorexia, vomiting, excessive thirst, fatigue, and confusion, may become evident. Kidney stones may occur, and bones may fracture easily.

PROTOTYPE DRUG	Calcitriol (Calcijet, Rocaltrol)

Classification: **Therapeutic:** Vitamin D
Pharmacologic: Bone resorption inhibitor

Therapeutic Effects and Uses: Calcitriol is the active form of vitamin D. This medication is used in cases of hypocalcemia and for patients who have hypoparathyroidism. Calcitriol reduces bone resorption and is useful in treating rickets. Patients with chronic kidney disease are unable to synthesize sufficient calcitriol and thus will receive this drug as replacement therapy.

The effectiveness of calcitriol depends on having an adequate amount of calcium; therefore, it is usually prescribed in combination with calcium supplements. It is available for administration via the oral (PO) route in the form of tablets and solutions. An IV solution for injection is available to treat dialysis-associated hypocalcemia.

Mechanism of Action: Calcitriol elevates serum calcium levels, decreases elevated blood levels of phosphate, and decreases bone resorption and demineralization by promoting the intestinal absorption and renal reabsorption of calcium. The rising calcium levels provide negative feedback to the parathyroid glands, reducing the secretion of PTH. Calcitriol itself also provides negative feedback to the parathyroid glands.

Pharmacokinetics:

Route(s)	PO (tablets, capsules, or solution), IV
Absorption	Readily absorbed from the GI tract
Distribution	Widely distributed; crosses the placenta; small amounts are secreted in breast milk; 99% bound to vitamin D–binding protein
Primary metabolism	Hepatic
Primary excretion	Mostly feces with small amounts in urine
Onset of action	2–6 h
Duration of action	3–5 days

Adverse Effects: The adverse effects of vitamin D therapy include symptoms of hypercalcemia, such as palpitations, anorexia, nausea, vomiting, blurred vision, photophobia, constipation, abdominal cramps, metallic taste, headache, weakness, dry mouth, thirst, increased urination, and muscle or bone pain.

Contraindications/Precautions: This drug should not be given to patients with hypercalcemia or those who have evidence of vitamin D toxicity. Caution must be used in patients with renal failure who are at increased risk for vitamin D–induced hypercalcemia.

Drug Interactions: Thiazide diuretics may enhance the effects of vitamin D, causing hypercalcemia. Too much vitamin D may cause dysrhythmias in patients who are receiving digoxin. Magnesium antacids or supplements should not be given concurrently owing to an increased risk of hypermagnesemia. Orlistat (Xenical) may prevent the absorption of fat-soluble nutrients such as vitamin D. Corticosteroids inhibit the absorption of calcium, which is a major effect of vitamin D. **Herbal/Food**: Unknown.

Pregnancy: Category C.

Treatment of Overdose: Vitamin D overdose results in hypercalcemia, hypercalciuria, and hyperphosphatemia. If the overdosage was recent, emesis should be induced to remove any remaining drug from the stomach. All vitamin D and calcium supplements are discontinued and the patient is placed on a low-calcium diet until the hypercalcemia resolves.

Nursing Responsibilities: Key nursing implications for patients receiving calcitriol are included in the Nursing Practice Application for Patients Receiving Pharmacotherapy for Osteoporosis.

Drugs Similar to Calcitriol (Calcijet, Rocaltrol)

Other forms of vitamin D for therapy include cholecalciferol, dihydrotachysterol, doxercalciferol, ergocalciferol, and paricalcitol. Doses for the vitamin D preparations are given in Table 72.4.

Cholecalciferol (Delta-D): Cholecalciferol (vitamin D_3) is the form of vitamin D that is produced in the skin after exposure to ultraviolet (UV) light. It is activated by the liver and kidneys to form calcitriol. Once activated, cholecalciferol produces identical actions and adverse effects as calcitriol. It is an oral dietary supplement for the prophylaxis and treatment of vitamin D deficiency. Fosamax plus D is a combination drug containing alendronate and cholecalciferol.

Dihydrotachysterol (DHT, Hytakerol): Dihydrotachysterol is an oral analog of vitamin D. This drug does not require kidney enzymes for activation and thus is useful in patients with renal impairment. Several weeks of therapy are required for maximum effect. Adverse effects are the same as those of calcitriol. Dihydrotachysterol is excreted primarily in the bile. Its indications include hypocalcemia, hypoparathyroidism, hypophosphatemia, and tetany.

Doxercalciferol (Hectorol): Doxercalciferol is an analog of vitamin D that is given by either the PO or IV route. This drug is activated by the liver alone: No kidney metabolism is necessary. Adverse effects are the same as those of calcitriol. However, caution must be taken to avoid the rapid development of hypercalcemia when this drug is administered by the IV route. Its only approved indication is for the treatment of secondary hyperparathyroidism and resultant bone disease.

Ergocalciferol (Calciferol, Drisdol): Ergocalciferol (vitamin D_2) is a natural vitamin D analog found in plants, fortified milk, eggs, and cereals. Once activated, ergocalciferol produces actions and adverse effects identical to those of calcitriol. Bile is required for its

---

TABLE 72.4   Vitamin D Preparations

Drug	Route and Adult Dose (Maximum Dose Where Indicated)	Adverse Effects
calcitriol (Calcijex, Rocaltrol)	PO: 0.25–0.50 mcg/day IV: Begin with 1–4 mcg three times weekly	*Diarrhea, infection, hypertension, dizziness* <u>Hypercalcemia, bone pain, lethargy, anorexia, nausea, vomiting, increased urination, hallucinations, dysrhythmias</u>
cholecalciferol (Delta-D)	PO: 400–1,000 international units/day	
dihydrotachysterol (DHT, Hytakerol)	PO: 0.75–2.5 mg/day for several days then 0.2–1 mg/day	
doxercalciferol (Hectorol)	PO: 10 mcg, 3 times/week IV: 4 mcg, 3 times/week (max: 60 mcg/week [PO]; 18 mcg/week [IV])	
ergocalciferol (Calciferol, Drisdol)	PO: 15–25 mcg once daily IV: 4 mcg three times weekly	
paricalcitol (Zemplar)	IV: 0.04–0.1 mcg/kg, every other day (max: 24 mcg/kg) PO: 1–4 mcg every other day or three times per week	

Note: *Italics* indicate common adverse effects. <u>Underline</u> indicates serious adverse effects.

absorption, and the drug requires adequate kidney function to be metabolized to its active form. Indications for therapy with ergocalciferol are the same as those for calcitriol.

Paricalcitol (Zemplar): Paricalcitol is an analog of vitamin D that is given by either the PO or IV route. Adverse effects are the same as those of calcitriol; however, caution must be taken to avoid the rapid development of hypercalcemia when this drug is administered by the IV route. The only indication for paricalcitol is for the treatment of secondary hyperparathyroidism and resultant bone disease.

72.6 Bisphosphonates increase bone density and are used to treat osteoporosis.

The most frequently prescribed drug class for osteoporosis is the **bisphosphonates**. These drugs are structural analogs of pyrophosphate, which is a natural substance that inhibits bone resorption. Bisphosphonates bind to hydroxyapatite in bone and suppress osteoclast activity, thus increasing bone mass density and reducing the incidence of fractures by about 50%. Examples include etidronate (Didronel), alendronate (Fosamax), tiludronate (Skelid), zoledronate (Zometa), risedronate (Actonel), and pamidronate (Aredia), which is available as an injectable drug. Etidronate also inhibits bone demineralization that could lead to osteomalacia; the other bisphosphonates do not have this effect. In addition to treating postmenopausal osteoporosis, some of the bisphosphonates are approved to treat corticosteroid-induced osteoporosis. A summary of the indications for bisphosphonates is given in Table 72.5 and their doses are listed in Table 72.6.

The beneficial effects of bisphosphonates on bone mass density increase rapidly during the first year of therapy and plateau after 2 to 3 years. Even after discontinuation of therapy, bone density will remain increased for up to a year. For optimum effects, the patient must have adequate dietary consumption of calcium and vitamin D; any deficiencies should be corrected prior to initiating bisphosphonate therapy. Studies suggest that once-weekly dosing with bisphosphonates may give the same bone density benefits as daily dosing because of their extended duration of drug action.

Bisphosphonates are also preferred drugs for the pharmacotherapy of Paget's disease. For this disorder, therapy is usually cyclic, with bisphosphonates administered until serum ALP levels return to normal followed by several months without drugs. When the serum ALP level becomes elevated, therapy is begun again. The pharmacologic goals are to slow the rate of bone reabsorption and encourage the deposition of strong bone.

Several bisphosphonates are used to treat bone metastases and malignant hypercalcemia. Bone metastases are characterized by osteoclast hyperactivity, which creates "punched-out," osteolytic lesions that release large amounts of calcium into the blood. Bisphosphonates suppress osteoclast activity, thus slowing the rate of bone resorption and the rate of calcium release. Thus some of these drugs are approved for treating hypercalcemia due to malignancy. It is important to note that bisphosphonates are not antineoplastics; they have no effect on tumor cells and are only given as a palliative measure.

The most frequent adverse effects of bisphosphonates include GI symptoms such as nausea, vomiting, abdominal pain, dyspepsia, and esophageal irritation. Because these drugs are poorly absorbed from the intestinal tract, they must be taken on an empty stomach with plain water, at least 30 minutes before any other fluid, food, or medications. To avoid esophageal irritation, the patient should stay in an upright position for at least 30 minutes following the dose. Bisphosphonates are not metabolized and are excreted in the urine.

Patients taking the bisphosphonates are evaluated on a regular basis to determine if the drug is still necessary. To avoid the possibility of long-term adverse effects, these drugs are usually discontinued after several years of therapy in patients who have a low risk for fracture.

One unusual adverse effect that may occur during bisphosphonate therapy is osteonecrosis of the jaw. Symptoms include local

TABLE 72.5 Indications for Bisphosphonates

Drug	Osteoporosis in Postmenopausal Women	Osteoporosis in Men	Glucocorticoid-Induced Osteoporosis	Paget's Disease	Hypercalcemia of Malignancy	Breast Cancer Metastases	Multiple Myeloma/Bone Metastases
alendronate (Fosamax)	X	X	X	X			
etidronate (Didronel)				X			
ibandronate (Boniva)	X						
pamidronate (Aredia)				X	X	X	
risedronate (Actonel, Atelvia)	X	X	X	X			
tiludronate (Skelid)				X			
zoledronate (Reclast, Zometa)	X	X		X	X		X

TABLE 72.6   Selected Drugs for Osteoporosis and Other Bone Disorders

Drug	Route and Adult Dose (Maximum Dose Where Indicated)	Adverse Effects
Bisphosphonates		
alendronate (Fosamax)	Osteoporosis: PO: 10 mg/day or 70 mg once weekly Paget's disease: PO: 40 mg/day for 6 months	*Nausea, dyspepsia, diarrhea, bone pain, back pain* Bone fractures, nephrotoxicity, hypocalcemia, hypophosphatemia, gastric ulcer, esophageal perforation, dysrhythmias, anemia, osteonecrosis of the jaw, atrial fibrillation
etidronate (Didronel)	PO: 5–10 mg/kg/day for 6 months or 11–20 mg/kg/day for 3 months	
ibandronate (Boniva)	PO: 2.5 mg/day or one 150-mg tablet per month, taken on the same date each month IV: 3 mg every 3 months	
pamidronate (Aredia)	IV: 15–90 mg in 1,000 mL normal saline or D₅W over 4–24 h	
risedronate (Actonel, Atelvia)	PO: 5 mg/day or 35 mg once weekly at least 30 min before the first drink or meal of the day	
tiludronate (Skelid)	PO: 400 mg/day taken with 6–8 oz of water 2 h before or after food for 3 months	
zoledronate (Reclast, Zometa)	IV (Zometa): 4-mg single dose infused over at least 15 min. May be repeated every 3–4 weeks for cancer IV (Reclast): one 5-mg single dose per year, infused over at least 15 min	
Miscellaneous Drugs		
calcitonin-salmon (Fortical, Miacalcin)	Hypercalcemia: subcutaneous/IM: salmon, 4 international units/kg bid Osteoporosis: intranasal: 1 spray/day (200 international units) in one nostril, alternating nostrils each day	*Rhinitis, flushing of the face and hands, pain at the injection site* Anaphylaxis
cinacalcet (Sensipar)	PO: Start with 30 mg once daily; may increase every 2–4 weeks until target PTH of 150–300 mg/mL (max: 300 mg/day) for secondary hyperparathyroidism	*Dizziness, noncardiac chest pain, HTN, nausea, anorexia, hypocalcemia, myalgia* Hypocalcemia, seizures
denosumab (Prolia, Xgen)	Subcutaneous (Prolia): 60 mg every 6 months Subcutaneous (Xgen): 120 mg every 4 weeks	*Fatigue, asthenia, hypophosphatemia, nausea, hypercholesterolemia, musculoskeletal pain, and cystitis* Hypocalcemia, serious infections, osteonecrosis of jaw
raloxifene (Evista)	PO: 60 mg/day	*Hot flashes, leg cramps, peripheral edema, flu syndrome, arthralgia, sweating* Breast pain, vaginal bleeding, pneumonia, chest pain, venous thromboembolism, stroke
teriparatide (Forteo)	Subcutaneous: 20 mcg/day	*Dizziness, depression, insomnia, vertigo, rhinitis, increased cough, leg cramps, nausea, arthralgia* Syncope, angina, transient hypercalcemia

Note: Italics indicate common adverse effects. <u>Underline</u> indicates serious adverse effects.

pain and swelling, loosening of teeth, and infection at the site of the lesion. It is not clear what causes the necrosis. Discontinuing the bisphosphonate does not resolve the lesion because the drugs are incorporated in bone for many months and perhaps years.

PROTOTYPE DRUG   Alendronate (Fosamax)

Classification: **Therapeutic:** Drug for osteoporosis and Paget's disease
Pharmacologic: Bisphosphonate, bone resorption inhibitor

Therapeutic Actions and Uses: First approved in 1995, alendronate is the best studied drug in this class. Alendronate is approved for the following indications:

- Prevention and treatment of osteoporosis in postmenopausal women
- Treatment of glucocorticoid-induced osteoporosis in both women and men
- Treatment to increase bone mass in men with osteoporosis
- Treatment of symptomatic Paget's disease in both women and men

Alendronate is also used off-label for treating hypercalcemia due to malignancy. Several regimens for alendronate are available: once daily (10 mg), twice weekly (35 mg), or once weekly (70 mg). Although the once weekly is more convenient, higher doses can produce more GI-related adverse effects. All doses must be taken on an empty stomach, preferably in a fasting state 2 hours before breakfast.

Therapeutic effects of alendronate may take 1 to 3 months to appear and may continue for several months after therapy is discontinued. This drug lowers serum alkaline phosphatase, which is the enzyme associated with bone turnover, without major adverse effects.

The safety and effectiveness of long-term therapy with alendronate is still being investigated. Patients should be regularly evaluated to determine the need for continued therapy and those at low risk for fracture should be discontinued after 3 to 5 years of use.

Mechanism of Action: Alendronate inhibits osteoclast-mediated bone resorption to minimize loss of bone density. Its effects appear to be localized to resorption sites of active bone turnover and it does not interfere with bone mineralization.

Pharmacokinetics:

Route(s)	PO
Absorption	Less than 1% (significantly decreased by food or beverages)
Distribution	Rapid skeletal uptake; unknown if secreted in breast milk; 78% bound to plasma protein
Primary metabolism	Not metabolized
Primary excretion	50% excreted unchanged in the urine
Onset of action	3–6 weeks
Duration of action	12 weeks or more after discontinuation

Adverse Effects: The most common adverse effect of alendronate is hypocalcemia, which is usually transient and mild. Other adverse effects include diarrhea, constipation, flatulence, nausea, vomiting, GI irritation, a metallic or altered taste perception, hypocalcemia, hypophosphatemia, abdominal pain, dyspepsia, myalgias, and headache. Pathologic fractures may occur if the drug is taken longer than 3 months or in cases of chronic overdose. Although rare, this drug may cause serious esophagitis, which is why patients should remain in an upright position at least 30 minutes after receiving a dose. Osteonecrosis of the jaw has occurred spontaneously in patients taking bisphosphonates.

Contraindications/Precautions: Contraindications include patients with osteomalacia or who have hypersensitivity to this drug. Caution should be used in patients with renal impairment, heart failure, hyperphosphatemia, liver disease, fever or infection, active upper GI problems, and pregnancy. This drug is contraindicated in patients with abnormalities of the esophagus that delay esophageal emptying, such as stricture or achalasia, and in those who are unable to stand or sit upright for at least 30 minutes following administration of the drug.

Drug Interactions: Calcium, iron, antacids containing aluminum or magnesium, and certain mineral supplements interfere with the absorption of alendronate and have the potential to decrease its effectiveness. Patients should wait at least 30 minutes after taking alendronate before taking any other supplements or other medications. **Herbal/Food**: The patient's diet must have adequate amounts of vitamin D, calcium, and phosphates. Excessive amounts of calcium supplements or dairy products reduce alendronate absorption.

Pregnancy: Category C.

Treatment of Overdose: Hypocalcemia is an expected effect of overdose and may be treated with PO or IV calcium compounds.

Nursing Responsibilities: Key nursing implications for patients receiving alendronate are included in the Nursing Practice Application for Patients Receiving Pharmacotherapy for Osteoporosis.

Drugs Similar to Alendronate (Fosamax)

Other bisphosphonates include clodronate, etidronate, ibandronate, pamidronate, risedronate, tiludronate, and zoledronate.

Etidronate disodium (Didronel): Etidronate was the first bisphosphonate approved in the United States in 1977. It is less selective for bone than some of the other medications in this class and is not a first-line drug. It is approved for moderate to severe Paget's disease and for hypertrophic ossification following total hip replacement or spinal cord injury. It is used off-label as an alternative to other bisphosphonates for prevention of postmenopausal and corticosteroid-induced osteoporosis. It is available only PO; the IV preparation was withdrawn from the market in 2005. Like all bisphosphonates, etidronate causes GI mucosa irritation and bone and joint pain. This drug is nephrotoxic and may increase the risk of dysrhythmias. This drug is pregnancy category C.

Ibandronate (Boniva): Ibandronate was approved in 2003 for the prevention and treatment of postmenopausal osteoporosis. In addition to its oral formulation, it is the only IV bisphosphonate approved for the prophylaxis of postmenopausal osteoporosis. When administered IV, injections are spaced 3 months apart. Off-label indications include Paget's disease, bone metastases from prostate cancer, and malignant hypercalcemia. Adverse effects are similar to those of other drugs in this class. This drug is pregnancy category C.

Pamidronate (Aredia): Approved in 1991, pamidronate is available by slow IV infusion for hypercalcemia, moderate to severe Paget's disease, and bone metastases due to breast cancer or multiple myeloma. It may be used off-label to treat osteoporosis and osteogenesis imperfecta. Caution must be used when treating patients with renal impairment or who are receiving nephrotoxic drugs because significant renal function deterioration can occur with pamidronate, even after a single dose. Other common adverse effects are nausea, fever, constipation, and dyspnea. Pamidronate is pregnancy category D.

Risedronate (Actonel, Atelvia): Approved in 1998, risedronate is FDA approved to prevent and treat glucocorticoid-induced and postmenopausal osteoporosis and symptomatic Paget's disease. It may be used off-label to treat osteolytic lesions due to multiple myeloma. Available by the PO route, it is reported to cause less GI distress than other bisphosphonates. Like other oral bisphosphonates, it is contraindicated in patients who are unable to sit upright for at least 30 minutes after drug administration or who have disorders that cause delayed esophageal emptying. Atelvia is a delayed release form of the drug that can be taken once weekly. Arthralgia, back pain, diarrhea, abdominal pain, and dyspepsia are common adverse effects. This drug is pregnancy category C.

Tiludronate (Skelid): Tiludronate was approved in 1997 to treat symptomatic Paget's disease. It is administered PO and has a similar adverse effect profile to that of other drugs in this class. This drug is pregnancy category C.

Zoledronate (Reclast, Zometa): Originally approved in 2001, zoledronate (also called zoledronic acid) is available by the IV route to treat hypercalcemia of malignancy, multiple myeloma, and bone metastases. One advantage of Zometa is that it can be infused over 15 to 20 minutes compared to 2 to 4 hours for pamidronate. Frequent adverse effects include nausea, fatigue, anemia, bone pain, constipation, fever, vomiting, and dyspnea.

In 2007, the FDA expanded the indications for zoledronate (Reclast) to include prevention or treatment of postmenopausal osteoporosis, osteoporosis in men, and Paget's disease. A major advantage of Reclast is that its prolonged duration of action results in a once-yearly dose for Paget's disease and osteoporosis prophylaxis. Reclast is available by IV infusion, administered over at least 15 minutes. Common adverse effects include bone pain, pyrexia, nausea, headache, arthralgia, fatigue, and constipation.

Reclast and Zometa are not interchangeable and the drugs should not be administered concurrently. Zoledronate is nephrotoxic and should be used with caution in patients with renal impairment. Like pamidronate, zoledronate is pregnancy category D and should not be used during pregnancy.

72.7 Selective estrogen receptor modulators increase bone mass density and prevent fractures in postmenopausal women.

Selective estrogen receptor modulators (SERMs) are drugs that bind to estrogen receptors (ERs). Estrogen exerts its effects on target tissues by interacting with ERs and causing either activation or inhibition of specific cellular actions. ERs are found in the reproductive organs of both males and females where they enhance the development of reproductive tissues. But ERs are found in more than just reproductive tissues. In the cardiovascular system, ERs are responsible for lowering blood cholesterol, and in the brain, these receptors influence behavior and mood. In bone, ERs help to maintain bone mineral density.

Certain estrogens are produced by plants. These substances, called phytoestrogens, mimic the effects of natural estrogen and are thought to exert beneficial effects on the cardiovascular system and possibly protection from cancer. For example, soybeans, flax seed, and tofu are rich sources of phytoestrogens.

SERMs are medications that may activate or inhibit ERs. Thus, SERMs may be estrogen agonists or antagonists, depending on the specific drug and the tissue involved. For example, raloxifene (Evista) blocks estrogen receptors in the uterus and breast; it has no estrogen-like proliferative effects on these tissues that might promote cancer. Raloxifene does, however, have estrogen-like effects that reduce bone resorption, thus increasing bone density and reducing the likelihood of fractures. It is most effective in preventing vertebral fractures. The dose for raloxifene is shown in Table 72.6.

The other SERMs include tamoxifen, toremifene (Rareston), and bazedoxifene (Duavee). Tamoxifen and toremifene are used to treat metastatic breast cancer in postmenopausal women (see Chapter 57). Bazedoxifene is formulated in a fixed-dose combination with conjugated estrogens to manage symptoms of menopause as well as to prevent bone fractures (see Chapter 69).

PROTOTYPE DRUG	Raloxifene (Evista)

Classification: Therapeutic: Drug for osteoporosis prophylaxis
Pharmacologic: Selective estrogen receptor modifier

Therapeutic Effects and Uses: Approved in 1997, raloxifene is primarily used for the prevention or treatment of osteoporosis in postmenopausal women. In 2007, it was approved for the prophylaxis of invasive breast cancer in postmenopausal women at high risk for breast cancer. High risk of breast cancer is defined as at least one breast biopsy showing carcinoma or atypical hyperplasia or having a first-degree relative with breast cancer. Other factors considered are current age, number of breast biopsies, age at menarche, nulliparity, or age of first live birth. It is important for nurses and patients to understand that this drug is for the prevention, not treatment, of breast carcinoma.

Raloxifene increases bone mass density, reducing vertebral fractures. It does not appear to reduce the incidence of fractures at nonvertebral sites. Raloxifene also reduces serum total cholesterol and low-density lipoproteins (LDLs) without lowering high-density lipoproteins (HDLs) or triglycerides. Unlike estrogen, which causes proliferation of uterine and breast tissue, causing adverse effects, raloxifene is an estrogen antagonist on these tissues. Raloxifene has been used off-label to treat uterine leiomyomas, for pubertal gynecomastia, and for the prevention of bone loss in men with prostate cancer.

Mechanism of Action: As a selective estrogen receptor antagonist or agonist, raloxifene decreases bone resorption while increasing bone mass and density by activating estrogen receptors.

Pharmacokinetics:

Route(s)	PO
Absorption	60% absorbed
Distribution	Crosses the placenta; unknown if secreted in breast milk; 95% bound to plasma protein
Primary metabolism	Hepatic; extensive first-pass metabolism
Primary excretion	Primarily in feces
Onset of action	8 weeks
Duration of action	Half-life: 28 h

Adverse Effects: The most common adverse effects of raloxifene therapy are hot flashes, leg cramps, and weight gain. Less common adverse effects include fever, arthralgia, myalgia, arthritis, depression, insomnia, chest pain, peripheral edema, decreased serum cholesterol, nausea, dyspepsia, vomiting, flatulence, GI disorders, gastroenteritis, cystitis, migraine headache, flulike symptoms, endometrial disorder, breast pain, and vaginal bleeding. Raloxifene may cause fetal harm when administered to a pregnant woman. **Black Box Warning**: Raloxifene increases the risk of venous thromboembolism and death from strokes. Women with a history of venous thromboembolism should not take this drug.

Contraindications/Precautions: This drug is contraindicated during lactation and pregnancy and in women who may become pregnant. Patients with a history of venous thromboembolism and those who are hypersensitive to raloxifene should not take this drug.

Raloxifene should be discontinued 72 hours before prolonged immobilization is anticipated due to risk of thromboembolic events.

Drug Interactions: Concurrent use with warfarin may decrease prothrombin time (PT). Decreased raloxifene absorption will result from concurrent use with ampicillin or cholestyramine. Use of raloxifene with other highly protein-bound drugs (ibuprofen, indomethacin, diazepam, etc.) may interfere with binding sites. Patients should not take cholesterol-lowering drugs or ERT concurrently with this medication. **Herbal/Food**: Black cohosh has estrogenic effects and may interfere with the actions of raloxifene.

Pregnancy: Category X.

Treatment of Overdose: Overdose with raloxifene is uncommon and symptoms are given supportive treatment.

Nursing Responsibilities: Key nursing implications for patients receiving raloxifene are included in the Nursing Practice Application for Patients Receiving Pharmacotherapy for Osteoporosis.

Drugs Similar to Raloxifene (Evista)

The other SERMs are discussed in previous chapters: tamoxifen and toremifene in Chapter 57 and bazedoxifene with conjugated estrogens in Chapter 69.

CONNECTION Checkpoint 72.2

From what you learned in Chapter 57, what are the indications for pharmacotherapy with tamoxifen (Nolvadex)? *See Answer to Connection Checkpoint 72.2 on student resource website.*

72.8 Calcitonin and several miscellaneous drugs are used for osteoporosis and other metabolic bone diseases.

Several miscellaneous drugs are used to treat MBDs. Although they act by different mechanisms, they are presented together in this section because each is the only drug in its class.

Calcitonin (Fortical, Miacalcin): Calcitonin is a hormone that is produced and secreted by the thyroid gland in response to elevated serum calcium levels. This hormone directly inhibits osteoclasts. The function of calcitonin is to lower serum calcium levels by decreasing bone resorption and increasing the urinary excretion of calcium. It acts in direct opposition to PTH and vitamin D.

As a drug calcitonin is approved for the treatment of osteoporosis in women who are more than 5 years postmenopause. Calcitonin increases bone mass density and reduces the risk of vertebral fractures when the diet is adequate for calcium and vitamin D. Because calcitonin is less effective for reducing osteoporosis-related fractures than the bisphosphonates, it is considered a second-line treatment. The dose for calcitonin is given in Table 72.6.

In addition to treating osteoporosis, calcitonin is indicated for Paget's disease and hypercalcemia. In Paget's disease calcitonin slows the rate of bone turnover and decreases the incidence of bone pain. It is most effective in treating hypercalcemia caused by hyperparathyroidism, prolonged immobility, or that accompanies certain malignancies. Calcitonin may be used off-label to reduce neuropathic pain and bone pain associated with metastatic bone cancer and osteoporosis.

CONNECTIONS ⟨ Evidence-Based Practice

◀ Outcome Differences in Osteoporosis and Low Bone Density Treatment

Clinical Question

Do all patients respond to osteoporosis or low bone density treatment in the same way?

Evidence

With over 50 million people in the United States living with osteoporosis (National Osteoporosis Foundation, n.d.) and over one and a half million fractures attributed to osteoporosis, the Agency for Healthcare Research and Quality (AHRQ) conducted a systematic review of the comparative effectiveness of the various treatments for osteoporosis and low bone density in 2007 and updated it again in 2012 after the bisphosphonates became available in longer acting formulations (Levis & Theodore, 2012). The review found high strength of evidence for a reduction in risk for hip, vertebral, and nonvertebral fractures in postmenopausal women treated with alendronate, risendronate, zoledronic acid, or denosumab, and also high strength of evidence for risk reduction of vertebral fractures when ibandronate, teripatratide, or raloxifene was used. Likewise, estrogen therapy resulted in reduction of vertebral and hip fractures in postmenopausal women, but not in women with existing osteoporosis. Risk reduction was noted for hip fractures when calcium was used, and reductions in vertebral fractures when vitamin D therapy was used in patients with existing osteoporosis, but combining calcium with vitamin C did not demonstrate the same results. Calcium plus vitamin D had different results in men and women, with women experiencing reduction of fracture risk, but not men. Adherence to osteoporosis therapy was improved by the use of the weekly treatment strategies. However, there was insufficient strong evidence to suggest that monthly treatments resulted in better adherence than weekly. It was recognized that routine screening for bone mineral density has not been studied in large randomized controlled trials, although outcomes of the systematic review suggested that ongoing screening did not help to predict fracture risk in patients taking anti-osteoporotic drugs.

Implications

Both women and men are at risk for low bone density and osteoporosis, although women are 50% more likely to experience a fracture from osteoporosis than men (National Osteoporosis Foundation, n.d.). From the results of the AHRQ's systematic review of low bone density and osteoporosis treatments, adherence to treatment, and screening, high strength evidence demonstrated that not all populations respond in the same way to the different treatments. It also showed that some treatments were more effective for certain populations than others. Discussing population-specific osteoporosis treatment with the health care provider, weight-bearing exercise, and adequate intake of calcium and vitamin D are strategies to lower the risk of low bone density and osteoporosis. In the case of drug therapy, "one size does not fit all."

Critical Thinking Question

A 68-year-old woman who has been taking raloxifene for osteoporosis risk reduction asks if her husband, also age 68, should take it too. How should the nurse respond?

See Answers to Critical Thinking Questions on student resource website.

Calcitonin-salmon is available by nasal spray (Fortical) or subcutaneous injection (Miacalcin). Subcutaneous injections are initially given as a daily dose then decreased to two to three times per week. Calcitonin is also available as an IV injection. Because parenteral forms cause more nausea and vomiting than the intranasal form, they are rarely used except in patients with severe, acute hypercalcemia. When given IV, calcitonin decreases serum calcium levels in approximately 2 hours, with its effects lasting up to 8 hours. Adverse effects of calcitonin-salmon are generally minor; the nasal formulation may irritate the nasal mucosa and cause rhinitis or epistaxis. Generalized flushing of the face and hands may occur and anaphylaxis has been reported. This drug is pregnancy category C.

Cinacalcet (Sensipar): Cinacalcet is a calcium modifier approved in 2004 for the treatment of hypercalcemia caused by parathyroid gland cancer or for secondary hyperparathyroidism due to chronic kidney disease. Cinacalcet is a calcium mimic; it is recognized as calcium by the parathyroid glands. The parathyroid glands are tricked into sensing high levels of calcium and they shut down the production of PTH. With decreased levels of PTH, bone resorption diminishes and serum calcium falls.

Cinacalcet is an oral drug. Its dose is slowly escalated until serum PTH and calcium levels return to normal values. Overtreatment may cause hypocalcemia. Nausea, vomiting, and diarrhea are common during therapy. This drug is a strong inhibitor of CYP450 enzymes and should be used with caution in patients who are receiving other drugs that are CYP450 substrates or inhibitors. This drug is pregnancy category C.

Denosumab (Prolia, Xgen): Approved in 2010, denosumab is used to prevent bone fractures in postmenopausal women and to prevent skeletal-related events in patients with bone metastases with solid tumors. Denosumab is given by subcutaneous injection, either every 4 weeks (Xgen) or every 6 months (Prolia). The drug is a monoclonal antibody classified as a RANKL inhibitor. RANKL is a protein that binds to the RANK receptor on osteoblasts. Once bound, RANKL promotes the removal of calcium from bone. By inhibiting this action, denosumab helps to maintain bone mineral density and prevent fractures due to osteoporosis or bone metastases. Common adverse effects include fatigue, asthenia, hypophosphatemia, nausea, hypercholesterolemia, musculoskeletal pain, and cystitis. Because the drug can cause severe hypocalcemia, serum calcium levels should be monitored regularly and calcium supplements and vitamin D administered as necessary. Some patients also experience osteonecrosis of the jaw. This drug is pregnancy category C.

Teriparatide (Forteo): Approved in 2002, teriparatide is a form of human PTH produced by recombinant DNA technology. Its only approved indication is for the treatment of osteoporosis in men and postmenopausal women. This drug is usually reserved for patients with a high risk of bone fractures. Teriparatide is used off-label to treat hypoparathyroidism and corticosteroid-induced osteoporosis.

The actions of teriparatide are identical to those of endogenous PTH. It is the only drug that will increase bone formation. Unlike other medications that simply reduce bone resorption, teriparatide reduces resorption and stimulates the production of new bone. These actions increase bone mass density and reduce the incidence of fractures. A disadvantage of this drug is that it must be given daily

by the subcutaneous route. It is available as a prefilled pen injector. Teriparatide is well tolerated, with dizziness and leg cramps being the most frequent adverse effects. This drug should be avoided in patients with an increased risk of bone cancer because it may increase the risks for acquiring osteosarcoma. Because patients with Paget's disease have an increased risk of osteosarcoma, they should not receive teriparatide. Although this drug is rated as pregnancy category C, it has been shown to cause cancer in laboratory animals at 60 times the doses used in patients.

Pathophysiology and Pharmacotherapy of Joint Disorders

72.9 Osteoarthritis is treated with a combination of analgesics and nonpharmacologic therapies.

A simple classification of joint disorders places them into two categories: noninflammatory and inflammatory. The most common of the noninflammatory disorders is osteoarthritis. Common inflammatory joint disorders such as rheumatoid arthritis and gout are covered in Sections 72.10 and 72.11, respectively. These joint conditions are frequent indications for pharmacotherapy, with joint pain being common to all disorders. Analgesics and anti-inflammatory drugs are important components of pharmacotherapy. A few additional drugs are specific to the particular joint pathology. Pharmacotherapy Illustrated 72.1 shows the types of joint pathology and their drug therapy.

Osteoarthritis (OA) is a progressive, degenerative joint disease caused by the breakdown of articular cartilage. It is the most common type of arthritis and the second most common cause of disability in the United States, affecting between 20 and 40 million persons. Weight-bearing joints such as the knee, vertebral column, and hip are most commonly affected. The hands are also affected because they are frequently used. OA may be classified as idiopathic or secondary. Idiopathic OA, the most common type, has no known cause but is associated with increasing age. The causes of secondary OA include trauma, mechanical stress, inflammation of the joint structures, neurologic disorders, use of certain medications, and joint instability. Excessive weight contributes to the development of OA, particularly in the knee and hip. Other risk factors associated with OA include decreased estrogen in menopausal women, excessive growth hormone, and increased PTH.

As cartilage thins in the affected joints, there is less padding and, eventually, the underlying bone is exposed. The bone thickens in the exposed areas, forming bone spurs and cysts that narrow the joint space. As these growths enlarge, small pieces may break off, leading to inflammation of the synovial membrane and a loss of lubricating fluid. This leads to further pain, inflammation, and destruction of the synovial membrane lining the joint. The affected joint becomes unstable and more susceptible to injury, with partial joint dislocations and other deformities that are common in advanced disease being seen.

The onset of OA is usually gradual, with pain and stiffness in one or more joints being the first manifestations. The patient with OA typically describes a deep, aching, localized pain, which is usually aggravated by movement and relieved by rest. Pain at night may be

PHARMACOTHERAPY ILLUSTRATED 72.1

Joint Disorders

Periosteum — Cortical bone

Joint capsule — Cancellous bone

Synovial membrane

Meniscus — Articular cartilage

(a) Normal

Bone cysts

Osteophytes (bone spurs) — Loose fragments of cartilage — Pannus

Loss of cartilage — Masses of uric acid (tophi)

Calcified cartilage — Sclerotic bone — Proliferative synovitis — Uric acid crystals

Worn cartilage — Inflamed synovium — Swollen and inflamed joint

Erosion of cartilage

Periarticular fibrosis — Erosion of bone

(b) Advanced osteoarthritis **(c) Rheumatoid arthritis** **(d) Gout**

Acetaminophen
NSAIDs
Tramadol
Topical ointments
Intra-articular
  corticosteroids

NSAIDs
Corticosteroids
Hydroxychloroquine
  (or other DMARD)
Biologic response
  modifiers

Colchicine
Probenecid
Allopurinol
NSAIDs
Sulfinpyrazone

accompanied by paresthesias. As the disease advances, the range of motion (ROM) of the joint decreases; this is often accompanied by complaints of progressive pain. Bone enlargement can increase joint size; flexion contractures contribute to joint instability. It is important to note that OA is not accompanied by the degree of inflammation associated with other forms of arthritis. The joints of a patient with OA are characteristically hard and cool to palpation. A patient

with OA is shown in Figure 72.4. The diagnosis of OA is typically made using a detailed history and physical examination. Routine x-rays may be useful in determining structural joint changes.

Nonpharmacologic therapies are an essential component of OA management. Walking, nonimpact aerobics, and passive ROM exercises are important to maintain joint flexibility. Improving muscle strength, especially of the quadriceps muscle, will help patients

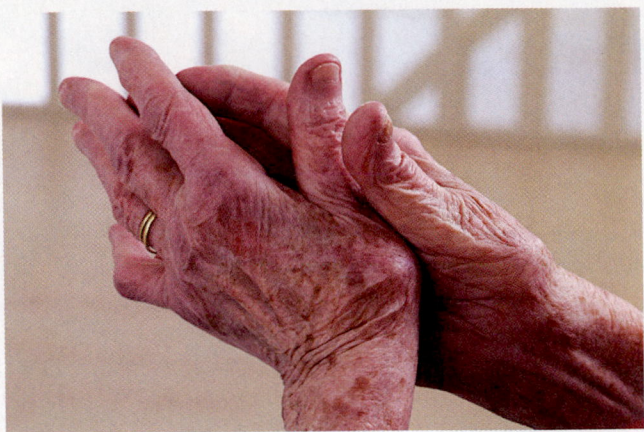

Figure 72.4 Patient with osteoarthritis.
Courtesy of JPC-PROD/Shutterstock.

improve their ability to perform ADLs. Bracing may help keep joints positioned correctly and relieve pain. Knowledge of proper body mechanics and posture may offer some benefit. Patients who are obese should consider a weight loss program, especially if weight-bearing joints such as the hip and knee are affected. Weight loss has been associated with decreased pain and disability. Surgical procedures such as joint replacement and reconstructive surgery may become necessary when other methods are ineffective.

Drugs should be considered as additions to nonpharmacologic therapies in the overall management of OA. The goals of pharmacotherapy for OA include reducing pain and inflammation and minimizing disability. The initial treatment of choice for most patients is acetaminophen. Acetaminophen is inexpensive, participates in few drug–drug interactions, and has fewer serious adverse effects than other analgesics. For patients whose pain is unrelieved by acetaminophen, nonsteroidal anti-inflammatory drugs (NSAIDs), including naproxen and ibuprofen derivatives, are usually given. Because high doses of NSAIDs can result in GI bleeding and affect platelet aggregation, patients must be carefully monitored. Aspirin is no longer recommended because the high doses needed to produce pain relief in patients with OA may cause GI bleeding. Tramadol (Ultram) has become a popular drug for the treatment of moderate to severe pain. Although classified as an opioid, tramadol does not have abuse potential and is not a scheduled drug. Opioids such as codeine may be combined with acetaminophen for severe pain. The student should refer to Chapter 25 for a complete discussion of the actions and adverse effects of analgesics.

In acute cases, intra-articular corticosteroid injections may be used. With intra-articular injections, a long-acting corticosteroid such as triamcinolone is injected directly into the joint space of the affected joint. Pain relief generally lasts 3 months following the injection. Although this procedure relieves pain on a temporary basis, it can speed the destruction of cartilage if it is performed more frequently than every 4 to 6 months.

Many patients use topical medications, including salicylates (Aspercreme and Sportscreme), capsaicin (Capzasin), and counterirritants (Bengay and Icy Hot), which are sold OTC as creams, gels, sprays, patches, or ointments, to relieve OA pain. These therapies are well tolerated and produce few adverse effects. These products should not be used more than four times daily and should be discontinued if irritation occurs.

A newer drug therapy for patients with moderate OA who do not respond adequately to analgesics includes hyaluronate sodium (Hyalgan), a chemical normally found in high amounts within the synovial fluid. Administered by injection directly into the knee joint, this drug replaces or supplements the body's natural hyaluronic acid, which deteriorates as a result of the inflammation of OA. Treatment consists of one injection per week for three to five injections. Hyalgan helps provide a barrier that prevents friction and further inflammation of the joint by coating the articulating cartilage surface. Information that is given to the patient prior to administration should include adverse effects such as pain or swelling at the injection site and the avoidance of any strenuous activities for approximately 48 hours after injection.

PharmFACT

Genetic factors account for 50% of the risk for developing rheumatoid arthritis. Disease concordance in identical twins is 15% to 20%. The primary environmental risk is smoking (Temprano, 2014).

72.10 Pharmacotherapy for rheumatoid arthritis includes analgesics, anti-inflammatory drugs, corticosteroids, and disease-modifying antirheumatic drugs.

Rheumatoid arthritis (RA) is a chronic, progressive autoimmune disease that causes inflammation of the joints. It is characterized by disfigurement and inflammation of multiple joints. RA is less common than OA, with RA affecting about 2.1 million persons in the United States. Typically RA occurs at an earlier age than OA, with the incidence of RA increasing up to age 70. It is important to differentiate between the two types of arthritis because the treatments vary greatly.

In RA, autoantibodies known as rheumatoid factors attack the person's tissues, activating complement and drawing leukocytes into the area, where they attack the cells of the synovial membranes and blood. Inflammation first occurs in the synovial membranes, which line joint cavities, then progresses to the surrounding articular cartilage. The damaged synovial membrane swells and the persistent inflammation spreads and damages the surrounding blood vessels, ligaments, and tendons. The swelling also causes hemorrhage, coagulation, and deposits of fibrin within the joints. This ultimately leads to scar tissue formation that immobilizes the joint.

The exact etiology of RA is not known, but it is likely a combination of environmental and genetic factors. Female reproductive hormones may influence the development of RA because it affects women three to five times more frequently than men. Infectious organisms, such as the Epstein-Barr virus, may play a role in a person developing the autoimmune processes seen with RA.

The course of RA is variable and the rate at which joint deformities develop is not consistent. Disease progression is typically fastest during the first 6 years, slowing thereafter. The onset is typically insidious, though it may be acute if precipitated by a stressor, such as infection. The patient with early RA typically experiences morning joint stiffness, swelling, pain, and generalized fatigue. The joints may be slightly reddened, warm, and tender to palpation. The pattern of joints involved is usually symmetric. The upper extremity joints are often involved, beginning with the hands and wrists, as well as the joints of the toes, ankles, and knees. As the disease worsens, the

Glucosamine and Chondroitin for Osteoarthritis

Description
Many patients use OTC herbal medicines to relieve the pain and inflammation associated with OA. Two of the most commonly used agents are glucosamine and chondroitin.

History and Claims
Glucosamine is a natural substance that is an important building block of cartilage. With aging, glucosamine is lost with the natural thinning of cartilage. As cartilage wears down, the joints lose their normal cushioning ability, resulting in the pain and inflammation of OA. Chondroitin is another substance that forms part of the matrix between cartilage cells.

The use of glucosamine is thought to reduce cartilage breakdown and improve cartilage production and repair. Chondroitin is another dietary supplement purported to repair cartilage damaged by inflammation or injury.

Standardization
Glucosamine is made from the crushed shells of shrimps, lobsters, and crabs, although non-shellfish forms are available for patients allergic to shellfish. It

is available as oral tablets, capsules, or in powder form, with a typical dose being 1.5 g/day. Chondroitin is derived from bovine or shark cartilage and is also taken orally, with doses in the range of 800 to 1,200 mg/day.

Evidence
Typical of many other specialty supplements, research regarding the effectiveness of chondroitin and glucosamine has delivered mixed results. In most European countries, these two supplements are prescribed for the symptomatic treatment of knee OA (Henrotin, Marty, & Mobasheri, 2014). On the other hand, the American College of Rheumatology recommends that patients not use glucosamine or chondroitin for knee OA (Hochberg et al., 2012). Concurrent use of these supplements with conventional pharmacotherapy may allow for lower dose NSAIDs and the potential for fewer adverse effects from those drugs.

morning stiffness can extend several hours into the day and occur with any periods of prolonged rest. The persistent inflammation causes deformities of the joints and the supporting ligaments, tendons, and muscles, making activity painful. Muscle weakness and decreased ROM may be apparent. Most or all synovial joints are eventually affected. A patient with RA is shown in Figure 72.5.

Joint manifestations in RA typically precede systemic manifestations, which are associated with advancing disease. Extreme fatigue, anorexia, weight loss, anemia, and low-grade fever are common. Rheumatoid nodules may develop in the subcutaneous tissue of the forearm, toes, and fingers and in the viscera surrounding the heart, lungs, dura, and intestinal tract. Inflammation of the blood vessels can result in vasculitis. Respiratory complications, including pleurisy, pneumonitis, and fibrosis, are common as well as cardiac complications such as pericarditis and myocarditis.

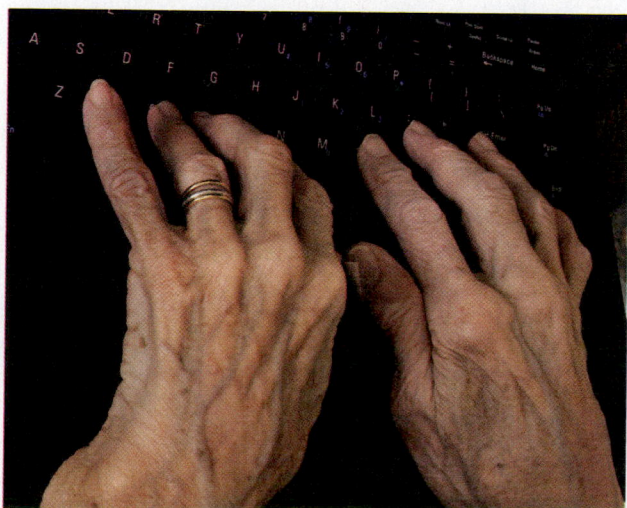

Figure 72.5 Patient with rheumatoid arthritis.
American College of Rheumatology.

Diagnosis of RA is based on the patient's history, physical examination, and diagnostic tests. Laboratory tests that are helpful in supporting a diagnosis of RA include elevations in the serum rheumatoid factor, erythrocyte sedimentation rate (ESR), antinuclear antibody titers, and serum immunoglobulin levels. Routine x-rays are used to determine the degree of structural joint damage.

Like OA, nonpharmacologic therapies are an essential component of RA management. ROM and joint and muscle strengthening exercises are important if the patient is to continue performing normal ADLs. Psychological counseling may be helpful to help the patient deal with a potentially debilitating disease. Braces, splints, canes, and walkers can assist in ambulation. Loss of excess weight can help take the stress off inflamed joints. Proper rest helps reduce pain.

The primary goals of RA pharmacotherapy are to manage inflammation, reduce pain, and maximize physical abilities. Pharmacotherapy for the relief of pain associated with RA includes the same classes of analgesics used for OA. Therapy is begun with NSAIDs, because these drugs relieve both pain and inflammation. NSAIDs that are used to treat RA are usually given in doses that are higher than those for the patient with OA. Aspirin is not recommended for long-term therapy due to its adverse effects on the GI system and platelet aggregation. Acetaminophen is effective at relieving pain and fever but has no anti-inflammatory actions. Although the analgesics relieve symptomatic pain, they have little effect on disease progression.

Corticosteroids may be considered for moderate or severe RA. Because of their potent anti-inflammatory action, the goal of therapy with corticosteroids is to relieve the symptoms associated with RA flare-ups. They are not used for long-term therapy because of their adverse effects, including a greater susceptibility to infections, poor wound healing, and osteoporosis. Severe rebound symptoms can occur when these medicines are discontinued. For these reasons, corticosteroids, when used, are given at the lowest daily doses possible.

The progression of tissue damage characteristic of RA can be slowed or modified with a diverse group of drugs called **disease-modifying antirheumatic drugs (DMARDs)**. These drugs include gold salts, antimalarial agents, D-penicillamine, and drugs that modify immune and inflammatory responses. They have been found to reduce mortality rates, improve symptoms, and enhance the quality of life in patients with RA. Most health care providers begin therapy with a DMARD within 3 months of a confirmed diagnosis of RA. It would not be unusual for a patient to be taking several DMARDs and analgesics. The maximum therapeutic effects from DMARDs often take several months to achieve. All of these drugs can be toxic and close monitoring of patients is required during the course of therapy. Doses of DMARDs are listed in Table 72.7.

The choice of a specific DMARD depends on the experiences of the health care provider and the response of the patient to therapy. Therapy often begins with hydroxychloroquine (Plaquenil), methotrexate (Otrexup, Rheumatrex, Trexall), or sulfasalazine (Azulfidine) because these drugs have the most research-based evidence for reducing mortality. Many rheumatologists consider methotrexate to be the first-line treatment for patients with aggressive RA. It acts quickly, has a relatively favorable safety profile, is low cost, and slows the progression of the disease. A once-weekly subcutaneous formulation of methotrexate (Otrexup) was approved in 2013 for severe RA that has not responded to other forms of therapy. Hydroxychloroquine therapy for 3 to 6 months is required to achieve therapeutic effects. Risks of toxicity with this drug are among the lowest associated with DMARDs.

Gold salts, D-penicillamine (Cuprimine), azathioprine (Azasan, Imuran), cyclosporine (Neoral), and cyclophosphamide (Cytoxan) have been used in the past but are more toxic than many other DMARDs.

TABLE 72.7 Selected Disease-Modifying Antirheumatic Drugs

Drug	Route and Adult Dose (Maximum Dose Where Indicated)	Adverse Effects
Biologic Therapies		
abatacept (Orencia)	IV: 500–1,000 mg given at 0, 2, and 4 weeks, then every 4 weeks thereafter	*Local reactions at the injection site (pain, erythema, myalgia), nasopharyngitis* Serious infections, sepsis, and invasive fungal infections, lupus-like syndrome, positive antinuclear antibodies, tumor lysis syndrome, heart failure exacerbations, Stevens–Johnson syndrome, increased malignancies, neutropenia, malignancies (tofacitinib)
adalimumab (Humira)	Subcutaneous: 40 mg every other week	
anakinra (Kineret)	Subcutaneous: 100 mg/day	
certolizumab pegol (Cimzia)	Subcutaneous: 400 mg initially and at weeks 2 and 4, followed by 200 mg every other week	
etanercept (Enbrel)	Subcutaneous: 25 mg twice weekly; or 0.08 mg/kg or 50 mg once weekly	
golimumab (Simponi)	Subcutaneous: 50 mg once monthly (for RA) or 100 mg every 4 weeks (for ulcerative colitis)	
infliximab (Remicade)	IV: 3 mg/kg at weeks 0, 2, and 6, then every 8 weeks	
rituximab (Rituxan)	IV: 1,000 mg every 2 weeks for a total of two doses (give a corticosteroid 30 min prior to infusion)	
tocilzumab (Actemra)	IV: 4–8 mg/kg every other week Subcutaneous: 162 mg every week or every other week	
tofacitinib (Xeljanz)	PO: 5 mg bid	
Nonbiologic Therapies		
apremilast (Otezla)	PO: start with 10 mg once daily and gradually increase to 30 mg bid	*Diarrhea, nausea, headache* Depression with possible suicidal thoughts, weight loss
azathioprine (Azasan, Imuran)	PO: 1 mg/kg/day once or in divided doses bid for 6–8 weeks (max: 2.5 mg/kg/day) Maintenance dose: 1–2.5 mg/kg/day as a single dose or divided	*Chills, fever, malaise, myalgia* Myelosuppression, hepatotoxicity, lymphoproliferative disorders
hydroxychloroquine (Plaquenil)	PO: 400–600 mg/day for 4–12 weeks, then 200–400 mg once daily Maintenance dose: 10–20 mg/day	*Anorexia, nausea, vomiting, headache, and personality changes* Retinopathy, agranulocytosis, aplastic anemia, seizures
leflunomide (Arava)	PO: 100-mg loading dose for 3 days, then 20 mg/day	*Diarrhea, elevated hepatic enzymes, alopecia and rash* Hepatotoxicity, immunosuppression
methotrexate (Otrexup, Rheumatrex, Trexall)	PO: 7.5 mg once/week or 2.5 mg every 12 h for three doses once/week (max: 20 mg/week) Subcutaneous (Otrexup): 10–25 mg once weekly	*Headache, glossitis, gingivitis, mild leukopenia, nausea* Ulcerative stomatitis, myelosuppression, aplastic anemia, hepatic cirrhosis, nephrotoxicity, sudden death, pulmonary fibrosis, teratogenicity
sulfasalazine (Azulfidine)	PO: 500–1,000 mg/day (max: 3 g/day)	*Headache, anorexia, nausea, vomiting* Anaphylaxis, Stevens–Johnson syndrome, agranulocytosis, leukopenia, reversible oligospermia

Note: Italics indicate common adverse effects. Underline indicates serious adverse effects.

Biologic therapies are the newest DMARD therapy for the treatment of RA. These biologic drugs block steps in the inflammatory response, reduce joint inflammation, and slow the progression of joint damage. Adalimumab (Humira), etanercept (Enbrel), cerolizumab (Cimzia), golimumab (Simponi), and infliximab (Remicade) are tumor necrosis factor (TNF) antagonists. TNF is a naturally occurring cytokine produced by macrophages and activated T cells that mediates inflammation and modulates cellular immune responses. Elevated levels of TNF are found in the synovial fluid of patients with RA. Certolizumab (Cimzia) and golimumab (Simponi) are newer generation TNF blockers. Anakinra (Kineret) and abatacept (Orencia) are biologic agents that block actions of interleukins in inflammatory pathways. The biologic agents appear to be effective and relatively nontoxic but they are expensive (about $20,000 per year) when compared to first-line therapies; thus they are normally not prescribed until conventional therapy has been attempted and failed. Combinations of biologic and nonbiologic drugs may be effective for patients unresponsive to monotherapy.

| PROTOTYPE DRUG | Hydroxychloroquine (Plaquenil) |

Classification: Therapeutic: Antirheumatic drug, antimalarial **Pharmacologic:** Disease-modifying antirheumatic drug

Therapeutic Effects and Uses: Approved in 1955, hydroxychloroquine is approved for the treatment of RA for which it is a first-line drug. This drug is also used for the prophylaxis and treatment of malaria, but chloroquine (Aralen) is the preferred drug for this parasitic infection (see Chapter 53). It may be used to treat systemic lupus erythematosus in patients who have not responded well to other anti-inflammatory drugs. This drug relieves the severe inflammation characteristic of these disorders.

For full effectiveness, hydroxychloroquine is most often prescribed concurrently with salicylates and glucocorticoids. The major advantage of hydroxychloroquine is that it exhibits less bone marrow, renal, and hepatic toxicity than other DMARDs.

Mechanism of Action: The exact mechanism of action of hydroxychloroquine in reducing the symptoms of RA is unknown. This drug reduces the migration of neutrophils and eosinophils and likely inhibits the synthesis of histamine and prostaglandins.

Pharmacokinetics:

Route(s)	PO
Absorption	Rapidly and almost completely absorbed
Distribution	Widely distributed; concentrated in the lungs, liver, erythrocytes, eyes, skin, and kidneys; crosses the placenta; secreted in breast milk
Primary metabolism	Partially in the liver to active metabolite
Primary excretion	Renal
Onset of action	4–6 weeks for antirheumatic response
Duration of action	Unknown

Adverse Effects: The primary adverse effects of hydroxychloroquine are GI related, such as anorexia, weight loss, nausea, and vomiting. Possible ocular effects include blurred vision, photophobia, diminished ability to read, and blacked-out areas in the visual field. With high doses or prolonged therapy, these retinal changes may be irreversible in some patients. Other adverse effects of hydroxychloroquine include fatigue, anxiety, vertigo, skin rash, itching, bleaching or loss of hair, headache, and mood and mental changes.

Contraindications/Precautions: Patients with known hypersensitivity to this drug or who exhibit retinal or visual field changes associated with quinoline drugs should not receive hydroxychloroquine. Caution should be used in patients with hepatic impairment, alcoholism, impaired renal function, porphyria, metabolic acidosis, and those with a tendency for dermatitis.

Drug Interactions: Antacids that contain aluminum or magnesium may prevent the absorption of hydroxychloroquine. Hydroxychloroquine may increase the risk of liver damage when administered with other hepatotoxic drugs. Alcohol use should be eliminated during therapy. This drug may increase digoxin levels and may interfere with the patient's response to the rabies vaccine. Concurrent administration with cimetidine may increase hydroxychloroquine levels. **Herbal/Food**: None known.

Pregnancy: Category C.

Treatment of Overdose: Overdose may be life threatening, especially in children. Therapy with anticonvulsants, vasopressors, and antidysrhythmics may be necessary.

Nursing Responsibilities: Key nursing implications for patients receiving hydroxychloroquine are included in the Nursing Practice Application for Patients Receiving Pharmacotherapy for Rheumatoid Arthritis and Osteoarthritis.

Drugs Similar to Hydroxychloroquine (Plaquenil)

The first- and second-choice DMARDs are described next. Gold salts (Auranofin, Aurothioglucose, and gold sodium thiomalate) and penicillamine (Cuprimine, Depen) are DMARDs that are rarely used and the student should refer to a drug guide for information. Cyclosporine and azathioprine are immunosuppressants that occasionally are used as DMARDs. They are described in Chapter 42.

TNF Blockers: The TNF blockers include the monoclonal antibodies adalimumab, certolizumab, etanercept, golimumab, and infliximab. Although each of these drugs is unique, they have similar actions and adverse effects. The most common adverse effects are injection-site reactions such as pain, swelling, and bruising. Other adverse effects include upper respiratory tract infection, neutropenia, and rare cases of central nervous system (CNS) demyelinating disorders such as multiple sclerosis. Also, some of these medications may worsen or cause heart failure. Because they are potent immunosuppressants, all pose an increased risk for serious infections and malignancy. These drugs carry a black box warning that reactivation of latent infections such as tuberculosis may occur. The warning also includes an increased risk for lymphoma and other malignancies, especially when used in children and adolescents treated for juvenile RA. All TNF blockers are pregnancy category B.

- **Adalimumab (Humira).** Approved in 2002, adalimumab is approved for moderate to severe RA, psoriatic RA in adults, polyarticular juvenile RA in children age 2 and older, ankylosing spondylitis, Crohn's disease, and plaque psoriasis. Adalimumab is administered by the subcutaneous route twice a week.

- **Certolizumab pegol (Cimzia).** Certolizumab was approved in 2008 for the treatment of moderate to severe RA and Crohn's disease unresponsive to safer medications. The drug is given as a subcutaneous injection, usually every other week.

- **Etanercept (Enbrel).** Approved in 1998, etanercept is approved for the treatment of moderate to severe RA, psoriatic RA in adults, polyarticular juvenile RA in children age 2 and older, ankylosing spondylitis, and plaque psoriasis. Etanercept is administered by the subcutaneous route twice a week. Concurrent use of etanercept with sulfasalazine may result in leukopenia.

- **Golimumab (Simponi).** Golimumab was approved in 2009 for the management of moderate to severe RA, active psoriatic RA in adults, and active ankylosing spondylitis in adults. More recently, the drug was approved to treat moderate to severe ulcerative colitis that cannot be managed by first-line medications. Golimumab is usually combined with methotrexate and is given as a subcutaneous injection once a month.

- **Infliximab (Remicade).** Originally approved in 1998, infliximab is indicated for moderate to severe RA, psoriatic RA, ankylosing spondylitis, Crohn's disease, ulcerative colitis, and plaque psoriasis. For RA infliximab is usually combined with methotrexate and is given as an IV infusion over several hours, followed by subsequent injections in weeks 2 and 6 and every 8 weeks thereafter. Acetaminophen and diphenhydramine (Benadryl) are given prior to infusion to decrease the symptoms of infusion reaction such as chest pain, tachycardia, shortness of breath, and light-headedness.

Abatacept (Orencia): Abatacept was approved in 2005 for the treatment of moderate to severe RA in adults and for juvenile idiopathic RA in children age 6 and older. The drug acts by inhibiting the actions of T cells, which are often hyperactive in patients with RA. It is administered as an IV infusion, usually every other week. Headache, upper respiratory tract infection, and nausea are common adverse effects. Like other immunosuppressants, there is an increased risk of serious infections, or reactivation of latent infections. The risk for malignancies may also be increased. Although abatacept is sometimes used in combination with other DMARDs, it should not be administered concurrently with TNF blockers due to a high incidence of serious infections. This drug is pregnancy category C.

Anakinra (Kineret): Approved in 2001, anakinra inhibits interleukin-1 (IL-1), an important chemical mediator of inflammation. It is approved for RA that has not responded to one or more DMARDs. A major disadvantage of this drug is that it must be given daily by the subcutaneous route. Injection-site reactions such as pain, swelling, edema, and bruising occur more often than with the other drugs in its class. Ice and hydrocortisone cream are recommended to diminish the pain, along with site rotation. Upper respiratory infections and influenza symptoms occur in many patients. The manufacturer recommends that anakinra not be administered concurrently with TNF inhibitors such as etanercept due to an increased risk of infections. Anakinra is pregnancy category B.

Apremilast (Otezla): One of the newest DMARDs, apremilast is the first drug in this class to inhibit the enzyme phosphodiesterase-4 (PDE-4). Unlike the biologic therapies that target specific inflammatory molecules, apremilast affects a larger number of inflammatory mediators, including TNF and several interleukins. Approved in 2014 to treat psoriatic arthritis, apremilast has the advantage of being administered by the oral route. The drug is well tolerated, with the most common adverse effects being diarrhea, nausea, and headache. The drug has been associated with an increased incidence of depression and weight loss. Apremilast is pregnancy category C.

Leflunomide (Arava): Approved in 1998, leflunomide is a DMARD with a unique mechanism of action. It inhibits an enzyme in mitochondria that is responsible for the synthesis of pyrimidines, which are building blocks for DNA and ribonucleic acid (RNA). The result is an inhibition in B-cell and T-cell function. Reduced cytokine and antibody production by these cells reduces inflammation and joint destruction. After a loading dose for 3 days, this drug is given PO once daily. Leflunomide has an exceptionally long half-life, and it can be detected in the blood as long as 2 years after discontinuation. If toxicity occurs, the administration of cholestyramine for 11 days can clear most leflunomide from the body. Common adverse effects include diarrhea, nausea, vomiting, headache, and alopecia. Leflunomide is hepatotoxic and liver function must be regularly monitored during therapy. The possibility of pregnancy should be excluded before therapy is begun because this drug is pregnancy category X.

Methotrexate (Rheumatrex, Trexall): Methotrexate is a drug used for a number of proliferative and inflammatory diseases, including various carcinomas and leukemias, immunosuppression following kidney transplantation, severe psoriasis, and RA. Methotrexate acts as a folic acid antagonist, and it is a potent immunosuppressant. Gastric irritation and stomatitis are the most frequent adverse effects; these are minimized by the concurrent use of folic acid. Patients, particularly those who are older, obese, or have diabetes or renal disease, need to be monitored for hepatotoxicity, bone marrow suppression, and pneumonitis. The possibility of pregnancy should be excluded before therapy is begun because this drug is pregnancy category X. A prototype feature for methotrexate may be found in Chapter 57.

Rituximab (Rituxan): Rituximab (Rituxan) is a monoclonal antibody originally approved in 1997 as an antineoplastic drug. The drug binds to CD20, a surface protein present on B lymphocytes involved in certain leukemias and lymphomas. Once bound, rituximab lyses the tumor cells. Later, it was discovered that B lymphocytes also play a major role in producing the severe inflammation associated with RA. In 2006, rituximab was approved to treat moderate to severe RA that has not responded to therapy with TNF blockers. For RA, the drug is administered concurrently with methotrexate. Common adverse effects include upper respiratory tract infection, urinary tract infection, and bronchitis. Rituximab can produce adverse effects such as serious infections, life-threatening dysrhythmias, and tumor lysis syndrome. This drug is pregnancy category C.

Sulfasalazine (Azulfidine): Sulfasalazine is a sulfonamide and, having been approved in 1950, one of the oldest drugs for RA. It is also approved for juvenile RA, Crohn's disease, and ulcerative colitis. It is available as an enteric-coated tablet that must be taken three to four times daily. Its beneficial effects are noted quickly, often after 4 weeks of therapy. GI complaints such as nausea, vomiting, anorexia, diarrhea, and abdominal pain occur in a significant number of patients taking this drug, and these may cause discontinuation of therapy. The adverse GI effects are better tolerated if therapy starts with a low dose that is gradually increased. Headache; blood dyscrasias, especially leukopenia; and skin rashes are also frequent. Regular monitoring of CBCs for bone marrow suppression should be conducted. Patients with allergies to sulfur or other sulfonamides should not receive sulfasalazine. Concurrent administration with iron supplements or antibiotics should be avoided because doing so diminishes the absorption of sulfasalazine. Sulfasalazine is pregnancy category B.

Tocilizumab (Actemra): One of the newer biologic therapies, tocilizumab was approved in 2010 for the treatment of moderate to severe RA in adults and for juvenile idiopathic arthritis in children age 2 and older. It may be used as monotherapy or in combination with other DMARDs such as methotrexate. Tocilizumab acts by inhibiting interleukin-6 (IL-6), a substance secreted by immune cells that promotes inflammation and activates the immune response. It is administered by either the IV or subcutaneous route. The IV is given once every 4 weeks, whereas the subcutaneous dose is given every other week. Headache, upper respiratory tract infection, hypertension (HTN), and increased liver enzymes are common adverse effects. Like other immunosuppressants, the risk of serious infections or reactivation of latent infections is increased. Tocilizumab therapy should not be initiated if the absolute neutrophil count (ANC) is less than 2,000/mm^3, if the platelet count is below 100,000/mm^3, or if liver enzymes are elevated (1.5 times normal). This drug is pregnancy category C.

CONNECTIONS: NURSING PRACTICE APPLICATION

Patients Receiving Pharmacotherapy for Rheumatoid Arthritis and Osteoarthritis

Assessment	Potential Nursing Diagnoses*
Baseline assessment prior to administration: • Obtain a complete health history including musculoskeletal, GI, cardiovascular, neurologic, endocrine, hepatic, or renal disease. Obtain a drug history including allergies, current prescription and OTC drugs, and herbal preparations, alcohol use, or smoking. Be alert to possible drug interactions. • Obtain a history of any current symptoms or pain and their effect on ADLs. Assess for inflammation, nodules, deformities, as well as location, and note the presence of pain or discomfort, time of day of occurrence, on movement, or at rest. Assess effects on sleep. • Obtain a dietary history and the effect of the disease on the ability to obtain food sources, cooking, and eating. Assess adequacy of fluid intake. • Obtain baseline weight and vital signs. • Evaluate appropriate laboratory findings (e.g., CBC, sedimentation rate, hepatic and renal function studies, rheumatoid factor, coagulation panels, bleeding time, electrolytes, glucose, lipid profile). • Assess the patient's ability to receive and understand instructions. Include the family or caregiver as needed.	• *Acute Pain* • *Chronic Pain* • *Activity Intolerance* • *Fatigue* • *Disturbed Body Image* • *Impaired Physical Mobility* • *Ineffective Role Performance* • *Deficient Knowledge* (Drug Therapy) • *Risk for Injury*, related to adverse drug effects
Assessment throughout administration: • Assess for desired therapeutic effects dependent on the reason for the drug (e.g., symptoms of acute inflammation are diminished or absent, pain is diminished or absent, ability to carry out ROM and ADLs has increased). • Continue monitoring vital signs and level of pain. • Continue to monitor laboratory studies as ordered. • Assess for and promptly report adverse effects: symptoms of GI bleeding (dark or tarry stools, hematemesis, coffee-ground emesis, or blood in the stool), abdominal pain, severe tinnitus, dizziness, drowsiness, light-headedness, palpitations, tachycardia, HTN, increased respiratory rate and depth, pulmonary congestion, edema, diminished urine output, fever, infections, visual effects (blurred vision, photophobia, blacked-out areas in the vision field).	

Implementation

Interventions and (Rationales)	Patient-Centered Care
Ensuring therapeutic effects: • Continue assessments as above for therapeutic effects. (Diminished inflammation, pain, stiffness, improved ROM, and ability to carry out ADLs should continue to improve.)	• Teach the patient to supplement drug therapy with nonpharmacologic measures, e.g., a balance between low-impact activity and rest, application of warm or cool compresses, or warm showers prior to activity. • Teach the patient to promptly report increasing pain, stiffness, and decreased ability to carry out ADLs. Hospitalization may be required during acute exacerbations dependent on the severity of symptoms.

(continued)

CONNECTIONS: NURSING PRACTICE APPLICATION (continued)

• Continue to assess fluid and nutrition intake. (Inflammation, pain, and deformities may make eating and drinking difficult. Dietitian consultation may be required.)	• Encourage the patient to eat small, nutrient-dense foods with adequate fluids frequently throughout the day to maintain nutrition and hydration as well as to conserve energy. The family or caregiver may need to prepare meals, and a dietary consult may be useful.
• Continue to monitor CBC, sedimentation rate, RA factor, hepatic and renal laboratory values, glucose, electrolytes, and lipid levels.	• Instruct the patient on the need to return for periodic laboratory testing.
Minimizing adverse effects: • Instruct the patient to promptly report any worsening inflammation, pain, increased joint involvement, or overall worsening of symptoms. (Drugs for RA treat the symptoms and slow the progression of the disease but are not a cure. Acute exacerbations may require hospitalization and a change in the medication regimen.)	• Instruct the patient to promptly report any continued inflammation, pain, increased joint involvement, or general worsening of symptoms.
• Continue to monitor periodic laboratory work: CBC, coagulation panels, bleeding time, electrolytes, glucose, hepatic and renal function tests, and lipid levels. (Aspirin, salicylates, and NSAIDs affect platelet aggregation and should be monitored when used long term or if excessive bleeding or bruising is noted. Corticosteroids may affect electrolytes, glucose, and lipid levels. DMARDs may cause hemolysis, agranulocytosis, or aplastic anemia. **Lifespan:** Age-related physiological differences may place the older adult at greater risk for adverse hepatic, renal, or cardiac effects.)	• Instruct the patient on the need to return periodically for laboratory work.
• Monitor for abdominal pain, black or tarry stools, blood in the stool, hematemesis, coffee-ground emesis, dizziness, light-headedness, or hypotension, especially if associated with tachycardia. (NSAIDs and glucocorticoids may cause GI irritation and bleeding.)	• Instruct the patient to immediately report any signs or symptoms of GI bleeding. • Teach the patient to take the drug with food or milk to decrease GI irritation. Enteric-coated tablets should be swallowed whole without chewing, crushing, or breaking. Alcohol use should be avoided or eliminated.
• Monitor for tinnitus, difficulty hearing, light-headedness, or difficulty with balance and report promptly. (NSAIDs and salicylates may be ototoxic and cause hearing loss.)	• Instruct the patient to immediately report any signs or symptoms of ringing, humming, buzzing in ears, difficulty with balance, dizziness, vertigo, or nausea.
• Monitor urine output and renal function studies periodically. Weigh the patient on corticosteroids daily and report weight gain of 1 kg (2 lb) or more in a 24-h period or more than 2 kg (5 lb) per week, or increasing peripheral edema. (NSAIDs and salicylates may be renal toxic. Patients on long-term or high-dose therapy should monitor urine output and have periodic renal function studies. Daily weight is an accurate measure of fluid status and takes into account intake, output, and insensible losses.)	• Instruct the patient on NSAIDs and salicylates to report any changes in the quantity of urine output, darkening of urine, or edema promptly. • Teach the patient on NSAIDs and salicylates to increase fluid intake, especially if fever is present. • Instruct the patient to weigh self daily, ideally at the same time of day. The patient should report a weight gain of more than 1 kg (2 lb) in a 24-h period or more than 2 kg (5 lb) per week, or increasing peripheral edema.
• Observe for skin rashes, fever, stomatitis, flulike symptoms, or general malaise. (Bone marrow suppression may occur with corticosteroids or DMARDs and result in an increased risk of infection.)	• Teach the patient to immediately report any flulike symptoms, fever, mouth irritation or soreness, or skin rashes.
• Periodically monitor vision in patients on NSAIDs or DMARDs. Immediately report unusual changes in visual acuity, blurred or diminished vision, reports of spots in vision, difficulty reading, blacked-out areas of the vision field, or changes to color sense to the provider. (NSAIDs may cause blurred or diminished vision, decreased color sense, diplopia, or scotomas. DMARDs may cause significant retinal changes with blurred vision, difficulty reading, photophobia, or blacked-out areas of the vision field.)	• Teach the patient on NSAIDs or DMARDs to obtain eye exams twice yearly or more frequently as instructed by the provider. Immediately report any sudden changes in vision.
Patient understanding of drug therapy: • Use opportunities during administration of medications and during assessments to discuss the rationale for the drug therapy, desired therapeutic outcomes, commonly observed adverse effects, parameters for when to call the health care provider, and any necessary monitoring or precautions. (Using time during nursing care helps to optimize and reinforce key teaching areas.)	• The patient should be able to state the reason for the drug, appropriate dose and scheduling, what adverse effects to observe for and when to report them, and the anticipated length of medication therapy.
Patient self-administration of drug therapy: • When administering the medication, instruct the patient, family, or caregiver in proper self-administration of the drug, e.g., taken with food or meals or with additional fluids, followed by teach-back. (Utilizing time during nurse-administration of these drugs helps to reinforce teaching.)	• The patient, family, or caregiver is able to discuss appropriate dosing and administration needs.

Chloroquine (Aralen) and hydroxychloroquine (Plaquenil) are very similar, and both may be used to treat malaria. From what you learned in Chapter 53, what organism causes malaria? Describe how these drugs are used for prophylaxis of malaria. *See Answer to Connection Checkpoint 72.3 on student resource website.*

Pharmacotherapy of Gout and Hyperuricemia

72.11 Gout is treated with drugs that decrease joint pain and inflammation and lower uric acid levels.

Gout is a form of acute arthritis caused by an accumulation of uric acid (urate) crystals in the joints and other body tissues, causing inflammation. Between 1% and 3% of the U.S. population are affected by gout. Of patients with gout 90% are men, who first manifest symptoms between the age of 30 and 60; women are affected after menopause.

Gout may be classified as primary or secondary. Primary gout is caused by genetic errors in the metabolism of purines. Uric acid is a waste product created by the metabolic breakdown of the nucleic acids DNA and RNA. The kidneys are responsible for excreting uric acid. High levels of uric acid crystals may result from an increased metabolism of nucleic acids or the reduced excretion of uric acid by the kidneys. Primary gout may therefore be viewed as an imbalance in the handling of uric acid by the body. The production of uric acid crystals exceeds the excretion capability of the kidneys. Primary gout is inherited as an X-linked trait; males inherit the disorder through female carriers.

Secondary gout is caused by diseases or drugs that increase the metabolic turnover of nucleic acids or that interfere with the excretion of uric acid. Some examples of drugs that may cause gout include thiazide diuretics, aspirin, cyclosporine, and alcohol, when ingested on a chronic basis. Conditions that can cause secondary gout include diabetic ketoacidosis, hypothyroidism, multiple myeloma, renal impairment, and diseases associated with a rapid cell turnover such as leukemia, hemolytic anemia, and polycythemia.

The primary diagnostic criterion for gout is the serum uric acid level. **Hyperuricemia** is defined as a serum uric acid level of 7 mg/dL. Patients with mild hyperuricemia are asymptomatic. Once the level of uric acid rises to saturation levels in body fluids, urate crystals form and symptoms appear, usually with a sudden onset.

Acute gouty arthritis occurs when needle-shaped uric acid crystals accumulate in joints, resulting in extremely painful, red, and inflamed tissue. Attacks have a sudden onset, often occur at night, and may be triggered by ingestion of alcohol, dehydration, stress, injury to the joint, or fever. Gouty arthritis most often occurs in the big toes, heels, ankles, wrists, fingers, knees, or elbows and may be accompanied by an elevated temperature. With chronic gout, bumps called tophi, or deposits of sodium urate crystals in the subcutaneous tissue, may be present, particularly on the outer ear, arms, and fingers. Deposits of urate crystals in the kidneys may lead to the development of urinary calculi and renal failure. Nephrolithiasis occurs in 10% to 25% of patients with gout and is more likely to occur in patients with low fluid intake and when the urine is acidic.

Gout may be difficult to diagnose because early symptoms may be vague. Although most people with gout have hyperuricemia, the serum levels of uric acid may be normal even during an acute attack. To confirm a diagnosis, a synovial fluid analysis may be performed to evaluate for the presence of uric acid crystals or to rule out synovial fluid infection as the cause of the symptoms.

In its early phases, treatment of gout is very successful. The goals of gout pharmacotherapy are threefold:

- Termination of acute episodes
- Prevention of future gout attacks
- Avoidance of the formation of gout complications, such as tophi and kidney stones

Combination therapy using anti-inflammatory drugs such as colchicine and uric acid inhibitors such as probenecid (Probalan) and allopurinol (Lopurin, Zyloprim) is the mainstay of gout therapy. Uric acid inhibitors block the accumulation of uric acid in the blood or uric acid crystals within the joints. When uric acid accumulation is blocked, the symptoms associated with gout diminish. These drugs are most effective when taken within the first 12 hours of an acute attack. About 80% of the patients using uric acid inhibitors experience GI complaints such as abdominal cramping, nausea, vomiting, and diarrhea. Drugs for gout are listed in Table 72.8.

NSAIDs are the preferred drugs for treating the pain and inflammation of acute episodes of gout. Commonly used NSAIDs include indomethacin (Indocin) and naproxen (Naprosyn), which are taken PO every day. Aspirin should be avoided because it can increase uric acid levels and worsen symptoms. Corticosteroids may be used to treat exacerbations of acute gout, particularly when the symptoms are in a single joint and the medication can be delivered intra-articularly. The most commonly used corticosteroid is prednisone. Most patients report that symptoms improve within a few hours of treatment and that an acute episode terminates within a week.

Prophylaxis of gout includes dietary management, avoidance of drugs that worsen the condition, and therapy with antigout medications. Patients should avoid high-purine foods such as organ meats, legumes, alcoholic beverages, mushrooms, and oatmeal because these foods form nucleic acids when they are metabolized. Patients should avoid aspirin, niacin, and diuretics because their use can precipitate an acute episode of gout. Renal complications may be avoided by adequate fluid intake and consumption of a low-protein diet.

PROTOTYPE DRUG | **Colchicine (Colcrys)**

Classification: Therapeutic: Antigout drug
Pharmacologic: Anti-inflammatory drug

Therapeutic Effects and Uses: Colchicine is a natural product obtained from the autumn crocus, which is grown in gardens and found in meadows throughout the United States and Canada. It has been used for centuries as a natural product. Although first available by prescription prior to 1938, colchicine was not officially approved by the FDA until 2009. The brand name form, Colcrys, is approved for the treatment and prophylaxis of acute gout flares and for familial Mediterranean fever.

Although NSAIDs have largely replaced colchicine as first-line therapy, it is prescribed for some patients with acute gouty arthritis. It is much more effective if taken within 24 hours of the onset

TABLE 72.8 Drugs for Gout

Drug	Route and Adult Dose (Maximum Dose Where Indicated)	Adverse Effects
allopurinol (Lopurin, Zyloprim)	PO (primary): 100 mg/day; may increase by 100 mg/week (max: 800 mg/day) PO (secondary): 200–800 mg/day	*Drowsiness, skin rash, diarrhea* <u>Severe skin reactions, bone marrow depression, hepatotoxicity, renal failure</u>
colchicine (Colcrys)	PO for prophylaxis: 0.5 mg once or twice daily PO for gout flare: 1.2 mg followed by another dose of 0.6 mg 1 h later	*Nausea, vomiting, diarrhea, GI upset* <u>Bone marrow depression, aplastic anemia, leukopenia, thrombocytopenia, agranulocytosis, severe diarrhea, nephrotoxicity</u>
febuxostat (Uloric)	PO: 40–80 mg once daily	*Liver enzyme elevation, nausea, arthralgia, and rash* <u>Thromboembolism, gout flare</u>
pegloticase (Krystexxa)	IV: 8 mg every 2 weeks by IV infusion	*Gout flare, nausea, ecchymosis, nasopharyngitis* <u>Anaphylaxis, infusion reaction, worsening heart failure</u>
probenecid (Probalan)	PO: 250 mg bid for 1 week, then 500 mg bid (max: 3 g/day)	*Nausea, vomiting, headache, anorexia, flushed face* <u>Anaphylaxis, severe skin reactions, hepatotoxicity, anemia, aplastic anemia, leukopenia</u>
sulfinpyrazone (Anturane)	PO: 100–200 mg bid for 1 week, then increase to 200–400 mg bid	*GI distress, rash* <u>Blood dyscrasias, nephrolithiasis</u>

Note: *Italics* indicate common adverse effects. <u>Underline</u> indicates serious adverse effects.

of symptoms. Colchicine has several off-label indications that include amyloidosis, Paget's disease, hepatic cirrhosis, and Mediterranean fever.

Although colchicine has no analgesic properties, patients experience pain relief due to the reduction in inflammation. Low doses of colchicine may be used as prophylactic therapy for gouty arthritis in patients with normal or slightly elevated serum uric acid levels. Should the patient note the onset of an acute episode, the dose can be increased until symptoms subside. It is important to understand, however, that colchicine does not inhibit uric acid synthesis and does not promote uric acid excretion. Thus, if the patient has escalating serum uric acid levels, allopurinol and sulfinpyrazone are the preferred drugs for prophylaxis (see Section 72.12). Patients who are on colchicine prophylaxis therapy may discontinue the drug after they have been symptom free for a year and have normal serum uric acid levels. In some patients, discontinuation may precipitate an acute gout episode.

Mechanism of Action: Colchicine inhibits the migration of neutrophils into the area of inflammation. This drug reduces the inflammation associated with acute gouty arthritis by inhibiting the synthesis of microtubules, which are the subcellular structures responsible for helping white blood cells infiltrate an area.

Pharmacokinetics:

Route(s)	PO
Absorption	Rapidly absorbed
Distribution	Widely distributed, concentrated in leukocytes, kidney, liver, spleen, and intestinal tract
Primary metabolism	Hepatic
Primary excretion	Feces
Onset of action	12 h
Duration of action	Half-life: variable (1.7–20.9 h)

Adverse Effects: The most significant adverse effects of colchicine are GI related and these may occur in up to 80% of patients. Adverse effects include nausea, vomiting, abdominal pain, anorexia, and diarrhea. This drug may cause bone marrow toxicity, and aplastic anemia, leukopenia, thrombocytopenia, or agranulocytosis may occur. Additional adverse effects include hepatotoxicity, mental confusion, azotemia, proteinuria, hematuria, and oliguria. Severe irritation and tissue damage may occur if the IV formulation leaks around the injection site.

Contraindications/Precautions: This drug is contraindicated in patients with a known hypersensitivity to colchicine, and in those with serious GI, renal, hepatic, pregnancy, or cardiac impairment. Patients with blood dyscrasias should not receive colchicine. Colchicine should be used with caution in older adults and debilitated patients, or in patients with an early manifestation of GI, renal, hepatic, or cardiac disease.

Drug Interactions: Concurrent use with NSAIDs may increase the risk of serious GI symptoms. Colchicine may exhibit additive bone marrow toxicity with cyclosporine, phenylbutazone, and other drugs that adversely affect bone marrow. Erythromycin may increase serum colchicine levels. Loop diuretics may decrease colchicine effects. Alcohol or products that contain alcohol may cause skin rashes and result in additive liver damage. Colchicine may increase a patient's sensitivity to CNS depressants. Colchicine may also directly interfere with the absorption of vitamin B_{12}. **Herbal/Food**: Alcohol and foods that are rich in purines, including salmon, sardines, and organ meats, should be avoided. Foods that cause the urine to become more alkaline, such as milk, fruits, carbonated drinks, most vegetables, molasses, and baking soda, may increase the risk of kidney stones.

Pregnancy: Category C (PO) or D (IV).

Treatment of Overdose: Overdoses (including accidental ingestion of autumn crocus) may cause severe GI distress, shock, paralysis, delirium, respiratory failure, and death. Treatment is symptomatic and may include gastric lavage and hemodialysis.

Nursing Responsibilities: Key nursing implications for patients receiving colchicine are included in the Nursing Practice Application for Patients Receiving Pharmacotherapy for Gout.

Drugs Similar to Colchicine (Colcrys)

Colchicine is the only drug in this class.

PharmFACT

Pseudogout is a type of arthritis that can cause symptoms similar to gout but involves accumulation of a different type of crystal: calcium pyrophosphate. The patient is treated with analgesics or anti-inflammatory drugs: There is no therapy available to dissolve these types of crystals (American College of Rheumatology, 2012).

72.12 Hyperuricemia is treated with drugs that reduce serum levels of uric acid.

Many patients with increased uric acid levels are asymptomatic. In most cases, pharmacotherapy is not indicated for asymptomatic patients. For patients with repeated acute episodes of chronic gout, however, prophylactic pharmacotherapy should be used to lower serum uric acid levels. Prophylaxis may be obtained by blocking the formation of uric acid or by increasing its excretion.

Allopurinol (Lopurin, Zyloprim) is a preferred drug for gout *prophylaxis*. Allopurinol acts by inhibiting **xanthine oxidase**, which is the enzyme responsible for the formation of uric acid. Blocking the synthesis of uric acid will lower serum uric acid levels, thus preventing gout. It is also used in patients with renal impairment or those who have renal obstruction caused by uric acid stones.

Uricosurics are drugs that increase the rate of excretion of uric acid by blocking its reabsorption in the kidney. These drugs are most effective in preventing hyperuricemia and tophi associated with chronic gout and should not be used to treat acute attacks of gouty arthritis. The uricosuric drugs have no analgesic or anti-inflammatory properties. The uricosuric drugs used for gout prophylaxis include probenecid (Probalan) and sulfinpyrazone (Anturane). These drugs may precipitate acute gout during the period of initial therapy because they mobilize the uric acid that has been stored in the body. Concurrent administration of colchicine can help prevent this adverse effect. The mobilization of uric acid may also cause or worsen kidney stones due to the increased amount of uric acid being excreted by the kidneys. To prevent these adverse effects of early therapy, the uricosurics are started at low doses and increased gradually over several weeks. During this initial therapy, the urine may be made more alkaline by the administration of sodium bicarbonate to prevent uric acid crystals from forming. Drugs for hyperuricemia and gout are listed in Table 72.8.

Acute hyperuricemia can occur following antineoplastic therapy as part of a serious condition called tumor lysis syndrome when cancer cells are broken down. The massive load of uric acid crystals can result in acute renal failure and possibly death. Rasburicase

(Elitek) is a recombinant form of the enzyme urate oxidase, which can lower serum uric acid levels when given IV to patients receiving antineoplastic therapy.

PROTOTYPE DRUG	Allopurinol (Lopurin, Zyloprim)

Classification: **Therapeutic:** Antigout drug
Pharmacologic: Xanthine oxidase inhibitor

Therapeutic Effects and Uses: Allopurinol is an older drug that was approved in 1966 for gout and its complications. It is used to control the hyperuricemia that causes severe gout and to reduce the possibility of flare-ups of acute gouty attacks. It is also approved to prevent recurrent nephrolithiasis due to calcium oxalate stones in patients with elevated uric acid levels. It may be used prophylactically to reduce the severity of the hyperuricemia associated with antineoplastic and radiation therapies, both of which increase plasma uric acid levels by promoting nucleic acid degradation. This drug takes 1 to 3 weeks to bring serum uric acid levels to within the normal range.

Allopurinol is available by the PO and IV routes. IV administration is usually reserved for patients with high uric acid levels resulting from cancer chemotherapy.

Mechanism of Action: Allopurinol reduces uric acid formation by selectively inhibiting the action of xanthine oxidase, which is the enzyme responsible for the formation of uric acid. Lowering the formation of uric acid prevents hyperuricemia. Unlike the uricosuric drugs, allopurinol does not increase the renal excretion of uric acid.

Pharmacokinetics:

Route(s)	PO, IV
Absorption	80–90% absorbed in the GI tract
Distribution	Widely distributed; secreted in breast milk; less than 1% bound to plasma proteins
Primary metabolism	Hepatic to the active metabolite oxypurinol
Primary excretion	Primarily renal
Onset of action	24–48 h
Duration of action	1–3 weeks after drug is discontinued

Adverse Effects: The most frequent and serious adverse effects are dermatologic, including micropapular rash, rare cases of fatal toxic epidermal necrolysis, and Stevens–Johnson syndrome. A rare, sometimes fatal, hypersensitivity syndrome may occur and includes a skin rash, fever, hepatitis, leukocytosis, eosinophilia, and progressive renal failure. Other adverse effects include drowsiness, headache, vertigo, nausea, vomiting, malaise, diarrhea, cataracts, retinopathy, and thrombocytopenia.

Contraindications/Precautions: Contraindications include hypersensitivity to allopurinol and idiopathic hemochromatosis. Use cautiously in patients with impaired hepatic or renal function, history of peptic ulcers, lower GI tract disease, bone marrow depression, and pregnancy.

Drug Interactions: Alcohol may inhibit the renal excretion of uric acid. Ampicillin and amoxicillin may increase the risk of skin rashes. An enhanced anticoagulant effect may be seen with the use of warfarin, and toxicity risks increase for azathioprine, mercaptopurine, cyclophosphamide, and cyclosporine. An increased hypoglycemic effect may be seen with chlorpropamide. The risk of ototoxicity is increased when allopurinol is used with thiazides and angiotensin-converting enzyme (ACE) inhibitors. Aluminum antacids taken concurrently with allopurinol may decrease its effects. An increased effect may be seen with phenytoin, theophylline, and anticancer drugs, necessitating the need for altered doses of these medications. **Herbal/Food**: Unknown.

Pregnancy: Category C.

Treatment of Overdose: Overdose with allopurinol is rare. There is no specific treatment for an overdose and the patient is treated symptomatically.

Nursing Responsibilities: Key nursing implications for patients receiving allopurinol are included in the Nursing Practice Application for Patients Receiving Pharmacotherapy for Gout.

Drugs Similar to Allopurinol (Lopurin, Zyloprim)

Additional drugs for gout prophylaxis include febuxostat, pegloticase, probenecid, and sulfinpyrazone.

Febuxostat (Uloric): An alternative to allopurinol, febuxostat was approved in 2009 for the chronic management of hyperuricemia in patients with gout. The drug acts by inhibiting xanthine oxidase. It offers the convenience of once-daily dosing. Unlike some of the other medications in this class, febuxostat exhibits little dermatologic or renal toxicity. Liver function tests should be monitored periodically to prevent the development of hepatotoxicity. It should not be administered concurrently with drugs metabolized by xanthine oxidase such as mercaptopurine or azathioprine because these drugs could accumulate to toxic levels. Febuxostat is pregnancy category C.

Pegloticase (Krystexxa): Approved in 2010, pegloticase is a synthetic enzyme that metabolizes uric acid to an inert substance. It is used to lower uric acid levels in patients with chronic gout who have not responded well to conventional therapies. It is

administered over a 2-hour period by IV infusion, once every 2 weeks. The drug has a black box warning that anaphylaxis may occur during and after the infusion, and emergency equipment should be readily available to address such a reaction. Patients should also be pretreated with antihistamines and corticosteroids. Other common adverse effects include gout flares at the initiation of therapy, infusion reactions, nausea, ecchymosis, nasopharyngitis, and worsening of heart failure. This drug is pregnancy category C.

Probenecid (Probalan): Probenecid is an older drug approved in 1951 that inhibits the reabsorption of uric acid in the renal tubules, thus increasing its excretion. Given PO, it is effective for prophylaxis but will not terminate acute gout episodes. Probenecid should be taken with meals to decrease gastric irritation. It should be used cautiously when given with other drugs that are highly protein bound. Several combination drugs that contain probenecid and colchicine are available for long-term maintenance therapy. Adverse effects are generally minor and include headache, nausea, vomiting, and anorexia. This drug is pregnancy category C.

Unrelated to its use in treating gout, probenecid blocks the transport of organic acids in the renal tubule. When given concurrently with antibiotics such as penicillins or cephalosporins, the serum levels of antibiotics will be boosted, making them more effective. Because of its effect on renal transport mechanisms, probenecid has the potential to interact with virtually any acidic drug. A drug guide should be consulted when administering probenecid to patients who are taking multiple medications.

Sulfinpyrazone (Anturane): Approved in 1959, sulfinpyrazone is another oral uricosuric drug that is very similar to probenecid. Sulfinpyrazone reduces uric acid levels in patients with chronic gout conditions but is not effective in treating acute episodes. It is more potent than probenecid and its use is generally reserved for patients with symptoms that are resistant to other drugs. Although rare, severe blood dyscrasias have been known to occur with its use and should therefore be given with extreme caution to those patients who have a history of hematologic disorders. Sulfinpyrazone also has the potential to cause serious gastric distress, and it should be taken with meals or with antacids to decrease irritation. It is contraindicated in patients with peptic ulcer disease. This drug is pregnancy category C.

CONNECTIONS: NURSING PRACTICE APPLICATION

Patients Receiving Pharmacotherapy for Gout

Assessment	Potential Nursing Diagnoses*
Baseline assessment prior to administration: <ul><li>Understand the reason the drug has been prescribed in order to assess for therapeutic effects (e.g., decreasing acute inflammatory stage, preventing recurrence).</li><li>Obtain a complete health history including musculoskeletal, GI, cardiovascular, neurologic, endocrine, hepatic, or renal disease. Obtain a drug history including allergies, current prescription and OTC drugs, herbal preparations, alcohol use, or smoking. Be alert to possible drug interactions.</li><li>Obtain a history of any current symptoms and their effect on ADLs. Assess for inflammation and location, and note any pain or discomfort on movement or at rest.</li><li>Obtain a dietary history, noting correlations between food intake and increase in symptoms. Assess fluid intake.</li><li>Obtain baseline weight and vital signs.</li><li>Evaluate appropriate laboratory findings (e.g., uric acid level, CBC, hepatic and renal function studies, urinalysis).</li><li>Assess the patient's ability to receive and understand instructions. Include the family or caregiver as needed.</li></ul> **Assessment throughout administration:** <ul><li>Assess for desired therapeutic effects dependent on the reason for the drug (e.g., symptoms of acute inflammation are diminished or absent, no return of symptoms).</li><li>Continue monitoring vital signs and urine output.</li><li>Continue to monitor uric acid level, CBC, hepatic and renal studies.</li><li>Assess for and promptly report adverse effects: nausea, vomiting, abdominal pain, skin rash, pruritus, paresthesia, diminished urine output, fever, or infections.</li></ul>	<ul><li>*Acute Pain*</li><li>*Activity Intolerance*</li><li>*Disturbed Body Image*</li><li>*Deficient Knowledge* (Drug Therapy)</li><li>*Risk for Injury,* related to adverse drug effects or acute inflammatory condition</li></ul>

Implementation

Interventions and (Rationales)	Patient-Centered Care
Ensuring therapeutic effects: <ul><li>Review the dietary history with the patient, noting any correlation between diet and symptoms, especially after ingestion of purine-containing foods (e.g., salmon, sardines, organ meats, alcohol, mushrooms, legumes, oatmeal). Avoid large doses of vitamin C. (Gout may occur due to overproduction or underexcretion of uric acid or a combination of both. Correlating symptoms to intake of high-purine foods assists in determining the most effective drug therapy. Large doses of vitamin C may acidify the urine, leading to formation of uric acid stones.)</li></ul>	<ul><li>Encourage the patient to keep a food diary, noting any occurrence or increasing of symptoms related to food or beverage intake.</li><li>Teach the patient to limit intake of high-purine foods and to limit or eliminate alcohol consumption.</li></ul>
<ul><li>Increase fluid intake to 2–4 L/day. Monitor urine output and obtain periodic urinalysis. (Increased fluid intake will help increase uric acid excretion and prevent urinary uric acid crystal formation or renal calculi.)</li></ul>	<ul><li>Teach the patient to increase fluid intake to 2–4 L/day, taken throughout the day.</li></ul>
<ul><li>Continue to monitor serum and urinary uric acid levels, and note improvement in symptoms of acute inflammation, gouty tophi, and improved movement with less pain of affected joints. (As uric acid levels decrease, inflammation due to uric acid crystals should improve.)</li></ul>	<ul><li>Encourage the patient to maintain consistent drug dosing to ensure that uric acid levels are diminishing.</li><li>Instruct the patient on the need to return for periodic laboratory testing and urinalysis.</li></ul>
Minimizing adverse effects: <ul><li>Monitor serum and urinary uric acid levels and symptoms associated with acute inflammatory period. (Decreased uric acid levels should decrease the amount of inflammation. Continued or increasing inflammation may indicate a need for additional antigout or anti-inflammatory medication.)</li></ul>	<ul><li>Instruct the patient to promptly report any continued inflammation, pain, increased joint involvement, or general worsening of symptoms.</li></ul>
<ul><li>Monitor daily weight and urinary output. Record intake and output in the hospitalized patient. Immediately report any flank pain to the provider. (Uric acid excretion may cause urate crystal formation in the kidneys with resulting renal impairment. Daily weight is an accurate measure of overall body fluid volume and any gain of over 1 kg [2 lb] per day should be reported. Flank pain may indicate the presence of renal calculi.)</li></ul>	<ul><li>Instruct the patient to report any diminished urine output or changes in urine appearance, and to return periodically for urinalysis.</li><li>Have the patient weigh self daily at the same time each day and report any weight gain of over 1 kg (2 lb) in a 24-h period to the health care provider.</li><li>Instruct the patient to immediately report any flank pain to the provider.</li></ul>

(continued)

CONNECTIONS: NURSING PRACTICE APPLICATION (continued)

• Continue to monitor periodic hepatic and renal laboratory work. (**Lifespan:** Age-related physiological differences may place the older adult at greater risk for hepatic and renal toxicity.)	• Instruct the patient on the need to return periodically for laboratory work.
• Decrease intake of purine-containing foods (e.g., salmon, sardines, organ meat, mushrooms, legumes, oatmeal, and alcohol). Avoid large doses of vitamin C. (Intake of high-purine foods and alcohol may increase production of uric acid. Large doses of vitamin C may acidify the urine, leading to formation of uric acid stones.)	• Teach the patient to avoid high-purine foods, decrease or eliminate alcohol consumption, and avoid increased vitamin C intake or supplementation. Provide dietitian consult as needed.
• Observe for skin rashes, fever, stomatitis, flulike symptoms, or general malaise. (Bone marrow suppression may occur with antigout drugs and result in leukopenia and an increased risk of infection. Severe dermatologic reactions are possible and any skin rashes, especially with the appearance of blisters and discoloration, should be reported immediately.)	• Teach the patient to immediately report any flulike symptoms, fever, mouth irritation or soreness, or skin rashes.
Patient understanding of drug therapy: • Use opportunities during administration of medications and during assessments to discuss the rationale for drug therapy, desired therapeutic outcomes, commonly observed adverse effects, parameters for when to call the health care provider, and any necessary monitoring or precautions. (Using time during nursing care helps to optimize and reinforce key teaching areas.)	• The patient should be able to state the reason for the drug, appropriate dose and scheduling, what adverse effects to observe for and when to report them, and the anticipated length of medication therapy.
Patient self-administration of drug therapy: • When administering the medication, instruct the patient, family, or caregiver in proper self-administration of the drug, e.g., taken on an empty stomach or with meals or additional fluids, followed by teach-back. (Utilizing time during nurse-administration of these drugs helps to reinforce teaching.)	• The patient, family, or caregiver is able to discuss appropriate dosing and administration needs including taking medications at the first sign of a gout attack. • Colchicine should be taken on an empty stomach. Other antigout medications should be taken with food or meals.

*Nursing Diagnoses—Definitions and Classification 2015–2017. Copyright © 2014, 1994–2014 by NANDA International. Used by arrangement with John Wiley & Sons Limited.

CHAPTER

72

Understanding the Chapter

Key Concepts Summary

72.1 Adequate levels of calcium in the body are necessary to transmit nerve impulses, to prevent muscle spasms, and for proper bone health.

72.2 Calcium balance is regulated by parathyroid hormone, calcitonin, and vitamin D.

72.3 Hypocalcemia is a condition that requires therapy with calcium supplements, often concurrently with vitamin D.

72.4 Metabolic bone disease is characterized by abnormal bone structure.

72.5 Vitamin D therapy is indicated for treating osteomalacia, hypoparathyroidism, and osteoporosis.

72.6 Bisphosphonates increase bone density and are used to treat osteoporosis.

72.7 Selective estrogen receptor modulators increase bone mass density and prevent fractures in postmenopausal women.

72.8 Calcitonin and several miscellaneous drugs are used for osteoporosis and other metabolic bone diseases.

72.9 Osteoarthritis is treated with a combination of analgesics and nonpharmacologic therapies.

72.10 Pharmacotherapy for rheumatoid arthritis includes analgesics, anti-inflammatory drugs, corticosteroids, and disease-modifying antirheumatic drugs.

72.11 Gout is treated with drugs that decrease joint pain and inflammation and lower uric acid levels.

72.12 Hyperuricemia is treated with drugs that reduce serum levels of uric acid.

Case Study: Making the Patient Connection

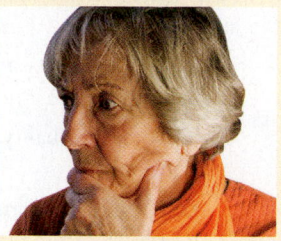

Remember the patient "Darlene Coleman" at the beginning of the chapter? Now read the remainder of the case study. Based on the information presented within this chapter, respond to the critical thinking questions that follow.

Darlene Coleman is a 65-year-old woman who is generally in good health. She has a checkup visit with her gynecologist annually. While assessing Darlene's vital signs, height, and weight, the nurse notes a significant deviation from the data recorded during last year's visit. Apparently, the patient has lost 2.5 cm (1 in.) in height during the last year. The nurse then shares this information with Darlene. The patient states, "I have always been short. You should see my mother who is much shorter than I am. But lately, my clothes just don't seem to fit. I haven't lost any weight, but my pant legs drag on the ground. Is it possible that I'm actually getting shorter?"

Critical Thinking Questions

1. As the nurse, how would you respond to the patient's statement?
2. As you talk with Ms. Coleman, she asks you, "Is there any way to slow my declining height?" What could you recommend?

See Answers to Critical Thinking Questions on student resource website.

Additional Case Study

A female patient, age 56, has been ordered methotrexate (Rheumatrex, Trexall) and etanercept (Enbrel) for treatment of severe rheumatoid arthritis. She wants her daughter to administer the etanercept because of limitations due to arthritis-related deformities in her hands. The daughter is worried about giving her mother the medication.

1. How is etanercept (Enbrel) given? How often?
2. What instructions should the nurse give the daughter about administering this medication?

3. What potential adverse effects may occur in addition to those related to the injection itself?
4. What is the drug classification for methotrexate? What are potential adverse effects for this drug?

See Answers to Additional Case Study on student resource website.

Chapter Review

1 The patient who has been prescribed alendronate (Fosamax) demonstrates an understanding of how to correctly take the medication when stating:

1. "I will take my medication prior to eating my lunch or dinner."
2. "I will take my medication immediately before bedtime or at 9 p.m."
3. "I will take my medication with a full glass of water 30 minutes before breakfast."
4. "I should lie flat for at least 30 minutes after I take this medication."

2 Which of the following symptoms would alert the nurse to the possibility of the development of toxicity to methotrexate (Rheumatrex, Trexall)?

1. Headache, dizziness, and blurred vision
2. Hematuria, hiccoughs, and jaundice
3. Stomatitis, constipation, and dyspepsia
4. Jaundice, ascites, and edema formation

3 The patient asks the nurse to explain how colchicine (Colcrys) works. The nurse would base the response on which physiological principle?

1. It increases the deposits of uric acid in the synovial spaces of the joints.
2. It reduces the pain associated with joint inflammation from gouty arthritis.
3. It prevents the accumulation of uric acid crystals in the joints.
4. It increases renal excretion of uric acid crystals.

4 Which laboratory findings would the nurse monitor to determine if pharmacotherapy is helping a patient taking calcium supplementation for osteomalacia?

1. Increasing serum calcium and increasing phosphate levels
2. Increasing serum calcium and decreasing phosphate levels
3. Decreasing serum calcium and increasing phosphate levels
4. Decreasing serum calcium and decreasing phosphate levels

5 Which assessment findings in a patient who is receiving calcitriol (Rocaltrol) should the nurse immediately report to the prescriber?

1. Muscle weakness, nausea, and vomiting
2. Diarrhea, abdominal pain, and stomatitis
3. Bone pain, joint stiffness, and fever
4. Photosensitivity, tinnitus, and bone pain

6 Disease-modifying antirheumatic drugs (DMARDs) are prescribed for patients with rheumatoid arthritis. Which statement related to this therapy is correct? Select all that apply. DMARDs:

1. Include gold salts, antimalarial drugs, and medications that modify the immune response.
2. Enhance the quality of life in patients with rheumatoid arthritis.
3. Often take several months to achieve maximum therapeutic effects.
4. Are very safe and require very little monitoring during therapy.
5. Are not accepted in modern pharmacotherapy as a viable treatment option.

See Answers to Chapter Review in Appendix A.

References

American College of Rheumatology. (2012). *Calcium pyrophosphate deposition (CPPD) (formerly called pseudogout).* Retrieved from http://www.rheumatology.org/practice/clinical/patients/diseases_and_conditions/pseudogout.asp

Henrotin, Y., Marty, M., & Mobasheri, A. (2014). What is the current status of chondroitin sulfate and glucosamine for the treatment of knee osteoarthritis? *Maturitas, 78,* 184–187. doi:10.1016/j.maturitas.2014.04.015

Hochberg, M. C., Altman, R. D., April, K. T., Benkhalti, M., Guyatt, G., McGowan, J., . . .

Tugwell, P. (2012). American College of Rheumatology 2012 recommendations for the use of nonpharmacologic and pharmacologic therapies in osteoarthritis of the hand, hip, and knee. *Arthritis Care & Research, 64,* 465–474. doi:10.1002/acr.21596

Jacobs-Kosmin, D. (2013). *Osteoporosis.* Retrieved from http://emedicine.medscape.com/article/330598-overview#a0156

Levis, S., & Theodore, G. (2012). AHRQ's comparative effectiveness review of treatments to prevent fractures in men and women with low bone density or osteoporosis: A summary of

key findings. *Journal of Managed Care Pharmacy, 18*(4 Suppl. B), S1–S15.

National Osteoporosis Foundation. (n.d.). *What is osteoporosis?* Retrieved from http://nof.org/articles/7

Temprano, K. (2014). *Rheumatoid arthritis.* Retrieved from http://emedicine.medscape.com/article/331715-overview

Selected Bibliography

Allaart, C. F., & Huizinga, T. (2011). Treatment strategies in recent onset rheumatoid arthritis. *Current Opinion in Rheumatology, 23,* 241–244. doi:10.1097/BOR.0b013e3283454111

Black, D. M., Bauer, D. C., Schwartz, A. V., Cummings, S. R., & Rosen, C. J. (2012). Continuing bisphosphonate treatment for osteoporosis— for whom and for how long? *New England Journal of Medicine, 366,* 2051–2053. doi:10.1056/NEJMp1202623

Britton, C., & Walsh, J. (2012). Paget disease of bone: An update. *Australian Family Physician, 41*(3), 100–103.

Buch, M. H., & Emery, P. (2011). New therapies in the management of rheumatoid arthritis. *Current Opinion in Rheumatology, 23,* 245–251. doi:10.1097/BOR.0b013e3283454124

Donahue, K. E., Jonas, D. E., Hansen, R. A., Roubey, R., Jonas, B., Lux, L. J., . . . Van Noord, M. (2012). Drug therapy for rheumatoid arthritis in adults: An update. *Comparative Effectiveness Review, 55.*

Eriksen, E. F., Díez-Pérez, A., & Boonen, S. (2014). Update on long-term treatment with bisphosphonates for postmenopausal osteoporosis: A systematic review. *Bone, 58,* 126–135. doi:10.1016/j.bone.2013.09.023

Herdman, T. H., & Kamitsuru, S. (Eds.). (2014). *NANDA International nursing diagnoses: Definitions and classification, 2015–2017.* Oxford, United Kingdom: Wiley-Blackwell.

Rothschild, B. M. (2014). *Gout and pseudogout.* Retrieved from http://emedicine.medscape.com/article/329958-overview

Singh, J. A., Furst, D. E., Bharat, A., Curtis, J. R., Kavanaugh, A. F., Kremer, J. M., . . . Saag, K. G. (2012). 2012 update of the 2008 American College of Rheumatology recommendations for the use of disease-modifying antirheumatic drugs and biologic agents in the treatment of rheumatoid arthritis. *Arthritis Care & Research, 64,* 625–639. doi:10.1002/acr.21641

U.S. Food and Drug Administration. (2010). *FDA drug safety communication: Safety update for osteoporosis drugs, bisphosphonates, and atypical fractures.* Retrieved from http://www.fda.gov/drugs/drugsafety/ucm229009.htm

Warriner, A. H., & Saag, K. G. (2013). Osteoporosis diagnosis and medical treatment. *Orthopedic Clinics of North America, 44,* 125–135. doi:10.1016/j.ocl.2013.01.005

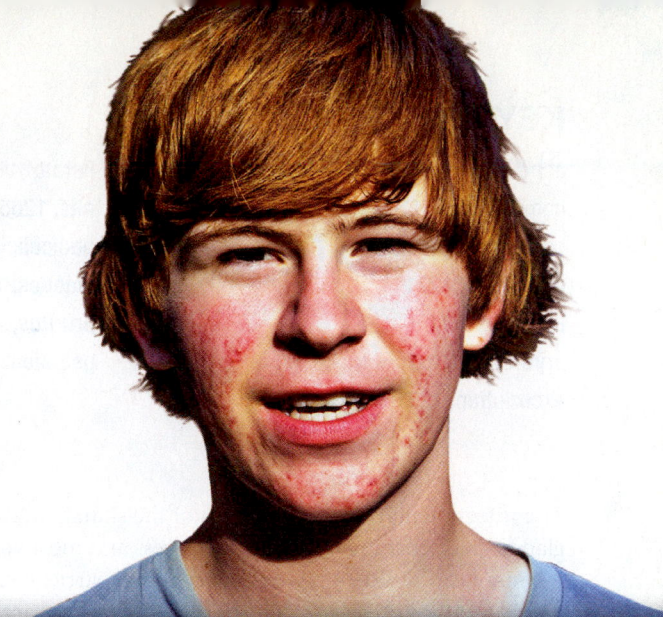

"I hate the way my skin looks. I know people are just staring at my face and not really listening to me."

Patient "Danny McBride"

Pharmacotherapy of Dermatologic Disorders

LEARNING OUTCOMES

After reading this chapter, the student should be able to:

1. Identify the structure and functions of the skin and associated structures.
2. Explain the process by which superficial skin cells are replaced.
3. Explain how skin diseases are classified.
4. Describe the drug therapies for bacterial, fungal, viral, and parasitic infections of the skin.
5. Explain the etiology, pathogenesis, and pharmacotherapy for acne vulgaris, rosacea, dermatitis, and psoriasis.
6. Outline the stepwise approach to treating psoriasis.
7. Describe the prevention and management of minor burns.
8. Explain the pharmacotherapy of alopecia.
9. Describe the nurse's role in the pharmacologic management of skin disorders.
10. For each of the classes shown in the chapter outline, identify the prototype and representative drugs and explain the mechanism(s) of drug action, primary indications, contraindications, significant drug interactions, pregnancy category, and important adverse effects.
11. Apply the nursing process to the care of patients who are receiving pharmacotherapy for skin disorders.

CHAPTER OUTLINE

▶ **Anatomy of the Integumentary System**

▶ **Classification of Skin Disorders**

▶ **Pharmacotherapy of Skin Infections**
  Scabicides and Pediculicides
  PROTOTYPE Permethrin (Acticin, Elimite, Nix), *p. 1265*

▶ **Pharmacotherapy of Acne and Rosacea**
  PROTOTYPE Tretinoin (Avita, Retin-A, Others), *p. 1269*

▶ **Pharmacotherapy of Dermatitis**

▶ **Pharmacotherapy of Psoriasis**

▶ **Pharmacotherapy of Minor Skin Burns**
  PROTOTYPE Benzocaine (Americaine, Anbesol, Others), *p. 1278*

▶ **Pharmacotherapy of Alopecia**

KEY TERMS

acne vulgaris, 1267

comedolytics, 1269

comedones, 1268

dermatitis, 1271

eczema, 1271

erythema, 1263

excoriation, 1271

keratolytic, 1269

nits, 1265

pediculicides, 1265

plaques, 1274

pruritus, 1263

psoralens, 1277

retinoids, 1269

rhinophyma, 1269

rosacea, 1269

scabicides, 1265

seborrhea, 1267

urticaria, 1263

The integumentary system consists of the skin, hair, nails, sweat glands, and sebaceous glands. The largest and most visible of all organs, healthy skin provides an effective barrier between the outside environment and the body's internal tissues, helps to regulate body temperature, and assists in maintaining fluid and electrolyte balance. At times, however, environmental conditions damage the skin, or conditions within the body change, resulting in unhealthy skin. Some of these changes can even lead to systemic changes that affect tissues outside the integumentary system. When this occurs, pharmacotherapy may be utilized to improve the skin's condition. The purpose of this chapter is to examine the broad scope of skin disorders and the drugs used for skin pharmacotherapy.

Anatomy of the Integumentary System

73.1 Three layers of skin, known as the epidermis, dermis, and subcutaneous layers, provide effective barrier defenses for the body.

To understand the actions of dermatologic drugs, it is necessary to have a thorough knowledge of the structure of the skin. The skin comprises three primary layers: the epidermis, dermis, and subcutaneous layers, as illustrated in Figure 73.1. The epidermis is the visible, outermost layer that constitutes only about 5% of the skin depth. The middle layer is the dermis, which accounts for about

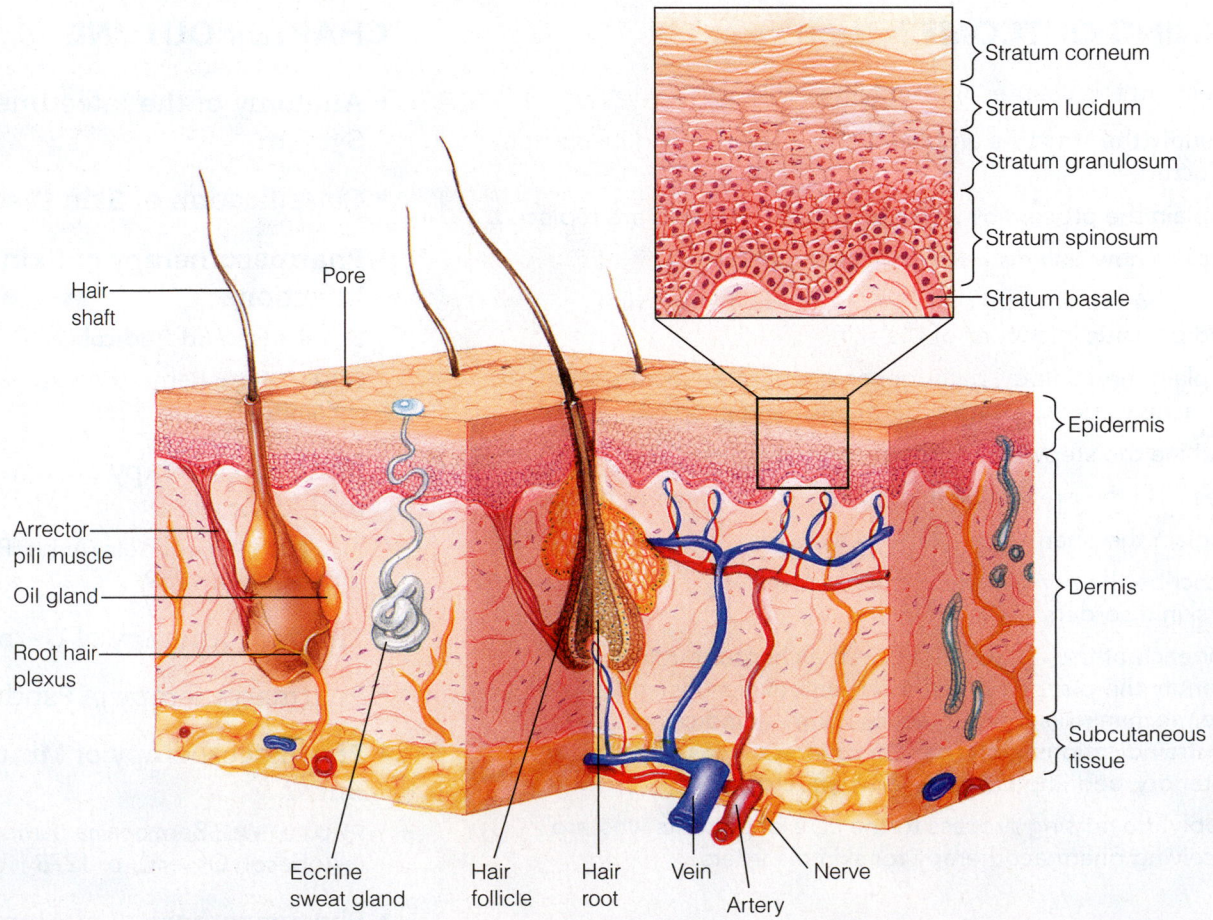

Figure 73.1 Anatomy of the skin.

95% of the entire skin thickness. The subcutaneous layer lies beneath the dermis. Some textbooks consider the subcutaneous layer as being separate from the skin and not one of its layers. Each layer of skin is distinct in form and function and provides the basis for how drugs are injected or topically applied.

Epidermis: The epidermis consists of epithelial cells with either four or five sublayers depending on its location. The five layers from the innermost to outermost are the stratum basale (also referred to as the stratum germinativum), stratum spinosum, stratum granulosum, stratum lucidum, and the strongest layer, the stratum corneum. The stratum corneum is referred to as the "horny layer" because of the abundance of the protein keratin, a water-insoluble material secreted by keratinocytes, which is also found in the hair, hooves, and horns of many mammals. Keratin gives the skin its tough, protective seal, forming a barrier that repels bacteria and foreign matter. Most substances cannot penetrate it. The largest amount of keratin is found in those areas subject to mechanical stress, for example, the soles of the feet and the palms of the hands.

The deepest epidermal sublayer, the stratum basale, supplies the epidermis with new cells after older superficial cells have been damaged or lost through normal wear. Over time, these newly created cells migrate from the stratum basale to the outermost layers of the skin. As these cells are pushed to the surface they are flattened and covered with keratin. The outermost skin layer, called the stratum corneum, is composed of these dead cells. On average, it takes a cell about 2 to 3 weeks to move from the stratum basale to the body surface.

Specialized cells within the deeper layers of the epidermis, called melanocytes, secrete the dark pigment melanin. Melanin forms a protective shield, which protects the keratinocytes and the nerve endings in the dermis from the sun's ultraviolet (UV) rays. The number and type of melanocytes determine the overall pigment of the skin and determine racial differences in skin tone. Darker skin tones are not caused by an increased number of melanocytes, but by the amount of the pigment melanin that is contained in each cell. The more melanin, the darker the skin color. Freckles, birthmarks, and age spots are caused by the production of melanin. In areas where the melanocytes are destroyed, there are milk-white areas of depigmented skin referred to as vitiligo.

The junction of the epidermis and the dermis is an area of many ridges and furrows called the rete ridges. This area anchors the epidermis to the dermis. The epidermis does not have a separate blood supply. It receives its nutrients by diffusion in the rete ridges from the many blood vessels in the dermis. This surface also provides for the ripples seen on the skin surface, which on the fingertips are called fingerprints.

Dermis: The second primary layer of skin, called the dermis, is a layer of connective tissue that contains no cells. The dermis is composed of collagen fibers and elastic fibers that give the skin both flexibility and strength. It provides a foundation for the epidermis and accessory structures such as hair and nails. Most sensory nerves that transmit the sensations of touch, pressure, temperature, pain, and itch are located within the dermis, as well as the oil glands and sweat glands. A vast network of lymph and capillary vessels is found within the dermis.

Subcutaneous tissue: Beneath the dermis is the subcutaneous tissue, or hypodermis, which lies over muscle and bone. It consists mainly of adipose tissue, which cushions, insulates, and serves as an energy reserve in the event that extra calories are needed to fuel the body. The amount of subcutaneous tissue varies in an individual and is determined by body area, sex, age, nutritional status, and heredity. Many blood vessels pass through the fatty layer and extend into the dermis, forming capillary networks that supply nutrients and remove wastes.

Skin appendages: Hair follicles are located in the dermis. Hair growth varies by race, gender, age, and heredity. Individual hairs vary in both structure and rate of growth, depending on their location. Composed primarily of dead cells, hair consists of a root that begins in the bulb of the hair follicle and grows from the dermis outward. The hair shaft is the portion that projects through the epidermis and exits the skin. Hair growth occurs in cycles; a growth phase is followed by a resting phase during which hair is shed from the body. Stressors can alter the growth cycle and cause temporary hair loss. Permanent baldness is genetic in origin and is seldom influenced by stressors. Hair color is genetically determined by a person's rate of melanin production within the hair shaft.

The sebaceous glands are distributed over the entire skin surface, except for the palms of the hand and the soles of the feet. Most sebaceous glands are directly connected to the hair follicles; the glands of the eyelids, nipple areolae, and genitalia are freestanding. Sebaceous glands produce sebum, which is emptied into the space between the hair follicle and shaft. Sebum lubricates and softens the skin and hair and reduces water loss from the skin surface in low humidity. Sebum also is mildly bacteriostatic. The secretion of sebum is stimulated by hormones, especially androgens.

The skin has two types of sweat glands: apocrine and eccrine. The apocrine glands are directly connected to the hair follicles and are mainly found in the axillary, perineal, nipple areolae, and umbilical areas. The interaction of skin bacteria with the milky secretions of apocrine glands causes distinct body odor. The eccrine glands are found over the entire skin surface. Their ducts open directly onto the skin surface and are not associated with hair follicles. The secretions of the eccrine glands are an important factor in the regulation of body temperature. Sweat is released from the eccrine glands in response to elevated body temperature or ambient temperature and is under control of the sympathetic nervous system.

Classification of Skin Disorders

73.2 The etiology of skin disorders may be classified as infectious, inflammatory, or neoplastic.

Of the many types of skin disorders, some have vague, generalized signs and symptoms, and others have specific and easily identifiable causes. **Urticaria** is a hypersensitivity response that is characterized by hives and is often accompanied by pruritus, or itching. Allergies to foods often manifest as urticaria. **Pruritus** is a general condition that is associated with dry, scaly skin or a parasite infestation. Pruritus may also be a sign of serious systemic pathology, such as cholestatic disease and uremia. A substantial number of drugs have urticaria or pruritus listed as potential adverse effects. Local **erythema** or redness accompanies inflammation and many other skin disorders. Inflammation is a characteristic of burns and trauma to the skin.

TABLE 73.1	Classification of Skin Disorders
Type	**Examples**
Infectious	Bacterial infections: boils, impetigo, infected hair follicles
	Fungal infections: ringworm, athlete's foot, jock itch, nail infection
	Parasitic infections: ticks, mites, lice
	Viral infections: cold sores, fever blisters (herpes simplex), chickenpox, warts, shingles (herpes zoster), measles (rubeola), and German measles (rubella)
Inflammatory	Injury and exposure to the sun
	Combination of overactive glands, increased hormone production, and/or infection such as acne and rosacea
	Disorders with itching, cracking, and discomfort such as atopic dermatitis, contact dermatitis, seborrheic dermatitis, stasis dermatitis, and psoriasis
Neoplastic	Skin cancers: squamous cell carcinoma, basal cell carcinoma, and malignant melanoma
	Benign neoplasms include keratosis and keratoacanthoma

Skin disorders are diverse and difficult to classify because some conditions have overlapping components. For example, lesions that are characteristic of acne may be inflamed and become infected. One simple method, which is summarized in Table 73.1, is to group the disorders into the following categories:

- **Infectious.** Bacterial, fungal, viral, and parasitic infections of the skin and mucous membranes are relatively common and are frequent indications for anti-infective pharmacotherapy. A brief overview of anti-infectives most frequently prescribed for skin conditions is presented in Section 73.3, with further emphasis on parasitic infections in Section 73.4. Greater detail on the individual anti-infective drugs may be found in Chapters 46 through 54.

- **Inflammatory.** Inflammatory disorders encompass a broad range of pathology that includes acne, dermatitis, burns, and psoriasis. The pharmacotherapy of inflammatory skin disorders includes many of the drugs discussed in Chapter 41, such as corticosteroids.

- **Neoplastic.** Malignant tumors include malignant melanoma and basal cell carcinoma, which are treated with the therapies described in Chapter 57. Warts are a type of benign tumor.

Systemic disease processes that occur in the body may manifest as dermatologic signs and symptoms. Skin abnormalities, including color, sizes, types, and character of surface lesions, and skin turgor and moisture may have systemic causes such as liver or renal impairment, cardiovascular insufficiency, metastatic tumors, recent injury, and poor nutritional status.

Although there are many skin disorders, some warrant only localized or short-term pharmacotherapy. Examples include lice infestation, sunburn with minor irritation, and acne. Eczema, dermatitis, and psoriasis are more serious disorders that require extensive and more prolonged therapy.

Pharmacotherapy of Skin Infections

73.3 When the integrity of the skin is compromised, microbes can gain entrance and cause infections that require anti-infective therapy.

The skin is normally populated with microorganisms or flora that includes a diverse collection of bacteria, fungi, and viruses. The skin provides an effective barrier against infection from these organisms as long as it remains healthy and intact. The skin is very dry, and keratin is a poor energy source for microbes. Although perspiration provides a wet environment, its high-salt content discourages microbial growth. Furthermore, the outer layer is continually being sloughed off, and the microorganisms leave with the dead skin.

Bacterial skin diseases can occur when the skin is punctured or cut, or when the outer layer is abraded through trauma or removed through severe burns. Some bacteria also infect hair follicles. The most common bacterial infections of the skin are caused by *Staphylococcus* and *Streptococcus,* which are normal skin inhabitants. *Staphylococcus aureus* is responsible for furuncles (boils), carbuncles (abscesses), and other pus-containing lesions of the skin. Both *S. aureus* and *Streptococcus pyogenes* can cause impetigo, which is a superficial skin disorder that commonly occurs in school-age children. Cellulitis is an acute skin and subcutaneous tissue infection caused by *Staphylococcus* and *Streptococcus.* Folliculitis, an infection of hair follicles usually caused by *S. aureus,* is often called a "hot-tub" infection because it is acquired when water in these tubs is not adequately treated with chlorine.

Although many skin bacterial infections are self-limiting, others may be serious enough to require pharmacotherapy. When possible, topical agents are applied directly to the infection site. Topical drugs offer the advantage of causing fewer adverse effects, and many are available over the counter (OTC) for self-treatment. If the infection is deep within the skin, affects large regions of the body, or has the potential to enter the systemic circulation, oral (PO) or parenteral therapy is indicated. Furthermore, the incidence of methicillin-resistant *S. aureus* (MRSA) skin infections is increasing. MRSA often requires pharmacotherapy with two or more antibiotics. Some of the more common topical antibiotics for skin infections include the following:

- Bacitracin ointment
- Erythromycin ointment (Eryderm, Others)
- Gentamicin cream and ointment
- Metronidazole cream and lotion
- Mupirocin (Bactroban)
- Neomycin with polymyxin B (Neosporin), cream and ointment
- Tetracycline

Fungal infections of the skin or nails such as tinea pedis (athlete's foot) and tinea cruris (jock itch) commonly occur in warm, moist areas covered by clothing. Tinea capitis (ringworm of the scalp) and tinea unguium (ringworm of the nails) are also common. These pathogens are responsive to therapy with topical OTC antifungals such as undecylenic acid (Cruex, Desenex, Others). More serious fungal infections of the skin and mucous membranes, such as *Candida albicans* infections that occur in immunocompromised patients, require systemic antifungals (see Chapter 52). Clotrimazole (Lotrimin, Mycelex, Others) and miconazole (Micatin) are common antifungals available as creams and lotions that are used for a variety of dermatologic mycoses. Oral fluconazole (Diflucan) is indicated for more serious fungal infections of the skin.

Certain viral infections can manifest with skin lesions. Childhood viral infections that affect the skin include varicella (chickenpox), rubeola (measles), and rubella (German measles). Usually, these infections are self-limiting and nonspecific, so treatment is directed at controlling the extent of skin lesions. Viral infections with skin lesions in adults include herpes zoster (shingles) and herpes simplex (cold sores and genital lesions). Pharmacotherapy of severe or persistent viral skin lesions may include topical or PO antiviral therapy with acyclovir (Zovirax) or other antivirals.

CONNECTION Checkpoint 73.1

From what you learned in Chapter 52, what is onychomycosis and what types of drugs are used to treat it? *See Answer to Connection Checkpoint 73.1 on student resource website.*

Scabicides and Pediculicides

73.4 Scabicides and pediculicides are used to treat parasitic skin infestations.

Common skin parasites include mites and lice. Scabies is an eruption of the skin caused by the female mite *Sarcoptes scabiei*, which burrows into the skin to lay eggs that hatch after about 5 days. Scabies mites are barely visible without magnification. Scabies lesions most commonly occur between the fingers, on the extremities, in axillary and gluteal folds, around the trunk, and in the genital area. The major symptom is intense pruritus; vigorous scratching may lead to secondary infections. Scabies is easily spread through skin-to-skin contact and from mites living in upholstery, shared beds, and bath linens. Diagnosis is made by visual inspection of the burrows and confirmed by microscopic scrapings of the mite's ova or fecal pellets.

Over 3 million new cases of lice infestation or pediculosis are treated each year in the United States. Lice are larger than mites, measuring from 1 to 4 mm in length. They are readily spread by sharing infected hats, hairbrushes, bedding, or clothes, or by close personal contact. These parasites require human blood for survival and die within 24 hours without the blood of a human host. Lice (singular: louse) often infest the pubic area or the scalp and lay eggs, referred to as **nits**, which attach to body hairs. Head lice are referred to as *Pediculus humanus capitis*, body lice as *Pediculus humanus corporis*, and pubic lice as *Phthirus pubis*. The pubic louse is referred to as a "crab louse," because it looks like a tiny crab when viewed under the microscope. Individuals with pubic lice will sometimes say that they have "crabs." Pubic lice may produce sky-blue macules on the inner thighs or lower abdomen. The bite of the louse and the release of its saliva into the wound both lead to intense pruritus, followed by vigorous scratching. Secondary infections can result from scratching.

The treatment of skin parasites consists of using **scabicides**, which are drugs that kill mites, or **pediculicides**, which are drugs that kill lice. Some drugs are effective against both mites and lice. The choice of drug depends on where the infestation is located as well as other factors such as age, pregnancy, or breast-feeding.

The traditional drug of choice for both mites and lice was lindane. Lindane was also widely used as an agricultural pesticide in the 1950s and 1960s, causing pollution of waterways and prompting restrictions on its use. Because lindane has the potential to cause serious nervous system toxicity, its use is now limited to cases where less toxic drugs have failed to produce an adequate therapeutic response.

The preferred drug for lice is now permethrin, a chemical derived from chrysanthemum flowers and formulated as a 1% liquid (Nix). This drug is considered the safest agent, especially for infants and children. Pyrethrin (RID, Others) is a related product that also is obtained from the chrysanthemum plant. Permethrin and pyrethrin, which are also widely used as insecticides on crops and livestock, kill lice and their eggs on contact. These drugs are effective in 97% to 99% of patients, although a repeat application may be needed. Adverse effects are generally minor and include stinging, itching, or tingling. If two treatments of pyrethrin-based medications fail to eliminate the infestation, lindane or malathion (Ovide) may be prescribed. Resistant lice are most likely to appear in patients who have received multiple treatments with pyrethrin-based shampoos.

Permethrin is also a first-line drug for scabies. The 5% cream (Elimite) is applied to the entire skin surface and allowed to remain for 8 to 14 hours before bathing. A single application cures 95% of patients, although itching may continue for several weeks as the dead mites are removed from the skin. Crotamiton (Eurax) is an alternative scabicide that is available by prescription as a 10% cream. If the scabies is unresponsive to topical agents, the antiparasitic drug ivermectin (Sklice) may be administered as a single oral dose.

All scabicides and pediculicides must be used strictly as directed, because excessive use can cause serious systemic effects and skin irritation. Drugs for the treatment of lice or mites must not be applied to the mouth, open skin lesions, or eyes, because this will cause severe irritation.

PROTOTYPE DRUG | Permethrin (Acticin, Elimite, Nix)

Classification: Therapeutic: Antiparasitic
Pharmacologic: Scabicide, pediculicide

Therapeutic Effects and Uses: Nix is marketed as a cream, lotion, or shampoo to kill head and crab lice and mites and to eradicate their ova. A 1% lotion is approved for lice and a 5% lotion for mites. The medication should be allowed to remain on the hair and scalp 10 minutes before removal. Patients should be aware that penetration of the skin by mites causes itching, which lasts up to 2 or 3 weeks even after the parasites have been killed.

Successful elimination of parasitic infections should include removing the nits with a nit comb, washing bedding, and cleaning or removing objects that have been in contact with the head or hair.

Mechanism of Action: Permethrin affects the nervous system of the parasite, causing paralysis. Because lice are dependent on blood for survival, they die within 24 to 28 hours. It has ectoparasitic and ovicidal activity against *P. humanus capitis*, *P. pubis*, *S. scabiei* (scabies), ticks, mites, and fleas.

Pharmacokinetics:

Route(s)	Topical: 5% and 1% formulations
Absorption	Less than 2% is absorbed through intact skin
Distribution	Stored in body fat
Primary metabolism	Hepatic
Primary excretion	Urine
Onset of action	10 min
Duration of action	14 days

Adverse Effects: Permethrin causes few systemic effects. Local reactions may occur and include pruritus, rash, transient tingling, burning, stinging, erythema, and edema of the affected area.

Contraindications/Precautions: Contraindications include hypersensitivity to pyrethrins, chrysanthemums, sulfites, or other preservatives. Permethrin should be used cautiously on inflamed skin, in those with asthma, or in lactating women.

Drug Interactions: No clinically significant interactions have been documented.

Pregnancy: Category B.

Treatment of Overdose: No specific treatment for overdose with permethrin has been reported. Flush eyes well with water if the medicine accidentally gets into the eyes.

Nursing Responsibilities: Key nursing implications for patients receiving permethrin are included in the Nursing Practice Application for Patients Receiving Pharmacotherapy for Lice or Mite Infestation.

Drugs Similar to Permethrin (Acticin, Elimite, Nix)

Other drugs for parasitic skin infections include crotamiton, ivermectin, lindane, malathion, and pyrethrin.

Crotamiton (Eurax): Crotamiton is a scabicide and antipruritic that is used to eradicate *S. scabiei* and relieve itching. Available as a 10% cream or lotion, this drug should not be applied to skin that is acutely inflamed, raw, or has weeping surfaces. It should not be instilled into the eyes or mouth. If this drug comes in contact with the eyes, they must be flushed thoroughly with water. Adverse effects may include skin irritation, rash, and erythema. This drug is pregnancy category C.

Ivermectin (Sklice): Ivermectin is a drug that was approved in 1996 and has been widely used to treat helminthic infections. It is a drug of choice for treating river blindness, a debilitating infection in many developing countries. In 2012, ivermectin (Sklice) was approved as a 0.5% lotion for a new indication: head lice in patients 6 months of age and older. Sklice is applied to dry hair and rinsed off with water after 10 minutes. A single application is usually sufficient. Side effects are minor and include dry scalp and eye irritation if the eyes are exposed to the drug. This drug is pregnancy category C.

Lindane: Lindane is a scabicide and pediculicide in a 1% lotion or shampoo form that is applied directly to the skin to be absorbed by parasites and ova (nits), resulting in their death. This drug is used for treatment of head and crab lice and scabies infestations.

Lindane should not be applied to skin that has open cuts or to mucous membranes, eyes, or face. It should be used cautiously in infants and patients with a history of seizures, human immunodeficiency virus (HIV) infections, and alcoholism. Disposable or rubber gloves should be worn when applying the medication to reduce exposure to the skin. Although effective, this drug penetrates the skin and may cause significant adverse effects. Lindane has a black box warning that states that the drug is only indicated for patients who are unresponsive to safer therapies because seizures and deaths have been reported with repeated applications. The warning also states that the drug is contraindicated in premature infants and in individuals with uncontrolled seizure disorders. Additional adverse effects include dizziness, tremors, seizures, and death. This drug is pregnancy category C.

Malathion (Ovide): Available as a 0.5% lotion, malathion kills lice and ova by poisoning the nervous system of the parasite. It is contraindicated in children under the age of 6. Care must be taken to keep this drug out of the eyes during treatment because it can cause conjunctivitis. One treatment is all that is needed when using this medication. Because the solution contains alcohol, it is flammable and needs to be kept away from any heat source such as hair dryers or cigarettes. Malathion is very toxic if swallowed. This drug is pregnancy category B.

Pyrethrin (RID): Pyrethrin is a pediculicide solution or shampoo that poisons the parasite's nervous system, resulting in paralysis and death. Pyrethrin may require a repeat application a week after the first dose. Contraindications include skin infections, abrasions, lactation, and sensitivity to the solution components. Pyrethrin is usually formulated with 4% piperonyl butoxide because this combination results in greater parasite killing. Pyrethrin should be used with caution in ragweed-sensitized patients, infants, and children. This medication is applied to infested areas that are wet, allowing it to stay in place for at least 10 minutes. The areas are then washed and rinsed with warm water. For shampoo applications, the hair is shampooed as usual then a fine-toothed comb is used to remove the lice and eggs from the hair. This drug is pregnancy category C.

PharmFACT

Although many young people believe that indoor tanning helps to clear up acne, there is no scientific evidence to support this claim. Indoor tanning is responsible for hundreds of thousands of cases of non-melanoma skin cancer in the United States each year (Wehner et al., 2012).

Pharmacotherapy of Acne and Rosacea

73.5 The pharmacotherapy of acne includes treatment with benzoyl peroxide, retinoids, and antibiotics; pharmacotherapy for rosacea includes retinoids and metronidazole.

Acne vulgaris and rosacea are two disorders that produce similar appearing lesions on the face. Although the two conditions have some visual similarities and share a few common treatments, the pharmacotherapy of the disorders is very different.

Acne Vulgaris

Acne vulgaris, a disorder of the hair follicles and sebaceous glands, is a common condition that affects 80% of adolescents. Although acne occurs most often in teenagers, it is not unusual to find patients with acne who are older than 30 years, which is a condition referred to as mature acne or acne tardive. Acne vulgaris is more common in men but tends to persist longer in women. Acne affects approximately 17 million persons in the United States, making it one of the most common skin conditions encountered by the nurse.

Although the precise cause of acne is unknown, several factors that are associated with acne vulgaris include abnormal formation of keratin that blocks oil glands and **seborrhea**, the overproduction of sebum by oil glands. The bacterium *Propionibacterium*

CONNECTIONS: NURSING PRACTICE APPLICATION

Patients Receiving Pharmacotherapy for Lice or Mite Infestation

Assessment	Potential Nursing Diagnoses*
Baseline assessment prior to administration: • Obtain a complete health history including dermatologic and social history of recent exposure. • Obtain a drug history including allergies, current prescription and OTC drugs, herbal preparations, alcohol use, and smoking. Be alert to possible drug interactions. • Assess skin areas to be treated for signs of infestation (e.g., lice or nits in hair, reddened track areas between webs of fingers, around belt, or elastic lines), irritation, excoriation, or drainage. • Obtain baseline height, weight, and vital signs. • Assess the patient's ability to receive and understand instructions. Include the family or caregiver as needed.	• *Disturbed Body Image* • *Impaired Skin Integrity* • *Deficient Knowledge* (Drug Therapy) • *Risk for Poisoning*, related to incorrect use of the drug or adverse drug effects
Assessment throughout administration: • Assess for desired therapeutic effects dependent on the reason the drug is given (e.g., decreased visible infestation, nits are removed, skin healing is visible). • Assess for adverse effects: localized tingling, pruritus, stinging, or burning. Promptly report any severe skin reactions or edema.	

Implementation

Interventions and (Rationales)	Patient-Centered Care
Ensuring therapeutic effects: • Monitor the appropriate medication administration for optimum results. Monitor the affected area after treatment over the next 1 to 2 weeks to ensure that the infestation has been eliminated. (Appropriate administration will optimize therapeutic effects and limit the need for re-treatment.)	• Teach the patient, family, or caregiver the appropriate administration techniques.
Minimizing adverse effects: • Monitor the area of infestation over the next 1 to 2 weeks. Reinfestations will usually appear within 1 week and need to be re-treated at that time. (Most treatments are highly effective when administered correctly. Re-treatment may be needed dependent on the type of infestation.)	• Instruct the patient, family, or caregiver to continue to assess the area daily for 1 to 2 weeks and contact the health care provider for a second prescription if reinfestation is noted.
• Monitor family members, caregivers, or sexual contacts for infestation. Bedding and personal objects should be cleansed before reuse. (Reinfestation may recur if those in close contact with the patient are infested. Close contacts should be treated at the same time as the patient. Brushes, combs, and bedding should be washed before reuse. Vacuum cloth that cannot be washed. Children's toys that cannot be washed may be placed in a plastic bag and sealed for 2 weeks. Lice and mites perish quickly once separated from a human host food source.)	• Instruct the patient, family, or caregiver to wash bedding, clothing used currently, combs, and brushes in soapy water and dry thoroughly. Vacuum furniture or fabric that cannot be cleaned to remove any errant vermin. Dry clean hats or caps that cannot be washed. Seal children's toys in plastic bags for 2 weeks if they cannot be washed.
• Monitor skin condition in areas that have been treated. Promptly report any irritation, broken skin, erythema, rashes, or edema. (Skin reactions are relatively uncommon but may occur. Allergic reactions should be reported promptly.)	• Teach the patient, family, or caregiver to report any redness, swelling, itching, excoriation, or burning to the health care provider.
Patient understanding of drug therapy: • Use opportunities during administration of medications and during assessments to discuss the rationale for the drug therapy, desired therapeutic outcomes, commonly observed adverse effects, parameters for when to call the health care provider, and any necessary monitoring or precautions. (Using time during nursing care helps to optimize and reinforce key teaching areas.)	• The patient should be able to state the reason for the drug, appropriate dose and scheduling, what adverse effects to observe for, and when to report them.

(continued)

CONNECTIONS: NURSING PRACTICE APPLICATION (continued)

Patient self-administration of drug therapy:

- When administering the medication, instruct the patient, family, or caregiver in proper self-administration of the drug, e.g., use exactly as directed or per package directions. (Utilizing time during nurse-administration of these drugs helps to reinforce teaching.)

- Teach the patient to take the drug following appropriate guidelines:
  - Wash hair or shower to remove any residual creams or gels before applying the drug. Dry thoroughly.
  - Apply the drug per package directions and allow it to remain in the hair or on the skin for the prescribed length of time (usually approximately 10 min). Most packages contain enough drug for one treatment, although a second package may be required if the hair is long. Do not allow the drug to come in contact with eyes.
  - Dry thoroughly after showering or shampooing the drug out of the hair or skin.
  - Comb through the hair with a small-toothed comb to remove any remaining dead lice, nits, or nit casings.
  - If eyelashes are infested, apply a thin coat of petroleum jelly to eyelashes once a day for 1 week. Comb through using a small-toothed comb to remove any dead lice, nits, or nit casings.
  - Check hair, webbings of fingers and toes, belt, or elastic waist bands for signs of reinfestation over the next week. If needed, a second application of the drug can be used after 1 week.

*Nursing Diagnoses—Definitions and Classification 2015–2017. Copyright © 2014, 1994–2014 by NANDA International. Used by arrangement with John Wiley & Sons Limited.

acnes grows within oil gland openings and changes sebum to an acidic and irritating substance. As a result, small inflamed bumps appear on the surface of the skin. Other factors associated with acne include androgens, which stimulate the sebaceous glands to produce more sebum. This is clearly evident in teenage boys and in patients who are administered testosterone. Studies have indicated that dietary factors do not promote acne. Remissions tend to occur in the summer, perhaps due to more exposure of the skin to the UV rays from sunlight.

The lesions of acne are most frequently distributed on the face, chest, and back. Acne lesions include open and closed **comedones**. Blackheads, or open comedones, occur when sebum has plugged the oil gland, causing it to become black because of the presence of melanin granules. Whiteheads, or closed comedones, develop just beneath the surface of the skin and appear white rather than black. Some closed comedones may rupture, resulting in an inflammatory response. The result is seen as papules, inflammatory pustules, and cysts. Mild papules and cysts drain on their own without treatment. Deeper lesions can cause scarring of the skin. Acne is graded as mild, moderate, or severe, depending on the number and type of lesions present.

The goals of acne therapy are to treat existing lesions and to prevent or lessen the severity of future recurrences. Severe acne can cause permanent scarring of the face. Treatment for acne is directed toward the pathogenesis of the lesion and there are multiple treatment options. The regimen used depends on the extent and severity of the acne and the response of each individual patient. Mechanisms of action of antiacne medications include the following:

- Inhibit sebaceous gland overactivity
- Reduce bacterial colonization
- Prevent follicles from becoming plugged with keratin
- Reduce inflammation of lesions

Many of the medications used for acne and related disorders are available OTC. Mild acne is treated by topical therapy with drugs such as benzoyl peroxide, topical antibiotics, and salicylic acid. Moderate to severe acne is treated with increasing strengths of tretinoin and the use of systemic antibiotics. Because of their increased toxicity, prescription medications are reserved for more severe, persistent cases. These drugs are listed in Table 73.2.

TABLE 73.2 Drugs for Acne

Drug	Remarks
adapalene (Differin)	Retinoid-like compound used to treat acne formation
azelaic acid (Azelex, Finacea)	For mild to moderate inflammatory acne
benzoyl peroxide (Clearasil, Fostex, Others)	Keratinolytic available OTC: sometimes combined with erythromycin (Benzamycin) or clindamycin (BenzaClin) for acne caused by *P. acnes*
clindamycin and tretinoin (Veltin, Ziana)	Combination product with an antibiotic and a retinoid in a gel base; for mild to moderate acne
ethinyl estradiol (Estinyl)	Oral contraceptives are sometimes used for acne; for example, ethinyl estradiol plus norgestimate (Ortho Tri-Cyclen-28)
isotretinoin (Accutane)	For severe acne with cysts or acne formed in small, rounded masses; pregnancy category X
sulfacetamide sodium (Cetamide, Klaron, Others)	For sensitive skin; sometimes combined with sulfur to promote peeling, as in the condition rosacea; also used for conjunctivitis
tazarotene (Avage, Tazorac)	A retinoid drug that may also be used for plaque psoriasis; has antiproliferative and anti-inflammatory effects
tetracyclines	Antibiotics; refer to Chapter 48
tretinoin (Avita, Retin-A, Others)	To prevent clogging of pore follicles; also used for the treatment of acute promyelocytic leukemia and wrinkles

Benzoyl peroxide (Clearasil, Fostex, Others) is the most common topical OTC medication for acne. Benzoyl peroxide has a **keratolytic** effect, which helps to treat acne by loosening dry skin and causing an increased shedding of the outer layer of the epidermis. In addition, this drug suppresses sebum production and exhibits antibacterial effects against *P. acnes*. Benzoyl peroxide is available as a topical lotion, cream, or gel in various percentage concentrations. Typically the patient applies benzoyl peroxide once daily and, in many instances, this is the only treatment needed. The drug is very safe, with local redness, irritation, and drying being the most common adverse effects. Although the symptoms might worsen during the early weeks of therapy, the skin usually adjusts quickly to its use. Other keratolytic agents that are available by prescription are used for severe acne and include benzoyl peroxide with erythromycin (Benzamycin) and benzoyl peroxide with sulfur (Sulfoxyl).

Retinoids are a class of drug closely related to vitamin A. They are used in the treatment of inflammatory skin conditions, dermatologic malignancies, and acne. The topical formulations are often the first-line drugs for mild to moderate acne characterized by inflammatory cysts. Drugs in this class are called **comedolytics** because they prevent and break up the formation of clogged pores. Tretinoin (Avita, Retin-A, Others) is an older drug with comedolytic action that decreases comedone formation and increases extrusion of comedones from the skin. Tretinoin also has the ability to improve photodamaged skin and is used for wrinkle removal. Other retinoids include isotretinoin (Accutane), a PO vitamin A metabolite medication that aids in reducing the size of sebaceous glands, thereby decreasing oil production and the occurrence of clogged pores. Therapy with retinoids may require 8 to 12 weeks to achieve maximum effectiveness. Common reactions to retinoids include burning, stinging, and sensitivity to sunlight. Adapalene (Differin) is a third-generation retinoid that causes less irritation than the older drugs. Epiduo is a topical drug that contains both adapalene and benzoyl peroxide. Additional retinoid-like agents and the related compounds that are used to treat acne are listed in Table 73.2.

Antibiotics are prescribed to lessen the severe redness and inflammation associated with moderate to severe acne, especially when the acne is inflammatory and results in cysts and pustules. Oral doxycycline (Vibramycin, Others), minocycline, and tetracycline, which are administered in small doses over a long period, have been the traditional antibiotics used in acne therapy. Due to their effects on teeth formation, tetracyclines should not be used in children younger than age 8. Erythromycin and clindamycin are frequently used topically and have a low incidence of adverse effects. Antibiotics are not comedolytic and resistance can develop with continued therapy. To lessen the possibility of resistance, topical antibiotics are often combined with benzoyl peroxide.

Oral contraceptives that contain ethinyl estradiol and norgestimate are also used in pubertal females to help clear the skin of acne by suppressing sebum production and reducing skin oiliness. Hormonal therapy is used when antibiotic therapy has proved ineffective. They are most effective for young women when the acne begins somewhat later than usual and tends to flare up at certain times in the menstrual cycle. Estrogen is not administered to male patients because of undesirable adverse effects, such as breast enlargement and decrease in body hair. For the actions and contraindications of oral contraceptives, see Chapter 70.

CONNECTION Checkpoint 73.2

Retinoids are derivatives of vitamin A. From what you learned in Chapter 61, what type of vitamin is vitamin A? What are some signs of toxicity due to excess amounts of this vitamin? *See Answers to Connection Checkpoint 73.2 on student resource website.*

Rosacea

Rosacea is an inflammatory skin disorder of unknown etiology with lesions affecting mainly the face. Unlike acne, which most commonly affects teenagers, rosacea is a progressive disorder with an onset between 30 and 50 years of age. Rosacea is characterized by small papules or inflammatory bumps without pus that swell, thicken, and become painful. These lesions typically occur in the middle third of the face, including the forehead, nose, cheeks, and chin. The face takes on a reddened or flushed appearance with accompanying telangiectasia (dilation of small blood vessels). With time the redness becomes more permanent, and lesions resembling acne appear. The soft tissues of the nose may thicken, resulting in a reddened, bulbous, irregular swelling called **rhinophyma**. Disorders of the eye frequently accompany rosacea, particularly conjunctivitis, itching, edema, and keratitis.

Rosacea is exacerbated by factors such as sunlight, stress, increased temperature, and medications that dilate facial blood vessels, including alcohol, spicy foods, skin care products, and hot beverages. Rosacea affects more women than men, although men more often develop rhinophyma. Learning and avoiding the environmental triggers that worsen the symptoms of the condition may prevent mild rosacea.

The two most effective treatments for rosacea are topical metronidazole (MetroGel, MetroCream) and azelaic acid (Azelex, Finacea). Benzoyl peroxide may be applied as needed. Alternative medications include topical tretinoin (Avita, Retin-A, Others), clindamycin (Cleocin-T, ClindaMax), and sulfacetamide. Tetracycline antibiotics are of benefit to patients with rosacea who have multiple pustules or ocular involvement. Severe, resistant cases may respond to isotretinoin (Accutane). In 2013, brimonidine (Mirvaso) was approved as a topical treatment to reduce the persistent redness of facial rosacea. In addition to medications, some patients receive vascular or carbon dioxide laser surgery to reduce the excessive tissue associated with rhinophyma.

PROTOTYPE DRUG	Tretinoin (Avita, Retin-A, Others)

Classification: Therapeutic: Antiacne drug
Pharmacologic: Retinoid

Therapeutic Effects and Uses: Approved as a topical drug in 1971, tretinoin is a natural derivative of vitamin A. This drug is indicated for the early treatment and control of mild to moderate acne vulgaris. Renova is a topical form of tretinoin that has been approved to treat fine facial wrinkles and hyperpigmentation associated with photodamaged skin. Tretinoin has antineoplastic actions; a PO form (Vesanoid) is approved to treat acute promyelocytic leukemia (APL) and may be prescribed off-label for skin malignancies.

Symptoms take 4 to 8 weeks to improve, and maximum therapeutic benefit may take 5 to 6 months. Because of potentially serious adverse effects, this drug is most often reserved for cystic acne or severe keratinization disorders.

Mechanism of Action: The principal action of tretinoin is regulation of skin growth and turnover. As cells from the stratum germinativum grow toward the surface, skin cells are lost from the stratum pore openings, and their replacement is slowed. Tretinoin reverses retention hyperkeratosis and comedone formation, which are the primary events in acne pathology. The drug increases the permeability of the skin and supports conversion of follicular epithelium into a less sturdy and almost fragile condition. Tretinoin also decreases oil production by reducing the size and number of oil glands.

Pharmacokinetics:

Route(s)	Topical, PO
Absorption	Minimally absorbed from intact skin; well absorbed PO
Distribution	Secreted in breast milk; more than 95% bound to plasma protein
Primary metabolism	Hepatic
Primary excretion	Renal; small amounts in feces
Onset of action	Unknown
Duration of action	Half-life: 0.5–2 h

Adverse Effects: Nearly all patients who use topical tretinoin will experience local effects such as redness, scaling, erythema, crusting, and peeling of the skin with temporary hypopigmentation or hyperpigmentation. Skin irritation can be severe and cause discontinuation of therapy; a lower strength solution may be necessary to limit the severity of these adverse effects. Dermatologic adverse effects resolve once therapy is discontinued. Oral therapy can also cause adverse skin effects.

For treatment of APL, very high oral doses are used and adverse effects are more serious than with topical therapy. The most common effects with PO therapy include bone pain, fever, headache, nausea, vomiting, rash, stomatitis, pruritus, sweating, and ocular disorders. Other adverse effects may include hyperlipidemia, shivering, hemorrhage, pain, dizziness, paresthesias, anxiety, insomnia, depression, cerebral hemorrhage, intracranial hypertension (HTN), hallucinations, dysrhythmias, flushing, hypotension or HTN, heart failure, visual disturbances, abdominal pain, diarrhea, constipation, dyspepsia, gastrointestinal (GI) hemorrhage, renal insufficiency, dysuria, and acute kidney failure. **Black Box Warning**: Patients with APL are at high risk for serious adverse effects. About 25% of patients develop retinoic acid-APL syndrome, which is a serious condition characterized by fever, weakness, fatigue, dyspnea, weight gain, peripheral edema, respiratory insufficiency, and pneumonia. About 40% of patients develop a rapidly evolving leukocytosis, which is associated with a high risk of life-threatening complications. There is a high risk that infants will be severely deformed if this drug is administered during pregnancy.

Contraindications/Precautions: Contraindications for topical administration include eczema, exposure to sunlight or UV rays, sunburn, hypersensitivity to this drug or vitamin A preparation, and children less than 12 years of age. This drug should be used cautiously in patients who are in an occupation necessitating considerable sun exposure or weather extremes or in patients with hepatic disease. This drug may cause birth defects and is contraindicated during lactation, pregnancy, or suspected pregnancy. Pregnancy testing is advised before starting therapy in female patients of childbearing age. Oral tretinoin is contraindicated in patients who have hepatic disease, leukopenia or neutropenia, or who are hypersensitive to the drug.

Drug Interactions: Topical acne keratolytics (sulfur, resorcinol, benzoyl peroxide, and salicylic acid) may increase inflammation and peeling; topical products that contain alcohol or menthol may cause stinging. Additive phototoxicity can occur if tretinoin is used concurrently with other phototoxic drugs such as tetracyclines, fluoroquinolone, or sulfonamides. Use of this drug with hypoglycemic agents may lead to a loss of glycemic control and cardiovascular risk, because tretinoin raises serum triglyceride levels. Hepatotoxic drugs may cause additive liver impairment if used concurrently with PO tretinoin. **Herbal/Food**: The PO absorption of tretinoin is increased if taken with a high-fat meal.

Pregnancy: Category C (topical) and D (PO).

Treatment of Overdose: Overuse of the topical drug will lead to excessive skin drying and peeling. Symptoms of PO overdose are nonspecific and resolve with symptomatic treatment.

Nursing Responsibilities: Key nursing implications for patients receiving tretinoin are included in the Nursing Practice Application for Patients Receiving Pharmacotherapy for Acne and Related Skin Conditions.

Drugs Similar to Tretinoin (Avita, Retin-A, Others)

Other antiacne drugs include adapalene, azelaic acid, isotretinoin, and tazarotene.

Adapalene (Differin): Approved in 1996, adapalene is a topical acne drug that modulates the inflammation, epithelial keratinization, and differentiation of follicular cells. It is very similar to the retinoids but is reported to produce less skin irritation. Optimum results may take up to 12 weeks of therapy. Patients must take caution with sun exposure because this drug can increase the potential for sunburn. Other adverse effects include local burning, pruritus, scaling, and peeling. Only minimal amounts of adapalene are absorbed through the skin. Safety of this drug in patients under age 12 has not been established. This drug is pregnancy category C.

Azelaic acid (Azelex, Finacea): Approved in 1995, azelaic acid is a natural product found in wheat, rye, and barley. Azelaic acid is a topical therapy that is effective for the treatment of mild to moderate acne by suppressing the growth of *P. acnes* and decreasing the proliferation of keratinocytes. It is also approved for the topical treatment of inflammatory pustules associated with rosacea. Only 4% is absorbed systemically. Adverse effects are typical of other topical antiacne drugs: local burning, pruritus, scaling, and peeling. Safety of this drug in patients under age 12 has not been established. This drug is pregnancy category B.

Isotretinoin (Accutane): Approved in 1982, isotretinoin is a PO retinoid that is the most effective drug for severe, inflammatory acne. Therapy may require several months for optimum benefit. Off-label uses include rosacea, psoriasis, and the treatment of squamous cell carcinoma of the skin. Because of potentially serious adverse effects, this drug is usually used when other therapies fail to produce satisfactory results. Isotretinoin carries a black box warning that the drug causes birth defects (category X), which can occur after even short courses of isotretinoin therapy. The warning further states that the drug has special requirements for distribution that require patients, physicians, and pharmacists to register and adhere to the iPledge Program, a pregnancy risk management program. Before starting therapy, the patient must submit to two negative pregnancy tests and sign a statement of understanding about the drug's adverse effects. Each subsequent month, the pharmacist must document receipt of a negative pregnancy test and verify that two forms of effective contraception are being utilized by the patient. Males must also register with the iPledge Program because small amounts of isotretinoin are found in semen and could potentially cause birth defects in a pregnant partner. Other common adverse effects include cheilitis, epistaxis, xerostomia, hair loss, eczema, elevated serum lipid levels, myalgia, and arthralgia. Clinical depression, psychosis, and aggression have been reported.

Tazarotene (Avage, Tazorac): Approved in 1997, tazarotene is a topical retinoid derivative of vitamin A that is used for the treatment of acne, fine facial wrinkles, and psoriasis. Patients become sensitive to the sun's UV light and need to wear protective sunscreen and clothing when using this drug. Adverse effects are similar to those of topical tretinoin: local burning, stinging, erythema, and general skin irritation. This drug is metabolized in the skin to an active metabolite; small amounts are absorbed systemically. Safety of this drug in patients under age 12 has not been established. Tazarotene is pregnancy category X.

Pharmacotherapy of Dermatitis

73.6 The most effective treatment for dermatitis is topical corticosteroids, which are classified by their potency.

Dermatitis is a general term that refers to superficial inflammatory disorders of the skin. General symptoms include local redness, pain, and pruritus. Intense scratching may lead to **excoriation**, which are scratches that break the skin surface and fill with blood or serous fluid to form crusty scales. A wide variety of factors can cause dermatitis, with different types of symptoms occurring depending on the causative agent. The three most common types that respond to topical pharmacotherapy are atopic, contact, and seborrheic. Dermatitis may be acute or chronic.

PharmFACT

About 27% of children who have a food allergy also have eczema or a skin allergy. More than 3,700 substances have been identified as contact allergens (American Academy of Allergy, Asthma and Immunology, n.d.).

Atopic dermatitis, or **eczema**, is a chronic, inflammatory skin disorder with a genetic predisposition. Patients who present with eczema often have a family history of asthma and hay fever as well as allergies to a variety of irritants such as cosmetics, lotions, soaps, pollens, food, pet dander, and dust. About 75% of patients with atopic dermatitis have had an initial onset before 1 year of age. In those babies predisposed to eczema, breast-feeding seems to offer protection, because it is rare for a breast-fed child to develop eczema before the introduction of other foods. In infants and small children, lesions usually begin on the face and scalp, and then progress to other parts of the body. A frequent and prominent symptom in infants is the appearance of red cheeks.

Contact dermatitis can be caused by a hypersensitivity response, resulting from exposure to specific natural or synthetic allergens such as plants, chemicals, latex, drugs, metals, or foreign proteins. Accompanying the allergic reaction may be various degrees of cracking, bleeding, or small blisters. See Figure 73.2.

CONNECTIONS: NURSING PRACTICE APPLICATION

Patients Receiving Pharmacotherapy for Acne and Related Skin Conditions

Assessment	Potential Nursing Diagnoses*
Baseline assessment prior to administration: • Obtain a complete health history including dermatologic, hepatic, or renal disease; psychiatric disorders; pregnancy; or breast-feeding. • Obtain a drug history including allergies, current prescription and OTC drugs, herbal preparations, alcohol use, and smoking. Be alert to possible drug interactions. • Evaluate appropriate laboratory findings (e.g., CBC, lipid profiles, hepatic or renal function laboratory tests). • Obtain baseline vital signs. • Assess the patient's ability to receive and understand instructions. Include the family or caregiver as needed.	• *Disturbed Body Image* • *Impaired Skin Integrity*, related to adverse drug effects • *Deficient Knowledge* (Drug Therapy) • *Risk for Injury*, related to adverse drug effects
Assessment throughout administration: • Assess for desired therapeutic effects dependent on the reason drug is given (e.g., skin is clearing of acne lesions). • Continue periodic monitoring of CBC, lipid profiles, glucose, and hepatic function tests if on a PO drug. • Monitor vital signs at each health care visit. • Monitor eye health periodically with eye examinations every 6 months while on PO drug therapy. • Assess for adverse effects: localized skin irritation, erythema, pruritus, dry or peeling skin; dry mouth, eyes, or nose may occur if on the PO drug. Immediately report any sudden or significant changes in mood, especially depression or suicidal thoughts in patients on PO isotretinoin.	

(continued)

CONNECTIONS: NURSING PRACTICE APPLICATION (continued)

Implementation

Interventions and (Rationales)	Patient-Centered Care
Ensuring therapeutic effects: • Monitor appropriate medication administration for optimum results. (Topical treatment areas should show signs of improvement within 2 to 4 weeks but may require up to 3 or 4 months of treatment. PO treatment is usually successful within one course and a second course may be delayed for several weeks to monitor continuing improvement.)	• Teach the patient appropriate administration techniques. • Advise the patient that significant improvement may take several weeks but some improvement should be noticed within a few days of treatment.
Minimizing adverse effects: • Monitor the area under topical treatment for excessive dryness and irritation. (Overcleansing or overdrying of the skin may make the condition worse. If other drying products such as benzoyl peroxide were used before treatment, a brief recovery period may be needed to avoid excessive skin irritation.)	• Teach the patient to gently cleanse the skin using a non-oily soap and avoiding vigorous scrubbing. If excessive dryness occurs, use a non-oily lotion to areas of dryness.
• Monitor patients on isotretinoin for emotional health or changes in mood. (Depression, including with suicidal ideations, has been noted as an adverse effect.)	• Instruct the patient, family, or caregiver to immediately report any signs of decreased mood, affect, depression, or expressed suicidal thoughts to the health care provider.
• Monitor CBC, lipid levels, and hepatic function laboratory values periodically for patients on PO medication. (Lipid levels may increase in up to 70% of patients on PO acne therapy. Hepatic toxicity is an adverse effect of PO drugs.)	• Instruct the patient to return periodically for laboratory tests. • Teach the patient to report any symptoms of abdominal or right upper quadrant discomfort or pain, yellowing of the skin or sclera, fatigue, anorexia, darkened urine, or clay-colored stools immediately.
• Monitor for vision changes. (Corneal opacities or cataracts are an adverse effect of PO antiacne medications. Dryness of eyes during treatment is common. Night vision may be diminished during treatment.)	• Instruct the patient to maintain regular eye exams and to report any changes in visual acuity, especially with night driving. • Teach the patient that artificial tear solutions may assist in relieving eye dryness. Consult the health care provider if dryness is severe or increases.
• Monitor the patient's exposure to sun and UV light. Use oil-free sunscreen of SPF 15 or higher prior to any sun exposure. (Drying, skin sensitivity, and peeling skin are possible adverse effects of antiacne and antiwrinkle medications, especially for patients on tretinoin. Protection from sun exposure is essential to prevent increasing skin damage.)	• Teach the patient to use sunscreens of SPF 15 or higher and to wear protective clothing and hats to avoid sun exposure to areas under treatment for acne or wrinkles. • Teach the patient that UV light therapy from a health care provider is monitored, and tanning beds are not a substitute. Tanning beds should be avoided unless specifically ordered by the health care provider.

• Monitor adherence with iPledge requirements for patients on isotretinoin. (iPledge is required of all patients on isotretinoin before receiving a prescription or refills of the drug. It includes educational information and requires the patient to ensure that all requirements to prevent teratogenic effects have been met.)	• Instruct the patient on isotretinoin of the requirements of the iPledge mandatory program to ensure continued prescriptions, including:
	  • Females of childbearing age must use two methods of birth control while on the drug.
	  • Females of childbearing age must have two negative pregnancy tests 1 month before, during, and after drug therapy, conducted at certified laboratories. The results of these tests are submitted by the health care provider, along with a description of the two types of birth control used by the patient.
	  • Male patients must verify that they will use a barrier method of birth control and will not donate blood while on the drug.

Patient understanding of drug therapy: • Use opportunities during administration of medications and during assessments to discuss the rationale for drug therapy, desired therapeutic outcomes, commonly observed adverse effects, parameters for when to call the health care provider, and any necessary monitoring or precautions. (Using time during nursing care helps to optimize and reinforce key teaching areas.)	• The patient should be able to state the reason for the drug, appropriate dose and scheduling, what adverse effects to observe for, and when to report them.

Patient self-administration of drug therapy:
• When administering the medication, instruct the patient, family, or caregiver in proper self-administration of the drug, e.g., topical drug used appropriately, iPledge program is followed. (Utilizing time during nurse-administration of these drugs helps to reinforce teaching.)
	• Teach the patient to take the drug following appropriate guidelines:
	  • Gently cleanse the affected skin twice daily with non-oily soap, avoiding excessive or vigorous scrubbing.
	  • Apply a thin layer of topical cream or lotion to the affected area after cleansing the skin. Keep the drug out of the eyes. Allow to dry and avoid contact with clothing, towels, or bedding to avoid staining or bleaching.
	  • For oral medications, take in the morning, and if twice-a-day dosing is ordered, take the second dose approximately 8 h after the first.

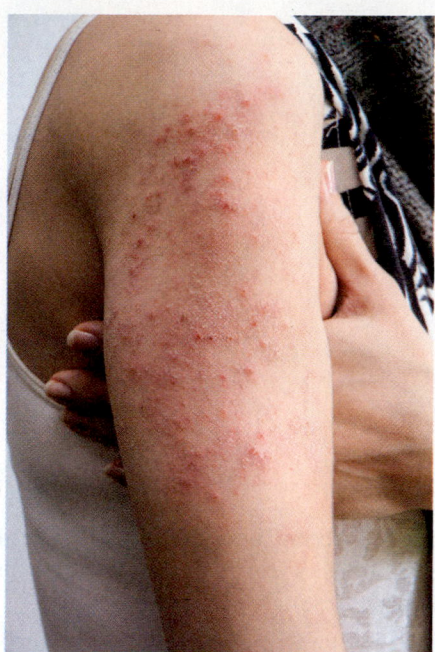

Figure 73.2 Dermatitis.
Courtesy of librakv/Fotolia.

TABLE 73.3 Selected Topical Corticosteroids for Dermatitis and Related Symptoms

Generic Name	Strength (%)	Trade Name
Very High Potency		
betamethasone dipropionate, augmented, cream	0.05	Diprolene
clobetasol propionate	0.05	Temovate
diflorasone diacetate	0.05	Maxiflor
halobetasolol	0.05	Ultravate
High Potency		
amcinonide	0.1	Cyclocort
fluocinonide	0.025	Lidex
halcinonide	0.1	Halog
Medium Potency		
betamethasone benzoate	0.025	Uticort
betamethasone valerate	0.1	Valisone
clocortolone pivalate	0.1	Cloderm
desoximetasone, cream	0.025	Topicort
fluocinolone acetonide	0.025	Synalar
flurandrenolide, cream	0.025	Cordran
fluticasone propionate, cream	0.05	Cutivate
hydrocortisone valerate	0.2	Westcort
mometasone furoate	0.1	Elocon
prednicarbate	0.1	Dermatop
triamcinolone acetonide	0.025–0.1	Aristocort, Kenalog
Low Potency		
alclometasone dipropionate	0.05	Aclovate
desonide	0.05	Desonate, DesOwen, Verdeso
dexamethasone	0.1	Decaspray
hydrocortisone	0.25–1	Cortizone, Hycort

Seborrheic dermatitis is a form of eczema that can affect patients at any age. The exact cause of seborrheic dermatitis is unknown, but hormone levels, coexisting fungal infections, nutritional deficiencies, and immunodeficiency states are associated with the disease. Seborrheic dermatitis presents as greasy, not dry, scales that affect the scalp, central face, and anterior chest, often presenting as scalp scaling, or dandruff. Other symptoms may include redness of the nasolabial fold, particularly during times of stress; blepharitis; otitis externa; and acne vulgaris. In infants, thick, greasy scales on the vertex of the scalp, commonly known as cradle cap, are seen. These scales can become more widespread, with the central face, forehead, and ears being affected.

Pharmacotherapy of dermatitis is symptomatic and involves lotions and ointments to control itching and skin flaking. Antihistamines may be used to control inflammation and reduce itching, and analgesics or topical anesthetics may be prescribed for pain relief. Atopic dermatitis can be controlled, but not cured, by medications. Part of the management plan must include the identification and elimination of allergic triggers that cause flare-ups.

Topical corticosteroids are the most effective treatment for controlling the inflammation and itching of dermatitis. Creams, lotions, solutions, gels, and pads that contain corticosteroids are specially formulated to penetrate deep into the skin layers. These dermatologic drugs are classified by potency, as listed in Table 73.3. The high-potency agents are used to treat acute flare-ups and are limited to 2 to 3 weeks of therapy. The medium-potency formulations are for more prolonged therapy of chronic dermatitis. The low-potency corticosteroids are prescribed for children.

Long-term corticosteroid use may lead to irritation, redness, hypopigmentation, and thinning of the skin. High-potency formulations are not advised for the head or neck regions because of potential adverse effects. If absorption occurs, topical corticosteroids may produce undesirable systemic effects, including adrenal insufficiency, mood changes, serum imbalances, and loss of bone mass, as discussed in Chapter 68. To avoid serious adverse effects, careful attention must be given to the amount of corticosteroid applied, the frequency of application, and how long it should be used. For most patients with dermatitis, topical corticosteroids have minimal adverse effects.

Several alternatives to the corticosteroids are available. Patients with persistent atopic dermatitis that does not respond to corticosteroids may benefit from PO immunosuppressants, such as cyclosporine. This drug is generally used for the short-term treatment of severe disease. The topical calcineurin inhibitors pimecrolimus 1% (Elidel) and tacrolimus 0.03%, 0.1% (Protopic) are available for patients older than 2 years of age. These medications may be used on all skin surfaces (including the face and neck) because they have fewer adverse effects than the topical corticosteroids. Adverse effects include burning and stinging on broken skin. Pimecrolimus and tacrolimus are not approved for long-term therapy because of a small risk of skin cancer and lymphoma. They are reserved for patients who have not responded to topical corticosteroids. When using these drugs, occlusive dressings should not be used because this promotes absorption of the drug and can increase the risk of systemic toxicity. The immunosuppressants are presented in Chapter 42.

Another alternative to corticosteroids for atopic dermatitis is doxepin (Zonalon). When given PO this drug is used to treat depression; however, Zonalon cream is indicated for atopic dermatitis. The mechanism by which doxepin reduces itching is unknown. Some of the drug is absorbed across the skin, causing drowsiness in about 20% of patients.

Topical therapy for seborrheic dermatitis primarily consists of antifungals and low-dose topical corticosteroids, depending on the location affected. The first-line therapy for seborrheic dermatitis that affects the scalp should be topical corticosteroids. These may be administered as a shampoo, topical solution, or a lotion applied to the scalp. A typical regimen for an adult would be to use a topical corticosteroid once or twice daily with the use of a medicated shampoo two to three times per week. Shampoos that contain selenium sulfide (Selsun), salicylic acid, zinc pyrithione, or an antifungal azole are most often used. Once-daily antifungal medication with fluconazole (Diflucan), ketoconazole (Nizoral), or ciclopirox (Loprox) combined with 2 weeks of once-daily desonide (DesOwen) is recommended for seborrheic dermatitis of the face and ears.

CONNECTION Checkpoint 73.3

Topical applications of corticosteroids are used for a variety of conditions. What are some indications for corticosteroids given by the following routes of administration: aerosol inhalation (see Chapter 44), intranasal (see Chapter 45), and intra-articular (see Chapter 72)? *See Answer to Connection Checkpoint 73.3 on student resource website.*

Pharmacotherapy of Psoriasis

73.7 Psoriasis is a chronic, inflammatory disease that is treated with topical and systemic medications.

Psoriasis is a chronic, inflammatory skin disorder that affects 1% to 2% of the population and appears with greater frequency in people of European ancestry. The onset of psoriasis is generally established by 20 years of age, although it may occur throughout the lifespan.

Although the etiology of psoriasis is incompletely understood, it appears to have both genetic and autoimmune components. About 33% to 50% of the cases have a genetic basis, with a close family member also having the disorder. When one identical twin presents with psoriasis, the other twin has a 70% probability of also acquiring the disease. The immune nature of psoriasis is supported by the discovery that activated T lymphocytes (T cells) migrate to the dermis and release cytokines such as tumor necrosis factor (TNF) that increase the production of skin cells and cause inflammation. Furthermore, suppressing T-cell function through the use of immunosuppressants or biologic therapies improves symptoms of psoriasis.

Specific environmental triggers worsen psoriasis, including stress, smoking, alcohol, climate changes, and infections. In addition, certain drugs, including angiotensin-converting enzyme (ACE) inhibitors, beta-adrenergic blockers, tetracyclines, and nonsteroidal anti-inflammatory drugs (NSAIDs), act as triggers. People with psoriasis seem to improve in warmer climates, where there is more exposure to sunlight.

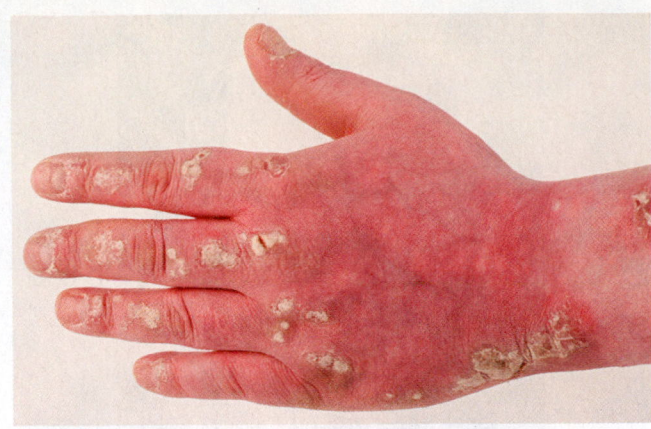

Figure 73.3 Psoriasis.
Courtesy of Casi/Fotolia.

When psoriasis occurs, both the dermis and epidermis become thickened from an extremely fast skin turnover rate, with skin cells reaching the surface in 4 to 7 days instead of the normal 2 to 3 weeks. This rapid proliferation time does not allow for cell maturation and keratinization to occur, giving the skin lesions their characteristic appearance. The typical psoriatic lesions are characterized by red, raised patches of skin covered with flaky, thick, silver scales called **plaques**. Plaques are ultimately shed from the surface while the underlying skin becomes inflamed and irritated. If the scales are scraped away, the dark-red base of the lesion is exposed, producing multiple bleeding points. Lesions vary in size and are usually present on the scalp, elbows, knees, extensor surfaces of the arms and legs, sacrum, hands, and occasionally around the nails (Figure 73.3). The face is rarely affected. When psoriasis affects the nails, a yellow or brown discoloration may result, and the nail itself may separate from the nail bed, thicken, and crumble. The various forms of psoriasis are described in Table 73.4.

The goal of psoriasis pharmacotherapy is to reduce erythema, plaques, and scales to improve the cosmetic appearance of the patient, leading to the ability to perform normal lifestyle activities. This is accomplished by reducing epidermal cell turnover and promoting healing of the psoriatic lesions. The choice of therapy depends on the type and extent of the disease and the history of response to a previous treatment of psoriasis. A number of prescription and OTC drugs are available for the treatment of psoriasis and are listed in Table 73.5. Therapy is often conducted in a stepwise manner. Psoriasis is a lifelong disease and there is no pharmacologic cure.

PharmFACT

Psoriasis affects almost 7.5 million Americans. More than 30% of these patients will experience their first episode before age 20 (National Psoriasis Foundation, 2014).

Topical Drugs

Corticosteroids: Topical corticosteroids are a first-line therapy for the initial treatment of psoriasis. These drugs are effective, inexpensive, and relatively safe. When they are applied to psoriatic lesions, topical corticosteroids suppress cell division, reduce inflammation, relieve pruritus, and delay the movement of keratinocytes that are associated with fast skin turnover. Choosing the correct strength of corticosteroid and the most effective vehicle base are important aspects of treatment because the effectiveness of

TABLE 73.4 Types of Psoriasis

Form of Psoriasis	Description	Most Common Location of Lesions	Comments
Guttate (droplike) or eruptive psoriasis	Lesions smaller than those of psoriasis vulgaris	Upper trunk and extremities	More common in early-onset psoriasis; can appear and resolve spontaneously a few weeks following a streptococcal respiratory infection
Psoriatic arthritis	Resembles rheumatoid arthritis	Fingers and toes at the distal interphalangeal joints; can affect the skin and nails	About 20% of patients with psoriasis also have arthritis
Psoriasis vulgaris	Lesions are papules that form into erythematous plaques with thick, silver or gray plaques that bleed when removed; plaques in dark-skinned individuals often appear purple	Skin over scalp, elbows, and knees; lesions possible anywhere on the body	Most common form; requires long-term specialized management
Psoriatic erythroderma or exfoliative dermatitis	Generalized scaling; erythema without lesions	All body surfaces	Least common form
Pustular psoriasis	Eruption of pustules; presence of fever	Trunk and extremities; can appear on the palms, soles, and nail beds	Average age of onset is 50 years

a topical steroid depends on its potency and ability to be absorbed into the skin. Initial therapy may begin with a high-potency agent to obtain rapid clearing of the lesions. High-potency drugs are also used for acute flare-ups for 2 to 3 weeks. The high-potency formulations are best applied to the areas thickest with plaque, such as the hands or feet, and should not be used on the face and genital areas. For chronic maintenance therapy, the patient is switched to moderate- and low-potency corticosteroids because they have a lower potential for adverse effects.

Occlusive dressings may be applied to increase the effectiveness of the corticosteroid. A simple way to enhance drug penetration is to apply the steroid directly to the skin followed by warm, moist dressings and an occlusive outer wrap. Wraps may be large plastic bags, vinyl jogging suits, or rolls of tubular plastic. Care should be taken that the wraps not be left in place longer than 8 hours. The skin should be inspected for atrophy, striae, hypopigmentation, and telangiectasias, which are all adverse effects of topical corticosteroid therapy.

Repeated use of topical corticosteroids will result in tolerance. To delay tolerance, doses of the high-potency drugs are kept as low as possible. Some health care providers discontinue corticosteroids after an adequate response has been obtained and switch to a different therapy such as coal tar for several weeks.

When large areas of the body have psoriatic lesions, topical corticosteroid therapy can be expensive and involve some systemic risk. The larger the area treated, the greater the absorbed doses. The student should refer to Chapter 68 for a discussion of the adverse effects of systemic corticosteroid therapy.

Coal tar: Coal tar may be used as monotherapy or in combination with other psoriasis medications. The drug inhibits deoxyribonucleic acid (DNA) synthesis, arrests abnormal cell growth, and reduces inflammation. Coal tar is inexpensive and available as a solution, gel, lotion, and shampoo. Coal tar preparations, however, are messy, staining, and have a foul odor. The use of coal tar is considered a second-line therapy except for shampoos, which can treat scalp lesions.

Calcipotriene (Dovonex): Approved in 1993, calcipotriene is a derivative of vitamin D that is available as a cream for use on the body and as a solution for the scalp. The drug binds to vitamin D receptors in the skin, suppresses cellular proliferation, and decreases cellular turnover in the psoriatic plaques. Symptomatic improvement is seen in 2 to 3 weeks. Calcipotriene is an effective alternative to topical corticosteroids. Only about 6% of a topical dose is absorbed systemically. Its most common adverse effect is local irritation. It is not recommended for use by patients over age 65, who have an increased incidence of adverse effects with the drug, or by pregnant and lactating women (category C). Its use may produce hypercalcemia if applied over large areas of the body or if used in higher than recommended doses. Phototherapy of excessive exposure to UV light should be avoided due to the potential for increased tumor incidence. This drug is pregnancy category C.

Tazarotene (Tazorac): Approved in 1997, tazarotene (Tazorac) is a vitamin A retinoid that causes sloughing of the scales covering the psoriatic plaques. Available as an ointment or gel to psoriatic regions, this drug is applied once daily in the evening. Tazarotene is also approved for facial wrinkles and acne. Because this drug is pregnancy category X, its use is contraindicated during pregnancy.

Systemic Drugs

Some patients have severe psoriasis that is resistant to topical therapy. Because these drugs have the potential to cause serious adverse effects, they are generally used when topical agents and phototherapy fail to produce an adequate response. In some cases, systemic drugs may be used for a few weeks to produce a rapid improvement in symptoms before beginning topical therapy.

Acitretin (Soriatane): Acitretin is a PO retinoid that is approved for severe, resistant psoriasis. Two to three months of therapy may be required for significant symptomatic improvement. Approved in 1997, acitretin acts like other retinoids to inhibit keratin formation and skin inflammation. This drug is very effective at eliminating psoriatic lesions. However, the lesions return soon after therapy is discontinued. The most serious adverse effect is teratogenicity (category X). At least two negative pregnancy tests should be obtained before beginning therapy, and the patient should use

TABLE 73.5 Selected Drugs for Psoriasis and Related Disorders

Drug	Route and Adult Dose (Maximum Dose Where Indicated)	Adverse Effects
Topical Medications		
calcipotriene (Dovonex)	Topical: Apply a thin layer to the lesions 1–2 times/day up to 8 weeks	*Burning, stinging, folliculitis, itching, dry skin, hyperpigmentation* No serious adverse effects
coal tar (Balnetar, Cutar, Others)	Topical: Apply to affected areas once–qid	*Folliculitis, irritation, photosensitivity* No serious adverse effects
salicylic acid (Salex, Neutrogena, others)	Topical: Apply to affected areas tid–qid in concentrations ranging from 2% to 10%	*Erythema, pruritus, stinging of the skin* No serious adverse effects
tazarotene (Tazorac)	Acne: Apply a thin film to the clean, dry area daily Plaque psoriasis: Apply thin film daily in the evening	*Pruritus, burning, stinging, skin irritation, transient worsening of psoriasis, skin peeling, photosensitivity* Hypertriglyceridemia, teratogenicity
Systemic Medications		
acitretin (Soriatane)	PO: 25–50 mg/day with the main meal	*Dry mouth, alopecia, cheilitis, dry skin, dry mucous membranes* Increased triglycerides and cholesterol, paresthesias, rigors, arthralgia, skin peeling, pseudotumor cerebri, depression, elevated liver function tests, teratogenicity
adalimumab (Humira)	Subcutaneous: 40 mg every other week	*Upper respiratory infection, local reactions at the injection site (pain, erythema, myalgia)* Malignancies, serious infections, worsening heart failure
alefacept (Amevive)	IM: 15 mg once weekly for 12 weeks	*Nausea, vomiting, diarrhea, pharyngitis, dizziness, cough, pruritus* Malignancies, serious infection, hepatotoxicity, lymphopenia
apremilast (Otezia)	PO: Begin with 10 mg/day and increase over a 6 day period to 30 mg bid	*Diarrhea, nausea, headache* Depression, weight loss
cyclosporine (Neoral, Gengraf, Sandimmune)	PO: 1.25 mg/kg bid (max: 4 mg/kg/day)	*Hirsutism, tremor, vomiting, headache, pruritus, nausea, diarrhea* HTN, myocardial infarction (MI), nephrotoxicity, hyperkalemia, gingival enlargement, paresthesias, hepatotoxicity, infection
etanercept (Enbrel)	Subcutaneous: 50 mg twice weekly (given 3–4 days apart) Maintenance dose: 50 mg/week	*Local reactions at the injection site (pain, erythema, myalgia), abdominal pain, vomiting, nasopharyngitis* Serious infections, lupus-like syndrome, positive antinuclear antibodies, heart failure exacerbations
infliximab (Remicade)	IV: 5 mg/kg given as an induction dose at 0, 2, and 6 weeks followed by a maintenance dose of 5 mg/kg every 8 weeks thereafter	*Infections, headache, abdominal pain* Infusion-related reactions, invasive fungal infections, malignancies, hepatotoxicity, lupus-like syndrome
methotrexate (Otrexup, Rheumatrex, Trexall)	PO: 2.5–5 mg bid for three doses each week (max: 25–30 mg/week) Subcutaneous (Otrexup): 10–25 mg once weekly	*Headache, glossitis, gingivitis, mild leukopenia, nausea* Ulcerative stomatitis, myelosuppression, aplastic anemia, hepatic cirrhosis, nephrotoxicity, sudden death, pulmonary fibrosis, acute renal failure, teratogenicity
ustekinumab (Stelara)	Subcutaneous: 45–90 mg initially and 4 weeks later, followed by 45–90 mg every 12 weeks	*Nasopharyngitis, upper respiratory tract infection, headache, and fatigue* Malignancies, serious infections

Note: Italics indicate common adverse effects. Underline indicates serious adverse effects.

effective birth control for 3 years after discontinuing the drug. Many adverse effects occur frequently during therapy, including cheilitis, hair loss, dry skin, pruritus, rash, epistaxis, bleeding gums, and joint pain. The active metabolite of acitretin, etretinate (Tegison), was withdrawn from the market in 1998 due to high toxicity. The patient should refrain from drinking alcohol during acitretin therapy because this converts more of the drug to its toxic metabolite.

Apremilast (Otezia): Approved in 2014, apremilast is a newer drug approved to treat psoriatic arthritis and plaque psoriasis. The drug inhibits the enzyme phosphodiesterase-4, which results in a reduction in several different pro-inflammatory mediators. It is the first drug approved for psoriasis that acts by this mechanism.

Apremilast is considered an option for patients who have not responded to phototherapy or systemic therapy with other drugs. Patients with a history of depression, suicidal behavior, or weight loss should be monitored regularly while on apremilast therapy. This drug is pregnancy category C.

Cyclosporine (Gengraf, Neoral): Cyclosporine is an immunosuppressant that is presented as a prototype drug in Chapter 42. The drug acts by suppressing T-cell functions. It is effective at providing rapid relief from the symptoms of psoriasis and is often combined with other drugs, such as calcipotriene, to provide for a lower dose and reduced toxicity. Due to the potential for serious adverse effects such as nephrotoxicity, hepatotoxicity, and increased risk for infections and neoplasia, cyclosporine is only used for extensive psoriasis when other treatment methods have failed.

Methotrexate (Otrexup, Rheumatrex, Trexall): Methotrexate is one of the most frequently prescribed systemic drugs for severe psoriasis. An older drug approved in 1953, methotrexate is used in the treatment of a variety of disorders, including carcinomas and rheumatoid arthritis, in addition to being prescribed for psoriasis. For psoriasis, methotrexate inhibits the rapid proliferation of cells in the skin. It is administered either once weekly or bid for 3 days each week. In 2013 a new formulation of the drug, Otrexup, was approved that permits a once-weekly subcutaneous injection for patients with severe psoriasis. Improvement is noted after several weeks of therapy but maximum effects may take 2 to 3 months. For resistant lesions, methotrexate may be combined with phototherapy or alternated with other systemic drugs. Methotrexate is discussed as a prototype drug in Chapter 57.

Biologic therapies: An understanding of the role of the immune system in the pathogenesis of psoriasis has led to the use of biologic therapies to treat patients with moderate to severe disease. Biologic agents suppress the hyperactive inflammatory and immune responses characteristic of psoriasis. Approved biologic drugs include adalimumab (Humira), alefacept (Amevive), etanercept (Enbrel), infliximab (Remicade), tocilizumab (Actrema), and ustekinumab (Stelara). These medications induce general immunosuppression, and patients are at an increased risk for infection, including reactivation of latent infections such as tuberculosis. In fact, efalizumab (Raptiva) was removed from the market in 2009 due to incidences of progressive multifocal leukoencephalopathy, a rare and fatal brain infection caused by reactivation of a latent virus. Major disadvantages of biologic drugs are that they are not available in PO formulations and their annual costs may exceed $10,000 per year.

Nonpharmacologic therapy: Phototherapy with ultraviolet-A (UVA) and ultraviolet-B (UVB) light is used in cases of severe debilitating psoriasis. Phototherapy with UVA is combined with methoxsalen, a drug from a chemical family known as the psoralens.

The concurrent use of UVA and the drug is called PUVA therapy. **Psoralens** are PO or topical agents that produce a photosensitive reaction when exposed to UV light. This reaction reduces the number of psoriatic lesions, but unpleasant adverse effects such as headache, nausea, and skin sensitivity occur that may limit the effectiveness of PUVA therapy. Treatments are limited to two to three times per week, and an interim period of 48 hours between treatments is necessary. Because of the strong photosensitizing properties of the psoralens, patients must wear dark glasses during treatment and for the remainder of the day. The use of PUVA has been associated with an increased risk for cataract development.

The second type of phototherapy is with narrow-band UVB light, which is less hazardous than UVA therapy. The wavelength of UVB is similar to that of sunlight, and it reduces the lesions that cover a large area of the body that normally resist topical treatments. It is usually used in conjunction with topical coal tar. If access to a light treatment unit is not feasible, natural sunlight may be used. The use of commercial tanning beds is not recommended for the patient with psoriasis.

All UV treatments may cause acute sunburn reactions, including generalized redness with edema and tenderness as well as the development of long-term effects of actinic keratosis, premature aging of the skin, and skin cancers. Immunosuppressant drugs such as cyclosporine are not used in conjunction with PUVA therapy, because they increase the risk of skin cancer.

Pharmacotherapy of Minor Skin Burns

73.8 The pharmacotherapy of sunburn includes prevention with sunscreens and treatment with lotions, topical anesthetics, and analgesics.

Sunburn results from overexposure of the skin to UV light and is associated with light skin complexions, prolonged exposure to the sun during the more hazardous hours of the day (10 a.m. until 3 p.m.), and lack of protective clothing when outdoors. Chronic

---

CONNECTIONS | Complementary and Alternative Therapies

◄ Aloe Vera

Description
There are numerous products on the market, including soaps, lotions, creams, and sunscreens, that are aimed at the consumer who is seeking the healing properties of aloe vera gel. Health care providers have also recommended aloe vera gel to treat dermatitis, burns, and a variety of skin disorders.

History and Claims
Aloe vera is derived from the gel inside the leaf of the aloe plant, which is a member of the lily family. Aloe vera contains over 70 active substances, including antioxidants, minerals, vitamins, and enzymes. These substances are supposed to kill a variety of microorganisms, decrease pain, and reduce localized inflammation. Aloe vera also has value for its moisturizing and wound healing properties. It has been used medicinally for thousands of years. Early mention is made of aloe's use in ancient Sumaria in 2200 B.C., where it was proclaimed a plant of great healing power.

Standardization
Aloe vera has not been evaluated by the FDA for safety, effectiveness, or purity.

Evidence
Like other herbal products, controlled research studies demonstrating the effectiveness are lacking. There are some components of aloe that produce a strong laxative effect, although intense cramping may occur, and the drug is not recommended for this indication (National Center for Complementary and Alternative Medicine, 2012). The antimicrobial actions of aloe vera extracts have been clearly demonstrated (Stanley, Ifeanyi, & Eziokwu, 2014). A meta-analysis of seven clinical trials could not find convincing evidence that the application of topical aloe vera improved healing of acute or chronic wounds (Dat, Poon, Pham, & Doust, 2012). Until more rigorous clinical trials have been conducted, nurses should advise patients wanting to use aloe vera, particularly the PO form, to discuss its use with their health care provider.

sun exposure can result in serious conditions, including eye injury, cataracts, and skin cancer.

Minor, first-degree burns affect only the outer layers of the epidermis. Excessive exposure to UV light, however, injures the dermis and dilates the capillaries, leading to redness, tenderness, edema, and occasional blister formation. In addition to producing local skin damage, sun overexposure releases toxins that may produce systemic effects. The signs and symptoms of sunburn include erythema, intense pain, nausea, vomiting, chills, edema, and headache. These symptoms usually resolve within a matter of hours or days, depending on the severity of the exposure. Once sunburn has occurred, medications can only alleviate the symptoms; they do not speed recovery time.

The best treatment for sunburn is prevention. Sunscreens are liquids or lotions applied for chemical or physical protection. Chemical sunscreens absorb the spectrum of UV light that is responsible for most sunburns. Chemical sunscreens include those that contain benzophenone for protection against UVA rays; those that work against UVB rays include cinnamates, p-aminobenzoic acid (PABA), and salicylates. Physical sunscreens such as zinc oxide, talc, and titanium dioxide reflect or scatter light to prevent the penetration of both UVA and UVB rays. Parsol is another sunscreen product that is being used more frequently as a key ingredient in lip balm.

The effectiveness of a sunscreen is indicated by its SPF. An SPF of 8 means the product offers eight times more protection than using no sunscreen. Patients with skin that sunburns easily should use products with an SPF of 15 or greater. Waterproof sunscreens are meant to withstand 8 minutes of exposure to water. People tend to apply sunscreen too infrequently and in layers that are too thin. To be effective, sunscreen must be applied generously and often during the exposure period.

Treatment for sunburn consists of addressing symptoms with soothing lotions, rest, prevention of dehydration, and topical anesthetics, if needed. Treatment is usually done on an outpatient basis. Topical anesthetics for minor burns include benzocaine (Solarcaine), dibucaine (Nupercainal), lidocaine (Xylocaine), and tetracaine HCl (Pontocaine). Aloe vera is a popular natural therapy for minor skin irritations and burns. Hydrocortisone cream may decrease pain and swelling and assist in the healing of damaged tissue. These same agents may also provide relief from minor pain due to insect bites and pruritus. In more severe cases, PO analgesics and anti-inflammatory agents such as aspirin or ibuprofen may be indicated.

| PROTOTYPE DRUG | **Benzocaine (Americaine, Anbesol, Others)** |

Classification: Therapeutic: Topical anesthetic
Pharmacologic: Local anesthetic (ester type), antipruritic

Therapeutic Effects and Uses: Approved in 1938, benzocaine inhibits the conduction of nerve impulses from sensory nerve endings, producing surface anesthesia. It is indicated for the temporary relief of pain and discomfort in patients with pruritic skin problems, minor burns and wounds, and insect bites. It is available in a variety of delivery forms, including sprays, lotions, gels, and lozenges. Several products are available OTC to treat pain

due to toothaches, dentures, or canker sores. Because of its short duration of action, it must be applied three to four times a day.

Mechanism of Action: Benzocaine produces surface anesthesia by inhibiting the conduction of nerve endings.

Pharmacokinetics:

Route(s)	Topical
Absorption	Minimally absorbed from intact skin
Distribution	Unknown
Primary metabolism	Hepatic
Primary excretion	Renal
Onset of action	1 min
Duration of action	15–20 min

Adverse Effects: Adverse effects include sensitization in susceptible individuals, allergic reactions, and anaphylaxis. Because it is poorly absorbed, systemic adverse effects are rarely observed.

Contraindications/Precautions: Contraindications include hypersensitivity to benzocaine or other PABA derivatives or to any of the components in the formulation. Caution should be used in patients with a history of drug sensitivity to ester-type anesthetics, denuded skin, or severely traumatized mucosa, and in children under 6 years.

Drug Interactions: Benzocaine may antagonize the antibacterial activity of sulfonamides.

Pregnancy: Category C.

Treatment of Overdose: Overdose with topical benzocaine is unlikely.

Nursing Responsibilities:

- Assess the sunburn, including the location, portion of body surface area, edema, erythema, and blistering.

- Assess for systemic symptoms such as fever, chills, weakness, and shock. These may occur following severe exposure, or when the sunburn affects a large portion of the body surface area.

- Obtain a thorough history, including sunburn and tanning history, the amount of time the patient usually spends in the sun, how easily the patient burns, and the type of sun protection used. If the patient uses a sunscreen, obtain the SPF rating.

- Obtain an allergy history and use of OTC products or home remedies to treat the sunburn.

- If topical anesthetics or ointments are ordered, assess the skin for secondary infections for which these medications are contraindicated.

- For patients using the medication for the first time, conduct a trial application on a small area of skin to assess for an allergic reaction. If no adverse effects occur within 30 to 60 minutes, the medication may be applied to the entire area of sunburn.

- Report any serious sunburn in children under age 6 to the health care provider.

Lifespan and Diversity Considerations:

- The drug should not be used for children under 1 year of age except on direction of the health care provider.

Patient and Family Education:

- Avoid applying the medication to open or infected areas of skin.

- Report severe, persistent pain.

- Avoid additional sun exposure while receiving treatment.

- Prevent sunburn in the future by wearing protective clothing such as long-sleeved shirts and large-brim hats, and by using sunscreen with an SPF of 15 or greater.

- Follow the directions regarding use and reapplication of sunscreen after swimming or sweating.

- Refrigerate topical lotions so they will provide a soothing, cooling effect when applied.

- Increase hydration after sunburning to aid in cooling the skin. Avoid excessive cool bathing, which may dry the skin further.

- Do not apply benzocaine to infants and young children.

Drugs Similar to Benzocaine (Americaine, Anbesol, Others)

Benzocaine is the only drug in its class that is used for minor burns.

Pharmacotherapy of Alopecia

73.9 Several drugs are able to stimulate moderate hair regrowth in patients with male- and female-pattern alopecia.

Alopecia is the loss of hair, resulting in baldness. Male-pattern baldness is the most common cause of hair loss in men and is genetically determined. Males affected by this type of alopecia typically experience a loss of hair at the temples, followed by a recession of the hairline and baldness at the crown.

Two drugs are currently available to promote hair regrowth in patients with male-pattern baldness: topical minoxidil (Rogaine) and PO finasteride (Propecia, Proscar). Neither drug was originally developed for baldness. Although their exact mechanisms of action are unknown, it is thought that these drugs work by stimulating the epithelial cells within the hair follicle. They are most successful in patients with recent onset of symptoms or who are less than 50 years of age. About 40% of patients who are treated two to three times daily for a year will experience moderate regrowth of hair. For both drugs, hair regrowth stops when the drug is discontinued.

Female hair loss differs from hair loss in males and varies by ethnicity. A common type of alopecia in Caucasian women, female-pattern hair loss, typically begins in the early 20s and 30s, with progressive thinning and loss of hair on the top of the scalp but not the back. These females typically do not have a receding hairline. The hair also becomes finer as individual hairs become smaller, resulting in less dense hair. Some females with this pattern of hair loss may have elevated androgen levels or diabetes that requires treatment. Topical minoxidil is currently the only hair regrowth treatment approved for women by the U.S. Food and Drug Administration (FDA). Applied to the scalp twice daily, it stimulates hairs that are actively growing to have more robust growth.

Women of African descent have a different type of alopecia called central centrifugal alopecia. This type also results in hair loss on the top of the scalp, but it is different from the female-pattern hair loss in that the hair follicles are destroyed. Topical minoxidil is used in this group to stimulate growth in the unaffected hair follicles, whereas anti-inflammatory medications are used to decrease the destruction of the hair follicles.

CONNECTIONS | Treating the Diverse Patient

❰ Not All Skin Reactions Are Alike

Dermatologic symptoms are sometimes caused by systemic reactions to medications. Some reactions, while annoying or distressing to the patient, are self-limiting and benign. Other reactions may be severe and potentially life-threatening. While all dermatologic symptoms that may signal potential systemic drug reactions should be reported, benign reactions may have significant differences than more severe ones (Treat, 2012):

- Benign reactions tend to be maculopapular or "measles-like," itchy, blanch upon pressure, and do not involve mucous membranes. No fever is associated with these reactions and they tend to occur 5 to 10 days after the first exposure (dose) of a drug. If the drug is vital to treatment, providers may opt to continue the medication as long as a fever is not present, because the reaction tends to be self-limiting.

- Drug-induced hypersensitivity syndrome reactions have dermatologic symptoms but include systemic involvement. Although a reaction of this type may occur more quickly, these reactions tend to occur 2 to 6 weeks after a drug is started. A measles-like rash, facial edema, fever, mucous membrane involvement, and a general feeling of malaise occur. Other causes such as viral infections must be ruled out, and stopping the drug therapy and possible treatment with corticosteroids may be needed.

- Stevens–Johnson syndrome (SJS) and toxic epidermal necrosis (TEN) are severe dermatologic reactions with systemic involvement. These reactions are almost consistently related to drug reactions, and pharmacotherapy is stopped and aggressive treatment required to prevent complications. Skin necrosis, including of mucous membranes, can occur.

- Acute generalized exanthematous pustulosis is a reaction most often caused by antibiotics that results in multiple pustular eruptions that become generalized, causing skin sloughing. Pharmacotherapy that may be causing the reaction must be stopped, and treatments with corticosteroids and antihistamines are often needed.

- Drug-induced systemic lupus erythematosus is a relatively rare drug reaction that causes symptoms similar to the actual disease condition. Plaques on the trunk and arms rather than on the face may be present, and the offending drug should be stopped, with possible corticosteroid treatment considered.

Any suspicious skin reaction should be reported to the health care provider. Certain drug classes are known to have a higher incidence of dermatologic reactions than others, including antibiotics, cardiovascular drugs (e.g., CCBs, hydralazine, procainamide), and CNS drugs (e.g., carbamazepine, lamotrigene, phenytoin). Evaluating the extent of systemic involvement (e.g., mucous membrane involvement, fever, presence or absence of other systemic symptoms), the time since drug therapy began, and whether a drug that is known to be at high risk for causing skin and systemic reactions may be the cause, should also be considered.

Minoxidil (Rogaine): Oral minoxidil (Loniten) was first approved for HTN in 1979. Approval to market the topical solution for hair loss occurred in 1996. The drug is rubbed onto the scalp twice daily. Although the drug is a potent vasodilator, this mechanism is likely not involved in its effectiveness as a hair regrowth agent. The exact mechanism of action is unknown. Only 2% of a topical dose is absorbed systemically; therefore, this route does not affect blood pressure. Various brands of minoxidil include 2% Rogaine for Women, 2% Rogaine for Men Regular Strength, and 5% Rogaine for Men Extra Strength. An off-label use is to treat chemotherapy-induced alopecia. Response rates vary and over half of patients treated do not experience significant regrowth. In patients who are receiving chemotherapy, hair regrowth occurs at a faster rate with minoxidil use. The drug has no significant adverse effects. This drug is pregnancy category C. Caution should be taken to keep the solution out of the reach of children. One teaspoon of the solution contains the amount of a daily adult antihypertensive dose.

Finasteride (Propecia, Proscar): Proscar was approved for benign prostatic hyperplasia (BPH) in 1992. Propecia was later approved to treat male-pattern baldness in 1997. The dose used for treating BPH is five times higher than that used for baldness. Unlike minoxidil, finasteride is a PO medication. This drug is thought to act by reducing the amounts of dihydroxytestosterone (DHT) in hair follicles, thus slowing hair loss. It is less effective than minoxidil at promoting hair regrowth. At the low doses used for hair regrowth, adverse effects are uncommon. It is not approved for use in women. This drug is pregnancy category X. Pregnant women should not touch this drug because it may harm a male fetus if absorbed.

CONNECTION Checkpoint 73.4

From what you learned in Chapter 71, describe the mechanism by which finasteride reduces symptoms of BPH. *See Answer to Connection Checkpoint 73.4 on student resource website.*

CHAPTER

73

Understanding the Chapter

Key Concepts Summary

73.1 Three layers of skin, known as the epidermis, dermis, and subcutaneous layers, provide effective barrier defenses for the body.

73.2 The etiology of skin disorders may be classified as infectious, inflammatory, or neoplastic.

73.3 When the integrity of the skin is compromised, microbes can gain entrance and cause infections that require anti-infective therapy.

73.4 Scabicides and pediculicides are used to treat parasitic skin infestations.

73.5 The pharmacotherapy of acne includes treatment with benzoyl peroxide, retinoids, and antibiotics; pharmacotherapy for rosacea includes retinoids and metronidazole.

73.6 The most effective treatment for dermatitis is topical corticosteroids, which are classified by their potency.

73.7 Psoriasis is a chronic, inflammatory disease that is treated with topical and systemic medications.

73.8 The pharmacotherapy of sunburn includes prevention with sunscreens and treatment with lotions, topical anesthetics, and analgesics.

73.9 Several drugs are able to stimulate moderate hair regrowth in patients with male- and female-pattern alopecia.

Case Study: Making the Patient Connection

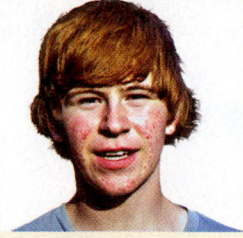

Remember the patient "Danny McBride" at the beginning of the chapter? Now read the remainder of the case study. Based on the information presented within this chapter, respond to the critical thinking questions that follow.

Danny McBride is a 17-year-old high school student in his senior year. He is active in lacrosse and baseball but is finding that his skin is breaking out more often lately and is becoming discouraged at the increase. He feels it has started to affect his social life and his parents make an appointment with a dermatologist. The health care provider diagnoses Danny's skin condition as acne vulgaris and prescribes tretinoin (Retin-A).

Critical Thinking Questions

1. What would you tell Danny about his condition? Include what acne is, who is prone to develop it, and what methods of treatment have been found to be beneficial.

2. What are some reasons why Danny's acne outbreaks may have increased at this time?

3. What will you teach Danny about the application of tretinoin and adverse effects that may occur?

See Answers to Critical Thinking Questions on student resource website.

Additional Case Study

Stephanie Caldera, age 36, is seen by her provider for scaling patches on her forearms, elbows, and lower legs. She is diagnosed with psoriasis vulgaris and the provider prescribes betamethasone cream (Diprosone). Stephanie asks the nurse, "What is psoriasis? I look so awful! Is it contagious?"

1. How should the nurse respond?

2. What specific instructions should Stephanie be given about the application of the betamethasone cream?

3. Stephanie's psoriasis has not been responsive to betamethasone and she is prescribed calcipotriene (Dovonex). What teaching does Stephanie receive about this new prescription?

See Answers to Additional Case Study on student resource website.

Chapter Review

1 An important inclusion in a teaching plan prepared for the patient who is taking permethrin (Nix) is:

1. Nix can be applied after body lotion is applied.
2. All body hair, including eyelashes and eyebrows, can be treated with lindane.
3. Lice cannot live outside the body.
4. In addition to hair shafts, examine the inner thigh areas, gluteal folds, and pubic areas for lice.

2 A patient is being treated with a course of topical desoximetasone (Topicort) for atopic dermatitis. In planning teaching for this patient, which adverse effects would the nurse anticipate?

1. Burning and stinging of the skin in the affected area
2. Development of localized pruritus and hives
3. Hair loss in the application area
4. Worsening of acne vulgaris

3 The patient reports using benzoyl peroxide (Benzac) for treatment of acne. The nurse notes that the action of this drug includes which of the following? Select all that apply.

1. Sebum suppression
2. Antimicrobial effect
3. Keratolytic effect
4. Microdermal abrasion
5. Sunscreen activity

4 A patient has been prescribed topical tretinoin (Retin-A) for treatment of acne unresponsive to over-the-counter products. What essential information should the nurse include in the patient's teaching?

1. Wash the face thoroughly three times a day with an antiacne soap while using this medication.
2. Plan to expose the involved skin areas to sunlight for a minimum of 15 minutes each day.
3. Use only mild soaps, warm water, and pat the skin dry to avoid excessive irritation.
4. Alternate the topical tretinoin (Retin-A) with benzoyl peroxide on an every-other-day rotation for best results.

5 Benzocaine (Americaine) has been recommended to a 17-year-old patient for treatment of a mild sunburn. What should the patient be taught about using this product?

1. It may be used on superficial and partial-thickness sunburns.

2. Warming the lotion under warm water will prevent a chilled sensation when applied.

3. A small test area should be used if the drug has not been used before to assess for allergy.

4. Cover the treated area with a light dressing wrapped in plastic wrap to keep it from rubbing off.

6 A patient who has been prescribed isotretinoin (Accutane) must comply with the iPledge Program because of the risk of _____ effects.

See Answers to Chapter Review in Appendix A.

References

American Academy of Allergy, Asthma and Immunology. (n.d.). *Allergy statistics.* Retrieved from http://www.aaaai.org/about-the-aaaai/newsroom/allergy-statistics.aspx

Dat, A. D., Poon, F., Pham, K. B., & Doust, J. (2012). Aloe vera for treating acute and chronic wounds. *Cochrane Database of Systematic Reviews, 2*, CD008762. doi:10.1002/14651858.CD008762.pub2

National Center for Complementary and Alternative Medicine. (2012). *Aloe vera.* Retrieved from http://nccam.nih.gov/health/aloevera

National Psoriasis Foundation. (2014). *Facts about psoriasis.* Retrieved from http://www.psoriasis.org/learn_forteens_facts

Stanley, M. C., Ifeanyi, O. E., & Eziokwu, O. G. (2014). Antimicrobial effects of aloe vera on some human pathogens. *International Journal of Current Microbiology and Applied Science, 3*(3), 1022–1028.

Treat, J. R. (2012). Skin signs of severe systemic medication reactions. *Current Problems in Pediatric and Adolescent Health Care, 42*(8), 193–197. doi:10.1016/j.cppeds.2012.02.001

Wehner, M. R., Shive, M. L., Chren, M. M., Han, J., Qureshi, A. A., & Linos, E. (2012). Indoor tanning and non-melanoma skin cancer: Systematic review and meta-analysis. *BMJ: British Medical Journal, 345*, e5909. doi:10.1136/bmj.e5909

Selected Bibliography

Baldwin, H. E. (2012). Diagnosis and treatment of rosacea: State of the art. *Journal of Drugs in Dermatology, 11*(6), 725–730.

Banasikowska, A. K. (2013). *Rosacea.* Retrieved from http://emedicine.medscape.com/article/1071429-overview

Del Rosso, J. Q., Thiboutot, D., Gallo, R., Webster, G., Tanghetti, E., Eichenfield, L., … Zaenglein, A. (2013). Consensus recommendations from the American Acne & Rosacea Society on the management of rosacea, part 2: A status report on topical agents. *Cutis, 92*(6), 277–284.

Rao, J. (2014). *Acne vulgaris.* Retrieved from http://emedicine.medscape.com/article/1069804-overview

Hall, B. J., & Hall, J. C. (2010). *Sauer's manual of skin diseases* (10th ed.). Philadelphia, PA: Lippincott, Williams & Wilkins.

Herdman, T. H., & Kamitsuru, S. (Eds.). (2014). *NANDA International nursing diagnoses:*

Definitions and classification, 2015-2017. Oxford, United Kingdom: Wiley-Blackwell.

Meffert, J. (2014). *Psoriasis.* Retrieved from http://emedicine.medscape.com/article/1943419-overview

Rahman, M., Alam, K., Zaki Ahmad, M., Gupta, G., Afzal, M., Akhter, S., … Anwar, F. (2012). Classical to current approach for treatment of psoriasis: A review. *Endocrine, Metabolic & Immune Disorders-Drug Targets, 12*(3), 287–302. doi:10.2174/187153012802002901

Ring, J., Alomar, A., Bieber, T., Deleuran, M., Fink-Wagner, A., Gelmetti, C., … Darsow, U. (2012). Guidelines for treatment of atopic eczema (atopic dermatitis) part I. *Journal of the European Academy of Dermatology and Venereology, 26*, 1045–1060. doi:10.1111/j.1468-3083.2012.04635.x

Roebuck, H. (2011). Treatment options for rosacea with concomitant conditions. *Nurse*

Practitioner, 36(2), 24–31. doi:10.1097/01.NPR.0000392794.17007.36

Rustin, M. H. A. (2012). Long-term safety of biologics in the treatment of moderate-to-severe plaque psoriasis: Review of current data. *British Journal of Dermatology, 167*(Suppl. 3), 3–11. doi:10.1111/j.1365-2133.2012.11208.x

Samarasekera, E. J., Sawyer, L., Wonderling, D., Tucker, R., & Smith, C. H. (2013). Topical therapies for the treatment of plaque psoriasis: Systematic review and network meta-analyses. *British Journal of Dermatology, 168*, 954–967. doi:10.1111/bjd.12276

Williams, H. C., Dellavalle, R. P., & Garner, S. (2012). Acne vulgaris. *The Lancet, 379*(9813), 361–372. doi:10.1016/S0140-6736(11)60321-8

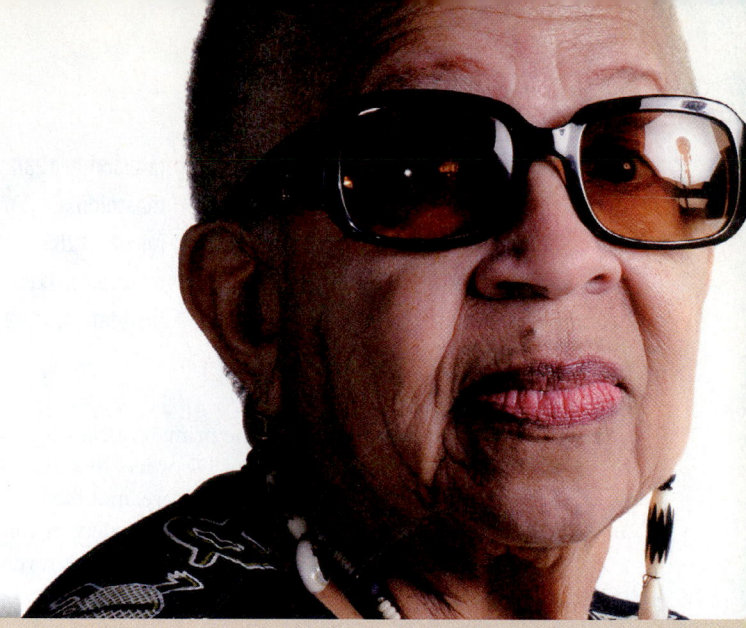

"*I just cannot see clearly while driving at nighttime anymore. All I see are halos around the other cars' headlights.*"

Patient "Therese Duclos"

LEARNING OUTCOMES

After reading this chapter, the student should be able to:

1. Identify the major anatomic structures of the eye.
2. Identify the primary risk factors associated with glaucoma.
3. Compare and contrast open-angle and closed-angle glaucoma.
4. Explain the two major mechanisms by which drugs reduce intraocular pressure.
5. Describe the nurse's role in the nonpharmacologic and pharmacologic management of eye and ear disorders.
6. For each of the classes shown in the chapter outline, identify the prototype and representative drugs and explain the mechanism(s) of drug action, primary indications, contraindications, significant drug interactions, pregnancy category, and important adverse effects.
7. Identify examples of drugs that dilate or constrict pupils, relax ciliary muscles, constrict ocular blood vessels, or moisten eye membranes.
8. Identify the types of ear conditions that could benefit from pharmacotherapy.
9. Apply the nursing process to the care of patients who are receiving pharmacotherapy for eye and ear disorders.

CHAPTER OUTLINE

▶ Anatomy of the Eye
▶ Pathophysiology of Glaucoma
▶ Pharmacotherapy of Glaucoma
   Prostaglandins
   PROTOTYPE Latanoprost (Xalatan), *p. 1287*
   Autonomic Drugs
   PROTOTYPE Timolol (Betimol, Timoptic, Others), *p. 1290*
   Miscellaneous Drugs for Glaucoma
   Carbonic Anhydrase Inhibitors
   Osmotic Diuretics
▶ Pharmacotherapy for Eye Examinations
   Anticholinergics
   Sympathomimetics
▶ Pharmacotherapy for Other Eye Conditions
   Lubricants
   Vasoconstrictors
▶ Anatomy of the Ear
▶ Pharmacotherapy with Otic Preparations
   Antibiotics
   Cerumenolytics

KEY TERMS

aqueous humor, 1285

cerumenolytics, 1297

closed-angle glaucoma, 1286

cycloplegics, 1292

external otitis, 1295

glaucoma, 1286

mastoiditis, 1297

miosis, 1289

mydriasis, 1289

mydriatics, 1292

open-angle glaucoma, 1286

otitis interna, 1297

otitis media, 1296

tonometry, 1286

The senses of vision and hearing are the primary means for us to communicate with the world around us. Disorders that affect the eye and ear can result in problems with self-care, mobility, safety, and communication. The eye is vulnerable to a variety of conditions, many of which can be prevented, controlled, or reversed with proper pharmacotherapy. The first part of this chapter covers drugs that are used for the treatment of glaucoma and those used routinely by ophthalmic health care providers. The remaining part of this chapter presents drugs that are used for the treatment of common ear disorders, including infections, inflammation, and the buildup of earwax.

Anatomy of the Eye

74.1 Knowledge of basic eye anatomy is fundamental to understanding eye disorders and their pharmacotherapy.

Knowledge of basic ocular anatomy is required to understand eye disorders and their pharmacotherapy. The important structures of the eye are shown in Figures 74.1 and 74.2.

The wall of the eye contains three layers, known as tunics. The outermost fibrous tunic is composed of the cornea and the sclera. The cornea is the transparent layer that covers the anterior portion part of the eye. It has no blood vessels and receives nutrients from

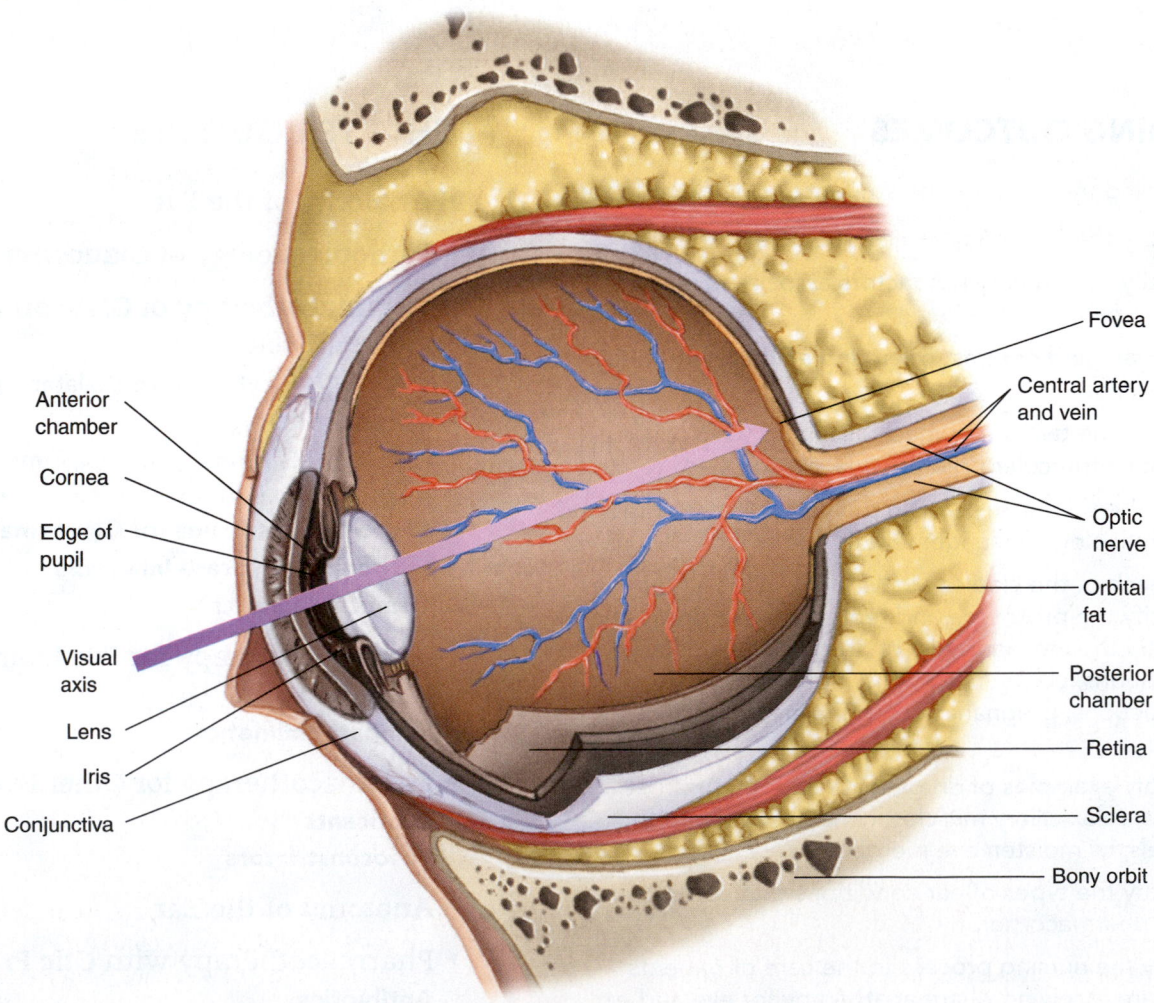

Figure 74.1 Anatomy of the interior of the eye.

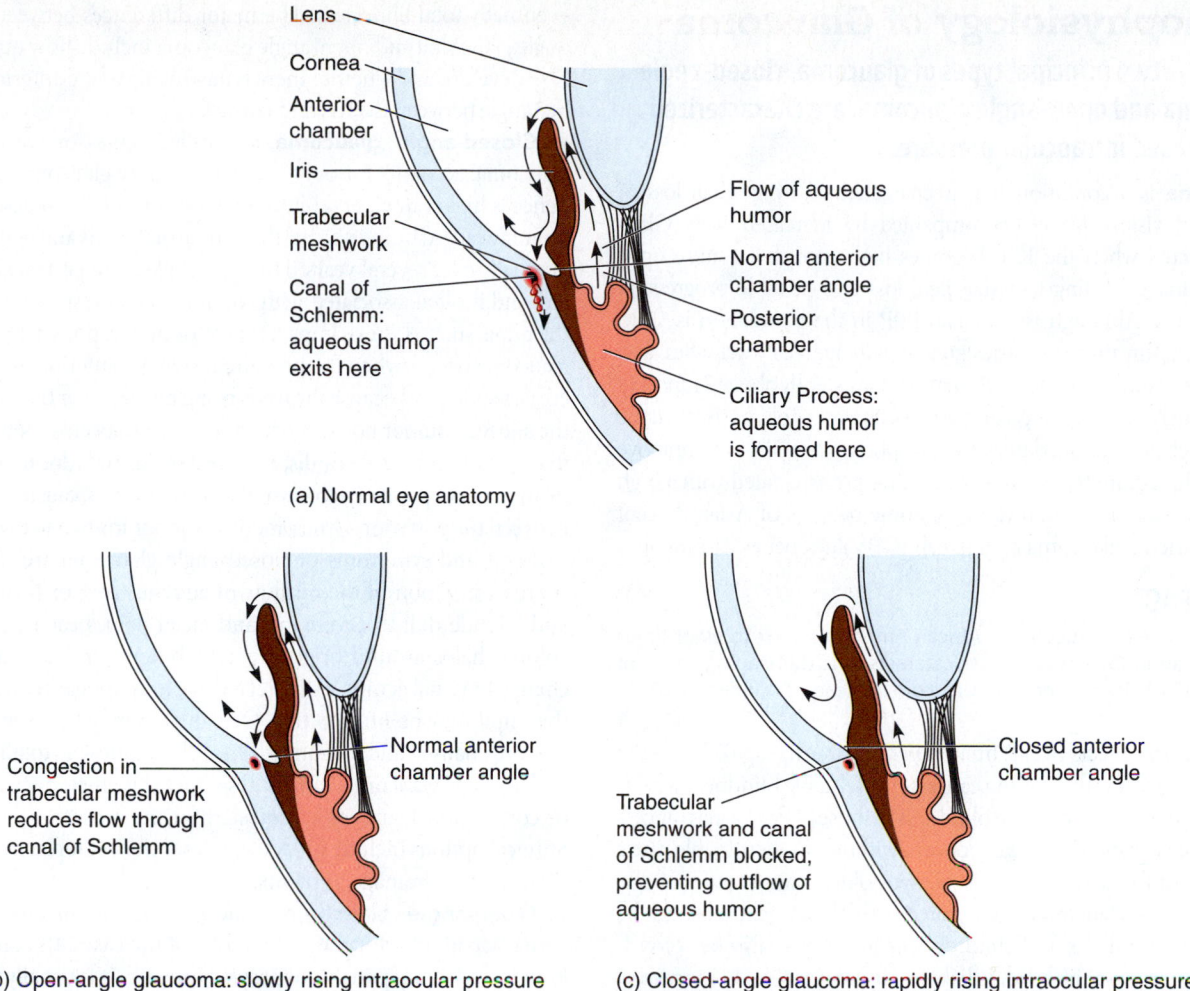

Figure 74.2 (a) In a healthy eye, aqueous humor is formed in the ciliary process and drains through the canal of Schlemm. (b) In chronic open-angle glaucoma, the anterior chamber angle remains open, but drainage of aqueous humor through the canal of Schlemm is impaired. (c) In acute closed-angle glaucoma, the angle of the iris and anterior chamber narrows, obstructing the drainage of aqueous humor through the canal of Schlemm.

the fluid lying behind the cornea, or aqueous humor. It is continuous with the sclera, which is the thick, white, opaque portion covering the posterior portion of the eye. The vascular tunic is the middle layer of the eye, which is rich in blood vessels. The vascular tunic contains specialized structures that include the iris and ciliary body. The innermost layer is the neural tunic or retina, which contains the photoreceptors for vision.

The interior of the eye is divided into two cavities. The largest portion of the interior of the eye is the posterior cavity, which is filled with a gel-like substance called vitreous humor that helps the eyeball to maintain its shape and keep the retina in place.

The anterior cavity is smaller but is very important from a pharmacologic perspective. This cavity is separated into two chambers by the lens. The anterior chamber extends from the cornea to the iris; the posterior chamber lies between the iris and the lens. In front of the lens is the pigmented iris, which is made up of smooth muscle fibers that change the diameter of the pupil. The pupil is the central opening that allows light to enter. These muscle fibers are under control of the sympathetic nervous system. Pupil constriction is the result of parasympathetic stimulation, and its dilation is a sympathetic response.

The anterior cavity is filled with a thin fluid called **aqueous humor** that slowly circulates to bring nutrients to the area and remove wastes. The aqueous humor is secreted by cells in a muscular structure called the ciliary body. Once secreted, the aqueous humor flows from the posterior chamber through the pupil and into the anterior chamber. Within the anterior chamber and around the periphery is a network of spongy connective tissue, or trabecular meshwork, that contains an opening called the canal of Schlemm (scleral venous sinus). The aqueous humor drains into the canal of Schlemm and out of the anterior chamber into the venous system, thus completing its circulation. Under normal circumstances, the rate of aqueous humor production is equal to its outflow, maintaining intraocular pressure (IOP) within a normal range. Interference with either the production or outflow of aqueous humor, however, can lead to an increase in IOP.

The conjunctiva, eyebrows, eyelashes, eyelids, and lacrimal apparatus that produce tears all serve to protect the eye. Infection and inflammatory responses are common conditions in these supporting structures. Redness, edema, and itching are common symptoms.

Pathophysiology of Glaucoma

74.2 The two principal types of glaucoma, closed-angle glaucoma and open-angle glaucoma, are characterized by increased intraocular pressure.

Glaucoma is a condition that is characterized by gradual loss of peripheral vision, usually accompanied by increased IOP. Glaucoma occurs when the IOP becomes high enough to cause optic nerve damage, leading to visual field loss and possible progression to blindness. Although the median IOP in the population is 15 to 16 mmHg, this pressure varies greatly with age, daily activities, and even time of day. As a rule, IOPs that are consistently above 21 mmHg are considered abnormal. Many patients, however, tolerate IOPs in the mid to high 20s without damage to the optic nerve. IOPs that are above 30 mmHg require treatment because they are associated with a high risk for permanent vision changes. Some patients of Asian descent may experience glaucoma at "normal" IOP values, below 21 mmHg.

PharmFACT

The incidence of glaucoma in African Americans is six to eight times higher than in Caucasians. After cataracts, it is the leading cause of blindness in African Americans (Glaucoma Research Foundation, 2011).

Glaucoma affects over 2 million people over the age of 40 in the United States. It is the leading cause of preventable blindness worldwide and the leading cause of blindness in those of Far Eastern ancestry. Primary glaucoma usually occurs without an identifiable cause and is most frequently found in persons older than 60 years of age. In some cases, glaucoma is associated with genetic factors; it can be congenital in infants and children. Glaucoma can also be secondary to eye trauma, infection, diabetes, inflammation, hemorrhage, tumor, or cataracts. Some medications may contribute to the development or progression of glaucoma, including the long-term use of corticosteroids, some antihypertensives, antihistamines, and antidepressants. Other major risk factors associated with glaucoma include hypertension (HTN), migraine headaches, refractive disorders with high degrees of nearsightedness or farsightedness, and normal aging.

Diagnosis of glaucoma can be difficult because it sometimes occurs so gradually that patients do not experience symptoms or seek medical attention until late in the disease process. **Tonometry** is a primary ophthalmic technique that tests for glaucoma by measuring IOP. Patients with unusually thick or thin corneas may have false negatives or false positives during tonometry. Patients who have had Lasik surgery, which removes corneal tissue to correct myopia, may appear to have normal IOPs, yet have glaucoma. Gonioscopy uses a gonioscope to measure the depth of the anterior chamber and is useful in distinguishing between open-angle and closed-angle glaucoma. Visual field testing assesses the degree of central visual field narrowing and peripheral vision loss. Funduscopic exams look at retinal field changes that accompany glaucoma.

The two major types of primary glaucoma are closed-angle glaucoma and open-angle glaucoma, as shown in Figure 74.2. Both disorders result from the same problem: a buildup of aqueous humor in the anterior cavity. This buildup is caused either by an excessive production of aqueous humor or by a blockage of its outflow. In either case, IOP increases, leading to progressive damage to the optic nerve. As the optic nerve degenerates, the patient will first notice a loss of visual field, then a loss of central visual acuity, and

eventually total blindness. The major differences between closed-angle glaucoma and open-angle glaucoma include how quickly the IOP develops and whether there is narrowing of the anterior chamber angle between the iris and cornea.

Closed-angle glaucoma, also called acute- or narrow-angle glaucoma, accounts for only 5% of all primary glaucoma. The incidence is higher in older adults and in persons of Asian descent. It is typically caused by the normal thickening of the lens and may develop gradually over several years. This type of glaucoma is usually unilateral and is often associated with conditions that result in dilation of the pupil, such as stress, impact injury, or medications. Closed-angle glaucoma occurs when the pressure inside the anterior chamber increases suddenly because the iris is being pushed over the area where the aqueous humor normally drains into the trabecular network and the canal of Schlemm. The displacement of the iris is due in part to the dilation of the pupil or accommodation of the lens, causing the angle between the posterior cornea and the anterior iris to narrow or close.

Signs and symptoms of closed-angle glaucoma are caused by acute obstruction of the outflow of aqueous humor from the eye and include dull to severe eye and facial pain, headaches, seeing colored halos around bright lights, a bulging iris, and a sudden change in visual acuity. The affected eye may appear reddened and the pupil may be nonreactive. Ocular pain may be so severe that it causes nausea and vomiting. Once the outflow is totally closed, closed-angle glaucoma constitutes a medical emergency and laser or conventional surgery is indicated for the preservation of sight. Surgical options include iridectomy, laser trabeculoplasty, trabeculectomy, and drainage implants.

Open-angle glaucoma is the most common type of glaucoma, accounting for more than 90% of the cases. Its cause is not known and many patients are asymptomatic. It is usually bilateral, with the elevated IOP developing over years. Open-angle glaucoma is named as such because the anterior chamber angle is normal; the iris does not completely cover the trabecular meshwork and canal of Schlemm. They remain open with their flow being partially obstructed. This leads to the gradual development of increased IOP with slow degeneration of the optic nerve, resulting in a gradual loss of vision. Most patients with open-angle glaucoma can be successfully treated with medications.

Pharmacotherapy of Glaucoma

74.3 The primary goal of glaucoma pharmacotherapy is to prevent damage to the optic nerve by lowering intraocular pressure.

When glaucoma is diagnosed and treated early in the course of the disease, permanent vision disability can usually be prevented. Some health care providers initiate pharmacotherapy in all patients with an IOP greater than 21 mmHg. Because of the expense of pharmacotherapy and potential adverse drug effects, other health care providers will instead carefully monitor the patient through regular follow-up exams and wait until the IOP rises to 28 to 30 mmHg before initiating treatment. If signs of optic nerve damage or visual field changes are evident, the patient is treated regardless of the IOP.

Once pharmacotherapy has been initiated, reevaluation is performed after 2 to 4 months to assess for therapeutic effectiveness. Some of the antiglaucoma drugs take 6 to 8 weeks to reach peak effect.

If the therapeutic goals are not achieved with a single agent, it is common to add a second drug from a different class to the regimen to produce an additive decrease in IOP. Some of the agents may continue to have effects on the eye for 2 to 4 weeks after being discontinued.

Maintaining patient adherence with the medication regimen is a key factor in preventing progressive vision impairment. It is essential for the nurse to determine any factors that could decrease adherence, such as insufficient financial resources, lack of knowledge about the disease, inability to properly instill the medication, or difficulty remembering the dosing schedule. The patient diagnosed with glaucoma may experience fear and anxiety about potential blindness and disability. Accurate and thorough teaching for the patient and family or caregiver should be directed at how the disease can be managed with the correct use of the medications.

Many drugs are available to treat glaucoma. These agents work by one of two mechanisms: increasing the outflow of aqueous humor at the canal of Schlemm or decreasing the formation of aqueous humor at the ciliary body. Many antiglaucoma agents produce these effects by modifying actions of the autonomic nervous system.

Although topical drugs are most commonly prescribed, oral (PO) medications may be used for severe glaucoma. Agents for glaucoma, which are listed in Table 74.1, include the following classes:

- Prostaglandins
- Autonomic agents, including beta-adrenergic blockers, nonselective sympathomimetics, alpha$_2$-adrenergic agonists, and cholinergic agonists
- Carbonic anhydrase inhibitors
- Osmotic diuretics

74.4 Prostaglandin analogs are the first-line drugs for treating high intraocular pressure because of their long durations of action and high safety profiles.

Prostaglandin analogs are often the preferred drugs for glaucoma because they have long durations of action, allowing for once-daily dosing, and produce fewer adverse effects than the beta-adrenergic blockers. They may be used as monotherapy or combined with drugs from other classes to produce an additive reduction in IOP in patients with resistant glaucoma.

Prostaglandin analogs lower IOP by increasing the outflow of aqueous humor. Latanoprost (Xalatan), which is available as a 0.005% eyedrop solution, is one of the most commonly used prostaglandin analogs. Several newer ocular prostaglandins include bimatoprost (Lumigan) and travoprost (Travatan). An occasional adverse effect of these medications is heightened pigmentation, which turns a blue iris to a more brown color. Many patients experience thicker and longer eyelashes. These drugs cause local irritation, stinging of the eyes, and redness during the first month of therapy. Because of these effects, prostaglandins are normally administered just before bedtime.

PROTOTYPE DRUG | **Latanoprost (Xalatan)**

Classification: Therapeutic: Drug for glaucoma
Pharmacologic: Prostaglandin analog

Therapeutic Effects and Uses: Approved in 1996, latanoprost is a prostaglandin analog believed to reduce IOP by increasing the outflow of aqueous humor for patients with open-angle glaucoma and ocular HTN. The recommended dose is one drop in the affected eye(s) in the evening. It is used to treat open-angle glaucoma.

Mechanism of Action: Latanoprost reduces elevated IOP in patients with open-angle glaucoma. Latanoprost is a prodrug that is metabolized to its active form in the cornea, reaching its peak effect in about 12 hours.

Pharmacokinetics:

Route(s)	Ophthalmic solution
Absorption	Through the cornea
Distribution	Enters systemic distribution in small amounts
Primary metabolism	Metabolized in the aqueous humor to its active form
Primary excretion	Renal
Onset of action	3–4 h with peak effect at 8–12 h
Duration of action	Unknown

Adverse Effects: Adverse effects include ocular symptoms such as conjunctival edema, tearing, dryness, burning, pain, irritation, itching, sensation of a foreign body in the eye, photophobia, or visual disturbances. The eyelashes on the treated eye may grow thicker or darker. Changes may occur in the pigmentation of the iris of the treated eye and in the periocular skin. Rare, systemic adverse effects include headaches, rashes, flulike symptoms, and abnormal liver function tests.

Contraindications/Precautions: Contraindications include hypersensitivity to the drug or another component in the solution, pregnancy, lactation, intraocular infection, or conjunctivitis. It should not be administered to patients with closed-angle glaucoma. The safety of this drug has not been demonstrated in children.

Drug Interactions: Latanoprost interacts with the preservative thimerosal: If used concurrently with other eyedrops that contain thimerosal, precipitation may occur. **Herbal/Food**: Unknown.

Pregnancy: Category C.

Treatment of Overdose: Overdose with the ophthalmic solution is unlikely.

Nursing Responsibilities: Key nursing implications for patients receiving latanoprost are included in the Nursing Practice Application for Patients Receiving Pharmacotherapy for Glaucoma.

Drugs Similar to Latanoprost (Xalatan)

Bimatoprost, tafluprost, and travoprost are other prostaglandin analogs used for glaucoma.

Bimatoprost (Lumigan): Approved in 2001, bimatoprost is a synthetic prostaglandin analog indicated for the treatment of open-angle glaucoma. It is usually used when the patient has not responded adequately to other antiglaucoma drugs. In 2008, a newer formulation of this drug, Latisse, was approved to treat hypotrichosis, a condition of having too few eyelashes. Use of bimatoprost can cause a gradual increase in the development of brown pigmentation in the iris, which may be irreversible, and includes an increase in pigmentation of the eyelid. Other adverse effects include blurred vision, eye discomfort, ocular pruritus, conjunctivitis, dry eye, light

TABLE 74.1	Selected Drugs for Glaucoma	
Drug	**Route and Adult Dose (Maximum Dose Where Indicated)**	**Adverse Effects**
Prostaglandins		
bimatoprost (Lumigan)	1 drop of 0.03% solution daily in the evening	*Increased length and thickness of eyelashes, darkening of the iris, stinging, sensation of foreign body in the eye*
latanoprost (Xalatan)	1 drop of 0.005% solution daily in the evening	
tafluprost (Zioptan)	1 drop of 0.0015% solution daily in the evening	<u>Respiratory infection, flu, angina, muscle or joint pain</u>
travoprost (Travatan)	1 drop of 0.004% solution daily in the evening	
Beta-Adrenergic Blockers		
betaxolol (Betoptic)	1 drop of 0.5% solution bid	*Local burning and stinging, blurred vision, headache*
carteolol (Ocupress)	1 drop of 1% solution bid	<u>Conjunctival hyperemia, angina, anxiety, bronchoconstriction, hypotension, dysrhythmias</u>
levobunolol (Betagan)	1–2 drops of 0.25–0.5% solution 1–2 times/day	
metipranolol (OptiPranolol)	1 drop of 0.3% solution bid	
timolol (Betimol, Timoptic, Others)	1–2 drops of 0.25–0.5% solution 1–2 times/day Gel (salve): apply daily	
Alpha₂-Adrenergic Agonists		
apraclonidine (Iopidine)	1 drop of 0.5% solution bid	*Local itching and burning, blurred vision, dry mouth, headache, eye discharge*
brimonidine (Alphagan P)	1 drop of 0.1–0.15% solution in the affected eye tid, 8 h apart	<u>Allergic conjunctivitis, conjunctival hyperemia, hypotension, bulbar conjunctival follicles</u>
Cholinergic Agonists		
carbachol (Isopto Carbachol)	1–2 drops of 0.75–3% solution in the lower conjunctival sac up to 3 times/day	*Induced myopia, reduced visual acuity in low light, eye redness, headache*
echothiophate iodide (Phospholine Iodide)	1 drop of 0.03–0.25% solution 1–2 times/day	<u>Salivation, tachycardia, hypotension, bronchospasm, sweating, nausea, vomiting, retinal detachment (pilocarpine)</u>
pilocarpine (Isopto Carpine, Pilopine)	Acute glaucoma: 1 drop of 1–2% solution every 5–10 min for three to six doses Chronic glaucoma: 1 drop of 0.5–4% solution every 4–12 h	
Sympathomimetics		
dipivefrin (Propine)	1 drop of 0.1% solution every 12 h	*Local burning and stinging, blurred vision, headache, photosensitivity* <u>Tachycardia, HTN</u>
Carbonic Anhydrase Inhibitors		
acetazolamide (Diamox)	PO: 250 mg 1–4 times/day	*For topical agents: blurred vision, bitter taste, dry eye, blepharitis, local itching, sensation of foreign body in the eye, headache*
brinzolamide (Azopt)	1 drop of 1% solution tid	
dorzolamide (Trusopt)	1 drop of 2% solution in the affected eye(s) tid	<u>For PO agents: diuresis, electrolyte imbalances, blood dyscrasias, flaccid paralysis, hepatic impairment</u>
methazolamide (Neptazane)	PO: 50–100 mg bid–tid	
Osmotic Diuretics		
isosorbide (Ismotic)	PO: 1–3 g/kg 1–2 times/day	*Orthostatic hypotension, facial flushing, headache, palpitations, anxiety, nausea*
mannitol (Osmitrol)	IV: 1.5–2 mg/kg as a 15–25% solution over 30–60 min	<u>Severe headache, electrolyte imbalances, edema</u>

Note: *Italics* indicate common adverse effects. <u>Underline</u> indicates serious adverse effects.

intolerance, and tearing. It is available as a 0.01% or 0.03% solution applied once daily in the evening. This drug is pregnancy category C.

Tafluprost (Zioptan): Tafluprost is one of the newer medications for open-angle glaucoma. When approved in 2012, tafluprost became the first antiglaucoma prostaglandin completely free of preservatives. Preservatives sometimes cause allergic reactions in susceptible patients and may worsen ocular surface disorders such

as dry eye syndrome. The actions, effectiveness, and side effects of tafluprost are equivalent to those of other prostaglandins.

Travoprost (Travatan): Approved in 2001, travoprost is approved for the treatment of open-angle glaucoma. Travoprost has been found to be more effective in African Americans than in non–African Americans. Like bimatoprost, travoprost is usually used when other drugs have failed to produce a satisfactory response.

Use of this drug can cause a gradual increase in the development of brown pigmentation in the iris, which may be irreversible, and includes an increase in pigmentation of the eyelid and growth of the eyelashes. Conjunctival hyperemia has been reported in 35% to 50% of patients treated with travoprost. Some other adverse effects include blurred vision, eye discomfort, ocular pruritus, dry eye, light intolerance, and tearing. It is available as a 0.004% solution, applied once daily in the evening. This drug is pregnancy category C.

CONNECTION Checkpoint 74.1

Several prostaglandins are used for their actions on uterine smooth muscle. From what you learned in Chapter 70, what are the primary indications for the prostaglandins carboprost (Hemabate), dinoprostone (Cervidil), and mifepristone (Mifeprex)? *See Answer to Connection Checkpoint 74.1 on student resource website.*

74.5 Drugs that affect the autonomic nervous system are sometimes prescribed to treat glaucoma.

Several structures within the eye are activated by the sympathetic and parasympathetic divisions of the autonomic nervous system. As such, a significant number of autonomic agents have been used to treat glaucoma and to aid in ophthalmic examinations of the eyeball.

- Sympathetic activation (or parasympathetic division blockade): Muscles of the iris contract to dilate the pupil; the ciliary muscle relaxes to enhance distance vision.

- Parasympathetic activation (or sympathetic division blockade): Muscles of the iris contract to constrict the pupil; the ciliary muscle contracts to enhance near vision.

The most frequently used autonomic drugs are the beta-adrenergic antagonists or blockers. Alpha$_2$-adrenergic agonists, nonselective sympathomimetics, and cholinergic agonists play minor roles, as discussed next. Prior to reading this section, the student may want to review Chapter 12 to brush up on the terminology and anatomy of the autonomic nervous system.

Beta-adrenergic blockers: Before the discovery of the prostaglandin analogs, beta-adrenergic blockers were the drugs of choice for open-angle glaucoma. These drugs decrease the production of aqueous humor by the ciliary body in the affected eye and can lower IOP by 20% to 30%. Five beta-adrenergic blockers are available as ophthalmic solutions: betaxolol (Betoptic), carteolol (Ocupress), levobunolol (Betagan), metipranolol (OptiPranolol), and timolol (Betimol, Timoptic, Others). These agents generally produce fewer adverse ocular effects than cholinergic agonists or sympathomimetics. In most patients, the topical administration of beta blockers does not result in significant systemic absorption. Should absorption occur, however, adverse systemic effects may include bronchoconstriction, dysrhythmias, and hypotension. Because of the potential for adverse systemic effects, these drugs should be used with caution in patients with asthma, bradycardia, or heart failure. Tolerance will develop with long-term use in about 25% of patients who take these drugs.

Alpha2-adrenergic agonists: Alpha$_2$-adrenergic agonists lower IOP by decreasing the production of aqueous humor and increasing its absorption. Only two alpha$_2$-adrenergic agonists are currently approved for use: apraclonidine and brimonidine. Apraclonidine (Iopidine) is infrequently used but may be prescribed for the prevention or short-term therapy of postoperative increases in IOP. Brimonidine (Alphagan) is more commonly prescribed,

either as monotherapy or as an adjunct in combination with a beta-adrenergic blocker, for the long-term treatment of open-angle glaucoma or glaucoma secondary to uveitis, which is an inflammation of the middle layer of the eyeball. Alpha$_2$-adrenergic agonists may be used in combination with other antiglaucoma drugs to cause additive reduction in IOP. In 2007, the U.S. Food and Drug Administration (FDA) approved Combigan, an ophthalmic solution that consists of brimonidine and timolol to treat glaucoma.

Alpha$_2$-adrenergic agonists are contraindicated in closed-angle glaucoma because the pupil dilation that results would worsen the condition. The most significant adverse effect, and one that is a frequent cause for discontinuation of therapy, is an allergic-type reaction that causes sensation of a foreign body, itching, and hyperemia. Other adverse effects include headache, drowsiness, dry mucosal membranes, blurred vision, and irritated eyelids. These drugs produce few cardiovascular or pulmonary adverse effects. Rare systemic adverse effects may occur, including nervousness, anxiety, and muscle tremors. Patients should immediately notify their health care provider if they experience acute eye pain, because this may signal the onset of closed-angle glaucoma.

Cholinergic agonists (miotics): Drugs that directly activate cholinergic receptors in the eye produce **miosis**, or constriction of the pupil, and contraction of the ciliary muscle. These actions physically stretch the trabecular meshwork to allow greater outflow of aqueous humor and a lowering of IOP. Pilocarpine (Isopto Carpine, Pilopine) is the most commonly prescribed antiglaucoma drug in this class. The cholinergic agonists are applied topically to the eye four times daily. Because of their greater toxicity and frequent dosing, these drugs are normally used only in patients with open-angle glaucoma who do not respond to other agents. Local effects include headache, induced myopia, and decreased vision in low light. Systemic absorption can result in hypotension, vomiting, diuresis, bronchoconstriction, diaphoresis, and abdominal pain with diarrhea. Toxic effects include vertigo, bradycardia, tremors, syncope, and cardiac dysrhythmias. Other actions of the cholinergic agonists are presented in Chapter 13.

A second group of cholinergic agonists, the cholinesterase inhibitors, act indirectly to lower IOP. They produce essentially the same actions as the direct-acting agents but exhibit a higher incidence of adverse effects. Cholinesterase inhibitors such as echothiophate cause cataracts in a significant percentage of patients and are only used in those who are resistant to therapy with other agents.

CONNECTION Checkpoint 74.2

Cholinergic agonists such as pilocarpine activate muscarinic receptors. From what you learned in Chapter 13, what effect do muscarinic agonists have on lacrimation and how is this used therapeutically? *See Answer to Connection Checkpoint 74.2 on student resource website.*

Nonselective sympathomimetics: Nonselective sympathomimetics activate the sympathetic nervous system to produce **mydriasis** (pupil dilation) and increase the outflow of aqueous humor, resulting in a lower IOP. They are not as effective as the beta-adrenergic blockers or the prostaglandin analogs. Agents in this class include epinephrine and dipivefrin, which is converted to epinephrine in the eye. Both are administered topically for open-angle glaucoma and are contraindicated in closed-angle glaucoma. Epinephrine will increase blood pressure and the heart rate if it reaches the systemic circulation; thus the drug is contraindicated in patients with unstable cardiovascular disease. Sympathomimetics also produce a high frequency of ocular adverse effects, including tearing, burning, hyperemia, and stenosis of the nasolacrimal duct. Because of the potential for systemic adverse effects, these agents are third-choice drugs for glaucoma.

PROTOTYPE DRUG	Timolol (Betimol, Timoptic, Others)

Classification: **Therapeutic:** Drug for glaucoma
Pharmacologic: Miotic, beta-adrenergic antagonist

Therapeutic Effects and Uses: Approved in 1978, timolol is a nonselective beta-adrenergic blocker available as a 0.25% or 0.5% ophthalmic solution. Its primary indication is chronic open-angle glaucoma. It may also be used for aphakic glaucoma (high IOP in patients with no lens), secondary glaucoma, and ocular HTN. The usual dose is one drop in the affected eye(s) twice a day. Timoptic XE allows for once-daily dosing. Treatment may require 2 to 4 weeks to reach the maximum therapeutic effect.

Timolol is available in several formulations. Cosopt is an antiglaucoma drug that combines timolol with dorzolamide, a topical carbonic anhydrase inhibitor. Combigan is an ophthalmic solution of timolol with brimonidine, an alpha-adrenergic agonist. Timolol is also available in tablets (Blocadren), which are prescribed to treat mild HTN.

Mechanism of Action: Timolol topically lowers the elevated and normal IOP by reducing the formation of aqueous humor and possibly increasing outflow. It affects both beta$_1$ and beta$_2$ receptors.

Pharmacokinetics:

Route(s)	Eye solution or gel
Absorption	Small amounts reach the systemic circulation from topical application
Distribution	Secreted in breast milk
Primary metabolism	80% metabolized in the liver to inactive metabolites
Primary excretion	Renal
Onset of action	30 min
Duration of action	12–24 h

Adverse Effects: The most common adverse effects from ophthalmic administration are local burning and stinging on instillation. Vision may become temporarily blurred. In most patients absorption is not significant enough to cause adverse systemic effects as long as timolol is applied correctly. If absorption occurs, hypotension or dysrhythmias are possible.

Contraindications/Precautions: Although little is absorbed through ocular administration, this drug should be used with caution in certain patients. Timolol is contraindicated in patients with asthma, severe chronic obstructive pulmonary disease (COPD), sinus bradycardia, second- or third-degree atrioventricular block, heart failure, cardiogenic shock, or hypersensitivity to the drug. Safety in children has not been established.

Drug Interactions: Drug interactions may result if significant systemic absorption occurs. Timolol should be used with caution in patients who are taking other beta blockers owing to additive cardiac effects. Concurrent use with anticholinergics, nitrates, reserpine, methyldopa, or verapamil could lead to hypotension and

bradycardia. Epinephrine use could lead to HTN followed by severe bradycardia. When given by the ocular route, timolol will produce additive lowering of IOP when given concurrently with other antiglaucoma agents. **Herbal/Food:** There are no known herbal or food interactions with this drug.

Pregnancy: Category C.

Treatment of Overdose: Overdose with ophthalmic solution is unlikely but could result in systemic symptoms such as reduced heart rate and bronchospasm.

Nursing Responsibilities: Key nursing implications for patients receiving timolol are included in the Nursing Practice Application for Patients Receiving Pharmacotherapy for Glaucoma.

Drugs Similar to Timolol (Betimol, Timoptic, Others)

Other beta-adrenergic blockers with ophthalmic indications include betaxolol, carteolol, levobunolol, and metipranolol. Levobetaxolol (Betaxon) is an ophthalmic beta blocker that has been discontinued in the United States.

Betaxolol (Betoptic): Approved in 1985, betaxolol is a selective beta$_1$-adrenergic receptor blocker. This drug reduces IOP by decreasing the production of aqueous humor. Betaxolol is indicated for intraocular HTN and chronic open-angle glaucoma. A tablet form of this drug (Kerlone) is available to treat HTN. Although only small amounts are absorbed from ophthalmic administration, this drug should be used cautiously in patients with heart failure and if used concurrently with a systemic beta-adrenergic blocker. Ocular irritation and tearing are frequent adverse effects. This drug is pregnancy category C.

Carteolol (Ocupress): Carteolol is a nonselective beta-adrenergic blocker that competes for available beta receptor sites and is used for the treatment of chronic open-angle glaucoma. Both beta$_1$ and beta$_2$ receptors are inhibited. Carteolol (Cartrol) was also available as tablets to treat HTN, but it has been discontinued for this indication in the United States. Adverse effects and contraindications are the same as those of other ophthalmic beta blockers. This drug is pregnancy category C.

Levobunolol (Betagan): Approved in 1985, levobunolol is a nonselective beta-adrenergic blocker that is indicated for the treatment of intraocular HTN and chronic open-angle glaucoma. Because small amounts may reach the systemic circulation, caution needs to be practiced when using this drug in patients with asthma, COPD, bradycardia, thyroid conditions, diabetes, and abnormal blood glucose levels. Tolerance can develop with long-term use. Ocular irritation is a frequent, transient adverse effect. This drug is pregnancy category C.

Metipranolol (OptiPranolol): Approved in 1989, this drug is a nonselective beta-adrenergic blocker used for the treatment of elevated IOP and chronic open-angle glaucoma. It is available as a 0.3% solution that is applied to the affected eye(s) twice daily. Small amounts may be absorbed systemically. Contraindications are the same as those of other ophthalmic beta blockers. Ocular irritation is a frequent, transient adverse effect. Although rare, uveitis has been associated with metipranolol use. If this occurs, this drug should be discontinued because uveitis can cause an increase in IOP. This drug is pregnancy category C.

CONNECTIONS: NURSING PRACTICE APPLICATION

Patients Receiving Pharmacotherapy for Glaucoma

Assessment	Potential Nursing Diagnoses*
Baseline assessment prior to administration: • Obtain a complete health history including ophthalmologic, respiratory, cardiovascular, and endocrine disease. • Assess visual acuity and visual fields. Assess for the presence of eye pain, visual disturbances such as halos around lights, diminished foggy vision, or loss of peripheral vision. • Assess for history of recent eye trauma or infection. • Obtain a drug history including allergies, current prescription and OTC drugs, herbal preparations, alcohol use, and smoking. Be alert to possible drug interactions. • Obtain baseline vital signs. • Assess the patient's ability to receive and understand instructions. Include the family or caregiver as needed.	• *Anxiety* • *Acute Pain* • *Self-Care Deficit: Bathing, Dressing, Feeding* • *Deficient Knowledge* (Drug Therapy) • *Risk for Injury*, related to condition or adverse drug effects
Assessment throughout administration: • Assess for desired therapeutic effects dependent on the reason the drug is given (e.g., IOP remains below 21 mmHg, no changes in visual acuity or fields). • Assess for adverse effects: conjunctival edema, tearing, dryness, burning, pain, irritation, itching, sensation of foreign body in the eye, or photophobia. Severe visual disturbances or eye pain should be reported to the health care provider.	

Implementation

Interventions and (Rationales)	Patient-Centered Care
Ensuring therapeutic effects: • Monitor visual acuity, vision fields, and IOP. (IOP should remain less than 21 mmHg or per parameters set by health care provider. Visual acuity and fields remain intact.)	• Instruct the patient to immediately report changes in vision, eye pain, light sensitivity, halos around lights, or headache to the health care provider.
Minimizing adverse effects: • Monitor appropriate administration of the drug to avoid extraocular effects. (Eyedrops should be instilled into the conjunctival sac and the lacrimal duct area held with gentle pressure for one full minute to prevent drug leakage into the nasopharynx with possible systemic effects. PO drugs should be taken consistently throughout the day with no doses omitted.)	• Teach the patient the proper administration techniques for eyedrops. PO medications should be taken as regularly throughout the day as possible and with consistent dosing.
• Monitor IOP periodically. (Consistent readings above 21 mmHg may indicate worsening disease or improper use of drug therapy.)	• Instruct the patient of the importance to return for and maintain regular eye exams.
• Monitor for increasing eye redness, pain, light sensitivity, or changes in visual acuity. (Eye changes or pain may indicate worsening disease, infection, or adverse drug effects.)	• Instruct the patient to avoid touching the eyedrop tip to the conjunctival sac when instilling eyedrops. Immediately report any increasing redness, eye pain, eye drainage, or changes in vision.
• Remove contact lenses before administering ophthalmic solutions. Avoid use of other eyedrops or ointments unless approved by the health care provider. (Contact lenses may hinder eye solution from fully reaching all eye surfaces or may absorb solution, resulting in higher than expected amounts in the eye over time. Other eye solutions may interact with or counteract the effects of the prescribed solution.)	• Instruct the patient to remove contact lenses prior to administering eyedrops and wait at least 15 min before reinserting them. • Instruct the patient to seek the health care provider's advice before using any other eye solution.
• Monitor vital signs periodically for signs of systemic absorption of ophthalmic preparations. (Ophthalmic drugs such as beta blockers or cholinergic drugs may result in hypotension, bradycardia, or respiratory distress due to bronchospasm if the drug is absorbed systemically. Ensure that the patient is administering drops appropriately if changes in blood pressure are noted. **Lifespan:** Monitor older adults frequently for hypotension related to systemic absorption to prevent falls.)	• Teach the patient to return to the health care provider periodically for monitoring. Assess blood pressure once per week (e.g., at supermarket pharmacy counter sphygmomanometer) and report any blood pressure less than 90/60 mmHg or per parameters set by the health care provider. Immediately report any dizziness, light-headedness, headache, palpitations, syncope, or difficulty breathing.
• Provide for eye comfort such as an adequately lighted room. (Ophthalmic drugs such as beta blockers used in the treatment of glaucoma can cause miosis and difficulty seeing in low light levels.)	• Caution the patient about driving or other activities in low-light conditions or at night until the effects of the drug are known.
• Monitor adherence to the treatment regimen. (Nonadherence with drug therapy may result in the total loss of vision.)	• Teach the patient the importance of adhering to the medication schedule as prescribed. • Address any concerns the patient may have about cost or discomfort related to drug therapy, and provide appropriate referrals (e.g., social service agency) as needed.

(continued)

CONNECTIONS: NURSING PRACTICE APPLICATION (continued)

Patient understanding of drug therapy: • Use opportunities during administration of medications and during assessments to discuss the rationale for the drug therapy, desired therapeutic outcomes, commonly observed adverse effects, parameters for when to call the health care provider, and any necessary monitoring or precautions. (Using time during nursing care helps to optimize and reinforce key teaching areas.)	• The patient should be able to state the reason for the drug, appropriate dose and scheduling, what adverse effects to observe for, and when to report them.

Patient self-administration of drug therapy:
• When administering the medication, instruct the patient, family, or caregiver in proper self-administration of the drug, e.g., appropriate instillation of eyedrops followed by teach-back. (Utilizing time during nurse-administration of these drugs helps to reinforce teaching.)
	• Teach the patient to take the drug following appropriate guidelines:
	  • Remove contact lenses if worn.
	  • Gently pull down on the lower eyelid, anchoring the hand against the cheekbone.
	  • Tilt the head back; steadying the hand on the forehead as needed, drop prescribed numbers of drops into the conjunctival sac. Do not drop solution directly onto the eye surface.
	  • Close the eye gently. Hold light pressure on the tear duct for one full minute to retain the solution.
	  • Do not reinsert contact lenses for a minimum of 15 min after eyedrop instillation, or as directed.

*Nursing Diagnoses—Definitions and Classification 2015–2017. Copyright © 2014, 1994–2014 by NANDA International. Used by arrangement with John Wiley & Sons Limited.

Miscellaneous Drugs for Treating Glaucoma

74.6 Carbonic anhydrase inhibitors and osmotic diuretics are occasionally used for treating glaucoma.

Although prostaglandin analogs and beta-adrenergic blockers are the two most frequently prescribed classes for lowering IOP, some patients may experience adverse effects from these agents or have particularly resistant glaucoma. Two additional classes, the carbonic anhydrase inhibitors and the osmotic diuretics, are not routinely prescribed.

Carbonic anhydrase inhibitors: Carbonic anhydrase inhibitors interfere with the synthesis of carbonic acid, which decreases the production of aqueous humor and reduces IOP. They are used as long-term therapy in patients with open-angle glaucoma when prostaglandin inhibitors, beta blockers, and other autonomic agents have not been effective.

Drugs in this class are divided into topical or oral formulations. Dorzolamide (Trusopt) is used topically to treat open-angle glaucoma, either as monotherapy or in combination with other agents. Dorzolamide and other topical carbonic anhydrase inhibitors, including brinzolamide (Azopt), are well tolerated and produce few significant adverse effects other than photosensitivity. PO formulations such as acetazolamide (Diamox) are very effective at lowering IOP in both open-angle and closed-angle glaucoma but are rarely used because they produce more adverse systemic effects than drugs from other classes. These adverse effects include lethargy, nausea, vomiting, depression, paresthesias, and drowsiness. Patients must be cautioned when taking these medications because they contain sulfur and may cause allergic reactions. Because the oral formulations are diuretics and can reduce IOP quickly, serum electrolytes should be monitored during treatment. A prototype feature for acetazolamide is presented in Chapter 32.

Osmotic diuretics: Osmotic diuretics are occasionally used preoperatively and postoperatively with ocular surgery or as emergency treatment of acute closed-angle glaucoma attacks. Examples include isosorbide (Ismotic), urea, and mannitol (Osmitrol). Because they have the ability to quickly reduce plasma volume, these drugs are effective in reducing the formation of aqueous humor, thereby reducing IOP. Adverse effects include headache, tremors, dizziness, dry mouth, fluid and electrolyte imbalances, and thrombophlebitis or venous clot formation near the site of intravenous (IV) administration. A prototype feature for mannitol is presented in Chapter 32.

CONNECTION Checkpoint 74.3

Mannitol is given by the IV route under controlled conditions. From what you learned in Chapter 32, describe the mechanism of action of osmotic diuretics. *See Answer to Connection Checkpoint 74.3 on student resource website.*

Pharmacotherapy for Eye Examinations

74.7 Drugs that are routinely used for eye examinations include mydriatics, cycloplegics, diagnostic dyes, and local anesthetics.

Various drugs are used to enhance diagnostic eye examinations and during ophthalmic surgery. Mydriatic drugs cause sympathetic activation that relaxes the ciliary muscle, causing dilation of the pupil and thus allowing for better visualization of retinal structures. Cycloplegic drugs not only dilate the pupil but also paralyze the ciliary muscle and prevent the lens from moving during assessment. Mydriatics and cycloplegics are often used in combination to achieve the maximum pupil dilation needed for surgery or during funduscopic exams. Examples of agents used for eye examinations include anticholinergics, such as atropine (Isopto Atropine) and tropicamide (Mydriacyl, Tropicacyl), and sympathomimetics, such as phenylephrine (Mydfrin, Neo-Synephrine). Mydriatic, cycloplegic, and other drugs for eye conditions are listed in Table 74.2.

Mydriatics cause intense photophobia and pain in response to bright light. Mydriatics can worsen glaucoma by impairing aqueous humor outflow and thereby increasing IOP. In addition, strong concentrations of anticholinergics have the potential to have systemic effects on the central nervous system (CNS) and cause confusion, unsteadiness, or drowsiness. **Cycloplegics** can cause severe

◀ Bilberry for Eye Health

Description

Bilberry (*Vaccinium myrtillus*), a close relative of the blueberry, is a perennial ornamental shrub whose leaves and fruit are used medicinally. It is found throughout central and northern Europe, Asia, and North America.

History and Claims

Bilberry has been used for nearly 1,000 years in traditional European medicine to treat diarrhea, scurvy, and other conditions. Today, the fruit is used in a tea to treat nonspecific diarrhea, menstrual cramps, varicose veins, venous insufficiency, and, most importantly, a number of conditions associated with disorders of the eye, including glaucoma, poor night vision, and eye inflammation. A widely circulated story is that bilberry jam was used by pilots in the Royal Air Force during World War II to improve their night vision. Bilberry and blueberries contain high concentrations of compounds called anthocyanins, which are thought to assist in the functioning of the rods in the retina for night vision. Bilberry is believed to have factors that stabilize blood vessels, decreasing blood vessel leakage associated with diabetic retinopathy and macular degeneration. Bilberry has also been used to reduce eye inflammation and to lower the increased IOP associated with glaucoma.

Standardization

Preparations of available bilberry extract are standardized to contain 25% anthocyanidin.

Evidence

Although bilberry is widely used as a supplement to protect or improve eye health, large-scale, controlled studies are lacking. Some clinical studies have shown an association between bilberry intake and improvement in night vision or in disease conditions such as retinitis pigmentosa (Kiser & Dagnelie, 2007) and uveitis (Yao, Lan, He, & Kurlhara, 2010). Anthocyanin extracts from bilberry also appear to improve visual function in certain types of glaucoma (Shim, Kim, Choi, Kim, & Park, 2012). Bilberry is generally believed to be safe in recommended doses for short periods based on its history as a foodstuff. There are no known reports of serious adverse effects, although when taken in large doses, there is an increased risk of bleeding, upset stomach, or hydroquinone poisoning. Further research is needed to identify the active compounds in bilberry and to assess its effects on vision health.

TABLE 74.2 Miscellaneous Agents Used for the Eye

Drug	Route and Adult Dose (Maximum Dose Where Indicated)	Adverse Effects
Mydriatics: Sympathomimetics		
phenylephrine (Mydfrin, Neo-Synephrine)	1 drop of 2.5% or 10% solution before eye examination	*Eye pain, photosensitivity, eye irritation, headache* <u>HTN, tremor, dysrhythmias</u>
Cycloplegics: Anticholinergics		
atropine (Isopto Atropine, Others)	Uveitis: 1–2 drops of 1% solution up to 4 times daily; also give 1–2 drops 1 h prior to eye examination	*Eye irritation and redness, dry mouth, local burning or stinging, headache, blurred vision, photosensitivity, eczematoid dermatitis (scopolamine and tropicamide)* <u>Somnolence, tachycardia, convulsions, mental changes, keratitis, increased IOP (homatropine)</u>
cyclopentolate (Cyclogyl, Pentolair)	1 drop of 0.5–2% solution 40–50 min before eye examination	
homatropine (Isopto Homatropine, Others)	1–2 drops of 2% or 5% solution before eye examination Uveitis: 1–2 drops of 2–5% solution bid–tid up to every 3–4 h as needed	
scopolamine (Isopto Hyoscine)	1–2 drops of 0.25% solution 1 h before eye examination	
tropicamide (Mydriacyl, Tropicacyl)	1–2 drops of 0.5–1% solution before eye examination	
Anesthetics		
lidocaine (Akten)	2 drops of 3.5% gel in affected eye, reapplied as needed	*Stinging, corneal erosion, headache, slowed healing of corneal abrasions* <u>Anaphylactic reactions</u>
proparacaine (Alcaine, Ophthaine)	1 drop of 0.5% solution in affected eye every 5–10 min for five to seven doses	
tetracaine	1–2 drops of a 0.5% solution or 1.25–2.5 cm of ointment in the lower conjunctival sac	
Lubricants		
lanolin alcohol (Lacril-lube)	Apply a thin film to the inside of the eyelid	*Temporary burning or stinging, eye itching or redness, headache* <u>No serious adverse effects</u>
polyvinyl alcohol (Liquifilm, Others)	1–2 drops tid–qid prn	
Vasoconstrictors		
naphazoline (Albalon Allerest, Clear Eyes, Others)	1–3 drops of 0.1% solution every 3–4 h prn	*Temporary burning or stinging, eye itching or redness, headache* <u>No serious adverse effects</u>
oxymetazoline (OcuClear, Visine LR)	1–2 drops of 0.025% solution qid	
phenylephrine (Neo-Synephrine)	1–2 drops of 0.12% solution up to 4 times daily	
tetrahydrozoline (Murine Plus, Visine, Others)	1–2 drops of 0.05% solution bid–tid	

Note: Italics indicate common adverse effects. <u>Underline</u> indicates serious adverse effects.

blurred vision and loss of near vision. Scopolamine, an anticholinergic often used to prevent motion sickness, can cause blurred vision due to cycloplegia, as well as angle-closure glaucoma attacks. The response to mydriatics and cycloplegics can last from 3 hours up to several days. The patient should be taught to wear sunglasses and that the ability to drive, read, and perform visual tasks may be affected during treatment.

Diagnostic agents are used to help locate lesions or foreign bodies within the eye and to provide some local anesthesia. Fluorescein sodium is a dye used in assessing the cornea and fitting contact lenses. Scratches may turn bright green; foreign bodies are surrounded by a green halo. Areas where the conjunctiva is damaged show an orange-yellow discoloration. Fluorescein sodium with benoxinate (Fluress) adds local anesthesia, making it useful for the identification and removal of foreign bodies from the cornea.

Local anesthetic agents are used to prevent the pain associated with diagnostic and surgical procedures, suturing and removal of foreign bodies, and ocular injections. The agents used include proparacaine (Alcaine, Ophthaine) and tetracaine. Application consists of one to two drops applied to the affected eye. Anesthesia typically occurs within 20 seconds and lasts for 10 to 20 minutes. Adverse effects of their use include local irritation, including conjunctivitis. Systemic effects are rarer, but CNS excitation has been known to occur. The nurse must be careful to protect the patient's eye from injury while anesthetized, or corneal damage may occur.

PharmFACT

Steroid-induced open-angle glaucoma is common, occurring in 75% of patients who receive steroid implants. Elevated IOP may begin immediately or as late as 12 weeks after initiating therapy. Even after discontinuation of the steroid, the IOP may remain elevated for 2 to 4 weeks (Razeghinejad & Katz, 2011).

Pharmacotherapy for Other Eye Conditions

74.8 Numerous pharmacologic agents are used to treat minor eye irritation and redness.

Drugs for minor eye irritation and dryness come from a broad range of classes. Some agents lubricate only the eye's surface, whereas others are designed to penetrate and affect a specific area of the eye.

Lubricants are used to lessen the discomfort associated with dryness and maintain the patency of the cornea. They are used as artificial tears in persons who have dry eye syndrome, during anesthesia with acute or chronic nervous system disorders that result in decreased blinking, and as extra moisture for those who have contact lenses or artificial eyes. Artificial tear agents are topical preparations of methyl or vinyl cellulose. These drops can be instilled as often as every hour. A wide variety of over-the-counter (OTC) preparations are available, including eyedrop solutions, ointments, and inserts. There is currently only one prescription drug for dry eye and that is cyclosporine ophthalmic emulsion (Restasis). Restasis is the only drug available that actually stimulates the production of tears. It is most effective when used in combination with artificial tear replacement and is administered as one drop in the affected eye(s) twice daily. Cyclosporine is presented as a prototype immunosuppressant in Chapter 42.

Vasoconstrictors are commonly used to treat minor eye irritation. Common vasoconstrictors include phenylephrine (Neo-Synephrine), naphazoline (Clear Eyes, Others), and tetrahydrozoline (Murine Plus, Visine, Others). The adverse effects of the vasoconstrictors are usually minor and include blurred vision, tearing, headache, and rebound vasodilation with redness.

Infection and inflammatory responses are common conditions in the supporting structures of the eye and may result from foreign bodies, bacteria, or viruses. Allergies and irritants such as tobacco smoke are also common sources of inflammation. Redness, edema, and itching are common symptoms. The anti-infectives used to treat eye infections are the same agents used to treat infections in other areas of the body. Applied topically they carry the common adverse effects of conjunctivitis and local skin and eye irritation. Examples of eye infections that are treated with anti-infective medications include:

- **Blepharitis.** Inflammation of the edges of the eyelids that is commonly seen in older adults and those with dry eyes.
- **Conjunctivitis.** Inflammation or infection of the lining of the eyelids. Bacterial conjunctivitis is often caused by *Staphylococcus aureus*, *Streptococcus pneumoniae*, and *Haemophilus influenzae*. Viral conjunctivitis is highly contagious and treatment is symptomatic.
- **Chalazion and styes.** A chalazion is a lump or cyst along the edge of an eyelid. Hordeolum, or an external stye, is a blockage of the sebaceous glands at the base of the eyelashes. A chalazion or hordeolum may become infected and require the use of ocular antibiotics.
- **Keratitis.** An inflammation of the cornea that may also be caused by trauma or dryness of the cornea from decreased lubrication. If left untreated, corneal scarring with impaired vision may result.

Nonsteroidal anti-inflammatory drugs (NSAIDs), such as ketorolac (Acular, Acuvail), can be used to treat conjunctivitis and other inflammatory conditions. They are also used to reduce inflammation postoperatively and the symptoms associated with seasonal allergies. Topical corticosteroids are also very effective at reducing inflammation in the eye, although they should not be administered if an infection is suspected. The most common adverse effects of topical corticosteroids are cataracts, glaucoma, mydriasis, and ptosis. Cycloplegics can also be used to treat ocular pain caused by almost any inflammatory condition, except glaucoma.

Several medications, including antihistamines, mast cell stabilizers, and combination antihistamine–mast cell stabilizers, are used to decrease the redness and itching associated with allergic conjunctivitis. Systemic antihistamines may be used but they may cause ocular dryness, which could aggravate symptoms. Topical mast cell stabilizers, with or without an antihistamine, are the preferred treatment for allergic conjunctivitis because they do not cause further drying of the eyes. Two new drugs, olopatadine (Patanol) and pemirolast (Alamast), provide for once-daily dosing for allergic conjunctivitis. Azelastine (Optivar) and epinastine (Elestat) are combination antihistamine–mast cell stabilizers that are indicated for twice-daily dosing. Drugs for the treatment of allergic conjunctivitis are listed in Table 74.3.

TABLE 74.3 Drugs for the Treatment of Allergic Conjunctivitis

Drug	Route and Adult Dose (Maximum Dose Where Indicated)	Adverse Effects
Mast Cell Stabilizers		
cromolyn (Crolom)	1–2 drops of 4% solution every 4–6 h	*Dry mouth, headache, nausea, sneezing, nasal symptoms, and transient eye stinging and burning*
lodoxamide (Alomide)	1–2 drops of 0.1% solution qid	
nedocromil (Alocril)	1–2 drops of 2% solution bid	Bronchospasm, angioedema, anaphylaxis
pemirolast (Alamast)	1–2 drops of 0.1% solution qid	
Antihistamines		
azelastine (Optivar)	1 drop of 0.05% solution bid	*Fatigue, dizziness, dry mouth, headache, pharyngitis, cough, bitter taste, rhinitis*
bepotastine (Bepreve)	1 drop of 1.5% solution bid	No serious adverse effects
emedastine (Emadine)	1 drop of 0.05% solution qid	
epinastine (Elestat)	1 drop of 0.05% solution bid	
ketotifen (Alaway, Zaditor)	1 drop of 0.025% solution every 8–12 h	
olopatadine (Patanol)	1 drop of 0.1% solution bid	

Note: Italics indicate common adverse effects. Underline indicates serious adverse effects.

Anatomy of the Ear

74.9 Knowledge of basic ear anatomy is fundamental to understanding ear disorders and pharmacotherapy.

The ear has two major sensory functions: hearing and maintenance of equilibrium and balance. The three structural areas of the ear—the external, middle, and inner ear—carry out these functions, as shown in Figure 74.3.

The external ear consists of the pinna, which is the visible portion of the ear, and the external auditory canal. The external auditory canal transmits sound waves to the tympanic membrane, or eardrum. This canal is lined with numerous ceruminous glands that protect the canal and help keep the tympanic membrane pliable. The tympanic membrane separates the external ear from the middle ear. The middle ear consists of a bony cavity containing the three ossicles, called the malleus, incus, and stapes, which transmit sound waves to the inner ear. The eustachian tube provides a connection between the middle ear and the nasopharynx. It permits equalization of pressure in the middle ear by allowing air to enter or leave the middle ear cavity and for the drainage of secretions. Its mucosa is continuous with the mucosal lining of the throat, providing a means for infectious organisms to enter the middle ear from the nose and throat. The inner ear consists of the semicircular canals, the vestibule, and the cochlea. The cochlea is the main organ of hearing, whereas the semicircular canals and vestibule are responsible for balance and equilibrium.

Pharmacotherapy with Otic Preparations

74.10 Otic preparations treat infections, inflammation, and earwax buildup.

Otitis, or inflammation of the ear, is a common indication for pharmacotherapy. **External otitis**, commonly called swimmer's ear, is an inflammation with or without infection of the outer ear. The acute form is bacterial in origin and most often due to *Pseudomonas aeruginosa* or *S. aureus*. It is associated with water exposure, high humidity, and a history of ear trauma generally from sharp or small objects. Chronic external otitis is most often caused by a fungal infection or an allergic response usually associated with cosmetics, hair products, or devices placed within the ear canal. The typical presentation is that of acute-onset ear pain associated with pruritus, swelling, and tenderness to the touch or with movement. A greenish white drainage may accompany symptoms. Hearing impairment may result if the swelling is sufficient to obstruct the auditory canal.

Treatment of external otitis focuses on reducing pain and inflammation, usually with topical corticosteroids, antibiotics, and analgesics, as needed. Neomycin, gentamicin, and ciprofloxacin (Cipro otic) are the most commonly used topical otic antibiotics. Mild fungal infections can be treated with a 90% to 95% alcohol solution; more advanced disease may be treated with topical 1% clotrimazole (Lotrimin) or tolnaftate (Tinactin). If swelling

CONNECTIONS | Patient Safety

◄ Reaction to Eyedrops

A 22-year-old female is given a prescription for levofloxacin (Quixin) ophthalmic drops for treatment of bacterial conjunctivitis. Immediately after instilling the drops, she experiences eye itching, periorbital edema, rhinitis, and sneezing. She has a friend drive her to the emergency department where it is noted that she has mild dyspnea and wheezing, facial edema, and a pruritic rash on her cheeks and neck. She is treated with corticosteroids and after a period of observation, discharged home. When providing discharge instructions to this patient, what should the nurse include in the teaching?

See Answers to Patient Safety Question on student resource website.

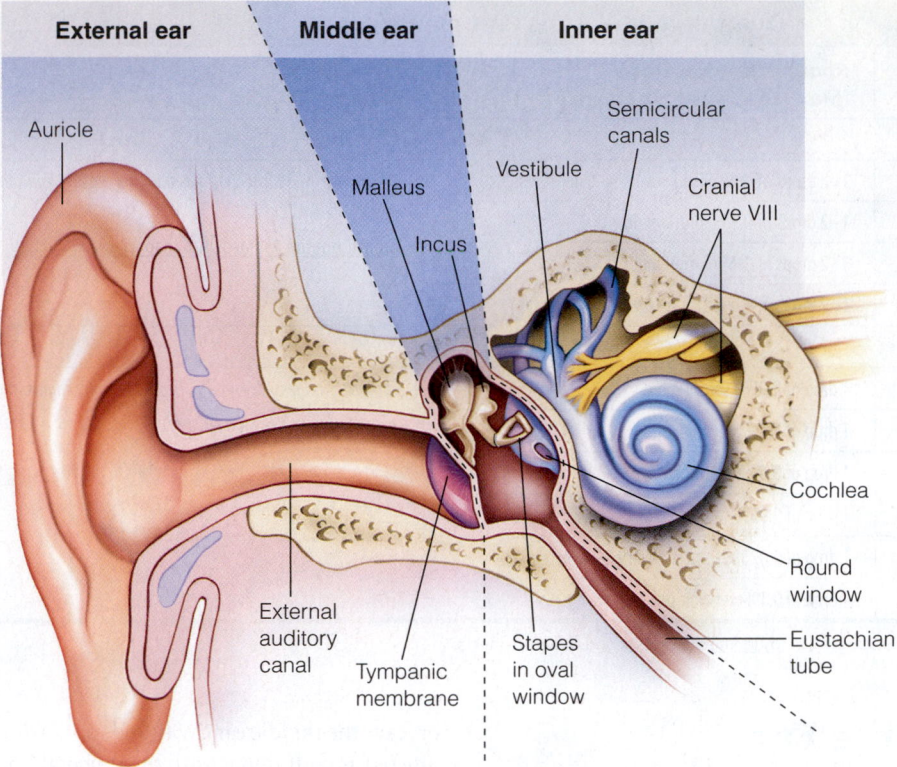

Figure 74.3 Anatomy of the ear.

obstructs the external canal, an ear wick may be placed past the blockage and the drops applied to the end. The use of systemic antibiotics may be necessary in cases when outer ear infections are extensive, such as with cellulitis or lymph node involvement.

Otitis media, which is inflammation of the middle ear, is a common disorder that affects infants and young children, although people of any age may be affected. Among children 75% experience at least one episode of otitis media by their third birthday, and almost half of these children will have three or more ear infections during that time.

There are three common types of otitis media: acute, chronic, and serous. Acute otitis media and chronic otitis media are similar. An infectious agent, most often a viral upper respiratory infection, results in pathogens being introduced into the middle ear through the eustachian tube, leading to swelling and inflammation of the ossicles of the middle ear. Bacterial infection with *S. pneumoniae*, *H. influenzae*, and *Streptococcus pyogenes* cause most cases. Otitis media may also be associated with allergies or eustachian tube dysfunction. Acute otitis has a duration of less than 3 weeks; chronic otitis follows repeated episodes and has a longer duration of symptoms. Sometimes the eardrum ruptures, and pus drains out of the ear. More commonly, the pus and mucus remain in the middle ear due to the swollen and inflamed eustachian tube. This is called middle ear effusion or serous otitis media. After the acute infection has passed, the effusion may remain and become chronic, lasting for weeks, months, or even years.

The chief symptom of otitis media is ear pain with an accompanying sense of fullness in the ear. Headaches are common, along with malaise and nausea. The patient may experience tinnitus or popping sounds when yawning or swallowing. Otitis media is often

difficult to detect because most children affected by this disorder do not yet have sufficient speech and language skills to tell someone what is bothering them. Common signs include the following:

- Unusual irritability
- Difficulty sleeping
- Tugging or pulling at one or both ears
- Fever
- Purulent or bloody drainage from the ear
- Loss of balance
- Unresponsiveness to quiet sounds, or other signs of hearing difficulty such as sitting too close to the television or being inattentive

The American Academy of Pediatrics and the American Academy of Family Physicians released clinical practice guidelines for the treatment of otitis media. The management of pain, especially during the first 24 hours of an episode of acute otitis media, should be part of the plan of care, regardless of the use of antibacterial agents. Whether or not to place a patient on antibiotics or to observe is based on a child's age, diagnostic certainty, and illness severity. The observation option is defined as deferring antibacterial treatment of selected children for 48 to 72 hours and limiting management to symptomatic relief. This option should be limited to otherwise healthy children 6 months to 2 years of age with nonsevere illness at presentation and an uncertain diagnosis and to children 2 years of age and older without severe symptoms at presentation or with an uncertain diagnosis. All children under 6 months of age should receive antibiotic therapy.

TABLE 74.4   Otic Preparations

Drug	Route and Adult Dose (Maximum Dose Where Indicated)	Adverse Effects
acetic acid and hydrocortisone (VoSoL HC)	3–5 drops every 4 h–qid for 24 h, then 5 drops tid–qid	*Ear irritation, local stinging or burning, dizziness*
benzocaine and antipyrine (Auralgan)	Fill the ear canal with solution tid for 2–3 days	
carbamide peroxide (Debrox)	1–5 drops of 6.5% solution bid for 4 days	<u>Allergic reactions (antibiotics)</u>
ciprofloxacin/dexamethasone (Ciprodex)	4 drops in the affected ear bid for 7 days	
ciprofloxacin/hydrocortisone (Cipro HC)	3 drops of the suspension instilled into the ear bid for 7 days	
polymyxin B, neomycin, and hydrocortisone (Cortisporin)	3 drops in the ear tid–qid	

Note: *Italics* indicate common adverse effects. <u>Underline</u> indicates serious adverse effects.

Otitis media is treated with a course of systemic, rather than topical, antibiotics. Amoxicillin, at a dose of 80 to 90 mg/kg/day, is prescribed for most children. For patients who have symptoms of a more severe illness and in those for whom additional coverage for β-lactamase-positive *H. influenzae* and *Moraxella catarrhalis* is desired, therapy is initiated with high-dose amoxicillin-clavulanate. For patients with mild penicillin allergy, a cephalosporin may be considered. If the penicillin allergy is more severe, azithromycin or clarithromycin can be used. In the patient who is vomiting or cannot otherwise tolerate oral medication, a single dose of parenteral ceftriaxone has been shown to be effective.

Symptomatic relief for otitis externa and otitis media involves the use of analgesics, such as acetaminophen, or NSAIDs, such as ibuprofen, to relieve pain and reduce fever. Patients with severe pain may require therapy with opioid analgesics such as codeine. A 7-day course of a corticosteroid is often combined with antibiotics when severe inflammation is present. Antihistamines or decongestants may be used to decrease mucus production and fluid levels in the middle ear. Examples of these drugs are listed in Table 74.4.

Otitis interna, or labyrinthitis, may occur as the result of chronic otitis media or as part of a viral systemic infection, including mononucleosis or an upper respiratory infection. Of all ear infections, otitis interna is the most difficult to treat because the blood–labyrinth barrier makes it difficult for systemic medications to reach the affected areas. **Mastoiditis**, or inflammation of the mastoid sinus, is frequently the result of chronic or inadequately treated bacterial otitis media or inner ear infection. The infection moves into the bone and surrounding structures of the ear. Symptoms of pain, hearing loss, and tenderness typically appear 2 to 3 weeks after an episode of otitis media. Mastoiditis can be a serious problem. If left untreated, it can result in hearing loss.

The treatment of acute mastoiditis involves aggressive antibiotic therapy. IV gentamicin or ticarcillin may be used initially. Therapy may be adjusted once culture and sensitivity results are obtained. Therapy is continued for at least 14 days. If the antibiotics are not effective and symptoms persist, surgery such as a mastoidectomy or meatoplasty may be indicated.

Cerumen (earwax) softeners are also used for proper ear health. When cerumen accumulates, it narrows the ear canal and may interfere with hearing. **Cerumenolytics** may be needed to loosen and remove impacted cerumen from the ear canal. Use of these agents usually involves the instillation of an earwax softener and then a gentle lavage of the wax-impacted ear with tepid water using an irrigating syringe to gently insert the water. An instrument called an ear loop may be used to help remove earwax but should be used only by health care providers who are skilled in using it. There are three types of cerumen-softening preparations: water based, oil based, and nonwater oil based. Water-based preparations include solutions of triethanolamine, 3% hydrogen peroxide, 10% sodium bicarbonate, and saline or water. The nonwater oil-based preparation available in the United States includes the OTC drug carbamide peroxide (Debrox). Oil-based preparations include household olive, mineral, and almond oils and commercially prepared combinations, such as Cerumol, Earex, and Otocerol. Research has shown that the water-based and nonwater oil-based agents have equal effectiveness.

PharmFACT

Viral labyrinthitis is the most common cause of labyrinthitis, which occurs most frequently in adults age 30 to 60. The condition usually presents with severe vertigo, nausea, and vomiting. Permanent hearing loss is common in adults and may occur in up to 20% of pediatric cases (Boston, 2012).

Patients Receiving Pharmacotherapy for Otitis

Assessment	Potential Nursing Diagnoses*
Baseline assessment prior to administration: • Obtain a complete health history including neurologic disease. • Assess hearing and balance. Obtain audiology screening as needed. • Assess for history of recent infections, swimming, condition of external ear canal, presence of drainage, and tympanic membrane assessment. • Obtain a drug history including allergies, current prescription and OTC drugs, herbal preparations, alcohol use, and smoking. Be alert to possible drug interactions. • Obtain baseline vital signs. • Assess the patient's ability to receive and understand instructions. Include the family or caregiver as needed.	• *Acute Pain*, related to adverse drug effects • *Activity Intolerance* • *Deficient Knowledge* (Drug Therapy) • *Risk for Injury*, related to condition or adverse drug effects • *Risk for Falls*, related to condition or adverse drug effects • *Risk for Impaired Verbal Communication*
Assessment throughout administration: • Assess for desired therapeutic effects dependent on the reason the drug is given (e.g., infection is clearing, or hearing is maintained). • Assess for adverse effects: localized irritation or burning, dizziness, vertigo, nausea, or vomiting. Severe ear pain, increased drainage, fever, increasing dizziness, vertigo, nausea, and vomiting should be immediately reported to the health care provider.	

Implementation

Interventions and (Rationales)	Patient-Centered Care
Ensuring therapeutic effects: • Monitor hearing and balance. Obtain audiology screening periodically as needed. (Hearing remains within the patient's baseline assessment parameters, no dizziness or vertigo is noted.)	• Instruct the patient to immediately report severe ear pain, increased drainage, fever, increasing dizziness, vertigo, nausea, vomiting, or tenderness in or around the ear to the health care provider.
Minimizing adverse effects: • Monitor appropriate administration of the drug to avoid adverse effects. (Eardrops should be administered into the ear canal without dropping the solution directly on the tympanic membrane, which may induce vertigo.)	• Teach the patient the proper administration techniques for eardrops.
• Monitor hearing periodically in patients with chronic otitis with effusion. (Otitis media with effusion may lead to hearing loss and speech or language impairment, especially in young children.)	• Instruct the patient, family, or caregiver on the importance of returning for and maintaining regular hearing exams.
• Monitor balance and for changes in gait or ambulation. (Dizziness or vertigo may cause an intolerance to activity and increase the risk for falls. **Lifespan:** Monitor older adults more frequently for dizziness to prevent falls.)	• Instruct the patient to immediately report any increasing dizziness or vertigo. Assist the patient with ambulation if dizziness is present to prevent falls. If dizziness occurs at home, the patient should sit or lie down and not attempt to stand or walk, until the sensation passes.
• Provide for ear comfort such as warm, moist compresses to the outer ear. (Warm, moist compresses to the outer ear may increase circulation to the local area and ease ear discomfort.)	• Teach the patient to apply warm but not hot compresses to the external ear for approximately 15–20 min as needed for discomfort.
Patient understanding of drug therapy: • Use opportunities during administration of medications and during assessments to discuss the rationale for the drug therapy, desired therapeutic outcomes, commonly observed adverse effects, parameters for when to call the health care provider, and any necessary monitoring or precautions. (Using time during nursing care helps to optimize and reinforce key teaching areas.)	• The patient should be able to state the reason for the drug, appropriate dose and scheduling, what adverse effects to observe for, and when to report them.

Patient self-administration of drug therapy:
• When administering the medication, instruct the patient, family, or caregiver in proper self-administration of the drug, e.g., appropriate instillation of eardrops, followed by teach-back. (Utilizing time during nurse-administration of these drugs helps to reinforce teaching.)
	• Teach the patient to take the drug following appropriate guidelines:
	  • Warm eardrop solution by placing in or under warm but not hot water. The bottle may be placed in a plastic bag to protect the label before warming. *Never* warm eardrops in the microwave.
	  • Have the patient lie supine with the ear to be treated uppermost. Gently pull the pinna down and back for children under age 3, up and back for children over age 3, adolescents, and adults.
	  • Instill the number of drops ordered into the ear canal, taking care not to drop the solution directly onto the eardrum but allowing it to slide down the side of the ear canal.
	  • Gently massage the area in front of the ear (tragus) to promote thorough administration of the drop unless pain is severe.
	  • Have the patient continue lying down for 5–10 min to ensure complete absorption of the eardrop. A small piece of cotton may be placed at the entrance to the ear canal if any solution returns upon arising.

*Nursing Diagnoses—Definitions and Classification 2015–2017. Copyright © 2014, 1994–2014 by NANDA International. Used by arrangement with John Wiley & Sons Limited.

CHAPTER 74

Understanding the Chapter

Key Concepts Summary

74.1 Knowledge of basic eye anatomy is fundamental to understanding eye disorders and their pharmacotherapy.

74.2 The two principal types of glaucoma, closed-angle glaucoma and open-angle glaucoma, are characterized by increased intraocular pressure.

74.3 The primary goal of glaucoma pharmacotherapy is to prevent damage to the optic nerve by lowering intraocular pressure.

74.4 Prostaglandin analogs are the first-line drugs for treating high intraocular pressure because of their long durations of action and high safety profiles.

74.5 Drugs that affect the autonomic nervous system are sometimes prescribed to treat glaucoma.

74.6 Carbonic anhydrase inhibitors and osmotic diuretics are occasionally used for treating glaucoma.

74.7 Drugs that are routinely used for eye examinations include mydriatics, cycloplegics, diagnostic dyes, and local anesthetics.

74.8 Numerous pharmacologic agents are used to treat minor eye irritation and redness.

74.9 Knowledge of basic ear anatomy is fundamental to understanding ear disorders and pharmacotherapy.

74.10 Otic preparations treat infections, inflammation, and earwax buildup.

Case Study: Making the Patient Connection

Remember the patient "Therese Duclos" from the beginning of the chapter? Now read the remainder of the case study. Based on the information presented within this chapter, respond to the critical thinking questions that follow.

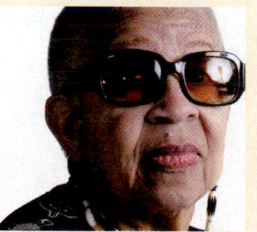

Therese Duclos, a 65-year-old African American woman, visits her ophthalmologist with reports of blurry vision and not being able to see well at night while driving. Her health history includes adult-onset diabetes for the past 10 years and osteoporosis since age 55. Her medical regimen includes diet control for the diabetes and Boniva monthly. She denies any injury to her eyes and last had an eye checkup 1 year ago.

Critical Thinking Questions

1. What factors are present in Mrs. Duclos's health history that you identify as predisposing conditions for the development of primary open-angle glaucoma?

2. Therese needs to learn the proper administration of eyedrops. What teaching would you provide to ensure that the skill will be performed correctly?

3. What would be possible effects from systemic absorption if the patient were taking beta-adrenergic drops (e.g., timolol, carteolol)? Prostaglandin drops (e.g., latanoprost, bimatoprost)? Cholinergic agonists (e.g., carbachol, pilocarpine)?

See Answers to Critical Thinking Questions on student resource website.

Additional Case Study

Zachary, a 4-year-old boy, is experiencing pain in his right ear. His mother takes him to the health care provider and he is diagnosed with otitis media. Zachary is prescribed ciprofloxacin with dexamethasone (Ciprodex) otic drops to be instilled in his right ear two times a day for a week. To ensure that the mother is knowledgeable in this form of administration, the nurse will teach her about the proper technique. Create a patient information sheet for a parent who needs to administer eardrops.

See Answers to Additional Case Study on student resource website.

Chapter Review

1 The nurse is teaching a patient about a new eyedrop prescription for timolol (Timoptic) for treatment of open-angle glaucoma. The patient has a history of seasonal allergies and hypertension. What is an important administration technique to stress for this patient?

1. Take any eyedrops for allergies 5 minutes before administering the timolol drops.
2. Do not use the timolol drops while concurrently taking allergy medication.
3. The timolol drops may temporarily worsen seasonal allergies.
4. Gently put pressure on the inner canthus (tear duct) for 1 minute after instilling the timolol drop.

2 The nurse is providing health teaching to a patient who has been prescribed latanoprost (Xalatan) for open-angle glaucoma. While harmless, the nurse would caution the patient about which potential nonocular effects of the drug? Select all that apply.

1. Darkening and thickening of the upper eyelid
2. Darkening and thickening of eyelashes
3. A lightening of iris color and a slight darkening of the sclera
4. A slight darkening of the iris color
5. A permanent bluish tint to the conjunctiva

3 Pilocarpine (Isopto Carpine) has been ordered for a patient with closed-angle glaucoma who has not responded well to other drugs. Pilocarpine causes _____, which stretches the trabecular meshwork, allowing a greater outflow of aqueous humor and lowering intraocular pressure.

4 The nurse is teaching a 25-year-old patient about the administration of ciprofloxacin with hydrocortisone (Cipro) for otitis. In which order will the nurse instruct the patient to use the drug?

1. Gently massage the area in front of the ear.
2. Pull the earlobe upward and back.
3. Allow the drop to fall into the ear canal flowing down the side.
4. Remain with the treated ear in an uppermost position for 5 minutes.

5 The nurse is teaching a patient with otitis about a prescription for polymyxin B, neomycin, with hydrocortisone (Cortisporin). The patient should be instructed to immediately report which symptom?

1. Mild itching in the outer ear canal
2. Gradually decreasing pain
3. Slight dizziness after instilling the eardrop
4. Increasing pain, particularly in the area around the ear

6 The nurse is instilling drops of phenylephrine (Neo-Synephrine) into the patient's eye before cataract surgery. Phenylephrine is used prior to cataract surgery because it causes _____, allowing visualization of the operative area.

See Answers to Chapter Review in Appendix A.

References

Boston, M. E. (2012). *Labyrinthitis*. Retrieved from http://emedicine.medscape.com/article/856215-overview

Glaucoma Research Foundation. (2011). *Are you at risk for glaucoma?* Retrieved from http://www.glaucoma.org/glaucoma/are-you-at-risk-for-glaucoma.php

Kiser, A. K., & Dagnelie, G. (2007). Reported effects of non-traditional treatments and complementary and alternative medicine by retinitis pigmentosa patients. *Clinical and Experimental Optometry, 91,* 166–176. doi:10.1111/j.1444-0938.2007.00224.x

Razeghinejad, M. R., & Katz, L. J. (2011). Steroid-induced iatrogenic glaucoma. *Ophthalmic Research, 47,* 66–80. doi:10.1159/000328630

Shim, S. H., Kim, J. M., Choi, C. Y., Kim, C. Y., & Park, K. H. (2012). Ginkgo biloba extract and bilberry anthocyanins improve visual function in patients with normal tension glaucoma. *Journal of Medicinal Food, 15,* 818–823. doi:10.1089/jmf.2012.2241

Yao, N., Lan, F., He, R. R., & Kurlhara, H. (2010). Protective effects of bilberry (*Vaccinium myrtillus* L.) extract against endotoxin-induced uveitis in mice. *Journal of Agricultural and Food Chemistry, 58,* 4731–4736. doi:10.1021/jf904572a

Selected Bibliography

Herdman, T. H., & Kamitsuru, S. (Eds.). (2014). *NANDA International nursing diagnoses: Definitions and classification, 2015–2017.* Oxford, United Kingdom: Wiley-Blackwell.

Huber, M., Kölzsch, M., Stahlmann, R., Hofmann, W., Bolbrinker, J., Dräger, D., & Kreutz, R. (2013). Ophthalmic drugs as part of polypharmacy in nursing home residents with glaucoma. *Drugs & Aging, 30,* 31–38. doi:10.1007/s40266-012-0036-x

Kaufman, P. L., & Rasmussen, C. A. (2012). Advances in glaucoma treatment and management: Outflow drugs. *Investigative Ophthalmology & Visual Science, 53,* 2495–2500. doi:10.1167/iovs.12-9483m

Kopczynski, C. C., & Epstein, D. L. (2013). Emerging trabecular outflow drugs. *Journal* of *Ocular Pharmacology and Therapeutics, 30*, 85–87. doi:10.1089/jop.2013.0197

Lieberthal, A. S., Carroll, A. E., Chonmaitree, T., Ganiats, T. G., Hoberman, A., Jackson, M. A.,...Tunkel, D. E. (2013). The diagnosis and management of acute otitis media. *Pediatrics, 131*(3), e963–e999. doi:10.1542/peds.2012-3488

Oron, Y., Zwecker-Lazar, I., Levy, D., Kreitler, S., & Roth, Y. (2010). Cerumen removal: Comparison of cerumenolytic agents and effect on cognition among the elderly. *Archives of Gerontology and Geriatrics, 52*(2), 228–232. doi:10.1016/j.archger.2010.03.025

Saito, M., & Nakada, T. (2013). Contact urticarial syndrome from eye drops: Levofloxacin hydrate ophthalmic solution. *The Journal of Dermatology, 40*(2), 130–131. doi:10.1111/1346-8138.12019

Saxby, C., Williams, R., & Hickey, S. (2013). Finding the most effective cerumenolytic. *The Journal of Laryngology & Otology, 127*, 1067–1070. doi.10.1017/S0022215113002375

Shields, M. B. (2010). *Textbook of glaucoma* (6th ed.). Philadelphia, PA: Lippincott, Williams and Wilkins.

Venekamp, R. P., Sanders, S., Glasziou, P. P., Del Mar, C. B., & Rovers, M. M. (2013). Antibiotics for acute otitis media in children. *Cochrane Database Systematic Reviews, 1,* CD000219. doi:10.1002/14651858.CD000219.pub3

Yumori, J. W., & Cadogan, M. P. (2011). Primary open-angle glaucoma: Clinical update. *Journal of Gerontological Nursing, 37*(3), 10–15. doi:10.3928/00989134-20110210-01

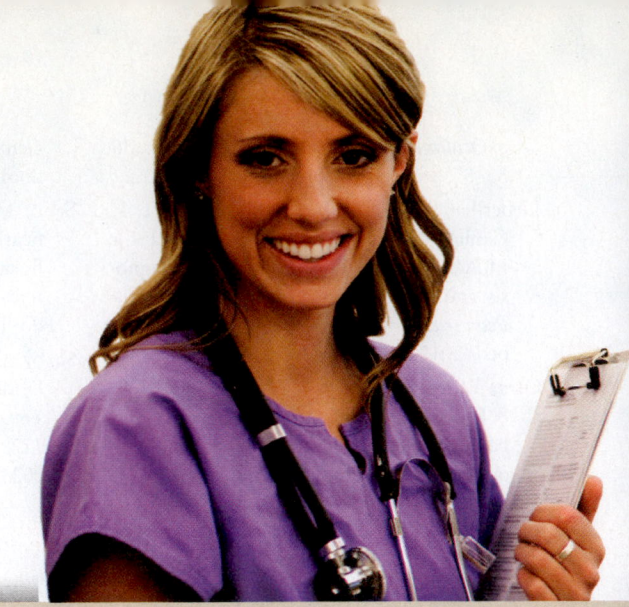

"I don't know if you can ever be completely prepared, but that's why we keep practicing and running drills. If something occurs, we'll be ready."

Emergency department nurse "Carol Boler"

Emergency Preparedness: Bioterrorism and Management of Poisoning

LEARNING OUTCOMES

After reading this chapter, the student should be able to:

1. Discuss the role of professional nursing in emergency preparedness and the management of poisoning.
2. Discuss the purpose, function, and components of the Strategic National Stockpile.
3. Identify the types of agents that might be used for a bioterrorist attack.
4. Compare and contrast the various chemical agents that can be used as poisons.
5. Explain the risks associated with ionizing radiation emitted from a nuclear terrorist attack.
6. Describe the five general principles of treating acute poisoning.
7. Identify the drugs important in emergency preparedness and management of poisoning.
8. Compare the pharmacologic management of biologic, chemical, radiologic, nuclear, and explosive agents in emergency preparedness.
9. Discuss the management of poisoning by the poison control center, including minimizing poison absorption and enhancing poison removal.
10. Apply the nursing process to the care of patients who are receiving pharmacotherapy for poisoning or overdose.

CHAPTER OUTLINE

▸ **Emergency Preparedness, Bioterrorism, and Nursing**

▸ **Biologic Agents**
 Anthrax
 Botulism
 Pneumonic Plague
 Tularemia
 Viruses

▸ **Chemical and Physical Agents**
 Chemical Toxins
 Ionizing Radiation

▸ **Management of Poisoning**
 Drugs Used in the Management of Poisoning
 PROTOTYPE Activated Charcoal (CharcoAid), *p. 1309*
 Ion Trapping
 Chelating Drugs
 PROTOTYPE Edetate Calcium Disodium (Calcium EDTA), *p. 1310*
 PROTOTYPE Dimercaprol (BAL in Oil), *p. 1311*

KEY TERMS

anthrax, 1305

bioterrorism, 1303

botulism, 1306

chelation therapy, 1310

emergency preparedness, 1303

pneumonic plague, 1306

radiation sickness, 1307

smallpox, 1306

Strategic National Stockpile (SNS), 1304

tularemia, 1306

Emergency preparedness is the ability to respond swiftly and effectively to an unexpected event that may impact human health. The unexpected event may be a natural disaster caused by severe weather, an accidental chemical spill, or a purposeful terrorist attack on the public. Nurses have an essential role in assessing and recognizing poisoning and taking appropriate interventions to save lives. Sometimes, specific drugs are necessary to counter the effects of biologic hazards and minimize the loss of life in emergency situations. This chapter focuses on the role of pharmacology in emergency preparedness as related to bioterrorism and management of poisoning.

Emergency Preparedness, Bioterrorism, and Nursing

75.1 Emergency preparedness has become an essential competency for all health care professionals.

Emergency preparedness has been an emerging role of professional nursing for many years. In the past, however, most training focused on emergency management for natural disasters, catastrophic accidents, or infectious epidemics. Often nurses responded to victims at the location of the disaster or accident. Today, nurses must learn how to respond to mass casualty incidents and potential disasters that can result from agents that are biologic, chemical, radiologic, nuclear, or explosive in nature. Standard emergency triage may be reversed, focusing on patients with the best chance to live.

Nurses may be among the first responders to victims who arrive at emergency departments, clinics, health care provider offices, or school health settings. They must be prepared to assess and recognize when someone has been exposed to potential hazards and to take appropriate actions. Failure to do so could lead to an epidemic or major loss of life. Examples include patients who present to the health care setting with symptoms of anthrax, avian flu, or severe acute respiratory syndrome (SARS).

Since the terrorist attacks of September 11, 2001, Americans are more concerned with threats of terrorism and are more aware of emergency preparedness than ever before. Increased efforts to safeguard the general populace remain at an all-time high. Health care providers must continually update their knowledge of emergency management and think more globally in dealing with patients whose illness presents in a less typical way. Knowledge of treatment modalities related to bioterrorism has become a basic competency required of all health care providers.

75.2 Bioterrorism is the intentional release of a virus or microorganism to cause human harm.

The last decade has brought the acts and effects of terrorism to the forefront of discussion in this and other countries. Terrorism is generally defined as the systematic use of terror, violence, or intimidation to achieve a desired purpose or end. The U.S. Federal Criminal Code describes terrorism as activities that involve life-threatening acts intended to coerce or intimidate a given population. Terrorists use chemical, nuclear, radiologic, explosive, or biologic hazards to commit violent and intimidating crimes against general and special targeted populations.

Bioterrorism is the intentional release of an infectious agent for the purpose of causing harm to a large number of people. In the United States, governmental agencies such as the Centers for Disease Control and Prevention (CDC) and the Department of Defense provide education to prepare the general public for possible bioterrorism events. In the wrong hands, simple and easily obtained toxic agents could be disseminated for public harm. However, of greatest concern is the use of highly infectious diseases such as anthrax, smallpox, hemorrhagic viruses, and plague, or toxic agents such as nerve gas, cyanide, and chlorinated agents as well as nuclear and radiation threats. Table 75.1 provides the CDC list of biologic threats and their potential impact on the health of the general public.

75.3 Nurses may have the first opportunity to recognize and initiate a response to bioterrorism.

Nursing has a rich history in emergency preparedness. Florence Nightingale began defining the role of nursing in emergency preparedness as early as the Crimean War. Throughout many wars and disasters, nurses have honed their assessment and critical care skills to support people in need and improve health care outcomes. The Civil War was a time when nurses worked together with leaders like Clara Barton to establish the American Red Cross, with nursing becoming a special service in 1909. In World War II, nurses became a defined group within the military, and the Cadet Nurse Corps was established. These wartime nurses learned triage, provided trauma care, and administered penicillin to save many lives. Nurses have played a major role in providing emergency assistance in natural disasters such as earthquakes, tornados, hurricanes, floods, and tsunamis. The challenges have now expanded to include bioterrorism, toxins, radiation, and mass casualty emergencies.

Today emergency preparedness has come to the forefront of professional nursing practice. Established through a grant in 2004 in collaboration with the U.S. Department of Homeland Security, the National Nurse Emergency Preparedness Initiative (NNEPI) advances the education and policy related to emergency preparedness for professional nurses.

In 2001, the International Nursing Coalition for Mass Casualty Education was established, defining emergency preparedness competencies for registered nurses responding to mass casualty incidents (MCIs). Now known as the Nursing Emergency Preparedness Education Coalition (NEPEC), the coalition identified a set of general core competencies that provides guidelines for the role of

TABLE 75.1	Categories of Infectious Agents	
Category	**Description**	**Examples**
A	Agents that pose a significant risk to national security because they • can easily be disseminated or transmitted person to person; • result in high mortality rates with potential for major public health impact; • might cause public panic and social disruption; and • require special action for public health preparedness.	Anthrax (*Bacillus anthracis*) Botulism (*Clostridium botulinum toxin*) Plague (*Yersinia pestis*) Smallpox (*Variola major*) Tularemia (*Francisella tularensis*) Viral hemorrhagic fevers such as Marburg, Ebola, Lassa, and Machupo
B	Second highest priority agents include those that • are moderately easy to disseminate; • result in moderate morbidity and low mortality rates; and • require specific enhancements of CDC's diagnostic capacity and enhanced disease surveillance.	Brucellosis (Brucella species) Epsilon toxin of *Clostridium perfringens* Food safety threats such as salmonella, Shigella, and *Escherichia coli* Glanders (*Burkholderia mallei*) Melioidosis (*Burkholderia pseudomallei*) Psittacosis (*Chlamydia psittaci*) Q fever (*Coxiella burnetii*) Ricin toxin from *Ricinus communis* Staphylococcal enterotoxin B Typhus fever (*Rickettsia prowazekii*) Viral encephalitis Water safety threats such as *Vibrio cholerae* and *Cryptosporidium parvum*
C	Third highest priority agents include emerging pathogens that could be engineered for mass dissemination in the future because of • availability; • ease of production and dissemination; and • potential for high morbidity and high mortality rates and major health impact.	Hantaviruses Nipah virus (NiV)

From *Emergency Preparedness & Response: Bioterrorism Agent/Diseases,* Centers for Disease Control and Prevention, n.d. Retrieved from http://www.bt.cdc.gov/agent/agentlist-category.asp

professional nurses in responding to mass casualty events. Competencies identified included the ability to adequately assess the situation and victims of an MCI and to have the technical and communication skills required to function as an effective member of the response team. Under technical skills, nurses must demonstrate safe administration of medications and immunizations and have knowledge of nursing interventions for adverse medication events. This is but one area of professional nursing practice where knowledge of pharmacology is important to nursing emergency preparedness.

For more than 30 years The Joint Commission, formerly called the Joint Commission for Accreditation of Healthcare Organizations (JCAHO), has required accredited hospitals to meet standards in disaster planning. In the late 1990s, The Joint Commission added standards that address possible bioterrorism and emergency management. State and federal agencies have developed updated emergency preparedness plans that include bioterrorism. Nurses are part of the collaborative developed by health care professionals to respond immediately to a community emergency. Key roles for nurses include education, resources, referrals, diagnosis, treatment, and planning. Pharmacology for emergency preparedness has a role in each of these.

75.4 The Strategic National Stockpile has large quantities of medicine to protect the public if there is a health emergency.

When a health emergency such as a biologic or chemical attack, flu outbreak, or earthquake occurs, the response must be rapid to minimize health consequences and protect the American public. Due to the unexpected nature of such an incident, shortages in medical supplies, equipment, and drugs may occur. The **Strategic National Stockpile (SNS)** is a national repository of antibiotics, chemical antidotes, antitoxins, antiviral drugs, life support medications, intravenous (IV) administration equipment, airway maintenance supplies, and surgical material for use in a declared biologic or terrorism incident or other major health emergency. The CDC manages the SNS to ensure immediate availability and deployment of essentials to any state. These antibiotics, vaccines, and medical supplies are free to the population affected by the adverse event.

One of the two components of the SNS is the Push Packages, which include preassembled caches of drugs, antidotes, and medical supplies that broadly cover a nonspecific emergency for use in early hours. Stored strategically, deployment can be accomplished within 12 hours. The SNS program ensures that the medical materials stock is rotated and kept within potency shelf-life limits. The second component is vendor-managed inventory (VMI) packages that contain additional supplies that can be more event specific and ship within 24 to 36 hours. This plan is designed to minimize local hospital stockpiling of bioterrorism pharmaceuticals that have expiration dates and can be costly.

Parts of the SNS were deployed for relatively recent health threats. In 2005, SNS response teams were sent to support state efforts in responding to hurricanes Rita and Katrina on the Gulf Coast. Part of the SNS antiviral inventory was used to help state efforts to control the H1N1 swine influenza outbreak in 2009.

Biologic Agents

75.5 Highly infectious bacteria or viruses could be used as bioterrorist threats.

The U.S. government takes the threat of bioterrorism seriously and has implemented a program to prepare the public for such catastrophes. Six biologic agents are considered category A threats (see Table 75.1), meaning they could cause enough mortality and morbidity damage to interfere with the social functioning of a large city or populated area. Included in these are anthrax, botulism toxin, pneumonic plague, smallpox, tularemia, and viral hemorrhagic fevers. Knowing the agents most likely to be used in a terrorist event allows the professional nurse to plan and to prepare for emergencies of this nature. The nurse can be an effective member of the emergency team who is responding to the widespread panic and life-threatening illnesses caused by an attack of bioterrorism.

Anthrax is an acute infectious disease that results from exposure to the spore-forming bacterium *Bacillus anthracis*. The spore produces a toxin that can be fatal to the host. Although microbiologist Robert Koch confirmed the bacterial nature of anthrax in 1876, anthrax has plagued the world for many centuries, even in biblical times. Anthrax infection is found among hoofed animals such as cattle, sheep, goats, pigs, bison, antelopes, and elephants. It was recognized as a potential biologic weapon in World War I, and several countries were suspected of experimentation with the use of the bacterium as a weapon in World War II. In 1995, Iraq admitted production of anthrax as a biologic weapon. U.S. military personnel were vaccinated before deployment to the Gulf War areas.

In the fall of 2001, following the terrorist attacks on the World Trade Center, five people died from exposure to anthrax in what most believe were purposeful acts of bioterrorism. In total there were 19 confirmed and 4 suspected cases occurring across the United States in Florida, Pennsylvania, Maryland, New York, Virginia, Connecticut, New Jersey, and the District of Columbia. Over 32,000 people were treated for possible exposure, many of whom were postal workers, between October 8 and November 9, 2001. Lives were lost, government workers and U.S. citizens were critically threatened, and agency operations such as the U.S. Postal Service were interrupted for weeks.

Anthrax poisoning can occur by ingestion, absorption through an open wound on the skin, or inhalation, which is the most dangerous route. The method of transmission affects the symptoms demonstrated. Table 75.2 summarizes the clinical picture of anthrax. Anthrax infects by releasing two toxins, edema toxin and lethal toxin, which cause necrosis and exudate accumulation and cause symptoms such as pain, edema, and restricted activity. The anthrax-binding receptor binds with a human cell, allowing the bacterial toxins to enter. Anthrax produces heat and chemically resistant spores, which can remain viable in soil for many years. These are dangerous because they have the potential for inhalation infection for humans. Left untreated inhalation anthrax is usually deadly. In the anthrax attacks in the United States in fall 2001, anthrax was delivered as a fine powder. This form of anthrax is easily inhaled and adheres to almost any surface.

Several drugs can be used to treat anthrax. Ciprofloxacin (Cipro) is the primary antibiotic used with a prophylaxis oral (PO) dose of 500 mg every 12 hours for 60 days. If anthrax exposure is confirmed, the patient is immediately administered IV treatment with 400 mg every 12 hours. Anthrax can also be treated with other antibiotics such as penicillin, ampicillin, vancomycin, erythromycin, tetracycline, and doxycycline. Inhalation anthrax exposure may necessitate the combined use of ciprofloxacin and doxycycline but must be done immediately to avoid death. The public should be discouraged from seeking the prophylactic use of antibiotics in cases where anthrax exposure has not been confirmed. Indiscriminate, unnecessary use of antibiotics can be expensive, can cause significant adverse effects, and can promote the appearance of resistant bacterial strains. A prototype feature for ciprofloxacin can be found in Chapter 49.

CONNECTION Checkpoint 75.1

From what you learned in Chapter 49, name the antibiotic class to which ciprofloxacin belongs and describe its mechanism of bacteriocidal action. *See Answer to Connection Checkpoint 75.1 on student resource website.*

Although anthrax immunization was approved by the U.S. Food and Drug Administration (FDA) 30 years ago, it has not been widely used because of the extremely low incidence of this disease in the United States. The vaccine is prepared from proteins from the anthrax bacteria, dubbed "protective antigens." The anthrax vaccine causes the body to make protective antibodies, thus preventing the onset of disease and its symptoms. Immunization for anthrax consists of three subcutaneous injections given 2 weeks apart, followed by three additional subcutaneous injections given at 6, 12, and 18 months. Annual booster injections of the vaccine are recommended. At this time, the CDC recommends vaccination for only select populations such as laboratory personnel who work with anthrax, military personnel who are deployed to high-risk areas, and those who deal with animal products imported from areas with a high incidence of the disease.

TABLE 75.2 Clinical Manifestations of Anthrax

Type	Description	Symptoms
Cutaneous anthrax	Most common but least complicated form of anthrax; almost always curable if treated within the first few weeks of exposure; results from direct contact of contaminated products with an open wound or cut	Small skin lesions develop and turn into black scabs; inoculation takes less than 1 week; cannot be spread by person-to-person contact
Gastrointestinal anthrax	Rare form of anthrax; without treatment, can be lethal in up to 50% of cases; results from eating anthrax-contaminated food, usually meat	Sore throat, difficulty swallowing, cramping, diarrhea, and abdominal swelling
Inhalation anthrax	Least common but the most dangerous form of anthrax; can be successfully treated if identified within the first few days after exposure; results from inhaling anthrax spores	Initially, fatigue and fever for several days, followed by persistent cough and shortness of breath; without treatment, death can result within 4–6 days

There is an ongoing controversy regarding the safety of the anthrax vaccine and whether it is truly effective in preventing the disease. Until these issues are resolved, the use of anthrax immunization will likely remain limited to select groups. Vaccines and the immune response are discussed in more detail in Chapter 43.

Botulism is caused by *Clostridium botulinum*, an organism that secretes a potent toxin that paralyzes the muscles after a person is poisoned. Respiratory failure and paralysis may force a patient to be on a ventilator for weeks or months. As a biologic weapon, botulism could be transmitted in air, food, or water. Treatment includes immediate administration of an antitoxin and assisted ventilation until patients are able to function independently. The antitoxin should be given as soon as possible and never delayed pending the microbiologic testing. Trivalent botulinum antitoxin is available through state departments of health or the CDC. A pentavalent toxoid vaccine for botulism prophylaxis is available as an investigation drug through the Department of Defense.

Pneumonic plague is a life-threatening infectious lung disease that occurs after breathing *Yersinia pestis*, a bacterium found on rodents and their fleas that is responsible for the bubonic plague. It is highly contagious and can be deadly if untreated within 24 hours of contact. As a biologic agent, *Y. pestis* could be spread by aerosol over the population. Within 1 to 6 days of exposure, the patient would be infectious to everyone he or she has come in contact with during that time. This makes the plague difficult to contain. Symptoms include fever and weakness, rapid development of pneumonia, chest pain with shortness of breath, cough, and bloody sputum. Without immediate treatment, respiratory failure will result followed by shock and death. Treatment with antibiotics must occur within 24 hours and last for at least 7 days to prevent death from the infection. The primary antibiotic for *Y. pestis* infection is doxycycline 100 mg twice a day or ciprofloxacin 500 mg twice a day for 7 days. There is no vaccine approved in the United States for this bacterium at the present time.

Caused by the organism *Francisella tularensis*, **tularemia** is a serious infectious disease found in rodents, rabbits, and hares. Cases have been reported in almost every state, although overall the infection is rare in the United States. *F. tularensis* is one of the most infectious bacteria known and survives at low temperatures for weeks in hay, straw, moist soil, or in the bodies of decaying animals. As a biologic weapon the most casualties would be with aerosol release in an area of high population, causing hemorrhagic inflammation of the respiratory airway. Treatment includes IV therapy with streptomycin as the drug of choice, with parenteral gentamicin being an alternative. Aminoglycosides should be used for 10 days. Tetracyclines and chloramphenicol can be used for at least 14 days but have a higher rate of relapse and treatment failure. In mass casualty incidents, oral doxycycline for 14 to 21 days and ciprofloxacin for 10 days are preferred for adults and children. Antibiotics for treating tularemia are included in the SNS. A live attenuated vaccine is available as an investigational drug and is under review by the FDA.

A major viral biologic threat is the variola virus, better known as **smallpox**. This serious, contagious disease is fatal in up to 30% of cases. Although believed to be eradicated, with the last case in the United States occurring in 1949 and in Somalia in 1977, the virus may still be stockpiled in laboratories across the world for use as a biologic weapon. Generally personal contact is needed to spread this disease, but only a few viral droplets spread through the air or on contaminated objects are needed to produce the disease. Humans are the only carriers. Unvaccinated populations are at risk.

Vaccination is the only known treatment for smallpox. The vaccination gives immunity for 3 to 5 years and is effective if given prior to exposure to the virus or up to 3 days postexposure. Smallpox vaccinations are contraindicated for certain groups such as pregnant or lactating women, children under 1 year old, persons with impaired immune systems (such as with human immunodeficiency virus [HIV] or leukemia), persons with atopic dermatitis or eczema, or anyone with an allergy to a component in the vaccine. Although serious adverse effects are very rare, vaccines can cause death. A mutation in the virus would render the vaccine ineffective, so mass vaccinations for smallpox are not considered prudent at this time. Persons at risk such as law enforcement, health care professionals, or military personnel might need vaccination if exposed to the virus. The U.S. government maintains enough vaccinations for the public in the event of an outbreak.

Viral hemorrhagic fevers, which are caused by a number of virus families, can cause severe physical damage affecting multiple organ systems. Usually these viruses damage the circulatory system, resulting in hemorrhage. The host can be the cotton rat and deer mouse but some, such as Ebola or Marburg, have unknown hosts. There is no cure or vaccine for these viruses and patients are treated with supportive therapy, such as fluid and electrolytes, and management of complications. Ribavirin is an antiviral drug that has shown some success in treating Lassa fever. CDC researchers in the Special Pathogens Branch work with these hemorrhagic fever viruses, which are considered a biosafety level 4. This class consists of exotic agents that can be transmitted by aerosol and pose a high risk of life-threatening disease.

PharmFACT

Humans are not the natural hosts for the viruses that cause hemorrhagic fevers and only become infected when contacted by the urine, feces, saliva, or other body excretions from infected rodents and other carriers. Most cases are geographically restricted to the regions where the carriers exist (CDC, 2013b).

Chemical and Physical Agents

75.6 There are 13 categories of toxic chemicals that could cause mass casualties if released into the environment.

Chemical warfare agents have been used since World War I, but few drug antidotes exist today. Many treatments provide minimal help other than to relieve some symptoms and provide comfort following exposure. Whether a chemical is released by terrorists, enemy military, or by industry in a chemical accident, the result is the same: A hazardous chemical is released into the environment that may harm the health of the public. The CDC has classified hazardous chemicals into categories that include:

- **Biotoxins.** Poisons from plants or animals
- **Vesicants and blister agents.** Severely blister the skin, respiratory tract, or eyes on contact

- **Blood agents.** Poisons that are absorbed into the circulation
- **Acids and caustics.** Chemicals that burn the eyes, skin, or lining of the respiratory tract on contact
- **Pulmonary and choking agents.** Chemicals that irritate the lung and cause swelling and choking
- **Incapacitating agents.** Chemicals that alter consciousness, making it difficult for the patient to think clearly
- **Long-acting anticoagulants.** Chemicals that produce uncontrolled bleeding by preventing clotting
- **Metals.** Agents that are metallic poisons
- **Nerve agents.** Poisons that impair nervous system functioning
- **Organic solvents.** Chemicals that damage living tissue by dissolving fats and oils
- **Tear gas or mace.** Used for riot or crowd control by law enforcement or for self-defense; irritates the eyes and the respiratory tract, resulting in incapacitation
- **Toxic alcohols.** Chemicals that damage vital organs such as the heart, kidneys, and nervous system
- **Vomiting agents.** Chemicals that induce nausea and vomiting

Table 75.3 lists well-known chemical agents and their symptoms and treatments. The primary chemical hazards related to pharmacology are nerve agents. Persons who breathe nerve gas experience convulsions and loss of consciousness, which result in respiratory failure within minutes. The antidote for nerve gas is the anticholinergic drug atropine.

75.7 Ionizing radiation produces immediate and long-term effects on human tissue.

Bioterrorists may use nuclear bombs or attack nuclear facilities that could cause mass casualty deaths at the point of impact and create residual ionizing radiation for miles around the site. Some radioisotopes emit radiation for decades and even centuries. Smaller scale radiation could occur with the release of solid or liquid nuclear material into public areas or a dirty bomb, which explodes with radioactive powder or pellets, contaminating the area.

Radiation sickness occurs after exposure to ionizing radiation and can last from hours to days. Initial symptoms include nausea, vomiting, and diarrhea with later symptoms of weight loss, anorexia, fatigue, and suppression of the bone marrow. When exposed to large amounts of radiation or to small amounts over many decades, patients tend to develop certain malignancies such as leukemia or thyroid cancer.

Except for supportive therapies, the only recognized treatment available to counter the thyroid uptake of radiation is ingestion of potassium iodine (KI) before or immediately after exposure. One of the radioisotopes produced by a nuclear explosion is iodine 131 (I-131). Because iodine is naturally concentrated in the thyroid gland, I-131 will immediately enter the thyroid and damage thyroid cells. For example, following the Chernobyl nuclear disaster, the incidence of thyroid cancer in the Ukraine jumped from 4 to 6 cases per million people to 45 cases per million. If taken prior to, or immediately following, a nuclear incident, KI can prevent up to 100% of the radioactive iodine from entering the thyroid gland. It is

TABLE 75.3 Chemical Agents and Treatments

Agent	Signs and Symptoms	Decontamination	Persistence
Nerve Agents			
Tabun (GA)	Salivation Lacrimation Urination Defecation Gastric disturbances Emesis	Remove contaminated clothing. Flush with a soap and water solution for patients. Flush with large amounts of a 5% bleach and water solution for objects.	1–2 days if heavy concentration
Sarin (GB)			1–2 days will evaporate with water
Soman (GD)			Moderate, 1–2 days
V agents (VX)			High, 1 week if heavy concentration; as volatile as motor oil
Vesicants (Blister Agents)			
Sulfur mustard (H)	Acts first as a cell irritant, then as a cell poison. Conjunctivitis, reddened skin, blisters, nasal irritation, inflammation of throat and lungs.	Remove contaminated clothing. Flush with soap and water solution for patients. Flush with large amounts of a 5% bleach and water solution for objects.	Very high, days to weeks
Distilled mustard (HD)			
Nitrogen mustard (HN 1,3)			
Mustargen (HN 2)			Moderate
Lewisite (L)	Immediate pain with blisters later.		Days, rapid hydrolysis with humidity
Phosgene oxime (CX)	Immediate pain with blisters later—necrosis equivalent to second- and third-degree burns.		Low, 2 h in soil
Chemical Asphyxiants (Blood agents)			
Hydrogen cyanide (AC)	Cherry red skin or ~ 30% cyanosis. Patients may appear to be gasping for air. Seizures prior to death. Effect is similar to asphyxiation but is more sudden.	Remove contaminated clothing. Flush with a soap and water solution for patients. Flush with large amounts of 5% bleach and water solution for objects.	Extremely volatile, 1–2 days
Cyanogen chloride (CK)			Rapidly evaporates and disperses
Arsine (SA)			Low

From *Biological and Chemical Agent Quick Reference Tables*, Edgewood Chemical Biological Center, n.d. Retrieved from http://www.ecbc.army.mil/hld/ip/bca_qr.htm.

effective even if taken 3 to 4 hours after radiation exposure. Generally, a single 130-mg dose is necessary for adults.

Unfortunately, KI protects only the thyroid gland from I-131. It has no protective effects on other body tissues, and it offers no protection against the dozens of other harmful radioisotopes generated by a nuclear explosion. As with vaccines and antibiotics, the stockpiling of KI by local health care agencies or individuals is not recommended.

CONNECTION Checkpoint 75.2

From what you learned in Chapter 67, describe the therapeutic use of I-131 in treating thyroid disease. *See Answer to Connection Checkpoint 75.2 on student resource website.*

PharmFACT

The most serious nuclear accident in the United States occurred at the Three Mile Island nuclear plant in Pennsylvania in 1979. No injuries or deaths occurred and the average estimated dose of radiation to the public around the plant was 1 millirem, which is an amount equivalent to one sixth of a chest x-ray (U.S. Nuclear Regulatory Commission, 2013).

Management of Poisoning

75.8 The general management of poisoning includes contacting the poison control center or emergency medical services as soon as possible.

Virtually any chemical may cause poisoning if taken in excessive amounts. The body has a remarkable capacity to tolerate a wide variety of chemicals and has physiological mechanisms to detoxify and rapidly eliminate many of them. Toxicity results when the body's abilities for detoxification and excretion are exceeded. Toxic effects may appear immediately or they may appear decades after the initial exposure.

PharmFACT

About 100 people die every day in the United States from drug overdoses, most of which are caused by prescription medications. Prescription opioids cause more deaths each year than deaths from heroin and cocaine combined (CDC, 2013a).

Medications are the most frequently involved substances in poisonings for all age groups. Household cleaning compounds comprise a second large group of poisonings, with cosmetics being close behind. Although exposure to poisons may occur by any route, ingestion accounts for over 75% of all poisoning cases. Swallowing dangerous substances is common among children with curious minds who naturally put strange substances into their mouths. Most poisonings present with low levels of toxicity, but some can result in fatalities, such as the ingestion of gun-bluing agents used to maintain the color of gun barrels. Signs and symptoms of ingested poisons include abdominal cramping or stomach pain, nausea, vomiting, diarrhea, sleepiness or loss of consciousness, bottles or containers of poisons close by, or odor, stains, or burns around the oral cavity.

Poisoning from medications may be unintentional or intentional (suicide). Acetaminophen is a common toxin because so many analgesic medications contain this drug. Although legal for adults, alcohol is a potential poison and its abuse is a major health problem in the United States. Ingestion of alcohol, along with

certain prescribed medications, amphetamines, hallucinogens, barbiturates, tranquilizers, opiates, or inhaled substances such as solvents or glue can create life-threatening situations. Whether the overdose of alcohol is intentional or unintentional, the result is the same. Symptoms of drug overdose include confusion, elevated heart rate, drowsiness, enlarged or dilated pupils, and hallucinations. Other medications that cause frequent poisonings include iron, calcium channel blockers, and tricyclic antidepressants.

CONNECTION Checkpoint 75.3

From what you learned in Chapter 14, identify the cholinergic antagonist used to treat organophosphate poisoning. *See Answer to Connection Checkpoint 75.3 on student resource website.*

When a specific antidote is available, it is administered as soon as the poisoning is diagnosed (Table 75.4). In the vast majority of poisoning cases, there is no specific antidote. General therapies such as activated charcoal, peritoneal dialysis, and gastric lavage have only limited effectiveness. In some cases, they are totally ineffective. Emergency physicians and nurses are generally faced with treating individual symptoms either because the poison is unknown or because there is no antidote. The strategy for treatment of acute poisoning consists of five general principles:

- **Topical decontamination.** Removal of contaminated clothing, flushing of the skin or eyes
- **Prevention of absorption.** Administration of adsorbents (activated charcoal), whole-bowel irrigation, induction of vomiting, and gastric lavage

TABLE 75.4	**Specific Antidotes**
Poison	**Antidote**
acetaminophen	acetylcysteine (Mucomyst)
anticholinergic drugs	physostigmine (Antilirium)
benzodiazepines	flumazenil (Romazicon)
beta-adrenergic blockers	glucagon
calcium channel blockers	calcium, IV insulin in high doses with IV glucose
carbamates	atropine, pralidoxime (Protopam)
digoxin (Lanoxin)	digoxin immune Fab (Digibind)
ethylene glycol (antifreeze, brake fluid, coolants)	ethanol, fomepizole (Antizol)
heavy metals	chelating drugs
iron	deferoxamine (Desferal)
isoniazid (INH)	pyridoxine (vitamin B_6)
methanol	ethanol, fomepizole (Antizol)
methemoglobin-forming drugs (some local anesthetics, nitrates, nitrites, phenacetin, sulfonamides)	methylene blue
opioids	naloxone (Narcan)
organophosphates	atropine, pralidoxime (Protopam)
tricyclic antidepressants	sodium bicarbonate

- **Neutralization.** Administration of acids or bases
- **Increase in the rate of excretion.** Administration of diuretics, peritoneal or extracorporeal dialysis, and ion trapping
- **Antidotes and symptomatic therapy.** Administration of specific antidotes and support of vital functions

Treatment for ingested poisons depends on the age of the patient, physical size of the patient, and the time between swallowing and presenting for medical intervention. Any information about the poisoning that can be obtained from the patient, family, or caregiver can be helpful, such as the type of poison that was swallowed, when it was ingested, and how much was swallowed. Following are some specific interventions for managing the patient poisoned by ingestion:

- Do not implement the package instructions for poisoning without consulting the American Association of Poison Control Centers or an appropriate health care provider. Preferred therapy may have changed since the packaging was printed.

- Contact the poison control center if the poisoning is the result of taking too much or the wrong medication was taken.

- Provide fresh air to the person if the poison was inhaled.

- Remove contaminated clothes if the poison came in contact with the person's skin. Take care not to spread contamination from the poisoned clothes to the surrounding environment. Flush the skin with water for 15 to 20 minutes to dilute or remove the poison.

- Rinse the eyes with running water for 15 to 20 minutes if contacted by poison.

- Do not induce vomiting by gagging or tickling the back of the throat.

- Do not give ipecac syrup. Though once considered a routine procedure, this method of poison management is now considered ineffective. Discourage parents from keeping ipecac syrup in the home. There is no evidence that syrup of ipecac actually helps improve the outcome in poisoning cases. Furthermore,

the administration of syrup of ipecac can delay the administration of more effective treatments, such as activated charcoal or antidotes.

- Do not give milk or water unless directed to do so by the poison center. Though once thought to dilute the poison, fluids can liquefy dry poison and send it more rapidly to the small intestine. The exception to this is caustic or corrosive poisons.

75.9 Activated charcoal is effective at adsorbing (binding) most poisons if administered within 60 minutes of ingestion.

Activated charcoal has been used as an adsorbent for acute poisoning for almost 200 years. Activated charcoal is the only FDA-approved poison adsorbent drug. Although activated charcoal is effective in the treatment of many poisons, it is not beneficial when given to individuals with lithium, iron, or cyanide poisoning or strong acid or alkali ingestion.

PROTOTYPE DRUG	Activated Charcoal (CharcoAid)

Classification: Therapeutic: Antidote
Pharmacologic: Adsorbent drug

Therapeutic Effect and Uses: Activated charcoal consists of organic material such as coal, wood, or vegetables that have been carbonized, reduced, and dried to a charcoal-like substance. It is then activated by exposing it to steam, carbon dioxide, or other oxidizing chemicals at extremely high temperatures. The activation drives off impurities and reduces the particle size so that the surface area of the charcoal is very large.

This drug effectively adsorbs toxins in the intestinal tract, thus preventing their systemic absorption. Adsorption is the process of a drug physically binding to the charcoal. As a general-purpose emergency antidote, it is used in the treatment of poisonings of most drugs and chemicals. To be most effective the charcoal should be administered within 1 hour of oral ingestion. Normally, a single dose is administered, although some poisons benefit from multiple doses. The general dosage is 5 to 10 times the estimated weight of the poison ingested.

Activated charcoal can also be used off-label to adsorb intestinal gases in the treatment of dyspepsia, flatulence, and distention. It is sometimes used topically as a deodorant for foul-smelling wounds and ulcers.

Mechanism of Action: Activated charcoal (carbon) is a chemically inert, odorless, tasteless, fine black powder. It acts by binding (adsorbing) toxic substances, thereby inhibiting their gastric absorption, enterohepatic circulation, and bioavailability.

Pharmacokinetics:

Route(s)	PO or via nasogastric tube
Absorption	Not absorbed
Distribution	Not distributed systemically
Primary metabolism	Not metabolized
Primary excretion	Fecal
Onset of action	Rapid
Duration of action	Unknown

CONNECTIONS · Patient Safety

◀ Treating Accidental Poisonings in the Home

Luke, a 3-year-old boy, is rushed to the local emergency department after ingesting unknown quantities of medication while visiting his grandparents and cousins. When the child was found in the home by his mother, a multiday pill container was found nearby with four of the 7-day compartments open. In the panic and rush, no one is sure how many pills Luke consumed. He is oriented and talking but drowsy. While waiting for the rescue squad to arrive, a neighbor recommends that they give Luke 15 mL of syrup of ipecac followed by 240 mL of water. The family locates an old bottle of ipecac given by their pediatrician some years ago to "have on hand, just in case," but the rescue squad arrives before a dose is given.

What potential error was prevented by the timely arrival of the rescue squad? Should syrup of ipecac be given for accidental poisonings? Why or why not?

See Answers to Patient Safety Questions on student resource website.

Adverse Effects: Vomiting may occur when given by rapid ingestion and at high doses. Constipation and diarrhea have also been reported.

Contraindications/Precautions: Activated charcoal is not effective for poisonings by cyanide, mineral acids, caustic alkalis, organic solvents, iron, ethanol, or methanol ingestion. This drug should not be used in patients at a decreased level of consciousness or with a diminished gag reflex due to the risk of pulmonary aspiration. Activated charcoal also should not be used in individuals with central nervous system depression, coma, or gastrointestinal (GI) obstruction.

Drug Interactions: Activated charcoal will decrease absorption of all other oral medications. Oral medication should not be given for at least 2 hours after administration of activated charcoal. **Herbal/Food**: Milk and dairy products may decrease the effectiveness of activated charcoal.

Pregnancy: Category C.

Nursing Responsibilities: Key nursing implications for patients receiving activated charcoal are included in the Nursing Practice Application for Patients Receiving Pharmacotherapy for Poisoning or Overdose.

Drugs Similar to Activated Charcoal (CharcoAid)

Activated charcoal is the only drug in this class.

75.10 Ion trapping with forced diuresis may be helpful for some poisonings.

One procedure that is occasionally used in acute poisoning is ion trapping through forced diuresis. Because most drugs are either weak acids or weak bases, changing the urine pH can be used to enhance the elimination of some drugs. For example, if the urine is made alkaline the acidic drugs are trapped in the renal tubules and their elimination in urine is increased. The opposite effect applies for alkaline drugs.

Forced alkaline diuresis may be used to increase the excretion of acidic drugs like salicylates and phenobarbital, and forced acid diuresis has been used to eliminate amphetamines, quinine, and strychnine. When forced alkaline diuresis is employed, a diuretic such as furosemide along with IV sodium bicarbonate will make the urine more alkaline. Forced alkaline diuresis is specifically recommended when rhabdomyolysis (the rapid breakdown of skeletal muscle tissue) occurs.

Ascorbic acid is used for forced acid diuresis. In past decades, ammonium chloride was used for forced acid diuresis; however, due to the toxicity its use has greatly diminished. Research studies indicate that ion trapping through forced diuresis produces only a slight increase in the renal clearance of the drug and is rarely done in practice.

75.11 Chelating agents are capable of forming bonds with heavy metals.

Human exposure to metals has risen dramatically in the past 50 years as a result of an increase in the use of heavy metals in industrial processes and products. **Chelation therapy** is the use of drugs to detoxify poisonous metals such as mercury, arsenic, and lead by converting them to a chemically inert form that can be easily excreted. The compound formed by a chelating agent and a metal is called a chelate. Chelating agents are most frequently administered intravenously or intramuscularly depending on the agent and the type of poisoning. Chelation was introduced during World War I originally as an antidote to arsenic-based poison gas.

The mechanism of action of chelation therapies involves the chelating agent "latching onto" and removing positively charged metals from the body. Once the amino acid binds with the metal or poison, it can be eliminated from the body by the kidneys. Two chelating agents are described in this chapter. Many times both agents are given to the individual who is experiencing heavy metal poisoning.

PROTOTYPE DRUG	Edetate Calcium Disodium (Calcium EDTA)

Classification: **Therapeutic:** Drug for heavy metal poisoning **Pharmacologic:** Chelating agent

Therapeutic Effects and Uses: Approved in 1953, edetate calcium disodium is a chelating agent that binds with heavy metals such as lead to form a soluble complex that can be excreted by the kidneys, thereby ridding the body of the poisonous substance. Although usually used for acute poisoning, this drug can also remove lead that is stored in fat, bone, or other locations. Edetate calcium disodium is administered by the IV or intramuscular (IM) routes. This drug is generally used in combination with dimercaprol (BAL) in the treatment of lead encephalopathy or when the blood lead level exceeds 100 mcg/dL.

The off-label uses of edetate calcium disodium include the treatment of poisoning from other heavy metals such as chromium, manganese, nickel, zinc, and possibly vanadium, and removal of radioactive and nuclear fission products such as plutonium, yttrium, and uranium. However, this drug is not effective in treating poisoning from arsenic, gold, or mercury.

Mechanism of Action: As a chelating agent, Calcium EDTA combines with metals to form stable, nonionizing soluble complexes that can be readily excreted by the kidneys. Action is dependent on the ability of the heavy metal to displace the weakly bound calcium in the drug molecules.

Pharmacokinetics:

Route(s)	IV/IM
Absorption	Rapidly absorbed
Distribution	Distributed to extracellular fluid; does not enter the cerebrospinal fluid
Primary metabolism	Not metabolized
Primary excretion	Chelated lead is excreted in urine; 50% is excreted in 1 h
Onset of action	Peak chelation: 24–48 h
Duration of action	Half-life: 20–60 min IV, 90 min IM

Adverse Effects: Calcium EDTA may produce renal damage such as proteinuria and microscopic hematuria. Treatment-induced nephrotoxicity is dose dependent and may be reduced by ensuring adequate diuresis before therapy begins. Patients should be monitored for cardiac rhythm irregularities and other electrocardiogram (ECG) changes during IV therapy. Additional cardiovascular effects include hypotension and thrombophlebitis.

Many patients experience febrile reaction (excessive thirst, fever, chills, severe myalgia, arthralgia, GI distress) or histamine-like reactions (flushing, throbbing headache, sweating, sneezing, nasal congestion, lacrimation, postural hypotension, tachycardia). **Black Box Warning**: Patients with lead encephalopathy and cerebral edema may experience a lethal increase in intracranial pressure if the drug is given by IV infusion. The IM route is preferred for these patients.

Contraindications/Precautions: Edetate calcium disodium is contraindicated in patients with severe kidney disease, anuria, or oliguria. IV administration is contraindicated in patients with lead encephalopathy because of a possible increase in intracranial pressure.

Drug Interactions: No clinically significant interactions have been identified. **Herbal/Food**: None known.

Pregnancy: Category C.

Nursing Responsibilities: Key nursing implications for patients receiving edetate calcium disodium are included in the Nursing Practice Application for Patients Receiving Pharmacotherapy for Poisoning or Overdose.

PROTOTYPE DRUG	Dimercaprol (BAL in Oil)

Classification: Therapeutic: Antidote
Pharmacologic: Chelating agent

Therapeutic Effects and Uses: Given by the IM route, dimercaprol is a chelating agent that neutralizes the effects of various heavy metals such as arsenic, gold, and mercury. The drug forms stable, nontoxic intermediates with these metals so they are more easily excreted in the urine and bile. Dimercaprol is also used as an adjunct to EDTA in the treatment of lead encephalopathy. Off-label uses include chromium dermatitis and ocular and dermatologic manifestations of arsenic poisoning. Some studies indicate that dimercaprol may be used as an adjunct to penicillamine to increase the rate of copper excretion in Wilson's disease. Wilson's disease is a rare genetic disorder in which copper builds up in the liver and is released into other parts of the body.

Mechanism of Action: Dimercaprol forms ring complexes with some heavy metals, such as arsenic, gold, and mercury, preventing or reversing the binding of metallic cations to body proteins.

Pharmacokinetics:

Route(s)	IM only
Absorption	Well absorbed
Distribution	Distributed mainly in intracellular spaces, including the brain; highest concentration is in the liver and kidneys
Primary metabolism	Unknown
Primary excretion	Urine and feces
Onset of action	Peak: 30–60 min
Duration of action	Half-life: unknown

Adverse Effects: About 50% of patients who receive high therapeutic doses have minor reactions, which include nausea, vomiting, fatigue, restlessness, apprehension, headache, burning sensation of the mouth, throat, and eyes, lacrimation, blepharospasm, salivation, tingling of extremities, a feeling of constriction in the chest muscle, diffuse pain and muscle spasm, hypertension (systolic and diastolic), and tachycardia. Most patients report pain at the injection site.

Contraindications/Precautions: Dimercaprol is contraindicated in individuals with hepatic insufficiency (with the exception of postarsenic jaundice); severe renal insufficiency; or poisoning due to cadmium, iron, selenium, or uranium. Because dimercaprol is formulated in peanut oil, patients with a hypersensitivity to peanut products should not receive this drug. This drug should be used cautiously in patients with hypertension, oliguria, G6PD deficiency, and preexisting renal disease.

Drug Interactions: Dimercaprol should not be given when iron, cadmium, selenium, or uranium poisoning is suspected. When this drug is given in the presence of these poisonings, it forms toxic complexes. **Herbal/Food**: Unknown.

Pregnancy: Category C.

Nursing Responsibilities: Key nursing implications for patients receiving dimercaprol are included in the Nursing Practice Application for Patients Receiving Pharmacotherapy for Poisoning or Overdose.

CONNECTIONS: NURSING PRACTICE APPLICATION

Patients Receiving Pharmacotherapy for Poisoning or Overdose

Assessment	Potential Nursing Diagnoses*
Baseline assessment prior to administration: • Obtain a complete health history including musculoskeletal, GI, cardiovascular, neurologic, endocrine, hepatic, or renal disease. • Obtain a drug history including allergies, current prescription and OTC drugs, herbal preparations, alcohol use, or smoking. Be alert to possible drug interactions. • Obtain baseline weight, vital signs, and assessment of cardiopulmonary status. • Evaluate appropriate laboratory findings (e.g., hepatic and renal function studies, CBC, and urinalysis). • Assess the patient's ability to receive and understand instructions. Include the family or caregiver as needed. **Assessment throughout administration and care:** • Assess for desired therapeutic effects dependent on the reason for the drug (e.g., cardiopulmonary status is maintained, symptoms related to poison or drug overdose are diminishing, level of consciousness is maintained or improving). • Continue monitoring vital signs and urine output. • Continue to monitor hepatic and renal studies, CBC, urinalysis, and other drug-specific laboratory values. • Assess for and promptly report adverse effects: worsening respiratory distress, decreasing level of consciousness, agitation, confusion, vomiting, diminished urine output, or dysrhythmias.	• *Contamination* • *Decreased Cardiac Output*, related to cardiotoxicity of poison, overdose, or adverse drug effects • *Ineffective Breathing Pattern* • *Deficient Knowledge* (Health or Home Maintenance) • *Risk for Poisoning* • *Risk for Self-Directed Violence*

Implementation

Interventions and (Rationales)	Patient-Centered Care
Ensuring therapeutic effects: • Administer antidotes, activated charcoal, or chelating agents as appropriate for drug overdose or poisoning once the substance is identified. (Commonly known antidotes include acetylcysteine for acetaminophen, flumazenil for benzodiazepines, sodium bicarbonate for cyclic antidepressants, amyl nitrate for cyanide, naloxone for opioids, and osmotic diuretics for methanol and ethylene glycol.)	• Explain the purpose and expected outcome of antidotes administered to the patient, family, or caregiver. • When no antidote exists for the poisonous substance, inform the patient, family, or caregiver what supportive care will be provided.
Minimizing adverse effects: • Maintain airway and provide supplemental oxygen as needed. (Patients with an overdose or poisoning may be unable to maintain a patent airway, leading to respiratory arrest and death. Intubation also protects against possible aspiration.)	• Instruct the patient to notify the health care provider at the onset of difficulty breathing or swallowing.
• Monitor cardiopulmonary status. (Cardiac dysrhythmias and pulmonary edema may result from overdose of many poisons, including barbiturates, sedatives, hypnotics, and tranquilizers. **Lifespan:** Age-related physiological differences or undetected cardiac disease may place the older adult at greater risk for adverse effects from Calcium EDTA.)	• To allay possible anxiety, teach the patient, family, or caregiver the rationale for all equipment used and the need for frequent monitoring.
• Administer IV fluids as ordered. (Crystalloid solutions are used to treat hypovolemia, which may occur because of compromised circulatory status.)	• Instruct the patient, family, or caregiver to report burning, swelling, or discomfort at the IV site.
• Continue to monitor hepatic and renal function laboratory values, CBC, electrolytes, and glucose. Administer concentrated dextrose solution (D_5W) as ordered. (Hypoglycemia may occur due to acute poisoning or overdose with agents such as ethanol and salicylates. Renal and hepatic toxicities may occur related to the poisoning or overdose or related to adverse effects of the treatment. **Lifespan:** Age-related physiological differences may place older adults at greater risk for hepatic and renal toxicity.)	• Explain to the patient, family, or caregiver the need for frequent laboratory work. • Instruct the patient, family, or caregiver to report symptoms of hypoglycemia such as nervousness, anxiety, hunger, shakiness, perspiration, dizziness, or light-headedness.
• Monitor urinary output. (Observe for changes in urine character and color. Myoglobin may be present if rhabdomyolysis occurs as a result of overdose, causing a cola-colored or rust-brown appearance to the urine. Immediately report these changes or oliguria.)	• Instruct the patient, family, or caregiver to report any diminished urine output or changes in urine appearance.
• If ordered, insert a nasogastric tube, aspirate fluid for analysis, and perform gastric lavage. (Aspiration and lavage removes drugs that may remain in the stomach, preventing further absorption. Aspirate may be sent to the laboratory for analysis of the drugs ingested to provide identification for appropriate treatment.)	• To allay possible anxiety, teach the patient, family, or caregiver the rationale for the nasogastric tube and procedure.

CONNECTIONS: NURSING PRACTICE APPLICATION (continued)

• Continue administration of activated charcoal, chelating agents, or antidotes as ordered. (Activated charcoal absorbs drugs from gastric content to prevent systemic absorption. Chelating agents bind heavy metal toxins to remove them from the body.)	• Explain the purpose and expected outcome of activated charcoal, chelating agent, or antidote if administered. • Inform the patient, family, or caregiver that stools may become temporarily black if activated charcoal has been used.
• Prepare the patient for dialysis procedures as ordered. (Hemodialysis or hemoperfusion removes poisons from the system and is used when levels are potentially lethal; otherwise the toxin may be metabolized to a more lethal substance.)	• Explain the rationale for hemodialysis or hemoperfusion to the patient, family, or caregiver.
• Assess for suicidal ideation and refer to a mental health professional as appropriate. (A psychiatric consultation should be ordered for patients who demonstrate suicidal ideations or behaviors.)	• When suicidal ideation is present and poisoning is self-inflicted, explain the reason for referral to a mental health professional.
• Assess learning needs and provide education related to poisoning and overdose. (Poisoning may often be prevented by personal and public education efforts.)	• Instruct the patient, family, or caregiver on the importance of maintaining a safe environment to prevent recurrence of accidental poisonings.
Patient understanding of drug therapy: • Use opportunities during administration of medications and during assessments to discuss the rationale for the drug therapy, desired therapeutic outcomes, commonly observed adverse effects, and any necessary monitoring or precautions. (Using time during nursing care helps to optimize and reinforce key teaching areas.)	• The patient, family, or caregiver should be able to state the reason for the drug, appropriate dose and scheduling, what adverse effects to observe for and when to report them, and the anticipated length of the medication therapy.

*Nursing Diagnoses—Definitions and Classification 2015–2017. Copyright © 2014, 1994–2014 by NANDA International. Used by arrangement with John Wiley & Sons Limited.

CHAPTER
75
Understanding the Chapter

Key Concepts Summary

75.1 Emergency preparedness has become an essential competency for all health care professionals.

75.2 Bioterrorism is the intentional release of a virus or microorganism to cause human harm.

75.3 Nurses may have the first opportunity to recognize and initiate a response to bioterrorism.

75.4 The Strategic National Stockpile has large quantities of medicine to protect the public if there is a health emergency.

75.5 Highly infectious bacteria or viruses could be used as bioterrorist threats.

75.6 There are 13 categories of toxic chemicals that could cause mass casualties if released into the environment.

75.7 Ionizing radiation produces immediate and long-term effects on human tissue.

75.8 The general management of poisoning includes contacting the poison control center or emergency medical services as soon as possible.

75.9 Activated charcoal is effective at adsorbing (binding) most poisons if administered within 60 minutes of ingestion.

75.10 Ion trapping with forced diuresis may be helpful for some poisonings.

75.11 Chelating agents are capable of forming bonds with heavy metals.

Case Study: Making the Patient Connection

Remember the nurse manager "Carol Boler" at the beginning of the chapter? Now read the remainder of the case study. Based on the information presented within this chapter, respond to the critical thinking questions that follow.

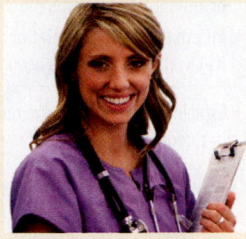

As an emergency department nurse in a busy urban hospital, Carol Boler participates in frequent emergency practice drills to be prepared for mass casualty events and acts of bioterrorism. Although there have been no incidents yet, she knows that with a military base nearby, there is a chance that such

an incident could occur. She is working with unit staff to plan a series of staff education meetings to discuss bioterrorism threats.

Critical Thinking Questions

1. When discussing the bioterrorism threat with a group of staff nurses, which information regarding smallpox should be included?

2. Identify the nursing assessments and interventions that the nurse should initiate when a patient is exposed to anthrax.

3. Discuss the mode of transmission and symptoms associated with *Y. pestis* exposure.

See Answers to Critical Thinking Questions on student resource website.

Additional Case Study

As a school nurse, you have been asked to speak to a group of mothers about accidental poisonings in young children.

1. Outline the information you need to present to this audience.

2. What recommendations should you give to the group about the use of ipecac syrup?

See Answers to Additional Case Study on student resource website.

Chapter Review

1 The patient is suspected of being exposed to ionizing radiation. Which nursing intervention would have the greatest priority?

1. Provide supportive care for nausea, vomiting, and diarrhea.
2. Limit the patient's exposure to ultraviolet light.
3. Avoid contamination of self through limited exposure to the patient.
4. Administer antiradiation medications as indicated.

2 The patient is exhibiting the symptoms of *Yersinia pestis* exposure. Which pharmacologic therapy would most likely be used in the treatment of this patient?

1. Doxycycline
2. Trivalent botulinum antitoxin
3. Ribavirin
4. Atropine sulfate

3 The nurse has received a telephone call from an anxious mother of an 18-month-old child. In a panicked voice, the mother states, "I just discovered that my baby has swallowed an unknown amount of household cleanser." Which instruction would be appropriate for the nurse to give?

1. "Consult the package instructions for information concerning poisoning."
2. "Force your child to vomit using a mixture of warm water and raw eggs."
3. "Call 911 to take your child immediately to the nearest emergency department or health care agency."
4. "If your child develops seizures or difficulty breathing, call the health provider."

4 Activated charcoal is ordered for a patient who accidentally overdosed on prescription medications. The nurse would question the order for activated charcoal for the patient with which condition?

1. Acute hepatitis and cirrhosis
2. Impairment of renal function
3. Decreased level of consciousness
4. Anxiety and nervousness

5 The nurse knows that the mechanism of action for chelating therapy is:

1. Removal of positively charged metals.
2. Deactivation of chemical reaction.
3. Increased liver metabolism.
4. Decreased glomerular filtration.

6 Which of the preadministration assessment parameters would the nurse consider before administering edetate calcium disodium (Calcium EDTA) to a patient?

1. Bowel sounds
2. Urinary output
3. Visual acuity
4. Skin turgor

See Answers to Chapter Review in Appendix A.

References

Centers for Disease Control and Prevention. (n.d.). *Emergency preparedness and response: Bioterrorism agents/diseases*. Retrieved from http://www.bt.cdc.gov/agent/agentlist-category.asp

Centers for Disease Control and Prevention. (2013a). *Policy impact: Prescription pain killer overdoses*. Retrieved from http://www.cdc.gov/homeandrecreationalsafety/rxbrief/

Centers for Disease Control and Prevention. (2013b). *Viral hemorrhagic fevers*. Retrieved from http://www.cdc.gov/ncidod/dvrd/spb/mnpages/dispages/vhf.htm

Edgewood Chemical Biological Center. (n.d.). *Biological and chemical agent quick reference tables*. Retrieved from http://www.ecbc.army.mil/hld/ip/bca_qr.htm

U.S. Nuclear Regulatory Commission. (2013). *Backgrounder on the Three Mile Island accident*. Retrieved from http://www.nrc.gov/reading-rm/doc-collections/fact-sheets/3mile-isle.html

Selected Bibliography

Biddinger, P. D., Savoia, E., Massin-Short, S. B., Preston, J., & Stoto, M. A. (2010). Public health emergency preparedness exercises: Lessons learned. *Public Health Reports, 125*(Suppl. 5), 100–106.

Cao, Y., Skaug, M. A., Andersen, O., & Aaseth, J. (2014). Chelation therapy in intoxications with mercury, lead and copper. *Journal of Trace Elements in Medicine and Biology*. doi:10.1016/j.jtemb.2014.04.010

Chandran, L., & Cataldo, R. (2010). Lead poisoning: Basics and new developments. *Pediatrics in Review, 31*, 399–406. doi:10.1542/pir.31-10-399

Danzig, R. (2012). A decade of countering bioterrorism: Incremental progress, fundamental failings. *Biosecurity and Bioterrorism: Biodefense Strategy, Practice, and Science, 10*, 49–54. doi:10.1089/bsp.2011.0104

Elder, G. M. (2010). Activated charcoal: To give or not to give? *International Emergency Nursing, 18*, 154–157. doi:10.1016/j.ienj.2009.10.005

Herdman, T. H., & Kamitsuru, S. (Eds.). (2014). *NANDA International nursing diagnoses: Definitions and classification, 2015-2017*. Oxford, United Kingdom: Wiley-Blackwell.

McHugh, M. (2010). Hospital nurse staffing and public health emergency preparedness: Implications for policy. *Public Health Nursing, 27*, 442–449. doi:10.1111/j.1525-1446.2010.00877.x

Mitchell, C. J., Kernohan, W. G., & Higginson, R. (2012). Are emergency care nurses prepared for chemical, biological, radiological, nuclear or explosive incidents? *International Emergency Nursing, 20*, 151–161. doi:10.1016/j.ienj.2011.10.001

Smith, C., & Hewison, A. (2012). Are nurses prepared to respond to a bioterrorist attack: A narrative synthesis. *Journal of Advanced Nursing, 68*, 2597–2609. doi:10.1111/j.1365-2648.2012.06061.x

Spain, K. M., Clements, P. T., DeRanieri, J. T., & Holt, K. (2012). When disaster happens: Emergency preparedness for nurse practitioners. *The Journal for Nurse Practitioners, 8*, 38–44. doi:10.1016/j.nurpra.2011.07.024

Stokowski, L. A. (2012). *Ready, willing and able: Preparing nurses to respond to disasters*. Retrieved from http://www.medscape.com/viewarticle/579888_8

Strangeland, P. A. (2010). Disaster nursing: A retrospective review. *Critical Care Nursing Clinics of North America, 22*(4), 421–436. doi:10.1016/j.ccell.2010.09.003

Appendix A

Answers to Chapter Review

Chapter 1

1 Answer: 3 Rationale: Indications are the conditions for which a particular drug is approved. Options 1, 2, and 4 are incorrect. A description of how a drug works on its target organs and cells is called the mechanism of action. The dosage is the amount of the drug that is given. The conditions whereby the drug should be avoided are contraindications. Cognitive Level: Applying; Client Need: Safe and Effective Care Environment; Nursing Process: Implementation

2 Answer: 3 Rationale: Trade names or proprietary names are designed to help the patient remember the name of the drug. Options 1, 2, and 4 are incorrect. The chemical name refers to the chemical substances that comprise the drug. A drug's generic name is assigned by the U.S. Adopted Name Council, and each drug has only one generic name. There is no category that is referred to as "standard" in the categories of drug names. Cognitive Level: Applying; Client Need: Physiological Integrity; Nursing Process: Assessment

3 Answer: 1 Rationale: Drugs are only tools that are part of the overall therapeutic treatment plan. Other treatment options and the nurse–patient relationship are also important to the care of the patient as an individual. Options 2, 3, and 4 are incorrect. Drug therapy alone is usually insufficient to correct and cure human illness. Nurses play a major role in the drug therapy of patients by administering, educating, monitoring, and assessing the response to drugs. Too much reliance on drug therapy can diminish the importance of the nurse–patient relationship. Cognitive Level: Applying; Client Need: Physiological Integrity; Nursing Process: Implementation

4 Answer: 1, 2, 3, 4 Rationale: Physiological responses to drug therapy are affected by a patient's age, gender, race, body mass, and health status. Many diseases such as diabetes have genetic origins. Familial history of disease conditions may reflect potential problems in the patient. Option 5 is incorrect because not having medical insurance is not a physiological variable that would affect drug therapy. Cognitive Level: Applying; Client Need: Physiological Integrity; Nursing Process: Evaluation

5 Answer: 2 Rationale: Antihypertensive indicates the therapeutic classification of the drug by describing its usefulness in lowering blood pressure. Options 1, 3, and 4 are incorrect. Beta-adrenergic antagonists, diuretics, and calcium channel blockers all focus on how the drug works, rather than on what therapeutic effects occur. Cognitive Level: Applying; Client Need: Physiological Integrity; Nursing Process: Implementation

6 Answer: 4 Rationale: Motrin and Advil are trade names for the generic drug ibuprofen. Options 1, 2, and 3 are incorrect. No error is noted because "ibuprofen" is the generic name for Advil and Motrin, both trade names. Each drug has only one generic name but may have different trade names, depending on the company that manufactures the drug. Cognitive Level: Applying; Client Need: Health Promotion and Maintenance; Nursing Process: Implementation

Chapter 2

1 Answer: 2 Rationale: The FDA requires that drug manufacturers demonstrate both the safety and effectiveness of pharmaceutical products. Options 1, 3, and 4 are incorrect. All drugs have potential reactions and adverse effects. Many factors determine the cost of a drug and newly approved drugs may be the most expensive and not fully covered by health care insurance plans. Not all drugs have been tested in diverse populations and women, minority ethnic groups, children, and the older adults are often underrepresented in drug research studies. Cognitive Level: Applying; Client Need: Safe and Effective Care Environment; Nursing Process: Implementation

2 Answer: 2 Rationale: Phase 2 of the clinical investigation relies on studying patients with the disease to be treated. Options 1, 3, and 4 are incorrect. Phase 1 studies use small groups of healthy subjects. Phase 3 studies use large numbers of subjects with the condition being treated by the drug. Phase 4 is considered postmarketing surveillance after the drug has been approved. Cognitive Level: Applying; Client Need: Safe and Effective Care Environment; Nursing Process: Implementation

3 Answer: 2 Rationale: Most drug testing occurs using adult, white, non-Hispanic males, which may limit the generalization of the results to other populations. Options 1, 3, and 4 are incorrect. Drug testing is seldom performed on children, women, or older adults. Although many drugs are tested using animals, effectiveness in animals does not always verify that the drug will be effective in humans. Cognitive Level: Applying; Client Need: Safe and Effective Care Environment; Nursing Process: Implementation

4 Answer: 4 Rationale: Telephone orders are not permissible under federal law for Schedule II controlled substances. Options 1, 2, and 3 are incorrect. Refill prescriptions are usually not any more or less expensive than the original prescription. The number of listeners is irrelevant. Prescriptions are not confirmed or verified by the DEA. Cognitive Level: Applying; Client Need: Safe and Effective Care Environment; Nursing Process: Implementation

5 Answer: 1 Rationale: The more likely a drug's potential for abuse and dependency, the stricter the regulation to control access to the substance. Options 2, 3, and 4 are incorrect. The cost and production difficulty do not influence the degree of regulation. Adverse effects and drug or food interactions do not dictate the level of regulatory control. The length of time taken to confirm that a drug is effective does not affect the degree of regulation. Cognitive Level: Applying; Client Need: Safe and Effective Care Environment; Nursing Process: Implementation

6 Answer: 1, 2, 3 Rationale: Adverse drug reactions may continue to be discovered well after the FDA approval process as larger groups of patients take the drug. Any reaction should be noted in the patient's chart, the provider notified, and an Adverse Event Report filed with the FDA when adverse reactions are noted. Options 4 and 5 are incorrect. Health care providers are responsible for reporting adverse reactions as they occur and should not wait for the FDA to send a recall notice. Many factors influence a patient's reaction to medications and each patient may not have the same exact reaction to the medication. Cognitive Level: Applying; Client Need: Safe and Effective Care Environment; Nursing Process: Implementation

Chapter 3

1 Answer: 2 Rationale: Although taking a larger dose of a medication usually results in a greater therapeutic response, the response also depends on the drug's plasma concentration. If a toxic level is reached from too large a dose, the drug will have adverse effects instead of a better therapeutic response. Options 1, 3, and 4 are incorrect because they are true statements. The liquid form of a drug will be absorbed faster than its tablet form. Food decreases the absorption rate of most drugs. Patients should always consult a health care provider if unexpected adverse effects develop. Cognitive Level: Applying; Client Need: Physiological Integrity; Nursing Process: Evaluation

2 Answer: 1 Rationale: Infants do not develop a mature microsomal enzyme system until they are a year old and therefore do not metabolize drugs very efficiently. Options 2, 3, and 4 are incorrect. Pregnancy does not significantly affect drug metabolism. The concern with pregnant patients is primarily focused on alterations in distribution due to the fetal–placental barrier. The presence of kidney stones would not influence drug metabolism. Hypertension is not a factor that directly results in abnormal metabolism. Cognitive Level: Applying; Client Need: Physiological Integrity; Nursing Process: Implementation

3 Answer: 3 Rationale: Peristalsis is the wavelike muscular contraction of the gastrointestinal tract that propels stomach and intestinal content through the system. An increase in this activity would decrease the time that drugs would remain in the GI system and therefore decrease absorption. Options 1, 2, and 4 are incorrect. Excretion for most drugs occurs mostly through the kidneys, lungs, and glands. Peristalsis would not reduce excretions of medications. A delay in peristalsis would prolong absorption time, and peristalsis is not involved in the distribution of drugs to their target sites. Cognitive Level: Applying; Patient Need: Physiological Integrity; Nursing Process: Evaluation

4 Answer: 3 Rationale: Inhaled drugs produce an immediate therapeutic response. Options 1, 2, and 4 are incorrect. Inhaled medication can be used at any time during the day and is not restricted to the morning. Doses for inhaled drugs are small compared to orally ingested medications, and because these drugs go directly to the lung surface area and are readily absorbed, very little of the substance is lost due to metabolism. Cognitive Level: Applying; Client Need: Physiological Integrity; Nursing Process: Evaluation

5 Answer: 4 Rationale: The length of time a drug concentration remains in the therapeutic range is its duration of action. Patients with hepatic impairment do not effectively metabolize drugs, which increases the duration of action. Options 1, 2, and 3 are incorrect. In patients with hepatic disease, the duration of action most likely will increase since drug metabolism is impaired. Although the duration of action is extended, the effects of the drug are not improved. Cognitive Level: Applying; Client Need: Physiological Integrity; Nursing Process: Evaluation

6 Answer: 2, 4 Rationale: A therapeutic drug level that is in the acceptable range indicates that the drug is at a minimally effective concentration but not at a toxic level. Because each patient response to a drug is unique, the nurse should continue monitoring the patient throughout the drug's use. Options 1, 3, and 5 are incorrect. Because individual patient responses to drugs can be highly variable, adverse effects, toxicities, or even no effect may occur at levels within the therapeutic range. For that reason, the drug dose may need to be adjusted throughout therapy. Therapeutic effectiveness of a drug depends on many factors and the therapeutic range of a drug is the level between minimally effective and toxic levels. It is not an indicator of how effective a drug will be in treating an individual condition. Cognitive Level: Applying; Client Need: Physiological Integrity; Nursing Process: Evaluation

Chapter 4

1 Answer: 1, 2, 3, 5 Rationale: One of the critical determinants of the effectiveness of drug therapy is a physical examination. Nurses will utilize assessment skills to ascertain whether the drug is being effective. In many cases, a patient's vital signs may indicate the effectiveness of a drug such as a decrease in body temperature, a change in blood pressure and pulse, or improved respiratory status. The effects of many drugs are monitored by diagnostic laboratory values such as white blood cell counts, cultures, and various electrolyte values. *Efficacy* is the term that describes the ability of a drug to produce the desired therapeutic effect. Option 4 is incorrect. The dosage time does not directly evaluate the effectiveness of drug therapy. Cognitive Level: Applying; Client Need: Physiological Integrity; Nursing Process: Implementation

2 Answer: 1 Rationale: Therapeutic index is the ratio between therapeutic dose of a drug and the toxic dose and is used as a measure of the relative safety of the drug. The higher the therapeutic index, the greater the safety of the drug. Options 2, 3, and 4 are incorrect. A drug may be labeled "dangerous" for many reasons other than the therapeutic index, including potential for abuse. The higher the therapeutic index, the less risk of drug toxicity. A high degree of safety does not signify the degree of effectiveness. Cognitive Level: Applying; Client Need: Physiological Integrity; Nursing Process: Assessment

3 Answer: 1 Rationale: A dose response curve is a graphic representation that shows the relation between the amount of a drug administered and the extent of response it produces. Options 2, 3, and 4 are incorrect. A dose response curve does not illustrate the toxic effects related to a drug or any specific

population or graphically present the duration of action of a drug. Serum drug levels must be measured to determine the peak serum drug level. It is unique to each patient and the dose response curve only represents a maximum (toxic) dose level. Cognitive Level: Applying; Client Need: Physiological Integrity; Nursing Process: Assessment

4 Answer: 4 Rationale: The TD_{50} measures the median toxicity dose. This information indicates the dose that will produce a given toxicity in 50% of a group of patients. Options 1, 2, and 3 are incorrect. Effectiveness, dose response, and receptor subtypes are not represented by the TD_{50} level. Cognitive Level: Applying; Client Need: Physiological Integrity; Nursing Process: Implementation

5 Answer: 2 Rationale: Antagonists bind to receptors and block the effects of an endogenous chemical or another drug by competing with receptor binding sites or inhibiting the drug effect. As an antagonist, benztropine would block the effects of neostigmine and the neostigmine would exhibit a lesser effect. Options 1, 3, and 4 are incorrect. A drug that produces an effect after binding with a receptor is an agonist. Cognitive Level: Analyzing; Client Need: Physiological Integrity; Nursing Process: Implementation

6 Answer: 1 Rationale: Potency is a reflection of a drug's ability to bind to a receptor. Options 2, 3, and 4 are incorrect. Efficacy and the affinity of a drug to bind to a receptor are separate variables from potency. Metabolism is a function of pharmacokinetics, not pharmacodynamics. First-pass effect is a phenomenon that occurs during enteral absorption and does not affect drug affinity. Cognitive Level: Applying; Client Need: Safe and Effective Care Environment; Nursing Process: Implementation

Chapter 5

1 Answer: 1 Rationale: Collecting additional information will provide the prescriber with knowledge about the type and severity of the reaction to that specific drug and will assist in determining the appropriateness of the order. Options 2, 3, and 4 are incorrect. The nurse should gather additional information from the patient or family member before notifying the prescriber. A medication is never administered to a patient when allergic sensitivity is suspected until further investigation into the type and severity of the reaction has been completed. Although documentation of the event may be in the patient's medical record, the reaction may not have been documented or may have occurred after the last health care visit. Cognitive Level: Applying; Client Need: Physiological Integrity; Nursing Process: Implementation

2 Answer: 1 Rationale: As the dose increases, the risk for adverse effects also increases. The patient should be closely observed for the onset of adverse effects whenever the dose of the drug is increased. Options 2, 3, and 4 are incorrect. Although adverse effects are sometimes noted after the first dose, they may occur at any time during drug administration. Although some adverse effects are common when a drug is given PO, others are more common when given by other routes, such as IV or IM. The timing of medication is not a factor associated with dose-related adverse effects. Cognitive Level: Applying; Client Need: Physiological Integrity; Nursing Process: Implementation

3 Answer: 4 Rationale: Promoting adequate hydration may significantly reduce the risk of renal damage produced by drug therapies. Options 1, 2, and 3 are incorrect. Avoiding direct sunlight is appropriate teaching to provide to patients receiving drugs that cause photosensitivity or phototoxicity. The consumption of potassium-enriched foods will not reduce the risk of drug-induced nephrotoxicity, nor will avoiding alcohol consumption. Cognitive Level: Applying; Client Need: Physiological Integrity; Nursing Process: Implementation

4 Answer: 3 Rationale: Urticaria or hives, with raised, itchy areas of skin, is often a sign of an allergic reaction. Options 1, 2, and 4 are incorrect. Angioedema is a notable swelling around the eyes and lips and sometimes of the hands and feet that occurs beneath the skin instead of on the surface. SJS is characterized by a flulike period of fever, sore throat, and headache followed by the sudden development of circular lesions that cover the majority of the skin. Photosensitivity occurs when a drug renders the skin susceptible to damage by sunlight. Cognitive Level: Applying; Client Need: Physiological Integrity; Nursing Process: Evaluation

5 Answer: 2 Rationale: The function of the bone marrow is to produce blood cells. When drugs cause bone marrow toxicity, the condition manifests as a decrease in all blood cell types. Options 1, 3, and 4 are incorrect. Muscle and bone pain are most often associated with muscle toxicity. Bone marrow toxicity is not related to a decline in an individual's range of motion. Liver enzymes are not typically affected by bone marrow toxicity. Cognitive Level: Applying; Client Need: Physiological Integrity; Nursing Process: Evaluation

6 Answer: 3 Rationale: The presence of right upper quadrant pain and anorexia are early symptoms often associated with drug-induced liver damage. Options 1, 2, and 4 are incorrect. Black, "furry" tongue or infections elsewhere are not related to liver damage. A sudden drop in BP is orthostatic hypotension. Unusual and uncontrolled movements are neurologic-related effects. Cognitive Level: Analyzing; Client Need: Physiological Integrity; Nursing Process: Evaluation

Chapter 6

1 Answer: 4 Rationale: When medication orders are given via telephone, it is critical for the nurse to repeat the order verbatim to the prescriber. Options 1, 2, and 3 are incorrect. Whenever possible it is best for the prescriber to write an order for medication, but this is not always possible. It is correct for the nurse to attempt to comfort the patient using a number of nursing interventions for pain. However, the nurse is required to consult the prescriber when a change in the patient's status occurs, regardless of the time. The nurse is responsible for contacting the prescriber and it is the nurse who can relay clinical findings and assessment. Cognitive Level: Applying; Client Need: Safe and Effective Care Environment; Nursing Process: Planning

2 Answer: 1 Rationale: Whenever a medication order is unclear, the nurse should always contact the prescriber, and then have the order rewritten to prevent errors. Options 2, 3, and 4 are incorrect. Having another nurse read the order will not necessarily ensure that the dosage is correct for the patient's condition. Whereas the pharmacist or a drug guide may provide the nurse with the usual dose for most patients, they do not take into consideration the patient's weight, disease condition, and other variables that influence the drug's pharmacokinetic and pharmacodynamic actions. Cognitive Level: Applying; Client Need: Safe and Effective Care Environment; Nursing Process: Implementation

3 Answer: 2 Rationale: Pharmacies maintain records of medication dispensed to individuals. If a pharmacist can conduct a medication reconciliation by reviewing the patient's drug history on each subsequent visit, serious potential drug–drug interactions may be identified. Options 1, 3, and 4 are incorrect. Insisting on acquiring a brand name drug rather than a generic does not ensure the safety of a medication. For safety reasons, drugs are dispensed in containers that are sometimes difficult to open. Unless there is a specific reason (such as impaired hand dexterity), medications should be stored in their original safety bottles. Information found on the Internet may vary in quality and may be provided by non–health care-related sources. When in doubt, the prescriber or pharmacist can provide the most accurate information about expected effects. Cognitive Level: Applying; Client Need: Health Promotion and Maintenance; Nursing Process: Implementation

4 Answer: 3 Rationale: The nurse should always validate a questionable order when a patient or a family member verbalizes concern. Options 1, 2, and 4 are incorrect. Medications purchased by a clinical agency vary in appearance depending on the manufacturer from which the drug is purchased. The nurse should withhold the medication and then confirm that it is the correct drug as ordered before administering. If a patient questions a change in medication or procedure, the nurse should verify the order and obtain validation from the prescriber. Cognitive Level: Applying; Client Need: Safe and Effective Care Environment; Nursing Process: Implementation

5 Answer: 1 Rationale: The nurse's first priority is always the patient. The nurse should first determine the patient's baseline assessment data in order to determine if any adverse effects are occurring. Options 2, 3, and 4 are incorrect. The health care provider should be notified of the medication error; however, it is also important to report the patient's assessment data at the same time. All health care agencies have reporting mechanisms for drug errors, and the nurse is responsible for completing this process after assessing the patient and notifying the provider. If the patient experiences an adverse reaction to the drug, further assessment is needed before confirming that the drug itself, rather than

a patient variable (e.g., allergy), was behind the reaction before filing an Adverse Drug Reaction report (see Chapter 5). Cognitive Level: Applying; Client Need: Safe and Effective Care Environment; Nursing Process: Implementation

6 Answer: 3 Rationale: Returning when the patient is available ensures that the patient takes the medication and offers opportunity for the nurse to assess for effects or provide teaching related to the medication. Options 1, 2, and 4 are incorrect. A nurse must ensure that the patient takes the medication. By leaving the medication at the bedside or with visitors, the nurse will not know with certainty that the patient took the medication. When a patient refuses a medication, the nurse should document reasons for the refusal so that appropriate follow-up may be carried out. In this situation, the patient did not refuse the medication but was not available to take it at that moment. Cognitive Level: Applying; Client Need: Safe and Effective Care Environment; Nursing Process: Implementation

Chapter 7

1 Answer: 1 Rationale: Although CAM medications have been used for thousands of years, many of these substances lack adequate scientific clinical studies to verify their effectiveness. Most health care providers are hesitant to recommend a substance that has questionable effectiveness. Options 2, 3, and 4 are incorrect. CAM has a rich history of use over thousands of years in treating certain diseases and conditions. To imply that all alternative therapies are nothing more than fable is incorrect. There is no evidence that response to CAM therapies is related to the placebo effect. In many cases the CAM therapy may be less expensive than prescription medications. Cognitive Level: Applying; Client Need: Safe and Effective Care Environment; Nursing Process: Implementation

2 Answer: 3 Rationale: It is best to advise the patient to take small amounts of a new supplement to determine any initial intolerance. Options 1, 2, and 4 are incorrect. Doubling dosages can be extremely dangerous and is seldom, if ever, advisable. There is no indication that fluid intake should be reduced with echinacea. Allergic reactions are possible with natural supplements. Patients should be taught to read the label carefully and avoid any supplement that contains any known allergy-provoking substances. Cognitive Level: Applying; Client Need: Physiological Integrity; Nursing Process: Implementation

3 Answer: 1 Rationale: Older adults with hepatic disease are at higher risk of developing serious drug reactions when taking herbal supplements. Options 2, 3, and 4 are incorrect. Patients with cardiac irregularities, pneumonia, or acne may require traditional medications and should be encouraged to consult their health care provider. If the patient prefers to use CAM, this can also be discussed with the provider at the time of the health care visit. Cognitive Level: Applying; Client Need: Physiological Integrity; Nursing Process: Evaluation

4 Answer: 1, 2, 3, 5 Rationale: Herbal supplements can be found in almost every supermarket, pharmacy, and health food store. Due to aggressive marketing, herbal supplements are also extremely popular. Most herbal supplements are less expensive than prescribed medications and are therefore more appealing to individuals for whom cost is a critical issue. Older patients may also seek therapeutic alternatives for chronic health conditions. Option 4 is incorrect. Natural substances are not necessarily safer than synthetic products and do not undergo the same rigorous testing as synthetic products. Cognitive Level: Applying; Client Need: Safe and Effective Care Environment; Nursing Process: Implementation

5 Answer: 1 Rationale: The USP verified dietary supplement mark is awarded to dietary supplements that pass verification processes. The mark represents that USP has tested the supplement to verify that the label accurately reflects the product in the bottle and that the supplement does not contain harmful levels of contaminants. Options 2, 3, and 4 are incorrect. A DEA number is assigned to a health care provider and allows him or her to write prescriptions for controlled substances such as a narcotic. The FDA does not control herbal supplements and this code does not exist. U.S. Customs is not responsible for ensuring that herbal supplements are pure. Cognitive Level: Applying; Client Need: Safe and Effective Care Environment; Nursing Process: Implementation

6 Answer: 4 Rationale: Changes in liver or kidney function in the older adult may lead to changes in metabolism or excretion for herbal as well as synthetic medications. Options 1, 2, and 3 are incorrect. Older adults are no more likely to have difficulty taking herbal medications or to spend more money on these products than the younger adult population. These difficulties are patient specific at any age. Due to aggressive marketing campaigns by the herbal and dietary supplement industry, all age groups are as likely to hold unrealistic expectations for herbal products. Cognitive Level: Applying; Client Need: Physiological Integrity; Nursing Process: Evaluation

Chapter 8

1 Answer: 2   Rationale: It is recommended that all drugs be avoided as much as possible during pregnancy due to the potential effect on the fetus or infant. Options 1, 3, and 4 are incorrect. Drugs that are available OTC may also be hazardous and may affect the unborn fetus and nursing infant. Drugs used for treating medical conditions such as asthma, hypertension, diabetes, and epilepsy should be continued throughout pregnancy after review by the health care provider for the safety of both mother and infant. There must be close monitoring during this time. In such cases the benefits may outweigh the risks. The woman should consult with her health care provider regarding any drugs taken during pregnancy and lactation. Cognitive Level: Applying; Client Need: Physiological Integrity; Nursing Process: Implementation

2 Answer: 4   Rationale: Drugs in category X are clearly contraindicated because they pose serious risk to the fetus. Options 1, 2, and 3 are incorrect. Category A drugs are safe for the pregnant woman because they demonstrate no risk of injury to the unborn fetus. Category B consists of drugs that may be given to the mother during pregnancy. Drugs in category C represent those whereby there is insufficient evidence that the drug is either safe or dangerous to the fetus, and these drugs will be evaluated by the provider to determine if the benefit outweighs the risk. Cognitive Level: Applying; Client Need: Physiological Integrity; Nursing Process: Implementation

3 Answer: 1   Rationale: Although multiple factors affect the transfer of drugs across the placenta, highly lipid soluble drugs will cross the placental barrier more easily than water-soluble drugs. Options 2, 3, and 4 are incorrect. Small molecules such as alcohol easily cross the placental barrier, whereas larger molecules are slower to cross. When drugs are highly protein bound, they are too large to cross the placental membrane. Cognitive Level: Applying; Client Need: Health Promotion and Maintenance; Nursing Process: Implementation

4 Answer: 1   Rationale: Weeks 1–2 of the first trimester are known as the preimplantation phase. Before implantation, the developing embryo has not yet established a blood supply with the mother. This is sometimes called the "all-or-none" period because exposure to a teratogen either causes death of the embryo or has no effect. Drugs are less likely to cause congenital malformations during this period because the baby's organ systems have not yet begun to form. Options 2, 3, and 4 are incorrect because the embryonic period is 3 to 8 weeks postconception. During the embryonic period there is rapid development of internal structures and maximum sensitivity to teratogens. Teratogenic agents taken during this phase can lead to structural malformation and spontaneous abortion. The specific abnormality depends on which organ is forming at the time of exposure. Cognitive Level: Analyzing; Client Need: Physiological Integrity; Nursing Process: Planning

5 Answer: 1, 3, 4, and 5   Rationale: OTC drugs are generally safe when taken as directed but any drug taken by the mother should be discussed with the health care provider first. Lowering the dose will not alter the safety profile of an unsafe OTC drug. Medications are found in breast milk and may be ingested by the infant. The provider will review any prescription medications the mother is taking and will plan for alternatives if any are unsafe during breast-feeding. The form of the medication does not affect the passage of the drug into the breast milk. Option 2 is incorrect. It is true that the higher the dose, the more likely it is that the drug will enter the breast milk and the patient has understood that part of the teaching. Cognitive Level: Analyzing; Client Need: Health Promotion and Maintenance; Nursing Process: Evaluation

6 Answer: 3   Rationale: Increased levels of progesterone cause a decrease in gastric tone and intestinal motility, resulting in delayed gastric emptying. This leads to extended time for drug absorption. Options 1, 2, and 4 are incorrect. Medications may take a longer time to be absorbed and distributed, thus delaying their onset and prolonging their duration of action. Due to the changes in

body fluid volume associated with pregnancy, there is greater hemodilution, not hemoconcentration, of drugs. Of all pharmacokinetic factors, drug metabolism is least affected by pregnancy. Cognitive Level: Applying; Client Need: Physiological Integrity; Nursing Process: Implementation

Chapter 9

1 Answer: 1, 3   Rationale: In young children, delayed gastric emptying causes oral medications to remain in the stomach longer, resulting in slowed absorption and an increased risk for adverse drug reactions. Between age 3 and 5, the liver's metabolic rate reaches adult levels. Before age 5, extra caution and dosage adjustments may be required, particularly for drugs that are metabolized primarily in the liver. Options 2, 4, and 5 are incorrect. Before 6 months of age, there are very small amounts of plasma proteins, and drugs that are normally protein bound remain as free drugs, increasing drug distribution and increasing the risk for adverse effects. Drug excretion through the kidneys increases with age, and standard pediatric doses may be used between 3 and 5 months of age. Cautious monitoring should be continued even after this age, especially with drugs known to be nephrotoxic. The blood–brain barrier is not well developed at birth and drugs can easily penetrate the CNS, causing heightened effects. Cognitive Level: Applying; Client Need: Physiological Integrity; Nursing Process: Planning

2 Answer: 1   Rationale: The vastus lateralis muscle mass is the most developed in infants and toddlers and therefore most appropriate for IM injections. Options 2, 3, and 4 are incorrect. The deltoid, dorsogluteal, and ventrogluteal sites have very little muscle tissue available for injection and may have erratic blood flow, leading to decreased medication absorption. Cognitive Level: Applying; Client Need: Physiological Integrity; Nursing Process: Implementation

3 Answer: 1   Rationale: IM injections in infants are absorbed slowly due to low blood flow to skeletal muscles. Options 2, 3, and 4 are incorrect because children experience delayed absorption and distribution of IM drugs and IM medications may be absorbed slowly and erratically in children. Children have very weak muscle contractions that contribute to this delayed absorption and distribution. Cognitive Level: Analyzing; Client Need: Physiological Integrity; Nursing Process: Evaluation

4 Answer: 3   Rationale: At 3 years of age the child begins seeking control and independence. Giving the patient a choice of liquid with which to combine the medicine will give the child a feeling of control and independence and at the same time encourage cooperation. Options 1, 2, and 4 are incorrect. At age 3 years the child does not yet associate medicine with getting better. Threatening patients to get them to take medicine is never appropriate in any situation. Three-year-olds do not imitate actions unless they want to, and saying that a roommate took the medicine may not result in the child doing the same. Cognitive Level: Applying; Client Need: Physiological Integrity; Nursing Process: Implementation

5 Answer: 3   Rationale: Drugs with extensive protein binding compete for binding sites, resulting in increased absorption and high potential for drug interactions. Options 1, 2, and 4 are incorrect. Low-potency drugs, drugs with a wide therapeutic index, and drugs applied to the skin are at low risk for drug interactions. Cognitive Level: Applying; Client Need: Physiological Integrity; Nursing Process: Evaluation

6 Answer: 1   Rationale: Children and their parents are most likely to adhere if their medication regimen is simple and inexpensive. Options 2, 3, and 4 are incorrect. Patients are less likely to adhere to the regimen if the medications are costly, they have to be taken over an extended period of time, or they have to be taken at varying times during the day. Cognitive Level: Analyzing; Client Need: Physiological Integrity; Nursing Process: Planning

Chapter 10

1 Answer: 1, 2   Rationale: Increased gastric pH is a common physiological condition of aging that can affect absorption by increasing the time it takes for oral medications to dissolve. Decreased blood flow to the GI tract decreases the amount of absorption as well as distribution. Options 3, 4, and 5 are incorrect. GI motility slows in the older adult and increased body surface area does not directly impact the area of absorption of oral drugs. The older adult may have decreased cardiac output, but this will not affect the absorption of a drug. Cognitive Level: Understanding; Client Need: Physiological Integrity; Nursing Process: Implementation

2 Answer: 2 Rationale: A patient who is functioning independently in all ADLs should be encouraged to take full responsibility for self-administering medications. Options 1, 3, and 4 are incorrect. Teaching the daughter to administer the insulin may become an option if the patient does not want to or cannot self-administer the drug, but that is not noted at this time. There is no reason for recommending a home health aide if the patient is competent in self-administering. Since the provider's original order was to treat the patient's condition with insulin, there may be a reason that an oral antidiabetic medication is not appropriate for this patient or not appropriate at this time. Cognitive Level: Applying; Client Need: Health Promotion and Maintenance; Nursing Process: Implementation

3 Answer: 2 Rationale: In the older adult, renal blood flow decreases and excretion of drugs also decreases, requiring dosage or frequency adjustments for many drugs. Options 1, 3, and 4 are incorrect. Total body fat increases rather than decreases, which may increase storage of fat-soluble drugs. Liver function declines and the amount of plasma proteins decreases. There is a decrease in total body water, and water-soluble drug concentration may increase. Cognitive Level: Applying; Client Need: Physiological Integrity; Nursing Process: Evaluation

4 Answer: 1, 2, 3 Rationale: Excessive prescribing, multiple drug therapy, and increased drug sensitivity are all reasons for adverse effects in older adults. As a person ages, renal function decreases, leading to alterations in pharmacokinetics and pharmacodynamics. Coupled with multiple drug therapy and increased sensitivity, it is not unusual for adverse effects to develop. Options 4 and 5 are incorrect. Body mass decreases as age increases. Exercise engagement does not influence the frequency of adverse effects. Cognitive Level: Applying; Client Need: Health Promotion and Maintenance; Nursing Process: Evaluation

5 Answer: 2 Rationale: 31% of older adult patients report that they did not take their medication because they did not have it on hand when it was time to take it. Options 1, 3, and 4 are incorrect. These are other reasons cited for nonadherence but they are not the most frequently cited answer. Cognitive Level: Analyzing; Client Need: Health Promotion and Maintenance; Nursing Process: Evaluation

6 Answer: 1 Rationale: Older adults may comply with prescribed drug regimens because of confidence in the ability of their provider. Making the statement "It doesn't matter if the medication works as long as the doctor prescribed it" indicates that the patient is not aware of how to monitor the drug's effectiveness or for its adverse effects, and more teaching is required. Options 2, 3, and 4 are positive responses by the patient that indicate that teaching has been effective toward increasing the potential for adherence. Cognitive Level: Analyzing; Client Need: Health Promotion and Maintenance; Nursing Process: Evaluation

Chapter 11

1 Answer: 2 Rationale: The statement reflects an attempt to understand the patient holistically. The nurse understands that multiple contributing factors may contribute to illness and involving the patient helps elicit possible factors. Options 1, 3, and 4 are incorrect. Tylenol should not be recommended initially because it may not address the possible causative factors related to the headaches. Monitoring the patient's pupil response to light, although eventually appropriate, should not be performed initially. An ophthalmology referral may be inevitable; however, making such a referral should be done after ruling out other possible sources of the headaches. Cognitive Level: Applying; Client Need: Health Promotion and Maintenance; Nursing Process: Implementation

2 Answer: 3 Rationale: Factors associated with a drug's expense and the patient's ability to purchase or access needed medication are considered psychosocial variables that may influence adherence to drug therapy. Options 1, 2, and 4 are incorrect. Unpleasant taste or medications that are difficult to swallow may hinder patient adherence; however, the problem is physiological rather than psychosocial. Liver damage (hepatotoxicity) is also a physiological factor. Cognitive Level: Analyzing; Client Need: Health Promotion and Maintenance; Nursing Process: Evaluation

3 Answer: 2 Rationale: Cultural beliefs refer to the cumulative ideas of knowledge, experiences, values, attitudes, meanings, and roles acquired by a group of people. A preference for traditional healers, such as a Shaman, reflects these beliefs. Options 1, 3, and 4 are incorrect. Ethnicity is a population of human beings whose members identify with each other either on the basis of common genealogy or ancestry. Genetic polymorphisms are changes in enzyme structure and DNA function that occur within a specific subset of the population. A health-related bias is a prejudice or a sense of preference for one particular point of view and is not specifically culturally related. Cognitive Level: Analyzing; Client Need: Health Promotion and Maintenance; Nursing Process: Evaluation

4 Answer: 1 Rationale: Patients who are known as slow acetylators have reduced hepatic metabolism and reduced clearance by the kidney. These patients have a greater potential for drug toxicity. Options 2, 3, and 4 are incorrect. Acetylation is a metabolic process that does not influence absorption. The route or form of administration is not associated with acetylation, and protein intake does not affect the rate of acetylation. Cognitive Level: Applying; Client Need: Physiological Integrity; Nursing Process: Implementation

5 Answer: 1, 2, 3, 4 Rationale: All of these factors—fat-to-muscle ratio, cerebral blood flow, limited drug research on women, and health beliefs—may be considered gender factors that influence pharmacotherapy. Option 5 is incorrect. Dietary considerations are a potential ethnic or cultural consideration. Cognitive Level: Applying; Client Need: Physiological Integrity; Nursing Process: Evaluation

6 Answer: 4 Rationale: Drug response is unique to each individual. The nurse should observe the responses and exercise caution with all medications. Options 1, 2, and 3 are incorrect. Patient self-report may not be a reliable method, and the patient may not have taken a particular drug before. Learning more about genetic effects on pharmacotherapy is important, but each patient response is unique. Other patients' responses to a drug will not help predict the response in another patient and there are many genetic variations, even within racial groups. Cognitive Level: Applying; Client Need: Physiological Integrity; Nursing Process: Implementation

Chapter 13

1 Answer: 1 Rationale: Muscarinic agonists may cause reflex tachycardia, which is precipitated by a drop in the patient's blood pressure. When this occurs, the baroreceptors recognize the decline in pressure and alert the medulla to increase the heart rate as a compensatory mechanism. Options 2, 3, and 4 are incorrect. Although the heart rate increases, muscarinic agonists do not directly affect the sinoatrial node. Hypertension is not a problem with this drug therapy; however, hypotension may occur. Muscarinic agents stimulate bronchial smooth muscles; however, this does not impact the heart rate. Cognitive Level: Applying; Client Need: Physiological Integrity; Nursing Process: Implementation

2 Answer: 3 Rationale: Pyridostigmine is used primarily for myasthenia gravis, a neurologic disorder characterized by muscle weakness and ptosis. A decrease in these symptoms is an expected therapeutic outcome for this drug. Options 1, 2, and 4 are incorrect because the symptoms listed are not usual problems faced by the patient with myasthenia gravis and would therefore be inappropriate outcome statements. Cognitive Level: Applying; Client Need: Physiological Integrity; Nursing Process: Planning

3 Answer: 4 Rationale: Bethanechol works on the muscles needed for urination by increasing ureteral peristalsis and promoting urinary bladder elimination. Options 1, 2, and 3 are incorrect. Bethanechol does not cause changes to urinary structures, nor does it increase urine production or renal blood flow. Cognitive Level: Applying; Client Need: Physiological Integrity; Nursing Process: Implementation

4 Answer: 1, 2, 3, 5 Rationale: Common adverse effects of bethanechol include abdominal discomfort, sweating, flushed skin, and blurred vision. Option 4 is incorrect because bethanechol increases GI peristalsis and promotes bowel evacuation. Cognitive Level: Analyzing; Client Need: Physiological Integrity; Nursing Process: Evaluation

5 Answer: 3 Rationale: Because of the potential for bronchoconstriction, patients with COPD should be treated cautiously with cholinergic agonists.

Options 1, 2, and 4 are incorrect. Neostigmine is used to reduce postoperative abdominal distention. Urinary retention may also be relieved with the administration of neostigmine. Neostigmine may be used to reverse the effects of nondepolarizing muscle relaxants. Cognitive Level: Applying; Client Need: Physiological Integrity; Nursing Process: Evaluation

6 Answer: 1   Rationale: If the heart rate falls below 60 beats/min or other established parameter, the nurse should notify the prescriber. Atropine may be ordered to restore heart rate. Options 2, 3, and 4 are incorrect. Miosis and increased salivation are expected adverse effects of this drug therapy. A respiratory rate of 16 is normal, so there is no need to notify the prescriber. Cognitive Level: Analyzing; Client Need: Physiological Integrity; Nursing Process: Evaluation

Chapter 14

1 Answer: 2   Rationale: Anticholinergic drugs such as tolterodine can cause constipation by slowing GI motility. Therefore, increases in dietary fiber and water intake will help avoid constipation. Options 1, 3, and 4 are incorrect. Daily exercise helps in avoiding muscle atrophy and anticholinergic drugs are not related to muscle atrophy. Consuming foods high in iron to increase red blood cell production is not related to the effects of anticholinergic drugs. Anticholinergic drugs cause tachycardia, not bradycardia. Cognitive Level: Applying; Client Need: Health Promotion and Maintenance; Nursing Process: Implementation

2 Answer: 1, 2, 3, 4   Rationale: These drugs cause mydriasis and paralysis of the ciliary muscle, which is useful in ophthalmic examinations. These drugs are therapeutic in correcting cardiac rhythm abnormalities such as bradycardia. Muscarinic antagonists, most notably ipratropium and tiotropium, are useful in treating asthma due to their ability to dilate the bronchi. These drugs are used to reverse the symptoms of overdose of organophosphate insecticides or ingestion of poison mushrooms. Option 5 is incorrect. Urinary retention is an adverse effect of these drugs. Cognitive Level: Applying; Client Need: Physiological Integrity; Nursing Process: Evaluation

3 Answer: 2   Rationale: Atropine causes urinary retention to worsen in patients with BPH. Options 1, 3, and 4 are incorrect because these are not contraindications for using atropine. Cognitive Level: Analyzing; Client Need: Physiological Integrity; Nursing Process: Evaluation

4 Answer: 1   Rationale: Muscarinic drugs affect the intraocular pressure by causing mydriasis and paralysis of the ciliary muscle. Options 2, 3, and 4 are incorrect because the drug does not promote infections, cause miosis, or affect the retina. Cognitive Level: Applying; Client Need: Safe and Effective Care Environment; Nursing Process: Implementation

5 Answer: 3   Rationale: Cholinergic antagonists typically cause dry eyes and the patient should be encouraged to use lubricating eyedrops. Options 1, 2, and 4 are incorrect. These statements suggest that the patient has understood the teaching. Patients receiving anticholinergic antagonists frequently complain of extreme dry mouth discomfort and increased fluid intake may ease this symptom. Many anticholinergic antagonists may cause drowsiness initially. Women receiving anticholinergic therapy should be advised to avoid breastfeeding until the medication is discontinued. Cognitive Level: Analyzing; Client Need: Health Promotion and Maintenance; Nursing Process: Evaluation

6 Answer: 1   Rationale: The therapeutic effect of succinylcholine is to paralyze skeletal muscles. However, this drug does not produce anesthesia or a loss of consciousness. Options 2, 3, and 4 are incorrect. Succinylcholine produces no change in the patient's sensorium (consciousness) and the patient can still experience pain. The effect of succinylcholine is total muscle paralysis, not muscle relaxation. Cognitive Level: Applying; Client Need: Physiological Integrity; Nursing Process: Implementation

Chapter 15

1 Answer: 1   Rationale: Phenylephrine causes vasoconstriction, reducing the swelling in the nasal passages. Options 2, 3, and 4 are incorrect. The drug does not destroy organisms or coat nasal passages. Whereas some drugs may be swallowed via the nasopharynx, localized action is predominant, and excessive

drug use and swallowing may result in adverse effects. Cognitive Level: Applying; Client Need: Physiological Integrity; Nursing Process: Implementation

2 Answer: 1, 2, 4   Rationale: Adrenergic agonist nasal sprays should not be shared among individuals due to the risk of spreading infection. Individuals should be taught the dangers of using adrenergic nasal sprays for longer than 3 days. These medications can cause increased blood pressure, increased heart rate, and insomnia. Habitual use of nasal adrenergic drugs can also cause rebound congestion as well as necrosis of the nasal mucosa due to the severe vasoconstriction caused by the drug. Due to the CNS stimulation, nasal adrenergic agents are not indicated in children and infants. Options 3 and 5 are incorrect. The drug causes CNS stimulation rather than depression. People with diabetes must use caution when using adrenergic drugs and must monitor their blood glucose levels more frequently for hyperglycemia. They are also at higher risk for adverse cardiac effects. Cognitive Level: Applying; Client Need: Health Promotion and Maintenance; Nursing Process: Implementation

3 Answer: 4   Rationale: Epinephrine is used during anaphylaxis to prevent hypotension and bronchoconstriction. Options 1, 2, and 3 are incorrect because the administration of epinephrine for anaphylaxis does not prevent the formation of histamine or antibodies in response to an invading antigen nor does it affect white blood cell function. Cognitive Level: Applying; Client Need: Physiological Integrity; Nursing Process: Evaluation

4 Answer: 1   Rationale: When beta$_2$-adrenergic agonists such as albuterol are taken too close to bedtime, the patient may experience insomnia. Options 2, 3, and 4 are incorrect because all adrenergic agonists act as stimulators, and urticaria and tinnitus are not adverse effects associated with this drug therapy. Cognitive Level: Applying; Client Need: Physiological Integrity; Nursing Process: Evaluation

5 Answer: 2   Rationale: At high dosage, dopamine stimulates alpha$_1$-adrenergic receptors, causing vasodilation and increased blood pressure. Options 1, 3, and 4 are incorrect. Dopamine does not affect the reflexes responsible for pupillary response or the patient's gag reflex, and it does not directly affect the patient's level of consciousness. Cognitive Level: Applying; Client Need: Physiological Integrity; Nursing Process: Evaluation

6 Answer: 1, 4   Rationale: The nurse should consult with the prescriber when adrenergic drugs are prescribed for individuals with hyperthyroid disease or dysrhythmias. The medication will further increase the already overactive metabolic system in hyperthyroidism and may increase the risk for dysrhythmias due to the cardiac stimulation caused by these medications. Options 2, 3, and 5 are incorrect. These are therapeutic indications for the administration of adrenergic agonists. Cognitive Level: Analyzing; Client Need: Physiological Integrity; Nursing Process: Implementation

Chapter 16

1 Answer: 1   Rationale: With beta-adrenergic blockers such as propranolol, the most important action is to monitor the patient for adverse effects associated with the cardiovascular system such as changes in pulse and blood pressure. Options 2, 3, and 4 are incorrect. Elevation of the head of the bed is not specifically required for this drug regimen. Inderal can be taken anytime regardless of meals, and its therapeutic action is not contingent on serum K$^+$ levels. Cognitive Level: Applying; Client Need: Physiological Integrity; Nursing Process: Planning

2 Answer: 4   Rationale: Beta-adrenergic antagonists may cause hypoglycemic episodes in patients with diabetes. The patient should be instructed to monitor blood glucose levels frequently initially and to notify the prescriber of a decrease. Options 1, 2, and 3 are incorrect. Insulin dosages are never arbitrarily increased without checking with a health care provider. Patients with diabetes should remain on their normal diabetic diets even though they may be taking antihypertensive medications. Elevation of the extremities is not relevant to a patient with diabetes taking beta-adrenergic blocker drugs. Cognitive Level: Applying; Client Need: Health Promotion and Maintenance; Nursing Process: Implementation

3 Answer: 1   Rationale: Initial doses of drugs that cause a "first-dose phenomenon" should be very low doses and administered at bedtime. The decline in blood pressure due to prazosin is often marked when beginning pharmacotherapy and when increasing the dose. This "first-dose phenomenon" can lead to syncope due to reduced blood flow to the brain. Options 2, 3, and 4 are incorrect. Doses of antihypertensive medications should never be doubled but should be gradually increased to avoid hypotension, and the best time to give prazosin in the initial phases of therapy is at bedtime. Cognitive Level: Applying; Client Need: Physiological Integrity; Nursing Process: Implementation

4 Answer: 1 Rationale: The nurse should suspect that the patient is describing orthostatic hypotension induced by the medication. Most patients find it helpful to move slowly from a recumbent position to avoid dizziness and syncope. Options 2, 3, and 4 are incorrect. Although drinking a full glass of water with the medication is a health promotion activity that the nurse might suggest, this action does not eliminate orthostatic hypotension. Sleeping positions do not influence the presence of orthostatic hypotension. The patient should never abruptly stop taking antihypertensive medication. Such action could result in hypertensive crisis, stroke, or heart attack. Cognitive Level: Applying; Client Need: Physiological Integrity; Nursing Process: Implementation

5 Answer: 4 Rationale: One adverse effect of alpha$_1$-adrenergic antagonists is tachycardia. Patients experiencing tachycardia should not receive alpha$_1$-adrenergic antagonists. Options 1, 2, and 3 are incorrect. Alpha$_1$-adrenergic antagonists are often prescribed for BPH because they relax muscles in the prostate. A pheochromocytoma is a benign tumor of the adrenal medulla that secretes catecholamines. Alpha$_1$-adrenergic antagonists help to reduce the HTN associated with these tumors. Alpha$_1$-adrenergic antagonists diminish the vasospasms associated with Raynaud's disease. Cognitive Level: Applying; Client Need: Physiological Integrity; Nursing Process: Implementation

6 Answer: 2, 3, 4 Rationale: Beta-adrenergic blockers can have dramatic metabolic effects that produce an increase in serum triglycerides and hypoglycemia. Additionally, these drugs can affect the sexual function of men by producing a decreased libido. Options 1 and 5 are incorrect. Anorexia and thrombocytopenia are not adverse effects associated with beta-adrenergic antagonists. Cognitive Level: Analyzing; Client Need: Physiological Integrity; Nursing Process: Evaluation

Chapter 18

1 Answer: 3 Rationale: Ataxia, weakness, restlessness, dizziness, and other motor problems can occur with lorazepam. Options 1, 2, and 4 are incorrect. These are not adverse effects associated with lorazepam. Cognitive Level: Applying; Client Need: Physiological Integrity; Nursing Process: Implementation

2 Answer: 4 Rationale: Sleeping for 7 hours is the desired effect of temazepam. Options 1, 2, and 3 are incorrect. The patient should experience periods of sleep lasting longer than 3 hours and should obtain a full night's sleep. The patient will be taking temazepam to assist with insomnia, not to treat anxiety related to everyday stress or to help control panic attacks. Cognitive Level: Applying; Client Need: Physiological Integrity; Nursing Process: Evaluation

3 Answer: 3 Rationale: This medication must be gradually reduced, not abruptly terminated. Abrupt termination may cause withdrawal symptoms (nausea, vomiting, abdominal cramps, diaphoresis, confusion, tremors, seizures). Options 1, 2, and 4 are incorrect. These are appropriate statements, and indicate that the patient understands the teaching. Cognitive Level: Analyzing; Client Need: Health Promotion and Maintenance; Nursing Process: Evaluation

4 Answer: 2 Rationale: Panic disorder is not an appropriate use for phenobarbital. Options 1, 3, and 4 are incorrect. Treatment of status epilepticus, use prior to diagnostic testing, and use prior to receiving general anesthesia are all appropriate for phenobarbital. Cognitive Level: Applying; Client Need: Physiological Integrity; Nursing Process: Implementation

5 Answer: 3 Rationale: Patient safety is the major concern with sedative–hypnotics, so prevention of falls is the highest priority. Options 1, 2, and 4 are incorrect. The patient may experience urinary incontinence, activity intolerance, or poor nutritional intake related to drug therapy or other reasons. Safety, however, is the priority concern. Cognitive Level: Analyzing; Client Need: Physiological Integrity; Nursing Process: Evaluation

6 Answer: 1 Rationale: Smoking enhances the metabolism of benzodiazepines, so the medication is broken down and removed from the body more quickly if the patient is a smoker. Therefore, a smoker may require a larger dose of a benzodiazepine to get the same effect as that of a nonsmoker. Options 2, 3, and 4 are incorrect. A smaller or half dose, or a single extra dose, may not adequately help relieve the patient's symptoms. Cognitive Level: Applying; Client Need: Physiological Integrity; Nursing Process: Implementation

Chapter 19

1 Answer: 1 Rationale: Imipramine should not be used by patients with seizure disorders because it lowers the seizure threshold. Options 2, 3, and 4 are incorrect. Imipramine is a drug that is effective in treating depression and is one of only two drugs approved for enuresis (bedwetting) in children. Like other TCAs, imipramine has a number of off-label indications. These include the adjuvant treatment of cancer or neuropathic pain. Cognitive Level: Applying; Client Need: Physiological Integrity; Nursing Process: Implementation

2 Answer: 3 Rationale: Full therapeutic effects of fluoxetine may take up to 1 month. Options 1, 2, and 4 are incorrect. Normal water and sodium intake do not affect fluoxetine. The patient cannot take an MAOI or other CNS depressant concurrently. The use of other drugs or CNS depressants such as alcohol could increase the risk of adverse effects or increased depression. Cognitive Level: Analyzing; Client Need: Physiological Integrity; Nursing Process: Evaluation

3 Answer: 1, 2 Rationale: Persistent GI upset and confusion are signs of elevated lithium levels between 1.5 and 2, which signify early toxicity. Options 3, 4, and 5 are incorrect. Polyuria is an adverse effect that may occur in early therapy but is not associated with early toxicity. Convulsions may occur at serum levels above 2.5 but not in early stages of toxicity. Ataxia is also not a sign of early lithium toxicity. Cognitive Level: Analyzing; Client Need: Physiological Integrity; Nursing Process: Evaluation

4 Answer: 1 Rationale: The patient taking lithium must be conscious of maintaining normal sodium intake. Because lithium is a salt, if sodium intake is low the body will replace the sodium with lithium, leading to lithium toxicity. Options 2, 3, and 4 are incorrect. The patient taking lithium must have regular blood studies, and toxicity is a very real concern; hence the necessity for routine blood studies. Women should refrain from breast-feeding while taking lithium. Cognitive Level: Analyzing; Client Need: Physiological Integrity; Nursing Process: Evaluation

5 Answer: 3 Rationale: A typical antidepressant such as venlafaxine may take up to 3 weeks or longer to reach full therapeutic effect. Therefore, the patient must continue taking the medication as ordered so that therapeutic drug levels can be reached and maintained. Options 1, 2, and 4 are incorrect. It is not within a nurse's scope of practice to suggest changes in medication routine without consulting the prescriber, and these comments are not helpful to maintaining a therapeutic nurse–patient relationship. Cognitive Level: Analyzing; Client Need: Health Promotion and Maintenance; Nursing Process: Evaluation

6 Answer: 2, 3 Rationale: Fluoxetine causes weight loss in some patients, while other patients experience weight gain or fluctuations in weight. A healthy diet and adequate exercise will help maintain normal weight while on this drug. While rare, an increased risk of suicide has been noted in patients up to age 24, and the patient should be carefully monitored, especially during the early initiation of therapy. Options 1, 4, and 5 are incorrect. Fluoxetine may cause insomnia but not sedation. Abrupt withdrawal of fluoxetine may lead to withdrawal symptoms. If the drug needs to be discontinued, gradually tapering the dose is recommended. Fluoxetine is not known to cause excessive thirst. Cognitive Level: Analyzing; Client Need: Physiological Integrity; Nursing Process: Evaluation

Chapter 20

1 Answer: 4 Rationale: Antipsychotic medications treat the symptoms associated with mental illness but do not cure these disorders. Without the medication, the symptoms will return. Options 1, 2, and 3 are incorrect. These are not symptoms associated with abrupt withdrawal of an antipsychotic medication. Cognitive Level: Analyzing; Client Need: Physiological Integrity; Nursing Process: Evaluation

2   Answer: 2   Rationale: Acute dystonia, or severe muscle spasms, especially of the back, neck, face, or tongue, may appear within hours or days of the first dose of a phenothiazine and should be reported immediately. Options 1, 3, and 4 are incorrect. Social withdrawal is a symptom of the disease, and slowed activity may occur as a result of the medication. However, the patient's body will become adjusted to the medication in a short time period and it will disappear. TD occurs late in therapy and is more common in the older adult. The phenothiazine medications usually cause adverse effects even when taken as prescribed. Cognitive Level: Analyzing; Client Need: Physiological Integrity; Nursing Process: Implementation

3   Answer: 1   Rationale: Benztropine is classified as an autonomic nervous system drug and an anticholinergic. It suppresses tremor and rigidity by decreasing the excess cholinergic effect associated with dopamine deficiency. Options 2, 3, and 4 are incorrect. Diazepam and lorazepam are antianxiety medications that will not improve the patient's symptoms. Haloperidol is an antipsychotic medication that may cause these symptoms. Cognitive Level: Analyzing; Client Need: Physiological Integrity; Nursing Process: Planning

4   Answer: 2, 4   Rationale: EPS occurs frequently, especially at the beginning of therapy with haloperidol. A person with Parkinson's disease, seizure disorders, alcoholism, or severe mental depression should not take haloperidol because they are all disorders that affect the CNS. Dementia, seizures, depression, and severe CNS depression are known to occur with the use of haloperidol in these patients. Options 1, 3, and 5 are incorrect. Haloperidol and antacids may be given simultaneously; there are no known interactions between these two medications. Haloperidol must be taken as ordered, on a regular schedule. Taking the drug prn will not reduce symptoms of psychosis because it takes several weeks of regular administration before therapeutic levels are reached. Sustained release medications should never be crushed. If the patient cannot take the medication, another form should be used. Cognitive Level: Applying; Client Need: Physiological Integrity; Nursing Process: Implementation

5   Answer: 4   Rationale: The patient taking risperidone or any antipsychotic medication should refrain from consuming alcohol. Concurrent use of alcohol with antipsychotic medications will increase CNS depression. Because there is an increased risk of hyperglycemia or diabetes in patients taking risperidone, alcohol should also be avoided because it may affect blood sugar levels. Options 1, 2, and 3 are incorrect. Weight gain may occur, and obtaining a weekly weight will help the patient track any gain. Increasing fluids and fiber may help to limit GI adverse effects. Hypotension is related to adverse reactions the patient may experience and must be monitored and reported if it occurs. Cognitive Level: Analyzing; Client Need: Physiological Integrity; Nursing Process: Evaluation

6   Answer: 1   Rationale: Fever, tachycardia, stupor, and incontinence are symptoms of neuroleptic malignant syndrome (NMS), a potentially fatal adverse effect of antipsychotics that must be diagnosed and treated immediately. Options 2, 3, and 4 are possible adverse reactions, but are not life threatening, and therefore do not need to be reported with the same urgency as symptoms of NMS. Cognitive Level: Analyzing; Client Need: Physiological Integrity; Nursing Process: Evaluation

Chapter 21

1   Answer: 2   Rationale: Benztropine, a cholinergic antagonist, is frequently used as combination therapy with other antiparkinson drugs to decrease tremors. Options 1, 3, and 4 are incorrect. Amantadine acts to increase dopamine's release, but only as long as dopamine is available. Haloperidol is a phenothiazine antipsychotic that may lead to pseudo-Parkinson's disease in many persons. Donepezil prolongs the time between diagnosis and the institutionalization of the patient with Alzheimer's disease and is not used for Parkinson's disease. Cognitive Level: Analyzing; Client Need: Physiological Integrity; Nursing Process: Implementation

2   Answer: 3   Rationale: Being independent with ADLs shows an improvement in physical abilities. Options 1, 2, and 4 are incorrect. Drowsiness is a common adverse effect of anti-Parkinson's medications. Anorexia or loss of appetite is a common adverse effect, not an expected therapeutic effect. Itchy

skin is not directly related to PD symptoms or to the medications used. Cognitive Level: Applying; Client Need: Health Promotion and Maintenance; Nursing Process: Evaluation

3   Answer: 3   Rationale: It is important that the caregivers understand that there is no cure for AD, but that the medication may delay the worsening of symptoms. Options 1, 2, and 4 are incorrect. The medication should be given continuously and not only when the symptoms are present. The patient may become constipated but does not require emergency treatment. The drug may cause bradycardia or atrial fibrillation and the pulse rate should be checked weekly, but it is not necessary to take the patient's vital signs before each dose of medication. Cognitive Level: Applying; Client Need: Health Promotion and Maintenance; Nursing Process: Evaluation

4   Answer: 1, 4   Rationale: It is difficult to remember to take a medication four times a day, and as the patient's cognitive functioning declines, it may be increasingly difficult to administer it. Potentially life-threatening cardiac dysrhythmias, including atrial fibrillation and sinus bradycardia, are possible adverse effects associated with donepezil. Options 2, 3, and 5 are incorrect. Donepezil may cause diarrhea, rather than constipation, and does not cause vision difficulties. Donepezil is available by prescription only and cannot be purchased over the counter. Cognitive Level: Applying; Client Need: Physiological Integrity; Nursing Process: Planning

5   Answer: 1   Rationale: Rivastigmine has no significant drug interactions. This is thought to be true because there is no interaction with enzymes in the liver that metabolize drugs. Options 2, 3, and 4 are incorrect because they do not apply to rivastigmine. Cognitive Level: Applying; Client Need: Physiological Integrity; Nursing Process: Planning

6   Answer: 1, 2, 4   Rationale: Flulike symptoms with general malaise, body aches, fever, and headache are common. Insomnia and rashes may also occur and may be treated symptomatically after conferral with the provider. Options 3 and 5 are incorrect. Depression should never be ignored and should be reported immediately. Significant pain with darkening or blackening of the skin at the injection site indicates that tissue necrosis may be occurring and requires prompt treatment. Cognitive Level: Analyzing; Client Need: Psychosocial Integrity; Nursing Process: Evaluation

Chapter 22

1   Answer: 3   Rationale: GI effects such as nausea, anorexia, and abdominal pain are common with ethosuximide. Because the patient is still growing, improper nutrition may affect normal growth. Monitoring height and weight weekly will assist in tracking normal growth. Options 1, 2, and 4 are incorrect. Physical activity will not affect the drug's metabolism and activity is normal and needed for healthy growth and development. Ethosuximide is not known to cause bone loss or dehydration. Cognitive Level: Applying; Client Need: Health Promotion and Maintenance; Nursing Process: Planning

2   Answer: 4   Rationale: Oxcarbazepine is excreted by the kidneys, and renal function laboratory studies will be monitored to detect adverse renal effects. Because hyponatremia may develop during treatment, serum sodium levels should also be monitored. Options 1, 2, and 3 are incorrect. Oxcarbazepine does not affect CBC, platelets, sedimentation rate, or albumin or serum glucose levels. Cognitive Level: Applying; Client Need: Physiological Integrity; Nursing Process: Planning

3   Answer: 4   Rationale: Sedation and an increased risk of falls are associated with carbamazepine. Options 1, 2, and 3 are incorrect. Carbamazepine is used off-label to treat dementia with aggressiveness and agitation. The drug is not associated with insomnia and has not been demonstrated to increase the risk of stroke. Cognitive Level: Applying; Client Need: Physiological Integrity; Nursing Process: Implementation

4   Answer: 2   Rationale: Slurred speech, diplopia, sedation, and dyspnea are symptoms of gabapentin overdose. Options 1, 3, and 4 are incorrect. Seizure activity is likely to recur if the drug is stopped abruptly. Neither grapefruit juice nor smoking is known to affect drug level. Cognitive Level: Analyzing; Client Need: Physiological Integrity; Nursing Process: Evaluation

5   Answer: 1   Rationale: High doses of phenytoin can cause nystagmus, confusion, ataxia, coma, and seizures and the dosage should be reduced.

Options 2, 3, and 4 are incorrect. Increasing or maintaining the same dose will continue or exacerbate the symptoms of toxicity. The drug should not be discontinued abruptly because seizure activity may occur. Cognitive Level: Analyzing; Client Need: Physiological Integrity; Nursing Process: Planning

6 Answer: 3 Rationale: Carbamazepine is associated with an increased risk of SJS and toxic epidermal necrosis in genetically susceptible individuals. Sunburning and a reddish-purple rash, especially associated with blisters, are possible symptoms of severe dermatologic reactions and should be evaluated immediately. Options 1, 2, and 4 are incorrect. Blurred vision, leg cramping, and lethargy are all possible side effects of carbamazepine but tolerance to these effects usually develops over time. Cognitive Level: Applying; Client Need: Physiological Integrity; Nursing Process: Evaluation

Chapter 23

1 Answer: 1, 4, 5 Rationale: Cyclobenzaprine may cause tachycardia, and any palpitations or rapid heart rate should be reported. Drowsiness may also occur, and driving or other hazardous activities should be avoided until the effects of the drug are known. Swelling of the face or tongue may occur and must be reported immediately to the provider. Options 2 and 3 are incorrect. Patients with severe muscle spasms are encouraged to rest affected muscle groups until acute spasms subside. Cyclobenzaprine may cause dry mouth, and alcohol-based mouth rinses may exacerbate the condition. Cognitive Level: Applying; Client Need: Physiological Integrity; Nursing Process: Planning

2 Answer: 3 Rationale: Abruptly discontinuing baclofen may result in fever, seizures, rebound spasticity, and hallucinations. Options 1, 2, and 4 are incorrect. Baclofen may cause weakness, and like other muscle relaxants and antispasmodics, may cause constipation. Being cautious with activities and increasing fluid and fiber intake will help to limit the adverse effects caused by baclofen. It may take several months before the full effects of baclofen are reached. Cognitive Level: Analyzing; Client Need: Physiological Integrity; Nursing Process: Evaluation

3 Answer: 2 Rationale: Capsaicin should be applied to the site of pain with a gloved hand to prevent irritation of the skin on the hands and to avoid introducing the capsaicin to the eyes or other parts of the body not under treatment. Options 1, 3, and 4 are incorrect. Capsaicin should only be applied to the site of pain, not proximal or distal to the pain. If capsaicin begins to irritate and cause redness and inflammation, it should be discontinued. Capsaicin should not be applied with a bare hand. Cognitive Level: Applying; Client Need: Physiological Integrity; Nursing Process: Implementation

4 Answer: 2 Rationale: Dysphagia, blurred vision, and ptosis are all symptoms of possible botulism toxicity and should be reported immediately. Options 1, 3, and 4 are incorrect. Fever, aches, and chills are not anticipated adverse effects of this drug, and while they should be evaluated, they do not require immediate reporting. Moderate levels of muscle weakness may occur after the drug is administered, and strengthening exercises may be needed on the affected side. Continuous muscle spasms and pain should not occur because the drug blocks muscle contraction. Cognitive Level: Analyzing; Client Need: Physiological Integrity; Nursing Process: Evaluation

5 Answer: 4 Rationale: Physostigmine may be administered to reverse serious anticholinergic adverse effects. Options 1, 2, and 3 are incorrect. Naloxone is often used to decrease the effects of opioids on the CNS but is not the drug of choice in the treatment of CNS depression with cyclobenzaprine. Meperidine is a CNS depressant and should not be administered with cyclobenzaprine. Diazepam is a skeletal muscle relaxant and should not be administered with cyclobenzaprine. Cognitive Level: Applying; Client Need: Physiological Integrity; Nursing Process: Planning

6 Answer: 2, 3, 5 Rationale: Dantrolene may cause hepatotoxicity with the greatest risk occurring in women over age 35. Estrogen taken concurrently with dantrolene may increase this risk. The drug may cause xerostomia, and sucking on hard candy or sipping water or ice chips may relieve the dryness. Options 1 and 4 are incorrect. Fluids and fiber may also help diarrhea, but dantrolene may cause diarrhea, not constipation. Dantrolene may cause photosensitivity, so patients taking the drug should avoid direct exposure to the sun. Cognitive Level: Applying; Client Need: Health Promotion and Maintenance; Nursing Process: Implementation

Chapter 24

1 Answer: 4 Rationale: ADHD drugs are Schedule II through IV drugs that require tight controls. Because they can be abused, they should be kept under lock and tightly monitored with only the minimal number of doses kept at the school as per school policy. Options 1, 2, and 3 are incorrect. Keeping the drug in a lunch bag may lead to the child forgetting to take it or to other children taking the drug. Because it is a highly regulated drug, additional prescriptions or dosages are not allowed under the Schedule because they could result in the misuse of the drug by people other than the student for whom it is prescribed. Cognitive Level: Applying; Client Need: Health Promotion and Maintenance; Nursing Process: Implementation

2 Answer: 2 Rationale: Atomoxetine should decrease hyperactivity. Options 1, 3, and 4 are incorrect. Atomoxetine should increase attention, not decrease it. Mydriasis and elevated liver enzymes are adverse effects associated with atomoxetine; they are not therapeutic effects. Cognitive Level: Applying; Client Need: Health Promotion and Maintenance; Nursing Process: Evaluation

3 Answer: 1 Rationale: Chlorpromazine is the preferred drug to assist in counteracting amphetamine overdosage. It has strong alpha-adrenergic blocking actions that treat the effects of amphetamine. Options 2, 3, and 4 are incorrect. Phenytoin is an antiepileptic drug; propofol is a nonbarbiturate sedative–hypnotic; and dexamethasone is a corticosteroid. None of these drugs would counteract the effects of an amphetamine overdose. Cognitive Level: Applying; Client Need: Physiological Integrity; Nursing Process: Planning

4 Answer: 3 Rationale: Atomoxetine has been linked to suicidal ideations and an increased risk of suicide. These symptoms should be reported immediately to the family or caregiver for assessment and treatment by the health care provider. Options 1, 2, and 4 are incorrect. The need for drug withdrawal will be determined by the provider after assessing the patient. The drug may take up to 4 weeks to achieve maximum therapeutic effects, but this patient is experiencing an adverse effect linked to the drug. Caffeine will not counteract depressive effects and may increase the risk of CNS adverse effects. Cognitive Level: Analyzing; Client Need: Psychosocial Integrity; Nursing Process: Evaluation

5 Answer: 2 Rationale: Palpitations, dysrhythmias, and facial tingling are all symptoms of a caffeine overdose. Options 1, 3, and 4 are incorrect. Zolpidem and gabapentin are associated with CNS depressant-type effects such as drowsiness, dizziness, and bradycardia. Some herbal teas may contain stimulant properties, but many have calming effects and are not as likely as caffeine to cause these symptoms. Cognitive Level: Analyzing; Client Need: Physiological Integrity; Nursing Process: Evaluation

6 Answer: 3 Rationale: Taking the medication before late afternoon ensures that peak drug activity will occur during waking hours. Options 1, 2, and 4 are incorrect. Drinking wine with dinner should not have a noticeable effect on sleep unless taken directly before bedtime when the metabolism of the alcohol may actually diminish sleep as the blood glucose rises and falls. Chocolate contains caffeine, and also sugar, which may cause additional wakefulness. Decaffeinated coffee will limit the intake of the additional stimulant of caffeine but will not significantly improve the patient's sleep if the methylphenidate is taken later in the afternoon or evening. Cognitive Level: Applying; Client Need: Health Promotion and Maintenance; Nursing Process: Implementation

Chapter 25

1 Answer: 1, 3, 4, 5 Rationale: Common adverse effects of opioids include respiratory depression, urinary retention, constipation, and nausea. Option 2 is incorrect. Hypotension, not hypertension, is an adverse effect of opioids. Cognitive Level: Analyzing; Client Need: Physiological Integrity; Nursing Process: Evaluation

2 Answer: 4 Rationale: Opioids decrease peristalsis, and bowel surgery may produce a temporary cessation of peristalsis (paralytic ileus). Both lead to constipation. Once bowel function has returned enough for the patient to start eating, constipation is still likely and needs to be prevented by increased dietary fiber and fluids as well as taking a stool softener. Options 1, 2, and 3 are incorrect. Respiratory depression and urinary retention are not likely after several days with decreasing opioid use. Addiction is not a concern in the treatment of

acute pain in this scenario. Cognitive Level: Applying; Client Need: Physiological Integrity; Nursing Process: Planning

3 Answer: 3   Rationale: Chest pain is a serious adverse effect of sumatriptan and needs to be differentiated from angina, which can also be caused by the drug. Options 1, 2, and 4 are incorrect. The patient should not use the drug again until being evaluated by the provider and should report the chest pain immediately. Reclining in a quiet room with cold packs is a nondrug treatment for migraines, but reporting the chest pain is most important at this time. Cognitive Level: Applying; Client Need: Physiological Integrity; Nursing Process: Implementation

4 Answer: 2   Rationale: The patient is describing neuropathic pain, which is most likely to respond to the adjuvant analgesic gabapentin, an antiseizure drug used for neuropathic pain. Options 1, 3, and 4 are incorrect. Nonopioids such as ibuprofen, or opioids such as methadone, are less effective at relieving pain that is of neurologic origin. Naloxone is an opioid antagonist and will not relieve the patient's pain. Cognitive Level: Applying; Client Need: Physiological Integrity; Nursing Process: Planning

5 Answer: 2   Rationale: Ergot alkaloids such as dihydroergotamine (Migranal) are one of the two drug classes for aborting migraines. Options 1, 3, and 4 are incorrect. Morphine is an opioid agonist and is not effective in aborting migraines. Propranolol is a beta blocker and is used to prevent migraines. Ibuprofen is a nonopioid analgesic that is used to treat mild to moderate pain. Cognitive Level: Applying; Client Need: Physiological Integrity; Nursing Process: Planning

6 Answer: 4   Rationale: Older adult patients are at highest risk for hypotension, respiratory depression, and increased incidence of adverse CNS effects such as confusion. Options 1, 2, and 3 are incorrect. Most 23-year-old patients can tolerate opioids without adverse effects. Individuals who suffer from traumatic injury may receive narcotic analgesia. However, caution should be taken if the individual has also experienced any type of head injury. Opioids are often used with individuals who suffer MI. No adverse effects such as hypotension or respiratory depression are usually present if the dose is appropriate for the size of the patient. Cognitive Level: Analyzing; Client Need: Physiological Integrity; Nursing Process: Evaluation

Chapter 26

1 Answer: 2   Rationale: In stage 2 the patient becomes excitable with hyperactivity and irregular heart and respiratory rates. Options 1, 3, and 4 are incorrect. In stage 1, the patient loses general sensation but remains awake. In stage 3, the patient's skeletal muscles become relaxed, and delirium stabilizes. In stage 4, the patient has paralysis of the medulla with possible adverse effects on respiratory and cardiac function. Cognitive Level: Analyzing; Client Need: Physiological Integrity; Nursing Process: Evaluation

2 Answer: 1   Rationale: Patients who have an allergy to eggs or soy products may have an allergic reaction to the propofol emulsion, which contains these products. Options 2, 3, and 4 are incorrect. Patients with allergies to iodine, kidney disease, or Addison's disease may be administered propofol cautiously. Cognitive Level: Analyzing; Client Need: Physiological Integrity; Nursing Process: Implementation

3 Answer: 4   Rationale: Anxiety, excitement, and combativeness are signs that the dose of nitrous oxide is high and the patient is exhibiting signs of the second stage of anesthesia. Lowering the dose may reduce these symptoms. Options 1, 2, and 3 are incorrect. The dose of nitrous oxide would be lowered, not increased. Propofol would cause additional CNS depression and is not advised. Succinylcholine is a neuromuscular blocking agent that will increase the risk of significant respiratory adverse effects due to its muscle-paralyzing actions. Cognitive Level: Analyzing; Client Need: Physiological Integrity; Nursing Process: Planning

4 Answer: 3   Rationale: Ketamine produces dissociation anesthesia, which is a feeling of being separated from the environment. Options 1, 2, and 4 are incorrect because anxiety and dry mouth are not significant adverse effects of ketamine. Ketamine may cause decreased energy. Cognitive Level: Applying; Client Need: Physiological Integrity; Nursing Process: Evaluation

5 Answer: 1   Rationale: Epinephrine is administered with lidocaine to increase the duration of the anesthetic action at the site by causing vasoconstriction, keeping the anesthetic localized. Options 2, 3, and 4 are incorrect because epinephrine will cause vasoconstriction, not vasodilation at the site; may increase blood pressure if the drug enters the systemic circulation; and neither lidocaine nor epinephrine has any antibacterial properties. Cognitive Level: Applying; Client Need: Physiological Integrity; Nursing Process: Evaluation

6 Answer: 2, 3, 4   Rationale: Alfentanil is a parenteral opioid agent that promotes general anesthesia. Sufentanil is also a parenteral opioid agent. Regimental is an opioid agent that is used to induce and maintain general anesthesia. Options 1 and 5 are incorrect. Nitrous oxide is not an opioid agent and it is administered by inhalation. Succinylcholine is a neuromuscular blocking agent. Cognitive Level: Applying; Client Need: Physiological Integrity; Nursing Process: Implementation

Chapter 27

1 Answer: 1   Rationale: Addiction is not a problem for the majority of patients who receive narcotic analgesia in the postoperative period. The nurse should administer the dose to treat the pain. Options 2, 3, and 4 are incorrect. Reviewing the patient's past medical history is an important assessment that should guide nursing practice, but a patient's past tendencies toward substance abuse are not appropriate criteria to consider in the nurse's decision to treat the pain with analgesia. Pain is best treated in the early stage. If a nurse waits to treat pain until it becomes intolerable, the patient may require a higher dose of the analgesia. There is no evidence that patients request medication when it is not needed. Cognitive Level: Applying; Client Need: Physiological Integrity; Nursing Process: Implementation

2 Answer: 3   Rationale: Patients with a substance use disorder tend to revert back to drug-seeking behavior when they return to the company of other substance abusers. Options 1, 2, and 4 are incorrect. A good support system can be extremely beneficial when an individual is attempting to withdraw from physiologically and psychologically addictive substances. Patients with substance use disorder may experience the desire to use drugs long after the drug has physiologically cleared the body. Generally speaking, individuals who share a common experience will be perceived as being most helpful to an individual undergoing the same or similar experience. Cognitive Level: Analyzing; Client Need: Health Promotion and Maintenance; Nursing Process: Evaluation

3 Answer: 1, 4, 5   Rationale: Varenicline (Chantix) doses are increased over an 8-day period and maintained for 12 to 24 weeks, reducing withdrawal symptoms and craving for smoking. Serious dermatologic reactions have been noted and any unusual skin reactions or angioedema should be reported to the provider immediately and the drug stopped. Varenicline carries a black box warning for serious neuropsychiatric events, and any changes in behavior, depression, hostility, or thoughts of suicide should be immediately reported. Options 2 and 3 are incorrect. Varenicline (Chantix) activates nicotinic acetylcholine receptors in the brain and blocks nicotine from reaching the receptors. It does not prevent nicotine's harmful effects on body systems from occurring. It has several adverse effects, including serious dermatologic and neuropsychiatric effects. Cognitive Level: Applying; Client Need: Physiological Integrity; Nursing Process: Evaluation

4 Answer: 2   Rationale: Sedatives cause a profound suppression of the respiratory system through direct action with the CNS. Patients who have experienced an overdose of sedatives are at high risk for respiratory arrest. Options 1, 3, and 4 are incorrect. Sedatives do not typically cause any type of stimulation. Long-term effects of overdose will most likely manifest through liver and kidney dysfunction, but the immediate need is to determine the current status of the patient. Level of consciousness is one of the assessments to be made with a patient receiving sedatives, but the nurse would expect a decrease in consciousness with an overdose of sedatives. Cognitive Level: Applying; Client Need: Physiological Integrity; Nursing Process: Assessment

5 Answer: 4   Rationale: Typical symptoms of heroin withdrawal include chills, dilated pupils, diarrhea, runny nose, muscle spasms, goose bumps, abdominal pain, sweating, and agitation. Options 1, 2, and 3 are incorrect. Heroin is an opiate that depresses the CNS, and the patient may exhibit hyperactive behavior during withdrawal. Dermatologic effects are not common during heroin withdrawal. Paranoia, delusions, or hallucinations are more typical effects. Cognitive Level: Applying; Client Need: Physiological Integrity; Nursing Process: Evaluation

6 Answer: 1   Rationale: Disulfiram is a drug used in the rehabilitation of alcoholism. When patients are taking this drug, even small amounts of alcohol, such as found in mouthwash and many OTC medications, can produce flushing, throbbing in the head and neck, respiratory difficulty, nausea, vomiting, sweating, thirst, chest pain, blurred vision, and confusion. Options 2, 3, and 4 are incorrect. There is no reason for a patient to avoid dairy products or foods high in iron. Disulfiram should not directly impact the patient's driving or level of alertness. Cognitive Level: Applying; Client Need: Health Promotion and Maintenance; Nursing Process: Implementation

Chapter 29

1 Answer: 1   Rationale: Rhabdomyolysis is a serious adverse effect of the statins. Early signs include unexplained fatigue or muscle weakness, pain in joints or muscles, and an increase in CK level. Options 2, 3, and 4 are incorrect. The weakness, fatigue, and pain that the patient is experiencing are not symptoms of renal failure or hepatic insufficiency. In rheumatoid arthritis, pain is often present but tends to be greatest in the mornings and associated with red, hot, swollen joints. Cognitive Level: Analyzing; Client Need: Physiological Integrity; Nursing Process: Evaluation

2 Answer: 2   Rationale: One of the most serious adverse effects of cholestyramine is obstruction of the GI tract. Options 1, 3, and 4 are incorrect. Cholestyramine does not cause orange urine, sore throat, and fever, or affect capillary refill. Cognitive Level: Applying; Client Need: Physiological Integrity; Nursing Process: Planning

3 Answer: 1   Rationale: Although there are few contraindications to using bile acid sequestrants such as colestipol, they should be used cautiously in patients with GI disorders such as peptic ulcer disease. Options 2, 3, and 4 are incorrect. MI is not a contraindication for the use of bile acid sequestrants. Bile acid sequestrant agents do not affect serum sodium levels, and patients allergic to foods high in tyramine may be prescribed bile acid sequestrants. Cognitive Level: Applying; Client Need: Physiological Integrity; Nursing Process: Implementation

4 Answer: 2, 3   Rationale: Intense flushing and hot flashes occur in almost every patient who is taking niacin. Tingling of the extremities may also occur. Options 1, 4, and 5 are incorrect. Neither fever and chills nor dry mucous membranes are associated adverse effects of niacin therapy. Niacin may cause an *increase* in fasting blood glucose, especially in people with diabetes. Cognitive Level: Analyzing; Client Need: Physiological Integrity; Nursing Process: Evaluation

5 Answer: 4   Rationale: Grapefruit juice inhibits the metabolism of statins such as lovastatin, allowing them to reach high serum levels. Options 1, 2, and 3 are incorrect. Most patients with lipid disorders are asymptomatic. A patient should be instructed that maintenance of optimal body weight will help reduce unhealthy lipid levels. Because cholesterol biosynthesis in the liver is higher at night, statins are usually best taken in the evening. Cognitive Level: Applying; Client Need: Health Promotion and Maintenance; Nursing Process: Evaluation

6 Answer: 1, 4, 5   Rationale: Fibric acid agents (fibrates) such as gemfibrozil may cause or worsen gallbladder disease and may enhance the hypoglycemic effects of antidiabetes drugs. Because it is excreted through the kidneys, it may be used cautiously in patients with renal impairment, but the order should be validated with the provider before giving if the patient has a history of renal impairment. Options 2 and 3 are incorrect. Angina and hypertension may indicate the existence of atherosclerosis and arteriosclerosis, both of which are indications for a lipid-lowering drug. Cognitive Level: Applying; Client Need: Physiological Integrity; Nursing Process: Implementation

Chapter 30

1 Answer: 1   Rationale: A major complication associated with the administration of CCBs such as nifedipine is HF. Daily weighing will alert the patient to signs of fluid retention, which may indicate cardiac dysfunction. A weight gain of 1 kg or more in 24 hours indicates possible fluid retention and may signal impending HF. Options 2, 3, and 4 are incorrect. Nifedipine does not affect the immune system, and there is no reason to avoid crowds. The intake of oral or dietary calcium and CCBs has not been shown to be problematic. HTN is asymptomatic, and patients should be instructed to take the medication even when feeling healthy. Cognitive Level: Applying; Client Need: Health Promotion and Maintenance; Nursing Process: Implementation

2 Answer: 4   Rationale: Felodipine may cause hypotension with associated reflex tachycardia. Options 1, 2, and 3 are incorrect. Rash and chills, increased urine output, and weight loss are not adverse effects of CCBs. Cognitive Level: Applying; Client Need: Physiological Integrity; Nursing Process: Planning

3 Answer: 4   Rationale: An adverse effect of verapamil is HF, which will be reflected in the patient's intake and output ratio and weight gain of more than 1 kg per 24 hours. Options 1, 2, and 3 are incorrect. Verapamil does not affect coagulation or affect thrombocytes. Verapamil is usually given during hours that the patient is awake; however, it can be administered at any time. Cognitive Level: Applying; Client Need: Physiological Integrity; Nursing Process: Implementation

4 Answer: 2   Rationale: Grapefruit juice will enhance the absorption of nifedipine. Options 1, 3, and 4 are incorrect. Nifedipine should not be taken with antacids since this will affect the absorption rate of the drug. Patients should never double the dose of nifedipine because life-threatening hypotension could result. Nifedipine does not affect the efficacy of birth control pills. Cognitive Level: Analyzing; Client Need: Health Promotion and Maintenance; Nursing Process: Evaluation

5 Answer: 1, 2, 3, 4   Rationale: Diltiazem reduces the patient's blood pressure, which may result in syncope or dizziness. Until the effects of the medication are known the patient should avoid driving or other activities requiring mental alertness. One of the adverse effects associated with diltiazem and CCBs is constipation, which can be reduced by increasing fluid and dietary fiber intake. Diltiazem may cause orthostatic hypotension. To ensure safety, patients should be instructed to rise slowly from sitting or lying positions. Patients should be taught to report a weight gain of 1 kg (2 lb) per day or 2 kg (5 lb) per week. Option 5 is incorrect. Sudden discontinuation could cause the patient to experience hypertensive crisis. Cognitive Level: Applying; Client Need: Physiological Integrity; Nursing Process: Implementation

6 Answer: 3   Rationale: Nifedipine is a negative inotropic drug and symptoms of pulmonary edema call for discontinuation of the drug. The nurse should also monitor a patient more closely for congestive HF and pulmonary edema if the patient has a medical history of pulmonary edema. Options 1, 2, and 4 are incorrect. An appendectomy does not warrant monitoring the patient any more than usual. Patients receiving renal dialysis should be closely monitored during therapy with nifedipine due to a reduction in renal function. However, these patients are not as high risk as a patient with pulmonary edema. Psychotropic drugs are not known to interact negatively with this drug. Cognitive Level: Analyzing; Client Need: Physiological Integrity; Nursing Process: Evaluation

Chapter 31

1 Answer: 4   Rationale: Lisinopril does not affect serum calcium levels and, thus, would not cause an elevated blood pressure. Options 1, 2, and 3 are incorrect. Common adverse effects for lisinopril are cough, headache, dizziness, and orthostatic hypotension. These symptoms should be reported to the prescriber. Salt substitutes usually contain potassium chloride and should be avoided to reduce the risk of hyperkalemia. Patients on this medication should be instructed to stay on regular doses of blood pressure medication. If a dose is missed, take it as soon as possible but not too close to the next dose. Never take a double dose. Cognitive Level: Analyzing; Client Need: Health Promotion and Maintenance; Nursing Process: Evaluation

2 Answer: 1   Rationale: Lisinopril should be stored in a dry place at room temperature, because heat and moisture may cause drug breakdown. Options 2, 3, and 4 are incorrect. Heat and moisture do not enhance the strength of the drug, crystallize the medication, or convert the medication to toxic metabolites. Cognitive Level: Analyzing; Client Need: Health Promotion and Maintenance; Nursing Process: Evaluation

3 Answer: 3   Rationale: ACE inhibitors such as enalapril also prevent the breakdown of bradykinin. Accumulation of bradykinin in certain tissues such as the lungs can cause adverse effects, as manifested by a nonproductive cough, and may require an antihistamine for treatment. Options 1, 2, and 4 are incorrect. Dry mucous membranes are not adverse effects related to ACE inhibitors. The expected outcome associated with ACE inhibitors is a decline in blood pressure, and the nurse should expect both systolic and diastolic pressures to be reduced. Cognitive Level: Applying; Client Need: Physiological Integrity; Nursing Process: Implementation

4 Answer: 2 Rationale: The most common adverse effects of losartan are headache, dizziness, nasal congestion, and insomnia. Options 1, 3, and 4 are incorrect. Irritability, tremors, sleepiness, slurred speech, pruritus, or rash are not common adverse effects associated with losartan. Cognitive Level: Analyzing; Client Need: Physiological Integrity; Nursing Process: Evaluation

5 Answer: 1 Rationale: Patients with severe dehydration may experience hypovolemia and are at high risk of life-threatening hypotension. Options 2, 3, and 4 are incorrect. Irbesartan may be prescribed for the prevention of diabetic nephropathy, HTN, and as an off-label use for heart failure. Cognitive Level: Applying; Client Need: Physiological Integrity; Nursing Process: Implementation

6 Answer: 3 Rationale: Patients receiving benazepril should avoid driving or engaging in other potentially hazardous activities until the effects of the drug are known. Benazepril may cause adverse effects that impair thinking and reaction time. Options 1, 2, and 4 are incorrect. The patient or family should be taught methods of home blood pressure measurement and maintenance of a blood pressure log while taking benazepril. OTC medications for colds, sinus, fever, asthma, or appetite control should be avoided because they may increase blood pressure. The consumption of alcohol while taking benazepril can lower blood pressure, which will lead to dizziness and fainting. Cognitive Level: Analyzing; Client Need: Health Promotion and Maintenance; Nursing Process: Evaluation

Chapter 32

1 Answer: 2 Rationale: As a diuretic, furosemide may dramatically reduce the patient's circulating blood volume, thus producing episodes of orthostatic hypotension. Patients may minimize this effect by rising slowly from sitting or lying positions. Options 1, 3, and 4 are incorrect. Cabbage, cauliflower, and kale are high in vitamin K, but furosemide does not require restricted consumption of these foods. Monitoring pulse rate during administration of furosemide for reflex tachycardia secondary to hypotension is advised, but it is not required that it be taken before the dose or for 1 full minute. Due to the potential for significant diuresis, fluids should not be restricted unless ordered by the health care provider. Cognitive Level: Applying; Client Need: Physiological Integrity; Nursing Process: Implementation

2 Answer: 2 Rationale: Loop diuretics such as bumetanide cause a significant loss of potassium. Hypokalemia is often the most predominant electrolyte imbalance. Options 1, 3, and 4 are incorrect. Hypernatremia is unlikely with the administration of bumetanide because it promotes sodium loss. Hyperkalemia is inconsistent with the administration of bumetanide due to the increase in potassium excretion. If elevated potassium levels are present in these patients, other etiologies should be investigated. Bumetanide does not cause hypocalcemia but may cause hypercalciuria with an increased risk of calcium-based kidney stones. Cognitive Level: Analyzing; Client Need: Physiological Integrity; Nursing Process: Evaluation

3 Answer: 3 Rationale: Muscle cramps and weakness may indicate hypokalemia and should be reported to the health care provider. Options 1, 2, and 4 are incorrect. Many patients taking diuretic therapy are instructed to monitor the intake of both sodium and water to maintain adequate but not excessive amounts. Patients should ingest foods high in potassium, not vitamin K. Thiazide diuretics and antihypertensive drugs are not known to cause sleepiness when taken together. Cognitive Level: Applying; Client Need: Physiological Integrity; Nursing Process: Implementation

4 Answer: 1 Rationale: Spironolactone is a potassium-sparing diuretic and may cause hyperkalemia. Options 2, 3, and 4 are incorrect. This drug does not have a direct effect on magnesium and does not cause hypokalemia. It does not have calcium-binding effects. Cognitive Level: Applying; Client Need: Physiological Integrity; Nursing Process: Assessment

5 Answer: 4 Rationale: In the early stages of the administration of mannitol, fluid is drawn into extracellular spaces and vascular compartments. Pulmonary and peripheral edema may occur, and increased intracranial pressure may also occur along with an early change in level of consciousness. Options 1, 2, and 3 are incorrect. Keeping a urinal or bedpan nearby; monitoring electrolytes, including potassium; and recording I&O and daily weight are important nursing interventions but are not the main nursing priority in the early administration of mannitol. Cognitive Level: Applying; Client Need: Physiological Integrity; Nursing Process: Implementation

6 Answer: 1 Rationale: Patients receiving acetazolamide are at risk for metabolic acidosis due to excess bicarbonate loss. Options 2, 3, and 4 are incorrect. Metabolic alkalosis is characterized by a deficit of bicarbonate and is not an adverse effect of acetazolamide (Diamox). Acetazolamide does not cause respiratory acidosis. Respiratory alkalosis is also not an expected adverse effect of acetazolamide. Cognitive Level: Analyzing; Client Need: Physiological Integrity; Nursing Process: Evaluation

Chapter 33

1 Answer: 1 Rationale: The serum pH is a measure of alkalinity or acidity in the blood. The administration of bicarbonate neutralizes acidic conditions and causes the patient's serum to become more alkaline. Options 2, 3, and 4 are incorrect. Changes in the pH can affect the ability of RBCs to release oxygen, but administration of sodium bicarbonate will not influence the number of circulating RBCs. The liver does not metabolize sodium bicarbonate; it is naturally occurring in the body and does not metabolize. Liver function tests are not indicators of the drug's effectiveness. Although sodium bicarbonate excretion occurs in the kidneys, the blood urea nitrogen level will not reflect the effectiveness of this drug. Cognitive Level: Applying; Client Need: Physiological Integrity; Nursing Process: Evaluation

2 Answer: 2 Rationale: Liquid preparations are very irritating to the gastric mucosa and should always be diluted with juice or water. Options 1, 3, and 4 are incorrect. Salt substitutes are high in potassium and should be avoided by patients on potassium supplementation. Symptoms such as weakness or fatigue may be the first indicators of potassium imbalances. The GI secretions are rich in potassium. Episodes of persistent vomiting may lead to hypokalemia and should be reported to the health care provider. Cognitive Level: Applying; Client Need: Physiological Integrity; Nursing Process: Evaluation

3 Answer: 4 Rationale: Dextran 40 interferes with coagulation and reduces blood viscosity. Bleeding, potentially severe, is associated with these effects. Options 1, 2, and 3 are incorrect. Dextran solutions are used to correct low circulating blood volume states. This solution does not cause dehydration. Dextran increases the circulating volume and thereby increases urine output, which is a therapeutic effect of the solution. Dextran is used for shock (hypovolemia); it does not cause shock. Cognitive Level: Analyzing; Client Need: Physiological Integrity; Nursing Process: Evaluation

4 Answer: 2 Rationale: This solution is often used to dilute (reconstitute) powdered forms of drugs that are intended to be given parenterally. Options 1, 3, and 4 are incorrect. This solution can cause hyperglycemia in the patient with diabetes due to the dextrose content. D_5W is considered a crystalloid solution. One liter of this solution supplies only 170 calories, which is not enough to supply the metabolic nutritional needs of adult patients. Cognitive Level: Applying; Client Need: Physiological Integrity; Nursing Process: Implementation

5 Answer: 4 Rationale: Magnesium sulfate toxicity may cause significant neuromuscular depression as noted by changes in level of consciousness and diminished deep tendon reflexes. Options 1, 2, and 3 are incorrect. Pupillary constriction to bright light is a normal physiological response. The nurse should notify the prescriber when the patient develops chest congestion and coughing, but they are not directly associated with magnesium sulfate toxicity. Elevated blood pressure is common in preeclampsia but it is not associated with magnesium toxicity. Cognitive Level: Applying; Client Need: Physiological Integrity; Nursing Process: Implementation

6 Answer: 1, 3, 4 Rationale: Normal serum albumin is a product derived from blood. Although rare, transfusion reactions can still occur with normal serum albumin. Albumin causes intercellular and interstitial fluid to move into the intravascular compartment. This movement of fluid will cause increases in the patient's blood pressure and heart rate. The nurse should monitor the patient for fluid overload with this solution. As the circulating fluid volume is corrected, the patient's urinary output will increase. Options 2 and 5 are incorrect. Patients receiving normal serum albumin typically do not have any dietary restrictions while receiving this solution. Serum albumin is not administered for potassium imbalances. Cognitive Level: Applying; Client Need: Physiological Integrity; Nursing Process: Planning

Chapter 34

1. Answer: 1 Rationale: Hot baths and showers, prolonged standing in one position, and strenuous exercise may enhance orthostatic hypotension. Options 2, 3, and 4 are incorrect. Methyldopa does not discolor the urine. Bloating and weight gain are not typical adverse effects of methyldopa, and methyldopa can be taken without food. Cognitive Level: Applying; Client Need: Physiological Integrity; Nursing Process: Implementation

2. Answer: 4 Rationale: Orthostatic hypotension is a common adverse effect of vasodilators such as hydralazine. Options 1, 2, and 3 are incorrect. Hydralazine does not typically cause atelectasis. Crystalluria is not an adverse effect of hydralazine and it does not cause photosensitivity. Cognitive Level: Applying; Client Need: Physiological Integrity; Nursing Process: Planning

3. Answer: 1 Rationale: Patients who have recently been prescribed hydralazine may experience dizziness initially and should be instructed not to engage in activities that may be hazardous. Options 2, 3, and 4 are incorrect. Patients should always consult their health care providers before discontinuing antihypertensive medications. Patients should report dizziness to the health care provider and should not adjust the dosage until the etiology of the problem is determined. Patients on this drug have no restriction on air travel. Cognitive Level: Analyzing; Client Need: Health Promotion and Maintenance; Nursing Process: Evaluation

4. Answer: 4 Rationale: The nurse will titrate (adjust) the rate of infusion based on the patient's blood pressure. Options 1, 2, and 3 are incorrect. Listening for bowel sounds in the patient with hypertensive crisis is not a nursing priority. Urine specific gravity and glucose levels may be obtained but are not associated with hypertensive crisis or the administration of this drug. Observing skin pressure points is a nursing intervention that does not directly relate to hypertensive crisis or nitroprusside therapy. Cognitive Level: Applying; Client Need: Physiological Integrity; Nursing Process: Implementation

5. Answer: 2, 3, 4 Rationale: New guidelines in the JNC-8 report recommend ACEIs or ARBs, CCBs, and thiazide diuretics as primary treatment options for most patients. Options 1 and 5 are incorrect. Beta blockers may still be used for some patients but are no longer recommended for primary treatment of HTN. Direct-acting vasodilators are used to treat hypertensive crisis and for patients who have not responded adequately to other antihypertensive drugs. Cognitive Level: Analyzing; Client Need: Physiological Integrity; Nursing Process: Planning

6. Answer: 1, 2, 4 Rationale: Thiocyanate poisoning may develop more quickly in patients with impaired renal function. Renal function and creatinine levels should be evaluated before starting the drug. Signs of thiocyanate poisoning include hypotension, lethargy, unconsciousness, and faint heart sounds. Options 3 and 5 are incorrect. Past alcohol use will not determine whether thiocyanate poisoning develops or influences its symptoms. While flushing of the skin may occur with nitroprusside administration, skin color and turgor are not reliable indicators of thiocyanate poisoning. Cognitive Level: Analyzing; Client Need: Physiological Integrity; Nursing Process: Evaluation

Chapter 35

1. Answer: 3 Rationale: Patients should be taught to remove the old ointment before applying the next dose. Options 1, 2, and 4 are incorrect. Nitroglycerin should be kept at room temperature, not in the refrigerator. Patients should take the medication before chest pain becomes severe. Nitroglycerin can be applied to any skin surface. However, absorption is decreased when applied to hairy areas, soles of feet, and palms. Cognitive Level: Applying; Client Need: Health Promotion and Maintenance; Nursing Process: Implementation

2. Answer: 4 Rationale: A decline in blood pressure is an expected adverse effect. The nurse should always assess the blood pressure prior to and 5 minutes after administering nitroglycerin. Options 1, 2, and 3 are incorrect. Photosensitivity, vomiting, and diarrhea are not expected adverse effects. Nitroglycerin will cause a decline in blood pressure, not an increase. Cognitive Level: Applying; Client Need: Physiological Integrity; Nursing Process: Planning

3. Answer: 4 Rationale: Skin irritation due to the nitroglycerin ointment can occur if the same site is used repeatedly. Options 1, 2, and 3 are incorrect. Patients should be instructed to rotate the site of application when using nitroglycerin ointment. Repeated use of the same application site may actually decrease absorption. Rebound phenomenon is not an expected occurrence with nitroglycerin. Cognitive Level: Applying; Client Need: Health Promotion and Maintenance; Nursing Process: Implementation

4. Answer: 3 Rationale: Patients may experience light-headedness or dizziness as a result of the hypotensive effects of isosorbide. Options 1, 2, and 4 are incorrect. Because the oral form of isosorbide has a slower onset than sublingual forms, a flushing sensation and headache are not usually experienced as they are with nitroglycerin sublingual. Tremors and anxiety are not associated adverse effects with this drug. Isosorbide does not usually cause sleepiness or lethargy, and if these occur they should be evaluated. Cognitive Level: Analyzing; Client Need: Physiological Integrity; Nursing Process: Evaluation

5. Answer: 1 Rationale: Atenolol increases blood flow to the myocardium, thereby increasing oxygen supply by reducing the heart rate and decreasing the contractility. Options 2, 3, and 4 are incorrect. Atenolol is a beta-adrenergic antagonist, which decreases heart rate. This drug does not affect the sodium channels. Although this drug reduces blood pressure, the mechanism of action is not by blocking the alpha$_2$ receptors. Cognitive Level: Applying; Client Need: Physiological Integrity; Nursing Process: Implementation

6. Answer: 1, 3 Rationale: Verapamil decreases blood pressure and heart rate. The administration of this drug may cause significant hypotension and bradycardia in some patients. Options 2, 4, and 5 are incorrect. Verapamil may be used to treat fast heart rates and HTN in addition to angina. Tinnitus and hearing loss are not adverse effects associated with verapamil. Cognitive Level: Analyzing; Client Need: Physiological Integrity; Nursing Process: Evaluation

Chapter 36

1. Answer: 2 Rationale: ACE inhibitors such as enalapril lower peripheral resistance through the inhibition of angiotensin II formation, and reduce blood volume through inhibition of aldosterone secretion. This reduces arterial blood pressure, decreasing afterload and increasing cardiac output. Options 1, 3, and 4 are incorrect. Enalapril is not a positive inotropic agent and does not strengthen the force of myocardial contraction. It does not slow heart rate (negative chronotropic and dromotropic effects) and it does not have diuretic effects. Cognitive Level: Analyzing; Client Need: Physiological Integrity; Nursing Process: Evaluation

2. Answer: 2 Rationale: The patient will be taught to take the pulse daily and to contact the prescriber if the pulse rate is less than 60 or greater than 100 beats per minute. Options 1, 3, and 4 are incorrect. The medication should be taken at the same time each day, but preferably after the patient has been active for a period of time (midmorning). Typically, the pulse rate will be lower in the morning before the patient rises. Digoxin should be withheld if the pulse rate is below 60 beats per minute. A high-fiber diet may decrease the absorption of digoxin, and the drug should not be taken along with meals high in fiber. Furthermore, foods high in calcium may create hypercalcemia, which will potentiate the possibility of digoxin toxicity. Cognitive Level: Applying; Client Need: Health Promotion and Maintenance; Nursing Process: Implementation

3. Answer: 1 Rationale: Milrinone is a positive inotropic drug and is given to increase the force of the contraction of the heart, which improves cardiac output. Options 2, 3, and 4 are incorrect. Inotropic effects increase the volume of the cardiac output rather than decrease it and do not relax the myocardial muscle. Milrinone may cause cardiac dysrhythmias as an adverse effect. Cognitive Level: Analyzing; Client Need: Physiological Integrity; Nursing Process: Evaluation

4 Answer: 4   Rationale: Hydralazine with isosorbide may cause hypotension with reflex tachycardia, resulting in dizziness and rapid heart rate. Options 1, 2, and 3 are incorrect. Hydralazine with isosorbide does not cause confusion, agitation, bleeding, or tingling of the extremities. If these occur, other causes should be investigated. Cognitive Level: Analyzing; Client Need: Physiological Integrity; Nursing Process: Evaluation

5 Answer: 1   Rationale: Beta-adrenergic blockers such as carvedilol must be started at 1/10 to 1/20 of a usual dose and gradually increased to a target dosage. Options 2, 3, and 4 are incorrect. Because lower dosages are required, a higher loading dose will not be given, and beta-adrenergic blockers are often combined with ACE inhibitors, although dosage will not be directly related to the ACE inhibitor. While caution is required if beta-adrenergic blockers are used to treat HF, they are an important drug group used to treat heart failure. Cognitive Level: Applying; Client Need: Physiological Integrity; Nursing Process: Implementation

6 Answer: 1, 2, 4   Rationale: Beta-adrenergic blockers require gradual increases in dosage amount approximately every 2 weeks to a target dosage. Significant improvement may not be noticed in early therapy and the patient may feel worse during initiation of therapy. Overall, however, the therapy has been proven to reduce the number of HF-related hospitalizations and mortalities. Options 3 and 5 are incorrect. Beta-adrenergic blocker therapy may require alterations in dosage for other cardiac drugs but not all drugs will be affected. Lifestyle changes may be advisable in HF but are not necessarily directly related to beta-adrenergic blocker use. Cognitive Level: Applying; Client Need: Health Promotion and Maintenance; Nursing Process: Planning

Chapter 37

1 Answer: 4   Rationale: Procainamide should be avoided in patients suffering from severe HF since this drug can worsen the condition. Options 1, 2, and 3 are incorrect. Ventricular tachycardia, paroxysmal atrial tachycardia, and atrial fibrillation are indications for the use of procainamide. Cognitive Level: Applying; Client Need: Physiological Integrity; Nursing Process: Implementation

2 Answer: 3   Rationale: Early signs of lidocaine toxicity include CNS effects such as paresthesias, drowsiness, confusion, anxiety, or tremors. Options 1, 2, and 4 are incorrect. Decreased platelet levels are not related to the administration of lidocaine. Unless the patient experiences hypotension, there is no need to routinely keep the patient supine. Although coughing and deep breathing are effective nursing strategies to maintain pulmonary function, they are not pertinent for the administration of IV lidocaine. Cognitive Level: Applying; Client Need: Physiological Integrity; Nursing Process: Implementation

3 Answer: 3   Rationale: The therapeutic goal of verapamil is to stabilize the dysrhythmia by slowing the conduction. While the atrial dysrhythmia may continue, the rate should return to a normal range (e.g., 60–100 in an adult). Options 1, 2, and 4 are incorrect. Verapamil may cause hypotension, but as an adverse rather than a therapeutic effect. It should not cause increases in potassium levels or reduction in urine output. Cognitive Level: Analyzing; Client Need: Physiological Integrity; Nursing Process: Evaluation

4 Answer: 4   Rationale: Adenosine has an extremely short half-life and must be administered by rapid IV push, over 1 to 2 seconds. Options 1, 2, and 3 are incorrect. Adenosine is not given by IV infusion or slowly. While potassium is an important electrolyte to monitor in patients with dysrhythmias, adenosine does not cause hypo- or hyperkalemia. Cognitive Level: Applying; Client Need: Physiological Integrity; Nursing Process: Implementation

5 Answer: 3   Rationale: Beta blockers such as propranolol are negative inotropic drugs and reduce myocardial contractility. In patients with existing HF, this may result in less cardiac output and worsening of symptoms. Options 1, 2, and 4 are incorrect. Propranolol does not cause sodium retention and its adverse effects include hypotension rather than HTN. It may cause bronchoconstriction because it is a nonselective beta-adrenergic antagonist (blocker), but this effect does not worsen HF. It warrants caution or is contraindicated in patients with COPD and other respiratory conditions. Cognitive Level: Analyzing; Client Need: Physiological Integrity; Nursing Process: Evaluation

6 Answer: 3   Rationale: An adverse effect associated with amiodarone is photosensitivity. The patient should be instructed to avoid direct sunlight, wear protective clothing, and use adequate sunscreen lotions of SPF 15 or higher. Options 1, 2, and 4 are incorrect. Amiodarone is not known to cause immunosuppression or to interact with oral contraceptives. Increased bleeding tendencies are not an adverse effect of amiodarone. Cognitive Level: Applying; Client Need: Health Promotion and Maintenance; Nursing Process: Implementation

Chapter 38

1 Answer: 1   Rationale: An activated partial thromboplastin time (aPTT) is the appropriate laboratory value that should be monitored with heparin infusions. When the patient is receiving this drug, the results should be 1.5 to 2 times that patient's baseline, or 60 to 80 seconds. Options 2, 3, and 4 are incorrect. A prothrombin time or INR is used to monitor the effectiveness of warfarin. Platelets are not affected by anticoagulants and are therefore not used in the monitoring of these drugs. Cognitive Level: Analyzing; Client Need: Physiological Integrity; Nursing Process: Evaluation

2 Answer: 1, 2, 3   Rationale: The patient should be taught proper injection technique, including the need to inject the heparin into the deep subcutaneous fat layer. A soft toothbrush should be used for oral hygiene. Puncture wounds or cuts will require longer than normal pressure held at the site to stop bleeding—15 minutes or longer. Options 4 and 5 are incorrect. Dental flossing should be avoided while the patient is receiving anticoagulants. The flossing can cause gum irritation and excessive bleeding. Aspirin has antiplatelet effects and concurrent use may increase the risk of bleeding or hemorrhage. Cognitive Level: Applying; Client Need: Health Promotion and Maintenance; Nursing Process: Planning

3 Answer: 3   Rationale: Many drugs such as aspirin and ibuprofen have strong anticoagulant effects. When the patient on warfarin takes these drugs, the increased risk of bleeding can be hazardous. Options 1, 2, and 4 are incorrect. Drugs such as aspirin and ibuprofen do not neutralize the effect of an anticoagulant. Anticoagulants do not influence the half-life of any drugs. The pain associated with arthritis is not worsened by the combination of these drugs. Cognitive Level: Applying; Client Need: Physiological Integrity; Nursing Process: Implementation

4 Answer: 2   Rationale: Because of the risk of hemorrhage, dysrhythmias, and hypotension, the patient should remain supine during and for up to 8 hours post–drug infusion. Options 1, 3, and 4 are incorrect. The patient will remain in the hospital for a minimum of 24 hours or longer postprocedure for monitoring per agency protocol. The risk of bleeding remains elevated for 2 to 4 days postinfusion. Oral anticoagulants such as warfarin or antiplatelet drugs will be ordered after the infusion; increasing vitamin K in the diet or by supplement may increase the risk of clotting. Cognitive Level: Applying; Client Need: Physiological Integrity; Nursing Process: Implementation

5 Answer: 1   Rationale: Clopidogrel is an antiplatelet drug used to prevent blood clots from forming inside arteries by inhibiting platelet aggregation. Options 2, 3, and 4 are incorrect. Heparin is an anticoagulant that blocks the formation of blood clots by activating antithrombin III. Warfarin is a vitamin K antagonist used to prevent the blood from clotting. The drug alteplase is a tissue plasminogen activator that dissolves fibrin clots. Cognitive Level: Applying; Client Need: Physiological Integrity; Nursing Process: Implementation

6 Answer: 1, 3, 4, 5   Rationale: Ginger, garlic, and green tea may all increase the risk of bleeding. Dabigatran may be used for DVT and is monitored by aPTT, similar to heparin. The drug is contraindicated in patients with gastritis because of the increased risk of bleeding. Option 2 is incorrect. Vitamin B_{12} does not enhance the response of dabigatran. Cognitive Level: Applying; Client Need: Physiological Integrity; Nursing Process: Planning

Chapter 39

1 Answer: 2   Rationale: The patient who receives epoetin alfa has anemia. This reduction in RBCs produces cellular oxygen deficiency, which causes severe fatigue and weakness. Patients receiving this drug should be taught to take scheduled rest periods to avoid overexertion. Options 1, 3, and 4 are incorrect. Avoiding fresh fruits and vegetables or uncooked meat would be instructions more appropriate for an individual with neutropenia. Limiting exposure to direct sunlight and using sunscreen would be appropriate instructions for a patient who is receiving a drug that causes photosensitivity, but epoetin alfa is not associated with this adverse effect. Patients with anemia are not necessarily thrombocytopenic and do not routinely need to avoid activities that may cause injury. Cognitive Level: Applying; Client Need: Health Promotion and Maintenance; Nursing Process: Planning

2 Answer: 2 Rationale: Darbepoetin should not be given to patients with uncontrolled HTN because hematopoietic growth factors can increase blood pressure. Options 1, 3, and 4 are incorrect. HIV patients may receive hematopoietic growth factors such as epoetin alfa to correct anemia caused by their HIV drug therapy. Patients with chronic renal failure often suffer from anemia because they are unable to secrete sufficient endogenous erythropoietin. Hematopoietic growth factors are often prescribed for these patients. Chemotherapy also causes anemia and patients may require hematopoietic growth factors if the anemia is severe. Cognitive Level: Applying; Client Need: Physiological Integrity; Nursing Process: Implementation

3 Answer: 3 Rationale: Neupogen increases WBC counts. The nurse would monitor for effectiveness by examining this laboratory value. Options 1, 2, and 4 are incorrect. Epoetin alfa is the drug that increases RBC count. Oprelvekin may be given to increase platelet levels. Reticulocytes are immature RBCs and mean cell volume is a measure of the volume of RBCs. Cognitive Level: Analyzing; Client Need: Physiological Integrity; Nursing Process: Evaluation

4 Answer: 4 Rationale: Oprelvekin does not affect iron levels and there would be no reason to instruct the patient to increase dietary intake of it. Options 1, 2, and 3 are incorrect. Oprelvekin is used to stimulate the production of platelets in patients who are at risk for severe thrombocytopenia. Oprelvekin may cause severe fluid retention that may lead to pulmonary edema, pericardial effusion, and ascites. Patients should monitor weight gain and report significant increases to the health care provider. Visual impairment, including blurred vision, papilledema, and optic neuropathy, may occur with oprelvekin, and vision changes should be reported. Cognitive Level: Analyzing; Client Need: Physiological Integrity; Nursing Process: Evaluation

5 Answer: 1 Rationale: Patients who regularly consume large amounts of alcohol often suffer from a nutritional deficit of vitamin B_{12}, which can manifest as abnormal neurologic symptoms. Options 2, 3, and 4 are incorrect. Alcohol interferes with folate metabolism in the liver, but lack of folate does not cause destruction of vitamin B_{12}. Pernicious anemia is caused by a lack of intrinsic factor, a substance needed to absorb vitamin B_{12} from the GI tract, which may lead to the anemia, not neutropenia. Vitamin B_{12} is a water-soluble vitamin and is not stored in the body. Cognitive Level: Applying; Client Need: Physiological Integrity; Nursing Process: Implementation

6 Answer: 1, 2, 3 Rationale: Ferrous preparations bind to many substances including food and other drugs. To ensure complete absorption of the drug, iron supplements should be taken 1 hour before or 2 hours after eating. Liquid iron preparations are often given to children. Such preparations should be given with a straw to prevent contact with the teeth, which can produce staining. After swallowing, the patient should be instructed to brush the teeth or thoroughly rinse the mouth to prevent staining. The patient should be informed that iron preparations can cause dark tarry-like or green-tinged stools and may cause constipation. When patients take iron preparations, increased fiber and water intake are measures to take to decrease constipation. Options 4 and 5 are incorrect. Vitamin C increases the absorption of iron preparations, not vitamin E. Caffeinated beverages inhibit the absorption of this drug. Cognitive Level: Applying; Client Need: Physiological Integrity; Nursing Process: Planning

Chapter 41

1 Answer: 2 Rationale: Acetaminophen overdose is treated with PO or IV acetylcysteine. For maximum effectiveness, the antidote should be administered within 8 hours of acetaminophen ingestion. Options 1, 3, and 4 are incorrect. The administration of 1,000 mL per hour of normal saline IV would place the patient at risk for fluid volume overload. The patient will not require cardioversion to treat acetaminophen poisoning. The patient's hepatic enzymes will be assessed; however, these enzymes only provide information as to the extent of liver damage. They do not treat acute acetaminophen overdose; they merely

monitor for the effectiveness of the treatment and any effects of the overdose itself. Cognitive Level: Applying; Client Need: Physiological Integrity; Nursing Process: Planning

2 Answer: 3 Rationale: Acetaminophen is the drug of choice for reduction of fever in the event the patient has a hypersensitivity to aspirin. Options 1, 2, and 4 are incorrect. A patient who has hypersensitivity to aspirin should not be administered ibuprofen or celecoxib due to the risk of hypersensitivity with the NSAIDs. Ketorolac is not administered for reduction of fever; it is administered for pain control. Cognitive Level: Applying; Client Need: Physiological Integrity; Nursing Process: Planning

3 Answer: 1 Rationale: Ketorolac is administered parenterally for pain. Options 2, 3, and 4 are incorrect. Ketoprofen, ibuprofen, and celecoxib are all administered PO. Cognitive Level: Applying; Client Need: Physiological Integrity; Nursing Process: Implementation

4 Answer: 4 Rationale: Ibuprofen should be discontinued 7 to 14 days before surgery to reduce the risk of bleeding. Options 1, 2, and 3 are incorrect. Ibuprofen should not be continued until surgery and the patient should continue her anti-inflammatory agent until 7 to 14 days before surgery to maintain its antiarthritis effects. Cognitive Level: Applying; Client Need: Physiological Integrity; Nursing Process: Implementation

5 Answer: 1 Rationale: Acetaminophen is metabolized in the liver. The patient with cirrhosis of the liver has impaired liver function and should not receive acetaminophen for pain or fever reduction. Options 2, 3, and 4 are incorrect. A patient who has COPD, breast cancer, or who is taking warfarin can be administered acetaminophen for fever and analgesia. Cognitive Level: Applying; Client Need: Physiological Integrity; Nursing Process: Implementation

6 Answer: 1, 2, 3, 4 Rationale: A patient who is experiencing toxic effects from aspirin may experience tinnitus, hyperventilation, GI bleeding, or decreased urine output related to renal impairment. Option 5 is incorrect. A patient with salicylate toxicity does not tend to experience peripheral neuropathy. Cognitive Level: Analyzing; Client Need: Physiological Integrity; Nursing Process: Evaluation

Chapter 42

1 Answer: 1 Rationale: Interferon alpha-2b causes flulike symptoms in up to 50% of patients receiving the drug. Options 2, 3, and 4 are incorrect. While depression with suicidal thoughts has been reported, it is not a common effect. Hypotension or hypertension, edema, fluid volume overload, tachycardia, and renal insufficiency are not adverse effects commonly associated with this drug. Cognitive Level: Analyzing; Client Need: Physiological Integrity; Nursing Process: Assessment

2 Answer: 2 Rationale: The patient's high fever (103°F; 39.4°C) and chills are indicative of an infectious process. The use of two immunosuppressant drugs (i.e., basiliximab and cyclosporine) increases the risk of infection related to the additional immunosuppressant effects. Options 1, 3, and 4 are incorrect. Basiliximab (Simulect) has fewer significant adverse effects than other monoclonal antibodies; however, GI effects (nausea, vomiting, abdominal pain) are common and anaphylaxis has been reported. Capillary leak syndrome is a condition in which fluid and protein leak out of tiny blood vessels and flow into surrounding tissue. This complication is not associated with basiliximab administration. Graft vs. host rejection is a type of transplant rejection, and androgen insensitivity is a genetically linked syndrome. Both are unrelated to the drug. Cognitive Level: Analyzing; Client Need: Physiological Integrity; Nursing Process: Assessment

3 Answer: 2 Rationale: Cyclosporine is toxic to bone marrow although less so than other immunosuppressants. A decrease in WBCs to below 4,000/mm³ should be reported to the provider. Options 1, 3, and 4 are incorrect. Cyclosporine does not cause an elevation in RBCs. The provider should be notified if platelet counts drop below 75,000/mm³, but a count of 100,000/mm³ is within acceptable limits. A creatinine level of less than 1 mg/100 mL is within normal limits. Cognitive Level: Applying; Client Need: Physiological Integrity; Nursing Process: Assessment

4 Answer: 3 Rationale: Azathioprine should be used with extreme caution in patients with a previous history of varicella zoster (chickenpox, shingles)

because the immunosuppression may cause the virus to reactivate and cause a serious infection. Options 1, 2, and 4 are incorrect. Benign prostatic hyperplasia and cataracts are not contraindications for the drug. Azathioprine may be used as a treatment for severe RA. Cognitive Level: Applying; Client Need: Physiological Integrity; Nursing Process: Assessment

5 Answer: 4   Rationale: Tacrolimus is a potent immunosuppressant and patients should decrease their risk for infection by taking precautions such as avoiding raw fruits and vegetables that may harbor pathogens on the skin or inside, and by eating only fully cooked meats after the heat of cooking has destroyed pathogens. Options 1, 2, and 3 are incorrect. Aspirin may increase GI irritation, placing the patient at risk for GI infections gaining entry through the inflamed mucosa. Physical activity is important to overall health, but this drug has no direct connection with weight gain. Tacrolimus is not known to have significant cardiac effects, although HTN is a possible adverse effect and the blood pressure should be monitored. Cognitive Level: Applying; Client Need: Health Promotion and Maintenance; Nursing Process: Planning

6 Answer: 3   Rationale: Aldesleukin causes capillary leak syndrome, which causes fluid to exit the capillary beds and vasculature, decreasing the circulating blood volume. As many as 70% of patients will develop hypotension. With the drop in blood pressure, organs may not perfuse adequately, and urine output will assess the adequacy of renal blood flow. Options 1, 2, and 4 are incorrect. Altered skin condition, rashes, increased pancreatic enzymes such as amylase and lipase, and alterations in vision and hearing are not symptoms of capillary leak syndrome. Cognitive Level: Analyzing; Client Need: Physiological Integrity; Nursing Process: Assessment

Chapter 43

1 Answer: 2   Rationale: A parent's preconceived ideas or reservations about accepting vaccinations will be most influential on whether the infant receives the scheduled injections. This also presents an excellent teaching opportunity for the nurse to answer questions, allay any fears the mother may have, and teach post-vaccine care. Options 1, 3, and 4 are incorrect. An allergy history will be taken, but unless the infant has demonstrated an allergy to the components in the vaccine, allergies to other medications will not necessarily increase the risk of reaction, nor will the parents' allergies increase the risk. Nurses working with pediatric patients should be knowledgeable about the recommended schedule and, when in doubt, verify the necessary immunizations needed. Cognitive Level: Analyzing; Client Need: Physiological Integrity; Nursing Process: Assessment

2 Answer: 3   Rationale: The MMR vaccination is an attenuated (live) virus and there is a slight risk that the virus could be transmitted to the child's father because he is immunocompromised from the chemotherapy. The nurse would check with the provider about delaying the vaccine until the father is finished with the chemotherapy. Options 1, 2, and 4 are incorrect. The nurse would teach the mother the signs of reaction and when to report them, and the family can safely go out of town if health care is available at their destination. Although additional teaching may be required to allay the mother's fears of reaction, the mother's reaction to MMR will not necessarily result in a reaction in the child. As long as the brother's immune system is healthy, he should not have any adverse effects from his sister's MMR because of his cold. Cognitive Level: Applying; Client Need: Physiological Integrity; Nursing Process: Implementation

3 Answer: 3, 4   Rationale: This child would need to receive rabies immunoglobulin to provide passive immunity to the potential exposure. A series of five rabies vaccines will be started over a 28-day period unless it is confirmed that the dog did not have rabies. If the dog is shown not to have rabies, the series can be stopped. Options 1, 2, and 5 are incorrect. Tetanus and DTaP would not be required as long as the child was current on her vaccination schedule. Rabies is a viral disease and the use of rabies toxoid would be ineffective. Cognitive Level: Applying; Client Need: Physiological Integrity; Nursing Process: Planning

4 Answer: 4   Rationale: Acetaminophen (Tylenol) or ibuprofen (Advil) is an appropriate analgesic to treat the soreness that occurs post–tetanus toxoid vaccination. Options 1, 2, and 3 are incorrect. There is no requirement to keep the arm still; in fact, motion may help disperse the medication and help it to absorb. There is no need to restrict fluids or to avoid crowds with a toxoid vaccination. Cognitive Level: Analyzing; Client Need: Health Promotion and Maintenance; Nursing Process: Evaluation

5 Answer: 3   Rationale: Known hypersensitivity to yeast is an absolute contraindication for hepatitis B vaccine. Options 1, 2, and 4 are incorrect. Smoking and HTN are not contraindications for the vaccine and present an opportunity for health teaching. Hepatitis B is only available by injection and the nurse would explore methods to help the patient be less fearful of the injection prior to administration. Cognitive Level: Analyzing; Client Need: Physiological Integrity; Nursing Process: Assessment

6 Answer: 1   Rationale: Hypersensitivity reactions are likely to occur within the first 20 minutes of administration. The nurse should closely monitor the patient's vital signs during the initial period. Options 2, 3, and 4 are incorrect. RhoGAM does not cause thrombocytopenia or anemia or increase liver enzymes. There is no need for a low-saturated-fat, low-cholesterol diet after receiving Rh_o immune globulin, and RhoGAM does not cause a cough. Cognitive Level: Applying; Client Need: Physiological Integrity; Nursing Process: Implementation

Chapter 44

1 Answer: 1   Rationale: A quick-acting inhaled beta agonist such as albuterol is used to abort bronchospasm. Options 2, 3, and 4 are incorrect. Beclomethasone, ipratropium, and zafirlukast are drugs used to prevent and control bronchospastic attacks and will not cause bronchodilation quickly enough to abort an attack. Cognitive Level: Applying; Client Need: Physiological Integrity; Nursing Process: Implementation

2 Answer: 3   Rationale: Corticosteroids can decrease the beneficial oral flora that will allow for an overgrowth of fungal infections such as *Candida*. Rinsing the mouth removes any corticosteroid drug deposited there and prevents it from being swallowed, decreasing the likelihood of systemic absorption. Options 1, 2, and 4 are incorrect. Inhaled corticosteroids such as beclomethasone do not cause tachycardia, nervousness, or tremors, and caffeine does not need to be avoided while the drug is used. Cognitive Level: Applying; Client Need: Health Promotion and Maintenance; Nursing Process: Implementation

3 Answer: 1   Rationale: Bronchodilators such as albuterol may have an adverse effect on heart rate elevation and palpitations related to dosage. Options 2, 3, and 4 are incorrect. Bronchodilators do not decrease the immune response or increase alertness. While some bronchodilators have been known to cause unexpected problems and paradoxical bronchospasm, this is uncommon. Cognitive Level: Applying; Client Need: Physiological Integrity; Nursing Process: Implementation

4 Answer: 1, 2   Rationale: Because corticosteroids such as beclomethasone decrease the immune response, the risk for infections is increased. Corticosteroids also increase blood glucose, thus increasing the possibility of hyperglycemia. Options 3, 4, and 5 are incorrect. Corticosteroids do not cause urinary retention, do not increase the likelihood of tachycardia, and do not cause photophobia. Cognitive Level: Applying; Client Need: Physiological Integrity; Nursing Process: Assessment

5 Answer: 1   Rationale: Beta agonists are agents that may be given to children younger than age 5 to manage asthma. They are available in formulations suitable for nebulizer treatments. Options 2, 3, and 4 are incorrect. Beta antagonists, corticosteroids, and leukotriene modifiers will not cause the rapid bronchodilation required in an acute asthma attack. Cognitive Level: Applying; Client Need: Physiological Integrity; Nursing Process: Planning

6 Answer: 3   Rationale: Some patients have difficulty mastering the coordination between inhalation and activation of the medication. In these instances, a spacer will hold the medication cloud so that this is not a concern. The spacer has additional advantages because it results in more effective delivery of the drug to the site of action and less drug deposition in the mouth and oropharynx. Options 1, 2, and 4 are incorrect. Additional practice may help in the long term, but it is not the priority for an immediate solution to the problem and may only serve to frustrate the patient further. The health care provider would not need to be contacted because the patient has difficulty learning, provided that a solution is readily available. Substitution of an oral form of the drug is not within the nursing scope of practice. Cognitive Level: Analyzing; Client Need: Health Promotion and Maintenance; Nursing Process: Planning

Chapter 45

1 Answer: 2, 5 Rationale: Priming any inhaler prior to first use ensures that the correct dosage is delivered. Corticosteroids take about 3 weeks to become fully effective. Options 1, 3, and 4 are incorrect. The medication is inhaled so water is not important, although any liquid that drips into the oral pharynx should be spit out. Corticosteroids are used primarily for prophylaxis of allergic rhinitis. Unlike inhaled sympathomimetics, corticosteroids do not cause rebound congestion. Cognitive Level: Applying; Client Need: Physiological Integrity; Nursing Process: Planning

2 Answer: 4 Rationale: Pseudoephedrine is a sympathomimetic and is used only for nasal decongestion. Options 1, 2, and 3 are incorrect. Dextromethorphan and diphenhydramine are both effective for some coughs associated with allergic rhinitis and the common cold. Mucolytics are found in some OTC cough preparations used in colds but are best used to treat chronic productive coughs. Cognitive Level: Applying; Client Need: Health Promotion and Maintenance; Nursing Process: Implementation

3 Answer: Because diphenhydramine may cause dizziness and drowsiness, an increased risk of **falls** is possible, particularly in the older adult. Cognitive Level: Applying; Client Need: Safe and Effective Care Environment; Nursing Process: Implementation

4 Answer: 4 Rationale: Second-generation (nonsedating) antihistamines such as fexofenadine have been associated with dysrhythmias in the sensitive individual. Options 1, 2, and 3 are incorrect. A history of osteoporosis, peptic ulcer disease, or psoriasis is not a contraindication for the drug. Cognitive Level: Analyzing; Client Need: Physiological Integrity; Nursing Process: Assessment

5 Answer: 3, 2, 1, 4 Rationale: When an intranasal inhaler is used, the device should be primed prior to the first use; the nasal passages should be cleared by blowing; the drug should be instilled by spray directed high into the nasal passages; and any liquid that drains into the mouth should be spit out. Level: Applying; Client Need: Health Promotion and Maintenance; Nursing Process: Implementation

6 Answer: 4 Rationale: The syrup base of an antitussive cough syrup such as dextromethorphan will help to soothe throat irritation, and the patient should avoid drinking fluids immediately following drug administration. Increasing overall fluid intake throughout the day will help moisten irritated mucous membranes as well as loosen secretions for better effects from the expectorant, guaifenesin. Options 1, 2, and 3 are incorrect. The patient does not have to remain supine after administration, and taking the drug with food will not enhance the effects. Avoiding fluid intake will not prevent cough and may cause additional respiratory tract dryness. Cognitive Level: Applying; Client Need: Physiological Integrity; Nursing Process: Implementation

Chapter 47

1 Answer: 3 Rationale: Ampicillin may decrease the effectiveness of oral contraceptives, and the patient should be instructed to use a barrier method to avoid unwanted pregnancies while on the antibiotic and until the next cycle of oral contraceptives is started. Options 1, 2, and 4 are incorrect. The combination of ampicillin and oral contraceptives will not increase the risk of adverse effects related to the antibiotic. Oral contraceptive effectiveness may be reduced during ampicillin therapy, and ampicillin will not create serious toxicity related to the use of oral contraceptives. Cognitive Level: Applying; Client Need: Health Promotion and Maintenance; Nursing Process: Implementation

2 Answer: 3 Rationale: Ototoxicity is associated with serum concentrations of vancomycin above 60 to 80 mcg/mL and manifests with tinnitus, dizziness, or balance and coordination effects. Options 1, 2, and 4 are incorrect. Redness of the ears, itching of the ears, and ocular pain are not symptoms related to ototoxicity caused by vancomycin. Cognitive Level: Analyzing; Client Need: Physiological Integrity; Nursing Process: Evaluation

3 Answer: 2 Rationale: A vaginal yeast infection with discharge may be a symptom of a superinfection. Superinfection is a possible adverse effect associated with all antibiotics and particularly with fungal and viral infections. Options 1, 3, and 4 are incorrect. A hypersensitivity reaction is not usually manifested by vaginal discharge. The symptoms associated with PMC are

significant GI effects. Vaginal discharge is not a symptom of antibiotic toxicity. Cognitive Level: Applying; Client Need: Physiological Integrity; Nursing Process: Evaluation

4 Answer: 4 Rationale: Watery diarrhea containing mucus, blood, or pus is symptomatic of CDAD and must be monitored closely for progressing to PMC; both are adverse effects related to antibiotic use. Options 1, 2, and 3 are incorrect. These symptoms are not related to peptic ulcers, malabsorption, or hypersensitivity reactions. Cognitive Level: Analyzing; Client Need: Physiological Integrity; Nursing Process: Evaluation

5 Answer: 1 Rationale: Shortness of breath, mouth and tongue swelling, and generalized itching are signs of hypersensitivity reaction. Options 2, 3, and 4 are incorrect. Blood dyscrasias include such problems as thrombocytopenia and neutropenia, and the drug does not cause these symptoms. Beta lactamase is a substance secreted by some bacteria that renders the antibiotic ineffective. Drug toxicity may result from an excessive level of the medication or adverse effects on body organ systems related to age or other changes. Hypersensitivity is associated with antigen and antibody reactions. Cognitive Level: Analyzing; Client Need: Physiological Integrity; Nursing Process: Assessment

6 Answer: 1 Rationale: Ampicillin should be taken on an empty stomach to ensure adequate absorption. Options 2, 3, and 4 are incorrect. A black and furry tongue is the symptom of an oral superinfection and should be reported. The patient should be taught to take the full prescription even if the symptoms subside. Patients should never take two doses because this will place them at risk for toxicity. Cognitive Level: Analyzing; Client Need: Health Promotion and Maintenance; Nursing Process: Evaluation

Chapter 48

1 Answer: 4 Rationale: This drug potentially causes photosensitivity. Options 1, 2, and 3 are incorrect. Calcium products should not be taken at the same time as tetracycline but taken 1 hour before or 2 hours after the dose. Brushing will not remove teeth staining caused by the drug. The staining of the teeth due to medication can only be removed by a dental specialist. Ototoxicity is not associated with tetracycline use, and any tinnitus or dizziness may be related to other causes. Cognitive Level: Applying; Client Need: Health Promotion and Maintenance; Nursing Process: Implementation

2 Answer: 1 Rationale: Longer duration of action is one of the benefits of azithromycin therapy. Options 2, 3, and 4 are incorrect. There is no evidence that azithromycin causes any more nausea than other antibiotics. Azithromycin is not affected by the gastric content and can be taken any time. Azithromycin is not affected by calcium-based foods. Cognitive Level: Analyzing; Client Need: Physiological Integrity; Nursing Process: Evaluation

3 Answer: 1 Rationale: Weight gain may be an early sign associated with renal damage secondary to amikacin toxicity. Options 2, 3, and 4 are incorrect. Adverse effects of amikacin are not manifested by visual disturbances, mental depression, or urinary frequency. Cognitive Level: Applying; Client Need: Physiological Integrity; Nursing Process: Planning

4 Answer: 1 Rationale: Drug-induced renal toxicity would cause an elevated serum creatinine level and should be reported to the health care provider. Options 2, 3, and 4 are incorrect. BUN level is more commonly associated with hepatic toxicity but would be elevated and not decreased if renal toxicity is present. Nephrotoxicity is not typically indicated via the WBC levels or changes in serum iron levels. Cognitive Level: Analyzing; Client Need: Physiological Integrity; Nursing Process: Assessment

5 Answer: Rationale: Tetracycline antibiotics should not be taken concurrently with **dairy products**, **iron-containing preparations** such as multivitamins, or with **antacids**. If these products are to be consumed, they should be taken 1 hour before or 2 hours after the tetracycline. Cognitive Level: Applying; Client Need: Health Promotion and Maintenance; Nursing Process: Implementation

6 Answer: 1, 2, 4, 5 Rationale: Aminoglycosides are renal, oto-, and neurotoxic. They may also cause neuromuscular blockade. Increases in serum creatinine may indicate renal toxicity. Urine output should also be monitored. Dizziness, vertigo, or tinnitus may be signs of ototoxicity. Muscle weakness may indicate neuromuscular blockade and may last for several days. Option 3 is incorrect. Gentamicin is not metabolized, and changes in liver function tests would not be drug related. Cognitive Level: Analyzing; Client Need: Physiological Integrity; Nursing Process: Assessment

Chapter 49

1 Answer: 2 Rationale: Because pathogens grow rapidly and are constantly proliferating, all antibiotic therapies should be taken around the clock. Taking the drug as evenly spaced apart during the day as possible will help ensure a steady serum drug level to fight the bacteria. Options 1, 3, and 4 are incorrect. Ciprofloxacin is not known to cause problems with patients' sleep patterns. Superinfections occur when an antibiotic eradicates normal flora and an opportunistic organism invades. This is a problem associated with antibiotic therapy in general and is not caused by not adhering to the prescribed schedule. Allergic reactions are very common with antibiotic therapy, but they do not result from failing to adhere to the medication schedule. Cognitive Level: Applying; Client Need: Physiological Integrity; Nursing Process: Implementation

2 Answer: 3, 4, 5 Rationale: Itching, even without the presence of a rash, may indicate histamine release from a drug allergy. Swelling of the face, lips, or tongue, known as angioedema, is also a symptom of allergy. Nervousness or anxiety may indicate an adrenergic response secondary to an allergic reaction, and, while they may have other causes, should be investigated further to rule out a developing allergic reaction. Options 1 and 2 are incorrect. Common adverse effects of ofloxacin are headache, nausea, and vomiting. Cognitive Level: Analyzing; Client Need: Physiological Integrity; Nursing Process: Assessment

3 Answer: 1, 2 Rationale: Ciprofloxacin is excreted renally and increasing fluid intake will help to prevent drug accumulation in the kidneys. Dairy products and antacids taken concurrently may inhibit absorption of the ciprofloxacin. Options 3, 4, and 5 are incorrect. Vitamin C does not need to be avoided while on ciprofloxacin; however, products containing iron or zinc should be avoided. An antihistamine does not need to be taken concurrently and may mask the symptoms of adverse effects such as allergy. Excessive caffeine intake may increase the chance of nervousness or anxiety and should be avoided. Cognitive Level: Applying; Client Need: Physiological Integrity; Nursing Process: Implementation

4 Answer: 1 Rationale: Fluoroquinolones such as levofloxacin have been associated with tendonitis and tendon rupture, especially in patients over age 65. Any unusual joint or tendon pain or difficulty moving or walking should be reported to the provider. Options 2, 3, and 4 are incorrect. Many multivitamins may contain iron and zinc, and concurrent administration with levofloxacin will impair the antibiotic's absorption. Fluoroquinolones do not impair vitamin D absorption and may cause dermatologic toxicities such as photosensitivity and photoallergy. Sunscreens and protective clothing should be used if sun exposure is anticipated. Fluoroquinolones may be renal toxic and *increased* fluid intake is advised. Cognitive Level: Applying; Client Need: Physiological Integrity; Nursing Process: Implementation

5 Answer: 4 Rationale: Fluoroquinolones such as ciprofloxacin may cause profound muscle weakness in patients with myasthenia gravis. Options 1, 2, and 3 are incorrect. Anxiety and nervousness do not require cautious use and are not contraindications to ciprofloxacin. While the incidence of tendonitis and tendon rupture is higher in the adult over age 65, the drug is not contraindicated in this population. However, more frequent monitoring may be needed. Cross-allergy to penicillins is not known for the fluoroquinolones and a history of penicillin is not a contraindication to ciprofloxacin. Cognitive Level: Analyzing; Client Need: Physiological Integrity; Nursing Process: Assessment

6 Answer: 1 Rationale: Polymyxin B is a topical antibiotic used to promote wound healing. Options 2, 3, and 4 are incorrect. Skin and mucous membranes cannot be made sterile. Polymyxin B will cause cell death of the invading pathogenic bacteria but will not completely sterilize the skin. Polymyxin B does not prevent allergic reaction, nor does it provide pain relief to wounds. Cognitive Level: Applying; Client Need: Physiological Integrity; Nursing Process: Planning

Chapter 50

1 Answer: 3 Rationale: Crystalluria is the excretion of crystals in the urine. To prevent this adverse effect, patients are instructed to consume approximately 2 to 3 L of fluid per day. This action will flush the crystal from the renal system. Options 1, 2, and 4 are incorrect. Limiting foods high in calcium will not prevent crystalluria. Positional changes are not related to the adverse effects of crystalluria. Alcohol should be avoided when taking most medications. However, the effects attributed to alcohol consumption do not include crystalluria. Cognitive Level: Applying; Client Need: Physiological Integrity; Nursing Process: Implementation

2 Answer: 1 Rationale: Nitrofurantoin is prescribed most commonly for the prophylaxis of recurrent UTIs. Options 2, 3, and 4 are incorrect. Furadantin has no analgesic effect. The excretion of urine is not affected by this drug, and the drug is not used for pyelonephritis. Cognitive Level: Applying; Client Need: Physiological Integrity; Nursing Process: Planning

3 Answer: 2, 4, 5 Rationale: Trimethoprim-sulfamethoxazole (TMP-SMZ) is a sulfonamide and would be contraindicated in a patient with a previous history of allergy. The drug is pregnancy category C (D in the third trimester), and the use of the drug may result in kernicterus in the newborn. For people with diabetes who are taking oral sulfonylureas, an increased risk of hypoglycemia is possible when TMP-SMZ is used; hence, blood sugars must be monitored closely. Options 1 and 3 are incorrect. The occurrence of migraine headaches is not affected by TMP-SMZ. While it is an important teaching point, urinating before or after sexual intercourse will not affect the use of TMP-SMZ. Cognitive Level: Applying; Client Need: Physiological Integrity; Nursing Process: Assessment

4 Answer: 3 Rationale: Nausea and vomiting are the most common adverse effects of oral sulfonamide therapy but should not occur with topical use. If they occur, the patient should be evaluated for possible systemic effects and for the proper self-administration of the topical drug. This statement indicates that the patient has understood the teaching and when to report potential adverse effects. Options 1, 2, and 4 are incorrect. The drug should be applied topically only to affected areas. Stinging and burning are common effects of the topical application of this drug. Excess potassium consumption should be avoided with the oral forms of sulfonamides but is not necessary with the topical drug. Cognitive Level: Analyzing; Client Need: Physiological Integrity; Nursing Process: Evaluation

5 Answer: 1 Rationale: Nitrofurantoin is associated with pulmonary toxicities such as interstitial pneumonitis and pulmonary fibrosis. The drug should be used with extreme caution or not at all in the patient with preexisting pulmonary disease. Options 2, 3, and 4 are incorrect. Diabetes, rheumatoid arthritis, or angina and hypertension are not contraindications for the drug. Cognitive Level: Applying; Client Need: Physiological Integrity; Nursing Process: Assessment

6 Answer: 3 Rationale: TMP-SMZ causes dermatologic toxicities including Stevens–Johnson syndrome. Unusual, blistering-type rashes with purplish-red discoloration should be immediately reported to the provider. Options 1, 2, and 4 are incorrect. Fungal superinfections may be wet or dry and are reddened, possibly denuded areas. Viral eruptions are most often vesicular rashes. Nonadherence with drug therapy would not result in a rash. Cognitive Level: Applying; Client Need: Physiological Integrity; Nursing Process: Implementation

Chapter 51

1 Answer: 2 Rationale: For some antituberculosis drugs such as isoniazid (INH), peripheral neuropathy is problematic. This is due to a decrease in the activity of pyridoxine on the nervous tissue. Often supplemental vitamin B_6 is prescribed to prevent this adverse effect. Options 1, 3, and 4 are incorrect. Isoniazid does not cause an increase in the nerve ending sensitivity or accelerate the excretion of neurotransmitters. Isoniazid does not affect ascorbic acid. Cognitive Level: Analyzing; Client Need: Physiological Integrity; Nursing Process: Evaluation

2 Answer: 2, 3, 4, 5 Rationale: Once the diagnosis of pulmonary tuberculosis is verified, sputum specimens are routinely collected to determine the effectiveness of the drug therapy. Ethambutol (Myambutol) may cause hepatotoxicity and decreases renal excretion of uric acid. Hepatic function tests and uric acid levels will be monitored before beginning the drug and routinely thereafter. It may also cause optic neuritis and vision acuity, and color vision sense will be tested before starting the drug and periodically while the drug is used. Option 1 is incorrect. Coagulation studies are not affected by ethambutol. Cognitive Level: Applying; Client Need: Physiological Integrity; Nursing Process: Assessment

3 Answer: To ensure that the patient is not experiencing adverse effects related to the acetylation process, both **hepatic function** and **serum drug level** will be monitored frequently. Cognitive Level: Applying; Client Need: Physiological Integrity; Nursing Process: Planning

4 Answer: 4 Rationale: Treatment of MAC infections in patients who are HIV positive is prolonged and relapse rates are as high as 20%. Options 1, 2, and 3 are incorrect. MAC is not considered a contagious infection. Treatment is prolonged and is indicated when CD4 counts drop below 50 cells/mL. Cognitive Level: Applying; Client Need: Physiological Integrity; Nursing Process: Implementation

5 Answer: 1 Rationale: The nurse should observe for any reddish-brown discoloration of skin, cornea, conjunctiva, and body fluids. This adverse effect occurs in 75% to 90% of patients within a few weeks of treatment. Even after discontinuation of therapy, skin discoloration may take months or years to fade. Options 2, 3, and 4 are incorrect. The drug does not cause constipation, chills, dehydration, hypoglycemia, impaired memory, impotence, memory loss, nervousness, or pruritus. Cognitive Level: Analyzing; Client Need: Physiological Integrity; Nursing Process: Evaluation

6 Answer: 3 Rationale: Isoniazid may increase glucose levels and more frequent monitoring is required. Options 1, 2, and 4 are incorrect. Isoniazid does not cause a decrease or rapid rises and falls of glucose level. Cognitive Level: Applying; Client Need: Physiological Integrity; Nursing Process: Evaluation

Chapter 52

1 Answer: 2, 3, 4 Rationale: When administered too rapidly, amphotericin B may cause hypotension, hypokalemia, and shock. Options 1 and 5 are incorrect. Amphotericin is not known to cause laryngeal spasms or hypoglycemia. Cognitive Level: Analyzing; Client Need: Physiological Integrity; Nursing Process: Evaluation

2 Answer: 1 Rationale: Patients who take fluconazole (Diflucan) may experience nausea, vomiting, and diarrhea. Nutritional intake is especially important to maintain optimum health in a patient with AIDS. Keeping a food diary will assist the provider in determining overall calorie and fluid intake. Antinausea medication may be helpful if nausea or vomiting is severe. Options 2, 3, and 4 are incorrect. Loss of muscle mass is not related to fluconazole therapy. The decision to wear a high-filtration mask is not related to fluconazole, and patients on this drug do not need to avoid fat-based soaps. Allowing adequate air circulation to body areas will help prevent surface fungal infections but is not required as part of fluconazole therapy. Cognitive Level: Applying; Client Need: Physiological Integrity; Nursing Process: Implementation

3 Answer: 1, 2 Rationale: Unless otherwise directed by the provider, small amounts of water after a feeding will rinse the mouth of milk proteins and sugars that can provide an ideal medium for *Candida* to grow. The suspension should be applied to all surfaces of the mouth and tongue, by syringe or applicator, and the infant should swallow the remainder to treat possible GI *Candida*. Options 3, 4, and 5 are incorrect. Nystatin (Mycostatin) suspension does not require chilling before administration. The suspension should not be added to formula or given before feedings and should be administered after feedings so that it can be retained in the mouth to treat the area of infection. Cognitive Level: Applying; Client Need: Physiological Integrity; Nursing Process: Implementation

4 Answer: 4 Rationale: Nails grow very slowly and lengthy treatment may be required to adequately treat the infection. Options 1, 2, and 3 are incorrect. The infection will be evaluated during the treatment period but it will take many months to adequately treat the infection. Purchasing more pills at one time does not necessarily reduce the cost of the prescription. Toxic doses are never administered, even to shorten treatment cycles. Cognitive Level: Applying; Client Need: Health Promotion and Maintenance; Nursing Process: Implementation

5 Answer: 3 Rationale: Amphotericin B can cause a number of serious adverse effects including fever, chills, and headache. Pretreatment with corticosteroids, antihistamines, and antipyretics may reduce the severity of these distressing adverse effects. Options 1, 2, and 4 are incorrect. Pretreatment does not enhance the effectiveness of this antifungal agent. The by-products of amphotericin are not affected by the pretreatment of the patient, and pretreatment does not affect the half-life of the drug. Cognitive Level: Applying; Client Need: Physiological Integrity; Nursing Process: Planning

6 Answer: 3 Rationale: Dependent on which oral antidiabetes medication is used (e.g., glyburide), fluconazole (Diflucan) may decrease blood sugar levels, and an adjustment in antidiabetes treatments may be required. Options 1, 2, and 4 are incorrect. Fluconazole (Diflucan) has an effect when given concurrently with some antidiabetes drugs (e.g., glyburide) and may cause hypoglycemia. It does not antagonize the effect of antidiabetes medications and does not cause an increase in blood sugar level. Cognitive Level: Applying; Client Need: Physiological Integrity; Nursing Process: Implementation

Chapter 53

1 Answer: 1 Rationale: Chloroquine therapy begins 1 to 2 weeks before travel and continues once a week during travel and for 4 weeks after returning. Options 2, 3, and 4 are incorrect. Once the prophylaxis is initiated, it should be continued for 4 weeks following departure from the site of malaria. Three days is not a sufficient amount of time to ensure that the patient has adequate protection against malaria infection. If the patient develops symptoms of malaria, prophylaxis is no longer indicated, but the drug may be continued as part of the treatment regimen. Cognitive Level: Applying; Client Need: Health Promotion and Maintenance; Nursing Process: Evaluation

2 Answer: 1, 4 Rationale: Hydroxychloroquine has anti-inflammatory effects and is used in the treatment of systemic lupus erythematosus, rheumatoid arthritis, and other inflammatory diseases. Options 2, 3, and 5 are incorrect. Hydroxychloroquine is not used to treat roundworm, leishmaniasis, or urinary tract infections. Cognitive Level: Applying; Client Need: Physiological Integrity; Nursing Process: Assessment

3 Answer: 3 Rationale: Many patients complain of an unpleasant metallic taste that can be caused by metronidazole. Options 1, 2, and 4 are incorrect. Flatus and intestinal bloating are not characteristic adverse effects of metronidazole. Metronidazole does not cause bad breath (halitosis) and if it occurs, other causes should be considered. Alopecia (hair loss) is not associated with metronidazole. Cognitive Level: Applying; Client Need: Health Promotion and Maintenance; Nursing Process: Implementation

4 Answer: 2 Rationale: The use of pyrimethamine is associated with megaloblastic anemia, leukopenia, thrombocytopenia, and pancytopenia as possible adverse effects. Unusual bleeding or fatigue, sores that do not heal, or low-grade fevers may indicate that blood cell counts are low and should be assessed by the health care provider. Options 1, 3, and 4 are incorrect. Pyrimethamine is associated with nausea, vomiting, and abdominal cramping as adverse effects, and increasing fiber-rich foods will not affect these. Increasing fluid intake is important with most anti-infective drugs but 3 L per day is not required for this drug. Adverse eye effects are not associated with pyrimethamine and sulfadiazine. Cognitive Level: Applying; Client Need: Physiological Integrity; Nursing Process: Implementation

5 Answer: 4 Rationale: To reduce the risk of reinfection, bed linens and undergarments should be washed thoroughly after treatment is given. Options 1, 2, and 3 are incorrect. Mebendazole is usually given as a single dose but may be repeated for up to 3 days. Family members are also at risk and should be evaluated or treated empirically. While consuming citrus products may increase the risk of GI adverse effects, citrus and dairy do not need to be eliminated from the diet. Cognitive Level: Applying; Client Need: Health Promotion and Maintenance; Nursing Process: Implementation

6 Answer: 1 Rationale: An acute onset of any CNS abnormality may indicate metronidazole toxicity. If ataxia and confusion suddenly develop after the initiation of metronidazole, the nurse should discontinue the medication and contact the health care provider. Options 2, 3, and 4 are incorrect. Adverse effects to metronidazole are rare; however, nausea and diarrhea can occur. Anorexia and dryness of the mouth are common adverse effects with metronidazole. However, these adverse effects will usually disappear as the therapy continues. Weight gain and irritability are not typical adverse effects associated with metronidazole. Cognitive Level: Analyzing; Client Need: Physiological Integrity; Nursing Process: Evaluation

Chapter 54

1 Answer: 1   Rationale: Acyclovir is associated with renal toxicity, especially when given IV. The drug should be administered IV over a minimum of 1 hour and increased fluid intake encouraged throughout the day to prevent adverse renal effects. Options 2, 3, and 4 are incorrect. Acyclovir is not associated with an increased risk of fungal infections or eye discomfort. Itching and skin irritation may occur with topical use but if it occurs with IV drug administration, drug allergy should be questioned and the administration stopped until evaluated. Cognitive Level: Applying; Client Need: Physiological Integrity; Nursing Process: Implementation

2 Answer: 1   Rationale: Individuals with herpes must understand that transferring the virus remains a possibility even if drug therapies are used. Options 2, 3, and 4 are incorrect. Patients with herpes lesions should gently cleanse affected areas with soap and water three to four times daily and dry well prior to application of the topical medication. With application of medication to the genitals, the patient should wear loose-fitting clothes over affected areas for comfort. For best results, the patient should be instructed to start the antiviral therapy as soon as possible after the onset of signs and symptoms. Cognitive Level: Applying; Client Need: Health Promotion and Maintenance; Nursing Process: Evaluation

3 Answer: 2, 3, 5   Rationale: Amantadine is associated with renal toxicity, possible severe CNS effects including seizures, psychosis and suicidal ideation, and peripheral edema and heart failure. Options 1 and 4 are incorrect. Amantadine is not known to interfere or affect the white blood cell or platelet count. Potassium and sodium levels are not affected by amantadine. Cognitive Level: Applying; Client Need: Physiological Integrity; Nursing Process: Assessment

4 Answer: 4   Rationale: Zanamivir must be started within 48 hours after the onset of symptoms to be effective. Options 1, 2, and 3 are incorrect. Waiting to take the drug longer than 48 hours will not shorten the infection period. It should not be saved because any future infection should be evaluated at that time to ascertain it is the flu and that it will respond to the zanamivir. Cognitive Level: Applying; Client Need: Health Promotion and Maintenance; Nursing Process: Implementation

5 Answer: 2   Rationale: Tenofovir is known to cause lactic acidosis. Symptoms such as anxiety, fatigue, nausea, vomiting, palpitations, lethargy, rapid breathing and heart rate, weakness, chest pain or tightening, hypotension, or shortness of breath should be immediately reported to the provider. Options 1, 3, and 4 are incorrect. Tenofovir is not associated with systemic yeast infections, heart failure, or ventricular dysrhythmias. Cognitive Level: Applying; Client Need: Physiological Integrity; Nursing Process: Implementation

6 Answer: 4   Rationale: Ribavirin is associated with an increased risk of hemolytic anemia. Increased fatigue, dizziness, headache, abdominal pain, pallor, and chest pain are associated with this anemia. Options 1, 2, and 3 are incorrect. Respiratory, dermatologic, or neurologic adverse effects may occur but are not as severe as the hemolytic anemia associated with this drug. Cognitive Level: Analyzing; Client Need: Physiological Integrity; Nursing Process: Evaluation

Chapter 55

1 Answer: 2   Rationale: This is a false statement. No vaccine currently exists to provide immunity to this disease, although testing is ongoing. Options 1, 3, and 4 are incorrect. The patient should be informed that therapy for HIV will require lifelong treatment since there is not a cure. Since treatment is often complex and lifelong, whenever possible, the patient should be taught how to adjust the daily schedule so as to not interfere with ADLs. With recent advances in pharmacotherapy for HIV infection, many individuals are able to live symptom-free lives. Cognitive Level: Applying; Client Need: Health Promotion and Maintenance; Nursing Process: Evaluation

2 Answer: 2, 3, 5   Rationale: Hyperglycemia, pancreatitis, and hepatic failure are adverse effects associated with lopinavir with ritonavir. Options 1 and 4

are incorrect. Renal failure and bone marrow suppression are not adverse effects associated with lopinavir with ritonavir. Cognitive Level: Analyzing; Client Need: Physiological Integrity; Nursing Process: Evaluation

3 Answer: 4   Rationale: Lactic acidosis is known to occur with all NRTIs, although the risk with emtricitabine is less than that of some drugs. It is one of the preferred drugs for initial HIV therapy. Options 1, 2, and 3 are incorrect. Ventricular cardiac dysrhythmias, pulmonary fibrosis, and necrotic bowel syndrome are not associated with emtricitabine. Cognitive Level: Applying; Client Need: Physiological Integrity; Nursing Process: Evaluation

4 Answer: 3   Rationale: Myelosuppression is the declining ability of the bone marrow to produce blood cells such as platelets, red blood cells, and white blood cells. Options 1, 2, and 4 are incorrect. Myelosuppression is not reflected in an increase in the serum blood urea nitrogen level. Myelosuppression causes a decrease in white blood cells rather than an increase. A decline in blood pressure is not indicative of myelosuppression. Cognitive Level: Analyzing; Client Need: Physiological Integrity; Nursing Process: Evaluation

5 Answer: 1, 2, 3   Rationale: Patients receiving antiretroviral therapy are immunocompromised and should avoid sources of infection such as crowds and individuals who have infections. The patient should be instructed to notify the health care provider at the first sign of a rash. Several antiretroviral medications may cause Stevens–Johnson syndrome, a dermatologic adverse effect that can be fatal. Current research has shown that HAART, especially when started early in HIV infection, significantly reduces viral load, reducing the chance of transmission. Transmission is still possible and infection control measures should still be practiced. Options 4 and 5 are incorrect. Total discontinuation of medication is not recommended because viral load increases when drug therapy is discontinued. Some herbal supplements, such as St. John's wort, interfere with antiretroviral therapy. Cognitive Level: Applying; Client Need: Health Promotion and Maintenance; Nursing Process: Planning

6 Answer: 4   Rationale: Tenofovir is known to lower bone mineral density, which may increase the risk for osteopenia or bone fractures. The patient should alert the chiropractor to this drug and possible risk before beginning any treatments. Options 1, 2, and 3 are incorrect. Many patients will turn to alternative therapy when faced with HIV infection. These activities provide the patient with a sense of control and comfort and should be supported as long as they are not contraindicated with the prescribed drug therapy. Yoga, guided imagery, massage therapy, meditation, and journaling are low-impact alternative therapies that may be tried. Cognitive Level: Applying; Client Need: Health Promotion and Maintenance; Nursing Process: Planning

Chapter 56

1 Answer: 3   Rationale: Stage 1 suggests that the tumor is relatively small in size, has not invaded the surrounding tissue, and has not been detected in surrounding lymph nodes; thus it has been detected at an early stage. Options 1, 2, and 4 are incorrect. Stage 1 is the earliest staging and has the best prognosis. Cell differentiation refers to grading of cancer cells, not staging of cancer cells. Stage 1 suggests that the tumor is small and has not begun to invade surrounding tissue. Cognitive Level: Analyzing; Client Need: Physiological Integrity; Nursing Process: Evaluation

2 Answer: 4, 5   Rationale: Patients and family members should avoid receiving live virus vaccination or exposure to chickenpox. Varicella (chickenpox) vaccination is usually given to children between the age of 12 and 18 months and the patient should not care for her granddaughter if immunization with live virus vaccines is planned. The patient should also avoid crowds, especially in enclosed areas, to minimize the risk of infection. Options 1, 2, and 3 are incorrect. Attending a support group, maintaining normal activities when possible, and eating small, frequent meals with sufficient protein are routine care measures during chemotherapy. Cognitive Level: Analyzing; Client Need: Physiological Integrity; Nursing Process: Evaluation

3 Answer: 1   Rationale: The use of multiple drugs affects different stages of the cancer cell's life cycle and attacks the various clones within the tumor via several mechanisms of action, thus increasing the percentage of cell kill. Combination chemotherapy also allows lower dosages of each individual agent, thus reducing toxicity and slowing the development of resistance. Options 2, 3, and 4 are incorrect. Staging describes the process of determining the extent of cancer in the body and where the cancer is located. Antineoplastic drugs may kill only a small portion of the tumor, leaving some clones unaffected and able to repopulate the tumor with resistant cells. Combination chemotherapy also allows lower dosages of each individual agent, thus reducing toxicity and slowing the development of resistance. Cognitive Level: Applying; Client Need: Physiological Integrity; Nursing Process: Evaluation

4 Answer: 3 Rationale: Mucositis is the painful inflammation and ulceration of the mucous membranes lining the digestive tract, an adverse effect of chemotherapy and radiation treatment for cancer. Patients experiencing this adverse effect should be instructed to eat a bland diet with low roughage and to use a soft toothbrush or plain water rinses for oral care if the mucositis is severe. Options 1, 2, and 4 are incorrect. Most OTC mouthwashes contain a significant amount of alcohol, which will further inflame the oral tissue and should be avoided. Citrus foods and beverages should be avoided because the acidic nature of these foods would cause the patient pain. Mucositis can last the duration of the chemotherapy treatment and should be treated rather than ignored. This condition will prevent intake of adequate nutrition to build new cells. Cognitive Level: Applying; Client Need: Physiological Integrity; Nursing Process: Implementation

5 Answer: 1 Rationale: Myelosuppression is the most common dose-limiting adverse effect of chemotherapy and the one that most often causes discontinuation or delays of chemotherapy. Options 2, 3, and 4 are incorrect. Although alopecia may be distressing for the patient, its presence does not determine when the next round of chemotherapy can be administered. Mucositis is not a reason that subsequent rounds of chemotherapy should be delayed. Cachexia is the physical wasting with loss of weight and muscle mass caused by disease. Although it is considered, it is not the most common reason for delaying chemotherapy. Cognitive Level: Applying; Client Need: Physiological Integrity; Nursing Process: Planning

6 Answer: 4 Rationale: Many antineoplastics are classified as vesicant agents that can cause serious tissue injury if they leak into the surrounding tissue from an artery or vein during an infusion or injection. The nurse should closely monitor the infusion site for swelling and pain. Options 1, 2, and 3 are incorrect. Vesicants do not necessarily cause nausea. It would be inappropriate for the nurse to monitor the patient's intake of calcium-rich foods because this is not related to receiving a chemotherapy classified as a vesicant. Respiratory status is not related to the administration of a vesicant-type chemotherapy agent. Cognitive Level: Applying; Client Need: Physiological Integrity; Nursing Process: Implementation

Chapter 57

1 Answer: 2 Rationale: The nadir indicates that myelosuppression has occurred and is indicated by decreased blood cell counts. WBC and ANC are sensitive indicators of the nadir. Options 1, 3, and 4 are incorrect. BUN, creatinine, ionized calcium, and serum albumin are not indicators of the nadir and myelosuppression. Cognitive Level: Analyzing; Client Need: Physiological Integrity; Nursing Process: Evaluation

2 Answer: 1, 3, 4 Rationale: The main dose-limiting toxicity to occur with vincristine is neurotoxicity. Numbness of the hands and feet, constipation related to decreased peristalsis, and diminished reflexes are all signs of neurotoxicity. Options 2 and 5 are incorrect. Cardiac and pulmonary toxicities are not associated with vincristine. Cognitive Level: Analyzing; Client Need: Physiological Integrity; Nursing Process: Evaluation

3 Answer: 4 Rationale: Tamoxifen is associated with an increased risk of endometrial cancer and monitoring will be necessary to detect early changes that may indicate that this adverse effect has occurred. Options 1, 2, and 3 are incorrect. Paralytic ileus and pulmonary fibrosis are not associated with tamoxifen. Alopecia is a common adverse effect of many chemotherapy drugs but will not require long-term monitoring. Cognitive Level: Applying; Client Need: Physiological Integrity; Nursing Process: Implementation

4 Answer: 3 Rationale: As with many chemotherapy drugs, doxorubicin is associated with mucositis. Daily mouth rinses will be prescribed to decrease the risk of opportunistic infections from yeast and mouth bacteria. Options 1, 2, and 4 are incorrect. Performing active or assisted ROM is an important intervention associated with drugs that cause neurotoxicities. Controlling pain is associated with chemotherapy that may cause pain as an adverse effect.

Maintaining bed rest is not related to the use of chemotherapy but may be required for other reasons. Cognitive Level: Applying; Client Need: Physiological Integrity; Nursing Process: Implementation

5 Answer: 1 Rationale: NSAIDs may cause severe and fatal myelosuppression when taken concurrently with methotrexate. Options 2, 3, and 4 are incorrect. Antihistamines, laxatives, and cough suppressants may be used with methotrexate. However, the provider should be consulted if they are needed because symptoms associated with these drugs may indicate a more serious condition that requires additional treatment. Cognitive Level: Applying; Client Need: Physiological Integrity; Nursing Process: Implementation

6 Answer: 3 Rationale: Filgrastim increases neutrophil production and decreases the duration of neutropenia with associated infection risk. Options 1, 2, and 4 are incorrect. Filgrastim does not boost the action of carboplatin, prevent the formation of additional cancers, or prevent bone loss. Cognitive Level: Applying; Client Need: Physiological Integrity; Nursing Process: Implementation

Chapter 59

1 Answer: 2 Rationale: Magnesium compounds, especially in higher doses, often cause diarrhea. Options 1, 3, and 4 are incorrect. Aluminum compounds and calcium compounds may cause constipation. Sodium compounds may cause flatulence. Cognitive Level: Applying; Client Need: Physiological Integrity; Nursing Process: Evaluation

2 Answer: 1, 2, 4, 5 Rationale: Symptoms of GERD include dysphagia, dyspepsia, nausea, belching, heartburn, and chest pain. Option 3 is incorrect. The nurse would not expect a decrease in the patient's appetite due to this medication. Cognitive Level: Applying; Client Need: Physiological Integrity; Nursing Process: Evaluation

3 Answer: 3 Rationale: The proton pump is activated by food intake. Thus, administering it about 20 to 30 minutes before the first major meal of the day allows peak serum levels to coincide with when the maximum levels of pumps are activated, allowing maximum efficiency of the PPI. Options 1, 2, and 4 are incorrect. The proton pumps are less active at night, in the fasting state, or between meals. Cognitive Level: Applying; Client Need: Physiological Integrity; Nursing Process: Planning

4 Answer: 2 Rationale: Blood dyscrasias have been reported, especially neutropenia and thrombocytopenia, with long-term use. Periodic blood counts should be performed. Options 1, 3, and 4 are incorrect. Ranitidine does not cause photophobia and skin irritations. Dyspnea and productive cough are not expected adverse effects for this medication. Ranitidine is not known to cause these symptoms. Cognitive Level: Applying; Client Need: Physiological Integrity; Nursing Process: Planning

5 Answer: 4 Rationale: Concurrent use of aluminum salts and sucralfate poses a risk for aluminum toxicity. Options 1, 2, and 3 are incorrect. There is no risk of aluminum toxicity with PPIs, other antacids, or H_2-receptor antagonists. Cognitive Level: Applying; Client Need: Physiological Integrity; Nursing Process: Implementation

6 Answer: 3 Rationale: Antibiotics have no role in the treatment of GERD although certain antibiotics are used in treating PUD to eradicate the *H. pylori* organism. Options 1, 2, and 4 are incorrect. H_2-receptor antagonists and PPIs are used routinely to relieve symptoms of GERD. OTC antacids provide intermittent relief for mild cases. Cognitive Level: Applying; Client Need: Physiological Integrity; Nursing Process: Implementation

Chapter 60

1 Answer: 3 Rationale: Diphenoxylate with atropine is given for diarrhea. The patient should report a decrease in the number of loose, watery stools after administration. Options 1, 2, and 4 are incorrect. Although diphenoxylate with atropine may decrease abdominal cramping and gas as a result of slowed peristalsis, it is not the main therapeutic effect desired from this drug. Slowing peristalsis may cause a decrease in bowel sounds rather than an increase. Cognitive Level: Analyzing; Client Need: Physiological Integrity; Nursing Process: Evaluation

2 Answer: 2   Rationale: One adverse effect of sulfasalazine is blood dyscrasias, which may include anemia, leukopenia, and thrombocytopenia. Fever, an increase in bruising, and sore throat are all possible symptoms of these decreased cell counts. Options 1, 3, and 4 are incorrect. Stevens–Johnson syndrome results in inflammation of the skin and mucous membranes and includes a sunburn-like appearance, blisters, and possible exfoliation of the dermis. Idiosyncratic reactions are aberrant reactions that cannot be explained by the known pharmacologic action of the drug and occur only in a small percentage of the population. This patient's symptoms are well documented as adverse effects. Hypersensitivity responses are due to stimulation of the immune system and are invoked by an antigen or antibody response. The symptoms presented do not reflect hypersensitivity to the drug. Cognitive Level: Analyzing; Client Need: Physiological Integrity; Nursing Process: Evaluation

3 Answer: 4   Rationale: Ondansetron is known to prolong the QT interval and may cause cardiac dysrhythmias. Options 1, 2, and 3 are incorrect. An allergy to soy or soy products, chronic constipation, or glaucoma does not present contraindications to the drugs. Cognitive Level: Analyzing; Client Need: Physiological Integrity; Nursing Process: Evaluation

4 Answer: 1   Rationale: The enzymes in pancrelipase come from pork. If the patient is allergic to or has religious restrictions on pork, the drug is contraindicated. Options 2, 3, and 4 are incorrect. Pancrelipase is not contraindicated for individuals with HTN or coronary artery disease. Pancrelipase is not an iodine-based agent. There is no expected cross sensitivity. Cognitive Level: Applying; Client Need: Physiological Integrity; Nursing Process: Implementation

5 Answer: 4   Rationale: Because magnesium hydroxide will stimulate peristalsis, it is important that the nurse assess for bowel sounds before giving the drug. If blockage or an ileus is suspected, the drug should be held and the provider notified. Options 1, 2, and 3 are incorrect. Blood pressure is an important vital sign to monitor postoperatively, but the magnesium hydroxide should not have direct effects. The dosage of the opioid drug and the patient's ability to ambulate to the bathroom will not impact the drug's use or action. Cognitive Level: Applying; Client Need: Physiological Integrity; Nursing Process: Assessment

6 Answer: 1, 3   Rationale: The nurse should explore possible causes for the diarrhea with the mother before making a recommendation because if diarrhea is caused by infections, slowing motility may allow the infection to increase. Salicylates, including bismuth subsalicylate, are contraindicated in children under the age of 19 because of an increased risk for Reye's syndrome. Options 2, 4, and 5 are incorrect. Activity level and weight are important growth and development parameters to assess but are unrelated to the drug's use. The school schedule would not have a direct impact on which drug is recommended. Cognitive Level: Applying; Client Need: Physiological Integrity; Nursing Process: Implementation

Chapter 61

1 Answer: 2   Rationale: Oral contraceptives may increase the serum levels of vitamin A. Options 1, 3, and 4 are incorrect. Vitamins D and E are also fat-soluble vitamins and may be taken along with vitamin A. Mineral oil may decrease the fat-soluble vitamins, including vitamin A. Antibiotics are not known to have an effect on the serum levels of vitamin A. Cognitive Level: Applying; Client Need: Physiological Integrity; Nursing Process: Assessment

2 Answer: Vitamin C may cause a false-negative result in **occult blood** if taken within 48 to 72 hours of the stool collection. Cognitive Level: Remembering; Client Need: Physiological Integrity; Nursing Process: Implementation

3 Answer: 4   Rationale: Pyridoxine (vitamin B_6) may reverse or antagonize the effects of anti-Parkinson's drugs. Options 1, 2, and 3 are incorrect. INH, oral contraceptives, and hydralazine (Apresoline) may increase the need for pyridoxine. Cognitive Level: Applying; Client Need: Physiological Integrity; Nursing Process: Assessment

4 Answer: 1   Rationale: Zinc is found in protein foods such as beans, lentils, nuts, meats, and dairy. Options 2, 3, and 4 are incorrect. Vegetables such as leafy greens, carrots, squash, cruciferous vegetables, or citrus fruits are not high in zinc. Cognitive Level: Applying; Client Need: Health Promotion and Maintenance; Nursing Process: Implementation

5 Answer: 1, 3   Rationale: Vitamin K is routinely given to newborn infants to prevent bleeding postdelivery. Vitamin K decreases the anticoagulant effects of the drug warfarin. Options 2, 4, and 5 are incorrect. Vitamin K is not indicated for visual disturbances, or in the treatment of hypothyroidism or chronic acne. Cognitive Level: Applying; Client Need: Physiological Integrity; Nursing Process: Planning

6 Answer: 3   Rationale: Muscle cramping and spasms may be early signs of hypocalcemia. Options 1, 2, and 4 are incorrect. Night blindness is a sign of possible vitamin A deficiency. Anemia may indicate an iron deficiency. Bleeding abnormalities may signal a deficiency in vitamin K. Cognitive Level: Analyzing; Client Need: Physiological Integrity; Nursing Process: Evaluation

Chapter 62

1 Answer: 3   Rationale: A patient receiving enteral feedings can be at risk for dehydration caused by an inadequate intake of free water. It is important to irrigate the tube with water as ordered, or per protocol (before and after an intermittent feeding or medication, or every 4 to 6 hours for continuous feedings), and to include additional free water throughout the day unless contraindicated. Options 1, 2, and 4 are incorrect. Daily weights are important to track fluid balance, but they do not maintain fluid balance. The NG tube should be irrigated more than just once a day. While assessment of the skin around a PEG tube site is important, it will not indicate the patient's fluid balance. This patient is receiving the feeding via an NG tube, which is passed through the nose. Cognitive Level: Applying; Client Need: Physiological Integrity; Nursing Process: Assessment

2 Answer: 1, 3, 5   Rationale: In addition to the base solution, TPN contains electrolytes (sodium, potassium, chloride), trace minerals, and multivitamins. Options 2 and 4 are incorrect. If diuretics are needed because of an underlying medical condition, they should be administered separately and not added to the TPN solution. Regular insulin may be added to the bag, but not NPH insulin. Cognitive Level: Applying; Client Need: Physiological Integrity; Nursing Process: Assessment

3 Answer: 4   Rationale: 10% dextrose in water contains the highest concentration of glucose and should be hung until the new TPN bag is available. The solution selected should minimize the risk of hypoglycemia. Options 1, 2, and 3 are incorrect. They will not be effective in preventing hypoglycemia. Cognitive Level: Applying; Client Need: Physiological Integrity; Nursing Process: Implementation

4 Answer: 2   Rationale: The patient's temperature should be monitored for signs of infection and subsequent sepsis, which are complications of TPN therapy. The weight is monitored to assess the nutritional effectiveness of the TPN and to detect signs of fluid overload. Options 1, 3, and 4 are incorrect. Blood pressure and pulse are important assessments but do not relate specifically to the effects of TPN. Cognitive Level: Applying; Client Need: Physiological Integrity; Nursing Process: Assessment

5 Answer: 4   Rationale: The nurse should not hang the lipids if separation of the emulsion or fat globules is visible in the solution. The solution should be returned to the pharmacy. Options 1, 2, and 3 are incorrect. Rolling or shaking the container or running the container under warm water will not correct the separation and may increase the risk of harm if the solution is used after separation has occurred. Cognitive Level: Applying; Client Need: Physiological Integrity; Nursing Process: Implementation

6 Answer: 1, 2   Rationale: Refrigerating unused enteral feeding solutions and limiting the length of time the solution is not refrigerated will prevent the growth of pathogens. Options 3, 4, and 5 are incorrect. Feeding bags and tubings are used for a limited length of time, most for 24 hours, and washing out the bag and tubing will not prevent the growth of harmful pathogens. Using plain water to irrigate the feeding tube is an accepted technique. Sterile technique is not needed when working with enteral feedings because the solution enters the GI tract. Clean technique is adequate except in severely immunocompromised patients. Cognitive Level: Applying; Client Need: Physiological Integrity; Nursing Process: Implementation

Chapter 63

1 Answer: 1 Rationale: It is recommended that if a 5% weight loss is not achieved after 12 weeks of therapy with lorcaserin, the drug be discontinued and other options considered. Options 2, 3, and 4 are incorrect. It is not known whether there are long-term adverse effects that arise after the time lorcaserin is taken or whether the risk continues after the drug is discontinued. Monthly visits to a cardiologist may be cost prohibitive and will not necessarily determine conclusively that a cardiovascular risk from the drug is present. Because health care is an individual's choice based on personal preference, insurance coverage, and other factors, the drug company would not be the best source for a follow-up program. Cognitive Level: Applying; Client Need: Health Promotion and Maintenance; Nursing Process: Implementation

2 Answer: 4 Rationale: Phentermine is a pregnancy category X drug and should not be used if the patient is pregnant or there is a possibility of pregnancy. Options 1, 2, and 3 are incorrect. Phentermine is used for short-term treatment of obesity and the presence of extreme obesity may be an indication for the drug. The drug is used cautiously in patients with diabetes and HTN, but neither is an absolute contraindication for the drug. Careful monitoring will be required if either of these conditions exist. Cognitive Level: Applying; Client Need: Physiological Integrity; Nursing Process: Assessment

3 Answer: 4 Rationale: Typically, orlistat is taken just prior to meals containing fats so that the drug can inhibit lipase and thus the absorption of lipids in the meal. Options 1, 2, and 3 are incorrect. Orlistat is taken throughout the day with each meal. It does not decrease appetite; it interferes with the absorption of fat in the diet. Although exercise is a part of the treatment plan for obesity, orlistat does not have to be administered before exercise. Cognitive Level: Applying; Client Need: Health Promotion and Maintenance; Nursing Process: Implementation

4 Answer: 4 Rationale: Intake of the proper amount and type of vitamins and nutrients is important in a healthy weight loss program. Because orlistat interferes with lipid absorption, the patient should be taught to supplement the diet with a product that contains all the essential fat-soluble vitamins. The supplement should be taken at least 2 hours before or after the orlistat. Options 1, 2, and 3 are incorrect. While increasing fluid intake may assist in a weight loss program, diet soda may contain sodium, citric acid, or other ingredients not necessary to a balanced diet. Orlistat does not cause photosensitivity, and additional sunscreen is not needed. Orlistat does not cause orthostatic hypotension, and no dizziness should be noted when rising from a lying or sitting position. Cognitive Level: Applying; Client Need: Health Promotion and Maintenance; Nursing Process: Implementation

5 Answer: 1 Rationale: Flatus and oily stools are adverse effects that are often troubling to the patient. The nurse should inform the patient that these often occur when taking orlistat. Options 2, 3, and 4 are incorrect. Heartburn and dyspepsia (indigestion), constipation, and nausea and vomiting are not common adverse effects associated with orlistat. Cognitive Level: Applying; Client Need: Physiological Integrity; Nursing Process: Implementation

6 Answer: 1, 2, 3 Rationale: Body weight, body mass index (BMI), and waist circumference are all indicators used to assess levels of obesity. Options 4 and 5 are incorrect. A treadmill test assesses physical fitness, not necessarily obesity. Buoyancy analysis is not a test used to determine the degree of obesity. Cognitive Level: Applying; Client Need: Physiological Integrity; Nursing Process: Assessment

Chapter 65

1 Answer: 2 Rationale: GH cannot be given PO; it can only be administered subcutaneously by injections. Options 1, 3, and 4 are incorrect. A lack of GH is not associated with mental retardation. Children whose epiphyseal plates have closed are not candidates for GH therapy; therefore, most adolescents would see minimal gain in height. Periodic testing for blood hormone levels is required during therapy. Cognitive Level: Applying; Client Need: Physiological Integrity; Nursing Process: Planning

2 Answer: 1, 2, 3 Rationale: GH increases the length and width of long bones; promotes organ, muscle, and connective tissue growth; and increases the synthesis of proteins. Options 4 and 5 are incorrect. GH may cause an increase in serum glucose levels, not a decrease. It may improve and decrease fat deposits around the abdomen and improve lipid levels. Cognitive Level: Applying; Client Need: Physiological Integrity; Nursing Process: Evaluation

3 Answer: 3 Rationale: Patients on desmopressin need to obtain a daily weight and should monitor for the presence of any peripheral edema. Options 1, 2, and 4 are incorrect. Desmopressin must be given in regular doses for continued therapeutic effects. Increasing the dosage may cause an increased risk of vasoconstriction and other adverse effects. Leg cramping when walking may indicate adverse peripheral vascular effects and should be assessed by the provider. Taking NSAIDs concurrently may increase the antidiuretic effect, leading to adverse effects. Cognitive Level: Applying; Client Need: Health Promotion and Maintenance; Nursing Process: Planning

4 Answer: 1 Rationale: Octreotide prolongs intestinal transit time and stimulates reabsorption of fluids and electrolytes from the GI tract. These effects would have the therapeutic action of decreasing diarrhea related to the cancer or treatment. Options 2, 3, and 4 are incorrect. Octreotide will not slow cancer growth or metastasis or improve lean body mass or fat deposits. Hypo- and hyperglycemia are possible adverse effects of octreotide, not therapeutic effects. Cognitive Level: Analyzing; Client Need: Physiological Integrity; Nursing Process: Evaluation

5 Answer: 4 Rationale: Vasopressin is a potent vasoconstrictor and may precipitate angina or myocardial infarction. Options 1, 2, and 3 are incorrect. Glaucoma, COPD, or alcoholism would not be contraindications for this drug. Cognitive Level: Applying; Client Need: Physiological Integrity; Nursing Process: Assessment

6 Answer: 1 Rationale: A patient with diabetes insipidus (DI) who is responding to therapy with desmopressin would have decreasing signs of dehydration. Options 2, 3, and 4 are incorrect. DI is characterized by large volumes of urine output with a very low urine specific gravity accompanied by signs of dehydration, including complaints of thirst and an increased pulse rate. The patient responding to desmopressin therapy would see a lowered pulse rate related to an increase in circulating volume secondary to the decrease in urine output. Desmopressin therapy would also cause the urine specific gravity to increase, not decrease. Blood glucose levels are not affected by desmopressin. Cognitive Level: Analyzing; Client Need: Physiological Integrity; Nursing Process: Evaluation

Chapter 66

1 Answer: 2 Rationale: Insulin peaks are the times of maximum insulin utilization with the greatest risk of hypoglycemia. Options 1, 3, and 4 are incorrect. Because the risk for hypoglycemia is highest at peak serum insulin levels, exercise or additional insulin may increase the risk further. Insulin schedules for the patient are developed by the provider and the patient should not self-select a schedule for insulin use. Cognitive Level: Applying; Client Need: Physiological Integrity; Nursing Process: Implementation

2 Answer: 2, 3, 5 Rationale: The blood glucose level should be checked prior to administering any type of insulin. Because lispro is a rapid-acting insulin, the nurse should ensure that a meal is available and that the patient will be able to eat shortly after receiving a dose. If signs of hypoglycemia are present, the insulin dose should be held and the patient treated for hypoglycemia. The provider should be notified. Options 1 and 4 are incorrect. Urine testing for glucose and ketones does not give exact information, and patients vary on the degree to which glucose and ketones will "spill" into the urine. While a check of the pulse or blood pressure may be included in routine vital signs or to further assess symptoms of hypoglycemia, they do not provide information directly pertinent to the administration of insulin. Cognitive Level: Applying; Client Need: Physiological Integrity; Nursing Process: Implementation

3 Answer: 3 Rationale: A serious adverse effect of metformin is the risk for developing lactic acidosis. Renal insufficiency and failure, excess alcohol use, and IV contrast agents increase the risk for lactic acidosis and are contraindications to the use of metformin. Options 1, 2, and 4 are incorrect. Hypoglycemia, GI distress, and weight loss are common adverse effects to most oral antidiabetic drugs and are not specific to metformin. Cognitive Level: Analyzing; Client Need: Physiological Integrity; Nursing Process: Evaluation

4 Answer: 2   Rationale: It can take several weeks for rosiglitazone to provide full therapeutic effects, so the appropriate response would be to give it more time to reach effectiveness. Options 1, 3, and 4 are incorrect. It is not within a nurse's scope of practice to prescribe additional drugs or change the dosage. The health care provider should be consulted about any change to the patient's drug regimen. Cognitive Level: Applying; Client Need: Health Promotion and Maintenance; Nursing Process: Implementation

5 Answer: 4   Rationale: Glucagon injections can be repeated if one dose is not effective. Hypoglycemia is a medical emergency, and because this woman has not fully recovered, medical attention is needed. Options 1, 2, and 3 are incorrect. The patient is still experiencing symptoms of hypoglycemia, and continued treatment is indicated. Because she is still groggy and disoriented, it would not be safe to give this patient anything by mouth. Cognitive Level: Applying; Client Need: Physiological Integrity; Nursing Process: Implementation

6 Answer: 4   Rationale: Insulin glargine has no definite peak, so there is a minimal risk for hypoglycemic reaction. Options 1, 2, and 3 are incorrect. Insulin glargine must be given by subcutaneous injection, it cannot be given by IM injection, and blood glucose monitoring is required for all patients taking any insulin. Cognitive Level: Applying; Client Need: Physiological Integrity; Nursing Process: Implementation

Chapter 67

1 Answer: 4   Rationale: The administration of too much levothyroxine may cause hyperthyroidism, characterized by nervousness, palpitations, weight loss, diarrhea, and muscle tremors. Before altering the dosage, thyroid function studies will be performed to verify this condition. Options 1, 2, and 3 are incorrect. Nervousness, palpitations, and tremors are not symptoms of hypothyroidism or normal thyroid states. While these symptoms may occur with diabetes and hyperglycemia, other symptoms would dominate and would be noted before these symptoms occurred. Cognitive Level: Analyzing; Client Need: Physiological Integrity; Nursing Process: Evaluation

2 Answer: 3, 4, 5   Rationale: A euthyroid (normal) state is indicated by a return to normal performance of ADLs without fatigue, normalizing cholesterol levels, and vital signs within normal limits with a pulse rate between 60 and 100 beats/minute. Options 1 and 2 are incorrect. Constipation and weight gain are symptoms of hypothyroidism. Decreased blinking and exophthalmos are symptoms of hyperthyroidism. Cognitive Level: Applying; Client Need: Physiological Integrity; Nursing Process: Evaluation

3 Answer: 1   Rationale: Low-grade fever, sore throat, and chills are symptoms of a possible infection. Because propylthiouracil may cause agranulocytosis, these symptoms should be reported to the provider. Options 2, 3, and 4 are incorrect. Increased appetite and caloric intake signal a return to a more euthyroid state. Tinnitus, altered taste, thickened saliva, insomnia, nightmares, and night sweats are not effects usually associated with propylthiouracil and if they occur, other causes should be investigated. Cognitive Level: Analyzing; Client Need: Physiological Integrity; Nursing Process: Implementation

4 Answer: 3   Rationale: A heart rate of 110 beats/minute would cause the nurse to hold the scheduled dose of levothyroxine, because it could indicate too high a level of thyroid hormone. Options 1, 2, and 4 are incorrect. A low level of thyroid hormone could cause weight gain or decreased blood pressure. These are symptoms of hypothyroidism and would not cause the nurse to hold the medication. An elevated temperature without other signs of hyperthyroidism would not warrant withholding the medication. Cognitive Level: Analyzing; Client Need: Physiological Integrity; Nursing Process: Implementation

5 Answer: 2   Rationale: The high levels of iodine found in potassium iodide solution will inhibit the synthesis and release of thyroid hormone. The effectiveness decreases over time so it is only used short term before more definitive treatment can be accomplished. Options 1, 3, and 4 are incorrect. Iodine deficiency is rare and does not cause symptoms of hyperthyroidism, the indication for the patient's potassium iodide solution. High-dose iodine is not always used prior to thyroid surgery and the thyroidectomy is not related to a loss of iodine. High doses of iodine will not prevent diabetes. Cognitive Level: Applying; Client Need: Physiological Integrity; Nursing Process: Implementation

6 Answer: 3   Rationale: To closely approximate the body's own hormone levels, levothyroxine should be taken in the morning, ideally at the same time each day. Options 1, 2, and 4 are incorrect. Taking levothyroxine along with food or meals containing high fiber may affect the absorption of the drug. Foods such as strawberries, spinach, and kale may inhibit thyroid secretion, reducing the effectiveness of the levothyroxine. If diarrhea occurs, the provider should be notified to determine the need to alter the dose. Cognitive Level: Applying; Client Need: Health Promotion and Maintenance; Nursing Process: Implementation

Chapter 68

1 Answer: 1, 3, 5   Rationale: Edema, eye pain or vision changes, and abdominal pain are symptoms of possible adverse effects from the methylprednisolone. Options 2 and 4 are incorrect. Tinnitus is not an adverse effect commonly associated with methylprednisolone and if it occurs, other causes should be investigated. Dizziness upon standing indicates possible *hypo*tension. *Hyper*tension is a possible adverse effect from methylprednisolone. Cognitive Level: Analyzing; Client Need: Physiological Integrity; Nursing Process: Implementation

2 Answer: 1   Rationale: An irregular heart rate and rhythm is a symptom of hypokalemia. Hydrocortisone given concurrently with diuretics such as thiazides, which cause loss of potassium, increases the risk of hypokalemia. Options 2, 3, and 4 are incorrect. While these are common adverse effects of hydrocortisone, they do not require immediate attention. Cognitive Level: Analyzing; Client Need: Physiological Integrity; Nursing Process: Evaluation

3 Answer: 1, 2   Rationale: Weight-bearing exercise three to four times weekly and increased dietary intake of calcium and vitamin D may help to prevent bone loss and osteoporosis. Options 3, 4, and 5 are incorrect. Remaining sedentary is not advisable and may increase the risk of osteoporosis and other adverse effects such as thrombophlebitis. Increased fluid intake and avoidance of alcohol are advised, but carbonated sodas should also be avoided because they have been linked to an increased risk of osteoporosis. While a bisphosphonate may be needed if bone density studies indicate the development of osteoporosis, it is not necessarily required at this time. Cognitive Level: Applying; Client Need: Health Promotion and Maintenance; Nursing Process: Implementation

4 Answer: 4   Rationale: The patient should obtain a daily weight, ideally at the same time each day to assess for excessive fluid retention. Fludrocortisone is a mineralocorticoid and may cause fluid retention, edema, and HTN. Options 1, 2, and 3 are incorrect. Abdominal pain and changes to the stool color may indicate GI bleeding, which is an adverse effect associated with glucocorticoids. Increased lipid levels and mood changes are also associated with glucocorticoids. Cognitive Level: Applying; Client Need: Physiological Integrity; Nursing Process: Implementation

5 Answer: 3   Rationale: The patient is experiencing symptoms of acute adrenal insufficiency related to the inability to take the prescribed drug for several days and will require immediate IV administration of hydrocortisone. Options 1, 2, and 4 are incorrect. Fludrocortisone is a mineralocorticoid and is not indicated in this emergency situation. Ketoconazole and metyrapone have antiadrenal effects and would worsen the situation. Cognitive Level: Analyzing; Client Need: Physiological Integrity; Nursing Process: Planning

6 Answer: 4   Rationale: Patients receiving replacement therapy for chronic adrenal insufficiency should carry PO and parenteral forms of the drugs they are prescribed in case of emergencies where the drugs may not be readily available. Options 1, 2, and 3 are incorrect. Checking BP, avoiding crowds and infections, and monitoring for visual changes are appropriate interventions when hyperphysiological doses are given to treat disease and other conditions. Patients on replacement therapy for adrenal insufficiency receive physiological doses to maintain normal levels of the hormones in their body and should not experience adverse effects unless the dosage is inappropriate. Cognitive Level: Applying; Client Need: Health Promotion and Maintenance; Nursing Process: Implementation

Chapter 69

1 Answer: 2, 3, 4   Rationale: A history of thromboembolic conditions, breast cancer, or hyperlipidemia may be contraindications for the use of HRT for this patient and will require further assessment by the health care provider before prescribing conjugated estrogen. Options 1 and 5 are incorrect. Because conjugated estrogen is metabolized through the P450 pathways and the drug may have hepatic effects, women with diabetes may need to more closely monitor their blood glucose to ensure that their diabetes medications are effective, but this is not considered a contraindication to the drug. A past history of cesarean section is also not a contraindication. Cognitive Level: Analyzing; Client Need: Physiological Integrity; Nursing Process: Assessment

2 Answer: 3 Rationale: Regular contractions increasing in occurrence indicate that the oxytocin is exerting a therapeutic effect. Options 1, 2, and 4 are incorrect. Control of postpartum hemorrhage is a therapeutic effect of oxytocin but would not be considered a therapeutic effect during labor. Sustained contractions are an adverse effect of oxytocin and immediate intervention is needed to prevent serious injury to the mother or baby should they occur. Oxytocin stimulates the milk letdown reflex in nursing, but this would not be considered a therapeutic effect during labor. Cognitive Level: Analyzing; Client Need: Physiological Integrity; Nursing Process: Evaluation

3 Answer: 4 Rationale: Clomiphene is given over six ovulatory-menstrual cycles in increasing doses with HCG added as needed. If no pregnancy has occurred after six cycles, other treatment options will be considered. Options 1, 2, and 3 are incorrect. The drug will not be continued for 1 year if pregnancy has not occurred, and the dosage may be increased after each cycle. Clomiphene is a category X drug and should be stopped if pregnancy occurs. Cognitive Level: Applying; Client Need: Health Promotion and Maintenance; Nursing Process: Implementation

4 Answer: 3 Rationale: Medroxyprogesterone is known to decrease bone density over time. The patient should be taught to report any bone, joint, or musculoskeletal pain and to report any difficulty or pain with movement or ambulation. Options 1, 2, and 4 are incorrect. Insomnia or sleep difficulty and mouth, eye, or vaginal dryness are not related adverse effects. The drug may cause breakthrough spotting between menstrual cycles but this is a common effect and does not require evaluation unless the bleeding is heavy or continuous. Cognitive Level: Analyzing; Client Need: Physiological Integrity; Nursing Process: Implementation

5 Answer: 2 Rationale: The standard treatment with clomiphene is to begin with a low dose for 5 days beginning on the fifth day of the menstrual cycle. Options 1, 3, and 4 are incorrect. Starting therapy on the first day of the menstrual cycle would not be as effective in stimulating ovulation because this usually occurs closer to midcycle. Because women experience menstrual periods of varying length, starting the drug on the "last day" would vary, and the drug might be started sooner or later than the recommended fifth day of the menstrual cycle. Many women do not know when ovulation occurs to be able to take it based on an ovulatory cycle and there is likelihood that this patient is not experiencing ovulation. Cognitive Level: Applying; Client Need: Health Promotion and Maintenance; Nursing Process: Implementation

6 Answer: 4 Rationale: Sedation, intense thirst, flushing of the skin, confusion, and muscle weakness are early symptoms of magnesium toxicity and should be immediately reported to the provider. Options 1, 2, and 3 are incorrect. The drug decreases deep tendon reflexes and CNS stimulation, and hyperactivity or seizure activity would not be expected. Chest congestion and cough are not associated with the drug and other causes should be explored. Cognitive Level: Analyzing; Client Need: Physiological Integrity; Nursing Process: Evaluation

Chapter 70

1 Answer: 3, 4 Rationale: Smokers have a significantly increased risk of serious thromboembolic events when taking OCs. Mood disorders, including depression, may worsen in patients taking OCs, and additional monitoring may be advised. Options 1, 2, and 5 are incorrect. Obesity is a risk factor for both treatment failure and thromboembolic events; however, this patient is considered overweight and is not in the high-risk category. Patients with asthma are not high risk, and a healthy 42-year-old woman with no significant health history is not considered high risk. Cognitive Level: Analyzing; Client Need: Physiological Integrity; Nursing Process: Assessment

2 Answer: 1 Rationale: If two consecutive days are missed, the patient should take two pills on the day it is discovered, two pills the following day, then resume the normal one pill per day routine. A second method of contraception should be used for 7 days after resuming the pills. Options 2, 3, and 4 are incorrect. Taking only one pill, skipping additional doses, or stopping the drug will not allow continued contraception. If the patient is concerned about pregnancy due to the missed pills, a pregnancy test may be conducted. Cognitive Level: Applying; Client Need: Health Promotion and Maintenance; Nursing Process: Implementation

3 Answer: 4 Rationale: Levonorgestrel/estradiol is taken for 84 days followed by a lower dose of estrogen included in the pill package for 7 days. Options 1, 2, and 3 are incorrect. Taking levonorgestrel/estradiol for 3 weeks, year-round, or for 2 months would be incorrect administration cycles. Cognitive Level: Applying; Client Need: Health Promotion and Maintenance; Nursing Process: Implementation

4 Answer: 3 Rationale: The patient takes mifepristone, followed by an assessment by the health care provider 2 days later. If abortion has not occurred, the misoprostol is taken. The patient returns to the health care provider in 14 days to confirm that abortion is complete. Options 1, 2, and 4 are incorrect. Two doses of mifepristone are not taken and the patient must be assessed by the provider before taking the misoprostol dose. Bleeding is a common effect of both drugs and is not an indication of when or whether to take the misoprostol. Cognitive Level: Applying; Client Need: Health Promotion and Maintenance; Nursing Process: Implementation

5 Answer: 2 Rationale: Patients should be informed that spermicidal agents have relatively low levels of efficacy when used alone and should therefore be used only in conjunction with barrier methods such as condoms and diaphragms. Options 1, 3, and 4 are incorrect. Spermicides such as nonoxynol-9 are not extremely effective in preventing pregnancy, do not cause or protect against HIV or PID, and do not prevent ectopic pregnancies. Cognitive Level: Applying; Client Need: Health Promotion and Maintenance; Nursing Process: Implementation

6 Answer: 5, 1, 4, 3, 2 The correct ranking from most effective to least effective with *typical* use of the method is

1. Transdermal (Ortho-Evra): 95% effective
2. Depo-Provera: 94% effective
3. Oral contraceptives: 91% effective
4. Calendar rhythm: 76% effective
5. Spermicides: 71% effective

Cognitive Level: Applying; Client Need: Health Promotion and Maintenance; Nursing Process: Assessment

Chapter 71

1 Answer: 2 Rationale: Primary hypogonadism results in patients with normal pituitary function and testes that are either diseased or unresponsive to FSH and LH. A primary goal of therapy would be an increased sperm count with an increase in male masculinization. Options 1, 3, and 4 are incorrect. Testosterone should not affect RBC count. Administering testosterone to the patient will not increase FSH or LH levels. Cognitive Level: Applying; Client Need: Physiological Integrity; Nursing Process: Evaluation

2 Answer: 1 Rationale: The use of nitrates is contraindicated with sildenafil because dangerous hypotension may result. Options 2, 3, and 4 are incorrect. A history of diabetes would not be of concern and may be an indication for treatment if ED occurs. An allergy to penicillin products is not a contraindication for use of sildenafil. There are no expected adverse reactions with sildenafil and the use of antiulcer medication. Cognitive Level: Applying; Client Need: Physiological Integrity; Nursing Process: Assessment

3 Answer: 2, 3, 5 Rationale: Women and children should avoid skin contact with areas where testosterone gels or creams have been applied to avoid drug absorption. Testosterones may trigger sodium and water retention and a weight gain of 2 kg (5 lb) or more per week should be reported to the provider. They may also increase blood lipid levels. Therefore, the patient should follow a low-fat diet and have periodic blood lipid level assessments. Options 1 and 4 are incorrect. Testosterone gel should be applied to the upper arms, shoulders, or abdomen and never to the scrotum, perineal area, or on broken or irritated skin. Showering or swimming should be avoided for several hours after application to allow drug absorption, but a wait of 12 to 14 hours is excessive. Cognitive Level: Applying; Client Need: Physiological Integrity; Nursing Process: Implementation

4 Answer: 2 Rationale: For sildenafil to be effective, the ED must be physiological in nature. It is not effective if the dysfunction has solely psychological origins and therefore does not always cause an erection. Options 1, 3, and 4 are incorrect. Sildenafil simply enhances, rather than causes, an erection. Prolonged use does not result in less intense feelings over time. Use of sildenafil by men will not have effects on female sexual function. Cognitive Level: Applying; Client Need: Health Promotion and Maintenance; Nursing Process: Implementation

5 Answer: 1, 2, 4 Rationale: Finasteride promotes shrinkage of enlarged prostates and subsequently helps restore urinary function. Women should avoid handling crushed medication because it may be absorbed through the skin and have teratogenic effects. Maximum benefit may take 6 to 12 months to be achieved. Options 3 and 5 are incorrect. Dizziness is a possible adverse effect but significant dizziness or orthostatic hypotension should not occur and should be reported to the health care provider. Finasteride does not affect vision. Cognitive Level: Applying; Client Need: Physiological Integrity; Nursing Process: Implementation

6 Answer: 4 Rationale: Full effects of finasteride are realized within 6 to 12 months of therapy. Because the symptoms of dysuria have suddenly increased, the patient should be assessed for possible prostate cancer. Options 1, 2, and 3 are incorrect. Continuing to take the drug after full therapeutic results should have been realized is not appropriate, given the sudden increase in symptoms. Decreasing fluid irritants such as caffeine and alcohol may help overall but will not cause the sudden symptoms. A low-dose diuretic may not be appropriate in this situation and may worsen the dysuria. Cognitive Level: Analyzing; Client Need: Physiological Integrity; Nursing Process: Evaluation

Chapter 72

1 Answer: 3 Rationale: Alendronate may cause severe GI adverse effects. To decrease this risk, particularly for esophageal irritation, and to promote the absorption of the medication, alendronate should be taken with a full glass of water after rising in the morning. The patient should not eat or drink anything or lie down for 30 minutes after administration. Options 1, 2, and 4 are incorrect. The medication should be taken before breakfast, not before lunch or at bedtime. The patient should not lie down after taking alendronate for at least 30 minutes, preferably longer. Cognitive Level: Applying; Client Need: Health Promotion and Maintenance; Nursing Process: Evaluation

2 Answer: 1 Rationale: Headache, dizziness, and blurred vision are all early symptoms of toxicity to methotrexate. Options 2, 3, and 4 are incorrect. Hematuria, jaundice, and ascites are not associated with the use of methotrexate. While stomatitis may occur, constipation would be unrelated to methotrexate. Cognitive Level: Analyzing; Client Need: Physiological Integrity; Nursing Process: Evaluation

3 Answer: 2 Rationale: Colchicine prevents the migration of neutrophils (WBCs) into the area of inflammation caused by uric acid crystals, reducing further inflammation and relieving the symptoms of gout and gouty arthritis. Options 1, 3, and 4 are incorrect. Colchicine does not increase uric acid deposits in the synovial spaces of the joints, prevent accumulation of uric acid crystals in the joints, or increase renal excretion of uric acid crystals. Patients feel better from decreased inflammation secondary to fewer uric acid crystal deposits. Renal excretion of uric acid is not a mechanism of action of colchicine. Cognitive Level: Applying; Client Need: Physiological Integrity; Nursing Process: Implementation

4 Answer: 1 Rationale: The patient with osteomalacia has low serum calcium and low phosphate levels. An indicator that replacement therapy is achieving therapeutic benefits would be increasing serum calcium and phosphate levels. Options 2, 3, and 4 are incorrect. Increasing or decreasing actions of the serum calcium and phosphate levels are incorrectly stated. Cognitive Level: Analyzing; Client Need: Physiological Integrity; Nursing Process: Evaluation

5 Answer: 1 Rationale: Vitamin D toxicity may occur in the patient receiving calcitriol. Symptoms to assess include muscle weakness, fatigue, nausea, vomiting, and changes in the color or amount of urine. Options 2, 3, and 4 are incorrect. Diarrhea, stomatitis, and photosensitivity are not symptoms that would be associated with the effects of vitamin D therapy. Bone pain and fever are symptoms of vitamin D deficiency. Cognitive Level: Analyzing; Client Need: Physiological Integrity; Nursing Process: Evaluation

6 Answer: 1, 2, 3 Rationale: DMARDs include gold salts, antimalarial agents, D-penicillamine, and drugs that modify immune and inflammatory responses and have been found to reduce mortality rate, improve symptoms, and enhance the quality of life in patients with RA. Maximum therapeutic effects from DMARDs often take several months to achieve. Options 4 and 5 are incorrect. These drugs can be toxic and close monitoring of patients is required during the course of therapy. DMARDs are well accepted in medical practice because they have been found to reduce mortality rate and improve symptoms of RA. Cognitive Level: Applying; Client Need: Physiological Integrity; Nursing Process: Evaluation

Chapter 73

1 Answer: 4 Rationale: Lice and nits can live in areas of the body other than the hair on the patient's head. Options 1, 2, and 3 are incorrect. Permethrin should not be applied after body lotions and should not be used on eyelashes or eyebrows. Lice can survive for up to 24 to 48 hours on inanimate objects. Cognitive Level: Applying; Client Need: Health Promotion and Maintenance; Nursing Process: Implementation

2 Answer: 1 Rationale: Patients taking topical corticosteroids for the treatment of atopic dermatitis may expect to experience a degree of burning and stinging of the skin in the affected area. Options 2, 3, and 4 are incorrect. Localized pruritus and hives, a loss of hair in the application area, or a worsening of acne vulgaris are not symptoms that would be related specifically to the effects of therapy. Cognitive Level: Applying; Client Need: Physiological Integrity; Nursing Process: Assessment

3 Answer: 1, 2, 3 Rationale: Benzoyl peroxide suppresses sebum production and has antimicrobial action against the bacteria that cause acne. It also has a keratolytic effect, drying and encouraging more rapid cell turnover in the outer layer of the epidermis. Options 4 and 5 are incorrect. Microdermal abrasion is not a primary mechanism of action of the drug and benzoyl peroxide does not have sunscreening activity. Cognitive Level: Applying; Client Need: Physiological Integrity; Nursing Process: Evaluation

4 Answer: 3 Rationale: Tretinoin may cause dryness, irritation, and erythema. Mild soaps, gentle cleansing, warm but not hot water, and gentle drying should be used while tretinoin therapy is used. Options 1, 2, and 4 are incorrect. Antiacne soaps often contain compounds that dry and desquamate the skin and may cause further irritation. Sunscreens with an SPF of 15 and coverings should be used while on tretinoin to avoid sunburn. Alternating tretinoin with benzoyl peroxide may cause excessive dryness and irritation and increase the risk of adverse effects. Cognitive Level: Applying; Client Need: Health Promotion and Maintenance; Nursing Process: Implementation

5 Answer: 3 Rationale: A small test area should be used if benzocaine has not been used before to assess for allergy. If no symptoms are noted within 30 to 60 minutes, it may be used on a wider area. Options 1, 2, and 4 are incorrect. Benzocaine should not be used on partial-thickness burns because of the risk of open blistered areas. The solution should not be warmed to avoid further heat and damage to the area of the burn. The burn should not be covered with plastic wrap to avoid heat trapping, potentially increasing the damage. Cognitive Level: Applying; Client Need: Health Promotion and Maintenance; Nursing Process: Implementation

6 Answer: A patient who has been prescribed isotretinoin must comply with the iPledge Program because of the risk of **teratogenic** effects. Cognitive Level: Applying; Client Need: Physiological Integrity; Nursing Process: Assessment

Chapter 74

1 Answer: 4 Rationale: Timolol is a beta-adrenergic blocker. To prevent swallowing and systemic absorption, pressure is to be applied to the inner canthus of the eye for 1 minute after instilling the drop. Options 1, 2, and 3 are incorrect. No other eyedrops or ointments should be used when taking timolol or other drops for glaucoma without the approval of the provider. Eye solutions for allergies may contain adrenergic drugs that may worsen glaucoma. Timolol is not contraindicated during seasonal allergies. It is not known to worsen seasonal allergies although it may cause bronchoconstriction in the sensitive individual or if swallowed and systemic effects occur. Cognitive Level: Applying; Client Need: Physiological Integrity; Nursing Process: Planning

2 Answer: 1, 2, 4   Rationale: Latanoprost (Xalatan) may cause thickening and darkening of the eyelashes and upper eyelid and may cause darkening of the iris, especially noticeable in patients with light eye colors. Options 3 and 5 are incorrect. Latanoprost will not cause lightening of the iris or darkening of the sclera or a permanent bluish tint to the conjunctiva. Cognitive Level: Applying; Client Need: Physiological Integrity; Nursing Process: Implementation

3 Answer: Pilocarpine causes miosis, which stretches the trabecular meshwork, allowing greater outflow of aqueous humor and decreasing the IOP. Cognitive Level: Applying; Client Need: Physiological Integrity; Nursing Process: Implementation

4 Answer: 2, 3, 1, 4   Rationale: The ear should be pulled gently upward and back and the drop instilled, allowing it to flow down the side of the canal. Dropping the solution directly on the tympanic membrane may cause dizziness or nausea. The area in front of the ear (the tragus) should be gently massaged. The patient should remain in a side-lying position or with the treated ear uppermost for 5 minutes to allow complete absorption of the solution. If needed, a dry cotton ball may be placed in the outer ear area to prevent leakage of solution. Cognitive Level: Applying; Client Need: Health Promotion and Maintenance; Nursing Process: Implementation

5 Answer: 4   Rationale: Increasing pain, particularly around the ear area, may indicate worsening infection or mastoiditis and should be immediately reported. Options 1, 2, and 3 are incorrect. Mild itching and irritation may occur, but severe itching or swelling should be reported. Gradually decreasing pain is a therapeutic effect as the infection clears. Dizziness may occur if the eardrop is instilled directly onto the tympanic membrane. Cognitive Level: Applying; Client Need: Physiological Integrity; Nursing Process: Planning

6 Answer: Phenylephrine causes **mydriasis,** allowing better visualization of the area of the lens during cataract surgery. Cognitive Level: Applying; Client Need: Physiological Integrity; Nursing Process: Implementation

Chapter 75

1 Answer: 1   Rationale: No antidote or specific treatment exists for radiation poisoning. Supportive therapy for the associated symptoms is the only treatment available. Options 2, 3, and 4 are incorrect. Ultraviolet light does not affect individuals who experience radiation poisoning. An individual with radiation toxicity is incapable of contaminating other individuals. No antiradiation medications exist. Cognitive Level: Applying; Client Need: Physiological Integrity; Nursing Process: Implementation

2 Answer: 1   Rationale: The drug of choice for *Y. pestis* exposure is doxycycline. Options 2, 3, and 4 are incorrect. Trivalent botulinum antitoxin is one of the two available treatments for botulism. The other antitoxin for botulism is heptavalent botulinum antitoxin. Ribavirin is an antiviral agent that may be used to treat serious virus infections. Atropine sulfate is a cholinergic antagonist used for organophosphate poisoning and other health problems. Cognitive Level: Applying; Client Need: Physiological Integrity; Nursing Process: Implementation

3 Answer: 3   Rationale: Time is a critical factor in acute poisonings. The emergency should be called into 911 and the rescue squad should transport the child to the nearest health care facility immediately. Options 1, 2, and 4 are incorrect. Instructions for poisoning may have changed since the packaging was printed. Based on the information provided in the question, the nurse does not know what chemicals the child has ingested. Forced vomiting is contraindicated for most poisonings. Waiting for the child to develop seizures or shortness of breath is too late since the development of these symptoms most likely represents a toxic level of the poison. Cognitive Level: Applying; Client Need: Physiological Integrity; Nursing Process: Implementation

4 Answer: 3   Rationale: Patients with decreased sensorium are at high risk for pulmonary aspiration. Activated charcoal should only be given to these patients if the airway is maintained with an endotracheal tube. Options 1, 2, and 4 are incorrect. Activated charcoal is not absorbed in the GI tract and therefore would not be contraindicated in patients with liver pathology. Activated charcoal is eliminated in the feces and therefore would not be contraindicated in patients with renal impairment. Anxiety and nervousness are not reasons to withhold the administration of activated charcoal. Cognitive Level: Applying; Client Need: Physiological Integrity; Nursing Process: Assessment

5 Answer: 1   Rationale: Chelating agents capture the toxic metal through a bonding process. The kidneys remove both the chelator and the metal bound to it from the body. Options 2, 3, and 4 are incorrect. A chelator binds heavy metals but does not deactivate any chemical reactions. Chelation therapy is not involved in metabolism. Glomerular filtration is not affected by chelation therapy. Cognitive Level: Applying; Client Need: Physiological Integrity; Nursing Process: Assessment

6 Answer: 2   Rationale: Edetate calcium disodium may produce renal damage that may be reduced by ensuring adequate diuresis before therapy begins. Options 1, 3, and 4 are incorrect. Bowel function is not a critical parameter to consider prior to giving this drug. Edetate calcium disodium administration is not based on visual acuity. Skin integrity is not a critical parameter to consider prior to giving edetate calcium disodium. Cognitive Level: Applying; Client Need: Physiological Integrity; Nursing Process: Assessment

Appendix B

ISMP List of *High-Alert* Medications in Acute Care Settings

High-alert medications are drugs that bear a heightened risk of causing significant patient harm when they are used in error. Although mistakes may or may not be more common with these drugs, the consequences of an error are clearly more devastating to patients. We hope you will use this list to determine which medications require special safeguards to reduce the risk of errors. This may include strategies such as standardizing the ordering, storage, preparation, and administration of these products; improving access to information about these drugs; limiting access to high-alert medications; using auxiliary labels and automated alerts; and employing redundancies such as automated or independent double-checks when necessary. (Note: Manual independent double-checks are not always the optimal error-reduction strategy and may not be practical for all of the medications on the list.)

Classes/Categories of Medications
adrenergic agonists, IV (e.g., **EPINEPH**rine, phenylephrine, norepinephrine)
adrenergic antagonists, IV (e.g., propranolol, metoprolol, labetalol)
anesthetic agents, general, inhaled and IV (e.g., propofol, ketamine)
antiarrhythmics, IV (e.g., lidocaine, amiodarone)
antithrombotic agents, including: • anticoagulants (e.g., warfarin, low molecular weight heparin, IV unfractionated heparin)   • Factor Xa inhibitors (e.g., fondaparinux, apixaban, rivaroxaban)   • direct thrombin inhibitors (e.g., argatroban, bivalirudin, dabigatran etexilate)   • thrombolytics (e.g., alteplase, reteplase, tenecteplase)   • glycoprotein IIb/IIIa inhibitors (e.g., eptifibatide)
cardioplegic solutions
chemotherapeutic agents, parenteral and oral
dextrose, hypertonic, 20% or greater
dialysis solutions, peritoneal and hemodialysis
epidural or intrathecal medications
hypoglycemics, oral
inotropic medications, IV (e.g., digoxin, milrinone)
insulin, subcutaneous and IV
liposomal forms of drugs (e.g., liposomal amphotericin B) and conventional counterparts (e.g., amphotericin B desoxycholate)
moderate sedation agents, IV (e.g., dexmedetomidine, midazolam)
moderate sedation agents, oral, for children (e.g., chloral hydrate)
narcotics/opioids   • IV   • transdermal   • oral (including liquid concentrates, immediate and sustained-release formulations)
neuromuscular blocking agents (e.g., succinylcholine, rocuronium, vecuronium)
parenteral nutrition preparations
radiocontrast agents, IV
sterile water for injection, inhalation, and irrigation (excluding pour bottles) in containers of 100 mL or more
sodium chloride for injection, hypertonic, greater than 0.9% concentration

Specific Medications
EPINEPHrine, subcutaneous
epoprostenol (Flolan), IV
insulin U-500 (special emphasis)*
magnesium sulfate injection
methotrexate, oral, non-oncologic use
opium tincture
oxytocin, IV
nitroprusside sodium for injection
potassium chloride for injection concentrate
potassium phosphates injection
promethazine, IV
vasopressin, IV or intraosseous

*All forms of insulin, subcutaneous and IV, are considered a class of high-alert medications. Insulin U-500 has been singled out for special emphasis to bring attention to the need for distinct strategies to prevent the types of errors that occur with this concentrated form of insulin.

Background

Based on error reports submitted to the ISMP National Medication Errors Reporting Program, reports of harmful errors in the literature, studies that identify the drugs most often involved in harmful errors, and input from practitioners and safety experts, ISMP created and periodically updates a list of potential high-alert medications. During May and June 2014, practitioners responded to an ISMP survey designed to identify which medications were most frequently considered high-alert drugs by individuals and organizations. Further, to assure relevance and completeness, the clinical staff at ISMP, members of the ISMP advisory board, and safety experts throughout the US were asked to review the potential list. This list of drugs and drug categories reflects the collective thinking of all who provided input.

Glossary

A

Abortifacients drugs used to induce abortion

Absence seizures seizures with a loss or reduction of normal activity, including staring and transient loss of responsiveness

Absorption the process by which drug molecules move from their site of administration to the blood; movement of nutrients and other substances from the alimentary canal to the circulation

Accessory organs of digestion include the salivary glands, liver, gallbladder, and pancreas

Acetylation a general biochemical process that adds a two-carbon chain to a drug molecule, which usually renders the drug less effective

Acetylcholine (Ach) primary neurotransmitter of the autonomic nervous system

Acetylcholinesterase (AchE) enzyme that resides in the synaptic cleft and catalyzes the destruction of Ach

Acetylcholinesterase (AchE) inhibitors indirect-acting cholinergic agonists that are nonselective and affect all Ach synapses

Acidosis condition of having too much acid in the blood; plasma pH below 7.35

Acne vulgaris disorder of the hair follicles and sebaceous glands characterized by small inflamed bumps that appear on the surface of the skin

Acquired immunodeficiency syndrome (AIDS) infection caused by the human immunodeficiency virus (HIV)

Acquired resistance ability of an organism to become unresponsive over time to the effects of an anti-infective

Acromegaly excessive growth hormone disorder in which bones become deformed

Activated partial thromboplastin time (aPTT) laboratory test used to measure blood coagulation

Active immunity resistance resulting from a previous exposure to an antigen

Acute dystonia occurs during early pharmacotherapy with antipsychotics and involves severe muscle spasms, particularly of the back, neck, tongue, and face

Acute gouty arthritis condition in which uric acid crystals accumulate in the joints of the big toes, ankles, wrists, fingers, knees, or elbows, resulting in extremely painful and red, inflamed tissue

Acute retroviral syndrome symptoms during the initial phase of HIV infection

Adaptive defenses defenses that are specific to certain threats; the immune response

Addiction the continued use of a substance despite serious health and social consequences

Addison's disease hyposecretion of glucocorticoids and mineralocorticoids by the adrenal cortex

Additive effect type of drug interaction in which two agents combine to produce a summation response

Adherence taking medications in the manner prescribed by the health care provider, or in the case of OTC drugs, following the instructions on the label or as provided by the prescriber; also called compliance

Adhesins chemicals produced by *H. pylori* that allow the organism to penetrate the GI mucosa and cause inflammation

Adipocytes fat cells

Adjuvant analgesics drugs that have indications other than pain but are used to enhance analgesia

Adjuvant chemotherapy administration of antineoplastic drugs *after* surgery or radiation therapy

Adrenal atrophy condition in which the adrenal cortex shrinks and stops secreting endogenous corticosteroids due to lack of stimulation by adrenocorticotropic hormone (ACTH)

Adrenal crisis condition that occurs when corticosteroid medication is abruptly withdrawn

Adrenergic receptors at the ends of postganglionic sympathetic neurons

Adrenergic agonists agents that activate adrenergic receptors in the sympathetic nervous system; also known as sympathomimetics

Adrenergic antagonists drugs that block norepinephrine from reaching its receptors

Adrenocortical insufficiency lack of adequate corticosteroid secretion by the adrenal cortex

Adrenocorticotropic hormone (ACTH) hormone secreted by the anterior pituitary that stimulates the release of glucocorticoids by the adrenal cortex

Adverse drug effect an undesirable and potentially harmful action caused by the administration of medication

Adverse event reporting system (FAERS) voluntary program that encourages health care providers and consumers to report suspected adverse effects directly to the FDA or the product manufacturer

Aerobic pertaining to an oxygen environment

Aerosol suspension of minute liquid droplets or fine solid particles in a gas

Affinity the ability of some tissues to attract, accumulate, and store drugs in high concentrations relative to other tissues

Afterload pressure in the aorta that must be overcome for blood to be ejected from the left ventricle

Agonist drug that activates a receptor and produces the same type of response as the endogenous substance

Agoraphobia an extreme avoidance of closed places where a panic attack might occur such as airplanes, public meetings, or elevators

Akathisia inability to rest or relax; constantly moving

Alimentary canal a long, continuous, hollow tube that extends from the mouth to the anus; the GI tract

Alkalosis plasma pH above 7.45

Alkylating agents agents that kill cancer cells by altering the shape of the DNA double helix and preventing the DNA from duplicating during cell division

Allergen anything that is recognized as foreign by the body's defense system; also called antigen

Allergic rhinitis inflammation of the nasal mucosa due to exposure to allergens

Alopecia hair loss

Alpha-adrenergic antagonists drugs that block alpha-adrenergic receptors in the sympathetic nervous system

Alzheimer's disease (AD) neurodegenerative disease that involves a chronic progressive loss of cognitive function

Amide local anesthetic that has the same mechanism of action as esters but has less effect on myocardial contraction and lower allergic reaction

Amygdala a key part of the limbic system that helps determine the emotional significance of the conscious or unconscious signals received from the cerebral cortex

Anabolic effects testosterone hormone's ability to accelerate the growth of RBCs, muscle, bone, and neural tissues

Anabolic steroids testosterone-like substances with hormonal activity that are commonly abused by athletes

Anaerobic pertaining to an environment without oxygen

Analgesics drugs used to relieve pain

Anaphylaxis life-threatening allergic response that may cause cardiovascular shock and death

Androgens steroid sex hormones that promote the appearance of masculine characteristics

Anemia decreased oxygen-carrying capacity of the blood

Angina pectoris acute chest pain caused by myocardial ischemia

Angioedema rapid swelling of the throat, face, larynx, and tongue that can lead to airway obstruction and death

Angiogenesis the formation of new blood vessels

Angiotensin I a precursor to the formation of angiotensin II that is produced when angiotensinogen is split by the enzyme renin

Angiotensin II vasopressor substance released in response to falling blood pressure that causes vasoconstriction and release of aldosterone

Angiotensin-converting enzyme (ACE) inhibitor enzyme that blocks the formation of angiotensin II, decreasing blood pressure

Angiotensinogen protein synthesized by the liver that is continuously circulating in the bloodstream

Anorexiants drugs used to suppress appetite

Anovulatory cycles menstrual cycles without ovulation

Antacids inorganic compounds containing aluminum, magnesium, sodium, or calcium that neutralize gastric acid and inactivate pepsin

Antagonist agent that blocks the response of another drug

Antagonistic effect type of drug interaction in which adding a second drug results in a diminished pharmacologic response

Anterior pituitary gland (adenohypophysis) consists of glandular tissue that manufactures and secretes hormones that control major body functions and systems

Anterograde amnesia type of short-term memory loss where the user cannot remember events that occurred while under the influence of a drug

Anthrax an acute infectious disease that results from exposure to the spore-forming bacterium *Bacillus anthracis*

Antibiotic natural substance produced by a microorganism that can kill other microorganisms

Antibodies proteins produced by the body in response to an antigen; used interchangeably with the term *immunoglobulin*

Anticholinergic syndrome symptoms such as dry mouth, blurred vision, photophobia, visual changes, difficulty swallowing, agitation, and hallucinations, caused by an overdose of anticholinergic substances

Anticoagulants natural substances that inhibit the formation of blood clots

Antidepressants drugs used to enhance, elevate, or stabilize mood

Antidiuretic hormone (ADH) hormone released by the posterior pituitary gland when blood pressure falls or when the osmotic pressure of the blood increases; most important means the body uses to maintain fluid homeostasis

Antiflatulent agent that reduces gas

Antigens microbes and foreign substances that elicit an immune response

Anti-infective general term for any medication that is effective against pathogens

Antipyretics medications used to reduce body temperature

Antiretrovirals drugs that are effective against retroviruses

Antithrombin III (AT-III) protein that prevents abnormal clotting by inhibiting thrombin and other clotting factors

Antitussives medications that control cough

Anxiety state of apprehension, tension, or uneasiness that stems from the anticipation of danger, the source of which is largely unknown or unrecognized

Anxiolytic drugs that relieve anxiety

Apoprotein protein component of a lipoprotein

Apothecary system of measurement older system of measurement developed in ancient Greece; rarely used in modern medicine

Appetite a psychological response that drives food intake based on associations and memory

Aqueous humor fluid that fills the anterior and posterior chambers of the eye

Assessment appraisal of a patient's condition that involves gathering and interpreting subjective and objective data

Asthma chronic inflammatory disease of the lungs characterized by airway obstruction

Atherosclerosis condition characterized by the presence of plaque within the walls of arteries

Atonic seizures very short-lasting seizures during which the patient may stumble and fall for no apparent reason

Atrial natriuretic peptide (ANP) hormone secreted by specialized cells in the right atrium when large increases in blood volume produce excessive stretch on the atrial wall

Atrial reflex causes the heart rate and CO to increase until the backlog of venous blood (or IV fluid) is distributed throughout the body

Attention deficit/hyperactivity disorder (ADHD) disorder typically diagnosed in childhood characterized by hyperactivity as well as attention, organization, and behavior control issues

Attenuated organisms that have been rendered less able to cause disease through the application of heat or chemicals from which effective vaccines can be developed

Atypical antidepressants diverse class of drugs that act by mechanisms other than those of the selective serotonin reuptake inhibitors (SSRIs), tricyclic antidepressants, and monoamine oxidase inhibitors

Atypical mycobacterial infections (AMIs) nontuberculosis opportunistic diseases caused by mycobacteria

Auras sensory warnings such as flashing lights, visual blind spots, and arm or leg tingling that precede a migraine

Automaticity ability of certain myocardial cells to spontaneously generate an action potential without an outside signal from the nervous system

Automatisms repetitive arm movements, leg movements, head rolling, chewing, lip smacking, or swallowing that occur in complex partial seizures

Autonomic nervous system (ANS) portion of the peripheral nervous system that provides for the involuntary control of vital functions of the cardiovascular, digestive, respiratory, and genitourinary systems

Autonomic tone the background level of autonomic activity that occurs even in the absence of stimuli

Azole term for the major class of drugs used to treat mycoses

Azoospermia complete absence of sperm in an ejaculate

B

B cell lymphocyte responsible for humoral immunity

β-glucan an essential component that shapes and strengthens the cell walls of fungi

Bacteriocidal drug that kills bacteria

Bacteriostatic drug that inhibits the growth of bacteria

Bacteriuria uropathogens

Balanced anesthesia use of multiple medications to produce general anesthesia, provide sedation, rapid induction of unconsciousness, muscle relaxation, and analgesia

Baroreceptors receptors in the aorta and carotid artery that sense changes in blood pressure

Barrett's esophagus precancerous condition of the esophagus

Basal nuclei area of the brain responsible for starting and stopping synchronized motor activity such as leg and arm motions during walking; also called basal ganglia

Baseline data data gathered during the initial assessment that is compared with data gathered during later interactions

Beers criteria list of drugs compiled by the American Geriatrics Society that have produced a high incidence of adverse effects in older adults

Belladonna natural source of alkaloids with anticholinergic activity acquired from the deadly nightshade plant, *Atropa belladonna*, which grows throughout the world

Benign prostatic hyperplasia (BPH) nonmalignant abnormal enlargement of the prostate gland

Best Pharmaceuticals for Children Act authorizes the FDA to contract for the testing of already approved pediatric drugs, or when the pharmaceutical company declines the option of exclusivity

Beta-adrenergic antagonists drugs that block beta-adrenergic receptors; may be nonselective or selective; also called beta blockers

Beta-lactamase enzyme produced by certain bacteria that are able to render certain antibiotics ineffective

Beta-lactam ring portion of the chemical structure of penicillin and some other antibiotics that is responsible for their antibacterial activity

Bioavailability the rate and extent to which the active ingredient is absorbed from a drug product and becomes available at the site of drug action to produce its effect

Biologic response modifiers natural cytokines that boost specific functions of the immune system

Bioterrorism intentional release of an infectious agent for the purpose of causing harm to a large number of people

Bipolar disorder syndrome characterized by extreme and opposite moods, such as euphoria and depression

Bisphosphonates class of drugs for treating osteoporosis that inhibit bone resorption by suppressing osteoclast activity

Black box warning in some drug inserts, a requirement by the FDA that warns prescribers that the drug carries a risk for serious or fatal adverse effects

Blood–brain barrier network of capillaries in the CNS that inhibits many chemicals and drugs from gaining access to the brain

Body mass index (BMI) measurement of obesity determined by dividing body weight (in kilograms) by the square of height (in meters)

Body surface area (BSA) method method of calculating pediatric dosages using an estimate of the child's BSA

Body weight method method of calculating pediatric dosages that requires a calculation of the number of milligrams of drug, based on the child's weight in kilograms (mg/kg)

Bolus feedings method of enteral feeding that typically delivers 250 to 400 mL of formula every 4 to 6 hours via a syringe or funnel

Bone deposition opposite of bone resorption; bone building

Bone resorption process of bone demineralization or the breaking down of bone into mineral components

Boosters follow-up doses of vaccines that are required to provide prolonged protection

Botanical plant extract used to treat or prevent illness

Botulism condition caused by *Clostridium botulinum*, an organism that secretes a potent toxin that paralyzes the muscles after a person is poisoned

Bradydysrhythmias disorders characterized by a heart rate of less than 60 beats/minute

Bradykinesia difficulty initiating movement and controlling fine muscle movements

Bradykinin chemical released by cells during inflammation that produces pain and side effects similar to those of histamine

Broad-spectrum antibiotic an anti-infective that is effective against a wide variety of different microbial species

Bronchospasm sudden contraction of the smooth muscle of the airways that causes acute dyspnea

Buffers chemicals that help maintain normal body pH by neutralizing strong acids or bases

C

Cachexia general wasting of muscle and other tissue

Calcineurin intracellular messenger enzyme that is activated when a T cell encounters an antigen

Calcitonin hormone secreted by the thyroid gland that decreases plasma levels of calcium by inhibiting resorption of calcium from bone and increasing excretion of calcium by the kidneys

Calcitriol the active form of vitamin D

Calcium channel type of voltage-gated channel in cardiac muscle and smooth muscles

Cancer malignant disease characterized by abnormal, uncontrolled cell division

Capillary leak syndrome a serious condition in which plasma proteins and other substances leave the blood and enter the interstitial spaces because of porous capillaries

Capsid protein coat that surrounds a virus

Carbonic anhydrase enzyme that forms carbonic acid by combining carbon dioxide and water

Carcinogens agents that cause cancer

Cardiac output (CO) amount of blood pumped by a ventricle per minute

Cardiac remodeling change in the size, shape, and structure of the myocardial cells (myocytes) that occurs over time in heart failure

Cardiotonic drugs agents that increase the force of cardiac contraction; also called inotropic agents

Cardioversion electrical shock of the heart that under ideal conditions will allow the return to a normal heart rhythm; also called defibrillation

Cataplexy sudden loss of muscle strength manifested as slurred speech, sagging of the jaw, head nodding, or even complete collapse of the body

Catecholamine class of endogenous hormones involved in neurotransmission that include epinephrine (adrenalin), norepinephrine, and dopamine

Catechol-O-methyltransferase (COMT) enzyme that destroys catecholamines such as norepinephrine in kidney and liver cells

Cathartic substance that causes accelerated, stronger, and more complete bowel emptying

CD4 receptor protein that accepts HIV and allows entry of the virus into the T_4 lymphocyte

Cell-kill hypothesis theoretical model that predicts the ability of antineoplastic drugs to eliminate cancer cells

Central nervous system (CNS) stimulants agents that raise the general alertness level of the brain

Central vein total parenteral nutrition the administration of enteral feeding solution through a central vein

Cerumenolytics agents used to loosen and remove impacted cerumen from the ear canal

Chelation therapy use of agents to detoxify poisonous metals such as mercury, arsenic, and lead by converting them to a chemically inert form that can be easily excreted

Chemical names standard nomenclature for drugs assigned by the International Union of Pure and Applied Chemistry (IUPAC)

Chemoreceptors sensory receptors in the aorta and carotid artery that recognize levels of oxygen, pH, or carbon dioxide in the blood

Chemoreceptor trigger zone (CTZ) location in the cerebral cortex that sends sensory signals to the vomiting center

Chemotherapy pharmacotherapy of cancer

Chief cells cells located in the mucosa of the stomach that secrete pepsinogen, an inactive form of the enzyme pepsin that chemically breaks down proteins

Chloasma darkened pigmentation found on the forehead, temples, cheeks, and upper lips

Cholecalciferol inactive form of vitamin D

Cholestatic hepatitis type of liver inflammation caused by obstruction of the bile ducts

Cholinergic relating to neurons that release acetylcholine (Ach)

Cholinergic agonists drugs and chemicals that increase the action of acetylcholine (Ach) at a cholinergic receptor; also called parasympathomimetics

Cholinergic crisis caused by an overdosage with acetylcholinesterase (AchE) inhibitors or poisoning with organophosphate insecticides or toxic nerve gases; characterized by intense signs of parasympathetic stimulation such as miosis, nausea, vomiting, urinary incontinence, increased exocrine secretions, abdominal cramping, and diarrhea

Cholinesterase inhibitors the most widely prescribed drug class for treating Alzheimer's disease

Chronic bronchitis recurrent disease of the lungs characterized by excess mucus production, inflammation, and coughing

Chronic obstructive pulmonary disease (COPD) progressive pulmonary disorder characterized by chronic obstructive airflow

Chyme partly digested food that is passed from the stomach to the small intestine

Cinchonism syndrome with symptoms such as tinnitus, headache, diarrhea, blurred vision, hearing loss, and dysrhythmias, caused by high doses of quinidine

Circadian rhythm cyclic basis by which body temperature, blood pressure, hormone levels, and respiration all fluctuate throughout the 24-hour day

Climacteric the period of endocrine, somatic, and psychological changes occurring in the transition to menopause

Clinical phase trials the second stage of drug testing in a clinical investigation; involves the testing of a new drug in selected patients

Closed-angle glaucoma acute glaucoma that is caused by obstruction of drainage of aqueous humor through the canal of Schlemm

Club drug a diverse group of abused substances taken by people at dance clubs, all-night parties, and raves

Coagulation formation of an insoluble clot

Colloids proteins, starches, or other large molecules that remain in the blood for a long time because they are too large to easily cross the capillary membranes

Colony-stimulating factors (CSFs) hormones that activate existing white blood cells to fight an infection and stimulate the growth and differentiation of one or more types of leukocytes

Combination drugs drug products with more than one active generic ingredient

Comedolytics drugs that prevent and break up the formation of clogged pores

Comedones types of acne lesions that develop just beneath the surface of the skin (whitehead) or as a result of a plugged oil gland (blackhead)

Complement system a cluster of 20 plasma proteins that combine in a specific sequence and order when an infection occurs

Complementary and alternative medicine (CAM) diverse set of therapies and healing systems that are considered to be outside of mainstream health care

Complex partial seizures seizures that originate from a single focus, usually in the temporal lobe of the brain, and involve sensory, motor, or autonomic symptoms with some degree of altered or impaired consciousness

COMT inhibitors drugs that prevent the destruction of catechol-O-methyltransferase (COMT) in peripheral tissues, thus increasing the amount of levodopa available to enter the brain

Conjugation the direct transfer of small pieces of DNA from one bacterium to another

Constipation infrequent passage of abnormally hard and dry stools

Continuous infusion feedings enteral feedings delivered by an infusion pump at a slow rate over a 16- to 24-hour period

Contraception the use of devices, drugs, or surgery to prevent pregnancy

Contractility the strength with which the myocardial fibers contract

Controlled substance in the United States, a drug whose use is restricted by the Comprehensive Drug Abuse Prevention and Control Act

Convulsions involuntary violent spasms of the face, neck, arms, and legs

Coronary artery disease (CAD) a narrowing or occlusion of one or more coronary arteries

Corpora cavernosa tissue in the penis that fills with blood during an erection

Corpus luteum endocrine tissue formed from a ruptured follicle that remains in the ovary after ovulation and secretes progesterone

Council for Responsible Nutrition (CRN) trade association representing ingredient suppliers and manufacturers in the dietary supplement industry

Cretinism condition marked by profound mental retardation and impaired growth that results from untreated congenital hypothyroidism

Cross-tolerance situation in which tolerance to one drug makes the patient tolerant to another drug

Crystalloids IV solutions that contain electrolytes and other agents in concentrations that mimic the body's extracellular fluid

Crystalluria crystals that form in the urine and potentially obstruct the kidneys or ureters

Culture set of beliefs, values, religious rituals, language, customs, and behavioral expectations that provide meaning for an individual or group

Culture and sensitivity (C&S) testing a laboratory test used to identify bacteria and the most effective antibiotic

Curare the first neuromuscular blocker, which was initially extracted from several different plant species native to the rain forests of South America

Cushing's syndrome condition of high levels of corticosteroids in the body over a prolonged period of time

Cyclic feedings enteral feedings that are commonly infused over 8 to 16 hours daily (day or night)

Cyclooxygenase (COX) key enzyme in the synthesis of prostaglandin that is blocked by aspirin and other NSAIDs

Cycloplegics drugs that relax or temporarily paralyze ciliary muscles and cause blurred vision

Cystitis bladder infection

Cysts protective capsules formed by some protozoa that allow the organisms to survive in harsh environments in a dormant state for prolonged time periods

Cytokine release syndrome an acute inflammatory response that occurs 30 to 60 minutes following the initial IV administration of muromonab due to massive cytokine release

Cytokines proteins produced by T cells, such as interleukins, leukotrienes, interferon, and tumor necrosis factor, that guide the immune response

D

Deep venous thrombosis (DVT) thrombosis that occurs in the legs

Defecation elimination of the indigestible substances from the body

Defibrillation electrical shock of the heart that under ideal conditions will allow the return to a normal heart rhythm; also called cardioversion

Delirium tremens a syndrome of intense agitation, confusion, terrifying hallucinations, uncontrollable tremors, panic attacks, and paranoia caused by alcohol withdrawal

Delusions false ideas and beliefs not founded in reality

Dementia degenerative disorder characterized by progressive memory loss, confusion, and the inability to think or communicate effectively

Dependence a powerful physiological or psychological need for a substance

Depolarization loss of membrane potential in a cell

Depression characterized by a sad or despondent mood that becomes out of proportion to actual life events

Dermatitis superficial inflammatory disorders of the skin characterized by redness, pain, and pruritus

Dermatomycosis fungal infections of the skin and hair

Diabetes insipidus (DI) disorder marked by production of large volumes of urine, usually accompanied by increased thirst

Diabetes mellitus metabolic disorder characterized by an imbalance between insulin availability and insulin need

Diabetic ketoacidosis (DKA) acute condition that occurs primarily in patients with type 1 diabetes characterized by hyperglycemia, metabolic acidosis, and osmotic diuresis

Diarrhea increase in the frequency and fluidity of bowel movements

Dietary Supplement and Nonprescription Drug Consumer Protection Act law that requires companies that market herbal and dietary supplements to include their address and phone number on the product labels so consumers can report adverse events

Dietary Supplement Health and Education Act of 1994 (DSHEA) primary law in the United States regulating herbal and dietary supplements

Dietary supplements nondrug substances regulated by the DSHEA

Diffusion the movement of a chemical from an area of higher concentration to an area of lower concentration

Digestion the mechanical and chemical breakdown of food into a form that may be absorbed into the systemic circulation

Digestive system body system consisting of the alimentary canal and the accessory organs

Digitalization procedure in which the dose of digoxin is gradually increased until tissues become saturated with the drug, and the symptoms of heart failure diminish

Dihydropyridines the largest class of CCBs that bind reversibly to closed-type (inactivated) calcium channels to make them unresponsive to depolarization

Directly observed therapy (DOT) requires that a health care provider directly observe the patient swallowing the pills, whether it is in the hospital, office, or home care setting

Disease-modifying antirheumatic drugs (DMARDs) drugs that slow or modify the progression of rheumatoid arthritis

Dissociative anesthesia a trance-like feeling of being separated from the environment produced by an anesthetic agent

Distribution the transport of drugs throughout the body after they are absorbed

Diuretic substance that increases the rate of urine flow

Diuretic resistance phenomenon in some patients who become less responsive as therapy continues with loop diuretics

DNA gyrase (topoisomerase II) in bacterial DNA replication, the enzyme that relaxes the supercoil

DNA helicase in bacterial DNA replication, the enzyme that unwinds the two DNA strands after the supercoil is relaxed

DNA polymerase in bacterial DNA replication, the enzyme that adds the precursor bases to replicate the original DNA and form new DNA strands

Dopamine chemical precursor in the synthesis of norepinephrine; classified as a catecholamine

Dopamine system stabilizers (DSSs) drugs that exhibit both antagonist and partial agonist activities on dopamine receptors

Dopamine type 2 (D_2) receptors receptors for dopamine in the basal nuclei of the brain that are associated with schizophrenia and anti-psychotic drugs

Dose–response relationship the way a patient responds to varying doses of a drug

Down-regulation the process by which cells make fewer receptors on their surface

Drug any substance that is taken to prevent, cure, or reduce symptoms of a medical condition

Drug allergies a hyperresponse of body defenses to a particular drug that may result in a diverse range of patient symptoms

Drug interaction occurs when a medication interacts with another substance such as another drug, a dietary supplement, an herbal product, or food that is taken concurrently with the medication, and the drug's actions are affected

Drug misuse improper use of drugs that includes overuse, underuse, or, in some cases, erratic use

Drug–protein complexes formed when a drug that binds reversibly to a plasma protein, particularly albumin, that makes the drug unavailable for distribution to its site of action

Dry powder inhaler (DPI) device used to convert a solid drug to a fine powder for the purpose of inhalation

Dumping syndrome the result of a sudden influx of enteral feeding into the GI tract and the creation of a high osmotic gradient within the small intestine

Dwarfism a growth hormone deficiency disorder in children associated with normal birth length followed by a slowing of the growth rate

Dysfunctional uterine bleeding hemorrhage that occurs on a noncyclic basis or in abnormal amounts

Dyslipidemia abnormal (excess or deficient) level of lipoproteins in the blood

Dysrhythmias disorders of cardiac rhythm characterized by an abnormal heart rate or irregular contractions

Dystonia chronic neurologic disorder that is characterized by involuntary muscle contraction that forces body parts into abnormal painful movements or postures

E

Eclampsia pregnancy-induced hypertensive disorder

Ectopic foci regions of the heart outside the normal cardiac conduction pathway that may send impulses across the myocardium

Ectopic pregnancy the development of the fetus elsewhere rather than in the uterus

Eczema chronic, inflammatory skin disorder

Efficacy the maximal response that can be produced from a particular drug

Electrocardiogram (ECG) graphic recording of the wave of electrical conduction across the myocardium

Electroconvulsive therapy (ECT) treatment used for serious and life-threatening mood disorders in patients who are unresponsive to pharmacotherapy and psychotherapy

Electrolyte charged substance in the blood such as sodium, potassium, calcium, chloride, and phosphate

Elemental (monomeric) formulas enteral products that are usually lactose free and contain only a small percentage of calories from fat

Emergency contraception (EC) the prevention of implantation following unprotected intercourse or contraceptive failure

Emergency preparedness the ability to respond quickly and effectively to an unexpected event that may impact human health

Emetic potential usually applied to antineoplastic agents; degree to which an agent is likely to trigger the vomiting center in the medulla, resulting in nausea and vomiting

Emetogenic potential the capacity of a chemotherapeutic drug to cause vomiting

Emphysema lung disease characterized by loss of bronchiolar elasticity and destruction of alveolar walls

Endocrine system body system that consists of various glands that secrete hormones

Endometriosis presence of endometrial tissue in nonuterine locations such as the pelvis and ovaries; a common cause of infertility

Endorphins a group of neurotransmitters that function as endogenous opioids or natural pain modifiers in the CNS

Endotoxins harmful nonproteins that are part of the normal cell wall of gram-negative bacteria

Enteral nutrition (EN) nutritional support used for patients with functioning GI tracts but who are unable to orally ingest adequate amounts of nutrients to meet their metabolic needs

Enteral route administration of drugs orally or through nasogastric or gastrostomy tubes

Enteric-coated tablets that have a hard, waxy coating designed to dissolve in the alkaline environment of the small intestine

Enteric nervous system (ENS) network of neurons in the submucosa of the alimentary canal that has sensory and motor functions that regulate the GI tract

Enteroendocrine cells cells that secrete hormones that modify the digestive processes

Enterohepatic recirculation recycling of drugs and other substances by the circulation of bile through the intestine and liver

Enzyme induction process by which a drug increases the activity of the hepatic microsomal enzymes

Epilepsy disruption of the activity of clusters of neurons in the brain that is characterized by two or more seizures

Erectile dysfunction (ED) consistent inability to either attain an erection or to sustain an erection long enough to achieve satisfactory sexual intercourse

Ergosterol lipid substance in fungal cell membranes

Erythema redness associated with skin irritation

Erythrocytic stage phase in malaria during which infected red blood cells rupture, releasing more merozoites and causing acute symptoms

Erythropoietin hormone secreted by the kidney that stimulates the body's production of erythrocytes (red blood cells)

Esters local anesthetics that act by decreasing the amount of sodium that enters the neuron

Estrogen general term that refers to several female sex hormones

Ethnicity groups of people with biologic and genetic similarities

Euphoria an intense sense of happiness and well-being

Evaluation systematic objective assessment of the effectiveness and impact of interventions

Evaluation criteria specific and measurable achievements that will be used to determine if a particular goal has been met

Evidence-based practice use of research, observations, nursing practice, and clinical judgment to determine care

Exclusivity after approval of a drug application by the U.S. Food and Drug Administration, a period of time when competing companies are not allowed to market generic versions of a drug

Excoriation scratches that break the skin surface and fill with blood or serous fluid to form crusty scales

Excretion the process of removing substances from the body

Exophthalmos an outward bulging of the eyes

Exotoxins proteins released by bacteria into surrounding tissues that have the ability to inactivate or kill host cells

Expectorants drugs used to increase bronchial secretions

Expiration date approximation of when a drug will begin to lose its effectiveness

Extended release tablets or capsules designed to dissolve very slowly, resulting in a longer duration of action for the medication; also called long-acting sustained release

External otitis an inflammation of the outer ear; commonly called swimmer's ear

Extracellular fluid (ECF) compartment of body fluid lying outside cells, which includes plasma and interstitial fluid

Extrapyramidal symptoms (EPS) symptoms of acute dystonia, akathisia, parkinsonism, and tardive dyskinesia often caused by antipsychotic drugs

Extrapyramidal system part of the CNS that controls locomotion, complex muscular movements, and posture

Extrinsic pathway activated in response to injury when blood leaks out of a vessel and enters tissue spaces; the pathway takes several seconds to complete

F

Fasting plasma glucose (FPG) test a primary blood test for diagnosing diabetes

Fat-soluble vitamins group of vitamins stored in the liver and fatty tissue that includes A, D, E, and K

Febrile seizures tonic–clonic motor activity lasting 1 to 2 minutes with rapid return of consciousness that occurs in conjunction with fever

Ferritin one of two protein complexes that maintain iron stores inside cells (hemosiderin is the other)

Fetal–placental barrier special anatomic barrier that inhibits many chemicals and drugs from entering the fetus

Fibrin an insoluble protein formed from fibrinogen by the action of thrombin in the blood clotting process

Fibrinogen blood protein that is converted to fibrin by the action of thrombin in the blood coagulation process

Fibrinolysis physiological process that limits clot formation and removes existing clots

Fight-or-flight response characteristic set of actions produced when the sympathetic nervous system is activated that prepares the body for heightened activity and for an immediate response to a threat

Filtrate fluid in the nephron that is filtered into the Bowman's capsule

First-dose phenomenon serious orthostatic hypotension that occurs with the initial doses of alpha$_1$-adrenergic blockers

First-pass effect mechanism whereby drugs are absorbed, enter into the hepatic portal circulation, and are inactivated by the liver before they reach the general circulation

Folic acid B vitamin that is essential for normal DNA and RNA synthesis; also called folate

Food and Drug Administration (FDA) U.S. agency responsible for the evaluation and approval of new drugs

Food and Drug Administration (FDA) Modernization Act act that gave financial incentives to pharmaceutical companies to conduct pediatric research in pharmacology; in exchange for providing pediatric labeling, the legislation gives drug companies the ability to exclusively market the drug for an additional 6 months with no competition

Formulary list of drug and drug recipes commonly used by pharmacists

Frequency distribution curve a graphic representation of the actual number of patients responding to a particular drug action at different doses

Fungi kingdom of organisms that includes mushrooms, yeasts, and molds

G

Gamma aminobutyric acid (GABA) neurotransmitter in the CNS

Ganglia collection of neuron cell bodies located outside the central nervous system

Ganglionic blockers drugs that inhibit transmission at the ganglia in the sympathetic and parasympathetic nervous systems

Gastroesophageal reflux disease (GERD) regurgitation of acidic stomach contents into the esophagus

Gate control theory proposes a gating mechanism for the transmission of pain in the spinal cord

General anesthesia medical procedure that produces unconsciousness and loss of sensation throughout the entire body

Generalized anxiety disorder (GAD) difficult-to-control, excessive anxiety that lasts for 6 months or longer

Generalized seizures seizures that travel throughout the entire brain

Generic name name assigned to a drug by the U.S. Adopted Name Council

Genetic polymorphism changes in enzyme structure and function due to mutation of the encoding gene

Gestational diabetes condition resulting from glucose intolerance with an onset, or first recognition, during pregnancy

Gigantism unusual tallness

Glaucoma condition that is characterized by optic neuropathy with gradual loss of peripheral vision and usually accompanied by increased intraocular pressure

Glomerular filtration rate (GFR) the volume of water filtered through the Bowman's capsules per minute

Glomerulus a specialized capillary in the Bowman's capsule of the kidney that filters the blood during urine formation

Glucocorticoids class of hormones secreted by the adrenal cortex that prepare the body for long-term stress; also called corticosteroids

Gluconeogenesis the production of new glucose from noncarbohydrate molecules

Glutamate amino acid that is the most common neurotransmitter in the CNS

Glycogenolysis the process of glycogen breaking down

Glycoprotein IIb/IIIa receptor found on the surface of platelets

Goal what the patient should be able to achieve and do, based on the problem or nursing diagnosis established from the assessment data

Goiter refers to an increase in the size of the thyroid gland

Gonadocorticoids sex hormones secreted by the adrenal cortex

Gout form of acute arthritis caused by an accumulation of uric acid (urate) crystals in the joints and other body tissues

Grading process that examines potential cancer cells under a microscope and compares their appearance to normal parent cells

Gram-negative bacteria that do not retain a purple stain because they have thinner cell walls

Gram-positive bacteria that contain a thick cell wall composed of peptidoglycan and retain the violet color after staining

Graves' disease syndrome caused by hypersecretion of thyroid hormone

Gray baby syndrome serious condition seen most often in premature or newborn infants that occurs when the baby's liver is unable to metabolize or excrete chloramphenicol

Growth fraction the ratio of the number of replicating cells to resting cells in a tissue or tumor

Growth hormone (GH) hormone that is produced and secreted by the anterior pituitary gland; also called somatotropin or somatropin

H

H⁺, K⁺-ATPase enzyme secreting hydrochloride acid in the stomach

H₁ receptors histamine receptors that, when activated, produce allergy symptoms

H₂-receptor antagonists drugs that suppress gastric acid by blocking histamine receptors in the stomach

Hallucinations seeing, hearing, or feeling things that are not there

Hallucinogens chemicals that have the ability to produce an altered, dreamlike state of consciousness

Hashimoto's thyroiditis an autoimmune disorder that is the most common cause of hypothyroidism

Health care-associated infections (HAIs) infections acquired in a health care setting that are often resistant to common antibiotics

Health care failure mode and effect analysis (HFMEA) a tool that helps health care agencies identify processes where errors may occur related to prescription, dispensing, and administration

Heart failure (HF) inability of the heart to pump enough blood to meet the body's metabolic needs

Helminths various species of multicell parasitic worms

Hemagglutinin an enzyme that facilitates the attachment of the virus to host cells

Hematopoiesis production and maturation of blood cells that occurs in red bone marrow; also called hemopoiesis

Hematopoietic growth factors drugs that promote the formation of specific blood cells and enhance the ability of the immune system to reduce some of the myelosuppression caused by antineoplastic medications

Hemoglobin A1C (HbA1C) a laboratory test used in diabetic management; also called glycosylated hemoglobin

Hemophilia series of coagulation disorders caused by genetic insufficiencies

Hemopoiesis production and maturation of blood cells that occurs in red bone marrow; also called hematopoiesis

Hemosiderin one of two protein complexes that maintain iron stores inside cells (ferritin is the other)

Hemostasis the slowing or stopping of blood flow

Hepatic microsomal enzyme system as it relates to pharmacotherapy, liver enzymes that metabolize drugs as well as nutrients and other endogenous substances; sometimes called the P-450 system

Hepatic portal system a network of venous vessels that collects blood draining from the stomach, small intestine, and most of the large intestine

Hepatitis inflammation of the liver

Herb plant with a soft stem that is used for healing or as a seasoning

High-alert medications drugs that have a high risk of causing significant harm to the patient when used in error

High-density lipoprotein (HDL) lipid-carrying particle in the blood that transports excess cholesterol away from body tissues or back to the liver for metabolism

Highly active antiretroviral therapy (HAART) drug therapy for HIV infection that includes high doses of multiple medications given concurrently

Histamine chemical released by mast cells in response to foreign agents or injury that initiates the inflammatory response within seconds

HMG-CoA reductase primary enzyme in the biochemical pathway for the synthesis of cholesterol

Home care nurse monitors the patient's condition, including medication adherence and reports any adverse effects, and works with the health care provider and pharmacist to achieve optimal therapeutic outcomes

Hormone replacement therapy (HRT) supplies physiological doses of estrogen, sometimes combined with progestin, to treat unpleasant symptoms of menopause and to prevent long-term consequences of estrogen loss

Hormones chemicals secreted by endocrine glands that act as chemical messengers to maintain homeostasis

Hospice nursing the care of terminally ill patients in their homes or in a health care facility that involves effective pain management

Host flora microorganisms that normally inhabit the human body

Household system of measurement older system of measurement that uses teaspoons, tablespoons, and cups

Human immunodeficiency virus (HIV) the causative agent for AIDS

Hyperaldosteronism excessive secretion of aldosterone

Hypercholesterolemia high levels of cholesterol in the blood

Hyperemesis gravidarum condition of continual vomiting during pregnancy

Hyperkalemia serum potassium level above 5 mEq/L

Hyperlipidemia high levels of lipids in the blood

Hypernatremia high sodium level in the blood

Hyperosmolar hyperglycemic state (HHS) acute complication seen in persons with type 2 diabetes that is characterized by extreme hyperglycemia, hyperosmolarity with dehydration, the absence of ketoacidosis, and CNS dysfunction

Hypertension (HTN) consistent elevation of systemic arterial blood pressure

Hypertensive emergency (HTN-E) a diastolic pressure of greater than 120 mmHg, with evidence of target-organ system damage; also called hypertensive crisis

Hypertensive urgency severe hypertension, but with no evidence of target-organ damage

Hypertrichosis the elongation, thickening, and increased pigmentation of body hair

Hypertriglyceridemia refers to an increase in triglyceride levels

Hyperuricemia serum uric acid level 7 mg/dL or higher

Hypervitaminosis intake of toxic levels of vitamins

Hypnagogic hallucinations vivid, fearful illusions that may be experienced at the onset of sleep or on awakening

Hypoaldosteronism lack of adequate aldosterone secretion

Hypogonadism lack of sufficient testosterone by the testes

Hypokalemia serum potassium level below 3.5 mEq/L

Hypomania characterized by the same symptoms as bipolar disorder, but they are less severe and do not cause impaired functioning

Hyponatremia low sodium level in the blood

I

Idiosyncratic response unpredictable and unexplained drug reaction

Immunity ability to resist injury and infections

Immunization process of disease prevention in which the body produces its own antibodies in response to initial exposure to antigens

Immunomodulator general term referring to any drug or therapy that affects body defenses

Immunostimulants drugs that increase the ability of the immune system to fight infection and disease

Immunosuppressants drugs that diminish the ability of the immune system to fight infection and disease

Implementation when the nurse applies the knowledge, skills, and principles of nursing care to help move the patient toward the desired goal and optimal wellness

Impotence inability to obtain or sustain an erection; also called erectile dysfunction

Incretins hormones released by the mucosa of the small intestine in response to meals

Incubation period following the first exposure to an antigen, the time needed for the body to process the antigen and mount an effective response

Indications the medical conditions for which a drug is approved

Infantile spasm usually occurs in the first year of life and is characterized by a sudden bending forward, body stiffening, or arching of the torso; also called West syndrome

Infertility inability to become pregnant after at least 1 year of frequent, unprotected intercourse

Inflammation nonspecific body defense that occurs in response to an injury or antigen

Inflammatory bowel disease (IBD) disease characterized by the presence of ulcers in the distal portion of the small intestine (Crohn's disease) or mucosal erosions in the large intestine (ulcerative colitis)

Influenza a viral infection characterized by acute symptoms that include sore throat, sneezing, coughing, fever, and chills; also called flu

Ingestion the process of taking food into the body by mouth

Innate body defenses those that are present even before an infection occurs and which provide the first line of protection from pathogens

Inoculation the placement of a foreign substance on or in an individual for the purpose of disease prevention using "live" virus particles obtained from an infected patient

Inotropic agents drugs or chemicals that increase the force of contraction of the heart; also called cardiotonic drugs

Insomnia inability to fall asleep or stay asleep

Insulin pancreatic hormone that acts to decrease blood glucose levels

Insulin resistance occurs in type 2 diabetes mellitus; cells become unresponsive to insulin due to a defect in insulin receptor function

Insulin-like growth factor (IGF) a family of peptides that promote cartilage and bone growth

Integrase an enzyme unique to HIV that incorporates the viral DNA into the host's chromosomes

Interferons (IFNs) type of cytokine secreted by T cells in response to antigens to protect uninfected cells

Interleukins (ILs) class of cytokines synthesized by lymphocytes, monocytes, macrophages, and certain other cells in response to antigen exposure

Intermittent claudication (IC) pain or cramping in the lower legs that worsens with walking or exercise

Intermittent feedings enteral feedings that are administered every 3 to 6 hours

Intervention nursing action that produces an effect or that is intended to alter the course of a disease or condition designed to move the patient toward the desired goal

Intracellular fluid (ICF) compartment contains water that is inside cells

Intracellular parasites infectious microbes that live inside host cells

Intrinsic activity the ability of a drug to bind to a receptor and produce a strong action

Intrinsic factor chemical substance secreted by stomach cells that is essential for the absorption of vitamin B_{12}

Intrinsic pathway coagulation pathway activated in response to injury; it takes several minutes to complete

Intrinsic sympathomimetic activity (ISA) low level of beta-agonist activity possessed by certain beta-adrenergic blockers

Invasiveness the ability of a pathogen to grow extremely rapidly and cause direct damage to surrounding tissues by virtue of sheer numbers

Investigational New Drug (IND) application to the FDA that contains all the animal and cell testing data

Iodism toxicity to Lugol's iodine solution therapy

Ion trapping phenomenon in which alkalinizing agents are used to aid in the renal excretion of toxic substances

Irritable bowel syndrome (IBS) disease of the lower GI tract, characterized by abdominal pain, bloating, gas, cramping, and alternating diarrhea and constipation

Irritative voiding symptoms cluster of complaints that accompanies cystitis

Isozymes multiple, similar forms of an enzyme that perform slightly different metabolic functions

J

Juxtaglomerular (JG) cells specialized smooth muscle cells found in the afferent arteriole that sense blood pressure and release renin

K

Kappa receptors one of two major receptors in the CNS where opioids act

Keratolytic action that promotes shedding of the outer layer of the epidermis

Ketolides class of antibiotics that block bacterial protein synthesis by binding to two different sites on the 50S ribosomal subunit

L

Laxatives drugs that promote defecation

Lecithins phospholipids that are an important component of plasma membranes

Lennox-Gestaut syndrome mixed seizure that has characteristics of tonic–clonic, atonic, and atypical absence seizures

Leprosy a chronic infection caused by *Mycobacterium leprae*

Leptin hormone that regulates hunger and weight balance

Leucovorin rescue therapy drug therapy administered following chemotherapy with toxic folic acid analogs such as methotrexate to rescue normal cells

Leukotrienes chemical mediators of inflammation stored and released by mast cells

Leydig cells the primary cells in the testes that are responsible for androgen secretion

Libido interest in sexual activity

Limbic system area in the brain responsible for emotional expression, learning, and memory

Lipodystrophy a disorder in which fat is redistributed in specific areas in the body

Lipoproteins substances that carry lipids in the bloodstream that are composed of fat bound to carrier proteins

Loading dose relatively large dose of a drug given at the beginning of treatment to rapidly obtain a therapeutic response

Local anesthesia loss of sensation to a limited part of the body without loss of consciousness

Locus coeruleus within the brainstem, an area in the pons that has been associated with fear responses and panic attacks

Low-density lipoprotein (LDL) lipoprotein that carries the highest amount of cholesterol

Lymph nodes the principal lymphoid organs in the body

Lymphatic system consists of a network of cells, vessels, and tissues that provide immune surveillance

M

Macrominerals inorganic compound needed by the body in amounts of 100 mg or more daily

Macula densa specialized cells in the distal convoluted tubule of the nephron that sense the flow rate and osmolality in the filtrate and send a message to the juxtaglomerular cells to release more renin

Maintenance dose amount of drug that keeps the plasma drug concentration in the therapeutic range

Major depressive disorder a depressed mood lasting for a minimum of 2 weeks that is present for most of the day, every day, or almost every day

Malaria disease characterized by severe fever and chills caused by the protozoan *Plasmodium*

Malignant hyperthermia rare but potentially fatal condition that is an adverse effect of some general anesthetics characterized by a rapid onset of extremely high fever with muscle rigidity

Mania condition characterized by an inflated self-esteem, decreased need for sleep or food, distractibility, increased activity, excessive pursuit of pleasurable activities, increased talkativeness, delusions, paranoia, hallucinations, and bizarre behavior

Margin of safety (MOS) the amount of drug that is lethal to 1% of animals (LD_1) divided by the amount of drug that produces a therapeutic effect in 99% of the animals (ED_{99})

Mast cell stabilizers drugs that inhibit the release of inflammatory mediators from mast cells

Mastoiditis inflammation of the mastoid sinus

Median effective dose (ED_{50}) the dose of a drug required to produce a specific therapeutic response in 50% of a group of patients

Median lethal dose (LD_{50}) the dose of a drug that will kill 50% of a group of animals

Median toxicity dose (TD_{50}) the dose that will produce a given toxicity in 50% of a group of patients

Medication administration record (MAR) legal documentation of all pharmacotherapies received by the patient

Medication error any preventable event that may cause or lead to inappropriate medication use or patient harm while the medication is in the control of the health care provider, patient, or consumer

Medication error index categorization of medication errors according to the degree of harm an error can cause

Medication reconciliation the process of keeping track of a patient's medications as the patient's care proceeds from one health care provider to another

Menopause progressive decrease in estrogen secretion by the ovaries resulting in the permanent cessation of menses

Merozoites transformation of sporozoites carried by the blood to the liver inside the human host where they multiply into millions of progeny

Metabolic bone disease (MBD) refers to a cluster of disorders that have in common defects in the structure of bone

Metabolic syndrome a group of abnormalities that tend to occur together that places the patient at increased risk for developing diabetes and vascular complications

Metabolism the process used by the body to chemically change a drug molecule; also called biotransformation

Metastasis travel of cancer cells from their original site to a distant site

Metered-dose inhaler (MDI) inhaler device used to deliver a precise amount of medicine to the respiratory system

Methylxanthines chemical class for theophylline and caffeine and theobromine

Metric system of measurement the most common system of drug measurement that uses liters, milliliters, and grams

Microbial antagonism condition of various host flora in competition with each other for physical space and nutrients that helps protect the host from being overrun by pathogenic organisms

Microminerals inorganic compound needed by the body in amounts of 20 mg or less daily

Migraine severe headache preceded by auras and that may include nausea and vomiting

Milk-alkali syndrome syndrome caused by the administration of calcium carbonate antacids with milk or food containing vitamin D; symptoms include headache, urinary frequency, anorexia, nausea, and fatigue

Mineralocorticoids hormones secreted by the adrenal glands that affect the secretion of sodium and water

Minerals essential substances that constitute about 4% of a person's body weight and serve many diverse functions

Minimum alveolar concentration describes the potency of inhalation anesthetics

Minimum effective concentration amount of drug required to produce a therapeutic effect

Miosis constriction of the pupil

Mitochondrial toxicity specific type of adverse effects resulting from a drug's toxic actions on mitochondria

Modular formulas enteral feedings that contain nutrients that are designed to meet a specific nutrient deficiency or disease state

Monitored anesthesia care (MAC) use of sedatives, analgesics, and other low-dose drugs that allow patients to remain responsive and breathe without assistance

Monoamine oxidase (MAO) enzyme that destroys catecholamines such as norepinephrine in the nerve terminal

Monoamine oxidase inhibitor (MAOI) drug inhibiting monoamine oxidase, an enzyme that slows the destruction of norepinephrine, dopamine, and serotonin

Monoclonal antibody (MAB) antibody produced by a single B cell that targets a single type of cell or receptor

Mood disorder change in emotion that impairs the patient's ability to effectively deal with normal ADLs

Mood stabilizers drugs for bipolar disorder that can moderate extreme shifts in emotions and relieve symptoms of mania and depression during acute episodes

Motor end plate cholinergic synapse on skeletal muscle that allows for communication between the nervous system and skeletal muscle

Mu receptors one of two types of opioid receptors in the CNS

Mucolytics drugs used to remove mucus by loosening thick bronchial secretions

Mucositis inflammation of the epithelial lining of the digestive tract

Multipotent stem cells cells that are capable of maturing (differentiating) into any blood cell type depending on the internal needs of the body

Muscarinic type of cholinergic receptor found at postganglionic nerve endings in the parasympathetic nervous system that, when activated, result in stimulation

Muscarinic agonist drug that is selective for muscarinic receptors

Muscarinic antagonists drugs that block receptors at cholinergic synapses in the parasympathetic nervous system and at a few target organs in the sympathetic nervous system

Muscle rigidity stiffness occurring in Parkinson's disease that causes difficulty bending over and moving limbs, changes in facial expression, or a lack of facial expression

Muscle spasms involuntary contractions of muscles that cause sudden, intense pain, which slowly diminishes after a few minutes

Muscle spasticity condition caused by damage to the CNS in which certain muscle groups remain in a continuous state of contraction

Mutations errors made by bacteria while duplicating their genetic code

Myasthenia gravis (MG) muscular disorder caused by a destruction of nicotinic synapses on skeletal muscles and characterized by extreme fatigue, double vision, speech impairment, and difficulty chewing or swallowing

Myasthenic crisis extreme muscular weakness and symptoms similar to those of cholinergic crisis; caused by abrupt discontinuation of medication for myasthenia gravis

Mycobacterium avium complex (MAC) infection that usually arises as a secondary infection due to the immunosuppression caused by HIV-AIDS

Mycolic acid a complex lipid that covers the cell surfaces of the genus *Mycobacterium*, which protects them and makes them resistant to many disinfectants

Mycoses diseases caused by fungi

Mydriasis pupil dilation

Mydriatics drugs that cause pupil dilation

Myocardial infarctions (MIs) blood clots blocking a portion of a coronary artery that cause necrosis of cardiac muscle

Myocardial ischemia condition in which the heart is receiving an insufficient amount of oxygen to meet its metabolic needs

Myocardium the muscular layer of the heart, responsible for its physical pumping action

Myoclonic seizures seizures characterized by brief, sudden contractions of major muscle groups

Myxedema mucous type of edema caused by accumulation of hydrophilic substances in connective tissues

Myxedema coma a life-threatening end-stage condition of hypothyroidism

N

Nadir lowest values of erythrocyte, leukocyte, and platelet counts caused by chemotherapy

Narcolepsy sleep disorder that is characterized by severe daytime sleepiness and inability to stay awake

Narcotic natural or synthetic drug related to morphine; may be used as a broader legal term referring to hallucinogens, CNS stimulants, marijuana, and other illegal drugs

Narrow-spectrum antibiotic an anti-infective that is effective against only one or a small number of organisms

Natriuresis sodium excretion in the urine

Natriuretic peptides substances secreted in response to increased pressure in the heart

Nausea unpleasant feeling of the need to vomit accompanied by weakness, diaphoresis, dizziness, and hyperproduction of saliva

Nebulizer machine that delivers medication as a fine mist for the purpose of inhalation; also called small-volume nebulizer

Negative chronotropic effect the property of slowing the speed of electrical conduction across the myocardium

Negative feedback controls secretion and release of hormones by signaling the endocrine system once homeostasis is restored

Negative inotropic effect the reduction in the force of myocardial contraction

Negative symptoms in schizophrenia, symptoms associated with a loss of normal functioning, including a lack of interest, motivation, responsiveness, or pleasure in daily activities

Neoadjuvant chemotherapy the administration of antineoplastic drugs before surgery or radiation therapy with the goal of shrinking a large tumor to a more manageable size

Neoplasm swelling, abnormal enlargement or mass; same as *tumor*

Nephrons structural and functional units of the kidney

Neuraminidase an enzyme that assists the virus in exiting the host cell

Neurodegenerative diseases degenerative diseases of the CNS that include a diverse set of disorders differing in their causes and outcomes

Neuroeffector junction specialized synapse where the postganglionic neuron terminates on smooth muscle, cardiac muscle, or a gland

Neurofibrillary tangles bundles of nerve fibers found in the brain of patients with Alzheimer's disease on autopsy

Neurolept analgesia type of general anesthesia that combines fentanyl with droperidol to produce a state in which patients are conscious though insensitive to pain and unconnected with surroundings

Neuroleptic malignant syndrome (NMS) potentially fatal condition caused by certain antipsychotic medications characterized by high fever, sweating, fluctuating blood pressure, tachycardia, and muscle rigidity

Neuromuscular blockers drugs that inhibit transmission at the neuromuscular junctions on skeletal muscles in the somatic nervous system

Neuron the primary functional cell in all portions of the nervous system; its purpose is to communicate messages through conduction of an action potential

Neuropathic pain is caused by injury or irritation to nerve tissue described as burning, shooting, or numbing pain

Neurotransmitters chemicals utilized in the communication of a message from one cell to another, or synaptic transmission

New Drug Application (NDA) application submitted to the FDA that signals that the pharmaceutical company is ready to sell the new drug

New molecular entities medications that are truly unique and structurally different from existing drugs

Nicotinic receptor for acetylcholine in the ganglia of both the sympathetic and parasympathetic nervous systems

Nicotinic agonist drug that selectively activates nicotinic receptors

Nicotinic antagonists drugs that block receptors at cholinergic synapses in the ganglia or in the somatic nervous system at the neuromuscular junction

Nitric oxide in vascular smooth muscle, an important cell signaling molecule and a potent vasodilator causing relaxation of both arterial and venous smooth muscle

Nits eggs of the louse parasite

Nociceptor pain pain produced by injury to body tissue

Nociceptors sensory nerve receptors located throughout the body that initiate pain transmission when stimulated

Nomogram chart used to plot a child's height and weight to determine body surface area

Nondepolarizing neuromuscular blocker (NDNB) class of nicotinic antagonists that bind to Ach receptors at motor end plates in skeletal muscle and prevent Ach from reaching its receptors

Nonopioid analgesics analgesics that have a peripheral site of action, no dependence potential, and provide the baseline pharmacotherapy for pain management; include NSAIDs, acetaminophen, and a few centrally acting agents

Non–rapid eye movement (NREM) sleep phase of sleep during which respirations slow, heart rate and blood pressure decrease, oxygen consumption by muscles decreases, and urine formation decreases

Norepinephrine (NE) primary neurotransmitter in the sympathetic and autonomic nervous systems

Nursing diagnoses list of problems that address the patient's responses to health and life processes

Nursing process five-part decision-making system that includes assessment, nursing diagnosis, planning, implementation, and evaluation

O

Obsessive–compulsive disorder (OCD) recurrent, intrusive thoughts or repetitive behaviors that interfere with normal activities or relationships

Occupational health nurse (OHN) addresses the health and safety of workers on the job

Oligospermia presence of less than 20 million sperm per milliliter of ejaculate

Oncology nurse nurse who has received special training to care for patients with cancer and to administer chemotherapy

On–off syndrome occurs when a patient with Parkinson's disease alternates between symptom-free periods (on) and times when the drugs stop working and symptoms abruptly reappear (off)

Onychomycosis the invasion of the nail plate by a fungus; also called tinea unguium

Open-angle glaucoma common form of glaucoma caused by the partial obstruction of the outflow of aqueous humor through the canal of Schlemm

Opiates natural substances obtained from opium, such as morphine and codeine

Opioid class of drugs that includes natural substances obtained from the seeds of the poppy plant such as opium, morphine, and codeine, and synthetic drugs such as meperidine, oxycodone, fentanyl, methadone, and heroin

Opium a milky substance extracted from the unripe seeds of the poppy plant that contains over 20 different chemicals having pharmacologic activity

Oral glucose tolerance test (OGTT) a primary blood test for diagnosing diabetes

Orphan disease serious, though rare, disease that affects less than 200,000 people in the United States

Orthostatic hypotension fall in blood pressure that occurs when changing position from recumbent to upright

Osmolality number of dissolved particles, or solutes, in 1 kg (1 L) of water

Osmosis process by which water moves from areas of low solute concentration (low osmolality) to areas of high solute concentration (high osmolality)

Osmotic pressure creates a force that moves substances between body compartments or across a membrane

Osteoarthritis (OA) progressive, degenerative joint disease caused by the breakdown of articular cartilage

Osteomalacia rickets in children; caused by vitamin D deficiency and characterized by softening of the bones without alteration of basic bone structure

Osteoporosis metabolic bone disease characterized by bone demineralization, decreased bone density, and subsequent fractures

Otitis interna condition that may occur as the result of chronic otitis media or as an upper respiratory infection; also called labyrinthitis

Otitis media inflammation of the middle ear

Ototoxity drug-induced hearing impairment

Outcome statement that includes specific measurable evaluation criteria

Ovarian hyperstimulation syndrome (OHS) serious complication of certain fertility drugs characterized by rapid, massive enlargement of the ovaries accompanied by physical symptoms

Ovulation release of an oocyte (egg) by the ovary

Ovulatory dysfunction the presence of abnormal, irregular, or absent ovulation

Oxazolidinones class of antibiotics that act by binding to a part of the bacterial 50S ribosome

Oxytocics drugs that stimulate uterine contractions and promote the induction of labor

P

Paget's disease chronic progressive condition characterized by accelerated remodeling of the bone, producing enlarged and softened bones; also called osteitis deformans

Palliation form of cancer chemotherapy intended to alleviate symptoms rather than cure the disease

Pancreatitis inflammation of the pancreas

Panic disorder anxiety disorder characterized by intense feelings of immediate apprehension, fearfulness, terror, or impending doom, accompanied by increased autonomic nervous system activity

Para-aminobenzoic acid (PABA) precursor molecule used by bacteria to make their own folic acid

Parasympathetic nervous system portion of the autonomic nervous system that is activated during nonstressful conditions and produces a set of symptoms known as the rest-and-digest response

Parenteral nutrition the administration of high-calorie nutrients via a central vein, such as the subclavian vein

Parietal cells cells in the stomach mucosa that secrete hydrochloric acid

Parish nursing refers to a specialty practice that emphasizes health and healing within a faith community

Parkinsonism having tremor, loss of fine motor skills, muscle rigidity, stooped posture, and a shuffling gait

Parkinson's disease (PD) degenerative disorder of the nervous system characterized by tremor, muscle rigidity, hypokinesia, masklike faces, and a slow, shuffling gait

Paroxysmal supraventricular tachycardia (PSVT) occurs when episodes of atrial tachycardia alternate with periods of normal rhythm; also called paroxysmal atrial tachycardia (PAT)

Partial agonist medication that produces a weaker, or less efficacious, response than an agonist

Partial fatty-acid oxidation inhibitors a class of drugs used in the treatment of CAD

Partial (focal) seizures seizures that start on one side of the brain and travel a short distance before stopping

Partial parenteral nutrition a parenteral solution that lacks an essential element, usually fats or lipids

Passive immunity immune defense that lasts 2 to 3 weeks; obtained by administering antibodies

Patent medicines in early America before drug regulation, products that contained an easily identified brand name that claimed to cure just about any symptom or disease

Pathogenicity ability of an organism to cause disease in humans

Pathogens microbes that are capable of causing disease

Pediatric Research Equity Act of 2003 act that authorizes the FDA to require research of pediatric uses for new drugs

Pediculicides drugs that kill lice

Pegylation process that attaches polyethylene glycol to a drug molecule to extend its duration of activity

Penicillinase enzyme present in certain bacteria that is able to make penicillin ineffective

Penicillin-binding proteins (PBPs) enzymes used by bacteria to build bacterial cell walls that are targets for penicillins and related antibiotics

Pepsin digestive enzyme that breaks down proteins from food

Peptic ulcer erosion of the mucosa in the stomach or small intestine

Peptidoglycan substance containing sugars bound to peptides that is only found in bacteria

Peripheral resistance amount of friction encountered by blood in the arteries

Peripherally inserted central catheter (PICC) line a central catheter that is threaded into the vena cava for administration of chemotherapy

Peripheral vein total parenteral nutrition delivery system used when a central venous line cannot be accessed or when it is not appropriate for the patient

Peristalsis contractions of layers of smooth muscle

Pernicious anemia type of anemia usually caused by a deficiency of vitamin B_{12}

Phagocytes cells that engulf and destroy pathogens and other foreign substances

Pharmacodynamics study of the mechanisms of drug action and how the body responds to drugs

Pharmacogenetics the study of genetic variations that alter patients' responses to medications; branch of pharmacology that examines the role of genetics in drug response

Pharmacokinetics study of drug movement throughout the body

Pharmacologic classification method of organizing drugs on the basis of their mechanisms of action

Pharmacology the study of medicines, ranging from how drugs are administered, to where they travel in the body, to the actual responses they produce

Pharmacopoeia a medical reference summarizing standards of drug purity, strength, and directions for synthesis

Pharmacotherapy the application of drugs for the purpose of disease prevention and treatment of suffering; also called pharmacotherapeutics

Pheochromocytoma a tumor, usually benign, arising from the adrenal medulla that is characterized by excessive secretion of catecholamines

Phobia fearful feeling attached to situations or objects such as snakes, spiders, crowds, or heights

Phosphodiesterase III enzyme in cardiac and smooth muscle; inhibition increases cardiac output due to an increase in myocardial contractility and a decrease in left ventricular afterload

Phospholipids type of lipid that contains two fatty acids, a phosphate group, and a chemical backbone of glycerol

Phototherapy therapy used for persons suffering from seasonal affective disorder that consists of artificial lighting approximately 5 to 20 times brighter than normal indoor lighting

Physical dependence condition of experiencing unpleasant withdrawal symptoms when a substance is discontinued after repeated use

Pill rolling common behavior in Parkinson's disease, in which patients rub the thumb and forefinger together in a circular motion, resembling the motion of rolling a tablet between two fingers

Placebo in drug testing, an inert substance that serves as a control "nontreatment" group used to compare the effectiveness of the new drug

Placenta organ that allows for nutrition and gas exchange between the mother and fetus

Planning phase of the nursing process in which appropriate goals and outcomes are developed and nursing interventions that will help the patient achieve them are determined

Plaque fibrous, fatty material that builds up in the walls of arteries

Plaques psoriatic lesions characterized by red, raised patches of skin covered with flaky, thick, silver scales

Plasma cells cells derived from B lymphocytes that secrete antibodies

Plasma half-life ($t_{1/2}$) the length of time required for the plasma concentration of a drug to decrease by one half after administration

Plasminogen inactive protein that is present in fibrin clot formation; precursor of plasmin

Pluripotent stem cell cell that is capable of maturing (differentiating) into any blood cell type

Pneumonic plague life-threatening infectious lung disease that occurs after breathing *Yersinia pestis*, a bacterium found on rodents and their fleas that is responsible for the bubonic plague

Polarized describes a cell that has negative membrane potential

Polyclonal antibodies contain a wide mixture of different antibodies that attack the T cells or T-cell receptors

Polycystic ovary syndrome a condition in which the ovaries are filled with follicular cysts and the patient has elevated levels of androgens and estrogen

Polydipsia excessive thirst

Polyherbacy use of multiple herbal and other supplements

Polymeric formulas solutions that contain various mixtures of proteins, lipids, and carbohydrates in high-molecular-weight form and are considered the most common enteral preparation

Polyphagia excessive appetite

Polypharmacy taking multiple drugs concurrently

Polyuria excessive urine production

Positive symptoms in schizophrenia, symptoms associated with an excess of distortion of normal function, including hallucinations, delusions, disorganized thought or speech patterns, and movement disorders

Postantibiotic effect antimicrobial activity that continues for a time after discontinuation of a drug

Posterior pituitary gland (neurohypophysis) consists of nervous tissue and is an extension of the hypothalamus that secretes antidiuretic hormone and oxytocin

Postherpetic neuralgia a serious form of the shingles in which the pain lasts for years

Postictal state period immediately following a seizure

Postmarketing surveillance stage 4 of the drug approval process during which testing is done to survey for harmful drug effects in a larger population

Postpartum onset depression major depression experienced by new mothers following delivery, which is related to hormonal shifts and situational stresses that occur during that period

Post-traumatic stress disorder (PTSD) type of anxiety that develops in response to reexperiencing a previous life event that was psychologically traumatic

Potency the strength of a drug at a specified concentration or dose

Potentially inappropriate medications (PIMs) medications that comprise the Beers criteria that are of special concern for older adults

Preclinical research first stage of drug development that involves extensive laboratory testing by the pharmaceutical company on human and microbial cells

Prediabetes condition in which serum glucose levels are elevated but are not high enough to be diagnosed as diabetes

Preeclampsia occurs during pregnancy when blood pressure increases to 140/90 mmHg or higher on two separate occasions, and 300 mg of protein is found in the urine over a 24-hour period

Pregnancy categories five classifications developed by the U.S. Food and Drug Administration (FDA) that rate medication risks during pregnancy

Preload degree of stretch of the cardiac muscle fibers just before they contract

Preterm labor the initiation of labor prior to week 37 of gestation

Primary hypertension hypertension having no identifiable cause

Procoagulants natural substances that promote the formation of blood clots

Prodrugs drugs that become more active after they are metabolized

Prodysrhythmics conditions that promote the formation of cardiac rhythm abnormalities

Progesterone a natural progestin secreted by the corpus luteum

Progestins synthetic hormones that have actions identical to natural endogenous progesterone

Prostaglandin E$_2$ hormone that stimulates the secretion of mucus and bicarbonate, promotes repair of damaged gastric mucosal cells, and increases blood flow to the mucosa to help maintain optimal mucosal conditions

Prostaglandins local hormones that have diverse functions depending on the location

Prostatitis bacterial infection of the prostate gland

Protease viral enzyme that is responsible for the final assembly of the HIV virions

Prothrombin blood clotting factor that is converted to the enzyme thrombin

Prothrombin time (PT) laboratory test used to measure blood coagulation

Proton pump inhibitors (PPIs) drugs that inhibit the enzyme H^+, K^+-ATPase

Prototype drug well-understood model drug to which other drugs in a pharmacologic class are compared

Protozoan single-celled organism that inhabits water, soil, and animal hosts

Provirus stage of a virus in which the viral DNA integrates into the host chromosome

Pruritus itching associated with dry, scaly skin or a parasite infection

Pseudocholinesterase enzyme that rapidly destroys certain drugs in the plasma

Pseudomembranous colitis (PMC) caused by *Clostridium difficile*, a rare though potentially severe disorder resulting from therapy with tetracyclines and other classes of antibiotics

Psoralens agents used along with phototherapy for the treatment of severe psoriasis

Psychological dependence desire to continue using a drug despite obvious negative economic, physical, or social consequences

Psychosis general term used in medicine to describe a loss of contact with reality

Psychosocial describes a person's psychological development in the context of one's social environment

Public health nurse has a primary focus on population-level outcomes to promote health and prevent disease for entire population groups

Pulmonary embolism condition that occurs when a venous clot dislodges, migrates to the pulmonary vessels, and blocks arterial circulation to the lungs

Pulmonary perfusion blood flow through the lung

Purified protein derivative (PPD) tuberculin skin test

Pyelonephritis an inflammation of the kidney, pelvis, and other renal cells

R

Radiation sickness occurs after exposure to ionizing radiation; symptoms include nausea, vomiting, and diarrhea, weight loss, anorexia, fatigue, and suppression of the bone marrow

Rapid eye movement (REM) sleep stage of sleep characterized by diminished muscle tone, movements of the eyes, and irregular heart rate and breathing

Raynaud's disease vasospasms of vessels serving the fingers and toes that can lead to intermittent pain and cyanosis of the digits

Reabsorption movement of filtered substances from the kidney tubule back into the blood

Rebound congestion adverse effect of intranasal decongestants; prolonged use causes hypersecretion of mucus and worsening nasal congestion once the drug effects wear off

Rebound effects symptoms of lethargy and fatigue caused by withdrawal of methamphetamine and other stimulants

Rebound insomnia increased sleeplessness that occurs when long-term sedative medication is discontinued abruptly

Receptor cellular molecule to which a drug binds to produce its effects

Recommended dietary allowances (RDAs) minimum amount of vitamins and minerals needed each day to prevent disease

Rectal route administration of drugs into the rectum for either local or systemic delivery

Refeeding syndrome metabolic complications that can occur when nutritional support, including enteral nutrition therapy, is introduced to severely malnourished patients

Reflex tachycardia temporary increase in heart rate that occurs when blood pressure falls

Refractory period time during which the myocardial cells rest and are not able to contract

Regional anesthesia similar to local anesthesia except that it encompasses a larger body area, such as an entire limb

Renal failure a condition characterized by a decrease in the kidneys' ability to maintain electrolyte and fluid balance and excrete waste products

Renin an enzyme that is synthesized, stored, and secreted by juxtaglomerular cells in the kidney

Renin-angiotensin-aldosterone system (RAAS) series of enzymatic steps by which the body raises blood pressure

Replacement therapy hormones administered to patients who are unable to secrete sufficient quantities of their own endogenous hormones

Repolarization return of a negative resting membrane potential to the cell

Rest-and-digest response signs and symptoms produced when the parasympathetic nervous system is activated that promote relaxation and maintenance activities

Reticular activating system (RAS) responsible for sleeping and wakefulness and performs an alerting function for the cerebral cortex

Reticular formation portion of the brain affecting awareness and wakefulness

Retinoids drug class related to vitamin A used in the treatment of inflammatory skin conditions, dermatologic malignancies, and acne

Reverse cholesterol transport the process by which cholesterol is transported away from body tissues to the liver

Reverse remodeling occurs after several months of therapy with beta-adrenergic antagonists, when heart size, shape, and function return to normal

Reverse transcriptase viral enzyme that converts RNA to DNA

Rhabdomyolysis breakdown of muscle fibers usually due to muscle trauma or ischemia

Rheumatoid arthritis (RA) chronic, progressive, autoimmune disease that causes inflammation of the joints

Rhinophyma reddened, bulbous, irregular swelling of the nose

Rifamycin derivatives include rifampin, rifabutin, and rifapentine, used in combination with other antituberculosis medications

Risk management system of reducing medication errors by modifying policies and procedures within the institution

Risk–benefit ratio determination of whether the risks from a drug outweigh the potential benefits received by taking the medication

Root-cause analysis (RCA) attempts to focus attention on the causes of the medication error, rather than on the person responsible for the error

Rosacea inflammatory skin disorder affecting mainly the face, characterized by small papules that swell, thicken, and become painful

S

Salicylates the chemical family to which aspirin belongs

Salicylism acute or chronic overdose of aspirin

Sarcolemma the muscle membrane

Sarcoplasmic reticula structures within cells that store the calcium ions that are released by depolarization

Satiety the psychological feeling of fullness or satisfaction following a meal

Satiety center region of the hypothalamus that recognizes satiety

Scabicides drugs that kill scabies mites

Schizoaffective disorder psychosis with symptoms of both schizophrenia and mood disorders

Schizophrenia psychosis characterized by abnormal thoughts and thought processes, withdrawal from people and the outside environment, an inability to independently perform ADLs, and a high risk of suicide

Sclerosing abnormal tissue hardening of the veins

Seasonal affective disorder a type of depression experienced during the dark winter months

Seborrhea skin condition characterized by overproduction of sebum by the oil glands

Secondary hypertension hypertension having a specific identifiable cause

Second messenger cascade of biochemical events that initiates a drug's action by either stimulating or inhibiting a normal activity of the cell

Secretion in the kidney, movement of substances from the blood into the tubule after filtration has occurred

Sedative–hypnotic drug with the ability to produce a calming effect at lower doses and sleep at higher doses

Sedatives substances that depress the CNS and cause drowsiness or sleep

Seizure symptom of epilepsy characterized by abnormal neuronal discharges within the brain

Selective estrogen receptor modulators (SERMs) drugs that produce an action similar to estrogen in body tissues; used for the treatment of osteoporosis in postmenopausal women

Semielemental (oligomeric) formulas enteral solutions that contain larger molecules than elemental products and a higher percentage of fat

Sentinel event an unexpected death or injury, or the risk of death or injury from medication errors

Serotonin a natural neurotransmitter that is found in high concentrations in the hypothalamus, limbic system, medulla, and spinal cord

Serotonin syndrome (SES) set of signs and symptoms associated with overmedication with antidepressants that includes altered mental status, fever, hypertension, tremors, sweating, and lack of muscular coordination

Shingles herpes zoster infection caused by reactivation of the varicella-zoster virus or chickenpox

Short stature height below the fifth percentile for age and gender, or more than two standard deviations below the mean (average) for age and gender

Side effects types of drug effects that are less serious than adverse effects, are predictable, and may occur even at therapeutic doses

Silent angina myocardial ischemia that occurs in the absence of pain

Simple partial seizures seizures that have an onset that may begin as a small, regional focus, and subsequently progress to a generalized seizure

Sinus rhythm number of beats per minute normally generated by the SA node

Situational anxiety anxiety experienced by people faced with a temporarily stressful environment

Sjögren's syndrome chronic autoimmune disorder characterized by excessive dryness of mucous membranes

Sleep attacks sudden bouts of sleep that last 10 to 30 minutes and may occur during the daytime without warning

Sleep paralysis the temporary inability to move after waking up from sleep

Smallpox serious, contagious potentially fatal disease that is caused by the variola virus

Small volume nebulizer machine that delivers medication as a fine mist for the purpose of inhalation; also called nebulizer

Social anxiety disorder unreasonable and persistent fear of crowds or of being judged, ridiculed, or embarrassed by others; also called social phobia

Somatic nervous system nerves that provide for voluntary control of the skeletal muscle

Somatostatin hormone released by the hypothalamus, stomach, intestine, and pancreas that inhibits the effects of growth hormone and lowers acid secretion; also known as growth hormone-inhibiting hormone

Specialty supplements nonherbal dietary products used to enhance a wide variety of body functions

Spermicides agents that kill sperm

Sporozoite mature and infective form of *Plasmodium* that resides in the gut of the female *Anopheles* mosquito

Stable angina type of angina that occurs in a predictable pattern of frequency, intensity, and duration, usually relieved by rest

Staging the process of determining where a cancer is located and the extent of its invasion

Status asthmaticus emergency situation in which acute asthma attacks are unresponsive to drug treatment; may lead to respiratory failure

Status epilepticus medical emergency that occurs when a seizure continues for more than 30 minutes or when two successive seizures occur without full recovery of consciousness between seizures

Steatorrhea the passing of bulky, foul-smelling fatty stools

Steroids types of lipids consisting of a ring structure

Sterol nucleus ring structure common to all steroids

Strategic National Stockpile (SNS) national repository of antibiotics, chemical antidotes, antitoxins, antiviral agents, and other essential medical supplies for use in a major health emergency

Striatum location in the brain, where dopamine encounters its receptors and produces multiple actions

Stroke volume amount of blood pumped by a ventricle in a single contraction

Substance abuse self-administration of a drug that does not conform to the medical or social norms within the patient's given culture or society

Substantia nigra location in the brain where dopamine is produced that is responsible for regulation of unconscious muscle movement

Substrate drug that is metabolized by a CYP enzyme

Suicide the intentional act of ending one's life

Supercoil the highly twisted arrangement of the helix in bacterial DNA

Superinfections new infections caused when an antibiotic kills the host's normal flora, making additional space and nutrients available for pathogenic organisms to grow unchecked

Supplements additional vitamins or minerals that some people take to supplement their diets

Surgical anesthesia stage 3 of anesthesia, in which most major surgery occurs

Svedberg unit a unit of measurement represented by the letter "S" that indicates the size or sedimentation rate of the bacterial 70S ribosome

Sympathetic nervous system portion of the autonomic nervous system that is activated under emergency conditions or stress and produces a set of actions called the fight-or-flight response

Sympathomimetics drugs that activate adrenergic receptors in the sympathetic nervous system

Symporter a membrane protein that transports two molecules at the same time

Synapse a junction between two neurons or a neuron and a muscle

Synaptic cleft space where neurotransmitters enter that must be crossed for the impulse to reach the postganglionic neuron or organ

Syndrome of inappropriate antidiuretic hormone (SIADH) condition characterized by marked fluid retention, elevated urine osmolality, low serum osmolality, and sodium loss in the urine

Synergistic effect type of drug interaction in which two drugs produce an effect that is much greater than would be expected from simply adding the two individual drugs' responses

T

T cells types of lymphocytes that are essential for the cell-mediated immune response

Tachydysrhythmias disorders exhibiting a heart rate greater than 100 beats/minute

Tachyphylaxis the rapid development of tolerance to any action of a drug, either adverse or therapeutic effects

Tardive dyskinesia (TD) unusual tongue and face movements such as lip smacking, rapid eye blinking, and wormlike motions of the tongue that occur during pharmacotherapy with certain antipsychotics

Target cells cells affected by hormones

Targeted therapy drug that has been specifically engineered to attack cancer-specific antigens, such as those on cancer cells

Telomerase an enzyme contained in certain human stem cells that can lengthen the DNA chains and allow continued replication

Telomeres regions in chromosomes that prevent the vital sequences of DNA from being destroyed each time a cell divides

Tension headache common type of head pain caused by stress and relieved by OTC analgesics

Teratogen agent that causes birth defects

Tetrahydrocannabinol (THC) the active chemical in marijuana

Therapeutic classification method of organizing drugs on the basis of what condition is being treated by the drug

Therapeutic drug monitoring practice of monitoring plasma levels of drugs that have low safety profiles and using the data to predict drug action or toxicity

Therapeutic index (TI) the ratio of a drug's LD_{50} to its ED_{50}

Therapeutic range dosage that produces the desired effects of a drug

Threshold potential an action potential triggered by the membrane potential during myocardial electrical conduction

Thrombin enzyme that causes clotting by catalyzing the conversion of fibrinogen to fibrin

Thrombocytopenia coagulation disorder in which there is a deficiency of platelets

Thromboembolic disorder condition in which the body forms undesirable clots

Thrombopoietin hormone that promotes the formation of platelets in the blood

Thyroid crisis a rare, life-threatening form of thyrotoxicosis; also called thyroid storm

Thyroid storm a rare, life-threatening form of thyrotoxicosis; also called thyroid crisis

Thyroid-stimulating hormone (TSH) hormone secreted by the anterior pituitary when stimulated by thyrotropin-releasing hormone

Thyroid-stimulating immunoglobulins (TSIs) stimulate the thyroid gland in Graves' disease

Thyrotoxicosis an acute condition caused by very high levels of circulating thyroid hormone

Thyrotropin-releasing hormone (TRH) hormone secreted by the hypothalamus when blood levels of thyroid hormone are low

Thyroxine (T_4) thyroid hormone that is synthesized from the amino acid tyrosine and 4 atoms of iodine

Thyroxine-binding globulin (TBG) a plasma protein produced in the liver

Tocolytics drugs used to delay preterm labor

Tolerance process of adapting to a drug over a period of time and subsequently requiring higher doses to achieve the same effect

Tonic–clonic seizures seizures characterized by intense muscle contractions and loss of consciousness

Tonicity the ability of a solution to cause a change in water movement across a membrane owing to osmotic forces

Tonometry technique that tests for glaucoma by measuring intraocular pressure

Topical route medications applied to the skin or the membranous linings of the eye, ear, nose, respiratory tract, urinary tract, vagina, and rectum

Topoisomerase IV in DNA replication, the enzyme that frees the newly formed interlocked strands, allowing them to migrate into the two daughter cells

Torsades de pointe type of ventricular tachycardia that is characterized by rates between 200 and 250 beats/minute and "twisting of the points" of the QRS complex on the ECG

Total parenteral nutrition (TPN) nutrition provided through a peripheral or central vein

Toxic concentration level of drug that results in serious adverse effects

Toxoids type of vaccine that uses bacterial toxins that have been chemically modified to be incapable of causing disease

Trade name name assigned by the pharmaceutical company marketing a drug; sometimes called the proprietary, product, or brand name

Transdermal patches topical delivery method that uses patches that contain a specified amount of medication that is released over a specified time period

Transferrin protein complex that transports iron to sites in the body where it is needed

Translation basic steps in protein synthesis

Transplant rejection recognition by the immune system of a transplanted tissue as foreign and subsequent attack on the tissue

Tricyclic antidepressants (TCAs) class of drugs used in the pharmacotherapy of depression

Triglycerides types of lipids that contain three fatty acids attached to a chemical backbone of glycerol

Tri-iodothyronine (T_3) thyroid hormone that is synthesized from the amino acid tyrosine and 3 atoms of iodine

Troches drugs in lozenge format formulated to slowly dissolve in the mouth

Trophozoite the active, growing stage during which a protozoan organism feeds, often at the expense of its host

Tropic hormones ability of the anterior pituitary gland hormones to regulate the secretory actions of other endocrine glands

Tubercles cavity-like lesions in the lung characteristic of infection by *Mycobacterium tuberculosis*

Tuberculosis (TB) a highly contagious infection caused by the organism *Mycobacterium tuberculosis*

Tularemia serious infectious disease found in rodents, rabbits, and hares that is caused by the organism *Francisella tularensis*

Tumor abnormal swelling, enlargement, or mass; also called neoplasm

Type 1 diabetes metabolic disorder characterized by hyperglycemia caused by a lack of secretion of insulin by the pancreas in which glucose cannot enter cells and fatty acids are used as the primary energy source

Type 2 diabetes chronic metabolic disease characterized by hyperglycemia and insulin resistance

Tyramine form of the amino acid tyrosine that is found in foods such as cheese, beer, wine, and yeast products

U

Unstable angina angina that occurs suddenly, has added intensity, and occurs during periods of rest

Up-regulation process by which cells create more receptors on their surface to capture hormone molecules

Urethritis infection of the urethra

Uricosurics drugs that increase the rate of excretion of uric acid by blocking its reabsorption in the kidney

Uropathogens harmful microorganisms that invade the urinary system

Urticaria hypersensitivity response that is characterized by hives and is often accompanied by pruritus (itching)

U.S. Food and Drug Administration (FDA) U.S. regulatory agency responsible for ensuring that drugs and medical devices are safe and effective

USP verification program mark on the label of a dietary supplement that indicates to consumers that the product has been manufactured under acceptable standards of purity, has been tested for active ingredients stated on the label, and is free of harmful contaminants

V

Vaccination process of introducing foreign proteins or inactive cells (vaccines) into the body to trigger immune activation before the patient is exposed to the real pathogen

Vaginal route administration of drugs into the vagina to treat local conditions such as infections, pain, and itching

Vasomotor center cluster of neurons in the medulla that controls baseline blood pressure

Vasospastic (Prinzmetal's) angina type of angina in which the decreased myocardial blood flow is caused by spasms of the coronary arteries

Vectors organisms that harbor pathogens and spread several major protozoan infections by carrying them from one host to another

Venous return the volume of blood returning to the heart from the veins

Venous thromboembolism (VTE) occurs when blood flow through a vein is very slow (stasis)

Ventilation process of moving air into and out of the lungs

Very low-density lipoprotein (VLDL) primary carrier of triglycerides in the blood that is converted to LDL in the liver

Vesicants agents that can cause serious tissue injury if they escape from an artery or vein during an infusion or injection; many antineoplastics are vesicants

Viral load a measurement of HIV RNA levels in the blood that provides an estimate of how rapidly the virus is replicating

Virilization appearance of the male sex characteristics

Virion mature infective virus particle

Virulence quantitative measure of an organism's pathogenicity

Viruses nonliving agents that do not contain any of the cellular organelles that are present in living organisms that are able to cause disease

Vitamins organic nutrient substances required for the health of the human body

Vomiting emesis in which the stomach contents are forced upward into the esophagus and out of the mouth

Vomiting center area in the medulla that controls the vomiting reflex

von Willebrand's disease (vWD) decrease in quantity or quality of von Willebrand factor

W

Water-soluble vitamins group of vitamins stored briefly in the body and then excreted in the urine, including the C and B-complex vitamins

Wearing-off effect appears gradually near the end of a dosing interval; symptoms become worse because the concentration of the drug has fallen below the therapeutic level

Withdrawal syndrome symptoms that result when a patient discontinues taking a substance on which he or she was dependent

X

Xanthine oxidase enzyme responsible for the formation of uric acid

Xerostomia dry mouth

Z

Zollinger-Ellison syndrome (ZES) disorder of excess acid secretion in the stomach resulting in peptic ulcer disease

Credits

Unit Opener Sources

1. Diego Cervo/Shutterstock; Pearson Education, Inc.; Pearson Education, Thinkstock Images/Getty Images
2. Dorling Kindersley, Ltd.; Stokmen/Shutterstock, Lisa F. Young/Shutterstock; Anantha Vardhan/Getty Images
3. StudioSmart/Shutterstock; fotorobs/Shutterstock; Image Point Fr/Shutterstock; Steve Gorton/Dorling Kindersley
4. Ladida/Getty Images; Bassittart/Shutterstock; Imagesbybarbara/Getty Images; Upthebanner/Shutterstock
5. hfng/Shutterstock; Nadino/Shutterstock; Pearson Education; Inc., T. Design/Shutterstock
6. Maya2008/Shutterstock; Lakov Filimonov/Shutterstock; Shutterstock; Christo/Shutterstock
7. Carol Urban; marinaks/Shutterstock
8. Andrey Popov/Shutterstock; wavebreakmedia/Shutterstock; Kim Reinick/Shutterstock; Carol Urban
9. Alexander Raths/Shutterstock; michaeljung/Shutterstock; Carol Urban; Pearson Education, Inc.
10. Omer N. Raja/Shutterstock; Carol Urban; Juanmonino/Getty Images; Yuri Arcurs/Shutterstock
11. Mary Hope/Getty Images; Jorg HackemannShutterstock; Jeff Banke/Shutterstock; Andrew Rich/Getty Images

Chapter Opener Sources

1. Diego Cervo/Shutterstock
2. Aletia/Shutterstock
3. Tyler Olson/Shutterstock
4. Pearson Education, Inc.
5. Pearson Education
6. Thinkstock Images/Getty Images
7. Alexander Raths/Shutterstock
8. Dorling Kindersley, Ltd.
9. Stokmen/Shutterstock
10. Lisa F. Young/Shutterstock
11. Anantha Vardhan/Getty Images
12. StudioSmart/Shutterstock
13. Pearson Education
14. fotorobs/Shutterstock
15. Image Point Fr/Shutterstock
16. Steve Gorton/Dorling Kindersley
17. Storm/Fotolia
18. Ladida/Getty Images
19. Palmer Kane LLC/Shutterstock
20. Kevin Russ/Getty Images
21. Jack Cronkhite/Shutterstock
22. Bassittart/Shutterstock
23. Valua Vitaly/Shutterstock
24. Imagesbybarbara/Getty Images
25. Upthebanner/Shutterstock
26. holbox/Shutterstock
27. Stock Shop Photography LLC/Getty Images
28. Sebastian Kaulitzki/Shutterstock
29. hfng/Shutterstock
30. Elena Elisseeva/Shutterstock
31. Real Deal Photo/Shutterstock
32. Ocskay Mark/Shutterstock
33. michaeljung/Shutterstuck
34. Nadino/Shutterstock
35. Pearson Education, Inc.
36. Pearson Education, Inc.
37. Carol Urban
38. Elena Elisseeva/Shutterstock
39. T. Design/Shutterstock
40. Maya2008/Shutterstock
41. Lakov Filimonov/Shutterstock
42. Shutterstock
43. Christo/Shutterstock
44. Carol Urban
45. marinaks/Shutterstock
46. Tishenko Irina/Shutterstock
47. Ragne Kabanova/Shutterstock
48. Andrey Popov/Shutterstock
49. Pearson Education, Inc.
50. wavebreakmedia/Shutterstock
51. Kim Reinick/Shutterstock
52. Image Point Fr/Shutterstock
53. oliveromg/Shutterstock
54. Pearson Education, Inc.
55. Rui Vale Sousa/Shutterstock
56. Sharon Dominick/Getty Images
57. Carol Urban
58. decade3d/Shutterstock
59. wavebreakmedia/Shutterstock
60. Alexander Raths/Shutterstock
61. michaeljung/Shutterstock
62. Carol Urban
63. Pearson Education, Inc.
64. Designua/Shutterstock
65. Omer N. Raja/Shutterstock
66. Carol Urban
67. Tracy WhitesideShutterstock
68. Juanmonino/Getty Images
69. Yuri Arcurs/Shutterstock
70. Yuri Arcurs/Shutterstock
71. David Hanover/Getty Images
72. Mary Hope/Getty Images
73. Jorg HackemannShutterstock
74. Jeff Banke/Shutterstock
75. Andrew Rich/Getty Images

Index

Page numbers followed by *f* indicate figures. Those followed by *t* indicate tables, boxes, or special features. The titles of special features (e.g., Nursing Practice Applications, Pharmacotherapy Illustrated, Treating the Diverse Patient) are also first-letter capitalized.

Prototype drug names appear in red, drug classifications are in SMALL CAPS, and trade names are first-letter capitalized and cross-referenced to their generic names.

A

A fibers, 369–370
abacavir, 932*t*, 934
abarelix, 978
abatacept, 1248*t*, 1249, 1250
abbreviations, medication errors and, 69
abciximab, 571, 626*t*, 629–630
Abel, John Jacob, 3, 144*t*
Abelcet. *See* amphotericin B lipid complex
Abilify. *See* aripiprazole
abiraterone, 976*t*, 979
abnormal foci, in seizure activity, 313
abobotulinumtoxinA, 341*t*, 343, 343*t*
ABORTIFACIENTS, 1202–1205, 1203*t*. *See also* methotrexate; mifepristone
Abreva. *See* docosanol
abscesses (carbuncles), 1264
absence seizures, 311, 313, 313*t*, 325
absorption
  blood flow at site of administration and, 31
  concentrations and dosages, impact on, 30
  defined, 27, 997
  drug interactions and, 31, 58–59, 59*f*
  gastrointestinal tract environment and, 30–31
  in geriatric patients, 118–119
  ionization and, 31, 31*f*
  in pediatric patients, 106
  during pregnancy, 93–94
  route of administration and, 27–30
  surface area and, 31
Abstral. *See* fentanyl
acai, 81*t*
acarbose, 1122*t*, 1129
ACC (American College of Cardiology), 457, 459, 582
accessory organs of digestion, 997, 1000–1001
Accolate. *See* zafirlukast
Accupril. *See* quinapril
Accuretic, 493, 546*t*
Accutane. *See* isotretinoin
ACE (angiotensin-converting enzyme), 487, 489
ACE inhibitors. *See* ANGIOTENSIN-CONVERTING ENZYME INHIBITORS
acebutolol, 198*t*, 603*t*, 606
Aceon. *See* perindopril
acesulfame, 1085
Acetadote. *See* acetylcysteine
acetaldehyde dehydrogenase, 426
acetaminophen, 683–684
  adverse effects, 616*t*, 684
  breast-feeding and, 98*t*
  in combination products, 683, 757*t*, 766*t*
  cultural differences in metabolism of, 684*t*
  drug interactions, 424, 425*t*, 618*t*, 622*t*, 684

  lactation risk categories, 99*t*
  mechanism of action, 683
  metabolism of, 33
  nursing responsibilities, 684
  overdoses/poisoning, 684, 1000*t*, 1308, 1308*t*
  with oxycodone, 378, 422
  pharmacokinetics, 684
  pregnancy category, 95*t*
  routes and dosages, 112*t*, 371–372, 680*t*
  for seizures, 313*t*
  therapeutic effects and uses, 379, 682*t*, 683, 1246
  toxicity, 33
  with tramadol, 382
acetazolamide, 513*t*, 515–516, 839, 1041, 1288*t*, 1292
acetic acid and hydrocortisone, 1297*t*
acetylation, 129, 855, 856*f*
acetylcholine (Ach)
  Alzheimer's disease and, 296, 297, 298*f*
  discovery of, 142*t*
  effects and clinical applications, 140, 141*t*, 210*t*
  life cycle of, 144*f*
  Parkinson's disease and, 287
  receptors, 142–143, 144*t*, 150–151*f*, 150–152, 151*t*
  synthesis and release of, 142, 143*f*
  termination of action, 143–144
acetylcholinesterase (AchE), 143–144, 151
ACETYLCHOLINESTERASE (AchE) INHIBITORS, 154–158
  adverse effects, 297
  for Alzheimer's disease, 154, 296–297
  drugs in class
    ambenonium, 152*t*, 158
    donepezil, 152*t*, 154, 296–297, 297*t*, 298–299
    edrophonium, 152*t*, 155, 157, 158
    galantamine, 152*t*, 154, 297*t*, 299–300
    neostigmine, 151, 152*t*, 158, 173
    physostigmine, 152*t*, 154, 166
    pyridostigmine, 152*t*, 154, 155, 157
    rivastigmine, 152*t*, 297, 297*t*, 300
    tacrine, 152*t*, 299
  glaucoma, 154, 1289
  mechanism of action, 154
  for nerve gas poisoning prophylaxis, 154–155
  overdoses of, 155
acetylcysteine, 766*t*, 767, 1308*t*
acetylsalicylic acid. *See* aspirin
acetyltransferase, 129
Ach. *See* acetylcholine
AchE (acetylcholinesterase), 143–144, 151
AchE inhibitors. *See* ACETYLCHOLINESTERASE INHIBITORS
acid. *See* lysergic acid diethylamide
acid–base imbalances
  acidosis, 533–535, 534*f*, 534*t*
  alkalosis, 534*f*, 534*t*, 535–536
  buffers and, 533
acidosis, 533–535, 534*f*, 534*t*
AcipHex. *See* rabeprazole
acitretin, 1275–1276, 1276*t*
ACK. *See* acesulfame
aclidinium, 165*t*, 166, 168, 740
Aclovate. *See* alclometasone dipropionate
acne vulgaris, 807, 809, 1267–1271, 1271–1272*t*

Acomplia. *See* rimonabant
Acova. *See* argatroban
acquired immunodeficiency syndrome (AIDS). *See* HIV-AIDS
acquired resistance, 779–782, 779*t*, 781*f*
acrivastine and pseudoephedrine, 756*t*, 758
acromegaly, 1102
Actemra. *See* tocilizumab
ACTH (adrenocorticotropic hormone), 315, 1153, 1210
Acticin. *See* permethrin
Actifed, 757*t*
actigraphy, 222
Actimmune. *See* INTERFERON(s), IFN gamma-1b
Actinomycin-D. *See* dactinomycin
action potentials, 445
Actiq. *See* fentanyl
Activase. *See* alteplase
activated charcoal, 1309–1310
activated partial thromboplastin time (aPTT), 617
active immunity, 710, 711, 722*f*
active transport, 27
Activella. *See* estradiol and norethindrone
Actonel. *See* risedronate
Actoplus Met, 1125*t*
Actos. *See* pioglitazone
Acular. *See* ketorolac
acupuncture, 336, 389*t*, 953*t*
acute dystonia, 270
acute gouty arthritis, 1253. *See also* gout
acute otitis media (AOM), 108*t*, 1296
acute pain, 367. *See also* pain
acute pancreatitis, 1041
acute psychosis, 265
acute retroviral syndrome, 928
acute stress disorder, 219
acute uncomplicated cystitis (AUC), 834–836, 835*t*
Acuvail. *See* ketorolac
acyclovir, 911–912
  adverse effects, 56*t*, 616*t*, 912
  breast-feeding and, 98*t*
  clinical applications, 719, 823, 910, 911, 1265
  drug interactions, 58, 912
  mechanism of action, 911
  Nursing Responsibilities, 912
  routes and dosages, 112*t*, 911*t*
Aczone. *See* dapsone
AD. *See* Alzheimer's disease
Adalat/Adalat CC. *See* nifedipine
adalimumab
  clinical applications, 702*t*, 1033, 1249, 1250, 1277
  routes and dosages, 1248*t*, 1276*t*
adapalene, 1268*t*, 1269, 1270
adaptive (specific) body defenses, 668–671
Adcetris. *See* brentuximab
Adcirca. *See* tadalafil
Adderall/Adderall XR. *See* amphetamine and dextroamphetamine
addiction, 369, 418. *See also* substance abuse
Addison's disease, 1155–1156, 1156*t*
additive effects, 60–61, 61*f*
adefovir dipivoxil, 917*t*, 918, 919, 933

Adenocard. *See* adenosine
Adenoscan. *See* adenosine
adenosine, 603*t*, 609
ADENOSINE DIPHOSPHATE RECEPTOR BLOCKERS, 571, 627–629
adenoviruses, 908*t*
ADH. *See* antidiuretic hormone
ADHD. *See* attention deficit/hyperactivity disorder
adherence
  to antihypertensives, 546
  defined, 73
  factors impacting, 73–74, 74*t*, 268
  in geriatric patients, 120, 120*t*
  in pediatric patients, 113
adhesins, 1017
Adipex-P. *See* phentermine
adipocytes, 1080
ADJUVANT ANALGESICS, 383–384, 384*t*
  antidepressants. *See* ANTIDEPRESSANTS
  antiseizure agents. *See* ANTIEPILEPTIC DRUGS
  benzodiazepines. *See* BENZODIAZEPINES
  bisphosphonates, 384, 384*t*, 1239–1240*t*, 1239–1242
  corticosteroids. *See* CORTICOSTEROIDS
adjuvant chemotherapy, 951. *See also* ANTINEOPLASTIC AGENTS
adolescents, 109, 110, 422, 653. *See also* pediatric patients
ado-trastuzumab, 987*t*
adrenal atrophy, 1156, 1157*f*
adrenal crisis, 1156
adrenal gland, physiology of, 1152–1153, 1152–1153*f*
adrenal medulla, 146, 489
Adrenalin. *See* epinephrine
adrenaline, 144*t*
ADRENERGIC AGONISTS, 177–191
  catecholamines *vs.* noncatecholamines, 179, 180*f*
  classification of, 179
  for glaucoma, 1289–1290
  mechanism of action, 147, 178–179, 179*f*
  nonselective, 180–183, 181*t*
    amphetamines. *See* AMPHETAMINES
    dopamine. *See* dopamine
    ephedrine, 178, 179, 181*t*, 183
    epinephrine. *See* epinephrine
    norepinephrine. *See* norepinephrine
  Nursing Practice Applications, 187–189*t*
  selective. *See* ALPHA-ADRENERGIC AGONISTS; BETA-ADRENERGIC AGONISTS
ADRENERGIC ANTAGONISTS, 192–206
  alpha. *See* ALPHA-ADRENERGIC ANTAGONISTS
  beta. *See* BETA-ADRENERGIC ANTAGONISTS
  mechanism of action, 147, 193, 194*f*, 548
  Nursing Practice Applications, 203–204*t*
ADRENERGIC NEURON BLOCKERS, 550
adrenergic receptors, 144
adrenergic synapses, 211
adrenergic transmission, 144–146, 145*f*
  alpha$_1$-adrenergic receptors, 144, 144*t*, 145, 180
  alpha$_2$-adrenergic receptors, 144, 144*t*, 145, 180
  beta$_1$-adrenergic receptors, 144, 144*t*, 145, 180
  beta$_2$-adrenergic receptors, 144, 144*t*, 145, 180
  norepinephrine. *See* norepinephrine
adrenocortical insufficiency, 1155–1158, 1157*f*
adrenocorticotropic hormone (ACTH), 313*t*, 315, 1094*t*, 1153, 1210
Adriamycin. *See* doxorubicin
Adrucil. *See* fluorouracil
advanced practice registered nurses (APRNs), 20–21
adverse drug effects, 53–58. *See also* Black Box Warnings
  allergic reactions, 54–55, 86–87

cancer-causing drugs, 55–56, 55*t*
  defined, 53
  drug-induced myopathies, 335, 335*t*
  drugs most associated with, 54*t*
  fetal, 56, 96, 97
  in geriatric patients, 121–122, 122*t*
  herbal and dietary supplements, 84–85
  idiosyncratic reactions, 48, 55
  interactions. *See* drug interactions
  monitoring of, 18, 54
  nursing role in, 53–54
  organ-specific, 56–58, 56*t*, 85
  in pediatric patients, 106, 110–113, 112*t*
  prevention of, 53–54
Adverse Event Reporting System (AERS), 18, 54
Advicor, 463, 465
Advil. *See* ibuprofen
AEDs. *See* ANTIEPILEPTIC DRUGS
aerobic bacteria, 776
AeroBid. *See* flunisolide
aerosols, 733
AERS (Adverse Event Reporting System), 18, 54
affinity, 32
Affordable Care Act. *See* Patient Protection and Affordable Care Act of 2010
Afinitor. *See* everolimus
African Americans
  antihypertensive therapy in, 131*t*, 197*t*, 544, 546
  diabetes mellitus and, 1113
  G6PD deficiency in, 49*t*
  genetic polymorphisms in, 129
  renal failure among, 504*t*
African trypanosomiasis (sleeping sickness), 895
Afrin. *See* oxymetazoline
Afrin 4-6 Hour. *See* phenylephrine
Aftate. *See* tolnaftate
afterload, 448, 448*f*
Agenerase. *See* amprenavir
Aggrastat. *See* tirofiban
aging. *See* geriatric patients
agonists, 48, 48*f*
agoraphobia, 218
agranulocytosis, 57
Agrylin. *See* anagrelide
AHA (American Heart Association), 457, 459, 582
AIDS. *See* HIV-AIDS
air embolism, 1071*t*
akathisia, 270, 270*t*
Akineton. *See* biperiden
Akten. *See* lidocaine
Alamast. *See* pemirolast
Alaska Natives. *See* Native Americans and Alaska Natives
alatrofloxacin, 826
Albalon. *See* naphazoline
albendazole, 897, 898, 899*t*, 900
Albenza. *See* albendazole
albiglutide, 1122*t*, 1131
albumin, 442, 502
Albuminar. *See* normal serum albumin
albuterol, 736–737
  adverse effects, 351, 736–737
  for asthma, 187, 736–737, 737*t*
  drug interactions, 200, 737
  duration of action, 186
  mechanism of action, 736
  nursing responsibilities, 737
  routes and dosages, 181*t*
Alcaine. *See* proparacaine
alclometasone dipropionate, 1273*t*
alcohol
  abuse of, 417, 423, 424
  adolescent use of, 109

adverse effects, 1215*t*
  dependence and, 419
  drug interactions, 58, 86*t*, 424–425, 425*t*
  metabolism of, 423, 424*f*
  pharmacologic management of, 58, 227, 425, 426
  during pregnancy, 94, 95–96, 425
  pregnancy category, 95*t*
  vitamin metabolism impacted by, 1050
  withdrawal from, 420*t*, 425
Aldactazide, 506, 546*t*
Aldactone. *See* spironolactone
aldesleukin, 692*t*, 693, 694–695, 988
Aldomet. *See* methyldopa
Aldoril, 546*t*
aldosterone
  excessive secretion of, 1162
  in fluid balance, 523, 529, 529*f*
  functions of, 1153
  inadequate secretion, 1162
  reabsorption, effects on, 503
  regulation of, 1094*t*
  release of, 489–490, 1152
ALDOSTERONE ANTAGONISTS, 490, 494*t*, 495–496, 511–512
alefacept, 1276*t*, 1277
alemtuzumab, 987*t*
alendronate, 32, 1239–1240*t*, 1240–1241
Aleve. *See* naproxen
Alfenta. *See* alfentanil
alfentanil, 377, 396, 397*t*, 398
Alferon N. *See* INTERFERON(s), IFN alfa-n3
alfuzosin, 193, 194*t*, 196, 1221*t*
alimentary canal, 997. *See also* gastrointestinal tract
Alimta. *See* pemetrexed
Alinia. *See* nitazoxanide
aliskiren, 479, 490, 495, 546*t*, 548
alkalosis, 534*f*, 534*t*, 535–536
Alka-Seltzer. *See* sodium bicarbonate
Alkeran. *See* melphalan
ALKYLATING AGENTS, 963–968, 964*t*, 965*f*
  bendamustine, 964*t*, 966
  busulfan, 964*t*, 966
  carboplatin, 504*t*, 616*t*, 964*t*, 966
  carmustine, 958, 964*t*, 966
  chlorambucil, 55*t*, 964*t*, 966
  cisplatin, 55–56*t*, 504*t*, 958, 964*t*, 966
  cyclophosphamide. *See* cyclophosphamide
  dacarbazine, 55*t*, 964*t*, 967
  estramustine, 964*t*, 967
  ifosfamide, 964*t*, 967
  lomustine, 964*t*, 967
  mechlorethamine, 963, 964*t*, 967
  melphalan, 964*t*, 967
  oxaliplatin, 964*t*, 967
  procarbazine, 964*t*, 967–968
  streptozocin, 964*t*, 968
  temozolomide, 105*t*, 964*t*, 967
  thiotepa, 964*t*, 968
Allegra. *See* fexofenadine
Allerest. *See* naphazoline
allergens, 754
allergic reactions, 54–55, 86–87
allergic rhinitis, 754–764
  decongestants. *See* NASAL DECONGESTANTS
  goals of, 754–755
  mast cell stabilizers, 762–763
  pathophysiology, 754, 755*f*
  pharmacotherapy, 755–764
    antihistamines, 755–761, 756*t*
    corticosteroids, 759, 759*t*, 762, 1159. *See also under* CORTICOSTEROIDS

cromolyn, 94, 741*t*, 742–743, 759*t*, 763, 1295*t*
ipratropium. *See* ipratropium
montelukast, 741*t*, 744, 759*t*, 763
prevalence of, 754*t*
allergy testing, 754
Alli. *See* orlistat
Allium sativum. *See* garlic
allopurinol, 622*t*, 674, 1253, 1254*t*, 1255–1256, 1334*t*
almotriptan, 387*t*, 388
Alocril. *See* nedocromil
aloe, 81*t*
aloe vera, 85, 1026, 1277*t*, 1278
alogliptin, 1122*t*, 1125*t*, 1131
Alomide. *See* lodoxamide
alopecia, 958, 963, 1279–1280
Alora. *See* estradiol
alosetron, 1033*t*, 1036
Aloxi. *See* palonosetron
alpha$_1$-adrenergic receptors, 144, 144*t*, 145, 180
alpha$_2$-adrenergic receptors, 144, 144*t*, 145, 180
ALPHA-ADRENERGIC AGONISTS
adverse effects, 184, 549
clinical applications, 183–184
for glaucoma, 1289
for hypertension, 544*t*, 549–550
mechanism of action, 184
for nasal congestion, 183, 184–185, 763–764.
See also NASAL DECONGESTANTS
ocular decongestants/vasoconstrictors,
185, 1293*t*, 1294
ophthalmic applications, 183
ALPHA-ADRENERGIC ANTAGONISTS, 193–197
adverse effects, 194*t*, 195, 549, 1215*t*
for benign prostatic hyperplasia, 1221
clinical applications, 193–197
drugs in class
alfuzosin, 193, 194*t*, 196, 1221*t*
doxazosin, 193, 194*t*, 196, 1221, 1221*t*
phenoxybenzamine, 193, 194*t*, 196
phentolamine. *See* phentolamine
prazosin, 98*t*, 193, 194*t*, 196, 546*t*, 549
tamsulosin, 193, 194*t*, 197, 549, 1221*t*
terazosin, 193, 194*t*, 197, 549, 1221, 1221*t*
for hypertension, 193, 195, 196–197, 544*t*, 549
routes and dosages, 194*t*
alpha-blockers. *See* ALPHA-ADRENERGIC ANTAGONISTS
Alphagan P. *See* brimonidine
ALPHA-GLUCOSIDASE INHIBITORS, 1129–1130
acarbose, 1122*t*, 1129
miglitol, 1122*t*, 1130
5-ALPHA REDUCTASE INHIBITORS, 1221–1222, 1221*t*
dutasteride, 1221*t*, 1222
finasteride, 1215*t*, 1221–1222, 1221*t*, 1279, 1280
alprazolam, 7, 95*t*, 225–226*t*, 227, 417, 425*t*
alprostadil, 1217
ALS (amyotrophic lateral sclerosis), 304, 336
Alsuma. *See* sumatriptan
Altace. *See* ramipril
alteplase, 632, 632*t*
AlternaGel. *See* aluminum hydroxide
alternative medicine. *See* Complementary and
Alternative Therapies
Altoprev. *See* lovastatin
altretamine, 988–989, 990*t*
aluminum antacids, 1016
aluminum hydroxide, 98*t*, 1015*t*, 1016–1017
alveoli, 731
Alvesco. *See* ciclesonide
alvimopan, 385, 423
Alzheimer's disease (AD), 295–300
epilepsy and, 311*t*
etiology of, 295–296, 296*f*
gender differences in, 130

genetic influences on, 296
pharmacotherapy, 152*t*, 154, 296–300, 297*t*, 298*f*
prevalence of, 295*t*
symptoms of, 210*t*, 295, 296*t*
Amanita muscaria, 143, 153, 153*t*
amantadine, 290*t*, 293, 913, 914–915, 914*t*
Amaryl. *See* glimepiride
ambenonium, 152*t*, 158
Ambenyl Cough Syrup, 766*t*
Ambien/Ambien CR. *See* zolpidem
AmBisome. *See* liposomal amphotericin B
amcinonide, 1273*t*
amebiasis, 885*t*, 890, 890*t*, 891*f*
amenorrhea, 1171
Amerge. *See* naratriptan
Americaine. *See* benzocaine
American Academy of Family Physicians, 1296
American Academy of Neurology, 337–338
American Academy of Pain Management, 368*t*
American Academy of Pediatrics, 109, 463*t*, 1296
American Cancer Society, 951
American College of Cardiology (ACC), 457, 459, 582
American College of Gastroenterology, 1018
American Heart Association (AHA), 457, 459, 582
American Indians. *See* Native Americans and Alaska
Natives
American Pain Society, 368*t*
American Pharmaceutical Association (APhA), 15
American Society of Clinical Oncology (ASCO), 975
American Thoracic Society, 852
American trypanosomiasis (Chagas' disease), 894–895
Amevive. *See* alefacept
Amicar. *See* aminocaproic acid
Amidate. *See* etomidate
amide-type local anesthesia, 406*t*, 409–411
Amigesic. *See* salsalate
amikacin, 812, 812*t*, 814, 853*t*, 857, 863
Amikin. *See* amikacin
amiloride, 506, 511, 511*t*, 513
amino acids, 87, 87*t*, 1070–1071
aminocaproic acid, 635–636, 635*t*, 637
AMINOGLYCOSIDES, 812–814
adverse effects, 56*t*, 504*t*, 813
breast-feeding and, 98*t*, 784
clinical applications, 812–814, 857, 1306
drugs in class
amikacin, 812, 812*t*, 814, 853*t*, 857, 863
gentamicin. *See* gentamicin
kanamycin, 812*t*, 814, 853*t*, 857, 1072
neomycin, 812, 812*t*, 814, 830, 1264, 1295
paromomycin. *See* paromomycin
streptomycin. *See* streptomycin
tobramycin, 812*t*, 814
mechanism of action, 812
Nursing Practice Applications, 816–817*t*
resistance to, 812
types of, 812*t*
aminopenicillins, 791–792
aminophylline, 737*t*, 745
aminosalicylic acid, 853*t*, 858, 1032
amiodarone, 607–608
adverse effects, 607
clinical applications, 572, 607
half-life of, 38
interactions with, 86*t*, 622*t*
mechanism of action, 607
Nursing Responsibilities, 608
routes and dosages, 603*t*
AMIs (atypical mycobacterial infections), 849
Amitiza. *See* lubiprostone
amitriptyline
adverse effects, 247
for anxiety, 231*t*

for depression, 1036
drug interactions, 425*t*
for insomnia, 231*t*
mechanism of action, 247
for migraine prophylaxis, 389, 389*t*
in pain management, 303, 383
routes and dosages, 245*t*
amlodipine
aliskiren with, 546*t*
benazepril with, 492, 546*t*
clinical applications, 45, 477*t*, 479, 548
hydrochlorothiazide with, 495, 546*t*
olmesartan with, 495, 546*t*
routes and dosages, 478*t*, 568*t*
telmisartan with, 495
valsartan with, 495, 546*t*
ammonium chloride, 60, 535–536
amnesia, anterograde, 421
amobarbital, 234
amoxapine, 251–252
amoxicillin, 111, 112*t*, 789*t*, 792, 1017, 1297
Amoxil. *See* amoxicillin
amphetamine and dextroamphetamine, 34, 354*t*,
355–356, 1082
AMPHETAMINES
abuse of, 353, 430
for ADHD, 353–356, 354*t*
adverse effects, 180, 353
drug interactions, 1016
drugs in class
benzphetamine, 356
dexmethylphenidate, 354*t*, 356
lisdexamphetamine, 354*t*, 356
methylphenidate. *See* methylphenidate
mechanism of action, 178, 353, 429–430
for narcolepsy, 222
during pregnancy, 96*t*
withdrawal symptoms and treatment, 420*t*
Amphotec. *See* amphotericin B cholesteryl sulfate
complex
amphotericin B cholesteryl sulfate complex, 870
amphotericin B deoxycholate, 868–871
adverse effects, 56*t*, 504*t*, 616*t*, 871
clinical applications, 869–870, 895
drug interactions, 1072
mechanism of action, 868, 871
Nursing Responsibilities, 871
routes and dosages, 870*t*
amphotericin B lipid complex, 870
ampicillin, 792
absorption of, 106
adverse effects, 616*t*, 792
clinical applications, 792, 836
drug interactions, 1072
mechanism of action, 792
Nursing Responsibilities, 792
routes and dosages, 112*t*, 789*t*
Amplified *Mycobacterium Tuberculosis* Direct
Test, 851
amprenavir, 937
Ampyra. *See* dalfampridine
Amrix. *See* cyclobenzaprine
Amturnide, 479, 546*t*
amygdala, 220
amyotrophic lateral sclerosis (ALS), 304, 336
Amytal. *See* amobarbital
anabolic effects, 1212
Anabolic Steroid Control Act of 2004, 434, 1214
ANABOLIC STEROIDS, 1212
abuse of, 434
adverse effects, 55*t*, 1214, 1215*t*
clinical applications, 1212, 1214
drugs in class

ANABOLIC STEROIDS (*continued*)
danazol, 622*t*, 1182*t*, 1183, 1185
nandrolone, 1210*t*, 1214
oxandrolone, 1210*t*, 1214
oxymetholone, 1210*t*, 1214
interactions with, 86*t*, 622*t*
routes and dosages, 1210*t*
withdrawal symptoms and treatment, 420*t*
Anacin. *See* aspirin
Anadrol-50. *See* oxymetholone
anaerobic bacteria, 776
Anafranil. *See* clomipramine
anagrelide, 626*t*
anakinra, 696*t*, 701, 1248*t*, 1249, 1250
analgesics, 368. *See also* pain management
anaphylaxis, 45, 53, 673
Anaprox. *See* naproxen
Anaspaz. *See* hyoscyamine
anastrozole, 976*t*, 978
Anbesol. *See* benzocaine
Ancef. *See* cefazolin
Ancobon. *See* flucytosine
Ancylostoma duodenale, 897
Andro. *See* androstenedione
Androderm patch, 1211
AndroGel, 1211
ANDROGEN(s), 1209, 1210–1212
adverse effects, 1210*t*, 1212
drugs in class
fluoxymesterone, 976*t*, 1210*t*, 1212
methyltestosterone, 1210*t*, 1212
testosterone. *See* testosterone
testosterone cypionate, 1210*t*, 1211
testosterone enanthate, 1210*t*, 1211
for hypogonadism, 1210
nonreproductive uses, 1211
Nursing Practice Applications, 1213–1214
ANDROGEN RECEPTOR BLOCKERS, 976, 979
abiraterone, 976*t*, 979
bicalutamide, 976*t*, 979
flutamide, 976*t*, 979
nilutamide, 976*t*, 979
Android. *See* methyltestosterone
androstenedione, 434, 1209
Anectine. *See* succinylcholine
anemias, 505*t*, 652–653, 653*t*, 957. *See also*
ANTIANEMIC AGENTS
Anestacon. *See* lidocaine
anesthesia, 394–415
adjunctive agents for, 411, 413
deaths related to, 404*t*
drug interactions with, 425*t*
general. *See* general anesthesia
local. *See* local anesthesia
Nursing Practice Applications, 407–408*t*,
412–413*t*
types of, 395
angina pectoris
pathophysiology of, 561–562
pharmacotherapy, 562–567
beta-adrenergic antagonists, 198, 199, 563,
563*f*, 566–567, 568*t*
calcium channel blockers, 476–481, 563,
563*f*, 567, 568*t*
goals of, 562–563
organic nitrates, 563, 563*f*, 564–566, 564*t*, 568*t*
partial fatty-acid oxidation inhibitors, 563
prevalence of, 562*t*
symptoms of, 445
angioedema, 57, 490*t*, 491
angiogenesis, 950. *See also* VASCULAR ENDOTHELIAL
GROWTH FACTOR (VEGF) INHIBITORS
Angiomax. *See* bivalirudin

angiotensin I, 487, 489
angiotensin II, 451, 487, 488–490
ANGIOTENSIN II RECEPTOR BLOCKERS (ARBs)
adverse effects, 493, 548
drugs in class
azilsartan medoxomil, 494*t*, 495, 546*t*
candesartan, 494*t*, 495, 546*t*, 548, 584*t*
eprosartan, 494*t*, 495, 546*t*, 548
irbesartan, 494*t*, 495, 546*t*, 548
losartan, 33, 493–495, 494*t*, 546*t*, 548
olmesartan medoxomil, 479, 494*t*, 495,
546*t*, 548
telmisartan, 479, 494*t*, 495, 546*t*, 548
valsartan, 479, 494*t*, 495, 546*t*, 548, 584*t*
for heart failure, 493–495, 494*t*, 584*t*, 585
for hypertension, 493–495, 494*t*, 544*t*, 548
mechanism of action, 490
for myocardial infarction, 493
Nursing Practice Applications, 496–497*t*
pregnancy category, 95*t*
angiotensin-converting enzyme (ACE), 487, 489
ANGIOTENSIN-CONVERTING ENZYME (ACE) INHIBITORS
adverse effects, 56*t*, 488*t*, 490*t*, 491, 504*t*, 548,
585, 1215*t*
angioedema and, 490*t*, 491
Black Box Warning, 491
breast-feeding and, 98*t*
for diabetes, 491*t*
drugs in class
benazepril, 33, 479, 491*t*, 492, 546*t*, 548
captopril. *See* captopril
enalapril, 33, 491*t*, 492, 546*t*, 548, 584*t*
enalaprilat, 33, 492, 553*t*
fosinopril, 491*t*, 492, 548, 584*t*
lisinopril, 491–492, 491*t*, 548, 572, 584*t*
moexipril, 491*t*, 492–493, 548
perindopril, 491*t*, 493, 548
quinapril, 491*t*, 493, 548, 584*t*
ramipril, 491*t*, 493, 548, 584*t*
trandolapril, 491*t*, 493, 546*t*, 548
for heart failure, 490–493, 491*t*, 583–585, 584*t*
hyperkalemia and, 488*t*, 491
for hypertension, 490–493, 491*t*, 544*t*, 548
mechanism of action, 490, 491, 583–584
for myocardial infarction, 490–491, 572
Nursing Practice Applications, 496–497*t*
pregnancy category, 95, 95*t*
angiotensinogen, 487
anidulafungin, 870*t*, 872
animal-derived products, refusal based on religious
grounds, 128*t*
anions, 528
Anopheles mosquito, 886
anora ellipta, 746
anorexia, 957
ANOREXIANTS, 353, 1082, 1085
diethylpropion, 1083*t*, 1085
phentermine, 1082, 1083*t*, 1085
rimonabant, 1082
anovulatory cycles, 1171
ANPs (atrial natriuretic peptides), 451, 581
ANS. *See* autonomic nervous system
Ansaid. *See* flurbiprofen
Antabuse. *See* disulfiram
ANTACIDS, 1015–1017
aluminum hydroxide, 98*t*, 1015*t*, 1016–1017
calcium carbonate, 1015*t*, 1233–1234*t*
clinical applications, 59, 200, 1037
magaldrate, 1015*t*
magnesium hydroxide, 98*t*, 533, 1015*t*, 1025*t*,
1027, 1057
sodium bicarbonate. *See* sodium bicarbonate
antagonistic effects, 61, 61*f*, 782

antagonists, 48, 48*f*
Antara. *See* fenofibrate
anterior pituitary gland, 1098
anterograde amnesia, 421
anthracyclines, 56*t*, 973, 974
anthrax, 711, 777*t*, 824, 1305–1306, 1305*t*
antiadrenal drugs, 1163
ANTIANEMIC AGENTS
cyanocobalamin. *See* cyanocobalamin
folic acid. *See* folic acid
iron salts, 98*t*, 653–657, 654*f*, 656*t*
routes and dosages, 653*t*
antianxiety medications. *See* NONBENZODIAZEPINE
ANXIOLYTICS
ANTIBIOTICS
adverse effects, 57, 783–784, 1028
broad-spectrum, 782, 784, 791–792
cell wall inhibitors
aztreonam, 797*t*, 799
carbapenems, 797–798, 797*t*
cephalosporins, 778, 790, 794–797, 794*t*
fosfomycin, 797*t*, 799, 836, 838*t*, 842
miscellaneous agents, 797*t*, 798–799
penicillins. *See* PENICILLIN(s)
telavancin, 797*t*, 799
vancomycin, 37, 616*t*, 778, 797*t*, 798–799,
800–801*t*
combination therapy with, 782–783
cyclic lipopeptides, 827
defined, 776
drug interactions with, 425*t*
fluoroquinolones. *See* FLUOROQUINOLONES
in geriatric patients, 794*t*
ketolides, 818, 830
mechanisms of action, 776, 778, 779*f*
miscellaneous
bacitracin, 827, 827*t*, 830, 1264
metronidazole. *See* metronidazole
polymyxin B, 827, 827*t*, 830, 1264
rifampin. *See* rifampin
narrow-spectrum, 782
photosensitivity and, 808, 808*t*
in pregnancy and lactation, 784
prophylactic therapy with, 783
protein synthesis inhibitors
aminoglycosides. *See* AMINOGLYCOSIDES
chloramphenicol, 56*t*, 98*t*, 814–815,
815*t*, 1306
clindamycin, 815, 815*t*, 886, 1268*t*, 1269
lincomycin, 815, 815*t*
linezolid, 616*t*, 782, 815, 815*t*
macrolides. *See* MACROLIDES
mechanism of action, 806, 806*f*
quinupristin-dalfopristin, 61, 782, 815,
815*t*, 818
telithromycin, 815*t*, 818, 827*t*, 830
tetracyclines. *See* TETRACYCLINES
resistance to, 779–782, 779*t*, 781*f*
selection of, 782–784
sulfonamides. *See* SULFONAMIDES
superinfections and, 784
ANTIBODIES, 442, 669–670, 670*f*, 702–703. *See also*
MONOCLONAL ANTIBODIES
anticholinergic syndrome, 166
anticholinergics. *See* MUSCARINIC ANTAGONISTS
anticholinesterase agents. *See* ACETYLCHOLINESTERASE
INHIBITORS
ANTICOAGULANTS, 617–626
direct thrombin inhibitors. *See* direct thrombin
inhibitors
indirect thrombin inhibitors, 617–622. *See also*
heparin; warfarin
interactions with, 62*t*, 425*t*

low-molecular-weight heparins. *See* low-molecular-weight heparins
mechanism of action, 615, 617, 617*t*
for myocardial infarction, 571
Nursing Practice Applications, 624–626*t*
routes and dosages, 618*t*
anticonvulsants. *See* ANTIEPILEPTIC DRUGS
ANTIDEPRESSANTS
   for ADHD, 357
   as adjuvant analgesics, 383
   for anxiety, 223, 224, 230–232, 231*t*
   atypical. *See* ATYPICAL ANTIDEPRESSANTS
   Black Box Warnings, 234*t*, 242
   for cataplexy, 358
   classification of, 244, 245*t*
   defined, 244
   for insomnia, 223, 224, 230–232, 231*t*
   interactions with, 425*t*
   for irritable bowel syndrome, 1036
   MAOIs. *See* MONOAMINE OXIDASE INHIBITORS
   mechanism of action, 230–231
   metabolism of, 275*t*
   for migraine prophylaxis, 389
   Nursing Practice Applications for, 255–256*t*
   SSRIs. *See* selective serotonin reuptake inhibitors
   suicide risk and, 234*t*, 242–243
   tricyclic. *See* TRICYCLIC ANTIDEPRESSANTS
ANTIDIABETIC AGENTS, 1121–1134
   adverse effects, 1121
   alpha-glucosidase inhibitors, 1122*t*, 1129–1130
   biguanides, 1122*t*, 1125*t*, 1126–1127, 1131
   classification of, 1121, 1121*t*
   combination agents, 1125, 1125*t*
   drug interactions, 86*t*
   incretin enhancers, 1130–1131
   meglitinides, 1122*t*, 1125*t*, 1127–1128
   principles of therapy, 1121
   routes and dosages of, 1122*t*, 1125*t*
   sulfonylureas, 425*t*, 839, 1125–1126
   thiazolidinediones, 1122*t*, 1125*t*, 1126, 1128–1129, 1131
ANTIDIARRHEALS, 1028–1030, 1028*t*, 1030–1031*t*
   bismuth subsalicylate, 1017, 1018, 1028, 1028*t*, 1029
   furazolidone, 425*t*, 893
   octreotide, 616*t*, 1028*t*, 1029, 1100*t*, 1102–1103
   opioids. *See* OPIOID(s)
antidiuretic hormone (ADH)
   blood pressure and, 450–451
   deficiencies in, 1105
   drugs affecting secretion of, 1105, 1105*t*
   excess of, 1105–1106
   in fluid balance regulation, 1103, 1105
   in heart failure, 581
   mechanism of action, 503, 523
   Nursing Practice Applications, 1107–1108*t*
   regulation of, 1094*t*
   secretion of, 1098
ANTIDYSRHYTHMICS, 600–609
   adverse effects, 600–601
   beta-adrenergic antagonists, 198, 199, 200, 603*t*, 606–607
     acebutolol, 198*t*, 603*t*, 606
     esmolol, 198*t*, 202, 553*t*, 603*t*, 606–607
     propranolol. *See* propranolol
   calcium channel blockers, 603*t*, 609
     diltiazem. *See* diltiazem
     verapamil. *See* verapamil
   mechanisms of action, 601, 602*t*
   miscellaneous agents, 609
   Nursing Practice Applications, 610–611*t*
   potassium channel blockers, 603*t*, 607–609
     amiodarone. *See* amiodarone
     dofetilide, 603*t*, 608
     dronedarone, 603*t*, 608
     ibutilide, 603*t*, 608
     sotalol, 198*t*, 200, 603*t*, 608–609
   sodium channel blockers, 601, 602*f*, 603*t*, 604–606
     disopyramide, 603*t*, 604, 605
     flecainide, 603*t*, 606
     lidocaine. *See* lidocaine
     mexiletine, 384, 603*t*, 605
     phenytoin. *See* phenytoin
     procainamide, 603*t*, 604–605, 616*t*
     propafenone, 603*t*, 606, 622*t*
     quinidine sulfate, 603*t*
   treatment guidelines, 601
ANTIEMETICS, 1037–1041
   as anesthesia adjuncts, 413
   antihistamines/anticholinergics, 1037
     cyclizine, 757, 1039*t*
     dimenhydrinate, 756*t*, 757, 1037, 1039*t*
     diphenhydramine. *See* diphenhydramine
     hydroxyzine, 228–229, 1039*t*
     meclizine, 757, 1037, 1039*t*
     scopolamine, 29, 165*t*, 168, 1037, 1039*t*, 1293*t*
   benzodiazepines, 1038. *See also* lorazepam
   cannabinoids, 1038, 1040
     dronabinol, 1038, 1039*t*
     nabilone, 1038, 1039*t*
   as chemotherapy adjuncts, 957, 991
   corticosteroids, 1040
     dexamethasone. *See* dexamethasone
     methylprednisolone, 303, 705, 1040, 1156*t*
   herbal products as, 1037
   mechanisms of action, 1037, 1038*f*
   neurokinin receptor antagonists, 1039*t*, 1040
     aprepitant, 1039*t*, 1040
   Nursing Practice Applications, 1042–1043*t*
   phenothiazines, 1038
     metoclopramide, 98*t*, 386, 413, 1018, 1039*t*
     perphenazine, 271*t*, 273, 1039*t*
     prochlorperazine, 29, 271*t*, 273, 386, 957, 1039*t*
     promethazine. *See* promethazine
     trimethobenzamide, 292, 1039*t*
   routes and dosages, 1039*t*
   serotonin antagonists, 1036, 1037, 1040–1041
     dolasetron, 1037, 1039*t*, 1041
     granisetron, 1037, 1039*t*, 1041
     ondansetron. *See* ondansetron
     palonosetron, 1037, 1039*t*, 1041
ANTIEPILEPTIC DRUGS (AEDs)
   adherence issues, 315
   as adjuvant analgesics, 383–384, 384*t*
   adverse effects, 56*t*, 311, 383–384
   for bipolar disorder, 260
   breast-feeding and, 98–99*t*
   classification of, 317, 318–319*t*
   drug interactions, 86*t*, 311, 425*t*
   drugs in class
     barbiturates, 317, 319–320. *See also under* BARBITURATES
     benzodiazepines, 320–321. *See also under* BENZODIAZEPINES
     dibenzazepines, 323–325
     ezogabine, 319*t*, 327
     felbamate, 313*t*, 317, 319*t*, 327
     gabapentin. *See* gabapentin
     hydantoins, 322–323. *See also under* HYDANTOINS
     lacosamide, 319*t*
     lamotrigine. *See* lamotrigine
     levetiracetam, 313*t*, 319*t*, 328
     miscellaneous agents, 325–329
     pregabalin, 313*t*, 316, 319*t*, 328
     rufinamide, 313*t*, 319*t*, 328
     succinimides, 325. *See also under* SUCCINIMIDES
     tiagabine, 312, 313*t*, 319*t*, 328
     valproic acid. *See* valproic acid
     vigabatrin, 319*t*, 329
     zonisamide, 313*t*, 319*t*, 329
   for geriatric patients, 312, 314*t*
   mechanism of action, 315–317, 316–317*f*
   for migraine prophylaxis, 389, 389*t*
   Nursing Practice Applications, 329–331*t*
   for pediatric patients, 312
   selection of, 313*t*, 315
antifibrinolytics. *See* HEMOSTATICS
ANTIFUNGALS
   β-glucan synthesis inhibitors, 872
   mechanisms of action, 868–869, 868*f*
   Nursing Practice Applications, 879–880*t*
   for superficial infections, 872–878, 875*t*
     azoles. *See* AZOLES
     butenafine, 875*t*
     ciclopirox, 875*t*, 1274
     griseofulvin. *See* griseofulvin
     naftifine, 875*t*
     nystatin, 112*t*, 868, 875*t*, 876, 877–878
     terbinafine, 868, 874, 875, 875*t*, 876, 878
     tolnaftate, 875*t*, 1295
     undecylenic acid, 875*t*, 1265
   for systemic infections, 869–874, 870*t*
     amphotericin B. *See* amphotericin B deoxycholate
     anidulafungin, 870*t*, 872
     azoles. *See* AZOLES
     caspofungin, 868, 870, 870*t*, 872
     flucytosine, 868, 869–870, 870*t*, 872
antigen-presenting cells (APCs), 671*t*
antigens, 669, 710
ANTIHELMINTHICS, 899–900, 899*t*
ANTIHISTAMINES
   adverse effects of, 351, 756
   clinical applications, 755–756, 757, 758–759
   for dermatitis, 1273
   first-generation, 756*t*
   in geriatric patients, 122*t*, 757*t*
   interactions with, 425*t*
   lactation risk categories, 99*t*
   mechanism of action, 755, 756
   for nausea and vomiting, 1037, 1039*t*
   Nursing Practice Applications, 760–761*t*
   for ocular conditions, 1294, 1295*t*
   over-the-counter combinations of, 755–756, 757*t*
   routes and dosages, 756–757, 756*t*
   second-generation, 756*t*
   sedative effects of, 221*t*, 223
Antihypertensive and Lipid-Lowering Treatment to Prevent Heart Attack Trial, 197*t*
ANTIHYPERTENSIVES
   ACE inhibitors, 490–493, 491*t*, 548
   adherence to, 546
   adrenergic neuron blockers, 550
   adverse effects, 130, 545–546
   alpha-adrenergic agonists, 549–550
   alpha-adrenergic antagonists, 193, 195, 196–197*, 549
   angiotensin II receptor blockers, 493–495, 548
   ARBs, 494*t*
   beta-adrenergic antagonists, 197, 199, 200, 201–202, 549
   calcium channel blockers, 476–481, 547–548
   classification of, 544, 544*t*
   combination therapy, 545, 546*t*

ANTIHYPERTENSIVES (*continued*)
    cultural differences in response to, 131*t*, 197*t*,
      544, 546
    diuretics, 505, 509, 546–547
    mechanism of action, 545*f*
    pregnancy category, 95, 95*t*
    selection of, 544–546
    vasodilators, 550–552
anti-infectives
    adverse effects, 778
    antibiotics. *See* ANTIBIOTICS
    antifungals. *See* ANTIFUNGALS
    breast-feeding and, 98*t*
    classification of, 776, 778*t*
    mechanisms of action, 776, 778, 779*f*
    prophylactic therapy with, 783
    resistance to, 779–782, 779*t*, 781*f*
    selection of, 782–784
    superinfections and, 784
ANTI-INFLAMMATORY AGENTS, 673–683, 741*t*. *See also*
    NONSTEROIDAL ANTI-INFLAMMATORY DRUGS
Antilirium. *See* physostigmine
ANTIMALARIALS, 56*t*, 886–890, 888*t*
ANTIMETABOLITES
    in cancer treatment, 969–972
    folic acid analogs
      methotrexate. *See* methotrexate
      pemetrexed, 968, 969*t*, 972
      pralatrexate, 968, 969*t*, 972
      pyrimethamine, 838*t*, 839, 892*t*, 894,
        895–896, 968
      trimethoprim, 98*t*, 616*t*, 841, 968
      trimetrexate, 968
    as immunosuppressants, 700–702
    mechanisms of action, 788, 968–969, 968*f*
    purine analogs
      cladribine, 969*t*, 970–971
      clofarabine, 969*t*, 971
      fludarabine, 969*t*, 971
      nelarabine, 969*t*, 972
      pentostatin, 969*t*, 972
      thioguanine, 969*t*, 972
    pyrimidine analogs
      capecitabine, 969*t*, 970
      cytarabine, 822–823, 969*t*, 971
      floxuridine, 969*t*, 971
      fluorouracil, 95*t*, 822–823, 868, 954, 969*t*, 971
      gemcitabine, 969*t*, 971
    routes and dosages, 969*t*
Antiminth. *See* pyrantel pamoate
ANTINEOPLASTIC AGENTS, 962–994
    adjuncts for managing adverse effects,
      991, 1160
    adverse effects, 55–56*t*, 55–57, 643, 956–959,
      956*t*, 1037, 1215*t*
    alkylating agents. *See* ALKYLATING AGENTS
    antimetabolites. *See* ANTIMETABOLITES
    antitumor antibiotics. *See* ANTITUMOR
      ANTIBIOTICS
    biologic response modifiers. *See* BIOLOGIC
      RESPONSE MODIFIERS
    breast-feeding and, 99*t*
    cell cycle and growth fraction, 952–954, 953*f*
    cell kill hypothesis and, 954, 955*f*
    classification of, 963
    combination therapy, 955
    dosing schedules, 955
    geriatric patients, effects on, 977*t*
    hormone antagonists. *See* HORMONE
      ANTAGONISTS
    hormones as, 55–56, 55*t*, 975–979, 980*t*,
      1093, 1095
    mechanisms of action, 954

miscellaneous agents, 988–991, 990*t*
    altretamine, 988–989, 990*t*
    arsenic trioxide, 989, 990*t*
    asparaginase, 989–990, 990*t*
    bexarotene, 990, 990*t*
    hydroxyurea, 990*t*, 991
    ixabepilone, 990*t*, 991
    lenalidomide, 988, 990*t*
    mitotane, 990*t*, 991, 1163
    pegaspargase, 989–990, 990*t*
    romidepsin, 990, 990*t*
    sipuleucel-T, 990*t*, 991
    thalidomide. *See* thalidomide
    vorinostat, 990, 990*t*
    zoledronate (zoledronic acid), 384, 990*t*, 991,
      1239–1240*t*, 1242
monoclonal antibodies. *See* MONOCLONAL
    ANTIBODIES
natural products, 980–983, 980*t*
Nursing Practice Applications, 983–986*t*
preparation and administration of, 992
routes of administration, 29, 955–956
targeted therapies, 691, 983, 987*t*, 988
ANTIPLATELET AGENTS
    adenosine diphosphate receptor blockers,
      627–629
      clopidogrel, 571, 616*t*, 617, 622*t*, 626*t*, 627–628
      prasugrel, 626*t*, 627, 628
      ticagrelor, 626*t*, 628
      ticlopidine, 571, 622*t*, 626*t*, 627, 628–629
    aspirin. *See* aspirin
    dipyridamole, 626*t*, 628
    glycoprotein IIb/IIIa receptor inhibitors,
      629–630, 629*f*
      abciximab, 571, 626*t*, 629–630
      eptifibatide, 626*t*, 630
      tirofiban, 626*t*, 630
    interactions with, 62*t*
    mechanism of action, 617*t*, 626–627
    for myocardial infarction, 571
    routes and dosages, 626*t*
antipseudomonal penicillins, 792–793
ANTIPSYCHOTICS
    adverse effects, 269–270, 270*t*
    classification of, 269
    first-generation. *See* FIRST-GENERATION
      ANTIPSYCHOTICS
    interactions with, 425*t*
    mechanism of action, 267*f*
    metabolism of, 275*t*
    nonadherence issues with, 268
    Nursing Practice Applications, 279–281*t*
    second-generation. *See* SECOND-GENERATION
      (ATYPICAL) ANTIPSYCHOTICS
    selection of, 269
ANTIPYRETICS, 674. *See also* acetaminophen;
    NONSTEROIDAL ANTI-INFLAMMATORY DRUGS
antipyrine, 1297*t*
ANTIRETROVIRALS, 931–939
    adherence issues, 930
    adverse effects, 930
    classification of, 931, 932*t*
    entry inhibitors, 938–939
      enfuvirtide, 932*t*, 939
      maraviroc, 932*t*, 939
    initiation of therapy, 929
    integrase inhibitors (raltegravir), 932*t*, 939
    mechanism of action, 778
    monitoring progress of, 929–930, 930*f*
    nonnucleoside reverse transcriptase inhibitors,
      935–936
      delavirdine, 932*t*, 933, 936
      efavirenz, 86*t*, 932*t*, 935–936

      etravirine, 932*t*, 936
      nevirapine, 931, 932*t*, 933, 936
      rilpivirine, 932*t*, 936
    nucleoside/nucleotide reverse transcriptase
      inhibitors, 933–935
      abacavir, 932*t*, 934
      didanosine, 932*t*, 934
      emtricitabine, 932*t*, 933, 934–935, 943
      lamivudine, 917*t*, 918, 920, 931, 932*t*, 935
      stavudine, 932*t*, 935
      tenofovir. *See* tenofovir
      zidovudine. *See* zidovudine
    Nursing Practice Applications, 940–942*t*
    pharmacokinetics of, 933
    protease inhibitors, 936–938
      atazanavir, 932*t*, 937–938
      darunavir, 932*t*, 937, 938
      fosamprenavir, 932*t*, 938
      indinavir, 86*t*, 616*t*, 932*t*, 938
      lopinavir with ritonavir, 58, 932*t*, 937
      nelfinavir, 932*t*, 938
      ritonavir, 58, 60, 932*t*, 937, 938
      saquinavir, 86*t*, 932*t*, 938
      tipranavir, 932*t*, 938
    regimens for therapy, 931
    resistance to, 930, 931
    sexual lifestyle adjustments with, 931
    structured treatment interruptions, 931
    treatment failures, 930–931
antisecretory agents, 167
antiseizure medications. *See* ANTIEPILEPTIC DRUGS
antispasmodic agents, 167, 341, 342*f*, 1036. *See also*
    MUSCLE RELAXANTS
antistaphylococcal penicillins, 793–794
antithrombin, recombinant, 618*t*, 620
antithrombin III (AT-III), 618
antithymocyte globulin, 696*t*, 702, 703
ANTITHYROID AGENTS, 56*t*, 1145–1146, 1145*t*,
    1147–1148*t*
ANTITUMOR ANTIBIOTICS, 57, 972–975, 972*t*
    anthracyclines, 973, 974
      daunorubicin, 56*t*, 57, 823, 972*t*, 974
      daunorubicin liposomal, 972*t*, 974
      doxorubicin, 55–56*t*, 57, 958, 972*t*, 973–974
      doxorubicin liposomal, 973
      epirubicin, 56*t*, 57, 972*t*, 974
      idarubicin, 56*t*, 57, 972, 972*t*, 974
      mitoxantrone, 56*t*, 57, 302*t*, 303, 972*t*, 974
    nonanthracyclines, 973
      bleomycin, 823, 958, 972*t*, 974
      dactinomycin, 972*t*, 975
      mitomycin, 95*t*, 972*t*, 975
      plicamycin, 972
ANTITUSSIVES, 765–767, 766*t*
    nonopioids, 351, 429, 766–767, 766*t*
    opioids, 374*t*, 377, 765, 766*t*. *See also* codeine
Antivert. *See* meclizine
ANTIVIRALS. *See also* ANTIRETROVIRALS
    for hepatitis viruses, 915–921, 917*t*
    for herpes simplex viruses, 910–913, 911*t*
    for influenza viruses, 717, 913–915, 914*t*
    mechanism of action, 909–910
    Nursing Practice Applications, 921–922*t*
Antizol. *See* fomepizole
Anturane. *See* sulfinpyrazone
anxiety. *See also* anxiety disorders
    definition and model of, 217, 217*f*
    medical conditions and medications
      associated with, 217, 218*f*
    situational, 218
    sleep disorders and, 222–223
anxiety disorders
    brain regions responsible for, 219–220, 219*f*

categories of, 218–219
comorbidities with, 218t
complementary and alternative medicine
  for, 217, 223, 223t
diagnosing, 217
gender differences in, 219t
generalized anxiety disorder, 218, 224, 227, 228,
  230, 231
Nursing Practice Applications, 234–235t
obsessive-compulsive disorder, 218–219, 232
panic disorder, 218, 227
in pediatric patients, 234t
pharmacological management of, 223–234
  antidepressants, 223, 224, 230–232, 231t
  barbiturates, 224, 232–234, 233t
  benzodiazepines, 223, 224–228, 225–226t, 297
  nonbenzodiazepine anxiolytics, 223, 224,
    225t, 228–230
post-traumatic stress disorder, 219, 232, 258t
prevalence of, 218t
social anxiety disorder, 218, 232
anxiolysis, 395
anxiolytics, 224, 297. See also NONBENZODIAZEPINE
  ANXIOLYTICS
Anzemet. See dolasetron
AOM (acute otitis media), 108t, 1296
APCs (antigen-presenting cells), 671t
APhA (American Pharmaceutical Association), 15
Apidra. See insulin glulisine
apixaban, 618t, 621, 622
aplastic anemia, 57
Aplenzin. See bupropion hydrobromide
apocrine glands, 1263
Apokyn. See apomorphine
apomorphine, 290t, 292
apoproteins, 454
apoptosis, 691
appetite, regulation of, 1079–1080
appetite suppressants. See ANOREXIANTS
Approved Drug Products with Therapeutic Equivalence
  Evaluations. See "Orange Book" (FDA)
apraclonidine, 1288t, 1289
apremilast, 1248t, 1250, 1276, 1276t
aprepitant, 1039t, 1040
Apresazide, 506, 546t
Apresoline. See hydralazine
APRNs (advanced practice registered nurses), 20–21
aprotinin, 636
Aptiom. See eslicarbazepine
Aptivus. See tipranavir
aPTT (activated partial thromboplastin time), 617
AquaMEPHYTON. See vitamin K
Aquasol A. See vitamin A
Aquasol E. See vitamin E
Aquatensen. See methyclothiazide
aqueous humor, 1285
Aralen. See chloroquine
Aranesp. See darbepoetin alfa
Arava. See leflunomide
ARBs. See ANGIOTENSIN II RECEPTOR BLOCKERS
Arcapta Neohaler. See indacaterol
ardeparin, 620
Aredia. See pamidronate
arenaviruses, 908t
Arestin. See minocycline
arformoterol, 187, 737t, 738
argatroban, 618t, 623
Argesic. See salsalate
Aricept/Aricept ODT. See donepezil
Arimidex. See anastrozole
aripiprazole, 258t, 260, 275t, 277–279
Aristocort. See triamcinolone
Aristospan. See triamcinolone

Arixtra. See fondaparinux
armodafinil, 354t, 359
Armour. See desiccated thyroid
Aromasin. See exemestane
AROMATASE INHIBITORS, 975, 978
  anastrozole, 976t, 978
  exemestane, 976t, 978
  letrozole, 976t, 978
Arranon. See nelarabine
arrhythmias. See dysrhythmias
arsenic trioxide, 989, 990t
arsine, 1307t
Arsobal. See melarsoprol
Artane. See trihexyphenidyl
artemether-lumefantrine, 887, 888t, 889
arterial thromboembolism, 616
arthritis, defined, 1159. See also osteoarthritis;
  rheumatoid arthritis
articaine, 406t, 410
artificial sweeteners, 1085–1086
Arzerra. See ofatumumab
ASA. See aspirin
Asacol. See mesalamine
Ascarel. See pyrantel
ascariasis, 897, 898f
Ascaris lumbricoides, 897, 898f
ascending infections, 834
ASCO (American Society of Clinical Oncology), 975
ascorbic acid. See vitamin C
Ascorbicap. See vitamin C
asenapine, 258t, 260, 275t, 276
Asendin. See amoxapine
Asian populations
  alcohol metabolism in, 423
  antihypertensive response in, 197t
  complementary and alternative medicine use
    among, 128
  debrisoquin hydroxylase and, 275t
  diabetes mellitus and, 1113
  genetic polymorphisms in, 129
  propranolol, sensitivity to, 606t
Asmanex. See mometasone
asparaginase, 989–990, 990t
aspartame, 1085
Aspercreme, 1326
aspergillosis, 867, 867t
Aspergillus flavus, 867
aspiration, during enteral nutrition therapy, 1065, 1066t
aspirin
  absorption of, 31, 31f
  adverse effects, 111, 569, 616t, 675–676, 678
  analgesic properties of, 379, 674, 675
  anticoagulant activity of, 627, 676
  antipyretic effects of, 674, 675
  breast-feeding and, 98t
  in combination drugs, 7t
  drug interactions, 59, 86t, 425t, 622t, 678, 1016
  excretion of, 35, 36
  gender differences in effectiveness, 130
  history of, 674
  indications for use, 674
  mechanism of action, 617, 627, 674–675,
    675f, 677
  for myocardial infarction, 569, 571
  nursing responsibilities, 678
  overdose treatment, 36, 60, 676t, 678
  with oxycodone, 378, 422
  pharmacokinetics, 678
  plasma half-life, 38
  potency and efficacy of, 45–46
  with pravastatin, 463
  routes and dosages, 626t, 676t
  therapeutic effects and uses, 676–677

Astelin. See azelastine
Astepro. See azelastine
asthma, 732–745
  assessment of, 733, 733t
  Nursing Practice Applications, 746–748t
  pathophysiology, 732–733, 732–733f
  in pediatric patients, 1155t
  pharmacotherapy, 734–745
    anticholinergics, 166, 735t, 737t, 738–740
    beta-adrenergic agonists, 735–738, 735t, 737t
    corticosteroids, 735t, 740–742, 741t, 1159
    immunomodulators, 735t
    leukotriene modifiers, 735t, 741t, 743–744
    mast cell stabilizers, 735t, 741t, 742–743
    methylxanthines, 359–360, 735t, 737t,
      744–745
    monoclonal antibodies, 745
    overview, 735t
    routes of administration, 733–734
    stepwise approach to, 734–735, 734f
  prevalence of, 732, 733t, 735t
Astramorph PF. See morphine sulfate
Atacand. See candesartan
Atacand HCT, 495, 546t
Atarax. See hydroxyzine
atazanavir, 932t, 937–938
Atelvia. See risedronate
atenolol
  adverse effects, 567
  for angina and myocardial infarction, 568t
  breast-feeding and, 98t
  for hypertension, 202, 228, 546t
  for migraine prophylaxis, 389t
  Nursing Responsibilities, 567
  routes and dosages, 198t
  therapeutic effects and uses, 566
Atgam. See antithymocyte globulin
atherosclerosis, 445, 454, 561, 561f. See also
  coronary artery disease
athlete's foot. See tinea pedis
Ativan. See lorazepam
Atolone. See triamcinolone
atomoxetine, 354t, 356, 357
atonic seizures, 313–314, 313t
atopic dermatitis, 1271, 1273, 1274
atorvastatin
  adverse events, 462, 616t
  amlodipine with, 479
  ezetimibe with, 467
  interactions with, 425t
  mechanism of action, 462
  Nursing Responsibilities, 462
  routes and dosages, 459–460, 461t
  therapeutic effects and uses, 462
atovaquone, 62t, 889
atovaquone-proguanil, 886, 887, 888t, 889
atracurium, 169t, 173, 411
atrial fibrillation, 600
atrial flutter, 600
atrial natriuretic peptides (ANPs), 451, 581
atrial reflex, 450
atrial tachycardia, 600
Atridox. See doxycycline
atrioventricular conduction block, 600
atrioventricular (AV) node, 445, 476
Atripla, 934
Atropa belladonna, 165
Atropen. See atropine
atropine
  in anesthesia, 411
  for cholinergic crisis, 153, 155, 157
  clinical applications and considerations,
    166–167

atropine (*continued*)
  difenoxin with, 1028*t*, 1029
  diphenoxylate with, 1028, 1028*t*, 1029
  example, 6*f*
  history of, 166*t*
  as overdose treatment, 199, 201, 202, 1308*t*
  routes and dosages, 165*t*, 1293*t*
Atrovent. *See* ipratropium
ATryn. *See* antithrombin, recombinant
attention deficit/hyperactivity disorder (ADHD)
  etiology and pathophysiology of, 352
  gender differences in, 352, 353*t*
  pharmacotherapy, 353–358, 354*t*, 430
  prevalence of, 352, 352*t*
  symptoms of, 352, 352*t*
attenuated (live) vaccines, 711, 711*t*
ATYPICAL ANTIDEPRESSANTS, 250–253. *See also*
    SEROTONIN-NOREPINEPHRINE REUPTAKE
    INHIBITORS
  for anxiety disorders, 232
  for depression, 250–253
  drugs in class
    amoxapine, 251–252
    bupropion, 250, 252, 260, 357, 432, 1083*t*
    mirtazapine, 250, 252
    nefazodone, 250, 252–253
    reboxetine, 250
    trazodone, 86*t*, 231*t*, 250, 253, 1215*t*
    vilazodone, 253
  mechanism of action, 250
  Nursing Practice Application, 255–256*t*
atypical antipsychotics. *See* SECOND-GENERATION
    (ATYPICAL) ANTIPSYCHOTICS
atypical mycobacterial infections (AMIs), 849
Aubagio. *See* teriflunomide
AUC (acute uncomplicated cystitis), 834–836, 835*t*
auditory canal, 1295
Augmentin, 789*t*, 792
Auralgan, 1297*t*
Auranofin. *See* gold salts
auras
  in migraines, 385
  in seizures, 313, 314
Aurothioglucose. *See* gold salts
autoimmune disorders
  immunosuppressants for, 695, 697
  multiple sclerosis, 301*f*, 302*t*, 304*t*
  Raynaud's disease and, 195*t*
automaticity, 445
automatisms, 314
autonomic nervous system (ANS), 136–148
  adrenergic transmission in, 144–146, 145*f*
  cholinergic transmission in, 142–144,
    143–144*f*, 144*t*
  drugs affecting
    adrenergic agonists, 177–191. *See also*
      ADRENERGIC AGONISTS
    adrenergic antagonists, 192–206. *See also*
      ADRENERGIC ANTAGONISTS
    cholinergic agonists, 149–162. *See also*
      cholinergic agonists
    cholinergic antagonists, 163–176. *See also*
      cholinergic antagonists
    classifications for, 147, 147*t*
  overview, 137, 138*f*
  parasympathetic division of, 138–140, 139*f*
  regulation of functions, 146–147, 146*f*
  sites of action in, 142
  structure and function of, 138–140, 139*f*
  sympathetic division of, 138–140, 139*f*, 146, 489,
    580–581
  synaptic transmission in, 140–141*f*, 140–142
autonomic tone, 139

AV (atrioventricular) node, 445, 476
Avage. *See* tazarotene
Avalide, 495, 546*t*
avanafil, 1217, 1217*t*, 1218–1219
Avandamet, 1125*t*
Avandaryl, 1125*t*, 1126
Avandia. *See* rosiglitazone
Avapro. *See* irbesartan
Avastin. *See* bevacizumab
Aveed. *See* testosterone undecanoate
Avelox. *See* moxifloxacin
Aventyl. *See* nortriptyline
avian flu, 913
Avinza. *See* morphine sulfate
Avita. *See* tretinoin
Avodart. *See* dutasteride
Avonex. *See* INTERFERON(s), IFN beta-1a
Axert. *See* almotriptan
Axid. *See* nizatidine
axitinib, 987*t*
Aygestin. *See* norethindrone
Azactam. *See* aztreonam
Azasan. *See* azathioprine
AzaSite. *See* azithromycin
azathioprine
  adverse effects, 55*t*, 700–701, 1041*t*
  clinical applications, 156, 696*t*, 700, 1033
  mechanism of action, 700
  Nursing Responsibilities, 701
  routes and dosages, 1248*t*
azelaic acid, 1268*t*, 1269, 1270
azelastine, 756–757, 756*t*, 758, 1294, 1295*t*
Azelex. *See* azelaic acid
Azilect. *See* rasagiline
azilsartan medoxomil, 494*t*, 495, 546*t*
azithromycin
  clinical applications, 811, 863, 891, 894
  half-life of, 810
  interactions with, 62*t*
  pregnancy category rating, 95*t*
  routes and dosages, 112*t*, 810*t*
Azmacort. *See* triamcinolone
AZOLES, 872–874, 878
  classification, 872
  drugs in class
    butoconazole, 875*t*, 877
    clotrimazole, 875*t*, 877, 1265, 1295
    econazole, 875*t*
    fluconazole. *See* fluconazole
    itraconazole. *See* itraconazole
    ketoconazole. *See* ketoconazole
    miconazole, 875*t*, 877, 1265
    oxiconazole, 875*t*
    sulconazole, 875*t*
    terconazole, 875*t*
    tioconazole, 875*t*
    voriconazole, 870*t*, 872, 874
  mechanism of action, 868–869
azoospermia, 1215
Azopt. *See* brinzolamide
Azor, 479, 495, 546*t*
AZT. *See* zidovudine
aztreonam, 797*t*, 799
Azulfidine. *See* sulfasalazine

B

B cells, 669–670
bacilli, 776
Bacillus anthracis. See anthrax
bacillus Calmette-Guérin (BCG) vaccine,
    692*t*, 693, 695
bacitracin, 827, 827*t*, 830, 1264

baclofen, 303, 304, 336, 337*t*, 339*t*, 340
Bacteremia, 781*t*
bacteria
  cell walls, 787–788, 787*f*
  classification of, 776, 777*t*
  DNA replication, 822–823, 822*f*
  on skin, 667*t*
bacterial immunizations, 712–715
bacteriocidal agents, 776
bacteriostatic agents, 776
bacteriuria, 834, 835, 836, 837
Bacteroides fragilis, 796
Bactine Antibiotic, 830
Bactrim. *See* trimethoprim-sulfamethoxazole
Bactroban. *See* mupirocin
baking soda. *See* sodium bicarbonate
BAL in Oil. *See* dimercaprol
balanced anesthesia, 395, 396
Balnetar. *See* coal tar
balsalazide, 1032, 1033*t*, 1035
Banflex. *See* orphenadrine
Banzel. *See* rufinamide
Baraclude. *See* entecavir
BARBITURATES
  abuse of, 421
  adverse effects, 317
  for anxiety, 224, 232–234, 233*t*
  dependence with, 421
  drug interactions, 86*t*, 622*t*
  drugs in class
    amobarbital, 234
    butabarbital, 233*t*, 234
    mephobarbital, 234, 318*t*, 320
    methohexital, 233, 397*t*, 399–400
    pentobarbital, 233*t*
    phenobarbital. *See* phenobarbital
    secobarbital, 233–234, 233*t*
    thiopental sodium, 400
  excretion of, 36
  for insomnia, 224, 232–234, 233*t*
  mechanism of action, 232, 317
  overdose, 232
  for seizures, 317, 319–320
  tolerance to, 232
  withdrawal symptoms and treatment, 420*t*
barley grass, 81*t*
baroreceptors, 449, 450
Barrett's esophagus, 1008
basal nuclei (ganglia), 214, 215*f*, 287
basiliximab, 696*t*, 702, 702*t*, 703
BayRab. *See* rabies immune globulin
bazedoxifene, 1175
BCG (bacillus Calmette-Guérin) vaccine, 693, 695
beclomethasone, 740–741, 741*t*, 759*t*
Beconase AQ. *See* beclomethasone
bedaquiline, 853*t*, 858
Beers criteria, 121, 122*t*
behavior modification programs, in weight
    management, 1081–1082
belatacept, 696*t*, 701
Beleodaq. *See* belinostat
belimumab, 702*t*
belinostat, 990, 990*t*
belladonna, 165–166
Belsomra. *See* suvorexant
Belviq. *See* lorcaserin
Benadryl. *See* diphenhydramine
benazepril, 33, 479, 491*t*, 492, 546*t*, 548
bendamustine, 964*t*, 966
bendroflumethiazide and nadolol, 510*t*, 511, 546*t*
Ben-Gay, 1326
Benicar. *See* olmesartan medoxomil
Benicar HCT, 495, 546*t*

benign prostatic hyperplasia (BPH)
  complementary and alternative therapies for, 1222*t*
  Nursing Practice Applications, 1223–1224*t*
  pathophysiology of, 1219–1220
  pharmacotherapy for, 193, 196–197, 1220–1222, 1220*f*, 1221*t*
benign tumors, 949, 949*t*
Benlysta. *See* belimumab
benoxinate, 1294
Bentyl. *See* dicyclomine
Benzalin. *See* benzoyl peroxide
Benzamycin, 1269
benzimidazole, 894
benzocaine, 406*t*, 409, 1278–1279, 1297*t*
BENZODIAZEPINES
  abuse of, 421
  as adjuvant analgesics, 384*t*
  adverse effects, 225–226
  in anesthesia, 398–399, 411
  for anxiety, 223, 224–228, 225–226*t*, 297
  breast-feeding and, 99*t*
  drug interactions, 62, 86*t*
  drugs in class
    alprazolam, 7, 95*t*, 225–226*t*, 227, 417, 425*t*
    chlordiazepoxide, 224, 225–226*t*, 227–228
    clonazepam, 225–226*t*, 260, 313*t*, 318*t*, 320, 321
    clorazepate, 225–226*t*, 228, 313*t*, 318*t*, 320, 321
    diazepam. *See* diazepam
    estazolam, 225–226*t*, 228
    flurazepam, 225–226*t*, 228
    halazepam, 225
    lorazepam. *See* lorazepam
    midazolam, 225, 226, 226*t*, 397*t*, 398–399, 411
    oxazepam, 225–226*t*, 228, 384, 419
    quazepam, 225–226*t*, 228
    temazepam, 95*t*, 225–226*t*, 228
    triazolam, 225–226*t*, 228
  for dystonia, 336
  in geriatric patients, 122*t*
  for insomnia, 223, 224–228, 225–226*t*
  mechanism of action, 225, 317, 320
  for muscle spasms, 338, 384
  for nausea and vomiting, 1038, 1039*t*
  overdose/poisoning, 226, 1308*t*
  for seizures, 313*t*, 320–321
  withdrawal symptoms and treatment, 420*t*
benzonatate, 766*t*, 767
benzoyl peroxide, 1268, 1268*t*, 1269
benzphetamine, 356
benztropine
  adverse effects, 295
  in ALS, 304
  for dystonia, 270, 336
  mechanism of action, 294
  nursing responsibilities, 295
  for Parkinson's disease, 294–295
  routes and dosages, 165*t*, 294*t*
  therapeutic effects and uses, 166, 168
benzyl alcohol, 106
bepotastine, 1295*t*
beriberi, 1048
besifloxacin, 823*t*, 826
Besivance. *See* besifloxacin
Best Pharmaceuticals for Children Act of 2002 (BPCA), 105
beta lactamase, 779, 788, 790*f*
beta$_1$-adrenergic receptors, 144, 144*t*, 145, 180
beta$_2$-adrenergic receptors, 144, 144*t*, 145, 180
beta$_3$-adrenergic receptors, 187

BETA-ADRENERGIC AGONISTS
  adverse effects, 589, 736
  for asthma, 735–738, 735*t*, 737*t*
  for heart failure, 587*t*, 589
  mechanisms of action, 185–187, 735
  nonselective (isoproterenol). *See* isoproterenol
  selective
    albuterol. *See* albuterol
    arformoterol, 187, 737*t*, 738
    bitolterol mesylate, 737
    dopamine. *See* dopamine
    epinephrine. *See* epinephrine
    formoterol, 186, 187, 737*t*, 738
    indacaterol, 181*t*, 187, 737*t*, 738
    levalbuterol, 181*t*, 187, 737*t*, 738
    norepinephrine. *See* norepinephrine
    pirbuterol, 186, 187, 737*t*, 738
    salmeterol, 187, 737*t*, 738
    terbutaline. *See* terbutaline
  tocolytics, 186, 187, 1179
BETA-ADRENERGIC ANTAGONISTS
  adverse effects, 198–199, 198*t*, 201, 549, 566, 606, 1215*t*
  for angina pectoris, 198, 199, 563, 563*f*, 566–567, 568*t*
  Black Box Warnings for, 199
  breast-feeding and, 99*t*
  drug interactions with, 425*t*
  for dysrhythmias, 198, 199, 200, 603*t*, 606–607
  for glaucoma, 198, 200, 202, 1289
  for heart failure, 198, 584*t*, 586
  for hypertension, 197, 199, 200, 201–202, 544*t*, 549
  metoprolol. *See* metoprolol
  for migraine prophylaxis, 389, 389*t*
  for myocardial infarction, 198, 199, 572
  nonselective, 197–200
    betaxolol, 198*t*, 202, 549, 1288*t*, 1289, 1290
    carteolol, 1288*t*, 1289, 1290
    carvedilol. *See* carvedilol
    labetalol, 198*t*, 200, 549, 552, 553*t*
    levobunolol, 1288*t*, 1289, 1290
    metipranolol, 1288*t*, 1289, 1290
    penbutolol, 198*t*, 200
    pindolol, 197, 198*t*, 200
    propranolol. *See* propranolol
    sotalol, 198*t*, 200, 603*t*, 608–609
    timolol. *See* timolol
  overdose/poisoning, 199, 201, 1308*t*
  routes and dosages, 198*t*
  selective, 197, 201–202
    acebutolol, 198*t*, 603*t*, 606
    atenolol. *See* atenolol
    betaxolol, 198*t*, 202, 549, 1288*t*, 1289, 1290
    bisoprolol, 198*t*, 202, 546*t*, 549, 586
    esmolol, 198*t*, 202, 553*t*, 603*t*, 606–607
    nebivolol, 198*t*, 202
beta-blockers. *See* BETA-ADRENERGIC ANTAGONISTS
Betagan. *See* levobunolol
β-glucan, 868
β-GLUCAN SYNTHESIS INHIBITORS, 872
beta-lactam ring, 788, 789*f*, 794, 797
Betalin 12. *See* cyanocobalamin
betamethasone, 1156*t*, 1273*t*
betamethasone benzoate, 1273*t*
betamethasone valerate, 1273*t*
Betapace/Betapace AF. *See* sotalol
Betaseron. *See* INTERFERON(s), IFN beta-1b
betaxolol, 198*t*, 202, 549, 1288*t*, 1289, 1290
Betaxon. *See* levobetaxolol
bethanechol, 150, 152*t*, 153–154
Betimol. *See* timolol

Betoptic. *See* betaxolol
bevacizumab, 987*t*, 988
bexarotene, 990, 990*t*
Bextra. *See* valdecoxib
Bexxar. *See* tositumomab
Biaxin. *See* clarithromycin
bicalutamide, 976*t*, 979
bicarbonate, in antacids, 1016
Bicillin. *See* PENICILLIN(s), penicillin G benzathine
BiCNU. *See* carmustine
BiDil, 131*t*, 584*t*, 586
BIGUANIDES, 1122*t*, 1125*t*, 1126–1127, 1131
bilberry, 81*t*, 1293*t*
bile, 35
BILE ACID SEQUESTRANTS (RESINS), 460*f*, 461*t*, 463–465, 622*t*
  adverse effects, 463, 464
  drugs in class
    cholestyramine, 58, 62*t*, 461*t*, 464–465
    colesevelam, 461*t*, 465
    colestipol, 461*t*, 465
  mechanism of action, 460*f*
  Nursing Practice Application, 468
  therapeutic effects and uses, 463, 464
biliary excretion, 36
Biltricide. *See* praziquantel
bimatoprost, 1287–1288, 1288*t*
bioavailability, 8
biofeedback, 389*t*
BIOLOGIC RESPONSE MODIFIERS, 691, 983, 987*t*, 988
  interferons. *See* INTERFERON(s)
  interleukins, 693–695
    aldesleukin, 692*t*, 693, 694–695, 988
    oprelvekin. *See* oprelvekin
  monoclonal antiboes. *See* MONOCLONAL ANTIBODIES
Biologics Control Act of 1902, 13
Bio-Statin. *See* nystatin
bioterrorism
  biologic agents for, 1305–1306
  categories of infectious agents, 1304*t*
  chemical and physical agents for, 1306–1308, 1307*t*
  defined, 1303
  ionizing radiation, 1307–1308
  role of nurses in, 1303–1304
biotoxins, 1306
biotransformation. *See* metabolism
biperiden, 294*t*
bipolar disorder
  defined, 240, 257
  nonpharmacologic therapies for, 257
  pathophysiology, 257
  in pediatric patients, 258*t*
  pharmacotherapy for, 257–260, 258*t*
  symptoms of, 257
bird flu, 717, 913
birth control. *See* contraception and contraceptive methods
birth defects, 56, 96, 97, 311
bisacodyl, 1025*t*, 1027
bismuth compounds, 1018
bismuth subsalicylate, 1017, 1018, 1028, 1028*t*, 1029
bisoprolol, 198*t*, 202, 546*t*, 549, 586
BISPHOSPHONATES, 384, 1239–1242
  adverse effects, 1239–1240, 1241
  drug interactions, 1241
  drugs in class
    alendronate, 32, 1239–1240*t*, 1240–1241
    etidronate disodium, 62*t*, 1239–1240*t*, 1241
    ibandronate, 1239–1240*t*, 1241
    pamidronate, 384, 1239–1240*t*, 1241
    risedronate, 1239–1240*t*, 1241

BISPHOSPHONATES (*continued*)
    tiludronate, 1239–1240t, 1241
    zoledronate (zoledronic acid), 384, 990t, 991,
        1239–1240t, 1242
  mechanism of action, 1241
  therapeutic uses and effects, 1239, 1241
bithionol, 900
Bitin. *See* bithionol
bitolterol mesylate, 737
bivalirudin, 618t, 623, 626
Black Box Warnings
  abilify, 278
  abiraterone, 979
  ACE inhibitors, 491
  acetaminophen, 684
  adefovir dipivoxil, 919
  albiglutide, 1131
  aldesleukin, 694
  alosetron, 1036
  amiodarone, 607
  amphetamine-containing products, 355–356
  amphotericin B, 871
  antidepressants, 234t, 242
  apixaban, 622
  atenolol, 567
  atomoxetine, 357
  azathioprine, 701
  bacitracin, 827
  basiliximab, 703
  bedaquiline, 858
  beta-adrenergic antagonists, 199
  bleomycin, 974
  botulinum toxin, 344, 344t
  bupropion, 432
  busulfan, 966
  cabazitaxel, 982
  capecitabine, 970
  capreomycin, 858
  carbamazepine, 324
  carbidopa/levodopa, 291
  carboplatin, 966
  chloramphenicol, 815
  chlorpromazine, 272
  cidofovir, 912
  cladribine, 971
  clonidine, 383
  clopidogrel, 628
  conjugated estrogens, 1169
  cyclosporine, 698
  dabigatran, 623
  dacarbazine, 967
  dactinomycin, 975
  dantrolene, 343
  darbepoetin alfa, 646
  defined, 54
  docetaxel, 982
  doxorubicin, 973
  droxidopa, 182
  edetate calcium disodium, 1311
  epoetin alfa, 645
  estradiol and norethindrone, 1195
  etanercept, 701
  etoposide, 983
  everolimus, 699
  fentanyl, 397
  ferrous sulfate, 655
  flecainide, 606
  floxuridine, 971
  flucytosine, 872
  fludarabine, 971
  fluoroquinolones, 825, 826–827
  fluorouracil, 971
  fluoxetine, 249

flutamide, 979
foscarnet, 912
furosemide, 508
ganciclovir, 912
gentamicin, 813
haloperidol, 274
heparin, 619
hydroxyurea, 991
ibuprofen, 680–681
imipramine, 247
indacaterol, 738
interferon alfa-2b, 691
irinotecan, 982
isoniazid, 855–856
ixabepilone, 991
ketoconazole, 874
levothyroxine, 1141
linaclotide, 1036
liraglutide, 1131
lisinopril, 492
lithium carbonate, 259
lomitapide, 467
lomustine, 967
losartan, 494
mechlorethamine, 967
medroxyprogesterone, 1173
melphalan, 967
metformin, 1127
methotrexate, 701, 970
metoclopramide, 1018
metoprolol, 201
metronidazole, 830, 893
midazolam, 399
midodrine, 185
mifepristone, 1204
mipomersen, 467
misoprostol, 1018
mitomycin, 975
mitotane, 991
mitoxantrone, 974
morphine sulfate, 376
mycophenolate, 701
natalizumab, 303
nefazodone, 252
nelarabine, 972
nitroprusside sodium, 553
oprelvekin, 651
oxaliplatin, 967
oxycodone, 378
oxytocin, 1178
paclitaxel, 982
pentostatin, 972
phenelzine, 254
phenytoin, 322
pramlintide, 1119
procainamide, 604
propranolol, 199
propylthiouracil, 1146
quinidine, 605
quinine, 338, 889
quinupristin-dalfopristin, 818
raloxifene, 1242
risperidone, 276
rivaroxaban, 622
rosiglitazone, 1128
sirolimus, 699
sotalol, 608
spironolactone, 512
streptomycin, 857
streptozocin, 968
succinylcholine, 171
tamoxifen, 977
telithromycin, 818

teniposide, 983
tenofovir, 919
terbutaline, 738
teriflunomide, 303
testosterone, 1212
thalidomide, 702
ticagrelor, 628
ticlopidine, 628–629
tigecycline, 809
tinidazole, 893–894
tipranavir, 938
tolvaptan, 529–530
topotecan, 982
toremifene, 978
tretinoin, 1270
tumor necrosis factor inhibitors, 1249
valganciclovir, 913
valproic acid, 327
varenicline, 432
venlafaxine, 251
vinblastine, 981
vincristine, 981
vinorelbine, 982
vitamin K, 1053
vorapaxar, 629
warfarin, 622
zidovudine, 934
zolpidem, 229
black cohosh, 81t, 83t, 336, 1192t
bladder cancer, 950
blastomycosis, 867, 867t
Blenoxane. *See* bleomycin
bleomycin, 823, 958, 972t, 974
Blephamide, 839
blepharitis, 1294
blister agents, 1306
Blocadren. *See* timolol
blood
  donations, 524t
  functions and properties of, 441–444, 443–444f
  glucose regulation. *See* diabetes mellitus
blood doping, 653t
blood pressure. *See also* hypertension
  factors influencing, 448–449, 449f, 488
  hormones and, 450–451, 451f
  neural regulation of, 449–450, 450f
BLOOD PRODUCTS, 523–525, 524t
blood thinners. *See* ANTICOAGULANTS
blood vessels, 449t
blood–brain barrier, 32, 106, 213, 213f
Bloxiverz. *See* neostigmine
BMI (body mass index), 1080, 1081f, 1081t
BNPs (B-type natriuretic peptides), 581
boceprevir, 917t, 918, 919
body defenses
  adaptive (specific), 668–671
  innate (nonspecific), 665–668, 667t
body mass index (BMI), 1080, 1081f, 1081t
body surface area (BSA) method, for dosage
    calculations, 110, 111f
body weight method, for dosage calculations, 110
boils (furuncles), 1264
bolus administration, 30
bolus feedings, in enteral nutrition, 1064
bone deposition, 1231
bone marrow toxicity, 56t, 57
bone pain, 384
bone resorption, 1231
Bonine. *See* meclizine
Boniva. *See* ibandronate
boosters, 710
Bordetella pertussis. See pertussis
Borrelia burgdorferi, Se Lyme disease

bortezomib, 987t
Bosulif. See bosutinib
bosutinib, 987t
botanicals, defined, 81
Botox/Botox Cosmetic. See onabotulinumtoxinA
botulinum antitoxin, 1306
botulinum toxin, 343–344, 343t
botulism, 775, 1306
Bowman's capsule, 502
BPCA (Best Pharmaceuticals for Children Act of 2002), 105
BPH. See benign prostatic hyperplasia
bradydysrhythmias, 599–600
bradykinesia, 287
bradykinin, 489, 491, 668, 668t
brain. See also central nervous system
    anxiety disorders, regions responsible for, 219–220, 219f
    injuries to, 336, 352
    structures of, 211–213, 212–213f
brand name drugs, 7, 8
Bravelle. See urofollitropin
breakthrough bleeding, 1171
breast cancer, 56, 950, 952, 972t, 1174, 1197
breast-feeding. See lactation
brentuximab, 987t
breo ellipta, 746
Brethaire. See terbutaline
Brethine. See terbutaline
Brevibloc. See esmolol
Brevital. See methohexital
Brilinta. See ticagrelor
brimonidine, 1269, 1288t, 1289
Brintellix. See vortioxetine
brinzolamide, 515, 1288t, 1292
broad-spectrum antibiotics, 782, 784, 791–792
bromocriptine
    adverse effects, 292, 1185
    clinical applications, 292, 1131, 1185
    routes and dosages, 290t, 1100t, 1122t, 1182t
bromodiphenhydramine, 766t
brompheniramine, 756–757t
BRONCHODILATORS
    anticholinergics, 737t, 738–740
        ipratropium. See ipratropium
        tiotropium, 165t, 166, 168, 737t, 740
    beta-adrenergic agonists, 187, 735–738, 737t
    methylxanthines, 359–360, 735t, 737t, 744–745
    muscarinic antagonists, 168
bronchospasm, 732, 733
Brovana. See arformoterol
brucellosis, 824
BSA (body surface area) method, for dosage calculations, 110, 111f
B-type natriuretic peptides (BNPs), 581
bubonic plague, 787, 809t, 1306
buccal route of administration, 28–29
budesonide
    adverse effects, 742
    clinical applications, 742, 1032
    labeling changes, 105t
    routes and dosages, 112t, 741t, 759t, 1156t
buffers, 533
bulk-forming laxatives, 1026
bumetanide, 508t, 509, 547, 584t, 585
Bumex. See bumetanide
bundle of His, 445
bupivacaine, 406t, 410
Buprenex. See buprenorphine
buprenorphine, 374t, 378
buprenorphine/naloxone, 385, 422–423
bupropion, 250, 252, 260, 357, 432, 1083t
bupropion hydrobromide, 252

Burkitt's lymphoma, 910
burns, 1277–1279
BuSpar. See buspirone
buspirone, 225t, 230, 297
busulfan, 964t, 966
Busulfex. See busulfan
butabarbital, 233t, 234
butenafine, 875t
Butisol. See butabarbital
butoconazole, 875t, 877
butorphanol, 374t, 378
Butrans. See buprenorphine
Byetta. See exenatide
Bystolic. See nebivolol

C

C fibers, 369–370
cabazitaxel, 980, 980t, 982
cabozantinib, 987t
cachexia, 958
CAD (coronary artery disease), 560–562. See also angina pectoris; myocardial infarctions
Caduet, 479
Cafcit. See caffeine
Cafergot, 360
caffeine, 354t, 359–360, 360t, 431
Calan/Calan SR. See verapamil
Calcidrine Syrup, 766t
Calciferol. See ergocalciferol
Calcijet. See calcitriol
Calcijex. See vitamin D
calcineurin, 698
CALCINEURIN INHIBITORS, 697f, 698–700
    cyclosporine. See cyclosporine
    tacrolimus, 56t, 504t, 696t, 698, 699, 1273–1274
calcipotriene, 1275, 1276t
calcitonin, 29, 384, 1138, 1231, 1243–1244
calcitonin-salmon, 1240t, 1243–1244
calcitriol, 1232, 1237–1238, 1238t. See also vitamin D
calcium
    in antacids, 1016
    in body homeostasis, 1229–1230
    deficiencies in, 528t, 1056
    function of, 1056, 1057t
    as overdose treatment, 1308t
    recommended intake, 1057t, 1229, 1229t
    regulation of, 1230–1231f, 1230–1232
calcium acetate, 1233–1234t
calcium carbonate, 1015t, 1233–1234t
CALCIUM CHANNEL BLOCKERS (CCBs), 473–485
    adverse effects, 477, 479t, 480, 481t, 548, 567
    for angina pectoris, 476–481, 563, 563f, 567, 568t
    cardiac conduction, effects on, 476
    classification of, 476
    dihydropyridines, 476–479, 477–478t. See also dihydropyridines
    drug interactions, 62, 62t, 199, 201–202, 476t
    for dysrhythmias, 603t, 609
    heart failure and, 481t
    for hypertension, 476–481, 544t, 547–548
    for migraine prophylaxis, 389, 389t
    for muscle spasms, 337–338
    myocardium, effects on, 476
    nondihydropyridines, 477–478t, 479–481. See also diltiazem; verapamil
    Nursing Practice Applications, 482–483t
    overdose/poisoning, 1308, 1308t
    physiological role in muscle contraction, 474, 474f
    vascular smooth muscle, effects on, 475–476
calcium channels, 474–475, 474–475f
calcium chloride, 531, 1233–1234t

calcium citrate, 1233–1234t
Calcium EDTA. See edetate calcium disodium
calcium gluconate, 531, 1233–1234t
calcium iodide, 766t
calcium lactate, 1233–1234t
calcium phosphate tribasic, 1233–1234t
calcium polycarbophil, 1025t
calcium salts, 1232–1233, 1233–1234t
Cal-Lac. See calcium lactate
Camila. See norethindrone
camphorated opium tincture, 1028t, 1030
Camptosar. See irinotecan
Camptotheca acuminata, 980, 982
camptothecins. See TOPOISOMERASE INHIBITORS
canagliflozin, 1122t, 1131
canal of Schlemm, 1285
Canasa. See mesalamine
cancer, 949–961. See also specific types of cancer
    cell cycle and growth fraction, 952–954, 953f
    characteristics of, 949–950, 950f
    chemotherapy, 951–952
    clotting factors and, 616t
    cultural differences in, 959t
    detection and prevention of, 950–951
    drug-induced, 55–56, 55t, 958–959
    etiology of, 950
    gender differences in, 950
    pain management strategies in, 372, 383
    pharmacotherapy. See ANTINEOPLASTIC AGENTS
    prevalence of, 949, 949t
    radiation therapy for, 951
    staging and grading of, 952, 952t
    surgeries for, 951
    survival rates, 951t
    tumors, classification and naming of, 949, 949t
Cancidas. See caspofungin
candesartan, 494t, 495, 546t, 548, 584t
Candida albicans, 808, 876, 877, 1265
Candida glabrata, 877
candidiasis, 867, 867t, 876–877, 944t
CANNABINOID RECEPTOR (CB1) BLOCKERS, 1082
CANNABINOIDS, 426–427, 1038, 1039t, 1040
cannabis. See marijuana
Cantil. See mepenzolate
Capastat. See capreomycin
capecitabine, 969t, 970
capillary leak syndrome, 694
Capoten. See captopril
Capozide, 492, 546t
Caprelsa. See vandetanib
capreomycin, 853t, 858
capsaicin, 336, 384, 1246
capsids, 907
capsules, 28
captopril
    adverse effects, 492, 616t
    clinical applications, 492, 548, 572
    onset of action, 552
    routes and dosages, 491t, 584t
Capzasin. See capsaicin
Carac. See fluorouracil
Carafate. See sucralfate
carbachol, 152t, 154, 1288t
carbamazepine
    adverse effects, 56t, 260, 324, 616t, 1215t
    for bipolar disorder, 260
    breast-feeding and, 98t
    drug interactions, 324, 622t
    excretion of, 36
    mechanism of action, 316, 324
    for neuropathic pain, 303, 383
    nursing responsibilities, 324
    pregnancy category, 95t

carbamazepine (*continued*)
    routes and dosages, 258*t*
      for seizures, 313*t*, 318*t*, 323–324
carbamide peroxide, 1297, 1297*t*
carbapenem-resistant *Enterobacteriaceae* (CRE), 797
CARBAPENEMS, 797–798
    doripenem, 797, 797*t*, 798
    ertapenem, 797, 797*t*, 798
    imipenem-cilastatin, 797–798, 797*t*
    meropenem, 797, 797*t*, 798
Carbatrol/Carbatrol CR. *See* carbamazepine
carbenicillin, 792
carbidopa. *See* levodopa/carbidopa
Carbocaine. *See* mepivacaine
carbohydrates, 1065, 1070
carbonic anhydrase, 515
CARBONIC ANHYDRASE INHIBITORS, 505, 506*f*, 515–516
    acetazolamide, 513*t*, 515–516, 839, 1041,
      1288*t*, 1292
    brinzolamide, 515, 1288*t*, 1292
    dorzolamide, 515, 1288*t*, 1292
    methazolamide, 513*t*, 515, 516, 1288*t*
carbonyl iron, 656, 656*t*
carboplatin, 504*t*, 616*t*, 964*t*, 966
carboprost, 1177, 1177*t*, 1179, 1203, 1203–1204*t*
carbuncles (abscesses), 1264
carcinogens, 950
carcinomas, 949, 949*t*
Cardene/Cardene SR. *See* nicardipine
cardiac action potential, 597–598*f*, 597–599
cardiac conduction system, 445, 447*f*
CARDIAC GLYCOSIDES, 584*t*, 587–588. *See also* digoxin
cardiac output (CO), 447–448, 448*f*
cardiac remodeling, 489, 579–580
cardiopulmonary resuscitation (CPR), 572
cardiopulmonary toxicity, 958
cardiotonic drugs, 185
cardiotoxicity, 56*t*, 57–58, 824
cardiovascular disease (CVD), 547*t*, 562. *See also*
    angina pectoris; coronary artery disease;
    dysrhythmias; heart failure; myocardial
    infarctions
cardiovascular system, 440–452
    age-related changes, 118, 119*t*
    blood and blood pressure. *See* blood; blood
      pressure
    heart. *See* heart
    heart, structure and functions of, 444–448,
      446–448*f*
    structure and function of, 441, 442*f*
cardioversion, 601
Cardizem. *See* diltiazem
Cardura/Cardura XL. *See* doxazosin
carfilzomib, 987*t*
Carimune. *See* intravenous immune globulin
carisoprodol, 339*t*, 340
carmustine, 958, 964*t*, 966
carnitine (L-carnitine), 84, 84*f*, 87*t*, 589*t*
carteolol, 1288*t*, 1289, 1290
Cartia XT. *See* diltiazem
cartilage toxicity, 824
Cartrol. *See* carteolol
carvedilol
    antagonistic effects of, 61
    for heart failure, 584*t*, 586
    for hypertension, 549
    mechanism of action, 197
    routes and dosages, 198*t*
    therapeutic applications, 200
cascara sagrada, 83*t*, 1026
Casodex. *See* bicalutamide
caspofungin, 868, 870, 870*t*, 872
castor oil, 336, 1025*t*, 1027

cataplexy, 222, 358
Catapres. *See* clonidine
catecholamines, 144, 179, 180*f*
catechol-O-methyltransferase (COMT), 145, 179
CATECHOL-O-METHYLTRANSFERASE (COMT)
    INHIBITORS, 290*t*, 293
category ratings, for medications during pregnancy,
    95, 95*t*
cathartic, 1025. *See also* LAXATIVES
catheter ablation, 601
catheter-associated urinary tract infections, 837
cations, 528
caustic chemicals, 1307
Caverject. *See* alprostadil
Cayston. *See* aztreonam
CB1 (CANNABINOID RECEPTOR) BLOCKERS, 1082
CBER (Center for Biologics Evaluation and Research),
    16–17
CCBs. *See* CALCIUM CHANNEL BLOCKERS
CCNU. *See* lomustine
CD4 receptors, 927
CDAD (*Clostridium difficile*–associated diarrhea),
    796*t*, 809, 824
CDC (Centers for Disease Control and Prevention),
    712, 780, 852, 886, 1196
CDER (Center for Drug Evaluation and Research),
    16, 54
Cebid. *See* vitamin C
Ceclor. *See* cefaclor
Cedax. *See* ceftibuten
CeeNU. *See* lomustine
cefaclor, 794*t*, 796
cefadroxil, 794*t*, 796
cefazolin, 794*t*, 795–796
cefdinir, 794*t*, 796
cefditoren, 794*t*, 796
cefepime, 794*t*, 796
cefixime, 794*t*, 796
Cefizox. *See* ceftizoxime
Cefobid. *See* cefoperazone
cefoperazone, 796
Cefotan. *See* cefotetan
cefotaxime, 794*t*, 796
cefotetan, 794*t*, 795, 796
cefoxitin, 794*t*, 796
cefpodoxime, 794*t*, 796
cefprozil, 794*t*, 796
ceftaroline, 794*t*, 795, 796–797
ceftazidime, 794*t*, 796
ceftibuten, 794*t*, 796
Ceftin. *See* cefuroxime
ceftizoxime, 794*t*, 796
ceftriaxone, 112*t*, 794*t*, 796, 836
cefuroxime, 794*t*, 796
Cefzil. *See* cefprozil
Celebrex. *See* celecoxib
celecoxib, 680–681*t*, 682–683
Celestone. *See* betamethasone
Celexa. *See* citalopram
cell kill hypothesis, 954, 955*f*
cell wall inhibitors
    carbapenems, 797–798, 797*t*
    cephalosporins, 778, 790, 794–797, 794*t*
    miscellaneous agents, 797*t*, 798–799
    penicillins. *See* PENICILLIN(S)
CellCept. *See* mycophenolate
cell-mediated immune response, 670–671
cellular receptors. *See* receptors
cellulitits, 1264
Celontin. *See* methsuximide
Cenestin. *See* conjugated estrogens
Center for Biologics Evaluation and Research (CBER),
    16–17

Center for Drug Evaluation and Research
    (CDER), 16, 54
Center for Food Safety and Applied Nutrition
    (CFSAN), 17
Center for Tobacco Products, 17
Centers for Disease Control and Prevention (CDC),
    712, 780, 852, 886, 1196
central centrifugal alopecia, 1279
central nervous system (CNS), 208–215
    age-related changes, 118, 119*t*
    degenerative diseases. *See* neurodegenerative
      diseases
    depressants. *See* CENTRAL NERVOUS SYSTEM
      DEPRESSANTS
    drug mechanisms in, 209
    functional systems of, 213–214, 213–215*f*
    muscle spasticity and damage to, 335
    neurons and neurotransmission in, 210–211,
      210*f*, 210*t*
    organ-specific toxicity and, 56*t*, 57
    overview, 137, 138*f*
    stimulants. *See* CENTRAL NERVOUS SYSTEM
      STIMULANTS
    structural divisions of, 211–213, 212–213*f*
    toxicity to, 824–825
CENTRAL NERVOUS SYSTEM DEPRESSANTS, 420–429. *See*
    also ANTIDEPRESSANTS
    alcohol. *See* alcohol
    dependence and, 419
    drug interactions, 86*t*
    hallucinogens, 427–429
    interactions with, 62*t*
    marijuana, 417, 418, 421*t*, 426–427
    opioids. *See* opioid(s)
    sedatives and antianxiety drugs. *See*
      BARBITURATES; BENZODIAZEPINES;
      NONBENZODIAZEPINE ANXIOLYTICS
CENTRAL NERVOUS SYSTEM STIMULANTS, 350–365
    abuse of, 351, 429
    for ADHD, 353–356, 354*t*
    adverse effects of, 351, 358
    amphetamines. *See* AMPHETAMINES
    caffeine, 354*t*, 359–360, 360*t*, 431
    cocaine. *See* cocaine
    methylphenidate, 222, 356, 358, 417, 430
    methylxanthines, 359–360
    for narcolepsy, 358–359
    Nursing Practice Applications, 361–362*t*
    regulation of, 351, 351*t*
central vein total parenteral nutrition, 1069
central-line associated bloodstream infections, 798*t*
cephalexin, 112*t*, 794*t*, 796
CEPHALOSPORINS
    adverse effects, 56*t*, 795
    breast-feeding and, 98*t*
    classification of, 795, 796–797
    clinical applications, 795–796
    cross-sensitivity with penicillins, 790, 795
    drug interactions, 622*t*
    first generation, 794*t*, 795
    second generation, 794*t*, 795
    third generation, 794*t*, 795
    fourth generation, 794*t*, 795
    fifth generation, 794*t*, 795
    lactation risk categories, 99*t*
    mechanism of action, 778, 794
    Nursing Practice Applications, 800–801*t*
    pregnancy category, 95*t*, 836
    resistance to, 779, 795
    routes and dosages, 794*t*
cephradine, 796
cerebellum, 212*f*, 213
cerebral malaria, 886

cerebral palsy (CP), 336, 337t, 341t

cerebrum, 211, 212f

Cerebyx. See fosphenytoin

Cerespan. See papaverine-phentolamine

ceritinib, 987t

certolizumab pegol, 702t, 1033, 1248t, 1249, 1250

Cerubidine. See daunorubicin

cerumenolytics, 1297

Cervarix, 720

cervical cancer, 950, 1197

Cervidil. See dinoprostone

Cesamet. See nabilone

Cetamide. See sulfacetamide sodium

cetirizine, 425t, 756t, 758

cetrorelix, 1182t, 1183, 1185

Cetrotide. See cetrorelix

cetuximab, 987t, 988

cevimeline, 152t, 154

CFSAN (Center for Food Safety and Applied
    Nutrition), 17

cGMP (current Good Manufacturing Practice)
    regulations, 1049–1050

Chagas' disease (American trypanosomiasis), 894–895

chalazion, 1294

chamomile, 82, 233

Chantix. See varenicline

CharcoAid. See activated charcoal

chelation therapy, 1310–1311

chemical names, 7

chemical warfare agents, 1306–1308, 1307t

chemoreceptor trigger zone (CTZ), 1036–1037

chemoreceptors, 449, 450

chemotaxis, 667

chemotherapy, 951–952. See also ANTINEOPLASTIC
    AGENTS

Chernobyl nuclear disaster (1986), 1307

chest pain. See angina pectoris

chest radiography, 851

chewable medications, 28

CHF (congestive heart failure), 579. See also heart
    failure

chickenpox (varicella), 719–720, 910, 1265

chief cells, 998

Childhood Vaccine Act of 1986, 16

children. See pediatric patients

Chirocaine. See levobupivacaine

chiropractic therapy, 389t

chlamdia, 777t, 807

chloasma, 1197

chloral hydrate, 223, 228

chlorambucil, 55t, 964t, 966

chloramphenicol, 56t, 98t, 814–815, 815t, 1306

chlordiazepoxide, 224, 225–226t, 227–228

chloride, 528t, 1056, 1057t

chlorophyll/chlorella, 81t

chloroprocaine, 406t, 409

chloroquine, 783, 886, 887–889, 888t

chlorothiazide, 509, 510t, 511, 547

chlorpheniramine, 756–757t, 766t

chlorpromazine, 56t, 265, 271t, 272, 425t, 616t

chlorpropamide, 56t, 1122t, 1126

chlorthalidone, 202, 509, 510t, 511, 546t, 547

Chlor-Trimeton. See chlorpheniramine

chlorzoxazone, 339t, 340

choking agents, 1307

cholecalciferol, 1232, 1238, 1238t. See also vitamin D

cholecystokinin, 1000

cholera, 713t, 775, 777t, 807

cholestatic hepatitis, 811

cholesterol, 454, 458–459, 459f. See also dyslipidemia

CHOLESTEROL ABSORPTION INHIBITORS, 461t, 467

cholestyramine, 58, 62t, 461t, 464–465

choline magnesium trisalicylate, 676t, 678

cholinergic agonists, 149–162. See also
    ACETYLCHOLINESTERASE INHIBITORS;
    MUSCARINIC AGONISTS
    adverse effects of, 152t
    for glaucoma, 154, 1289
    mechanism of action, 150–151f, 150–152
    nicotinic agonists, 158, 160
    Nursing Practice Applications, 159–160t
    receptors, 142–143, 144t, 150–151f,
        150–152, 151t
    routes and dosages, 152t

cholinergic antagonists, 163–176. See also MUSCARINIC
    ANTAGONISTS; NICOTINIC ANTAGONISTS
    classification of, 164–165
    mechanism of action, 164–165, 164f
    Nursing Practice Applications, 173–174t

cholinergic crisis, 153, 155, 157

cholinergic nerves, 142

cholinergic receptors, 142–143, 144t, 150–151f,
    150–152, 151t

cholinergic synapses, 211

cholinergic transmission, 142–144, 143–144f, 144t

cholinesterase. See acetylcholinesterase

cholinesterase inhibitors. See ACETYLCHOLINESTERASE
    INHIBITORS

chondroitin, 87, 87t, 1247t

chorionic gonadotropin-HCG, 1182t, 1185

Christmas disease, 637

chromium, 87t, 1057t, 1132t

chromoblastomycosis, 867t

chronic bronchitis, 745–746

chronic obstructive pulmonary disease (COPD)
    Nursing Practice Applications, 746–748t
    pathophysiology, 745–746
    pharmacotherapy, 166, 359, 746

chronic opioid therapy (COT), 368t

chronic pain, 367, 368t. See also pain

chronic pancreatitis, 1041

chronic psychosis, 265

chyme, 997–998, 1000

Cialis. See tadalafil

ciclesonide, 741t, 742, 759t

ciclopirox, 875t, 1274

ciclopirox nail lacquer, 876

cidofovir, 911t, 912

cilastatin. See imipenem-cilastatin

cilostazol, 626t, 630–631

Ciloxan. See ciprofloxacin

cimetidine
    adverse effects, 56t, 616t, 622t, 1015, 1215t
    breast-feeding and, 98t
    clinical applications, 1015, 1041
    routes and dosages, 1014t

Cimzia. See certolizumab pegol

cinacalcet, 1240t, 1244

cinchonism, 605, 889–890

cinnamates, 1278

Cinobac. See cinoxacin

cinoxacin, 826

Cipro HC otic, 825, 1297t

Cipro XR. See ciprofloxacin

Cipro/Cipro XR. See ciprofloxacin

Ciprodex otic, 825, 1297t

ciprofloxacin
    adverse effects, 825
    for anthrax, 1305
    breast-feeding and, 98t
    clinical applications, 824, 825, 835, 858–859
    dexamethasone with, 825, 1297t
    drug interactions, 825–826
    for external otitis, 1295
    hydrocortisone with, 825, 1297t
    labeling changes, 105t

mechanism of action, 34, 825

nursing responsibilities, 826

for pneumonic plague, 1306

routes and dosages, 823t, 853t

for tularemia, 1306

circadian dysrhythm, 221

circadian rhythm, 221

cirrhosis, 424

cisatracurium, 169t, 173, 411

cisplatin, 55–56t, 504t, 958, 964t, 966

citalopram, 231t, 245t, 250, 297

Citanest. See prilocaine

Citracal. See calcium citrate

Citrucel. See methylcellulose

CK (creatine kinase), 460

cladribine, 969t, 970–971

Claforan. See cefotaxime

Clarinex. See desloratadine

clarithromycin
    adverse effects, 616t
    clinical applications, 809, 811, 859, 863,
        894, 1017
    pregnancy category rating, 95t
    routes and dosages, 112t, 810t

Claritin. See loratadine

claudication, 335

clavulanate, 789t, 792, 793

Clear Eyes. See naphazoline

Clearasil. See benzoyl peroxide

clemastine, 756, 756–757t

Cleocin/Cleocin-T. See clindamycin

clevidipine, 477–478t, 479, 548, 553t

Cleviprex. See clevidipine

climacteric, 1174

Climara. See estradiol

ClindaMax. See clindamycin

clindamycin, 815, 815t, 886, 1268t, 1269

Clindesse. See clindamycin

clinical phase trials, 17–18, 127–128

Clinoril. See sulindac

clobazam, 318t, 321

clobetasol propionate, 1273t

clocortolone pivalate, 1273t

Cloderm. See clocortolone pivalate

clofarabine, 969t, 971

clofazimine, 859, 862

Clolar. See clofarabine

Clomid. See clomiphene

clomiphene, 95t, 1181–1182, 1182t, 1183–1185, 1216

clomipramine, 231t, 232, 245t, 247

clonal division, 669

clonazepam, 225–226t, 260, 313t, 318t, 320, 321

clonidine
    for ADHD, 356, 357–358
    adverse effects, 550
    for anxiety, 228
    for hypertension, 184, 550, 552
    off-label indications, 550
    for pain, 383, 411
    routes and dosages, 354t, 379t

clopidogrel, 571, 616t, 617, 622t, 626t, 627–628

clorazepate, 225–226t, 228, 313t, 318t, 320, 321

closed-angle glaucoma, 1285f, 1286

Clostridium albicans, 784

Clostridium botulinum, 343, 775, 1306

Clostridium difficile, 779t, 781t, 784, 808, 1028

Clostridium difficile–associated diarrhea (CDAD),
    796t, 809, 824

Clostridium tetani. See tetanus

clotrimazole, 875t, 877, 1265, 1295

clotting. See coagulation

clotting factors, for hemophilia, 637–638

cloxacillin, 793

Cloxapen. *See* cloxacillin
clozapine, 275*t*, 276
Clozaril. *See* clozapine
club drugs, 96*t*, 427, 428–429
CMV (cytomegalovirus), 723, 910
CNPs (C-type natriuretic peptides), 581
CNS. *See* central nervous system
CO (cardiac output), 447–448, 448*f*
coagulation, 614–636
    disorders, 616–617, 636–638
    modifiers, 617–636
        anticoagulants. *See* ANTICOAGULANTS
        antiplatelets. *See* ANTIPLATELET AGENTS
        hemostatics, 617, 617*t*, 635–636, 635*t*
        for intermittent claudication, 630–631
        mechanisms of action, 617, 617*f*, 617*t*
        thrombolytics. *See* THROMBOLYTICS
    process of, 443–444, 443–444*f*
    regulation of, 615
coal tar, 1275, 1276*t*
Coartem. *See* artemether-lumefantrine
cobalt, 1057*t*
Cobex. *See* cyanocobalamin
cocaine
    abuse of, 417, 430
    adverse effects, 56*t*
    as anesthetic, 405
    lactation risk categories, 99*t*
    mechanism of action, 178
    during pregnancy, 96, 96*t*
    similarities with amphetamines, 353–354
    withdrawal symptoms and treatment, 420*t*
cocci, 776
coccidioidomycosis, 867, 867*t*
cochlea, 1295
Codamine Syrup, 766*t*
codeine
    adverse effects, 375
    as antitussive, 765, 766, 766*t*
    breast-feeding and, 98*t*
    clinical applications, 377, 1028
    dosing schedule, 39
    drug interactions, 425*t*
    metabolism of, 33
    routes and dosages, 374*t*
    as substrate, 34
Codiclear DH Syrup, 766*t*
Codimal DH, 766*t*
coenzyme Q10, 87*t*, 389*t*, 464*t*
Cogentin. *See* benztropine
Cognex. *See* tacrine
cognitive dysfunction, after noncardiac
    surgery, 405*t*
cognitive symptoms, of schizophrenia, 266, 266*t*
cognitive–behavioral therapy, 243*t*
Colace. *See* docusate; glycerin
Colazal. *See* balsalazide
colchicine, 674, 1253–1255, 1254*t*
Colcrys. *See* colchicine
colds. *See* cough and colds
colesevelam, 461*t*, 465
Colestid. *See* colestipol
colestipol, 461*t*, 465
collagenase, 336
COLLOIDS, 527, 527*t*
colonoscopies, 951
COLONY-STIMULATING FACTORS (CSFs), 646,
    648–649
    adverse effects, 646, 648, 651
    drugs in class
        filgrastim, 645*t*, 646, 648, 694, 957, 991
        pegfilgrastim, 645*t*, 648–649
        sargramostim, 645*t*, 649, 694, 957

mechanism of action, 646, 648
    Nursing Practice Application, 649–651*t*
    therapeutic effects and uses, 646, 648, 651
colorectal cancer, 462
Combigan, 1289
combination drugs, 7, 7*t*, 371–372
Combivent. *See* ipratropium
Combivir, 934
COMEDOLYTICS, 1269
comedones, 1268
Cometriq. *See* cabozantinib
comfrey, 85
common cold. *See* cough and colds
community-acquired infections, 781, 867
Community-Oriented Practice
    ACE inhibitors and angioedema, 490*t*
    ACE inhibitors and hyperkalemia, 488*t*
    antihistamines, sedative effects of, 221*t*
    botox, 344*t*
    calcium supplements and calcium channel
        blockers, 476*t*
    diuretics as banned substances, 509*t*
    epoetin alfa for blood doping, 653*t*
    fever in patients on immunosuppressants, 694*t*
    fluid balance during exercise, 530*t*
    food–drug interactions, 62*t*
    home care of patients on total parenteral
        nutrition, 1073*t*
    laxative abuse, 1027*t*
    lifestyle modifications for hypertension, 195*t*
    macular edema in women on oral
        contraceptives, 1199*t*
    medication errors in geriatric patients, 117*t*
    myasthenia gravis, 158*t*
    NSAIDs for Alzheimer's disease, 300*t*
    pseudomembranous colitis, 796*t*
    self-administration of growth hormone by pen
        device, 1100*t*
    sleep, cardiovascular disease, and timing of anti-
        hypertensives, 547*t*
    soy, effects on drug treatment for hypothyroid-
        ism, 1141*t*
    test and treat prevention strategies, 943*t*
    travel and tuberculosis risk, 854*t*
comorbidities
    anxiety disorders and, 218*t*
    epilepsy and, 320*t*
    in geriatric patients, 117
comorbidities, in geriatric patients, 121–122
Compazine. *See* prochlorperazine
Compazine Spansule. *See* prochlorperazine
complement system, 667, 668*t*
Complementary and Alternative Therapies, 79–90
    acupuncture, 336, 389*t*, 953*t*
    aloe vera, 85, 1026, 1277*t*, 1278
    for anxiety disorders, 217, 223, 223*t*
    bilberry, 1293*t*
    black cohosh, 336, 1192*t*
    chromium, 1132*t*
    coenzyme Q10, 389*t*, 464*t*
    cranberry, 841*t*
    cultural considerations in, 128
    dandelion, 516*t*, 1026
    defined, 80
    for dementia, 299*t*
    dietary supplements. *See* dietary supplements
    echinacea, 700*t*
    galactogogues, 99*t*
    garlic, 81, 627*t*
    ginger, 82, 82*t*, 85, 1011*t*, 1037
    glucosamine and chondroitin, 87, 1247*t*
    goldenseal, 674*t*
    grape seed extract, 543*t*

    green tea, 1083*t*
    hawthorn, 196, 200, 496*t*
    herbal therapies. *See* herbal supplements
    for insomnia, 223, 223*t*
    ketogenic diet, 312, 312*t*, 315
    Lactobacillus acidophilus, 1040*t*
    melatonin, 171, 220, 223, 224*t*, 227, 229
    for migraines, 389*t*
    for muscle spasms and spasticity, 336–337
    omega-3 fatty acids, 87, 467, 562*t*, 1154*t*
    for pain management, 370
    patient education on, 87
    St. John's wort. *See* St. John's wort
    saw palmetto, 82, 1222*t*
    for seizures, 312, 312*t*
    soy, 1141*t*, 1178*t*
    specialty supplements, 87, 87*t*
    types of, 80, 80*t*
    vitamin C, 765*t*
complex partial seizures, 313*t*, 314
compliance. *See* adherence
complicated urinary tract infections (C-UTIs),
    835*t*, 836
Comprehensive Drug Abuse Prevention and Control
    Act of 1970, 14, 20, 418
compulsions. *See* obsessive-compulsive disorder
COMT (catechol-O-methyltransferase), 145, 179
COMT (CATECHOL-O-METHYLTRANSFERASE)
    INHIBITORS, 290, 290*t*, 293
Comtan. *See* entacapone
Comvax, 917
Concerta. *See* methylphenidate
congestive heart failure (CHF), 579. *See also* heart
    failure
conivaptan, 1106
conjugated estrogens, 1168–1171, 1170*t*, 1174
conjugated estrogens with medroxyprogesterone,
    1170*t*, 1174
conjugation, 780
conjunctivitis, 1294, 1295*t*
conscious sedation, 395
constipation
    antineoplastic agents and, 957–958, 991
    etiology of, 1024–1025, 1024*t*
    opioids and, 375, 385
    pharmacotherapy. *See* LAXATIVES
consumption. *See* tuberculosis
contact dermatitis, 1271
continuous infusion feedings, in enteral
    nutrition, 1064
contraception and contraceptive methods, 1189–1207
    defined, 1190
    depot injections, 1198
    effectiveness of, 1191*t*
    emergency, 1200, 1202, 1203*t*
    intrauterine devices, 1199
    long-term, 1197–1199
    mechanisms of action, 1192*f*
    Nursing Practice Applications, 1201–1202*t*
    oral. *See* ORAL CONTRACEPTIVES
    prevalence of use, 1190*t*, 1193*t*
    selection of, 1190
    spermicides, 1199–1200
    sponges, 1199, 1199*f*
    subdermal implants, 1198–1199
    transdermal, 1197
    vaginal, 1197–1198
Contrave, 1083*t*, 1085
controlled substance(s), 14, 20, 20*t*, 418
Controlled Substances Act. *See* Comprehensive Drug
    Abuse Prevention and Control Act of 1970
convulsions, 310–311. *See also* seizures
Conzip. *See* tramadol

Copaxone. *See* glatiramer
COPD. *See* chronic obstructive pulmonary disease
Copegus. *See* ribavirin
copper, 1057*t*
Copper T380A, 1199
Cordarone. *See* amiodarone
Cordran. *See* flurandrenolide
Coreg. *See* carvedilol
Corgard. *See* nadolol
Corlopam. *See* fenoldopam
cornea, 1284–1285
coronary arteries, 445, 446*f*, 476
coronary artery disease (CAD), 560–562. *See also*
     angina pectoris; myocardial infarctions
coronaviruses, 908*t*
corpora cavernosa, 1216
corpus luteum, 1167
corpus striatum, 287
Correctol. *See* bisacodyl
Cortef. *See* hydrocortisone
CORTICOSTEROIDS
    as adjuvant analgesics, 384, 384*t*
    adverse effects of, 156, 158*t*, 705, 740,
        1154–1155
    for allergic rhinitis, 759, 759*t*, 762, 1159
    as antineoplastic adjuncts, 1160
    for arthritis, 1159, 1246, 1247
    for asthma, 735*t*, 740–742, 741*t*, 1159
    classification of, 1154
    for dermatitis, 1273, 1273*t*
    drug interactions, 233, 622*t*, 1155
    drugs in class
        beclomethasone, 740–741, 741*t*, 759
        betamethasone, 1156*t*, 1273*t*
        budesonide. *See* budesonide
        ciclesonide, 741*t*, 742, 759*t*
        cortisone, 1156*t*
        dexamethasone. *See* dexamethasone
        flunisolide, 741*t*, 742
        fluticasone, 105*t*, 112*t*, 741*t*, 742, 759*t*, 762
        hydrocorisone. *See* hydrocortisone
        methylprednisolone, 303, 705, 1040, 1156*t*
        mometasone, 741*t*, 742, 759*t*, 1273*t*
        prednisolone, 839, 1156*t*
        prednisone. *See* prednisone
        triamcinolone, 741*t*, 742, 759*t*, 1156*t*, 1273*t*
    for edema, 1160
    for gout, 1253
    as immunosuppressants, 703, 705, 1158–1159
    for inflammatory bowel disease, 1032, 1159
    intranasal, 759, 759*t*, 762
    lactation risk categories, 99*t*
    mechanism of action, 740, 762
    mechanisms of action, 1154, 1154*t*
    for multiple sclerosis, 303
    for myasthenia gravis, 155–156
    for nausea and vomiting, 1039*t*, 1040
    Nursing Practice Applications, 1160–1161*t*
    for ocular conditions, 1294
    pregnancy category, 95*t*
    preterm labor risk and, 1159*t*
    prevalence of use, 1153–1154
    for psoriasis, 1274–1275
    regulation of, 1094*t*
    replacement therapy with, 1155–1158
    routes and dosages of, 1156*t*
    routes of administration, 29
    topical, 1160
    for transplant rejection prophylaxis, 1159–1160
corticotropin-releasing hormone (CRH), 1098
cortisone, 1156*t*
Cortisporin. *See* hydrocortisone; neomycin;
    polymyxin B

Cortizone. *See* hydrocortisone
Cortrosyn. *See* cosyntropin
Corvert. *See* ibutilide
Corynebacterium diphtheriae. *See* diphtheria
Corzide, 511, 546*t*. *See also* bendroflumethiazide
    and nadolol
Cosmegen. *See* dactinomycin
cosmetics, 14, 17
cosyntropin, 1156
COT (chronic opioid therapy), 368*t*
Cotazym S. *See* pancrelipase
cough and colds
    nonpharmacologic therapies for, 765*t*
    Nursing Practice Applications for, 768–769*t*
    pharmacotherapy
        antihistamines. *See* ANTIHISTAMINES
        antitussives, 765–767, 766*t*
        combination products, 765
        decongestants. *See* NASAL DECONGESTANTS
        expectorants, 766*t*, 767
        first-generation antipsychotics, 271
        mucolytics, 746, 766*t*, 767, 769
    prevalence of, 765*t*
    symptoms of, 765
Coumadin. *See* warfarin
Council for Responsible Nutrition (CRN), 1049
Covera-HS. *See* verapamil
COX (cyclooxygenase), 379, 675, 675*f*
COX-2 (CYCLOOXYGENASE-2) INHIBITORS, 682–683
Cozaar. *See* losartan
CP (cerebral palsy), 336, 337*t*, 341*t*
CPR (cardiopulmonary resuscitation), 572
crab louse, 1265
cranberry, 81*t*, 622*t*, 841*t*
CRE (carbapenem-resistant *Enterobacteriaceae*), 797
C-reactive protein, 668*t*
creatine kinase (CK), 460
Creon. *See* pancrelipase
Crestor. *See* rosuvastatin
cretinism, 1140
CRH (corticotropin-releasing hormone), 1098
Crinone. *See* progesterone
Crixivan. *See* indinavir
crizotinib, 987*t*, 988
CRN (Council for Responsible Nutrition), 1049
Crohn's disease, 1030, 1032, 1033, 1035
Crolom. *See* cromolyn
cromolyn, 94, 741*t*, 742–743, 759*t*, 763, 1295*t*
cross-allergies, 55
cross-tolerance, 420
crotamiton, 1265, 1266
Cruex. *See* undecylenic acid
crushing medications, 28
cryoprecipitate, 524*t*, 525
cryptococcosis, 867, 867*t*, 944*t*
cryptosporidiosis, 885*t*, 891, 944*t*
Cryptosporidium parvum, 885*t*, 891
CRYSTALLOIDS, 525–527, 526*t*
crystalluria, 839
CSFs. *See* COLONY-STIMULATING FACTORS
C-type natriuretic peptides (CNPs), 581
CTZ (chemoreceptor trigger zone), 1036–1037
Cubicin. *See* daptomycin
cultural differences. *See also* Treating the Diverse
    Patient; *specific racial and ethnic groups*
    in acetaminophen metabolism, 684*t*
    in acetylation of isoniazid, 855, 856*f*
    in antihypertensive response, 131*t*, 197*t*,
        544, 546
    in cancer, 959*t*
    in diabetes, 128*t*, 1113
    in glaucoma, 1286*t*
    health insurance coverage and, 128*t*

    in obesity, 1080*t*
    in pharmacotherapy, 127–128
    in renal failure, 504*t*
    in substance abuse, 429*t*
culture and sensitivity (C&S) testing, 782, 836, 837, 852
Cuprimine. *See* D-penicillamine
curare, 172, 335
current Good Manufacturing Practice (cGMP)
    regulations, 1049–1050
Cushing's syndrome, 1163, 1163*t*
cutaneous anthrax, 1305*t*
cutaneous fungal infections, 868
cutaneous larva migrans, 898, 900
Cutaneous leishmaniasis, 895
Cutar. *See* coal tar
C-UTIs (complicated urinary tract infections),
    835*t*, 836
Cutivate. *See* fluticasone propionate
Cuvposa. *See* glycopyrrolate
CVD. *See* cardiovascular disease
cyanocobalamin (vitamin B$_{12}$), 657–658, 657*f*
    clinical applications, 1055–1056
    functions of, 1049*t*
    routes and dosages, 29, 653*t*, 1050*t*
cyanogen chloride, 1307*t*
cyclic feedings, in enteral nutrition, 1064
cyclic guanosine monophosphate, 1216
CYCLIC LIPOPEPTIDES, 827, 827*t*
cyclizine, 757, 1039*t*
cyclobenzaprine, 338–340, 339*t*
Cyclocort. *See* amcinonide
Cyclogyl. *See* cyclopentolate
cycloheptadine, 248
cyclooxygenase (COX), 379, 675, 675*f*
CYCLOOXYGENASE-2 (COX-2) INHIBITORS, 682–683.
    See also celecoxib
cyclopentolate, 165*t*, 168, 1293*t*
cyclophosphamide
    adverse effects, 55*t*, 701, 965
    clinical applications, 701, 964, 1248
    mechanism of action, 954, 964
    Nursing Responsibilities, 966
    pregnancy rating category, 95*t*
    routes and dosages, 696*t*, 964*t*
CYCLOPLEGICS, 167, 168, 1292, 1294
    atropine. *See* atropine
    cyclopentolate, 165*t*, 168, 1293*t*
    homatropine, 766*t*, 1293*t*
    scopolamine, 29, 165*t*, 168, 1037, 1039*t*, 1293*t*
    tropicamide, 165*t*, 168, 1293*t*
cycloserine, 853*t*, 858
Cycloset. *See* bromocriptine
cyclosporine
    adverse effects, 55–56*t*, 504*t*, 698
    drug interactions with, 62*t*, 86*t*, 622*t*, 699
    as immunosuppressant, 156, 696*t*, 1273,
        1276–1277
    mechanism of action, 698
    Nursing Responsibilities, 699
    routes and dosages, 1276*t*
    therapeutic effects and uses, 698
cyclosporine ophthalmic emulsion, 1294
cyclothymic disorder, 240
Cyklokapron. *See* tranexamic acid
Cymbalta. *See* duloxetine
Cynapin. *See* cyanocobalamin
CYP (cytochrome P450) isozymes, 33–34, 33*t*, 94, 106
cyproheptadine, 756*t*
Cyramza. *See* ramucirumab
cystic fibrosis, 767, 769
cystitis, 834
Cystospaz. *See* hyoscyamine
cysts, 885

cytarabine, 822–823, 969*t*, 971
cytochrome P450 (CYP) isozymes, 33–34, 33*t*, 94, 106
CytoGam. *See* cytomegalovirus immune globulin
cytokine(s), 670–671, 690–691, 983, 988
cytokine release syndrome, 703
cytomegalovirus (CMV), 723, 910
cytomegalovirus immune globulin, 721*t*, 723
Cytomel. *See* liothyronine
Cytosar-U. *See* cytarabine
Cytotec. *See* misoprostol
CYTOTOXIC AGENTS, 98*t*, 700–702
    anakinra, 696*t*, 701, 1248*t*, 1249, 1250
    azathioprine. *See* azathioprine
    belatacept, 696*t*, 701
    cyclophosphamide. *See* cyclophosphamide
    etanercept. *See* etanercept
    mycophenolate, 156, 696*t*, 701
    thalidomide. *See* thalidomide
cytotoxic (CD8) T cells, 670
Cytovene. *See* ganciclovir
Cytoxan. *See* cyclophosphamide

D

D₅W. *See* 5% dextrose in water
dabigatran, 618*t*, 621, 623
dacarbazine, 55*t*, 964*t*, 967
daclizumab, 753
dactinomycin, 972*t*, 975
Dale, Henry, 142*t*
Dale, Samuel, 3
dalfampridine, 302*t*, 303
dalfopristin. *See* quinupristin-dalfopristin
Daliresp. *See* roflumilast
Dalmane. *See* flurazepam
dalteparin, 618*t*, 620
danaparoid, 620
danazol, 622*t*, 1182*t*, 1183, 1185
Danocrine. *See* danazol
dandelion, 516*t*, 1026
Dantrium. *See* dantrolene sodium
dantrolene sodium, 341*t*, 342–343
dapagliflozin, 1122*t*, 1131
dapsone, 129, 859, 861–862
daptomycin, 782, 827, 827*t*
Daraprim. *See* pyrimethamine
darbepoetin alfa, 643, 645*t*, 646
darunavir, 932*t*, 937, 938
Darvocet. *See* propoxyphene
Darvon. *See* propoxyphene
dasatinib, 987*t*, 988
DASH (Dietary Approaches to Stop Hypertension) diet, 195*t*
date-rape drugs, 421
daunorubicin, 56*t*, 57, 823, 972*t*, 974
daunorubicin liposomal, 972*t*, 974
DaunoXome. *See* daunorubicin liposomal
Daypro. *See* oxaprozin
Daytrana. *See* methylphenidate
DBS (deep brain stimulation), 288, 288*t*
DDAVP. *See* desmopressin
ddC. *See* zalcitabine
ddI. *See* didanosine
DDS. *See* dapsone
DEA (Drug Enforcement Administration), 20
debrisoquin hydroxylase, 129, 275*t*
Debrox. *See* carbamide peroxide
debulking, 951, 954
Decadron. *See* dexamethasone
Decaspray. *See* dexamethasone
Declomycin. *See* demeclocycline

DECONGESTANTS
    nasal. *See* NASAL DECONGESTANTS
    ocular. *See* OCULAR DECONGESTANTS/ VASOCONSTRICTORS
deep brain stimulation (DBS), 288, 288*t*
deep sedation/analgesia, 395
deep vein thrombosis (DVT), 615, 1072
defecation, 997
deferoxamine, 1308*t*
defibrillation, 601
degarelix, 976*t*, 978–979
dehydration
    causes and interventions, 1067*t*
    fluid replacement therapy for, 523, 524*t*. *See also* FLUID REPLACEMENT AGENTS
    in geriatric patients, 528*t*
dehydroepiandrosterone (DHEA), 87*t*, 434, 1209
Delatest. *See* testosterone
Delatestryl. *See* testosterone enanthate
delavirdine, 932*t*, 933, 936
delayed release drugs, 1016
Delestrogen. *See* estradiol valerate
delirium tremens, 425
Delsym. *See* dextromethorphan
Delta-D. *See* cholecalciferol
Deltasone. *See* prednisone
delusions, 265, 266*t*
Demadex. *See* torsemide
demeclocycline, 807*t*, 809, 1106
dementia, 295, 299*t*, 461. *See also* Alzheimer's disease
Demerol. *See* meperidine
Denavir. *See* penciclovir
Dendrid. *See* idoxuridine
dendritic cells, 667
denosumab, 991, 1240*t*, 1244
dental health, dysrhythmias and, 601*t*
DentiPatch. *See* lidocaine
deoxyribonucleic acid. *See* DNA
Depacon. *See* valproic acid
Depakene. *See* valproic acid
Depakote. *See* valproic acid
Depakote ER. *See* divalproex sodium
Depen. *See* D-penicillamine
dependence, 20, 375, 418–419
DepoDur. *See* morphine sulfate
depolarization, 598
depolarizing neuromuscular blockers, 168–172, 170*f*
Depo-Medrol. *See* methylprednisolone
Depo-Provera. *See* medroxyprogesterone
Depo-subQ-Provera. *See* medroxyprogesterone
Depot-Cyt. *See* cytarabine
Depo-Testosterone. *See* testosterone cypionate
depressants. *See* CENTRAL NERVOUS SYSTEM DEPRESSANTS
depression
    assessment and diagnosis, 242
    defined, 240
    drug-induced, 242
    gender differences in, 241*t*
    genetic influences on, 241
    in geriatric patients, 242, 242*t*
    multiple sclerosis and, 303
    nonpharmacologic therapies for, 243–244, 243*t*
    pathophysiology of, 241
    pharmacotherapy. *See* ANTIDEPRESSANTS
    postpartum, 241
    prevalence of, 240*t*, 241*t*
    seasonal affective disorder, 241, 243
    suicide risk and, 242–243
    symptoms of, 230, 240–241, 241*t*
dermatitis, 1160, 1271, 1273–1274, 1273*t*
dermatologic disorders, 1261–1282
    acne vulgaris, 807, 809, 1267–1269, 1268*t*

alopecia, 958, 963, 1279–1280
anatomy of skin and, 1262–1263, 1262*f*
burns, 1277–1279
classification of, 1263–1264, 1264*t*
dermatitis, 1160, 1271, 1273–1274, 1273*t*
psoriasis, 1274–1276*t*, 1274–1277, 1274*f*
rosacea, 1269
skin infections, 1264–1266
dermatologic toxicity, 56*t*, 57, 958
dermatomycoses, 874–876
Dermatop. *See* prednicarbate
dermis, 1262, 1262*f*, 1263
Desenex. *See* undecylenic acid
Desferal. *See* deferoxamine
desflurane, 403, 403*t*, 404
desiccated thyroid, 1141*t*, 1142
desipramine, 231*t*, 244, 245*t*, 246, 357, 1036
desirudin, 618*t*, 623, 626
desloratadine, 756*t*, 758–759
desmopressin, 636–637, 638, 1100*t*, 1105, 1106, 1107*t*
Desogen, 1193*t*
desogestrel, 1193*t*
Desonate. *See* desonide
desonide, 1273*t*, 1274
DesOwen. *See* desonide
desoximetasone, 1273*t*
Desoxyn. *See* methamphetamines
desvenlafaxine, 245*t*, 250, 252
Desyrel. *See* trazodone
detachment, 266*t*
Detrol. *See* tolterodine
development, defined, 107
DEXA (dual-energy x-ray absorptiometry), 1236
dexamethasone
    for adrenal insufficiency, 1156, 1158
    in cancer treatment, 978
    ciprofloxacin with, 825, 1297*t*
    for dermatitis, 1273*t*
    for hyperthyroid states, 1145
    for nausea and vomiting, 1040
    in pain management, 384
    routes and dosages, 976*t*, 1039*t*, 1156*t*
Dexchlor. *See* dexchlorpheniramine
dexchlorpheniramine, 756*t*
Dexedrine. *See* dextroamphetamine
Dexferrum. *See* iron dextran
Dexilant. *See* dexlansoprazole
dexlansoprazole, 1013
dexmethylphenidate, 354*t*, 356
dexrazoxane, 958, 973
dextran 40, 527
dextroamphetamine, 353, 354*t*, 358, 430, 1082
dextromethorphan, 351, 429, 766–767, 766*t*
5% dextrose in water, 526
d4T. *See* stavudine
DHA (docosahexaenoic acid), 467
DHE 45. *See* dihydroergotamine
DHEA. *See* dehydroepiandrosterone
DHT. *See* dihydrotachysterol
DiaBeta. *See* glyburide
diabetes insipidus (DI), 1105, 1105*t*
diabetes mellitus, 1111–1136
    ACE inhibitors for, 491*t*
    complications of, 1114–1116, 1215
    cultural considerations and, 128*t*, 1113
    diagnosis of, 1114
    gestational, 1114
    heart failure and, 582*t*
    nonpharmacologic therapies for, 1132*t*
    Nursing Practice Applications, 1132–1134*t*
    obesity and, 1113
    pathophysiology of, 1113–1114, 1113*t*

pharmacotherapy. *See* ANTIDIABETIC AGENTS; insulin therapy
prevalence of, 1112, 1112*t*
risk factors for, 1113
in school-age children, 1121*t*
sleep and, 230*t*
symptoms of, 1114
type 1, 1113, 1113*t*
type 2, 1113, 1113*t*
diabetic ketoacidosis (DKA), 1114–1115
Diabinese. *See* chlorpropamide
Diagnostic and Statistical Manual of Mental Disorders, 5th edition (DSM-5), 417
Dialose. *See* docusate
Diamox. *See* acetazolamide
diarrhea
antibiotic-related, 796*t*, 808, 1028
antineoplastic agents and, 957–958, 991
in enteral nutrition therapy, 1065, 1066*t*, 1068
etiology, 1028
pathophysiology of, 1027–1028
pharmacotherapy for, 1028–1030, 1028*t*, 1030–1031*t*
traveler's, 807*t*
diastolic heart failure, 579
diazepam
adverse effects, 225–226, 321, 616*t*
in anesthesia, 397*t*, 398, 399
breast-feeding and, 98*t*
clinical applications, 226*t*, 228
for delirium tremens, 425
distribution of, 32, 119
drug interactions, 59, 321, 425*t*
for dystonia, 270
excretion of, 35, 36
genetic polymorphisms and actions of, 129
mechanism of action, 320
for muscle spasms, 338, 384
nursing responsibilities, 321
routes and dosages, 225*t*
for seizures, 313*t*, 318*t*, 320–321
diazoxide, 550, 552
DIBENZAZEPINES, 323–325
carbamazepine. *See* carbamazepine
eslicarbazepine, 318*t*, 324
oxcarbazepine, 105*t*, 112*t*, 260, 313*t*, 318*t*, 324–325
Dibenzyline. *See* phenoxybenzamine
dibucaine, 406*t*, 410–411, 1278
diclofenac, 616*t*, 680–681*t*
dicloxacillin, 622*t*, 789*t*, 793
dicyclomine, 165*t*, 167, 1033*t*, 1036, 1041
didanosine, 932*t*, 934
Didrex. *See* benzphetamine
Didronel. *See* etidronate disodium
dienogest, 1193*t*
Dietary Approaches to Stop Hypertension (DASH) diet, 195*t*
dietary reference intake (DRI), 1050
Dietary Supplement and Nonprescription Drug Consumer Protection Act of 2007, 84
Dietary Supplement Health and Education Act of 1994 (DSHEA), 14, 84, 1049
dietary supplements. *See also* vitamin(s)
adverse effects, 84–85
defined, 84
drug interactions with, 61–62, 62*t*
regulation of, 14, 17, 20, 84–85
diethyl ether, 401
diethylcarbamazine, 900
diethylpropion, 1083*t*, 1085
diethylstilbestrol (DES), 976*t*, 978
dieting, 1080–1082

difenoxin with atropine, 1028*t*, 1029
Differin. *See* adapalene
diffusion, 26–27, 27*f*
Dificid. *See* fidaxomicin
diflorasone diacetate, 1273*t*
Diflucan. *See* fluconazole
diflunisal, 680–681*t*
digestion and digestive system. *See also* gastrointestinal tract
accessory organs of, 997, 1000–1001
defined, 1060
enzymes in, 1002, 1002*t*
liver and, 1000–1001
regulation of, 1001–1002
structures and functions of, 997, 998*f*
digitalization, 587
digitoxin, 587
digoxin
adverse effects, 588, 616*t*, 1215*t*
breast-feeding and, 98*t*
drug interactions, 61, 86*t*, 233, 588, 1016
for dysrhythmias, 603*t*, 609
in geriatric patients, 122*t*
for heart failure, 584*t*, 587–588
mechanism of action, 588
nursing responsibilities, 588
as overdose treatment, 199, 201, 1308*t*
overdose/poisoning, 1308*t*
dihydroergotamine, 387, 387*t*
DIHYDROPYRIDINES, 476–479
amlodipine. *See* amlodipine
clevidipine, 477–478*t*, 479, 548, 553*t*
felodipine. *See* felodipine
isradipine, 477–478*t*, 479, 548
nicardipine/nicardipine SR, 477–478*t*, 479, 548, 553*t*, 568*t*
nifedipine. *See* nifedipine
nimodipine, 389*t*, 477–478*t*, 479
nisoldipine, 477–478*t*, 479, 548
dihydrotachysterol, 1238, 1238*t*. *See also* vitamin D
Dilacor/Dilacor XR. *See* diltiazem
Dilantin. *See* phenytoin
Dilatrate. *See* isosorbide dinitrate
Dilatrate SR. *See* isosorbide dinitrate
Dilaudid. *See* hydromorphone
Dilocaine. *See* lidocaine
diltiazem
absorption of, 30
for angina pectoris, 477*t*
drug interactions, 199–200
for dysrhythmias, 603*t*, 609
for hypertension, 477*t*, 481, 548
mechanism of action, 476
for muscle spasms, 337
routes and dosages, 478*t*, 568*t*
dimenhydrinate, 756*t*, 757, 1037, 1039*t*
dimercaprol, 1311
Dimetapp. *See* brompheniramine
dimethyl fumarate, 302, 302*t*
dimethyltryptamine (DMT), 428
dinoprostone, 1177, 1177*t*, 1179, 1203, 1203–1204*t*
Diovan. *See* valsartan
Diovan HCT, 495, 546*t*
Dipentum. *See* olsalazine
diphenhydramine
adverse effects, 756
antitussive actions of, 766
in combination drugs, 757*t*7*t*
drug interactions, 425*t*
for dystonia, 270
for nausea and vomiting, 1037
routes and dosages, 294*t*, 756*t*, 1039*t*
sedative effects of, 221*t*, 223, 228–229

therapeutic effects and uses, 759
trade names, 7
diphenoxylate with atropine, 112*t*, 1028, 1028*t*, 1029
diphtheria, 713–714, 713*t*, 814*t*
dipivefrin, 1288*t*, 1289
Diprivan. *See* propofol
Diprolene. *See* betamethasone
dipyridamole, 626*t*, 628
DIRECT THROMBIN INHIBITORS, 623, 626
argatroban, 618*t*, 623
bivalirudin, 618*t*, 623, 626
dabigatran, 618*t*, 621, 623
desirudin, 618*t*, 623, 626
lepirudin, 623
direct vasodilators. *See* VASODILATORS
directly observed therapy (DOT), 113, 851, 852, 854*t*
dirithromycin, 811
DISEASE-MODIFYING ANTIRHEUMATIC DRUGS (DMARDs), 1247–1251
abatacept, 1248*t*, 1249, 1250
adalimumab. *See* adalimumab
anakinra, 696*t*, 701, 1248*t*, 1249, 1250
azathioprine. *See* azathioprine
etanercept. *See* etanercept
hydroxychloroquine, 888*t*, 889, 1248, 1248*t*, 1249
infliximab. *See* infliximab
leflunomide, 105*t*, 1248*t*, 1250
methotrexate. *See* methotrexate
rituximab, 987*t*, 988, 1248*t*, 1250
sulfasalazine. *See* sulfasalazine
disopyramide, 603*t*, 604, 605
dissociative anesthesia, 400
distilled mustard, 1307*t*
distribution
defined, 31
drug interactions and, 59, 59*f*
factors influencing, 31–32
in geriatric patients, 119
in pediatric patients, 106
during pregnancy, 94
disulfiram, 58, 227, 425, 426, 622*t*
Ditropan. *See* oxybutynin chloride
Diulo. *See* metolazone
DIURETIC(s), 505–518
adverse effects, 547, 585–586
as banned substances, 509*t*
carbonic anhydrase inhibitors, 505, 506*f*, 513*t*, 515–516
clinical applications, 505
combination therapy, 505–506
drug interactions, 86*t*
in geriatric patients, 507*t*
for heart failure, 505, 584*t*, 585–586
for hypertension, 505, 509, 544*t*, 546–547
loop (high-ceiling), 56*t*, 505, 506–507*f*, 506–509, 508*t*, 547
mechanisms of action, 505, 506*f*
Nursing Practice Applications, 516–518*t*
osmotic, 505, 506*f*, 513–515, 513*t*, 1292
in pediatric patients, 110
potassium-sparing, 505, 506*f*, 511–513, 511*t*, 547
thiazide. *See* THIAZIDE DIURETICS
diuretic resistance, 585
Diurigen. *See* chlorothiazide
Diuril. *See* chlorothiazide
divalproex. *See* valproic acid
divalproex sodium, 260
diversity. *See* Treating the Diverse Patient; *specific racial and ethnic groups*
Divigel. *See* estradiol

DMARDs (DISEASE-MODIFYING ANTIRHEUMATIC DRUGS), 1247–1251, 1248t
DMT. *See* dimethyltryptamine
DNA (deoxyribonucleic acid)
  bacterial DNA replication, 822–823, 822f
  genetic polymorphisms and, 128–129, 129f, 129t
  gyrase, 822
  helicase, 822
  polymerase, 822
Doan's Pills. *See* magnesium salicylate
dobutamine, 179, 181t, 187, 587t, 589
Dobutrex. *See* dobutamine
docetaxel, 980, 980t, 982
docosahexaenoic acid (DHA), 467
docosanol, 911t, 912
docusate, 1025t, 1027
dofetilide, 603t, 608
dolasetron, 1037, 1039t, 1041
Dolophine. *See* methadone
dolutegravir, 932t
donepezil, 152t, 154, 296–297, 297t, 298–299
dopamine
  chemical structure of, 179, 180f
  effects and clinical applications, 141t, 210t
  for heart failure, 587t, 589
  mechanism of action, 178
  as overdose treatment, 196, 201
  Parkinson's disease and, 287
  routes and dosages, 181t
DOPAMINE AGONISTS, 288, 291–293, 386. *See also* ERGOT ALKALOIDS
  adverse effects, 292
  classification, 291
  drug interactions, 292
  drugs in class
    apomorphine, 290t, 292
    bromocriptine. *See* bromocriptine
    fenoldopam, 553t
    pramipexole, 290t, 291–292
    ropinirole, 290t, 292
  versus levodopa, 291
  mechanism of action, 291, 292
  therapeutic effects and uses, 291–292
dopamine receptors, 145
DOPAMINE REPLACEMENT AGENTS, 271, 288–291, 289f, 290t
dopamine system stabilizers (DSS), 277. *See also* aripiprazole
dopamine type 2 (D₂) receptors, 267
dopaminergic agonists. *See* DOPAMINE AGONISTS
dopaminergic synapses, 211
Dopar. *See* levodopa
Dopastat. *See* dopamine
Doral. *See* quazepam
Doribax. *See* doripenem
Doriglute. *See* glutethimide
doripenem, 797, 797t, 798
dornase alfa, 766t, 769
Doryx. *See* doxycycline
dorzolamide, 515, 1288t, 1292
dosage calculations, for pediatric patients, 110, 111f
dose dependent adverse effects, 53
dose–response relationship, 44–45, 45f
DOT (directly observed therapy), 113, 851, 852, 854t
Dovonex. *See* calcipotriene
down-regulation, 1091
doxazosin, 193, 194t, 196, 1221, 1221t
doxepin
  for anxiety disorders, 232
  for depression, 247
  for dermatitis, 1274
  indications for, 231t
  for irritable bowel syndrome, 1036

for neuropathic pain, 383
  routes and dosages, 245t
doxercalciferol, 1238, 1238t. *See also* vitamin D
Doxil. *See* doxorubicin liposomal
doxorubicin, 55–56t, 57, 958, 972t, 973–974
doxorubicin liposomal, 973
doxycycline
  breast-feeding and, 99t
  clinical applications, 809, 886, 887, 1269, 1306
  routes and dosages, 807t
doxylamine, 223, 1037, 1039t
D-penicillamine, 1248
DPIs (dry powder inhalers), 734
Dramamine. *See* dimenhydrinate
Drisdol. *See* ergocalciferol
dronabinol, 1038, 1039t
dronedarone, 603t, 608
drop attacks. *See* atonic seizures
droperidol, 396
drospirenone, 1193t
Droxia. *See* hydroxyurea
droxidopa, 182
drug(s)
  of abuse. *See* substance abuse
  administration. *See* routes of administration
  approval process, 17–19, 17f
  classification of, 5–6, 5–6t
  defining, 4, 5
  errors. *See* medication error(s)
  ideal drugs, characteristics of, 5
  interactions. *See* drug interactions
  labeling. *See* labeling
  marketing rights, 7
  naming, 7
  off-label indications, 5, 18, 106t
  over-the-counter. *See* over-the-counter products
  pharmacokinetics. *See* pharmacokinetics
  prototypes, 6
  regulations. *See* laws and regulations
  scheduled, 20, 20t
drug abuse. *See* substance abuse
drug allergies, 54–55
Drug Enforcement Administration (DEA), 20
Drug Importation Act of 1848, 13
drug interactions
  absorption and, 31
  defined, 58
  drug–drug, 31, 32, 33–34, 58–60
  food–drug, 31, 32, 59, 61–62, 62t
  in geriatric patients, 121–122, 122t
  with herbal products, 61–62, 62t, 85–87, 86t
  mechanisms of, 58
  patient teaching, 62t
  pharmacodynamic, 60–61, 61f
  pharmacokinetic, 58–60, 59f
  preventing, 5t
drug misuse, defined, 153. *See also* substance abuse
drug-protein complexes, 32, 32f
dry mouth. *See* xerostomia
dry powder inhalers (DPIs), 734
DSHEA (Dietary Supplement Health and Education Act of 1994), 14, 84, 1049
DSM-5 (*Diagnostic and Statistical Manual of Mental Disorders*, 5th edition), 417
DSS (dopamine system stabilizers), 277
DTaP vaccine, 713, 714
DTIC-Dome. *See* dacarbazine
dual-energy x-ray absorptiometry (DEXA), 1236
Duavee, 1175
Duetact, 1125t, 1126
dulaglutide, 1122t, 1131
Dulcolax. *See* bisacodyl
Dulcolax Stool Softener. *See* docusate

duloxetine, 231t, 232, 245t, 250, 252, 383
dumping syndrome, 1064
duodenal ulcers, 1006, 1007, 1013. *See also* peptic ulcer disease
duodenum, 999
Duodote, 155
Dupuytren's contracture, 336
Duraclon. *See* clonidine
Duragesic. *See* fentanyl
Duramorph RF. *See* morphine sulfate
Duranest. *See* etidocaine
duration of action, 38
Durham-Humphrey Amendment of 1951, 14, 19
Duricef. *See* cefadroxil
dutasteride, 1221t, 1222
Duvoid. *See* bethanechol
DVT (deep vein thrombosis), 615, 1072
dwarfism, 1098–1099
Dyazide, 506, 513, 546t
Dymista. *See* azelastine
Dynabac. *See* dirithromycin
DynaCirc. *See* isradipine
dyphylline, 737t, 745
Dyrenium. *See* triamterene
dysfunctional uterine bleeding, 1171, 1171t
dyslipidemia, 453–472
  defined, 455
  diagnostic tools, 456–457, 457t
  factors influencing, 456
  Nursing Practice Applications, 468–469t
  in pediatric patients, 458t
  pharmacotherapy, 458–467
    bile acid sequestrants, 460f, 461t, 463–465, 622t
    cholesterol absorption inhibitors, 467
    for familial hypercholesterolemia, 467
    fibric acid agents, 460f, 461t, 465–467
    mechanisms of action, 459, 460f
    niacin, 460f, 461t, 465
    statins, 458–463. *See also* STATINS
  primary vs. secondary prevention of, 459
  screening for, 463t
  therapeutic lifestyle changes for, 457–458
  treatment guidelines, 457, 459
  types of, 457, 458t
Dysport. *See* abobotulinumtoxinA
dysrhythmias, 596–613
  acute, 601
  asymptomatic, 601
  bradydysrhythmias, 599–600
  classification of, 599–600
  consequences of, 445
  dental health and, 601t
  drugs causing, 597t
  etiology of, 597
  long QT syndrome, 599t
  nonpharmacologic treatment, 601
  pharmacotherapy. *See* ANTIDYSRHYTHMICS
  phases and measurement of cardiac action potential, 597–598f, 597–599
  prophylaxis, 601
  tachydysrhythmias, 600, 606
dysthymic disorder, 240
dystonia, 270, 270t, 336, 336t
dysuria, 834

E

eardrum, 1295
ears
  anatomy of, 1295, 1296f
  infections. *See* otitis media
  Nursing Practice Applications, 1298t

pharmacotherapy for, 1295–1297, 1297*t*
as route of administration, 29
eating disorders, 109
Eber's papyrus, 3
Ebola, 1306
EBV (Epstein-Barr virus), 910
EC (emergency contraception), 1200, 1202, 1203*t*
eccrine glands, 1263
ECF (extracellular fluid) compartment, 522, 522*f*
ECGs (electrocardiograms), 445, 568, 598–599, 599*f*, 600*t*
echinacea, 81*t*, 83*t*, 86*t*, 700*t*
Echinacea angustifolia. See echinacea
Echinacea purpurea. See echinacea
echinocandins. *See* β-GLUCAN SYNTHESIS INHIBITORS
echothiophate iodide, 154, 1288*t*
eclampsia, 311
econazole, 875*t*
ecstasy, 417, 428
ECT (electroconvulsive therapy), 243, 257
ectopic foci, 445
ectopic pregnancy, 1194
eculizumab, 702*t*
eczema, 1271, 1271*t*
ED (erectile dysfunction), 1214, 1216–1219, 1217*t*
Edarbi. *See* azilsartan medoxomil
Edarbyclor, 546*t*
Edecrin. *See* ethacrynic acid
edema, corticosteroids for, 1160
edetate calcium disodium, 1310–1311
Edluar. *See* zolpidem
Edronax. *See* reboxetine
edrophonium, 152*t*, 155, 157, 158
Edurant. *See* rilpivirine
EEGs (electroencephalograms), 222, 310
EF (erythroblastosis fetalis), 722
efalizumab, 1277
efavirenz, 86*t*, 932*t*, 935–936
Efedron. *See* ephedrine
Effexor. *See* venlafaxine
efficacy, 45–46, 46*f*
Effient. *See* prasugrel
eflornithine, 892*t*, 895, 896
Efudex. *See* fluorouracil
EGFR (EPIDERMAL GROWTH FACTOR RECEPTOR) INHIBITORS, 988
Egrifta. *See* tesamorelin
eicosapentaenoic acid (EPA), 467
ejaculation disorders, 1214
Elavil. *See* amitriptyline
Eldepryl. *See* selegiline
elderberry, 81*t*
elderly patients. *See* geriatric patients
electrocardiograms (ECGs), 445, 568, 598–599, 599*f*, 600*t*
electroconvulsive therapy (ECT), 243, 243*t*, 257
electroencephalograms (EEGs), 222, 310
electrolyte, defined, 528
electrolyte imbalances
calcium, 1230, 1232–1233
magnesium, 528*t*, 532–533
Nursing Practice Applications for, 536–537*t*
phosphate, 528*t*
potassium, 528*t*, 529*f*, 530–532
sodium, 528–530, 528*t*, 529*f*
types of, 528, 528*t*
elemental formulas, for enteral nutrition, 1064
Elestat. *See* epinastine
Elestrin. *See* estradiol
eletriptan, 387*t*, 388
Eleutherococcus senticosus. See ginseng; goldenseal
Elidel. *See* pimecrolimus
Eligard. *See* leuprolide

Elimite. *See* permethrin
Eliquis. *See* apixaban
Elitek. *See* rasburicase
Ella. *See* ulipristal
Ellence. *See* epirubicin
Elocon. *See* mometasone
Eloxatin. *See* oxaliplatin
Elspar. *See* asparaginase
eltrombopag, 645*t*, 649, 652
elvitegravir, 932*t*
embolus, 615
embryonic period, of fetal development, 97
Emcyt. *See* estramustine
emedastine, 1295*t*
Emend. *See* aprepitant
emergency contraception (EC), 1200, 1202, 1203*t*
emergency preparedness, 1303–1304
emesis. *See* nausea and vomiting
emetic potential, 957
emetogenic potential, 1037
empagliflozin, 1122*t*, 1131
emphysema, 745–746
Emsam. *See* selegiline
emtricitabine, 932*t*, 933, 934–935, 943
Emtriva. *See* emtricitabine
Emulsoil. *See* castor oil
E-mycin. *See* erythromycin
EN. *See* enteral nutrition
enalapril, 33, 491*t*, 492, 546*t*, 548, 584*t*
enalaprilat, 33, 492, 553*t*
Enbrel. *See* etanercept
encephalitis, 910
endocannabinoids, 427
Endocet, 378
endocrine system
age-related changes, 118, 119*t*
functions of, 1091
hormone secretions and, 1091, 1092*f*, 1094*t. See also* HORMONE(S)
endometrial carcinoma, 1171
Endometrin. *See* progesterone
endometriosis, 1171, 1183
endorphins, 210*t*, 211, 370
endotoxins, 775
end-stage renal disease (ESRD), 504
Enduron. *See* methyclothiazide
energy drinks, 999*t*
enflurane, 403*t*, 404, 425*t*
enfuvirtide, 932*t*, 939
Engerix-B. *See* hepatitis B vaccine
Enjuvia. *See* conjugated estrogens
enkephalins, 210*t*, 211, 370
Enlon. *See* edrophonium
enoxacin, 826
enoxaparin, 571, 618*t*, 620
ENS (enteric nervous system), 1002
entacapone, 290, 290*t*, 293
Entamoeba histolytica, 885*t*, 890, 891*f*
entecavir, 917*t*, 918, 919–920
enteral nutrition (EN), 1063–1069
administration of, 1063–1064
complications of, 1065–1068, 1066–1067*t*
drug administration guidelines with, 1068*t*
food and drug interactions with, 1068–1069, 1069*t*
formulations of, 1064–1065
Nursing Practice Applications, 1073–1075*t*
enteral route of administration, 27–29
Entereg. *See* alvimopan
enteric nervous system (ENS), 1002
enteric-coated tablets, 28, 1016
enterobiasis, 897
Enterobius vermicularis, 897

enterococci, vancomycin-resistant, 782
Enterococcus faecium, 782
enteroendocrine cells, 998
enterohepatic circulation, 463
enterohepatic recirculation, 36, 36*f*, 1001
Entocort/Entocort-EC. *See* budesonide
ENTRY INHIBITORS, 938–939
enfuvirtide, 932*t*, 939
maraviroc, 932*t*, 939
Entyvio. *See* vedolizumab
enzalutamide, 976*t*, 979
enzyme induction, 34
enzyme inhibition, 34
enzymes, in digestion, 1002, 1002*t*
EPA (eicosapentaenoic acid), 467
ephedra, 82*t*, 84, 182
ephedrine, 178, 179, 181*t*, 183
EPIDERMAL GROWTH FACTOR RECEPTOR (EGFR) INHIBITORS, 988
cetuximab, 987*t*, 988
trastuzumab, 987*t*, 988
epidermis, 1262, 1262*f*, 1263
Epidermophyton, 876
Epiduo, 1269
epidural anesthesia, 396*t*, 404, 405*f*
epilepsy, 310, 311, 323*t. See also* seizures
epinastine, 1294, 1295*t*
epinephrine
adrenal secretion of, 146, 1152
adverse effects, 182
in anesthesia, 404–405, 408
chemical structure of, 179, 180*f*
classification of, 6
clinical applications and considerations, 181–182, 186
for glaucoma, 1289–1290
for heart failure, 587*t*, 589
history of, 144*t*, 179
mechanism of action, 178, 182
nursing responsibilities, 182
routes and dosages, 181*t*
EpiPen⁻, 183*t*
epirubicin, 56*t*, 57, 972*t*, 974
Epivir. *See* lamivudine
eplerenone
adverse effects, 513
chemical structure of, 496
clinical applications, 513
mechanism of action, 495, 511–512
routes and dosages, 494*t*, 511*t*, 584*t*
epoetin alfa, 643, 644–646, 645*t*, 653*t*, 957, 991
Epogen. *See* epoetin alfa
eprosartan, 494*t*, 495, 546*t*, 548
EPS (extrapyramidal symptoms), 214, 269–270, 270*t*, 288
Epstein-Barr virus (EBV), 910
eptifibatide, 626*t*, 630
Epzicom, 934
Equal⁻. *See* aspartame
Equalactin. *See* calcium polycarbophil
Equanil. *See* meprobamate
equianalgesic doses, 374*t*, 376
Eraxis. *See* anidulafungin
Erbitux. *See* cetuximab
erectile dysfunction (ED), 1214, 1216–1219, 1217*t*
Ergamisol. *See* levamisole
ergocalciferol, 1238–1239, 1238*t*
Ergostat. *See* ergotamine
ergosterol, 868
ERGOT ALKALOIDS, 99*t*, 291, 387
dihydroergotamine, 387, 387*t*
ergotamine, 98*t*, 360, 387, 387*t*
methylergonovine, 1176–1177, 1177*t*, 1179

ergotamine, 98*t*, 360, 387, 387*t*
eribulin, 980*t*
Erivedge. *See* vismodegib
erlotinib, 987*t*, 988
Errin. *See* norethindrone
errors. *See* medication error(s)
ertapenem, 797, 797*t*, 798
eruptive psoriasis, 1275*t*
EryC. *See* erythromycin
Eryderm. *See* erythromycin
EryPed. *See* erythromycin
erythema, 1263
erythroblastosis fetalis (EF), 722
Erythrocin. *See* erythromycin
erythrocytes, 441, 443*t*, 643
erythrocytic stage, of malaria, 886
erythromycin
    adverse effects, 56*t*, 811
    clinical applications, 810, 1264, 1269
    history of, 809
    mechanism of action, 810
    Nursing Responsibilities, 811
    routes and dosages, 112*t*, 810*t*
ERYTHROPOIETIC GROWTH FACTORS, 441, 643–646
    darbepoetin alfa, 643, 645*t*, 646
    epoetin alfa, 643, 644–646, 645*t*, 653*t*, 957, 991
    mechanism of action, 643
    Nursing Practice Application, 647–648*t*
Erythroxylum coca, 405
Escherichia coli, 777*t*, 780, 781*t*, 835, 836
escitalopram, 231*t*, 245*t*, 250
Eskalith/Eskalith CR. *See* lithium carbonate
eslicarbazepine, 318*t*, 324
esmolol, 198*t*, 202, 553*t*, 603*t*, 606–607
esomeprazole, 1011*t*, 1013
esophageal cancer, 950
ESRD (end-stage renal disease), 504
estazolam, 225–226*t*, 228
ester-type local anesthesia, 405, 406*t*, 408–409
Estinyl. *See* ethinyl estradiol
Estrace. *See* estradiol
Estraderm. *See* estradiol
estradiol, 1167, 1170*t*
estradiol and norethindrone, 1170*t*, 1194–1195, 1269
estradiol and norgestimate, 1170*t*
estradiol valerate, 1170*t*
estramustine, 964*t*, 967
ESTROGEN(s)
    adverse effects, 1167
    breast-feeding and, 98*t*
    drugs in class
        conjugated estrogens, 1168–1171, 1170*t*, 1174
        estradiol, 1167, 1170*t*
        estradiol and norethindrone, 1170*t*, 1194–1195, 1269
        estradiol and norgestimate, 1170*t*
        estradiol valerate, 1170*t*
        ethinyl estradiol, 976*t*, 1193*t*, 1268*t*
        progestins. *See* PROGESTINS
    Nursing Practice Applications, 1172–1173*t*
    in oral contraceptives, 1190
    therapeutic effects and uses, 1167–1168
    types of, 1168, 1170*t*
estrogen receptor antagonists. *See* SELECTIVE
         ESTROGEN RECEPTOR MODULATORS
eszopiclone, 225*t*, 230
etanercept
    adverse effects, 701
    clinical applications, 701, 1249, 1250, 1277
    routes and dosages, 696*t*, 1248*t*, 1276*t*
ethacrynic acid, 508*t*, 509, 547
ethambutol, 616*t*, 852, 853*t*, 854, 856, 863
ethanol, 56*t*, 200, 223, 622*t*, 1308*t*. *See also* alcohol

ethchlorvynol, 228
ethinyl estradiol, 976*t*, 1193*t*, 1268*t*
ethinyl estradiol with norethindrone acetate. *See*
    estradiol and norethindrone
ethinyl valerate, 1193*t*
ethionamide, 853*t*, 858
ethnicity, influence on pharmacotherapy, 127–128.
        See also Treating the Diverse Patient; *specific*
        ethnic groups
ethosuximide, 98*t*, 313*t*, 316, 318*t*, 325
Ethrane. *See* enflurane
ethylene glycol, 1308*t*
ethynodiol diacetate, 1193*t*
etidocaine, 410
etidronate disodium, 62*t*, 1239–1240*t*, 1241
etodolac, 680–681*t*
etomidate, 397*t*, 399, 400
etoposide, 55*t*, 823, 980, 980*t*, 983
etravirine, 932*t*, 936
eucalyptus, 233
Eulexin. *See* flutamide
euphoria, 351
Eurax. *See* crotamiton
eustachian tubes, 1295
Evacet. *See* doxorubicin liposomal
evening primrose, 81*t*
everolimus, 696*t*, 699, 988
Evidence-Based Practice
    acute otitis media vs. otitis media with
        effusion, 108*t*
    asthma management, 736*t*
    bipolar disorder in pediatric patients, 258*t*
    calcium channel blockers and heart failure, 481*t*
    cerebral palsy, 337*t*
    diabetes and heart failure, 582*t*
    directly observed therapy and multidrug-
        resistant tuberculosis, 854*t*
    diuretic use as risk for falls in geriatric
        patients, 507*t*
    fever in pediatric patients, 682*t*
    malignant hyperthermia, 401*t*
    neurodegeneration prevention in Parkinson's
        disease, 293*t*
    neutropenic patient exposure to fungal
        pathogens, 869*t*
    nitroglycerin and chest pain, 571*t*
    opioids for pain management, 368*t*
    outcome differences in osteoporosis and low
        bone density treatment, 1243*t*
    seizures in geriatric patients, 314*t*
    traveler's diarrhea, 807*t*
    urinary tract infection in geriatric patients, 835*t*
    weight gain in children using atypical
        antipsychotics, 278*t*
Evista. *See* raloxifene
Evithrom. *See* thrombin, topical
Evoclin. *See* clindamycin
Evoxac. *See* cevimeline
Evzio. *See* naloxone
Exalgo. *See* hydromorphone
excitation-contraction coupling, 169
exclusivity period, 7
excretion
    defined, 35
    drug interactions and, 59*f*, 60
    in geriatric patients, 120
    methods of, 35–36
    in pediatric patients, 106–107
    during pregnancy, 94
Exelderm. *See* sulconazole
Exelon. *See* rivastigmine
exemestane, 976*t*, 978
exenatide, 293*t*, 1122*t*, 1131

exercise
    asthma caused by, 733
    fluid balance during, 530*t*
    weight management and, 1081
exfoliative dermatitis, 1275*t*
Exforge/Exforge HCT, 479, 495, 546*t*
Ex-Lax. *See* senna
exophthalmos, 1142, 1144
exotoxins, 775
Exparel. *See* bupivacaine
EXPECTORANTS, 766*t*, 767
Extavia. *See* INTERFERON(s), IFN beta-1b
extended release formulations, 28, 39
extended-spectrum penicillins, 792–793
external otitis, 1295
extracellular fluid (ECF) compartment, 522, 522*f*
extrapyramidal symptoms (EPS), 214, 269–270,
    270*t*, 288
extravasation, 180, 183, 184, 342
extrinsic pathway, in coagulation, 443, 444*f*
eyes
    anatomy of, 1284–1285, 1284–1285*f*
    complementary and alternative therapies
        for, 1293*t*
    pharmacotherapy
        anticholinergics, 168, 183
        for examinations, 1292, 1294
        for glaucoma. *See* glaucoma
        for irritation and redness, 1294, 1295*t*
        routes and dosages of, 1293*t*
    as route of administration, 29
ezetimibe, 461*t*, 467
ezogabine, 319*t*, 327

F

facilitated diffusion, 27
Factive. *See* gemifloxacin
factor VIII, 637
factor IX, 637
factor X, 637
factor XI deficiency, 638
famciclovir, 910, 911*t*, 912
famotidine, 411, 1014*t*, 1015
Famvir. *See* famciclovir
Fanapt. *See* iloperidone
Fansidar, 839, 840, 889
Fareston. *See* toremifene
Farxiga. *See* dapagliflozin
Fasciola hepatica, 900
Faslodex. *See* fulvestrant
Fastin. *See* phentermine
fasting plasma glucose (FPG) tests, 1114
fat substitutes, 1085–1086
fatigue, antineoplastic agents and, 958
fat-soluble vitamins, 1048, 1049*t*, 1051–1053. *See also*
        specific vitamins
FazaClo. *See* clozapine
FDA. *See* Food and Drug Administration
FDCA (Food, Drug, and Cosmetic Act of 1938), 14, 84
febrile seizures, 312, 313*t*, 314–315
febuxostat, 1254*t*, 1256
fecal excretion, 36
feeding tubes, 1064, 1068. *See also* enteral nutrition
felbamate, 313*t*, 317, 319*t*, 327
Felbatol. *See* felbamate
Feldene. *See* piroxicam
felodipine
    drug interactions, 62
    enalapril and, 546*t*
    for hypertension, 477*t*, 479, 548
    plasma half-life, 38
    routes and dosages, 478*t*

female infertility, 1181–1186
    causes of, 1181, 1181t
    pharmacotherapy for, 1181–1186, 1182t, 1184t
female reproductive system, regulation of, 1167, 1168–1169f
females. See gender differences; pregnancy
Femara. See letrozole
Femstat. See butoconazole
fenamates, 682
fenfluramine/phentermine, 1082
fenofibrate, 461t, 466–467
fenofibric acid, 461t, 466–467
fenoldopam, 553t
fenoprofen, 680–681t
Fen-Phen. See fenfluramine/phentermine
fentanyl, 105t, 374t, 377, 396–398, 397t
Fentora. See fentanyl
fenugreek, 99t
Feosol. See ferrous sulfate
Feosol-caps. See carbonyl iron
Feostat. See ferrous fumarate
Feraheme. See ferumoxytol
Fergon. See ferrous gluconate
Ferralet. See ferrous gluconate
ferric gluconate, 656
ferritin, 654
Ferrlecit. See ferric gluconate
Ferronyl. See carbonyl iron
ferrous fumarate, 653t, 656, 656t
ferrous gluconate, 653t, 656, 656t
ferrous sulfate, 112t, 653t, 655–656, 656t
ferumoxytol, 653t, 656
fesoterodine, 168
fetal alcohol syndrome, 425
fetal period, 97
fetal tissue transplantation, 288, 288t
fetal–placental barrier, 32
fetus, 94, 96–97. See also pregnancy
fever
    as body defense, 667
    Nursing Practice Applications, 685–686t
    pathophysiology of, 673
    in patients on immunosuppressants, 694t
    in pediatric patients, 682t
feverfew, 86t, 622t
fexofenadine, 756t, 758
FFP (fresh frozen plasma), 524t, 525, 637
fiber, in enteral nutrition, 1065
FiberCon. See calcium polycarbophil
FIBRIC ACID AGENTS, 460f, 465–467
    adverse effects, 466
    drug interactions, 466
    drugs in class
        fenofibrate, 461t, 466–467
        fenofibric acid, 461t, 466–467
        gemfibrozil, 461t, 466
    Nursing Practice Application, 469t
Fibricor. See fenofibric acid
fibrin, 444
fibrinogen, 442, 444
fibrinolysis, 631, 631f
fibrinolytics. See THROMBOLYTICS
fidaxomicin, 809, 810t, 811–812
fight-or-flight response, 138, 178, 220
filgrastim, 645t, 646, 648, 694, 957, 991
filtrate, 502, 503
Finacea. See azelaic acid
finasteride, 1215t, 1221–1222, 1221t, 1279, 1280
fingolimod, 302–303, 302t
Firmagon. See degarelix
first-dose phenomenon, 195, 549
FIRST-GENERATION ANTIPSYCHOTICS
    adverse effects, 271, 273

for Alzheimer's disease, 297
    nonphenothiazines. See nonphenothiazines
    phenothiazines. See PHENOTHIAZINES
first-pass effect, 28, 34–35, 34f, 1000–1001
fish oil. See omega-3 fatty acids
5-hydroxytryptamine (5-HT). See serotonin
5-FU. See fluorouracil
FLACC scale for pain assessment, 370t
Flagyl. See metronidazole
flaxseed, 81t, 85, 86t, 87, 1026
flecainide, 603t, 606
Fleet Phospho-Soda, 1025t
Flexeril. See cyclobenzaprine
Flomax. See tamsulosin
Flonase. See fluticasone
Flovent. See fluticasone
Floxin. See ofloxacin
Floxin Otic. See ofloxacin
floxuridine, 969t, 971
flu. See influenza
fluconazole
    adverse effects, 616t, 872–873
    breast-feeding and, 98t
    clinical applications, 873, 874, 875–877, 1265, 1274
    mechanism of action, 873
    Nursing Responsibilities, 873
    routes and dosages, 112t, 870t, 875t
flucytosine, 868, 869–870, 870t, 872
Fludara. See fludarabine
fludarabine, 969t, 971
fludrocortisone, 1162
fluid balance
    during exercise, 530t
    Nursing Practice Applications for, 536–537t
    principles of, 522–523, 522f
fluid deficit disorders, 523
fluid excess disorders, 523
FLUID REPLACEMENT AGENTS
    blood products, 523–525, 524t
    colloids, 527, 527t
    crystalloids, 525–527, 526t
    for dehydration, 523, 524t
Flumadine. See rimantadine
flumazenil, 226, 321, 1308t
flunisolide, 741t, 742
flunitrazepam, 421
fluocinolone acetonide, 1273t
fluocinonide, 1273t
fluorescein sodium, 1294
fluoride, 1057–1058, 1057t
5-fluorocytosine. See flucytosine
FLUOROQUINOLONES, 823–827
    adverse effects, 56t, 58, 824–825, 825t
    clinical applications, 823–824, 835–836, 858–859, 1018
    drug interactions, 62t, 1069
    drugs in class
        besifloxacin, 823t, 826
        cinoxacin, 826
        ciprofloxacin. See ciprofloxacin
        gatifloxacin, 823t, 824, 826
        gemifloxacin, 823t, 826
        levofloxacin, 823t, 826, 826t, 835, 863
        moxifloxacin, 823t, 824, 826
        nalidixic acid, 622t, 823, 823t, 838t, 842
        norfloxacin, 823t, 826, 835
        ofloxacin, 823t, 826–827, 835, 853t, 858–859
    generations of, 823, 824t
    mechanism of action, 778, 823
    Nursing Practice Applications, 828–829t
    pregnancy category, 95t

resistance to, 825
    routes and dosages, 823t
fluorouracil, 95t, 822–823, 868, 954, 969t, 971
Fluothane. See halothane
fluoxetine
    adverse effects, 249–250
    for anxiety, 232, 297
    for cataplexy, 358
    for depression, 248–250
    drug interactions, 425t
    indications for, 231t
    labeling changes, 105t
    mechanism of action, 249
    for migraine prophylaxis, 389
    nursing responsibilities, 250
    routes and dosages, 245t
fluoxymesterone, 976t, 1210t, 1212
fluphenazine, 271, 271t, 273
fluphenazine decanoate, 269
flurandrenolide, 1273t
flurazepam, 225–226t, 228
flurbiprofen, 680–681t
Fluress. See fluorescein sodium
flushing effects, of niacin, 465
flutamide, 976t, 979
fluticasone, 105t, 112t, 741t, 742, 759t, 762
fluticasone propionate, 1273t
fluvastatin, 459, 461t, 462
fluvoxamine, 230, 231t, 232, 250
focal (partial) seizures, 313t, 314
Focalin/Focalin XR. See dexmethylphenidate
folate. See folic acid
Foley catheters, 956
folic acid (folate; vitamin B$_9$), 95, 657–658, 968
    clinical applications, 1055
    functions of, 1049t
    metabolism, drug inhibition of, 837, 838f
    pregnancy category, 95t
    routes and dosages, 653t, 1050t
folic acid analogs, 968–969
    methotrexate. See methotrexate
    pemetrexed, 968, 969t, 972
    pralatrexate, 968, 969t, 972
    pyrimethamine, 838t, 839, 892t, 894, 895–896, 968
    trimethoprim, 98t, 616t, 841, 968
    trimetrexate, 968
folic acid deficiency, 311, 657–658
folinic acid. See leucovorin
follicle-stimulating hormone (FSH), 975, 1094t, 1167, 1193, 1209
follicular cells, 1138
folliculitis, 1264
Follistim. See follitropin beta
follitropin alfa, 1182t
follitropin beta, 1182t
follitropins, 1185
Folotyn. See pralatrexate
fomepizole, 1308t
fondaparinux, 618t, 620
Food, Drug, and Cosmetic Act of 1938 (FDCA), 14, 84
Food and Drug Administration (FDA)
    adverse event monitoring, 18, 54
    on antibacterial additives, 790t
    drug approval process, 17–19, 17f
    exclusivity period granted by, 7
    on long-acting beta agonists, 735
    medication error prevention and reporting, 69, 70–71
    "Orange Book," 5, 7
    on pregnancy risk categories, 56, 95–96, 95–96t
    role of, 16

Food and Drug Administration (FDA) (*continued*)
structural organization of, 16–17, 16*f*
on supplement safety, 1049–1050
Food and Drug Administration Modernization
Act of 1997, 14, 104–105
food–drug interactions, 31, 32, 59, 61–62, 62*t*
foot ulcers, 1116
Foradil. *See* formoterol
Forane. *See* isoflurane
forced alkaline diuresis, 1310
formoterol, 186, 187, 737*t*, 738
formularies, 15
Fortamet. *See* metformin
Fortaz. *See* ceftazidime
Forteo. *See* teriparatide
Fortesta, 1211
Fortical. *See* calcitonin-salmon
Fosamax. *See* alendronate
fosamprenavir, 932*t*, 938
foscarnet, 504*t*, 911*t*, 912
Foscavir. *See* foscarnet
fosfomycin, 797*t*, 799, 836, 838*t*, 842
fosinopril, 491*t*, 492, 548, 584*t*
fosphenytoin, 318*t*, 323
fospropofol, 397*t*, 399, 400
Fostex. *See* benzoyl peroxide
FPG (fasting plasma glucose) tests, 1114
Fragmin. *See* dalteparin
Francisella tularensis, 824, 1306
frequency distribution curves, 43, 43*f*
fresh frozen plasma (FFP), 524*t*, 525, 637
Frova. *See* frovatriptan
frovatriptan, 387*t*, 388
FSH (follicle-stimulating hormone), 975, 1167,
1193, 1209
FUDR. *See* floxuridine
fulvestrant, 976*t*, 978
Fulvicin. *See* griseofulvin
fungal infections, 866–883. *See also* specific infections
characteristics of, 867
classification of, 868
cutaneous and subcutaneous, 868
in HIV/AIDS patients, 869
neutropenia and, 869*t*
pathogens involved in, 867, 867*t*
pharmacotherapy. *See* ANTIFUNGALS
superficial, 868, 872–878, 875*t*
systemic, 868, 869–874, 870*t*
fungi, defined, 867
Fungi-Nail. *See* undecylenic acid
Fungizone. *See* amphotericin B deoxycholate
Furadantin. *See* nitrofurantoin
furanocoumarins, 62
furazolidone, 425*t*, 893
furosemide
adverse effects, 56*t*, 508
breast-feeding and, 98*t*
mechanism of action, 508
Nursing Responsibilities, 509
routes and dosages, 508*t*
therapeutic effects and uses, 508, 531, 547,
584*t*, 585, 1106
Furoxone. *See* furazolidone
furuncles (boils), 1264
Fusilev. *See* levoleucovorin
Fuzeon. *See* enfuvirtide

G

GABA. *See* gamma aminobutyric acid
gabapentin
adverse effects, 326
for bipolar disorder, 260

drug interactions, 326
mechanism of action, 316, 326
for migraine prophylaxis, 389*t*
for muscle spasms, 303
for neuropathic pain, 383, 384
nursing responsibilities, 326
for seizures, 313–314*t*, 319*t*, 326
Gabitril. *See* tiagabine
GAD (generalized anxiety disorder), 218, 224, 227,
228, 230, 231
galactagogues, 99*t*
galantamine, 152*t*, 154, 297*t*, 299–300
galega, 99*t*
Galen, 3
gamma aminobutyric acid (GABA)
antiepileptic drugs and, 316–317, 317*f*
effects and clinical applications, 141*t*, 210*t*
mechanism of action, 210
synapses, 211
gamma globulin, 303
gamma hydroxybutyrate (GHB). *See* sodium oxybate
Gammagard. *See* intravenous immune globulin
ganciclovir, 911*t*, 912–913
ganglia, 140
GANGLIONIC BLOCKERS, 165, 168, 169*t*
ganirelix, 1182*t*, 1183, 1185
Gantrisin. *See* sulfisoxazole
Garamycin. *See* gentamicin
Gardasil, 720
garlic, 81, 81*t*, 86*t*, 627*t*
gaseous anesthetics, 401–402
gasping syndrome, 106
gastric bypass surgery, 1082
gastric cancer, 950
gastric ulcers, 379, 1006, 1007, 1013. *See also* peptic
ulcer disease
gastrin, 1005, 1007
Gastrocrom. *See* cromolyn
gastroesophageal reflux disease (GERD)
etiology and pathogenesis, 1008, 1009*f*
gender differences in, 1008*t*
nonpharmacologic management of, 1008
pharmacotherapy, 1008–1018
adverse effects, 1009
antacids, 59, 200, 1015–1017, 1015*t*
goals of, 1008
histamine (H₂) receptor antagonists, 411,
1013–1015, 1014*t*
mechanisms of action, 1008–1009, 1010*f*
miscellaneous agents, 1018
proton pump inhibitors, 724, 1010–1013,
1011–1013*t*
symptoms of, 1008
gastrointestinal anthrax, 1305*t*
gastrointestinal tract
absorption in, 30–31
age-related changes, 118, 119*t*
digestion. *See* digestion and digestive system
drug excretion in, 35–36
ginger's effect on, 1011*t*
lower, 999–1000
physiology of, 997–1000
toxicity to, 824, 957–958
upper, 997–998, 1005
Gastrosed. *See* hyoscyamine
gastrostomy tubes, 27, 29, 1064
gate control theory, 369–370
gatifloxacin, 823*t*, 824, 826
Gavison. *See* magnesium trisilicate and aluminum
hydroxide
Gazyva. *See* obinutuzumab
gefitinib, 987*t*
gemcitabine, 969*t*, 971

gemfibrozil, 461*t*, 466
gemifloxacin, 823*t*, 826
gemtuzumab ozogamicin, 987*t*, 988
Gemzar. *See* gemcitabine
Genabid. *See* papaverine-phentolamine
gender differences
in ADHD, 352, 353*t*
in anxiety disorder incidence, 219*t*
in cancer, 950
in depression, 241*t*
in desmopressin dose for nocturia, 1107*t*
in gastroesophageal reflux disease, 1008*t*
in hemophilia, 637
in pharmacotherapy response, 130–131
in urinary tract infections, 834, 836*t*, 837*t*
general anesthesia, 395–404
defined, 395
inhalation agents, 401–404, 403*t*
intravenous agents, 396–401, 397*t*
Nursing Practice Applications, 407–408*t*
stages of, 395, 396*t*
generalized anxiety disorder (GAD), 218, 224, 227,
228, 230, 231
generalized seizures, 313–314, 313*t*
generic drugs, 7, 8, 8*t*
genetic influences
in ADHD, 352
in Alzheimer's disease, 296
in depression, 241
in hypertension, 542
in metabolism, 35
in narcolepsy, 358
in obesity, 1079
in pharmacotherapy, 128–130, 129–130*f*, 129*t*
in rheumatoid arthritis, 1246*t*
in schizophrenia, 267
genetic polymorphisms, 128–129, 129*f*, 129*t*
Gengraf. *See* cyclosporine
genital herpres, 910*t*
Genotropin. *See* somatropin
gentamicin
adverse effects, 813
clinical applications, 813
drug interactions, 58, 814
in geriatric patients, 119
mechanism of action, 813
nursing responsibilities, 814
for otitis, 1295, 1297
in pediatric patients, 107
pregnancy category, 95*t*
routes and dosages, 112*t*, 812*t*
for skin infections, 1264
Gentran 40. *See* dextran 40
Geodon. *See* ziprasidone
GERD. *See* gastroesophageal reflux disease
geriatric patients, 116–125
adherence and drug misuse among, 120, 120*t*
adverse drug reactions in, 121–122, 122*t*
antibiotic use in, 794*t*
antihistamines in, 757*t*
chemotherapy effects in, 977*t*
comorbidities in, 117, 121–122
defined, 117
dehydration in, 528*t*
dental health and dysrhythmias in, 601*t*
depression in, 242, 242*t*
diuretic therapy in, 507*t*
drug interactions in, 121–122, 122*t*
drug monitoring in, 120*t*
growth of, 117
herbal supplements and, 85*t*, 86
high-risk medications for, 121, 122*t*
inhaler use in, 740*t*

insomnia in, 242*t*
medication costs and, 19*t*
medication errors and, 117*t*
metabolism in, 35
pain management in, 382*t*
pharmacodynamic changes, 120
pharmacokinetic changes in, 118–120
physiologic changes related to aging, 118, 118*f*, 119*t*
polypharmacy and, 117–118
proton pump inhibitors and osteoporosis risk in, 1013*t*
seizures in, 312, 314*t*
sleep-wake patterns in, 220*t*
substance abuse in, 429*t*
thrombolytics in, 632
urinary tract infections in, 835*t*, 837
German measles. *See* rubella
Germanin. *See* suramin
gestational diabetes, 1114
gestational epilepsy, 311
GFR (glomerular filtration rate), 60, 94, 504
GH. *See* growth hormone
GHB (gamma hydroxybutyrate). *See* sodium oxybate
GHIH (growth hormone-inhibiting hormone), 1098
GHRH (growth hormone-releasing hormone), 1098
Giardia lamblia, 885*t*, 890
giardiasis, 885*t*, 890, 890*t*
Giazo. *See* balsalazide
gigantism, 1102–1103
Gilenya. *See* fingolimod
ginger, 81–83*t*, 82, 85, 86*t*, 1011*t*, 1037
gingival hyperplasia, 479*t*, 480
ginkgo biloba
for dementia, 299*t*
drug interactions, 62, 85, 86*t*, 622*t*
primary uses, 81*t*
standardization, 83*t*
standardized formulations of, 83, 83*f*
ginseng, 81*t*, 82, 83*t*, 86*t*, 622*t*
glandular excretion, 36
glatiramer, 301, 302*t*, 303
glaucoma
cultural differences in, 1286*t*
Nursing Practice Applications, 1291–1292*t*
pathophysiology of, 1286
pharmacotherapy
adherence to, 1287
alpha-adrenergic agonists, 1289
beta-adrenergic antagonists, 198, 200, 202, 1289
carbonic anhydrase inhibitors, 1292
cholinergic agonists, 154, 1289
goals of, 1286–1287
muscarinic agonists for, 153
osmotic diuretics, 1292
prostaglandins. *See* PROSTAGLANDIN(S)
routes and dosages, 1288*t*
sympathomimetics, 1289–1290
prevalence of, 1286
types of, 1285*f*, 1286, 1294*t*
Gleevec. *See* imatinib
Gliadel. *See* carmustine
glimepiride, 1122*t*, 1125*t*, 1126
gliomas, 949*t*
glipizide, 1122*t*, 1125*t*, 1126
glomerular filtration rate (GFR), 60, 94, 504
glomerulus, 502, 503*f*
GLP-1 agonists
liraglutide, 1122*t*, 1131
GlucaGen. *See* glucagon
glucagon, 1115–1116, 1308*t*

glucocorticoids, 1153. *See also* CORTICOSTEROIDS
gluconeogenesis, 1112
Glucophage/Glucophage XR. *See* metformin
glucosamine, 87, 87*t*, 1247*t*
glucose-6-phosphate dehydrogenase (G6PD) deficiencies, 49*t*, 784
Glucotrol/Glucotrol XL. *See* glipizide
Glucovance, 1125*t*
Glumetza. *See* metformin
glutamate
Alzheimer's disease and, 297
antiepileptic drugs and, 317
effects and clinical applications, 141*t*, 210*t*
mechanism of action, 210
in pain transmission, 370
synapses, 211
glutamic acid. *See* glutamate
glutethimide, 228
glyburide, 1122*t*, 1125–1126, 1125*t*
glycerin, 513*t*, 514
glycogenolysis, 1112
GLYCOPROTEIN IIB/IIIA RECEPTOR INHIBITORS, 629–630, 629*f*
abciximab, 571, 626*t*, 629–630
eptifibatide, 626*t*, 630
tirofiban, 626*t*, 630
glycopyrrolate, 165*t*, 167
Glynase. *See* glyburide
Glyset. *See* miglitol
GnRH (gonadotropin-releasing hormone), 1097, 1098, 1167
GnRH ANALOGS/AGONISTS. *See* GONADOTROPIN-RELEASING HORMONE (GnRH) ANALOGS/AGONISTS
GnRH ANTAGONISTS. *See* GONADOTROPIN-RELEASING HORMONE (GnRH) ANTAGONISTS
goat's rue, 99*t*
goiters, 1138
gold salts, 1248, 1249
gold sodium thiomalate. *See* gold salts
goldenseal, 86*t*, 674*t*
golimumab, 702*t*, 1033, 1248*t*, 1249, 1250
gonadocorticoids, 1153. *See also* ANDROGEN(S); ESTROGEN(S)
gonadotropin-releasing hormone (GnRH), 1097, 1098, 1167
GONADOTROPIN-RELEASING HORMONE (GnRH) ANALOGS/AGONISTS, 975–976, 978–979, 1097–1098
goserelin, 976*t*, 979, 1182*t*, 1186
histrelin, 976*t*, 979
leuprolide. *See* leuprolide
nafarelin, 95*t*, 1182*t*, 1183, 1186
triptorelin, 976*t*, 979
GONADOTROPIN-RELEASING HORMONE (GnRH) ANTAGONISTS, 1098
cetrorelix, 1182*t*, 1183, 1185
degarelix, 976*t*, 978–979
ganirelix, 1182*t*, 1183, 1185
Gonal-F. *See* follitropin alfa
gonorrhea, 777*t*, 825
Gordochom. *See* undecylenic acid
goserelin, 976*t*, 979, 1182*t*, 1186
gout, 674, 1253–1255, 1254*t*, 1257–1258*t*
graded dose–response curves, 45
grading, of cancer, 952, 952*t*
Gralise. *See* gabapentin
gram negative bacteria, 776, 787
gram positive bacteria, 776, 787
grand mal seizures. *See* tonic–clonic seizures
granisetron, 1037, 1039*t*, 1041
grape seed extract, 81*t*, 543*t*
grapefruit juice, 62, 62*t*, 227, 230, 250, 479

Graves' disease, 1142, 1144, 1144*t*. *See also* hyperthyroidism
gray baby syndrome, 815
green tea, 86*t*, 622*t*, 1083*t*
Grifulvin V. *See* griseofulvin
griseofulvin
adverse effects, 878
clinical applications, 874, 875, 876
interactions with, 425*t*
mechanism of action, 778, 869
routes and dosages, 875*t*
Gris-PEG. *See* griseofulvin
Groshong catheters, 956
growth, defined, 107
growth fraction, 952–954
growth hormone (GH)
deficiencies of, 1098–1101
defined, 1098
factors affecting release of, 1098, 1099*t*
in HIV/AIDS patients, 1101*t*
Nursing Practice Applications, 1104–1105*t*
overproduction of, 1102–1103
physiological and pharmacologic effects of, 1098, 1099*f*
regulation of, 1094*t*
self-administration by pen device, 1100*t*
growth hormone-inhibiting hormone (GHIH), 1098
growth hormone-releasing hormone (GHRH), 1098
guaifenesin, 766*t*, 767
guanethidine, 550
guanfacine, 354*t*, 356, 358
Guttate psoriasis, 1275*t*
Gynazole. *See* butoconazole
gynecomastia, 130, 512, 585
Gyne-Lotrimin. *See* clotrimazole

H

H⁺, K⁺-ATPase, 1010
H₁-RECEPTOR ANTAGONISTS. *See* ANTIHISTAMINES
H₂-RECEPTOR ANTAGONISTS. *See* HISTAMINE (H₂) RECEPTOR ANTAGONISTS
HAART. *See* highly active antiretroviral therapy
Habitrol. *See* nicotine replacement therapy
Haemophilus influenzae, 777*t*, 913
HAIg (hepatitis A immunoglobulin), 916
hair follicles, 1263
hair loss. *See* alopecia
HAIs (health care–associated infections), 780–782, 781*t*, 792, 798*t*
Halaven, 980*t*
halazepam, 225
halcinonide, 1273*t*
Halcion. *See* triazolam
Haldol. *See* haloperidol
Haldol LA. *See* haloperidol decanoate
Hale's lactation risk categories, 99*t*
half-life, 38
hallucinations, 265, 266*t*
hallucinogens, 427–429
halobetasol, 1273*t*
halofantrine, 889
Halog. *See* halcinonide
haloperidol, 119, 271*t*, 273–274, 297, 616*t*, 1215*t*
haloperidol decanoate, 273
Halotestin. *See* fluoxymesterone
halothane, 404
Hansen's disease. *See* leprosy
Harrison Narcotic Act of 1914, 14
Hashimoto's thyroiditis, 1140
hashish, 426
HAV (hepatitis A virus), 717, 915–916, 916*f*
Havrix. *See* hepatitis A vaccine

hawthorn, 196, 200, 496t
hay fever. *See* allergic rhinitis
HBIG. *See* hepatitis B immune globulin
HBIG (hepatitis B immune globulin), 723, 917
HBV. *See* hepatitis B virus
HCG (human chorionic gonadotropin), 1216
HCTZ. *See* hydrochlorothiazide
HCV (hepatitis C virus), 916t, 918, 920, 921
HDL (high-density lipoprotein), 454–455, 456,
        456f, 457t
HDV (hepatitis D virus), 916t, 918
headaches, 45–46, 385. *See also* migraines
health care agencies, medication error prevention
        strategies for, 74–75, 75f
health care failure mode and effect analysis
        (HFMEA), 74
health care–associated infections (HAIs), 780–782,
        781t, 792, 798t
health insurance coverage, cultural differences in, 128t
hearing impairment, 57
heart
        cardiac output, 445t, 447–448, 448f
        organ-specific toxicity and, 56t, 57–58, 824
        structure and functions of, 444–446,
                446–447f
Heart and Estrogen/Progestin Replacement Study
        (HERS), 1174
heart attacks. *See* myocardial infarctions
heart failure (HF), 578–595
        calcium channel blockers and, 481t
        diabetes and, 582t
        drugs that worsen, 581, 581t
        etiology of, 579
        nonpharmacologic therapies, 589t
        Nursing Practice Applications for, 591–592t
        pathophysiology of, 579–581, 580f
        pharmacotherapy, 582–590
                ACE inhibitors, 490–493, 491t, 583–585, 584t
                angiotensin II receptor blockers, 493–495,
                        494t, 584t, 585
                ARBs, 494t
                beta-adrenergic agonists, 587t, 589
                beta-adrenergic antagonists, 198, 584t, 586
                cardiac glycosides, 584t, 587–588
                diuretics, 505, 584t, 585–586
                goals of, 582–583
                mechanisms of action, 583f
                phosphodiesterase III inhibitors, 587t,
                        589–590
                vasodilators, 584t, 586, 587t
        prevalence of, 579t
        stages for treating, 581–582, 582t
        sympathetic nervous system and, 580–581
        symptoms of, 581
        ventricular hypertrophy and, 579–580
heart rate, 448
heartburn. *See* gastroesophageal reflux disease
heavy metals poisoning, 1308t
Hectorol. *See* doxercalciferol
Helicobacter pylori, 950, 1006, 1016t, 1017–1018
Helidac, 892, 1018
helminthic infections, 897–902
        ascariasis, 897, 898f
        enterobiasis, 897
        hookworms, 897–898
        Nursing Practice Applications, 901–902t
        pathogenesis, 897–898
        pharmacotherapy, 899–900, 899t
        tapeworms, 898
helminths, defined, 897
helper (CD4) T cells, 670
Hemabate. *See* carboprost
hemagglutinin, 913

hematogenous infections, 834
hematologic toxicity, 957
hematopoiesis, 643, 644f
HEMATOPOIETIC GROWTH FACTORS, 643–652
        with cancer chemotherapy, 988
        colony-stimulating factors, 646, 648–649,
                649–651t, 957, 991
        erythropoietin, 441, 643–646, 647–648t
        platelet enhancers, 649, 651–652
        routes and dosages of, 645t
hemoglobin A1C (HbA1C), 1114
hemophilia, 616, 617, 636–638, 637t
hemopoiesis (hematopoiesis), 442
hemorrhagic fevers, 1306, 1306t
hemosiderin, 654
hemostasis, 443–444, 443f, 615. *See also* coagulation
HEMOSTATICS, 617, 617t, 635–636
        aminocaproic acid, 635–636, 635t, 637
        desmopressin, 636–637, 638, 1100t, 1105,
                1106, 1107t
        thrombin, topical, 636
        tranexamic acid, 635, 635t, 636, 637
hemothorax, 1071t
hepadnaviruses, 908t
heparin
        adverse effects, 616t, 619
        breast-feeding and, 98t
        chemical structure of, 617–618
        clinical applications, 619
        drug interactions, 86t, 622t
        low-molecular-weight heparins, 618–619, 620
        mechanism of action, 617, 618, 619
        for myocardial infarction, 571
        nursing responsibilities, 620
        routes and dosages, 618t
heparin-induced thrombocytopenia (HIT), 619
hepatic microsomal enzyme system, 33–34, 33t
hepatic portal system, 1000, 1001f
hepatitis A immunoglobulin (HAIg), 916
hepatitis A vaccine, 717, 916
hepatitis A virus (HAV), 713t, 717, 915–916, 916t
hepatitis B immune globulin (HBIG), 721t, 723, 917
hepatitis B vaccine, 712, 716–717, 723, 917
hepatitis B virus (HBV)
        epidemiology, 713t
        immunization for, 712, 716–717, 723, 917
        overview, 916t
        pathophysiology, 715–716
        pharmacotherapy, 918, 919–921
        prevalence of, 918t
        risk factors, 918t
        symptoms of, 917
        transmission, 917
hepatitis C virus (HCV), 916t, 918, 920, 921
hepatitis D virus (HDV), 916t, 918
hepatitis E virus (HEV), 916t, 918
hepatitis viruses, 424, 910, 915–921, 916–917t. *See also*
        specific types
hepatotoxicity, 56t, 57, 60, 85, 825
Hepsera. *See* adefovir dipivoxil
herbal supplements
        adverse effects, 84–85
        drug interactions with, 61–62, 62t, 85–87, 86t
        formulations of, 83, 83t
        geriatric patients and, 85t, 86
        history of, 3, 81–82
        as laxatives, 1026
        for muscle spasms, 336
        for nausea and vomiting, 1037
        popularity of, 82
        regulation, 84–85
        standardization of, 82–84, 83f, 83t
        types of, 81t

herbs, defined, 81
Herceptin. *See* trastuzumab
heroin, 61, 96t, 99t, 384–385, 419
herpes simplex viruses (HSVs), 910–911t, 910–913,
        944t, 1265
herpes zoster. *See* shingles
Herplex. *See* idoxuridine
HERS (Heart and Estrogen/Progestin Replacement
        Study), 1174
Hespan. *See* hetastarch
Hespera. *See* adefovir
hetastarch, 527
Hetlioz. *See* tasimelteon
Hetrazan. *See* diethylcarbamazine
HEV (hepatitis E virus), 916t, 918
Hexa-Betalin. *See* pyridoxine
Hexalen. *See* altretamine
HF. *See* heart failure
HFMEA (health care failure mode and effect
        analysis), 74
HHS (hyperosmolar hyperglycemic state), 1115
high blood pressure. *See* hypertension
high-alert medications, 70
HIGH-CEILING DIURETICS. *See* LOOP DIURETICS
high-density lipoprotein (HDL), 454–455,
        456, 456f, 457t
highly active antiretroviral therapy (HAART),
        931, 935, 936–937, 1101t. *See also*
        ANTIRETROVIRALS
hippurate. *See* methenamine hippurate
Hiprex. *See* methenamine hippurate
hirudotherapy, 623
Hispanic populations
        complementary and alternative medicine use
                among, 128
        diabetes mellitus and, 1113
histamine, 668, 668t
HISTAMINE (H₁) RECEPTOR ANTAGONISTS. *See*
        ANTIHISTAMINES
HISTAMINE (H₂) RECEPTOR ANTAGONISTS, 411,
        1013–1015, 1014t
Histerone. *See* testosterone
histoplasmosis, 867, 867t, 944t
histrelin, 976t, 979
HIT (heparin-induced thrombocytopenia), 619
HIV-AIDS, 926–947
        growth hormone in, 1101t
        hemophilia and, 637t
        opportunistic infections in
                fungal, 869
                M. avium complex, 849, 863
                pharmacotherapy, 944, 944t
                tuberculosis, 849, 852
        pathogenesis of, 927–928, 928f
        pharmacotherapy, 929–944
                antiretrovirals. *See* ANTIRETROVIRALS
                general principles of, 929–931
                Nursing Practice Applications, 940–942t
                prophylaxis, 939, 942–944
        prevalence of, 927t
        prevention strategies, 943t
        replication cycle of, 927–928, 928f
        symptoms of, 928
        transmission of, 927, 943–944
        vaccine development, 711, 939
hives. *See* urticaria
Hivid. *See* zalcitabine
HMG (human menopausal gonadotropin), 1183
HMG-CoA reductase, 458–459
HoFH (homozygous familial hypercholesterolemia), 467
homatropine, 766t, 1293t
homeopathic medicine. *See* Complementary
        and Alternative Therapies

homeostasis, 443*t*, 489, 502
homocysteine, 657*t*
homozygous familial hypercholesterolemia (HoFH), 467
hookworms, 897–898
Horizont. *See* gabapentin
HORMONE(s). *See also specific hormones*
  adverse effects, 55, 55*t*, 56
  as antineoplastic agents, 55–56, 55*t*, 975–979, 980*t*, 1093, 1095
  blood pressure and, 450–451, 451*f*
  breast-feeding and, 98*t*
  for cancer treatment, 975–979, 980*t*
  defined, 1091
  endocrine system secretion of, 1091, 1092*f*, 1094*t*
  hypothalamus secretion of, 1097, 1097*t*
  negative feedback mechanisms and, 1091–1093, 1093*f*
  pharmacotherapy with, 1093, 1094*t*, 1095
  target cells and, 1091, 1093*f*
HORMONE ANTAGONISTS, 55–56, 55*t*, 975–979, 980*t*
  androgen receptor blockers, 976, 979
  aromatase inhibitors, 975, 976*t*, 978
  GnRH analogs. *See* GONADOTROPIN-RELEASING HORMONE (GnRH) ANALOGS/AGONISTS
  selective estrogen receptor modulators, 975, 978, 1175, 1242–1243
hormone replacement therapy (HRT), 1093, 1174–1175
horny goat weed, 81*t*
host flora, 782, 784
HPV (human papillomavirus), 712, 720, 720*t*, 950, 1197
HSVs (herpes simplex viruses), 910–911*t*, 910–913, 1265
HTN. *See* hypertension
HTN-E (hypertensive emergency), 552–553, 553*t*
Humalog. *See* insulin lispro
Humalog Mix 75/25, 1119, 1120*t*
human beta-type natriuretic peptide (hBNP), 586
human chorionic gonadotropin (HCG), 1216
human immunodeficiency virus (HIV). *See* HIV-AIDS
human menopausal gonadotropin (HMG), 1183
human papillomavirus (HPV), 712, 720, 720*t*, 950, 1197
human regular insulin, 1118*t*, 1119
Humatin. *See* paromomycin
Humatrope. *See* somatropin
Humira. *See* adalimumab
humoral immune response, 669–670
Humulin 50/50, 1119, 1120*t*
Humulin 70/30, 1119, 1120*t*
Humulin N. *See* isophane insulin suspension
Humulin R. *See* human regular insulin
hunger, regulation of, 1079–1080
Huntington's disease, 286
Hyalgan. *See* hyaluronate sodium
hyaluronate sodium, 1246
hyaluronidase, 775
Hycamtin. *See* topotecan
Hycodan. *See* hydrocodone
Hycomine Compound, 766*t*
Hycort. *See* hydrocortisone
Hycotuss Expectorant, 766*t*
HYDANTOINS, 322–323
  fosphenytoin, 318*t*, 323
  phenytoin. *See* phenytoin
hydralazine
  adverse effects, 551
  drug interactions, 551
  genetic polymorphisms and actions of, 129

for heart failure, 584*t*, 586
hydrochlorothiazide with, 506, 546*t*
for hypertension, 551, 553*t*
mechanism of action, 551
nursing responsibilities, 551
Hydrastis canadensis, 674*t*
Hydrea. *See* hydroxyurea
hydrochloric acid, 536
hydrochlorothiazide
  adverse effects, 510, 616*t*
  aliskiren with, 546*t*, 548
  amiloride with, 506, 513
  amlodipine with, 495, 546*t*
  benazepril with, 492, 546*t*
  bendroflumethiazide and nadolol with, 546*t*
  bisoprolol with, 202, 546*t*
  breast-feeding and, 98*t*
  candesartan with, 495, 546*t*
  captopril with, 492, 546*t*
  clinical applications, 510, 547, 584*t*
  drug interactions, 510–511
  enalapril with, 492, 546*t*
  eprosartan with, 495, 546*t*
  fosinopril with, 492
  hydralazine with, 506, 546*t*
  irbesartan with, 495, 546*t*
  lisinopril with, 491, 546*t*
  losartan with, 494, 546*t*
  mechanism of action, 510
  methyldopa and, 546*t*
  metoprolol with, 202, 546*t*
  moexipril with, 493, 546*t*
  nursing responsibilities, 511
  olmesartan with, 479, 495, 546*t*
  overdose treatment, 511
  propranolol and, 546*t*
  quinapril with, 493, 546*t*
  routes and dosages, 510*t*
  spironolactone with, 506, 546*t*
  telmisartan with, 495, 546*t*
  timolol and, 546*t*
  triamterene with, 506, 513, 546*t*
  valsartan with, 479, 495, 546*t*
hydrocodone, 374*t*, 377, 765, 766*t*
hydrocortisone
  acetic acid and, 1297*t*
  adverse effects, 1158
  breast-feeding and, 98*t*
  ciprofloxacin with, 825, 1297*t*
  clinical applications, 1095, 1145, 1156, 1157, 1273*t*
  mechanism of action, 1158
  Nursing Responsibilities, 1158
  routes and dosages, 1156*t*
hydrocortisone valerate, 1273*t*
hydrogen cyanide, 1307*t*
hydromorphone, 374*t*, 375, 377, 1041
hydrothorax, 1071*t*
hydroxychloroquine, 888*t*, 889, 1248, 1248*t*, 1249
hydroxyurea, 990*t*, 991
hydroxyzine, 228–229, 1039*t*
Hygroton. *See* chlorthalidone
Hyoscine. *See* scopolamine
hyoscyamine, 165*t*, 167, 1033*t*, 1036
Hyperab. *See* rabies immune globulin
hyperaldosteronism, 512, 1162
hyperalimentation. *See* parenteral nutrition
hypercalcemia, 1230, 1232
hypercholesterolemia, 455, 465*t*, 467. *See also* dyslipidemia
hyperemesis gravidarum, 1037
hyperglycemia, 1067*t*, 1071*t*, 1132*t*
Hypericum perforatum. *See* St. John's wort

hyperkalemia, 488*t*, 491, 505*t*, 530, 531, 1067*t*
hyperlipidemia, 455, 456. *See also* dyslipidemia
hypermagnesemia, 532
hypernatremia, 529
hyperosmolar hyperglycemic state (HHS), 1115
hyperphosphatemia, 505*t*, 1067*t*
hypersensitivity reactions, 824
Hyperstat IV. *See* diazoxide
hypertension (HTN), 541–558
  consequences of, 542–543, 542*t*, 1215
  defined, 543
  eclampsia and preeclampsia, 311
  etiology and pathogenesis of, 542–543
  genetic influences in, 542
  guidelines for treatment of, 543–544, 544*t*
  lifestyle modifications for, 195*t*
  nonpharmacologic management of, 543
  in pediatric patients, 480*t*
  pharmacotherapy. *See* ANTIHYPERTENSIVES
hypertensive emergency (HTN-E), 552–553, 553*t*
hypertensive urgency, 552
hyperthyroidism, 1142, 1144–1146, 1145*t*
hypertonia. *See* muscle spasticity
hypertonic solutions, 523, 525–526
hypertrichosis, 552
hypertriglyceridemia, 455, 465–466, 1072. *See also* dyslipidemia
hyperuricemia, 507, 959, 1253, 1255–1256. *See also* gout
hypervitaminosis, 1049
hypervolemia, 505*t*
hypnagogic hallucinations, 222, 358
hypnotics, defined, 224. *See also* BARBITURATES; BENZODIAZEPINES; NONBENZODIAZEPINE ANXIOLYTICS
hypoaldosteronism, 1162
hypocalcemia, 505*t*, 1232–1233
hypoglycemia, 1067*t*, 1071*t*, 1115
hypogonadism, 1210–1212
hypokalemia, 507, 511, 531, 1067*t*
hypomagnesemia, 532, 1067*t*
hypomania, 240, 257
hyponatremia, 529–530, 1067*t*
hypoperfusion, 504
hypophosphatemia, 1067*t*
hypotension. *See* orthostatic hypotension
hypothalamus
  adrenergic synapses in, 211
  functions of, 146, 213, 220, 1097–1098
  hormones secreted by, 1097, 1097*t*, 1167
  pharmacotherapy for, 1100*t*
  thirst and, 523
hypothyroidism, 241, 1140–1142, 1141*t*
hypotonic solutions, 523, 526
Hytakerol. *See* dihydrotachysterol
Hytrin. *See* terazosin
Hyzaar, 494, 546*t*

I

[131]I. *See* radioactive iodide
ibandronate, 1239–1240*t*, 1241
IBD. *See* inflammatory bowel disease
ibritumomab, 987*t*
ibrutinib, 987*t*
IBS. *See* irritable bowel syndrome
ibuprofen
  adverse effects, 616*t*, 680–681
  breast-feeding and, 98*t*
  in combination drugs, 7*t*
  cost considerations, 679
  drug interactions, 425*t*, 681
  history of, 679

ibuprofen (*continued*)
mechanism of action, 679
nursing responsibilities, 681
overdose treatment, 681
for pain management, 379
pharmacokinetics, 679
potency and efficacy of, 45–46
pregnancy category, 95*t*
routes and dosages, 112*t*, 680–681*t*
therapeutic effects and uses, 679, 682*t*
ibuprofen-like drugs, 679–682, 680–681*t*
ibutilide, 603*t*, 608
IC (intermittent claudication), 630–631
ICDs (implantable cardioverter defibrillators), 601
ICF (intracellular fluid) compartment, 522, 522*f*
icosapent, 461*t*, 467
ICSH (interstitial cell-stimulating hormone), 975, 1209
Icy Hot, 1326
Idamycin. *See* idarubicin
idarubicin, 56*t*, 57, 972, 972*t*, 974
ideal drugs, 5
idiopathic parkinsonism, 287
idiosyncratic responses, 48, 55
idoxuridine, 910, 911*t*
Ifex. *See* ifosfamide
IFNs. *See* INTERFERON(S)
ifosfamide, 964*t*, 967
IGF (insulin-like growth factor), 1098
IGRA (interferon gamma release assay), 851
ileum, 999–1000
illusions, 266*t*
iloperidone, 275*t*, 276
ILs. *See* INTERLEUKIN(S)
imatinib, 987*t*, 988
Imbruvica. *See* ibrutinib
Imdur. *See* isosorbide mononitrate
imidazoles, 872
imipenem-cilastatin, 797–798, 797*t*
imipramine
for ADHD, 357
adverse effects, 247
for cataplexy, 358
for depression, 246–247
indications for, 231*t*
mechanism of action, 178, 246
for migraine prophylaxis, 389*t*
for neuropathic pain, 383
nursing responsibilities, 247
overdose treatment, 247
routes and dosages, 112*t*, 245*t*
imipramine pamoate, 246
Imitrex. *See* sumatriptan
immune globulins, 524*t*, 525, 721*t*
immune response, 668–671, 1155
immune thrombocytopenia purpura (ITP), 649
immunity
active, 710, 711, 722*f*
defined, 665
passive, 710–711, 721–723, 722*f*
immunization. *See* VACCINE(S)
immunoglobulins, 442, 669, 670*f*
IMMUNOMODULATORS, 689–708
for asthma, 735*t*
immunostimulants, 690–695. *See also*
IMMUNOSTIMULANTS
immunosuppressants, 695–703. *See also*
IMMUNOSUPPRESSANTS
Nursing Practice Applications, 704–705*t*
overview, 301, 690, 690*f*
IMMUNOSTIMULANTS, 690–695
colony-stimulating factors. *See* COLONY-
STIMULATING FACTORS
interferons. *See* INTERFERON(S)

interleukins, 693–695, 988
overview, 690, 690*f*
routes and dosages, 692*t*
vaccines. *See* VACCINE(S)
IMMUNOSUPPRESSANTS, 695–703
adverse effects, 55, 55*t*, 56
antibodies. *See* ANTIBODIES
for autoimmune disorders, 695, 697
breast-feeding and, 98*t*
calcineurin inhibitors. *See* CALCINEURIN
INHIBITORS
corticosteroids. *See* CORTICOSTEROIDS
cytotoxic agents and antimetabolites, 700–702.
See also CYTOTOXIC AGENTS
for dermatitis, 1273
for inflammatory bowel disease, 1033
kinase inhibitors. *See* KINASE INHIBITORS
mechanism of action, 697, 697*f*
for myasthenia gravis, 156
for organ transplantation, 695
overview, 690, 690*f*
in pediatric patients, 698*t*
routes and dosages, 696*t*
immunotherapy, 690
Imodium. *See* loperamide
Imogam Rabies-HT. *See* rabies immune globulin
Impavido. *See* miltefosine
impetigo, 1264
Implanon, 1198–1199
implantable cardioverter defibrillators (ICDs), 601
impotence, 1216. *See also* erectile dysfunction
Imuran. *See* azathioprine
inactivated polio vaccine (IPV), 719
inactivated (killed) vaccines, 711, 711*t*
inamrinone, 587*t*, 589, 590, 616*t*
Incivek. *See* telaprevir
incobotulinumtoxinA, 341*t*, 343, 343*t*
incontinence, 166, 168, 187, 343–344
increased intracranial pressure (ICP), 375
Increlex. *See* mecasermin
INCRETIN ENHANCERS, 1130–1131
DPP-4 inhibitors
linagliptin, 1122*t*, 1125*t*, 1131
saxagliptin, 1122*t*, 1131
sitagliptin, 1122*t*, 1125*t*, 1130
GLP-1 agonists
exenatide, 293*t*, 1122*t*, 1131
liraglutide, 1122*t*, 1131
mechanism of action, 1130
Nursing Practice Application, 1123–1124
incretins, 1130
incruse ellipta, 746
incubation period, 710
IND (Investigational New Drug) applications, 17
indacaterol, 181*t*, 187, 737*t*, 738
indapamide, 509, 510*t*, 511, 547
Inderal/Inderal LA. *See* propranolol
Inderide, 546*t*
Indians. *See* Native Americans and Alaska Natives
indications, 5
indinavir, 86*t*, 616*t*, 932*t*, 938
INDIRECT THROMBIN INHIBITORS, 617–622
heparin. *See* heparin
rivaroxaban, 618*t*, 621, 622
warfarin. *See* warfarin
Indocin/Indocin SR. *See* indomethacin
indole acetic acids, 682
indomethacin, 616*t*, 680–681*t*, 1253
indoor tanning, 1052*t*, 1266*t*
infantile spasms, 313*t*, 315
infants, 107. *See also* pediatric patients
infectious diseases, 775, 775*t*. *See also* anti-infectives;
specific diseases

Infectious Diseases Society of America, 852
Infergen. *See* INTERFERON(s), IFN alfacon-1
infertility
defined, 1181
female. *See* female infertility
male, 1214, 1215–1216
infiltration anesthesia, 404, 405*f*
inflammation
acute, 668, 669*f*, 673
as body defense, 667–668
chemical mediators, 668, 668*t*
chronic, 673
defined, 667, 673
nonpharmacologic therapies, 673, 1154*t*
Nursing Practice Applications, 685–686*t*
pathophysiology of, 673
pharmacotherapy, 673–683, 741*t*. *See also*
NONSTEROIDAL ANTI-INFLAMMATORY DRUGS
inflammatory bowel disease (IBD)
etiology of, 1030
pharmacotherapy, 674, 1032–1035, 1032*f*,
1033*t*, 1159
symptoms of, 1030, 1032
infliximab
clinical applications, 1033, 1249, 1250, 1277
routes and dosages, 702*t*, 1248*t*, 1276*t*
influenza viruses, 713*t*, 717, 913–915, 914*t*
infusion calculations, 1035*t*
ingestion, 997
INH. *See* isoniazid
inhalants, 96*t*, 422*t*, 432
INHALATION ANESTHETICS, 401–404
desflurane, 403, 403*t*, 404
enflurane, 403*t*, 404, 425*t*
halothane, 404
isoflurane, 403–404, 403*t*
nitrous oxide, 141*t*, 401, 402, 403*t*
sevoflurane, 403, 403*t*, 404
inhalation anthrax, 1305*t*
inhalation route, in drug administration, 733–734
inhalers, 733–734, 740*t*
innate (nonspecific) body defenses, 665–668, 667*t*
Innohep. *See* tinzaparin
InnoPran XL. *See* propranolol
Inocor. *See* inamrinone
inoculation, 710
inotropic agents, 185, 448
insomnia
anxiety and, 222–223
causes of, 222, 222*t*
complementary and alternative medicine for,
223, 223*t*
defined, 221–222
in geriatric patients, 242*t*
pharmacological management of, 223–234
antidepressants, 223, 224, 230–232, 231*t*
antihistamines, 757
barbiturates, 224, 232–234, 233*t*
benzodiazepines, 223, 224–228, 225–226*t*
nonbenzodiazepine anxiolytics, 223, 224,
225*t*, 228–230
types of, 221–222
Inspra. *See* eplerenone
Institute for Safe Medication Practice (ISMP), 69,
70, 71
insulin aspart, 1118*t*, 1119–1120
insulin detemir, 1118*t*, 1120
insulin glargine, 1118*t*, 1120
insulin glulisine, 1118*t*, 1120
insulin lispro, 1118*t*, 1120
insulin pumps, 1117–1118, 1118*f*
insulin regular. *See* human regular insulin
insulin resistance, 1113

insulin therapy
  actions and administration, 1118*t*
  adjuncts, 1118–1119
  adverse effects, 1118
  breast-feeding and, 98*t*
  drug interactions, 86*t*, 122
  errors in administration, 1121*t*
  Nursing Practice Applications, 1123–1124*t*
  pregnancy category, 95*t*
  principles of therapy, 1117, 1117*f*
  subcutaneous infusion, 1117, 1118*f*
  types of, 1117, 1118*t*, 1119–1120, 1120*t*
insulin-like growth factor (IGF), 1098
insurance coverage, cultural differences in, 128*t*
Intal. *See* cromolyn
integrase, 927
INTEGRASE INHIBITORS, 932*t*, 939
Integrilin. *See* eptifibatide
INTEGRIN INHIBITORS, 1033
  natalizumab, 302*t*, 303, 702*t*, 1033
  vedolizumab, 1033
integumentary system, anatomy of, 1262–1263, 1262*f*
Intelence. *See* etravirine
interactions. *See* drug interactions
INTERFERON(s) (IFNs)
  as biologic response modifiers, 691, 983
  in body defense, 667
  drugs in class
    IFN alfa-2a, 692
    IFN alfa-2b, 691–692, 692*t*, 917*t*, 920, 983
    IFN alfacon-1, 692, 917*t*, 920
    IFN alfa-n 1, 692
    IFN alfa-n3, 692*t*, 693
    IFN beta-1a, 301, 302*t*, 303, 692*t*, 693
    IFN beta-1b, 301–302, 302*t*, 692*t*, 693
    IFN gamma-1b, 692*t*, 693
    pegIFN alfa-2a, 692*t*, 693, 917*t*, 920–921, 983, 988
    pegIFN alfa-2b, 692*t*, 693, 917*t*, 920–921, 983, 988
  as immunostimulants, 690–693
  pegylation, 691
  in viral infections, 715, 918, 920–921
interferon gamma release assay (IGRA), 851
INTERLEUKIN(s) (ILs), 693–695, 988
interleukin-2. *See* aldesleukin
interleukin-11. *See* oprelvekin
intermenstrual bleeding, 1171
Intermezzo. *See* zolpidem
intermittent claudication (IC), 630–631
intermittent feedings, in enteral nutrition, 1064
intermittent infusions, 30
International Union of Pure and Applied Chemistry (IUPAC), 7
Internet pharmacies, 8
interpatient variability, 43, 43*f*
interpersonal therapy, 243*t*
interstitial cell-stimulating hormone (ICSH), 975, 1209
intra-arterial route of administration, 956
intracellular fluid (ICF) compartment, 522, 522*f*
intracellular parasites, 907
intradermal route of administration, 30
Intralipid, 1070
intramuscular route of administration, 30, 31, 106
INTRANASAL DECONGESTANTS, 185
  oxymetazoline, 185, 763, 764*t*, 1293*t*
  pseudoephedrine. *See* pseudoephedrine
  tetrahydrozoline, 183, 185, 764*t*, 1293*t*
  xylometazoline, 185, 764*t*
intranasal route of administration, 29
intraperitoneal route of administration, 956
intrathecal baclofen (ITB), 336, 337*t*
intrathecal route of administration, 956

intrauterine devices (IUDs), 1199
INTRAVENOUS ANESTHETICS, 396–401
  benzodiazepines, 398–399
    diazepam. *See* diazepam
    midazolam, 225, 226, 226*t*, 397*t*, 398–399, 411
  miscellaneous agents, 399–401
    etomidate, 397*t*, 399, 400
    fospropofol, 397*t*, 399, 400
    ketamine, 96*t*, 397*t*, 399, 400, 429
    methohexital, 233, 397*t*, 399–400
    propofol, 397*t*, 399–400, 425*t*
  opioids, 396–398, 397*t*
    alfentanil, 377, 396, 397*t*, 398
    fentanyl, 105*t*, 374*t*, 377, 396–398, 397*t*
    remifentanil, 377, 396, 397*t*, 398
    sufentanil, 377, 396, 397*t*, 398
intravenous gamma globulin, 303
intravenous immune globulin (IVIG), 721*t*, 723
intravenous route of administration, 26, 30, 956
intravesicular route of administration, 956
intrinsic activity, 47
intrinsic factor, 657
intrinsic pathway, in coagulation, 443, 444*f*
intrinsic sympathomimetic activity (ISA), 197
Intron-A. *See* INTERFERON(s), IFN alfa-2b
Intropin. *See* dopamine
Intuniv. *See* guanfacine
Invanz. *See* ertapenem
invasiveness, 775
Invega/Invega Sustenna. *See* paliperidone
Inversine. *See* mecamylamine
Investigational New Drug (IND) applications, 17
Invirase. *See* saquinavir
Invokana. *See* canagliflozin
iodide, 1057*t*, 1058, 1146
iodism, 1146
iodoquinol, 890, 892*t*, 893
ion trapping, 94, 534, 1310
ionization
  absorption and, 31, 31*f*
  drug transfer across the placenta and, 94
ionizing radiation, 1307–1308
Iopidine. *See* apraclonidine
ipilimumab, 987*t*
iPledge Program, 1271
ipratropium
  adverse effects, 739
  clinical applications, 166, 168, 739, 759*t*, 763
  mechanism of action, 739
  Nursing Responsibilities, 739
  routes and dosages, 165*t*, 737*t*
Iprivask. *See* desirudin
Iquix. *See* levofloxacin
irbesartan, 494*t*, 495, 546*t*, 548
Iressa. *See* gefitinib
irinotecan, 105*t*, 980, 980*t*, 982
iris, 1285
iron
  deficiencies in, 653–657
  functions of, 1057*t*, 1058
  metabolism, 653, 654*f*
  overdose/poisoning, 1308, 1308*t*
  recommended intake, 643*t*, 1057*t*
iron deficiency anemia, 653–657
iron dextran, 653*t*, 656–657
iron poisoning, 654*t*
IRON SALTS, 98*t*, 653–657, 654*f*
  oral
    carbonyl iron, 656, 656*t*
    ferrous fumarate, 653*t*, 656, 656*t*
    ferrous gluconate, 653*t*, 656, 656*t*
    ferrous sulfate, 112*t*, 653*t*, 655–656, 656*t*
    polysaccharide iron complex, 656, 656*t*

  parenteral
    ferric gluconate, 656
    ferumoxytol, 653*t*, 656
    iron dextran, 653*t*, 656–657
    iron sucrose, 653*t*, 656
iron sucrose, 653*t*, 656
irreversible cholinesterase inhibitors, 152
irritable bowel syndrome (IBS)
  nonpharmacologic therapies, 1035
  pharmacotherapy, 166, 167, 1033*t*, 1035–1036
  prevalence of, 1035*t*
  symptoms of, 1035
irritative voiding symptoms, 834
ISA (intrinsic sympathomimetic activity), 197
Isentress. *See* raltegravir
Ismelin. *See* guanethidine
Ismo. *See* isosorbide mononitrate
Ismotic. *See* isosorbide
ISMP (Institute for Safe Medication Practice), 69, 70, 71
Isocaine. *See* mepivacaine
isocarboxazid, 255
isoflurane, 403–404, 403*t*
isonarif, 857
isoniazid
  acetylation of, 855, 856*f*
  adverse effects, 616*t*, 855–856
  breast-feeding and, 98*t*
  clinical applications, 778, 851, 852, 855
  drug interactions, 425*t*, 622*t*
  genetic polymorphisms and actions of, 129
  mechanism of action, 855
  nursing responsibilities, 856
  overdose/poisoning, 859*t*, 1308*t*
  routes and dosages, 853*t*
isophane insulin suspension, 1118*t*, 1120
isoproterenol
  chemical structure of, 179
  clinical applications and considerations, 186–187
  for heart failure, 587*t*, 589
  as overdose treatment, 199, 201, 202
  routes and dosages, 181*t*
Isoptin/Isoptin SR. *See* verapamil
Isopto Atropine. *See* atropine
Isopto Carbachol. *See* carbachol
Isopto Carpine. *See* pilocarpine
Isordil. *See* isosorbide dinitrate
isosorbide, 1288*t*, 1292
isosorbide dinitrate, 425*t*, 564, 566, 568*t*, 584*t*, 586
isosorbide mononitrate, 566, 568*t*
isotonic solutions, 522–523, 525
isotretinoin
  adverse effects, 95, 616*t*, 1270–1271
  clinical applications, 1268*t*, 1269, 1270
  pregnancy category rating, 95*t*
  prescribing requirements, 56
isozymes, 33–34, 33*t*
isradipine, 477–478*t*, 479, 548
Istalol. *See* timolol
Istodax. *See* romidepsin
Isuprel. *See* isoproterenol
ITB (intrathecal baclofen), 336, 337*t*
ITP (immune thrombocytopenia purpura), 649
itraconazole
  adverse effects, 616*t*
  clinical applications, 872–873, 874, 875–876, 877
  routes and dosages, 870*t*, 875*t*
IUDs (intrauterine devices), 1199
IUPAC (International Union of Pure and Applied Chemistry), 7
ivermectin, 898, 899*t*, 900, 1265, 1266

IVIG (intravenous immune globulin), 723
ixabepilone, 990t, 991
Ixempra. See ixabepilone

J

Janumet, 1125t
Januvia. See sitagliptin
Jehovah's Witnesses, 128t
jejunostomy tubes, 1064
jejunum, 999
Jenner, Edward, 710
Jentadueto, 1125t, 1131
jet lag, 221
Jevtana. See cabazitaxel
JG (juxtaglomerular) cells, 487–488, 488f
jock itch. See tinea cruris
Joint Commission, 67, 73, 1304
joint disorders, 1228–1260
    arthritis. See osteoarthritis; rheumatoid
        arthritis
    gout, 674, 1253–1255, 1254t, 1257–1258t
    hyperuricemia, 507, 959, 1253, 1255–1256
    pathophysiology, 1245f
Jolivette. See norethindrone
Juvisync, 1125t, 1130
juxtaglomerular (JG) cells, 487–488, 488f
Juxtapid. See lomitapide

K

Kadcycla. See ado-trastuzumab
Kadian. See morphine sulfate
Kalcinate. See calcium gluconate
Kaletra. See lopinavir with ritonavir
kanamycin, 812t, 814, 853t, 857, 1072
Kantrex. See kanamycin
Kaon CL. See potassium chloride
Kaopectate. See bismuth subsalicylate
Kaposi's sarcoma, 951
kappa receptors, 372, 373f, 373t
Kapvay. See clonidine
kava, 85, 86t, 223, 227, 229, 233
Kavatrol. See kava
Kayexalate. See polystyrene sulfonate
Kazano, 1125t, 1131
KCl. See potassium chloride
K-Dur 20. See potassium chloride
Kefauver-Harris Amendment of 1962, 14
Keflex. See cephalexin
Kefzol. See cefazolin
Kenalog. See triamcinolone
Keppra. See levetiracetam
keratin, 1263
keratitis, 1294
keratolytic effects, 1269
Kerlone. See betaxolol
Kerydin. See tavaborole
Ketalar. See ketamine
ketamine, 96t, 397t, 399, 400, 429
Ketek. See telithromycin
ketoconazole
    clinical applications, 872, 873–874, 1163, 1274
    interactions with, 86t
    routes and dosages, 870t, 875t
ketogenic diet, 312, 312t, 315
KETOLIDES, 818, 830
ketones, 682
ketoprofen, 680–681t
ketorolac, 680–681t, 1294
ketotifen, 1295t
kidney(s)
    age-related changes, 118
    excretion and homeostasis, 48–49, 502

function improvement from thyroid hormone
        replacement, 1142t
    organ-specific toxicity and, 56–57, 56t, 60,
        106–107, 504, 504t
    physiology, 502–503, 502–503f, 504t
    reabsorption and secretion, 503
    renal failure, 36, 504–505, 504–505t
    transplantation, 502t
KINASE INHIBITORS
    everolimus, 696t, 699, 988
    sirolimus, 616t, 696t, 699
    temsirolimus, 696t, 699–700
    vemurafenib, 987t, 988
Kineret. See anakinra
kininase, 489
Klebsiella pneumoniae, 777t, 781t
Klonopin. See clonazepam
Klor-Con. See potassium chloride
Klotrix. See potassium chloride
Koch, Robert, 849
Krystexxa. See pegloticase
K-Tab. See potassium chloride
Kynamro. See mipomersen
Kyprolis. See carfilzomib
Kytril. See granisetron

L

LABAs (long-acting beta agonists), 735
labeling
    of pediatric medications, 104–105, 105t
    regulations regarding, 14
    USP-NF standards for, 16, 16f
labetalol, 198t, 200, 549, 552, 553t
labyrinthitis, 1297t
lacosamide, 319t
Lacril-lube. See lanolin alcohol
lactated Ringer's solution, 525, 526
lactation. See also pregnancy
    galactagogues for improving, 99t
    oxytocin and, 1176, 1177f
    pharmacotherapy during
        adverse effects and, 98, 99t
        antibiotics, 784
        Hale's risk categories for, 99, 99t
        rationale for, 93
        transfer of drugs through breast milk, 97–98,
            97f, 98t
    seizures in, 311–312
LACTIN-V, 837t
Lactobacillus, 1028
Lactobacillus acidophilus, 87t, 1040t
Lactobacillus crispatus, 837t
LAIV (live attenuated intranasal vaccine), 717
Lamictal. See lamotrigine
Lamisil. See terbinafine
lamivudine, 917t, 918, 920, 931, 932t, 935
lamotrigine
    adverse effects, 328
    for bipolar disorder, 258t, 260
    for seizures, 313–314t, 314, 316, 319t, 327–328
Lampit. See nifurtimox
Lamprene. See clofazimine
lanolin alcohol, 1293t
Lanoxicaps. See digoxin
Lanoxin. See digoxin
lanreotide, 1100t, 1103
lansoprazole, 1010, 1011t, 1013
Lantus. See insulin glargine
lapatinib, 987t
large intestine, 1000
large volume infusions, 30
Larodopa. See levodopa

Lasix. See furosemide
Lassa fever, 1306
latanoprost, 910, 1287, 1288t
Latinos/Latinas. See Hispanic populations
Latisse. See bimatoprost
Latuda. See lurasidone
laws and regulations, 12–23. See also Food and Drug
        Administration
    approval process for drugs, 17–19, 17f
    controlled substances, 14, 20, 418
    dietary supplements, 14, 17, 20, 84–85
    on drug standards, 15–16
    herbal supplements, 84–85
    history of, 13–14, 15t
    labeling, 14
    patent medicines, 13, 13f
    prescription vs. OTC drugs, 19–20
    prescriptive authority, 20–21
    scheduled drugs, 20, 20t
    vitamins, 1049–1050
LAXATIVES
    abuse of, 1027t
    adverse effects, 1026
    bulk-forming, 1025t, 1026–1027
    classification of, 1026
    for constipation, 1025–1027
    drug interactions, 58
    herbal agents, 336, 1025t, 1026, 1027
    miscellaneous agents, 385, 1025t, 1026,
        1033t, 1036
    Nursing Practice Applications, 1030–1031t
    routes and dosages, 1025t
    saline/osmotic, 98t, 533, 691, 1015t, 1025t,
        1027, 1057
    stimulant, 336, 1025t, 1027
    surfactant, 1025t, 1027
L-carnitine. See carnitine
LDL (low-density lipoprotein), 454, 456–457,
        456f, 457t
L-dopa. See levodopa/carbidopa
lecithins, 454
leeches, 623
leflunomide, 105t, 1248t, 1250
left ventricular hypertrophy, 445
Leishmania, 885t, 895
leishmaniasis, 885t, 895
lemon balm, 233
lenalidomide, 988, 990t
Lennox-Gastaut syndrome, 312t, 313t, 315, 321
lens, of eye, 1285
lepirudin, 623
lepromatous leprosy, 859
leprosy, 777t, 849, 859, 859t, 861–862
leptin, 1080
Lescol/Lescol-XL. See fluvastatin
letrozole, 976t, 978
leucovorin, 894, 969
leucovorin rescue therapy, 969
leukemias, 56, 949t
Leukeran. See chlorambucil
Leukine. See sargramostim
leukocytes, 441, 643
LEUKOTRIENE MODIFIERS, 735t, 743–744
    montelukast, 741t, 744, 759t, 763
    zafirlukast, 741t, 743–744
    zileuton, 741t, 744
leukotrienes, 668, 668t, 743
leuprolide
    adverse effects, 979, 1186
    clinical applications, 1183, 1186, 1210
    pregnancy category rating, 95t
    routes and dosages, 976t, 1182t
Leustatin. See cladribine

levalbuterol, 181*t*, 187, 737*t*, 738
levamisole, 695
Levaquin. *See* levofloxacin
levarterenol, 196
Levatol. *See* penbutolol
Levemir. *See* insulin detemir
levetiracetam, 313*t*, 319*t*, 328
Levitra. *See* vardenafil
levobetaxolol, 1290
levobunolol, 1288*t*, 1289, 1290
levobupivacaine, 410
levocetirizine, 756*t*, 758
levodopa, 271, 288–289, 289*f*
levodopa/carbidopa, 86*t*, 289–291, 290*t*
Levo-Dromoran. *See* levorphanol
levofloxacin, 823*t*, 826, 826*t*, 835, 863
levoleucovorin, 969
levonorgestrel, 27, 1193*t*, 1200, 1203*t*
Levophed. *See* norepinephrine
levorphanol, 374*t*, 377
Levothroid. *See* levothyroxine
levothyroxine, 1140, 1141–1142, 1141*t*
Levoxyl. *See* levothyroxine
Levsin. *See* hyoscyamine
Lewisite, 1307*t*
Lexapro. *See* escitalopram
Lexiva. *See* fosamprenavir
Lexxel, 546*t*
Leydig cells, 1209
LH. *See* luteinizing hormone
LH (luteinizing hormone), 1167, 1193, 1209
Lialda. *See* mesalamine
libido, 1210, 1214
Librium. *See* chlordiazepoxide
lice, 1265, 1267–1268*t*
Lidex. *See* fluocinonide
lidocaine
    adverse effects, 410
    breast-feeding and, 98*t*
    for dysrhythmias, 572, 603*t*, 604, 605
    as local anesthetic, 384, 406*t*, 1278
    mechanism of action, 410
    Nursing Responsibilities, 410
    routes and dosages, 1293*t*
    therapeutic effects and uses, 410
Lidoderm. *See* lidocaine
Lifespan and Diversity Considerations. *See also*
    Treating the Diverse Patient
    aminocaproic acid, 636
    antibiotic use in geriatric patients, 794*t*
    antihistamines in geriatric patients, 757*t*
    asthma in pediatric patients, 1155*t*
    benzocaine, 1278
    chemotherapy effects in geriatric patients, 977*t*
    childhood anxiety disorders, 234*t*
    cost of medications, 19*t*
    cyanocobalamin (vitamin B$_{12}$), 658
    dapsone, 862
    dehydration in geriatric patients, 528*t*
    dental health and dysrhythmias in geriatric
        patients, 601*t*
    depression in geriatric patients, 242*t*
    diabetes in school-aged children, 1121*t*
    drug monitoring in geriatric patients, 120*t*
    ferrous sulfate, 656
    glucagon, 1116
    hypertension in pediatric patients, 480*t*
    immunosuppressants in pediatric patients, 698*t*
    inhalant abuse by children, 422*t*
    inhaler use in geriatric patients, 740*t*
    insomnia in geriatric patients, 242*t*
    lithium carbonate, 259
    mifepristone, 1205

octreotide, 1103
oprelvekin, 652
orlistat, 1084
oropharyngeal candidiasis in infants, 876*t*
pain assessment in pediatric patients, 370*t*
pain expression and management in geriatric
    patients, 382*t*
pancrelipase, 1043
parental role in medication error prevention, 70*t*
pediatric dyslipidemias and lipid-lowering
    drugs, 458*t*
polyherbacy, 85*t*
proton pump inhibitors and osteoporosis
    risk, 1013*t*
shingles vaccine, 720*t*
sildenafil, 1218
succinylcholine, 172
sulfasalazine, 1034
light therapy. *See* phototherapy
limbic system, 211, 213, 213*f*, 219–220, 219*f*
linaclotide, 1033*t*, 1036
linagliptin, 1122*t*, 1125*t*, 1131
Lincocin. *See* lincomycin
lincomycin, 815, 815*t*
lindane, 1265, 1266
linezolid, 616*t*, 782, 815, 815*t*
Linum usitatissimum. *See* flaxseed
Linzess. *See* linaclotide
Lioresal. *See* baclofen
liothyronine, 1140, 1141*t*, 1142
liotrix, 1141*t*, 1142
LIPASE INHIBITORS, 1082–1085
lipid(s). *See also* dyslipidemia
    cardiovascular disease and, 454–456
    chemical structure of, 455*f*
    classification of, 454
    in enteral nutrition, 1065
    measurement of, 456–458, 457*t*
    in parenteral nutrition, 1070
    storage capacity for, 1080
Lipitor. *See* atorvastatin
lipodystrophy, 933
lipoproteins, 454–457, 456*f*
liposomal amphotericin B, 870, 871*f*. *See also*
    amphotericin B deoxycholate
Liposyn, 1070
Liptruzet, 467
liquid medications, 28
Liquifilm. *See* polyvinyl alcohol
liraglutide, 1122*t*, 1131
lisdexamphetamine, 354*t*, 356
lisinopril, 491–492, 491*t*, 548, 572, 584*t*
lithium carbonate
    adverse effects, 259, 616*t*, 1105, 1215*t*
    breast-feeding and, 98–99*t*
    clinical applications, 257, 258–259
    Lifespan and Diversity Considerations, 259
    mechanism of action, 259
    Nursing Responsibilities, 259
    Patient and Family Education, 259–260
    pregnancy category rating, 95*t*
    routes and dosages, 258*t*
Lithobid. *See* lithium carbonate
Livalo. *See* pitavastatin
live attenuated intranasal vaccine (LAIV), 717
liver
    acetaminophen and liver failure, 1000*t*
    age-related changes, 119
    in digestive process, 1000–1001
    drug metabolism in, 1000
    functions of, 1000
    hepatic portal circulation and, 1000, 1001*f*
    organ-specific toxicity and, 56*t*, 57, 60, 85, 825

liver cancer, 950, 951*t*
LMWHs. *See* LOW-MOLECULAR-WEIGHT
      HEPARINS
loading doses, 39
local anesthesia
    as adjuvant analgesic, 384
    amide-type, 406*t*, 409–411
      articaine, 406*t*, 410
      bupivacaine, 406*t*, 410
      dibucaine, 406*t*, 410–411, 1278
      lidocaine. *See* lidocaine
      mepivacaine, 406*t*, 411
      prilocaine, 406*t*, 411
      ropivacaine, 406*t*, 411
    defined, 395
    ester-type, 405, 406*t*, 408–409
      benzocaine, 406*t*, 409, 1278–1279, 1297*t*
      chloroprocaine, 406*t*, 409
      procaine, 38, 406*t*, 408–409
      tetracaine, 406*t*, 409, 1278, 1293*t*, 1294
    Nursing Practice Applications, 412–413*t*
    for ocular procedures, 1294
    onset and duration of, 404–405
    techniques for applying, 404, 405*f*
locus coeruleus, 220
lodoxamide, 1295*t*
Loestrin, 1193*t*
Loewi, Otto, 142*t*
Lofibra. *See* fenofibrate
lomefloxacin, 826
lomitapide, 461*t*, 467
Lomotil. *See* diphenoxylate with atropine
lomustine, 964*t*, 967
long QT syndrome (LQTS), 599*t*
long-acting beta agonists (LABAs), 735
long-acting formulations, 28
Loniten. *See* minoxidil
look-alike drug names, 70, 71*t*
LOOP (HIGH-CEILING) DIURETICS, 56*t*, 505,
      506–507*f*, 506–509, 508*t*, 547
    adverse effects, 507–508
    drug interactions, 508
    drugs in class
      bumetanide, 508*t*, 509, 547, 584*t*, 585
      ethacrynic acid, 508*t*, 509, 547
      furosemide. *See* furosemide
      torsemide, 508*t*, 509, 547, 584*t*, 585
    mechanism of action, 506, 508
    therapeutic effects and uses, 506–507, 508
loperamide, 1028, 1028*t*, 1029, 1036
Lopid. *See* gemfibrozil
lopinavir with ritonavir, 58, 932*t*, 937
Lopressor. *See* metoprolol
Lopressor HCT, 201, 546*t*
Loprox. *See* ciclopirox
Lopurin. *See* allopurinol
Lorabid. *See* loracarbef
loracarbef, 112*t*
loratadine, 425*t*, 756*t*, 759
lorazepam
    adverse effects, 227
    in anesthesia, 398
    for anxiety and insomnia, 226–227
    for bipolar disorder, 260
    for delirium tremens, 425
    drug interactions, 227, 425*t*
    indications for, 226*t*
    mechanism of action, 227
    for muscle spasms, 384
    for nausea and vomiting, 957, 1038
    nursing responsibilities, 227
    routes and dosages, 225*t*, 1039*t*
    for seizures, 313*t*, 318*t*, 320, 321

lorcaserin, 1083*t*, 1085
losartan, 33, 493–495, 494*t*, 546*t*, 548
LoSeasonique, 1194
Lotensin. *See* benazepril
Lotensin HCT, 492, 546*t*
Lotrel, 479, 492, 546*t*
Lotrimin AF. *See* clotrimazole
Lotronex. *See* alosetron
Lou Gehrig's disease. *See* amyotrophic lateral sclerosis
lovastatin, 62*t*, 459, 460–461, 461*t*, 463, 465
Lovaza. *See* omega-3 fatty acids
Lovenox. *See* enoxaparin
low back pain, 368*t*
low-density lipoprotein (LDL), 454, 456–457, 456*f*, 457*t*
LOW-MOLECULAR-WEIGHT HEPARINS (LMWHs), 618–619, 620
    dalteparin, 618*t*, 620
    enoxaparin, 571, 618*t*, 620
    tinzaparin, 618*t*, 620
loxapine, 271*t*, 274
Loxitane. *See* loxapine
Lozol. *See* indapamide
LQTS (long QT syndrome), 599*t*
LSD (lysergic acid diethylamide), 96*t*, 417, 427–428, 428*f*
L-type calcium channels, 475, 475*f*
lubiprostone, 1025*t*, 1026, 1033*t*, 1036
LUBRICANTS, OCULAR, 1293*t*, 1294
Ludiomil. *See* maprotiline
Lufyllin. *See* dyphylline
Lugol's solution. *See* potassium iodide and iodine
luliconazole, 875*t*
lumefantrine-artemether, 887, 888*t*, 889
Lumigan. *See* bimatoprost
Luminal. *See* phenobarbital
Lunesta. *See* eszopiclone
lung(s). *See* respiratory system
lung cancer, 951*t*, 954, 983*t*
Lupron. *See* leuprolide
lupus, 195*t*, 551, 616, 668
lurasidone, 275*t*, 276–277
Lusedra. *See* fospropofol
luteinizing hormone (LH), 1094*t*, 1167, 1193, 1209
Luvox/Luvox CR. *See* fluvoxamine
Luzu. *See* luliconazole
Lyme disease, 777*t*, 807
lymph nodes, 665
lymphangiogenesis, 665*t*
lymphatic system, organization of, 665
lymphocytes, 441, 668, 673
lymphomas, 56, 949*t*
Lyrica. *See* pregabalin
lysergic acid diethylamide (LSD), 96*t*, 417, 427–428, 428*f*
Lysodren. *See* mitotane
lysosomes, 667
Lysteda. *See* tranexamic acid

M

m̃a huang, 183
Maalox Plus, 1015*t*
MABs. *See* MONOCLONAL ANTIBODIES
MAC (monitored anesthesia care), 395
mace, 1307
Macrobid. *See* nitrofurantoin
Macrodantin. *See* nitrofurantoin
MACROLIDES, 809–812
    adverse effects, 810
    breast-feeding and, 98*t*
    clinical applications, 809, 863
    drug interactions, 622*t*, 810

drugs in class
    azithromycin. *See* azithromycin
    clarithromycin. *See* clarithromycin
    erythromycin. *See* erythromycin
    fidaxomicin, 809, 810*t*, 811–812
    lactation risk categories, 99*t*
    mechanism of action, 809–810
    Nursing Practice Applications, 816–817*t*
    pregnancy category, 95
    resistance to, 780, 810
    routes and dosages, 810*t*
macrominerals, 1056–1057, 1057*t*. *See also* specific minerals
macula densa, 488, 488*f*
macular edema, 1199*t*
mafenide, 839
magaldrate, 1015*t*
Magan. *See* magnesium salicylate
magnesium
    in antacids, 1016
    deficiencies in, 528*t*, 1057
    function of, 1056–1057, 1057*t*
    imbalances, 528*t*, 532–533
    for migraines, 389*t*
    recommended intake of, 533*t*, 1057*t*
magnesium antacids. *See* ANTACIDS
magnesium citrate, 533, 1057
magnesium hydroxide, 98*t*, 533, 1015*t*, 1025*t*, 1027, 1057
magnesium oxide, 533
magnesium salicylate, 533, 676*t*, 678, 1057
magnesium sulfate (MgSO₄), 311, 532–533, 1057, 1177*t*, 1179
magnesium trisilicate and aluminum hydroxide, 1015*t*
magnetic resonance imaging (MRI), 296
Mag-Ox. *See* magnesium oxide
maintenance doses, 39
major depressive disorder, 230, 240. *See also* depression
major tranquilizers, 269. *See also* FIRST-GENERATION ANTIPSYCHOTICS
malaria
    etiology and pathogenesis, 885*t*, 886, 887*f*
    pharmacotherapy, 886–890, 888*t*
    prevalence of, 886, 886*t*
Malarone. *See* atovaquone-proguanil
malathion, 1265, 1266
male reproductive system, regulation of, 1209–1210, 1209*f*
male sexual dysfunction
    erectile dysfunction, 1214, 1216–1219, 1217*t*
    etiology of, 1214–1215, 1215*t*
    infertility, 1214, 1215–1216
male-pattern baldness, 1279
males. *See* gender differences
malignant hyperthermia, 171, 342, 401*t*
malignant tumors, 949. *See also* cancer
malnutrition, 1063. *See also* nutritional considerations
mammograms, 951
mandrake, 980
manganese, 1057*t*
mania, 240, 257
manic-depression. *See* bipolar disorder
mannitol, 513*t*, 514, 1106, 1288*t*, 1292
MAO (monoamine oxidase), 145, 178, 179, 253
MAO-B inhibitors. *See* MONOAMINE OXIDASE-B (MAO-B) INHIBITORS
MAOIs. *See* MONOAMINE OXIDASE INHIBITORS
maprotiline, 244, 245*t*, 247
maraviroc, 932*t*, 939
Marburg fever, 1306
Marcaine. *See* bupivacaine
Marezine. *See* cyclizine

margin of safety (MOS), 44
marijuana, 96*t*, 417, 418, 420*t*, 421*t*, 426–427
Marinol. *See* dronabinol
marketing rights, 7
Marplan. *See* isocarboxazid
Marquibo. *See* vincristine
MARs (medication administration records), 71
mass casualty incidents (MCIs), 1303–1304
massage, 389*t*
MAST CELL STABILIZERS
    for allergic rhinitis, 762–763
    for asthma, 735*t*, 741*t*, 742–743
    drugs in class
        cromolyn, 94, 741*t*, 742–743, 759*t*, 763, 1295*t*
        lodoxamide, 1295*t*
        nedocromil, 741*t*, 743, 763, 1295*t*
        pemirolast, 1294, 1295*t*
    for ocular conditions, 1294, 1295*t*
mastoiditis, 1297
Materia Medica, 3
Matulane. *See* procarbazine
Mavik. *See* trandolapril
Maxair. *See* pirbuterol
Maxalt. *See* rizatriptan
Maxaquin. *See* lomefloxacin
Maxiflor. *See* diflorasone diacetate
Maxipime. *See* cefepime
MBD. *See* metabolic bone disease
MCIs (mass casualty incidents), 1303–1304
MCV (meningococcal conjugate vaccine), 715
MDIs (metered-dose inhalers), 733–734
MDMA (ecstasy), 417, 428
MDR-TB (multidrug-resistant tuberculosis), 854*t*, 857, 858
measles (rubeola), 713*t*, 718–719, 1265
Mebaral. *See* mephobarbital
mebendazole, 36, 778, 897, 898, 899–900, 899*t*
mecamylamine, 168, 169*t*
mecasermin, 1100*t*, 1101
mechlorethamine, 963, 964*t*, 967
meclizine, 757, 1037, 1039*t*
meclofenamate, 680–681*t*
median effective dose (ED₅₀), 43, 43*f*
median lethal dose (LD₅₀), 44, 44*f*
median toxicity dose (TD₅₀), 44
Medicare Prescription Drug Improvement and Modernization Act of 2003, 14
medicated urethral system for erection (MUSE), 1217
medication administration records (MARs), 71
medication error(s), 66–78
    abbreviations and, 69
    categorization of, 67, 68–69*f*
    defined, 67
    documentation and reporting, 70–71
    drug names and, 69, 70, 71*t*
    factors contributing to, 67, 69
    frequency of, 67*t*, 70*t*
    geriatric patients and, 117*t*
    impact on health care, 67
    during interunit hospital transfers, 172*t*
    patient education on, 73–74
    pediatric patients and, 70*t*, 109–110, 110*t*
    prevention strategies, 70*t*, 72–75
medication error index, 67, 68–69*f*
medication reconciliation, 72–73
medication refusal, 128*t*
MEDMARX, 71
Medrol. *See* methylprednisolone
medroxyprogesterone
    adverse effects, 1173
    breast-feeding and, 99*t*
    clinical applications, 978, 1171, 1198
    mechanism of action, 1171

Nursing Responsibilities, 1173
routes and dosages, 976t, 1170t
MedWatch Safety Information program, 54, 70–71
mefenamic acid, 680–681t
mefloquine, 886, 887, 888t, 889
Mefoxin. See cefoxitin
Megace. See megestrol
megakaryocytes, 442, 649
megaloblastic anemia. See pernicious anemia
megestrol, 976t
MEGLITINIDES, 1127–1128
nateglinide, 1122t, 1128
repaglinide, 1122t, 1125t, 1127–1128
melanocytes, 1263
melarsoprol, 892t, 895, 896
melatonin, 87t, 171, 220, 223, 224t
Mellaril. See thioridazine
meloxicam, 680–681t
melphalan, 964t, 967
memantine, 297, 297t
men. See gender differences
meningococcal conjugate vaccine (MCV), 715
meningococcal infection, 713t, 715, 775, 777t, 796
meningococcal polysaccharide vaccine (MPSV), 715
menopause, 1174, 1174t
Menopur. See menotropins
menorrhagia, 1171
menotropins, 95t, 1182t, 1183, 1186, 1216
menstrual cycle, 1167
Mentax. See butenafine
Menveo. See meningococcal conjugate vaccine
mepenzolate, 165t
meperidine, 374t, 375, 377–378, 425t
mephobarbital, 234, 318t, 320
mepivacaine, 406t, 411
meprobamate, 223, 228
Mepron. See atovaquone
mercaptopurine, 969t, 971–972, 1033
Meridia. See sibutramine
meropenem, 797, 797t, 798
merozoites, 886
Merrem. See meropenem
mesalamine, 1032, 1033t, 1035
mesalazine, 1041t
mescaline, 428, 428f
mesna, 958, 967
Mesnex. See mesna
Mestinon. See pyridostigmine
metabolic acidosis, 505t
metabolic bone disease (MBD)
defined, 1233
pharmacotherapy, 1237–1244
bisphosphonates, 1239–1240t, 1239–1242
miscellaneous agents, 1243–1244
selective estrogen receptor modulators,
1242–1243
vitamin D therapy, 1237–1239, 1238t
types of, 1236–1237
metabolic syndrome, 1114
metabolism
of alcohol, 423, 424f
of antipsychotics and antidepressants, 275t
defined, 33
drug interactions and, 59–60, 59f
first-pass effect, 28, 34–35, 34f
in geriatric patients, 118, 119
hepatic microsomal enzyme system
and, 33–34, 33t
nutrient categories and, 1002, 1002t
patient variations in, 35
in pediatric patients, 106
during pregnancy, 94
Metadate. See methylphenidate

Metaglip, 1125t, 1126
Metamucil. See psyllium mucilloid
metaproterenol, 737t, 738
metastasis, 950, 950f
metaxalone, 339t, 340
metered-dose inhalers (MDIs), 733–734
metformin, 1122t, 1125t, 1126–1127, 1131
methadone, 374t, 378, 419, 422
methamphetamines, 96t, 430
methanol, 1308t
methaqualone, 223, 224
methazolamide, 513t, 515, 516, 1288t
methemoglobin-forming drugs, 1308t
methenamine hippurate, 838t, 842
Methergine. See methylergonovine
methicillin, 793
methicillin-resistant Staphylococcus aureus (MRSA),
781–782, 782t, 793, 1264
methimazole, 95t, 1145, 1145t, 1146
Methitest. See methyltestosterone
methocarbamol, 339t, 340
methohexital, 233, 397t, 399–400
methotrexate
for abortion, 1203
adverse effects, 616t, 1215t
as antineoplastic agent, 968–970
drug interactions, 86t
as immunosuppressant, 696t, 701
for inflammatory bowel disease, 1033
misoprostol with, 1203t
pregnancy category, 95t
for psoriasis, 1277
for rheumatoid arthritis, 1248, 1250
routes and dosages, 969t, 1248t, 1276t
methoxamine, 185
methscopolamine, 165t, 167
methsuximide, 318t, 325
methyclothiazide, 510t, 511, 547
methyl sulfonyl methane (MSM), 87t
methylcellulose, 1025t
methyldopa, 56t, 184, 546t, 550, 1215t
methylene blue, 1308t
methylergonovine, 1176–1177, 1177t, 1179
Methylin. See methylphenidate
methylnaltrexone, 385, 1025t, 1026
methylphenidate
abuse of, 417, 430
for ADHD, 356
labeling changes, 105t
for narcolepsy, 222, 358
routes and dosages, 112t, 354t, 1039t
methylprednisolone, 303, 705, 1040, 1156t
methyltestosterone, 1210t, 1212
METHYLXANTHINES, 735t, 744–745
aminophylline, 737t, 745
caffeine, 354t, 359–360, 360t, 431
dyphylline, 737t, 745
theobromine, 359
theophylline, 359, 360, 737t, 744–745
methysergide, 389, 389t
metipranolol, 1288t, 1289, 1290
metoclopramide, 98t, 386, 413, 1018, 1039t
metolazone, 509, 510t, 511, 547
Metopirone. See metyrapone
metoprolol
adverse effects, 201–202
clinical applications, 201, 228, 389t, 584t, 586
hydrochlorothiazide with, 546t
mechanism of action, 201
Nursing Responsibilities, 202
routes and dosages, 198t, 568t
MetroCream. See metronidazole
MetroGel. See metronidazole

MetroLotion. See metronidazole
metronidazole
adverse effects, 55t, 827, 893
breast-feeding and, 98t
clinical applications, 830, 891–892, 892t, 1017,
1264, 1269
drug interactions, 425t, 622t, 893
effectiveness of, 894
mechanism of action, 893
Nursing Responsibilities, 893
resistance to, 827
routes and dosages, 827t
metyrapone, 1163
Mevacor. See lovastatin
mexiletine, 384, 603t, 605
Mexitil. See mexiletine
MG. See myasthenia gravis
MgSO₄. See magnesium sulfate
Miacalcin. See calcitonin-salmon
mibefradil, 475
micafungin, 870t, 872
Micardis. See telmisartan
Micardis HCT, 495, 546t
Micatin. See miconazole
miconazole, 875t, 877, 1265
microbial antagonism, 784
Micro-K. See potassium chloride
microminerals, 1057–1058, 1057t. See also specific
minerals
Micronase. See glyburide
Micronor. See PROGESTINS
Microsporum, 874
Microzide. See hydrochlorothiazide
Midamor. See amiloride
midazolam, 225, 226, 226t, 397t, 398–399, 411
midodrine, 181t, 185
Mifeprex. See mifepristone
mifepristone, 1202–1205, 1203t
miglitol, 1122t, 1130
migraines, 385–391
characteristics of, 385, 386t
complementary and alternative therapies
for, 389t
ergot alkaloids for, 291
Nursing Practice Applications, 390–391t
pharmacotherapy, 198, 199, 386–388, 387t
prophylaxis, 388–389, 389t
statistics, 386t
triggers for, 386, 388–389
Migranal. See dihydroergotamine
Milk of Magnesia. See magnesium hydroxide
milk thistle, 81t, 83t, 99t
milk-alkali syndrome, 1016
milnacipran, 384
Milontin. See phensuximide
Milophene. See clomiphene
milrinone, 587t, 589–590
miltefosine, 892t, 895
Miltown. See meprobamate
mineral oil, 1025t, 1026
MINERALOCORTICOIDS, 1152–1153, 1162
minerals. See also specific minerals
functions of, 1056
macrominerals, 1056–1057, 1057t
microminerals, 1057–1058, 1057t
Nursing Practice Applications, 1058–1059t
in parenteral nutrition, 1071
minimal sedation (anxiolysis), 395
Mini-Mental State Exam (MMSE), 296
minimum alveolar concentration, 401
minimum effective concentrations, 37
Minipress. See prazosin
Minizide. See polythiazide and prazosin

Minocin. *See* minocycline
minocycline, 112*t*, 807*t*, 809, 859
minorities. *See* Treating the Diverse Patient;
  specific racial and ethnic groups
minoxidil, 552, 1279, 1280
Mintezol. *See* thiabendazole
miosis, 153, 1289
Miostat. *See* carbachol
mipomersen, 461*t*, 467
mirabegron, 181*t*, 187
MiraLAX. *See* polyethylene glycol
Mirapex. *See* pramipexole
Mircette, 1193*t*
Mirena. *See* levonorgestrel
mirtazapine, 250, 252
Mirvaso. *See* brimonidine
MIs. *See* myocardial infarctions
misoprostol
  adverse effects, 95, 1018, 1202–1203
  clinical applications, 676, 1018, 1177,
    1202, 1204*t*
  pregnancy category rating, 95*t*
  routes and dosages, 1203*t*
mites, 1265, 1267–1268*t*
Mithramycin. *See* plicamycin
mitochondrial toxicity, 933
mitomycin, 95*t*, 972*t*, 975
mitosis, 954
mitotane, 990*t*, 991, 1163
mitoxantrone, 56*t*, 57, 302*t*, 303, 972*t*, 974
Mivacron. *See* mivacurium
mivacurium, 169*t*, 173
MIXED OPIOID AGONIST-ANTAGONISTS, 372, 373*f*,
    378–379
  buprenorphine, 374*t*, 378
  butorphanol, 374*t*, 378
  nalbuphine, 374*t*, 378
  pentazocine, 374*t*, 378–379
MMR vaccine, 616*t*, 718–719
MMSE (Mini-Mental State Exam), 296
Moban. *See* molindone
Mobic. *See* meloxicam
Mobidin. *See* magnesium salicylate
modafinil, 222, 354*t*, 358–359
moderate (conscious) sedation, 395
modular formulas, for enteral nutrition, 1065
Moduretic, 506, 513
moexipril, 491*t*, 492–493, 548
molindone, 274
molybdenum, 1057*t*
MOM. *See* magnesium hydroxide
mometasone, 741*t*, 742, 759*t*, 1273*t*
Monistat-1, 875*t*, 877
monitored anesthesia care (MAC), 395
monoamine oxidase (MAO), 145, 178,
    179, 253
MONOAMINE OXIDASE INHIBITORS (MAOIs)
  adverse effects, 253
  for anxiety disorders, 232
  for depression, 253–255, 257
  drug interactions, 62*t*, 86*t*, 200, 247
  drugs in class
    isocarboxazid, 255
    phenelzine, 178, 254–255
    selegiline, 257, 290*t*, 294, 358
    tranylcypromine, 257
  mechanism of action, 178, 253
MONOAMINE OXIDASE-B (MAO-B) INHIBITORS,
    290*t*, 294
  adverse effects, 294
  rasagiline, 290*t*, 294
  selegiline, 257, 290*t*, 294, 358
MONOBACTAMS, 799

MONOCLONAL ANTIBODIES (MABs), 702, 745, 988, 989*f*
  adalimumab. *See* adalimumab
  alemtuzumab, 987*t*
  basiliximab, 696*t*, 702, 702*t*, 703
  belimumab, 702*t*
  bevacizumab, 987*t*, 988
  bortezomib, 987*t*
  brentuximab, 987*t*
  certolizumab pegol, 702*t*, 1033, 1248*t*, 1249, 1250
  daclizumab, 753
  eculizumab, 702*t*
  erlotinib, 987*t*, 988
  gefitinib, 987*t*
  gemtuzumab ozogamicin, 987*t*, 988
  golimumab, 702*t*, 1033, 1248*t*, 1249, 1250
  ibritumomab, 987*t*
  infliximab. *See* infliximab
  ipilimumab, 987*t*
  lapatinib, 987*t*
  muromonab-CD3, 702
  natalizumab, 302*t*, 303, 702*t*, 1033
  nilotinib, 987*t*
  ofatumumab, 987*t*
  omalizumab, 745
  panitumumab, 987*t*
  plerixafor, 987*t*
  rituximab, 987*t*, 988, 1248*t*, 1250
  sorafenib, 987*t*
  sunitinib, 987*t*
  tocilizumab, 702*t*, 1248*t*, 1251, 1277
  tositumomab, 987*t*, 988
  vandetanib, 987*t*
Mono-gesic. *See* salsalate
Monoket. *See* isosorbide mononitrate
monomeric formulas, for enteral nutrition, 1064
Monopril. *See* fosinopril
Monopril HCT, 492
montelukast, 741*t*, 744, 759*t*, 763
Monurol. *See* fosfomycin
mood disorders, defined, 240. *See also* bipolar disorder;
    depression
MOOD STABILIZERS, 257, 260, 297. *See also* lithium
    carbonate
Morbillivirus. *See* measles
moricizine, 605
morning sickness, 1037, 1037*t*
morphine sulfate
  adverse effects, 375–376, 419, 616*t*
  breast-feeding and, 98*t*
  clinical applications, 376
  drug interactions, 376, 425*t*
  mechanism of action, 376
  Nursing Responsibilities, 377
  routes and dosages, 374*t*
MOS (margin of safety), 44
motion sickness, 168, 757, 1037
Motofen. *See* difenoxin with atropine
motor end plate, 168, 170*f*
Motrin. *See* ibuprofen
Movantik. *See* naloxegol
Moxatag. *See* amoxicillin
Moxeza. *See* moxifloxacin
moxifloxacin, 823*t*, 824, 826
Mozobil. *See* plerixafor
MPSV (meningococcal polysaccharide vaccine), 715
MRI (magnetic resonance imaging), 296
MRSA (methicillin-resistant *Staphylococcus aureus*),
    781–782, 782*t*, 793, 1264
MS. *See* multiple sclerosis
MS Contin. *See* morphine sulfate
MSM (methyl sulfonyl methane), 87*t*
MTX. *See* methotrexate
mu receptors, 372, 373*f*, 373*t*

Mucinex. *See* guaifenesin
Mucocutaneous leishmaniasis, 895
MUCOLYTICS, 746, 767, 769
  acetylcysteine, 766*t*, 767, 1308*t*
  dornase alfa, 766*t*, 769
Mucomyst. *See* acetylcysteine
mucormycosis, 867, 867*t*
mucositis, 957
mucous colitis. *See* irritable bowel syndrome
mucous membranes, as body defense, 666–667
Multaq. *See* dronedarone
multidrug-resistant tuberculosis (MDR-TB), 854*t*,
    857, 858
multiple sclerosis (MS)
  depression and, 303
  muscle spasticity in, 336
  pain in, 303
  pathophysiology, 300–301, 301*f*
  in pediatric patients, 304*t*
  pharmacotherapy, 300–303, 302*t*
multipotent stem cells, 643
multivitamins. *See* vitamin(s)
mumps, 713*t*, 718–719
mupirocin, 1264
Murine Plus. *See* tetrahydrozoline
muromonab-CD3, 702
MUSCARINIC AGONISTS
  adverse effects of, 152*t*, 153
  bethanechol, 150, 153–154
  carbachol, 154
  cevimeline, 154
  clinical applications, 153
  direct acting
    bethanechol, 150, 152*t*, 153–154
    carbachol, 152*t*, 154, 1288*t*
    cevimeline, 152*t*, 154
    pilocarpine, 152*t*, 153, 154, 1288*t*, 1289
  indirect acting. *See* ACETYLCHOLINESTERASE
    (AchE) INHIBITORS
  mechanism of action, 147, 152–153
  pilocarpine, 153, 154
  routes and dosages, 152*t*
MUSCARINIC ANTAGONISTS
  as adjuncts to anesthesia, 411
  adverse effects, 165*t*, 166, 739
  for ALS, 304
  antisecretory agents, 167
    glycopyrrolate, 165*t*, 167
    mepenzolate, 165*t*
    methscopolamine, 165*t*, 167
    propantheline, 165*t*, 167
  antispasmodic agents, 167
    dicyclomine, 165*t*, 167, 1033*t*, 1036, 1041
    hyoscyamine, 165*t*, 167, 1033*t*, 1036
  asthma agents/bronchodilators, 166, 735*t*, 737*t*,
    738–740
    ipratropium. *See* ipratropium
    tiotropium, 165*t*, 166, 168, 737*t*, 740
  atropine. *See* atropine
  bronchodilators, 168
  centrally acting agents, 168
    benztropine. *See* benztropine
    trihexyphenidyl, 165*t*, 168, 294, 294*t*, 295, 304
  for dystonia, 336
  incontinence agents, 168
  mechanism of action, 164–165, 164*f*, 739
  for nausea and vomiting, 1037, 1039*t*
  Nursing Practice Applications, 173–174*t*
  ophthalmic agents, 168
    cyclopentolate, 165*t*, 168, 1293*t*
    tropicamide, 165*t*, 168, 1293*t*
  overdoses/poisoning, 1308*t*
  for Parkinson's disease, 288, 294–295, 294*t*

routes and dosages, 165t
scopolamine, 29, 165t, 168, 1037, 1039t, 1293t
therapeutic applications, 165–166
urge incontinence agents
fesoterodine, 168
oxybutynin chloride, 165t, 166, 168
tolterodine tartrate, 105t, 165t, 168
muscarinic receptors, 142, 143, 144t, 150, 151t
muscle contraction, 474, 474f
MUSCLE RELAXANTS, 337–345
as adjuvant analgesics, 384
adverse effects, 337
centrally acting, 337–341, 338f, 339t
baclofen, 303, 304, 336, 337t, 339t, 340
carisoprodol, 339t, 340
chlorzoxazone, 339t, 340
cyclobenzaprine, 338–340, 339t
diazepam. See diazepam
metaxalone, 339t, 340
methocarbamol, 339t, 340
orphenadrine, 339t, 341
tizanidine, 339t, 341
direct-acting, 341–344, 341t, 342f
abobotulinumtoxinA, 341t, 343, 343t
dantrolene sodium, 341t, 342–343
incobotulinumtoxinA, 341t, 343, 343t
onabotulinumtoxinA, 341t, 343–344,
343–344t, 344f, 389
rimabotulinumtoxinB, 304, 341t, 343, 343t
dosages, 339t, 341t
in geriatric patients, 122t
mechanism of action, 337, 338f
for muscle spasms, 337–341, 339t
for muscle spasticity, 304, 341–344, 341t
as surgical adjuncts, 345
muscle rigidity, 287
muscle spasms
etiology, 335
nonpharmacologic therapies for, 336–337
Nursing Practice Applications, 345–346t
pain caused by, 303, 384
pharmacotherapy, 337–341, 338f, 339t
muscle spasticity
etiology, 335–336, 337t
nonpharmacologic therapies for, 336–337
Nursing Practice Applications, 345–346t
pain caused by, 304
pharmacotherapy, 304, 341–344, 341t, 342f
muscle toxicity, 56t, 58
MUSE (medicated urethral system for erection), 1217
mustargen, 1307t
Mustargen. See mechlorethamine
Mutamycin. See mitomycin
mutations, 780
Myambutol. See ethambutol
myasthenia gravis (MG)
nutritional considerations in, 158t
pharmacotherapy for, 155–158, 156f
symptoms and risk factors for, 155, 155t
myasthenic crisis, 156–157
Mycamine. See micafungin
Mycelex. See clotrimazole
Mycobacterial infections, 848–865
leprosy, 849, 859, 859t, 861–862
M. avium, 849, 862–863
tuberculosis. See tuberculosis
types of, 849
Mycobacterium abscessus, 849
Mycobacterium avium complex, 849, 862–863
Mycobacterium bovis, 693, 849
Mycobacterium chelonae, 849
Mycobacterium kansasii, 849
Mycobacterium leprae. See leprosy

Mycobacterium scrofulaceum, 849
Mycobacterium tuberculosis. See tuberculosis
Mycobutin. See rifabutin
mycolic acid, 849
mycophenolate, 156, 696t, 701
Mycoplasma pneumoniae. See pneumonia
mycoses. See fungal infections
Mycostatin. See nystatin
Mydfrin. See phenylephrine
Mydriacyl. See tropicamide
mydriasis, 1289
MYDRIATICS, 1292, 1293t. See also phenylephrine
myelosuppression, 442, 957, 980, 981, 991
Myfortic. See mycophenolate
Mykrox. See metolazone
Mylanta, 1015t
Myleran. See busulfan
Mylocel. See hydroxyurea
Mylotarg. See gemtuzumab ozogamicin
Myobloc. See rimabotulinumtoxinB
myocardial infarctions (MIs)
angina pectoris and, 561–562
blood test values and, 568, 569t
coronary artery disease and, 560–561
pathophysiology, 567–568
pharmacotherapy
ACE inhibitors, 490–491, 572
anticoagulant and antiplatelet agents, 571
ARBs, 493
aspirin, 569, 571
beta-adrenergic antagonists, 198, 199, 572
goals of, 568–569
nitrates, 572
pain management, 572
thrombolytics, 569, 570f
vasopressors, 572
prevalence and mortality, 572t
symptoms of, 568
myocardial ischemia, 560, 561
myocardium, 444–445
myoclonic seizures, 313t, 314
Myophen. See orphenadrine
Myrbetriq. See mirabegron
Mysoline. See primidone
Mytelase. See ambenonium
myxedema, 1140
myxedematous coma, 1140, 1140t
myxoviruses, 908t

N

nabilone, 1038, 1039t
nabumetone, 680–681t
NaCl. See sodium chloride
nadir, 957
nadolol, 198t, 200, 511, 546t, 549
NAEPP (National Asthma Education and Prevention Program), 734, 735
nafarelin, 95t, 1182t, 1183, 1186
nafcillin, 789t, 793
naftifine, 875t
Naftin. See naftifine
nalbuphine, 374t, 378
Nalfon. See fenoprofen
nalidixic acid, 622t, 823, 823t, 838t, 842
naloxegol, 1025t, 1026
naloxone, 61, 327, 377, 385, 385t, 1308t
naloxone/buprenorphine, 385, 422–423
naltrexone, 385t, 426, 1083t
Namenda/Namenda XR. See memantine
nandrolone, 1210t, 1214
naphazoline, 185, 764t, 1293t
Naphcon. See naphazoline

Naprosyn. See naproxen
naproxen, 34, 379, 425t, 616t, 680–681t, 1253
naratriptan, 387t, 388
Narcan. See naloxone
narcolepsy, 222, 358–359
narcotic analgesics. See OPIOID ANALGESICS
narcotics, defined, 372
Nardil. See phenelzine
Naropin. See ropivacaine
narrow-spectrum antibiotics, 782
Nasacort. See triamcinolone
NASAL DECONGESTANTS
adverse effects, 763
alpha-adrenergic agonists, 183, 184–185, 763–764
anticholinergic. See ipratropium
routes and dosages, 29, 763, 764t
sympathomimetics
naphazoline, 185, 764t, 1293t
oxymetazoline, 185, 763, 764t, 1293t
phenylephrine. See phenylephrine
pseudoephedrine. See pseudoephedrine
tetrahydrozoline, 183, 185, 764t, 1293t
xylometazoline, 185, 764t
NasalCrom. See cromolyn
Nasalide. See flunisolide
Nasarel. See flunisolide
Nascobal. See cyanocobalamin
nasogastric (NG) tubes, 27, 29, 1064
Nasonex. See mometasone
natalizumab, 302t, 303, 702t, 1033
Nataxia, 1191
Natazia, 1193t, 1194
nateglinide, 1122t, 1128
Natesto, 1211
National Asthma Education and Prevention Program (NAEPP), 734, 735
National Center for Complementary and Alternative Medicine (NCCAM), 82, 254t
National Coordinating Council for Medication Error Reporting and Prevention (NCC MERP), 67, 68–69f, 71
National Formulary (NF), 15
National Nurse Emergency Preparedness Initiative (NNEPI), 1303
Native Americans and Alaska Natives
complementary and alternative medicine use among, 128
diabetes among, 128t
diabetes mellitus and, 1113
infant mortality rates among, 128t
Natrecor. See nesiritide
natriuresis, 505
natriuretic peptides, 581
Naturacil. See psyllium mucilloid
natural killer (NK) cells, 667
natural penicillins, 790–791
nausea and vomiting
with antineoplastic agents, 957, 991, 1037
in enteral nutrition therapy, 1065, 1066t
first-generation antipsychotics for, 271
pathophysiology of, 1036–1037
pharmacotherapy. See ANTIEMETICS
postanesthesia, 413
in pregnancy, 1037, 1037t
Navane. See thiothixene
Navelbine. See vinorelbine
NCC MERP (National Coordinating Council for Medication Error Reporting and Prevention), 67, 68–69f, 71
NCCAM (National Center for Complementary and Alternative Medicine), 82, 254t
NDAs (New Drug Applications), 18

NDNBs (nondepolarizing neuromuscular blockers), 172–173
NDRIs (NOREPINEPHRINE AND DOPAMINE REUPTAKE INHIBITORS), 250. *See also* bupropion
NE. *See* norepinephrine
nebivolol, 198*t*, 202
nebulizers, 734
NebuPent. *See* pentamidine
Necator americanus, 897
nedocromil, 741*t*, 743, 763, 1295*t*
nefazodone, 250, 252–253
negative chronotropic effect, 476
negative feedback mechansims, 1091–1093, 1093*f*
negative inotropic effect, 476, 480
negative symptoms, of schizophrenia, 266, 266*t*
NegGram. *See* nalidixic acid
Neisseria gonorrhoeae. See gonorrhea
Neisseria meningitidis. See meningococcal infection
nelarabine, 969*t*, 972
nelfinavir, 932*t*, 938
neoadjuvant chemotherapy, 951
Neoloid. *See* castor oil
neomycin, 812, 812*t*, 814, 830, 1264, 1295
neonates, 107. *See also* pediatric patients
neoplasms, 949. *See also* cancer
Neoral. *See* cyclosporine
Neosporin, 827, 830, 1264
neostigmine, 151, 152*t*, 158, 173
Neo-Synephrine. *See* phenylephrine
Neo-Synephrine 12 Hour. *See* oxymetazoline
Neo-Synephrine II, Long-Acting. *See* xylometazoline
NEPEC (Nursing Emergency Preparedness Education Coalition), 1303–1304
nephrons, 502, 502*f*
nephropathy, diabetic, 1116
nephrotoxicity, 56–57, 56*t*, 60, 106–107, 504, 504*t*
Neptazane. *See* methazolamide
nerve agents, 1307
nerve blocks, 372, 404, 405*f*
nerve gas poisoning, 154–155
nervous system. *See also* central nervous system; peripheral nervous system
    functional divisions of, 137, 138*f*
    toxicity to, 824–825, 958
Nesacaine. *See* chloroprocaine
Nesina. *See* alogliptin
nesiritide, 581, 586, 587*t*
Nestrex. *See* pyridoxine
Neulasta. *See* pegfilgrastim
Neumega. *See* oprelvekin
Neupogen. *See* filgrastim
Neupro. *See* rotigotine
neuraminidase, 913
NEURAMINIDASE INHIBITORS, 913–914
    oseltamivir, 914, 914*t*, 915
    zanamivir, 914, 914*t*, 915
neurodegenerative diseases, 285–308
    Alzheimer's disease, 295–300. *See also* Alzheimer's disease
    amyotrophic lateral sclerosis, 304, 336
    etiology of, 286
    Huntington's disease, 286
    multiple sclerosis, 300–303, 301*f*, 302*t*, 304*t*
    muscle spasticity in, 335–336
    myasthenia gravis, 155–158, 155*t*, 156*f*, 158*t*
    Nursing Practice Applications for, 304–305*t*
    overview, 286, 286*t*
    Parkinson's disease, 286–295. *See also* Parkinson's disease
neuroeffector junction, 140
neurofibrillary tangles, 295, 296*f*
NEUROKININ RECEPTOR ANTAGONISTS, 1039*t*, 1040
neurolept analgesia, 396

neuroleptic malignant syndrome (NMS), 249, 270
neuroleptics, 269. *See also* ANTIPSYCHOTICS
NEUROMUSCULAR BLOCKERS
    as adjuncts to anesthesia, 411
    depolarizing, 168–172, 170*f*. *See also* succinylcholine
    mechanism of action, 165
    nondepolarizing, 172–173
        atracurium, 169*t*, 173, 411
        cisatracurium, 169*t*, 173, 411
        mivacurium, 169*t*, 173
        pancuronium, 169*t*, 173
        rocuronium, 169*t*, 173
        tubocurarine, 169*t*, 172, 345
        vecuronium, 169*t*, 173
neurons, 210–211, 210*f*, 210*t*
Neurontin. *See* gabapentin
neuropathic pain, 303, 368, 383
neuropathy, diabetic, 1116
neuropeptide Y (NPY), 1080
neurotoxicity, 56*t*, 57, 977*t*
neurotransmitters. *See also specific neurotransmitters*
    in appetite suppression, 1080
    defined, 140
    effects and clinical applications, 140, 141*t*
    in synaptic transmission, 140, 142, 210–211, 210*f*, 210*t*
Neutrexin. *See* trimetrexate
Neutrogena. *See* salicylic acid
neutropenia, 57, 643, 646, 869*t*, 957
neutrophils, 441, 646, 957
nevirapine, 931, 932*t*, 933, 936
New Drug Applications (NDAs), 18
new molecular entities, 18
New York Heart Association (NYHA), 581–582
Nexavar. *See* sorafenib
Nexiclon XR. *See* clonidine
Nexium. *See* esomeprazole
NF (*National Formulary*), 15
NG (nasogastric) tubes, 27, 29, 1064
niacin (nicotinic acid; vitamin B$_3$)
    adverse effects, 465
    clinical applications, 1054
    for dyslipidemia, 461*t*, 465
    functions of, 1049*t*
    with lovastatin, 463, 465
    mechanism of action, 460*f*
    routes and adult dosages for, 1050*t*
Niaspan. *See* niacin
nicardipine/nicardipine SR, 477–478*t*, 479, 548, 553*t*, 568*t*
Nicobid. *See* niacin
NicoDerm. *See* nicotine replacement therapy
Nicorette. *See* nicotine replacement therapy
nicotinamide, 465
nicotine
    addiction to, 417, 431–432
    dependence and, 419
    mechanism of action, 150, 158
    pharmacologic treatment for, 432
    polycyclic aromatic hydrocarbons and, 60*t*
    during pregnancy, 94, 95–96, 95*t*, 431
    prevalence of use, 431*t*
    withdrawal symptoms and treatment, 420*t*
nicotine replacement therapy (NRT), 97*t*, 158, 160, 419, 431–432, 431*f*
nicotinic acid. *See* niacin
NICOTINIC AGONISTS, 158, 160. *See also* nicotine
NICOTINIC ANTAGONISTS
    ganglionic blockers, 165, 168, 169*t*
    mechanism of action, 164, 164*f*, 165
    neuromuscular blockers. *See* NEUROMUSCULAR BLOCKERS

nicotinic receptors, 142–143, 144*t*, 150, 151*t*
Nicotrol NS. *See* nicotine replacement therapy
nifedipine
    adverse effects, 478
    breast-feeding and, 98*t*
    drug interactions, 60, 478–479
    for hypertension, 477–478, 477*t*, 548
    mechanism of action, 478
    for migraine prophylaxis, 389*t*
    nursing responsibilities, 479
    potency of, 45
    for Raynaud's disease, 195
    routes and dosages, 478*t*, 568*t*, 1177*t*
    as tocolytic, 1179
Niferex PN Forte, 656
nifurtimox, 892*t*, 894, 896
Nilandron. *See* nilutamide
nilotinib, 987*t*
Nilstat. *See* nystatin
nilutamide, 976*t*, 979
Nimbex. *See* cisatracurium
nimodipine, 389*t*, 477–478*t*, 479
Nimotop. *See* nimodipine
Nipent. *See* pentostatin
Nipride. *See* nitroprusside sodium
Niravam. *See* alprazolam
Nisocor. *See* nisoldipine
nisoldipine, 477–478*t*, 479, 548
nitazoxanide, 890, 891, 892*t*, 893
nitrates. *See* ORGANIC NITRATES
nitric oxide, 564
Nitro-Bid. *See* nitroglycerin
Nitro-Dur. *See* nitroglycerin
nitrofurantoin, 836, 838*t*, 841–842
nitrogen mustards
    bendamustine, 964*t*, 966
    chlorambucil, 55*t*, 964*t*, 966
    cyclophosphamide. *See* cyclophosphamide
    estramustine, 964*t*, 967
    ifosfamide, 964*t*, 967
    mechlorethamine, 963, 964*t*, 967
    melphalan, 964*t*, 967
nitroglycerin
    adverse effects, 565, 616*t*
    chest pain and, 571*t*, 572
    clinical applications, 564, 565
    interactions with, 425*t*, 565
    mechanism of action, 565
    Nursing Responsibilities, 565
    routes and dosages, 29, 564, 568*t*
Nitropress. *See* nitroprusside sodium
nitroprusside sodium, 550, 552–553, 553*t*
nitrosoureas
    carmustine, 958, 964*t*, 966
    lomustine, 964*t*, 967
    streptozocin, 964*t*, 968
Nitrostat. *See* nitroglycerin
nitrous oxide, 141*t*, 401, 402, 403*t*
nits, 1265
Nix. *See* permethrin
nizatidine, 1014*t*, 1015
Nizoral. *See* ketoconazole
NK (natural killer) cells, 667
NMDA (N-methyl-D-aspartate) receptors, 211, 297
N-methyl-D-aspartate (NMDA) receptors, 211, 297
NMS (neuroleptic malignant syndrome), 249, 270
NNEPI (National Nurse Emergency Preparedness Initiative), 1303
NNRTIs (NONNUCLEOSIDE REVERSE TRANSCRIPTASE INHIBITORS), 935–936
nociceptor pain, 368
nociceptors, 368
nocturia, 1107*t*

nocturnal penile tumescence and rigidity (NPTR) test, 1217
Nolvadex. *See* tamoxifen
nomograms, 110, 111*f*
NONBENZODIAZEPINE ANXIOLYTICS, 223, 224, 228–230
    buspirone, 225*t*, 230, 297
    doxepin. *See* doxepin
    eszopiclone, 225*t*, 230
    ramelteon, 220, 225*t*, 230
    zaleplon, 225*t*, 230
    zolpidem, 225*t*, 229
noncatecholamines, 179
nondepolarizing neuromuscular blockers (NDNBs), 172–173
NONDIHYDROPYRIDINES, 477–478*t*, 479–481. *See also*
    diltiazem; verapamil
nonmalarial protozoan infections, 890–896
    amebiasis, 890, 890*t*, 891*f*
    cryptosporidiosis, 891
    giardiasis, 890, 890*t*
    leishmaniasis, 895
    pharmacotherapy, 891–894, 892*t*, 895–896
    toxoplasmosis, 894
    trichomoniasis, 894
    trypanosomiasis, 894–895
NONNUCLEOSIDE REVERSE TRANSCRIPTASE INHIBITORS (NNRTIs), 935–936
    delavirdine, 932*t*, 933, 936
    efavirenz, 86*t*, 932*t*, 935–936
    etravirine, 932*t*, 936
    nevirapine, 931, 932*t*, 933, 936
    rilpivirine, 932*t*, 936
NONOPIOID ANALGESICS, 98*t*, 379, 379*t*, 382–383
    acetaminophen. *See* acetaminophen
    clonidine. *See* clonidine
    nonsteroidal anti-inflammatory drugs. *See*
        NONSTEROIDAL ANTI-INFLAMMATORY DRUGS
    tramadol, 379, 379*t*, 382, 1246
    ziconotide, 379*t*, 383
nonoxynol-9, 1200
nonphenothiazines, 273–274
    haloperidol, 119, 271*t*, 273–274, 297, 616*t*, 1215*t*
    loxapine, 271*t*, 274
    molindone, 274
    pimozide, 271*t*, 274
    thiothixene, 271*t*, 274
non–rapid eye movement (NREM) sleep, 220, 221, 221*t*
nonrestorative sleep, 222
nonspecific body defenses. *See* innate body defenses
NONSTEROIDAL ANTI-INFLAMMATORY DRUGS (NSAIDs), 674–683
    adverse effects, 56*t*, 379, 504*t*, 676, 679, 682*t*, 1006–1007
    for Alzheimer's disease, 300*t*
    breast-feeding and, 99*t*
    for conjunctivitis, 1294
    COX-2 inhibitors, 682–683. *See also* celecoxib
    drug interactions, 59–60, 62*t*, 86*t*, 122, 424, 425*t*, 622*t*
    in geriatric patients, 122*t*
    for gout, 1253
    ibuprofen-like drugs, 679–682, 680–681*t*
    mechanism of action, 379, 674–675
    for migraines, 386
    for muscle spasms, 337, 338*f*
    nonaspirin NSAIDs, 679–682, 680–681*t*
    for osteoarthritis, 1246
    for pain management, 379
    for pediatric patients, 379
    pregnancy category, 95*t*
    salicylates, 674–679, 676*t*
    similarities among, 679
    usage statistics, 674*t*

Nora-BE. *See* norethindrone
Norcuron. *See* vecuronium
Norditropin. *See* somatropin
norepinephrine (NE)
    adrenal medulla secretion of, 146
    in appetite control, 1080
    chemical structure of, 179, 180*f*
    effects and clinical applications, 140, 141*t*, 183, 210*t*
    for heart failure, 587*t*, 589
    life cycle of, 145*f*
    mechanism of action, 178, 179*f*, 210
    receptors, 144, 144*t*, 145
    routes and dosages, 181*t*
    synthesis and release of, 143*f*, 144
    termination of action, 145–146
NOREPINEPHRINE AND DOPAMINE REUPTAKE INHIBITORS (NDRIs), 250. *See also*
    bupropion
NOREPINEPHRINE REUPTAKE INHIBITORS (NRIs), 250
norethindrone, 1193*t*, 1194–1195, 1196, 1269
Norflex. *See* orphenadrine
norfloxacin, 823*t*, 826, 835
norgestimate, 1193*t*
normal serum albumin, 525
Normiflo. *See* ardeparin
Normodyne. *See* labetalol
Noroxin. *See* norfloxacin
Norpace. *See* disopyramide
Norpramin. *See* desipramine
Nor-QD. *See* PROGESTINS
Northera. *See* droxidopa
nortriptyline, 231*t*, 245*t*, 247, 357
Norvasc. *See* amlodipine
Norvir. *See* ritonavir
nosocomial infections. *See* health care–associated infections
Novahistine DH, 766*t*
Novantrone. *See* mitoxantrone
Novarel. *See* chorionic gonadotropin-HCG
Novastan. *See* argatroban
Novocaine. *See* procaine
Novolin 70/30, 1119, 1120*t*
Novolin R. *See* human regular insulin
NovoLog. *See* insulin aspart
NovoLog Mix 70/30, 1119, 1120*t*
Noxafil. *See* posaconazole
NPH. *See* isophane insulin suspension
Nplate. *See* romiplostim
NPTR (nocturnal penile tumescence and rigidity) test, 1217
NPY (neuropeptide Y), 1080
NREM (non–rapid eye movement) sleep, 220, 221, 221*t*
NRIs (NOREPINEPHRINE REUPTAKE INHIBITORS), 250
NRT (nicotine replacement therapy), 97*t*, 158, 160, 419, 431–432, 431*f*
NRTIs and NtRTIs. *See* NUCLEOSIDE/NUCLEOTIDE REVERSE TRANSCRIPTASE INHIBITORS
NSAIDs. *See* NONSTEROIDAL ANTI-INFLAMMATORY DRUGS
N-type calcium channels, 475
Nubain. *See* nalbuphine
nuclear accidents, 1307, 1308*t*
nucleic acid amplification tests, 851
NUCLEOSIDE/NUCLEOTIDE REVERSE TRANSCRIPTASE INHIBITORS (NRTIs/NtRTIs), 933–935
    abacavir, 932*t*, 934
    didanosine, 932*t*, 934
    emtricitabine, 932*t*, 933, 934–935, 943
    lamivudine, 917*t*, 918, 920, 931, 932*t*, 935
    stavudine, 932*t*, 935

    tenofovir. *See* tenofovir
    zidovudine. *See* zidovudine
Nucynta. *See* tapentadol
Nulojix. *See* belatacept
Nupercainal. *See* dibucaine
nurse anesthetists, 396*t*
Nursing Emergency Preparedness Education Coalition (NEPEC), 1303–1304
Nursing Practice Applications
    ACE inhibitors, 496–497*t*
    acne vulgaris, 1271–1272*t*
    adrenergic agonists, 187–189*t*
    aminoglycosides, 816–817*t*
    androgens, 1213–1214*t*
    anticoagulants, 624–626*t*
    antidiarrheals, 1030–1031*t*
    antidiuretic hormone, 1107–1108*t*
    antidysrhythmics, 610–611*t*
    antiemetics, 1042–1043*t*
    antiepileptic drugs, 329–331*t*
    antifungals, 879–880*t*
    antihistamines, 760–761*t*
    antineoplastic agents, 983–986*t*
    antipsychotics, 279–281*t*
    antivirals, 921–922*t*
    ARBs, 496–497*t*
    arthritis, 1251–1252*t*
    asthma, 746–748*t*
    benign prostatic hyperplasia, 1223–1224*t*
    calcium channel blockers, 482–483*t*
    central nervous system stimulants, 361–362*t*
    cephalosporins, 800–801*t*
    cholinergic agonists, 159–160*t*
    cholinergic antagonists, 173–174*t*
    colony-stimulating factors, 646, 648–649, 649–651*t*
    contraceptives, 1201–1202*t*
    COPD, 746–748*t*
    corticosteroids, 1160–1161*t*
    cough and colds, 768–769*t*
    diabetes mellitus, 1132–1134*t*
    direct vasodilators, 554–555*t*
    diuretics, 516–518*t*
    dyslipidemia, 468–469*t*
    enteral and parenteral nutrition, 1073–1075*t*
    erythropoietin, 647–648*t*
    estrogens, 1172–1173*t*
    fluid and electrolyte imbalances, 536–537*t*
    fluoroquinolones, 828–829*t*
    general anesthesia, 407–408*t*
    glaucoma, 1291–1292*t*
    growth hormone, 1104–1105*t*
    heart failure, 591–592*t*
    helminthic infections, 901–902*t*
    immunomodulators, 704–705*t*
    inflammation and fever, 685–686*t*
    insulin therapy, 1123–1124*t*
    laxatives, 1030–1031*t*
    lice or mite infestations, 1267–1268*t*
    local anesthesia, 412–413*t*
    macrolides, 816–817*t*
    migraines, 390–391*t*
    minerals, 1058–1059*t*
    muscle spasms and spasticity, 345–346*t*
    neurodegenerative diseases, 304–305*t*
    organic nitrates, 573–574*t*
    osteoporosis, 1234–1235*t*
    pain management, 380–381*t*
    penicillins, 800–801*t*
    peptic ulcer disease, 1019–1020*t*
    pharmacology and, 8–9
    poisonings, 1312–1313*t*
    progestins, 1175–1176*t*
    protozoan infections, 901–902*t*

Nursing Practice Applications (*continued*)
    substance abuse, 433*t*, 434
    tetracyclines, 816–817*t*
    thrombolytics, 633–634*t*
    thyroid disorders, 1143–1144*t*, 1147–1148*t*
    tuberculosis, 860–861*t*
    urinary tract infections, 843–844*t*
    vaccines, 724–725*t*
    vancomycin, 800–801*t*
    vitamins, 1058–1059*t*
nursing process, in medication error prevention, 72
Nursing Responsibilities
    abciximab, 630
    abilify, 279
    acarbose, 1129
    acetaminophen, 684
    acetazolamide, 516
    activated charcoal, 1310
    acyclovir, 912
    albuterol, 737
    aldesleukin, 695
    alendronate, 1241
    allopurinol, 1256
    alteplase, 632
    aluminum hydroxide, 1017
    amantadine, 915
    aminocaproic acid, 636
    amiodarone, 608
    ammonium chloride, 536
    amphetamine and dextroamphetamine, 356
    amphotericin B, 871
    ampicillin, 792
    aspirin, 678
    atenolol, 567
    atomoxetine, 357
    atorvastatin, 462
    atropine, 167
    azathioprine, 701
    basiliximab, 703
    beclomethasone, 741
    benzocaine, 1278
    benztropine, 295
    bethanechol, 154
    caffeine, 360
    calcitriol, 1238
    calcium salts, 1233
    carbamazepine, 324
    carbidopa/levodopa, 291
    celecoxib, 683
    cephalosporins, 796
    chloroquine, 889
    chlorpromazine, 272
    cholestyramine, 465
    ciprofloxacin, 826
    clomiphene, 1184
    clopidogrel, 628
    colchicine, 1255
    conjugated estrogens, 1171
    cromolyn, 743
    cyanocobalamin (vitamin B_{12}), 658, 1056
    cyclobenzaprine, 340
    cyclophosphamide, 966
    cyclosporine, 699
    dabigatran, 623
    dantrolene, 343
    dapsone, 862
    desmopressin, 1106
    dextran 40, 527
    dextromethorphan, 767
    5% dextrose in water, 526
    diazepam, 321
    digoxin, 588
    dimercaprol, 1311

diphenoxylate with atropine, 1029
disulfiram, 426
donepezil, 299
doxorubicin, 974
edetate calcium disodium, 1311
efavirenz, 936
epinephrine, 182
epoetin alfa, 646
erythromycin, 811
estradiol and norethindrone, 1195
ethosuximide, 325
fentanyl, 398
ferrous sulfate, 655
fexofenadine, 758
filgrastim, 648
finasteride, 1222
fluconazole, 873
fludrocortisone, 1162
fluoxetine, 250
fluticasone, 762
folic acid (vitamin B_9), 1055
furosemide, 509
gabapentin, 326
gemfibrozil, 466
gentamicin, 814
glucagon, 1116
glyburide, 1126
haloperidol, 274
heparin, 620
hepatitis B vaccine, 717
human regular insulin, 1119
hydralazine, 551
hydrochlorothiazide, 511
hydrocortisone, 1158
hydroxychloroquine, 1249
ibuprofen, 681
imipenem-cilastatin, 798
imipramine, 247
interferon alfa-2b, 692
interferon beta-1b, 302
ipratropium, 739
isoflurane, 404
isoniazid, 856
isoproterenol, 187
latanoprost, 1287
levothyroxine, 1142
lidocaine, 410
lisinopril, 492
lopinavir with ritonavir, 937
lorazepam, 227
losartan, 495
magnesium sulfate, 533
mannitol, 514
mebendazole, 900
medroxyprogesterone, 1173
metformin, 1127
methotrexate, 970
metoprolol, 202
metronidazole, 893
midazolam, 399
mifepristone, 1204–1205
milrinone, 590
modafinil, 359
morphine sulfate, 377
naloxone/buprenorphine, 385, 422–423
nifedipine, 479
nitrofurantoin, 842
nitroglycerin, 565
nitroprusside sodium, 553
nitrous oxide, 402
nonoxynol-9, 1200
normal serum albumin, 525
nystatin, 878

octreotide, 1102–1103
omeprazole, 1013
ondansetron, 1041
oprelvekin, 651–652
orlistat, 1084
oxytocin, 1179
pancrelipase, 1043
penicillin G, 791
permethrin, 1266
phenelzine, 255
phenobarbital, 233
phenylephrine, 185
phenytoin, 323
potassium chloride, 532
pramipexole, 292
prazosin, 196
procainamide, 605
procaine, 409
propofol, 400
propranolol, 200
propylthiouracil, 1146
pseudoephedrine, 764
psyllium mucilloid, 1027
pyridostigmine, 157
pyridoxine (vitamin B_6), 1055
pyrimethamine, 896
raloxifene, 1243
ranitidine, 1015
repaglinide, 1128
Rh$_o$ D immune globulin, 723
riboflavin (vitamin B_2), 1054
risperidone, 276
rosiglitazone, 1129
sildenafil, 1218
sitagliptin, 1130
sodium bicarbonate, 535
sodium chloride, 530
somatotropin, 1101
spironolactone, 513
succinylcholine, 172
sulfasalazine, 1034
sumatriptan, 388
tamoxifen, 978
tenofovir, 919
testosterone, 1212
tetracycline, 809
theophylline, 745
thiamine (vitamin B_1), 1054
timolol, 1290
tramadol, 382
tretinoin, 1270
trimethoprim-sulfamethoxazole, 840
valproic acid, 327
vancomycin, 799
varenicline, 432
venlafaxine, 251
verapamil, 481
vincristine, 981
vitamin A, 1051
vitamin C, 1056
vitamin D, 1052
vitamin E, 1053
vitamin K, 1053
warfarin, 622
zafirlukast, 744
zidovudine, 934
zolpidem, 229
nursing roles
    adverse drug effects and, 53–54, 122, 122*t*
    in bioterrorism, 1303–1304
    medication safety and error prevention, 72–74, 109–110
    prescriptive authority, 20–21

NutraSweet. *See* aspartame
nutritional considerations
  culture and, 128
  DASH diet, 195*t*
  dyslipidemia and, 457–458
  iron requirements during pregnancy, 643*t*
  ketogenic diet, 312, 312*t*, 315
  myasthenia gravis and, 158*t*
  supplemental, 1062–1077. *See also* enteral
      nutrition; parenteral nutrition
Nutropin. *See* somatropin
NuvaRing, 29, 1197–1198, 1198*f*
Nuvigil. *See* armodafinil
NYHA (New York Heart Association), 581–582
NyQuil, 765
nystatin, 112*t*, 868, 875*t*, 876, 877–878
Nystex. *See* nystatin
Nystop. *See* nystatin
Nytol. *See* diphenhydramine

O

OA. *See* osteoarthritis
obesity, 1078–1088
  adjuncts to therapy for, 1085–1086
  cultural differences in, 1080*t*
  diabetes mellitus and, 1113
  etiology of, 1079
  genetic influences in, 1079
  measurement of, 1080, 1081*f*, 1081*t*
  nonpharmacologic therapies for,
      1080–1082, 1083*t*
  pathogenesis of, 1079–1080
  pharmacotherapy, 1082–1085, 1083*t*
  prevalence of, 1079, 1079*t*
obinutuzumab, 987*t*
OBS (organic brain syndrome), 271
obsessive-compulsive disorder (OCD), 218–219, 232
Octagam. *See* intravenous immune globulin
octreotide, 616*t*, 1028*t*, 1029, 1100*t*, 1102–1103
OcuClear. *See* oxymetazoline
Ocuflox. *See* ofloxacin
OCULAR DECONGESTANTS/VASOCONSTRICTORS, 185,
      1293*t*, 1294
  naphazoline, 185, 764*t*, 1293*t*
  oxymetazoline, 185, 763, 764*t*, 1293*t*
  phenylephrine. *See* phenylephrine
  tetrahydrozoline, 183, 185, 764*t*, 1293*t*
ocular herpes, 910
OCULAR LUBRICANTS, 1294
  lanolin alcohol, 1293*t*
  polyvinyl alcohol, 1293*t*
Ocupress. *See* carteolol
Ocusert. *See* pilocarpine
ODTs (orally disintegrating tablets), 28, 28*t*
ofatumumab, 987*t*
off-label indications, 5, 18, 106*t*
ofloxacin, 823*t*, 826–827, 835, 853*t*, 858–859
Ogen. *See* stropipate
OGTTs (oral glucose tolerance tests), 1114
OHS (ovarian hyperstimulation syndrome), 1183
OKT3. *See* muromonab-CD3
olanzapine
  adverse effects, 277
  clinical applications, 248, 260, 277, 297
  fluoxetine and, 249
  routes and dosages, 258*t*, 275*t*
older adults. *See* geriatric patients
Oleptro. *See* trazodone
Olestra, 1085
oligomenorrhea, 1171
oligomeric formulas, for enteral nutrition, 1064
oligospermia, 1215

olmesartan medoxomil, 479, 494*t*, 495, 546*t*, 548
olopatadine, 756–757, 756*t*, 759, 1294, 1295*t*
olsalazine, 1032, 1033*t*, 1035
Olysia. *See* simeprevir
omacetaxine, 980*t*
omalizumab, 745
OME (otitis media with effusion), 108*t*
omega-3 fatty acids, 87, 87*t*, 461*t*, 467, 562*t*, 1154*t*
omeprazole
  adverse effects, 1012
  clinical applications, 1011–1012, 1017, 1041
  in combination products, 379
  interactions with, 86*t*, 622*t*, 1012
  mechanism of action, 1012
  Nursing Responsibilities, 1013
  over-the-counter availability of, 1010
  routes and dosages, 1011*t*
Omnaris. *See* ciclesonide
Omnicef. *See* cefdinir
Omontys. *See* peginesatide
onabotulinumtoxinA, 341*t*, 343–344, 343–344*t*,
      344*f*, 389
Oncaspar. *See* pegaspargase
oncology nurses, 992
Oncovin. *See* vincristine
ondansetron
  adverse effects, 292, 1040
  clinical applications, 271, 375, 413, 957, 1040
  mechanism of action, 1040
  Nursing Responsibilities, 1041
  routes and dosages, 1039*t*
Onfi. *See* clobazam
Onglyza. *See* saxagliptin
on–off syndrome, 288
Onsolis. *See* fentanyl
onychomycosis, 876, 876*t*
Opana. *See* oxymorphone
OPC (oropharyngeal candidiasis), 876, 876*t*, 877
open-angle glaucoma, 1285*f*, 1286, 1294*t*
Ophthaine. *See* proparacaine
ophthalmic route of administration, 29.
      See also eyes
opioid(s). *See also* OPIOID ANALGESICS
  addiction to, 421–423
  as anesthetics, 396–398, 397*t*
  in antitussives, 765–766, 766*t*
  defined, 372, 421
  for diarrhea, 1028–1030, 1028*t*
  drug interactions, 86*t*, 425*t*
  overdose/poisoning, 1308*t*
  withdrawal symptoms and treatment, 420*t*
OPIOID ANALGESICS
  abuse of, 375, 384–385
  adverse effects of, 373, 374–375*t*, 375–376, 385
  breast-feeding and, 98–99*t*
  classification of, 373, 374*t*
  dependence on, 375
  drug interactions, 58
  equianalgesic doses, 374*t*, 376
  in geriatric patients, 122*t*
  mechanism of action, 372–373, 373*f*, 373*t*
  mixed opioid agonist-antagonists. *See* MIXED
      OPIOID AGONIST-ANTAGONISTS
  opioid agonists, 372, 373*f*, 376–379
      codeine. *See* codeine
      fentanyl, 105*t*, 374*t*, 377, 396–398, 397*t*
      hydrocodone, 374*t*, 377, 765, 766*t*
      hydromorphone, 374*t*, 375, 377, 1041
      levorphanol, 374*t*, 377
      meperidine, 374*t*, 375, 377–378, 425*t*
      methadone, 374*t*, 378, 419, 422
      morphine sulfate. *See* morphine sulfate
      oxycodone, 374*t*, 378, 385, 417, 422

overdoses, 384–385
tolerance to, 375, 385
OPIOID ANTAGONISTS, 372, 373*f*, 384–385, 385*t*
  drugs in class
      naloxone, 61, 327, 377, 385,
          385*t*, 1308*t*
      naltrexone, 385*t*, 426, 1083*t*
  indications, 384–385
  mechanism of action, 372, 373*f*
opioid receptors, 372, 373, 373*f*
opium, 223, 372
opportunistic infections, in HIV/AIDS patients
  fungal, 869
  M. avium complex, 849, 863
  pharmacotherapy, 944, 944*t*
  tuberculosis, 849, 852
oprelvekin
  adverse effects, 651
  clinical applications, 649, 651, 693,
      957, 991
  Lifespan and Diversity Considerations, 652
  mechanism of action, 651
  Nursing Responsibilities, 651–652
  Patient and Family Education, 652
  routes and dosages, 645*t*
OptiPranolol. *See* metipranolol
Optivar. *See* azelastine
OPV (oral polio vaccine), 719
Oracea. *See* doxycycline
oral antidiabetics. *See* ANTIDIABETIC AGENTS
oral cancer, 950
ORAL CONTRACEPTIVES
  adverse effects of, 55*t*, 130, 1196–1197, 1196*t*
  breast-feeding and, 98*t*
  drug interactions, 86*t*, 202, 227, 233, 622*t*
  estrogen-progestin combinations, 1190,
      1193–1195
  excretion of, 36
  macular edema and, 1199*t*
  for men, 1195*t*
  Nursing Practice Applications, 1201–1202*t*
  pregnancy category, 95*t*
  prevalence of use, 1190*t*, 1193*t*
  progestin-only, 1195–1196
  types of, 1193*t*, 1194*f*
oral glucose tolerance tests (OGTTs), 1114
oral iron salts, 656, 656*t*
oral polio vaccine (OPV), 719
oral route of administration
  absorption and, 28–29
  for antineoplastic agents, 955–956
  barriers encountered in, 25, 25*f*
  in pediatric patients, 106
oral soluble films, 28
orally disintegrating tablets (ODTs), 28, 28*t*
Oramorph SR. *See* morphine sulfate
"Orange Book" (FDA), 5, 7
Orap. *See* pimozide
Oravig. *See* miconazole
Orencia. *See* abatacept
OREXIN RECEPTOR ANTAGONISTS, 225*t*, 230
organ transplantation, 695, 695*t*, 698
organic brain syndrome (OBS), 271
ORGANIC NITRATES
  for angina pectoris, 563, 563*f*, 564–566,
      564*t*, 568*t*
  drugs in class
      isosorbide dinitrate, 425*t*, 564, 566, 568*t*,
          584*t*, 586
      isosorbide mononitrate, 566, 568*t*
      nitroglycerin. *See* nitroglycerin
  for myocardial infarction, 572
  Nursing Practice Applications, 573–574*t*

organic solvents, 1307

organophosphate pesticide poisoning, 155, 166, 1308*t*

organ-specific toxicity, 56–58, 56*t*, 85

Orgaran. *See* danaparoid

Orinase. *See* tolbutamide

orlistat, 1082–1085, 1083*t*

Ornidyl. *See* eflornithine

oropharyngeal candidiasis (OPC), 876, 876*t*, 877

orphan diseases, defined, 14

Orphan Drug Act of 1983, 14

orphenadrine, 339*t*, 341

Ortho Micronor, 1196

Ortho Tri-Cyclen, 1193*t*

Orthoclone. *See* muromonab-CD3

Ortho-Cyclen-28, 1193*t*

Ortho-Evra, 1197

orthomyxoviruses, 908*t*

Ortho-Novum. *See* estradiol and norethindrone

orthostatic hypotension

    in ACE inhibitors, 491

    in carvedilol, 200

    defined, 195

    in doxazosin, 196

    in opioids, 375

    in organic nitrates, 565

    in tricyclic antidepressants, 246

oseltamivir, 914, 914*t*, 915

Oseni, 1125*t*, 1131

Osmitrol. *See* mannitol

Osmoglyn. *See* glycerin

osmolality, 522, 1103, 1105

osmosis, 523

OSMOTIC DIURETICS, 505, 506*f*, 513–515

    glycerin, 513*t*, 514

    isosorbide, 1288*t*, 1292

    mannitol, 513*t*, 514, 1106, 1288*t*, 1292

    urea, 513*t*, 515

osmotic laxatives, 1026

osmotic pressure, 442

ospemiphene, 1175

Osphema. *See* ospemiphene

osteoarthritis (OA)

    nonpharmacologic therapies, 1245–1246, 1247*t*

    Nursing Practice Applications, 1251–1252*t*

    pathophysiology, 1244–1245, 1246*f*

    pharmacotherapy for, 1246

osteomalacia, 1236–1237

osteoporosis

    Nursing Practice Applications, 1234–1235*t*

    pathophysiology, 1236, 1236*f*

    pharmacotherapy, 1236, 1240*t*, 1243*t*

    prevalence of, 1230*t*

    proton pump inhibitors and, 1013*t*

    risk factors for, 1155

osteosarcomas, 951

OTC products. *See* over-the-counter products

Otezla. *See* apremilast

otic route of administration, 29. *See also* ears

otitis interna, 1297

otitis media, 1296–1297

otitis media with effusion (OME), 108*t*

ototoxicity, 57, 507–508

Otrexup. *See* methotrexate

Otrivin. *See* xylometazoline

ovarian cycle, 1167, 1168*f*, 1174

ovarian hyperstimulation syndrome (OHS), 1183

overactive bladder. *See* incontinence

overhydration, 1067*t*

overseas pharmacies, 8

over-the-counter (OTC) products. *See also specific products*

    dietary supplements. *See* dietary supplements

    herbal supplements. *See* herbal supplements

prescription vs., 19

    regulation of, 14

overweight concerns. *See* obesity

Ovide. *See* malathion

Ovidrel. *See* chorionic gonadotropin-HCG

ovulation, 1167

ovulatory dysfunction, 1181

oxacillin, 616*t*, 789*t*, 793

oxaliplatin, 964*t*, 967

Oxandrin. *See* oxandrolone

oxandrolone, 1210*t*, 1214

oxaprozin, 680–681*t*

oxazepam, 225–226*t*, 228, 384, 419

OXAZOLIDINONES, 815. *See also* linezolid

oxcarbazepine, 105*t*, 112*t*, 260, 313*t*, 318*t*, 324–325

oxicams, 682

oxiconazole, 875*t*

Oxistat. *See* oxiconazole

Oxtellar XR. *See* oxcarbazepine

oxybutynin chloride, 165*t*, 166, 168

oxycodone, 374*t*, 378, 385, 417, 422

OxyContin. *See* oxycodone

oxymetazoline, 185, 763, 764*t*, 1293*t*

oxymetholone, 1210*t*, 1214

oxymorphone, 374*t*

OXYTOCICS, 1176–1179. *See also* UTERINE STIMULANTS

oxytocin

    breast-feeding and, 98*t*, 1177*f*

    clinical applications, 1176, 1177–1178

    Nursing Practice Applications, 1180–1181*t*

    regulation of, 1094*t*

    release of, 1092, 1098

    routes and dosages, 1177*t*

Oxytrol. *See* oxybutynin chloride

P

P waves, 599, 599*f*, 600*t*

PABA (para-aminobenzoic acid), 778, 837, 839*f*, 1278

pacemakers, 601

Pacerone. *See* amiodarone

Pacific yew, 980

packed red blood cells, 524*t*, 525

paclitaxel, 963, 980, 980*t*, 982

Paget's disease, 1237

PAHs (polycyclic aromatic hydrocarbons), 60*t*

pain

    classification and assessment of, 367–368, 370*t*

    gate control theory of, 369–370

    in low back, 368*t*

    management of. *See* pain management

    in multiple sclerosis, 303

    in pediatric patients, 370*t*

    phases of pain physiology, 369–370, 369*f*

pain management, 367–385

    in geriatric patients, 382*t*

    goals of, 367

    in multiple sclerosis, 303

    in myocardial infarction, 572

    myths regarding, 368–369

    nonpharmacologic therapies for, 370

    Nursing Practice Applications, 380–381*t*

    pharmacologic therapies, 370–385

        adjuvant analgesics, 383–384, 384*t*

        for cancer pain, 372, 383

        combination drugs, 371–372

        mechanism of action, 371, 371*f*

        nonopioid analgesics, 379, 379*t*, 382–383

        opioids. *See* OPIOID ANALGESICS

        patient-controlled analgesia, 372

        selection of, 370–371

    in surgery, 411

paliperidone, 269, 275*t*, 277

palliation, 951

pallidotomy, 288, 288*t*

palonosetron, 1037, 1039*t*, 1041

Pamelor. *See* nortriptyline

pamidronate, 384, 1239–1240*t*, 1241

Pamine. *See* methscopolamine

Panax quinquefolius. See ginseng

pancreas, 1001

pancreatic cancer, 951, 951*t*

pancreatic islet cells, 1092, 1112

pancreatitis, 1041, 1041*t*, 1043–1044

Pancreaze. *See* pancrelipase

pancrelipase, 1041, 1043–1044, 1068

pancuronium, 169*t*, 173

pancytopenia, 57

panic attacks, 218, 220

panic disorder, 218, 227

panitumumab, 987*t*

pantoprazole, 1011*t*, 1013

Papanicolaou (Pap) smears, 951

Papaver somniferum, 372

papaverine-phentolamine, 1217

papovaviruses, 908*t*

para-aminobenzoic acid (PABA), 778, 837, 839*f*, 1278

Paracetaldehyde. *See* paraldehyde

Paraflex. *See* chlorzoxazone

parafollicular cells, 1138

Parafon Forte. *See* chlorzoxazone

ParaGard, 1277

paraldehyde, 228

paramyxoviruses, 908*t*

paranoia, 266*t*

Paraplatin. *See* carboplatin

parasympathetic nervous system, structure and function of, 138–140, 139*f*

parasympathomimetics. *See* cholinergic agonists

parathyroid hormone (PTH), 1092, 1094*t*, 1230–1231

Parcopa. *See* levodopa/carbidopa

Paregoric. *See* camphorated opium tincture

parenteral iron salts, 656–657

parenteral nutrition

    administration of, 1063, 1069, 1070*f*

    complications, 1071–1072, 1071*t*

    components of, 1070–1071

    food and drug interactions with, 1072

    home care for patients on, 1073*t*

    indications for, 1069, 1069*t*

    Nursing Practice Applications, 1073–1075*t*

parenteral route of administration, 30

parents, role in medication error prevention, 70*t*

paricalcitol, 1238*t*, 1239

parietal cells, 998

Parjeta. *See* pertuzumab

Parkinson's disease (PD), 286–295

    characteristics of, 286, 286*t*

    etiologies of, 287

    neurodegeneration prevention in, 293*t*

    nonpharmacologic therapies for, 288, 288*t*

    pathophysiology, 287

    pharmacotherapy, 288–295

        amantadine, 293

        anticholinergics, 288, 294–295, 294*t*

        antihistamines, 757

        COMT inhibitors, 290*t*, 293

        dopamine agonists, 288, 290*t*, 291–293

        levodopa replacement therapy, 288–291, 289*f*, 290*t*

        loss of drug effect, 288

        MAO-B inhibitors, 290*t*, 294

        muscarinic antagonists, 166, 168

    prevalence of, 286*t*

    symptoms of, 287

Parlodel. *See* bromocriptine

Parnate. *See* tranylcypromine

paromomycin

    adverse effects, 814, 893

    clinical applications, 812, 814, 890, 891, 893, 895

    routes and dosages, 812*t*, 892*t*

paroxetine

    for anxiety disorders, 231, 232

    for depression, 250

    drug interactions, 5*t*, 425*t*, 622*t*

    indications for, 231*t*

    for irritable bowel syndrome, 1036

    for neuropathic pain, 383

    routes and dosages, 245*t*

paroxysmal supraventricular tachycardia (PSVT), 600

partial agonists, 48, 48*f*

PARTIAL FATTY-ACID OXIDATION INHIBITORS, 563

partial parenteral nutrition, 1069

partial (focal) seizures, 313*t*, 314, 323

Paser. *See* aminosalicylic acid

pasireotide, 1163

passive immunity, 710–711, 721–723, 722*f*

passive transport, 26–27, 27*f*

Patanase. *See* olopatadine

Patanol. *See* olopatadine

patent medicines, 13, 13*f*

pathogenicity, 775

pathogens, 775

Patient and Family Education

    aminocaproic acid, 636

    benzocaine, 1279

    clomiphene, 1185

    cyanocobalamin (vitamin B$_{12}$), 658

    dapsone, 862

    ferrous sulfate, 656

    glucagon, 1116

    lithium carbonate, 259–260

    mifepristone, 1205

    nonoxynol-9, 1200

    octreotide, 1103

    oprelvekin, 652

    orlistat, 1084–1085

    pancrelipase, 1043–1044

    sildenafil, 1218

    succinylcholine, 172

    sulfasalazine, 1034

Patient Education

    complementary and alternative medicine, 87

    food–drug interactions, 62*t*

    medication errors, 73–74

Patient Protection and Affordable Care Act of 2010, 21

Patient Safety

    accidental poisonings at home, 1309*t*

    concentrated electrolyte solutions, 532*t*

    concurrent medication administration, 466*t*

    EpiPen⁻ autoinjectors, 183*t*

    eyedrops, reactions to, 1295*t*

    incomplete medication orders, 1178*t*

    infusion calculations, 1035*t*

    insulin dosages, 1121*t*

    interaction prevention, 5*t*

    iron poisoning in pediatric patients, 654*t*

    isoniazid overdose, 859*t*

    levofloxacin, 826*t*

    medication errors, 110*t*, 172*t*

    MMR vaccine, 719*t*

    packaging, 620*t*

    photosensitivity and antibiotics, 808*t*

    plasma drug concentrations, 1219*t*

    similar drug names, 1237*t*

    trimethoprim-sulfamethoxazole, 839*t*

patient-controlled analgesia (PCA), 372

Pavabid. *See* papaverine-phentolamine

Pavulon. *See* pancuronium

Paxil/Paxil CR. *See* paroxetine

Paxipam. *See* halazepam

pazopanib, 987*t*

PBPs (penicillin-binding proteins), 787, 788

PCA (patient-controlled analgesia), 372

PCI (percutaneous coronary intervention), 571

PCP (phencyclidine), 96*t*, 417, 428–429

PCV (pneumococcal conjugate vaccine), 715

PD. *See* Parkinson's disease

PDUFA (Prescription Drug User Fee Act of 1992), 14, 19

Pediamycin. *See* erythromycin

pediatric patients, 103–115

    ADHD in, 352, 352–353*t*

    adherence issues in, 113

    adverse drug effects in, 106, 110–113, 112*t*

    anxiety disorders in, 234*t*

    asthma in, 1155*t*

    bipolar disorder in, 258*t*

    cerebral palsy in, 337*t*

    cholesterol screening for, 463*t*

    commonly prescribed medications for, 104, 104*t*

    defined, 107

    diabetes mellitus in, 1121*t*

    dosage calculations for, 110, 111*f*

    dwarfism in, 1098–1099

    dyslipidemia in, 458*t*

    fever in, 682*t*

    Graves' disease in, 1144*t*

    herpesviruses in, 910

    hypertension in, 480*t*

    immunosuppressants in, 698*t*

    inhalant abuse and, 422*t*

    iron poisoning in, 654*t*

    medication errors and, 70*t*, 109–110, 110*t*

    metabolism in, 35

    multiple sclerosis in, 304*t*

    NSAIDs for, 379

    off-label prescribing for, 106*t*

    oropharyngeal candidiasis in, 876*t*, 877

    pain in, 370*t*

    pharmacokinetic variables in, 106–107

    pharmacologic implications associated with development, 107–109

    routes of administration for, 28

    schizophrenia in, 268*t*

    seizures in, 312, 313, 314–315

    suicide risk in, 244*t*

    testing and labeling of drugs for, 104–105, 105*t*

    urinary tract infections in, 836

    vaccines for, 712

    weight gain with atypical antipsychotic use, 278*t*

Pediatric Research Equity Act of 2003 (PREA), 105

Pediatrix, 917

PEDICULICIDES, 1265

    lindane, 1265, 1266

    malathion, 1265, 1266

    Nursing Practice Application, 1267–1268*t*

    permethrin, 1265–1266

    pyrethrin, 1265, 1266

Pediculus humanus capitis, 1265

Pediculus humanus corporis, 1265

PEG (percutaneous endoscopic gastrostomy) tubes, 1064

pegaspargase, 989–990, 990*t*

Pegasys. *See* pegIFN alfa-2a

pegfilgrastim, 645*t*, 648–649

pegIFN alfa-2a, 692*t*, 693, 917*t*, 920–921, 983, 988

pegIFN alfa-2b, 692*t*, 693, 917*t*, 920–921, 983, 988

peginesatide, 646

Pegintron. *See* pegIFN alfa-2b

pegloticase, 1254*t*, 1256

pegvisomant, 1100*t*, 1103

pegylation, 691

pemetrexed, 968, 969*t*, 972

pemirolast, 1294, 1295*t*

Pen Tsao (Great Herbal), 3

penbutolol, 198*t*, 200

penciclovir, 911*t*, 913

Penetrex. *See* enoxacin

PENICILLIN(s), 788–793

    adverse effects, 56*t*, 783, 790

    breast-feeding and, 98*t*

    broad-spectrum (aminopenicillins), 791–792

        amoxicillin, 111, 112*t*, 789*t*, 792, 1017, 1297

        ampicillin. *See* ampicillin

    characteristics of, 789

    cross-sensitivity with cephalosporins, 790, 795

    extended-spectrum (antipseudomonal), 792–793

        piperacillin, 616*t*, 789*t*, 792, 793

        ticarcillin, 789*t*, 792, 793, 1297

    history of, 788

    interactions with, 62*t*, 622*t*

    lactation risk categories, 99*t*

    mechanism of action, 778, 787–788, 788*f*

    natural, 790–791

        penicillin G, 112*t*, 790–791

        penicillin G benzathine, 789*t*, 791

        penicillin G potassium, 789*t*, 791

        penicillin G procaine, 789*t*, 791

        penicillin V, 789*t*, 791

    Nursing Practice Applications, 800–801*t*

    penicillinase-resistant (antistaphylococcal), 793–794

        dicloxacillin, 622*t*, 789*t*, 793

        nafcillin, 789*t*, 793

        oxacillin, 616*t*, 789*t*, 793

    pregnancy category, 95, 95*t*

    resistance to, 779, 780, 788, 790*f*

    routes and dosages of, 789*t*

penicillinase, 788

penicillin-binding proteins (PBPs), 787, 788

penis, 1216, 1216*f*

Penlac. *See* ciclopirox nail lacquer

Pentacarinat. *See* pentamidine

Pentam. *See* pentamidine

pentamidine, 504*t*, 892*t*, 895

pentazocine, 374*t*, 378–379

pentobarbital, 233*t*

Pentostam. *See* sodium stibogluconate

pentostatin, 969*t*, 972

Pentothal. *See* thiopental sodium

pentoxifylline, 626*t*, 630–631

Pepcid. *See* famotidine

peppermint, 1037

pepsin, 1005

peptic ulcer disease (PUD)

    etiology and pathogenesis of, 1005–1007

    nonpharmacologic management of, 1008

    Nursing Practice Applications, 1019–1020*t*

    pharmacotherapy, 1008–1018

        adverse effects, 1009

        antacids, 59, 200, 1015–1017, 1015*t*

        goals of, 1008

        histamine (H$_2$) receptor antagonists, 411, 1013–1015, 1014*t*

        for *H.pylori* infections, 1017–1018

        macrolides, 809

        mechanisms of action, 1008–1009, 1010*f*

        miscellaneous agents, 1018

        proton pump inhibitors, 724, 1010–1013, 1011–1013*t*

        tetracyclines, 807

    prevalence of, 1006*t*

peptic ulcer disease (PUD) (*continued*)
 risk factors for, 1005–1006, 1007, 1155
 symptoms of, 1007
peptidoglycan, 778, 787
Pepto-Bismol. *See* bismuth subsalicylate
Percocet, 378, 422
Percodan, 378, 422
percutaneous coronary intervention (PCI), 571
percutaneous endoscopic gastrostomy (PEG)
 tubes, 1064
perennial allergic rhinitis, 754
Perforomist. *See* formoterol
Periactin. *See* cycloheptadine
perindopril, 491*t*, 493, 548
Periostat. *See* doxycycline
peripheral nervous system (PNS), 137, 138*f*. *See also*
 autonomic nervous system; somatic
 nervous system
peripheral resistance, 449
peripheral vascular disease (PVD), 630
peripheral vein parenteral nutrition (PPN), 1069
peripherally inserted central catheter (PICC)
 lines, 956
peristalsis, 997
periwinkle, 980
permethrin, 1265–1266
pernicious anemia, 657–658
perphenazine, 271*t*, 273, 1039*t*
Persantine. *See* dipyridamole
personalized medicine, 131*t*
pertussis (whooping cough), 713*t*, 714
pertussis immunization, 712
pertuzumab, 987*t*
petit mal seizures. *See* absence seizures
Pexeva. *See* paroxetine
peyote, 428, 428*f*
PFDA (Pure Food and Drug Act of 1906), 13–14
pH, 533
phagocytes, 667
pharmacodynamics, 42–51
 agonists and antagonists, 48, 48*f*
 defined, 43
 dose–response relationship, 44–45, 45*f*
 drug interactions and, 60–61, 61*f*
 in geriatric patients, 120
 interpatient variability and, 43, 43*f*
 pharmacogenetics, 48–49, 130, 130*f*
 potency and efficacy, 45–46, 46*f*
 receptor theory, 46–48, 47*f*
 therapeutic index, 44, 44*f*
pharmacogenetics, 48–49, 130, 130*f*
pharmacokinetics, 24–41
 defined, 25
 drug interactions and, 58–60, 59*f*
 in geriatric patients, 118–120
 in pediatric patients, 106–107
 pregnancy, alteration of responses
 during, 93–94, 93*f*
 processes, 26–36
 absorption, 27–31, 31*f*
 active transport, 27
 diffusion, 26–27, 27*f*
 distribution, 31–32, 32*f*
 excretion, 35–36, 36*f*
 metabolism, 33–35, 33*t*, 34*f*
 overview, 26, 26*f*
 time-response relationships, 36–39, 37*f*
pharmacologic classification, 5, 6, 6*t*
pharmacology
 clinical nursing practice and, 8–9
 defined, 4
 history of, 3
pharmacopeias, 15

pharmacotherapy
 alternative therapies. *See* Complementary and
 Alternative Therapies
 cultural and ethnic variables in, 127–128
 defined, 4
 gender influences on, 130–131
 genetic influences on, 128–130, 129–130*f*, 129*t*
 in geriatric patients. *See* geriatric patients
 in pediatric patients. *See* pediatric patients
 during pregnancy and lactation. *See* lactation;
 pregnancy
 psychosocial influences on, 177
 rationale for, 4–5, 4*f*
Pharmacotherapy Illustrated
 active and passive immunity, 722*f*
 alcohol metabolism, 424*f*
 Alzheimer's drugs, 298*f*
 analgesics, 371*f*
 angina medications, 563*f*
 antiemetics, 1038*f*
 antiepileptic drugs, 316*f*
 antihypertensives, 545*f*
 antimicrobial drugs, 779*f*
 antiparkinson drugs, 289*f*
 antiprostatic drugs, 1220*f*
 antipsychotic drugs, 267*f*
 antiulcer drugs, 1010*f*
 anxiety disorders, brain regions responsible for,
 219–220, 219*f*
 contraceptives, 1192*f*
 corticosteroids and adrenal atrophy, 1157*f*
 diuretics, 506*f*
 first-pass effect, 34*f*
 gastroesophageal reflux disease, 1009*f*
 heart failure drugs, 583*f*
 HIV/AIDS replication, 928*f*
 immunosuppressants, 697*f*
 infertility agents, 1184*t*
 inflammatory bowel disease, 1032*f*
 joint disorders, 1245*f*
 lipid-lowering drugs, 460*f*
 monoclonal antibodies, 989*f*
 myasthenia gravis, 156*f*
 NSAID-induced ulcer formation, 677*f*
 synaptic transmission, 141*f*
 thrombolytic therapy, 570*f*
PharmFacts
 ACE inhibitors in diabetes, 491*t*
 acetaminophen and liver failure, 1000*t*
 Addison's disease, 1156*t*
 ADHD, 352*t*
 adherence to medications, 74*t*
 adrenaline/epinephrine, 144*t*
 adverse drug reactions, 54*t*, 55
 allergic rhinitis, 754*t*
 Alzheimer's disease, 210*t*, 295*t*, 311*t*
 Amanita mushroom poisoning, 153*t*
 amebiasis, 890*t*
 anabolic steroids, 1214*t*
 anesthesia-related deaths, 404*t*
 angina pectoris, 562*t*
 antibacterial additives, 790*t*
 antibiotic resistance, 779*t*
 antidepressant use in pregnancy, 95*t*
 antigen-presenting cells, 671*t*
 anxiety disorders, 218*t*, 219*t*
 arthritis, 1246*t*
 asthma, 733*t*, 735*t*
 bacterial population of skin, 667*t*
 Beers criteria, 122*t*
 blood donations, 524*t*
 blood vessels, 449*t*
 bubonic plague, 809*t*

caffeine intake during pregnancy, 360*t*
cancer, 949*t*, 951*t*, 959*t*, 972*t*, 983*t*
cardiac output, 445*t*
central-line associated bloodstream infections, 798*t*
cerebral palsy, 341*t*
cholesterol screening for pediatric patients, 463*t*
colds, 765*t*
conduction of nerve impulses, 211*t*
Corynebacterium diphtheriae, 814*t*
cultural differences in obesity, 1080*t*
Cushing's syndrome, 1163*t*
depression, 240*t*, 241*t*
diabetes, cultural differences in, 128*t*
diabetes insipidus, 1105*t*
diabetes mellitus, 1112*t*
drug approval process, 18*t*, 19*t*
drug poisoning in pediatric patients, 113*t*
dysfunctional uterine bleeding, 1171*t*
dystonia, 336*t*
eczema, 1271*t*
emergency room visits due to drugs, 20*t*
energy drinks, 999*t*
epidural anesthesia, 396*t*
epilepsy, 311*t*
fluoroquinolones, 825*t*
gastroesophageal reflux disease, 1008*t*
generic drug perceptions, 8*t*
genital herpes, 910*t*
geriatric population growth, 117*t*
giardiasis, 890*t*
gingival hyperplasia, 479*t*
glaucoma, 1286*t*
Graves' disease, 1144*t*
health insurance, cultural differences in, 128*t*
heart failure, 579*t*
hemophilia, 637*t*
hemorrhagic fevers, 1306*t*
hepatitis B, 918*t*
HIV/AIDS, 927*t*
homeostasis, 443*t*
homocysteine, 657*t*
human papillomavirus, 720*t*
hypercholesterolemia, 465*t*
hypertension, 542*t*
hypertensive crisis, 553*t*
indoor tanning, 1052*t*, 1266*t*
infectious diseases as cause of death, 775*t*
iron, 643*t*
kidney transplants, 502*t*
labyrinthitis, 1297*t*
leprosy, 859*t*
long QT syndrome (LQTS), 599*t*
low back pain, 368*t*
lymphangiogenesis, 665*t*
magnesium, 533*t*
malaria, 886*t*
marijuana, 421*t*
medication errors, 67*t*, 70*t*
medication overdoses, 1308*t*
menopause, 1174*t*
migraine statistics, 386*t*
morning sickness, 1037*t*
multiple sclerosis, 304*t*
muscle spasticity after spinal cord injury, 337*t*
myasthenia gravis, 155*t*
myocardial infarction, 572*t*
neurons, 214*t*
nicotine, prevalence of use, 431*t*
nicotine replacement therapy in pregnancy, 97*t*
NSAIDs, 674*t*, 682*t*
nuclear accidents, 1308*t*
nurse anesthetists, 396*t*
obesity, 1079*t*

off-label prescribing in pediatrics, 106t
onychomycosis, 876t
oral contraceptives, 1190t, 1193t
orally disintegrating tablets, 28t
organ transplants, 695t
osteoporosis, 1230t
pancreatitis, 1041t
Parkinson's disease, 286t
peptic ulcer disease, 1006t
pheochromocytomas, 178t
pneumonia, 913t
polycyclic aromatic hydrocarbons, 60t
prescription use, 3t
prostate cancer, 1219t
pseudoephedrine, 763t
pseudogout, 1255t
in psoriasis, 1274t
renal failure, 504t
salicylate poisoning, 676t
schizophrenia, 265t, 268t
seizures, 315t, 320t
sleep and diabetes, relationship between, 230t
sleep disorders, 223t, 358t
sleep-wake patterns, 220t
Staphylococcus aureus, 782t
steroid-induced open-angle glaucoma, 1294t
stomach size, 997t
substance abuse, 417t, 418t
sudden cardiac arrest, 609t
suicide risk in pediatric patients, 244t
T cells, 670–671t
thyroid gland in pregnancy, 1139t
tuberculosis, 849t
undernourished patients, assessment of, 1069t
urinary tract infections, 836t
varicella zoster virus, 720t
venous thrombosis, 616t
vitamin toxicity, 1050t
vulvovaginal candidiasis, 877t
Phenazine. See perphenazine
phencyclidine (PCP), 96t, 417, 428–429
phenelzine, 178, 254–255
Phenergan. See promethazine
Phenergan with Codeine. See promethazine
phenobarbital
adverse effects, 56t, 233, 616t
clinical applications, 232–233, 320
distribution of, 119
drug interactions, 60, 320, 425t
enzyme induction and, 34
mechanism of action, 233
nursing responsibilities, 233
overdose treatment, 233
routes and dosages, 233t
for seizures, 313t, 318t
PHENOTHIAZINES, 270–273
adverse effects, 1215t
antipsychotic, 270–273, 271t
breast-feeding and, 99t
chlorpromazine, 56t, 265, 271t, 272, 425t, 616t
drug interactions, 86t, 200, 247
fluphenazine, 271, 271t, 273
for nausea and vomiting, 1038, 1039t
perphenazine, 271t, 273, 1039t
prochlorperazine, 29, 271t, 273, 386, 957, 1039t
thioridazine, 271, 271t, 273
trifluoperazine, 271t, 273
phenoxybenzamine, 193, 194t, 196
phensuximide, 325
phentermine, 1082, 1083t, 1085
phentolamine
adverse effects, 193
for extravasation, 180, 183, 184, 342

for hypertension, 196–197, 356, 553t
with papaverine, 1217
routes and dosages, 194t
phenylacetic acids, 681
phenylbutazone, 56t, 59
phenylephrine
adverse effects, 184–185
chemical structure of, 179
clinical applications and considerations, 183, 184–185, 763
in combination products, 757t, 766t
mechanism of action, 184
nursing responsibilities, 185
routes and dosages, 181t, 764t, 1293t
phenylpropanolamine, 766t, 1082
Phenytek. See phenytoin
phenytoin
adverse effects, 55–56t, 616t
breast-feeding and, 98t
clinical applications and considerations, 322–323
drug interactions, 59, 425t, 622t, 1069
for dysrhythmias, 603t, 605
in geriatric patients, 122t
mechanism of action, 316
for neuropathic pain, 383
pregnancy category, 95t
protein binding in, 106, 119, 312
for seizures, 313t, 318t
pheochromocytoma, 178t, 193, 195
phobias, 218
phosgene oxime, 1307t
PhosLo. See calcium acetate
phosphate, deficiencies in, 528t
PHOSPHODIESTERASE III INHIBITORS, 587t, 589–590
inamrinone, 587t, 589, 590, 616t
milrinone, 587t, 589–590
PHOSPHODIESTERASE 5 INHIBITORS, 1216, 1217–1219
sildenafil, 196, 1217, 1217t, 1218
tadalafil, 1217, 1217t, 1219, 1221, 1221t
vardenafil, 1217, 1217t, 1219
Phospholine Iodide. See echothiophate iodide
phospholipids, 454, 455f, 907
phosphorus (phosphate), 1057, 1057t
photophobia, 166
photosensitivity, 808, 808t
phototherapy, 243, 243t, 1277
phototoxicity, 57, 825
Phthirus pubis, 1265
physical dependence, 419
physostigmine, 152t, 154, 166, 340, 1308t
phytonadione. See vitamin K
PICC (peripherally inserted central catheter) lines, 956
picornaviruses, 908t
PIH (prolactin-inhibiting hormone), 1098
pill rolling, 287
pilocarpine, 152t, 153, 154, 1288t, 1289
Pilopine. See pilocarpine
pimecrolimus, 1273–1274
pimozide, 271t, 274
PIMs (potentially inappropriate medications), 121, 122t
pindolol, 197, 198t, 200
pinna, 1295
Pin-Rid. See pyrantel pamoate
Pinworm Caplets. See pyrantel
Pin-X. See pyrantel
pioglitazone, 1122t, 1125t, 1126, 1129, 1131
Piper methysticum. See kava
piperacillin, 616t, 789t, 792, 793
pirbuterol, 186, 187, 737t, 738
piroxicam, 680–681t
PIs (PROTEASE INHIBITORS), 936–938

pitavastatin, 459, 461t, 463
Pitocin. See oxytocin
pituitary gland, 1097t, 1098, 1100t
placebos, 17, 54
placenta, 94
Placidyl. See ethchlorvynol
Plan B, 1193t, 1200, 1202
Plaquenil. See hydroxychloroquine
plaques
in atherosclerosis, 561
in multiple sclerosis, 300, 301
in psoriasis, 1274
Plasbumin. See normal serum albumin
plasma cells, 669
plasma cholinesterase. See pseudocholinesterase
plasma half-life (t1/2), 38
Plasma-Lyte, 525, 527
plasminogen, 631
Plasmodium, 886, 887, 887f. See also malaria
plateau drug plasma levels, 38, 38f
PLATELET ENHANCERS, 649, 651–652
eltrombopag, 645t, 649, 652
oprelvekin. See oprelvekin
romiplostim, 645t, 649, 652
platelets, 441–442, 525, 616
Platinol. See cisplatin
platinum compounds
carboplatin, 504t, 616t, 964t, 966
cisplatin, 55–56t, 504t, 958, 964t, 966
oxaliplatin, 964t, 967
Plavix. See clopidogrel
Plenaxis. See abarelix
Plendil. See felodipine
plerixafor, 987t
Pletal. See cilostazol
plicamycin, 972
PMC (pseudomembranous colitis), 796t, 808
PML (progressive multifocal leukoencephalopathy), 303, 1033
PMS (premenstrual syndrome), 1171
pneumococcal conjugate vaccine (PCV), 715
pneumococcal infection, 714–715
pneumococcal polysaccharide vaccine (PPV), 714–715
pneumonia, 777t, 781t, 867t, 913t, 944t
pneumonic plague, 1306
pneumothorax, 1071t
PNS. See peripheral nervous system
POCD (postoperative cognitive dysfunction), 405t
Podophyllum peltatum, 980
poisonings
at home, 1309t
management of, 1308–1311, 1308t
medication overdoses, 1308, 1308t
Nursing Practice Applications, 1312–1313t
Poladex. See dexchlorpheniramine
Polaramine. See dexchlorpheniramine
polarized cells, 597
poliomyelitis, 713t, 719
Polocaine. See mepivacaine
POLYCLONAL ANTIBODIES, 702. See also antithymocyte globulin
polycyclic aromatic hydrocarbons (PAHs), 60t
polycystic ovary syndrome, 1181
polydipsia, 1105, 1114
polyethylene glycol, 691, 1025t
polyherbacy, 85t
polymeric formulas, for enteral nutrition, 1064
polymyxin B, 827, 827t, 830, 1264
polypeptides, 805
polyphagia, 1114
polypharmacy, 73, 117–118
polysaccharide iron complex, 656, 656t
polysomnography, 222

Polysporin, 827, 830
polystyrene sulfonate, 531
polythiazide and prazosin, 546t
polyuria, 1105, 1114
polyvinyl alcohol, 1293t
pomalidomide, 990t
Pomalyst. *See* pomalidomide
Ponstel. *See* mefenamic acid
Pontocaine. *See* tetracaine
poppy plant, 372
posaconazole, 870t, 872, 874
positive symptoms, of schizophrenia, 266, 266t
postantibiotic effect, 812, 824
posterior pituitary gland, 1098
postexposure prophylaxis, for HIV, 942–943
postganglionic neurons, 140
postherpetic neuralgia, 719
postictal state, 313
postmarketing surveillance, 18
postmenopausal bleeding, 1171
postoperative cognitive dysfunction (POCD), 405t
postoperative medications, 413
postpartum depression, 241
post-traumatic epilepsy (PTE), 323t
post-traumatic stress disorder (PTSD), 219, 232, 258t
Posture. *See* calcium phosphate tribasic
potassium acetate, 532
potassium bicarbonate, 532
POTASSIUM CHANNEL BLOCKERS, 603t, 607–609
    adverse effects, 607
    drugs in class
        amiodarone. *See* amiodarone
        dofetilide, 603t, 608
        ibutilide, 603t, 608
        sotalol, 198t, 200, 603t, 608–609
    mechanism of action, 602f, 607
potassium chloride (KCl), 531–532, 1057t
potassium citrate, 532
potassium gluconate, 532
potassium imbalances, 528t, 529f, 530–532
potassium iodide (KI), 1146, 1307–1308
potassium iodide and iodine, 1145t, 1146
POTASSIUM-SPARING DIURETICS, 505, 506f, 511–513
    adverse effects, 512
    doses and routes, 511t
    drugs in class
        amiloride, 506, 511, 511t, 513
        eplerenone. *See* eplerenone
        spironolactone. *See* spironolactone
        triamterene, 506, 511, 511t, 513, 546t, 547
    mechanism of action, 506f, 511
    therapeutic effects and uses, 512
potency, 45–46, 46f
potentially inappropriate medications (PIMs), 121, 122t
Potiga. *See* ezogabine
poxvirus, 908t
PPDs (purified protein derivatives), 851
PPIs. *See* PROTON PUMP INHIBITORS
PPN (peripheral vein parenteral nutrition), 1069
PPV (pneumococcal polysaccharide vaccine), 714–715
PQ intervals, 600t
PQ segments, 600t
Pradaxa. *See* dabigatran
pralatrexate, 968, 969t, 972
pralidoxime, 155, 1308t
pramipexole, 290t, 291–292
pramlintide, 1118–1119
PrandiMet, 1125t
Prandin. *See* repaglinide
prasugrel, 626t, 627, 628
Pravachol. *See* pravastatin

pravastatin, 60, 459, 461t, 463
Pravigard PAC, 463
praziquantel, 898, 899t, 900
prazosin, 98t, 193, 194t, 196, 546t, 549
preclinical research, 17
Precose. *See* acarbose
prediabetes, 1114
prednicarbate, 1273t
prednisolone, 839, 1156t
prednisone
    for adrenal insufficiency, 1158
    breast-feeding and, 98t
    in cancer treatment, 978
    for gout, 1253
    for infantile spasms, 315
    lactation risk categories, 99t
    for multiple sclerosis, 303
    for myasthenia gravis, 155–156
    in pain management, 384
    routes and dosages, 976t, 1156t
    for transplant rejection, 705
preeclampsia, 311
preexposure prophylaxis, for HIV, 943
Prefest. *See* estradiol and norgestimate
pregabalin, 313t, 316, 319t, 328
preganglionic neurons, 140
pregnancy. *See also* lactation
    alcohol use during, 94, 95–96, 425
    caffeine intake during, 360t
    cocaine use during, 430
    corticosteroid use for women at risk of preterm labor, 1159t
    eclampsia during, 311
    epidural anesthesia for delivery, 396t
    gestational diabetes and, 1114
    herbal supplement use during, 82t, 85–86
    iron requirements during, 643t
    nausea and vomiting during, 1037, 1037t
    nicotine during, 94, 95–96, 95t, 431
    nicotine use during, 94, 95–96
    perinatal transmission of HIV/AIDS, 943–944
    pharmacotherapy during
        antibiotics, 784
        antidepressants, 95t
        drug transfer across placenta, 94
        fetal stage of development and, 96–97
        physiologic changes altering pharmacokinetic responses, 93–94, 93f
        pregnancy risk categories, 56, 95–96, 95–96t
        rationale for, 93
    preeclampsia during, 311
    preterm labor, 1179
    seizures in, 311
    substance abuse during, 95–96, 96t
    thyroid gland in, 1139t
    tuberculosis and, 854
    urinary tract infections during, 836
    vaccines during, 712
    vitamins during, 95, 1051t
pregnancy categories, 56, 95–96, 95–96t
Pregnyl. *See* chorionic gonadotropin-HCG
preimplantation phase, of fetal development, 96–97
preload, 447, 448f
Premarin. *See* conjugated estrogens
premenstrual syndrome (PMS), 1171
Premphase. *See* conjugated estrogens with medroxyprogesterone
Prempro. *See* conjugated estrogens with medroxyprogesterone
prenatal multivitamins, 95t
preoperative medications, 411
Prepidil. *See* dinoprostone

preschoolers, 108. *See also* pediatric patients
Prescription Drug User Fee Act of 1992 (PDUFA), 14, 19
prescription drugs. *See* drug(s)
prescriptive authority, 20–21
preterm labor, 1179
Prevacid/Prevacid SoluTab. *See* lansoprazole
Prezista. *See* darunavir
PRH (prolactin-releasing hormone), 1098
Prialt. *See* ziconotide
Priftin. *See* rifapentine
prilocaine, 406t, 411
Prilosec. *See* omeprazole
Primacor. *See* milrinone
primaquine, 886, 887, 888t, 889
primary hypertension, 542. *See also* hypertension
Primaxin. *See* imipenem-cilastatin
primidone, 318t, 320
Primsol. *See* trimethoprim
Principen. *See* ampicillin
Prinivil. *See* lisinopril
Prinzide, 491
Prinzmetal's (vasospastic) angina, 561
Pristiq. *See* desvenlafaxine
Privine. *See* naphazoline
ProAmatine. *See* midodrine
Probalan. *See* probenecid
Pro-Banthine. *See* propantheline
probenecid, 1253, 1254t, 1255, 1256
procainamide, 603t, 604–605, 616t
procaine, 38, 406t, 408–409
procarbazine, 964t, 967–968
Procardia/Procardia XL. *See* nifedipine
Prochieve. *See* progesterone
prochlorperazine, 29, 271t, 273, 386, 957, 1039t
procoagulants, 615
Procrit. *See* epoetin alfa
prodrugs, 33
prodysrhythmics, 597, 597t
Pro-Fast. *See* phentermine
progesterone, 55t, 93–94, 1170t, 1173–1174, 1190. *See also* PROGESTINS
PROGESTINS. *See also* medroxyprogesterone
    Nursing Practice Applications, 1175–1176t
    in oral contraceptives, 1190
    therapeutic effects and uses, 1171
    types of, 1171t
Proglycem. *See* diazoxide
Prograf. *See* tacrolimus
progressive multifocal leukoencephalopathy (PML), 303, 1033
proguanil-atovaquone, 886, 887, 888t, 889
proinflammatory substances, 668
prolactin-inhibiting hormone (PIH), 1098
prolactin-releasing hormone (PRH), 1098
Proleukin. *See* aldesleukin
Prolia. *See* denosumab
Promacta. *See* eltrombopag
promethazine
    breast-feeding and, 98t
    clinical applications, 271, 272, 375, 413
    in combination products, 766t
    routes and dosages, 756t, 1038, 1039t
Prometrium. *See* progesterone
propafenone, 603t, 606, 622t
propantheline, 165t, 167
proparacaine, 1293t, 1294
Propecia. *See* finasteride
Propine. *See* dipivefrin
Propionibacterium acnes, 1267–1268
propionic acids, 681
propofol, 397t, 399–400, 425t
propoxyphene, 377

propranolol
adverse effects, 199–200
breast-feeding and, 98t
clinical applications and considerations, 198, 199–200, 228
drug interactions, 425t
for dysrhythmias, 603t, 607
genetic polymorphisms and actions of, 129
hydrochlorothiazide and, 546t
for hypertension, 549
mechanism of action, 199
for migraine prophylaxis, 389, 389t
protein binding in, 106
routes and dosages, 198t, 568t
sensitivity in Asian patients, 606t
proprietary drugs. See trade name drugs
propylthiouracil, 55t, 95t, 1095, 1145–1146, 1145t
Proquin XR. See ciprofloxacin
Proscar. See finasteride
ProSom. See estazolam
PROSTAGLANDIN(S)
as abortifacient, 1203, 1204t
for glaucoma, 1287–1289
bimatoprost, 1287–1288, 1288t
latanoprost, 910, 1287, 1288t
travoprost, 1288–1289, 1288t
for inflammation, 668t
physiological properties of, 674–675
as uterine stimulant, 1177
carboprost, 1177, 1177t, 1179, 1203, 1203–1204t
dinoprostone, 1177, 1177t, 1179, 1203, 1203–1204t
misoprostol. See misoprostol
prostaglandin E$_2$, 1005
prostate cancer, 951t, 963t, 1219t. See also benign prostatic hyperplasia
prostatitis, 834
Prostigmin. See neostigmine
Prostin E$_2$. See dinoprostone
protease, 928
PROTEASE INHIBITORS (PIs), 936–938
atazanavir, 932t, 937–938
darunavir, 932t, 937, 938
fosamprenavir, 932t, 938
indinavir, 86t, 616t, 932t, 938
lopinavir with ritonavir, 58, 932t, 937
nelfinavir, 932t, 938
ritonavir, 58, 60, 932t, 937, 938
saquinavir, 86t, 932t, 938
tipranavir, 932t, 938
PROTEASE-ACTIVATED RECEPTOR-1 ANTAGONISTS, 571
protein synthesis, 778, 805–806, 805f
protein synthesis inhibitors
aminoglycosides. See AMINOGLYCOSIDES
macrolides. See MACROLIDES
mechanism of action, 806, 806f
miscellaneous agents, 814–815, 815t, 818
tetracyclines. See TETRACYCLINES
proteins, in enteral nutrition, 1065
Proteus mirabilis, 775, 777t
prothrombin, 444
prothrombin time (PT), 617
PROTON PUMP INHIBITORS (PPIs), 724, 1010–1013, 1011–1013t
adverse effects, 1011, 1012
doses and routes, 1011t
drugs in class
dexlansoprazole, 1013
esomeprazole, 1011t, 1013
lansoprazole, 1010, 1011t, 1013
omeprazole. See omeprazole
pantoprazole, 1011t, 1013
rabeprazole, 1011t, 1013

mechanism of action, 1010–1011, 1010f, 1012
Nursing Practice Application, 1019–1020t
nursing responsibilities, 1013
therapeutic effects and use, 1011–1012
Protonix. See pantoprazole
Protopam. See pralidoxime
Protopic. See tacrolimus
prototype drugs, 6
protozoan infections, 885–896
classification and pathogenesis of, 885–886, 885t
malarial, 886–890. See also malaria
nonmalarial, 890–896. See also nonmalarial protozoan infections
Nursing Practice Applications, 901–902t
protozoans, defined, 885
protriptyline, 244, 245t, 247, 389t
Provenge. See sipuleucel-T
Proventil. See albuterol
Proventil Repetabs. See albuterol
Provera. See medroxyprogesterone
Provigil. See modafinil
proviruses, 909
Prozac. See fluoxetine
pruritus, 57, 1263
pseudocholinesterase, 144, 170
pseudoephedrine
acrivastine with, 756t, 758
adverse effects, 764
breast-feeding and, 99t
clinical applications, 185, 763–764
in combination products, 757t, 766t
drug interactions, 764
illegal uses of, 184, 185, 430, 763t
mechanism of action, 764
nursing responsibilities, 764
restrictions on sale, 184, 763–764
routes and dosages, 764t
pseudogout, 1255t
pseudomembranous colitis (PMC), 796t, 808
Pseudomonas aeruginosa, 777t, 781t, 792–793, 796, 807, 824
psilocybin, 428, 428f
psoralens, 1277
psoriasis, 1274–1276t, 1274–1277, 1274f
psoriasis vulgaris, 1275t
psoriatic arthritis, 1275t
psoriatic erythroderma, 1275t
PSVT (paroxysmal supraventricular tachycardia), 600
psychodynamic therapy, 243t
psychological dependence, 419
psychomotor seizures. See complex partial seizures
psychosis, 265, 268. See also schizophrenia
psychosocial influences, on pharmacotherapy, 177
psychostimulants. See CENTRAL NERVOUS SYSTEM STIMULANTS
psyllium (herbal), 85
psyllium mucilloid, 1025t, 1026–1027
PT (prothrombin time), 617
PTE (post-traumatic epilepsy), 323t
PTH (parathyroid hormone), 1092, 1230–1231
PTSD (post-traumatic stress disorder), 219, 232, 258t
PTU. See propylthiouracil
pubic lice, 1265
PUD. See peptic ulcer disease
Pulmicort. See budesonide
pulmonary edema, 579, 581
pulmonary embolism, 615–616
pulmonary excretion, 36
pulmonary perfusion, 731
Pulmozyme. See dornase alfa
pupil, of eye, 1285
Pure Food and Drug Act of 1906 (PFDA), 13–14
purified protein derivatives (PPDs), 851

purine analogs, 969
cladribine, 969t, 970–971
clofarabine, 969t, 971
fludarabine, 969t, 971
mercaptopurine, 969t, 971–972, 1033
nelarabine, 969t, 972
pentostatin, 969t, 972
thioguanine, 969t, 972
Purinethol. See mercaptopurine
Purkinje fibers, 445
Push Packages, 1304
pustular psoriasis, 1275t
PUVA therapy, 1277
PVD (peripheral vascular disease), 630
pyelonephritis, 834, 836
Pylera, 1018
pyramidal tracts, 214
pyrantel pamoate, 897, 898, 899t, 900
pyrazinamide, 851, 852, 853t, 854, 857
pyrethrin, 1265, 1266
pyridostigmine, 152t, 154, 155, 157
pyridoxine (vitamin B$_6$), 337, 854, 1049–1050t, 1054–1055, 1308t
pyrilamine, 766t
pyrimethamine, 838t, 839, 892t, 894, 895–896, 968
pyrimidine analogs, 969
capecitabine, 969t, 970
cytarabine, 822–823, 969t, 971
floxuridine, 969t, 971
fluorouracil, 95t, 822–823, 868, 954, 969t, 971
gemcitabine, 969t, 971
PZA. See pyrazinamide

Q

QRS complex, 599, 599f, 600t
Qsymia, 1083t, 1085
QT intervals, 58, 600t
Quaalude. See methaqualone
Qualaquin. See quinine
quazepam, 225–226t, 228
Qudexy XR. See topiramate
Quelicin. See succinylcholine
Questran. See cholestyramine
quetiapine fumarate, 258t, 260, 275t, 277
QuickCaps. See diphenhydramine
Quillivant XR. See methylphenidate
quinapril, 491t, 493, 548, 584t
quinidine, 604, 605, 616t, 622t
quinidine gluconate, 603t, 887
quinidine sulfate, 603t
quinine, 338, 887, 888t, 889–890
quinolones. See FLUOROQUINOLONES
quinupristin-dalfopristin, 61, 782, 815, 815t, 818
Quixin. See levofloxacin
Qutenza. See capsaicin
Qvar. See beclomethasone

R

RA. See rheumatoid arthritis
RAAS. See renin-angiotensin-aldosterone system
rabeprazole, 1011t, 1013
rabies, 713t, 717–718
rabies immune globulin, 721, 721t
race, influence on pharmacotherapy, 127–128. See also Treating the Diverse Patient; specific racial groups
racemic amphetamine, 353
radiation sickness, 1307–1308
radiation therapy, 951
radioactive iodide, 1145t, 1146
radiologic contrast media, 56t, 504t
raloxifene, 95t, 976t, 978, 1240t, 1242–1243

raltegravir, 932t, 939
ramelteon, 220, 225t, 230
ramipril, 491t, 493, 548, 584t
ramucirumab, 987t, 988
Ranexa. See ranolazine
ranitidine, 411, 616t, 1014–1015, 1014t
ranolazine, 563, 568t
Rapaflow. See silodosin
Rapamune. See sirolimus
rapid eye movement (REM) sleep, 220, 221, 221t
RAS (reticular activating system), 211, 214, 214f,
        219, 219f, 220
rasagiline, 290t, 294
rasburicase, 1255
rashes, drug-induced, 57
Raynaud's disease, 193, 195, 195t
Razadyne. See galantamine
RCA (root-cause analysis), 74–75, 75f
RDAs (recommended dietary allowances), 1050
reabsorption, 503
Rebetol. See ribavirin
Rebif. See INTERFERON(s), IFN beta-1a
rebound cardiac excitation, 199
rebound congestion, 185, 763
rebound depression, 246
rebound effects, in substance abuse, 419
rebound insomnia, 223, 226
reboxetine, 250
receptors
        genetic polymorphisms and, 129
        in geriatric patients, 120
        pharmacodynamic theory of, 46–48
        types of, 47f
Reclast. See zoledronate
recombinant technology vaccines, 711, 711t
Recombivax HB. See hepatitis B vaccine
recommended dietary allowances (RDAs), 1050
Recothrom. See thrombin, topical
rectal route of administration, 30
red blood cells. See erythrocytes
refeeding syndrome, 1068
reflex tachycardia, 153, 195, 449–450, 550–551, 565
Refludan. See lepirudin
refractory period, 598
refusal of medication, 128t
regional anesthesia, 395
Regitine. See phentolamine
Reglan. See metoclopramide
Regonol. See pyridostigmine
regorafenib, 987t
regulations. See laws and regulations
Relafen. See nabumetone
relaxation training, 389t
Relaxin. See methocarbamol
Relenza. See zanamivir
religion, medication refusal based on, 128t
Relistor. See methylnaltrexone
Relpax. See eletriptan
REM (rapid eye movement) sleep, 220, 221, 221t
Remeron. See mirtazapine
Remicade. See infliximab
remifentanil, 377, 396, 397t, 398
Reminyl. See galantamine
renal corpuscle, 502
renal excretion, 35–36
renal failure, 36, 504–505, 504–505t
renal physiology, 502–503, 502–503f, 504t
renin, 487–488
RENIN INHIBITORS, 490, 494t, 544t. See also aliskiren
renin-angiotensin-aldosterone system (RAAS),
        486–500
        blood pressure and, 451, 488
        components of, 487–489, 487–489f
        drugs affecting, 490–496
                ACE inhibitors, 490–493, 491t
                aldosterone antagonists, 490, 494t, 495–496
                ARBs, 493–495, 494t
                renin inhibitors, 490, 494t
        physiological actions of, 489–490
        points for drug intervention, 490
Renova. See tretinoin
ReoPro. See abciximab
reoviruses, 908t
repaglinide, 1122t, 1125t, 1127–1128
repetitive transcranial magnetic stimulation (rTMS)
        therapy, 243t
replacement therapies
        corticosteroids, 1155–1158
        hormones, 1093, 1174–1175
        nicotine, 97t, 158, 160, 419, 431–432, 431f
        thyroid hormones, 1140–1142, 1142t, 1143–1144t
replication cycle, of viral infections, 907–909, 909f
repolarization, 598
reproductive system regulation
        female, 1167, 1168–1169f
        male, 1209–1210, 1209f
reproductive system toxicity, 958
Repronex. See menotropins
Requip. See ropinirole
Rescriptor. See delavirdine
reserpine, 550
resistance, to antibiotics, 779–782, 779t, 781f
respiratory depression, with opioids, 373, 375, 385
respiratory system
        drug excretion by, 36
        lower, 731–732, 731f
        upper, 753–754, 753f
rest-and-digest response, 138–139, 193
Restasis. See cyclosporine ophthalmic emulsion
Restoril. See temazepam
Retavase. See reteplase
rete ridges, 1263
reteplase, 632t, 634
reticular activating system (RAS), 211, 214, 214f, 219,
        219f, 220
reticular formation, 429
Retin-A. See tretinoin
RETINOIDS, 1269
        adapalene, 1268t, 1269, 1270
        isotretinoin. See isotretinoin
        tazarotene, 1268t, 1271, 1275, 1276t
        tretinoin, 1268t, 1269–1270
retinopathy, diabetic, 1116
retrograde infections, 834
Retrovir. See zidovudine
retroviruses, 908t, 927. See also HIV/AIDS
reuptake, 145
reverse cholesterol transport, 454
reverse remodeling, 586
reverse transcriptase, 927
REVERSE TRANSCRIPTASE INHIBITORS, 933–935
reversible cholinesterase inhibitors. See
                NONNUCLEOSIDE REVERSE TRANSCRIPTASE
                INHIBITORS; NUCLEOSIDE/NUCLEOTIDE
                REVERSE TRANSCRIPTASE INHIBITORS
ReVia. See naltrexone
Revlimid. See lenalidomide
Revonto. See dantrolene sodium
Reyataz. See atazanavir
Reye's syndrome, 111, 676
Rezulin. See troglitazone
rhabdomyolysis, 58, 335, 460
rheumatoid arthritis (RA)
        genetic influences in, 1246t
        inflammation in, 668
        nonpharmacologic therapies, 1247
        Nursing Practice Applications, 1251–1252t
        pathophysiology, 1246–1247, 1247f
        pharmacotherapy, 1159, 1247–1251, 1248t
Rheumatrex. See methotrexate
Rhinocort/Rhinocort Aqua. See budesonide
rhinophyma, 1269
$Rh_o[D]$ immune globulin, 721–723, 721t
RhoGAM. See $Rh_o[D]$ immune globulin
rhubarb, 1026
ribavirin, 95t, 917t, 918, 920, 921, 1306
riboflavin (vitamin B_2), 389t, 1049–1050t, 1054
ribosomes, 806
Rickettsia rickettsii. See Rocky Mountain spotted fever
RID. See pyrethrin
rifabutin, 852, 853t, 857, 863, 1018
Rifadin. See rifampin
Rifamate, 857
rifampin
        adverse effects, 616t, 830
        clinical applications, 830, 852, 859
        in combination products, 857
        drug interactions, 425t, 622t
        excretion of, 36
        routes and dosages, 827t, 853t
rifamycin derivatives, 857
rifapentine, 853t, 857
Rifater, 857
rilpivirine, 932t, 936
Rilutek. See riluzole
riluzole, 304
rimabotulinumtoxinB, 304, 341t, 343, 343t
Rimactane. See rifampin
rimantadine, 913, 914t, 915
rimonabant, 1082
Ringer's solution, 525, 526
ringworm. See tinea capitis
Riomet. See metformin
Riopan, 1015t
risedronate, 1239–1240t, 1241
risk management, 74
risk-benefit ratio, 55
Risperdal/Risperdal Consta/Risperdal M-TAB. See
                risperidone
risperidone
        adverse effects, 258t, 275–276
        for bipolar disorder, 258t, 260
        clinical applications and considerations,
                274–276, 297
        long-acting preparation, 269
        mechanism of action, 275
        for organic brain syndrome, 271
        routes and dosages, 258t, 275t
Ritalin/Ritalin SR. See methylphenidate
ritodrine, 186, 1179
ritonavir, 58, 60, 932t, 937, 938. See also lopinavir
                with ritonavir
Rituxan. See rituximab
rituximab, 987t, 988, 1248t, 1250
rivaroxaban, 618t, 621, 622
rivastigmine, 152t, 297, 297t, 300
rizatriptan, 387t, 388
Robaxin. See methocarbamol
Robinul. See glycopyrrolate
Robitussin A-C, 766t
Robitussin DM. See dextromethorphan
Rocaltrol. See calcitriol; vitamin D
Rocephin. See ceftriaxone
Rocky Mountain spotted fever, 777t, 807
rocuronium, 169t, 173
rofecoxib, 682
roflumilast, 741t, 746
Rogaine. See minoxidil

Rohypnol. *See* flunitrazepam
Rolaids, 1015*t*
Romazicon. *See* flumazenil
romidepsin, 990, 990*t*
romiplostim, 645*t*, 649, 652
root-cause analysis (RCA), 74–75, 75*f*
ropinirole, 290*t*, 292
ropivacaine, 406*t*, 411
rosacea, 1269
roseola, 910
rosiglitazone, 1122*t*, 1125*t*, 1126, 1128–1129
rosuvastatin, 459, 460, 461*t*, 463
Rotarix, 721
RotaShield, 721
RotaTeq, 721
rotavirus, 720–721
rotigotine, 290*t*, 292–293
routes of administration
    absorption, impact on, 27–30
    buccal, 28–29
    enteral, 27–29
    inhalation, 733–734
    intra-arterial, 956
    intradermal, 30
    intramuscular, 30, 31, 106
    intranasal, 29
    intraperitoneal, 956
    intrathecal, 956
    intravenous, 26, 30, 956
    intravesicular, 956
    ophthalmic, 29
    oral, 25, 25*f*, 28–29, 106, 955–956
    otic, 29
    parenteral, 30
    for pediatric patients, 28
    rectal, 30
    subcutaneous, 30, 106
    sublingual, 28
    topical, 29–30, 31, 106
    vaginal, 29
Roxanol. *See* morphine sulfate
Rozerem. *See* ramelteon
rTMS (repetitive transcranial magnetic stimulation)
    therapy, 243*t*
rubella (German measles), 713*t*, 718–719, 1265
rubeola. *See* measles
rufinamide, 313*t*, 319*t*, 328
Rythmol/Rythmol SR. *See* propafenone
Ryzolt. *See* tramadol

S

Sabril. *See* vigabatrin
saccharin, 1085
safety. *See* Patient Safety
safflower oil, 1070
Saizen. *See* somatropin
Salagen. *See* pilocarpine
Salex. *See* salicylic acid
SALICYLATES, 56*t*, 674–679. *See also* aspirin
    adverse effects, 675–676, 678
    doses and routes, 676*t*
    drugs in class
        aspirin. *See* aspirin
        choline magnesium trisalicylate, 676*t*, 678
        magnesium salicylate, 533, 676*t*, 678, 1057
        salsalate, 676*t*, 678–679
    mechanism of action, 674–675, 675*f*, 677
    therapeutic effects and uses, 676–677
salicylic acid, 674, 1268, 1276*t*
salicylism, 678
saline/osmotic cathartics, 1026
Salk, Jonas, 719

salmeterol, 187, 737*t*, 738
Salmonella, 777*t*
salsalate, 676*t*, 678–679
Salsitab. *See* salsalate
Samsca. *See* tolvaptan
Sancuso. *See* granisetron
Sandimmune. *See* cyclosporine
Sandostatin. *See* octreotide
Sansert. *See* methysergide
Saphris. *See* asenapine
saquinavir, 86*t*, 932*t*, 938
Sarafem. *See* fluoxetine
sarcolemma, 474
sarcomas, 949, 949*t*
sarcoplasmic reticula, 474
sargramostim, 645*t*, 649, 694, 957
sarin, 1307*t*
satiety, 1079
satiety center, 1079, 1080
Savella. *See* milnacipran
saw palmetto, 81*t*, 82, 83*t*, 1222*t*
saxagliptin, 1122*t*, 1131
SCA (sudden cardiac arrest), 609*t*
scabies, 1265
Schedule I drugs, 222, 427–428
Schedule II drugs, 20, 232, 353
Schedule III drugs, 222
Schedule IV drugs, 222, 225
scheduled drugs, 20, 20*t*, 418
schizoaffective disorder, 266
schizophrenia
    etiology of, 267
    genetic influences on, 267
    nonpharmacologic therapies for, 268–269
    in pediatric patients, 268*t*
    pharmacotherapy. *See* ANTIPSYCHOTICS
    prevalence of, 265*t*
    prognosis, 269
    symptoms of, 265–266, 266*t*
school-age children, 108. *See also* pediatric patients
sclera, 1284, 1285
scleroderma, 195*t*
sclerosing, 956
scopolamine, 29, 165*t*, 168, 1037, 1039*t*, 1293*t*
scurvy, 1048
seasonal affective disorder, 241, 243
seasonal allergic rhinitis, 754
Seasonale, 1194
Seasonique, 1194
sebaceous glands, 1263
seborrhea, 1267
seborrheic dermatitis, 1273, 1274
secobarbital, 233–234, 233*t*
Seconal. *See* secobarbital
second messenger events, 47
secondary hypertension, 542. *See also* hypertension
secondary parkinsonism, 270, 287
SECOND-GENERATION (ATYPICAL) ANTIPSYCHOTICS
    adverse effects, 274, 275*t*
    for Alzheimer's disease, 297
    for bipolar disorder, 260
    dopamine system stabilizers, 277
    drugs in class
        aripiprazole, 258*t*, 260, 275*t*, 277–279
        asenapine, 258*t*, 260, 275*t*, 276
        clozapine, 275*t*, 276
        iloperidone, 275*t*, 276
        lurasidone, 275*t*, 276–277
        olanzapine. *See* olanzapine
        paliperidone, 269, 275*t*, 277
        quetiapine fumarate, 258*t*, 260, 275*t*, 277
        risperidone. *See* risperidone
        ziprasidone, 258*t*, 260, 275*t*, 277

    mechanism of action, 274
    route and dosages for, 275*t*
    for schizophrenia, 274–279
    weight gain in children using, 278*t*
secretion, 503
Sectral. *See* acebutolol
sedatives, 224, 421, 425*t*. *See also* BARBITURATES; BENZODIAZEPINES; NONBENZODIAZEPINE ANXIOLYTICS
seizures, 309–333
    Alzheimer's disease and, 311*t*
    classification of, 313–315
    convulsions vs., 310–311
    defined, 310
    etiology of, 310, 310*t*
    generalized, 313–314, 313*t*
    in geriatric patients, 312, 314*t*
    impact on quality of life, 311
    nonpharmacologic therapies, 312, 312*t*, 315
    partial, 313*t*, 314, 323
    in pediatric patients, 312, 313, 314–315
    pharmacotherapy. *See* ANTIEPILEPTIC DRUGS
    in pregnancy and lactation, 311–312
    psychiatric comorbidities with, 320*t*
SELECTIVE ESTROGEN RECEPTOR MODULATORS (SERMs), 975, 978, 1175, 1242–1243
    fulvestrant, 976*t*, 978
    raloxifene, 95*t*, 976*t*, 978, 1240*t*, 1242–1243
    tamoxifen. *See* tamoxifen
    toremifene, 976*t*, 978
SELECTIVE SEROTONIN REUPTAKE INHIBITORS (SSRIs)
    as adjuvant analgesics, 383, 384*t*
    adverse effects, 231, 248, 1215*t*
    for bipolar disorder, 260
    for cataplexy, 222
    clinical applications for, 231–232, 231*t*
    for depression, 245*t*, 248–250, 248*f*
    drug interactions, 62*t*, 86*t*, 229, 247
    drugs in class
        citalopram, 231*t*, 245*t*, 250, 297
        escitalopram, 231*t*, 245*t*, 250
        fluoxetine. *See* fluoxetine
        fluvoxamine, 230, 231*t*, 232, 250
        paroxetine. *See* paroxetine
        sertraline. *See* sertraline
    history of, 248
    for irritable bowel syndrome, 1036
    lactation risk categories, 99*t*
    for migraine prophylaxis, 389
    during pregnancy, 95*t*
    pregnancy category, 95*t*
selegiline, 257, 290*t*, 294, 358
selenium, 87*t*, 1057*t*
Selzentry. *See* maraviroc
semielemental formulas, for enteral nutrition, 1064
Semprex-D, 758
senna, 1025*t*, 1026
Senokot. *See* senna
Sensipar. *See* cinacalcet
Sensorcaine. *See* bupivacaine
sentinel events, 67
sepsis, 1071*t*
Septocaine. *See* articaine
Septra. *See* trimethoprim-sulfamethoxazole
Serax. *See* oxazepam
Serevent. *See* salmeterol
SERMs. *See* SELECTIVE ESTROGEN RECEPTOR MODULATORS
Seromycin. *See* cycloserine
Serophene. *See* clomiphene
Seroquel/Seroquel XR. *See* quetiapine fumarate
Serostim. *See* somatropin

serotonin
actions and effects of, 248, 248f
in appetite control, 1080
effects and clinical applications, 141t, 210t
in migraines, 386
synapses, 211
SEROTONIN (5-HT) AGONISTS, 386–388. See also
ERGOT ALKALOIDS; TRIPTANS
SEROTONIN (5-HT) ANTAGONISTS, 1036, 1037, 1039t,
1040–1041
alosetron, 1033t, 1036
dolasetron, 1037, 1039t, 1041
granisetron, 1037, 1039t, 1041
ondansetron. See ondansetron
palonosetron, 1037, 1039t, 1041
serotonin syndrome (SES), 247, 248, 249, 250
SEROTONIN-NOREPINEPHRINE REUPTAKE INHIBITORS
(SNRIs), 232, 250
desvenlafaxine, 245t, 250, 252
duloxetine, 231t, 232, 245t, 250, 252, 383
venlafaxine. See venlafaxine
Serpalan. See reserpine
Serratia, 777t
sertraline
adverse effects, 250
clinical applications, 231–232, 231t, 250, 297
interactions with, 425t
routes and dosages, 245t
Sertürner, Friedrich, 3
serum, 442–443
serum glucose control, 1112, 1113f. See also diabetes
mellitus
Serzone. See nefazodone
SES (serotonin syndrome), 247, 248, 249, 250
sevoflurane, 403, 403t, 404
sexual dysfunction. See male sexual dysfunction
Sherley Amendment of 1912, 14
Shigella, 777t
shingles (herpes zoster), 719, 720, 720t, 910, 1265
short stature, defined, 1099
SIADH (syndrome of inappropriate diuretic
hormone), 809, 1105–1106
sibutramine, 1082
sick sinus syndrome, 599–600
sickle cell anemia, 652
side effects, defined, 53. See also adverse drug effects
Signifor. See pasireotide
sildenafil, 196, 1217, 1217t, 1218
Silenor. See doxepin
silent angina, 561
silodosin, 193, 194t, 197, 1221t
Silvadene. See silver sulfadiazine
silver sulfadiazine, 838t, 839
silymarin, 99t
Simcor, 465
simeprevir, 917t, 918, 920
simple partial seizures, 313t, 314
Simplesse, 1085
Simponi. See golimumab
Simulect. See basiliximab
simvastatin
adverse effects, 616t, 1041t
chemical structure of, 459
ezetimibe and, 467
interactions with, 425t
niacin and, 465
pregnancy category rating, 463
routes and dosages, 461t
sitagliptin with, 1130
Sinemet/Sinemet SR. See levodopa/carbidopa
Sinequan. See doxepin
Singulair. See montelukast
sinoatrial (SA) node, 445, 475, 476

sinoatrial node dysfunction, 599–600
sinus bradycardia, 599
sinus rhythm, 445
sipuleucel-T, 990t, 991
sirolimus, 616t, 696t, 699
Sirturo. See bedaquiline
sitagliptin, 1122t, 1125t, 1130
situational anxiety, 218
6-MP. See mercaptopurine
Sjögren's syndrome, 153, 154
SJS (Stevens–Johnson syndrome), 53, 57, 260,
321, 839
Skelaxin. See metaxalone
skeletal muscle relaxants. See MUSCLE RELAXANTS
skeletal muscle toxicity, 56t, 58
Skelid. See tiludronate
skin. See also dermatologic disorders
anatomy of, 1262–1263, 1262f
bacteria population on, 667t
as body defense, 665–666
cancer, 950
dermatologic toxicity, 56t, 57
infections, 1264–1266
Sklice. See ivermectin
Skyla, 1199
sleep. See also sleep disorders
cardiovascular disease and, 547t
diabetes and, 230t
stages of, 220–221, 221t
sleep apnea, 547t
sleep attacks, 222, 358
sleep disorders. See also insomnia
narcolepsy, 222, 358–359
Nursing Practice Applications, 234–235t
prevalence of, 221, 358t
types of, 221–222, 222t
sleep paralysis, 358
sleeping sickness (African trypanosomiasis), 895
sleep-maintenance insomnia, 222
sleep-offset insomnia, 222
sleep-onset insomnia, 221
sleep-wake patterns, 220, 220t, 221
Slow-K. See potassium chloride
small intestine, 999–1000, 999f
small volume nebulizers, 734
smallpox, 713t, 1306
smoking. See nicotine
SNRIs. See SEROTONIN-NOREPINEPHRINE REUPTAKE
INHIBITORS
SNS. See sympathetic nervous system
SNS (Strategic National Stockpile), 1304
social anxiety disorder, 218, 232
sodium
in antacids, 1016
as fluid replacement agent, 525
functions and recommended dietary
allowance, 1057t
imbalances, 528–530, 528t, 529f
sodium bicarbonate
adverse effects, 535
clinical applications, 531, 534–535
drug interactions, 59, 60, 535
Nursing Responsibilities, 535
as overdose treatment, 36, 1308t
routes and dosages, 1015t
sodium biphosphate, 1025t
SODIUM CHANNEL BLOCKERS, 601, 602f, 603t,
604–606
class IA
disopyramide, 603t, 604, 605
procainamide, 603t, 604–605, 616t
quinidine gluconate, 603t, 887
quinidine sulfate, 603t

class IB
lidocaine. See lidocaine
mexiletine, 384, 603t, 605
phenytoin. See phenytoin
class IC
flecainide, 603t, 606
propafenone, 603t, 606, 622t
mechanism of action, 602f, 604
sodium chloride (NaCl), 530
SODIUM ION CHANNEL INHIBITORS, 511
amiloride, 506, 511, 511t, 513
triamterene, 506, 511, 511t, 513, 546t, 547
sodium nitroprusside. See nitroprusside sodium
sodium oxybate, 222, 354t, 358, 359, 418, 421
sodium stibogluconate, 892t, 895, 896
sofosbuvir, 917t, 918, 920
Solarcaine. See benzocaine
Soliris. See eculizumab
Solodyn. See minocycline
solubility, impact on distribution, 32
soluble films, 28
Solu-Cortef. See hydrocortisone
Solu-Medrol. See methylprednisolone
Soma. See carisoprodol
soman, 1307t
somatic nervous system, 137, 138f
somatic pain, 368
somatostatin, 1005
somatotropin. See growth hormone
somatropin, 1099–1101, 1100t
Somatuline Depot. See lanreotide
Somavert. See pegvisomant
Sominex. See diphenhydramine
Somogyi phenomenon, 1118
Sonata. See zaleplon
sorafenib, 987t
Soriatane. See acitretin
Sorine. See sotalol
sotalol, 198t, 200, 603t, 608–609
soundalike drug names, 70, 71t
Sovaldi. See sofosbuvir
soy, 81t, 86t, 1141t, 1178t
soybean oil, 1070
spacers, 734
sparfloxacin, 826
spasms. See muscle spasms
spastic colon. See irritable bowel syndrome
spasticity. See muscle spasticity
specialty supplements, 87, 87t
specific defenses. See adaptive body defenses
Spectazole. See econazole
spectinomycin, 814
Spectracef. See cefditoren
SPERMICIDES, 1199–1200
SPF, 1278
spinal anesthesia, 404, 405f
spinal cord, 212f, 213
spirilla, 776
Spiriva. See tiotropium
spironolactone
adverse effects, 512, 585, 1215t
breast-feeding and, 98t
as diuretic, 511–513
for heart failure, 584t, 585
hydrochlorothiazide and, 506, 546t
for hypertension, 495–496, 547
mechanism of action, 512
nursing responsibilities, 585
routes and dosages, 494t, 511t
Splenda®. See sucralose
Sporanox. See itraconazole
sporotrichosis, 867, 867t
sporozoites, 886

Sportscreme, 1326
Sprix. *See* ketorolac
Sprycel. *See* dasatinib
sputum cultures, 851
SSRIs. *See* SELECTIVE SEROTONIN REUPTAKE
    INHIBITORS
St. John's wort
    for depression, 254*t*
    drug interactions, 5*t*, 20, 86*t*, 185, 229, 247
    as enzyme inducer, 35
    primary uses, 81*t*
    serotonin syndrome and, 250
    standardization, 83*t*
ST segments, 600*t*
stable angina, 561
Stadol. *See* butorphanol
staging, of cancer, 952, 952*t*
Stalevo, 290
Staphylococcus aureus
    characteristics of, 777*t*
    health-care associated infections and, 781*t*
    invasiveness of, 775
    methicillin-resistant, 781–782, 782*t*, 793
    in skin infections, 1264
Staphylococcus saprophyticus, 835, 836
Starling's law of the heart, 447
Starlix. *See* nateglinide
STATINS
    adverse effects, 56*t*, 335, 460, 461*t*
    breast-feeding and, 98*t*
    for colorectal cancer, 462
    for dementia, 461
    drug interactions, 62, 460, 622*t*
    drugs in class
        atorvastatin. *See* atorvastatin
        fluvastatin, 459, 461*t*, 462
        lovastatin, 62*t*, 459, 460–461, 461*t*, 463, 465
        pitavastatin, 459, 461*t*, 463
        pravastatin, 60, 459, 461*t*, 463
        rosuvastatin, 459, 460, 461*t*, 463
        simvastatin. *See* simvastatin
    for dyslipidemia, 458–463, 461*t*
    mechanism of action, 458–459, 460*f*
    for pediatric patients, 458*t*
    pregnancy category, 95*t*
    routes and dosages, 461*t*
status asthmaticus, 733
status epilepticus, 227, 313*t*, 315, 320
stavudine, 932*t*, 935
Stavzor. *See* valproic acid
Staxyn. *See* vardenafil
steatorrhea, 1041
Stelara. *See* ustekinumab
Stendra. *See* avanafil
steroids, 434, 454, 455*f*
sterol nucleus, 454
Stevens–Johnson syndrome (SJS), 53, 57, 260, 321, 839
stevia, 81*t*, 1085
Stilbestrol. *See* diethylstilbestrol
Stimate. *See* desmopressin
stimulant laxatives, 1026
stimulants. *See* CENTRAL NERVOUS SYSTEM STIMULANTS
Stivarga. *See* regorafenib
stomach, 997–998, 997*t*, 1005, 1006–1007*f*
stool softeners, 1026
Strategic National Stockpile (SNS), 1304
Strattera. *See* atomoxetine
stratum basale, 1263
stratum corneum, 1263
Streptase. *See* streptokinase
Streptococcus pneumoniae. *See* pneumococcal infection
Streptococcus pyogenes, 1264
streptokinase, 632, 632*t*, 634

streptomycin
    adverse effects, 812, 814, 854, 857
    clinical applications, 814, 852, 857
    pregnancy category rating, 95*t*
    routes and dosages, 812*t*, 853*t*
streptozocin, 964*t*, 968
stress ulcers, 1007. *See also* peptic ulcer disease
Striant, 1211
striatum, 287
stroke, 542
stroke volume, 447–448
Stromectol. *See* ivermectin
stropipate, 1170*t*
styes, 1294
subcutaneous fungal infections, 868
subcutaneous layer, of skin, 1262*f*, 1263
subcutaneous route of administration, 30, 106
Sublimaze. *See* fentanyl
sublingual route of administration, 28
Suboxone. *See* naloxone/buprenorphine
substance abuse, 416–437. *See also specific substances*
    addiction and, 369, 418
    adolescents and, 109
    anabolic steroids, 434
    cultural differences in, 429*t*
    defined, 417
    dependence and, 20, 375, 418–419
    depressants. *See* CENTRAL NERVOUS SYSTEM
        DEPRESSANTS
    diagnosis of, 417
    in geriatric patients, 429*t*
    inhalants, 422*t*, 432
    nicotine. *See* nicotine
    Nursing Practice Applications, 433*t*, 434
    during pregnancy, 95–96, 96*t*
    prescription drugs and, 418
    prevalence of, 417*t*, 418*t*
    stimulants. *See* CENTRAL NERVOUS SYSTEM
        STIMULANTS
    tolerance and, 375, 385, 419–420
    withdrawal syndrome and, 419, 420*t*
substance P, 141*t*
substantia gelatinosa, 369
substantia nigra, 287
substrates, 34
subunit vaccines, 711
Subutex. *See* buprenorphine
SUCCINIMIDES, 325
    ethosuximide, 98*t*, 313*t*, 316, 318*t*, 325
    methsuximide, 318*t*, 325
succinylcholine, 144, 169–172, 169*t*, 342, 345, 411
sucralfate, 62*t*, 1018
sucralose, 1085
Sudafed. *See* pseudoephedrine
sudden cardiac arrest (SCA), 609*t*
Sufenta. *See* sufentanil
sufentanil, 377, 396, 397*t*, 398
Sugar-Twin. *See* saccharin
suicide and suicide risk, 219, 242–243, 244*t*
Sular. *See* nisoldipine
sulbactam, 789*t*, 792
sulconazole, 875*t*
sulfa drugs. *See* SULFONAMIDES
sulfacetamide sodium, 839, 1268*t*
sulfadiazine, 838*t*, 839, 840
sulfadoxine-pyrimethamine, 838*t*, 840
sulfamethoxazole. *See* trimethoprim-sulfamethoxazole
Sulfamylon. *See* mafenide
sulfanilamide, 14
sulfasalazine
    adverse effects, 839, 1034, 1251
    clinical applications, 839, 1032, 1033–1034,
        1248*t*, 1251

    Lifespan and Diversity Considerations, 1034
    mechanism of action, 1034
    Nursing Responsibilities, 1034
    Patient and Family Education, 1034
    routes and dosages, 1033*t*, 1248*t*
sulfinpyrazone, 1254*t*, 1255, 1256
sulfisoxazole, 98*t*, 838*t*, 839, 840–841
SULFONAMIDES, 837–841
    adverse effects, 56*t*, 111, 616*t*, 839
    classification of, 838–839
    clinical applications, 835, 837, 839–841, 894
    drug interactions, 59
    drugs in class
        mafenide, 839
        silver sulfadiazine, 838*t*, 839
        sulfacetamide sodium, 839, 1268*t*
        sulfadiazine, 838*t*, 839, 840
        sulfadoxine-pyrimethamine, 838*t*, 840
        sulfasalazine. *See* sulfasalazine
        sulfisoxazole, 98*t*, 838*t*, 839, 840–841
        trimethoprim, 98*t*, 838*t*, 616*t*, 841, 968
        trimethoprim-sulfamethoxazole. *See*
           trimethoprim-sulfamethoxazole
    genetic polymorphisms and actions of, 129
    mechanism of action, 778, 837
    resistance to, 780, 835, 838
    routes and dosages, 838*t*
SULFONYLUREAS, 425*t*, 839, 1125–1126
    adverse effects, 1125–1126
    drug interactions, 1126
    first generation
        chlorpropamide, 56*t*, 1122*t*, 1126
        tolazamide, 1122*t*, 1126
        tolbutamide, 1122*t*, 1126
    mechanism of action, 1125
    nursing responsibilities, 1126
    second generation
        glimepiride, 1122*t*, 1125*t*, 1126
        glipizide, 1122*t*, 1125*t*, 1126
        glyburide, 1122*t*, 1125–1126, 1125*t*
    therapeutic effects and uses, 1125
Sulfoxyl, 1269
sulfur, 1057*t*
sulfur mustard, 1307*t*
sulindac, 680–681*t*
sumatriptan, 105*t*, 386, 387–388, 387*t*
Sumavel DosePro. *See* sumatriptan
Sumycin. *See* tetracycline
sunburns, 1277–1279
Sunett¯. *See* acesulfame
sunitinib, 987*t*
sunscreens, 1278
supercoils, 822
superficial fungal infections, 868, 872–878, 875*t*
superinfections, 784
supplemental nutrition, 1062–1077. *See also* enteral
    nutrition; parenteral nutrition
supplements
    dietary. *See* dietary supplements
    herbal. *See* herbal supplements
    minerals. *See* minerals
    specialty, 87, 87*t*
    vitamins. *See* vitamin(s)
Supprelin LA. *See* histrelin
suprachiasmatic nucleus, 220
Suprane. *See* desflurane
Suprax. *See* cefixime
Suprenza. *See* phentermine
suramin, 892*t*, 895, 896
surface (topical) anesthesia, 404, 405*f*
surface area, impact on absorption, 31
surfactant laxatives, 1026
surgical anesthesia, 395

Surmontil. *See* trimipramine
sustained release formulations, 28, 39
Sustiva. *See* efavirenz
Sutent. *See* sunitinib
suvorexant, 225*t*, 230
Svedberg unit, 806
sweat glands, 1263
Sweet One. *See* acesulfame
Sweet'N Low. *See* saccharin
swimmer's ear, 1295
Syaxyn. *See* vardenafil
Sylatron. *See* pegIFN alfa-2b
Symbyax, 249
Symlin. *See* pramlintide
Symmetrel. *See* amantadine
sympathetic nervous system (SNS)
      adrenal medulla and, 146
      angiotensin II and, 489
      in heart failure, 580–581
      structure and function of, 138–140, 139*f*
sympathomimetics. *See* ADRENERGIC AGONISTS
symporter, 506, 507*f*
Synalar. *See* fluocinolone acetonide
synapses, 140, 210
synaptic cleft, 140
synaptic transmission, 140–141*f*, 140–142,
      210–211, 210*f*, 210*t*
Synarel. *See* nafarelin
syndrome of inappropriate diuretic hormone
      (SIADH), 809, 1105–1106
Synercid. *See* quinupristin-dalfopristin
synergistic effects, 61, 61*f*
Synribo, 980*t*
Synthroid. *See* levothyroxine
syphilis, 777*t*, 807, 944*t*
systemic fungal infections, 868, 869–874, 870*t*
systemic lupus erythematosus, 195*t*, 551, 616, 668
systolic heart failure, 579

T

T cells, 670–671, 670–671*t*
T waves, 599, 599*f*, 600*t*
tablets, 28
Tabloid. *See* thioguanine
tabun, 1307*t*
tachydysrhythmias, 600, 606
tachyphylaxis, 420
tacrine, 152*t*, 299
tacrolimus, 56*t*, 504*t*, 696*t*, 698, 699, 1273–1274
tadalafil, 1217, 1217*t*, 1219, 1221, 1221*t*
Taenia saginata, 898
tafluprost, 1288, 1288*t*
Tagamet. *See* cimetidine
talc, 1278
Talwin. *See* pentazocine
Tambocor. *See* flecainide
Tamiflu. *See* oseltamivir
tamoxifen
      adverse effects, 55*t*, 977
      clinical applications, 952, 976–977, 1095, 1216
      excretion of, 36
      interactions with, 622*t*, 977–978
      mechanism of action, 977
      Nursing Responsibilities, 978
      routes and dosages, 976*t*
tamsulosin, 193, 194*t*, 197, 549, 1221*t*
tanning devices, 1052*t*, 1266*t*
Tanzeum. *See* albiglutide
Tapazole. *See* methimazole
tapentadol, 378
tapeworms, 898
Tarceva. *See* erlotinib

tardive dyskinesia (TD), 270, 270*t*
target cells, 1091, 1093*f*
targeted therapies, 691, 983, 987*t*, 988
Targretin. *See* bexarotene
Tarka, 493, 546*t*
Tasigna. *See* nilotinib
tasimelteon, 220, 225*t*, 230
Tasmar. *See* tolcapone
tavaborole, 875*t*
Tavist. *See* clemastine
TAXANES, 980, 982
      cabazitaxel, 980, 980*t*, 982
      docetaxel, 980, 980*t*, 982
      paclitaxel, 963, 980, 980*t*, 982
Taxol. *See* paclitaxel
Taxotere. *See* docetaxel
tazarotene, 1268*t*, 1271, 1275, 1276*t*
Tazicef. *See* ceftazidime
tazobactam, 789*t*, 793
Tazorac. *See* tazarotene
Taztia XT. *See* diltiazem
TB. *See* tuberculosis
TBG (thyroxine-binding globulin), 1138
TCAs. *See* TRICYCLIC ANTIDEPRESSANTS
TD (tardive dyskinesia), 270
Tdap. *See* pertussis immunization
tear gas, 1307
Tecfidera. *See* dimethyl fumarate
Teflaro. *See* ceftaroline
Tega-Tussin Syrup, 766*t*
Tegretol/Tegretol XR. *See* carbamazepine
Tekamlo, 479, 546*t*
Tekturna. *See* aliskiren
Tekturna HCT, 546*t*, 548
telaprevir, 917*t*, 918, 920
telavancin, 797*t*, 799
telbivudine, 917*t*, 920
telithromycin, 815*t*, 818, 827*t*, 830
telmisartan, 479, 494*t*, 495, 546*t*, 548
telomerase, 950
telomeres, 950
temazepam, 95*t*, 225–226*t*, 228
Temodar. *See* temozolomide
temozolomide, 105*t*, 964*t*, 967
Temovate. *See* clobetasol propionate
temporal lobe seizures. *See* complex partial seizures
temsirolimus, 696*t*, 699–700
Tenckhoff catheters, 956
tendon toxicity, 56*t*, 58
tenecteplase, 632, 632*t*, 634–635
teniposide, 55*t*, 823, 980, 980*t*, 983
tenofovir
      adverse effects, 919, 935
      clinical applications, 918, 919, 933, 935, 943
      mechanism of action, 919
      Nursing Responsibilities, 919
      routes and dosages, 917*t*, 932*t*
Tenoretic, 202, 546*t*
Tenormin. *See* atenolol
Tensilon. *See* edrophonium
tension headaches, 385, 386*t*
Tepanil. *See* diethylpropion
Terazol. *See* terconazole
terazosin, 193, 194*t*, 197, 549, 1221, 1221*t*
terbinafine, 868, 874, 875, 875*t*, 876, 878
terbutaline
      as bronchodilator, 186, 187, 737*t*, 738
      chemical structure of, 179
      routes and dosages, 1177*t*
      as tocolytic, 1179
terconazole, 875*t*
teriflunomide, 302*t*, 303

teriparatide, 1240*t*, 1244
terrorism. *See* bioterrorism
tesamorelin, 933
Tessalon Perles. *See* benzonatate
test and treat prevention strategies, 943*t*
testicular cancer, 951*t*
Testim, 1211
Testopel, 1211
testosterone. *See also* ANDROGEN(s)
      adverse effects, 1212
      breast-feeding and, 98*t*
      clinical applications, 978, 1211
      mechanism of action, 1212
      Nursing Responsibilities, 1212
      pregnancy category rating, 95*t*
      routes and dosages, 29, 976*t*, 997, 1210*t*
testosterone cypionate, 1210*t*, 1211
testosterone enanthate, 1210*t*
testosterone undecanoate, 1210*t*, 1211
Testred. *See* methyltestosterone
tetanus, 713*t*, 714
tetanus immune globulin, 721*t*
tetanus toxoid, 714
tetracaine, 406*t*, 409, 1278, 1293*t*, 1294
tetracycline
      adverse effects, 111, 808
      clinical applications, 808, 887, 1017
      distribution of, 32
      drug interactions, 58, 1072
      mechanism of action, 808
      nursing responsibilities, 809
      routes and dosages, 807*t*
      for skin infections, 1264
TETRACYCLINES
      adverse effects, 56*t*, 95, 784, 808
      breast-feeding and, 98*t*
      clinical applications, 806–807, 808–809,
            1268*t*, 1306
      drug interactions, 31, 62*t*, 622*t*, 1016
      drugs in class
            demeclocycline, 807*t*, 809, 1106
            doxycycline. *See* doxycycline
            minocycline, 112*t*, 807*t*, 809, 859
            tetracycline. *See* tetracycline
            tigecycline, 807*t*, 809
      mechanism of action, 778, 807–808
      Nursing Practice Applications, 816–817*t*
      pregnancy category, 95, 95*t*
      resistance to, 780, 806, 807
      routes and dosages, 807*t*
tetrahydrocannabinol (THC), 426
tetrahydrozoline, 183, 185, 764*t*, 1293*t*
Teveten. *See* eprosartan
Teveten HCT, 495, 546*t*
6-TG. *See* thioguanine
thalamotomy, 288, 288*t*
thalamus, 211, 212*f*
thalassemia, 652
thalidomide
      adverse effects, 14, 96, 702
      clinical applications, 702, 988
      as immunosuppressant, 696*t*
      pregnancy category rating, 95, 95*t*, 702
      routes and dosages, 990*t*
Thalomid. *See* thalidomide
THC (tetrahydrocannabinol), 426
theobromine, 359
Theo-Dur. *See* theophylline
theophylline, 359, 360, 737*t*, 744–745
TheraCys. *See* bacillus Calmette-Guérin vaccine
therapeutic classification, 5–6, 5*t*
therapeutic drug monitoring, 37
therapeutic index (TI), 44, 44*f*

therapeutic lifestyle changes (TLCs), 457–458, 543, 562
therapeutic range, 37
Thermazene. *See* silver sulfadiazine
thiabendazole, 898, 899*t*, 900
thiamine (vitamin B₁), 1049–1050*t*, 1053–1054
THIAZIDE DIURETICS
    adverse effects, 509, 547, 1215*t*
    clinical applications, 509, 510–511
    drug interactions, 122, 839
    drugs in class
        bendroflumethiazide and nadolol, 510*t*,
            511, 546*t*
        chlorothiazide, 509, 510*t*, 511, 547
        chlorthalidone, 202, 509, 510*t*, 511, 546*t*, 547
        hydrochlorothiazide. *See* hydrochlorothiazide
        indapamide, 509, 510*t*, 511, 547
        methyclothiazide, 510*t*, 511, 547
        metolazone, 509, 510*t*, 511, 547
    mechanism of action, 505, 506*f*, 509
    routes and dosages, 510*t*
THIAZOLIDINEDIONES (TZDs), 1128–1129
    pioglitazone, 1122*t*, 1125*t*, 1126, 1129, 1131
    rosiglitazone, 1122*t*, 1125*t*, 1126, 1128–1129
thioguanine, 969*t*, 972
thiopental sodium, 400
thioridazine, 271, 271*t*, 273
thiotepa, 964*t*, 968
thiothixene, 271*t*, 274
thirst center, 523
Thorazine. *See* chlorpromazine
Three Mile Island nuclear accident (1979), 1308*t*
3TC. *See* lamivudine
threshold potential, 597–598
thrombin, 444, 635*t*
thrombin, topical, 636
Thrombinar. *See* thrombin, topical
thrombocytes. *See* platelets
thrombocytopenia, 442, 616, 616*t*, 649, 957
thromboembolic disorders, 615–616
THROMBOLYTICS
    adverse effects, 569, 631–632
    for clot dissolving, 631–632, 634–635
    drugs in class
        alteplase, 632, 632*t*
        reteplase, 632*t*, 634
        streptokinase, 632, 632*t*, 634
        tenecteplase, 632, 632*t*, 634–635
    in geriatric patients, 632
    mechanism of action, 617*t*, 631
    for myocardial infarction, 569, 570*f*
    Nursing Practice Applications, 633–634*t*
    routes and dosages, 632*t*
thrombopoietin, 442, 649
thrush, 876, 876*t*
Thymoglobulin. *See* antithymocyte globulin
Thyro-Block. *See* potassium iodide
thyroid cancer, 951*t*
thyroid crisis (thyroid storm), 1140, 1140*t*, 1144
thyroid disorders
    diagnosis of, 1139, 1139*t*
    emergencies, 1140, 1140*t*
    hyperthyroidism, 1142, 1144–1146, 1145*t*
    hypothyroidism, 241, 1140–1142, 1141*t*
    Nursing Practice Applications, 1143–1144*t*,
        1147–1148*t*
    signs and symptoms of, 1140*t*
thyroid gland, 1138, 1139*f*, 1139*t*
thyroid hormone, 98*t*, 622*t*, 1092–1093, 1094*t*, 1138
thyroid hormone replacement, 1140–1142, 1142*t*,
    1143–1144*t*
thyroid storm. *See* thyroid crisis
Thyroid USP. *See* desiccated thyroid
thyroid-stimulating hormone (TSH), 1092

thyroid-stimulating immunoglobulins (TSI), 1144
Thyrolar. *See* liotrix
thyrotoxicosis, 1144
thyrotropin-releasing hormone (TRH),
    1092, 1093, 1098, 1138
thyrotropin-stimulating hormone (TSH), 1138
thyroxine (T₄), 95*t*, 1138
thyroxine-binding globulin (TBG), 1138
TI (therapeutic index), 44, 44*f*
tiagabine, 312, 313*t*, 319*t*, 328
Tiazac. *See* diltiazem
ticagrelor, 626*t*, 628
ticarcillin, 789*t*, 792, 793, 1297
Tice. *See* bacillus Calmette-Guérin vaccine
Ticlid. *See* ticlopidine
ticlopidine, 571, 622*t*, 626*t*, 627, 628–629
ticonazole, 877
Tigan. *See* trimethobenzamide
tigecycline, 807*t*, 809
TIIV (trivalent inactivated influenza vaccine), 717
Tikosyn. *See* dofetilide
Tilade. *See* nedocromil
tiludronate, 1239–1240*t*, 1241
Timentin, 789*t*, 793
time-response relationships, 36–39, 37*f*
Timolide, 546*t*
timolol
    adverse effects, 200, 1290
    clinical applications, 200, 389*t*, 568*t*, 1290
    in combination products, 546*t*, 1289
    mechanism of action, 1290
    Nursing Responsibilities, 1290
    routes and dosages, 198*t*, 1288*t*
Timoptic/Timoptic XE. *See* timolol
Tinactin. *See* tolnaftate
Tindamax. *See* tinidazole
tinea capitis, 867*t*, 874, 876, 1265
tinea corporis, 874
tinea cruris, 867*t*, 874–875, 1264–1265
tinea pedis, 867*t*, 874, 875, 1264–1265
tinea unguium, 876, 1265
tinidazole, 890, 892*t*, 893–894
tinzaparin, 618*t*, 620
tioconazole, 875*t*
tiotropium, 165*t*, 166, 168, 737*t*, 740
tipranavir, 932*t*, 938
tirofiban, 626*t*, 630
titanium dioxide, 1278
Titralac. *See* calcium carbonate
Tivicay. *See* dolutegravir
tizanidine, 339*t*, 341
TLCs (therapeutic lifestyle changes), 457–458,
    543, 562
TMP-SMZ. *See* trimethoprim-sulfamethoxazole
TMS (transcranial magnetic stimulation), 243
TNF. *See* TUMOR NECROSIS FACTOR (TNF) INHIBITORS
TNKase. *See* tenecteplase
tobacco use. *See* nicotine
tobramycin, 812*t*, 814
Tobrex. *See* tobramycin
tocainide, 605
tocilizumab, 702*t*, 1248*t*, 1251, 1277
TOCOLYTICS, 186, 187, 1179
    magnesium sulfate (MgSO₄), 311, 532–533,
        1057, 1177*t*, 1179
    nifedipine. *See* nifedipine
    ritodrine, 186, 1179
    terbutaline. *See* terbutaline
Today Sponge, 1199, 1199*f*
toddlers, 107. *See also* pediatric patients
tofacitinib, 702*t*, 1248*t*
Tofranil. *See* imipramine
Tofranil PM. *See* imipramine pamoate

tolazamide, 1122*t*, 1126
tolbutamide, 1122*t*, 1126
tolcapone, 290*t*, 293
Tolectin. *See* tolmetin
tolerance, 375, 385, 419–420
Tolinase. *See* tolazamide
tolmetin, 680–681*t*
tolnaftate, 875*t*, 1295
tolterodine tartrate, 105*t*, 165*t*, 168
tolvaptan, 529–530, 1106
tonic–clonic seizures, 311, 313, 313*t*, 317, 323
tonicity, 522–523
tonometry, 1286
Topamax. *See* topiramate
topical (surface) anesthesia, 404, 405*f*
topical route of administration, 29–30, 31, 106
Topicort. *See* desoximetasone
topiramate
    adverse effects, 329
    in combination products, 1085
    mechanism of action, 317
    for migraine prophylaxis, 389*t*
    phentermine with, 1083*t*
    for seizures, 260, 313*t*, 314, 328–329
topoisomerase II (DNA gyrase), 822
TOPOISOMERASE INHIBITORS, 980–981, 982–983
    etoposide, 55*t*, 823, 980, 980*t*, 983
    irinotecan, 105*t*, 980, 980*t*, 982
    teniposide, 55*t*, 823, 980, 980*t*, 983
    topotecan, 980, 980*t*, 982–983
topoisomerase IV, 822
topotecan, 980, 980*t*, 982–983
Toprol/Toprol XL. *See* metoprolol
Toradol. *See* ketorolac
toremifene, 976*t*, 978
Torisel. *See* temsirolimus
torsades de pointes, 58, 600
torsemide, 508*t*, 509, 547, 584*t*, 585
tositumomab, 987*t*, 988
total parenteral nutrition (TPN), 1069. *See also*
    parenteral nutrition
Totect. *See* dexrazoxane
Tourette's syndrome, 168, 271
Toviaz. *See* fesoterodine
toxic concentrations, 37
toxoid vaccines, 711, 711*t*
toxoids, 711, 711*t*
Toxoplasma gondii, 885*t*, 894, 944*t*
toxoplasmosis, 885*t*, 894
TPN (total parenteral nutrition), 1069. *See also*
    parenteral nutrition
trace minerals. *See* microminerals
Tracrium. *See* atracurium
trade name drugs, 7, 8
Tradjenta. *See* linagliptin
tramadol, 379, 379*t*, 382, 1246
Trandate. *See* labetalol
trandolapril, 491*t*, 493, 546*t*, 548
tranexamic acid, 635, 635*t*, 636, 637
tranquilizers, 224, 421. *See also* BARBITURATES;
    BENZODIAZEPINES; NONBENZODIAZEPINE
    ANXIOLYTICS
transcranial magnetic stimulation (TMS), 243
transdermal patches, 29
Transderm-Scop. *See* scopolamine
transferrin, 654
transfusions
    blood products, 523–525, 524*t*
    fluid. *See* FLUID REPLACEMENT AGENTS
transient ischemic attacks, 542
translation. *See* protein synthesis
transplant rejection, 695, 698, 1159–1160
Tranxene. *See* clorazepate

tranylcypromine, 257

trastuzumab, 987*t*, 988

Trasylol. *See* aprotinin

Travatan. *See* travoprost

traveler's diarrhea, 807*t*

travoprost, 1288–1289, 1288*t*

trazodone, 86*t*, 231*t*, 250, 253, 1215*t*

Treanda. *See* bendamustine

Treating the Diverse Patient. *See also* Lifespan
 and Diversity Considerations

 antihypertensive response, ethnic differences
  in, 197*t*

 attention deficit/hyperactivity disorder in girls, 353*t*

 cognitive dysfunction after noncardiac
  surgery, 405*t*

 corticosteroid use by mothers at risk for
  preterm labor, 1159*t*

 debrisoquin hydroxylase, 275*t*

 drug and alcohol abuse, 429*t*

 enzyme deficiencies, 49*t*

 ethnic differences in acetaminophen
  metabolism, 684*t*

 gender differences in desmopressin dose
  for nocturia, 1107*t*

 global health implications of *H.Pylori*
  infection, 1016*t*

 growth hormone in HIV/AIDS patients
  on antiretroviral therapy, 1101*t*

 improved kidney function from thyroid
  hormone replacement, 1142*t*

 lithium carbonate, 259

 male birth control pills, 1195*t*

 medication refusal on religious grounds, 128*t*

 personalized medicine, 131*t*

 post-traumatic epilepsy in veterans, 323*t*

 propranolol sensitivity in Asian patients, 606*t*

 responses to medications, 35*t*

 skin reactions, 1279*t*

 succinylcholine, 225

 vitamins during pregnancy, 1051*t*

 weight loss and diabetes treatment, 1084*t*

Trecator-SC. *See* ethionamide

Trelstar. *See* triptorelin

tremors, in Parkinson's disease, 287, 294

Trental. *See* pentoxifylline

Treponema pallidum. See syphilis

tretinoin, 1268*t*, 1269–1270

Trexall. *See* methotrexate

Treximet. *See* sumatriptan

TRH (thyrotropin-releasing hormone), 1092, 1093,
  1098, 1138

triamcinolone, 741*t*, 742, 759*t*, 1156*t*, 1273*t*

Triaminic, 757*t*

Triaminic Expectorant DH, 766*t*

triamterene, 506, 511, 511*t*, 513, 546*t*, 547

triazolam, 225–226*t*, 228

triazoles, 872

Tribenzor, 479, 495, 546*t*

Trichomonas vaginalis, 885*t*, 894

trichomoniasis, 885*t*, 894

Trichophyton, 874, 876

TriCor. *See* fenofibrate

Tricosal. *See* choline magnesium trisalicylate

TRICYCLIC ANTIDEPRESSANTS (TCAs)

 for ADHD, 357

 as adjuvant analgesics, 383, 384*t*

 advantages of, 244

 adverse effects, 244, 246, 357, 1215*t*

 for anxiety disorders, 232

 breast-feeding and, 98*t*

 for cataplexy, 222

 for depression, 245*t*, 246–247

 drug interactions, 86*t*, 233

drugs in class

 amitriptyline. *See* amitriptyline

 clomipramine, 231*t*, 232, 245*t*, 247

 desipramine, 231*t*, 244, 245*t*, 246, 357, 1036

 doxepin. *See* doxepin

 imipramine. *See* imipramine

 maprotiline, 244, 245*t*, 247

 nortriptyline, 231*t*, 245*t*, 247, 357

 protriptyline, 244, 245*t*, 247, 389*t*

 trimipramine, 245*t*, 247

 in geriatric patients, 122*t*

 for irritable bowel syndrome, 1036

 mechanism of action, 244, 246*f*

 for migraine prophylaxis, 389, 389*t*

 overdose/poisoning, 1308, 1308*t*

Triesence. *See* triamcinolone

trifluoperazine, 271*t*, 273

trifluridine, 910, 911*t*, 913

Triglide. *See* fenofibrate

triglycerides, 454, 455*f*

trihexyphenidyl, 165*t*, 168, 294, 294*t*, 295, 304

tri-iodothyronine (T₃), 1138

Trilafon. *See* perphenazine

Trileptal. *See* oxcarbazepine

Trilipix. *See* fenofibric acid

Trilisate. *See* choline magnesium trisalicylate

trimethobenzamide, 292, 1039*t*

trimethoprim, 98*t*, 616*t*, 841, 968

trimethoprim-sulfamethoxazole

 absorption of, 839

 adverse effects, 840

 clinical applications, 835, 836, 839–840

 lactation risk categories, 99*t*

 mechanism of action, 840

 nursing responsibilities, 840

 patient safety and, 839*t*

 pregnancy category, 95*t*

 resistance to, 835, 838

 routes and dosages, 112*t*, 838*t*

 synergistic effects of, 61

trimetrexate, 968

trimipramine, 245*t*, 247

Trimox. *See* amoxicillin

Tri-Norinyl-28, 1193*t*

Triostat. *See* liothyronine

Tri-pak. *See* azithromycin

triprolidine, 756–757*t*

TRIPTANS, 386–387, 387*t*

triptorelin, 976*t*, 979

Trisenox. *See* arsenic trioxide

trivalent inactivated influenza vaccine (TiIV), 717

Trivora-28, 1193*t*

Trizivir, 934

Trobicin. *See* spectinomycin

troglitazone, 18, 1129

Trokendi XR. *See* topiramate

trophozoite stage, 885

tropic hormones, 1098

Tropicacyl. *See* tropicamide

tropicamide, 165*t*, 168, 1293*t*

trovafloxacin, 825, 826

Trovan. *See* trovafloxacin

Trovan IV, 826

Trulicity. *See* dulaglutide

Truphylline. *See* aminophylline

Trusopt. *See* dorzolamide

Truvada, 934

Truvia. *See* stevia

Trypanosoma brucei, 885*t*, 895

Trypanosoma cruzi, 885*t*, 894

trypanosomiasis, 885*t*, 894–895

TSH (thyroid-stimulating hormone), 1092

TSH (thyrotropin-stimulating hormone), 1138

TSI (thyroid-stimulating immunoglobulins), 1144

T-type calcium channels, 475

tubercles, 850

tuberculin skin tests, 851

tuberculoid leprosy, 859

tuberculosis (TB), 849–859

 in chemoprophylaxis patients, 854–855

 diagnosis of, 851

 in HIV/AIDS patients, 849, 852

 inflammation from, 673

 multidrug-resistant, 854*t*, 857, 858

 Nursing Practice Applications, 860–861*t*

 pathogenesis of, 777*t*, 849–851, 850*f*

 pharmacotherapy, 851–859

  adherence issues, 851, 854*t*

  combination therapy, 851, 852*f*, 857

  first-line drugs, 851–852, 853*t*, 854–857

  in HIV/AIDS patients, 944*t*

  mechanisms of action, 778

  prophylactic therapy, 851

  regimens, 851, 852, 855

  routes and dosages, 853*t*

  second-line agents, 853*t*, 857–859

 pregnancy and, 854

 prevalence of, 849, 849*t*

 travel and risk of, 854*t*

tubocurarine, 169*t*, 172, 345

Tudorza Pressair. *See* aclidinium

tularemia, 824, 1306

TUMOR NECROSIS FACTOR (TNF) INHIBITORS, 668*t*,
  1033, 1249–1250

 adalimumab. *See* adalimumab

 certolizumab pegol, 702*t*, 1033, 1248*t*, 1249, 1250

 etanercept. *See* etanercept

 golimumab, 702*t*, 1033, 1248*t*, 1249, 1250

 infliximab. *See* infliximab

tumors, classification and naming of, 949, 949*t*. *See
  also* cancer

Tums. *See* calcium carbonate

Tussionex, 766*t*

Twinrix, 917

Twynsta, 479, 495

Tygacil. *See* tigecycline

Tykerb. *See* lapatinib

Tylenol. *See* acetaminophen

tympanic membrane, 1295

type 1 diabetes, 1113, 1113*t*. *See also* diabetes mellitus

type 2 diabetes, 1113, 1113*t*. *See also* diabetes mellitus

typhus, 807

tyramine, 253, 253*t*, 254

TYROSINE KINASE INHIBITORS, 988

 crizotinib, 987*t*, 988

 dasatinib, 987*t*, 988

 imatinib, 987*t*, 988

Tysabri. *See* natalizumab

Tyzeka. *See* telbivudine

Tyzine. *See* tetrahydrozoline

TZDs. *See* THIAZOLIDINEDIONES

U

ulcerative colitis. *See* inflammatory bowel disease

ulcers. *See* peptic ulcer disease

uliprista, 1200, 1202, 1203*t*

Uloric. *See* febuxostat

Ultane. *See* sevoflurane

Ultiva. *See* remifentanil

Ultracet, 382

Ultram. *See* tramadol

Ultravate. *See* halobetasolol

ultraviolet light therapy, 243, 1277

Unasyn, 789*t*, 792

undecylenic acid, 875*t*, 1265

Uniretic, 493, 546t
Unisom. *See* diphenhydramine
United States Adopted Name Council, 7
United States Pharmacopeia (USP), 15, 71, 85
United States Pharmacopeia-National Formulary
    (USP-NF), 16, 16f
Unithroid. *See* levothyroxine
Univasc. *See* moexipril
unlabeled indications, 5
unstable angina, 561
up-regulation, 1091
urea, 513t, 515
Ureaphil. *See* urea
Urecholine. *See* bethanechol
urethritis, 834
Urex. *See* methenamine hippurate
URIC ACID INHIBITORS, 1253. *See also* colchicine
URICOSURICS, 1255
    probenecid, 1253, 1254t, 1255, 1256
    sulfinpyrazone, 1254t, 1255, 1256
urinalysis, 504, 834
URINARY ANTISEPTICS, 836, 841–842
    fosfomycin, 797t, 799, 836, 838t, 842
    nitrofurantoin, 836, 838t, 841–842
urinary retention, 150, 153–154, 375
urinary system toxicity, 958
urinary tract infections (UTIs), 833–847
    acute uncomplicated, 834–836, 835t
    complicated, 835t, 836
    gender differences in, 834, 836t, 837t
    in geriatric patients, 835t, 837
    Nursing Practice Applications, 843–844t
    pathogens causing, 775
    pathophysiology of, 834
    in pediatric patients, 836
    pharmacotherapy, 837–842
        fluoroquinolones, 835–836
        sulfonamides. *See* SULFONAMIDES
        urinary antiseptics, 836, 838t, 841–842
    during pregnancy, 836
    prevalence of, 834
    recurring, 837
urofollitropin, 1182t
uropathogens, 834, 835t
Uroxatral. *See* alfuzosin
urticaria, 57, 757, 1263
U.S. Food and Drug Administration. *See* Food and
    Drug Administration
USP (*United States Pharmacopeia*), 15, 71, 85
USP-NF (*United States Pharmacopeia-National
    Formulary*), 16, 16f
ustekinumab, 1276t, 1277
uterine cancer, 1174
uterine relaxants. *See* TOCOLYTICS
UTERINE STIMULANTS, 1176–1179, 1177t
    egot alkaloids
        methylergonovine, 1176–1177, 1177t, 1179
    oxytocin. *See* oxytocin
    prostaglandins
        carboprost, 1177, 1177t, 1179, 1203, 1203–1204t
        dinoprostone, 1177, 1177t, 1179, 1203,
            1203–1204t
        misoprostol. *See* misoprostol
Uticort. *See* betamethasone benzoate
UTIs. *See* urinary tract infections

V

V agents, 1307t
vaccination, defined, 710
VACCINE(s), 709–727
    administration principles, 712
    adverse effects, 712

anthrax, 711, 1305–1306
bacillus Calmette-Guérin, 692t, 693, 695
bacterial, 712–715
chickenpox, 719–720
diphtheria, 714
discovery of, 710
disease epidemiology, 713t
hepatitis A, 717, 916
hepatitis B, 712, 716–717, 723, 917
for HIV/AIDS patients, 711, 939
human papillomavirus, 712, 720, 950
immune globulin preparations, 721–723, 721t
immune system and, 694, 710–711
influenza, 717, 913
measles, 718–719
meningococcal, 715
mumps, 718–719
Nursing Practice Applications, 724–725t
for pediatric patients, 712
pertussis, 712, 714
pneumococcal, 714–715
poliomyelitis, 719
during pregnancy, 712
rabies, 718
rotavirus, 720–721
rubella, 718–719
shingles, 720, 720t
smallpox, 1306
tetanus, 714
types of, 711, 711t
varicella zoster virus, 719–720
viral, 715–721
Vaccine Adverse Event Reporting System
    (VAERS), 712
vaccine-associated paralytic polio (VAPP), 719
vagal nerve stimulators, 312
vaginal route of administration, 29
Vagistat-1, 875t, 877
vagus nerve stimulation (VNS), 243–244, 243t
valacyclovir, 910, 911t, 913
Valcyte. *See* valganciclovir
valdecoxib, 682
valerian, 81t, 85, 86t, 223
Valeriana officinalis. See valerian
valganciclovir, 911t, 913
Valisone. *See* betamethasone valerate
Valium. *See* diazepam
valproate. *See* valproic acid
valproic acid
    adverse effects, 260, 327, 616t
    for bipolar disorder, 257, 260
    breast-feeding and, 98t
    clinical applications, 228
    drug interactions, 227, 233, 327
    mechanism of action, 327
    for migraine prophylaxis, 389, 389t
    for neuropathic pain, 383
    nursing responsibilities, 327
    pregnancy category, 95t
    protein binding in, 312
    routes and dosages, 112t, 258t
    for seizures, 313t, 314, 319t, 326–327
valrubicin, 974
valsartan, 479, 494t, 495, 546t, 548, 584t
Valstar. *See* valrubicin
Valtrex. *See* valacyclovir
Vancocin. *See* vancomycin
vancomycin, 37, 616t, 778, 797t, 798–799, 800–801t
vancomycin-resistant enterococci (VRE), 782
vandetanib, 987t
Vantas. *See* histrelin
Vantin. *See* cefpodoxime
VAPP (vaccine-associated paralytic polio), 719

VAQTA. *See* hepatitis A vaccine
vardenafil, 1217, 1217t, 1219
varenicline, 432
varicella zoster immune globulin, 721t
varicella zoster virus (VZV), 719–720, 720t, 910, 1265
variola virus, 1306
Varivax, 719–720
vascular disease, diabetes and, 1116
VASCULAR ENDOTHELIAL GROWTH FACTOR
    (VEGF) INHIBITORS, 988
    bevacizumab, 987t, 988
    ramucirumab, 987t, 988
vascular headache. *See* migraines
Vaseretic, 492, 546t
vasoconstrictors, ocular. *See* OCULAR DECONGESTANTS/
    VASOCONSTRICTORS
VASODILATORS
    adverse effects, 551
    drugs in class
        diazoxide, 550, 552
        hydralazine. *See* hydralazine
        minoxidil, 552, 1279, 1280
        nesiritide, 581, 586, 587t
        nitroprusside sodium, 550, 552–553, 553t
    for heart failure, 584t, 586, 587t
    for hypertension, 544t, 550–552
    Nursing Practice Applications, 554–555t
vasomotor center, 449
vasopressin, 1100t, 1106. *See also* antidiuretic
    hormone
VASOPRESSORS, 572
vasospastic (Prinzmetal's) angina, 561
Vasotec. *See* enalapril
Vasotec IV. *See* enalaprilat
Vasoxyl. *See* methoxamine
Vaughan Williams classification, 601
Vecamyl. *See* mecamylamine
Vectibix. *See* panitumumab
vectors, 885–886
vecuronium, 169t, 173
vedolizumab, 1033
VEGF. *See* VASCULAR ENDOTHELIAL GROWTH
    FACTOR INHIBITORS
Velban. *See* vinblastine
Velcade. *See* bortezomib
Velosef. *See* cephradine
Veltin, 1268t
vemurafenib, 987t, 988
vendor-managed inventory (VMI) packages, 1304
venlafaxine
    adverse effects, 251
    clinical applications, 231t, 232, 251, 260, 383
    labeling changes, 105t
    mechanism of action, 250, 251
    Nursing Responsibilities, 251
    routes and dosages, 245t
Venofer. *See* iron sucrose
venous return, 447–448
venous thromboembolism (VTE), 615
venous thrombosis. *See* deep vein thrombosis
ventilation, 731
Ventolin. *See* albuterol
ventricular fibrillation (VF), 58, 600, 609t
ventricular hypertrophy, 579–580
ventricular tachycardia, 600
VePesid. *See* etoposide
Veramyst. *See* fluticasone
verapamil
    adverse effects, 480–481
    for angina pectoris, 477t
    breast-feeding and, 98t
    drug interactions, 199–200, 201, 481
    for dysrhythmias, 477t, 603t, 609

verapamil (*continued*)
    for hypertension, 477*t*, 480–481, 548
    mechanism of action, 476, 480
    for migraine prophylaxis, 389*t*
    for muscle spasms, 337
    nursing responsibilities, 481
    routes and dosages, 478*t*, 568*t*
    trandolapril and, 493, 546*t*
Verdeso. *See* desonide
Verelan. *See* verapamil
Verification Program (USP), 85
Vermox. *See* mebendazole
Versed. *See* midazolam
vertigo, 757
very low-density lipoprotein (VLDL), 454, 456*f*
Vesanoid. *See* tretinoin
vesicants, 958, 1306
Vestra. *See* reboxetine
veterans, post-traumatic epilepsy in, 323*t*
VF (ventricular fibrillation), 58, 600, 609*t*
Vfend. *See* voriconazole
Viadur. *See* leuprolide
Viagra. *See* sildenafil
Vibativ. *See* telavancin
Vibramycin. *See* doxycycline
Vibrio cholerae. See cholera
Victoza. *See* liraglutide
Victrelis. *See* boceprevir
Videx EC. *See* didanosine
vigabatrin, 319*t*, 329
Vigamox. *See* moxifloxacin
Viibryd. *See* vilazodone
vilazodone, 253
Vimovo, 379
Vimpat. *See* lacosamide
vinblastine, 980, 980*t*, 981
VINCA ALKALOIDS, 980, 980*t*, 981–982
    vinblastine, 980, 980*t*, 981
    vincristine, 56*t*, 954, 958, 980, 980*t*, 981
    vinorelbine, 980, 980*t*, 981–982
vincristine, 56*t*, 954, 958, 980, 980*t*, 981
vinorelbine, 980, 980*t*, 981–982
Vioxx. *See* rofecoxib
Viprostol. *See* conivaptan
Viracept. *See* nelfinavir
Viractin. *See* tetracaine
viral immunizations, 715–721
viral infections, 906–925. *See also specific infections*
    characteristics of, 907, 907*f*
    hepatitis viruses, 424, 910, 915–921,
        916–917*t*
    herpes simplex viruses, 910–911*t*, 910–913
    HIV/AIDS. *See* HIV/AIDS
    influenza viruses, 717, 913–915, 914*t*
    pharmacotherapy principles, 909–910. *See also*
        ANTIVIRALS
    replication cycle of, 907–909, 909*f*
    types of, 908*t*
viral labyrinthitis, 1297*t*
viral load, 929–930
Viramune. *See* nevirapine
Virazole. *See* ribavirin
Viread. *See* tenofovir
virilization, 1209
virions, 907
Viroptic. *See* trifluridine
virulence, 775
viruses, defined, 907. *See also* viral infections
Visceral leishmaniasis, 895
visceral pain, 368
Visine. *See* tetrahydrozoline
Visine LR. *See* oxymetazoline
Visken. *See* pindolol

vismodegib, 987*t*
Vistaril. *See* hydroxyzine
Vistide. *See* cidofovir
Vita-C. *See* vitamin C
vitamin(s), 1047–1056. *See also specific vitamins*
    deficiencies, 1050
    defined, 1048
    fat-soluble, 1048, 1049*t*, 1051–1053
    functions of, 1048, 1049*t*
    history of, 1048
    metabolism, factors impacting, 1050
    Nursing Practice Applications, 1058–1059*t*
    in parenteral nutrition, 1071
    during pregnancy, 95, 1051*t*
    prenatal, 95*t*
    recommended dietary allowances, 1050
    regulation of, 1049–1050
    role in health and disease, 1048
    toxicity, 1049, 1050*t*
    water-soluble, 1048, 1050*t*, 1053–1056
vitamin A, 1049*t*, 1051
vitamin B$_1$ (thiamine), 1049–1050*t*, 1053–1054
vitamin B$_2$ (riboflavin), 389*t*, 1049–1050*t*, 1054
vitamin B$_3$. *See* niacin
vitamin B$_6$ (pyridoxine), 337, 854, 1049–1050*t*,
    1054–1055
vitamin B$_9$. *See* folic acid
vitamin B$_{12}$. *See* cyanocobalamin
vitamin C (ascorbic acid)
    clinical applications, 1056
    as dietary supplement, 765*t*
    drug interactions, 87*t*, 200
    functions of, 1049*t*
    for poisonings, 1310
    routes and adult dosages for, 1050*t*
vitamin D
    functions of, 1049*t*1051–1052, 1052*t*,
        1231–1232, 1231*f*
    indoor tanning as source of, 1052*t*
    for metabolic bone disease, 1237–1239, 1238*t*
    pathway for activation of, 1231–1232, 1231*f*
    therapeutic effects and uses, 1051–1052
vitamin E, 622*t*, 1049*t*, 1052–1053
vitamin K, 61, 311, 444, 622*t*, 1049*t*, 1053
vita-Plus E. *See* vitamin E
Vitrasert. *See* ganciclovir
vitreous humor, 1285
Vivactil. *See* protriptyline
Vivitrol. *See* naltrexone
VLDL (very low-density lipoprotein), 454, 456*f*
VMI (vendor-managed inventory) packages, 1304
VNS (vagus nerve stimulation), 243–244, 243*t*
Vogelxo, 1211
volatile liquid anesthetics, 402–404
vomiting and vomiting center, 957, 1036. *See also*
    nausea and vomiting
von Willebrand's disease (vWD), 638
vorapaxar, 571, 626*t*, 629
voriconazole, 870*t*, 872, 874
vorinostat, 990, 990*t*
vortioxetine, 245*t*, 250
VoSol HC. *See* acetic acid and hydrocortisone
VoSpire/VoSpire ER. *See* albuterol
Votrient. *See* pazopanib
VRE (vancomycin-resistant enterococci), 782
VTE (venous thromboembolism), 615
vulvovaginal candidiasis (VVC), 876, 877, 877*t*
Vumon. *See* teniposide
vWD (von Willebrand's disease), 638
Vytorin, 467
Vyvanse. *See* lisdexamphetamine
VZV (varicella zoster virus), 719–720, 720*t*,
    910, 1265

W

waist circumference, 1080, 1081*t*
warfarin
    adverse effects, 620, 621–622
    breast-feeding and, 98*t*
    clinical applications, 621
    drug interactions, 34, 62*t*, 86*t*, 122, 622,
        810, 1069
    genetic polymorphisms and actions of, 129
    mechanism of action, 617, 621
    for myocardial infarction, 571
    nursing responsibilities, 622
    pregnancy category, 95*t*
    protein binding in, 32, 119
    routes and dosages, 618*t*
    as substrate, 34
    transition to, 620–621
water-soluble vitamins, 1048, 1050*t*, 1053–1056. *See
    also specific vitamins*
wearing-off effect, 288
weight management, 1080–1082, 1083–1084*t*,
    1085–1086. *See also* obesity
WelChol. *See* colesevelam
Wellbutrin/Wellbutrin SR/Wellbutrin XL. *See*
    bupropion
Wellferon. *See* INTERFERON(s), IFN alfa-n 1
West nomograms, 110, 111*f*
West syndrome. *See* infantile spasms
Westcort. *See* hydrocortisone valerate
wheat grass, 81*t*
WHI (Women's Health Initiative), 1174
white blood cells. *See* leukocytes
WHO (World Health Organization), 371, 1196
whole blood, 524–525, 524*t*
whole-agent vaccines, 711
whooping cough (pertussis), 713*t*, 714
withdrawal syndrome, 419, 420*t*
women. *See* gender differences; pregnancy
Women's Health Initiative (WHI), 1174
Wong-Baker Faces scale, 382*t*
World Fellowship for Schizophrenia and Allied
    Disorders, 269
World Health Organization (WHO), 371, 1196
Wycillin. *See* PENICILLIN(s), penicillin G procaine

X

Xalatan. *See* latanoprost
Xalkori. *See* crizotinib
Xanax/Xanax XR. *See* alprazolam
xanthine oxidase, 1255
xanthine oxidase inhibitors. *See* allopurinol
Xarelto. *See* rivaroxaban
Xeljanz. *See* tofacitinib
Xeloda. *See* capecitabine
Xenical. *See* orlistat
Xeomin. *See* incobotulinumtoxinA
xerostomia, 153, 154, 166
Xgen. *See* denosumab
Xgeva. *See* denosumab
Xiaflex. *See* collagenase
Xolair. *See* omalizumab
Xopenex. *See* levalbuterol
Xtandi. *See* enzalutamide
Xylocaine. *See* lidocaine
xylometazoline, 185, 764*t*
Xyrem. *See* sodium oxybate
Xyzal. *See* levocetirizine

Y

Yasmin, 1193*t*
Yersinia pestis, 787, 809*t*, 824, 1306
Yervoy. *See* ipilimumab

Yodoxin. *See* iodoquinol
yohimbe, 195
Yutopar. *See* ritodrine

Z

zafirlukast, 741*t*, 743–744
Zagam. *See* sparfloxacin
zalcitabine, 934
zaleplon, 225*t*, 230
Zaltrap. *See* ziv-aflibercept
Zanaflex. *See* tizanidine
zanamivir, 914, 914*t*, 915
Zanosar. *See* streptozocin
Zantac. *See* ranitidine
Zarontin. *See* ethosuximide
Zaroxolyn. *See* metolazone
Zebeta. *See* bisoprolol
Zelapar. *See* selegiline
Zelboraf. *See* vemurafenib
Zemplar. *See* paricalcitol
Zemuron. *See* rocuronium
Zenapax. *See* daclizumab
Zenpep. *See* pancrelipase
Zerit. *See* stavudine
ZES (Zollinger-Ellison syndrome), 1007
Zestoretic, 491, 546*t*
Zestril. *See* lisinopril
Zetia. *See* ezetimibe
Zevalin. *See* ibritumomab
Ziac, 202, 546*t*
Ziagen. *See* abacavir

Ziana, 1268*t*
ziconotide, 379*t*, 383
zidovudine
    adverse effects, 934
    clinical applications, 783, 933–934, 943
    interactions with, 62*t*
    mechanism of action, 778, 934
    Nursing Responsibilities, 934
    routes and dosages, 932*t*
zileuton, 741*t*, 744
Zimulti. *See* rimonabant
Zinacef. *See* cefuroxime
zinc, 1057*t*, 1058
zinc oxide, 1278
Zinecard. *See* dexrazoxane
Zingiber officinale. See ginger
Zingo. *See* lidocaine
Zioptan. *See* tafluprost
ziprasidone, 258*t*, 260, 275*t*, 277
Zirgan. *See* ganciclovir
Zithromax. *See* azithromycin
ziv-aflibercept, 987*t*
Zmax. *See* azithromycin
Zocor. *See* simvastatin
Zofran. *See* ondansetron
Zoladex. *See* goserelin
zoledronate (zoledronic acid), 384, 990*t*, 991,
        1239–1240*t*, 1242
Zolinza. *See* vorinostat
Zollinger-Ellison syndrome (ZES), 1007
zolmitriptan, 387*t*, 388

Zoloft. *See* sertraline
zolpidem, 225*t*, 229
Zolpimist. *See* zolpidem
Zometa. *See* zoledronate
Zomig. *See* zolmitriptan
Zonalon. *See* doxepin
Zonegran. *See* zonisamide
zonisamide, 313*t*, 319*t*, 329
Zontivity. *See* vorapaxar
Zorbtive. *See* somatropin
Zorcaine. *See* articaine
Zortress. *See* everolimus
Zostavax, 720
Zosyn, 789*t*, 793
Zovia 1/50E-28, 1193*t*
Zovirax. *See* acyclovir
Z-pak. *See* azithromycin
Zubsolv. *See* naloxone/buprenorphine
Zuplenz. *See* ondansetron
Zyban. *See* bupropion
Zyflo CR. *See* zileuton
Zykadia, 987*t*
Zyloprim. *See* allopurinol
Zymar. *See* gatifloxacin
Zymaxid. *See* gatifloxacin
Zyprexa. *See* olanzapine
Zyrtec. *See* cetirizine
Zytiga. *See* abiraterone
Zyvox. *See* linezolid